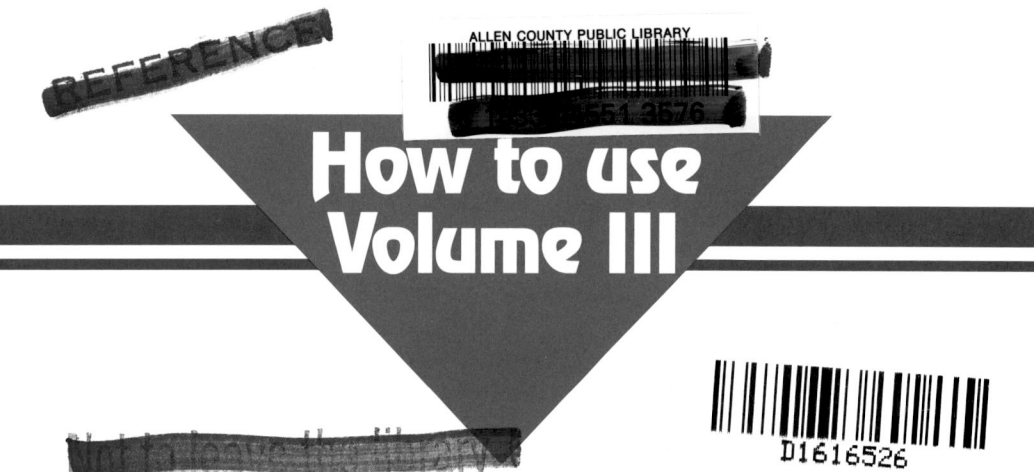

How to use Volume III

This book has important information about the therapeutic equivalence of prescription drugs. It also includes selected federal legal requirements that affect the prescribing and dispensing of drugs.

This unique combination makes *USP DI Volume III, Approved Drug Products and Legal Requirements*, a reliable and time saving reference for health care professionals.

On this page, you'll find general information about how to use the two main parts of this book. An illustration showing how the product list for prescription drugs is organized appears on the back of this page. For more detailed information about USP and this book, see *Preface* (page v).

About part 1

In this section, you'll find a copy of the FDA's complete listing of approved drug products and their therapeutic equivalence evaluations—commonly known as the "Orange Book." It lists the following:

▶ *Prescription Drug Products*

▶ *OTC Drug Products*

▶ *Drug Products with Approval Under Section 505 of the Act Administered by the Center for Biologics Evaluation and Research*

▶ *Discontinued Drug Products*

▶ *Orphan Drug Product Designations and Approvals*

▶ *Drug Products Which Must Demonstrate in vivo Bioavailability only if Product Fails to Achieve Adequate Dissolution*

▶ *Product Name Index* **Appendix A**

▶ *Product Name Index* **Appendix B** *Listed by Applicant*

▶ *Uniform Terms* **Appendix C**

▶ *Patent and Exclusivity Information Addendum*

Part 1 also has the following lists developed by USP.

▶ Listing of B-rated Drugs

▶ Listing of "Pre-1938" Products

About part 2

The second half of this book includes chemistry information, abstracted *USP* and *NF* drug standards, and dispensing requirements, as well as relevant federal legal requirements.

Part 2 also has information about Poison Control Centers, the USP Practitioners' Reporting Network, and a Medicine Chart, showing actual-size photographs of more than 1,600 widely used capsules and tablets. You'll find a separate index for the part 2 information at the back of the book.

See "Orange Book" illustration on the back of this sheet.

Sample list

Single-ingredient product
Active ingredient
> Dosage form; route of administration
>> Trade or generic names
>>> Applicant and available strengths
>>>> Application number, product number, and approval date

Multiple-ingredient product
Active ingredients, listed alphabetically
> To find information about multiple-ingredient products, look under the ingredient that is first alphabetically. For example, if you looked for this drug combination under either Butalbital or Caffeine, you would find a cross reference that says "see Acetaminophen; Butalbital; Caffeine."

> Product information—see *Single-ingredient product* listing

PRESCRIPTION DRUG PRODUCTS

ACARBOSE
TABLET; ORAL
> PRECOSE
>> BAYER 50MG N020482 001 SEP 06, 1995
>> 100MG N020482 002 SEP 06, 1995

ACEBUTOLOL HYDROCHLORIDE
CAPSULE; ORAL
> ACEBUTOLOL HCL
>> AB MYLAN EQ 200MG BASE N074288 001 APR 24, 1995
>> AB   EQ 400MG BASE N074288 002 APR 24, 1995
>> AB WATSON LABS EQ 200MG BASE N074007 001 OCT 18, 1995
>> AB   EQ 400MG BASE N074007 002 OCT 18, 1995
> SECTRAL
>> AB WYETH AYERST EQ 200MG BASE N018917 001 DEC 28, 1984
>> AB * EQ 400MG BASE N018917 003 DEC 28, 1984

ACETAMINOPHEN; ASPIRIN; CODEINE PHOSPHATE
CAPSULE; ORAL
> ACETAMINOPHEN, ASPIRIN, AND CODEINE PHOSPHATE
>> * MIKART 150MG;180MG;15MG N081095 001 OCT 26, 1990
>> * 150MG;180MG;30MG N081096 001 OCT 26, 1990
>> * 150MG;180MG;60MG N081097 001 OCT 26, 1990

ACETAMINOPHEN; BUTALBITAL
CAPSULE; ORAL
> BUTALBITAL AND ACETAMINOPHEN
>> AB GRAHAM 650MG;50MG N088991 001 JUN 28, 1985
> CONTEN
>> AB GRAHAM 650MG;50MG N089405 001 MAY 15, 1990
> PHRENILIN FORTE
>> AB + CARNRICK 650MG;50MG N088831 001 JUN 19, 1985
> TRIAPRIN
>> DUNHALL 325MG;50MG N089268 001 JUL 02, 1987

ACETAMINOPHEN; BUTALBITAL (continued)
TABLET; ORAL
> BUTALBITAL AND ACETAMINOPHEN
>> AB DANBURY PHARMA 325MG;50MG N087550 001 OCT 19, 1984
> BUTAPAP
>> AB MIKART 325MG;50MG N089987 001 OCT 26, 1992
>> AB   650MG;50MG N089988 001 OCT 26, 1992
> PHRENILIN
>> AB + CARNRICK 325MG;50MG N087811 001 JUN 19, 1985
> SEDAPAP
>> AB + MAYRAND 650MG;50MG N088964 001 OCT 17, 1985

ACETAMINOPHEN; BUTALBITAL; CAFFEINE
CAPSULE; ORAL
> ACETAMINOPHEN, BUTALBITAL AND CAFFEINE
>> AB + GILBERT LABS 325MG;50MG;40MG N088825 001 DEC 05, 1984
> ACETAMINOPHEN, BUTALBITAL, AND CAFFEINE
>> AB MIKART 325MG;50MG;40MG N089007 001 MAR 17, 1986
> ANOQUAN
>> AB ROBERTS AND HAUCK 325MG;50MG;40MG N087628 001 OCT 01, 1986
> BUTALBITAL, ACETAMINOPHEN, CAFFEINE
>> AB GRAHAM 325MG;50MG;40MG N088743 001 JUL 18, 1985
>> AB   325MG;50MG;40MG N088758 001 MAR 27, 1985
>> AB   325MG;50MG;40MG N088765 001 MAR 27, 1985
>> AB   325MG;50MG;40MG N089023 001 JUN 19, 1985
>> AB   325MG;50MG;40MG N089067 001 APR 19, 1985
>> AB   325MG;50MG;40MG N089102 001 JUN 19, 1985
> ESGIC-PLUS
>> + MIKART 500MG;50MG;40MG N040085 001 MAR 28, 1996

Therapeutic equivalence codes (TE)
Therapeutically equivalent drug products have TE codes beginning with an **"A,"** such as **AB**. Drug products that are not therapeutically equivalent have codes that begin with a **"B,"** such as **BP**.

Drug products offered by a single source do not have TE codes.

THOMSON

MICROMEDEX

Volume III

Approved Drug Products

and Legal Requirements

FREE MONTHLY UPDATES
on the Internet!
See inside front cover
for more details.

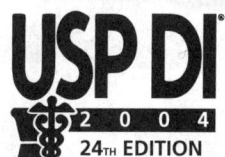
USP DI
2 0 0 4
24TH EDITION

Content reviewed by the United States Pharmacopeial Convention, Inc.

Contents

USP DI—Volume III
Approved Drug Products and Legal Requirements

USP DI—Volume III
Approved Drug Products and Legal Requirements

Preface

Volume III is not a product of the USP Council of Experts, although some of the Committee determinations in *USP–NF* are reproduced in it. Rather, Volume III is intended as a service to those who need a convenient source of the legal requirements that affect prescribing/dispensing activities—more convenient, and considerably less expensive than tracking them all down and purchasing them separately.

Volume III contains federal and state requirements relevant to the dispensing situation, including:
- the FDA's "Orange Book," *Approved Drug Products with Therapeutic Equivalence Evaluations.*
- a separate listing of B-rated drugs.
- a list of pre-1938 ("grandfathered") products.
- abstracted *USP–NF* monograph requirements relating to strength, quality, purity, packaging, labeling, and storage.
- selected *USP–NF* General Chapters and General Notices particularly applicable to the practice situation.
- selected portions of the Federal Food, Drug and Cosmetic Act relating to drugs for human and animal use, and to dietary supplements.
- the FDA's Current Good Manufacturing Practice Regulations for Finished Pharmaceuticals.

The entire Orange Book and those supplements issued up to our printing deadline are directly reproduced in this 2004 Volume III.

Inclusion of these selected federal statutes and regulations should assist in voluntary compliance. However, pharmacists should consult with official versions of the laws (United States Code) and regulations (Code of Federal Regulations) for complete information. Inclusion of drug standards information from the *United States Pharmacopeia* and the *National Formulary* should assist practitioners in obtaining a better understanding of drug product quality requirements overall.

The Orange Book—The FDA list, *Approved Drug Products with Therapeutic Equivalence Evaluations,* serves two basic purposes:
(1) it identifies the prescription and nonprescription drug products formally approved by the FDA on the basis of safety and effectiveness; and
(2) it provides the FDA's therapeutic equivalence evaluations for those approved multi-source prescription drug products.

In 1984, the Food, Drug and Cosmetic Act (FFDC) was amended by the Drug Price Competition and Patent Term Restoration Act. This law requires the FDA to publish a list of all currently approved drug products and to update it on a monthly basis. The Orange Book and its supplements satisfy this statutory requirement. An addendum providing patent information and identifying those drugs which qualify under this Act for periods of exclusivity is also included.

The Orange Book is referenced in numerous state laws and regulations governing drug substitution in prescribing/dispensing.

USP–NF requirements—The United States Pharmacopeial Convention is the publisher of the *United States Pharmacopeia* and the *National Formulary*. These texts are recognized as official compendia under federal law and by the pharmacy and medical professions. They contain standards, specifications, and other requirements relating to drugs and other articles used in medical and pharmacy practice that may be enforceable under various statutes. These requirements are applicable not only when drugs are in the possession of the manufacturer, but at the practice level as well.

Although the standards continue to be applicable when drugs are dispensed or sold, it must also be recognized that most prescriptions today are filled with manufactured products and for the most part physicians and pharmacists do not routinely compound or analyze drug products. On the other hand, dispensers need to be aware of the quality attributes of products, their packaging and storage requirements, and the other applicable standards to which legal consequences may attach.

In recognition of this need, Volume III presents abstracts of the applicable *USP–NF* standards. Similarly, selected portions of the *USP–NF* General Notices and Chapters that are deemed to be especially relevant are reprinted in Volume III. These extracts have been taken from *USP 27–NF 22*, as it appeared on January 1, 2004.

The incorporation of these official *USP–NF* materials into *USP DI* is for informational purposes only. Because of varying publication schedules, there may occasionally be a time difference between publication of revisions in the *USP–NF* and the appearance of these changes in *USP DI*. Readers are advised that only the standards as written in the *USP–NF* are official.

The *USP–NF* material included in *USP DI* is not intended to represent nor shall it be interpreted to be the equivalent of or a substitute for the official *United States Pharmacopeia* and/or *National Formulary*. In the event of any difference or discrepancy between the current official *USP* or *NF* standards and the information contained herein, the context and effect of the official compendia shall prevail.

Acknowledgments—The efforts of the USP Legal Department, in particular those of F. Gail Bormel, Lynn Lang, and Joseph G. Valentino, in abstracting the various statutes and regulations, should be noted.

USP PEOPLE 2000 – 2005

Ronald J. Callahan, Ph.D., Boston, MA;
Edward M. Cohen, Ph.D., Danbury, CT;
Mark G. Papich, DVM, Raleigh, NC;
Stephen G. Schulman, Ph.D., Gainesville, FL;
James T. Stewart, Ph.D., Athens, GA;
Henry S. I. Tan, Ph.D., Cincinnati, OH;
Timothy J. Wozniak, Ph.D., Indianapolis, IN

Nomenclature and Labeling Expert Committee (2000 – 2005)

Herbert S. Carlin, D.Sc., *Chair*, Califon, NJ;
Loyd V. Allen, Jr., Ph.D., Edmond, OK;

Joseph M. Betz, Ph.D., Bethesda, MD;
Dawn M. Boothe, DVM, College Station, TX;
Daniel L. Boring, Ph.D., Silver Spring, MD;
Edward M. Cohen, Ph.D., Danbury, CT;
Stephanie Y. Crawford, Ph.D., Chicago, IL;
Thomas S. Foster, Pharm.D., Lexington, KY;
Douglas D. Glover, M.D., Morgantown, WV;
Michael J. Groves, Ph.D., Deerfield, IL;
R. David Lauper, Pharm.D., Dublin, CA;
Keith Marshall, Ph.D., Brick, NJ;
Jerry Phillips, BS, Rockville, MD;
Thomas P. Reinders, Pharm.D., Richmond, VA;

2000 – 2005 INFORMATION EXPERT COMMITTEES

Members who serve as Chairs are listed first.

The information presented in this text represents an ongoing review of the drugs contained herein and represents a consensus of various viewpoints expressed. The individuals listed below have served on the USP Expert Committees for the 2000-2005 revision period and have contributed to the development of the 2004 USP DI database. Such listing does not imply that these individuals have reviewed all of the material in this text or that they individually agree with all statements contained therein.

Jan F. Towers, Ph.D., Biglerville, PA;
Philip D. Walson, M.D., Cincinnati, OH

Anesthesiology
Carl E. Rosow, M.D., *Chair*, Boston, MA; Charles J. Cote, M.D., Chicago, IL; Peter Glass, M.D., Stoneybrook, NY; Michele E. Gold, Ph.D., Los Angeles, CA; Thomas K. Henthorn, M.D., Denver, CO; Michael B. Howie, M.D., Columbus, OH; Robert Hudson, M.D., Winnipeg, MB, Canada; Susan K. Palmer, M.D., West Linn, OR; Mark A. Schumacher, Ph.D., M.D., San Francisco, CA; Peter S. Sebel, Ph.D., Atlanta, GA; Theodore W. Striker, M.D., Cincinnati, OH; Mehernoor F. Watcha, M.D., Philadelphia, PA; David H. Wong, M.D., Long Beach, CA

Cardiovascular and Renal Drugs
Alexander M. Shepherd, M.D., Ph.D., *Chair*, San Antonio, TX; Ellon D. Burgess, M.D., Calgary, Alberta, Canada; Moses S.S. Chow, Pharm.D., Shatin, Hong Kong; Ross D. Feldman, M.D., London, ON, Canada; Jean D. Gray, M.D., Halifax, NS, Canada; Brian B. Hoffman, M.D., Palo Alto, CA; Joseph Izzo, M.D., Buffalo, NY; Howard R. Knapp, M.D., Ph.D., Billings, MT; Peter Kowey, M.D., Wynnewood, PA; Barry Massie, M.D., San Francisco, CA; Jean M. Nappi, Pharm.D., Charleston, SC; Cynthia L. Raehl, Pharm.D., Amarillo, TX; Addison A. Taylor, M.D., Ph.D., Houston, TX; Gerald J. Wilson, MA, M.B.A., Potomac, MD

Clinical Toxicology and Substance Abuse
Edward P. Krenzelok, Pharm.D., *Chair*, Pittsburgh, PA; Bruce D. Anderson, Pharm.D., Baltimore, M.D.; Donald G. Barceloux, M.D., Topanga, CA; Neal L. Benowitz, M.D., San Francisco, CA; Jeffrey Brent, M.D., Denver, CO; Gregory G. Gaar, M.D., Tampa, FL; Robert S. Hoffman, M.D., New York, NY; Jude McNally, R.Ph., Tucson, AZ; Elizabeth Scharman, Pharm.D., Charleston, WV; Rose Ann G. Soloway, MS, Washington, DC; Christine M. Stork, Pharm.D., Syracuse, NY; Milton Tenenbein, M.D., Winnipeg, MB, Canada; J. Allister Vale, M.D., Birmingham, England; William A. Watson, Pharm.D., San Antonio, TX

Critical Care and Emergency Medicine
Daniel A. Notterman, M.D., *Chair*, New Brunswick, NJ; Philip Barie, M.D., New York, NY; Joseph Carcillo, M.D., Pittsburgh, PA; Eugene Y. Cheng, M.D., San Jose, CA; George Foltin, M.D., New York, NY; Louis J. Ling, M.D., Minneapolis, MN; Steven Lowry, M.D., New Brunswick, NJ; Catherine MacLeod, M.D., East Hanover, NJ; Gail McCarver, M.D., Milwaukee, WI; Mary McCready, RN, New York, NY; Elena Mendez-Rico, Pharm.D., New York, NY; Lewis Nelson, M.D., New York, NY; Arthur Slutsky, M.D., Toronto, ON, Canada

Dentistry
Bridget E. Byrne, R.Ph., DDS, Ph.D., *Chair*, Richmond, VA; Gary C. Armitage, DDS, San Francisco, CA; Sebastian G. Ciancio, DDS, Buffalo, NY; Frederick A. Curro, D.M.D., Ph.D., Emerson, NJ; Raymond A. Dionne, DDS, Bethesda, MD; Tommy W. Gage, Ph.D., Rockwall, TX; Michael Glick, M.D., Newark, NJ; Daniel A. Haas, Ph.D., Toronto, ON, Canada; Arthur H. Jeske, D.M.D., Ph.D., Houston, TX; Christopher L. Maestrello, DDS, Richmond, VA; Barbara Regua-Clark, Pharm.D., Kansas City, MO; Joel M. Weaver, DDS, Ph.D., Columbus, OH; Clifford W. Whall, Ph.D., Chicago, IL; John A. Yagiela, DDS, Ph.D., Los Angeles, CA

Dermatology
Michael E. Bigby, M.D., *Chair*, Boston, MA; Robert B. Armstrong, M.D., Raritan, NJ; Mary-Margaret Chren, M.D., San Francisco, CA; Vincent Falanga, M.D., Providence, RI; Gordon L. Flynn, Ph.D., Ann Arbor, MI; Aditya K. Gupta, M.D., London, ON, Canada; Vincent Ho, M.D., Vancouver, BC, Canada; Sewon Kang, M.D., Ann Arbor, MI; David Margolis, M.D., Ph.D., Philadelphia, PA; Scott Norton, M.D., MPH, Washington, D.C.; Jean-Claude Roujeau, M.D., Creteil, France; Matthew Stiller, M.D., New York, NY; Dennis P. West, Ph.D., Chicago, IL

Diagnostic Agents – Nonradioactive
Sachiko T. Cochran, M.D., *Chair*, Los Angeles, CA; Max D. Adams, Ph.D., St. Charles, MO; Michael A. Bettmann, M.D., Lebanon, NH; Martin J.K. Blomley, MBBS, London, England; Robert C. Brasch, M.D., San Francisco, CA; Henry Bryant, Ph.D., Bethesda, M.D.; Richard W. Katzberg, M.D., Sacramento, CA; Elliott C. Lasser, M.D., La Jolla, CA; Maythem Saeed, DVM, Ph.D., San Francisco, CA; Udo P. Schmiedl, M.D., Seattle, WA; Jovitas Skucas, M.D., Rochester, NY; David B. Spring, M.D., Oakland, CA; Michael F. Tweedle, Ph.D., Princeton, NJ

Dietary Supplements
Tieraona Low Dog, M.D., *Chair*, Corrales, NM; Marilyn L. Barrett, Ph.D., San Carlos, CA; Werner R. Busse, Ph.D., Karlsruhe, Germany; Elaine Chiquette, Pharm.D., San Antonio, TX; Cynthia T. Culmo, RPh, Austin, TX; Adriane J. Fugh-Berman, M.D., Washington, DC; Kathryn L. Grant, Pharm.D., Tucson, AZ; Gail B. Mahady, Ph.D., Chicago, IL; Paolo Morazzoni, Ph.D., Milano, Italy; Harold H. Sandstead, M.D., Galveston, TX; Judith S. Stern, ScD, Lafayette, CA

Endocrinology
Lawrence A. Frohman, M.D., *Chair*, Chicago, IL; Stuart J. Brink, M.D., Waltham, MA; Karim Anton Calis, Pharm.D., Bethesda, M.D.; David S. Cooper, M.D., Baltimore, M.D.; Betty J. Dong, Pharm.D., San Francisco, CA; Selna L. Kaplan, M.D., San Francisco, CA; Michael Kleerekoper, M.D., Detroit, MI; James Liu, M.D., Cleveland, OH; Shlomo Melmed, M.D., Los Angeles, CA; John E. Morley, M.D., St. Louis, MO; Paul Saenger, M.D., Bronx, NY; Arthur B. Schneider, M.D., Chicago, IL; Ronald Swerdloff, M.D., Torrance, CA

Gastroenterology
Karl E. Anderson, M.D., *Chair*, Galveston, TX; Jeffrey P. Baker, M.D., Toronto, ON, Canada; Paul Bass, Ph.D., Madison, WI; Gerald Friedman, M.D., New York, NY; Flavio M. Habal, M.D., Toronto, ON, Canada; Melvin B. Heyman, M.D., San Francisco, CA; Karen C. Hobdy-Henderson, Pharm.D., Nashville, TN; Alan F. Hofmann, M.D., La Jolla, CA; Paul E. Hyman, M.D., Kansas City, KS; Gordon L. Klein, M.D., Galveston, TX; William J. Snape Jr., M.D., San Francisco, CA; Keith G. Tolman, M.D., Salt Lake City, UT

Gerontology
Darrell R. Abernethy, M.D., *Chair*, Baltimore, M.D.; Larry A. Bauer, Pharm.D., Seattle, WA; John C. Beck, M.D., Pacific Palisades, CA; James W. Cooper, Ph.D., Athens, GA; Barry J. Cusack, M.D., Boise, ID; Joseph T. Hanlon, Pharm.D., Minneapolis, MN; Patricia D. Kroboth, Ph.D., Pittsburgh, PA; Shari M. Ling, M.D., Baltimore, MD; Paul A. Mitenko, M.D., Nanaimo, BC, Canada; Maureen J. Osis, RN, MN, Calgary, Alberta, Canada; Bruce G. Pollock, M.D., Pittsburgh, PA; Janice B. Schwartz, M.D., San Francisco, CA; Joanne G. Schwartzberg, M.D., Chicago, IL; Brian L. Strom, M.D., Philadelphia, PA; Alastair J. Wood, M.D., Nashville, TN

Hematology, Blood and Blood Products
Patrick A. McKee, M.D., *Chair*, Oklahoma City, OK; Morris A. Blajchman, M.D., Hamilton, ON, Canada; Kenneth Bridges, M.D., Boston, MA; Ronald O. Gilcher, M.D., Oklahoma City, OK; Naomi Luban, M.D., Washington, DC; Joe Moake, M.D., Houston, TX; Kevin Moore, M.D., Oklahoma City, OK; Margaret Pierce, MSN, MPH, Knoxville, TN; David S. Rosenthal, M.D., Cambridge, MA

Immunizing Agents
Cheston M. Berlin Jr., M.D., *Chair*, Hershey, PA; Ron Dagan, M.D., Beersheva, Israel; John D. Grabenstein, Ph.D., Falls Church, VA; Jill Hackell, Pearl River, NY; Barbara J. Howe, M.D., King of Prussia, PA; Karen Kaplan, M.D., West Point, PA; Benjamin Levi, M.D., Ph.D., Hershey, PA; Carlton Meschievitz,

INFORMATION DIVISION
ADDITIONAL CONTRIBUTORS

The information presented in the USP DI database represents ongoing review and the consensus of various viewpoints expressed. In addition to the individuals listed elsewhere many schools, associations, pharmaceutical companies, and governmental agencies have provided comment or otherwise contributed to the development of the 2004 USP DI database.

MEMBERS OF THE UNITED STATES
PHARMACOPEIAL CONVENTION
as of May 2003

U.S. Colleges and Schools of Medicine
Boston University School of Medicine, Carol T. Walsh, Ph.D.
Brown University School of Medicine, Edward Hawrot, Ph.D.
Creighton University School of Medicine, Peter W. Abel, Ph.D.
Duke University Medical Center School of Medicine, Michael J. Gabriel, Ph.D.
East Carolina University Brody School of Medicine, Donald W. Barnes, Ph.D.
East Tennessee State University Quillen College of Medicine, Peter J. Rice, Ph.D.
Harvard Medical School, David E. Golan, M.D., Ph.D.
Indiana University School of Medicine, David R. Jones, Ph.D.
Johns Hopkins University School of Medicine, Daniel M. Ashby, M.S., FASHP
Loma Linda University School of Medicine, W. William Hughes, Ph.D.
Loyola University Stritch School of Medicine, Stanley A. Lorens, Ph.D.
Mayo Medical School, Andre Terzic, M.D., Ph.D.
MCP-Hahnemann School of Medicine, Michael M. White, Ph.D.
Morehouse School of Medicine, David E. Potter, Ph.D.
New York Medical College, Mario A. Inchiosa, Ph.D.
Oregon Health Sciences University School of Medicine, George D. Olsen, M.D.
Pennsylvania State University College of Medicine, Charles D. Smith, M.D.
Ponce School of Medicine, Manuel Martinez-Maldonado, M.D.
Stanford University School of Medicine, Edward D. Harris, Jr., M.D.
SUNY at Buffalo School of Medicine and Biomedical Sciences, Paul J. Kostyniak, Ph.D.
The Medical College of Georgia School of Medicine, Anthony L. Mulloy, DO
The University of Iowa College of Medicine, John E. Kasik, M.D., Ph.D.
Tufts University School of Medicine, William Gouveia, M.S.
Universidad Central del Caribe School of Medicine, Carmen M. Suarez, M.D.
University of California Davis School of Medicine, Timothy E. Albertson, M.D., Ph.D.
University of California Irvine College of Medicine, Gregory Prouty, Pharm.D.
University of California San Diego School of Medicine, Harold J. Simon, M.D., Ph.D.
University of California San Francisco School of Medicine, Linda L. Liu, M.D.
University of Chicago Pritzker School of Medicine, Mark J. Ratain, MD
University of Colorado School of Medicine, Joseph Gal, Ph.D.
University of Connecticut Health Center School of Medicine, Paul F. Davern, M.B.A.
University of Florida College of Medicine, Lal C. Garg, Ph.D.
University of Hawaii John A. Burns School of Medicine, Bert K.B. Lum, Ph.D., M.D.
University of Louisville School of Medicine, Peter P. Rowell, Ph.D.
University of Maryland School of Medicine, Jordan E. Warnick, Ph.D.
University of Medicine and Dentistry of New Jersey–Robert Wood Johnson Medical School, Alice B. Gottlieb, M.D., Ph.D.
University of Nebraska College of Medicine, Terry D. Hexum, Ph.D.
University of New Mexico School of Medicine, Ellen M. Cosgrove, M.D.
University of North Dakota School of Medicine and Health Sciences, Manuchair Ebadi, Ph.D.

University of Oklahoma College of Medicine, Gary E. Raskob, Ph.D.
University of Pittsburgh School of Medicine, Carl A. Sirio, M.D.
University of Rochester School of Medicine and Dentistry, Richard C. Reichman, M.D.
University of South Alabama College of Medicine, Samuel J. Strada, Ph.D.
University of South Florida College of Medicine, Joseph J. Krzanowski, Ph.D.
University of Southern California Keck School of Medicine, Paul D. Holtom, M.D.
University of Texas-Houston Medical School, Gary C. Rosenfeld, PhD
University of Washington School of Medicine, Georgiana K. Ellis, M.D.
Wake Forest University School of Medicine, Jack W. Strandhoy, Ph.D.
West Virginia University Robert C. Byrd Health Sciences Center, Douglas D. Glover, MD
Wright State University School of Medicine, Robert L. Koerker, Ph.D.

State Medical Societies
California Medical Association, Rene H. Bravo, M.D.
Idaho Medical Association, Lawrence L. Knight, M.D.
Indiana State Medical Association, Daria Schooler, M.D., R.Ph.
Iowa Medical Society, Harold W. Miller, M.D.
Kentucky Medical Association, Donald R. Neel, M.D.
Louisiana State Medical Society, Merlin H. Allen, M.D.
Massachusetts Medical Society, Bruce G. Karlin, M.D.
Medical Association of Georgia, John S. Antalis, M.D.
Medical Society of New Jersey, Joseph N. Micale, M.D.
Medical Society of the District of Columbia, Kim A. Bullock, M.D.
Medical Society of the State of New York, Richard S. Blum, M.D.
Missouri State Medical Association, C.C. Swarens
Nebraska Medical Association, Fred H. Ayers, M.D.
North Carolina Medical Society, Carl K. Rust, II, M.D.
Oklahoma State Medical Association, Carl Manion, M.D.
State Medical Society of Wisconsin, Melvin Rosen, M.D., Ph.D.
Washington State Medical Association, William O. Robertson, M.D.

U.S. Colleges and Schools of Pharmacy
Albany College of Pharmacy, Mary Andritz, Pharm.D.
Auburn University School of Pharmacy, Kenneth N. Barker, Ph.D.
Butler University College of Pharmacy and Health Sciences, LeRoy Salerni, Ph.D.
Creighton University School of Pharmacy and Allied Health Professions, Kenneth R. Keefner, Ph.D.
Drake University College of Pharmacy and Health Sciences, Sidney L. Finn, Ph.D.
Duquesne University Mylan School of Pharmacy, Lawrence H. Block, Ph.D.
Ferris State University College of Pharmacy, Kim E. Hancock, Ph.D.
Howard University College of Pharmacy, Nursing & AHS, Pedro J. Lecca, Ph.D.
Idaho State University College of Pharmacy, Thomas R. LaHann, Ph.D.
Massachusetts College of Pharmacy and Health Sciences, David A. Williams, Ph.D.

Mercer University Southern School of Pharmacy, J. Grady Strom, Ph.D.

Midwestern University Chicago College of Pharmacy, Thomas J. Reutzel, Ph.D.

Midwestern University College of Pharmacy - Glendale, Edward Fisher, Ph.D.

NOVA Southeastern University College of Pharmacy, William D. Hardigan, Ph.D.

North Dakota State University College of Pharmacy, Jagdish Singh, Ph.D.

Northeastern University Bouve College of Pharmacy, Mansoor A. Amiji, Ph.D.

Ohio Northern University College of Pharmacy, Kimberly Broedel-Zaugg, Ph.D.

Oregon State University College of Pharmacy, Wayne A. Kradjan, Pharm.D.

Purdue University School of Pharmacy & Pharmacal Sciences, Stephen R. Byrn, PhD

Rutgers University College of Pharmacy, Thomas Medwick, PhD

Samford University McWhorter School of Pharmacy, H. Anthony McBride, Ph.D.

Shenandoah University Bernard J. Dunn School of Pharmacy, Regina F. Peacock, Ph.D.

South Dakota State University College of Pharmacy, Yadhu N. Singh, Ph.D.

Southwestern Oklahoma State University School of Pharmacy, Keith W. Reichmann, Ph.D.

St. Louis College of Pharmacy, Thomas F. Patton, Ph.D.

State University of New York at Buffalo School of Pharmacy, Wayne K. Anderson, Ph.D.

Texas Southern University College of Pharmacy and Health Sciences, Dong Liang, Ph.D.

Texas Tech University School of Pharmacy, Arthur A. Nelson, Ph.D.

The University of Arizona College of Pharmacy, Michael Mayersohn, PhD

The University of Georgia College of Pharmacy, James T. Stewart, PhD

The University of Iowa College of Pharmacy, Dale E. Wurster, Ph.D.

The University of Toledo College of Pharmacy, Laurie S. Mauro, Pharm.D.

University of Arkansas for Medical Sciences College of Pharmacy, Jonathan J. Wolfe, Ph.D.

University of California San Francisco School of Pharmacy, Emil T. Lin, Ph.D.

University of Cincinnati College of Pharmacy, Arthur R. Buckley, Ph.D.

University of Colorado School of Pharmacy, Louis Diamond, Ph.D.

University of Connecticut School of Pharmacy, Michael C. Gerald, Ph.D.

University of Florida College of Pharmacy, Michael W. McKenzie, Ph.D.

University of Houston College of Pharmacy, Mustafa F. Lokhandwala, Ph.D.

University of Illinois College of Pharmacy, John F. Fitzloff, Ph.D.

University of Kansas School of Pharmacy, J. Howard Rytting, Ph.D.

University of Kentucky College of Pharmacy, Kelly M. Smith, Pharm.D.

University of Maryland School of Pharmacy, Larry L. Augsburger, PhD

University of Michigan College of Pharmacy, Duane M. Kirking, PhD

University of Minnesota College of Pharmcy, Marilyn K. Speedie, Ph.D.

University of Mississippi School of Pharmacy, Christy M. Wyandt, Ph.D.

University of Missouri-Kansas City School of Pharmacy, Patrick J. Bryant, Pharm D.

University of Montana School of Pharmacy and Allied Health Sciences, David S. Forbes, Ph.D.

University of Nebraska College of Pharmacy, Clarence T. Ueda, Pharm.D., Ph.D.

University of New Mexico College of Pharmacy, John A. Pieper, Pharm.D.

University of North Carolina School of Pharmacy, Anthony J. Hickey, Ph.D.

University of Oklahoma College of Pharmacy, Loyd V. Allen, Jr., PhD

University of Pittsburgh School of Pharmacy, Dennis P. Swanson, MS

University of Puerto Rico, Medical Sciences Campus School of Pharmacy, Ilia I. Oquendo, Ph.D.

University of Rhode Island College of Pharmacy, Hossein Zia, Ph.D.

University of South Carolina College of Pharmacy, L. Clifton Fuhrman, Ph.D.

University of Southern California School of Pharmacy, Wei-Chiang Shen, Ph.D.

University of Tennessee College of Pharmacy, Dick R. Gourley, Pharm.D.

University of Texas at Austin College of Pharmacy, Salomon Stavchansky, Ph.D.

University of the Pacific School of Pharmacy, William Chan, Ph.D.

University of the Sciences in Philadelphia, Daniel A. Hussar, Ph.D.

University of Utah College of Pharmacy, John W. Mauger, Ph.D.

University of Washington School of Pharmacy, Gary W. Elmer, Ph.D.

University of Wisconsin School of Pharmacy, Melvin H. Weinswig, Ph.D.

University of Wyoming School of Pharmacy, Kurt Dolence, Ph.D.

Virginia Commonwealth University/Medical College of Virginia School of Pharmacy, Mary Ann Kirkpatrick, Ph.D.

Washington State University College of Pharmacy, Danial E. Baker, Pharm.D.

Wayne State University College of Pharmacy and Allied Health Professions Craig K. Svensson, Pharm.D., Ph.D.

West Virginia University School of Pharmacy, Arthur I. Jacknowitz, Pharm.D.

Western University of Health Sciences College of Pharmacy, Sunil Prabhu, Ph.D.

Xavier University of Louisiana College of Pharmacy, Tarun K. Mandal, Ph.D.

State Pharmacy Associations

Alaska Pharmacy Association, Roger Penrod, R.Ph.

Arizona Pharmacy Association, Edward P. Armstrong, PharmD

California Pharmacists Association, R. David Lauper, Pharm.D.

Colegio de Farmaceuticos de Puerto Rico, Benjamin Perez

Connecticut Pharmacists Association, Henry A. Palmer, Ph.D.

Delaware Pharmacists Society, Kenneth Musto, R.Ph.

Florida Pharmacy Association, Michael A. Mone, B.S., J.D.

Georgia Pharmacists Association, Oren "Buddy" Harden, R.Ph.

Hawaii Pharmacists Association, Ronald T. Taniguchi, Pharm.D.

Idaho State Pharmacy Association, Edward Reddish, B.S.

Illinois Pharmacists Association, Ronald W. Gottrich, R.Ph.

Indiana Pharmacists Alliance, Bonnie K. Brown, Pharm.D.

Iowa Pharmacists Association, Thomas R. Temple, R.Ph., M.S.

Kentucky Pharmacists Association, Robert L. Barnett, R.Ph.

Maryland Pharmacists Association, Matthew G. Shimoda, Pharm.D.

Massachusetts Pharmacists Association, Steven D. Geoffroy, R.Ph.

Michigan Pharmacists Association, Joseph Ringer, M.B.A.

Mississippi Pharmacists Association, Ronnie Bagwell

Montana Pharmacy Association, Lori Morin, M.B.A., R.Ph.

Nebraska Pharmacists Association, Maurice L. Russell, B.S.

New Hampshire Pharmacists Association, Elizabeth A. Gower, R.Ph.

New Jersey Pharmacists Association, Steve H. Zlotnick, Pharm.D.

New Mexico Pharmaceutical Association, William G. Troutman, Pharm.D

North Carolina Association of Pharmacists, Stephen F. Eckel, Pharm.D.

North Dakota Pharmaceutical Association, Galen D. Jordre, R.Ph.

Ohio Pharmacists Association, Amelia S. Bennett, R.Ph.

Oregon State Pharmacists Association, Tom Holt

Pharmacy Society of Wisconsin, Judith E. Thompson, R.Ph., M.S.

South Carolina Pharmacy Association, James R. Bracewell

South Dakota Pharmacists Association, Monica Jones

Texas Pharmacy Association, Eric H. Frankel, Pharm.D., MSE.

Utah Pharmaceutical Association, Reid L. Barker

Virginia Pharmacists Association, Marianne R. Rollings, R.Ph.

Washington D.C. Pharmaceutical Association, Herbert Kwash, R.Ph.

Washington State Pharmacists Association, Rodney D. Shafer, R.Ph.

National and State Professional and Scientific Organizations

Academy of Managed Care Pharmacy, Marissa Schlaifer, M.S., R.Ph.

American Academy of Allergy, Asthma and Immunology, Lanny J. Rosenwasser, M.D.

American Academy of Clinical Toxicology, Inc., Edward P. Krenzelok, PharmD

American Academy of Family Physicians, Charles E. Driscoll, M.D.

American Academy of Neurology, Thomas N. Chase, M.D.

American Academy of Nurse Practitioners, Jan Towers, Ph.D., NP-C

American Academy of Ophthalmology, Joel S. Mindel, MD

American Academy of Pediatrics, Richard L. Gorman, M.D.

American Academy of Physician Assistants, Robert J. McNellis, MPH, PA-C

American Academy of Veterinary Pharmacology and Therapeutics, Cory Langston, DVM, Ph.D.

American Association of Colleges of Nursing, Ellen Rudy, Ph.D.

American Association of Colleges of Osteopathic Medicine, Anthony J. Silvagni, D.O., Pharm.D.

American Association of Colleges of Pharmacy, Kenneth W. Miller, Ph.D.

American Association of Critical-Care Nurses, Barbara A. Johnston, Ph.D.

American Association of Pharmaceutical Scientists, Eugene F. Fiese, Ph.D.

American Association of Pharmacy Technicians, Inc., Douglas E. Scribner

American Association of Poison Control Centers, Rose Ann G. Soloway, BSN, MS

American Chemical Society, David A. Fay, Ph.D.

American College of Cardiology, William E. Boden, M.D., FACC

American College of Clinical Pharmacy, C. Edwin Webb, Pharm.D.

American College of Obstetricians and Gynecologists, Marilynn C. Frederiksen, M.D.
American College of Physicians-American Society of Internal Medicine, David A. Flockhart, M.D., Ph.D.
American Dental Association, Clifford W. Whall, Ph.D
American Dental Education Association, Vahn A. Lewis, Ph.D.
American Gastroenterological Association, Elizabeth A. Adams, MPH
American Geriatrics Society, Jerry Gurwitz, M.D.
American Medical Association, Joseph W. Cranston, Ph.D.
American Nurses Association, Inc., Rita Munley Gallagher, PhD, RN, C
American Optometric Association, Jimmy D. Bartlett, O.D.
American Osteopathic Association, Max T. McKinney, D.O.
American Pharmaceutical Association, Robert D. Gibson, Pharm.D.
American Podiatric Medical Association, Pamela J. Colman, DPM
American Psychiatric Association, Lloyd I. Sederer, M.D.
American Society for Clinical Pharmacology and Therapeutics, Sally U. Yasuda, Pharm.D.
American Society for Healthcare Risk Management, Monica Berry, J.D.
American Society for Pharmacology and Experimental Therapeutics, Kenneth L. Dretchen, Ph.D.
American Society of Clinical Oncology, Michael B. Troner, M.D.
American Society of Consultant Pharmacists, Thomas R. Clark, R.Ph,
American Society of Gene Therapy, Kenneth Cornetta, M.D.
American Society of Health-System Pharmacists, Henri R. Manasse, Jr., Ph.D., Sc.D.
American Type Culture Collection, Frank P. Simione, M.S.
American Veterinary Medical Association, Dawn M. Boothe, DVM
Association of American Medical Colleges, Raymond L. Woosley, M.D., Ph.D.
Association of Food and Drug Officials, Cynthia T. Culmo, RPh
Drug Information Association, Judith Weissinger, Ph.D.
Federation of State Medical Boards of the United States, Inc., Dale L. Austin, M.A.
Infusion Nurses Society, Mary Alexander, CRNI
International Academy of Compounding Pharmacists, E. Eldon Armstrong
National Association of Boards of Pharmacy, Carmen A. Catizone, M.S., R.Ph.
National Community Pharmacists Association (formerly NARD), Jack Dease, B.S.
National Medical Association, Randall W. Maxey, M.D., Ph.D.
National Pharmaceutical Association, Barry A. Bleidt, Ph.D.
New Jersey Pharmaceutical Quality Control Association, Herbert Letterman, Ph.D.
Oncology Nursing Society, Barbara B. Rogers, CRNP, MN, AOCN
Regulatory Affairs Professionals Society, Sherry L. Keramidas, Ph.D., CAE

Governmental Bodies

Agency for Healthcare Research and Quality, Lynn A. Bosco, M.D.
Centers for Disease Control and Prevention, John A. Becher
Centers for Medicare and Medicaid Services (formerly HCFA), Sean R. Tunis, M.D., M.Sc.
Department of Veterans Affairs Veterans Health Administration, John E. Ogden
FDA Center for Biologics Evaluation and Research, Jerome A. Donlon, M.D., Ph.D.
FDA Center for Devices and Radiological Health, Marilyn M. Lightfoote, M.D., Ph.D.
FDA Center for Drug Evaluation and Research, Yana R. Mille
FDA Center for Food Safety and Applied Nutrition, Elizabeth A. Yetley, Ph.D.
FDA Center for Veterinary Medicine, Claire M. Lathers, Ph.D.
Health Canada, Sultan Ghani, B.S., M.Ph.
National Institute of Standards and Technology, John R. Rumble, Ph.D.
National Institutes of Health, Joseph F. Gallelli, Ph.D.
United States Air Force, Ardis Meier
United States Army Office of the Surgeon General, W. Michael Heath, M.B.A., B.S.
United States Department of Health and Human Services, Arthur J. Lawrence, Ph.D., R.Ph.,
United States Navy Bureau of Medicine and Surgery, Elizabeth A. Nolan
United States Public Health Service, Patrick J. McNeilly, Ph.D.

Health Science and other Foreign Organizations and Pharmacopeias

Association of Faculties of Pharmacy of Canada, Colin J. Briggs, Ph.D.
Canadian Nurses Association, Sharon Nield
Canadian Pharmacists Association, Jeff Poston, Ph.D.
European Federation of Pharmaceutical Scientists, Hendrik de Jong, Ph.D.
Federation Internationale Pharmaceutique, Daan J.A. Crommelin, Ph.D.
Pan American Health Organization, A. David Brandling-Bennett, M.D.
Permanent Commission of the Mexican United States Pharmacopeia, Carmen Becerril, Chemist
Royal College of Physicians and Surgeons of Canada, Michel Brazeau, M.D.
Russian Center for Pharmaceutical and Medical Technical Information (PHARMEDINFO), Galina Shashkova

Consumer Organizations and Individuals Representing Public Interests

Center for Science in the Public Interest, David G. Schardt, MS
Citizens for Public Action on Blood Pressure and Cholesterol, Inc., Gerald J. Wilson, M.A., M.B.A.
Consumers Union, Christopher J. Hendel
National Consumers League, Rebecca Burkholder, J.D.
National Organization for Rare Disorders, Diane E. Dorman

Domestic, Foreign, and International Manufacturers, Trade, and Affiliated Associations

American Herbal Products Association, Steven J. Dentali, Ph.D.
American Hospital Association, Donald M. Nielsen, M.D.
Council for Responsible Nutrition, V. Annette Dickinson, Ph.D.
Generic Pharmaceutical Association, Steve Bende, Ph.D.
Healthcare Distribution Management Association (formerly NWDA), Lisa D. Clowers
International Pharmaceutical Excipients Council of the Americas, David R. Schoneker, M.S.
Joint Commission on Accreditation of Healthcare Organizations, Jerod M. Loeb, Ph.D.
National Association of Chain Drug Stores, Mary Ann Wagner, B.S.
Nonprescription Drug Manufacturers Association of Canada, David S. Skinner
Parenteral Drug Association, Russell E. Madsen, M.S.
Pharmaceutical Care Management Association, M. John Coburn, Pharm.M.S.
Pharmaceutical Research and Manufacturers of America Science and Regulatory Section, Thomas X. White
The Cosmetic, Toiletry and Fragrance Association, Gerald N. McEwen, Ph.D., J.D.
World Self-Medication Industry, Jerome A. Reinstein, Ph.D.

Committee Members

Barbara A. Durand, Ed.D.
John H. Block, Ph.D.
Thomas M. Schafer, M.B.A.
Gillian R. Woollett, D.Phil., M.A.

Honorary Members

Lloyd E. Davis, D.V.M., Ph.D.
J. Richard Crout, M.D.
Joseph F. Gallelli, Ph.D.
John V. Bergen, Ph.D.
Herbert S. Carlin, DSc
Thomas Medwick, PhD
Lee Anderson, Ph.D.
Klaus G. Florey, Ph.D.
Mary Griffiths
Lester Chafetz, Ph.D.
William M. Heller, Ph.D.
William J. Kinnard, Ph.D.
John H. Moyer, M.D., D.Sc.
John A. Owen, M.D.
Murray S. Cooper, Ph.D.
Salomon Stavchansky, Ph.D.
Donald R. Bennett, M.D., Ph.D.
Kenneth N. Barker, Ph.D.
Enrique Fefer, Ph.D.
Frederick Mahaffey, Pharm.D.

Section I

USP DI VOLUME III REPRODUCTION OF
FDA'S APPROVED DRUG PRODUCTS
WITH THERAPEUTIC EQUIVALENCE EVALUATIONS

24th EDITION
incorporating supplements issued
through June 30, 2003

The products in this list have been approved under sections
505 and 507 of the Federal Food, Drug, and Cosmetic Act.
This information is current through June 30, 2003.

FOOD AND DRUG ADMINISTRATION
CENTER FOR DRUG EVALUATION AND RESEARCH
APPROVED DRUG PRODUCTS
with
Therapeutic Equivalence Evaluations

CONTENTS

Food and Drug Administration
Center for Drug Evaluation and Research
Approved Drug Products
with
Therapeutic Equivalence Evaluations

PREFACE TO TWENTY FOURTH EDITION

The publication, *Approved Drug Products with Therapeutic Equivalence Evaluations* (the List), identifies drug products approved on the basis of safety and effectiveness by the Food and Drug Administration (FDA) under the Federal Food, Drug, and Cosmetic Act (the Act). Drugs on the market approved only on the basis of safety (covered by the ongoing Drug Efficacy Study Implementation [DESI] review [e.g., Donnatal® Tablets and Librax® Capsules] or pre-1938 drugs [e.g., Phenobarbital Tablets]) are not included in this publication. The main criterion for the inclusion of any product is that the product is the subject of an application with an effective approval that has not been withdrawn for safety or efficacy reasons. Inclusion of products on the List is independent of any current regulatory action through administrative or judicial means against a drug product. In addition, the List contains therapeutic equivalence evaluations for approved multisource prescription drug products. These evaluations have been prepared to serve as public information and advice to state health agencies, prescribers, and pharmacists to promote public education in the area of drug product selection and to foster containment of health care costs. Therapeutic equivalence evaluations in this publication are not official FDA actions affecting the legal status of products under the Act.

Background of the Publication. To contain drug costs, virtually every state has adopted laws and/or regulations that encourage the substitution of drug products. These state laws generally require either that substitution be limited to drugs on a specific list (the positive formulary approach) or that it be permitted for all drugs except those prohibited by a particular list (the negative formulary approach). Because of the number of requests in the late 1970s for FDA assistance in preparing both positive and negative formularies, it became apparent that FDA could not serve the needs of each state on an individual basis. The Agency also recognized that providing a single list based on common criteria would be preferable to evaluating drug products on the basis of differing definitions and criteria in various state laws. As a result, on May 31, 1978, the Commissioner of the Food and Drug Administration sent a letter to officials of each state stating FDA's intent to provide a list of all prescription drug products that are approved by FDA for safety and effectiveness, along with therapeutic equivalence determinations for multisource prescription products.

The List was distributed as a proposal in January 1979. It included only currently marketed prescription drug products approved by FDA through new drug applications (NDAs) and abbreviated new drug applications (ANDAs) under the provisions of Section 505 of the Act.

The therapeutic equivalence evaluations in the List reflect FDA's application of specific criteria to the approved multisource prescription drug products on the List. These evaluations are presented in the form of code letters that indicate the basis for the evaluation made. An explanation of the code appears in the *Introduction*.

A complete discussion of the background and basis of FDA's therapeutic equivalence evaluation policy was published in the *Federal Register* on January 12, 1979 (44 FR 2932). The final rule, which includes FDA's responses to the public comments on the proposal, was published in the *Federal Register* on October 31, 1980 (45 FR 72582). The first publication, October 1980, of the final version of the List incorporated appropriate corrections and additions. Each subsequent edition has included the new approvals and made appropriate changes in data.

On September 24, 1984, the President signed into law the Drug Price Competition and Patent Term Restoration Act (1984 Amendments). The 1984 Amendments require that FDA, among other things, make publicly available a list of approved drug products that is updated monthly. The *Approved Drug Products with Therapeutic Equivalence Evaluations* publication satisfies this requirement. The *Addendum* to this publication identifies drugs that qualify under the 1984 Amendments for periods of exclusivity (during which ANDAs or applications described in Section 505(b)(2) of the Act for those drugs may not be submitted for a specified period of time and, if allowed to be submitted, would be tentatively approved) and provides patent information concerning the listed drugs which also may delay the approval of ANDAs or Section 505(b)(2) applications. The *Addendum* also provides additional information that may be helpful to those submitting a new drug application to the Agency.

The Agency intends to use this publication to further its objective of obtaining input and comment on the publication itself and related Agency procedures. Therefore, if you have comments on how the publication can be improved, please send them to the Director, Division of Data Management and Services, Office of Information Technology, Center for Drug and Evaluation and Research, HFD-90, 5600 Fishers Lane, Rockville, MD 20857. Comments received are publicly available to the extent allowable under the Freedom of Information regulations.

INTRODUCTION

1.1 Content and Exclusion

The List is composed of four parts: (1) approved prescription drug products with therapeutic equivalence evaluations; (2) approved over-the-counter (OTC) drug products for those drugs that may not be marketed without NDAs or ANDAs because they are not covered under existing OTC monographs; (3) drug products with approval under Section 505 of the Act administered by the Center for Biologics Evaluation and Research; and (4) a cumulative list of approved products that have never been marketed, have been discontinued from marketing, or have had their approvals withdrawn for other than safety or efficacy reasons subsequent to being discontinued from marketing. All established names for active ingredients generally conform to official compendial names or *United States Adopted Names* (USAN) as prescribed in (21 CFR 299.4(e)). In addition, a list of uniform terms is provided. An *Addendum* contains drug patent and exclusivity information for the Prescription and OTC Drug Product Lists, and for the Drug Products with Approval under Section 505 of the Act Administered by the Center for Biologics Evaluation and Research.

This publication also includes additional information such as Orphan Drug Product Designations and other data that the Agency deems appropriate to disseminate.

Prior to the 6th Edition, the publication had excluded OTC drug products and drug products with approval under Section 505 of the Act Administered by the Center for Biologics Evaluation and Research because the main purpose of the publication was to provide information to states regarding FDA's recommendation as to which generic prescription drug products were acceptable candidates for drug product selection. The 1984 Amendments required the Agency to begin publishing an up-to-date list of all marketed drug products, OTC as well as prescription, that have been approved for safety and efficacy and for which new drug applications are required.

Under the 1984 Amendments, some drug products were given tentative approvals. Prior to the effective date, the Agency will not include drug products with tentative approval in the List; however, they are available in the *FDA Drug Product Approvals List* on the Internet World Wide Web. When the tentative approval becomes a full approval through a subsequent action letter to the application holder, the Agency will list the drug product and the final, effective approval date in the appropriate approved drug product list.

Distributors or repackagers of products on the List are not identified. Because distributors or repackagers are not required to notify FDA when they shift their sources of supply from one approved manufacturer to another, it is not possible to maintain complete information linking product approval with the distributor or repackager handling the products.

1.2 Therapeutic Equivalence-Related Terms

Pharmaceutical Equivalents. Drug products are considered pharmaceutical equivalents if they contain the same active ingredient(s), are of the same dosage form, route of administration and are identical in strength or concentration (e.g., chlordiazepoxide hydrochloride, 5mg capsules). Pharmaceutically equivalent drug products are formulated to contain the same amount of active ingredient in the same dosage form and to meet the same or compendial or other applicable standards (i.e., strength, quality, purity, and identity), but they may differ in characteristics such as shape, scoring configuration, release mechanisms, packaging, excipients (including colors, flavors, preservatives), expiration time, and, within certain limits, labeling.

Pharmaceutical Alternatives. Drug products are considered pharmaceutical alternatives if they contain the same therapeutic moiety, but are different salts, esters, or complexes of that moiety,

or are different dosage forms or strengths (e.g., tetracycline hydrochloride, 250mg capsules vs. tetracycline phosphate complex, 250mg capsules; quinidine sulfate, 200mg tablets vs. quinidine sulfate, 200mg capsules). Data are generally not available for FDA to make the determination of tablet to capsule bioequivalence. Different dosage forms and strengths within a product line by a single manufacturer are thus pharmaceutical alternatives, as are extended-release products when compared with immediate- or standard-release formulations of the same active ingredient.

Therapeutic Equivalents. Drug products are considered to be therapeutic equivalents only if they are pharmaceutical equivalents and if they can be expected to have the same clinical effect and safety profile when administered to patients under the conditions specified in the labeling.

FDA classifies as therapeutically equivalent those products that meet the following general criteria: (1) they are approved as safe and effective; (2) they are pharmaceutical equivalents in that they (a) contain identical amounts of the same active drug ingredient in the same dosage form and route of administration, and (b) meet compendial or other applicable standards of strength, quality, purity, and identity; (3) they are bioequivalent in that (a) they do not present a known or potential bioequivalence problem, and they meet an acceptable *in vitro* standard, or (b) if they do present such a known or potential problem, they are shown to meet an appropriate bioequivalence standard; (4) they are adequately labeled; and (5) they are manufactured in compliance with Current Good Manufacturing Practice regulations. *The concept of therapeutic equivalence, as used to develop the List, applies only to drug products containing the same active ingredient(s) and does not encompass a comparison of different therapeutic agents used for the same condition (e.g., propoxyphene hydrochloride vs. pentazocine hydrochloride for the treatment of pain).* Any drug product in the List repackaged and/or distributed by other than the application holder is considered to be therapeutically equivalent to the application holder's drug product even if the application holder's drug product is single source or coded as non-equivalent (e.g., **BN**). Also, distributors or repackagers of an application holder's drug product are considered to have the same code as the application holder. Therapeutic equivalence determinations are not made for unapproved, off-label indications.

FDA considers drug products to be therapeutically equivalent if they meet the criteria outlined above, even though they may differ in certain other characteristics such as shape, scoring configuration, release mechanisms, packaging, excipients (including colors, flavors, preservatives), expiration date/time and minor aspects of labeling (e.g., the presence of specific pharmacokinetic information) and storage conditions. When such differences are important in the care of a particular patient, it may be appropriate for the prescribing physician to require that a particular brand be dispensed as a medical necessity. With this limitation, however, FDA believes that products classified as therapeutically equivalent can be substituted with the full expectation that the substituted product will produce the same clinical effect and safety profile as the prescribed product.

Bioavailability. This term means the rate and extent to which the active ingredient or active moiety is absorbed from a drug product and becomes available at the site of action. For drug products that are not intended to be absorbed into the bloodstream, bioavailability may be assessed by measurements intended to reflect the rate and extent to which the active ingredient or active moiety becomes available at the site of action.

Bioequivalent Drug Products. This term describes pharmaceutical equivalent or pharmaceutical alternative products that display comparable bioavailability when studied under similar ex-

perimental conditions. Section 505 (j)(7)(B) of the Act describes one set of conditions under which a test and reference listed drug shall be considered bioequivalent:

the rate and extent of absorption of the test drug do not show a significant difference from the rate and extent of absorption of the reference drug when administered at the same molar dose of the therapeutic ingredient under similar experimental conditions in either a single dose or multiple doses; or

the extent of absorption of the test drug does not show a significant difference from the extent of absorption of the reference drug when administered at the same molar dose of the therapeutic ingredient under similar experimental conditions in either a single dose or multiple doses and the difference from the reference drug in the rate of absorption of the drug is intentional, is reflected in its proposed labeling, is not essential to the attainment of effective body drug concentrations on chronic use, and is considered medically insignificant for the drug.

Where these above methods are not applicable (e.g., for drug products that are not intended to be absorbed into the bloodstream), other *in vivo* or *in vitro* test methods to demonstrate bioequivalence may be appropriate.

Bioequivalence may sometimes be demonstrated using an *in vitro* bioequivalence standard, especially when such an *in vitro* test has been correlated with human *in vivo* bioavailability data. In other situations, bioequivalence may sometimes be demonstrated through comparative clinical trials or pharmacodynamic studies.

1.3 Statistical Criteria for Bioequivalence

Under the Drug Price Competition and Patent Term Restoration Act of 1984, manufacturers seeking approval to market a generic drug product must submit data demonstrating that the drug product is bioequivalent to the pioneer (innovator) drug product. A major premise underlying the 1984 law is that bioequivalent drug products are therapeutically equivalent and, therefore, interchangeable.

Bioavailability refers to the rate and extent to which the active ingredient or therapeutic ingredient is absorbed from a drug product and becomes available at the site of drug action (Federal Food, Drug and Cosmetic Act, section 505(j)(8)). Bioequivalence refers to equivalent release of the same drug substance from two or more drug products or formulations. This leads to an equivalent rate and extent of absorption from these formulations. Underlying the concept of bioequivalence is the thesis that, if a drug product contains a drug substance that is chemically identical and is delivered to the site of action at the same rate and extent as another drug product, then it is equivalent and can be substituted for that drug product. Methods used to define bioequivalence can be found in 21 CFR 320.24, and include (1) pharmacokinetic (PK) studies, (2) pharmacodynamic (PD) studies, (3) comparative clinical trials, and (4) in-vitro studies. The choice of study used is based on the site of action of the drug and the ability of the study design to compare drug delivered to that site by the two products.

The standard bioequivalence (PK) study is conducted using a two-treatment crossover study design in a limited number of volunteers, usually 24 to 36 adults. Alternately, a four-period, replicate design crossover study may also be used. Single doses of the test and reference drug products are administered and blood or plasma levels of the drug are measured over time. Pharmacokinetic parameters characterizing rate and extent of drug absorption are evaluated statistically. The PK parameters of interest are the resulting area under the plasma concentration-time curve (AUC), calculated to the last measured concentration ($AUC_{(0-t)}$) and extrapolated to infinity ($AUC_{(0-inf)}$), for extent of absorption; and the maximum or peak drug concentrations (Cmax), for rate of absorption. Crossover studies may not be practical in drugs with a long half-life in the body, and a parallel study design may be used instead. Alternate study methods, such as in-vitro studies or equivalence studies with clinical or pharmacodynamic endpoints, are used for drug products where plasma concentrations are not useful to determine delivery of the drug substance to the site of activity (such as inhalers, nasal sprays and topical products applied to the skin).

The statistical methodology for analyzing these bioequivalence studies is called the two one-sided test procedure. Two situations are tested with this statistical methodology. The first of the two one-sided tests determines whether a generic product (test), when substituted for a brand-name product (reference) is significantly less bioavailable. The second of the two one-sided tests determines whether a brand-name product when substituted for a generic product is significantly less bioavailable. Based on the opinions of FDA medical experts, a difference of greater than 20% for each of the above tests was determined to be significant, and therefore, undesirable for all drug products. Numerically, this is expressed as a limit of test-product average/reference-product average of 80% for the first statistical test and a limit of reference-product average/test-product average of 80% for the second statistical test. By convention, all data is expressed as a ratio of the average response (AUC and Cmax) for test/reference, so the limit expressed in the second statistical test is 125% (reciprocal of 80%).

For statistical reasons, all data is log-transformed prior to conducting statistical testing. In practice, these statistical tests are carried out using an analysis of variance procedure (ANOVA) and calculating a 90% confidence interval for each pharmacokinetic parameter (Cmax and AUC). The confidence interval for both pharmacokinetic parameters, AUC and Cmax, must be entirely within the 80% to 125% boundaries cited above. Because the mean of the study data lies in the center of the 90% confidence interval, the mean of the data is usually close to 100% (a test/reference ratio of 1). Different statistical criteria are sometimes used when bioequivalence is demonstrated through comparative clinical trials, pharmacodynamic studies, or comparative in-vitro methodology.

The bioequivalence methodology and criteria described above simultaneously control for both, differences in the average response between test and reference, as well as the precision with which the average response in the population is estimated. This precision depends on the within-subject (normal volunteer or patient) variability in the pharmacokinetic parameters (AUC and Cmax) of the two products and on the number of subjects in the study. The width of the 90% confidence interval is a reflection in part of the within-subject variability of the test and reference products in the bioequivalence study. A test product with no differences in the average response when compared to the reference might still fail to pass the bioequivalence criteria if the variability of one or both products is high and the bioequivalence study has insufficient statistical power (i.e., insufficient number of subjects). Likewise, a test product with low variability may pass the bioequivalence criteria, when there are somewhat larger differences in the average response.

This system of assessing bioequivalence of generic products assures that these substitutable products do not deviate substantially in in-vivo performance from the reference product. The Office of Generic Drugs has conducted two surveys to quantify the differences between generic and brand name products. The first survey included 224 bioequivalence studies submitted in approved applications during 1985 and 1986. The observed average differences between reference and generic products for AUC was 3.5% (JAMA, Sept. 4, 1987, Vol. 258, No. 9). The second survey included 127 bioequivalence studies submitted to the agency in 273 ANDAs approved in 1997. The three measures reviewed include $AUC_{(0-t)}$, $AUC_{(0-inf)}$, and Cmax. The observed average differences between the reference and generic products were ± 3.47% (SD 2.84) for $AUC_{(0-t)}$, ± 3.25% (SD 2.97) for $AUC_{(0-inf)}$, and ± 4.29% (SD 3.72) for Cmax (JAMA, Dec. 1, 1999, Vol. 282, No. 21).

The primary concern from the regulatory point of view is the protection of the patient against approval of products that are not bioequivalent. The current practice of carrying out two one-sided tests at the 0.05 level of significance ensures that there is no more than a 5% chance that a generic product that is not truly equivalent to the reference will be approved.

1.4 Reference Listed Drug

A reference listed drug (21 CFR 314.94(a)(3)) means the listed drug identified by FDA as the drug product upon which an applicant relies in seeking approval of its ANDA.

FDA has identified in the Prescription Drug Product and OTC Drug Product Lists those reference listed drugs to which the *in vivo* bioequivalence and, in some instances, the *in vitro* bioequivalence of the applicant's product is compared. By designating a single reference listed drug as the standard to which all generic versions must be shown to be bioequivalent, FDA hopes to avoid possible significant variations among generic drugs and their brand name counterpart. Such variations could result if generic drugs were compared to different reference listed drugs. However, in some instances when multiple NDAs are approved for a single drug product, a product not designated as the reference listed drug and not shown to be bioequivalent to the reference listed drug may be shielded from generic competition. A firm wishing to market a generic version of an NDA listed drug that is not designated as the reference listed may petition the Agency through the Citizen Petition procedure (see 21 CFR 10.25(a) and CFR 10.30). When the Citizen Petition is approved, the second NDA will be designated as an additional reference listed drug and the petitioner may submit an Abbreviated New Drug Application citing the designated reference listed drug. *Therapeutic Equivalence Evaluations Codes—Products meeting necessary bioequivalence requirements* explains the *AB, AB1, AB2, AB3* coding system for multisource drug products listed under the same heading with two reference listed drugs.

In addition, there are two situations in which two listed drugs that have been shown to be bioequivalent to each other may both be designated as reference listed drugs. The first situation occurs when the *in vivo* determination of bioequivalence is self-evident and a waiver of *in vivo* determination of bioequivalence may be granted. The second situation occurs when the bioequivalence of two NDA drug products may be determined through *in vitro* methodology. The reference listed drug is identified by a "Yes" in the Prescription and Over-the-Counter (OTC) Drug Product Lists and is identified in the printed version by a "+". These identified reference listed drugs represent the best judgment of the Division of Bioequivalence at this time. The Prescription and OTC Drug Product Lists identify reference drugs for oral dosage forms, injectables, ophthalmics, otics, and topical products. It is recommended that a firm planning to conduct an *in vivo* bioequivalence study, or planning to manufacture a batch of a drug product for which an *in vivo* waiver of bioequivalence will be requested, contact the Division of Bioequivalence, Office of Generic Drugs, to confirm the appropriate reference listed drug.

Acyclovir 200mg Tablet-Reference Listed Drug. Novopharm's single source acyclovir tablets have been declared to be a reference listed drug for the 200 mg tablet in addition to the acylcovir (Zovirax) 800 mg tablet of the innovator. A generic firm wishing to submit an ANDA for a duplicate of the 200 mg acyclovir tablet will be eligible for a waiver of the *in vivo* determination of bioequivalence (1) if their product is proportionally similar in its active and inactive ingredients to their own 800 mg acyclovir tablet and (2) by doing an acceptable comparative dissolution test (dissolution profile) against Novopharm's 200 mg acyclovir reference listed drug.

Before a waiver of the *in vivo* determination of bioequivalence can be granted for the 200 mg acyclovir tablet, the generic firm must have completed an acceptable fasting and fed study comparing their acyclovir 800 mg tablet against the Zovirax 800 mg tablet.

For further information on the study designs, you should contact the Division of Bioequivalence, Office of Generic Drugs.

1.5 General Policies and Legal Status

The List contains public information and advice. It does not mandate the drug products which may be purchased, prescribed, dispensed, or substituted for one another, nor does it, conversely, mandate the products that should be avoided. To the extent that the List sets forth FDA's evaluations of the therapeutic equivalence of drug products that have been approved, it contains FDA's advice to the public, to practitioners and to the states regarding drug product selection. These evaluations do not constitute determinations that any product is in violation of the Act or that any product is preferable to any other. Therapeutic equivalence evaluations are a scientific judgment based upon evidence, while generic substitution may involve social and economic policy administered by the states, intended to reduce the cost of drugs to consumers. To the extent that the List identifies drug products approved under Section 505 of the Act, it sets forth information that the Agency is required to publish and that the public is entitled to under the Freedom of Information Act. Exclusion of a drug product from the List does not necessarily mean that the drug product is either in violation of Section 505 of the Act, or that such a product is not safe or effective, or that such a product is not therapeutically equivalent to other drug products. Rather, the exclusion is based on the fact that FDA has not evaluated the safety, effectiveness, and quality of the drug product.

1.6 Practitioner/User Responsibilities

Professional care and judgment should be exercised in using the List. Evaluations of therapeutic equivalence for prescription drugs are based on scientific and medical evaluations by FDA. Products evaluated as therapeutically equivalent can be expected, in the judgment of FDA, to have equivalent clinical effect and no difference in their potential for adverse effects when used under the conditions of their labeling. However, these products may differ in other characteristics such as shape, scoring configuration, release mechanisms, packaging, excipients (including colors, flavors, preservatives), expiration date/time, and, in some instances, labeling. If products with such differences are substituted for each other, there is a potential for patient confusion due to differences in color or shape of tablets, inability to provide a given dose using a partial tablet if the proper scoring configuration is not available, or decreased patient acceptance of certain products because of flavor. There may also be better stability of one product over another under adverse storage conditions, or allergic reactions in rare cases due to a coloring or a preservative ingredient, as well as differences in cost to the patient.

FDA evaluation of therapeutic equivalence in no way relieves practitioners of their professional responsibilities in prescribing and dispensing such products with due care and with appropriate information to individual patients. In those circumstances where the characteristics of a specific product, other than its active ingredient, are important in the therapy of a particular patient, the physician's specification of that product is appropriate. Pharmacists must also be familiar with the expiration dates/times and labeling directions for storage of the different products, particularly for reconstituted products, to assure that patients are properly advised when one product is substituted for another.

Multisource and single-source drug products. FDA has evaluated for therapeutic equivalence only multisource prescription drug products, which in most instances means those pharmaceutical equivalents available from more than one manufacturer. A therapeutic equivalence code is included for such products. Those products with approved applications that are single-source (i.e., there is only one approved product available for that active ingredient, dosage form and route of administration) are also included on the List, but no therapeutic equivalence code is included with such products. Any drug product in the List repackaged and/or distributed by other than the application holder is considered to be therapeutically equivalent to the application holder's drug product even if the application holder's drug product is single source or coded as non-equivalent (e.g., **BN**). Also, although not identified in the List, distributors or repackagers of an application holder's drug product are considered to have the same code as the application holder. The details of these codes and the policies underlying them are discussed in *Therapeutic Equivalence Evaluations Codes.*

Products on the List are identified by the names of the holders of approved applications (applicants) who may not necessarily be the manufacturer of the product. The applicant may have had its product manufactured by a contract manufacturer and may simply be distributing the product for which it has obtained approval. In most instances, however, the manufacturer of the product is also the applicant. The name of the manufacturer is permitted by regulation to appear on the label, even when the manufacturer is not the marketer.

Although the products on the List are identified by the names of the applicants, circumstances, such as changing corporate ownership, have sometimes made identification of the applicant difficult. The Agency believes, based on continuing document review and communication with firms, that the applicant designations on the List are, in most cases, correct.

To relate firm name information on a product label to that on the List, the following should be noted: the applicant's name always appears on the List. This applies whether the applicant (firm name on the Form FDA 356h in the application) is the marketer (firm name in largest letters on the label) or not. However, the applicant's name may not always appear on the label of the product.

If the applicant is the marketer, its name appears on the List and on the label; if the applicant is not the marketer, and the Agency is aware of a corporate relationship (e.g., parent and subsidiary) between the applicant and the marketer, the name of the applicant appears on the List and both firm names may appear on the label. If there is no known corporate relationship between the applicant and the marketer, the applicant's name appears on the List; however, unless the applicant is the manufacturer, packager, or distributor, the applicant's name may not appear on the label. In this case, the practitioner, from labeling alone, will not be able to relate the marketed product to an applicant cited in the List, and hence to a specific approved drug product. In such cases, to assure that the product in question is the subject of an approved application, the firm named on the label should be contacted.

To relate trade name (proprietary name) information on a product label to that on the List, the following should be noted: if the applicant is the marketer, its name appears on the List and on the label; if the Agency is aware of a corporate relationship between the applicant and the marketer, the trade name (proprietary name) of the drug product (established drug name if no trade name exists) appears on the List. If a corporate relationship exists between an application holder and a marketer and both firms are distributing the drug product, the FDA reserves the right to select the trade name of either the marketer or the application holder to appear on the List. If there is no known corporate relationship between the applicant and the marketer, the established drug name appears on the List.

Every product on the List is subject at all times to regulatory action. From time to time, approved products may be found in violation of one or more provisions of the Act. In such circumstances, the Agency will commence appropriate enforcement action to correct the violation, if necessary, by securing removal of the product from the market by voluntary recall, seizure,or other enforcement actions. Such regulatory actions are, however, independent of the inclusion of a product on the List. The main criterion for inclusion of a product is that it has an application with an effective approval that has not been withdrawn for safety or efficacy reasons. FDA believes that retention of a violative product on the List will not have any significant adverse health consequences, because other legal mechanisms are available to the Agency to prevent the product's actual marketing. FDA may however, change a product's therapeutic equivalence rating if the circumstances giving rise to the violation change or otherwise call into question the data upon which the Agency's assessment of whether a product meets the criteria for therapeutic equivalence was made.

1.7 Therapeutic Equivalence Evaluations Codes

The coding system for therapeutic equivalence evaluations is constructed to allow users to determine quickly whether the Agency has evaluated a particular approved product as therapeutically equivalent to other pharmaceutically equivalent products (first letter) and to provide additional information on the basis of FDA's evaluations (second letter). With few exceptions, the therapeutic equivalence evaluation date is the same as the approval date.

The two basic categories into which multisource drugs have been placed are indicated by the first letter as follows:

A—Drug products that FDA considers to be therapeutically equivalent to other pharmaceutically equivalent products, i.e., drug products for which:

(1) there are no known or suspected bioequivalence problems. These are designated **AA, AN, AO, AP,** or **AT,** depending on the dosage form; or

(2) actual or potential bioequivalence problems have been resolved with adequate *in vivo* and/or *in vitro* evidence supporting bioequivalence. These are designated **AB.**

B—Drug products that FDA at this time, considers not to be therapeutically equivalent to other pharmaceutically equivalent products, i.e.,

drug products for which actual or potential bioequivalence problems have not been resolved by adequate evidence of bioequivalence. Often the problem is with specific dosage forms rather than with the active ingredients. These are designated **BC, BD, BE, BN, BP, BR, BS, BT, BX,** or **B*.**

Individual drug products have been evaluated as therapeutically equivalent to the reference product in accordance with the definitions and policies outlined below:

"A" CODES

Drug products that are considered to be therapeutically equivalent to other pharmaceutically equivalent products.

"**A**" products are those for which actual or potential bioequivalence problems have been resolved with adequate *in vivo* and/or *in vitro* evidence supporting bioequivalence. Drug products designated with an "A" code fall under one of two main policies:

(1) for those active ingredients or dosage forms for which no *in vivo* bioequivalence issue is known or suspected, the information necessary to show bioequivalence between pharmaceutically equivalent products is presumed and considered self-evident based on other data in the application for some dosage forms (e.g., solutions) or satisfied for solid oral dosage forms by a showing that an acceptable *in vitro* dissolution standard is met. A therapeutically equivalent rating is assigned such products so long as they are manufactured in accordance with Current Good Manufacturing Practice regulations and meet the other requirements of their approved applications (these are designated **AA, AN, AO, AP,** or **AT,** depending on the dosage form, as described below); or

(2) for those DESI drug products containing active ingredients or dosage forms that have been identified by FDA as having actual or potential bioequivalence problems, and for post-1962 drug products in a dosage form presenting a potential bioequivalence problem, an evaluation of therapeutic equivalence is assigned to pharmaceutical equivalents only if the approved application contains adequate scientific evidence establishing through *in vivo* and/or *in vitro* studies the bioequivalence of the product to a selected reference product (these products are designated as **AB**).

There are some general principles that may affect the substitution of pharmaceutically equivalent products in specific cases. Prescribers and dispensers of drugs should be alert to these principles so as to deal appropriately with situations that require professional judgment and discretion.

There may be labeling differences among pharmaceutically equivalent products that require attention on the part of the health professional. For example, pharmaceutically equivalent powders to be reconstituted for administration as oral or injectable liquids may vary with respect to their expiration time or storage conditions after reconstitution. An FDA evaluation that such products are therapeutically equivalent is applicable only when each product is reconstituted, stored, and used under the conditions specified in the labeling of that product.

The Agency will use notes in this publication to point out special situations such as potential differences between two drug products that have been evaluated as bioequivalent and otherwise therapeutically equivalent, when they should be brought to the attention of health professionals. These notes are contained in Section 1.8, *Description of Special Situations.*

For example, in rare instances, there may be variations among therapeutically equivalent products in their use or in conditions of administration. Such differences may be due to patent or exclusivity rights associated with such use. When such variations may, in the Agency's opinion, affect prescribing or substitution decisions by health professionals, a note will be added to Section 1.8, *Description of Special Situations.*

Also, occasionally a situation may arise in which changes in a listed drug product after its approval (for example, a change in dosing interval) may have an impact on the substitutability of already approved generic versions of that product that were rated by the Agency as therapeutically equivalent to the listed product. When such changes in the listed drug product are considered by the Agency to have a significant impact on therapeutic equivalence, the Agency will change the therapeutic equivalence ratings for other versions of the drug product unless the manufacturers of those other versions of the product provide additional information to assure equivalence under the changed conditions. Pending receipt of the additional data, the Agency may add a note to Section 1.8, *Description of Special Situations,* or, in rare cases, may even change the therapeutic equivalence rating.

In some cases (e.g., Isolyte® S w/ Dextrose 5% in Plastic Container and Plasma-Lyte® 148 and Dextrose 5% in Plastic Container), closely related products are listed as containing the same active ingredients, but in somewhat different amounts. In determining which of these products are pharmaceutically equivalent, the Agency has considered products to be pharmaceutically equivalent with labeled strengths of an ingredient that do not vary by more than 1%.

Different salts and esters of the same therapeutic moiety are regarded as pharmaceutical alternatives. For the purpose of this publication, such products are not considered to be therapeutically equivalent. There are no instances in this List where pharmaceutical alternatives are evaluated or coded with regard to therapeutic equivalence. Anhydrous and hydrated entities, as well as different polymorphs, are considered pharmaceutical equivalents and must meet the same standards and, where necessary, as in the case of ampicillin/ampicillin trihydrate, their equivalence is supported by appropriate bioavailability/bioequivalence studies.

The codes in this book are not intended to preclude health care professionals from converting pharmaceutically different concentrations into pharmaceutical equivalents using accepted professional practice.

Where package size variations have therapeutic implications, products so packaged have not been considered pharmaceutically equivalent. For example, some oral contraceptives are supplied in 21-tablet and 28-tablet packets; the 28-tablet packets contain 7 placebo or iron tablets. These two packaging configurations are not regarded as pharmaceutically equivalent; thus, they are not designated as therapeutically equivalent.

Preservatives may differ among some therapeutically equivalent drug products. Differences in preservatives and other inactive ingredients do not affect FDA's evaluation of therapeutic equivalence except in cases where these components may influence bioequivalence or routes of administration.

The specific sub-codes for those drugs evaluated as therapeutically equivalent and the policies underlying these sub-codes follow:

AA

Products in conventional dosage forms not presenting bioequivalence problems

Products coded as **AA** contain active ingredients and dosage forms that are not regarded as presenting either actual or potential bioequivalence problems or drug quality or standards issues. However, all oral dosage forms must, nonetheless, meet an appropriate *in vitro* bioequivalence standard that is acceptable to the Agency in order to be approved.

AB, AB1, AB2, AB3 . . .

Products meeting necessary bioequivalence requirements

Multisource drug products listed under the same heading (i.e., identical active ingredients(s), dosage form, and route(s) of administration) and having the same strength (see *Therapeutic Equivalence-Related Terms, Pharmaceutical Equivalents*) generally will be coded **AB** if a study is submitted demonstrating bioequivalence.

In certain instances, a number is added to the end of the **AB** code to make a three character code (i.e., **AB1, AB2, AB3,** etc.). Three-character codes are assigned only in situations when more than one reference listed drug of the same strength has been designated under the same heading. Two or more reference listed drugs are generally selected only when there are at least two potential reference drug products which are not bioequivalent to each other. If a study issubmitted that demonstrates bioequivalence to a specific listed drug product, the generic product will be given the same three-character code as the reference listed drug it was compared against. For example, Adalat® CC (Miles) and Procardia XL® (Pfizer), extended-release tablets, are listed under the active ingredient nifedipine. These drug products, listed under the same heading, are not bioequivalent to each other. Once generic drug products deemed by FDA to be bioequivalent to either Adalat® CC or Procardia XL® are approved, Adalat® CC and Procardia XL® would be assigned ratings of **AB1** and **AB2**, respectively. The generic drug products bioequivalent to Adalat® CC would be assigned a rating of **AB1** and those bioequivalent to Procardia XL® would be assigned a rating of **AB2**. (The assignment of an **AB1** or **AB2** rating to a specific product does not imply product preference.) Even though drug products of distributors and/or repackagers are not included in the List, they are considered therapeutically equivalent to the application holder's drug product if the application holder's drug product is rated either with an **AB** or three-character code or is single source in the List. Drugs coded as **AB** under a heading are considered therapeutically equivalent only to other drugs coded as **AB** under that heading. Drugs coded with a three-character code under a heading are considered therapeutically equivalent only to other drugs coded with the same three-character code under that heading.

AN

Solutions and powders for aerosolization

Uncertainty regarding the therapeutic equivalence of aerosolized products arises primarily because of differences in the drug delivery system. Solutions and powders intended

for aerosolization that are marketed for use in any of several delivery systems are considered to be pharmaceutically and therapeutically equivalent and are coded **AN**. Those products that are compatible only with a specific delivery system or those products that are packaged in and with a specific delivery system are coded **BN**, unless they have met an appropriate bioequivalence standard. Solutions or suspensions in a specific delivery system will be coded **AN** if the bioequivalence standard is based upon *in vitro* methodology, if bioequivalence needs to be demonstrated by *in vivo* methodology then the drug products will be coded **AB**.

AO

Injectable oil solutions

The absorption of drugs in injectable (parenteral) oil solutions may vary substantially with the type of oil employed as a vehicle and the concentration of the active ingredient. Injectable oil solutions are therefore considered to be pharmaceutically and therapeutically equivalent only when the active ingredient, its concentration, and the type of oil used as a vehicle are all identical.

AP

Injectable aqueous solutions and, in certain instances, intravenous non-aqueous solutions

It should be noted that even though injectable (parenteral) products under a specific listing may be evaluated as therapeutically equivalent, there may be important differences among the products in the general category, *Injectable; Injection*. For example, some injectable products that are rated therapeutically equivalent are labeled for different routes of administration. In addition, some products evaluated as therapeutically equivalent may have different preservatives or no preservatives at all. Injectable products available as dry powders for reconstitution, concentrated sterile solutions for dilution, or sterile solutions ready for injection are all considered to be pharmaceutically and therapeutically equivalent provided they are designed to produce the same concentration prior to injection and are similarly labeled. Consistent with accepted professional practice, it is the responsibility of the prescriber, dispenser, or individual administering the product to be familiar with a product's labeling to assure that it is given only by the route(s) of administration stated in the labeling.

Certain commonly used large volume intravenous products in glass containers are not included on the List (e.g., dextrose injection 5%, dextrose injection 10%, sodium chloride injection 0.9%) since these products are on the market without FDA approval and the FDA has not published conditions for marketing such parenteral products under approved NDAs. When packaged in plastic containers, however, FDA regulations require approved applications prior to marketing. Approval then depends on, among other things, the extent of the available safety data involving the specific plastic component of the product. All large volume parenteral products are manufactured under similar standards, regardless of whether they are packaged in glass or plastic. Thus, FDA has no reason to believe that the packaging container of large volume parenteral drug products that are pharmaceutically equivalent would have any effect on their therapeutic equivalence.

AT

Topical products

There are a variety of topical dosage forms available for dermatologic, ophthalmic, otic, rectal, and vaginal administration, including solutions, creams, ointments, gels, lotions, pastes, sprays, and suppositories. Even though different topical dosage forms may contain the same active ingredient and potency, these dosage forms are not considered pharmaceutically equivalent. Therefore, they are not considered therapeutically equivalent. All solutions and DESI drug products containing the same active ingredient in the same topical dosage form for which a waiver of *in vivo* bioequivalence has been granted and for which chemistry and manufacturing processes are adequate to demonstrate bioequivalence, are considered therapeutically equivalent and coded **AT**. Pharmaceutically equivalent topical products that raise questions of bioequivalence, including all post-1962 non-solution topical drug products, are coded **AB** when supported by adequate bioequivalence data, and **BT** in the absence of such data.

"B" CODES

Drug products that FDA, at this time, considers not to be therapeutically equivalent to other pharmaceutically equivalent products.

"B" products, for which actual or potential bioequivalence problems have not been resolved by adequate evidence of bioequivalence, often have a problem with specific dosage forms rather than with the active ingredients. Drug products designated with a "B" code fall under one of three main policies:

(1)   the drug products contain active ingredients or are manufactured in dosage forms that have been identified by the Agency as having documented bioequivalence problems or a significant potential for such problems and for which no adequate studies demonstrating bioequivalence have been submitted to FDA; or

(2)   the quality standards are inadequate or FDA has an insufficient basis to determine therapeutic equivalence; or

(3)   the drug products are under regulatory review.

The specific coding definitions and policies for the "B" subcodes are as follows:

B*

Drug products requiring further FDA investigation and review to determine therapeutic equivalence

The code **B*** is assigned to products previously assigned an **A** or **B** code when FDA receives new information that raises a significant question regarding therapeutic equivalence that can be resolved only through further Agency investigation and/or review of data and information submitted by the applicant. The **B*** code signifies that the Agency will take no position regarding the therapeutic equivalence of the product until the Agency completes its investigation and review.

BC

Extended-release dosage forms (capsules, injectables and tablets)

An extended-release dosage form is defined by the official compendia as one that allows at least a twofold reduction in dosing frequency as compared to that drug presented as a conventional dosage form (e.g., as a solution or a prompt drug-releasing, conventional solid dosage form).

Although bioavailability studies have been conducted on these dosage forms, they may be subject to bioavailability differences, primarily because firms developing extended-release products for the same active ingredient rarely em-

ploy the same formulation approach. FDA, therefore, does not consider different extended-release dosage forms containing the same active ingredient in equal strength to be therapeutically equivalent unless equivalence between individual products in both rate and extent has been specifically demonstrated through appropriate bioequivalence studies. Extended-release products for which such bioequivalence data have not been submitted are coded **BC**, while those for which such data are available have been coded **AB**.

BD

Active ingredients and dosage forms with documented bioequivalence problems

The **BD** code denotes products containing active ingredients with known bioequivalence problems and for which adequate studies have not been submitted to FDA demonstrating bioequivalence. Where studies showing bioequivalence have been submitted, the product has been coded **AB**.

BE

Delayed-release oral dosage forms

A delayed-release dosage form is defined by the official compendia as one that releases a drug (or drugs) at a time other than promptly after administration. Enteric-coated articles are delayed-release dosage forms.

Drug products in delayed-release dosage forms containing the same active ingredients are subject to significant differences in absorption. Unless otherwise specifically noted, the Agency considers different delayed-release products containing the same active ingredients as presenting a potential bioequivalence problem and codes these products **BE** in the absence of *in vivo* studies showing bioequivalence. If adequate *in vivo* studies have demonstrated the bioequivalence of specific delayed-release products, such products are coded **AB**.

BN

Products in aerosol-nebulizer drug delivery systems

This code applies to drug solutions or powders that are marketed only as a component of, or as compatible with, a specific drug delivery system. There may, for example, be significant differences in the dose of drug and particle size delivered by different products of this type. Therefore, the Agency does not consider different metered aerosol dosage forms containing the same active ingredient(s) in equal strengths to be therapeutically equivalent unless the drug products meet an appropriate bioequivalence standard.

BP

Active ingredients and dosage forms with potential bioequivalence problems

FDA's bioequivalence regulations (21 CFR 320.33) contain criteria and procedures for determining whether a specific active ingredient in a specific dosage form has a potential for causing a bioequivalence problem. It is FDA's policy to consider an ingredient meeting these criteria as having a potential bioequivalence problem even in the absence of positive data demonstrating inequivalence. Pharmaceutically equivalent products containing these ingredients in oral dosage forms are coded **BP** until adequate *in vivo* bioequivalence data are submitted. Injectable suspensions containing an active ingredient suspended in an aqueous or oleaginous vehicle have also been coded **BP**. Injectable suspensions are subject to bioequivalence problems because differences in particle size, polymorphic structure of the suspended ac-

tive ingredient, or the suspension formulation can significantly affect the rate of release and absorption. FDA does not consider pharmaceutical equivalents of these products bioequivalent without adequate evidence of bioequivalence.

BR

Suppositories or enemas that deliver drugs for systemic absorption

The absorption of active ingredients from suppositories or enemas that are intended to have a systemic effect (as distinct from suppositories administered for local effect) can vary significantly from product to product. Therefore, FDA considers pharmaceutically equivalent systemic suppositories or enemas bioequivalent only if *in vivo* evidence of bioequivalence is available. In those cases where *in vivo* evidence is available, the product is coded **AB**. If such evidence is not available, the products are coded **BR**.

BS

Products having drug standard deficiencies

If the drug standards for an active ingredient in a particular dosage form are found by FDA to be deficient so as to prevent an FDA evaluation of either pharmaceutical or therapeutic equivalence, all drug products containing that active ingredient in that dosage form are coded **BS**. For example, if the standards permit a wide variation in pharmacologically active components of the active ingredient such that pharmaceutical equivalence is in question, all products containing that active ingredient in that dosage form are coded **BS**.

BT

Topical products with bioequivalence issues

This code applies mainly to post-1962 dermatologic, ophthalmic, otic, rectal, and vaginal products for topical administration, including creams, ointments, gels, lotions, pastes, and sprays, as well as suppositories not intended for systemic drug absorption. Topical products evaluated as having acceptable clinical performance, but that are not bioequivalent to other pharmaceutically equivalent products or that lack sufficient evidence of bioequivalence, will be coded **BT**.

BX

Drug products for which the data are insufficient to determine therapeutic equivalence

The code **BX** is assigned to specific drug products for which the data that have been reviewed by the Agency are insufficient to determine therapeutic equivalence under the policies stated in this document. In these situations, the drug products are presumed to be therapeutically inequivalent until the Agency has determined that there is adequate information to make a full evaluation of therapeutic equivalence.

1.8 Description of Special Situations

Certain drugs listed in the Orange Book present special situations that merit further discussion. Following is a description of those special situations.

Amino Acid and Protein Hydrolysate Injections. These products differ in the amount and kinds of amino acids they contain and, therefore, are not considered pharmaceutical equivalents. For this reason, these products are not considered therapeutically equivalent. At the same time, the Agency believes that it is appropriate to point out that where nitrogen balance is the sole thera-

peutic objective and individual amino acid content is not a consideration, pharmaceutical alternatives with the same total amount of nitrogen content may be considered therapeutically equivalent.

Follitropin Alfa and Beta. Based on available data derived from physico-chemical tests and bioassay, follitropin alfa and follitropin beta are indistinguishable.

Gaviscon®. Gaviscon® is an OTC product which has been marketed since September 1970. The active ingredients in this product, aluminum hydroxide and magnesium trisilicate, were reviewed by the Agency's OTC Antacid Panel and were considered to be safe and effective ingredients (Category I) by that Panel. However, the tablet failed to pass the antacid test which is required of all antacid products. The Agency, therefore, placed the tablet in Category III for lack of effectiveness. A full NDA with clinical studies was submitted by Marion Laboratories, Inc., and approved by FDA on December 9, 1983. Gaviscon® 's activity in treating reflux acidity is made possible by the physical-chemical properties of the inactive ingredients, sodium bicarbonate and alginic acid. Therefore, *all ANDAs which cite Gaviscon® tablets as the listed drug must contain the inactive ingredients sodium bicarbonate and alginic acid.* A full NDA will be required to support the effectiveness of the drug product if different inactive ingredients are to be substituted for sodium bicarbonate or alginic acid or if different proportions of these ingredients are to be used.

Metaxalone Tablets. In Cumulative Supplement 6 of the *Approved Drug Products with Therapeutic Equivalence Evaluations, 21st Edition,* (the Orange Book), the Agency proposed to reclassify metaxalone tablets from a drug product not presenting bioequivalence problems to one that has a known or potential bioequivalence problem that requires an *in vivo* demonstration of bioequivalence as a condition of approval for an ANDA. The Agency solicited comments from interested persons to be received no later than November 30, 2001. No comments were received. Accordingly, the therapeutic equivalence category for metaxalone tablets will be changed from a "nonbioproblem drug" to a "bioproblem drug." An ANDA for metaxalone tablets must include acceptable *in vivo* bioequivalence study or studies. As long as metaxalone tablets are a single source drug product, no therapeutic equivalence code will be assigned to the product in the Orange Book. If the Agency approves an ANDA for metaxalone tablets, the innovator's NDA for metaxalone (Skelaxin) tablets and the approved ANDA will both be coded as **AB**.

Patent Certification(s) Reference Listed Drug based upon a suitability petition. An abbreviated new drug application that refers to a Reference Listed Drug (RLD) approved pursuant to a suitability petition must demonstrate that the proposed product is bioequivalent to the RLD, and it must include appropriate patent certification(s) and an exclusivity statement with respect to the listed drug which served as the basis for the approved suitability petition.

Ribavirin 200mg Oral Capsule. Indicated for use and comarketed with interferon alfa-2b, recombinant (Intron A), as Rebetron Combination Therapy.

Tramadol Hydrochloride 50 mg tablet. Products approved under section 505(j) are marked with (*) because there are special considerations governing the substitution of these products. The tramadol hydrochloride 50 mg tablets marked with a (*) are therapeutically equivalent (AB) to RW Johnson's Ultram (Tramadol Hydrochloride) 50 mg tablets. However, because of RW Johnson's exclusivity and patent protection for the 25 mg titration dosing regimen, tramadol hydrochloride drug products approved under section 505(j) may not carry the labeling for the 25 mg titration dosing regimen. Ultram 50 mg tablets are scored for use in the 25 mg titration schedule; tramadol hydrochloride 50 mg tablets approved under 505(j) are not scored. Prescribers and dispensers should be aware of this scoring difference between Ultram and other tramadol hydrochloride tablets and take it into account when writing a prescription or practicing drug product selection.

Waived exclusivity. If a new drug application (NDA) submitted under section 505(b) of the Federal Food, Drug, and Cosmetic Act (Act) qualifies for exclusivity under sections 505(c) (3) (D) and 505(j) (5) (D), the exclusivity is listed in the Patent and Exclusivity Section of the Orange Book. If a drug product has received this exclusivity, the FDA wil delay the approval of a 505(b) (2) application or an abbreviated new drug application (ANDA) under section 505(j) of the Act until the expiration of the exclusivity. If the listed drug is also protected by one or more patents, the approval date for the 505(b) (2) application or ANDA will be determined by the latest expiring patent or exclusivity listed in the Orange Book.

However, the holder of the NDA may waiver its exclusivity as to any or all 505(b) (2) and ANDA applications referencing the protected drug product. If an NDA sponsor waivers its right to the exclusivity protection, qualified 505(b) (2) or ANDA applications may be approved without regard to the NDA holder's exclusivity. An NDA for which the holder has waived its exclusivity as to all 505(b) (2) and ANDA applications will be coded with a W in the Patent and Exclusivity Section of the Orange Book and be referred to this section. The applicant referencing this listed drug should indicate in the exclusivity statement that the holder of the listed drug has waived its exclusivity.

1.9 Therapeutic Equivalence Code Change for a Drug Entity

The Agency will use the following procedures when, in response to a petition or on its own initiative, it is considering a change in the therapeutic equivalence code for approved multisource drug products. Such changes will generally occur when the Agency becomes aware of new scientific information affecting the therapeutic equivalence of an entire category of drug products in the List (e.g., information concerning the active ingredient or the dosage form), rather than information concerning a single drug product within the category. These procedures will be used when a change in therapeutic equivalence code is under consideration for all drug products found in the Prescription Drug Product List under a specific drug entity and dosage form. The change may be from the code signifying that the drug does not present a bioequivalence problem (e.g., **AA**) to a code signifying a bioequivalence problem (e.g., **BP**), or vice versa. This procedure does not apply to a change of a particular product code (e.g., a change from **BP** to **AB** or from **AB** to **BX**).

Before making a change in a therapeutic equivalence code for an entire category of drugs, the Agency will announce in the *Introduction* that it is considering the change, and will invite comment. Comments, along with scientific data, may be sent to the Director, Division of Bioequivalence, Office of Generic Drugs, Center for Drug Evaluation and Research, (MPN-2) HFD-650, 7500 Standish Place, Rockville, MD 20855. The comment period will generally be 60 days in length, and the closing date for comments will be listed in the description of the proposed change for each drug entity.

The most useful type of scientific data submission is an *in vivo* bioavailability/bioequivalence study conducted on batches of the subject drug products. These submissions should present a full description of the analytical procedures and equipment used, a validation of the analytical methodology, including the standard curve, a description of the method of calculating results, and a description of the pharmacokinetic and statistical models used in analyzing the data. Anecdotal or testimonial information is the least useful to the Agency, and such submissions are discouraged. Copies of supporting reports published in the scientific literature or unpublished material, however, are welcome.

1.10 Change of the Therapeutic Equivalence Evaluation for a Single Product

The aforementioned procedure does not apply to a change in a single drug product code. For example, a change in a single drug product's code from **BP** to **AB** as a result of the submission of a bioequivalence study ordinarily will not be the subject of notice and comment. Likewise, a change in a single drug product's code from **AB** to **BX** (e.g., as a result of new information raising a significant question as to bioequivalence) does not require notice and comment. The Agency's responsibility to provide the public with the Agency's most current information related to therapeutic equivalence may require a change in a drug product's code prior to any formal notice and opportunity for the applicant to be heard. The publication in the *Federal Register* of a proposal to withdraw approval of a drug product will ordinarily result in a change in a product's code from **AB** to **BX** if this action has not already been taken.

1.11 Availability of Internal Policy and Procedure Guides

The Office of Generic Drugs maintains internal policy and procedure guides. Although these guides are designed for Office personnel and are subject to change without public notice, they are available to members of the public who may wish to know more about the Office's policies and procedures. Copies of these guides may be obtained from the FDA, Center for Drug Evaluation and Research, HFD-210, Division of Communications Management, Drug Information Branch, 5600 Fishers Lane, Rockville, MD 20857. The Agency welcomes public comment on the policies, procedures, and practices employed in the approval of generic drugs. Such comments may be sent to the Director, Office of Generic Drugs, (MPN-2) HFD-600, 7500 Standish Place, Rockville, MD 20855.

1.12 Discontinued Section

Those drug products in the Discontinued Section of the Orange Book in which a determination has already been made that the products were not marketed or withdrawn for safety or efficacy reasons have been designated by the symbol "*". Those drug products with the symbol "*" are only reflective of citizen petitions approved since 1995.

The identification of these drug products in the Discontinued Section of the Orange Book with the symbol "*" should avoid the submission of multiple citizen petitions for the same drug product.

2. HOW TO USE THE DRUG PRODUCT LISTS

2.1 Key Sections for Using the Drug Product Lists

This publication contains illustrations, along with Drug Product Lists, indices, and lists of abbreviations and terms which facilitate their use.

Illustrations. The annotated *Drug Product Illustration*, see Section 2.2, and the *Therapeutic Equivalence Evaluations Illustration*, see Section 2.3, are offered to provide further clarification. These depict the format found in the Prescription Drug Product List (the only list in which therapeutic equivalence evaluation codes are displayed).

Drug Product Lists. The Drug Product Lists, arranged alphabetically by active ingredient, contain product identification information (active ingredients, dosage forms, routes of administration, product names, application holders, strengths) for single and multiple ingredient drug products. Also shown are the application number and drug product number (FDA internal computer data use only) and approval dates for those drug products approved on or after January 1, 1982.

The abridged Discontinued Product List, arranged alphabetically by active ingredient(s), contain product identification information (dosage form, product name, strength, and application number).

If a prescription drug product is available from more than one source (multisource), a therapeutic equivalence code will appear in front of the applicant's name. If a product is therapeutically equivalent to one or more products or to an appropriate reference, it will be designated with a code beginning with "**A**" and the entry will be underlined and printed in bold font for emphasis.

Active ingredient headings for multiple ingredient (combination) drug products are arranged alphabetically. For purposes of this publication, this alphabetical sort takes precidence over United States Pharmacopeia official monograph order (i.e., Reserpine, Hydralazine Hydrochloride, Hydrochlorthiazide). For example, product information labeled as Reserpine, Hydrochlorothiazide and Hydralazine Hydrochloride appears under the active ingredient heading *Hydralazine Hydrochloride; Hydrochlorothiazide; Reserpine*. A cross-reference to the product information (for prescription and OTC products) appears for each additional active ingredient in the product. For combination drug products, the ingredient strengths are separated by semicolons and appear in the same relative sequence as the ingredients in the heading. Available strengths of the dosage form from an applicant appear on separate lines.

To use the Drug Product Lists, determine by alphabetical order the ingredient under which the product information is listed, using the Product Name Index, if necessary. Then, find the ingredient in the applicable Drug Product List. Proceed to the dosage form and route of administration and compare products within that ingredient heading only. Therapeutic equivalence or inequivalence for prescription products is determined on the basis of the therapeutic equivalence codes provided within that specific dosage form heading. The OTC Drug Product List, Discontinued Drug Product List, and Drug Products with Approval under Section 505 of the Act Administered by the Center for Biologics Evaluation and Research List have their data arranged similarly. The Discontinued Drug Product List contains approved products that have never been marketed, have been discontinued from marketing, or have had their approvals withdrawn for other than safety or efficacy reasons subsequent to being discontinued from marketing. All products having a "@" in the 12th Cumulative Supplement of the 22nd Edition List have been added to the Discontinued Drug Product List appearing in the 23rd Edition. In addition, approved drug products that are not in the commercial distribution channel e.g. approved drug products in applications for export only are also listed in the Discontinued Section of the Orange Book.

Orphan Drug Product Designations. Drugs and biologics that have been granted Orphan Designation pursuant to Section 526 as amended by the Orphan Drug Act [P.L. 97-414, January 4, 1983] are listed in Section 3.5.

Product Name Index (Prescription and OTC Drug Product Lists). This is an index of drug products by established or trade name. The second term of each entry indicates the active ingredient name under which product information can be found in the appropriate Drug Product List. For those drug products with multiple active ingredients, only the first active ingredient (in alphabetical order) will appear. OTC products are so designated.

Product Name Index Listed by Applicant (Prescription and OTC Drug Product Lists). This is an index that cross-refereences applicants to drug products. The bolded and underlined entry represents the applicant name abbreviation used in this publication. Each complete applicant name that is represented by the abbreviated name is marked with an asterisk (*). Listed under each complete applicant name is the first alphabetically arranged ingredient under which product information can be found in the appropriate Drug Product List. OTC products are so designated. To use the Drug Product Lists, determine by alphabetical order the ingredient under which the product information is listed, using the Product Name Index, if appropriate.

Uniform Terms. To improve readability, uniform terms are used to designate dosage forms, routes of administration, and abbreviations used to express strengths. These terms are listed in Appendix C. In some cases, the terms used may differ from those used in product labels and other labeling.

2.2 DRUG PRODUCT ILLUSTRATION

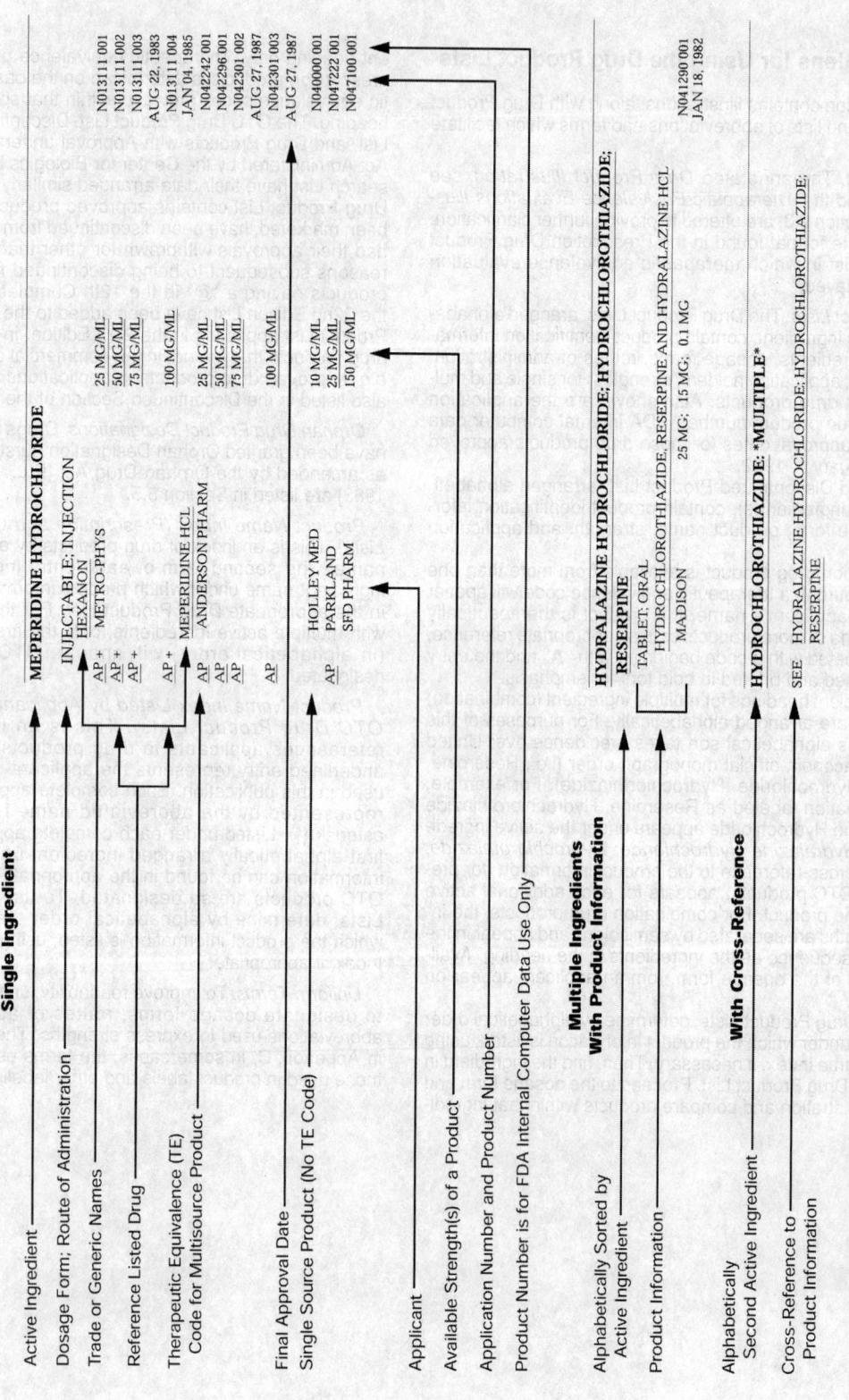

Single Ingredient

Active Ingredient

Dosage Form; Route of Administration

Trade or Generic Names

Reference Listed Drug

Therapeutic Equivalence (TE)
Code for Multisource Product

Final Approval Date

Single Source Product (No TE Code)

Applicant

Available Strength(s) of a Product

Application Number and Product Number

Product Number is for FDA Internal Computer Data Use Only

Multiple Ingredients
With Product Information

Alphabetically Sorted by
Active Ingredient

Product Information

With Cross-Reference

Alphabetically
Second Active Ingredient

Cross-Reference to
Product Information

MEPERIDINE HYDROCHLORIDE

INJECTABLE; INJECTION
  HEXANON
  METRO-PHYS

  AP +   25 MG/ML   N013111 001
  AP +   50 MG/ML   N013111 002
  AP +   75 MG/ML   N013111 003
                                                      AUG 22, 1983
  AP +   100 MG/ML   N013111 004
                                                      JAN 04, 1985
  MEPERIDINE HCL
  ANDERSON PHARM

  AP   25 MG/ML   N04242 001
  AP   50 MG/ML   N042296 001
  AP   75 MG/ML   N042301 002
                                                      AUG 27, 1987
  AP   100 MG/ML   N042301 003
                                                      AUG 27, 1987

  HOLLEY MED   10 MG/ML   N040000 001
  PARKLAND   25 MG/ML   N047222 001
  AP SFD PHARM   150 MG/ML   N047100 001

**HYDRALAZINE HYDROCHLORIDE; HYDROCHLOROTHIAZIDE;
RESERPINE**

TABLET; ORAL
  HYDROCHLOROTHIAZIDE, RESERPINE AND HYDRALAZINE HCL
  MADISON   25 MG; 15 MG; 0.1 MG   N041290 001
                                                     JAN 18, 1982

HYDROCHLOROTHIAZIDE: *MULTIPLE*

SEE HYDRALAZINE HYDROCHLORIDE; HYDROCHLOROTHIAZIDE;
    RESERPINE

This example is for purposes of illustration only. It does not represent actual products from the Prescription Drug Product list.

2.3 THERAPEUTIC EQUIVALENCE EVALUATIONS ILLUSTRATION

Drug products coded **AB** (or any code beginning with an "**A**") under an ingredient and dosage form heading are considered therapeutically equivalent only to other products coded **AB** (or any code beginning with an "**A**") and **NOT** to those coded **BP** (or any code beginning with a "**B**") and any products not listed. Drug products coded **BP** (or any code beginning with a "**B**") are **NOT** considered therapeutically equivalent to any other product. For a complete explanation of the TE codes refer to Section 1.7 of the *Introduction.*

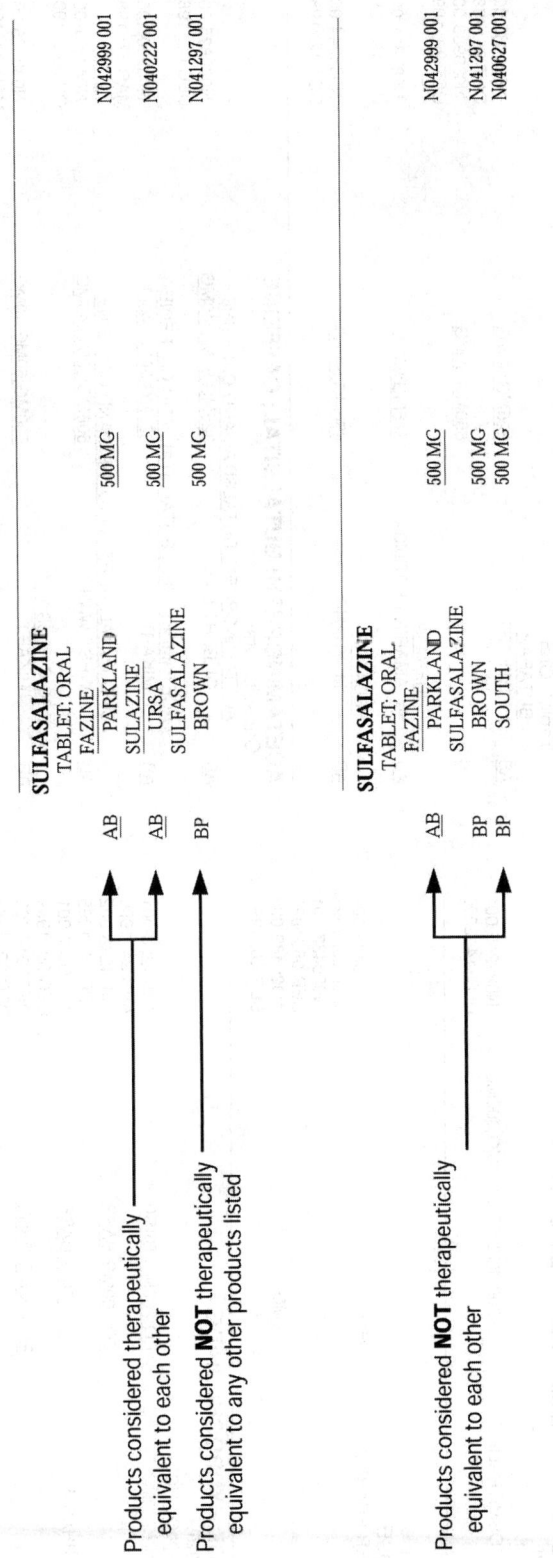

SULFASALAZINE
TABLET; ORAL

AB	FAZINE PARKLAND	500 MG	N042999 001
AB	SULAZINE URSA	500 MG	N040222 001
BP	SULFASALAZINE BROWN	500 MG	N041297 001

Products considered therapeutically equivalent to each other

Products considered **NOT** therapeutically equivalent to any other products listed

SULFASALAZINE
TABLET; ORAL

AB	FAZINE PARKLAND	500 MG	N042999 001
BP	SULFASALAZINE BROWN	500 MG	N041297 001
BP	SOUTH	500 MG	N040627 001

Products considered **NOT** therapeutically equivalent to each other

NOTE: Underlining denotes multisource products which are considered therapeutically equivalent.
This example is for purposes of illustration only. It does not represent actual products from the Prescription Drug Product list.

PRESCRIPTION DRUG PRODUCTS

ABACAVIR SULFATE
Solution; Oral
ZIAGEN
+ GLAXOSMITHKLINE   EQ 20MG BASE/ML   N020978 001 DEC 17, 1998

Tablet; Oral
ZIAGEN
+ GLAXOSMITHKLINE   EQ 300MG BASE   N020977 001 DEC 17, 1998

ABACAVIR SULFATE; LAMIVUDINE; ZIDOVUDINE
Tablet; Oral
TRIZIVIR
+ GLAXOSMITHKLINE   EQ 300MG BASE;150MG;300MG   N021205 001 NOV 14, 2000

ACARBOSE
Tablet; Oral
PRECOSE
BAYER PHARMS   25MG   N020482 004 MAY 29, 1997
   50MG   N020482 001 SEP 06, 1995
   100MG   N020482 002 SEP 06, 1995

ACEBUTOLOL HYDROCHLORIDE
Capsule; Oral
ACEBUTOLOL HCL
AB   MYLAN   EQ 200MG BASE   N074288 001 APR 24, 1995
AB   EQ 400MG BASE   N074288 002 APR 24, 1995
AB   PAR PHARM   EQ 200MG BASE   N075047 001 DEC 30, 1999
AB   EQ 400MG BASE   N075047 002 DEC 30, 1999
AB   WATSON LABS   EQ 200MG BASE   N074007 001 OCT 18, 1995
AB   EQ 400MG BASE   N074007 002 OCT 18, 1995
SECTRAL
AB   ESP PHARMA   EQ 200MG BASE   N018917 001 DEC 28, 1984
AB +   EQ 400MG BASE   N018917 003 DEC 28, 1984

ACETAMINOPHEN; ASPIRIN; CODEINE PHOSPHATE
Capsule; Oral
ACETAMINOPHEN, ASPIRIN, AND CODEINE PHOSPHATE
+ MIKART   150MG;180MG;30MG   N081096 001 OCT 26, 1990

ACETAMINOPHEN; BUTALBITAL
Capsule; Oral
BUCET
AB   MALLINCKRODT   650MG;50MG   N088991 001 JUN 28, 1985
PHRENILIN FORTE
AB + AMARIN PHARMS   650MG;50MG   N088831 001 JUN 19, 1985
TENCON
AB   MALLINCKRODT   650MG;50MG   N089405 001 MAY 15, 1990

Tablet; Oral
BUTAPAP
AB   MIKART   325MG;50MG   N089987 001 OCT 26, 1992
AB   650MG;50MG   N089988 001 OCT 26, 1992
PHRENILIN
AB + AMARIN PHARMS   325MG;50MG   N087811 001 JUN 19, 1985
SEDAPAP
AB + MAYRAND   650MG;50MG   N088944 001 OCT 17, 1985

ACETAMINOPHEN; BUTALBITAL; CAFFEINE
Capsule; Oral
ACETAMINOPHEN, BUTALBITAL AND CAFFEINE
AB + GILBERT LABS   325MG;50MG;40MG   N088825 001 DEC 05, 1984
ACETAMINOPHEN, BUTALBITAL, AND CAFFEINE
AB   MIKART   325MG;50MG;40MG   N089007 001 MAR 17, 1986
BUTALBITAL, ACETAMINOPHEN AND CAFFEINE
AB   WEST WARD   500MG;50MG;40MG   N040261 001 OCT 28, 1998
ESGIC-PLUS
AB + MIKART   500MG;50MG;40MG   N040085 001 MAR 28, 1996

Solution; Oral
ACETAMINOPHEN AND BUTALBITAL AND CAFFEINE
AB + MIKART   325MG/15ML;50MG/15ML;40MG/15ML   N040387 001 JAN 31, 2003

Tablet; Oral
BUTALBITAL, ACETAMINOPHEN AND CAFFEINE
AB   ABLE   325MG;50MG;40MG   N040390 001 JUL 23, 2001
                              N040394 001 JUL 23, 2001
AB   MALLINCKRODT   500MG;50MG;40MG   N087804 001 JAN 24, 1985
AB   MIKART   325MG;50MG;40MG   N089175 001 JAN 21, 1987
                               N089451 001 MAY 23, 1988
AB +   500MG;50MG;40MG   N040267 001 JUL 30, 1998
AB   WATSON LABS   500MG;50MG;40MG

Prescription Drug Products (continued)

ACETAMINOPHEN; BUTALBITAL; CAFFEINE (continued)

Tablet; Oral

BUTALBITAL, ACETAMINOPHEN AND CAFFEINE
- AB WEST WARD 325MG;50MG;40MG N089718 001 JUN 12, 1995

BUTALBITAL, ACETAMINOPHEN, AND CAFFEINE
- AB WEST WARD 500MG;50MG;40MG N040336 001 AUG 18, 1999

BUTALBITAL, APAP, AND CAFFEINE
- AB AXIOM PHARM 325MG;50MG;40MG N089536 001 FEB 16, 1988

FIORICET
- AB + WATSON PHARMS 325MG;50MG;40MG N088616 001 NOV 09, 1984

ACETAMINOPHEN; BUTALBITAL; CAFFEINE; CODEINE PHOSPHATE

Capsule; Oral

ACETAMINOPHEN, BUTALBITAL, CAFFEINE, AND CODEINE PHOSPHATE
- AB VINTAGE PHARMS 325MG;50MG;40MG;30MG N075929 001 APR 22, 2002

BUTALBITAL; ACETAMINOPHEN; AND CAFFEINE WITH CODEINE PHOSPHATE
- AB WEST WARD 325MG;50MG;40MG;30MG N075618 001 MAR 23, 2001

FIORICET W/ CODEINE
- AB + WATSON PHARMS 325MG;50MG;40MG;30MG N020232 001 JUL 30, 1992

PHRENILIN WITH CAFFEINE AND CODEINE
- AB AMARIN PHARMS 325MG;50MG;40MG;30MG N074911 001 AUG 22, 2001

ACETAMINOPHEN; CAFFEINE; DIHYDROCODEINE BITARTRATE

Capsule; Oral

ACETAMINOPHEN, CAFFEINE, AND DIHYDROCODEINE BITARTRATE
- AA + MIKART 356.4MG;30MG;16MG N040109 001 AUG 26, 1997

Tablet; Oral

ACETAMINOPHEN, CAFFEINE, AND DIHYDROCODEINE BITARTRATE
- AA + MIKART 712.8MG;60MG;32MG N040316 001 APR 28, 1999

ACETAMINOPHEN; CODEINE PHOSPHATE

Solution; Oral

ACETAMINOPHEN AND CODEINE PHOSPHATE
- AA + ALPHARMA 120MG/5ML;12MG/5ML N085861 001 FEB 10, 1988
- AA CLONMEL 120MG/5ML;12MG/5ML N040098 001 SEP 20, 1996
- AA HI TECH PHARMA 120MG/5ML;12MG/5ML N040119 001 APR 26, 1996
- AA MIKART 120MG/5ML;12MG/5ML N089450 001 OCT 27, 1992
- AA MORTON GROVE 120MG/5ML;12MG/5ML N087006 001
- AA PHARM ASSOC 120MG/5ML;12MG/5ML N087508 001

ACETAMINOPHEN W/ CODEINE
- AA ROXANE 120MG/5ML;12MG/5ML N086366 001

ACETAMINOPHEN; CODEINE PHOSPHATE (continued)

Suspension; Oral

ACETAMINOPHEN AND CODEINE PHOSPHATE
- AA AMARIN PHARMS 120MG/5ML;12MG/5ML N086024 001

CAPITAL AND CODEINE
- AA ALPHARMA 120MG/5ML;12MG/5ML N085883 001

Tablet; Oral

ACETAMINOPHEN AND CODEINE PHOSPAHTE
- AA ANDRX PHARMS 300MG;15MG N040443 001 JAN 22, 2003
- AA   300MG;30MG N040443 002 JAN 22, 2003
- AA   300MG;60MG N040443 003 JAN 22, 2003

ACETAMINOPHEN AND CODEINE PHOSPHATE
- AA ABLE 300MG;30MG N040452 001 AUG 01, 2002
- AA   300MG;60MG N040459 001 AUG 01, 2002
- AA DURAMED PHARM BARR 300MG;15MG N040223 001 NOV 18, 1997
- AA   300MG;30MG N040223 002 NOV 18, 1997
- AA   300MG;60MG N040223 003 NOV 18, 1997
- AA GENEVA PHARMS 300MG;60MG N081249 001 JUL 16, 1992
- AA   300MG;30MG N081250 001 JUL 16, 1992
- AA MALLINCKRODT 300MG;15MG N040419 001 MAY 31, 2001
- AA   300MG;30MG N040419 002 MAY 31, 2001
- AA   300MG;60MG N040419 003 MAY 31, 2001
- AA   650MG;30MG N089231 001 MAR 03, 1986
- AA + MIKART 300MG;30MG N089238 001 FEB 25, 1986
- AA +   650MG;60MG N089363 001 SEP 09, 1991
- AA + 300MG;15MG N089671 001 FEB 10, 1988
- AA MUTUAL PHARM 300MG;30MG N089672 001 FEB 10, 1988
- AA   300MG;60MG N089673 001 FEB 10, 1988
- AA PHARMERAL 300MG;30MG N087762 001 DEC 10, 1982
- AA PUREPAC PHARM 300MG;30MG N086681 001
- AA RANBAXY 300MG;60MG N087083 001
- AA TEVA 300MG;15MG N088627 001 MAR 06, 1985
- AA   300MG;30MG N088628 001 MAR 06, 1985
- AA   300MG;60MG N088629 001 MAR 06, 1985

Prescription Drug Products (continued)

ACETAMINOPHEN; CODEINE PHOSPHATE (continued)

Tablet; Oral

ACETAMINOPHEN AND CODEINE PHOSPHATE

TE	Strength	Applicant	Appl. No.	Approval Date
AA	300MG;30MG	VINTAGE PHARMS	N089805 001	SEP 30, 1988
AA	300MG;60MG		N089828 001	SEP 30, 1988
AA	300MG;15MG		N089990 001	SEP 30, 1988
AA	300MG;15MG	WATSON LABS	N089997 001	DEC 28, 1994
AA	300MG;30MG		N089998 001	DEC 28, 1994
AA	300MG;60MG		N089999 001	DEC 28, 1994

ACETAMINOPHEN AND CODEINE PHOSPHATE #2

TE	Strength	Applicant	Appl. No.	Approval Date
AA	300MG;15MG	SUPERPHARM	N089183 001	OCT 18, 1985

ACETAMINOPHEN W/ CODEINE NO. 3

TE	Strength	Applicant	Appl. No.	Approval Date
AA	300MG;30MG	ROXANE	N084656 001	

ACETAMINOPHEN W/ CODEINE PHOSPHATE #3

TE	Strength	Applicant	Appl. No.	Approval Date
AA	300MG;30MG	RANBAXY	N085868 001	

CODRIX

TE	Strength	Applicant	Appl. No.	Approval Date
+	500MG;15MG	ANDRX PHARMS	N040447 001	FEB 26, 2003
+	500MG;30MG		N040441 001	MAR 27, 2003
+	500MG;60MG		N040488 001	MAR 28, 2003

TYLENOL W/ CODEINE NO. 1

TE	Strength	Applicant	Appl. No.	Approval Date
+	300MG;7.5MG	ORTHO MCNEIL PHARM		

TYLENOL W/ CODEINE NO. 2

TE	Strength	Applicant	Appl. No.	Approval Date
+	300MG;15MG	ORTHO MCNEIL PHARM		

TYLENOL W/ CODEINE NO. 3

TE	Strength	Applicant	Appl. No.	Approval Date
+	300MG;30MG	ORTHO MCNEIL PHARM		

TYLENOL W/ CODEINE NO. 4

TE	Strength	Applicant	Appl. No.	Approval Date
+	300MG;60MG	ORTHO MCNEIL PHARM		

ACETAMINOPHEN; HYDROCODONE BITARTRATE

Capsule; Oral

ACETAMINOPHEN AND HYDROCODONE BITARTRATE

TE	Strength	Applicant	Appl. No.	Approval Date
AA	500MG;5MG	CENT PHARMS	N088898 001	MAR 27, 1985

ALLAY

TE	Strength	Applicant	Appl. No.	Approval Date
AA	500MG;5MG	IVAX PHARMS	N089907 001	JAN 13, 1989

HYDROCET

TE	Strength	Applicant	Appl. No.	Approval Date
AA	500MG;5MG	MALLINCKRODT	N089006 001	AUG 09, 1985

HYDROCODONE BITARTRATE AND ACETAMINOPHEN

TE	Strength	Applicant	Appl. No.	Approval Date
AA	500MG;5MG	MALLINCKRODT	N088956 001	JUL 19, 1985

MIKART

TE	Strength	Applicant	Appl. No.	Approval Date
AA	500MG;5MG	MIKART	N081067 001	NOV 30, 1989
AA	500MG;5MG		N081068 001	NOV 30, 1989
AA	500MG;5MG		N081069 001	NOV 30, 1989

ACETAMINOPHEN; HYDROCODONE BITARTRATE (continued)

Capsule; Oral

HYDROCODONE BITARTRATE AND ACETAMINOPHEN

MIKART

TE	Strength	Applicant	Appl. No.	Approval Date
AA	500MG;5MG	MIKART	N081070 001	NOV 30, 1989
AA	500MG;5MG		N089008 001	NOV 30, 1989

LORCET-HD

TE	Strength	Applicant	Appl. No.	Approval Date
AA	+	500MG;5MG	MALLINCKRODT	FEB 21, 1986

Solution; Oral

HYDROCODONE BITARTRATE AND ACETAMINOPHEN

TE	Strength	Applicant	Appl. No.	Approval Date
AA	500MG/15ML;7.5MG/15ML	KV PHARM	N087336 001	JUL 08, 1982
AA	500MG/15ML;7.5MG/15ML	MALLINCKRODT	N040366 001	JAN 23, 2002
AA	500MG/15ML;7.5MG/15ML		N040418 001	JUN 27, 2001
AA	+ MIKART	500MG/15ML;7.5MG/15ML		N081051 001	AUG 28, 1992
AA	500MG/15ML;5MG/15ML		N081226 001	OCT 27, 1992
AA	500MG/15ML;5MG/15ML		N089557 001	APR 29, 1992
AA	+ PHARM ASSOC	500MG/15ML;7.5MG/15ML		N040182 001	MAR 13, 1998

Tablet; Oral

ACETAMINOPHEN AND HYDROCODONE BITARTRATE

TE	Strength	Applicant	Appl. No.	Approval Date
AA	650MG;7.5MG	ABLE	N040474 001	JAN 02, 2003

ANEXSIA

TE	Strength	Applicant	Appl. No.	Approval Date
AA	500MG;5MG	MALLINCKRODT	N089160 001	APR 23, 1987

ANEXSIA 5/325

TE	Strength	Applicant	Appl. No.	Approval Date
AA	325MG;5MG	MALLINCKRODT	N040409 001	OCT 20, 2000

ANEXSIA 7.5/325

TE	Strength	Applicant	Appl. No.	Approval Date
AA	325MG;7.5MG	MALLINCKRODT	N040405 001	SEP 08, 2000

ANEXSIA 7.5/650

TE	Strength	Applicant	Appl. No.	Approval Date
AA	650MG;7.5MG	MALLINCKRODT	N089725 001	SEP 30, 1987

CO-GESIC

TE	Strength	Applicant	Appl. No.	Approval Date
AA	500MG;5MG	SCHWARZ PHARMA	N087757 001	MAY 03, 1982

HY-PHEN

TE	Strength	Applicant	Appl. No.	Approval Date
AA	500MG;5MG	ASCHER	N087677 001	MAY 03, 1982

HYDROCODONE BITARTRATE AND ACETAMINOPHEN

TE	Strength	Applicant	Appl. No.	Approval Date
AA	325MG;7.5MG	ABLE	N040464 001	OCT 23, 2002
AA	325MG;10MG		N040464 002	OCT 23, 2002
AA	750MG;7.5MG		N040469 001	OCT 23, 2002
AA	500MG;10MG		N040473 001	OCT 25, 2002
AA	650MG;10MG		N040476 001	NOV 06, 2002

Prescription Drug Products (continued)

ACETAMINOPHEN; HYDROCODONE BITARTRATE (continued)

Tablet; Oral

HYDROCODONE BITARTRATE AND ACETAMINOPHEN

Firm	TE	Strength	Approval Date	Appl. No.
ABLE	AA	500MG;5MG	OCT 23, 2002	N040477 001
	AA	325MG;5MG	NOV 06, 2002	N040478 001
	AA	500MG;7.5MG	NOV 08, 2002	N040490 001
ANDRX PHARMS	AA	500MG;5MG	MAY 21, 2003	N040493 001
	AA	750MG;7.5MG	MAY 28, 2003	N040494 001
	AA	660MG;10MG	MAY 28, 2003	N040495 001
AXIOM PHARM	AA	500MG;5MG	SEP 25, 1997	N040236 001
	AA	750MG;7.5MG	SEP 25, 1997	N040236 002
	AA	650MG;10MG	NOV 26, 1997	N040240 001
	AA	650MG;7.5MG	NOV 26, 1997	N040240 002
BARR	AA	500MG;2.5MG	NOV 26, 1997	N040307 001
	AA	500MG;7.5MG	JUL 26, 2000	N040307 002
	AA	650MG;7.5MG	JUL 26, 2000	N040307 003
	AA	650MG;10MG	JUL 26, 2000	N040307 004
	AA	500MG;5MG	JUL 26, 2000	N040308 001
	AA	750MG;7.5MG	JUL 26, 2000	N040308 002
	AA	500MG;10MG	JUL 26, 2000	N040309 001
ENDO PHARMS	AA	500MG;7.5MG	JUL 26, 2000	N040280 001
	AA	650MG;7.5MG	SEP 30, 1998	N040280 002
	AA	650MG;10MG	SEP 30, 1998	N040280 003
	AA	500MG;5MG	SEP 30, 1998	N040281 001
	AA	750MG;7.5MG	SEP 30, 1998	N040281 002
	AA	400MG;5MG	SEP 30, 1998	N040288 001
	AA+	400MG;7.5MG	NOV 27, 1998	N040288 002
	AA+	400MG;10MG	NOV 27, 1998	N040288 003
EON	AA+	500MG;5MG	NOV 27, 1998	N040149 001
	AA	750MG;7.5MG	JAN 27, 1997	N040149 002

ACETAMINOPHEN; HYDROCODONE BITARTRATE (continued)

Tablet; Oral

HYDROCODONE BITARTRATE AND ACETAMINOPHEN

Firm	TE	Strength	Approval Date	Appl. No.
EON	AA	500MG;5MG	JAN 27, 1997	N089696 001
IVAX PHARMS	AA	750MG;7.5MG	APR 21, 1988	N040084 001
MALLINCKRODT	AA	500MG;5MG	JUN 01, 1995	N040084 001
	AA+	660MG;10MG	JUN 01, 1995	N040084 002
	AA	650MG;10MG	JUN 01, 1995	N040084 003
	AA	500MG;7.5MG	JUL 29, 1996	N040084 004
	AA	500MG;10MG	OCT 16, 1996	N040201 001
	AA	325MG;10MG	FEB 27, 1998	N040201 002
	AA	750MG;10MG	FEB 27, 1998	N040400 001
	AA	325MG;7.5MG	JUL 26, 2000	N040468 001
	AA	650MG;10MG	OCT 31, 2002	N040432 001
	AA	500MG;5MG	JAN 22, 2003	N081223 001
MIKART	AA+	650MG;7.5MG	MAY 29, 1992	N089271 001
	AA	500MG;5MG	JUL 16, 1986	N089689 001
	AA	500MG;2.5MG	JUN 29, 1988	N089697 001
	AA+	500MG;7.5MG	JAN 28, 1992	N089698 001
	AA+	650MG;7.5MG	AUG 25, 1989	N089699 001
UCB	AA+	500MG;10MG	AUG 25, 1989	N040134 001
	AA	650MG;10MG	AUG 25, 1989	N040210 001
VINTAGE PHARMS	AA	500MG;7.5MG	NOV 21, 1996	N040143 001
	AA	500MG;2.5MG	AUG 13, 1997	N040144 001
	AA	650MG;7.5MG	FEB 22, 1996	N040144 002
	AA	750MG;7.5MG	FEB 22, 1996	N040155 001
	AA	325MG;10MG	APR 25, 1997	N040157 001
	AA	500MG;10MG	APR 14, 1997	N040355 001
	AA	660MG;10MG	APR 12, 1996	N040356 001
	AA	500MG;5MG	MAY 31, 2000	N040358 001
	AA		MAY 31, 2000	N089831 001

Prescription Drug Products *(continued)*

ACETAMINOPHEN; HYDROCODONE BITARTRATE *(continued)*

Tablet; Oral

HYDROCODONE BITARTRATE AND ACETAMINOPHEN

TE	Firm / Tradename	Strength	Appl No	Approval Date
	VINTAGE PHARMS			
AA		500MG;5MG		SEP 07, 1988
	WATSON LABS			
AA		650MG;7.5MG	N089971 001	DEC 02, 1988
AA		650MG;10MG	N040094 001	SEP 29, 1995
AA		660MG;10MG	N040094 002	SEP 29, 1995
AA		750MG;10MG	N040094 003	AUG 08, 2000
AA	+	500MG;5MG	N040094 004	MAR 22, 1999
AA		750MG;7.5MG	N040122 001	MAR 04, 1996
AA		650MG;7.5MG	N040122 002	MAR 04, 1996
AA		650MG;10MG	N040123 001	MAR 04, 1996
AA		500MG;2.5MG	N040123 002	MAR 04, 1996
AA		500MG;7.5MG	N040123 003	MAR 04, 1996
AA		500MG;10MG	N040123 004	MAR 04, 1996
AA		325MG;10MG	N040148 002	FEB 14, 1997
AA		500MG;2.5MG	N040248 002	APR 28, 2000
AA		500MG;7.5MG	N081079 001	AUG 30, 1991
AA		750MG;7.5MG	N081080 001	AUG 30, 1991
AA		500MG;5MG	N081083 001	AUG 30, 1991
	LORTAB			
AA	MALLINCKRODT	500MG;5MG	N089883 001	DEC 01, 1988
AA	+ UCB	500MG;5MG	N087722 001	JUL 09, 1982
AA	+ UCB	500MG;10MG	N040100 001	JAN 26, 1996
	NORCO			
AA	+ WATSON LABS	325MG;5MG	N040099 001	JUN 25, 1997
AA	+	325MG;7.5MG	N040148 003	SEP 12, 2000
AA	+	325MG;10MG	N040148 001	FEB 14, 1997
	VICODIN			
AA	+ ABBOTT	500MG;5MG	N088058 001	JAN 07, 1983
	VICODIN ES			
AA	+ ABBOTT	750MG;7.5MG	N089736 001	DEC 09, 1988

ACETAMINOPHEN; HYDROCODONE BITARTRATE *(continued)*

Tablet; Oral

VICODIN HP

TE	Firm	Strength	Appl No	Approval Date
	ABBOTT			
AA		660MG;10MG	N040117 001	SEP 23, 1996

ACETAMINOPHEN; OXYCODONE HYDROCHLORIDE

Capsule; Oral

OXYCODONE AND ACETAMINOPHEN

TE	Firm / Tradename	Strength	Appl No	Approval Date
	AMIDE PHARM			
AA		500MG;5MG	N040199 001	DEC 30, 1998
	AXIOM PHARM			
AA		500MG;5MG	N040219 001	JAN 22, 1998
	BARR			
AA		500MG;5MG	N040304 001	OCT 02, 2000
	DURAMED PHARM BARR			
AA		500MG;5MG	N040289 001	MAR 16, 1999
	ENDO PHARMS			
AA		500MG;5MG	N040303 001	DEC 30, 1999
	MALLINCKRODT			
AA		500MG;5MG	N040257 001	AUG 04, 1998
	VINTAGE PHARMS			
AA		500MG;5MG	N040106 001	JUL 30, 1996
	WATSON LABS			
AA		500MG;5MG	N040234 001	OCT 30, 1997
	ROXILOX			
AA	ROXANE	500MG;5MG	N040061 001	JUL 03, 1995
	TYLOX			
AA	+ ORTHO MCNEIL PHARM	500MG;5MG	N088790 001	DEC 12, 1984

Solution; Oral

ROXICET

TE	Firm	Strength	Appl No	Approval Date
	ROXANE			
AA		325MG/5ML;5MG/5ML	N089351 001	DEC 03, 1986

Tablet; Oral

OXYCET

TE	Firm / Tradename	Strength	Appl No	Approval Date
	MALLINCKRODT			
AA		325MG;5MG	N087463 001	DEC 07, 1983
	OXYCODONE AND ACETAMINOPHEN			
	AMIDE PHARM			
AA		325MG;5MG	N040203 001	MAR 15, 1999
	BARR			
AA		325MG;5MG	N087406 001	
	DURAMED PHARM BARR			
AA		325MG;5MG	N040272 001	JUN 30, 1998
	VINTAGE PHARMS			
AA		325MG;5MG	N040105 001	JUL 30, 1996
	WATSON LABS			
AA		325MG;5MG	N040171 001	OCT 30, 1997
AA		500MG;7.5MG	N040371 001	DEC 29, 2000
AA		650MG;10MG	N040371 002	DEC 29, 2000
	PERCOCET			
AA	+ ENDO PHARMS	325MG;2.5MG	N040330 001	JUN 25, 1999
AA		325MG;5MG	N040330 002	

ACETAMINOPHEN; PROPOXYPHENE NAPSYLATE (continued)

Tablet; Oral

PROPOXYPHENE NAPSYLATE AND ACETAMINOPHEN

TE	Manufacturer	Strength	Appl. No.	Date
AB	HALSEY	650MG;100MG	N070771 001	MAR 21, 1986
			N070775 001	MAR 21, 1986
AB	IVAX PHARMS	650MG;100MG	N070146 001	AUG 02, 1985
AB	MALLINCKRODT	650MG;100MG	N075738 001	FEB 02, 2001
AB	MYLAN	650MG;100MG	N070145 001	JUN 12, 1985
			N072195 001	FEB 16, 1988
AB	PUREPAC PHARM	650MG;100MG	N070910 001	JAN 02, 1987
AB	TEVA	650MG;100MG	N074119 001	DEC 19, 1994
AB	VINTAGE PHARMS	650MG;100MG	N074843 001	FEB 12, 1997
AB		325MG;50MG	N074843 002	FEB 15, 2001

ACETAMINOPHEN; TRAMADOL HYDROCHLORIDE

Tablet; Oral

ULTRACET

TE	Manufacturer	Strength	Appl. No.	Date
+	ORTHO MCNEIL PHARM	325MG;37.5MG	N021123 001	AUG 15, 2001

ACETAZOLAMIDE

Capsule, Extended Release; Oral

DIAMOX

TE	Manufacturer	Strength	Appl. No.	Date
+	DURAMED PHARM BARR	500MG	N012945 003	APR 25, 1995

Tablet; Oral

ACETAZO_AMIDE

TE	Manufacturer	Strength	Appl. No.	Date
	LANNETT	250MG	N084840 001	
AB	MUTUAL PHARM	125MG	N089752 001	JUN 22, 1988
AB		250MG	N089753 001	JUN 22, 1988
AB	TARO	125MG	N040195 001	MAY 28, 1997
AB		250MG	N040195 002	MAY 28, 1997
AB	WATSON LABS	250MG	N088882 001	OCT 22, 1985

DIAMOX

TE	Manufacturer	Strength	Appl. No.	Date
AB	DURAMED PHARM BARR	125MG	N008943 001	
AB +		250MG	N008943 002	

ACETAZOLAMIDE SODIUM

Injectable; Injection

ACETAZOLAMIDE SODIUM

TE	Manufacturer	Strength	Appl. No.	Date
AP	ABBOTT	EQ 500MG BASE/VIAL	N040108 001	

Prescription Drug Products (continued)

ACETAMINOPHEN; OXYCODONE HYDROCHLORIDE (continued)

Tablet; Oral

PERCOCET — ENDO PHARMS

TE	Strength	Appl. No.	Date
AA +	325MG;5MG	N085106 002	JUN 25, 1999
+	325MG;7.5MG	N040434 001	NOV 23, 2001
+	325MG;10MG	N040434 002	NOV 23, 2001
AA +	500MG;7.5MG	N040341 001	JUL 26, 1999
AA +	650MG;10MG	N040341 002	JUL 26, 1999

ROXICET — ROXANE

TE	Strength	Appl. No.	Date
AA +	325MG;5MG	N087003 001	

ROXICET 5/500

TE	Strength	Appl. No.	Date
+ ROXANE	500MG;5MG	N089775 001	JAN 12, 1989

ACETAMINOPHEN; PENTAZOCINE HYDROCHLORIDE

Tablet; Oral

ACETAMINOPHEN AND PENTAZOCINE HCL

TE	Manufacturer	Strength	Appl. No.	Date
AB	AMIDE PHARM	650MG;EQ 25MG BASE	N076202 001	AUG 02, 2002

PENTAZOCINE HCL AND ACETAMINOPHEN

TE	Manufacturer	Strength	Appl. No.	Date
AB	WATSON LABS	650MG;EQ 25MG BASE	N074699 001	MAR 24, 2000

TALACEN

TE	Manufacturer	Strength	Appl. No.	Date
AB +	SANOFI SYNTHELABO	650MG;EQ 25MG BASE	N018458 001	SEP 23, 1982

ACETAMINOPHEN; PROPOXYPHENE HYDROCHLORIDE

Tablet; Oral

PROPOXYPHENE HCL AND ACETAMINOPHEN

TE	Manufacturer	Strength	Appl. No.	Date
AA	GENEVA PHARMS	650MG;65MG	N089959 001	JUL 18, 1989
AA	MYLAN	650MG;65MG	N083978 001	
AA	WATSON LABS	650MG;65MG	N040139 001	DEC 16, 1996

WYGESIC

TE	Manufacturer	Strength	Appl. No.	Date
AA +	WOMEN FIRST HLTHCARE	650MG;65MG	N084999 001	

ACETAMINOPHEN; PROPOXYPHENE NAPSYLATE

Tablet; Oral

DARVOCET-N 50

TE	Manufacturer	Strength	Appl. No.	Date
AB	AAIPHARMA LLC	325MG;50MG	N017122 001	

DARVOCET-N 100

TE	Manufacturer	Strength	Appl. No.	Date
AB +	AAIPHARMA LLC	650MG;100MG	N017122 002	

PROPOXYPHENE NAPSYLATE AND ACETAMINOPHEN

TE	Manufacturer	Strength	Appl. No.	Date
AB +	ABLE	650MG;100MG	N075838 001	JUL 11, 2001
AB	GENEVA PHARMS	650MG;100MG	N070443 001	JAN 23, 1986
AB	HALSEY	650MG;100MG	N070615 001	MAR 21, 1986

Prescription Drug Products (continued)

ACETAZOLAMIDE SODIUM (continued)
Injectable; Injection

ACETAZOLAMIDE SODIUM

AP	ABBOTT		N040089 001	OCT 30, 1995
AP	BEDFORD	EQ 500MG BASE/VIAL		FEB 28, 1995

DIAMOX

AP	+ DURAMED PHARM BARR	EQ 500MG BASE/VIAL	N009388 001	DEC 05, 1990

ACETIC ACID, GLACIAL
Solution/Drops; Otic

ACETASOL

AT	ALPHARMA	2%	N087146 001	

ACETIC ACID

AT	MORTON GROVE	2%	N040166 001	JUL 26, 1996
			N088638 001	SEP 06, 1984
AT	TARO	2%	N012179 001	

VOSOL

AT	+ MEDPOINTE PHARM HLC	2%	

Solution; Irrigation, Urethral

ACETIC ACID 0.25% IN PLASTIC CONTAINER

AT	ABBOTT	250MG/100ML	N017656 001	
AT	B BRAUN	250MG/100ML	N018161 001	
AT	BAXTER HLTHCARE	250MG/100ML	N018523 001	FEB 19, 1982

ACETIC ACID, GLACIAL; ALUMINUM ACETATE
Solution/Drops; Otic

ACETIC ACID 2% IN AQUEOUS ALUMINUM ACETATE

AT	BAUSCH AND LOMB	2%;0.79%	N040063 001	FEB 25, 1994

DOMEBORO

AT	+ BAYER PHARMS	2%;0.79%	N084476 001	

ACETIC ACID, GLACIAL; HYDROCORTISONE
Solution/Drops; Otic

ACETASOL HC

AT	ALPHARMA	2%;1%	N087143 001	JAN 13, 1982

HYDROCORTISONE AND ACETIC ACID

AT	MORTON GROVE	2%;1%	N040168 001	AUG 30, 1996
			N088759 001	MAR 04, 1985
AT	TARO	2%;1%	N012770 001	

VOSOL HC

AT	+ MEDPOINTE PHARM HLC	2%;1%	

ACETOHEXAMIDE
Tablet; Oral

ACETOHEXAMIDE

AB	BARR	250MG	N070869 001	FEB 09, 1987
AB	+	500MG	N070870 001	FEB 09, 1987

ACETOHEXAMIDE (continued)
Tablet; Oral

ACETOHEXAMIDE

AB	WATSON LABS	250MG	N071893 001	NOV 25, 1987
AB		500MG	N071894 001	NOV 25, 1987

ACETOHYDROXAMIC ACID
Tablet; Oral

LITHOSTAT

+ MISSION PHARMA	250MG	N018749 001	MAY 31, 1983

ACETYLCHOLINE CHLORIDE
For Solution; Ophthalmic

MIOCHOL

+ NOVARTIS	20MG/VIAL	N016211 001	

MIOCHOL-E

+ NOVARTIS	20MG/VIAL	N020213 001	SEP 22, 1993

ACETYLCYSTEINE
Solution; Inhalation, Oral

ACETYLCYSTEINE

AN	ABBOTT	10%	N073664 001	AUG 30, 1994
AN		20%	N074037 001	AUG 30, 1994
AN	BEDFORD	10%	N072323 001	APR 30, 1992
AN		20%	N072324 001	APR 30, 1992
AN	FAULDING	10%	N071364 001	MAY 01, 1989
AN		10%	N071365 002	JAN 18, 2002
AN		20%	N071364 002	JAN 18, 2002
AN	LUITPOLD	10%	N071365 001	MAY 01, 1989
AN		20%	N072489 001	JUL 28, 1995
AN	ROXANE	10%	N072547 001	JUL 28, 1995
AN		20%	N072621 001	SEP 30, 1992
			N072622 001	SEP 30, 1992

MUCOMYST

AN	+ APOTHECON	10%	N013601 002
AN	+	20%	N013601 001

MUCOSIL-10

AN	DEY	10%	N070575 001	OCT 14, 1986

Prescription Drug Products *(continued)*

ACETYLCYSTEINE *(continued)*
Solution; Inhalation, Oral
MUCOSIL-20

TE	Manufacturer	Strength	Appl. No.	Date
AN	DEY	20%	N070576 001	OCT 14, 1986

ACITRETIN
Capsule; Oral
SORIATANE

TE	Manufacturer	Strength	Appl. No.	Date
	HLR	10MG	N019821 001	OCT 28, 1996
+		25MG	N019821 002	OCT 28, 1996

ACRIVASTINE; PSEUDOEPHEDRINE HYDROCHLORIDE
Capsule; Oral
SEMPREX-D

TE	Manufacturer	Strength	Appl. No.	Date
+	CELLTECH PHARMS	8MG;60MG	N019806 001	MAR 25, 1994

ACYCLOVIR
Capsule; Oral
ACYCLOVIR

TE	Manufacturer	Strength	Appl. No.	Date
AB	AAIPHARMA	200MG	N074833 001	APR 22, 1997
AB	APOTHECON	200MG	N074889 001	OCT 31, 1997
AB	CLONMEL HLTHCARE	200MG	N074872 001	APR 22, 1997
AB	COPLEY PHARM	200MG	N074914 001	NOV 26, 1997
AB	GENPHARM	200MG	N074977 001	APR 13, 1998
AB	IVAX PHARMS	200MG	N074674 001	APR 22, 1997
AB	MYLAN	200MG	N074727 001	APR 22, 1997
AB	PUREPAC PHARM	200MG	N074906 001	AUG 26, 1997
AB	RANBAXY	200MG	N074975 001	SEP 30, 1998
AB	STASON	200MG	N075090 001	JAN 26, 1999
AB	TEVA	200MG	N074578 001	APR 22, 1997
AB	WATSON LABS	200MG	N074828 001	APR 22, 1997
AB		200MG	N075101 001	APR 15, 1998

ZOVIRAX

TE	Manufacturer	Strength	Appl. No.	Date
AB	+ GLAXOSMITHKLINE	200MG	N018828 001	JAN 25, 1985

Cream; Topical
ZOVIRAX

TE	Manufacturer	Strength	Appl. No.	Date
	+ GLAXOSMITHKLINE	5%	N021478 001	DEC 30, 2002

ACYCLOVIR *(continued)*
Ointment; Topical
ZOVIRAX

TE	Manufacturer	Strength	Appl. No.	Date
AB	+ GLAXOSMITHKLINE	5%	N018604 001	MAR 29, 1982

Suspension; Oral
ACYCLOVIR

TE	Manufacturer	Strength	Appl. No.	Date
AB	ALPHARMA	200MG/5ML	N074738 001	APR 28, 1997

ZOVIRAX

TE	Manufacturer	Strength	Appl. No.	Date
AB	+ GLAXOSMITHKLINE	200MG/5ML	N019909 001	DEC 22, 1989

Tablet; Oral
ACYCLOVIR

TE	Manufacturer	Strength	Appl. No.	Date
AB	APOTHECON	400MG	N074891 001	OCT 31, 1997
AB		800MG	N074891 002	OCT 31, 1997
AB	CARLSBAD	400MG	N075382 001	APR 30, 1999
AB		800MG	N075382 002	APR 30, 1999
AB	CLONMEL HLTHCARE	400MG	N074834 001	APR 24, 1997
AB		800MG	N074834 002	APR 24, 1997
AB	COPLEY PHARM	400MG	N075021 001	MAR 18, 1998
AB		800MG	N075021 002	MAR 18, 1998
AB	GENPHARM	400MG	N074976 001	APR 13, 1998
AB		800MG	N074976 002	APR 13, 1998
AB	IVAX PHARMS	400MG	N074836 001	APR 22, 1997
AB		800MG	N074836 002	APR 22, 1997
AB	MYLAN	400MG	N075211 001	SEP 28, 1998
AB		800MG	N075211 002	SEP 28, 1998
AB	NEOSAN PHARMS	400MG	N074946 001	NOV 19, 1997
AB		800MG	N074946 002	NOV 19, 1997
AB	PUREPAC PHARM	400MG	N074870 001	JUN 05, 1997
AB		800MG	N074870 002	JUN 05, 1997
AB	RANBAXY	400MG	N074980 001	SEP 30, 1998
AB		800MG	N074980 002	SEP 30, 1998
AB	TEVA	400MG	N074556 002	APR 22, 1997
AB		800MG	N074556 003	

Prescription Drug Products *(continued)*

ACYCLOVIR *(continued)*

Tablet; Oral

ACYCLOVIR

TE	Applicant	Strength	Appl No	Date
	TEVA			APR 22, 1997

ZOVIRAX

TE	Applicant	Strength	Appl No	Date
AB	GLAXOSMITHKLINE	400MG	N020089 001	APR 30, 1991
AB +	GLAXOSMITHKLINE	800MG	N020089 002	APR 30, 1991

ACYCLOVIR SODIUM

Injectable; Injection

ACYCLOVIR

TE	Applicant	Strength	Appl No	Date
AP	ABBOTT	EQ 50MG BASE/ML	N075114 001	JUL 26, 1999
AP	GENSIA SICOR PHARMS	EQ 50MG BASE/ML	N075627 001	MAR 28, 2001

ACYCLOVIR IN SODIUM CHLORIDE 0.9% PRESERVATIVE FREE

TE	Applicant	Strength	Appl No	Date
AP +	ESI LEDERLE	EQ 500MG BASE/VIAL	N074885 001	DEC 19, 1997
		EQ 1GM BASE/VIAL	N074885 002	DEC 19, 1997

ACYCLOVIR SODIUM

TE	Applicant	Strength	Appl No	Date
AP	ABBOTT	EQ 1GM BASE/VIAL	N074663 002	APR 22, 1997
		EQ 1GM BASE/VIAL	N074758 002	APR 22, 1997
		EQ 500MG BASE/VIAL	N074663 001	APR 22, 1997
AP		EQ 500MG BASE/VIAL	N074758 001	APR 22, 1997
AP +	AM PHARM PARTNERS	EQ 50MG BASE/ML	N074930 001	APR 22, 1997
AP		EQ 500MG BASE/VIAL	N075015 001	MAY 13, 1998
AP	BEDFORD	EQ 1GM BASE/VIAL	N074596 001	APR 30, 1998
AP		EQ 500MG BASE/VIAL	N074596 002	APR 22, 1997
AP	ESI LEDERLE	EQ 1GM BASE/VIAL	N074913 002	APR 22, 1997
AP		EQ 500MG BASE/VIAL	N074913 001	OCT 15, 1997
AP +	FAULDING	EQ 25MG BASE/ML	N074720 001	OCT 15, 1997
AP	GENSIA SICOR PHARMS	EQ 1GM BASE/VIAL	N074969 002	APR 22, 1997
AP		EQ 500MG BASE/VIAL	N074969 001	AUG 26, 1997
AP	MERIDIAN MEDCL TECHN	EQ 50MG BASE/ML	N075065 001	AUG 26, 1997

ZOVIRAX

TE	Applicant	Strength	Appl No	Date
AP +	GLAXOSMITHKLINE	EQ 1GM BASE/VIAL	N075065 001	FEB 25, 1999
AP +		EQ 500MG BASE/VIAL	N018603 002	JUN 29, 1989
			N018603 001	OCT 22, 1982

ADAPALENE

Cream; Topical

DIFFERIN

TE	Applicant	Strength	Appl No	Date
+	GALDERMA LABS LP	0.1%	N020748 001	MAY 26, 2000

Gel; Topical

DIFFERIN

TE	Applicant	Strength	Appl No	Date
+	GALDERMA LABS LP	0.1%	N020380 001	MAY 31, 1996

Solution; Topical

DIFFERIN

TE	Applicant	Strength	Appl No	Date
+	GALDERMA LABS LP	0.1%	N020338 001	MAY 31, 1996

ADEFOVIR DIPIVOXIL

Tablet; Oral

HEPSERA

TE	Applicant	Strength	Appl No	Date
+	GILEAD	10MG	N021449 001	SEP 20, 2002

ADENOSINE

Injectable; Injection

ADENOCARD

TE	Applicant	Strength	Appl No	Date
+	FUJISAWA HLTHCARE	3MG/ML	N019937 002	OCT 30, 1989

ADENOSCAN

TE	Applicant	Strength	Appl No	Date
+	FUJISAWA HLTHCARE	3MG/ML	N020059 001	MAY 18, 1995

ALATROFLOXACIN MESYLATE

Injectable; Injection

TROVAN PRESERVATIVE FREE

TE	Applicant	Strength	Appl No	Date
	PFIZER	EQ 200MG BASE/VIAL	N020760 001	DEC 18, 1997
+		EQ 300MG BASE/VIAL	N020760 002	DEC 18, 1997

ALBENDAZOLE

Tablet; Oral

ALBENZA

TE	Applicant	Strength	Appl No	Date
+	GLAXOSMITHKLINE	200MG	N020666 001	JUN 11, 1996

ALBUMIN HUMAN

Injectable; Injection

OPTISON

TE	Applicant	Strength	Appl No	Date
+	AMERSHAM HLTH	10MG/ML	N020899 001	DEC 31, 1997

ALBUMIN IODINATED I-125 SERUM

Injectable; Injection

RADIOIODINATED SERUM ALBUMIN (HUMAN) IHSA I 125

TE	Applicant	Strength	Appl No	Date
	MALLINCKRODT	10uCi/ML	N017844 001	

Prescription Drug Products *(continued)*

ALBUMIN IODINATED I-131 SERUM
Injectable; Injection

TE	Applicant	Strength	NDA	Date
	MEGATOPE			
	ISO TEX	0.5mCi/VIAL	N017837 001	
		1mCi/VIAL	N017837 002	

ALBUTEROL
Aerosol, Metered; Inhalation

TE	Applicant	Strength	NDA	Date
	ALBUTEROL			
AB	ARMSTRONG PHARMS	0.09MG/INH	N072273 001	AUG 14, 1996
AB	GENPHARM	0.09MG/INH	N073045 001	AUG 19, 1997
AB	IVAX PHARMS	0.09MG/INH	N073272 001	DEC 28, 1995
AB	PLIVA	0.09MG/INH	N074072 001	AUG 01, 1996
	PROVENTIL			
BN	+ SCHERING	0.09MG/INH	N017559 001	
	VENTOLIN			
AB	+ GLAXOSMITHKLINE	0.09MG/INH	N018473 001	

ALBUTEROL SULFATE
Aerosol, Metered; Inhalation

TE	Applicant	Strength	NDA	Date
	PROVENTIL-HFA			
BX	+ 3M	EQ 0.09MG BASE/INH	N020503 001	AUG 15, 1996
	VENTOLIN HFA			
BX	+ GLAXOSMITHKLINE	EQ 0.09MG BASE/INH	N020983 001	APR 19, 2001

Solution; Inhalation

TE	Applicant	Strength	NDA	Date
	ACCUNEB			
	+ DEY	EQ 0.021% BASE	N020949 002	APR 30, 2001
	+	EQ 0.042% BASE	N020949 001	APR 30, 2001
	ALBUTEROL SULFATE			
AN	ALPHARMA	EQ 0.083% BASE	N073533 001	SEP 26, 1995
AN	BAUSCH AND LOMB	EQ 0.5% BASE	N075050 001	JUN 18, 1998
AN		EQ 0.083% BASE	N075358 001	MAR 29, 2000
AN	DEY	EQ 0.083% BASE	N072652 001	FEB 21, 1992
AN	HI TECH PHARMA	EQ 0.5% BASE	N074543 001	JAN 15, 1998
AN		EQ 0.083% BASE	N075063 001	FEB 09, 1999
AN	IVAX PHARMS	EQ 0.083% BASE	N075343 001	NOV 09, 1999
AN	MORTON GROVE	EQ 0.083% BASE	N075394 001	NOV 22, 1999
AN	NEPHRON	EQ 0.5% BASE	N075664 001	JUN 26, 2001
AN		EQ 0.083% BASE	N074880 001	

ALBUTEROL SULFATE *(continued)*
Solution; Inhalation

TE	Applicant	Strength	NDA	Date
	ALBUTEROL SULFATE			
AN	NEPHRON	EQ 0.5% BASE	N076391 001	SEP 17, 1997
AN	NOVEX	EQ 0.083% BASE	N075129 001	APR 01, 2003
AN	ROXANE	EQ 0.083% BASE		FEB 13, 2001
	PROVENTIL			
AN	+ SCHERING	EQ 0.5% BASE	N019243 001	JAN 14, 1987
AN	+	EQ 0.083% BASE	N019243 002	JAN 14, 1987

Syrup; Oral

TE	Applicant	Strength	NDA	Date
	ALBUTEROL SULFATE			
AA	ALPHARMA	EQ 2MG BASE/5ML	N074454 001	SEP 25, 1995
AA	HI TECH PHARMA	EQ 2MG BASE/5ML	N074749 001	JAN 30, 1998
AA	TEVA	EQ 2MG BASE/5ML	N073419 001	MAR 30, 1992
AA	UDL	EQ 2MG BASE/5ML	N075262 001	MAR 30, 1999
	PROVENTIL			
AA	+ SCHERING	EQ 2MG BASE/5ML	N018062 001	JAN 19, 1983

Tablet, Extended Release; Oral

TE	Applicant	Strength	NDA	Date
	ALBUTEROL SULFATE			
AB	PLIVA	EQ 4MG BASE	N076130 002	SEP 26, 2002
AB		EQ 8MG BASE	N076130 003	SEP 26, 2002
	PROVENTIL			
BC	SCHERING	EQ 4MG BASE	N019383 001	JUL 13, 1987
	VOLMAX			
AB	+ MURO	EQ 4MG BASE	N019604 002	DEC 23, 1992
AB	+	EQ 8MG BASE	N019604 001	DEC 23, 1992

Tablet; Oral

TE	Applicant	Strength	NDA	Date
	ALBUTEROL SULFATE			
AB	GENEVA PHARMS	EQ 2MG BASE	N072151 001	DEC 05, 1989
AB		EQ 4MG BASE	N072152 001	DEC 05, 1989
AB	MUTUAL PHARM	EQ 2MG BASE	N072636 001	DEC 05, 1989
AB		EQ 4MG BASE	N072637 001	DEC 05, 1989
AB	MYLAN	EQ 2MG BASE	N072893 001	JAN 17, 1991
AB		EQ 4MG BASE	N072894 001	JAN 17, 1991
AB	PLIVA	EQ 2MG BASE	N072316 001	DEC 05, 1989
AB		EQ 4MG BASE	N072317 001	

Prescription Drug Products (continued)

ALBUTEROL SULFATE (continued)
Tablet; Oral

ALBUTEROL SULFATE

	Firm	Strength	Appl. No.	Date
AB	PLIVA / TEVA	EQ 2MG BASE	N072619 001	DEC 05, 1989
AB		EQ 2MG BASE	N072779 001	DEC 05, 1989
AB		EQ 2MG BASE	N072938 001	JUN 25, 1993
AB		EQ 2MG BASE	N072620 001	MAR 30, 1990
AB		EQ 4MG BASE	N072780 001	DEC 05, 1989
AB		EQ 4MG BASE	N072939 001	JUN 25, 1993
AB		EQ 4MG BASE	N072629 001	MAR 30, 1990
AB	WATSON LABS	EQ 2MG BASE	N072764 001	JAN 31, 1991
AB		EQ 2MG BASE	N072630 001	AUG 28, 1991
AB		EQ 4MG BASE	N072765 001	JAN 31, 1991
AB		EQ 4MG BASE		AUG 28, 1991
AB	PROVENTIL SCHERING	EQ 2MG BASE	N017853 001	MAY 07, 1982
AB	+	EQ 4MG BASE	N017853 002	MAY 07, 1982

ALBUTEROL SULFATE; IPRATROPIUM BROMIDE
Aerosol, Metered; Inhalation

COMBIVENT
	Firm	Strength	Appl. No.	Date
+	BOEHRINGER INGELHEIM	EQ 0.09MG BASE/INH;0.018MG/INH	N020291 001	OCT 24, 1996

Solution; Inhalation

DUONEB
	Firm	Strength	Appl. No.	Date
+	DEY	EQ 0.083% BASE;0.017%	N020950 001	MAR 21, 2001

ALCLOMETASONE DIPROPIONATE
Cream; Topical

ACLOVATE
	Firm	Strength	Appl. No.	Date
+	GLAXOSMITHKLINE	0.05%	N018707 001	DEC 14, 1982

Ointment; Topical

ACLOVATE
	Firm	Strength	Appl. No.	Date
+	GLAXOSMITHKLINE	0.05%	N018702 001	DEC 14, 1982

ALCOHOL; DEXTROSE
Injectable; Injection

ALCOHOL 5% AND DEXTROSE 5%
	Firm	Strength	Appl. No.
AP	+ B BRAUN	5ML/100ML;5GM/100ML	N004589 004

ALCOHOL; DEXTROSE (continued)
Injectable; Injection

ALCOHOL 5% IN D5-W
	Firm	Strength	Appl. No.
AP	ABBOTT	5ML/100ML;5GM/100ML	N083263 001

ALCOHOL 10% AND DEXTROSE 5%
	Firm	Strength	Appl. No.
	+ B BRAUN	10ML/100ML;5GM/100ML	N004589 006

ALENDRONATE SODIUM
Tablet; Oral

FOSAMAX
Firm	Strength	Appl. No.	Date
MERCK	EQ 5MG BASE	N020560 003	APR 25, 1997
	EQ 10MG BASE	N020560 001	SEP 29, 1995
	EQ 35MG BASE	N020560 004	OCT 20, 2000
	EQ 40MG BASE	N020560 002	SEP 29, 1995
+	EQ 70MG BASE	N020560 005	OCT 20, 2000

ALFENTANIL HYDROCHLORIDE
Injectable; Injection

ALFENTA
	Firm	Strength	Appl. No.	Date
AP	+ AKORN	EQ 0.5MG BASE/ML	N019353 001	DEC 29, 1986

ALFENTANIL
	Firm	Strength	Appl. No.	Date
AP	ABBOTT	EQ 0.5MG BASE/ML	N075221 001	OCT 28, 1999

ALFUZOSIN HYDROCHLORIDE
Tablet, Extended Release; Oral

UROXATRAL
	Firm	Strength	Appl. No.	Date
+	SANOFI SYN RES	10MG	N021287 001	JUN 12, 2003

ALGLUCERASE
Injectable; Injection

CEREDASE
	Firm	Strength	Appl. No.	Date
+	GENZYME	80 UNITS/ML	N020057 003	APR 05, 1991

ALITRETINOIN
Gel; Topical

PANRETIN
	Firm	Strength	Appl. No.	Date
+	LIGAND	EQ 0.1% BASE	N020886 001	FEB 02, 1999

ALLOPURINOL
Tablet; Oral

ALLOPURINOL
	Firm	Strength	Appl. No.	Date
AB	GENEVA PHARMS	100MG	N070268 001	DEC 31, 1985
AB		300MG	N070269 001	DEC 31, 1985

Prescription Drug Products (continued)

ALLOPURINOL (continued)
Tablet; Oral
ALLOPURINOL

		Strength	NDA	Date
AB	MUTUAL PHARM	100MG	N071449 001	JAN 09, 1987
AB		300MG	N071450 001	JAN 09, 1987
AB	MYLAN	100MG	N018659 001	OCT 24, 1986
AB		300MG	N018659 002	OCT 24, 1986
AB	PAR PHARM	100MG	N070150 001	DEC 10, 1985
AB		300MG	N070147 001	DEC 10, 1985
AB	SUPERPHARM	300MG	N070951 001	NOV 30, 1988
AB	VINTAGE PHARMS	100MG	N075798 001	JUN 27, 2003
AB		300MG	N075798 002	JUN 27, 2003
AB	WATSON LABS	100MG	N018832 002	SEP 28, 1984
AB		300MG	N018877 001	SEP 28, 1984

LOPURIN

		Strength	NDA	Date
AB	BASF	100MG	N071586 001	APR 02, 1987
AB		300MG	N071587 001	APR 02, 1987

ZYLOPRIM

		Strength	NDA
AB +	PROMETHEUS LABS	100MG	N016084 001
AB		300MG	N016084 002

ALLOPURINOL SODIUM
Injectable; Injection
ALOPRIM

		Strength	NDA	Date
AB +	DSM PHARMS	EQ 500MG BASE/VIAL	N020298 001	MAY 17, 1996

ALMOTRIPTAN MALATE
Tablet; Oral
AXERT

	Strength	NDA	Date
JANSSEN ORTHO	EQ 6.25MG BASE	N021001 001	MAY 07, 2001
+	EQ 12.5MG BASE	N021001 002	MAY 07, 2001

ALOSETRON HYDROCHLORIDE
Tablet; Oral
LOTRONEX

		Strength	NDA	Date
+	GLAXOSMITHKLINE	EQ 1MG BASE	N021107 001	FEB 09, 2000

ALPHA-TOCOPHEROL ACETATE; ASCORBIC ACID; BIOTIN; CHOLECALCIFEROL; CYANOCOBALAMIN; DEXPANTHENOL; FOLIC ACID; NIACINAMIDE; PYRIDOXINE HYDROCHLORIDE; RIBOFLAVIN PHOSPHATE SODIUM; THIAMINE HYDROCHLORIDE; VITAMIN A PALMITATE; VITAMIN K
Injectable; Injection
INFUVITE ADULT

		Strength	NDA	Date
+	SABEX 2302	2 IU/ML;40MG/ML;12UGM/ML;40 IU/ML;1UGM/ML;3MG/ML;120UGM/ML;8MG/ML;1.2MG/ML;0.72MG/ML;1.2MG/ML;660 IU/ML;0.03MG/ML	N021163 001	MAY 18, 2000

Injectable; Iv (Infusion)
INFUVITE ADULT

		Strength	NDA	Date
+	SABEX 2002	2 IU/ML;40MG/ML;12UGM/ML;40 IU/ML;1UGM/ML;3MG/ML;120UGM/ML;8MG/ML;1.2MG/ML;0.72MG/ML;1.2MG/ML;660 IU/ML;30UGM/ML	N021559 001	JUN 16, 2003

ALPRAZOLAM
Concentrate; Oral
ALPRAZOLAM

		Strength	NDA	Date
+	ROXANE	1MG/ML	N074312 001	OCT 31, 1993

Tablet, Extended Release; Oral
XANAX XR

	Strength	NDA	Date
PHARMACIA AND UPJOHN	0.5MG	N021434 001	JAN 17, 2003
	1MG	N021434 002	JAN 17, 2003
	2MG	N021434 003	JAN 17, 2003
+	3MG	N021434 004	JAN 17, 2003

Tablet; Oral
ALPRAZOLAM

		Strength	NDA	Date
AB	ALPHAPHARM	0.5MG	N074046 002	OCT 19, 1993
AB		0.25MG	N074046 001	OCT 19, 1993
AB		1MG	N074046 003	OCT 19, 1993
AB		2MG	N074046 004	MAY 07, 1997
AB	GENEVA PHARMS	0.5MG	N074112 002	DEC 29, 1995
AB		0.25MG	N074112 001	DEC 29, 1995
AB		1MG	N074112 003	DEC 29, 1995
AB		2MG	N074909 001	

Prescription Drug Products *(continued)*

ALPRAZOLAM *(continued)*

Tablet; Oral

ALPRAZOLAM

TE Code	Manufacturer	Strength	Appl. No.	Approval Date
	GENEVA PHARMS / IVAX PHARMS			
AB		0.5MG		MAR 25, 1998
AB		0.25MG	N074294 002	JUL 29, 1994
AB			N074294 001	JUL 29, 1994
AB		1MG	N074294 003	JUL 29, 1994
AB		2MG	N074294 004	JUL 29, 1994
	MYLAN			
AB		0.5MG	N074215 002	JUL 06, 1995
AB		0.25MG	N074215 001	JAN 27, 1994
AB		1MG	N074215 003	JAN 27, 1994
AB		2MG	N074215 004	JAN 27, 1994
	PUREPAC PHARM			
AB		0.5MG	N074342 002	OCT 31, 1993
AB		0.25MG	N074342 001	OCT 31, 1993
AB		1MG	N074342 003	OCT 31, 1993
AB		2MG	N074342 004	OCT 31, 1993
	TEVA			
AB		0.5MG	N074085 002	FEB 16, 1994
AB		0.25MG	N074085 001	FEB 16, 1994
AB		1MG	N074085 003	FEB 16, 1994
AB		2MG	N074085 004	FEB 16, 1994
	WATSON LABS			
AB		0.5MG	N074456 002	AUG 31, 1995
AB		0.5MG	N074479 002	JAN 21, 1997
AB		0.25MG	N074456 001	AUG 31, 1995
AB		0.25MG	N074479 001	JAN 21, 1997
AB		1MG	N074456 003	AUG 31, 1995
AB		1MG	N074479 003	JAN 21, 1997
	XANAX			
AB +	PHARMACIA AND UPJOHN	0.5MG	N018276 002	
AB		0.25MG	N018276 001	
AB		1MG	N018276 003	
AB		2MG	N018276 004	NOV 27, 1985

ALPROSTADIL

Injectable; Injection

TE Code	Manufacturer	Strength	Appl. No.	Approval Date
	ALPROSTADIL			
AP	BEDFORD	0.5MG/ML	N074815 001	JAN 20, 1998
AP	GENSIA SICOR PHARMS	0.5MG/ML	N075196 001	APR 30, 1999
	CAVERJECT			
	PHARMACIA AND UPJOHN			
AP		0.01MG/ML	N020755 002	OCT 01, 1997
AP		0.01MG/VIAL	N020379 001	JUL 06, 1995
		0.01MG/VIAL	N021212 001	JUN 11, 2002
		0.02MG/ML	N020755 003	OCT 01, 1997
AP +		0.02MG/VIAL	N020379 002	JUL 06, 1995
		0.02MG/VIAL	N021212 002	JUN 11, 2002
AP +		0.04MG/VIAL	N020379 004	MAY 19, 1997
AP		0.005MG/VIAL	N020379 003	JUN 27, 1996
	EDEX			
	SCHWARZ PHARMA			
AP		0.01MG/VIAL	N020649 002	JUN 12, 1997
		0.01MG/VIAL	N020649 005	JUL 30, 1998
AP +		0.02MG/VIAL	N020649 003	JUN 12, 1997
		0.02MG/VIAL	N020649 006	JUL 30, 1998
AP +		0.04MG/VIAL	N020649 004	JUN 12, 1997
		0.04MG/VIAL	N020649 007	JUL 30, 1998
	PROSTIN VR PEDIATRIC			
AP	+ PHARMACIA AND UPJOHN	0.5MG/ML	N018484 001	

Suppository; Urethral

TE Code	Manufacturer	Strength	Appl. No.	Approval Date
	MUSE			
	VIVUS			
		0.5MG	N020700 003	NOV 19, 1996
		0.25MG	N020700 002	NOV 19, 1996
		0.125MG	N020700 001	NOV 19, 1996
	+	1MG	N020700 004	NOV 19, 1996

ALTRETAMINE

Capsule; Oral

TE Code	Manufacturer	Strength	Appl. No.	Approval Date
	HEXALEN			
	+ MGI PHARMA INC	50MG	N019926 001	DEC 26, 1990

Prescription Drug Products *(continued)*

ALUMINUM ACETATE *MULTIPLE*
SEE ACETIC ACID, GLACIAL; ALUMINUM ACETATE

AMANTADINE HYDROCHLORIDE
Capsule; Oral
AMANTADINE HCL

AB	GENEVA PHARMS	100MG	N071293 001	FEB 18, 1987
AB	+ USL PHARMA	100MG	N070589 001	AUG 05, 1986

Syrup; Oral
AMANTADINE HCL

AA	ALPHARMA	50MG/5ML	N072655 001	OCT 30, 1990
AA	CAROLINA MEDCL	50MG/5ML	N075819 001	SEP 11, 2002
AA	COPLEY PHARM	50MG/5ML	N073115 001	AUG 23, 1991
AA	HI TECH PHARMA	50MG/5ML	N074170 001	OCT 28, 1994
AA	MIKART	50MG/5ML	N074028 001	JUN 28, 1993
AA	MORTON GROVE	50MG/5ML	N075060 001	DEC 24, 1998
AA	PHARM ASSOC	50MG/5ML	N074509 001	JUL 17, 1995
AA	SYMMETREL + ENDO PHARMS	50MG/5ML	N016023 002	

Tablet; Oral
AMANTADINE HCL

AB	USL PHARMA	100MG	N076186 001	DEC 16, 2002
AB	SYMMETREL + ENDO PHARMS	100MG	N018101 001	

AMBENONIUM CHLORIDE
Tablet; Oral

	MYTELASE + SANOFI SYNTHELABO	10MG	N010155 002	

AMCINONIDE
Cream; Topical
AMCINONIDE

AB	ALTANA	0.1%	N076065 001	MAY 15, 2003
AB	TARO PHARM INDS	0.1%	N076229 001	MAY 31, 2002
AB	CYCLOCORT + FUJISAWA HLTHCARE	0.1%	N018116 002	

Lotion; Topical
AMCINONIDE

AB	ALTANA	0.1%	N076329 001	NOV 06, 2002
AB	CYCLOCORT + FUJISAWA HLTHCARE	0.1%	N019729 001	JUN 13, 1988

AMCINONIDE *(continued)*
Ointment; Topical
AMCINONIDE

AB	ALTANA	0.1%	N076096 001	NOV 19, 2002
AB	TARO PHARM INDS	0.1%	N076367 001	MAR 19, 2003
AB	CYCLOCORT + FUJISAWA HLTHCARE	0.1%	N018498 001	

AMIFOSTINE
Injectable; Injection

	ETHYOL + MEDIMMUNE ONCOLOGY	500MG/VIAL	N020221 001	DEC 08, 1995

AMIKACIN SULFATE
Injectable; Injection
AMIKACIN SULFATE

AP	ABBOTT	EQ 50MG BASE/ML	N063263 001	NOV 30, 1994
		EQ 62.5MG BASE/ML	N063283 001	OCT 31, 1994
AP		EQ 250MG BASE/ML	N063264 001	NOV 30, 1994
AP		EQ 250MG BASE/ML	N064098 001	JUN 26, 1995
AP	BEDFORD	EQ 50MG BASE/ML	N063313 001	APR 11, 1994
AP		EQ 250MG BASE/ML	N063315 001	APR 11, 1994
AP	FAULDING	EQ 50MG BASE/ML	N063350 001	JUL 30, 1993
AP		EQ 250MG BASE/ML	N063350 002	JUL 30, 1993
AP	GENSIA SICOR PHARMS	EQ 50MG BASE/ML	N064045 001	SEP 28, 1993
AP		EQ 250MG BASE/ML	N064045 002	SEP 28, 1993

AMIKACIN SULFATE IN SODIUM CHLORIDE 0.9% IN PLASTIC CONTAINER

AP	ABBOTT	EQ 500MG BASE/100ML	N064146 001	APR 02, 1997

AMIKIN

AP	+ APOTHECON	EQ 50MG BASE/ML	N062311 001	
AP	+	EQ 250MG BASE/ML	N062311 002	

AMILORIDE HYDROCHLORIDE
Tablet; Oral
AMILORIDE HCL

AB	PAR PHARM	5MG	N070346 001	JAN 22, 1986

MIDAMOR

AB	+ MERCK	5MG	N018200 001	

Prescription Drug Products (continued)

AMILORIDE HYDROCHLORIDE; HYDROCHLOROTHIAZIDE
Tablet; Oral

AMILORIDE HCL AND HYDROCHLOROTHIAZIDE

AB	BARR	EQ 5MG ANHYDROUS;50MG	N071111 001 MAY 10, 1988
AB	GENEVA PHARMS	EQ 5MG ANHYDROUS;50MG	N073357 001 NOV 27, 1991
AB	MYLAN	EQ 5MG ANHYDROUS;50MG	N073209 001 OCT 31, 1991
AB	TEVA	EQ 5MG ANHYDROUS;50MG	N070795 001 APR 17, 1988
AB	WATSON LABS	EQ 5MG ANHYDROUS;50MG	N073334 001 JUL 19, 1991

HYDRO-RIDE

AB	PAR PHARM	EQ 5MG ANHYDROUS;50MG	N070347 001 DEC 25, 1990

MODURETIC 5-50

AB +	MERCK	EQ 5MG ANHYDROUS;50MG	N018201 001

AMINO ACIDS
Injectable; Injection

AMINESS 5.2% ESSENTIAL AMINO ACIDS W/ HISTADINE

	FRESENIUS KABI	5.2% (5.2GM/100ML)	N018901 001 APR 06, 1984

AMINOSYN 3.5%

	ABBOTT	3.5% (3.5GM/100ML)	N017789 004

AMINOSYN 5%

	ABBOTT	5% (5GM/100ML)	N017673 001

AMINOSYN 7% (PH6)

	ABBOTT	7% (7GM/100ML)	N017673 006 NOV 18, 1985

AMINOSYN 8.5% (PH6)

	ABBOTT	8.5% (8.5GM/100ML)	N017673 007 NOV 18, 1985

AMINOSYN 10%

	ABBOTT	10% (10GM/100ML)	N017673 003

AMINOSYN 10% (PH6)

	ABBOTT	10% (10GM/100ML)	N017673 008 NOV 18, 1985

AMINOSYN II 7%

	ABBOTT	7% (7GM/100ML)	N019438 003 APR 03, 1986

AMINOSYN II 8.5%

	ABBOTT	8.5% (8.5GM/100ML)	N019438 004 APR 03, 1986

AMINOSYN II 10%

	ABBOTT	10% (10GM/100ML)	N019438 005 APR 03, 1986

AMINOSYN II 10% IN PLASTIC CONTAINER

	ABBOTT	10% (10GM/100ML)	N020015 001 DEC 19, 1991

AMINOSYN II 15% IN PLASTIC CONTAINER

	ABBOTT	15% (15GM/100ML)	N020041 001 DEC 19, 1991

AMINO ACIDS (continued)
Injectable; Injection

AMINOSYN-HBC 7%

	ABBOTT	7% (7GM/100ML)	N019374 001 JUL 12, 1985

AMINOSYN-HF 8%

	ABBOTT	8% (8GM/100ML)	N020345 001 APR 04, 1996

AMINOSYN-PF 7%

	ABBOTT	7% (7GM/100ML)	N019398 001 SEP 06, 1985

AMINOSYN-PF 10%

	ABBOTT	10% (10GM/100ML)	N019492 002 OCT 17, 1986

AMINOSYN-RF 5.2%

	ABBOTT	5.2% (5.2GM/100ML)	N018429 001

BRANCHAMIN 4% IN PLASTIC CONTAINER

	BAXTER HLTHCARE	4% (4GM/100ML)	N018684 001 SEP 28, 1984

CLINISOL 15% SULFITE FREE IN PLASTIC CONTAINER

	CLINTEC NUTR	15% (15GM/100ML)	N020512 001 AUG 30, 1996

FREAMINE HBC 6.9%

	B BRAUN	6.9% (6.9GM/100ML)	N016822 006 MAY 17, 1983

FREAMINE III 8.5%

	B BRAUN	8.5% (8.5GM/100ML)	N016822 004

FREAMINE III 10%

	B BRAUN	10% (10GM/100ML)	N016822 005

HEPATAMINE 8%

	B BRAUN	8% (8GM/100ML)	N018676 001 AUG 03, 1982

HEPATASOL 8%

	BAXTER HLTHCARE	8% (8GM/100ML)	N020360 001 APR 04, 1996

NEPHRAMINE 5.4%

	B BRAUN	5.4% (5.4GM/100ML)	N017766 001

NOVAMINE 11.4%

	FRESENIUS KABI	11.4% (11.4GM/100ML)	N017957 003 AUG 09, 1982

NOVAMINE 15%

	FRESENIUS KABI	15% (15GM/100ML)	N017957 004 NOV 28, 1986

PREMASOL 6% IN PLASTIC CONTAINER

	BAXTER HLTHCARE	EQ 6% (6GM/100ML)	N075880 001 JUN 19, 2003

PREMASOL 10% IN PLASTIC CONTAINER

	BAXTER HLTHCARE	EQ 10% (10GM/100ML)	N075880 002 JUN 19, 2003

PROSOL 20% SULFITE FREE IN PLASTIC CONTAINER

+	BAXTER HLTHCARE	20% (20GM/100ML)	N020849 001 AUG 26, 1998

RENAMIN W/O ELECTROLYTES

	BAXTER HLTHCARE	6.5% (6.5GM/100ML)	N017493 007 OCT 15, 1982

Prescription Drug Products (continued)

AMINO ACIDS (continued)
Injectable; Injection

TRAVASOL 5.5% IN PLASTIC CONTAINER
BAXTER HLTHCARE   5.5% (5.5GM/100ML)   N018931 001   AUG 23, 1984

TRAVASOL 5.5% W/O ELECTROLYTES
BAXTER HLTHCARE   5.5% (5.5GM/100ML)   N017493 004

TRAVASOL 8.5% IN PLASTIC CONTAINER
BAXTER HLTHCARE   8.5% (8.5GM/100ML)   N018931 002   AUG 23, 1984

TRAVASOL 8.5% W/O ELECTROLYTES
BAXTER HLTHCARE   8.5% (8.5GM/100ML)   N017493 005

TRAVASOL 10% IN PLASTIC CONTAINER
BAXTER HLTHCARE   10% (10MG/100ML)   N018931 003   AUG 23, 1984

TRAVASOL 10% W/O ELECTROLYTES
BAXTER HLTHCARE   10% (10GM/100ML)   N017493 006

TROPHAMINE
+ B BRAUN   6% (6GM/100ML)   N019018 001   JUL 20, 1984

TROPHAMINE 10%
+ B BRAUN   10% (10GM/100ML)   N019018 003   SEP 07, 1988

AMINO ACIDS; CALCIUM ACETATE; GLYCERIN; MAGNESIUM ACETATE; PHOSPHORIC ACID; POTASSIUM CHLORIDE; SODIUM ACETATE; SODIUM CHLORIDE
Injectable; Injection

PROCALAMINE
B BRAUN   3%;26MG/100ML;3GM/ 100ML;54MG/100ML;41MG/ 100ML;150MG/100ML;200MG/ 100ML;120MG/100ML   N018582 001   MAY 08, 1982

AMINO ACIDS; CALCIUM CHLORIDE; DEXTROSE; MAGNESIUM CHLORIDE; POTASSIUM CHLORIDE; POTASSIUM PHOSPHATE, DIBASIC; SODIUM CHLORIDE
Injectable; Injection

AMINOSYN II 3.5% W/ ELECTROLYTES IN DEXTROSE 25% W/ CALCIUM IN PLASTIC CONTAINER
ABBOTT   3.5%;36.8MG/100ML;25GM/ 100ML;51MG/100ML;22.4MG/ 100ML;261MG/100ML;205MG/ 100ML   N019683 001   NOV 07, 1988

AMINOSYN II 4.25% W/ ELECTROLYTES IN DEXTROSE 20% W/ CALCIUM IN PLASTIC CONTAINER
ABBOTT   4.25%;36.8MG/100ML;20GM/ 100ML;51MG/100ML;22.4MG/ 100ML;261MG/100ML;205MG/ 100ML   N019683 002   NOV 07, 1988

AMINO ACIDS; CALCIUM CHLORIDE; DEXTROSE; MAGNESIUM CHLORIDE; POTASSIUM CHLORIDE; POTASSIUM PHOSPHATE, DIBASIC; SODIUM CHLORIDE (continued)
Injectable; Injection

AMINOSYN II 4.25% W/ ELECTROLYTES IN DEXTROSE 25% W/ CALCIUM IN PLASTIC CONTAINER
ABBOTT   4.25%;36.8MG/100ML;25GM/ 100ML;51MG/100ML;22.4MG/ 100ML;261MG/100ML;205MG/ 100ML   N019683 003   NOV 07, 1988

AMINO ACIDS; CALCIUM CHLORIDE; DEXTROSE; MAGNESIUM CHLORIDE; POTASSIUM PHOSPHATE, DIBASIC; SODIUM ACETATE; SODIUM CHLORIDE
Injectable; Injection

CLINIMIX E 2.75/5 SULFITE-FREE W/ ELECT IN DEXTROSE 5% W/ CALCIUM IN PLASTIC CONTAINER
+ BAXTER HLTHCARE   2.75%;33MG/100ML;5GM/ 100ML;51MG/100ML;261MG/ 100ML;217MG/100ML;112MG/ 100ML   N020678 001   MAR 26, 1997

CLINIMIX E 2.75/10 SULFITE-FREE W/ ELECT IN DEXTROSE 10% W/ CALCIUM IN PLASTIC CONTAINER
+ BAXTER HLTHCARE   2.75%;33MG/100ML;10GM/ 100ML;51MG/100ML;261MG/ 100ML;217MG/100ML;112MG/ 100ML   N020678 002   MAR 26, 1997

CLINIMIX E 2.75/25 SULFITE-FREE W/ ELECT IN DEXTROSE 25% W/ CALCIUM IN PLASTIC CONTAINER
+ BAXTER HLTHCARE   2.75%;33MG/100ML;25GM/ 100ML;51MG/100ML;261MG/ 100ML;217MG/100ML;112MG/ 100ML   N020678 005   MAR 26, 1997

CLINIMIX E 4.25/5 SULFITE-FREE W/ ELECT IN DEXTROSE 5% W/ CALCIUM IN PLASTIC CONTAINER
+ BAXTER HLTHCARE   4.25%;33MG/100ML;5GM/ 100ML;51MG/100ML;261MG/ 100ML;297MG/100ML;77MG/ 100ML   N020678 008   MAR 26, 1997

CLINIMIX E 4.25/10 SULFITE-FREE W/ ELECT IN DEXTROSE 10% W/ CALCIUM IN PLASTIC CONTAINER
+ BAXTER HLTHCARE   4.25%;33MG/100ML;10GM/ 100ML;51MG/100ML;261MG/ 100ML;297MG/100ML;77MG/ 100ML   N020678 009   MAR 26, 1997

Prescription Drug Products (continued)

AMINO ACIDS; CALCIUM CHLORIDE; DEXTROSE; MAGNESIUM CHLORIDE; POTASSIUM PHOSPHATE, DIBASIC; SODIUM ACETATE; SODIUM CHLORIDE (continued)
Injectable; Injection

CLINIMIX E 4.25/20 SULFITE-FREE W/ ELECT IN DEXTROSE 20% W/ CALCIUM IN PLASTIC CONTAINER
+ BAXTER HLTHCARE   4.25%;33MG/100ML;20GM/100ML;51MG/100ML;261MG/100ML;297MG/100ML;77MG/100ML   N020678 011 MAR 26, 1997

CLINIMIX E 4.25/25 SULFITE-FREE W/ ELECT IN DEXTROSE 25% W/ CALCIUM IN PLASTIC CONTAINER
+ BAXTER HLTHCARE   4.25%;33MG/100ML;25GM/100ML;51MG/100ML;261MG/100ML;297MG/100ML;77MG/100ML   N020678 012 MAR 26, 1997

CLINIMIX E 5/10 SULFITE-FREE W/ ELECT IN DEXTROSE 10% W/ CALCIUM IN PLASTIC CONTAINER
+ BAXTER HLTHCARE   5%;33MG/100ML;10GM/100ML;51MG/100ML;261MG/100ML;340MG/100ML;59MG/100ML   N020678 016 MAR 26, 1997

CLINIMIX E 5/15 SULFITE-FREE W/ ELECT IN DEXTROSE 15% W/ CALCIUM IN PLASTIC CONTAINER
+ BAXTER HLTHCARE   5%;33MG/100ML;15GM/100ML;51MG/100ML;261MG/100ML;340MG/100ML;59MG/100ML   N020678 017 MAR 26, 1997

CLINIMIX E 5/20 SULFITE-FREE W/ ELECT IN 20% DEXTROSE W/ CALCIUM IN PLASTIC CONTAINER
+ BAXTER HLTHCARE   5%;33MG/100ML;20GM/100ML;51MG/100ML;261MG/100ML;340MG/100ML;59MG/100ML   N020678 018 MAR 26, 1997

CLINIMIX E 5/25 SULFITE-FREE W/ ELECT IN DEXTROSE 25% W/ CALCIUM IN PLASTIC CONTAINER
+ BAXTER HLTHCARE   5%;33MG/100ML;25GM/100ML;51MG/100ML;261MG/100ML;340MG/100ML;59MG/100ML   N020678 019 MAR 26, 1997

CLINIMIX E 5/35 SULFITE FREE W/ ELECT IN DEXTROSE 35% W/ CALCIUM IN PLASTIC CONTAINER
+ BAXTER HLTHCARE   5%;33MG/100ML;35GM/100ML;51MG/100ML;261MG/100ML;340MG/100ML;59MG/100ML   N020678 021 MAR 26, 1997

AMINO ACIDS; DEXTROSE
Injectable; Injection

AMINOSYN II 3.5% IN DEXTROSE 5% IN PLASTIC CONTAINER
ABBOTT   3.5%;5GM/100ML   N019681 002 NOV 01, 1988

AMINOSYN II 3.5% IN DEXTROSE 25% IN PLASTIC CONTAINER
ABBOTT   3.5%;25GM/100ML   N019681 001 NOV 01, 1988

AMINOSYN II 4.25% IN DEXTROSE 10% IN PLASTIC CONTAINER
ABBOTT   4.25%;10GM/100ML   N019681 004 NOV 01, 1988

AMINOSYN II 4.25% IN DEXTROSE 20% IN PLASTIC CONTAINER
ABBOTT   4.25%;20GM/100ML   N019681 005 NOV 01, 1988

AMINOSYN II 4.25% IN DEXTROSE 25% IN PLASTIC CONTAINER
ABBOTT   4.25%;25GM/100ML   N019681 003 NOV 01, 1988

AMINOSYN II 5% IN DEXTROSE 25% IN PLASTIC CONTAINER
ABBOTT   5%;25GM/100ML   N019681 006 NOV 01, 1988

CLINIMIX 2.75/5 SULFITE FREE IN DEXTROSE 5% IN PLASTIC CONTAINER
BAXTER HLTHCARE   2.75%;5GM/100ML   N020734 001 SEP 29, 1997

CLINIMIX 2.75/10 SULFITE FREE IN DEXTROSE 10% IN PLASTIC CONTAINER
BAXTER HLTHCARE   2.75%;10GM/100ML   N020734 002 SEP 29, 1997

CLINIMIX 2.75/25 SULFITE FREE IN DEXTROSE 25% IN PLASTIC CONTAINER
BAXTER HLTHCARE   2.75%;25GM/100ML   N020734 005 SEP 29, 1997

CLINIMIX 4.25/5 SULFITE FREE IN DEXTROSE 5% IN PLASTIC CONTAINER
BAXTER HLTHCARE   4.25%;5GM/100ML   N020734 007 SEP 29, 1997

CLINIMIX 4.25/10 SULFITE FREE IN DEXTROSE 10% IN PLASTIC CONTAINER
BAXTER HLTHCARE   4.25%;10GM/100ML   N020734 008 SEP 29, 1997

CLINIMIX 4.25/20 SULFITE FREE IN DEXTROSE 20% IN PLASTIC CONTAINER
BAXTER HLTHCARE   4.25%;20GM/100ML   N020734 010 SEP 29, 1997

CLINIMIX 4.25/25 SULFITE FREE IN DEXTROSE 25% IN PLASTIC CONTAINER
BAXTER HLTHCARE   4.25%;25GM/100ML   N020734 011 SEP 29, 1997

CLINIMIX 5/10 SULFITE FREE IN DEXTROSE 10% IN PLASTIC CONTAINER
BAXTER HLTHCARE   5%;10GM/100ML   N020734 014 SEP 29, 1997

CLINIMIX 5/15 SULFITE FREE IN DEXTROSE 15% IN PLASTIC CONTAINER
BAXTER HLTHCARE   5%;15GM/100ML   N020734 015 SEP 29, 1997

Prescription Drug Products *(continued)*

AMINO ACIDS; DEXTROSE *(continued)*

Injectable; Injection

CLINIMIX 5/20 SULFITE FREE IN DEXTROSE 20% IN PLASTIC CONTAINER
BAXTER HLTHCARE   5%;20GM/100ML   N020734 016   SEP 29, 1997

CLINIMIX 5/25 SULFITE FREE IN DEXTROSE 25% IN PLASTIC CONTAINER
BAXTER HLTHCARE   5%;25GM/100ML   N020734 017   SEP 29, 1997

CLINIMIX 5/35 SULFITE FREE IN DEXTROSE 35% IN PLASTIC CONTAINER
BAXTER HLTHCARE   5%;35GM/100ML   N020734 018   SEP 29, 1997

TRAVASOL 2.75% IN DEXTROSE 5% IN PLASTIC CONTAINER
BAXTER HLTHCARE   2.75%;5GM/100ML   N019520 001   SEP 23, 1988

TRAVASOL 2.75% IN DEXTROSE 10% IN PLASTIC CONTAINER
BAXTER HLTHCARE   2.75%;10GM/100ML   N019520 002   SEP 23, 1988

TRAVASOL 2.75% IN DEXTROSE 15% IN PLASTIC CONTAINER
BAXTER HLTHCARE   2.75%;15GM/100ML   N019520 003   SEP 23, 1988

TRAVASOL 2.75% IN DEXTROSE 20% IN PLASTIC CONTAINER
BAXTER HLTHCARE   2.75%;20GM/100ML   N019520 004   SEP 23, 1988

TRAVASOL 2.75% IN DEXTROSE 25% IN PLASTIC CONTAINER
BAXTER HLTHCARE   2.75%;25GM/100ML   N019520 005   SEP 23, 1988

TRAVASOL 4.25% IN DEXTROSE 5% IN PLASTIC CONTAINER
BAXTER HLTHCARE   4.25%;5GM/100ML   N019520 006   SEP 23, 1988

TRAVASOL 4.25% IN DEXTROSE 10% IN PLASTIC CONTAINER
BAXTER HLTHCARE   4.25%;10GM/100ML   N019520 007   SEP 23, 1988

TRAVASOL 4.25% IN DEXTROSE 15% IN PLASTIC CONTAINER
BAXTER HLTHCARE   4.25%;15GM/100ML   N019520 008   SEP 23, 1988

TRAVASOL 4.25% IN DEXTROSE 20% IN PLASTIC CONTAINER
BAXTER HLTHCARE   4.25%;20GM/100ML   N019520 009   SEP 23, 1988

TRAVASOL 4.25% IN DEXTROSE 25% IN PLASTIC CONTAINER
BAXTER HLTHCARE   4.25%;25GM/100ML   N019520 010   SEP 23, 1988

AMINO ACIDS; DEXTROSE; MAGNESIUM CHLORIDE; POTASSIUM CHLORIDE; SODIUM CHLORIDE; SODIUM PHOSPHATE, DIBASIC, HEPTAHYDRATE

Injectable; Injection

AMINOSYN II 3.5% M IN DEXTROSE 5% IN PLASTIC CONTAINER
ABBOTT   3.5%;5GM/100ML;30MG/100ML;97MG/100ML;120MG/100ML;49.3MG/100ML   N019682 001   NOV 01, 1988

AMINO ACIDS; DEXTROSE; MAGNESIUM CHLORIDE; POTASSIUM CHLORIDE; SODIUM CHLORIDE; SODIUM PHOSPHATE, DIBASIC, HEPTAHYDRATE *(continued)*

Injectable; Injection

AMINOSYN II 4.25% M IN DEXTROSE 10% IN PLASTIC CONTAINER
ABBOTT   4.25%;5GM/100ML;30MG/100ML;97MG/100ML;120MG/100ML;49.3MG/100ML   N019682 002   NOV 01, 1988

AMINO ACIDS; DEXTROSE; MAGNESIUM CHLORIDE; POTASSIUM PHOSPHATE, DIBASIC; SODIUM ACETATE; SODIUM CHLORIDE

Injectable; Injection

TRAVASOL 2.75% SULFITE FREE W/ ELECTROLYTES IN DEXTROSE 5% IN PLASTIC CONTAINER
BAXTER HLTHCARE   2.75%;5GM/100ML;51MG/100ML;261MG/100ML;216MG/100ML;112MG/100ML   N020147 001   OCT 23, 1995

TRAVASOL 2.75% SULFITE FREE W/ ELECTROLYTES IN DEXTROSE 10%
BAXTER HLTHCARE   2.75%;10GM/100ML;51MG/100ML;261MG/100ML;216MG/100ML;112MG/100ML   N020147 002   OCT 23, 1995

TRAVASOL 2.75% SULFITE FREE W/ ELECTROLYTES IN DEXTROSE 15% IN PLASTIC CONTAINER
BAXTER HLTHCARE   2.75%;15GM/100ML;51MG/100ML;261MG/100ML;216MG/100ML;112MG/100ML   N020147 003   OCT 23, 1995

TRAVASOL 2.75% SULFITE FREE W/ ELECTROLYTES IN DEXTROSE 20% IN PLASTIC CONTAINER
BAXTER HLTHCARE   2.75%;20GM/100ML;51MG/100ML;261MG/100ML;216MG/100ML;112MG/100ML   N020147 004   OCT 23, 1995

TRAVASOL 2.75% SULFITE FREE W/ ELECTROLYTES IN DEXTROSE 25% IN PLASTIC CONTAINER
BAXTER HLTHCARE   2.75%;25GM/100ML;51MG/100ML;261MG/100ML;216MG/100ML;112MG/100ML   N020147 005   OCT 23, 1995

TRAVASOL 4.25% SULFITE FREE W/ ELECTROLYTES IN DEXTROSE 5% IN PLASTIC CONTAINER
BAXTER HLTHCARE   4.25%;5GM/100ML;51MG/100ML;261MG/100ML;297MG/100ML;77MG/100ML   N020147 006   OCT 23, 1995

TRAVASOL 4.25% SULFITE FREE W/ ELECTROLYTES IN DEXTROSE 10% IN PLASTIC CONTAINER
BAXTER HLTHCARE   4.25%;10GM/100ML;51MG/100ML;261MG/100ML;297MG/100ML;77MG/100ML   N020147 007

Prescription Drug Products (continued)

AMINO ACIDS; DEXTROSE; MAGNESIUM CHLORIDE; POTASSIUM PHOSPHATE, DIBASIC; SODIUM ACETATE; SODIUM CHLORIDE (continued)
Injectable; Injection

TRAVASOL 4.25% SULFITE FREE W/ ELECTROLYTES IN DEXTROSE 10% IN PLASTIC CONTAINER
BAXTER HLTHCARE
4.25%;15GM/100ML;51MG/100ML;261MG/100ML;297MG/100ML;77MG/100ML
N020147 008 OCT 23, 1995

TRAVASOL 4.25% SULFITE FREE W/ ELECTROLYTES IN DEXTROSE 15% IN PLASTIC CONTAINER
BAXTER HLTHCARE
4.25%;20GM/100ML;51MG/100ML;261MG/100ML;297MG/100ML;77MG/100ML
N020147 009 OCT 23, 1995

TRAVASOL 4.25% SULFITE FREE W/ ELECTROLYTES IN DEXTROSE 20% IN PLASTIC CONTAINER
BAXTER HLTHCARE
4.25%;25GM/100ML;51MG/100ML;261MG/100ML;297MG/100ML;77MG/100ML
N020147 010 OCT 23, 1995

AMINO ACIDS; MAGNESIUM ACETATE; PHOSPHORIC ACID; POTASSIUM ACETATE; POTASSIUM CHLORIDE; SODIUM ACETATE
Injectable; Injection

FREAMINE III 8.5% W/ ELECTROLYTES
8.5%;110MG/100ML;230MG/100ML;10MG/100ML;440MG/100ML;690MG/100ML
B BRAUN
N016822 007 JUL 01, 1988

AMINO ACIDS; MAGNESIUM ACETATE; PHOSPHORIC ACID; POTASSIUM ACETATE; SODIUM CHLORIDE
Injectable; Injection

AMINOSYN 3.5% M
3.5%;21MG/100ML;40MG/100ML;128MG/100ML;234MG/100ML
ABBOTT
N017789 003

AMINO ACIDS; MAGNESIUM ACETATE; PHOSPHORIC ACID; POTASSIUM CHLORIDE; SODIUM ACETATE; SODIUM CHLORIDE
Injectable; Injection

FREAMINE III 3% W/ ELECTROLYTES
3%;54MG/100ML;40MG/100ML;150MG/100ML;200MG/100ML;120MG/100ML
B BRAUN
N016822 003

AMINO ACIDS; MAGNESIUM CHLORIDE; POTASSIUM CHLORIDE; POTASSIUM PHOSPHATE, DIBASIC; SODIUM CHLORIDE
Injectable; Injection

AMINOSYN II 10% W/ ELECTROLYTES
10%;102MG/100ML;45MG/100ML;522MG/100ML;410MG/100ML
ABBOTT
N019437 004 APR 03, 1986

AMINOSYN II 8.5% W/ ELECTROLYTES
8.5%;102MG/100ML;45MG/100ML;522MG/100ML;410MG/100ML
ABBOTT
N019437 005 APR 03, 1986

AMINO ACIDS; MAGNESIUM CHLORIDE; POTASSIUM CHLORIDE; POTASSIUM PHOSPHATE, DIBASIC; SODIUM ACETATE; SODIUM CHLORIDE
Injectable; Injection

TRAVASOL 5.5% W/ ELECTROLYTES
5.5%;102MG/100ML;522MG/100ML;431MG/100ML;224MG/100ML
BAXTER HLTHCARE
N017493 001

TRAVASOL 8.5% W/ ELECTROLYTES
8.5%;102MG/100ML;522MG/100ML;594MG/100ML;154MG/100ML
BAXTER HLTHCARE
N017493 002

TRAVASOL 3.5% W/ ELECTROLYTES
3.5%;51MG/100ML;131MG/100ML;218MG/100ML;35MG/100ML
BAXTER HLTHCARE
N017493 003

TRAVASOL 5.5% SULFITE FREE W/ ELECTROLYTES IN PLASTIC CONTAINER
5.5%;102MG/100ML;522MG/100ML;431MG/100ML;224MG/100ML
BAXTER HLTHCARE
N020173 001 OCT 27, 1995

TRAVASOL 8.5% SULFITE FREE W/ ELECTROLYTES IN PLASTIC CONTAINER
8.5%;102MG/100ML;522MG/100ML;594MG/100ML;154MG/100ML
BAXTER HLTHCARE
N020173 002 OCT 27, 1995

TRAVASOL 3.5% SULFITE FREE W/ ELECTROLYTES IN PLASTIC CONTAINER
3.5%;51MG/100ML;131MG/100ML;218MG/100ML;35MG/100ML
BAXTER HLTHCARE
N020177 001 OCT 23, 1995

AMINO ACIDS; MAGNESIUM CHLORIDE; POTASSIUM CHLORIDE; POTASSIUM PHOSPHATE, DIBASIC; SODIUM CHLORIDE
Injectable; Injection

AMINOSYN 8.5% W/ ELECTROLYTES
8.5%;102MG/100ML;522MG/100ML;410MG/100ML
ABBOTT
N017673 005

Prescription Drug Products *(continued)*

AMINO ACIDS; MAGNESIUM CHLORIDE; POTASSIUM PHOSPHATE, DIBASIC; SODIUM CHLORIDE *(continued)*

Injectable; Injection
AMINOSYN 7% W/ ELECTROLYTES
ABBOTT   7%;102MG/100ML;522MG/100ML;410MG/100ML   N017789 002

AMINOCAPROIC ACID

Injectable; Injection
AMICAR
AP + XANODYNE PHARM   250MG/ML   N015229 002
AMINOCAPROIC ACID
AP + ABBOTT   250MG/ML   N070888 001   JUN 16, 1988
AP   LUITPOLD   250MG/ML   N071192 001   DEC 01, 1987
AMINOCAPROIC ACID IN PLASTIC CONTAINER
AP   ABBOTT   250MG/ML   N070010 001   MAR 09, 1987

Syrup; Oral
AMICAR
AA + XANODYNE PHARM   1.25GM/5ML   N015230 002
AMINOCAPROIC ACID
AA   MIKART   1.25GM/5ML   N074759 001   SEP 02, 1998

Tablet; Oral
AMICAR
AB + XANODYNE PHARM   500MG   N015197 001
AMINOCAPROIC
AB   MIKART   500MG   N075602 001   MAY 24, 2001

AMINOGLUTETHIMIDE

Tablet; Oral
CYTADREN
+ NOVARTIS   250MG   N018202 001

AMINOHIPPURATE SODIUM

Injectable; Injection
AMINOHIPPURATE SODIUM
+ MERCK   20%   N005619 001

AMINOLEVULINIC ACID HYDROCHLORIDE

Solution; Topical
LEVULAN
+ DUSA   20%   N020965 001   DEC 03, 1999

AMINOPHYLLINE

Injectable; Injection
AMINOPHYLLINE
AP   ABBOTT   25MG/ML   N087242 001   OCT 26, 1983
AP +   25MG/ML   N087601 001   JUL 23, 1982

AMINOPHYLLINE *(continued)*

Injectable; Injection
AMINOPHYLLINE
AP   GENSIA SICOR PHARMS   25MG/ML   N081142 001   SEP 25, 1991
AP   INTL MEDICATION   25MG/ML   N087209 001   FEB 01, 1982
AP   LUITFOLD   25MG/ML   N087240 001
AP   25MG/ML   N087600 001
AP   PHARMA SERVE NY   25MG/ML   N087392 001   DEC 15, 1983

AMINOPHYLLINE IN SODIUM CHLORIDE 0.45%
+ ABBOTT   100MG/100ML   N088147 002   MAY 03, 1983
+   100MG/100ML   N088147 001
+   200MG/100ML   N088147 003   MAY 03, 1983

Solution; Oral
AMINOPHYLLINE
AA + ROXANE   105MG/5ML   N088126 001   AUG 19, 1983

AMINOPHYLLINE DYE FREE
AA + ALPHARMA   105MG/5ML   N087727 001   APR 16, 1982

Suppository; Rectal
TRUPHYLLINE
G AND W LABS   250MG   N085498 001   MAR 23, 1983
+   500MG   N085498 002   JAN 03, 1983

Tablet; Oral
AMINOPHYLLINE
AB + GENEVA PHARMS   100MG   N085262 002
AB   200MG   N085261 002
AB + ROXANE   100MG   N087500 001   FEB 09, 1982
AB +   200MG   N087501 001   FEB 09, 1982
AB   WEST WARD   100MG   N084540 001
AB   200MG   N085003 001

AMINOSALICYLATE SODIUM

Tablet; Oral
SODIUM P.A.S.
+ LANNETT   500MG   N080138 002

AMINOSALICYLIC ACID

Granule, Delayed Release; Oral
PASER
+ JACOBUS   4GM/PACKET   N074346 001   JUN 30, 1994

AMIODARONE HYDROCHLORIDE

Injectable; Injection
AMIODARONE HCL
AP   ABBOTT   50MG/ML   N075955 001   OCT 18, 2002

Prescription Drug Products *(continued)*

AMIODARONE HYDROCHLORIDE *(continued)*

Injectable; Injection
AMIODARONE HCL

AP	AM PHARM PARTNERS	50MG/ML	N075761 001	OCT 15, 2002
AP	APOTEX	50MG/ML	N076394 001	APR 25, 2003
AP	BEDFORD	50MG/ML	N076018 001	OCT 15, 2002
AP	BEDFORD LABS	50MG/ML	N076299 001	OCT 24, 2002
AP	BEN VENUE	50MG/ML	N076088 001	OCT 15, 2002
AP	BIONICHE (CANADA)	50MG/ML	N076217 001	OCT 15, 2002
AP	FAULDING	50MG/ML	N076108 001	OCT 15, 2002
	CORDARONE			
AP	+ WYETH PHARMS INC	50MG/ML	N020377 001	AUG 03, 1995

Tablet; Oral
AMIODARONE HCL

AB	ALPHAPHARM	200MG	N075188 001	FEB 24, 1999
AB	BARR	200MG	N075389 001	JAN 25, 2001
AB	COPLEY PHARM	200MG	N074739 001	NOV 30, 1998
AB	EON	200MG	N075315 001	DEC 23, 1998
AB	+	400MG	N075315 002	JUN 30, 2000
AB	+ TARO	100MG	N075424 002	DEC 18, 2002
AB		200MG	N075424 001	MAR 30, 2001
AB		400MG	N076362 001	NOV 29, 2002
AB	TEVA	200MG	N074895 001	APR 16, 1999
	CORDARONE			
AB	WYETH PHARMS INC	200MG	N018972 001	DEC 24, 1985
	PACERONE			
AB	UPSHER SMITH	200MG	N075135 001	APR 30, 1998

AMITRIPTYLINE HYDROCHLORIDE

Injectable; Injection
ELAVIL

+	ASTRAZENECA	10MG/ML	N012704 001

Tablet; Oral
AMITRIPTYLINE HCL

AB	GENEVA PHARMS	10MG	N085969 001
AB		25MG	N085966 001
AB		50MG	N085968 001
AB		75MG	N085971 001

AMITRIPTYLINE HYDROCHLORIDE *(continued)*

Tablet; Oral
AMITRIPTYLINE HCL

AB	GENEVA PHARMS	100MG	N085967 001	
AB		150MG	N085970 001	
AB	MUTUAL PHARM	10MG	N089398 001	JUL 14, 1987
AB		25MG	N089399 001	JUL 14, 1987
AB		50MG	N089400 001	JUL 14, 1987
AB		75MG	N089401 001	JUL 14, 1987
AB		100MG	N089402 001	JUL 14, 1987
AB		150MG	N089403 001	JUL 14, 1987
AB	MYLAN	10MG	N086157 001	
AB		25MG	N086010 001	
AB		50MG	N086009 001	
AB		75MG	N086011 001	
AB		100MG	N086158 001	
AB		150MG	N086153 001	
AB	PLIVA	10MG	N088883 001	SEP 26, 1984
AB		25MG	N088884 001	SEP 26, 1984
AB		50MG	N088885 001	SEP 26, 1984
AB		75MG	N088886 001	SEP 26, 1984
AB		100MG	N088887 001	SEP 26, 1984
AB		150MG	N088888 001	SEP 26, 1984
AB	SUPERPHARM	10MG	N088853 001	NOV 13, 1984
AB		25MG	N088854 001	NOV 13, 1984
AB		50MG	N088855 001	NOV 13, 1984
AB		75MG	N088856 001	NOV 13, 1984
AB		100MG	N088857 001	NOV 13, 1984
AB	TEVA	10MG	N084910 003	
AB		25MG	N085031 001	
AB		50MG	N085032 001	
AB		100MG	N085836 001	

AMITRIPTYLINE HYDROCHLORIDE

AB	VINTAGE PHARMS	10MG	N040218 001	SEP 11, 1997
AB		25MG	N040218 002	SEP 11, 1997
AB		50MG	N040218 003	SEP 11, 1997
AB		75MG	N040218 004	

Prescription Drug Products (continued)

AMITRIPTYLINE HYDROCHLORIDE (continued)

Tablet; Oral

AMITRIPTYLINE HYDROCHLORIDE

		Strength		
	VINTAGE PHARMS	100MG	N040218 005	SEP 11, 1997
		150MG	N040218 006	SEP 11, 1997

ELAVIL

		Strength		
AB	ASTRAZENECA	10MG	N012703 001	
AB +		25MG	N012703 003	
AB		50MG	N012703 004	
AB		75MG	N012703 005	
AB		100MG	N012703 006	
AB		150MG	N012703 007	

AMITRIPTYLINE HYDROCHLORIDE; CHLORDIAZEPOXIDE

Tablet; Oral

CHLORDIAZEPOXIDE AND AMITRIPTYLINE HCL

		Strength		
AB	MYLAN	EQ 12.5MG BASE;5MG	N071296 001	DEC 10, 1986
AB		EQ 25MG BASE;10MG	N071297 001	DEC 10, 1986
AB	PAR PHARM	EQ 12.5MG BASE;5MG	N072277 001	MAY 09, 1988
AB		EQ 25MG BASE;10MG	N072278 001	MAY 09, 1988
AB	WATSON LABS	EQ 12.5MG BASE;5MG	N072052 001	DEC 16, 1988
AB		EQ 25MG BASE;10MG	N072053 001	DEC 16, 1988

LIMBITROL

		Strength		
AB	ICN	EQ 12.5MG BASE;5MG	N016949 001	

LIMBITROL DS

		Strength		
AB +	ICN	EQ 25MG BASE;10MG	N016949 002	

AMITRIPTYLINE HYDROCHLORIDE; PERPHENAZINE

Tablet; Oral

PERPHENAZINE AND AMITRIPTYLINE HCL

		Strength		
AB	GENEVA PHARMS	10MG;2MG	N071062 001	NOV 27, 1987
AB		25MG;2MG	N071063 001	NOV 27, 1987
AB		25MG;4MG	N071064 001	NOV 27, 1987
AB		10MG;4MG	N071862 001	NOV 27, 1987
AB		50MG;4MG	N071863 001	DEC 21, 1987
AB	MYLAN	10MG;2MG	N070336 001	DEC 21, 1987
AB		25MG;2MG	N070337 001	NOV 10, 1988
AB +		25MG;4MG	N070338 001	NOV 10, 1988
AB		10MG;4MG	N071442 001	NOV 10, 1988

AMITRIPTYLINE HYDROCHLORIDE; PERPHENAZINE (continued)

Tablet; Oral

PERPHENAZINE AND AMITRIPTYLINE HCL

		Strength		
AB +	MYLAN	50MG;4MG	N071443 001	NOV 10, 1988
AB	WATSON LABS	10MG;2MG	N073007 001	OCT 17, 1991
AB		25MG;2MG	N073008 001	OCT 17, 1991
AB		10MG;4MG	N073009 001	OCT 17, 1991
AB		25MG;4MG	N073010 001	OCT 17, 1991

AMLEXANOX

Paste; Dental

APHTHASOL

		Strength		
+	GLAXOSMITHKLINE CONS	5%	N020511 001	DEC 17, 1996

AMLODIPINE BESYLATE

Tablet; Oral

NORVASC

		Strength		
	PFIZER	EQ 2.5MG BASE	N019787 001	JUL 31, 1992
		EQ 5MG BASE	N019787 002	JUL 31, 1992
+		EQ 10MG BASE	N019787 003	JUL 31, 1992

AMLODIPINE BESYLATE; BENAZEPRIL HYDROCHLORIDE

Capsule; Oral

LOTREL

		Strength		
	NOVARTIS	EQ 2.5MG BASE;10MG	N020364 002	MAR 03, 1995
		EQ 5MG BASE;10MG	N020364 003	MAR 03, 1995
		EQ 5MG BASE;20MG	N020364 004	MAR 03, 1995
+		EQ 10MG BASE;20MG	N020364 005	JUN 20, 2002

AMMONIUM CHLORIDE

Injectable; Injection

AMMONIUM CHLORIDE IN PLASTIC CONTAINER

		Strength		
+	ABBOTT	5MEQ/ML	N088366 001	JUN 13, 1984

AMMONIUM LACTATE

Cream; Topical

AMMONIUM LACTATE

		Strength		
AB	CLAY PARK	EQ 12% BASE	N075774 001	MAY 01, 2002
AB	TARO	EQ 12% BASE	N075883 001	

Prescription Drug Products (continued)

AMMONIUM LACTATE (continued)

Cream; Topical

AMMONIUM LACTATE

	TARO			APR 10, 2003

LAC-HYDRIN

AB	+ WESTWOOD SQUIBB	EQ 12% BASE	N020508 001	AUG 29, 1996

Lotion; Topical

AMMONIUM LACTATE

AB	PADDOCK	EQ 12% BASE	N075575 001	JUN 11, 2002

LAC-HYDRIN

AB	+ WESTWOOD SQUIBB	EQ 12% BASE	N019155 001	APR 24, 1985

AMOXAPINE

Tablet; Oral

AMOXAPINE

AB	GENEVA PHARMS	25MG	N072943 001	JUN 28, 1991
AB		50MG	N072944 001	JUN 28, 1991
AB		100MG	N072878 001	JUN 28, 1991
AB		150MG	N072879 001	JUN 28, 1991
AB	WATSON LABS	25MG	N072418 001	JUN 28, 1991
AB		25MG	N072688 001	MAY 11, 1989
AB		50MG	N072419 001	AUG 28, 1992
AB		50MG	N072689 001	MAY 11, 1989
AB		100MG	N072420 001	AUG 28, 1992
AB		100MG	N072690 001	MAY 11, 1989
AB	+	150MG	N072421 001	AUG 28, 1992
AB		150MG	N072691 001	MAY 11, 1989
				AUG 28, 1992

AMOXICILLIN

Capsule; Oral

AMOXICILLIN

AB	BIOCHEMIE	250MG	N064076 001	SEP 30, 1994
AB		500MG	N064076 002	SEP 30, 1994
AB	CLONMEL	250MG	N062884 001	FEB 25, 1988
AB		500MG	N062881 001	FEB 25, 1988
AB	CONSOLIDATED PHARM	250MG	N062058 001	
AB		500MG	N062058 002	
AB	RANBAXY	250MG	N065016 001	

AMOXICILLIN (continued)

Capsule; Oral

AMOXICILLIN

	RANBAXY	500MG	N065016 002	APR 08, 1999
				APR 08, 1999
AB	TEVA	250MG	N061926 001	
AB		250MG	N062853 001	DEC 22, 1987
AB		500MG	N061926 003	
AB		500MG	N062854 001	DEC 22, 1987

AMOXIL

AB	GLAXOSMITHKLINE	250MG	N062216 001	
AB		500MG	N062216 004	

TRIMOX

AB	+ APOTHECON	250MG	N061885 001	
AB		500MG	N061885 002	

For Suspension; Oral

AMOXICILLIN

AB	CLONMEL	125MG/5ML	N062927 001	NOV 25, 1988
AB		250MG/5ML	N062927 002	NOV 25, 1988
AB	CONSOLIDATED PHARM	125MG/5ML	N062059 001	
AB		250MG/5ML	N062059 002	
AB		200MG/5ML	N065113 001	NOV 29, 2002
AB	RANBAXY	400MG/5ML	N065113 002	NOV 29, 2002
AB	TEVA	125MG/5ML	N061931 001	
AB		125MG/5ML	N062946 001	NOV 01, 1988
AB		200MG/5ML	N065119 001	DEC 04, 2002
AB		250MG/5ML	N061931 002	
AB		250MG/5ML	N063001 001	JAN 06, 1989
AB		400MG/5ML	N065119 002	DEC 04, 2002

AMOXICILLIN PEDIATRIC

AB	TEVA	50MG/ML	N061931 003	DEC 01, 1982

AMOXIL

AB	+ GLAXOSMITHKLINE	50MG/ML	N062226 005	
AB		125MG/5ML	N062226 001	
AB		200MG/5ML	N050760 001	APR 15, 1999
AB	+	250MG/5ML	N062226 002	
AB	+	400MG/5ML	N050760 002	APR 15, 1999

LAROTID

AB	GLAXOSMITHKLINE	125MG/5ML	N062226 003	
AB		250MG/5ML	N062226 004	

TRIMOX

AB	APOTHECON	125MG/5ML	N062885 001	MAR 08, 1988

Prescription Drug Products *(continued)*

AMOXICILLIN *(continued)*

For Suspension; Oral

TE	Applicant	Strength	Appl. No.	Date
	TRIMOX			
AB	APOTHECON	250MG/5ML	N062885 002	MAR 08, 1988

Tablet, Chewable; Oral

TE	Applicant	Strength	Appl. No.	Date
	AMOXICILLIN			
	CLONMEL			
AB		125MG	N064139 001	JAN 29, 1996
AB		250MG	N064139 002	JAN 29, 1996
	AMOXICILLIN			
	RANBAXY			
AB		125MG	N065021 001	DEC 23, 1999
AB		200MG	N065060 001	NOV 29, 2000
AB		250MG	N065021 002	DEC 23, 1999
AB		400MG	N065060 002	NOV 29, 2000
	TEVA			
AB		125MG	N064013 002	SEP 11, 1995
AB		125MG	N064031 001	DEC 19, 1996
AB		250MG	N064013 001	DEC 22, 1992
AB		250MG	N064031 002	DEC 19, 1996
	AMOXIL			
	GLAXOSMITHKLINE			
AB		125MG	N050542 002	APR 15, 1999
AB		200MG	N050761 001	APR 15, 1999
AB	+	250MG	N050542 001	APR 15, 1999
AB		400MG	N050761 002	APR 15, 1999

Tablet; Oral

TE	Applicant	Strength	Appl. No.	Date
	AMOXICILLIN			
	RANBAXY			
AB		500MG	N065059 001	NOV 24, 2000
AB		875MG	N065059 002	NOV 24, 2000
	TEVA			
AB		500MG	N065056 001	SEP 18, 2000
AB		875MG	N065056 002	SEP 18, 2000
	AMOXIL			
	GLAXOSMITHKLINE			
AB		500MG	N050754 002	JUL 10, 1998
AB	+	875MG	N050754 001	JUL 10, 1998

AMOXICILLIN; CLARITHROMYCIN; LANSOPRAZOLE

Capsule, Tablet, Capsule, Delayed Rel Pellets; Oral

TE	Applicant	Strength	Appl. No.	Date
	PREVPAC			
	+ TAP PHARM	500MG;500MG;30MG	N050757 001	DEC 02, 1997

AMOXICILLIN; CLAVULANATE POTASSIUM

For Suspension; Oral

AMOXICILLIN AND CLAVULANATE POTASSIUM

TE	Applicant	Strength	Appl. No.	Date
	GENEVA PHARMS			
AB		200MG/5ML;EQ 28.5MG BASE/5ML	N065066 001	JUN 05, 2002
AB		400MG/5ML;EQ 57MG BASE/5ML	N065066 002	JUN 05, 2002
	LEK PHARMS			
AB		200MG/5ML;EQ 28.5MG BASE/5ML	N065098 001	DEC 16, 2002
AB		400MG/5ML;EQ 57MG BASE/5ML	N065098 002	DEC 16, 2002
	RANBAXY			
AB		200MG/5ML;EQ 28.5MG BASE/5ML	N065132 001	MAR 19, 2003
AB		400MG/5ML;EQ 57MG BASE/5ML	N065132 002	MAR 19, 2003
	AUGMENTIN '125'			
	GLAXOSMITHKLINE			
AB		125MG/5ML;EQ 31.25MG BASE/5ML	N050575 001	AUG 06, 1984
	AUGMENTIN '200'			
	GLAXOSMITHKLINE			
AB		200MG/5ML;EQ 28.5MG BASE/5ML	N050725 001	MAY 31, 1996
	AUGMENTIN '250'			
	+ GLAXOSMITHKLINE			
AB		250MG/5ML;EQ 62.5MG BASE/5ML	N050575 002	AUG 06, 1984
	AUGMENTIN '400'			
	GLAXOSMITHKLINE			
AB		400MG/5ML;EQ 57MG BASE/5ML	N050725 002	MAY 31, 1996
	AUGMENTIN ES-600			
	+ GLAXOSMITHKLINE	600MG/5ML;EQ 42.9MG BASE/5ML	N050755 001	JUN 22, 2001

Tablet, Chewable; Oral

AMOXICILLIN AND CLAVULANATE POTASSIUM

TE	Applicant	Strength	Appl. No.	Date
	GENEVA PHARMS			
AB		200MG;EQ 28.5MG BASE	N065065 001	APR 18, 2002
AB		400MG;EQ 57MG BASE	N065065 002	APR 18, 2002
	AUGMENTIN '125'			
	+ GLAXOSMITHKLINE			
AB		125MG;EQ 31.25MG BASE	N050597 001	JUL 22, 1985
	AUGMENTIN '200'			
	GLAXOSMITHKLINE			
AB		200MG;EQ 28.5MG BASE	N050726 001	MAY 31, 1996
	AUGMENTIN '250'			
	+ GLAXOSMITHKLINE			
AB		250MG;EQ 62.5MG BASE	N050597 002	JUL 22, 1985
	AUGMENTIN '400'			
	+ GLAXOSMITHKLINE			
AB		400MG;EQ 57MG BASE	N050726 002	MAY 31, 1996

Prescription Drug Products (continued)

AMOXICILLIN; CLAVULANATE POTASSIUM (continued)

Tablet, Extended Release; Oral

AUGMENTIN XR

+	GLAXOSMITHKLINE	1GM;62.5MG	N050785 001	SEP 25, 2002

Tablet; Oral

AMOXICILLIN AND CLAVULANATE POTASSIUM

AB	GENEVA PHARMS	875MG;EQ 125MG BASE	N065063 001	MAR 14, 2002
AB		500MG;EQ 125MG BASE	N065064 001	MAR 15, 2002
AB	LEK PHARMS	875MG;EQ 125MG BASE	N065093 001	NOV 21, 2002
AB	RANBAXY	875MG;EQ 125MG BASE	N065102 001	SEP 17, 2002
AB		500MG;EQ 125MG BASE	N065109 001	NOV 04, 2002
AB	TEVA	875MG;EQ 125MG BASE	N065096 001	OCT 29, 2002
AB		500MG;EQ 125MG BASE	N065101 001	OCT 30, 2002

AMOXICILLIN AND CLAVULANATE POTSSSIUM

AB	LEK PHARMS	500MG;EQ 125MG BASE	N065117 001	NOV 27, 2002

AUGMENTIN '250'

AB	GLAXOSMITHKLINE	250MG;EQ 125MG BASE	N050564 001	AUG 06, 1984

AUGMENTIN '500'

AB	GLAXOSMITHKLINE	500MG;EQ 125MG BASE	N050564 002	AUG 06, 1984

AUGMENTIN '875'

AB	+ GLAXOSMITHKLINE	875MG;EQ 125MG BASE	N050720 001	FEB 13, 1996

AMPHETAMINE ASPARTATE; AMPHETAMINE SULFATE; DEXTROAMPHETAMINE SACCHARATE; DEXTROAMPHETAMINE SULFATE

Capsule, Extended Release; Oral

ADDERALL XR 10

AB	SHIRE LABS	2.5MG;2.5MG;2.5MG;2.5MG	N021303 001	OCT 11, 2001

ADDERALL XR 20

AB	SHIRE LABS	5MG;5MG;5MG;5MG	N021303 002	OCT 11, 2001

ADDERALL XR 30

AB	+ SHIRE LABS	7.5MG;7.5MG;7.5MG;7.5MG	N021303 003	OCT 11, 2001

ADDERALL XR 25

AB	SHIRE LABS	6.25MG;6.25MG;6.25MG;6.25MG	N021303 004	MAY 22, 2002

ADDERALL XR 5

AB	SHIRE LABS	1.25MG;1.25MG;1.25MG;1.25MG	N021303 005	MAY 22, 2002

ADDERALL XR 15

AB	SHIRE LABS	3.75MG;3.75MG;3.75MG;3.75MG	N021303 006	

AMPHETAMINE ASPARTATE; AMPHETAMINE SULFATE; DEXTROAMPHETAMINE SACCHARATE; DEXTROAMPHETAMINE SULFATE (continued)

Capsule, Extended Release; Oral

ADDERALL XR 15

	SHIRE LABS			MAY 22, 2002

Tablet; Oral

ADDERALL 10

AB	SHIRE LABS	2.5MG;2.5MG;2.5MG;2.5MG	N011522 007	FEB 13, 1996

ADDERALL 20

AB	SHIRE LABS	5MG;5MG;5MG;5MG	N011522 008	FEB 13, 1996

ADDERALL 5

AB	SHIRE LABS	1.25MG;1.25MG;1.25MG;1.25MG	N011522 009	MAY 12, 1997

ADDERALL 30

AB	+ SHIRE LABS	7.5MG;7.5MG;7.5MG;7.5MG	N011522 010	MAY 12, 1997

ADDERALL 7.5

AB	SHIRE LABS	1.875MG;1.875MG;1.875MG;1.875MG	N011522 011	AUG 31, 2000

ADDERALL 12.5

AB	SHIRE LABS	3.125MG;3.125MG;3.125MG;3.125MG	N011522 012	AUG 31, 2000

ADDERALL 15

AB	SHIRE LABS	3.75MG;3.75MG;3.75MG;3.75MG	N011522 013	AUG 31, 2000

DEXTROAMP SACCHARATE, AMP ASPARTATE, DEXTROAMP SULFATE AND AMP SULFATE

AB	BARR	1.25MG;1.25MG;1.25MG;1.25MG	N040422 001	FEB 11, 2002
AB		2.5MG;2.5MG;2.5MG;2.5MG	N040422 002	FEB 11, 2002
AB		5MG;5MG;5MG;5MG	N040422 003	FEB 11, 2002
AB		7.5MG;7.5MG;7.5MG;7.5MG	N040422 004	FEB 11, 2002
AB		1.875MG;1.875MG;1.875MG;1.875MG	N040422 005	MAR 19, 2003
AB		3.125MG;3.125MG;3.125MG;3.125MG	N040422 006	MAR 19, 2003
AB		3.75MG;3.75MG;3.75MG;3.75MG	N040422 007	MAR 19, 2003
AB	EON	2.5MG;2.5MG;2.5MG;2.5MG	N040439 001	JUN 14, 2002
AB		5MG;5MG;5MG;5MG	N040439 002	JUN 14, 2002
AB		7.5MG;7.5MG;7.5MG;7.5MG	N040439 003	JUN 14, 2002
AB	COREPHARMA	1.25MG;1.25MG;1.25MG;1.25MG	N040444 001	JUN 19, 2002
AB		2.5MG;2.5MG;2.5MG;2.5MG	N040444 002	

Prescription Drug Products (continued)

AMPHETAMINE ASPARTATE; AMPHETAMINE SULFATE; DEXTROAMPHETAMINE SACCHARATE; DEXTROAMPHETAMINE SULFATE (continued)

Tablet; Oral

DEXTROAMP SACCHARATE, AMP ASPARTATE, DEXTROAMP SULFATE AND AMP SULFATE

COREPHARMA

AB	5MG;5MG;5MG;5MG	N040444 003	JUN 19, 2002
AB	7.5MG;7.5MG;7.5MG;7.5MG	N040444 004	JUN 19, 2002

DEXTROAMP SACCHARATE, AMP ASPARTATE, DEXTROAMP SULFATE AND AMP SULFATE

WATSON LABS

AB	1.25MG;1.25MG;1.25MG;1.25MG	N040456 001	MAY 06, 2003
AB	2.5MG;2.5MG;2.5MG;2.5MG	N040456 002	MAY 06, 2003
AB	5MG;5MG;5MG;5MG	N040456 003	MAY 06, 2003
AB	7.5MG;7.5MG;7.5MG;7.5MG	N040456 004	MAY 06, 2003

DEXTROAMP SACCHARATE, AMP ASPARTATE, DEXTROAMP SULFATE AND AMP SULFATE

EON

AB	1.25MG;1.25MG;1.25MG;1.25MG	N040470 001	SEP 27, 2002

AMPHETAMINE SULFATE *MULTIPLE*

SEE   AMPHETAMINE ASPARTATE; AMPHETAMINE SULFATE; DEXTROAMPHETAMINE SACCHARATE; DEXTROAMPHETAMINE SULFATE

AMPHOTERICIN B

Cream; Topical

FUNGIZONE

	+ APOTHECON	3%	N050314 001	

Injectable, Lipid Complex; Injection

ABELCET

	+ ENZON	5MG/ML	N050724 001	NOV 20, 1995

AMPHOTEC

	+ INTERMUNE PHARMS	50MG/VIAL	N050729 001	NOV 22, 1996
	+	100MG/VIAL	N050729 002	NOV 22, 1996

Injectable, Liposomal; Injection

AMBISOME

	+ FUJISAWA HLTHCARE	50MG/VIAL	N050740 001	AUG 11, 1997

Injectable; Injection

AMPHOTERICIN B

AP	GENSIA SICOR PHARMS	50MG/VIAL	N064062 001	MAR 31, 1995
AP	PHARMA TEK	50MG/VIAL	N063206 001	APR 29, 1992

FUNGIZONE

AP	+ APOTHECON	50MG/VIAL	N060517 001	

AMPHOTERICIN B (continued)

Lotion; Topical

FUNGIZONE

	+ APOTHECON	3%	N060570 001

AMPICILLIN SODIUM

Injectable; Injection

AMPICILLIN SODIUM

APOTHECON

AP		EQ 1GM BASE/VIAL	N061395 004	
AP		EQ 1GM BASE/VIAL	N062738 001	FEB 19, 1987
AP		EQ 1GM BASE/VIAL	N062860 004	FEB 05, 1988
AP		EQ 2GM BASE/VIAL	N061395 005	
AP		EQ 2GM BASE/VIAL	N062738 002	FEB 19, 1987
AP		EQ 2GM BASE/VIAL	N062860 005	FEB 05, 1988
AP		EQ 10GM BASE/VIAL	N061395 006	
AP		EQ 125MG BASE/VIAL	N061395 001	
AP		EQ 125MG BASE/VIAL	N062860 001	FEB 05, 1988
AP		EQ 250MG BASE/VIAL	N061395 002	
AP		EQ 250MG BASE/VIAL	N062860 002	FEB 05, 1988
AP		EQ 500MG BASE/VIAL	N061395 003	
AP		EQ 500MG BASE/VIAL	N062860 003	FEB 05, 1988

IBI

AP		EQ 1GM BASE/VIAL	N062719 002	MAY 12, 1987
AP		EQ 250MG BASE/VIAL	N062719 001	MAY 12, 1987
AP		EQ 500MG BASE/VIAL	N062719 003	MAY 12, 1987

MARSAM PHARMS LLC

AP		EQ 1GM BASE/VIAL	N062816 004	OCT 24, 1988
AP		EQ 2GM BASE/VIAL	N062816 005	OCT 24, 1988
AP		EQ 125MG BASE/VIAL	N062816 001	OCT 24, 1988
AP		EQ 250MG BASE/VIAL	N062816 002	OCT 24, 1988
AP		EQ 500MG BASE/VIAL	N062816 003	OCT 24, 1988

TOTACILLIN-N

AP	+ GLAXOSMITHKLINE	EQ 1GM BASE/VIAL	N060677 004
AP	+	EQ 2GM BASE/VIAL	N060677 005
AP	+	EQ 10GM BASE/VIAL	N060677 006
AP	+	EQ 125MG BASE/VIAL	N060677 001
AP	+	EQ 250MG BASE/VIAL	N060677 002
AP	+	EQ 500MG BASE/VIAL	N060677 003

Prescription Drug Products (continued)

AMPICILLIN SODIUM; SULBACTAM SODIUM
Injectable; Injection
AMPICILLIN AND SULBACTAM

AP	ESI LEDERLE	EQ 1GM BASE/VIAL;EQ 500MG BASE/VIAL	N065074 001	MAR 19, 2002
AP		EQ 2GM BASE/VIAL;EQ 1GM BASE/VIAL	N065074 002	MAR 19, 2002
AP		EQ 10GM BASE/VIAL;EQ 5GM BASE/VIAL	N065076 001	MAR 19, 2002

UNASYN

AP	+ PFIZER	EQ 1GM BASE/VIAL;EQ 500MG BASE/VIAL	N050608 002	DEC 31, 1986
		EQ 1GM BASE/VIAL;EQ 500MG BASE/VIAL	N062901 001	NOV 23, 1988
AP	+	EQ 2GM BASE/VIAL;EQ 1GM BASE/VIAL	N050608 001	DEC 31, 1986
AP	+	EQ 10GM BASE/VIAL;EQ 5GM BASE/VIAL	N050608 005	DEC 10, 1993

AMPICILLIN/AMPICILLIN TRIHYDRATE
Capsule; Oral
AMPICILLIN TRIHYDRATE

AB	CLONMEL	EQ 250MG BASE	N062883 001	FEB 25, 1988
AB		EQ 500MG BASE	N062882 001	FEB 25, 1988
AB	CONSOLIDATED PHARM	EQ 250MG BASE	N061602 001	
AB		EQ 500MG BASE	N061602 002	
AB	PUREPAC PHARM	EQ 250MG BASE	N061853 002	
AB	TEVA	EQ 250MG BASE	N061502 001	
AB		EQ 500MG BASE	N061502 002	

PRINCIPEN

AB	APOTHECON	EQ 250MG BASE	N061392 001	
AB		EQ 250MG BASE	N062888 001	MAR 04, 1988
AB	+	EQ 500MG BASE	N061392 002	
AB	+	EQ 500MG BASE	N062888 002	MAR 04, 1988

TOTACILLIN

AB	GLAXOSMITHKLINE	EQ 250MG BASE	N062212 001	
AB		EQ 500MG BASE	N062212 002	

For Suspension; Oral
AMPICILLIN TRIHYDRATE

AB	CLONMEL	EQ 125MG BASE/5ML	N062982 001	FEB 10, 1989
AB		EQ 250MG BASE/5ML	N062982 002	FEB 10, 1989
AB	CONSOLIDATED PHARM	EQ 125MG BASE/5ML	N061601 001	
AB		EQ 250MG BASE/5ML	N061601 002	
AB	PUREPAC PHARM	EQ 250MG BASE/5ML	N061980 002	

AMPICILLIN/AMPICILLIN TRIHYDRATE (continued)
For Suspension; Oral
AMPICILLIN TRIHYDRATE

AB	TEVA	EQ 125MG BASE/5ML	N061370 001	
AB		EQ 250MG BASE/5ML	N061370 002	

PRINCIPEN

AB	APOTHECON	EQ 100MG BASE/ML	N061394 001	
AB	+	EQ 125MG BASE/5ML	N061394 002	
AB	+	EQ 250MG BASE/5ML	N061394 003	

AMPRENAVIR
Capsule; Oral
AGENERASE

	GLAXOSMITHKLINE	50MG	N021007 001	APR 15, 1999
+		150MG	N021007 002	APR 15, 1999

Solution; Oral
AGENERASE

+	GLAXOSMITHKLINE	15MG/ML	N021039 001	APR 15, 1999

ANAGRELIDE HYDROCHLORIDE
Capsule; Oral
AGRYLIN

	SHIRE LABS	EQ 0.5MG BASE	N020333 001	MAR 14, 1997
+		EQ 1MG BASE	N020333 002	MAR 14, 1997

ANASTROZOLE
Tablet; Oral
ARIMIDEX

+	ASTRAZENECA	1MG	N020541 001	DEC 27, 1995

ANISINDIONE
Tablet; Oral
MIRADON

+	SCHERING	50MG	N010909 003	

APRACLONIDINE HYDROCHLORIDE
Solution/Drops; Ophthalmic
IOPIDINE

+	ALCON	EQ 0.5% BASE	N020258 001	JUL 30, 1993
+		EQ 1% BASE	N019779 001	DEC 31, 1987

APREPITANT
Capsule; Oral
EMEND

	MERCK	80MG	N021549 001	MAR 26, 2003

Prescription Drug Products (continued)

APREPITANT (continued)
Capsule; Oral
  EMEND
  + MERCK   125MG   N021549 002   MAR 26, 2003

APROTININ BOVINE
Injectable; Injection
  TRASYLOL
  + BAYER PHARMS   10,000KIU/ML   N020304 001   DEC 29, 1993

ARGATROBAN
Injectable; Injection
  ARGATROBAN
  + ENCYSIVE   100MG/ML   N020883 001   JUN 30, 2000

ARGININE HYDROCHLORIDE
Injectable; Injection
  R-GENE 10
  + PHARMACIA AND UPJOHN   10GM/100ML   N016931 001

ARIPIPRAZOLE
Tablet; Oral
  ABILIFY
  OTSUKA   2MG   N021436 006   NOV 15, 2002
          5MG   N021436 005   NOV 15, 2002
          10MG   N021436 001   NOV 15, 2002
          15MG   N021436 002   NOV 15, 2002
          20MG   N021436 003   NOV 15, 2002
  +   30MG   N021436 004   NOV 15, 2002

ARSENIC TRIOXIDE
Injectable; Injection
  TRISENOX
  + CELL THERAP   1MG/ML   N021248 001   SEP 25, 2000

ARTICAINE HYDROCHLORIDE; EPINEPHRINE
Injectable; Injection
  SEPTOCAINE
  + DEPROCO   4%;EQ 0.01MG BASE/ML   N020971 001   APR 03, 2000

ASCORBIC ACID; BIOTIN; CHOLECALCIFEROL; CYANOCOBALAMIN; DEXPANTHENOL; FOLIC ACID; NIACINAMIDE; PYRIDOXINE; RIBOFLAVIN; THIAMINE; TOCOPHEROL ACETATE; VITAMIN A; VITAMIN K
Injectable; Iv 'Infusion)
  INFUVITE PEDIATRIC
  + SABEX 2002   80MG/VIAL;0.02MG/VIAL;400 IU/VIAL;0.001MG/VIAL;5MG/VIAL;0.14MG/VIAL;17MG/VIAL;1MG/VIAL;1.4MG/VIAL;1.2MG/VIAL;7 IU/VIAL;2,300 IU/VIAL;0.2MG/VIAL   N021265 001   FEB 21, 2001

ASCORBIC ACID; BIOTIN; CYANOCOBALAMIN; DEXPANTHENOL; ERGOCALCIFEROL; FOLIC ACID; NIACINAMIDE; PHYTONADIONE; PYRIDOXINE HYDROCHLORIDE; RIBOFLAVIN PHOSPHATE SODIUM; THIAMINE HYDROCHLORIDE; VITAMIN A; VITAMIN E
For Solution; Iv (Infusion)
  M.V.I. PEDIATRIC
  + AAIPHARMA   80MG/VIAL;0.02MG/VIAL;0.001MG/VIAL;5MG/VIAL;0.01MG/VIAL;0.14MG/VIAL;17MG/VIAL;0.2MG/VIAL;1MG/VIAL;1.4MG/VIAL;EQ 1.2MG BASE/VIAL;0.7MG/VIAL;7MG/VIAL   N018920 001   SEP 21, 2000

ASCORBIC ACID; BIOTIN; CYANOCOBALAMIN; DEXPANTHENOL; ERGOCALCIFEROL; FOLIC ACID; NIACINAMIDE; PYRIDOXINE HYDROCHLORIDE; RIBOFLAVIN PHOSPHATE SODIUM; THIAMINE HYDROCHLORIDE; VITAMIN A; VITAMIN E
Injectable; Injection
  M.V.I.-12
  + AAIPHARMA   10MG/ML;0.006MG/ML;0.5UGM/ML;1.5MG/ML;20 IU/ML;0.04MG/ML;4MG/ML;0.4MG/ML;0.36MG/ML;0.3MG/ML;330 UNITS/ML;1 IU/ML   N008809 004   AUG 08, 1985

ASCORBIC ACID *MULTIPLE*
SEE   ALPHA-TOCOPHEROL ACETATE; ASCORBIC ACID; BIOTIN; CHOLECALCIFEROL; CYANOCOBALAMIN; DEXPANTHENOL; FOLIC ACID; NIACINAMIDE; PYRIDOXINE HYDROCHLORIDE; RIBOFLAVIN PHOSPHATE SODIUM; THIAMINE HYDROCHLORIDE; VITAMIN A PALMITATE; VITAMIN K

ASPIRIN; BUTALBITAL; CAFFEINE
Capsule; Oral
  FIORINAL
AB + WATSON PHARMS   325MG;50MG;40MG   N017534 005   APR 16, 1986

Prescription Drug Products (continued)

ASPIRIN; BUTALBITAL; CAFFEINE (continued)

Capsule; Oral

LANORINAL

AB	LANNETT	325MG;50MG;40MG	N086996 002	OCT 11, 1985

Tablet; Oral

ASPIRIN AND CAFFEINE W/ BUTALBITAL

AB	PUREPAC PHARM	325MG;50MG;40MG	N086710 002	AUG 23, 1983

BUTAL COMPOUND

AB	GENEVA PHARMS	325MG;50MG;40MG	N086398 002	APR 06, 1984

BUTALBITAL W/ ASPIRIN 50MG;40MG

			N087048 002	DEC 09, 1983

BUTALBITAL, ASPIRIN AND CAFFEINE

AB	WEST WARD	325MG;50MG;40MG	N086162 002	FEB 16, 1984

FIORINAL

AB +	WATSON PHARMS	325MG;50MG;40MG	N017534 003	APR 16, 1986

ASPIRIN; BUTALBITAL; CAFFEINE; CODEINE PHOSPHATE

Capsule; Oral

BUTALBITAL, ASPIRIN, CAFFEINE, AND CODEINE PHOSPHATE

AB	WATSON LABS	325MG;50MG;40MG;30MG	N074359 001	AUG 31, 1995
AB	STEVENS J	325MG;50MG;40MG;30MG	N074951 001	AUG 31, 1998
AB	ANABOLIC	325MG;50MG;40MG;30MG	N075231 001	NOV 30, 2001
AB	ENDO PHARMS	325MG;50MG;40MG;30MG	N075351 001	MAR 05, 1999

FIORINAL W/CODEINE NO 3

AB +	WATSON PHARMS	325MG;50MG;40MG;30MG	N019429 003	OCT 26, 1990

ASPIRIN; CAFFEINE; DIHYDROCODEINE BITARTRATE

Capsule; Oral

SYNALGOS-DC

AB +	WOMEN FIRST HLTHCARE	356.4MG;30MG;16MG	N011483 004	SEP 06, 1983

ASPIRIN; CAFFEINE; ORPHENADRINE CITRATE

Tablet; Oral

INVAGESIC

AB	GENEVA PHARMS TECH	385MG;30MG;25MG	N074817 001	NOV 27, 1996

INVAGESIC FORTE

AB	GENEVA PHARMS TECH	770MG;60MG;50MG	N074817 002	NOV 27, 1996

NORGESIC

AB	3M	385MG;30MG;25MG	N013416 002	OCT 27, 1982

ASPIRIN; CAFFEINE; ORPHENADRINE CITRATE (continued)

Tablet; Oral

NORGESIC FORTE

AB +	3M	770MG;60MG;50MG	N013416 004	OCT 27, 1982

ORPHENADRINE CITRATE, ASPIRIN, AND CAFFEINE

AB	EON	385MG;30MG;25MG	N074654 001	DEC 31, 1996
AB	EON	770MG;60MG;50MG	N074654 002	DEC 31, 1996
AB	STEVENS J	385MG;30MG;25MG	N074988 001	APR 30, 1999
AB	STEVENS J	770MG;60MG;50MG	N074988 002	APR 30, 1999

ORPHENGESIC

AB	PAR PHARM	385MG;30MG;25MG	N075141 001	MAY 29, 1998

ORPHENGESIC FORTE

AB	PAR PHARM	770MG;60MG;50MG	N075141 002	MAY 29, 1998

ASPIRIN; CAFFEINE; PROPOXYPHENE HYDROCHLORIDE

Capsule; Oral

DARVON COMPOUND

AB +	AAIPHARMA LLC	389MG;32.4MG;32MG	N010996 006	MAR 08, 1983

DARVON COMPOUND-65

AA +	AAIPHARMA LLC	389MG;32.4MG;65MG	N010996 007	MAR 08, 1983

PROPOXYPHENE COMPOUND 65

AA	TEVA	389MG;32.4MG;65MG	N089025 001	MAR 29, 1985

ASPIRIN; CARISOPRODOL

Tablet; Oral

CARISOPRODOL AND ASPIRIN

AB	AMIDE PHARM	325MG;200MG	N040252 001	DEC 10, 1997
AB	EON	325MG;200MG	N040116 001	APR 25, 1996
AB	PAR PHARM	325MG;200MG	N089594 001	MAR 31, 1989

SOMA COMPOUND

AB +	MEDPOINTE PHARM HLC	325MG;200MG	N012365 005	JUL 11, 1983

ASPIRIN; CARISOPRODOL; CODEINE PHOSPHATE

Tablet; Oral

CARISOPRODOL, ASPIRIN AND CODEINE PHOSPHATE

AB	AMIDE PHARM	325MG;200MG;16MG	N040283 001	DEC 29, 1998
AB	EON	325MG;200MG;16MG	N040118 001	APR 16, 1996

SOMA COMPOUND W/ CODEINE

AB +	MEDPOINTE PHARM HLC	325MG;200MG;16MG	N012366 002	JUL 11, 1983

Prescription Drug Products (continued)

ASPIRIN; DIPYRIDAMOLE
Capsule, Extended Release; Oral
AGGRENOX
+ BOEHRINGER INGELHEIM   25MG;200MG   N020884 001   NOV 22, 1999

ASPIRIN; HYDROCODONE BITARTRATE
Tablet; Oral
AZDONE
+ CENT PHARMS   500MG;5MG   N089420 001   JAN 25, 1988

ASPIRIN; MEPROBAMATE
Tablet; Oral
EQUAGESIC
+ WOMEN FIRST HLTHCARE   325MG;200MG   N011702 003   DEC 29, 1983

ASPIRIN; METHOCARBAMOL
Tablet; Oral
METHOCARBAMOL AND ASPIRIN
AB + IVAX PHARMS   325MG;400MG   N087211 001   DEC 22, 1982
AB PAR PHARM   325MG;400MG   N089657 001   NOV 04, 1988
AB STEVENS J   325MG;400MG   N081145 001   JAN 31, 1995

ASPIRIN; OXYCODONE HYDROCHLORIDE; OXYCODONE TEREPHTHALATE
Tablet; Oral
OXYCODONE AND ASPIRIN
AA AXIOM PHARM   325MG;4.5MG;0.38MG   N040260 001   JUL 17, 1998
AA HALSEY   325MG;4.5MG;0.38MG   N087794 001   MAY 26, 1982
AA WATSON LABS   325MG;4.5MG;0.38MG   N040255 001   FEB 27, 1998
PERCODAN
AA + ENDO PHARMS   325MG;4.5MG;0.38MG   N007337 006
PERCODAN-DEMI
AA + ENDO PHARMS   325MG;2.25MG;0.19MG   N007337 005

ASPIRIN; PRAVASTATIN SODIUM
Tablet; Oral
PRAVIGARD PAC (COPACKAGED)
BRISTOL MYERS SQUIBB   81MG;20MG   N021387 001   JUN 24, 2003
  81MG;40MG   N021387 002   JUN 24, 2003
  81MG;80MG   N021387 003   JUN 24, 2003

ASPIRIN; PRAVASTATIN SODIUM (continued)
Tablet; Oral
PRAVIGARD PAC (COPACKAGED)
BRISTOL MYERS SQUIBB   325MG;20MG   N021387 004   JUN 24, 2003
  325MG;40MG   N021387 005   JUN 24, 2003
  325MG;80MG   N021387 006   JUN 24, 2003

ASPIRIN; PROPOXYPHENE HYDROCHLORIDE
Capsule; Oral
DARVON W/ ASA
+ AAIPHARMA LLC   325MG;65MG   N010996 005

ASPIRIN *MULTIPLE*
SEE ACETAMINOPHEN; ASPIRIN; CODEINE PHOSPHATE

ATAZANAVIR SULFATE
Capsule; Oral
REYATAZ
BRISTOL MYERS SQUIBB   EQ 100MG BASE   N021567 001   JUN 20, 2003
  EQ 150MG BASE   N021567 002   JUN 20, 2003
+   EQ 200MG BASE   N021567 003   JUN 20, 2003

ATENOLOL
Injectable; Injection
TENORMIN
+ ASTRAZENECA   0.5MG/ML   N019058 001   SEP 13, 1989

Tablet; Oral
ATENOLOL
AB CLONMEL HLTHCARE   25MG   N074099 001   APR 28, 1992
AB   50MG   N073542 001   DEC 19, 1991
AB   100MG   N073543 001   DEC 19, 1991
AB COPLEY PHARM   50MG   N074120 001   FEB 24, 1995
AB   100MG   N074120 002   FEB 24, 1995
AB GENEVA PHARMS   25MG   N074052 001   MAY 01, 1992
AB   50MG   N073025 001   SEP 17, 1991
AB   100MG   N073026 001   SEP 17, 1991
AB GENEVA PHARMS TECH   25MG   N074265 001   FEB 28, 1994
AB   50MG   N074265 002

Prescription Drug Products *(continued)*

ATENOLOL *(continued)*
Tablet; Oral

ATENOLOL

TE Code	Firm / Product	Strength	Approval Date	Appl. No.
AB	GENEVA PHARMS TECH	100MG	FEB 28, 1994	N074265 003
AB	IPR	25MG	FEB 28, 1994	N073646 001
AB		50MG	JUL 31, 1992	N072303 001
AB		100MG	JUL 15, 1988	N072304 001
AB	MARTEC	50MG	JUL 15, 1988	N074127 001
AB		100MG	FEB 21, 1995	N074127 002
AB	MUTUAL PHARM	25MG	FEB 21, 1995	N074499 001
AB		50MG	JUL 30, 1997	N073475 001
AB		100MG	MAR 30, 1993	N073476 001
AB	MYLAN	25MG	MAR 30, 1993	N073457 002
AB		50MG	APR 26, 1999	N073456 001
AB		100MG	JAN 24, 1992	N073457 001
AB	PLIVA	25MG	JAN 24, 1992	N074101 001
AB		50MG	JUL 17, 1997	N074101 002
AB		100MG	JUL 17, 1997	N074101 003
AB	SCS	50MG	JUL 17, 1997	N073676 001
AB		100MG	OCT 30, 1992	N073676 002
AB	TEVA	50MG	OCT 30, 1992	N073315 001
AB		50MG	MAY 28, 1993	N074056 001
AB		100MG	JAN 18, 1995	N073316 001
AB		100MG	MAY 28, 1993	N074056 002
AB	WATSON LABS	50MG	JAN 18, 1995	N073352 001
AB		100MG	DEC 27, 1991	N073353 001

TENORMIN

TE Code	Firm	Strength	Approval Date	Appl. No.
AB	ASTRAZENECA	25MG	DEC 27, 1991	N018240 004
AB		50MG	APR 09, 1990	N018240 001
AB +		100MG		N018240 002

ATENOLOL; CHLORTHALIDONE
Tablet; Oral

ATENOLOL AND CHLORTHALIDONE

TE Code	Firm / Product	Strength	Approval Date	Appl. No.
AB	IPR	50MG;25MG	MAY 31, 1990	N072301 001
AB		100MG;25MG	MAY 31, 1990	N072302 001
AB	MARTEC	50MG;25MG	MAY 14, 1998	N074404 001
AB		100MG;25MG	MAY 14, 1998	N074404 002
AB	MUTUAL PHARM	50MG;25MG	APR 29, 1993	N073581 001
AB		100MG;25MG	APR 29, 1993	N073582 001
AB	MYLAN	50MG;25MG	OCT 31, 1993	N074203 001
AB		100MG;25MG	OCT 31, 1993	N074203 002
AB	PLIVA	50MG;25MG	SEP 24, 1997	N074107 001
AB		100MG;25MG	SEP 24, 1997	N074107 002
AB	WATSON LABS	50MG;25MG	JUL 02, 1992	N073665 001
AB		100MG;25MG	JUL 02, 1992	N073665 002

TENORETIC 50

TE Code	Firm	Strength	Approval Date	Appl. No.
AB	ASTRAZENECA	50MG;25MG	JUN 08, 1984	N018760 002

TENORETIC 100

TE Code	Firm	Strength	Approval Date	Appl. No.
AB +	ASTRAZENECA	100MG;25MG	JUN 08, 1984	N018760 001

ATOMOXETINE HYDROCHLORIDE
Capsule; Oral

STRATTERA

Firm / Product	Strength	Approval Date	Appl. No.
LILLY	10MG	NOV 26, 2002	N021411 002
	18MG	NOV 26, 2002	N021411 003
	25MG	NOV 26, 2002	N021411 004
	40MG	NOV 26, 2002	N021411 005
+	60MG	NOV 26, 2002	N021411 006

ATORVASTATIN CALCIUM
Tablet; Oral

LIPITOR

Firm	Strength	Approval Date	Appl. No.
PFIZER	EQ 10MG BASE	DEC 17, 1996	N020702 001
	EQ 20MG BASE	DEC 17, 1996	N020702 002
	EQ 40MG BASE	DEC 17, 1996	N020702 003

Prescription Drug Products (continued)

ATORVASTATIN CALCIUM (continued)
Tablet; Oral

LIPITOR

TE	Firm	Strength	Appl. No.	Date
+	PFIZER	EQ 80MG BASE	N020702 004	DEC 17, 1996 / APR 07, 2000

ATOVAQUONE
Suspension; Oral

MEPRON

TE	Firm	Strength	Appl. No.	Date
+	GLAXOSMITHKLINE	750MG/5ML	N020500 001	FEB 08, 1995

Tablet; Oral

MEPRON

TE	Firm	Strength	Appl. No.	Date
+	GLAXOSMITHKLINE	250MG	N020259 001	NOV 25, 1992

ATOVAQUONE; PROGUANIL HYDROCHLORIDE
Tablet; Oral

MALARONE

TE	Firm	Strength	Appl. No.	Date
+	GLAXOSMITHKLINE	250MG;100MG	N021078 001	JUL 14, 2000

MALARONE PEDIATRIC

TE	Firm	Strength	Appl. No.	Date
+	GLAXOSMITHKLINE	62.5MG;25MG	N021078 002	JUL 14, 2000

ATRACURIUM BESYLATE
Injectable; Injection

ATRACURIUM BESYLATE

TE	Firm	Strength	Appl. No.	Date
AP	ABBOTT	10MG/ML	N074632 001	DEC 23, 1996
AP	BAXTER HLTHCARE CORP	10MG/ML	N074753 001	JAN 23, 1997
AP	BEDFORD	10MG/ML	N074901 001	JUL 18, 1997
AP	ESI LEDERLE	10MG/ML	N074824 001	SEP 30, 1997
AP	FAULDING	10MG/ML	N074740 001	MAR 28, 1997
AP	GENSIA SICOR PHARMS	10MG/ML	N074784 001	JUN 11, 1997
AP	MARSAM PHARMS LLC	10MG/ML	N074945 001	JUL 28, 1998

ATRACURIUM BESYLATE PRESERVATIVE FREE

TE	Firm	Strength	Appl. No.	Date
AP	ABBOTT	10MG/ML	N074633 001 / N074639 001	DEC 23, 1996 / MAR 25, 1997
AP	BAXTER HLTHCARE CORP	10MG/ML	N074768 001 / N074900 001	JAN 23, 1997 / JUL 18, 1997
AP	BEDFORD	10MG/ML	N074825 001	SEP 30, 1997
AP	ESI LEDERLE	10MG/ML		

ATRACURIUM BESYLATE (continued)
Injectable; Injection

ATRACURIUM BESYLATE PRESERVATIVE FREE

TE	Firm	Strength	Appl. No.	Date
AP	FAULDING	10MG/ML	N074741 001 / N074944 001	MAR 28, 1997 / JUL 28, 1998
AP	MARSAM PHARMS LLC	10MG/ML		

TRACRIUM

TE	Firm	Strength	Appl. No.	Date
AP	+ ABBOTT	10MG/ML	N018831 002	JUN 20, 1985

TRACRIUM PRESERVATIVE FREE

TE	Firm	Strength	Appl. No.	Date
AP	+ ABBOTT	10MG/ML	N018831 001	NOV 23, 1983

ATROPINE
Injectable; Injection

ATROPEN

TE	Firm	Strength	Appl. No.
+	MERIDIAN MEDCL TECHN	EQ 2MG SULFATE/0.7ML	N017106 001

ATROPINE SULFATE
Injectable; Im-Iv-Sc

ATROPINE SULFATE ANSYR PLASTIC SYRINGE

TE	Firm	Strength	Appl. No.	Date
+	ABBOTT	0.1MG/ML	N021146 001	JUL 09, 2001
		0.05MG/ML	N021146 002	JUL 09, 2001

ATROPINE SULFATE; DIFENOXIN HYDROCHLORIDE
Tablet; Oral

MOTOFEN

TE	Firm	Strength	Appl. No.
+	AMARIN PHARMS	0.025MG;1MG	N017744 002

ATROPINE SULFATE; DIPHENOXYLATE HYDROCHLORIDE
Capsule; Oral

DIPHENOXYLATE HCL W/ ATROPINE SULFATE

TE	Firm	Strength	Appl. No.
	SCHERER RP	0.025MG;2.5MG	N086440 001

Solution; Oral

DIPHENOXYLATE HCL AND ATROPINE SULFATE

TE	Firm	Strength	Appl. No.	Date
AA	ROXANE	0.025MG/5ML;2.5MG/5ML	N087708 001	MAY 03, 1982

LOMOTIL

TE	Firm	Strength	Appl. No.
AA	+ GD SEARLE LLC	0.025MG/5ML;2.5MG/5ML	N012699 001

Tablet; Oral

DIPHENOXYLATE HCL AND ATROPINE SULFATE

TE	Firm	Strength	Appl. No.	Date
AA	ABLE	0.025MG;2.5MG	N040395 001	NOV 27, 2000
AA	LANNETT	0.025MG;2.5MG	N085372 001	
AA	MY_AN	0.025MG;2.5MG	N085762 001	
AA	PAR PHARM	0.025MG;2.5MG	N040357 001	MAY 02, 2000

DIPHENOXYLATE HCL W/ ATROPINE SULFATE

TE	Firm	Strength	Appl. No.
AA	EON	0.025MG;2.5MG	N086173 001
AA	IVAX PHARMS	0.025MG;2.5MG	N086727 001

Prescription Drug Products (continued)

ATROPINE SULFATE; DIPHENOXYLATE HYDROCHLORIDE (continued)

Tablet; Oral

		LOMOTIL			
AA	+	GD SEARLE LLC	0.025MG;2.5MG	N012462 001	
		LONOX			
AA		GENEVA PHARMS	0.025MG;2.5MG	N085311 002	

ATROPINE SULFATE; EDROPHONIUM CHLORIDE

Injectable; Injection

		ENLON-PLUS			
	+	BAXTER HLTHCARE CORP	0.14MG/ML;10MG/ML	N019677 001	NOV 06, 1991
	+		0.14MG/ML;10MG/ML	N019678 001	NOV 06, 1991

ATROPINE SULFATE; MEPERIDINE HYDROCHLORIDE

Injectable; Injection

		ATROPINE AND DEMEROL			
	+	ABBOTT	0.4MG/ML;75MG/ML	N087847 001	NOV 26, 1982
	+		0.4MG/ML;100MG/ML	N087848 001	NOV 26, 1982
	+		0.4MG/ML;50MG/ML	N087853 001	NOV 26, 1982

AURANOFIN

Capsule; Oral

		RIDAURA			
	+	PROMETHEUS LABS	3MG	N018689 001	MAY 24, 1985

AZATADINE MALEATE

Tablet; Oral

		OPTIMINE			
	+	SCHERING	1MG	N017601 001	

AZATADINE MALEATE; PSEUDOEPHEDRINE SULFATE

Tablet, Extended Release; Oral

		TRINALIN			
	+	SCHERING	1MG;120MG	N018506 001	MAR 23, 1982

AZATHIOPRINE

Tablet; Oral

		AZASAN			
		AAIPHARMA LLC	25MG	N075252 002	FEB 03, 2003
			50MG	N075252 001	JUN 07, 1999
			75MG	N075252 003	FEB 03, 2003
AB			100MG	N075252 004	FEB 03, 2003

AZATHIOPRINE (continued)

Tablet; Oral

		AZATHIOPRINE			
AB	+	GENPHARM	50MG	N075568 001	DEC 13, 1999
AB		ROXANE	50MG	N074069 001	FEB 16, 1996
		IMURAN			
AB	+	PROMETHEUS LABS	50MG	N016324 001	

AZATHIOPRINE SODIUM

Injectable; Injection

		AZATHIOPRINE SODIUM			
AP		BEDFORD	EQ 100MG BASE/VIAL	N074419 001	MAR 31, 1995
		IMURAN			
AP	+	PROMETHEUS LABS	EQ 100MG BASE/VIAL	N017391 001	

AZELAIC ACID

Cream; Topical

		AZELEX			
	+	ALLERGAN	20%	N020428 001	SEP 13, 1995

Gel; Topical

		FINACEA			
	+	BERLEX	15%	N021470 001	DEC 24, 2002

AZELASTINE HYDROCHLORIDE

Solution/Drops; Ophthalmic

		OPTIVAR			
	+	MEDPOINTE PHARM HLC	0.05%	N021127 001	MAY 22, 2000

Spray, Metered; Nasal

		ASTELIN			
	+	MEDPOINTE PHARM HLC	EQ 0.125MG BASE/SPRAY	N020114 001	NOV 01, 1996

AZITHROMYCIN DIHYDRATE

Capsule; Oral

		ZITHROMAX			
	+	PFIZER	EQ 250MG BASE	N050670 001	NOV 01, 1991

For Suspension; Oral

		ZITHROMAX			
	+	PFIZER	EQ 1GM BASE/PACKET	N050693 001	SEP 28, 1994
			EQ 100MG BASE/5ML	N050710 001	OCT 19, 1995
	+		EQ 200MG BASE/5ML	N050710 002	OCT 19, 1995

Injectable; Injection

		ZITHROMAX			
	+	PFIZER	EQ 500MG BASE/VIAL	N050733 001	JAN 30, 1997

Prescription Drug Products (continued)

AZITHROMYCIN DIHYDRATE (continued)
Tablet; Oral
ZITHROMAX

	PFIZER	EQ 250MG BASE	N050711 001	JUL 18, 1996
	+	EQ 500MG BASE	N050784 001	MAY 24, 2002
	+	EQ 600MG BASE	N050730 001	JUN 12, 1996

AZTREONAM
Injectable; Injection
AZACTAM IN PLASTIC CONTAINER

	+ BRISTOL MYERS SQUIBB	20MG/ML	N050632 002	MAY 24, 1989
	+	40MG/ML	N050632 001	MAY 24, 1989

BACAMPICILLIN HYDROCHLORIDE
For Suspension; Oral
SPECTROBID

	+ PFIZER	125MG/5ML	N050556 001	MAR 23, 1982

Tablet; Oral
SPECTROBID

	+ PFIZER	400MG	N050520 001

BACITRACIN
Injectable; Injection
BACIM

AP	PHARMA TEK	50,000 UNITS/VIAL	N064153 001	MAY 09, 1997

BACITRACIN

AP	AM PHARM PARTNERS	50,000 UNITS/VIAL	N065116 001	DEC 03, 2002
AP	PHARMACIA AND UPJOHN	10,000 UNITS/VIAL	N060733 001	
	+	50,000 UNITS/VIAL	N060733 002	

Ointment; Ophthalmic
BACITRACIN

	+ ALTANA	500 UNITS/GM	N061212 001

Powder; For Rx Compounding
BACI-RX

AA	PHARMA TEK	5,000,000 UNITS/BOT	N061580 001

BACITRACIN

AA	APOTHEKERNES	5,000,000 UNITS/BOT	N061699 001

BACITRACIN; HYDROCORTISONE ACETATE; NEOMYCIN SULFATE; POLYMYXIN B SULFATE
Ointment; Ophthalmic
BACITRACIN-NEOMYCIN-POLYMYXIN W/ HYDROCORTISONE ACETATE

	+ PHARMADERM	400 UNITS/GM;1%;EQ 3.5MG BASE/GM:10,000 UNITS/GM	N062166 002

BACITRACIN ZINC; HYDROCORTISONE; NEOMYCIN SULFATE; POLYMYXIN B SULFATE
Ointment; Ophthalmic
CORTISPORIN

AT	+ MONARCH PHARMS	400 UNITS/GM;GM:1%;EQ 3.5MG BASE/GM:10,000 UNITS/GM	N050416 002	

NEOMYCIN AND POLYMYXIN B SULFATES, BACITRACIN ZINC AND HYDROCORTISONE

AT	BAUSCH AND LOMB	400 UNITS/GM;GM:1%;EQ 3.5MG BASE/GM:10,000 UNITS/GM	N064068 001	OCT 30, 1995

Ointment; Topical
CORTISPORIN

	+ MONARCH PHARMS	400 UNITS/GM;1%;EQ 3.5MG BASE/GM:5,000 UNITS/GM	N050168 002	MAY 04, 1984

BACITRACIN ZINC; NEOMYCIN SULFATE; POLYMYXIN B SULFATE
Ointment; Ophthalmic
BACITRACIN-NEOMYCIN-POLYMYXIN

AT	ALTANA	400 UNITS/GM;EQ 3.5MG BASE/GM:10,000 UNITS/GM	N060764 002	

NEOMYCIN AND POLYMYXIN B SULFATES AND BACITRACIN ZINC

AT	BAUSCH AND LOMB	400 UNITS/GM;EQ 3.5MG BASE/GM:10,000 UNITS/GM	N064064 001	OCT 30, 1995

NEOSPORIN

AT	+ MONARCH PHARMS	400 UNITS/GM;EQ 3.5MG BASE/GM:10,000 UNITS/GM	N050417 001

BACITRACIN ZINC; POLYMYXIN B SULFATE
Ointment; Ophthalmic
BACITRACIN ZINC AND POLYMYXIN B SULFATE

AT	AKORN	500 UNITS/GM;GM:10,000 UNITS/GM	N064028 001	JAN 30, 1995
AT	ALTANA	500 UNITS/GM;GM:10,000 UNITS/GM	N065022 001	FEB 27, 2002
AT	BAUSCH AND LOMB	500 UNITS/GM;GM:10,000 UNITS/GM	N064046 001	JAN 26, 1995

POLYSPORIN

AT	+ MONARCH PHARMS	500 UNITS/GM;GM:10,000 UNITS/GM	N061229 001

BACLOFEN
Injectable; Intrathecal
LIORESAL

	+ MEDTRONIC	0.5MG/ML	N020075 001	JUN 17, 1992
	+	0.05MG/ML	N020075 003	NOV 07, 1996
	+	2MG/ML	N020075 002	JUN 17, 1992

Tablet; Oral
BACLOFEN

AB	IVAX PHARMS	10MG	N072234 001	JUL 21, 1988
AB		20MG	N072235 001	

Prescription Drug Products (continued)

BACLOFEN (continued)
Tablet; Oral

BACLOFEN

TE	Firm	Strength	Appl. No.	Date
AB	IVAX PHARMS		N074584 001	JUL 21, 1988
AB	USL PHARMA	10MG	N074584 002	AUG 19, 1996
AB		20MG	N072824 001	AUG 19, 1996
AB	WATSON LABS	10MG	N073092 001	SEP 18, 1991
AB		10MG	N074698 001	JAN 28, 1994
AB		10MG	N072825 001	AUG 20, 1996
AB		20MG	N073093 001	SEP 18, 1991
AB	+	20MG	N074698 002	JAN 28, 1994
AB		20MG		AUG 20, 1996

BALSALAZIDE DISODIUM
Capsule; Oral

	Firm	Strength	Appl. No.	Date
	COLAZAL			
+	SALIX PHARMS	750MG	N020610 001	JUL 18, 2000

BECLOMETHASONE DIPROPIONATE
Aerosol, Metered; Inhalation

TE	Firm	Strength	Appl. No.	Date
	QVAR 40			
+	3M	0.04MG/INH	N020911 002	SEP 15, 2000
	QVAR 80			
+	3M	0.08MG/INH	N020911 001	SEP 15, 2000
	VANCERIL			
BN	+ SCHERING	0.042MG/INH	N017573 001	
	VANCERIL DOUBLE STRENGTH			
	+ SCHERING	0.084MG/INH	N020486 001	DEC 24, 1996

BECLOMETHASONE DIPROPIONATE MONOHYDRATE
Spray, Metered; Nasal

TE	Firm	Strength	Appl. No.	Date
	BECONASE AQ			
BN	+ GLAXOSMITHKLINE	EQ 0.042MG DIPROP/SPRAY	N019389 001	JUL 27, 1987
	VANCENASE AQ			
BN	+ SCHERING	EQ 0.042MG DIPROP/SPRAY	N019589 001	DEC 23, 1987

BENAZEPRIL HYDROCHLORIDE
Tablet; Oral

Firm	Strength	Appl. No.	Date
LOTENSIN			
NOVARTIS	5MG	N019851 001	JUN 25, 1991

BENAZEPRIL HYDROCHLORIDE (continued)
Tablet; Oral

LOTENSIN

Firm	Strength	Appl. No.	Date
NOVARTIS	10MG	N019851 002	JUN 25, 1991
	20MG	N019851 003	JUN 25, 1991
+	40MG	N019851 004	JUN 25, 1991

BENAZEPRIL HYDROCHLORIDE; HYDROCHLOROTHIAZIDE
Tablet; Oral

LOTENSIN HCT

Firm	Strength	Appl. No.	Date
NOVARTIS	5MG;6.25MG	N020033 001	MAY 19, 1992
	10MG;12.5MG	N020033 002	MAY 19, 1992
	20MG;25MG	N020033 003	MAY 19, 1992
+	20MG;12.5MG	N020033 004	MAY 19, 1992

BENAZEPRIL HYDROCHLORIDE *MULTIPLE*
SEE   AMLODIPINE BESYLATE; BENAZEPRIL HYDROCHLORIDE

BENDROFLUMETHIAZIDE
Tablet; Oral

Firm	Strength	Appl. No.
NATURETIN-5		
+ APOTHECON	5MG	N012164 002

BENDROFLUMETHIAZIDE; NADOLOL
Tablet; Oral

CORZIDE

Firm	Strength	Appl. No.	Date
KING PHARMS	5MG;40MG	N018647 001	MAY 25, 1983
+	5MG;80MG	N018647 002	MAY 25, 1983

BENZONATATE
Capsule; Oral

TE	Firm	Strength	Appl. No.	Date
	BENZONATATE			
AA	BANNER PHARMACAPS	100MG	N081297 001	JAN 29, 1993
	TESSALON			
AA	+ FOREST LABS	100MG	N011210 001	
	+	200MG	N011210 003	JUN 25, 1999

BENZOYL PEROXIDE; CLINDAMYCIN PHOSPHATE
Gel; Topical

Firm	Strength	Appl. No.	Date
BENZACLIN			
+ DERMIK LABS	5%;EQ 1% BASE	N050756 001	DEC 21, 2000
DUAC			
+ STIEFEL	5%;EQ 1% BASE	N050741 001	

Prescription Drug Products (continued)

BENZOYL PEROXIDE; CLINDAMYCIN PHOSPHATE (continued)
Gel; Topical

DUAC			
STIEFEL			AUG 26, 2002

BENZOYL PEROXIDE; ERYTHROMYCIN
Gel; Topical

BENZAMYCIN			
+ DERMIK LABS	5%;3%	N050557 001	OCT 26, 1984
BENZAMYCIN PAK			
+ DERMIK LABS	5%;3%	N050769 001	NOV 27, 2000

BENZPHETAMINE HYDROCHLORIDE
Tablet; Oral

DIDREX		
+ PHARMACIA AND UPJOHN	50MG	N012427 002

BENZQUINAMIDE HYDROCHLORIDE
Injectable; Injection

EMETE-CON		
+ PFIZER	EQ 50MG BASE/VIAL	N016820 001

BENZTROPINE MESYLATE
Injectable; Injection

COGENTIN		
+ MERCK	1MG/ML	N012015 001

Tablet; Oral
BENZTROPINE MESYLATE

	COREPHARMA			
AA		0.5MG	N072264 001	FEB 27, 1989
AA		1MG	N072265 001	FEB 27, 1989
AA		2MG	N072266 001	FEB 27, 1989
	MUTUAL PHARM			
AA		1MG	N081264 001	JAN 23, 1992
AA		2MG	N081265 001	JAN 23, 1992
AA	+ PAR PHARM	0.5MG	N088877 001	APR 11, 1985
AA	+	1MG	N088894 001	APR 11, 1985
AA	+	2MG	N088895 001	APR 11, 1985
AA	PLIVA	0.5MG	N089058 001	AUG 10, 1988
AA		1MG	N089059 001	AUG 10, 1988
AA		2MG	N089060 001	AUG 10, 1988
AA	USL PHARMA	0.5MG	N040103 001	DEC 12, 1996

BENZTROPINE MESYLATE (continued)
Tablet; Oral
BENZTROPINE MESYLATE

	USL PHARMA			
AA		1MG	N040103 002	DEC 12, 1996
AA		2MG	N040103 003	DEC 12, 1996

BENZYL PENICILLOYL-POLYLYSINE
Injectable; Injection

PRE-PEN			
+ SCHWARZ PHARMA	60UMOLAR	N050114 001	

BEPRIDIL HYDROCHLORIDE
Tablet; Oral

VASCOR			
ORTHO MCNEIL PHARM	200MG	N019002 001	DEC 28, 1990
+	300MG	N019002 002	DEC 28, 1990

BERACTANT
Suspension; Intratracheal

SURVANTA			
+ ROSS LABS	25MG/ML	N020032 001	JUL 01, 1991

BETAINE, ANHYDROUS
For Solution; Oral

CYSTADANE			
+ ORPHAN MEDCL	1GM/SCOOPFUL	N020576 001	OCT 25, 1996

BETAMETHASONE
Syrup; Oral

CELESTONE		
+ SCHERING	0.6MG/5ML	N014215 002

BETAMETHASONE ACETATE; BETAMETHASONE SODIUM PHOSPHATE
Injectable; Injection

CELESTONE SOLUSPAN		
+ SCHERING	3MG/ML;EQ 3MG BASE/ML	N014602 001

BETAMETHASONE DIPROPIONATE
Cream, Augmented; Topical

DIPROLENE AF			
+ SCHERING	EQ 0.05% BASE	N019555 001	APR 27, 1987

Cream; Topical

	ALPHATREX			
AB	+ SAVAGE LABS	EQ 0.05% BASE	N019138 001	JUN 26, 1984

Prescription Drug Products (continued)

BETAMETHASONE DIPROPIONATE (continued)

Cream; Topical
 BETAMETHASONE DIPROPIONATE
AB　ALPHARMA US PHARM　EQ 0.05% BASE　N070885 001　FEB 03, 1987
AB　FOUGERA　EQ 0.05% BASE　N019137 001　JUN 26, 1984
AB　TARO　EQ 0.05% BASE　N071143 001　JUN 17, 1987
　　　　　　　　　　　N073552 001　APR 30, 1992
AB　TEVA　EQ 0.05% BASE　N071476 001　AUG 10, 1987

Gel, Augmented; Topical
 BETAMETHASONE DIPROPIONATE
AB　ALTANA　EQ 0.05% BASE　N075276 001　MAY 13, 2003
　DIPROLENE
AB + SCHERING　EQ 0.05% BASE　N019408 002　NOV 22, 1991

Lotion, Augmented; Topical
 DIPROLENE
AB + SCHERING　EQ 0.05% BASE　N019716 001　AUG 01, 1988

Lotion; Topical
 ALPHATREX
AB　SAVAGE LABS　EQ 0.05% BASE　N070273 001　AUG 12, 1985
 BETAMETHASONE DIPROPIONATE
AB　ALPHARMA　EQ 0.05% BASE　N070281 001　JUL 31, 1985
AB　CLAY PARK　EQ 0.05% BASE　N072538 001　JAN 31, 1990
AB　COPLEY PHARM　EQ 0.05% BASE　N071882 001　JUN 06, 1988
AB　FOUGERA　EQ 0.05% BASE　N070275 001　AUG 12, 1985
AB　TARO　EQ 0.05% BASE　N072276 001　AUG 24, 1988
AB　TEVA　EQ 0.05% BASE　N074272 001　SEP 30, 1994
　　　　　　　　　　　N071467 001　AUG 10, 1987
　DIPROSONE
AB + SCHERING　EQ 0.05% BASE　N017781 001

Ointment, Augmented; Topical
 BETAMETHASONE DIPROPIONATE
AB　ALPHARMA US PHARM　EQ 0.05% BASE　N074304 001　AUG 31, 1995
AB　ALTANA　EQ 0.05% BASE　N075373 001　JUN 22, 1999
　DIPROLENE
AB + SCHERING　EQ 0.05% BASE　N018741 001　JUL 27, 1983

Ointment; Topical
 ALPHATREX
AB　SAVAGE LABS　EQ 0.05% BASE　N019143 001

BETAMETHASONE DIPROPIONATE (continued)

Ointment; Topical
 ALPHATREX
　　SAVAGE LABS　　　　　　　　　SEP 04, 1984
 BETAMETHASONE DIPROPIONATE
AB　ALPHARMA US PHARM　EQ 0.05% BASE　N071012 001　FEB 03, 1987
　　　　　　　　　　　　　　　　　　N019141 001　SEP 04, 1984
AB + FOUGERA　EQ 0.05% BASE　N074271 001　SEP 04, 1984
AB　TARO　EQ 0.05% BASE　N071477 001　SEP 15, 1994
AB　TEVA　EQ 0.05% BASE　　　　　　AUG 10, 1987

BETAMETHASONE DIPROPIONATE; CLOTRIMAZOLE

Cream; Topical
 CLOTRIMAZOLE AND BETAMETHASONE DIPROPIONATE
AB　ALPHARMA US PHARM　EQ 0.05% BASE;1%　N076002 001　AUG 02, 2002
AB　ALTANA　EQ 0.05% BASE;1%　N075502 001　JUN 05, 2001
AB　TARO　EQ 0.05% BASE;1%　N075673 001　MAY 29, 2001
 LOTRISONE
AB + SCHERING　EQ 0.05% BASE;1%　N018827 001　JUL 10, 1984

Lotion; Topical
 LOTRISONE
AB + SCHERING PLOUGH RES　EQ 0.05% BASE;1%　N020010 001　DEC 08, 2000

BETAMETHASONE SODIUM PHOSPHATE

Injectable; Injection
 BETAMETHASONE SODIUM PHOSPHATE
AP　STERIS　EQ 3MG BASE/ML　N085738 001
 CELESTONE
AP + SCHERING　EQ 3MG BASE/ML　N017561 001

BETAMETHASONE SODIUM PHOSPHATE *MULTIPLE*
SEE　BETAMETHASONE ACETATE; BETAMETHASONE SODIUM PHOSPHATE

BETAMETHASONE VALERATE

Aerosol; Topical
 LUXIQ
AB + CONNETICS　EQ 0.12% BASE　N020934 001　FEB 28, 1999

Cream; Topical
 BETA-VAL
AB　TEVA　EQ 0.1% BASE　N018642 001　MAR 24, 1983
 BETADERM
AB　ROACO　EQ 0.1% BASE　N018839 001　JUN 30, 1983
 BETAMETHASONE VALERATE
AB + FOUGERA　EQ 0.1% BASE　N018861 001　AUG 31, 1983

Prescription Drug Products *(continued)*

BETAMETHASONE VALERATE *(continued)*

Cream; Topical

TE	Product / Firm	Strength	Appl. No.	Date
	BETAMETHASONE VALERATE			
AB	TARO	EQ 0.1% BASE	N070062 001	MAY 14, 1985
AB	BETATREX SAVAGE LABS	EQ 0.1% BASE	N018862 001	AUG 31, 1983
AB	DERMABET TARO	EQ 0.1% BASE	N072041 001	JAN 06, 1988
AB	VALNAC ALPHARMA US PHARM	EQ 0.1% BASE	N070050 001	OCT 10, 1984

Lotion; Topical

TE	Product / Firm	Strength	Appl. No.	Date
AB	BETA-VAL TEVA	EQ 0.1% BASE	N070072 001	JUN 27, 1985
	BETAMETHASONE VALERATE			
AB	ALPHARMA	EQ 0.1% BASE	N070052 001	JUL 31, 1985
AB	COPLEY PHARM	EQ 0.1% BASE	N071883 001	APR 22, 1988
AB +	FOUGERA	EQ 0.1% BASE	N018866 001	AUG 31, 1983
AB	BETATREX SAVAGE LABS	EQ 0.1% BASE	N018867 001	AUG 31, 1983

Ointment; Topical

TE	Product / Firm	Strength	Appl. No.	Date
AB	BETA-VAL TEVA	EQ 0.1% BASE	N070069 001	DEC 19, 1985
	BETAMETHASONE VALERATE			
AB	ALPHARMA US PHARM	EQ 0.1% BASE	N070051 001	OCT 10, 1984
AB +	FOUGERA	EQ 0.1% BASE	N018865 001	AUG 31, 1983
AB	BETATREX SAVAGE LABS	EQ 0.1% BASE	N018863 001	AUG 31, 1983

BETAXOLOL HYDROCHLORIDE

Solution/Drops; Ophthalmic

TE	Product / Firm	Strength	Appl. No.	Date
	BETAXOLOL			
AT	AKORN	EQ 0.5% BASE	N075386 001	JUN 30, 2000
AT	NOVEX	EQ 0.5% BASE	N075446 001	SEP 28, 2000
	BETAXOLOL HCL			
AT	BAUSCH AND LOMB	EQ 0.5% BASE	N075630 001	APR 12, 2001
	BETOPTIC			
AT +	ALCON	EQ 0.5% BASE	N019270 001	AUG 30, 1985

Suspension/Drops; Ophthalmic

TE	Product / Firm	Strength	Appl. No.	Date
	BETOPTIC S			
+	ALCON	EQ 0.25% BASE	N019845 001	

BETAXOLOL HYDROCHLORIDE *(continued)*

Suspension/Drops; Ophthalmic

TE	Product / Firm	Strength	Appl. No.	Date
	BETOPTIC S ALCON			DEC 29, 1989

Tablet; Oral

TE	Product / Firm	Strength	Appl. No.	Date
	BETAXOLOL HCL			
AB	AMIDE PHARM	10MG	N075541 001	OCT 22, 1999
AB		20MG	N075541 002	OCT 22, 1999
	KERLONE			
AB	LOREX	10MG	N019507 001	OCT 27, 1989
AB +		20MG	N019507 002	OCT 27, 1989

BETHANECHOL CHLORIDE

Tablet; Oral

TE	Product / Firm	Strength	Appl. No.	Date
	URECHOLINE			
AB	ODYSSEY PHARMS	5MG	N089095 001	DEC 19, 1985
AB		10MG	N088440 001	MAY 29, 1984
AB		25MG	N088441 001	MAY 29, 1984
AB		50MG	N089096 001	DEC 19, 1985

BEXAROTENE

Capsule; Oral

TE	Product / Firm	Strength	Appl. No.	Date
	TARGRETIN			
+	LIGAND	75MG	N021055 001	DEC 29, 1999

Gel; Topical

TE	Product / Firm	Strength	Appl. No.	Date
	TARGRETIN			
+	LIGAND	1%	N021056 001	JUN 28, 2000

BICALUTAMIDE

Tablet; Oral

TE	Product / Firm	Strength	Appl. No.	Date
	CASODEX			
+	ASTRAZENECA	50MG	N020498 001	OCT 04, 1995

BIMATOPROST

Solution/Drops; Ophthalmic

TE	Product / Firm	Strength	Appl. No.	Date
	LUMIGAN			
+	ALLERGAN	0.03%	N021275 001	MAR 16, 2001

BIOTIN *MULTIPLE*

SEE   ALPHA-TOCOPHEROL ACETATE; ASCORBIC ACID; BIOTIN; CHOLECALCIFEROL; CYANOCOBALAMIN; DEXPANTHENOL; FOLIC ACID; NIACINAMIDE; PYRIDOXINE HYDROCHLORIDE; RIBOFLAVIN PHOSPHATE SODIUM; THIAMINE HYDROCHLORIDE; VITAMIN A PALMITATE; VITAMIN K

Prescription Drug Products (continued)

BIOTIN *MULTIPLE* (continued)

SEE ASCORBIC ACID: BIOTIN: CHOLECALCIFEROL: CYANOCOBALAMIN: DEXPANTHENOL: FOLIC ACID: NIACINAMIDE: PYRIDOXINE: RIBOFLAVIN: THIAMINE: TOCOPHEROL ACETATE: VITAMIN A: VITAMIN K

SEE ASCORBIC ACID: BIOTIN: CYANOCOBALAMIN: DEXPANTHENOL: ERGOCALCIFEROL: FOLIC ACID: NIACINAMIDE: PHYTONADIONE: PYRIDOXINE HYDROCHLORIDE: RIBOFLAVIN: VITAMIN A: VITAMIN E

SEE ASCORBIC ACID: BIOTIN: CYANOCOBALAMIN: DEXPANTHENOL: ERGOCALCIFEROL: FOLIC ACID: NIACINAMIDE: PYRIDOXINE HYDROCHLORIDE: RIBOFLAVIN PHOSPHATE SODIUM: THIAMINE HYDROCHLORIDE: VITAMIN A: VITAMIN E

BIPERIDEN HYDROCHLORIDE
Tablet; Oral

AKINETON				
+	ABBOTT	2MG	N012003 001	

BISMUTH SUBSALICYLATE; METRONIDAZOLE; TETRACYCLINE HYDROCHLORIDE
Tablet, Chewable, Tablet, Capsule; Oral

HELIDAC				
+	PROMETHEUS LABS	262.4MG:250MG:500MG	N050719 001	AUG 15, 1996

BISOPROLOL FUMARATE
Tablet; Oral
BISOPROLOL FUMARATE

	COPLEY PHARM	5MG	N075644 001	JUN 26, 2001
AB		10MG	N075644 002	JUN 26, 2001
	EON	5MG	N075643 001	NOV 16, 2000
AB		10MG	N075643 002	NOV 16, 2000
	MUTUAL PHARM	5MG	N075474 001	OCT 25, 2002
AB		10MG	N075474 002	OCT 25, 2002
	ZEBETA			
	DURAMED PHARM BARR	5MG	N019982 002	JUL 31, 1992
AB +		10MG	N019982 001	JUL 31, 1992

BISOPROLOL FUMARATE; HYDROCHLOROTHIAZIDE
Tablet; Oral
BISOPROLOL FUMARATE AND HYDROCHLOROTHIAZIDE

AB	EON	2.5MG:6.25MG	N075579 001	SEP 25, 2000
AB		5MG:6.25MG	N075579 002	SEP 25, 2000
AB		10MG:6.25MG	N075579 003	SEP 25, 2000

BISOPROLOL FUMARATE; HYDROCHLOROTHIAZIDE (continued)
Tablet; Oral
BISOPROLOL FUMARATE AND HYDROCHLOROTHIAZIDE

AB	GENEVA PHARMS TECH	2.5MG:6.25MG	N075527 001	SEP 25, 2000
AB		10MG:6.25MG	N075527 002	SEP 25, 2000
AB		5MG:6.25MG	N075527 003	SEP 25, 2000
AB	IVAX PHARMS	2.5MG:6.25MG	N075632 001	SEP 27, 2000
AB		5MG:6.25MG	N075632 002	SEP 27, 2000
AB		10MG:6.25MG	N075632 003	SEP 27, 2000
AB	MYLAN	2.5MG:6.25MG	N075768 001	SEP 25, 2000
AB		5MG:6.25MG	N075768 002	SEP 25, 2000
AB		10MG:6.25MG	N075768 003	SEP 25, 2000
AB	PUREPAC PHARM	2.5MG:6.25MG	N075672 001	SEP 25, 2000
AB		5MG:6.25MG	N075672 002	SEP 25, 2000
AB		10MG:6.25MG	N075672 003	SEP 25, 2000
AB	TEVA	2.5MG:6.25MG	N075686 001	JAN 19, 2001
AB		5MG:6.25MG	N075686 002	JAN 19, 2001
AB		10MG:6.25MG	N075686 003	JAN 19, 2001
AB	WATSON LABS	2.5MG:6.25MG	N075469 001	SEP 25, 2000
AB		5MG:6.25MG	N075469 002	SEP 25, 2000
AB		10MG:6.25MG	N075469 003	SEP 25, 2000
	ZIAC			
AB	DURAMED PHARM BARR	2.5MG:6.25MG	N020186 003	MAR 26, 1993
AB		5MG:6.25MG	N020186 001	MAR 26, 1993
AB +		10MG:6.25MG	N020186 002	MAR 26, 1993

BIVALIRUDIN
Injectable; Intravenous

ANGIOMAX				
+	MEDS (TMC)	250MG/VIAL	N020873 001	DEC 15, 2000

Prescription Drug Products (continued)

BLEOMYCIN SULFATE
Injectable; Injection

BLENOXANE
+ BRISTOL MYERS SQUIBB

AP	+	EQ 15 UNITS BASE/VIAL	N050443 001	
AP	+	EQ 30 UNITS BASE/VIAL	N050443 002	SEP 07, 1995

BLEOMYCIN
BEDFORD

AP	EQ 15 UNITS BASE/VIAL	N065042 002	OCT 17, 2001
AP	EQ 30 UNITS BASE/VIAL	N065042 001	OCT 17, 2001
AP	FAULDING EQ 15 UNITS BASE/VIAL	N065031 001	MAR 10, 2000
AP	EQ 30 UNITS BASE/VIAL	N065031 002	MAR 10, 2000
AP	GENSIA SICOR PHARMS EQ 15 UNITS BASE/VIAL	N065033 001	JUN 27, 2000
AP	EQ 30 UNITS BASE/VIAL	N065033 002	JUN 27, 2000

BLEOMYCIN SULFATE
PHARMACIA AND UPJOHN

AP	EQ 15 UNITS BASE/VIAL	N064084 001	JUN 01, 1996
AP	EQ 30 UNITS BASE/VIAL	N064084 002	JUN 01, 1996

BORTEZOMIB
Injectable; Intravenous

VELCADE

	+ MILLENNIUM PHARMS	3.5MG/VIAL	N021602 001	MAY 13, 2003

BOSENTAN
Tablet; Oral

TRACLEER
ACTELION

+	62.5MG	N021290 001	NOV 20, 2001
+	125MG	N021290 002	NOV 20, 2001

BRETYLIUM TOSYLATE
Injectable; Injection

BRETYLIUM TOSYLATE

AP	+ ABBOTT	50MG/ML	N019033 001	APR 29, 1986
AP	+ INTL MEDICATION	50MG/ML	N070119 001	APR 29, 1986
AP	+ LUITPOLD	50MG/ML	N070891 001	JUL 26, 1988

BRETYLIUM TOSYLATE IN DEXTROSE 5% IN PLASTIC CONTAINER

AP	+ ABBOTT	200MG/100ML	N019008 002	APR 29, 1986
AP	+	400MG/100ML	N019008 003	APR 29, 1986
AP	+ B BRAUN	100MG/100ML	N019121 001	

BRETYLIUM TOSYLATE (continued)
Injectable; Injection

BRETYLIUM TOSYLATE IN DEXTROSE 5% IN PLASTIC CONTAINER
B BRAUN

AP	+	200MG/100ML	N019121 002	APR 29, 1986
AP	+	400MG/100ML	N019121 003	APR 29, 1986

BRETYLIUM TOSYLATE IN PLASTIC CONTAINER

AP	+ ABBOTT	50MG/ML	N019030 001	APR 29, 1986

BRIMONIDINE TARTRATE
Solution/Drops; Ophthalmic

ALPHAGAN P

AP	+ ALLERGAN	0.15%	N021262 001	MAR 16, 2001

BRIMONIDINE TARTRATE

AP	+ BAUSCH AND LOMB	0.2%	N076260 001	MAY 28, 2003

BRINZOLAMIDE
Suspension/Drops; Ophthalmic

AZOPT

AP	+ ALCON	1%	N020816 001	APR 01, 1998

BROMOCRIPTINE MESYLATE
Capsule; Oral

PARLODEL

	+ NOVARTIS	EQ 5MG BASE	N017962 002	MAR 01, 1982

Tablet; Oral

BROMOCRIPTINE MESYLATE

AB	LEK PHARMS	EQ 2.5MG BASE	N074631 001	JAN 13, 1998

PARLODEL

AB	+ NOVARTIS	EQ 2.5MG BASE	N017962 001	

BROMODIPHENHYDRAMINE HYDROCHLORIDE; CODEINE PHOSPHATE
Syrup; Oral

AMBENYL

AA	+ FORREST LABS	12.5MG/5ML;10MG/5ML	N009319 006	JAN 10, 1984

MYBANIL

AA	MORTON GROVE	12.5MG/5ML;10MG/5ML	N088626 001	OCT 12, 1984

BROMPHENIRAMINE MALEATE
Elixir; Oral

BROMPHENIRAMINE MALEATE

	+ KV PHARM	2MG/5ML	N085466 001	

Prescription Drug Products (continued)

BROMPHENIRAMINE MALEATE (continued)

Injectable; Injection
BROMPHENIRAMINE MALEATE

TE	Firm	Strength	Appl. No.	Date
	+ STERIS	10MG/ML	N083821 001	

BROMPHENIRAMINE MALEATE; CODEINE PHOSPHATE; PHENYLPROPANOLAMINE HYDROCHLORIDE

Syrup; Oral

TE	Firm	Strength	Appl. No.	Date
	BROMANATE DC			
AA	ALPHARMA	2MG/5ML;10MG/5ML;12.5MG/5ML	N088723 001	FEB 25, 1985
	MYPHETANE DC			
AA	+ MORTON GROVE	2MG/5ML;10MG/5ML;12.5MG/5ML	N088904 001	FEB 21, 1985

BROMPHENIRAMINE MALEATE; DEXTROMETHORPHAN HYDROBROMIDE; PSEUDOEPHEDRINE HYDROCHLORIDE

Syrup; Oral

TE	Firm	Strength	Appl. No.	Date
	BROMFED-DM			
AA	VERUM PHARMS	2MG/5ML;10MG/5ML;30MG/5ML	N089681 001	DEC 22, 1988
	MYPHETANE DX			
AA	+ MORTON GROVE	2MG/5ML;10MG/5ML;30MG/5ML	N088811 001	JUN 07, 1985

BUDESONIDE

TE	Firm	Strength	Appl. No.	Date
	Aerosol, Metered; Nasal			
	RHINOCORT			
	+ ASTRAZENECA	0.032MG/INH	N020233 001	FEB 14, 1994
	Capsule; Oral			
	ENTOCORT EC			
	+ ASTRAZENECA	3MG	N021324 001	OCT 02, 2001
	Powder, Metered; Inhalation			
	PULMICORT			
	+ ASTRAZENECA	0.16MG/INH	N020441 002	JUN 24, 1997
	Spray, Metered; Nasal			
	RHINOCORT			
	ASTRAZENECA	0.032MG/INH	N020746 001	OCT 01, 1999
	+	0.064MG/INH	N020746 002	OCT 01, 1999
	Suspension; Inhalation			
	PULMICORT RESPULES			
	+ ASTRAZENECA	0.5MG/2ML	N020929 002	AUG 08, 2000
		0.25MG/2ML	N020929 001	AUG 08, 2000

BUMETANIDE

Injectable; Injection

TE	Firm	Strength	Appl. No.	Date
	BUMETANIDE			
AP	ABBOTT	0.25MG/ML	N074160 001	OCT 30, 1997
AP	BEDFORD	0.25MG/ML	N074332 001	OCT 31, 1994
AP		0.25MG/ML	N074441 001	JAN 27, 1995
AP	GENSIA SICOR PHARMS	0.25MG/ML	N074613 001	NOV 18, 1997
	BUMEX			
AP	+ ROCHE	0.25MG/ML	N018226 001	FEB 28, 1983

Tablet; Oral

TE	Firm	Strength	Appl. No.	Date
	BUMETANIDE			
AB	EON	0.5MG	N074700 001	NOV 21, 1996
AB		1MG	N074700 002	NOV 21, 1996
AB		2MG	N074700 003	NOV 21, 1996
AB	IVAX PHARMS	0.5MG	N074225 001	APR 24, 1995
AB		1MG	N074225 002	APR 24, 1995
AB		2MG	N074225 003	APR 24, 1995
	BUMEX			
AB	ROCHE	0.5MG	N018225 002	FEB 28, 1983
AB		1MG	N018225 001	FEB 28, 1983
AB	+	2MG	N018225 003	JUN 14, 1985

BUPIVACAINE HYDROCHLORIDE

Injectable; Injection

TE	Firm	Strength	Appl. No.	Date
	BUPIVACAINE HCL			
AP	ABBOTT	0.5%	N018053 001	
AP		0.5%	N070584 001	FEB 17, 1986
AP		0.5%	N070597 001	MAR 03, 1987
AP		0.5%	N070609 001	MAR 03, 1987
AP		0.25%	N018053 002	
AP		0.25%	N070583 001	FEB 17, 1987
AP		0.25%	N070586 001	MAR 03, 1987
AP		0.25%	N070590 001	FEB 17, 1987
AP		0.75%	N018053 003	
AP		0.75%	N070585 001	MAR 03, 1987
AP		0.75%	N070587 001	MAR 03, 1987

Prescription Drug Products (continued)

BUPIVACAINE HYDROCHLORIDE (continued)

Injectable; Injection

		Strength	NDC	Date
BUPIVACAINE HCL				
	ABBOTT			MAR 03, 1987
BUPIVACAINE HCL PRESERVATIVE FREE				
	INTL MEDICATED			
AP		0.5%	N076012 002	JAN 09, 2002
AP		0.25%	N076012 001	JAN 09, 2002
AP		0.75%	N076012 003	JAN 09, 2002
MARCAINE HCL				
AP	+ ABBOTT	0.5%	N016964 006	
AP	+ ABBOTT	0.25%	N016964 001	
MARCAINE HCL PRESERVATIVE FREE				
AP	+ ABBOTT	0.5%	N016964 005	
AP	+ ABBOTT	0.25%	N016964 012	
AP	+ ABBOTT	0.75%	N016964 009	
SENSORCAINE				
AP	ASTRAZENECA	0.5%	N018304 002	
AP		0.5%	N070553 001	MAY 21, 1986
AP		0.25%	N018304 001	
AP		0.25%	N070552 001	
AP		0.75%	N018304 003	MAY 21, 1986
AP		0.75%	N070554 001	
AP		0.75%		MAY 21, 1986

Injectable; Spinal

		Strength	NDC	Date
BUPIVACAINE				
AP	ABBOTT	0.75%	N071810 001	DEC 11, 1987
MARCAINE				
AP	+ ABBOTT	0.75%	N018692 001	MAY 04, 1984
SENSORCAINE				
AP	ASTRAZENECA	0.75%	N071202 001	APR 15, 1987

BUPIVACAINE HYDROCHLORIDE; EPINEPHRINE

Injectable; Injection

		Strength	NDC	Date
BUPIVACAINE HCL AND EPINEPHRINE				
AP	+ ABBOTT	0.25%;0.005MG/ML	N071165 001	JUN 16, 1988
		0.25%;0.005MG/ML	N071166 001	JUN 16, 1988
		0.25%;0.005MG/ML	N071167 001	JUN 16, 1988
		0.5%;0.005MG/ML	N071168 001	JUN 16, 1988
+		0.5%;0.005MG/ML	N071169 001	JUN 16, 1988
		0.5%;0.005MG/ML	N071170 001	JUN 16, 1988
+		0.75%;0.005MG/ML	N071171 001	JUN 16, 1988

BUPIVACAINE HYDROCHLORIDE; EPINEPHRINE BITARTRATE

Injectable; Injection

		Strength	NDC	Date
MARCAINE HCL W/ EPINEPHRINE				
AP	+ ABBOTT	0.25%;0.0091MG/ML	N016964 004	
AP	+ ABBOTT	0.5%;0.0091MG/ML	N016964 008	
MARCAINE HCL W/ EPINEPHRINE PRESERVATIVE FREE				
AP	+ ABBOTT	0.5%;0.0091MG/ML	N016964 007	
AP	+ ABBOTT	0.75%;0.0091MG/ML	N016964 010	
AP	+ ABBOTT	0.25%;0.0091MG/ML	N016964 013	
SENSORCAINE				
AP	ASTRAZENECA	0.5%;0.0091MG/ML	N018304 004	SEP 02, 1983
AP		0.75%;0.0091MG/ML	N018304 005	SEP 02, 1983
			N070966 001	OCT 13, 1987
AP		0.25%;0.0091MG/ML	N070967 001	OCT 13, 1987
			N070968 001	OCT 13, 1987
AP		0.5%;0.0091MG/ML		

BUPIVACAINE HYDROCHLORIDE; LIDOCAINE HYDROCHLORIDE

Injectable; Injection

		Strength	NDC	Date
DUOCAINE				
	+ AMPAHSTAR	EQ 0.375% (37.5MG/10ML);EQ 1% (100MG/10ML)	N021496 001	MAY 23, 2003

BUPRENORPHINE HYDROCHLORIDE

Injectable; Injection

		Strength	NDC	Date
BUPRENEX				
AP	+ RECKITT BENCKISER	EQ 0.3MG BASE/ML	N018401 001	
BUPRENORPHINE HCL				
AP	ABBOTT	EQ 0.3MG BASE/ML	N074137 001	JUN 03, 1996

Tablet; Sublingual

		Strength	NDC	Date
SUBUTEX				
	RECK TT BENCKISER	EQ 2MG BASE	N020732 002	OCT 08, 2002
+		EQ 8MG BASE	N020732 003	OCT 08, 2002

BUPRENORPHINE HYDROCHLORIDE; NALOXONE HYDROCHLORIDE

Tablet; Sublingual

		Strength	NDC	Date
SUBOXONE				
	RECKITT BENCKISER	2MG;0.5MG	N020733 001	OCT 08, 2002
+		8MG;2MG	N020733 002	OCT 08, 2002

BUPROPION HYDROCHLORIDE

Tablet, Extended Release; Oral

		Strength	NDC	Date
WELLBUTRIN SR				
	GLAXOSMITHKLINE	50MG	N020358 001	OCT 04, 1996

Prescription Drug Products *(continued)*

BUPROPION HYDROCHLORIDE *(continued)*
Tablet, Extended Release; Oral
WELLBUTRIN SR

	GLAXOSMITHKLINE	100MG	N020358 002
			OCT 04, 1996
		150MG	N020358 003
			OCT 04, 1996
+		200MG	N020358 004
			JUN 14, 2002
	ZYBAN		
+	GLAXOSMITHKLINE	150MG	N020711 003
			MAY 14, 1997

Tablet; Oral
BUPROPION HCL

AB	EON	75MG	N075613 002
			OCT 10, 2000
AB		100MG	N075613 001
			OCT 10, 2000
AB	GENEVA PHARMS TECH	75MG	N075584 001
			FEB 07, 2000
AB		100MG	N075584 002
			FEB 07, 2000
AB	MYLAN	75MG	N075491 001
			APR 17, 2000
AB		100MG	N075491 002
			APR 17, 2000
AB	TEVA	75MG	N075310 001
			NOV 29, 1999
AB		100MG	N075310 002
			NOV 29, 1999
	WELLBUTRIN		
AB	GLAXOSMITHKLINE	75MG	N018644 002
			DEC 30, 1985
AB +		100MG	N018644 003
			DEC 30, 1985

BUSPIRONE HYDROCHLORIDE
Tablet; Oral
BUSPAR

AB	BRISTOL MYERS SQUIBB	5MG	N018731 001
			SEP 29, 1986
AB		10MG	N018731 002
			SEP 29, 1986
AB		15MG	N018731 003
			APR 22, 1996
AB +		30MG	N018731 004
			APR 22, 1996

BUSPIRONE HCL

AB	EGIS	5MG	N075119 001
			MAR 14, 2002
AB		10MG	N075119 002
			MAR 14, 2002
AB		15MG	N075119 003
			JAN 23, 2003
AB	GENEVA PHARMS	5MG	N075413 001
			MAR 19, 2002

BUSPIRONE HYDROCHLORIDE *(continued)*
Tablet; Oral
BUSPIRONE HCL

AB	GENEVA PHARMS	10MG	N075413 002
			MAR 19, 2002
AB		15MG	N075413 003
			MAR 19, 2002
AB	KV PHARM	5MG	N075572 001
			FEB 27, 2002
AB		10MG	N075572 002
			FEB 27, 2002
AB		15MG	N075572 003
			FEB 27, 2002
AB	MYLAN	5MG	N075272 001
			MAR 01, 2002
AB		10MG	N075272 002
			MAR 01, 2002
AB		15MG	N075272 003
			MAR 28, 2001
AB		30MG	N076008 001
			JUN 28, 2001
AB	PAR PHARM	5MG	N075467 001
			FEB 28, 2002
AB		7.5MG	N075467 002
			MAR 28, 2001
AB		10MG	N075467 003
			FEB 28, 2002
AB		15MG	N075467 004
			FEB 28, 2002
AB	PHARMEX PRODS	5MG	N075388 001
			MAY 09, 2002
AB		10MG	N075388 002
			MAY 09, 2002
AB		15MG	N075388 003
			MAY 09, 2002
AB	TEVA	5MG	N075022 001
			FEB 28, 2002
AB		10MG	N075022 002
			FEB 28, 2002
AB		15MG	N075022 003
			FEB 28, 2002
AB	TORPHARM	5MG	N075521 001
			APR 05, 2002
AB		10MG	N075521 002
			APR 05, 2002
AB		15MG	N075521 003
			APR 05, 2002
AB	WATSON LABS	5MG	N074253 001
			MAR 28, 2001
AB		10MG	N074253 002
			MAR 28, 2001
AB		15MG	N074253 003
			MAR 13, 2002
AB	ZENITH GOLDLINE	5MG	N075385 001
			MAR 01, 2002
AB		10MG	N075385 002
			MAR 01, 2002

Prescription Drug Products (continued)

BUSPIRONE HYDROCHLORIDE (continued)
Tablet; Oral

	BUSPIRONE HCL			
AB	ZENITH GOLDLINE	15MG	N075385 003	MAR 01, 2002

BUSULFAN
Injectable; Injection

	BUSULFEX			
	+ ESP PHARMA	6MG/ML	N020954 001	FEB 04, 1999

Tablet; Oral

	MYLERAN			
	+ GLAXOSMITHKLINE	2MG	N009386 001	

BUTABARBITAL SODIUM
Elixir; Oral

	BUTISOL SODIUM			
	+ MEDPOINTE PHARM HLC	30MG/5ML	N085380 001	

Tablet; Oral

	BUTABARBITAL			
AA	BUNDY	30MG	N085550 001	
	BUTISOL SODIUM			
AA	+ MEDPOINTE PHARM HLC	30MG	N000793 004	
		50MG	N000793 003	
	SODIUM BUTABARBITAL			
	MARSHALL PHARMA	16.2MG	N083524 001	
		32.4MG	N083858 001	

BUTALBITAL *MULTIPLE*
SEE	ACETAMINOPHEN; BUTALBITAL
SEE	ACETAMINOPHEN; BUTALBITAL; CAFFEINE
SEE	ACETAMINOPHEN; BUTALBITAL; CAFFEINE; CODEINE PHOSPHATE
SEE	ASPIRIN; BUTALBITAL; CAFFEINE
SEE	ASPIRIN; BUTALBITAL; CAFFEINE; CODEINE PHOSPHATE

BUTENAFINE HYDROCHLORIDE
Cream; Topical

	MENTAX			
	+ BERTEK PHARMS	1%	N020524 001	OCT 18, 1996
	MENTAX-TC			
	+ BERTEK	1%	N021408 001	OCT 17, 2002

BUTOCONAZOLE NITRATE
Cream; Vaginal

	GYNAZOLE-1			
	+ KV PHARM	2%	N019881 001	FEB 07, 1997

BUTORPHANOL TARTRATE
Injectable; Injection

	BUTORPHANOL TARTRATE			
AP	ABBOTT	1MG/ML	N075559 001	MAR 20, 2000
		2MG/ML	N075559 002	MAR 20, 2000
AP	APOTEX	2MG/ML	N075697 001	OCT 23, 2001
AP	BEDFORD	2MG/ML	N075046 001	AUG 12, 1998
AP	MERIDIAN MEDCL TECHN	1MG/ML	N075342 001	NOV 04, 1999
AP		2MG/ML	N075342 002	NOV 04, 1999

	BUTORPHANOL TARTRATE PRESERVATIVE FREE			
AP	ABBOTT	1MG/ML	N074620 001	JAN 22, 1997
AP		1MG/ML	N074626 001	JAN 23, 1997
AP		2MG/ML	N074620 002	JAN 22, 1997
AP		2MG/ML	N074626 002	JAN 23, 1997
AP	APOTEX	1MG/ML	N075695 001	OCT 23, 2001
AP		2MG/ML	N075695 002	OCT 23, 2001
AP	BEDFORD	1MG/ML	N075045 001	AUG 12, 1998
AP		2MG/ML	N075045 002	AUG 12, 1998
AP	FAULDING	1MG/ML	N075170 001	SEP 28, 1998
AP		2MG/ML	N075170 002	SEP 28, 1998

	STADOL			
AP	+ APOTHECON	2MG/ML	N017857 004	
	STADOL PRESERVATIVE FREE			
AP	+ APOTHECON	1MG/ML	N017857 001	
AP		2MG/ML	N017857 002	

Spray, Metered; Nasal

	BUTORPHANOL TARTRATE			
AB	MYLAN	1MG/SPRAY	N075759 001	AUG 08, 2001
AB	NOVEX	1MG/SPRAY	N075499 001	DEC 04, 2002
AB	ROXANE	1MG/SPRAY	N075824 001	MAR 12, 2002
	STADOL			
AB	+ BRISTOL MYERS SQUIBB	1MG/SPRAY	N019890 001	DEC 12, 1991

Prescription Drug Products (continued)

CABERGOLINE
Tablet; Oral
DOSTINEX
+ PHARMACIA AND UPJOHN — 0.5MG — N020664 001 — DEC 23, 1996

CAFFEINE; ERGOTAMINE TARTRATE
Suppository; Rectal
CAFERGOT
+ NOVARTIS — 100MG;2MG — N009000 002

Tablet; Oral
ERCATAB
+ GENEVA PHARMS — 100MG;1MG — N084294 001

CAFFEINE *MULTIPLE*
SEE ACETAMINOPHEN; BUTALBITAL; CAFFEINE
SEE ACETAMINOPHEN; BUTALBITAL; CAFFEINE; CODEINE PHOSPHATE
SEE ACETAMINOPHEN; CAFFEINE; DIHYDROCODEINE BITARTRATE
SEE ASPIRIN; BUTALBITAL; CAFFEINE
SEE ASPIRIN; BUTALBITAL; CAFFEINE; CODEINE PHOSPHATE
SEE ASPIRIN; CAFFEINE; DIHYDROCODEINE BITARTRATE
SEE ASPIRIN; CAFFEINE; ORPHENADRINE CITRATE
SEE ASPIRIN; CAFFEINE; PROPOXYPHENE HYDROCHLORIDE

CAFFEINE CITRATE
Solution; Intravenous, Oral
CAFCIT
+ MEAD JOHNSON — EQ 10MG BASE/ML — N020793 001 — SEP 21, 1999

CALCIPOTRIENE
Cream; Topical
DOVONEX
+ BRISTOL MYERS SQUIBB — 0.005% — N020554 001 — JUL 22, 1996

Ointment; Topical
DOVONEX
+ BRISTOL MYERS SQUIBB — 0.005% — N020273 001 — DEC 29, 1993

Solution; Topical
DOVONEX
+ BRISTOL MYERS SQUIBB — 0.005% — N020611 001 — MAR 03, 1997

CALCITONIN, SALMON
Injectable; Injection
CALCIMAR
AP + AVENTIS — 200 IU/ML — N017769 001
MIACALCIN
AP + NOVARTIS — 200 IU/ML — N017808 002 — MAR 29, 1991

CALCITONIN, SALMON (continued)
Spray, Metered; Nasal
MIACALCIN
+ NOVARTIS — 200 IU/SPRAY — N020313 002 — AUG 17, 1995

CALCITRIOL
Capsule; Oral
CALCITRIOL
AB TEVA — 0.5UGM — N075765 002 — OCT 12, 2001
AB — 0.25UGM — N075765 001 — OCT 12, 2001
ROCALTROL
AB + ROCHE — 0.5UGM — N018044 002
AB — 0.25UGM — N018044 001

Injectable; Injection
CALCIJEX
AP + ABBOTT — 0.001MG/ML — N018874 001 — SEP 25, 1986
AP — 0.002MG/ML — N018874 002 — SEP 25, 1986
CALCITRIOL
AP AAIPHARMA — 0.001MG/ML — N075766 001 — FEB 20, 2003
AP — 0.002MG/ML — N075766 002 — FEB 20, 2003
AP AM PHARM PARTNERS — 0.001MG/ML — N075836 001 — DEC 31, 2002
AP — 0.002MG/ML — N075836 002 — DEC 31, 2002
AP GENSIA SICOR PHARMS — 0.001MG/ML — N075823 001 — MAR 31, 2003
AP — 0.002MG/ML — N075823 002 — MAR 31, 2003

Solution; Oral
ROCALTROL
AP + ROCHE — 1UGM/ML — N021068 001 — NOV 20, 1998

CALCIUM ACETATE
Capsule; Oral
PHOSLO GELCAPS
+ BRAINTREE — EQ 169MG CALCIUM — N021160 003 — APR 02, 2001

Tablet; Oral
PHOSLO
+ BRAINTREE — EQ 169MG CALCIUM — N019976 001 — DEC 10, 1990

CALCIUM ACETATE *MULTIPLE*
SEE AMINO ACIDS; CALCIUM ACETATE; GLYCERIN; MAGNESIUM ACETATE; PHOSPHORIC ACID; POTASSIUM CHLORIDE; SODIUM ACETATE; SODIUM CHLORIDE

Prescription Drug Products *(continued)*

CALCIUM CHLORIDE
Injectable; Injection
  CALCIUM CHLORIDE 10% IN PLASTIC CONTAINER
+ ABBOTT   100MG/ML   N021117 001
                                          JAN 28, 2000

CALCIUM CHLORIDE; DEXTROSE; GLUTATHIONE DISULFIDE; MAGNESIUM CHLORIDE; POTASSIUM CHLORIDE; SODIUM BICARBONATE; SODIUM CHLORIDE; SODIUM PHOSPHATE
Solution; Irrigation
  BSS PLUS
AT   ALCON   0.154MG/ML;0.92MG/   N018469 001
                    ML;0.184MG/ML;0.2MG/
                    ML;0.38MG/ML;2.1MG/
                    ML;7.14MG/ML;0.42MG/ML

  ENDOSOL EXTRA
AT   AKORN   0.154MG/ML;0.92MG/   N020079 001
                    ML;0.184MG/ML;0.2MG/   NOV 27, 1991
                    ML;0.38MG/ML;2.1MG/
                    ML;7.14MG/ML;0.42MG/ML

CALCIUM CHLORIDE; DEXTROSE; MAGNESIUM CHLORIDE; POTASSIUM CHLORIDE; SODIUM ACETATE; SODIUM CHLORIDE
Injectable; Injection
  ISOLYTE R IN DEXTROSE 5% IN PLASTIC CONTAINER
  B BRAUN   37MG/100ML;5GM/100ML;31MG/   N019864 001
               100ML;120MG/100ML;330MG/   JUN 10, 1993
               100ML;88MG/100ML

CALCIUM CHLORIDE; DEXTROSE; MAGNESIUM CHLORIDE; POTASSIUM CHLORIDE; SODIUM ACETATE; SODIUM CHLORIDE; SODIUM CITRATE
Injectable; Injection
  ISOLYTE E IN DEXTROSE 5% IN PLASTIC CONTAINER
  B BRAUN   35MG/100ML;5GM/100ML;30MG/   N019867 001
               100ML;74MG/100ML;640MG/   DEC 20, 1993
               100ML;500MG/100ML;74MG/
               100ML

CALCIUM CHLORIDE; DEXTROSE; MAGNESIUM CHLORIDE; POTASSIUM CHLORIDE; SODIUM ACETATE; SODIUM CHLORIDE; SODIUM LACTATE
Injectable; Injection
  PLASMA-LYTE M AND DEXTROSE 5% IN PLASTIC CONTAINER
  BAXTER HLTHCARE   37MG/100ML;5GM/100ML;30MG/   N017390 001
                        100ML;119MG/100ML;161MG/
                        100ML;94MG/100ML;138MG/
                        100ML

CALCIUM CHLORIDE; DEXTROSE; MAGNESIUM CHLORIDE; SODIUM ACETATE; SODIUM CHLORIDE
Solution; Intraperitoneal
  DIALYTE CONCENTRATE W/ DEXTROSE 30% IN PLASTIC CONTAINER
  B BFAUN   510MG/100ML;30GM/   N018807 001
             100ML;200MG/100ML;9.2GM/   AUG 26, 1983
             100ML;9.6GM/100ML

  DIALYTE CONCENTRATE W/ DEXTROSE 50% IN PLASTIC CONTAINER
  B BFAUN   510MG/100ML;50GM/   N018807 002
             100ML;200MG/100ML;9.2GM/   AUG 26, 1983
             100ML;9.6GM/100ML

  DIALYTE CONCENTRATE W/ DEXTROSE 30% IN PLASTIC CONTAINER
  B BRAUN   510MG/100ML;30GM/   N018807 003
             100ML;200MG/100ML;9.4GM/   AUG 26, 1983
             100ML;11GM/100ML

  DIALYTE CONCENTRATE W/ DEXTROSE 50% IN PLASTIC CONTAINER
  B BRAUN   510MG/100ML;50GM/   N018807 004
             100ML;200MG/100ML;9.4GM/   AUG 26, 1983
             100ML;11GM/100ML

CALCIUM CHLORIDE; DEXTROSE; MAGNESIUM CHLORIDE; SODIUM CHLORIDE; SODIUM LACTATE
Solution; Intraperitoneal
  DELFLEX W/ DEXTROSE 4.25% IN PLASTIC CONTAINER
AT   FRESENIUS MEDCL   25.7MG/100ML;4.25GM/   N018379 001
                         100ML;15.2MG/100ML;567MG/
                         100ML;392MG/100ML

  DELFLEX W/ DEXTROSE 1.5% IN PLASTIC CONTAINER
AT   FRESENIUS MEDCL   25.7MG/100ML;1.5GM/   N018379 002
                         100ML;15.2MG/100ML;567MG/
                         100ML;392MG/100ML

  DELFLEX W/ DEXTROSE 2.5% IN PLASTIC CONTAINER
AT   FRESENIUS MEDCL   25.7MG/100ML;2.5GM/   N018379 003
                         100ML;15.2MG/100ML;567MG/
                         100ML;392MG/100ML

  DELFLEX W/ DEXTROSE 3.5% IN PLASTIC CONTAINER
AT   FRESENIUS MEDCL   25.7MG/100ML;3.5GM/   N018379 007
                         100ML;15.2MG/100ML;567MG/   JUN 24, 1988
                         100ML;392MG/100ML

  DELFLEX W/ DEXTROSE 1.5% IN PLASTIC CONTAINER
AT   FRESENIUS MEDCL   25.7MG/100ML;1.5GM/   N018883 001
                         100ML;15.2MG/100ML;567MG/   NOV 30, 1984
                         100ML;392MG/100ML

  DELFLEX W/ DEXTROSE 2.5% IN PLASTIC CONTAINER
AT   FRESENIUS MEDCL   25.7MG/100ML;2.5GM/   N018883 002
                         100ML;15.2MG/100ML;567MG/   NOV 30, 1984
                         100ML;392MG/100ML

Prescription Drug Products *(continued)*

CALCIUM CHLORIDE; DEXTROSE; MAGNESIUM CHLORIDE; SODIUM CHLORIDE; SODIUM LACTATE *(continued)*
Solution; Intraperitoneal

DELFLEX W/ DEXTROSE 4.25% IN PLASTIC CONTAINER
FRESENIUS MEDCL
AT 25.7MG/100ML;4.25GM/100ML;15.2MG/100ML;567MG/100ML;392MG/100ML   N018883 003 NOV 30, 1984

DELFLEX W/ DEXTROSE 1.5% LOW MAGNESIUM IN PLASTIC CONTAINER
FRESENIUS MEDCL
AT 25.7MG/100ML;1.5GM/100ML;5.08MG/100ML;538MG/100ML;448MG/100ML   N018883 004 NOV 30, 1984

DELFLEX W/ DEXTROSE 2.5% LOW MAGNESIUM IN PLASTIC CONTAINER
FRESENIUS MEDCL
AT 25.7MG/100ML;2.5GM/100ML;5.08MG/100ML;538MG/100ML;448MG/100ML   N018883 005 NOV 30, 1984

DELFLEX W/ DEXTROSE 4.25% LOW MAGNESIUM IN PLASTIC CONTAINER
FRESENIUS MEDCL
AT 25.7MG/100ML;4.25GM/100ML;5.08MG/100ML;538MG/100ML;448MG/100ML   N018883 006 NOV 30, 1984

DELFLEX W/ DEXTROSE 1.5% LOW MAGNESIUM LOW CALCIUM IN PLASTIC CONTAINER
FRESENIUS MEDCL
AT 18.4MG/100ML;1.5GM/100ML;5.08MG/100ML;538MG/100ML;448MG/100ML   N020171 001 AUG 19, 1992

DELFLEX W/ DEXTROSE 2.5% LOW MAGNESIUM LOW CALCIUM IN PLASTIC CONTAINER
FRESENIUS MEDCL
AT 18.4MG/100ML;2.5GM/100ML;5.08MG/100ML;538MG/100ML;448MG/100ML   N020171 002 AUG 19, 1992

DELFLEX W/ DEXTROSE 4.25% LOW MAGNESIUM LOW CALCIUM IN PLASTIC CONTAINER
FRESENIUS MEDCL
AT 18.4MG/100ML;4.25GM/100ML;5.08MG/100ML;538MG/100ML;448MG/100ML   N020171 003 AUG 19, 1992

DELFLEX-LM W/ DEXTROSE 1.5% IN PLASTIC CONTAINER
FRESENIUS MEDCL
AT 25.7MG/100ML;1.5GM/100ML;5.08MG/100ML;538MG/100ML;448MG/100ML   N018379 004 JUL 07, 1982

DELFLEX-LM W/ DEXTROSE 2.5% IN PLASTIC CONTAINER
FRESENIUS MEDCL
AT 25.7MG/100ML;2.5GM/100ML;5.08MG/100ML;538MG/100ML;448MG/100ML   N018379 005 JUL 07, 1982

DELFLEX-LM W/ DEXTROSE 4.25% IN PLASTIC CONTAINER
FRESENIUS MEDCL
AT 25.7MG/100ML;4.25GM/100ML;5.08MG/100ML;538MG/100ML;448MG/100ML   N018379 006 JUL 07, 1982

CALCIUM CHLORIDE; DEXTROSE; MAGNESIUM CHLORIDE; SODIUM CHLORIDE; SODIUM LACTATE *(continued)*
Solution; Intraperitoneal

DELFLEX-LM W/ DEXTROSE 3.5% IN PLASTIC CONTAINER
FRESENIUS MEDCL
AT 25.7MG/100ML;3.5GM/100ML;5.08MG/100ML;538MG/100ML;448MG/100ML   N018379 008 JUN 24, 1988

DIALYTE LM/ DEXTROSE 2.5% IN PLASTIC CONTAINER
B BRAUN
26MG/100ML;2.5GM/100ML;5MG/100ML;530MG/100ML;450MG/100ML   N018460 005 NOV 02, 1983

DIALYTE LM/ DEXTROSE 1.5% IN PLASTIC CONTAINER
B BRAUN
26MG/100ML;1.5GM/100ML;5MG/100ML;530MG/100ML;450MG/100ML   N018460 007 JAN 29, 1986

DIALYTE LM/ DEXTROSE 4.25% IN PLASTIC CONTAINER
B BRAUN
26MG/100ML;4.25GM/100ML;5MG/100ML;530MG/100ML;450MG/100ML   N018460 009 JAN 29, 1986

DIANEAL 137 W/ DEXTROSE 1.5% IN PLASTIC CONTAINER
BAXTER HLTHCARE
AT 25.7MG/100ML;1.5GM/100ML;15.2MG/100ML;567MG/100ML;392MG/100ML   N017512 001

DIANEAL 137 W/ DEXTROSE 4.25% IN PLASTIC CONTAINER
BAXTER HLTHCARE
AT 25.7MG/100ML;4.25GM/100ML;15.2MG/100ML;567MG/100ML;392MG/100ML   N017512 002

DIANEAL 137 W/ DEXTROSE 2.5% IN PLASTIC CONTAINER
BAXTER HLTHCARE
AT 25.7MG/100ML;2.5GM/100ML;15.2MG/100ML;567MG/100ML;392MG/100ML   N017512 003

DIANEAL LOW CALCIUM W/ DEXTROSE 1.5% IN PLASTIC CONTAINER
BAXTER HLTHCARE
AT 18.3MG/100ML;1.5GM/100ML;5.08MG/100ML;538MG/100ML;448MG/100ML   N020183 001 DEC 04, 1992

DIANEAL LOW CALCIUM W/ DEXTROSE 2.5% IN PLASTIC CONTAINER
BAXTER HLTHCARE
AT 18.3MG/100ML;2.5GM/100ML;5.08MG/100ML;538MG/100ML;448MG/100ML   N020183 002 DEC 04, 1992

DIANEAL LOW CALCIUM W/ DEXTROSE 3.5% IN PLASTIC CONTAINER
BAXTER HLTHCARE
AT 18.3MG/100ML;3.5GM/100ML;5.08MG/100ML;538MG/100ML;448MG/100ML   N020183 003 DEC 04, 1992

DIANEAL LOW CALCIUM W/ DEXTROSE 4.25% IN PLASTIC CONTAINER
BAXTER HLTHCARE
AT 18.3MG/100ML;4.25GM/100ML;5.08MG/100ML;538MG/100ML;448MG/100ML   N020183 004 DEC 04, 1992

Prescription Drug Products *(continued)*

CALCIUM CHLORIDE; DEXTROSE; MAGNESIUM CHLORIDE; SODIUM CHLORIDE; SODIUM LACTATE *(continued)*

Solution; Intraperitoneal

INPERSOL-LC/LM W/ DEXTROSE 1.5% IN PLASTIC CONTAINER
FRESENIUS   18.4MG/100ML;1.5GM/100ML;5.08MG/100ML;538MG/100ML;448MG/100ML
AT   N020374 001   JUN 13, 1994

INPERSOL-LC/LM W/ DEXTROSE 2.5% IN PLASTIC CONTAINER
FRESENIUS   18.4MG/100ML;2.5GM/100ML;5.08MG/100ML;538MG/100ML;448MG/100ML
AT   N020374 002   JUN 13, 1994

INPERSOL-LC/LM W/ DEXTROSE 3.5% IN PLASTIC CONTAINER
FRESENIUS   18.4MG/100ML;3.5GM/100ML;5.08MG/100ML;538MG/100ML;448MG/100ML
AT   N020374 003   JUN 13, 1994

INPERSOL-LC/LM W/ DEXTROSE 4.25% IN PLASTIC CONTAINER
FRESENIUS   18.4MG/100ML;4.25GM/100ML;5.08MG/100ML;538MG/100ML;448MG/100ML
AT   N020374 004   JUN 13, 1994

CALCIUM CHLORIDE; DEXTROSE; MAGNESIUM SULFATE; POTASSIUM CHLORIDE; SODIUM BICARBONATE; SODIUM CHLORIDE; SODIUM PHOSPHATE, DIBASIC, HEPTAHYDRATE

Injectable; Intrathecal
ELLIOTTS B SOLUTION   0.2MG/ML;0.8MG/ML;0.3MG/ML;0.3MG/ML;1.9MG/ML;7.3MG/ML;0.2MG/ML
+ QOL MEDCL   N020577 001   SEP 27, 1996

CALCIUM CHLORIDE; DEXTROSE; POTASSIUM CHLORIDE; SODIUM ACETATE; SODIUM CHLORIDE

Injectable; Injection
DEXTROSE 5% IN ACETATED RINGER'S IN PLASTIC CONTAINER
B BRAUN   20MG/100ML;5GM/100ML;30MG/100ML;380MG/100ML;600MG/100ML
N018258 001

CALCIUM CHLORIDE; DEXTROSE; POTASSIUM CHLORIDE; SODIUM CHLORIDE

Injectable; Injection
DEXTROSE 5% AND RINGER'S IN PLASTIC CONTAINER
ABBOTT   33MG/100ML;5GM/100ML;30MG/100ML;860MG/100ML
AP   N018254 001

DEXTROSE 5% IN RINGER'S IN PLASTIC CONTAINER
BAXTER HLTHCARE   33MG/100ML;5GM/100ML;30MG/100ML;860MG/100ML
AP   N016695 001

B BRAUN   33MG/100ML;5GM/100ML;30MG/100ML;860MG/100ML
AP   N018256 001

AP   N020000 001

CALCIUM CHLORIDE; DEXTROSE; MAGNESIUM CHLORIDE; SODIUM CHLORIDE; SODIUM LACTATE *(continued)*

Solution; Intraperitoneal

DIANEAL PD-2 W/ DEXTROSE 1.5% IN PLASTIC CONTAINER
BAXTER HLTHCARE   18.3MG/100ML;1.5GM/100ML;5.08MG/100ML;538MG/100ML;448MG/100ML
AT   N017512 004

DIANEAL PD-2 W/ DEXTROSE 2.5% IN PLASTIC CONTAINER
BAXTER HLTHCARE   25.7MG/100ML;2.5GM/100ML;5.08MG/100ML;538MG/100ML;448MG/100ML
AT   N017512 005

DIANEAL PD-2 W/ DEXTROSE 4.25% IN PLASTIC CONTAINER
BAXTER HLTHCARE   25.7MG/100ML;4.25GM/100ML;5.08MG/100ML;538MG/100ML;448MG/100ML
AT   N017512 006

DIANEAL PD-1 W/ DEXTROSE 1.5% IN PLASTIC CONTAINER
BAXTER HLTHCARE   25.7MG/100ML;1.5GM/100ML;15.2MG/100ML;567MG/100ML;392MG/100ML
AT   N017512 007   JUL 09, 1984

DIANEAL PD-1 W/ DEXTROSE 2.5% IN PLASTIC CONTAINER
BAXTER HLTHCARE   25.7MG/100ML;2.5GM/100ML;15.2MG/100ML;567MG/100ML;392MG/100ML
AT   N017512 008   JUL 09, 1984

DIANEAL PD-1 W/ DEXTROSE 4.25% IN PLASTIC CONTAINER
BAXTER HLTHCARE   25.7MG/100ML;4.25GM/100ML;15.2MG/100ML;567MG/100ML;392MG/100ML
AT   N017512 009   JUL 09, 1984

DIANEAL PD-1 W/ DEXTROSE 3.5% IN PLASTIC CONTAINER
BAXTER HLTHCARE   25.7MG/100ML;3.3GM/100ML;15.2MG/100ML;567MG/100ML;392MG/100ML
AT   N017512 010   NOV 18, 1985

DIANEAL PD-2 W/ DEXTROSE 3.5% IN PLASTIC CONTAINER
BAXTER HLTHCARE   25.7MG/100ML;3.5GM/100ML;5.08MG/100ML;538MG/100ML;448MG/100ML
AT   N017512 011   NOV 18, 1985

DIANEAL PD-2 W/ DEXTROSE 1.5% IN PLASTIC CONTAINER
BAXTER HLTHCARE   25.7MG/100ML;1.5GM/100ML;5.08MG/100ML;538MG/100ML;448MG/100ML
AT   N020163 001   DEC 04, 1992

DIANEAL PD-2 W/ DEXTROSE 2.5% IN PLASTIC CONTAINER
BAXTER HLTHCARE   25.7MG/100ML;2.5GM/100ML;5.08MG/100ML;538MG/100ML;448MG/100ML
AT   N020163 002   DEC 04, 1992

DIANEAL PD-2 W/ DEXTROSE 4.25% IN PLASTIC CONTAINER
BAXTER HLTHCARE   25.7MG/100ML;4.25GM/100ML;5.08MG/100ML;538MG/100ML;448MG/100ML
AT   N020163 003   DEC 04, 1992

Prescription Drug Products *(continued)*

CALCIUM CHLORIDE; DEXTROSE; POTASSIUM CHLORIDE; SODIUM CHLORIDE *(continued)*
Injectable; Injection
DEXTROSE 5% IN RINGER'S IN PLASTIC CONTAINER
B BRAUN   APR 17, 1992

CALCIUM CHLORIDE; DEXTROSE; POTASSIUM CHLORIDE; SODIUM CHLORIDE; SODIUM LACTATE
Injectable; Injection
DEXTROSE 5% AND LACTATED RINGER'S IN PLASTIC CONTAINER
AP   ABBOTT   20MG/100ML;5GM/100ML;30MG/100ML;600MG/100ML;310MG/100ML   N017608 001

DEXTROSE 2.5% IN HALF-STRENGTH LACTATED RINGER'S IN PLASTIC CONTAINER
B BRAUN   10MG/100ML;2.5GM/100ML;15MG/100ML;300MG/100ML;160MG/100ML   N019634 001 FEB 24, 1988

DEXTROSE 5% IN LACTATED RINGER'S IN PLASTIC CONTAINER
AP   B BRAUN   20MG/100ML;5GM/100ML;30MG/100ML;600MG/100ML;310MG/100ML   N019634 003 FEB 24, 1988

LACTATED RINGER'S AND DEXTROSE 5% IN PLASTIC CONTAINER
AP   BAXTER HLTHCARE   20MG/100ML;5GM/100ML;30MG/100ML;600MG/100ML;310MG/100ML   N016679 001

POTASSIUM CHLORIDE 5MEQ IN DEXTROSE 5% AND LACTATED RINGER'S IN PLASTIC CONTAINER
BAXTER HLTHCARE   20MG/100ML;5GM/100ML;105MG/100ML;600MG/100ML;310MG/100ML   N019367 001 APR 05, 1985

POTASSIUM CHLORIDE 10MEQ IN DEXTROSE 5% AND LACTATED RINGER'S IN PLASTIC CONTAINER
BAXTER HLTHCARE   20MG/100ML;5GM/100ML;105MG/100ML;600MG/100ML;310MG/100ML   N019367 002 APR 05, 1985
20MG/100ML;5GM/100ML;179MG/100ML;600MG/100ML;310MG/100ML   N019367 003 APR 05, 1985

POTASSIUM CHLORIDE 20MEQ IN DEXTROSE 5% AND LACTATED RINGER'S IN PLASTIC CONTAINER
AP   BAXTER HLTHCARE   20MG/100ML;5GM/100ML;179MG/100ML;600MG/100ML;310MG/100ML   N019367 004 APR 05, 1985
AP   20MG/100ML;5GM/100ML;328MG/100ML;600MG/100ML;310MG/100ML   N019367 005 APR 05, 1985

CALCIUM CHLORIDE; DEXTROSE; POTASSIUM CHLORIDE; SODIUM CHLORIDE; SODIUM LACTATE *(continued)*
Injectable; Injection
POTASSIUM CHLORIDE 15MEQ IN DEXTROSE 5% AND LACTATED RINGER'S IN PLASTIC CONTAINER
AP   BAXTER HLTHCARE   20MG/100ML;5GM/100ML;254MG/100ML;600MG/100ML;310MG/100ML   N019367 006 APR 05, 1985

POTASSIUM CHLORIDE 30MEQ IN DEXTROSE 5% AND LACTATED RINGER'S IN PLASTIC CONTAINER
AP   BAXTER HLTHCARE   20MG/100ML;5GM/100ML;254MG/100ML;600MG/100ML;310MG/100ML   N019367 007 APR 05, 1985

POTASSIUM CHLORIDE 40MEQ IN DEXTROSE 5% AND LACTATED RINGER'S IN PLASTIC CONTAINER
AP   BAXTER HLTHCARE   20MG/100ML;5GM/100ML;328MG/100ML;600MG/100ML;310MG/100ML   N019367 008 APR 05, 1985

POTASSIUM CHLORIDE 20MEQ IN DEXTROSE 5% AND LACTATED RINGER'S IN PLASTIC CONTAINER
AP   ABBOTT   20MG/100ML;5GM/100ML;179MG/100ML;600MG/100ML;310MG/100ML   N019685 002 OCT 17, 1988

POTASSIUM CHLORIDE 40MEQ IN DEXTROSE 5% AND LACTATED RINGER'S IN PLASTIC CONTAINER
AP   ABBOTT   20MG/100ML;5GM/100ML;328MG/100ML;600MG/100ML;310MG/100ML   N019685 004 OCT 17, 1988

POTASSIUM CHLORIDE 20MEQ IN DEXTROSE 5% AND LACTATED RINGER'S IN PLASTIC CONTAINER
AP   ABBOTT   20MG/100ML;5GM/100ML;328MG/100ML;600MG/100ML;310MG/100ML   N019685 008 OCT 17, 1988

CALCIUM CHLORIDE; ICODEXTRIN; MAGNESIUM CHLORIDE; SODIUM CHLORIDE; SODIUM LACTATE
Solution; Intraperitoneal
EXTRANEAL
+   BAXTER HLTHCARE   25.7MG/100ML;7.5GM/100ML;5.08MG/100ML;535MG/100ML;448MG/100ML   N021321 001 DEC 20, 2002

CALCIUM CHLORIDE; MAGNESIUM CHLORIDE; POTASSIUM CHLORIDE; SODIUM ACETATE; SODIUM CHLORIDE
Injectable; Injection
TPN ELECTROLYTES IN PLASTIC CONTAINER
AP   ABBOTT   16.5MG/ML;25.4MG/ML;74.6MG/ML;121MG/ML;16.1MG/ML   N018895 001 JUL 20, 1984

Prescription Drug Products (continued)

CALCIUM CHLORIDE; MAGNESIUM CHLORIDE; POTASSIUM CHLORIDE; SODIUM ACETATE; SODIUM CHLORIDE; SODIUM CITRATE
Injectable; Injection
ISOLYTE E IN PLASTIC CONTAINER

	Firm	Strength	Appl No	Date
	B BRAUN	35MG/100ML;30MG/100ML;74MG/100ML;640MG/100ML;500MG/100ML;74MG/100ML	N019718 001	SEP 29, 1989

Solution; Irrigation
BSS

	Firm	Strength	Appl No	Date
+	ALCON	0.48MG/ML;0.3MG/ML;0.75MG/ML;3.9MG/ML;6.4MG/ML;1.7MG/ML	N020742 001	DEC 10, 1997

CALCIUM CHLORIDE; MAGNESIUM CHLORIDE; POTASSIUM CHLORIDE; SODIUM ACETATE; SODIUM CHLORIDE; SODIUM LACTATE
Injectable; Injection
PLASMA-LYTE R IN PLASTIC CONTAINER

	Firm	Strength	Appl No	Date
	BAXTER HLTHCARE	36.8MG/100ML;30.5MG/100ML;74.6MG/100ML;640MG/100ML;496MG/100ML;89.6MG/100ML	N017438 001	

CALCIUM CHLORIDE; MAGNESIUM CHLORIDE; POTASSIUM CHLORIDE; SODIUM CHLORIDE
Solution; Perfusion, Cardiac
CARDIOPLEGIC IN PLASTIC CONTAINER

		Firm	Strength	Appl No	Date
AT		BAXTER HLTHCARE	17.6MG/100ML;119.3MG/100ML;325.3MG/100ML;643MG/100ML	N075323 001	APR 21, 2000

PLEGISOL IN PLASTIC CONTAINER

		Firm	Strength	Appl No	Date
AT	+	ABBOTT	17.6MG/100ML;119.3MG/100ML;325.3MG/100ML;643MG/100ML	N018608 001	FEB 26, 1982

CALCIUM CHLORIDE; POTASSIUM CHLORIDE; SODIUM CHLORIDE
Injectable; Injection
RINGER'S IN PLASTIC CONTAINER

	Firm	Strength	Appl No	Date
AP	ABBOTT	33MG/100ML;30MG/100ML;860MG/100ML	N018251 001	
AP	B BRAUN	33MG/100ML;30MG/100ML;860MG/100ML	N018721 001	NOV 09, 1982
AP		33MG/100ML;30MG/100ML;860MG/100ML	N020002 001	APR 17, 1992
AP	BAXTER HLTHCARE	33MG/100ML;30MG/100ML;860MG/100ML	N016693 001	

CALCIUM CHLORIDE; POTASSIUM CHLORIDE; SODIUM CHLORIDE (continued)
Solution; Irrigation
RINGER'S IN PLASTIC CONTAINER

	Firm	Strength	Appl No	Date
AT	ABBOTT	33MG/100ML;30MG/100ML;860MG/100ML	N017635 001	
AT	B BRAUN	33MG/100ML;30MG/100ML;860MG/100ML	N018156 001	
AT	BAXTER HLTHCARE	33MG/100ML;30MG/100ML;860MG/100ML	N018495 001	FEB 19, 1982

CALCIUM CHLORIDE; POTASSIUM CHLORIDE; SODIUM CHLORIDE; SODIUM LACTATE
Injectable; Injection
LACTATED RINGER'S IN PLASTIC CONTAINER

	Firm	Strength	Appl No	Date
AP	BAXTER HLTHCARE	20MG/100ML;30MG/100ML;600MG/100ML;310MG/100ML	N016682 001	
AP	ABBOTT	20MG/100ML;30MG/100ML;600MG/100ML;310MG/100ML	N017641 001	
AP	B BRAUN	20MG/100ML;30MG/100ML;600MG/100ML;310MG/100ML	N019632 001	FEB 29, 1988

Solution; Irrigation
LACTATED RINGER'S IN PLASTIC CONTAINER

	Firm	Strength	Appl No	Date
AT	BAXTER HLTHCARE	20MG/100ML;30MG/100ML;600MG/100ML;310MG/100ML	N018494 001	FEB 19, 1982
AT	B BRAUN	20MG/100ML;30MG/100ML;600MG/100ML;310MG/100ML	N018681 001	DEC 27, 1982
AT	BAXTER HLTHCARE	20MG/100ML;30MG/100ML;600MG/100ML;310MG/100ML	N018921 001	APR 03, 1984
AT	ABBOTT	20MG/100ML;30MG/100ML;600MG/100ML;310MG/100ML	N019416 001	JAN 17, 1986
AT	BAXTER HLTHCARE	20MG/100ML;30MG/100ML;600MG/100ML;310MG/100ML	N019933 001	AUG 29, 1989

CALCIUM CHLORIDE *MULTIPLE*
SEE   AMINO ACIDS: CALCIUM CHLORIDE: DEXTROSE: MAGNESIUM CHLORIDE: POTASSIUM CHLORIDE: POTASSIUM PHOSPHATE, DIBASIC: SODIUM CHLORIDE

SEE   AMINO ACIDS: CALCIUM CHLORIDE: DEXTROSE: MAGNESIUM CHLORIDE: POTASSIUM PHOSPHATE, DIBASIC: SODIUM ACETATE: SODIUM CHLORIDE

Prescription Drug Products (continued)

CALFACTANT
Suspension; Intratracheal

TE Code	Product / Firm	Strength	Appl. No.	Date
	INFASURF PRESERVATIVE FREE			
+	ONY	35MG/ML	N020521 001	JUL 01, 1998

CANDESARTAN CILEXETIL
Tablet; Oral

TE Code	Product / Firm	Strength	Appl. No.	Date
	ATACAND			
	ASTRAZENECA	4MG	N020838 001	JUN 04, 1998
		8MG	N020838 002	JUN 04, 1998
		16MG	N020838 003	JUN 04, 1998
+		32MG	N020838 004	JUN 04, 1998

CANDESARTAN CILEXETIL; HYDROCHLOROTHIAZIDE
Tablet; Oral

TE Code	Product / Firm	Strength	Appl. No.	Date
	ATACAND HCT			
	ASTRAZENECA	16MG;12.5MG	N021093 001	SEP 05, 2000
+		32MG;12.5MG	N021093 002	SEP 05, 2000

CAPECITABINE
Tablet; Oral

TE Code	Product / Firm	Strength	Appl. No.	Date
	XELODA			
	HLR	150MG	N020896 001	APR 30, 1998
+		500MG	N020896 002	APR 30, 1998

CAPREOMYCIN SULFATE
Injectable; Injection

TE Code	Product / Firm	Strength	Appl. No.	Date
	CAPASTAT SULFATE			
+	LILLY	EQ 1GM BASE/VIAL	N050095 001	

CAPTOPRIL
Tablet; Oral

TE Code	Product / Firm	Strength	Appl. No.	Date
	CAPOTEN			
AB	PAR PHARM	12.5MG	N018343 005	JAN 17, 1985
AB		25MG	N018343 002	
AB		50MG	N018343 001	
AB		100MG	N018343 003	
+	CAPTOPRIL			
	APOTHECON			
AB		12.5MG	N074472 001	MAR 31, 1995
AB		25MG	N074472 002	MAR 31, 1995
AB		50MG	N074472 003	MAR 31, 1995
AB		100MG	N074472 004	MAR 31, 1995

CAPTOPRIL (continued)
Tablet; Oral
CAPTOPRIL

TE Code	Firm	Strength	Appl. No.	Date
AB	APOTHECON CLONMEL HLTHCARE	12.5MG	N074423 001	MAR 31, 1995
AB		25MG	N074423 002	FEB 13, 1996
AB		50MG	N074423 003	FEB 13, 1996
AB		100MG	N074423 004	FEB 13, 1996
AB	COPLEY PHARM	12.5MG	N074462 001	FEB 13, 1996
AB		25MG	N074462 002	FEB 13, 1996
AB		50MG	N074462 003	FEB 13, 1996
AB		100MG	N074462 004	FEB 13, 1996
AB	EGIS PHARMS	12.5MG	N074748 004	FEB 13, 1996
AB		25MG	N074748 002	MAY 29, 1997
AB		50MG	N074748 001	MAY 29, 1997
AB		100MG	N074748 003	MAY 29, 1997
AB	ENDO LABS	12.5MG	N074418 001	MAY 29, 1997
AB		25MG	N074418 002	FEB 13, 1996
AB		50MG	N074418 003	FEB 13, 1996
AB		100MG	N074418 004	FEB 13, 1996
AB	EON	12.5MG	N074519 001	FEB 13, 1996
AB		25MG	N074519 002	FEB 13, 1996
AB		50MG	N074519 003	FEB 13, 1996
AB		100MG	N074519 004	FEB 13, 1996
AB	GENEVA PHARMS	12.5MG	N074363 001	NOV 09, 1995
AB		25MG	N074363 002	NOV 09, 1995
AB		50MG	N074363 003	NOV 09, 1995
AB		100MG	N074363 004	NOV 09, 1995
AB	GENEVA PHARMS TECH	12.5MG	N074481 001	FEB 13, 1996
AB		25MG	N074481 002	FEB 13, 1996
AB		50MG	N074481 003	FEB 13, 1996

Prescription Drug Products *(continued)*

CAPTOPRIL *(continued)*
Tablet; Oral
CAPTOPRIL

TE	Manufacturer	Strength	Approval Date	Appl. No.
AB	GENEVA PHARMS TECH	100MG	FEB 13, 1996	N074481 004
AB	HALLMARK PHARMS	12.5MG	FEB 13, 1996	N074477 001
AB		25MG	FEB 13, 1996	N074477 002
AB		50MG	FEB 13, 1996	N074477 003
AB		100MG	FEB 13, 1996	N074477 004
AB	IVAX PHARMS	12.5MG	FEB 13, 1996	N074590 004
AB		25MG	AUG 30, 1996	N074590 002
AB		50MG	AUG 30, 1996	N074590 001
AB		100MG	AUG 30, 1996	N074590 003
AB	MYLAN	12.5MG	FEB 13, 1996	N074434 001
AB		25MG	FEB 13, 1996	N074434 002
AB		50MG	FEB 13, 1996	N074434 003
AB		100MG	FEB 13, 1996	N074434 004
AB	PAR PHARM	12.5MG	FEB 13, 1996	N074493 001
AB		25MG	FEB 13, 1996	N074493 002
AB		50MG	FEB 13, 1996	N074493 003
AB		100MG	FEB 13, 1996	N074493 004
AB	STASON	12.5MG	FEB 13, 1996	N074677 004
AB		25MG	MAY 30, 1997	N074677 002
AB		50MG	MAY 30, 1997	N074677 001
AB		100MG	MAY 30, 1997	N074677 003
AB	TEVA	12.5MG	MAY 30, 1997	N074322 001
AB		12.5MG	FEB 13, 1996	N074433 001
AB		12.5MG	FEB 13, 1996	N074483 001
AB		25MG	FEB 13, 1996	N074322 002
AB		25MG	FEB 13, 1996	N074433 002
AB		25MG	FEB 13, 1996	N074483 002

CAPTOPRIL *(continued)*
Tablet; Oral
CAPTOPRIL

TE	Manufacturer	Strength	Approval Date	Appl. No.
AB	TEVA	50MG	FEB 13, 1996	N074322 003
AB		50MG	FEB 13, 1996	N074433 003
AB		50MG	FEB 13, 1996	N074483 003
AB		100MG	FEB 13, 1996	N074322 004
AB		100MG	FEB 13, 1996	N074433 004
AB		100MG	FEB 13, 1996	N074483 004
AB	TORPHARM	12.5MG	OCT 28, 1998	N074737 001
AB		25MG	OCT 28, 1998	N074737 002
AB		50MG	OCT 28, 1998	N074737 003
AB		100MG	OCT 28, 1998	N074737 004
AB	WATSON LABS	12.5MG	OCT 28, 1998	N074386 001
AB		12.5MG	MAY 23, 1996	N074451 001
AB		12.5MG	FEB 13, 1996	N074576 001
AB		25MG	APR 23, 1996	N074386 002
AB		25MG	MAY 23, 1996	N074451 002
AB		25MG	FEB 13, 1996	N074576 002
AB		50MG	APR 23, 1996	N074386 003
AB		50MG	MAY 23, 1996	N074451 003
AB		50MG	FEB 13, 1996	N074576 003
AB		100MG	APR 23, 1996	N074386 004
AB		100MG	MAY 23, 1996	N074451 004
AB		100MG	FEB 13, 1996	N074576 004
AB	WEST WARD	12.5MG	APR 23, 1996	N074505 001
AB		25MG	FEB 13, 1996	N074505 002
AB		50MG	FEB 13, 1996	N074505 003
AB		100MG	FEB 13, 1996	N074505 004
AB	WOCKHARDT	12.5MG	FEB 13, 1996	N074532 001

Prescription Drug Products (continued)

CAPTOPRIL (continued)
Tablet; Oral

CAPTOPRIL
  WOCKHARDT
AB	25MG	MAR 28, 1997	N074532 002
AB	50MG	MAR 28, 1997	N074532 003
AB	100MG	MAR 28, 1997	N074532 004

CAPTOPRIL; HYDROCHLOROTHIAZIDE
Tablet; Oral

CAPOZIDE 25/15
  APOTHECON
AB	25MG;15MG	N018709 001	OCT 12, 1984

CAPOZIDE 25/25
+ APOTHECON
AB	25MG;25MG	N018709 002	OCT 12, 1984

CAPOZIDE 50/15
+ APOTHECON
AB	50MG;15MG	N018709 004	OCT 12, 1984

CAPOZIDE 50/25
  APOTHECON
AB	50MG;25MG	N018709 003	OCT 12, 1984

CAPTOPRIL AND HYDROCHLOROTHIAZIDE
  ENDO LABS
AB	25MG;15MG	N074788 001	DEC 29, 1997
AB	25MG;25MG	N074788 002	DEC 29, 1997
AB	50MG;25MG	N074788 003	DEC 29, 1997
AB	50MG;15MG	N074788 004	DEC 29, 1997

  IVAX PHARMS
AB	25MG;15MG	N075055 001	JUN 18, 1998
AB	25MG;25MG	N075055 002	JUN 18, 1998
AB	50MG;25MG	N075055 003	JUN 18, 1998
AB	50MG;15MG	N075055 004	JUN 18, 1998

  MYLAN
AB	25MG;15MG	N074896 001	DEC 29, 1997
AB	25MG;25MG	N074896 002	DEC 29, 1997
AB	50MG;15MG	N074896 003	DEC 29, 1997
AB	50MG;25MG	N074896 004	DEC 29, 1997

  TEVA
AB	25MG;15MG	N074827 001	DEC 29, 1997
AB	25MG;25MG	N074827 002	DEC 29, 1997
AB	50MG;25MG	N074827 003	DEC 29, 1997
AB	50MG;15MG	N074827 004	DEC 29, 1997

CAPTOPRIL; HYDROCHLOROTHIAZIDE (continued)
Tablet; Oral

CAPTOPRIL AND HYDROCHLOROTHIAZIDE
  TEVA
	DEC 29, 1997	

CARBACHOL
Solution; Intraocular

CARBASTAT
  NOVARTIS
AT	0.01%	N073677 001	APR 28, 1995

MIOSTAT
+ ALCON
AT	0.01%	N016968 001	

CARBAMAZEPINE
Capsule, Extended Release; Oral

CARBATROL
+ SHIRE PHARM
AB	100MG	N020712 003	SEP 30, 1997
+	200MG	N020712 001	SEP 30, 1997
+	300MG	N020712 002	SEP 30, 1997

Suspension; Oral

CARBAMAZEPINE
  MORTON GROVE
AB	100MG/5ML	N075714 001	JUN 05, 2002

  TARO
AB	100MG/5ML	N075875 001	DEC 21, 2000

TEGRETOL
+ NOVARTIS
AB	100MG/5ML	N018927 001	DEC 18, 1987

Tablet, Chewable; Oral

CARBAMAZEPINE
  CARACO
AB	100MG	N075712 001	JUL 05, 2001

  TARO PHARM INDS
AB	100MG	N075687 001	OCT 24, 2000
+	200MG	N075687 002	JUL 29, 2002

  WARNER CHILCOTT
AB	100MG	N071940 001	FEB 01, 1988

EPITOL
  TEVA
AB	100MG	N073524 001	JUL 29, 1992

TEGRETOL
+ NOVARTIS
AB	100MG	N018281 001	

Tablet, Extended Release; Oral

TEGRETOL-XR
  NOVARTIS
AB	100MG	N020234 001	MAR 25, 1996
+	200MG	N020234 002	MAR 25, 1996
	400MG	N020234 003	MAR 25, 1996

Prescription Drug Products *(continued)*

CARBAMAZEPINE *(continued)*
Tablet; Oral
  CARBAMAZEPINE
AB	APOTEX	200MG	N075948 001 FEB 27, 2002
AB	INWOOD LABS	200MG	N070231 001 AUG 14, 1986
AB	PLIVA	200MG	N071479 001 JUL 24, 1987
AB	PUREPAC PHARM	200MG	N071696 001 NOV 09, 1987
AB	TARO	200MG	N074649 001 OCT 03, 1996

  EPITOL
AB	TEVA	200MG	N070541 001 SEP 17, 1986

  TEGRETOL
AB +	NOVARTIS	200MG	N016608 001

CARBENICILLIN INDANYL SODIUM
Tablet; Oral
  GEOCILLIN
+	PFIZER	EQ 382MG BASE	N050435 001

CARBIDOPA
Tablet; Oral
  LODOSYN
+	BRISTOL MYERS SQUIBB	25MG	N017830 001

CARBIDOPA; ENTACAPONE; LEVODOPA
Tablet; Oral
  STALEVO 50
AB	ORION PHARMA INC	12.5MG;200MG;50MG	N021485 001 JUN 11, 2003

  STALEVO 100
AB	ORION PHARMA INC	25MG;200MG;100MG	N021485 002 JUN 11, 2003

  STALEVO 150
AB	ORION PHARMA INC	37.5MG;200MG;150MG	N021485 003 JUN 11, 2003

CARBIDOPA; LEVODOPA
Tablet, Extended Release; Oral
  CARBIDOPA AND LEVODOPA
AB	MYLAN	25MG;100MG	N075091 002 APR 21, 2000
AB		50MG;200MG	N075091 001 SEP 30, 1999

  SINEMET CR
AB	BRISTOL MYERS SQUIBB	25MG;100MG	N019856 002 DEC 24, 1992
AB +		50MG;200MG	N019856 001 MAY 30, 1991

CARBIDOPA; LEVODOPA *(continued)*
Tablet; Oral
  CARBIDOPA AND LEVODOPA
AB	GENEVA PHARMS	10MG;100MG	N073586 001 JUN 29, 1995
AB		25MG;100MG	N073587 001 JUN 29, 1995
AB		25MG;250MG	N073620 001 JUN 29, 1995
AB	PUREPAC PHARM	10MG;100MG	N074260 001 SEP 03, 1993
AB		25MG;100MG	N074260 002 SEP 03, 1993
AB		25MG;250MG	N074260 003 SEP 03, 1993
AB	TEVA	10MG;100MG	N073618 001 AUG 28, 1992
AB		25MG;100MG	N073589 001 AUG 28, 1992
AB		25MG;250MG	N073607 001 AUG 28, 1992

  SINEMET
AB	BRISTOL MYERS SQUIBB	10MG;100MG	N017555 001
AB		25MG;100MG	N017555 003
AB +		25MG;250MG	N017555 002

CARBINOXAMINE MALEATE
Solution; Oral
  CARBINOXAMINE MALEATE
+	MIKART	4MG/5ML	N040458 001 APR 25, 2003

Tablet; Oral
  CARBINOXAMINE MALEATE
+	MIKART	4MG	N040442 001 MAR 19, 2003

CARBOPLATIN
Injectable; Injection
  PARAPLATIN
+	BRISTOL MYERS SQUIBB	50MG/VIAL	N019880 001 MAR 03, 1989
+		150MG/VIAL	N019880 002 MAR 03, 1989
+		450MG/VIAL	N019880 003 MAR 03, 1989

CARBOPROST TROMETHAMINE
Injectable; Injection
  HEMABATE
+	PHARMACIA AND UPJOHN	EQ 0.25MG BASE/ML	N017989 001

Prescription Drug Products (continued)

CARISOPRODOL
Tablet; Oral

		CARISOPRODOL			
AA	ABLE	350MG	N040421 001	JUN 21, 2001
AA	AMIDE PHARM	350MG	N040188 001	MAR 07, 1997
AA	COREPHARMA	350MG	N040397 001	SEP 21, 2000
AA	GENEVA PHARMS	350MG	N081025 001	APR 13, 1989
AA	MUTUAL PHARM	350MG	N089346 001	OCT 17, 1991
AA	VINTAGE PHARMS	350MG	N040245 001	SEP 08, 1997
AA	WATSON LABS	350MG	N040152 001	DEC 03, 1996
AA		350MG	N086179 001	
AA		350MG	N087499 001	APR 20, 1982
AA	WEST WARD	350MG	N040124 001	JAN 24, 1996

SOMA

AA	+ MEDPOINTE PHARM HLC	350MG	N011792 001

CARISOPRODOL *MULTIPLE*
SEE   ASPIRIN; CARISOPRODOL
SEE   ASPIRIN; CARISOPRODOL; CODEINE PHOSPHATE

CARMUSTINE
Implant; Intracranial

GLIADEL

	+ GUILFORD PHARMS	7.7MG	N020637 001	SEP 23, 1996

Injectable; Injection

BICNU

	+ BRISTOL	100MG/VIAL	N017422 001

CARTEOLOL HYDROCHLORIDE
Solution/Drops; Ophthalmic

		CARTEOLOL HCL			
AT	ALCON	1%	N075476 001	JAN 03, 2000
AT	BAUSCH AND LOMB	1%	N075546 001	JAN 20, 2000
AT	NOVEX	1%	N076097 001	FEB 06, 2002

OCUPRESS

AT	+ NOVARTIS	1%	N019972 001	MAY 23, 1990

Tablet; Oral

CARTROL

	ABBOTT	2.5MG	N019204 001	DEC 28, 1988
	+	5MG	N019204 002	DEC 28, 1988

CARVEDILOL
Tablet; Oral

COREG

	GLAXOSMITHKLINE	3.125MG	N020297 004	MAY 29, 1997
		6.25MG	N020297 003	SEP 14, 1995
		12.5MG	N020297 002	SEP 14, 1995
	+	25MG	N020297 001	SEP 14, 1995

CASPOFUNGIN ACETATE
Injectable; Iv (Infusion)

CANCIDAS

	+ MERCK RES	50MG/VIAL	N021227 001	JAN 26, 2001
	+	70MG/VIAL	N021227 002	JAN 26, 2001

CEFACLOR
Capsule; Oral

CECLOR

AB	CEPH INTL	EQ 250MG BASE	N062205 001	APR 27, 1995
AB		EQ 500MG BASE	N062205 002	APR 27, 1995
AB	LILLY	EQ 250MG BASE	N050521 001	
AB	+	EQ 500MG BASE	N050521 002	

CEFACLOR

AB	IVAX PHARMS	EQ 250MG BASE	N064061 001	APR 27, 1995
AB		EQ 500MG BASE	N064061 002	APR 27, 1995
AB	MARSAM PHARMS LLC	EQ 250MG BASE	N064148 001	MAY 23, 1996
AB		EQ 500MG BASE	N064148 002	MAY 23, 1996
AB	RANBAXY	EQ 250MG BASE	N064156 001	AUG 28, 1997
AB		EQ 500MG BASE	N064156 002	AUG 28, 1997
AB	TEVA	EQ 250MG BASE	N064145 001	JUN 24, 1996
AB		EQ 500MG BASE	N064145 002	JUN 24, 1996

For Suspension; Oral

CECLOR

AB	LILLY	EQ 125MG BASE/5ML	N050522 001	
AB		EQ 125MG BASE/5ML	N062206 001	
AB		EQ 187MG BASE/5ML	N062206 003	APR 20, 1988

CEFACLOR

AB	+	EQ 250MG BASE/5ML	N050522 002	
AB	+	EQ 250MG BASE/5ML	N062206 002	
AB		EQ 375MG BASE/5ML	N062206 004	APR 20, 1988

CEFACLOR

AB	IVAX PHARMS	EQ 375MG BASE/5ML	N064070 001

Prescription Drug Products (continued)

CEFACLOR (continued)

For Suspension; Oral
CEFACLOR
  IVAX PHARMS
    MARSAM PHARMS LLC

TE	Strength	Appl. No.	Date
AB	EQ 125MG BASE/5ML	N064204 001	APR 28, 1995
AB	EQ 187MG BASE/5ML	N064205 001	FEB 18, 1998
AB	EQ 250MG BASE/5ML	N064206 001	FEB 18, 1998
AB	EQ 375MG BASE/5ML	N064207 001	FEB 18, 1998

  RANBAXY

TE	Strength	Appl. No.	Date
AB	EQ 125MG BASE/5ML	N064166 001	FEB 18, 1998
AB	EQ 187MG BASE/5ML	N064165 001	OCT 02, 1997
AB	EQ 250MG BASE/5ML	N064164 001	OCT 02, 1997
AB	EQ 375MG BASE/5ML	N064155 001	OCT 02, 1997

Tablet, Extended Release; Oral
CECLOR CD
  + LILLY

TE	Strength	Appl. No.	Date
AB	EQ 500MG BASE	N050673 002	JUN 28, 1996

CEFACLOR
  IVAX PHARMS

TE	Strength	Appl. No.	Date
AB	EQ 500MG BASE	N065057 001	JAN 05, 2001
AB	EQ 375MG BASE	N065058 001	SEP 04, 2002

  TEVA

TE	Strength	Appl. No.	Date
AB	EQ 500MG BASE	N065058 002	SEP 04, 2002

CEFADROXIL/CEFADROXIL HEMIHYDRATE

Capsule; Oral
CEFADROXIL
  APOTHECON
  BARR

TE	Strength	Appl. No.	Date
AB	EQ 500MG BASE	N062291 001	
AB	EQ 500MG BASE	N065015 001	JUN 22, 1999

  IVAX PHARMS

TE	Strength	Appl. No.	Date
AB	EQ 500MG BASE	N062766 001	MAR 03, 1987

DURICEF
  + WARNER CHILCOTT

TE	Strength	Appl. No.	Date
AB	EQ 500MG BASE	N050512 001	

For Suspension; Oral
CEFADROXIL
  RANBAXY

TE	Strength	Appl. No.	Date
AB	EQ 125MG BASE/5ML	N065115 001	MAR 26, 2003
AB	EQ 250MG BASE/5ML	N065115 002	MAR 26, 2003
AB	EQ 500MG BASE/5ML	N065115 003	MAR 26, 2003

DURICEF
  WARNER CHILCOTT

TE	Strength	Appl. No.
AB	EQ 125MG BASE/5ML	N050527 002
AB	EQ 250MG BASE/5ML	N050527 003
AB	EQ 500MG BASE/5ML	N050527 001

Tablet; Oral
CEFADROXIL
  + RANBAXY

TE	Strength	Appl. No.
AB	EQ 1GM BASE	N065018 001

CEFADROXIL/CEFADROXIL HEMIHYDRATE (continued)

Tablet; Oral
CEFADROXIL
  RANBAXY
DURICEF
  + WARNER CHILCOTT

TE	Strength	Appl. No.	Date
AB	EQ 1GM BASE	N050528 001	APR 23, 1999

CEFAMANDOLE NAFATE

Injectable; Injection
MANDOL
  + LILLY
  +

Strength	Appl. No.
EQ 1GM BASE/VIAL	N050504 002
EQ 2GM BASE/VIAL	N050504 003

CEFAZOLIN SODIUM

Injectable; Injection
ANCEF
  + GLAXOSMITHKLINE

TE	Strength	Appl. No.
AP	EQ 1GM BASE/VIAL	N050461 003
AP	EQ 5GM BASE/VIAL	N050461 004
AP	EQ 10GM BASE/VIAL	N050461 005
AP	EQ 500MG BASE/VIAL	N050461 002

ANCEF IN PLASTIC CONTAINER
  + BAXTER HLTHCARE
  +

TE	Strength	Appl. No.	Date
AP	EQ 10MG BASE/ML	N063002 001	MAR 28, 1991
AP	EQ 20MG BASE/ML	N063002 002	MAR 28, 1991

CEFAZOLIN AND DEXTROSE
  + B BRAUN
  +

TE	Strength	Appl. No.	Date
AP	EQ 1GM BASE/VIAL	N050779 002	JUL 27, 2000
AP	EQ 500MG BASE/VIAL	N050779 001	JUL 27, 2000

CEFAZOLIN SODIUM
  AM PHARM PARTNERS

TE	Strength	Appl. No.	Date
AP	EQ 1GM BASE/VIAL	N064169 002	AUG 14, 1998
AP	EQ 10GM BASE/VIAL	N064170 001	AUG 14, 1998
AP	EQ 20GM BASE/VIAL	N064170 002	MAR 18, 1998
AP	EQ 500MG BASE/VIAL	N064169 001	MAR 18, 1998

  APOTHECON

TE	Strength	Appl. No.	Date
AP	EQ 1GM BASE/VIAL	N062831 002	AUG 14, 1998
AP	EQ 10GM BASE/VIAL	N062831 003	DEC 09, 1988
AP	EQ 500MG BASE/VIAL	N062831 001	SEP 25, 1992

  GLAXCSMITHKLINE

TE	Strength	Appl. No.	Date
AP	EQ 1GM BASE/VIAL	N064033 001	DEC 09, 1988

  HANFORD GC

TE	Strength	Appl. No.	Date
AP	EQ 1GM BASE/VIAL	N063207 001	OCT 31, 1993
AP	EQ 1GM BASE/VIAL	N063208 001	DEC 27, 1991
AP	EQ 10GM BASE/VIAL	N063209 001	DEC 27, 1991
AP	EQ 500MG BASE/VIAL	N063214 001	DEC 27, 1991
AP	EQ 500MG BASE/VIAL	N063216 001	DEC 27, 1991

Prescription Drug Products (continued)

CEFAZOLIN SODIUM (continued)
Injectable; Injection

CEFAZOLIN SODIUM
HANFORD GC
MARSAM PHARMS LLC

TE	Strength	Appl. No.	Date
AP	EQ 1GM BASE/VIAL	N062988 003	DEC 27, 1991
AP	EQ 5GM BASE/VIAL	N062989 001	DEC 29, 1989
AP	EQ 10GM BASE/VIAL	N062989 002	DEC 29, 1989
AP	EQ 20GM BASE/VIAL	N062989 003	DEC 29, 1989
AP	EQ 250MG BASE/VIAL	N062988 001	DEC 29, 1989
AP	EQ 500MG BASE/VIAL	N062988 002	DEC 29, 1989

TEVA

TE	Strength	Appl. No.	Date
AP	EQ 5GM BASE/VIAL	N063018 001	MAR 05, 1990
AP	EQ 10GM BASE/VIAL	N063018 002	MAR 05, 1990

WESTWARD

TE	Strength	Appl. No.	Date
AP	EQ 1GM BASE/VIAL	N065047 002	SEP 18, 2001
AP	EQ 500MG BASE/VIAL	N065047 001	SEP 18, 2001

KEFZOL
LILLY

TE	Strength	Appl. No.	Date
AP	EQ 1GM BASE/VIAL	N061773 003	
AP	EQ 10GM BASE/VIAL	N061773 004	
AP	EQ 20GM BASE/VIAL	N061773 005	SEP 08, 1987
+ AP	EQ 250MG BASE/VIAL	N061773 001	
+ AP	EQ 500MG BASE/VIAL	N061773 002	

CEFDINIR
Capsule; Oral

OMNICEF

TE	Strength	Appl. No.	Date
+	ABBOTT — 300MG	N050739 001	DEC 04, 1997

For Suspension; Oral

OMNICEF

TE	Strength	Appl. No.	Date
+	ABBOTT — 125MG/5ML	N050749 001	DEC 04, 1997

CEFDITOREN PIVOXIL
Tablet; Oral

SPECTRACEF

TE	Strength	Appl. No.	Date
+	PURDUE PHARMA LP — 200MG	N021222 001	AUG 29, 2001

CEFEPIME HYDROCHLORIDE (ARGININE FORMULATION)
Injectable; Injection

MAXIPIME
+ BRISTOL MYERS SQUIBB

TE	Strength	Appl. No.	Date
	EQ 1GM BASE/VIAL	N050679 002	JAN 18, 1996
+	EQ 2GM BASE/VIAL	N050679 003	JAN 18, 1996

CEFEPIME HYDROCHLORIDE (ARGININE FORMULATION) (continued)
Injectable; Injection

MAXIPIME
+ BRISTOL MYERS SQUIBB

TE	Strength	Appl. No.	Date
	EQ 500MG BASE/VIAL	N050679 001	JAN 18, 1996

CEFOPERAZONE SODIUM
Injectable; Injection

CEFOBID
+ PFIZER

TE	Strength	Appl. No.	Date
+	EQ 1GM BASE/VIAL	N050551 001	NOV 18, 1982
+	EQ 2GM BASE/VIAL	N050551 002	NOV 18, 1982
+	EQ 10GM BASE/VIAL	N050551 003	MAR 05, 1990

CEFOBID IN PLASTIC CONTAINER
+ PFIZER

TE	Strength	Appl. No.	Date
+	EQ 20MG BASE/ML	N050613 002	JUL 31, 1987
+	EQ 40MG BASE/ML	N050613 001	JUL 23, 1986

CEFOTAXIME SODIUM
Injectable; Injection

CEFOTAXIME
AM PHARM PARTNERS

TE	Strength	Appl. No.	Date
AP	EQ 1GM BASE/VIAL	N064200 002	MAR 24, 2000
AP	EQ 2GM BASE/VIAL	N064200 003	MAR 24, 2000
AP	EQ 10GM BASE/VIAL	N064201 002	MAR 24, 2000
AP	EQ 20GM BASE/VIAL	N064201 001	MAR 24, 2000
+ AP	EQ 500MG BASE/VIAL		

HIKMA

TE	Strength	Appl. No.	Date
AP	EQ 1GM BASE/VIAL	N065072 002	NOV 20, 2002
AP	EQ 2GM BASE/VIAL	N065072 003	NOV 20, 2002
AP	EQ 10GM BASE/VIAL	N065071 001	NOV 20, 2002
AP	EQ 500MG BASE/VIAL	N065072 001	NOV 20, 2002

CLAFORAN
+ AVENTIS PHARMS

TE	Strength	Appl. No.	Date
AP	EQ 1GM BASE/VIAL	N050547 002	
+	EQ 1GM BASE/VIAL	N062659 001	JAN 13, 1987
AP	EQ 2GM BASE/VIAL	N050547 003	
+	EQ 2GM BASE/VIAL	N062659 002	JAN 13, 1987
AP	EQ 10GM BASE/VIAL	N050547 004	DEC 29, 1983
AP	EQ 500MG BASE/VIAL	N050547 001	

CLAFORAN IN DEXTROSE 5% IN PLASTIC CONTAINER
+ AVENTIS PHARMS

TE	Strength	Appl. No.	Date
AP	EQ 20MG BASE/ML	N050596 002	MAY 20, 1985

Prescription Drug Products *(continued)*

CEFOTAXIME SODIUM *(continued)*

Injectable; Injection

CLAFORAN IN DEXTROSE 5% IN PLASTIC CONTAINER

+	AVENTIS PHARMS	EQ 40MG BASE/ML	N050596 004	MAY 20, 1985

CLAFORAN IN SODIUM CHLORIDE 0.9% IN PLASTIC CONTAINER

+	AVENTIS PHARMS	EQ 20MG BASE/ML	N050596 001	MAY 20, 1985
+		EQ 40MG BASE/ML	N050596 003	MAY 20, 1985

CEFOTETAN DISODIUM

Injectable; Injection

CEFOTAN

+	ASTRAZENECA	EQ 1GM BASE/VIAL	N050588 001	DEC 27, 1985
		EQ 1GM BASE/VIAL	N063293 001	APR 29, 1993
+		EQ 2GM BASE/VIAL	N050588 002	DEC 27, 1985
		EQ 2GM BASE/VIAL	N063293 002	APR 29, 1993
+		EQ 10GM BASE/VIAL	N050588 003	APR 25, 1988

CEFOTAN IN PLASTIC CONTAINER

+	ASTRAZENECA	EQ 20MG BASE/ML	N050694 002	JUL 30, 1993
		EQ 40MG BASE/ML	N050694 001	JUL 30, 1993

CEFOXITIN SODIUM

Injectable; Injection

CEFOXITIN

AP	AM PHARM PARTNERS	EQ 1GM BASE/VIAL	N065012 001	JUL 03, 2000
AP		EQ 2GM BASE/2VIAL	N065012 002	JUL 03, 2000
AP		EQ 10GM BASE/VIAL	N065011 001	JUL 03, 2000
AP	ESI LEDERLE	EQ 1GM BASE/VIAL	N065051 001	SEP 11, 2000
AP		EQ 2GM BASE/VIAL	N065051 002	SEP 11, 2000
AP		EQ 10GM BASE/VIAL	N065050 001	SEP 11, 2000

MEFOXIN

AP	+ MERCK	EQ 1GM BASE/VIAL	N050517 001	
AP		EQ 1GM BASE/VIAL	N062757 001	JAN 08, 1987
AP	+	EQ 2GM BASE/VIAL	N050517 002	
AP		EQ 2GM BASE/VIAL	N062757 002	JAN 08, 1987
AP	+	EQ 10GM BASE/VIAL	N050517 003	JAN 08, 1987

MEFOXIN IN PLASTIC CONTAINER

+	MERCK	EQ 20MG BASE/ML	N063182 001	JAN 25, 1993

CEFOXITIN SODIUM *(continued)*

Injectable; Injection

MEFOXIN IN PLASTIC CONTAINER

+	MERCK	EQ 40MG BASE/ML	N063182 002	JAN 25, 1993

CEFPODOXIME PROXETIL

For Suspension; Oral

CEFPODOXIME PROXETIL

AB	RANBAXY	EQ 50MG BASE/5ML	N065082 001	MAY 31, 2002
AB		EQ 100MG BASE/5ML	N065082 002	MAY 31, 2002

VANTIN

AB	PHARMACIA AND UPJOHN	EQ 50MG BASE/5ML	N050675 001	AUG 07, 1992
AB	+	EQ 100MG BASE/5ML	N050675 002	AUG 07, 1992

Tablet; Oral

VANTIN

	PHARMACIA AND UPJOHN	EQ 100MG BASE	N050674 001	AUG 07, 1992
	+	EQ 200MG BASE	N050674 002	AUG 07, 1992

CEFPROZIL

For Suspension; Oral

CEFZIL

	BRISTOL MYERS SQUIBB	125MG/5ML	N050665 001	DEC 23, 1991
	+	250MG/5ML	N050665 002	DEC 23, 1991

Tablet; Oral

CEFZIL

	BRISTOL MYERS SQUIBB	250MG	N050664 001	DEC 23, 1991
	+	500MG	N050664 002	DEC 23, 1991

CEFTAZIDIME

Injectable; Injection

FORTAZ

AP	+ GLAXOSMITHKLINE	1GM/VIAL	N050578 001	JUL 19, 1985
AP		1GM/VIAL	N062757 001	JUL 19, 1985
AP	+	2GM/VIAL	N050578 003	JUL 19, 1985
AP	+	6GM/VIAL	N050578 004	JUL 19, 1985
AP	+	500MG/VIAL	N050578 001	JUL 19, 1985

TAZICEF

AP	ABBOTT	1GM/VIAL	N062662 002	JAN 25, 1993

Prescription Drug Products *(continued)*

CEFTAZIDIME *(continued)*
Injectable; Injection

TAZICEF
ABBOTT

TE	Strength	Appl. No.	Date
AP	1GM/VIAL	N064032 001	MAR 06, 1986
AP	2GM/VIAL	N062662 003	OCT 31, 1993
AP	2GM/VIAL	N064032 002	MAR 06, 1986
AP	6GM/VIAL	N062662 004	OCT 31, 1993
AP	500MG/VIAL	N062662 001	MAR 06, 1986

TAZIDIME
LILLY

TE	Strength	Appl. No.	Date
AP	1GM/VIAL	N062640 002	NOV 20, 1985
AP	1GM/VIAL	N062655 001	NOV 20, 1985
AP	2GM/VIAL	N062640 003	NOV 20, 1985
AP	2GM/VIAL	N062655 002	NOV 20, 1985
AP	500MG/VIAL	N062640 001	NOV 20, 1985

CEFTAZIDIME (ARGININE FORMULATION)
Injectable; Injection

CEPTAZ

TE	Mfr	Strength	Appl. No.	Date
+	GLAXOSMITHKLINE	1GM/VIAL	N050646 002	SEP 27, 1990
+		2GM/VIAL	N050646 003	SEP 27, 1990
+		10GM/VIAL	N050646 004	SEP 27, 1990

CEFTAZIDIME SODIUM
Injectable; Injection

CEFTAZIDIME SODIUM IN PLASTIC CONTAINER

TE	Mfr	Strength	Appl. No.	Date
+	BAXTER HLTHCARE	EQ 10MG BASE/ML	N063221 001	APR 29, 1993
AP		EQ 20MG BASE/ML	N063221 002	APR 29, 1993
AP		EQ 40MG BASE/ML	N063221 003	APR 29, 1993

FORTAZ IN PLASTIC CONTAINER

TE	Mfr	Strength	Appl. No.	Date
AP +	GLAXOSMITHKLINE	EQ 20MG BASE/ML	N050634 002	APR 28, 1989
AP +		EQ 40MG BASE/ML	N050634 003	APR 28, 1989

CEFTIBUTEN DIHYDRATE
Capsule; Oral

CEDAX

TE	Mfr	Strength	Appl. No.	Date
+	BIOVAIL	EQ 400MG BASE	N050685 002	DEC 20, 1995

CEFTIBUTEN DIHYDRATE *(continued)*
For Suspension; Oral

CEDAX

Mfr	Strength	Appl. No.	Date
BIOVAIL	EQ 90MG BASE/5ML	N050686 001	DEC 20, 1995
+	EQ 180MG BASE/5ML	N050686 002	DEC 20, 1995

CEFTIZOXIME SODIUM
Injectable; Injection

CEFIZOX

Mfr	Strength	Appl. No.	Date
AM PHARM PARTNERS	EQ 1GM BASE/VIAL	N063294 002	MAR 31, 1994
	EQ 2GM BASE/VIAL	N063294 003	MAR 31, 1994
+ FUJISAWA HLTHCARE	EQ 1GM BASE/VIAL	N050560 002	SEP 15, 1983
+	EQ 2GM BASE/VIAL	N050560 003	SEP 15, 1983
+	EQ 10GM BASE/VIAL	N050560 005	SEP 15, 1983
			MAR 19, 1993

CEFIZOX IN PLASTIC CONTAINER

Mfr	Strength	Appl. No.	Date
+ FUJISAWA HLTHCARE	EQ 20MG BASE/ML	N050589 003	APR 13, 1995
+	EQ 40MG BASE/ML	N050589 004	APR 13, 1995

CEFTRIAXONE SODIUM
Injectable; Injection

ROCEPHIN

Mfr	Strength	Appl. No.	Date
+ HLR	EQ 1GM BASE/VIAL	N050585 003	DEC 21, 1984
	EQ 1GM BASE/VIAL	N062654 002	APR 30, 1987
	EQ 1GM BASE/VIAL	N063239 003	AUG 13, 1993
+	EQ 2GM BASE/VIAL	N050585 004	DEC 21, 1984
	EQ 2GM BASE/VIAL	N062654 003	APR 30, 1987
+	EQ 10GM BASE/VIAL	N050585 005	DEC 21, 1984
+	EQ 250MG BASE/VIAL	N050585 001	DEC 21, 1984
	EQ 250MG BASE/VIAL	N063239 001	AUG 13, 1993
+	EQ 500MG BASE/VIAL	N050585 002	DEC 21, 1984
+	EQ 500MG BASE/VIAL	N063239 002	AUG 13, 1993

ROCEPHIN W/ DEXTROSE IN PLASTIC CONTAINER

Mfr	Strength	Appl. No.	Date
+ HLR	EQ 20MG BASE/ML	N050624 002	FEB 11, 1987
+	EQ 40MG BASE/ML	N050624 003	FEB 11, 1987

Prescription Drug Products (continued)

CEFUROXIME AXETIL

For Suspension; Oral

TE	Brand / Firm	Strength	Appl. No.	Date
	CEFTIN			
	GLAXOSMITHKLINE	EQ 125MG BASE/5ML	N050672 001	JUN 30, 1994
	+	EQ 250MG BASE/5ML	N050672 002	APR 29, 1997

Tablet; Oral

TE	Brand / Firm	Strength	Appl. No.	Date
	CEFTIN			
AB	GLAXOSMITHKLINE	EQ 125MG BASE	N050605 001	DEC 28, 1987
AB		EQ 250MG BASE	N050605 002	DEC 28, 1987
AB	+	EQ 500MG BASE	N050605 003	DEC 28, 1987
	CEFUROXIME AXETIL			
AB	APOTEX	EQ 250MG BASE	N065069 001	OCT 02, 2002
AB		EQ 500MG BASE	N065069 002	OCT 02, 2002
AB	RANBAXY	EQ 125MG BASE	N065043 003	FEB 15, 2002
AB		EQ 125MG BASE	N065118 001	APR 25, 2003
AB		EQ 250MG BASE	N065043 002	FEB 15, 2002
AB		EQ 250MG BASE	N065118 002	APR 25, 2003
AB		EQ 500MG BASE	N065043 001	FEB 15, 2002
AB		EQ 500MG BASE	N065118 003	APR 25, 2003

CEFUROXIME SODIUM

Injectable; Im-Iv

TE	Brand / Firm	Strength	Appl. No.	Date
	CEFUROXIME			
AB	AM PHARM PARTNERS	EQ 750MG BASE/VIAL	N065001 001	MAY 30, 2001
AB	TEVA	EQ 750MG BASE/VIAL	N064192 002	APR 16, 1998
	CEFUROXIME SODIUM			
AB	HANFORD GC	EQ 750MG BASE/VIAL	N064125 001	MAY 30, 1997
AB	MARSAM PHARMS LLC	EQ 750MG BASE/VIAL	N064035 001	FEB 26, 1993
	KEFUROX			
AB	LILLY	EQ 750MG BASE/VIAL	N062591 001	JAN 10, 1986
	ZINACEF			
AB	+ GLAXOSMITHKLINE	EQ 750MG BASE/VIAL	N050558 002	OCT 19, 1983

Injectable; Injection

TE	Brand / Firm	Strength	Appl. No.	Date
	CEFUROXIME			
AP	AM PHARM PARTNERS	EQ 1.5GM BASE/VIAL	N065001 002	MAY 30, 2001
AP	TEVA	EQ 1.5GM BASE/VIAL	N064192 001	APR 16, 1998

CEFUROXIME SODIUM (continued)

Injectable; Injection

TE	Brand / Firm	Strength	Appl. No.	Date
	CEFUROXIME			
AP	TEVA	EQ 7.5GM BASE/VIAL	N064191 001	APR 16, 1998
	CEFUROXIME AND DEXTROSE IN DUPLEX CONTAINER			
	+ B BRAUN	EQ 15MG BASE/ML	N050780 001	FEB 21, 2001
	+	EQ 30MG BASE/ML	N050780 002	FEB 21, 2001
	CEFUROXIME SODIUM			
AP	AM PHARM PARTNERS	EQ 7.5GM BASE/VIAL	N065002 001	SEP 28, 1998
AP	HANFORD GC	EQ 1.5GM BASE/VIAL	N064125 002	MAY 30, 1997
AP		EQ 7.5GM BASE/VIAL	N064124 001	MAY 30, 1997
AP	MARSAM PHARMS LLC	EQ 1.5GM BASE/VIAL	N064035 002	FEB 26, 1993
AP		EQ 7.5GM BASE/VIAL	N064036 001	FEB 26, 1993
	KEFUROX			
AP	LILLY	EQ 1.5GM BASE/VIAL	N062591 002	JAN 10, 1986
AP		EQ 1.5GM BASE/VIAL	N062592 002	JAN 10, 1986
AP		EQ 7.5GM BASE/VIAL	N062591 003	DEC 17, 1987
	ZINACEF			
AP	+ GLAXOSMITHKLINE	EQ 1.5GM BASE/VIAL	N050558 003	OCT 19, 1983
AP	+	EQ 7.5GM BASE/VIAL	N050558 004	OCT 23, 1986
	ZINACEF N PLASTIC CONTAINER			
	+ GLAXOSMITHKLINE	EQ 15MG BASE/ML	N050643 001	APR 28, 1989
	+	EQ 30MG BASE/ML	N050643 002	APR 28, 1989

Injectable; Intravenous

TE	Brand / Firm	Strength	Appl. No.	Date
	KEFUROX			
AP	LILLY	EQ 750MG BASE/VIAL	N062592 001	JAN 10, 1986

CELECOXIB

Capsule; Oral

TE	Brand / Firm	Strength	Appl. No.	Date
	CELEBREX			
	GD SEARLE LLC	100MG	N020998 001	DEC 31, 1998
		200MG	N020998 002	DEC 31, 1998
	+	400MG	N020998 003	AUG 29, 2002

Prescription Drug Products (continued)

CELLULOSE SODIUM PHOSPHATE

Powder; Oral

TE	Applicant	Strength	Appl. No.	Approval
	CALCIBIND			
+	MISSION PHARMA	300GM/BOT	N018757 003	OCT 16, 1984

CEPHALEXIN

Capsule; Oral
CEPHALEXIN

TE	Applicant	Strength	Appl. No.	Approval
AB	APOTHECON	EQ 250MG BASE	N063063 001	SEP 29, 1989
AB		EQ 250MG BASE	N063186 001	DEC 30, 1994
AB		EQ 500MG BASE	N063063 002	SEP 29, 1989
AB		EQ 500MG BASE	N063186 002	DEC 30, 1994
AB	BARR	EQ 250MG BASE	N062773 001	JUN 26, 1987
AB		EQ 500MG BASE	N062775 001	APR 22, 1987
AB	IVAX PHARMS	EQ 250MG BASE	N061969 001	
AB		EQ 500MG BASE	N061969 002	
AB	LABS ATRAL	EQ 250MG BASE	N062713 001	JUL 15, 1988
AB		EQ 500MG BASE	N062713 002	JUL 15, 1988
AB	MJ PHARMS	EQ 250MG BASE	N062791 001	JUN 11, 1987
AB		EQ 500MG BASE	N062791 002	JUN 11, 1987
AB	RANBAXY	EQ 250MG BASE	N065007 001	SEP 16, 1999
AB		EQ 500MG BASE	N065007 002	SEP 16, 1999
AB	STEVENS J	EQ 250MG BASE	N062870 001	MAR 17, 1988
AB	TEVA	EQ 250MG BASE	N062702 001	FEB 13, 1987
AB		EQ 250MG BASE	N062760 001	APR 24, 1987
AB		EQ 250MG BASE	N062821 001	FEB 05, 1988
AB		EQ 500MG BASE	N062702 002	FEB 13, 1987
AB		EQ 500MG BASE	N062761 001	APR 24, 1987
	KEFLEX			
AB	+ CEPH INTL	EQ 250MG BASE	N062118 001	
AB		EQ 500MG BASE	N062118 002	
AB	+ LILLY	EQ 250MG BASE	N050405 002	
AB		EQ 500MG BASE	N050405 003	

For Suspension; Oral
CEPHALEXIN

TE	Applicant	Strength	Appl. No.	Approval
AB	APOTHECON	EQ 125MG BASE/5ML	N062986 001	APR 18, 1991
AB		EQ 250MG BASE/5ML	N062987 001	

CEPHALEXIN (continued)

For Suspension; Oral
CEPHALEXIN

TE	Applicant	Strength	Appl. No.	Approval
AB	APOTHECON	EQ 250MG BASE/5ML	N062777 001	JUL 25, 1989
AB	BARR	EQ 125MG BASE/5ML	N065081 001	AUG 06, 1987
AB		EQ 250MG BASE/5ML	N065081 002	JUL 27, 2001
AB	RANBAXY	EQ 125MG BASE/5ML	N062703 001	JUL 27, 2001
AB		EQ 250MG BASE/5ML	N062703 002	FEB 13, 1987
AB	TEVA	EQ 125MG BASE/5ML	N062767 001	JUN 16, 1987
AB		EQ 250MG BASE/5ML	N062768 001	FEB 13, 1987
	KEFLEX			
AB	+ CEPH INTL	EQ 100MG BASE/ML	N062117 001	JUN 16, 1987
AB		EQ 125MG BASE/5ML	N062117 002	
AB		EQ 250MG BASE/5ML	N062117 003	

Tablet; Oral
CEPHALEXIN

TE	Applicant	Strength	Appl. No.	Approval
AB	TEVA	EQ 250MG BASE	N063023 001	JAN 12, 1989
AB		EQ 500MG BASE	N063024 001	JAN 12, 1989
	KEFLET			
AB	+ LILLY	EQ 250MG BASE	N050440 003	FEB 26, 1987

CEPHALEXIN HYDROCHLORIDE

Tablet; Oral

TE	Applicant	Strength	Appl. No.	Approval
	KEFTAB			
AB	+ LILLY	EQ 500MG BASE	N050614 002	OCT 29, 1987

CEPHALOTHIN SODIUM

Injectable; Injection
CEPHALOTHIN SODIUM

TE	Applicant	Strength	Appl. No.	Approval
+	BRISTOL	EQ 1GM BASE/VIAL	N062464 001	MAY 07, 1984
+		EQ 2GM BASE/VIAL	N062464 002	MAY 07, 1984
+		EQ 4GM BASE/VIAL	N062464 003	MAY 07, 1984

CEPHAPIRIN SODIUM

Injectable; Injection

TE	Applicant	Strength	Appl. No.	Approval
	CEFADYL			
	+ APOTHECON	EQ 1GM BASE/VIAL	N061769 001	
		EQ 2GM BASE/VIAL	N061769 002	
		EQ 4GM BASE/VIAL	N061769 003	

Prescription Drug Products (continued)

CEPHRADINE
Capsule; Oral

		Strength	Appl. No.	Date
	ANSPOR			
AB	GLAXOSMITHKLINE	250MG	N061859 001	
AB		500MG	N061859 002	
	CEPHRADINE			
AB	TEVA	250MG	N062683 001	JAN 09, 1987
AB		500MG	N062683 002	JAN 09, 1987
	VELOSEF			
AB	+ APOTHECON	250MG	N061764 001	
AB	+	500MG	N061764 002	

For Suspension; Oral

		Strength	Appl. No.	Date
	ANSPOR			
AB	GLAXOSMITHKLINE	125MG/5ML	N061866 001	
AB		250MG/5ML	N061866 002	
	CEPHRADINE			
AB	TEVA	125MG/5ML	N062693 001	JAN 09, 1987
AB		250MG/5ML	N062693 002	JAN 09, 1987
AB	VELOSEF '125' + APOTHECON	125MG/5ML	N061763 001	
AB	VELOSEF '250' + APOTHECON	250MG/5ML	N061763 002	

CETIRIZINE HYDROCHLORIDE
Syrup; Oral

		Strength	Appl. No.	Date
	ZYRTEC			
	+ PFIZER	5MG/5ML	N020346 001	SEP 27, 1996

Tablet; Oral

		Strength	Appl. No.	Date
	ZYRTEC			
	+ PFIZER	5MG	N019835 001	DEC 08, 1995
	+	10MG	N019835 002	DEC 08, 1995

CETIRIZINE HYDROCHLORIDE; PSEUDOEPHEDRINE HYDROCHLORIDE
Tablet, Extended Release; Oral

		Strength	Appl. No.	Date
	ZYRTEC-D 12 HOUR			
	+ PFIZER	5MG;120MG	N021150 001	AUG 10, 2001

CETRORELIX
Injectable; Injection

		Strength	Appl. No.	Date
	CETROTIDE			
	+ SERONO INC	EQ 0.25MG BASE/ML	N021197 001	AUG 11, 2000
	+	EQ 3MG BASE/ML	N021197 002	AUG 11, 2000

CETYL ALCOHOL; COLFOSCERIL PALMITATE; TYLOXAPOL
For Suspension; Intratracheal

		Strength	Appl. No.	Date
	EXOSURF NEONATAL			
	+ GLAXOSMITHKLINE	12MG/VIAL;108MG/VIAL;8MG/VIAL	N020044 001	AUG 02, 1990

CEVIMELINE HYDROCHLORIDE
Capsule; Oral

		Strength	Appl. No.	Date
	EVOXAC			
	+ DAIICHI	EQ 30MG BASE	N020989 002	JAN 11, 2000

CHLORAMBUCIL
Tablet; Oral

		Strength	Appl. No.	Date
	LEUKERAN			
	+ GLAXOSMITHKLINE	2MG	N010669 002	

CHLORAMPHENICOL
Capsule; Oral

		Strength	Appl. No.	Date
	MYCHEL			
	+ ARMENPHARM	250MG	N060851 001	

Ointment; Ophthalmic

		Strength	Appl. No.	Date
	CHLORAMPHENICOL			
AT	+ ALTANA	1%	N060133 001	

CHLORAMPHENICOL; DESOXYRIBONUCLEASE; FIBRINOLYSIN
Ointment; Topical

		Strength	Appl. No.	Date
	ELASE-CHLOROMYCETIN			
	+ PARKE DAVIS	10MG/GM;666 UNITS/GM;1 UNITS/GM	N050294 001	

CHLORAMPHENICOL SODIUM SUCCINATE
Injectable; Injection

		Strength	Appl. No.	Date
	CHLORAMPHENICOL SODIUM SUCCINATE			
AP	AM PHARM PARTNERS	EQ 1GM BASE/VIAL	N062365 001	AUG 25, 1982
			N062278 001	
	CHLOROMYCETIN			
AP	+ GRUPPO LEPETIT	EQ 1GM BASE/VIAL		
AP	+ PARKEDALE	EQ 1GM BASE/VIAL	N050155 001	

CHLORDIAZEPOXIDE *MULTIPLE*
SEE AMITRIPTYLINE HYDROCHLORIDE; CHLORDIAZEPOXIDE: CHLORDIAZEPOXIDE

CHLORDIAZEPOXIDE HYDROCHLORIDE
Capsule; Oral

		Strength	Appl. No.	Date
	CHLORDIAZEPOXIDE HCL			
AB	BARR	5MG	N084768 001	
AB		10MG	N083116 001	
AB		25MG	N084769 001	
AB	IMPAX LABS	10MG	N085113 001	
AB	USL PHARMA	10MG	N084623 001	
AB	WATSON LABS	5MG	N086383 001	
AB		10MG	N086294 001	

Prescription Drug Products *(continued)*

CHLORDIAZEPOXIDE HYDROCHLORIDE *(continued)*

Capsule; Oral

CHLORDIAZEPOXIDE HCL

AB	WATSON LABS	25MG		N086382 001
	LIBRIUM			
AB	ICN	5MG		N085461 001
AB		10MG		N085472 001
AB		25MG		N085475 001
	+			

Injectable; Injection

LIBRIUM

	+ ICN	100MG/AMP		N012301 001

CHLORHEXIDINE GLUCONATE

Solution; Dental

CHLORHEXIDINE GLUCONATE

AT	ALPHARMA	0.12%		N074291 001 DEC 28, 1995
AT	HI TECH PHARMA	0.12%		N074356 001 MAY 07, 1996
AT	NOVEX	0.12%		N075561 001 NOV 14, 2000
AT	TEVA	0.12%		N074522 001 DEC 15, 1995
	PERIDEX			
AT	+ ZILA	0.12%		N019028 001 AUG 13, 1986
	PERIOGARD			
AT	COLGATE	0.12%		N073695 001 JAN 14, 1994

Tablet; Dental

PERIOCHIP

	+ DEXCEL PHARMA	2.5MG		N020774 001 MAY 15, 1998

CHLOROPROCAINE HYDROCHLORIDE

Injectable; Injection

CHLOROPROCAINE HCL

AP	ABBOTT	2%		N087447 001 APR 16, 1982
AP		3%		N087446 001 APR 16, 1982
AP	BEDFORD	2%		N040273 001 SEP 09, 1998
AP		3%		N040273 002 SEP 09, 1998
	NESACAINE			
	ASTRAZENECA	1%		N009435 001
		2%		N009435 002
	NESACAINE-MPF			
AP	+ ASTRAZENECA	2%		N009435 006 MAY 02, 1996
AP	+	3%		N009435 007 MAY 02, 1996

CHLOROQUINE PHOSPHATE

Tablet; Oral

ARALEN

AA	+ SANOFI SYNTHELABO	EQ 300MG BASE		N006002 001
	CHLOROQUINE PHOSPHATE			
AA	IMPAX LABS	EQ 150MG BASE		N080880 001
AA	+ WATSON LABS	EQ 150MG BASE		N087979 001 DEC 21, 1982
AA		EQ 300MG BASE		N088030 001 DEC 21, 1982
AA	WEST WARD	EQ 150MG BASE		N083082 001
AA		EQ 300MG BASE		N083082 002 SEP 17, 1999

CHLOROTHIAZIDE

Suspension; Oral

DIURIL

	+ MERCK	250MG/5ML		N011870 001

Tablet; Oral

CHLOROTHIAZIDE

AB	MYLAN	250MG		N084388 001
AB		500MG		N084217 001
AB	WEST WARD	250MG		N086028 001 JUL 14, 1982
AB		500MG		N087736 001 JUL 14, 1982
	DIURIL			
AB	MERCK	250MG		N011145 004
AB	+	500MG		N011145 002

CHLOROTHIAZIDE; RESERPINE

Tablet; Oral

DIUPRES-250

BP	MERCK	250MG;0.125MG		N011635 003 AUG 26, 1987
	DIUPRES-500			
BP	+ MERCK	500MG;0.125MG		N011635 006 AUG 26, 1987

CHLOROTHIAZIDE SODIUM

Injectable; Injection

DIURIL

	+ MERCK	EQ 500MG BASE/VIAL		N011145 005

CHLOROXINE

Shampoo; Topical

CAPITROL

	+ WESTWOOD SQUIBB	2%		N017594 001

CHLORPHENIRAMINE MALEATE

Tablet; Oral

CHLORPHENIRAMINE MALEATE

AA	+ ICN	4MG		N080598 001
AA	MARSHALL PHARMA	4MG		N083286 001
AA	PHOENIX LABS NY	4MG		N085522 001

Prescription Drug Products *(continued)*

CHLORPHENIRAMINE MALEATE *(continued)*
Tablet; Oral
  CHLORPHENIRAMINE MALEATE

AA	SUPERPHARM	4MG	N087747 001	APR 20, 1982
AA	TABLICAPS	4MG	N083394 001	

CHLORPHENIRAMINE POLISTIREX; HYDROCODONE POLISTIREX
Suspension, Extended Release; Oral
  TUSSIONEX   EQ 8MG MALEATE/5ML;EQ 10MG BITARTRATE/5ML

+	CELLTECH PHARMS	N019111 001	DEC 31, 1987

CHLORPROMAZINE
Suppository; Rectal
  THORAZINE

+	GLAXOSMITHKLINE	25MG	N009149 024
+		100MG	N009149 033

CHLORPROMAZINE HYDROCHLORIDE
Capsule, Extended Release; Oral
  THORAZINE

+	GLAXOSMITHKLINE	200MG	N011120 019
+		300MG	N011120 020

Concentrate; Oral
  CHLORPROMAZINE HCL

AA	ALPHARMA	100MG/ML	N086863 001	
AA	PHARM ASSOC	30MG/ML	N040231 001	DEC 30, 1999
			N040224 001	JAN 26, 1999
AA		100MG/ML		

  CHLORPROMAZINE HCL INTENSOL

AA	ROXANE	30MG/ML	N088157 001	APR 27, 1983
AA		100MG/ML	N088158 001	APR 27, 1983

  SONAZINE

AA	GENEVA PHARMS	30MG/ML	N080983 004
AA		100MG/ML	N080983 005

  THORAZINE

AA	+ GLAXOSMITHKLINE	30MG/ML	N009149 032
AA	+	100MG/ML	N009149 043

Injectable; Injection
  CHLORPROMAZINE HCL

AP	BAXTER HLTHCARE	25MG/ML	N083329 001

  THORAZINE

AP	+ GLAXOSMITHKLINE	25MG/ML	N009149 011

Syrup; Oral
  SONAZINE

AA	GENEVA PHARMS	10MG/5ML	N083040 001

  THORAZINE

AA	+ GLAXOSMITHKLINE	10MG/5ML	N009149 022

Tablet; Oral
  CHLORPROMAZINE HCL

BP	GENEVA PHARMS	10MG	N080439 001

CHLORPROMAZINE HYDROCHLORIDE *(continued)*
Tablet; Oral
  CHLORPROMAZINE HCL

BP	GENEVA PHARMS	25MG	N080439 002
BP		50MG	N080439 003
BP		100MG	N080439 004
BP		200MG	N080439 005
BP	USL PHARMA	10MG	N083386 001
BP		25MG	N084112 001
BP		50MG	N084113 001
BP		100MG	N084114 001
BP		200MG	N084115 001

  THORAZINE

BP	+ GLAXOSMITHKLINE	10MG	N009149 002
BP		25MG	N009149 007
BP		50MG	N009149 013
BP		100MG	N009149 018
BP	+	200MG	N009149 020

CHLORPROPAMIDE
Tablet; Oral
  CHLORPROPAMIDE

AB	GENEVA PHARMS	100MG	N088725 001	AUG 31, 1984
AB		250MG	N088726 001	AUG 31, 1984
AB	MYLAN	100MG	N088548 001	JUN 01, 1984
AB		250MG	N088549 001	JUN 01, 1984
AB	PAR PHARM	100MG	N088175 001	FEB 27, 1984
AB		250MG	N088176 001	FEB 27, 1984
AB	PLIVA	100MG	N088921 001	APR 12, 1985
AB		250MG	N088922 001	APR 12, 1985
AB	SUPERPHARM	100MG	N086694 001	SEP 17, 1984
AB	WATSON LABS	100MG	N088852 001	SEP 26, 1984
AB		250MG	N088826 001	SEP 26, 1984

  DIABINESE

AB	+ PFIZER	100MG	N011641 003
AB	+	250MG	N011641 006

CHLORTHALIDONE
Tablet; Oral
  CHLORTHALIDONE

AB	GENEVA PHARMS	50MG	N087381 001	
AB	IVAX PHARMS	25MG	N088164 001	JAN 09, 1984
AB	MUTUAL PHARM	50MG	N087176 001	
AB		25MG	N089285 001	

Prescription Drug Products (continued)

CHLORTHALIDONE (continued)
Tablet; Oral

CHLORTHALIDONE

	Firm	Strength	NDA	Date
AB	MUTUAL PHARM	50MG	N089286 001	JUL 21, 1986
AB	MYLAN	25MG	N087180 001	JUL 21, 1986
AB		50MG	N086831 001	
AB	PLIVA	25MG	N088902 001	
		50MG	N088903 001	SEP 19, 1985
AB	USL PHARMA	50MG	N089051 001	SEP 19, 1985
AB	WATSON LABS	25MG	N087100 001	JUN 01, 1987

HYGROTON

	Firm	Strength	NDA	Date
AB	AVENTIS PHARMS	25MG	N012283 004	
AB		50MG	N012283 003	

THALITONE

	Firm	Strength	NDA	Date
+	MONARCH PHARMS	15MG	N019574 001	DEC 20, 1988

CHLORTHALIDONE; CLONIDINE HYDROCHLORIDE
Tablet; Oral

CLORPRES

	Firm	Strength	NDA	Date
AB	MYLAN	15MG;0.1MG	N071323 001	FEB 09, 1987
AB		15MG;0.2MG	N071324 001	FEB 09, 1987
+		15MG;0.3MG	N071325 001	FEB 09, 1987

CHLORTHALIDONE *MULTIPLE*
SEE ATENOLOL; CHLORTHALIDONE

CHLORZOXAZONE
Tablet; Oral

CHLORZOXAZONE

	Firm	Strength	NDA	Date
AA	AMIDE PHARM	250MG	N088928 001	MAY 08, 1987
AA		500MG	N040113 001	SEP 29, 1995
AA	BARR	500MG	N089895 001	MAY 04, 1988
AA	GENEVA PHARMS	250MG	N089852 001	MAY 04, 1988
AA		500MG	N089853 001	MAY 04, 1988
AA	MUTUAL PHARM	500MG	N089970 001	SEP 27, 1990
AA	OHM LABS	250MG	N081298 001	DEC 29, 1993
AA		500MG	N081299 001	DEC 29, 1993
AA	PAR PHARM	250MG	N087981 001	SEP 20, 1983

CHLORZOXAZONE (continued)
Tablet; Oral

CHLORZOXAZONE

	Firm	Strength	NDA	Date
AA	TEVA	500MG	N089859 001	MAY 04, 1988
AA	WATSON LABS	500MG	N040137 001	AUG 09, 1996
AA		500MG	N081040 001	AUG 22, 1989

PARAFON FORTE DSC

	Firm	Strength	NDA	Date
AA	+ ORTHO MCNEIL PHARM	500MG	N011529 002	JUN 15, 1987

STRIFON FORTE DSC

	Firm	Strength	NDA	Date
AA	FERNDALE LABS	500MG	N081008 001	DEC 23, 1988

CHOLECALCIFEROL *MULTIPLE*
SEE ALPHA-TOCOPHEROL ACETATE; ASCORBIC ACID; BIOTIN; CHOLECALCIFEROL; CYANOCOBALAMIN; DEXPANTHENOL; FOLIC ACID; NIACINAMIDE; PYRIDOXINE HYDROCHLORIDE; RIBOFLAVIN PHOSPHATE SODIUM; THIAMINE HYDROCHLORIDE; VITAMIN A PALMITATE; VITAMIN K

SEE ASCORBIC ACID; BIOTIN; CHOLECALCIFEROL; CYANOCOBALAMIN; DEXPANTHENOL; FOLIC ACID; NIACINAMIDE; PYRIDOXINE; RIBOFLAVIN; THIAMINE; TOCOPHEROL ACETATE; VITAMIN A; VITAMIN K

CHOLESTYRAMINE
Powder; Oral

CHOLESTYRAMINE

	Firm	Strength	NDA	Date
AB	COPLEY PHARM	EQ 4GM RESIN/PACKET	N074554 001	OCT 02, 1996
AB		EQ 4GM RESIN/SCOOPFUL	N074554 002	OCT 02, 1996
AB	EON	EQ 4GM RESIN/PACKET	N074557 001	AUG 15, 1996
AB		EQ 4GM RESIN/SCOOPFUL	N074557 002	AUG 15, 1996
AB	IVAX PHARMS	EQ 4GM RESIN/PACKET	N074771 001	JUL 09, 1997
AB		EQ 4GM RESIN/SCOOPFUL	N074771 002	JUL 09, 1997
AB	TEVA	EQ 4GM RESIN/PACKET	N074347 001	MAY 28, 1998
AB		EQ 4GM RESIN/SCOOPFUL	N074347 002	MAY 28, 1998

CHOLESTYRAMINE LIGHT

	Firm	Strength	NDA	Date
AB	COPLEY PHARM	EQ 4GM RESIN/PACKET	N074555 001	SEP 30, 1998
AB		EQ 4GM RESIN/SCOOPFUL	N074555 002	SEP 30, 1998
AB	EON	EQ 4GM RESIN/PACKET	N074558 001	AUG 15, 1996
AB		EQ 4GM RESIN/SCOOPFUL	N074558 002	AUG 15, 1996
AB	TEVA	EQ 4GM RESIN/PACKET	N074348 001	MAY 28, 1998
AB		EQ 4GM RESIN/SCOOPFUL	N074348 002	MAY 28, 1998

Prescription Drug Products (continued)

CHOLESTYRAMINE (continued)

Powder; Oral

TE	Manufacturer	Strength	Appl No	Date
LOCHOLEST				
AB	EON	EQ 4GM RESIN/PACKET	N074561 001	AUG 15, 1996
AB		EQ 4GM RESIN/SCOOPFUL	N074561 002	AUG 15, 1996
LOCHOLEST LIGHT				
AB	EON	EQ 4GM RESIN/PACKET	N074562 001	AUG 15, 1996
AB		EQ 4GM RESIN/SCOOPFUL	N074562 002	AUG 15, 1996
PREVALITE				
AB	UPSHER SMITH	EQ 4GM RESIN/PACKET	N073263 001	FEB 22, 1996
QUESTRAN				
AB	+ BRISTOL MYERS	EQ 4GM RESIN/PACKET	N016640 001	
AB		EQ 4GM RESIN/SCOOPFUL	N016640 003	
QUESTRAN LIGHT				
AB	BRISTOL MYERS	EQ 4GM RESIN/PACKET	N019669 001	DEC 05, 1988
AB		EQ 4GM RESIN/SCOOPFUL	N019669 003	DEC 05, 1988

CHORIOGONADOTROPIN ALFA

Injectable; Injection

TE	Manufacturer	Strength	Appl No	Date
OVIDREL				
	+ SERONO INC	0.25MG/VIAL	N021149 001	SEP 20, 2000

CHROMIC CHLORIDE

Injectable; Injection

TE	Manufacturer	Strength	Appl No	Date
CHROMIC CHLORIDE IN PLASTIC CONTAINER				
	+ ABBOTT	EQ 0.004MG CHROMIUM/ML	N018961 001	JUN 26, 1986

CHROMIC PHOSPHATE, P-32

Injectable; Injection

TE	Manufacturer	Strength	Appl No	Date
PHOSPHOCOL P32				
	+ MALLINCKRODT	5mCi/ML	N017084 001	

CICLOPIROX

TE	Manufacturer	Strength	Appl No	Date
Cream; Topical				
LOPROX				
	+ MEDICIS	0.77%	N018748 001	DEC 30, 1982
Gel; Topical				
LOPROX				
	+ MEDICIS	0.77%	N020519 001	JUL 21, 1997
Lotion; Topical				
LOPROX				
	+ MEDICIS	0.77%	N019824 001	DEC 30, 1988

CICLOPIROX (continued)

TE	Manufacturer	Strength	Appl No	Date
Shampoo; Topical				
LOPROX				
	+ MEDICIS	1%	N021159 001	FEB 28, 2003
Solution; Topical				
PENLAC				
	+ DERMIK LABS	8%	N021022 001	DEC 17, 1999

CIDOFOVIR

Injectable; Injection

TE	Manufacturer	Strength	Appl No	Date
VISTIDE				
	+ GILEAD	EQ 75MG BASE/ML	N020638 001	JUN 26, 1996

CILASTATIN SODIUM; IMIPENEM

Injectable; Injection

TE	Manufacturer	Strength	Appl No	Date
PRIMAXIN				
	+ MERCK	EQ 250MG BASE/VIAL;250MG/VIAL	N050587 001	NOV 26, 1985
		EQ 250MG BASE/VIAL;250MG/VIAL	N062756 001	JAN 08, 1987
	+	EQ 500MG BASE/VIAL;500MG/VIAL	N050587 002	NOV 26, 1985
		EQ 500MG BASE/VIAL;500MG/VIAL	N050630 001	DEC 14, 1990
		EQ 500MG BASE/VIAL;500MG/VIAL	N062756 002	JAN 08, 1987
	+	EQ 750MG BASE/VIAL;750MG/VIAL	N050630 002	DEC 14, 1990

CILOSTAZOL

Tablet; Oral

TE	Manufacturer	Strength	Appl No	Date
PLETAL				
	OTSUKA	50MG	N020863 001	JAN 15, 1999
	+	100MG	N020863 002	JAN 15, 1999

CIMETIDINE

TE	Manufacturer	Strength	Appl No	Date
Solution; Oral				
CIMETIDINE HCL				
AA	DURAMED PHARM BARR	300MG/5ML	N075110 001	JUN 18, 1998
Tablet; Oral				
CIMETIDINE				
AB	CLONMEL HLTHCARE	300MG	N074340 001	JUN 23, 1995

Prescription Drug Products *(continued)*

CIMETIDINE *(continued)*
Tablet; Oral
CIMETIDINE

AB	CLONMEL HLTHCARE	400MG	N074340 002	JUN 23, 1995
AB		800MG	N074339 001	JUN 23, 1995
AB	ENDO PHARMS	200MG	N074281 001	MAY 17, 1994
AB		300MG	N074281 002	MAY 17, 1994
AB		400MG	N074281 003	MAY 17, 1994
AB		800MG	N074329 001	MAY 17, 1994
AB	GENEVA PHARMS	200MG	N074100 001	JAN 31, 1995
AB		300MG	N074100 002	JAN 31, 1995
AB		400MG	N074100 003	JAN 31, 1995
AB		800MG	N074100 004	JAN 31, 1995
AB	GENEVA PHARMS TECH	200MG	N074506 001	JAN 24, 1996
AB		300MG	N074506 002	JAN 24, 1996
AB		400MG	N074506 003	JAN 24, 1996
AB		800MG	N074506 004	JAN 24, 1996
AB	IVAX PHARMS	200MG	N074401 001	MAY 30, 1995
AB		200MG	N074424 001	JUL 28, 1995
AB		300MG	N074401 002	MAY 30, 1995
AB		300MG	N074424 002	JUL 28, 1995
AB		400MG	N074401 003	MAY 30, 1995
AB		400MG	N074424 003	JUL 28, 1995
AB		800MG	N074402 001	MAY 30, 1995
AB		800MG	N074424 004	JUL 28, 1995
AB	LEK PHARMS	300MG	N074250 002	JUN 29, 1995
AB		400MG	N074250 003	JUN 29, 1995
AB		800MG	N074250 004	JUN 29, 1995
AB	MYLAN	200MG	N074246 001	MAY 17, 1994
AB		300MG	N074246 002	MAY 17, 1994

CIMETIDINE *(continued)*
Tablet; Oral
CIMETIDINE

AB	MYLAN	400MG	N074246 003	MAY 17, 1994
AB		800MG	N074246 004	MAY 17, 1994
AB	PLIVA	200MG	N074568 001	FEB 27, 1997
AB		300MG	N074568 002	FEB 27, 1997
AB		400MG	N074568 003	FEB 27, 1997
AB		800MG	N074566 001	FEB 27, 1997
AB	TEVA	200MG	N074151 001	MAY 17, 1994
AB		200MG	N074365 001	FEB 28, 1995
AB		300MG	N074151 002	MAY 17, 1994
AB		300MG	N074365 002	FEB 28, 1995
AB		400MG	N074151 003	MAY 17, 1994
AB		400MG	N074365 003	FEB 28, 1995
AB		800MG	N074365 004	FEB 28, 1995
AB		800MG	N074463 001	MAY 17, 1994
AB	TORPHARM	200MG	N074890 001	DEC 18, 1998
AB		300MG	N074890 002	DEC 18, 1998
AB		400MG	N074890 003	DEC 18, 1998
AB		800MG	N074890 004	DEC 18, 1998
AB	WATSON LABS	200MG	N074349 001	AUG 30, 1996
AB		300MG	N074349 002	AUG 30, 1996
AB		400MG	N074349 003	AUG 30, 1996
AB		800MG	N074316 001	FEB 28, 1996
	TAGAMET			
AB	GLAXOSMITHKLINE	200MG	N017920 002	
AB		300MG	N017920 003	
AB		400MG	N017920 004	DEC 14, 1983
AB +		800MG	N017920 005	APR 30, 1986

Prescription Drug Products (continued)

CIMETIDINE HYDROCHLORIDE

Injectable; Injection

CIMETIDINE HCL

AP	ABBOTT	EQ 300MG BASE/2ML	N074296 001 MAR 28, 1997
AP		EQ 300MG BASE/2ML	N074344 001 JAN 31, 1995
AP		EQ 300MG BASE/2ML	N074345 001 JAN 31, 1995
AP		EQ 300MG BASE/2ML	N074412 001 MAR 28, 1997
AP		EQ 300MG BASE/2ML	N074422 001 JAN 31, 1995
AP	CLONMEL HLTHCARE	EQ 300MG BASE/2ML	N074428 001 APR 25, 1996
AP	ENDO PHARMS	EQ 300MG BASE/2ML	N074005 001 AUG 31, 1994
AP	GENSIA SICOR PHARMS	EQ 300MG BASE/2ML	N074252 001 NOV 26, 1997
AP	LUITPOLD	EQ 300MG BASE/2ML	N074353 001 DEC 20, 1994

CIMETIDINE HCL IN SODIUM CHLORIDE 0.9% IN PLASTIC CONTAINER

AP	ABBOTT	EQ 6MG BASE/ML	N074269 001 DEC 27, 1994
+		EQ 360MG BASE/100ML	N074468 001 DEC 29, 1994
+		EQ 480MG BASE/100ML	N074468 002 DEC 29, 1994
+		EQ 180MG BASE/100ML	N074468 003 DEC 29, 1994
+		EQ 240MG BASE/100ML	N074468 004 DEC 29, 1994
+		EQ 90MG BASE/100ML	N074468 005 DEC 29, 1994
+		EQ 120MG BASE/100ML	N074468 006 DEC 29, 1994

TAGAMET

AP	+ GLAXOSMITHKLINE	EQ 300MG BASE/2ML	N017939 002

TAGAMET HCL IN SODIUM CHLORIDE 0.9% IN PLASTIC CONTAINER

AP	+ GLAXOSMITHKLINE	EQ 6MG BASE/ML	N019434 001 OCT 31, 1985

Solution; Oral

CIMETIDINE HCL

AA	ALPHARMA	EQ 300MG BASE/5ML	N074176 001 JUN 01, 1994
AA	COPLEY PHARM	EQ 300MG BASE/5ML	N074859 001 JUL 09, 1998
AA	ENDO PHARMS	EQ 300MG BASE/5ML	N074251 001 DEC 22, 1994
AA	HI TECH PHARMA	EQ 300MG BASE/5ML	N074664 001 OCT 28, 1997
AA	MORTON GROVE	EQ 300MG BASE/5ML	N074757 001 OCT 17, 1997
AA	NOVEX	EQ 300MG BASE/5ML	N075560 001 MAR 15, 2000
AA	PHARM ASSOC	EQ 300MG BASE/5ML	N074553 001 JAN 27, 1997

CIMETIDINE HYDROCHLORIDE (continued)

Solution; Oral

CIMETIDINE HCL

AA	ROXANE	EQ 300MG BASE/5ML	N074541 001 AUG 05, 1997
AA	TEVA	EQ 300MG BASE/5ML	N074610 001 SEP 26, 1996

TAGAMET

AA	+ GLAXOSMITHKLINE	EQ 300MG BASE/5ML	N017924 001

CIPROFLOXACIN

For Suspension; Oral

CIPRO

	BAYER PHARMS	250MG/5ML	N020780 001 SEP 26, 1997
+		500MG/5ML	N020780 002 SEP 26, 1997

Injectable; Injection

CIPRO

+	BAYER PHARMS	10MG/ML	N019847 001 DEC 26, 1990

CIPRO IN DEXTROSE 5% IN PLASTIC CONTAINER

+	BAYER PHARMS	200MG/100ML	N019857 001 DEC 26, 1990

CIPROFLOXACIN; CIPROFLOXACIN HYDROCHLORIDE

Tablet, Extended Release; Oral

CIPRO XR

+	BAYER PHARMS	212.6MG;EQ 287.5MG BASE	N021473 001 DEC 13, 2002

CIPROFLOXACIN HYDROCHLORIDE

Ointment; Ophthalmic

CILOXAN

+	ALCON	EQ 0.3% BASE	N020369 001 MAR 30, 1998

Solution/Drops; Ophthalmic

CILOXAN

+	ALCON	EQ 0.3% BASE	N019992 001 DEC 31, 1990

Tablet; Oral

CIPRO

	BAYER PHARMS	EQ 100MG BASE	N019537 001 APR 08, 1996
		EQ 250MG BASE	N019537 002 OCT 22, 1987
		EQ 500MG BASE	N019537 003 OCT 22, 1987
+		EQ 750MG BASE	N019537 004 OCT 22, 1987

CIPROFLOXACIN HYDROCHLORIDE; HYDROCORTISONE

Suspension/Drops; Otic

CIPRO HC

+	ALCON	EQ 0.2% BASE;1%	N020805 001

CITRIC ACID; GLUCONOLACTONE; MAGNESIUM CARBONATE
Solution; Irrigation
RENACIDIN
  UNITED GUARDIAN   6.602GM/100ML;198MG/100ML;3.177GM/100ML   N019481 001   OCT 02, 1990

CITRIC ACID; MAGNESIUM OXIDE; SODIUM CARBONATE
Solution; Irrigation
IRRIGATING SOLUTION G IN PLASTIC CONTAINER
AT BAXTER HLTHCARE   3.24GM/100ML;380MG/100ML;430MG/100ML   N018519 001   JUN 22, 1982
UROLOGIC G IN PLASTIC CONTAINER
AT ABBOTT   3.24GM/100ML;380MG/100ML;430MG/100ML   N018904 001   MAY 27, 1983

CITRIC ACID; UREA, C-13
For Solution, Tablet, For Solution; Oral
IDKIT:HP
+ ORIDION   4GM;75MG   N021314 001   DEC 17, 2002

CLADRIBINE
Injectable; Injection
CLADRIBINE
AP BEDFORD   1MG/ML   N075405 001   FEB 28, 2000
LEUSTATIN
AP + ORTHO BIOTECH   1MG/ML   N020229 001   FEB 26, 1993

CLARITHROMYCIN
For Suspension; Oral
BIAXIN
+ ABBOTT   125MG/5ML   N050698 001   DEC 23, 1993
+   250MG/5ML   N050698 002   DEC 23, 1993
Tablet, Extended Release; Oral
BIAXIN XL
+ ABBOTT   500MG   N050775 001   MAR 03, 2000
Tablet; Oral
BIAXIN
+ ABBOTT   250MG   N050662 001   OCT 31, 1991
+   500MG   N050662 002   OCT 31, 1991

CLARITHROMYCIN *MULTIPLE*
SEE AMOXICILLIN; CLARITHROMYCIN; LANSOPRAZOLE

Prescription Drug Products *(continued)*

CIPROFLOXACIN HYDROCHLORIDE; HYDROCORTISONE *(continued)*
Suspension/Drops; Otic
CIPRO HC
  ALCON   FEB 10, 1998

CIPROFLOXACIN HYDROCHLORIDE *MULTIPLE*
SEE CIPROFLOXACIN; CIPROFLOXACIN HYDROCHLORIDE

CISATRACURIUM BESYLATE
Injectable; Injection
NIMBEX
+ ABBOTT   EQ 2MG BASE/ML   N020551 001   DEC 15, 1995
NIMBEX PRESERVATIVE FREE
+ ABBOTT   EQ 2MG BASE/ML   N020551 003   DEC 15, 1995
             EQ 2MG BASE/ML   N020551 002   DEC 15, 1995
+   EQ 10MG BASE/ML

CISPLATIN
Injectable; Injection
CISPLATIN
AP AM PHARM PARTNERS   1MG/ML   N074735 001   JUL 16, 1999
AP BEDFORD   1MG/ML   N075036 001   NOV 07, 2000
AP   10MG/VIAL   N074713 001   NOV 14, 2000
AP   50MG/VIAL   N074713 002   NOV 14, 2000
AP GENSIA SICOR PHARMS   1MG/ML   N074814 001   NOV 14, 2000
AP PHARMACHEMIE   1MG/ML   N074656 001   MAY 16, 2000
PLATINOL
AP + BRISTOL MYERS   10MG/VIAL   N018057 001   MAY 16, 2000
AP +   50MG/VIAL   N018057 002
PLATINOL-AQ
AP + BRISTOL MYERS   1MG/ML   N018057 004   NOV 08, 1988

CITALOPRAM HYDROBROMIDE
Solution; Oral
CELEXA
+ FOREST LABS   EQ 10MG BASE/5ML   N021046 001   DEC 22, 1999
Tablet; Oral
CELEXA
+ FOREST LABS   EQ 10MG BASE   N020822 001   APR 27, 2000
                  EQ 20MG BASE   N020822 002   JUL 17, 1998
+   EQ 40MG BASE   N020822 003   JUL 17, 1998

Prescription Drug Products *(continued)*

CLAVULANATE POTASSIUM; TICARCILLIN DISODIUM
Injectable; Injection

TIMENTIN

+	GLAXOSMITHKLINE	EQ 1GM BASE/VIAL;EQ 30GM BASE/VIAL	N050590 003	AUG 18, 1987
+		EQ 100MG BASE/VIAL;EQ 3GM BASE/VIAL	N050590 001	APR 01, 1985
		EQ 100MG BASE/VIAL;EQ 3GM BASE/VIAL	N062691 001	DEC 19, 1986
+		EQ 200MG BASE/VIAL;EQ 3GM BASE/VIAL	N050590 002	APR 01, 1985

TIMENTIN IN PLASTIC CONTAINER

+	GLAXOSMITHKLINE	EQ 100MG BASE/100ML;EQ 3GM BASE/100ML	N050658 001	DEC 15, 1989

CLAVULANATE POTASSIUM *MULTIPLE*
SEE   AMOXICILLIN: CLAVULANATE POTASSIUM

CLEMASTINE FUMARATE
Syrup; Oral

CLEMASTINE FUMARATE

AA	ALPHARMA	EQ 0.5MG BASE/5ML	N074075 001	OCT 31, 1993
AA	COPLEY PHARM	EQ 0.5MG BASE/5ML	N073095 001	APR 21, 1992
AA	MORTON GROVE	EQ 0.5MG BASE/5ML	N074863 001	MAR 13, 1998
AA	NOVEX	EQ 0.5MG BASE/5ML	N075703 001	NOV 27, 2000
AA	SILARX	EQ 0.5MG BASE/5ML	N074884 001	DEC 17, 1997
AA	+ TEVA	EQ 0.5MG BASE/5ML	N073399 001	JUN 30, 1994

Tablet; Oral

CLEMASTINE FUMARATE

AB	GENEVA PHARMS	2.68MG	N073459 001	OCT 31, 1993
AB	TEVA	2.68MG	N073283 001	JAN 31, 1992

TAVIST

AB	+ NOVARTIS	2.68MG	N017661 001	

CLINDAMYCIN HYDROCHLORIDE
Capsule; Oral

CLEOCIN HCL

AB	PHARMACIA AND UPJOHN	EQ 75MG BASE	N050162 001	
AB		EQ 150MG BASE	N050162 002	
AB	+	EQ 300MG BASE	N050162 003	APR 14, 1988

CLINDAMYCIN HYDROCHLORIDE *(continued)*
Capsule; Oral

CLINDAMYCIN HCL

AB	RANBAXY	EQ 150MG BASE	N065061 001	FEB 02, 2001
AB		EQ 300MG BASE	N065061 002	FEB 02, 2001
AB	TEVA	EQ 75MG BASE	N063027 001	SEP 20, 1989
AB		EQ 150MG BASE	N063029 001	SEP 20, 1989
AB	WATSON LABS	EQ 150MG BASE	N063083 001	JUL 31, 1991
AB		EQ 300MG BASE	N063083 002	MAR 18, 2003

CLINDAMYCIN PALMITATE HYDROCHLORIDE
For Solution; Oral

CLEOCIN

	PHARMACIA AND UPJOHN	EQ 75MG BASE/5ML	N062644 001	APR 07, 1986

CLINDAMYCIN PHOSPHATE
Cream; Vaginal

CLEOCIN

	+ PHARMACIA AND UPJOHN	EQ 2% BASE	N050680 002	MAR 02, 1998

Gel; Topical

CLEOCIN T

AB	+ PHARMACIA AND UPJO-IN	EQ 1% BASE	N050615 001	JAN 07, 1987

CLINDAGEL

BT	GALDERMA LABS LP	EQ 1% BASE	N050782 001	NOV 27, 2000

CLINDAMYCIN PHOSPHATE

AB	ALTANA	EQ 1% BASE	N064160 001	JAN 28, 2000

Injectable; Injection

CLEOCIN PHOSPHATE

AP	+ PHARMACIA AND UPJOHN	EQ 150MG BASE/ML	N050441 001	
AP		EQ 150MG BASE/ML	N062803 001	OCT 16, 1987

CLEOCIN PHOSPHATE IN DEXTROSE 5% IN PLASTIC CONTAINER

AP	+ PHARMACIA AND UPJCHN	EQ 6MG BASE/ML	N050639 001	AUG 30, 1989
AP	+	EQ 12MG BASE/ML	N050639 002	AUG 30, 1989
AP	+	EQ 18MG BASE/ML	N050639 003	APR 10, 1991

CLINDAMYCIN PHOSPHATE

AP	ABBOTT	EQ 150MG BASE/ML	N062800 001	

Prescription Drug Products (continued)

CLINDAMYCIN PHOSPHATE (continued)

Injectable; Injection

CLINDAMYCIN PHOSPHATE

TE	Firm	Strength	Appl No	Date
AP	ABBOTT	EQ 150MG BASE/ML	N062801 001	JUL 24, 1987
AP	LEDERLE	EQ 150MG BASE/ML	N062889 001	JUL 24, 1987
AP	LOCH	EQ 150MG BASE/ML	N062905 001	APR 25, 1988
AP		EQ 150MG BASE/ML		MAY 09, 1988

CLINDAMYCIN PHOSPHATE IN DEXTROSE 5%

TE	Firm	Strength	Appl No	Date
AP	+ AM PHARM PARTNERS	EQ 900MG BASE/100ML	N050635 001	DEC 22, 1989

CLINDAMYCIN PHOSPHATE IN DEXTROSE 5% IN PLASTIC CONTAINER

TE	Firm	Strength	Appl No	Date
AP	ABBOTT	EQ 6MG BASE/ML	N065027 001	JUN 29, 2001
AP		EQ 12MG BASE/ML	N065027 002	JUN 29, 2001
AP		EQ 18MG BASE/ML	N065027 003	JUN 29, 2001
AP	+ BAXTER HLTHCARE	EQ 6MG BASE/ML	N050648 001	DEC 29, 1989
AP	+	EQ 12MG BASE/ML	N050648 002	DEC 29, 1989
AP	+	EQ 900MG BASE/100ML	N050648 003	DEC 29, 1989

Lotion; Topical

CLEOCIN T

TE	Firm	Strength	Appl No	Date
AB	+ PHARMACIA AND UPJOHN	EQ 1% BASE	N050600 001	MAY 31, 1989

CLINDAMYCIN PHOSPHATE

TE	Firm	Strength	Appl No	Date
AB	ALTANA	EQ 1% BASE	N065067 001	JAN 31, 2002

Solution; Topical

CLEOCIN T

TE	Firm	Strength	Appl No	Date
AT	+ PHARMACIA AND UPJOHN	EQ 1% BASE	N050537 001	

CLINDA-DERM

TE	Firm	Strength	Appl No	Date
AT	PADDOCK	EQ 1% BASE	N063329 001	SEP 30, 1992

CLINDAMYCIN PHOSPHATE

TE	Firm	Strength	Appl No	Date
AT	ALPHARMA	EQ 1% BASE	N062811 001	SEP 01, 1988
AT	CLAY PARK	EQ 1% BASE	N064050 001	NOV 30, 1995
AT	FOUGERA	EQ 1% BASE	N064159 001	JUN 05, 1997
AT	MORTON GROVE	EQ 1% BASE	N063304 001	JUL 15, 1997
AT	STIEFEL	EQ 1% BASE	N064108 001	SEP 27, 1996

Suppository; Vaginal

CLEOCIN

TE	Firm	Strength	Appl No	Date
	+ PHARMACIA AND UPJOHN	100MG	N050767 001	AUG 13, 1999

CLINDAMYCIN PHOSPHATE (continued)

Swab; Topical

CLEOCIN

TE	Firm	Strength	Appl No	Date
AT	PHARMACIA AND UPJOHN	EQ 1% BASE	N050537 002	FEB 22, 1994

CLINDAMYCIN PHOSPHATE

TE	Firm	Strength	Appl No	Date
AT	CLAY PARK	EQ 1% BASE	N065049 001	MAY 25, 2000

CLINDETS

TE	Firm	Strength	Appl No	Date
AT	STIEFEL	EQ 1% BASE	N064136 001	SEP 30, 1996

CLINDAMYCIN PHOSPHATE *MULTIPLE*

SEE BENZOYL PEROXIDE; CLINDAMYCIN PHOSPHATE

CLOBETASOL PROPIONATE

Aerosol; Topical

OLUX FOAM

TE	Firm	Strength	Appl No	Date
	+ CONNETICS	0.05%	N021142 001	MAY 26, 2000

Cream; Topical

CLOBETASOL PROPIONATE

TE	Firm	Strength	Appl No	Date
AB1	ALPHARMA US PHARM	0.05%	N074139 001	AUG 03, 1994
AB1	COPLEY PHARM	0.05%	N074087 001	FEB 16, 1994
AB1	FOUGERA	0.05%	N074392 001	SEP 30, 1996
AB1	STIEFEL	0.05%	N075338 001	FEB 09, 2001
AB2	TARO	0.05%	N075733 001	AUG 22, 2001
AB1	TARO	0.05%	N074249 001	JUL 08, 1996

CLOBETASOL PROPIONATE (EMOLLIENT)

TE	Firm	Strength	Appl No	Date
AB2	ALTANA	0.05%	N075430 001	MAY 26, 1999
AB2	TARO	0.05%	N075633 001	MAY 17, 2000

CORMAX

TE	Firm	Strength	Appl No	Date
AB1	HEALTHPOINT	0.05%	N074220 001	MAY 16, 1997

EMBELINE E

TE	Firm	Strength	Appl No	Date
AB2	HEALTHPOINT	0.05%	N075325 001	DEC 24, 1998

TEMOVATE

TE	Firm	Strength	Appl No	Date
AB1	+ GLAXOSMITHKLINE	0.05%	N019322 001	DEC 27, 1985

TEMOVATE E

TE	Firm	Strength	Appl No	Date
AB2	+ GLAXOSMITHKLINE	0.05%	N020340 001	JUN 17, 1994

Gel; Topical

CLOBETASOL PROPIONATE

TE	Firm	Strength	Appl No	Date
AB	ALTANA	0.05%	N075368 001	FEB 15, 2000

Prescription Drug Products (continued)

CLOBETASOL PROPIONATE (continued)

Gel; Topical

CLOBETASOL PROPIONATE

TE	Firm	Strength	Appl. No.	Date
AB	STIEFEL	0.05%	N075027 001	OCT 31, 1997
			N075279 001	MAY 28, 1999
AB	TARO	0.05%	N076141 001	APR 12, 2002

EMBELINE

TE	Firm	Strength	Appl. No.	Date
AB	HEALTHPOINT	0.05%	N020337 001	APR 29, 1994

TEMOVATE

TE	Firm	Strength	Appl. No.	Date
AB	+ GLAXOSMITHKLINE	0.05%	N074128 001	AUG 03, 1994

Ointment; Topical

CLOBETASOL PROPIONATE

TE	Firm	Strength	Appl. No.	Date
AB	ALPHARMA US PHARM	0.05%	N074089 001	FEB 16, 1994
AB	COPLEY PHARM	0.05%	N074407 001	FEB 23, 1996
AB	FOUGERA	0.05%	N075057 001	AUG 12, 1998
AB	STIEFEL	0.05%	N074248 001	JUL 12, 1996
AB	TARO	0.05%	N074221 001	MAR 31, 1995

EMBELINE

TE	Firm	Strength	Appl. No.	Date
AB	HEALTHPOINT	0.05%	N019323 001	DEC 27, 1985

TEMOVATE

TE	Firm	Strength	Appl. No.	Date
AB	+ GLAXOSMITHKLINE	0.05%	N074331 001	DEC 15, 1995

Solution; Topical

CLOBETASOL PROPIONATE

TE	Firm	Strength	Appl. No.	Date
AT	ALPHARMA US PHARM	0.05%	N075391 001	FEB 08, 1999
AT	ALTANA	0.05%	N075205 001	NOV 13, 1998
AT	MORTON GROVE	0.05%	N075224 001	NOV 16, 1998
AT	TARO	0.05%	N075363 001	DEC 29, 2000

EMBELINE

TE	Firm	Strength	Appl. No.	Date
AT	DPT	0.05%	N074222 001	DEC 06, 1995

TEMOVATE

TE	Firm	Strength	Appl. No.	Date
AT	+ GLAXOSMITHKLINE	0.05%	N019966 001	FEB 22, 1990

CLOCORTOLONE PIVALATE

Cream; Topical

CLODERM

Firm	Strength	Appl. No.	Date
+ HEALTHPOINT	0.1%	N017765 001	

CLOFAZIMINE

Capsule; Oral

LAMPRENE

Firm	Strength	Appl. No.	Date
NOVARTIS	50MG	N019500 002	DEC 15, 1986

CLOFIBRATE

Capsule; Oral

CLOFIBRATE

TE	Firm	Strength	Appl. No.	Date
AB	BANNER PHARMACAPS	500MG	N073396 001	MAR 20, 1992
AB	TEVA	500MG	N072600 001	JUL 25, 1991
AB	USL PHARMA	500MG	N070531 001	JUN 16, 1986

CLOMIPHENE CITRATE

Tablet; Oral

CLOMID

TE	Firm	Strength	Appl. No.	Date
AB	+ AVENTIS PHARMS	50MG	N016131 002	

CLOMIPHENE CITRATE

TE	Firm	Strength	Appl. No.	Date
AB	PAR PHARM	50MG	N075528 001	AUG 30, 1999

MILOPHENE

TE	Firm	Strength	Appl. No.	Date
AB	MILEX	50MG	N072196 001	DEC 20, 1988

SEROPHENE

TE	Firm	Strength	Appl. No.	Date
AB	SERONO	50MG	N018361 001	MAR 22, 1982

CLOMIPRAMINE HYDROCHLORIDE

Capsule; Oral

ANAFRANIL

TE	Firm	Strength	Appl. No.	Date
AB	TYCC HLTHCARE	25MG	N019906 001	DEC 29, 1989
AB	+	50MG	N019906 002	DEC 29, 1989
AB		75MG	N019906 003	DEC 29, 1989

CLOMIPRAMINE HCL

TE	Firm	Strength	Appl. No.	Date
AB	GENEVA PHARMS	25MG	N074364 001	MAR 29, 1996
AB		50MG	N074364 002	MAR 29, 1996
AB		75MG	N074364 003	MAR 29, 1996
AB	GENEVA PHARMS TECH	25MG	N074953 001	JUN 25, 1997
AB		50MG	N074953 002	JUN 25, 1997
AB		75MG	N074953 003	JUN 25, 1997
AB	MYLAN	25MG	N074947 001	APR 30, 1998
AB		50MG	N074947 002	APR 30, 1998

Prescription Drug Products *(continued)*

CLOMIPRAMINE HYDROCHLORIDE *(continued)*
Capsule; Oral

CLOMIPRAMINE HCL

AB	MYLAN	75MG	N074947 003	APR 30, 1998
AB	TARO	25MG	N074694 001	DEC 31, 1996
AB		50MG	N074694 002	DEC 31, 1996
AB		75MG	N074694 003	DEC 31, 1996
AB	TEVA	25MG	N074849 001	APR 04, 1997
AB		25MG	N074958 001	AUG 26, 1997
AB		50MG	N074849 002	APR 04, 1997
AB		50MG	N074958 002	AUG 26, 1997
AB		75MG	N074849 003	APR 04, 1997
AB		75MG	N074958 003	AUG 26, 1997
AB	WATSON LAB	25MG	N074600 001	NOV 27, 1996
AB		50MG	N074600 002	NOV 27, 1996
AB		75MG	N074600 003	NOV 27, 1996
AB	WATSON LABS	25MG	N074751 001	SEP 30, 1998
AB		50MG	N074751 002	SEP 30, 1998
AB		75MG	N074751 003	SEP 30, 1998

CLONAZEPAM
Tablet, Orally Disintegrating; Oral

KLONOPIN RAPIDLY DISINTEGRATING

	ROCHE	0.5MG	N020813 003	DEC 23, 1997
		0.25MG	N020813 002	DEC 23, 1997
		0.125MG	N020813 001	DEC 23, 1997
+		1MG	N020813 004	DEC 23, 1997
		2MG	N020813 005	DEC 23, 1997

Tablet; Oral

CLONAZEPAM

AB	ALPHAPHARM	0.5MG	N074940 001	OCT 30, 1997
AB		1MG	N074940 002	OCT 30, 1997
AB		2MG	N074940 003	OCT 30, 1997

CLONAZEPAM *(continued)*
Tablet; Oral

CLONAZEPAM

AB	CARACO	0.5MG	N075423 001	APR 27, 2001
AB		1MG	N075423 002	APR 27, 2001
AB		2MG	N075423 003	APR 27, 2001
AB	EON	0.5MG	N074979 001	AUG 29, 1997
AB		1MG	N074979 002	AUG 29, 1997
AB		2MG	N074979 003	AUG 29, 1997
AB	GENEVA PHARMS TECH	0.5MG	N074925 001	SEP 30, 1997
AB		1MG	N074925 002	SEP 30, 1997
AB		2MG	N074925 003	SEP 30, 1997
AB	MYLAN	0.5MG	N075150 001	OCT 05, 1998
AB		1MG	N075150 002	OCT 05, 1998
AB		2MG	N075150 003	OCT 05, 1998
AB	PUREPAC PHARM	0.5MG	N074869 001	OCT 31, 1996
AB		1MG	N074869 002	OCT 31, 1996
AB		2MG	N074869 003	OCT 31, 1996
AB	TEVA	0.5MG	N074569 001	SEP 10, 1996
AB		0.5MG	N074920 001	AUG 04, 1998
AB		1MG	N074569 002	SEP 10, 1996
AB		1MG	N074920 002	AUG 04, 1998
AB		2MG	N074569 003	SEP 10, 1996
AB		2MG	N074920 003	AUG 04, 1998
AB	TORPHARM	0.5MG	N075468 001	OCT 06, 2000
AB		1MG	N075468 002	OCT 06, 2000
AB		2MG	N075468 003	OCT 06, 2000
AB	WATSON LABS	0.5MG	N074964 001	DEC 30, 1997
AB		1MG	N074964 002	DEC 30, 1997
AB		2MG	N074964 003	DEC 30, 1997

Prescription Drug Products *(continued)*

CLONAZEPAM *(continued)*

Tablet; Oral

KLONOPIN
+ ROCHE

Code	Strength	Appl No	Date
AB	0.5MG	N017533 001	
AB	1MG	N017533 002	
AB	2MG	N017533 003	

CLONIDINE

Film, Extended Release; Transdermal

CATAPRES-TTS-1
+ BOEHRINGER INGELHEIM

Code	Strength	Appl No	Date
	0.1MG/24HR	N018891 001	OCT 10, 1984

CATAPRES-TTS-2
BOEHRINGER INGELHEIM

Code	Strength	Appl No	Date
	0.2MG/24HR	N018891 002	OCT 10, 1984

CATAPRES-TTS-3
+ BOEHRINGER INGELHEIM

Code	Strength	Appl No	Date
	0.3MG/24HR	N018891 003	OCT 10, 1984

CLONIDINE HYDROCHLORIDE

Injectable; Injection

DURACLON
+ ELAN PHARMS

Code	Strength	Appl No	Date
	0.1MG/ML	N020615 001	OCT 02, 1996

Tablet; Oral

CATAPRES
CATAPRES
BOEHRINGER INGELHEIM

Code	Strength	Appl No	Date
AB	0.1MG	N017407 001	
AB	0.2MG	N017407 002	
AB	0.3MG	N017407 003	

CLONIDINE HCL
+ CLONMEL HLTHCARE

Code	Strength	Appl No	Date
AB	0.1MG	N071783 001	APR 05, 1988
AB	0.2MG	N071784 001	APR 05, 1988
AB	0.3MG	N071785 001	APR 05, 1988

GENEVA PHARMS

Code	Strength	Appl No	Date
AB	0.1MG	N070887 001	APR 05, 1988
AB	0.2MG	N070886 001	AUG 31, 1988
AB	0.3MG	N071294 001	AUG 31, 1988

HALSEY

Code	Strength	Appl No	Date
AB	0.1MG	N070925 001	SEP 04, 1987

MYLAN

Code	Strength	Appl No	Date
AB	0.1MG	N070315 001	JUN 09, 1987
AB	0.2MG	N070316 001	JUN 09, 1987
AB	0.3MG	N070317 001	JUN 09, 1987

PUREPAC PHARM

Code	Strength	Appl No	Date
AB	0.1MG	N070974 001	DEC 16, 1986

CLONIDINE HYDROCHLORIDE *(continued)*

Tablet; Oral

CLONIDINE HCL
PUREPAC PHARM

Code	Strength	Appl No	Date
AB	0.2MG	N070975 001	DEC 16, 1986
AB	0.3MG	N070976 001	DEC 16, 1986

WATSON LABS

Code	Strength	Appl No	Date
AB	0.1MG	N070965 001	JUL 08, 1986
AB	0.2MG	N070964 001	JUL 08, 1986
AB	0.3MG	N070963 001	JUL 08, 1986

CLONIDINE HYDROCHLORIDE *MULTIPLE*

SEE CHLORTHALIDONE; CLONIDINE HYDROCHLORIDE

CLOPIDOGREL BISULFATE

Tablet; Oral

PLAVIX
+ SANOFI SYNTHELABO

Code	Strength	Appl No	Date
	EQ 75MG BASE	N020839 001	NOV 17, 1997

CLORAZEPATE DIPOTASSIUM

Capsule; Oral

CLORAZEPATE DIPOTASSIUM
GENEVA PHARMS

Code	Strength	Appl No	Date
AB	3.75MG	N072219 001	AUG 26, 1988
AB	7.5MG	N072220 001	AUG 26, 1988
AB	15MG	N072112 001	AUG 26, 1988

MYLAN

Code	Strength	Appl No	Date
AB	3.75MG	N071509 001	OCT 19, 1987
AB	7.5MG	N071510 001	OCT 19, 1987
AB +	15MG	N071511 001	OCT 19, 1987

Tablet; Oral

CLORAZEPATE DIPOTASSIUM
ABLE

Code	Strength	Appl No	Date
AB	3.75MG	N071780 001	JUN 26, 1987
AB	7.5MG	N071781 001	JUN 26, 1987
AB	15MG	N071782 001	JUN 26, 1987

GENEVA PHARMS

Code	Strength	Appl No	Date
AB	7.5MG	N072513 001	MAY 11, 1990
AB	15MG	N072514 001	MAY 11, 1990

MYLAN

Code	Strength	Appl No	Date
AB	3.75MG	N071856 001	JUL 17, 1987
AB	7.5MG	N071857 001	JUL 17, 1987
AB	15MG	N071858 001	JUL 17, 1987

Prescription Drug Products *(continued)*

CLORAZEPATE DIPOTASSIUM *(continued)*
Tablet; Oral

TE	Firm	Strength	Appl. No.	Date
	CLORAZEPATE DIPOTASSIUM			
AB	TARO	3.75MG	N075731 003	APR 27, 2000
AB		7.5MG	N075731 002	APR 27, 2000
AB		15MG	N075731 001	APR 27, 2000
AB	WATSON LABS	3.75MG	N071852 001	FEB 09, 1988
AB		7.5MG	N071853 001	FEB 09, 1988
AB		15MG	N071854 001	FEB 09, 1988
	GEN-XENE			
AB	ALRA	3.75MG	N071787 001	APR 26, 1988
AB		7.5MG	N071788 001	APR 26, 1988
AB		15MG	N071789 001	APR 26, 1988
	TRANXENE			
AB	OVATION PHARMS	3.75MG	N017105 006	
AB		7.5MG	N017105 007	
AB		15MG	N017105 008	
	+ **TRANXENE SD**			
AB	OVATION PHARMS	11.25MG	N017105 005	
		22.5MG	N017105 004	

CLOTRIMAZOLE
Cream; Topical

TE	Firm	Strength	Appl. No.	Date
	CLOTRIMAZOLE			
AB	TARO	1%	N072640 001	AUG 31, 1993
	LOTRIMIN			
AB	+ SCHERING PLOUGH	1%	N017619 001	
	MYCELEX			
BT	+ BAYER PHARMS	1%	N018183 001	

Lotion; Topical

TE	Firm	Strength	Appl. No.	Date
	LOTRIMIN			
	+ SCHERING	1%	N018813 001	FEB 17, 1984

Solution; Topical

TE	Firm	Strength	Appl. No.	Date
	CLOTRIMAZOLE			
AT	TARO	1%	N074580 001	JUL 29, 1996
AT	TEVA	1%	N073306 001	FEB 28, 1995
	LOTRIMIN			
AT	+ SCHERING PLOUGH	1%	N017613 001	
	MYCELEX			
AT	+ BAYER PHARMS	1%	N018181 001	

Troche/Lozenge; Oral

TE	Firm	Strength	Appl. No.	Date
	MYCELEX			
	+ BAYER PHARMS	10MG	N018713 001	

CLOTRIMAZOLE *(continued)*
Troche/Lozenge; Oral

TE	Firm	Strength	Appl. No.	Date
	MYCELEX			
	BAYER PHARMS			JUN 17, 1983

CLOTRIMAZOLE *MULTIPLE*
SEE BETAMETHASONE DIPROPIONATE; CLOTRIMAZOLE

CLOXACILLIN SODIUM
Capsule; Oral

TE	Firm	Strength	Appl. No.
	CLOXACILLIN SODIUM		
AB	TEVA	EQ 250MG BASE	N062240 001
AB		EQ 500MG BASE	N062240 002
	CLOXAPEN		
AB	GLAXOSMITHKLINE	EQ 250MG BASE	N061806 001
AB		EQ 500MG BASE	N061806 002

For Solution; Oral

TE	Firm	Strength	Appl. No.
	CLOXACILLIN SODIUM		
	+ TEVA	EQ 125MG BASE/5ML	N062268 001

CLOZAPINE
Tablet; Oral

TE	Firm	Strength	Appl. No.	Date
	CLOZAPINE			
AB	CARACO	25MG	N075713 001	NOV 15, 2002
AB		100MG	N075713 002	NOV 15, 2002
AB	IVAX PHARMS	25MG	N074949 001	NOV 26, 1997
AB		100MG	N074949 002	NOV 26, 1997
AB	MYLAN	25MG	N075417 001	MAY 27, 1999
AB		100MG	N075417 002	MAY 27, 1999
	CLOZARIL			
AB	NOVARTIS	25MG	N019758 001	SEP 26, 1989
AB	+	100MG	N019758 002	SEP 26, 1989

COBALT CHLORIDE, CO-57; CYANOCOBALAMIN; CYANOCOBALAMIN, CO-57; INTRINSIC FACTOR
N/A; N/A

TE	Firm	Strength	Appl. No.
	RUBRATOPE-57 KIT		
	BRACCO	N/A;N/A;N/A;N/A	N016089 001

CODEINE PHOSPHATE; PHENYLEPHRINE HYDROCHLORIDE; PROMETHAZINE HYDROCHLORIDE
Syrup; Oral

TE	Firm	Strength	Appl. No.	Date
	PROMETH VC W/ CODEINE			
AA	+ ALPHARMA	10MG/5ML;5MG/5ML;6.25MG/5ML	N088764 001	OCT 31, 1984

Prescription Drug Products *(continued)*

CODEINE PHOSPHATE; PHENYLEPHRINE HYDROCHLORIDE; PROMETHAZINE HYDROCHLORIDE *(continued)*

Syrup; Oral

PROMETHAZINE VC W/ CODEINE

AA MORTON GROVE 10MG/5ML;5MG/5ML;6.25MG/5ML N088896 001 JAN 04, 1985

CODEINE PHOSPHATE; PROMETHAZINE HYDROCHLORIDE

Syrup; Oral

PROMETH W/ CODEINE

AA + ALPHARMA 10MG/5ML;6.25MG/5ML N088763 001 OCT 31, 1984

PROMETHAZINE HCL AND CODEINE PHOSPHATE

AA HI TECH PHARMA 10MG/5ML;6.25MG/5ML N040151 001 AUG 26, 1997

AA PHARM ASSOC 10MG/5ML;6.25MG/5ML N089647 001 DEC 22, 1988

PROMETHAZINE W/ CODEINE

AA MORTON GROVE 10MG/5ML;6.25MG/5ML N088875 001 DEC 17, 1984

CODEINE PHOSPHATE; PSEUDOEPHEDRINE HYDROCHLORIDE; TRIPROLIDINE HYDROCHLORIDE

Syrup; Oral

TRIACIN-C

AA ALPHARMA 10MG/5ML;30MG/5ML;1.25MG/5ML N088704 001 MAR 22, 1985

TRIPROLIDINE HCL, PSEUDOEPHEDRINE HCL AND CODEINE PHOSPHATE

AA + MORTON GROVE 10MG/5ML;30MG/5ML;1.25MG/5ML N088833 001 NOV 16, 1984

CODEINE PHOSPHATE *MULTIPLE*

SEE ACETAMINOPHEN; ASPIRIN; CODEINE PHOSPHATE
SEE ACETAMINOPHEN; BUTALBITAL; CAFFEINE; CODEINE PHOSPHATE
SEE ACETAMINOPHEN; CODEINE PHOSPHATE
SEE ASPIRIN; BUTALBITAL; CAFFEINE; CODEINE PHOSPHATE
SEE ASPIRIN; CARISOPRODOL; CODEINE PHOSPHATE
SEE BROMODIPHENHYDRAMINE HYDROCHLORIDE; CODEINE PHOSPHATE
SEE BROMPHENIRAMINE MALEATE; CODEINE PHOSPHATE; PHENYLPROPANOLAMINE HYDROCHLORIDE

COLCHICINE; PROBENECID

Tablet; Oral

COL-PROBENECID

BP + WATSON LABS 0.5MG;500MG N084279 001

PROBENECID AND COLCHICINE

BP IVAX PHARMS 0.5MG;500MG N083734 001

COLESEVELAM HYDROCHLORIDE

Tablet; Oral

WELCHOL

\+ SANKYO 625MG N021176 001

COLESEVELAM HYDROCHLORIDE *(continued)*

Tablet; Oral

WELCHOL

SANKYO MAY 26, 2000

COLESTIPOL HYDROCHLORIDE

Granule; Oral

COLESTID

\+ PHARMACIA AND UPJOHN 5GM/PACKET N017563 004 SEP 22, 1995

5GM/SCOOPFUL N017563 003 SEP 22, 1995

FLAVORED COLESTID

\+ PHARMACIA AND UPJOHN 5GM/PACKET N017563 001

5GM/SCOOPFUL N017563 002

Tablet; Oral

COLESTID

\+ PHARMACIA AND UPJOHN 1GM N020222 001 JUL 19, 1994

COLFOSCERIL PALMITATE *MULTIPLE*

SEE CETYL ALCOHOL; COLFOSCERIL PALMITATE; TYLOXAPOL

COLISTIMETHATE SODIUM

Injectable; Injection

COLISTIMETHATE

AP PHARMA TEK EQ 150MG BASE/VIAL N064216 001 FEB 26, 1999

COLY-MYCIN M

AP + PARKEDALE EQ 150MG BASE/VIAL N050108 002

COLISTIN SULFATE; HYDROCORTISONE ACETATE; NEOMYCIN SULFATE; THONZONIUM BROMIDE

Suspension/Drops; Otic

COLY-MYCIN S

\+ PARKEDALE EQ 3MG BASE/ML;10MG/ML;EQ 3.3MG BASE/ML;0.5MG/ML N050356 001

COPPER

Intrauterine Device; Intrauterine

COPPER T MODEL TCU 380A

\+ FEI 309MG/COPPER N018680 001 NOV 15, 1984

CORTICORELIN OVINE TRIFLUTATE

Injectable; Injection

ACTHREL

\+ FERRING EQ 0.1MG BASE/VIAL N020162 001 MAY 23, 1996

Prescription Drug Products *(continued)*

CORTICOTROPIN
Injectable; Injection
CORTICOTROPIN

	Firm	Strength	Appl. No.	Date
BC	+ ORGANICS LAGRANGE	40 UNITS/ML	N010831 001	
		80 UNITS/ML	N010831 002	

H.P. ACTHAR GEL

	Firm	Strength	Appl. No.	Date
BC	+ QUESTCOR PHARMS	80 UNITS/ML	N008372 008	

CORTISONE ACETATE
Tablet; Oral
CORTISONE ACETATE

	Firm	Strength	Appl. No.	Date
	PHARMACIA AND UPJOHN	5MG	N008126 003	
		10MG	N008126 004	
BP	+	25MG	N008126 001	
BP	+ WEST WARD	25MG	N080776 002	

COSYNTROPIN
Injectable; Injection
CORTROSYN

Firm	Strength	Appl. No.	Date
+ AMPAHSTAR	0.25MG/VIAL	N016750 001	

CROMOLYN SODIUM
Aerosol, Metered; Inhalation
INTAL

Firm	Strength	Appl. No.	Date
+ AVENTIS	0.8MG/INH	N018887 001	DEC 05, 1985

Solution, Concentrate; Oral
GASTROCROM

Firm	Strength	Appl. No.	Date
+ CELLTECH PHARMS	100MG/5ML	N020479 001	FEB 29, 1996

Solution/Drops; Ophthalmic
CROLOM

	Firm	Strength	Appl. No.	Date
AT	BAUSCH AND LOMB	4%	N074443 001	JAN 30, 1995

CROMOLYN SODIUM

	Firm	Strength	Appl. No.	Date
AT	AKORN	4%	N074706 001	APR 29, 1998
AT	ALCON	4%	N075282 001	JUN 16, 1999
AT	NOVEX	4%	N075615 001	JAN 26, 2001

OPTICROM

	Firm	Strength	Appl. No.	Date
AT	+ ALLERGAN	4%	N018155 001	OCT 03, 1984

Solution; Inhalation
CROMOLYN SODIUM

	Firm	Strength	Appl. No.	Date
AN	ALPHARMA	10MG/ML	N075067 001	JUL 19, 1999
AN	BAUSCH AND LOMB	10MG/ML	N075585 001	DEC 21, 2000
AN	DEY	10MG/ML	N074209 001	APR 26, 1994
AN	IVAX PHARMS	10MG/ML	N075271 001	JAN 18, 2000

CROMOLYN SODIUM *(continued)*
Solution; Inhalation
CROMOLYN SODIUM

	Firm	Strength	Appl. No.	Date
AN	MORTON GROVE	10MG/ML	N075346 001	OCT 25, 1999
AN	NOVEX	10MG/ML	N075333 001	APR 30, 2002
AN	ROXANE	10MG/ML	N075175 001	SEP 30, 1999
AN	WARRICK PHARMS	10MG/ML	N075437 001	APR 21, 2000

INTAL

	Firm	Strength	Appl. No.	Date
AN	+ AVENTIS PHARMS	10MG/ML	N018596 001	MAY 28, 1982

CROTAMITON
Cream; Topical
EURAX

	Firm	Strength	Appl. No.	Date
	+ WESTWOOD SQUIBB	10%	N006927 001	

Lotion; Topical
CROTAN

	Firm	Strength	Appl. No.	Date
AT	SUMMERS	10%	N087204 001	

EURAX

	Firm	Strength	Appl. No.	Date
AT	+ WESTWOOD SQUIBB	10%	N009112 003	

CUPRIC CHLORIDE
Injectable; Injection
CUPRIC CHLORIDE IN PLASTIC CONTAINER

	Firm	Strength	Appl. No.	Date
	+ ABBOTT	EQ 0.4MG COPPER/ML	N018960 001	JUN 26, 1986

CYANOCOBALAMIN
Gel, Metered; Nasal
NASCOBAL

Firm	Strength	Appl. No.	Date
+ QUESTCOR PHARMS	0.5MG/INH	N019722 001	NOV 05, 1996

Injectable; Injection
CYANOCOBALAMIN

	Firm	Strength	Appl. No.	Date
AP	AM PHARM PARTNERS	0.1MG/ML	N080557 002	
AP	LUITPOLD	1MG/ML	N080737 001	
AP	STERIS	0.1MG/ML	N080573 002	
AP		1MG/ML	N080573 001	
AP		1MG/ML	N083120 002	

RUBRAMIN PC

	Firm	Strength	Appl. No.	Date
AP	+ BRISTOL MYERS SQUIBB	1MG/ML	N006799 010	APR 28, 1988

VIBISONE

	Firm	Strength	Appl. No.	Date
AP	AM PHARM PARTNERS	1MG/ML	N080557 003	

Tablet; Oral
CYANOCOBALAMIN

Firm	Strength	Appl. No.	Date
+ WEST WARD	1MG	N084264 001	

Prescription Drug Products (continued)

CYANOCOBALAMIN *MULTIPLE*
SEE ALPHA-TOCOPHEROL ACETATE; ASCORBIC ACID; BIOTIN; CHOLECALCIFEROL; CYANOCOBALAMIN; DEXPANTHENOL; FOLIC ACID; NIACINAMIDE; PYRIDOXINE HYDROCHLORIDE; RIBOFLAVIN PHOSPHATE SODIUM; THIAMINE HYDROCHLORIDE; VITAMIN A PALMITATE; VITAMIN K

SEE ASCORBIC ACID; BIOTIN; CHOLECALCIFEROL; CYANOCOBALAMIN; DEXPANTHENOL; FOLIC ACID; NIACINAMIDE; PYRIDOXINE; RIBOFLAVIN; THIAMINE; TOCOPHEROL ACETATE; VITAMIN A; VITAMIN K

SEE ASCORBIC ACID; BIOTIN; CYANOCOBALAMIN; DEXPANTHENOL; ERGOCALCIFEROL; FOLIC ACID; NIACINAMIDE; PHYTONADIONE; PYRIDOXINE HYDROCHLORIDE; RIBOFLAVIN PHOSPHATE SODIUM; THIAMINE HYDROCHLORIDE; VITAMIN A; VITAMIN E

SEE ASCORBIC ACID; BIOTIN; CYANOCOBALAMIN; DEXPANTHENOL; ERGOCALCIFEROL; FOLIC ACID; NIACINAMIDE; PYRIDOXINE HYDROCHLORIDE; RIBOFLAVIN PHOSPHATE SODIUM; THIAMINE HYDROCHLORIDE; VITAMIN A; VITAMIN E

SEE COBALT CHLORIDE, CO-57; CYANOCOBALAMIN; CYANOCOBALAMIN, CO-57; INTRINSIC FACTOR

CYANOCOBALAMIN, CO-57
Capsule; Oral

	RUBRATOPE-57			
	BRACCO	0.5-1uCi	N016089 002	

CYANOCOBALAMIN, CO-57 *MULTIPLE*
SEE COBALT CHLORIDE, CO-57; CYANOCOBALAMIN; CYANOCOBALAMIN, CO-57; INTRINSIC FACTOR

CYCLOBENZAPRINE HYDROCHLORIDE
Tablet; Oral

	CYCLOBENZAPRINE HCL			
AB	GENEVA PHARMS	10MG	N072854 001	NOV 19, 1991
AB	GENEVA PHARMS TECH	10MG	N073683 001	FEB 26, 1993
			N073541 001	MAY 23, 1995
AB	HALSEY	10MG	N073144 001	MAY 30, 1991
AB	MYLAN	10MG	N074421 001	SEP 29, 1995
AB	PLIVA	10MG	N071611 001	MAY 03, 1989
AB	WATSON LABS	10MG	N073143 001	NOV 27, 1991
AB		10MG	N074436 001	NOV 30, 1994
	FLEXERIL			
AB +	MCNEIL CONS SPECLT	5MG	N017821 001	
		10MG	N017821 002	

CYCLOPENTOLATE HYDROCHLORIDE
Solution/Drops; Ophthalmic

	AKPENTOLATE			
AT	AKORN	1%	N040164 001	JAN 13, 1997

CYCLOPENTOLATE HYDROCHLORIDE (continued)
Solution/Drops; Ophthalmic

	AKPENTOLATE			
AT	AKORN	2%	N040165 001	JAN 13, 1997
	CYCLOGYL			
AT +	ALCON	0.5%	N084109 001	
AT +		1%	N084110 001	
AT +		2%	N084108 001	
	CYCLOPENTOLATE HCL			
AT	ALCON UNIVERSAL	1%	N089162 001	JAN 24, 1991
	PENTOLAR			
AT	BAUSCH AND LOMB	1%	N040075 001	APR 29, 1994

CYCLOPENTOLATE HYDROCHLORIDE; PHENYLEPHRINE HYDROCHLORIDE
Solution/Drops; Ophthalmic

	CYCLOMYDRIL			
	+ ALCON	0.2%,1%	N084300 001	

CYCLOPHOSPHAMIDE
Injectable; Injection

	CYCLOPHOSPHAMIDE			
AP	BAXTER HLTHCARE	1GM/VIAL	N088374 001	SEP 24, 1986
AP		100MG/VIAL	N088371 001	JUL 03, 1986
AP		200MG/VIAL	N088372 001	JUL 03, 1986
AP		500MG/VIAL	N088373 001	JUL 03, 1986
	LYOPHILIZED CYTOXAN			
AP +	BRISTOL MYERS SQUIBB	1GM/VIAL	N012142 010	SEP 24, 1985
AP +		2GM/VIAL	N012142 009	DEC 10, 1984
AP +		100MG/VIAL	N012142 006	DEC 05, 1985
AP +		200MG/VIAL	N012142 007	DEC 10, 1985
AP +		500MG/VIAL	N012142 008	JAN 04, 1984
	NEOSAR			
AP	PHARMACIA AND UPJOHN	1GM/VIAL	N040015 004	APR 29, 1993
AP		1GM/VIAL	N087442 004	JUL 08, 1983
AP		2GM/VIAL	N040015 005	APR 29, 1993
AP		2GM/VIAL	N087442 005	MAR 30, 1989
AP		100MG/VIAL	N040015 001	

Prescription Drug Products *(continued)*

CYCLOPHOSPHAMIDE *(continued)*

Injectable; Injection
NEOSAR
PHARMACIA AND UPJOHN

TE	Strength	Appl. No.	Date
AP	100MG/VIAL	N087442 001	APR 29, 1993
AP	200MG/VIAL	N040015 002	FEB 16, 1982
AP	200MG/VIAL	N087442 002	APR 29, 1993
AP	500MG/VIAL	N040015 003	FEB 16, 1982
AP	500MG/VIAL	N087442 003	APR 29, 1993

Tablet; Oral
CYCLOPHOSPHAMIDE
ROXANE

TE	Strength	Appl. No.	Date
AB	25MG	N040032 001	AUG 17, 1999
AB	50MG	N040032 002	AUG 17, 1999

CYTOXAN
BRISTOL MYERS SQUIBB

TE	Strength	Appl. No.
AB	25MG	N012141 002
AB +	50MG	N012141 001

CYCLOSERINE

Capsule; Oral
SEROMYCIN
+ LILLY

Strength	Appl. No.
250MG	N060593 001

CYCLOSPORINE

Capsule; Oral
CYCLOSPORINE
EON

TE	Strength	Appl. No.	Date
AB1	25MG	N065017 002	JAN 13, 2000
AB1	100MG	N065017 001	JAN 13, 2000

PLIVA

TE	Strength	Appl. No.	Date
AB1	25MG	N065044 002	DEC 20, 2000
AB1	100MG	N065044 001	DEC 20, 2000

TORPHARM

TE	Strength	Appl. No.	Date
AB2	25MG	N065040 001	MAY 09, 2002
AB2	100MG	N065040 002	MAY 09, 2002

GENGRAF
ABBOTT

TE	Strength	Appl. No.	Date
AB1	25MG	N065003 001	MAY 12, 2000
BX	50MG	N065003 002	MAY 12, 2000
AB1	100MG	N065003 003	MAY 12, 2000

NEORAL
NOVARTIS

TE	Strength	Appl. No.	Date
AB1	25MG	N050715 001	JUL 14, 1995

CYCLOSPORINE *(continued)*

Capsule; Oral
NEORAL
+ NOVARTIS

TE	Strength	Appl. No.	Date
AB1	100MG	N050715 002	JUL 14, 1995

SANDIMMUNE
NOVARTIS

TE	Strength	Appl. No.	Date
AB2	25MG	N050625 001	MAR 02, 1990
BX	50MG	N050625 003	NOV 23, 1992
AB2 +	100MG	N050625 002	MAR 02, 1990

Emulsion; Ophthalmic
RESTASIS
+ ALLERGAN

Strength	Appl. No.	Date
0.05%	N050790 001	DEC 23, 2002

Injectable; Injection
CYCLOSPORINE
BEDFORD

TE	Strength	Appl. No.	Date
AP	50MG/ML	N065004 001	OCT 29, 1999

SANDIMMUNE
+ NOVARTIS

TE	Strength	Appl. No.	Date
AP	50MG/ML	N050573 001	NOV 14, 1983

Solution; Oral
CYCLOSPORINE
ABBOTT

TE	Strength	Appl. No.	Date
AB	100MG/ML	N065025 001	MAR 03, 2000

PLIVA

TE	Strength	Appl. No.	Date
AB	100MG/ML	N065054 001	DEC 18, 2001

NEORAL
+ NOVARTIS

TE	Strength	Appl. No.	Date
AB	100MG/ML	N050716 001	JUL 14, 1995

SANDIMMUNE
+ NOVARTIS

TE	Strength	Appl. No.	Date
BX	100MG/ML	N050574 001	NOV 14, 1983

CYPROHEPTADINE HYDROCHLORIDE

Syrup; Oral
CYPROHEPTADINE HCL
ALPHARMA

TE	Strength	Appl. No.
AA	2MG/5ML	N086833 001

PERIACTIN
+ MERCK

TE	Strength	Appl. No.
AA	2MG/5ML	N013220 002

Tablet; Oral
CYPROHEPTADINE HCL
ABC HOLDING

TE	Strength	Appl. No.	Date
AA	4MG	N088212 001	MAY 26, 1983

+ IVAX PHARMS

TE	Strength	Appl. No.
AA	4MG	N087056 001

PAR PHARM

TE	Strength	Appl. No.
AA	4MG	N087129 001

PLIVA

TE	Strength	Appl. No.	Date
AA	4MG	N088205 001	JUL 26, 1983

CYSTEAMINE BITARTRATE

Capsule; Oral
CYSTAGON
MYLAN

Strength	Appl. No.	Date
EQ 50MG BASE	N020392 001	AUG 15, 1994

Prescription Drug Products (continued)

CYSTEAMINE BITARTRATE (continued)

Capsule; Oral

TE	Product / Applicant	Strength	Application No.	Date
	CYSTAGON			
	+ MYLAN	EQ 150MG BASE	N020392 002	AUG 15, 1994

CYTARABINE

Injectable, Liposomal; Injection

TE	Product / Applicant	Strength	Application No.	Date
	DEPOCYT			
	+ SKYEPHARMA	10MG/ML	N021041 001	APR 01, 1999

Injectable; Injection

TE	Product / Applicant	Strength	Application No.	Date
	CYTARABINE			
AP	BEDFORD	1GM/VIAL	N074245 001	AUG 31, 1994
AP		2GM/VIAL	N074245 002	AUG 31, 1994
AP		100MG/VIAL	N071471 001	AUG 02, 1989
AP		500MG/VIAL	N071472 001	AUG 02, 1989
AP	+ FAULDING	20MG/ML	N071868 001	JUN 04, 1990
AP	+	20MG/ML	N072168 001	AUG 31, 1990
AP	+	20MG/ML	N072945 001	FEB 28, 1994
AP	+	100MG/ML	N075383 001	NOV 22, 1999
AP	GENSIA SICOR PHARMS	1GM/VIAL	N075206 004	DEC 30, 1998
AP		2GM/VIAL	N075206 003	DEC 30, 1998
AP		100MG/VIAL	N075206 001	DEC 30, 1998
AP	+	500MG/VIAL	N075206 002	DEC 30, 1998
	CYTOSAR-U			
AP	+ GENSIA SICOR PHARMS	1GM/VIAL	N016793 003	DEC 21, 1987
AP	+	2GM/VIAL	N016793 004	DEC 21, 1987
AP	+	100MG/VIAL	N016793 001	DEC 21, 1987
AP	+	500MG/VIAL	N016793 002	DEC 21, 1987

DACARBAZINE

Injectable; Injection

TE	Product / Applicant	Strength	Application No.	Date
	DACARBAZINE			
AP	AM PHARM PARTNERS	100MG/VIAL	N075371 001	AUG 27, 1999
AP		200MG/VIAL	N075371 002	AUG 27, 1999
AP	BEDFORD	200MG/VIAL	N075812 001	JUN 15, 2001
AP		500MG/VIAL	N075812 002	OCT 31, 2002

DACARBAZINE (continued)

Injectable; Injection

TE	Product / Applicant	Strength	Application No.	Date
	DACARBAZINE			
AP	FAULDING	200MG/VIAL	N075940 001	OCT 18, 2001
AP	GENSIA SICOR PHARMS	200MG/VIAL	N075259 002	AUG 27, 1998
AP	+	500MG/VIAL	N075259 001	SEP 22, 2000
	DTIC-DOME			
AP	+ BAYER PHARMS	100MG/VIAL	N017575 001	
AP	+	200MG/VIAL	N017575 002	

DACTINOMYCIN

Injectable; Injection

TE	Product / Applicant	Strength	Application No.	Date
	COSMEGEN			
	+ MERCK	0.5MG/VIAL	N050682 001	

DALFOPRISTIN; QUINUPRISTIN

Injectable; Iv (Infusion)

TE	Product / Applicant	Strength	Application No.	Date
	SYNERCID			
	+ KING PHARMS	350MG/VIAL;150MG/VIAL	N050748 001	SEP 21, 1999

DALTEPARIN SODIUM

Injectable; Injection

TE	Product / Applicant	Strength	Application No.	Date
	FRAGMIN			
	+ PHARMACIA AND UPJOHN	2,500 IU/0.2ML	N020287 001	DEC 22, 1994
			N020287 003	
	+	5,000 IU/0.2ML	N020287 002	MAR 18, 1996
	+	10,000 IU/ML	N020287 004	JAN 30, 1998

DANAZOL

Capsule; Oral

TE	Product / Applicant	Strength	Application No.	Date
	DANAZOL			
AB	BARR	50MG	N074582 003	MAY 29, 1998
AB		100MG	N074582 002	MAY 29, 1998
AB		200MG	N074582 001	AUG 09, 1996
	DANOCRINE			
AB	+ SANOFI SYNTHELABO	50MG	N017557 003	
AB		100MG	N017557 004	
AB		200MG	N017557 002	

DANTROLENE SODIUM

Capsule; Oral

TE	Product / Applicant	Strength	Application No.	Date
	DANTRIUM			
	+ PROCTER AND GAMBLE	25MG	N017443 001	
		50MG	N017443 003	
	+	100MG	N017443 002	

Prescription Drug Products (continued)

DANTROLENE SODIUM (continued)
Injectable; Injection
DANTRIUM

+ PROCTER AND GAMBLE	20MG/VIAL	N018264 001	

DAPIPRAZOLE HYDROCHLORIDE
Solution/Drops; Ophthalmic
REV-EYES

+ ANGELINI	0.5%	N019849 001	DEC 31, 1990

DAPSONE
Tablet; Oral
DAPSONE

JACOBUS	25MG	N086841 001	
+	100MG	N086842 001	

DAUNORUBICIN CITRATE
Injectable, Liposomal; Injection
DAUNOXOME

+ GILEAD	EQ 2MG BASE/ML	N050704 002	APR 08, 1996

DAUNORUBICIN HYDROCHLORIDE
Injectable; Injection
CERUBIDINE

AP	+ BEDFORD	EQ 20MG BASE/VIAL	N064103 001	FEB 03, 1995

DAUNORUBICIN HCL

AP	+ BEDFORD	EQ 5MG BASE/ML	N050731 001	JAN 30, 1998
AP	BIGMAR	EQ 20MG BASE/VIAL	N065000 001	MAY 25, 1999
AP	GENSIA SICOR PHARMS	EQ 5MG BASE/ML	N065035 001	JAN 24, 2000
AP		EQ 20MG BASE/VIAL	N064212 001	JUN 23, 1998
AP	+	EQ 50MG BASE/VIAL	N064212 002	MAY 03, 1999
AP	SUPERGEN	EQ 5MG BASE/VIAL	N065034 001	NOV 20, 2001

DEFEROXAMINE MESYLATE
Injectable; Injection
DESFERAL

+ NOVARTIS	2GM/VIAL	N016267 002	MAY 25, 2000
+	500MG/VIAL	N016267 001	

DELAVIRDINE MESYLATE
Tablet; Oral
RESCRIPTOR

AGOURON	100MG	N020705 001	APR 04, 1997
+	200MG	N020705 002	

DELAVIRDINE MESYLATE (continued)
Tablet; Oral
RESCRIPTOR

AGOURON		JUL 14, 1999

DEMECLOCYCLINE HYDROCHLORIDE
Tablet; Oral
DECLOMYCIN

WYETH PHARMS INC	150MG	N050261 002
+	300MG	N050261 003

DESERPIDINE; METHYCLOTHIAZIDE
Tablet; Oral
ENDURONYL

ABBOTT	0.25MG;5MG	N012775 001

ENDURONYL FORTE

+ ABBOTT	0.5MG;5MG	N012775 002

DESFLURANE
Liquid; Inhalation
SUPRANE

BAXTER HLTHCARE CORP	99.9%	N020118 001	SEP 18, 1992

DESIPRAMINE HYDROCHLORIDE
Tablet; Oral
DESIPRAMINE HCL

AB	EON	10MG	N074430 001	FEB 09, 1996
AB		25MG	N071601 001	JUN 05, 1987
AB		50MG	N071588 001	JUN 05, 1987
AB		75MG	N071602 001	OCT 05, 1987
AB		100MG	N071766 001	OCT 05, 1987
AB		150MG	N074430 002	FEB 09, 1996
AB	GENEVA PHARMS	10MG	N072099 001	MAY 24, 1988
AB		25MG	N072100 001	MAY 24, 1988
AB		50MG	N072101 001	MAY 24, 1988
AB		75MG	N072102 001	JUN 20, 1988
AB		100MG	N072103 001	JUN 20, 1988
AB		150MG	N072104 001	JUN 20, 1988
AB	PLIVA	25MG	N071800 001	DEC 08, 1987
AB		50MG	N071801 001	

Prescription Drug Products (continued)

DESIPRAMINE HYDROCHLORIDE (continued)

Tablet; Oral

DESIPRAMINE HCL

TE Code	Firm	Strength	Appl No	Date
	PLIVA			
AB		75MG	N071802 001	DEC 08, 1987
AB		100MG	N071803 001	DEC 08, 1987
AB		150MG	N071804 001	MAY 29, 1997
				MAY 29, 1997

NORPRAMIN

TE Code	Firm	Strength	Appl No	Date
	AVENTIS PHARMS			
AB		10MG	N014399 007	FEB 11, 1982
AB		25MG	N014399 001	
AB		50MG	N014399 003	
AB +		75MG	N014399 004	
AB +		100MG	N014399 005	
AB +		150MG	N014399 006	

DESIRUDIN

Injectable; Subcutaneous

IPRIVASK

TE Code	Firm	Strength	Appl No	Date
+	AVENTIS PHARMS	15MG/VIAL	N021271 001	APR 04, 2003

DESLORATADINE

Tablet, Orally Disintegrating; Oral

CLARINEX

TE Code	Firm	Strength	Appl No	Date
+	SCHERING	5MG	N021312 001	JUN 26, 2002

Tablet; Oral

CLARINEX

TE Code	Firm	Strength	Appl No	Date
+	SCHERING PLOUGH	5MG	N021165 001	DEC 21, 2001

DESMOPRESSIN ACETATE

Injectable; Injection

DDAVP

TE Code	Firm	Strength	Appl No	Date
AP +	AVENTIS	0.004MG/ML	N018938 001	MAR 30, 1984
		0.015MG/ML	N018938 002	APR 25, 1995

DESMOPRESSIN ACETATE

TE Code	Firm	Strength	Appl No	Date
AP	ABBOTT	0.004MG/ML	N075220 001	AUG 28, 2000
AP	BEDFORD	0.004MG/ML	N074575 001	FEB 18, 2000
AP	GENSIA SICOR PHARMS	0.004MG/ML	N074888 001	OCT 15, 1997

DESMOPRESSIN ACETATE PRESERVATIVE FREE

TE Code	Firm	Strength	Appl No	Date
AP	BEDFORD	0.004MG/ML	N074574 001	FEB 18, 2000

Solution; Nasal

DDAVP

TE Code	Firm	Strength	Appl No	Date
+	AVENTIS	0.01%	N017922 001	

DESMOPRESSIN ACETATE (continued)

Spray, Metered; Nasal

DDAVP (NEEDS NO REFRIGERATION)

TE Code	Firm	Strength	Appl No	Date
AB +	AVENTIS	0.01MG/SPRAY	N017922 003	AUG 07, 1996

DESMOPRESSIN ACETATE

TE Code	Firm	Strength	Appl No	Date
AB +	BAUSCH AND LOMB	0.01MG/SPRAY	N074830 001	JAN 25, 1999

MINIRIN

TE Code	Firm	Strength	Appl No	Date
AB +	FERRING	0.01MG/SPRAY	N021333 001	SEP 16, 2002

STIMATE

TE Code	Firm	Strength	Appl No	Date
+	AVENT S BEHRING	0.15MG/SPRAY	N020355 001	MAR 07, 1994

Tablet; Oral

DDAVP

TE Code	Firm	Strength	Appl No	Date
	AVENTIS	0.1MG	N019955 001	SEP 06, 1995
+		0.2MG	N019955 002	SEP 06, 1995

DESOGESTREL; ETHINYL ESTRADIOL

Tablet; Oral-21

DESOGESTREL AND ETHINYL ESTRADIOL

TE Code	Firm	Strength	Appl No	Date
AB	DURAMED PHARM BARR	0.15MG;0.03MG	N075256 001	AUG 12, 1999

Tablet; Oral-28

CYCLESSA

TE Code	Firm	Strength	Appl No	Date
+	ORGANON USA INC	0.1MG,0.125MG,0.15MG;0.025MG-G,0.025MG,0.025MG	N021090 001	DEC 20, 2000

DESOGEN

TE Code	Firm	Strength	Appl No	Date
AB	ORGANON USA INC	0.15MG;0.03MG	N020071 002	DEC 10, 1992

DESOGESTREL AND ETHINYL ESTRADIOL

TE Code	Firm	Strength	Appl No	Date
AB	DURAMED PHARM BARR	0.15MG;0.03MG	N075256 002	AUG 12, 1999

KARIVA

TE Code	Firm	Strength	Appl No	Date
AB	BARR	0.15MG;0.02MG;0.01MG	N075863 001	APR 05, 2002

MIRCETTE

TE Code	Firm	Strength	Appl No	Date
AB +	ORGANON USA INC	0.15MG;0.02MG;0.01MG	N020713 001	APR 22, 1998

ORTHO-CEPT

TE Code	Firm	Strength	Appl No	Date
AB +	ORTHO MCNEIL PHARM	0.15MG;0.03MG	N020301 002	DEC 14, 1992

DESONIDE

Cream; Topical

DESONIDE

TE Code	Firm	Strength	Appl No	Date
AB	COPLEY PHARM	0.05%	N074027 001	SEP 28, 1992
AB	TARO	0.05%	N073548 001	JUN 30, 1992

DESOWEN

TE Code	Firm	Strength	Appl No	Date
AB	GALDERMA LABS LP	0.05%	N019048 001	

Prescription Drug Products *(continued)*

DESONIDE *(continued)*

Cream; Topical
DESOWEN
  GALDERMA LABS LP — 0.05% — DEC 14, 1984
TRIDESILON
  + CLAY PARK — 0.05% — N017010 001

Lotion; Topical
DESONIDE
AB ALTANA — 0.05% — N075860 001 / MAR 19, 2002
DESOWEN
AB + GALDERMA LABS LP — 0.05% — N072354 001 / JAN 24, 1992

Ointment; Topical
DESONIDE
AB ALTANA — 0.05% — N075751 001 / MAR 12, 2001
AB TARO — 0.05% — N074254 001 / AUG 03, 1994
DESOWEN
AB + GALDERMA LABS LP — 0.05% — N071425 001 / JUN 15, 1988
TRIDESILON
AB + CLAY PARK — 0.05% — N017426 001

DESOXIMETASONE

Cream; Topical
DESOXIMETASONE
AB TARO — 0.05% — N073210 001 / NOV 30, 1990
AB   — 0.25% — N073193 001 / NOV 30, 1990
TOPICORT
AB + MEDICIS — 0.25% — N017856 001
TOPICORT LP
AB + MEDICIS — 0.05% — N018309 001

Gel; Topical
DESOXIMETASONE
AB TARO — 0.05% — N074904 001 / JUL 14, 1998
TOPICORT
AB + MEDICIS — 0.05% — N018586 001 / MAR 29, 1982

Ointment; Topical
DESOXIMETASONE
AB TARO — 0.25% — N074286 001 / JUN 07, 1996
TOPICORT
AB + MEDICIS — 0.25% — N018763 001 / SEP 30, 1983

DESOXYRIBONUCLEASE *MULTIPLE*
SEE CHLORAMPHENICOL; DESOXYRIBONUCLEASE; FIBRINOLYSIN

DEXAMETHASONE

Concentrate; Oral
DEXAMETHASONE INTENSOL
  + ROXANE — 1MG/ML — N088252 001 / SEP 01, 1983

Elixir; Oral
DEXAMETHASONE
AA ALPHARMA — 0.5MG/5ML — N084754 001
AA HEXADROL + ORGANON USA INC — 0.5MG/5ML — N012674 001
AA MYMETHASONE + MORTON GROVE — 0.5MG/5ML — N088254 001 / JUL 27, 1983

Solution; Oral
DEXAMETHASONE
  + ROXANE — 0.5MG/5ML — N088248 001 / SEP 01, 1983

Suspension/Drops; Ophthalmic
MAXIDEX
  + ALCON — 0.1% — N013422 001

Tablet; Oral
DECADRON
  + MERCK
AB — 0.5MG — N011664 001
BP — 0.25MG — N011664 004
AB — 0.75MG — N011664 002
AB — 1.5MG — N011664 003
BP — 4MG — N011664 005
BP — 6MG — N011664 006 / JUL 30, 1982

DEXAMETHASONE
  PAR PHARM
BP — 0.5MG — N088148 001 / APR 28, 1983
BP — 0.25MG — N088149 001
BP — 0.75MG — N088160 001 / APR 28, 1983
BP — 1.5MG — N088237 001
BP — 4MG — N088238 001 / APR 28, 1983
BP — 6MG — N088481 001

  ROXANE
AB — 0.5MG — N084611 001 / NOV 28, 1983
AB — 0.75MG — N084613 001
AB — 1.5MG — N084610 001
  — 1MG — N088306 001 / SEP 15, 1983
  — 2MG — N087916 001
AB — 4MG — N084612 001 / AUG 26, 1982
BP — 6MG — N088316 001 / SEP 15, 1983

HEXADROL
BP ORGANON USA — 4MG — N012675 010

Prescription Drug Products (continued)

DEXAMETHASONE; NEOMYCIN SULFATE; POLYMYXIN B SULFATE

Ointment; Ophthalmic

MAXITROL

TE	Firm	Strength	Appl. No.	Date
AT	+ FALCON PHARMS	0.1%;EQ 3.5MG BASE/GM;10,000 UNITS/GM	N050065 002	

NEOMYCIN AND POLYMYXIN B SULFATES AND DEXAMETHASONE

TE	Firm	Strength	Appl. No.	Date
AT	FOUGERA	0.1%;EQ 3.5MG BASE/GM;10,000 UNITS/GM	N062938 001	JUL 31, 1989
AT	BAUSCH AND LOMB	0.1%;EQ 3.5MG BASE/GM;10,000 UNITS/GM	N064063 001	JUL 25, 1994

Suspension/Drops; Ophthalmic

DEXACIDIN

TE	Firm	Strength	Appl. No.	Date
AT	NOVARTIS	0.1%;EQ 3.5MG BASE/ML;10,000 UNITS/ML	N062544 001	OCT 29, 1984

DEXASPORIN

TE	Firm	Strength	Appl. No.	Date
AT	BAUSCH AND LOMB	0.1%;EQ 3.5MG BASE/ML;10,000 UNITS/ML	N064135 001	SEP 13, 1995

MAXITROL

TE	Firm	Strength	Appl. No.	Date
AT	ALCON	0.1%;EQ 3.5MG BASE/ML;10,000 UNITS/ML	N062341 001	MAY 22, 1984
AT	+ FALCON PHARMS	0.1%;EQ 3.5MG BASE/ML;10,000 UNITS/ML	N050023 002	

NEOMYCIN AND POLYMYXIN B SULFATES AND DEXAMETHASONE

TE	Firm	Strength	Appl. No.	Date
AT	ALCON UNIVERSAL	0.1%;EQ 3.5MG BASE/ML;10,000 UNITS/ML	N062721 001	NOV 17, 1986

DEXAMETHASONE; TOBRAMYCIN

Ointment; Ophthalmic

TOBRADEX

TE	Firm	Strength	Appl. No.	Date
AB	+ ALCON	0.1%;0.3%	N050616 001	SEP 28, 1988

Suspension/Drops; Ophthalmic

TOBRADEX

TE	Firm	Strength	Appl. No.	Date
AB	+ ALCON	0.1%;0.3%	N050592 001	AUG 18, 1988

TOBRAMYCIN AND DEXAMETHASONE

TE	Firm	Strength	Appl. No.	Date
AB	BAUSCH AND LOMB	0.1%;0.3%	N064134 001	OCT 27, 1999

DEXAMETHASONE SODIUM PHOSPHATE

Injectable; Injection

DEXAMETHASONE

TE	Firm	Strength	Appl. No.	Date
AP	ELKINS SINN	EQ 4MG PHOSPHATE/ML	N084282 001	
AP		EQ 10MG PHOSPHATE/ML	N087702 001	SEP 07, 1982

DEXAMETHASONE SODIUM PHOSPHATE

TE	Firm	Strength	Appl. No.	Date
AP	AM PHARM	EQ 10MG PHOSPHATE/ML	N040491 001	APR 11, 2003
AP	AM PHARM PARTNERS	EQ 4MG PHOSPHATE/ML	N084916 001	
AP	+ GENSIA SICOR PHARMS	EQ 10MG PHOSPHATE/ML	N081126 001	

DEXAMETHASONE SODIUM PHOSPHATE (continued)

Injectable; Injection

DEXAMETHASONE SODIUM PHOSPHATE

TE	Firm	Strength	Appl. No.	Date
AP	GENSIA SICOR PHARMS			AUG 31, 1990
	+ LUITPOLD	EQ 4MG PHOSPHATE/ML	N087440 001	JUL 21, 1982

Solution/Drops; Ophthalmic, Otic

DECADRON

TE	Firm	Strength	Appl. No.	Date
	+ MERCK		N011984 001	

DEXAMETHASONE SODIUM PHOSPHATE

TE	Firm	Strength	Appl. No.	Date
AT	ALCON UNIVERSAL	EQ 0.1% PHOSPHATE	N088771 001	JAN 16, 1985
AT		EQ 0.1% PHOSPHATE	N040069 001	JUL 26, 1996
AT	BAUSCH AND LOMB	EQ 0.1% PHOSPHATE		

DEXCHLORPHENIRAMINE MALEATE

Syrup; Oral

MYLARAMINE

TE	Firm	Strength	Appl. No.	Date
AA	MORTON GROVE	2MG/5ML	N088251 001	MAR 23, 1984

POLARAMINE

TE	Firm	Strength	Appl. No.	Date
AA	SCHERING	2MG/5ML	N086837 001	JUL 19, 1982

Tablet; Oral

DEXCHLORPHENIRAMINE MALEATE

TE	Firm	Strength	Appl. No.	Date
AA	PLIVA	2MG	N088682 001	JAN 17, 1986

POLARAMINE

TE	Firm	Strength	Appl. No.	Date
AA	+ SCHERING	2MG	N086835 001	

DEXMEDETOMIDINE

Injectable; Injection

PRECEDEX

TE	Firm	Strength	Appl. No.	Date
	+ ABBOTT	EQ 100UGM BASE/ML	N021038 001	DEC 17, 1999

DEXMETHYLPHENIDATE HYDROCHLORIDE

Tablet; Oral

FOCALIN

TE	Firm	Strength	Appl. No.	Date
	NOVARTIS	2.5MG	N021278 001	NOV 13, 2001
		5MG	N021278 002	NOV 13, 2001
+		10MG	N021278 003	NOV 13, 2001

DEXPANTHENOL *MULTIPLE*

SEE ALPHA-TOCOPHEROL ACETATE; ASCORBIC ACID; BIOTIN; CHOLECALCIFEROL; CYANOCOBALAMIN; DEXPANTHENOL; FOLIC ACID; NIACINAMIDE; PYRIDOXINE HYDROCHLORIDE; RIBOFLAVIN PHOSPHATE SODIUM; THIAMINE HYDROCHLORIDE; VITAMIN A PALMITATE; VITAMIN K

SEE ASCORBIC ACID; BIOTIN; CHOLECALCIFEROL; CYANOCOBALAMIN; DEXPANTHENOL; FOLIC ACID; NIACINAMIDE; PYRIDOXINE; RIBOFLAVIN; THIAMINE; TOCOPHEROL ACETATE; VITAMIN A; VITAMIN K

Prescription Drug Products (continued)

DEXPANTHENOL *MULTIPLE* (continued)
SEE ASCORBIC ACID: BIOTIN: CYANOCOBALAMIN: DEXPANTHENOL: ERGOCALCIFEROL: FOLIC ACID: NIACINAMIDE: PHYTONADIONE: PYRIDOXINE HYDROCHLORIDE: RIBOFLAVIN PHOSPHATE SODIUM: THIAMINE HYDROCHLORIDE: VITAMIN A: VITAMIN E
SEE ASCORBIC ACID: BIOTIN: CYANOCOBALAMIN: DEXPANTHENOL: ERGOCALCIFEROL: FOLIC ACID: NIACINAMIDE: PYRIDOXINE HYDROCHLORIDE: RIBOFLAVIN PHOSPHATE SODIUM: THIAMINE HYDROCHLORIDE: VITAMIN A: VITAMIN E

DEXRAZOXANE HYDROCHLORIDE
Injectable; Injection
ZINECARD

	+	PHARMACIA AND UPJOHN	EQ 250MG BASE/VIAL	N020212 001 MAY 26, 1995
	+		EQ 500MG BASE/VIAL	N020212 002 MAY 26, 1995

DEXTROAMPHETAMINE SACCHARATE *MULTIPLE*
SEE AMPHETAMINE ASPARTATE: AMPHETAMINE SULFATE: DEXTROAMPHETAMINE SACCHARATE: DEXTROAMPHETAMINE SULFATE

DEXTROAMPHETAMINE SULFATE
Capsule, Extended Release; Oral
DEXEDRINE

AB	+	GLAXOSMITHKLINE	5MG	N017078 001
AB	+		10MG	N017078 002
AB	+		15MG	N017078 003

DEXTROAMPHETAMINE SULFATE

AB	BARR	5MG	N076137 001	JAN 18, 2002
AB		10MG	N076137 002	JAN 18, 2002
AB		15MG	N076137 003	JAN 18, 2002
AB	MALLINCKRODT	5MG	N076353 001	MAY 06, 2003
AB		10MG	N076353 002	MAY 06, 2003
AB		15MG	N076353 003	MAY 06, 2003

Tablet; Oral
DEXEDRINE

AA	GLAXOSMITHKLINE	5MG	N084935 001

DEXTROAMPHETAMINE SULFATE

AA	BARR	5MG	N040361 001	JAN 31, 2001
AA		10MG	N040361 002	JAN 31, 2001
AA	ENDO PHARMS	5MG	N040299 001	MAY 13, 1999
AA	KV PHARM	5MG	N040365 001	OCT 31, 2002
AA		10MG	N040367 001	OCT 31, 2002

DEXTROAMPHETAMINE SULFATE (continued)
Tablet; Oral
DEXTROAMPHETAMINE SULFATE

AA		MALLINCKRODT	5MG	N040436 001 JAN 29, 2002
AA			10MG	N040436 002 JAN 29, 2002

DEXTROSTAT

AA	+	SHIRE RICHWOOD	5MG	N084051 001
AA	+		10MG	N084051 002

DEXTROAMPHETAMINE SULFATE *MULTIPLE*
SEE AMPHETAMINE ASPARTATE: AMPHETAMINE SULFATE: DEXTROAMPHETAMINE SACCHARATE: DEXTROAMPHETAMINE SULFATE

DEXTROMETHORPHAN HYDROBROMIDE; PROMETHAZINE HYDROCHLORIDE
Syrup; Oral
PROMETH W/ DEXTROMETHORPHAN

AA	+	ALPHARMA	15MG/5ML;6.25MG/5ML	N088762 001 OCT 31, 1984

PROMETHAZINE HCL AND DEXTROMETHORPHAN HYDROBROMIDE

AA	HI TECH PHARMA	15MG/5ML;6.25MG/5ML	N040027 001 JUL 31, 1996

PROMETHAZINE W/ DEXTROMETHORPHAN

AA	MORTON GROVE	15MG/5ML;6.25MG/5ML	N088864 001 JAN 04, 1985

DEXTROMETHORPHAN HYDROBROMIDE *MULTIPLE*
SEE BROMPHENIRAMINE MALEATE: DEXTROMETHORPHAN HYDROBROMIDE: PSEUDOEPHEDRINE HYDROCHLORIDE

DEXTROSE
Injectable; Injection
DEXTROSE 2.5% IN PLASTIC CONTAINER

AP	B BRAUN	2.5GM/100ML	N018358 001

DEXTROSE 5% IN PLASTIC CONTAINER

AP	ABBOTT	5GM/100ML	N019466 001	JUL 15, 1985
AP		5GM/100ML	N019479 001	SEP 17, 1985
AP		50MG/ML	N016367 002	
AP		50MG/ML	N019222 001	JUL 13, 1984
AP	B BRAUN	5GM/100ML	N016730 001	
AP		5GM/100ML	N019626 002	FEB 02, 1988
AP	BAXTER HLTHCARE	50MG/ML	N016730 002	
AP		5GM/100ML	N016673 001	
AP		5GM/100ML	N020179 001	DEC 07, 1992
AP		50MG/ML	N016673 003	OCT 30, 1985
AP	DHL	50MG/ML	N020179 002	DEC 07, 1992
AP		5GM/100ML	N019971 001	

Prescription Drug Products *(continued)*

DEXTROSE *(continued)*
Injectable; Injection

DEXTROSE 5% IN PLASTIC CONTAINER
- DHL — SEP 28, 1995

DEXTROSE 10% IN PLASTIC CONTAINER
- AP ABBOTT 10GM/100ML N018080 001
- AP B BRAUN 10GM/100ML N018046 001
- AP 10GM/100ML N019626 004 FEB 02, 1988
- AP BAXTER HLTHCARE 10GM/100ML N016694 001

DEXTROSE 20% IN PLASTIC CONTAINER
- AP ABBOTT 20GM/100ML N018564 001 MAR 23, 1982
- AP BAXTER HLTHCARE 20GM/100ML N017521 004

DEXTROSE 25%
- AP ABBOTT 250MG/ML N019445 002 NOV 23, 1998

DEXTROSE 30% IN PLASTIC CONTAINER
- AP ABBOTT 30GM/100ML N019345 001 JAN 26, 1985
- AP BAXTER HLTHCARE 30GM/100ML N017521 003

DEXTROSE 40% IN PLASTIC CONTAINER
- AP ABBOTT 40GM/100ML N018562 001 MAR 23, 1982
- AP BAXTER HLTHCARE 40GM/100ML N017521 002

DEXTROSE 50% IN PLASTIC CONTAINER
- AP ABBOTT 50GM/100ML N018563 001 MAR 23, 1982
- AP 50GM/100ML N019894 001 DEC 26, 1989
- AP BAXTER HLTHCARE 50GM/100ML N017521 001
- AP 50GM/100ML N020047 001 JUL 02, 1991

DEXTROSE 60% IN PLASTIC CONTAINER
- AP ABBOTT 60GM/100ML N019346 001 JAN 25, 1985
- AP BAXTER HLTHCARE 60GM/100ML N017521 005 MAR 26, 1982

DEXTROSE 70% IN PLASTIC CONTAINER
- AP ABBOTT 70GM/100ML N018561 001 MAR 23, 1982
- AP 70GM/100ML N019893 001 DEC 26, 1989
- AP BAXTER HLTHCARE 70GM/100ML N017521 006 MAR 26, 1982
- AP 70GM/100ML N020047 003 JUL 02, 1991

DEXTROSE; MAGNESIUM ACETATE; POTASSIUM ACETATE; SODIUM CHLORIDE
Injectable; Injection

NORMOSOL-M AND DEXTROSE 5% IN PLASTIC CONTAINER
- ABBOTT 5GM/100ML;21MG/100ML;128MG/100ML;234MG/100ML N017610 001

DEXTROSE; MAGNESIUM ACETATE TETRAHYDRATE; POTASSIUM ACETATE; SODIUM CHLORIDE
Injectable; Injection

PLASMA-LYTE 56 AND DEXTROSE 5% IN PLASTIC CONTAINER
- BAXTER HLTHCARE 5GM/100ML;32MG/100ML;128MG/100ML;234MG/100ML N017385 001

DEXTROSE; MAGNESIUM CHLORIDE; POTASSIUM CHLORIDE; POTASSIUM PHOSPHATE, DIBASIC; SODIUM ACETATE
Injectable; Injection

ISOLYTE P W/ DEXTROSE 5% IN PLASTIC CONTAINER
- B BRAUN 5GM/100ML;31MG/100ML;130MG/100ML;26MG/100ML;320MG/100ML N019025 001 DEC 27, 1984

ISOLYTE P IN DEXTROSE 5% IN PLASTIC CONTAINER
- B BRAUN 5GM/100ML;31MG/100ML;130MG/100ML;26MG/100ML;320MG/100ML N019873 001 JUN 10, 1993

DEXTROSE; MAGNESIUM CHLORIDE; POTASSIUM CHLORIDE; POTASSIUM PHOSPHATE, DIBASIC; SODIUM CHLORIDE; SODIUM LACTATE; SODIUM PHOSPHATE, MONOBASIC, ANHYDROUS
Injectable; Injection

IONOSOL B AND DEXTROSE 5% IN PLASTIC CONTAINER
- ABBOTT 5GM/100ML;53MG/100ML;100MG/100ML;100MG/100ML;180MG/100ML;280MG/100ML;16MG/100ML N019515 001 MAY 08, 1986

DEXTROSE; MAGNESIUM CHLORIDE; POTASSIUM CHLORIDE; POTASSIUM PHOSPHATE, MONOBASIC; SODIUM CHLORIDE; SODIUM LACTATE
Injectable; Injection

DEXTROSE 5% AND ELECTROLYTE NO.48 IN PLASTIC CONTAINER
- BAXTER HLTHCARE 5GM/100ML;31MG/100ML;141MG/100ML;20MG/100ML;12MG/100ML;260MG/100ML N017484 001

DEXTROSE; MAGNESIUM CHLORIDE; POTASSIUM CHLORIDE; POTASSIUM PHOSPHATE, MONOBASIC; SODIUM LACTATE; SODIUM PHOSPHATE, MONOBASIC, ANHYDROUS
Injectable; Injection

IONOSCL MB AND DEXTROSE 5% IN PLASTIC CONTAINER
- ABBCTT 5GM/100ML;30MG/100ML;141MG/100ML;15MG/100ML;260MG/100ML;25MG/100ML N019513 001 MAY 08, 1986

Prescription Drug Products *(continued)*

DEXTROSE; MAGNESIUM CHLORIDE; POTASSIUM CHLORIDE; SODIUM ACETATE; SODIUM CHLORIDE
Injectable; Injection

ISOLYTE H W/ DEXTROSE 5% IN PLASTIC CONTAINER
B BRAUN   5GM/100ML;30MG/100ML;97MG/100ML;220MG/100ML;140MG/100ML   N018273 001

ISOLYTE H IN DEXTROSE 5% IN PLASTIC CONTAINER
B BRAUN   5GM/100ML;30MG/100ML;97MG/100ML;220MG/100ML;140MG/100ML   N019844 001   JUN 10, 1993

DEXTROSE; MAGNESIUM CHLORIDE; POTASSIUM CHLORIDE; SODIUM ACETATE; SODIUM CHLORIDE; SODIUM GLUCONATE
Injectable; Injection

PLASMA-LYTE 148 AND DEXTROSE 5% IN PLASTIC CONTAINER
AP   BAXTER HLTHCARE   5GM/100ML;30MG/100ML;37MG/100ML;368MG/100ML;526MG/100ML;502MG/100ML   N017451 001

NORMOSOL-R AND DEXTROSE 5% IN PLASTIC CONTAINER
ABBOTT   5GM/100ML;30MG/100ML;37MG/100ML;222MG/100ML;526MG/100ML;502MG/100ML   N017609 001

ISOLYTE S W/ DEXTROSE 5% IN PLASTIC CONTAINER
AP   B BRAUN   5GM/100ML;30MG/100ML;37MG/100ML;370MG/100ML;530MG/100ML;500MG/100ML   N018274 001

ISOLYTE S IN DEXTROSE 5% IN PLASTIC CONTAINER
AP   B BRAUN   5GM/100ML;30MG/100ML;37MG/100ML;370MG/100ML;530MG/100ML;500MG/100ML   N019843 001   AUG 09, 1993

DEXTROSE; POTASSIUM CHLORIDE
Injectable; Injection

DEXTROSE 5% AND POTASSIUM CHLORIDE 0.3% IN PLASTIC CONTAINER
AP   BRISTOL MYERS SQUIBB   5GM/100ML;300MG/100ML   N017634 002

DEXTROSE 5% AND POTASSIUM CHLORIDE 0.15% IN PLASTIC CONTAINER
AP   BRISTOL MYERS SQUIBB   5GM/100ML;150MG/100ML   N017634 001

DEXTROSE 5% AND POTASSIUM CHLORIDE 0.075% IN PLASTIC CONTAINER
AP   BRISTOL MYERS SQUIBB   5GM/100ML;75MG/100ML   N017634 004

DEXTROSE 5% AND POTASSIUM CHLORIDE 0.224% IN PLASTIC CONTAINER
AP   BRISTOL MYERS SQUIBB   5GM/100ML;224MG/100ML   N017634 003

POTASSIUM CHLORIDE 0.3% IN DEXTROSE 5% IN PLASTIC CONTAINER
AP   B BRAUN   5GM/100ML;300MG/100ML   N018744 004   NOV 09, 1982
     B BRAUN   5GM/100ML;300MG/100ML   N019699 006   SEP 29, 1989

POTASSIUM CHLORIDE 0.15% IN DEXTROSE 5% IN PLASTIC CONTAINER
AP   B BRAUN   5GM/100ML;150MG/100ML   N018744 002   NOV 09, 1982

DEXTROSE; POTASSIUM CHLORIDE *(continued)*
Injectable; Injection

POTASSIUM CHLORIDE 0.15% IN DEXTROSE 5% IN PLASTIC CONTAINER
AP   B BRAUN   5GM/100ML;150MG/100ML   N019699 004   SEP 29, 1989

POTASSIUM CHLORIDE 0.22% IN DEXTROSE 5% IN PLASTIC CONTAINER
B BRAUN   5GM/100ML;220MG/100ML   N018744 003   NOV 09, 1982

POTASSIUM CHLORIDE 0.075% IN DEXTROSE 5% IN PLASTIC CONTAINER
AP   B BRAUN   5GM/100ML;75MG/100ML   N018744 001   NOV 09, 1982

POTASSIUM CHLORIDE 20MEQ IN DEXTROSE 5% IN PLASTIC CONTAINER
ABBOTT   5GM/100ML;149MG/100ML   N018371 001

POTASSIUM CHLORIDE 30MEQ IN DEXTROSE 5% IN PLASTIC CONTAINER
ABBOTT   5GM/100ML;224MG/100ML   N018371 003

POTASSIUM CHLORIDE 40MEQ IN DEXTROSE 5% IN PLASTIC CONTAINER
AP   ABBOTT   5GM/100ML;298MG/100ML   N018371 002

DEXTROSE; POTASSIUM CHLORIDE; POTASSIUM LACTATE; SODIUM CHLORIDE; SODIUM PHOSPHATE, MONOBASIC, ANHYDROUS
Injectable; Injection

IONOSOL T AND DEXTROSE 5% IN PLASTIC CONTAINER
ABBOTT   5GM/100ML;111MG/100ML;256MG/100ML;146MG/100ML;207MG/100ML   N019514 001   MAY 08, 1986

DEXTROSE; POTASSIUM CHLORIDE; POTASSIUM PHOSPHATE, DIBASIC; SODIUM ACETATE; SODIUM CHLORIDE
Injectable; Injection

ISOLYTE M W/ DEXTROSE 5% IN PLASTIC CONTAINER
B BRAUN   5GM/100ML;150MG/100ML;130MG/100ML;280MG/100ML;91MG/100ML   N018270 001

ISOLYTE M IN DEXTROSE 5% IN PLASTIC CONTAINER
B BRAUN   5GM/100ML;150MG/100ML;130MG/100ML;280MG/100ML;91MG/100ML   N019870 001   JUN 10, 1993

DEXTROSE; POTASSIUM CHLORIDE; POTASSIUM PHOSPHATE, MONOBASIC; SODIUM CHLORIDE; SODIUM LACTATE
Injectable; Injection

DEXTROSE 5% AND ELECTROLYTE NO 75 IN PLASTIC CONTAINER
BAXTER HLTHCARE   5GM/100ML;205MG/100ML;100MG/100ML;120MG/100ML;220MG/100ML   N018840 001   JUN 29, 1983

Prescription Drug Products (continued)

DEXTROSE; POTASSIUM CHLORIDE; SODIUM CHLORIDE
Injectable; Injection

DEXTROSE 5%, SODIUM CHLORIDE 0.2% AND POTASSIUM CHLORIDE 20MEQ (K)
AP   BAXTER HLTHCARE   5GM/100ML;300MG/100ML;200MG/100ML   N018037 001

DEXTROSE 5%, SODIUM CHLORIDE 0.2% AND POTASSIUM CHLORIDE 5MEQ
AP   BAXTER HLTHCARE   5GM/100ML;75MG/100ML;200MG/100ML   N018037 002

DEXTROSE 5%, SODIUM CHLORIDE 0.2% AND POTASSIUM CHLORIDE 5MEQ (K)
AP   BAXTER HLTHCARE   5GM/100ML;150MG/100ML;200MG/100ML   N018037 003

DEXTROSE 5%, SODIUM CHLORIDE 0.2% AND POTASSIUM CHLORIDE 15MEQ (K)
AP   BAXTER HLTHCARE   5GM/100ML;224MG/100ML;200MG/100ML   N018037 004

DEXTROSE 5%, SODIUM CHLORIDE 0.2% AND POTASSIUM CHLORIDE 30MEQ
AP   BAXTER HLTHCARE   5GM/100ML;224MG/100ML;200MG/100ML   N018037 005   APR 13, 1982

DEXTROSE 5%, SODIUM CHLORIDE 0.2% AND POTASSIUM CHLORIDE 10MEQ
AP   BAXTER HLTHCARE   5GM/100ML;75MG/100ML;200MG/100ML   N018037 006   APR 13, 1982
    BAXTER HLTHCARE   5GM/100ML;150MG/100ML;200MG/100ML   N018037 007   APR 13, 1982

DEXTROSE 5%, SODIUM CHLORIDE 0.2% AND POTASSIUM CHLORIDE 20MEQ
AP   BAXTER HLTHCARE   5GM/100ML;150MG/100ML;200MG/100ML   N018037 008   APR 13, 1982

DEXTROSE 5%, SODIUM CHLORIDE 0.33% AND POTASSIUM CHLORIDE 40MEQ
AP   BAXTER HLTHCARE   5GM/100ML;300MG/100ML;200MG/100ML   N018037 009   APR 13, 1982

DEXTROSE 5%, SODIUM CHLORIDE 0.33% AND POTASSIUM CHLORIDE 5MEQ IN
PLASTIC CONTAINER
AP   BAXTER HLTHCARE   5GM/100ML;75MG/100ML;330MG/100ML   N018629 001   MAR 23, 1982

DEXTROSE 5%, SODIUM CHLORIDE 0.33% AND POTASSIUM CHLORIDE 10MEQ IN
PLASTIC CONTAINER
AP   BAXTER HLTHCARE   5GM/100ML;150MG/100ML;330MG/100ML   N018629 002   MAR 23, 1982

DEXTROSE 5%, SODIUM CHLORIDE 0.33% AND POTASSIUM CHLORIDE 15MEQ IN
PLASTIC CONTAINER
AP   BAXTER HLTHCARE   5GM/100ML;224MG/100ML;330MG/100ML   N018629 003   MAR 23, 1982

DEXTROSE 5%, SODIUM CHLORIDE 0.33% AND POTASSIUM CHLORIDE 20MEQ IN
PLASTIC CONTAINER
AP   BAXTER HLTHCARE   5GM/100ML;150MG/100ML;330MG/100ML   N018629 004   MAR 23, 1982

DEXTROSE 5%, SODIUM CHLORIDE 0.33% AND POTASSIUM CHLORIDE 10MEQ IN
PLASTIC CONTAINER
AP   BAXTER HLTHCARE   5GM/100ML;75MG/100ML;330MG/100ML   N018629 005

DEXTROSE; POTASSIUM CHLORIDE; SODIUM CHLORIDE (continued)
Injectable; In ection

DEXTROSE 5%, SODIUM CHLORIDE 0.33% AND POTASSIUM CHLORIDE 10MEQ IN
PLASTIC CONTAINER
    BAXTER HLTHCARE   MAR 23, 1982

DEXTROSE 5%, SODIUM CHLORIDE 0.33% AND POTASSIUM CHLORIDE 20MEQ IN
PLASTIC CONTAINER
    BAXTER HLTHCARE   5GM/100ML;300MG/100ML;330MG/100ML   N018629 006   MAR 23, 1982

DEXTROSE 5%, SODIUM CHLORIDE 0.33% AND POTASSIUM CHLORIDE 30MEQ
AP   BAXTER HLTHCARE   5GM/100ML;224MG/100ML;330MG/100ML   N018629 007   MAR 23, 1982

DEXTROSE 5%, SODIUM CHLORIDE 0.33% AND POTASSIUM CHLORIDE 40MEQ IN
AP   BAXTER HLTHCARE   5GM/100ML;300MG/100ML;330MG/100ML   N018629 008   MAR 23, 1982

DEXTROSE 5%, SODIUM CHLORIDE 0.45% AND POTASSIUM CHLORIDE 20MEQ (K)
IN PLASTIC CONTAINER
AP   BAXTER HLTHCARE   5GM/100ML;450MG/100ML   N018008 010

POTASSIUM CHLORIDE 0.3% IN DEXTROSE 5% AND SODIUM CHLORIDE
0.11% IN PLASTIC CONTAINER
AP   B BRAUN   5GM/100ML;300MG/100ML;110MG/100ML   N019630 006   FEB 17, 1988

POTASSIUM CHLORIDE 0.3% IN DEXTROSE 5% AND SODIUM CHLORIDE 0.2% IN
PLASTIC CONTAINER
AP   B BRAUN   5GM/100ML;300MG/100ML;200MG/100ML   N019630 012   FEB 17, 1988

POTASSIUM CHLORIDE 0.3% IN DEXTROSE 5% AND SODIUM CHLORIDE 0.33% IN
PLASTIC CONTAINER
AP   B BRAUN   5GM/100ML;300MG/100ML;330MG/100ML   N019630 018   FEB 17, 1988

POTASSIUM CHLORIDE 0.3% IN DEXTROSE 5% AND SODIUM CHLORIDE 0.45% IN
PLASTIC CONTAINER
AP   B BRAUN   5GM/100ML;450MG/100ML;330MG/100ML   N019630 024   FEB 17, 1988

POTASS UM CHLORIDE 0.3% IN DEXTROSE 5% AND SODIUM CHLORIDE 0.9% IN
PLAST C CONTAINER
AP   B BRAUN   5GM/100ML;300MG/100ML;900MG/100ML   N019630 030   FEB 17, 1988

POTASSIUM CHLORIDE 0.3% IN DEXTROSE 10% AND SODIUM
CHLORIDE 0.2% IN PLASTIC CONTAINER
    B BRAUN   10GM/100ML;300MG/100ML;200MG/100ML   N019630 036   FEB 17, 1988

Prescription Drug Products *(continued)*

DEXTROSE; POTASSIUM CHLORIDE; SODIUM CHLORIDE *(continued)*
Injectable; Injection

POTASSIUM CHLORIDE 0.3% IN DEXTROSE 10% AND SODIUM CHLORIDE 0.45% IN PLASTIC CONTAINER
B BRAUN
10GM/100ML;300MG/100ML;450MG/100ML
N019630 042
FEB 17, 1988

POTASSIUM CHLORIDE 0.3% IN DEXTROSE 10% AND SODIUM CHLORIDE 0.9% IN PLASTIC CONTAINER
B BRAUN
10GM/100ML;300MG/100ML;900MG/100ML
N019630 048
FEB 17, 1988

POTASSIUM CHLORIDE 0.3% IN DEXTROSE 3.3% AND SODIUM CHLORIDE 0.3% IN PLASTIC CONTAINER
B BRAUN
3.3GM/100ML;300MG/100ML;300MG/100ML
N019630 053
MAY 07, 1992

POTASSIUM CHLORIDE 0.11% IN DEXTROSE 5% AND SODIUM CHLORIDE 0.11% IN PLASTIC CONTAINER
B BRAUN
5GM/100ML;110MG/100ML;110MG/100ML
N019630 003
FEB 17, 1988

POTASSIUM CHLORIDE 0.11% IN DEXTROSE 5% AND SODIUM CHLORIDE 0.2% IN PLASTIC CONTAINER
B BRAUN
5GM/100ML;110MG/100ML;200MG/100ML
N019630 009
FEB 17, 1988

POTASSIUM CHLORIDE 0.11% IN DEXTROSE 5% AND SODIUM CHLORIDE 0.33% IN PLASTIC CONTAINER
B BRAUN
5GM/100ML;110MG/100ML;330MG/100ML
N019630 015
FEB 17, 1988

POTASSIUM CHLORIDE 0.11% IN DEXTROSE 5% AND SODIUM CHLORIDE 0.45% IN PLASTIC CONTAINER
B BRAUN
5GM/100ML;110MG/100ML;450MG/100ML
N019630 021
FEB 17, 1988

POTASSIUM CHLORIDE 0.11% IN DEXTROSE 5% AND SODIUM CHLORIDE 0.9% IN PLASTIC CONTAINER
B BRAUN
5GM/100ML;110MG/100ML;900MG/100ML
N019630 027
FEB 17, 1988

POTASSIUM CHLORIDE 0.11% IN DEXTROSE 10% AND SODIUM CHLORIDE 0.2% IN PLASTIC CONTAINER
B BRAUN
10GM/100ML;110MG/100ML;200MG/100ML
N019630 033
FEB 17, 1988

POTASSIUM CHLORIDE 0.11% IN DEXTROSE 10% AND SODIUM CHLORIDE 0.45% IN PLASTIC CONTAINER
B BRAUN
10GM/100ML;110MG/100ML;450MG/100ML
N019630 039
FEB 17, 1988

DEXTROSE; POTASSIUM CHLORIDE; SODIUM CHLORIDE *(continued)*
Injectable; Injection

POTASSIUM CHLORIDE 0.11% IN DEXTROSE 10% AND SODIUM CHLORIDE 0.9% IN PLASTIC CONTAINER
B BRAUN
10GM/100ML;110MG/100ML;900MG/100ML
N019630 045
FEB 17, 1988

POTASSIUM CHLORIDE 0.11% IN DEXTROSE 3.3% AND SODIUM CHLORIDE 0.3% IN PLASTIC CONTAINER
B BRAUN
3.3GM/100ML;110MG/100ML;300MG/100ML
N019630 050
MAY 07, 1992

POTASSIUM CHLORIDE 0.15% IN DEXTROSE 5% AND SODIUM CHLORIDE 0.11% IN PLASTIC CONTAINER
B BRAUN
5GM/100ML;150MG/100ML;110MG/100ML
N019630 004
FEB 17, 1988

POTASSIUM CHLORIDE 0.15% IN DEXTROSE 5% AND SODIUM CHLORIDE 0.2% IN PLASTIC CONTAINER
B BRAUN
5GM/100ML;150MG/100ML;200MG/100ML
N019630 010
FEB 17, 1988
AP

POTASSIUM CHLORIDE 0.15% IN DEXTROSE 5% AND SODIUM CHLORIDE 0.33% IN PLASTIC CONTAINER
B BRAUN
5GM/100ML;150MG/100ML;330MG/100ML
N019630 016
FEB 17, 1988
AP

POTASSIUM CHLORIDE 0.15% IN DEXTROSE 5% AND SODIUM CHLORIDE 0.45% IN PLASTIC CONTAINER
B BRAUN
5GM/100ML;150MG/100ML;450MG/100ML
N019630 022
FEB 17, 1988
AP

POTASSIUM CHLORIDE 0.15% IN DEXTROSE 5% AND SODIUM CHLORIDE 0.9% IN PLASTIC CONTAINER
B BRAUN
5GM/100ML;150MG/100ML;900MG/100ML
N019630 028
FEB 17, 1988
AP

POTASSIUM CHLORIDE 0.15% IN DEXTROSE 10% AND SODIUM CHLORIDE 0.2% IN PLASTIC CONTAINER
B BRAUN
10GM/100ML;150MG/100ML;200MG/100ML
N019630 034
FEB 17, 1988

POTASSIUM CHLORIDE 0.15% IN DEXTROSE 10% AND SODIUM CHLORIDE 0.45% IN PLASTIC CONTAINER
B BRAUN
10GM/100ML;150MG/100ML;450MG/100ML
N019630 040
FEB 17, 1988

POTASSIUM CHLORIDE 0.15% IN DEXTROSE 10% AND SODIUM CHLORIDE 0.9% IN PLASTIC CONTAINER
B BRAUN
10GM/100ML;150MG/100ML;900MG/100ML
N019630 046
FEB 17, 1988

Prescription Drug Products (continued)

DEXTROSE; POTASSIUM CHLORIDE; SODIUM CHLORIDE (continued)

Injectable; Injection

POTASSIUM CHLORIDE 0.15% IN DEXTROSE 3.3% AND SODIUM CHLORIDE 0.3% IN PLASTIC CONTAINER
B BRAUN — 3.3GM/100ML;150MG/100ML;300MG/100ML — N019630 051 — MAY 07, 1992

POTASSIUM CHLORIDE 0.22% IN DEXTROSE 5% AND SODIUM CHLORIDE 0.11% IN PLASTIC CONTAINER
B BRAUN — 5GM/100ML;220MG/100ML;110MG/100ML — N019630 005 — FEB 17, 1988

POTASSIUM CHLORIDE 0.22% IN DEXTROSE 5% AND SODIUM CHLORIDE 0.2% IN PLASTIC CONTAINER
B BRAUN — 5GM/100ML;220MG/100ML;200MG/100ML — N019630 011 — FEB 17, 1988

POTASSIUM CHLORIDE 0.22% IN DEXTROSE 5% AND SODIUM CHLORIDE 0.33% IN PLASTIC CONTAINER
B BRAUN — 5GM/100ML;220MG/100ML;330MG/100ML — N019630 017 — FEB 17, 1988

POTASSIUM CHLORIDE 0.22% IN DEXTROSE 5% AND SODIUM CHLORIDE 0.45% IN PLASTIC CONTAINER
B BRAUN — 5GM/100ML;220MG/100ML;450MG/100ML — N019630 023 — FEB 17, 1988

POTASSIUM CHLORIDE 0.22% IN DEXTROSE 5% AND SODIUM CHLORIDE 0.9% IN PLASTIC CONTAINER
B BRAUN — 5GM/100ML;220MG/100ML;900MG/100ML — N019630 029 — FEB 17, 1988

POTASSIUM CHLORIDE 0.22% IN DEXTROSE 10% AND SODIUM CHLORIDE 0.2% IN PLASTIC CONTAINER
B BRAUN — 10GM/100ML;220MG/100ML;200MG/100ML — N019630 035 — FEB 17, 1988

POTASSIUM CHLORIDE 0.22% IN DEXTROSE 10% AND SODIUM CHLORIDE 0.45% IN PLASTIC CONTAINER
B BRAUN — 10GM/100ML;220MG/100ML;450MG/100ML — N019630 041 — FEB 17, 1988

POTASSIUM CHLORIDE 0.22% IN DEXTROSE 10% AND SODIUM CHLORIDE 0.9% IN PLASTIC CONTAINER
B BRAUN — 10GM/100ML;220MG/100ML;900MG/100ML — N019630 047 — FEB 17, 1988

POTASSIUM CHLORIDE 0.22% IN DEXTROSE 3.3% AND SODIUM CHLORIDE 0.3% IN PLASTIC CONTAINER
B BRAUN — 3.3GM/100ML;220MG/100ML;300MG/100ML — N019630 052 — MAY 07, 1992

DEXTROSE; POTASSIUM CHLORIDE; SODIUM CHLORIDE (continued)

Injectable; Injection

POTASSIUM CHLORIDE 0.037% IN DEXTROSE 5% AND SODIUM CHLOR DE 0.11% IN PLASTIC CONTAINER
B BRAUN — 5GM/100ML;37MG/100ML;110MG/100ML — N019630 001 — FEB 17, 1988

POTASSIUM CHLORIDE 0.037% IN DEXTROSE 5% AND SODIUM CHLORIDE 0.2% IN PLASTIC CONTAINER
B BRAJN — 5GM/100ML;37MG/100ML;200MG/100ML — N019630 007 — FEB 17, 1988

POTASSIUM CHLORIDE 0.037% IN DEXTROSE 5% AND SODIUM CHLORIDE 0.33% IN PLASTIC CONTAINER
B BRAUN — 5GM/100ML;37MG/100ML;330MG/100ML — N019630 013 — FEB 17, 1988

POTASS UM CHLORIDE 0.037% IN DEXTROSE 5% AND SODIUM CHLORIDE 0.45% IN PLASTIC CONTAINER
B BRAUN — 5GM/100ML;37MG/100ML;450MG/100ML — N019630 019 — FEB 17, 1988

POTASSIUM CHLORIDE 0.037% IN DEXTROSE 5% AND SODIUM CHLOFIDE 0.9% IN PLASTIC CONTAINER
B BRAUN — 5GM/100ML;37MG/100ML;900MG/100ML — N019630 025 — FEB 17, 1988

POTASSIUM CHLORIDE 0.037% IN DEXTROSE 10% AND SODIUM CHLORIDE 0.2% IN PLASTIC CONTAINER
B BRAJN — 10GM/100ML;37MG/100ML;200MG/100ML — N019630 031 — FEB 17, 1988

POTASSIUM CHLORIDE 0.037% IN DEXTROSE 10% AND SODIUM CHLORIDE 0.45% IN PLASTIC CONTAINER
B BRAUN — 10GM/100ML;37MG/100ML;450MG/100ML — N019630 037 — FEB 17, 1988

POTASSIUM CHLORIDE 0.037% IN DEXTROSE 10% AND SODIUM CHLORIDE 0.9% IN PLASTIC CONTAINER
B BRAUN — 10GM/100ML;37MG/100ML;900MG/100ML — N019630 043 — FEB 17, 1988

POTASSIUM CHLORIDE 0.075% IN DEXTROSE 5% AND SODIUM CHLORIDE 0.11% IN PLASTIC CONTAINER
B BRAUN — 5GM/100ML;75MG/100ML;110MG/100ML — N019630 002 — FEB 17, 1988

POTASSIUM CHLORIDE 0.075% IN DEXTROSE 5% AND SODIUM CHLORIDE 0.2% IN PLASTIC CONTAINER
AP — B BRAUN — 5GM/100ML;75MG/100ML;200MG/100ML — N019630 008 — FEB 17, 1988

Prescription Drug Products *(continued)*

DEXTROSE; POTASSIUM CHLORIDE; SODIUM CHLORIDE *(continued)*
Injectable; Injection

POTASSIUM CHLORIDE 0.075% IN DEXTROSE 5% AND SODIUM CHLORIDE 0.33% IN PLASTIC CONTAINER
AP   B BRAUN   5GM/100ML;75MG/100ML;330MG/100ML   N019630 014   FEB 17, 1988

POTASSIUM CHLORIDE 0.075% IN DEXTROSE 5% AND SODIUM CHLORIDE 0.45% IN PLASTIC CONTAINER
AP   B BRAUN   5GM/100ML;75MG/100ML;450MG/100ML   N019630 020   FEB 17, 1988

POTASSIUM CHLORIDE 0.075% IN DEXTROSE 5% AND SODIUM CHLORIDE 0.9% IN PLASTIC CONTAINER
AP   B BRAUN   5GM/100ML;75MG/100ML;900MG/100ML   N019630 026   FEB 17, 1988

POTASSIUM CHLORIDE 0.075% IN DEXTROSE 10% AND SODIUM CHLORIDE 0.2% IN PLASTIC CONTAINER
B BRAUN   10GM/100ML;75MG/100ML;200MG/100ML   N019630 032   FEB 17, 1988

POTASSIUM CHLORIDE 0.075% IN DEXTROSE 10% AND SODIUM CHLORIDE 0.45% IN PLASTIC CONTAINER
B BRAUN   10GM/100ML;75MG/100ML;450MG/100ML   N019630 038   FEB 17, 1988

POTASSIUM CHLORIDE 0.075% IN DEXTROSE 10% AND SODIUM CHLORIDE 0.9% IN PLASTIC CONTAINER
B BRAUN   10GM/100ML;75MG/100ML;900MG/100ML   N019630 044   FEB 17, 1988

POTASSIUM CHLORIDE 0.075% IN DEXTROSE 3.3% AND SODIUM CHLORIDE 0.3% IN PLASTIC CONTAINER
B BRAUN   3.3GM/100ML;75MG/100ML;300MG/100ML   N019630 049   MAY 07, 1992

POTASSIUM CHLORIDE 5MEQ IN DEXTROSE 5% AND SODIUM CHLORIDE 0.45% IN PLASTIC CONTAINER
AP   BAXTER HLTHCARE   5GM/100ML;150MG/100ML;450MG/100ML   N018008 004
AP   ABBOTT   5GM/100ML;149MG/100ML;450MG/100ML   N018362 004   MAR 28, 1988
AP   5GM/100ML;74.5MG/100ML;450MG/100ML   N018362 008   MAR 28, 1988

POTASSIUM CHLORIDE 5MEQ IN DEXTROSE 5% AND SODIUM CHLORIDE 0.225% IN PLASTIC CONTAINER
ABBOTT   5GM/100ML;74.5MG/100ML;225MG/100ML   N018365 005   MAR 28, 1988
5GM/100ML;149MG/100ML;225MG/100ML   N018365 007   MAR 28, 1988

DEXTROSE; POTASSIUM CHLORIDE; SODIUM CHLORIDE *(continued)*
Injectable; Injection

POTASSIUM CHLORIDE 5MEQ IN DEXTROSE 5% AND SODIUM CHLORIDE 0.3% IN PLASTIC CONTAINER
ABBOTT   5GM/100ML;74.5MG/100ML;300MG/100ML   N018876 005   MAR 28, 1988
5GM/100ML;149MG/100ML;300MG/100ML   N018876 009   MAR 28, 1988

POTASSIUM CHLORIDE 5MEQ IN DEXTROSE 5% AND SODIUM CHLORIDE 0.9% IN PLASTIC CONTAINER
AP   BAXTER HLTHCARE   5GM/100ML;150MG/100ML;900MG/100ML   N019308 001   APR 05, 1985
AP   ABBOTT   5GM/100ML;74.5MG/100ML;900MG/100ML   N019691 001   MAR 24, 1988
AP   5GM/100ML;149MG/100ML;900MG/100ML   N019691 003   MAR 24, 1988

POTASSIUM CHLORIDE 10MEQ IN DEXTROSE 5% AND SODIUM CHLORIDE 0.45% IN PLASTIC CONTAINER
AP   BAXTER HLTHCARE   5GM/100ML;75MG/100ML;450MG/100ML   N018008 005   APR 28, 1982
AP   5GM/100ML;150MG/100ML;450MG/100ML   N018008 006   APR 28, 1982
AP   ABBOTT   5GM/100ML;74.5MG/100ML;450MG/100ML   N018362 005   MAR 28, 1988
AP   5GM/100ML;74.5MG/100ML;450MG/100ML   N018362 009   JUL 05, 1983

POTASSIUM CHLORIDE 10MEQ IN DEXTROSE 5% AND SODIUM CHLORIDE 0.225% IN PLASTIC CONTAINER
ABBOTT   5GM/100ML;74.5MG/100ML;225MG/100ML   N018365 002   JUL 05, 1983
5GM/100ML;149MG/100ML;225MG/100ML   N018365 006   MAR 28, 1988

POTASSIUM CHLORIDE 10MEQ IN DEXTROSE 5% AND SODIUM CHLORIDE 0.3% IN PLASTIC CONTAINER
ABBOTT   5GM/100ML;74.5MG/100ML;300MG/100ML   N018876 001   JAN 17, 1986
5GM/100ML;149MG/100ML;300MG/100ML   N018876 006   MAR 28, 1988

POTASSIUM CHLORIDE 10MEQ IN DEXTROSE 5% AND SODIUM CHLORIDE 0.9% IN PLASTIC CONTAINER
BAXTER HLTHCARE
AP   5GM/100ML;150MG/100ML;900MG/100ML   N019308 002   APR 05, 1985

Prescription Drug Products *(continued)*

DEXTROSE; POTASSIUM CHLORIDE; SODIUM CHLORIDE *(continued)*
Injectable; Injection

POTASSIUM CHLORIDE 10MEQ IN DEXTROSE 5% AND SODIUM CHLORIDE 0.9% IN PLASTIC CONTAINER
BAXTER HLTHCARE
AP 5GM/100ML;75MG/100ML;900MG/100ML N019308 004 APR 05, 1985
AP 5GM/100ML;74.5MG/100ML;900MG/100ML N019691 002 MAR 24, 1988
AP 5GM/100ML;149MG/100ML;900MG/100ML N019691 004 MAR 24, 1988

POTASSIUM CHLORIDE 15MEQ IN DEXTROSE 5% AND SODIUM CHLORIDE 0.45% IN PLASTIC CONTAINER
ABBOTT
AP 5GM/100ML;224MG/100ML;450MG/100ML N018362 006 MAR 28, 1988

POTASSIUM CHLORIDE 15MEQ IN DEXTROSE 5% AND SODIUM CHLORIDE 0.225% IN PLASTIC CONTAINER
ABBOTT 5GM/100ML;224MG/100ML;225MG/100ML N018365 008 MAR 28, 1988

POTASSIUM CHLORIDE 15MEQ IN DEXTROSE 5% AND SODIUM CHLORIDE 0.3% IN PLASTIC CONTAINER
ABBOTT 5GM/100ML;224MG/100ML;300MG/100ML N018876 007 MAR 28, 1988

POTASSIUM CHLORIDE 15MEQ IN DEXTROSE 5% AND SODIUM CHLORIDE 0.9% IN PLASTIC CONTAINER
BAXTER HLTHCARE
AP 5GM/100ML;224MG/100ML;900MG/100ML N019691 006 MAR 24, 1988

POTASSIUM CHLORIDE 20MEQ IN DEXTROSE 5% AND SODIUM CHLORIDE 0.45% IN PLASTIC CONTAINER
BAXTER HLTHCARE
AP 5GM/100ML;150MG/100ML;450MG/100ML N018008 007 APR 28, 1982
AP 5GM/100ML;298MG/100ML;450MG/100ML N018362 007 MAR 28, 1988
AP 5GM/100ML;149MG/100ML;450MG/100ML N018362 010 JUL 05, 1983

POTASSIUM CHLORIDE 20MEQ IN DEXTROSE 5% AND SODIUM CHLORIDE 0.225% IN PLASTIC CONTAINER
ABBOTT 5GM/100ML;149MG/100ML;225MG/100ML N018365 001
        5GM/100ML;298MG/100ML;225MG/100ML N018365 009 MAR 28, 1988

POTASSIUM CHLORIDE 20MEQ IN DEXTROSE 5% IN SODIUM CHLORIDE 0.3% IN PLASTIC CONTAINER
ABBOTT 5GM/100ML;149MG/100ML;300MG/100ML N018876 002 JAN 17, 1986

DEXTROSE; POTASSIUM CHLORIDE; SODIUM CHLORIDE *(continued)*
Injectable; Injection

POTASSIUM CHLORIDE 20MEQ IN DEXTROSE 5% AND SODIUM CHLORIDE 0.3% IN PLASTIC CONTAINER
ABBOTT 5GM/100ML;298MG/100ML;300MG/100ML N018876 008 MAR 28, 1988

POTASSIUM CHLORIDE 20MEQ IN DEXTROSE 5% AND SODIUM CHLORIDE 0.9% IN PLASTIC CONTAINER
BAXTER HLTHCARE
AP 5GM/100ML;300MG/100ML;900MG/100ML N019308 003 APR 05, 1985
AP 5GM/100ML;150MG/100ML;900MG/100ML N019308 005 APR 05, 1985
AP 5GM/100ML;149MG/100ML;900MG/100ML N019691 005 MAR 24, 1988
AP 5GM/100ML;298MG/100ML;900MG/100ML N019691 008 MAR 24, 1988

POTASSIUM CHLORIDE 30MEQ IN DEXTROSE 5% AND SODIUM CHLORIDE 0.45% IN PLASTIC CONTAINER
BAXTER HLTHCARE
AP 5GM/100ML;224MG/100ML;450MG/100ML N018008 008 APR 28, 1982
AP 5GM/100ML;224MG/100ML;450MG/100ML N018362 002

POTASSIUM CHLORIDE 30MEQ IN DEXTROSE 5% AND SODIUM CHLORIDE 0.225% IN PLASTIC CONTAINER
ABBOTT 5GM/100ML;224MG/100ML;225MG/100ML N018365 003 JUL 05, 1983

POTASSIUM CHLORIDE 30MEQ IN DEXTROSE 5% AND SODIUM CHLORIDE 0.3% IN PLASTIC CONTAINER
ABBOTT 5GM/100ML;224MG/100ML;300MG/100ML N018876 003 JAN 17, 1986

POTASSIUM CHLORIDE 30MEQ IN DEXTROSE 5% AND SODIUM CHLORIDE 0.9% IN PLASTIC CONTAINER
BAX'ER HLTHCARE
AP 5GM/100ML;224MG/100ML;900MG/100ML N019308 006 APR 05, 1985
AP 5GM/100ML;224MG/100ML;900MG/100ML N019691 007 MAR 24, 1988

POTASSIUM CHLORIDE 40MEQ IN DEXTROSE 5% AND SODIUM CHLORIDE 0.45% IN PLASTIC CONTAINER
BAXTER HLTHCARE
AP 5GM/100ML;300MG/100ML;450MG/100ML N018008 009 APR 28, 1982
AP 5GM/100ML;298MG/100ML;450MG/100ML N018362 003

Prescription Drug Products (continued)

DEXTROSE; POTASSIUM CHLORIDE; SODIUM CHLORIDE (continued)
Injectable; Injection

POTASSIUM CHLORIDE 40MEQ IN DEXTROSE 5% AND SODIUM CHLORIDE 0.225% IN PLASTIC CONTAINER
ABBOTT   5GM/100ML;298MG/100ML;225MG/100ML   N018365 004 JUL 05, 1983

POTASSIUM CHLORIDE 40MEQ IN DEXTROSE 5% AND SODIUM CHLORIDE 0.3% IN PLASTIC CONTAINER
ABBOTT   5GM/100ML;298MG/100ML;300MG/100ML   N018876 004 MAR 28, 1988

POTASSIUM CHLORIDE 40MEQ IN DEXTROSE 5% AND SODIUM CHLORIDE 0.9% IN PLASTIC CONTAINER
AP   BAXTER HLTHCARE   5GM/100ML;300MG/100ML;900MG/100ML   N019308 007 APR 05, 1985
AP   ABBOTT   5GM/100ML;298MG/100ML;900MG/100ML   N019691 009 MAR 24, 1988

DEXTROSE; SODIUM CHLORIDE
Injectable; Injection

DEXTROSE 2.5% AND SODIUM CHLORIDE 0.2% IN PLASTIC CONTAINER
B BRAUN   2.5GM/100ML;200MG/100ML   N019631 002 FEB 24, 1988

DEXTROSE 2.5% AND SODIUM CHLORIDE 0.9% IN PLASTIC CONTAINER
B BRAUN   2.5GM/100ML;900MG/100ML   N019631 005 FEB 24, 1988

DEXTROSE 2.5% AND SODIUM CHLORIDE 0.11% IN PLASTIC CONTAINER
B BRAUN   2.5GM/100ML;110MG/100ML   N019631 001 FEB 24, 1988

DEXTROSE 2.5% AND SODIUM CHLORIDE 0.33% IN PLASTIC CONTAINER
B BRAUN   2.5GM/100ML;330MG/100ML   N019631 003 FEB 24, 1988

DEXTROSE 2.5% AND SODIUM CHLORIDE 0.45% IN PLASTIC CONTAINER
AP   BAXTER HLTHCARE   2.5GM/100ML;450MG/100ML   N016697 001
AP   ABBOTT   2.5GM/100ML;450MG/100ML   N018096 001
AP   B BRAUN   2.5GM/100ML;450MG/100ML   N019631 004 FEB 24, 1988

DEXTROSE 3.3% AND SODIUM CHLORIDE 0.3% IN PLASTIC CONTAINER
B BRAUN   3.3GM/100ML;300MG/100ML   N019631 016 JAN 19, 1990

DEXTROSE 5% AND SODIUM CHLORIDE 0.2% IN PLASTIC CONTAINER
AP   B BRAUN   5GM/100ML;200MG/100ML   N019631 007 FEB 24, 1988

DEXTROSE 5% AND SODIUM CHLORIDE 0.3% IN PLASTIC CONTAINER
B BRAUN   5GM/100ML;300MG/100ML   N017799 001

DEXTROSE 5% AND SODIUM CHLORIDE 0.9% IN PLASTIC CONTAINER
AP   ABBOTT   5GM/100ML;900MG/100ML   N017585 001
AP   B BRAUN   5GM/100ML;900MG/100ML   N019631 010 FEB 24, 1988

DEXTROSE; SODIUM CHLORIDE (continued)
Injectable; Injection

DEXTROSE 5% AND SODIUM CHLORIDE 0.11% IN PLASTIC CONTAINER
B BRAUN   5GM/100ML;110MG/100ML   N019631 006 FEB 24, 1988

DEXTROSE 5% AND SODIUM CHLORIDE 0.33% IN PLASTIC CONTAINER
AP   B BRAUN   5GM/100ML;330MG/100ML   N019631 008 FEB 24, 1988

DEXTROSE 5% AND SODIUM CHLORIDE 0.45% IN PLASTIC CONTAINER
AP   ABBOTT   5GM/100ML;450MG/100ML   N017607 001
AP   B BRAUN   5GM/100ML;450MG/100ML   N019631 009 FEB 24, 1988

DEXTROSE 5% AND SODIUM CHLORIDE 0.225% IN PLASTIC CONTAINER
ABBOTT   5GM/100ML;225MG/100ML   N017606 001

DEXTROSE 5% IN SODIUM CHLORIDE 0.2% IN PLASTIC CONTAINER
AP   BAXTER HLTHCARE   5GM/100ML;200MG/100ML   N016689 001

DEXTROSE 5% IN SODIUM CHLORIDE 0.9% IN PLASTIC CONTAINER
AP   BAXTER HLTHCARE   5GM/100ML;900MG/100ML   N016678 001

DEXTROSE 5% IN SODIUM CHLORIDE 0.33% IN PLASTIC CONTAINER
AP   BAXTER HLTHCARE   5GM/100ML;330MG/100ML   N016687 001

DEXTROSE 5% IN SODIUM CHLORIDE 0.45% IN PLASTIC CONTAINER
AP   BAXTER HLTHCARE   5GM/100ML;450MG/100ML   N016683 001

DEXTROSE 10% AND SODIUM CHLORIDE 0.2% IN PLASTIC CONTAINER
B BRAUN   10GM/100ML;200MG/100ML   N019631 012 FEB 24, 1988

DEXTROSE 10% AND SODIUM CHLORIDE 0.9% IN PLASTIC CONTAINER
AP   BAXTER HLTHCARE   10GM/100ML;900MG/100ML   N016696 001
AP   B BRAUN   10GM/100ML;900MG/100ML   N019631 015 FEB 24, 1988

DEXTROSE 10% AND SODIUM CHLORIDE 0.11% IN PLASTIC CONTAINER
B BRAUN   10GM/100ML;110MG/100ML   N019631 011 FEB 24, 1988

DEXTROSE 10% AND SODIUM CHLORIDE 0.33% IN PLASTIC CONTAINER
B BRAUN   10GM/100ML;330MG/100ML   N019631 013 FEB 24, 1988

DEXTROSE 10% AND SODIUM CHLORIDE 0.45% IN PLASTIC CONTAINER
B BRAUN   10GM/100ML;450MG/100ML   N019631 014 FEB 24, 1988

DEXTROSE *MULTIPLE*
SEE   ALCOHOL; DEXTROSE
SEE   AMINO ACIDS; CALCIUM CHLORIDE; DEXTROSE; MAGNESIUM CHLORIDE; POTASSIUM CHLORIDE; POTASSIUM PHOSPHATE, DIBASIC; SODIUM CHLORIDE
SEE   AMINO ACIDS; CALCIUM CHLORIDE; DEXTROSE; MAGNESIUM CHLORIDE; POTASSIUM PHOSPHATE, DIBASIC; SODIUM ACETATE; SODIUM CHLORIDE
SEE   AMINO ACIDS; DEXTROSE
SEE   AMINO ACIDS; DEXTROSE; MAGNESIUM CHLORIDE; SODIUM PHOSPHATE, DIBASIC, HEPTAHYDRATE
SEE   AMINO ACIDS; DEXTROSE; MAGNESIUM CHLORIDE; POTASSIUM PHOSPHATE, DIBASIC; SODIUM CHLORIDE
SEE   CALCIUM CHLORIDE; DEXTROSE; GLUTATHIONE DISULFIDE; MAGNESIUM CHLORIDE; POTASSIUM CHLORIDE; SODIUM BICARBONATE; SODIUM CHLORIDE; SODIUM PHOSPHATE
SEE   CALCIUM CHLORIDE; DEXTROSE; MAGNESIUM CHLORIDE; POTASSIUM CHLORIDE; SODIUM ACETATE; SODIUM CHLORIDE

Prescription Drug Products (continued)

DEXTROSE *MULTIPLE* (continued)

SEE CALCIUM CHLORIDE; DEXTROSE; MAGNESIUM CHLORIDE; POTASSIUM CHLORIDE; SODIUM ACETATE; DEXTROSE; SODIUM CHLORIDE; SODIUM CITRATE

SEE CALCIUM CHLORIDE; DEXTROSE; MAGNESIUM CHLORIDE; POTASSIUM CHLORIDE; SODIUM ACETATE; SODIUM CHLORIDE; SODIUM LACTATE

SEE CALCIUM CHLORIDE; DEXTROSE; MAGNESIUM CHLORIDE; SODIUM ACETATE; SODIUM CHLORIDE

SEE CALCIUM CHLORIDE; DEXTROSE; MAGNESIUM CHLORIDE; SODIUM CHLORIDE; SODIUM

SEE CALCIUM CHLORIDE; DEXTROSE; MAGNESIUM CHLORIDE; SODIUM LACTATE

SEE CALCIUM CHLORIDE; DEXTROSE; MAGNESIUM SULFATE; POTASSIUM

SEE CALCIUM CHLORIDE; DEXTROSE; SODIUM BICARBONATE; SODIUM PHOSPHATE, DIBASIC, HEPTAHYDRATE

SEE CALCIUM CHLORIDE; DEXTROSE; POTASSIUM CHLORIDE; SODIUM ACETATE; SODIUM CHLORIDE

SEE CALCIUM CHLORIDE; DEXTROSE; POTASSIUM CHLORIDE; SODIUM CHLORIDE

SEE CALCIUM CHLORIDE; DEXTROSE; POTASSIUM CHLORIDE; SODIUM CHLORIDE; SODIUM LACTATE

DIATRIZOATE MEGLUMINE

Injectable; Injection

TE	Firm	Strength	Appl. No.	Date
	HYPAQUE			
AP	+ AMERSHAM HLTH	30%	N016403 002	
AP	+	60%	N016403 001	
	RENO-60			
AP	+ BRACCO	60%	N010040 016	
	RENO-DIP			
AP	+ BRACCO	30%	N010040 012	

Solution; Ureteral

TE	Firm	Strength	Appl. No.	Date
	RENO-30			
	BRACCO	30%	N010040 021	

Solution; Urethral

TE	Firm	Strength	Appl. No.	Date
	CYSTOGRAFIN			
AT	BRACCO	30%	N010040 018	
	CYSTOGRAFIN DILUTE			
	BRACCO	18%	N010040 022	NOV 09, 1982
	HYPAQUE-CYSTO			
AT	AMERSHAM HLTH	30%	N016403 003	

DIATRIZOATE MEGLUMINE; DIATRIZOATE SODIUM

Injectable; Injection

TE	Firm	Strength	Appl. No.	Date
	HYPAQUE-76			
AP	+ AMERSHAM HLTH	66%;10%	N086505 001	
	MD-76R			
AP	+ MALLINCKRODT	66%;10%	N019292 001	SEP 29, 1989
	RENOCAL-76			
AP	+ BRACCO	66%;10%	N089347 001	JUN 01, 1988
	RENOGRAFIN-60			
	+ BRACCO	52%;8%	N010040 006	
	RENOGRAFIN-76			
AP	+ BRACCO	66%;10%	N010040 001	

Solution; Oral, Rectal

TE	Firm	Strength	Appl. No.	Date
	GASTROGRAFIN			
AA	+ BRACCO	66%;10%	N011245 003	

DIATRIZOATE MEGLUMINE; DIATRIZOATE SODIUM (continued)

Solution; Oral, Rectal

TE	Firm	Strength	Appl. No.	Date
	MD-GASTROVIEW			
AA	MALLINCKRODT	66%;10%	N087388 001	

DIATRIZOATE MEGLUMINE; IODIPAMIDE MEGLUMINE

Solution; Intrauterine

TE	Firm	Strength	Appl. No.	Date
	SINOGRAFIN			
	BRACCO	52.7%;26.8%	N011324 002	

DIATRIZOATE SODIUM

For Solution; Oral, Rectal

TE	Firm	Strength	Appl. No.	Date
	HYPAQUE			
	AMERSHAM HLTH	100%	N011386 001	

Injectable; Injection

TE	Firm	Strength	Appl. No.	Date
	HYPAQUE			
	+ AMERSHAM HLTH	50%	N009561 001	

DIATRIZOATE SODIUM *MULTIPLE*

SEE DIATRIZOATE MEGLUMINE; DIATRIZOATE SODIUM

DIAZEPAM

Concentrate; Oral

TE	Firm	Strength	Appl. No.	Date
	DIAZEPAM INTENSOL			
	+ ROXANE	5MG/ML	N071415 001	APR 03, 1987

Gel; Rectal

TE	Firm	Strength	Appl. No.	Date
	DIASTAT			
	+ XCEL PHARMS	2.5MG/0.5ML	N020648 001	JUL 29, 1997
		5MG/ML	N020648 002	JUL 29, 1997
			N020648 003	JUL 29, 1997
		10MG/2ML	N020648 004	JUL 29, 1997
		15MG/3ML	N020648 005	JUL 29, 1997
	+	20MG/4ML		JUL 29, 1997

Injectable; Injection

TE	Firm	Strength	Appl. No.	Date
	DIAZEPAM			
AP	+ ABBOTT	5MG/ML	N071583 001	OCT 13, 1987
AP		5MG/ML	N071584 001	OCT 13, 1987
AP		5MG/ML	N072079 001	DEC 20, 1988
AP	LEDERLE	5MG/ML	N071309 001	JUL 17, 1987
AP		5MG/ML	N071310 001	JUL 17, 1987
AP	MARSAM PHARMS LLC	5MG/ML	N072370 001	JAN 29, 1993
AP		5MG/ML	N072397 001	JAN 29, 1993
AP	STERIS	5MG/ML	N070296 001	

Prescription Drug Products *(continued)*

DIAZEPAM *(continued)*

Injectable; Injection

DIAZEPAM

TE	Firm	Strength	Appl. No.	Date
	STERIS			FEB 12, 1986

Solution; Oral

DIAZEPAM

TE	Firm	Strength	Appl. No.	Date
	+ ROXANE	5MG/5ML	N070928 001	APR 03, 1987

Tablet; Oral

DIAZEPAM

TE	Firm	Strength	Appl. No.	Date
AB	BARR	2MG	N070152 001	NOV 01, 1985
AB		5MG	N070153 001	NOV 01, 1985
AB		10MG	N070154 001	NOV 01, 1985
AB	CLONMEL HLTHCARE	2MG	N070226 001	NOV 01, 1985
AB		5MG	N070227 001	SEP 26, 1985
AB		10MG	N070228 001	SEP 26, 1985
AB	GENEVA PHARMS	2MG	N070302 001	SEP 26, 1985
AB		5MG	N070303 001	DEC 20, 1985
AB		10MG	N070304 001	DEC 20, 1985
AB	IVAX PHARMS	2MG	N071307 001	DEC 10, 1986
AB		5MG	N071321 001	DEC 10, 1986
AB		10MG	N071322 001	DEC 10, 1986
AB	MYLAN	2MG	N070323 001	DEC 10, 1986
AB		5MG	N070324 001	SEP 04, 1985
AB		10MG	N070325 001	SEP 04, 1985
AB	PAR PHARM	2MG	N070462 001	SEP 04, 1985
AB		5MG	N070463 001	FEB 25, 1986
AB		10MG	N070464 001	FEB 25, 1986
AB	PUREPAC PHARM	2MG	N070781 001	FEB 25, 1986
AB		5MG	N070706 001	MAR 19, 1986
AB		10MG	N070707 001	MAR 19, 1986
AB	WATSON LABS	2MG	N071134 001	MAR 19, 1986
AB		5MG	N071135 001	FEB 03, 1987
AB		10MG	N071136 001	FEB 03, 1987

DIAZEPAM *(continued)*

Tablet; Oral

DIAZEPAM

TE	Firm	Strength	Appl. No.	Date
	WATSON LABS			

VALIUM

TE	Firm	Strength	Appl. No.	Date
AB	ROCHE	2MG	N013263 002	FEB 03, 1987
AB		5MG	N013263 004	
AB		10MG	N013263 006	

DIAZOXIDE

Injectable; Injection

HYPERSTAT

TE	Firm	Strength	Appl. No.	Date
	+ SCHERING	15MG/ML	N016996 001	

Suspension; Oral

PROGLYCEM

TE	Firm	Strength	Appl. No.	Date
	+ BAKER NORTON	50MG/ML	N017453 001	

DICLOFENAC POTASSIUM

Tablet; Oral

CATAFLAM

TE	Firm	Strength	Appl. No.	Date
AB	+ NOVARTIS	50MG	N020142 002	NOV 24, 1993

DICLOFENAC POTASSIUM

TE	Firm	Strength	Appl. No.	Date
AB	EON	50MG	N075582 001	FEB 23, 2001
AB	GENEVA PHARMS TECH	50MG	N075229 001	NOV 20, 1998
AB	MUTUAL PHARM	50MG	N075470 001	FEB 21, 2002
AB	MYLAN	50MG	N075463 001	JUL 26, 1999
AB	TEVA	50MG	N075219 001	AUG 06, 1998
AB	WATSON LABS	50MG	N075152 001	NOV 27, 1998

DICLOFENAC SODIUM

Gel; Topical

SOLARAZE

TE	Firm	Strength	Appl. No.	Date
	+ BIOGLAN PHARMA	3%	N021005 001	OCT 16, 2000

Solution/Drops; Ophthalmic

VOLTAREN

TE	Firm	Strength	Appl. No.	Date
	+ NOVARTIS	0.1%	N020037 001	MAR 28, 1991

Tablet, Delayed Release; Oral

DICLOFENAC SODIUM

TE	Firm	Strength	Appl. No.	Date
AB	ALPHAPHARM	50MG	N075281 002	FEB 12, 2002
AB		75MG	N075281 003	FEB 12, 2002
AB	CARLSBAD	25MG	N075185 002	NOV 13, 1998
AB		50MG	N075185 003	NOV 13, 1998
AB		75MG	N075185 001	NOV 13, 1998

Prescription Drug Products *(continued)*

DICLOFENAC SODIUM *(continued)*

Tablet, Delayed Release; Oral

DICLOFENAC SODIUM

TE	Applicant	Strength	Appl. No.	Approval Date
	CARLSBAD COPLEY PHARM	25MG	N074459 001	NOV 13, 1998
AB		50MG	N074459 002	JUN 25, 1997
AB		75MG	N074459 003	JUN 25, 1997
AB	GENEVA PHARMS	25MG	N074376 001	JUN 25, 1997
AB		50MG	N074376 002	SEP 28, 1995
AB		75MG	N074394 001	SEP 28, 1995
AB	MARTEC	50MG	N074986 001	NOV 30, 1995
AB		75MG	N074986 002	FEB 26, 1999
AB	PLIVA	50MG	N074432 002	FEB 26, 1999
AB		75MG	N074432 003	JUL 29, 1999
AB	PUREPAC PHARM	50MG	N074514 001	JUL 29, 1999
AB		75MG	N074514 002	MAR 26, 1996
AB	ROXANE	25MG	N074391 001	MAR 26, 1996
AB		50MG	N074391 002	JUN 29, 1995
AB		75MG	N074391 003	JUN 29, 1995
AB	TEVA	50MG	N074723 001	JUN 29, 1995
AB		75MG	N074390 001	MAR 30, 1999
AB	VOLTAREN + NOVARTIS	25MG	N019201 001	AUG 15, 1996
AB	+	50MG	N019201 002	JUL 28, 1988
AB	+	75MG	N019201 003	JUL 28, 1988

Tablet, Extended Release; Oral

DICLOFENAC SODIUM

TE	Applicant	Strength	Appl. No.	Approval Date
AB	BIOVAIL	100MG	N075492 001	FEB 11, 2000
AB	DEXCEL LTD	100MG	N076201 001	NOV 06, 2002
AB	MYLAN	100MG	N076152 001	DEC 13, 2001
AB	PUREPAC PHARM	100MG	N075910 001	JAN 07, 2002
AB	VOLTAREN-XR + NOVARTIS	100MG	N020254 001	MAR 08, 1996

DICLOFENAC SODIUM *(continued)*

Tablet, Extended Release; Oral

VOLTAREN-XR
NOVARTIS — MAR 08, 1996

DICLOFENAC SODIUM; MISOPROSTOL

Tablet, Delayed Release; Oral

ARTHROTEC

TE	Applicant	Strength	Appl. No.	Approval Date
	+ GD SEARLE LLC	50MG;0.2MG	N020607 001	DEC 24, 1997
	+	75MG;0.2MG	N020607 002	DEC 24, 1997

DICLOXACILLIN SODIUM

Capsule; Oral

DICLOXACILLIN SODIUM

TE	Applicant	Strength	Appl. No.	Approval Date
AB	APOTHECON	EQ 125MG BASE	N061454 002	
AB		EQ 250MG BASE	N061454 001	
AB		EQ 500MG BASE	N061454 003	
AB	+ TEVA	EQ 250MG BASE	N062286 001	JUN 03, 1982
AB		EQ 500MG BASE	N062286 002	JUN 03, 1982

For Suspension; Oral

DICLOXACILLIN SODIUM

TE	Applicant	Strength	Appl. No.	Approval Date
AB	+ APOTHECON	EQ 62.5MG BASE/5ML	N061455 001	JUN 03, 1982

DICYCLOMINE HYDROCHLORIDE

Capsule; Oral

TE	Applicant	Strength	Appl. No.	Approval Date
AB	BENTYL + AVENTIS PHARMS	10MG	N007409 003	OCT 15, 1984
AB	DICYCLOMINE HCL LANNETT	10MG	N084285 001	
AB	MYLAN	10MG	N040319 001	SEP 07, 1999
AB	WATSON LABS	10MG	N085082 001	JUN 19, 1986
AB	WEST WARD	10MG	N040204 001	FEB 28, 1997

Injectable; Injection

TE	Applicant	Strength	Appl. No.	Approval Date
AP	BENTYL + AVENTIS PHARMS	10MG/ML	N008370 001	OCT 15, 1984
AP	BENTYL PRESERVATIVE FREE + AVENTIS PHARMS	10MG/ML	N008370 002	OCT 15, 1984
AP	DICYCLOMINE HCL (PRESERVATIVE-FREE) BEDFORD	10MG/ML	N040465 001	JUN 30, 2003

Syrup; Oral

TE	Applicant	Strength	Appl. No.	Approval Date
AB	BENTYL + AVENTIS PHARMS	10MG/5ML	N007961 002	OCT 15, 1984

Prescription Drug Products (continued)

DICYCLOMINE HYDROCHLORIDE (continued)
Tablet; Oral

	BENTYL			
AB	+ AVENTIS PHARMS	20MG	N007409 001	OCT 15, 1984
	DICYCLOMINE HCL			
AB	LANNETT	20MG	N040230 001	FEB 26, 1999
AB	MYLAN	20MG	N040317 001	SEP 07, 1999
AB	WATSON LABS	20MG	N085223 001	JUL 30, 1986
AB	WEST WARD	20MG	N040161 001	OCT 01, 1996

DIDANOSINE
Capsule, Delayed Rel Pellets; Oral

	VIDEX EC			
	+ BRISTOL MYERS SQUIBB	125MG	N021183 001	OCT 31, 2000
	+	200MG	N021183 002	OCT 31, 2000
	+	250MG	N021183 003	OCT 31, 2000
	+	400MG	N021183 004	OCT 31, 2000

For Solution; Oral

	VIDEX			
	+ BRISTOL MYERS SQUIBB	10MG/ML	N020156 001	OCT 09, 1991
		100MG/PACKET	N020155 003	OCT 09, 1991
		167MG/PACKET	N020155 004	OCT 09, 1991
		250MG/PACKET	N020155 005	OCT 09, 1991

Tablet, Chewable; Oral

	VIDEX			
	+ BRISTOL MYERS SQUIBB	25MG	N020154 002	OCT 09, 1991
		50MG	N020154 003	OCT 09, 1991
		100MG	N020154 004	OCT 09, 1991
	+	150MG	N020154 005	OCT 09, 1991
		200MG	N020154 006	OCT 28, 1999

DIENESTROL
Cream; Vaginal

	DIENESTROL			
	+ ORTHO MCNEIL	0.01%	N006110 005	

DIETHYLPROPION HYDROCHLORIDE
Tablet, Extended Release; Oral

	TENUATE DOSPAN			
	+ AVENTIS PHARMS	75MG	N012546 001	

Tablet; Oral

	DIETHYLPROPION HCL			
AA	ABC HOLDING	25MG	N088267 001	AUG 25, 1983
AA		25MG	N088268 001	AUG 25, 1983
	TENUATE			
AA	+ AVENTIS PHARMS	25MG	N011722 002	

DIFENOXIN HYDROCHLORIDE *MULTIPLE*
SEE ATROPINE SULFATE; DIFENOXIN HYDROCHLORIDE

DIFLORASONE DIACETATE
Cream; Topical

	DIFLORASONE DIACETATE			
AB1	ALTANA	0.05%	N075187 001	MAR 30, 1998
AB2		0.05%	N076263 001	DEC 20, 2002
AB1	TARO	0.05%	N075508 001	APR 24, 2000
	FLORONE			
BX	+ PHARMACIA AND UPJOHN	0.05%	N017741 001	
	FLORONE E			
AB2	+ PHARMACIA AND UPJOHN	0.05%	N019259 001	AUG 28, 1985
	PSORCON			
AB1	+ DERMIK LABS	0.05%	N020205 001	NOV 20, 1992

Ointment; Topical

	DIFLORASONE DIACETATE			
AB	ALTANA	0.05%	N075374 001	APR 27, 1999
AB	TARO	0.05%	N075331 001	MAY 14, 1999
	FLORONE			
	+ PHARMACIA AND UPJOHN	0.05%	N017994 001	
	PSORCON			
AB	+ PHARMACIA AND UPJOHN	0.05%	N019260 001	AUG 28, 1985

DIFLUNISAL
Tablet; Oral

	DIFLUNISAL			
AB	GENEVA PHARMS	500MG	N074604 001	JUN 10, 1996
AB	ROXANE	250MG	N073562 001	NOV 27, 1992

Prescription Drug Products *(continued)*

DIFLUNISAL *(continued)*
Tablet; Oral

DIFLUNISAL

			Strength	Appl. No.	Date
	ROXANE				
AB			500MG	N073563 001	NOV 27, 1992
AB	TEVA		250MG	N073679 001	JUL 31, 1992
AB			500MG	N073673 001	JUL 31, 1992
	WATSON LABS				
AB			250MG	N074400 001	JUL 17, 1997
AB			500MG	N074400 002	JUL 17, 1997

DOLOBID

			Strength	Appl. No.	Date
	MERCK				
AB			250MG	N018445 001	APR 19, 1982
AB	+		500MG	N018445 002	APR 19, 1982

DIGOXIN
Capsule; Oral

LANOXICAPS

			Strength	Appl. No.	Date
	GLAXO WELLCOME				
AB			0.1MG	N018118 003	JUL 26, 1982
AB			0.2MG	N018118 001	JUL 26, 1982
AB	+		0.05MG	N018118 002	JUL 26, 1982

Injectable; Injection

DIGOXIN

			Strength	Appl. No.	Date
	ABBOTT				
AP			0.25MG/ML	N040093 001	MAY 16, 1996
AP			0.25MG/ML	N040206 001	AUG 28, 1998
	ELKINS SINN				
AP			0.25MG/ML	N083391 001	

DIGOXIN PEDIATRIC

			Strength	Appl. No.	Date
	ABBOTT				
AP			0.1MG/ML	N040092 001	APR 25, 1996

LANOXIN

			Strength	Appl. No.	Date
AP	+	GLAXOSMITHKLINE	0.25MG/ML	N009330 002	

LANOXIN PEDIATRIC

			Strength	Appl. No.	Date
AP	+	GLAXOSMITHKLINE	0.1MG/ML	N009330 004	

Tablet; Oral

DIGOXIN

			Strength	Appl. No.	Date
	AMIDE PHARM				
AB			0.25MG	N040282 002	DEC 23, 1999
AB			0.125MG	N040282 001	DEC 23, 1999
	CARACO				
AB			0.25MG	N076363 002	JAN 31, 2003
AB			0.125MG	N076363 001	JAN 31, 2003
	STEVENS J				
AB			0.25MG	N076268 002	JUL 26, 2002
AB			0.125MG	N076268 001	JUL 26, 2002

DIGOXIN *(continued)*
Tablet; Oral

LANOXIN

			Strength	Appl. No.	Date
AB	+	GLAXO WELLCOME	0.25MG	N020405 004	SEP 30, 1997
AB			0.125MG	N020405 002	SEP 30, 1997

DIHYDROCODEINE BITARTRATE *MULTIPLE*
SEE ACETAMINOPHEN; CAFFEINE; DIHYDROCODEINE BITARTRATE
SEE ASPIRIN; CAFFEINE; DIHYDROCODEINE BITARTRATE

DIHYDROERGOTAMINE MESYLATE
Injectable; Injection

D.H.E. 45

			Strength	Appl. No.	Date
AP	+	XCEL PHARMS	1MG/ML	N005929 001	

DIHYDROERGOTAMINE MESYLATE

			Strength	Appl. No.	Date
AP		BEDFORD	1MG/ML	N040453 001	JUN 09, 2003

DIHYDROERGOTAMINE MESYLATE

			Strength	Appl. No.	Date
AP		PADDOCK	1MG/ML	N040475 001	APR 28, 2003

Spray, Metered; Nasal

MIGRANAL

			Strength	Appl. No.	Date
AP	+	XCEL PHARM	0.5MG/INH	N020148 001	DEC 08, 1997

DILTIAZEM HYDROCHLORIDE
Capsule, Extended Release; Oral

CARDIZEM CD

			Strength	Appl. No.	Date
AB3	+	AVENTIS PHARMS	120MG	N020062 001	AUG 10, 1992
AB3	+		180MG	N020062 002	DEC 27, 1991
AB3	+		240MG	N020062 003	DEC 27, 1991
AB3	+		300MG	N020062 004	DEC 27, 1991

CARDIZEM SR

			Strength	Appl. No.	Date
AB1	+	AVENTIS PHARMS	60MG	N019471 001	JAN 23, 1989
AB1	+		90MG	N019471 002	JAN 23, 1989
AB1	+		120MG	N019471 003	JAN 23, 1989

CARTIA XT

			Strength	Appl. No.	Date
AB3		ANDRX PHARMS	120MG	N074752 002	JUL 09, 1998
AB3			180MG	N074752 001	JUL 09, 1998
AB3			240MG	N074752 003	JUL 09, 1998
AB3			300MG	N074752 004	JUL 09, 1998

DILACOR XR

			Strength	Appl. No.	Date
AB2	+	WATSON LABS	120MG	N020092 001	

Prescription Drug Products *(continued)*

DILTIAZEM HYDROCHLORIDE *(continued)*
Capsule, Extended Release; Oral

DILACOR XR
WATSON LABS

TE		Strength	Appl No	Date
AB2	+	180MG	N020092 002	MAY 29, 1992
AB2	+	240MG	N020092 003	MAY 29, 1992

DILTIAZEM HCL
ANDRX

TE	Strength	Appl No	Date
AB2	120MG	N074852 001	OCT 10, 1997
AB2	180MG	N074852 002	OCT 10, 1997
AB2	240MG	N074852 003	OCT 10, 1997

BIOVAIL

TE	Strength	Appl No	Date
AB1	60MG	N074845 001	SEP 15, 1999
AB1	90MG	N074845 002	SEP 15, 1999
AB3	120MG	N020939 001	JAN 28, 2000
AB1	120MG	N074845 003	SEP 15, 1999
AB3	120MG	N075116 001	DEC 23, 1999
AB3	180MG	N020939 002	JAN 28, 2000
AB3	180MG	N075116 002	DEC 23, 1999
AB3	240MG	N020939 003	JAN 28, 2000
AB3	240MG	N075116 003	DEC 23, 1999
AB3	300MG	N020939 004	JAN 28, 2000
AB3	300MG	N075116 004	DEC 23, 1999

MYLAN

TE	Strength	Appl No	Date
AB1	60MG	N074910 001	MAY 02, 1997
AB1	90MG	N074910 002	MAY 02, 1997
AB1	120MG	N074910 003	MAY 02, 1997
AB2	120MG	N075124 002	MAR 18, 1998
AB2	180MG	N075124 003	MAR 18, 1998
AB2	240MG	N075124 001	MAR 18, 1998

PUREPAC PHARM

TE	Strength	Appl No	Date
AB3	120MG	N074984 001	DEC 20, 1999
AB3	180MG	N074984 002	DEC 20, 1999
AB3	240MG	N074984 003	DEC 20, 1999
AB3	300MG	N074984 004	DEC 20, 1999

DILTIAZEM HYDROCHLORIDE *(continued)*
Capsule, Extended Release; Oral

DILTIAZEM HCL
TEVA

TE	Strength	Appl No	Date
AB1	60MG	N074079 001	NOV 30, 1993
AB1	90MG	N074079 002	NOV 30, 1993
AB1	120MG	N074079 003	NOV 30, 1993

TORPHARM

TE	Strength	Appl No	Date
AB2	120MG	N074943 003	DEC 19, 2000
AB2	180MG	N074943 002	DEC 19, 2000
AB2	240MG	N074943 001	AUG 06, 1998

TAZTIA XT
ANDRX PHARMS

TE	Strength	Appl No	Date
AB4	120MG	N075401 001	APR 10, 2003
AB4	180MG	N075401 002	APR 10, 2003
AB4	240MG	N075401 003	APR 10, 2003
AB4	300MG	N075401 004	APR 10, 2003
AB4	360MG	N075401 005	APR 10, 2003

TIAZAC
BIOVAIL

TE		Strength	Appl No	Date
AB4	+	120MG	N020401 001	SEP 11, 1995
AB4	+	180MG	N020401 002	SEP 11, 1995
AB4	+	240MG	N020401 003	SEP 11, 1995
AB4	+	300MG	N020401 004	SEP 11, 1995
AB4	+	360MG	N020401 005	SEP 11, 1995
	+	420MG	N020401 006	OCT 16, 1998

Injectable; Injection

CARDIZEM
AVENTIS PHARMS

TE		Strength	Appl No	Date
AP	+	100MG/VIAL	N020792 001	SEP 05, 1997
AP	+	5MG/ML	N020027 001	OCT 24, 1991

BIOVAIL

TE		Strength	Appl No	Date
AP	+	25MG/VIAL	N020027 003	AUG 18, 1995

DILTIAZEM HCL
ABBOTT

TE	Strength	Appl No	Date
AP	5MG/ML	N074941 001	APR 15, 1998

APOTEX

TE	Strength	Appl No	Date
AP	5MG/ML	N075004 001	FEB 16, 2000
AP	100MG/VIAL	N075853 001	DEC 17, 2002

BEDFORD

TE	Strength	Appl No	Date
AP	5MG/ML	N075375 001	SEP 30, 1999
AP	5MG/ML	N074617 001	

Prescription Drug Products (continued)

DILTIAZEM HYDROCHLORIDE (continued)

Injectable; Injection

DILTIAZEM HCL

TE	Applicant	Strength	Approval Date	Appl. No.
	BEDFORD			
AP	GENSIA SICOR PHARMS	5MG/ML	FEB 28, 1996	N074894 001
	+	10MG/ML	AUG 26, 1997	N074894 002
AP	+ INTL MEDICATION	5MG/ML	APR 19, 2002	N075749 001
AP	MERIDIAN MEDCL TECHN	5MG/ML	NOV 21, 2001	N075106 001
AP	TAYLOR PHARMA	5MG/ML	APR 29, 1999	N075086 001
			APR 09, 1998	

Tablet, Extended Release; Oral

CARDIZEM LA

TE	Applicant	Strength	Appl. No.	Approval Date
AB	+ BIOVAIL	120MG	N021392 001	FEB 06, 2003
AB	+	180MG	N021392 002	FEB 06, 2003
AB	+	240MG	N021392 003	FEB 06, 2003
AB	+	300MG	N021392 004	FEB 06, 2003
AB	+	360MG	N021392 005	FEB 06, 2003
AB	+	420MG	N021392 006	FEB 06, 2003

Tablet; Oral

CARDIZEM

TE	Applicant	Strength	Appl. No.	Approval Date
AB	AVENTIS PHARMS	30MG	N018602 001	NOV 05, 1982
AB		60MG	N018602 002	NOV 05, 1982
AB		90MG	N018602 003	DEC 08, 1986
AB		120MG	N018602 004	DEC 08, 1986

DILTIAZEM HCL

TE	Applicant	Strength	Appl. No.	Approval Date
AB	APOTHECON	30MG	N074051 001	MAR 31, 1993
AB		60MG	N074051 002	MAR 31, 1993
AB		90MG	N074051 003	MAR 31, 1993
AB		120MG	N074051 004	MAR 31, 1993
AB	CLONMEL HLTHCARE	30MG	N074093 001	MAR 31, 1993
AB		60MG	N074093 002	NOV 05, 1992
AB		90MG	N074093 003	NOV 05, 1992
AB		120MG	N074093 004	NOV 05, 1992
AB	COPLEY PHARM	30MG	N074067 001	NOV 05, 1992

DILTIAZEM HYDROCHLORIDE (continued)

Tablet; Oral

DILTIAZEM HCL

TE	Applicant	Strength	Approval Date	Appl. No.
	COPLEY PHARM			
AB		60MG	NOV 05, 1992	N074067 002
AB		90MG	NOV 05, 1992	N074067 003
AB		120MG	NOV 05, 1992	N074067 004
AB	IVAX PHARMS	30MG	NOV 05, 1992	N074168 001
AB		60MG	MAR 03, 1995	N074168 002
AB		90MG	MAR 03, 1995	N074168 003
AB		120MG	MAR 03, 1995	N074168 004
AB	MYLAN	30MG	MAR 03, 1995	N073185 001
AB		60MG	NOV 05, 1992	N073186 001
AB		90MG	NOV 05, 1992	N072837 001
AB		120MG	NOV 05, 1992	N072838 001
AB	TEVA	30MG	NOV 05, 1992	N074185 001
AB		60MG	MAY 31, 1995	N074185 002
AB		90MG	MAY 31, 1995	N074185 003
AB		120MG	MAY 31, 1995	N074185 004

DILTIAZEM MALATE; ENALAPRIL MALEATE

Tablet, Extended Release; Oral

TECZEM

TE	Applicant	Strength	Appl. No.	Approval Date
	+ BIOVAIL	EQ 180MG HCL;5MG	N020507 001	OCT 04, 1996

DIMENHYDRINATE

Injectable; Injection

DIMENHYDRINATE

Applicant	Strength	Appl. No.
+ STERIS	50MG/ML	N080615 001

DIMERCAPROL

Injectable; Injection

BAL

Applicant	Strength	Appl. No.
+ AKORN	10%	N005939 001

DIMETHYL SULFOXIDE

Solution; Intravesical

DIMETHYL SULFOXIDE

TE	Applicant	Strength	Appl. No.	Approval Date
AT	BIONICHE (CANADA)	50%	N076185 001	NOV 29, 2002

Prescription Drug Products (continued)

DIMETHYL SULFOXIDE (continued)
Solution; Intravesical
RIMSO-50

	Firm	Strength	Appl. No.	Date
AT	+ RES INDS	50%	N017788 001	

DIMYRISTOYL LECITHIN; PERFLEXANE
Injectable; Intravenous
IMAGENT

	Firm	Strength	Appl. No.	Date
	+ ALLIANCE PHARM	0.92MG/VIAL;0.092MG/VIAL	N021191 001	MAY 31, 2002

DINOPROSTONE
Gel; Endocervical
PREPIDIL

	Firm	Strength	Appl. No.	Date
	+ PHARMACIA AND UPJOHN	0.5MG/3GM	N019617 001	DEC 09, 1992

Insert, Extended Release; Vaginal
CERVIDIL

	Firm	Strength	Appl. No.	Date
	+ CONTROLLED THERAP	10MG	N020411 001	MAR 30, 1995

Suppository; Vaginal
PROSTIN E2

	Firm	Strength	Appl. No.	Date
	+ PHARMACIA AND UPJOHN	20MG	N017810 001	

DIPHENHYDRAMINE HYDROCHLORIDE
Capsule; Oral
DIPHENHYDRAMINE HCL

	Firm	Strength	Appl. No.	Date
AA	BARR	50MG	N080738 001	
AA	+ GENEVA PHARMS	25MG	N080832 001	
AA		50MG	N080832 002	
AA	+ HALSEY	25MG	N084506 001	
AA	ICN	25MG	N080596 001	
AA		50MG	N080592 001	
AA	LNK	25MG	N087977 001	JAN 27, 1983
AA		50MG	N087978 001	JAN 27, 1983
AA	MK LABS	25MG	N083087 001	
AA		50MG	N083087 002	
AA	MUTUAL PHARM	25MG	N089488 001	JAN 02, 1987
AA		50MG	N089489 001	JAN 02, 1987
AA	PVT FORM	25MG	N083027 001	
AA		50MG	N083027 002	
AA	SUPERPHARM	25MG	N089040 001	MAY 15, 1985
AA	WATSON LABS	25MG	N080728 001	
AA		50MG	N080727 001	

Elixir; Oral
DIPHENHYDRAMINE HCL

	Firm	Strength	Appl. No.	Date
AA	LANNETT	12.5MG/5ML	N080939 002	
AA	MK LABS	12.5MG/5ML	N083088 002	
AA	PHARM ASSOC	12.5MG/5ML	N087513 001	

DIPHENHYDRAMINE HYDROCHLORIDE (continued)
Elixir; Oral
DIPHENHYDRAMINE HCL
PHARM ASSOC

	Firm	Strength	Appl. No.	Date
AA	+ ROXANE	12.5MG/5ML	N080643 001	FEB 10, 1982

Injectable; Injection
BENADRYL

	Firm	Strength	Appl. No.	Date
AP	+ PARKE DAVIS	50MG/ML	N006146 002	

BENADRYL PRESERVATIVE FREE

	Firm	Strength	Appl. No.	Date
AP	+ PARKE DAVIS	50MG/ML	N009486 001	

DIPHENHYDRAMINE HCL

	Firm	Strength	Appl. No.	Date
AP	ABBOTT	50MG/ML	N040140 001	NOV 20, 1998
AP	AM PHARM PARTNERS	50MG/ML	N040466 001	MAY 28, 2002
AP	BAXTER HLTHCARE	50MG/ML	N080817 002	
		10MG/ML	N080873 001	
AP	+ STERIS	50MG/ML	N080873 002	

DIPHENHYDRAMINE HCL PRESERVATIVE FREE

	Firm	Strength	Appl. No.	Date
AP	INTL MEDICATION	50MG/ML	N084094 001	
AP	STERIS	50MG/ML	N080873 003	

DIPHENOXYLATE HYDROCHLORIDE *MULTIPLE*
SEE   ATROPINE SULFATE; DIPHENOXYLATE HYDROCHLORIDE

DIPIVEFRIN HYDROCHLORIDE
Solution/Drops; Ophthalmic
AKPRO

	Firm	Strength	Appl. No.	Date
AT	AKORN	0.1%	N074382 001	SEP 29, 1995

DIPIVEFRIN HCL

	Firm	Strength	Appl. No.	Date
AT	BAUSCH AND LOMB	0.1%	N074188 001	MAY 19, 1995
AT	FALCON PHARMS	0.1%	N073636 001	JUN 30, 1994

PROPINE

	Firm	Strength	Appl. No.	Date
AT	+ ALLERGAN	0.1%	N018239 001	

DIPYRIDAMOLE
Injectable; Injection
DIPYRIDAMOLE

	Firm	Strength	Appl. No.	Date
AP	ABBOTT	5MG/ML	N074601 001	DEC 19, 1997
AP	AM PHARM PARTNERS	5MG/ML	N074956 001	SEP 30, 1998
AP	APOTEX	5MG/ML	N075769 001	NOV 27, 2002
AP	BEDFORD	5MG/ML	N074939 001	APR 13, 1998
AP	ELKINS SINN	5MG/ML	N074521 001	OCT 18, 1996
AP	GENSIA SICOR PHARMS	5MG/ML	N074952 001	NOV 26, 1997

IV PERSANTINE

	Firm	Strength	Appl. No.	Date
AP	+ BOEHRINGER INGELHEIM	5MG/ML	N019817 001	

Prescription Drug Products (continued)

DIPYRIDAMOLE (continued)

Injectable; Injection
IV PERSANTINE
  BOEHRINGER INGELHEIM   DEC 13, 1990

Tablet; Oral
DIPYRIDAMOLE

AB	BARR	25MG	N087184 001	OCT 03, 1990
AB		50MG	N087716 001	OCT 03, 1990
AB		75MG	N087717 001	OCT 03, 1990
AB	CLONMEL HLTHCARE	25MG	N088999 001	FEB 05, 1991
AB		50MG	N089000 001	FEB 05, 1991
AB		75MG	N089001 001	FEB 05, 1991
AB	GENEVA PHARMS	25MG	N086944 002	APR 16, 1991
AB		50MG	N087562 001	FEB 25, 1992
AB		75MG	N087561 001	FEB 25, 1992
AB	PUREPAC PHARM	25MG	N089425 001	JUL 12, 1990
AB	WATSON LABS	50MG	N087160 001	JUN 07, 1996

PERSANTINE
BOEHRINGER INGELHEIM

AB	25MG	N012836 003	DEC 22, 1986
AB	50MG	N012836 004	FEB 06, 1987
AB +	75MG	N012836 005	FEB 06, 1987

DIPYRIDAMOLE *MULTIPLE*
SEE ASPIRIN; DIPYRIDAMOLE

DIRITHROMYCIN
Tablet, Delayed Release; Oral
DYNABAC

+	LILLY RES LABS	250MG	N050678 001	JUN 19, 1995

DISOPYRAMIDE PHOSPHATE
Capsule, Extended Release; Oral
DISOPYRAMIDE PHOSPHATE

AB	KV PHARM	EQ 150MG BASE	N071200 001	DEC 15, 1987

NORPACE CR
GD SEARLE LLC

AB	EQ 100MG BASE	N018655 001	JUL 20, 1982
AB +	EQ 150MG BASE	N018655 002	

DISOPYRAMIDE PHOSPHATE (continued)
Capsule, Extended Release; Oral
NORPACE CR
  GD SEARLE LLC   JUL 20, 1982

Capsule; Oral
DISOPYRAMIDE PHOSPHATE

AB	GENEVA PHARMS	EQ 100MG BASE	N070470 001	DEC 10, 1985
AB		EQ 150MG BASE	N070471 001	DEC 10, 1985
AB	IVAX PHARMS	EQ 100MG BASE	N070186 001	NOV 18, 1985
AB		EQ 150MG BASE	N070187 001	NOV 18, 1985
AB	SUPERPHARM	EQ 100MG BASE	N070940 001	FEB 09, 1987
AB	TEVA	EQ 100MG BASE	N070101 001	FEB 22, 1985
AB		EQ 150MG BASE	N070102 001	FEB 22, 1985
AB	WATSON LABS	EQ 100MG BASE	N070173 001	MAY 31, 1985
AB		EQ 150MG BASE	N070174 001	MAY 31, 1985

NORPACE

AB	GD SEARLE LLC	EQ 100MG BASE	N017447 001	
AB +		EQ 150MG BASE	N017447 002	

DISULFIRAM
Tablet; Oral
ANTABUSE

+	ODYSSEY PHARMS	250MG	N008482 001	DEC 08, 1983

DIVALPROEX SODIUM
Capsule, Delayed Rel Pellets; Oral
DEPAKOTE

+	ABBOTT	EQ 125MG VALPROIC ACID	N019680 001	SEP 12, 1989

Tablet, Delayed Release; Oral
DEPAKOTE

+	ABBOTT	EQ 125MG VALPROIC ACID	N018723 003	OCT 26, 1984
+		EQ 250MG VALPROIC ACID	N018723 001	MAR 10, 1983
+		EQ 500MG VALPROIC ACID	N018723 002	MAR 10, 1983

Tablet, Extended Release; Oral
DEPAKOTE ER

	ABBOTT	EQ 250MG VALPROIC ACID	N021168 002	MAY 31, 2002
+		EQ 500MG VALPROIC ACID	N021168 001	AUG 04, 2000

Prescription Drug Products *(continued)*

DOBUTAMINE HYDROCHLORIDE
Injectable; Injection
  DOBUTAMINE HCL

AP	+ ABBOTT	EQ 1.25GM BASE/100ML	N074634 001	SEP 27, 1996
AP		EQ 12.5MG BASE/ML	N074086 001	NOV 29, 1993
AP		EQ 12.5MG BASE/ML	N074292 001	FEB 16, 1995
AP	ASTRAZENECA	EQ 12.5MG BASE/ML	N074098 001	FEB 21, 1995
AP	BEDFORD	EQ 12.5MG BASE/ML	N074277 001	OCT 31, 1994
AP	GENSIA SICOR PHARMS	EQ 12.5MG BASE/ML	N074206 001	OCT 19, 1993
AP	LUITPOLD	EQ 12.5MG BASE/ML	N074545 001	JUN 25, 1998
AP	MARSAM PHARMS LLC	EQ 12.5MG BASE/ML	N074279 001	FEB 18, 1998
AP	STERIS	EQ 12.5MG BASE/ML	N074995 001	MAR 31, 1998
AP		EQ 12.5MG BASE/ML	N074114 001	NOV 30, 1993

  DOBUTAMINE HCL IN DEXTROSE 5%

AP	+ ABBOTT	EQ 50MG BASE/100ML	N020269 001	OCT 19, 1993
AP	+	EQ 100MG BASE/100ML	N020269 002	OCT 19, 1993
AP	+	EQ 200MG BASE/100ML	N020269 003	OCT 19, 1993

  DOBUTAMINE HCL IN DEXTROSE 5% IN PLASTIC CONTAINER

AP	+ ABBOTT	EQ 200MG BASE/100ML	N020201 001	OCT 19, 1993
AP	+	EQ 100MG BASE/100ML	N020201 002	OCT 19, 1993
AP	+	EQ 50MG BASE/100ML	N020201 003	OCT 19, 1993
AP	+	EQ 400MG BASE/100ML	N020201 006	JUL 07, 1994
AP	+ BAXTER HLTHCARE	EQ 50MG BASE/100ML	N020255 001	OCT 19, 1993
AP	+	EQ 100MG BASE/100ML	N020255 003	OCT 19, 1993
AP	+	EQ 200MG BASE/100ML	N020255 004	OCT 19, 1993
AP	+	EQ 400MG BASE/100ML	N020255 005	OCT 19, 1993

  DOBUTREX

AP	+ LILLY	EQ 12.5MG BASE/ML	N017820 002	

DOCETAXEL
Injectable; Injection
  TAXOTERE

	+ AVENTIS PHARMS	EQ 40MG BASE/ML	N020449 001	MAY 14, 1996

DOFETILIDE
Capsule; Oral
  TIKOSYN

	+ PFIZER	0.5MG	N020931 003	OCT 01, 1999
		0.25MG	N020931 002	OCT 01, 1999
		0.125MG	N020931 001	OCT 01, 1999

DOLASETRON MESYLATE MONOHYDRATE
Injectable; Injection
  ANZEMET

	AVENTIS PHARMS	EQ 12.5MG BASE/ML	N020624 002	SEP 11, 1997
	+	EQ 20MG BASE/ML	N020624 001	SEP 11, 1997

Tablet; Oral
  ANZEMET

	AVENTIS PHARMS	EQ 50MG BASE	N020623 001	SEP 11, 1997
	+	EQ 100MG BASE	N020623 002	SEP 11, 1997

DONEPEZIL HYDROCHLORIDE
Tablet; Oral
  ARICEPT

	EISAI MEDCL RES	5MG	N020690 002	NOV 25, 1996
	+	10MG	N020690 001	NOV 25, 1996

DOPAMINE HYDROCHLORIDE
Injectable; Injection
  DOPAMINE HCL

AP	+ ABBOTT	40MG/ML	N018132 001	
AP		40MG/ML	N074403 001	MAY 23, 1996
AP	+	80MG/100ML	N018132 002	FEB 04, 1982
AP	+	80MG/ML	N018132 004	JUL 09, 1982
AP	+	160MG/100ML	N018132 003	FEB 04, 1982
AP	+	80MG/ML	N070013 001	JUN 12, 1985
AP	+ AM PHARM PARTNERS	80MG/ML	N018656 001	JUN 28, 1983
AP	+ ASTRAZENECA	40MG/ML	N070091 001	OCT 23, 1985
AP		80MG/ML	N070092 001	OCT 23, 1985
AP		160MG/ML	N072999 001	OCT 23, 1991
AP	GENSIA SICOR PHARMS	40MG/ML	N073000 001	OCT 23, 1991
AP		80MG/ML		

Prescription Drug Products (continued)

DOPAMINE HYDROCHLORIDE (continued)
Injectable; Injection

DOPAMINE HCL

TE		Applicant	Strength	Appl No	Date
AP	+	INTL MEDICATION	40MG/ML	N018014 001	
AP		LUITPOLD	40MG/ML	N070799 001	FEB 11, 1987
AP			80MG/ML	N070820 001	FEB 11, 1987
AP			160MG/ML	N070826 001	FEB 11, 1987

DOPAMINE HCL AND DEXTROSE 5%

TE		Applicant	Strength	Appl No	Date
AP	+	B BRAUN	80MG/100ML	N019099 002	OCT 15, 1986
AP	+		320MG/100ML	N019099 004	OCT 15, 1986

DOPAMINE HCL AND DEXTROSE 5% IN PLASTIC CONTAINER

TE		Applicant	Strength	Appl No	Date
AP	+	B BRAUN	40MG/100ML	N019099 001	OCT 15, 1986
AP	+		160MG/100ML	N019099 003	OCT 15, 1986

DOPAMINE HCL IN DEXTROSE 5%

TE		Applicant	Strength	Appl No	Date
AP	+	ABBOTT	1.6MG/ML	N020542 001	AUG 30, 1995

DOPAMINE HCL IN DEXTROSE 5% IN PLASTIC CONTAINER

TE		Applicant	Strength	Appl No	Date
AP	+	ABBOTT	80MG/100ML	N018826 001	SEP 30, 1983
AP	+		160MG/100ML	N018826 002	SEP 30, 1983
AP	+		320MG/100ML	N018826 003	SEP 30, 1983
AP	+	BAXTER HLTHCARE	80MG/100ML	N019615 001	MAR 27, 1987
AP	+		160MG/100ML	N019615 002	MAR 27, 1987
AP	+		320MG/100ML	N019615 003	MAR 27, 1987
AP	+		640MG/100ML	N019615 004	MAR 27, 1987

INTROPIN

TE		Applicant	Strength	Appl No	Date
AP	+	FAULDING	40MG/ML	N017395 001	
AP	+		80MG/ML	N017395 002	
AP	+		160MG/ML	N017395 003	

DORZOLAMIDE HYDROCHLORIDE
Solution/Drops; Ophthalmic

TRUSOPT

	Applicant	Strength	Appl No	Date
+	MERCK	EQ 2% BASE	N020408 001	DEC 09, 1994

DORZOLAMIDE HYDROCHLORIDE; TIMOLOL MALEATE
Solution/Drops; Ophthalmic

COSOPT

	Applicant	Strength	Appl No	Date
+	MERCK	EQ 2% BASE;EQ 0.5% BASE	N020869 001	APR 07, 1998

DOXACURIUM CHLORIDE
Injectable; Injection

NUROMAX

	Applicant	Strength	Appl No	Date
+	ABBOTT	EQ 1MG BASE/ML	N019946 001	MAR 07, 1991

DOXAPRAM HYDROCHLORIDE
Injectable; Injection

DOPRAM

TE		Applicant	Strength	Appl No	Date
AP	+	BAXTER HLTHCARE CORP	20MG/ML	N014879 001	

DOXAPRAM HCL

TE		Applicant	Strength	Appl No	Date
AP	+	BEDFORD	20MG/ML	N076266 001	JAN 10, 2003
AP		STERIS	20MG/ML	N073529 001	JAN 30, 1992

DOXAZOSIN MESYLATE
Tablet; Oral

CARDURA

TE		Applicant	Strength	Appl No	Date
AB	+	PFIZER	EQ 1MG BASE	N019668 001	NOV 02, 1990
AB			EQ 2MG BASE	N019668 002	NOV 02, 1990
AB			EQ 4MG BASE	N019668 003	NOV 02, 1990
AB			EQ 8MG BASE	N019668 004	NOV 02, 1990

DOXAZOSIN MESYLATE

TE	Applicant	Strength	Appl No	Date
AB	EON	EQ 1MG BASE	N075646 001	OCT 18, 2000
AB		EQ 2MG BASE	N075646 002	OCT 18, 2000
AB		EQ 4MG BASE	N075646 003	OCT 18, 2000
AB		EQ 8MG BASE	N075646 004	OCT 18, 2000
AB	GENEVA PHARMS TECH	EQ 1MG BASE	N075432 001	OCT 18, 2000
AB		EQ 2MG BASE	N075432 002	OCT 18, 2000
AB		EQ 4MG BASE	N075432 003	OCT 18, 2000
AB		EQ 8MG BASE	N075432 004	OCT 18, 2000
AB	GENPHARM	EQ 1MG BASE	N075466 001	OCT 18, 2000
AB		EQ 2MG BASE	N075466 002	OCT 18, 2000
AB		EQ 4MG BASE	N075466 003	OCT 18, 2000
AB		EQ 8MG BASE	N075466 004	OCT 18, 2000
AB	IVAX PHARMS	EQ 1MG BASE	N075453 001	OCT 18, 2000
AB		EQ 2MG BASE	N075453 002	

Prescription Drug Products (continued)

DOXAZOSIN MESYLATE (continued)
Tablet; Oral

DOXAZOSIN MESYLATE

TE Code	Firm	Strength	Approval Date	Appl. No.
AB	IVAX PHARMS	EQ 4MG BASE	OCT 18, 2000	N075453 003
AB		EQ 8MG BASE	OCT 18, 2000	N075453 004
AB	KV PHARM	EQ 1MG BASE	OCT 18, 2000	N075609 001
AB		EQ 2MG BASE	OCT 18, 2000	N075609 002
AB		EQ 4MG BASE	OCT 18, 2000	N075609 003
AB		EQ 8MG BASE	OCT 18, 2000	N075609 004
AB	MYLAN	EQ 1MG BASE	OCT 18, 2000	N075509 001
AB		EQ 2MG BASE	OCT 19, 2000	N075509 002
AB		EQ 4MG BASE	OCT 19, 2000	N075509 003
AB		EQ 8MG BASE	OCT 19, 2000	N075509 004
AB	PLIVA	EQ 1MG BASE	JUN 08, 2001	N075750 001
AB		EQ 2MG BASE	JUN 08, 2001	N075750 002
AB		EQ 4MG BASE	JUN 08, 2001	N075750 003
AB		EQ 8MG BASE	JUN 08, 2001	N075750 004
AB	PUREPAC PHARM	EQ 1MG BASE	OCT 18, 2000	N075574 001
AB		EQ 2MG BASE	OCT 18, 2000	N075574 002
AB		EQ 4MG BASE	OCT 18, 2000	N075574 003
AB		EQ 8MG BASE	OCT 18, 2000	N075574 004
AB	TEVA	EQ 1MG BASE	JAN 12, 2001	N075536 001
AB		EQ 1MG BASE	OCT 18, 2000	N075353 001
AB		EQ 2MG BASE	OCT 18, 2000	N075536 002
AB		EQ 2MG BASE	JAN 12, 2001	N075353 002
AB		EQ 4MG BASE	OCT 18, 2000	N075536 003
AB		EQ 4MG BASE	JAN 12, 2001	N075353 003
AB		EQ 8MG BASE	OCT 18, 2000	N075536 004
AB		EQ 8MG BASE	JAN 12, 2001	N075353 004
AB	TORPHARM	EQ 1MG BASE	OCT 18, 2000	N075580 001
AB		EQ 2MG BASE	OCT 18, 2000	N075580 002
AB		EQ 4MG BASE	OCT 18, 2000	N075580 003
AB		EQ 8MG BASE	OCT 18, 2000	N075580 004
AB	WATSON LABS	EQ 1MG BASE	OCT 18, 2000	N075426 001
AB		EQ 2MG BASE	OCT 18, 2000	N075426 002
AB		EQ 4MG BASE	OCT 18, 2000	N075426 003
AB		EQ 8MG BASE	OCT 18, 2000	N075426 004

DOXEPIN HYDROCHLORIDE
Capsule; Oral

DOXEPIN HCL

TE Code	Firm	Strength	Approval Date	Appl. No.
AB	GENEVA PHARMS	EQ 10MG BASE		N071487 001
AB		EQ 25MG BASE	MAR 02, 1987	N070827 001
AB		EQ 50MG BASE	MAY 15, 1986	N070828 001
AB		EQ 75MG BASE	MAY 15, 1986	N070825 001
AB		EQ 100MG BASE	MAY 15, 1986	N071562 001
AB	MYLAN	EQ 10MG BASE	MAR 02, 1987	N070789 001
AB		EQ 25MG BASE	MAY 13, 1986	N070790 001
AB		EQ 50MG BASE	MAY 13, 1986	N070791 001
AB		EQ 75MG BASE	MAY 13, 1986	N070792 001
AB		EQ 100MG BASE	MAY 13, 1986	N070793 001
AB	PAR PHARM	EQ 10MG BASE	MAY 13, 1986	N071697 001
AB		EQ 25MG BASE	NOV 09, 1987	N071437 001
AB		EQ 50MG BASE	NOV 09, 1987	N071595 001
AB		EQ 75MG BASE	NOV 09, 1987	N071608 001
AB		EQ 100MG BASE	NOV 09, 1987	N071422 001
AB		EQ 150MG BASE	NOV 09, 1987	N071669 001
AB	WATSON LABS	EQ 10MG BASE	NOV 09, 1987	N071485 001
AB		EQ 10MG BASE	APR 30, 1987	N072985 001

Prescription Drug Products (continued)

DOXEPIN HYDROCHLORIDE (continued)

Capsule; Oral
DOXEPIN HCL

TE	Firm	Strength	Appl. No.	Date
AB	WATSON LABS	EQ 25MG BASE	N071486 001	MAR 29, 1991
AB		EQ 25MG BASE	N072986 001	APR 30, 1987
AB		EQ 50MG BASE	N071238 001	MAR 29, 1991
AB		EQ 50MG BASE	N072987 001	APR 30, 1987
AB		EQ 75MG BASE	N071326 001	MAR 29, 1991
AB		EQ 100MG BASE	N071239 001	APR 30, 1987

SINEQUAN

TE	Firm	Strength	Appl. No.
AB	PFIZER	EQ 10MG BASE	N016798 003
AB +		EQ 25MG BASE	N016798 001
AB		EQ 50MG BASE	N016798 002
AB +		EQ 75MG BASE	N016798 006
AB		EQ 100MG BASE	N016798 005
AB		EQ 150MG BASE	N016798 007

Concentrate; Oral
DOXEPIN HCL

TE	Firm	Strength	Appl. No.	Date
AA	COPLEY PHARM	EQ 10MG BASE/ML	N071609 001	NOV 09, 1987
AA	MORTON GROVE	EQ 10MG BASE/ML	N071918 001	JUL 20, 1988
AA	SILARX	EQ 10MG BASE/ML	N074721 001	DEC 29, 1998

SINEQUAN

TE	Firm	Strength	Appl. No.
AA +	PFIZER	EQ 10MG BASE/ML	N017516 001

Cream; Topical
ZONALON

TE	Firm	Strength	Appl. No.	Date
AA +	BIOGLAN PHARMS	5%	N020126 001	APR 01, 1994

DOXERCALCIFEROL

Capsule; Oral
HECTOROL

TE	Firm	Strength	Appl. No.	Date
+	BONE CARE	2.5UGM	N020862 001	JUN 09, 1999

Injectable; Injection
HECTOROL

TE	Firm	Strength	Appl. No.	Date
+	BONE CARE	2UGM/ML	N021027 001	APR 06, 2000

DOXORUBICIN HYDROCHLORIDE

Injectable, Liposomal; Injection
DOXIL

TE	Firm	Strength	Appl. No.	Date
+	ALZA	2MG/ML	N050718 001	NOV 17, 1995

DOXORUBICIN HYDROCHLORIDE (continued)

Injectable; Injection
ADRIAMYCIN PFS

TE	Firm	Strength	Appl. No.	Date
AP +	PHARMACIA AND UPJOHN	2MG/ML	N050629 001	DEC 23, 1987
			N063165 001	JAN 30, 1991
AP		2MG/ML	N050629 002	MAY 03, 1988
AP +		200MG/100ML	N063165 002	JAN 30, 1991
AP +		200MG/100ML		

ADRIAMYCIN RDF

TE	Firm	Strength	Appl. No.	Date
AP +	PHARMACIA AND UPJOHN	10MG/VIAL	N050467 001	
AP +		20MG/VIAL	N050467 003	MAY 20, 1985
AP +		50MG/VIAL	N050467 002	
AP +		150MG/VIAL	N050467 004	JUL 22, 1987

DOXORUBICIN HCL

TE	Firm	Strength	Appl. No.	Date
AP	AM PHARM PARTNERS	2MG/ML	N063277 001	
AP	BEDFORD	2MG/ML	N062975 001	OCT 26, 1995
AP		10MG/VIAL	N062921 001	MAR 17, 1989
AP		20MG/VIAL	N062921 002	MAR 17, 1989
AP		50MG/VIAL	N062921 003	MAR 17, 1989
AP		200MG/100ML	N064097 001	MAR 17, 1989
AP	GENSIA SICOR PHARMS	2MG/ML	N064140 001	SEP 13, 1994
AP		200MG/100ML	N064140 002	JUL 28, 1995
AP	PHARMACHEMIE	2MG/ML	N063336 001	JUL 28, 1995
AP		10MG/VIAL	N063097 001	FEB 28, 1995
AP		20MG/VIAL	N063097 002	MAY 21, 1990
AP		50MG/VIAL	N063097 003	MAY 21, 1990
AP		200MG/100ML	N063336 004	MAY 21, 1990 / FEB 28, 1995

RUBEX

TE	Firm	Strength	Appl. No.	Date
AP	BRISTOL MYERS SQUIBB	10MG/VIAL	N062926 001	APR 13, 1989
AP		50MG/VIAL	N062926 002	APR 13, 1989
AP		100MG/VIAL	N062926 003	APR 13, 1989

Prescription Drug Products (continued)

DOXYCYCLINE

Capsule; Oral

DOXYCYCLINE

TE	Applicant	Strength	Appl No	Date
AB	AXIOM PHARM	EQ 50MG BASE	N065041 001	APR 28, 2000
AB		EQ 100MG BASE	N065041 002	APR 28, 2000
AB	EON	EQ 50MG BASE	N065032 001	JUN 30, 2000
AB		EQ 100MG BASE	N065032 002	JUN 30, 2000
AB	PAR PHARM	EQ 50MG BASE	N065055 001	DEC 01, 2000
AB		EQ 100MG BASE	N065055 002	DEC 01, 2000
AB	RANBAXY	EQ 50MG BASE	N065053 001	NOV 22, 2000
AB		EQ 100MG BASE	N065053 002	NOV 22, 2000

MONODOX

TE	Applicant	Strength	Appl No	Date
AB	OCLASSEN	EQ 50MG BASE	N050641 002	FEB 10, 1992
AB +		EQ 100MG BASE	N050641 001	DEC 29, 1989

For Suspension; Oral

VIBRAMYCIN

TE	Applicant	Strength	Appl No	Date
AB +	PFIZER	EQ 25MG BASE/5ML	N050006 001	

Tablet; Oral

DOXYCYCLINE

TE	Applicant	Strength	Appl No	Date
	PAR PHARM	EQ 50MG BASE	N065070 001	DEC 15, 2000
		EQ 75MG BASE	N065070 003	DEC 30, 2002
+		EQ 100MG BASE	N065070 002	DEC 15, 2000

DOXYCYCLINE CALCIUM

Suspension; Oral

VIBRAMYCIN

TE	Applicant	Strength	Appl No	Date
+	PFIZER	EQ 50MG BASE/5ML	N050480 001	

DOXYCYCLINE HYCLATE

Capsule, Coated Pellets; Oral

DORYX

TE	Applicant	Strength	Appl No	Date
	FAULDING	EQ 75MG BASE	N050582 002	AUG 13, 2001
+		EQ 100MG BASE	N050582 001	JUL 22, 1985
AB	WARNER CHILCOTT	EQ 100MG BASE	N062653 001	OCT 30, 1985

Capsule; Oral

DOXYCYCLINE HYCLATE

TE	Applicant	Strength	Appl No	Date
AB	AXIOM PHARM	EQ 50MG BASE	N061717 001	
AB		EQ 100MG BASE	N061717 002	
AB	IVAX PHARMS	EQ 50MG BASE	N062500 001	SEP 11, 1984

DOXYCYCLINE HYCLATE (continued)

Capsule; Oral

DOXYCYCLINE HYCLATE

TE	Applicant	Strength	Appl No	Date
AB	IVAX PHARMS	EQ 100MG BASE	N062500 002	SEP 11, 1984
AB	MUTUAL PHARM	EQ 50MG BASE	N062675 001	JUL 10, 1986
AB		EQ 100MG BASE	N062676 001	JUL 10, 1986
AB	MYLAN	EQ 50MG BASE	N062337 001	MAR 29, 1982
AB		EQ 100MG BASE	N062337 002	MAR 29, 1982
AB	WATSON LABS	EQ 50MG BASE	N062031 002	OCT 13, 1982
AB		EQ 100MG BASE	N062031 001	
AB	WEST WARD	EQ 50MG BASE	N062396 002	NOV 07, 1984
AB		EQ 100MG BASE	N062396 001	MAY 07, 1984

VIBRAMYCIN

TE	Applicant	Strength	Appl No	Date
AB +	PFIZER	EQ 50MG BASE	N050007 001	
AB		EQ 100MG BASE	N050007 002	

Injectable; Injection

DOXY 100

TE	Applicant	Strength	Appl No	Date
AB +	AM PHARM PARTNERS	EQ 100MG BASE/VIAL	N062475 001	DEC 09, 1983

DOXY 200

TE	Applicant	Strength	Appl No	Date
+	AM PHARM PARTNERS	EQ 200MG BASE/VIAL	N062475 002	DEC 09, 1983

Liquid, Extended Release; Periodontal

ATRIDOX

TE	Applicant	Strength	Appl No	Date
+	ATRIX	EQ 10% W/W	N050751 001	SEP 03, 1998

Tablet; Oral

DOXYCYCLINE HYCLATE

TE	Applicant	Strength	Appl No	Date
AB	AXIOM PHARM	EQ 100MG BASE	N062269 002	NOV 08, 1982
AB	IVAX PHARMS	EQ 100MG BASE	N062505 001	SEP 11, 1984
AB	MUTUAL PHARM	EQ 100MG BASE	N062677 001	JUL 10, 1986
AB	MYLAN	EQ 100MG BASE	N062432 001	FEB 15, 1983
AB	VINTAGE PHARMS	EQ 100MG BASE	N062538 001	APR 07, 1986
AB	WATSON LABS	EQ 100MG BASE	N062421 001	FEB 02, 1983

PERIOSTAT

TE	Applicant	Strength	Appl No	Date
+	COLLAGENEX PHARMS	20MG	N050783 001	FEB 02, 2001

VIBRA-TABS

TE	Applicant	Strength	Appl No	Date
AB +	PFIZER	EQ 100MG BASE	N050533 001	

Prescription Drug Products (continued)

DRONABINOL
Capsule; Oral
  MARINOL

		Strength	Appl. No.	Date
	UNIMED	2.5MG	N018651 001	MAY 31, 1985
		5MG	N018651 002	MAY 31, 1985
+		10MG	N018651 003	MAY 31, 1985

DROPERIDOL
Injectable; Injection
  DROPERIDOL

		Strength	Appl. No.	Date
AP	ABBOTT	2.5MG/ML	N071981 001	FEB 29, 1988
AP		2.5MG/ML	N072272 001	AUG 31, 1995
AP	FAULDING	2.5MG/ML	N071645 001	APR 07, 1988
AP	LUITPOLD	2.5MG/ML	N072123 001	OCT 24, 1988
AP		2.5MG/ML	N072335 001	OCT 24, 1988

  INAPSINE

		Strength	Appl. No.
AP	+ AKORN	2.5MG/ML	N016796 001

DROPERIDOL; FENTANYL CITRATE
Injectable; Injection
  FENTANYL CITRATE AND DROPERIDOL

		Strength	Appl. No.	Date
AP	+ ABBOTT	2.5MG/ML;EQ 0.05MG BASE/ML	N071982 001	MAY 04, 1988

DROSPIRENONE; ETHINYL ESTRADIOL
Tablet; Oral-28
  YASMIN

		Strength	Appl. No.	Date
+	BERLEX LABS	3MG;0.03MG	N021098 001	MAY 11, 2001

DUTASTERIDE
Capsule; Oral
  AVODART

		Strength	Appl. No.	Date
+	GLAXOSMITHKLINE	0.5MG	N021319 001	NOV 20, 2001

DYPHYLLINE
Tablet; Oral
  DILOR

		Strength	Appl. No.
BP	SAVAGE LABS	200MG	N084514 001

  DILOR-400

		Strength	Appl. No.
BP	+ SAVAGE LABS	400MG	N084751 001

  LUFYLLIN

		Strength	Appl. No.
BP	MEDPOINTE PHARM HLC	200MG	N084566 001
BP		400MG	N084566 002

ECHOTHIOPHATE IODIDE
For Solution; Ophthalmic
  PHOSPHOLINE IODIDE

		Strength	Appl. No.
+	AYERST	0.125%	N011963 001

ECONAZOLE NITRATE
Cream; Topical
  ECONAZOLE NITRATE

		Strength	Appl. No.	Date
AB	ALTANA	1%	N076075 001	NOV 26, 2002
AB	TARO	1%	N076005 001	NOV 26, 2002

  SPECTAZOLE

		Strength	Appl. No.	Date
AB	+ JOHNSON AND JOHNSON	1%	N018751 001	DEC 23, 1982

EDETATE CALCIUM DISODIUM
Injectable; Injection
  CALCIUM DISODIUM VERSENATE

		Strength	Appl. No.
+	3M	200MG/ML	N008922 001

EDETATE DISODIUM
Injectable; Injection
  EDETATE DISODIUM

		Strength	Appl. No.	Date
AP	APOTEX	150MG/ML	N040376 001	NOV 04, 2002
AP	BIONICHE (CANADA)	150MG/ML	N040437 001	JUL 09, 2002
AP	STERIS	150MG/ML	N080391 001	

  ENDRATE

		Strength	Appl. No.
AP	+ ABBOTT	150MG/ML	N011355 001

EDROPHONIUM CHLORIDE
Injectable; Injection
  EDROPHONIUM CHLORIDE

		Strength	Appl. No.	Date
AP	ABBOTT	10MG/ML	N040131 001	FEB 24, 1998

  ENLON

		Strength	Appl. No.	Date
AP	BAXTER HLTHCARE CORP	10MG/ML	N088873 001	AUG 06, 1985

  TENSILON

		Strength	Appl. No.
AP	+ ICN	10MG/ML	N007959 001

  TENSILON PRESERVATIVE FREE

		Strength	Appl. No.
AP	+ ICN	10MG/ML	N007959 002

EDROPHONIUM CHLORIDE *MULTIPLE*
SEE   ATROPINE SULFATE; EDROPHONIUM CHLORIDE

EFAVIRENZ
Capsule; Oral
  SUSTIVA

		Strength	Appl. No.
	BRISTOL MYERS SQUIBB	50MG	N020972 001

Prescription Drug Products *(continued)*

EFAVIRENZ *(continued)*
Capsule; Oral
SUSTIVA
BRISTOL MYERS SQUIBB

	Strength	Application	Date
			SEP 17, 1998
	100MG		
	200MG	N020972 002	SEP 17, 1998
		N020972 003	SEP 17, 1998
+			

Tablet; Oral
SUSTIVA
BRISTOL MYERS SQUIBB

	Strength	Application	Date
	300MG	N021360 001	FEB 01, 2002
+	600MG	N021360 002	FEB 01, 2002

EFLORNITHINE HYDROCHLORIDE
Cream; Topical
VANIQA

	Strength	Application	Date
+ WOMEN FIRST HLTHCARE	13.9%	N021145 001	JUL 27, 2000

ELETRIPTAN HYDROBROMIDE
Tablet; Oral
RELPAX

	Strength	Application	Date
PFIZER IRELAND	EQ 20MG BASE	N021016 001	DEC 26, 2002
+	EQ 40MG BASE	N021016 002	DEC 26, 2002

EMEDASTINE DIFUMARATE
Solution/Drops; Ophthalmic
EMADINE

	Strength	Application	Date
+ ALCON	0.05%	N020706 001	DEC 29, 1997

ENALAPRIL MALEATE
Tablet; Oral
ENALAPRIL MALEATE

TE Code	Firm	Strength	Application	Date
AB	APOTHECON	2.5MG	N075583 001	AUG 22, 2000
AB		5MG	N075583 002	AUG 22, 2000
AB		10MG	N075583 003	AUG 22, 2000
AB		20MG	N075583 004	AUG 22, 2000
AB	EON	2.5MG	N075621 001	AUG 22, 2000
AB		5MG	N075621 002	AUG 22, 2000
AB		10MG	N075621 003	AUG 22, 2000

ENALAPRIL MALEATE *(continued)*
Tablet; Oral
ENALAPRIL MALEATE

TE Code	Firm	Strength	Application	Date
AB	EON	20MG	N075621 004	AUG 22, 2000
AB	GENEVA PHARMS	2.5MG	N075048 001	AUG 22, 2000
AB		5MG	N075048 002	AUG 22, 2000
AB		10MG	N075048 003	AUG 22, 2000
AB		20MG	N075048 004	AUG 22, 2000
AB	GENPHARM	2.5MG	N075472 001	AUG 22, 2000
AB		5MG	N075472 002	AUG 22, 2000
AB		10MG	N075472 003	AUG 22, 2000
AB		20MG	N075472 004	AUG 22, 2000
AB	IVAX PHARMS	2.5MG	N075482 001	AUG 22, 2000
AB		5MG	N075482 002	AUG 22, 2000
AB		10MG	N075482 003	AUG 22, 2000
AB		20MG	N075482 004	AUG 22, 2000
AB	KRKA DD NOVO MESTO	2.5MG	N075370 001	AUG 22, 2000
AB		5MG	N075370 002	AUG 22, 2000
AB		10MG	N075369 001	AUG 22, 2000
AB		20MG	N075369 002	AUG 22, 2000
AB	LEK PHARMS	2.5MG	N075496 001	AUG 22, 2000
AB		5MG	N075496 002	AUG 22, 2000
AB		10MG	N075459 001	AUG 22, 2000
AB		20MG	N075459 002	AUG 22, 2000
AB	MYLAN	2.5MG	N075480 001	AUG 22, 2000
AB		5MG	N075480 002	AUG 22, 2000
AB		10MG	N075480 003	AUG 22, 2000
AB		20MG	N075480 004	AUG 22, 2000
AB	RANBAXY	2.5MG	N075556 001	AUG 22, 2000
AB		5MG	N075556 002	AUG 22, 2000

Prescription Drug Products *(continued)*

ENALAPRIL MALEATE *(continued)*
Tablet; Oral
ENALAPRIL MALEATE

	RANBAXY	Strength	Appl. No.	Date
AB	RANBAXY	10MG	N075556 003	AUG 22, 2000
AB		20MG	N075556 004	AUG 22, 2000
AB	TARO	2.5MG	N075657 001	JAN 23, 2001
AB		5MG	N075657 002	JAN 23, 2001
AB		10MG	N075657 003	JAN 23, 2001
AB		20MG	N075657 004	JAN 23, 2001
AB	TEVA	2.5MG	N075479 001	AUG 22, 2000
AB		5MG	N075479 002	AUG 22, 2000
AB		10MG	N075479 003	AUG 22, 2000
AB		20MG	N075479 004	AUG 22, 2000
AB	TORPHARM	2.5MG	N075178 002	MAR 23, 2001
AB		5MG	N075178 001	MAR 23, 2001
AB		10MG	N075178 003	MAR 23, 2001
AB		20MG	N075178 004	MAR 23, 2001
AB	WATSON LABS	2.5MG	N075501 001	AUG 22, 2000
AB		5MG	N075501 002	AUG 22, 2000
AB		10MG	N075501 003	AUG 22, 2000
AB		20MG	N075501 004	AUG 22, 2000
AB	WOCKHARDT	2.5MG	N075483 001	AUG 22, 2000
AB		5MG	N075483 002	AUG 22, 2000
AB		10MG	N075483 003	AUG 22, 2000
AB		20MG	N075483 004	AUG 22, 2000

VASOTEC

	BIOVAIL	Strength	Appl. No.	Date
AB	BIOVAIL	2.5MG	N018998 005	JUL 26, 1988
AB		5MG	N018998 001	DEC 24, 1985
AB		10MG	N018998 002	DEC 24, 1985
AB +		20MG	N018998 003	DEC 24, 1985

ENALAPRIL MALEATE; FELODIPINE
Tablet, Extended Release; Oral
LEXXEL

		Strength	Appl. No.	Date
+	ASTRAZENECA	5MG;2.5MG	N020668 002	OCT 28, 1998
+		5MG;5MG	N020668 001	DEC 27, 1996

ENALAPRIL MALEATE; HYDROCHLOROTHIAZIDE
Tablet; Oral
ENALAPRIL MALEATE AND HYDROCHLOROTHIAZIDE

		Strength	Appl. No.	Date
AB	DR REDDYS LABS LTD	5MG;12.5MG	N075909 001	OCT 15, 2001
AB		10MG;25MG	N075909 002	OCT 15, 2001
AB	EON	5MG;12.5MG	N076116 001	SEP 19, 2001
AB		10MG;25MG	N076116 002	SEP 19, 2001
AB	IVAX PHARMS	5MG;12.5MG	N075736 001	MAR 25, 2003
AB		10MG;25MG	N075736 002	MAR 25, 2003
AB	MYLAN	5MG;12.5MG	N075624 001	SEP 18, 2001
AB		10MG;25MG	N075624 002	SEP 18, 2001
AB	TARO PHARM INDS	5MG;12.5MG	N075788 001	SEP 18, 2001
AB		10MG;25MG	N075788 002	SEP 18, 2001
AB	TEVA	5MG;12.5MG	N075727 001	SEP 18, 2001
AB		10MG;25MG	N075727 002	SEP 18, 2001

VASERETIC

	BIOVAIL	Strength	Appl. No.	Date
AB	BIOVAIL	5MG;12.5MG	N019221 003	JUL 12, 1995
AB +		10MG;25MG	N019221 001	OCT 31, 1986

ENALAPRIL MALEATE *MULTIPLE*
SEE DILTIAZEM MALATE; ENALAPRIL MALEATE

ENALAPRILAT
Injectable; Injection
ENALAPRILAT

		Strength	Appl. No.	Date
AP	ABBOTT	1.25MG/ML	N075456 001	AUG 22, 2000
AP	BEDFORD	1.25MG/ML	N075458 001	AUG 22, 2000
AP	FAULDING	1.25MG/ML	N075634 001	AUG 22, 2000
AP	GENSIA SICOR PHARMS	1.25MG/ML	N075571 001	AUG 22, 2000
AP		1.25MG/ML	N075578 001	AUG 22, 2000

Prescription Drug Products (continued)

ENALAPRILAT (continued)
Injectable; Injection
ENALAPRILAT
  GENSIA SICOR PHARMS   AUG 22, 2000
VASOTEC
AP + BIOVAIL   1.25MG/ML   N019309 001 FEB 09, 1988

ENFLURANE
Liquid; Inhalation
ENFLURANE
AN   ABBOTT   99.9%   N070803 001 SEP 08, 1987
AN   MINRAD   99.9%   N074396 001 JUL 29, 1994
ETHRANE
AN + BAXTER HLTHCARE CORP   99.9%   N017087 001

ENFUVIRTIDE
Injectable; Subcutaneous
FUZEON
  + ROCHE   90MG/VIAL   N021481 001 MAR 13, 2003

ENOXAPARIN SODIUM
Injectable; Subcutaneous
LOVENOX
  + AVENTIS   30MG/0.3ML   N020164 001 MAR 29, 1993
  +   40MG/0.4ML   N020164 002 JAN 30, 1998
  +   60MG/0.6ML   N020164 003 MAR 27, 1998
  +   80MG/0.8ML   N020164 004 MAR 27, 1998
  +   100MG/ML   N020164 005 MAR 27, 1998
  +   120MG/0.8ML   N020164 007 JUN 02, 2000
  +   150MG/ML   N020164 008 JUN 02, 2000
  +   300MG/3ML   N020164 009 JAN 23, 2003

ENTACAPONE
Tablet; Oral
COMTAN
  + ORION   200MG   N020796 001 OCT 19, 1999

ENTACAPONE *MULTIPLE*
SEE   CARBIDOPA; ENTACAPONE; LEVODOPA

EPINEPHRINE
Injectable; Im-Sc
TWINJECT
  + HOLLISTER STIER LABS   EQ 0.3MG /DELIVERY   N020800 001 MAY 30, 2003
Injectable, Intramuscular
EPIPEN
  + MERIDIAN MEDCL TECHN   0.3MG/DELIVERY   N019430 001 DEC 22, 1987
EPIPEN JR.
  + MERIDIAN MEDCL TECHN   0.15MG/DELIVERY   N019430 002 DEC 22, 1987

EPINEPHRINE; LIDOCAINE HYDROCHLORIDE
Injectable; Injection
LIDOCAINE HCL AND EPINEPHRINE
AP   ABBOTT   0.005MG/ML;1.5%   N088571 001 SEP 13, 1985
AP   0.005MG/ML;0.5%   N089635 001 JUN 21, 1988
AP   0.01MG/ML;1%   N089644 001 JUN 21, 1988
AP   0.005MG/ML;1.5%   N089645 001 JUN 21, 1988
AP   0.01MG/ML;2%   N089646 001 JUN 21, 1988
AP   0.005MG/ML;1%   N089649 001 JUN 21, 1988
AP   0.005MG/ML;1.5%   N089650 001 JUN 21, 1988
AP   0.005MG/ML;2%   N089651 001 JUN 21, 1988
AP   EASTMAN KODAK   0.02MG/ML;2%   N040057 001 FEB 26, 1993
AP   0.01MG/ML;2%   N040057 002 FEB 26, 1993
AP   GRAHAM CHEM   0.01MG/ML;2%   N080504 004 OCT 19, 1983
AP   0.02MG/ML;2%   N080504 005 OCT 19, 1983
LIDOCAINE HCL W/ EPINEPHRINE
   DELL LABS
AP   0.01MG/ML;1%   N083389 001
AP   0.01MG/ML;2%   N083390 001
LIDOCATON
AP   PHARMATON   0.01MG/ML;2%   N084729 001 AUG 17, 1983
OCTOCAINE
   SEPTODONT
AP   0.01MG/ML;2%   N084048 001
AP   0.02MG/ML;2%   N084048 002
XYLOCAINE W/ EPINEPHRINE
   ASTRAZENECA
AP + 0.01MG/ML;1%   N006488 004
AP + 0.005MG/ML;0.5%   N006488 012
AP + 0.005MG/ML;1.5%   N006488 017
AP + 0.005MG/ML;1%   N006488 018

Prescription Drug Products (continued)

EPINEPHRINE; LIDOCAINE HYDROCHLORIDE (continued)
Injectable; Injection
XYLOCAINE W/ EPINEPHRINE
AP	+ ASTRAZENECA	0.005MG/ML;2%		NOV 13, 1986 / N006488 019
	+ DENTSPLY PHARM	0.01MG/ML;2%		NOV 13, 1986 / N021381 001
		0.02MG/ML;2%		N021381 002

Solution; Iontophoresis
IONTOCAINE
+ IOMED   2%   N020530 001   DEC 21, 1995

EPINEPHRINE *MULTIPLE*
SEE ARTICAINE HYDROCHLORIDE: EPINEPHRINE
SEE BUPIVACAINE HYDROCHLORIDE: EPINEPHRINE

EPINEPHRINE BITARTRATE; ETIDOCAINE HYDROCHLORIDE
Injectable; Injection
DURANEST
+ ASTRAZENECA   0.005MG/ML;1%   N017751 006

EPINEPHRINE BITARTRATE; LIDOCAINE HYDROCHLORIDE
Injectable; Injection
LIGNOSPAN FORTE
+ DEPROCO   EQ 0.02MG BASE/ML;2%   N088389 001   JAN 22, 1985
LIGNOSPAN STANDARD
+ DEPROCO   EQ 0.01MG BASE/ML;2%   N088390 001   JAN 22, 1985

EPINEPHRINE BITARTRATE; PRILOCAINE HYDROCHLORIDE
Injectable; Injection
CITANEST FORTE
+ DENTSPLY PHARM   0.005MG/ML;4%   N021383 001

EPINEPHRINE BITARTRATE *MULTIPLE*
SEE BUPIVACAINE HYDROCHLORIDE: EPINEPHRINE BITARTRATE

EPIRUBICIN HYDROCHLORIDE
Injectable; Injection
ELLENCE
BX + PHARMACIA AND UPJOHN   2MG/ML   N050778 001   SEP 15, 1999

EPLERENONE
Tablet; Oral
INSPRA
GD SEARLE LLC	25MG	N021437 001	SEP 27, 2002
	50MG	N021437 002	SEP 27, 2002
+	100MG	N021437 003	

EPLERENONE (continued)
Tablet; Oral
INSPRA
  GD SEARLE LLC   SEP 27, 2002

EPOPROSTENOL SODIUM
Injectable; Injection
FLOLAN
+ GLAXOSMITHKLINE   EQ 0.5MG BASE/VIAL   N020444 001   SEP 20, 1995
+   EQ 1.5MG BASE/VIAL   N020444 002   SEP 20, 1995

EPROSARTAN MESYLATE
Tablet; Oral
TEVETEN
BIOVAIL PHARMS	EQ 300MG BASE	N020738 004	DEC 22, 1997
	EQ 400MG BASE	N020738 005	DEC 22, 1997
+	EQ 600MG BASE	N020738 006	MAY 27, 1999

EPROSARTAN MESYLATE; HYDROCHLOROTHIAZIDE
Tablet; Oral
TEVETEN HCT
BIOVAIL PHARMS	600MG;12.5MG	N021268 001	NOV 01, 2001
+	600MG;25MG	N021268 002	NOV 01, 2001

EPTIFIBATIDE
Injectable; Injection
INTEGRILIN
+ MILLENNIUM PHARMS   2MG/ML   N020718 001   MAY 18, 1998
+   75MG/100ML   N020718 002   MAY 18, 1998

ERGOCALCIFEROL
Capsule; Oral
DRISDOL
AA + SANOFI SYNTHELABO   50,000 IU   N003444 001
VITAMIN D
AA   BANNER PHARMACAPS   50,000 IU   N080704 001

ERGOCALCIFEROL *MULTIPLE*
SEE ASCORBIC ACID: BIOTIN: CYANOCOBALAMIN: DEXPANTHENOL: ERGOCALCIFEROL: FOLIC ACID: NIACINAMIDE: PHYTONADIONE: PYRIDOXINE HYDROCHLORIDE: RIBOFLAVIN PHOSPHATE SODIUM: THIAMINE HYDROCHLORIDE: VITAMIN A: VITAMIN E
SEE ASCORBIC ACID: BIOTIN: CYANOCOBALAMIN: DEXPANTHENOL: ERGOCALCIFEROL: FOLIC ACID: NIACINAMIDE: PYRIDOXINE HYDROCHLORIDE: RIBOFLAVIN PHOSPHATE SODIUM: THIAMINE HYDROCHLORIDE: VITAMIN A: VITAMIN E

Prescription Drug Products (continued)

ERGOLOID MESYLATES

Tablet; Oral

TE	Brand / Firm	Strength	Appl. No.	Date
	ERGOLOID MESYLATES			
AB	MUTUAL PHARM	1MG	N081113 001	OCT 31, 1991
	HYDERGINE			
AB	+ NOVARTIS	1MG	N017993 001	

Tablet; Sublingual

TE	Brand / Firm	Strength	Appl. No.	Date
	ERGOLOID MESYLATES			
AA	WATSON LABS	0.5MG	N087233 001	JUL 03, 1985
	GERIMAL			
AA	WATSON LABS	0.5MG	N086189 001	
AA		1MG	N086188 001	
	HYDERGINE			
AA	+ NOVARTIS	0.5MG	N009087 002	
AA	+	1MG	N009087 001	
	+ HYDROGENATED ERGOT ALKALOIDS			
AA	IVAX PHARMS	1MG	N087185 001	

ERGOTAMINE TARTRATE

Tablet; Sublingual

TE	Brand / Firm	Strength	Appl. No.	Date
	ERGOMAR			
	+ HARVEST PHARMS	2MG	N087693 001	FEB 24, 1983

ERGOTAMINE TARTRATE *MULTIPLE*

SEE   CAFFEINE; ERGOTAMINE TARTRATE

ERTAPENEM SODIUM

Injectable; Intramuscular, Iv (Infusion)

TE	Brand / Firm	Strength	Appl. No.	Date
	INVANZ			
	+ MERCK	EQ 1GM BASE/VIAL	N021337 001	NOV 21, 2001

ERYTHROMYCIN

Capsule, Delayed Rel Pellets; Oral

TE	Brand / Firm	Strength	Appl. No.	Date
	ERYC			
AB	+ FAULDING	250MG	N050536 001	
	ERYTHROMYCIN			
AB	ABBOTT	250MG	N062746 001	DEC 22, 1986
			N063098 001	MAY 04, 1989
AB	BARR	250MG		

Gel; Topical

TE	Brand / Firm	Strength	Appl. No.	Date
	E-GLADES			
AT	GLADES PHARMS	2%	N065009 001	MAR 18, 2002
	EMGEL			
AT	GLAXOSMITHKLINE	2%	N063107 001	AUG 23, 1991
	ERYGEL			
AT	+ ALLERGAN HERBERT	2%	N050617 001	OCT 21, 1987
	ERYTHROMYCIN			
AT	ALTANA	2%	N064184 001	SEP 30, 1997

ERYTHROMYCIN (continued)

Gel; Topical

TE	Brand / Firm	Strength	Appl. No.	Date
	ERYTHROMYCIN			
AT	STIEFEL	2%	N063211 001	JAN 29, 1993

Lotion; Topical

TE	Brand / Firm	Strength	Appl. No.	Date
	E-SOLVE 2			
	+ SYOSSET	2%	N062467 001	JUL 03, 1985

Ointment; Ophthalmic

TE	Brand / Firm	Strength	Appl. No.	Date
	ERYTHROMYCIN			
AT	AKORN	0.5%	N064030 001	JUL 18, 1996
AT	BAUSCH AND LOMB	0.5%	N064067 001	JUL 29, 1994
AT	FOUGERA	0.5%	N062447 001	SEP 26, 1983
	ILOTYCIN			
	+ DISTA	0.5%	N050368 001	

Ointment; Topical

TE	Brand / Firm	Strength	Appl. No.	Date
	AKNE-MYCIN			
	+ HEALTHPOINT	2%	N050584 001	JAN 10, 1985

Solution; Topical

TE	Brand / Firm	Strength	Appl. No.	Date
	A/T/S			
AT	AVENTIS PHARMS	2%	N062405 001	NOV 18, 1982
	C-SOLVE-2			
AT	BIOGLAN PHARMA	2%	N062468 001	JUL 03, 1985
	ERYDERM			
AT	ABBOTT	2%	N062290 001	
	ERYMAX			
AT	ALLERGAN HERBERT	2%	N062508 002	JUL 11, 1985
	ERYTHRA-DERM			
AT	PADDOCK	2%	N062687 001	FEB 05, 1988
	ERYTHRO-STATIN			
AT	HI TECH PHARMA	2%	N064101 001	OCT 22, 1996
	ERYTHROMYCIN			
AT	ALPHARMA	2%	N062326 001	APR 19, 1982
AT	ALTANA	2%	N064187 001	SEP 30, 1997
AT	BAUSCH AND LOMB	2%	N064039 001	JAN 27, 1994
AT	CLAY PARK	2%	N063038 001	JAN 11, 1991
AT	MORTON GROVE	2%	N062825 001	OCT 23, 1987
AT	STIEFEL	2%	N064127 001	FEB 14, 1997
	SANSAC			
AT	HEALTHPOINT	2%	N062522 001	JAN 24, 1985

Prescription Drug Products (continued)

ERYTHROMYCIN (continued)

Solution; Topical

	STATICIN		
	+ WESTWOOD SQUIBB	1.5%	N050526 001
	T-STAT		
AT	+ WESTWOOD SQUIBB	2%	N062436 001 MAR 09, 1983

Swab; Topical

	C-SOLVE-2		
AT	IVAX PHARMS	2%	N062751 001 JUL 30, 1993
	ERYCETTE		
AT	+ J AND J	2%	N050594 001 FEB 15, 1985
	ERYTHROMYCIN		
AT	STIEFEL	2%	N064126 001 JUL 03, 1996
AT		2%	N064128 001 JUL 03, 1996
	T-STAT		
AT	WESTWOOD SQUIBB	2%	N062748 001 JUL 23, 1987

Tablet, Coated Particles; Oral

	PCE		
	ABBOTT	333MG	N050611 001 SEP 09, 1986
	+	500MG	N050611 002 AUG 22, 1990

Tablet, Delayed Release; Oral

	E-BASE		
AB	BARR	333MG	N063086 001 MAY 15, 1990
AB		500MG	N062999 001 NOV 25, 1988
	E-MYCIN		
AB	ABBOTT	250MG	N060272 001
AB		333MG	N060272 002
	ERY-TAB		
AB	+ ABBOTT	250MG	N062298 001
AB	+	333MG	N062298 003 MAR 29, 1982
AB	+	500MG	N062298 002

Tablet; Oral

	ERYTHROMYCIN		
	ABBOTT	250MG	N061621 001
	+	500MG	N061621 002

ERYTHROMYCIN *MULTIPLE*
SEE   BENZOYL PEROXIDE; ERYTHROMYCIN

ERYTHROMYCIN ESTOLATE

Capsule; Oral

	ERYTHROMYCIN ESTOLATE		
	+ BARR	EQ 250MG BASE	N062162 002

ERYTHROMYCIN ESTOLATE (continued)

Suspension; Oral

	ERYTHROMYCIN ESTOLATE		
AB	ALPHARMA	EQ 125MG BASE/5ML	N062353 001 NOV 18, 1982
AB		EQ 250MG BASE/5ML	N062409 001 DEC 16, 1982
	ILOSONE		
AB	LILLY	EQ 125MG BASE/5ML	N050010 001
AB	+	EQ 250MG BASE/5ML	N050010 002

ERYTHROMYCIN ETHYLSUCCINATE

Granule; Oral

	E.E.S.		
AB	ABBOTT	EQ 200MG BASE/5ML	N050207 001
	ERYPED		
AB	ABBOTT	EQ 200MG BASE/5ML	N050207 003 MAR 30, 1987
AB		EQ 400MG BASE/5ML	N050207 002
	ERYTHROMYCIN ETHYLSUCCINATE		
AB	+ BARR	EQ 200MG BASE/5ML	N062055 001

Suspension; Oral

	E.E.S. 200		
AB	ABBOTT	EQ 200MG BASE/5ML	N061639 001
	E.E.S. 400		
AB	+ ABBOTT	EQ 400MG BASE/5ML	N061639 002
	ERYTHROMYCIN ETHYLSUCCINATE		
AB	ALPHARMA	EQ 200MG BASE/5ML	N062200 001
AB		EQ 400MG BASE/5ML	N062200 002
	PEDIAMYCIN		
AB	ROSS LABS	EQ 200MG BASE/5ML	N062304 001
	PEDIAMYCIN 400		
AB	ROSS LABS	EQ 400MG BASE/5ML	N062304 002

Tablet, Chewable; Oral

	E.E.S.		
AB	+ ABBCTT	EQ 200MG BASE	N050297 002
	ERYPED		
AB	ABBCTT	EQ 200MG BASE	N050297 003 JUL 05, 1988

Tablet; Oral

	E.E.S. 400		
AB	+ ABBCTT	EQ 400MG BASE	N061905 002 AUG 12, 1982
	ERYTHROMYCIN ETHYLSUCCINATE		
AB	MYLAN	EQ 400MG BASE	N062847 001 SEP 14, 1988

ERYTHROMYCIN ETHYLSUCCINATE; SULFISOXAZOLE ACETYL

Granule; Oral

	ERYTHROMYCIN ETHYLSUCCINATE AND SULFISOXAZOLE ACETYL		
AB	BARR	EQ 200MG BASE/5ML;EQ 600MG BASE/5ML	N062759 001 MAY 20, 1988
	ERYZOLE		
AB	ALRA	EQ 200MG BASE/5ML;EQ 600MG BASE/5ML	N062758 001 JUN 15, 1988

Prescription Drug Products *(continued)*

ERYTHROMYCIN ETHYLSUCCINATE; SULFISOXAZOLE ACETYL *(continued)*
Granule; Oral

	PEDIAZOLE			
AB	+ ROSS LABS	EQ 200MG BASE/5ML;EQ 600MG BASE/5ML	N050529 001	

ERYTHROMYCIN LACTOBIONATE
Injectable; Injection

	ERYTHROCIN			
AP	+ ABBOTT	EQ 1GM BASE/VIAL	N050182 003	
AP		EQ 1GM BASE/VIAL	N050609 002	SEP 24, 1986
AP		EQ 1GM BASE/VIAL	N062638 002	OCT 31, 1986
AP	+	EQ 500MG BASE/VIAL	N050182 002	
AP		EQ 500MG BASE/VIAL	N050609 001	SEP 24, 1986
AP		EQ 500MG BASE/VIAL	N062638 001	OCT 31, 1986
	ERYTHROMYCIN LACTOBIONATE			
	GENSIA SICOR PHARMS			
AP		EQ 1GM BASE/VIAL	N063253 002	JUL 30, 1993
AP		EQ 500MG BASE/VIAL	N063253 001	JUL 30, 1993
AP	LEDERLE	EQ 1GM BASE/VIAL	N062993 002	MAY 09, 1989
AP		EQ 500MG BASE/VIAL	N062993 001	MAY 09, 1989

ERYTHROMYCIN STEARATE
Tablet; Oral

	ERYTHROCIN STEARATE			
	ABBOTT			
AB		EQ 250MG BASE	N060359 001	
AB		EQ 500MG BASE	N060359 003	
	+ ERYTHROMYCIN STEARATE			
	BARR			
AB		EQ 250MG BASE	N061591 001	
	MYLAN			
AB		EQ 250MG BASE	N061505 001	
AB		EQ 500MG BASE	N061505 002	
	WATSON LABS			
AB		EQ 250MG BASE	N062121 002	
AB		EQ 500MG BASE	N062121 001	

ESCITALOPRAM OXALATE
Solution; Oral

	LEXAPRO			
	+ FOREST LABS	EQ 5MG BASE/5ML	N021365 001	NOV 27, 2002

Tablet; Oral

	LEXAPRO			
	FOREST LABS	5MG	N021323 001	AUG 14, 2002
		10MG	N021323 002	AUG 14, 2002
	+	20MG	N021323 003	AUG 14, 2002

ESMOLOL HYDROCHLORIDE
Injectable; Injection

	BREVIBLOC			
	+ BAXTER HLTHCARE CORP	10MG/ML	N019386 006	FEB 25, 2003
		20MG/ML	N019386 007	MAY 28, 2003
	+	250MG/ML	N019386 002	DEC 31, 1986
	BREVIBLOC DOUBLE STRENGTH IN PLASTIC CONTAINER			
	+ BAXTER HLTHCARE CORP	2GM/100ML	N019386 005	JAN 27, 2003
	BREVIBLOC IN PLASTIC CONTAINER			
	+ BAXTER HLTHCARE CORP	1GM/100ML	N019386 004	FEB 16, 2001

ESOMEPRAZOLE MAGNESIUM
Capsule, Delayed Rel Pellets; Oral

	NEXIUM			
	+ ASTRAZENECA	EQ 20MG BASE	N021153 001	FEB 20, 2001
	+	EQ 40MG BASE	N021153 002	FEB 20, 2001

ESTAZOLAM
Tablet; Oral

	ESTAZOLAM			
AB	IVAX PHARMS	1MG	N074826 001	JUL 03, 1997
AB		2MG	N074826 002	JUL 03, 1997
AB	TEVA	1MG	N074921 001	JUL 10, 1997
AB		2MG	N074921 002	JUL 10, 1997
AB	WATSON LABS	1MG	N074818 001	AUG 19, 1997
AB		2MG	N074818 002	AUG 19, 1997
	PROSOM			
AB	ABBOTT	1MG	N019080 001	DEC 26, 1990
AB	+	2MG	N019080 002	DEC 26, 1990

ESTRADIOL
Cream; Vaginal

	ESTRACE			
	+ WARNER CHILCOTT	0.01%	N086069 001	JAN 31, 1984

Prescription Drug Products (continued)

ESTRADIOL (continued)

Film, Extended Release; Transdermal

ALORA
WATSON LABS

TE		Strength	Appl. No.	Date
BX		0.1MG/24HR	N020655 003	DEC 20, 1996
BX		0.05MG/24HR	N020655 001	DEC 20, 1996
BX		0.025MG/24HR	N020655 004	APR 05, 2002
BX		0.075MG/24HR	N020655 002	DEC 20, 1996

CLIMARA
BERLEX LABS

TE		Strength	Appl. No.	Date
AB2	+	0.1MG/24HR	N020375 002	DEC 22, 1994
AB2	+	0.05MG/24HR	N020375 001	DEC 22, 1994
	+	0.06MG/24HR	N020375 006	MAY 27, 2003
BX	+	0.025MG/24HR	N020375 004	MAR 05, 1999
BX	+	0.075MG/24HR	N020375 003	MAR 23, 1998
BX	+	0.0375MG/24HR	N020375 005	MAY 27, 2003

ESCLIM
WOMEN FIRST HLTHCARE

TE		Strength	Appl. No.	Date
BX		0.1MG/24HR	N020847 005	AUG 04, 1998
BX		0.05MG/24HR	N020847 003	AUG 04, 1998
BX		0.025MG/24HR	N020847 001	AUG 04, 1998
BX		0.075MG/24HR	N020847 004	AUG 04, 1998
BX		0.0375MG/24HR	N020847 002	AUG 04, 1998

ESTRADERM
NOVARTIS

TE		Strength	Appl. No.	Date
BX	+	0.1MG/24HR	N019081 003	SEP 10, 1986
BX	+	0.05MG/24HR	N019081 002	SEP 10, 1986

ESTRADIOL
MYLAN TECHNOLOGIES

TE		Strength	Appl. No.	Date
AB2		0.1MG/24HR	N075182 001	FEB 24, 2000
AB2		0.05MG/24HR	N075233 001	FEB 24, 2000

VIVELLE
NOVARTIS

TE		Strength	Appl. No.	Date
AB1	+	0.1MG/24HR	N020323 004	OCT 28, 1994
AB1	+	0.05MG/24HR	N020323 002	OCT 28, 1994
	+	0.025MG/24HR	N020323 005	AUG 16, 2000
AB1	+	0.075MG/24HR	N020323 003	OCT 28, 1994
AB1	+	0.0375MG/24HR	N020323 001	OCT 28, 1994

ESTRADIOL (continued)

Cream; Vaginal

VIVELLE-DOT
NOVARTIS

TE	Strength	Appl. No.	Date
AB1	0.1MG/24HR	N020538 008	JAN 08, 1999
AB1	0.05MG/24HR	N020538 006	JAN 08, 1999
AB1	0.075MG/24HR	N020538 007	JAN 08, 1999
AB1	0.0375MG/24HR	N020538 005	JAN 08, 1999

Insert, Extended Release; Vaginal

ESTRING
+ PHARMACIA AND UPJOHN

Strength	Appl. No.	Date
0.0075MG/24HR	N020472 001	APR 26, 1996

Tablet; Oral

ESTRACE
BRISTOL MYERS SQU BB

TE	Strength	Appl. No.	Date
AB	0.5MG	N081295 001	JUN 30, 1993
AB	1MG	N084499 001	
AB	2MG	N084500 001	

+ ESTRADIOL
APPLIED ANAL

TE	Strength	Appl. No.	Date
AB	0.5MG	N040138 001	JAN 30, 1998
AB	1MG	N040138 002	JAN 30, 1998
AB	2MG	N040138 003	JAN 30, 1998

BARR

TE	Strength	Appl. No.	Date
AB	0.5MG	N040197 001	OCT 22, 1997
AB	1MG	N040197 002	OCT 22, 1997
AB	2MG	N040197 003	OCT 22, 1997

CLONMEL HLTHCARE

TE	Strength	Appl. No.	Date
AB	0.5MG	N040275 001	DEC 29, 1998
AB	1MG	N040275 002	DEC 29, 1998
AB	2MG	N040275 003	DEC 29, 1998

MYLAN

TE	Strength	Appl. No.	Date
AB	0.5MG	N040326 001	APR 21, 1999
AB	1MG	N040326 002	APR 21, 1999
AB	2MG	N040326 003	APR 21, 1999

USL PHARMA

TE	Strength	Appl. No.	Date
AB	0.5MG	N040297 001	APR 17, 2002
AB	1MG	N040297 002	APR 17, 2002
AB	2MG	N040297 003	APR 17, 2002

WATSON LABS

TE	Strength	Appl. No.	Date
AB	0.5MG	N040114 003	MAR 14, 1996
AB	1MG	N040114 001	

Prescription Drug Products *(continued)*

ESTRADIOL *(continued)*

Tablet; Oral

TE	Applicant	Strength	Appl. No.	Date
	ESTRADIOL			
	WATSON LABS			MAR 14, 1996
AB	2MG		N040114 002	MAR 14, 1996
	GYNODIOL			
	DURAMED PHARM BARR			
AB	0.5MG		N040212 001	DEC 29, 1997
	1.5MG		N040212 003	DEC 29, 1997
AB	1MG		N040212 002	DEC 29, 1997
AB	2MG		N040212 004	DEC 29, 1997
	INNOFEM			
	NOVO NORDISK			
AB	0.5MG		N040312 001	NOV 19, 1999
AB	1MG		N040312 002	NOV 19, 1999
AB	2MG		N040312 003	NOV 19, 1999

Tablet; Vaginal

TE	Applicant	Strength	Appl. No.	Date
	VAGIFEM			
+	NOVO NORDISK	25UGM	N020908 001	MAR 26, 1999

ESTRADIOL; NORETHINDRONE ACETATE

Film, Extended Release; Transdermal

TE	Applicant	Strength	Appl. No.	Date
	COMBIPATCH			
	NOVARTIS	0.05MG/24HR;0.14MG/24HR	N020870 001	AUG 07, 1998
+		0.05MG/24HR;0.25MG/24HR	N020870 002	AUG 07, 1998

Tablet; Oral

TE	Applicant	Strength	Appl. No.	Date
	ACTIVELLA			
+	NOVO NORDISK	1MG;0.5MG	N020907 001	NOV 18, 1998

ESTRADIOL; NORGESTIMATE

Tablet; Oral

TE	Applicant	Strength	Appl. No.	Date
	PREFEST			
+	KING PHARMS	1MG;1MG;0.09MG	N021040 001	OCT 22, 1999

ESTRADIOL ACETATE

Insert, Extended Release; Vaginal

TE	Applicant	Strength	Appl. No.	Date
	FEMRING			
+	GALEN LTD	0.1MG/24HR	N021367 002	MAR 20, 2003
		0.05MG/24HR	N021367 001	MAR 20, 2003

ESTRADIOL CYPIONATE

Injectable; Injection

TE	Applicant	Strength	Appl. No.	Date
	DEPO-ESTRADIOL			
AO	+ PHARMACIA AND UPJOHN	5MG/ML	N085470 003	
	ESTRADIOL CYPIONATE			
AO	STERIS	5MG/ML	N085620 001	

ESTRADIOL CYPIONATE; MEDROXYPROGESTERONE ACETATE

Injectable; Intramuscular

TE	Applicant	Strength	Appl. No.	Date
	LUNELLE			
	+ PHARMACIA AND UPJOHN	5MG/0.5ML;25MG/0.5ML	N020874 001	OCT 05, 2000

ESTRADIOL VALERATE

Injectable; Injection

TE	Applicant	Strength	Appl. No.	Date
	DELESTROGEN			
	+ KING PHARMS	10MG/ML	N009402 002	
		20MG/ML	N009402 004	
		40MG/ML	N009402 003	
	ESTRADIOL VALERATE			
AO	STERIS	20MG/ML	N083547 001	
AO		40MG/ML	N083714 001	

ESTRAMUSTINE PHOSPHATE SODIUM

Capsule; Oral

TE	Applicant	Strength	Appl. No.	Date
	EMCYT			
	+ PHARMACIA AND UPJOHN	EQ 140MG PHOSPHATE	N018045 001	

ESTROGENS, CONJUGATED

Cream; Topical, Vaginal

TE	Applicant	Strength	Appl. No.	Date
	PREMARIN			
	+ WYETH PHARMS INC	0.625MG/GM	N020216 001	

Injectable; Injection

TE	Applicant	Strength	Appl. No.	Date
	PREMARIN			
	+ WYETH PHARMS INC	25MG/VIAL	N010402 001	

Tablet; Oral

TE	Applicant	Strength	Appl. No.	Date
	PREMARIN			
	WYETH PHARMS INC	0.3MG	N004782 003	
		0.9MG	N004782 005	JAN 26, 1984
		0.625MG	N004782 004	
	+	1.25MG	N004782 001	
	+	2.5MG	N004782 002	

ESTROGENS, CONJUGATED; MEDROXYPROGESTERONE ACETATE

Tablet; Oral-28

TE	Applicant	Strength	Appl. No.	Date
	PREMPHASE 14/14			
	+ WYETH PHARMS INC	0.625MG;0.625MG;5MG	N020527 002	NOV 17, 1995
	PREMPRO			
	+ WYETH PHARMS INC	0.3MG;1.5MG	N020527 005	JUN 04, 2003

Prescription Drug Products *(continued)*

ESTROGENS, CONJUGATED; MEDROXYPROGESTERONE ACETATE *(continued)*

Tablet; Oral-28

PREMPRO

TE	Firm	Strength	Appl. No.	Date
+	WYETH PHARMS INC	0.45MG;1.5MG	N020527 004	MAR 12, 2003
+		0.625MG;0.625MG;2.5MG;2.5MG	N020527 001	NOV 17, 1995
+		0.625MG;0.625MG;5MG;5MG	N020527 003	JAN 09, 1998

ESTROGENS, CONJUGATED SYNTHETIC A

Tablet; Oral

CENESTIN

TE	Firm	Strength	Appl. No.	Date
	DURAMED	0.3MG	N020992 001	JUN 21, 2002
		0.9MG	N020992 003	MAR 24, 1999
		0.625MG	N020992 002	MAR 24, 1999
+		1.25MG	N020992 004	MAR 13, 2000

ESTROGENS, ESTERIFIED

Tablet; Oral

MENEST

TE	Firm	Strength	Appl. No.
	MONARCH PHARMS	0.3MG	N084951 001
		0.625MG	N084948 001
		1.25MG	N084950 001
+		2.5MG	N084949 001

ESTRONE

Injectable; Injection

ESTRONE

TE	Firm	Strength	Appl. No.
+	STERIS	5MG/ML	N085239 001

ESTROPIPATE

Cream; Vaginal

OGEN

TE	Firm	Strength	Appl. No.
+	PHARMACIA AND UPJOHN	1.5MG/GM	N084710 001

Tablet; Oral

ESTROPIPATE

TE	Firm	Strength	Appl. No.	Date
AB	BARR	0.75MG	N040135 001	NOV 27, 1996
AB		1.5MG	N040135 002	NOV 27, 1996
AB		3MG	N040135 003	NOV 27, 1996
AB	DURAMED PHARM BARR	0.75MG	N040296 001	NOV 01, 1999
AB		1.5MG	N040296 002	NOV 01, 1999
AB		3MG	N040296 003	NOV 01, 1999

ESTROPIPATE *(continued)*

Tablet; Oral

ESTROPIPATE

TE	Firm	Strength	Appl. No.	Date
AB	MYLAN	0.75MG	N040359 001	AUG 26, 1999
AB		1.5MG	N040359 002	AUG 26, 1999
AB		3MG	N040359 003	AUG 26, 1999
AB	WATSON LABS	0.75MG	N081213 001	SEP 23, 1993
AB		1.5MG	N081214 001	SEP 23, 1993
AB		3MG	N081215 001	SEP 23, 1993
AB		6MG	N081216 001	SEP 23, 1993

OGEN .625

TE	Firm	Strength	Appl. No.
AB	PHARMACIA AND UPJOHN	0.75MG	N083220 001

OGEN 1.25

| AB | PHARMACIA AND UPJOHN | 1.5MG | N083220 002 |

OGEN 2.5

| AB + | PHARMACIA AND UPJOHN | 3MG | N083220 003 |

OGEN 5

| AB | PHARMACIA AND UPJOHN | 6MG | N083220 004 |

ORTHO-EST

TE	Firm	Strength	Appl. No.	Date
AB	WOMEN FIRST HLTHCARE	0.75MG	N089567 001	FEB 27, 1991
AB		1.5MG	N089582 001	JUL 17, 1991

ETHACRYNATE SODIUM

Injectable; Injection

EDECRIN

TE	Firm	Strength	Appl. No.
+	MERCK	EQ 50MG BASE/VIAL	N016093 001

ETHACRYNIC ACID

Tablet; Oral

EDECRIN

TE	Firm	Strength	Appl. No.
+	MERCK	25MG	N016092 001

ETHAMBUTOL HYDROCHLORIDE

Tablet; Oral

ETHAMBUTOL HCL

TE	Firm	Strength	Appl. No.	Date
AB	BARR	400MG	N076057 001	NOV 26, 2001
AB	WEST WARD	100MG	N075095 001	NOV 30, 1999
AB +		400MG	N075095 002	NOV 30, 1999

Prescription Drug Products *(continued)*

ETHANOLAMINE OLEATE
Injectable; Injection

	ETHAMOLIN		
	+ QUESTCOR PHARMS	50MG/ML	N019357 001 DEC 22, 1988

ETHINYL ESTRADIOL
Tablet; Oral

	ESTINYL		
	SCHERING	0.02MG	N005292 001
		0.05MG	N005292 002
		0.5MG	N005292 003
	+		

ETHINYL ESTRADIOL; ETHYNODIOL DIACETATE
Tablet; Oral-21

AB	DEMULEN 1/35-21		
	+ GD SEARLE LLC	0.035MG;1MG	N018168 001
AB	DEMULEN 1/50-21		
	+ GD SEARLE LLC	0.05MG;1MG	N016927 001
AB	ZOVIA 1/35E-21		
	WATSON LABS	0.035MG;1MG	N072720 001 DEC 30, 1991
AB	ZOVIA 1/50E-21		
	WATSON LABS	0.05MG;1MG	N072722 001 DEC 30, 1991

Tablet; Oral-28

AB	DEMULEN 1/35-28		
	+ GD SEARLE LLC	0.035MG;1MG	N018160 001
AB	DEMULEN 1/50-28		
	+ GD SEARLE LLC	0.05MG;1MG	N016936 001
AB	ZOVIA 1/35E-28		
	WATSON LABS	0.035MG;1MG	N072721 001 DEC 30, 1991
AB	ZOVIA 1/50E-28		
	WATSON LABS	0.05MG;1MG	N072723 001 DEC 30, 1991

ETHINYL ESTRADIOL; ETONOGESTREL
Ring; Vaginal

	NUVARING		
	+ ORGANON USA INC	0.015MG;0.12MG	N021187 001 OCT 03, 2001

ETHINYL ESTRADIOL; LEVONORGESTREL
Tablet; Oral

	PREVEN EMERGENCY CONTRACEPTIVE KIT		
	+ GYNETICS	0.05MG;0.25MG	N020946 001 SEP 01, 1998

Tablet; Oral-21

AB1	ALESSE		
	+ WYETH PHARMS INC	0.02MG;0.1MG	N020683 001 MAR 27, 1997
AB1	AVIANE-21		
	DURAMED PHARM BARR	0.02MG;0.1MG	N075796 002 APR 30, 2001

ETHINYL ESTRADIOL; LEVONORGESTREL *(continued)*
Tablet; Oral-21

	ENPRESSE-21		
AB	DURAMED PHARM BARR	0.03MG;0.05MG;0.075MG;0.04M-G;0.03MG;0.125MG	N075809 001 JUL 16, 2001
AB2	LESSINA-21		
	BARR	0.02MG;0.1MG	N075803 001 MAR 20, 2002
AB2	LEVLITE		
	+ BERLEX LABS	0.02MG;0.1MG	N020860 001 JUL 13, 1998
	LEVONORGESTREL AND ETHINYL ESTRADIOL		
AB1	BARR	0.02MG;0.1MG	N075862 001 APR 29, 2003
AB	LEVORA 0.15/30-21		
	WATSON LABS	0.03MG;0.15MG	N073592 001 DEC 13, 1993
AB	NORDETTE-21		
	+ WYETH PHARMS INC	0.03MG;0.15MG	N018668 001 MAY 10, 1982
AB2	PORTIA-21		
	BARR	0.03MG;0.15MG	N075866 001 MAY 23, 2002
AB	TRIPHASIL-21		
	+ WYETH PHARMS INC	0.03MG;0.04MG;0.03MG;0.05M-G;0.125MG;0.075MG	N019192 001 NOV 01, 1984
AB	TRIVORA-21		
	WATSON LABS	0.03MG;0.04MG;0.03MG;0.05M-G;0.125MG;0.075MG	N074538 001 DEC 18, 1997

Tablet; Oral-28

	ALESSE		
AB1	WYETH PHARMS INC	0.02MG;0.1MG	N020683 002 MAR 27, 1997
AB1	AVIANE-28		
	DURAMED PHARM BARR	0.02MG;0.1MG	N075796 001 APR 30, 2001
	ENPRESSE-28		
AB	DURAMED PHARM BARR	0.03MG;0.03MG;0.075MG;0.04M-G;0.05MG;0.125MG	N075809 002 JUL 16, 2001
AB	LESSINA-28		
	BARR	0.02MG;0.1MG	N075803 002 MAR 20, 2002
AB	LEVLITE		
	BERLEX LABS	0.02MG;0.1MG	N020860 002 JUL 13, 1998
	LEVONORGESTREL AND ETHINYL ESTRADIOL		
AB1	BARR	0.02MG;0.1MG	N075862 002 APR 29, 2003
AB	LEVORA 0.15/30-28		
	WATSON LABS	0.03MG;0.15MG	N073594 001 DEC 13, 1993
AB	NORDETTE-28		
	WYETH PHARMS INC	0.03MG;0.15MG	N018782 001

Prescription Drug Products *(continued)*

ETHINYL ESTRADIOL; LEVONORGESTREL *(continued)*
Tablet; Oral-28

NORDETTE-28
- WYETH PHARMS INC — JUL 21, 1982

PORTIA-28
- AB BARR — 0.03MG;0.15MG — N075866 002 — MAY 23, 2002

TRIPHASIL-28
- WYETH PHARMS INC
- AB 0.03MG;0.04MG;0.03MG;0.05M-G;0.125MG;0.075MG — N019190 001 — NOV 01, 1984

TRIVORA-28
- AB WATSON LABS — 0.03MG;0.04MG;0.03MG;0.05M-G;0.125MG;0.075MG — N074538 002 — DEC 18, 1997

ETHINYL ESTRADIOL; NORELGESTROMIN
Film, Extended Release; Transdermal

ORTHO EVRA
- + ORTHO MCNEIL PHARM — 0.02MG/24HR;0.015MG/24HR — N021180 001 — NOV 20, 2001

ETHINYL ESTRADIOL; NORETHINDRONE
Tablet; Oral-21

BREVICON 21-DAY
- AB WATSON LABS — 0.035MG;0.5MG — N017566 001

GENCEPT 10/11-21
- AB BARR — 0.035MG;0.035MG;0.5MG;1MG — N072694 001 — FEB 28, 1992

MODICON 21
- + ORTHO MCNEIL PHARM
- AB 0.035MG;0.5MG — N017488 001

NORCEPT-E 1/35 21
- AB GYNOPHARMA — 0.035MG;1MG — N071545 001 — FEB 09, 1989

NORETHIN 1/35E-21
- AB WATSON LABS — 0.035MG;1MG — N071480 001 — APR 12, 1988

NORETHINDRONE AND ETHINYL ESTRADIOL
- AB WATSON LABS — 0.035MG;0.5MG — N070684 001 JAN 29, 1987 — N070685 001 JAN 29, 1987
- AB WATSON LABS — 0.035MG;1MG — N071041 001 — SEP 24, 1991

NORETHINDRONE AND ETHINYL ESTRADIOL (7/14)
- + WATSON LABS — 0.035MG;0.035MG;0.5MG;1MG

NORETHINDRONE AND ETHINYL ESTRADIOL (10/11)
- AB WATSON LABS — 0.035MG;0.035MG;0.5MG;1MG — N071043 001 — APR 01, 1988

NORINYL 1+35 21-DAY
- AB WATSON LABS — 0.035MG;1MG — N017565 001

NORTREL 0.5/35-21
- AB BARR — 0.035MG;0.5MG — N072692 001 — FEB 28, 1992

NORTREL 1/35-21
- AB BARR — 0.035MG;1MG — N072693 001 — FEB 28, 1992

ETHINYL ESTRADIOL; NORETHINDRONE *(continued)*
Tablet; Oral-21

NORTREL 7/7/7
- AB BARR — 0.035MG,0.035MG,0.035MG;0.5-MG,1MG,0.75MG — N075478 001 — AUG 30, 2002

ORTHO-NOVUM 1/35-21
- + ORTHO MCNEIL PHARM — 0.035MG;1MG — N017489 002

ORTHO-NOVUM 7/7/7-21
- + ORTHO MCNEIL PHARM — 0.035MG,0.035MG,0.035MG;0.5-MG,1MG,0.75MG — N019985 001 — APR 04, 1984

ORTHO-NOVUM 10/11-21
- + ORTHO MCNEIL PHARM — 0.035MG;0.035MG;0.5MG;1MG — N018354 001 — JAN 11, 1982

OVCON-35
- + WARNER CHILCOTT — 0.035MG;0.4MG — N018127 001

Tablet; Oral-28

BREVICON 28-DAY
- AB WATSON LABS — 0.035MG;0.5MG — N017743 001

GENCEPT 10/11-28
- AB BARR — 0.035MG;0.035MG;0.5MG;1MG — N072697 001 — FEB 28, 1992

MODICON 28
- + ORTHO MCNEIL PHARM — 0.035MG;0.5MG — N017735 001

NORCEPT-E 1/35 28
- AB GYNCPHARMA — 0.035MG;1MG — N071546 001 — FEB 09, 1989

NORETHIN 1/35E-28
- AB WATSON LABS — 0.035MG;1MG — N071481 001 — APR 12, 1988

NORETHINDRONE AND ETHINYL ESTRADIOL
- AB WATSON LABS — 0.035MG;0.5MG — N070686 001 JAN 29, 1987 — N070687 001 JAN 29, 1987
- AB WATSON LABS — 0.035MG;1MG — N071042 001 — SEP 24, 1991

NORETHINDRONE AND ETHINYL ESTRADIOL (7/14)
- AB WATSON LABS — 0.035MG;0.035MG;0.035MG;0.5MG;1MG — N071044 001 — APR 01, 1988

NORETHINDRONE AND ETHINYL ESTRADIOL (10/11)
- AB WATSON LABS — 0.035MG;0.035MG;0.5MG;1MG

NORINYL 1+35 28-DAY
- AB WATSON LABS — 0.035MG;1MG — N017565 002

NORTREL 0.5/35-28
- AB BARR — 0.035MG;0.5MG — N072695 001 — FEB 28, 1992

NORTREL 1/35-28
- AB BARR — 0.035MG;1MG — N072696 001 — FEB 28, 1992

NORTREL 7/7/7
- AB BARR — 0.035MG,0.035MG,0.035MG;0.05-MG,0.75MG,1MG — N075478 002 — AUG 30, 2002

ORTHO-NOVUM 1/35-28
- AB ORTHO MCNEIL PHARM — 0.035MG;1MG — N017919 002

Prescription Drug Products *(continued)*

ETHINYL ESTRADIOL; NORETHINDRONE *(continued)*
Tablet; Oral-28

ORTHO-NOVUM 7/7/7-28
AB + ORTHO MCNEIL PHARM | 0.035MG,0.035MG,0.035MG;0.5-MG,1MG,0.75MG | N018985 002 APR 04, 1984

ORTHO-NOVUM 7/14-28
AB + ORTHO MCNEIL PHARM | 0.035MG;0.035MG;0.5MG;1MG | N019004 002 APR 04, 1984

ORTHO-NOVUM 10/11-28 IN PLASTIC CONTAINER
AB ORTHO MCNEIL PHARM | 0.035MG;0.035MG;0.5MG;1MG | N018354 002 JAN 11, 1982

OVCON-35
+ WARNER CHILCOTT | 0.035MG;0.4MG | N017716 001

OVCON-50
+ WARNER CHILCOTT | 0.05MG;1MG | N017576 001

TRI-NORINYL 28-DAY
+ WATSON LABS | 0.035MG,0.035MG,0.035MG;0.5-MG,1MG,0.5MG | N018977 002 APR 13, 1984

ETHINYL ESTRADIOL; NORETHINDRONE ACETATE
Tablet; Oral
FEMHRT
AB + GALEN CHEM | 0.005MG;1MG | N021065 002 OCT 15, 1999

Tablet; Oral-21
JUNEL 1.5/30
AB BARR | 0.03MG;1.5MG | N076381 001 MAY 30, 2003

JUNEL 1/20
AB BARR | 0.02MG;1MG | N076380 001 MAY 30, 2003

LOESTRIN 21 1.5/30
AB + GALEN CHEM | 0.03MG;1.5MG | N017875 001

LOESTRIN 21 1/20
AB + GALEN CHEM | 0.02MG;1MG | N017876 001

Tablet; Oral-28
ESTROSTEP FE
AB + GALEN CHEM | 0.02MG;0.03MG;0.035MG;1MG;1-MG;1MG | N020130 002 OCT 09, 1996

LOESTRIN FE 1.5/30
AB + GALEN CHEM | 0.03MG;1.5MG | N017355 001

LOESTRIN FE 1/20
AB + GALEN CHEM | 0.02MG;1MG | N017354 001

MICROGESTIN FE 1.5/30
AB WATSON LABS | 0.03MG;1.5MG | N075548 001 FEB 05, 2001

MICROGESTIN FE 1/20
AB WATSON LABS | 0.02MG;1MG | N075647 001 FEB 05, 2001

ETHINYL ESTRADIOL; NORGESTIMATE
Tablet; Oral-28

ORTHO CYCLEN-28
AB + ORTHO MCNEIL PHARM | 0.035MG;0.25MG | N019653 002 DEC 29, 1989

ORTHO TRI-CYCLEN
AB + ORTHO MCNEIL PHARM | 0.035MG,0.035MG,0.035MG;0.18-MG,0.215MG;0.25MG | N019697 001 JUL 03, 1992

ORTHO TRI-CYCLEN LO
+ JOHNSON AND JOHNSON | 0.025MG,0.025MG,0.25MG;0.18-MG,0.25MG,0.215MG | N021241 001 AUG 22, 2002

SPRINTEC
AB BARR | 0.035MG;0.25MG | N075804 001 SEP 25, 2002

TRI-SPRINTEC
AB BARR | 0.035MG,0.035MG,0.035MG;0.18-MG,0.215MG,0.25MG | N075808 001 DEC 18, 2002

ETHINYL ESTRADIOL; NORGESTREL
Tablet; Oral-21

CRYSELLE
AB DURAMED PHARM BARR | 0.03MG;0.3MG | N075840 001 NOV 30, 2001

LO/OVRAL
AB + WYETH PHARMS INC | 0.03MG;0.3MG | N017612 001

LOW-OGESTREL-21
AB WATSON LABS | 0.03MG;0.3MG | N075288 001 JUL 28, 1999

OGESTREL 0.5/50-21
AB WATSON LABS | 0.05MG;0.5MG | N075406 001 DEC 15, 1999

OVRAL
AB + WYETH PHARMS INC | 0.05MG;0.5MG | N016672 001

Tablet; Oral-28
CRYSELLE
AB DURAMED PHARM BARR | 0.03MG;0.3MG | N075840 002 NOV 30, 2001

LO/OVRAL-28
AB + WYETH PHARMS INC | 0.03MG;0.3MG | N017802 001

LOW-OGESTREL-28
AB WATSON LABS | 0.03MG;0.3MG | N075288 002 JUL 28, 1999

OGESTREL 0.5/50-28
AB WATSON LABS | 0.05MG;0.5MG | N075406 002 DEC 15, 1999

OVRAL-28
AB + WYETH PHARMS INC | 0.05MG;0.5MG | N016806 001

ETHINYL ESTRADIOL *MULTIPLE*
SEE DESOGESTREL; ETHINYL ESTRADIOL
SEE DROSPIRENONE; ETHINYL ESTRADIOL *(continued)*

Prescription Drug Products (continued)

ETHIODIZED OIL
Oil; Intralymphatic, Intrauterine
ETHIODOL
  SAVAGE LABS — 99% — N009190 001

ETHIONAMIDE
Tablet; Oral
TRECATOR-SC
  + WYETH PHARMS INC — 250MG — N013026 002

ETHOSUXIMIDE
Capsule; Oral
ETHOSUXIMIDE
  AB BANNER PHARMACAPS — 250MG — N040430 001 OCT 28, 2002
ZARONTIN
  AB PARKE DAVIS — 250MG — N012380 001
Syrup; Oral
ETHOSUXIMIDE
  AA COPLEY PHARM — 250MG/5ML — N081306 001 JUL 30, 1993
  AA PHARM ASSOC — 250MG/5ML — N040253 001 NOV 22, 2000
ZARONTIN
  AA PARKE DAVIS — 250MG/5ML — N080258 001

ETHOTOIN
Tablet; Oral
PEGANONE
  AB OVATION PHARMS — 250MG — N010841 001

ETHYNODIOL DIACETATE *MULTIPLE*
  SEE ETHINYL ESTRADIOL; ETHYNODIOL DIACETATE

ETIDOCAINE HYDROCHLORIDE *MULTIPLE*
  SEE EPINEPHRINE BITARTRATE; ETIDOCAINE HYDROCHLORIDE

ETIDRONATE DISODIUM
Injectable; Injection
DIDRONEL
  + MGI PHARMA INC — 50MG/ML — N019545 001 APR 20, 1987
Tablet; Oral
DIDRONEL
  PROCTER AND GAMBLE — 200MG — N017831 001
       — 400MG — N017831 002
ETIDRONATE DISODIUM
  GENPHARM — 200MG — N075800 001 JAN 24, 2003
  AB — 400MG — N075800 002 JAN 24, 2003
  AB

ETODOLAC
Capsule; Oral
ETODOLAC
  AB ENDO PHARMS — 200MG — N074842 001 JUL 17, 1997
  AB — 300MG — N074842 002 JUL 17, 1997
  AB GENEVA PHARMS — 200MG — N074840 001 AUG 29, 1997
  AB — 300MG — N074840 002 AUG 29, 1997
  AB GENEVA PHARMS TECH — 200MG — N074942 001 SEP 30, 1997
  AB — 300MG — N074942 002 SEP 30, 1997
  AB GENPHARM — 200MG — N075071 001 SEP 30, 1998
  AB — 300MG — N075071 002 SEP 30, 1998
  AB IVAX PHARMS — 200MG — N074899 001 JUL 08, 1997
  AB — 300MG — N074899 002 JUL 08, 1997
  AB MYLAN — 200MG — N074932 001 MAY 16, 1997
  AB — 300MG — N074932 002 MAY 16, 1997
  AB NEOSAN PHARMS — 300MG — N074929 001 JAN 30, 1998
  AB TARO — 200MG — N075078 001 APR 30, 1998
  AB — 300MG — N075078 002 APR 30, 1998
  AB TEVA — 200MG — N075126 001 SEP 16, 1999
  AB — 300MG — N075126 002 SEP 16, 1999
  AB TORPHARM — 200MG — N075419 001 SEP 16, 1999
  AB — 300MG — N075419 002 JUL 28, 2000
  AB WATSON LABS — 200MG — N074844 001 JUL 28, 2000
  AB — 300MG — N074844 002 DEC 23, 1997
LODINE
WYETH PHARMS INC
  AB + — 200MG — N018922 002 DEC 23, 1997
  AB + — 300MG — N018922 003 JAN 31, 1991
Tablet, Extended Release; Oral
ETODOLAC
  AB ANDRX PHARM — 400MG — N075829 001 JAN 31, 1991
  AB — 500MG — N075829 002 NOV 30, 2001
  AB EON — 400MG — N075943 001 NOV 30, 2001

Prescription Drug Products (continued)

ETODOLAC (continued)

Tablet, Extended Release; Oral

ETODOLAC

TE	Firm	Strength	Appl. No.	Approval
AB	EON	400MG	N075943 001	JUL 26, 2002
AB		500MG	N075943 002	JUL 26, 2002
AB		600MG	N075943 003	JUL 26, 2002
AB	POINT HOLDINGS	400MG	N075696 001	JUL 26, 2002
AB	TARO	400MG	N076174 001	JUL 31, 2000
AB		500MG	N076174 002	MAR 13, 2003
AB		600MG	N076174 003	MAR 13, 2003
AB	TEVA	400MG	N075665 001	JUL 31, 2000
AB		500MG	N075665 002	FEB 05, 2001
AB		600MG	N075665 003	MAR 13, 2003

LODINE XL

TE	Firm	Strength	Appl. No.	Approval
AB +	WYETH PHARMS INC	400MG	N020584 001	OCT 25, 1996
AB +		500MG	N020584 002	JAN 20, 1998
AB +		600MG	N020584 003	OCT 25, 1996

Tablet; Oral

ETODOLAC

TE	Firm	Strength	Appl. No.	Approval
AB	APOTEX	400MG	N076004 001	DEC 03, 2002
AB		500MG	N076004 002	DEC 03, 2002
AB	ENDO PHARMS	400MG	N074841 001	JUN 27, 1997
AB	EON	400MG	N074903 001	APR 11, 1997
AB		500MG	N074903 002	APR 19, 1999
AB	GENEVA PHARMS	400MG	N074839 001	JUL 11, 1997
AB	GENEVA PHARMS TECH	400MG	N074846 001	FEB 28, 1997
AB	GENPHARM	400MG	N075012 001	SEP 30, 1998
AB		500MG	N075012 002	SEP 30, 1998
AB	IVAX PHARMS	400MG	N074883 001	FEB 28, 1997
AB		500MG	N074883 002	NOV 20, 1998
AB	MYLAN	400MG	N075104 001	FEB 06, 1998
AB		500MG	N075104 002	NOV 20, 1998
AB	NEOSAN PHARMS	400MG	N074927 001	OCT 30, 1997
AB	PUREPAC PHARM	400MG	N074819 001	FEB 28, 1997
AB	RANBAXY	400MG	N075226 001	NOV 24, 1998
AB		500MG	N075226 002	NOV 24, 1998
AB	TARO PHARM INDS	400MG	N075074 001	MAR 11, 1998
AB		500MG	N075074 002	APR 25, 2000
AB	TEVA	400MG	N074847 001	APR 23, 1999
AB		400MG	N075009 001	NOV 26, 1997
AB		500MG	N074847 002	APR 23, 1999
AB		500MG	N075009 002	DEC 28, 1999
AB	WATSON LABS	400MG	N074892 001	APR 16, 1997
AB		500MG	N075069 001	APR 16, 1998
AB		500MG	N074892 002	OCT 29, 1998

LODINE

TE	Firm	Strength	Appl. No.	Approval
AB	WYETH PHARMS INC	400MG	N018922 004	JUL 29, 1993
AB +		500MG	N018922 005	JUN 28, 1996

ETOMIDATE

Injectable; Injection

AMIDATE

TE	Firm	Strength	Appl. No.	Approval
AP +	ABBOTT	2MG/ML	N018227 001	SEP 07, 1982

ETOMIDATE

TE	Firm	Strength	Appl. No.	Approval
AP	BEDFORD	2MG/ML	N074593 001	NOV 04, 1996

ETONOGESTREL *MULTIPLE*

SEE ETHINYL ESTRADIOL; ETONOGESTREL

ETOPOSIDE

Capsule; Oral

ETOPOSIDE

TE	Firm	Strength	Appl. No.	Approval
AB	GENPHARM	50MG	N075635 001	SEP 19, 2001

VEPESID

TE	Firm	Strength	Appl. No.	Approval
AB +	BRISTOL	50MG	N019557 001	DEC 30, 1986

Prescription Drug Products (continued)

ETOPOSIDE (continued)

Injectable; Injection

ETOPOSIDE

TE	Applicant	Strength	Appl. No.	Approval
AP	ABBOTT	20MG/ML	N074320 001	AUG 30, 1995
AP		20MG/ML	N074351 001	AUG 30, 1995
AP	AM PHARM PARTNERS	20MG/ML	N074983 001	SEP 30, 1998
AP	BEDFORD	20MG/ML	N074290 001	JUL 17, 1995
AP	GENSIA SICOR PHARMS	20MG/ML	N074284 001	FEB 10, 1994
AP		20MG/ML	N074529 001	JUL 24, 1996
AP	MARSAM PHARMS LLC	20MG/ML	N074968 001	JAN 09, 1998
AP	PHARMACHEMIE	20MG/ML	N074227 001	FEB 22, 1996
AP	SUPERGEN	20MG/ML	N074513 001	MAR 14, 1996

TOPOSAR

TE	Applicant	Strength	Appl. No.	Approval
AP	PHARMACIA AND UPJOHN	20MG/ML	N074166 001	FEB 27, 1995

VEPESID

TE	Applicant	Strength	Appl. No.	Approval
AP	+ BRISTOL MYERS SQUIBB	20MG/ML	N018768 001	NOV 10, 1983

ETOPOSIDE PHOSPHATE

Injectable; Injection

ETOPOPHOS PRESERVATIVE FREE

TE	Applicant	Strength	Appl. No.	Approval
	+ BRISTOL MYERS SQUIBB	EQ 100MG BASE/VIAL	N020457 001	MAY 17, 1996

EXEMESTANE

Tablet; Oral

AROMASIN

TE	Applicant	Strength	Appl. No.	Approval
	+ PHARMACIA AND UPJOHN	25MG	N020753 001	OCT 21, 1999

EZETIMIBE

Tablet; Oral

ZETIA

TE	Applicant	Strength	Appl. No.	Approval
	+ MSP SINGAPORE	10MG	N021445 001	OCT 25, 2002

FAMCICLOVIR

Tablet; Oral

FAMVIR

TE	Applicant	Strength	Appl. No.	Approval
	NOVARTIS	125MG	N020363 003	DEC 11, 1995

FAMCICLOVIR (continued)

Tablet; Oral

FAMVIR

TE	Applicant	Strength	Appl. No.	Approval
	NOVARTIS	250MG	N020363 001	APR 26, 1996
	+	500MG	N020363 002	JUN 29, 1994

FAMOTIDINE

For Suspension; Oral

PEPCID

TE	Applicant	Strength	Appl. No.	Approval
	+ MERCK	40MG/5ML	N019527 001	FEB 02, 1987

Injectable; Injection

FAMOTIDINE

TE	Applicant	Strength	Appl. No.	Approval
AP	ABBOTT	10MG/ML	N075870 001	NOV 23, 2001
AP		10MG/ML	N075905 001	NOV 23, 2001
AP	AM PHARM PARTNERS	10MG/ML	N075709 001	APR 16, 2001
AP		10MG/ML	N075942 001	AUG 02, 2002
AP	APOTEX	10MG/ML	N075799 001	APR 30, 2002
AP	BAXTER HLTHCARE	10MG/ML	N075651 001	APR 16, 2001
AP	BEDFORD	10MG/ML	N075684 001	APR 16, 2001
AP		10MG/ML	N075488 001	APR 16, 2001
AP	ESI LEDERLE	10MG/ML	N075705 001	APR 16, 2001
AP	FAULDING	10MG/ML	N075813 001	APR 16, 2001

FAMOTIDINE PRESERVATIVE FREE

TE	Applicant	Strength	Appl. No.	Approval
AP	AM PHARM PARTNERS	10MG/ML	N076324 001	NOV 27, 2002
AP	APOTEX	10MG/ML	N075486 001	APR 16, 2001
AP	BAXTER HLTHCARE	10MG/ML	N075789 001	APR 30, 2002
AP	BEDFORD	10MG/ML	N075622 001	APR 16, 2001
AP	BEN VENUE	10MG/ML	N075825 001	APR 17, 2001
AP	FAULDING	10MG/ML	N075669 001	APR 16, 2001

FAMOTIDINE PRESERVATIVE FREE (PHARMACY BULK)

TE	Applicant	Strength	Appl. No.	Approval
AP	APOTEX	10MG/ML	N076322 001	NOV 27, 2002

FAMOTIDINE PRESERVATIVE FREE IN PLASTIC CONTAINER

TE	Applicant	Strength	Appl. No.	Approval
AP	ABBOTT	0.4MG/ML	N075729 001	DEC 17, 2001
AP	BAXTER HLTHCARE	0.4MG/ML	N075591 001	MAY 10, 2001

Prescription Drug Products (continued)

FAMOTIDINE (continued)

Injectable; Injection

PEPCID

TE	Firm	Strength	Appl. No.	Date
AP	+ MERCK	10MG/ML	N019510 001	NOV 04, 1986

PEPCID PRESERVATIVE FREE

TE	Firm	Strength	Appl. No.	Date
AP	+ MERCK	10MG/ML	N019510 004	NOV 04, 1986

PEPCID PRESERVATIVE FREE IN PLASTIC CONTAINER

TE	Firm	Strength	Appl. No.	Date
AP	+ MERCK	0.4MG/ML	N020249 001	FEB 18, 1994

Tablet; Oral

FAMOTIDINE

TE	Firm	Strength	Appl. No.	Date
AB	CARLSBAD	20MG	N075805 001	APR 16, 2001
AB		40MG	N075805 002	APR 16, 2001
AB	DR REDDYS LABS LTD	20MG	N075718 001	APR 16, 2001
AB		40MG	N075718 002	APR 16, 2001
AB	EON	20MG	N075793 001	APR 16, 2001
AB		40MG	N075793 002	APR 16, 2001
AB	GENEVA PHARMS	20MG	N075302 001	APR 16, 2001
AB		40MG	N075302 002	APR 16, 2001
AB	GENPHARM	20MG	N075457 001	APR 16, 2001
AB		40MG	N075457 002	APR 18, 2001
AB	INVAMED	20MG	N075607 001	MAY 10, 2001
AB		40MG	N075607 002	MAY 10, 2001
AB	IVAX PHARMS	20MG	N075511 001	APR 16, 2001
AB		40MG	N075511 002	APR 16, 2001
AB	MUTUAL PHARM	20MG	N075639 002	DEC 12, 2001
AB		40MG	N075639 001	DEC 12, 2001
AB	MYLAN	20MG	N075704 001	APR 16, 2001
AB		40MG	N075704 002	APR 16, 2001
AB	PUREPAC PHARM	20MG	N075650 001	SEP 14, 2001
AB		40MG	N075650 002	SEP 14, 2001
AB	TEVA	20MG	N075311 001	APR 16, 2001
AB		40MG	N075311 002	APR 16, 2001

FAMOTIDINE (continued)

Tablet; Oral

FAMOTIDINE

TE	Firm	Strength	Appl. No.	Date
AB	TORPHARM	20MG	N075611 001	JUL 23, 2001
AB		40MG	N075611 002	JUL 23, 2001
AB	WATSON LABS	20MG	N075062 002	APR 16, 2001
AB		40MG	N075062 001	APR 16, 2001
AB	WOCKHARDT	20MG	N075786 001	APR 16, 2001
AB		40MG	N075786 002	APR 16, 2001

PEPCID

TE	Firm	Strength	Appl. No.	Date
AB	MERCK	20MG	N019462 001	OCT 15, 1986
AB	+	40MG	N019462 002	OCT 15, 1986

FELBAMATE

Suspension; Oral

FELBATOL

TE	Firm	Strength	Appl. No.	Date
	+ MEDPOINTE	600MG/5ML	N020189 003	JUL 29, 1993

Tablet; Oral

FELBATOL

TE	Firm	Strength	Appl. No.	Date
	MEDPOINTE	400MG	N020189 001	JUL 29, 1993
	+	600MG	N020189 002	JUL 29, 1993

FELODIPINE

Tablet, Extended Release; Oral

PLENDIL

TE	Firm	Strength	Appl. No.	Date
	ASTRAZENECA	2.5MG	N019834 004	SEP 22, 1994
		5MG	N019834 001	JUL 25, 1991
	+	10MG	N019834 002	JUL 25, 1991

FELODIPINE *MULTIPLE*

SEE ENALAPRIL MALEATE; FELODIPINE

FENOFIBRATE

Capsule; Oral

FENOFIBRATE (MICRONIZED)

TE	Firm	Strength	Appl. No.	Date
	TEVA	67MG	N075753 001	SEP 03, 2002
		134MG	N075753 002	APR 09, 2002
	+	200MG	N075753 003	APR 09, 2002

Prescription Drug Products (continued)

FENOFIBRATE (continued)
Tablet; Oral

TRICOR

	ABBOTT	54MG	N021203 001	SEP 04, 2001
+		160MG	N021203 003	SEP 04, 2001

FENOLDOPAM MESYLATE
Injectable; Injection

CORLOPAM

+	ABBOTT	EQ 10MG BASE/ML	N019922 001	SEP 23, 1997

FENOPROFEN CALCIUM
Capsule; Oral

FENOPROFEN CALCIUM

AB	GENEVA PHARMS	EQ 200MG BASE	N072394 001	OCT 17, 1988
AB		EQ 300MG BASE	N072395 001	OCT 17, 1988
AB	PAR PHARM	EQ 200MG BASE	N072437 001	AUG 22, 1988
AB		EQ 300MG BASE	N072438 001	AUG 22, 1988

NALFON
+ RANBAXY

NALFON 200
RANBAXY

AB		EQ 300MG BASE	N017604 002	
AB		EQ 200MG BASE	N017604 003	

Tablet; Oral

FENOPROFEN CALCIUM

AB	CLONMEL HLTHCARE	EQ 600MG BASE	N072326 001	AUG 17, 1988
AB	GENEVA PHARMS	EQ 600MG BASE	N072396 001	OCT 17, 1988
AB		EQ 600MG BASE	N072557 001	
AB	IVAX PHARMS	EQ 600MG BASE	N072429 001	AUG 29, 1988
AB	MUTUAL PHARM	EQ 600MG BASE	N072902 001	DEC 21, 1990
AB	+ MYLAN	EQ 600MG BASE	N072267 001	AUG 17, 1988
AB	PAR PHARM	EQ 600MG BASE	N072429 001	AUG 17, 1988
AB	PUREPAC PHARM	EQ 600MG BASE	N072274 001	MAY 02, 1988
AB	WATSON LABS	EQ 600MG BASE	N072407 001	AUG 17, 1988
AB		EQ 600MG BASE	N072602 001	OCT 11, 1988

FENTANYL
Film, Extended Release; Transdermal

DURAGESIC

+	ALZA	0.6MG/24HR	N019813 004	AUG 07, 1990
		1.2MG/24HR	N019813 003	AUG 07, 1990
	ALZA	1.8MG/24HR	N019813 002	AUG 07, 1990
+		2.4MG/24HR	N019813 001	AUG 07, 1990

FENTANYL CITRATE
Injectable; Injection

FENTANYL CITRATE

AP	ABBOTT	EQ 0.05MG BASE/ML	N019115 001	JAN 12, 1985

FENTANYL CITRATE PRESERVATIVE FREE

AP	ABBOTT	EQ 0.05MG BASE/ML	N072786 001	SEP 24, 1991
AP	+ ELKINS SINN	EQ 0.05MG BASE/ML	N019101 001	JUL 11, 1984

SUBLIMAZE PRESERVATIVE FREE

AP	+ AKORN MFG	EQ 0.05MG BASE/ML	N016619 001	

Troche/Lozenge; Oral

ACTIQ

	ANESTA	EQ 0.2MG BASE	N020747 001	NOV 04, 1998
		EQ 0.4MG BASE	N020747 002	NOV 04, 1998
		EQ 0.6MG BASE	N020747 003	NOV 04, 1998
		EQ 0.8MG BASE	N020747 004	NOV 04, 1998
		EQ 1.2MG BASE	N020747 005	NOV 04, 1998
		EQ 1.6MG BASE	N020747 006	NOV 04, 1998

FENTANYL CITRATE *MULTIPLE*
SEE DROPERIDOL; FENTANYL CITRATE

+

FERUMOXIDES
Injectable; Injection

FERIDEX I.V.

+	ADV MAGNETICS	EQ 11.2MG IRON/ML	N020416 001	AUG 30, 1996

FERUMOXSIL
Suspension; Oral

GASTROMARK

+	ADV MAGNETICS	EQ 0.175MG IRON/ML	N020410 001	DEC 06, 1996

FEXOFENADINE HYDROCHLORIDE
Capsule; Oral

ALLEGRA

+	AVENTIS PHARMS	60MG	N020625 001	

Prescription Drug Products *(continued)*

FEXOFENADINE HYDROCHLORIDE *(continued)*
Capsule; Oral
  ALLEGRA
    AVENTIS PHARMS   JUL 25, 1996
Tablet; Oral
  ALLEGRA
    AVENTIS PHARMS   30MG   N020872 001   FEB 25, 2000
                     60MG   N020872 002   FEB 25, 2000
  +   180MG   N020872 004   FEB 25, 2000

FEXOFENADINE HYDROCHLORIDE; PSEUDOEPHEDRINE HYDROCHLORIDE
Tablet, Extended Release; Oral
  ALLEGRA-D
  + AVENTIS PHARMS   60MG;120MG   N020786 001   DEC 24, 1997

FIBRINOLYSIN *MULTIPLE*
SEE CHLORAMPHENICOL; DESOXYRIBONUCLEASE; FIBRINOLYSIN

FINASTERIDE
Tablet; Oral
  PROPECIA
  + MERCK   1MG   N020788 001   DEC 19, 1997
  PROSCAR
  + MERCK   5MG   N020180 001   JUN 19, 1992

FLAVOXATE HYDROCHLORIDE
Tablet; Oral
  URISPAS
  + ORTHO MCNEIL PHARM   100MG   N016769 001

FLECAINIDE ACETATE
Tablet; Oral
  FLECAINIDE ACETATE
AB ALPHAPHARM   50MG   N075442 001   JUL 31, 2001
AB   100MG   N075442 002   JUL 31, 2001
AB   150MG   N075442 003   JUL 31, 2001
AB BARR   50MG   N075882 001   OCT 28, 2002
AB   100MG   N075882 002   OCT 28, 2002
AB   150MG   N075882 003   OCT 28, 2002
AB GENEVA PHARMS   50MG   N076030 001   OCT 28, 2002
AB   100MG   N076030 002   OCT 28, 2002

FLECAINIDE ACETATE *(continued)*
Tablet; Oral
  FLECAINIDE ACETATE
    GENEVA PHARMS 150MG   N076030 003   OCT 28, 2002
AB RANBAXY   50MG   N076421 001   MAR 28, 2003
AB   100MG   N076421 002   MAR 28, 2003
AB   150MG   N076421 003   MAR 28, 2003
AB ROXANE   50MG   N076278 001   JAN 14, 2003
AB   100MG   N076278 002   JAN 14, 2003
AB   150MG   N076278 003   JAN 14, 2003
  TAMBOCOR
AB 3M   50MG   N018830 004   AUG 23, 1988
AB   100MG   N018830 001   OCT 31, 1985
AB   150MG   N018830 003   JUN 03, 1988

FLOXURIDINE
Injectable; Injection
  FLOXURIDINE
AP AM PHARM PARTNERS   500MG/VIAL   N075837 001   FEB 22, 2001
AP BEDFORD   500MG/VIAL   N075387 001   APR 16, 2000
  FUDR
AP + FAULDING   500MG/VIAL   N016929 001

FLUCONAZOLE
For Suspension; Oral
  DIFLUCAN
    PFIZER   50MG/5ML   N020090 001   DEC 23, 1993
  +   200MG/5ML   N020090 002   DEC 23, 1993

Injectable; Injection
  DIFLUCAN IN DEXTROSE 5% IN PLASTIC CONTAINER
  + PFIZER   200MG/100ML N019950 003   SEP 29, 1992
  DIFLUCAN IN SODIUM CHLORIDE 0.9%
  + PFIZER   200MG/100ML N019950 001   JAN 29, 1990
  DIFLUCAN IN SODIUM CHLORIDE 0.9% IN PLASTIC CONTAINER
  + PFIZER   200MG/100ML N019950 002   JAN 29, 1990
Tablet; Oral
  DIFLUCAN
    PFIZER   50MG   N019949 001

Prescription Drug Products (continued)

FLUCONAZOLE (continued)
Tablet; Oral
DIFLUCAN
PFIZER
- 100MG — JAN 29, 1990 / N019949 002
- 150MG — JAN 29, 1990 / N019949 004 — JUN 30, 1994 / N019949 003
- + 200MG — JAN 29, 1990

FLUCYTOSINE
Capsule; Oral
ANCOBON
ICN
- 250MG — N017001 001
- + 500MG — N017001 002

FLUDARABINE PHOSPHATE
Injectable; Injection
FLUDARA
- + BERLEX — 50MG/VIAL — N020038 001 — APR 18, 1991

FLUDEOXYGLUCOSE, F-18
Injectable; Injection
FLUDEOXYGLUCOSE F 18
- + DOWNSTATE CLINCL — 4-90mCi/ML — N020306 002 — SEP 25, 2001

FLUDROCORTISONE ACETATE
Tablet; Oral
FLORINEF
- AB + KING PHARMS — 0.1MG — N010060 001

FLUDROCORTISONE ACETATE
- AB BARR — 0.1MG — N040425 001 — JAN 21, 2003 / N040431 001 — MAR 18, 2002
- AB IMPAX LABS — 0.1MG

FLUMAZENIL
Injectable; Injection
ROMAZICON
- + HLR — 0.1MG/ML — N020073 001 — DEC 20, 1991

FLUNISOLIDE
Aerosol, Metered; Inhalation
AEROBID
- + ROCHE PALO — 0.25MG/INH — N018340 001 — AUG 17, 1984

Spray, Metered; Nasal
FLUNISOLIDE
- AB BAUSCH AND LOMB — 0.025MG/SPRAY — N074805 001 — FEB 20, 2002

FLUNISOLIDE (continued)
Spray, Metered; Nasal
NASALIDE
- AB + IVAX RES — 0.025MG/SPRAY — N018148 001

NASAREL
- BX + IVAX RES — 0.025MG/SPRAY — N020409 001 — MAR 08, 1995

FLUOCINOLONE ACETONIDE
Cream; Topical
FLUOCINOLONE ACETONIDE
- AT FOUGERA — 0.01% — N088170 001 — DEC 16, 1982 / N088169 001 — DEC 16, 1982
- AT — 0.025% — N089526 001 — JUL 26, 1988
- AT G AND W LABS — 0.01% — N089525 001 — JUL 26, 1988 / N040035 001
- AT — 0.025% — OCT 31, 1994 / N087102 001 — APR 27, 1982
- AT TARO — 0.01% — N040042 001 — OCT 31, 1994 / N087104 001 — APR 27, 1982
- AT — 0.01%
- AT — 0.025%
- AT — 0.025%

SYNALAR
- AT + MEDICIS — 0.01% — N012787 004
- AT + — 0.025% — N012787 002
- AT + — 0.025% — N012787 005

Oil; Topical
DERMA-SMOOTHE/FS
- + HILL DERMAC — 0.01% — N019452 001 — FEB 03, 1988

Ointment; Topical
FLUOCINOLONE ACETONIDE
- AT FOUGERA — 0.025% — N088168 001 — DEC 16, 1982 / N089524 001
- AT G AND W LABS — 0.025% — JUL 26, 1988 / N040041 001
- AT TARO — 0.025% — SEP 15, 1994

SYNALAR
- AT + MEDICIS — 0.025% — N013960 001

Shampoo; Topical
FS SHAMPOO
- + GALDERMA LABS LP — 0.01% — N020001 001 — AUG 27, 1990

Solution; Topical
FLUOCINOLONE ACETONIDE
- AT ALPHARMA — 0.01% — N087159 001 — JUN 16, 1982
- AT FOUGERA — 0.01% — N088167 001 — DEC 16, 1982
- AT TARO — 0.01% — N089124 001

Prescription Drug Products *(continued)*

FLUOCINOLONE ACETONIDE *(continued)*
Solution; Topical

FLUOCINOLONE ACETONIDE
SYNALAR
TARO

TE	Product / Applicant	Strength	Appl. No.	Date
AT	+ MEDICIS	0.01%	N015296 001	SEP 11, 1985

FLUOCINOLONE ACETONIDE; HYDROQUINONE; TRETINOIN
Cream; Topical

TRI-LUMA

TE	Product / Applicant	Strength	Appl. No.	Date
	+ HILL DERMAC	0.01%;4%;0.05%	N021112 001	JAN 18, 2002

FLUOCINONIDE
Cream; Topical

FLUOCINONIDE

TE	Applicant	Strength	Appl. No.	Date
AB1	ALPHARMA US PHARM	0.05%	N073085 001	FEB 14, 1992
AB1	FOUGERA	0.05%	N073030 001	OCT 17, 1994
AB1	TARO	0.05%	N019117 001	JUN 26, 1984
AB1		0.05%	N071500 001	JUN 10, 1987
AB1	TEVA	0.05%	N072488 001	FEB 06, 1989

FLUOCINONIDE EMULSIFIED BASE

TE	Applicant	Strength	Appl. No.	Date
AB2	ALPHARMA US PHARM	0.05%	N074204 001	JUN 13, 1995
AB2	TARO	0.05%	N072494 001	JAN 19, 1989
AB2	TEVA	0.05%	N072490 001	FEB 07, 1989

LIDEX

TE	Applicant	Strength	Appl. No.	Date
AB1	+ MEDICIS	0.05%	N016908 002	

LIDEX-E

TE	Applicant	Strength	Appl. No.	Date
AB2	+ MEDICIS	0.05%	N016908 003	

Gel; Topical

FLUOCINONIDE

TE	Applicant	Strength	Appl. No.	Date
AB	FOUGERA	0.05%	N072933 001	DEC 30, 1994
AB	TARO	0.05%	N074935 001	JUL 29, 1997
AB	TEVA	0.05%	N072537 001	FEB 07, 1989

LIDEX

TE	Applicant	Strength	Appl. No.	Date
AB	+ MEDICIS	0.05%	N017373 001	

Ointment; Topical

FLUOCINONIDE

TE	Applicant	Strength	Appl. No.	Date
AB	ALTANA	0.05%	N074905 001	AUG 26, 1997
AB	TARO	0.05%	N075008 001	JUN 30, 1999
AB	TEVA	0.05%	N073481 001	DEC 27, 1991

FLUOCINONIDE *(continued)*
Ointment; Topical

LIDEX

TE	Applicant	Strength	Appl. No.	Date
AB	+ MEDICIS	0.05%	N016909 002	

Solution; Topical

FLUOCINONIDE

TE	Applicant	Strength	Appl. No.	Date
	ALPHARMA	0.05%	N071535 001	DEC 02, 1988
AT	COPLEY PHARM	0.05%	N072522 001	SEP 28, 1990
AT	FOUGERA	0.05%	N072934 001	FEB 27, 1995
AT	TARO	0.05%	N072857 001	AUG 02, 1989
AT		0.05%	N074799 001	DEC 31, 1996
AT	TEVA	0.05%	N072511 001	FEB 07, 1989

LIDEX

TE	Applicant	Strength	Appl. No.	Date
AT	+ MEDICIS	0.05%	N018849 001	APR 06, 1984

FLUOROMETHOLONE
Ointment; Ophthalmic

FML

TE	Applicant	Strength	Appl. No.	Date
	+ ALLERGAN	0.1%	N017760 001	SEP 04, 1985

Suspension/Drops; Ophthalmic

FML

TE	Applicant	Strength	Appl. No.	Date
AB	+ ALLERGAN	0.1%	N016851 002	JUL 28, 1982

FML FORTE

TE	Applicant	Strength	Appl. No.	Date
	ALLERGAN	0.25%	N019216 001	APR 23, 1986

Suspension; Ophthalmic

FLUOR-OP

TE	Applicant	Strength	Appl. No.	Date
AB	NOVARTIS	0.1%	N070185 001	FEB 27, 1986

FLUOROMETHOLONE; SULFACETAMIDE SODIUM
Suspension/Drops; Ophthalmic

FML-S

TE	Applicant	Strength	Appl. No.	Date
AB	+ ALLERGAN	0.1%;10%	N019525 001	SEP 29, 1989

FLUOROMETHOLONE ACETATE
Suspension/Drops; Ophthalmic

FLAREX

TE	Applicant	Strength	Appl. No.	Date
	+ ALCON	0.1%	N019079 001	FEB 11, 1986

FLUOROMETHOLONE ACETATE; TOBRAMYCIN
Suspension/Drops; Ophthalmic

TOBRASONE

TE	Applicant	Strength	Appl. No.	Date
	+ ALCON	0.1%;0.3%	N050628 001	

Prescription Drug Products (continued)

FLUOROMETHOLONE ACETATE; TOBRAMYCIN (continued)
Suspension/Drops; Ophthalmic

	Firm	Strength	NDA	Date
	TOBRASONE			
	ALCON			JUL 21, 1989

FLUOROURACIL
Cream; Topical

	Firm	Strength	NDA	Date
	CARAC			
+	DERMIK LABS	0.5%	N020985 001	OCT 27, 2000
	EFUDEX			
+	ICN	5%	N016831 003	
	FLUOROPLEX			
+	ALLERGAN HERBERT	1%	N016988 001	

Injectable; Injection

	Firm	Strength	NDA	Date
	ADRUCIL			
AP	PHARMACIA AND UPJOHN	50MG/ML	N040023 001	OCT 18, 1991
AP +		50MG/ML	N081225 001	AUG 28, 1991
	FLUOROURACIL			
AP	AM PHARM PARTNERS	50MG/ML	N040278 001	SEP 30, 1998
AP		50MG/ML	N040279 001	SEP 30, 1998
AP	BEDFORD	50MG/ML	N089508 001	JAN 26, 1988
AP	BIGMAR	50MG/ML	N040291 001	MAR 24, 1999
AP		50MG/ML	N040379 001	NOV 15, 2000
AP	GENSIA SICOR PHARMS	50MG/ML	N040333 001	JAN 27, 2000
AP		50MG/ML	N040334 001	FEB 25, 2000
AP +	ICN PUERTO RICO	50MG/ML	N012209 001	
AP	STERIS	50MG/ML	N087792 001	OCT 13, 1982

Solution; Topical

	Firm	Strength	NDA	Date
	EFUDEX			
+	ICN	2%	N016831 001	
+ +		5%	N016831 002	

FLUOXETINE HYDROCHLORIDE
Capsule, Delayed Rel Pellets; Oral

	Firm	Strength	NDA	Date
	PROZAC WEEKLY			
+	LILLY	EQ 90MG BASE	N021235 001	FEB 26, 2001

Capsule; Oral

	Firm	Strength	NDA	Date
	FLUOXETINE			
AB	ALPHAPHARM	EQ 10MG BASE	N075577 001	JAN 29, 2002
AB		EQ 20MG BASE	N075577 002	JAN 29, 2002
AB	BARR	EQ 10MG BASE	N074803 002	JAN 29, 2002

FLUOXETINE HYDROCHLORIDE (continued)
Capsule; Oral

	Firm	Strength	NDA	Date
	FLUOXETINE			
AB	BARR	EQ 20MG BASE	N074803 001	JAN 30, 2002
AB	CARLSBAD	EQ 10MG BASE	N076022 001	AUG 02, 2001
AB		EQ 20MG BASE	N076022 002	JAN 30, 2002
AB	DR REDDYS LABS INC	EQ 10MG BASE	N075465 001	JAN 30, 2002
AB		EQ 20MG BASE	N075465 002	JAN 29, 2002
AB		EQ 40MG BASE	N075465 003	JAN 29, 2002
AB	EON	EQ 10MG BASE	N075807 001	AUG 02, 2001
AB		EQ 20MG BASE	N075807 002	JAN 29, 2002
AB	GENEVA PHARMS	EQ 10MG BASE	N075049 001	JAN 29, 2002
AB		EQ 20MG BASE	N075245 002	AUG 02, 2001
AB	IVAX PHARMS	EQ 20MG BASE	N075245 001	JAN 31, 2002
AB	MALLINCKRODT	EQ 10MG BASE	N075658 001	JAN 31, 2002
AB		EQ 20MG BASE	N075658 002	JAN 29, 2002
AB	MUTUAL PHARMA	EQ 10MG BASE	N075787 001	JAN 29, 2002
AB		EQ 20MG BASE	N075787 002	JAN 29, 2002
AB	MYLAN	EQ 10MG BASE	N075207 001	JAN 29, 2002
AB		EQ 20MG BASE	N075207 002	JAN 30, 2002
AB	PLIVA	EQ 10MG BASE	N076001 001	JAN 30, 2002
AB		EQ 20MG BASE	N076001 002	JAN 29, 2002
AB	RANBAXY	EQ 10MG BASE	N076165 001	JAN 29, 2002
AB		EQ 20MG BASE	N076165 002	FEB 01, 2002
AB	SIEGFRIED	EQ 10MG BASE	N075464 001	FEB 01, 2002
AB		EQ 20MG BASE	N075464 002	JAN 30, 2002
AB	TEVA	EQ 10MG BASE	N075452 001	JAN 30, 2002
AB		EQ 20MG BASE	N075452 002	JAN 29, 2002
AB		EQ 40MG BASE	N075452 003	JAN 29, 2002
AB	WATSON LABS	EQ 10MG BASE	N075662 001	JAN 29, 2002

Prescription Drug Products *(continued)*

FLUOXETINE HYDROCHLORIDE *(continued)*

Capsule; Oral

TE	Product / Firm	Strength	Appl. No.	Date
	FLUOXETINE			
AB	WATSON LABS	EQ 20MG BASE	N075662 002	JAN 29, 2002
	FLUOXETINE HCL			
AB	GENEVA PHARMS	EQ 20MG BASE	N075049 002	JAN 29, 2002
AB		EQ 40MG BASE	N075049 003	JAN 29, 2002
	PROZAC			
AB	LILLY	EQ 10MG BASE	N018936 006	DEC 23, 1992
AB		EQ 20MG BASE	N018936 001	DEC 29, 1987
AB		EQ 40MG BASE	N018936 003	JUN 15, 1999
	SARAFEM			
+	LILLY	EQ 10MG BASE	N018936 007	JUL 06, 2000
		EQ 20MG BASE	N018936 008	JUL 06, 2000

Solution; Oral

TE	Product / Firm	Strength	Appl. No.	Date
	FLUOXETINE			
AA	ALPHARMA	EQ 20MG BASE/5ML	N075690 001	JAN 31, 2002
AA	MALLINCKRODT	EQ 20MG BASE/5ML	N075920 001	JAN 29, 2002
AA	NOVEX	EQ 20MG BASE/5ML	N075292 001	FEB 07, 2002
AA	PHARM ASSOC	EQ 20MG BASE/5ML	N076015 001	JAN 30, 2002
AA	TEVA	EQ 20MG BASE/5ML	N075506 001	AUG 02, 2001
	FLUOXETINE HCL			
AA	HI TECH PHARMA	EQ 20MG BASE/5ML	N075525 001	JUN 27, 2002
AA	MORTON GROVE	EQ 20MG BASE/5ML	N075514 001	AUG 29, 2002
	PROZAC			
AA	+ LILLY	EQ 20MG BASE/5ML	N020101 001	APR 24, 1991

Tablet; Oral

TE	Product / Firm	Strength	Appl. No.	Date
	FLUOXETINE HCL			
AB	ALPHAPHARM	EQ 10MG BASE	N075755 001	AUG 02, 2001
AB	+	EQ 20MG BASE	N075755 002	AUG 02, 2001
AB	BARR	EQ 10MG BASE	N075810 001	FEB 01, 2002
AB	DR REDDYS LABS INC	EQ 10MG BASE	N076006 001	JAN 30, 2002
AB	EON	EQ 10MG BASE	N076024 001	JAN 29, 2002
AB	TEVA	EQ 10MG BASE	N075872 001	JAN 29, 2002

FLUOXETINE HYDROCHLORIDE *(continued)*

Tablet; Oral

TE	Product / Firm	Strength	Appl. No.	Date
	FLUOXETINE HCL			
AB	ZENITH GOLDLINE	EQ 10MG BASE	N075865 001	FEB 28, 2002
	PROZAC			
AB	+ LILLY	EQ 10MG BASE	N020974 001	MAR 09, 1999

FLUOXYMESTERONE

Tablet; Oral

TE	Product / Firm	Strength	Appl. No.	Date
	FLUOXYMESTERONE			
BP	USL PHARMA	10MG	N088342 001	OCT 21, 1983
	HALOTESTIN			
BP	+ PHARMACIA AND UPJOHN	2MG	N010611 002	
		5MG	N010611 006	
		10MG	N010611 010	

FLUPHENAZINE DECANOATE

Injectable; Im-Sc

TE	Product / Firm	Strength	Appl. No.	Date
	FLUPHENAZINE DECANOATE			
AO	APOTEX	25MG/ML	N075918 001	AUG 17, 2001

Injectable; Injection

TE	Product / Firm	Strength	Appl. No.	Date
	FLUPHENAZINE DECANOATE			
AO	AM PHARM PARTNERS	25MG/ML	N071413 001	JUL 14, 1987
AO	BEDFORD	25MG/ML	N074531 001	AUG 30, 1996
AO	GENSIA SICOR PHARMS	25MG/ML	N074795 001	SEP 10, 1996
	PROLIXIN DECANOATE			
AO	+ BRISTOL MYERS SQUIBB	25MG/ML	N016727 001	

FLUPHENAZINE HYDROCHLORIDE

Concentrate; Oral

TE	Product / Firm	Strength	Appl. No.	Date
	FLUPHENAZINE HCL			
AA	COPLEY PHARM	5MG/ML	N073058 001	AUG 30, 1991
AA	PHARM ASSOC	5MG/ML	N074725 001	SEP 16, 1996
	PERMITIL			
AA	+ SCHERING	5MG/ML	N016008 001	
	PROLIXIN			
AA	APOTHECON	5MG/ML	N070533 001	NOV 07, 1985

Elixir; Oral

TE	Product / Firm	Strength	Appl. No.	Date
	FLUPHENAZINE HCL			
AA	COPLEY PHARM	2.5MG/5ML	N081310 001	APR 29, 1993
AA	PHARM ASSOC	2.5MG/5ML	N040146 001	AUG 21, 1996

Prescription Drug Products (continued)

FLUPHENAZINE HYDROCHLORIDE (continued)

Elixir; Oral

TE	Product	Strength	Appl. No.	Date
	PROLIXIN			
AA	+ APOTHECON	2.5MG/5ML	N012145 003	

Injectable; Injection

TE	Product	Strength	Appl. No.	Date
	FLUPHENAZINE HCL			
AP	AM PHARM PARTNERS	2.5MG/ML	N089556 001	APR 16, 1987
	PROLIXIN			
AP	+ APOTHECON	2.5MG/ML	N011751 005	

Tablet; Oral

TE	Product	Strength	Appl. No.	Date
	FLUPHENAZINE HCL			
	GENEVA PHARMS			
AB		1MG	N089583 001	OCT 16, 1987
AB		2.5MG	N089584 001	OCT 16, 1987
AB		5MG	N089585 001	OCT 16, 1987
AB		10MG	N089586 001	OCT 16, 1987
	MYLAN			
AB		1MG	N089801 001	AUG 12, 1988
AB		2.5MG	N089802 001	AUG 12, 1988
AB		5MG	N089803 001	AUG 12, 1988
AB		10MG	N089804 001	AUG 12, 1988
	PAR PHARM			
AB		1MG	N089740 001	AUG 25, 1988
AB		2.5MG	N088741 001	AUG 25, 1988
AB		5MG	N089742 001	AUG 25, 1988
AB		10MG	N089743 001	AUG 25, 1988
	PROLIXIN			
	APOTHECON			
AB		1MG	N011751 004	
AB		2.5MG	N011751 001	
AB		5MG	N011751 003	
AB		10MG	N011751 002	

FLURANDRENOLIDE

Cream; Topical

TE	Product	Strength	Appl. No.
	CORDRAN SP		
	+ OCLASSEN	0.05%	N012806 002
		0.025%	N012806 003

Lotion; Topical

TE	Product	Strength	Appl. No.
	CORDRAN		
	+ OCLASSEN	0.05%	N013790 001

Ointment; Topical

TE	Product	Strength	Appl. No.
	CORDRAN		
	+ OCLASSEN	0.05%	N012806 001
		0.025%	N012806 004

FLURANDRENOLIDE (continued)

Tape; Topical

TE	Product	Strength	Appl. No.
	CORDRAN		
AA	+ OCLASSEN	0.004MG/SQ CM	N016455 001

FLURAZEPAM HYDROCHLORIDE

Capsule; Oral

TE	Product	Strength	Appl. No.	Date
	DALMANE			
AB	ICN	15MG	N016721 001	
AB		30MG	N016721 002	
	FLURAZEPAM HCL			
	GENEVA PHARMS			
AB		15MG	N071716 001	JUL 31, 1991
AB		30MG	N071717 001	JUL 31, 1991
	MYLAN			
AB		15MG	N070344 001	NOV 27, 1985
AB		30MG	N070345 001	NOV 27, 1985
	PAR PHARM			
AB		15MG	N070444 001	MAR 20, 1986
AB		30MG	N070445 001	MAR 20, 1986
	WATSON LABS			
AB		15MG	N071205 001	NOV 25, 1986
AB		30MG	N071068 001	NOV 25, 1986
AB		30MG	N072369 001	MAR 30, 1989
	WEST WARD			
AB		15MG	N071107 001	DEC 08, 1986
AB		30MG	N071108 001	DEC 08, 1986

FLURBIPROFEN

Tablet; Oral

TE	Product	Strength	Appl. No.	Date
	ANSAID			
	PHARMACIA AND UPJOHN			
AB		50MG	N018766 002	OCT 31, 1988
AB	+	100MG	N018766 003	OCT 31, 1988
	FLURBIPROFEN			
	CARACO			
AB		50MG	N075058 001	APR 27, 2001
AB		100MG	N075058 002	APR 27, 2001
	GENEVA PHARMS			
AB		50MG	N074448 001	JUL 28, 1995
AB		100MG	N074448 002	JUL 28, 1995
	IVAX PHARMS			
AB		50MG	N074411 001	MAY 31, 1995
AB		100MG	N074411 002	MAY 31, 1995
	MYLAN			
AB		50MG	N074358 001	MAY 31, 1995

Prescription Drug Products (continued)

FLURBIPROFEN (continued)

Tablet; Oral

FLURBIPROFEN

	MYLAN		
AB	100MG	N019958 001	JUN 20, 1994
		N074358 002	JUN 20, 1994
	PLIVA		
AB	50MG	N074647 001	APR 01, 1997
AB	100MG	N074647 002	APR 01, 1997
	TEVA		
AB	50MG	N074405 002	MAY 24, 1995
AB	100MG	N074405 001	MAY 24, 1995
AB	100MG	N074431 001	MAY 31, 1995
	WARNER CHILCOTT		
AB	100MG	N074560 002	MAY 16, 1997

FLURBIPROFEN SODIUM

Solution/Drops; Ophthalmic

FLURBIPROFEN SODIUM

	AVENTIS BEHRING		
AT	0.03%	N074447 001	JAN 04, 1995
	OCUFEN		
AT +	ALLERGAN 0.03%	N019404 001	DEC 31, 1986

FLUTAMIDE

Capsule; Oral

EULEXIN

AB +	SCHERING 125MG	N018554 001	JAN 27, 1989
	FLUTAMIDE		
	BARR		
AB	125MG	N075820 001	SEP 18, 2001
	EON		
AB	125MG	N075818 001	SEP 18, 2001
	GENPHARM		
AB	125MG	N076224 001	MAY 09, 2003
	IVAX PHARMS		
AB	125MG	N075780 001	SEP 19, 2001
	TEVA		
AB	125MG	N075298 001	SEP 18, 2001

FLUTICASONE PROPIONATE

Aerosol, Metered; Inhalation

FLOVENT

	GLAXOSMITHKLINE	0.11MG/INH
+		0.22MG/INH
		0.044MG/INH

FLUTICASONE PROPIONATE (continued)

Cream; Topical

CUTIVATE

+	GLAXOSMITHKLINE 0.05%	N019958 001	DEC 18, 1990

Ointment; Topical

CUTIVATE

+	GLAXOSMITHKLINE 0.005%	N019957 001	DEC 14, 1990

Powder; Inhalation

FLOVENT

+	GLAXOSMITHKLINE 0.22MG/INH	N020549 003	NOV 07, 1997
+	0.044MG/INH	N020549 001	NOV 07, 1997
+	0.088MG/INH	N020549 002	NOV 07, 1997

FLOVENT DISKUS 50

+	GLAXOSMITHKLINE 0.05MG/INH	N020833 001	SEP 29, 2000

FLOVENT DISKUS 100

+	GLAXOSMITHKLINE 0.1MG/INH	N020833 002	SEP 29, 2000

FLOVENT DISKUS 250

+	GLAXOSMITHKLINE 0.25MG/INH	N020833 003	SEP 29, 2000

Spray, Metered; Nasal

FLONASE

+	GLAXOSMITHKLINE 0.05MG/SPRAY	N020121 001	OCT 19, 1994

FLUTICASONE PROPIONATE; SALMETEROL XINAFOATE

Powder; Inhalation

ADVAIR DISKUS 100/50

+	GLAXOSMITHKLINE 0.1MG/INH;EQ 0.05MG BASE/INH	N021077 001	AUG 24, 2000

ADVAIR DISKUS 250/50

+	GLAXOSMITHKLINE 0.25MG/INH;EQ 0.05MG BASE/INH	N021077 002	AUG 24, 2000

ADVAIR DISKUS 500/50

+	GLAXOSMITHKLINE 0.5MG/INH;EQ 0.05MG BASE/INH	N021077 003	AUG 24, 2000

FLUVASTATIN SODIUM

Capsule; Oral

LESCOL

	NOVARTIS EQ 20MG BASE	N020261 001	DEC 31, 1993
+	EQ 40MG BASE	N020261 002	DEC 31, 1993

Tablet, Extended Release; Oral

LESCOL XL

+	NOVARTIS 80MG	N021192 001	OCT 06, 2000

Prescription Drug Products (continued)

FLUVOXAMINE MALEATE
Tablet; Oral

FLUVOXAMINE MALEATE

	Manufacturer	Strength	Number	Date
	BARR			
AB		25MG	N075897 001	JAN 25, 2001
AB		50MG	N075897 002	JAN 25, 2001
AB		100MG	N075897 003	JAN 25, 2001
	EON			
AB		25MG	N075888 001	NOV 29, 2000
AB		50MG	N075888 002	NOV 29, 2000
AB		100MG	N075888 003	NOV 29, 2000
	GENEVA PHARMS			
AB +		25MG	N075887 001	JAN 05, 2001
AB		50MG	N075887 002	JAN 05, 2001
AB		100MG	N075887 003	JAN 05, 2001
	GENPHARM			
AB		50MG	N075950 001	OCT 15, 2001
AB		100MG	N075950 002	OCT 15, 2001
	IVAX PHARMS			
AB		25MG	N075898 001	MAR 12, 2001
AB		50MG	N075898 002	MAR 12, 2001
AB		100MG	N075898 003	MAR 12, 2001
	MUTUAL PHARM			
AB		25MG	N076125 001	APR 29, 2002
AB		50MG	N076125 002	APR 29, 2002
AB		100MG	N076125 003	APR 29, 2002
	MYLAN			
AB		25MG	N075889 001	NOV 29, 2000
AB		50MG	N075889 002	NOV 29, 2000
AB		100MG	N075889 003	NOV 29, 2000
	PUREPAC PHARM			
AB		25MG	N075901 001	DEC 28, 2000
AB		50MG	N075901 002	DEC 28, 2000
AB		100MG	N075901 003	DEC 28, 2000
	SYNTHON PHARMS			
AB		25MG	N075899 001	JAN 17, 2001
AB		50MG	N075899 002	JAN 17, 2001
AB		100MG	N075899 003	JAN 17, 2001
	TEVA			
AB		25MG	N075893 001	SEP 10, 2002

FLUVOXAMINE MALEATE (continued)
Tablet; Oral

FLUVOXAMINE MALEATE

	Manufacturer	Strength	Number	Date
	TEVA			
AB		50MG	N075893 002	SEP 10, 2002
AB		100MG	N075893 003	SEP 10, 2002
	TORPHARM			
AB		25MG	N075902 001	MAY 07, 2001
AB		50MG	N075902 002	MAY 07, 2001
AB		100MG	N075902 003	MAY 07, 2001
	WATSON LABS			
AB		25MG	N075894 001	APR 18, 2001
AB		50MG	N075894 002	APR 18, 2001
AB		100MG	N075894 003	APR 18, 2001

FOLIC ACID
Injectable; Injection

FOLIC ACID

	Manufacturer	Strength	Number	Date
AP +	AM PHARM PARTNERS	5MG/ML	N089202 001	FEB 18, 1986
AP	LOCH	5MG/ML	N081066 001	DEC 29, 1993

Tablet; Oral

FOLIC ACID

	Manufacturer	Strength	Number
AA	ICN	1MG	N080903 001
AA	IVAX PHARMS	1MG	N083000 001
AA	MK LABS	1MG	N083526 001
AA	PVT FORM	1MG	N085061 001
AA	TABLICAPS	1MG	N083133 002
AA +	WATSON LABS	1MG	N080680 001
AA	WEST WARD	1MG	N080600 001

FOLICET

	Manufacturer	Strength	Number
AA	MISSION PHARMA	1MG	N087438 001

FOLIC ACID *MULTIPLE*
SEE ALPHA-TOCOPHEROL ACETATE; ASCORBIC ACID; BIOTIN; CHOLECALCIFEROL; CYANOCOBALAMIN; DEXPANTHENOL; FOLIC ACID; NIACINAMIDE; PYRIDOXINE HYDROCHLORIDE; RIBOFLAVIN PHOSPHATE SODIUM; THIAMINE HYDROCHLORIDE; VITAMIN A PALMITATE; VITAMIN K

SEE ASCORBIC ACID; BIOTIN; CHOLECALCIFEROL; CYANOCOBALAMIN; DEXPANTHENOL; FOLIC ACID; NIACINAMIDE; PYRIDOXINE; RIBOFLAVIN; THIAMINE; TOCOPHEROL ACETATE; VITAMIN A; VITAMIN K

SEE ASCORBIC ACID; BIOTIN; CYANOCOBALAMIN; DEXPANTHENOL; ERGOCALCIFEROL; FOLIC ACID; NIACINAMIDE; PHYTONADIONE; PYRIDOXINE HYDROCHLORIDE; RIBOFLAVIN PHOSPHATE SODIUM; THIAMINE HYDROCHLORIDE; VITAMIN A; VITAMIN E

SEE ASCORBIC ACID; BIOTIN; CYANOCOBALAMIN; DEXPANTHENOL; ERGOCALCIFEROL; FOLIC ACID; NIACINAMIDE; PYRIDOXINE HYDROCHLORIDE; RIBOFLAVIN PHOSPHATE SODIUM; THIAMINE HYDROCHLORIDE; VITAMIN A; VITAMIN E

Prescription Drug Products (continued)

FOLLITROPIN ALFA
Injectable; Injection
 GONAL-F
+ SERONO   1,200 IU/VIAL   N020378 004   FEB 28, 2001

FOLLITROPIN ALFA/BETA
Injectable; Injection
 FOLLISTIM
BX ORGANON USA INC   75 IU/VIAL   N020582 001   SEP 29, 1997
BX   150 IU/VIAL   N020582 002   SEP 29, 1997
 GONAL-F
BX SERONO   75 IU/VIAL   N020378 001   SEP 29, 1997
BX   150 IU/VIAL   N020378 002   SEP 29, 1997

FOMEPIZOLE
Injectable; Injection
 ANTIZOL
+ ORPHAN MEDCL   1GM/ML   N020696 001   DEC 04, 1997

FOMIVIRSEN SODIUM
Injectable; Injection
 VITRAVENE PRESERVATIVE FREE
+ NOVARTIS   6.6MG/ML   N020961 001   AUG 26, 1998

FONDAPARINUX SODIUM
Injectable; Subcutaneous
 ARIXTRA
+ FONDA BV   2.5MG/0.5ML   N021345 001   DEC 07, 2001

FORMOTEROL FUMARATE
Capsule; Inhalation
 FORADIL
+ NOVARTIS   0.012MG/INH   N020831 001   FEB 16, 2001

FOSCARNET SODIUM
Injectable; Injection
 FOSCAVIR
+ ASTRAZENECA   2.4GM/100ML   N020068 001   SEP 27, 1991

FOSFOMYCIN TROMETHAMINE
For Suspension; Oral
 MONUROL
+ ZAMBON   EQ 3GM BASE/PACKET   N050717 001   DEC 19, 1996

FOSINOPRIL SODIUM
Tablet; Oral
 MONOPRIL
   BRISTOL MYERS SQUIBB   10MG   N019915 002   MAY 16, 1991
                          20MG   N019915 003   MAY 16, 1991
+   40MG   N019915 004   MAR 28, 1995

FOSINOPRIL SODIUM; HYDROCHLOROTHIAZIDE
Tablet; Oral
 MONOPRIL-HCT
   BRISTOL MYERS SQUIBB   10MG;12.5MG   N020286 002   NOV 30, 1994
                          20MG;12.5MG   N020286 001   NOV 30, 1994
+   N020286 001   NOV 30, 1994

FOSPHENYTOIN SODIUM
Injectable; Injection
 CEREBYX
+ PARKE DAVIS   EQ 50MG PHENYTOIN NA/ML   N020450 001   AUG 05, 1996

FROVATRIPTAN SUCCINATE
Tablet; Oral
 FROVA
+ ELAN PHARMS   EQ 2.5MG BASE   N021006 001   NOV 08, 2001

FULVESTRANT
Injectable; Intramuscular
 FASLODEX
+ ASTRAZENECA   50MG/ML   N021344 001   APR 25, 2002

FUROSEMIDE
Injectable; Injection
 FUROSEMIDE
AP   ABBOTT   10MG/ML   N018667 001   MAY 28, 1982
AP   10MG/ML   N070578 001   JUL 08, 1987
AP   10MG/ML   N072080 001   AUG 13, 1991
AP   10MG/ML   N074337 001   OCT 31, 1994
AP   10MG/ML   N075241 001   MAY 28, 1999
AP   AM PHARM PARTNERS   10MG/ML   N018902 001   MAY 22, 1984
AP   INTL MEDICATION   10MG/ML   N018025 001
AP   LEDERLE   10MG/ML   N071439 001

Prescription Drug Products (continued)

FUROSEMIDE (continued)

Injectable; Injection

FUROSEMIDE
LEDERLE
AP	LUITPOLD	10MG/ML	SEP 14, 1990	N018579 001
AP		10MG/ML	NOV 30, 1983	N074017 001
AP	MARSAM PHARMS LLC	10MG/ML	JUN 30, 1994	N016363 001

LASIX
+ AVENTIS PHARMS

Solution; Oral

FUROSEMIDE
AA	MORTON GROVE	10MG/ML		N070655 001
			OCT 02, 1987	N070434 001
AA	ROXANE	10MG/ML	APR 22, 1987	N070433 001
		40MG/5ML	APR 22, 1987	

LASIX
+ AVENTIS PHARMS

Tablet; Oral

FUROSEMIDE
AA	CLONMEL HLTHCARE	10MG/ML		N017688 001
AB		20MG	JUL 27, 1982	N018415 001
AB		40MG	JUL 27, 1982	N018415 002
AB		80MG	NOV 26, 1984	N018415 003
AB	GENEVA PHARMS	20MG		N018569 002
AB		40MG		N018569 001
AB		80MG	AUG 14, 1984	N018569 005
AB	INTL MEDICATION	20MG	FEB 28, 1984	N018753 001
AB		40MG	FEB 28, 1984	N018753 002
AB	IVAX PHARMS	20MG	NOV 30, 1983	N018413 001
AB		40MG	NOV 30, 1983	N018413 002
AB	KALAPHARM	20MG	NOV 30, 1983	N018868 001
AB		40MG	JUN 28, 1983	N018868 002
AB	MYLAN	20MG	JUN 28, 1983	N018487 001
AB		40MG	JUN 28, 1983	N018487 002
AB		80MG	OCT 29, 1986	N070082 001
AB	ROXANE	20MG	NOV 10, 1983	N018823 001
AB		40MG	NOV 10, 1983	N018823 002
AB		80MG	JAN 24, 1986	N070086 001
AB	WATSON LABS	20MG	FEB 26, 1986	N070412 001
AB		20MG		N070449 001

FUROSEMIDE
WATSON LABS
AB		20MG	NOV 22, 1985	N071379 001
AB		40MG	JAN 02, 1987	N070413 001
			FEB 26, 1986	N070450 001
AB		40MG	NOV 22, 1985	N070528 001
AB		80MG	JAN 07, 1986	N071594 001
AB		80MG	FEB 09, 1988	

LASIX
AVENTIS PHARMS
AB	20MG		N016273 002
AB	40MG		N016273 001
AB	80MG		N016273 003
+			

GABAPENTIN

Capsule; Oral

NEURONTIN
	PFIZER PHARMS	100MG	N020235 001	DEC 30, 1993
		300MG	N020235 002	DEC 30, 1993
+		400MG	N020235 003	DEC 30, 1993

Solution; Oral

NEURONTIN
+	PARKE DAVIS	250MG/5ML	N021129 001	MAR 02, 2000

Tablet; Oral

NEURONTIN
	PFIZER PHARMS	600MG	N020882 001	OCT 09, 1998
+		800MG	N020882 002	OCT 09, 1998

GADODIAMIDE

Injectable; Injection

OMNISCAN
+	AMERSHAM HLTH	287MG/ML	N020123 001	JAN 08, 1993

GADOPENTETATE DIMEGLUMINE

Injectable; Injection

MAGNEVIST
+	BER-EX	469.01MG/ML	N019596 001	JUN 02, 1988
+	BERLEX LABS	469.01MG/ML	N021037 001	MAR 10, 2000

Prescription Drug Products (continued)

TE	Drug / Form / Applicant	Strength	Appl. No.	Date
GADOTERIDOL	Injectable; Injection			
	PROHANCE			
	+ BRACCO	279.3MG/ML	N020131 001	NOV 16, 1992
GADOVERSETAMIDE	Injectable; Injection			
	OPTIMARK			
	+ MALLINCKRODT	330.9MG/ML	N020937 001	DEC 08, 1999
	+	330.9MG/ML	N020975 001	DEC 08, 1999
	OPTIMARK IN PLASTIC CONTAINER			
	+ MALLINCKRODT	330.9MG/ML	N020976 001	DEC 08, 1999
GALANTAMINE HYDROBROMIDE	Solution; Oral			
	REMINYL			
	+ JANSSEN PHARMA	4MG/ML	N021224 001	JUN 22, 2001
	Tablet; Oral			
	REMINYL			
	+ JANSSEN PHARMA	EQ 4MG BASE	N021169 001	FEB 28, 2001
	+	EQ 8MG BASE	N021169 002	FEB 28, 2001
		EQ 12MG BASE	N021169 003	FEB 28, 2001
GALLIUM CITRATE, GA-67	Injectable; Injection			
	GALLIUM CITRATE GA 67			
BS	BRISTOL MYERS SQUIBB	2mCi/ML	N017478 001	
BS	MALLINCKRODT	2mCi/ML	N018058 001	
GALLIUM NITRATE	Injectable; Injection			
	GANITE			
	+ GENTA	25MG/ML	N019961 002	JAN 17, 1991
GANCICLOVIR	Capsule; Oral			
	CYTOVENE			
AB	ROCHE PALO	250MG	N020460 001	DEC 22, 1994
AB	+	500MG	N020460 002	DEC 12, 1997
	GANCICLOVIR			
AB	RANBAXY	250MG	N076457 001	JUN 27, 2003
AB		500MG	N076457 002	

TE	Drug / Form / Applicant	Strength	Appl. No.	Date
GANCICLOVIR *(continued)*	Capsule; Oral			
	GANCICLOVIR			
	RANBAXY			JUN 27, 2003
	Implant; Implantation			
	VITRASERT			
	+ BAUSCH AND LOMB	4.5MG	N020569 001	MAR 04, 1996
GANCICLOVIR SODIUM	Injectable; Injection			
	CYTOVENE IV			
	+ ROCHE PALO	EQ 500MG BASE/VIAL	N019661 001	JUN 23, 1989
GANIRELIX ACETATE	Injectable; Injection			
	ANTAGON			
	+ ORGANON USA INC	EQ 250UGM BASE/0.5ML	N021057 001	JUL 29, 1999
GATIFLOXACIN	Injectable; Injection			
	TEQUIN			
	+ BRISTOL MYERS SQUIBB	EQ 2MG /ML(200MG/100ML)	N021062 001	DEC 17, 1999
		EQ 2MG /ML(400MG/200ML)	N021062 002	DEC 17, 1999
	+	EQ 10MG /ML(200MG)	N021062 003	DEC 17, 1999
	+	EQ 10MG /ML(400MG)	N021062 004	DEC 17, 1999
	Solution/Drops; Ophthalmic			
	ZYMAR			
	+ ALLERGAN	0.3%	N021493 001	MAR 28, 2003
	Tablet; Oral			
	TEQUIN			
	+ BRISTOL MYERS SQUIBB	200MG	N021061 001	DEC 17, 1999
	+	400MG	N021061 002	DEC 17, 1999
GEFITINIB	Tablet; Oral			
	IRESSA			
	+ ASTRAZENECA	250MG	N021399 001	MAY 05, 2003
GEMCITABINE HYDROCHLORIDE	Injectable; Injection			
	GEMZAR			
	+ LILLY	EQ 1GM BASE/VIAL	N020509 002	

Prescription Drug Products (continued)

GEMCITABINE HYDROCHLORIDE (continued)

Injectable; Injection

TE	Firm	Strength	Appl No	Date
	GEMZAR			
+	LILLY	EQ 200MG BASE/VIAL	N020509 001	MAY 15, 1996

GEMFIBROZIL

Tablet; Oral

TE	Firm	Strength	Appl No	Date
	GEMFIBROZIL			
AB	CLONMEL HLTHCARE	600MG	N074270 001	SEP 27, 1993
AB	GENEVA PHARMS TECH	600MG	N074615 001	SEP 29, 1995
AB	MYLAN	600MG	N074452 001	FEB 16, 1995
AB	TEVA	600MG	N074256 001	OCT 31, 1993
AB	TORPHARM	600MG	N075034 001	JUL 20, 1998
AB	WATSON LABS	600MG	N074442 001	APR 28, 1995
	LOPID			
AB	+ PFIZER PHARMS	600MG	N018422 003	NOV 20, 1986

GEMIFLOXACIN MESYLATE

Tablet; Oral

TE	Firm	Strength	Appl No	Date
	FACTIVE			
+	GENESOFT PHARMS	EQ 320MG BASE	N021158 001	APR 04, 2003

GEMTUZUMAB OZOGAMICIN

Injectable; Injection

TE	Firm	Strength	Appl No	Date
	MYLOTARG			
+	WYETH PHARMS INC	5MG/VIAL	N021174 001	MAY 17, 2000

GENTAMICIN SULFATE

Cream; Topical

TE	Firm	Strength	Appl No	Date
	GENTAMICIN			
AT	CLAY PARK	EQ 0.1% BASE	N062307 001	
	GENTAMICIN SULFATE			
AT	+ FOUGERA	EQ 0.1% BASE	N062531 001	JUL 05, 1984
AT	TARO	EQ 0.1% BASE	N062427 001	MAY 26, 1983

Injectable; Injection

TE	Firm	Strength	Appl No	Date
	GARAMYCIN			
AP	+ SCHERING	EQ 1MG BASE/ML	N061716 002	
AP	+	EQ 40MG BASE/ML	N061716 001	
	GENTAMICIN SULFATE			
AP	ABBOTT	EQ 10MG BASE/ML	N062420 001	AUG 15, 1983
AP		EQ 10MG BASE/ML	N062612 004	FEB 20, 1986

GENTAMICIN SULFATE (continued)

Injectable; Injection

TE	Firm	Strength	Appl No	Date
	GENTAMICIN SULFATE			
	ABBOTT			
AP		EQ 40MG BASE/ML	N062420 002	AUG 15, 1983
AP	+ AM PHARM PARTNERS	EQ 10MG BASE/ML	N062356 001	MAR 04, 1982
AP		EQ 40MG BASE/ML	N062356 002	MAR 04, 1982
AP	KALAP-IARM	EQ 40MG BASE/ML	N062366 001	AUG 04, 1983
AP	PHARM SPEC	EQ 40MG BASE/ML	N062354 001	APR 05, 1982
AP		EQ 40MG BASE/ML	N062340 001	MAR 28, 1983
	GENTAMICIN SULFATE IN SODIUM CHLORIDE 0.9% IN PLASTIC CONTAINER			
	ABBOTT			
AP		EQ 1.2MG BASE/ML	N062414 001	AUG 15, 1983
AP		EQ 1.4MG BASE/ML	N062414 002	AUG 15, 1983
AP		EQ 1.6MG BASE/ML	N062414 003	AUG 15, 1983
AP		EQ 1.8MG BASE/ML	N062414 004	AUG 15, 1983
AP		EQ 2MG BASE/ML	N062414 005	AUG 15, 1983
AP		EQ 60MG BASE/100ML	N062414 006	AUG 15, 1983
AP		EQ 70MG BASE/100ML	N062414 007	AUG 15, 1983
AP		EQ 80MG BASE/100ML	N062414 008	AUG 15, 1983
AP		EQ 90MG BASE/100ML	N062414 009	AUG 15, 1983
AP		EQ 100MG BASE/100ML	N062414 010	AUG 15, 1983
AP	B BRAUN	EQ 0.8MG BASE/ML	N062814 001	AUG 28, 1987
AP		EQ 1.2MG BASE/ML	N062814 002	AUG 28, 1987
AP		EQ 1.4MG BASE/ML	N062814 003	AUG 28, 1987
AP		EQ 1.6MG BASE/ML	N062814 004	AUG 28, 1987
AP		EQ 1.8MG BASE/ML	N062814 005	AUG 28, 1987
AP		EQ 2MG BASE/ML	N062814 006	AUG 28, 1987
AP		EQ 2.4MG BASE/ML	N062814 007	AUG 28, 1987
AP		EQ 40MG BASE/100ML	N062814 008	AUG 28, 1987
AP		EQ 60MG BASE/100ML	N062814 009	AUG 28, 1987
AP		EQ 70MG BASE/100ML	N062814 010	AUG 28, 1987
AP		EQ 80MG BASE/100ML	N062814 011	AUG 28, 1987

Prescription Drug Products (continued)

GENTAMICIN SULFATE (continued)
Injectable; Injection

GENTAMICIN SULFATE IN SODIUM CHLORIDE 0.9% IN PLASTIC CONTAINER

TE	Firm	Strength	Appl No	Date
	B BRAUN			
AP		EQ 90MG BASE/100ML	N062814 012	AUG 28, 1987
AP		EQ 100MG BASE/100ML	N062814 013	AUG 28, 1987
AP		EQ 120MG BASE/100ML	N062814 014	AUG 28, 1987

ISOTONIC GENTAMICIN SULFATE IN PLASTIC CONTAINER

TE	Firm	Strength	Appl No	Date
	BAXTER HLTHCARE			
AP		EQ 0.8MG BASE/ML	N062373 001	SEP 07, 1982
AP		EQ 80MG BASE/100ML	N062373 002	SEP 07, 1982
AP		EQ 40MG BASE/100ML	N062373 003	SEP 07, 1982
AP		EQ 60MG BASE/100ML	N062373 004	SEP 07, 1982
AP		EQ 100MG BASE/100ML	N062373 005	SEP 07, 1982
AP		EQ 120MG BASE/100ML	N062373 006	SEP 07, 1982
AP		EQ 1.2MG BASE/ML	N062373 007	SEP 07, 1982
AP		EQ 1.6MG BASE/ML	N062373 008	SEP 07, 1982
AP		EQ 2MG BASE/ML	N062373 009	SEP 07, 1982
AP		EQ 2.4MG BASE/ML	N062373 010	SEP 07, 1982

Ointment; Ophthalmic

TE	Firm	Strength	Appl No	Date
	GENTAMICIN SULFATE			
	+ AKORN			
AP		EQ 0.3% BASE	N064093 001	AUG 31, 1995

Ointment; Topical

TE	Firm	Strength	Appl No	Date
	GENTAMICIN			
	+ CLAY PARK			
AT		EQ 0.1% BASE	N062351 001	FEB 18, 1982
	GENTAMICIN SULFATE			
	FOUGERA			
AT		EQ 0.1% BASE	N062533 001	OCT 05, 1984
	TARO			
AT		EQ 0.1% BASE	N062477 001	DEC 23, 1983

Solution/Drops; Ophthalmic

TE	Firm	Strength	Appl No	Date
	GENOPTIC			
	ALLERGAN			
AT		EQ 0.3% BASE	N062452 001	OCT 10, 1984
	GENTACIDIN			
	NOVARTIS			
AT		EQ 0.3% BASE	N062480 001	MAR 30, 1984
	GENTAK			
	AKORN			
AT		EQ 0.3% BASE	N064163 001	OCT 12, 2001
	GENTAMICIN SULFATE			
	AKORN			
AT		EQ 0.3% BASE	N062635 001	JAN 08, 1987

GENTAMICIN SULFATE (continued)
Solution/Drops; Ophthalmic

TE	Firm	Strength	Appl No	Date
	GENTAMICIN SULFATE			
	BAUSCH AND LOMB			
AT		EQ 0.3% BASE	N064048 001	MAY 11, 1994
	FALCON PHARMS			
AT		EQ 0.3% BASE	N062196 001	

Solution; Ophthalmic

TE	Firm	Strength	Appl No	Date
	GARAMYCIN			
	+ SCHERING			
AT		EQ 0.3% BASE	N050039 002	

GENTAMICIN SULFATE; PREDNISOLONE ACETATE
Ointment; Ophthalmic

TE	Firm	Strength	Appl No	Date
	PRED-G			
	+ ALLERGAN			
		EQ 0.3% BASE;0.6%	N050612 001	DEC 01, 1989

Suspension/Drops; Ophthalmic

TE	Firm	Strength	Appl No	Date
	PRED-G			
	+ ALLERGAN			
		EQ 0.3% BASE;1%	N050586 001	JUN 10, 1988

GENTIAN VIOLET
Suppository; Vaginal

TE	Firm	Strength	Appl No	Date
	GVS			
	+ SAVAGE LABS			
		0.4%	N083513 001	

GLATIRAMER ACETATE
For Solution; Subcutaneous

TE	Firm	Strength	Appl No	Date
	COPAXONE			
	+ TEVA			
		20MG/VIAL	N020622 001	DEC 20, 1996

Injectable: Subcutaneous

TE	Firm	Strength	Appl No	Date
	COPAXONE			
	+ TEVA			
		20MG/ML	N020622 002	FEB 12, 2002

GLIMEPIRIDE
Tablet; Oral

TE	Firm	Strength	Appl No	Date
	AMARYL			
	+ AVENTIS PHARMS			
		1MG	N020496 001	NOV 30, 1995
		2MG	N020496 002	NOV 30, 1995
		4MG	N020496 003	NOV 30, 1995

GLIPIZIDE
Tablet, Extended Release; Oral

TE	Firm	Strength	Appl No	Date
	GLUCOTROL XL			
	PFIZER			
		2.5MG	N020329 003	AUG 10, 1999
		5MG	N020329 001	APR 26, 1994
		10MG	N020329 002	APR 26, 1994
	+			

Prescription Drug Products *(continued)*

GLIPIZIDE *(continued)*
Tablet; Oral

GLIPIZIDE

TE	Manufacturer	Strength	Appl No	Date
AB	ALPHAPHARM	5MG	N074438 001	JUN 20, 1995
AB		10MG	N074438 002	JUN 20, 1995
AB	DURAMED PHARM BARR	5MG	N074550 001	SEP 11, 1997
AB		10MG	N074550 002	SEP 11, 1997
AB	ENDO PHARMS	5MG	N074378 001	NOV 28, 1994
AB		10MG	N074378 002	NOV 28, 1994
AB	GENEVA PHARMS	5MG	N074305 001	APR 07, 1995
AB		10MG	N074305 002	APR 07, 1995
AB	GENEVA PHARMS TECH	5MG	N074542 001	JUN 20, 1995
AB		10MG	N074542 002	JUN 20, 1995
AB	IVAX PHARMS	5MG	N074497 001	AUG 31, 1995
AB		10MG	N074497 002	AUG 31, 1995
AB	MYLAN	5MG	N074226 001	MAY 10, 1994
AB		10MG	N074226 002	MAY 10, 1994
AB	PLIVA	5MG	N074619 001	APR 04, 1997
AB		10MG	N074619 002	APR 04, 1997
AB	TEVA	5MG	N074387 001	MAR 04, 1996
AB		10MG	N074387 002	MAR 04, 1996
AB	TORPHARM	5MG	N075795 001	JUN 13, 2001
AB		10MG	N075795 002	JUN 13, 2001
AB	WATSON LAB	5MG	N074370 001	NOV 22, 1994
AB		10MG	N074370 002	NOV 22, 1994
AB	WATSON LABS	5MG	N074223 001	FEB 27, 1995
AB		10MG	N074223 002	FEB 27, 1995

GLUCOTROL

TE	Manufacturer	Strength	Appl No	Date
AB	PFIZER	5MG	N017783 001	MAY 08, 1984
AB +		10MG	N017783 002	MAY 08, 1984

GLIPIZIDE; METFORMIN HYDROCHLORIDE
Tablet; Oral

METAGLIP

TE	Manufacturer	Strength	Appl No	Date
	BRISTO_MYERS SQUIBB	2.5MG;250MG	N021460 001	OCT 21, 2002
		2.5MG;500MG	N021460 002	OCT 21, 2002
+		5MG;500MG	N021460 003	OCT 21, 2002

GLUCAGON HYDROCHLORIDE RECOMBINANT
Injectable; Injection

GLUCAGEN

TE	Manufacturer	Strength	Appl No	Date
+	NOVO NORDISK	EQ 1MG BASE/VIAL	N020918 001	JUN 22, 1998

GLUCAGON RECOMBINANT
Injectable; Injection

GLUCAGON

TE	Manufacturer	Strength	Appl No	Date
+	LILLY	1MG/VIAL	N020928 001	SEP 11, 1998

GLUCONOLACTONE *MULTIPLE*
SEE CITRIC ACID; GLUCONOLACTONE; MAGNESIUM CARBONATE

GLUTATHIONE DISULFIDE *MULTIPLE*
SEE CALCIUM CHLORIDE; DEXTROSE; GLUTATHIONE DISULFIDE; MAGNESIUM CHLORIDE; POTASSIUM CHLORIDE; SODIUM BICARBONATE; SODIUM CHLORIDE; SODIUM PHOSPHATE

GLYBURIDE
Tablet; Oral

DIABETA

TE	Manufacturer	Strength	Appl No	Date
BX	AVENTIS PHARMS	1.25MG	N017532 001	MAY 01, 1984
BX		2.5MG	N017532 002	MAY 01, 1984
BX		5MG	N017532 003	MAY 01, 1984

GLYBURIDE

TE	Manufacturer	Strength	Appl No	Date
AB	AMIDE PHARM	1.5MG	N075947 001	NOV 14, 2002
AB		3MG	N075947 002	NOV 14, 2002
AB		6MG	N075947 003	NOV 14, 2002
AB	COREPHARMA	1.25MG	N076257 001	JUN 27, 2002
AB		2.5MG	N076257 002	JUN 27, 2002
AB		5MG	N076257 003	JUN 27, 2002
AB	TEVA	1.25MG	N074388 001	AUG 29, 1995

Prescription Drug Products *(continued)*

GLYBURIDE *(continued)*
Tablet; Oral

GLYBURIDE

AB	TEVA	2.5MG	N074388 002	AUG 29, 1995
AB		5MG	N074388 003	AUG 29, 1995

GLYBURIDE (MICRONIZED)

AB	AVENTIS PHARMS	1.5MG	N020055 001	APR 17, 1992
AB		3MG	N020055 002	APR 17, 1992
AB		6MG	N020055 003	MAR 08, 2000
AB	CLONMEL HLTHCARE	1.5MG	N074591 001	DEC 22, 1997
AB		3MG	N074591 002	DEC 22, 1997
AB		4.5MG	N074591 003	DEC 22, 1997
AB		6MG	N074591 004	DEC 22, 1997
AB	GENEVA PHARMS TECH	1.5MG	N075174 001	JUN 22, 1998
AB		3MG	N075174 002	JUN 22, 1998
AB	MYLAN	1.5MG	N074792 001	JUN 26, 1998
AB		3MG	N074792 002	JUN 26, 1998
AB		6MG	N074792 003	AUG 17, 1999
AB	TEVA	1.5MG	N074686 001	APR 20, 1999
AB		3MG	N074686 002	APR 20, 1999
AB		4.5MG	N074686 003	APR 20, 1999
AB		6MG	N074686 004	APR 20, 1999

GLYNASE

AB	PHARMACIA AND UPJOHN	1.5MG	N020051 001	MAR 04, 1992
AB		3MG	N020051 002	MAR 04, 1992
AB +		6MG	N020051 004	SEP 24, 1993

MICRONASE

AB	PHARMACIA AND UPJOHN	1.25MG	N017498 001	MAY 01, 1984
AB		2.5MG	N017498 002	MAY 01, 1984
AB +		5MG	N017498 003	MAY 01, 1984

GLYBURIDE; METFORMIN HYDROCHLORIDE
Tablet; Oral

GLUCOVANCE
BRISTOL MYERS SQUIBB

	1.25MG;250MG	N021178 001	JUL 31, 2000
	2.5MG;500MG	N021178 002	JUL 31, 2000
+	5MG;500MG	N021178 003	JUL 31, 2000

GLYCERIN *MULTIPLE*
SEE AMINO ACIDS; CALCIUM ACETATE; GLYCERIN; MAGNESIUM ACETATE; PHOSPHORIC ACID; POTASSIUM CHLORIDE; SODIUM ACETATE; SODIUM CHLORIDE

GLYCINE
Solution; Irrigation

AMINOACETIC ACID 1.5% IN PLASTIC CONTAINER

AT	BAXTER HLTHCARE	1.5GM/100ML	N017865 001

GLYCINE 1.5% IN PLASTIC CONTAINER

AT	ABBOTT	1.5GM/100ML	N017633 001
AT		1.5GM/100ML	N018315 001
AT	B BRAUN	1.5GM/100ML	N016784 001

GLYCOPYRROLATE
Injectable; Injection

GLYCOPYRROLATE

AP	LUITPOLD	0.2MG/ML	N089335 001	JUL 23, 1986

ROBINUL

AP +	ROBINS AH	0.2MG/ML	N017558 001

Tablet; Oral

ROBINUL

+	FIRST HORIZON	1MG	N012827 001

ROBINUL FORTE

+	FIRST HORIZON	2MG	N012827 002

GONADORELIN HYDROCHLORIDE
Injectable; Injection

FACTREL

+	BAXTER HLTHCARE CORP	EQ 0.1MG BASE/VIAL	N018123 001	SEP 30, 1982

GONADOTROPIN, CHORIONIC
Injectable; Injection

CHORIONIC GONADOTROPIN

AP +	AM PHARM PARTNERS	10,000 UNITS/VIAL	N017067 002
AP +	STERIS	5,000 UNITS/VIAL	N017016 006
AP		10,000 UNITS/VIAL	N017016 007

PREGNYL

AP +	ORGANON USA INC	10,000 UNITS/VIAL	N017692 001

Prescription Drug Products (continued)

GOSERELIN ACETATE
Implant; Implantation

ZOLADEX

TE	Firm	Strength	NDA	Date
+	ASTRAZENECA	EQ 3.6MG BASE	N019726 001	DEC 29, 1989
+		EQ 10.8MG BASE	N020578 001	JAN 11, 1996

GRAMICIDIN; NEOMYCIN SULFATE; POLYMYXIN B SULFATE
Solution/Drops; Ophthalmic

NEOMYCIN AND POLYMYXIN B SULFATES AND GRAMICIDIN

TE	Firm	Strength	NDA	Date
AT	BAUSCH AND LOMB	0.025MG/ML;EQ 1.75MG BASE/ML;10,000 UNITS/ML	N064047 001	JAN 31, 1996

NEOSPORIN

TE	Firm	Strength	NDA	Date
AT	+ MONARCH PHARMS	0.025MG/ML;EQ 1.75MG BASE/ML;10,000 UNITS/ML	N060582 001	

GRANISETRON HYDROCHLORIDE
Injectable; Injection

KYTRIL

TE	Firm	Strength	NDA	Date
	+ ROCHE	EQ 1MG BASE/ML	N020239 002	MAR 11, 1994

Tablet; Oral

KYTRIL

TE	Firm	Strength	NDA	Date
	+ ROCHE	EQ 1MG BASE	N020305 001	MAR 16, 1995

GRISEOFULVIN, MICROCRYSTALLINE
Suspension; Oral

GRIFULVIN V

TE	Firm	Strength	NDA	Date
	+ J AND J	125MG/5ML	N062483 001	JAN 26, 1984

Tablet; Oral

FULVICIN-U/F

TE	Firm	Strength	NDA	Date
AB	SCHERING	250MG	N060569 002	
AB	+	500MG	N060569 001	

GRIFULVIN V

TE	Firm	Strength	NDA	Date
AB	J AND J	125MG	N062279 001	
AB		250MG	N062279 002	
AB		500MG	N062279 003	

GRISEOFULVIN, ULTRAMICROCRYSTALLINE
Tablet; Oral

FULVICIN P/G

TE	Firm	Strength	NDA	Date
AB	SCHERING	125MG	N061996 001	
AB		250MG	N061996 002	

FULVICIN P/G 165

TE	Firm	Strength	NDA	Date
AB	+ SCHERING	165MG	N061996 003	APR 06, 1982

FULVICIN P/G 330

TE	Firm	Strength	NDA	Date
AB	+ SCHERING	330MG	N061996 004	APR 06, 1982

GRIS-PEG

TE	Firm	Strength	NDA	Date
AB	PEDINOL	125MG	N050475 001	

GRISEOFULVIN, ULTRAMICROCRYSTALLINE (continued)
Tablet; Oral

GRIS-PEG

TE	Firm	Strength	NDA	Date
AB	+ PEDINOL	250MG	N050475 002	

GUANABENZ ACETATE
Tablet; Oral

GUANABENZ ACETATE

TE	Firm	Strength	NDA	Date
AB	COPLEY PHARM	EQ 4MG BASE	N074267 001	JUN 01, 1994
AB		EQ 8MG BASE	N074267 002	JUN 01, 1994
AB	EON	EQ 4MG BASE	N074517 001	SEP 30, 1998
AB		EQ 8MG BASE	N074517 002	SEP 30, 1998
AB	IVAX PHARMS	EQ 4MG BASE	N074149 001	APR 07, 1995
AB		EQ 8MG BASE	N074149 002	APR 07, 1995
AB	WATSON LABS	EQ 4MG BASE	N074025 001	FEB 28, 1994
AB	+	EQ 8MG BASE	N074025 002	FEB 28, 1994

GUANFACINE HYDROCHLORIDE
Tablet; Oral

GUANFACINE HCL

TE	Firm	Strength	NDA	Date
AB	AMIDE PHARM	EQ 1MG BASE	N074673 001	FEB 28, 1997
AB		EQ 2MG BASE	N074673 002	FEB 28, 1997
AB	GENPHARM	EQ 1MG BASE	N075109 001	NOV 25, 1998
AB		EQ 2MG BASE	N075109 002	NOV 25, 1998
AB	MYLAN	EQ 1MG BASE	N074796 001	JAN 27, 1997
AB		EQ 2MG BASE	N074796 002	JAN 27, 1997
AB	WATSON LABS	EQ 1MG BASE	N074145 001	OCT 17, 1995
AB		EQ 1MG BASE	N074762 001	JUN 25, 1997
AB		EQ 2MG BASE	N074145 002	OCT 17, 1995
AB		EQ 2MG BASE	N074762 002	JUN 25, 1997

TENEX

TE	Firm	Strength	NDA	Date
AB	ESP PHARMA	EQ 1MG BASE	N019032 001	OCT 27, 1986
AB	+	EQ 2MG BASE	N019032 002	NOV 07, 1988

Prescription Drug Products (continued)

GUANIDINE HYDROCHLORIDE
Tablet; Oral

TE	Brand / Manufacturer	Strength	Appl. No.	Date
	GUANIDINE HCL			
	SCHERING	125MG	N001546 001	

HALAZEPAM
Tablet; Oral

TE	Brand / Manufacturer	Strength	Appl. No.	Date
	PAXIPAM			
	SCHERING	20MG	N017736 003	
+	SCHERING	40MG	N017736 004	

HALCINONIDE
Cream; Topical

TE	Brand / Manufacturer	Strength	Appl. No.	Date
	HALOG			
+	WESTWOOD SQUIBB	0.1%	N017556 001	
	HALOG-E			
	WESTWOOD SQUIBB	0.1%	N018234 001	

Ointment; Topical

TE	Brand / Manufacturer	Strength	Appl. No.	Date
	HALOG			
+	WESTWOOD SQUIBB	0.1%	N017824 001	

Solution; Topical

TE	Brand / Manufacturer	Strength	Appl. No.	Date
	HALOG			
	WESTWOOD SQUIBB	0.1%	N017823 001	

HALOBETASOL PROPIONATE
Cream; Topical

TE	Brand / Manufacturer	Strength	Appl. No.	Date
	ULTRAVATE			
+	WESTWOOD SQUIBB	0.05%	N019967 001	DEC 27, 1990

Ointment; Topical

TE	Brand / Manufacturer	Strength	Appl. No.	Date
	ULTRAVATE			
+	WESTWOOD SQUIBB	0.05%	N019968 001	DEC 17, 1990

HALOPERIDOL
Tablet; Oral

TE	Brand / Manufacturer	Strength	Appl. No.	Date
	HALOPERIDOL			
	GENEVA PHARMS			
AB		0.5MG	N071206 001	NOV 17, 1986
AB		1MG	N071207 001	NOV 17, 1986
AB		2MG	N071208 001	NOV 17, 1986
AB		5MG	N071209 001	NOV 17, 1986
AB		10MG	N071210 001	MAR 11, 1988
AB		20MG	N071211 001	MAR 11, 1988
	+ MYLAN			
AB		0.5MG	N070276 001	JUN 10, 1986
AB		1MG	N070277 001	JUN 10, 1986
AB		2MG	N070278 001	JUN 10, 1986

HALOPERIDOL (continued)
Tablet; Oral

TE	Brand / Manufacturer	Strength	Appl. No.	Date
	HALOPERIDOL			
	MYLAN			
AB		5MG	N070279 001	JUN 10, 1986
	PAR PHARM			
AB		0.5MG	N071233 001	NOV 03, 1986
AB		1MG	N071234 001	NOV 03, 1986
AB		2MG	N071235 001	NOV 03, 1986
AB		5MG	N071236 001	NOV 03, 1986
AB		10MG	N071237 001	JUL 20, 1987
	WATSON LABS			
AB		0.5MG	N070981 001	MAR 06, 1987
AB		2MG	N070983 001	MAR 06, 1987
AB		5MG	N070984 001	MAR 06, 1987

HALOPERIDOL DECANOATE
Injectable; Injection

TE	Brand / Manufacturer	Strength	Appl. No.	Date
	HALDOL			
AO	+ ORTHO MCNEIL	EQ 50MG BASE/ML	N018701 001	JAN 14, 1986
AO	+	EQ 100MG BASE/ML	N018701 002	JAN 31, 1997
	HALOPERIDOL DECANOATE			
	AM PHARM PARTNERS			
AO		EQ 50MG BASE/ML	N074893 001	DEC 19, 1997
AO		EQ 100MG BASE/ML	N074893 002	DEC 19, 1997
	APOTEX			
AO		EQ 50MG BASE/ML	N075440 001	DEC 19, 1997
AO		EQ 100MG BASE/ML	N075440 002	FEB 28, 2000
	BEDFORD			
AO		EQ 50MG BASE/ML	N074811 001	FEB 28, 2000
AO		EQ 100MG BASE/ML	N075305 001	JAN 30, 1998
	GENSIA SICOR PHARMS			
AO		EQ 50MG BASE/ML	N075393 001	SEP 28, 1998
AO		EQ 100MG BASE/ML	N075393 002	MAY 11, 1999

HALOPERIDOL LACTATE
Concentrate; Oral

TE	Brand / Manufacturer	Strength	Appl. No.	Date
	HALOPERIDOL			
AA	COPLEY PHARM	EQ 2MG BASE/ML	N071617 001	DEC 01, 1988
AA	PHARM ASSOC	EQ 2MG BASE/ML	N073037 001	FEB 26, 1993
AA	SILARX	EQ 2MG BASE/ML	N073364 001	SEP 28, 1993
AA	+ TEVA	EQ 2MG BASE/ML	N071015 001	

Prescription Drug Products (continued)

HALOPERIDOL LACTATE (continued)

Concentrate; Oral

HALOPERIDOL
	Applicant	Strength	NDC	Date
	TEVA			AUG 25, 1987

Injectable; Injection

HALDOL
	Applicant	Strength	NDC	Date
AP	+ ORTHO MCNEIL	EQ 5MG BASE/ML	N015923 001	

HALOPERIDOL
	Applicant	Strength	NDC	Date
AP	AM PHARM PARTNERS	EQ 5MG BASE/ML	N075689 001	MAR 09, 2001
		EQ 5MG BASE/ML	N075858 001	APR 28, 1983
AP	BEDFORD	EQ 5MG BASE/ML	N076035 001	JUN 18, 2001
AP	GENSIA SICOR PHARMS	EQ 5MG BASE/ML	N070714 001	AUG 29, 2001
AP	STERIS	EQ 5MG BASE/ML		MAY 17, 1988

Solution; Oral

HALOPERIDOL LACTATE
	Applicant	Strength	NDC	Date
AP	UDL	EQ 1MG BASE/ML	N074536 001	NOV 02, 1995

HALOTHANE

Liquid; Inhalation

HALOTHANE
	Applicant	Strength	NDC
AN	+ ABBOTT	99.99%	N083254 001
AN	+ HALOCARBON	99.99%	N080810 001

HEPARIN SODIUM

Injectable; Injection

HEP-LOCK
	Applicant	Strength	NDC
AP	+ BAXTER HLTHCARE	10 UNITS/ML	N017037 007
AP	+	100 UNITS/ML	N017037 006

HEP-LOCK U/P
	Applicant	Strength	NDC	Date
AP	BAXTER HLTHCARE	10 UNITS/ML	N017037 010	JUN 10, 1983
		100 UNITS/ML	N017037 011	JUN 10, 1983

HEPARIN LOCK FLUSH
	Applicant	Strength	NDC	Date
AP	ABBOTT	10 UNITS/ML	N005264 001	
AP		10 UNITS/ML	N040082 001	FEB 28, 1995
		10 UNITS/ML	N088097 001	APR 28, 1983
AP		10 UNITS/ML	N088346 001	MAY 18, 1983
AP		100 UNITS/ML	N040082 002	FEB 28, 1995
AP		100 UNITS/ML	N088098 001	APR 28, 1983
AP		100 UNITS/ML	N088347 001	MAY 18, 1983
AP	AM PHARM PARTNERS	100 UNITS/ML	N017029 007	MAY 06, 1982
		100 UNITS/ML	N017029 006	

HEPARIN LOCK FLUSH IN PLASTIC CONTAINER
	Applicant	Strength	NDC
AP	ABBOTT	10 UNITS/ML	N005264 015

HEPARIN SODIUM (continued)

Injectable; Injection

HEPARIN LOCK FLUSH IN PLASTIC CONTAINER
	Applicant	Strength	NDC	Date
	ABBOTT	100 UNITS/ML		MAY 21, 1985
AP			N005264 016	MAY 21, 1985

HEPARIN SODIUM
	Applicant	Strength	NDC	Date
AP	+ ABBOTT	2,500 UNITS/ML	N088099 001	APR 28, 1983
AP		5,000 UNITS/ML	N088100 001	APR 28, 1983
AP	AM PHARM PARTNERS	1,000 UNITS/ML	N017029 001	
AP		1,000 UNITS/ML	N017979 001	
AP		5,000 UNITS/ML	N017651 006	
AP		10,000 UNITS/ML	N017029 003	
AP		10,000 UNITS/ML	N017979 002	
AP		20,000 UNITS/ML	N017029 004	
AP	+ BAXTER HLTHCARE	1,000 UNITS/ML	N017037 001	
AP		5,000 UNITS/0.5ML	N017037 013	APR 07, 1986
AP	LILLY	5,000 UNITS/ML	N017037 002	
AP	MARSAM PHARMS LLC	10,000 UNITS/ML	N017037 003	
AP	+	1,000 UNITS/ML	N005521 002	
AP		1,000 UNITS/ML	N040007 001	JUN 07, 1996
AP	+ PHARMACIA AND UPJOHN	1,000 UNITS/ML	N040008 001	OCT 10, 1995
AP	+	5,000 UNITS/ML	N004570 001	
AP	+	10,000 UNITS/ML	N004570 002	
AP			N004570 003	

HEPARIN SODIUM 1,000 UNITS AND SODIUM CHLORIDE 0.9% IN PLASTIC CONTAINER
	Applicant	Strength	NDC	Date
AP	BAXTER HLTHCARE	200 UNITS/100ML	N018609 001	APR 28, 1982

HEPARIN SODIUM 1,000 UNITS IN SODIUM CHLORIDE 0.9% IN PLASTIC CONTAINER
	Applicant	Strength	NDC	Date
AP	ABBOTT	200 UNITS/100ML	N018916 010	JUN 23, 1989
			N019953 001	JUL 20, 1992
AP	B BRAUN	200 UNITS/100ML		

HEPARIN SODIUM 2,000 UNITS AND SODIUM CHLORIDE 0.9% IN PLASTIC CONTAINER
	Applicant	Strength	NDC	Date
AP	BAXTER HLTHCARE	200 UNITS/100ML	N018609 002	APR 28, 1982

HEPARIN SODIUM 2,000 UNITS IN SODIUM CHLORIDE 0.9% IN PLASTIC CONTAINER
	Applicant	Strength	NDC	Date
AP	ABBOTT	200 UNITS/100ML	N018916 011	JUN 23, 1989

HEPARIN SODIUM 10,000 UNITS IN DEXTROSE 5% IN PLASTIC CONTAINER
	Applicant	Strength	NDC	Date
AP	ABBOTT	10,000 UNITS/100ML	N019339 003	MAR 27, 1985

HEPARIN SODIUM 12,500 UNITS IN DEXTROSE 5% IN PLASTIC CONTAINER
	Applicant	Strength	NDC	Date
AP	ABBOTT	5,000 UNITS/100ML	N019339 001	MAR 27, 1985

Prescription Drug Products (continued)

HEPARIN SODIUM (continued)
Injectable; Injection
HEPARIN SODIUM 12,500 UNITS IN SODIUM CHLORIDE 0.45% IN PLASTIC CONTAINER

	ABBOTT	5,000 UNITS/100ML	N018916 006 JAN 31, 1984

HEPARIN SODIUM 20,000 UNITS AND DEXTROSE 5% IN PLASTIC CONTAINER

AP	BAXTER HLTHCARE	4,000 UNITS/100ML	N018814 001 OCT 31, 1983

HEPARIN SODIUM 20,000 UNITS IN DEXTROSE 5% IN PLASTIC CONTAINER

AP	ABBOTT	4,000 UNITS/100ML	N019805 001 JAN 25, 1989
AP	B BRAUN	4,000 UNITS/100ML	N019952 001 JUL 20, 1992

HEPARIN SODIUM 25,000 UNITS AND DEXTROSE 5% IN PLASTIC CONTAINER

AP	BAXTER HLTHCARE	5,000 UNITS/100ML	N018814 003 JUL 09, 1985
AP		10,000 UNITS/100ML	N018814 004 JUL 02, 1987

HEPARIN SODIUM 25,000 UNITS IN DEXTROSE 5% IN PLASTIC CONTAINER

AP	ABBOTT	10,000 UNITS/100ML	N019339 002 MAR 27, 1985
AP		5,000 UNITS/100ML	N019339 004 MAR 27, 1985
AP		5,000 UNITS/100ML	N019805 002 JAN 25, 1989
AP	B BRAUN	5,000 UNITS/100ML	N019952 004 JUL 20, 1992
AP		10,000 UNITS/100ML	N019952 005 JUL 20, 1992

HEPARIN SODIUM 25,000 UNITS IN SODIUM CHLORIDE 0.45% IN PLASTIC CONTAINER

AP	ABBOTT	5,000 UNITS/100ML	N018916 007 JAN 31, 1984
		10,000 UNITS/100ML	N018916 008 JAN 31, 1984

HEPARIN SODIUM IN PLASTIC CONTAINER

AP	AM PHARM PARTNERS	1,000 UNITS/ML	N017029 013 DEC 05, 1985
AP		5,000 UNITS/ML	N017029 014 DEC 05, 1985
AP		10,000 UNITS/ML	N017029 015 DEC 05, 1985
AP		20,000 UNITS/ML	N017029 016 DEC 05, 1985

HEPARIN SODIUM PRESERVATIVE FREE

AP	+ ABBOTT	2,000 UNITS/ML	N005264 013 APR 07, 1986
AP	+	2,500 UNITS/ML	N005264 014 APR 07, 1986
AP	+	10,000 UNITS/ML	N089522 001 MAY 04, 1987
AP	+ AM PHARM PARTNERS	1,000 UNITS/ML	N017029 010 APR 28, 1986
AP	MARSAM PHARMS LLC	1,000 UNITS/ML	N089464 001 JUN 03, 1986

HEPARIN SODIUM (continued)
Injectable; Injection
HEPFLUSH-10

AP	AM PHARM PARTNERS	10 UNITS/ML	N017651 009 JUN 26, 1984

SODIUM HEPARIN

AP	BAXTER HLTHCARE	1,000 UNITS/ML	N017036 001

HEXACHLOROPHENE
Emulsion; Topical
PHISOHEX

	+ SANOFI SYNTHELABO	3%	N006882 001

Sponge; Topical
PRE-OP

AT	+ DAVIS AND GECK	480MG	N017433 001

PRE-OP II

AT	+ DAVIS AND GECK	480MG	N017433 002

HOMATROPINE METHYLBROMIDE; HYDROCODONE BITARTRATE
Syrup; Oral
HYCODAN

AA	+ ENDO PHARMS	1.5MG/5ML;5MG/5ML	N005213 002 JUL 26, 1988

HYDROCODONE BITARTRATE AND HOMATROPINE METHYLBROMIDE

AA	AXIOM PHARM	1.5MG/5ML;5MG/5ML	N040285 001 JUL 19, 1999

HYDROCODONE COMPOUND

AA	ALPHARMA	1.5MG/5ML;5MG/5ML	N088017 001 JUL 05, 1983

MYCODONE

AA	MORTON GROVE	1.5MG/5ML;5MG/5ML	N088008 001 MAR 03, 1983

Tablet; Oral
HOMATROPINE METHYLBROMIDE AND HYDROCODONE BITARTRATE

AA	AMIDE PHARM	1.5MG;5MG	N040295 001 DEC 01, 2000

HYCODAN

AA	+ ENDO PHARMS	1.5MG;5MG	N005213 001 JUL 26, 1988

TUSSIGON

AA	JONES PHARMA	1.5MG;5MG	N088508 001 JUL 30, 1985

HYDRALAZINE HYDROCHLORIDE
Injectable; Injection
HYDRALAZINE HCL

AP	AM PHARM PARTNERS	20MG/ML	N040388 001 MAR 13, 2001
AP	GENSIA SICOR PHARMS	20MG/ML	N040373 001 FEB 23, 2000
AP	+ LUITPOLD	20MG/ML	N040136 001 JUN 30, 1997

Tablet; Oral
APRESOLINE

AA	+ NOVARTIS	10MG	N008303 004
AA	+	25MG	N008303 001

Prescription Drug Products *(continued)*

HYDRALAZINE HYDROCHLORIDE *(continued)*
Tablet; Oral

APRESOLINE

TE	Firm	Strength	Appl. No.	Date
AA	+ NOVARTIS	50MG	N008303 002	
AA		100MG	N008303 005	

+

HYDRALAZINE HCL

TE	Firm	Strength	Appl. No.	Date
AA	ABC HOLDING	10MG	N088846 001	FEB 26, 1985
AA		25MG	N088847 001	FEB 26, 1985
AA		50MG	N088848 001	FEB 26, 1985
AA		100MG	N088849 001	FEB 26, 1985
AA	CLONMEL HLTHCARE	25MG	N086243 001	
AA		50MG	N086242 002	
AA	GENEVA PHARMS	10MG	N083241 001	
AA		25MG	N083560 001	
AA	IMPAX LABS	50MG	N083561 001	
AA	MUTUAL PHARM	50MG	N084923 001	
AA		10MG	N089359 001	JUL 25, 1986
AA	PAR PHARM	25MG	N089258 001	MAY 05, 1986
AA		50MG	N089259 001	MAY 05, 1986
AA		10MG	N087836 001	OCT 05, 1982
AA		25MG	N086961 002	
AA		50MG	N086962 001	
AA		100MG	N088391 001	SEP 27, 1983
AA	PLIVA	10MG	N089097 001	DEC 18, 1985
AA		25MG	N088467 001	MAY 01, 1984
AA		50MG	N088468 001	MAY 01, 1984
AA		100MG	N089098 001	DEC 18, 1985
AA	WATSON LABS	25MG	N084504 001	
AA		50MG	N084503 001	

HYDRALAZINE HYDROCHLORIDE; HYDROCHLOROTHIAZIDE
Capsule; Oral

APRESAZIDE

TE	Firm	Strength	Appl. No.	Date
AB	NOVARTIS	25MG;25MG	N084735 001	
AB		50MG;50MG	N084810 001	

HYDRA-ZIDE

TE	Firm	Strength	Appl. No.	Date
AB	PAR PHARM	25MG;25MG	N088957 001	OCT 21, 1985
AB		50MG;50MG	N088946 001	OCT 21, 1985
		100MG;50MG	N088961 001	OCT 21, 1985

+

HYDRALAZINE HCL AND HYDROCHLOROTHIAZIDE

TE	Firm	Strength	Appl. No.	Date
AB	SUPERPHARM	50MG;50MG	N089201 001	

HYDRALAZINE HYDROCHLORIDE; HYDROCHLOROTHIAZIDE *(continued)*
Capsule; Oral

HYDRALAZINE HCL AND HYDROCHLOROTHIAZIDE

TE	Firm	Strength	Appl. No.	Date
	SUPERPHARM			FEB 09, 1987

HYDROCHLOROTHIAZIDE
Capsule; Oral

HYDROCHLOROTHIAZIDE

TE	Firm	Strength	Appl. No.	Date
AB	MYLAN	12.5MG	N075640 001	JAN 28, 2000
AB	VINTAGE PHARMS	12.5MG	N075907 001	SEP 17, 2002

MICROZIDE

TE	Firm	Strength	Appl. No.	Date
AB	+ WATSON LABS	12.5MG	N020504 001	DEC 27, 1996

Solution; Oral

HYDROCHLOROTHIAZIDE

TE	Firm	Strength	Appl. No.	Date
	+ ROXANE	50MG/5ML	N088587 001	JUL 02, 1984

Tablet; Oral

ESIDRIX

TE	Firm	Strength	Appl. No.	Date
AB	NOVARTIS	25MG	N011793 005	
AB		50MG	N011793 008	

HYDROCHLOROTHIAZIDE

TE	Firm	Strength	Appl. No.	Date
AB	ABC HOLDING	25MG	N085683 001	
AB		50MG	N083965 001	
AB		50MG	N085672 001	
AB	CLONMEL HLTHCARE	25MG	N087059 001	
AB	EON	50MG	N085219 001	
AB	GENEVA PHARMS	25MG	N087565 001	MAR 09, 1982
AB	IVAX PHARMS	50MG	N084912 001	
AB		25MG	N083177 001	
AB		50MG	N083177 002	
AB		100MG	N085022 001	
AB	+ LEDEFLE	50MG	N087068 001	
AB	PUREPAC PHARM	25MG	N085054 002	
AB		50MG	N085208 001	
AB	PVT FORM	25MG	N085181 001	
AB		50MG	N085182 001	
AB	ROXANE	50MG	N084536 002	
AB	VINTAGE PHARMS	25MG	N040412 001	MAR 29, 2002
AB		50MG	N040412 002	MAR 29, 2002
AB	WATSON LABS	25MG	N081189 001	JAN 24, 1992

ORETIC

TE	Firm	Strength	Appl. No.	Date
AB	ABBOTT	50MG	N011971 002	

HYDROCHLOROTHIAZIDE; IRBESARTAN
Tablet; Oral

AVALIDE

TE	Firm	Strength	Appl. No.	Date
AB	SANOFI SYNTHELABO	12.5MG;150MG	N020758 002	SEP 30, 1997

Prescription Drug Products (continued)

HYDROCHLOROTHIAZIDE; IRBESARTAN (continued)
Tablet; Oral

AVALIDE

	Strength	Appl. No.	Date
+ SANOFI SYNTHELABO	12.5MG;300MG	N020758 003	AUG 31, 1998

HYDROCHLOROTHIAZIDE; LISINOPRIL
Tablet; Oral

LISINOPRIL AND HYDROCHLOROTHIAZIDE

		Strength	Appl. No.	Date
	EON			
AB		12.5MG;10MG	N076262 001	JUL 01, 2002
AB		12.5MG;20MG	N076262 002	JUL 01, 2002
AB		25MG;20MG	N076262 003	JUL 01, 2002
	GENEVA PHARMS TECH			
AB		12.5MG;10MG	N075926 001	JUL 01, 2002
AB		12.5MG;20MG	N075926 002	JUL 01, 2002
AB		25MG;20MG	N075926 003	JUL 01, 2002
	IVAX PHARMS			
AB		12.5MG;10MG	N075776 001	JUL 01, 2002
AB		12.5MG;20MG	N075776 002	JUL 01, 2002
AB		25MG;20MG	N075776 003	JUL 01, 2002
	MYLAN			
AB		12.5MG;10MG	N076113 001	JUL 01, 2002
AB		12.5MG;20MG	N076113 002	JUL 01, 2002
AB		25MG;20MG	N076113 003	JUL 01, 2002
	PUREPAC PHARM			
AB		12.5MG;10MG	N076230 001	JUL 01, 2002
AB		12.5MG;20MG	N076230 002	JUL 01, 2002
AB		25MG;20MG	N076230 003	JUL 01, 2002
	RANBAXY			
AB		12.5MG;10MG	N076007 001	JUL 01, 2002
AB		12.5MG;20MG	N076007 002	JUL 01, 2002
AB		25MG;20MG	N076007 003	JUL 01, 2002
	TEVA			
AB		12.5MG;10MG	N075869 001	JUL 01, 2002
AB		12.5MG;20MG	N075869 002	JUL 01, 2002
AB		25MG;20MG	N075869 003	JUL 01, 2002
	WATSON LABS			
AB		12.5MG;20MG	N076194 001	JUL 01, 2002
AB		25MG;20MG	N076194 002	JUL 01, 2002
AB		12.5MG;10MG	N076194 003	JUL 01, 2002

HYDROCHLOROTHIAZIDE; LISINOPRIL (continued)
Tablet; Oral

LISINOPRIL AND HYDROCHLOROTHIAZIDE

		Strength	Appl. No.	Date
	WEST WARD			
AB		12.5MG;10MG	N076265 001	JUL 08, 2002
AB		12.5MG;20MG	N076265 002	JUL 08, 2002
AB		25MG;20MG	N076265 003	JUL 08, 2002
	PRINZIDE			
	MERCK			
AB		12.5MG;10MG	N019778 003	NOV 18, 1993
AB		12.5MG;20MG	N019778 001	FEB 16, 1989
AB		25MG;20MG	N019778 002	FEB 16, 1989
	ZESTORETIC			
	ASTRAZENECA			
AB		12.5MG;10MG	N019888 003	NOV 18, 1993
AB		12.5MG;20MG	N019888 001	SEP 20, 1990
AB +		25MG;20MG	N019888 002	JUL 20, 1989

HYDROCHLOROTHIAZIDE; LOSARTAN POTASSIUM
Tablet; Oral

HYZAAR

		Strength	Appl. No.	Date
	MERCK			
AB		12.5MG;50MG	N020387 001	APR 28, 1995
AB +		25MG;100MG	N020387 002	NOV 10, 1998

HYDROCHLOROTHIAZIDE; METHYLDOPA
Tablet; Oral

		Strength	Appl. No.	Date
	ALDORIL 15			
	MERCK			
AB		15MG;250MG	N013402 001	
	ALDORIL 25			
	MERCK			
AB		25MG;250MG	N013402 002	
	ALDORIL D30			
	MERCK			
AB		30MG;500MG	N013402 003	
	ALDORIL D50			
AB +	MERCK	50MG;500MG	N013402 004	
	METHYLDOPA AND HYDROCHLOROTHIAZIDE			
AB	GENEVA PHARMS	15MG;250MG	N070182 001	JAN 15, 1986
AB		25MG;250MG	N070183 001	JAN 15, 1986
AB		30MG;500MG	N070543 001	JAN 15, 1986
AB		50MG;500MG	N070544 001	JAN 15, 1986
AB	LEDERLE	15MG;250MG	N072507 001	JUN 02, 1989
AB		25MG;250MG	N072508 001	JUN 02, 1989
AB		30MG;500MG	N072509 001	JUN 02, 1989

Prescription Drug Products *(continued)*

HYDROCHLOROTHIAZIDE; METHYLDOPA *(continued)*
Tablet; Oral

METHYLDOPA AND HYDROCHLOROTHIAZIDE

TE	Applicant	Strength	Appl. No.	Date
AB	LEDERLE	50MG;500MG	N072510 001	JUN 02, 1989
AB	MYLAN	15MG;250MG	N070264 001	JUN 02, 1989
AB		25MG;250MG	N070265 001	JAN 23, 1986
AB	PAR PHARM	25MG;250MG	N070612 001	JAN 23, 1986
AB		30MG;500MG	N070613 001	FEB 02, 1987
AB		50MG;500MG	N070614 001	FEB 02, 1987
AB		15MG;250MG	N070616 001	FEB 02, 1987
AB	WATSON LABS	15MG;250MG	N070958 001	FEB 06, 1989
AB		25MG;250MG	N070959 001	JAN 19, 1989
AB		50MG;500MG	N070960 001	JAN 19, 1989
AB		30MG;500MG	N071069 001	FEB 06, 1989
				JAN 19, 1989

HYDROCHLOROTHIAZIDE; METOPROLOL TARTRATE
Tablet; Oral

LOPRESSOR HCT

Applicant	Strength	Appl. No.	Date
NOVARTIS	25MG;50MG	N018303 001	DEC 31, 1984
	25MG;100MG	N018303 002	DEC 31, 1984
+	50MG;100MG	N018303 003	DEC 31, 1984
			DEC 31, 1984

HYDROCHLOROTHIAZIDE; MOEXIPRIL HYDROCHLORIDE
Tablet; Oral

UNIRETIC

Applicant	Strength	Appl. No.	Date
SCHWARZ PHARMA	12.5MG;7.5MG	N020729 001	JUN 27, 1997
	12.5MG;15MG	N020729 003	JUN 27, 1997
+	25MG;15MG	N020729 002	FEB 14, 2002
			JUN 27, 1997

HYDROCHLOROTHIAZIDE; OLMESARTAN MEDOXOMIL
Tablet; Oral

BENICAR HCT

Applicant	Strength	Appl. No.	Date
SANKYO	12.5MG;20MG	N021532 002	JUN 05, 2003
	12.5MG;40MG	N021532 003	JUN 05, 2003
+	25MG;40MG	N021532 005	JUN 05, 2003
			JUN 05, 2003

HYDROCHLOROTHIAZIDE; PROPRANOLOL HYDROCHLORIDE
Tablet; Oral

INDERIDE-40/25

TE	Applicant	Strength	Appl. No.
AB	WYETH PHARMS INC	25MG;40MG	N018031 001

INDERIDE-80/25

TE	Applicant	Strength	Appl. No.
+	WYETH PHARMS INC	25MG;80MG	N018031 002

PROPRANOLOL HCL AND HYDROCHLOROTHIAZIDE

TE	Applicant	Strength	Appl. No.	Date
AB	BARR	25MG;40MG	N070704 001	OCT 01, 1986
AB		25MG;80MG	N070705 001	OCT 01, 1986
AB	GENEVA PHARMS	25MG;40MG	N071060 001	OCT 01, 1986
AB		25MG;80MG	N071061 001	AUG 26, 1987
AB	MYLAN	25MG;40MG	N070946 001	AUG 26, 1987
AB		25MG;80MG	N070947 001	MAR 04, 1987
AB	PLIVA	25MG;40MG	N072042 001	APR 01, 1987
AB		25MG;80MG	N072043 001	MAR 14, 1988
AB	PUREPAC PHARM	25MG;40MG	N070851 001	MAR 14, 1988
AB		25MG;80MG	N070852 001	MAY 15, 1986
AB	WATSON LABS	25MG;40MG	N070301 001	MAY 15, 1986
AB		25MG;80MG	N070305 001	APR 18, 1986
				APR 18, 1986

HYDROCHLOROTHIAZIDE; QUINAPRIL HYDROCHLORIDE
Tablet; Oral

ACCURETIC

TE	Applicant	Strength	Appl. No.	Date
AB	PFIZER PHARMS	12.5MG;EQ 10MG BASE	N020125 001	DEC 28, 1999
		12.5MG;EQ 20MG BASE	N020125 002	DEC 28, 1999
+		25MG;EQ 20MG BASE	N020125 003	DEC 28, 1999
				DEC 28, 1999

HYDROCHLOROTHIAZIDE; SPIRONOLACTONE
Tablet; Oral

ALDACTAZIDE

TE	Applicant	Strength	Appl. No.	Date
AB	GD SEARLE LLC	25MG;25MG	N012616 004	DEC 30, 1982
+		50MG;50MG	N012616 005	DEC 30, 1982
				DEC 30, 1982

SPIRONOLACTONE AND HYDROCHLOROTHIAZIDE

TE	Applicant	Strength	Appl. No.	Date
AB	GENEVA PHARMS	25MG;25MG	N086881 001	
AB	HALSEY	25MG;25MG	N087267 001	
AB	MUTUAL PHARM	25MG;25MG	N089534 001	JUL 02, 1987
AB	MYLAN	25MG;25MG	N086513 001	

Prescription Drug Products (continued)

HYDROCHLOROTHIAZIDE; SPIRONOLACTONE (continued)
Tablet; Oral

SPIRONOLACTONE W/ HYDROCHLOROTHIAZIDE
AB	PARKE DAVIS	25MG;25MG	N087948 001	FEB 22, 1983

SPIRONOLACTONE/HYDROCHLOROTHIAZIDE
AB	WATSON LABS	25MG;25MG	N087398 001

HYDROCHLOROTHIAZIDE; TELMISARTAN
Tablet; Oral

MICARDIS HCT
	BOEHRINGER INGELHEIM	12.5MG;40MG	N021162 001	NOV 17, 2000
+		12.5MG;80MG	N021162 002	NOV 17, 2000

HYDROCHLOROTHIAZIDE; TIMOLOL MALEATE
Tablet; Oral

TIMOLIDE 10-25
+	MERCK	25MG;10MG	N018061 001

HYDROCHLOROTHIAZIDE; TRIAMTERENE
Capsule; Oral

DYAZIDE
AB +	GLAXOSMITHKLINE	25MG;37.5MG	N016042 003	MAR 03, 1994

TRIAMTERENE AND HYDROCHLOROTHIAZIDE
AB	BARR	25MG;37.5MG	N074970 001	JAN 06, 1998
AB	DURAMED PHARM BARR	25MG;37.5MG	N075052 001	JUN 18, 1999
AB +	GENEVA PHARMS	25MG;50MG	N073191 001	JUL 31, 1991
AB		25MG;37.5MG	N074821 001	JUN 05, 1997
AB	IVAX PHARMS	25MG;50MG	N074259 001	MAR 30, 1995
AB	MYLAN	25MG;37.5MG	N074701 001	JUN 07, 1996

Tablet; Oral

MAXZIDE
AB +	MYLAN	50MG;75MG	N019129 001	OCT 22, 1984

MAXZIDE-25
AB	MYLAN	25MG;37.5MG	N019129 003	MAY 13, 1988

TRIAMTERENE AND HYDROCHLOROTHIAZIDE
AB	BARR	50MG;75MG	N071251 001	APR 17, 1988
		25MG;37.5MG	N071251 002	APR 17, 1988
AB	GENEVA PHARMS	50MG;75MG	N072011 001	MAY 05, 1998
AB		25MG;37.5MG	N073281 001	JUN 17, 1988 / APR 30, 1992

HYDROCHLOROTHIAZIDE; TRIAMTERENE (continued)
Tablet; Oral

TRIAMTERENE AND HYDROCHLOROTHIAZIDE
AB	PLIVA	50MG;75MG	N073467 001	JAN 31, 1996
AB		25MG;37.5MG	N074026 001	APR 26, 1996
AB	WATSON LABS	50MG;75MG	N071851 001	NOV 30, 1988
AB		50MG;75MG	N071969 001	APR 17, 1988
AB		25MG;37.5MG	N073449 001	SEP 23, 1993

HYDROCHLOROTHIAZIDE; VALSARTAN
Tablet; Oral

DIOVAN HCT
	NOVARTIS	12.5MG;80MG	N020818 001	MAR 06, 1998
+		12.5MG;160MG	N020818 002	MAR 06, 1998

HYDROCHLOROTHIAZIDE *MULTIPLE*
SEE	AMILORIDE HYDROCHLORIDE; HYDROCHLOROTHIAZIDE
SEE	BENAZEPRIL HYDROCHLORIDE; HYDROCHLOROTHIAZIDE
SEE	BISOPROLOL FUMARATE; HYDROCHLOROTHIAZIDE
SEE	CANDESARTAN CILEXETIL; HYDROCHLOROTHIAZIDE
SEE	CAPTOPRIL; HYDROCHLOROTHIAZIDE
SEE	ENALAPRIL MALEATE; HYDROCHLOROTHIAZIDE
SEE	EPROSARTAN MESYLATE; HYDROCHLOROTHIAZIDE
SEE	FOSINOPRIL SODIUM; HYDROCHLOROTHIAZIDE
SEE	HYDRALAZINE HYDROCHLORIDE; HYDROCHLOROTHIAZIDE

HYDROCODONE BITARTRATE; IBUPROFEN
Tablet; Oral

HYDROCODONE BITARTRATE AND IBUPROFEN
AB	TEVA	7.5MG;200MG	N076023 001	APR 11, 2003

VICOPROFEN
AB +	ABBOTT	7.5MG;200MG	N020716 001	SEP 23, 1997

HYDROCODONE BITARTRATE *MULTIPLE*
SEE	ACETAMINOPHEN; HYDROCODONE BITARTRATE
SEE	ASPIRIN; HYDROCODONE BITARTRATE
SEE	HOMATROPINE METHYLBROMIDE; HYDROCODONE BITARTRATE

HYDROCODONE POLISTIREX *MULTIPLE*
SEE	CHLORPHENIRAMINE POLISTIREX; HYDROCODONE POLISTIREX

HYDROCORTISONE
Cream; Topical

ALA-CORT
AT	DEL RAY LABS	1%	N080706 006	

Prescription Drug Products *(continued)*

HYDROCORTISONE *(continued)*

Cream; Topical

TE	Product / Applicant	Strength	Appl. No.	Approval Date
	ANUSOL HC			
AT	PARKEDALE	2.5%	N088250 001	JUN 06, 1984
	HI-COR			
AT	C AND M PHARMA	2.5%	N080483 001	
	HYDROCORTISONE			
AT	ALPHARMA	2.5%	N089682 001	MAR 10, 1988
AT	ALPHARMA US PHARM	1%	N087795 001	MAY 03, 1983
AT	ALTANA	0.5%	N080848 002	
AT	ALTANA	1%	N080848 003	
AT	ALTANA	2.5%	N085025 001	
AT	CLAY PARK	1%	N080452 002	
AT	EVERYLIFE	2.5%	N080693 003	
AT	FOUGERA	1%	N089414 001	DEC 16, 1986
AT	INGRAM PHARM	0.5%	N080456 002	
AT	INGRAM PHARM	1%	N080456 003	
AT	PHARMADERM	2.5%	N089413 001	DEC 16, 1986
AT	SYOSSET	0.5%	N085527 001	
AT	TARO	1%	N086155 001	
AT	TARO	2.5%	N088799 001	NOV 09, 1984
	HYTONE			
AT	+ DERMIK LABS	1%	N080472 003	
AT	+	2.5%	N080472 004	
	PENECORT			
AT	+ ALLERGAN HERBERT	1%	N088216 001	JUN 06, 1984
	SYNACORT			
AT	MEDICIS	1%	N087458 001	
AT	MEDICIS	2.5%	N087457 001	

Enema; Rectal

TE	Product / Applicant	Strength	Appl. No.	Approval Date
	COLOCORT			
AB	PADDOCK	100MG/60ML	N075172 001	DEC 03, 1999
	CORTENEMA			
AB	+ SOLVAY	100MG/60ML	N016199 001	
	HYDROCORTISONE			
AB	COPLEY PHARM	100MG/60ML	N074171 001	MAY 27, 1994

Lotion; Topical

TE	Product / Applicant	Strength	Appl. No.	Approval Date
	ALA-CORT			
AT	DEL RAY LABS	1%	N083201 001	
	ALA-SCALP			
	DEL RAY LABS	2%	N083231 001	
	CETACORT			
AT	HEALTHPOINT	0.5%	N080426 002	
AT	HEALTHPOINT	1%	N080426 001	
	EPICORT			
AT	BLULINE	0.5%	N083219 002	
	HYDROCORTISONE			
AT	ALTANA	2.5%	N040351 001	JUL 25, 2000
AT	TARO	2.5%	N040247 001	JUL 23, 1999
	HYTONE			
AT	+ DERMIK LABS	1%	N080473 003	
AT	+	2.5%	N080473 004	NOV 30, 1982
	NUTRACORT			
AT	HEALTHPOINT	1%	N080443 003	
AT	HEALTHPOINT	2.5%	N087644 001	AUG 24, 1982
	STIE-CORT			
AT	STIEFEL	1%	N089066 001	NOV 25, 1985
AT	STIEFEL	2.5%	N089074 001	NOV 26, 1985

Ointment; Topical

TE	Product / Applicant	Strength	Appl. No.	Approval Date
	CORTRIL			
AT	+ PFIPHARMECS	1%	N009176 001	
AT	+	2.5%	N009176 002	
	HYDROCORTISONE			
AT	ALPHARMA US PHARM	1%	N087796 001	OCT 13, 1982
AT	ALTANA	1%	N080489 003	
AT	ALTANA	1%	N080692 001	
AT	CLAY PARK	2.5%	N085027 001	
AT	FOUGERA	2.5%	N081203 001	MAY 28, 1993
AT	TARO	1%	N086257 001	
AT	TARO	2.5%	N040310 001	DEC 29, 2000
	HYDROCORTISONE IN ABSORBASE			
AT	CAROLINA MEDCL	1%	N088138 001	SEP 06, 1985

Powder; For Rx Compounding

TE	Product / Applicant	Strength	Appl. No.	Approval Date
	HYDROCORTISONE			
AA	PADDOCK	100%	N088082 001	APR 08, 1983
AA	PHARMA TEK	100%	N085982 001	

Solution; Topical

TE	Product / Applicant	Strength	Appl. No.	Approval Date
	PENECORT			
AT	ALLERGAN HERBERT	1%	N088214 001	JUN 06, 1984
	TEXACORT			
AT	+ SIRIUS LABS	1%	N080425 001	
AT	+	2.5%	N081271 001	APR 17, 1992

Tablet; Oral

TE	Product / Applicant	Strength	Appl. No.	Approval Date
	CORTEF			
BP	PHARMACIA AND UPJOHN	5MG	N008697 003	
BP		10MG	N008697 001	
BP	+	20MG	N008697 002	

Prescription Drug Products *(continued)*

HYDROCORTISONE *(continued)*
Tablet; Oral
HYDROCORTISONE
BP   WEST WARD   20MG   N083365 001
HYDROCORTONE
BP   MERCK   10MG   N008506 007
BP +   20MG   N008506 011

HYDROCORTISONE; NEOMYCIN SULFATE; POLYMYXIN B SULFATE
Solution/Drops; Otic
CORTISPORIN
AT + MONARCH PHARMS   1%;EQ 3.5MG BASE/ML;10,000 UNITS/ML   N050479 001
NEOMYCIN AND POLYMYXIN B SULFATES AND HYDROCORTISONE
AT   ALCON   1%;EQ 3.5MG BASE/ML;10,000 UNITS/ML   N062423 001 AUG 25, 1983
AT   BAUSCH AND LOMB   1%;EQ 3.5MG BASE/ML;10,000 UNITS/ML   N064053 001 DEC 29, 1995

Suspension/Drops; Ophthalmic
CORTISPORIN
AT + MONARCH PHARMS   1%;EQ 3.5MG BASE/ML;10,000 UNITS/ML   N050169 001
NEOMYCIN AND POLYMYXIN B SULFATES AND HYDROCORTISONE
AT   ALCON UNIVERSAL   1%;EQ 3.5MG BASE/ML;10,000 UNITS/ML   N062874 001 MAY 11, 1988

Suspension/Drops; Otic
CORTISPORIN
AT + MONARCH PHARMS   1%;EQ 3.5MG BASE/ML;10,000 UNITS/ML   N060613 001
NEOMYCIN AND POLYMYXIN B SULFATES AND HYDROCORTISONE
AT   ALCON UNIVERSAL   1%;EQ 3.5MG BASE/ML;10,000 UNITS/ML   N062488 001 NOV 06, 1985
OTICAIR
AT   BAUSCH AND LOMB   1%;EQ 3.5MG BASE/ML;10,000 UNITS/ML   N064065 001 AUG 28, 1996
PEDIOTIC
AT   MONARCH PHARMS   1%;EQ 3.5MG BASE/ML;10,000 UNITS/ML   N062822 001 SEP 29, 1987

HYDROCORTISONE; POLYMYXIN B SULFATE
Solution/Drops; Otic
OTOBIOTIC
+   SCHERING   5MG/ML;EQ 10,000 UNITS BASE/ML   N062302 001

HYDROCORTISONE *MULTIPLE*
SEE   ACETIC ACID, GLACIAL; HYDROCORTISONE
SEE   BACITRACIN ZINC; HYDROCORTISONE; NEOMYCIN SULFATE; POLYMYXIN B SULFATE
SEE   CIPROFLOXACIN HYDROCHLORIDE; HYDROCORTISONE

HYDROCORTISONE ACETATE
Aerosol, Metered; Rectal
CORTIFOAM
+   SCHWARZ PHARMA   10%   N017351 001 FEB 10, 1982

Cream; Topical
HYDROCORTISONE ACETATE
+   FERNDALE LABS   2.5%   N040259 001 JUL 29, 1999
MICORT-HC
+   FERNDALE LABS   2%   N040398 001 MAR 29, 2002
                           2.5%   N040396 001 FEB 27, 2001

Lotion; Topical
DRICORT
+   INGRAM PHARM   0.5%   N086207 001

Ointment; Ophthalmic
HYDROCORTISONE ACETATE
+   ALTANA   0.5%   N080828 001

Paste; Topical
ORABASE HCA
COLGATE   0.5%   N083205 001

Powder; For Rx Compounding
HYDROCORTISONE ACETATE
PHARMA TEK   100%   N085981 001

HYDROCORTISONE ACETATE; NEOMYCIN SULFATE; POLYMYXIN B SULFATE
Cream; Topical
CORTISPORIN
+   MONARCH PHARMS   0.5%;EQ 3.5MG BASE/GM;10,000 UNITS/GM   N050218 001 AUG 09, 1985

HYDROCORTISONE ACETATE; OXYTETRACYCLINE HYDROCHLORIDE
Suspension/Drops; Ophthalmic
TERRA-CORTRIL
+   PFIZER   1.5%;EQ 5MG BASE/ML   N061016 001

HYDROCORTISONE ACETATE; PRAMOXINE HYDROCHLORIDE
Aerosol, Metered; Topical
EPIFOAM
BX   SCHWARZ PHARMA   1%;1%   N086457 001
HYDROCORTISONE ACETATE 1% AND PRAMOXINE HCL 1%
BX   COPLEY PHARM   1%;1%   N089440 001 MAY 17, 1988
PROCTOFOAM HC
BX   SCHWARZ PHARMA   1%;1%   N086195 001

Cream; Topical
PRAMOSONE
FERNDALE LABS   0.5%;1%   N083778 001
                           1%;1%   N085368 001

Prescription Drug Products (continued)

HYDROCORTISONE ACETATE; PRAMOXINE HYDROCHLORIDE (continued)

Lotion; Topical
PRAMOSONE
FERNDALE LABS

	1%;1%	N085980 001	
	2.5%;1%	N085979 001	

HYDROCORTISONE ACETATE; UREA

Cream; Topical
CARMOL HC

AT	+ KENWOOD LABS	1%;10%	N080505 001	

U-CORT

AT	TARO	1%;10%	N089472 001	JUN 13, 1988

HYDROCORTISONE ACETATE *MULTIPLE*

SEE   BACITRACIN; HYDROCORTISONE ACETATE; NEOMYCIN SULFATE; POLYMYXIN B SULFATE

SEE   COLISTIN SULFATE; HYDROCORTISONE ACETATE; NEOMYCIN SULFATE; THONZONIUM BROMIDE

HYDROCORTISONE BUTYRATE

Cream; Topical
LOCOID

	+ FERNDALE LABS	0.1%	N018514 001	MAR 31, 1982

LOCOID LIPOCREAM

	+ FERNDALE LABS	0.1%	N020769 001	SEP 08, 1997

Ointment; Topical
LOCOID

	+ FERNDALE LABS	0.1%	N018652 001	OCT 29, 1982

Solution; Topical
LOCOID

	+ FERNDALE LABS	0.1%	N019116 001	FEB 25, 1987

HYDROCORTISONE CYPIONATE

Suspension; Oral
CORTEF

	+ PHARMACIA AND UPJOHN	EQ 10MG BASE/5ML	N009900 001

HYDROCORTISONE PROBUTATE

Cream; Topical
PANDEL

	+ SAVAGE LABS	0.1%	N020453 001	FEB 28, 1997

HYDROCORTISONE SODIUM SUCCINATE

Injectable; Injection
A-HYDROCORT
ABBOTT

AP	EQ 1GM BASE/VIAL	N085932 001

HYDROCORTISONE SODIUM SUCCINATE (continued)

Injectable; Injection
A-HYDROCORT
ABBOTT

AP	EQ 100MG BASE/VIAL	N085929 001	
AP	EQ 250MG BASE/VIAL	N085930 001	
AP	EQ 500MG BASE/VIAL	N085931 001	

HYDROCORTISONE SODIUM SUCCINATE
INTL MEDICATION

AP	EQ 100MG BASE/VIAL	N087532 001	MAR 19, 1982

SOLU-CORTEF
+ PHARMACIA AND UPJOHN

AP	EQ 1GM BASE/VIAL	N009866 004	
AP +	EQ 100MG BASE/VIAL	N009866 001	
AP +	EQ 250MG BASE/VIAL	N009866 002	
AP +	EQ 500MG BASE/VIAL	N009866 003	

HYDROCORTISONE VALERATE

Cream; Topical
HYDROCORTISONE VALERATE

AB	CLAY PARK	0.2%	N075666 001	MAY 24, 2000
AB	COPLEY PHARM	0.2%	N074489 001	AUG 12, 1998
AB	TARO	0.2%	N075042 001	AUG 25, 1998

WESTCORT
+ WESTWOOD SQUIBB

AB	0.2%	N017950 001

Ointment; Topical
HYDROCORTISONE VALERATE

AB	ALTANA	0.2%	N075085 001	JUL 31, 2001
AB	TARO	0.2%	N075043 001	AUG 25, 1998

WESTCORT
+ WESTWOOD SQUIBB

AB	0.2%	N018726 001	AUG 08, 1983

HYDROFLUMETHIAZIDE

Tablet; Oral
HYDROFLUMETHIAZIDE

AB	PAR PHARM	50MG	N088850 001	MAY 31, 1985

SALURON
+ SHIRE LABS

AB	50MG	N011949 001

HYDROFLUMETHIAZIDE; RESERPINE

Tablet; Oral
SALUTENSIN
+ SHIRE LABS

	50MG;0.125MG	N012359 003

HYDROMORPHONE HYDROCHLORIDE

Injectable; Injection
DILAUDID-HP
+ ABBOTT

AP	10MG/ML	N019034 001	JAN 11, 1984
	250MG/VIAL	N019034 002	

Prescription Drug Products (continued)

HYDROMORPHONE HYDROCHLORIDE (continued)

Injectable; Injection

DILAUDID-HP
	ABBOTT			AUG 04, 1994

HYDROMORPHONE HCL
AP	ABBOTT	10MG/ML	N074598 001	JUN 19, 1997
AP	FAULDING	10MG/ML	N076444 001	APR 25, 2003
AP	STERIS	10MG/ML	N074317 001	AUG 23, 1995

Solution; Oral

DILAUDID
AA +	ABBOTT	5MG/5ML	N019891 001	DEC 07, 1992

HYDROMORPHONE HCL
AA	ROXANE	5MG/5ML	N074653 001	JUL 29, 1998

Tablet; Oral

DILAUDID
AB +	ABBOTT	8MG	N019892 001	DEC 07, 1992

HYDROMORPHONE HCL
AB	ROXANE	8MG	N074597 001	JUL 29, 1998

HYDROQUINONE *MULTIPLE*

SEE FLUOCINOLONE ACETONIDE; HYDROQUINONE; TRETINOIN

HYDROXOCOBALAMIN

Injectable; Injection

HYDROXOCOBALAMIN
+	STERIS	1MG/ML	N085998 001

HYDROXYAMPHETAMINE HYDROBROMIDE; TROPICAMIDE

Solution/Drops; Ophthalmic

PAREMYD
+	AKORN	1%;0.25%	N019261 001	JAN 30, 1992

HYDROXYCHLOROQUINE SULFATE

Tablet; Oral

HYDROXYCHLOROQINE SULFATE
AB	MYLAN	200MG	N040274 001	MAY 29, 1998

HYDROXYCHLOROQUINE SULFATE
AB	COPLEY PHARM	200MG	N040081 001	SEP 30, 1994
AB	GENEVA PHARMS	200MG	N040104 001	NOV 30, 1995
AB	GENEVA PHARMS TECH	200MG	N040150 001	JAN 27, 1996
AB	WATSON LABS	200MG	N040133 001	NOV 30, 1995

PLAQUENIL
AB +	SANOFI SYNTHELABO	200MG	N009768 001	

HYDROXYPROPYL CELLULOSE

Insert; Ophthalmic

LACRISERT
+	MERCK	5MG	N018771 001

HYDROXYUREA

Capsule; Oral

DROXIA
	BRISTOL MYERS SQUIBB	200MG	N016295 002	FEB 25, 1998
		300MG	N016295 003	FEB 25, 1998
+		400MG	N016295 004	FEB 25, 1998

HYDREA
AB +	BRISTOL MYERS SQUIBB	500MG	N016295 001	

HYDROXYUREA
AB	BARR	250MG	N075143 002	SEP 21, 2000
AB	BARR	500MG	N075143 001	OCT 16, 1998
AB +	DURAMED PHARM BARR	250MG	N075020 002	JUN 26, 2000
AB		500MG	N075020 001	JUL 30, 1998
AB	PAR PHARM	500MG	N075340 001	FEB 24, 1999
AB	ROXANE	500MG	N074476 001	AUG 18, 1995

Tablet; Oral

HYDROXYUREA
AB +	BARR	1GM	N075734 001	AUG 29, 2000

HYDROXYZINE HYDROCHLORIDE

Injectable; Injection

HYDROXYZINE HCL
AP	ABBOTT	25MG/ML	N087416 001
AP		50MG/ML	N087546 001
AP	AM PHARM PARTNERS	25MG/ML	N087329 001
AP		50MG/ML	N087329 002
AP	LUITPOLD	25MG/ML	N087408 001
AP		50MG/ML	N087408 002
AP	STERIS	50MG/ML	N085779 001

VISTARIL
AP +	PFIZER	25MG/ML	N011111 001
AP		50MG/ML	N011111 002

Syrup; Oral

ATARAX
AA +	ROERIG	10MG/5ML	N010485 001

HYDROXYZINE HCL
AA	ALPHARMA	10MG/5ML	N086880 001	
AA	HI TECH PHARMA	10MG/5ML	N040010 001	OCT 28, 1994

Prescription Drug Products (continued)

HYDROXYZINE HYDROCHLORIDE (continued)

Syrup; Oral
HYDROXYZINE HCL

TE	Firm	Strength	Appl. No.	Date
AA	MORTON GROVE	10MG/5ML	N087294 001	APR 12, 1982
AA	VINTAGE PHARMS	10MG/5ML	N040391 001	APR 10, 2002

Tablet; Oral
HYDROXYZINE HCL

TE	Firm	Strength	Appl. No.	Date
AB	GENEVA PHARMS	10MG	N087869 001	DEC 20, 1982
AB		25MG	N087870 001	DEC 20, 1982
AB		50MG	N087871 001	DEC 20, 1982
AB	MUTUAL PHARM	10MG	N089381 001	MAY 19, 1986
AB		25MG	N089382 001	MAY 19, 1986
AB		50MG	N089383 001	MAY 19, 1986
AB	+ PLIVA	10MG	N088617 001	JAN 10, 1986
AB	+	25MG	N088618 001	JAN 10, 1986
AB	+	50MG	N088619 001	JAN 10, 1986
AB	WATSON LABS	10MG	N081149 001	MAR 18, 1994
AB		10MG	N088348 001	SEP 15, 1983
AB		25MG	N081150 001	MAR 18, 1994
AB		25MG	N088349 001	SEP 15, 1983
AB		50MG	N081151 001	MAR 18, 1994
AB		50MG	N088350 001	SEP 15, 1983

HYDROXYZINE PAMOATE

Capsule; Oral
HYDROXYZINE PAMOATE

TE	Firm	Strength	Appl. No.	Date
AB	BARR	EQ 25MG HCL	N088496 001	JUN 15, 1984
AB		EQ 50MG HCL	N088487 001	JUN 15, 1984
AB		EQ 100MG HCL	N088488 001	JUN 15, 1984
AB	EON	EQ 25MG HCL	N087479 001	
AB		EQ 50MG HCL	N086183 001	
AB	GENEVA PHARMS	EQ 25MG HCL	N081127 001	JUN 28, 1991
AB	IVAX PHARMS	EQ 25MG HCL	N087761 001	MAR 05, 1982
AB		EQ 50MG HCL	N087760 001	MAR 05, 1982

HYDROXYZINE PAMOATE (continued)

Capsule; Oral
HYDROXYZINE PAMOATE

TE	Firm	Strength	Appl. No.	Date
AB	WATSON LABS	EQ 25MG HCL	N040156 001	JUL 15, 1996
AB		EQ 25MG HCL	N081165 001	JUL 31, 1991
AB		EQ 50MG HCL	N040156 002	JUL 15, 1996

+ VISTARIL

TE	Firm	Strength	Appl. No.	Date
AB	PFIZER	EQ 25MG HCL	N011459 002	
AB	+	EQ 50MG HCL	N011459 004	
AB	+	EQ 100MG HCL	N011459 006	

Suspension; Oral
VISTARIL

TE	Firm	Strength	Appl. No.	Date
AB	PFIZER	EQ 25MG HCL/5ML	N011795 001	

IBANDRONATE SODIUM

Tablet; Oral
BONIVA

TE	Firm	Strength	Appl. No.	Date
	+ ROCHE	EQ 2.5MG BASE	N021455 001	MAY 16, 2003

IBUPROFEN

Suspension; Oral
CHILDREN'S ADVIL

TE	Firm	Strength	Appl. No.	Date
BX	WYETH CONS	100MG/5ML	N019833 002	SEP 19, 1989

IBUPROFEN

TE	Firm	Strength	Appl. No.	Date
AB	ALPHARMA	100MG/5ML	N074978 001	MAR 25, 1998

MOTRIN

TE	Firm	Strength	Appl. No.	Date
AB	+ MCNEIL CONS SPECLT	100MG/5ML	N019842 001	SEP 19, 1989

Tablet; Oral
IBU

TE	Firm	Strength	Appl. No.	Date
AB	BASF	400MG	N018197 001	
AB		400MG	N070083 001	FEB 22, 1985
AB		600MG	N070088 001	FEB 08, 1985
AB		600MG	N070099 001	MAR 29, 1985
AB		800MG	N070745 001	JUL 23, 1986

IBU-TAB

TE	Firm	Strength	Appl. No.	Date
AB	ALRA	400MG	N071058 001	AUG 11, 1988
AB		600MG	N071059 001	AUG 11, 1988

IBUPROFEN

TE	Firm	Strength	Appl. No.	Date
AB	BASF	400MG	N075682 001	NOV 14, 2001
AB		600MG	N075682 002	NOV 14, 2001
AB		800MG	N075682 003	

Prescription Drug Products *(continued)*

IBUPROFEN *(continued)*
Tablet; Oral

IBUPROFEN

BASF

TE	Firm	Strength	Approval Date	Appl. No.
	DR REDDYS LABS INC			
AB		400MG	NOV 14, 2001	N076112 001
AB		600MG	OCT 31, 2001	N076112 002
AB		800MG	OCT 31, 2001	N076112 003
	GENEVA PHARMS			
AB		300MG	OCT 31, 2001	N070734 001
AB		400MG	JUN 12, 1986	N070735 001
AB		600MG	JUN 12, 1986	N070736 001
AB		800MG	JUN 12, 1986	N072169 001
	INTERPHARM			
AB		400MG	DEC 11, 1987	N071334 001
AB		600MG	NOV 25, 1986	N071335 001
AB		800MG	NOV 25, 1986	N071935 001
	IVAX PHARMS			
AB		400MG	OCT 13, 1987	N071145 001
AB		600MG	SEP 23, 1986	N071146 001
AB		800MG	SEP 23, 1986	N071769 001
	MUTUAL PHARM			
AB		300MG	MAY 08, 1987	N071230 001
AB		400MG	OCT 22, 1986	N071231 001
AB		600MG	OCT 22, 1986	N071232 001
AB		800MG	OCT 22, 1986	N072004 001
	MYLAN			
AB		400MG	NOV 18, 1987	N070045 001
AB		600MG	SEP 24, 1985	N070057 001
AB		800MG	SEP 24, 1985	N071999 001
	OHM LABS			
AB		400MG	DEC 03, 1987	N070818 001
	PAR PHARM			
AB		400MG	DEC 26, 1985	N070329 001
AB		600MG	AUG 06, 1985	N070330 001
AB		800MG	AUG 06, 1985	N070986 001
	PLIVA			
AB		400MG	JUL 25, 1986	N071666 001
AB		600MG	JUN 18, 1987	N071667 001
AB		800MG	JUN 18, 1987	N071668 001

IBUPROFEN *(continued)*
Tablet; Oral

IBUPROFEN

PLIVA

TE	Firm	Strength	Approval Date	Appl. No.
	PVT FORM			
AB		300MG	JUN 18, 1987	N071266 001
AB		400MG	OCT 15, 1986	N071267 001
AB		600MG	OCT 15, 1986	N071268 001
AB		800MG	OCT 15, 1986	N072300 001
	VINTAGE PHARMS			
AB		400MG	JUL 01, 1988	N071644 001
	WATSON LABS			
AB		400MG	FEB 01, 1988	N070436 001
AB		600MG	AUG 21, 1985	N070437 001
AB		800MG	AUG 21, 1985	N071547 001
	IBUPROHM			
	OHM LABS			
AB		400MG	JUL 02, 1987	N070469 001
	MOTRIN			
	MCNEIL CONS SPECLT			
AB		300MG	AUG 29, 1985	N017463 003
AB		400MG		N017463 002
AB		600MG		N017463 004
AB+		800MG	MAY 22, 1985	N017463 005

IBUPROFEN *MULTIPLE*
SEE HYDROCODONE BITARTRATE; IBUPROFEN

IBUTILIDE FUMARATE
Injectable; Injection

CORVERT
+ PHARMACIA AND UPJOHN

TE	Strength	Appl. No.	Approval Date
AP	0.1MG/ML	N020491 001	DEC 28, 1995

ICODEXTRIN *MULTIPLE*
SEE CALCIUM CHLORIDE; ICODEXTRIN; MAGNESIUM CHLORIDE; SODIUM CHLORIDE; SODIUM LACTATE

IDARUBICIN HYDROCHLORIDE
Injectable; Injection

IDAMYCIN PFS
+ PHARMACIA AND UPJOHN

TE	Strength	Appl. No.	Approval Date
AP	1MG/ML	N050734 001	FEB 17, 1997

IDARUBICIN HCL
GENSIA SICOR PHARMS

TE	Strength	Appl. No.	Approval Date
AP	5MG/VIAL	N065037 003	MAY 01, 2002
AP	10MG/VIAL	N065037 002	MAY 01, 2002
AP+	20MG/VIAL	N065037 001	MAY 01, 2002

Prescription Drug Products (continued)

IDARUBICIN HYDROCHLORIDE (continued)
Injectable; Injection

IDARUBICIN HCL
  GENSIA SICOR PHARMS

IDARUBICIN HCL PFS

TE	Firm	Strength	Appl. No.	Date
AP	GENSIA SICOR PHARMS	1MG/ML	N065036 001	MAY 01, 2002

IDOXURIDINE
Solution/Drops; Ophthalmic

TE		Firm	Strength	Appl. No.
		DENDRID		
AT	+	ALCON	0.1%	N014169 001
		HERPLEX		
AT	+	ALLERGAN	0.1%	N013935 002

IFOSFAMIDE
Injectable; Injection

	Firm	Strength	Appl. No.	Date
	IFOSFAMIDE			
+	AM PHARM PARTNERS	1GM/VIAL	N076078 001	MAY 28, 2002
+		3GM/VIAL	N076078 002	MAY 28, 2002

IFOSFAMIDE; MESNA
Injectable; Injection

	Firm	Strength	Appl. No.	Date
	IFEX/MESNEX KIT			
+	BRISTOL MYERS SQUIBB	100MG/ML	N019763 003	OCT 10, 1992
+		100MG/ML	N019763 004	OCT 10, 1992

Injectable; Intravenous

	Firm	Strength	Appl. No.	Date
	IFOSFAMIDE/MESNA KIT			
+	GENSIA SICOR PHARMS	1GM /20ML(50MG/ML);1GM /10ML(100MG/ML)	N075874 001	FEB 26, 2002
+		3GM /60ML(50MG/ML);1GM /10ML(100MG/ML)	N075874 002	FEB 26, 2002

IMATINIB MESYLATE
Capsule; Oral

	Firm	Strength	Appl. No.	Date
	GLEEVEC			
+	NOVARTIS	100MG	N021335 002	MAY 10, 2001

Tablet; Oral

	Firm	Strength	Appl. No.	Date
	GLEEVEC			
	NOVARTIS	100MG	N021588 001	APR 18, 2003
+		400MG	N021588 002	APR 18, 2003

IMIGLUCERASE
Injectable; Injection

	Firm	Strength	Appl. No.	Date
	CEREZYME			
	GENZYME	200 UNITS/VIAL	N020367 001	MAY 23, 1994
+		400 UNITS/VIAL	N020367 002	SEP 22, 1999

IMIPENEM *MULTIPLE*
SEE CILASTATIN SODIUM; IMIPENEM

IMIPRAMINE HYDROCHLORIDE
Concentrate; Oral

	Firm	Strength	Appl. No.
	IMIPRAMINE HCL		
	NOVARTIS	25MG/ML	N086765 001

Tablet; Oral

TE	Firm	Strength	Appl. No.	Date
	IMIPRAMINE HCL			
AB	GENEVA PHARMS	10MG	N084936 002	JUN 05, 1990
AB		25MG	N083745 001	JUN 05, 1990
AB		50MG	N084937 001	JUN 05, 1990
AB	MUTUAL PHARM	10MG	N081048 001	
		25MG	N081049 001	
AB		50MG	N081050 001	JUN 05, 1990
AB	PAR PHARM	10MG	N088292 001	OCT 21, 1983
AB		10MG	N089422 001	JUL 14, 1987
AB		25MG	N088262 001	OCT 21, 1983
AB		25MG	N089497 001	JUL 14, 1987
AB		50MG	N088276 001	OCT 21, 1983
AB	ROXANE	10MG	N083799 001	
AB	TEVA	10MG	N083729 001	
AB		25MG	N083729 004	
AB		50MG	N083729 003	
	TOFRANIL			
AB	TYCO HLTHCARE	10MG	N087844 001	MAY 22, 1984
AB		25MG	N087845 001	MAY 22, 1984
AB +		50MG	N087846 001	MAY 22, 1984

IMIPRAMINE PAMOATE
Capsule; Oral

	Firm	Strength	Appl. No.
	TOFRANIL-PM		
	TYCO HLTHCARE	EQ 75MG HCL	N017090 001
+		EQ 100MG HCL	N017090 004
+		EQ 125MG HCL	N017090 003
+		EQ 150MG HCL	N017090 002

Prescription Drug Products (continued)

IMIQUIMOD
Cream; Topical

	Firm	Strength	Appl No	Date
	ALDARA			
+	3M	5%	N020723 001	FEB 27, 1997

INAMRINONE LACTATE
Injectable; Injection

	Firm	Strength	Appl No	Date
	AMRINONE			
AP +	ABBOTT	EQ 5MG BASE/ML	N074616 001	AUG 03, 1998
AP	BEDFORD	EQ 5MG BASE/ML	N075513 001	MAY 09, 2000
	AMRINONE LACTATE			
AP	BAXTER HLTHCARE CORP	EQ 5MG BASE/ML	N075542 001	MAY 10, 2000

INDAPAMIDE
Tablet; Oral

	Firm	Strength	Appl No	Date
	INDAPAMIDE			
AB	ALPHAPHARM	1.25MG	N075105 001	JUL 23, 1998
AB		2.5MG	N075105 002	JUL 23, 1998
AB	GENEVA PHARMS TECH	1.25MG	N074594 001	MAY 23, 1996
AB		2.5MG	N074594 002	MAY 23, 1996
AB	IVAX PHARMS	1.25MG	N074299 002	APR 29, 1996
AB		2.5MG	N074299 001	JUL 27, 1995
AB	MYLAN	1.25MG	N074461 002	MAR 26, 1997
AB		2.5MG	N074461 001	MAR 27, 1996
AB	PUREPAC PHARM	1.25MG	N074722 001	JUN 17, 1996
AB		2.5MG	N074722 002	JUN 17, 1996
AB	TEVA	1.25MG	N074498 002	FEB 12, 1998
AB		2.5MG	N074498 001	OCT 31, 1996
AB	TRIGEN	1.25MG	N075201 001	DEC 04, 1998
AB		2.5MG	N075201 002	DEC 04, 1998
AB	WATSON LABS	1.25MG	N074585 001	SEP 26, 1996
AB		2.5MG	N074585 002	SEP 26, 1996
	LOZOL			
AB	AVENTIS	1.25MG	N018538 002	APR 29, 1993

INDAPAMIDE (continued)
Tablet; Oral

	Firm	Strength	Appl No	Date
	LOZOL			
AB +	AVENTIS	2.5MG	N018538 001	JUL 06, 1983

INDINAVIR SULFATE
Capsule; Oral

	Firm	Strength	Appl No	Date
	CRIXIVAN			
	MERCK	EQ 100MG BASE	N020685 006	APR 19, 2000
		EQ 200MG BASE	N020685 003	MAR 13, 1996
			N020685 005	DEC 17, 1998
+		EQ 333MG BASE		
		EQ 400MG BASE	N020685 001	MAR 13, 1996

INDIUM IN-111 OXYQUINOLINE
Injectable; Injection

	Firm	Strength	Appl No	Date
	INDIUM IN-111 OXYQUINOLINE			
	AMERSHAM HLTH	1mCi/ML	N019044 001	DEC 24, 1985

INDIUM IN-111 PENTETATE DISODIUM
Injectable; Intrathecal

	Firm	Strength	Appl No	Date
	MPI INDIUM DTPA IN 111			
	AMERSHAM HLTH	1mCi/ML	N017707 001	FEB 18, 1982

INDIUM IN-111 PENTETREOTIDE KIT
Injectable; Injection

	Firm	Strength	Appl No	Date
	OCTREOSCAN			
	MALLINCKRODT	3mCi/ML	N020314 001	JUN 02, 1994

INDOCYANINE GREEN
Injectable; Injection

	Firm	Strength	Appl No	Date
	CARDIO-GREEN			
+	AKORN	25MG/VIAL	N011525 001	

INDOMETHACIN
Capsule, Extended Release; Oral

	Firm	Strength	Appl No	Date
	INDOCIN SR			
AB +	EON	75MG	N074464 001	MAY 28, 1998
	INDOMETHACIN			
AB	ABLE	75MG	N076114 001	FEB 06, 2002
AB	INWOOD LABS	75MG	N072410 001	MAR 15, 1989

Capsule; Oral

	Firm	Strength	Appl No	Date
	INDO-LEMMON			
AB	TEVA	25MG	N070266 001	NOV 07, 1985

Prescription Drug Products (continued)

INDOMETHACIN (continued)

Capsule; Oral

TE	Brand / Manufacturer	Strength	Appl. No. / Date
AB	INDO-LEMMON — TEVA	50MG	N070267 001 NOV 07, 1985
AB	INDOCIN + MERCK	25MG	N016059 001
AB	INDOCIN + MERCK	50MG	N016059 002
AB	INDOMETHACIN — GENEVA PHARMS	25MG	N070673 001 APR 29, 1987
AB	GENEVA PHARMS	50MG	N070674 001 APR 29, 1987
AB	IVAX PHARMS	25MG	N070719 001 FEB 12, 1986
AB	IVAX PHARMS	50MG	N070756 001 FEB 12, 1986
AB	LEDERLE	25MG	N018851 001 MAY 18, 1984
AB	LEDERLE	50MG	N018851 002 MAY 18, 1984
AB	MUTUAL PHARM	25MG	N070899 001 FEB 09, 1987
AB	MUTUAL PHARM	50MG	N070900 001 FEB 09, 1987
AB	MYLAN	25MG	N018858 001 APR 20, 1984
AB	MYLAN	50MG	N018858 002 APR 20, 1984
AB	MYLAN	50MG	N070624 001 SEP 04, 1985
AB	PAR PHARM	25MG	N018829 002 AUG 06, 1984
AB	PAR PHARM	50MG	N018829 001 AUG 06, 1984
AB	PAR PHARM	50MG	N070651 001 MAR 05, 1986
AB	PLIVA	25MG	N071148 001 MAR 18, 1987
AB	PLIVA	50MG	N071149 001 MAR 18, 1987
AB	TEVA	25MG	N071342 001 APR 18, 1988
AB	TEVA	50MG	N071343 001 APR 18, 1988

Suppository; Rectal

TE	Brand / Manufacturer	Strength	Appl. No. / Date
	INDOMETHACIN + INDOMETHEGAN — G AND W LABS	50MG	N073314 001 AUG 31, 1992

Suspension; Oral

TE	Brand / Manufacturer	Strength	Appl. No. / Date
AB	INDOCIN + MERCK	25MG/5ML	N018332 001 OCT 10, 1985
AB	INDOMETHACIN — ROXANE	25MG/5ML	N071412 001 MAR 18, 1987

INDOMETHACIN SODIUM

Injectable; Injection

TE	Brand / Manufacturer	Strength	Appl. No. / Date
	INDOCIN I.V. + MERCK	EQ 1MG BASE/VIAL	N018878 001 JAN 30, 1985

INSULIN ASPART

Injectable; Subcutaneous

TE	Brand / Manufacturer	Strength	Appl. No. / Date
	NOVOLOG + NOVO NORDISK	100 UNITS/ML	N020986 001 JUN 07, 2000

INSULIN ASPART; INSULIN ASPART PROTAMINE

Injectable; Subcutaneous

TE	Brand / Manufacturer	Strength	Appl. No. / Date
	NOVOLOG MIX 70/30 + NOVO NORDISK	30 UNITS/ML;70 UNITS/ML	N021172 001 NOV 01, 2001

INSULIN ASPART PROTAMINE *MULTIPLE*

SEE INSULIN ASPART; INSULIN ASPART PROTAMINE

INSULIN GLARGINE

Injectable; Injection

TE	Brand / Manufacturer	Strength	Appl. No. / Date
	LANTUS + AVENTIS PHARMS	100 UNITS/ML	N021081 001 APR 20, 2000

INSULIN LISPRO

Injectable; Injection

TE	Brand / Manufacturer	Strength	Appl. No. / Date
	HUMALOG + LILLY	100 UNITS/ML	N020563 001 JUN 14, 1996
	HUMALOG PEN + LILLY	100 UNITS/ML	N020563 002 AUG 06, 1998

INSULIN LISPRO; INSULIN LISPRO PROTAMINE

Injectable; Injection

TE	Brand / Manufacturer	Strength	Appl. No. / Date
	HUMALOG MIX 50/50 + LILLY	50 UNITS/ML;50 UNITS/ML	N021018 001 DEC 22, 1999
	HUMALOG MIX 75/25 + LILLY	25 UNITS/ML;75 UNITS/ML	N021017 001 DEC 22, 1999

INSULIN LISPRO PROTAMINE *MULTIPLE*

SEE INSULIN LISPRO; INSULIN LISPRO PROTAMINE

INSULIN PURIFIED PORK

Injectable; Injection

TE	Brand / Manufacturer	Strength	Appl. No. / Date
	ILETIN II + LILLY	500 UNITS/ML	N018344 002

Prescription Drug Products (continued)

INSULIN RECOMBINANT HUMAN
Injectable: Injection

HUMULIN R				
+ LILLY	500 UNITS/ML		N018780 004	MAR 31, 1994

INTRINSIC FACTOR *MULTIPLE*
SEE   COBALT CHLORIDE, CO-57; CYANOCOBALAMIN; CYANOCOBALAMIN, CO-57; INTRINSIC FACTOR

INULIN
Injectable: Injection

INULIN AND SODIUM CHLORIDE			
+ QUESTCOR PHARMS	100MG/ML	N002282 001	

IOBENGUANE SULFATE I 131
Injectable: Injection

IOBENGUANE SULFATE I 131			
CIS	2.3mCi/ML	N020084 001	MAR 25, 1994

IODIPAMIDE MEGLUMINE
Injectable: Injection

CHOLOGRAFIN MEGLUMINE			
+ BRACCO	52%	N009321 003	

IODIPAMIDE MEGLUMINE *MULTIPLE*
SEE   DIATRIZOATE MEGLUMINE; IODIPAMIDE MEGLUMINE

IODIXANOL
Injectable: Injection

VISIPAQUE 270				
+ AMERSHAM HLTH	55%		N020351 001	MAR 22, 1996
VISIPAQUE 320				
+ AMERSHAM HLTH	65.2%		N020351 002	MAR 22, 1996

IOHEXOL
Injectable: Injection

OMNIPAQUE 140				
+ AMERSHAM HLTH	30.2%		N018956 005	NOV 30, 1988

Solution; Injection, Oral

OMNIPAQUE 350				
+ AMERSHAM HLTH	75.5%		N018956 004	DEC 26, 1985
			N020608 003	OCT 24, 1995

Solution; Injection, Oral, Rectal

OMNIPAQUE 180				
+ AMERSHAM HLTH	38.8%		N018956 001	DEC 26, 1985

IOHEXOL (continued)
Solution; Injection, Oral, Rectal

OMNIPAQUE 240				
+ AMERSHAM HLTH	51.8%		N018956 002	DEC 26, 1985
			N020608 001	OCT 24, 1995
OMNIPAQUE 300				
+ AMERSHAM HLTH	64.7%		N018956 003	DEC 26, 1985
			N020608 002	OCT 24, 1995

IOPAMIDOL
Injectable: Injection

TE	Firm	Strength	Appl. No.	Approval Date
IOPAMIDOL-200				
AP	ABBOTT	41%	N074898 001	DEC 30, 1997
AP	COOK IMAGING	41%	N074881 001	JUL 28, 2000
IOPAMIDOL-200 IN PLASTIC CONTAINER				
AP	ABBOTT	41%	N074636 001	DEC 30, 1997
IOPAMIDOL-250				
AP	ABBOTT	51%	N074898 002	DEC 30, 1997
			N075005 001	FEB 24, 1998
AP	AM PHARM PARTNERS	51%	N074679 001	APR 02, 1997
			N074881 002	JUL 28, 2000
AP	COOK IMAGING	51%		
IOPAMIDOL-250 IN PLASTIC CONTAINER				
AP	ABBOTT	51%	N074636 002	DEC 30, 1997
IOPAMIDOL-300				
AP	ABBOTT	61%	N074898 003	DEC 30, 1997
			N075005 002	FEB 24, 1998
AP	AM PHARM PARTNERS	61%	N074679 002	APR 02, 1997
			N074881 003	JUL 28, 2000
IOPAMIDOL-300 IN PLASTIC CONTAINER				
AP	ABBOTT	61%	N074636 003	DEC 30, 1997
AP		61%	N074637 001	APR 03, 1997
IOPAMIDOL-370				
AP	ABBOTT	76%	N074898 004	DEC 30, 1997
			N075005 003	DEC 30, 1997
AP	AM PHARM PARTNERS	76%	N074679 003	FEB 24, 1998
			N074881 004	APR 02, 1997
AP	COOK IMAGING	76%		

Prescription Drug Products *(continued)*

IOPAMIDOL *(continued)*

Injectable; Injection

IOPAMIDOL-370

	COOK IMAGING			JUL 28, 2000

IOPAMIDOL-370 IN PLASTIC CONTAINER

AP	ABBOTT	76%	N074636 004	DEC 30, 1997

ISOVUE-200

AP	+ BRACCO	41%	N018735 006	JUL 07, 1987

ISOVUE-250

AP	+ BRACCO	51%	N018735 007	JUL 06, 1992
AP	+	51%	N020327 002	OCT 12, 1994

ISOVUE-300

AP	+ BRACCO	61%	N018735 002	DEC 31, 1985
AP	+	61%	N020327 003	OCT 12, 1994

ISOVUE-370

AP	+ BRACCO	76%	N018735 003	DEC 31, 1985
AP	+	76%	N020327 004	OCT 12, 1994

ISOVUE-M 200

	+ BRACCO	41%	N018735 001	DEC 31, 1985

ISOVUE-M 300

	+ BRACCO	61%	N018735 004	DEC 31, 1985

IOPANOIC ACID

Tablet; Oral

TELEPAQUE

	+ AMERSHAM HLTH	500MG	N008032 001	

IOPROMIDE

Injectable; Injection

ULTRAVIST (PHARMACY BULK)

	+ BERLEX LABS	300MG/ML	N021425 001	SEP 20, 2002
	+	370MG/ML	N021425 002	SEP 20, 2002

ULTRAVIST 150

	+ BERLEX LABS	31.2%	N020220 004	MAY 10, 1995

ULTRAVIST 240

	+ BERLEX LABS	49.9%	N020220 003	MAY 10, 1995

ULTRAVIST 300

	+ BERLEX LABS	62.3%	N020220 002	MAY 10, 1995

ULTRAVIST 370

	+ BERLEX LABS	76.9%	N020220 001	MAY 10, 1995

IOTHALAMATE MEGLUMINE

Injectable; Injection

CONRAY

	+ MALLINCKRODT	60%	N013295 001	

CONRAY 30

	+ MALLINCKRODT	30%	N016983 001	

CONRAY 43

	+ MALLINCKRODT	43%	N013295 002	

Solution; Intravesical

CYSTO-CONRAY II

	MALLINCKRODT	17.2%	N017057 002	

IOTHALAMATE MEGLUMINE; IOTHALAMATE SODIUM

Injectable; Injection

VASCORAY

	+ MALLINCKRODT	52%;26%	N016783 001	

IOTHALAMATE SODIUM

Injectable; Injection

CONRAY 400

	+ MALLINCKRODT	66.8%	N014295 001	

IOTHALAMATE SODIUM *MULTIPLE*

SEE IOTHALAMATE MEGLUMINE; IOTHALAMATE SODIUM

IOTHALAMATE SODIUM, I-125

Injectable; Injection

GLOFIL-125

	QUESTCOR PHARMS	250-300uCi/ML	N017279 001	

IOVERSOL

Injectable; Injection

OPTIRAY 160

	+ MALLINCKRODT	34%	N019710 003	DEC 30, 1988

OPTIRAY 240

	+ MALLINCKRODT	51%	N019710 002	DEC 30, 1988

OPTIRAY 300

	+ MALLINCKRODT	64%	N019710 004	JAN 22, 1992
	+	64%	N020923 004	MAY 13, 1999

OPTIRAY 320

	+ MALLINCKRODT	68%	N019710 001	DEC 30, 1988

OPTIRAY 350

	+ MALLINCKRODT	74%	N019710 005	JAN 22, 1992
	+	74%	N020923 003	MAY 28, 1998

Prescription Drug Products *(continued)*

IOXAGLATE MEGLUMINE; IOXAGLATE SODIUM
Injectable; Injection
	HEXABRIX			
+	MALLINCKRODT	39.3%;19.6%	N018905 002	JUL 26, 1985

IOXAGLATE SODIUM *MULTIPLE*
SEE IOXAGLATE MEGLUMINE; IOXAGLATE SODIUM

IOXILAN
Injectable; Injection
	OXILAN-300			
	GUERBET	62%	N020316 001	DEC 21, 1995
	OXILAN-350			
	GUERBET	73%	N020316 002	DEC 21, 1995

IPRATROPIUM BROMIDE
Aerosol, Metered; Inhalation
	ATROVENT			
+	BOEHRINGER INGELHEIM	0.018MG/INH	N019085 001	DEC 29, 1986

Solution; Inhalation
	ATROVENT			
AN +	BOEHRINGER INGELHEIM	0.02%	N020228 001	SEP 29, 1993
	IPRATROPIUM BROMIDE			
AN	ROXANE	0.02%	N075867 001	JUL 22, 2002
	IPRATROPIUM BROMIDE			
AN	ALPHARMA	0.02%	N075111 001	APR 22, 1999
AN	ASLUNG PHARM	0.02%	N075693 001	JAN 26, 2001
AN	BAUSCH AND LOMB	0.02%	N075835 001	OCT 15, 2001
AN	DEY	0.02%	N074755 001	JAN 10, 1997
AN	IVAX PHARMS	0.02%	N075313 001	FEB 07, 2000
AN	NEPHRON	0.02%	N075562 001	SEP 27, 2001
AN	NOVEX	0.02%	N075441 001	MAR 28, 2001
AN	WARRICK PHARMS	0.02%	N075507 001	JAN 19, 2001

Spray, Metered; Nasal
	ATROVENT			
AB +	BOEHRINGER INGELHEIM	0.021MG/SPRAY	N020393 001	OCT 20, 1995
AB +		0.042MG/SPRAY	N020394 001	OCT 20, 1995

IPRATROPIUM BROMIDE *(continued)*
Spray, Metered; Nasal
	IPRATROPIUM BROMIDE			
AB	BAUSCH AND LOMB	0.021MG/SPRAY	N076025 001	MAR 31, 2003
AB		0.042MG/SPRAY	N076103 001	MAR 31, 2003
AB	DEY	0.021MG/SPRAY	N075552 001	MAR 31, 2003
AB		0.042MG/SPRAY	N075553 001	MAR 31, 2003
AB	NOVEX	0.021MG/SPRAY	N076156 001	APR 18, 2003
AB		0.042MG/SPRAY	N076155 001	APR 18, 2003

IPRATROPIUM BROMIDE *MULTIPLE*
SEE ALBUTEROL SULFATE; IPRATROPIUM BROMIDE

IRBESARTAN
Tablet; Oral
	AVAPRO			
AB	SANOFI SYNTHELABO	75MG	N020757 001	SEP 30, 1997
		150MG	N020757 002	SEP 30, 1997
		300MG	N020757 003	SEP 30, 1997

IRBESARTAN *MULTIPLE*
SEE HYDROCHLOROTHIAZIDE; IRBESARTAN

IRINOTECAN HYDROCHLORIDE
Injectable; Injection
	CAMPTOSAR			
+	PHARMACIA AND UPJOHN	20MG/ML	N020571 001	JUN 14, 1996

IRON DEXTRAN
Injectable; Injection
	DEXFERRUM			
BP	LUITPOLD	EQ 50MG IRON/ML	N040024 001	FEB 23, 1996
	INFED			
BP +	SCHEIN	EQ 50MG IRON/ML	N017441 001	
	PROFERDEX			
BP +	NEW RIVER	EQ 50MG IRON/ML	N017807 001	

IRON SUCROSE
Injectable; Intravenous
	VENOFER			
+	LUITPOLD	EQ 20MG BASE/ML	N021135 001	NOV 06, 2000

Prescription Drug Products (continued)

ISOCARBOXAZID
Tablet; Oral

	MARPLAN		
	+ OXFORD PHARM	10MG	N011961 001

ISOETHARINE HYDROCHLORIDE
Solution; Inhalation

	BETA-2		
AN	NEPHRON	1%	N086711 001
	ISOETHARINE HCL		
	DEY	0.1%	N087389 001
	INTL MEDICATION	0.08%	N086651 002
		0.143%	N086651 004
	+ ROXANE	0.2%	N087324 001
		0.167%	N088226 001
			SEP 16, 1983
AN	+	1%	N086899 001

ISOFLURANE
Liquid; Inhalation

	FORANE		
AN	+ BAXTER HLTHCARE CORP	99.9%	N017624 001
	ISOFLURANE		
AN	ABBOTT	99.9%	N074097 001
			JAN 25, 1993
AN	HALOCARBON PRODS	99.9%	N075225 001
			OCT 20, 1999
AN	MARSAM PHARMS LLC	99.9%	N074393 001
			MAY 12, 1995
AN	MINRAD	99.9%	N074416 001
			SEP 30, 1994
AN	RHODIA	99.9%	N074502 001
			JUN 27, 1995

ISONIAZID
Injectable; Injection

	NYDRAZID		
	+ APOTHECON	100MG/ML	N008662 001

Syrup; Oral

	ISONIAZID		
	CAROLINA MEDCL	50MG/5ML	N088235 001
			NOV 10, 1983

Tablet; Oral

	ISONIAZID		
AA	AXIOM PHARM	300MG	N083633 001
AA	BARR	100MG	N080936 001
AA		300MG	N080937 002
AA	DURAMED PHARM BARR	300MG	N088119 001
			MAR 17, 1983
AA	+ EON	100MG	N008678 002
AA		300MG	N008678 003
AA	+ MIKART	100MG	N040090 001
			JUN 26, 1997
AA		300MG	N040090 002
			JUN 26, 1997

ISONIAZID (continued)
Tablet; Oral

	ISONIAZID		
AA	WATSON LABS	300MG	N080521 001
AA	WEST WARD	100MG	N080212 001
AA		300MG	N087425 001
	LANIAZID		
AA	LANNETT	50MG	N080140 001
AA		100MG	N080140 002
		300MG	N089776 001
			JUN 13, 1988

ISONIAZID; PYRAZINAMIDE; RIFAMPIN
Tablet; Oral

	RIFATER		
	+ AVENTIS PHARMS	50MG;300MG;120MG	N050705 001
			MAY 31, 1994

ISONIAZID; RIFAMPIN
Capsule; Oral

	RIFAMATE		
	+ AVENTIS PHARMS	150MG;300MG	N061884 001

ISOPROTERENOL HYDROCHLORIDE
Injectable; Injection

	ISOPROTERENOL HCL		
	ABBOTT	0.02MG/ML	N083283 001
AP		0.2MG/ML	N083346 001
AP		0.2MG/ML	N083724 001
	INTL MEDICATION		
	ISUPREL		
AP	+ ABBOTT	0.2MG/ML	N010515 001

ISOSORBIDE DINITRATE
Capsule, Extended Release; Oral

	DILATRATE-SR		
BC	+ SCHWARZ PHARMA	40MG	N019790 001
			SEP 02, 1988

Tablet, Chewable; Oral

	SORBITRATE		
	+ ASTRAZENECA	10MG	N016776 003
			APR 01, 1996

Tablet, Extended Release; Oral

	ISOSORBIDE DINITRATE		
	+ INWOOD LABS	40MG	N040009 001
			DEC 30, 1998

Tablet; Oral

	ISORDIL		
AB	BIOVAIL	5MG	N012093 007
			JUL 29, 1988
AB		10MG	N012093 002
			JUL 29, 1988
AB		20MG	N012093 006
			JUL 29, 1988
AB	+	30MG	N012093 005
			JUL 29, 1988

Prescription Drug Products *(continued)*

ISOSORBIDE DINITRATE *(continued)*

Tablet; Oral

ISORDIL

AB	BIOVAIL	40MG	N012093 001	JUL 29, 1988

ISOSORBIDE DINITRATE

	GENEVA PHARMS			
AB		5MG	N086221 001	JAN 07, 1988
AB		10MG	N086223 001	JAN 07, 1988
AB		20MG	N089367 001	APR 07, 1988
AB	PAR PHARM	5MG	N086923 001	MAR 12, 1987
AB		10MG	N086925 001	MAR 12, 1987
AB		20MG	N087537 001	OCT 02, 1987
AB		30MG	N087946 001	JAN 12, 1988
AB	WATSON LABS	5MG	N086034 001	JAN 06, 1988
AB		10MG	N086032 001	JAN 07, 1988
AB	WEST WARD	5MG	N086067 001	OCT 29, 1987
AB		10MG	N086066 001	OCT 29, 1987
AB		20MG	N088088 001	NOV 02, 1987

SORBITRATE

AB	ASTRAZENECA	20MG	N086405 002	AUG 21, 1990
AB		40MG	N088125 001	AUG 21, 1990

Tablet; Sublingual

ISORDIL

AB	BIOVAIL	2.5MG	N012940 004	JUL 29, 1988
AB		5MG	N012940 003	JUL 29, 1988
AB +		10MG	N012940 005	JUL 29, 1988

ISOSORBIDE DINITRATE

	GENEVA PHARMS			
AB		2.5MG	N086225 001	FEB 19, 1988
AB		5MG	N086222 001	FEB 19, 1988
AB	WATSON LABS	2.5MG	N086033 001	FEB 26, 1988
AB		5MG	N086031 001	SEP 29, 1987
AB	WEST WARD	2.5MG	N086054 001	OCT 29, 1987
AB		5MG	N086055 001	NOV 02, 1987

ISOSORBIDE MONONITRATE

Tablet, Extended Release; Oral

IMDUR

AB +	SCHERING	30MG	N020225 001	AUG 12, 1993
AB +		60MG	N020225 002	AUG 12, 1993
AB +		120MG	N020225 003	MAR 30, 1995

ISOSORBIDE MONONITRATE

AB	BRIGHTSTONE	60MG	N075166 001	OCT 07, 1999
AB	DEXCEL LTD	60MG	N075522 001	APR 17, 2000
AB	ELAN PHARM	60MG	N075041 001	SEP 22, 1998
AB	IVAX PHARMS	30MG	N075448 002	AUG 07, 2001
AB		60MG	N075448 001	JUN 19, 2000
AB		120MG	N075448 003	AUG 07, 2001
AB	KREMERS URBAN	30MG	N075155 002	JAN 13, 2000
AB		60MG	N075155 001	OCT 30, 1998
AB		120MG	N075155 003	AUG 04, 2000
AB	KV PHARM	30MG	N075395 001	MAR 16, 2000
AB		60MG	N075395 002	MAR 16, 2000
AB		120MG	N075395 003	MAR 16, 2000
AB	PUREPAC PHARM	30MG	N075306 001	DEC 31, 1998
AB		60MG	N075306 002	DEC 31, 1998

Tablet; Oral

ISMO

AB	ESP PHARMA	20MG	N019091 001	DEC 30, 1991

ISOSORBIDE MONONITRATE

AB	PUREPAC PHARM	10MG	N075037 002	OCT 30, 1998
AB		20MG	N075037 001	OCT 30, 1998
AB	TEVA	20MG	N075147 001	NOV 27, 1998
AB	WEST WARD	20MG	N075361 001	OCT 05, 2000

MONOKET

AB	SCHWARZ	10MG	N020215 002	JUN 30, 1993
AB +	ISD *(continued)*	20MG	N020215 001	JUN 30, 1993

Prescription Drug Products (continued)

ISOSULFAN BLUE
Injectable; Injection
  LYMPHAZURIN
  + US SURGCL   1%   N018310 001

ISOTRETINOIN
Capsule; Oral
  ACCUTANE
AB   HLR   10MG   N018662 002   MAY 07, 1982
AB +   20MG   N018662 004   MAR 28, 1983
AB +   40MG   N018662 003   MAY 07, 1982
  AMNESTEEM
AB   GENPHARM   10MG   N075945 001   NOV 08, 2002
AB   20MG   N075945 002   NOV 08, 2002
AB   40MG   N075945 003   NOV 08, 2002
  CLARAVIS
AB   BARR   10MG   N076356 001   APR 11, 2003
AB   20MG   N076135 002   APR 11, 2003
AB   40MG   N076135 001   APR 11, 2003
  ISOTRETINOIN
AB   RANBAXY   10MG   N076041 001   DEC 24, 2002
AB   20MG   N076041 002   DEC 24, 2002
AB   40MG   N076041 003   DEC 24, 2002
  SOTRET
AB   RANBAXY   30MG   N076503 001   JUN 20, 2003

ISRADIPINE
Capsule; Oral
  DYNACIRC
    RELIANT PHARMS   2.5MG   N019546 001   DEC 20, 1990
  +   5MG   N019546 002   DEC 20, 1990
Tablet, Extended Release; Oral
  DYNACIRC CR
  + RELIANT PHARMS   5MG   N020336 001   JUN 01, 1994
  +   10MG   N020336 002   JUN 01, 1994

ITRACONAZOLE
Capsule; Oral
  SPORANOX
  + JANSSEN PHARMA   100MG   N020083 001   SEP 11, 1992
Injectable; Injection
  SPORANOX
  + JANSSEN PHARMA   10MG/ML   N020966 001   MAR 30, 1999
Solution; Oral
  SPORANOX
  + JANSSEN PHARMA   10MG/ML   N020657 001   FEB 21, 1997

IVERMECTIN
Tablet; Ora
  STROMECTOL
    MERCK   3MG   N050742 002   OCT 08, 1998
  +   6MG   N050742 001   NOV 22, 1996

KANAMYCIN SULFATE
Capsule; Oral
  KANTREX
  + APOTHECON   EQ 500MG BASE   N062726 001   MAR 06, 1987
Injectable; Injection
  KANAMYCIN
AP   AM FHARM PARTNERS   EQ 1GM BASE/3ML   N065111 002   DEC 17, 2002
AP   EQ 500MG BASE/2ML N065111 001   DEC 17, 2002
  KANTREX
AP + APOTHECON   EQ 1GM BASE/3ML   N061901 002
AP +   EQ 75MG BASE/2ML   N061901 003
AP +   EQ 500MG BASE/2ML N061901 001

KETAMINE HYDROCHLORIDE
Injectable; Injection
  KETALAR
AP + PARKEDALE   EQ 10MG BASE/ML   N016812 001
AP +   EQ 50MG BASE/ML   N016812 002
  +   EQ 100MG BASE/ML   N016812 003
  KETAMINE HCL
AP   ABBOTT   EQ 50MG BASE/ML   N074549 001   JUN 27, 1996
                                             EQ 100MG BASE/ML   N074549 002   JUN 27, 1996
AP   BEDFORD   EQ 50MG BASE/ML   N074524 001   MAR 22, 1996
                                             EQ 100MG BASE/ML   N074524 002   MAR 22, 1996
AP   BIONICHE (CANADA)   EQ 50MG BASE/ML   N076092 002   DEC 28, 2001
AP   EQ 100MG BASE/ML   N076092 003

Prescription Drug Products (continued)

KETAMINE HYDROCHLORIDE (continued)
Injectable; Injection
KETAMINE HCL

	BIONICHE (CANADA)		OCT 25, 2002

KETOCONAZOLE
Cream; Topical
KETOCONAZOLE

AB	TEVA	2%	N075581 001	APR 25, 2000

KETOZOLE

AB	TARO	2%	N075638 001	DEC 18, 2002

NIZORAL

AB +	JANSSEN PHARMA	2%	N019084 001	DEC 31, 1985

Shampoo; Topical
NIZORAL

AB +	MCNEIL CONS SPECLT	2%	N019927 001	AUG 31, 1990

Tablet; Oral
KETOCONAZOLE

AB	MUTUAL PHARMA	200MG	N075314 001	JUN 15, 1999
AB	MYLAN	200MG	N075597 001	DEC 23, 1999
AB	NEOSAN PHARMS	200MG	N075341 001	JUL 27, 1999
AB	PLIVA	200MG	N075362 001	JUN 15, 1999
AB	TARO	200MG	N075319 001	JUN 15, 1999
AB	TEVA	200MG	N074971 001	JUN 15, 1999
AB		200MG	N075273 001	JUN 15, 1999
AB	TORPHARM	200MG	N075912 001	JAN 10, 2002

NIZORAL

AB +	JANSSEN	200MG	N018533 001	

KETOPROFEN
Capsule, Extended Release; Oral
KETOPROFEN

AB	ANDRX PHARMS	100MG	N075270 002	MAR 24, 1999
AB		150MG	N075270 003	MAR 24, 1999
AB		200MG	N075270 001	MAR 24, 1999
AB	ELAN PHARM	200MG	N074879 001	DEC 10, 1997
AB	MYLAN	100MG	N075679 003	FEB 20, 2002
AB		150MG	N075679 002	FEB 20, 2002

KETOPROFEN (continued)
Capsule, Extended Release; Oral
KETOPROFEN

AB	MYLAN	200MG	N075679 001	FEB 20, 2002

ORUVAIL

AB	WYETH PHARMS INC	100MG	N019816 003	FEB 08, 1995
AB		150MG	N019816 002	FEB 08, 1995
AB +		200MG	N019816 001	SEP 24, 1993

Capsule; Oral
KETOPROFEN

AB	GENEVA PHARMS	50MG	N074024 001	DEC 29, 1995
AB		75MG	N074024 002	DEC 29, 1995
AB	LEDERLE	25MG	N074014 001	JAN 29, 1993
AB		50MG	N074014 002	JAN 29, 1993
AB		75MG	N074014 003	JAN 29, 1993
AB	MYLAN	50MG	N074035 002	DEC 31, 1996
AB		75MG	N074035 003	DEC 31, 1996
AB	TEVA	25MG	N073515 001	DEC 22, 1992
AB		50MG	N073516 001	DEC 22, 1992
AB +		75MG	N073517 001	DEC 22, 1992

KETOROLAC TROMETHAMINE
Injectable; Injection
KETOROLAC TROMETHAMINE

AP	ABBOTT	15MG/ML	N074801 001	JUN 05, 1997
AP		15MG/ML	N074802 001	JUN 05, 1997
AP		30MG/ML	N074993 001	JAN 27, 1999
AP		30MG/ML	N074801 002	JUN 05, 1997
AP		30MG/ML	N074802 002	JUN 05, 1997
AP		30MG/ML	N074993 002	JAN 27, 1999
AP	AM PHARM PARTNERS	15MG/ML	N075784 001	JAN 11, 2002
AP		30MG/ML	N075784 002	JAN 11, 2002
AP	APOTEX	15MG/ML	N075631 002	JUN 29, 2001
AP		30MG/ML	N075626 001	

Prescription Drug Products (continued)

KETOROLAC TROMETHAMINE (continued)

Injectable; Injection

KETOROLAC TROMETHAMINE

TE Code	Firm	Strength	Appl. No.	Date
AP	APOTEX	30MG/ML	N075631 001	JUL 24, 2001 / JUN 29, 2001
AP	BAXTER HLTHCARE CORP	15MG/ML	N075299 001	NOV 03, 1999
AP		30MG/ML	N075299 002	NOV 03, 1999
AP	BEDFORD	15MG/ML	N075222 001	APR 26, 1999
AP		30MG/ML	N075222 002	APR 26, 1999
AP		30MG/ML	N075228 001	APR 26, 1999
AP	TORADOL + ROCHE PALO	15MG/ML	N019698 001	NOV 30, 1989
AP	+	30MG/ML	N019698 002	NOV 30, 1989

Solution/Drops; Ophthalmic

TE Code	Firm	Strength	Appl. No.	Date
AB	ACULAR + ALLERGAN	0.5%	N019700 001	NOV 09, 1992
AB	ACULAR LS + ALLERGAN	0.4%	N021528 001	MAY 30, 2003
AB	ACULAR PRESERVATIVE FREE + ALLERGAN	0.5%	N020811 001	NOV 03, 1997

Tablet; Oral

KETOROLAC TROMETHAMINE

TE Code	Firm	Strength	Appl. No.	Date
AB	MYLAN	10MG	N074761 001	MAY 16, 1997
AB	PLIVA	10MG	N075284 001	JUN 23, 1999
AB	TEVA	10MG	N074754 001	MAY 16, 1997
AB	WATSON LABS	10MG	N074955 001	SEP 19, 1997
AB	TORADOL + ROCHE PALO	10MG	N019645 001	DEC 20, 1991

KETOTIFEN FUMARATE

Solution/Drops; Ophthalmic

TE Code	Firm	Strength	Appl. No.	Date
	ZADITOR + NOVARTIS	EQ 0.025% BASE	N021066 001	JUL 02, 1999

LABETALOL HYDROCHLORIDE

Injectable; Injection

LABETALOL HCL

TE Code	Firm	Strength	Appl. No.	Date
AP	ABBOTT	5MG/ML	N075239 001	

LABETALOL HYDROCHLORIDE (continued)

Injectable; Injection

LABETALOL HCL

TE Code	Firm	Strength	Appl. No.	Date
AP	ABBOTT	5MG/ML	N075240 001	NOV 29, 1999 / NOV 29, 1999
AP	APOTEX	5MG/ML	N076051 001	JUL 05, 2002
AP	BEDFORD	5MG/ML	N075303 001	MAY 28, 1999
AP	FAULDING	5MG/ML	N075242 001	SEP 30, 1999
AP	TAYLOR	5MG/ML	N075431 001	NOV 29, 1999
AP		5MG/ML	N075524 001	NOV 29, 1999
AP	NORMODYNE + SCHERING	5MG/ML	N018686 001	AUG 01, 1984
AP	TRANDATE + PROMETHEUS LABS	5MG/ML	N019425 001	DEC 31, 1985

Tablet; Oral

LABETALOL HCL

TE Code	Firm	Strength	Appl. No.	Date
AB	APOTHECON	100MG	N075223 001	NOV 20, 1998
AB		200MG	N075223 002	NOV 20, 1998
AB		300MG	N075223 003	NOV 20, 1998
AB	EON	100MG	N075113 001	AUG 04, 1998
AB		200MG	N075113 002	AUG 04, 1998
AB		300MG	N075113 003	AUG 04, 1998
AB	IVAX PHARMS	100MG	N074787 001	AUG 03, 1998
AB		200MG	N074787 002	AUG 03, 1998
AB		300MG	N074787 003	AUG 03, 1998
AB	MUTUAL PHARM	100MG	N075215 001	JUL 29, 1999
AB		200MG	N075215 002	JUL 29, 1999
AB		300MG	N075215 003	JUL 29, 1999
AB	TEVA	100MG	N074989 001	SEP 30, 1998
AB		200MG	N074989 002	SEP 30, 1998
AB		300MG	N074989 003	SEP 30, 1998
AB	WATSON LABS	100MG	N075133 001	AUG 03, 1998
AB		200MG	N075133 002	

Prescription Drug Products *(continued)*

LABETALOL HYDROCHLORIDE *(continued)*

Tablet; Oral

Code	Name / Firm	Strength	Number	Date
	LABETALOL HCL			
	WATSON LABS	300MG		AUG 03, 1998
AB			N075133 003	AUG 03, 1998
	NORMODYNE			
	SCHERING	100MG	N018687 001	AUG 31, 1987
AB		200MG	N018687 002	AUG 01, 1984
AB		300MG	N018687 003	AUG 01, 1984
AB +				
	TRANDATE			
	PROMETHEUS LABS	100MG	N018716 001	MAY 24, 1985
AB		200MG	N018716 002	AUG 01, 1984
AB		300MG	N018716 003	AUG 01, 1984
AB				

LACTULOSE

For Solution; Oral

Code	Name / Firm	Strength	Number	Date
	LACTULOSE			
AA	+ INALCO	10GM/PACKET	N074712 001	DEC 10, 1997
AA	+	20GM/PACKET	N074712 002	DEC 10, 1997

Solution; Oral

Code	Name / Firm	Strength	Number	Date
	CHRONULAC			
AA	+ AVENTIS PHARMS	10GM/15ML	N017884 001	
	CONSTILAC			
AA	ALRA	10GM/15ML	N071054 001	JUL 26, 1988
	CONSTULOSE			
AA	ALPHARMA	10GM/15ML	N070288 001	AUG 15, 1988
	EVALOSE			
AA	COPLEY PHARM	10GM/15ML	N073497 001	MAY 28, 1993
	LACTULOSE			
AA	HI TECH PHARMA	10GM/15ML	N074076 001	JUL 03, 1995
AA	MORTON GROVE	10GM/15ML	N074602 001	NOV 14, 1996
AA	NOVEX	10GM/15ML	N075911 001	FEB 21, 2002
AA	PHARM ASSOC	10GM/15ML	N074623 001	JUL 30, 1996
AA	ROXANE	10GM/15ML	N073591 001	MAY 29, 1992
AA	VINTAGE PHARMS	10GM/15ML	N075993 001	JUL 26, 2001
AA	VISTAPHARM	10GM/15ML	N074138 001	SEP 30, 1992
	LAXILOSE			
AA	TECHNILAB	10GM/15ML	N073686 001	MAY 28, 1993

Solution; Oral, Rectal

Code	Name / Firm	Strength	Number	Date
	ACILAC			
AA	TECHNILAB	10GM/15ML	N073685 001	MAY 28, 1993
	CHOLAC			
AA	ALRA	10GM/15ML	N071331 001	JUL 26, 1988
	ENULOSE			
AA	+ ALPHARMA	10GM/15ML	N071548 001	AUG 15, 1988
	GENERLAC			
AA	MORTON GROVE	10GM/15ML	N074603 001	OCT 31, 1996
	HEPTALAC			
AA	COPLEY PHARM	10GM/15ML	N073504 001	MAY 28, 1993
	LACTULOSE			
AA	HI TECH PHARMA	10GM/15ML	N074077 001	JUL 03, 1995

LAMIVUDINE

Solution; Oral

Code	Name / Firm	Strength	Number	Date
	EPIVIR			
AA	+ GLAXOSMITHKLINE	10MG/ML	N020596 001	NOV 17, 1995
	EPIVIR-HBV			
AA	+ GLAXOSMITHKLINE	5MG/ML	N021004 001	DEC 08, 1998

Tablet; Oral

Code	Name / Firm	Strength	Number	Date
	EPIVIR			
AA	+ GLAXOSMITHKLINE	150MG	N020564 001	NOV 17, 1995
	EPIVIR-HBV			
AA	+ GLAXOSMITHKLINE	100MG	N021003 001	DEC 08, 1998

LAMIVUDINE; ZIDOVUDINE

Tablet; Oral

Code	Name / Firm	Strength	Number	Date
	COMBIVIR			
AA	+ GLAXOSMITHKLINE	150MG;300MG	N020857 001	SEP 26, 1997

LAMIVUDINE *MULTIPLE*

SEE ABACAVIR SULFATE; LAMIVUDINE; ZIDOVUDINE

LAMOTRIGINE

Tablet, Chewable; Oral

Code	Name / Firm	Strength	Number	Date
	LAMICTAL CD			
	GLAXOSMITHKLINE	2MG	N020764 004	SEP 08, 2000
		5MG	N020764 001	

Prescription Drug Products (continued)

LAMOTRIGINE (continued)

Tablet, Chewable; Oral

LAMICTAL CD

	Firm	Strength	NDA	Date
	GLAXOSMITHKLINE	25MG	N020764 002	AUG 24, 1998
+				AUG 24, 1998

Tablet; Oral

LAMICTAL

	Firm	Strength	NDA	Date
	GLAXOSMITHKLINE	25MG	N020241 005	DEC 27, 1994
		100MG	N020241 001	DEC 27, 1994
			N020241 002	DEC 27, 1994
		150MG	N020241 002	DEC 27, 1994
+		200MG	N020241 003	DEC 27, 1994

LANSOPRAZOLE

Capsule, Delayed Rel Pellets; Oral

PREVACID

	Firm	Strength	NDA	Date
	TAP PHARM	15MG	N020406 001	MAY 10, 1995
+		30MG	N020406 002	MAY 10, 1995

For Suspension, Extended Release; Oral

PREVACID

	Firm	Strength	NDA	Date
	TAP PHARM	15MG/PACKET	N021281 001	MAY 03, 2001
+		30MG/PACKET	N021281 002	MAY 03, 2001

Tablet, Orally Disintegrating; Oral

PREVACID

	Firm	Strength	NDA	Date
	TAP PHARM	15MG	N021428 001	AUG 30, 2002
+		30MG	N021428 002	AUG 30, 2002

LANSOPRAZOLE *MULTIPLE*

SEE   AMOXICILLIN; CLARITHROMYCIN; LANSOPRAZOLE

LATANOPROST

Solution/Drops; Ophthalmic

XALATAN

	Firm	Strength	NDA	Date
+	PHARMACIA AND UPJOHN	0.005%	N020597 001	JUN 05, 1996

LEFLUNOMIDE

Tablet; Oral

ARAVA

	Firm	Strength	NDA	Date
	AVENTIS PHARMS	10MG	N020905 001	SEP 10, 1998
+		20MG	N020905 002	SEP 10, 1998

LEPIRUDIN

Injectable; Injection

REFLUDAN

	Firm	Strength	NDA	Date
+	BERLEX LABS	50MG/VIAL	N020807 001	MAR 06, 1998

LETROZOLE

Tablet; Oral

FEMARA

	Firm	Strength	NDA	Date
+	NOVARTIS	2.5MG	N020726 001	JUL 25, 1997

LEUCOVORIN CALCIUM

Injectable; Injection

LEUCOVORIN CALCIUM

TE		Firm	Strength	NDA	Date
AP		BEDFORD	EQ 50MG BASE/VIAL	N089384 001	SEP 14, 1987
AP			EQ 100MG BASE/VIAL	N089717 001	MAR 28, 1988
AP		GENSIA SICOR PHARMS	EQ 50MG BASE/VIAL	N081278 001	SEP 28, 1993
AP			EQ 100MG BASE/VIAL	N081277 001	SEP 28, 1993
AP			EQ 350MG BASE/VIAL	N040174 001	JUN 12, 1997
AP		PHARMACHEMIE	EQ 350MG BASE/VIAL	N040262 001	DEC 15, 1999
AP		PHARMACHEMIE USA	EQ 50MG BASE/VIAL	N089628 001	APR 17, 1997
AP			EQ 100MG BASE/VIAL	N089915 001	APR 17, 1997
AP	+	XANODYNE PHARM	EQ 50MG BASE/VIAL	N008107 002	APR 17, 1997
AP	+		EQ 100MG BASE/VIAL	N008107 004	MAY 23, 1988
AP			EQ 350MG BASE/VIAL	N008107 005	APR 05, 1989

LEUCOVORIN CALCIUM PRESERVATIVE FREE

TE		Firm	Strength	NDA	Date
AP	+	ABBOTT	EQ 10MG BASE/ML	N040147 001	JUN 25, 1997
AP		BEDFORD	EQ 10MG BASE/ML	N040347 001	APR 25, 2000
AP	+		EQ 200MG BASE/VIAL	N040056 001	MAY 23, 1995
AP			EQ 350MG BASE/VIAL	N040335 001	APR 20, 2000
AP	+	BIGMAR	EQ 200MG BASE/VIAL	N040258 001	FEB 26, 1999
AP	+		EQ 500MG BASE/VIAL	N040286 001	FEB 26, 1999
AP		GENSIA SICOR PHARMS	EQ 10MG BASE/ML	N040332 001	JUN 28, 1999
AP		LUITPOLD	EQ 50MG BASE/VIAL	N040338 001	JAN 31, 2001

WELLCOVORIN

	Firm	Strength	NDA	Date
+	GLAXOSMITHKLINE	EQ 5MG BASE/ML	N087439 001	OCT 19, 1982

Prescription Drug Products (continued)

LEUCOVORIN CALCIUM (continued)
Tablet; Oral

LEUCOVORIN CALCIUM

TE	Firm	Strength	Appl No	Date
AB	BARR	EQ 5MG BASE	N071198 001	SEP 24, 1987
AB		EQ 25MG BASE	N071199 001	SEP 24, 1987
AB	GENEVA PHARMS TECH	EQ 15MG BASE	N075327 001	MAR 24, 1999
AB	PAR PHARM	EQ 5MG BASE	N074544 001	AUG 28, 1997
AB		EQ 25MG BASE	N074544 002	AUG 28, 1997
AB	PHARMACHEMIE	EQ 5MG BASE	N073099 001	MAR 28, 1997
AB		EQ 25MG BASE	N073101 001	MAR 28, 1997
AB	ROXANE	EQ 5MG BASE	N072733 001	FEB 22, 1993
AB		EQ 10MG BASE	N072734 001	FEB 22, 1993
AB		EQ 15MG BASE	N072735 001	FEB 22, 1993
AB		EQ 25MG BASE	N072736 001	FEB 22, 1993
BX	XANODYNE PHARM	EQ 5MG BASE	N018459 001	JAN 30, 1986
AB		EQ 10MG BASE	N071962 001	NOV 19, 1987
AB		EQ 15MG BASE	N071104 001	MAR 04, 1987

LEUPROLIDE ACETATE
Implant; Implantation

VIADUR

TE	Firm	Strength	Appl No	Date
+	ALZA	EQ 65MG BASE	N021088 001	MAR 03, 2000

Injectable; Injection

LEUPROLIDE ACETATE

TE	Firm	Strength	Appl No	Date
AP	BEDFORD LABS	1MG/0.2ML	N074728 001	AUG 04, 1998
AP	GENSIA SICOR PHARMS	1MG/0.2ML	N075471 001	OCT 25, 2000
AP	GENZYME	1MG/0.2ML	N075721 001	NOV 29, 2001

LUPRON

TE	Firm	Strength	Appl No	Date
AP	+ TAP PHARM	1MG/0.2ML	N019010 001	APR 09, 1985

LUPRON DEPOT

TE	Firm	Strength	Appl No	Date
	+ TAP PHARM	3.75MG/VIAL	N020011 001	OCT 22, 1990
	+	7.5MG/VIAL	N019732 001	JAN 26, 1989
	+	22.5MG/VIAL	N020517 001	DEC 22, 1995

LEUPROLIDE ACETATE (continued)
Injectable; Injection

LUPRON DEPOT-3

TE	Firm	Strength	Appl No	Date
	+ TAP PHARM	11.25MG/VIAL	N020708 001	MAR 07, 1997

LUPRON DEPOT-4

TE	Firm	Strength	Appl No	Date
	+ TAP PHARM	30MG/VIAL	N020517 002	MAY 30, 1997

LUPRON DEPOT-PED

TE	Firm	Strength	Appl No	Date
	+ TAP PHARM	7.5MG/VIAL	N020263 002	APR 16, 1993
	+	11.25MG/VIAL	N020263 005	AUG 28, 1997
	+	15MG/VIAL	N020263 006	JAN 21, 1994
	+	15MG/VIAL	N020263 006	JAN 21, 1994

Injectable; Subcutaneous

ELIGARD

TE	Firm	Strength	Appl No	Date
	+ ATRIX	7.5MG/VIAL	N021343 001	JAN 23, 2002
	+	22.5MG/VIAL	N021379 001	JUL 24, 2002
	+	30MG/VIAL	N021488 001	FEB 13, 2003

LEVALBUTEROL HYDROCHLORIDE
Solution; Inhalation

XOPENEX

TE	Firm	Strength	Appl No	Date
	+ SEPRACOR	EQ 0.021% BASE	N020837 001	MAR 25, 1999
	+	EQ 0.042% BASE	N020837 002	MAR 25, 1999
	+	EQ 0.0105% BASE	N020837 003	JAN 30, 2002

LEVAMISOLE HYDROCHLORIDE
Tablet; Oral

ERGAMISOL

TE	Firm	Strength	Appl No	Date
	+ JANSSEN PHARMA	EQ 50MG BASE	N020035 001	JUN 18, 1990

LEVETIRACETAM
Tablet; Oral

KEPPRA

TE	Firm	Strength	Appl No	Date
	UCB	250MG	N021035 001	NOV 30, 1999
		500MG	N021035 002	NOV 30, 1999
		750MG	N021035 003	NOV 30, 1999
	+		N021035 003	NOV 30, 1999

LEVOBETAXOLOL HYDROCHLORIDE
Suspension/Drops; Ophthalmic

BETAXON

TE	Firm	Strength	Appl No	Date
	+ MEDPOINTE	EQ 0.5% BASE	N021114 001	FEB 23, 2000

Prescription Drug Products (continued)

LEVOBUNOLOL HYDROCHLORIDE
Solution/Drops; Ophthalmic

	AKBETA			
AT	AKORN	0.5%	N074780 001	OCT 29, 1996
AT		0.25%	N074779 001	OCT 29, 1996
	BETAGAN			
AT	+ ALLERGAN	0.5%	N019219 002	DEC 19, 1985
AT	+	0.25%	N019814 001	JUN 28, 1989
	LEVOBUNOLOL HCL			
AT	BAUSCH AND LOMB	0.5%	N074326 001	MAR 04, 1994
AT		0.25%	N074307 001	MAR 04, 1994
AT	FALCON PHARMS	0.5%	N074850 001	OCT 28, 1996
AT		0.25%	N074851 001	OCT 28, 1996
AT	NOVEX	0.5%	N075475 001	AUG 03, 2000
AT		0.25%	N075473 001	AUG 03, 2000

LEVOBUPIVACAINE HYDROCHLORIDE
Injectable; Injection

	CHIROCAINE			
	PURDUE PHARMA LP	EQ 2.5MG BASE/ML	N020997 001	AUG 05, 1999
		EQ 5MG BASE/ML	N020997 002	AUG 05, 1999
		EQ 7.5MG BASE/ML	N020997 002	AUG 05, 1999
	+		N020997 003	AUG 05, 1999

LEVOCABASTINE HYDROCHLORIDE
Suspension/Drops; Ophthalmic

	LIVOSTIN			
AT	+ NOVARTIS	EQ 0.05% BASE	N020219 001	NOV 10, 1993

LEVOCARNITINE
Injectable; Injection

	CARNITOR			
AP	+ SIGMA TAU	200MG/ML	N020182 001	DEC 16, 1992
	LEVOCARNITINE			
AP	BEDFORD	200MG/ML	N075567 001	MAR 29, 2001
			N075881 001	MAR 29, 2001
AP	GENSIA SICOR PHARMS	200MG/ML	N075861 001	JUN 22, 2001
AP	LUITPOLD	200MG/ML		

LEVOCARNITINE (continued)
Solution; Oral

	CARNITOR			
	+ SIGMA TAU	1GM/10ML	N019257 001	APR 10, 1986

Tablet; Oral

	CARNITOR			
	+ SIGMA TAU	330MG	N018948 001	DEC 27, 1985

LEVODOPA *MULTIPLE*
SEE   CARBIDOPA; ENTACAPONE; LEVODOPA
SEE   CARBIDOPA; LEVODOPA

LEVOFLOXACIN
Injectable; Injection

LEVAQUIN			
+ ORTHO MCNEIL PHARM	25MG/ML	N020635 001	DEC 20, 1996

LEVAQUIN IN DEXTROSE 5% IN PLASTIC CONTAINER

+ ORTHO MCNEIL PHARM	5MG/ML	N020635 002	DEC 20, 1996
+	500MG/100ML	N020635 003	DEC 20, 1996

Solution/Drops; Ophthalmic

QUIXIN			
+ SANTEN	0.5%	N021199 001	AUG 18, 2000

Tablet; Oral

LEVAQUIN			
ORTHO MCNEIL PHARM	250MG	N020634 001	DEC 20, 1996
	500MG	N020634 002	DEC 20, 1996
+	750MG	N020634 003	SEP 08, 2000

LEVOMETHADYL ACETATE HYDROCHLORIDE
Concentrate; Oral

	ORLAAM			
	+ ROXANE	10MG/ML	N020315 001	JUL 09, 1993

LEVONORDEFRIN; MEPIVACAINE HYDROCHLORIDE
Injectable; Injection

	CARBOCAINE W/ NEO-COBEFRIN			
AP	+ EASTMAN KODAK	0.05MG/ML :2%	N012125 002	
	ISOCAINE HCL W/ LEVONORDEFRIN			
AP	NOVOCOL	0.05MG/ML :2%	N084697 001	
	MEPIVACAINE HCL W/ LEVONORDEFRIN			
AP	GRAHAM CHEM	0.05MG/ML :2%	N084850 002	OCT 21, 1983
	POLOCAINE W/ LEVONORDEFRIN			
AP	DENTSPLY PHARM	0.05MG/ML :2%	N089517 001	APR 14, 1988

Prescription Drug Products (continued)

LEVONORDEFRIN; MEPIVACAINE HYDROCHLORIDE (continued)
Injectable; Injection
SCANDONEST L

AP	DEPROCO	0.05MG/ML;2%	N088388 001	OCT 10, 1984

LEVONORGESTREL
Implant; Implantation
NORPLANT II

BX	+ POPULATION COUNCIL	75MG/IMPLANT	N020544 001	NOV 01, 1996

Intrauterine Device; Intrauterine
MIRENA

	+ BERLEX LABS	52MG	N021225 001	DEC 06, 2000

Tablet; Oral
PLAN B

	+ WOMENS CAPITAL	0.75MG	N021045 001	JUL 28, 1999

LEVONORGESTREL *MULTIPLE*
SEE ETHINYL ESTRADIOL; LEVONORGESTREL

LEVORPHANOL TARTRATE
Injectable; Injection
LEVO-DROMORAN

	+ ICN	2MG/ML	N008719 001	DEC 19, 1991

Tablet; Oral
LEVORPHANOL TARTRATE

	+ ROXANE	2MG	N074278 001	MAR 31, 2000

LEVOTHYROXINE SODIUM
Tablet; Oral
LEVO-T

BX	ALARA PHARM	0.1MG	N021342 005	
BX		0.2MG	N021342 010	MAR 01, 2002
BX		0.3MG	N021342 011	MAR 01, 2002
BX		0.05MG	N021342 002	MAR 01, 2002
BX		0.15MG	N021342 008	MAR 01, 2002
BX		0.025MG	N021342 001	MAR 01, 2002
BX		0.075MG	N021342 003	MAR 01, 2002
BX		0.088MG	N021342 004	MAR 01, 2002
BX		0.112MG	N021342 006	MAR 01, 2002
BX		0.125MG	N021342 007	MAR 01, 2002

LEVOTHYROXINE SODIUM (continued)
Tablet; Oral
LEVO-T

BX	ALARA PHARM	0.175MG	N021342 009	MAR 01, 2002

LEVOLET
VINTAGE PHARMS

BX		0.1MG	N021137 005	JUN 06, 2003
BX		0.2MG	N021137 011	JUN 06, 2003
BX		0.3MG	N021137 012	JUN 06, 2003
BX		0.05MG	N021137 002	JUN 06, 2003
BX		0.15MG	N021137 009	JUN 06, 2003
BX		0.025MG	N021137 001	JUN 06, 2003
BX		0.075MG	N021137 003	JUN 06, 2003
BX		0.088MG	N021137 004	JUN 06, 2003
BX		0.112MG	N021137 006	JUN 06, 2003
BX		0.125MG	N021137 007	JUN 06, 2003
BX		0.137MG	N021137 008	JUN 06, 2003
BX		0.175MG	N021137 010	JUN 06, 2003

LEVOTHYROXINE SODIUM
MYLAN

AB		0.1MG	N076187 005	JUN 05, 2002
AB		0.2MG	N076187 010	JUN 05, 2002
AB		0.3MG	N076187 011	JUN 05, 2002
AB		0.05MG	N076187 002	JUN 05, 2002
AB		0.15MG	N076187 008	JUN 05, 2002
AB		0.025MG	N076187 001	JUN 05, 2002
AB		0.075MG	N076187 003	JUN 05, 2002
AB		0.088MG	N076187 004	JUN 05, 2002
AB		0.112MG	N076187 006	JUN 05, 2002
AB		0.125MG	N076187 007	JUN 05, 2002
AB		0.175MG	N076187 009	JUN 05, 2002

LEVOXYL
JONES PHARMA

BX		0.1MG	N021301 005	MAY 25, 2001

Prescription Drug Products *(continued)*

LEVOTHYROXINE SODIUM *(continued)*
Tablet; Oral

LEVOXYL
JONES PHARMA

TE		Strength	NDC	Date
BX		0.2MG	N021301 011	MAY 25, 2001
BX	+	0.3MG	N021301 012	MAY 25, 2001
BX		0.05MG	N021301 002	MAY 25, 2001
BX		0.15MG	N021301 009	MAY 25, 2001
BX		0.025MG	N021301 001	MAY 25, 2001
BX		0.075MG	N021301 003	MAY 25, 2001
BX		0.088MG	N021301 004	MAY 25, 2001
BX		0.112MG	N021301 006	MAY 25, 2001
BX		0.125MG	N021301 007	MAY 25, 2001
BX		0.137MG	N021301 008	MAY 25, 2001
BX		0.175MG	N021301 010	MAY 25, 2001

NOVOTHYROX
GENPHARM

TE		Strength	NDC	Date
BX		0.1MG	N021292 005	MAY 31, 2002
BX		0.2MG	N021292 011	MAY 31, 2002
BX	+	0.3MG	N021292 012	MAY 31, 2002
BX		0.05MG	N021292 002	MAY 31, 2002
BX		0.15MG	N021292 009	MAY 31, 2002
BX		0.025MG	N021292 001	MAY 31, 2002
BX		0.075MG	N021292 003	MAY 31, 2002
BX		0.088MG	N021292 004	MAY 31, 2002
BX		0.112MG	N021292 006	MAY 31, 2002
BX		0.125MG	N021292 007	MAY 31, 2002
BX		0.137MG	N021292 008	MAY 31, 2002
BX		0.175MG	N021292 010	MAY 31, 2002

SYNTHROID
ABBOTT

TE		Strength	NDC	Date
BX		0.1MG	N021402 005	JUL 24, 2002
BX		0.2MG	N021402 012	JUL 24, 2002
BX	+	0.3MG	N021402 011	JUL 24, 2002

LEVOTHYROXINE SODIUM *(continued)*
Tablet; Oral

SYNTHROID
ABBOTT

TE		Strength	NDC	Date
BX		0.05MG	N021402 002	JUL 24, 2002
BX		0.15MG	N021402 009	JUL 24, 2002
BX		0.025MG	N021402 001	JUL 24, 2002
BX		0.075MG	N021402 003	JUL 24, 2002
BX		0.088MG	N021402 004	JUL 24, 2002
BX		0.112MG	N021402 006	JUL 24, 2002
BX		0.125MG	N021402 007	JUL 24, 2002
BX		0.137MG	N021402 008	JUL 24, 2002
BX		0.175MG	N021402 010	JUL 24, 2002

THYRO-TABS
LLOYD

TE		Strength	NDC	Date
BX		0.1MG	N021116 004	OCT 24, 2002
BX		0.2MG	N021116 008	OCT 24, 2002
BX	+	0.3MG	N021116 009	OCT 24, 2002
BX		0.05MG	N021116 002	OCT 24, 2002
BX		0.15MG	N021116 006	OCT 24, 2002
BX		0.025MG	N021116 001	OCT 24, 2002
BX		0.075MG	N021116 003	OCT 24, 2002
BX		0.088MG	N021116 010	OCT 24, 2002
BX		0.112MG	N021116 011	OCT 24, 2002
BX		0.125MG	N021116 005	OCT 24, 2002
BX		0.175MG	N021116 007	OCT 24, 2002

UNITHROID
STEVENS J

TE		Strength	NDC	Date
AB		0.1MG	N021210 005	AUG 21, 2000
AB		0.2MG	N021210 010	AUG 21, 2000
AB	+	0.3MG	N021210 011	AUG 21, 2000
AB		0.05MG	N021210 002	AUG 21, 2000
AB		0.15MG	N021210 008	AUG 21, 2000
AB		0.025MG	N021210 001	AUG 21, 2000

Prescription Drug Products *(continued)*

LEVOTHYROXINE SODIUM *(continued)*

Tablet; Oral
UNITHROID

		Strength	Appl. No.	Date
AB	STEVENS J	0.075MG	N021210 003	AUG 21, 2000
AB		0.088MG	N021210 004	AUG 21, 2000
AB		0.112MG	N021210 006	AUG 21, 2000
AB		0.125MG	N021210 007	AUG 21, 2000
AB		0.175MG	N021210 009	AUG 21, 2000

LIDOCAINE

Film, Extended Release; Buccal
LIDOCAINE

		Strength	Appl. No.	Date
	+ NOVEN	46.1MG/PATCH	N020575 002	MAY 21, 1996

Film, Extended Release; Topical
LIDODERM

		Strength	Appl. No.	Date
	+ TEIKOKU PHARMA USA	700MG/12HR	N020612 001	MAR 19, 1999

Ointment; Topical
ALPHACAINE

		Strength	Appl. No.
AT	CARLISLE	5%	N084947 001

LIDOCAINE

		Strength	Appl. No.
AT	+ FOUGERA	5%	N080198 001
AT	+ GRAHAM CHEM	5%	N080210 001
AT	TARO	5%	N086724 001

Solution; Topical
XYLOCAINE

		Strength	Appl. No.
	+ ASTRAZENECA	5%	N014127 001

LIDOCAINE; PRILOCAINE

Cream; Topical
EMLA

		Strength	Appl. No.	Date
	+ ASTRAZENECA	2.5%;2.5%	N019941 001	DEC 30, 1992

Disc; Topical
EMLA

		Strength	Appl. No.	Date
	+ ASTRAZENECA	2.5%;2.5%	N020962 001	FEB 04, 1998

LIDOCAINE HYDROCHLORIDE

Injectable; Injection
LIDOCAINE HCL

		Strength	Appl. No.	Date
AP	ABBOTT	0.5%	N088328 001	MAY 17, 1984
AP		1%	N040013 001	JUN 23, 1995
AP		1%	N083158 001	
AP		1%	N088329 001	MAY 17, 1984
AP		2%	N040078 001	JUN 23, 1995

LIDOCAINE HYDROCHLORIDE *(continued)*

Injectable; Injection
LIDOCAINE HCL

		Strength	Appl. No.	Date
AP	ABBOTT	2%	N083158 002	
AP		2%	N088294 001	MAY 17, 1984
AP		2%	N088331 001	MAY 17, 1984
	GRAHAM CHEM	20%	N083158 003	
AP	INTL MEDICATION	2%	N080504 001	
AP		1%	N083173 001	
AP	LUITPOLD	2%	N083173 002	
AP		1%	N080850 001	
AP		2%	N083198 001	

LIDOCAINE HCL 0.2% AND DEXTROSE 5% IN PLASTIC CONTAINER
BAXTER HLTHCARE

		Strength	Appl. No.	Date
AP		200MG/100ML	N018461 002	
AP		200MG/100ML	N018967 001	MAR 30, 1984
	B BRAUN			
AP		200MG/100ML	N019830 002	APR 08, 1992

LIDOCAINE HCL 0.2% IN DEXTROSE 5%
ABBOTT

		Strength	Appl. No.
AP		200MG/100ML	N083158 005

LIDOCAINE HCL 0.2% IN DEXTROSE 5% IN PLASTIC CONTAINER
ABBOTT

		Strength	Appl. No.
AP		200MG/100ML	N018388 001

LIDOCAINE HCL 0.4% AND DEXTROSE 5% IN PLASTIC CONTAINER
BAXTER HLTHCARE

		Strength	Appl. No.	Date
AP		400MG/100ML	N018461 003	
AP		400MG/100ML	N018967 002	MAR 30, 1984
	B BRAUN			
AP		400MG/100ML	N019830 003	APR 08, 1992

LIDOCAINE HCL 0.4% IN DEXTROSE 5%
ABBOTT

		Strength	Appl. No.
AP		400MG/100ML	N083158 006

LIDOCAINE HCL 0.4% IN DEXTROSE 5% IN PLASTIC CONTAINER
ABBOTT

		Strength	Appl. No.
AP		400MG/100ML	N018388 002

LIDOCAINE HCL 0.8% AND DEXTROSE 5% IN PLASTIC CONTAINER
BAXTER HLTHCARE

		Strength	Appl. No.	Date
AP		800MG/100ML	N018461 004	FEB 22, 1982
AP		800MG/100ML	N018967 003	MAR 30, 1984
	B BRAUN			
AP		800MG/100ML	N019830 004	APR 08, 1992

LIDOCAINE HCL 0.8% IN DEXTROSE 5% IN PLASTIC CONTAINER
ABBOTT

		Strength	Appl. No.	Date
AP		800MG/100ML	N018388 003	NOV 05, 1982

LIDOCAINE HCL IN PLASTIC CONTAINER
ABBOTT

		Strength	Appl. No.	Date
AP		0.5%	N088325 001	JUL 31, 1984
			N088299 001	
AP		1%	N088326 001	JUL 31, 1984
AP		1.5%	N088327 001	JUL 31, 1984
AP		2%	N088367 001	JUL 31, 1984
AP		10%	N088368 001	JUL 31, 1984
AP		20%		

Prescription Drug Products (continued)

LIDOCAINE HYDROCHLORIDE (continued)

Injectable; Injection

LIDOCAINE HCL IN PLASTIC CONTAINER

AP	AM PHARM PARTNERS	1%	N088586 001	JUL 24, 1985

LIDOCAINE HCL PRESERVATIVE FREE

	ABBOTT	1%	N080408 001	
AP		1.5%	N080408 002	
AP		4%	N088295 001	MAY 17, 1984
AP	AM PHARM PARTNERS	1%	N080404 002	
AP		2%	N017584 001	
AP		2%	N080404 003	
AP		4%	N017584 002	
AP		20%	N017702 001	
	INTL MEDICATION			

LIDOCAINE HCL PRESERVATIVE FREE IN PLASTIC CONTAINER

AP	ABBOTT	1%	N040302 001	SEP 28, 1998
AP		2%	N040302 002	SEP 28, 1998

LIDOPEN

AP	MERIDIAN MEDCL TECHN	10%	N017549 001	

XYLOCAINE

AP	+ ASTRAZENECA	0.5%	N006488 008	
AP	+	1%	N006488 007	
AP	+	1.5%	N006488 010	
AP	+ DENTSPLY PHARM	2%	N021380 001	

XYLOCAINE 4% PRESERVATIVE FREE

AP	ASTRAZENECA	4%	N010417 001	

XYLOCAINE PRESERVATIVE FREE

AP	ASTRAZENECA	1%	N016801 005	JAN 19, 1988
AP		2%	N016801 001	
AP		4%	N016801 002	
AP		10%	N016801 003	
AP		20%	N016801 004	

Injectable; Spinal

LIDOCAINE HCL 5% AND DEXTROSE 7.5%

AP	+ ABBOTT	5%	N083914 001	

XYLOCAINE 1.5% W/ DEXTROSE 7.5%

AP	+ ASTRAZENECA	1.5%	N016297 001	

Jelly; Topical

LIDOCAINE HCL

AT	AKORN	2%	N040433 001	FEB 12, 2003
AT	COPLEY PHARM	2%	N081318 001	APR 29, 1993
AT	INTL MEDICATION	2%	N086283 001	

XYLOCAINE

AT	+ ASTRAZENECA	2%	N008816 001	

Solution; Oral

LIDOCAINE HCL

AT	HI TECH PHARMA	2%	N040014 001	JUL 10, 1995
AT	MORTON GROVE	2%	N087872 001	NOV 18, 1982

LIDOCAINE HYDROCHLORIDE (continued)

Solution; Oral

LIDOCAINE HCL VISCOUS

AT	ALPHARMA	2%	N086578 001	

LIDOCAINE VISCOUS

AT	ROXANE	2%	N088802 001	APR 26, 1985

XYLOCAINE VISCOUS

AT	+ ASTRAZENECA	2%	N009470 001	

Solution; Topical

ANESTACON

AT	+ POLYMEDICA	2%	N080429 001	

LARYNG-O-JET KIT

AT	INTL MEDICATION	4%	N086364 001	

LIDOCAINE HCL

AT	MORTON GROVE	4%	N087881 001	NOV 18, 1982
AT	ROXANE	4%	N088803 001	APR 03, 1985

LTA II KIT

AT	ABBOTT	4%	N080409 001	
AT		4%	N088542 001	JUL 31, 1984

PEDIATRIC LTA KIT

AT	ABBOTT	2%	N085995 001	

XYLOCAINE 4% PRESERVATIVE FREE

AT	+ ASTRAZENECA	4%	N010417 002	

LIDOCAINE HYDROCHLORIDE; OXYTETRACYCLINE

Injectable; Injection

TERRAMYCIN

	PFIZER	2%;50MG/ML	N060567 001
		2%;125MG/ML	N060567 002

LIDOCAINE HYDROCHLORIDE *MULTIPLE*

SEE BUPIVACAINE HYDROCHLORIDE; LIDOCAINE HYDROCHLORIDE
SEE EPINEPHRINE; LIDOCAINE HYDROCHLORIDE
SEE EPINEPHRINE BITARTRATE; LIDOCAINE HYDROCHLORIDE

LINCOMYCIN HYDROCHLORIDE

Injectable; Injection

LINCOCIN

	PHARMACIA AND UPJOHN	EQ 300MG BASE/ML	N050317 001

LINDANE

Lotion; Topical

LINDANE

AT	+ ALPHARMA	1%	N087313 001	
AT	MORTON GROVE	1%	N088190 001	AUG 16, 1984

Shampoo; Topical

LINDANE

AT	+ ALPHARMA	1%	N087266 001	
AT	MORTON GROVE	1%	N088191 001	SEP 18, 1984

Prescription Drug Products *(continued)*

LINEZOLID

For Suspension; Oral

ZYVOX
+ PHARMACIA AND UPJOHN — 100MG/5ML — N021132 001 — APR 18, 2000

Injectable; Injection

ZYVOX
+ PHARMACIA AND UPJOHN — 200MG/100ML — N021131 001 — APR 18, 2000

Tablet; Oral

ZYVOX
+ PHARMACIA AND UPJOHN — 600MG — N021130 002 — APR 18, 2000

LIOTHYRONINE SODIUM

Injectable; Injection

TRIOSTAT
+ JONES PHARMA — EQ 0.01MG BASE/ML — N020105 001 — DEC 31, 1991

Tablet; Oral

CYTOMEL
JONES PHARMA
+

Strength	Appl. No.
EQ 0.005MG BASE	N010379 001
EQ 0.05MG BASE	N010379 003
EQ 0.025MG BASE	N010379 002

LIOTRIX (T4;T3)

Tablet; Oral

Product	Manufacturer	Strength	Appl. No.
THYROLAR-0.5	FORREST LABS	0.025MG;0.0063MG	N016807 005
THYROLAR-0.25	FORREST LABS	0.0125MG;0.0031MG	N016807 001
THYROLAR-1	FORREST LABS	0.05MG;0.0125MG	N016807 004
THYROLAR-2	FORREST LABS	0.1MG;0.025MG	N016807 002
THYROLAR-3 +	FORREST LABS	0.15MG;0.0375MG	N016807 003

LISINOPRIL

Tablet; Oral

LISINOPRIL
APOTEX

TE	Strength	Appl. No.	Date
AB	2.5MG	N076102 001	SEP 30, 2002
AB	5MG	N076102 002	SEP 30, 2002
AB	10MG	N076102 003	SEP 30, 2002
AB	20MG	N076102 004	SEP 30, 2002
AB	30MG	N076102 005	SEP 30, 2002
AB	40MG	N076102 006	SEP 30, 2002

LISINOPRIL *(continued)*

Tablet; Oral

LISINOPRIL
APOTEX

TE	Manufacturer	Strength	Appl. No.	Date
AB	EON	2.5MG	N075994 001	SEP 30, 2002
AB		5MG	N075994 002	JUL 01, 2002
AB		10MG	N075994 003	JUL 01, 2002
AB		20MG	N075994 004	JUL 01, 2002
AB		30MG	N075994 005	JUL 01, 2002
AB		40MG	N075994 006	JUL 01, 2002
AB	GENEVA PHARMS TECH	2.5MG	N075903 001	JUL 01, 2002
AB		5MG	N075903 002	JUL 01, 2002
AB		10MG	N075903 003	JUL 01, 2002
AB		20MG	N075903 004	JUL 01, 2002
AB		30MG	N075903 005	JUL 01, 2002
AB		40MG	N075903 006	JUL 01, 2002
AB	IVAX PHARMS	2.5MG	N075752 001	JUL 01, 2002
AB		5MG	N075752 002	JUL 01, 2002
AB		10MG	N075752 003	JUL 01, 2002
AB		20MG	N075752 004	JUL 01, 2002
AB		30MG	N075752 005	JUL 01, 2002
AB		40MG	N075752 006	JUL 01, 2002
AB	LEK PHARMS	2.5MG	N075999 001	JUL 01, 2002
AB		5MG	N075999 002	JUL 01, 2002
AB		10MG	N075999 003	JUL 01, 2002
AB		20MG	N075999 004	JUL 01, 2002
AB		30MG	N075999 005	JUL 01, 2002
AB		40MG	N075999 006	JUL 01, 2002
AB	MYLAN	2.5MG	N076071 001	JUL 01, 2002
AB		5MG	N076071 002	JUL 01, 2002
AB		10MG	N076071 003	JUL 01, 2002

Prescription Drug Products (continued)

LISINOPRIL (continued)
Tablet; Oral

LISINOPRIL

MYLAN

TE Code	Strength	Appl No	Date
AB	20MG	N076071 004	JUL 01, 2002
AB	30MG	N076071 005	JUL 01, 2002
AB	40MG	N076071 006	JUL 01, 2002

PAR PHARM

TE Code	Strength	Appl No	Date
AB	2.5MG	N075743 001	JUL 01, 2002
AB	5MG	N075743 002	JUL 01, 2002
AB	10MG	N075743 003	JUL 01, 2002
AB	20MG	N075743 004	JUL 01, 2002
AB	30MG	N075743 005	JUL 01, 2002
AB	40MG	N075743 006	JUL 01, 2002

PUREPAC PHARM

TE Code	Strength	Appl No	Date
AB	2.5MG	N076180 001	JUL 01, 2002
AB	5MG	N076180 002	JUL 01, 2002
AB	10MG	N076180 003	JUL 01, 2002
AB	20MG	N076164 001	JUL 01, 2002
AB	30MG	N076164 002	JUL 01, 2002
AB	40MG	N076164 003	JUL 01, 2002

RANBAXY

TE Code	Strength	Appl No	Date
AB	2.5MG	N075944 001	JUL 01, 2002
AB	5MG	N075944 002	JUL 01, 2002
AB	10MG	N075944 003	JUL 01, 2002
AB	20MG	N075944 004	JUL 01, 2002
AB	30MG	N075944 006	JUL 01, 2002
AB	40MG	N075944 005	FEB 11, 2003

TEVA

TE Code	Strength	Appl No	Date
AB	2.5MG	N075783 001	JUL 01, 2002
AB	5MG	N075783 002	JUL 01, 2002
AB	10MG	N075783 003	JUL 01, 2002
AB	20MG	N075783 004	JUL 01, 2002
AB	30MG	N075783 005	JUL 01, 2002
AB	40MG	N075783 006	JUL 01, 2002

LISINOPRIL (continued)
Tablet; Oral

LISINOPRIL

WATSON LABS

TE Code	Strength	Appl No	Date
AB	2.5MG	N076059 001	JUL 01, 2002
AB	5MG	N076059 002	JUL 01, 2002
AB	10MG	N076059 003	JUL 01, 2002
AB	20MG	N076059 004	JUL 01, 2002
AB	30MG	N076059 005	JUL 01, 2002
AB	40MG	N076059 006	JUL 01, 2002

WEST WARD

TE Code	Strength	Appl No	Date
AB	2.5MG	N076063 001	JUL 01, 2002
AB	5MG	N076063 002	JUL 01, 2002
AB	10MG	N076063 003	JUL 01, 2002
AB	20MG	N076063 004	JUL 01, 2002
AB	30MG	N076063 006	JUL 01, 2002
AB	40MG	N076063 005	JUN 27, 2003

PRINIVIL
MERCK

TE Code	Strength	Appl No	Date
AB	2.5MG	N019558 006	JAN 28, 1994
AB	5MG	N019558 001	DEC 29, 1987
AB	10MG	N019558 002	DEC 29, 1987
AB	20MG	N019558 003	DEC 29, 1987
AB	40MG	N019558 004	OCT 25, 1988

ZESTRIL
ASTRAZENECA

TE Code	Strength	Appl No	Date
AB	2.5MG	N019777 005	APR 29, 1993
AB	5MG	N019777 001	MAY 19, 1988
AB	10MG	N019777 002	MAY 19, 1988
AB	20MG	N019777 003	MAY 19, 1988
AB	30MG	N019777 006	JAN 20, 1999
AB +	40MG	N019777 004	MAY 19, 1988

LISINOPRIL *MULTIPLE*
SEE HYDROCHLOROTHIAZIDE; LISINOPRIL

Prescription Drug Products (continued)

LITHIUM CARBONATE

Capsule; Oral

TE	Brand/Manufacturer	Strength	NDA	Date
	ESKALITH			
	GLAXOSMITHKLINE	300MG	N016860 001	
	LITHIUM CARBONATE			
AB	ABLE	300MG	N076121 001	SEP 27, 2001
AB	ROXANE	150MG	N017812 002	JAN 28, 1987
AB		300MG	N017812 001	JAN 28, 1987
AB	+	600MG	N017812 003	JAN 28, 1987
AB	WEST WARD	150MG	N076243 002	FEB 24, 2003
AB		300MG	N076243 001	JUN 27, 2002

Tablet, Extended Release; Oral

TE	Brand/Manufacturer	Strength	NDA	Date
	ESKALITH CR			
AB	+ GLAXOSMITHKLINE	450MG	N018152 001	MAR 29, 1982
	LITHIUM CARBONATE			
AB	ABLE	300MG	N076382 001	APR 21, 2003
AB	BARR	300MG	N076170 001	JUN 10, 2002
AB	WEST WARD	450MG	N076490 001	JUN 17, 2003
	LITHOBID			
AB	+ SOLVAY	300MG	N018027 001	

Tablet; Oral

TE	Brand/Manufacturer	Strength	NDA	Date
	LITHIUM CARBONATE			
AB	+ PFIZER	300MG	N016834 001	
AB	ROXANE	300MG	N018558 001	JAN 29, 1982

LITHIUM CITRATE

Syrup; Oral

TE	Brand/Manufacturer	Strength	NDA	Date
	LITHIUM CITRATE			
AA	MORTON GROVE	EQ 300MG CARBONATE/5ML	N070755 001	MAY 21, 1986
AA	+ ROXANE	EQ 300MG CARBONATE/5ML	N018421 001	

LODOXAMIDE TROMETHAMINE

Solution/Drops; Ophthalmic

TE	Brand/Manufacturer	Strength	NDA	Date
	ALOMIDE			
	+ ALCON	EQ 0.1% BASE	N020191 001	SEP 23, 1993

LOMEFLOXACIN HYDROCHLORIDE

Tablet; Oral

TE	Brand/Manufacturer	Strength	NDA	Date
	MAXAQUIN			
	+ PHARMACIA	EQ 400MG BASE	N020013 001	FEB 21, 1992

LOMUSTINE

Capsule; Oral

TE	Brand/Manufacturer	Strength	NDA	Date
	CEENU			
	BRISTOL MYERS SQUIBB	10MG	N017588 001	
		40MG	N017588 002	
		100MG	N017588 003	

LOPERAMIDE HYDROCHLORIDE

Capsule; Oral

TE	Brand/Manufacturer	Strength	NDA	Date
	IMODIUM			
AB	+ MCNEIL CONS SPECLT	2MG	N017694 001	
	LOPERAMIDE HCL			
AB	GENEVA PHARMS	2MG	N072993 001	AUG 28, 1992
AB	MYLAN	2MG	N072741 001	SEP 18, 1991
AB		2MG	N073122 001	AUG 30, 1991
AB	TEVA	2MG	N073192 001	APR 30, 1992

LOPINAVIR; RITONAVIR

Capsule; Oral

TE	Brand/Manufacturer	Strength	NDA	Date
	KALETRA			
	+ ABBOTT	133.3MG;33.3MG	N021226 001	SEP 15, 2000

Solution; Oral

TE	Brand/Manufacturer	Strength	NDA	Date
	KALETRA			
	+ ABBOTT	80MG/ML;20MG/ML	N021251 001	SEP 15, 2000

LORACARBEF

Capsule; Oral

TE	Brand/Manufacturer	Strength	NDA	Date
	LORABID			
	KING PHARMS	200MG	N050668 001	DEC 31, 1991
		400MG	N050668 002	APR 05, 1996

For Suspension; Oral

TE	Brand/Manufacturer	Strength	NDA	Date
	LORABID			
	KING PHARMS	100MG/5ML	N050667 001	DEC 31, 1991
	+	200MG/5ML	N050667 002	DEC 31, 1991

LORAZEPAM

Concentrate: Oral

TE	Brand/Manufacturer	Strength	NDA	Date
	LORAZEPAM INTENSOL			
	+ ROXANE	2MG/ML	N072755 001	JUN 28, 1991

Injectable; Injection

TE	Brand/Manufacturer	Strength	NDA	Date
	ATIVAN			
AP	+ BAXTER HLTHCARE CORP	2MG/ML	N018140 001	

Prescription Drug Products *(continued)*

LORAZEPAM *(continued)*

Injectable; Injection

TE	Firm / Product	Strength	Appl. No.	Date
	ATIVAN			
AP +	BAXTER HLTHCARE CORP	4MG/ML	N018140 002	
	LORAZEPAM			
	ABBOTT			
AP		2MG/ML	N074243 001	APR 12, 1994
AP		2MG/ML	N074280 001	MAY 27, 1994
AP		2MG/ML	N074282 001	MAY 27, 1994
AP		2MG/ML	N074300 001	APR 12, 1994
AP		4MG/ML	N074243 002	APR 12, 1994
AP		4MG/ML	N074280 002	MAY 27, 1994
AP		4MG/ML	N074282 002	MAY 27, 1994
AP		4MG/ML	N074300 003	MAR 19, 1997
	AKORN			
AP		2MG/ML	N074974 001	JUL 23, 1998
	CLONMEL HLTHCARE			
AP		2MG/ML	N074793 001	MAR 16, 2000
AP		4MG/ML	N074793 002	MAR 16, 2000
	ELKINS SINN			
AP		2MG/ML	N074496 001	SEP 28, 1998
AP		4MG/ML	N074496 002	SEP 28, 1998
	MARSAM PHARMS LLC			
AP		1MG/0.5ML	N074551 003	SEP 12, 1996
AP		2MG/ML	N074535 001	SEP 12, 1996
AP		2MG/ML	N074551 001	SEP 12, 1996
AP		4MG/ML	N074535 002	SEP 12, 1996
AP		4MG/ML	N074551 002	SEP 12, 1996
	STERIS			
AP		2MG/ML	N074276 001	APR 15, 1994
AP		4MG/ML	N074276 002	APR 15, 1994
	TAYLOR			
AP		2MG/ML	N075025 001	JUL 23, 1998

Solution; Oral

TE	Firm / Product	Strength	Appl. No.	Date
	LORAZEPAM			
+	ROXANE	0.5MG/5ML	N074648 001	MAR 18, 1997

Tablet; Oral

TE	Firm / Product	Strength	Appl. No.	Date
	ATIVAN			
	BIOVAIL			
AB		0.5MG	N017794 001	
AB		1MG	N017794 002	
AB +		2MG	N017794 003	
	LORAZEPAM			
	GENEVA PHARMS			
AB		0.5MG	N071193 001	APR 15, 1988
AB		1MG	N071194 001	APR 15, 1988
AB		2MG	N071195 001	APR 15, 1988
	MUTUAL PHARM			
AB		0.5MG	N072553 001	MAR 29, 1991
AB		1MG	N072554 001	MAR 29, 1991
AB		2MG	N072555 001	MAR 29, 1991
	MYLAN			
AB		0.5MG	N071589 001	OCT 13, 1987
AB		1MG	N071590 001	OCT 13, 1987
AB		2MG	N071591 001	OCT 13, 1987
	PUREPAC PHARM			
AB		0.5MG	N071403 001	APR 21, 1987
AB		1MG	N071404 001	APR 21, 1987
AB		2MG	N071141 001	APR 21, 1987
	RANBAXY			
AB		0.5MG	N076045 001	AUG 29, 2001
AB		1MG	N076045 002	AUG 29, 2001
AB		2MG	N076045 003	AUG 29, 2001
	WATSON LABS			
AB		0.5MG	N071117 001	JUL 24, 1986
AB		0.5MG	N072926 001	OCT 31, 1991
AB		1MG	N071087 001	MAR 23, 1987
AB		1MG	N071118 001	JUL 24, 1986
AB		1MG	N072927 001	OCT 31, 1991
AB		2MG	N071088 001	MAR 23, 1987
AB		2MG	N071110 001	JUL 24, 1986
AB		2MG	N072928 001	OCT 31, 1991

LOSARTAN POTASSIUM

Tablet; Oral

TE	Firm / Product	Strength	Appl. No.	Date
	COZAAR			
	MERCK			
		25MG	N020386 001	APR 14, 1995
		50MG	N020386 002	APR 14, 1995

Prescription Drug Products (continued)

LOSARTAN POTASSIUM (continued)
Tablet; Oral

		Strength		Appl. No.	Date
	COZAAR				
+	MERCK	100MG		N020386 003	OCT 13, 1998

LOSARTAN POTASSIUM *MULTIPLE*
SEE HYDROCHLOROTHIAZIDE; LOSARTAN POTASSIUM

LOTEPREDNOL ETABONATE
Suspension/Drops; Ophthalmic

		Strength	Appl. No.	Date
	ALREX			
+	BAUSCH AND LOMB	0.2%	N020803 001	MAR 09, 1998
	LOTEMAX			
+	BAUSCH AND LOMB	0.5%	N020583 001	MAR 09, 1998

LOVASTATIN
Tablet, Extended Release; Oral

		Strength	Appl. No.	Date
	ALTOCOR			
	ANDRX	10MG	N021316 001	JUN 26, 2002
		20MG	N021316 002	JUN 26, 2002
		40MG	N021316 003	JUN 26, 2002
		60MG	N021316 004	JUN 26, 2002

Tablet; Oral

		Strength	Appl. No.	Date
	LOVASTATIN			
	CARLSBAD			
AB		10MG	N075991 001	JUN 05, 2002
AB		20MG	N075991 002	JUN 05, 2002
AB		40MG	N075991 003	JUN 05, 2002
	EON			
AB		10MG	N075636 001	DEC 17, 2001
AB		20MG	N075636 002	DEC 17, 2001
AB		40MG	N075636 003	DEC 17, 2001
	GENEVA PHARMS			
AB		10MG	N075300 001	DEC 17, 2001
AB		20MG	N075300 002	DEC 17, 2001
AB		40MG	N075300 003	DEC 17, 2001
	GENPHARM			
AB		10MG	N075935 001	DEC 17, 2001
AB		20MG	N075935 002	DEC 17, 2001
AB		40MG	N075935 003	DEC 17, 2001
	MYLAN			
AB		10MG	N075451 001	DEC 17, 2001

LOVASTATIN (continued)
Tablet; Oral

		Strength	Appl. No.	Date
	LOVASTATIN			
	MYLAN			
AB		20MG	N075451 002	DEC 17, 2001
AB		40MG	N075451 003	DEC 17, 2001
	PUREPAC PHARM			
AB		10MG	N075828 001	DEC 17, 2001
AB		20MG	N075828 002	DEC 17, 2001
AB		40MG	N075828 003	DEC 17, 2001
	TEVA			
AB		10MG	N075551 003	DEC 17, 2001
AB		20MG	N075551 002	DEC 17, 2001
AB		40MG	N075551 001	DEC 17, 2001
	MEVACOR			
	MERCK			
AB		10MG	N019643 002	MAR 28, 1991
AB		20MG	N019643 003	AUG 31, 1987
AB +		40MG	N019643 004	DEC 14, 1988

LOVASTATIN; NIACIN
Tablet, Extended Release; Oral

		Strength	Appl. No.	Date
	ADVICOR			
+	KOS	20MG;1GM	N021249 003	DEC 17, 2001
		20MG;500MG	N021249 001	DEC 17, 2001
		20MG;750MG	N021249 002	DEC 17, 2001

LOXAPINE SUCCINATE
Capsule; Oral

		Strength	Appl. No.	Date
	LOXAPINE SUCCINATE			
	WATSON LABS			
AB		EQ 5MG BASE	N072204 001	JUN 15, 1988
AB		EQ 10MG BASE	N072205 001	JUN 15, 1988
AB		EQ 25MG BASE	N072206 001	JUN 15, 1988
AB		EQ 50MG BASE	N072062 001	JUN 15, 1988
	LOXITANE			
	WATSON LABS			
AB		EQ 5MG BASE	N017525 001	
AB		EQ 10MG BASE	N017525 002	
AB		EQ 25MG BASE	N017525 003	
AB +		EQ 50MG BASE	N017525 004	

Prescription Drug Products (continued)

MAFENIDE ACETATE
Cream; Topical
  SULFAMYLON
  + BERTEK PHARMS   EQ 85MG BASE/GM   N016763 001
For Solution; Topical
  SULFAMYLON
  + MYLAN   5%   N019832 003   JUN 05, 1998

MAGNESIUM ACETATE *MULTIPLE*
SEE AMINO ACIDS: CALCIUM ACETATE: GLYCERIN: MAGNESIUM ACETATE: PHOSPHORIC ACID: POTASSIUM CHLORIDE: SODIUM ACETATE: SODIUM CHLORIDE

SEE AMINO ACIDS: MAGNESIUM ACETATE: PHOSPHORIC ACID: POTASSIUM ACETATE: POTASSIUM CHLORIDE: SODIUM ACETATE

SEE AMINO ACIDS: MAGNESIUM ACETATE: PHOSPHORIC ACID: POTASSIUM ACETATE: SODIUM CHLORIDE

SEE AMINO ACIDS: MAGNESIUM ACETATE: PHOSPHORIC ACID: POTASSIUM CHLORIDE: SODIUM ACETATE: SODIUM CHLORIDE

SEE DEXTROSE: MAGNESIUM ACETATE: POTASSIUM ACETATE: SODIUM CHLORIDE

MAGNESIUM ACETATE TETRAHYDRATE; POTASSIUM ACETATE; SODIUM CHLORIDE
Injectable; Injection
  PLASMA-LYTE 56 IN PLASTIC CONTAINER
  BAXTER HLTHCARE   32MG/100ML;128MG/100ML;234MG/100ML   N019047 001   JUN 15, 1984

MAGNESIUM ACETATE TETRAHYDRATE *MULTIPLE*
SEE DEXTROSE: MAGNESIUM ACETATE TETRAHYDRATE: POTASSIUM ACETATE: SODIUM CHLORIDE

MAGNESIUM CARBONATE *MULTIPLE*
SEE CITRIC ACID: GLUCONOLACTONE: MAGNESIUM CARBONATE

MAGNESIUM CHLORIDE; POTASSIUM CHLORIDE; POTASSIUM PHOSPHATE, MONOBASIC; SODIUM ACETATE; SODIUM CHLORIDE; SODIUM GLUCONATE; SODIUM PHOSPHATE, DIBASIC, HEPTAHYDRATE
Injectable; Injection
  ISOLYTE S PH 7.4 IN PLASTIC CONTAINER
  B BRAUN   30MG/100ML;37MG/100ML;0.82MG/100ML;370MG/100ML;530MG/100ML;500MG/100ML;12MG/100ML   N019696 001   SEP 29, 1989

MAGNESIUM CHLORIDE; POTASSIUM CHLORIDE; SODIUM ACETATE; SODIUM CHLORIDE; SODIUM GLUCONATE
Injectable; Injection
  ISOLYTE S IN PLASTIC CONTAINER
  B BRAUN   30MG/100ML;37MG/100ML;530MG/100ML   N018252 001
AP
    30MG/100ML;37MG/100ML;530MG/100ML   N019711 001   SEP 29, 1989
AP

  NORMOSOL-R IN PLASTIC CONTAINER
  ABBOTT   30MG/100ML;37MG/100ML;222MG/100ML;526MG/100ML;502MG/100ML   N017586 001

  PLASMA-LYTE 148 IN WATER IN PLASTIC CONTAINER
  BAXTER HLTHCARE   30MG/100ML;37MG/100ML;368MG/100ML;526MG/100ML;502MG/100ML   N017378 001
AP

  PLASMA-LYTE A IN PLASTIC CONTAINER
  BAXTER HLTHCARE   30MG/100ML;37MG/100ML;368MG/100ML;526MG/100ML;502MG/100ML   N017378 002   NOV 22, 1982
AP

Solution; Irrigation
  PHYSIOSOL IN PLASTIC CONTAINER
  ABBOTT   30MG/100ML;37MG/100ML;222MG/100ML;526MG/100ML;502MG/100ML   N017637 002   JUL 08, 1982

  PHYSIOSOL PH 7.4 IN PLASTIC CONTAINER
  ABBOTT   30MG/100ML;37MG/100ML;222MG/100ML;526MG/100ML;502MG/100ML   N018406 002   JUL 08, 1982

  PHYSICLYTE IN PLASTIC CONTAINER
  B BRAUN   30MG/100ML;37MG/100ML;370MG/100ML;530MG/100ML;500MG/100ML   N019024 001   JUN 08, 1984

MAGNESIUM CHLORIDE *MULTIPLE*
SEE AMINO ACIDS: CALCIUM CHLORIDE: DEXTROSE: MAGNESIUM CHLORIDE: POTASSIUM CHLORIDE: POTASSIUM PHOSPHATE, DIBASIC: SODIUM CHLORIDE

SEE AMINO ACIDS: CALCIUM CHLORIDE: DEXTROSE: MAGNESIUM CHLORIDE: POTASSIUM PHOSPHATE, DIBASIC: SODIUM ACETATE: SODIUM CHLORIDE

SEE AMINO ACIDS: DEXTROSE: MAGNESIUM CHLORIDE: POTASSIUM CHLORIDE: SODIUM CHLORIDE

SEE AMINO ACIDS: DEXTROSE: MAGNESIUM CHLORIDE: POTASSIUM PHOSPHATE, DIBASIC: SODIUM PHOSPHATE, HEPTAHYDRATE

SEE AMINO ACIDS: DEXTROSE: MAGNESIUM CHLORIDE: POTASSIUM PHOSPHATE, DIBASIC: SODIUM ACETATE: SODIUM CHLORIDE

SEE AMINO ACIDS: MAGNESIUM CHLORIDE: POTASSIUM CHLORIDE: POTASSIUM PHOSPHATE, DIBASIC: SODIUM CHLORIDE

SEE AMINO ACIDS: MAGNESIUM CHLORIDE: POTASSIUM PHOSPHATE, DIBASIC: SODIUM ACETATE: SODIUM CHLORIDE

Prescription Drug Products (continued)

MAGNESIUM CHLORIDE *MULTIPLE* (continued)

SEE AMINO ACIDS; MAGNESIUM CHLORIDE; POTASSIUM PHOSPHATE, DIBASIC; SODIUM CHLORIDE
SEE CALCIUM CHLORIDE; DEXTROSE; GLUTATHIONE DISULFIDE; MAGNESIUM CHLORIDE; POTASSIUM CHLORIDE; SODIUM BICARBONATE; SODIUM CHLORIDE; SODIUM PHOSPHATE
SEE CALCIUM CHLORIDE; DEXTROSE; MAGNESIUM CHLORIDE; POTASSIUM CHLORIDE; SODIUM CHLORIDE
SEE CALCIUM CHLORIDE; DEXTROSE; MAGNESIUM CHLORIDE; POTASSIUM CHLORIDE; SODIUM CITRATE
SEE CALCIUM CHLORIDE; DEXTROSE; MAGNESIUM CHLORIDE; POTASSIUM CHLORIDE; SODIUM ACETATE; SODIUM CHLORIDE
SEE CALCIUM CHLORIDE; DEXTROSE; MAGNESIUM CHLORIDE; POTASSIUM CHLORIDE; SODIUM ACETATE; SODIUM CHLORIDE; SODIUM LACTATE
SEE CALCIUM CHLORIDE; DEXTROSE; MAGNESIUM CHLORIDE; SODIUM ACETATE; SODIUM CHLORIDE
SEE CALCIUM CHLORIDE; DEXTROSE; MAGNESIUM CHLORIDE; SODIUM CHLORIDE; SODIUM LACTATE
SEE CALCIUM CHLORIDE; ICODEXTRIN; MAGNESIUM CHLORIDE; SODIUM CHLORIDE; SODIUM LACTATE
SEE CALCIUM CHLORIDE; MAGNESIUM CHLORIDE; POTASSIUM CHLORIDE; SODIUM ACETATE; SODIUM CHLORIDE
SEE CALCIUM CHLORIDE; MAGNESIUM CHLORIDE; POTASSIUM CHLORIDE; SODIUM CITRATE
SEE CALCIUM CHLORIDE; MAGNESIUM CHLORIDE; POTASSIUM CHLORIDE; SODIUM LACTATE
SEE CALCIUM CHLORIDE; MAGNESIUM CHLORIDE; POTASSIUM CHLORIDE; SODIUM CHLORIDE
SEE DEXTROSE; MAGNESIUM CHLORIDE; POTASSIUM CHLORIDE; SODIUM ACETATE
SEE DEXTROSE; MAGNESIUM CHLORIDE; POTASSIUM CHLORIDE; SODIUM CHLORIDE; SODIUM ACETATE; SODIUM
PHOSPHATE, DIBASIC; SODIUM CHLORIDE; SODIUM LACTATE; SODIUM
PHOSPHATE, MONOBASIC, ANHYDROUS
SEE DEXTROSE; MAGNESIUM CHLORIDE; POTASSIUM CHLORIDE; POTASSIUM
PHOSPHATE, DIBASIC; SODIUM CHLORIDE; SODIUM LACTATE; SODIUM
PHOSPHATE, MONOBASIC, ANHYDROUS
SEE DEXTROSE; MAGNESIUM CHLORIDE; POTASSIUM CHLORIDE; SODIUM LACTATE
SEE DEXTROSE; MAGNESIUM CHLORIDE; POTASSIUM CHLORIDE; SODIUM LACTATE; SODIUM
PHOSPHATE, MONOBASIC; SODIUM CHLORIDE; POTASSIUM
PHOSPHATE, MONOBASIC; SODIUM CHLORIDE; SODIUM PHOSPHATE,
MONOBASIC, ANHYDROUS
SEE DEXTROSE; MAGNESIUM CHLORIDE; POTASSIUM CHLORIDE; SODIUM
ACETATE; SODIUM CHLORIDE
SEE DEXTROSE; MAGNESIUM CHLORIDE; POTASSIUM CHLORIDE; SODIUM
ACETATE; SODIUM CHLORIDE; SODIUM GLUCONATE

MAGNESIUM OXIDE *MULTIPLE*

SEE CITRIC ACID; MAGNESIUM OXIDE; SODIUM CARBONATE

MAGNESIUM SULFATE

Injectable; Injection
MAGNESIUM SULFATE

AP	ABBOTT	500MG/ML	N075151 001	APR 25, 2000
AP +	AM PHARM PARTNERS	500MG/ML	N019316 001	SEP 08, 1986

MAGNESIUM SULFATE IN DEXTROSE 5% IN PLASTIC CONTAINER

+	ABBOTT	1GM/100ML	N020488 001	JUL 11, 1995
+		2GM/100ML	N020488 002	JUL 11, 1995

MAGNESIUM SULFATE (continued)

Injectable; Injection
MAGNESIUM SULFATE IN PLASTIC CONTAINER

+	ABBOTT	4GM/100ML	N020309 001	JUN 24, 1994
+		80MG/ML	N020309 002	JUN 24, 1994

MAGNESIUM SULFATE; POTASSIUM CHLORIDE; POTASSIUM PHOSPHATE, MONOBASIC; SODIUM CHLORIDE; SODIUM PHOSPHATE

Solution; Irrigation
TIS-U-SOL IN PLASTIC CONTAINER

AT	BAXTER HLTHCARE	20MG/100ML;40MG/100ML;6.25MG/100ML;800MG/100ML;8.75MG/100ML	N018336 001

TIS-U-SOL

AT	BAXTER HLTHCARE	20MG/100ML;40MG/100ML;6.25MG/100ML;800MG/100ML;8.75MG/100ML	N018508 001	FEB 19, 1982

MAGNESIUM SULFATE *MULTIPLE*

SEE CALCIUM CHLORIDE; DEXTROSE; MAGNESIUM SULFATE; POTASSIUM CHLORIDE; SODIUM BICARBONATE; SODIUM CHLORIDE; SODIUM PHOSPHATE, DIBASIC, HEPTAHYDRATE

MALATHION

Lotion; Topical
OVIDE

+	MEDICIS	0.5%	N018613 001	AUG 02, 1982

MANGAFODIPIR TRISODIUM

Injectable; Injection
TESLASCAN

+	AMERSHAM HLTH	37.9MG/ML	N020652 001	NOV 26, 1997

MANGANESE CHLORIDE

Injectable; Injection
MANGANESE CHLORIDE IN PLASTIC CONTAINER

ABBOTT	EQ 0.1MG MANGANESE/ML	N018962 001	JUN 26, 1986

MANNITOL

Injectable; Injection
MANNITOL 5%

AP	B BRAUN	5GM/100ML	N016080 001

MANNITOL 5% IN PLASTIC CONTAINER

AP	ABBOTT	5GM/100ML	N019603 001	JAN 08, 1987
AP	B BRAUN	5GM/100ML	N020006 001	JUL 26, 1993

Prescription Drug Products *(continued)*

MANNITOL *(continued)*
Injectable; Injection

TE	Manufacturer	Strength	Appl. No.
MANNITOL 5% W/ DEXTROSE 5% IN SODIUM CHLORIDE 0.12%			
AP	B BRAUN	5GM/100ML	N016080 007
MANNITOL 10%			
AP	B BRAUN	10GM/100ML	N016080 002
MANNITOL 10% IN PLASTIC CONTAINER			
AP	ABBOTT	10GM/100ML	N019603 002 JAN 08, 1987 / N020006 002 JUL 26, 1993
AP	B BRAUN	10GM/100ML	N016080 006
MANNITOL 10% W/ DEXTROSE 5% IN DISTILLED WATER			
AP	B BRAUN	10GM/100ML	N016080 003
MANNITOL 15%			
AP	B BRAUN	15GM/100ML	N019603 003 JAN 08, 1990 / N020006 003 JUL 26, 1993
MANNITOL 15% IN PLASTIC CONTAINER			
AP	ABBOTT	15GM/100ML	
AP	B BRAUN	15GM/100ML	N016080 005
MANNITOL 15% W/ DEXTROSE 5% IN SODIUM CHLORIDE 0.45%			
AP	B BRAUN	15GM/100ML	N014738 001
MANNITOL 20%			
AP	B BRAUN	20GM/100ML	N016080 004
AP	B BRAUN	20GM/100ML	
MANNITOL 20% IN PLASTIC CONTAINER			
AP	ABBOTT	20GM/100ML	N019603 004 JAN 08, 1990 / N020006 004 JUL 26, 1993
AP	B BRAUN	20GM/100ML	
MANNITOL 25%			
AP	ABBOTT	12.5GM/50ML	N016269 006 AUG 25, 1994
AP	AM PHARM PARTNERS	12.5GM/50ML	N080677 001
AP	INTL MEDICATION	12.5GM/50ML	N083051 001
AP	LUITPOLD	12.5GM/50ML	N087409 001 JAN 21, 1982
OSMITROL 5% IN WATER			
AP	BAXTER HLTHCARE	5GM/100ML	N013684 001
OSMITROL 5% IN WATER IN PLASTIC CONTAINER			
AP	BAXTER HLTHCARE	5GM/100ML	N013684 005
OSMITROL 10% IN WATER			
AP	BAXTER HLTHCARE	10GM/100ML	N013684 002
OSMITROL 10% IN WATER IN PLASTIC CONTAINER			
AP	BAXTER HLTHCARE	10GM/100ML	N013684 006
OSMITROL 15% IN WATER			
AP	BAXTER HLTHCARE	15GM/100ML	N013684 004
OSMITROL 15% IN WATER IN PLASTIC CONTAINER			
AP	BAXTER HLTHCARE	15GM/100ML	N013684 008
OSMITROL 20% IN WATER			
AP	BAXTER HLTHCARE	20GM/100ML	N013684 003
OSMITROL 20% IN WATER IN PLASTIC CONTAINER			
AP	BAXTER HLTHCARE	20GM/100ML	N013684 007
Solution; Irrigation			
RESECTISOL IN PLASTIC CONTAINER			
AP	B BRAUN	5GM/100ML	N016772 002

MANNITOL; SORBITOL
Solution; Irrigation

TE	Manufacturer	Strength	Appl. No.
SORBITOL-MANNITOL IN PLASTIC CONTAINER			
AT	ABBOTT	540MG/100ML;2.7GM/100ML	N017636 001
AT	ABBOTT	540MG/100ML;2.7GM/100ML	N018316 001

MAPROTILINE HYDROCHLORIDE
Tablet; Oral

TE	Manufacturer	Strength	Appl. No.
LUDIOMIL			
AB	NOVARTIS	25MG	N017543 001
AB	+	50MG	N017543 002
AB	+	75MG	N017543 003 SEP 30, 1982
MAPROTILINE HCL			
AB	MYLAN	25MG	N072284 001 OCT 03, 1988
AB	MYLAN	50MG	N072285 001 OCT 03, 1988
AB	MYLAN	75MG	N072286 001 OCT 03, 1988
AB	WATSON LABS	25MG	N072162 001 JUN 01, 1988
AB	WATSON LABS	50MG	N072163 001 JUN 01, 1988
AB	WATSON LABS	75MG	N072164 001 JUN 01, 1988

MEBENDAZOLE
Tablet, Chewable; Oral

TE	Manufacturer	Strength	Appl. No.
MEBENDAZOLE			
AB	COPLEY PHARM	100MG	N073580 001 JAN 04, 1995
VERMOX			
AB	+ MCNEIL CONS SPECLT	100MG	N017481 001

MECAMYLAMINE HYDROCHLORIDE
Tablet; Oral

TE	Manufacturer	Strength	Appl. No.
INVERSINE			
	+ TARGACEPT	2.5MG	N010251 001

MECHLORETHAMINE HYDROCHLORIDE
Injectable; Injection

TE	Manufacturer	Strength	Appl. No.
MUSTARGEN			
	+ MERCK	10MG/VIAL	N006695 001

MECLIZINE HYDROCHLORIDE
Tablet, Chewable; Oral

TE	Manufacturer	Strength	Appl. No.
ANTIVERT			
AA	+ PFIZER	25MG	N010721 005
MECLIZINE HCL			
AA	PLIVA	25MG	N088733 001 DEC 11, 1985
Tablet; Oral			
ANTIVERT			
AA	+ PFIZER	12.5MG	N010721 006

Prescription Drug Products (continued)

MECLIZINE HYDROCHLORIDE (continued)
Tablet; Oral

ANTIVERT

AA	+ PFIZER	25MG	N010721 004
AA	+	50MG	N010721 001
			JAN 20, 1982

MECLIZINE HCL

AA	ABC HOLDING	12.5MG	N085253 001
AA		25MG	N085252 001
AA	BUNDY	12.5MG	N084382 001
AA	GENEVA PHARMS	12.5MG	N084872 001
AA		25MG	N084843 002 MAY 22, 1989
AA		25MG	N084092 003 MAY 22, 1989
AA	IVAX PHARMS	12.5MG	N084975 001
AA	PAR PHARM	25MG	N084657 001
AA		12.5MG	N087127 001
AA		25MG	N087128 001
AA		50MG	N089674 001 MAR 31, 1988
AA	PLIVA	12.5MG	N088732 001 DEC 11, 1985
AA		25MG	N088734 001 DEC 11, 1985
AA	VINTAGE PHARMS	12.5MG	N040179 001 JAN 30, 1997
AA		25MG	N040179 002 JAN 30, 1997
AA	WATSON LABS	25MG	N085740 001

MECLOFENAMATE SODIUM
Capsule; Oral

MECLOFENAMATE SODIUM

AB	GENEVA PHARMS	EQ 50MG BASE	N072262 001 NOV 29, 1988
AB		EQ 100MG BASE	N072263 001 NOV 29, 1988
AB	MYLAN	EQ 50MG BASE	N071080 001 SEP 03, 1986
AB		EQ 100MG BASE	N071081 001 SEP 03, 1986
AB	+ WATSON LABS	EQ 50MG BASE	N071468 001 APR 15, 1987
AB		EQ 100MG BASE	N071469 001 APR 15, 1987

MEDROXYPROGESTERONE ACETATE
Injectable; Injection

DEPO-PROVERA

	+ PHARMACIA AND UPJOHN	150MG/ML	N020246 001 OCT 29, 1992
		400MG/ML	N012541 003

MEDROXYPROGESTERONE ACETATE (continued)
Tablet; Oral

MEDROXYPROGESTERONE ACETATE

AB	BARR	2.5MG	N040159 001 AUG 09, 1996
AB		5MG	N040159 002 AUG 09, 1996
AB		10MG	N040159 003 AUG 09, 1996
AB	DURAMED PHARM BARR	2.5MG	N040311 001 DEC 01, 1999
AB		5MG	N040311 002 DEC 01, 1999
AB		10MG	N040311 003 DEC 01, 1999
BP	USL PHARMA	10MG	N088484 001 JUL 26, 1984

PROVERA

AB	PHARMACIA AND UPJOHN	2.5MG	N011839 001
AB		5MG	N011839 003
AB	+	10MG	N011839 004

MEDROXYPROGESTERONE ACETATE *MULTIPLE*
SEE ESTRADIOL CYPIONATE; MEDROXYPROGESTERONE ACETATE
SEE ESTROGENS, CONJUGATED; MEDROXYPROGESTERONE ACETATE

MEDRYSONE
Suspension; Ophthalmic

HMS

	+ ALLERGAN	1%	N016624 003

MEFENAMIC ACID
Capsule; Oral

PONSTEL

	+ FIRST HORIZON	250MG	N015034 003

MEFLOQUINE HYDROCHLORIDE
Tablet; Oral

LARIAM

AB	+ ROCHE	250MG	N019591 001 MAY 02, 1989

MEFLOQUINE HCL

AB	GENEVA PHARMS	250MG	N076175 001 FEB 20, 2002

MEGESTROL ACETATE
Suspension; Oral

MEGACE

AB	+ BRISTOL MYERS SQUIBB	40MG/ML	N020264 001 SEP 10, 1993

MEGESTROL ACETATE

AB	COPLEY PHARM	40MG/ML	N075681 001 MAY 05, 2003

Prescription Drug Products (continued)

MEGESTROL ACETATE (continued)

Suspension; Oral

MEGESTROL ACETATE

TE	Firm	Strength	Appl No	Date
AB	PAR PHARM	40MG/ML	N075671 001	JUL 25, 2001
			N075997 001	FEB 15, 2002
AB	ROXANE	40MG/ML		

Tablet; Oral

MEGACE

TE	Firm	Strength	Appl No	Date
AB	BRISTOL MYERS SQUIBB	20MG	N016979 001	
AB +		40MG	N016979 002	

MEGESTROL ACETATE

TE	Firm	Strength	Appl No	Date
AB	BARR	20MG	N074621 002	AUG 16, 1996
AB		40MG	N074621 001	NOV 30, 1995
AB	PAR PHARM	20MG	N072422 001	AUG 08, 1988
AB		40MG	N072423 001	AUG 08, 1988
AB	ROXANE	20MG	N074458 001	SEP 29, 1995
AB		40MG	N074458 002	SEP 29, 1995
AB	TEVA	40MG	N074745 001	FEB 27, 1998

MELOXICAM

Tablet; Oral

MOBIC

TE	Firm	Strength	Appl No	Date
	BOEHRINGER INGELHEIM	7.5MG	N020938 001	APR 13, 2000
+		15MG	N020938 002	AUG 23, 2000

MELPHALAN

Tablet; Oral

ALKERAN

TE	Firm	Strength	Appl No	Date
AB +	GLAXOSMITHKLINE	2MG	N014691 002	

MELPHALAN HYDROCHLORIDE

Injectable; Injection

ALKERAN

TE	Firm	Strength	Appl No	Date
+	GLAXOSMITHKLINE	EQ 50MG BASE/VIAL	N020207 001	NOV 18, 1992

MENOTROPINS (FSH;LH)

Injectable; Injection

PERGONAL

TE	Firm	Strength	Appl No	Date
BX +	SERONO	75 IU/AMP;75 IU/AMP	N017646 001	

REPRONEX

TE	Firm	Strength	Appl No	Date
BX +	FERRING	75 IU/VIAL;75 IU/VIAL	N021047 001	AUG 27, 1999

MEPENZOLATE BROMIDE

Tablet; Oral

CANTIL

TE	Firm	Strength	Appl No
+	AVENT'S PHARMS	25MG	N010679 003

MEPERIDINE HYDROCHLORIDE

Injectable; Injection

DEMEROL

TE	Firm	Strength	Appl No
AP +	ABBOTT	25MG/ML	N021171 001
AP +		50MG/ML	N021171 002
AP +		75MG/ML	N021171 003
AP +		100MG/ML	N021171 004

MEPERIDINE HCL

TE	Firm	Strength	Appl No	Date
AP	BAXTER HLTHCARE CORP	25MG/ML	N080455 007	
AP		50MG/ML	N080455 008	
AP		75MG/ML	N080455 009	
AP		100MG/ML	N080455 010	
AP	ELKINS SINN	25MG/ML	N080445 001	
AP		50MG/ML	N080445 002	
AP		75MG/ML	N080445 003	
AP		100MG/ML	N080445 004	
AP	STERIS	50MG/ML	N073444 001	MAR 17, 1992
AP		100MG/ML	N073445 001	MAR 17, 1992

MEPERIDINE HCL PRESERVATIVE FREE

TE	Firm	Strength	Appl No	Date
AP +	ABBOTT	10MG/ML	N088432 001	AUG 16, 1984
AP	ASTRAZENECA	10MG/ML	N081002 001	JUL 30, 1993
AP	FAULDING	10MG/ML	N040305 001	MAR 10, 1999
AP	INTL MEDICATION	10MG/ML	N081309 001	AUG 30, 1993
AP	MALLINCKRODT	10MG/ML	N040163 001	MAY 12, 1997
AP	STERIS	10MG/ML	N073443 001	MAR 17, 1992

Syrup; Oral

DEMEROL

TE	Firm	Strength	Appl No
AA +	SANOFI SYNTHELABO	50MG/5ML	N005010 005

MEPERIDINE HCL

TE	Firm	Strength	Appl No	Date
AA	ROXANE	50MG/5ML	N088744 001	JAN 30, 1985

Tablet; Ora[l]

DEMEROL

TE	Firm	Strength	Appl No
AA +	SANOFI SYNTHELABO	50MG	N005010 001
AA		100MG	N005010 004

MEPERIDINE HCL

TE	Firm	Strength	Appl No	Date
AA	AMIDE PHARM	50MG	N040331 001	MAY 28, 1999
AA		100MG	N040331 002	MAY 28, 1999
AA	AXIOM PHARM	50MG	N080448 001	
AA		100MG	N080448 002	
AA	BARR	50MG	N088639 001	

Prescription Drug Products (continued)

MEPERIDINE HYDROCHLORIDE (continued)
Tablet; Oral

MEPERIDINE HCL

TE	Applicant	Strength	Appl. No.	Date
AA	BARR	100MG		JUL 02, 1984
AA		100MG	N088640 001	SEP 19, 1984
AA	CARACO	50MG	N040446 001	AUG 08, 2002
AA		100MG	N040446 002	AUG 08, 2002
AA	DURAMED PHARM BARR	50MG	N040318 001	OCT 05, 1999
AA		100MG	N040318 002	OCT 05, 1999
AA	MALLINCKRODT	50MG	N040352 001	JUN 13, 2000
AA		100MG	N040352 002	JUN 13, 2000
AA	ROXANE	50MG	N040110 001	MAR 12, 1997
AA		100MG	N040110 002	MAR 12, 1997
AA	VINTAGE PHARMS	50MG	N040191 001	DEC 17, 1998
AA		100MG	N040191 002	DEC 17, 1998
AA	WATSON LABS	50MG	N040186 001	JUN 30, 1997
AA		100MG	N040186 002	JUN 30, 1997

MEPERIDINE HYDROCHLORIDE *MULTIPLE*
SEE ATROPINE SULFATE; MEPERIDINE HYDROCHLORIDE

MEPIVACAINE HYDROCHLORIDE
Injectable; Injection

CARBOCAINE

TE	Applicant	Strength	Appl. No.	Date
AP	+ EASTMAN KODAK	3%	N012125 003	
AP	+ STERLING WINTHROP	1%	N012250 001	
AP	+	1.5%	N012250 005	
AP	+	2%	N012250 002	

ISOCAINE HCL

TE	Applicant	Strength	Appl. No.	Date
AP	NOVOCOL	3%	N080925 001	

MEPIVACAINE HCL

TE	Applicant	Strength	Appl. No.	Date
AP	GRAHAM CHEM	3%	N083559 001	
AP	STERIS	1%	N088769 001	NOV 20, 1984
AP		2%	N088770 001	NOV 20, 1984

POLOCAINE

TE	Applicant	Strength	Appl. No.	Date
AP	ASTRAZENECA	1%	N089407 001	DEC 01, 1986
AP		2%	N089410 001	DEC 01, 1986
AP	DENTSPLY PHARM	3%	N088653 001	AUG 21, 1984

MEPIVACAINE HYDROCHLORIDE (continued)
Injectable; Injection

POLOCAINE-MPF

TE	Applicant	Strength	Appl. No.	Date
AP	ASTRAZENECA	1%	N089406 001	DEC 01, 1986
AP		1.5%	N089408 001	DEC 01, 1986
AP		2%	N089409 001	DEC 01, 1986
AP	SCANDONEST PLAIN DEPROCO	3%	N088387 001	OCT 10, 1984

MEPIVACAINE HYDROCHLORIDE *MULTIPLE*
SEE LEVONORDEFRIN; MEPIVACAINE HYDROCHLORIDE

MEPROBAMATE
Tablet; Oral

MEPROBAMATE

TE	Applicant	Strength	Appl. No.
AA	EON	200MG	N014547 002
AA		400MG	N014547 001
AA	GENEVA PHARMS	400MG	N080655 001
AA	MYLAN	400MG	N083618 001
AA	+ ROXANE	600MG	N084332 001
AA	SCHERER LABS	400MG	N083343 001
AA	TABLICAPS	400MG	N083494 001
AA	WATSON LABS	200MG	N083304 001
AA		400MG	N085720 001
AA		200MG	N083308 001
AA		400MG	N085721 001
AA	WEST WARD	200MG	N015417 003
AA		400MG	N015417 002

MILTOWN

TE	Applicant	Strength	Appl. No.
AA	+ MEDPOINTE PHARM HLC	200MG	N009698 004
AA		400MG	N009698 002

TRANMEP

TE	Applicant	Strength	Appl. No.
AA	+ SOLVAY	400MG	N016249 001

MEPROBAMATE *MULTIPLE*
SEE ASPIRIN; MEPROBAMATE

MEQUINOL; TRETINOIN
Solution; Topical

SOLAGE

TE	Applicant	Strength	Appl. No.	Date
	+ GALDERMA LABS	2%;0.01%	N020922 001	DEC 10, 1999

MERCAPTOPURINE
Tablet; Oral

PURINETHOL

TE	Applicant	Strength	Appl. No.
	+ GLAXOSMITHKLINE	50MG	N009053 002

Prescription Drug Products *(continued)*

MEROPENEM
Injectable; Injection
MERREM I.V.

TE	Firm	Strength	Appl. No.	Date
	+ ASTRAZENECA	1GM/VIAL	N050706 001	JUN 21, 1996
	+	500MG/VIAL	N050706 003	JUN 21, 1996

MESALAMINE
Capsule, Extended Release; Oral
PENTASA

TE	Firm	Strength	Appl. No.	Date
	+ SHIRE LABS	250MG	N020049 001	MAY 10, 1993

Enema; Rectal
ROWASA

TE	Firm	Strength	Appl. No.	Date
	+ SOLVAY	4GM/60ML	N019618 001	DEC 24, 1987

Suppository; Rectal
CANASA

TE	Firm	Strength	Appl. No.	Date
	+ AXCAN SCANDIPHARM	500MG	N021252 001	JAN 05, 2001

Tablet, Delayed Release; Oral
ASACOL

TE	Firm	Strength	Appl. No.	Date
	+ PROCTER AND GAMBLE	400MG	N019651 001	JAN 31, 1992

MESNA
Injectable; Intravenous
MESNA

TE	Firm	Strength	Appl. No.	Date
AP	AM PHARM PARTNERS	100MG/ML	N075811 001	APR 26, 2001
AP	GENSIA SICOR PHARMS	100MG/ML	N075764 001	APR 27, 2001

MESNEX

TE	Firm	Strength	Appl. No.	Date
AP	+ BAXTER HLTHCARE	100MG/ML	N019884 001	DEC 30, 1988

Tablet; Oral
MESNEX

TE	Firm	Strength	Appl. No.	Date
	+ BAXTER HLTHCARE	400MG	N020855 001	MAR 21, 2002

MESNA *MULTIPLE*
SEE IFOSFAMIDE; MESNA

MESORIDAZINE BESYLATE
Concentrate; Oral
SERENTIL

TE	Firm	Strength	Appl. No.	Date
	+ NOVARTIS	EQ 25MG BASE/ML	N016997 001	

Tablet; Oral
SERENTIL

TE	Firm	Strength	Appl. No.	Date
	NOVARTIS	EQ 25MG BASE	N016774 002	
	+	EQ 100MG BASE	N016774 004	

MESTRANOL; NORETHINDRONE
Tablet; Oral-21
NORETHIN 1/50M-21

TE	Firm	Strength	Appl. No.	Date
AB	WATSON LABS	0.05MG;1MG	N071539 001	APR 12, 1988

NORETHINDRONE AND MESTRANOL

TE	Firm	Strength	Appl. No.	Date
AB	WATSCN LABS	0.05MG;1MG	N070758 001	JUL 01, 1988

NORINYL 1+50 21-DAY

TE	Firm	Strength	Appl. No.	Date
AB	WATSON LABS	0.05MG;1MG	N013625 002	

ORTHO-NOVUM 1/50 21

TE	Firm	Strength	Appl. No.	Date
AB	+ ORTHO MCNEIL PHARM	0.05MG;1MG	N012728 004	

Tablet; Oral-28
NORETHIN 1/50M-28

TE	Firm	Strength	Appl. No.	Date
AB	WATSON LABS	0.05MG;1MG	N071540 001	APR 12, 1988

NORETHINDRONE AND MESTRANOL

TE	Firm	Strength	Appl. No.	Date
AB	WATSON LABS	0.05MG;1MG	N070759 001	JUL 01, 1988

NORINYL 1+50 28-DAY

TE	Firm	Strength	Appl. No.	Date
AB	WATSON LABS	0.05MG;1MG	N016659 001	

ORTHO-NOVUM 1/50 28

TE	Firm	Strength	Appl. No.	Date
AB	+ ORTHO MCNEIL PHARM	0.05MG;1MG	N016709 001	

METAPROTERENOL SULFATE
Aerosol, Metered; Inhalation
ALUPENT

TE	Firm	Strength	Appl. No.	Date
	+ BOEHRINGER INGELHEIM	0.65MG/INH	N016402 001	

Solution; Inhalation
ALUPENT

TE	Firm	Strength	Appl. No.	Date
AN	+ BOEHRINGER INGELHEIM	0.4%	N018761 002	OCT 10, 1986
AN	+	0.6%	N018761 001	JUN 30, 1983

METAPROTERENOL SULFATE

TE	Firm	Strength	Appl. No.	Date
AN	DEY	0.4%	N071786 001	AUG 05, 1988
AN		0.6%	N070804 001	AUG 17, 1987
AN	MORTON GROVE	0.4%	N075586 001	MAY 30, 2002
AN		0.6%	N075586 002	MAY 30, 2002
AN	NEPHRON	0.4%	N071855 001	JUL 14, 1988
AN		0.6%	N071726 001	JUL 14, 1988
AN	NOVEX	0.4%	N075402 001	FEB 28, 2001
AN		0.6%	N075403 001	FEB 28, 2001

Syrup; Oral
METAPROTERENOL SULFATE

TE	Firm	Strength	Appl. No.	Date
AA	+ MORTON GROVE	10MG/5ML	N074702 001	MAR 24, 1997

Prescription Drug Products (continued)

METAPROTERENOL SULFATE (continued)

Syrup; Oral

METAPROTERENOL SULFATE

TE	Applicant	Strength	Appl. No.	Date
AA	NOVEX	10MG/5ML	N075235 001	JAN 27, 2000
AA	SILARX	10MG/5ML	N073632 001	JUL 22, 1992

Tablet; Oral

METAPROTERENOL SULFATE

TE	Applicant	Strength	Appl. No.	Date
AB	PAR PHARM	10MG	N072024 001	JUN 28, 1988
AB +		20MG	N072025 001	JUN 28, 1988
AB	TEVA	10MG	N072519 001	MAR 30, 1990
AB		20MG	N072520 001	MAR 30, 1990
AB	WATSON LABS	10MG	N073013 001	JAN 31, 1991
AB		20MG	N072795 001	JAN 31, 1991

METARAMINOL BITARTRATE

Injectable; Injection

ARAMINE

TE	Applicant	Strength	Appl. No.	Date
AP +	MERCK	EQ 10MG BASE/ML	N009509 002	DEC 22, 1987

METARAMINOL BITARTRATE

TE	Applicant	Strength	Appl. No.	Date
AP	AM PHARM PARTNERS	EQ 10MG BASE/ML	N080722 001	

METAXALONE

Tablet; Oral

SKELAXIN

TE	Applicant	Strength	Appl. No.	Date
	JONES PHARMA INC	400MG	N013217 001	
+		800MG	N013217 003	AUG 30, 2002

METFORMIN HYDROCHLORIDE

Tablet, Extended Release; Oral

GLUCOPHAGE XR

TE	Applicant	Strength	Appl. No.	Date
AB +	BRISTOL MYERS SQUIBB	500MG	N021202 001	OCT 13, 2000
AB +		750MG	N021202 004	APR 11, 2003

Tablet; Oral

GLUCOPHAGE

TE	Applicant	Strength	Appl. No.	Date
AB +	BRISTOL MYERS SQUIBB	1GM	N020357 005	NOV 05, 1998
AB		500MG	N020357 001	MAR 03, 1995
AB		850MG	N020357 002	MAR 03, 1995

METFORMIN HCL

TE	Applicant	Strength	Appl. No.	Date
AB	ALPHAPHARM	1GM	N075969 003	

METFORMIN HYDROCHLORIDE (continued)

Tablet; Oral

METFORMIN HCL

TE	Applicant	Strength	Appl. No.	Date
	ALPHAPHARM			
AB		500MG	N075969 001	JAN 29, 2002
AB		850MG	N075969 002	JAN 29, 2002
	ANDRX PHARMS			
AB		1GM	N075961 003	JAN 29, 2002
AB		500MG	N075961 001	JAN 25, 2002
AB		850MG	N075961 002	JAN 25, 2002
	BARR			
AB		1GM	N075971 003	JAN 25, 2002
AB		500MG	N075971 001	JAN 25, 2002
AB		850MG	N075971 002	JAN 25, 2002
	CARACO			
AB		1GM	N075967 003	JAN 25, 2002
AB		500MG	N075967 001	JAN 29, 2002
AB		850MG	N075967 002	JAN 29, 2002
	EON			
AB		1GM	N075965 003	JAN 29, 2002
AB		500MG	N075965 001	JAN 25, 2002
AB		850MG	N075965 002	JAN 25, 2002
	GENEVA PHARMS			
AB		1GM	N075985 003	JAN 25, 2002
AB		500MG	N075985 001	JAN 25, 2002
AB		850MG	N075985 002	JAN 25, 2002
	GENPHARM			
AB		1GM	N075973 003	JAN 25, 2002
AB		500MG	N075973 001	JAN 25, 2002
AB		850MG	N075973 002	JAN 25, 2002
	GOLDLINE			
AB		1GM	N075972 003	JAN 25, 2002
AB		500MG	N075972 001	JAN 24, 2002
AB		625MG	N075972 005	JAN 24, 2002
AB		750MG	N075972 004	JAN 24, 2002
AB		850MG	N075972 002	JAN 24, 2002
	MUTUAL PHARMA			
AB		1GM	N076038 003	FEB 21, 2002
AB		500MG	N076038 001	

Prescription Drug Products (continued)

METFORMIN HYDROCHLORIDE (continued)
Tablet; Oral

METFORMIN HCL

TE	Firm	Strength	Appl. No.	Date
	MUTUAL PHARMA			
AB		850MG	N076038 002	FEB 21, 2002
	MYLAN			
AB		1GM	N075976 003	FEB 21, 2002
AB		500MG	N075976 001	JAN 24, 2002
AB		850MG	N075976 002	JAN 24, 2002
	PUREPAC PHARM			
AB		1GM	N076033 003	JAN 24, 2002
AB		500MG	N076033 001	JAN 24, 2002
AB		850MG	N076033 002	JAN 24, 2002
	TEVA			
AB		1GM	N075978 003	JAN 24, 2002
AB		1GM	N076328 003	NOV 05, 2002
AB		500MG	N075978 001	DEC 16, 2002
AB		500MG	N076328 001	JAN 25, 2002
AB		850MG	N075978 002	DEC 16, 2002
AB		850MG	N076328 002	JAN 25, 2002
	TORPHARM			
AB		1GM	N075984 003	DEC 16, 2002
AB		500MG	N075984 001	APR 23, 2002
AB		850MG	N075984 002	APR 23, 2002
	WATSON LABS			
AB		1GM	N075979 003	APR 23, 2002
AB		500MG	N075979 001	JAN 24, 2002
AB		850MG	N075979 002	JAN 24, 2002
	ZENITH GOLDLINE			
AB		1GM	N075975 003	JAN 24, 2002
AB		500MG	N075975 001	JAN 24, 2002
AB		625MG	N075975 004	JAN 24, 2002
AB		750MG	N075975 005	JAN 24, 2002
AB		850MG	N075975 002	JAN 24, 2002

METFORMIN HYDROCHLORIDE; ROSIGLITAZONE MALEATE
Tablet; Oral

TE	Firm	Strength	Appl. No.
	AVANDAMET SB PHARMCO	500MG;EQ 1MG BASE	N021410 001

METFORMIN HYDROCHLORIDE; ROSIGLITAZONE MALEATE (continued)
Tablet; Oral

TE	Firm	Strength	Appl. No.	Date
	AVANDAMET SB PHARMCO	500MG;EQ 2MG BASE	N021410 002	OCT 10, 2002
		500MG;EQ 4MG BASE	N021410 003	OCT 10, 2002
+				OCT 10, 2002

METFORMIN HYDROCHLORIDE *MULTIPLE*
SEE GLIPIZIDE; METFORMIN HYDROCHLORIDE
SEE GLYBURIDE; METFORMIN HYDROCHLORIDE

METHACHOLINE CHLORIDE
For Solution; Inhalation

PROVOCHOLINE

TE	Firm	Strength	Appl. No.	Date
	METHAPHARM	100MG/VIAL	N019193 001	OCT 31, 1986

METHADONE HYDROCHLORIDE
Concentrate; Oral

METHADONE HCL

TE	Firm	Strength	Appl. No.	Date
AA	ROXANE	10MG/ML	N040180 001	APR 30, 1998
AA	UDL	10MG/ML	N040088 001	NOV 30, 1994

METHADONE HCL INTENSOL

TE	Firm	Strength	Appl. No.	Date
AA	ROXANE	10MG/ML	N089897 001	SEP 06, 1988

METHADOSE

TE	Firm	Strength	Appl. No.
AA +	MALLINCKRODT	10MG/ML	N017116 002

Injectable; Injection

DOLOPHINE HCL

TE	Firm	Strength	Appl. No.
+	AAIPHARMA	10MG/ML	N021624 001

Powder; For Rx Compounding

METHADONE HCL

TE	Firm	Strength	Appl. No.
	MALLINCKRODT	50GM/BOT	N006383 002
		100GM/BOT	N006383 003
		500GM/BOT	N006383 004

Solution; Oral

METHADONE HCL

TE	Firm	Strength	Appl. No.
+	ROXANE	5MG/5ML	N087393 001
+		10MG/5ML	N087997 001

Tablet; Oral

DOLOPHINE HCL

TE	Firm	Strength	Appl. No.	Date
AA +	ROXANE	5MG	N006134 002	AUG 30, 1982
AA +		10MG	N006134 010	

METHADONE HCL

TE	Firm	Strength	Appl. No.	Date
AA	EON	5MG	N040241 001	MAY 29, 1998
AA		10MG	N040241 002	MAY 29, 1998
AA		40MG	N075082 001	MAR 25, 1998

Prescription Drug Products (continued)

METHADONE HYDROCHLORIDE (continued)
Tablet; Oral

METHADONE HCL

TE	Firm	Strength	Appl. No.	Date
AA	ROXANE	5MG	N088108 001	MAR 08, 1983
AA		10MG	N088109 001	MAR 08, 1983
AA +		40MG	N017058 001	
AA		40MG	N074081 001	APR 28, 1995

METHADOSE

TE	Firm	Strength	Appl. No.	Date
AA	MALLINCKRODT	5MG	N040050 001	APR 15, 1993
AA		10MG	N040050 002	APR 15, 1993
AA		40MG	N074184 001	APR 29, 1993

METHAMPHETAMINE HYDROCHLORIDE
Tablet; Oral

DESOXYN

TE	Firm	Strength	Appl. No.
+	OVATION PHARMS	5MG	N005378 002

METHAZOLAMIDE
Tablet; Oral

METHAZOLAMIDE

TE	Firm	Strength	Appl. No.	Date
AB	COPLEY PHARM	25MG	N040001 001	JUN 30, 1993
AB		50MG	N040001 002	JUN 30, 1993
AB	GENEVA PHARMS	25MG	N040036 001	JUN 30, 1993
AB		50MG	N040036 002	JUN 30, 1993
AB	INVAMED	25MG	N040102 001	AUG 28, 1996
AB		50MG	N040102 002	AUG 28, 1996
AB	MIKART	25MG	N040062 001	JAN 27, 1994
AB +		50MG	N040062 002	JAN 27, 1994

METHENAMINE HIPPURATE
Tablet; Oral

HIPREX

TE	Firm	Strength	Appl. No.
AB +	AVENTIS PHARMS	1GM	N017681 001

METHENAMINE HIPPURATE

TE	Firm	Strength	Appl. No.	Date
AB	COREPHARMA	1GM	N076411 001	JUN 20, 2003

UREX

TE	Firm	Strength	Appl. No.
AB	3M	1GM	N016151 001

METHIMAZOLE
Tablet; Oral

METHIMAZOLE

TE	Firm	Strength	Appl. No.	Date
AB	EON	5MG	N040411 001	MAR 27, 2001
AB		10MG	N040411 002	MAR 27, 2001
AB	GENPHARM	5MG	N040350 001	MAR 29, 2000
AB		10MG	N040350 002	MAR 29, 2000
AB		20MG	N040350 003	JUN 07, 2001
AB	JONES PHARMA	5MG	N040320 001	MAR 31, 2000
AB		10MG	N040320 002	MAR 31, 2000

TAPAZOLE

TE	Firm	Strength	Appl. No.
AB	LILLY	5MG	N007517 002
AB		10MG	N007517 004

METHOCARBAMOL
Injectable; Injection

METHOCARBAMOL

TE	Firm	Strength	Appl. No.
AP	STERIS	100MG/ML	N086459 001
AP +	ROBINS AH	100MG/ML	N011790 001

Tablet; Oral

METHOCARBAMOL

TE	Firm	Strength	Appl. No.	Date
AA	ABLE	500MG	N040413 001	MAR 17, 2003
AA		750MG	N040413 002	MAR 17, 2003
AA	EON	500MG	N087283 001	
AA		750MG	N087282 001	
AA	GENEVA PHARMS	500MG	N084616 001	
AA		750MG	N084615 001	
AA	IMPAX LABS	500MG	N084927 001	
AA		750MG	N084928 001	
AA	LANNETT	750MG	N084756 002	MAR 31, 2003
AA	NYLOS	750MG	N084756 001	
AA	PAR PHARM	500MG	N085033 001	
AA		750MG	N086989 001	
AA	SUPERPHARM	500MG	N086988 001	
AA		750MG	N087589 001	
AA	TABLICAPS	750MG	N087590 001	JAN 22, 1982
AA	VINTAGE PHARMS	500MG	N084846 001	JAN 22, 1982
AA		500MG	N040489 001	
AA		750MG	N040489 002	JAN 29, 2003
AA	WATSON LABS	500MG	N084277 001	JAN 29, 2003
AA		500MG	N085180 001	
AA		750MG	N084276 002	

Prescription Drug Products (continued)

METHOCARBAMOL (continued)
Tablet; Oral

TE	METHOCARBAMOL	Strength	Appl. No.
AA	WATSON LABS	750MG	N085192 001
AA	WEST WARD	500MG	N085159 001
AA		750MG	N085123 001
	ROBAXIN		
AA	+ SCHWARZ PHARMA	500MG	N011011 004
	ROBAXIN-750		
AA	+ SCHWARZ PHARMA	750MG	N011011 006

METHOCARBAMOL *MULTIPLE*
SEE ASPIRIN; METHOCARBAMOL

METHOHEXITAL SODIUM
Injectable; Injection

	BREVITAL SODIUM	Strength	Appl. No.
	+ KING PHARMS	2.5GM/VIAL	N011559 002
	+	5GM/VIAL	N011559 003
	+	500MG/VIAL	N011559 001

METHOTREXATE SODIUM
Injectable; Injection

TE	FOLEX	Strength	Appl. No.	Date
	PHARMACIA AND UPJOHN	EQ 25MG BASE/VIAL	N087695 001	APR 08, 1983
		EQ 50MG BASE/VIAL	N087695 002	APR 08, 1983
	+	EQ 100MG BASE/VIAL	N087695 003	APR 08, 1983
	+	EQ 250MG BASE/VIAL	N088954 001	OCT 24, 1985
	METHOTREXATE			
AP	BIGMAR	EQ 25MG BASE/ML	N040263 001	FEB 26, 1999
	METHOTREXATE LPF			
AP	+ WYETH PHARMS INC	EQ 25MG BASE/ML	N011719 007	MAR 31, 1982
	METHOTREXATE PRESERVATIVE FREE			
AP	BIGMAR	EQ 1GM BASE/VIAL	N040266 001	FEB 26, 1999
AP		EQ 25MG BASE/ML	N040265 001	FEB 26, 1999
	METHOTREXATE SODIUM			
AP	BEDFORD	EQ 25MG BASE/ML	N089340 001	SEP 16, 1986
AP		EQ 25MG BASE/ML	N089341 001	SEP 16, 1986
AP		EQ 25MG BASE/ML	N089342 001	SEP 16, 1986
AP		EQ 25MG BASE/ML	N089343 001	SEP 16, 1986
AP	NORBROOK	EQ 25MG BASE/ML	N088648 001	MAY 09, 1986
AP	PHARMACHEMIE USA	EQ 25MG BASE/ML	N089158 001	

METHOTREXATE SODIUM (continued)
Injectable; Injection

TE	METHOTREXATE SODIUM	Strength	Appl. No.	Date
	PHARMACHEMIE USA			
	+ WYETH PHARMS INC	EQ 20MG BASE/VIAL	N011719 001	JUL 08, 1988
	+	EQ 25MG BASE/ML	N011719 005	
	METHOTREXATE SODIUM PRESERVATIVE FREE			
AP	+ WYETH PHARMS INC	EQ 1GM BASE/VIAL	N011719 009	APR 07, 1988
	MEXATE-AQ			
AP	BRISTOL MYERS	EQ 25MG BASE/ML	N088760 001	FEB 14, 1985

Tablet; Oral

TE	METHOTREXATE SODIUM	Strength	Appl. No.	Date
AB	BARR	EQ 2.5MG BASE	N081099 001	OCT 15, 1990
AB	+ CLONMEL HLTHCARE	EQ 2.5MG BASE	N008085 002	
AB	DURAMED PHARM BARR	EQ 2.5MG BASE	N040233 001	JUN 17, 1999
AB	MYLAN	EQ 2.5MG BASE	N081235 001	MAY 15, 1992
AB	ROXANE	EQ 2.5MG BASE	N040054 001	AUG 01, 1994
	TREXALL			
AB	BARR	EQ 5MG BASE	N040385 001	MAR 21, 2001
		EQ 7.5MG BASE	N040385 002	MAR 21, 2001
		EQ 10MG BASE	N040385 003	MAR 21, 2001
	+	EQ 15MG BASE	N040385 004	MAR 21, 2001

METHOXSALEN
Capsule; Oral

	8-MOP	Strength	Appl. No.	Date
	+ ICN	10MG	N009048 001	
	OXSORALEN-ULTRA			
	+ ICN	10MG	N019600 001	OCT 30, 1986

Injectable; Injection

	UVADEX	Strength	Appl. No.	Date
	+ THERAKOS	0.02MG/ML	N020969 001	FEB 25, 1999

Lotion; Topical

	OXSORALEN	Strength	Appl. No.
	+ ICN	1%	N009048 002

METHSCOPOLAMINE BROMIDE
Tablet; Oral

	PAMINE	Strength	Appl. No.	Date
	+ BRACLEY PHARMS	2.5MG	N008848 001	
	PAMINE FORTE			
	+ BRACLEY PHARMS	5MG	N008848 002	MAR 25, 2003

Prescription Drug Products *(continued)*

METHSUXIMIDE
Capsule; Oral
  CELONTIN
    PARKE DAVIS
    +   150MG   N010596 007
       300MG   N010596 008

METHYCLOTHIAZIDE
Tablet; Oral
  ENDURON
    +   ABBOTT
  AB   2.5MG   N012524 001
  AB   5MG   N012524 004
  METHYCLOTHIAZIDE
    GENEVA PHARMS
  AB   2.5MG   N089835 001   AUG 18, 1988
       5MG   N089837 001   AUG 18, 1988
  AB   2.5MG   N087913 001   JUN 03, 1982
    IVAX PHARMS
  AB   5MG   N087672 001   AUG 17, 1982
    MYLAN
  AB   5MG   N088724 001   SEP 06, 1984
    WATSON LABS

METHYCLOTHIAZIDE *MULTIPLE*
  SEE   DESERPIDINE; METHYCLOTHIAZIDE

METHYLDOPA
Tablet; Oral
  ALDOMET
    +   MERCK
  AB   500MG   N013400 002
  METHYLDOPA
    GENEVA PHARMS
  AB   125MG   N071700 001   MAR 02, 1988
  AB   250MG   N018934 001   JUN 29, 1984
  AB   500MG   N018934 002   JUN 29, 1984
    IVAX PHARMS
  AB   250MG   N070098 001   FEB 20, 1986
  AB   500MG   N070343 001   FEB 20, 1986
    LEDERLE
  AB   250MG   N070084 001   OCT 15, 1985
  AB   500MG   N070085 001   OCT 15, 1985
    MYLAN
  AB   250MG   N070075 001   APR 18, 1985
  AB   500MG   N070076 001   APR 18, 1985
    PAR PHARM
  AB   125MG   N070535 001   JAN 02, 1987
  AB   250MG   N070536 001   JAN 02, 1987
  AB   500MG   N070537 001   JAN 02, 1987
    PLIVA
  AB   125MG   N072126 001   JUL 07, 1988

METHYLDOPA *(continued)*
Tablet; Oral
  METHYLDOPA
    PLIVA
  AB   250MG   N072127 001   JUL 07, 1988
  AB   500MG   N072128 001   JUL 07, 1988
    SUPERPHARM
  AB   250MG   N070669 001   JUN 23, 1989
  AB   500MG   N070670 001   JUN 23, 1989
    WATSON LABS
  AB   250MG   N070703 001   JUN 06, 1986
  AB   500MG   N070625 001   JUN 06, 1986

METHYLDOPA *MULTIPLE*
  SEE   HYDROCHLOROTHIAZIDE; METHYLDOPA

METHYLDOPATE HYDROCHLORIDE
Injectable; Injection
  ALDOMET
    +   MERCK
  AP   50MG/ML   N013401 001
  METHYLDOPATE HCL
    ABBOTT
  AP   50MG/ML   N070698 001   JUN 15, 1987
  AP   50MG/ML   N070699 001   JUN 15, 1987
    GENSIA SICOR PHARMS
  AP   50MG/ML   N072974 001   NOV 22, 1991
    LUITPOLD
  AP   50MG/ML   N071279 001   OCT 02, 1987

METHYLERGONOVINE MALEATE
Injectable; Injection
  METHERGINE
    +   NOVARTIS
       0.2MG/ML   N006035 004
Tablet; Oral
  METHERGINE
    NOVARTIS
       0.2MG   N006035 003

METHYLPHENIDATE HYDROCHLORIDE
Capsule, Extended Release; Oral
  METADATE CD
  BX   +   CELLTECH PHARMS
       20MG   N021259 001   APR 03, 2001
    +   30MG   N021259 002   JUN 19, 2003
  RITALIN LA
  BX   NOVARTIS
       20MG   N021284 001   JUN 05, 2002
       30MG   N021284 002   JUN 05, 2002
    +   40MG   N021284 003   JUN 05, 2002

Prescription Drug Products (continued)

METHYLPHENIDATE HYDROCHLORIDE (continued)

Capsule, Extended Release; Oral

RITALIN LA
NOVARTIS .... JUN 05, 2002

Solution; Oral

METHYLIN

	Manufacturer	Strength	NDA	Date
	+ MALLINCKRODT BAKER	5MG/5ML	N021419 001	DEC 19, 2002
		10MG/5ML	N021419 002	DEC 19, 2002

Tablet, Chewable; Oral

METHYLIN

	Manufacturer	Strength	NDA	Date
	MALLINCKRODT	2.5MG	N021475 001	APR 15, 2003
		5MG	N021475 002	APR 15, 2003
		10MG	N021475 003	APR 15, 2003

Tablet, Extended Release; Oral

CONCERTA

	Manufacturer	Strength	NDA	Date
	+ MCNEIL CONS SPECLT	18MG	N021121 001	AUG 01, 2000
	+	27MG	N021121 004	APR 01, 2002
	+	36MG	N021121 002	AUG 01, 2000
	+	54MG	N021121 003	DEC 08, 2000

METADATE ER

	Manufacturer	Strength	NDA	Date
AB	+ CELLTECH MFG	20MG	N089601 001	JUN 01, 1988
AB	CELLTECH PHARMS	10MG	N040306 001	OCT 20, 1999

METHYLIN ER

	Manufacturer	Strength	NDA	Date
AB	MALLINCKRODT	10MG	N075629 001	MAY 09, 2000
AB		20MG	N075629 002	MAY 09, 2000

METHYLPHENIDATE HCL

	Manufacturer	Strength	NDA	Date
AB	ABLE	20MG	N076032 001	MAY 09, 2001
AB	PUREPAC PHARM	20MG	N075450 001	DEC 21, 2001
AB	WATSON LABS	20MG	N040410 001	FEB 09, 2001

RITALIN-SR

	Manufacturer	Strength	NDA	Date
AB	NOVARTIS	20MG	N018029 001	MAR 30, 1982

Tablet; Oral

METHYLPHENIDATE HCL

	Manufacturer	Strength	NDA	Date
AB	ABLE	5MG	N040404 001	MAR 29, 2001
AB		10MG	N040404 002	MAR 29, 2001
AB		20MG	N040404 003	MAR 29, 2001
AB	CELLTECH MFG	5MG	N086429 001	

METHYLPHENIDATE HYDROCHLORIDE (continued)

Tablet; Oral

METHYLPHENIDATE HCL

	Manufacturer	Strength	NDA	Date
AB	CELLTECH MFG	10MG	N085799 001	
AB		20MG	N086428 001	
AB	MALLINCKRODT	5MG	N040300 001	NOV 27, 1998
AB		10MG	N040300 002	NOV 27, 1998
AB		20MG	N040300 003	NOV 27, 1998
AB	PUREPAC PHARM	5MG	N040321 001	FEB 05, 2002
AB		10MG	N040321 002	FEB 05, 2002
AB		20MG	N040321 003	FEB 05, 2002
AB	WATSON LABS	5MG	N040220 001	AUG 29, 1997
AB		10MG	N040220 002	AUG 29, 1997
AB		20MG	N040220 003	AUG 29, 1997

RITALIN

	Manufacturer	Strength	NDA	Date
AB	NOVARTIS	5MG	N010187 003	
AB		10MG	N010187 006	
AB	+	20MG	N010187 010	

METHYLPREDNISOLONE

Tablet; Oral

MEDROL

	Manufacturer	Strength	NDA	Date
AB	PHARMACIA AND UPJOHN	2MG	N011153 002	
AB		4MG	N011153 001	
AB		8MG	N011153 004	
AB		16MG	N011153 003	
		24MG	N011153 005	
		32MG	N011153 006	

METHYLPREDNISOLONE

	Manufacturer	Strength	NDA	Date
	+ DURAMED PHARM BARR	4MG	N088497 001	FEB 21, 1984
AB	GENEVA PHARMS	4MG	N040194 001	OCT 31, 1997
AB	PAR PHARM	16MG	N089207 001	APR 25, 1988
AB		24MG	N089208 001	APR 25, 1988
AB		32MG	N089209 001	APR 25, 1988
AB	TRIGEN	4MG	N040189 001	OCT 31, 1997
AB		8MG	N040189 002	OCT 31, 1997
AB	VINTAGE PHARMS	4MG	N040183 001	DEC 22, 1998
AB	WATSON LABS	4MG	N040232 001	OCT 16, 1997

Prescription Drug Products (continued)

METHYLPREDNISOLONE ACETATE

Injectable; Injection

DEPO-MEDROL

	Firm	Strength	Appl. No.	Date
BP	PHARMACIA AND UPJOHN	20MG/ML	N011757 002	
		40MG/ML	N011757 001	
+		80MG/ML	N011757 004	

METHYLPREDNISOLONE SODIUM SUCCINATE

Injectable; Injection

A-METHAPRED

	Firm	Strength	Appl. No.	Date
AP	ABBOTT	EQ 1GM BASE/VIAL	N085852 001	
AP		EQ 1GM BASE/VIAL	N089174 001	AUG 18, 1987
AP		EQ 40MG BASE/VIAL	N085853 001	
AP		EQ 125MG BASE/VIAL	N085855 001	
AP		EQ 500MG BASE/VIAL	N085854 001	
AP		EQ 500MG BASE/VIAL	N089173 001	AUG 18, 1987

METHYLPREDNISOLONE SODIUM SUCCINATE

	Firm	Strength	Appl. No.	Date
AP	GENSIA SICOR PHARMS	EQ 125MG BASE/VIAL	N081266 001	NOV 30, 1992

SOLU-MEDROL

	Firm	Strength	Appl. No.	Date
AP +	PHARMACIA AND UPJOHN	EQ 1GM BASE/VIAL	N011856 006	
+		EQ 2GM BASE/VIAL	N011856 007	FEB 27, 1985
+		EQ 40MG BASE/VIAL	N011856 003	
AP +		EQ 125MG BASE/VIAL	N011856 004	
AP +		EQ 500MG BASE/VIAL	N011856 005	

METHYLTESTOSTERONE

Capsule; Oral

TESTRED

	Firm	Strength	Appl. No.	Date
BP +	ICN	10MG	N083976 001	

VIRILON

	Firm	Strength	Appl. No.	Date
BP	STAR PHARMS FL	10MG	N087750 001	NOV 24, 1982

Tablet; Oral

ANDROID 10

	Firm	Strength	Appl. No.	Date
AB	ICN	10MG	N086450 001	

ANDROID 25

	Firm	Strength	Appl. No.	Date
AB +	ICN	25MG	N087147 001	

METHYLTESTOSTERONE

	Firm	Strength	Appl. No.	Date
BP	IMPAX LABS	10MG	N080767 002	
BP		25MG	N084310 001	

METIPRANOLOL HYDROCHLORIDE

Solution/Drops; Ophthalmic

METIPRANOLOL

	Firm	Strength	Appl. No.	Date
AT	FALCON PHARMS	0.3%	N075720 001	AUG 06, 2001

OPTIPRANOLOL

	Firm	Strength	Appl. No.	Date
AT +	BAUSCH AND LOMB	0.3%	N019907 001	DEC 29, 1989

METOCLOPRAMIDE HYDROCHLORIDE

Concentrate: Oral

METOCLOPRAMIDE INTENSOL

	Firm	Strength	Appl. No.	Date
	ROXANE	EQ 10MG BASE/ML	N072995 001	JAN 30, 1992

Injectable; Injection

METOCLOPRAMIDE HCL

	Firm	Strength	Appl. No.	Date
AP	ABBOTT	EQ 5MG BASE/ML	N070505 001	JUN 23, 1989
			N073117 001	JAN 17, 1991
AP		EQ 5MG BASE/ML	N073118 001	JAN 17, 1991
AP		EQ 5MG BASE/ML	N074147 001	AUG 02, 1996
AP	FAULDING	EQ 5MG BASE/ML	N070847 001	NOV 07, 1988
AP		EQ 5MG BASE/ML	N071291 001	MAR 03, 1989
AP	GENSIA SICOR PHARMS	EQ 5MG BASE/ML	N073135 001	NOV 27, 1991

REGLAN

	Firm	Strength	Appl. No.	Date
AP +	ROBINS AH	EQ 5MG BASE/ML	N017862 001	

Solution; Oral

METOCLOPRAMIDE

	Firm	Strength	Appl. No.	Date
AA	JVL	EQ 5MG BASE/5ML	N074703 001	OCT 31, 1997
AA	VISTAPHARM	EQ 5MG BASE/5ML	N075051 001	JAN 26, 2001

METOCLOPRAMIDE HCL

	Firm	Strength	Appl. No.	Date
AA	ALPHARMA	EQ 5MG BASE/5ML	N071340 001	AUG 18, 1988
AA	PHARM ASSOC	EQ 5MG BASE/5ML	N072744 001	MAY 28, 1991
AA	PHARM VENTURES	EQ 5MG BASE/5ML	N071402 001	JUN 25, 1993
AA	ROXANE	EQ 5MG BASE/5ML	N072038 001	DEC 05, 1988
AA	SILARX	EQ 5MG BASE/5ML	N073680 001	OCT 27, 1992
AA +	TEVA	EQ 5MG BASE/5ML	N070819 001	JUL 10, 1987
AA		EQ 5MG BASE/5ML	N071315 001	JUN 30, 1993

Tablet; Oral

METOCLOPRAMIDE HCL

	Firm	Strength	Appl. No.	Date
AB	GENEVA PHARMS	EQ 10MG BASE	N072215 001	JAN 30, 1990
AB	GENEVA PHARMS TECH	EQ 5MG BASE	N074478 001	OCT 05, 1995
AB		EQ 10MG BASE	N074478 002	OCT 05, 1995
AB	PLIVA	EQ 5MG BASE	N072750 001	DEC 28, 1995
AB	PUREPAC PHARM	EQ 10MG BASE	N071250 001	FEB 03, 1988
AB			N070581 001	

Prescription Drug Products *(continued)*

METOCLOPRAMIDE HYDROCHLORIDE *(continued)*

Tablet; Oral

METOCLOPRAMIDE HCL

TE	Firm	Strength	Appl. No.	Date
AB	PUREPAC PHARM	EQ 5MG BASE		OCT 17, 1985
AB	TEVA	EQ 5MG BASE	N072801 001	JUN 15, 1993
AB		EQ 10MG BASE	N070184 001	JUL 29, 1985
AB	WATSON LABS	EQ 10MG BASE	N070511 001	JAN 22, 1986

REGLAN

TE	Firm	Strength	Appl. No.	Date
AB	SCHWARZ PHARMA	EQ 5MG BASE	N017854 002	MAY 05, 1987
AB +		EQ 10MG BASE	N017854 001	

METOLAZONE

Tablet; Oral

MYKROX

TE	Firm	Strength	Appl. No.	Date
AB +	CELLTECH PHARMS	0.5MG	N019532 001	OCT 30, 1987

ZAROXOLYN

TE	Firm	Strength	Appl. No.	Date
AB +	CELLTECH PHARMS	2.5MG	N017386 001	
		5MG	N017386 002	
AB +		10MG	N017386 003	

METOPROLOL SUCCINATE

Tablet, Extended Release; Oral

TOPROL-XL

TE	Firm	Strength	Appl. No.	Date
	ASTRAZENECA	EQ 25MG TARTRATE	N019962 004	FEB 05, 2001
		EQ 50MG TARTRATE	N019962 001	JAN 10, 1992
			N019962 002	JAN 10, 1992
+		EQ 100MG TARTRATE	N019962 002	JAN 10, 1992
+		EQ 200MG TARTRATE	N019962 003	JAN 10, 1992

METOPROLOL TARTRATE

Injectable; Injection

LOPRESSOR

TE	Firm	Strength	Appl. No.	Date
AP +	NOVARTIS	1MG/ML	N018704 001	MAR 30, 1984

METOPROLOL TARTRATE

TE	Firm	Strength	Appl. No.	Date
AP	ABBOTT	1MG/ML	N074133 001	DEC 21, 1993
AP		1MG/ML	N075160 001	JUL 06, 1998
AP	STERIS	1MG/ML	N074032 001	DEC 21, 1993

Tablet; Oral

LOPRESSOR

TE	Firm	Strength	Appl. No.	Date
AB	NOVARTIS	50MG	N017963 001	
AB +		100MG	N017963 002	

METOPROLOL TARTRATE

TE	Firm	Strength	Appl. No.	Date
AB	APOTHECON	50MG	N074258 001	JAN 27, 1994

METOPROLOL TARTRATE *(continued)*

Tablet; Oral

METOPROLOL TARTRATE

TE	Firm	Strength	Appl. No.	Date
AB	APOTHECON	100MG	N074258 002	JAN 27, 1994
AB	CARACO	50MG	N074644 001	DEC 10, 1996
AB		100MG	N074644 002	DEC 10, 1996
AB	COPLEY PHARM	50MG	N074333 001	JAN 27, 1994
AB		100MG	N074333 002	JAN 27, 1994
AB	GENEVA PHARMS	50MG	N073288 001	MAR 25, 1994
AB		100MG	N073289 001	MAR 25, 1994
AB	MUTUAL PHARM	50MG	N073653 001	DEC 21, 1993
AB		100MG	N073654 001	DEC 21, 1993
AB	MYLAN	50MG	N073666 001	DEC 21, 1993
AB		100MG	N073666 002	DEC 21, 1993
AB	PAR PHARM	50MG	N074453 001	APR 27, 1995
AB		100MG	N074453 002	APR 27, 1995
AB	TEVA	50MG	N074141 001	JAN 31, 1995
AB		50MG	N074143 001	SEP 30, 1994
AB		100MG	N074141 002	JAN 31, 1995
AB		100MG	N074143 002	SEP 30, 1994
AB	WATSON LABS	50MG	N074217 001	MAY 27, 1994
AB		100MG	N074217 002	MAY 27, 1994

METOPROLOL TARTRATE *MULTIPLE*

SEE HYDROCHLOROTHIAZIDE; METOPROLOL TARTRATE

METRONIDAZOLE

Capsule; Oral

FLAGYL

TE	Firm	Strength	Appl. No.	Date
+	GD SEARLE LLC	375MG	N020334 001	MAY 03, 1995

Cream; Topical

METROCREAM

TE	Firm	Strength	Appl. No.	Date
+	GALDERMA LABS LP	0.75%	N020531 001	SEP 20, 1995

NORITATE

TE	Firm	Strength	Appl. No.	Date
+	DERMIK LABS	1%	N020743 001	

Prescription Drug Products *(continued)*

METRONIDAZOLE *(continued)*

Cream; Topical
  NORITATE
    DERMIK LABS   SEP 26, 1997

Gel; Topical
  METROGEL
  + GALDERMA LABS LP   0.75%   N019737 001   NOV 22, 1988

Gel; Vaginal
  METROGEL-VAGINAL
  + 3M   0.75%   N020208 001   AUG 17, 1992

Injectable; Injection
  FLAGYL I.V. RTU IN PLASTIC CONTAINER
  AP + BAXTER HLTHCARE   500MG/100ML
  AP + GD SEARLE LLC   500MG/100ML
  METRO I.V. IN PLASTIC CONTAINER
  AP + B BRAUN   500MG/100ML   N018900 001   SEP 29, 1983
  METRONIDAZOLE IN PLASTIC CONTAINER
  AP + ABBOTT   500MG/100ML   N018890 002   NOV 18, 1983

Lotion; Topical
  METROLOTION
  + GALDERMA LABS LP   0.75%   N020901 001   NOV 24, 1998

Tablet, Extended Release; Oral
  FLAGYL ER
  AB + GD SEARLE LLC   750MG   N020868 001   NOV 26, 1997
  METRONIDAZOLE
  AB ABLE   750MG   N076462 001   JUN 25, 2003

Tablet; Oral
  FLAGYL
  AB + GD SEARLE LLC   250MG   N012623 001
  AB   500MG   N012623 003
  METRONIDOL
  + LABS AF   250MG   N074523 001   OCT 24, 1996
  AB   500MG   N074523 002   OCT 24, 1996
  METRONIDAZOLE
  AB ABLE   250MG   N076519 001   JUN 27, 2003
  AB   500MG   N076519 002   JUN 27, 2003
  AB EON   250MG   N018620 001   MAR 04, 1982
  AB   500MG   N018620 002   JUN 02, 1983
  AB GENEVA PHARMS   250MG   N018740 001   OCT 22, 1982
  AB   500MG   N018740 002   OCT 22, 1982
  AB IVAX PHARMS   250MG   N018517 001
  AB   500MG   N018517 002

METRONIDAZOLE *(continued)*

Tablet; Oral
  METRONIDAZOLE
    IVAX PHARMS
  AB LNK   250MG   N019029 001   MAY 05, 1982
  AB MUTUAL PHARM   250MG   N070772 001   APR 10, 1984
  AB   500MG   N070773 001   JUL 16, 1986
  AB PAR PHARM   250MG   N018845 001   JUL 16, 1986
  AB   250MG   N070040 001   AUG 18, 1983
  AB   500MG   N018930 001   JAN 29, 1985
  AB   500MG   N070039 001   AUG 18, 1983
  AB PLIVA   250MG   N070027 001   JAN 29, 1985
  AB   500MG   N070033 001   NOV 06, 1984
  AB TEVA   250MG   N070035 001   DEC 06, 1984
  AB   500MG   N070044 001   DEC 20, 1984
  AB WATSON LABS   250MG   N018764 001   FEB 08, 1985
  AB   500MG   N018764 002   SEP 17, 1982
     DEC 20, 1982

METRONIDAZOLE *MULTIPLE*
  SEE BISMUTH SUBSALICYLATE; METRONIDAZOLE; TETRACYCLINE HYDROCHLORIDE

METRONIDAZOLE HYDROCHLORIDE
Injectable; Injection
  FLAGYL I.V.
  + GD SEARLE LLC   EQ 500MG BASE/VIAL   N018353 001

METYRAPONE
Capsule; Oral
  METOPIRONE
  + NOVARTIS   250MG   N012911 002   AUG 09, 1996

METYROSINE
Capsule; Oral
  DEMSER
  + MERCK   250MG   N017871 001

MEXILETINE HYDROCHLORIDE
Capsule; Oral
  MEXILETINE HCL
  AB GENEVA PHARMS   150MG   N074450 001

Prescription Drug Products (continued)

MEXILETINE HYDROCHLORIDE (continued)

Capsule; Oral

MEXILETINE HCL

TE Code	Firm	Strength	Appl. No.	Date
	GENEVA PHARMS			
AB		200MG	N074450 002	MAY 16, 1996
AB		250MG	N074450 003	MAY 16, 1996
	TEVA			
AB		150MG	N074377 001	MAY 16, 1996
AB		200MG	N074377 002	MAY 16, 1995
AB		250MG	N074377 003	MAY 16, 1995
	WATSON LABS			
AB		150MG	N074711 001	MAY 16, 1995
AB		150MG	N074865 001	FEB 26, 1997
AB		200MG	N074711 002	APR 13, 1998
AB		200MG	N074865 002	FEB 26, 1997
AB		250MG	N074711 003	APR 13, 1998
AB		250MG	N074865 003	FEB 26, 1997

MEXITIL

TE Code	Firm	Strength	Appl. No.	Date
	BOEHRINGER INGELHEIM			
AB		150MG	N018873 002	DEC 30, 1985
AB		200MG	N018873 003	DEC 30, 1985
AB +		250MG	N018873 004	DEC 30, 1985

MICONAZOLE NITRATE

Cream; Topical

MONISTAT-DERM

TE Code	Firm	Strength	Appl. No.	Date
+	JOHNSON AND JOHNSON	2%	N017494 001	

Suppository; Vaginal

MICONAZOLE NITRATE

TE Code	Firm	Strength	Appl. No.	Date
	ALPHARMA US PHARM			
AB		200MG	N073508 001	NOV 19, 1993

MONISTAT 3

TE Code	Firm	Strength	Appl. No.	Date
AB +	ORTHO MCNEIL PHARM	200MG	N018888 001	AUG 15, 1984

MIDAZOLAM HYDROCHLORIDE

Injectable; Injection

MIDAZOLAM HCL

TE Code	Firm	Strength	Appl. No.	Date
	+ ABBOTT			
AP		EQ 1MG BASE/ML	N075293 001	JUN 20, 2000
AP		EQ 1MG BASE/ML	N075409 002	JUN 20, 2000
AP		EQ 1MG BASE/ML	N075857 001	JUN 20, 2000

MIDAZOLAM HYDROCHLORIDE (continued)

Injectable; Injection

MIDAZOLAM HCL

TE Code	Firm	Strength	Appl. No.	Date
	ABBOTT			
AP +		EQ 5MG BASE/ML	N075293 002	JUL 22, 2002
AP		EQ 5MG BASE/ML	N075409 001	JUN 20, 2000
AP		EQ 5MG BASE/ML	N075857 002	JUN 20, 2000
	AM PHARM PARTNERS			
AP		EQ 1MG BASE/ML	N075154 002	JUL 22, 2002
AP		EQ 5MG BASE/ML	N075154 001	JUN 20, 2000
	APOTEX			
AP		EQ 1MG BASE/ML	N075637 001	JUN 20, 2000
AP		EQ 5MG BASE/ML	N075637 002	OCT 31, 2000
	BAXTER HLTHCARE			
AP		EQ 1MG BASE/ML	N075243 001	OCT 31, 2000
AP		EQ 5MG BASE/ML	N075243 002	JUN 20, 2000
	BAXTER HLTHCARE CORP			
AP		EQ 1MG BASE/ML	N075324 001	JUN 20, 2000
AP		EQ 5MG BASE/ML	N075324 002	JUN 20, 2000
	BEDFORD			
AP		EQ 1MG BASE/ML	N075247 002	JUN 20, 2000
AP		EQ 5MG BASE/ML	N075247 001	JUN 23, 2000
	BEN VENUE			
AP		EQ 1MG BASE/ML	N075421 002	JUN 23, 2000
AP		EQ 5MG BASE/ML	N075421 001	JUN 20, 2000
	FAULDING			
AP		EQ 1MG BASE/ML	N075396 001	JUN 20, 2000
AP		EQ 5MG BASE/ML	N075396 002	JUN 20, 2000
	ROSS LABS			
AP		EQ 5MG BASE/ML	N075484 001	JUN 20, 2000
AP		EQ 1MG BASE/ML	N075856 001	JUN 20, 2000
	TAYLOR			
AP		EQ 5MG BASE/ML	N075856 002	JUN 13, 2002
	TAYLOR PHARMA			
AP		EQ 1MG BASE/ML	N075481 001	JUN 13, 2002
AP		EQ 5MG BASE/ML	N075494 001	JUN 30, 2000
AP		EQ 5MG BASE/ML	N075494 002	JUN 30, 2000

Syrup; Oral

MIDAZOLAM HCL

TE Code	Firm	Strength	Appl. No.	Date
	RANBAXY			
AA		EQ 2MG BASE/ML	N076058 001	MAR 15, 2002
	ROXANE			
AA +		EQ 2MG BASE/ML	N075873 001	APR 30, 2002

Prescription Drug Products (continued)

MIDODRINE HYDROCHLORIDE
Tablet; Oral

	PROAMATINE			
	SHIRE PHARM	2.5MG	N019815 001	SEP 06, 1996
		5MG	N019815 002	SEP 06, 1996
+		10MG	N019815 003	MAR 20, 2002

MIFEPRISTONE
Tablet; Oral

	MIFEPREX			
+	DANCO LABS LLC	200MG	N020687 001	SEP 28, 2000

MIGLITOL
Tablet; Oral

	GLYSET			
	PHARMACIA AND UPJOHN	25MG	N020682 001	DEC 18, 1996
		50MG	N020682 002	DEC 18, 1996
+		100MG	N020682 003	DEC 18, 1996

MILRINONE LACTATE
Injectable; Injection

MILRINONE LACTATE

AP	ABBOTT	EQ 1MG BASE/ML	N075884 001	MAY 28, 2002
AP	AM PHARM PARTNERS	EQ 1MG BASE/ML	N075936 001	MAY 28, 2002
AP	BAXTER HLTHCARE	EQ 1MG BASE/ML	N075530 001	MAY 28, 2002
AP	BAXTER HLTHCARE CORP	EQ 1MG BASE/ML	N075852 001	MAY 28, 2002
AP	BEDFORD	EQ 10MG BASE /10ML (10MG/ML)	N075660 001	MAY 28, 2002
AP	BIONICHE (CANADA)	EQ 1MG BASE/ML	N076428 001	JUN 16, 2003
AP	FAULDING	EQ 1MG BASE/ML	N075830 001	MAY 28, 2002
AP	INTL MEDICATED	EQ 1MG BASE/ML	N076013 001	AUG 02, 2002

MILRINONE LACTATE IN DEXTROSE 5% IN PLASTIC CONTAINER

AP	ABBOTT	EQ 20MG BASE/100ML	N075885 001	MAY 28, 2002
AP	BAXTER HLTHCARE	EQ 20MG BASE/100ML	N075834 001	MAY 28, 2002
AP		EQ 40MG BASE/200ML	N075834 002	MAY 28, 2002
AP	ESI LEDERLE	EQ 20MG BASE/100ML	N075510 001	MAY 28, 2002

MILRINONE LACTATE (continued)
Injectable; Injection

MILRINONE LACTOSE IN 5% DEXTROSE

AP	ESI LEDERLE	EQ 20MG BASE/100ML	N076259 001	AUG 08, 2002

PRIMACOR

AP	+ SANOFI SYNTHELABO	EQ 1MG BASE/ML	N019436 001	DEC 31, 1987

PRIMACOR IN DEXTROSE 5% IN PLASTIC CONTAINER

AP	+ SANOFI SYNTHELABO	EQ 20MG BASE/100ML	N020343 003	AUG 09, 1994
AP	+	EQ 40MG BASE/200ML	N020343 004	AUG 09, 1994

MINOCYCLINE HYDROCHLORIDE
Capsule; Oral

MINOCIN

AB	WYETH PHARMS INC	EQ 50MG BASE	N050649 001	MAY 31, 1990
AB		EQ 75MG BASE	N050649 003	FEB 12, 2001
AB		EQ 100MG BASE	N050649 002	MAY 31, 1990

MINOCYCLINE HCL

AB	IMPAX LABS	EQ 50MG BASE	N065005 001	MAR 23, 1999
AB		EQ 75MG BASE	N065005 003	APR 18, 2001
AB		EQ 100MG BASE	N065005 002	MAR 23, 1999
AB	RANBAXY	EQ 50MG BASE	N065062 001	NOV 30, 2000
AB		EQ 75MG BASE	N065062 002	NOV 30, 2000
AB		EQ 100MG BASE	N065062 003	NOV 30, 2000
AB	TEVA	EQ 50MG BASE	N063011 001	MAR 02, 1992
AB		EQ 100MG BASE	N063009 001	MAR 02, 1992
AB	WATSON LABS	EQ 50MG BASE	N063181 001	DEC 30, 1991
AB		EQ 75MG BASE	N063065 002	JUN 10, 1999
AB		EQ 100MG BASE	N063065 001	DEC 30, 1991

VECTRIN

AB	MEDICIS	EQ 50MG BASE	N063066 001	AUG 14, 1990

Injectable; Injection

MINOCIN

	+ WYETH PHARMS INC	EQ 100MG BASE/VIAL	N050444 001	

Powder, Extended Release; Dental

ARESTIN

	+ ORAPHARMA	EQ 1MG BASE	N050781 001	FEB 16, 2001

Prescription Drug Products (continued)

MINOCYCLINE HYDROCHLORIDE (continued)

Tablet; Oral

TE	Applicant	Strength	Appl No	Approval
	MINOCYCLINE HCL			
	PAR PHARM	EQ 50MG BASE	N065131 001	APR 16, 2003
		EQ 75MG BASE	N065131 002	APR 16, 2003
+		EQ 100MG BASE	N065131 003	APR 16, 2003

MINOXIDIL

Tablet; Oral

TE	Applicant	Strength	Appl No	Approval
	LONITEN			
AB	PHARMACIA AND UPJOHN	2.5MG	N018154 001	
		10MG	N018154 003	
	+ MINOXIDIL			
AB	MUTUAL PHARM	2.5MG	N072708 001	DEC 14, 1995
		10MG	N072709 001	DEC 14, 1995
AB	PAR PHARM	2.5MG	N071826 001	NOV 14, 1988
		10MG	N071839 001	NOV 14, 1988
AB	WATSON LABS	2.5MG	N071344 001	MAR 03, 1987
AB		10MG	N071345 001	MAR 03, 1987

MIRTAZAPINE

Tablet, Orally Disintegrating; Oral

TE	Applicant	Strength	Appl No	Approval
	REMERON SOLTAB			
	+ ORGANON USA INC	15MG	N021208 001	JAN 12, 2001
		30MG	N021208 002	JAN 12, 2001
		45MG	N021208 003	JAN 12, 2001

Tablet; Oral

TE	Applicant	Strength	Appl No	Approval
	MIRTAZAPINE			
AB	ALPHAPHARM	15MG	N076176 001	JUN 19, 2003
AB		30MG	N076176 002	JUN 19, 2003
AB		45MG	N076176 003	JUN 19, 2003
AB	AMIDE PHARM	15MG	N076241 001	JUN 25, 2003
AB		30MG	N076241 002	JUN 25, 2003
AB		45MG	N076241 003	JUN 25, 2003
AB	ANDRX PHARMS	15MG	N076336 001	JUN 20, 2003
AB		30MG	N076336 002	JUN 20, 2003

MIRTAZAPINE (continued)

Tablet; Oral

TE	Applicant	Strength	Appl No	Approval
	MIRTAZAPINE			
AB	ANDRx PHARMS	45MG	N076336 003	JUN 20, 2003
AB	EON	15MG	N076219 001	JUN 20, 2003
AB		30MG	N076219 002	JUN 19, 2003
AB		45MG	N076219 003	JUN 19, 2003
AB	GENEVA PHARMS	15MG	N076189 001	JUN 19, 2003
AB		30MG	N076189 002	JUN 19, 2003
AB		45MG	N076189 003	JUN 19, 2003
AB	MYLAN	15MG	N076122 001	JUN 19, 2003
AB		30MG	N076122 002	JUN 19, 2003
AB		45MG	N076122 003	JUN 19, 2003
AB	PUREPAC PHARM	15MG	N076308 001	JUN 20, 2003
AB		30MG	N076308 002	JUN 20, 2003
AB		45MG	N076308 003	JUN 20, 2003
AB	ROXANE	15MG	N076270 001	JUN 19, 2003
AB		30MG	N076270 002	JUN 19, 2003
AB		45MG	N076270 003	JUN 19, 2003
AB	TEVA	15MG	N076119 001	JUN 19, 2003
AB		30MG	N076119 002	JAN 24, 2003
AB		45MG	N076119 003	JAN 24, 2003
AB	WATSON LABS	15MG	N076312 001	JUN 19, 2003
AB		30MG	N076312 002	JUN 19, 2003
AB		45MG	N076312 003	JUN 19, 2003
	REMERON			
	+ ORGANON USA INC	15MG	N020415 001	JUN 14, 1996
AB		30MG	N020415 002	JUN 14, 1996
AB		45MG	N020415 003	MAR 17, 1997

Prescription Drug Products *(continued)*

MISOPROSTOL
Tablet; Oral
CYTOTEC
AB	GD SEARLE LLC	0.1MG	N019268 003	SEP 21, 1990
AB	+	0.2MG	N019268 001	DEC 27, 1988

MISOPROSTOL
AB	IVAX PHARMS	0.1MG	N076095 001	JUL 10, 2002
AB		0.2MG	N076095 002	JUL 10, 2002

MISOPROSTOL *MULTIPLE*
SEE DICLOFENAC SODIUM; MISOPROSTOL

MITOMYCIN
Injectable; Injection
MITOMYCIN
AP	BEDFORD	5MG/VIAL	N064117 001	APR 19, 1995
AP		20MG/VIAL	N064117 002	APR 19, 1995
AP	ESI LEDERLE	5MG/VIAL	N064180 001	DEC 23, 1999
AP		20MG/VIAL	N064180 002	DEC 23, 1999
AP	FAULDING	20MG/VIAL	N064106 001	NOV 29, 1995
AP	SUPERGEN	5MG/VIAL	N064144 001	APR 30, 1998
AP		20MG/VIAL	N064144 002	APR 30, 1998

MUTAMYCIN
AP	+ BRISTOL MYERS	5MG/VIAL	N062336 001	
AP	+	20MG/VIAL	N062336 002	
		40MG/VIAL	N062336 003	MAR 10, 1988

MYTOZYTREX
AP	+ SUPERGEN	5MG/VIAL	N050763 001	NOV 14, 2002

MITOTANE
Tablet; Oral
LYSODREN
+ BRISTOL	500MG	N016885 001	

MITOXANTRONE HYDROCHLORIDE
Injectable; Injection
NOVANTRONE
+ SERONO INC	EQ 2MG BASE/ML	N019297 001	DEC 23, 1987

MIVACURIUM CHLORIDE
Injectable; Injection
MIVACRON
+ ABBOTT	EQ 2MG BASE/ML	N020098 001	JAN 22, 1992

MIVACRON IN DEXTROSE 5% IN PLASTIC CONTAINER
+ ABBOTT	EQ 50MG BASE/100ML	N020098 003	JAN 22, 1992

MODAFINIL
Tablet; Oral
PROVIGIL
CEPHALON	100MG	N020717 001	DEC 24, 1998
+	200MG	N020717 002	DEC 24, 1998

MOEXIPRIL HYDROCHLORIDE
Tablet; Oral
MOEXIPRIL HCL
AB	TEVA	7.5MG	N076204 001	MAY 08, 2003
AB		15MG	N076204 002	MAY 08, 2003

UNIVASC
AB	SCHWARZ PHARMA	7.5MG	N020312 001	APR 19, 1995
AB	+	15MG	N020312 002	APR 19, 1995

MOEXIPRIL HYDROCHLORIDE *MULTIPLE*
SEE HYDROCHLOROTHIAZIDE; MOEXIPRIL HYDROCHLORIDE

MOLINDONE HYDROCHLORIDE
Concentrate; Oral
MOBAN
+ ENDO PHARMS	20MG/ML	N017938 001

Tablet; Oral
MOBAN
ENDO PHARMS	5MG	N017111 004
	10MG	N017111 005
	25MG	N017111 006
	50MG	N017111 007
+	100MG	N017111 008

MOMETASONE FUROATE
Cream; Topical
ELOCON
+ SCHERING	0.1%	N019625 001	MAY 06, 1987

Lotion; Topical
ELOCON
+ SCHERING	0.1%	N019796 001	MAR 30, 1989

Prescription Drug Products *(continued)*

MOMETASONE FUROATE *(continued)*
Ointment; Topical

TE	Firm	Strength	Appl. No.	Date
	ELOCON			
AB	+ SCHERING	0.1%	N019543 001	APR 30, 1987
	MOMETASONE FUROATE			
AB	CLAY PARK	0.1%	N076067 001	MAR 18, 2002

MOMETASONE FUROATE MONOHYDRATE
Spray, Metered; Nasal

TE	Firm	Strength	Appl. No.	Date
	NASONEX			
	+ SCHERING PLOUGH	EQ 0.05MG BASE/SPRAY	N020762 001	OCT 01, 1997

MONOBENZONE
Cream; Topical

TE	Firm	Strength	Appl. No.	Date
	BENOQUIN			
	+ ICN	20%	N008173 003	

MONTELUKAST SODIUM
Granule; Oral

TE	Firm	Strength	Appl. No.	Date
	SINGULAIR			
	+ MERCK	EQ 4MG BASE/PACKET	N021409 001	JUL 26, 2002

Tablet, Chewable; Oral

TE	Firm	Strength	Appl. No.	Date
	SINGULAIR			
	+ MERCK	EQ 4MG BASE	N020830 002	MAR 03, 2000
	+	EQ 5MG BASE	N020830 001	

Tablet; Oral

TE	Firm	Strength	Appl. No.	Date
	SINGULAIR			
	+ MERCK	EQ 10MG BASE	N020829 002	FEB 20, 1998

MORICIZINE HYDROCHLORIDE
Tablet; Oral

TE	Firm	Strength	Appl. No.	Date
	ETHMOZINE			
	SHIRE LABS	200MG	N019753 001	JUN 19, 1990
		250MG	N019753 002	JUN 19, 1990
		300MG	N019753 003	JUN 19, 1990

MORPHINE SULFATE
Capsule, Extended Release; Oral

TE	Firm	Strength	Appl. No.	Date
	AVINZA			
BX	+ LIGAND	30MG	N021260 001	MAR 20, 2002
BX	+	60MG	N021260 002	MAR 20, 2002
	+	90MG	N021260 003	MAR 20, 2002

MORPHINE SULFATE *(continued)*
Capsule, Extended Release; Oral

TE	Firm	Strength	Appl. No.	Date
	AVINZA			
	+ LIGAND	120MG	N021260 004	MAR 20, 2002
	KADIAN			
	+ FAULDING PHARMS	20MG	N020616 001	JUL 03, 1996
		30MG	N020616 004	MAR 09, 2001
BX	+	50MG	N020616 002	JUL 03, 1996
	+	60MG	N020616 005	MAR 09, 2001
BX	+	100MG	N020616 003	JUL 03, 1996

Injectable; Injection

TE	Firm	Strength	Appl. No.	Date
	ASTRAMORPH PF			
	ASTRAZENECA			
AP		0.5MG/ML	N071050 001	OCT 07, 1986
AP		0.5MG/ML	N071051 001	OCT 07, 1986
AP		1MG/ML	N071052 001	OCT 07, 1986
AP		1MG/ML	N071053 001	OCT 07, 1986
	DURAMORPH PF			
AP	+ ELKINS SINN	0.5MG/ML	N018565 001	SEP 18, 1984
AP	+	1MG/ML	N018565 002	SEP 18, 1984
	INFUMORPH			
AP	+ ELKINS SINN	10MG/ML	N018565 003	JUL 19, 1991
AP	+	25MG/ML	N018565 004	JUL 19, 1991
	MORPHINE SULFATE			
AP	+ ABBOTT	0.5MG/ML	N019917 001	OCT 30, 1992
AP		0.5MG/ML	N071849 001	MAY 11, 1988
AP		0.5MG/ML	N073509 001	SEP 30, 1992
AP		1MG/ML	N019916 001	OCT 30, 1992
AP		1MG/ML	N071850 001	MAY 11, 1988
AP		1MG/ML	N073510 001	SEP 30, 1992
AP	+ MALLINCKRODT	1MG/ML	N020631 001	JUL 03, 1996
AP	+	2MG/ML	N020631 002	JUL 03, 1996
AP	+ MERIDIAN MEDCL TECHN	15MG/ML	N019999 001	JUL 12, 1990
AP	STERIS	0.5MG/ML	N073373 001	

Prescription Drug Products (continued)

MORPHINE SULFATE (continued)

Injectable; Injection

MORPHINE SULFATE
  STERIS

AP	0.5MG/ML	N073375 001	SEP 30, 1991
AP	1MG/ML	N073374 001	SEP 30, 1991
AP	1MG/ML	N073376 001	SEP 30, 1991

Tablet, Extended Release; Oral

MORPHINE SULFATE
  AB GENERICS

AB	15MG	N074862 001	JUL 07, 1998
AB	30MG	N074862 002	JUL 07, 1998
AB	60MG	N074862 003	JUL 07, 1998
AB	100MG	N074769 001	JUL 02, 1998
AB	200MG	N074769 002	JUL 02, 1998

  ENDO PHARMS

AB	15MG	N075295 001	OCT 28, 1998
AB	30MG	N075295 002	OCT 28, 1998
AB	60MG	N075295 003	OCT 28, 1998
AB	100MG	N075295 004	SEP 15, 2000
AB	200MG	N075295 005	SEP 15, 2000

  ESI LEDERLE

AB	15MG	N075407 001	JAN 28, 2000

  WATSON LABS

AB	100MG	N075656 001	JAN 30, 2001

MS CONTIN
  PURDUE FREDERICK

AB	15MG	N019516 003	SEP 12, 1989
AB	30MG	N019516 001	MAY 29, 1987
AB +	60MG	N019516 002	APR 08, 1988
AB	100MG	N019516 004	JAN 16, 1990
AB	200MG	N019516 005	NOV 08, 1993

ORAMORPH SR
  ELAN PHARMS

BC	15MG	N019977 004	NOV 23, 1994
BC	30MG	N019977 001	AUG 15, 1991
BC	60MG	N019977 002	AUG 15, 1991
BC	100MG	N019977 003	AUG 15, 1991

MOXIFLOXACIN HYDROCHLORIDE

Injectable; Iv (Infusion)

AVELOX IN SODIUM CHLORIDE 0.8% IN PLASTIC CONTAINER

+ BAYER PHARMS	160MG/100ML	N021277 001	NOV 30, 2001

Solution/Drops; Ophthalmic

VIGAMOX

+ ALCON	0.5%	N021598 001	APR 15, 2003

Tablet; Oral

AVELOX

+ BAYER PHARMS	EQ 400MG BASE	N021085 001	DEC 10, 1999

MUPIROCIN

Ointment; Topical

BACTROBAN

BX	+ GLAXOSMITHKLINE	2%	N050591 001	DEC 31, 1987

MUPIROCIN

BX	JOHNSON AND JOHNSON	2%	N050788 001	DEC 04, 2002

MUPIROCIN CALCIUM

Cream, Augmented; Topical

BACTROBAN

+ GLAXOSMITHKLINE	2%	N050746 001	DEC 11, 1997

Ointment; Nasal

BACTROBAN

+ GLAXOSMITHKLINE	EQ 2% BASE	N050703 001	SEP 18, 1995

MYCOPHENOLATE MOFETIL

Capsule; Oral

CELLCEPT

+ ROCHE PALO	250MG	N050722 001	MAY 03, 1995

Suspension; Oral

CELLCEPT

+ ROCHE PALO	200MG/ML	N050759 001	OCT 01, 1998

Tablet; Oral

CELLCEPT

+ ROCHE PALO	500MG	N050723 001	JUN 19, 1997

MYCOPHENOLATE MOFETIL HYDROCHLORIDE

Injectable; Injection

CELLCEPT

+ ROCHE PALO	500MG/VIAL	N050758 001	AUG 12, 1998

Prescription Drug Products (continued)

NABUMETONE
Tablet; Oral

NABUMETONE

TE	Firm	Strength	Appl. No.	Date
AB	COPLEY PHARM	750MG	N075179 001	JUN 06, 2000
AB	EON	500MG	N075280 001	FEB 25, 2002
AB		750MG	N075280 002	FEB 25, 2002
AB	INVAMED	500MG	N075590 001	FEB 25, 2002
AB		750MG	N075590 002	FEB 25, 2002
AB	IVAX PHARMS	500MG	N076009 001	JAN 24, 2003
AB		750MG	N076009 002	JAN 24, 2003
AB	TEVA	500MG	N075189 001	MAY 26, 2000
AB		750MG	N075189 002	SEP 24, 2001

RELAFEN

TE	Firm	Strength	Appl. No.	Date
AB +	GLAXOSMITHKLINE	500MG	N019583 001	DEC 24, 1991
AB		750MG	N019583 002	DEC 24, 1991

NADOLOL
Tablet; Oral

CORGARD

TE	Firm	Strength	Appl. No.	Date
AB	APOTHECON	20MG	N018063 005	OCT 28, 1986
AB		40MG	N018063 001	
AB		80MG	N018063 002	
AB		120MG	N018063 003	
AB		160MG	N018063 004	

NADOLOL

TE	Firm	Strength	Appl. No.	Date
AB +	COPLEY PHARM	80MG	N074368 001	AUG 31, 1994
AB		120MG	N074368 002	AUG 31, 1994
AB		160MG	N074368 003	AUG 31, 1994
AB	GENEVA PHARMS TECH	20MG	N074501 001	AUG 31, 1994
AB		40MG	N074501 002	NOV 09, 1995
AB		80MG	N074501 003	NOV 09, 1995
AB	IVAX PHARMS	20MG	N074229 001	NOV 09, 1995
AB		40MG	N074229 002	AUG 30, 1996
AB		80MG	N074255 001	AUG 30, 1996
AB		120MG	N074255 002	JAN 24, 1996

NADOLOL (continued)
Tablet; Oral

NADOLOL

TE	Firm	Strength	Appl. No.	Date
AB	IVAX PHARMS	160MG	N074255 003	JAN 24, 1996
AB	MYLAN	20MG	N074172 001	OCT 31, 1993
AB		40MG	N074172 002	OCT 31, 1993
AB		80MG	N074172 003	OCT 31, 1993

NADOLOL *MULTIPLE*
SEE BENDROFLUMETHIAZIDE; NADOLOL

NAFARELIN ACETATE
Spray, Metered; Nasal

SYNAREL

TE	Firm	Strength	Appl. No.	Date
+	GD SEARLE LLC	EQ 0.2MG BASE/SPRAY	N019886 001	FEB 13, 1990

NAFCILLIN SODIUM
Injectable; Injection

NAFCILLIN SODIUM

TE	Firm	Strength	Appl. No.	Date
AP	APOTHECON	EQ 1GM BASE/VIAL	N062527 002	AUG 02, 1984
AP		EQ 1GM BASE/VIAL	N062732 001	DEC 23, 1986
AP		EQ 2GM BASE/VIAL	N062527 003	AUG 02, 1984
AP		EQ 2GM BASE/VIAL	N062732 002	DEC 23, 1986
AP		EQ 10GM BASE/VIAL	N062527 004	AUG 02, 1984
+		EQ 500MG BASE/VIAL	N062527 001	AUG 02, 1984

NALLPEN IN PLASTIC CONTAINER

TE	Firm	Strength	Appl. No.	Date
+	BAXTER HLTHCARE	EQ 2GM BASE/100ML	N050655 002	OCT 31, 1989
+		EQ 20MG BASE/ML	N050655 001	OCT 31, 1989

NALBUPHINE HYDROCHLORIDE
Injectable; Injection

NALBUP-IINE HCL

TE	Firm	Strength	Appl. No.	Date
AP	ABBOTT	10MG/ML	N070914 001	FEB 03, 1989
AP		10MG/ML	N070915 001	FEB 03, 1989
AP		20MG/ML	N070916 001	FEB 03, 1989
AP		20MG/ML	N070917 001	FEB 03, 1989
AP		20MG/ML	N070918 001	FEB 03, 1989

Prescription Drug Products *(continued)*

NALBUPHINE HYDROCHLORIDE *(continued)*
Injectable; Injection

NUBAIN

AP	+ ENDO PHARMS	10MG/ML	N018024 001	
AP	+	20MG/ML	N018024 002	MAY 27, 1982

NALIDIXIC ACID
Tablet; Oral

NALIDIXIC ACID

AB	WATSON LABS	1GM	N071919 001	JUN 29, 1988
		250MG	N071936 001	JUN 29, 1988
AB		500MG	N072061 001	JUN 29, 1988

NEGGRAM

AB	+ SANOFI SYNTHELABO	1GM	N014214 005	
AB		250MG	N014214 002	
AB		500MG	N014214 004	

NALMEFENE HYDROCHLORIDE
Injectable; Injection

REVEX

AP	+ BAXTER HLTHCARE CORP	EQ 0.1MG BASE/ML	N020459 001	APR 17, 1995
AP	+	EQ 1MG BASE/ML	N020459 002	APR 17, 1995

NALOXONE HYDROCHLORIDE
Injectable; Injection

NALOXONE HCL

AP	ABBOTT	0.02MG/ML	N070171 001	SEP 24, 1986
AP		0.02MG/ML	N070252 001	JAN 16, 1987
AP		0.02MG/ML	N070253 001	JAN 16, 1987
AP		0.4MG/ML	N070254 001	JAN 07, 1987
AP		0.4MG/ML	N070255 001	JAN 07, 1987
AP		0.4MG/ML	N070256 001	JAN 07, 1987
AP		0.4MG/ML	N070257 001	JAN 07, 1987

INTL MEDICATION

AP		0.4MG/ML	N070639 001	SEP 24, 1986
AP		1MG/ML	N072076 001	MAR 24, 1988

NARCAN

AP	+ ENDO PHARMS	0.02MG/ML	N016636 002	
AP	+	0.4MG/ML	N016636 001	
AP	+	1MG/ML	N016636 003	JUN 14, 1982

NALOXONE HYDROCHLORIDE; PENTAZOCINE HYDROCHLORIDE
Tablet; Oral

NALOXONE HCL AND PENTAZOCINE

AB	AMIDE PHARM	EQ 0.5MG BASE;EQ 50MG BASE	N075735 001	JUL 11, 2001

PENTAZOCINE AND NALOXONE HYDROCHLORIDES

AB	RANBAXY	EQ 0.5MG BASE;EQ 50MG BASE	N075523 001	MAR 17, 2000
AB	WATSON LABS	EQ 0.5MG BASE;EQ 50MG BASE	N074736 001	JAN 21, 1997

TALWIN NX

AB	+ SANOFI SYNTHELABO	EQ 0.5MG BASE;EQ 50MG BASE	N018733 001	DEC 16, 1982

NALOXONE HYDROCHLORIDE *MULTIPLE*
SEE BUPRENORPHINE HYDROCHLORIDE; NALOXONE HYDROCHLORIDE

NALTREXONE HYDROCHLORIDE
Tablet; Oral

NALTREXONE HCL

AB	AMIDE PHARM	50MG	N075274 001	MAY 26, 1999
AB	BARR	50MG	N074918 001	MAY 08, 1998
AB	EON	50MG	N075434 001	MAR 08, 2000
	MALLINCKRODT	25MG	N076264 001	MAR 22, 2002
		50MG	N076264 002	MAR 22, 2002
AB	+	100MG	N076264 003	MAR 22, 2002

REVIA

AB	+ BARR PHARMS	50MG	N018932 001	NOV 20, 1984

NANDROLONE DECANOATE
Injectable; Injection

NANDROLONE DECANOATE

	+ STERIS	50MG/ML	N086385 001	JAN 13, 1984
	+	100MG/ML	N086598 001	JAN 13, 1984
	+	200MG/ML	N088128 001	JAN 13, 1984

NAPHAZOLINE HYDROCHLORIDE
Solution/Drops; Ophthalmic

ALBALON

AT	+ ALLERGAN	0.1%	N080248 001	

NAFAZAIR

AT	BAUSCH AND LOMB	0.1%	N040073 001	MAY 25, 1994

NAPHAZOLINE HCL

AT	TAYLOR	0.1%	N083590 001	

Prescription Drug Products (continued)

NAPHAZOLINE HYDROCHLORIDE (continued)
Solution/Drops; Ophthalmic

	VASOCON			
AT	NOVARTIS	0.1%	N080235 002	MAR 24, 1983

NAPROXEN
Suspension; Oral

	NAPROSYN			
AB +	ROCHE PALO	25MG/ML	N018965 001	MAR 23, 1987

	NAPROXEN			
	ROXANE			
AB		25MG/ML	N074190 001	MAR 30, 1994

Tablet, Delayed Release; Oral

	EC-NAPROSYN			
AB +	ROCHE PALO	375MG	N020067 002	OCT 14, 1994
AB +		500MG	N020067 003	OCT 14, 1994

	NAPROXEN			
	GENEVA PHARMS TECH			
AB		375MG	N075061 001	FEB 18, 1998
AB		500MG	N075061 002	FEB 18, 1998
AB	PLIVA	375MG	N075337 001	FEB 18, 1998
AB		500MG	N075337 002	MAY 26, 1999
				MAY 26, 1999
AB	PUREPAC PHARM	375MG	N074936 001	FEB 24, 1998
AB		500MG	N074936 002	FEB 24, 1998
AB	TEVA	375MG	N075227 001	JUN 30, 1998
AB		500MG	N075227 002	JUN 30, 1998

Tablet, Extended Release; Oral

	NAPROXEN			
	ALPHAPHARM			
AB +		375MG	N075390 001	APR 19, 2001
AB +		500MG	N075390 002	APR 19, 2001

Tablet; Oral

	NAPROSYN			
	ROCHE PALO			
AB +		250MG	N017581 002	
AB +		375MG	N017581 003	
AB +		500MG	N017581 004	APR 15, 1982

	NAPROXEN			
	CLONMEL HLTHCARE			
AB		250MG	N074410 001	APR 28, 1995
AB		375MG	N074410 002	APR 28, 1995
AB		500MG	N074410 003	APR 28, 1995
AB	COPLEY PHARM	250MG	N074207 001	APR 28, 1995

NAPROXEN (continued)
Tablet; Oral

	NAPROXEN			
	COPLEY PHARM			
AB		375MG	N074207 002	DEC 21, 1993
AB		500MG	N074207 003	DEC 21, 1993
AB	GENEVA PHARMS	250MG	N074140 001	DEC 21, 1993
AB		375MG	N074140 002	DEC 21, 1993
AB		500MG	N074140 003	DEC 21, 1993
AB	INTERPHARM	250MG	N075927 001	DEC 18, 2001
AB		375MG	N075927 002	DEC 18, 2001
AB		500MG	N075927 003	DEC 18, 2001
AB	IVAX PHARMS	250MG	N074111 001	DEC 18, 2001
AB		375MG	N074111 002	FEB 28, 1995
AB		500MG	N074111 003	FEB 28, 1995
AB	LEDERLE	250MG	N074105 001	FEB 28, 1995
AB		375MG	N074105 002	DEC 21, 1993
AB		500MG	N074105 003	DEC 21, 1993
AB	MYLAN	250MG	N074121 001	DEC 21, 1993
AB		375MG	N074121 002	DEC 21, 1993
AB		500MG	N074121 003	DEC 21, 1993
AB	PLIVA	250MG	N074182 001	DEC 21, 1993
AB		375MG	N074182 002	JUN 27, 1996
AB		500MG	N074182 003	JUN 27, 1996
AB	PUREPAC PHARM	250MG	N074263 001	JUN 27, 1996
AB		375MG	N074263 002	DEC 21, 1993
AB		500MG	N074263 003	DEC 21, 1993
AB	ROXANE	250MG	N074211 001	DEC 21, 1993
AB		375MG	N074211 002	FEB 28, 1994
AB		500MG	N074211 003	FEB 28, 1994
AB	TEVA	250MG	N074129 001	FEB 28, 1994

Prescription Drug Products (continued)

NAPROXEN (continued)
Tablet; Oral
NAPROXEN

TE	Firm	Strength	Approval Date	Appl. No.
	TEVA			
AB		250MG	DEC 21, 1993	N074201 001
AB		250MG	DEC 21, 1993	N074216 001
AB		375MG	APR 11, 1996	N074129 002
AB		375MG	DEC 21, 1993	N074201 002
AB		375MG	DEC 21, 1993	N074216 002
AB		500MG	APR 11, 1996	N074129 003
AB		500MG	DEC 21, 1993	N074201 003
AB		500MG	DEC 21, 1993	N074216 003
	WATSON LABS			
AB		250MG	APR 11, 1996	N074163 001
AB		250MG	FEB 10, 1995	N074457 001
AB		375MG	MAY 31, 1995	N074163 002
AB		375MG	FEB 10, 1995	N074457 002
AB		500MG	MAY 31, 1995	N074163 003
AB		500MG	FEB 10, 1995	N074457 003
AB		500MG	MAY 31, 1995	

NAPROXEN SODIUM
Tablet, Extended Release; Oral

TE	Firm	Strength	Appl. No.	Approval Date
	NAPRELAN			
AB	+ ELAN PHARMA	EQ 375MG BASE	N020353 001	JAN 05, 1996
AB	+	EQ 500MG BASE	N020353 002	JAN 05, 1996
	NAPROXEN SODIUM			
	ANDRX PHARMS			
AB		EQ 375MG BASE	N075416 002	APR 23, 2003
AB		EQ 500MG BASE	N075416 001	AUG 27, 2002

Tablet; Oral

TE	Firm	Strength	Appl. No.	Approval Date
	ANAPROX			
AB	ROCHE PALO	EQ 250MG BASE	N018164 001	
	ANAPROX DS			
AB	+ ROCHE PALO	EQ 500MG BASE	N018164 003	SEP 30, 1987
	NAPROXEN SODIUM			
	AL HIKMA			
AB		EQ 250MG BASE	N074480 002	FEB 18, 1998
AB		EQ 500MG BASE	N074480 001	MAY 14, 1996
	COPLEY PHARM			
AB		EQ 250MG BASE	N074289 001	

NAPROXEN SODIUM (continued)
Tablet; Oral
NAPROXEN SODIUM

TE	Firm	Strength	Approval Date	Appl. No.
	COPLEY PHARM			
AB		EQ 500MG BASE	JAN 27, 1994	N074289 002
	GENEVA PHARMS			
AB		EQ 250MG BASE	JAN 27, 1994	N074162 001
AB		EQ 500MG BASE	DEC 21, 1993	N074162 002
	GENEVA PHARMS TECH			
AB		EQ 250MG BASE	DEC 21, 1993	N074495 001
AB		EQ 500MG BASE	DEC 05, 1994	N074495 002
	IVAX PHARMS			
AB		EQ 250MG BASE	DEC 05, 1994	N074230 001
AB		EQ 500MG BASE	MAR 14, 1995	N074230 002
	MYLAN			
AB		EQ 250MG BASE	MAR 14, 1995	N074367 001
AB		EQ 500MG BASE	AUG 31, 1994	N074367 002
	PLIVA			
AB		EQ 250MG BASE	AUG 31, 1994	N074242 001
AB		EQ 500MG BASE	JUN 20, 1996	N074242 002
	ROXANE			
AB		EQ 250MG BASE	JUN 20, 1996	N074257 001
AB		EQ 500MG BASE	DEC 21, 1993	N074257 002
	TEVA			
AB		EQ 250MG BASE	DEC 21, 1993	N074142 001
AB		EQ 500MG BASE	DEC 21, 1993	N074142 002
AB		EQ 250MG BASE	DEC 21, 1993	N074198 001
AB		EQ 500MG BASE	DEC 21, 1993	N074198 002
	WATSON LABS			
AB		EQ 250MG BASE	DEC 21, 1993	N074195 001
AB		EQ 250MG BASE	DEC 21, 1993	N074455 001
AB		EQ 500MG BASE	MAY 31, 1995	N074195 002
AB		EQ 500MG BASE	DEC 21, 1993	N074455 002
			MAY 31, 1995	

NARATRIPTAN HYDROCHLORIDE
Tablet; Oral

TE	Firm	Strength	Appl. No.	Approval Date
	AMERGE			
	GLAXOSMITHKLINE			
	+	EQ 1MG BASE	N020763 002	FEB 10, 1998
		EQ 2.5MG BASE	N020763 001	FEB 10, 1998

Prescription Drug Products (continued)

NATAMYCIN
Suspension; Ophthalmic
NATACYN
+ ALCON   5%   N050514 001

NATEGLINIDE
Tablet; Oral
STARLIX
NOVARTIS   60MG   N021204 001   DEC 22, 2000
+   120MG   N021204 002   DEC 22, 2000

NEDOCROMIL SODIUM
Aerosol, Metered; Inhalation
TILADE
+ AVENTIS   1.75MG/INH   N019660 001   DEC 30, 1992

Solution/Drops; Ophthalmic
ALOCRIL
+ ALLERGAN   2%   N021009 001   DEC 08, 1999

NEFAZODONE HYDROCHLORIDE
Tablet; Oral
SERZONE
BRISTOL MYERS SQUIBB   50MG   N020152 001   DEC 22, 1994
   100MG   N020152 002   DEC 22, 1994
   150MG   N020152 003   DEC 22, 1994
   200MG   N020152 004   DEC 22, 1994
+   250MG   N020152 005   DEC 22, 1994

NELFINAVIR MESYLATE
For Suspension; Oral
VIRACEPT
+ AGOURON   EQ 50MG BASE/SCOOPFUL   N020778 001   MAR 14, 1997

Tablet; Oral
VIRACEPT
+ AGOURON   EQ 250MG BASE   N020779 001   MAR 14, 1997
+   EQ 625MG BASE   N021503 001   APR 30, 2003

NEOMYCIN SULFATE
Powder; For Rx Compounding
NEO-RX
AA   PHARMA TEK   100%   N061579 001

NEOMYCIN SULFATE (continued)
Solution; Oral
NEO-FRADIN
+ PHARMATEK   EQ 87.5MG BASE/5ML   N065010 001   MAY 23, 2002

Tablet; Oral
NEOMYCIN SULFATE
+ TEVA   EQ 350MG BASE   N060304 001

NEOMYCIN SULFATE; POLYMYXIN B SULFATE
Solution; Irrigation
NEOSPORIN G.U. IRRIGANT
+ MONARCH PHARMS   EQ 40MG BASE/ML;200,000 UNITS/ML   N060707 001

NEOMYCIN SULFATE; POLYMYXIN B SULFATE; PREDNISOLONE ACETATE
Suspension/Drops; Ophthalmic
POLY-PRED
+ ALLERGAN   EQ 0.35% BASE;10,000 UNITS/ML;0.5%   N050081 002

NEOMYCIN SULFATE *MULTIPLE*
SEE BACITRACIN; HYDROCORTISONE ACETATE; NEOMYCIN SULFATE; POLYMYXIN B SULFATE
SEE BACITRACIN ZINC; HYDROCORTISONE; NEOMYCIN SULFATE; POLYMYXIN B SULFATE
SEE BACITRACIN ZINC; NEOMYCIN SULFATE; POLYMYXIN B SULFATE
SEE COLISTIN SULFATE; HYDROCORTISONE ACETATE; NEOMYCIN SULFATE; THONZONIUM BROMIDE
SEE DEXAMETHASONE; NEOMYCIN SULFATE; POLYMYXIN B SULFATE
SEE GRAMICIDIN; NEOMYCIN SULFATE; POLYMYXIN B SULFATE
SEE HYDROCORTISONE; NEOMYCIN SULFATE; POLYMYXIN B SULFATE
SEE HYDROCORTISONE ACETATE; NEOMYCIN SULFATE; POLYMYXIN B SULFATE

NESIRITIDE
For Solution; Intravenous
NATRECOR
+ SCIOS   1.5MG/VIAL   N020920 001   AUG 10, 2001

NEVIRAPINE
Suspension; Oral
VIRAMUNE
+ BOEHRINGER INGELHEIM   50MG/5ML   N020933 001   SEP 11, 1998

Tablet; Oral
VIRAMUNE
+ BOEHRINGER INGELHEIM   200MG   N020636 001   JUN 21, 1996

Prescription Drug Products (continued)

NIACIN

Tablet, Extended Release; Oral

NIASPAN

+	KOS	1GM	N020381 004 JUL 28, 1997
+		500MG	N020381 002 JUL 28, 1997
+		750MG	N020381 003 JUL 28, 1997

Tablet; Oral

NIACIN

AA	MK LABS	500MG	N083525 001
AA	TABLICAPS	500MG	N084237 001
AA	WOCKHARDT	500MG	N081134 001 APR 28, 1992

NIACOR

AA	UPSHER SMITH	500MG	N040378 001 MAY 03, 2000

NICOLAR

AA	+ AVENTIS	500MG	N083823 001

NIACIN *MULTIPLE*
SEE   LOVASTATIN; NIACIN

NIACINAMIDE *MULTIPLE*
SEE   ALPHA-TOCOPHEROL ACETATE; ASCORBIC ACID; BIOTIN; CHOLECALCIFEROL; CYANOCOBALAMIN; DEXPANTHENOL; FOLIC ACID; NIACINAMIDE; PYRIDOXINE HYDROCHLORIDE; RIBOFLAVIN PHOSPHATE SODIUM; THIAMINE HYDROCHLORIDE; VITAMIN A PALMITATE; VITAMIN K

SEE   ASCORBIC ACID; BIOTIN; CHOLECALCIFEROL; CYANOCOBALAMIN; DEXPANTHENOL; FOLIC ACID; NIACINAMIDE; PYRIDOXINE; RIBOFLAVIN; THIAMINE; TOCOPHEROL ACETATE; VITAMIN A; VITAMIN K

SEE   ASCORBIC ACID; BIOTIN; CYANOCOBALAMIN; DEXPANTHENOL; ERGOCALCIFEROL; FOLIC ACID; NIACINAMIDE; PHYTONADIONE; PYRIDOXINE HYDROCHLORIDE; RIBOFLAVIN PHOSPHATE SODIUM; THIAMINE HYDROCHLORIDE; VITAMIN A; VITAMIN E

SEE   ASCORBIC ACID; BIOTIN; CYANOCOBALAMIN; DEXPANTHENOL; ERGOCALCIFEROL; FOLIC ACID; NIACINAMIDE; PYRIDOXINE HYDROCHLORIDE; RIBOFLAVIN PHOSPHATE SODIUM; THIAMINE HYDROCHLORIDE; VITAMIN A; VITAMIN E

NICARDIPINE HYDROCHLORIDE

Capsule, Extended Release; Oral

CARDENE SR

+	ROCHE PALO	30MG	N020005 001 FEB 21, 1992
+		45MG	N020005 002 FEB 21, 1992
+		60MG	N020005 003 FEB 21, 1992

Capsule; Oral

CARDENE

AB	+ ROCHE PALO	20MG	N019488 001 DEC 21, 1988
AB	+	30MG	N019488 002 DEC 21, 1988

NICARDIPINE HYDROCHLORIDE (continued)

Capsule; Oral

NICARDIPINE HCL

AB	GENPHARM	20MG	N074928 001 MAR 19, 1998
AB		30MG	N074928 002 MAR 19, 1998
AB	IVAX PHARMS	20MG	N074439 001 DEC 10, 1996
AB		30MG	N074439 002 DEC 10, 1996
AB	MYLAN	20MG	N074642 001 JUL 18, 1996
AB		30MG	N074642 002 JUL 18, 1996
AB	TEVA	20MG	N074540 001 OCT 28, 1996
AB		30MG	N074540 002 OCT 28, 1996
AB	WATSON LABS	20MG	N074670 001 OCT 28, 1996
AB		30MG	N074670 002 OCT 28, 1996

Injectable; Injection

CARDENE

+	ROCHE PALO	2.5MG/ML	N019734 001 JAN 30, 1992

NICOTINE

Film, Extended Release; Transdermal

NICOTINE

	SANO	7MG/24HR	N074645 001 OCT 20, 1997
		14MG/24HR	N074611 001 OCT 20, 1997
		21MG/24HR	N074612 001 OCT 20, 1997

Spray, Metered; Nasal

NICOTROL

+	PHARMACIA AND UPJOHN	0.5MG/SPRAY	N020385 001 MAR 22, 1996

NIFEDIPINE

Capsule; Oral

NIFEDIPINE

AB	FLEMINGTON PHARM	10MG	N072781 001 JUL 30, 1993
AB	PUREPAC PHARM	10MG	N072579 001 JAN 08, 1991
AB		20MG	N072556 001 SEP 20, 1990
AB	SCHERER RP	10MG	N073250 001 OCT 08, 1991
AB		20MG	N074045 001 APR 30, 1992

Prescription Drug Products (continued)

NIFEDIPINE (continued)

Capsule; Oral

TE Code	Brand	Firm	Strength	Appl No	Date
	NIFEDIPINE				
AB		TEVA	10MG	N072651 001	FEB 19, 1992
	PROCARDIA				
AB		PFIZER	10MG	N018482 001	
AB	+		20MG	N018482 002	JUL 24, 1986

Tablet, Extended Release; Oral

TE Code	Brand	Firm	Strength	Appl No	Date
	ADALAT CC	BAYER PHARMS			
AB1			30MG	N020198 001	APR 21, 1993
AB1	+		60MG	N020198 002	APR 21, 1993
AB1	+		90MG	N020198 003	APR 21, 1993
	NIFEDIPINE	BIOVAIL			
AB1			30MG	N075269 001	DEC 04, 2000
AB2			30MG	N075289 002	FEB 06, 2001
AB1			60MG	N075269 002	DEC 04, 2000
AB2			60MG	N075289 001	SEP 27, 2000
AB1			90MG	N076070 001	AUG 16, 2002
	ELAN PHARM				
AB1			30MG	N075128 001	MAR 10, 2000
AB1			60MG	N075659 001	OCT 26, 2001
	PROCARDIA XL				
AB2	+	PFIZER	30MG	N019684 001	SEP 06, 1989
AB2	+		60MG	N019684 002	SEP 06, 1989
BC	+		90MG	N019684 003	SEP 06, 1989

NILUTAMIDE

Tablet; Oral

TE Code	Brand	Firm	Strength	Appl No	Date
	NILANDRON				
	+	AVENTIS PHARMS	150MG	N020169 002	APR 30, 1999

NIMODIPINE

Capsule; Oral

TE Code	Brand	Firm	Strength	Appl No	Date
	NIMOTOP				
	+	BAYER PHARMS	30MG	N018869 001	DEC 28, 1988

NISOLDIPINE

Tablet, Extended Release; Oral

TE Code	Brand	Firm	Strength	Appl No	Date
	SULAR				
	+	FIRST HORIZON	10MG	N020356 001	

NISOLDIPINE (continued)

Tablet, Extended Release; Oral

TE Code	Brand	Firm	Strength	Appl No	Date
	SULAR	FIRST HORIZON			
			20MG	N020356 002	FEB 02, 1995
	+		30MG	N020356 003	FEB 02, 1995
	+		40MG	N020356 004	FEB 02, 1995

NITAZOXANIDE

For Suspension; Oral

TE Code	Brand	Firm	Strength	Appl No	Date
	ALINIA				
	+	ROMARK	100MG/5ML	N021498 001	NOV 22, 2002

NITISINONE

Capsule; Oral

TE Code	Brand	Firm	Strength	Appl No	Date
	ORFADIN	SWEDISH ORPHAN			
			2MG	N021232 001	JAN 18, 2002
			5MG	N021232 002	JAN 18, 2002
	+		10MG	N021232 003	JAN 18, 2002

NITRIC OXIDE

Gas; Inhalation

TE Code	Brand	Firm	Strength	Appl No	Date
	INOMAX	INO	100PPM	N020845 002	DEC 23, 1999
	+		800PPM	N020845 003	DEC 23, 1999

NITROFURANTOIN

Suspension; Oral

TE Code	Brand	Firm	Strength	Appl No	Date
	FURADANTIN				
	+	FIRST HORIZON	25MG/5ML	N009175 001	

NITROFURANTOIN; NITROFURANTOIN, MACROCRYSTALLINE

Capsule; Oral

TE Code	Brand	Firm	Strength	Appl No	Date
	MACROBID				
	+	PROCTER AND GAMBLE	75MG;25MG	N020064 001	DEC 24, 1991

NITROFURANTOIN, MACROCRYSTALLINE

Capsule; Oral

TE Code	Brand	Firm	Strength	Appl No	Date
	MACRODANTIN	PROCTER AND GAMBLE			
AB			25MG	N016620 003	
AB			50MG	N016620 001	
AB			100MG	N016620 002	
	NITROFURANTION				
AB	+	MYLAN	100MG	N074967 002	JUL 09, 1997

Prescription Drug Products (continued)

NITROFURANTOIN, MACROCRYSTALLINE (continued)

Capsule; Oral

NITROFURANTOIN

TE	Firm	Strength	Appl No	Date
AB	GENEVA PHARMS	25MG	N074336 001	JAN 25, 1995
AB		50MG	N074336 002	JAN 25, 1995
AB		100MG	N074336 003	JAN 25, 1995
AB	IVAX PHARMS	50MG	N073671 001	JAN 28, 1993
AB		100MG	N073652 001	JAN 28, 1993
AB	MYLAN	50MG	N074967 001	JUL 09, 1997
AB	WATSON LABS	25MG	N073696 001	DEC 31, 1992
AB		50MG	N073696 002	DEC 31, 1992
AB		100MG	N073696 003	DEC 31, 1992

NITROFURANTOIN, MACROCRYSTALLINE *MULTIPLE*
SEE NITROFURANTOIN; NITROFURANTOIN, MACROCRYSTALLINE

NITROFURAZONE

Ointment; Topical

NITROFURAZONE

TE	Firm	Strength	Appl No
AT	TARO	0.2%	N086156 001
AT	WENDT	0.2%	N086766 001

Solution; Topical

NITROFURAZONE

TE	Firm	Strength	Appl No
+	WENDT	0.2%	N087081 001

NITROGLYCERIN

Film, Extended Release; Transdermal

MINITRAN
3M

TE	Strength	Appl No	Date
AB1	0.1MG/HR	N089771 001	AUG 30, 1996
AB1	0.2MG/HR	N089772 001	AUG 30, 1996
AB1	0.4MG/HR	N089773 001	AUG 30, 1996
AB1	0.6MG/HR	N089774 001	AUG 30, 1996

NITRO-DUR
+ KEY PHARMS

TE	Strength	Appl No	Date
AB1	0.1MG/HR	N020145 001	APR 04, 1995
AB1	0.2MG/HR	N020145 002	APR 04, 1995
+	0.3MG/HR	N020145 003	APR 04, 1995
+	0.4MG/HR	N020145 004	APR 04, 1995
+	0.6MG/HR	N020145 005	APR 04, 1995

NITROGLYCERIN (continued)

Film, Extended Release; Transdermal

NITRO-DUR

TE	Firm	Strength	Appl No	Date
BX	+ KEY PHARMS	0.8MG/HR	N020145 006	APR 04, 1995

NITROGLYCERIN
HERCON LABS

TE	Strength	Appl No	Date
AB2	0.2MG/HR	N089884 001	OCT 30, 1998
AB2	0.4MG/HR	N089885 001	OCT 30, 1998
AB2	0.6MG/HR	N089886 001	OCT 30, 1998

MYLAN TECHNOLOGIES

TE	Strength	Appl No	Date
AB2	0.1MG/HR	N075033 001	FEB 06, 1998
AB1	0.1MG/HR	N075076 001	NOV 12, 1999
AB2	0.2MG/HR	N074609 001	AUG 30, 1996
AB1	0.2MG/HR	N075073 001	NOV 12, 1999
AB2	0.4MG/HR	N074607 001	AUG 30, 1996
AB1	0.4MG/HR	N075075 001	NOV 12, 1999
AB2	0.6MG/HR	N074559 001	AUG 30, 1996
AB1	0.6MG/HR	N074992 001	NOV 12, 1999

TRANSDERM-NITRO
NOVARTIS

TE	Strength	Appl No	Date
AB2	0.1MG/HR	N020144 001	FEB 27, 1996
AB2	0.2MG/HR	N020144 002	FEB 27, 1996
AB2	0.4MG/HR	N020144 003	FEB 27, 1996
AB2	0.6MG/HR	N020144 004	FEB 27, 1996
BX	0.8MG/HR	N020144 005	FEB 27, 1996

Injectable; Injection

NITRO-BID

TE	Firm	Strength	Appl No	Date
AP	+ AVENTIS PHARMS	5MG/ML	N018621 001	JAN 05, 1982

NITROGLYCERIN

TE	Firm	Strength	Appl No	Date
AP	+ ABBOTT	5MG/ML	N018531 001	
AP	LUITPOLD	5MG/ML	N072034 001	MAY 24, 1988

NITROGLYCERIN IN DEXTROSE 5%

TE	Firm	Strength	Appl No	Date
AP	ABBOTT	0.1MG/ML	N074083 001	OCT 26, 1994
AP		10MG/100ML	N071846 001	AUG 31, 1990
AP		20MG/100ML	N071847 001	AUG 31, 1990
AP		40MG/100ML	N071848 001	AUG 31, 1990
AP	+ BAXTER HLTHCARE	10MG/100ML	N019970 001	AUG 31, 1990

Prescription Drug Products (continued)

NITROGLYCERIN (continued)

Injectable; Injection
NITROGLYCERIN IN DEXTROSE 5%
BAXTER HLTHCARE

		Strength	Date	Number
AP	+	20MG/100ML	DEC 29, 1989	N019970 002
AP	+	40MG/100ML	DEC 29, 1989	N019970 003

Ointment; Transdermal
NITROGLYCERIN

	Strength	Date	Number
+ FOUGERA	2%	JUL 08, 1988	N087355 001

Spray, Metered; Sublingual
NITROLINGUAL PUMPSPRAY

	Strength	Date	Number
+ POHL BOSKAMP	0.4MG/SPRAY	JAN 10, 1997	N018705 002

Tablet; Sublingual
NITROSTAT
PFIZER PHARMS

	Strength	Date	Number
	0.3MG	MAY 01, 2000	N021134 001
+	0.4MG	MAY 01, 2000	N021134 002
+	0.6MG	MAY 01, 2000	N021134 003

NIZATIDINE

Capsule; Oral
AXID
RELIANT PHARMS

		Strength	Date	Number
AB		150MG	APR 12, 1988	N019508 001
AB	+	300MG	APR 12, 1988	N019508 002

NIZATIDINE
EON

	Strength	Date	Number
AB	150MG	JUL 05, 2002	N076178 001
AB	300MG	JUL 05, 2002	N076178 002

GENPHARM

	Strength	Date	Number
AB	150MG	JUL 09, 2002	N075934 001
AB	300MG	JUL 09, 2002	N075934 002

MYLAN

	Strength	Date	Number
AB	150MG	JUL 05, 2002	N075806 001
AB	300MG	JUL 05, 2002	N075806 002

TEVA

	Strength	Date	Number
AB	150MG	SEP 12, 2002	N075668 001
AB	300MG	SEP 12, 2002	N075668 002

TORPHARM

	Strength	Date	Number
AB	150MG	JAN 23, 2003	N076383 001
AB	300MG	JAN 23, 2003	N076383 002

WATSON LABS

	Strength	Date	Number
AB	150MG	JUL 09, 2002	N075616 001
AB	300MG		N075616 002

NIZATIDINE (continued)

Capsule; Oral
NIZATIDINE
WATSON LABS
ZENITH- GOLDLINE

	Strength	Date	Number
AB	150MG	JUL 09, 2002	N075461 001
AB	300MG	JUL 08, 2002	N075461 002
		JUL 08, 2002	

NORELGESTROMIN *MULTIPLE*
SEE ETHINYL ESTRADIOL; NORELGESTROMIN

NOREPINEPHRINE BITARTRATE

Injectable; Injection
LEVOPHED

	Strength	Number
AP	+ ABBOTT	EQ 1MG BASE/ML	N007513 001

NOREPINEPHRINE BITARTRATE
GENSIA SICOR PHARMS

	Strength	Date	Number
AP	EQ 1MG BASE/ML	MAR 03, 2003	N040455 001

NORETHINDRONE

Tablet; Oral-28
CAMILA
BARR

	Strength	Date	Number
AB1	0.35MG	OCT 21, 2002	N076177 001

ERRIN
BARR

	Strength	Date	Number
AB2	0.35MG	OCT 21, 2002	N076225 001

MICRONOR

	Strength	Number
AB2	+ ORTHO MCNEIL PHARM	0.35MG	N016954 001

NOR-QD

	Strength	Number
AB1	+ WATSON LABS (UTAH)	0.35MG	N017060 001

NORETHINDRONE *MULTIPLE*
SEE ETHINYL ESTRADIOL; NORETHINDRONE
SEE MESTRANOL; NORETHINDRONE

NORETHINDRONE ACETATE

Tablet; Oral
AYGESTIN

	Strength	Date	Number
AB	+ DURAMED PHARM BARR	5MG	APR 21, 1982	N018405 001

NORETH-INDRONE ACETATE
BARR

	Strength	Date	Number
AB	5MG	MAY 25, 2001	N075951 001

NORETHINDRONE ACETATE *MULTIPLE*
SEE ESTRADIOL; NORETHINDRONE ACETATE
SEE ETHINYL ESTRADIOL; NORETHINDRONE ACETATE

NORFLOXACIN

Tablet; Oral
NOROXIN

	Strength	Date	Number
	+ MERCK	400MG	OCT 31, 1986	N019384 002

Prescription Drug Products (continued)

NORGESTIMATE *MULTIPLE*
SEE ESTRADIOL; NORGESTIMATE
SEE ETHINYL ESTRADIOL; NORGESTIMATE

NORGESTREL
Tablet; Oral

OVRETTE

	Manufacturer	Strength	Appl. No.	Date
	+ WYETH PHARMS INC	0.075MG	N017031 001	

NORGESTREL *MULTIPLE*
SEE ETHINYL ESTRADIOL; NORGESTREL

NORTRIPTYLINE HYDROCHLORIDE
Capsule; Oral

AVENTYL HCL

TE	Manufacturer	Strength	Appl. No.	Date
BD	LILLY	EQ 10MG BASE	N014684 001	
BD		EQ 25MG BASE	N014684 002	

NORTRIPTYLINE HCL

TE	Manufacturer	Strength	Appl. No.	Date
AB	GENEVA PHARMS	EQ 10MG BASE	N074054 001	DEC 31, 1992
AB		EQ 25MG BASE	N074054 002	DEC 31, 1992
AB		EQ 50MG BASE	N074054 003	DEC 31, 1992
AB		EQ 75MG BASE	N074054 004	DEC 31, 1992
AB	GENEVA PHARMS TECH	EQ 10MG BASE	N074835 001	JUN 30, 1997
AB		EQ 25MG BASE	N074835 002	JUN 30, 1997
AB		EQ 50MG BASE	N074835 003	JUN 30, 1997
AB		EQ 75MG BASE	N074835 004	JUN 30, 1997
AB	MYLAN	EQ 10MG BASE	N074234 001	JUL 26, 1993
AB		EQ 25MG BASE	N074234 002	JUL 26, 1993
AB		EQ 50MG BASE	N074234 003	JUL 26, 1993
AB		EQ 75MG BASE	N074234 004	JUL 26, 1993
AB	TARO	EQ 10MG BASE	N075520 004	MAY 08, 2000
AB		EQ 25MG BASE	N075520 003	MAY 08, 2000
AB		EQ 50MG BASE	N075520 001	MAY 08, 2000
AB		EQ 75MG BASE	N075520 002	MAY 08, 2000
AB	TEVA	EQ 10MG BASE	N073667 001	APR 11, 1996
AB		EQ 10MG BASE	N074132 001	MAR 27, 1995
AB		EQ 25MG BASE	N073667 002	APR 11, 1996

NORTRIPTYLINE HYDROCHLORIDE (continued)
Capsule; Oral

NORTRIPTYLINE HCL

TE	Manufacturer	Strength	Appl. No.	Date
AB	TEVA	EQ 25MG BASE	N074132 002	MAR 27, 1995
AB		EQ 50MG BASE	N073667 003	APR 11, 1996
AB		EQ 50MG BASE	N074132 003	MAR 27, 1995
AB		EQ 75MG BASE	N073667 004	APR 11, 1996
AB		EQ 75MG BASE	N074132 004	APR 11, 1996
AB	WATSON LABS	EQ 10MG BASE	N073553 001	MAR 30, 1992
AB		EQ 25MG BASE	N073554 001	MAR 30, 1992
AB		EQ 50MG BASE	N073555 001	MAR 30, 1992
AB		EQ 75MG BASE	N073556 001	MAR 30, 1992

PAMELOR

TE	Manufacturer	Strength	Appl. No.	Date
AB	TYCO HLTHCARE	EQ 10MG BASE	N018013 001	
AB		EQ 25MG BASE	N018013 002	
AB		EQ 50MG BASE	N018013 003	
AB		EQ 75MG BASE	N018013 004	

Solution; Oral

AVENTYL HCL

TE	Manufacturer	Strength	Appl. No.	Date
AA	+ RANBAXY	EQ 10MG BASE/5ML	N014685 001	

NORTRIPTYLINE HCL

TE	Manufacturer	Strength	Appl. No.	Date
AA	PHARM ASSOC	EQ 10MG BASE/5ML	N075606 001	AUG 28, 2000

PAMELOR

TE	Manufacturer	Strength	Appl. No.	Date
AA	TYCO HLTHCARE	EQ 10MG BASE/5ML	N018012 001	

NYSTATIN
Cream; Topical

MYCOSTATIN

TE	Manufacturer	Strength	Appl. No.	Date
AT	+ WESTWOOD SQUIBB	100,000 UNITS/GM	N060575 001	

NYSTATIN

TE	Manufacturer	Strength	Appl. No.	Date
AT	ALPHARMA	100,000 UNITS/GM	N062949 001	JUN 13, 1988
AT	ALTANA	100,000 UNITS/GM	N062129 001	
AT	CLAY PARK	100,000 UNITS/GM	N062225 001	
AT	TARO	100,000 UNITS/GM	N062457 001	JUL 28, 1983
AT		100,000 UNITS/GM	N064022 001	JAN 29, 1993

Ointment; Topical

NYSTATIN

TE	Manufacturer	Strength	Appl. No.	Date
AT	ALPHARMA	100,000 UNITS/GM	N062840 001	NOV 13, 1987
AT	+ ALTANA	100,000 UNITS/GM	N062124 002	SEP 23, 1982
AT	CLAY PARK	100,000 UNITS/GM	N062472 001	FEB 13, 1984

Prescription Drug Products (continued)

NYSTATIN (continued)

TE Code	Product / Firm	Strength	Appl. No. / Date
	Pastille; Oral		
	MYCOSTATIN + BRISTOL MYERS SQUIBB	200,000 UNITS	N050619 001 APR 09, 1987
	Powder; Oral		
AA	NILSTAT + LEDERLE	100%	N050576 001 DEC 22, 1983
AA	NYSTATIN PADDOCK	100%	N062613 001 NOV 26, 1985
	Powder; Topical		
AT	MYCOSTATIN + WESTWOOD SQUIBB NYSTOP	100,000 UNITS/GM	N060578 001
AT	PADDOCK	100,000 UNITS/GM	N064118 001 AUG 16, 1996
	Suspension; Oral		
AA	MYCOSTATIN + APOTHECON	100,000 UNITS/ML	N061533 001
AA	NILSTAT + LEDERLE	100,000 UNITS/ML	N050299 001
AA	NYSTATIN ALPHARMA	100,000 UNITS/ML	N062349 001 JUL 14, 1982
AA		100,000 UNITS/ML	N064042 001 FEB 28, 1994
AA	BAUSCH AND LOMB	100,000 UNITS/ML	N062517 001 JUN 07, 1984
AA	FOUGERA	100,000 UNITS/ML	N062512 001 OCT 29, 1984
AA	MORTON GROVE	100,000 UNITS/ML	N064142 001 JUN 25, 1998
AA	UDL	100,000 UNITS/ML	
AA	NYSTEX SAVAGE LABS	100,000 UNITS/ML	N062519 001 JUL 06, 1984
	Tablet; Oral		
AA	MYCOSTATIN + APOTHECON	500,000 UNITS	N060574 001
AA	NYSTATIN MUTUAL PHARM	500,000 UNITS	N062838 001 DEC 22, 1988
AA	PAR PHARM	500,000 UNITS	N062474 001 DEC 22, 1983
AA	TEVA	500,000 UNITS	N062506 001 JAN 16, 1984
	Tablet; Vaginal		
AT	NYSTATIN FOUGERA	100,000 UNITS	N062459 001 NOV 09, 1983
AT	ODYSSEY PHARMS	100,000 UNITS	N062615 001 OCT 17, 1985
AT	PHARMADERM	100,000 UNITS	N062460 001 NOV 09, 1983

NYSTATIN; TRIAMCINOLONE ACETONIDE

TE Code	Product / Firm	Strength	Appl. No. / Date
	Cream; Topical		
AT	MYCO-TRIACET II TEVA	100,000 UNITS/GM;0.1%	N061954 002 SEP 20, 1985
AT	MYCOLOG-II + APOTHECON	100,000 UNITS/GM;0.1%	N062606 001 MAY 15, 1985
AT	MYKACET ALPHARMA US PHARM	100,000 UNITS/GM;0.1%	N062367 001 MAY 28, 1985
AT	MYTREX F SAVAGE LABS	100,000 UNITS/GM;0.1%	N062597 001 OCT 08, 1985
AT	NYSTATIN AND TRIAMCINOLONE ACETONIDE TARO	100,000 UNITS/GM;0.1%	N062347 001 MAR 30, 1987
AT		100,000 UNITS/GM;0.1%	N062364 001 DEC 22, 1987
AT	NYSTATIN-TRIAMCINOLONE ACETONIDE FOUGERA	100,000 UNITS/GM;0.1%	N062599 001 OCT 08, 1985
	Ointment; Topical		
AT	MYCOLOG-II + APOTHECON	100,000 UNITS/GM;0.1%	N060572 001 JUN 28, 1985
AT	MYKACE ALPHARMA US PHARM	100,000 UNITS/GM;0.1%	N062733 001 MAR 09, 1987
AT	MYTREX F SAVAGE LABS	100,000 UNITS/GM;0.1%	N062601 001 OCT 09, 1985
AT	NYSTATIN AND TRIAMCINOLONE ACETONIDE TARO	100,000 UNITS/GM;0.1%	N063305 001 MAR 29, 1993
AT	NYSTATIN-TRIAMCINOLONE ACETONIDE FOUGERA	100,000 UNITS/GM;0.1%	N062602 001 OCT 09, 1985

OCTREOTIDE ACETATE

Product / Firm	Strength	Appl. No. / Date
Injectable; Injection		
SANDOSTATIN + NOVARTIS	EQ 0.1MG BASE/ML	N019667 002 OCT 21, 1988
	EQ 0.2MG BASE/ML	N019667 004 JUN 12, 1991
+	EQ 0.05MG BASE/ML	N019667 001 OCT 21, 1988
+	EQ 0.5MG BASE/ML	N019667 003 OCT 21, 1988
+	EQ 1MG BASE/ML	N019667 005 JUN 12, 1991
SANDOSTATIN LAR NOVARTIS	EQ 10MG BASE/VIAL	N021008 001 NOV 25, 1998
	EQ 20MG BASE/VIAL	N021008 002 NOV 25, 1998

Prescription Drug Products (continued)

OCTREOTIDE ACETATE (continued)
Injectable; Injection

SANDOSTATIN LAR			
+ NOVARTIS	EQ 30MG BASE/VIAL	N021008 003	NOV 25, 1998

OFLOXACIN
Injectable; Injection

FLOXIN				
AP	+ ORTHO MCNEIL PHARM	40MG/ML	N020087 003	MAR 31, 1992
FLOXIN IN DEXTROSE 5%				
	+ ORTHO MCNEIL PHARM	400MG/100ML	N020087 001	MAR 31, 1992
FLOXIN IN DEXTROSE 5% IN PLASTIC CONTAINER				
	+ ORTHO MCNEIL PHARM	400MG/100ML	N020087 005	MAR 31, 1992
OFLOXACIN				
AP	BEDFORD	40MG/ML	N075762 001	JAN 16, 2002

Solution/Drops; Ophthalmic

OCUFLOX			
+ ALLERGAN	0.3%	N019921 001	JUL 30, 1993

Solution/Drops; Otic

FLOXIN			
+ DAIICHI	0.3%	N020799 001	DEC 16, 1997

Tablet; Oral

FLOXIN			
ORTHO MCNEIL PHARM	200MG	N019735 001	DEC 28, 1990
	300MG	N019735 002	DEC 28, 1990
+	400MG	N019735 003	DEC 28, 1990

OLANZAPINE
Tablet, Orally Disintegrating; Oral

ZYPREXA ZYDIS			
LILLY	5MG	N021086 001	APR 06, 2000
	10MG	N021086 002	APR 06, 2000
	15MG	N021086 003	APR 06, 2000
+	20MG	N021086 004	APR 06, 2000

Tablet; Oral

ZYPREXA			
LILLY	2.5MG	N020592 001	SEP 30, 1996
	5MG	N020592 002	SEP 30, 1996
+	7.5MG	N020592 003	SEP 30, 1996

OLANZAPINE (continued)
Tablet; Oral

ZYPREXA			
LILLY	10MG	N020592 004	SEP 30, 1996
	15MG	N020592 005	SEP 09, 1997
	20MG	N020592 006	SEP 09, 1997

OLMESARTAN MEDOXOMIL
Tablet; Oral

BENICAR			
SANKYO	5MG	N021286 001	APR 25, 2002
	20MG	N021286 003	APR 25, 2002
+	40MG	N021286 004	APR 25, 2002

OLMESARTAN MEDOXOMIL *MULTIPLE*
SEE HYDROCHLOROTHIAZIDE; OLMESARTAN MEDOXOMIL

OLOPATADINE HYDROCHLORIDE
Solution/Drops; Ophthalmic

PATANOL			
+ ALCON	EQ 0.1% BASE	N020688 001	DEC 18, 1996

OLSALAZINE SODIUM
Capsule; Oral

DIPENTUM			
+ PHARMACIA AND UPJOHN	250MG	N019715 001	JUL 31, 1990

OMEPRAZOLE
Capsule, Delayed Rel Pellets; Oral

OMEPRAZOLE				
AB	ANDRX PHARMS	10MG	N075347 001	NOV 16, 2001
AB		20MG	N075347 002	NOV 16, 2001
AB		40MG	N075347 003	NOV 16, 2001
AB	EON	10MG	N075791 001	DEC 23, 2002
AB		20MG	N075791 002	DEC 23, 2002
AB	IMPAX LABS	10MG	N075785 001	NOV 08, 2002
AB		20MG	N075785 002	NOV 08, 2002
AB	KREMERS URBAN DEV	10MG	N075410 001	NOV 01, 2002

Prescription Drug Products (continued)

OMEPRAZOLE (continued)

Capsule, Delayed Rel Pellets; Oral

OMEPRAZOLE

TE	Applicant	Strength	Appl. No.	Approval
AB	KREMERS URBAN DEV	20MG	N075410 002	NOV 01, 2002
AB	LEK PHARMS	10MG	N075757 001	JAN 28, 2003
AB		20MG	N075757 002	JAN 28, 2003
AB	MYLAN	10MG	N075876 001	MAY 29, 2003
AB		20MG	N075876 002	MAY 29, 2003

PRILOSEC

TE	Applicant	Strength	Appl. No.	Approval
AB	ASTRAZENECA	10MG	N019810 003	OCT 05, 1995
AB	+	20MG	N019810 001	SEP 14, 1989
AB	+	40MG	N019810 002	JAN 15, 1998

ONDANSETRON

Tablet, Orally Disintegrating; Oral

ZOFRAN ODT

TE	Applicant	Strength	Appl. No.	Approval
	GLAXOSMITHKLINE	EQ 4MG BASE	N020781 001	JAN 27, 1999
	+	EQ 8MG BASE	N020781 002	JAN 27, 1999

ONDANSETRON HYDROCHLORIDE

Injectable; Injection

ZOFRAN

TE	Applicant	Strength	Appl. No.	Approval
	+ GLAXOSMITHKLINE	EQ 2MG BASE/ML	N020007 001	JAN 04, 1991

ZOFRAN IN PLASTIC CONTAINER

TE	Applicant	Strength	Appl. No.	Approval
	+ GLAXOSMITHKLINE	EQ 0.64MG BASE/ML	N020403 001	JAN 31, 1995

ZOFRAN PRESERVATIVE FREE

TE	Applicant	Strength	Appl. No.	Approval
	+ GLAXOSMITHKLINE	EQ 2MG BASE/ML	N020007 003	DEC 10, 1993

Solution; Oral

ZOFRAN

TE	Applicant	Strength	Appl. No.	Approval
	+ GLAXOSMITHKLINE	EQ 4MG BASE/5ML	N020605 001	JAN 24, 1997

Tablet; Oral

ZOFRAN

TE	Applicant	Strength	Appl. No.	Approval
	GLAXOSMITHKLINE	EQ 4MG BASE	N020103 001	DEC 31, 1992
		EQ 8MG BASE	N020103 002	DEC 31, 1992
	+	EQ 24MG BASE	N020103 003	AUG 27, 1999

ORLISTAT

Capsule; Oral

XENICAL

TE	Applicant	Strength	Appl. No.	Approval
	+ HLR	120MG	N020766 001	APR 23, 1999

ORPHENADRINE CITRATE

Injectable; Injection

NORFLEX

TE	Applicant	Strength	Appl. No.	Approval
AP	+ 3M	30MG/ML	N013055 001	

ORPHENADRINE CITRATE

TE	Applicant	Strength	Appl. No.	Approval
AP	BEDFORD LABS	30MG/ML	N040463 001	MAR 04, 2003
AP	STERIS	30MG/ML	N084779 001	MAR 15, 1982
AP		30MG/ML	N087062 001	

Tablet, Extended Release; Oral

NORFLEX

TE	Applicant	Strength	Appl. No.	Approval
AP	+ 3M	100MG	N012157 001	

ORPHENADRINE CITRATE

TE	Applicant	Strength	Appl. No.	Approval
AB	EON	100MG	N040327 001	FEB 15, 2000
AB	GENEVA PHARMS TECH	100MG	N040284 001	JUN 19, 1998
AB	IMPAX PHARM	100MG	N040368 001	JUN 23, 2000
AB	KIEL	100MG	N040249 001	JAN 29, 1999

ORPHENADRINE CITRATE *MULTIPLE*

SEE ASPIRIN; CAFFEINE; ORPHENADRINE CITRATE

OSELTAMIVIR PHOSPHATE

Capsule; Oral

TAMIFLU

TE	Applicant	Strength	Appl. No.	Approval
	+ ROCHE	EQ 75MG BASE	N021087 001	OCT 27, 1999

For Suspension; Oral

TAMIFLU

TE	Applicant	Strength	Appl. No.	Approval
	+ ROCHE	EQ 12MG BASE/ML	N021246 001	DEC 14, 2000

OXACILLIN SODIUM

Capsule; Oral

BACTOCILL

TE	Applicant	Strength	Appl. No.	Approval
AB	GLAXOSMITHKLINE	EQ 250MG BASE	N061336 001	
AB		EQ 250MG BASE	N062241 001	
AB		EQ 500MG BASE	N061336 002	
AB		EQ 500MG BASE	N062241 002	

OXACILLIN SODIUM

TE	Applicant	Strength	Appl. No.	Approval
AB	+ TEVA	EQ 250MG BASE	N062222 001	
AB		EQ 500MG BASE	N062222 002	

For Solution; Oral

BACTOCILL

TE	Applicant	Strength	Appl. No.	Approval
AA	GLAXOSMITHKLINE	EQ 250MG BASE/5ML	N062321 001	

Prescription Drug Products (continued)

OXACILLIN SODIUM (continued)

For Solution; Oral

OXACILLIN SODIUM

TE	Firm	Strength	Appl No	Approval Date
AA	APOTHECON	EQ 250MG BASE/5ML	N061457 001	
AA	TEVA	EQ 250MG BASE/5ML	N062252 001	

Injectable; Injection

BACTOCILL IN PLASTIC CONTAINER

TE	Firm	Strength	Appl No	Approval Date
+	BAXTER HLTHCARE	EQ 20MG BASE/ML	N050640 001	OCT 26, 1989
+		EQ 40MG BASE/ML	N050640 002	OCT 26, 1989

OXACILLIN SODIUM

TE	Firm	Strength	Appl No	Approval Date
AP +	APOTHECON	EQ 1GM BASE/VIAL	N061490 003	
AP +		EQ 1GM BASE/VIAL	N062737 001	DEC 23, 1986
AP +		EQ 2GM BASE/VIAL	N062737 002	DEC 23, 1986
AP +		EQ 10GM BASE/VIAL	N061490 006	MAY 09, 1991
AP +		EQ 250MG BASE/VIAL	N061490 001	
AP +		EQ 500MG BASE/VIAL	N061490 002	
AP +		EQ 1GM BASE/VIAL	N062856 003	OCT 26, 1988
AP	MARSAM PHARMS LLC	EQ 2GM BASE/VIAL	N062856 004	OCT 26, 1988
AP		EQ 4GM BASE/VIAL	N062856 005	OCT 26, 1988
AP		EQ 10GM BASE/VIAL	N062984 001	SEP 29, 1988
AP		EQ 250MG BASE/VIAL	N062856 001	OCT 26, 1988
AP		EQ 500MG BASE/VIAL	N062856 002	OCT 26, 1988

OXALIPLATIN

Injectable; Iv (Infusion)

ELOXATIN

TE	Firm	Strength	Appl No	Approval Date
	SANOFI	50MG/VIAL	N021492 001	AUG 09, 2002
+		100MG/VIAL	N021492 002	AUG 09, 2002

OXAMNIQUINE

Capsule; Oral

VANSIL

TE	Firm	Strength	Appl No	Approval Date
+	PFIZER	250MG	N018069 001	

OXANDROLONE

Tablet; Oral

OXANDRIN

TE	Firm	Strength	Appl No	Approval Date
	BIO TECH GEN	2.5MG	N013718 001	
		10MG	N013718 002	NOV 05, 2001

OXAPROZIN

Tablet; Oral

DAYPRO

TE	Firm	Strength	Appl No	Approval Date
AB +	GD SEARLE LLC	600MG	N018841 004	OCT 29, 1992

OXAPROZIN

TE	Firm	Strength	Appl No	Approval Date
AB	CARACO	600MG	N075844 001	JAN 03, 2002
AB	DR REDDYS LABS LTD	600MG	N075855 001	JAN 31, 2001
AB	EON	600MG	N075845 001	JAN 31, 2001
AB	GENEVA PHARMS	600MG	N075850 001	APR 27, 2001
AB	GENPHARM	600MG	N075847 001	FEB 28, 2001
AB	INVAMED	600MG	N075842 001	APR 12, 2001
AB	IVAX PHARMS	600MG	N075846 001	MAY 13, 2002
AB	MYLAN	600MG	N075851 001	AUG 17, 2001
AB	PUREPAC PHARM	600MG	N075843 001	OCT 03, 2001
AB	TEVA	600MG	N075849 001	JUL 03, 2002
AB	WATSON LABS	600MG	N075848 001	FEB 09, 2001

OXAPROZIN POTASSIUM

Tablet; Oral

DAYPRO ALTA

TE	Firm	Strength	Appl No	Approval Date
+	PHARMACIA	600MG	N020776 001	OCT 17, 2002

OXAZEPAM

Capsule; Oral

OXAZEPAM

TE	Firm	Strength	Appl No	Approval Date
AB	GENEVA PHARMS	10MG	N071813 001	APR 19, 1988
AB		15MG	N071756 001	APR 19, 1988
AB		30MG	N071814 001	APR 19, 1988
AB	IVAX PHARMS	10MG	N070943 001	AUG 03, 1987
AB		15MG	N070944 001	AUG 03, 1987
AB		30MG	N070945 001	AUG 03, 1987
AB	PUREPAC PHARM	10MG	N072251 001	APR 14, 1988
AB		15MG	N072252 001	APR 14, 1988
AB		30MG	N072253 001	APR 14, 1988

Prescription Drug Products (continued)

OXAZEPAM (continued)

Capsule; Oral

OXAZEPAM

TE	Manufacturer	Strength	Appl. No.	Date
AB	WATSON LABS	10MG	N072952 001	SEP 28, 1990
AB		15MG	N072953 001	SEP 28, 1990
AB		30MG	N072954 001	SEP 28, 1990

SERAX

TE	Manufacturer	Strength	Appl. No.	Date
AB	FAULDING PHARMS	10MG	N015539 002	
AB		15MG	N015539 004	
AB		30MG	N015539 006	
+				

Tablet; Oral

SERAX

Manufacturer	Strength	Appl. No.
+ FAULDING PHARMS	15MG	N015539 008

OXCARBAZEPINE

Suspension; Oral

TRILEPTAL

Manufacturer	Strength	Appl. No.	Date
+ NOVARTIS	300MG/5ML	N021285 001	MAY 25, 2001

Tablet; Oral

TRILEPTAL

Manufacturer	Strength	Appl. No.	Date
NOVARTIS	150MG	N021014 001	JAN 14, 2000
	300MG	N021014 002	JAN 14, 2000
+	600MG	N021014 003	JAN 14, 2000

OXICONAZOLE NITRATE

Cream; Topical

OXISTAT

Manufacturer	Strength	Appl. No.	Date
+ GLAXOSMITHKLINE	EQ 1% BASE	N019828 001	DEC 30, 1988

Lotion; Topical

OXISTAT

Manufacturer	Strength	Appl. No.	Date
+ GLAXOSMITHKLINE	EQ 1% BASE	N020209 001	SEP 30, 1992

OXTRIPHYLLINE

Tablet, Extended Release; Oral

CHOLEDYL SA

Manufacturer	Strength	Appl. No.	Date
+ PARKE DAVIS	400MG	N087863 001	MAY 24, 1983
+ WARNER CHILCOTT	600MG	N086742 001	

OXYBUTYNIN

Film, Extended Release; Transdermal

OXYTROL

Manufacturer	Strength	Appl. No.	Date
+ WATSON LABS (UTAH)	3.9MG/24HR	N021351 002	FEB 26, 2003

OXYBUTYNIN CHLORIDE

Syrup; Oral

DITROPAN

TE	Manufacturer	Strength	Appl. No.
	+ ALZA	5MG/5ML	N018211 001

OXYBUTYNIN CHLORIDE

TE	Manufacturer	Strength	Appl. No.	Date
AA	MIKART	5MG/5ML	N075039 001	JAN 29, 1999
AA	MORTCN GROVE	5MG/5ML	N074868 001	FEB 12, 1997
AA	NOVEX	5MG/5ML	N074997 001	OCT 15, 1997
AA	PHARM ASSOC	5MG/5ML	N075137 001	DEC 18, 1998
AA	SILARx	5MG/5ML	N074520 001	MAR 29, 1996

Tablet, Extended Release; Oral

DITROPAN XL

Manufacturer	Strength	Appl. No.	Date
ALZA	5MG	N020897 001	DEC 16, 1998
	10MG	N020897 002	DEC 16, 1998
+	15MG	N020897 003	JUN 22, 1999

Tablet; Oral

DITROPAN

TE	Manufacturer	Strength	Appl. No.
	+ ALZA	5MG	N017577 001

OXYBUTYNIN CHLORIDE

TE	Manufacturer	Strength	Appl. No.	Date
AB	PLIVA	5MG	N071655 001	NOV 14, 1988
AB	USL PHARMA	5MG	N074625 001	JUL 31, 1996
AB	VINTAGE PHARMS	5MG	N075079 001	OCT 31, 1997

OXYCODONE HYDROCHLORIDE

Tablet, Extended Release; Oral

OXYCONTIN

Manufacturer	Strength	Appl. No.	Date
PURCUE PHARMA LP	10MG	N020553 001	DEC 12, 1995
	20MG	N020553 002	DEC 12, 1995
	40MG	N020553 003	DEC 12, 1995
+	80MG	N020553 004	JAN 06, 1997

Tablet; Oral

ROXICODONE

Manufacturer	Strength	Appl. No.	Date
ELAN PHARMS	15MG	N021011 001	AUG 31, 2000
	30MG	N021011 002	AUG 31, 2000
+			AUG 31, 2000

OXYCODONE HYDROCHLORIDE *MULTIPLE*

SEE   ACETAMINOPHEN; OXYCODONE HYDROCHLORIDE
SEE   ASPIRIN; OXYCODONE HYDROCHLORIDE; OXYCODONE TEREPHTHALATE

Prescription Drug Products (continued)

OXYCODONE TEREPHTHALATE *MULTIPLE*
SEE ASPIRIN; OXYCODONE HYDROCHLORIDE; OXYCODONE TEREPHTHALATE

OXYMETHOLONE
Tablet; Oral
ANADROL-50
+ UNIMED PHARMS — 50MG — N016848 001

OXYMORPHONE HYDROCHLORIDE
Injectable; Injection
NUMORPHAN
+ ENDO PHARMS — 1.5MG/ML — N011707 001
+ ENDO PHARMS — 1MG/ML — N011707 002
Suppository; Rectal
NUMORPHAN
+ ENDO PHARMS — 5MG — N011738 004

OXYTETRACYCLINE *MULTIPLE*
SEE LIDOCAINE HYDROCHLORIDE; OXYTETRACYCLINE

OXYTETRACYCLINE HYDROCHLORIDE
Capsule; Oral
TERRAMYCIN
+ PFIZER — EQ 250MG BASE — N050286 002

OXYTETRACYCLINE HYDROCHLORIDE; POLYMYXIN B SULFATE
Ointment; Ophthalmic
TERRAMYCIN W/ POLYMYXIN B SULFATE — EQ 5MG BASE/GM;10,000 UNITS/GM
+ PFIZER — N061015 001

OXYTETRACYCLINE HYDROCHLORIDE *MULTIPLE*
SEE HYDROCORTISONE ACETATE; OXYTETRACYCLINE HYDROCHLORIDE

OXYTOCIN
Injectable; Injection
OXYTOCIN
AP AM PHARM PARTNERS — 10USP UNITS/ML — N018248 001
PITOCIN
AP + PARKEDALE — 10USP UNITS/ML — N018261 001
SYNTOCINON
AP NOVARTIS — 10USP UNITS/ML — N018245 001

PACLITAXEL
Injectable; Injection
PACLITAXEL
AP ABBOTT — 6MG/ML — N076131 001 — MAY 08, 2002
AP BAKER NORTON — 6MG/ML — N075184 001 — JAN 25, 2002
                              N075190 001 — JAN 28, 2002
AP BEDFORD — 6MG/ML — N075297 001 — JAN 25, 2002
AP IVAX PHARMS — 6MG/ML

PACLITAXEL (continued)
Injectable; Injection
PACLITAXEL
AP MYLAN — 6MG/ML — N075278 001 — JAN 25, 2002
AP NAPRO — 6MG/ML — N076233 001 — AUG 01, 2002
TAXOL
AP + BRISTOL MYERS SQUIBB — 6MG/ML — N020262 001 — DEC 29, 1992

PAMIDRONATE DISODIUM
Injectable; Injection
AREDIA
AP + NOVARTIS — 30MG/VIAL — N020036 001 — OCT 31, 1991
                 60MG/VIAL — N020036 003 — MAY 06, 1993
AP + NOVARTIS — 90MG/VIAL — N020036 004 — MAY 06, 1993
PAMIDRONATE DISODIUM
AP AESGEN — 30MG/VIAL — N075594 001 — MAY 06, 2002
AP   90MG/VIAL — N075594 002 — MAY 06, 2002
AP AM PHARM PARTNERS — 30MG /10ML(3MG/ML) — N076207 001 — MAY 17, 2002
AP   30MG/VIAL — N075773 001 — MAY 06, 2002
AP   90MG /10ML(9MG/ML) — N076207 002 — MAY 17, 2002
AP   90MG/VIAL — N075773 002 — MAY 06, 2002
AP BEDFORD — 30MG /10ML(3MG/ML) — N021113 001 — MAR 04, 2002
AP   30MG/VIAL — N075290 001 — APR 30, 2001
AP   90MG /10ML(9MG/ML) — N021113 002 — MAR 04, 2002
AP   90MG/VIAL — N075290 003 — APR 30, 2001
AP FAULDING — 30MG /10ML(3MG/ML) — N075841 001 — JUN 27, 2002
AP   60MG /10ML(6MG/ML) — N075841 002 — JUN 27, 2002
AP   90MG /10ML(9MG/ML) — N075841 003 — JUN 27, 2002
AP GENSIA SICOR PHARMS — 30MG /10ML(3MG/ML) — N076153 001 — MAR 27, 2002
AP   90MG /10ML(9MG/ML) — N076153 002 — MAR 27, 2002

PANCURONIUM BROMIDE
Injectable; Injection
PANCURONIUM
AP ELKINS SINN — 1MG/ML — N072058 001

Prescription Drug Products *(continued)*

PANCURONIUM BROMIDE *(continued)*

Injectable; Injection

PANCURONIUM
ELKINS SINN

AP	2MG/ML	MAR 23, 1988	N072059 001
AP	2MG/ML	MAR 23, 1988	N072060 001

PANCURONIUM BROMIDE
ABBOTT

AP	1MG/ML	N072320 001	JAN 19, 1989
AP	2MG/ML	N072321 001	JAN 19, 1989
AP +	GENSIA SICOR PHARMS		
AP	1MG/ML	N072759 001	JUL 31, 1990
AP +	2MG/ML	N072760 001	JUL 31, 1990

PANTOPRAZOLE SODIUM

Injectable; Iv (Infusion)

PROTONIX IV
+ WYETH PHARMS INC

	EQ 40MG BASE/VIAL	N020988 001	MAR 22, 2001

Tablet, Delayed Release; Oral

PROTONIX
WYETH PHARMS INC

	EQ 20MG BASE	N020987 002	JUN 12, 2001
+	EQ 40MG BASE	N020987 001	FEB 02, 2000

PARICALCITOL

Injectable; Injection

ZEMPLAR
+ ABBOTT

	0.005MG/ML	N020819 001	APR 17, 1998

PAROMOMYCIN SULFATE

Capsule; Oral

HUMATIN

AA +	KING PHARMS	EQ 250MG BASE	N062310 001	

PAROMOMYCIN SULFATE

AA	CARACO	EQ 250MG BASE	N064171 001	JUN 30, 1997

PAROXETINE HYDROCHLORIDE

Suspension; Oral

PAXIL
+ GLAXOSMITHKLINE

	EQ 10MG BASE/5ML	N020710 001	JUN 25, 1997

Tablet, Extended Release; Oral

PAXIL CR
GLAXOSMITHKLINE

	EQ 12.5MG BASE	N020936 001	FEB 16, 1999
	EQ 25MG BASE	N020936 002	FEB 16, 1999

PAROXETINE HYDROCHLORIDE *(continued)*

Tablet, Extended Release; Oral

PAXIL CR
+ GLAXOSMITHKLINE

	EQ 37.5MG BASE	N020936 003	DEC 06, 2000

Tablet; Oral

PAXIL
GLAXOSMITHKLINE

	EQ 10MG BASE	N020031 001	DEC 29, 1992
	EQ 20MG BASE	N020031 002	DEC 29, 1992
	EQ 30MG BASE	N020031 003	DEC 29, 1992
+	EQ 40MG BASE	N020031 005	DEC 29, 1992

PEGADEMASE BOVINE

Injectable; Injection

ADAGEN
+ ENZON

	250 UNITS/ML	N019818 001	MAR 21, 1990

PEGVISOMANT

Injectable; Subcutaneous

SOMAVERT
+ PHARMACIA AND UPJOHN

	10MG/VIAL	N021106 001	MAR 25, 2003
	15MG/VIAL	N021106 002	MAR 25, 2003
+	20MG/VIAL	N021106 003	MAR 25, 2003

PEMIROLAST POTASSIUM

Solution/Drops; Ophthalmic

ALAMAST
+ SANTEN

	0.1%	N021079 001	SEP 24, 1999

PEMOLINE

Tablet, Chewable; Oral

CYLERT

AB +	ABBOTT	37.5MG	N017703 001	

PEMOLINE

AB	AMIDE PHARM	37.5MG	N075678 001	JUL 26, 2000
AB	COPLEY PHARM	37.5MG	N075555 001	FEB 18, 2000

Tablet; Oral

CYLERT

AB +	ABBOTT	18.75MG	N016832 001	
AB		37.5MG	N016832 002	
AB		75MG	N016832 003	

PEMOLINE

AB	AMIDE PHARM	18.75MG	N075595 001

Prescription Drug Products *(continued)*

PEMOLINE *(continued)*
Tablet; Oral
PEMOLINE

TE	Firm	Strength	Date	Appl. No.
	AMIDE PHARM			
AB		37.5MG	FEB 28, 2000	N075595 001
AB		75MG	FEB 28, 2000	N075595 002
	COPLEY PHARM			
AB		18.75MG	FEB 28, 2000	N075030 003
AB		37.5MG	FEB 22, 2000	N075030 001
AB		75MG	JAN 29, 1999	N075030 002
	GENEVA PHARMS TECH			
AB		18.75MG	JAN 29, 1999	N075286 001
AB		37.5MG	DEC 27, 1999	N075286 002
AB		75MG	JUN 30, 1999	N075286 003
	MALLINCKRODT			
AB		18.75MG	JUN 30, 1999	N075726 003
AB		37.5MG	JUN 30, 1999	N075726 002
AB		75MG	MAR 30, 2001	N075726 001
	VINTAGE PHARMS			
AB		18.75MG	MAR 30, 2001	N075328 001
AB		37.5MG	MAR 30, 2001	N075328 002
AB		75MG	APR 19, 2000	N075328 003
	WATSON LABS			
AB		18.75MG	APR 19, 2000	N075287 001
AB		37.5MG	APR 19, 2000	N075287 002
AB		75MG	JUN 13, 2001	N075287 003
			SEP 18, 2000	
			SEP 18, 2000	

PENBUTOLOL SULFATE
Tablet; Oral
LEVATOL
+ SCHWARZ PHARMA 20MG   JAN 05, 1989   N018976 004

PENCICLOVIR SODIUM
Cream; Topical
DENAVIR
+ NOVARTIS 1%   SEP 24, 1996   N020629 001

PENICILLAMINE
Capsule; Oral
CUPRIMINE
MERCK
+ 125MG N019853 002
+ 250MG N019853 001

PENICILLAMINE *(continued)*
Tablet; Oral
DEPEN
+ MEDPOINTE PHARM HLC 250MG N019854 001

PENICILLIN G BENZATHINE
Injectable; Injection
BICILLIN L-A
+ KING PHARMS 300,000 UNITS/ML N050141 003
BC + 600,000 UNITS/ML N050141 001
PERMAPEN
BC + PFIZER 600,000 UNITS/ML N060014 001

PENICILLIN G BENZATHINE; PENICILLIN G PROCAINE
Injectable; Injection
BICILLIN C-R
+ KING PHARMS 150,000 UNITS/ML;150,000 UNITS/ML N050138 002
300,000 UNITS/ML;300,000 UNITS/ML N050138 001
BICILLIN C-R 900/300
+ KING PHARMS 900,000 UNITS/2ML;300,000 UNITS/2ML N050138 003

PENICILLIN G POTASSIUM
Injectable; Injection
PENICILLIN G POTASSIUM

TE	Firm	Strength	Appl. No.	Date
	GENEVA PHARMS			
AP		1,000,000 UNITS/VIAL	N065079 001	AUG 30, 2002
AP		5,000,000 UNITS/VIAL	N065079 002	AUG 30, 2002
AP		20,000,000 UNITS/VIAL	N065079 003	AUG 30, 2002
	MARSAM PHARMS LLC			
AP		1,000,000 UNITS/VIAL	N062991 001	SEP 13, 1988
AP		5,000,000 UNITS/VIAL	N062991 002	SEP 13, 1988
AP		10,000,000 UNITS/VIAL	N062991 003	SEP 13, 1988
	PFIZER			
AP		20,000,000 UNITS/VIAL	N062991 004	SEP 13, 1988
	PENICILLIN G POTASSIUM IN PLASTIC CONTAINER			
AP	+ BAXTER HLTHCARE	20,000 UNITS/ML	N060074 003	SEP 13, 1988
	PFIZERPEN			
AP	+ PFIZER	40,000 UNITS/ML	N050638 001	JUN 25, 1990
AP	+	60,000 UNITS/ML	N050638 002	JUN 25, 1990
AP	+	1,000,000 UNITS/VIAL	N050638 003	JUN 25, 1990
AP	+	5,000,000 UNITS/VIAL	N060657 001	
AP	+	20,000,000 UNITS/VIAL	N060657 002	
AP	+		N060657 003	

Prescription Drug Products *(continued)*

PENICILLIN G PROCAINE
Injectable; Injection
WYCILLIN
+ KING PHARMS	300,000 UNITS/ML	N060101 002
	600,000 UNITS/ML	N060101 001

PENICILLIN G PROCAINE *MULTIPLE*
SEE   PENICILLIN G BENZATHINE; PENICILLIN G PROCAINE

PENICILLIN G SODIUM
Injectable; Im-Iv
PENICILLIN G SODIUM
+ BIOCHEMIE	5,000,000 UNITS/VIAL	N065068 001	FEB 26, 2001

PENICILLIN V POTASSIUM
For Solution; Oral
BEEPEN-VK
AA	GLAXOSMITHKLINE	EQ 125MG BASE/5ML	N062270 001	
AA		EQ 250MG BASE/5ML	N062270 002	
	PENICILLIN V POTASSIUM			
AA	CLONMEL	EQ 125MG BASE/5ML	N062981 001	FEB 10, 1989
AA		EQ 250MG BASE/5ML	N062981 002	FEB 10, 1989
AA		EQ 125MG BASE/5ML	N061529 001	
AA	CONSOLIDATED PHARM	EQ 250MG BASE/5ML	N061529 002	
	PENICILLIN-VK			
AA	TEVA	EQ 125MG BASE/5ML	N060456 001	
AA		EQ 250MG BASE/5ML	N060456 002	
	VEETIDS			
AA	APOTHECON	EQ 125MG BASE/5ML	N061410 001	
AA		EQ 250MG BASE/5ML	N061410 002	

Tablet; Oral
BEEPEN-VK
AB	GLAXOSMITHKLINE	EQ 250MG BASE	N062273 001	
AB		EQ 500MG BASE	N062273 002	
	BETAPEN-VK			
AB	BRISTOL	EQ 250MG BASE	N061150 001	
AB		EQ 500MG BASE	N061150 002	
	PENICILLIN V POTASSIUM			
AB	BIOCHEMIE	EQ 250MG BASE	N064071 001	NOV 30, 1995
AB		EQ 500MG BASE	N064071 002	NOV 30, 1995
AB	+	EQ 250MG BASE	N062936 001	NOV 30, 1995
	CLONMEL	EQ 500MG BASE	N062935 001	NOV 25, 1988
AB		EQ 250MG BASE	N061528 001	NOV 23, 1988
AB	CONSOLIDATED PHARM	EQ 250MG BASE	N061528 001	NOV 23, 1988
AB		EQ 500MG BASE	N061528 002	
	PENICILLIN-VK			
AB	TEVA	EQ 250MG BASE	N060711 002	
AB		EQ 500MG BASE	N060711 003	

PENICILLIN V POTASSIUM *(continued)*
Tablet; Oral
UTICILLIN VK
AB	PHARMACIA AND UPJOHN	EQ 250MG BASE	N061651 001
	VEETIDS		
AB	APOTHECON	EQ 250MG BASE	N061411 001
AB		EQ 500MG BASE	N061411 002

PENTAMIDINE ISETHIONATE
For Solution; Inhalation
NEBUPENT
+ AM PHARM PARTNERS	300MG/VIAL	N019887 001	JUN 15, 1989
	600MG/VIAL	N019887 002	MAR 22, 1996

Injectable; Injection
PENTAM
AP	+ AM PHARM PARTNERS	300MG/VIAL	N019264 001	OCT 16, 1984
	PENTAMIDINE ISETHIONATE			
AP	ABBOTT	300MG/VIAL	N073479 001	JUN 30, 1992
AP	STERIS	300MG/VIAL	N074303 001	AUG 17, 1995

PENTAZOCINE HYDROCHLORIDE *MULTIPLE*
SEE   ACETAMINOPHEN; PENTAZOCINE HYDROCHLORIDE
SEE   NALOXONE HYDROCHLORIDE; PENTAZOCINE HYDROCHLORIDE

PENTAZOCINE LACTATE
Injectable; Injection
TALWIN
+ ABBOTT	EQ 30MG BASE/ML	N016194 001

PENTOBARBITAL SODIUM
Capsule; Oral
NEMBUTAL SODIUM
AA	+ ABBOTT	30MG	N084095 001
		100MG	N083245 001
	SODIUM PENTOBARBITAL		
AA	ICN	100MG	N083264 001

Injectable; Injection
NEMBUTAL SODIUM
AA	+ ABBOTT	50MG/ML	N083246 001

PENTOSAN POLYSULFATE SODIUM
Capsule; Oral
ELMIRON
+ JOHNSON AND JOHNSON	100MG	N020193 001	SEP 26, 1996

Prescription Drug Products *(continued)*

PENTOSTATIN
Injectable; Injection

	NIPENT		
+	SUPERGEN	10MG/VIAL	N020122 001 OCT 11, 1991

PENTOXIFYLLINE
Tablet, Extended Release; Oral

	PENTOXIFYLLINE			
AB	BIOVAIL	400MG	N075028 001	JUL 20, 1998
AB	ESI LEDERLE	400MG	N074877 001	JUL 08, 1997
AB	IMPAX LABS	400MG	N075093 001	AUG 10, 1999
AB	MYLAN	400MG	N074425 001	JUL 08, 1997
AB	PLIVA	400MG	N074874 001	MAY 25, 1999
AB	PUREPAC PHARM	400MG	N074878 001	JUL 09, 1997
AB	TEVA	400MG	N075199 001	SEP 03, 1999
AB	TORPHARM	400MG	N075191 001	JUN 09, 1999
AB	WATSON LABS	400MG	N075107 001	SEP 04, 1998
	PENTOXIL			
AB	UPSHER SMITH	400MG	N074962 001	MAR 31, 1999
	TRENTAL			
AB	AVENTIS PHARMS	400MG	N018631 001	AUG 30, 1984

PERFLEXANE *MULTIPLE*
SEE DIMYRISTOYL LECITHIN; PERFLEXANE

PERFLUOROPOLYMETHYLISOPROPYL ETHER; POLYTETRAFLUOROETHYLENE
Paste; Topical

	SKIN EXPOSURE REDUCTION PASTE AGAINST CHEMICAL WARFARE AGENTS		
+	US ARMY	50%;50%	N021084 001 FEB 17, 2000

PERFLUTREN
Injectable; Intravenous

	DEFINITY		
+	BRISTOL MYERS SQUIBB	6.52MG/ML	N021064 001 JUL 31, 2001

PERGOLIDE MESYLATE
Tablet; Oral

	PERGOLIDE MESYLATE			
AB	TEVA	EQ 0.05MG BASE	N076061 001	NOV 27, 2002
AB		EQ 0.25MG BASE	N076061 002	NOV 27, 2002
AB		EQ 1MG BASE	N076061 003	NOV 27, 2002
	PERMAX			
AB	+ LILLY	EQ 0.05MG BASE	N019385 001	DEC 30, 1988
AB		EQ 0.25MG BASE	N019385 002	DEC 30, 1988
AB		EQ 1MG BASE	N019385 003	DEC 30, 1988

PERINDOPRIL ERBUMINE
Tablet; Oral

	ACEON			
	SOLVAY PHARMA	2MG	N020184 001	DEC 30, 1993
		4MG	N020184 002	DEC 30, 1993
		8MG	N020184 003	DEC 30, 1993

PERMETHRIN
Cream; Topical

	ELIMITE			
AB	+ ALLERGAN	5%	N019855 001	AUG 25, 1989
	PERMETHRIN			
AB	ALPHARMA	5%	N074806 001	JAN 23, 1998
AB	CLAY PARK	5%	N076369 001	APR 21, 2003

PERPHENAZINE
Concentrate; Oral

	PERPHENAZINE			
	+ PHARM ASSOC	16MG/5ML	N040360 001	MAY 25, 2001

Injectable; Injection

	TRILAFON		
	SCHERING	5MG/ML	N011213 002

Tablet; Oral

	PERPHENAZINE			
AB	GENEVA PHARMS	2MG	N089683 001	DEC 08, 1988
AB		4MG	N089684 001	DEC 08, 1988
AB		8MG	N089685 001	DEC 08, 1988
AB		16MG	N089686 001	DEC 08, 1988

Prescription Drug Products (continued)

PERPHENAZINE (continued)
Tablet; Oral
  PERPHENAZINE
    IVAX PHARMS

AB		2MG	N089707 001	SEP 10, 1987
AB		4MG	N089708 001	SEP 10, 1987
AB		8MG	N089456 001	SEP 10, 1987
AB		16MG	N089457 001	SEP 10, 1987
AB	+ VINTAGE PHARMS	2MG	N040226 001	DEC 31, 1998
AB		4MG	N040226 002	DEC 31, 1998
AB		8MG	N040226 003	DEC 31, 1998
AB		16MG	N040226 004	DEC 31, 1998

PERPHENAZINE *MULTIPLE*
  SEE AMITRIPTYLINE HYDROCHLORIDE; PERPHENAZINE

PHENDIMETRAZINE TARTRATE
Capsule, Extended Release; Oral
  BONTRIL

BC	MALLINCKRODT	105MG	N088021 001	SEP 21, 1982

  PHENDIMETRAZINE TARTRATE

BC	+ EON	105MG	N018074 001	

  X-TROZINE L.A.

BC	SHIRE RICHWOOD	105MG	N087371 001	AUG 24, 1982

Capsule; Oral
  PHENDIMETRAZINE TARTRATE

AA	+ EON	35MG	N085695 001	

  X-TROZINE

AA	SHIRE RICHWOOD	35MG	N087394 001	SEP 22, 1982

Tablet; Oral
  BONTRIL PDM

AA	AMARIN PHARMS	35MG	N085272 001	

  CAM-METRAZINE

AA	+ ABC HOLDING	35MG	N083922 001	
AA		35MG	N085318 001	
AA		35MG	N085320 001	
AA		35MG	N085321 001	
AA		35MG	N085511 001	
AA		35MG	N085756 001	

  CAMALL
  PHENDIMETRAZINE TARTRATE

AA	ABC HOLDING	35MG	N085761 001	
AA		35MG	N085941 001	JUN 27, 1983
AA	EON	35MG	N085588 001	
AA		35MG	N085830 001	
AA	MIKART	35MG	N089452 001	

PHENDIMETRAZINE TARTRATE (continued)
Tablet; Oral
  PHENDIMETRAZINE TARTRATE
    MIKART

				OCT 30, 1991

  X-TROZINE

AA	SHIRE RICHWOOD	35MG	N086553 001	
AA		35MG	N086554 001	

PHENELZINE SULFATE
Tablet; Oral
  NARDIL

	+ PARKE DAVIS	EQ 15MG BASE	N011909 002	

PHENOXYBENZAMINE HYDROCHLORIDE
Capsule; Oral
  DIBENZYLINE

	+ WELLSPRING PHARM	10MG	N008708 001	

PHENTERMINE HYDROCHLORIDE
Capsule; Oral
  ADIPEX-P

AA	+ TEVA	37.5MG	N088023 001	AUG 02, 1983

  ONA-MAST

AA	MAST MM	30MG	N086511 001	
AA		30MG	N086516 001	

  PHENTERMINE HCL

	ABC HOLDING	18.75MG	N088576 001	MAY 23, 1984
AA		30MG	N085417 001	
AA		30MG	N086732 002	
AA		30MG	N087215 001	
AA		37.5MG	N087915 001	DEC 22, 1983
AA		37.5MG	N087918 001	DEC 22, 1983
AA		37.5MG	N087930 001	OCT 14, 1983
AA		37.5MG	N086610 001	JUN 04, 1984
AA		37.5MG	N088611 001	JUN 04, 1984
AA		37.5MG	N088625 001	AUG 23, 1984
AA	ABLE	15MG	N040497 001	MAR 13, 2003
AA		30MG	N040403 001	AUG 30, 2001
AA		30MG	N040427 001	AUG 30, 2001
AA	AMBI PHARMS	30MG	N040083 001	MAR 07, 1997
AA	AMIDE PHARM	15MG	N040460 001	JAN 14, 2003
AA		30MG	N040227 001	JUN 18, 1997

Prescription Drug Products (continued)

PHENTERMINE HYDROCHLORIDE (continued)

Capsule; Oral

PHENTERMINE HCL

AA	+ AMIDE PHARM	30MG	N040448 001 JAN 22, 2003
AA		37.5MG	N040228 001 JUN 19, 1997
AA	CAMALL	15MG	N086735 001
AA		30MG	N087226 001
AA	+ EON	15MG	N087301 001
AA	+	30MG	N086945 001 JUL 20, 1983
AA		30MG	N087190 001
AA		30MG	N087208 001
AA		30MG	N087223 001
AA	USL PHARMA	30MG	N088797 001 DEC 10, 1984
AA	VINTAGE PHARMS	37.5MG	N040377 001 JAN 04, 2002

Tablet; Oral

ADIPEX-P

AA	+ TEVA	37.5MG	N085128 001

ONA MAST
MAST MM

AA		8MG	N086260 001

PHENTERMINE HCL

AA	+ ABC HOLDING	8MG	N083923 001
AA		8MG	N085319 001
AA		37.5MG	N087805 001 DEC 06, 1982
AA	ABLE	37.5MG	N088596 001 APR 04, 1984
AA	AMIDE PHARM	37.5MG	N040402 001 AUG 30, 2001
AA	+ EON	30MG	N040190 001 MAY 30, 1997
AA			N088605 001 SEP 28, 1987
AA	PUREPAC PHARM	37.5MG	N040276 001 NOV 25, 1998
AA	USL PHARMA	8MG	N083804 001
AA		37.5MG	N088910 001 JUL 17, 1985
AA		37.5MG	N088917 001 JUL 17, 1985

PHENTERMINE RESIN COMPLEX

Capsule, Extended Release; Oral

IONAMIN

	CELLTECH PHARMS	EQ 15MG BASE	N011613 004
	+	EQ 30MG BASE	N011613 002

PHENTOLAMINE MESYLATE

Injectable; Injection

PHENTOLAMINE MESYLATE

AP	BEDFORD	5MG/VIAL	N040235 001 MAR 11, 1998

PHENTOLAMINE MESYLATE (continued)

Injectable; Injection

REGITINE

AP	+ NOVARTIS	5MG/VIAL	N008278 003

PHENYLEPHRINE HYDROCHLORIDE; PROMETHAZINE HYDROCHLORIDE

Syrup; Oral

PROMETH VC PLAIN

AA	+ ALPHARMA	5MG/5ML;6.25MG/5ML	N088761 001 NOV 08, 1984

PROMETHAZINE VC PLAIN

AA	MORTON GROVE	5MG/5ML;6.25MG/5ML	N088897 001 JAN 04, 1985

PHENYLEPHRINE HYDROCHLORIDE *MULTIPLE*

SEE CODEINE PHOSPHATE; PHENYLEPHRINE HYDROCHLORIDE; PROMETHAZINE HYDROCHLORIDE

SEE CYCLOPENTOLATE HYDROCHLORIDE; PHENYLEPHRINE HYDROCHLORIDE

PHENYLPROPANOLAMINE HYDROCHLORIDE *MULTIPLE*

SEE BROMPHENIRAMINE MALEATE; CODEINE PHOSPHATE; PHENYLPROPANOLAMINE HYDROCHLORIDE

PHENYTOIN

Suspension; Oral

DILANTIN-125

AB	+ PARKE DAVIS	125MG/5ML	N008762 001

PHENYTOIN

AB	MORTON GROVE	125MG/5ML	N040420 001 APR 19, 2002

PHENYTOIN

AB	ALPHARMA	125MG/5ML	N089892 001 SEP 25, 1992
AB	VISTAPHARM	125MG/5ML	N040342 001 JAN 31, 2001

Tablet, Chewable; Oral

DILANTIN

AB	+ PFIZER PHARMS	50MG	N084427 001

PHENYTOIN SODIUM

Injectable; Injection

PHENYTOIN

AB	+ ELKINS SINN	50MG/ML	N084307 001

PHENYTOIN SODIUM, EXTENDED

Capsule; Oral

DILANTIN

AB	+ PARKE DAVIS	30MG	N084349 001
		100MG	N084349 002

EXTENDED PHENYTOIN SODIUM

AB	BARR	100MG	N040435 001 JUN 20, 2003
AB	MYLAN	100MG	N040298 001 DEC 28, 1998

Prescription Drug Products (continued)

PHENYTOIN SODIUM, EXTENDED (continued)

Capsule; Oral

PHENYTEK

+ MYLAN	200MG	N040298 002	DEC 06, 2001
+	300MG	N040298 003	DEC 06, 2001

PHENYTOIN SODIUM, PROMPT

Capsule; Oral

PROMPT PHENYTOIN SODIUM

+ IVAX PHARMS	100MG	N080259 001

PHOSPHORIC ACID *MULTIPLE*

SEE AMINO ACIDS: CALCIUM ACETATE: GLYCERIN: MAGNESIUM ACETATE: PHOSPHORIC ACID: POTASSIUM CHLORIDE: SODIUM ACETATE: SODIUM CHLORIDE

SEE AMINO ACIDS: MAGNESIUM ACETATE: PHOSPHORIC ACID: POTASSIUM CHLORIDE: SODIUM ACETATE

SEE AMINO ACIDS: MAGNESIUM ACETATE: PHOSPHORIC ACID: POTASSIUM ACETATE: SODIUM CHLORIDE

SEE AMINO ACIDS: MAGNESIUM ACETATE: PHOSPHORIC ACID: POTASSIUM CHLORIDE: SODIUM ACETATE: SODIUM CHLORIDE

PHYTONADIONE

Injectable; Injection

AQUAMEPHYTON

BP	+ MERCK	1MG/0.5ML	N012223 002	
BP	+	10MG/ML	N012223 001	

PHYTONADIONE

	INTL MEDICATION	1MG/0.5ML	N083722 001

VITAMIN K1

BP	ABBOTT	1MG/0.5ML	N087954 001	JUL 25, 1983
BP		10MG/ML	N087955 001	JUL 25, 1983

Tablet; Oral

MEPHYTON

BP	+ MERCK	5MG	N010104 003

PHYTONADIONE *MULTIPLE*

SEE ASCORBIC ACID: BIOTIN: CYANOCOBALAMIN: DEXPANTHENOL: ERGOCALCIFEROL: FOLIC ACID: NIACINAMIDE: PHYTONADIONE: PYRIDOXINE HYDROCHLORIDE: RIBOFLAVIN PHOSPHATE SODIUM: THIAMINE HYDROCHLORIDE: VITAMIN A: VITAMIN E

PILOCARPINE HYDROCHLORIDE

Gel; Ophthalmic

PILOPINE HS

+ ALCON	4%	N018796 001	OCT 01, 1984

Tablet; Oral

SALAGEN

MGI PHARMA INC	5MG	N020237 001	MAR 22, 1994

PILOCARPINE HYDROCHLORIDE (continued)

Tablet; Oral

SALAGEN

+ MGI PHARMA INC	7.5MG	N020237 002	APR 18, 2003

PIMECROLIMUS

Cream; Topical

ELIDEL

+ NOVARTIS	1%	N021302 001	DEC 13, 2001

PIMOZIDE

Tablet; Oral

ORAP

TEVA	1MG	N017473 003	AUG 27, 1997
+	2MG	N017473 001	JUL 31, 1984

PINDOLOL

Tablet; Oral

PINDOLOL

AB	GENEVA PHARMS	5MG	N073608 001	MAR 29, 1993
AB		10MG	N073609 001	MAR 29, 1993
AB	GENPHARM	5MG	N074013 001	SEP 24, 1992
AB		10MG	N074018 001	SEP 24, 1992
AB	IVAX PHARMS	5MG	N073687 001	FEB 26, 1993
AB		10MG	N073687 002	FEB 26, 1993
AB	MAR-TEC	5MG	N074474 001	OCT 28, 1996
AB		10MG	N074474 002	OCT 28, 1996
AB	MUTUAL PHARM	5MG	N074063 001	JAN 27, 1994
AB		10MG	N074063 002	JAN 27, 1994
AB	MYLAN	5MG	N074019 001	SEP 03, 1992
AB		10MG	N074019 002	SEP 03, 1992
AB	TEVA	5MG	N073661 001	OCT 31, 1993
AB		5MG	N074123 001	APR 17, 1997
AB		10MG	N073661 002	OCT 31, 1993
AB		10MG	N074123 002	APR 17, 1997
AB	WATSON LABS	5MG	N074437 001	

Prescription Drug Products (continued)

PINDOLOL (continued)
Tablet; Oral

PINDOLOL

Code	Strength	Firm	Appl No	Date
AB	10MG	WATSON LABS	N074437 002	FEB 27, 1995

VISKEN

Code	Strength	Firm	Appl No	Date
AB	5MG	NOVARTIS	N018285 001	SEP 03, 1982
AB +	10MG		N018285 002	SEP 03, 1982

PIOGLITAZONE HYDROCHLORIDE
Tablet; Oral

ACTOS

Code	Strength	Firm	Appl No	Date
	EQ 15MG BASE	TAKEDA PHARMS NA	N021073 001	JUL 15, 1999
	EQ 30MG BASE		N021073 002	JUL 15, 1999
+	EQ 45MG BASE		N021073 003	JUL 15, 1999

PIPERACILLIN SODIUM; TAZOBACTAM SODIUM
Injectable; Injection

ZOSYN

Code	Strength	Firm	Appl No	Date
+	EQ 2GM BASE/VIAL;EQ 250MG BASE/VIAL	WYETH PHARMS INC	N050684 001	OCT 22, 1993
+	EQ 3GM BASE/VIAL;EQ 375MG BASE/VIAL		N050684 002	OCT 22, 1993
+	EQ 4GM BASE/VIAL;EQ 500MG BASE/VIAL		N050684 003	OCT 22, 1993
+	EQ 36GM BASE/VIAL;EQ 4.5GM BASE/VIAL		N050684 004	OCT 22, 1993

ZOSYN IN PLASTIC CONTAINER

Code	Strength	Firm	Appl No	Date
+	EQ 40MG BASE/ML;EQ 5MG BASE/ML	WYETH PHARMS INC	N050750 001	FEB 24, 1998
+	EQ 60MG BASE/ML;EQ 7.5MG BASE/ML		N050750 002	FEB 24, 1998
+	EQ 4GM BASE/100ML;EQ 500MG BASE/100ML		N050750 003	FEB 24, 1998

PIPERAZINE CITRATE
Syrup; Oral

MULTIFUGE

Code	Strength	Firm	Appl No	Date
AA	EQ 500MG BASE/5ML	BLULINE	N009452 001	

PIPERAZINE CITRATE

Code	Strength	Firm	Appl No	Date
AA	EQ 500MG BASE/5ML	LUITPOLD	N080671 001	

PIRBUTEROL ACETATE
Aerosol, Metered; Inhalation

MAXAIR

Code	Strength	Firm	Appl No	Date
+	EQ 0.2MG BASE/INH	3M	N020014 001	NOV 30, 1992

PIROXICAM
Capsule; Oral

FELDENE

Code	Strength	Firm	Appl No	Date
AB	10MG	PFIZER	N018147 002	APR 06, 1982
AB +	20MG		N018147 003	APR 06, 1982

PIROXICAM

Code	Strength	Firm	Appl No	Date
AB	10MG	COPLEY PHARM	N074103 001	AUG 28, 1992
AB	20MG		N074103 002	AUG 28, 1992
AB	10MG	EGIS	N074808 001	JUL 08, 1997
AB	20MG		N074808 002	JUL 08, 1997
AB	10MG	GENPHARM	N074043 001	JUL 08, 1997
AB	20MG		N074043 002	SEP 22, 1992
AB	10MG	IVAX PHARMS	N074148 001	SEP 22, 1992
AB	20MG		N074148 002	JUN 03, 1996
AB	10MG	MEPHA	N074116 001	JUN 03, 1996
AB	20MG		N074118 001	JUN 15, 1993
AB	10MG	MUTUAL PHARM	N073535 001	JUN 15, 1993
AB	20MG		N073536 001	MAR 12, 1993
AB	10MG	MYLAN	N074102 001	MAR 12, 1993
AB	20MG		N074102 002	JUL 31, 1992
AB	10MG	SCS	N074036 001	JUL 31, 1992
AB	20MG		N074036 002	MAY 29, 1992
AB	10MG	TEVA	N073637 001	MAY 29, 1992
AB	20MG		N074131 001	JAN 28, 1994
AB	10MG	WATSON LABS	N073638 001	DEC 11, 1992
AB	20MG		N074131 002	JAN 28, 1994
AB	10MG		N074287 001	DEC 11, 1992
			N074460 001	MAY 16, 1996

Prescription Drug Products (continued)

PIROXICAM (continued)
Capsule; Oral
  PIROXICAM
    WATSON LABS

Code	Strength	Appl No	Date
AB	20MG	N074287 002	SEP 29, 1995
AB	20MG	N074460 002	MAY 16, 1996 / SEP 29, 1995

PLICAMYCIN
Injectable; Injection
  MITHRACIN
  + PFIZER

Code	Strength	Appl No
	2.5MG/VIAL	N050109 001

PODOFILOX
Gel; Topical
  CONDYLOX
  + OCLASSEN

Code	Strength	Appl No	Date
	0.5%	N020529 001	MAR 13, 1997

Solution; Topical
  CONDYLOX

Code	Strength	Appl No	Date
AT + PADDOCK	0.5%	N019795 001	DEC 13, 1990

  PODOFILOX

Code	Strength	Appl No	Date
AT + PADDOCK	0.5%	N075600 001	JAN 29, 2002

POLYETHYLENE GLYCOL 3350
For Solution; Oral
  MIRALAX
  + BRAINTREE

Code	Strength	Appl No	Date
	17GM/SCOOPFUL	N020698 001	FEB 18, 1999

POLYETHYLENE GLYCOL 3350; POTASSIUM CHLORIDE; SODIUM BICARBONATE; SODIUM CHLORIDE
For Solution; Oral
  NULYTELY
  + BRAINTREE

Code	Strength	Appl No	Date
	420GM/BOT;1.48GM/ BOT;5.72GM/BOT;11.2GM/BOT	N019797 001	APR 22, 1991

  NULYTELY-FLAVORED
  + BRAINTREE

Code	Strength	Appl No	Date
	420GM/BOT;1.48GM/ BOT;5.72GM/BOT;11.2GM/BOT	N019797 002	NOV 18, 1994

POLYETHYLENE GLYCOL 3350; POTASSIUM CHLORIDE; SODIUM BICARBONATE; SODIUM CHLORIDE; SODIUM SULFATE
Solution; Oral
  OCL
  + ABBOTT

Code	Strength	Appl No	Date
	6GM/100ML;75MG/ 100ML;168MG/100ML;146MG/ 100ML;1.29GM/100ML	N019284 001	APR 30, 1986

POLYETHYLENE GLYCOL 3350; POTASSIUM CHLORIDE; SODIUM BICARBONATE; SODIUM CHLORIDE; SODIUM SULFATE, ANHYDROUS
For Solution; Oral
  COLYTE

Code	Name	Strength	Appl No	Date
AA	+ SCHWARZ PHARMA	240GM/BOT;2.98GM/ BOT;6.72GM/BOT;5.84GM/ BOT;22.72GM/BOT	N018983 007	JUN 12, 1987

  COLYTE-FLAVORED

Code	Name	Strength	Appl No	Date
AA	+ SCHWARZ PHARMA	227.1GM/BOT;2.82GM/ BOT;6.36GM/BOT;5.53GM/ BOT;21.5GM/BOT	N018983 008	NOV 14, 1991
AA	+	240GM/BOT;2.98GM/ BOT;6.72GM/BOT;5.84GM/ BOT;22.72GM/BOT	N018983 009	NOV 14, 1991

  COLYTE

Code	Name	Strength	Appl No	Date
AA	+ SCHWARZ PHARMA	227.1GM/BOT;2.82GM/ BOT;6.36GM/BOT;5.53GM/ BOT;21.5GM/BOT	N018983 010	JAN 31, 1989

  COLYTE WITH FLAVOR PACKS

Code	Name	Strength	Appl No	Date
AA	+ SCHWARZ PHARMA	240GM/BOT;2.98GM/ BOT;6.72GM/BOT;5.84GM/ BOT;22.72GM/BOT	N018983 012	OCT 08, 1998

  GOLYTELY

Code	Name	Strength	Appl No	Date
AA	+ BRAINTREE	236GM/BOT;2.97GM/ BOT;6.74GM/BOT;5.86GM/ BOT;22.74GM/BOT	N019011 001	JUL 13, 1984
AA	+	227.1GM/PACKET;2.82GM/ PACKET;6.36GM/ PACKET;5.53GM/ PACKET;21.5GM/PACKET	N019011 002	JUN 02, 1992

For Suspension; Oral
  E-Z-EM PREP LYTE

Code	Name	Strength	Appl No	Date
AA	E Z EM	236GM/BOT;2.97GM/ BOT;6.74GM/BOT;5.86GM/ BOT;22.74GM/BOT	N071278 001	NOV 21, 1988

  COLOVAGE

Code	Name	Strength	Appl No	Date
AA	DYNAPHARM	227.1GM/PACKET;2.82GM/ PACKET;6.36GM/ PACKET;5.53GM/ PACKET;21.5GM/PACKET	N071320 001	APR 20, 1988

  GLYCOPREP

Code	Name	Strength	Appl No	Date
AA	GOLDLINE	236GM/BOT;2.97GM/ BOT;6.74GM/BOT;5.86GM/ BOT;22.74GM/BOT	N072319 001	DEC 23, 1988

Prescription Drug Products (continued)

POLYETHYLENE GLYCOL 3350; POTASSIUM CHLORIDE; SODIUM BICARBONATE; SODIUM CHLORIDE; SODIUM SULFATE, ANHYDROUS (continued)
For Suspension; Oral

	CO-LAV		
AA	COPLEY PHARM	240GM/BOT;2.98GM/BOT;6.72GM/BOT;5.84GM/BOT;22.72GM/BOT	N073428 001 JAN 28, 1992
	GO-EVAC		
AA	COPLEY PHARM	236GM/BOT;2.97GM/BOT;6.74GM/BOT;5.86GM/BOT;22.74GM/BOT	N073433 001 APR 28, 1992

POLYMYXIN B SULFATE
Injectable; Injection

	POLYMYXIN B SULFATE		
AP +	BEDFORD	EQ 500,000 U BASE/VIAL	N060716 001
AP	PHARMA TEK	EQ 500,000 U BASE/VIAL	N063000 001 SEP 30, 1994

Powder; For Rx Compounding

	POLY-RX		
+	PHARMA TEK	100,000,000 UNITS/BOT	N061578 001

POLYMYXIN B SULFATE; TRIMETHOPRIM
Solution/Drops; Ophthalmic

	TRIMETHOPRIM SULFATE AND POLYMYXIN B SULFATE		
AT	TAYLOR PHARMA	10,000 UNITS/ML;EQ 1MG BASE/ML	N065006 001 DEC 17, 1998

POLYMYXIN B SULFATE; TRIMETHOPRIM SULFATE
Solution/Drops; Ophthalmic

	POLYTRIM		
AT +	ALLERGAN	10,000 UNITS/ML;EQ 1MG BASE/ML	N050567 001 OCT 20, 1988
	TRIMETHOPRIM SULFATE AND POLYMYXIN B SULFATE		
AT	BAUSCH AND LOMB	10,000 UNITS/ML;EQ 1MG BASE/ML	N064120 001 FEB 14, 1997
AT	FALCON PHARMS	10,000 UNITS/ML;EQ 1MG BASE/ML	N064211 001 APR 13, 1998

POLYMYXIN B SULFATE *MULTIPLE*
SEE BACITRACIN: HYDROCORTISONE ACETATE: NEOMYCIN SULFATE: POLYMYXIN B SULFATE
SEE BACITRACIN ZINC: HYDROCORTISONE: NEOMYCIN SULFATE: POLYMYXIN B SULFATE
SEE BACITRACIN ZINC: NEOMYCIN SULFATE: POLYMYXIN B SULFATE
SEE DEXAMETHASONE: NEOMYCIN SULFATE: POLYMYXIN B SULFATE
SEE GRAMICIDIN: NEOMYCIN SULFATE: POLYMYXIN B SULFATE

POLYMYXIN B SULFATE *MULTIPLE* (continued)
SEE HYDROCORTISONE: NEOMYCIN SULFATE: POLYMYXIN B SULFATE
SEE HYDROCORTISONE: POLYMYXIN B SULFATE
SEE HYDROCORTISONE ACETATE: NEOMYCIN SULFATE: POLYMYXIN B SULFATE
SEE NEOMYCIN SULFATE: POLYMYXIN B SULFATE
SEE NEOMYCIN SULFATE: POLYMYXIN B SULFATE: PREDNISOLONE ACETATE
SEE OXYTETRACYCLINE HYDROCHLORIDE: POLYMYXIN B SULFATE

POLYTETRAFLUOROETHYLENE *MULTIPLE*
SEE PERFLUOROPOLYMETHYLISOPROPYL ETHER: POLYTETRAFLUOROETHYLENE

POLYTHIAZIDE
Tablet; Oral

	RENESE		
	PFIZER	1MG	N012845 001
		2MG	N012845 002
		4MG	N012845 003

POLYTHIAZIDE; PRAZOSIN HYDROCHLORIDE
Capsule; Oral

	MINIZIDE		
+	PFIZER	0.5MG;EQ 1MG BASE	N017986 001
		0.5MG;EQ 2MG BASE	N017986 002
		0.5MG;EQ 5MG BASE	N017986 003

POLYTHIAZIDE; RESERPINE
Tablet; Oral

	RENESE-R		
+	PFIZER	2MG;0.25MG	N013636 001

PORACTANT ALFA
Suspension; Intratracheal

	CUROSURF		
+	DEY	80MG/ML	N020744 001 NOV 18, 1999

PORFIMER SODIUM
Injectable; Injection

	PHOTOFRIN		
+	AXCAN SCANDIPHARM	75MG/VIAL	N020451 001 DEC 27, 1995

POTASSIUM ACETATE
Injectable; Injection

	POTASSIUM ACETATE IN PLASTIC CONTAINER		
+	ABBOTT	2MEQ/ML	N018896 001 JUL 20, 1984

POTASSIUM ACETATE *MULTIPLE*
SEE AMINO ACIDS: MAGNESIUM ACETATE: PHOSPHORIC ACID: POTASSIUM ACETATE: POTASSIUM CHLORIDE: SODIUM ACETATE
SEE AMINO ACIDS: MAGNESIUM ACETATE: PHOSPHORIC ACID: POTASSIUM ACETATE: SODIUM CHLORIDE

Prescription Drug Products (continued)

POTASSIUM ACETATE *MULTIPLE* (continued)

SEE   DEXTROSE; MAGNESIUM ACETATE; POTASSIUM ACETATE; SODIUM CHLORIDE
SEE   DEXTROSE; MAGNESIUM ACETATE TETRAHYDRATE; POTASSIUM ACETATE; SODIUM CHLORIDE
SEE   MAGNESIUM ACETATE TETRAHYDRATE; POTASSIUM ACETATE; SODIUM CHLORIDE

POTASSIUM AMINOSALICYLATE

Capsule; Oral

	PASKALIUM		
	+ GLENWOOD	500MG	N009395 004

Tablet; Oral

	PASKALIUM		
	+ GLENWOOD	1GM	N009395 003

POTASSIUM CHLORIDE

Capsule, Extended Release; Oral

	MICRO-K			
AB	KV PHARM	8MEQ	N018238 001	
	MICRO-K 10			
AB	+ KV PHARM	10MEQ	N018238 002	MAY 14, 1984
	POTASSIUM CHLORIDE			
AB	KV PHARM	10MEQ	N070980 001	FEB 17, 1987
AB	TEVA	8MEQ	N073531 001	APR 26, 1996
AB	TEVA	10MEQ	N073532 001	APR 26, 1996

Injectable; Injection

	POTASSIUM CHLORIDE			
AP	+ ABBOTT	1.5MEQ/ML	N083345 001	
AP	+	2MEQ/ML	N080205 001	
AP	AM PHARM PARTNERS	2MEQ/ML	N083345 002	
AP		2MEQ/ML	N080225 001	OCT 20, 1982
			N087817 001	
AP	+ B BRAUN	3MEQ/ML	N080225 003	
AP	+ BAXTER HLTHCARE	2MEQ/ML	N085870 001	
AP	+ INTL MEDICATION	2MEQ/ML	N083163 001	
AP	+ LUITPOLD	2MEQ/ML	N085499 001	
AP	+	2MEQ/ML	N087584 001	
AP	+ PHARMA SERVE NY	2MEQ/ML	N087585 001	
AP	+	2MEQ/ML	N086297 001	
			N087362 001	MAR 08, 1983
	POTASSIUM CHLORIDE 10MEQ IN PLASTIC CONTAINER			
AP	+ BAXTER HLTHCARE	14.9MG/ML	N019904 001	DEC 26, 1989
			N019904 005	DEC 17, 1990
AP	+	746MG/100ML	N020161 006	AUG 11, 1998
			N019904 002	
	POTASSIUM CHLORIDE 20MEQ IN PLASTIC CONTAINER			
AP	+ ABBOTT	29.8MG/ML		
AP	+ BAXTER HLTHCARE	29.8MG/ML		

POTASSIUM CHLORIDE (continued)

Injectable; Injection

	POTASSIUM CHLORIDE 20MEQ IN PLASTIC CONTAINER			
	BAXTER HLTHCARE	1.49GM/100ML		DEC 26, 1989
			N019904 006	DEC 17, 1990
	POTASSIUM CHLORIDE 30MEQ IN PLASTIC CONTAINER	2.24GM/100ML	N020161 003	AUG 11, 1998
AP	+ ABBOTT		N019904 003	DEC 26, 1989
AP	+ BAXTER HLTHCARE	2.24GM/100ML		
	POTASSIUM CHLORIDE 40MEQ IN PLASTIC CONTAINER	2.98GM/100ML	N020161 004	AUG 11, 1998
AP	+ ABBCTT		N019904 004	DEC 26, 1989
AP	+ BAXTER HLTHCARE	2.98GM/100ML		
	POTASSIUM CHLORIDE IN PLASTIC CONTAINER			
AP	+ AM PHARM PARTNERS	2MEQ/ML	N088901 001	JAN 25, 1985
			N088908 001	JAN 25, 1985
AP		2MEQ/ML		

Tablet, Extended Release; Oral

	K+8			
AB	ALRA	8MEQ	N070998 001	JAN 25, 1993
	K+10			
BC	ALRA	10MEQ	N070999 001	OCT 22, 1987
	K-DUR 10			
AB	+ KEY PHARMS	10MEQ	N019439 002	JUN 13, 1986
	K-DUR 20			
AB	+ KEY PHARMS	20MEQ	N019439 001	JUN 13, 1986
	K-TAB			
BC	ABBOTT	10MEQ	N018279 001	
	KLOR-CON			
AB	UPSHER SMITH	8MEQ	N019123 001	APR 17, 1986
BC	UPSHER SMITH	10MEQ	N019123 002	APR 17, 1986
	KLOR-CON M10			
AB	UPSHER SMITH	10MEQ	N074726 002	AUG 09, 2000
	KLOR-CON M15			
	UPSHER SMITH	15MEQ	N074726 003	JUN 06, 2003
	KLOR-CON M20			
AB	UPSHER SMITH	20MEQ	N074726 001	NOV 20, 1998
	KLOTRIX			
BC	APOTHECON	10MEQ	N017850 001	
	POTASSIUM CHLORIDE			
BC	ABBOTT	8MEQ	N018279 002	AUG 01, 1988
			N075604 001	
AB	ANDRX PHARMS	10MEQ		APR 10, 2002

Prescription Drug Products (continued)

POTASSIUM CHLORIDE (continued)
Tablet, Extended Release; Oral

POTASSIUM CHLORIDE

AB	ANDRX PHARMS	20MEQ	N075604 002	APR 10, 2002
AB	COPLEY PHARM	8MEQ	N070618 001	SEP 09, 1987
AB	KV PHARM	20MEQ	N076044 001	APR 05, 2002
AB	SLOW-K + NOVARTIS	8MEQ	N017476 002	

POTASSIUM CHLORIDE; SODIUM CHLORIDE
Injectable; Injection

AP POTASSIUM CHLORIDE 0.15% IN SODIUM CHLORIDE 0.9% IN PLASTIC CONTAINER

	B BRAUN	150MG/100ML;900MG/100ML	N019708 004	SEP 29, 1989

AP POTASSIUM CHLORIDE 20MEQ IN SODIUM CHLORIDE 0.9% IN PLASTIC CONTAINER

	ABBOTT	149MG/100ML;900MG/100ML	N019686 001	OCT 17, 1988

AP POTASSIUM CHLORIDE 40MEQ IN SODIUM CHLORIDE 0.9% IN PLASTIC CONTAINER

	ABBOTT	298MG/100ML;900MG/100ML	N019686 002	OCT 17, 1988

AP SODIUM CHLORIDE 0.9% AND POTASSIUM CHLORIDE 0.15% IN PLASTIC CONTAINER

	BAXTER HLTHCARE	150MG/100ML;900MG/100ML	N017648 001

AP SODIUM CHLORIDE 0.9% AND POTASSIUM CHLORIDE 0.3% IN PLASTIC CONTAINER

	BAXTER HLTHCARE	300MG/100ML;900MG/100ML	N017648 002

AP SODIUM CHLORIDE 0.9% AND POTASSIUM CHLORIDE 0.224%

	BAXTER HLTHCARE	224MG/100ML;900MG/100ML	N017648 003

POTASSIUM CHLORIDE *MULTIPLE*

SEE AMINO ACIDS; CALCIUM ACETATE; GLYCERIN; MAGNESIUM ACETATE; PHOSPHORIC ACID; POTASSIUM CHLORIDE; SODIUM ACETATE; SODIUM CHLORIDE

SEE AMINO ACIDS; CALCIUM CHLORIDE; DEXTROSE; MAGNESIUM CHLORIDE; POTASSIUM CHLORIDE; POTASSIUM PHOSPHATE, DIBASIC; SODIUM CHLORIDE

SEE AMINO ACIDS; DEXTROSE; MAGNESIUM CHLORIDE; POTASSIUM CHLORIDE; SODIUM CHLORIDE; SODIUM PHOSPHATE, DIBASIC, HEPTAHYDRATE

SEE AMINO ACIDS; MAGNESIUM ACETATE; PHOSPHORIC ACID; POTASSIUM ACETATE; POTASSIUM CHLORIDE; SODIUM ACETATE

SEE AMINO ACIDS; MAGNESIUM ACETATE; PHOSPHORIC ACID; POTASSIUM CHLORIDE; SODIUM ACETATE; SODIUM CHLORIDE

SEE AMINO ACIDS; MAGNESIUM CHLORIDE; POTASSIUM CHLORIDE; POTASSIUM PHOSPHATE, DIBASIC; SODIUM CHLORIDE

SEE CALCIUM CHLORIDE; DEXTROSE; GLUTATHIONE DISULFIDE; MAGNESIUM CHLORIDE; POTASSIUM CHLORIDE; SODIUM BICARBONATE; SODIUM CHLORIDE; SODIUM PHOSPHATE

SEE CALCIUM CHLORIDE; DEXTROSE; MAGNESIUM CHLORIDE; POTASSIUM CHLORIDE; SODIUM CHLORIDE

SEE CALCIUM CHLORIDE; DEXTROSE; MAGNESIUM CHLORIDE; POTASSIUM CHLORIDE; SODIUM CITRATE

POTASSIUM CHLORIDE *MULTIPLE* (continued)

SEE CALCIUM CHLORIDE; DEXTROSE; MAGNESIUM CHLORIDE; POTASSIUM CHLORIDE; SODIUM ACETATE; SODIUM CHLORIDE; SODIUM LACTATE; POTASSIUM CHLORIDE; SODIUM

SEE CALCIUM CHLORIDE; DEXTROSE; MAGNESIUM CHLORIDE; SODIUM CHLORIDE; SODIUM BICARBONATE; SODIUM CHLORIDE; SODIUM PHOSPHATE, DIBASIC, HEPTAHYDRATE

SEE CALCIUM CHLORIDE; DEXTROSE; POTASSIUM CHLORIDE; SODIUM ACETATE; SODIUM CHLORIDE

SEE CALCIUM CHLORIDE; DEXTROSE; POTASSIUM CHLORIDE; POTASSIUM CHLORIDE; SODIUM CHLORIDE; SODIUM

SEE CALCIUM CHLORIDE; DEXTROSE; POTASSIUM CHLORIDE; POTASSIUM CHLORIDE; SODIUM CHLORIDE; SODIUM LACTATE

SEE CALCIUM CHLORIDE; MAGNESIUM CHLORIDE; POTASSIUM CHLORIDE; POTASSIUM CHLORIDE; SODIUM

SEE CALCIUM CHLORIDE; MAGNESIUM CHLORIDE; POTASSIUM CHLORIDE; SODIUM ACETATE; SODIUM CHLORIDE; SODIUM CITRATE

SEE CALCIUM CHLORIDE; POTASSIUM CHLORIDE; SODIUM CHLORIDE; SODIUM LACTATE: SODIUM PHOSPHATE

SEE CALCIUM CHLORIDE; POTASSIUM CHLORIDE; SODIUM CHLORIDE; SODIUM LACTATE

SEE DEXTROSE; MAGNESIUM CHLORIDE; POTASSIUM CHLORIDE; POTASSIUM PHOSPHATE, DIBASIC; SODIUM ACETATE

SEE DEXTROSE; MAGNESIUM CHLORIDE; POTASSIUM CHLORIDE; POTASSIUM PHOSPHATE, DIBASIC; SODIUM CHLORIDE; SODIUM LACTATE; SODIUM PHOSPHATE, MONOBASIC, ANHYDROUS

SEE DEXTROSE; MAGNESIUM CHLORIDE; POTASSIUM CHLORIDE; POTASSIUM PHOSPHATE, MONOBASIC; SODIUM CHLORIDE; SODIUM LACTATE

SEE DEXTROSE; MAGNESIUM CHLORIDE; POTASSIUM CHLORIDE; POTASSIUM PHOSPHATE, MONOBASIC; SODIUM LACTATE; SODIUM PHOSPHATE, MONOBASIC, ANHYDROUS

SEE DEXTROSE; MAGNESIUM CHLORIDE; POTASSIUM CHLORIDE; SODIUM ACETATE; SODIUM CHLORIDE

SEE DEXTROSE; MAGNESIUM CHLORIDE; POTASSIUM CHLORIDE; SODIUM GLUCONATE

SEE DEXTROSE; POTASSIUM CHLORIDE

SEE DEXTROSE; POTASSIUM CHLORIDE; POTASSIUM LACTATE; SODIUM CHLORIDE; SODIUM PHOSPHATE, MONOBASIC, ANHYDROUS

SEE DEXTROSE; POTASSIUM CHLORIDE; POTASSIUM PHOSPHATE, DIBASIC; SODIUM ACETATE; SODIUM CHLORIDE

SEE DEXTROSE; POTASSIUM CHLORIDE; POTASSIUM PHOSPHATE, MONOBASIC; SODIUM CHLORIDE; SODIUM LACTATE

SEE DEXTROSE; POTASSIUM CHLORIDE; SODIUM CHLORIDE

SEE MAGNESIUM CHLORIDE; POTASSIUM CHLORIDE; POTASSIUM PHOSPHATE, MONOBASIC; SODIUM ACETATE; SODIUM CHLORIDE; SODIUM GLUCONATE; SODIUM PHOSPHATE, DIBASIC, HEPTAHYDRATE

SEE MAGNESIUM CHLORIDE; POTASSIUM CHLORIDE; SODIUM ACETATE; SODIUM CHLORIDE; SODIUM GLUCONATE

SEE MAGNESIUM SULFATE; POTASSIUM CHLORIDE; POTASSIUM PHOSPHATE, MONOBASIC; SODIUM CHLORIDE; SODIUM PHOSPHATE

SEE POLYETHYLENE GLYCOL 3350; POTASSIUM CHLORIDE; SODIUM BICARBONATE; SODIUM CHLORIDE; SODIUM SULFATE

SEE POLYETHYLENE GLYCOL 3350; POTASSIUM CHLORIDE; SODIUM SULFATE

SEE POLYETHYLENE GLYCOL 3350; POTASSIUM CHLORIDE; SODIUM BICARBONATE; SODIUM CHLORIDE; SODIUM SULFATE, ANHYDROUS

POVIDONE-IODINE
Solution/Drops; Ophthalmic

BETADINE	5%	N018634 001	
+ ALCON		DEC 17, 1986	

PRALIDOXIME CHLORIDE
Injectable; Injection

PRALIDOXIME CHLORIDE			
+ MERIDIAN MEDCL TECHN	300MG/ML	N019986 001	APR 26, 1983
PROTOPAM CHLORIDE			
+ WYETH AYERST	1GM/VIAL	N014134 001	

PRAMIPEXOLE DIHYDROCHLORIDE
Tablet; Oral

MIRAPEX			
PHARMACIA AND UPJOHN	0.5MG	N020667 006	FEB 12, 1998
	0.25MG	N020667 002	JUL 01, 1997
	0.125MG	N020667 001	JUL 01, 1997
+	1.5MG	N020667 005	JUL 01, 1997
+	1MG	N020667 003	JUL 01, 1997

PRAMOXINE HYDROCHLORIDE *MULTIPLE*
SEE   HYDROCORTISONE ACETATE; PRAMOXINE HYDROCHLORIDE

PRAVASTATIN SODIUM
Tablet; Oral

PRAVACHOL			
BRISTOL MYERS SQUIBB	10MG	N019898 002	OCT 31, 1991
	20MG	N019898 003	OCT 31, 1991
	40MG	N019898 004	MAR 22, 1993
+	80MG	N019898 008	DEC 18, 2001

PRAVASTATIN SODIUM *MULTIPLE*
SEE   ASPIRIN; PRAVASTATIN SODIUM

PRAZIQUANTEL
Tablet; Oral

BILTRICIDE			
+ BAYER PHARMS	600MG	N018714 001	DEC 29, 1982

Prescription Drug Products (continued)

POTASSIUM CITRATE
Tablet, Extended Release; Oral

POTASSIUM CITRATE			
MISSION PHARMA	5MEQ	N019071 001	AUG 30, 1985
+	10MEQ	N019071 002	AUG 31, 1992

POTASSIUM LACTATE *MULTIPLE*
SEE   DEXTROSE: POTASSIUM CHLORIDE: POTASSIUM LACTATE: SODIUM CHLORIDE: SODIUM PHOSPHATE, MONOBASIC, ANHYDROUS

POTASSIUM PERCHLORATE
Capsule; Oral

PERCHLORACAP		
+ MALLINCKRODT	200MG	N017551 001

POTASSIUM PHOSPHATE, DIBASIC *MULTIPLE*
SEE   AMINO ACIDS: CALCIUM CHLORIDE: DEXTROSE: MAGNESIUM CHLORIDE: POTASSIUM CHLORIDE: POTASSIUM PHOSPHATE, DIBASIC: SODIUM CHLORIDE

SEE   AMINO ACIDS: CALCIUM CHLORIDE: DEXTROSE: MAGNESIUM CHLORIDE: POTASSIUM PHOSPHATE, DIBASIC: SODIUM ACETATE: SODIUM CHLORIDE

SEE   AMINO ACIDS: DEXTROSE: MAGNESIUM CHLORIDE: POTASSIUM PHOSPHATE, DIBASIC: SODIUM ACETATE: SODIUM CHLORIDE

SEE   AMINO ACIDS: MAGNESIUM CHLORIDE: POTASSIUM CHLORIDE: POTASSIUM PHOSPHATE, DIBASIC: SODIUM CHLORIDE

SEE   AMINO ACIDS: MAGNESIUM CHLORIDE: POTASSIUM PHOSPHATE, DIBASIC: SODIUM ACETATE: SODIUM CHLORIDE

SEE   AMINO ACIDS: MAGNESIUM CHLORIDE: POTASSIUM CHLORIDE: POTASSIUM PHOSPHATE, DIBASIC: SODIUM CHLORIDE

SEE   DEXTROSE: MAGNESIUM CHLORIDE: POTASSIUM CHLORIDE: POTASSIUM PHOSPHATE, DIBASIC: SODIUM ACETATE

SEE   DEXTROSE: MAGNESIUM CHLORIDE: POTASSIUM CHLORIDE: SODIUM CHLORIDE: SODIUM LACTATE: SODIUM PHOSPHATE, MONOBASIC, ANHYDROUS

SEE   DEXTROSE: POTASSIUM CHLORIDE: POTASSIUM PHOSPHATE, DIBASIC: SODIUM ACETATE: SODIUM CHLORIDE

POTASSIUM PHOSPHATE, MONOBASIC *MULTIPLE*
SEE   DEXTROSE: MAGNESIUM CHLORIDE: POTASSIUM CHLORIDE: POTASSIUM PHOSPHATE, MONOBASIC: POTASSIUM PHOSPHATE, MONOBASIC: SODIUM CHLORIDE: SODIUM LACTATE

SEE   DEXTROSE: MAGNESIUM CHLORIDE: POTASSIUM CHLORIDE: POTASSIUM PHOSPHATE, MONOBASIC: SODIUM CHLORIDE: SODIUM LACTATE

SEE   DEXTROSE: MAGNESIUM CHLORIDE: POTASSIUM CHLORIDE: POTASSIUM PHOSPHATE, MONOBASIC: SODIUM PHOSPHATE, MONOBASIC, ANHYDROUS

SEE   DEXTROSE: POTASSIUM CHLORIDE: POTASSIUM PHOSPHATE, MONOBASIC: SODIUM CHLORIDE: SODIUM LACTATE

SEE   MAGNESIUM CHLORIDE: POTASSIUM CHLORIDE: POTASSIUM PHOSPHATE, MONOBASIC: SODIUM ACETATE: SODIUM CHLORIDE: SODIUM GLUCONATE: SODIUM PHOSPHATE, DIBASIC, HEPTAHYDRATE

SEE   MAGNESIUM SULFATE: POTASSIUM CHLORIDE: POTASSIUM PHOSPHATE, MONOBASIC: SODIUM CHLORIDE: SODIUM PHOSPHATE

Prescription Drug Products (continued)

PRAZOSIN HYDROCHLORIDE

Capsule; Oral
MINIPRESS

TE	Firm	Strength	Appl. No.	Date
AB	+ PFIZER	EQ 1MG BASE	N017442 002	
AB		EQ 2MG BASE	N017442 003	
AB		EQ 5MG BASE	N017442 001	

PRAZOSIN HCL

TE	Firm	Strength	Appl. No.	Date
AB	GENEVA PHARMS	EQ 1MG BASE	N072576 001	MAY 16, 1989
AB		EQ 2MG BASE	N072577 001	MAY 16, 1989
AB		EQ 5MG BASE	N072578 001	MAY 16, 1989
AB	IVAX PHARMS	EQ 1MG BASE	N071994 001	SEP 12, 1988
AB		EQ 2MG BASE	N071995 001	SEP 12, 1988
AB		EQ 5MG BASE	N071745 001	SEP 12, 1988
AB	LEDERLE	EQ 1MG BASE	N072705 001	MAY 16, 1989
AB		EQ 2MG BASE	N072706 001	MAY 16, 1989
AB		EQ 5MG BASE	N072707 001	MAY 16, 1989
AB	MYLAN	EQ 1MG BASE	N072573 001	MAY 16, 1989
AB		EQ 2MG BASE	N072574 001	MAY 16, 1989
AB		EQ 5MG BASE	N072575 001	MAY 16, 1989
AB	WATSON LABS	EQ 1MG BASE	N072352 001	MAY 16, 1989
AB		EQ 2MG BASE	N072333 001	MAY 16, 1989
AB		EQ 5MG BASE	N072609 001	MAY 16, 1989

Tablet, Extended Release; Oral
MINIPRESS XL

TE	Firm	Strength	Appl. No.	Date
	+ PFIZER	2.5MG	N019775 001	JAN 29, 1992
	+	5MG	N019775 002	JAN 29, 1992

PRAZOSIN HYDROCHLORIDE *MULTIPLE*
SEE POLYTHIAZIDE; PRAZOSIN HYDROCHLORIDE

PREDNICARBATE

Cream; Topical
DERMATOP E EMOLLIENT

TE	Firm	Strength	Appl. No.	Date
	+ DERMIK LABS	0.1%	N020279 001	OCT 29, 1993

Ointment; Topical
DERMATOP

TE	Firm	Strength	Appl. No.	Date
	+ DERMIK LABS	0.1%	N019568 001	SEP 23, 1991

PREDNISOLONE

Syrup; Oral
PREDNISOLONE

TE	Firm	Strength	Appl. No.	Date
AA	AXIOM PHARM	15MG/5ML	N040287 001	MAY 28, 1999
AA	COPLEY PHARM	15MG/5ML	N040322 001	JAN 19, 2000
AA	HI TECH PHARMA	15MG/5ML	N040401 001	FEB 27, 2003
AA	KV PHARM	5MG/5ML	N040423 001	OCT 22, 2001
AA		15MG/5ML	N040364 001	APR 10, 2002
AA	PHARM ASSOC	15MG/5ML	N040399 001	MAR 05, 2003
AA	UDL	15MG/5ML	N040323 001	MAY 13, 1999
AA	WE PHARMS	15MG/5ML	N040192 001	MAY 28, 1998

PRELONE

TE	Firm	Strength	Appl. No.	Date
AA	+ MURO	5MG/5ML	N089654 001	JAN 17, 1989
AA	+ TEVA	15MG/5ML	N089081 001	FEB 04, 1986

Tablet; Oral
PREDNISOLONE

TE	Firm	Strength	Appl. No.
BX	EVERYLIFE	2.5MG	N084439 002
BX		5MG	N084439 003
BX	LANNETT	5MG	N080531 002
BX	MARSHALL PHARMA	5MG	N080307 001
BX	SPERTI	1MG	N080358 001
BX		2.5MG	N080358 002
BX		5MG	N080358 003
BX	+ WATSON LABS	5MG	N080354 001

PREDNISOLONE ACETATE

Injectable; Injection
PREDNISOLONE ACETATE

TE	Firm	Strength	Appl. No.
	+ STERIS	25MG/ML	N083398 001
		50MG/ML	N083764 001
		50MG/ML	N085781 001

Suspension/Drops; Ophthalmic
ECONOPRED PLUS

TE	Firm	Strength	Appl. No.
AB	FALCON PHARMS	1%	N017469 001

PRED FORTE

TE	Firm	Strength	Appl. No.
AB	+ ALLERGAN	1%	N017011 001

PRED MILD

TE	Firm	Strength	Appl. No.
AB	+ ALLERGAN	0.12%	N017100 001

PREDNISOLONE ACETATE; SULFACETAMIDE SODIUM

Ointment; Ophthalmic
BLEPHAMIDE S.O.P.

Firm	Strength	Appl. No.	Date
+ ALLERGAN	0.2%;10%	N087748 001	DEC 03, 1986

VASOCIDIN

Firm	Strength	Appl. No.
+ NOVARTIS	0.5%;10%	N088791 001

Prescription Drug Products *(continued)*

PREDNISOLONE ACETATE; SULFACETAMIDE SODIUM *(continued)*

Ointment; Ophthalmic

TE	Applicant	Strength	Appl. No.	Date
	VASOCIDIN			OCT 05, 1984
	NOVARTIS			

Suspension; Ophthalmic

TE	Applicant	Strength	Appl. No.	Date
	BLEPHAMIDE			
	+ ALLERGAN	0.2%;10%	N012813 002	

PREDNISOLONE ACETATE *MULTIPLE*

SEE GENTAMICIN SULFATE; PREDNISOLONE ACETATE
SEE NEOMYCIN SULFATE; POLYMYXIN B SULFATE; PREDNISOLONE ACETATE

PREDNISOLONE SODIUM PHOSPHATE

Solution/Drops; Ophthalmic

TE	Applicant	Strength	Appl. No.	Date
	INFLAMASE FORTE			
AT	+ NOVARTIS	EQ 0.9% PHOSPHATE	N080751 002	
	INFLAMASE MILD			
AT	+ NOVARTIS	EQ 0.11% PHOSPHATE	N080751 001	
	PREDNISOLONE SODIUM PHOSPHATE			
AT	BAUSCH AND LOMB	EQ 0.11% PHOSPHATE	N040065 001	JUL 29, 1994
AT		EQ 0.9% PHOSPHATE	N040070 001	JUL 29, 1994

Solution; Oral

TE	Applicant	Strength	Appl. No.	Date
	ORAPRED			
AA	+ ASCENT PEDS	EQ 15MG BASE/5ML	N075117 001	DEC 14, 2000
	PEDIAPRED			
AA	+ CELLTECH PHARMS	EQ 5MG BASE/5ML	N019157 001	MAY 28, 1986
	PREDNISOLONE SODIUM PHOSPHATE			
AA	HI TECH PHARMA	EQ 5MG BASE/5ML	N075183 001	MAR 26, 2003
AA	MORTON GROVE	EQ 5MG BASE/5ML	N075099 001	JUN 28, 2002
AA	PHARM ASSOC	EQ 5MG BASE/5ML	N076123 001	DEC 23, 2002
AA	WE PHARMS	EQ 5MG BASE/5ML	N075181 001	DEC 23, 2002
AA		EQ 15MG BASE/5ML	N075250 001	JUL 12, 2002

PREDNISOLONE SODIUM PHOSPHATE; SULFACETAMIDE SODIUM

Solution/Drops; Ophthalmic
SULFACETAMIDE SODIUM AND PREDNISOLONE SODIUM PHOSPHATE

TE	Applicant	Strength	Appl. No.	Date
AT	ALCON	EQ 0.23% PHOSPHATE;10%	N073630 001	MAY 27, 1993
AT	BAUSCH AND LOMB	EQ 0.23% PHOSPHATE;10%	N074449 001	DEC 29, 1995
	VASOCIDIN			
AT	+ NOVARTIS	EQ 0.23% PHOSPHATE;10%	N018988 001	AUG 26, 1988

PREDNISONE

Solution; Oral

TE	Applicant	Strength	Appl. No.	Date
	PREDNISONE			
	+ ROXANE	5MG/5ML	N088703 001	NOV 08, 1984
	PREDNISONE INTENSOL			
	+ ROXANE	5MG/ML	N088810 001	FEB 20, 1985

Tablet; Oral

TE	Applicant	Strength	Appl. No.	Date
	DELTASONE			
	+ PHARMACIA AND UPJOHN			
AB		2.5MG	N009986 005	
AB		5MG	N009986 002	
AB		10MG	N009986 006	
AB		20MG	N009986 007	
		50MG	N009986 008	
	PREDNISONE			
AB	GENEVA PHARMS	10MG	N089983 001	JAN 12, 1989
AB		20MG	N085813 001	
AB		50MG	N089984 001	JAN 12, 1989
BX	MARSHALL PHARMA	5MG	N080301 001	
	MUTUAL PHARM	5MG	N089245 001	DEC 04, 1985
AB		10MG	N089246 001	DEC 04, 1985
AB		20MG	N089247 001	DEC 04, 1985
AB	+ PVT FORM	5MG	N080209 001	
AB	ROXANE	1MG	N087800 001	APR 22, 1982
AB		2.5MG	N087801 001	APR 22, 1982
AB		5MG	N080352 001	
AB		10MG	N084122 001	
AB		20MG	N087342 001	
AB		50MG	N084283 001	
AB	TRICEN	5MG	N040362 002	AUG 29, 2001
AB		10MG	N040362 001	AUG 29, 2001
AB	VINTAGE PHARMS	5MG	N040256 001	JUL 12, 2002
AB		10MG	N040256 002	JUL 12, 2002
AB		20MG	N040392 001	FEB 12, 2003
AB	WATSON LABS	5MG	N080356 001	
AB		10MG	N085162 001	
AB		10MG	N087773 001	JUL 13, 1982
AB	WEST WARD	20MG	N085161 001	
AB		20MG	N086813 001	
AB		50MG	N087772 001	JUL 13, 1982
AB		5MG	N080292 001	

Prescription Drug Products (continued)

PREDNISONE (continued)
Tablet; Oral
PREDNISONE
  WEST WARD
- AB 10MG N088832 001 DEC 04, 1985
- AB 20MG N083677 001
- AB 50MG N088465 001 JUN 01, 1984

PRILOCAINE *MULTIPLE*
  SEE LIDOCAINE; PRILOCAINE

PRILOCAINE HYDROCHLORIDE
Injectable; Injection
CITANEST PLAIN
+ DENTSPLY PHARM 4% N021382 001

PRILOCAINE HYDROCHLORIDE *MULTIPLE*
  SEE EPINEPHRINE BITARTRATE; PRILOCAINE HYDROCHLORIDE

PRIMAQUINE PHOSPHATE
Tablet; Oral
PRIMAQUINE
+ SANOFI SYNTHELABO EQ 15MG BASE N008316 001

PRIMIDONE
Tablet; Oral
MYSOLINE
  XCEL PHARMS
- AB 50MG N009170 003
- AB 250MG N009170 002
+
PRIMIDONE
  LANNETT
- AB 50MG N084903 002 MAY 24, 2001
- AB 250MG N084903 001
  WATSON LABS
- AB 250MG N083551 001

PROBENECID
Tablet; Oral
PROBALAN
  LANNETT
- AB 500MG N080966 001
PROBENECID
  IVAX PHARMS
- AB 500MG N083740 001 MAY 09, 1984
- + MYLAN 500MG N084211 002
  WATSON LABS
- AB 500MG N084442 004 MAR 29, 1983

PROBENECID *MULTIPLE*
  SEE COLCHICINE; PROBENECID

PROCAINAMIDE HYDROCHLORIDE
Capsule; Oral
PROCAINAMIDE HCL
  GENEVA PHARMS
- AB 250MG N089219 001

PROCAINAMIDE HYDROCHLORIDE (continued)
Capsule; Oral
PROCAINAMIDE HCL
  GENEVA PHARMS
- AB 375MG N089220 001 JUL 01, 1986
- AB 500MG N089221 001 JUL 01, 1986
  IVAX PHARMS
- AB 250MG N084604 001 JUL 01, 1986
- AB 375MG N084595 001
- AB 500MG N084606 001
  LANNETT
- AB 250MG N083693 001
  WATSON LABS
- AB 250MG N084280 001
- AB 375MG N083287 001
- AB 500MG N084403 001
PRONESTYL
  APOTHECON
- AB 250MG N007335 001
- AB 375MG N007335 004
- AB 500MG N007335 003
+

Injectable; Injection
PROCAINAMIDE HCL
  ABBOTT
- AP 100MG/ML N089069 001
-     500MG/ML N089070 001 FEB 12, 1986
                    FEB 12, 1986
  INTL MEDICATION
- AP 100MG/ML N089537 001 AUG 25, 1987
- AP 500MG/ML N088636 001 JUL 31, 1984
PRONESTYL
+ APOTHECON
- AP 100MG/ML N088637 001 JUL 31, 1984
- AP 500MG/ML N007335 002
-               N007335 005

Tablet, Extended Release; Oral
PROCAINAMIDE HCL
  COPLEY PHARM
- AB 1GM N040111 001
- AB 500MG N088974 001 DEC 13, 1996
- AB 750MG N089438 001 JUL 22, 1985
  GENEVA PHARMS
- AB 250MG N089369 001 MAR 23, 1987
- AB 500MG N089370 001 AUG 14, 1987
- AB 750MG N089371 001 JAN 09, 1987
  PLIVA
- AB 500MG N088959 001 AUG 14, 1987
  WATSON LABS
- AB 250MG N089026 001 DEC 02, 1985
- AB 500MG N089027 001 OCT 22, 1985
- AB 750MG N089042 001 OCT 22, 1985
                            OCT 22, 1985

Prescription Drug Products *(continued)*

PROCAINAMIDE HYDROCHLORIDE *(continued)*

Tablet, Extended Release; Oral

Code	Firm	Strength	NDA	Date
	PROCANBID			
	+ KING PHARMS	1GM	N020545 002	JAN 31, 1996
	+	500MG	N020545 001	JAN 31, 1996
	PRONESTYL-SR			
BC	APOTHECON	500MG	N087361 001	

Tablet; Oral

Code	Firm	Strength	NDA	Date
	PRONESTYL			
	APOTHECON	250MG	N017371 001	
		375MG	N017371 002	
	+	500MG	N017371 003	

PROCAINE HYDROCHLORIDE

Injectable; Injection

Code	Firm	Strength	NDA	Date
	NOVOCAIN			
AP	+ ABBOTT	1%	N085362 003	
AP	+	2%	N085362 004	
	+	10%	N086797 001	
	PROCAINE HCL			
AP	ABBOTT	1%	N080416 001	
AP		2%	N080416 002	
AP	AM PHARM PARTNERS	1%	N080421 001	
AP		2%	N080421 002	
AP	ELKINS SINN	1%	N083315 001	
AP		2%	N083315 002	
AP	STERIS	1%	N080658 001	
AP	+	2%	N080658 002	

PROCARBAZINE HYDROCHLORIDE

Capsule; Oral

Code	Firm	Strength	NDA	Date
	MATULANE			
	+ SIGMA TAU	EQ 50MG BASE	N016785 001	

PROCHLORPERAZINE

Suppository; Rectal

Code	Firm	Strength	NDA	Date
	COMPAZINE			
AB	GLAXOSMITHKLINE	2.5MG	N011127 003	
AB		5MG	N011127 001	
AB		25MG	N011127 002	
	+ **COMPRO**			
AB	PADDOCK	25MG	N040246 001	JUN 28, 2000
	PROCHLORPERAZINE			
AB	ABLE	2.5MG	N040407 001	JUL 11, 2001
		5MG	N040407 002	JUL 11, 2001
AB	MYLAN	25MG	N040407 003	JUL 11, 2001
AB	G AND W LABS	25MG	N040058 001	NOV 24, 1993

PROCHLORPERAZINE EDISYLATE

Injectable; Injection

Code	Firm	Strength	NDA	Date
	COMPAZINE			
AP	+ GLAXOSMITHKLINE	EQ 5MG BASE/ML	N010742 002	
	PROCHLORPERAZINE			
AP	ELKINS SINN	EQ 5MG BASE/ML	N087759 001	OCT 01, 1982
	PROCHLORPERAZINE EDISYLATE			
AP	ABBOTT	EQ 5MG BASE/ML	N089703 001	APR 07, 1988
AP	ELKINS SINN	EQ 5MG BASE/ML	N089903 001	AUG 29, 1989
AP	GENSIA SICOR PHARMS	EQ 5MG BASE/ML	N040505 001	MAY 30, 2003
AP	STERIS	EQ 5MG BASE/ML	N089530 001	JUL 08, 1987

Syrup; Oral

Code	Firm	Strength	NDA	Date
	COMPAZINE			
AP	GLAXOSMITHKLINE	EQ 5MG BASE/5ML	N011188 001	

PROCHLORPERAZINE MALEATE

Capsule, Extended Release; Oral

Code	Firm	Strength	NDA	Date
	COMPAZINE			
	+ GLAXOSMITHKLINE	EQ 10MG BASE	N021019 001	OCT 06, 1999
	+	EQ 15MG BASE	N021019 002	OCT 06, 1999

Tablet; Oral

Code	Firm	Strength	NDA	Date
	COMPAZINE			
AB	GLAXOSMITHKLINE	EQ 5MG BASE	N010571 001	
AB		EQ 10MG BASE	N010571 002	
AB		EQ 25MG BASE	N010571 003	
	PROCHLORPERAZINE MALEATE			
	+ COPLEY PHARM	EQ 5MG BASE	N040120 001	JUL 11, 1996
AB		EQ 10MG BASE	N040120 002	JUL 11, 1996
AB	DURAMED PHARM BARR	EQ 5MG BASE	N040207 001	MAY 01, 1997
		EQ 10MG BASE	N040207 002	MAY 01, 1997
AB	GENEVA PHARMS TECH	EQ 5MG BASE	N040101 001	JUL 19, 1996
		EQ 10MG BASE	N040101 002	JUL 19, 1996
AB		EQ 25MG BASE	N040101 003	JUL 19, 1996
AB	IVAX PHARMS	EQ 5MG BASE	N040162 001	JAN 20, 1998
AB		EQ 10MG BASE	N040162 002	JAN 20, 1998
AB	MYLAN	EQ 5MG BASE	N040185 002	OCT 28, 1996
AB		EQ 10MG BASE	N040185 001	OCT 28, 1996
AB	TRIGEN	EQ 5MG BASE	N040268 001	FEB 27, 1998

Prescription Drug Products (continued)

PROCHLORPERAZINE MALEATE (continued)
Tablet; Oral

PROCHLORPERAZINE MALEATE

AB	TRIGEN	EQ 10MG BASE	N040268 002	FEB 27, 1998

PROCYCLIDINE HYDROCHLORIDE
Tablet; Oral

KEMADRIN

+	MONARCH PHARMS	5MG	N009818 003

PROGESTERONE
Capsule; Oral

PROMETRIUM

	UNIMED PHARMS	100MG	N019781 001	MAY 14, 1998
+		200MG	N019781 002	OCT 15, 1999

Gel; Vaginal

CRINONE

	COLUMBIA RES LABS	4%	N020701 001	JUL 31, 1997
+		8%	N020701 002	JUL 31, 1997

Injectable; Injection

PROGESTERONE

AQ +	AM PHARM PARTNERS	50MG/ML	N075906 001	APR 25, 2001
AQ +	SCHEIN	50MG/ML	N017362 002	

PROGUANIL HYDROCHLORIDE *MULTIPLE*
SEE   ATOVAQUONE; PROGUANIL HYDROCHLORIDE

PROMETHAZINE HYDROCHLORIDE
Injectable; Injection

PROMETHAZINE HCL

AP	ABBOTT	25MG/ML	N040372 001	JUN 08, 2000
AP		50MG/ML	N040372 002	JUN 08, 2000
AP	BAXTER HLTHCARE	50MG/ML	N083838 002	JUN 08, 2000
AP		25MG/ML	N083312 001	
AP	GENSIA SICOR PHARMS	50MG/ML	N083312 002	
AP +		25MG/ML	N040454 001	AUG 22, 2002
AP +		50MG/ML	N040454 002	AUG 22, 2002
AP	PHARMAFORCE	25MG/ML	N040471 001	NOV 21, 2002
AP		25MG/ML	N040515 001	MAR 19, 2003
AP	STERIS	25MG/ML	N084591 001	
AP		50MG/ML	N080629 002	

Suppository; Rectal

PHENERGAN

AB	WYETH PHARMS INC	12.5MG	N010926 002

PROMETHAZINE HYDROCHLORIDE (continued)
Suppository; Rectal

PHENERGAN

AB +	WYETH PHARMS INC	25MG	N010926 001	
AB +		50MG	N011689 001	

PROMETHACON

+   POLYMEDICA

PROMETHAZINE HCL

BR	ABLE	25MG	N084901 001	
AB		12.5MG	N040504 001	APR 11, 2003
AB		25MG	N040504 002	APR 11, 2003
AB	CLAY PARK	50MG	N040449 001	FEB 27, 2003
AB		12.5MG	N040500 001	JUN 30, 2003
AB		25MG	N040500 002	JUN 30, 2003
AB	G AND W LABS	12.5MG	N040428 002	MAR 31, 2003
AB		25MG	N040428 001	FEB 05, 2002
AB	PADDOCK	12.5MG	N040479 001	JUN 24, 2003
AB		25MG	N040479 002	JUN 24, 2003

PROMETHEGAN

BR	G AND W LABS	50MG	N087165 001	AUG 14, 1987

Syrup; Oral

PROMETH PLAIN

AA +	ALPHARMA	6.25MG/5ML	N085953 001	

PROMETHAZINE HCL

AA	HI TECH PHARMA	6.25MG	N040026 001	SEP 25, 1998
AA	WHITEWORTH TOWN PLSN	6.25MG/5ML	N086395 001	

PROMETHAZINE PLAIN

AA	MORTON GROVE	6.25MG/5ML	N087953 001	NOV 15, 1982

Tablet; Oral

PHENERGAN

BP	WYETH PHARMS INC	12.5MG	N007935 002	
BP		25MG	N007935 003	
BP +		50MG	N007935 004	

PROMETHAZINE HCL

BP	GENEVA PHARMS	25MG	N084234 001	
BP		50MG	N084176 001	
BP	WATSON LABS	25MG	N083426 001	
BP		50MG	N083711 001	

PROMETHAZINE HYDROCHLORIDE *MULTIPLE*
SEE   CODEINE PHOSPHATE; PHENYLEPHRINE HYDROCHLORIDE; PROMETHAZINE HYDROCHLORIDE

SEE   CODEINE PHOSPHATE; PROMETHAZINE HYDROCHLORIDE

SEE   DEXTROMETHORPHAN HYDROBROMIDE; PROMETHAZINE HYDROCHLORIDE

Prescription Drug Products (continued)

PROMETHAZINE HYDROCHLORIDE *MULTIPLE* (continued)
SEE PHENYLEPHRINE HYDROCHLORIDE; PROMETHAZINE HYDROCHLORIDE

PROPAFENONE HYDROCHLORIDE
Tablet; Oral
PROPAFENONE HCL

AB	KV PHARM	150MG	N076193 001	FEB 07, 2002
AB		225MG	N076193 002	FEB 07, 2002
AB		300MG	N076193 003	FEB 07, 2002
AB	MUTUAL PHARM	150MG	N075998 001	NOV 29, 2001
AB		225MG	N075998 002	NOV 29, 2001
AB		300MG	N075998 003	NOV 29, 2001
AB	VINTAGE PHARMS	150MG	N075938 001	OCT 17, 2002
AB		225MG	N075938 002	OCT 17, 2002
AB		300MG	N075938 003	OCT 17, 2002
AB	WATSON LABS	150MG	N075203 001	OCT 24, 2000
AB		225MG	N075203 002	OCT 24, 2000

RYTHMOL

AB	ABBOTT	150MG	N019151 001	NOV 27, 1989
AB		225MG	N019151 003	NOV 20, 1992
AB	+	300MG	N019151 002	NOV 27, 1989

PROPANTHELINE BROMIDE
Tablet; Oral
PRO-BANTHINE

BP	+ SHIRE LABS	7.5MG	N008732 003
BP	+	15MG	N008732 002

PROPANTHELINE BROMIDE

BP	ROXANE	7.5MG	N080927 001
BP		15MG	N080927 002

PROPARACAINE HYDROCHLORIDE
Solution/Drops; Ophthalmic
ALCAINE

AT	ALCON	0.5%	N080027 001	
AT	OPHTHAINE + APOTHECON	0.5%	N008883 001	
AT	OPHTHETIC + ALLERGAN	0.5%	N012583 001	
AT	PARACAINE OPTOPICS	0.5%	N087681 001	AUG 05, 1982

PROPARACAINE HYDROCHLORIDE (continued)
Solution/Drops; Ophthalmic
PROPARACAINE HCL

AT	BAUSCH AND LOMB	0.5%	N040074 001	SEP 29, 1995

Solution; Ophthalmic
PROPARACAINE HCL

AT	TAYLOR PHARMA	0.5%	N040277 001	MAR 16, 2000

PROPOFOL
Injectable; Injection
DIPRIVAN

AB	+ ASTRAZENECA	10MG/ML	N019627 002	JUN 11, 1996

PROPOFOL

AB	GENSIA SICOR PHARMS	10MG/ML	N075102 001	JAN 04, 1999
AB		10MG/ML	N075392 001	SEP 19, 2000

PROPOXYPHENE HYDROCHLORIDE
Capsule; Oral
DARVON

AA	+ AAI PHARMA	32MG	N010997 001	
AA	+	65MG	N010997 003	

DOLENE

AA	+ CLONMEL HLTHCARE	65MG	N080530 001	

KESSO-GESIC
PROPOXYPHENE HCL

AA	MK LABS	65MG	N083544 001	
AA	ICN	65MG	N080783 001	
AA	IVAX PHARMS	65MG	N080269 001	
AA	MYLAN	32MG	N083528 001	
AA	TEVA	65MG	N088615 001	OCT 22, 1984
AA	WEST WARD	65MG	N083501 001	
AA	WHITEWORTH TOWN PLSN	65MG	N084551 001	

PROPOXYPHENE HYDROCHLORIDE *MULTIPLE*
SEE ACETAMINOPHEN; PROPOXYPHENE HYDROCHLORIDE
SEE ASPIRIN; CAFFEINE; PROPOXYPHENE HYDROCHLORIDE
SEE ASPIRIN; PROPOXYPHENE HYDROCHLORIDE

PROPOXYPHENE NAPSYLATE
Suspension; Oral
DARVON-N

	+ NEOSAN PHARMS	50MG/5ML	N016861 001

Tablet; Oral
DARVON-N

	+ AAIPHARMA LLC	100MG	N016862 002

PROPOXYPHENE NAPSYLATE *MULTIPLE*
SEE ACETAMINOPHEN; PROPOXYPHENE NAPSYLATE

Prescription Drug Products (continued)

PROPRANOLOL HYDROCHLORIDE

Capsule, Extended Release; Oral

INDERAL LA

TE	Firm	Strength	Appl. No.	Date
	WYETH PHARMS INC			
BX		60MG	N018553 004	MAR 18, 1987
BX		80MG	N018553 002	APR 19, 1983
BX		120MG	N018553 003	APR 19, 1983
+		160MG	N018553 001	APR 19, 1983

INNOPRAN XL

TE	Firm	Strength	Appl. No.	Date
	RELIANT PHARMS			
BX		80MG	N021438 001	MAR 12, 2003
BX		120MG	N021438 002	MAR 12, 2003

Concentrate; Oral

PROPRANOLOL HCL INTENSOL

TE	Firm	Strength	Appl. No.	Date
+	ROXANE	80MG/ML	N071388 001	MAY 15, 1987

Injectable; Injection

INDERAL

TE	Firm	Strength	Appl. No.	Date
AP	+ BAXTER HLTHCARE CORP	1MG/ML	N016419 001	

PROPRANOLOL HCL

TE	Firm	Strength	Appl. No.	Date
AP	BEDFORD	1MG/ML	N075792 001	AUG 29, 2000
AP	SABEX 2002	1MG/ML	N076400 001	FEB 26, 2003

Solution; Oral

PROPRANOLOL HCL

TE	Firm	Strength	Appl. No.	Date
AP	ROXANE	20MG/5ML	N070979 001	MAY 15, 1987
+		40MG/5ML	N070690 001	MAY 15, 1987

Tablet; Oral

INDERAL

TE	Firm	Strength	Appl. No.	Date
AB	+ WYETH PHARMS INC	10MG	N016418 001	
AB		20MG	N016418 003	
AB		40MG	N016418 002	
AB		60MG	N016418 009	OCT 18, 1982
AB	+	80MG	N016418 004	

PROPRANOLOL HCL

TE	Firm	Strength	Appl. No.	Date
AB	GENEVA PHARMS	10MG	N070663 001	JUN 13, 1986
AB		20MG	N070664 001	JUN 13, 1986
AB		40MG	N070665 001	JUN 13, 1986
AB		60MG	N070666 001	OCT 10, 1986
AB		80MG	N070667 001	JUN 13, 1986
AB	MYLAN	10MG	N070211 001	NOV 19, 1985
AB		20MG	N070212 001	NOV 19, 1985

PROPRANOLOL HYDROCHLORIDE (continued)

Tablet; Oral

PROPRANOLOL HCL

TE	Firm	Strength	Appl. No.	Date
	MYLAN			
AB		40MG	N070213 001	NOV 19, 1985
AB		80MG	N070214 001	NOV 19, 1985
	PAR PHARM			
AB		10MG	N070217 001	AUG 01, 1986
AB		20MG	N070218 001	AUG 01, 1986
AB		40MG	N070219 001	AUG 01, 1986
AB		60MG	N070220 001	SEP 24, 1986
AB		80MG	N070221 001	APR 14, 1986
AB		90MG	N071288 001	OCT 22, 1986
	PLIVA			
AB		10MG	N071972 001	APR 06, 1988
AB		20MG	N071973 001	APR 06, 1988
AB		40MG	N071974 001	APR 06, 1988
AB		60MG	N071975 001	APR 06, 1988
AB		80MG	N071976 001	APR 06, 1988
AB		90MG	N071977 001	APR 06, 1988
	TEVA			
AB		40MG	N070234 001	JUN 23, 1986
	WATSON LABS			
AB		10MG	N070175 001	MAY 13, 1986
AB		10MG	N070548 001	JUL 10, 1986
AB		20MG	N070176 001	MAY 13, 1986
AB		40MG	N070177 001	MAY 13, 1986
AB		40MG	N070550 001	APR 11, 1986
AB		60MG	N071791 001	JUL 15, 1987
AB		80MG	N070178 001	MAY 13, 1986
AB		80MG	N070551 001	JUL 10, 1986
AB		90MG	N071792 001	JUL 15, 1987

PROPRANOLOL HYDROCHLORIDE *MULTIPLE*

SEE HYDROCHLOROTHIAZIDE; PROPRANOLOL HYDROCHLORIDE

Prescription Drug Products (continued)

PROPYLTHIOURACIL
Tablet; Oral
PROPYLTHIOURACIL
BD	IMPAX LABS	50MG	N080159 001
BD +	LEDERLE	50MG	N006188 001
BD	PUREPAC PHARM	50MG	N080172 001
BD	WEST WARD	50MG	N080154 001

PROTAMINE SULFATE
Injectable; Injection
PROTAMINE SULFATE
AP	AM PHARM PARTNERS	10MG/ML	N089454 001 APR 07, 1987
AP +	LILLY	10MG/ML	N006460 002

PROTIRELIN
Injectable; Injection
THYREL TRH
+	FERRING	0.5MG/ML	N018087 001

PROTRIPTYLINE HYDROCHLORIDE
Tablet; Oral
VIVACTIL
AB	ODYSSEY PHARMS	5MG	N073644 001 AUG 24, 1995
AB +		10MG	N073645 001 AUG 24, 1995

PSEUDOEPHEDRINE HYDROCHLORIDE; TRIPROLIDINE HYDROCHLORIDE
Tablet; Oral
CORPHED
AA	GENEVA PHARMS	60MG;2.5MG	N088602 001 APR 11, 1985

PSEUDOEPHEDRINE HCL AND TRIPROLIDINE HCL
AA +	EON	60MG;2.5MG	N088193 001 MAY 17, 1983

TRILITRON
AA	NEWTRON PHARMS	60MG;2.5MG	N088515 001 JAN 09, 1985

TRIPROLIDINE HCL AND PSEUDOEPHEDRINE HCL
AA	SUPERPHARM	60MG;2.5MG	N088578 001 FEB 21, 1985

PSEUDOEPHEDRINE HYDROCHLORIDE *MULTIPLE*
SEE ACRIVASTINE: PSEUDOEPHEDRINE HYDROCHLORIDE
SEE BROMPHENIRAMINE MALEATE: DEXTROMETHORPHAN HYDROBROMIDE: PSEUDOEPHEDRINE HYDROCHLORIDE
SEE CETIRIZINE HYDROCHLORIDE: PSEUDOEPHEDRINE HYDROCHLORIDE
SEE CODEINE PHOSPHATE: PSEUDOEPHEDRINE HYDROCHLORIDE: TRIPROLIDINE HYDROCHLORIDE
SEE FEXOFENADINE HYDROCHLORIDE: PSEUDOEPHEDRINE HYDROCHLORIDE

PSEUDOEPHEDRINE SULFATE *MULTIPLE*
SEE AZATADINE MALEATE: PSEUDOEPHEDRINE SULFATE

PYRAZINAMIDE
Tablet; Oral
PYRAZINAMIDE
AB +	CLONMEL	500MG	N080157 001
AB	MIKART	500MG	N081319 001 JUN 30, 1992

PYRAZINAMIDE *MULTIPLE*
SEE ISONIAZID; PYRAZINAMIDE; RIFAMPIN

PYRIDOSTIGMINE BROMIDE
Injectable; Injection
MESTINON
AP +	ICN	5MG/ML	N009830 001

Syrup; Oral
MESTINON
+	ICN	60MG/5ML	N015193 001

Tablet, Extended Release; Oral
MESTINON
+	ICN	180MG	N011665 001

Tablet; Oral
MESTINON
AB +	ICN	60MG	N009829 002

PYRIDOSTIGMINE BROMIDE
AB	COREPHARMA	60MG	N040457 001 DEC 26, 2002
AB	IMPAX LABS	60MG	N040502 001 APR 24, 2003

PYRIDOXINE *MULTIPLE*
SEE ASCORBIC ACID: BIOTIN: CHOLECALCIFEROL: CYANOCOBALAMIN: DEXPANTHENOL: FOLIC ACID: NIACINAMIDE: PYRIDOXINE: RIBOFLAVIN: THIAMINE: TOCOPHEROL ACETATE: VITAMIN A: VITAMIN K

PYRIDOXINE HYDROCHLORIDE
Injectable; Injection
PYRIDOXINE HCL
AP	AM PHARM PARTNERS	100MG/ML	N080618 001
AP +	STERIS	100MG/ML	N080572 001

PYRIDOXINE HYDROCHLORIDE *MULTIPLE*
SEE ALPHA-TOCOPHEROL ACETATE: ASCORBIC ACID: BIOTIN: CHOLECALCIFEROL: CYANOCOBALAMIN: DEXPANTHENOL: FOLIC ACID: NIACINAMIDE: PYRIDOXINE HYDROCHLORIDE: RIBOFLAVIN PHOSPHATE SODIUM: THIAMINE: PYRIDOXINE HYDROCHLORIDE: VITAMIN A PALMITATE: VITAMIN K
SEE ASCORBIC ACID: BIOTIN: CYANOCOBALAMIN: DEXPANTHENOL: ERGOCALCIFEROL: FOLIC ACID: NIACINAMIDE: PHYTONADIONE: PYRIDOXINE HYDROCHLORIDE: RIBOFLAVIN PHOSPHATE SODIUM: THIAMINE HYDROCHLORIDE: VITAMIN A: VITAMIN E
SEE ASCORBIC ACID: BIOTIN: CYANOCOBALAMIN: DEXPANTHENOL: ERGOCALCIFEROL: FOLIC ACID: NIACINAMIDE: PYRIDOXINE HYDROCHLORIDE: RIBOFLAVIN PHOSPHATE SODIUM: THIAMINE HYDROCHLORIDE: VITAMIN A: VITAMIN E

Prescription Drug Products (continued)

PYRILAMINE MALEATE
Tablet; Oral
  PYRILAMINE MALEATE
  + IMPAX LABS   25MG   N080808 001

PYRIMETHAMINE
Tablet; Oral
  DARAPRIM
  + GLAXOSMITHKLINE   25MG   N008578 001

PYRIMETHAMINE; SULFADOXINE
Tablet; Oral
  FANSIDAR
  + ROCHE   25MG;500MG   N018557 001

QUAZEPAM
Tablet; Oral
  DORAL
    MEDPOINTE PHARM HLC   7.5MG   N018708 003   FEB 26, 1987
  +   15MG   N018708 001   DEC 27, 1985

QUETIAPINE FUMARATE
Tablet; Oral
  SEROQUEL
  + ASTRAZENECA   EQ 25MG BASE   N020639 001   SEP 26, 1997
     EQ 100MG BASE   N020639 002   SEP 26, 1997
     EQ 150MG BASE   N020639 004   DEC 20, 1998
     EQ 200MG BASE   N020639 003   SEP 26, 1997
     EQ 300MG BASE   N020639 005   JUL 26, 2000

QUINAPRIL HYDROCHLORIDE
Tablet; Oral
  ACCUPRIL
AB   PFIZER PHARMS   EQ 5MG BASE   N019885 001   NOV 19, 1991
AB   EQ 10MG BASE   N019885 002   NOV 19, 1991
AB   EQ 20MG BASE   N019885 003   NOV 19, 1991
AB   +   EQ 40MG BASE   N019885 004   NOV 19, 1991
  QUINAPRIL HCL
AB   TEVA   EQ 5MG BASE   N075504 001   MAY 30, 2003
AB   EQ 10MG BASE   N075504 002   MAY 30, 2003
AB   EQ 20MG BASE   N075504 003   MAY 30, 2003

QUINAPRIL HYDROCHLORIDE (continued)
Tablet; Oral
  QUINAPRIL HCL
AB   TEVA   EQ 40MG BASE   N075504 004   NOV 20, 1998

QUINAPRIL HYDROCHLORIDE *MULTIPLE*
  SEE   HYDROCHLOROTHIAZIDE; QUINAPRIL HYDROCHLORIDE

QUINIDINE GLUCONATE
Injectable; Injection
  QUINIDINE GLUCONATE
  + LILLY   80MG/ML   N007529 002   FEB 10, 1989

Tablet, Extended Release; Oral
  QUINIDINE GLUCONATE
  + MUTUAL PHARM   324MG   N089338 001   FEB 11, 1987

QUINIDINE SULFATE
Tablet, Extended Release; Oral
  QUINIDINE SULFATE
  + COPLEY PHARM   300MG   N040045 001   JUN 30, 1994

Tablet; Oral
  QUINIDINE SULFATE
AB   EON   200MG   N084631 001
AB   300MG   N088072 001   SEP 26, 1983
AB   GENEVA PHARMS   200MG   N084914 001
AB   300MG   N089839 001   SEP 29, 1988
AB   LANNETT   200MG   N083743 001
AB   LEDERLE   200MG   N087011 001
AB   MUTUAL PHARM   100MG   N081029 001   APR 14, 1989
AB   200MG   N081030 001   APR 14, 1989
AB   PVT FORM   200MG   N083808 001
AB   + ROXANE   200MG   N083640 001
AB   +   300MG   N085632 001
AB   SUPERPHARM   200MG   N088973 001   APR 10, 1985
AB   WATSON LABS   200MG   N083288 001
AB   200MG   N085140 002
AB   300MG   N085583 001

QUINUPRISTIN *MULTIPLE*
  SEE   DALFOPRISTIN; QUINUPRISTIN

RABEPRAZOLE SODIUM
Tablet, Delayed Release; Oral
  ACIPHEX
  + EISAI MEDCL RES   20MG   N020973 002   AUG 19, 1999

Prescription Drug Products (continued)

RALOXIFENE HYDROCHLORIDE
Tablet; Oral
EVISTA
+	LILLY	60MG		N020815 001	DEC 09, 1997

RAMIPRIL
Capsule; Oral
ALTACE
KING PHARMS	1.25MG	N019901 001	JAN 28, 1991
	2.5MG	N019901 002	JAN 28, 1991
	5MG	N019901 003	JAN 28, 1991
+	10MG	N019901 004	JAN 28, 1991

RANITIDINE HYDROCHLORIDE
Capsule; Oral
RANITIDINE HCL
AB	DR REDDYS LABS LTD	EQ 150MG BASE	N075742 001	NOV 29, 2000
AB		EQ 300MG BASE	N075742 002	NOV 29, 2000
AB	GENEVA PHARMS	EQ 150MG BASE	N074655 001	OCT 22, 1997
AB	+	EQ 300MG BASE	N074655 002	OCT 22, 1997
AB	GENPHARM	EQ 150MG BASE	N075564 001	OCT 27, 2000
AB		EQ 300MG BASE	N075564 002	OCT 27, 2000

Granule, Effervescent; Oral
ZANTAC 150
AB	+ GLAXOSMITHKLINE	EQ 150MG BASE/PACKET	N020251 002	MAR 31, 1994

Injectable; Injection
ZANTAC
AB	+ GLAXOSMITHKLINE	EQ 25MG BASE/ML	N019090 001	OCT 19, 1984

ZANTAC IN PLASTIC CONTAINER
AB	+ GLAXOSMITHKLINE	EQ 1MG BASE/ML	N019593 002	SEP 27, 1991

Syrup; Oral
ZANTAC
AB	+ GLAXOSMITHKLINE	EQ 15MG BASE/ML	N019675 001	DEC 30, 1988

Tablet, Effervescent; Oral
ZANTAC 150
AB	+ GLAXOSMITHKLINE	EQ 150MG BASE	N020251 001	MAR 31, 1994

Tablet; Oral
RANITIDINE
AB	RANBAXY	EQ 150MG BASE	N075439 001	APR 19, 2000

RANITIDINE HYDROCHLORIDE (continued)
Tablet; Oral
RANITIDINE
AB	RANBAXY	EQ 300MG BASE	N075439 002	APR 19, 2000

RANITIDINE HCL
AB	GENEVA PHARMS	EQ 150MG BASE	N074467 001	AUG 29, 1997
AB		EQ 300MG BASE	N074467 002	AUG 29, 1997
AB	GENPHARM	EQ 150MG BASE	N074023 001	AUG 22, 1997
AB		EQ 300MG BASE	N074023 002	AUG 22, 1997
AB	IVAX PHARMS	EQ 150MG BASE	N075165 001	SEP 30, 1998
AB		EQ 300MG BASE	N075165 002	SEP 30, 1998
AB	MYLAN	EQ 150MG BASE	N074552 001	JUL 30, 1998
AB		EQ 300MG BASE	N074552 002	JUL 30, 1998
AB	PAR PHARM	EQ 150MG BASE	N075180 001	JAN 28, 1999
AB		EQ 300MG BASE	N075180 002	JAN 28, 1999
AB	RANBAXY	EQ 150MG BASE	N075000 001	JAN 30, 1998
AB		EQ 300MG BASE	N075000 002	JAN 30, 1998
AB	TEVA	EQ 150MG BASE	N074488 001	JUL 31, 1997
AB		EQ 300MG BASE	N074488 002	JUL 31, 1997
AB	TORPHARM	EQ 150MG BASE	N074680 001	SEP 12, 1997
AB		EQ 300MG BASE	N074680 002	SEP 12, 1997
AB	WATSON LABS	EQ 150MG BASE	N074864 001	OCT 20, 1997
AB		EQ 300MG BASE	N074864 002	OCT 20, 1997
AB	WOCKHARDT	EQ 150MG BASE	N075208 001	DEC 17, 1998
AB		EQ 300MG BASE	N075208 002	DEC 17, 1998

ZANTAC 150
AB	+ GLAXOSMITHKLINE	EQ 150MG BASE	N018703 001	JUN 09, 1983

ZANTAC 300
AB	+ GLAXOSMITHKLINE	EQ 300MG BASE	N018703 002	DEC 09, 1985

REMIFENTANIL HYDROCHLORIDE
Injectable; Injection
ULTIVA
ABBOTT	EQ 1MG BASE/VIAL	N020630 001

Prescription Drug Products *(continued)*

REMIFENTANIL HYDROCHLORIDE *(continued)*
Injectable; Injection
ULTIVA

ABBOTT	EQ 2MG BASE/VIAL	N020630 002	JUL 12, 1996
+	EQ 5MG BASE/VIAL	N020630 003	JUL 12, 1996

REPAGLINIDE
Tablet; Oral
PRANDIN

NOVO NORDISK	0.5MG	N020741 001	DEC 22, 1997
	1MG	N020741 002	DEC 22, 1997
+	2MG	N020741 003	DEC 22, 1997

RESCINNAMINE
Tablet; Oral
MODERIL

+ PFIZER	0.5MG	N010686 006	
	0.25MG	N010686 003	

RESERPINE
Tablet; Oral
RESERPINE

BP	EON	0.1MG	N009838 001
BP		0.25MG	N009838 002

SERPALAN

BP	+ LANNETT	0.1MG	N010124 001
BP		0.25MG	N010124 002

RESERPINE *MULTIPLE*
SEE   CHLOROTHIAZIDE; RESERPINE
SEE   HYDROFLUMETHIAZIDE; RESERPINE
SEE   POLYTHIAZIDE; RESERPINE

RIBAVIRIN
Capsule; Oral
REBETOL

+ SCHERING PLOUGH RES	200MG	N020903 002	JUL 25, 2001
	200MG ***SEE 23RD ANNUAL OB SECTION 1.8 DESCRIPTION OF SPECIAL SITUATIONS: RIBAVIRIN ORAL 200MG CAPSULE***	N020903 001	JUN 03, 1998

For Solution; Inhalation
VIRAZOLE

+ ICN	6GM/VIAL	N018859 001	DEC 31, 1985

RIBAVIRIN *(continued)*
Tablet; Oral
COPEGUS

+ ROCHE	200MG	N021511 001	DEC 03, 2002

RIBOFLAVIN *MULTIPLE*
SEE   ASCORBIC ACID; BIOTIN; CHOLECALCIFEROL; CYANOCOBALAMIN; DEXPANTHENOL; FOLIC ACID; NIACINAMIDE; PYRIDOXINE; RIBOFLAVIN; THIAMINE; TOCOPHEROL ACETATE; VITAMIN A; VITAMIN K

RIBOFLAVIN PHOSPHATE SODIUM *MULTIPLE*
SEE   ALPHA-TOCOPHEROL ACETATE; ASCORBIC ACID; BIOTIN; CHOLECALCIFEROL; CYANOCOBALAMIN; DEXPANTHENOL; FOLIC ACID; NIACINAMIDE; PYRIDOXINE HYDROCHLORIDE; RIBOFLAVIN PHOSPHATE SODIUM; THIAMINE HYDROCHLORIDE; VITAMIN A PALMITATE; VITAMIN K

SEE   ASCORBIC ACID; BIOTIN; CYANOCOBALAMIN; DEXPANTHENOL; ERGOCALCIFEROL; FOLIC ACID; NIACINAMIDE; PHYTONADIONE; PYRIDOXINE HYDROCHLORIDE; RIBOFLAVIN PHOSPHATE SODIUM; THIAMINE HYDROCHLORIDE; VITAMIN A; VITAMIN E

SEE   ASCORBIC ACID; BIOTIN; CYANOCOBALAMIN; DEXPANTHENOL; ERGOCALCIFEROL; FOLIC ACID; NIACINAMIDE; PYRIDOXINE HYDROCHLORIDE; RIBOFLAVIN PHOSPHATE SODIUM; THIAMINE HYDROCHLORIDE; VITAMIN A; VITAMIN E

RIFABUTIN
Capsule; Oral
MYCOBUTIN

+ PHARMACIA AND UPJOHN	150MG	N050689 001	DEC 23, 1992

RIFAMPIN
Capsule; Oral
RIFADIN

AB	AVENTIS PHARMS	150MG	N062303 001	
AB		300MG	N050420 001	

RIFAMPIN

AB	EON	150MG	N064150 002	JAN 02, 1998
AB		300MG	N064150 001	MAY 28, 1997
AB	VERSAPHARM	150MG	N065028 001	MAR 14, 2001
AB		300MG	N065028 002	MAR 14, 2001

RIMACTANE

AB	GENEVA PHARMS	300MG	N050429 001	

Injectable; Injection
RIFADIN

AP	+ AVENTIS PHARMS	600MG/VIAL	N050627 001	MAY 25, 1989

RIFAMPIN

AP	BEDFORD	600MG/VIAL	N064217 001	OCT 29, 1999

Prescription Drug Products (continued)

RIFAMPIN *MULTIPLE*
SEE ISONIAZID: PYRAZINAMIDE: RIFAMPIN
SEE ISONIAZID: RIFAMPIN

RIFAPENTINE
Tablet; Oral
  PRIFTIN
  + AVENTIS PHARMS   150MG   N021024 001   JUN 22, 1998

RILUZOLE
Tablet; Oral
  RILUTEK
AB + AVENTIS   50MG   N020599 001   DEC 12, 1995
  RILUZOLE
AB IMPAX LABS   50MG   N076173 001   JAN 29, 2003

RIMANTADINE HYDROCHLORIDE
Syrup; Oral
  FLUMADINE
  + FOREST LABS   50MG/5ML   N019650 001   SEP 17, 1993
Tablet; Oral
  FLUMADINE
AB + FOREST LABS   100MG   N019649 001   SEP 17, 1993
  RIMANTADINE HCL
AB AMIDE PHARM   100MG   N076375 001   JAN 14, 2003
AB COREPHARMA   100MG   N075916 001   NOV 02, 2001
AB IMPAX LABS   100MG   N076132 001   AUG 30, 2002

RIMEXOLONE
Suspension/Drops; Ophthalmic
  VEXOL
  + ALCON   1%   N020474 001   DEC 30, 1994

RISEDRONATE SODIUM
Tablet; Oral
  ACTONEL
  PROCTER AND GAMBLE   5MG   N020835 002   APR 14, 2000
  30MG   N020835 001   MAR 27, 1998
  +   35MG   N020835 003   MAY 25, 2002

RISPERIDONE
Solution; Oral
  RISPERDAL
  + JANSSEN PHARMA   1MG/ML   N020588 001   JUN 10, 1996
Tablet, Orally Disintegrating; Oral
  RISPERDAL
  JOHNSON AND JOHNSON   0.5MG   N021444 001   APR 02, 2003
  1MG   N021444 002   APR 02, 2003
  +   2MG   N021444 003   APR 02, 2003
Tablet; Oral
  RISPERDAL
  JANSSEN PHARMA   0.5MG   N020272 007   JAN 27, 1999
  0.25MG   N020272 008   MAY 10, 1999
  1MG   N020272 001   DEC 29, 1993
  2MG   N020272 002   DEC 29, 1993
  +   3MG   N020272 003   DEC 29, 1993
  4MG   N020272 004   DEC 29, 1993

RITODRINE HYDROCHLORIDE
Injectable; Injection
  RITODRINE HCL
  + ABBOTT   10MG/ML   N071618 001   FEB 28, 1991
  +   15MG/ML   N071619 001   FEB 28, 1991
  RITODRINE HCL IN DEXTROSE 5% IN PLASTIC CONTAINER
  + ABBOTT   30MG/100ML   N071438 001   JAN 22, 1991

RITONAVIR
Capsule; Oral
  NORVIR
  + ABBOTT   100MG   N020945 001   JUN 29, 1999
Solution; Oral
  NORVIR
  + ABBOTT   80MG/ML   N020659 001   MAR 01, 1996

RITONAVIR *MULTIPLE*
SEE LOPINAVIR: RITONAVIR

Prescription Drug Products (continued)

RIVASTIGMINE TARTRATE
Capsule; Oral
EXELON

NOVARTIS	EQ 1.5MG BASE	N020823 003	APR 21, 2000
	EQ 3MG BASE	N020823 004	APR 21, 2000
	EQ 4.5MG BASE	N020823 005	APR 21, 2000
+	EQ 6MG BASE	N020823 006	APR 21, 2000

Solution; Oral
EXELON

+ NOVARTIS	EQ 2MG BASE/ML	N021025 001	APR 21, 2000

RIZATRIPTAN BENZOATE
Tablet, Orally Disintegrating; Oral
MAXALT-MLT

MERCK	EQ 5MG BASE	N020865 001	JUN 29, 1998
+	EQ 10MG BASE	N020865 002	JUN 29, 1998

Tablet; Oral
MAXALT

MERCK	EQ 5MG BASE	N020864 001	JUN 29, 1998
+	EQ 10MG BASE	N020864 002	JUN 29, 1998

ROCURONIUM BROMIDE
Injectable; Injection
ZEMURON (P/F)

+ ORGANON USA INC	10MG/ML	N020214 001	MAR 17, 1994

ROFECOXIB
Suspension; Oral
VIOXX

MERCK	12.5MG/5ML	N021052 001	MAY 20, 1999
+	25MG/5ML	N021052 002	MAY 20, 1999

Tablet; Oral
VIOXX

MERCK	12.5MG	N021042 001	MAY 20, 1999
	25MG	N021042 002	MAY 20, 1999
+	50MG	N021042 003	FEB 25, 2000

ROPINIROLE HYDROCHLORIDE
Tablet; Oral
REQUIP

GLAXOSMITHKLINE	EQ 0.5MG BASE	N020658 002	SEP 19, 1997
+	EQ 0.25MG BASE	N020658 001	SEP 19, 1997
	EQ 1MG BASE	N020658 003	SEP 19, 1997
	EQ 2MG BASE	N020658 004	SEP 19, 1997
	EQ 3MG BASE	N020658 006	SEP 19, 1997
		N020658 006	JAN 27, 1999
	EQ 4MG BASE	N020658 007	JAN 27, 1999
	EQ 5MG BASE	N020658 005	SEP 19, 1997

ROPIVACAINE HYDROCHLORIDE MONOHYDRATE
Injectable; Injection
NAROPIN

ASTRAZENECA	2MG/ML	N020533 001	SEP 24, 1996
	5MG/ML	N020533 003	SEP 24, 1996
	7.5MG/ML	N020533 004	SEP 24, 1996
+	10MG/ML	N020533 005	SEP 24, 1996

ROSIGLITAZONE MALEATE
Tablet; Oral
AVANDIA

SB PHARMCO	EQ 2MG BASE	N021071 002	MAY 25, 1999
	EQ 4MG BASE	N021071 003	MAY 25, 1999
+	EQ 8MG BASE	N021071 004	MAY 25, 1999

ROSIGLITAZONE MALEATE *MULTIPLE*
SEE METFORMIN HYDROCHLORIDE; ROSIGLITAZONE MALEATE

RUBIDIUM CHLORIDE RB-82
Injectable; Injection
CARDIOGEN-82

BRACCO	N/A	N019414 001	DEC 29, 1989
+			

SACROSIDASE
Solution; Oral
SUCRAID

+ QOL MEDCL	8,500 IU/ML	N020772 001	APR 09, 1998

Prescription Drug Products *(continued)*

SAFFLOWER OIL; SOYBEAN OIL
Injectable; Injection

	LIPOSYN II 10%			
	+ ABBOTT	5%;5% (5GM/100ML)	N018997 001	AUG 27, 1984
	LIPOSYN II 20%			
	+ ABBOTT	10%;10% (10GM/100ML)	N018991 001	AUG 27, 1984

SALMETEROL XINAFOATE
Aerosol, Metered; Inhalation

	SEREVENT			
	+ GLAXOSMITHKLINE	EQ 0.021MG BASE/INH	N020236 001	FEB 04, 1994

Powder; Inhalation

	SEREVENT			
	+ GLAXOSMITHKLINE	EQ 0.046MG BASE/INH	N020692 001	SEP 19, 1997

SALMETEROL XINAFOATE *MULTIPLE*
SEE   FLUTICASONE PROPIONATE; SALMETEROL XINAFOATE

SAMARIUM SM 153 LEXIDRONAM PENTASODIUM
Injectable; Injection

	QUADRAMET			
	+ CYTOGEN	50mCi/ML	N020570 001	MAR 28, 1997

SAQUINAVIR
Capsule; Oral

	FORTOVASE			
	+ HLR	200MG	N020828 001	NOV 07, 1997

SAQUINAVIR MESYLATE
Capsule; Oral

	INVIRASE			
	+ HLR	EQ 200MG BASE	N020628 001	DEC 06, 1995

SCOPOLAMINE
Film, Extended Release; Transdermal

	TRANSDERM SCOP			
	+ NOVARTIS	1MG/72HR	N017874 001	

SECOBARBITAL SODIUM
Capsule; Oral

	SECOBARBITAL SODIUM			
AA	EVERYLIFE	100MG	N085895 001	
	SECONAL SODIUM			
	+ RANBAXY	50MG	N086101 001	OCT 03, 1983
AA	+	100MG	N086101 002	OCT 03, 1983

SECOBARBITAL SODIUM *(continued)*
Capsule; Oral

	SODIUM SECOBARBITAL			
AA	WEST WARD	100MG	N084926 001	

Injectable; Injection

	SECOBARBITAL SODIUM			
	+ ELKINS SINN	100MG/VIAL	N083281 001	

SECRETIN
For Solution; Intravenous

	SECREFLO			
	+ CHIRHOCLIN	16UGM/VIAL	N021209 001	APR 04, 2002

SELEGILINE HYDROCHLORIDE
Capsule; Oral

	ELDEPRYL			
AB	+ SOMERSET	5MG	N020647 001	MAY 15, 1996
	SELEGILINE HCL			
AB	CLONMEL HLTHCARE	5MG	N075352 001	NOV 30, 1998
AB	TORPHARM	5MG	N075321 001	DEC 04, 1998

Tablet; Oral

	SELEGILINE HCL			
AB	ALPHAPHARM	5MG	N074866 001	NOV 26, 1997
			N074871 001	JUN 06, 1997
AB	APOTEX	5MG	N074641 001	AUG 02, 1996
AB	CLONMEL HLTHCARE	5MG	N074565 001	AUG 02, 1996
AB	ENDO PHARMS	5MG	N074756 001	NOV 25, 1998
AB	IVAX PHARMS	5MG	N074672 001	APR 01, 1997
AB	SIEGFRIED	5MG	N019334 001	JUN 05, 1989
AB	+ SOMERSET	5MG	N074912 001	APR 30, 1998
AB	STASON	5MG	N074537 001	AUG 02, 1996
AB	TEVA	5MG	N074744 001	JAN 27, 1997

SELENIUM SULFIDE
Lotion/Shampoo; Topical

	EXSEL			
AT	ALLERGAN HERBERT	2.5%	N083892 001	
	SELENIUM SULFIDE			
AT	ALPHARMA	2.5%	N084394 001	
AT	CLAY PARK	2.5%	N089996 001	JAN 10, 1991
AT	MORTON GROVE	2.5%	N088228 001	

Prescription Drug Products *(continued)*

SELENIUM SULFIDE *(continued)*
Lotion/Shampoo; Topical

SELENIUM SULFIDE
	MORTON GROVE			SEP 01, 1983

SELSUN
AT	+ CHATTEM	2.5%	N007936 001	

SERMORELIN ACETATE
Injectable; Injection

GEREF
+ SERONO	EQ 0.05MG BASE/AMP	N019863 001	DEC 28, 1990

SERTRALINE HYDROCHLORIDE
Concentrate; Oral

ZOLOFT
+ PFIZER	EQ 20MG BASE/ML	N020990 001	DEC 07, 1999

Tablet; Oral

ZOLOFT
PFIZER	EQ 25MG BASE	N019839 005	MAR 06, 1996
	EQ 50MG BASE	N019839 001	DEC 30, 1991
+	EQ 100MG BASE	N019839 002	DEC 30, 1991

SEVELAMER HYDROCHLORIDE
Capsule; Oral

RENAGEL
+ GENZYME	403MG	N020926 001	OCT 30, 1998

Tablet; Oral

RENAGEL
GENZYME	400MG	N021179 001	JUL 12, 2000
+	800MG	N021179 002	JUL 12, 2000

SEVOFLURANE
Liquid; Inhalation

SEVOFLURANE
AN	BAXTER HLTHCARE	100%	N075895 001	JUL 02, 2002

ULTANE
AN	+ ABBOTT	100%	N020478 001	JUN 07, 1995

SIBUTRAMINE HYDROCHLORIDE
Capsule; Oral

MERIDIA
ABBOTT	5MG	N020632 001	NOV 22, 1997
	10MG	N020632 002	NOV 22, 1997

SIBUTRAMINE HYDROCHLORIDE *(continued)*
Capsule; Oral

MERIDIA
+ ABBOTT	15MG	N020632 003	NOV 22, 1997

SILDENAFIL CITRATE
Tablet; Oral

VIAGRA
PFIZER	25MG	N020895 001	MAR 27, 1998
	50MG	N020895 002	MAR 27, 1998
+	100MG	N020895 003	MAR 27, 1998

SILVER SULFADIAZINE
Cream; Topical

SILVADENE
AB	+ KING PHARMS	1%	N017381 001	

SSD
AB	BASF	1%	N018578 001	FEB 25, 1982

SSD AF
BX	BASF	1%	N018578 003	JUL 11, 1990

THERMAZENE
AB	KENDALL LP	1%	N018810 001	DEC 23, 1985

SIMVASTATIN
Tablet; Oral

ZOCOR
MERCK	5MG	N019766 001	DEC 23, 1991
	10MG	N019766 002	DEC 23, 1991
	20MG	N019766 003	DEC 23, 1991
	40MG	N019766 004	DEC 23, 1991
+	80MG	N019766 005	JUL 10, 1998

SINCALIDE
Injectable; Injection

KINEVAC
+ BRACCO	0.005MG/VIAL	N017697 001	

SIROLIMUS
Solution; Oral

RAPAMUNE
+ WYETH PHARMS INC	1MG/ML	N021083 001	SEP 15, 1999

Prescription Drug Products (continued)

SIROLIMUS (continued)
Tablet; Oral
RAPAMUNE
WYETH PHARMS INC   1MG   N021110 001   AUG 25, 2000
   2MG   N021110 002   AUG 22, 2002
+

SODIUM ACETATE *MULTIPLE*
SEE AMINO ACIDS; CALCIUM ACETATE; GLYCERIN; MAGNESIUM ACETATE; PHOSPHORIC ACID; POTASSIUM CHLORIDE; SODIUM ACETATE; SODIUM CHLORIDE

SEE AMINO ACIDS; CALCIUM CHLORIDE; DEXTROSE; MAGNESIUM CHLORIDE; POTASSIUM PHOSPHATE, DIBASIC; SODIUM ACETATE; SODIUM CHLORIDE

SEE AMINO ACIDS; DEXTROSE; MAGNESIUM CHLORIDE; POTASSIUM PHOSPHATE, DIBASIC; SODIUM ACETATE; SODIUM CHLORIDE

SEE AMINO ACIDS; MAGNESIUM ACETATE; PHOSPHORIC ACID; POTASSIUM ACETATE; POTASSIUM CHLORIDE; SODIUM ACETATE

SEE AMINO ACIDS; MAGNESIUM ACETATE; PHOSPHORIC ACID; POTASSIUM CHLORIDE; SODIUM CHLORIDE

SEE AMINO ACIDS; MAGNESIUM CHLORIDE; POTASSIUM PHOSPHATE, DIBASIC; SODIUM ACETATE; SODIUM CHLORIDE

SEE CALCIUM CHLORIDE; DEXTROSE; MAGNESIUM CHLORIDE; POTASSIUM CHLORIDE; SODIUM ACETATE; SODIUM CHLORIDE

SEE CALCIUM CHLORIDE; DEXTROSE; MAGNESIUM CHLORIDE; POTASSIUM CHLORIDE; SODIUM ACETATE; SODIUM CITRATE

SEE CALCIUM CHLORIDE; DEXTROSE; MAGNESIUM CHLORIDE; POTASSIUM CHLORIDE; SODIUM ACETATE; SODIUM LACTATE

SEE CALCIUM CHLORIDE; DEXTROSE; MAGNESIUM CHLORIDE; SODIUM ACETATE; SODIUM CHLORIDE

SEE SODIUM CHLORIDE

SEE CALCIUM CHLORIDE; MAGNESIUM CHLORIDE; POTASSIUM CHLORIDE; SODIUM ACETATE; SODIUM CHLORIDE

SEE SODIUM ACETATE; SODIUM CHLORIDE

SEE CALCIUM CHLORIDE; MAGNESIUM CHLORIDE; SODIUM CHLORIDE; SODIUM CITRATE

SEE CALCIUM CHLORIDE; MAGNESIUM CHLORIDE; SODIUM CHLORIDE; SODIUM LACTATE

SEE DEXTROSE; MAGNESIUM CHLORIDE; POTASSIUM CHLORIDE; POTASSIUM PHOSPHATE, DIBASIC; SODIUM ACETATE

SEE DEXTROSE; MAGNESIUM CHLORIDE; POTASSIUM CHLORIDE; SODIUM ACETATE; SODIUM CHLORIDE

SEE ACETATE; SODIUM CHLORIDE

SEE DEXTROSE; MAGNESIUM CHLORIDE; POTASSIUM CHLORIDE; SODIUM GLUCONATE

SEE DEXTROSE; POTASSIUM CHLORIDE; POTASSIUM PHOSPHATE, DIBASIC; SODIUM ACETATE; SODIUM CHLORIDE

SEE MAGNESIUM CHLORIDE; POTASSIUM CHLORIDE; POTASSIUM PHOSPHATE, MONOBASIC; SODIUM CHLORIDE; SODIUM GLUCONATE; SODIUM PHOSPHATE, DIBASIC, HEPTAHYDRATE

SEE MAGNESIUM CHLORIDE; POTASSIUM CHLORIDE; SODIUM ACETATE; SODIUM CHLORIDE; SODIUM GLUCONATE

SODIUM ACETATE, ANHYDROUS
Injectable; Injection
SODIUM ACETATE IN PLASTIC CONTAINER
+ ABBOTT   2MEQ/ML   N018893 001

SODIUM ACETATE, ANHYDROUS (continued)
Injectable; Injection
SODIUM ACETATE IN PLASTIC CONTAINER
ABBOTT   MAY 04, 1983

SODIUM BICARBONATE; TARTARIC ACID
Granule, Effervescent; Oral
BAROS
LAFAYETTE PHARMS   460MG/GM;420MG/GM   N018509 001   AUG 07, 1985

SODIUM BICARBONATE *MULTIPLE*
SEE CALCIUM CHLORIDE; DEXTROSE; GLUTATHIONE DISULFIDE; MAGNESIUM CHLORIDE; POTASSIUM CHLORIDE; SODIUM BICARBONATE; SODIUM CHLORIDE; SODIUM PHOSPHATE

SEE CALCIUM CHLORIDE; DEXTROSE; MAGNESIUM SULFATE; POTASSIUM CHLORIDE; SODIUM BICARBONATE; SODIUM CHLORIDE; SODIUM CHLORIDE; SODIUM PHOSPHATE, DIBASIC, HEPTAHYDRATE

SEE POLYETHYLENE GLYCOL 3350; POTASSIUM CHLORIDE; SODIUM BICARBONATE; SODIUM CHLORIDE

SEE POLYETHYLENE GLYCOL 3350; POTASSIUM CHLORIDE; SODIUM BICARBONATE; SODIUM CHLORIDE; SODIUM SULFATE

SEE POLYETHYLENE GLYCOL 3350; POTASSIUM CHLORIDE; SODIUM BICARBONATE; SODIUM CHLORIDE; SODIUM SULFATE, ANHYDROUS

SODIUM CARBONATE *MULTIPLE*
SEE CITRIC ACID; MAGNESIUM OXIDE; SODIUM CARBONATE

SODIUM CHLORIDE
Injectable; Injection
BACTERIOSTATIC SODIUM CHLORIDE 0.9% IN PLASTIC CONTAINER
AP + ABBOTT   9MG/ML   N018800 001   OCT 29, 1982
AP   AM PHARM PARTNERS   9MG/ML   N088911 001   FEB 07, 1985
SODIUM CHLORIDE 0.9% IN PLASTIC CONTAINER
AP   ABBOTT   9MG/ML   N018803 001   OCT 29, 1982
AP   9MG/ML   N019217 001   JUL 13, 1984
AP   9MG/ML   N019465 002
AP   900MG/100ML   N016366 001
AP   900MG/100ML   N019465 001   JUL 15, 1985
AP   900MG/100ML   N019480 001   JUL 15, 1985
AP   AM PHARM PARTNERS   9MG/ML   N088912 001   SEP 17, 1985
AP   B BRAUN   900MG/100ML   N017464 001   JAN 10, 1985
AP   900MG/100ML   N019635 002
AP + BAXTER HLTHCARE   9MG/ML   N016677 004   MAR 09, 1988
AP   9MG/ML   N020178 002   OCT 30, 1985
   DEC 07, 1992

Prescription Drug Products *(continued)*

SODIUM CHLORIDE *(continued)*
Injectable; Injection

SODIUM CHLORIDE 0.9% IN PLASTIC CONTAINER

AP	BAXTER HLTHCARE	900MG/100ML	N016677 001
AP		900MG/100ML	N020178 001 DEC 07, 1992

SODIUM CHLORIDE 0.45% IN PLASTIC CONTAINER

AP	ABBOTT	450MG/100ML	N018090 001
AP		450MG/100ML	N019759 001 JUN 08, 1988
AP	B BRAUN	450MG/100ML	N019635 001 MAR 09, 1988
AP	BAXTER HLTHCARE	450MG/100ML	N018016 001

SODIUM CHLORIDE 3% IN PLASTIC CONTAINER

AP	BAXTER HLTHCARE	3GM/100ML	N019022 001 NOV 01, 1983

SODIUM CHLORIDE 5% IN PLASTIC CONTAINER

AP	BAXTER HLTHCARE	5GM/100ML	N019022 002 NOV 01, 1983

SODIUM CHLORIDE IN PLASTIC CONTAINER

AP	ABBOTT	2.5MEQ/ML	N018897 001 JUL 20, 1984

Solution For Slush; Irrigation

SODIUM CHLORIDE 0.9% IN STERILE PLASTIC CONTAINER

AP	BAXTER HLTHCARE	900MG/100ML	N019319 002 MAY 17, 1985

Solution; Irrigation

SODIUM CHLORIDE 0.9% IN PLASTIC CONTAINER

AT	ABBOTT	900MG/100ML	N017514 001
AT		900MG/100ML	N018314 001
AT	B BRAUN	900MG/100ML	N016733 001
AT	BAXTER HLTHCARE	900MG/100ML	N017427 001
AT		900MG/100ML	N017867 001

SODIUM CHLORIDE 0.45% IN PLASTIC CONTAINER

AT	ABBOTT	450MG/100ML	N017670 001
AT	BAXTER HLTHCARE	450MG/100ML	N017864 001

SODIUM CHLORIDE *MULTIPLE*
SEE AMINO ACIDS: CALCIUM ACETATE: GLYCERIN: MAGNESIUM ACETATE: PHOSPHORIC ACID: POTASSIUM CHLORIDE: SODIUM ACETATE: SODIUM CHLORIDE

SEE AMINO ACIDS: CALCIUM CHLORIDE: DEXTROSE: MAGNESIUM CHLORIDE: POTASSIUM CHLORIDE: POTASSIUM PHOSPHATE, DIBASIC: SODIUM CHLORIDE

SEE AMINO ACIDS: CALCIUM CHLORIDE: DEXTROSE: MAGNESIUM CHLORIDE: POTASSIUM PHOSPHATE, DIBASIC: SODIUM ACETATE: SODIUM CHLORIDE

SEE AMINO ACIDS: DEXTROSE: MAGNESIUM CHLORIDE: POTASSIUM CHLORIDE: POTASSIUM PHOSPHATE, DIBASIC: SODIUM PHOSPHATE, DIBASIC, HEPTAHYDRATE

SEE AMINO ACIDS: DEXTROSE: MAGNESIUM CHLORIDE: POTASSIUM PHOSPHATE, DIBASIC: SODIUM ACETATE: SODIUM CHLORIDE

SEE AMINO ACIDS: MAGNESIUM ACETATE: PHOSPHORIC ACID: POTASSIUM ACETATE: SODIUM CHLORIDE

SEE AMINO ACIDS: MAGNESIUM ACETATE: POTASSIUM CHLORIDE: SODIUM ACETATE: SODIUM CHLORIDE

SEE AMINO ACIDS: MAGNESIUM CHLORIDE: POTASSIUM CHLORIDE: POTASSIUM PHOSPHATE, DIBASIC: SODIUM CHLORIDE

SODIUM CHLORIDE *MULTIPLE* *(continued)*
SEE AMINO ACIDS: MAGNESIUM CHLORIDE: POTASSIUM PHOSPHATE, DIBASIC: SODIUM ACETATE: SODIUM CHLORIDE

SEE AMINO ACIDS: MAGNESIUM CHLORIDE: POTASSIUM PHOSPHATE, DIBASIC: SODIUM CHLORIDE

SEE CALCIUM CHLORIDE: DEXTROSE: GLUTATHIONE DISULFIDE: MAGNESIUM CHLORIDE: POTASSIUM CHLORIDE: SODIUM BICARBONATE: SODIUM CHLORIDE: SODIUM PHOSPHATE

SEE CALCIUM CHLORIDE: DEXTROSE: MAGNESIUM CHLORIDE: POTASSIUM CHLORIDE: SODIUM ACETATE: SODIUM CHLORIDE

SEE CALCIUM CHLORIDE: DEXTROSE: MAGNESIUM CHLORIDE: POTASSIUM CHLORIDE: SODIUM CITRATE

SEE CALCIUM CHLORIDE: SODIUM ACETATE: SODIUM CHLORIDE: SODIUM LACTATE

SEE CALCIUM CHLORIDE: SODIUM ACETATE: SODIUM CHLORIDE: SODIUM LACTATE

SEE CALCIUM CHLORIDE: DEXTROSE: MAGNESIUM CHLORIDE: SODIUM CHLORIDE: SODIUM ACETATE: SODIUM CHLORIDE

SEE CALCIUM CHLORIDE: DEXTROSE: MAGNESIUM CHLORIDE: SODIUM CHLORIDE: SODIUM LACTATE

SEE CALCIUM CHLORIDE: DEXTROSE: MAGNESIUM SULFATE: POTASSIUM CHLORIDE: SODIUM BICARBONATE: SODIUM CHLORIDE: SODIUM PHOSPHATE, DIBASIC, HEPTAHYDRATE

SEE CALCIUM CHLORIDE: DEXTROSE: POTASSIUM CHLORIDE: SODIUM ACETATE: SODIUM CHLORIDE

SEE CALCIUM CHLORIDE: DEXTROSE: POTASSIUM CHLORIDE: SODIUM CHLORIDE

SEE CALCIUM CHLORIDE: DEXTROSE: ICODEXTRIN: MAGNESIUM CHLORIDE: SODIUM CHLORIDE: SODIUM LACTATE

SEE CALCIUM CHLORIDE: MAGNESIUM CHLORIDE: POTASSIUM CHLORIDE: SODIUM ACETATE: SODIUM CHLORIDE

SEE CALCIUM CHLORIDE: MAGNESIUM CHLORIDE: POTASSIUM CHLORIDE: SODIUM CITRATE

SEE CALCIUM CHLORIDE: MAGNESIUM CHLORIDE: POTASSIUM CHLORIDE: SODIUM LACTATE

SEE CALCIUM CHLORIDE: MAGNESIUM CHLORIDE: POTASSIUM CHLORIDE: SODIUM CHLORIDE

SEE CALCIUM CHLORIDE: POTASSIUM CHLORIDE: SODIUM CHLORIDE

SEE CALCIUM CHLORIDE: POTASSIUM CHLORIDE: SODIUM CHLORIDE: SODIUM LACTATE

SEE DEXTROSE: MAGNESIUM ACETATE: POTASSIUM ACETATE: SODIUM CHLORIDE

SEE DEXTROSE: MAGNESIUM ACETATE TETRAHYDRATE: POTASSIUM ACETATE: SODIUM CHLORIDE

SEE DEXTROSE: MAGNESIUM CHLORIDE: POTASSIUM CHLORIDE: POTASSIUM PHOSPHATE, DIBASIC: SODIUM CHLORIDE: SODIUM LACTATE: SODIUM PHOSPHATE, MONOBASIC, ANHYDROUS

SEE DEXTROSE: MAGNESIUM CHLORIDE: POTASSIUM CHLORIDE: POTASSIUM PHOSPHATE, MONOBASIC: SODIUM CHLORIDE: SODIUM LACTATE

SEE DEXTROSE: MAGNESIUM CHLORIDE: POTASSIUM CHLORIDE: SODIUM ACETATE: SODIUM CHLORIDE

SEE DEXTROSE: MAGNESIUM CHLORIDE: POTASSIUM CHLORIDE: SODIUM GLUCONATE

SEE DEXTROSE: POTASSIUM CHLORIDE: POTASSIUM LACTATE: SODIUM CHLORIDE: SODIUM PHOSPHATE, MONOBASIC, ANHYDROUS

SEE DEXTROSE: POTASSIUM CHLORIDE: POTASSIUM PHOSPHATE, DIBASIC: SODIUM PHOSPHATE, DIBASIC: SODIUM CHLORIDE

Prescription Drug Products *(continued)*

SODIUM CHLORIDE *MULTIPLE* (continued)
SEE DEXTROSE: POTASSIUM CHLORIDE: POTASSIUM PHOSPHATE, MONOBASIC: SODIUM CHLORIDE: POTASSIUM PHOSPHATE, MONOBASIC: SODIUM CHLORIDE: SODIUM LACTATE
SEE DEXTROSE: POTASSIUM CHLORIDE: SODIUM CHLORIDE
SEE DEXTROSE: SODIUM CHLORIDE
SEE MAGNESIUM ACETATE TETRAHYDRATE: POTASSIUM ACETATE: SODIUM CHLORIDE
SEE MAGNESIUM CHLORIDE: POTASSIUM CHLORIDE: POTASSIUM PHOSPHATE, MONOBASIC: SODIUM ACETATE: SODIUM CHLORIDE: SODIUM GLUCONATE: SODIUM PHOSPHATE, DIBASIC, HEPTAHYDRATE
SEE MAGNESIUM CHLORIDE: POTASSIUM CHLORIDE: SODIUM ACETATE: SODIUM CHLORIDE: SODIUM GLUCONATE
SEE MAGNESIUM SULFATE: POTASSIUM CHLORIDE: POTASSIUM PHOSPHATE, MONOBASIC: SODIUM CHLORIDE: SODIUM PHOSPHATE
SEE POLYETHYLENE GLYCOL 3350: POTASSIUM CHLORIDE: SODIUM BICARBONATE: SODIUM CHLORIDE
SEE POLYETHYLENE GLYCOL 3350: POTASSIUM CHLORIDE: SODIUM BICARBONATE: SODIUM CHLORIDE: SODIUM SULFATE
SEE POLYETHYLENE GLYCOL 3350: POTASSIUM CHLORIDE: SODIUM BICARBONATE: SODIUM CHLORIDE: SODIUM SULFATE, ANHYDROUS
SEE POTASSIUM CHLORIDE: SODIUM CHLORIDE

SODIUM CHROMATE, CR-51
Injectable; Injection
CHROMITOPE SODIUM
  BRACCO 200uCi/ML N013993 001
SODIUM CHROMATE CR 51
  MALLINCKRODT 100uCi/ML N016708 001

SODIUM CITRATE *MULTIPLE*
SEE CALCIUM CHLORIDE: DEXTROSE: MAGNESIUM CHLORIDE: POTASSIUM CHLORIDE: DEXTROSE: SODIUM ACETATE: SODIUM CHLORIDE: SODIUM CITRATE
SEE CALCIUM CHLORIDE: MAGNESIUM CHLORIDE: POTASSIUM CHLORIDE: SODIUM ACETATE: SODIUM CHLORIDE: SODIUM CITRATE

SODIUM FERRIC GLUCONATE COMPLEX
Injectable; Injection
FERRLECIT
  + R AND D LABS 62.5MG/5ML N020955 001 FEB 18, 1999

SODIUM GLUCONATE *MULTIPLE*
SEE DEXTROSE: MAGNESIUM CHLORIDE: POTASSIUM CHLORIDE: SODIUM ACETATE: SODIUM CHLORIDE: SODIUM GLUCONATE
SEE MAGNESIUM CHLORIDE: POTASSIUM CHLORIDE: POTASSIUM PHOSPHATE, MONOBASIC: SODIUM ACETATE: SODIUM CHLORIDE: SODIUM GLUCONATE: SODIUM PHOSPHATE, DIBASIC, HEPTAHYDRATE
SEE MAGNESIUM CHLORIDE: POTASSIUM CHLORIDE: SODIUM ACETATE: SODIUM CHLORIDE: SODIUM GLUCONATE

SODIUM IODIDE, I-123
Capsule; Oral
SODIUM IODIDE I 123
AA AMERSHAM HLTH 100uCi N017630 001
AA MALLINCKRODT 100uCi N071909 001

SODIUM IODIDE, I-123 *(continued)*
Capsule; Oral
SODIUM IODIDE I 123
  MALLINCKRODT
AA 200uCi FEB 28, 1989 N071910 001
AA SYNCOR PHARMS 100uCi FEB 28, 1989 N018671 001
AA 200uCi MAY 27, 1982 N018671 002

Solution; Oral
SODIUM IODIDE I 123
  AMERSHAM HLTH 2mCi/ML MAY 27, 1982 N017630 002

SODIUM IODIDE, I-131
Capsule; Oral
IODOTOPE
  + BRACCO 1-130mCi N010929 001
SODIUM IODIDE I 131
  + MALLINCKRODT 0.8-100mCi N016517 001
                  15-100uCi N016517 002

Solution; Oral
SODIUM IODIDE I 131
  + CIS 50mCi/ML N017315 001
  + MALLINCKRODT 3.5-150mCi/VIAL N016515 001
SODIUM IODIDE I 131, KIT
  + DRAXIMAGE 1-250mCi/0.25ML N021305 002 JAN 24, 2003
                N021305 003 JAN 24, 2003
  + 1-500uCi/0.5ML

SODIUM LACTATE
Injectable; Injection
SODIUM LACTATE 0.167 MOLAR IN PLASTIC CONTAINER
AP ABBOTT 1.87GM/100ML N018249 001
AP BAXTER HLTHCARE 1.87GM/100ML N016692 001
SODIUM LACTATE 1/6 MOLAR IN PLASTIC CONTAINER
AP B BRAUN 1.87GM/100ML N020004 001 APR 21, 1992
SODIUM LACTATE IN PLASTIC CONTAINER
  ABBOTT 5MEQ/ML N018947 001 SEP 05, 1984

SODIUM LACTATE *MULTIPLE*
SEE CALCIUM CHLORIDE: DEXTROSE: MAGNESIUM CHLORIDE: POTASSIUM CHLORIDE: DEXTROSE: SODIUM CHLORIDE: SODIUM LACTATE
SEE CALCIUM CHLORIDE: DEXTROSE: MAGNESIUM CHLORIDE: SODIUM CHLORIDE: SODIUM LACTATE
SEE CALCIUM CHLORIDE: DEXTROSE: POTASSIUM CHLORIDE: SODIUM CHLORIDE: SODIUM LACTATE
SEE CALCIUM CHLORIDE: ICODEXTRIN: MAGNESIUM CHLORIDE: SODIUM CHLORIDE: SODIUM LACTATE
SEE CALCIUM CHLORIDE: MAGNESIUM CHLORIDE: POTASSIUM CHLORIDE: SODIUM CHLORIDE: SODIUM LACTATE
SEE SODIUM ACETATE: SODIUM CHLORIDE: SODIUM LACTATE

Prescription Drug Products (continued)

SODIUM LACTATE *MULTIPLE* (continued)
SEE CALCIUM CHLORIDE: POTASSIUM CHLORIDE: SODIUM CHLORIDE: SODIUM LACTATE
SEE DEXTROSE: MAGNESIUM CHLORIDE: POTASSIUM CHLORIDE: POTASSIUM PHOSPHATE, DIBASIC: SODIUM CHLORIDE: SODIUM LACTATE: SODIUM PHOSPHATE, MONOBASIC, ANHYDROUS
SEE DEXTROSE: MAGNESIUM CHLORIDE: POTASSIUM CHLORIDE: POTASSIUM PHOSPHATE, MONOBASIC: SODIUM CHLORIDE: SODIUM LACTATE
SEE DEXTROSE: MAGNESIUM CHLORIDE: POTASSIUM CHLORIDE: POTASSIUM PHOSPHATE, MONOBASIC: SODIUM LACTATE: SODIUM PHOSPHATE, MONOBASIC, ANHYDROUS
SEE DEXTROSE: POTASSIUM CHLORIDE: POTASSIUM PHOSPHATE, MONOBASIC: SODIUM CHLORIDE: SODIUM LACTATE

SODIUM NITROPRUSSIDE
Injectable; Injection
NITROPRESS
AP + ABBOTT   25MG/ML   N071961 001 AUG 01, 1988
AP +   50MG/VIAL N070566 001 JUN 09, 1986
SODIUM NITROPRUSSIDE
AP   GENSIA SICOR PHARMS   25MG/ML   N073465 001 MAR 30, 1992

SODIUM OXYBATE
Solution; Oral
XYREM
    + ORPHAN MEDCL   500MG/ML   N021196 001 JUL 17, 2002

SODIUM PHENYLBUTYRATE
Powder; Oral
BUPHENYL
    + MEDICIS   3GM/TEASPOONFUL N020573 001 APR 30, 1996
Tablet; Oral
BUPHENYL
    + MEDICIS   500MG   N020572 001 MAY 13, 1996

SODIUM PHOSPHATE, DIBASIC, ANHYDROUS *MULTIPLE*
SEE CALCIUM CHLORIDE: DEXTROSE: GLUTATHIONE DISULFIDE: MAGNESIUM CHLORIDE: POTASSIUM CHLORIDE: SODIUM BICARBONATE: SODIUM CHLORIDE: SODIUM PHOSPHATE
SEE MAGNESIUM SULFATE: POTASSIUM CHLORIDE: POTASSIUM PHOSPHATE, MONOBASIC: SODIUM CHLORIDE: SODIUM PHOSPHATE

SODIUM PHOSPHATE, DIBASIC, ANHYDROUS; SODIUM PHOSPHATE, MONOBASIC, MONOHYDRATE
Tablet; Oral
VISICOL   0.398GM;1.102GM
    + INKINE   N021097 001 SEP 21, 2000

SODIUM PHOSPHATE, DIBASIC, HEPTAHYDRATE; SODIUM PHOSPHATE, MONOBASIC, ANHYDROUS
Injectable; Injection
SODIUM PHOSPHATES IN PLASTIC CONTAINER   142MG/ML;276MG/ML
    ABBOTT   N018892 001 MAY 10, 1983

SODIUM PHOSPHATE, DIBASIC, HEPTAHYDRATE *MULTIPLE*
SEE AMINO ACIDS: DEXTROSE: MAGNESIUM CHLORIDE: POTASSIUM CHLORIDE: SODIUM CHLORIDE: SODIUM PHOSPHATE, DIBASIC, HEPTAHYDRATE
SEE CALCIUM CHLORIDE: DEXTROSE: MAGNESIUM SULFATE: POTASSIUM CHLORIDE: SODIUM BICARBONATE: SODIUM CHLORIDE: SODIUM PHOSPHATE, DIBASIC, HEPTAHYDRATE
SEE MAGNESIUM CHLORIDE: SODIUM ACETATE: SODIUM CHLORIDE: SODIUM GLUCONATE: SODIUM PHOSPHATE, DIBASIC, HEPTAHYDRATE

SODIUM PHOSPHATE, MONOBASIC, ANHYDROUS *MULTIPLE*
SEE DEXTROSE: MAGNESIUM CHLORIDE: POTASSIUM CHLORIDE: POTASSIUM PHOSPHATE, DIBASIC: SODIUM CHLORIDE: SODIUM LACTATE: SODIUM PHOSPHATE, MONOBASIC, ANHYDROUS
SEE DEXTROSE: MAGNESIUM CHLORIDE: POTASSIUM CHLORIDE: POTASSIUM PHOSPHATE, MONOBASIC: SODIUM LACTATE: SODIUM PHOSPHATE, MONOBASIC, ANHYDROUS
SEE DEXTROSE: POTASSIUM CHLORIDE: POTASSIUM LACTATE: SODIUM CHLORIDE: SODIUM PHOSPHATE, MONOBASIC, ANHYDROUS
SEE SODIUM PHOSPHATE, DIBASIC, HEPTAHYDRATE: SODIUM PHOSPHATE, MONOBASIC, ANHYDROUS

SODIUM PHOSPHATE, MONOBASIC, MONOHYDRATE *MULTIPLE*
SEE SODIUM PHOSPHATE, DIBASIC, ANHYDROUS: SODIUM PHOSPHATE, MONOBASIC, MONOHYDRATE

SODIUM PHOSPHATE, P-32
Solution; Injection, Oral
SODIUM PHOSPHATE P 32   0.67mCi/ML
    MALLINCKRODT   N011777 001

SODIUM POLYSTYRENE SULFONATE
Powder; Oral, Rectal
KAYEXALATE
AA + SANOFI SYNTHELABO   453.6GM/BOT   N011287 001
KIONEX
AA   PADDOCK   454GM/BOT   N040029 001 FEB 06, 1998
SODIUM POLYSTYRENE SULFONATE
AA   CAROLINA MEDCL   454GM/BOT   N089910 001 JAN 19, 1989
Suspension; Oral, Rectal
SODIUM POLYSTYRENE SULFONATE
AA   ROXANE   15GM/60ML   N089049 001 NOV 17, 1986
SPS
AA + CAROLINA MEDCL   15GM/60ML   N087859 001 DEC 08, 1982

Prescription Drug Products (continued)

SODIUM SULFATE *MULTIPLE*
SEE POLYETHYLENE GLYCOL 3350: POTASSIUM CHLORIDE: SODIUM BICARBONATE: SODIUM CHLORIDE: SODIUM SULFATE

SODIUM SULFATE, ANHYDROUS *MULTIPLE*
SEE POLYETHYLENE GLYCOL 3350: POTASSIUM CHLORIDE: SODIUM BICARBONATE: SODIUM CHLORIDE: SODIUM SULFATE, ANHYDROUS

SODIUM THIOSULFATE
Injectable; Injection

	SODIUM THIOSULFATE			
+	US ARMY	250MG/ML	N020166 001	FEB 14, 1992

SOMATREM
Injectable; Injection

	PROTROPIN			
+	GENENTECH	5MG/VIAL	N019107 001	OCT 17, 1985
+		10MG/VIAL	N019107 002	OCT 24, 1989

SOMATROPIN RECOMBINANT
Injectable; Injection

	GENOTROPIN			
+	PHARMACIA AND UPJOHN	5.8MG/VIAL	N020280 006	AUG 24, 1995
+		13.8MG/VIAL	N020280 007	OCT 23, 1996
	GENOTROPIN PRESERVATIVE FREE			
	PHARMACIA AND UPJOHN	0.2MG/VIAL	N020280 001	JAN 27, 1998
		0.4MG/VIAL	N020280 002	JAN 27, 1998
		0.6MG/VIAL	N020280 003	JAN 27, 1998
		0.8MG/VIAL	N020280 005	JAN 27, 1998
		1.2MG/VIAL	N020280 009	JAN 27, 1998
			N020280 010	JAN 27, 1998
		1.4MG/VIAL	N020280 004	JAN 27, 1998
		1.5MG/VIAL		AUG 24, 1995
		1.6MG/VIAL	N020280 011	JAN 27, 1998
		1.8MG/VIAL	N020280 012	JAN 27, 1998
		1MG/VIAL	N020280 008	JAN 27, 1998
+		2MG/VIAL	N020280 013	JAN 27, 1998

SOMATROPIN RECOMBINANT (continued)
Injectable; Injection

	HUMATROPE			
BX	+ LILLY	5MG/VIAL	N019640 004	MAR 08, 1987
BX		6MG/VIAL	N019640 005	FEB 04, 1999
	+	12MG/VIAL	N019640 006	FEB 04, 1999
	+	24MG/VIAL	N019640 007	FEB 04, 1999
	NORDITROPIN			
	NOVO NORDISK	5MG/1.5ML	N021148 001	JUN 20, 2000
		10MG/1.5ML	N021148 002	JUN 20, 2000
	+	15MG/1.5ML	N021148 003	JUN 20, 2000
	NUTROPIN			
BX	+ GENENTECH	5MG/VIAL	N020168 001	NOV 17, 1993
	+	10MG/VIAL	N020168 002	NOV 17, 1993
	NUTROPIN AQ			
	+ GENENTECH	5MG/ML	N020522 001	DEC 29, 1995
	NUTROPIN AQ PEN			
BX	+ GENENTECH	5MG/ML	N020522 002	APR 22, 2002
	NUTROPIN DEPOT			
	+ GENENTECH	13.5MG/VIAL	N021075 001	DEC 22, 1999
	+	18MG/VIAL	N021075 002	DEC 22, 1999
	+	22.5MG/VIAL	N021075 003	DEC 22, 1999
	SAIZEN			
BX	SERONO	5MG/VIAL	N019764 002	OCT 08, 1996
BX		6MG/VIAL	N019764 001	OCT 08, 1996
	+	8.8MG/VIAL	N019764 003	AUG 29, 2000
	SEROSTIM			
BX	+ SERONO	4MG/VIAL	N020604 003	JUL 25, 1997
BX		5MG/VIAL	N020604 002	AUG 23, 1996
BX		6MG/VIAL	N020604 001	AUG 23, 1996
	+	8.8MG/VIAL	N020604 004	SEP 06, 2001
	TEV-TROPIN			
BX	+ BIO TECH GEN	5MG/ML	N019774 002	JAN 04, 2002

Prescription Drug Products (continued)

SORBITOL
Solution; Irrigation

	Strength	Appl. No.	Date
SORBITOL 3% IN PLASTIC CONTAINER			
BAXTER HLTHCARE	3GM/100ML	N017863 001	
SORBITOL 3.3% IN PLASTIC CONTAINER			
B BRAUN	3.3GM/100ML	N016741 001	

SORBITOL *MULTIPLE*
SEE MANNITOL; SORBITOL

SOTALOL HYDROCHLORIDE
Tablet; Oral

TE		Strength	Appl. No.	Date
	BETAPACE			
	BERLEX LABS			
AB		80MG	N019865 001	OCT 30, 1992
AB		120MG	N019865 005	APR 20, 1994
AB +		160MG	N019865 002	OCT 30, 1992
AB		240MG	N019865 003	OCT 30, 1992
	BETAPACE AF			
	BERLEX LABS			
		80MG	N021151 001	FEB 22, 2000
		120MG	N021151 002	FEB 22, 2000
+		160MG	N021151 003	FEB 22, 2000
	SORINE			
	UPSHER SMITH			
AB		80MG	N075500 001	APR 27, 2001
AB		120MG	N075500 004	APR 27, 2001
AB		160MG	N075500 002	APR 27, 2001
AB		240MG	N075500 003	APR 27, 2001
	SOTALOL HCL			
	APOTEX			
AB		80MG	N076140 001	SEP 26, 2002
AB		120MG	N076140 002	SEP 26, 2002
AB		160MG	N076140 003	SEP 26, 2002
AB		240MG	N076140 004	SEP 26, 2002
	EON			
AB		80MG	N075366 001	MAY 01, 2000
AB		120MG	N075366 002	MAY 01, 2000
AB		160MG	N075366 003	MAY 01, 2000
AB		240MG	N075366 004	MAY 01, 2000
	GENPHARM			
AB		80MG	N075237 001	MAY 01, 2000

SOTALOL HYDROCHLORIDE (continued)
Tablet; Oral

TE		Strength	Appl. No.	Date
	SOTALOL HCL			
	GENPHARM			
AB		120MG	N075237 002	MAY 01, 2000
AB		160MG	N075237 003	MAY 01, 2000
AB		240MG	N075237 004	MAY 01, 2000
AB	IMPAX PHARM	80MG	N075663 001	NOV 07, 2000
AB		120MG	N075663 002	NOV 07, 2000
AB		160MG	N075663 003	NOV 07, 2000
AB		240MG	N075663 004	NOV 07, 2000
AB	MUTUAL PHARM	80MG	N075515 001	OCT 15, 2001
AB		120MG	N075515 004	OCT 15, 2001
AB		160MG	N075515 002	OCT 15, 2001
AB		240MG	N075515 003	OCT 15, 2001
AB	MYLAN	80MG	N075725 001	DEC 19, 2000
AB		120MG	N075725 002	DEC 19, 2000
AB		160MG	N075725 003	DEC 19, 2000
AB		240MG	N075725 004	DEC 19, 2000
AB	TEVA	80MG	N075429 001	MAY 01, 2000
AB		120MG	N075429 002	MAY 01, 2000
AB		160MG	N075429 003	MAY 01, 2000
AB		240MG	N075429 004	MAY 01, 2000
AB	WATSON LABS	80MG	N075238 001	JUL 13, 2000
AB		120MG	N075238 002	JUL 13, 2000
AB		160MG	N075238 003	JUL 13, 2000
AB		240MG	N075238 004	JUL 13, 2000

SOYBEAN OIL
Injectable; Injection

TE		Strength	Appl. No.
	INTRALIPID 10%		
AP	+ FRESENIUS KABI	10%	N017643 001
	INTRALIPID 20%		
AP	+ FRESENIUS KABI	20%	N018449 001
AP	+ FRESENIUS KABI	20%	N020248 001

Prescription Drug Products (continued)

SOYBEAN OIL (continued)

Injectable; Injection

INTRALIPID 20%

	FRESENIUS KABI				AUG 07, 1996

INTRALIPID 30%

AP	+	FRESENIUS KABI	30%	N019942 001	DEC 30, 1993

LIPOSYN III 10%

AP	+	ABBOTT	10%	N018969 001	SEP 24, 1984

LIPOSYN III 20%

AP	+	ABBOTT	20%	N018970 001	SEP 25, 1984

LIPOSYN III 30%

AP	+	ABBOTT	30%	N020181 001	JAN 13, 1998

NUTRILIPID 10%

AP	+	B BRAUN	10%	N019531 001	MAY 28, 1993

NUTRILIPID 20%

AP	+	B BRAUN	20%	N019531 002	MAY 28, 1993

SOYACAL 10%

AP	+	ALPHA THERA	10%	N018465 001	JUN 29, 1983

SOYACAL 20%

AP	+	ALPHA THERA	20%	N018786 001	JUN 29, 1983

SOYBEAN OIL *MULTIPLE*

SEE SAFFLOWER OIL: SOYBEAN OIL

SPARFLOXACIN

Tablet; Oral

ZAGAM

	+	MYLAN	200MG	N020677 001	DEC 19, 1996

SPECTINOMYCIN HYDROCHLORIDE

Injectable; Injection

TROBICIN

	+	PHARMACIA AND UPJOHN	EQ 2GM BASE/VIAL	N050347 001	

SPIRONOLACTONE

Tablet; Oral

ALDACTONE

AB	GD SEARLE LLC	25MG	N012151 009	DEC 30, 1983
AB		50MG	N012151 008	DEC 30, 1982
AB		100MG	N012151 010	DEC 30, 1983

SPIRONOLACTONE

AB	GENEVA PHARMS	25MG	N086809 001	
AB	HALSEY	25MG	N087265 001	

SPIRONOLACTONE (continued)

Tablet; Oral

SPIRONOLACTONE

AB	MUTUAL PHARM	25MG	N089424 001	JUL 23, 1986
AB		50MG	N089424 002	AUG 11, 1999
AB		100MG	N089424 003	AUG 11, 1999
AB	MYLAN	25MG	N040424 001	AUG 20, 2001
AB		25MG	N087086 001	AUG 20, 2001
AB		50MG	N040424 002	AUG 20, 2001
AB		100MG	N040424 003	AUG 20, 2001
AB	PUREPAC PHARM	50MG	N040353 001	JUL 29, 1999
AB		100MG	N040353 002	JUL 29, 1999
AB	SUPERPHARM	25MG	N089364 001	NOV 07, 1986

SPIRONOLACTONE *MULTIPLE*

SEE HYDROCHLOROTHIAZIDE: SPIRONOLACTONE

STANOZOLOL

Tablet; Oral

WINSTROL

	+	SANOFI SYNTHELABO	2MG	N012885 001	MAY 14, 1984

STAVUDINE

Capsule, Extended Release; Oral

ZERIT XR

	BRISTOL MYERS SQUIBB	37.5MG	N021453 001	DEC 31, 2002
		50MG	N021453 002	DEC 31, 2002
		75MG	N021453 003	DEC 31, 2002
+		100MG	N021453 004	DEC 31, 2002

Capsule; Oral

ZERIT

	BRISTOL MYERS SQUIBB	15MG	N020412 002	JUN 24, 1994
		20MG	N020412 003	JUN 24, 1994
		30MG	N020412 004	JUN 24, 1994
+		40MG	N020412 005	JUN 24, 1994

Prescription Drug Products *(continued)*

STAVUDINE *(continued)*
For Solution; Oral

	ZERIT			
	+ BRISTOL MYERS SQUIBB	1MG/ML	N020413 001	SEP 06, 1996

STREPTOMYCIN SULFATE
Injectable; Injection

	STREPTOMYCIN SULFATE			
	+ PFIZER	EQ 1GM BASE/2.5ML	N060111 001	
	+ PHARMA TEK	EQ 1GM BASE/VIAL	N064210 001	JUN 30, 1998

STREPTOZOCIN
Injectable; Injection

	ZANOSAR			
	+ GENSIA SICOR PHARMS	1GM/VIAL	N050577 001	MAY 07, 1982

STRONTIUM CHLORIDE, SR-89
Injectable; Injection

	METASTRON			
AP	+ AMERSHAM HLTH	1mCi/ML	N020134 001	JUN 18, 1993
	STRONTIUM CHLORIDE SR-89			
AP	+ BIO NUCLEONICS	1mCi/ML	N075941 001	JAN 06, 2003

SUCCIMER
Capsule; Oral

	CHEMET			
	+ SANOFI SYNTHELABO	100MG	N019998 002	JAN 30, 1991

SUCCINYLCHOLINE CHLORIDE
Injectable; Injection

	ANECTINE			
	+ GLAXOSMITHKLINE	1GM/VIAL	N008453 004	
		20MG/ML	N008453 002	
		500MG/VIAL	N008453 001	
	QUELICIN			
AP	+ ABBOTT	20MG/ML	N008845 006	
	QUELICIN PRESERVATIVE FREE			
AP	+ ABBOTT	20MG/ML	N008845 001	
		100MG/ML	N008845 004	
	SUCCINYLCHOLINE CHLORIDE			
AP	+ ORGANON USA INC	20MG/ML	N080997 001	

SUCRALFATE
Suspension; Oral

	CARAFATE			
	+ AVENTIS PHARMS	1GM/10ML	N019183 001	DEC 16, 1993

SUCRALFATE *(continued)*
Tablet; Oral

	CARAFATE			
AB	+ BLUE RIDGE	1GM	N018333 001	
	SUCRALFATE			
AB	+ RATIOPHARM	1GM	N074415 001	JUN 08, 1998
AB	TEVA	1GM	N070848 001	MAR 29, 1996

SUFENTANIL CITRATE
Injectable; Injection

	SUFENTA			
AP	+ AKORN	EQ 0.05MG BASE/ML	N019050 001	MAY 04, 1984
	SUFENTANIL CITRATE			
AP	+ ELKINS SINN	EQ 0.05MG BASE/ML	N074413 001	DEC 15, 1995
	SUFENTANIL CITRATE			
AP	+ ABBOTT	EQ 0.05MG BASE/ML	N074534 001	DEC 11, 1996

SULBACTAM SODIUM *MULTIPLE*
   SEE   AMPICILLIN SODIUM; SULBACTAM SODIUM

SULCONAZOLE NITRATE
Cream; Topical

	EXELDERM			
	+ WESTWOOD SQUIBB	1%	N018737 001	FEB 28, 1989

SULFACETAMIDE *MULTIPLE*
   SEE   TRIPLE SULFA (SULFABENZAMIDE;SULFACETAMIDE;SULFATHIAZOLE)

SULFACETAMIDE SODIUM
Lotion; Topical

	KLARON			
	+ DERMIK LABS	10%	N019931 001	DEC 23, 1996

Ointment; Ophthalmic

	CETAMIDE			
AT	+ ALCON	10%	N080021 001	
	SULFACETAMIDE SODIUM			
AT	+ ALTANA	10%	N080029 001	

Solution/Drops; Ophthalmic

	BLEPH-10			
AT	+ ALLERGAN	10%	N080028 001	
	BLEPH-30			
AT	+ ALLERGAN	30%	N080028 002	
	ISOPTO CETAMIDE			
AT	+ ALCON	15%	N080020 002	
	OCUSULF-10			
AT	+ MIZA PHARMS USA	10%	N080660 001	
	SULF-10			
AT	+ NOVARTIS	10%	N080025 001	

Prescription Drug Products (continued)

SULFACETAMIDE SODIUM (continued)
Solution/Drops; Ophthalmic

	Firm	Strength	Appl. No.	Date
	SULF-15			
AT	NOVARTIS	15%	N089047 001	OCT 31, 1995
	SULFACEL-15			
AT	OPTOPICS	15%	N080024 001	
	SULFACETAMIDE SODIUM			
AT	AKORN	10%	N040215 001	MAY 25, 1999
AT		30%	N040216 001	MAY 25, 1999
AT	ALCON UNIVERSAL	10%	N089560 001	OCT 18, 1988
AT	BAUSCH AND LOMB	10%	N040066 001	DEC 28, 1994
AT	STERIS	30%	N089068 001	MAY 05, 1987

SULFACETAMIDE SODIUM *MULTIPLE*
SEE   FLUOROMETHOLONE; SULFACETAMIDE SODIUM
SEE   PREDNISOLONE ACETATE; SULFACETAMIDE SODIUM
SEE   PREDNISOLONE SODIUM PHOSPHATE; SULFACETAMIDE SODIUM

SULFACYTINE
Tablet; Oral

	Firm	Strength	Appl. No.	Date
	RENOQUID			
+	GLENWOOD	250MG	N017569 001	

SULFADIAZINE
Tablet; Oral

	Firm	Strength	Appl. No.	Date
	SULFADIAZINE			
+	EON	500MG	N040091 001	JUL 29, 1994

SULFADOXINE *MULTIPLE*
SEE   PYRIMETHAMINE; SULFADOXINE

SULFAMERAZINE *MULTIPLE*
SEE   TRISULFAPYRIMIDINES (SULFADIAZINE;SULFAMERAZINE;SULFAMETHAZINE)

SULFAMETHOXAZOLE; TRIMETHOPRIM
Injectable; Injection

	Firm	Strength	Appl. No.	Date
	BACTRIM			
AP +	WOMEN FIRST HLTHCARE	80MG/ML;16MG/ML	N018374 001	
	SULFAMETHOXAZOLE AND TRIMETHOPRIM			
AP	ABBOTT	80MG/ML;16MG/ML	N073199 001	SEP 11, 1992
AP	ELKINS SINN	80MG/ML;16MG/ML	N070627 001	DEC 29, 1987
AP		80MG/ML;16MG/ML	N070628 001	DEC 29, 1987
AP	GENSIA SICOR PHARMS	80MG/ML;16MG/ML	N073303 001	OCT 31, 1991

SULFAMETHOXAZOLE; TRIMETHOPRIM (continued)
Suspension; Oral

	Firm	Strength	Appl. No.	Date
	SEPTRA			
AB +	MONARCH PHARMS	200MG/5ML;40MG/5ML	N017598 001	
	SEPTRA GRAPE			
AB	MONARCH PHARMS	200MG/5ML;40MG/5ML	N017598 002	FEB 12, 1986
	SULFAMETHOXAZOLE AND TRIMETHOPRIM			
AB	HI TECH PHARMA	200MG/5ML;40MG/5ML	N074650 001	DEC 29, 1997
AB	TEVA	200MG/5ML;40MG/5ML	N018812 001	JAN 28, 1983
AB		200MG/5ML;40MG/5ML	N018812 002	JUN 10, 1983
AB		200MG/5ML;40MG/5ML	N070028 001	JUN 02, 1987
	SULFATRIM			
AB	ALPHARMA	200MG/5ML;40MG/5ML	N018615 002	JAN 07, 1983
	SULFATRIM PEDIATRIC			
AB	ALPHARMA	200MG/5ML;40MG/5ML	N018615 001	JAN 07, 1983

Tablet; Oral

	Firm	Strength	Appl. No.	Date
	BACTRIM			
AB	WOMEN FIRST HLTHCARE	400MG;80MG	N017377 001	
	BACTRIM DS			
AB +	WOMEN FIRST HLTHCARE	800MG;160MG	N017377 002	
	COTRIM			
AB	TEVA	400MG;80MG	N070034 001	MAY 16, 1985
	COTRIM D.S.			
AB	TEVA	800MG;160MG	N070048 001	MAR 18, 1985
	SEPTRA			
AB	MONARCH PHARMS	400MG;80MG	N017376 001	
	SEPTRA DS			
AB	MONARCH PHARMS	800MG;160MG	N017376 002	
	SULFAMETHOPRIM			
AB	PAR PHARM	400MG;80MG	N070022 001	FEB 15, 1985
	SULFAMETHOPRIM-DS			
AB	PAR PHARM	800MG;160MG	N070032 001	FEB 15, 1985
	SULFAMETHOXAZOLE AND TRIMETHOPRIM			
AB	GENEVA PHARMS	400MG;80MG	N070889 001	NOV 13, 1986
AB		800MG;160MG	N070890 001	NOV 13, 1986
AB	MUTUAL PHARM	400MG;80MG	N071016 001	AUG 25, 1986
AB		800MG;160MG	N071017 001	AUG 25, 1986
AB	PLIVA	400MG;80MG	N070215 001	SEP 10, 1985
AB		800MG;160MG	N070216 001	

Prescription Drug Products *(continued)*

SULFAMETHOXAZOLE; TRIMETHOPRIM *(continued)*

Tablet; Oral

SULFAMETHOXAZOLE AND TRIMETHOPRIM

TE	Applicant	Strength	Appl. No.	Date
	PLIVA	400MG;80MG		SEP 10, 1985
AB	WATSON LABS	400MG;80MG	N018852 001	MAY 09, 1983

SULFAMETHOXAZOLE AND TRIMETHOPRIM DOUBLE STRENGTH

TE	Applicant	Strength	Appl. No.	Date
AB	EON	800MG;160MG	N018598 004	MAY 19, 1982
AB	TEVA	800MG;160MG	N070037 001	JUN 02, 1987
AB	WATSON LABS	800MG;160MG	N018854 001	MAY 09, 1983

SULFAMETHOXAZOLE AND TRIMETHOPRIM SINGLE STRENGTH

TE	Applicant	Strength	Appl. No.	Date
AB	PLANTEX	400MG;80MG	N070030 001	JUN 02, 1987

SULFANILAMIDE

Cream; Vaginal

AVC

TE	Applicant	Strength	Appl. No.	Date
AT	+ NOVAVAX	15%	N006530 003	JAN 27, 1987

SULFANILAMIDE

TE	Applicant	Strength	Appl. No.	Date
AT	TEVA	15%	N088718 001	SEP 19, 1985

Suppository; Vaginal

AVC

TE	Applicant	Strength	Appl. No.	Date
	+ NOVAVAX	1.05GM	N006530 004	JAN 27, 1987

SULFASALAZINE

Suspension; Oral

AZULFIDINE

TE	Applicant	Strength	Appl. No.	Date
	+ PHARMACIA AND UPJOHN	250MG/5ML	N086983 001	

Tablet, Delayed Release; Oral

AZULFIDINE EN-TABS

TE	Applicant	Strength	Appl. No.	Date
AB	+ PHARMACIA AND UPJOHN	500MG	N007073 002	APR 06, 1983

SULFASALAZINE

TE	Applicant	Strength	Appl. No.	Date
AB	VINTAGE PHARMS	500MG	N075339 001	JAN 11, 2002

Tablet; Oral

AZULFIDINE

TE	Applicant	Strength	Appl. No.	Date
AB	+ PHARMACIA AND UPJOHN	500MG	N007073 001	

SULFASALAZINE

TE	Applicant	Strength	Appl. No.	Date
AB	MUTUAL PHARM	500MG	N089590 001	OCT 19, 1987
AB	VINTAGE PHARMS	500MG	N040349 001	JAN 11, 2002
AB	WATSON LABS	500MG	N085828 001	
AB	WATSON LABS	500MG	N087197 001	

SULFINPYRAZONE

Capsule; Oral

ANTURANE

TE	Applicant	Strength	Appl. No.	Date
	+ NOVARTIS	200MG	N011556 004	

SULFINPYRAZONE

TE	Applicant	Strength	Appl. No.	Date
AB	BARR	200MG	N087666 001	SEP 17, 1982
AB	IVAX PHARMS	200MG	N087770 001	NOV 19, 1982
AB	PAR PHARM	200MG	N089934 001	SEP 06, 1985

Tablet; Oral

ANTURANE

TE	Applicant	Strength	Appl. No.	Date
	+ NOVARTIS	100MG	N011556 003	

SULFINPYRAZONE

TE	Applicant	Strength	Appl. No.	Date
AB	BARR	100MG	N087665 001	SEP 17, 1982
AB	PAR PHARM	100MG	N088933 001	SEP 06, 1985

SULFISOXAZOLE

Tablet; Oral

SOSOL

TE	Applicant	Strength	Appl. No.	Date
AB	MK LABS	500MG	N080036 001	

SULFISOXAZOLE

TE	Applicant	Strength	Appl. No.	Date
AB	ICN	500MG	N080268 002	
AB	+ IVAX PHARMS	500MG	N080142 001	
AB	ROXANE	500MG	N080082 001	

SULFISOXAZOLE ACETYL

Suspension; Oral

GANTRISIN PEDIATRIC

TE	Applicant	Strength	Appl. No.	Date
	+ ROCHE	EQ 500MG BASE/5ML	N009182 004	

SULFISOXAZOLE ACETYL *MULTIPLE*

SEE   ERYTHROMYCIN ETHYLSUCCINATE; SULFISOXAZOLE ACETYL

SULINDAC

Tablet; Oral

CLINORIL

TE	Applicant	Strength	Appl. No.	Date
AB	MERCK	150MG	N017911 001	
AB		200MG	N017911 002	

SULINDAC

TE	Applicant	Strength	Appl. No.	Date
AB	GENEVA PHARMS	150MG	N072712 001	AUG 30, 1991
AB		200MG	N072713 001	AUG 30, 1991
AB	LEDERLE	150MG	N073261 001	SEP 06, 1991
AB		200MG	N073262 001	SEP 06, 1991
AB	MUTUAL PHARM	150MG	N072050 001	APR 17, 1991
AB		200MG	N072051 001	APR 17, 1991
AB	MYLAN	150MG	N073038 001	

Prescription Drug Products (*continued*)

SULINDAC (*continued*)
Tablet; Oral

SULINDAC

TE	Manufacturer	Strength	NDA	Date
	MYLAN			
AB		200MG	N073039 001	JUN 22, 1993
AB	TEVA	150MG	N072972 001	JUN 22, 1993
AB		200MG	N072973 001	FEB 28, 1992
AB	WARNER CHILCOTT	150MG	N072710 001	FEB 28, 1992
AB		200MG	N072711 001	MAR 25, 1991
AB	WATSON LABS	150MG	N071891 001	MAR 25, 1991
AB		200MG	N071795 001	APR 03, 1990
				APR 03, 1990

SUMATRIPTAN
Spray; Nasal

IMITREX

TE	Manufacturer	Strength	NDA	Date
+	GLAXOSMITHKLINE	5MG/SPRAY	N020626 001	AUG 26, 1997
+		10MG/SPRAY	N020626 002	AUG 26, 1997
+		20MG/SPRAY	N020626 003	AUG 26, 1997

SUMATRIPTAN SUCCINATE
Injectable; Injection

IMITREX

TE	Manufacturer	Strength	NDA	Date
+	GLAXOSMITHKLINE	EQ 6MG BASE/0.5ML	N020080 001	DEC 28, 1992

Tablet; Oral

IMITREX

TE	Manufacturer	Strength	NDA	Date
	GLAXOSMITHKLINE	EQ 25MG BASE	N020132 002	JUN 01, 1995
		EQ 50MG BASE	N020132 003	JUN 01, 1995
+		EQ 100MG BASE	N020132 001	JUN 01, 1995

TACRINE HYDROCHLORIDE
Capsule; Oral

COGNEX

TE	Manufacturer	Strength	NDA	Date
	FIRST HORIZON	EQ 10MG BASE	N020070 001	SEP 09, 1993
		EQ 20MG BASE	N020070 002	SEP 09, 1993
		EQ 30MG BASE	N020070 003	SEP 09, 1993
+		EQ 40MG BASE	N020070 004	SEP 09, 1993

TACROLIMUS
Capsule; Oral

PROGRAF

TE	Manufacturer	Strength	NDA	Date
	FUJISAWA HLTHCARE	EQ 0.5MG BASE	N050708 003	AUG 24, 1998
		EQ 1MG BASE	N050708 001	APR 08, 1994
		EQ 5MG BASE	N050708 002	APR 08, 1994

Injectable; Injection

PROGRAF

TE	Manufacturer	Strength	NDA	Date
+	FUJISAWA HLTHCARE	EQ 5MG BASE/ML	N050709 001	APR 08, 1994

Ointment; Topical

PROTOPIC

TE	Manufacturer	Strength	NDA	Date
+	FUJISAWA HLTHCARE	0.1%	N050777 002	DEC 08, 2000
+	FUJISAWA HLTHCARE	0.03%	N050777 001	DEC 08, 2000

TALC
Aerosol, Metered; Intrapleural

SCLEROSOL

TE	Manufacturer	Strength	NDA	Date
+	BRYAN	400MG/SPRAY	N020587 001	DEC 24, 1997

TAMOXIFEN CITRATE
Tablet; Oral

NOLVADEX

TE	Manufacturer	Strength	NDA	Date
AB	ASTRAZENECA	EQ 10MG BASE	N017970 001	
AB		EQ 20MG BASE	N017970 002	
+				MAR 21, 1994

TAMOXIFEN CITRATE

TE	Manufacturer	Strength	NDA	Date
AB	AEGIS PHARMS	EQ 10MG BASE	N076398 001	MAR 31, 2003
AB		EQ 20MG BASE	N076398 002	MAR 31, 2003
AB	ANDRX PHARMS	EQ 10MG BASE	N076179 001	FEB 20, 2003
AB		EQ 20MG BASE	N076179 002	FEB 20, 2003
AB	BARR	EQ 10MG BASE	N070929 001	FEB 20, 2003
AB		EQ 20MG BASE	N070929 002	FEB 20, 2003
AB	IVAX PHARMS	EQ 10MG BASE	N075740 001	FEB 20, 2003
AB		EQ 20MG BASE	N075740 002	FEB 20, 2003
AB	MYLAN	EQ 10MG BASE	N074732 002	FEB 20, 2003
AB		EQ 20MG BASE	N074732 001	FEB 20, 2003
AB	PHARMACHEMIE	EQ 10MG BASE	N074539 001	MAR 31, 2003
AB		EQ 20MG BASE	N074858 001	

Prescription Drug Products *(continued)*

TAMOXIFEN CITRATE *(continued)*
Tablet; Oral

TAMOXIFEN CITRATE
PHARMACHEMIE

AB	ROXANE	EQ 10MG BASE	N076027 001	FEB 20, 2003
AB		EQ 20MG BASE	N076027 002	FEB 20, 2003
AB	TEVA	EQ 10MG BASE	N074504 001	FEB 20, 2003
AB		EQ 10MG BASE	N075797 001	APR 28, 2003
AB		EQ 20MG BASE	N074504 002	FEB 20, 2003
AB	+	EQ 20MG BASE		APR 28, 2003

TAMSULOSIN HYDROCHLORIDE
Capsule; Oral

FLOMAX

AB	+ BOEHRINGER INGELHEIM	0.4MG	N020579 001	APR 15, 1997

TARTARIC ACID *MULTIPLE*
SEE   SODIUM BICARBONATE; TARTARIC ACID

TAZAROTENE
Cream; Topical

AVAGE

	+ ALLERGAN	0.1%	N021184 003	SEP 30, 2002

TAZORAC

	+ ALLERGAN	0.1%	N021184 002	SEP 29, 2000
	+ ALLERGAN	0.05%	N021184 001	SEP 29, 2000

Gel; Topical

TAZORAC

	+ ALLERGAN	0.1%	N020600 002	JUN 13, 1997
	+	0.05%	N020600 001	JUN 13, 1997

TAZOBACTAM SODIUM *MULTIPLE*
SEE   PIPERACILLIN SODIUM; TAZOBACTAM SODIUM

TECHNETIUM TC-99M ALBUMIN AGGREGATED KIT
Injectable; Injection

MACROTEC

BS	BRACCO	N/A	N017833 001

PULMOLITE

BS	CIS	N/A	N017776 001

TECHNESCAN MAA

BS	MALLINCKRODT	N/A	N017842 001

TECHNETIUM TC 99M ALBUMIN AGGREGATED KIT

BS	DRAXIMAGE	N/A	N017881 001

TECHNETIUM TC-99M ALBUMIN AGGREGATED KIT *(continued)*
Injectable; Injection

TECHNETIUM TC 99M ALBUMIN AGGREGATED KIT

DRAXIMAGE		DEC 30, 1987

TECHNETIUM TC-99M APCITIDE
Injectable; Injection

ACUTECT

DIATIDE RES LABS	N/A	N020887 001	SEP 14, 1998

TECHNETIUM TC-99M BICISATE KIT
Injectable; Injection

NEUROLITE

BRISTOL MYERS SQUIBB	N/A/VIAL	N020256 001	NOV 23, 1994

TECHNETIUM TC-99M DEPREOTIDE
Injectable; Injection

NEO TECT KIT

+ DIATIDE RES LABS	N/A	N021012 001	AUG 03, 1999

TECHNETIUM TC-99M DISOFENIN KIT
Injectable; Injection

HEPATOLITE

CIS	N/A	N018467 001	MAR 16, 1982

TECHNETIUM TC-99M EXAMETAZIME KIT
Injectable; Injection

CERETEC

AMERSHAM HLTH	N/A	N019829 001	DEC 30, 1988

TECHNETIUM TC-99M GLUCEPTATE KIT
Injectable; Injection

TECHNESCAN GLUCEPTATE

DRAXIMAGE	N/A	N018272 001	JAN 27, 1982

TECHNETIUM TC-99M MEBROFENIN KIT
Injectable; Injection

CHOLETEC

BRACCO	N/A	N018963 001	JAN 21, 1987

TECHNETIUM TC-99M MEDRONATE KIT
Injectable; Injection

CIS-MDP

AP	CIS	N/A	N018124 001

MDP-BRACCO

AP	BRACCO	N/A	N018107 001

Prescription Drug Products *(continued)*

TECHNETIUM TC-99M MEDRONATE KIT *(continued)*
Injectable; Injection
OSTEOLITE
- AP CIS — N/A — N017972 001

TECHNESCAN MDP KIT
- AP + DRAXIMAGE — N/A — N018035 001

TECHNETIUM TC 99M MPI MDP
- AP AMERSHAM HLTH — N/A — N018141 001

TECHNETIUM TC-99M MERTIATIDE KIT
Injectable; Injection
TECHNESCAN MAG3
- MALLINCKRODT — N/A — N019882 001 — JUN 15, 1990

TECHNETIUM TC-99M OXIDRONATE KIT
Injectable; Injection
TECHNESCAN HDP
- MALLINCKRODT — N/A — N018321 001

TECHNETIUM TC-99M PENTETATE KIT
Injectable; Injection
AN-DTPA
- AP CIS — N/A — N017714 001

DTPA
- AP DRAXIMAGE — N/A — N018511 001 — DEC 29, 1989

TECHNETIUM TC-99M PENTETATE KIT
- AP AMERSHAM HLTH — N/A — N017264 002

TECHNETIUM TC-99M PYROPHOSPHATE KIT
Injectable; Injection
CIS-PYRO
- AP CIS — N/A — N019039 001 — JUN 30, 1987

PHOSPHOTEC
- AP BRACCO — N/A — N017680 001

TECHNESCAN PYP KIT
- AP MALLINCKRODT — N/A — N017538 001

TECHNETIUM TC-99M RED BLOOD CELL KIT
Injectable; Injection
ULTRATAG
- MALLINCKRODT — N/A — N019981 001 — JUN 10, 1991

TECHNETIUM TC-99M SESTAMIBI KIT
Injectable; Injection
CARDIOLITE
- BRISTOL MYERS SQUIBB — N/A — N019785 001 — DEC 21, 1990

MIRALUMA
- BRISTOL MYERS SQUIBB — N/A — N019785 003

TECHNETIUM TC-99M SESTAMIBI KIT *(continued)*
Injectable; Injection
MIRALUMA
- BRISTOL MYERS SQUIBB — MAY 23, 1997

TECHNETIUM TC-99M SODIUM PERTECHNETATE GENERATOR
Solution; Injection, Oral
TECHNELITE
- BRISTOL MYERS SQUIBB — 0.0083-2.7 CI/GENERATOR — N017771 001

ULTRA-TECHNEKOW FM
- MALLINCKRODT — 0.25-3 CI/GENERATOR — N017243 002

TECHNETIUM TC-99M SUCCIMER KIT
Injectable; Injection
MPI DMSA KIDNEY REAGENT
- AMERSHAM HLTH — N/A — N017944 001 — MAY 18, 1982

TECHNETIUM TC-99M SULFUR COLLOID KIT
Solution; Injection, Oral
AN-SULFUR COLLOID
- AP CIS — N/A — N017858 001

TECHNECOLL
- AP MALLINCKRODT — N/A — N017059 001

TECHNETIUM TC-99M TEBOROXIME KIT
Injectable; Injection
CARDIOTEC
- BRACCO — N/A — N019928 001 — DEC 19, 1990

TECHNETIUM TC-99M TETROFOSMIN KIT
Injectable; Injection
MYOVIEW
- AMERSHAM HLTH — N/A/VIAL — N020372 001 — FEB 09, 1996

TEGASEROD MALEATE
Tablet; Oral
ZELNORM
- NOVARTIS — EQ 2MG BASE — N021200 001 — JUL 24, 2002
- + — EQ 6MG BASE — N021200 002 — JUL 24, 2002

TELMISARTAN
Tablet; Oral
MICARDIS
- + BOEHRINGER INGELHEIM — 20MG — N020850 003 — APR 04, 2000
- 40MG — N020850 001

Prescription Drug Products *(continued)*

TELMISARTAN *(continued)*
Tablet; Oral
  MICARDIS
    BOEHRINGER INGELHEIM
    80MG — NOV 10, 1998
  + — N020850 002 NOV 10, 1998

TELMISARTAN *MULTIPLE*
  SEE HYDROCHLOROTHIAZIDE; TELMISARTAN

TEMAZEPAM
Capsule; Oral
  RESTORIL
    TYCO HLTHCARE
       7.5MG — N018163 003 OCT 25, 1991
  AB   15MG — N018163 001
  AB   30MG — N018163 002
  TEMAZEPAM
    GENEVA PHARMS
  AB   15MG — N071427 001 JAN 12, 1988
  AB   30MG — N071428 001 JAN 12, 1988
    MYLAN
  AB   15MG — N070919 001 JUL 07, 1986
  AB   30MG — N070920 001 JUL 10, 1986
    PAR PHARM
  AB   15MG — N071456 001 APR 21, 1987
  AB   30MG — N071457 001 APR 21, 1987
    PUREPAC PHARM
  AB   15MG — N071638 001 AUG 07, 1987
  AB   30MG — N071620 001 AUG 07, 1987
    WATSON LABS
  AB   15MG — N071446 001 MAY 21, 1993
  AB   30MG — N071447 001 MAY 21, 1993

TEMOZOLOMIDE
Capsule; Oral
  TEMODAR
    SCHERING
       5MG — N021029 001 AUG 11, 1999
       20MG — N021029 002 AUG 11, 1999
       100MG — N021029 003 AUG 11, 1999
  +   250MG — N021029 004 AUG 11, 1999

TENIPOSIDE
Injectable; Injection
  VUMON
  + BRISTOL MYERS SQUIBB
    10MG/ML — N020119 001 JUL 14, 1992

TENOFOVIR DISOPROXIL FUMARATE
Tablet; Oral
  VIREAD
  + GILEAD
    300MG — N021356 001 OCT 26, 2001

TERAZOSIN HYDROCHLORIDE
Capsule; Oral
  HYTRIN
    ABBOTT
  AB   EQ 1MG BASE — N020347 001 DEC 14, 1994
  AB + EQ 2MG BASE — N020347 002 DEC 14, 1994
  AB   EQ 5MG BASE — N020347 003 DEC 14, 1994
  AB   EQ 10MG BASE — N020347 004 DEC 14, 1994
  TERAZOSIN HCL
    GENEVA PHARMS
  AB   EQ 1MG BASE — N074823 001 MAR 30, 1998
  AB   EQ 2MG BASE — N074823 002 MAR 30, 1998
  AB   EQ 5MG BASE — N074823 003 MAR 30, 1998
  AB   EQ 10MG BASE — N074823 004 MAR 30, 1998
    INVAMED
  AB   EQ 1MG BASE — N075667 001 JUL 28, 2000
  AB   EQ 2MG BASE — N075667 002 JUL 28, 2000
  AB   EQ 5MG BASE — N075667 003 JUL 28, 2000
  AB   EQ 10MG BASE — N075667 004 JUL 28, 2000
    IVAX PHARMS
  AB   EQ 1MG BASE — N075614 002 JAN 30, 2001
  AB   EQ 2MG BASE — N075614 001 JAN 30, 2001
  AB   EQ 5MG BASE — N075614 003 JAN 30, 2001
  AB   EQ 10MG BASE — N075614 004 JAN 30, 2001
    MYLAN
  AB   EQ 1MG BASE — N075140 002 FEB 11, 2000
  AB   EQ 2MG BASE — N075140 003 FEB 11, 2000
  AB   EQ 5MG BASE — N075140 001 FEB 11, 2000
  AB   EQ 10MG BASE — N075140 004 FEB 11, 2000

Prescription Drug Products *(continued)*

TERAZOSIN HYDROCHLORIDE *(continued)*

Capsule; Oral

TERAZOSIN HCL

TE	Applicant	Strength	Appl No	Approval Date
	MYLAN			
	MYLAN TECHNOLOGIES			
AB		EQ 1MG BASE	N075384 001	FEB 11, 2000
AB		EQ 2MG BASE	N075384 002	DEC 01, 2000
AB		EQ 5MG BASE	N075384 003	DEC 01, 2000
AB		EQ 10MG BASE	N075384 004	DEC 01, 2000
AB	RANBAXY	EQ 1MG BASE	N076021 001	DEC 01, 2000
AB		EQ 2MG BASE	N076021 002	AUG 22, 2002
AB		EQ 5MG BASE	N076021 003	AUG 22, 2002
AB		EQ 10MG BASE	N076021 004	AUG 22, 2002
AB	TORPHARM	EQ 1MG BASE	N075498 001	AUG 22, 2002
AB		EQ 2MG BASE	N075498 002	APR 12, 2001
AB		EQ 5MG BASE	N075498 003	APR 12, 2001
AB		EQ 10MG BASE	N075498 004	APR 12, 2001

Tablet; Oral

HYTRIN

TE	Applicant	Strength	Appl No	Approval Date
	ABBOTT			
AB		EQ 1MG BASE	N019057 001	AUG 07, 1987
AB +		EQ 2MG BASE	N019057 002	AUG 07, 1987
AB		EQ 5MG BASE	N019057 003	AUG 07, 1987
AB		EQ 10MG BASE	N019057 004	AUG 07, 1987

TERAZOSIN HCL

TE	Applicant	Strength	Appl No	Approval Date
	GENEVA PHARMS			
AB		EQ 1MG BASE	N074315 001	DEC 31, 1998
AB		EQ 2MG BASE	N074315 002	DEC 31, 1998
AB		EQ 5MG BASE	N074315 003	DEC 31, 1998
AB		EQ 10MG BASE	N074315 004	DEC 31, 1998
AB	INVAMED	EQ 1MG BASE	N074657 001	APR 28, 2000
AB		EQ 2MG BASE	N074657 002	APR 28, 2000
AB		EQ 5MG BASE	N074657 003	APR 28, 2000
AB		EQ 10MG BASE	N074657 004	APR 28, 2000
AB	IVAX PHARMS	EQ 1MG BASE	N074530 001	APR 21, 2000
AB		EQ 2MG BASE	N074530 002	APR 21, 2000
AB		EQ 5MG BASE	N074530 003	APR 21, 2000
AB		EQ 10MG BASE	N074530 004	APR 21, 2000
AB	TEVA	EQ 1MG BASE	N074446 001	MAY 18, 2000
AB		EQ 2MG BASE	N074446 002	MAY 18, 2000
AB		EQ 5MG BASE	N074446 003	MAY 18, 2000
AB		EQ 10MG BASE	N074446 004	MAY 18, 2000

TERBINAFINE HYDROCHLORIDE

Cream; Topical

LAMISIL

TE	Applicant	Strength	Appl No	Approval Date
+	NOVARTIS	1%	N020192 001	DEC 30, 1992

Solution; Topical

LAMISIL

TE	Applicant	Strength	Appl No	Approval Date
+	NOVARTIS	1%	N020749 001	OCT 17, 1997

Tablet; Oral

LAMISIL

TE	Applicant	Strength	Appl No	Approval Date
+	NOVARTIS	EQ 250MG BASE	N020539 001	MAY 10, 1996

TERBUTALINE SULFATE

Injectable; Injection

BRETHINE

TE	Applicant	Strength	Appl No	Approval Date
+	AAIPHARMA	1MG/ML	N018571 001	

Tablet; Oral

BRETHINE

TE	Applicant	Strength	Appl No	Approval Date
AB +	AAIPHARMA	2.5MG	N017849 001	
AB		5MG	N017849 002	

TERBUTALINE SULFATE

TE	Applicant	Strength	Appl No	Approval Date
AB	IMPAX LABS	2.5MG	N075877 001	JUN 26, 2001
AB		5MG	N075877 002	JUN 26, 2001

TERCONAZOLE

Cream; Vaginal

TERAZOL 3

TE	Applicant	Strength	Appl No	Approval Date
+	ORTHO MCNEIL PHARM	0.8%	N019964 001	FEB 21, 1991

TERAZOL 7

TE	Applicant	Strength	Appl No	Approval Date
+	ORTHO MCNEIL PHARM	0.4%	N019579 001	DEC 31, 1987

Prescription Drug Products *(continued)*

TERCONAZOLE *(continued)*

Suppository; Vaginal

			Strength	NDA	Date
	TERAZOL 3				
	+ ORTHO MCNEIL PHARM		80MG	N019641 001	MAY 24, 1988

TERIPARATIDE ACETATE

Injectable; Subcutaneous

		Strength	NDA	Date
	FORTEO			
	+ LILLY	EQ 0.75MG 3ML(0.25MG/ML)	N021318 001	NOV 26, 2002

TESTOLACTONE

Tablet; Oral

		Strength	NDA
	TESLAC		
	+ BRISTOL MYERS SQUIBB	50MG	N016118 001

TESTOSTERONE

Film, Extended Release; Transdermal

TE		Strength	NDA	Date
	ANDRODERM			
	+ WATSON LABS	2.5MG/24HR	N020489 001	SEP 29, 1995
BX	+	5MG/24HR	N020489 002	MAY 02, 1997
	TESTODERM			
	+ ALZA	4MG/24HR	N019762 001	OCT 12, 1993
	+	6MG/24HR	N019762 002	OCT 12, 1993
	TESTODERM TTS			
BX	+ ALZA	5MG/24HR	N020791 001	DEC 18, 1997

Gel; Topical

TE		Strength	NDA	Date
	ANDROGEL			
BX	+ UNIMED PHARMS	1%	N021015 001	FEB 28, 2000
	TESTIM			
BX	+ AUXILIUM A2	1%	N021454 001	OCT 31, 2002

Injectable; Injection

		Strength	NDA	Date
	TESTOSTERONE			
	+ STERIS	100MG/ML	N086417 001	JUL 07, 1983

Pellet; Implantation

		Strength	NDA
	TESTOSTERONE		
	BARTOR	75MG	N080911 001

Tablet, Extended Release; Buccal

		Strength	NDA	Date
	STRIANT			
	+ COLUMBIA LABS	30MG	N021543 001	JUN 19, 2003

TESTOSTERONE CYPIONATE

Injectable; Injection

TE		Strength	NDA
	DEPO-TESTOSTERONE		
AO	+ PHARMACIA AND UPJOHN	100MG/ML	N085635 002
AO	+	200MG/ML	N085635 003
	TESTOSTERONE CYPIONATE		
AO	+ STERIS	100MG/ML	N086029 001
AO		200MG/ML	N086030 001

TESTOSTERONE ENANTHATE

Injectable; Injection

TE		Strength	NDA
	DELATESTRYL		
AO	+ BTG	200MG/ML	N009165 003
	TESTOSTERONE ENANTHATE		
AO	+ STERIS	200MG/ML	N085598 001

TESTOSTERONE PROPIONATE

Injectable; Injection

TE		Strength	NDA
	TESTOSTERONE PROPIONATE		
AO	+ STERIS	25MG/ML	N080188 001
AO		50MG/ML	N080188 002
AO		100MG/ML	N080188 003

TETRACYCLINE HYDROCHLORIDE

Capsule; Oral

TE		Strength	NDA	Date
	BRISTACYCLINE			
AB	+ BRISTOL	250MG	N061658 001	
AB		250MG	N061888 001	
AB		500MG	N061658 002	
AB		500MG	N061888 002	
	SUMYCIN			
AB	+ APOTHECON	250MG	N060429 001	
AB		500MG	N060429 003	
	TETRACYCLINE HCL			
AB	+ AXIOM PHARM	250MG	N060736 001	
AB		500MG	N060736 002	
AB	+ BARR	250MG	N061837 001	
AB		500MG	N061837 002	
AB	+ IMPAX LABS	100MG	N060469 001	
AB		250MG	N060469 002	
AB		500MG	N060469 003	
AB	+ IVAX PHARMS	250MG	N060704 001	
AB		500MG	N060704 002	
AB	+ LABS ATRAL	250MG	N062752 001	AUG 12, 1988
AB		500MG	N062752 002	AUG 12, 1988
AB	+ MAST MM	500MG	N062085 001	
AB	MYLAN	250MG	N060783 001	
AB		500MG	N060783 002	
AB	ROXANE	500MG	N061214 002	

Suspension; Oral

		Strength	NDA
	SUMYCIN		
	+ APOTHECON	125MG/5ML	N060400 001

Prescription Drug Products *(continued)*

TETRACYCLINE HYDROCHLORIDE *(continued)*

Tablet; Oral

		Strength	NDA	Date
	SUMYCIN			
+	PAR PHARM	250MG	N061147 001	
		500MG	N061147 004	

TETRACYCLINE HYDROCHLORIDE *MULTIPLE*

SEE BISMUTH SUBSALICYLATE; METRONIDAZOLE; TETRACYCLINE HYDROCHLORIDE

TETRACYCLINE PHOSPHATE COMPLEX

Capsule; Oral

		Strength	NDA	Date
	TETREX			
	BRISTOL	EQ 100MG HCL	N061653 001	
		EQ 250MG HCL	N061653 002	
		EQ 250MG HCL	N061889 002	
		EQ 500MG HCL	N061653 003	
+		EQ 500MG HCL	N061889 001	

TETRAHYDROZOLINE HYDROCHLORIDE

Solution; Nasal

		Strength	NDA	Date
	TYZINE			
+	KENWOOD LABS	0.1%	N086576 001	
		0.05%	N086576 002	

Spray; Nasal

		Strength	NDA	Date
	TYZINE			
+	KENWOOD LABS	0.1%	N086576 003	

THALIDOMIDE

Capsule; Oral

		Strength	NDA	Date
	THALOMID			
+	CELGENE	50MG	N020785 001	JUL 16, 1998
		100MG	N020785 002	JAN 17, 2003
		200MG	N020785 003	JAN 17, 2003

THALLOUS CHLORIDE, TL-201

Injectable; Injection

			Strength	NDA	Date
		THALLOUS CHLORIDE TL 201			
AP	+	AMERSHAM HLTH	1mCi/ML	N018110 002	FEB 27, 1996
AP	+	BRISTOL MYERS SQUIBB	1mCi/ML	N017806 001	
AP	+	MALLINCKRODT	1mCi/ML	N018150 001	
AP	+	MOUNT SINAI MEDCTR	1mCi/ML	N075569 001	NOV 21, 2001

THEOPHYLLINE

Capsule, Extended Release; Oral

		Strength	NDA	Date
	AEROLATE III			
+	FLEMING PHARMS	65MG	N085075 003	NOV 24, 1986

THEOPHYLLINE *(continued)*

Capsule, Extended Release; Oral

			Strength	NDA	Date
		AEROLATE JR			
BC		FLEMING PHARMS	130MG	N085075 002	NOV 24, 1986
		AEROLATE SR			
BC		FLEMING PHARMS	260MG	N085075 001	NOV 24, 1986
		SLO-BID			
BC	+	AVENTIS	50MG	N088269 001	JAN 31, 1985
			75MG	N089539 001	MAY 10, 1989
AB			100MG	N087892 001	JAN 31, 1985
AB			125MG	N089540 001	MAY 10, 1989
AB			200MG	N087893 001	JAN 31, 1985
AB	+		300MG	N087894 001	JAN 31, 1985
		THEO-24			
BC		UCB	100MG	N087942 001	AUG 22, 1983
BC			200MG	N087943 001	AUG 22, 1983
BC			300MG	N087944 001	AUG 22, 1983
BC			400MG	N081034 001	FEB 28, 1992
		THEOPHYLLINE			
AB		INWOOD LABS	100MG	N040052 001	FEB 14, 1994
AB			125MG	N040052 002	FEB 14, 1994
AB			200MG	N040052 003	FEB 14, 1994
AB			300MG	N040052 004	FEB 14, 1994

Elixir; Oral

		Strength	NDA	Date
	ELIXOPHYLLIN			
AA	FORREST LABS	80MG/15ML	N085186 001	
	THEOPHYLLINE			
AA	ALPH-ARMA	80MG/15ML	N085863 001	
AA	MORTON GROVE	80MG/15ML	N086748 001	
AA	PHARM ASSOC	80MG/15ML	N086720 001	
AA	TARO	80MG/15ML	N089626 001	OCT 28, 1988

Injectable; Injection

			Strength	NDA	Date
		THEOPHYLLINE 0.04% AND DEXTROSE 5% IN PLASTIC CONTAINER			
AP	+	B BRAUN	40MG/100ML	N019826 001	AUG 14, 1992
		THEOPHYLLINE 0.08% AND DEXTROSE 5% IN PLASTIC CONTAINER			
AP	+	B BRAUN	80MG/100ML	N019826 002	AUG 14, 1992
		THEOPHYLLINE 0.16% AND DEXTROSE 5% IN PLASTIC CONTAINER			
AP	+	B BRAUN	160MG/100ML	N019826 003	

Prescription Drug Products (continued)

THEOPHYLLINE (continued)

Injectable; Injection

	Product	Strength	NDA	Date
	THEOPHYLLINE 0.16% AND DEXTROSE 5% IN PLASTIC CONTAINER			
	B BRAUN			AUG 14, 1992
	THEOPHYLLINE 0.32% AND DEXTROSE 5% IN PLASTIC CONTAINER			
AP	+ B BRAUN	320MG/100ML	N019826 006	AUG 14, 1992
	THEOPHYLLINE AND DEXTROSE 5% IN PLASTIC CONTAINER			
AP	+ BAXTER HLTHCARE	40MG/100ML	N018649 001	
AP	+	80MG/100ML	N018649 002	JUL 26, 1982
AP	+	160MG/100ML	N018649 003	JUL 26, 1982
AP	+	200MG/100ML	N018649 004	JUL 26, 1982
AP	+	400MG/100ML	N018649 005	JUL 26, 1982
AP	+	320MG/100ML	N018649 006	JUL 26, 1982
AP	+	4MG/ML	N018649 007	NOV 13, 1985
	THEOPHYLLINE IN DEXTROSE 5% IN PLASTIC CONTAINER			
AP	+ ABBOTT	40MG/100ML	N019211 001	JUL 26, 1982
AP	+	80MG/100ML	N019211 002	DEC 14, 1984
AP	+	4MG/ML	N019211 007	DEC 14, 1984
AP	+	160MG/100ML	N019211 003	DEC 14, 1984
AP	+	200MG/100ML	N019211 004	DEC 14, 1984
AP	+	320MG/100ML	N019211 006	DEC 14, 1984
AP	+	400MG/100ML	N019211 005	JAN 20, 1988

Solution; Oral

	Product	Strength	NDA	Date
	AEROLATE			
AA	FLEMING PHARMS	150MG/15ML	N089141 001	DEC 03, 1986
	THEOLAIR			
AA	+ 3M	80MG/15ML	N086107 001	
	THEOPHYLLINE			
AA	ROXANE	80MG/15ML	N087449 001	SEP 15, 1983

Syrup; Oral

	Product	Strength	NDA	Date
	SLO-PHYLLIN			
AA	+ AVENTIS	80MG/15ML	N085187 001	

Tablet, Extended Release; Oral

	Product	Strength	NDA	Date
	QUIBRON-T/SR			
BC	MONARCH PHARMS	300MG	N087563 001	JUN 21, 1983
	T-PHYL			
BC	PURDUE FREDERICK	200MG	N088253 001	AUG 17, 1983

THEOPHYLLINE (continued)

Tablet, Extended Release; Oral

	Product	Strength	NDA	Date
	THEO-DUR			
AB	SCHERING	100MG	N085328 001	
AB		200MG	N086998 001	
AB		300MG	N085328 002	
AB		450MG	N089131 001	JUN 25, 1986
	THEOCHRON			
AB	INWOOD LABS	100MG	N088320 001	
AB		200MG	N088321 001	FEB 21, 1985
AB		300MG	N087400 002	FEB 21, 1985
				JAN 11, 1983
	THEOLAIR-SR			
BC	3M	200MG	N088369 001	JUL 16, 1987
		250MG	N086363 002	JUL 16, 1987
		300MG	N088364 001	JUL 16, 1987
BC		500MG	N089132 001	JUL 16, 1987
	THEOPHYLLINE			
AB	INWOOD LABS	450MG	N040034 001	APR 28, 1995
AB	+ PLIVA	100MG	N089807 001	APR 30, 1990
AB	+	200MG	N089808 001	APR 30, 1990
AB	+	300MG	N089763 001	APR 30, 1990
AB	+	450MG	N081236 001	NOV 09, 1992
	UNI-DUR			
BC	SCHERING	400MG	N089822 001	JAN 04, 1995
BC		600MG	N089823 001	JAN 04, 1995
	UNIPHYL			
BC	+ PURDUE FREDERICK	400MG	N087571 001	SEP 01, 1982
BC	+	600MG	N040086 001	APR 15, 1996

Tablet; Oral

	Product	Strength	NDA	Date
	QUIBRON-T			
	+ MONARCH PHARMS	300MG	N088656 001	AUG 22, 1985
	SLO-PHYLLIN			
	+ AVENTIS	100MG	N085202 001	
	+	200MG	N085204 001	
	THEOLAIR			
	+ 3M	125MG	N086399 001	
	+	250MG	N086399 002	

Prescription Drug Products (continued)

THIABENDAZOLE
Suspension; Oral

	MINTEZOL		
+	MERCK	500MG/5ML	N016097 001

Tablet, Chewable; Oral

	MINTEZOL		
+	MERCK	500MG	N016096 001

THIAMINE *MULTIPLE*
SEE ASCORBIC ACID; BIOTIN; CHOLECALCIFEROL; CYANOCOBALAMIN; DEXPANTHENOL; FOLIC ACID; NIACINAMIDE; PYRIDOXINE; RIBOFLAVIN; THIAMINE; TOCOPHEROL ACETATE; VITAMIN A; VITAMIN K

THIAMINE HYDROCHLORIDE
Injectable; Injection

	THIAMINE HCL			
AP		ABBOTT	100MG/ML	N040079 001 MAY 03, 1996
AP	+	AM PHARM PARTNERS	100MG/ML	N080556 001
AP		ELKINS SINN	100MG/ML	N080575 001
AP		STERIS	100MG/ML	N080571 001
	+		200MG/ML	N080571 002

THIAMINE HYDROCHLORIDE *MULTIPLE*
SEE ALPHA-TOCOPHEROL ACETATE; ASCORBIC ACID; BIOTIN; CHOLECALCIFEROL; CYANOCOBALAMIN; DEXPANTHENOL; FOLIC ACID; NIACINAMIDE; PYRIDOXINE HYDROCHLORIDE; RIBOFLAVIN PHOSPHATE SODIUM; THIAMINE HYDROCHLORIDE; VITAMIN A PALMITATE; VITAMIN K

SEE ASCORBIC ACID; BIOTIN; CYANOCOBALAMIN; DEXPANTHENOL; ERGOCALCIFEROL; FOLIC ACID; NIACINAMIDE; PHYTONADIONE; PYRIDOXINE HYDROCHLORIDE; RIBOFLAVIN PHOSPHATE SODIUM; THIAMINE HYDROCHLORIDE; VITAMIN A; VITAMIN E

SEE ASCORBIC ACID; BIOTIN; CYANOCOBALAMIN; DEXPANTHENOL; ERGOCALCIFEROL; FOLIC ACID; NIACINAMIDE; PYRIDOXINE HYDROCHLORIDE; RIBOFLAVIN PHOSPHATE SODIUM; THIAMINE HYDROCHLORIDE; VITAMIN A; VITAMIN E

THIETHYLPERAZINE MALEATE
Tablet; Oral

	TORECAN		
+	NOVARTIS	10MG	N012753 001

THIOGUANINE
Tablet; Oral

	THIOGUANINE		
+	GLAXOSMITHKLINE	40MG	N012429 001

THIORIDAZINE HYDROCHLORIDE
Concentrate; Oral

	THIORIDAZINE HCL			
AA		ALPHARMA	100MG/ML	N088229 001 AUG 23, 1983
AA	+	COPLEY PHARM	30MG/ML	N089602 001 NOV 09, 1987
AA	+		100MG/ML	N089603 001

THIORIDAZINE HYDROCHLORIDE (continued)
Concentrate; Oral

	THIORIDAZINE HCL			
		COPLEY PHARM		
AA		HI TECH PHARMA	30MG/ML	NOV 09, 1987 N040125 001 AUG 16, 1996
AA			100MG/ML	N040126 001 AUG 16, 1996
AA		PHARM ASSOC	30MG/ML	N040187 001 AUG 28, 1997
AA			100MG/ML	N040213 001 MAY 29, 1998
		THIORIDAZINE HCL INTENSOL		
AA		ROXANE	30MG/ML	N088941 001 DEC 16, 1985
AA			100MG/ML	N088942 001 DEC 16, 1985

Tablet; Oral

	THIORIDAZINE HCL			
AB		GENEVA PHARMS	10MG	N088131 001 AUG 30, 1983
AB			15MG	N088132 001 AUG 30, 1983
AB	+		25MG	N088133 001 AUG 30, 1983
AB			50MG	N088134 001 AUG 30, 1983
AB	+		100MG	N088135 001 NOV 20, 1984
AB			150MG	N088136 001 SEP 17, 1986
AB	+		200MG	N088137 001 SEP 17, 1986
AB	+	HALSEY	50MG	N088370 001 NOV 18, 1983
AB		IVAX PHARMS	10MG	N088270 001 APR 14, 1983
AB			15MG	N088271 001 APR 14, 1983
AB			25MG	N088272 001 APR 14, 1983
AB		MUTUAL PHARM	10MG	N089431 001 AUG 01, 1986
AB			25MG	N089432 001 AUG 01, 1986
AB			50MG	N089433 001 AUG 01, 1986
AB			100MG	N089953 001 OCT 07, 1988
AB		MYLAN	10MG	N088001 001 MAR 15, 1983
AB			25MG	N088002 001 MAR 15, 1983
AB			50MG	N088003 001 MAR 15, 1983
AB			100MG	N088004 001 NOV 18, 1983

Prescription Drug Products (continued)

THIORIDAZINE HYDROCHLORIDE (continued)
Tablet; Oral
THIORIDAZINE HCL

TE	Firm	Strength	Appl No	Date
AB	TEVA	100MG	N088456 001	MAY 17, 1985
AB	WATSON LABS	10MG	N088476 001	NOV 08, 1983
AB		15MG	N088477 001	NOV 08, 1983
AB		25MG	N088478 001	NOV 08, 1983
AB		25MG	N088567 001	MAY 11, 1984
AB		50MG	N088479 001	NOV 08, 1983
AB		50MG	N088563 001	NOV 08, 1983
AB		100MG	N088564 001	MAY 11, 1984
AB		100MG	N088736 001	JUL 24, 1984
AB		150MG	N088869 001	JUN 28, 1985
AB		200MG	N088872 001	APR 26, 1985

THIOTEPA
Injectable; Injection
THIOPLEX

TE	Firm	Strength	Appl No	Date
AP	+ IMMUNEX	15MG/VIAL	N020058 001	DEC 22, 1994

THIOTEPA

TE	Firm	Strength	Appl No	Date
AP	AM PHARM PARTNERS	15MG/VIAL	N075698 001	SEP 20, 2001
AP	BEDFORD	15MG/VIAL	N075547 001	APR 02, 2001
AP	GENSIA SICOR PHARMS	15MG/VIAL	N075730 001	APR 20, 2001
AP		30MG/VIAL	N075730 002	APR 20, 2001

THIOTHIXENE
Capsule; Oral
NAVANE

TE	Firm	Strength	Appl No	Date
AB	+ PFIZER	1MG	N016584 001	
AB		2MG	N016584 002	
AB		5MG	N016584 003	
AB		10MG	N016584 004	
AB		20MG	N016584 005	

THIOTHIXENE
GENEVA PHARMS

TE	Firm	Strength	Appl No	Date
AB		1MG	N071610 001	JUN 24, 1987
AB		2MG	N071570 001	JUN 24, 1987
AB		5MG	N071529 001	JUN 24, 1987
AB		10MG	N071530 001	JUN 24, 1987

THIOTHIXENE (continued)
Capsule; Oral
THIOTHIXENE
MYLAN

TE	Firm	Strength	Appl No	Date
AB		1MG	N071090 001	JUN 24, 1987
AB		2MG	N071091 001	JUN 23, 1987
AB		5MG	N071092 001	JUN 23, 1987
AB		10MG	N071093 001	JUN 23, 1987

WATSON LABS

TE	Firm	Strength	Appl No	Date
AB		1MG	N070600 001	JUN 05, 1987
AB		2MG	N070601 001	JUN 05, 1987
AB		5MG	N070602 001	JUN 05, 1987
AB		10MG	N070603 001	JUN 05, 1987

THIOTHIXENE HYDROCHLORIDE
Concentrate; Oral
NAVANE

TE	Firm	Strength	Appl No	Date
AA	+ PFIZER	EQ 5MG BASE/ML	N016758 001	

THIOTHIXENE HCL

TE	Firm	Strength	Appl No	Date
AA	COPLEY PHARM	EQ 5MG BASE/ML	N071554 001	OCT 16, 1987

Injectable; Injection
NAVANE

TE	Firm	Strength	Appl No	Date
AA	+ PFIZER	EQ 10MG BASE/VIAL	N016904 002	

THONZONIUM BROMIDE *MULTIPLE*
SEE   COLISTIN SULFATE; HYDROCORTISONE ACETATE; NEOMYCIN SULFATE; THONZONIUM BROMIDE

THYROTROPIN ALFA
Injectable; Injection
THYROGEN

TE	Firm	Strength	Appl No	Date
	+ GENZYME	1.1MG/VIAL	N020898 001	NOV 30, 1998

TIAGABINE HYDROCHLORIDE
Tablet; Oral
GABITRIL

TE	Firm	Strength	Appl No	Date
	+ CEPHALON	2MG	N020646 005	APR 16, 1999
		4MG	N020646 001	SEP 30, 1997
		12MG	N020646 002	SEP 30, 1997
		16MG	N020646 003	SEP 30, 1997

Prescription Drug Products (continued)

TICARCILLIN DISODIUM
Injectable; Injection

	TICAR			
+	GLAXOSMITHKLINE	EQ 1GM BASE/VIAL	N050497 001	
+		EQ 3GM BASE/VIAL	N050497 002	
+		EQ 20GM BASE/VIAL	N050497 004	
+		EQ 30GM BASE/VIAL	N050497 005	APR 04, 1984

TICARCILLIN DISODIUM *MULTIPLE*
SEE CLAVULANATE POTASSIUM; TICARCILLIN DISODIUM

TICLOPIDINE HYDROCHLORIDE
Tablet; Oral

	TICLID			
AB +	ROCHE PALO	250MG	N019979 002	OCT 31, 1991

	TICLOPIDINE HCL			
AB	CARACO	250MG	N075526 001	SEP 26, 2002
AB	EON	250MG	N075326 001	AUG 20, 1999
AB	GENEVA PHARMS TECH	250MG	N075318 001	AUG 20, 1999
AB	GENPHARM	250MG	N075161 001	SEP 13, 1999
AB	MYLAN	250MG	N075316 001	NOV 02, 1999
AB	PUREPAC PHARM	250MG	N075253 001	AUG 20, 1999
AB	TEVA	250MG	N075149 001	AUG 20, 1999
AB	TORPHARM	250MG	N075089 001	JUL 01, 1999
AB	WATSON LABS	250MG	N075309 001	APR 26, 2000

TILUDRONATE DISODIUM
Tablet; Oral

	SKELID			
+	SANOFI SYNTHELABO	EQ 200MG BASE	N020707 001	MAR 07, 1997

TIMOLOL
Solution/Drops; Ophthalmic

	BETIMOL			
+	SANTEN OY	EQ 0.5% BASE	N020439 002	MAR 31, 1995
+		EQ 0.25% BASE	N020439 001	MAR 31, 1995

TIMOLOL MALEATE
Solution, Gel Forming/Drops; Ophthalmic

	TIMOLOL MALEATE			
AB	FALCON PHARMS	EQ 0.5% BASE	N020963 002	

TIMOLOL MALEATE (continued)
Solution, Gel Forming/Drops; Ophthalmic

	TIMOLOL MALEATE			
	FALCON PHARMS			OCT 21, 1998
AB		EQ 0.25% BASE	N020963 001	OCT 21, 1998
	TIMOPTIC-XE			
AB +	MERCK	EQ 0.5% BASE	N020330 002	NOV 04, 1993
AB +		EQ 0.25% BASE	N020330 001	NOV 04, 1993

Solution/Drops; Ophthalmic

	TIMOLOL MALEATE			
AT	AKORN	EQ 0.5% BASE	N074466 001	MAR 25, 1997
AT		EQ 0.5% BASE	N074516 001	MAR 25, 1997
AT		EQ 0.25% BASE	N074465 001	MAR 25, 1997
AT		EQ 0.25% BASE	N074515 001	MAR 25, 1997
AT	BAUSCH AND LOMB	EQ 0.5% BASE	N074776 001	MAR 25, 1997
AT		EQ 0.25% BASE	N074778 001	MAR 25, 1997
AT	FOUGERA	EQ 0.5% BASE	N074668 001	MAR 25, 1997
AT		EQ 0.25% BASE	N074667 001	MAR 25, 1997
AT	NOVEX	EQ 0.5% BASE	N075412 001	SEP 08, 2000
AT		EQ 0.25% BASE	N075411 001	SEP 08, 2000
AT	PACIFIC PHARMA	EQ 0.5% BASE	N074747 001	MAR 25, 1997
AT		EQ 0.25% BASE	N074746 001	MAR 25, 1997
	TIMOPTIC			
AT +	MERCK	EQ 0.5% BASE	N018086 002	
AT +		EQ 0.25% BASE	N018086 001	
	TIMOPTIC IN OCUDOSE			
+	MERCK	EQ 0.5% BASE	N019463 002	NOV 05, 1986
+		EQ 0.25% BASE	N019463 001	NOV 05, 1986

Solution; Ophthalmic

	TIMOLOL MALEATE			
AT	HI TECH PHARMA	EQ 0.5% BASE	N075163 001	SEP 10, 2002

Tablet; Oral

	BLOCADREN			
AB	MERCK	5MG	N018017 001	
AB		10MG	N018017 002	
AB +		20MG	N018017 004	
	TIMOLOL MALEATE			
AB	GENEVA PHARMS	5MG	N072550 001	APR 13, 1989

Prescription Drug Products *(continued)*

TIMOLOL MALEATE *(continued)*
Tablet; Oral

TIMOLOL MALEATE

	GENEVA PHARMS			
AB		10MG	N072551 001	APR 13, 1989
AB		20MG	N072552 001	APR 13, 1989
AB	MYLAN	5MG	N072666 001	JUN 08, 1990
AB		10MG	N072667 001	JUN 08, 1990
AB		20MG	N072668 001	JUN 08, 1990
AB	WATSON LABS	5MG	N072917 001	JUL 31, 1991
AB		10MG	N072918 001	JUL 31, 1991
AB		20MG	N072919 001	JUL 31, 1991

TIMOLOL MALEATE *MULTIPLE*
SEE DORZOLAMIDE HYDROCHLORIDE; TIMOLOL MALEATE
SEE HYDROCHLOROTHIAZIDE; TIMOLOL MALEATE

TINZAPARIN SODIUM
Injectable; Injection

INNOHEP

+	PHARMION	20,000 IU/ML	N020484 001	JUL 14, 2000

TIOPRONIN
Tablet; Oral

TIOPRONIN

+	MISSION PHARMA	100MG	N019569 001	AUG 11, 1988

TIROFIBAN HYDROCHLORIDE
Injectable; Injection

AGGRASTAT

+	MERCK	EQ 0.05MG BASE/ML	N020913 001	MAY 14, 1998
+		EQ 0.25MG BASE/ML	N020912 001	MAY 14, 1998

TIZANIDINE HYDROCHLORIDE
Capsule; Oral

ZANAFLEX

	ELAN PHARMS	EQ 2MG BASE	N021447 001	AUG 29, 2002
		EQ 4MG BASE	N021447 002	AUG 29, 2002
+		EQ 6MG BASE	N021447 003	AUG 29, 2002

TIZANIDINE HYDROCHLORIDE *(continued)*
Tablet; Oral

TIZANIDINE HCL

	BARR			
AB		EQ 2MG BASE	N076371 001	APR 09, 2003
AB		EQ 4MG BASE	N076371 002	APR 09, 2003
AB	COREPHARMA	EQ 2MG BASE	N076347 001	OCT 11, 2002
AB		EQ 4MG BASE	N076347 002	OCT 11, 2002
AB	DR REDDYS LABS INC	EQ 2MG BASE	N076286 001	JUL 03, 2002
AB		EQ 4MG BASE	N076286 002	JUL 03, 2002
AB	EON	EQ 2MG BASE	N076399 001	NOV 26, 2002
AB		EQ 4MG BASE	N076280 002	JUN 27, 2002
AB	MYLAN	EQ 2MG BASE	N076354 001	MAR 28, 2003
AB		EQ 4MG BASE	N076354 002	MAR 28, 2003
AB	PUREPAC PHARM	EQ 2MG BASE	N076283 001	JUL 12, 2002
AB		EQ 4MG BASE	N076283 002	JUL 12, 2002
AB	TEVA	EQ 2MG BASE	N076284 001	JUL 03, 2002
AB		EQ 4MG BASE	N076284 002	JUL 03, 2002

ZANAFLEX

AB	ELAN PHARMS	EQ 2MG BASE	N020397 002	FEB 04, 2000
AB	+	EQ 4MG BASE	N020397 001	NOV 27, 1996

TOBRAMYCIN
Ointment; Ophthalmic

TOBREX

+	ALCON	0.3%	N050555 001

Solution/Drops; Ophthalmic

AKTOB

AT	AKORN	0.3%	N064096 001	JAN 31, 1996

TOBRAMYCIN

AT	ALTANA	0.3%	N065026 001	SEP 11, 2001
AT	BAUSCH AND LOMB	0.3%	N064052 001	NOV 29, 1993
AT	NOVEX	0.3%	N065087 001	FEB 25, 2002

TOBREX

AT	ALCON	0.3%	N062535 001	DEC 13, 1984
AT	+ FALCON PHARMS	0.3%	N050541 001	

Prescription Drug Products *(continued)*

TOBRAMYCIN *(continued)*

Solution; Inhalation

TOBI

+	CHIRON	300MG/5ML	N050753 001 DEC 22, 1997

TOBRAMYCIN *MULTIPLE*

SEE   DEXAMETHASONE; TOBRAMYCIN
SEE   FLUOROMETHOLONE ACETATE; TOBRAMYCIN

TOBRAMYCIN SULFATE

Injectable; Injection

NEBCIN

TE		Firm	Strength	Appl No	Date
AP	+	LILLY	EQ 1.2GM BASE/VIAL	N050519 001	
AP	+		EQ 10MG BASE/ML	N050477 005	
AP	+		EQ 10MG BASE/ML	N062008 004	
AP	+		EQ 10MG BASE/ML	N062707 001	APR 29, 1987
AP	+		EQ 40MG BASE/ML	N062008 001	

TOBRAMYCIN

TE	Firm	Strength	Appl No	Date
AP	AM PHARM PARTNERS	EQ 10MG BASE/ML	N065122 001	NOV 29, 2002
AP		EQ 40MG BASE/ML	N065122 002	NOV 29, 2002
AP	PHARMA TEK	EQ 1.2GM BASE/VIAL	N065013 001	AUG 17, 2001

TOBRAMYCIN (PHARMACY BULK)

TE	Firm	Strength	Appl No	Date
AP	AM PHARM PARTNERS	EQ 40MG BASE/ML	N065120 001	NOV 29, 2002

TOBRAMYCIN SULFATE

TE		Firm	Strength	Appl No	Date
AP		ABBOTT	EQ 10MG BASE/ML	N063080 001	APR 30, 1991
AP			EQ 10MG BASE/ML	N063112 001	APR 30, 1991
AP			EQ 40MG BASE/ML	N063111 001	APR 30, 1991
AP			EQ 40MG BASE/ML	N063116 001	MAY 18, 1992
AP	+		EQ 40MG BASE/ML	N063161 001	MAY 29, 1991
AP		APOTHECON	EQ 10MG BASE/ML	N064021 001	MAY 31, 1994
AP			EQ 40MG BASE/ML	N064021 002	MAY 31, 1994
AP		GENSIA SICOR PHARMS	EQ 40MG BASE/ML	N063100 001	JAN 30, 1992
AP		LEDERLE	EQ 40MG BASE/ML	N063117 001	APR 26, 1991
AP			EQ 40MG BASE/ML	N063118 001	JUL 29, 1991
AP		MARSAM PHARMS LLC	EQ 10MG BASE/ML	N062945 001	AUG 09, 1989
AP			EQ 40MG BASE/ML	N062945 002	AUG 09, 1989

TOBRAMYCIN SULFATE *(continued)*

Injectable; Injection

TOBRAMYCIN SULFATE IN SODIUM CHLORIDE 0.9% IN PLASTIC CONTA NER

TE		Firm	Strength	Appl No	Date
	+	ABBOTT	EQ 80MG BASE/100ML	N063081 001	JUL 31, 1990
	+		EQ 1.2MG BASE/ML	N063081 003	JUL 31, 1990
	+		EQ 1.6MG BASE/ML	N063081 006	JUN 02, 1993

TOCAINIDE HYDROCHLORIDE

Tablet; Oral

TONOCARD

	Firm	Strength	Appl No	Date
+	ASTRAZENECA	400MG	N018257 001	NOV 09, 1984
+		600MG	N018257 002	NOV 09, 1984

TOCOPHEROL ACETATE *MULTIPLE*

SEE   ASCORBIC ACID; BIOTIN; CHOLECALCIFEROL; CYANOCOBALAMIN; DEXPANTHENOL; FOLIC ACID; NIACINAMIDE; PYRIDOXINE; RIBOFLAVIN; THIAMINE; TOCOPHEROL ACETATE; VITAMIN A; VITAMIN K

TOLAZAMIDE

Tablet; Oral

TOLAZAMIDE

TE	Firm	Strength	Appl No	Date
AB	GENEVA PHARMS	100MG	N071633 001	DEC 09, 1987
AB		250MG	N070289 001	MAR 13, 1986
AB		500MG	N070290 001	MAR 13, 1986
AB	IVAX PHARMS	100MG	N018894 001	NOV 02, 1984
AB		250MG	N018894 002	NOV 02, 1984
AB		500MG	N018894 003	NOV 02, 1984
AB	MUTUAL PHARM	100MG	N071357 001	JUL 16, 1987
AB		250MG	N071358 001	JUL 16, 1987
AB		500MG	N071359 001	JUL 16, 1987
AB	MYLAN	250MG	N070259 001	JAN 02, 1986
AB		500MG	N070913 001	MAR 17, 1986
AB	PAR PHARM	100MG	N070159 001	JAN 06, 1986
AB		250MG	N070160 001	JAN 06, 1986
AB		500MG	N070161 001	JAN 06, 1986
AB	WATSON LABS	100MG	N070513 001	JAN 06, 1986

Prescription Drug Products *(continued)*

TOLAZAMIDE *(continued)*
Tablet; Oral

	Firm	Strength	Appl. No.	Date
	TOLAZAMIDE			
AB	WATSON LABS	250MG		JAN 09, 1986
			N070514 001	JAN 09, 1986
AB		500MG	N070515 001	JAN 09, 1986
	TOLINASE			
AB	PHARMACIA AND UPJOHN	100MG	N015500 002	
AB		250MG	N015500 004	
AB +		500MG	N015500 005	

TOLBUTAMIDE
Tablet; Oral

	Firm	Strength	Appl. No.	Date
	TOLBUTAMIDE			
AB	GENEVA PHARMS	500MG	N086574 001	
AB	IVAX PHARMS	500MG	N087093 001	
AB	LEDERLE	500MG	N086926 001	
AB	MYLAN	500MG	N086445 001	
AB	WATSON LABS	500MG	N086109 001	
AB +		500MG	N087318 001	

TOLCAPONE
Tablet; Oral

	Firm	Strength	Appl. No.	Date
	TASMAR			
AB	ROCHE	100MG	N020697 001	JAN 29, 1998
AB +		200MG	N020697 002	JAN 29, 1998

TOLMETIN SODIUM
Capsule; Oral

	Firm	Strength	Appl. No.	Date
	TOLECTIN DS			
AB +	ORTHO MCNEIL PHARM	EQ 400MG BASE	N018084 001	
	TOLMETIN SODIUM			
AB	IVAX PHARMS	EQ 400MG BASE	N073392 001	JAN 24, 1992
AB	MUTUAL PHARM	EQ 400MG BASE	N073311 001	NOV 27, 1991
AB	MYLAN	EQ 400MG BASE	N073393 001	MAY 27, 1993
AB	PUREPAC PHARM	EQ 400MG BASE	N073308 001	JAN 24, 1992
AB	TEVA	EQ 400MG BASE	N073290 001	NOV 27, 1991
AB		EQ 400MG BASE	N073519 001	MAY 29, 1992

Tablet; Oral

	Firm	Strength	Appl. No.	Date
	TOLECTIN			
AB	ORTHO MCNEIL PHARM	EQ 200MG BASE	N017628 001	
	TOLECTIN 600			
AB +	ORTHO MCNEIL PHARM	EQ 600MG BASE	N017628 002	MAR 08, 1989

TOLMETIN SODIUM *(continued)*
Tablet; Oral

	Firm	Strength	Appl. No.	Date
	TOLMETIN SODIUM			
AB	GENEVA PHARMS	EQ 200MG BASE	N073588 001	JUL 31, 1992
AB		EQ 600MG BASE	N074002 001	SEP 27, 1993
			N074399 001	MAR 28, 1996
AB	IVAX PHARMS	EQ 600MG BASE	N073310 001	NOV 27, 1991
AB	MUTUAL PHARM	EQ 200MG BASE	N074473 001	AUG 30, 1994
AB	MYLAN	EQ 600MG BASE	N073527 001	JUN 30, 1992
AB	PUREPAC PHARM	EQ 600MG BASE		

TOLTERODINE TARTRATE
Capsule, Extended Release; Oral

	Firm	Strength	Appl. No.	Date
	DETROL LA			
+	PHARMACIA AND UPJOHN	2MG	N021228 001	DEC 22, 2000
		4MG	N021228 002	DEC 22, 2000

Tablet; Oral

	Firm	Strength	Appl. No.	Date
	DETROL			
+	PHARMACIA AND UPJOHN	1MG	N020771 001	MAR 25, 1998
		2MG	N020771 002	MAR 25, 1998

TOPIRAMATE
Capsule; Oral

	Firm	Strength	Appl. No.	Date
	TOPAMAX SPRINKLE			
	ORTHO MCNEIL	15MG	N020844 001	OCT 26, 1998
+		25MG	N020844 002	OCT 26, 1998

Tablet; Oral

	Firm	Strength	Appl. No.	Date
	TOPAMAX			
+	ORTHO MCNEIL PHARM	25MG	N020505 004	DEC 24, 1996
		100MG	N020505 001	DEC 24, 1996
		200MG	N020505 002	DEC 24, 1996

TOPOTECAN HYDROCHLORIDE
Injectable; Injection

	Firm	Strength	Appl. No.	Date
	HYCAMTIN			
+	GLAXOSMITHKLINE	EQ 4MG BASE/VIAL	N020671 001	MAY 28, 1996

Prescription Drug Products (continued)

TOREMIFENE CITRATE
Tablet; Oral

		Strength	NDA	Date
	FARESTON			
+	ORION	EQ 60MG BASE	N020497 001	MAY 29, 1997

TORSEMIDE
Injectable; Injection

		Strength	NDA	Date
	DEMADEX			
+	ROCHE	10MG/ML	N020137 002	AUG 23, 1993

Tablet; Oral

		Strength	NDA	Date
	DEMADEX			
	ROCHE			
AB		5MG	N020136 001	AUG 23, 1993
AB		10MG	N020136 002	AUG 23, 1993
AB	+	20MG	N020136 003	AUG 23, 1993
AB		100MG	N020136 004	AUG 23, 1993
	TORSEMIDE			
	PAR PHARM			
AB		5MG	N076226 001	MAY 27, 2003
AB		10MG	N076226 002	MAY 27, 2003
AB		20MG	N076226 003	MAY 27, 2003
AB		100MG	N076226 004	MAY 27, 2003
	PLIVA PHARM IND			
AB		5MG	N076346 001	MAY 30, 2003
AB		10MG	N076346 002	MAY 30, 2003
AB		20MG	N076346 003	MAY 30, 2003
	TEVA			
AB		5MG	N076110 001	MAY 14, 2002
AB		10MG	N076110 002	MAY 14, 2002
AB		20MG	N076110 003	MAY 14, 2002
AB		100MG	N076110 004	MAY 14, 2002

TRAMADOL HYDROCHLORIDE
Tablet; Oral

		Strength	NDA	Date
	TRAMADOL HCL			
	ALPHAPHARM			
AB		50MG ***SEE 23RD ANNUAL OB SECTION 1.8 DESCRIPTION OF SPECIAL SITUATIONS: TRAMADOL HYDROCHLORIDE***	N075980 001	NOV 21, 2002

TRAMADOL HYDROCHLORIDE (continued)
Tablet; Oral

		Strength	NDA	Date
	TRAMADOL HCL			
	ASTA			
AB		50MG ***SEE 23RD ANNUAL OB SECTION 1.8 DESCRIPTION OF SPECIAL SITUATIONS: TRAMADOL HYDROCHLORIDE***	N075974 001	JUL 12, 2002
	CARACO			
AB		50MG ***SEE 23RD ANNUAL OB SECTION 1.8 DESCRIPTION OF SPECIAL SITUATIONS: TRAMADOL HYDROCHLORIDE***	N075964 001	JUN 19, 2002
	COREPHARMA			
AB		50MG ***SEE 23RD ANNUAL OB SECTION 1.8 DESCRIPTION OF SPECIAL SITUATIONS: TRAMADOL HYDROCHLORIDE***	N076003 001	JUN 20, 2002
	EON			
AB		50MG ***SEE 23RD ANNUAL OB SECTION 1.8 DESCRIPTION OF SPECIAL SITUATIONS: TRAMADOL HYDROCHLORIDE***	N075968 001	JUN 25, 2002
	IVAX PHARMS			
AB		50MG ***SEE 23RD ANNUAL OB SECTION 1.8 DESCRIPTION OF SPECIAL SITUATIONS: TRAMADOL HYDROCHLORIDE***	N075963 001	JUL 03, 2002
	MALLINCKRODT			
AB		50MG ***SEE 23RD ANNUAL OB SECTION 1.8 DESCRIPTION OF SPECIAL SITUATIONS: TRAMADOL HYDROCHLORIDE***	N075983 001	JUN 25, 2002
	MUTUAL PHARM			
AB		50MG ***SEE 23RD ANNUAL OB SECTION 1.8 DESCRIPTION OF SPECIAL SITUATIONS: TRAMADOL HYDROCHLORIDE***	N076100 001	JUN 20, 2002
	MYLAN			
AB		50MG ***SEE 23RD ANNUAL OB SECTION 1.8 DESCRIPTION OF SPECIAL SITUATIONS: TRAMADOL HYDROCHLORIDE***	N075986 001	JUN 21, 2002
	PLIVA			
AB		50MG ***SEE 23RD ANNUAL OB SECTION 1.8 DESCRIPTION OF SPECIAL SITUATIONS: TRAMADOL HYDROCHLORIDE***	N075982 001	JUL 01, 2002

Prescription Drug Products (continued)

TRAMADOL HYDROCHLORIDE (continued)
Tablet; Oral

TRAMADOL HCL

	Firm	Strength	NDA	Date
AB	PUREPAC PHARM	50MG ***SEE 23RD ANNUAL OB SECTION 1.8 DESCRIPTION OF SPECIAL SITUATIONS: TRAMADOL HYDROCHLORIDE***	N075960 001	JUN 19, 2002
AB	TEVA	50MG ***SEE 23RD ANNUAL OB SECTION 1.8 DESCRIPTION OF SPECIAL SITUATIONS: TRAMADOL HYDROCHLORIDE***	N075977 001	JUN 19, 2002
AB	TORPHARM	50MG ***SEE 23RD ANNUAL OB SECTION 1.8 DESCRIPTION OF SPECIAL SITUATIONS: TRAMADOL HYDROCHLORIDE***	N075981 001	JUL 10, 2002
AB	WATSON LABS	50MG ***SEE 23RD ANNUAL OB SECTION 1.8 DESCRIPTION OF SPECIAL SITUATIONS: TRAMADOL HYDROCHLORIDE***	N075962 001	JUN 24, 2002

ULTRAM

	Firm	Strength	NDA	Date
AB +	ORTHO MCNEIL PHARM	50MG	N020281 002	MAR 03, 1995

TRAMADOL HYDROCHLORIDE *MULTIPLE*
SEE ACETAMINOPHEN; TRAMADOL HYDROCHLORIDE

TRANDOLAPRIL
Tablet; Oral

MAVIK

	Firm	Strength	NDA	Date
	ABBOTT	1MG	N020528 001	APR 26, 1996
		2MG	N020528 002	APR 26, 1996
+		4MG	N020528 003	APR 26, 1996

TRANDOLAPRIL; VERAPAMIL HYDROCHLORIDE
Tablet, Extended Release; Oral

TARKA

	Firm	Strength	NDA	Date
+	ABBOTT	1MG;240MG	N020591 003	OCT 22, 1996
+		2MG;180MG	N020591 001	OCT 22, 1996
+		2MG;240MG	N020591 004	OCT 22, 1996
+		4MG;240MG	N020591 002	OCT 22, 1996

TRANEXAMIC ACID
Injectable; Injection

CYKLOKAPRON

	Firm	Strength	NDA	Date
+	PHARMACIA AND UPJOHN	100MG/ML	N019281 001	DEC 30, 1986

TRANYLCYPROMINE SULFATE
Tablet; Oral

PARNATE

	Firm	Strength	NDA	Date
+	GLAXOSMITHKLINE	EQ 10MG BASE	N012342 003	AUG 16, 1985

TRAVOPROST
Solution/Drops; Ophthalmic

TRAVATAN

	Firm	Strength	NDA	Date
+	ALCON UNIVERSAL	0.004%	N021257 001	MAR 16, 2001

TRAZODONE HYDROCHLORIDE
Tablet; Oral

DESYREL

	Firm	Strength	NDA	Date
AB	APOTHECON	50MG	N018207 001	MAR 25, 1987
AB		100MG	N018207 002	MAR 25, 1987
AB		150MG	N018207 003	MAR 25, 1985
AB		300MG	N018207 004	NOV 07, 1988

TRAZODONE HCL

	Firm	Strength	NDA	Date
AB	BARR	50MG	N071258 001	MAR 25, 1987
AB		100MG	N071196 001	MAR 25, 1987
AB		150MG	N071196 002	APR 26, 1999
AB		300MG	N071196 003	APR 26, 1999
AB	GENEVA PHARMS	50MG	N072484 001	APR 30, 1990
AB		100MG	N072483 001	APR 30, 1990
AB	MUTUAL PHARM	50MG	N073136 001	MAR 24, 1993
AB		100MG	N073137 001	MAR 24, 1993
AB		150MG	N073138 001	DEC 22, 1995
AB	MYLAN	50MG	N071405 001	FEB 27, 1991
AB		100MG	N071406 001	FEB 27, 1991
AB	PLIVA	50MG	N071523 001	DEC 11, 1987
AB		100MG	N071524 001	DEC 11, 1987
AB		150MG	N071525 001	

Prescription Drug Products (continued)

TRAZODONE HYDROCHLORIDE (continued)

Tablet; Oral

TRAZODONE HCL

TE	Firm	Strength	Appl No	Approval Date
AB	PUREPAC PHARM (PLIVA)	50MG	N071636 001	MAR 09, 1988
AB		100MG	N071514 001	APR 18, 1988
AB	TEVA	50MG	N072192 001	APR 18, 1988
AB		100MG	N072193 001	FEB 02, 1989
AB		150MG	N074357 001	FEB 02, 1989
AB	WATSON LABS	50MG	N070857 001	APR 30, 1997
AB		100MG	N070858 001	OCT 10, 1986

TREPROSTINIL SODIUM

Injectable; Subcutaneous

REMODULIN

TE	Firm	Strength	Appl No	Approval Date
	UNITED THERAP	1MG/ML	N021272 001	MAY 21, 2002
		2.5MG/ML	N021272 002	MAY 21, 2002
		5MG/ML	N021272 003	MAY 21, 2002
+		10MG/ML	N021272 004	MAY 21, 2002

TRETINOIN

Capsule; Oral

VESANOID

TE	Firm	Strength	Appl No	Approval Date
+	ROCHE	10MG	N020438 001	NOV 22, 1995

Cream, Augmented; Topical

RENOVA

TE	Firm	Strength	Appl No	Approval Date
+	JOHNSON AND JOHNSON	0.05%	N019963 001	DEC 29, 1995

Cream; Topical

AVITA

TE	Firm	Strength	Appl No	Approval Date
AB	BERTEK PHARMS	0.025%	N020404 003	JAN 14, 1997

RENOVA

TE	Firm	Strength	Appl No	Approval Date
+	JOHNSON AND JOHNSON	0.02%	N021108 001	AUG 31, 2000

RETIN-A

TE	Firm	Strength	Appl No	Approval Date
AB	+ JOHNSON AND JOHNSON	0.1%	N017340 001	
AB	+	0.05%	N017522 001	
AB	+	0.025%	N019049 001	SEP 16, 1988

TRETINOIN (continued)

Cream; Topical

TRETINOIN

TE	Firm	Strength	Appl No	Approval Date
AB	SPEAR PHARMS	0.1%	N075213 001	DEC 24, 1998
AB		0.05%	N075265 001	DEC 24, 1998
AB		0.025%	N075264 001	DEC 24, 1998

Gel; Topical

AVITA

TE	Firm	Strength	Appl No	Approval Date
BT	BERTEK PHARMS	0.025%	N020400 001	JAN 29, 1998

RETIN-A

TE	Firm	Strength	Appl No	Approval Date
AB	+ JOHNSON AND JOHNSON	0.01%	N017955 001	
AB	+ JOHNSON AND JOHNSON	0.025%	N017579 002	

RETIN-A MICRO

TE	Firm	Strength	Appl No	Approval Date
	+ JOHNSON AND JOHNSON	0.1%	N020475 001	FEB 07, 1997
	+	0.04%	N020475 002	MAY 10, 2002

TRETINOIN

TE	Firm	Strength	Appl No	Approval Date
AB	SPEAR PHARMS	0.01%	N075589 001	JUN 11, 2002
AB		0.025%	N075529 001	FEB 22, 2000

Solution; Topical

RETIN-A

TE	Firm	Strength	Appl No	Approval Date
AT	+ JOHNSON AND JOHNSON	0.05%	N016921 001	

TRETINOIN

TE	Firm	Strength	Appl No	Approval Date
AT	COPLEY PHARM	0.05%	N074873 001	JUN 19, 1998
AT	MORTON GROVE	0.05%	N075260 001	JAN 25, 1999

TRETINOIN *MULTIPLE*

SEE FLUOCINOLONE ACETONIDE; HYDROQUINONE; TRETINOIN
SEE MEQUINOL; TRETINOIN

TRIAMCINOLONE

Tablet; Oral

ARISTOCORT

TE	Firm	Strength	Appl No	Approval Date
BP	FUJISAWA HLTHCARE	4MG	N011161 007	

KENACORT

TE	Firm	Strength	Appl No	Approval Date
BP	BRISTOL MYERS SQUIBB	4MG	N011283 006	
BP		8MG	N011283 010	

TRIAMCINOLONE

TE	Firm	Strength	Appl No	Approval Date
BP	+ WATSON LABS	4MG	N084270 001	

Prescription Drug Products (continued)

TRIAMCINOLONE ACETONIDE

Aerosol, Metered; Inhalation

TE	Firm / Brand	Strength	Appl. No.	Approval
	AZMACORT			
+	AVENTIS	0.1MG/INH	N018117 001	APR 23, 1982

Aerosol, Metered; Nasal

TE	Firm / Brand	Strength	Appl. No.	Approval
	NASACORT			
+	AVENTIS	0.055MG/INH	N019798 001	JUL 11, 1991

Cream; Topical

TE	Firm / Brand	Strength	Appl. No.	Approval
	ARISTOCORT			
AT	FUJISAWA HLTHCARE	0.1%	N083016 004	
AT		0.5%	N083015 002	
AT		0.025%	N083017 003	
	ARISTOCORT A			
AT	FUJISAWA HLTHCARE	0.1%	N083016 005	
AT		0.1%	N088819 001	OCT 16, 1984
AT		0.5%	N083015 003	
AT		0.5%	N088820 001	OCT 16, 1984
AT		0.025%	N083017 004	
AT		0.025%	N088818 001	OCT 16, 1984
	KENALOG			
+	APOTHECON	0.1%	N011601 006	
+		0.5%	N083943 001	
+		0.025%	N011601 003	
	TRIACET			
AT	TEVA	0.1%	N084908 002	
AT		0.5%	N084908 003	
AT		0.025%	N084908 001	
	TRIAMCINOLONE ACETONIDE			
AT	ALPHARMA US PHARM	0.1%	N087798 001	JUN 04, 1982
AT	ALTANA	0.1%	N085692 003	
AT		0.5%	N085692 002	
AT		0.025%	N087932 001	
AT	AMBIX	0.1%	N086414 001	MAY 09, 1983
AT		0.5%	N086413 001	
AT		0.025%	N086415 001	
AT	CLAY PARK	0.1%	N089798 001	MAY 31, 1991
AT		0.5%	N089797 001	MAY 31, 1991
AT		0.025%	N040039 001	NOV 26, 1997
AT	G AND W LABS	0.1%	N086276 001	
AT		0.025%	N086275 001	
AT	TARO	0.1%	N086277 001	
	TRIDERM			
AT	DEL RAY LABS	0.1%	N088042 001	MAR 19, 1984
	TRYMEX			
AT	SAVAGE LABS	0.1%	N088197 001	

TRIAMCINOLONE ACETONIDE (continued)

Cream; Topical

TE	Firm / Brand	Strength	Appl. No.	Approval
	TRYMEX			
AT	SAVAGE LABS	0.025%	N088196 001	MAR 25, 1983

Injectable; Injection

TE	Firm / Brand	Strength	Appl. No.	Approval
	KENALOG-10			
+	APOTHECON	10MG/ML	N012041 001	
	KENALOG-40			
+	APOTHECON	40MG/ML	N014901 001	

Lotion; Topical

TE	Firm / Brand	Strength	Appl. No.	Approval
	KENALOG			
AT +	APOTHECON	0.1%	N084343 002	
AT		0.025%	N084343 001	
	TRIAMCINOLONE ACETONIDE			
AT	ALTANA	0.1%	N040467 002	APR 21, 2003
AT		0.025%	N040467 001	APR 21, 2003
AT	MORTON GROVE	0.1%	N088451 001	APR 03, 1985
AT		0.025%	N088450 001	APR 01, 1985
AT	TARO	0.1%	N089129 001	AUG 14, 1986

Ointment; Topical

TE	Firm / Brand	Strength	Appl. No.	Approval
	ARISTOCORT			
AT	FUJISAWA HLTHCARE	0.1%	N080750 004	
	ARISTOCORT A			
AT	FUJISAWA HLTHCARE	0.1%	N080750 003	
AT		0.1%	N088780 001	OCT 01, 1984
	KENALOG			
AT	APOTHECON	0.1%	N011600 001	
AT		0.025%	N011600 003	
	TRIAMCINOLONE ACETONIDE			
AT	ALPHARMA US PHARM	0.1%	N087799 001	JUN 07, 1982
AT	ALTANA	0.1%	N085691 003	
AT		0.5%	N085691 002	
AT		0.025%	N085691 001	
+	CLAY PARK	0.1%	N087357 001	
+		0.5%	N087385 001	
+		0.5%	N087356 001	
AT	TARO	0.1%	N040037 001	SEP 30, 1994
AT		0.1%	N087902 001	DEC 27, 1982
AT		0.5%	N040386 001	JUN 05, 2001
AT		0.025%	N040040 001	SEP 30, 1994
AT		0.025%	N040374 001	JUN 05, 2001

TRIAMCINOLONE ACETONIDE IN ABSORBASE

TE	Firm / Brand	Strength	Appl. No.	Approval
+	CAROLINA MEDCL	0.05%	N089595 001	

Prescription Drug Products (continued)

TRIAMCINOLONE ACETONIDE (continued)

Ointment; Topical

TRIAMCINOLONE ACETONIDE IN ABSORBASE

	CAROLINA MEDCL			MAR 23, 1995
	TRYMEX			
AT	SAVAGE LABS	0.1%	N088691 001	AUG 02, 1984
			N088693 001	AUG 02, 1984
AT		0.025%		AUG 02, 1984

Paste; Dental

KENALOG IN ORABASE

AT	+ APOTHECON	0.1%	N012097 001	
	ORACORT			
AT	TARO	0.1%	N070730 001	OCT 01, 1986
	ORALONE			
AT	TARO	0.1%	N071383 001	JUL 06, 1987

Spray, Metered; Nasal

	NASACORT AQ			
	+ AVENTIS	0.055MG/SPRAY	N020468 001	MAY 20, 1996

Spray; Topical

	KENALOG			
	+ APOTHECON	0.147MG/GM	N012104 001	

TRIAMCINOLONE ACETONIDE *MULTIPLE*
SEE NYSTATIN; TRIAMCINOLONE ACETONIDE

TRIAMCINOLONE DIACETATE

Injectable; Injection

ARISTOCORT

	+ FUJISAWA HLTHCARE	25MG/ML	N011685 003
		40MG/ML	N012802 001

TRIAMCINOLONE HEXACETONIDE

Injectable; Injection

ARISTOSPAN

	+ FUJISAWA HLTHCARE	5MG/ML	N016466 001
+		20MG/ML	N016466 002

TRIAMTERENE

Capsule; Oral

DYRENIUM

	WELLSPRING PHARM	50MG	N013174 001
		100MG	N013174 002

TRIAMTERENE *MULTIPLE*
SEE HYDROCHLOROTHIAZIDE; TRIAMTERENE

TRIAZOLAM

Tablet; Oral

HALCION

AB	+ PHARMACIA AND UPJOHN	0.25MG	N017892 001

TRIAZOLAM (continued)

Tablet; Oral

HALCION

	PHARMACIA AND UPJOHN	0.125MG	N017892 003	NOV 15, 1982
				APR 26, 1985
	TRIAZOLAM			
	ALPHAPHARM			
AB		0.25MG	N074031 002	MAR 25, 1994
AB		0.125MG	N074031 001	MAR 25, 1994
AB	ROXANE	0.25MG	N074224 002	JUN 01, 1994
AB		0.125MG	N074224 001	JUN 01, 1994
AB	WATSON LABS	0.25MG	N074445 002	OCT 20, 1995
AB		0.125MG	N074445 001	OCT 20, 1995

TRICHLORMETHIAZIDE

Tablet; Oral

NAQUA

BP	+ SCHERING	4MG	N012265 002
	TRICHLORMETHIAZIDE		
BP	ABC HOLDING	4MG	N085568 001
BP	PAR PHARM	2MG	N087007 001
BP		4MG	N087005 001

TRIENTINE HYDROCHLORIDE

Capsule; Oral

SYPRINE

	+ MERCK	250MG	N019194 001	NOV 08, 1985

TRIFLUOPERAZINE HYDROCHLORIDE

Concentrate; Oral

STELAZINE

AA	+ GLAXOSMITHKLINE	EQ 10MG BASE/ML	N011552 006

Injectable; Injection

STELAZINE

	+ GLAXOSMITHKLINE	EQ 2MG BASE/ML	N011552 005

Tablet; Oral

STELAZINE

	GLAXOSMITHKLINE			
AB		EQ 1MG BASE	N011552 001	
AB		EQ 2MG BASE	N011552 002	
AB		EQ 5MG BASE	N011552 003	
AB		EQ 10MG BASE	N011552 004	
	TRIFLUOPERAZINE HCL			
	GENEVA PHARMS			
AB		EQ 1MG BASE	N085785 001	
AB		EQ 2MG BASE	N085786 001	
AB		EQ 5MG BASE	N085789 001	
AB		EQ 10MG BASE	N085788 001	
AB	GENEVA PHARMS TECH	EQ 1MG BASE	N040153 001	OCT 25, 1996

Prescription Drug Products *(continued)*

TRIFLUOPERAZINE HYDROCHLORIDE *(continued)*

Tablet; Oral

TRIFLUOPERAZINE HCL

AB	GENEVA PHARMS TECH	EQ 2MG BASE	N040153 002	OCT 25, 1996
AB		EQ 5MG BASE	N040153 003	OCT 25, 1996
AB		EQ 10MG BASE	N040153 004	OCT 25, 1996
AB	MYLAN	EQ 1MG BASE	N040209 001	JUL 07, 1997
AB		EQ 2MG BASE	N040209 002	JUL 07, 1997
AB		EQ 5MG BASE	N040209 003	JUL 07, 1997
AB		EQ 10MG BASE	N040209 004	JUL 07, 1997

TRIFLURIDINE

Solution/Drops; Ophthalmic

TRIFLURIDINE

AT	ALCON	1%	N074311 001	OCT 06, 1995

VIROPTIC

AT	+ MONARCH PHARMS	1%	N018299 001	

TRIHEXYPHENIDYL HYDROCHLORIDE

Elixir; Oral

TRIHEXYPHENIDYL HCL

AA	MIKART	2MG/5ML	N040251 001	SEP 27, 1999
AA	PHARM ASSOC	2MG/5ML	N040177 001	APR 17, 1997
AA	+ PHARM VENTURES	2MG/5ML	N089514 001	APR 07, 1989

Tablet; Oral

TRIHEXYPHENIDYL HCL

AA	NYLOS	5MG	N085622 001	
AA	VINTAGE PHARMS	2MG	N040254 001	DEC 24, 1998
AA		5MG	N040254 002	DEC 24, 1998
AA	WATSON LAB	2MG	N040184 001	FEB 06, 1998
AA		5MG	N040184 002	FEB 06, 1998
AA	+ WATSON LABS	2MG	N084363 001	
AA	+	5MG	N084364 001	
AA		2MG	N040337 002	FEB 16, 2000
AA	WEST WARD	5MG	N040337 001	FEB 16, 2000

TRIMETHADIONE

Tablet; Oral

TRIDIONE

	+ ABBOTT	150MG	N005856 009	

TRIMETHOBENZAMIDE HYDROCHLORIDE

Capsule; Oral

TIGAN

	+ KING PHARMS	300MG	N017531 006	DEC 13, 2001

Injectable; Injection

TIGAN

AP	+ KING PHARMS	100MG/ML	N017530 001	

TRIMETHOBENZAMIDE HCL

AP	ABBOTT	100MG/ML	N088804 001	APR 03, 1987

TRIMETHOPRIM

Tablet; Oral

PROLOPRIM

AB	MONARCH PHARMS	100MG	N017943 001	

TRIMETHOPRIM

AB	TEVA	100MG	N018679 001	JUL 30, 1982
		200MG	N071259 001	JUN 18, 1987
AB	+ WATSON LABS	100MG	N070049 001	JUN 06, 1985

TRIMETHOPRIM *MULTIPLE*

SEE POLYMYXIN B SULFATE; TRIMETHOPRIM
SEE SULFAMETHOXAZOLE; TRIMETHOPRIM

TRIMETHOPRIM HYDROCHLORIDE

Solution; Oral

PRIMSOL

	+ ASCENT PEDS	EQ 50MG BASE/5ML	N074973 001	JAN 24, 2000

TRIMETHOPRIM SULFATE *MULTIPLE*

SEE POLYMYXIN B SULFATE: TRIMETHOPRIM SULFATE

TRIMETREXATE GLUCURONATE

Injectable; Injection

NEUTREXIN

	+ MEDIMMUNE ONCOLOGY	EQ 25MG BASE/VIAL	N020326 001	DEC 17, 1993
	+	EQ 200MG BASE/VIAL	N020326 002	JUL 31, 1998

Prescription Drug Products (continued)

TRIMIPRAMINE MALEATE
Capsule; Oral
SURMONTIL

PLIVA	EQ 25MG BASE	N016792 001
	EQ 50MG BASE	N016792 002
	EQ 100MG BASE	N016792 003
+		SEP 15, 1982

TRIPELENNAMINE HYDROCHLORIDE
Tablet; Oral
PBZ

	+ NOVARTIS	25MG	N083149 001
		50MG	N005914 002
	TRIPELENNAMINE HCL		
AA	LANNETT	50MG	N083557 001
AA	NYLOS	50MG	N085412 001
AA	WATSON LABS	50MG	N080713 001

TRIPLE SULFA
(SULFABENZAMIDE;SULFACETAMIDE;SULFATHIAZOLE)
Cream; Vaginal
GYNE-SULF

AT	G AND W LABS	3.7%;2.86%;3.42%	N088607 001
			JUN 09, 1986
	SULTRIN		
AT	+ ORTHO MCNEIL PHARM	3.7%;2.86%;3.42%	N005794 001
	TRIPLE SULFA		
AT	ALPHARMA	3.7%;2.86%;3.42%	N087864 001
			SEP 01, 1982
AT	CLAY PARK	3.7%;2.86%;3.42%	N087285 001
			NOV 15, 1982
	TRYSUL		
AT	SAVAGE LABS	3.7%;2.86%;3.42%	N087887 001
			JUL 23, 1982

TRIPROLIDINE HYDROCHLORIDE *MULTIPLE*
SEE CODEINE PHOSPHATE; PSEUDOEPHEDRINE HYDROCHLORIDE; TRIPROLIDINE HYDROCHLORIDE
SEE PSEUDOEPHEDRINE HYDROCHLORIDE; TRIPROLIDINE HYDROCHLORIDE

TRIPTORELIN PAMOATE
Injectable; Intramuscular
TRELSTAR

+ PHARMACIA AND UPJOHN	11.25MG/VIAL	N021288 001
		JUN 29, 2001

TRELSTAR DEPOT

+ PHARMACIA AND UPJOHN	EQ 3.75MG BASE/VIAL	N020715 001
		JUN 15, 2000

TRISULFAPYRIMIDINES
(SULFADIAZINE;SULFAMERAZINE;SULFAMETHAZINE)
Tablet; Oral
TRIPLE SULFOID

+ PAL PAK	167MG;167MG;167MG	N080094 001

TROLAMINE POLYPEPTIDE OLEATE CONDENSATE
Solution/Drops; Otic
CERUMENEX

+ PURDUE FREDERICK	10%	N011340 002

TROLEANDOMYCIN
Capsule; Oral
TAO

+ PFIZER	EQ 250MG BASE	N050336 002

TROMETHAMINE
Injectable; Injection
THAM

+ ABBOTT	3.6GM/100ML	N013025 002

TROPICAMIDE
Solution/Drops; Ophthalmic
MYDRIACYL

AT	+ ALCON	0.5%	N084305 001
AT		1%	N084306 001
	TROPICACYL		
AT	AKORN	0.5%	N040314 001
			SEP 29, 2000
AT		1%	N040315 001
			SEP 29, 2000
	TROPICAMIDE		
AT	ALCON UNIVERSAL	1%	N089172 001
			DEC 28, 1990
			N040067 001
			JUL 27, 1994
AT	BAUSCH AND LOMB	0.5%	N040064 001
			JUL 27, 1994
AT		1%	N087636 001
			JUL 30, 1982
AT	MIZA PHARMS USA	0.5%	N087637 001
			AUG 09, 1982
AT		1%	

TROPICAMIDE *MULTIPLE*
SEE HYDROXYAMPHETAMINE HYDROBROMIDE; TROPICAMIDE

TROVAFLOXACIN MESYLATE
Tablet; Oral
TROVAN

PFIZER	EQ 100MG BASE	N020759 001
		DEC 18, 1997
	EQ 200MG BASE	N020759 002
		DEC 18, 1997
+		

Prescription Drug Products (continued)

TUBOCURARINE CHLORIDE
Injectable; Injection
  TUBOCURARINE CHLORIDE
  AP + ABBOTT   3MG/ML   N006095 001
  AP + BRISTOL MYERS SQUIBB   3MG/ML   N005657 001

TYLOXAPOL *MULTIPLE*
  SEE CETYL ALCOHOL; COLFOSCERIL PALMITATE; TYLOXAPOL

UNOPROSTONE ISOPROPYL
Solution/Drops; Ophthalmic
  RESCULA
    + NOVARTIS   0.15%   N021214 001
                                                     AUG 03, 2000

UREA
Injectable; Injection
  UREAPHIL
    + ABBOTT   40GM/VIAL   N012154 001

UREA *MULTIPLE*
  SEE HYDROCORTISONE ACETATE; UREA

UREA, C-13
For Solution; Oral
  BREATHTEK UBT FOR H-PYLORI
    + MERETEK   EQ 75MG /POUCHE   N020586 002
                                                         MAY 10, 2001

UREA, C-13 *MULTIPLE*
  SEE CITRIC ACID; UREA, C-13

UREA, C-14
Capsule; Oral
  PYTEST
    + BALLARD MEDCL   1uCi   N020617 001
                                                     MAY 09, 1997
  PYTEST KIT
    + BALLARD MEDCL   1uCi   N020617 002
                                                     MAY 09, 1997

UROFOLLITROPIN
Injectable; Intramuscular, Subcutaneous
  BRAVELLE
  BX + FERRING   75 IU/VIAL   N021289 001
                                                     MAY 06, 2002
Injectable; Subcutaneous
  FERTINEX
  BX + SERONO   75 IU/AMP   N019415 005
                                                     AUG 23, 1996

URSODIOL
Capsule; Oral
  ACTIGALL
  AB + WATSON PHARMS   300MG   N019594 002
                                                     DEC 31, 1987
  URSODIOL
  AB   AMIDE PHARM   300MG   N075517 001
                                                     MAR 14, 2000
  AB + COPLEY PHARM   300MG   N075592 001
                                                     MAY 25, 2000
Tablet; Oral
  URSO
    + AXCAN SCANDIPHARM   250MG   N020675 001
                                                     DEC 10, 1997

VALACYCLOVIR HYDROCHLORIDE
Tablet; Oral
  VALTREX
  AB + GLAXOSMITHKLINE   EQ 1GM BASE   N020550 002
                                                         DEC 15, 1995
  AB   EQ 500MG BASE   N020550 001
                                                         DEC 15, 1995

VALDECOXIB
Tablet; Oral
  BEXTRA
    + GD SEARLE LLC   10MG   N021341 002
                                                     NOV 16, 2001
    +   20MG   N021341 003
                                                     NOV 16, 2001

VALGANCICLOVIR HYDROCHLORIDE
Tablet; Oral
  VALCYTE
    + ROCHE PALO   EQ 450MG BASE   N021304 001
                                                         MAR 29, 2001

VALPROATE SODIUM
Injectable; Injection
  DEPACON
  AP + ABBOTT   EQ 100MG BASE/ML N020593 001
                                                         DEC 30, 1996
  VALPROATE SODIUM
  AP   AM PHARM   EQ 100MG BASE/ML N076539 001
                                                         JUN 26, 2003
  AP   BEDFORD   EQ 100MG BASE/ML N076295 001
                                                         NOV 14, 2002

VALPROIC ACID
Capsule; Oral
  DEPAKENE
  AB + ABBOTT   250MG   N018081 001
  VALPROIC ACID
  AB   BANNER PHARMACAPS   250MG   N073484 001
                                                     JUN 29, 1993

Prescription Drug Products (continued)

VALPROIC ACID (continued)

Capsule; Oral

VALPROIC ACID

TE	Firm	Strength	Appl No	Date
AB	SCHERER RP	250MG	N073229 001	OCT 29, 1991
AB	USL PHARMA	250MG	N070631 001	JUN 11, 1987

Syrup; Oral

DEPAKENE

TE	Firm	Strength	Appl No	Date
AA +	ABBOTT	250MG/5ML	N018082 001	

MYPROIC ACID

TE	Firm	Strength	Appl No	Date
AA	MORTON GROVE	250MG/5ML	N070868 001	JUL 01, 1986

VALPROIC ACID

TE	Firm	Strength	Appl No	Date
AA	COPLEY PHARM	250MG/5ML	N073178 001	AUG 25, 1992
AA	HIGH TECH PHARMA	250MG/5ML	N074060 001	JAN 13, 1995
AA	PHARM ASSOC	250MG/5ML	N075379 001	DEC 15, 2000
AA	UDL	250MG/5ML	N075782 001	DEC 22, 2000

VALRUBICIN

Solution; Intravesical

VALSTAR PRESERVATIVE FREE

TE	Firm	Strength	Appl No	Date
+	ANTHRA	40MG/ML	N020892 001	SEP 25, 1998

VALSARTAN

Tablet; Oral

DIOVAN

TE	Firm	Strength	Appl No	Date
	NOVARTIS	80MG	N021283 001	JUL 18, 2001
		160MG	N021283 002	JUL 18, 2001
+		320MG	N021283 003	JUL 18, 2001

VALSARTAN *MULTIPLE*

SEE HYDROCHLOROTHIAZIDE; VALSARTAN

VANCOMYCIN HYDROCHLORIDE

Capsule; Oral

VANCOCIN HCL

TE	Firm	Strength	Appl No	Date
	LILLY	EQ 125MG BASE	N050606 001	APR 15, 1986
+		EQ 250MG BASE	N050606 002	APR 15, 1986

For Solution; Oral

VANCOCIN HCL

TE	Firm	Strength	Appl No	Date
+	LILLY	EQ 250MG BASE/5ML	N061667 002	JUL 13, 1983
+		EQ 500MG BASE/6ML	N061667 001	

VANCOMYCIN HYDROCHLORIDE (continued)

Injectable; Injection

VANCOCIN HCL

TE	Firm	Strength	Appl No	Date
AP +	LILLY	EQ 1GM BASE/VIAL	N060180 002	MAR 21, 1986
AP		EQ 1GM BASE/VIAL	N062476 002	MAR 21, 1986
AP		EQ 1GM BASE/VIAL	N062716 002	MAR 13, 1987
AP		EQ 1GM BASE/VIAL	N062812 002	NOV 17, 1987
AP +		EQ 10GM BASE/VIAL	N062812 003	NOV 17, 1987
AP +		EQ 500MG BASE/VIAL	N060180 001	MAR 15, 1984
AP +		EQ 500MG BASE/VIAL	N062476 001	MAR 15, 1984
AP		EQ 500MG BASE/VIAL	N062716 001	MAR 13, 1987
AP		EQ 500MG BASE/VIAL	N062812 001	NOV 17, 1987

VANCOCIN HCL IN PLASTIC CONTAINER

TE	Firm	Strength	Appl No	Date
+	BAXTER HLTHCARE	EQ 500MG BASE/100ML	N050671 001	APR 29, 1993

VANCOLED

TE	Firm	Strength	Appl No	Date
AP +	LEDERLE	EQ 1GM BASE/VIAL	N062682 002	MAR 30, 1988
AP +		EQ 2GM BASE/VIAL	N062682 003	MAY 11, 1988
AP		EQ 5GM BASE/VIAL	N062682 004	MAY 11, 1988
AP +		EQ 10GM BASE/VIAL	N062682 005	MAY 11, 1988
AP +		EQ 500MG BASE/VIAL	N062682 001	JUL 22, 1986

VANCOMYCIN HCL

TE	Firm	Strength	Appl No	Date
AP +	ABBOTT	EQ 1GM BASE/VIAL	N062912 001	AUG 04, 1988
AP		EQ 1GM BASE/VIAL	N062933 001	OCT 29, 1992
AP		EQ 5GM BASE/VIAL	N063076 001	DEC 21, 1990
AP +		EQ 500MG BASE/VIAL	N062911 001	AUG 04, 1988
AP		EQ 500MG BASE/VIAL	N062931 001	OCT 29, 1992
AP	AM PHARM PARTNERS	EQ 1GM BASE/VIAL	N062663 002	JUL 31, 1987
AP		EQ 5GM BASE/VIAL	N062663 003	JUN 03, 1988
AP		EQ 10GM BASE/VIAL	N062663 004	NOV 28, 1997
AP		EQ 500MG BASE/VIAL	N062663 001	MAR 17, 1987

Prescription Drug Products (continued)

VECURONIUM BROMIDE
Injectable; Injection

VECURONIUM BROMIDE

TE	Firm	Strength	Appl. No.	Date
	+ ABBOTT	4MG/VIAL	N075558 001	SEP 11, 2001
AP		10MG/VIAL	N075164 001	OCT 21, 1999
AP		20MG/VIAL	N075164 002	OCT 21, 1999
AP	+ BEDFORD	10MG/VIAL	N075549 001	JUN 13, 2000
AP		20MG/VIAL	N075549 002	JUN 13, 2000
AP	ESI LEDERLE	10MG/VIAL	N075218 001	AUG 23, 1999
AP		20MG/VIAL	N075218 002	AUG 23, 1999
AP	GENSIA	10MG/VIAL	N074688 001	AUG 25, 1999
AP		20MG/VIAL	N074688 002	AUG 25, 1999
AP	STERIS	10MG/VIAL	N074334 001	AUG 31, 1995
AP		20MG/VIAL	N074334 002	AUG 31, 1995

VENLAFAXINE HYDROCHLORIDE
Capsule, Extended Release; Oral

EFFEXOR XR

TE	Firm	Strength	Appl. No.	Date
	WYETH PHARMS INC	EQ 37.5MG BASE	N020699 001	OCT 20, 1997
		EQ 75MG BASE	N020699 002	OCT 20, 1997
		EQ 150MG BASE	N020699 004	OCT 20, 1997

Tablet; Oral

EFFEXOR

TE	Firm	Strength	Appl. No.	Date
	WYETH PHARMS INC	EQ 25MG BASE	N020151 002	DEC 28, 1993
		EQ 37.5MG BASE	N020151 006	DEC 28, 1993
		EQ 50MG BASE	N020151 003	DEC 28, 1993
		EQ 75MG BASE	N020151 004	DEC 28, 1993
+		EQ 100MG BASE	N020151 005	DEC 28, 1993

VERAPAMIL HYDROCHLORIDE
Capsule, Extended Release; Oral

VERAPAMIL HCL

TE	Firm	Strength	Appl. No.	Date
AB	MYLAN	120MG	N075138 001	APR 20, 1999
AB		180MG	N075138 002	APR 20, 1999
AB		240MG	N075138 003	APR 20, 1999

VERAPAMIL HYDROCHLORIDE (continued)
Capsule, Extended Release; Oral

VERAPAMIL HCL

TE	Firm	Strength	Appl. No.	Date
	MYLAN			APR 20, 1999

VERELAN

TE	Firm	Strength	Appl. No.	Date
AB	+ ELAN DRUG	120MG	N019614 001	MAY 29, 1990
AB	+	180MG	N019614 003	JAN 09, 1992
AB	+	240MG	N019614 002	MAY 29, 1990
	+	360MG	N019614 004	MAY 10, 1996

VERELAN PM

TE	Firm	Strength	Appl. No.	Date
	+ ELAN PHARM	100MG	N020943 001	NOV 25, 1998
	+	200MG	N020943 002	NOV 25, 1998
	+	300MG	N020943 003	NOV 25, 1998

Injectable; Injection

ISOPTIN

TE	Firm	Strength	Appl. No.	Date
AP	+ ABBOTT	2.5MG/ML	N018485 001	

VERAPAMIL HCL

TE	Firm	Strength	Appl. No.	Date
AP	+ ABBOTT	2.5MG/ML	N070577 001	FEB 02, 1987
AP		2.5MG/ML	N070737 001	MAY 06, 1987
AP		2.5MG/ML	N070738 001	MAY 06, 1987
AP		2.5MG/ML	N070739 001	MAY 06, 1987
AP		2.5MG/ML	N070740 001	MAY 06, 1987
AP	BEDFORD	2.5MG/ML	N075136 001	OCT 20, 1998
AP	INTL MEDICATION	2.5MG/ML	N072888 001	JUL 28, 1995
AP	LUITPOLD	2.5MG/ML	N070451 001	DEC 16, 1985
AP		2.5MG/ML	N070225 001	NOV 12, 1985
AP		2.5MG/ML	N070617 001	NOV 12, 1985

Tablet, Extended Release; Oral

COVERA-HS

TE	Firm	Strength	Appl. No.	Date
BC	+ GD SEARLE LLC	180MG	N020552 001	FEB 26, 1996
BC	+	240MG	N020552 002	FEB 26, 1996

ISOPTIN SR

TE	Firm	Strength	Appl. No.	Date
AB	+ ABBOTT	120MG	N019152 003	MAR 06, 1991
AB	+	180MG	N019152 002	DEC 15, 1989
AB	+	240MG	N019152 001	DEC 16, 1986

Prescription Drug Products (continued)

VERAPAMIL HYDROCHLORIDE (continued)

Tablet, Extended Release; Oral

VERAPAMIL HCL

IVAX PHARMS				
AB	120MG	N073568 002	OCT 10, 1997	
AB	180MG	N074330 001	JAN 31, 1994	
AB	240MG	N073568 001	JUL 31, 1992	
MYLAN				
AB	120MG	N074587 002	FEB 21, 1997	
AB	180MG	N074587 003	SEP 09, 1997	
AB	240MG	N074587 001	MAR 23, 1996	
PLIVA				
AB	240MG	N072922 001	MAR 01, 1996	

Tablet; Oral

CALAN

GD SEARLE LLC				
AB	40MG	N018817 003	FEB 23, 1988	
AB	80MG	N018817 001	SEP 10, 1984	
AB	120MG	N018817 002	SEP 10, 1984	

ISOPTIN

ABBOTT				
AB	40MG	N018593 003	NOV 23, 1987	
AB	80MG	N018593 001	MAR 08, 1982	
+ AB	120MG	N018593 002	MAR 08, 1982	

VERAPAMIL HCL

GENEVA PHARMS				
AB	40MG	N073168 001	JUL 31, 1992	
AB	80MG	N071423 001	MAY 24, 1988	
AB	120MG	N071424 001	MAY 25, 1988	
LEDERLE				
AB	80MG	N071880 001	APR 05, 1988	
AB	120MG	N071881 001	APR 05, 1988	
MUTUAL PHARM				
AB	80MG	N071488 001	JAN 13, 1988	
AB	120MG	N071489 001	JAN 13, 1988	
MYLAN				
AB	80MG	N071482 001	FEB 15, 1989	
AB	120MG	N071483 001	FEB 15, 1989	
PLIVA				
AB	40MG	N072751 001	FEB 23, 1996	
AB	80MG	N072124 001	JAN 26, 1989	
AB	120MG	N072125 001	JAN 26, 1989	

VERAPAMIL HYDROCHLORIDE (continued)

Tablet; Oral

VERAPAMIL HCL

PUREPAC PHARM				
AB	80MG	N071019 001	SEP 24, 1986	
AB	120MG	N070468 001	SEP 24, 1986	
WATSON LABS				
AB	40MG	N072923 001	JUN 29, 1993	
AB	40MG	N072924 001	JUN 29, 1993	
AB	80MG	N070855 001	SEP 24, 1986	
AB	80MG	N070995 001	OCT 01, 1986	
AB	80MG	N071366 001	OCT 01, 1986	
AB	120MG	N070856 001	SEP 24, 1986	
AB	120MG	N070994 001	OCT 01, 1986	
AB	120MG	N071367 001	OCT 01, 1986	

VERAPAMIL HYDROCHLORIDE *MULTIPLE*

SEE   TRANDOLAPRIL; VERAPAMIL HYDROCHLORIDE

VERTEPORFIN

Injectable; Injection

VISUDYNE

+	QLT	15MG/VIAL	N021119 001	APR 12, 2000

VINBLASTINE SULFATE

Injectable; Injection

VINBLASTINE SULFATE

+	AM PHARM PARTNERS	1MG/ML	N089515 001	APR 29, 1987
AP +	BEDFORD	10MG/VIAL	N089395 001	APR 09, 1987
AP	FAULDING	10MG/VIAL	N089565 001	AUG 18, 1987

VINCRISTINE SULFATE

Injectable; Injection

ONCOVIN

AP +	LILLY	1MG/ML	N014103 003	MAR 07, 1984
VINCASAR PFS				
AP	PHARMACIA AND UPJOHN	1MG/ML	N071426 001	JUL 17, 1987
VINCRISTINE SULFATE				
+	AM PHARM PARTNERS	1MG/ML	N076296 001	DEC 20, 2002

Prescription Drug Products *(continued)*

VINCRISTINE SULFATE *(continued)*
Injectable; Injection
VINCRISTINE SULFATE PFS
AP	FAULDING	1MG/ML	N071484 001	APR 19, 1988
AP	GENSIA SICOR PHARMS	1MG/ML	N075493 001	SEP 01, 1999

VINORELBINE TARTRATE
Injectable; Injection
NAVELBINE
AP	+ GLAXOSMITHKLINE	EQ 10MG BASE/ML	N020388 001	DEC 23, 1994

VINORELBINE TARTRATE
AP	ESI LEDERLE	EQ 10MG BASE/ML	N075992 001	JUN 10, 2003
AP	GENSIA SICOR PHARMS	EQ 10MG BASE/ML	N076028 001	FEB 03, 2003

VITAMIN A
Capsule; Oral
VITAMIN A
	+ WEST WARD	50,000 USP UNITS	N080985 001

VITAMIN A *MULTIPLE*
SEE ASCORBIC ACID; BIOTIN; CHOLECALCIFEROL; CYANOCOBALAMIN; DEXPANTHENOL; FOLIC ACID; NIACINAMIDE; PYRIDOXINE; RIBOFLAVIN; THIAMINE; TOCOPHEROL ACETATE; VITAMIN A; VITAMIN K

SEE ASCORBIC ACID; BIOTIN; CYANOCOBALAMIN; DEXPANTHENOL; ERGOCALCIFEROL; FOLIC ACID; NIACINAMIDE; PHYTONADIONE; PYRIDOXINE HYDROCHLORIDE; RIBOFLAVIN PHOSPHATE SODIUM; THIAMINE HYDROCHLORIDE; VITAMIN A; VITAMIN E

SEE ASCORBIC ACID; BIOTIN; CYANOCOBALAMIN; DEXPANTHENOL; ERGOCALCIFEROL; FOLIC ACID; NIACINAMIDE; PYRIDOXINE HYDROCHLORIDE; RIBOFLAVIN PHOSPHATE SODIUM; THIAMINE HYDROCHLORIDE; VITAMIN A; VITAMIN E

VITAMIN A PALMITATE
Capsule; Oral
VITAMIN A
AA	MK LABS	EQ 25,000 UNITS BASE	N083457 002
		EQ 50,000 UNITS BASE	N083457 001

VITAMIN A PALMITATE
AA	ARCUM	EQ 50,000 UNITS BASE	N083311 001
AA		EQ 50,000 UNITS BASE	N083321 001

Injectable; Injection
AQUASOL A
	+ AAIPHARMA	EQ 50,000 UNITS BASE/ML	N006823 001

VITAMIN A PALMITATE *MULTIPLE*
SEE ALPHA-TOCOPHEROL ACETATE; ASCORBIC ACID; BIOTIN; CHOLECALCIFEROL; CYANOCOBALAMIN; DEXPANTHENOL; FOLIC ACID; NIACINAMIDE; PYRIDOXINE HYDROCHLORIDE; RIBOFLAVIN PHOSPHATE SODIUM; THIAMINE HYDROCHLORIDE; VITAMIN A PALMITATE; VITAMIN K

VITAMIN E *MULTIPLE*
SEE ASCORBIC ACID; BIOTIN; CYANOCOBALAMIN; DEXPANTHENOL; ERGOCALCIFEROL; FOLIC ACID; NIACINAMIDE; PHYTONADIONE; PYRIDOXINE HYDROCHLORIDE; RIBOFLAVIN PHOSPHATE SODIUM; THIAMINE HYDROCHLORIDE; VITAMIN A; VITAMIN E

SEE ASCORBIC ACID; BIOTIN; CYANOCOBALAMIN; DEXPANTHENOL; ERGOCALCIFEROL; FOLIC ACID; NIACINAMIDE; PYRIDOXINE HYDROCHLORIDE; RIBOFLAVIN PHOSPHATE SODIUM; THIAMINE HYDROCHLORIDE; VITAMIN A; VITAMIN E

VITAMIN K *MULTIPLE*
SEE ALPHA-TOCOPHEROL ACETATE; ASCORBIC ACID; BIOTIN; CHOLECALCIFEROL; CYANOCOBALAMIN; DEXPANTHENOL; FOLIC ACID; NIACINAMIDE; PYRIDOXINE HYDROCHLORIDE; VITAMIN A PALMITATE; VITAMIN K

SEE ASCORBIC ACID; BIOTIN; CHOLECALCIFEROL; CYANOCOBALAMIN; DEXPANTHENOL; FOLIC ACID; NIACINAMIDE; PYRIDOXINE; RIBOFLAVIN; THIAMINE; TOCOPHEROL ACETATE; VITAMIN A; VITAMIN K

VORICONAZOLE
Injectable; Iv (Infusion)
VFEND
	+ PFIZER	200MG/VIAL	N021267 001	MAY 24, 2002

Tablet; Oral
VFEND
	PFIZER	50MG	N021266 001	MAY 24, 2002
		200MG	N021266 002	MAY 24, 2002

WARFARIN SODIUM
Injectable; Injection
COUMADIN
	+ BRISTOL MYERS SQUIBB	5MG/VIAL	N009218 024	FEB 07, 1995

Tablet; Oral
COUMADIN
	BRISTOL MYERS SQUIBB			
AB		1MG	N009218 022	MAR 01, 1990
AB		2.5MG	N009218 018	
AB		2MG	N009218 013	
AB		3MG	N009218 025	NOV 18, 1996
AB		4MG	N009218 023	AUG 24, 1993
AB		5MG	N009218 007	
AB		6MG	N009218 026	NOV 18, 1996
AB		7.5MG	N009218 016	
AB		10MG	N009218 005	

WARFARIN SODIUM
AB	BARR	1MG	N040145 001	MAR 26, 1997

Prescription Drug Products *(continued)*

WARFARIN SODIUM *(continued)*
Tablet; Oral

WARFARIN SODIUM

BARR

	Strength		Appl No	Date
AB	2.5MG		N040145 003	MAR 26, 1997
AB	2MG		N040145 002	MAR 26, 1997
AB	3MG		N040145 008	NOV 05, 1998
AB	4MG		N040145 004	MAR 26, 1997
AB	5MG		N040145 005	MAR 26, 1997
AB	6MG		N040145 009	NOV 05, 1998
AB	7.5MG		N040145 006	MAR 26, 1997
AB	10MG		N040145 007	MAR 26, 1997

GENEVA PHARMS TECH

	Strength		Appl No	Date
AB	1MG		N040196 001	SEP 30, 1997
AB	2.5MG		N040196 003	SEP 30, 1997
AB	2MG		N040196 002	SEP 30, 1997
AB	3MG		N040196 008	JUL 26, 2000
AB	4MG		N040196 004	SEP 30, 1997
AB	5MG		N040196 005	SEP 30, 1997
AB	6MG		N040196 009	JUL 26, 2000
AB	7.5MG		N040196 006	SEP 30, 1997
AB	10MG		N040196 007	SEP 30, 1997

TARO

	Strength		Appl No	Date
AB	1MG		N040301 002	JUL 15, 1999
AB	2.5MG		N040301 004	JUL 15, 1999
AB	2MG		N040301 003	JUL 15, 1999
AB	3MG		N040301 005	JUL 15, 1999
AB	4MG		N040301 006	JUL 15, 1999
AB	5MG		N040301 007	JUL 15, 1999
AB	6MG		N040301 008	JUL 15, 1999
AB	7.5MG		N040301 009	JUL 15, 1999
AB	10MG		N040301 001	JUL 15, 1999

WATER FOR INJECTION, STERILE
Liquid; N/A

BACTERIOSTATIC WATER FOR INJECTION IN PLASTIC CONTAINER

	Firm	Strength	Appl No	Date
AP	ABBOTT	100%	N018802 001	OCT 27, 1982

STERILE WATER FOR INJECTION IN PLASTIC CONTAINER

	Firm	Strength	Appl No	Date
AP	ABBOTT	100%	N018233 001	
AP		100%	N018801 001	OCT 27, 1982
AP		100%	N019869 001	DEC 26, 1989
AP	AM PHARM PARTNERS	100%	N088400 001	JAN 16, 1984
AP	B BRAUN	100%	N019077 001	MAR 02, 1984
AP		100%	N019633 001	FEB 29, 1988
AP	BAXTER HLTHCARE	100%	N018632 001	JUN 30, 1982
AP		100%	N018632 002	APR 19, 1988

WATER FOR IRRIGATION, STERILE
Liquid; Irrigation

STERILE WATER

	Firm	Strength	Appl No	Date
AT	BAXTER HLTHCARE	100%	N017428 001	

STERILE WATER IN PLASTIC CONTAINER

	Firm	Strength	Appl No	Date
AT	ABBOTT	100%	N017513 001	
AT	B BRAUN	100%	N016734 001	
AT	BAXTER HLTHCARE	100%	N017866 001	

XENON, XE-133
Gas; Inhalation

XENON XE 133

	Firm	Strength	Appl No	Date
AA	BRISTOL MYERS SQUIBB	10mCi/VIAL	N017284 001	
AA		20mCi/VIAL	N017284 002	
AA	GEN ELECTRIC	1-2.5 CI/AMP	N017550 003	
AA		5 CI/CYLINDER	N017550 001	
AA	MALLINCKRODT	10mCi/VIAL	N018327 001	MAR 09, 1982
AA		20mCi/VIAL	N018327 002	MAR 09, 1982

ZAFIRLUKAST
Tablet; Oral

ACCOLATE

ASTRAZENECA

	Strength	Appl No	Date
AB	10MG	N020547 003	SEP 17, 1999
+ AB	20MG	N020547 001	SEP 26, 1996

Prescription Drug Products (continued)

ZALCITABINE
Tablet; Oral
 HIVID
 + ROCHE
	0.75MG	N020199 002	JUN 19, 1992
	0.375MG	N020199 001	JUN 19, 1992

ZALEPLON
Capsule; Oral
 SONATA
 JONES PHARMA
 +
	5MG	N020859 001	AUG 13, 1999
	10MG	N020859 002	AUG 13, 1999

ZANAMIVIR
Capsule; Inhalation
 RELENZA
 + GLAXOSMITHKLINE
	5MG	N021036 001	JUL 26, 1999

ZIDOVUDINE
Capsule; Oral
 RETROVIR
 + GLAXOSMITHKLINE
	100MG	N019655 001	MAR 19, 1987

Injectable; Injection
 RETROVIR
 + GLAXOSMITHKLINE
	10MG/ML	N019951 001	FEB 02, 1990

Syrup; Oral
 RETROVIR
 GLAXOSMITHKLINE
	50MG/5ML	N019910 001	SEP 28, 1989

Tablet; Oral
 RETROVIR
 + GLAXOSMITHKLINE
	300MG	N020518 002	OCT 04, 1996

ZIDOVUDINE *MULTIPLE*
SEE ABACAVIR SULFATE; LAMIVUDINE; ZIDOVUDINE
SEE LAMIVUDINE; ZIDOVUDINE

ZILEUTON
Tablet; Oral
 ZYFLO
 + ABBOTT
	600MG	N020471 003	DEC 09, 1996

ZINC ACETATE
Capsule; Oral
 GALZIN
 TEVA
	EQ 25MG ZINC	N020458 001	

ZINC ACETATE *(continued)*
Capsule; Oral
 GALZIN
 TEVA
 +
	EQ 50MG ZINC	N020458 002	JAN 28, 1997
			JAN 28, 1997

ZINC CHLORIDE
Injectable; Injection
 ZINC CHLORIDE IN PLASTIC CONTAINER
 + ABBOTT
	EQ 1MG ZINC/ML	N018959 001	JUN 26, 1986

ZIPRASIDONE HYDROCHLORIDE
Capsule; Oral
 GEODON
 PFIZER
 +
	20MG	N020825 001	FEB 05, 2001
	40MG	N020825 002	FEB 05, 2001
	60MG	N020825 003	FEB 05, 2001
	80MG	N020825 004	FEB 05, 2001

ZIPRASIDONE MESYLATE
Injectable; Intramuscular
 GEODON
 + PFIZER
	EQ 20MG BASE/ML	N020919 001	JUN 21, 2002

ZOLEDRONIC ACID
Injectable; Iv (Infusion)
 ZOMETA
 + NOVARTIS
 +
	EQ 4MG BASE/5ML	N021223 002	MAR 07, 2003
	EQ 4MG BASE/VIAL	N021223 001	AUG 20, 2001

ZOLMITRIPTAN
Tablet; Orally Disintegrating; Oral
 ZOMIG-ZMT
 ASTRAZENECA
 +
	2.5MG	N021231 001	FEB 13, 2001
	5MG	N021231 002	SEP 17, 2001

Tablet; Oral
 ZOMIG
 IPR
 +
	2.5MG	N020768 001	NOV 25, 1997
	5MG	N020768 002	NOV 25, 1997

Prescription Drug Products *(continued)*

ZOLPIDEM TARTRATE
Tablet; Oral
AMBIEN
  LOREX

	5MG	N019908 001 DEC 16, 1992
+	10MG	N019908 002 DEC 16, 1992

ZONISAMIDE
Capsule; Oral
ZONEGRAN
+   DAINIPPON

	100MG	N020798 001 MAR 27, 2000

OTC DRUG PRODUCTS

ACETAMINOPHEN
Suppository; Rectal

ACEPHEN

	Strength	NDA	Date
G AND W LABS	120MG	N018060 001	
	120MG	N072218 001	MAR 27, 1992
	325MG	N018060 003	DEC 18, 1986
	325MG	N072344 001	MAR 27, 1992
	650MG	N018060 002	
	650MG	N072237 001	MAR 27, 1992

ACETAMINOPHEN

	Strength	NDA	Date
ALPHARMA US PHARM	120MG	N018337 003	SEP 12, 1983
+ SUPPOSITORIA	325MG	N018337 002	
	650MG	N018337 001	
	120MG	N070607 001	APR 06, 1987
	650MG	N070608 001	DEC 01, 1986

INFANTS' FEVERALL

	Strength	NDA	Date
ALPHARMA US PHARM	80MG	N018337 004	AUG 26, 1992

NEOPAP

	Strength	NDA	Date
POLYMEDICA	120MG	N016401 001	

Tablet, Extended Release; Oral

ACETAMINOPHEN

	Strength	NDA	Date
COREPHARMA	650MG	N076200 001	MAR 19, 2002
	650MG	N075077 001	FEB 25, 2000
PERRIGO	650MG	N019872 001	JUN 08, 1994

TYLENOL (CAPLET)

	Strength	NDA	Date
+ MCNEIL CONS SPECLT	650MG	N019872 002	JAN 11, 2001

TYLENOL (GELTAB)

	Strength	NDA	Date
+ MCNEIL CONS SPECLT	650MG		

ACETAMINOPHEN; ASPIRIN; CAFFEINE
Tablet; Oral

ACETAMINOPHEN, ASPIRIN AND CAFFEINE

	Strength	NDA	Date
PERRIGO	250MG;250MG;65MG	N075794 001	NOV 26, 2001

EXCEDRIN (MIGRAINE)

	Strength	NDA	Date
+ BRISTOL MYERS	250MG;250MG;65MG	N020802 001	JAN 14, 1998

ACETAMINOPHEN; CLEMASTINE FUMARATE; PSEUDOEPHEDRINE HYDROCHLORIDE
Tablet; Oral

TAVIST ALLERGY/SINUS/HEADACHE

	Strength	NDA	Date
+ NOVARTIS	500MG;EQ 0.25MG BASE;30MG	N021082 001	MAR 01, 2001

ACETAMINOPHEN; DEXBROMPHENIRAMINE MALEATE; PSEUDOEPHEDRINE SULFATE
Tablet, Extended Release; Oral

DRIXORAL PLUS

	Strength	NDA	Date
+ SCHERING PLOUGH	500MG;3MG;60MG	N019453 001	MAY 22, 1987

ALCOHOL; CHLORHEXIDINE GLUCONATE
Solution; Topical

AVAGARD

	Strength	NDA	Date
+ 3M	61%;1%	N021074 001	JUN 07, 2001

ALUMINUM HYDROXIDE; MAGNESIUM TRISILICATE
Tablet, Chewable; Oral

FOAMCOAT

	Strength	NDA	Date
GUARDIAN DRUG	80MG;20MG	N071793 001	SEP 04, 1987

FOAMICON

	Strength	NDA	Date
NOVARTIS	80MG;20MG	N072687 001	JUN 28, 1989

GAVISCON

	Strength	NDA	Date
AVENTIS PHARMS	80MG;20MG	N018685 001	DEC 09, 1983
+	160MG;40MG	N018685 002	DEC 09, 1983

ANTAZOLINE PHOSPHATE; NAPHAZOLINE HYDROCHLORIDE
Solution/Drops; Ophthalmic

VASOCON-A

	Strength	NDA	Date
+ NOVARTIS	0.5%;0.05%	N018746 002	JUL 11, 1994

ASPIRIN
Tablet; Oral

BAYER EXTRA STRENGTH ASPIRIN FOR MIGRAINE PAIN

	Strength	NDA	Date
+ BAYER	500MG	N021317 001	OCT 18, 2001

ASPIRIN *MULTIPLE*
SEE ACETAMINOPHEN; ASPIRIN; CAFFEINE

AVOBENZONE; OCTYL METHOXYCINNAMATE; OXYBENZONE
Lotion; Topical

SHADE UVAGUARD

	Strength	NDA	Date
+ SCHERING PLOUGH	3%;7.5%;3%	N020045 001	DEC 07, 1992

BACITRACIN
Ointment; Topical

BACITRACIN

	Strength	NDA	Date
+ NASKA	500 UNITS/GM	N062857 001	NOV 13, 1987

OTC Drug Products (continued)

BACITRACIN ZINC; NEOMYCIN SULFATE; POLYMYXIN B SULFATE
Ointment; Topical
BACITRACIN ZINC-NEOMYCIN SULFATE-POLYMYXIN B SULFATE
400 UNITS/GM;EQ 3.5MG BASE/GM;5,000 UNITS/GM
+ NASKA   N062833 001   NOV 09, 1987

BACITRACIN ZINC; POLYMYXIN B SULFATE
Ointment; Topical
BACITRACIN ZINC-POLYMYXIN B SULFATE
500 UNITS/GM;10,000 UNITS/GM
+ NASKA   N062849 001   NOV 13, 1987

BENTOQUATAM
Lotion; Topical
IVY BLOCK   5%
+ ENVIRODERM   N020532 001   AUG 26, 1996

BROMPHENIRAMINE MALEATE; PHENYLPROPANOLAMINE HYDROCHLORIDE
Elixir; Oral
DIMETAPP   2MG/5ML;12.5MG/5ML
+ WYETH CONS   N013087 003   MAR 29, 1984
Tablet, Extended Release; Oral
DIMETAPP   12MG;75MG
+ WYETH CONS   N012436 003   MAY 14, 1985

BROMPHENIRAMINE MALEATE; PSEUDOEPHEDRINE HYDROCHLORIDE
Tablet, Extended Release; Oral
EFIDAC 24 PSEUDOEPHEDRINE HCL/BROMPHENIRAMINE MALEATE
16MG;240MG
+ ALZA   N019672 001   MAR 29, 1996

BUTENAFINE HYDROCHLORIDE
Cream; Topical
LOTRIMIN ULTRA   1%
+ SCHERING PLOUGH   N021307 001   DEC 07, 2001

BUTOCONAZOLE NITRATE
Cream; Vaginal
FEMSTAT 3   2%
+ ROCHE PALO   N020421 001   DEC 21, 1995

CAFFEINE *MULTIPLE*
SEE   ACETAMINOPHEN; ASPIRIN; CAFFEINE

CALCIUM CARBONATE, PRECIPITATED; FAMOTIDINE; MAGNESIUM HYDROXIDE
Tablet, Chewable; Oral
PEPCID COMPLETE   800MG;10MG;165MG
+ MERCK   N020958 001   OCT 16, 2000

CHLORHEXIDINE GLUCONATE
Aerosol, Metered; Topical
EXIDINE   4%
+ XTTRIUM   N019127 001   DEC 24, 1984

Solution; Topical
BRIAN CARE   4%
SOAPCO   N071419 001   DEC 17, 1987
CHG SCRUB   4%
ECOLAB   N019258 002   JUL 22, 1986
CHLORAPREP ONE-STEP SEPP   2%
+ BECKLOFF   N021555 001   OCT 07, 2002
CIDA-STAT   2%
ECOLAB   N019258 001   JUL 22, 1986
DYNA-HEX   0.75%
XTTRIUM   N020111 001   SEP 11, 1997
EXIDINE   2%
+ XTTRIUM   N019422 001   DEC 17, 1985
    N019125 001   DEC 24, 1984
  4%
HIBICLENS   4%
+ SSL INTL   N017768 001
HIBISTAT   0.5%
+ SSL INTL   N018300 001
MICRODERM   4%
J AND J   N072255 001   APR 15, 1991
PREVACARE R   0.5%
J AND J   N072292 001   JAN 28, 1992
STERI-STAT   4%
MATRIX MEDCL   N070104 001   JUL 24, 1986

Sponge; Topical
BIOSCRUB   4%
GRIFFEN   N019822 001   MAR 31, 1989

CHLORHEXIDINE GLUCONATE*
DESERET   4%
    N072525 001   OCT 24, 1989
KENDALL IL   4%
    N019490 001   MAR 27, 1987

OTC Drug Products *(continued)*

CHLORHEXIDINE GLUCONATE *(continued)*
Sponge; Topical

HIBICLENS
+ SSL INTL   4%   N018423 001

MICRODERM
J AND J   4%   N072295 001
                                               FEB 28, 1991

PHARMASEAL SCRUB CARE
PHARMASEAL   4%   N019793 001
                                               DEC 02, 1988

CHLORHEXIDINE GLUCONATE; ISOPROPYL ALCOHOL
Sponge; Topical

CHLORAPREP
+ MEDI FLEX HOSP   2%;70%   N020832 001
                                               JUL 14, 2000

CHLORHEXIDINE GLUCONATE *MULTIPLE*
SEE ALCOHOL; CHLORHEXIDINE GLUCONATE

CHLORPHENIRAMINE MALEATE
Capsule, Extended Release; Oral

CHLORPHENIRAMINE MALEATE
+ GENEVA PHARMS   12MG   N070797 001
                                               AUG 12, 1988

Tablet, Extended Release; Oral

CHLOR-TRIMETON
+ SCHERING PLOUGH   8MG   N007638 001
                               12MG   N007638 002

EFIDAC 24 CHLORPHENIRAMINE MALEATE
ALZA   16MG   N019746 002
                                               NOV 18, 1994

CHLORPHENIRAMINE MALEATE; IBUPROFEN; PSEUDOEPHEDRINE HYDROCHLORIDE
Tablet; Oral

ADVIL ALLERGY SINUS
+ WYETH CONS   2MG;200MG;30MG N021441 001
                                               DEC 19, 2002

CHLORPHENIRAMINE MALEATE; PHENYLPROPANOLAMINE HYDROCHLORIDE
Tablet, Extended Release; Oral

CONTAC
+ NOVARTIS   12MG;75MG   N019613 001
                                               JUN 13, 1986

DEMAZIN
+ SCHERING PLOUGH   4MG;25MG   N018556 001
                                               MAY 14, 1984

CHLORPHENIRAMINE MALEATE; PSEUDOEPHEDRINE SULFATE
Tablet, Extended Release; Oral

CHLOR-TRIMETON
+ SCHERING PLOUGH   8MG;120MG   N018397 001

CIMETIDINE
Tablet; Oral

CIMETIDINE
IVAX PHARMS   200MG   N075345 001
                                               JUN 16, 1999
                                               N074961 001
LEINER   200MG   JUN 19, 1998
                                               N075122 002
LEK PHARMS   200MG   JUN 19, 1998
                                               N075285 001
PERRIGO   200MG   JUN 19, 1998
                                               OCT 29, 1998
PHARM FORM   200MG   N074963 001
                                               JUN 19, 1998
TORPHARM   100MG   N074948 001
                                               JUN 19, 1998
                               200MG   N074948 002
                                               JUL 26, 2002
WATSON LABS   200MG   N075425 001
                                               JUL 29, 1999
TAGAMET HB
+ GLAXOSMITHKLINE   200MG   N020238 002
                                               AUG 21, 1996

CLEMASTINE FUMARATE
Tablet; Oral

CLEMASTINE FUMARATE
GENEVA PHARMS   1.34MG   N073458 001
                                               OCT 31, 1993
PERRIGO   1.34MG   N074512 001
                                               NOV 22, 1995
TEVA   1.34MG   N073282 002
                                               DEC 03, 1992
TAVIST-1
+ NOVARTIS   1.34MG   N020925 001
                                               AUG 21, 1992

CLEMASTINE FUMARATE *MULTIPLE*
SEE ACETAMINOPHEN; CLEMASTINE FUMARATE; PSEUDOEPHEDRINE HYDROCHLORIDE

CLOTRIMAZOLE
Cream, Tablet; Topical, Vaginal

GYNE-LOTRIMIN 3 COMBINATION PACK
+ SCHERING PLOUGH   1%;200MG   N020526 002
                                               JUL 29, 1996
GYNE-LOTRIMIN COMBINATION PACK
+ SCHERING PLOUGH   1%;100MG   N020289 002
                                               APR 26, 1993
MYCELEX-7 COMBINATION PACK
BAYER PHARMS   1%;100MG   N020389 002

OTC Drug Products *(continued)*

CLOTRIMAZOLE *(continued)*

Cream, Tablet; Topical, Vaginal

MYCELEX-7 COMBINATION PACK
  BAYER PHARMS — JUN 23, 1994

Cream; Vaginal

CLOTRIMAZOLE
  ALPHARMA US PHARM — 1% — N074165 001 — JUL 16, 1993
  TARO — 1% — N072641 001 — DEC 04, 1995

GYNE-LOTRIMIN
  + SCHERING PLOUGH — 1% — N018052 002 — NOV 30, 1990

GYNE-LOTRIMIN 3
  + SCHERING PLOUGH — 2% — N020574 001 — NOV 24, 1998

MYCELEX-7
  BAYER PHARMS — 1% — N018230 002 — DEC 26, 1991

TRIVAGIZOLE 3
  TARO — 2% — N021143 001 — APR 12, 2000

Tablet; Vaginal

GYNE-LOTRIMIN
  + SCHERING PLOUGH — 100MG — N017717 002 — NOV 30, 1990

GYNE-LOTRIMIN 3
  + SCHERING PLOUGH — 200MG — N020525 001 — JUL 29, 1996

GYNIX
  COPLEY PHARM — 100MG — N073249 001 — FEB 13, 1998

MYCELEX-7
  BAYER PHARMS — 100MG — N018182 002 — DEC 26, 1991

CROMOLYN SODIUM

Spray, Metered; Nasal

CROMOLYN SODIUM
  ALPHARMA — 5.2MG/INH — N074800 001 — JUL 26, 2001
  BAUSCH AND LOMB — 5.2MG/SPRAY — N075702 001 — JUL 03, 2001
  PERRIGO — 5.2MG/SPRAY — N075427 001 — DEC 12, 2001

NASALCROM
  + PHARMACIA UPJOHN — 5.2MG/SPRAY — N020463 001 — JAN 03, 1997

DEXBROMPHENIRAMINE MALEATE; PSEUDOEPHEDRINE SULFATE

Tablet, Extended Release; Oral

BROMPHERIL
  COPLEY PHARM — 6MG;120MG — N089116 001 — JAN 22, 1987

DEXBROMPHENIRAMINE MALEATE; PSEUDOEPHEDRINE SULFATE *(continued)*

Tablet, Extended Release; Oral

DISOPHROL
  SCHERING PLOUGH — 6MG;120MG — N013483 004 — SEP 13, 1982

DRIXORAL
  + SCHERING PLOUGH — 6MG;120MG — N013483 003 — SEP 13, 1982

DEXBROMPHENIRAMINE MALEATE *MULTIPLE*

SEE ACETAMINOPHEN; DEXBROMPHENIRAMINE MALEATE; PSEUDOEPHEDRINE SULFATE

DEXTROMETHORPHAN POLISTIREX

Suspension, Extended Release; Oral

DELSYM
  + CELLTECH PHARMS — EQ 30MG HBR/5ML — N018658 001 — OCT 08, 1982

DOCOSANOL

Cream; Topical

ABREVA
  + GLAXOSMITHKLINE — 10% — N020941 001 — JUL 25, 2000

DOXYLAMINE SUCCINATE

Tablet; Oral

DOXYLAMINE SUCCINATE
  COPLEY PHARM — 25MG — N088900 002 — FEB 12, 1988
  PERRIGO — 25MG — N040167 001 — SEP 18, 1996

UNISOM
  + PFIZER — 25MG — N018066 001

EPINEPHRINE

Aerosol, Metered; Inhalation

EPINEPHRINE
  ALPHARMA — 0.2MG/INH — N087907 001 — MAY 23, 1984

PRIMATENE MIST
  + WHITEHALL ROBINS — 0.2MG/INH — N016126 001

EPINEPHRINE BITARTRATE

Aerosol, Metered; Inhalation

BRONITIN MIST
  WHITEHALL ROBINS — 0.3MG/INH — N016126 002

FAMOTIDINE

Tablet, Chewable; Oral

PEPCID AC
  + MERCK — 10MG — N020801 001 — SEP 24, 1998

OTC Drug Products (continued)

FAMOTIDINE (continued)

Tablet; Oral

FAMOTIDINE			
DR REDDYS LABS LTD	10MG	N075758 001	AUG 17, 2001
EON	10MG	N076101 001	OCT 21, 2002
GENPHARM	10MG	N075674 001	DEC 21, 2001
IVAX PHARMS	10MG	N075512 001	JUL 26, 2001
TEVA	10MG	N075312 001	MAY 31, 2001
TORPHARM	10MG	N076510 001	MAR 12, 2002
WATSON LABS	10MG	N075404 001	NOV 28, 2001
PEPCID AC			
+ MERCK	10MG	N020325 001	APR 28, 1995
	10MG	N020902 001	AUG 05, 1999

FAMOTIDINE *MULTIPLE*

SEE   CALCIUM CARBONATE, PRECIPITATED; FAMOTIDINE; MAGNESIUM HYDROXIDE

GUAIFENESIN

Tablet, Extended Release; Oral

MUCINEX			
+ ADAMS LABS	1.2GM	N021282 002	DEC 18, 2002
	600MG	N021282 001	JUL 12, 2002

IBUPROFEN

Capsule; Oral

IBUPROFEN			
BANNER PHARMACAPS	200MG	N021472 001	OCT 18, 2002
+ PHARM FORM	200MG	N074782 001	JUL 06, 1998

Suspension/Drops; Oral

CHILDREN'S MOTRIN			
+ MCNEIL	40MG/ML	N020603 001	JUN 10, 1996
IBUPROFEN			
PERRIGO	40MG/ML	N075217 001	DEC 16, 1998
PEDIATRIC ADVIL			
+ WYETH CONS	100MG/2.5ML	N020812 001	JAN 30, 1998

Suspension; Oral

CHILDREN'S ADVIL			
WYETH CONS	100MG/5ML	N020589 001	

IBUPROFEN (continued)

Suspension; Oral

CHILDREN'S ADVIL			
WYETH CONS			JUN 27, 1996
CHILDREN'S ADVIL-FLAVORED			
WYETH CONS	100MG/5ML	N020589 002	NOV 07, 1997
CHILDREN'S IBUPROFEN			
PERRIGO	100MG/5ML	N074937 001	DEC 22, 1998
CHILDREN'S MOTRIN			
+ MCNEIL	100MG/5ML	N020516 001	JUN 16, 1995
IBUPROFEN			
ALPHARMA	100MG/5ML	N074916 001	APR 30, 1999

Tablet, Chewable; Oral

CHILDREN'S ADVIL			
WYETH CONS	50MG	N020944 001	DEC 18, 1998
CHILDREN'S MOTRIN			
MCNEIL	50MG	N020601 001	NOV 15, 1996
JUNIOR STRENGTH ADVIL			
WYETH CONS	100MG	N020944 002	DEC 18, 1998
JUNIOR STRENGTH MOTRIN			
+ MCNEIL	100MG	N020601 003	NOV 15, 1996

Tablet; Oral

ADVIL			
WYETH CONS	200MG	N018989 001	MAY 18, 1984
CAP-PROFEN			
PERRIGO	200MG	N072097 001	DEC 08, 1987
IBU-TAB 200			
ALRA	200MG	N071057 001	AUG 11, 1988
IBUPROFEN			
BASF	200MG	N075661 001	DEC 12, 2001
DR REDDYS LABS INC	100MG	N076117 001	NOV 20, 2001
GENEVA PHARMS	200MG	N070733 001	SEP 19, 1986
INTERPHARM	200MG	N071333 001	FEB 17, 1987
	200MG	N072199 001	MAY 23, 1988
INVAMED	200MG	N071807 001	FEB 25, 1988
	200MG	N074525 001	DEC 15, 1995
	200MG	N074533 001	DEC 15, 1995

OTC Drug Products (continued)

IBUPROFEN (continued)

Tablet; Oral

IBUPROFEN

Firm	Strength	Application	Date
IVAX PHARMS	200MG	N071144 001	JAN 20, 1987
	200MG	N072901 001	DEC 19, 1991
	200MG	N072903 001	DEC 19, 1991
LEINER	200MG	N074931 001	JUL 20, 1998
LNK	200MG	N075010 001	MAR 01, 1999
	200MG	N075139 001	MAR 01, 1999
MCNEIL	200MG	N073019 001	MAR 30, 1994
MUTUAL PHARM	200MG	N071229 001	APR 01, 1987
	200MG	N072249 001	JAN 10, 1989
MYLAN	200MG	N071870 001	MAY 05, 1988
OHM	200MG	N071163 001	JUL 15, 1986
	200MG	N070481 001	SEP 24, 1986
PAR PHARM	200MG	N070985 001	OCT 02, 1987
	200MG	N071575 001	MAY 08, 1987
PERRIGO	200MG	N072096 001	DEC 08, 1987
	200MG	N072098 001	DEC 08, 1987
	200MG	N075995 001	MAR 14, 2002
PVT FORM	200MG	N071732 001	SEP 10, 1987
	200MG	N071735 001	SEP 10, 1987
	200MG	N072299 001	JUL 01, 1988
	200MG	N073691 001	FEB 25, 1994
VINTAGE PHARMS	200MG	N071639 001	FEB 02, 1988
WATSON LABS	200MG	N070435 001	MAR 05, 1986

IBUPROHM

Firm	Strength	Application	Date
OHM LABS	200MG	N071214 001	DEC 01, 1986

JUNIOR STRENGTH ADVIL

Firm	Strength	Application	Date
WYETH CONS	100MG	N020267 002	DEC 13, 1996

JUNIOR STRENGTH IBUPROFEN

Firm	Strength	Application	Date
PERRIGO	100MG	N075367 001	

IBUPROFEN (continued)

Tablet; Oral

JUNIOR STRENGTH IBUPROFEN

Firm	Strength	Application	Date
PERRIGO			APR 22, 1999

JUNIOR STRENGTH MOTRIN

Firm	Strength	Application	Date
MCNEIL	100MG	N020602 001	JUN 10, 1996

MEDIPREN

Firm	Strength	Application	Date
MCNEIL	200MG	N070475 001	FEB 06, 1986
MCNEIL	200MG	N071215 001	JUN 26, 1986

MOTRIN IB

Firm	Strength	Application	Date
+ MCNEIL	200MG	N019012 003	DEC 17, 1990

MOTRIN MIGRAINE PAIN

Firm	Strength	Application	Date
+ MCNEIL	200MG	N019012 004	FEB 25, 2000

PROFEN

Firm	Strength	Application	Date
PVT FORM	200MG	N071265 001	OCT 15, 1986

TAB-PROFEN

Firm	Strength	Application	Date
PERRIGO	200MG	N072095 001	DEC 08, 1987

IBUPROFEN; PSEUDOEPHEDRINE HYDROCHLORIDE

Capsule; Oral

ADVIL COLD AND SINUS

Firm	Strength	Application	Date
WYETH CONS	200MG;30MG	N021374 001	MAY 30, 2002

Suspension; Oral

CHILDREN'S ADVIL COLD

Firm	Strength	Application	Date
WYETH CONS	100MG/5ML;15MG/5ML	N021373 001	APR 18, 2002

CHILDREN'S MOTRIN COLD

Firm	Strength	Application	Date
+ MCNEIL CONS SPECLT	100MG/5ML;15MG/5ML	N021128 001	AUG 01, 2000

Tablet; Oral

ADVIL COLD AND SINUS

Firm	Strength	Application	Date
+ WYETH CONS	200MG;30MG	N019771 001	SEP 19, 1989

IBUPROFEN AND PSEUDOEPHEDRINE HCL

Firm	Strength	Application	Date
PHARM FORM	200MG;30MG	N075588 001	APR 08, 2002

IBUPROHM COLD AND SINUS

Firm	Strength	Application	Date
OHM LABS	200MG;30MG	N074567 001	APR 17, 2001

SINE-AID IB

Firm	Strength	Application	Date
MCNEIL CONS SPECLT	200MG;30MG	N019899 001	DEC 31, 1992

IBUPROFEN *MULTIPLE*

SEE CHLORPHENIRAMINE MALEATE; IBUPROFEN; PSEUDOEPHEDRINE HYDROCHLORIDE

OTC Drug Products *(continued)*

IBUPROFEN POTASSIUM
Capsule; Oral

ADVIL LIQUI-GELS	200MG	
+ WYETH CONS		N020402 001 APR 20, 1995
ADVIL MIGRAINE LIQUI-GELS	200MG	
+ WYETH CONS		N020402 002 MAR 16, 2000

INSULIN PURIFIED PORK
Injectable; Injection

REGULAR ILETIN II (PORK)		
+ LILLY	100 UNITS/ML	N018344 001

INSULIN RECOMBINANT HUMAN
Injectable; Injection

HUMULIN R		
+ LILLY	100 UNITS/ML	N018780 001 OCT 28, 1982
HUMULIN R PEN		
+ LILLY	100 UNITS/ML	N018780 005 AUG 06, 1998
NOVOLIN R		
+ NOVO NORDISK	100 UNITS/ML	N019938 001 JUN 25, 1991
VELOSULIN BR		
+ NOVO NORDISK	100 UNITS/ML	N021028 001 JUL 19, 1999

INSULIN RECOMBINANT HUMAN; INSULIN SUSP ISOPHANE RECOMBINANT HUMAN
Injectable; Injection

HUMULIN 50/50		
+ LILLY	50 UNITS/ML;50 UNITS/ML	N020100 001 APR 29, 1992
HUMULIN 70/30		
+ LILLY	30 UNITS/ML;70 UNITS/ML	N019717 001 APR 25, 1989
HUMULIN 70/30 PEN		
+ LILLY	30 UNITS/ML;70 UNITS/ML	N019717 002 AUG 06, 1998
NOVOLIN 70/30		
+ NOVO NORDISK	30 UNITS/ML;70 UNITS/ML	N019991 001 JUN 25, 1991

INSULIN SUSP ISOPHANE BEEF
Injectable; Injection

NPH INSULIN		
+ NOVO NORDISK	100 UNITS/ML	N017929 003

INSULIN SUSP ISOPHANE BEEF/PORK
Injectable; Injection

NPH ILETIN I (BEEF-PORK)		
+ LILLY	100 UNITS/ML	N017936 002

INSULIN SUSP ISOPHANE PURIFIED PORK
Injectable; Injection

NPH ILETIN II (PORK)		
+ LILLY	100 UNITS/ML	N018345 001

INSULIN SUSP ISOPHANE RECOMBINANT HUMAN
Injectable; Injection

HUMULIN N		
+ LILLY	100 UNITS/ML	N018781 001 OCT 28, 1982
NOVOLIN N		
+ NOVO NORDISK	100 UNITS/ML	N019959 001 JUL 01, 1991

INSULIN SUSP ISOPHANE RECOMBINANT HUMAN *MULTIPLE*
SEE INSULIN RECOMBINANT HUMAN; INSULIN SUSP ISOPHANE RECOMBINANT HUMAN

INSULIN ZINC SUSP EXTENDED RECOMBINANT HUMAN
Injectable; Injection

HUMULIN U		
+ LILLY	100 UNITS/ML	N019571 002 JUN 10, 1987

INSULIN ZINC SUSP PURIFIED PORK
Injectable; Injection

LENTE ILETIN II (PORK)		
+ LILLY	100 UNITS/ML	N018347 001

INSULIN ZINC SUSP RECOMBINANT HUMAN
Injectable; Injection

HUMULIN L		
+ LILLY	100 UNITS/ML	N019377 002 SEP 30, 1985
NOVOLIN L		
+ NOVO NORDISK	100 UNITS/ML	N019965 001 JUN 25, 1991

ISOPROPYL ALCOHOL *MULTIPLE*
SEE CHLORHEXIDINE GLUCONATE; ISOPROPYL ALCOHOL

KETOCONAZOLE
Shampoo; Topical

NIZORAL A-D	1%	
+ MCNEIL CONS SPECLT		N020310 001 OCT 10, 1997

KETOPROFEN
Tablet; Oral

ACTRON	12.5MG	
BAYER		N020499 001 OCT 06, 1995

OTC Drug Products (continued)

KETOPROFEN (continued)
Tablet; Oral

Product	Manufacturer	Strength	Application / Date
KETOPROFEN	PERRIGO	12.5MG	N075364 001 FEB 07, 2002
ORUDIS KT	+ WYETH CONS	12.5MG	N020429 001 OCT 06, 1995

LOPERAMIDE HYDROCHLORIDE
Solution; Oral

Product	Manufacturer	Strength	Application / Date
IMODIUM A-D	+ MCNEIL	1MG/5ML	N019487 001 MAR 01, 1988
LOPERAMIDE HCL	DURAMED PHARM BARR	1MG/5ML	N074991 001 DEC 29, 1997
	HI TECH PHARMA	1MG/5ML	N074352 001 NOV 17, 1995
	MORTON GROVE	1MG/5ML	N074730 001 AUG 28, 1997
	PERRIGO	1MG/5ML	N073243 001 JAN 21, 1992
	ROXANE	1MG/5ML	N073079 001 APR 30, 1992
	TEVA	1MG/5ML	N073478 001 JUN 23, 1995

Tablet, Chewable; Oral

Product	Manufacturer	Strength	Application / Date
IMODIUM A-D	+ MCNEIL	2MG	N020448 001 JUL 24, 1997

Tablet; Oral

Product	Manufacturer	Strength	Application / Date
IMODIUM A-D	+ MCNEIL	2MG	N019860 001 NOV 22, 1989
LOPERAMIDE HCL	LEINER	2MG	N073254 001 JUL 30, 1993
	LNK	2MG	N076497 001 JUN 10, 2003
	OHM LABS	2MG	N074091 001 DEC 10, 1992
	PERRIGO	2MG	N074194 001 OCT 30, 1992
		2MG	N075232 001 JAN 06, 2000

LOPERAMIDE HYDROCHLORIDE; SIMETHICONE
Tablet, Chewable; Oral

Product	Manufacturer	Strength	Application / Date
IMODIUM ADVANCED	+ MCNEIL	2MG;125MG	N020606 001 JUN 26, 1996
LOPERAMIDE HCL AND SIMETHICONE	PERRIGO	2MG;125MG	N076029 001 AUG 30, 2002

LOPERAMIDE HYDROCHLORIDE; SIMETHICONE (continued)
Tablet; Oral

Product	Manufacturer	Strength	Application / Date
IMODIUM ADVANCED	+ MCNEIL CONS SPECLT	2MG;125MG	N021140 001 NOV 30, 2000

LORATADINE
Syrup; Oral

Product	Manufacturer	Strength	Application / Date
CLARITIN	+ SCHERING	1MG/ML	N020641 002 NOV 27, 2002

Tablet, Orally Disintegrating; Oral

Product	Manufacturer	Strength	Application / Date
ALAVERT	WYETH CONS	10MG	N021375 001 DEC 19, 2002
CLARITIN REDITABS	+ SCHERING	10MG	N020704 002 NOV 27, 2002
LORATADINE	WYETH CONS	10MG	N075822 001 FEB 10, 2003

Tablet; Oral

Product	Manufacturer	Strength	Application / Date
CLARITIN	+ SCHERING	10MG	N019658 002 NOV 27, 2002
LORATADINE	GENEVA PHARMS	10MG	N075209 001 JAN 21, 2003

LORATADINE; PSEUDOEPHEDRINE SULFATE
Tablet, Extended Release; Oral

Product	Manufacturer	Strength	Application / Date
CLARITIN-D	+ SCHERING	5MG;120MG	N019670 002 NOV 27, 2002
CLARITIN-D 24 HOUR	+ SCHERING	10MG;240MG	N020470 002 NOV 27, 2002
LORATADINE AND PSEUDOEPHEDRINE HCL	ANDFX PHARMS	10MG;240MG	N075706 001 FEB 21, 2003
LORATADINE AND PSEUDOEPHEDRINE SULFATE	IMPAX LABS	5MG;120MG	N076050 001 JAN 30, 2003

MAGNESIUM HYDROXIDE *MULTIPLE*
SEE CALCIUM CARBONATE; PRECIPITATED; FAMOTIDINE; MAGNESIUM HYDROXIDE

MAGNESIUM TRISILICATE *MULTIPLE*
SEE ALUMINUM HYDROXIDE; MAGNESIUM TRISILICATE

OTC Drug Products *(continued)*

MICONAZOLE NITRATE
Cream, Suppository; Topical, Vaginal

Product / Firm	Strength	Appl. No.	Date
M-ZOLE 3 COMBINATION PACK			
ALPHARMA US PHARM	200MG;2%	N074926 001	APR 16, 1999
M-ZOLE 7 DUAL PACK			
ALPHARMA	2%;100MG	N074586 001	JUL 17, 1997
MICONAZOLE NITRATE COMBINATION PACK			
PERRIGO	2%;200MG	N075329 001	APR 20, 1999
MONISTAT 7 COMBINATION PACK			
+ ADV CARE	2%;100MG	N020288 002	APR 26, 1993
MONISTAT-3 COMBINATION PACK			
+ ADV CARE	2%;200MG	N020670 002	APR 16, 1996

Cream; Topical, Vaginal

Product / Firm	Strength	Appl. No.	Date
MONISTAT 3 COMBINATION PACK			
+ PERSONAL PRODS	2%;4%	N021261 003	JUN 17, 2003
MONISTAT 3 COMBINATION PACK (PREFILLED)			
+ PERSONAL PRODS	2%;4%	N021261 001	FEB 02, 2001

Cream; Vaginal

Product / Firm	Strength	Appl. No.	Date
MICONAZOLE 7			
ALPHARMA US PHARM	2%	N074164 001	MAR 29, 1996
MICONAZOLE NITRATE			
COPLEY PHARM	2%	N074030 001	OCT 30, 1992
G AND W LABS	2%	N074366 001	FEB 22, 1996
PERRIGO	2%	N074760 001	MAY 15, 1997
TARO	2%	N074444 001	JAN 13, 1997
TEVA	2%	N074136 001	JAN 04, 1995
MONISTAT 3			
+ ADVANCED CARE PRODS	4%	N020827 001	MAR 30, 1998

Suppository; Vaginal

Product / Firm	Strength	Appl. No.	Date
MONISTAT 7			
+ ADV CARE	2%	N017450 002	FEB 15, 1991
MICONAZOLE NITRATE			
ALPHARMA US PHARM	100MG	N073507 001	NOV 19, 1993
G AND W LABS	100MG	N074414 001	APR 30, 1997
+ PERRIGO	100MG	N074395 001	MAR 20, 1997

MICONAZOLE NITRATE *(continued)*
Suppository; Vaginal

Product / Firm	Strength	Appl. No.	Date
MONISTAT 7			
+ ADVANCED CARE PRODS	100MG	N018520 002	FEB 15, 1991

MINOXIDIL
Solution; Topical

Product / Firm	Strength	Appl. No.	Date
MINOXIDIL (FOR MEN)			
ALPHARMA	2%	N074588 001	APR 05, 1996
BAUSCH AND LOMB	2%	N074643 001	APR 09, 1996
COPLEY PHARM	2%	N074500 001	MAY 23, 1996
HI TECH PHARMA	2%	N074731 001	DEC 24, 1996
MORTON GROVE	2%	N074767 001	FEB 28, 1997
NOVEX	2%	N074924 001	APR 29, 1998
PERRIGO	2%	N075357 001	JUL 30, 1999
SIGHT PHARMS	2%	N074743 002	OCT 18, 1996
TEVA	2%	N074589 001	APR 05, 1996
MINOXIDIL (FOR WOMEN)			
NOVEX	2%	N074924 002	APR 29, 1998
PERRIGO	2%	N075357 002	JUL 30, 1999
SIGHT PHARMS	2%	N074743 001	OCT 18, 1996
MINOXIDIL EXTRA STRENGTH (FOR MEN)			
ALPHARMA	5%	N075518 001	NOV 17, 2000
CLAY PARK	5%	N075737 001	MAR 15, 2002
MORTON GROVE	5%	N075438 001	FEB 27, 2003
NOVEX	5%	N075839 001	OCT 01, 2001
PERRIGO	5%	N075598 001	JUN 13, 2001
TEVA	5%	N075619 001	NOV 17, 2000
ROGAINE (FOR MEN)			
+ PHARMACIA AND UPJOHN	2%	N019501 002	FEB 09, 1996
ROGAINE (FOR WOMEN)			
+ PHARMACIA AND UPJOHN	2%	N019501 003	FEB 09, 1996

OTC Drug Products (continued)

MINOXIDIL (continued)
Solution; Topical

ROGAINE EXTRA STRENGTH (FOR MEN)

+ PHARMACIA AND UPJOHN	5%	N020834 001	NOV 14, 1997

NAPHAZOLINE HYDROCHLORIDE; PHENIRAMINE MALEATE
Solution/Drops; Ophthalmic

NAPHCON-A			
+ ALCON	0.025%;0.3%	N020226 001	JUN 08, 1994
OPCON-A			
+ BAUSCH AND LOMB	0.0268%;0.315%	N020065 001	JUN 08, 1994
VISINE-A			
PFIZER	0.025%;0.3%	N020485 001	JAN 31, 1996

NAPHAZOLINE HYDROCHLORIDE *MULTIPLE*
SEE ANTAZOLINE PHOSPHATE; NAPHAZOLINE HYDROCHLORIDE

NAPROXEN SODIUM
Tablet; Oral

ALEVE			
+ BAYER	EQ 200MG BASE	N020204 002	JAN 11, 1994
NAPROXEN SODIUM			
DR REDDYS LABS INC	EQ 200MG BASE	N075168 001	JUL 28, 1998
INVAMED	EQ 200MG BASE	N074646 001	JAN 13, 1997
LEINER	EQ 200MG BASE	N074635 001	JAN 13, 1997
PERRIGO	EQ 200MG BASE	N074661 001	JAN 13, 1997
PVT FORM	EQ 200MG BASE	N074789 001	FEB 27, 1997

NAPROXEN SODIUM; PSEUDOEPHEDRINE HYDROCHLORIDE
Tablet, Extended Release; Oral

ALEVE COLD AND SINUS

+ BAYER	EQ 200MG BASE;120MG	N021076 001	NOV 29, 1999

NEOMYCIN SULFATE *MULTIPLE*
SEE BACITRACIN ZINC; NEOMYCIN SULFATE; POLYMYXIN B SULFATE

NICOTINE
Film, Extended Release; Transdermal

HABITROL

+ NOVARTIS	7MG/24HR	N020076 004	NOV 12, 1999
+	14MG/24HR	N020076 005	

NICOTINE (continued)
Film, Extended Release; Transdermal

HABITROL

NOVARTIS			
+	21MG/24HR	N020076 006	NOV 12, 1999
NICODERM CQ			
+ AVENTIS PHARMS	7MG/24HR	N020165 006	AUG 02, 1996
+	14MG/24HR	N020165 005	AUG 02, 1996
+	21MG/24HR	N020165 004	AUG 02, 1996
NICOTROL			
+ PHARMACIA AND UPJOHN	15MG/16HR	N020536 001	JUL 03, 1996
PROSTEP			
+ ELAN PHARM	11MG/24HR	N019983 003	DEC 23, 1998
+	22MG/24HR	N019983 004	DEC 23, 1998

NICOTINE POLACRILEX
Gum, Chewing; Buccal

NICORETTE			
+ GLAXOSMITHKLINE	EQ 2MG BASE	N018612 002	FEB 09, 1996
+	EQ 4MG BASE	N020066 002	FEB 09, 1996
NICORETTE (ORANGE)			
+ GLAXOSMITHKLINE	EQ 4MG BASE	N020066 004	SEP 25, 2000
NICORETTE (MINT)			
+ GLAXOSMITHKLINE	EQ 2MG BASE	N018612 003	DEC 23, 1998
+	EQ 4MG BASE	N020066 003	DEC 23, 1998
NICORETTE (ORANGE)			
+ GLAXOSMITHKLINE	EQ 2MG BASE	N018612 004	SEP 25, 2000
NICOTINE POLACRILEX			
WATSON LAB			
+	EQ 2MG BASE	N074507 001	MAR 15, 1999
+	EQ 4MG BASE	N074707 001	MAR 19, 1999

Troche/Lozenge; Oral

COMMIT			
GLAXOSMITHKLINE CONS	2MG	N021330 001	OCT 31, 2002
+	4MG	N021330 002	OCT 31, 2002

OTC Drug Products *(continued)*

NIZATIDINE
Tablet; Oral
AXID AR
+ WYETH CONS 75MG N020555 001 MAY 09, 1996

OCTYL METHOXYCINNAMATE *MULTIPLE*
SEE AVOBENZONE; OCTYL METHOXYCINNAMATE; OXYBENZONE

OMEPRAZOLE MAGNESIUM
Tablet, Delayed Release; Oral
PRILOSEC
+ ASTRAZENECA EQ 20MG BASE N021229 001 JUN 20, 2003

OXYBENZONE *MULTIPLE*
SEE AVOBENZONE; OCTYL METHOXYCINNAMATE; OXYBENZONE

OXYMETAZOLINE HYDROCHLORIDE
Solution/Drops; Ophthalmic
OCUCLEAR
SCHERING PLOUGH 0.025% N018471 001 MAY 30, 1986
VISINE L.R.
+ PFIZER 0.025% N019407 001 MAR 31, 1989

PERMETHRIN
Lotion; Topical
NIX
+ INSIGHT PHARMS 1% N019918 001 MAY 02, 1990
PERMETHRIN
ALPHARMA 1% N075014 001 MAR 28, 2000
                   N076090 001 DEC 20, 2001
CLAY PARK 1%

PHENIRAMINE MALEATE *MULTIPLE*
SEE NAPHAZOLINE HYDROCHLORIDE; PHENIRAMINE MALEATE

PHENYLPROPANOLAMINE HYDROCHLORIDE *MULTIPLE*
SEE BROMPHENIRAMINE MALEATE; PHENYLPROPANOLAMINE HYDROCHLORIDE
SEE CHLORPHENIRAMINE MALEATE; PHENYLPROPANOLAMINE HYDROCHLORIDE

PIPERONYL BUTOXIDE; PYRETHRINS
Aerosol; Topical
RID MOUSSE
+ PFIZER 4%:EQ 0.33% BASE N021043 001 MAR 07, 2000

POLYMYXIN B SULFATE *MULTIPLE*
SEE BACITRACIN ZINC; NEOMYCIN SULFATE; POLYMYXIN B SULFATE

POLYMYXIN B SULFATE *MULTIPLE* *(continued)*
SEE BACITRACIN ZINC; POLYMYXIN B SULFATE

POTASSIUM IODIDE
Tablet; Oral
IOSAT
ANBEX 130MG N018664 001 OCT 14, 1982
THYRO-BLOCK
+ MEDPOINTE PHARM HLC 130MG N018307 001
THYROSAFE
+ R R REGISTRATIONS 65MG N076350 001 SEP 10, 2002

POVIDONE-IODINE
Solution; Topical
E-Z PREP
+ BECTON DICKINSON 10% N019382 001 JUL 25, 1989
POVIDONE IODINE
+ ALLEGIANCE HLTHCARE 1% N019522 001 MAR 31, 1989
Sponge; Topical
E-Z PREP
+ BECTON DICKINSON 5% N019382 002 JUL 25, 1989
E-Z PREP 220
+ BECTON DICKINSON 5% N019382 003 JUL 25, 1989
E-Z SCRUB 201
+ BECTON DICKINSON 20% N019240 001 NOV 29, 1985
E-Z SCRUB 241
+ BECTON DICKINSON 10% N019476 001 JAN 07, 1987

PSEUDOEPHEDRINE HYDROCHLORIDE
Tablet, Extended Release; Oral
EFIDAC 24 PSEUDOEPHEDRINE HCL
+ ALZA 240MG N020021 002 DEC 15, 1992
PSEUDOEPHEDRINE HCL
PERRIGO 120MG N075153 001 FEB 26, 1999
SUDAFED 12 HOUR
+ WARNER LAMBERT 120MG N073585 001 OCT 31, 1991

PSEUDOEPHEDRINE HYDROCHLORIDE; TRIPROLIDINE HYDROCHLORIDE
Tablet, Extended Release; Oral
TRIPROLIDINE AND PSEUDOEPHEDRINE HYDROCHLORIDES
+ KV PHARM 120MG;5MG N072758 001 NOV 25, 1991

SODIUM CHLORIDE
Aerosol, Metered; Inhalation
BRONCHO SALINE
+ BLAIFEX   0.9%   N019912 001 SEP 03, 1992

SODIUM FLUORIDE; TRICLOSAN
Paste; Dental
COLGATE TOTAL
+ COLGATE PALMOLIVE   0.24%;0.3%   N020231 001 JUL 11, 1997

SODIUM MONOFLUOROPHOSPHATE
Gel; Dental
EXTRA-STRENGTH AIM
+ CHESEBROUGH PONDS   1.2%   N019518 002 AUG 06, 1986

Paste; Dental
EXTRA-STRENGTH AIM
+ CHESEBROUGH PONDS   1.2%   N019518 001 JUN 03, 1987

TERBINAFINE HYDROCHLORIDE
Cream; Topical
LAMISIL
+ NOVARTIS   1%   N020980 001 MAR 09, 1999

Solution; Topical
LAMISIL AT
+ NOVARTIS   1%   N021124 001 MAR 17, 2000

TRICLOSAN *MULTIPLE*
SEE SODIUM FLUORIDE; TRICLOSAN

TRIPROLIDINE HYDROCHLORIDE *MULTIPLE*
SEE PSEUDOEPHEDRINE HYDROCHLORIDE; TRIPROLIDINE HYDROCHLORIDE

OTC Drug Products (continued)

PSEUDOEPHEDRINE HYDROCHLORIDE *MULTIPLE*
SEE ACETAMINOPHEN; CLEMASTINE FUMARATE; PSEUDOEPHEDRINE HYDROCHLORIDE
SEE BROMPHENIRAMINE MALEATE; PSEUDOEPHEDRINE HYDROCHLORIDE
SEE CHLORPHENIRAMINE MALEATE; IBUPROFEN; PSEUDOEPHEDRINE HYDROCHLORIDE
SEE IBUPROFEN; PSEUDOEPHEDRINE HYDROCHLORIDE
SEE NAPROXEN SODIUM; PSEUDOEPHEDRINE HYDROCHLORIDE

PSEUDOEPHEDRINE SULFATE
Tablet, Extended Release; Oral
AFRINOL
+ SCHERING PLOUGH   120MG   N018191 001

PSEUDOEPHEDRINE SULFATE *MULTIPLE*
SEE ACETAMINOPHEN; DEXBROMPHENIRAMINE MALEATE; PSEUDOEPHEDRINE SULFATE
SEE CHLORPHENIRAMINE MALEATE; PSEUDOEPHEDRINE SULFATE
SEE DEXBROMPHENIRAMINE MALEATE; PSEUDOEPHEDRINE SULFATE
SEE LORATADINE; PSEUDOEPHEDRINE SULFATE

PYRETHRINS *MULTIPLE*
SEE PIPERONYL BUTOXIDE; PYRETHRINS

RANITIDINE HYDROCHLORIDE
Tablet; Oral
RANITIDINE

Firm	Strength	Appl. No.	Date
DR REDDYS LABS LTD	EQ 75MG BASE	N075294 001	MAR 28, 2000
GENEVA PHARMS	EQ 75MG BASE	N075519 001	SEP 26, 2002
	EQ 75MG BASE	N075497 001	JAN 14, 2000
GENPHARM	EQ 75MG BASE	N075296 001	JAN 14, 2000
IVAX PHARMS	EQ 75MG BASE	N075094 001	JUN 21, 1999
LEINER	EQ 75MG BASE	N076195 001	AUG 30, 2002
PERRIGO	EQ 75MG BASE	N075132 001	JAN 14, 2000
RANBAXY	EQ 75MG BASE	N075254 001	JAN 14, 2000
TORPHARM	EQ 75MG BASE	N075167 001	MAY 04, 2000
WATSON LABS	EQ 75MG BASE	N075212 001	JAN 14, 2000

ZANTAC 75
+ WARNER LAMBERT   EQ 75MG BASE   N020520 001 DEC 19, 1995

SIMETHICONE *MULTIPLE*
SEE LOPERAMIDE HYDROCHLORIDE; SIMETHICONE

DRUG PRODUCTS WITH APPROVAL UNDER SECTION 505 OF THE ACT ADMINISTERED BY THE CENTER FOR BIOLOGICS EVALUATION AND RESEARCH LIST

ANTICOAGULANT CITRATE DEXTROSE SOLUTION (ACD)
INJECTABLE; INJECTION
  ACD-A SOLUTION
    GAMBRO BCT, INC
      ANDA
      N010228
      FEB 25, 2002

ANTICOAGULANT CITRATE DEXTROSE SOLUTION (ACD)
INJECTABLE; INJECTION
  ANTICOAGULANT CITRATE DEXTROSE SOLUTION FORMULA A
    HAEMONETICS CORP
      ANDA
      N980728
      FEB 6, 2002

ANTICOAGULANT CITRATE DEXTROSE SOLUTION USP
INJECTABLE; INJECTION
  NONE
    MEDSEP CORPORATION
      ANDA
      N710497

ANTICOAGULANT CITRATE DEXTROSE SOLUTION USP
INJECTABLE; INJECTION
  NONE
    MILES, INC
      N100102
      DEC 14, 1961

ANTICOAGULANT CITRATE DEXTROSE SOLUTION USP
INJECTABLE; INJECTION
  NONE
    FRESENIUS USA, INC
      N110912
      SEP 02, 1959

ANTICOAGULANT CITRATE DEXTROSE SOLUTION USP
INJECTABLE; INJECTION
  NONE
    BAXTER HEALTHCARE
    CORP - FENWAL
    DIVISION
      N100855
      JUN 03, 1959

ANTICOAGULANT CITRATE DEXTROSE SOLUTION USP
INJECTABLE; INJECTION
  NONE
    BAXTER HEALTHCARE
    CORP - FENWAL
    DIVISION
      N160918
      MAR 17, 1978

ANTICOAGULANT CITRATE PHOSPHATE 2X DEXTROSE SOLUTION (CP2D)
INJECTABLE; INJECTION
  CITRATE PHOSPHATE DOUBLE DEXTROSE/ADDITIVE SOLUTION 3
    HAEMONETICS CORP
      N000127

ANTICOAGULANT CITRATE PHOSPHATE 2X DEXTROSE SOLUTION (CP2D) *(continued)*
INJECTABLE; INJECTION
  CITRATE PHOSPHATE DOUBLE DEXTROSE/ADDITIVE SOLUTION 3
    HAEMONETICS CORP
      JAN 18, 2002

ANTICOAGULANT CITRATE PHOSPHATE DEXTROSE ADENINE SOLUTION
INJECTABLE; INJECTION
  NONE
    FRESENIUS USA, INC
      N780519
      APR 23, 1980

ANTICOAGULANT CITRATE PHOSPHATE DEXTROSE ADENINE SOLUTION
INJECTABLE; INJECTION
  NONE
    TERUMO MEDICAL
    CORP
      N820528
      NOV 03, 1982

ANTICOAGULANT CITRATE PHOSPHATE DEXTROSE ADENINE SOLUTION
INJECTABLE; INJECTION
  NONE
    BAXTER HEALTHCARE
    CORP - FENWAL
    DIVISION
      N770420
      NAY 12, 1978

ANTICOAGULANT CITRATE PHOSPHATE DEXTROSE ADENINE SOLUTION USP
INJECTABLE; INJECTION
  BLOOD PACK UNIT CPDA-1 IN PLASTIC CONTAINER
    BAXTER HEALTHCARE -
    FENWAL DIVISION
      N940404
      JUL 28, 1994

ANTICOAGULANT CITRATE PHOSPHATE DEXTROSE ADENINE-1 SOLUTION
INJECTABLE; INJECTION
  NONE
    MEDSEP CORPORATION
      N800077
      NOV 06, 1980

ANTICOAGULANT CITRATE PHOSPHATE DEXTROSE SOLUTION USP
INJECTABLE; INJECTION
  NONE
    MILES, INC
      N160527
      JUN 22, 1970

Drug Products With Approval Under Section 505 of the Act Administered by the Center for Biologics Evaluation and Research List (continued)

ANTICOAGULANT CITRATE PHOSPHATE DEXTROSE SOLUTION USP
INJECTABLE; INJECTION
NONE
  MEDSEP CORPORATION
    N800222
    AUG 23, 1982

ANTICOAGULANT CITRATE PHOSPHATE DEXTROSE SOLUTION USP
INJECTABLE; INJECTION
NONE
  FRESENIUS USA, INC
    N160907
    MAY 16, 1973

ANTICOAGULANT CITRATE PHOSPHATE DEXTROSE SOLUTION USP
INJECTABLE; INJECTION
NONE
  TERUMO MEDICAL CORP
    N781211
    JUN 10, 1981

ANTICOAGULANT CITRATE PHOSPHATE DEXTROSE SOLUTION USP
INJECTABLE; INJECTION
NONE
  BAXTER HEALTHCARE CORP - FENWAL DIVISION
    N170401
    DEC 06, 1977

ANTICOAGULANT CITRATE PHOSPHATE DEXTROSE SOLUTION USP
INJECTABLE; INJECTION
NONE
  BAXTER HEALTHCARE CORP - FENWAL DIVISION
    N811012
    JUN 28, 1983

ANTICOAGULANT CITRATE PHOSPHATE DEXTROSE SOLUTION USP WITH: AS-1: DEXTROSE USP; SODIUM CHLORIDE USP; MANNITOL USP; ADENINE
INJECTABLE; INJECTION
ADSOL RED BLOOD CELL PRESERVATIVE SOLUTION
  BAXTER HEALTHCARE CORP - FENWAL DIVISION   2.2GM/100ML; 0.9GM/100ML; 0.75GM/100ML; 0.027GM/100ML
    N811104
    MAY 16, 1983

ANTICOAGULANT CITRATE PHOSPHATE DEXTROSE SOLUTION USP WITH: AS-5: DEXTROSE USP; SODIUM CHLORIDE USP; MANNITOL USP; ADENINE
INJECTABLE; INJECTION
OPTISOL RED BLOOD CELL PRESERVATIVE SOLUTION
  TERUMO MEDICAL CORP   0.9GM/100ML; 0.877GM/100ML; 0.525GM/100ML; 0.03GM/100ML
    N880217
    OCT 07, 1988

ANTICOAGULANT CITRATE PHOSPHATE DOUBLE DEXTROSE SOLUTION WITH: AS-2: CITRIC ACID USP; DIBASIC SODIUM PHOSPHATE USP; SODIUM CHLORIDE USP; ADENINE; DEXTROSE USP; SODIUM CITRATE USP
INJECTABLE; INJECTION
AS-2 NUTRICEL ADDITIVE SYSTEM
  MEDSEP CORP   0.042GM/100ML; 0.285GM/100ML; 0.718GM/100ML; 0.017GM/100ML; 0.396GM/100ML; 0.588GM/100ML
    N820915
    SEP 22, 1983

ANTICOAGULANT CITRATE PHOSPHATE DOUBLE DEXTROSE SOLUTION WITH: AS-3: CITRIC ACID USP; MONOBASIC SODIUM PHOSPHATE USP; SODIUM CHLORIDE USP; ADENINE; DEXTROSE USP; SODIUM CITRATE USP
INJECTABLE; INJECTION
AS-3 NUTRICEL ADDITIVE SYSTEM
  MEDSEP CORP   0.042GM/100ML; 0.276GM/100ML; 0.410GM/100ML; 0.30GM/100ML; 1.10GM/100ML; 0.588GM/100ML
    N820915
    OCT 19, 1984

ANTICOAGULANT CITRATE PHOSPHATE DEXTROSE SOLUTION
INJECTABLE; INJECTION
CDP BLOOD BAG UNIT IN PLASTIC CONTAINER
  BAXTER HEALTHCARE - FENWAL DIVISION
    N900224
    DEC 27, 1991

ANTICOAGULANT CITRATE PHOSPHATE DEXTROSE SOLUTION
INJECTABLE; INJECTION
ADSOL IN PLASTIC CONTAINER
  BAXTER HEALTHCARE - FENWAL DIVISION
    N900223
    DEC 27, 1991

Drug Products With Approval Under Section 505 of the Act Administered by the Center for Biologics Evaluation and Research List *(continued)*

ANTICOAGULANT HEPARIN SOLUTION USP
INJECTABLE; INJECTION
  NONE
    FRESENIUS USA, INC   N770822
                            MAY 17, 1978

ANTICOAGULANT 4% SODIUM CITRATE SOLUTION USP
INJECTABLE; INJECTION
  NONE
    MEDSEP CORPORATION   N760305
                            JUN 30, 1978

ANTICOAGULANT SODIUM CITRATE 4% SOLUTION
INJECTABLE; INJECTION
  NONE
    HAEMONETICS
      CORPORATION   N980123
                            MAR 3, 2000

ANTICOAGULANT SODIUM CITRATE SOLUTION USP
INJECTABLE; INJECTION
  NONE
    ALPHA THERPTC   N810416
                            APR 06, 1983

ANTICOAGULANT SODIUM CITRATE SOLUTION USP
INJECTABLE; INJECTION
  NONE
    FRESENIUS USA, INC   N160702
                            DEC 28, 1970

ANTICOAGULANT SODIUM CITRATE SOLUTION USP
INJECTABLE; INJECTION
  NONE
    TERUMO MEDICAL
      CORP   N781214
                            FEB 08, 1980

ANTICOAGULANT SODIUM CITRATE SOLUTION USP
INJECTABLE; INJECTION
  NONE
    BAXTER HEALTHCARE
      CORP - FENWAL
      DIVISION   N770923
                            JAN 20, 1978

DEXTRAN 1 IN SODIUM CHLORIDE 0.6%
INJECTABLE; INJECTION
  PROMIT   150MG/ML; 6MG/ML
    PHARMALINK
      BASLAKEMEDEL AB   N830715
                            OCT 30, 1984

DEXTRAN 40, 10% W/V DEXTRAN 40 IN 0.8% NACL 500 ML PVC BAGS
INJECTABLE; INJECTION
  RHEOMACRODEX
    PHARMALINK
      BASLAKEMEDEL AB   N830527
                            MAR 27, 1985

DEXTRAN 40, 10% W/V DEXTRAN 40 IN 5% DEXTROSE 500 ML PVC BAGS
INJECTABLE; INJECTION
  RHEOMACRODEX
    PHARMALINK
      BASLAKEMEDEL AB   N830627
                            MAR 27, 1985

DEXTRAN 40, 10% IN DEXTROSE 5%
INJECTABLE; INJECTION
  GENTRAN 40
    BAXTER HEALTHCARE -   10GM/100ML; 5GM/100ML
      IV SYSTEMS   N840619
                            FEB 22, 1985

DEXTRAN 40, 10% IN DEXTROSE 5%
INJECTABLE; INJECTION
  LMD IN PLASTIC CONTAINER
    ABBOTT LABS   10GM/100ML; 5GM/100ML
                            ANDA
                            N720563
                            OCT 30, 1992

DEXTRAN 40, 10% IN DEXTROSE 5%
INJECTABLE; INJECTION
  NONE
    ABBOTT LABS   10GM/100ML; 5GM/100ML
                            N160375
                            JUL 25, 1967

DEXTRAN 40, 10% IN DEXTROSE 5%
INJECTABLE; INJECTION
  NONE
    MCGAW, INC   10GM/100ML; 5GM/100ML
                            N160767
                            APR 6, 1970

DEXTRAN 40, 10% IN DEXTROSE 5%
INJECTABLE; INJECTION
  NONE
    MILES, INC   10GM/100ML; 5GM/100ML
                            N160653
                            SEP 23, 1969

Drug Products With Approval Under Section 505 of the Act Administered by the Center for Biologics Evaluation and Research List (continued)

DEXTRAN 40, 10% IN DEXTROSE 5%
INJECTABLE; INJECTION
NONE
    PHARMACHEM   10GM/100ML; 5GM/100ML   N160836 NOV 14, 1972

DEXTRAN 40, 10% IN DEXTROSE 5%
INJECTABLE; INJECTION
RHEOMACRODEX
    PHARMALINK
    BASLAKEMEDEL AB   10GM/100ML; 5GM/100ML   N140716 JAN 18, 1967

DEXTRAN 40, 10% IN SODIUM CHLORIDE 0.9%
INJECTABLE; INJECTION
GENTRAN 40
    BAXTER HEALTHCARE - IV SYSTEMS   10GM/100ML; 0.9GM/100ML   N840620 FEB 22, 1985

DEXTRAN 40, 10% IN SODIUM CHLORIDE 0.9%
INJECTABLE; INJECTION
LMD IN PLASTIC CONTAINER
    ABBOTT LABS   10GM/100ML; 0.9GM/100ML   ANDA N720562 OCT 30, 1992

DEXTRAN 40, 10% IN SODIUM CHLORIDE 0.9%
INJECTABLE; INJECTION
RHEOMACRODEX
    PHARMALINK
    BASLAKEMEDEL AB   10GM/100ML; 0.9GM/100ML   N140716 JAN 18, 1967

DEXTRAN 40, 10% IN SODIUM CHLORIDE 0.9%
INJECTABLE; INJECTION
NONE
    ABBOTT LABS   10GM/100ML; 0.9GM/100ML   N160375 JUL 25, 1967

DEXTRAN 40, 10% IN SODIUM CHLORIDE 0.9%
INJECTABLE; INJECTION
NONE
    MILES, INC   10GM/100ML; 0.9GM/100ML   N160653 SEP 23, 1969

DEXTRAN 40, 10% IN SODIUM CHLORIDE 0.9%
INJECTABLE; INJECTION
NONE
    PHARMACHEM   10GM/100ML; 0.9GM/100ML   N160836 NOV 14, 1972

DEXTRAN 40, 10% IN SODIUM CHLORIDE 0.9%
INJECTABLE; INJECTION
NONE
    MCGAW, INC   10GM/100ML; 0.9GM/100ML   N160767 APR 6, 1970

DEXTRAN 70, 6% W/V DEXTRAN 70 IN 0.9% NACL IN 50 ML PVC BAGS
INJECTABLE; INJECTION
MACRODEX
    PHARMALINK
    BASLAKEMEDEL AB   N830613 MAR 27, 1985

DEXTRAN 70, 6% W/V DEXTRAN 70 IN 5% DEXTROSE
INJECTABLE; INJECTION
MACRODEX
    PHARMALINK
    BASLAKEMEDEL AB   N830629 MAR 27, 1985

DEXTRAN 70, 6% IN DEXTROSE 5%
INJECTABLE; INJECTION
MACRODEX
    PHARMALINK
    BASLAKEMEDEL AB   6GM/100ML; 5GM/100ML   N060826 JUN 08, 1954

DEXTRAN 70, 6% IN SODIUM CHLORIDE 0.9%
INJECTABLE; INJECTION
MACRODEX
    PHARMALINK
    BASLAKEMEDEL AB   6GM/100ML; 0.9GM/100ML   N060826 JUN 08, 1954

DEXTRAN 70, 6% IN SODIUM CHLORIDE 0.9%
INJECTABLE; INJECTION
NONE
    MCGAW, INC   6GM/100ML; 0.9GM/100ML   N090024 AUG 18, 1969

Drug Products With Approval Under Section 505 of the Act Administered by the Center for Biologics Evaluation and Research List (continued)

DEXTRAN 70, 6% IN SODIUM CHLORIDE 0.9%
INJECTABLE; INJECTION
NONE
  MILES, INC   6GM/100ML; 0.9GM/100ML   N080716   MAR 13, 1953

DEXTRAN 70, 6% IN SODIUM CHLORIDE 0.9%
INJECTABLE; INJECTION
GENTRAN 70
  BAXTER HEALTHCARE - IV SYSTEMS   6GM/100ML; 0.9GM/100ML   N160607   JAN 26, 1970

DEXTRAN 70, 6% IN DEXTROSE 5%
INJECTABLE; INJECTION
NONE
  ABBOTT LABS   6GM/100ML; 5GM/100ML   N080819   MAR 31, 1953

DEXTRAN 75, 6% IN SODIUM CHLORIDE 0.9%
INJECTABLE; INJECTION
NONE
  PHARMACHEM   6GM/100ML; 0.9GM/100ML   N080564   SEP 19, 1952

DEXTRAN 75, 6% IN SODIUM CHLORIDE 0.9%
INJECTABLE; INJECTION
NONE
  PHARMACHEM   6GM/100ML; 0.9GM/100ML   N160579   AUG 19, 1970

DEXTRAN 75, 6% IN SODIUM CHLORIDE 0.9%
INJECTABLE; INJECTION
NONE
  ABBOTT LABS   6GM/100ML; 0.9GM/100ML   N18253   FEB 04, 1983

HETASTARCH 6% IN SODIUM CHLORIDE 0.9% NACL 500 ML GLASS BOTTLES
INJECTABLE; INJECTION
NONE
  ABBOTT LABORATORIES - HOSPITAL PRODUCTS DIV   ANDA N720746   FEB 07, 1996

HETASTARCH 6% IN SODIUM CHLORIDE 0.9%
INJECTABLE; INJECTION
HESPAN
  MCGAW, INC   6GM/100ML; 0.9GM/100ML   N160889   JUL 17, 1972

HETASTARCH 6% IN SODIUM CHLORIDE 0.9%
INJECTABLE; INJECTION
HESPAN IN PLASTIC CONTAINER
  MCGAW, INC   6GM/100ML; 0.9GM/100ML   N890105   APR 04, 1991

HETASTARCH 6% IN SODIUM CHLORIDE 0.9%
INJECTABLE; INJECTION
6% HETASTARCH IN SODIUM CHLORIDE 0.9% IN PLASTIC CONTAINER
  ABBOTT   6GM/100ML; 0.9GM/100ML   ANDA N740193   JAN 30, 1995

HETASTARCH 6% IN 0.9% NACL
INJECTABLE; INJECTION
NONE
  GENSIA LABS, INC   6GM/100ML; 0.9GM/100ML   ANDA N740592   NOV 12, 1998

HETASTARCH 6% IN 0.9% NACL
INJECTABLE; INJECTION
NONE
  MCGAW, INC   6GM/100ML; 0.9GM/100ML   ANDA N740283   OCT 21, 1998

HETASTARCH 6% IN LACTATED ELECTROLYTE INJECTION
INJECTABLE; INJECTION
HEXTEND
  BIOTIME, INC   6GM/100ML   N200952   MAR 31, 1999

INDIUM IN111 CHLORIDE
SOLUTION; INJECTION
INDICLOR
  AMERSHAM   N/A   N19862   DEC 29, 1992

Drug Products With Approval Under Section 505 of the Act Administered by the Center for Biologics Evaluation and Research List (continued)

INDIUM IN111 CHLORIDE STERILE SOLUTION
INJECTABLE; INJECTION
  ULTRAPURE   N/A
    MALLINCKRODT   N19841
                                                       SEP 27, 1994

PENTASTARCH 10% IN SODIUM CHLORIDE 0.9%
INJECTABLE; INJECTION
  PENTASPAN   10GM/100ML; 0.9GM/100ML
    MCGAW, INC   N841207
                                                       MAY 19, 1987

PENTASTARCH 10% IN SODIUM CHLORIDE 0.9%
INJECTABLE; INJECTION
  PENTASPAN IN PLASTIC CONTAINER   10GM/100ML; 0.9GM/100ML
    MCGAW, INC PHARM   N890104
                                                       APR 04, 1991

PERFLUORODECALIN; PERFLUOROTRI-N-PROPYLAMINE
INJECTABLE; INJECTION
  FLUOSOL   17.5GM/100ML; 7.5GM/100ML
    ALPHA THERPTC   N860909
                                                       DEC 26, 1989

RED BLOOD CELL PROCESSING SOLUTION
INJECTABLE; INJECTION
  REJUVESOL
    CYTOSOL LABS, INC   N950522
                                                       FEB 26, 1997

UROKINASE
INJECTABLE; INJECTION
  ABBOKINASE OPEN-CATHETER
    ABBOTT LABS   5,000 IU/VIAL   N761021
                                                       DEC 15, 1983

UROKINASE
INJECTABLE; INJECTION
  ABBOKINASE
    ABBOTT LABS   250,000 IU/VIAL   N761021

UROKINASE
INJECTABLE; INJECTION
  ABBOKINASE
    ABBOTT LABS   9,000 IU/VIAL   N761021

DISCONTINUED DRUG PRODUCTS

ACETAMINOPHEN

Injectable; Injection

INJECTAPAP
ORTHO MCNEIL PHARM	100MG/ML	N017785 001	MAR 07, 1986

Suppository; Rectal

ACETAMINOPHEN
ABLE	120MG	N073106 001	FEB 27, 1995
	325MG	N073107 001	FEB 27, 1995
	650MG	N073108 001	FEB 27, 1995
ROXANE	120MG	N071010 001	MAY 12, 1987
	650MG	N071011 001	MAY 12, 1987

TYLENOL
MCNEIL CONS SPECLT	120MG	N017756 002
	650MG	N017756 001

ACETAMINOPHEN; ASPIRIN; CODEINE PHOSPHATE

Capsule; Oral

ACETAMINOPHEN, ASPIRIN, AND CODEINE PHOSPHATE
MIKART	150MG;180MG;15MG	N081095 001	OCT 26, 1990
	150MG;180MG;60MG	N081097 001	OCT 26, 1990

CODEINE, ASPIRIN, APAP FORMULA NO. 2
SCHERER LABS	150MG;180MG;15MG	N085640 001

CODEINE, ASPIRIN, APAP FORMULA NO. 3
SCHERER LABS	150MG;180MG;30MG	N085639 001

CODEINE, ASPIRIN, APAP FORMULA NO. 4
SCHERER LABS	150MG;180MG;60MG	N085638 001

ACETAMINOPHEN; BUTALBITAL

Capsule; Oral

BANCAP
FOREST PHARMS	325MG;50MG	N088889 001	JAN 16, 1986

TRIAPRIN
DUNHALL	325MG;50MG	N089268 001	JUL 02, 1987

Tablet; Oral

BUTALBITAL AND ACETAMINOPHEN
HALSEY	325MG;50MG	N089568 001	OCT 05, 1988
WATSON LABS	325MG;50MG	N087550 001	OCT 19, 1984

ACETAMINOPHEN; BUTALBITAL; CAFFEINE

Capsule; Oral

ANOQUAN
SHIRE PHARM	325MG;50MG;40MG	N087628 001	OCT 01, 1986

ACETAMINOPHEN; BUTALBITAL; CAFFEINE (continued)

Capsule; Oral

BUTALBITAL, ACETAMINOPHEN, CAFFEINE
BUTALBITAL, ACETAMINOPHEN
GRAHAM DM	325MG;50MG;40MG	N088743 001	JUL 18, 1985
		N088765 001	MAR 27, 1985
		N089067 001	APR 19, 1985
MALLINCKRODT	325MG;50MG;40MG	N088758 001	MAR 27, 1985

FEMCET
MALLINCKRODT	325MG;50MG;40MG	N089102 001	JUN 19, 1985

MEDIGESIC PLUS
US CHEM	325MG;50MG;40MG	N089115 001	JAN 14, 1986

TRIAD
MALLINCKRODT	325MG;50MG;40MG	N089023 001	JUN 19, 1985

Tablet; Oral

ACETAMINOPHEN, BUTALBITAL, AND CAFFEINE
GILBERT LABS	325MG;50MG;40MG	N087629 001	NOV 13, 1984

ESGIC
FOREST PHARMS	325MG;50MG;40MG	N089660 001	DEC 23, 1988

ACETAMINOPHEN; CAFFEINE; DIHYDROCODEINE BITARTRATE

Capsule; Oral

DHC PLUS
PURDUE FREDERICK	356.4MG;30MG;16MG	N088584 001	MAR 04, 1986

SYNALGOS-DC-A
WOMEN FIRST HLTHCARE	356.4MG;30MG;16MG	N089166 001	MAY 14, 1986

ACETAMINOPHEN; CODEINE PHOSPHATE

Capsule; Oral

ACETAMINOPHEN AND CODEINE PHOSPHATE
TEVA	300MG;30MG	N088324 001	DEC 29, 1983

ACETAMINOPHEN W/ CODEINE #2
TEVA	300MG;15MG	N088537 001	JUN 04, 1984

ACETAMINOPHEN W/ CODEINE #4
TEVA	300MG;60MG	N088599 001	JUN 01, 1984

PHENAPHEN W/ CODEINE NO. 2
ROBINS AH	325MG;15MG	N084444 001

PHENAPHEN W/ CODEINE NO. 3
ROBINS AH	325MG;30MG	N084445 001

PHENAPHEN W/ CODEINE NO. 4
ROBINS AH	325MG;60MG	N084446 001

Discontinued Drug Products (continued)

ACETAMINOPHEN; CODEINE PHOSPHATE (continued)

Capsule; Oral

Product / Firm	Strength	Appl. No.	Date
PROVAL #3			
SOLVAY	325MG;30MG	N085685 001	
TYLENOL W/ CODEINE NO. 3			
ORTHO MCNEIL PHARM	300MG;30MG	N087422 001	
TYLENOL W/ CODEINE NO. 4			
ORTHO MCNEIL PHARM	300MG;60MG	N087421 001	

Solution; Oral

Product / Firm	Strength	Appl. No.	Date
TYLENOL W/ CODEINE			
ORTHO MCNEIL PHARM	120MG/5ML;12MG/5ML	N085057 001	

Tablet; Oral

Product / Firm	Strength	Appl. No.	Date
ACETAMINOPHEN AND CODEINE PHOSPHATE			
DURAMED PHARM BARR	300MG;15MG	N088353 001	FEB 06, 1984
	300MG;30MG	N088354 001	FEB 06, 1984
	300MG;60MG	N088355 001	FEB 06, 1984
EON	300MG;30MG	N085917 001	
	300MG;60MG	N087423 001	
	300MG;15MG	N087433 001	
GENEVA PHARMS	300MG;30MG	N085291 002	
	300MG;60MG	N085964 001	
HALSEY	300MG;30MG	N085794 001	
	300MG;15MG	N085795 001	
	300MG;60MG	N086549 001	
KV PHARM	300MG;30MG	N085288 001	
	325MG;45MG	*SEE ANNUAL PREFACE INTRODUCTION DISCONTINUED SECTION*	
	325MG;15MG	N085363 001	
	300MG;60MG	N085364 001	
	300MG;60MG	N085365 001	
MIKART	300MG;60MG	N089244 001	FEB 25, 1986
	300MG;60MG	N086683 001	
PUREPAC PHARM	300MG;60MG	N089511 001	APR 25, 1989
	500MG;15MG	*SEE ANNUAL PREFACE INTRODUCTION DISCONTINUED SECTION*	
ROXANE	500MG;30MG	*SEE ANNUAL PREFACE INTRODUCTION DISCONTINUED SECTION* — N089512 001	APR 25, 1989
	500MG;60MG	*SEE ANNUAL PREFACE INTRODUCTION DISCONTINUED SECTION*	
WARNER CHILCOTT	300MG;30MG	N089513 001	APR 25, 1989
	300MG;15MG	N085218 002	
		N085992 001	
ACETAMINOPHEN AND CODEINE PHOSPHATE #3			
PUREPAC PHARM	300MG;30MG	N089080 001	JUL 17, 1986
SUPERPHARM	300MG;30MG	N089184 001	OCT 18, 1985
	300MG;30MG	N089253 001	

ACETAMINOPHEN; CODEINE PHOSPHATE (continued)

Tablet; Oral

Product / Firm	Strength	Appl. No.	Date
ACETAMINOPHEN AND CODEINE PHOSPHATE #3			
SUPERPHARM	300MG;60MG	N089185 001	MAY 19, 1986
ACETAMINOPHEN AND CODEINE PHOSPHATE #4			
SUPERPHARM	300MG;60MG	N089254 001	OCT 18, 1985
SUPERPHARM	300MG;60MG	N089478 001	MAY 19, 1986
ACETAMINOPHEN AND CODEINE PHOSPHATE NO. 2			
AM THERAP	300MG;15MG	N089481 001	MAR 03, 1987
	300MG;15MG	N089479 001	MAR 03, 1987
ACETAMINOPHEN AND CODEINE PHOSPHATE NO. 3			
AM THERAP	300MG;30MG	N089482 001	MAR 03, 1987
	300MG;30MG	N089480 001	MAR 03, 1987
ACETAMINOPHEN AND CODEINE PHOSPHATE NO. 4			
AM THERAP	300MG;60MG	N089483 001	MAR 03, 1987
	300MG;60MG	N084667 001	MAR 03, 1987
ROXANE	300MG;60MG	N087653 001	
ACETAMINOPHEN W/ CODEINE			
HALSEY	300MG;60MG	N087141 001	APR 13, 1982
LEDERLE	300MG;30MG	N084659 001	
ACETAMINOPHEN W/ CODEINE NO. 2			
ROXANE	300MG;15MG	N083871 001	
ACETAMINOPHEN W/ CODEINE PHOSPHATE			
HALSEY	300MG;15MG	N083872 001	
	300MG;30MG	N087919 001	
	300MG;30MG	N087920 001	
USL PHARMA	300MG;60MG	N085676 001	JUN 22, 1982
VITARINE	300MG;30MG	N087306 001	JUN 22, 1982
WARNER CHILCOTT	300MG;60MG	N087275 001	
WATSON LABS	300MG;60MG	N087276 001	
	300MG;30MG	N087277 001	MAY 26, 1982
	300MG;15MG	N084360 001	MAY 26, 1982
WHITWORTH TOWN PLSN	300MG;30MG	N085607 001	MAY 26, 1982
	300MG;60MG	N085217 001	
APAP W/ CODEINE PHOSPHATE			
EVERYLIFE	325MG;30MG	N083643 001	
CAPITAL WITH CODEINE			
CARNRICK	325MG;30MG	N085896 001	
CODEINE PHOSPHATE AND ACETAMINOPHEN			
ICN	300MG;30MG		

Discontinued Drug Products *(continued)*

ACETAMINOPHEN; CODEINE PHOSPHATE *(continued)*

Tablet; Oral

EMPRACET W/ CODEINE PHOSPHATE #3
- GLAXOSMITHKLINE — 300MG;30MG — N083951 001

EMPRACET W/ CODEINE PHOSPHATE #4
- GLAXOSMITHKLINE — 300MG;60MG — N083951 002

PAPA-DEINE #3
- VANGARD — 300MG;30MG — N088037 001 — MAR 20, 1984

PAPA-DEINE #4
- VANGARD — 300MG;60MG — N088715 001 — MAR 20, 1984

PHENAPHEN-650 W/ CODEINE
- ROBINS AH — 650MG;30MG — N085856 001

TYLENOL W/ CODEINE
- ORTHO MCNEIL PHARM — 325MG;7.5MG — N085056 001
- 325MG;15MG — N085056 002
- 325MG;30MG — N085056 003
- 325MG;60MG — N085056 004

ACETAMINOPHEN; HYDROCODONE BITARTRATE

Capsule; Oral

BANCAP HC
- FOREST PHARMS — 500MG;5MG — N087961 001 — MAR 17, 1983

CO-GESIC
- CENT PHARMS — 500MG;5MG — N089360 001 — MAR 02, 1988

Tablet; Oral

DURADYNE DHC
- FOREST PHARMS — 500MG;5MG — N087809 001 — MAR 17, 1983

HYDROCODONE BITARTRATE AND ACETAMINOPHEN
- BARR — 500MG;5MG — N088577 001 — DEC 21, 1984
- HALSEY — 500MG;5MG — N089554 001 — JUN 12, 1987
- USL PHARMA — 500MG;5MG — N089290 001 — MAY 29, 1987
- 500MG;5MG — N089291 001 — MAY 29, 1987
- WATSON LABS — 325MG;7.5MG — N040248 001 — APR 28, 2000

NORCET
- ABANA — 500MG;5MG — N088871 001 — MAY 15, 1986

TYCOLET
- ORTHO MCNEIL PHARM — 500MG;5MG — N089385 001 — AUG 27, 1986

VICODIN
- ABBOTT — 500MG;5MG — N085667 001

ACETAMINOPHEN; OXYCODONE HYDROCHLORIDE

Capsule; Oral

OXYCODONE AND ACETAMINOPHEN
- HALSEY — 500MG;5MG — N089994 001 — MAY 04, 1989

TYLOX-325
- ORTHO MCNEIL PHARM — 325MG;5MG — N088246 001 — NOV 08, 1984

Tablet; Oral

OXYCODONE 2.5/APAP 500
- BRISTOL MYERS SQUIBB — 500MG;2.5MG — N085910 001

OXYCODONE 5/APAP 500
- BRISTOL MYERS SQUIBB — 500MG;5MG — N085911 001

ACETAMINOPHEN; OXYCODONE HYDROCHLORIDE; OXYCODONE TEREPHTHALATE

Capsule; Oral

TYLOX
- ORTHO MCNEIL PHARM — 500MG;4.5MG;0.38MG — N085375 001

ACETAMINOPHEN; PROPOXYPHENE HYDROCHLORIDE

Tablet; Oral

DARVOCET
- AAIPHARMA LLC — 325MG;32.5MG — N016844 001

DOLENE AP-65
- LEDERLE — 650MG;65MG — N085100 001

PROPOXYPHENE HCL AND ACETAMINOPHEN
- MYLAN — 325MG;32MG — N083689 001

ACETAMINOPHEN; PROPOXYPHENE NAPSYLATE

Tablet; Oral

PROPACET 100
- TEVA — 650MG;100MG — N070107 001 — JUN 12, 1985

PROPOXYPHENE NAPSYLATE AND ACETAMINOPHEN
- HALSEY — 325MG;50MG — N070115 001 — JUN 12, 1985
- 650MG;100MG — N070116 001 — JUN 12, 1985
- 325MG;50MG — N072105 001 — MAY 13, 1988
- 650MG;100MG — N072106 001 — MAY 13, 1988
- SUPERPHARM — 650MG;100MG — N071319 001 — JAN 06, 1987
- TEVA — 650MG;100MG — N070732 001 — JAN 03, 1986
- WATSON LAB — 325MG;50MG — N070398 001 — DEC 18, 1986
- 650MG;100MG — N070399 001 — DEC 18, 1986

Discontinued Drug Products (continued)

ACETAZOLAMIDE
Capsule, Extended Release; Oral
| DIAMOX | | | |
| DURAMED PHARM BARR | 500MG | N012945 001 | |

Tablet; Oral
ACETAZOLAMIDE			
ALRA	250MG	N083320 001	
ASCOT	250MG	N087686 001	OCT 20, 1982
VANGARD	250MG	N087654 001	FEB 05, 1982
WATSON LAB	250MG	N084498 002	

ACETAZOLAMIDE SODIUM
Injectable; Injection
| ACETAZOLAMIDE SODIUM | | | |
| QUAD PHARMS | EQ 500MG BASE/VIAL | N089619 001 | JAN 13, 1988 |

ACETIC ACID, GLACIAL
Solution/Drops; Otic
ACETIC ACID		
KV PHARM	2%	N085493 001
ORLEX		
PROCTER AND GAMBLE	2%	N086845 001

ACETIC ACID, GLACIAL; ALUMINUM ACETATE
Solution/Drops; Otic
| BOROFAIR | | | |
| PHARMAFAIR | 2%;0.79% | N088606 001 | AUG 21, 1985 |

ACETIC ACID, GLACIAL; DESONIDE
Solution/Drops; Otic
| TRIDESILON | | |
| BAYER PHARMS | 2%;0.05% | N017914 001 |

ACETIC ACID, GLACIAL; HYDROCORTISONE
Solution/Drops; Otic
ACETIC ACID W/ HYDROCORTISONE			
KV PHARM	2%;1%	N085492 001	
HYDROCORTISONE AND ACETIC ACID			
BAUSCH AND LOMB	2%;1%	N040097 001	OCT 31, 1994
ORLEX HC			
PROCTER AND GAMBLE	2%;1%	N086844 001	

ACETIC ACID, GLACIAL; HYDROCORTISONE; NEOMYCIN SULFATE
Suspension/Drops; Otic
| NEO-CORT-DOME | | |
| BAYER PHARMS | 2%;1%;EQ 0.35% BASE | N050238 001 |

ACETOHEXAMIDE
Tablet; Oral
ACETOHEXAMIDE			
USL PHARMA	250MG	N070753 001	NOV 03, 1986
	500MG	N070754 001	NOV 03, 1986
DYMELOR			
LILLY	250MG	N013378 002	
	500MG	N013378 001	

ACETOPHENAZINE MALEATE
Tablet; Oral
| TINDAL | | |
| SCHERING | 20MG | N012254 002 |

ACETRIZOATE SODIUM
Solution; Intrauterine
| SALPIX | | |
| ORTHO MCNEIL PHARM | 53% | N009008 001 |

ACETYLCYSTEINE
Solution; Inhalation, Oral
ACETYLCYSTEINE			
QUAD PHARMS	10%	N071740 001	AUG 11, 1987
	20%	N071741 001	AUG 11, 1987

ACETYLCYSTEINE; ISOPROTERENOL HYDROCHLORIDE
Solution; Inhalation
| MUCOMYST W/ ISOPROTERENOL | | |
| MEAD JOHNSON | 10%;0.05% | N017366 001 |

ACETYLDIGITOXIN
Tablet; Oral
| ACYLANID | | |
| NOVARTIS | 0.1MG | N009436 001 |

ACRISORCIN
Cream; Topical
| AKRINOL | | |
| SCHERING | 2MG/GM | N012470 001 |

ACYCLOVIR
Capsule; Oral
ACYCLOVIR			
LEK PHARM	200MG	N074750 001	APR 22, 1997
ROXANE	200MG	N074570 002	APR 22, 1997

Tablet; Oral
| ACYCLOVIR | | |
| LEK PHARM | 400MG | N074658 001 |

Discontinued Drug Products (continued)

ACYCLOVIR (continued)
Tablet; Oral

ACYCLOVIR			
LEK PHARM	800MG		APR 22, 1997
			N074658 002
			APR 22, 1997
TEVA	200MG *SEE ANNUAL PREFACE INTRODUCTION DISCONTINUED SECTION*		N074556 001
			APR 22, 1997

ACYCLOVIR SODIUM
Injectable; Injection

ACYCLOVIR SODIUM			
APOTHECON	EQ 1GM BASE/VIAL		N074897 002
			FEB 27, 1998
	EQ 500MG BASE/VIAL		N074897 001
			FEB 27, 1998
ZOVIRAX			
GLAXOSMITHKLINE	EQ 250MG BASE/VIAL		N018603 003
			AUG 30, 1983

ALBUMIN CHROMATED CR-51 SERUM
Injectable; Injection

CHROMALBIN			
ISO TEX	100uCi/VIAL		N017835 001
	250uCi/VIAL		N017835 002
	500uCi/VIAL		N017835 003

ALBUMIN IODINATED I-125 SERUM
Injectable; Injection

ALBUMOTOPE 125 I			
ISO TEX	5-50uCi/AMP		N017836 001
RADIO-IODINATED (I 125) SERUM ALBUMIN (HUMAN)			
BAYER PHARMS	2.5uCi/AMP		N017846 001
RADIOIODINATED SERUM ALBUMIN (HUMAN) IHSA I 125			
MALLINCKRODT	100uCi/ML		N017844 002
	6.67uCi/ML		N017844 003

ALBUMIN IODINATED I-131 SERUM
Injectable; Injection

MEGATOPE			
ISO TEX	2mCi/VIAL		N017837 003
	5uCi/AMP		N017837 004
	20uCi/AMP		N017837 005

ALBUTEROL SULFATE
Capsule; Inhalation

VENTOLIN ROTACAPS			
GLAXOSMITHKLINE	EQ 0.2MG BASE		N019489 001
			MAY 04, 1988

Solution; Inhalation

ALBUTEROL SULFATE			
COPLEY PHARM	EQ 0.5% BASE		N073307 001

ALBUTEROL SULFATE (continued)
Solution; Inhalation

ALBUTEROL SULFATE			
COPLEY PHARM	EQ 0.083% BASE		NOV 27, 1991
			N073495 001
			MAY 28, 1993
VENTOLIN			
GLAXOSMITHKLINE	EQ 0.5% BASE *SEE ANNUAL PREFACE INTRODUCTION DISCONTINUED SECTION*		N019269 002
			JAN 16, 1987
			N019773 001
	EQ 0.083% BASE		APR 23, 1992

Syrup; Oral

ALBUTEROL SULFATE			
MOVA	EQ 2MG BASE/5ML		N074302 001
			SEP 30, 1994
WATSON LABS	EQ 2MG BASE/5ML		N073165 001
			APR 29, 1993
VENTOLIN			
GLAXOSMITHKLINE	EQ 2MG BASE/5ML		N019621 001
			JUN 10, 1987

Tablet; Oral

ALBUTEROL SULFATE			
AM THERAP	EQ 2MG BASE		N072449 001
			DEC 05, 1989
	EQ 4MG BASE		N072450 001
			DEC 05, 1989
CELLTECH PHARMS	EQ 2MG BASE		N073120 001
			SEP 29, 1992
	EQ 4MG BASE		N073121 001
			SEP 29, 1992
CLONMEL HLTHCARE	EQ 2MG BASE		N072859 001
			DEC 20, 1989
	EQ 4MG BASE		N072860 001
			DEC 20, 1989
COPLEY PHARM	EQ 2MG BASE		N072966 001
			NOV 22, 1991
	EQ 4MG BASE		N072967 001
			NOV 22, 1991
WARNER CHILCOTT	EQ 2MG BASE		N072817 001
			JAN 09, 1990
	EQ 4MG BASE		N072818 001
			JAN 09, 1990
VENTOLIN			
GLAXOSMITHKLINE	EQ 2MG BASE		N019112 001
			JUL 10, 1986
	EQ 4MG BASE		N019112 002
			JUL 10, 1986

ALCOHOL
Injectable; Injection

ALCOHOL 5% IN DEXTROSE 5%			
MILES	5ML/100ML		N083483 001

ALPHA-TOCOPHEROL; ASCORBIC ACID; BIOTIN; CHOLECALCIFEROL; CYANOCOBALAMIN; FOLIC ACID; NIACINAMIDE; PANTOTHENIC ACID; PYRIDOXINE; RIBOFLAVIN; THIAMINE; VITAMIN A (continued)

Injectable; Injection
CERNEVIT-12
BAXTER HLTHCARE   APR 06, 1999

ALPRAZOLAM

Solution; Oral
ALPRAZOLAM
ROXANE   0.5MG/5ML   N074314 001   OCT 31, 1993

Tablet; Oral
ALPRAZOLAM

CLONMEL HLTHCARE	0.5MG	N074174 002	OCT 19, 1993
	0.25MG	N074174 001	OCT 19, 1993
	1MG	N074174 003	OCT 19, 1993
	2MG	N074174 004	OCT 19, 1993
ROXANE	0.5MG	N074199 002	OCT 19, 1993
	0.25MG	N074199 001	OCT 19, 1993
	1MG	N074199 003	OCT 19, 1993

ALPROSTADIL

Injectable; Injection
CAVERJECT
PHARMACIA AND UPJOHN   0.005MG/ML   N020755 001   OCT 31, 1997
EDEX
SCHWARZ PHARMA   0.005MG/VIAL   N020649 001   JUN 12, 1997

ALSEROXYLON

Tablet; Oral
RAUTENSIN
NOVARTIS   2MG   N009215 001
RAUWILOID
3M   2MG   N008867 001

ALUMINUM ACETATE *MULTIPLE*
SEE   ACETIC ACID, GLACIAL; ALUMINUM ACETATE

ALUMINUM HYDROXIDE AND MAGNESIUM TRISILICATE
Tablet, Chewable; Oral
ALUMINUM HYDROXIDE AND MAGNESIUM TRISILICATE
PENNEX   80MG;20MG   N089449 001

Discontinued Drug Products (continued)

ALCOHOL; DEXTROSE
Injectable; Injection
ALCOHOL 5% IN DEXTROSE 5% IN WATER
BAXTER HLTHCARE   5ML/100ML;5GM/100ML   N083256 001

ALGLUCERASE
Injectable; Injection
CEREDASE
GENZYME   10 UNITS/ML   N020057 004   MAY 08, 1992

ALKAVERVIR
Tablet; Oral
VERILOID
3M   2MG   N007336 002
    3MG   N007336 003

ALLOPURINOL
Tablet; Oral
ALLOPURINOL

HALSEY	100MG	N070466 001	DEC 24, 1985
	300MG	N070467 001	DEC 24, 1985
PUREPAC PHARM	100MG	N070579 001	APR 14, 1986
	300MG	N070580 001	APR 14, 1986
SUPERPHARM	100MG	N070950 001	NOV 30, 1988
WATSON LAB	100MG	N018241 001	NOV 16, 1984
	300MG	N018241 002	NOV 16, 1984
WATSON LABS	100MG	N018785 001	SEP 28, 1984
	300MG	N018785 002	SEP 28, 1984
LOPURIN			
ABBOTT	100MG	N018297 001	
	300MG	N018297 002	

ALPHA-TOCOPHEROL; ASCORBIC ACID; BIOTIN; CHOLECALCIFEROL; CYANOCOBALAMIN; FOLIC ACID; NIACINAMIDE; PANTOTHENIC ACID; PYRIDOXINE; RIBOFLAVIN; THIAMINE; VITAMIN A
Injectable; Injection
CERNEVIT-12
BAXTER HLTHCARE   11.2 IU/VIAL;125MG/VIAL;60UGM/VIAL;200 IU/VIAL;5.5MG/VIAL;414UGM/VIAL;46MG/VIAL;17.25MG/VIAL;4.53MG/VIAL;4.14MG/VIAL;3.51MG/VIAL;3,500 IU/VIAL   N020924 001

Discontinued Drug Products (continued)

ALUMINUM HYDROXIDE; MAGNESIUM TRISILICATE (continued)
Tablet, Chewable; Oral

ALUMINUM HYDROXIDE AND MAGNESIUM TRISILICATE
PENNEX			NOV 27, 1987

AMANTADINE HYDROCHLORIDE
Capsule; Oral

AMANTADINE HCL
WATSON LAB	100MG	N071382 001	JAN 21, 1987

SYMADINE
SOLVAY	100MG	N071000 001	SEP 04, 1986

SYMMETREL
ENDO PHARMS	100MG	N016020 001	

AMCINONIDE
Cream; Topical

CYCLOCORT
FUJISAWA HLTHCARE	0.025%	N018116 001	

AMDINOCILLIN
Injectable; Injection

COACTIN
ROCHE	1GM/VIAL	N050565 003	DEC 21, 1984
	250MG/VIAL	N050565 001	DEC 21, 1984
	500MG/VIAL	N050565 002	DEC 21, 1984

AMIFOSTINE
Injectable; Injection

ETHYOL
MEDIMMUNE ONCOLOGY	375MG/VIAL	N020221 002	SEP 10, 1999

AMIKACIN SULFATE
Injectable; Injection

AMIKACIN SULFATE
ABBOTT	EQ 250MG BASE/ML	N063265 001	NOV 30, 1994
	EQ 250MG BASE/ML	N063266 001	OCT 31, 1994
	EQ 250MG BASE/ML	N064099 001	JUN 20, 1995
ASTRAZENECA	EQ 50MG BASE/ML	N063167 001	DEC 14, 1995
	EQ 250MG BASE/ML	N063169 001	DEC 14, 1995
ELKINS SINN	EQ 50MG BASE/ML	N063274 001	MAY 18, 1992
	EQ 250MG BASE/ML	N063275 001	MAY 18, 1992

AMIKACIN SULFATE (continued)
Injectable; Injection

AMIKIN
APOTHECON	EQ 50MG BASE/ML	N050495 001	
	EQ 50MG BASE/ML	N062562 001	SEP 20, 1984
	EQ 250MG BASE/ML	N050495 002	
	EQ 250MG BASE/ML	N062562 002	SEP 20, 1984

AMIKIN IN SODIUM CHLORIDE 0.9% IN PLASTIC CONTAINER
APOTHECON	EQ 10MG BASE/ML	N050618 001	NOV 30, 1987
	EQ 5MG BASE/ML	N050618 002	NOV 30, 1987

AMINO ACIDS
Injectable; Injection

AMINOSYN 3.5% IN PLASTIC CONTAINER
ABBOTT	3.5% (3.5GM/100ML)	N018804 001	MAY 15, 1984
	3.5% (3.5GM/100ML)	N018875 001	AUG 08, 1984

AMINOSYN 7%
ABBOTT	7% (7GM/100ML)	N017673 002	

AMINOSYN 8.5%
ABBOTT	8.5% (8.5GM/100ML)	N017673 004	

AMINOSYN II 3.5%
ABBOTT	3.5% (3.5GM/100ML)	N019438 001	APR 03, 1986

AMINOSYN II 3.5% IN PLASTIC CONTAINER
ABBOTT	3.5% (3.5GM/100ML)	N019491 001	OCT 10, 1986

AMINOSYN II 5%
ABBOTT	5% (5GM/100ML)	N019438 002	APR 03, 1986

AMINOSYN-HBC 7% IN PLASTIC CONTAINER
ABBOTT	7% (7GM/100ML)	N019400 001	JUL 23, 1986

BRANCHAMIN 4%
BAXTER HLTHCARE	4% (4GM/100ML)	N018678 001	SEP 28, 1984

FREAMINE 8.5%
B BRAUN	8.5% (8.5GM/100ML)	N016822 001	

FREAMINE II 8.5%
B BRAUN	8.5% (8.5GM/100ML)	N016822 002	

NEOPHAM 6.4%
FRESENIUS KABI	6.4% (6.4GM/100ML)	N018792 001	JAN 17, 1984

NOVAMINE 8.5%
FRESENIUS KABI	8.5% (8.5GM/100ML)	N017957 002	AUG 09, 1982

NOVAMINE 15% SULFITE FREE IN PLASTIC CONTAINER
BAXTER HLTHCARE	15% (15GM/100ML)	N020107 001	FEB 05, 1993

Discontinued Drug Products (continued)

AMINO ACIDS; CALCIUM CHLORIDE; DEXTROSE; MAGNESIUM CHLORIDE; POTASSIUM CHLORIDE; POTASSIUM PHOSPHATE, DIBASIC; SODIUM CHLORIDE
Injectable; Injection

AMINOSYN II 5% W/ ELECTROLYTES IN DEXTROSE 25% W/ CALCIUM IN PLASTIC CONTAINER
ABBOTT 5%;.36.8MG/100ML;25GM/100ML;51MG/100ML;22.4MG/100ML;261MG/100ML;205MG/100ML N019683 004 NOV 07, 1988

AMINOSYN II 3.5% W/ ELECTROLYTES IN DEXTROSE 25% W/ CALCIUM IN PLASTIC CONTAINER
ABBOTT 3.5%;.36.8MG/100ML;25GM/100ML;51MG/100ML;22.4MG/100ML;261MG/100ML;205MG/100ML N019714 001 SEP 12, 1988

AMINOSYN II 4.25% W/ ELECTROLYTES IN DEXTROSE 20% W/ CALCIUM IN PLASTIC CONTAINER
ABBOTT 4.25%;.36.8MG/100ML;20GM/100ML;51MG/100ML;22.4MG/100ML;261MG/100ML;205MG/100ML N019714 002 SEP 12, 1988

AMINOSYN II 5% W/ ELECTROLYTES IN DEXTROSE 25% W/ CALCIUM IN PLASTIC CONTAINER
ABBOTT 5%;.36.8MG/100ML;25GM/100ML;51MG/100ML;22.4MG/100ML;261MG/100ML;205MG/100ML N019714 003 SEP 12, 1988

AMINOSYN II 4.25% W/ ELECTROLYTES IN DEXTROSE 25% W/ CALCIUM IN PLASTIC CONTAINER
ABBOTT 4.25%;.36.8MG/100ML;25GM/100ML;51MG/100ML;22.4MG/100ML;261MG/100ML;205MG/100ML N019714 004 SEP 12, 1988

AMINO ACIDS; DEXTROSE
Injectable; Injection

AMINOSYN 3.5% W/ DEXTROSE 5% IN PLASTIC CONTAINER
ABBOTT 3.5%;5GM/100ML N019120 001 OCT 11, 1984

AMINOSYN 3.5% W/ DEXTROSE 25% IN PLASTIC CONTAINER
ABBOTT 3.5%;25GM/100ML N019118 001 OCT 11, 1984

AMINOSYN 4.25% W/ DEXTROSE 25% IN PLASTIC CONTAINER
ABBOTT 4.25%;25GM/100ML N019119 001 OCT 11, 1984

AMINOSYN II 3.5% IN DEXTROSE 5% IN PLASTIC CONTAINER
ABBOTT 3.5%;5GM/100ML N019506 001 NOV 07, 1986
        3.5%;5GM/100ML N019713 002

AMINO ACIDS; DEXTROSE (continued)
Injectable; Injection

AMINOSYN II 3.5% IN DEXTROSE 5% IN PLASTIC CONTAINER SEP 09, 1988

AMINOSYN II 3.5% IN DEXTROSE 25% IN PLASTIC CONTAINER
ABBOTT 3.5%;25GM/100ML N019505 002 NOV 07, 1986
        3.5%;25GM/100ML N019713 006 SEP 09, 1988

AMINOSYN II 4.25% IN DEXTROSE 10% IN PLASTIC CONTAINER
ABBOTT 4.25%;10GM/100ML N019713 001 SEP 09, 1988

AMINOSYN II 4.25% IN DEXTROSE 20% IN PLASTIC CONTAINER
ABBOTT 4.25%;20GM/100ML N019713 004 SEP 09, 1988

AMINOSYN II 4.25% IN DEXTROSE 25% IN PLASTIC CONTAINER
ABBOTT 4.25%;25GM/100ML N019504 002 NOV 07, 1986
        4.25%;25GM/100ML N019713 005 SEP 09, 1988

AMINOSYN II 5% IN DEXTROSE 25% IN PLASTIC CONTAINER
ABBOTT 5%;25GM/100ML N019565 001 DEC 17, 1986
        5%;25GM/100ML N019713 003 SEP 09, 1988

AMINO ACIDS; DEXTROSE; MAGNESIUM CHLORIDE; POTASSIUM ACETATE; POTASSIUM CHLORIDE; POTASSIUM PHOSPHATE, DIBASIC; SODIUM CHLORIDE
Injectable; Injection

AMINOSYN II 4.25% W/ ELECT AND ADJUSTED PHOSPHATE IN DEXTROSE 10% IN PLASTIC CONTAINER
ABBOTT 4.25%;10GM/100ML;51MG/100ML;176.5MG/100ML;22.4MG/100ML;104.5MG/100ML;205MG/100ML N019682 003 NOV 01, 1988

        4.25%;10GM/100ML;51MG/100ML;176.5MG/100ML;22.4MG/100ML;104.5MG/100ML;205MG/100ML N019712 002 SEP 08, 1988

AMINO ACIDS; DEXTROSE; MAGNESIUM CHLORIDE; POTASSIUM CHLORIDE; POTASSIUM PHOSPHATE, DIBASIC; SODIUM CHLORIDE
Injectable; Injection

AMINOSYN II 3.5% W/ ELECTROLYTES IN DEXTROSE 25% IN PLASTIC CONTAINER
ABBOTT 3.5%;.25GM/100ML;22.4MG/100ML;261MG/100ML;205MG/100ML N019564 002 DEC 16, 1986

Discontinued Drug Products *(continued)*

AMINO ACIDS; DEXTROSE; MAGNESIUM CHLORIDE; POTASSIUM CHLORIDE; POTASSIUM PHOSPHATE, DIBASIC; SODIUM CHLORIDE *(continued)*
Injectable; Injection
AMINOSYN II 4.25% W/ ELECTROLYTES IN DEXTROSE 25% IN PLASTIC CONTAINER
ABBOTT   4.25%;.25GM/100ML;51MG/ 100ML;22.4MG/100ML;261MG/ 100ML;205MG/100ML   N019564 004   DEC 16, 1986

AMINO ACIDS; DEXTROSE; MAGNESIUM CHLORIDE; POTASSIUM CHLORIDE; SODIUM CHLORIDE; SODIUM PHOSPHATE, DIBASIC, HEPTAHYDRATE
Injectable; Injection
AMINOSYN II 3.5% M IN DEXTROSE 5% IN PLASTIC CONTAINER
ABBOTT   3.5%;.5GM/100ML;30MG/ 100ML;97MG/100ML;120MG/ 100ML;49.3MG/100ML   N019564 001   DEC 16, 1986

AMINOSYN II 4.25% M IN DEXTROSE 10% IN PLASTIC CONTAINER
ABBOTT   4.25%;10GM/100ML;30MG/ 100ML;97MG/100ML;120MG/ 100ML;49.3MG/100ML   N019564 003   DEC 16, 1986

AMINOSYN II 3.5% M IN DEXTROSE 5% IN PLASTIC CONTAINER
ABBOTT   3.5%;.5GM/100ML;30MG/ 100ML;97MG/100ML;120MG/ 100ML;49.3MG/100ML   N019712 001   SEP 08, 1988

AMINO ACIDS; MAGNESIUM ACETATE; PHOSPHORIC ACID; POTASSIUM ACETATE; SODIUM CHLORIDE
Injectable; Injection
AMINOSYN 3.5% M IN PLASTIC CONTAINER
ABBOTT   3.5%;21MG/100ML;40MG/ 100ML;128MG/100ML;234MG/ 100ML   N018804 002   MAY 15, 1984

    3.5%;21MG/100ML;40MG/ 100ML;128MG/100ML;234MG/ 100ML   N018875 002   AUG 08, 1984

AMINO ACIDS; MAGNESIUM ACETATE; POTASSIUM ACETATE; SODIUM CHLORIDE
Injectable; Injection
AMINOSYN 3.5% M
ABBOTT   3.5%;21MG/100ML;128MG/ 100ML;234MG/100ML   N017789 005

AMINO ACIDS; MAGNESIUM ACETATE; POTASSIUM ACETATE; SODIUM CHLORIDE; SODIUM PHOSPHATE, DIBASIC, HEPTAHYDRATE
Injectable; Injection
AMINOSYN II 3.5% M IN PLASTIC CONTAINER
ABBOTT   3.5%;32MG/100ML;128MG/ 100ML;222MG/100ML;49MG/ 100ML   N019493 001   OCT 16, 1986

AMINO ACIDS; MAGNESIUM CHLORIDE; POTASSIUM ACETATE; POTASSIUM CHLORIDE; SODIUM ACETATE
Injectable; Injection
VEINAMINE 8%
FRESENIUS KABI   8%;61MG/100ML;211MG/ 100ML;56MG/100ML;388MG/ 100ML   N017957 001

AMINO ACIDS; MAGNESIUM CHLORIDE; POTASSIUM CHLORIDE; POTASSIUM PHOSPHATE, DIBASIC; SODIUM CHLORIDE
Injectable; Injection
AMINOSYN II 7% W/ ELECTROLYTES
ABBOTT   7%;102MG/100ML;45MG/ 100ML;522MG/100ML;410MG/ 100ML   N019437 006   APR 03, 1986

AMINO ACIDS; MAGNESIUM CHLORIDE; POTASSIUM CHLORIDE; POTASSIUM PHOSPHATE, DIBASIC, SODIUM CHLORIDE; SODIUM PHOSPHATE, DIBASIC, HEPTAHYDRATE
Injectable; Injection
AMINOSYN II 3.5% M
ABBOTT   3.5%;30MG/100ML;97MG/ 100ML;120MG/100ML;49MG/ 100ML   N019437 007   APR 03, 1986

AMINOCAPROIC ACID
Injectable; Injection
AMINOCAPROIC ACID
AM PHARM PARTNERS   250MG/ML   N070522 001   JUN 17, 1986
ELKINS SINN   250MG/ML   N018590 001   OCT 29, 1982
QUAD PHARMS   250MG/ML   N070694 001   MAR 04, 1986

AMINOHIPPURATE SODIUM
Injectable; Injection
AMINOHIPPURATE SODIUM
QUAD PHARMS   20%   N089821 001   JUL 14, 1988

Discontinued Drug Products (continued)

AMINOPHYLLINE

Enema; Rectal

Brand / Firm	Strength	Appl No	Date
SOMOPHYLLIN — FISONS	300MG/5ML	N018232 001	APR 02, 1982

Injectable; Injection

Brand / Firm	Strength	Appl No	Date
AMINOPHYLLIN — GD SEARLE LLC	25MG/ML	N087243 001	MAY 24, 1982
	25MG/ML	N087621 001	MAY 24, 1982
AMINOPHYLLINE — AM PHARM PARTNERS	25MG/ML	N084568 001	
	25MG/ML	N087200 001	
	25MG/ML	N087250 001	JAN 06, 1982
	25MG/ML	N087431 001	
	25MG/ML	N087886 001	AUG 30, 1983
	25MG/ML	N088407 001	JAN 25, 1984
ELKINS SINN	25MG/ML	N087239 001	
INTL MEDICATION	25MG/ML	N087867 001	NOV 10, 1983
	25MG/ML	N087868 001	NOV 10, 1983
KING PHARMS	25MG/ML	N086606 001	
PHARMA SERVE NY	25MG/ML	N087387 001	JUN 03, 1983
SMITH AND NEPHEW	25MG/ML	N088429 001	MAY 30, 1985
	25MG/ML	N088749 001	MAY 30, 1985

AMINOPHYLLINE IN SODIUM CHLORIDE 0.45% IN PLASTIC CONTAINER

Brand / Firm	Strength	Appl No	Date
ABBOTT	100MG/100ML	N018924 001	DEC 12, 1984
	200MG/100ML	N018924 002	DEC 12, 1984
	400MG/100ML	N018924 003	DEC 12, 1984
	500MG/100ML	N018924 004	DEC 12, 1984

Solution; Oral

Brand / Firm	Strength	Appl No	Date
AMINOPHYLLINE — MORTON GROVE	105MG/5ML	N088156 001	DEC 05, 1983
SOMOPHYLLIN — FISONS	105MG/5ML	N086466 001	
SOMOPHYLLIN-DF — FISONS	105MG/5ML	N087045 001	

Tablet, Delayed Release; Oral

Brand / Firm	Strength	Appl No	Date
AMINOPHYLLINE — IMPAX LABS	100MG	N084577 001	
	200MG	N084575 001	
TABLICAPS	100MG	N084632 002	
VALE	100MG	N084531 001	

AMINOPHYLLINE (continued)

Tablet, Delayed Release; Oral

Brand / Firm	Strength	Appl No	Date
AMINOPHYLLINE — VALE	200MG	N084530 001	

Tablet, Extended Release; Oral

Brand / Firm	Strength	Appl No	Date
PHYLLOCONTIN — PURDUE FREDERICK	225MG	N086760 001	

Tablet; Oral

Brand / Firm	Strength	Appl No	Date
AMINOPHYLLIN — GD SEARLE LLC	100MG	N002386 002	
	200MG	N002386 003	
AMINOPHYLLINE — ASCOT	100MG	N087522 001	FEB 12, 1982
	200MG	N087523 001	FEB 12, 1982
BARR	100MG	N088297 001	AUG 19, 1983
	200MG	N088298 001	AUG 19, 1983
DURAMED PHARM BARR	100MG	N088182 001	MAR 31, 1983
	200MG	N088183 001	MAR 31, 1983
GENEVA PHARMS	100MG	N085261 003	
HALSEY	100MG	N084674 001	
ICN	200MG	N084563 001	
IMPAX LABS	100MG	N084574 001	
	200MG	N084576 001	
KV PHARM	100MG	N085284 001	
	200MG	N085289 001	
LANNETT	100MG	N084588 001	
	200MG	N084588 002	
PAL PAK	100MG	N084533 001	
PANRAY	100MG	N084552 001	
	200MG	N084552 002	
PUREPAC PHARM	100MG	N084699 001	
	200MG	N085333 001	
VANGARD	100MG	N088314 001	OCT 03, 1983
	200MG	N088319 001	OCT 03, 1983
VINTAGE PHARMS	100MG	N085409 001	
	200MG	N085410 001	
WATSON LABS	100MG	N085567 001	
	200MG	N085564 001	

AMINOSALICYLATE SODIUM

Powder; Oral

Brand / Firm	Strength	Appl No	Date
P.A.S. SODIUM — CENTURY PHARMS	4GM/PACKET	N080947 001	
SODIUM AMINOSALICYLATE — HEXCEL	100%	N080097 001	

Tablet; Oral

Brand / Firm	Strength	Appl No	Date
PARASAL SODIUM — PANRAY	1GM	N006811 011	

Discontinued Drug Products (continued)

AMINOSALICYLATE SODIUM (continued)
Tablet; Oral

Product / Manufacturer	Strength	Appl. No.	Date
PARASAL SODIUM			
PANRAY	500MG	N006811 006	
TEEBACIN			
CONSOLIDATED MIDLAND	500MG	N007320 002	

AMINOSALICYLATE SODIUM; AMINOSALICYLIC ACID
Tablet; Oral

Product / Manufacturer	Strength	Appl. No.	Date
NEOPASALATE			
MEDPOINTE PHARM HLC	846MG;112MG	N080059 002	

AMINOSALICYLIC ACID
Tablet; Oral

Product / Manufacturer	Strength	Appl. No.	Date
PARASAL			
PANRAY	1GM	N006811 002	
	500MG	N006811 001	

AMINOSALICYLIC ACID *MULTIPLE*
SEE   AMINOSALICYLATE SODIUM: AMINOSALICYLIC ACID

AMINOSALICYLIC ACID RESIN COMPLEX
Powder; Oral

Product / Manufacturer	Strength	Appl. No.	Date
REZIPAS			
BRISTOL MYERS SQUIBB	EQ 500MG BASE/GM	N009052 001	

AMITRIPTYLINE HYDROCHLORIDE
Concentrate; Oral

Product / Manufacturer	Strength	Appl. No.	Date
ENDEP			
ROCHE	40MG/ML	N085749 001	

Injectable; Injection

Product / Manufacturer	Strength	Appl. No.	Date
AMITRIPTYLINE HCL			
STERIS	10MG/ML	N085594 001	

Tablet; Oral

Product / Manufacturer	Strength	Appl. No.	Date
AMITID			
BRISTOL MYERS SQUIBB	10MG	N086454 001	
	25MG	N086454 002	
	50MG	N086454 003	
	75MG	N086454 004	
	100MG	N086454 005	
AMITRIL			
WARNER CHILCOTT	10MG	N083939 001	
	25MG	N083937 001	
	50MG	N083938 002	
	75MG	N084957 001	
	100MG	N085093 001	
	150MG	N086295 001	
AMITRIPTYLINE HCL			
AM THERAP	25MG	N088672 001	NOV 20, 1984
	50MG	N088673 001	

AMITRIPTYLINE HYDROCHLORIDE (continued)
Tablet; Oral

Product / Manufacturer	Strength	Appl. No.	Date
AMITRIPTYLINE HCL			
AM THERAP	75MG	N088674 001	NOV 20, 1984
	100MG	N088675 001	NOV 20, 1984
CELLTECH PHARMS	10MG	N085864 001	NOV 20, 1984
	25MG	N085935 001	
	50MG	N085936 001	
	75MG	N086337 001	
	100MG	N086336 001	
	150MG	N086335 001	
COPLEY PHARM	10MG	N088421 001	APR 30, 1984
	25MG	N088422 001	APR 30, 1984
	50MG	N088423 001	APR 30, 1984
	75MG	N088424 001	APR 30, 1984
	100MG	N088425 001	APR 30, 1984
	150MG	N088426 001	APR 30, 1984
HALSEY	10MG	N085744 001	
	10MG	N085923 001	
	25MG	N085627 001	
	25MG	N085922 001	
	50MG	N085745 001	
	50MG	N085925 001	
	50MG	N087557 001	
	75MG	N085743 001	MAR 05, 1982
	75MG	N085926 001	
	100MG	N085742 002	MAY 20, 1983
	100MG	N085927 001	MAY 11, 1982
	150MG	N089423 001	MAY 20, 1983
LEDERLE	10MG	N086744 001	FEB 17, 1987
	10MG	N087366 001	
	25MG	N086746 001	JAN 04, 1982
	25MG	N087367 001	
	50MG	N086743 001	MAY 03, 1982
	50MG	N087181 001	
	75MG	N086745 001	JAN 04, 1982
	75MG	N087369 001	
	100MG	N086747 001	JAN 04, 1982
	100MG	N087368 001	

Discontinued Drug Products *(continued)*

AMITRIPTYLINE HYDROCHLORIDE *(continued)*
Tablet; Oral
AMITRIPTYLINE HCL

Applicant	Strength	Date	Number
LEDERLE	150MG	MAY 03, 1982	N087370 001
PAR PHARM	10MG	JAN 04, 1982	N088697 001
	25MG	SEP 25, 1984	N088698 001
	50MG	SEP 25, 1984	N088699 001
	75MG	SEP 25, 1984	N088700 001
	100MG	SEP 25, 1984	N088701 001
	150MG	SEP 25, 1984	N088702 001
PUREPAC PHARM	10MG	SEP 16, 1983	N088075 001
	10MG	JUL 18, 1983	N088084 001
	25MG	MAY 20, 1983	N088076 001
	25MG	JUL 18, 1983	N088085 001
	50MG	JUL 18, 1983	N088077 001
	50MG	SEP 16, 1983	N088105 001
	75MG	JUL 18, 1983	N088078 001
	75MG	SEP 16, 1983	N088106 001
	100MG	SEP 16, 1983	N088079 001
	100MG	JUL 18, 1983	N088107 001
ROXANE	10MG		N086002 001
	10MG		N086144 001
	25MG		N085944 001
	25MG		N086145 001
	50MG		N085945 001
	50MG		N086143 001
	75MG		N086004 001
	75MG		N086147 001
	100MG		N086003 001
	100MG		N086146 001
	150MG		N086090 001
	150MG		N086148 001
TEVA	10MG		N086610 001
	25MG		N086859 001
	50MG		N086857 001
	75MG		N085030 001
	75MG		N086860 001
	100MG		N086854 001
	150MG		N086853 001

AMITRIPTYLINE HYDROCHLORIDE *(continued)*
Tablet; Oral
AMITRIPTYLINE HCL

Applicant	Strength	Date	Number
USL PHARMA	25MG	FEB 10, 1982	N087775 001
VANGARD	10MG	FEB 01, 1982	N087632 001
	50MG	FEB 08, 1982	N087616 001
	75MG	FEB 05, 1982	N087617 001
	100MG	FEB 08, 1982	N087639 001
WATSON LABS	10MG	FEB 08, 1982	N085816 001
	10MG	MAR 02, 1984	N088620 001
	25MG	MAR 02, 1984	N085817 001
	25MG	MAR 02, 1984	N088621 001
	50MG	MAR 02, 1984	N085815 001
	50MG	MAR 02, 1984	N088622 001
	75MG	MAR 02, 1984	N085819 001
	75MG	MAR 02, 1984	N088633 001
	100MG	MAR 02, 1984	N085820 001
	100MG	MAR 02, 1984	N088634 001
	150MG	MAR 02, 1984	N085821 001
	150MG	MAR 02, 1984	N088635 001
WEST WARD	10MG	MAR 05, 1982	N087647 001
	25MG		N087278 001
ENDEP			
ROCHE	10MG		N083639 001
	25MG		N083639 002
	50MG		N083639 003
	75MG		N083639 004
	100MG		N083639 005
	150MG		N085303 001

AMITRIPTYLINE HYDROCHLORIDE; CHLORDIAZEPOXIDE
Tablet; Oral
CHLORDIAZEPOXIDE AND AMITRIPTYLINE HCL

Applicant	Strength	Date	Number
HALSEY	EQ 12.5MG BASE;5MG	DEC 10, 1986	N070765 001
	EQ 25MG BASE;10MG	DEC 10, 1986	N070766 001
USL PHARMA	EQ 12.5MG BASE;5MG	JAN 12, 1988	N070477 001
	EQ 25MG BASE;10MG	JAN 12, 1988	N070478 001

Discontinued Drug Products *(continued)*

AMITRIPTYLINE HYDROCHLORIDE; PERPHENAZINE
Tablet; Oral

Product / Firm	Strength	Number	Date
ETRAFON 2-10			
SCHERING	10MG;2MG	N014713 007	
ETRAFON 2-25			
SCHERING	25MG;2MG	N014713 004	
ETRAFON-A			
SCHERING	10MG;4MG	N014713 002	
ETRAFON-FORTE			
SCHERING	25MG;4MG	N014713 006	
PERPHENAZINE AND AMITRIPTYLINE HCL			
HALSEY	25MG;2MG	N070297 001	NOV 12, 1986
	10MG;2MG	N071077 001	NOV 12, 1986
	10MG;4MG	N071078 001	NOV 12, 1986
	25MG;4MG	N071079 001	NOV 12, 1986
IVAX PHARMS	10MG;2MG	N070935 001	SEP 11, 1986
	25MG;2MG	N070936 001	SEP 11, 1986
	10MG;4MG	N070937 001	SEP 11, 1986
	25MG;4MG	N070938 001	SEP 11, 1986
	50MG;4MG	N070939 001	SEP 12, 1986
PAR PHARM	10MG;2MG	N070565 001	SEP 11, 1986
	50MG;4MG	N070574 001	SEP 11, 1986
	25MG;4MG	N070595 001	SEP 11, 1986
	10MG;4MG	N070620 001	SEP 11, 1986
	25MG;2MG	N070621 001	SEP 11, 1986
WATSON LAB	10MG;2MG	N070373 001	AUG 25, 1986
	25MG;2MG	N070374 001	AUG 25, 1986
	10MG;4MG	N070375 001	AUG 25, 1986
	25MG;4MG	N070376 001	AUG 25, 1986
	50MG;4MG	N070377 001	NOV 04, 1986
WATSON LABS	50MG;4MG	N071558 001	MAR 02, 1987
	25MG;4MG	N072134 001	FEB 15, 1989
	50MG;4MG	N072135 001	FEB 15, 1989
	10MG;2MG	N072539 001	FEB 15, 1989

AMITRIPTYLINE HYDROCHLORIDE; PERPHENAZINE *(continued)*
Tablet; Oral

Product / Firm	Strength	Number	Date
PERPHENAZINE AND AMITRIPTYLINE HCL			
WATSON LABS	10MG;4MG	N072540 001	FEB 15, 1989
	25MG;2MG	N072541 001	FEB 15, 1989
TRIAVIL 2-10			
NEW RIVER	10MG;2MG	N014715 004	
TRIAVIL 2-25			
NEW RIVER	25MG;2MG	N014715 002	
TRIAVIL 4-10			
NEW RIVER	10MG;4MG	N014715 003	
TRIAVIL 4-25			
NEW RIVER	25MG;4MG	N014715 005	
TRIAVIL 4-50			
NEW RIVER	50MG;4MG	N014715 006	

AMMONIUM CHLORIDE
Injectable; Injection

Product / Firm	Strength	Number
AMMONIUM CHLORIDE		
ABBOTT	5MEQ/ML	N083130 001
GD SEARLE LLC	3MEQ/ML	N066205 001
AMMONIUM CHLORIDE 0.9% IN NORMAL SALINE		
MCGAW	900MG/100ML	N006580 001
AMMONIUM CHLORIDE 2.14%		
B BRAUN	40MEQ/100ML	N085734 001

AMODIAQUINE HYDROCHLORIDE
Tablet; Oral

Product / Firm	Strength	Number
CAMOQUIN HCL		
PARKE DAVIS	EQ 200MG BASE	N006441 001

AMOXAPINE
Tablet; Oral

Product / Firm	Strength	Number
ASENDIN		
LEDERLE	25MG	N018021 001
	50MG	N018021 002
	100MG	N018021 003
	150MG	N018021 004

AMOXICILLIN
Capsule; Oral

Product / Firm	Strength	Number	Date
AMOXICILLIN			
LABS ATRAL	250MG	N062528 001	AUG 07, 1985
	500MG	N062528 002	AUG 07, 1985
MYLAN	250MG	N062067 001	
	500MG	N062067 002	
TEVA	250MG	N063030 001	FEB 28, 1989
	500MG	N063031 001	FEB 28, 1989

AMPHETAMINE ADIPATE; AMPHETAMINE SULFATE; DEXTROAMPHETAMINE ADIPATE; DEXTROAMPHETAMINE SULFATE

Capsule; Oral

DELCOBESE

TEVA	1.25MG;1.25MG;1.25MG;1.25MG	N083564 001
	2.5MG;2.5MG;2.5MG;2.5MG	N083564 002
	3.75MG;3.75MG;3.75MG;3.75MG	N083564 003
	5MG;5MG;5MG;5MG	N083564 004

Tablet; Oral

DELCOBESE

TEVA	5MG;5MG;5MG;5MG	N083563 001
	3.75MG;3.75MG;3.75MG;3.75MG	N083563 002
	2.5MG;2.5MG;2.5MG;2.5MG	N083563 003
	1.25MG;1.25MG;1.25MG;1.25MG	N083563 004

AMPHETAMINE RESIN COMPLEX; DEXTROAMPHETAMINE RESIN COMPLEX

Capsule, Extended Release; Oral

BIPHETAMINE 7.5

CELLTECH PHARMS	EQ 3.75MG BASE;EQ 3.75MG BASE	N010093 009

BIPHETAMINE 12.5

CELLTECH PHARMS	EQ 6.25MG BASE;EQ 6.25MG BASE	N010093 007

BIPHETAMINE 20

CELLTECH PHARMS	EQ 10MG BASE;EQ 10MG BASE	N010093 003

AMPHETAMINE SULFATE

Tablet; Oral

AMPHETAMINE SULFATE

LANNETT	5MG	N083901 001 AUG 31, 1984
	10MG	N083901 002 AUG 31, 1984

AMPHETAMINE SULFATE *MULTIPLE*

SEE AMPHETAMINE ADIPATE; AMPHETAMINE SULFATE; DEXTROAMPHETAMINE ADIPATE; DEXTROAMPHETAMINE SULFATE

AMPHOTERICIN B

Injectable; Injection

AMPHOTERICIN B

ABBCTT	50MG/VIAL	N064141 001 DEC 23, 1996
AM P-ARM PARTNERS	50MG/VIAL	N062728 001 APR 13, 1987

Ointment; Topical

FUNGIZONE

APOTHECON	3%	N050313 001

Suspension; Oral

FUNGIZONE

BRISTOL MYERS SQUIBB	100MG/ML	N050341 003

Discontinued Drug Products *(continued)*

AMOXICILLIN *(continued)*

Capsule; Oral

AMOXIL

GLAXOSMITHKLINE	250MG	N050459 001
	250MG	N062216 003
	500MG	N050459 002

TRIMOX

APOTHECON	250MG	N062098 001
	250MG	N062152 001
	250MG	N063099 001 MAR 20, 1992
	500MG	N062098 002
	500MG	N062152 002
	500MG	N063099 002 MAR 20, 1992

UTIMOX

PARKE DAVIS	250MG	N062107 001
	500MG	N062107 002

WYMOX

WYETH AYERST	250MG	N062120 001
	500MG	N062120 002

For Suspension; Oral

AMOXICILLIN

MYLAN	125MG/5ML	N062090 001
	250MG/5ML	N062090 002

AMOXIL

GLAXOSMITHKLINE	50MG/ML	N050460 005
	125MG/5ML	N050460 001
	250MG/5ML	N050460 002

LAROTID

GLAXOSMITHKLINE	50MG/ML	N050460 006

POLYMOX

APOTHECON	125MG/5ML	N061851 001
	125MG/5ML	N062323 001
	250MG/5ML	N061851 002
	250MG/5ML	N062323 002

TRIMOX

APOTHECON	50MG/ML	N061886 001
	125MG/5ML	N061886 002
	125MG/5ML	N062099 001
	125MG/5ML	N062154 001
	250MG/5ML	N061886 003
	250MG/5ML	N062099 002
	250MG/5ML	N062154 002

UTIMOX

PARKE DAVIS	125MG/5ML	N062127 001
	250MG/5ML	N062127 002

WYMOX

WYETH AYERST	125MG/5ML	N062131 001
	250MG/5ML	N062131 002

Tablet, Chewable; Oral

AMOXICILLIN

APOTHECON	125MG	N064131 001 MAY 06, 1996
	125MG	N064131 002 MAY 06, 1996
	250MG	N064131 003 MAY 06, 1996

Discontinued Drug Products (continued)

AMPICILLIN SODIUM
Injectable; Injection
AMPICILLIN SODIUM

CONSOLIDATED PHARM

Strength	Appl. No.	Date
EQ 1GM BASE/VIAL	N061936 003	
EQ 2GM BASE/VIAL	N061936 004	
EQ 125MG BASE/VIAL	N061936 005	
EQ 250MG BASE/VIAL	N061936 001	
EQ 500MG BASE/VIAL	N061936 002	

ELKINS SINN

Strength	Appl. No.	Date
EQ 1GM BASE/VIAL	N062692 004	
EQ 2GM BASE/VIAL	N062692 005	JUN 24, 1986
EQ 10GM BASE/VIAL	N062692 006	JUN 24, 1986
EQ 125MG BASE/VIAL	N062692 001	JUN 24, 1986
EQ 250MG BASE/VIAL	N062692 002	JUN 24, 1986
EQ 500MG BASE/VIAL	N062692 003	JUN 24, 1986

HANFORD GC

Strength	Appl. No.	Date
EQ 1GM BASE/VIAL	N062772 001	
EQ 1GM BASE/VIAL	N063139 001	APR 15, 1993
EQ 2GM BASE/VIAL	N063140 001	
EQ 2GM BASE/VIAL	N063141 001	APR 15, 1993
EQ 10GM BASE/VIAL	N063142 001	APR 15, 1993
EQ 125MG BASE/VIAL	N063143 001	APR 15, 1993
EQ 250MG BASE/VIAL	N063145 001	APR 15, 1993
EQ 500MG BASE/VIAL	N063146 001	APR 15, 1993
EQ 500MG BASE/VIAL	N063147 001	APR 15, 1993

IBI

Strength	Appl. No.	Date
EQ 2GM BASE/VIAL	N062797 001	JUL 12, 1993
EQ 125MG BASE/VIAL	N062797 001	JUL 12, 1993

INTL MEDICATION

Strength	Appl. No.	Date
EQ 1GM BASE/VIAL	N062634 002	JAN 09, 1987
EQ 2GM BASE/VIAL	N062634 003	JAN 09, 1987

LILLY

Strength	Appl. No.	Date
EQ 1GM BASE/VIAL	N062565 002	APR 04, 1985
EQ 2GM BASE/VIAL	N062565 003	JUN 24, 1986
EQ 500MG BASE/VIAL	N062565 001	APR 04, 1985

MARSAM PHARMS LLC

Strength	Appl. No.	Date
EQ 10GM BASE/VIAL	N062994 001	SEP 15, 1988

OMNIPEN-N
WYETH AYERST

Strength	Appl. No.	Date
EQ 1GM BASE/VIAL	N060626 004	
EQ 1GM BASE/VIAL	N062718 004	

AMPICILLIN SODIUM (continued)
Injectable; Injection
OMNIPEN-N
WYETH AYERST

Strength	Appl. No.	Date
EQ 2GM BASE/VIAL	N060626 005	DEC 16, 1986
EQ 2GM BASE/VIAL	N062718 005	DEC 16, 1986
EQ 125MG BASE/VIAL	N060626 001	DEC 16, 1986
EQ 125MG BASE/VIAL	N062718 001	DEC 16, 1986
EQ 250MG BASE/VIAL	N060626 002	DEC 16, 1986
EQ 250MG BASE/VIAL	N062718 002	DEC 16, 1986
EQ 500MG BASE/VIAL	N060626 003	DEC 16, 1986
EQ 500MG BASE/VIAL	N062718 003	DEC 16, 1986

PENBRITIN-S
WYETH AYERST

Strength	Appl. No.	Date
EQ 1GM BASE/VIAL	N050072 004	
EQ 2GM BASE/VIAL	N050072 005	
EQ 4GM BASE/VIAL	N050072 006	
EQ 125MG BASE/VIAL	N050072 001	
EQ 250MG BASE/VIAL	N050072 002	
EQ 500MG BASE/VIAL	N050072 003	

POLYCILLIN-N
BRISTOL

Strength	Appl. No.	Date
EQ 1GM BASE/VIAL	N050309 004	
EQ 2GM BASE/VIAL	N050309 005	
EQ 125MG BASE/VIAL	N050309 001	
EQ 250MG BASE/VIAL	N050309 002	
EQ 500MG BASE/VIAL	N050309 003	

TOTACILLIN-N
GLAXOSMITHKLINE

Strength	Appl. No.	Date
EQ 1GM BASE/VIAL	N062727 001	DEC 19, 1986
EQ 2GM BASE/VIAL	N062727 002	DEC 19, 1986

AMPICILLIN SODIUM; SULBACTAM SODIUM
Injectable; Injection
UNASYN
PFIZER

Strength	Appl. No.	Date
EQ 500MG BASE/VIAL;EQ 250MG BASE/VIAL	N050608 003	DEC 31, 1986

AMPICILLIN/AMPICILLIN TRIHYDRATE
Capsule; Oral
AMCILL
PARKE DAVIS

Strength	Appl. No.	Date
EQ 250MG BASE	N062041 001	
EQ 500MG BASE	N062041 002	

AMPICILLIN
LEDERLE

Strength	Appl. No.	Date
EQ 250MG BASE	N062208 001	
EQ 500MG BASE	N062208 002	

VITARINE

Strength	Appl. No.	Date
EQ 250MG BASE	N061387 001	
EQ 500MG BASE	N061387 003	

AMPICILLIN TRIHYDRATE
BIOCHEMIE

Strength	Appl. No.	Date
EQ 250MG BASE	N064082 001	AUG 29, 1995
EQ 500MG BASE	N064082 002	

AMPICILLIN/AMPICILLIN TRIHYDRATE *(continued)*

For Suspension; Oral

POLYCILLIN
- BRISTOL — EQ 500MG BASE/5ML — N050308 003

PRINCIPEN '125'
- APOTHECON — EQ 125MG BASE/5ML — N060127 002
- EQ 125MG BASE/5ML — N062151 001

PRINCIPEN '250'
- APOTHECON — EQ 250MG BASE/5ML — N060127 001
- EQ 250MG BASE/5ML — N062151 002

TOTACILLIN
- GLAXOSMITHKLINE — EQ 125MG BASE/5ML — N060666 001
- EQ 125MG BASE/5ML — N062223 001
- EQ 250MG BASE/5ML — N060666 002
- EQ 250MG BASE/5ML — N062223 002

Tablet, Chewable; Oral

POLYCILLIN
- BRISTOL — EQ 125MG BASE — N050093 001

AMPICILLIN/AMPICILLIN TRIHYDRATE; PROBENECID

Capsule; Oral

PRINCIPEN W/ PROBENECID
- APOTHECON — EQ 389MG BASE;111MG — N050488 001
- EQ 389MG BASE;111MG — N062150 001

For Suspension; Oral

POLYCILLIN-PRB
- APOTHECON — EQ 3.5GM BASE/BOT;1GM/BOT — N061898 001
- BRISTOL — EQ 3.5GM BASE/BOT;1GM/BOT — N050457 001

PROBAMPACIN
- TEVA — EQ 3.5GM BASE/BOT;1GM/BOT — N061741 001

ANILERIDINE HYDROCHLORIDE

Tablet; Oral

LERITINE
- MERCK — EQ 25MG BASE — N010585 002

ANILERIDINE PHOSPHATE

Injectable; Injection

LERITINE
- MERCK — 25MG/ML — N010520 003

ANISOTROPINE METHYLBROMIDE

Tablet; Oral

ANISOTROPINE METHYLBROMIDE
- WATSON LAB — 50MG — N086046 001

VALPIN 50
- ENDO PHARMS — 50MG — N013428 001

ARBUTAMINE HYDROCHLORIDE

Injectable; Injection

GENESA
- GENSIA AUTOMEDICS — 0.05MG/ML — N020420 001 — SEP 12, 1997

Discontinued Drug Products *(continued)*

AMPICILLIN/AMPICILLIN TRIHYDRATE *(continued)*

Capsule; Oral

AMPICILLIN TRIHYDRATE
- BIOCHEMIE — AUG 29, 1995
- IVAX PHARMS — EQ 250MG BASE — N060765 001
- EQ 500MG BASE — N060765 002
- MYLAN — EQ 250MG BASE — N061755 001
- EQ 500MG BASE — N061755 002
- PUREPAC PHARM — EQ 250MG BASE — N061853 001

OMNIPEN (AMPICILLIN)
- WYETH AYERST — 250MG — N060624 001
- 500MG — N060624 002

PENBRITIN
- WYETH AYERST — EQ 250MG BASE — N060908 001
- EQ 500MG BASE — N060908 002

PFIZERPEN-A
- PFIZER — EQ 250MG BASE — N062050 001
- EQ 500MG BASE — N062050 002

POLYCILLIN
- BRISTOL — EQ 250MG BASE — N050310 001
- EQ 500MG BASE — N050310 002

PRINCIPEN '250'
- APOTHECON — EQ 250MG BASE — N050056 001
- EQ 250MG BASE — N062157 002

PRINCIPEN '500'
- APOTHECON — EQ 500MG BASE — N050056 002
- EQ 500MG BASE — N062157 001

TOTACILLIN
- GLAXOSMITHKLINE — EQ 250MG BASE — N060060 001
- EQ 500MG BASE — N060060 002

For Suspension; Oral

AMCILL
- PARKE DAVIS — EQ 125MG BASE/5ML — N062030 001
- EQ 250MG BASE/5ML — N062030 002

AMPICILLIN TRIHYDRATE
- MYLAN — EQ 125MG BASE/5ML — N061829 002
- EQ 125MG BASE/5ML — N061829 001
- EQ 250MG BASE/5ML — N061980 001
- PUREPAC PHARM

OMNIPEN (AMPICILLIN)
- WYETH AYERST — 100MG/ML — N060625 001
- 125MG/5ML — N060625 002
- 250MG/5ML — N060625 003
- 500MG/5ML — N060625 004

PENBRITIN
- WYETH AYERST — EQ 100MG BASE/ML — N050019 001
- EQ 125MG BASE/5ML — N050019 002
- EQ 250MG BASE/5ML — N050019 003

PFIZERPEN-A
- PFIZER — EQ 125MG BASE/5ML — N062049 001
- EQ 250MG BASE/5ML — N062049 002

POLYCILLIN
- APOTHECON — EQ 125MG BASE/5ML — N062297 001
- EQ 250MG BASE/5ML — N062297 002
- EQ 100MG BASE/ML — N050308 004
- BRISTOL — EQ 125MG BASE/5ML — N050308 001
- EQ 250MG BASE/5ML — N050308 002

ASCORBIC ACID; BIOTIN; CYANOCOBALAMIN; DEXPANTHENOL; ERGOCALCIFEROL; FOLIC ACID; NIACINAMIDE; PYRIDOXINE HYDROCHLORIDE; RIBOFLAVIN PHOSPHATE SODIUM; THIAMINE HYDROCHLORIDE; VITAMIN A; VITAMIN E (continued)
Injectable; Injection
M.V.C. 9+3
  AM PHARM PARTNERS
  10MG/ML;0.006MG/ML;0.5UGM/ML;1.5MG/ML;20 IU/ML;0.04MG/ML;4MG/ML;0.4MG/ML;0.36MG/ML;0.3MG/ML;330 UNITS/ML;1 IU/ML
  N018440 002
  AUG 08, 1985

ASCORBIC ACID; BIOTIN; CYANOCOBALAMIN; ERGOCALCIFEROL; FOLIC ACID; NIACINAMIDE; PANTOTHENIC ACID; PYRIDOXINE; RIBOFLAVIN; THIAMINE; VITAMIN A PALMITATE; VITAMIN E
Injectable; Injection
VITAPED
  FRESENIUS KABI
  80 MG/VIAL;0.02MG/VIAL;0.001MG/VIAL;400 IU/10ML;0.14MG/VIAL;17MG/VIAL;5MG/VIAL;0.2MG/VIAL;1MG/VIAL;1.4MG/VIAL;1.2MG/VIAL;EQ 2,300 UNITS BASE/10ML;7 IU/10ML
  N020176 001
  DEC 29, 1993

ASCORBIC ACID *MULTIPLE*
SEE   ALPHA-TOCOPHEROL; ASCORBIC ACID; BIOTIN; CHOLECALCIFEROL; CYANOCOBALAMIN; FOLIC ACID; NIACINAMIDE; PANTOTHENIC ACID; PYRIDOXINE; RIBOFLAVIN; THIAMINE; VITAMIN A

ASPIRIN
Tablet, Extended Release; Oral
8-HOUR BAYER
  BAYER   650MG   N016030 001
MEASURIN
  BAYER   650MG   N016030 002

ASPIRIN; BUTALBITAL
Tablet; Oral
AXOTAL
  SAVAGE LABS   650MG;50MG   N088305 001   OCT 13, 1983

ASPIRIN; BUTALBITAL; CAFFEINE
Capsule; Oral
BUTALBITAL, ASPIRIN AND CAFFEINE
  WATSON LABS   325MG;50MG;40MG   N086231 002   FEB 12, 1985

Discontinued Drug Products (continued)

ARDEPARIN SODIUM
Injectable; Injection
NORMIFLO
  PHARMACIA AND UPJOHN
  5,000 UNITS/0.5ML *SEE ANNUAL PREFACE INTRODUCTION DISCONTINUED SECTION*
  N020227 002
  MAY 23, 1997
  10,000 UNITS/0.5ML *SEE ANNUAL PREFACE INTRODUCTION DISCONTINUED SECTION*
  N020227 001
  MAY 23, 1997

ASCORBIC ACID; BIOTIN; CYANOCOBALAMIN; DEXPANTHENOL; ERGOCALCIFEROL; FOLIC ACID; NIACINAMIDE; PYRIDOXINE; RIBOFLAVIN PHOSPHATE SODIUM; THIAMINE; VITAMIN A; VITAMIN E
Injectable; Injection
M.V.I.-12 LYOPHILIZED
  ASTRAZENECA
  100MG/VIAL;0.06MG/VIAL;0.005MG/VIAL;15MG/VIAL;5UGM/VIAL;0.4MG/VIAL;40MG/VIAL;4MG/VIAL;3.6MG/VIAL;3MG/VIAL;1MG/VIAL;10MG/VIAL
  N018933 002
  AUG 08, 1985

ASCORBIC ACID; BIOTIN; CYANOCOBALAMIN; DEXPANTHENOL; ERGOCALCIFEROL; FOLIC ACID; NIACINAMIDE; PYRIDOXINE HYDROCHLORIDE; RIBOFLAVIN PHOSPHATE SODIUM; THIAMINE; VITAMIN A PALMITATE; VITAMIN E
Injectable; Injection
BEROCCA PN
  ROCHE
  50MG/ML;0.03MG/ML;0.0025MG/ML;7.5MG/ML;100 IU/ML;0.2MG/ML;20MG/ML;2MG/ML;1.8MG/ML;1.5MG/ML;1,650 IU/ML;5 IU/ML
  N006071 003
  OCT 10, 1985

ASCORBIC ACID; BIOTIN; CYANOCOBALAMIN; DEXPANTHENOL; ERGOCALCIFEROL; FOLIC ACID; NIACINAMIDE; PYRIDOXINE HYDROCHLORIDE; RIBOFLAVIN PHOSPHATE SODIUM; THIAMINE HYDROCHLORIDE; VITAMIN A; VITAMIN E
Injectable; Injection
MVC PLUS
  STERIS
  10MG/ML;0.006MG/ML;0.5UGM/ML;1.5MG/ML;20 IU/ML;0.04MG/ML;4MG/ML;0.4MG/ML;0.36MG/ML;0.3MG/ML;330 UNITS/ML;1 IU/ML
  N018439 002
  AUG 08, 1985

Discontinued Drug Products (continued)

ASPIRIN; BUTALBITAL; CAFFEINE (continued)
Tablet; Oral

BUTALBITAL ASPIRIN AND CAFFEINE			
QUANTUM PHARMICS	325MG;50MG;40MG	N088972 001	JUN 18, 1985
BUTALBITAL COMPOUND			
IVAX PHARMS	325MG;50MG;40MG	N085441 002	OCT 31, 1984
BUTALBITAL, ASPIRIN CAFFEINE			
HALSEY	325MG;50MG;40MG	N089448 001	DEC 01, 1986
BUTALBITAL, ASPIRIN AND CAFFEINE			
WATSON LABS	325MG;50MG;40MG	N086237 002	MAR 23, 1984
LANORINAL			
LANNETT	325MG;50MG;40MG	N086986 002	OCT 18, 1985

ASPIRIN; CAFFEINE; PROPOXYPHENE HYDROCHLORIDE
Capsule; Oral

COMPOUND 65			
ALRA	389MG;32.4MG;65MG	N084553 002	AUG 17, 1983
PROPOXYPHENE COMPOUND 65			
EON	389MG;32.4MG;65MG	N080044 002	SEP 16, 1983
IVAX PHARMS	389MG;32.4MG;65MG	N083077 002	DEC 07, 1984
PROPOXYPHENE COMPOUND-65			
GENEVA PHARMS	389MG;32.4MG;65MG	N083101 002	JUN 24, 1985
PROPOXYPHENE HCL W/ ASPIRIN AND CAFFEINE			
WATSON LABS	389MG;32.4MG;65MG	N085732 002	SEP 03, 1984

ASPIRIN; CARISOPRODOL
Tablet; Oral

CARISOPRODOL COMPOUND			
WATSON LAB	325MG;200MG	N088809 001	OCT 03, 1985

ASPIRIN; HYDROCODONE BITARTRATE
Tablet; Oral

VICOPRIN			
ABBOTT	500MG;5MG	N086333 001	SEP 14, 1983

ASPIRIN; MEPROBAMATE
Tablet; Oral

MEPRO-ASPIRIN			
EON	325MG;200MG	N089127 001	MAR 02, 1987
MEPROBAMATE AND ASPIRIN			
PAR PHARM	325MG;200MG	N089126 001	

ASPIRIN; MEPROBAMATE (continued)
Tablet; Oral

MEPROBAMATE AND ASPIRIN			
PAR PHARM			AUG 19, 1986
MICRAININ			
MEDPOINTE PHARM HLC	325MG;200MG	N084978 001	
Q-GESIC			
QUANTUM PHARMICS	325MG;200MG	N088740 001	JUN 01, 1984

ASPIRIN; METHOCARBAMOL
Tablet; Oral

METHOCARBAMOL AND ASPIRIN			
MCNEIL	325MG;400MG	N089193 001	FEB 12, 1986
ROBAXISAL			
ROBINS AH	325MG;400MG	N012281 001	

ASPIRIN; OXYCODONE HYDROCHLORIDE; OXYCODONE TEREPHTHALATE
Tablet; Oral

CODOXY			
HALSEY	325MG;4.5MG;0.38MG	N087464 001	JUL 01, 1982
OXYCODONE AND ASPIRIN (HALF-STRENGTH)			
ROXANE	325MG;2.25MG;0.19MG	N087742 001	JUN 04, 1982
ROXIPRIN			
ROXANE	325MG;4.5MG;0.38MG	N087743 001	JUN 04, 1982

ASPIRIN; PENTAZOCINE HYDROCHLORIDE
Tablet; Oral

TALWIN COMPOUND			
SANOFI SYNTHELABO	325MG;EQ 12.5MG BASE	N016891 001	

ASPIRIN; PROPOXYPHENE NAPSYLATE
Capsule; Oral

DARVON-N W/ ASA			
AAIPHARMA LLC	325MG;100MG	N016829 001	

Tablet; Oral

DARVON-N W/ ASA			
AAIPHARMA LLC	325MG;100MG	N016863 001	

ASPIRIN *MULTIPLE*
SEE   ACETAMINOPHEN; ASPIRIN; CODEINE PHOSPHATE

ATENOLOL
Tablet; Oral

ATENOLOL			
APOTHECON	50MG	N073317 001	MAR 20, 1992
	100MG	N073318 001	MAR 20, 1992

Discontinued Drug Products *(continued)*

ATENOLOL *(continued)*
Tablet; Oral
ATENOLOL
GENPHARM	25MG	N074126 003	AUG 26, 1998
	50MG	N074126 001	MAR 23, 1994
	100MG	N074126 002	MAR 23, 1994

ATOMOXETINE HYDROCHLORIDE
Capsule; Oral
STRATTERA
LILLY	5MG	N021411 001	NOV 26, 2002

ATROPINE
Injectable; Injection
ATROPINE
SOLVAY	EQ 2MG SULFATE/0.7ML	N071295 001	JAN 30, 1987

ATROPINE; PRALIDOXIME CHLORIDE
Injectable; Intramuscular
ATNAA
US ARMY	2.1MG/0.7ML;600MG/2ML	N021175 001	JAN 17, 2002

ATROPINE SULFATE
Aerosol, Metered; Inhalation
ATROPINE SULFATE
US ARMY	EQ 0.36MG BASE/INH	N020056 001	SEP 19, 1990

ATROPINE SULFATE; DIFENOXIN HYDROCHLORIDE
Tablet; Oral
MOTOFEN HALF-STRENGTH
AMARIN PHARMS	0.025MG;0.5MG	N017744 001

ATROPINE SULFATE; DIPHENOXYLATE HYDROCHLORIDE
Solution; Oral
COLONAID
MEDPOINTE PHARM HLC	0.025MG/5ML;2.5MG/5ML	N085735 001

LOMANATE
ALPHARMA	0.025MG/5ML;2.5MG/5ML	N085746 001

Tablet; Oral
COLONAID
MEDPOINTE PHARM HLC	0.025MG;2.5MG	N085737 001

DI-ATRO
MD PHARM	0.025MG;2.5MG	N085266 001

DIPHENOXYLATE HCL AND ATROPINE SULFATE
ASCOT	0.025MG;2.5MG	N087934 001	JUL 19, 1983
HALSEY	0.025MG;2.5MG	N085506 001	

ATROPINE SULFATE; DIPHENOXYLATE HYDROCHLORIDE *(continued)*
Tablet; Oral
DIPHENOXYLATE HCL AND ATROPINE SULFATE
HEATHER	0.025MG;2.5MG	N086798 001	
INWOOD LABS	0.025MG;2.5MG	N085509 001	
LEDERLE	0.025MG;2.5MG	N086950 001	
PARKE DAVIS	0.025MG;2.5MG	N087131 001	
R AND S PHARMA	0.025MG;2.5MG	N085035 001	
ROXANE	0.025MG;2.5MG	N086057 001	
WATSON LABS	0.025MG;2.5MG	N085876 001	
WEST WARD	0.025MG;2.5MG	N087765 001	MAR 15, 1982

DIPHENOXYLATE HCL W/ ATROPINE SULFATE
ICN	0.025MG;2.5MG	N087195 001	FEB 16, 1982
KV PHARM	0.025MG;2.5MG	N085659 001	
PVT FORM	0.025MG;2.5MG	N085766 001	
USL PHARMA	0.025MG;2.5MG	N087842 001	MAR 29, 1982

LO-TROL
VANGARD	0.025MG;2.5MG	N088009 001	MAR 25, 1983

LOGEN
SUPERPHARM	0.025MG;2.5MG	N088962 001	MAY 10, 1985

LOW-QUEL
HALSEY	0.025MG;2.5MG	N085211 001

ATROPINE SULFATE; MEPERIDINE HYDROCHLORIDE
Injectable; Injection
MEPERIDINE AND ATROPINE SULFATE
WYETH AYERST	0.4MG/ML;50MG/ML	N085121 001
	0.4MG/ML;75MG/ML	N085121 002
	0.4MG/ML;100MG/ML	N085121 003

AZATHIOPRINE
Tablet; Oral
IMURAN
PROMETHEUS LABS	25MG	*SEE ANNUAL PREFACE INTRODUCTION DISCONTINUED SECTION*	N016324 002

AZATHIOPRINE SODIUM
Injectable; Injection
AZATHIOPRINE
QUAD PHARMS	EQ 100MG BASE/VIAL	N071056 001	JUN 08, 1988

AZITHROMYCIN DIHYDRATE; TROVAFLOXACIN MESYLATE
For Suspension, Tablet; Oral
TROVAN/ZITHROMAX COMPLIANCE PAK
PFIZER	EQ 1GM BASE;EQ 100MG BASE	N050762 001	DEC 18, 1998

Discontinued Drug Products (continued)

AZLOCILLIN SODIUM
Injectable; Injection
 AZLIN
  BAYER PHARMS
   EQ 2GM BASE/VIAL — N050562 001 SEP 03, 1982
   EQ 2GM BASE/VIAL — N062388 001 SEP 08, 1982
   EQ 2GM BASE/VIAL — N062417 001 OCT 12, 1982
   EQ 3GM BASE/VIAL — N050562 002 SEP 03, 1982
   EQ 3GM BASE/VIAL — N062388 002 SEP 08, 1982
   EQ 3GM BASE/VIAL — N062417 002 OCT 12, 1982
   EQ 4GM BASE/VIAL — N050562 003 SEP 03, 1982
   EQ 4GM BASE/VIAL — N062388 003 SEP 08, 1982
   EQ 4GM BASE/VIAL — N062417 003 OCT 12, 1982

AZTREONAM
Injectable; Injection
 AZACTAM
  BRISTOL MYERS SQUIBB
   1GM/VIAL — N050580 002 DEC 31, 1986
   2GM/VIAL — N050580 003 DEC 31, 1986
   500MG/VIAL — N050580 001 DEC 31, 1986
 AZACTAM IN PLASTIC CONTAINER
  BRISTOL MYERS SQUIBB
   10MG/ML — N050632 003 MAY 24, 1989

BACAMPICILLIN HYDROCHLORIDE
Tablet; Oral
 SPECTROBID
  PFIZER
   800MG — N050520 002 SEP 12, 1983

BACITRACIN
Injectable; Injection
 BACITRACIN
  PFIZER
   50,000 UNITS/VIAL — N060282 001
  QUAD PHARMS
   10,000 UNITS/VIAL — N062696 001 APR 17, 1987
   50,000 UNITS/VIAL — N062696 002 APR 17, 1987
Ointment; Ophthalmic
 BACIGUENT
  PHARMACIA AND UPJOHN
   500 UNITS/GM — N060734 001

BACITRACIN (continued)
Ointment; Ophthalmic
 BACITRACIN
  LILLY
   500 UNITS/GM — N060687 001
  PHARMADERM
   500 UNITS/GM — N062158 001
  PHARMAFAIR
   500 UNITS/GM — N062453 001 MAR 28, 1984
Ointment; Topical
 BACITRACIN
  COMBE
   500 UNITS/GM — N062799 001 MAY 14, 1987
Powder; For Rx Compounding
 BACITRACIN
  PADDOCK
   5,000,000 UNITS/BOT — N062456 001 JUL 27, 1983

BACITRACIN; HYDROCORTISONE ACETATE; NEOMYCIN SULFATE; POLYMYXIN B SULFATE
Ointment; Ophthalmic
 BACITRACIN-NEOMYCIN-POLYMYXIN W/ HYDROCORTISONE ACETATE
  ALTANA
   400 UNITS/GM;1%;EQ 3.5MG BASE/GM;10,000 UNITS/GM — N060731 002

BACITRACIN; NEOMYCIN SULFATE; POLYMYXIN B SULFATE
Ointment; Ophthalmic
 MYCITRACIN
  PHARMACIA AND UPJOHN
   500 UNITS/GM;EQ 3.5MG BASE/GM;10,000 UNITS/GM — N061048 001

BACITRACIN; POLYMYXIN B SULFATE
Disc; Topical
 LANABIOTIC
  COMBE
   500 UNITS/GM;5,000 UNITS/GM — N050598 001 SEP 22, 1986

BACITRACIN ZINC
Powder; For Rx Compounding
 ZIBA-RX
  PHARMA TEK
   500,000 UNITS/BOT — N061737 001

BACITRACIN ZINC; HYDROCORTISONE; NEOMYCIN SULFATE; POLYMYXIN B SULFATE
Ointment; Ophthalmic
 ZINC BACITRACIN,NEOMYCIN SULFATE,POLYMYXIN B SULFATE HYDROCORTISONE
  PHARMAFAIR
   400 UNITS/GM;1%;EQ 3.5MG BASE/GM;10,000 UNITS/GM — N062389 001 JUL 02, 1982
Ointment; Topical
 NEOMYCIN POLYMYXIN B SULFATES BACITRACIN ZINC HYDROCORTISONE
  PHARMAFAIR
   400 UNITS/GM;1%;EQ 3.5MG BASE/GM;5,000 UNITS/GM — N062381 001 SEP 06, 1985

Discontinued Drug Products (continued)

BACITRACIN ZINC; LIDOCAINE; NEOMYCIN SULFATE; POLYMYXIN B SULFATE
Ointment; Topical

LANABIOTIC			
COMBE	400 UNITS/GM;40MG/GM;EQ 5MG BASE/GM;5,000 UNITS/GM	N062499 001	JUN 03, 1985

BACITRACIN ZINC; NEOMYCIN SULFATE; POLYMYXIN B SULFATE
Ointment; Ophthalmic

BACITRACIN ZINC-NEOMYCIN SULFATE-POLYMYXIN B SULFATE			
PHARMAFAIR	400 UNITS/GM;EQ 3.5MG BASE/GM;10,000 UNITS/GM	N062386 001	SEP 09, 1982
BACITRACIN-NEOMYCIN-POLYMYXIN			
PHARMADERM	400 UNITS/GM;EQ 3.5MG BASE/GM;5,000 UNITS/GM	N062167 001	
NEO-POLYCIN			
DOW PHARM	500 UNITS/GM;EQ 3.5MG BASE/GM;10,000 UNITS/GM	N060647 001	

BACITRACIN ZINC; POLYMYXIN B SULFATE
Aerosol; Topical

POLYSPORIN			
GLAXOSMITHKLINE	10,000 UNITS/GM;2,000,000 UNITS/GM	N050167 002	MAR 01, 1985

Ointment; Ophthalmic

OCUMYCIN			
PHARMAFAIR	500 UNITS/GM;10,000 UNITS/GM	N062430 001	APR 08, 1983

BACLOFEN
Tablet; Oral

BACLOFEN			
TEVA	10MG	N073043 001	FEB 27, 1992
	20MG	N073044 001	FEB 27, 1992
USL PHARMA	10MG	N071260 001	MAY 06, 1988
	20MG	N071261 001	MAY 06, 1988
LIORESAL			
NOVARTIS	10MG	N017851 001	
	20MG	N017851 003	JAN 20, 1982

BECLOMETHASONE DIPROPIONATE
Aerosol, Metered; Inhalation

BECLOVENT			
GLAXOSMITHKLINE	0.042MG/INH	N018153 001	

BECLOMETHASONE DIPROPIONATE (continued)
Aerosol, Metered; Nasal

BECONASE			
GLAXOSMITHKLINE	0.042MG/INH	N018584 001	
VANCENASE			
SCHERING	0.042MG/INH	N018521 001	

BECLOMETHASONE DIPROPIONATE MONOHYDRATE
Spray, Metered; Nasal

VANCENASE AQ			
SCHERING	EQ 0.084MG DIPROP/SPRAY	N020469 001	JUN 26, 1996

BENDROFLUMETHIAZIDE
Tablet; Oral

NATURETIN-2.5			
APOTHECON	2.5MG	N012164 001	
NATURETIN-10			
APOTHECON	10MG	N012164 003	

BENOXINATE HYDROCHLORIDE
Solution/Drops; Ophthalmic

BENOXINATE HCL			
SOLA BARNES HIND	0.4%	N084149 001	

BENTIROMIDE
Solution; Oral

CHYMEX			
SAVAGE LABS	500MG/7.5ML	N018366 001	DEC 29, 1983

BENZPHETAMINE HYDROCHLORIDE
Tablet; Oral

DIDREX			
PHARMACIA AND UPJOHN	25MG	N012427 003	

BENZQUINAMIDE HYDROCHLORIDE
Suppository; Rectal

EMETE-CON			
ROERIG	EQ 100MG BASE	N016818 006	

BENZTHIAZIDE
Tablet; Oral

AQUATAG			
SOLVAY	25MG	N016001 001	
	50MG	N016001 002	
BENZTHIAZIDE			
PVT FORM	50MG	N083206 001	
EXNA			
AH ROBINS INC	50MG	N012489 001	
FOVANE			
PFIZER	50MG	N012128 002	

BETAMETHASONE (continued)

Tablet; Oral
CELESTONE
SCHERING — 0.6MG — N012657 003

BETAMETHASONE BENZOATE

Cream; Topical
UTICORT
PARKE DAVIS — 0.025% — N016998 002

Gel; Topical
UTICORT
PARKE DAVIS — 0.025% — N017244 001

Lotion; Topical
UTICORT
PARKE DAVIS — 0.025% — N017528 001

Ointment; Topical
UTICORT
PARKE DAVIS — 0.025% — N018089 001

BETAMETHASONE DIPROPIONATE

Cream, Augmented; Topical
DIPROLENE
SCHERING — EQ 0.05% BASE — N019408 001 JAN 31, 1986

Cream; Topical
BETAMETHASONE DIPROPIONATE
CLAY PARK — EQ 0.05% BASE — N072536 001 JAN 31, 1990 / N074579 001 NOV 26, 1997
PHARMADERM — EQ 0.05% BASE — N019136 001 JUN 26, 1984
DIPROSONE
SCHERING — EQ 0.05% BASE — N017536 001

Disc; Topical
DIPROSONE
SCHERING — EQ 0.1% BASE — N017829 001

Lotion; Topical
BETAMETHASONE DIPROPIONATE
ALPHARMA — EQ 0.05% BASE — N071085 001 FEB 03, 1987 / N070274 001 AUG 12, 1985
PHARMADERM — EQ 0.05% BASE —

Ointment; Topical
BETAMETHASONE DIPROPIONATE
CLAY PARK — EQ 0.05% BASE — N072526 001 JAN 31, 1990
PHARMADERM — EQ 0.05% BASE — N019140 001 SEP 04, 1984
DIPROSONE
SCHERING — EQ 0.05% BASE — N017691 001

Discontinued Drug Products (continued)

BENZTHIAZIDE (continued)

Tablet; Oral
URESE
PFIZER — 25MG — N012128 003

BENZTROPINE MESYLATE

Tablet; Oral
BENZTROPINE MESYLATE
QUANTUM PHARMICS — 0.5MG — N088514 001 JAN 31, 1984
— 1MG — N088510 001 JAN 31, 1984
— 2MG — N088511 001 JAN 31, 1984
USL PHARMA — 0.5MG — N089211 001 JUN 14, 1988
— 1MG — N089212 001 JUN 14, 1988
— 2MG — N089213 001 JUN 14, 1988
COGENTIN
MERCK — 0.5MG — N009193 004
— 1MG — N009193 003
— 2MG — N009193 002

BENZYL BENZOATE

Emulsion; Topical
BENZYL BENZOATE
LANNETT — 50% — N084535 001

BEPRIDIL HYDROCHLORIDE

Tablet; Oral
BEPADIN
MEDPOINTE PHARM HLC — 200MG — N019001 001 DEC 28, 1990
— 300MG — N019001 002 DEC 28, 1990
— 400MG — N019001 003 DEC 28, 1990
VASCOR
ORTHO MCNEIL PHARM — 400MG — N019002 003 DEC 28, 1990

BETA-CAROTENE

Capsule; Oral
SOLATENE
ROCHE — 30MG — N017589 001

BETAMETHASONE

Cream; Topical
CELESTONE
SCHERING — 0.2% — N014762 001

Discontinued Drug Products (continued)

BETAMETHASONE VALERATE

Cream; Topical

BETAMETHASONE VALERATE

CLAY PARK	EQ 0.1% BASE	N070053 001	JUN 10, 1986
PHARMADERM	EQ 0.1% BASE	N018860 002	AUG 31, 1983
PHARMAFAIR	EQ 0.1% BASE	N070485 001	MAY 29, 1987

VALISONE

SCHERING	EQ 0.1% BASE	N016322 001
	EQ 0.01% BASE	N016322 002

Lotion; Topical

BETAMETHASONE VALERATE

PHARMADERM	EQ 0.1% BASE	N018870 001	AUG 31, 1983
PHARMAFAIR	EQ 0.1% BASE	N070484 001	MAY 29, 1987

VALISONE

SCHERING	EQ 0.1% BASE	N016932 001

Ointment; Topical

BETAMETHASONE VALERATE

CLAY PARK	EQ 0.1% BASE	N071478 001	DEC 23, 1987
PHARMADERM	EQ 0.1% BASE	N018864 001	AUG 31, 1983
PHARMAFAIR	EQ 0.1% BASE	N070486 001	MAY 29, 1987

VALISONE

SCHERING	EQ 0.1% BASE	N016740 001

BETAXOLOL HYDROCHLORIDE; CHLORTHALIDONE

Tablet; Oral

KERLEDEX

LOREX	5MG;12.5MG	N019807 001	OCT 30, 1992
	10MG;12.5MG	N019807 002	OCT 30, 1992

BETAXOLOL HYDROCHLORIDE; PILOCARPINE HYDROCHLORIDE

Suspension/Drops; Ophthalmic

BETOPTIC PILO

ALCON	EQ 0.25% BASE;1.75%	N020619 001	APR 17, 1997

BETAZOLE HYDROCHLORIDE

Injectable; Injection

HISTALOG

LILLY	50MG/ML	N009344 001

BETHANECHOL CHLORIDE

Injectable; Injection

BETHANECHOL CHLORIDE

QUAD PHARMS	5MG/ML	N089815 001	APR 12, 1988

BETHANECHOL CHLORIDE (continued)

Injectable; Injection

URECHOLINE

PLIVA	5MG/ML *SEE ANNUAL PREFACE INTRODUCTION DISCONTINUED SECTION*	N006536 001

Tablet; Oral

BETHANECHOL CHLORIDE

ASCOT	10MG	N088288 001	JUN 08, 1983
	25MG	N088289 001	JUN 08, 1983
EON	5MG	N084353 001	
	10MG	N084378 001	
	10MG	N084379 001	
	25MG	N084383 001	
	25MG	N084384 001	
IVAX PHARMS	25MG	N084689 001	
LANNETT	5MG	N084702 001	
	10MG	N084712 001	
	25MG	N084074 001	
WATSON LAB	5MG	N085230 002	
	10MG	N085228 001	
	25MG	N085229 001	
	50MG	N087397 001	
WATSON LABS	5MG	N084402 001	
	5MG	N085841 001	
	10MG	N084408 001	
	10MG	N085842 001	
	25MG	N084441 001	
	25MG	N085839 001	
	50MG	N087444 001	

DUVOID

WELLSPRING PHARM	10MG	N086262 001
	25MG	N086263 001
	50MG	N085882 003

MYOTONACHOL

GLENWOOD	5MG	N084188 001
	10MG	N084188 003
	25MG	N084188 004

URECHOLINE

PLIVA	5MG *SEE ANNUAL PREFACE INTRODUCTION DISCONTINUED SECTION*	N006536 003
	10MG *SEE ANNUAL PREFACE INTRODUCTION DISCONTINUED SECTION*	N006536 002
	25MG *SEE ANNUAL PREFACE INTRODUCTION DISCONTINUED SECTION*	N006536 004
	50MG *SEE ANNUAL PREFACE INTRODUCTION DISCONTINUED SECTION*	N006536 005

BRETYLIUM TOSYLATE (continued)

Injectable; Injection

BRETYLIUM TOSYLATE

Firm	Strength	Number	Date
AM PHARM PARTNERS	100MG/ML	N071298 001	FEB 13, 1987
		N071151 001	AUG 10, 1987
ASTRAZENECA	50MG/ML	N071152 001	AUG 10, 1987
	50MG/ML	N071153 001	AUG 10, 1987
		N070545 001	MAY 14, 1986
ELKINS SINN	50MG/ML	N070546 001	MAY 14, 1986
	50MG/ML	N071181 001	FEB 16, 1988
QUAD PHARMS	50MG/ML		

BRETYLIUM TOSYLATE IN DEXTROSE 5%

Firm	Strength	Number	Date
ABBOTT	200MG/100ML	N019005 002	APR 29, 1986
	400MG/100ML	N019005 003	APR 29, 1986
	800MG/100ML	N019005 001	APR 29, 1986

BRETYLIUM TOSYLATE IN DEXTROSE 5% IN PLASTIC CONTAINER

Firm	Strength	Number	Date
ABBOTT	800MG/100ML	N019008 001	APR 29, 1986
		N019837 001	APR 12, 1989
BAXTER HLTHCARE	400MG/100ML	N019837 002	APR 12, 1989
	200MG/100ML		

BRETYLOL

Firm	Strength	Number	Date
FAULDING	50MG/ML	N017954 001	

BRIMONIDINE TARTRATE

Solution/Drops; Ophthalmic

ALPHAGAN

Firm	Strength	Number	Date
ALLERGAN	0.2% *SEE ANNUAL PREFACE INTRODUCTION DISCONTINUED SECTION*	N020613 001	SEP 06, 1996
		N020490 001	
	0.5%		MAR 13, 1997

BROMOCRIPTINE MESYLATE

Capsule; Oral

BROMOCRIPTINE MESYLATE

Firm	Strength	Number	Date
LEK PHARM	EQ 5MG BASE	N075100 001	DEC 10, 1998

BROMODIPHENHYDRAMINE HYDROCHLORIDE

Capsule; Oral

AMBODRYL

Firm	Strength	Number	Date
PARKE DAVIS	25MG	N007984 001	

Discontinued Drug Products (continued)

BETHANIDINE SULFATE

Tablet; Oral

TENATHAN

Firm	Strength	Number	Date
ROBINS AH	10MG	N017675 001	
	25MG	N017675 002	

BIOTIN *MULTIPLE*

SEE ALPHA-TOCOPHEROL; ASCORBIC ACID; BIOTIN; CHOLECALCIFEROL; CYANOCOBALAMIN; FOLIC ACID; NIACINAMIDE; PANTOTHENIC ACID; PYRIDOXINE; RIBOFLAVIN; THIAMINE; VITAMIN A

SEE ASCORBIC ACID; BIOTIN; CYANOCOBALAMIN; DEXPANTHENOL; ERGOCALCIFEROL; FOLIC ACID; NIACINAMIDE; PYRIDOXINE; RIBOFLAVIN PHOSPHATE SODIUM; THIAMINE; VITAMIN A; VITAMIN E

SEE ASCORBIC ACID; BIOTIN; CYANOCOBALAMIN; DEXPANTHENOL; ERGOCALCIFEROL; FOLIC ACID; NIACINAMIDE; PYRIDOXINE HYDROCHLORIDE; RIBOFLAVIN PHOSPHATE SODIUM; THIAMINE HYDROCHLORIDE; VITAMIN A PALMITATE; VITAMIN E

SEE ASCORBIC ACID; BIOTIN; CYANOCOBALAMIN; DEXPANTHENOL; ERGOCALCIFEROL; FOLIC ACID; NIACINAMIDE; PYRIDOXINE HYDROCHLORIDE; RIBOFLAVIN PHOSPHATE SODIUM; THIAMINE HYDROCHLORIDE; VITAMIN A; VITAMIN E

SEE ASCORBIC ACID; BIOTIN; CYANOCOBALAMIN; ERGOCALCIFEROL; FOLIC ACID; NIACINAMIDE; PANTOTHENIC ACID; PHYTONADIONE; PYRIDOXINE; RIBOFLAVIN; THIAMINE; VITAMIN A PALMITATE; VITAMIN E

BIPERIDEN LACTATE

Injectable; Injection

AKINETON

Firm	Strength	Number	Date
ABBOTT	5MG/ML	N012418 002	

BISOPROLOL FUMARATE; HYDROCHLOROTHIAZIDE

Tablet; Oral

BISOPROLOL FUMARATE AND HYDROCHLOROTHIAZIDE

Firm	Strength	Number	Date
APOTHECON	5MG;6.25MG	N075642 001	DEC 27, 2000
	2.5MG;6.25MG	N075642 002	DEC 27, 2000
	10MG;6.25MG	N075642 003	DEC 27, 2000

BITOLTEROL MESYLATE

Aerosol, Metered; Inhalation

TORNALATE

Firm	Strength	Number	Date
SANOFI SYNTHELABO	0.37MG/INH	N018770 001	DEC 28, 1984

Solution; Inhalation

TORNALATE

Firm	Strength	Number	Date
SANOFI SYNTHELABO	0.2%	N019548 001	FEB 19, 1992

BRETYLIUM TOSYLATE

Injectable; Injection

BRETYLIUM TOSYLATE

Firm	Strength	Number	Date
AM PHARM PARTNERS	50MG/ML	N070134 001	APR 29, 1986

Discontinued Drug Products *(continued)*

BROMODIPHENHYDRAMINE HYDROCHLORIDE; CODEINE PHOSPHATE
Syrup; Oral

Product	Strength	Appl. No.	Date
BROMANYL — ALPHARMA	12.5MG/5ML;10MG/5ML	N088343 001	AUG 15, 1984

BROMPHENIRAMINE MALEATE
Elixir; Oral

Product	Strength	Appl. No.	Date
BROMPHENIRAMINE MALEATE — ALPHARMA	2MG/5ML	N086936 001	
PHARM ASSOC	2MG/5ML	N087517 001	
USL PHARMA	2MG/5ML	N087964 001	JAN 25, 1983

Injectable; Injection

Product	Strength	Appl. No.	Date
BROMPHENIRAMINE MALEATE — STERIS	100MG/ML	N083820 001	
DIMETANE-TEN — WYETH AYERST	10MG/ML	N011418 002	

Tablet, Extended Release; Oral

Product	Strength	Appl. No.	Date
DIMETANE — WYETH CONS	8MG	N010799 010	JUN 10, 1983
		N010799 011	JUN 10, 1983
	12MG	N010799	JUN 10, 1983

Tablet; Oral

Product	Strength	Appl. No.	Date
BROMPHENIRAMINE MALEATE — ANABOLIC	4MG	N086187 001	
BARR	4MG	N084468 001	
GENEVA PHARMS	4MG	N083215 001	
IVAX PHARMS	4MG	N084351 001	
NEWTRON PHARMS	4MG	N086987 001	
PAR PHARM	4MG	N087009 001	
PIONEER PHARMS	4MG	N088604 001	JUL 13, 1984
VITARINE	4MG	N085850 001	
WATSON LABS	4MG	N083123 001	
	4MG	N085769 001	
DIMETANE — WYETH CONS	4MG	N010799 003	

BROMPHENIRAMINE MALEATE; CODEINE PHOSPHATE; PHENYLPROPANOLAMINE HYDROCHLORIDE
Syrup; Oral

Product	Strength	Appl. No.	Date
DIMETANE-DC — ROBINS AH	2MG/5ML;10MG/5ML;12.5MG/5ML	N011694 006	MAR 29, 1984

BROMPHENIRAMINE MALEATE; DEXTROMETHORPHAN HYDROBROMIDE; PSEUDOEPHEDRINE HYDROCHLORIDE
Syrup; Oral

Product	Strength	Appl. No.	Date
BROMANATE DM — ALPHARMA	2MG/5ML;10MG/5ML;30MG/5ML	N088722 001	

BROMPHENIRAMINE MALEATE; DEXTROMETHORPHAN HYDROBROMIDE; PSEUDOEPHEDRINE HYDROCHLORIDE *(continued)*
Syrup; Oral

Product	Strength	Appl. No.	Date
BROMANATE DM — ALPHARMA			MAR 07, 1985
DIMETANE-DX — ROBINS AH	2MG/5ML;10MG/5ML;30MG/5ML	N019279 001	AUG 24, 1984

BROMPHENIRAMINE MALEATE; PHENYLPROPANOLAMINE HYDROCHLORIDE
Elixir; Oral

Product	Strength	Appl. No.	Date
BIPHETAP — MORTON GROVE	4MG/5ML;25MG/5ML	N086687 001	SEP 26, 1984
BROMANATE — ALPHARMA	4MG/5ML;25MG/5ML	N086688 001	FEB 06, 1985

Tablet, Extended Release; Oral

Product	Strength	Appl. No.	Date
BROMATAPP — COPLEY PHARM	12MG;75MG	N071099 001	JUL 02, 1987

BUCLIZINE HYDROCHLORIDE
Tablet; Oral

Product	Strength	Appl. No.	Date
BUCLADIN-S — STUART PHARMS	50MG	N010911 006	

BUDESONIDE
Powder, Metered; Inhalation

Product	Strength	Appl. No.	Date
PULMICORT — ASTRAZENECA	0.32MG/INH	N020441 003	JUN 24, 1997

Suspension; Inhalation

Product	Strength	Appl. No.	Date
PULMICORT RESPULES — ASTRAZENECA	1MG/2ML	N020929 003	AUG 08, 2000

BUPIVACAINE HYDROCHLORIDE
Injectable; Injection

Product	Strength	Appl. No.	Date
BUPIVACAINE HCL KIT — ABBOTT	0.23%	N019978 003	SEP 03, 1992
	0.075%	N019978 001	SEP 03, 1992
	0.114%	N019978 002	SEP 03, 1992

BUPROPION HYDROCHLORIDE
Tablet, Extended Release; Oral

Product	Strength	Appl. No.	Date
ZYBAN — GLAXOSMITHKLINE	100MG	N020711 002	MAY 14, 1997

Discontinued Drug Products (continued)

BUPROPION HYDROCHLORIDE (continued)
Tablet; Oral

WELLBUTRIN			
GLAXOSMITHKLINE	50MG	N018644 001	DEC 30, 1985

BUSPIRONE HYDROCHLORIDE
Capsule; Oral

BUSPAR			
BRISTOL MYERS SQUIBB	5MG	N021190 001	DEC 20, 2000
	7.5MG	N021190 002	DEC 20, 2000
	10MG	N021190 003	DEC 20, 2000
	15MG	N021190 004	DEC 20, 2000

BUTABARBITAL SODIUM
Capsule; Oral

BUTICAPS		
MEDPOINTE PHARM HLC	15MG	N085381 001
	30MG	N085381 002
	50MG	N085381 003
	100MG	N085381 004

Elixir; Oral

BUTABARB		
ALPHARMA	30MG/5ML	N085873 001
BUTABARBITAL SODIUM		
MORTON GROVE	30MG/5ML	N085383 001
BUTALAN		
LANNETT	33.3MG/5ML	N085880 001
SARISOL		
HALSEY	30MG/5ML	N084723 001

Tablet; Oral

BUTABARBITAL SODIUM			
EON	15MG	N085938 001	
	30MG	N085934 001	
GENEVA PHARMS	15MG	N084292 003	FEB 09, 1982
SOLVAY	30MG	N084272 002	
	16.2MG	N083606 001	
	32.4MG	N083898 001	
	48.6MG	N083897 001	
	97.2MG	N083896 001	
TEVA	15MG	N088632 001	MAY 18, 1985
	30MG	N088631 001	MAY 01, 1985
WATSON LABS	15MG	N085764 001	
	30MG	N085772 001	
WHITEWORTH TOWN			
PLSN	15MG	N083325 002	
	30MG	N083337 001	

BUTABARBITAL SODIUM (continued)
Tablet; Oral

BUTISOL SODIUM		
MEDPOINTE PHARM HLC	15MG	N000793 002
	100MG	N000793 005
SARISOL NO. 1		
HALSEY	15MG	N084719 001
SARISOL NO. 2		
HALSEY	30MG	N084719 002
SODIUM BUTABARBITAL		
IVAX PHARMS	15MG	N083484 001
	30MG	N084040 001
LANNETT	15MG	N085849 001
	30MG	N085866 001
	100MG	N085881 001
WEST WARD	15MG	N085418 001
	30MG	N085432 001

BUTALBITAL *MULTIPLE*
SEE   ACETAMINOPHEN; BUTALBITAL
SEE   ACETAMINOPHEN; BUTALBITAL; CAFFEINE
SEE   ASPIRIN; BUTALBITAL
SEE   ASPIRIN; BUTALBITAL; CAFFEINE

BUTOCONAZOLE NITRATE
Cream; Vaginal

FEMSTAT			
ROCHE PALO	2%	N019215 001	NOV 25, 1985

Suppository; Vaginal

FEMSTAT			
ROCHE PALO	100MG	N019359 001	NOV 25, 1985

CAFFEINE; ERGOTAMINE TARTRATE
Suppository; Rectal

MIGERGOT			
G AND W LABS	100MG;2MG	N086557 001	OCT 04, 1983

Tablet; Oral

CAFERGOT		
NOVARTIS	100MG;1MG	N006620 001
WIGRAINE		
ORGANON USA INC	100MG;1MG	N086562 001

CAFFEINE *MULTIPLE*
SEE   ACETAMINOPHEN; BUTALBITAL; CAFFEINE
SEE   ACETAMINOPHEN; CAFFEINE; DIHYDROCODEINE BITARTRATE
SEE   ASPIRIN; BUTALBITAL; CAFFEINE
SEE   ASPIRIN; CAFFEINE; PROPOXYPHENE HYDROCHLORIDE

Discontinued Drug Products (continued)

CALCIFEDIOL
Capsule; Oral
CALDEROL
ORGANON USA INC   0.02MG   N018312 001
                   0.05MG   N018312 002

CALCITONIN HUMAN
Injectable; Injection
CIBACALCIN
NOVARTIS   0.5MG/VIAL   N018470 001
                          OCT 31, 1986

CALCITONIN, SALMON
Injectable; Injection
CALCIMAR
AVENTIS   400 IU/VIAL   N017497 001
CALCITONIN-SALMON
ASTRAZENECA   200 IU/ML   N073690 001
                            APR 14, 1995
MIACALCIN
NOVARTIS   100 IU/ML   N017808 001
                         JUL 03, 1986

CALCIUM; MEGLUMINE; METRIZOIC ACID
Injectable; Injection
ISOPAQUE 280
AMERSHAM HLTH   0.35MG/ML;140.1MG/ML;461.8MG/ML   N017506 001

CALCIUM ACETATE
Capsule; Oral
PHOSLO
BRAINTREE   EQ 84.5MG CALCIUM   N021160 001
                                  APR 02, 2001
             EQ 169MG CALCIUM   N021160 002
                                 APR 02, 2001

CALCIUM CHLORIDE; DEXTROSE; MAGNESIUM CHLORIDE; POTASSIUM CHLORIDE; SODIUM ACETATE; SODIUM CHLORIDE
Injectable; Injection
ISOLYTE R W/ DEXTROSE 5% IN PLASTIC CONTAINER
37MG/100ML;5GM/100ML;31MG/100ML;120MG/100ML;330MG/100ML;88MG/100ML
B BRAUN   N018271 001

CALCIUM CHLORIDE; DEXTROSE; MAGNESIUM CHLORIDE; POTASSIUM CHLORIDE; SODIUM ACETATE; SODIUM CHLORIDE; SODIUM CITRATE
Injectable; Injection
ISOLYTE E W/ DEXTROSE 5% IN PLASTIC CONTAINER
35MG/100ML;5GM/100ML;30MG/100ML;640MG/100ML;74MG/100ML;500MG/100ML;74MG/100ML
B BRAUN   N018269 002
           JAN 17, 1983

CALCIUM CHLORIDE; DEXTROSE; MAGNESIUM CHLORIDE; SODIUM ACETATE; SODIUM CHLORIDE
Solution; Intraperitoneal
DIALYTE LM/ DEXTROSE 2.5% IN PLASTIC CONTAINER
2.9MG/100ML;2.5GM/100ML;15MG/100ML;610MG/100ML;560MG/100ML
B BRAUN   N018460 006
           JAN 29, 1986

DIALYTE W/ DEXTROSE 1.5% IN PLASTIC CONTAINER
2.9MG/100ML;1.5GM/100ML;15MG/100ML;610MG/100ML;560MG/100ML
B BRAUN   N018460 001

DIALYTE W/ DEXTROSE 4.25% IN PLASTIC CONTAINER
2.9MG/100ML;4.25GM/100ML;15MG/100ML;610MG/100ML;560MG/100ML
B BRAUN   N018460 003

CALCIUM CHLORIDE; DEXTROSE; MAGNESIUM CHLORIDE; SODIUM CHLORIDE; SODIUM LACTATE
Solution; Intraperitoneal
DIALYTE LM/ DEXTROSE 1.5% IN PLASTIC CONTAINER
2.6MG/100ML;1.5GM/100ML;15MG/100ML;560MG/100ML;390MG/100ML
B BRAUN   N018460 002

DIALYTE LM/ DEXTROSE 4.25% IN PLASTIC CONTAINER
2.6MG/100ML;4.25GM/100ML;15MG/100ML;560MG/100ML;390MG/100ML
B BRAUN   N018460 004

DIALYTE LM/ DEXTROSE 2.5% IN PLASTIC CONTAINER
26MG/100ML;5GM/100ML;5MG/100ML;530MG/100ML;450MG/100ML
B BRAUN   N018460 008
           JAN 29, 1986

CALCIUM CHLORIDE; DEXTROSE; POTASSIUM CHLORIDE; SODIUM CHLORIDE; SODIUM LACTATE
Injectable; Injection
DEXTROSE 5% IN LACTATED RINGER'S IN PLASTIC CONTAINER
20MG/100ML;5GM/100ML;30MG/100ML;600MG/100ML;310MG/100ML
B BRAUN   N017510 001

CALCIUM CHLORIDE; DEXTROSE; SODIUM CHLORIDE; SODIUM LACTATE *(continued)*
Solution; Intraperitoneal
INPERSOL-ZM W/ DEXTROSE 4.25% IN PLASTIC CONTAINER
25.7MG/100ML;4.25GM/100ML;538MG/100ML;448MG/100ML
FRESENIUS MEDCL
N019395 003
MAR 26, 1986

CALCIUM CHLORIDE; MAGNESIUM CHLORIDE; POTASSIUM CHLORIDE; SODIUM ACETATE; SODIUM CHLORIDE
Injectable; Injection
TPN ELECTROLYTES IN PLASTIC CONTAINER
16.5MG/ML;25.4MG/ML;74.6MG/ML;121MG/ML;16.1MG/ML
ABBOTT
N019399 001
JUN 16, 1986

CALCIUM CHLORIDE; MAGNESIUM CHLORIDE; POTASSIUM CHLORIDE; SODIUM ACETATE; SODIUM CHLORIDE; SODIUM CITRATE
Injectable; Injection
ISOLYTE E IN PLASTIC CONTAINER
3.5MG/100ML;30MG/100ML;74MG/100ML;640MG/100ML;500MG/100ML;74MG/100ML
B BRAUN
N018899 001
OCT 31, 1983

CALCIUM CHLORIDE; POTASSIUM CHLORIDE; SODIUM ACETATE; SODIUM CHLORIDE
Injectable; Injection
ACETATED RINGER'S IN PLASTIC CONTAINER
20MG/100ML;30MG/100ML;380MG/100ML;600MG/100ML
B BRAUN
N018725 001
NOV 29, 1982

CALCIUM CHLORIDE; POTASSIUM CHLORIDE; SODIUM CHLORIDE
Solution; Irrigation
RINGER'S IN PLASTIC CONTAINER
33MG/100ML;30MG/100ML;860MG/100ML
ABBOTT
N018462 001

CALCIUM CHLORIDE; POTASSIUM CHLORIDE; SODIUM CHLORIDE; SODIUM LACTATE
Injectable; Injection
LACTATED RINGER'S IN PLASTIC CONTAINER
20MG/100ML;30MG/100ML;600MG/100ML;310MG/100ML
B BFAUN
N018023 001

20MG/100ML;30MG/100ML;600MG/100ML;310MG/100ML
MILES
N018417 001

Discontinued Drug Products *(continued)*

CALCIUM CHLORIDE; DEXTROSE; POTASSIUM CHLORIDE; SODIUM CHLORIDE; SODIUM LACTATE *(continued)*
Injectable; Injection
DEXTROSE 5% IN LACTATED RINGER'S IN PLASTIC CONTAINER
20MG/100ML;5GM/100ML;30MG/100ML;600MG/100ML;310MG/100ML
MILES
N018499 001

DEXTROSE 4% IN MODIFIED LACTATED RINGER'S IN PLASTIC CONTAINER
4MG/100ML;4GM/100ML;6MG/100ML;120MG/100ML;62MG/100ML
B BRAUN
N019634 002
FEB 24, 1988

POTASSIUM CHLORIDE 5MEQ IN DEXTROSE 5% AND LACTATED RINGER'S IN PLASTIC CONTAINER
20MG/100ML;5GM/100ML;104MG/100ML;600MG/100ML;310MG/100ML
ABBOTT
N019685 001
OCT 17, 1988

POTASSIUM CHLORIDE 30MEQ IN DEXTROSE 5% AND LACTATED RINGER'S IN PLASTIC CONTAINER
20MG/100ML;5GM/100ML;254MG/100ML;600MG/100ML;310MG/100ML
ABBOTT
N019685 005
OCT 17, 1988

20MG/100ML;5GM/100ML;179MG/100ML;600MG/100ML;310MG/100ML
N019685 006
OCT 17, 1988

POTASSIUM CHLORIDE 10MEQ IN DEXTROSE 5% AND LACTATED RINGER'S IN PLASTIC CONTAINER
20MG/100ML;5GM/100ML;104MG/100ML;600MG/100ML;310MG/100ML
ABBOTT
N019685 003
OCT 17, 1988

POTASSIUM CHLORIDE 15MEQ IN DEXTROSE 5% AND LACTATED RINGER'S IN PLASTIC CONTAINER
20MG/100ML;5GM/100ML;254MG/100ML;600MG/100ML;310MG/100ML
ABBOTT
N019685 007
OCT 17, 1988

CALCIUM CHLORIDE; DEXTROSE; SODIUM CHLORIDE; SODIUM LACTATE
Solution; Intraperitoneal
INPERSOL-ZM W/ DEXTROSE 1.5% IN PLASTIC CONTAINER
25.7MG/100ML;1.5GM/100ML;538MG/100ML;448MG/100ML
FRESENIUS MEDCL
N019395 001
MAR 26, 1986

INPERSOL-ZM W/ DEXTROSE 2.5% IN PLASTIC CONTAINER
25.7MG/100ML;2.5GM/100ML;538MG/100ML;448MG/100ML
FRESENIUS MEDCL
N019395 002
MAR 26, 1986

Discontinued Drug Products (continued)

CALCIUM CHLORIDE; POTASSIUM CHLORIDE; SODIUM CHLORIDE; SODIUM LACTATE (continued)
Injectable; Injection
  LACTATED RINGER'S IN PLASTIC CONTAINER
    ABBOTT 20MG/100ML;30MG/100ML;600MG/100ML;310MG/100ML N019485 001 OCT 24, 1985

CALCIUM CHLORIDE *MULTIPLE*
  SEE AMINO ACIDS; CALCIUM CHLORIDE; DEXTROSE; MAGNESIUM CHLORIDE; POTASSIUM CHLORIDE; POTASSIUM PHOSPHATE, DIBASIC; SODIUM CHLORIDE

CALCIUM GLUCEPTATE
Injectable; Injection
  CALCIUM GLUCEPTATE
    ABBOTT EQ 90MG CALCIUM/5ML N080001 001
             EQ 90MG CALCIUM/5ML N083159 001
    AM PHARM PARTNERS EQ 90MG CALCIUM/5ML N089373 001 APR 30, 1987
    LILLY EQ 90MG CALCIUM/5ML N006470 001

CALCIUM METRIZOATE; MEGLUMINE METRIZOATE; METRIZOATE MAGNESIUM; METRIZOATE SODIUM
Injectable; Injection
  ISOPAQUE 440
    AMERSHAM HLTH 0.78MG/ML;75.9MG/ML;0.15MG/ML;16.6MG/ML N016847 001

CANDICIDIN
Ointment; Vaginal
  VANOBID
    AVENTIS PHARMS 0.6MG/GM N061596 001
Tablet; Vaginal
  VANOBID
    AVENTIS PHARMS 3MG N061613 001

CAPTOPRIL
Tablet; Oral
  CAPOTEN
    PAR PHARM 37.5MG N018343 006 SEP 17, 1986
          75MG N018343 007 JUN 13, 1995
          150MG N018343 004 JUN 13, 1995
  CAPTOPRIL
    PUREPAC PHARM 12.5MG N074640 001 MAR 31, 1997
                25MG N074640 002 MAR 31, 1997
                50MG N074640 003 MAR 31, 1997

CAPTOPRIL (continued)
Tablet; Oral
  CAPTOPRIL
    PUREPAC PHARM 100MG N074640 004 MAR 31, 1997

CAPTOPRIL; HYDROCHLOROTHIAZIDE
Tablet; Oral
  CAPTOPRIL AND HYDROCHLOROTHIAZIDE
    WATSON LABS 50MG;25MG N074832 001 DEC 29, 1997

CARBACHOL
Solution; Intraocular
  CARBACHOL
    PHARMAFAIR 0.01% N070292 001 MAY 21, 1986

CARBAMAZEPINE
Tablet; Oral
  CARBAMAZEPINE
    USL PHARMA 200MG N070300 001 MAY 15, 1986
    WARNER CHILCOTT 200MG N070429 001 JAN 02, 1987

CARBENICILLIN DISODIUM
Injectable; Injection
  GEOPEN
    ROERIG EQ 1GM BASE/VIAL N050306 001
           EQ 2GM BASE/VIAL N050306 004
           EQ 5GM BASE/VIAL N050306 002
           EQ 10GM BASE/VIAL N050306 006
           EQ 30GM BASE/VIAL N050306 007
  PYOPEN
    GLAXOSMITHKLINE EQ 1GM BASE/VIAL N050298 001
                 EQ 2GM BASE/VIAL N050298 002
                 EQ 5GM BASE/VIAL N050298 003
                 EQ 10GM BASE/VIAL N050298 006
                 EQ 20GM BASE/VIAL N050298 007

CARBIDOPA; LEVODOPA
Tablet; Oral
  CARBIDOPA AND LEVODOPA
    SCS 10MG;100MG N074080 001 MAR 25, 1994
        25MG;100MG N074080 002 MAR 25, 1994
        25MG;250MG N074080 003 MAR 25, 1994
    WATSON LABS 10MG;100MG N073381 001 SEP 28, 1993
              25MG;100MG N073382 001 SEP 28, 1993
              25MG;250MG N073383 001

Discontinued Drug Products (continued)

CARBIDOPA; LEVODOPA (continued)
Tablet; Oral
CARBIDOPA AND LEVODOPA
WATSON LABS — SEP 28, 1993

CARBINOXAMINE MALEATE
Elixir; Oral
CLISTIN
MCNEIL — 4MG/5ML *SEE ANNUAL PREFACE INTRODUCTION DISCONTINUED SECTION* — N008955 001

Tablet; Oral
CLISTIN
ORTHO MCNEIL PHARM — 4MG *SEE ANNUAL PREFACE INTRODUCTION DISCONTINUED SECTION* — N008915 001

CARISOPRODOL
Capsule; Oral
SOMA
MEDPOINTE PHARM HLC — 250MG — N011792 003

Tablet; Oral
CARISOPRODOL
EON — 350MG — N089566 001 AUG 30, 1988
— N089390 001 OCT 13, 1988
PIONEER PHARMS — 350MG — N085433 001
WATSON LAB — 350MG
RELA
SCHERING — 350MG — N012155 001

CARISOPRODOL *MULTIPLE*
SEE <u>ASPIRIN; CARISOPRODOL</u>

CARPHENAZINE MALEATE
Concentrate; Oral
PROKETAZINE
WYETH AYERST — 50MG/ML — N014173 001

Tablet; Oral
PROKETAZINE
WYETH AYERST — 12.5MG — N012768 001
— 25MG — N012768 002
— 50MG — N012768 004

CARPROFEN
Tablet; Oral
RIMADYL
ROCHE — 100MG — N018550 002 DEC 31, 1987
— 150MG — N018550 003 DEC 31, 1987

CARTEOLOL HYDROCHLORIDE
Tablet; Oral
CARTROL
ABBOTT — 10MG — N019204 003 DEC 28, 1988

CEFACLOR
Capsule; Oral
CEFACLOR
CLONMEL HLTHCARE — EQ 250MG BASE — N064107 001 APR 27, 1995
— EQ 500MG BASE — N064107 002 APR 27, 1995
TEVA — EQ 250MG BASE — N064081 001 SEP 16, 1996
— EQ 500MG BASE — N064081 002 SEP 16, 1996

For Suspension; Oral
CEFACLOR
CLONMEL HLTHCARE — EQ 125MG BASE/5ML — N064114 001 APR 28, 1995
— EQ 187MG BASE/5ML — N064115 001 APR 28, 1995
— EQ 250MG BASE/5ML — N064116 001 APR 28, 1995
— EQ 375MG BASE/5ML — N064110 001 APR 28, 1995
IVAX PHARMS — EQ 125MG BASE/5ML — N064087 001 APR 28, 1995
— EQ 187MG BASE/5ML — N064086 001 APR 28, 1995
— EQ 250MG BASE/5ML — N064085 001 APR 28, 1995

Tablet, Extended Release; Oral
CECLOR CD
LILLY — EQ 375MG BASE — N050673 001 JUN 28, 1996

CEFADROXIL/CEFADROXIL HEMIHYDRATE
Capsule; Oral
CEFADROXIL
PUREPAC PHARM — EQ 500MG BASE — N063017 001 JAN 05, 1989
TEVA — EQ 500MG BASE — N062695 001 FEB 10, 1989
DURICEF
WARNER CHILCOTT — EQ 250MG BASE — N050512 002
ULTRACEF
BRISTOL — EQ 500MG BASE — N062378 001 MAR 16, 1982

For Suspension; Oral
CEFADROXIL
APOTHECON — EQ 125MG BASE/5ML — N062334 001
— EQ 250MG BASE/5ML — N062334 002
— EQ 500MG BASE/5ML — N062334 003
TEVA — EQ 125MG BASE/5ML — N062698 001

Discontinued Drug Products *(continued)*

CEFADROXIL/CEFADROXIL HEMIHYDRATE *(continued)*
For Suspension; Oral
CEFADROXIL

TEVA	EQ 250MG BASE/5ML	N062698 002	MAR 01, 1989
		N062698 002	MAR 01, 1989
	EQ 500MG BASE/5ML	N062698 003	MAR 01, 1989
		N062698 003	MAR 01, 1989

ULTRACEF

BRISTOL	EQ 125MG BASE/5ML	N062376 001	MAR 16, 1982
	EQ 250MG BASE/5ML	N062376 002	MAR 16, 1982
	EQ 500MG BASE/5ML	N062376 003	MAR 16, 1982

Tablet; Oral
CEFADROXIL

IVAX PHARMS	EQ 1GM BASE	N062774 001	APR 08, 1987

ULTRACEF

APOTHECON	EQ 1GM BASE	N062390 001	JUN 10, 1982
BRISTOL	EQ 1GM BASE	N062408 001	AUG 31, 1982

CEFAMANDOLE NAFATE
Injectable; Injection
MANDOL

LILLY	EQ 1GM BASE/VIAL	N062560 001	SEP 10, 1985
	EQ 2GM BASE/VIAL	N062560 002	SEP 10, 1985
	EQ 10GM BASE/VIAL	N050504 004	
	EQ 500MG BASE/VIAL	N050504 001	

CEFAZOLIN SODIUM
Injectable; Injection
ANCEF

GLAXOSMITHKLINE	EQ 250MG BASE/VIAL	N050461 001	

ANCEF IN DEXTROSE 5% IN PLASTIC CONTAINER

BAXTER HLTHCARE	EQ 10MG BASE/ML	N050566 003	JUN 08, 1983
	EQ 20MG BASE/ML	N050566 004	JUN 08, 1983

ANCEF IN SODIUM CHLORIDE 0.9% IN PLASTIC CONTAINER

BAXTER HLTHCARE	EQ 10MG BASE/ML	N050566 001	JUN 08, 1983
	EQ 20MG BASE/ML	N050566 002	JUN 08, 1983

CEFAZOLIN SODIUM

AM PHARM PARTNERS	EQ 1GM BASE/VIAL	N062688 003	NOV 17, 1986
	EQ 10GM BASE/VIAL	N062688 004	NOV 17, 1986
	EQ 20GM BASE/VIAL	N062688 005	AUG 03, 1987

CEFAZOLIN SODIUM *(continued)*
Injectable; Injection
CEFAZOLIN SODIUM

AM PHARM PARTNERS	EQ 500MG BASE/VIAL	N062688 002	NOV 17, 1986
BEDFORD	EQ 1GM BASE/VIAL	N062894 003	JUL 21, 1988
	EQ 5GM BASE/VIAL	N062894 004	JUL 21, 1988
	EQ 10GM BASE/VIAL	N062894 005	JUL 21, 1988
	EQ 250MG BASE/VIAL	N062894 001	JUL 21, 1988
	EQ 500MG BASE/VIAL	N062894 002	JUL 21, 1988
ELKINS SINN	EQ 1GM BASE/VIAL	N062807 003	JAN 12, 1988
		N062807 004	JAN 12, 1988
	EQ 5GM BASE/VIAL	N062807 005	JAN 12, 1988
	EQ 10GM BASE/VIAL	N062807 006	JAN 12, 1988
	EQ 20GM BASE/VIAL	N062807 001	JAN 12, 1988
	EQ 250MG BASE/VIAL	N062807 002	JAN 12, 1988
	EQ 500MG BASE/VIAL	N063016 003	MAR 14, 1989
TEVA	EQ 1GM BASE/VIAL	N063016 001	MAR 14, 1989
	EQ 250MG BASE/VIAL	N063016 002	MAR 14, 1989
	EQ 500MG BASE/VIAL		
KEFZOL			
LILLY	EQ 1GM BASE/VIAL	N062557 002	SEP 10, 1985
	EQ 500MG BASE/VIAL	N062557 001	SEP 10, 1985

CEFIXIME
For Suspension; Oral
SUPRAX

LEDERLE	100MG/5ML	N050622 001	APR 28, 1989

Tablet; Oral
SUPRAX

LEDERLE	200MG	N050621 001	APR 28, 1989
	400MG	N050621 002	APR 28, 1989

CEFMENOXIME HYDROCHLORIDE
Injectable; Injection
CEFMAX

TAP PHARM	EQ 1GM BASE/VIAL	N050571 002	DEC 30, 1987

CEFORANIDE (continued)

Injectable; Injection

PRECEF

APOTHECON	500MG/VIAL	N062579 001	NOV 26, 1984
			NOV 26, 1984
BRISTOL	1GM/VIAL	N050554 002	MAY 24, 1984
	2GM/VIAL	N050554 003	MAY 24, 1984
	10GM/VIAL	N050554 004	MAY 24, 1984
	20GM/VIAL	N050554 005	MAY 24, 1984
	500MG/VIAL	N050554 001	MAY 24, 1984

CEFOTIAM HYDROCHLORIDE

Injectable; Injection

CERADON

TAKEDA	EQ 1GM BASE/VIAL	N050601 001	DEC 30, 1988

CEFOXITIN SODIUM

Injectable; Injection

MEFOXIN IN DEXTROSE 5% IN PLASTIC CONTAINER

MERCK	EQ 20MG BASE/ML	N050581 003	SEP 20, 1984
	EQ 40MG BASE/ML	N050581 004	SEP 20, 1984

MEFOXIN IN SODIUM CHLORIDE 0.9% IN PLASTIC CONTAINER

MERCK	EQ 40MG BASE/ML	N050581 001	SEP 20, 1984
	EQ 20MG BASE/ML	N050581 002	SEP 20, 1984

CEFPIRAMIDE SODIUM

Injectable; Injection

CEFPIRAMIDE SODIUM

WYETH AYERST	EQ 1GM BASE/VIAL	N050633 002	JAN 31, 1989
	EQ 2GM BASE/VIAL	N050633 003	JAN 31, 1989
	EQ 10GM BASE/VIAL	N050633 005	JAN 31, 1989

CEFPODOXIME PROXETIL

For Suspension; Oral

BANAN

SANKYO	EQ 50MG BASE/5ML	N050688 002	AUG 07, 1992
	EQ 100MG BASE/5ML	N050688 001	AUG 07, 1992

Discontinued Drug Products (continued)

CEFMENOXIME HYDROCHLORIDE (continued)

Injectable; Injection

CEFMAX

TAP PHARM	EQ 2GM BASE/VIAL	N050571 003	DEC 30, 1987
	EQ 500MG BASE/VIAL	N050571 001	DEC 30, 1987

CEFMETAZOLE SODIUM

Injectable; Injection

ZEFAZONE

PHARMACIA AND UPJOHN	EQ 1GM BASE/VIAL	N050637 001	DEC 11, 1989
	EQ 2GM BASE/VIAL	N050637 002	DEC 11, 1989

ZEFAZONE IN PLASTIC CONTAINER

PHARMACIA AND UPJOHN	EQ 20MG BASE/ML	N050683 001	DEC 29, 1992
	EQ 40MG BASE/ML	N050683 002	DEC 29, 1992

CEFONICID SODIUM

Injectable; Injection

MONOCID

GLAXOSMITHKLINE	EQ 1GM BASE/VIAL	N050579 002	MAY 23, 1984
	EQ 1GM BASE/VIAL	N063295 001	JUL 26, 1993
	EQ 2GM BASE/VIAL	N050579 003	MAY 23, 1984
	EQ 10GM BASE/VIAL	N050579 004	MAY 23, 1984
	EQ 500MG BASE/VIAL	N050579 001	MAY 23, 1984

CEFOPERAZONE SODIUM

Injectable; Injection

CEFOBID

PFIZER	EQ 1GM BASE/VIAL	N063333 001	MAR 31, 1995
	EQ 2GM BASE/VIAL	N063333 002	MAR 31, 1995

CEFORANIDE

Injectable; Injection

PRECEF

APOTHECON	1GM/VIAL	N062579 002	NOV 26, 1984
	2GM/VIAL	N062579 003	NOV 26, 1984
	10GM/VIAL	N062579 004	NOV 26, 1984
	20GM/VIAL	N062579 005	NOV 26, 1984

Discontinued Drug Products *(continued)*

CEFPODOXIME PROXETIL *(continued)*
Tablet; Oral

BANAN

SANKYO	EQ 100MG BASE	N050687 001	AUG 07, 1992
	EQ 200MG BASE	N050687 002	AUG 07, 1992

CEFTAZIDIME
Injectable; Injection

TAZIDIME IN PLASTIC CONTAINER

LILLY	1GM/VIAL	N062739 001	JUL 10, 1986
	2GM/VIAL	N062739 002	JUL 10, 1986

CEFTAZIDIME (ARGININE FORMULATION)
Injectable; Injection

CEPTAZ

GLAXOSMITHKLINE	500MG/VIAL	N050646 001	SEP 27, 1990

PENTACEF

GLAXOSMITHKLINE	1GM/VIAL	N063322 001	NOV 07, 1995
	1GM/VIAL	N064006 001	MAR 31, 1992
	2GM/VIAL	N063322 002	NOV 07, 1995
	2GM/VIAL	N064006 002	MAR 31, 1992
	6GM/VIAL	N064008 001	MAR 31, 1992
	10GM/VIAL	N064008 002	MAR 31, 1992

CEFTAZIDIME SODIUM
Injectable; Injection

FORTAZ IN PLASTIC CONTAINER

GLAXOSMITHKLINE	EQ 10MG BASE/ML	N050634 001	APR 28, 1989

CEFTIZOXIME SODIUM
Injectable; Injection

CEFIZOX

FUJISAWA HLTHCARE	EQ 500MG BASE/VIAL	N050560 001	SEP 15, 1983

CEFIZOX IN DEXTROSE 5% IN PLASTIC CONTAINER

FUJISAWA HLTHCARE	EQ 20MG BASE/ML	N050589 001	OCT 03, 1984
	EQ 40MG BASE/ML	N050589 002	OCT 03, 1984

CEFTRIAXONE SODIUM
Injectable; Injection

ROCEPHIN

HLR	EQ 500MG BASE/VIAL	N062654 001	APR 30, 1987
	EQ 1GM BASE/VIAL	N062510 003	MAR 12, 1985
ROCHE	EQ 250MG BASE/VIAL	N062510 001	MAR 12, 1985
	EQ 500MG BASE/VIAL	N062510 002	MAR 12, 1985

ROCEPHIN W/ DEXTROSE IN PLASTIC CONTAINER

HLR	EQ 10MG BASE/ML	N050624 001	FEB 11, 1987

CEFTRIAXONE SODIUM; LIDOCAINE
Injectable; Injection

ROCEPHIN KIT

HLR	EQ 1GM BASE/VIAL;1%	N050585 006	MAY 08, 1996
	EQ 500MG BASE/VIAL,1%	N050585 007	MAY 08, 1996

CEFUROXIME SODIUM
Injectable; Injection

KEFUROX IN PLASTIC CONTAINER

LILLY	EQ 1.5GM BASE/VIAL	N062590 002	JAN 10, 1986

Injectable; Intravenous

KEFUROX IN PLASTIC CONTAINER

LILLY	EQ 750MG BASE/VIAL	N062590 001	JAN 10, 1986

CELLULOSE SODIUM PHOSPHATE
Powder; Oral

CALCIBIND

MISSION PHARMA	2.5GM/PACKET	N018757 002	DEC 28, 1982

CEPHALEXIN
Capsule; Oral

CEPHALEXIN

APOTHECON	EQ 250MG BASE	N062973 001	NOV 08, 1988
	EQ 500MG BASE	N062974 001	NOV 23, 1988
PUREPAC PHARM	EQ 250MG BASE	N062809 001	APR 22, 1987
	EQ 500MG BASE	N062809 002	APR 22, 1987
STEVENS J	EQ 500MG BASE	N062869 001	MAR 17, 1988
TEVA	EQ 500MG BASE	N062823 001	FEB 05, 1988
YOSHITOMI	EQ 250MG BASE	N062872 001	

Discontinued Drug Products *(continued)*

CEPHALEXIN *(continued)*

Capsule; Oral

CEPHALEXIN

Firm	Strength	Appl. No.	Date
YOSHITOMI	EQ 500MG BASE	N062871 001	JUN 20, 1988 / JUL 05, 1988

For Suspension; Oral

CEPHALEXIN

Firm	Strength	Appl. No.	Date
BARR	EQ 125MG BASE/5ML	N062778 001	AUG 06, 1987
TEVA	EQ 125MG BASE/5ML	N062873 001	MAY 23, 1988
TEVA	EQ 250MG BASE/5ML	N062867 001	APR 15, 1988
VITARINE	EQ 125MG BASE/5ML	N062779 001	DEC 22, 1987
VITARINE	EQ 250MG BASE/5ML	N062781 001	DEC 22, 1987

KEFLEX

Firm	Strength	Appl. No.	Date
LILLY	EQ 100MG BASE/ML	N050406 003	
LILLY	EQ 125MG BASE/5ML	N050406 001	
LILLY	EQ 250MG BASE/5ML	N050406 002	

Tablet; Oral

CEPHALEXIN

Firm	Strength	Appl. No.	Date
BARR	EQ 250MG BASE	N062826 001	AUG 17, 1987
BARR	EQ 500MG BASE	N062827 001	AUG 17, 1987
VITARINE	EQ 1GM BASE	N062863 003	AUG 11, 1988
VITARINE	EQ 250MG BASE	N062863 001	AUG 11, 1988
VITARINE	EQ 500MG BASE	N062863 002	AUG 11, 1988

KEFLET

Firm	Strength	Appl. No.	Date
LILLY	EQ 1GM BASE	N050440 002	
LILLY	EQ 250MG BASE	N062745 001	DEC 01, 1986
LILLY	EQ 500MG BASE	N050440 001	
LILLY	EQ 500MG BASE	N062745 002	DEC 01, 1986

CEPHALOTHIN SODIUM

Injectable; Injection

CEPHALOTHIN

Firm	Strength	Appl. No.	Date
INTL MEDICATION	EQ 1GM BASE/VIAL	N062426 002	MAY 03, 1985
INTL MEDICATION	EQ 2GM BASE/VIAL	N062426 003	MAY 03, 1985
INTL MEDICATION	EQ 4GM BASE/VIAL	N062426 004	MAY 03, 1985
INTL MEDICATION	EQ 500MG BASE/VIAL	N062426 001	MAY 03, 1985

CEPHALOTHIN SODIUM

Firm	Strength	Appl. No.	Date
ABBOTT	EQ 1GM BASE/VIAL	N062547 001	SEP 11, 1985
ABBOTT	EQ 1GM BASE/VIAL	N062548 001	SEP 11, 1985
ABBOTT	EQ 2GM BASE/VIAL	N062547 002	SEP 11, 1985
ABBOTT	EQ 2GM BASE/VIAL	N062548 002	SEP 11, 1985
AM PHARM PARTNERS	EQ 1GM BASE/VIAL	N062666 002	JUN 10, 1987
AM PHARM PARTNERS	EQ 2GM BASE/VIAL	N062666 001	JUN 10, 1987

CEPHALOTHIN SODIUM W/ DEXTROSE IN PLASTIC CONTAINER

Firm	Strength	Appl. No.	Date
BAXTER HLTHCARE	EQ 20MG BASE/ML	N062422 003	JAN 31, 1984
BAXTER HLTHCARE	EQ 40MG BASE/ML	N062422 004	JAN 31, 1984
BAXTER HLTHCARE	EQ 20MG BASE/ML	N062422 005	JUL 16, 1991
BAXTER HLTHCARE	EQ 40MG BASE/ML	N062422 006	JUL 16, 1991
BAXTER HLTHCARE	EQ 20MG BASE/ML	N062730 001	MAR 05, 1987
BAXTER HLTHCARE	EQ 40MG BASE/ML	N062730 002	MAR 05, 1987

CEPHALOTHIN SODIUM W/ SODIUM CHLORIDE IN PLASTIC CONTAINER

Firm	Strength	Appl. No.	Date
BAXTER HLTHCARE	EQ 20MG BASE/ML	N062422 001	JAN 31, 1984
BAXTER HLTHCARE	EQ 40MG BASE/ML	N062422 002	JAN 31, 1984

KEFLIN

Firm	Strength	Appl. No.	Date
LILLY	EQ 1GM BASE/VIAL	N050482 001	
LILLY	EQ 2GM BASE/VIAL	N050482 002	
LILLY	EQ 4GM BASE/VIAL	N050482 003	
LILLY	EQ 20GM BASE/VIAL	N050482 007	

KEFLIN IN PLASTIC CONTAINER

Firm	Strength	Appl. No.	Date
LILLY	EQ 1GM BASE/VIAL	N062549 001	SEP 10, 1985
LILLY	EQ 2GM BASE/VIAL	N062549 002	SEP 10, 1985

SEFFIN

Firm	Strength	Appl. No.	Date
GLAXOSMITHKLINE	EQ 1GM BASE/VIAL	N062435 001	NOV 15, 1983
GLAXOSMITHKLINE	EQ 2GM BASE/VIAL	N062435 002	

CEPHALEXIN HYDROCHLORIDE

Tablet; Oral

KEFTAB

Firm	Strength	Appl. No.	Date
LILLY	EQ 250MG BASE	N050614 001	OCT 29, 1987
LILLY	EQ 333MG BASE	N050614 003	MAY 16, 1988

CEPHALOGLYCIN

Capsule; Oral

KAFOCIN

Firm	Strength	Appl. No.	Date
LILLY	250MG	N050219 001	

CEPHRADINE (continued)

Capsule; Oral
CEPHRADINE

Company	Strength	Appl. No.	Date
IVAX PHARMS	500MG	N062762 002	MAR 06, 1987
	250MG	N062813 001	FEB 25, 1988
VITARINE	500MG	N062813 002	FEB 25, 1988
VELOSEF '250' ERSANA	250MG	N050548 001	
VELOSEF '500' ERSANA	500MG	N050548 002	

For Suspension; Oral
CEPHRADINE

Company	Strength	Appl. No.	Date
BARR	125MG/5ML	N062858 001	MAY 19, 1988
	250MG/5ML	N062859 001	MAY 19, 1988

Injectable; Injection
VELOSEF

Company	Strength	Appl. No.	Date
APOTHECON	1GM/VIAL	N061976 004	
	2GM/VIAL	N061976 003	
	4GM/VIAL	N061976 005	
	250MG/VIAL	N061976 001	
	500MG/VIAL	N061976 002	

Tablet; Oral
VELOSEF

Company	Strength	Appl. No.	Date
BRISTOL MYERS SQUIBB	1GM	N050530 001	

CERIVASTATIN SODIUM

Tablet; Oral
BAYCOL

Company	Strength	Appl. No.	Date
BAYER PHARMS	0.1MG	N020740 002	JUN 26, 1997
	0.2MG	N020740 003	JUN 26, 1997
	0.3MG	N020740 004	JUN 26, 1997
	0.4MG	N020740 005	MAY 24, 1999
	0.05MG	N020740 001	JUN 26, 1997
	0.8MG	N020740 006	JUL 24, 2000

CERULETIDE DIETHYLAMINE

Injectable; Injection
TYMTRAN

Company	Strength	Appl. No.	Date
PHARMACIA AND UPJOHN	0.02MG/ML	N018296 001	

Discontinued Drug Products (continued)

CEPHALOTHIN SODIUM (continued)

Injectable; Injection
SEFFIN

Company	Strength	Appl. No.	Date
GLAXOSMITHKLINE	EQ 10GM BASE/VIAL	N062435 003	NOV 15, 1983

CEPHAPIRIN SODIUM

Injectable; Injection
CEFADYL

Company	Strength	Appl. No.	Date
APOTHECON	EQ 1GM BASE/VIAL	N050446 001	
	EQ 1GM BASE/VIAL	N062724 001	DEC 23, 1986
	EQ 1GM BASE/VIAL	N062961 002	SEP 20, 1988
	EQ 2GM BASE/VIAL	N050446 002	
	EQ 2GM BASE/VIAL	N062724 002	DEC 23, 1986
	EQ 2GM BASE/VIAL	N062961 003	SEP 20, 1988
	EQ 4GM BASE/VIAL	N050446 003	
	EQ 4GM BASE/VIAL	N062961 004	SEP 20, 1988
	EQ 20GM BASE/VIAL	N050446 004	
	EQ 500MG BASE/VIAL	N050446 005	
	EQ 500MG BASE/VIAL	N062961 001	SEP 20, 1988

CEPHAPIRIN SODIUM

Company	Strength	Appl. No.	Date
AM PHARM PARTNERS	EQ 1GM BASE/VIAL	N062723 002	NOV 17, 1986
	EQ 2GM BASE/VIAL	N062723 003	NOV 17, 1986
	EQ 4GM BASE/VIAL	N062723 004	NOV 17, 1986
	EQ 20GM BASE/VIAL	N062723 005	NOV 17, 1986
	EQ 500MG BASE/VIAL	N062723 001	NOV 17, 1986
ELKINS SINN	EQ 1GM BASE/VIAL	N062720 002	JUL 02, 1987
	EQ 2GM BASE/VIAL	N062720 003	JUL 02, 1987
	EQ 20GM BASE/VIAL	N062720 004	JUL 02, 1987
	EQ 500MG BASE/VIAL	N062720 001	JUL 02, 1987

CEPHRADINE

Capsule; Oral
CEPHRADINE

Company	Strength	Appl. No.	Date
BARR	250MG	N062850 001	APR 22, 1988
	500MG	N062851 001	APR 22, 1988
IVAX PHARMS	250MG	N062762 001	MAR 06, 1987

Discontinued Drug Products (continued)

CHENODIOL
Tablet; Oral
CHENIX
| AXCAN SCANDIPHARM | 250MG | N018513 002 JUL 28, 1983 |

CHLOPHEDIANOL HYDROCHLORIDE
Syrup; Oral
ULO
| 3M | 25MG/5ML | N012126 001 |

CHLORAMPHENICOL
Capsule; Oral
AMPHICOL
| FERRANTE | 100MG | N060058 001 |
| | 250MG | N060058 002 |
CHLORAMPHENICOL
| IVAX PHARMS | 250MG | N062247 001 |
CHLOROMYCETIN
PARKEDALE	50MG	N060591 001
	100MG	N060591 003
	250MG	N060591 002

Cream; Topical
CHLOROMYCETIN
| PARKE DAVIS | 1% | N050183 001 |
For Solution; Ophthalmic
CHLOROMYCETIN
| PARKEDALE | 25MG/VIAL | N050143 001 |
Injectable; Injection
CHLOROMYCETIN
| PARKE DAVIS | 250MG/ML | N050153 001 |
Ointment; Ophthalmic
CHLOROFAIR
| PHARMAFAIR | 1% | N062439 001 APR 21, 1983 |
CHLOROMYCETIN
| PARKEDALE | 1% | N050156 001 |
CHLOROPTIC S.O.P.
| ALLERGAN | 1% | N061187 001 |
ECONOCHLOR
| ALCON | 1% | N061648 001 |
Solution/Drops; Ophthalmic
CHLORAMPHENICOL
| AKORN | 0.5% | N062042 001 |
| ALCON | 0.5% | N062628 001 SEP 25, 1985 |
CHLOROFAIR
| PHARMAFAIR | 0.5% | N062437 001 APR 14, 1983 |
CHLOROPTIC
| ALLERGAN | 0.5% | N050091 001 |
ECONOCHLOR
| ALCON | 0.5% | N061645 001 |

CHLORAMPHENICOL (continued)
Solution/Drops; Ophthalmic
OPHTHOCHLOR
| PARKEDALE | 0.5% | N061220 001 |
OPTOMYCIN
| OPTOPICS | 0.5% | N062171 001 MAR 31, 1982 |
CHLOROMYCETIN
| PARKEDALE | 0.5% | N050205 001 |
Solution/Drops; Otic
CHLOROMYCETIN
| PARKEDALE | 0.5% | |

CHLORAMPHENICOL; HYDROCORTISONE ACETATE
For Suspension; Ophthalmic
CHLOROMYCETIN HYDROCORTISONE
| PARKEDALE | 12.5MG/VIAL;25MG/VIAL | N050202 001 |

CHLORAMPHENICOL; HYDROCORTISONE ACETATE; POLYMYXIN B SULFATE
Ointment; Ophthalmic
OPHTHOCORT
| PARKEDALE | 10MG/GM;5MG/GM;10,000 UNITS/GM | N050201 002 |

CHLORAMPHENICOL; POLYMYXIN B SULFATE
Ointment; Ophthalmic
CHLOROMYXIN
| PARKE DAVIS | 1%;10,000 UNITS/GM | N050203 002 |

CHLORAMPHENICOL; PREDNISOLONE
Ointment; Ophthalmic
CHLOROPTIC-P S.O.P.
| ALLERGAN | 1%;0.5% | N061188 001 |

CHLORAMPHENICOL PALMITATE
Suspension; Oral
CHLOROMYCETIN PALMITATE
| PARKE DAVIS | EQ 150MG BASE/5ML | N050152 001 |
| | EQ 150MG BASE/5ML | N062301 001 |

CHLORAMPHENICOL SODIUM SUCCINATE
Injectable; Injection
CHLORAMPHENICOL
| ELKINS SINN | EQ 1GM BASE/VIAL | N062406 001 NOV 09, 1982 |
MYCHEL-S
| ANGUS | EQ 1GM BASE/VIAL | N060132 001 |

CHLORDIAZEPOXIDE
Capsule, Extended Release; Oral
LIBRELEASE
| ICN | 30MG | N017813 001 SEP 12, 1983 |

Discontinued Drug Products *(continued)*

CHLORDIAZEPOXIDE *(continued)*

Tablet; Oral

Product / Firm	Strength	Application No.	Date
LIBRITABS			
ICN	5MG	N085482 001	
	10MG	N085481 001	
	25MG	N085488 001	

CHLORDIAZEPOXIDE; ESTROGENS, ESTERIFIED

Tablet; Oral

Product / Firm	Strength	Application No.	Date
MENRIUM 5-2			
ROCHE	5MG;0.2MG	N014740 002	
MENRIUM 5-4			
ROCHE	5MG;0.4MG	N014740 004	
MENRIUM 10-4			
ROCHE	10MG;0.4MG	N014740 006	

CHLORDIAZEPOXIDE *MULTIPLE*

SEE AMITRIPTYLINE HYDROCHLORIDE; CHLORDIAZEPOXIDE

CHLORDIAZEPOXIDE HYDROCHLORIDE

Capsule; Oral

Product / Firm	Strength	Application No.	Date
A-POXIDE			
ABBOTT	5MG	N085447 001	
	5MG	N085517 001	JAN 07, 1982
	10MG	N085447 002	
	10MG	N085518 001	
	25MG	N085447 003	JAN 07, 1982
	25MG	N085513 001	
CHLORDIAZACHEL			
RACHELLE	5MG	N085086 001	
	10MG	N084639 001	
	25MG	N085087 001	
CHLORDIAZEPOXIDE HCL			
ASCOT	5MG	N087525 001	JAN 07, 1982
		N087524 001	JAN 07, 1982
	10MG	N087512 001	JAN 07, 1982
	25MG	N084919 001	
EON	5MG	N084920 001	
	10MG	N084823 001	
	25MG	N085118 001	
FERRANTE	5MG	N085119 001	
	10MG	N085120 001	
	25MG	N084678 001	
GENEVA PHARMS	5MG	N084041 001	
	10MG	N084679 002	
	25MG	N085340 001	
HALSEY	5MG	N085339 001	
	10MG	N084685 001	
	25MG	N086213 001	
IMPAX LABS	5MG	N086212 001	
	25MG	N083741 001	
IVAX PHARMS	5MG	N083742 001	
	10MG		

CHLORDIAZEPOXIDE HYDROCHLORIDE *(continued)*

Capsule; Oral

CHLORDIAZEPOXIDE HCL *(continued)*

Product / Firm	Strength	Application No.	Date
IVAX PHARMS	25MG	N083570 001	
LEDERLE	5MG	N086892 001	
	5MG	N087234 001	
	10MG	N086876 001	
	10MG	N087037 001	
	25MG	N086893 001	
	25MG	N087231 001	
MAST MM	10MG	N086217 001	
MYLAN	5MG	N084886 001	
	10MG	N084601 001	
	25MG	N084887 001	
PARKE DAVIS	5MG	N085163 001	
	10MG	N084598 001	
	25MG	N085164 001	
PIONEER PHARMS	10MG	N089533 001	JUL 15, 1988
	25MG	N089558 001	JUL 15, 1988
PUREPAC PHARM	5MG	N085155 001	
	10MG	N084939 002	
	25MG	N085144 001	
ROXANE	5MG	N084706 001	
	10MG	N084700 001	
	25MG	N084705 001	
SUPERPHARM	5MG	N088987 001	APR 25, 1985
	10MG	N088986 001	APR 25, 1985
	25MG	N088988 001	APR 25, 1985
TEVA	5MG	N088705 001	JAN 18, 1985
	10MG	N088706 001	JAN 18, 1985
	25MG	N086494 001	
	25MG	N088707 001	JAN 18, 1985
USL PHARMA	5MG	N084644 001	
	25MG	N084645 001	
VANGARD	5MG	N088129 001	MAR 28, 1983
	10MG	N088010 001	MAR 28, 1983
	25MG	N088130 001	MAR 28, 1983
WEST WARD	5MG	N085014 001	
	10MG	N085000 001	
	25MG	N085294 001	
LIBRIUM			
ICN	5MG	N012249 002	
	10MG	N012249 001	
	25MG	N012249 003	
LYGEN			
ALRA	5MG	N085107 001	

Discontinued Drug Products (continued)

CHLORDIAZEPOXIDE HYDROCHLORIDE (continued)
Capsule; Oral

LYGEN			
ALRA	10MG	N085009 001	
	25MG	N085108 001	

CHLORHEXIDINE GLUCONATE
Solution; Topical

EXIDINE			
XTTRIUM	2.5%	N019421 001	DEC 17, 1985

Sponge; Topical

E-Z SCRUB			
BECTON DICKINSON	4%	N073416 001	MAR 14, 2000

CHLORMERODRIN, HG-197
Injectable; Injection

CHLORMERODRIN HG 197		
BRACCO	0.6-1.4mCi/ML	N017269 001

CHLORMEZANONE
Tablet; Oral

TRANCOPAL		
SANOFI SYNTHELABO	100MG	N011467 003
	200MG	N011467 005

CHLOROPROCAINE HYDROCHLORIDE
Injectable; Injection

NESACAINE-MPF		
ASTRAZENECA	2%	N009435 003
	3%	N009435 004

CHLOROQUINE HYDROCHLORIDE
Injectable; Injection

ARALEN HCL		
SANOFI SYNTHELABO	EQ 40MG BASE/ML	N006002 002

CHLOROQUINE PHOSPHATE
Tablet; Oral

CHLOROQUINE PHOSPHATE			
MD PHARM	EQ 150MG BASE	N087228 001	
PUREPAC PHARM	EQ 150MG BASE	N080886 001	
TEVA	EQ 150MG BASE	N087504 001	JAN 13, 1982

CHLOROQUINE PHOSPHATE; PRIMAQUINE PHOSPHATE
Tablet; Oral

ARALEN PHOSPHATE W/ PRIMAQUINE PHOSPHATE		
SANOFI SYNTHELABO	EQ 300MG BASE;EQ 45MG BASE	N014860 002

CHLOROTHIAZIDE
Tablet; Oral

CHLOROTHIAZIDE			
ABC HOLDING	250MG	N085569 001	
EON	250MG	N085485 001	
LEDERLE	250MG	N086940 001	
	500MG	N086938 001	
WATSON LAB	250MG	N085165 001	
	500MG	N084026 001	SEP 01, 1982
WATSON LABS	250MG	N085173 001	
	250MG	N086795 001	AUG 15, 1983
	500MG	N086796 001	AUG 15, 1983

CHLOROTHIAZIDE; METHYLDOPA
Tablet; Oral

ALDOCLOR-150			
MERCK	150MG;250MG	N016016 001	
ALDOCLOR-250			
MERCK	250MG;250MG	N016016 002	
METHYLDOPA AND CHLOROTHIAZIDE			
PAR PHARM	150MG;250MG	N070783 001	NOV 06, 1987
	250MG;250MG	N070654 001	NOV 06, 1987

CHLOROTHIAZIDE; RESERPINE
Tablet; Oral

CHLOROTHIAZIDE AND RESERPINE			
WEST WARD	250MG;0.125MG	N088557 001	DEC 22, 1983
	500MG;0.125MG	N088365 001	DEC 22, 1983
CHLOROTHIAZIDE W/ RESERPINE			
WATSON LAB	250MG;0.125MG	N084853 001	
	500MG;0.125MG	N088151 001	JUN 09, 1983
CHLOROTHIAZIDE-RESERPINE			
MYLAN	250MG;0.125MG	N087744 001	MAY 06, 1982
	500MG;0.125MG	N087745 001	MAY 06, 1982

CHLOROTRIANISENE
Capsule; Oral

CHLOROTRIANISENE			
BANNER PHARMACAPS	12MG	N084652 001	
TACE			
AVENTIS PHARMS	12MG	N008102 004	
	25MG	N011444 001	
	72MG	N016235 001	

CHLORPHENIRAMINE MALEATE *(continued)*

Tablet; Oral

CHLORPHENIRAMINE MALEATE			
WATSON LABS	4MG	N085139 001	
WEST WARD	4MG	N083787 001	
KLOROMIN			
HALSEY	4MG	N083629 001	
PHENETRON			
LANNETT	4MG	N080846 001	

CHLORPHENIRAMINE MALEATE; PHENYLPROPANOLAMINE HYDROCHLORIDE

Capsule, Extended Release; Oral

CHLOROHENIRAMINE MALEATE AND PHENYLPROPANOLAMINE HCL			
WATSON LABS	12MG;75MG	N088681 001	SEP 29, 1987
CHLORPHENIRAMINE MALEATE AND PHENYLPROPANOLAMINE HCL			
GENEVA PHARMS	12MG;75MG	N088940 001	JAN 26, 1989
COLD CAPSULE IV			
GRAHAM DM	12MG;75MG	N018793 001	APR 25, 1985
COLD CAPSULE V			
GRAHAM DM	8MG;75MG	N018794 001	APR 23, 1985
CONTAC 12 HOUR			
GLAXOSMITHKLINE	8MG;75MG	N018099 001	
DRIZE			
ASCHER	12MG;75MG	N088359 001	FEB 13, 1986
ORNADE			
GLAXOSMITHKLINE	12MG;75MG	N012152 004	
PHENYLPROPANOLAMINE HCL W/ CHLORPHENIRAMINE MALEATE			
CENT PHARMS	8MG;75MG	N018809 001	MAY 07, 1984

Tablet, Extended Release; Oral

TRIAMINIC-12			
NOVARTIS	12MG;75MG	N018115 001	

CHLORPHENIRAMINE MALEATE; PSEUDOEPHEDRINE HYDROCHLORIDE

Capsule, Extended Release; Oral

CODIMAL-L.A. 12			
SCHWARZ PHARMA	12MG;120MG	N018935 001	APR 15, 1985
ISOCLOR			
FISONS	8MG;120MG	N018747 001	MAR 06, 1986
PSEUDOEPHEDRINE HCL AND CHLORPHENIRAMINE MALEATE			
CENT PHARMS	8MG;120MG	N019428 001	AUG 02, 1988
KV PHARM	12MG;120MG	N071455 001	MAR 01, 1989

Discontinued Drug Products *(continued)*

CHLORPHENESIN CARBAMATE

Tablet; Oral

MAOLATE			
PHARMACIA AND UPJOHN	400MG	N014217 002	

CHLORPHENIRAMINE MALEATE

Capsule, Extended Release; Oral

TELDRIN			
GLAXOSMITHKLINE	8MG	N017369 001	
	12MG	N017369 002	

Injectable; Injection

CHLOR-TRIMETON			
SCHERING PLOUGH	10MG/ML	N008826 001	
	100MG/ML	N008794 001	
CHLORPHENIRAMINE MALEATE			
BEL MAR	10MG/ML	N080821 001	
ELKINS SINN	10MG/ML	N080797 001	
STERIS	10MG/ML	N083593 001	
	10MG/ML	N086096 001	
	100MG/ML	N086095 001	
PYRIDAMAL 100			
BEL MAR	100MG/ML	N083733 001	

Syrup; Oral

CHLOR-TRIMETON			
SCHERING	2MG/5ML	N006921 006	
CHLORPHENIRAMINE MALEATE			
PHARM ASSOC	2MG/5ML	N087520 001	FEB 10, 1982

Tablet; Oral

ANTAGONATE			
BAYER PHARMS	4MG	N083381 001	
CHLOR-TRIMETON			
SCHERING	4MG	N006921 002	
CHLORPHENIRAMINE MALEATE			
ANABOLIC	4MG	N083078 001	
BELL PHARMA	4MG	N083062 001	
ELKINS SINN	4MG	N080938 001	
GENEVA PHARMS	4MG	N080961 001	
HALSEY	4MG	N080700 001	
IMPAX LABS	4MG	N080809 001	
IVAX PHARMS	4MG	N080779 001	
KV PHARM	4MG	N087164 001	
LEDERLE	4MG	N086941 001	
NEWTRON PHARMS	4MG	N086519 001	
PANRAY	4MG	N085104 001	
PHARMAVITE	4MG	N083243 001	
PHARMERAL	4MG	N083753 001	
PIONEER PHARMS	4MG	N088556 001	JUL 13, 1984
PUREPAC PHARM	4MG	N086306 001	
PVT FORM	4MG	N080786 001	
ROXANE	4MG	N080626 001	
VITARINE	4MG	N085837 001	
WATSON LAB	4MG	N080791 001	
WATSON LABS	4MG	N080696 001	

Discontinued Drug Products (continued)

CHLORPHENIRAMINE MALEATE; PSEUDOEPHEDRINE HYDROCHLORIDE (continued)
Capsule, Extended Release; Oral
PSEUDOEPHEDRINE HCL/CHLORPHENIRAMINE MALEATE

Applicant	Strength	Appl. No.	Date
GRAHAM DM	12MG;120MG	N018843 001	MAR 18, 1985
	8MG;120MG	N018844 001	MAR 20, 1985

CHLORPHENIRAMINE POLISTIREX; CODEINE POLISTIREX
Suspension, Extended Release; Oral
PENNTUSS

Applicant	Strength	Appl. No.	Date
FISONS	EQ 4MG MALEATE/5ML;EQ 10MG BASE/5ML	N018928 001	AUG 14, 1985

CHLORPHENIRAMINE POLISTIREX; PHENYLPROPANOLAMINE POLISTIREX
Suspension, Extended Release; Oral
CORSYM

Applicant	Strength	Appl. No.	Date
CELLTECH PHARMS	EQ 4MG MALEATE/5ML;EQ 37.5MG HCL/5ML	N018050 001	JAN 04, 1984

CHLORPHENTERMINE HYDROCHLORIDE
Tablet; Oral
PRE-SATE

Applicant	Strength	Appl. No.
PARKE DAVIS	EQ 65MG BASE	N014696 001

CHLORPROMAZINE HYDROCHLORIDE
Capsule, Extended Release; Oral
THORAZINE

Applicant	Strength	Appl. No.
GLAXOSMITHKLINE	30MG	N011120 016
	75MG	N011120 017
	150MG	N011120 018

Concentrate; Oral
CHLORPROMAZINE HCL

Applicant	Strength	Appl. No.	Date
MORTON GROVE	30MG/ML	N087032 001	JUL 08, 1982
	100MG/ML	N087053 001	

Injectable; Injection
CHLORPROMAZINE HCL

Applicant	Strength	Appl. No.	Date
AM PHARM PARTNERS	25MG/ML	N084911 001	
MARSAM PHARMS LLC	25MG/ML	N089563 001	APR 15, 1988
STERIS	25MG/ML	N080365 001	
	25MG/ML	N085591 001	
	25MG/ML	N080370 001	
WYETH AYERST			

Syrup; Oral
CHLORPROMAZINE HCL

Applicant	Strength	Appl. No.
ALPHARMA	10MG/5ML	N086712 001

Tablet; Oral
CHLORPROMAZINE HCL

Applicant	Strength	Appl. No.
ABBOTT	10MG	N084414 001

CHLORPROMAZINE HYDROCHLORIDE (continued)
Tablet; Oral
CHLORPROMAZINE HCL

Applicant	Strength	Appl. No.	Date
ABBOTT	25MG	N084415 001	
	50MG	N084411 001	
	100MG	N084412 001	
	200MG	N084413 001	
IVAX PHARMS	10MG	N083549 001	
	25MG	N083549 003	
	50MG	N083549 002	
	100MG	N083574 001	
	200MG	N083575 001	
KV PHARM	10MG	N085750 002	JAN 04, 1982
	25MG	N085751 001	
	50MG	N085484 001	
	100MG	N085752 001	
	200MG	N085748 002	
LEDERLE	10MG	N084803 001	JAN 04, 1982
	25MG	N084801 001	
	50MG	N084800 001	
	100MG	N084789 001	
	200MG	N084802 001	
PUREPAC PHARM	10MG	N080403 004	
	25MG	N080403 001	
	50MG	N080403 002	
	100MG	N080403 003	
	200MG	N080403 005	
PVT FORM	25MG	N080340 001	
	50MG	N080340 002	
	200MG	N080340 003	
ROXANE	10MG	N085331 001	
	25MG	N085331 002	
	50MG	N085331 003	
	100MG	N085331 004	
	200MG	N085331 005	
VANGARD	10MG	N088038 001	AUG 16, 1982
WATSON LABS	25MG	N087645 001	
	50MG	N087646 001	
	10MG	N085959 001	
	50MG	N085956 001	
	100MG	N085960 001	
	200MG	N085957 001	
WEST WARD	10MG	N085958 001	
	10MG	N087783 001	SEP 16, 1982
	25MG	N087865 001	SEP 16, 1982
	50MG	N087878 001	SEP 15, 1982
	100MG	N087884 001	SEP 15, 1982
	200MG	N087880 001	SEP 16, 1982

Discontinued Drug Products *(continued)*

CHLORPROMAZINE HYDROCHLORIDE *(continued)*
Tablet; Oral

PROMAPAR		
PARKE DAVIS	10MG	N086886 001
	25MG	N084423 001
	50MG	N086887 001
	100MG	N086888 001
	200MG	N086885 001

CHLORPROPAMIDE
Tablet; Oral

CHLORPROPAMIDE			
BARR	100MG	N088812 001	OCT 19, 1984
	100MG	N089446 001	NOV 17, 1986
	250MG	N088813 001	OCT 19, 1984
	250MG	N089447 001	NOV 17, 1986
CLONMEL HLTHCARE	100MG	N089561 001	SEP 04, 1987
	250MG	N089562 001	SEP 04, 1987
DURAMED PHARM BARR	100MG	N088918 001	OCT 16, 1984
	250MG	N088919 001	OCT 16, 1984
EON	250MG	N084669 001	
HALSEY	100MG	N089321 001	JAN 16, 1986
	250MG	N088662 001	JAN 09, 1986
IVAX PHARMS	100MG	N088840 001	OCT 25, 1984
	250MG	N087353 001	
SUPERPHARM	250MG	N088695 001	SEP 17, 1984
TEVA	100MG	N088768 001	OCT 11, 1984
USL PHARMA	100MG	N088708 001	AUG 30, 1984
	250MG	N088709 001	AUG 30, 1984
WATSON LAB	100MG	N088608 001	APR 12, 1984
	250MG	N088568 001	APR 12, 1984
WATSON LABS	100MG	N086865 001	SEP 24, 1984
	250MG	N086866 001	
GLUCAMIDE			
TEVA	250MG	N088641 001	OCT 11, 1984

CHLORPROTHIXENE
Concentrate; Oral

TARACTAN		
ROCHE	100MG/5ML	N016149 002

Injectable; Injection

TARACTAN		
ROCHE	12.5MG/ML	N012487 001

Tablet; Oral

TARACTAN		
ROCHE	10MG	N012486 005
	25MG	N012486 004
	50MG	N012486 003
	100MG	N012486 001

CHLORTETRACYCLINE HYDROCHLORIDE
Ointment; Ophthalmic

AUREOMYCIN		
LEDERLE	1%	N050404 001

CHLORTHALIDONE
Tablet; Oral

CHLORTHALIDONE			
ABBOTT	25MG	N087364 001	
	50MG	N087384 001	
ASCOT	25MG	N087698 001	OCT 20, 1982
	50MG	N087699 001	OCT 20, 1982
CLONMEL HLTHCARE	25MG	N087451 001	
	50MG	N087450 001	
EON	50MG	N087118 001	
GENEVA PHARMS	50MG	N087380 001	
HALSEY	25MG	N087292 001	
	50MG	N087293 001	
IVAX PHARMS	25MG	N087555 001	
	50MG	N087947 001	FEB 27, 1984
KV PHARM	25MG	N087311 001	
	50MG	N087312 001	
MUTUAL PHARM	25MG	N089738 001	SEP 19, 1988
	50MG	N089739 001	SEP 19, 1988
PIONEER PHARMS	50MG	N089591 001	JUL 21, 1988
PUREPAC PHARM	25MG	N088139 001	JUL 16, 1986
	50MG	N088140 001	AUG 11, 1983
SUPERPHARM	25MG	N087473 001	FEB 09, 1983
	50MG	N087247 001	FEB 09, 1983
TEVA	50MG	N088651 001	MAY 30, 1985
USL PHARMA	50MG	N089052 001	

Discontinued Drug Products (continued)

CHLORTHALIDONE (continued)

Tablet; Oral

CHLORTHALIDONE

USL PHARMA			
VANGARD	25MG	N088012 001	JUN 01, 1987
	50MG	N088073 001	JUL 14, 1982
WARNER CHILCOTT	25MG	N087515 001	MAR 25, 1983
	50MG	N087516 001	JAN 24, 1983
WATSON LAB	25MG	N087050 001	FEB 09, 1983
	50MG	N087029 001	
WATSON LABS	25MG	N087296 001	
	25MG	N087706 001	
	50MG	N087082 001	
	50MG	N087521 001	
	50MG	N087689 001	

THALITONE

MONARCH PHARMS	25MG	N019574 002	FEB 12, 1992
	25MG	N088051 001	NOV 12, 1982

CHLORTHALIDONE; CLONIDINE HYDROCHLORIDE

Tablet; Oral

CLONIDINE HCL AND CHLORTHALIDONE

PAR PHARM	15MG;0.3MG	N071142 001	DEC 16, 1987
	15MG;0.2MG	N071178 001	DEC 16, 1987
	15MG;0.1MG	N071179 001	DEC 16, 1987

COMBIPRES

BOEHRINGER INGELHEIM	15MG;0.1MG	N017503 001	
	15MG;0.2MG	N017503 002	
	15MG;0.3MG	N017503 003	APR 10, 1984

CHLORTHALIDONE; METOPROLOL TARTRATE

Capsule; Oral

LOPRESSIDONE

NOVARTIS	25MG;100MG	N019451 001	DEC 31, 1987
	25MG;200MG	N019451 002	DEC 31, 1987

CHLORTHALIDONE; RESERPINE

Tablet; Oral

DEMI-REGROTON

AVENTIS PHARMS	25MG;0.125MG	N015103 002

REGROTON

AVENTIS PHARMS	50MG;0.25MG	N015103 001

CHLORTHALIDONE *MULTIPLE*

SEE BETAXOLOL HYDROCHLORIDE; CHLORTHALIDONE

CHLORZOXAZONE

Tablet; Oral

CHLORZOXAZONE

PIONEER PHARMS	250MG	N089592 001	JAN 06, 1989
	500MG	N089948 001	JAN 06, 1989
WATSON LABS	250MG	N086901 001	
	250MG	N086948 001	AUG 09, 1982
	500MG	N081019 001	JUL 29, 1991

PARAFLEX

ORTHO MCNEIL PHARM	250MG	N011300 003

CHOLECALCIFEROL *MULTIPLE*

SEE ALPHA-TOCOPHEROL; ASCORBIC ACID; BIOTIN; CHOLECALCIFEROL; CYANOCOBALAMIN; FOLIC ACID; NIACINAMIDE; PANTOTHENIC ACID; PYRIDOXINE; RIBOFLAVIN; THIAMINE; VITAMIN A

CHOLESTYRAMINE

Bar, Chewable; Oral

CHOLYBAR

PARKE DAVIS	EQ 4GM RESIN/BAR	N071621 001	MAY 26, 1988
	EQ 4GM RESIN/BAR	N071739 001	MAY 26, 1988

Tablet; Oral

QUESTRAN

APOTHECON	EQ 1GM RESIN	N073403 001	APR 28, 1994
	EQ 800MG RESIN	N073403 002	DEC 27, 1999

CHROMIC CHLORIDE

Injectable; Injection

CHROMIC CHLORIDE

AM PHARM PARTNERS	EQ 0.004MG CHROMIUM/ML	N019271 001	MAY 05, 1987

CHYMOPAPAIN

Injectable; Injection

CHYMODIACTIN

ABBOTT	4,000 UNITS/VIAL	N018663 002	AUG 21, 1984
	10,000 UNITS/VIAL *SEE ANNUAL PREFACE INTRODUCTION DISCONTINUED SECTION*	N018663 001	NOV 10, 1982

DISCASE

ABBOTT	12,500 UNITS/VIAL	N018625 001

CIPROFLOXACIN (continued)

Injectable; Injection
CIPRO IN SODIUM CHLORIDE 0.9% IN PLASTIC CONTAINER
BAYER PHARMS — DEC 26, 1990

CISAPRIDE MONOHYDRATE

Suspension; Oral
PROPULSID
JANSSEN PHARMA — EQ 1MG BASE/ML — N020398 001 — SEP 15, 1995

Tablet, Orally Disintegrating; Oral
PROPULSID QUICKSOLV
JANSSEN PHARMA — EQ 20MG BASE — N020767 001 — NOV 07, 1997

Tablet; Oral
PROPULSID
JANSSEN PHARMA — EQ 10MG BASE — N020210 001 — JUL 29, 1993
EQ 20MG BASE — N020210 002 — DEC 23, 1993

CISPLATIN

Injectable; Injection
PLATINOL-AQ
BRISTOL MYERS — 0.5MG/ML — N018057 003 — JUL 18, 1984

CITALOPRAM HYDROBROMIDE

Tablet; Oral
CELEXA
FOREST LABS — EQ 60MG BASE — N020822 004 — JUL 17, 1998

CLARITHROMYCIN

For Suspension; Oral
BIAXIN
ABBOTT — 187MG/5ML — N050698 003 — SEP 30, 1998

CLEMASTINE FUMARATE

Syrup; Oral
TAVIST
NOVARTIS — EQ 0.5MG BASE/5ML — N018675 001 — JUN 28, 1985

Tablet; Oral
CLEMASTINE FUMARATE
TEVA — 1.34MG — N073282 001 — JAN 31, 1992
TAVIST-1
NOVARTIS — 1.34MG — N017661 002
1.34MG — N017661 003 — AUG 21, 1992

Discontinued Drug Products (continued)

CHYMOPAPAIN (continued)

Injectable; Injection
DISCASE
ABBOTT — JAN 18, 1984

CHYMOTRYPSIN

For Solution; Ophthalmic
ALPHA CHYMAR
SOLA BARNES HIND — 750 UNITS/VIAL — N011837 001
CATARASE
CIBA — 300 UNITS/VIAL — N016938 001
NOVARTIS — 150 UNITS/VIAL — N018121 001
ZOLYSE
ALCON — 750 UNITS/VIAL — N011903 001

CIMETIDINE

Suspension; Oral
TAGAMET HB 200
GLAXOSMITHKLINE — 200MG/20ML — N020951 001 — JUL 09, 1999

Tablet; Oral
CIMETIDINE
LEK PHARMS — 100MG — N075122 001 — JUN 19, 1998
200MG — N074250 001 — JUN 29, 1995
PERRIGO — 100MG — N074972 001 — JUN 19, 1998
ROXANE — 300MG — N074361 001 — DEC 23, 1994
400MG — N074361 002 — DEC 23, 1994
800MG — N074371 001 — DEC 23, 1994
TAGAMET HB
GLAXOSMITHKLINE — 100MG *SEE ANNUAL PREFACE INTRODUCTION DISCONTINUED SECTION* — N020238 001 — JUN 19, 1995

CINOXACIN

Capsule; Oral
CINOBAC
LILLY — 250MG — N018067 001
500MG — N018067 002
CINOXACIN
TEVA — 250MG — N073005 001 — FEB 28, 1992
500MG — N073006 001 — FEB 28, 1992

CIPROFLOXACIN

Injectable; Injection
CIPRO IN SODIUM CHLORIDE 0.9% IN PLASTIC CONTAINER
BAYER PHARMS — 200MG/100ML — N019858 001

Discontinued Drug Products (continued)

CLEMASTINE FUMARATE; PHENYLPROPANOLAMINE HYDROCHLORIDE

Tablet, Extended Release; Oral

Brand / Firm	Strength	Appl. No.	Approval Date
TAVIST D			
NOVARTIS	EQ 1MG BASE;75MG	N018298 001	DEC 15, 1982
TAVIST-D			
NOVARTIS	1.34MG;75MG	N018298 002	AUG 21, 1992
	1.34MG;75MG	N020640 001	AUG 09, 1996

CLIDINIUM BROMIDE

Capsule; Oral

Brand / Firm	Strength	Appl. No.	Approval Date
QUARZAN			
ROCHE	2.5MG	N010355 001	
	5MG	N010355 002	

CLINDAMYCIN HYDROCHLORIDE

Capsule; Oral

Brand / Firm	Strength	Appl. No.	Approval Date
CLEOCIN			
PHARMACIA AND UPJOHN	EQ 75MG BASE	N061809 001	
	EQ 150MG BASE	N061809 002	
CLINDAMYCIN HCL			
WATSON LABS	EQ 75MG BASE	N063082 001	JUL 31, 1991

CLINDAMYCIN PALMITATE HYDROCHLORIDE

For Solution; Oral

Brand / Firm	Strength	Appl. No.	Approval Date
CLEOCIN			
PHARMACIA AND UPJOHN	EQ 75MG BASE/5ML	N061827 001	

CLINDAMYCIN PHOSPHATE

Cream; Vaginal

Brand / Firm	Strength	Appl. No.	Approval Date
CLEOCIN			
PHARMACIA AND UPJOHN	EQ 2% BASE	N050680 001	AUG 11, 1992

Injectable; Injection

Brand / Firm	Strength	Appl. No.	Approval Date
CLEOCIN PHOSPHATE			
PHARMACIA AND UPJOHN	EQ 150MG BASE/ML	N061839 001	
CLINDAMYCIN PHOSPHATE			
ABBOTT	EQ 150MG BASE/ML	N062943 001	SEP 29, 1988
AM PHARM PARTNERS	EQ 150MG BASE/ML	N062747 001	JUN 03, 1988
ASTRAZENECA	EQ 150MG BASE/ML	N062928 001	FEB 13, 1989
BEDFORD	EQ 150MG BASE/ML	N063163 001	JUN 30, 1994
BRISTOL MYERS SQUIBB	EQ 150MG BASE/ML	N062908 001	

CLINDAMYCIN PHOSPHATE (continued)

Injectable; Injection

Brand / Firm	Strength	Appl. No.	Approval Date
CLINDAMYCIN PHOSPHATE			
BRISTOL MYERS SQUIBB		N062806 001	FEB 01, 1989
ELKINS SINN	EQ 150MG BASE/ML	N062953 001	OCT 15, 1987
	EQ 150MG BASE/ML	N063041 001	APR 21, 1988
GENSIA SICOR PHARMS	EQ 150MG BASE/ML	N063282 001	DEC 29, 1989
	EQ 150MG BASE/ML	N063068 001	MAY 29, 1992
LEDERLE	EQ 150MG BASE/ML	N062913 001	AUG 28, 1989
MARSAM PHARMS LLC	EQ 150MG BASE/ML	N062795 001	OCT 20, 1988
QUAD PHARMS	EQ 150MG BASE/ML	N062877 001	DEC 21, 1987
SOLOPAK	EQ 150MG BASE/ML	N062819 001	MAR 15, 1988
	EQ 150MG BASE/ML	N062852 001	MAR 15, 1988
STERIS	EQ 150MG BASE/ML	N062900 001	MAR 17, 1988
	EQ 150MG BASE/ML	N063079 001	JUN 08, 1988
			MAR 05, 1990

CLINDAMYCIN PHOSPHATE IN DEXTROSE 5%

Brand / Firm	Strength	Appl. No.	Approval Date
AM PHARM PARTNERS	EQ 12MG BASE/ML	N050636 001	DEC 22, 1989

Solution; Topical

Brand / Firm	Strength	Appl. No.	Approval Date
CLEOCIN T			
PHARMACIA AND UPJOHN	EQ 1% BASE	N062363 001	FEB 08, 1982
CLINDAMYCIN PHOSPHATE			
COPLEY PHARM	EQ 1% BASE	N062944 001	JAN 11, 1989
TEVA	EQ 1% BASE	N062930 001	JUN 28, 1989

CLIOQUINOL; NYSTATIN

Ointment; Topical

Brand / Firm	Strength	Appl. No.	Approval Date
NYSTAFORM			
BAYER PHARMS	10MG/GM;100,000 UNITS/GM	N050235 001	

CLOFAZIMINE

Capsule; Oral

Brand / Firm	Strength	Appl. No.	Approval Date
LAMPRENE			
NOVARTIS	100MG	N019500 001	DEC 15, 1986

Discontinued Drug Products (continued)

CLOFIBRATE
Capsule; Oral

ATROMID-S			
WYETH AYERST	500MG	N016099 002	
CLOFIBRATE			
GENEVA PHARMS	500MG	N072191 001	MAY 02, 1988
WATSON LABS	500MG	N071603 001	SEP 18, 1987

CLONAZEPAM
Tablet; Oral

KLONOPIN			
ROCHE	0.25MG	N017533 006	APR 09, 1997
	0.125MG	N017533 005	APR 09, 1997

CLONIDINE HYDROCHLORIDE
Tablet; Oral

CLONIDINE HCL			
AM THERAP	0.1MG	N070881 001	JUL 08, 1986
	0.2MG	N070882 001	JUL 08, 1986
	0.3MG	N070883 001	JUL 08, 1986
DURAMED PHARM BARR	0.1MG	N071103 001	AUG 14, 1986
	0.2MG	N071102 001	AUG 14, 1986
	0.3MG	N071101 001	AUG 14, 1986
HALSEY	0.2MG	N070924 001	SEP 04, 1987
	0.3MG	N070923 001	SEP 04, 1987
INTERPHARM	0.1MG	N071252 001	OCT 01, 1986
	0.2MG	N071253 001	OCT 01, 1986
	0.3MG	N071254 001	OCT 01, 1986
PAR PHARM	0.1MG	N070461 001	JUL 08, 1986
	0.2MG	N070460 001	JUL 08, 1986
	0.3MG	N070459 001	JUL 08, 1986
TEVA	0.1MG	N070747 001	JUL 08, 1986
	0.2MG	N070702 001	JUL 08, 1986
	0.3MG	N070659 001	JUL 08, 1986
WARNER CHILCOTT	0.1MG	N072138 001	

CLONIDINE HYDROCHLORIDE (continued)
Tablet; Oral

CLONIDINE HCL			
WARNER CHILCOTT	0.2MG	N072139 001	JUN 13, 1988
	0.3MG	N072140 001	JUN 13, 1988
WATSON LAB	0.1MG	N070395 001	JUN 13, 1988
	0.2MG	N070396 001	MAR 23, 1987
	0.3MG	N070397 001	MAR 23, 1987

CLONIDINE HYDROCHLORIDE *MULTIPLE*
SEE CHLORTHALIDONE; CLONIDINE HYDROCHLORIDE

CLORAZEPATE DIPOTASSIUM
Capsule; Oral

CLORAZEPATE DIPOTASSIUM			
ABLE	3.75MG	N071777 001	JUL 14, 1987
	7.5MG	N071778 001	JUL 14, 1987
	15MG	N071779 001	JUL 14, 1987
AM THERAP	3.75MG	N071429 001	JUN 23, 1987
	7.5MG	N071430 001	JUN 23, 1987
	15MG	N071431 001	JUN 23, 1987
CLONMEL HLTHCARE	3.75MG	N071742 001	DEC 14, 1987
	7.5MG	N071743 001	DEC 14, 1987
	15MG	N071744 001	DEC 14, 1987
GD SEARLE LLC	3.75MG	N071727 001	DEC 18, 1987
	7.5MG	N071728 001	DEC 18, 1987
	15MG	N071729 001	DEC 18, 1987
PUREPAC PHARM	3.75MG	N071924 001	APR 25, 1988
	7.5MG	N071925 001	APR 25, 1988
	15MG	N071926 001	APR 25, 1988
QUANTUM PHARMICS	3.75MG	N071549 001	SEP 12, 1988
	7.5MG	N071550 001	SEP 12, 1988
	15MG	N071522 001	

CLORAZEPATE DIPOTASSIUM (continued)

Tablet; Oral

CLORAZEPATE DIPOTASSIUM

Firm	Strength	Date	Appl. No.
WARNER CHILCOTT	15MG	MAR 03, 1988	N071830 001
		MAR 03, 1988	

CLOTRIMAZOLE

Tablet; Vaginal

MYCELEX-G

Firm	Strength	Appl. No.	Date
BAYER PHARMS	500MG	N019069 001	APR 19, 1985

CLOXACILLIN SODIUM

Capsule; Oral

CLOXACILLIN SODIUM

Firm	Strength	Appl. No.
APOTHECON	EQ 250MG BASE	N061452 001
	EQ 500MG BASE	N061452 002

CLOXAPEN

Firm	Strength	Appl. No.
GLAXOSMITHKLINE	EQ 250MG BASE	N062233 001
	EQ 500MG BASE	N062233 002

For Solution Oral

CLOXACILLIN SODIUM

Firm	Strength	Appl. No.	Date
TEVA	EQ 125MG BASE/5ML	N062978 001	APR 06, 1989

TEGOPEN

Firm	Strength	Appl. No.
APOTHECON	EQ 125MG BASE/5ML	N050192 001
	EQ 125MG BASE/5ML	N061453 001

CLOZAPINE

Tablet; Oral

CLOZAPINE

Firm	Strength	Appl. No.	Date
GENEVA PHARMS	25MG	N074546 001	AUG 30, 1996
	100MG	N074546 002	AUG 30, 1996

COBALT CHLORIDE, CO-60; CYANOCOBALAMIN; CYANOCOBALAMIN, CO-60; INTRINSIC FACTOR

N/A; N/A

RUBRATOPE-60 KIT

Firm	Strength	Appl. No.
BRACCO	N/A	N016090 001

CODEINE PHOSPHATE; PHENYLEPHRINE HYDROCHLORIDE; PROMETHAZINE HYDROCHLORIDE

Syrup; Oral

PHENERGAN VC W/ CODEINE

Firm	Strength	Appl. No.	Date
WYETH AYERST	10MG/5ML;5MG/5ML;6.25MG/5ML	N008306 005	APR 02, 1984

PHERAZINE VC W/ CODEINE

Firm	Strength	Appl. No.	Date
HALSEY	10MG/5ML;5MG/5ML;6.25MG/5ML	N088870 001	MAR 02, 1987

Discontinued Drug Products (continued)

CLORAZEPATE DIPOTASSIUM (continued)

Capsule; Oral

CLORAZEPATE DIPOTASSIUM

Firm	Strength	Date	Appl. No.
QUANTUM PHARMICS			
USL PHARMA	3.75MG	SEP 12, 1988	N071242 001
		JUN 23, 1987	N071243 001
	7.5MG	JUN 23, 1987	N071244 001
	15MG	JUN 23, 1987	N071774 001
WARNER CHILCOTT	3.75MG	MAR 01, 1988	N071775 001
	7.5MG	MAR 01, 1988	N071776 001
	15MG	MAR 01, 1988	N071878 001
WATSON LABS	3.75MG	MAR 15, 1988	N071879 001
	7.5MG	MAR 15, 1988	N071860 001
	15MG	MAR 15, 1988	N017105 001
TRANXENE			
OVATION PHARMS	3.75MG		N017105 002
	7.5MG		N017105 003
	15MG		N071747 001

Tablet; Oral

CLORAZEPATE DIPOTASSIUM

Firm	Strength	Date	Appl. No.
AM THERAP	3.75MG	JUN 23, 1987	N071748 001
	7.5MG	JUN 23, 1987	N071749 001
	15MG	JUN 23, 1987	N072512 001
GENEVA PHARMS	3.75MG	JUN 23, 1987	N072013 001
LEDERLE	3.75MG	MAY 11, 1990	N072014 001
	7.5MG	DEC 15, 1987	N072015 001
	15MG	DEC 15, 1987	N072330 001
PUREPAC PHARM	3.75MG	DEC 15, 1987	N072331 001
	7.5MG	AUG 08, 1988	N072332 001
	15MG	AUG 08, 1988	N071730 001
QUANTUM PHARMICS	3.75MG	AUG 08, 1988	N071731 001
	7.5MG	OCT 26, 1987	N071702 001
	15MG	OCT 26, 1987	N071828 001
WARNER CHILCOTT	3.75MG	OCT 26, 1987	N071829 001
	7.5MG	MAR 03, 1988	

Discontinued Drug Products (continued)

CODEINE PHOSPHATE; PHENYLEPHRINE HYDROCHLORIDE; PROMETHAZINE HYDROCHLORIDE (continued)
Syrup; Oral

PROMETHAZINE VC W/ CODEINE   10MG/5ML;5MG/5ML;6.25MG/5ML
- CENCI   N088816 001 NOV 22, 1985

CODEINE PHOSPHATE; PROMETHAZINE HYDROCHLORIDE
Syrup; Oral

PHENERGAN W/ CODEINE   10MG/5ML;6.25MG/5ML
- WYETH AYERST   N008306 004 APR 02, 1984

PHERAZINE W/ CODEINE   10MG/5ML;6.25MG/5ML
- HALSEY   N088739 001 DEC 23, 1988

PROMETHAZINE W/ CODEINE   10MG/5ML;6.25MG/5ML
- CENCI   N088814 001 NOV 22, 1985

CODEINE PHOSPHATE; PSEUDOEPHEDRINE HYDROCHLORIDE; TRIPROLIDINE HYDROCHLORIDE
Syrup; Oral

ACTIFED W/ CODEINE   10MG/5ML;30MG/5ML;1.25MG/5ML
- GLAXOSMITHKLINE   N012575 003 APR 04, 1984

TRIPROLIDINE AND PSEUDOEPHEDRINE HYDROCHLORIDES W/ CODEINE   10MG/5ML;30MG/5ML;1.25MG/5ML
- CENCI   N089018 001 JUL 23, 1986

CODEINE PHOSPHATE *MULTIPLE*
SEE   ACETAMINOPHEN; ASPIRIN; CODEINE PHOSPHATE
SEE   ACETAMINOPHEN; CODEINE PHOSPHATE
SEE   BROMODIPHENHYDRAMINE HYDROCHLORIDE; CODEINE PHOSPHATE
SEE   BROMPHENIRAMINE MALEATE; CODEINE PHOSPHATE; PHENYLPROPANOLAMINE HYDROCHLORIDE

CODEINE POLISTIREX *MULTIPLE*
SEE   CHLORPHENIRAMINE POLISTIREX; CODEINE POLISTIREX

COLCHICINE; PROBENECID
Tablet; Oral

COLBENEMID   0.5MG;500MG
- MERCK   N012383 001

PROBEN-C   0.5MG;500MG
- WATSON LABS   N085552 001

PROBENECID AND COLCHICINE   0.5MG;500MG
- BEECHAM   N084321 001
- EON   N086130 001
- IMPAX LABS   N083720 002

COLCHICINE; PROBENECID (continued)
Tablet; Oral

PROBENECID W/ COLCHICINE
- LEDERLE   0.5MG;500MG   N086954 001
- WATSON LAB   0.5MG;500MG   N083221 001

COLESEVELAM HYDROCHLORIDE
Capsule; Oral

WELCHOL   375MG
- SANKYO   N021141 001 MAY 26, 2000

COLISTIN SULFATE
Suspension; Oral

COLY-MYCIN S   EQ 25MG BASE/5ML
- PARKE DAVIS   N050355 001

COPPER
Intrauterine Device; Intrauterine

CU-7   89MG
- GD SEARLE LLC   N017408 001

TATUM-T   120MG
- GD SEARLE LLC   N018205 001

CORTICOTROPIN
Injectable; Injection

ACTH
- PARKEDALE   25 UNITS/VIAL   N008317 002
- PARKEDALE   40 UNITS/VIAL   N008317 004

ACTHAR
- AVENTIS   25 UNITS/VIAL   N007504 002
- AVENTIS   40 UNITS/VIAL   N007504 003

CORTICOTROPIN   40 UNITS/VIAL
- STERIS   N088772 001 NOV 21, 1984

H.P. ACTHAR GEL   40 UNITS/ML
- QUESTCOR PHARMS   N008372 006

PURIFIED CORTROPHIN GEL
- ORGANON USA INC   40 UNITS/ML   N008975 001
- ORGANON USA INC   80 UNITS/ML   N008975 002

CORTICOTROPIN-ZINC HYDROXIDE
Injectable; Injection

CORTROPHIN-ZINC   40 UNITS/ML
- ORGANON USA INC   N009854 001

CORTISONE ACETATE
Injectable; Injection

CORTISONE ACETATE
- PHARMACIA AND UPJOHN   25MG/ML   N008126 002
- PHARMACIA AND UPJOHN   25MG/ML   N083147 003
- STERIS   25MG/ML   N085677 001
- STERIS   50MG/ML   N083147 004

Discontinued Drug Products (continued)

CORTISONE ACETATE (continued)

Injectable; Injection

CORTISONE ACETATE	Strength	Appl. No.	Date
STERIS	50MG/ML	N085677 002	
CORTONE			
MERCK	25MG/ML	N007110 002	
	25MG/ML	N007110 003	

Tablet; Oral

CORTISONE ACETATE	Strength	Appl. No.
BARR	25MG	N083471 001
ELKINS SINN	25MG	N080836 001
EVERYLIFE	25MG	N084246 001
HEATHER	25MG	N085736 001
IMPAX LABS	25MG	N009458 001
INWOOD LABS	25MG	N080731 001
IVAX PHARMS	25MG	N080630 001
	25MG	N083536 001
	25MG	N080694 001
LANNETT	25MG	N008284 002
PANRAY	5MG	N008284 001
	25MG	N080493 001
PUREPAC PHARM	25MG	N080333 001
VITARINE	25MG	N085884 001
WATSON LABS	25MG	
WHITEWORTH TOWN PLSN	25MG	N080341 001
CORTONE		
MERCK	25MG	N007750 003

CROMOLYN SODIUM

Capsule; Inhalation

INTAL	Strength	Appl. No.	Date
AVENTIS	20MG	N016990 001	

Capsule; Oral

GASTROCROM	Strength	Appl. No.	Date
CELLTECH PHARMS	100MG	N019188 001	DEC 22, 1989

Solution/Drops; Ophthalmic

CROMOPTIC	Strength	Appl. No.	Date
KING PHARMS	4%	N075088 001	APR 27, 1999

CRYPTENAMINE ACETATES

Injectable; Injection

UNITENSEN	Strength	Appl. No.
MEDPOINTE PHARM HLC	260CSR UNIT/ML	N008814 001

CRYPTENAMINE TANNATES

Tablet; Oral

UNITENSEN	Strength	Appl. No.
MEDPOINTE PHARM HLC	260CSR UNIT	N009217 001

CUPRIC SULFATE

Injectable; Injection

CUPRIC SULFATE	Strength	Appl. No.
AM PHARM PARTNERS	EQ 0.4MG COPPER/ML	N019350 001

CUPRIC SULFATE (continued)

Injectable; Injection

CUPRIC SULFATE	Strength	Date
AM PHARM PARTNERS	50MG/ML	MAY 05, 1987

CYANOCOBALAMIN

Injectable; Injection

Product / Firm	Strength	Appl. No.	Date
BERUBIGEN			
PHARMACIA AND UPJOHN	1MG/ML	N006798 001	
BETALIN 12			
LILLY	0.1MG/ML	N080855 001	
	1MG/ML	N080855 002	
COBAVITE			
STERIS	0.1MG/ML	N083013 001	
	1MG/ML	N083064 001	
CYANOCOBALAMIN			
AKORN	1MG/ML	N087969 001	NOV 10, 1983
AM PHARM PARTNERS	0.1MG/ML	N080510 001	
	0.03MG/ML	N080510 003	
	1MG/ML	N080510 002	
	1MG/ML	N083075 001	
	1MG/ML	N080564 002	
AVENTIS PHARMS	0.03MG/ML	N080564 001	
DELL LABS	0.1MG/ML	N080689 002	
	1MG/ML	N080689 001	
	1MG/ML	N080689 003	
	1MG/ML	N080515 002	
ELKINS SINN	0.03MG/ML	N080668 001	
LUITPOLD	1MG/ML	N087551 001	
SOLOPAK			FEB 29, 1984
STERIS	0.1MG/ML	N083120 001	
WARNER CHILCOTT	1MG/ML	N007085 002	
WYETH AYERST	0.1MG/ML	N080554 001	
	1MG/ML	N080554 002	
REDISOL			
MERCK	1MG/ML	N006668 010	
RUBIVITE			
BEL MAR	0.1MG/ML	N010791 002	
	0.03MG/ML	N010791 004	
	0.05MG/ML	N010791 001	
	0.12MG/ML	N010791 005	
	1MG/ML	N010791 003	
RUBRAMIN PC			
BRISTOL MYERS SQUIBB	0.1MG/ML	N006799 002	
RUVITE	1MG/ML	*SEE ANNUAL PREFACE INTRODUCTION DISCONTINUED SECTION*	
SAVAGE LABS	1MG/ML	N006799 004	
VI-TWEL			
BERLEX	1MG/ML	N080570 002	
	1MG/ML	N007012 002	

Discontinued Drug Products (continued)

CYANOCOBALAMIN; CYANOCOBALAMIN, CO-57; CYANOCOBALAMIN, CO-58
N/A; N/A
DICOPAC KIT
AMERSHAM HLTH   N/A;N/A;N/A   N017406 001

CYANOCOBALAMIN; CYANOCOBALAMIN, CO-57; INTRINSIC FACTOR
N/A; N/A
CYANOCOBALAMIN CO 57 SCHILLING TEST KIT
MALLINCKRODT   0.1MG;0.5uCi;60MG   N016635 001

CYANOCOBALAMIN; TANNIC ACID; ZINC ACETATE
Injectable; Injection
DEPINAR
ARMOUR PHARM   0.5MG/ML;2.3MG/ML;1MG/ML   N011208 001

CYANOCOBALAMIN *MULTIPLE*
SEE ALPHA-TOCOPHEROL; ASCORBIC ACID; BIOTIN; CHOLECALCIFEROL; CYANOCOBALAMIN; FOLIC ACID; NIACINAMIDE; PANTOTHENIC ACID; PYRIDOXINE; RIBOFLAVIN; THIAMINE; VITAMIN A

SEE ASCORBIC ACID; BIOTIN; FOLIC ACID; NIACINAMIDE; PYRIDOXINE; RIBOFLAVIN; DEXPANTHENOL; ERGOCALCIFEROL; FOLIC ACID; NIACINAMIDE; PYRIDOXINE; RIBOFLAVIN PHOSPHATE SODIUM; THIAMINE; VITAMIN A; VITAMIN E

SEE ASCORBIC ACID; BIOTIN; CYANOCOBALAMIN; DEXPANTHENOL; ERGOCALCIFEROL; FOLIC ACID; NIACINAMIDE; PYRIDOXINE; HYDROCHLORIDE; RIBOFLAVIN PHOSPHATE SODIUM; THIAMINE; HYDROCHLORIDE; VITAMIN A PALMITATE; VITAMIN E

SEE ASCORBIC ACID; BIOTIN; CYANOCOBALAMIN; DEXPANTHENOL; ERGOCALCIFEROL; FOLIC ACID; NIACINAMIDE; PYRIDOXINE; HYDROCHLORIDE; RIBOFLAVIN PHOSPHATE SODIUM; THIAMINE; HYDROCHLORIDE; VITAMIN A; VITAMIN E

SEE ASCORBIC ACID; BIOTIN; CYANOCOBALAMIN; ERGOCALCIFEROL; FOLIC ACID; NIACINAMIDE; PANTOTHENIC ACID; PHYTONADIONE; PYRIDOXINE; RIBOFLAVIN; THIAMINE; VITAMIN A PALMITATE; VITAMIN E

SEE COBALT CHLORIDE, CO-60; CYANOCOBALAMIN; CYANOCOBALAMIN, CO-60; INTRINSIC FACTOR

CYANOCOBALAMIN, CO-57 *MULTIPLE*
SEE CYANOCOBALAMIN; CYANOCOBALAMIN, CO-57; CYANOCOBALAMIN, CO-58
SEE CYANOCOBALAMIN; CYANOCOBALAMIN, CO-57; INTRINSIC FACTOR

CYANOCOBALAMIN, CO-58 *MULTIPLE*
SEE CYANOCOBALAMIN; CYANOCOBALAMIN, CO-57; CYANOCOBALAMIN, CO-58

CYANOCOBALAMIN, CO-60
Capsule; Oral
RUBRATOPE-60
BRACCO   0.5-1uCi   N016090 002

CYANOCOBALAMIN, CO-60 *MULTIPLE*
SEE COBALT CHLORIDE, CO-60; CYANOCOBALAMIN; CYANOCOBALAMIN, CO-60; INTRINSIC FACTOR

CYCLACILLIN
For Suspension; Oral
CYCLAPEN-W
WYETH AYERST   125MG/5ML   N050508 001
                250MG/5ML   N050508 002
                500MG/5ML   N050508 003

Tablet; Oral
CYCLACILLIN
TEVA   250MG   N062895 001   AUG 04, 1988
        500MG   N062895 002   AUG 04, 1988

CYCLAPEN-W
WYETH AYERST   250MG   N050509 001
                500MG   N050509 002

CYCLIZINE LACTATE
Injectable; Injection
MAREZINE
GLAXOSMITHKLINE   50MG/ML   N009495 001

CYCLOPENTOLATE HYDROCHLORIDE
Solution/Drops; Ophthalmic
AK-PENTOLATE
AKORN   1%   N085555 001

CYCLOPENTOLATE HCL
SOLA BARNES HIND   1%   N084150 001
                    1%   N084863 001

PENTOLAIR
PHARMAFAIR   0.5%   N088643 001   FEB 09, 1987
              1%   N088150 001   FEB 25, 1983

CYCLOPHOSPHAMIDE
Injectable; Injection
CYTOXAN
BRISTOL MYERS SQUIBB   1GM/VIAL   N012142 004   AUG 30, 1982
                                    N012142 005   AUG 30, 1982
                        2GM/VIAL
                        100MG/VIAL   N012142 001
                        200MG/VIAL   N012142 002
                        500MG/VIAL   N012142 003

CYCLOSPORINE
Capsule; Oral
NEORAL
NOVARTIS   50MG *SEE ANNUAL PREFACE INTRODUCTION DISCONTINUED SECTION*   N050715 003   JUL 14, 1995

Discontinued Drug Products *(continued)*

CYCLOTHIAZIDE
Tablet; Oral
ANHYDRON
LILLY — 2MG — N013157 002
FLUIDIL
PHARMACIA AND
UPJOHN — 2MG — N018173 001

CYCRIMINE HYDROCHLORIDE
Tablet; Oral
PAGITANE
LILLY — 1.25MG — N008951 001
— 2.5MG — N008951 002

CYPROHEPTADINE HYDROCHLORIDE
Syrup; Oral
CYPROHEPTADINE HCL
HALSEY — 2MG/5ML — N089199 001
— JUL 03, 1986
MORTON GROVE — 2MG/5ML — N087001 001
— NOV 04, 1982
NASKA — 2MG/5ML — N089021 001
— DEC 21, 1987

Tablet; Oral
CYPROHEPTADINE HCL
AM THERAP — 4MG — N088798 001
— FEB 15, 1985
ASCOT — 4MG — N087685 001
— OCT 25, 1982
DURAMED PHARM BARR — 4MG — N088232 001
— OCT 25, 1983
GENEVA PHARMS — 4MG — N086808 001
HALSEY — 4MG — N089057 001
— JUL 03, 1986
KV PHARM — 4MG — N086737 001
MD PHARM — 4MG — N087566 001
— NOV 10, 1982
MYLAN — 4MG — N086678 001
PIONEER PHARMS — 4MG — N087839 001
— FEB 08, 1984
SUPERPHARM — 4MG — N087405 001
VITARINE — 4MG — N087284 001
WATSON LAB — 4MG — N085245 001
WATSON LABS — 4MG — N086165 001
— 4MG — N086580 001
PERIACTIN
MERCK — 4MG *SEE ANNUAL PREFACE — N012649 001
INTRODUCTION
DISCONTINUED SECTION*

CYSTEINE HYDROCHLORIDE
Injectable; Injection
CYSTEINE HCL
FRESENIUS KABI — 7.25% — N019523 001
— OCT 22, 1986

CYTARABINE
Injectable; Injection
CYTARABINE
QUAD PHARMS — 100MG/VIAL — N071248 001
— DEC 30, 1987
— 500MG/VIAL — N071249 001
— DEC 30, 1987

DACARBAZINE
Injectable; Injection
DACARBAZINE
AM PHARM PARTNERS — 100MG/VIAL — N070962 001
— AUG 28, 1986
— 200MG/VIAL — N070990 001
— AUG 28, 1986
QUAD PHARMS — 100MG/VIAL — N070821 001
— OCT 09, 1986
— 200MG/VIAL — N070822 001
— OCT 09, 1986
— 500MG/VIAL — N071563 001
— MAY 06, 1988

DALFOPRISTIN; QUINUPRISTIN
Injectable; Iv (Infusion)
SYNERCID
KING PHARMS — 420MG/VIAL;180MG/VIAL — N050748 002
— AUG 24, 2000

DANAPAROID SODIUM
Injectable; Injection
ORGARAN
ORGANON USA INC — 750 UNITS/0.6ML — N020430 001
— DEC 24, 1996

DANAZOL
Capsule; Oral
DANAZOL
AM THERAP — 200MG — N071569 001
— DEC 30, 1987

DAUNORUBICIN HYDROCHLORIDE
Injectable; Injection
CERUBIDINE
AVENTIS — EQ 20MG BASE/VIAL — N061876 001
WYETH AYERST — EQ 20MG BASE/VIAL — N050484 001

DECAMETHONIUM BROMIDE
Injectable; Injection
SYNCURINE
GLAXOSMITHKLINE — 1MG/ML — N006931 002

Discontinued Drug Products (continued)

DEMECARIUM BROMIDE
Solution/Drops; Ophthalmic
  HUMORSOL 0.25% MERCK N011860 001
  0.125% N011860 002

DEMECLOCYCLINE HYDROCHLORIDE
Capsule; Oral
  DECLOMYCIN 150MG LEDERLE N050262 001
Syrup; Oral
  DECLOMYCIN 75MG/5ML LEDERLE N050257 001
Tablet; Oral
  DECLOMYCIN 75MG WYETH PHARMS INC N050261 001

DESERPIDINE
Tablet; Oral
  HARMONYL 0.1MG ABBOTT N010796 001
  0.25MG N010796 002

DESERPIDINE; HYDROCHLOROTHIAZIDE
Tablet; Oral
  ORETICYL 25 0.125MG;25MG ABBOTT N012148 001
  ORETICYL 50 0.125MG;50MG ABBOTT N012148 003
  ORETICYL FORTE 0.25MG;25MG ABBOTT N012148 002

DESERPIDINE; METHYCLOTHIAZIDE
Tablet; Oral
  METHYCLOTHIAZIDE AND DESERPIDINE 0.5MG;5MG WATSON LAB N088452 001 AUG 10, 1984
  0.25MG;5MG N088486 001 AUG 10, 1984

DESIPRAMINE HYDROCHLORIDE
Capsule; Oral
  PERTOFRANE 25MG AVENTIS N013621 001
  50MG N013621 002
Tablet; Oral
  DESIPRAMINE HCL 25MG USL PHARMA N071864 001 SEP 09, 1987
  50MG N071865 001 SEP 09, 1987
  75MG N071866 001 SEP 09, 1987
  100MG N071867 001 SEP 09, 1987

DESIPRAMINE HYDROCHLORIDE (continued)
Tablet; Oral
  DESIPRAMINE HCL USL PHARMA SEP 09, 1987

DESLANOSIDE
Injectable; Injection
  CEDILANID-D 0.2MG/ML NOVARTIS N009282 002

DESMOPRESSIN ACETATE
Solution; Nasal
  CONCENTRAID 0.01% FERRING N019776 001 DEC 26, 1990
Spray, Metered; Nasal
  DDAVP 0.01MG/SPRAY AVENTIS N017922 002 FEB 06, 1989

DESOGESTREL; ETHINYL ESTRADIOL
Tablet; Oral-21
  DESOGEN 0.15MG;0.03MG ORGANON USA INC N020071 001 DEC 10, 1992
  ORTHO-CEPT 0.15MG;0.03MG ORTHO MCNEIL PHARM N020301 001 DEC 14, 1992

DESONIDE *MULTIPLE*
  SEE ACETIC ACID, GLACIAL; DESONIDE

DESOXIMETASONE
Ointment; Topical
  DESOXIMETASONE 0.25% ALTANA N073440 001 APR 01, 1998
  TOPICORT 0.05% MEDICIS N018594 001 JAN 17, 1985

DESOXYCORTICOSTERONE ACETATE
Injectable; Injection
  DOCA 5MG/ML ORGANON USA INC N001104 001
Pellet; Implantation
  PERCORTEN 125MG NOVARTIS N005151 001

DESOXYCORTICOSTERONE PIVALATE
Injectable; Injection
  PERCORTEN 25MG/ML NOVARTIS N008822 001

Discontinued Drug Products (continued)

DEXAMETHASONE

Aerosol; Topical

AEROSEB-DEX			
ALLERGAN HERBERT	0.01%	N083296 002	
DECASPRAY			
MERCK	0.04%	N012731 002	

Elixir; Oral

DECADRON			
MERCK	0.5MG/5ML	N012376 002	
DEXAMETHASONE			
ALPHARMA	0.5MG/5ML	N088997 001	OCT 10, 1986

Gel; Topical

DECADERM			
MERCK	0.1%	N013538 001	

Suspension/Drops; Ophthalmic

DEXAMETHASONE			
STERIS	0.1%	N089170 001	MAY 09, 1989

Tablet; Oral

DEXAMETHASONE		
GENEVA PHARMS	0.75MG	N080399 001
HALSEY	0.5MG	N084084 001
	0.5MG	N084766 001
	0.25MG	N084013 001
	0.25MG	N084764 001
	0.75MG	N084081 001
	0.75MG	N084765 001
	1.5MG	N084086 001
	1.5MG	N084763 001
IMPAX LABS	0.75MG	N085376 001
PHOENIX LABS NY	0.75MG	N083806 001
PVT FORM	0.75MG	N083420 001
ROXANE	0.25MG	N084614 001
UPSHER SMITH	0.75MG	N087534 001
	1.5MG	N087533 001
WATSON LAB	0.75MG	N084457 001
WATSON LABS	0.5MG	N085458 001
	0.25MG	N085455 001
	0.75MG	N080968 001
	0.75MG	N085818 001
	1.5MG	N085456 001
	1.5MG	N085840 001
WHITEWORTH TOWN PLSN	0.75MG	N084327 001
DEXONE 0.5		
SOLVAY	0.5MG	N084991 001
DEXONE 0.75		
SOLVAY	0.75MG	N084993 001
DEXONE 1.5		
SOLVAY	1.5MG	N084990 001
DEXONE 4		
SOLVAY	4MG	N084992 001
HEXADROL		
ORGANON USA	0.5MG	N012675 004
	0.75MG	N012675 007

DEXAMETHASONE (continued)

Tablet; Oral

HEXADROL		
ORGANON USA	1.5MG	N012675 009

DEXAMETHASONE; NEOMYCIN SULFATE; POLYMYXIN B SULFATE

Ointment; Ophthalmic

DEXACIDIN			
NOVARTIS	0.1%;EQ 3.5MG BASE/GM;10,000 UNITS/GM	N062566 001	FEB 22, 1985
DEXASPORIN			
PHARMAFAIR	0.1%;EQ 3.5MG BASE/GM;10,000 UNITS/GM	N062411 001	MAY 16, 1983

Suspension/Drops; Ophthalmic

DEXASPORIN			
PHARMAFAIR	0.1%;EQ 3.5MG BASE/ML;10,000 UNITS/ML	N062428 001	MAY 18, 1983

DEXAMETHASONE ACETATE

Injectable; Injection

DECADRON-LA			
MERCK	EQ 8MG BASE/ML	N016675 001	
DEXAMETHASONE ACETATE			
STEFIS	EQ 8MG BASE/ML	N084315 001	
	EQ 16MG BASE/ML	N087711 001	MAY 24, 1982

DEXAMETHASONE SODIUM PHOSPHATE

Aerosol, Metered; Inhalation

DEXACORT		
CELLTECH PHARMS	EQ 0.1MG PHOSPHATE/INH	N013413 001

Aerosol; Nasal

DEXACORT		
CELLTECH PHARMS	EQ 0.1MG PHOSPHATE/INH	N014242 001

Cream; Topical

DECADRON		
MERCK	EQ 0.1% PHOSPHATE	N011983 002

Injectable; Injection

DECADRON		
MERCK	EQ 4MG PHOSPHATE/ML	N012071 002
	EQ 24MG PHOSPHATE/ML	N012071 004
DEXACEN-4		
CENT PHARMS	EQ 4MG PHOSPHATE/ML	N084342 001
DEXAMETHASONE		
AM PHARM PARTNERS	EQ 4MG PHOSPHATE/ML	N088448 001 JAN 25, 1984
	EQ 10MG PHOSPHATE/ML	N088469 001 JAN 25, 1984
DEXAMETHASONE SODIUM PHOSPHATE		
AKORN	EQ 4MG PHOSPHATE/ML	N084493 001
AM PHARM PARTNERS	EQ 4MG PHOSPHATE/ML	N087065 001
BEL MAR	EQ 4MG PHOSPHATE/ML	N084752 001

Discontinued Drug Products *(continued)*

DEXAMETHASONE SODIUM PHOSPHATE *(continued)*

Injectable; Injection

DEXAMETHASONE SODIUM PHOSPHATE

DELL LABS	EQ 4MG PHOSPHATE/ML	N083161 001	
GENSIA SICOR PHARMS	EQ 4MG PHOSPHATE/ML	N081125 001	AUG 31, 1990
INTL MEDICATION	EQ 20MG PHOSPHATE/ML	N088522 001	FEB 17, 1984
QUAD PHARMS	EQ 4MG PHOSPHATE/ML	N089280 001	MAR 18, 1987
	EQ 10MG PHOSPHATE/ML	N089281 001	MAR 18, 1987
	EQ 20MG PHOSPHATE/ML	N089282 001	MAR 18, 1987
	EQ 24MG PHOSPHATE/ML	N089372 001	MAR 18, 1987
STERIS	EQ 4MG PHOSPHATE/ML	N083702 001	
	EQ 4MG PHOSPHATE/ML	N084355 001	
	EQ 4MG PHOSPHATE/ML	N089169 001	APR 09, 1986
	EQ 10MG PHOSPHATE/ML	N087668 001	JUL 01, 1982
	EQ 24MG PHOSPHATE/ML	N085606 001	
WYETH AYERST	EQ 4MG PHOSPHATE/ML	N085641 001	

HEXADROL

ORGANON USA INC	EQ 4MG PHOSPHATE/ML	N014694 002
	EQ 10MG PHOSPHATE/ML	N014694 003
	EQ 20MG PHOSPHATE/ML	N014694 004

Ointment; Ophthalmic

DECADRON

MERCK	EQ 0.05% PHOSPHATE	N011977 001	

DEXAIR

PHARMAFAIR	EQ 0.05% PHOSPHATE	N088071 001	DEC 28, 1982

MAXIDEX

ALCON	EQ 0.05% PHOSPHATE	N083342 001

Solution/Drops; Ophthalmic

DEXAIR

PHARMAFAIR	EQ 0.1% PHOSPHATE	N088433 001	DEC 15, 1983

DEXAMETHASONE SODIUM PHOSPHATE

SOLA BARNES HIND	EQ 0.1% PHOSPHATE	N084170 001
	EQ 0.1% PHOSPHATE	N084173 001

Solution/Drops; Otic

DEXAMETHASONE SODIUM PHOSPHATE

AKORN	EQ 0.1% PHOSPHATE	N084855 001

DEXAMETHASONE SODIUM PHOSPHATE; LIDOCAINE HYDROCHLORIDE

Injectable; Injection

DECADRON W/ XYLOCAINE

MERCK	EQ 4MG PHOSPHATE/ML;10MG/ML	N013334 002

DEXAMETHASONE SODIUM PHOSPHATE; NEOMYCIN SULFATE

Ointment; Ophthalmic

NEODECADRON

MERCK	EQ 0.05% PHOSPHATE;EQ 3.5MG BASE/GM	N050324 001

Solution/Drops; Ophthalmic

NEODECADRON

MERCK	EQ 0.1% PHOSPHATE;EQ 3.5MG BASE/ML	N050322 001

NEOMYCIN SULFATE AND DEXAMETHASONE SODIUM PHOSPHATE

BAUSCH AND LOMB	EQ 0.1% PHOSPHATE;EQ 3.5MG BASE/ML	N064055 001	OCT 30, 1995

NEOMYCIN SULFATE-DEXAMETHASONE SODIUM PHOSPHATE

PHARMAFAIR	EQ 0.1% PHOSPHATE;EQ 3.5MG BASE/ML	N062539 001	JAN 10, 1985
ALCON UNIVERSAL	EQ 0.1% PHOSPHATE;EQ 3.5MG BASE/ML	N062714 001	JUL 21, 1986

DEXBROMPHENIRAMINE MALEATE

Syrup; Oral

DISOMER

SCHERING	2MG/5ML	N011814 002

Tablet; Oral

DISOMER

SCHERING	2MG	N011814 001

DEXBROMPHENIRAMINE MALEATE; PSEUDOEPHEDRINE SULFATE

Tablet, Extended Release; Oral

DISOBROM

GENEVA PHARMS	6MG;120MG	N070770 001	SEP 30, 1991

RESPORAL

PIONEER PHARMS	6MG;120MG	N089139 001	JUN 16, 1988

Tablet; Oral

DISOPHROL

SCHERING	2MG;60MG	N012394 002

DEXPANTHENOL *MULTIPLE*

SEE   ASCORBIC ACID; BIOTIN; CYANOCOBALAMIN; DEXPANTHENOL; ERGOCALCIFEROL; FOLIC ACID; NIACINAMIDE; PYRIDOXINE; RIBOFLAVIN PHOSPHATE SODIUM; THIAMINE; VITAMIN A; VITAMIN E

SEE   ASCORBIC ACID; BIOTIN; CYANOCOBALAMIN; DEXPANTHENOL; ERGOCALCIFEROL; FOLIC ACID; NIACINAMIDE; PYRIDOXINE HYDROCHLORIDE; RIBOFLAVIN PHOSPHATE SODIUM; THIAMINE HYDROCHLORIDE; VITAMIN A PALMITATE; VITAMIN E

SEE   ASCORBIC ACID; BIOTIN; CYANOCOBALAMIN; DEXPANTHENOL; ERGOCALCIFEROL; FOLIC ACID; NIACINAMIDE; PYRIDOXINE HYDROCHLORIDE; RIBOFLAVIN PHOSPHATE SODIUM; THIAMINE HYDROCHLORIDE; VITAMIN A; VITAMIN E

Discontinued Drug Products (continued)

DEXTROAMPHETAMINE ADIPATE *MULTIPLE*
SEE   AMPHETAMINE ADIPATE; AMPHETAMINE SULFATE; DEXTROAMPHETAMINE ADIPATE; DEXTROAMPHETAMINE SULFATE

DEXTROAMPHETAMINE RESIN COMPLEX *MULTIPLE*
SEE   AMPHETAMINE RESIN COMPLEX; DEXTROAMPHETAMINE RESIN COMPLEX

DEXTROAMPHETAMINE SULFATE
Capsule; Oral
DEXAMPEX
TEVA   15MG   N085355 001
Elixir; Oral
DEXEDRINE
GLAXOSMITHKLINE   5MG/5ML   N083902 001
Tablet; Oral
DEXAMPEX
TEVA   5MG   N083735 001
                        10MG   N083735 002
DEXTROAMPHETAMINE SULFATE
GENEVA PHARMS   5MG   N085370 001
                        10MG   N085371 001
HALSEY   10MG   N083930 001
LANNETT   5MG   N083903 001
                        10MG   N083903 003
                        15MG *SEE ANNUAL PREFACE INTRODUCTION DISCONTINUED SECTION*
MAST MM   5MG   N085652 001
PUREPAC PHARM   5MG   N086521 001
VITARINE   5MG   N084125 001
                        10MG   N084986 001
                                          N085892 001
FERNDEX
FERNDALE LABS   5MG   N084001 001

DEXTROAMPHETAMINE SULFATE *MULTIPLE*
SEE   AMPHETAMINE ADIPATE; AMPHETAMINE SULFATE; DEXTROAMPHETAMINE ADIPATE; DEXTROAMPHETAMINE SULFATE

DEXTROMETHORPHAN HYDROBROMIDE; PROMETHAZINE HYDROCHLORIDE
Syrup; Oral
PHENERGAN W/ DEXTROMETHORPHAN
WYETH AYERST   15MG/5ML;6.25MG/5ML   N011265 002   APR 02, 1984
PHERAZINE DM
HALSEY   15MG/5ML;6.25MG/5ML   N088913 001   MAR 02, 1987

DEXTROMETHORPHAN HYDROBROMIDE *MULTIPLE*
SEE   BROMPHENIRAMINE MALEATE; DEXTROMETHORPHAN HYDROBROMIDE; PSEUDOEPHEDRINE HYDROCHLORIDE

DEXTROSE
Injectable; Injection
DEXTROSE 2.5% IN PLASTIC CONTAINER
B BRAUN   2.5GM/100ML   N019626 001   FEB 02, 1988
DEXTROSE 7.7% IN PLASTIC CONTAINER
B BRAUN   7.7GM/100ML   N019626 003   FEB 02, 1988
DEXTROSE 10% IN PLASTIC CONTAINER
MILES   10GM/100ML   N018504 001
DEXTROSE 38.5% IN PLASTIC CONTAINER
ABBOTT   38.5GM/100ML   N018923 001   SEP 19, 1984
DEXTROSE 50% IN PLASTIC CONTAINER
ABBOTT   500MG/ML   N019445 001   JUN 03, 1986
DEXTROSE 60%
B BRAUN   60GM/100ML   N017995 002   SEP 22, 1982
DEXTROSE 60% IN PLASTIC CONTAINER
B BRAUN   60GM/100ML   N017995 001
BAXTER HLTHCARE   60GM/100ML   N020047 002   JUL 02, 1991

DEXTROSE; POTASSIUM CHLORIDE
Injectable; Injection
POTASSIUM CHLORIDE 0.11% IN DEXTROSE 5% IN PLASTIC CONTAINER
B BRAUN   5GM/100ML,110MG/100ML   N019699 003   SEP 29, 1989
POTASSIUM CHLORIDE 0.22% IN DEXTROSE 5% IN PLASTIC CONTAINER
B BRAUN   5GM/100ML,220MG/100ML   N019699 005   SEP 29, 1989
POTASSIUM CHLORIDE 0.037% IN DEXTROSE 5% IN PLASTIC CONTAINER
B BRAUN   5GM/100ML,37MG/100ML   N019699 001   SEP 29, 1989
POTASSIUM CHLORIDE 0.075% IN DEXTROSE 5% IN PLASTIC CONTAINER
B BRAUN   5GM/100ML,75MG/100ML   N019699 002   SEP 29, 1989

DEXTROSE; POTASSIUM CHLORIDE; SODIUM CHLORIDE
Injectable; Injection
DEXTROSE 5%, SODIUM CHLORIDE 0.2% AND POTASSIUM CHLORIDE 0.15% IN PLASTIC CONTAINER
B BRAUN   5 G M / 1 0 0 M L ; 1 5 0 M G / 100ML ;200MG/100ML   N018268 004
DEXTROSE 5%, SODIUM CHLORIDE 0.2% AND POTASSIUM CHLORIDE 0.224% IN PLASTIC CONTAINER
B BRAUN   5 G M / 1 0 0 M L ; 2 2 0 M G / 100ML;200MG/100ML   N018268 005

DEXTROSE; POTASSIUM CHLORIDE; SODIUM CHLORIDE (continued)
Injectable; Injection
DEXTROSE 5%, SODIUM CHLORIDE 0.45% AND POTASSIUM CHLORIDE 0.075%
  B BRAUN   5 G M / 1 0 0 M L ; 7 5 M G /
             100ML,450MG/100ML   N018268 010

DEXTROSE; SODIUM CHLORIDE
Injectable; Injection
DEXTROSE 2.5% AND SODIUM CHLORIDE 0.9% IN PLASTIC CONTAINER
  B BRAUN   2.5GM/100ML,900MG/100ML   N018376 001
DEXTROSE 2.5% AND SODIUM CHLORIDE 0.45% IN PLASTIC CONTAINER
  B BRAUN   2.5GM/100ML,450MG/100ML   N018030 001
DEXTROSE 3.3% AND SODIUM CHLORIDE 0.3% IN PLASTIC CONTAINER
  ABBOTT   3.3GM/100ML,300MG/100ML   N018055 001
DEXTROSE 5% AND SODIUM CHLORIDE 0.2% IN PLASTIC CONTAINER
  B BRAUN   5GM/100ML,200MG/100ML   N018030 004
  MILES   5GM/100ML,200MG/100ML   N018399 001
DEXTROSE 5% AND SODIUM CHLORIDE 0.3% IN PLASTIC CONTAINER
  MILES   5GM/100ML,300MG/100ML   N018501 001
  ABBOTT   5GM/100ML,300MG/100ML   N019486 001   OCT 04, 1985
DEXTROSE 5% AND SODIUM CHLORIDE 0.9% IN PLASTIC CONTAINER
  B BRAUN   5GM/100ML,900MG/100ML   N018026 001
  MILES   5GM/100ML,900MG/100ML   N018500 001
  ABBOTT   5GM/100ML,900MG/100ML   N019483 001   OCT 04, 1985
DEXTROSE 5% AND SODIUM CHLORIDE 0.11% IN PLASTIC CONTAINER
  B BRAUN   5GM/100ML,110MG/100ML   N018030 005
DEXTROSE 5% AND SODIUM CHLORIDE 0.33% IN PLASTIC CONTAINER
  B BRAUN   5GM/100ML,330MG/100ML   N018030 003
DEXTROSE 5% AND SODIUM CHLORIDE 0.45% IN PLASTIC CONTAINER
  B BRAUN   5GM/100ML,450MG/100ML   N018030 002
  MILES   5GM/100ML,450MG/100ML   N018400 001
  ABBOTT   5GM/100ML,450MG/100ML   N019484 001   OCT 04, 1985
DEXTROSE 5% AND SODIUM CHLORIDE 0.225% IN PLASTIC CONTAINER
  ABBOTT   5GM/100ML,225MG/100ML   N019482 001   OCT 04, 1985
DEXTROSE 10% AND SODIUM CHLORIDE 0.2% IN PLASTIC CONTAINER
  B BRAUN   10GM/100ML,200MG/100ML   N018386 001
DEXTROSE 10% AND SODIUM CHLORIDE 0.9% IN PLASTIC CONTAINER
  B BRAUN   10GM/100ML,900MG/100ML   N018047 001
DEXTROSE 10% AND SODIUM CHLORIDE 0.45% IN PLASTIC CONTAINER
  B BRAUN   10GM/100ML,450MG/100ML   N018229 001

DEXTROSE *MULTIPLE*
SEE   ALCOHOL; DEXTROSE
SEE   AMINO ACIDS; CALCIUM CHLORIDE; DEXTROSE; MAGNESIUM CHLORIDE; POTASSIUM CHLORIDE; POTASSIUM PHOSPHATE, DIBASIC; SODIUM CHLORIDE
SEE   AMINO ACIDS; DEXTROSE

Discontinued Drug Products (continued)

DEXTROSE; POTASSIUM CHLORIDE; SODIUM CHLORIDE (continued)
Injectable; Injection
DEXTROSE 5%, SODIUM CHLORIDE 0.2% AND POTASSIUM CHLORIDE 0.3% IN PLASTIC CONTAINER
  B BRAUN   5 G M / 1 0 0 M L ; 3 0 0 M G /
             100ML,200MG/100ML   N018268 006
DEXTROSE 5%, SODIUM CHLORIDE 0.2% AND POTASSIUM CHLORIDE 0.075%
  B BRAUN   5 G M / 1 0 0 M L ; 7 5 M G /
             100ML,200MG/100ML   N018268 009
DEXTROSE 5%, SODIUM CHLORIDE 0.33% AND POTASSIUM CHLORIDE 0.075% IN PLASTIC CONTAINER
  B BRAUN   5 G M / 1 0 0 M L ; 7 5 M G /
             100ML,330MG/100ML   N018268 011   JAN 18, 1986
DEXTROSE 5%, SODIUM CHLORIDE 0.33% AND POTASSIUM CHLORIDE 0.15% IN PLASTIC CONTAINER
  B BRAUN   5 G M / 1 0 0 M L ; 1 5 0 M G /
             100ML,330MG/100ML   N018268 012   JAN 18, 1986
DEXTROSE 5%, SODIUM CHLORIDE 0.33% AND POTASSIUM CHLORIDE 0.22% IN PLASTIC CONTAINER
  B BRAUN   5 G M / 1 0 0 M L ; 2 2 0 M G /
             100ML,330MG/100ML   N018268 013   JAN 18, 1986
DEXTROSE 5%, SODIUM CHLORIDE 0.33% AND POTASSIUM CHLORIDE 0.30% IN PLASTIC CONTAINER
  B BRAUN   5 G M / 1 0 0 M L ; 3 0 0 M G /
             100ML,330MG/100ML   N018268 014   JAN 18, 1986
DEXTROSE 5%, SODIUM CHLORIDE 0.45% AND POTASSIUM CHLORIDE 20MEQ (K) IN PLASTIC CONTAINER
  BAXTER HLTHCARE   5 G M / 1 0 0 M L ; 3 0 0 M G /
             100ML,450MG/100ML   N018008 001
DEXTROSE 5%, SODIUM CHLORIDE 0.45% AND POTASSIUM CHLORIDE 5MEQ IN PLASTIC CONTAINER
  BAXTER HLTHCARE   5 G M / 1 0 0 M L ; 7 5 M G /
             100ML,450MG/100ML   N018008 002
DEXTROSE 5%, SODIUM CHLORIDE 0.45% AND POTASSIUM CHLORIDE 15MEQ IN PLASTIC CONTAINER
  BAXTER HLTHCARE   5 G M / 1 0 0 M L ; 2 2 4 M G /
             100ML,450MG/100ML   N018008 003
DEXTROSE 5%, SODIUM CHLORIDE 0.45% AND POTASSIUM CHLORIDE 0.15% IN PLASTIC CONTAINER
  B BRAUN   5 G M / 1 0 0 M L ; 1 5 0 M G /
             100ML,450MG/100ML   N018268 001
DEXTROSE 5%, SODIUM CHLORIDE 0.45% AND POTASSIUM CHLORIDE 0.22% IN PLASTIC CONTAINER
  B BRAUN   5 G M / 1 0 0 M L ; 2 2 0 M G /
             100ML,450MG/100ML   N018268 002
DEXTROSE 5%, SODIUM CHLORIDE 0.45% AND POTASSIUM CHLORIDE 0.3% IN PLASTIC CONTAINER
  B BRAUN   5 G M / 1 0 0 M L ; 3 0 0 M G /
             100ML,450MG/100ML   N018268 003

Discontinued Drug Products (continued)

DEXTROSE *MULTIPLE* (continued)

SEE AMINO ACIDS; DEXTROSE; MAGNESIUM CHLORIDE; POTASSIUM ACETATE; POTASSIUM CHLORIDE; POTASSIUM PHOSPHATE, DIBASIC; SODIUM CHLORIDE

SEE AMINO ACIDS; DEXTROSE; MAGNESIUM CHLORIDE; POTASSIUM CHLORIDE; POTASSIUM PHOSPHATE, DIBASIC; SODIUM CHLORIDE

SEE AMINO ACIDS; DEXTROSE; MAGNESIUM CHLORIDE; POTASSIUM CHLORIDE; SODIUM CHLORIDE; SODIUM PHOSPHATE, DIBASIC, HEPTAHYDRATE

SEE CALCIUM CHLORIDE; DEXTROSE; MAGNESIUM CHLORIDE; POTASSIUM CHLORIDE; SODIUM ACETATE; SODIUM CHLORIDE

SEE CALCIUM CHLORIDE; DEXTROSE; MAGNESIUM CHLORIDE; POTASSIUM CHLORIDE; SODIUM ACETATE; SODIUM CITRATE

SEE CALCIUM CHLORIDE; DEXTROSE; MAGNESIUM CHLORIDE; SODIUM ACETATE; SODIUM CHLORIDE

SEE CALCIUM CHLORIDE; DEXTROSE; MAGNESIUM CHLORIDE; SODIUM CHLORIDE; SODIUM LACTATE

SEE CALCIUM CHLORIDE; DEXTROSE; POTASSIUM CHLORIDE; SODIUM CHLORIDE; SODIUM LACTATE

SEE CALCIUM CHLORIDE; DEXTROSE; SODIUM CHLORIDE; SODIUM LACTATE

DEXTROTHYROXINE SODIUM

Tablet; Oral

CHOLOXIN
ABBOTT
1MG — N012302 005
2MG — N012302 002
4MG — N012302 004
6MG — N012302 006

DEZOCINE

Injectable; Injection

DALGAN
ASTRAZENECA
5MG/ML — N019082 001 — DEC 29, 1989
10MG/ML — N019082 002 — DEC 29, 1989
15MG/ML — N019082 003 — DEC 29, 1989

DIATRIZOATE MEGLUMINE

Injectable; Injection

ANGIOVIST 282
BERLEX — 60% — N087726 001 — SEP 23, 1982

CARDIOGRAFIN
BRACCO — 85% — N011620 002

DIATRIZOATE MEGLUMINE
BRACCO — 76% — N010040 017

UROVIST MEGLUMINE DIU/CT
BERLEX — 30% — N087739 001 — SEP 23, 1982

Solution; Ureteral

UROVIST CYSTO
BERLEX — 30% — N087729 001 — SEP 23, 1982

DIATRIZOATE MEGLUMINE (continued)

Solution; Ureteral

UROVIST CYSTO PEDIATRIC
BERLEX — 30% — N087731 001 — SEP 23, 1982

DIATRIZOATE MEGLUMINE; DIATRIZOATE SODIUM

Injectable; Injection

ANGIOVIST 292
BERLEX — 52%;8% — N087724 001 — SEP 23, 1982

ANGIOVIST 370
BERLEX — 66%;10% — N087723 001 — SEP 23, 1982

DIATRIZOATE-60
INTL MEDICATION — 52%;8% — N088166 001 — JUN 17, 1983

HYPAQUE-M,75%
AMERSHAM HLTH — 50%;25% — N010220 003

HYPAQUE-M,90%
AMERSHAM HLTH — 60%;30% — N010220 002

MD-60
MALLINCKRODT — 52%;8% — N087074 001

MD-76
MALLINCKRODT — 66%;10% — N087073 001

RENOVIST
BRACCO — 34.3%;35% — N010040 020

RENOVIST II
BRACCO — 28.5%;29.1% — N010040 019

Solution; Oral, Rectal

GASTROVIST
BERLEX — 66%;10% — N087728 001 — SEP 23, 1982

DIATRIZOATE SODIUM

Injectable; Injection

HYPAQUE
AMERSHAM HLTH — 25% — N009561 003

MD-50
MALLINCKRODT — 50% — N087075 001

UROVIST SODIUM 300
BERLEX — 50% — N087725 001 — SEP 23, 1982

Solution; Oral, Rectal

HYPAQUE
AMERSHAM HLTH — 40% — N011386 003

Solution; Ureteral

HYPAQUE SODIUM 20%
AMERSHAM HLTH — 20% — N009561 002

DIATRIZOATE SODIUM *MULTIPLE*

SEE DIATRIZOATE MEGLUMINE; DIATRIZOATE SODIUM

Discontinued Drug Products (continued)

DIAZEPAM

Capsule, Extended Release; Oral
VALRELEASE

Company	Strength	Appl. No.	Date
ROCHE	15MG	N018179 001	

Injectable; Injection
DIAZEPAM

Company	Strength	Appl. No.	Date
AM PHARM PARTNERS	5MG/ML	N070662 001	JUN 25, 1986
ELKINS SINN	5MG/ML	N070311 001	DEC 16, 1985
	5MG/ML	N070312 001	DEC 16, 1985
	5MG/ML	N070313 001	DEC 16, 1985
LEDERLE	5MG/ML	N071308 001	JUL 17, 1987
MARSAM PHARMS LLC	5MG/ML	N072371 001	JAN 29, 1993
STERIS	5MG/ML	N070911 001	AUG 28, 1986
	5MG/ML	N070912 001	AUG 28, 1986
	5MG/ML	N070930 001	DEC 01, 1986
US ARMY	5 MG/ML *SEE ANNUAL PREFACE INTRODUCTION DISCONTINUED SECTION*	N020124 001	DEC 05, 1990
WARNER CHILCOTT	5MG/ML	N071613 001	OCT 22, 1987
	5MG/ML	N071614 001	OCT 22, 1987

DIZAC

Company	Strength	Appl. No.	Date
PHARMACIA AND UPJOHN	5MG/ML	N019287 001	JUN 18, 1993

VALIUM

Company	Strength	Appl. No.	Date
ROCHE	5MG/ML	N016087 001	

Tablet; Oral
DIAZEPAM

Company	Strength	Appl. No.	Date
DURAMED PHARM BARR	2MG	N070894 001	AUG 27, 1986
	5MG	N070895 001	AUG 27, 1986
	10MG	N070896 001	AUG 27, 1986
FERNDALE LABS	2MG	N070903 001	APR 01, 1987
	5MG	N070904 001	APR 01, 1987
	10MG	N070905 001	APR 01, 1987
HALSEY	2MG	N070987 001	AUG 15, 1986
	5MG	N070996 001	AUG 15, 1986
	10MG	N070956 001	AUG 15, 1986

DIAZEPAM (continued)

Tablet; Oral
DIAZEPAM

Company	Strength	Appl. No.	Date
HALSEY			
IVAX PHARMS	2MG	N070360 001	SEP 04, 1985
	5MG	N070361 001	SEP 04, 1985
	10MG	N070362 001	SEP 04, 1985
MARTEC	10MG	N072402 001	APR 25, 1989
PIONEER PHARMS	2MG	N070787 001	AUG 02, 1988
	5MG	N070788 001	AUG 02, 1988
	10MG	N070776 001	AUG 02, 1988
ROXANE	2MG	N070356 001	JUN 17, 1986
	5MG	N070357 001	JUN 17, 1986
	10MG	N070358 001	JUN 17, 1986
WARNER CHILCOTT	2MG	N070209 001	SEP 04, 1985
	5MG	N070210 001	SEP 04, 1985
	10MG	N070222 001	SEP 04, 1985
WATSON LABS	2MG	N070456 001	NOV 01, 1985
	5MG	N070457 001	NOV 01, 1985
	10MG	N070458 001	NOV 01, 1985

Q-PAM

Company	Strength	Appl. No.	Date
QUANTUM PHARMICS	2MG	N070423 001	DEC 12, 1985
	2MG	N072431 001	APR 29, 1988
	5MG	N070424 001	DEC 12, 1985
	5MG	N072432 001	APR 29, 1988
	10MG	N070425 001	DEC 12, 1985
	10MG	N072433 001	APR 29, 1988

DIAZOXIDE

Capsule; Oral
PROGLYCEM

Company	Strength	Appl. No.	Date
BAKER NORTON	50MG	N017425 001	
	100MG	N017425 002	

Discontinued Drug Products (continued)

DIAZOXIDE (continued)
Injectable; Injection
  DIAZOXIDE
    AM PHARM PARTNERS 15MG/ML N071519 001 AUG 26, 1987
    QUAD PHARMS 15MG/ML N071908 001 JAN 26, 1988

DIBUCAINE HYDROCHLORIDE
Injectable; Injection
  HEAVY SOLUTION NUPERCAINE
    NOVARTIS 2.5MG/ML N006203 001

DICHLORPHENAMIDE
Tablet; Oral
  DARANIDE
    MERCK 50MG N011366 001

DICLOFENAC POTASSIUM
Tablet; Oral
  CATAFLAM
    NOVARTIS 25MG N020142 001 NOV 24, 1993

DICLOFENAC SODIUM
Solution/Drops; Ophthalmic
  DICLOFENAC SODIUM
    FALCON PHARMS 0.1% N020809 001 MAY 04, 1998

DICLOXACILLIN SODIUM
Capsule; Oral
  DYCILL
    GLAXOSMITHKLINE EQ 250MG BASE N060254 002
        EQ 250MG BASE N062238 001
        EQ 500MG BASE N060254 003
        EQ 500MG BASE N062238 002
  PATHOCIL
    WYETH AYERST EQ 250MG BASE N050011 002
        EQ 500MG BASE N050011 003 MAR 28, 1983
For Suspension; Oral
  DYNAPEN
    APOTHECON EQ 62.5MG BASE/5ML N050337 002
  PATHOCIL
    WYETH AYERST EQ 62.5MG BASE/5ML N050092 001

DICUMAROL
Capsule; Oral
  DICUMAROL
    LILLY 25MG N005509 003
        50MG N005509 001

DICUMAROL (continued)
Tablet; Oral
  DICUMAROL
    ABBOTT 25MG N005545 003
        50MG N005545 004
        100MG N005545 005

DICYCLOMINE HYDROCHLORIDE
Capsule; Oral
  DICYCLOMINE HCL
    HALSEY 10MG N084505 001 OCT 21, 1986
    PIONEER PHARMS 10MG N089361 001 JAN 10, 1989
    WATSON LAB 10MG N083179 001 FEB 12, 1986
Injectable; Injection
  DICYCLOMINE HCL
    STERIS 10MG/ML N080614 001 FEB 11, 1986
Syrup; Oral
  DICYCLOMINE HCL
    ALPHARMA 10MG/5ML N084479 001
Tablet; Oral
  DICYCLOMINE HCL
    HALSEY 20MG N084600 001 JUL 29, 1985
          N088585 001 AUG 20, 1986
    PIONEER PHARMS 20MG N084361 001 FEB 06, 1986
    WATSON LAB 20MG

DIDANOSINE
For Solution; Oral
  VIDEX
    BRISTOL MYERS SQUIBB 375MG/PACKET N020155 006 OCT 09, 1991

DIENESTROL
Cream; Vaginal
  DV
    AVENTIS PHARMS 0.01% N083518 001
  ESTRAGUARD
    SOLVAY 0.01% N084436 001
Suppository; Vaginal
  DV
    AVENTIS PHARMS 0.7MG N083517 001

DIETHYLCARBAMAZINE CITRATE
Tablet; Oral
  HETRAZAN
    LEDERLE 50MG N006459 001

Discontinued Drug Products (continued)

DIETHYLPROPION HYDROCHLORIDE
Tablet, Extended Release; Oral

TENUATE			
AVENTIS PHARMS	75MG	N017669 001	
TEPANIL TEN-TAB	75MG	N017956 001	
3M			

Tablet; Oral

DIETHYLPROPION HCL			
CELLTECH PHARMS	25MG	N085544 001	
EON	25MG	N085916 001	
TEVA	25MG	N088642 001	SEP 20, 1984
WATSON LABS	25MG	N085741 001	
TENUATE			
AVENTIS PHARMS	25MG	N017668 001	
TEPANIL	25MG	N011673 001	
3M			

DIETHYLSTILBESTROL
Injectable; Injection

STILBESTROL		
BRISTOL MYERS SQUIBB	0.2MG/ML	N004056 003
	0.5MG/ML	N004056 004
	1MG/ML	N004056 005
	5MG/ML	N004056 006

Suppository; Vaginal

DIETHYLSTILBESTROL		
LILLY	0.1MG	N004040 001
	0.5MG	N004040 002
STILBESTROL		
BRISTOL MYERS SQUIBB	0.1MG	N004056 001
	0.5MG	N004056 002

Tablet, Delayed Release; Oral

DIETHYLSTILBESTROL		
LILLY	0.1MG	N004039 002
	0.5MG	N004039 003
	0.25MG	N004039 005
	1MG	N004039 004
	5MG	N004039 006
STILBESTROL		
TABLICAPS	0.5MG	N083003 001
	1MG	N083005 001
	5MG	N083007 001
STILBETIN		
BRISTOL MYERS SQUIBB	0.1MG	N004056 011
	0.5MG	N004056 012
	1MG	N004056 013
	5MG	N004056 014

Tablet; Oral

DIETHYLSTILBESTROL		
LILLY	0.1MG	N004041 002
	0.5MG	N004041 003

DIETHYLSTILBESTROL (continued)
Tablet; Oral

DIETHYLSTILBESTROL		
LILLY	1MG	N004041 004
	5MG	N004041 005
STILBESTROL		
TABLICAPS	0.5MG	N083004 001
	1MG	N083002 001
	5MG	N083006 001
STILBETIN		
BRISTOL MYERS SQUIBB	0.1MG	N004056 007
	0.5MG	N004056 008
	0.25MG	N004056 017
	1MG	N004056 009
	5MG	N004056 010

DIETHYLSTILBESTROL DIPHOSPHATE
Injectable; Injection

STILPHOSTROL		
BAYER PHARMS	250MG/5ML	N010010 001

Tablet; Oral

STILPHOSTROL		
BAYER PHARMS	50MG	N010010 002

DIFENOXIN HYDROCHLORIDE *MULTIPLE*
SEE   ATROPINE SULFATE; DIFENOXIN HYDROCHLORIDE

DIFLUNISAL
Tablet; Oral

DIFLUNISAL			
PUREPAC PHARM	250MG	N074285 001	MAY 07, 1996
	500MG	N074285 002	MAY 07, 1996

DIGITOXIN
Injectable; Injection

CRYSTODIGIN		
LILLY	0.2MG/ML	N084100 005

DIGOXIN
Capsule; Oral

LANOXICAPS			
GLAXO WELLCOME	0.15MG	N018118 004	SEP 24, 1984

Injectable; Injection

DIGOXIN		
AM PHARM PARTNERS	0.25MG/ML	N083217 001
WYETH AYERST	0.25MG/ML	N084386 001

Tablet; Oral

LANOXIN			
GLAXO WELLCOME	0.5MG	N020405 006	SEP 30, 1997

Discontinued Drug Products (continued)

DIGOXIN (continued)
Tablet; Oral
DIGOXIN
  LANOXIN
    GLAXO WELLCOME   0.375MG   N020405 005 SEP 30, 1997
                      0.0625MG   N020405 001 SEP 30, 1997
                      0.1875MG   N020405 003 SEP 30, 1997

DIHYDROCODEINE BITARTRATE *MULTIPLE*
  SEE ACETAMINOPHEN; CAFFEINE; DIHYDROCODEINE BITARTRATE

DIHYDROERGOTAMINE MESYLATE; HEPARIN SODIUM; LIDOCAINE HYDROCHLORIDE
Injectable; Injection
EMBOLEX
  NOVARTIS   0.5MG/0.5ML;2,500 UNITS/0.5ML;5.33MG/0.5ML   N018885 001 NOV 30, 1984
             0.5MG/0.7ML;5,000 UNITS/0.7ML;7.46MG/0.7ML   N018885 002 NOV 30, 1984

DILTIAZEM HYDROCHLORIDE
Capsule, Extended Release; Oral
CARDIZEM SR
  AVENTIS PHARMS   180MG   N019471 004 JAN 23, 1989
Tablet; Oral
DILTIAZEM HCL
  TEVA   30MG   N074084 001 FEB 25, 1994
          60MG   N074084 002 FEB 25, 1994

DILTIAZEM MALATE
Tablet, Extended Release; Oral
TIAMATE
  MERCK   EQ 120MG HCL   N020506 001 OCT 04, 1996
          EQ 180MG HCL   N020506 002 OCT 04, 1996
          EQ 240MG HCL   N020506 003 OCT 04, 1996

DIMENHYDRINATE
Injectable; Injection
DIMENHYDRINATE
  ELKINS SINN   50MG/ML   N084767 001
  STERIS   50MG/ML   N083531 001
  WYETH AYERST   50MG/ML   N084316 001
Liquid; Oral
DIMENHYDRINATE
  ALRA   12.5MG/4ML   N080715 001

DIMENHYDRINATE (continued)
Tablet; Oral
DIMENHYDRINATE
  ANABOLIC   50MG   N085985 001
  HEATHER   50MG   N080841 001
  WATSON LABS   50MG   N085166 001

DINOPROST TROMETHAMINE
Injectable; Injection
PROSTIN F2 ALPHA
  PHARMACIA AND UPJOHN   EQ 5MG BASE/ML   N017434 001

DIPHEMANIL METHYLSULFATE
Tablet; Oral
PRANTAL
  SCHERING   100MG   N008114 004

DIPHENHYDRAMINE HYDROCHLORIDE
Capsule; Oral
BENADRYL
  PARKE DAVIS   25MG   N005845 007
                 50MG   N005845 001
DIPHENHYDRAMINE HCL
  ALRA   25MG   N080519 004
                 50MG   N080519 003
  ANABOLIC   25MG   N083634 001
                 50MG   N085701 001
  ELKINS SINN   25MG   N085701 002
                 50MG   N080845 002
  EON   25MG   N080845 001
                 50MG   N087914 001 JUN 04, 1984
  HALSEY   50MG   N084524 001
  HEATHER   25MG   N083953 001
                 50MG   N080807 001
  IMPAX LABS   25MG   N080807 002
                 50MG   N080762 001
  IVAX PHARMS   25MG   N080762 002
                 50MG   N080868 001
  LANNETT   25MG   N080868 002
                 50MG   N086874 001
  LEDERLE   25MG   N086875 001
                 50MG   N086543 001
  NEWTRON PHARMS 25MG   N086544 001
                 50MG   N083061 001
  PERRIGO   25MG   N083061 002
                 50MG   N089101 001
  PIONEER PHARMS 25MG   DEC 20, 1985
                         N088880 001 DEC 20, 1985
                 50MG
  PUREPAC PHARM 25MG   N085156 001
                 50MG   N085150 001
  ROXANE   50MG   N080635 001
  SUPERPHARM   50MG   N089041 001

DIPHENHYDRAMINE HYDROCHLORIDE (continued)

Syrup; Oral

ANTITUSSIVE

Firm	Strength	Appl No	Date
PERRIGO			APR 10, 1987

BELDIN

Firm	Strength	Appl No	Date
HALSEY	12.5MG/5ML	N089179 001	JUN 05, 1986

BENYLIN

Firm	Strength	Appl No	Date
PARKE DAVIS	12.5MG/5ML	N006514 004	

DIPHEN

Firm	Strength	Appl No	Date
MORTON GROVE	12.5MG/5ML	N070118 001	OCT 01, 1985

DIPHENHYDRAMINE HCL

Firm	Strength	Appl No	Date
ALPHARMA	12.5MG/5ML	N070497 001	APR 25, 1989
CUMBERLAND SWAN	12.5MG/5ML	N073611 001	AUG 20, 1992
HI TECH PHARMA	12.5MG/5ML	N072416 001	SEP 28, 1990

HYDRAMINE

Firm	Strength	Appl No	Date
ALPHARMA	12.5MG/5ML	N070205 001	JAN 28, 1986

SILPHEN

Firm	Strength	Appl No	Date
SILARX	12.5MG/5ML	N072646 001	FEB 27, 1992

VICKS FORMULA 44

Firm	Strength	Appl No	Date
PROCTER AND GAMBLE	12.5MG/5ML	N070524 001	JAN 14, 1987

DIPHENHYDRAMINE HYDROCHLORIDE; PSEUDOEPHEDRINE HYDROCHLORIDE

Solution; Oral

BENYLIN

Firm	Strength	Appl No	Date
PARKE DAVIS	12.5MG/5ML;30MG/5ML	N019014 001	JUN 11, 1985

DIPHENIDOL HYDROCHLORIDE

Tablet; Oral

VONTROL

Firm	Strength	Appl No
GLAXOSMITHKLINE	EQ 25MG BASE	N016033 001

DIPHENOXYLATE HYDROCHLORIDE *MULTIPLE*

SEE   ATROPINE SULFATE; DIPHENOXYLATE HYDROCHLORIDE

DIPHENYLPYRALINE HYDROCHLORIDE

Capsule, Extended Release; Oral

HISPRIL

Firm	Strength	Appl No
GLAXOSMITHKLINE	5MG	N011945 001

DIPYRIDAMOLE

Tablet; Oral

DIPYRIDAMOLE

Firm	Strength	Appl No	Date
PUREPAC PHARM	50MG	N089426 001	JUL 12, 1990

Discontinued Drug Products (continued)

DIPHENHYDRAMINE HYDROCHLORIDE (continued)

Capsule; Oral

DIPHENHYDRAMINE HCL

Firm	Strength	Appl No	Date
SUPERPHARM	25MG		MAY 15, 1985
TEVA	50MG	N085874 001	
	25MG	N085874 002	
VANGARD	25MG	N088034 001	OCT 27, 1982
WATSON LAB	50MG	N087630 001	
	25MG	N083797 001	
WATSON LABS	50MG	N083797 002	
	25MG	N085138 001	
WEST WARD	50MG	N085083 001	
WHITEWORTH TOWN	50MG	N083567 001	
PLSN	25MG	N083441 001	
	50MG	N080800 001	

Elixir; Oral

BELIX

Firm	Strength	Appl No	Date
HALSEY	12.5MG/5ML	N086586 001	OCT 03, 1983

BENADRYL

Firm	Strength	Appl No
PARKE DAVIS	12.5MG/5ML	N005845 004

DIBENIL

Firm	Strength	Appl No	Date
CENCI	12.5MG/5ML	N088304 001	DEC 16, 1983

DIPHEN

Firm	Strength	Appl No
USL PHARMA	12.5MG/5ML	N084640 001

DIPHENHYDRAMINE HCL

Firm	Strength	Appl No	Date
BUNDY	12.5MG/5ML	N083674 001	
CENCI	12.5MG/5ML	N087941 001	DEC 17, 1982
KV PHARM	12.5MG/5ML	N085621 001	
LEDERLE	12.5MG/5ML	N086937 001	
NASKA	12.5MG/5ML	N088680 001	MAY 31, 1985
PERRIGO	12.5MG/5ML	N083063 001	
PUREPAC PHARM	12.5MG/5ML	N083237 001	JAN 25, 1982
PVT FORM	12.5MG/5ML	N085287 001	

HYDRAMINE

Firm	Strength	Appl No
ALPHARMA	12.5MG/5ML	N080763 002

Injectable; Injection

BENADRYL

Firm	Strength	Appl No
PARKE DAVIS	10MG/ML	N006146 001

DIPHENHYDRAMINE HCL

Firm	Strength	Appl No
AM PHARM PARTNERS	10MG/ML	N087066 001
BEL MAR	10MG/ML	N080822 001
ELKINS SINN	50MG/ML	N083183 001
STERIS	10MG/ML	N083533 001
WYETH AYERST	50MG/ML	N080577 001

DIPHENHYDRAMINE HCL PRESERVATIVE FREE

Firm	Strength	Appl No
AM PHARM PARTNERS	50MG/ML	N080586 002

Syrup; Oral

ANTITUSSIVE

Firm	Strength	Appl No
PERRIGO	12.5MG/5ML	N071292 001

Discontinued Drug Products (continued)

DIPYRIDAMOLE (continued)
Tablet; Oral

DIPYRIDAMOLE

Manufacturer	Strength	NDC	Date
PUREPAC PHARM	75MG	N089427 001	JUL 12, 1990

DISOPYRAMIDE PHOSPHATE
Capsule; Oral

DISOPYRAMIDE PHOSPHATE

Manufacturer	Strength	NDC	Date
HALSEY	EQ 100MG BASE	N070351 001	DEC 17, 1985
	EQ 150MG BASE	N070352 001	DEC 17, 1985
INTERPHARM	EQ 100MG BASE	N071190 001	JAN 15, 1987
	EQ 150MG BASE	N071191 001	JAN 15, 1987
MYLAN	EQ 100MG BASE	N070138 001	JUN 14, 1985
	EQ 150MG BASE	N070139 001	JUN 14, 1985
SUPERPHARM	EQ 150MG BASE	N070941 001	FEB 09, 1987
WATSON LAB	EQ 100MG BASE	N070240 001	FEB 02, 1986
	EQ 150MG BASE	N070241 001	FEB 02, 1986

DISULFIRAM
Tablet; Oral

ANTABUSE

Manufacturer	Strength	NDC	Date
ODYSSEY PHARMS	500MG	N088483 001	DEC 08, 1983
PLIVA	250MG *SEE ANNUAL PREFACE INTRODUCTION DISCONTINUED SECTION*	N007883 003	
	500MG *SEE ANNUAL PREFACE INTRODUCTION DISCONTINUED SECTION*	N007883 002	

DISULFIRAM

Manufacturer	Strength	NDC	Date
PAR PHARM	250MG	N088792 001	AUG 14, 1984
	500MG	N088793 001	AUG 14, 1984
WATSON LABS	250MG	N086889 001	AUG 14, 1984
	250MG	N087973 001	AUG 05, 1983
	500MG	N086890 001	
	500MG	N087974 001	AUG 05, 1983

DIVALPROEX SODIUM
Tablet, Delayed Release; Oral

DEPAKOTE CP

Manufacturer	Strength	NDC	Date
ABBOTT	EQ 250MG BASE	N019794 001	JUL 11, 1990

DIVALPROEX SODIUM (continued)
Tablet, Delayed Release; Oral

DEPAKOTE CP

Manufacturer	Strength	NDC	Date
ABBOTT	EQ 500MG BASE	N019794 002	JUL 11, 1990

DOBUTAMINE HYDROCHLORIDE
Injectable; Injection

DOBUTAMINE HCL

Manufacturer	Strength	NDC	Date
ELKINS SINN	EQ 12.5MG BASE/ML	N074381 001	SEP 26, 1996

DOPAMINE HYDROCHLORIDE
Injectable; Injection

DOPAMINE HCL

Manufacturer	Strength	NDC	Date
ABBOTT	40MG/ML	N070656 001	JAN 24, 1989
	80MG/ML	N070657 001	JAN 24, 1989
	40MG/ML	N018549 001	MAR 11, 1983
AM PHARM PARTNERS	40MG/ML	N070012 001	JUN 12, 1985
	40MG/ML	N070058 001	MAR 20, 1985
	80MG/ML	N070059 001	MAR 20, 1985
	160MG/ML	N070364 001	MAR 20, 1985
	160MG/ML	N070087 001	DEC 04, 1985
ASTRAZENECA	40MG/ML	N070089 001	OCT 23, 1985
	80MG/ML	N070090 001	OCT 23, 1985
	160MG/ML	N070093 001	OCT 23, 1985
	160MG/ML	N070094 001	OCT 23, 1985
BAXTER HLTHCARE	40MG/ML	N018398 001	OCT 23, 1985
	80MG/ML	N018398 002	MAR 22, 1982
SMITH AND NEPHEW	40MG/ML	N070011 001	AUG 29, 1985
	40MG/ML	N070046 001	AUG 29, 1985
	80MG/ML	N070047 001	AUG 29, 1985
	40MG/ML	N018138 001	AUG 29, 1985
WARNER CHILCOTT	40MG/ML	N070558 001	SEP 20, 1985
	40MG/ML	N070559 001	SEP 20, 1985
	80MG/ML		

Discontinued Drug Products (continued)

DOXEPIN HYDROCHLORIDE
Capsule; Oral
DOXEPIN HCL

Applicant	Strength	Appl. No.	Date
CLONMEL HLTHCARE	EQ 10MG BASE	N071685 001	JAN 05, 1988
	EQ 25MG BASE	N071686 001	JAN 05, 1988
	EQ 50MG BASE	N071673 001	JAN 05, 1988
	EQ 75MG BASE	N071674 001	JAN 05, 1988
	EQ 100MG BASE	N071675 001	JAN 05, 1988
	EQ 150MG BASE	N071676 001	JAN 05, 1988
HALSEY	EQ 25MG BASE	N071502 001	FEB 18, 1988
	EQ 50MG BASE	N071653 001	FEB 18, 1988
	EQ 75MG BASE	N071654 001	FEB 18, 1988
	EQ 100MG BASE	N071521 001	FEB 18, 1988
NEW RIVER	EQ 10MG BASE	N016987 001	
	EQ 25MG BASE	N016987 002	
	EQ 50MG BASE	N016987 003	
	EQ 75MG BASE	N016987 006	
	EQ 100MG BASE	N016987 004	
	EQ 150MG BASE	N016987 007	APR 13, 1987
PUREPAC PHARM	EQ 10MG BASE	N073054 001	DEC 28, 1990
	EQ 25MG BASE	N072109 001	DEC 28, 1990
	EQ 50MG BASE	N073055 001	DEC 28, 1990
	EQ 75MG BASE	N072386 001	SEP 08, 1988
	EQ 100MG BASE	N072110 001	SEP 08, 1988
	EQ 150MG BASE	N072387 001	SEP 08, 1988
QUANTUM PHARMICS	EQ 10MG BASE	N070972 001	SEP 29, 1987
	EQ 25MG BASE	N070973 001	SEP 29, 1987
	EQ 50MG BASE	N070931 001	SEP 29, 1987
	EQ 75MG BASE	N070932 001	SEP 29, 1987
	EQ 100MG BASE	N072375 001	SEP 29, 1987
	EQ 150MG BASE	N072376 001	MAR 15, 1989
WATSON LABS	EQ 10MG BASE	N070952 001	MAR 15, 1989
	EQ 25MG BASE	N070953 001	MAR 04, 1987

DOXEPIN HYDROCHLORIDE (continued)
Capsule; Oral
DOXEPIN HCL

Applicant	Strength	Appl. No.	Date
WATSON LABS	EQ 50MG BASE	N070954 001	MAY 15, 1986
	EQ 75MG BASE	N071763 001	MAY 15, 1986
	EQ 100MG BASE	N070955 001	FEB 09, 1988
	EQ 150MG BASE	N071764 001	FEB 09, 1988

DOXYCYCLINE
For Suspension; Oral
DOXYCHEL

Applicant	Strength	Appl. No.	Date
RACHELLE	EQ 25MG BASE/5ML	N061720 001	

DOXYCYCLINE HYCLATE
Capsule, Coated Pellets; Oral
DOXYCYCLINE HYCLATE

Applicant	Strength	Appl. No.	Date
PLIVA	EQ 100MG BASE	N063187 001	JUN 30, 1992

Capsule; Oral
DOXY-LEMMON

Applicant	Strength	Appl. No.	Date
TEVA	EQ 50MG BASE	N062497 001	AUG 23, 1984
	EQ 100MG BASE	N062497 002	JUN 15, 1984

DOXYCYCLINE HYCLATE

Applicant	Strength	Appl. No.	Date
HALSEY	EQ 50MG BASE	N062119 002	MAY 24, 1985
	EQ 50MG BASE	N062418 001	JAN 28, 1983
	EQ 100MG BASE	N062119 001	MAY 24, 1985
	EQ 100MG BASE	N062418 002	JAN 28, 1983
HEATHER	EQ 50MG BASE	N062463 001	DEC 07, 1983
	EQ 100MG BASE	N062463 002	DEC 07, 1983
INTERPHARM	EQ 50MG BASE	N062763 001	SEP 02, 1988
	EQ 100MG BASE	N062763 002	SEP 02, 1988
PAR PHARM	EQ 50MG BASE	N062434 001	OCT 19, 1984
	EQ 100MG BASE	N062442 001	DEC 22, 1983
PVT FORM	EQ 50MG BASE	N062631 001	JUL 24, 1986
	EQ 100MG BASE	N062631 002	JUL 24, 1986
RANBAXY	EQ 50MG BASE	N062479 001	DEC 23, 1983

Discontinued Drug Products *(continued)*

DOXYCYCLINE HYCLATE *(continued)*

Capsule; Oral

DOXYCYCLINE HYCLATE

Applicant	Strength	Appl. No.	Date
RANBAXY	EQ 100MG BASE	N062479 002	DEC 23, 1983
		N062469 001	OCT 31, 1984
SUPERPHARM	EQ 50MG BASE	N062469 002	OCT 31, 1984
	EQ 100MG BASE	N062594 001	DEC 05, 1985
WARNER CHILCOTT	EQ 50MG BASE	N062594 002	DEC 05, 1985
	EQ 100MG BASE	N062142 001	DEC 05, 1985
WATSON LABS	EQ 50MG BASE	N062142 002	
	EQ 100MG BASE		

PERIOSTAT

Applicant	Strength	Appl. No.	Date
COLLAGENEX	EQ 20MG BASE	N050744 001	SEP 30, 1998

Injectable; Injection

DOXYCHEL HYCLATE

Applicant	Strength	Appl. No.	Date
RACHELLE	EQ 100MG BASE/VIAL	N061953 001	

DOXYCYCLINE

Applicant	Strength	Appl. No.	Date
BEDFORD	EQ 100MG BASE/VIAL	N062569 001	MAR 09, 1988
	EQ 100MG BASE/VIAL	N062569 002	MAR 09, 1988
	EQ 200MG BASE/VIAL	N062450 001	
ELKINS SINN	EQ 100MG BASE/VIAL	N062450 001	OCT 27, 1983
	EQ 200MG BASE/VIAL	N062450 002	OCT 27, 1983

DOXYCYCLINE HYCLATE

Applicant	Strength	Appl. No.	Date
LEDERLE	EQ 100MG BASE/VIAL	N062992 001	FEB 16, 1989
	EQ 200MG BASE/VIAL	N062992 002	FEB 16, 1989
QUAD PHARMS	EQ 100MG BASE/VIAL	N062643 001	FEB 13, 1986
	EQ 200MG BASE/VIAL	N062643 002	FEB 13, 1986

VIBRAMYCIN

Applicant	Strength	Appl. No.	Date
PFIZER	EQ 100MG BASE/VIAL	N050442 002	
	EQ 200MG BASE/VIAL	N050442 001	

Tablet; Oral

DOXY-LEMMON

Applicant	Strength	Appl. No.	Date
TEVA	EQ 100MG BASE	N062581 001	MAR 15, 1985

DOXYCYCLINE HYCLATE

Applicant	Strength	Appl. No.	Date
HALSEY	EQ 100MG BASE	N062391 001	SEP 30, 1982
HEATHER	EQ 100MG BASE	N062462 001	MAY 11, 1983
INTERPHARM	EQ 100MG BASE	N062764 001	SEP 02, 1988
SUPERPHARM	EQ 100MG BASE	N062494 001	FEB 20, 1985
WARNER CHILCOTT	EQ 100MG BASE	N062593 001	

DOXYCYCLINE HYCLATE *(continued)*

Tablet; Oral

DOXYCYCLINE HYCLATE

Applicant	Strength	Appl. No.	Date
WARNER CHILCOTT	EQ 50MG BASE	N062392 001	AUG 28, 1985
WATSON LABS	EQ 100MG BASE	N062392 002	MAR 31, 1983
			MAR 31, 1983

DOXYCYCLINE HYLATE

Applicant	Strength	Appl. No.	Date
AXIOM PHARM	EQ 50MG BASE	N062269 003	

DOXYLAMINE SUCCINATE

Capsule; Oral

UNISOM

Applicant	Strength	Appl. No.	Date
PFIZER	25MG	N019440 001	FEB 05, 1986

Tablet; Oral

DECAPRYN

Applicant	Strength	Appl. No.	Date
AVENTIS PHARMS	12.5MG	N006412 015	
	25MG	N006412 014	

DOXY-SLEEP-AID

Applicant	Strength	Appl. No.	Date
PAR PHARM	25MG	N070156 001	JUL 02, 1987

DOXYLAMINE SUCCINATE

Applicant	Strength	Appl. No.	Date
QUANTUM PHARMICS	25MG	N088603 001	AUG 07, 1984

DOXYLAMINE SUCCINATE; PYRIDOXINE HYDROCHLORIDE

Tablet, Extended Release; Oral

BENDECTIN

Applicant	Strength	Appl. No.	Date
AVENTIS PHARMS	10MG;10MG *SEE ANNUAL PREFACE INTRODUCTION DISCONTINUED SECTION*	N010598 002	

DROMOSTANOLONE PROPIONATE

Injectable; Injection

DROLBAN

Applicant	Strength	Appl. No.	Date
LILLY	50MG/ML	N012936 001	

DROPERIDOL

Injectable; Injection

DROPERIDOL

Applicant	Strength	Appl. No.	Date
AM PHARM PARTNERS	2.5MG/ML	N070992 001	NOV 17, 1986
	2.5MG/ML	N070993 001	NOV 17, 1986
ASTRAZENECA	2.5MG/ML	N072018 001	OCT 20, 1988
	2.5MG/ML	N072019 001	OCT 19, 1988
	2.5MG/ML	N072020 001	OCT 19, 1988
QUAD PHARMS	2.5MG/ML	N072021 001	OCT 19, 1988
	2.5MG/ML	N071941 001	

Discontinued Drug Products *(continued)*

DROPERIDOL *(continued)*
Injectable; Injection
DROPERIDOL

QUAD PHARMS	2.5MG/ML	AUG 17, 1988	N071942 001
	2.5MG/ML	AUG 17, 1988	N071750 001
SMITH AND NEPHEW	2.5MG/ML		
SOLOPAK	2.5MG/ML	SEP 06, 1988	N071754 001
	2.5MG/ML	SEP 06, 1988	N071755 001
STERIS	2.5MG/ML	SEP 06, 1988	N073520 001
	2.5MG/ML	NOV 27, 1991	N073521 001
	2.5MG/ML	NOV 27, 1991	N073523 001
	2.5MG/ML	NOV 27, 1991	

DROPERIDOL; FENTANYL CITRATE
Injectable; Injection
FENTANYL CITRATE AND DROPERIDOL

ASTRAZENECA	2.5MG/ML;EQ 0.05MG BASE/ML	N072026 001	APR 13, 1989
	2.5MG/ML;EQ 0.05MG BASE/ML	N072027 001	APR 13, 1989
	2.5MG/ML;EQ 0.05MG BASE/ML	N072028 001	APR 13, 1989
INNOVAR			
AKORN MFG	2.5MG/ML;EQ 0.05MG BASE/ML	N016049 001	

DYCLONINE HYDROCHLORIDE
Solution; Topical
DYCLONE

ASTRAZENECA	0.5%	N009925 002
	1%	N009925 001

DYDROGESTERONE
Tablet; Oral
GYNOREST

SOLVAY	5MG	N017388 001
	10MG	N017388 002

DYPHYLLINE
Elixir; Oral
NEOTHYLLINE

TEVA	160MG/15ML	N007794 003

Injectable; Injection
NEOTHYLLINE

TEVA	250MG/ML	N009088 001

Tablet; Oral
NEOTHYLLINE

TEVA	200MG	N007794 001
	400MG	N007794 002

ECHOTHIOPHATE IODIDE
For Solution; Ophthalmic
PHOSPHOLINE IODIDE

AYERST	0.03%	N011963 002
	0.06%	N011963 004
	0.25%	N011963 003

EDETATE CALCIUM DISODIUM
Tablet; Oral
CALCIUM DISODIUM VERSENATE

3M	500MG	N008922 002

EDETATE DISODIUM
Injectable; Injection
DISODIUM EDETATE

STERIS	150MG/ML	N084356 001

SODIUM VERSENATE

3M	200MG/ML	N010573 001

EDROPHONIUM CHLORIDE
Injectable; Injection
EDROPHONIUM CHLORIDE

STERIS	10MG/ML	N040044 001	MAR 20, 1996

EDROPHONIUM CHLORIDE PRESERVATIVE FREE

STERIS	10MG/ML	N040043 001	MAR 20, 1996

REVERSOL

ORGANON USA INC	10MG/ML	N089624 001	MAY 13, 1988

EFLORNITHINE HYDROCHLORIDE
Injectable; Injection
ORNIDYL

AVENTIS PHARMS	200MG/ML	N019879 002	NOV 28, 1990

ENOXACIN
Tablet; Oral
PENETREX

AVENTIS	200MG	N019616 004	DEC 31, 1991
	400MG	N019616 005	DEC 31, 1991

ENOXAPARIN SODIUM
Injectable; Subcutaneous
LOVENOX

AVENTIS	90MG/0.6ML	N020164 006	JUN 02, 2000

Discontinued Drug Products (continued)

EPINEPHRINE

Aerosol, Metered; Inhalation

BRONKAID MIST			
STERLING	0.25MG/INH	N016803 001	

Injectable; Injection

SUS-PHRINE SULFITE-FREE			
FORREST LABS	1.5MG/AMP	N007942 003	FEB 05, 1999
	5MG/ML	N007942 001	

Injectable; Intramuscular

EPI E Z PEN JR			
MERIDIAN MEDCL TECHN	0.15MG/DELIVERY	N019430 004	AUG 03, 1995

EPIPEN E Z PEN			
MERIDIAN MEDCL TECHN	0.3MG/DELIVERY	N019430 003	AUG 03, 1995

EPINEPHRINE; ETIDOCAINE HYDROCHLORIDE

Injectable; Injection

DURANEST		
ASTRAZENECA	0.005MG/ML;0.5%	N017751 004

EPINEPHRINE; LIDOCAINE HYDROCHLORIDE

Injectable; Injection

ALPHACAINE HCL W/ EPINEPHRINE		
CARLISLE	0.01MG/ML;2%	N084720 001
	0.02MG/ML;2%	N084732 001

LIDOCAINE HCL AND EPINEPHRINE		
ELKINS SINN	0.01MG/ML;1%	N080406 001
	0.01MG/ML;2%	N080406 002

LIDOCAINE HCL W/ EPINEPHRINE		
ABBOTT	0.01MG/ML;1%	N083154 001
	0.01MG/ML;2%	N080757 001
BEL MAR	0.01MG/ML;1%	N080820 001
	0.01MG/ML;1%	N086402 001
INTL MEDICATION	0.01MG/ML;1%	N080377 003
STERIS	0.01MG/ML;2%	N080377 004
	0.01MG/ML;1%	N085463 001

LIDOCATON			
PHARMATON	0.02MG/ML;2%	N084728 001	AUG 17, 1983

XYLOCAINE W/ EPINEPHRINE		
ASTRAZENECA	0.01MG/ML;2%	N006488 003
	0.02MG/ML;2%	N006488 005
	0.005MG/ML;1%	N010418 006
	0.005MG/ML;2%	N010418 008
	0.005MG/ML;1.5%	N010418 010

EPINEPHRINE; PROCAINE HYDROCHLORIDE

Injectable; Injection

PROCAINE HCL W/ EPINEPHRINE		
BEL MAR	0.02MG/ML;1%	N080758 001
	0.02MG/ML;2%	N080759 001

EPINEPHRINE BITARTRATE

Aerosol, Metered; Inhalation

MEDIHALER-EPI		
3M	0.3MG/INH	N010374 003

EPINEPHRINE BITARTRATE; ETIDOCAINE HYDROCHLORIDE

Injectable; Injection

DURANEST		
ASTRAZENECA	0.005MG/ML;1.5%	N017751 007
DENTSPLY PHARM	0.005MG/ML;1.5%	N021384 001

EPINEPHRINE BITARTRATE; PRILOCAINE HYDROCHLORIDE

Injectable; Injection

CITANEST FORTE		
ASTRAZENECA	0.005MG/ML;4%	N014763 008

ERGOCALCIFEROL

Capsule; Oral

DELTALIN		
LILLY	50,000 IU	N080884 001
VITAMIN D		
CHASE CHEM	50,000 IU	N080747 001
EVERYLIFE	50,000 IU	N080956 001
IMPAX LABS	50,000 IU	N080951 001
LANNETT	50,000 IU	N080825 001
VITARINE	50,000 IU	N084053 001
WEST WARD	50,000 IU	N083102 001

ERGOCALCIFEROL *MULTIPLE*

SEE ASCORBIC ACID; BIOTIN; CYANOCOBALAMIN; DEXPANTHENOL; ERGOCALCIFEROL; FOLIC ACID; NIACINAMIDE; PYRIDOXINE; RIBOFLAVIN PHOSPHATE SODIUM; THIAMINE; VITAMIN A; VITAMIN E

SEE ASCORBIC ACID; BIOTIN; CYANOCOBALAMIN; DEXPANTHENOL; ERGOCALCIFEROL; FOLIC ACID; NIACINAMIDE; PYRIDOXINE HYDROCHLORIDE; RIBOFLAVIN PHOSPHATE SODIUM; THIAMINE HYDROCHLORIDE; VITAMIN A PALMITATE; VITAMIN E

SEE ASCORBIC ACID; BIOTIN; CYANOCOBALAMIN; DEXPANTHENOL; ERGOCALCIFEROL; FOLIC ACID; NIACINAMIDE; PYRIDOXINE; RIBOFLAVIN PHOSPHATE SODIUM; THIAMINE HYDROCHLORIDE; VITAMIN A; VITAMIN E

SEE ASCORBIC ACID; BIOTIN; CYANOCOBALAMIN; ERGOCALCIFEROL; FOLIC ACID; NIACINAMIDE; PANTOTHENIC ACID; PHYTONADIONE; PYRIDOXINE; RIBOFLAVIN; THIAMINE; VITAMIN A PALMITATE; VITAMIN E

ERGOLOID MESYLATES

Capsule; Oral

HYDERGINE LC			
NOVARTIS	1MG	N018706 001	JAN 18, 1983

Solution; Oral

HYDERGINE		
NOVARTIS	1MG/ML	N018418 001

Tablet; Oral

ERGOLOID MESYLATES		
HALSEY	1MG	N088891 001

ERGOTAMINE TARTRATE (continued)

Tablet; Sublingual
WIGRETTES
ORGANON USA INC — JUL 29, 1982

ERGOTAMINE TARTRATE *MULTIPLE*

SEE CAFFEINE; ERGOTAMINE TARTRATE

ERYTHROMYCIN

Capsule, Delayed Rel Pellets; Oral
ERYC
PARKE DAVIS — 250MG — N062546 001
 — N062618 001 — JUL 25, 1985
 — N062338 001 — SEP 25, 1985
WARNER CHILCOTT — 250MG
ERYC 125
PARKE DAVIS — 125MG — N062648 001 — OCT 24, 1985
ERYC SPRINKLES
FAULDING — 125MG — N050593 001 — JUL 22, 1985

Ointment; Ophthalmic
ERYTHROMYCIN
PHARMADERM — 5MG/GM — N062446 001 — SEP 26, 1983
PHARMAFAIR — 5MG/GM — N062481 001 — APR 05, 1984

Powder; For Rx Compounding
ERYTHROMYCIN
PADDOCK — 100% — N050610 001 — NOV 07, 1986

Solution; Topical
ERYTHROMYCIN
ALPHARMA — 1.5% — N062328 001 — APR 19, 1982
 — 2% — N062327 001 — APR 19, 1982
 — 2% — N062342 001 — FEB 25, 1982
 — 2% — N062957 001 — JUL 21, 1988
LILLY — 2% — N050532 001
PHARMAFAIR — 1.5% — N062485 001 — JUL 11, 1984
 — 2% — N062616 001 — JUL 25, 1985

Tablet, Delayed Release; Oral
E-BASE
BARR — 333MG — N063028 001 — MAY 15, 1990
ILOTYCIN
DISTA — 250MG — N061910 001
R-P MYCIN
SOLVAY — 250MG — N061659 001

Discontinued Drug Products (continued)

ERGOLOID MESYLATES (continued)

Tablet; Oral
ERGOLOID MESYLATES
HALSEY
WATSON LAB — 1MG — N086433 001 — NOV 01, 1985
WATSON LABS — 1MG — N087244 001 — MAY 27, 1982
 — AUG 16, 1982
GERIMAL
WATSON LABS — 1MG — N088207 001 — MAR 22, 1984
HYDERGINE
NOVARTIS — 0.5MG — N017993 003

Tablet; Sublingual
ALKERGOT
EON — 0.5MG — N085153 001
 — 1MG — N087417 001
CIRCANOL
3M — 0.5MG — N084868 001
 — 1MG — N085809 001
DEAPRIL-ST
BRISTOL MYERS SQUIBB — 1MG — N085020 002
ERGOLOID MESYLATES
HALSEY — 0.5MG — N087407 001
 — 1MG — N087552 001
KV PHARM — 0.5MG — N085899 001
 — 0.5MG — N086265 001
 — 1MG — N085900 001
 — 1MG — N086264 001
LEDERLE — 0.5MG — N086984 001
 — 1MG — N086985 001
SUPERPHARM — 0.5MG — N089233 001 — SEP 23, 1986
 — 1MG — N089234 001 — SEP 23, 1986
VANGARD — 0.5MG — N088013 001 — SEP 20, 1982
 — 1MG — N088014 001 — SEP 20, 1982
WATSON LAB — 0.5MG — N084930 001
 — 1MG — N085177 001
 — 1MG — N087183 001
HYDROGENATED ERGOT ALKALOIDS
IVAX PHARMS — 0.5MG — N087186 001

ERGOTAMINE TARTRATE

Aerosol, Metered; Inhalation
MEDIHALER ERGOTAMINE
3M — 0.36MG/INH — N012102 001

Tablet; Sublingual
ERGOSTAT
PARKE DAVIS — 2MG — N088337 001 — JUN 08, 1984
WIGRETTES
ORGANON USA INC — 2MG — N086750 001

Discontinued Drug Products (continued)

ERYTHROMYCIN (continued)

Tablet, Delayed Release; Oral

Product / Firm	Strength	Appl. No.
ROBIMYCIN		
ROBINS AH	250MG	N061633 001

ERYTHROMYCIN ESTOLATE

Capsule; Oral

Product / Firm	Strength	Appl. No.
ERYTHROMYCIN ESTOLATE		
BARR	EQ 125MG BASE	N062162 001
IVAX PHARMS	EQ 250MG BASE	N062237 001
WATSON LABS	EQ 250MG BASE	N062087 001
ILOSONE		
LILLY	EQ 125MG BASE	N061897 001
	EQ 250MG BASE	N061897 002

For Suspension; Oral

Product / Firm	Strength	Appl. No.
ILOSONE		
DISTA	EQ 125MG BASE/5ML	N061893 001

Suspension/Drops; Oral

Product / Firm	Strength	Appl. No.
ILOSONE		
LILLY	EQ 100MG BASE/ML	N061894 003

Suspension; Oral

Product / Firm	Strength	Appl. No.	Date
ERYTHROMYCIN ESTOLATE			
BARR	EQ 125MG BASE/5ML	N062169 001	OCT 17, 1990
	EQ 250MG BASE/5ML	N062169 002	OCT 17, 1990
LIFE LABS	EQ 250MG BASE/5ML	N062362 001	DEC 17, 1982
ILOSONE			
LILLY	EQ 125MG BASE/5ML	N061894 001	
	EQ 250MG BASE/5ML	N061894 002	

Tablet, Chewable; Oral

Product / Firm	Strength	Appl. No.
ILOSONE		
DISTA	EQ 125MG BASE	N061895 001
	EQ 250MG BASE	N061895 002

Tablet; Oral

Product / Firm	Strength	Appl. No.
ILOSONE		
LILLY	EQ 500MG BASE	N061896 001

ERYTHROMYCIN ESTOLATE; SULFISOXAZOLE ACETYL

Suspension; Oral

Product / Firm	Strength	Appl. No.	Date
ILOSONE SULFA			
LILLY	EQ 125MG BASE/5ML;EQ 600MG BASE/5ML	N050599 001	SEP 29, 1989

ERYTHROMYCIN ETHYLSUCCINATE

Granule; Oral

Product / Firm	Strength	Appl. No.
PEDIAMYCIN		
ROSS LABS	EQ 200MG BASE/5ML	N062305 001

Suspension/Drops; Oral

Product / Firm	Strength	Appl. No.
PEDIAMYCIN		
ROSS LABS	EQ 100MG BASE/2.5ML	N062305 002

ERYTHROMYCIN ETHYLSUCCINATE (continued)

Suspension; Oral

Product / Firm	Strength	Appl. No.	Date
E-MYCIN E			
PHARMACIA AND UPJOHN	EQ 200MG BASE/5ML	N062198 001	
	EQ 400MG BASE/5ML	N062198 002	
ERYTHROMYCIN ETHYLSUCCINATE			
DISTA	EQ 200MG BASE/5ML	N062177 001	
	EQ 400MG BASE/5ML	N062177 002	
NASKA	EQ 400MG BASE/5ML	N062674 001	MAR 10, 1987
PARKE DAVIS	EQ 200MG BASE/5ML	N062231 001	
	EQ 400MG BASE/5ML	N062231 002	
PHARMAFAIR	EQ 200MG BASE/5ML	N062559 001	MAR 15, 1985
	EQ 400MG BASE/5ML	N062558 001	MAR 15, 1985
WYAMYCIN E			
WYETH AYERST	EQ 200MG BASE/5ML	N062123 002	
	EQ 400MG BASE/5ML	N062123 001	

Tablet, Chewable; Oral

Product / Firm	Strength	Appl. No.
PEDIAMYCIN		
ROSS LABS	EQ 200MG BASE	N062306 001

Tablet; Oral

Product / Firm	Strength	Appl. No.
E.E.S. 400		
ABBOTT	EQ 400MG BASE	N061905 001
ERYTHROMYCIN ETHYLSUCCINATE		
BARR	EQ 400MG BASE	N062256 001

ERYTHROMYCIN GLUCEPTATE

Injectable; Injection

Product / Firm	Strength	Appl. No.
ILOTYCIN GLUCEPTATE		
DISTA	EQ 1GM BASE/VIAL	N050370 003
	EQ 250MG BASE/VIAL	N050370 001
	EQ 500MG BASE/VIAL	N050370 002

ERYTHROMYCIN LACTOBIONATE

Injectable; Injection

Product / Firm	Strength	Appl. No.	Date
ERYTHROCIN			
ABBOTT	EQ 1GM BASE/VIAL	N062586 002	JAN 04, 1988
	EQ 500MG BASE/VIAL	N062586 001	JAN 04, 1988
ERYTHROMYCIN			
ELKINS SINN	EQ 1GM BASE/VIAL	N062563 002	MAR 28, 1985
	EQ 500MG BASE/VIAL	N062563 001	MAR 28, 1985
ERYTHROMYCIN LACTOBIONATE			
AM PHARM PARTNERS	EQ 1GM BASE/VIAL	N062604 002	NOV 24, 1986
	EQ 500MG BASE/VIAL	N062604 001	NOV 24, 1986
QUAD PHARMS	EQ 1GM BASE/VIAL	N062660 003	NOV 24, 1986

Discontinued Drug Products (continued)

ERYTHROMYCIN LACTOBIONATE (continued)
Injectable; Injection
ERYTHROMYCIN LACTOBIONATE
  QUAD PHARMS   EQ 500MG BASE/VIAL   N062660 001   NOV 24, 1986

ERYTHROMYCIN STEARATE
Tablet; Oral
BRISTAMYCIN
  BRISTOL   EQ 250MG BASE   N061304 001
             EQ 250MG BASE   N061887 001
ERYPAR
  PARKE DAVIS   EQ 250MG BASE   N062032 001
                 EQ 500MG BASE   N062032 002
  WARNER CHILCOTT   EQ 250MG BASE   N062322 001
ERYTHROCIN STEARATE
  ABBOTT   EQ 125MG BASE   N060359 002
ERYTHROMYCIN STEARATE
  BARR   EQ 500MG BASE   N063179 001   MAY 15, 1990
  IVAX PHARMS   EQ 250MG BASE   N061461 001
                 EQ 500MG BASE   N061461 002
  LEDERLE   EQ 250MG BASE   N062089 001
             EQ 500MG BASE   N062089 002
  PUREPAC PHARM   EQ 250MG BASE   N061743 001
ETHRIL 250
  BRISTOL MYERS SQUIBB   EQ 250MG BASE   N061605 001
ETHRIL 500
  BRISTOL MYERS SQUIBB   EQ 500MG BASE   N061605 002
PFIZER-E
  PFIZER   EQ 250MG BASE   N061791 001
            EQ 500MG BASE   N061791 002
WYAMYCIN S
  WYETH AYERST   EQ 250MG BASE   N061675 001
                  EQ 500MG BASE   N061675 002

ESMOLOL HYDROCHLORIDE
Injectable; Injection
BREVIBLOC
  BAXTER HLTHCARE CORP   100MG/ML   N019386 003   DEC 31, 1986

ESTRADIOL
Film, Extended Release; Transdermal
ESTRADIOL
  ORTHO MCNEIL PHARM   0.1MG/24HR   N021048 003   SEP 20, 1999
                        0.05MG/24HR   N021048 001   SEP 20, 1999
                        0.075MG/24HR   N021048 002   SEP 20, 1999

ESTRADIOL (continued)
Film, Extended Release; Transdermal
FEMPATCH
  PARKE DAVIS   0.025MG/24HR   N020417 001   DEC 03, 1996

ESTRADIOL CYPIONATE
Injectable; Injection
DEPO-ESTRADIOL
  PHARMACIA AND UPJOHN   1MG/ML   N085470 001
                          3MG/ML   N085470 002
ESTRADIOL CYPIONATE
  QUAD PHARMS   5MG/ML   N089310 001   FEB 09, 1987

ESTRADIOL CYPIONATE; TESTOSTERONE CYPIONATE
Injectable; Injection
DEPO-TESTADIOL
  PHARMACIA AND UPJOHN   2MG/ML;50MG/ML   N017968 001
TESTOSTERONE CYPIONATE-ESTRADIOL CYPIONATE
  STERIS   2MG/ML;50MG/ML   N085603 001   MAR 13, 1986

ESTRADIOL VALERATE
Injectable; Injection
ESTRADIOL VALERATE
  STERIS   10MG/ML   N083546 001

ESTRADIOL VALERATE; TESTOSTERONE ENANTHATE
Injectable; Injection
DITATE-DS
  SAVAGE LABS   8MG/ML;180MG/ML   N086423 001
TESTOSTERONE ENANTHATE AND ESTRADIOL VALERATE
  STERIS   8MG/ML;180MG/ML   N085860 001
            4MG/ML;90MG/ML   N085865 001

ESTROGENS, CONJUGATED; MEDROXYPROGESTERONE ACETATE
Tablet; Oral-28
PREMPHASE (PREMARIN;CYCRIN 14/14)
  WYETH PHARMS INC   0.625MG;0.625MG;5MG   N020303 002   DEC 30, 1994
PREMPRO (PREMARIN;CYCRIN)
  WYETH PHARMS INC   0.625MG;0.625MG;2.5MG;2.5MG   N020303 001   DEC 30, 1994

ESTROGENS, CONJUGATED; MEPROBAMATE
Tablet; Oral
MILPREM-200
  MEDPOINTE PHARM HLC   0.45MG;200MG   N011045 002
MILPREM-400
  MEDPOINTE PHARM HLC   0.45MG;400MG   N011045 001

ETHAMBUTOL HYDROCHLORIDE
Tablet; Oral

MYAMBUTOL		
LEDERLE	100MG	N016320 001
	200MG	N016320 002
	400MG	N016320 003
	500MG	N016320 004

ETHCHLORVYNOL
Capsule; Oral

ETHCHLORVYNOL		
BANNER PHARMACAPS	100MG	N084463 001
	200MG	N084463 002
	500MG	N084463 003
	750MG	N084463 004
PLACIDYL		
ABBOTT	100MG	N010021 004
	200MG	N010021 007
	500MG	N010021 002
	750MG	N010021 010

ETHINAMATE
Capsule; Oral

VALMID		
DISTA	500MG	N009750 001

ETHINYL ESTRADIOL
Tablet; Oral

FEMINONE		
PHARMACIA AND UPJOHN	0.05MG	N016649 001
LYNORAL		
ORGANON USA INC	0.01MG	N005490 003
	0.05MG	N005490 002

ETHINYL ESTRADIOL; FERROUS FUMARATE; NORETHINDRONE
Tablet; Oral-28

NORQUEST FE			
GD SEARLE LLC	0.035MG;75MG;1MG	N018926 001	JUL 18, 1986

ETHINYL ESTRADIOL; FERROUS FUMARATE; NORETHINDRONE ACETATE
Tablet; Oral-28

NORLESTRIN FE 1/50		
PARKE DAVIS	0.05MG;75MG;1MG	N016766 001
NORLESTRIN FE 2.5/50		
PARKE DAVIS	0.05MG;75MG;2.5MG	N016854 001

ETHINYL ESTRADIOL; NORETHINDRONE
Tablet; Oral-21

N.E. 1/35 21			
LPI	0.035MG;1MG	N071541 001	DEC 14, 1987

Discontinued Drug Products (continued)

ESTROGENS, CONJUGATED; MEPROBAMATE (continued)
Tablet; Oral

PMB 200		
WYETH AYERST	0.45MG;200MG	N010971 005
PMB 400		
WYETH AYERST	0.45MG;400MG	N010971 003

ESTROGENS, ESTERIFIED
Tablet; Oral

AMNESTROGEN		
BRISTOL MYERS SQUIBB	0.3MG	N083266 001
	0.625MG	N083266 002
	1.25MG	N083266 003
	2.5MG	N083266 004
ESTERIFIED ESTROGENS		
GENEVA PHARMS	1.25MG	N085302 001
PVT FORM	0.625MG	N083414 001
	1.25MG	N083765 001
	2.5MG	N085907 001
ESTRATAB		
SOLVAY	0.3MG	N086715 001
	0.625MG	N083209 001
	1.25MG	N083856 001
	2.5MG	N083857 001
EVEX		
ROCHE PALO	0.625MG	N084215 001
	1.25MG	N083376 002
FEMOGEN		
PVT FORM	0.625MG	N085076 001
	1.25MG	N085008 001
	2.5MG	N085007 001

ESTROGENS, ESTERIFIED *MULTIPLE*
SEE CHLORDIAZEPOXIDE; ESTROGENS, ESTERIFIED

ESTRONE
Injectable; Injection

ESTROGENIC SUBSTANCE			
WYETH AYERST	2MG/ML	N083488 001	
ESTRONE			
STERIS	2MG/ML	N083397 001	
NATURAL ESTROGENIC SUBSTANCE-ESTRONE			
STERIS	2MG/ML	N085237 001	NOV 23, 1982
THEELIN			
PARKEDALE	1MG/ML	N003977 001	
	2MG/ML	N003977 002	
	5MG/ML	N003977 003	

ETHACRYNIC ACID
Tablet; Oral

EDECRIN		
MERCK	50MG	N016092 002

Discontinued Drug Products (continued)

ETHINYL ESTRADIOL; NORETHINDRONE (continued)
Tablet; Oral-21
ORTHO-NOVUM 7/14-21
  ORTHO MCNEIL PHARM   0.035MG;0.035MG;0.5MG;1MG   N019004 001   APR 04, 1984
OVCON-50
  WARNER CHILCOTT   0.05MG;1MG   N018128 001
TRI-NORINYL 21-DAY
  WATSON LABS   0.035MG,0.035MG,0.035MG;0.5-MG,1MG,0.5MG   N018977 001   APR 13, 1984
Tablet; Oral-28
N.E.E. 1/35 28
  LPI   0.035MG;1MG   N071542 001   DEC 14, 1987

ETHINYL ESTRADIOL; NORETHINDRONE ACETATE
Tablet; Oral-21
ESTROSTEP 21
  GALEN CHEM   0.02MG;0.03MG;0.035MG;1MG;1-MG;1MG   N020130 001   OCT 09, 1996
NORLESTRIN 21 1/50
  PARKE DAVIS   0.05MG;1MG   N016749 001
NORLESTRIN 21 2.5/50
  PARKE DAVIS   0.05MG;2.5MG   N016852 001
Tablet; Oral-28
NORLESTRIN 28 1/50
  PARKE DAVIS   0.05MG;1MG   N016723 001

ETHINYL ESTRADIOL; NORGESTIMATE
Tablet; Oral-21
ORTHO CYCLEN-21
  ORTHO MCNEIL PHARM   0.035MG;0.25MG   N019653 001   DEC 29, 1989
ORTHO TRI-CYCLEN
  ORTHO MCNEIL PHARM   0.035MG;0.035MG;0.035MG;0.18-MG;0.215MG;0.25MG   N019697 002   JUL 03, 1992

ETHINYL ESTRADIOL *MULTIPLE*
SEE   DESOGESTREL; ETHINYL ESTRADIOL

ETHOPROPAZINE HYDROCHLORIDE
Tablet; Oral
PARSIDOL
  PARKE DAVIS   10MG   N009078 003
                 50MG   N009078 006
                 100MG   N009078 008

ETHOTOIN
Tablet; Oral
PEGANONE
  OVATION PHARMS   500MG   N010841 003

ETHOXZOLAMIDE
Tablet; Oral
CARDRASE
  PHARMACIA AND UPJOHN   62.5MG   N011047 002
                          125MG   N011047 001
ETHAMIDE
  ALLERGAN   125MG   N016144 001

ETHYLESTRENOL
Elixir; Oral
MAXIBOLIN
  ORGANON USA INC   2MG/5ML   N014006 002
Tablet; Oral
MAXIBOLIN
  ORGANON USA INC   2MG   N014005 002

ETHYNODIOL DIACETATE; MESTRANOL
Tablet; Oral-20
OVULEN
  GD SEARLE LLC   1MG;0.1MG   N016029 002
Tablet; Oral-21
OVULEN-21
  GD SEARLE LLC   1MG;0.1MG   N016029 003
Tablet; Oral-28
OVULEN-28
  GD SEARLE LLC   1MG;0.1MG   N016705 001

ETIDOCAINE HYDROCHLORIDE
Injectable; Injection
DURANEST
  ASTRAZENECA   0.5%   N017751 003
                 1%   N017751 005

ETIDOCAINE HYDROCHLORIDE *MULTIPLE*
SEE   EPINEPHRINE; ETIDOCAINE HYDROCHLORIDE
SEE   EPINEPHRINE BITARTRATE; ETIDOCAINE HYDROCHLORIDE

ETOPOSIDE
Capsule; Oral
VEPESID
  BRISTOL   100MG   N019557 002   DEC 30, 1986
Injectable; Injection
ETOPOSIDE
  GENSIA SICOR PHARMS   20MG/ML   N074510 001   JUN 29, 1995
  PIERRE FABRE   20MG/ML   N074813 001   JUL 09, 1997
  STERIS   20MG/ML   N074228 001   OCT 15, 1996

Discontinued Drug Products (continued)

ETOPOSIDE PHOSPHATE
Injectable; Injection
ETOPOPHOS PRESERVATIVE FREE
BRISTOL MYERS SQUIBB

Strength	NDA	Date
EQ 1GM BASE/VIAL	N020906 002	FEB 27, 1998
EQ 500MG BASE/VIAL	N020906 001	FEB 27, 1998

ETRETINATE
Capsule; Oral
TEGISON
ROCHE

Strength	NDA	Date
10MG	N019369 001	SEP 30, 1986
25MG	N019369 002	SEP 30, 1986

EVANS BLUE
Injectable; Injection
EVANS BLUE
PARKE DAVIS

Strength	NDA	Date
0.5% *SEE ANNUAL PREFACE INTRODUCTION DISCONTINUED SECTION*	N008041 001	

FAMOTIDINE
Injectable; Injection
FAMOTIDINE
APOTHECON

Strength	NDA	Date
10MG/ML	N075707 001	APR 16, 2001

FAMOTIDINE PRESERVATIVE FREE
APOTHECON

Strength	NDA	Date
10MG/ML	N075708 001	APR 16, 2001

Tablet, Orally Disintegrating; Oral
PEPCID RPD
MERCK

Strength	NDA	Date
20MG	N020752 001	MAY 28, 1998
40MG	N020752 002	MAY 28, 1998

FENOFIBRATE
Capsule; Oral
LIPIDIL
ABBOTT

Strength	NDA	Date
100MG	N019304 001	DEC 31, 1993

TRICOR (MICRONIZED)
ABBOTT

Strength	NDA	Date
67MG	N019304 002	FEB 09, 1998
134MG	N019304 003	JUN 30, 1999
200MG	N019304 004	JUN 30, 1999

FENOPROFEN CALCIUM
Capsule; Oral
FENOPROFEN CALCIUM
AM THERAP

Strength	NDA	Date
EQ 200MG BASE	N072307 001	AUG 22, 1988
EQ 300MG BASE	N072308 001	AUG 22, 1988

HALSEY

Strength	NDA	Date
EQ 200MG BASE	N072355 001	AUG 17, 1988
EQ 300MG BASE	N072356 001	AUG 17, 1988

QUANTUM PHARMICS

Strength	NDA	Date
EQ 200MG BASE	N072214 001	AUG 17, 1988
EQ 300MG BASE	N071738 001	AUG 17, 1988

WARNER CHILCOTT

Strength	NDA	Date
EQ 200MG BASE	N072946 001	APR 30, 1991
EQ 300MG BASE	N072472 001	APR 30, 1991

WATSON LABS

Strength	NDA	Date
EQ 200MG BASE	N072294 001	AUG 17, 1988
EQ 200MG BASE	N072981 001	AUG 19, 1991
EQ 300MG BASE	N072293 001	AUG 17, 1988
EQ 300MG BASE	N072982 001	AUG 19, 1991

Tablet; Oral
FENOPROFEN CALCIUM
AM TH-ERAP

Strength	NDA	Date
EQ 600MG BASE	N072309 001	AUG 17, 1988

HALSEY

Strength	NDA	Date
EQ 600MG BASE	N072357 001	AUG 17, 1988

QUANTUM PHARMICS

Strength	NDA	Date
EQ 600MG BASE	N072194 001	AUG 17, 1988

USL PHARMA

Strength	NDA	Date
EQ 600MG BASE	N072362 001	AUG 17, 1988

WATSON LABS

Strength	NDA	Date
EQ 600MG BASE	N072165 001	AUG 17, 1988

NALFON
DISTA

Strength	NDA	Date
EQ 600MG BASE	N017710 001	

FENTANYL CITRATE
Injectable; Injection
FENTANYL CITRATE
ABBCTT

Strength	NDA	Date
EQ 0.05MG BASE/ML	N070636 001	APR 30, 1990
EQ 0.05MG BASE/ML	N070637 001	APR 30, 1990

STERIS

Strength	NDA	Date
EQ 0.05MG BASE/ML	N073488 001	JUN 30, 1992

FENTANYL CITRATE PRESERVATIVE FREE
MARSAM PHARMS LLC

Strength	NDA	Date
EQ 0.05MG BASE/ML	N074917 001	FEB 03, 1998

Discontinued Drug Products *(continued)*

FENTANYL CITRATE *(continued)*
Troche/Lozenge; Oral
  FENTANYL
    ANESTA   EQ 0.1MG BASE   N020195 007   OCT 30, 1995
        EQ 0.2MG BASE   N020195 001   OCT 04, 1993
        EQ 0.3MG BASE   N020195 002   OCT 04, 1993
        EQ 0.4MG BASE   N020195 003   OCT 04, 1993

FENTANYL CITRATE *MULTIPLE*
  SEE   DROPERIDOL; FENTANYL CITRATE

FERRIC AMMONIUM CITRATE
For Solution; Oral
  FERRISELTZ
    AMERSHAM HLTH   600MG/PACKET   N020292 001   OCT 14, 1997

FERROUS CITRATE, FE-59
Injectable; Injection
  FERROUS CITRATE FE 59
    MALLINCKRODT   25uCi/ML   N016729 001

FERROUS FUMARATE *MULTIPLE*
  SEE   ETHINYL ESTRADIOL; FERROUS FUMARATE; NORETHINDRONE
  SEE   ETHINYL ESTRADIOL; FERROUS FUMARATE; NORETHINDRONE ACETATE

FERROUS SULFATE; FOLIC ACID
Capsule; Oral
  FOLVRON
    LEDERLE   182MG;0.33MG   N006012 003

FIBRINOGEN, I-125
Injectable; Injection
  IBRIN
    AMERSHAM HLTH   154uCi/VIAL   N017879 001
  RADIONUCLIDE-LABELED (125 I) FIBRINOGEN (HUMAN) SENSOR
    ABBOTT   140uCi/ML   N017787 001

FLECAINIDE ACETATE
Tablet; Oral
  TAMBOCOR
    3M   200MG   N018830 002   OCT 31, 1985

FLOXURIDINE
Injectable; Injection
  FLOXURIDINE
    QUAD PHARMS   500MG/VIAL   N071055 001   AUG 24, 1987

FLUCONAZOLE
Injectable; Injection
  DIFLUCAN IN DEXTROSE 5% IN PLASTIC CONTAINER
    PFIZER   2MG/ML   N019950 005   JUL 08, 1994
  DIFLUCAN IN SODIUM CHLORIDE 0.9% IN PLASTIC CONTAINER
    PFIZER   2MG/ML   N019950 004   JUL 08, 1994

FLUDEOXYGLUCOSE, F-18
Injectable; Injection
  FLUDEOXYGLUCOSE F 18
    DOWNSTATE CLINCL   4-40mCi/ML   N020306 001   AUG 19, 1994

FLUMETHASONE PIVALATE
Cream; Topical
  LOCORTEN
    NOVARTIS   0.03%   N016379 001

FLUOCINOLONE ACETONIDE
Cream; Topical
  FLUOCET
    ALPHARMA   0.025%   N088360 001   JAN 16, 1984
  FLUOCINOLONE ACETONIDE
    ALPHARMA   0.01%   N088361 001   JAN 16, 1984
    CLAY PARK   0.01%   N086810 001   MAR 04, 1982
        0.025%   N086811 001   MAR 04, 1982
    PHARMADERM   0.01%   N088047 001   MAR 04, 1982
        0.025%   N088045 001   DEC 16, 1982
    PHARMAFAIR   0.01%   N088499 001   DEC 16, 1982
        0.025%   N088506 001   AUG 02, 1984
    USL PHARMA   0.01%   N088757 001   AUG 02, 1984
        0.025%   N088756 001   FEB 11, 1985
           N088756 001   MAR 28, 1985
  FLUONID
    ALLERGAN HERBERT   0.025%   N087156 002   SEP 06, 1984
  FLUOTREX
    SAVAGE LABS   0.01%   N088174 001   MAY 06, 1983
        0.025%   N088173 001   MAR 09, 1983
  SYNALAR-HP
    MEDICIS   0.2%   N016161 002

FLUOROMETHOLONE

Cream; Topical

Product	Strength	Company	Application No.	Date
OXYLONE	0.025%	PHARMACIA AND UPJOHN	N011748 001	

FLUOROURACIL

Injectable; Injection

Product	Strength	Company	Application No.	Date
ADRUCIL	50MG/ML	PHARMACIA AND UPJOHN	N017959 001	
	50MG/ML		N081222 001	JUN 28, 1991
FLUOROURACIL	50MG/ML	ABIC	N088929 001	MAR 04, 1986
	50MG/ML	AM PHARM PARTNERS	N089152 001	MAR 21, 1986
	50MG/ML		N089428 001	JAN 12, 1987
	50MG/ML		N089519 001	MAR 12, 1987
	50MG/ML	MARCHAR	N087791 001	JAN 18, 1983
	50MG/ML	QUAD PHARMS	N089368 001	FEB 03, 1987
	50MG/ML		N089455 001	FEB 03, 1987
	50MG/ML	SMITH AND NEPHEW	N088766 001	DEC 28, 1984
	50MG/ML		N088767 001	DEC 28, 1984
	50MG/ML		N089434 001	MAR 26, 1987

Solution; Topical

Product	Strength	Company	Application No.	Date
FLUOROPLEX	1%	ALLERGAN HERBERT	N016765 001	

FLUOXETINE HYDROCHLORIDE

Capsule; Oral

Product	Strength	Company	Application No.	Date
PROZAC	EQ 60MG BASE	LILLY	N018936 004	JUN 15, 1999

Tablet; Oral

Product	Strength	Company	Application No.	Date
PROZAC	EQ 20MG BASE	LILLY	N020974 002	MAR 09, 1999

FLUOXYMESTERONE

Tablet; Oral

Product	Strength	Company	Application No.	Date
ANDROID-F	10MG	ICN	N087196 001	
FLUOXYMESTERONE	10MG	ICN	N088221 001	MAY 05, 1983

Discontinued Drug Products (continued)

FLUOCINOLONE ACETONIDE (continued)

Gel; Topical

Product	Strength	Company	Application No.	Date
FLUONID	0.025%	ALLERGAN HERBERT	N087300 001	MAY 27, 1982

Ointment; Topical

Product	Strength	Company	Application No.	Date
FLUOCINOLONE ACETONIDE				
PHARMADERM	0.025%		N088046 001	DEC 16, 1982
PHARMAFAIR	0.025%		N088507 001	FEB 27, 1984
USL PHARMA	0.025%		N088742 001	FEB 08, 1985
FLUONID	0.025%	ALLERGAN HERBERT	N087157 001	SEP 06, 1984
FLUOTREX	0.025%	SAVAGE LABS	N088172 001	MAR 09, 1983

Solution; Topical

Product	Strength	Company	Application No.	Date
FLUOCINOLONE ACETONIDE				
BAUSCH AND LOMB	0.01%		N040059 001	DEC 20, 1993
MORTON GROVE	0.01%		N088312 001	JAN 27, 1984
PHARMADERM	0.01%		N088048 001	DEC 16, 1982
PHARMAFAIR	0.01%		N088449 001	FEB 08, 1984
FLUONID	0.01%	ALLERGAN HERBERT	N087158 001	MAR 17, 1983
FLUOTREX	0.01%	SAVAGE LABS	N088171 001	MAR 09, 1983

FLUOCINOLONE ACETONIDE; NEOMYCIN SULFATE

Cream; Topical

Product	Strength	Company	Application No.	Date
NEO-SYNALAR	0.025%;EQ 3.5MG BASE/GM	MEDICIS	N060700 001	

FLUOCINONIDE

Cream; Topical

Product	Strength	Company	Application No.	Date
FLUOCINONIDE	0.05%	CLAY PARK	N071790 001	JUL 13, 1988

FLUORESCEIN SODIUM

Injectable; Injection

Product	Strength	Company	Application No.	Date
FUNDUSCEIN-25	25%	NOVARTIS	N017869 001	

Discontinued Drug Products (continued)

FLUOXYMESTERONE (continued)

Tablet; Oral

FLUOXYMESTERONE

Firm	Strength	Appl No	Date
WATSON LAB	2MG	N088260 001	DEC 06, 1983
	5MG	N088265 001	DEC 06, 1983
	10MG	N088309 001	DEC 06, 1983

ORA-TESTRYL

Firm	Strength	Appl No	Date
BRISTOL MYERS SQUIBB	2MG	N011359 001	
	5MG	N011359 002	

FLUPHENAZINE DECANOATE

Injectable; Injection

FLUPHENAZINE

Firm	Strength	Appl No	Date
QUAD PHARMS	25MG/ML	N070762 001	FEB 20, 1986

FLUPHENAZINE DECANOATE

Firm	Strength	Appl No	Date
KING PHARMS	25MG/ML	N074966 001	APR 16, 1998

FLUPHENAZINE ENANTHATE

Injectable; Injection

PROLIXIN ENANTHATE

Firm	Strength	Appl No	Date
APOTHECON	25MG/ML	N016110 001	

FLUPHENAZINE HYDROCHLORIDE

Injectable; Injection

FLUPHENAZINE HCL

Firm	Strength	Appl No	Date
QUAD PHARMS	2.5MG/ML	N089800 001	JUN 08, 1988

Tablet, Extended Release; Oral

PERMITIL

Firm	Strength	Appl No	Date
SCHERING	1MG	N012419 004	

Tablet; Oral

FLUPHENAZINE HCL

Firm	Strength	Appl No	Date
WATSON LAB	1MG	N088555 001	DEC 18, 1987
	2.5MG	N088544 001	DEC 18, 1987
	5MG	N088527 001	DEC 18, 1987
	10MG	N088550 001	DEC 18, 1987

PERMITIL

Firm	Strength	Appl No	Date
SCHERING	0.25MG	N012034 001	
	2.5MG	N012034 004	
	5MG	N012034 005	
	10MG	N012034 006	

FLUPREDNISOLONE

Tablet; Oral

ALPHADROL

Firm	Strength	Appl No	Date
PHARMACIA AND UPJOHN	1.5MG	N012259 002	

FLURANDRENOLIDE

Lotion; Topical

FLURANDRENOLIDE

Firm	Strength	Appl No	Date
ALPHARMA	0.05%	N087203 001	APR 29, 1982

FLURANDRENOLIDE; NEOMYCIN SULFATE

Cream; Topical

CORDRAN-N

Firm	Strength	Appl No	Date
LILLY	0.05%;EQ 3.5MG BASE/GM	N050346 001	

Ointment; Topical

CORDRAN-N

Firm	Strength	Appl No	Date
LILLY	0.05%;EQ 3.5MG BASE/GM	N050345 001	

FLURAZEPAM HYDROCHLORIDE

Capsule; Oral

FLURAZEPAM HCL

Firm	Strength	Appl No	Date
HALSEY	15MG	N070454 001	AUG 04, 1986
	15MG	N071808 001	JAN 07, 1988
	30MG	N070455 001	AUG 04, 1986
	30MG	N071809 001	JAN 07, 1988
PUREPAC PHARM	15MG	N071927 001	SEP 09, 1987
	30MG	N071551 001	SEP 09, 1987
SUPERPHARM	15MG	N071659 001	AUG 04, 1988
	30MG	N071660 001	AUG 04, 1988
USL PHARMA	15MG	N070562 001	JUL 09, 1987
	30MG	N070563 001	JUL 09, 1987
WARNER CHILCOTT	15MG	N071767 001	DEC 04, 1987
	30MG	N071768 001	DEC 04, 1987
WATSON LABS	15MG	N072368 001	MAR 30, 1989

FLUVOXAMINE MALEATE

Tablet; Oral

LUVOX

Firm	Strength	Appl No	Date
SOLVAY	25MG	N020243 001	DEC 05, 1994

Discontinued Drug Products (continued)

FLUVOXAMINE MALEATE (continued)
Tablet; Oral

LUVOX			
SOLVAY	50MG	N020243 002	DEC 05, 1994
	100MG	N020243 003	DEC 05, 1994
	150MG	N020243 004	DEC 05, 1994

FOLIC ACID
Injectable; Injection

FOLVITE			
WYETH PHARMS INC	5MG/ML	N005897 008	

Tablet; Oral

FOLIC ACID			
ANABOLIC	1MG	N084915 001	
BARR	1MG	N089177 001	
		N084472 001	JAN 08, 1986
EON	1MG	N080755 001	
EVERYLIFE	1MG	N083598 001	
HALSEY	1MG	N080686 001	
IMPAX LABS	1MG	N080816 001	
LANNETT	1MG	N006135 003	
LILLY	1MG	N084158 001	
PHARMERAL	1MG	N088949 001	
PIONEER PHARMS	1MG		SEP 13, 1985
PUREPAC PHARM	1MG	N080784 001	
UDL	1MG	N088199 001	MAR 29, 1983
USL PHARMA	1MG	N087828 001	MAY 13, 1982
VANGARD	1MG	N088730 001	MAR 23, 1984
VINTAGE PHARMS	1MG	N086296 001	
WATSON LAB	1MG	N083141 001	
WATSON LABS	1MG	N085141 002	
WHITEWORTH TOWN PLSN	1MG	N080691 002	
FOLVITE			
WYETH PHARMS INC	1MG	N005897 004	

FOLIC ACID *MULTIPLE*
SEE ALPHA-TOCOPHEROL; ASCORBIC ACID; BIOTIN; CHOLECALCIFEROL; CYANOCOBALAMIN; FOLIC ACID; NIACINAMIDE; PANTOTHENIC ACID; PYRIDOXINE; RIBOFLAVIN; THIAMINE; VITAMIN A

SEE ASCORBIC ACID; BIOTIN; CYANOCOBALAMIN; DEXPANTHENOL; ERGOCALCIFEROL; FOLIC ACID; NIACINAMIDE; PYRIDOXINE; RIBOFLAVIN PHOSPHATE SODIUM; THIAMINE; VITAMIN A; VITAMIN E

SEE ASCORBIC ACID; BIOTIN; CYANOCOBALAMIN; DEXPANTHENOL; ERGOCALCIFEROL; FOLIC ACID; NIACINAMIDE; PYRIDOXINE; HYDROCHLORIDE; RIBOFLAVIN PHOSPHATE SODIUM; THIAMINE; VITAMIN A PALMITATE; VITAMIN E

FOLIC ACID *MULTIPLE* (continued)
SEE ASCORBIC ACID; BIOTIN; CYANOCOBALAMIN; DEXPANTHENOL; ERGOCALCIFEROL; FOLIC ACID; NIACINAMIDE; PYRIDOXINE HYDROCHLORIDE; RIBOFLAVIN PHOSPHATE SODIUM; THIAMINE HYDROCHLORIDE; VITAMIN A; VITAMIN E

SEE ASCORBIC ACID; BIOTIN; CYANOCOBALAMIN; ERGOCALCIFEROL; FOLIC ACID; NIACINAMIDE; PANTOTHENIC ACID; PHYTONADIONE; PYRIDOXINE; RIBOFLAVIN; THIAMINE; VITAMIN A PALMITATE; VITAMIN E

SEE FERROUS SULFATE; FOLIC ACID

FOLLITROPIN ALFA/BETA
Injectable; Injection

GONAL-F			
SERONO	37.5 IU/VIAL	N020378 003	MAY 25, 2000

FURAZOLIDONE
Suspension; Oral

FUROXONE			
SHIRE LABS	50MG/15ML	N011323 002	

Tablet; Oral

FUROXONE			
SHIRE LABS	100MG	N011270 002	

FUROSEMIDE
Injectable; Injection

FUROSEMIDE			
AM PHARM PARTNERS	10MG/ML	N018507 001	JUL 30, 1982
		N019036 001	AUG 13, 1984
	10MG/ML	N070014 001	SEP 09, 1985
		N070095 001	SEP 09, 1985
ASTRAZENECA	10MG/ML	N070096 001	SEP 09, 1985
	10MG/ML	N018267 001	
		N070017 001	DEC 15, 1986
BAXTER HLTHCARE	10MG/ML	N070023 001	FEB 05, 1986
ORGANON USA INC	10MG/ML	N070078 001	FEB 05, 1986
SMITH AND NEPHEW	10MG/ML	N070019 001	SEP 22, 1986
		N070604 001	JAN 02, 1987
STERIS	10MG/ML	N018420 001	FEB 26, 1982
WARNER CHILCOTT	10MG/ML	N018670 001	JUL 20, 1982
WYETH AYERST	10MG/ML		

Tablet; Oral

FUROSEMIDE			
EON	40MG	N018750 002	JUL 30, 1984

Discontinued Drug Products (continued)

FUROSEMIDE (continued)

Tablet; Oral

FUROSEMIDE

Firm	Strength	Number	Date
HALSEY	20MG	N070043 001	SEP 26, 1985
	40MG	N018790 001	NOV 29, 1983
	80MG	N070100 001	
SUPERPHARM	20MG	N018370 001	JAN 26, 1988
	40MG	N018370 002	JUN 26, 1984
		N018370 001	
WARNER CHILCOTT	20MG	N018419 001	FEB 10, 1983
	40MG	N018419 002	JAN 31, 1983
		N018419 002	JAN 31, 1983
	80MG	N018419 003	NOV 13, 1984
WATSON LABS	20MG	N018369 001	MAY 14, 1982
	40MG	N018369 002	MAY 14, 1982

GALLAMINE TRIETHIODIDE

Injectable; Injection

FLAXEDIL

Firm	Strength	Number
DAVIS AND GECK	20MG/ML	N007842 001
	100MG/ML	N007842 002

GALLIUM CITRATE, GA-67

Injectable; Injection

GALLIUM CITRATE GA 67

Firm	Strength	Number
AMERSHAM HLTH	1mCi/ML	N017700 001

NEOSCAN

Firm	Strength	Number
AMERSHAM HLTH	2mCi/ML	N017655 001

GEMFIBROZIL

Capsule; Oral

GEMFIBROZIL

Firm	Strength	Number	Date
MYLAN	300MG	N073466 001	JAN 25, 1993
PUREPAC PHARM	300MG	N072929 001	JAN 29, 1993

LOPID

Firm	Strength	Number
PFIZER PHARMS	200MG	N018422 001
	300MG	N018422 002

Tablet; Oral

GEMFIBROZIL

Firm	Strength	Number	Date
PUREPAC PHARM	600MG	N074360 001	AUG 31, 1994
WATSON LABS	600MG	N074156 001	OCT 24, 1994

GENTAMICIN SULFATE

Cream; Topical

GARAMYCIN

Firm	Strength	Number
SCHERING	EQ 0.1% BASE	N060462 001

GENTAFAIR

Firm	Strength	Number	Date
PHARMAFAIR	EQ 0.1% BASE	N062458 001	SEP 01, 1983

GENTAMICIN SULFATE

Firm	Strength	Number	Date
ALPHARMA	EQ 0.1% BASE	N062471 001	SEP 27, 1983
BAUSCH AND LOMB	EQ 0.1% BASE	N064056 001	APR 29, 1994
PHARMADERM	EQ 1MG BASE/GM	N062530 001	JUL 05, 1984

Injectable; Injection

APOGEN

Firm	Strength	Number
KING PHARMS	EQ 10MG BASE/ML	N062289 001
	EQ 40MG BASE/ML	N062289 002

BRISTAGEN

Firm	Strength	Number
BRISTOL	EQ 40MG BASE/ML	N062288 001

GARAMYCIN

Firm	Strength	Number
SCHERING	EQ 10MG BASE/ML	N061739 001

GENTAFAIR

Firm	Strength	Number	Date
PHARMAFAIR	EQ 40MG BASE/ML	N062493 001	AUG 28, 1985

GENTAMICIN

Firm	Strength	Number	Date
INTL MEDICATION	EQ 1MG BASE/ML	N062325 003	JUN 23, 1982
	EQ 40MG BASE/ML	N062325 001	
	EQ 100MG BASE/100ML	N062325 004	JUN 23, 1982

GENTAMICIN SULFATE

Firm	Strength	Number	Date
ABBOTT	EQ 1.2MG BASE/ML	N062413 001	AUG 11, 1983
	EQ 1.4MG BASE/ML	N062413 002	AUG 11, 1983
	EQ 1.6MG BASE/ML	N062413 003	AUG 11, 1983
	EQ 1.8MG BASE/ML	N062413 004	AUG 11, 1983
	EQ 2MG BASE/ML	N062413 005	AUG 11, 1983
	EQ 60MG BASE/100ML	N062413 006	AUG 11, 1983
	EQ 70MG BASE/100ML	N062413 007	AUG 11, 1983
	EQ 80MG BASE/100ML	N062413 008	AUG 11, 1983
	EQ 90MG BASE/100ML	N062413 009	AUG 11, 1983
	EQ 100MG BASE/100ML	N062413 010	AUG 11, 1983
BAXTER HLTHCARE	EQ 10MG BASE/ML	N062251 002	
	EQ 40MG BASE/ML	N062251 001	
GENSIA SICOR PHARMS	EQ 10MG BASE/ML	N063149 001	NOV 21, 1991

Discontinued Drug Products *(continued)*

GENTAMICIN SULFATE *(continued)*

Injectable; Injection

GENTAMICIN SULFATE

GENSIA SICOR PHARMS	EQ 40MG BASE/ML	N063106 002	NOV 21, 1991
SOLOPAK	EQ 10MG BASE/ML	N062507 001	JUN 06, 1985
	EQ 40MG BASE/ML	N062507 002	JUN 06, 1985
STERIS	EQ 10MG BASE/ML	N062318 002	
	EQ 40MG BASE/ML	N062318 001	
WYETH AYERST	EQ 10MG BASE/ML	N062264 001	
	EQ 40MG BASE/ML	N062264 002	

GENTAMICIN SULFATE IN SODIUM CHLORIDE 0.9% IN PLASTIC CONTAINER

ABBOTT	EQ 1.2MG BASE/ML	N062588 001	JAN 06, 1986
	EQ 1.4MG BASE/ML	N062588 002	JAN 06, 1986
	EQ 1.6MG BASE/ML	N062588 003	JAN 06, 1986
	EQ 1.8MG BASE/ML	N062588 004	JAN 06, 1986
	EQ 2MG BASE/ML	N062588 005	JAN 06, 1986
	EQ 60MG BASE/100ML	N062588 006	JAN 06, 1986
	EQ 70MG BASE/100ML	N062588 007	JAN 06, 1986
	EQ 80MG BASE/100ML	N062588 008	JAN 06, 1986
	EQ 90MG BASE/100ML	N062588 009	JAN 06, 1986
	EQ 100MG BASE/100ML	N062588 010	JAN 06, 1986

U-GENCIN

PHARMACIA AND UPJOHN	EQ 10MG BASE/ML	N062248 001	
	EQ 40MG BASE/ML	N062248 002	

Injectable; Intrathecal

GARAMYCIN

SCHERING	EQ 2MG BASE/ML	N050505 001	

Ointment; Ophthalmic

GARAMYCIN

SCHERING	EQ 0.3% BASE	N050425 001	

GENTACIDIN

NOVARTIS	EQ 0.3% BASE	N062501 001	JUL 26, 1984

GENTAFAIR

PHARMAFAIR	EQ 3MG BASE/GM	N062443 001	MAY 26, 1983

Ointment; Topical

GARAMYCIN

SCHERING	EQ 0.1% BASE	N060463 001	

GENTAFAIR

PHARMAFAIR	EQ 0.1% BASE	N062444 001	

GENTAMICIN SULFATE *(continued)*

Ointment; Topical

GENTAFAIR

PHARMAFAIR			MAY 26, 1983

GENTAMICIN SULFATE

ALPHARMA	EQ 0.1% BASE	N062496 001	MAR 14, 1984
BAUSCH AND LOMB	EQ 0.1% BASE	N064054 001	APR 29, 1994
PHARMADERM	EQ 0.1% BASE	N062534 001	OCT 10, 1984

Solution/Drops; Ophthalmic

GENTAFAIR

PHARMAFAIR	EQ 0.3% BASE	N062440 001	MAY 03, 1983

GENTAMICIN SULFATE

ALCON UNIVERSAL	EQ 0.3% BASE	N062523 001	NOV 25, 1985
PACO	EQ 3MG BASE/ML	N062932 001	NOV 07, 1988

GENTIAN VIOLET

Tampon; Vaginal

GENAPAX

KEY PHARMS	5MG	N085017 001	

GLIPIZIDE

Tablet; Oral

GLUCOTROL

PFIZER	2.5MG	N017783 003	MAY 11, 1993

GLUCAGON HYDROCHLORIDE

Injectable; Injection

GLUCAGON

LILLY	EQ 1MG BASE/VIAL	N012122 001	
	EQ 10MG BASE/VIAL	N012122 002	
QUAD PHARMS	EQ 1MG BASE/VIAL	N071022 001	MAR 04, 1987
	EQ 10MG BASE/VIAL	N071023 001	MAR 04, 1987

GLUTETHIMIDE

Capsule; Oral

DORIDEN

AVENTIS	500MG	N009519 008	

Tablet; Oral

DORIDEN

AVENTIS	250MG	N009519 002	
	500MG	N009519 005	

GLUTETHIMIDE

CELLTECH PHARMS	500MG	N085171 001	
GENEVA PHARMS	500MG	N083234 002	
HALSEY	250MG	N089458 001	OCT 10, 1986

Discontinued Drug Products (continued)

GLUTETHIMIDE (continued)
Tablet; Oral
GLUTETHIMIDE
HALSEY
500MG — N089459 001 / OCT 10, 1986
LANNETT
250MG — N083475 001
500MG — N085571 001
500MG — N087297 001
VITARINE
500MG — N084362 001
WATSON LABS
500MG — N085763 001

GLYBURIDE
Tablet; Oral
GLYNASE
PHARMACIA AND UPJOHN
4.5MG *SEE ANNUAL PREFACE INTRODUCTION DISCONTINUED SECTION* — N020051 003 / SEP 24, 1993

GLYCINE
Solution; Irrigation
GLYCINE 1.5% IN PLASTIC CONTAINER
BAXTER HLTHCARE
1.5GM/100ML — N018522 001 / FEB 19, 1982

GLYCOPYRROLATE
Injectable; Injection
GLYCOPYRROLATE
ABBOTT
0.2MG/ML — N089393 001 / JUN 15, 1988
AM PHARM PARTNERS
0.2MG/ML — N088475 001 / JUN 12, 1984
GENSIA SICOR PHARMS
0.2MG/ML — N081169 001 / SEP 10, 1991
QUAD PHARMS
0.2MG/ML — N089397 001 / DEC 09, 1986
STERIS
0.2MG/ML — N086947 001 / JUN 24, 1983
ROBINUL
ROBINS AH
0.2MG/ML — N014764 001
Tablet; Oral
GLYCOPYRROLATE
WATSON LAB
1MG — N085562 001
2MG — N085563 001
WATSON LABS
1MG — N086902 001
2MG — N086178 001
2MG — N086900 001

GONADORELIN ACETATE
Injectable; Injection
LUTREPULSE KIT
FERRING
0.8MG/VIAL — N019687 001 / OCT 10, 1989
3.2MG/VIAL — N019687 002 / OCT 10, 1989

GONADORELIN HYDROCHLORIDE
Injectable; Injection
FACTREL
BAXTER HLTHCARE CORP
EQ 0.2MG BASE/VIAL — N018123 002 / SEP 30, 1982
EQ 0.5MG BASE/VIAL — N018123 003 / SEP 30, 1982

GONADOTROPIN, CHORIONIC
Injectable; Injection
A.P.L.
WYETH AYERST
5,000 UNITS/VIAL — N017055 001
10,000 UNITS/VIAL — N017055 002
20,000 UNITS/VIAL — N017055 003
CHORIONIC GONADOTROPIN
AM PHARM PARTNERS
5,000 UNITS/VIAL — N017067 001
15,000 UNITS/VIAL — N017067 004
20,000 UNITS/VIAL — N017067 003
BEL MAR
5,000 UNITS/VIAL — N017054 001
10,000 UNITS/VIAL — N017054 002
QUAD PHARMS
5,000 UNITS/VIAL — N089312 001
5,000 UNITS/VIAL — N089313 001 / DEC 04, 1986
10,000 UNITS/VIAL — N089314 001 / DEC 04, 1986
20,000 UNITS/VIAL — N089315 001 / DEC 04, 1986
— N089316 001 / DEC 04, 1986
STERIS
2,000 UNITS/VIAL — N017016 009 / DEC 27, 1984
2,000 UNITS/VIAL — N017016 011 / FEB 16, 1990
15,000 UNITS/VIAL — N017016 010 / FEB 15, 1985
20,000 UNITS/VIAL — N017016 004
FOLLUTEIN
BRISTOL MYERS SQUIBB
10,000 UNITS/VIAL — N017056 001

GRAMICIDIN; NEOMYCIN SULFATE; POLYMYXIN B SULFATE
Solution/Drops; Ophthalmic
NEO-POLYCIN
DOW PHARM
0.025MG/ML;EQ 1.75MG BASE/ML;10,000 UNITS/ML — N060427 001
NEOMYCIN AND POLYMYXIN B SULFATES AND GRAMICIDIN
STERIS
0.025MG/ML;EQ 1.75MG BASE/ML;10,000 UNITS/ML — N062788 001 / JUN 11, 1987
IPHARM
0.025MG/ML;EQ 1.75MG BASE/ML;10,000 UNITS/ML — N062818 001 / OCT 11, 1988

GRISEOFULVIN, ULTRAMICROCRYSTALLINE (continued)

Tablet; Oral

GRISACTIN ULTRA			
WYETH AYERST	250MG	N062178 002	
	330MG	N062438 002	NOV 17, 1983
ULTRAGRIS-165			
PLIVA	165MG	N062645 001	JUN 30, 1992
ULTRAGRIS-330			
PLIVA	330MG	N062646 001	JUN 30, 1992

GUANABENZ ACETATE

Tablet; Oral

WYTENSIN			
WYETH AYERST	EQ 4MG BASE	N018587 001	SEP 07, 1982
	EQ 8MG BASE	N018587 002	SEP 07, 1982
	EQ 16MG BASE	N018587 003	SEP 07, 1982

GUANADREL SULFATE

Tablet; Oral

HYLOREL			
PHARMACIA AND UPJOHN	10MG	N018104 001	DEC 29, 1982
	25MG	N018104 002	DEC 29, 1982

GUANETHIDINE MONOSULFATE

Tablet; Oral

GUANETHIDINE MONOSULFATE			
WATSON LAB	EQ 10MG SULFATE	N086113 001	MAR 26, 1985
	EQ 25MG SULFATE	N086114 001	MAR 26, 1985
ISMELIN			
NOVARTIS	EQ 10MG SULFATE	N012329 001	
	EQ 25MG SULFATE	N012329 002	

GUANETHIDINE MONOSULFATE; HYDROCHLOROTHIAZIDE

Tablet; Oral

ESIMIL		
NOVARTIS	10MG;25MG	N013553 001

GUANFACINE HYDROCHLORIDE

Tablet; Oral

TENEX			
ESP PHARMA	EQ 3MG BASE	N019032 003	NOV 07, 1988

Discontinued Drug Products (continued)

GRAMICIDIN; NEOMYCIN SULFATE; POLYMYXIN B SULFATE (continued)

Solution/Drops; Ophthalmic

NEOMYCIN SULFATE AND POLYMYXIN B SULFATE GRAMICIDIN			
PHARMAFAIR	0.025MG/ML;EQ 1.75MG BASE/ML;10,000 UNITS/ML	N062383 001	AUG 31, 1982

GRANISETRON HYDROCHLORIDE

Injectable; Injection

KYTRIL			
ROCHE	EQ 3MG BASE/ML	N020239 001	DEC 29, 1993

Solution; Oral

KYTRIL			
ROCHE	EQ 2MG BASE/10ML	N021238 001	JUN 27, 2001

Tablet; Oral

KYTRIL			
ROCHE	EQ 2MG BASE	N020305 002	JUN 15, 1998

GREPAFLOXACIN HYDROCHLORIDE

Tablet; Oral

RAXAR			
OTSUKA	EQ 200MG BASE	N020695 001	NOV 06, 1997
		N020695 002	MAY 14, 1998
	EQ 400MG BASE	N020695 003	MAY 14, 1998
	EQ 600MG BASE		

GRISEOFULVIN, MICROCRYSTALLINE

Capsule; Oral

GRISACTIN		
WYETH AYERST	125MG	N050051 002
	250MG	N050051 001

Suspension; Oral

GRIFULVIN V		
JOHNSON AND JOHNSON	125MG/5ML	N050448 001

Tablet; Oral

GRIFULVIN V		
J AND J	125MG	N060618 001
	250MG	N060618 002
	500MG	N060618 003
GRISACTIN		
WYETH AYERST	500MG	N060212 001

GRISEOFULVIN, ULTRAMICROCRYSTALLINE

Tablet; Oral

GRISACTIN ULTRA			
WYETH AYERST	125MG	N062178 001	
	165MG	N062438 001	NOV 17, 1983

Discontinued Drug Products (continued)

HALCINONIDE
Cream; Topical

Product / Firm	Strength	Appl. No.	Date
HALOG — WESTWOOD SQUIBB	0.025%	N017818 001	

Ointment; Topical

Product / Firm	Strength	Appl. No.	Date
HALOG — BRISTOL MYERS SQUIBB	0.025%	N018125 001	

HALOFANTRINE HYDROCHLORIDE
Tablet; Oral

Product / Firm	Strength	Appl. No.	Date
HALFAN — GLAXOSMITHKLINE	250MG	N020250 001	JUL 24, 1992

HALOPERIDOL
Tablet; Oral

HALDOL — ORTHO MCNEIL

Strength	Appl. No.	Date
0.5MG	N015921 001	
1MG	N015921 002	
2MG	N015921 003	
5MG	N015921 004	
10MG	N015921 005	
20MG	N015921 006	FEB 02, 1982

HALDOL SOLUTAB — ORTHO MCNEIL PHARM

Strength	Appl. No.	Date
1MG	N017079 001	

HALOPERIDOL — DURAMED PHARM BARR

Strength	Appl. No.	Date
0.5MG	N071216 001	DEC 04, 1986
1MG	N071217 001	DEC 04, 1986
2MG	N071218 001	DEC 04, 1986
5MG	N071219 001	DEC 04, 1986
10MG	N071220 001	
20MG	N071221 001	JUL 07, 1987

HALSEY

Strength	Appl. No.	Date
0.5MG	N071156 001	
1MG	N071157 001	JAN 02, 1987
2MG	N071172 001	JAN 02, 1987
5MG	N071212 001	
10MG	N071173 001	JAN 07, 1988
20MG	N071177 001	

LEDERLE

Strength	Appl. No.	Date
0.5MG	N072727 001	SEP 19, 1989
1MG	N072728 001	SEP 19, 1989

HALOPERIDOL (continued)
Tablet; Oral

HALOPERIDOL — LEDERLE

Strength	Appl. No.	Date
2MG	N072729 001	SEP 19, 1989
5MG	N072730 001	SEP 19, 1989
10MG	N072731 001	SEP 19, 1989
20MG	N072732 001	SEP 19, 1989

PAR PHARM

Strength	Appl. No.	Date
20MG	N071328 001	JUL 20, 1987

PUREPAC PHARM

Strength	Appl. No.	Date
0.5MG	N071071 001	NOV 03, 1986
1MG	N071072 001	NOV 03, 1986
2MG	N071073 001	NOV 03, 1986
5MG	N071074 001	NOV 03, 1986
10MG	N071075 001	AUG 04, 1987
20MG	N071076 001	AUG 04, 1987

QUANTUM PHARMICS

Strength	Appl. No.	Date
0.5MG	N071255 001	FEB 17, 1987
1MG	N071269 001	FEB 17, 1987
2MG	N071256 001	FEB 17, 1987
5MG	N071257 001	FEB 17, 1987

ROXANE

Strength	Appl. No.	Date
0.5MG	N071128 001	FEB 17, 1987
1MG	N071129 001	FEB 17, 1987
2MG	N071130 001	FEB 17, 1987
5MG	N071131 001	FEB 17, 1987
10MG	N071132 001	FEB 17, 1987
20MG	N071133 001	MAY 12, 1987

ROYCE LABS

Strength	Appl. No.	Date
0.5MG	N071722 001	MAY 12, 1987
1MG	N071723 001	DEC 24, 1987
2MG	N071724 001	DEC 24, 1987
5MG	N071725 001	DEC 24, 1987
10MG	N072121 001	DEC 24, 1987
20MG	N072122 001	DEC 24, 1987

Discontinued Drug Products (continued)

HALOPERIDOL (continued)
Tablet; Oral

HALOPERIDOL	Strength	Appl. No.	Date
SCS	0.5MG	N070720 001	JUN 10, 1986
	1MG	N070721 001	JUN 10, 1986
	2MG	N070722 001	JUN 10, 1986
	5MG	N070723 001	JUN 10, 1986
	10MG	N070724 001	JUN 10, 1986
	20MG	N070725 001	SEP 24, 1986
WATSON LAB	0.5MG	N071571 001	JUN 03, 1988
	1MG	N071572 001	JUN 03, 1988
	2MG	N071573 001	JUN 03, 1988
	5MG	N071374 001	JUN 03, 1988
	10MG	N071375 001	JUN 03, 1988
	20MG	N071376 001	JUN 03, 1988
WATSON LABS	1MG	N070982 001	MAR 06, 1987
	10MG	N072113 001	AUG 27, 1991
	20MG	N072353 001	AUG 27, 1991

HALOPERIDOL DECANOATE
Injectable; Injection

HALOPERIDOL DECANOATE	Strength	Appl. No.	Date
KING PHARMS	EQ 50MG BASE/ML	N075176 001	FEB 09, 2000
	EQ 100MG BASE/ML	N075176 002	FEB 09, 2000

HALOPERIDOL LACTATE
Concentrate; Oral

	Strength	Appl. No.	Date
HALDOL			
ORTHO MCNEIL	EQ 2MG BASE/ML	N015922 001	
HALOPERIDOL			
ALPHARMA	EQ 2MG BASE/ML	N070318 001	APR 11, 1986
MORTON GROVE	EQ 2MG BASE/ML	N070710 001	MAR 07, 1986
SCS	EQ 2MG BASE/ML	N070726 001	JUN 10, 1986
HALOPERIDOL INTENSOL			
ROXANE	EQ 2MG BASE/ML	N072045 001	APR 12, 1988

HALOPERIDOL LACTATE (continued)
Injectable; Injection

HALOPERIDOL	Strength	Appl. No.	Date
AM PHARM PARTNERS	EQ 5MG BASE/ML	N071187 001	JAN 20, 1987
MARSAM PHARMS LLC	EQ 5MG BASE/ML	N072516 001	FEB 25, 1993
	EQ 5MG BASE/ML	N072517 001	FEB 25, 1993
QUAD PHARMS	EQ 5MG BASE/ML	N071082 001	JAN 02, 1987
SMITH AND NEPHEW	EQ 5MG BASE/ML	N070802 001	DEC 14, 1987
SOLOPAK	EQ 5MG BASE/ML	N070800 001	DEC 14, 1987
	EQ 5MG BASE/ML	N070801 001	DEC 14, 1987
	EQ 5MG BASE/ML	N070864 001	DEC 14, 1987
STERIS	EQ 5MG BASE/ML	N070713 001	DEC 14, 1987
	EQ 5MG BASE/ML	N070744 001	MAY 17, 1988
	EQ 5MG BASE/ML		MAY 17, 1988

HALOPROGIN
Cream; Topical

HALOTEX	Strength	Appl. No.
WESTWOOD SQUIBB	1%	N016942 001

Solution; Topical

HALOTEX	Strength	Appl. No.
WESTWOOD SQUIBB	1%	N016943 001

HALOTHANE
Liquid; Inhalation

	Strength	Appl. No.
FLUOTHANE		
WYETH AYERST	99.99%	N011338 001
HALOTHANE		
BH	99.99%	N084977 001

HEPARIN CALCIUM
Injectable; Injection

CALCIPARINE	Strength	Appl. No.
SANOFI SYNTHELABO	25,000 UNITS/ML	N018237 001

HEPARIN SODIUM
Injectable; Injection

	Strength	Appl. No.	Date
HEP FLUSH KIT IN PLASTIC CONTAINER			
AM PHARM PARTNERS	10 UNITS/ML	N017029 017	DEC 05, 1985
	100 UNITS/ML	N017029 018	DEC 05, 1985
HEPARIN LOCK FLUSH			
ABBOTT	100 UNITS/ML	N005264 010	
AM PHARM PARTNERS	100 UNITS/ML	N017651 010	

Discontinued Drug Products (continued)

HEPARIN SODIUM (continued)
Injectable; Injection

HEPARIN LOCK FLUSH

BAXTER HLTHCARE CORP
- 10 UNITS/ML — N017007 008

INTL MEDICATION
- 100 UNITS/ML — N017007 009
- 100 UNITS/ML — N086357 001
- 500 UNITS/ML — N086357 002

LUITPOLD
- 10 UNITS/ML — N089063 001 — OCT 09, 1985
- 100 UNITS/ML — N089064 001 — OCT 09, 1985

PARKE DAVIS
- 10 UNITS/ML — N017346 006

SMITH AND NEPHEW
- 10 UNITS/ML — N087904 001 — APR 20, 1983
- 10 UNITS/ML — N087958 001 — APR 20, 1983
- 10 UNITS/ML — N088458 001 — JUL 26, 1984
- 10 UNITS/ML — N088580 001 — OCT 25, 1984
- 100 UNITS/ML — N087906 001 — APR 20, 1983
- 100 UNITS/ML — N087959 001 — APR 20, 1983
- 100 UNITS/ML — N088460 001 — APR 20, 1983
- 100 UNITS/ML — N088581 001 — JUL 26, 1984

SOLOPAK
- 10 UNITS/ML — N087903 001 — OCT 25, 1984
- 10 UNITS/ML — N088457 001 — APR 20, 1983
- 100 UNITS/ML — N087905 001 — OCT 25, 1984
- 100 UNITS/ML — N088459 001 — APR 20, 1983

STERIS
- 100 UNITS/ML — N017064 001 — JUL 26, 1984

HEPARIN LOCK FLUSH PRESERVATIVE FREE

AM PHARM PARTNERS
- 10 UNITS/ML — N017029 011 — SEP 22, 1987
- 100 UNITS/ML — N017029 012 — SEP 22, 1987

HEPARIN LOCK FLUSH PRESERVATIVE FREE IN PLASTIC CONTAINER

AM PHARM PARTNERS
- 10 UNITS/ML — N017029 008 — SEP 22, 1987
- 100 UNITS/ML — N017029 009 — SEP 22, 1987

HEPARIN SODIUM

ABBOTT
- 10,000 UNITS/ML — N040095 001 — JUL 26, 1996

AKORN
- 1,000 UNITS/ML — N017486 001
- 5,000 UNITS/ML — N017486 002
- 10,000 UNITS/ML — N017486 003
- 20,000 UNITS/ML — N017486 004
- 40,000 UNITS/ML — N017486 005

AM PHARM PARTNERS
- 1,000 UNITS/ML — N017033 001

HEPARIN SODIUM (continued)
Injectable; Injection

HEPARIN SODIUM

AM PHARM PARTNERS
- 1,000 UNITS/ML — N017651 005
- 5,000 UNITS/ML — N017029 002
- 5,000 UNITS/ML — N017979 003
- 10,000 UNITS/ML — N017651 003
- 20,000 UNITS/ML — N017651 008

BAXTER HLTHCARE CORP
- 1,000 UNITS/ML — N017007 001
- 2,500 UNITS/ML — N017007 007
- 5,000 UNITS/0.5ML — N017007 010
- 5,000 UNITS/ML — N017007 002
- 7,500 UNITS/ML — N017007 003
- 10,000 UNITS/ML — N017007 004
- 15,000 UNITS/ML — N017007 005
- 20,000 UNITS/ML — N017007 006

CHAMBERLIN PARENTERL
- 1,000 UNITS/ML — N017130 001
- 5,000 UNITS/ML — N017130 002
- 10,000 UNITS/ML — N017130 003
- 20,000 UNITS/ML — N017130 004

DELL LABS
- 1,000 UNITS/ML — N017540 001
- 5,000 UNITS/ML — N017540 002
- 10,000 UNITS/ML — N017540 003
- 20,000 UNITS/ML — N017540 004
- 40,000 UNITS/ML — N017540 005

LILLY
- 1,000 UNITS/ML — N005521 001
- 20,000 UNITS/ML — N005521 004

LUITPOLD
- 1,000 UNITS/ML — N087452 001 — OCT 31, 1983

ORGANON USA INC
- 1,000 UNITS/ML — N000552 008
- 5,000 UNITS/ML — N000552 009
- 10,000 UNITS/ML — N000552 010

PARKE DAVIS
- 1,000 UNITS/ML — N017346 001
- 5,000 UNITS/ML — N017346 002
- 7,500 UNITS/ML — N017346 003
- 10,000 UNITS/ML — N017346 004
- 20,000 UNITS/ML — N017346 005

PHARM SPEC
- 1,000 UNITS/ML — N017780 001
- 5,000 UNITS/ML — N017780 002
- 10,000 UNITS/ML — N017780 003
- 20,000 UNITS/ML — N017780 004
- 40,000 UNITS/ML — N017780 005

SMITH AND NEPHEW
- 1,000 UNITS/ML — N088239 001 — JUL 26, 1984

SOLOPAK
- 1,000 UNITS/ML — N087043 001
- 5,000 UNITS/0.5ML — N087363 001
- 10,000 UNITS/0.5ML — N087395 001
- 10,000 UNITS/ML — N087077 001

STERIS
- 1,000 UNITS/ML — N087107 001
- 2,500 UNITS/ML — N017064 015
- 3,000 UNITS/ML — N017064 016
- 4,000 UNITS/ML — N017064 017
- 5,000 UNITS/ML — N017064 003
- 6,000 UNITS/ML — N017064 018

Discontinued Drug Products (continued)

HEPARIN SODIUM (continued)
Injectable; Injection

HEPARIN SODIUM
  STERIS
    7,500 UNITS/ML N017064 019
    10,000 UNITS/ML N017064 004
    20,000 UNITS/ML N017064 005
    40,000 UNITS/ML N017064 006

HEPARIN SODIUM 1,000 UNITS IN DEXTROSE 5% IN PLASTIC CONTAINER
  MCGAW
    200 UNITS/100ML .... N019130 001   DEC 31, 1984

HEPARIN SODIUM 1,000 UNITS IN SODIUM CHLORIDE 0.9% IN PLASTIC CONTAINER
  B BRAUN
    200 UNITS/100ML .... N019042 001   MAR 29, 1985

HEPARIN SODIUM 2,000 UNITS IN DEXTROSE 5% IN PLASTIC CONTAINER
  MCGAW
    200 UNITS/100ML .... N019130 003   DEC 31, 1984

HEPARIN SODIUM 2,000 UNITS IN SODIUM CHLORIDE 0.9% IN PLASTIC CONTAINER
  B BRAUN
    200 UNITS/100ML .... N019042 002   MAR 29, 1985

HEPARIN SODIUM 5,000 UNITS AND SODIUM CHLORIDE 0.9% IN PLASTIC CONTAINER
  BAXTER HLTHCARE
    500 UNITS/100ML .... N018609 003   APR 28, 1982

HEPARIN SODIUM 5,000 UNITS IN DEXTROSE 5% IN PLASTIC CONTAINER
  MCGAW
    1,000 UNITS/100ML .... N019130 002   DEC 31, 1984

HEPARIN SODIUM 5,000 UNITS IN SODIUM CHLORIDE 0.9%
  ABBOTT
    1,000 UNITS/100ML .... N018916 001   JAN 31, 1984

HEPARIN SODIUM 5,000 UNITS IN SODIUM CHLORIDE 0.9% IN PLASTIC CONTAINER
  B BRAUN
    1,000 UNITS/100ML .... N019042 004   MAR 29, 1985

HEPARIN SODIUM 5,000 UNITS IN SODIUM CHLORIDE 0.45%
  ABBOTT
    100 UNITS/ML .... N018911 002   JAN 30, 1985
    100 UNITS/ML .... N018916 004   JAN 31, 1984

HEPARIN SODIUM 10,000 UNITS IN DEXTROSE 5%
  ABBOTT
    10,000 UNITS/100ML .... N018911 006   JAN 30, 1985

HEPARIN SODIUM 10,000 UNITS IN DEXTROSE 5% IN PLASTIC CONTAINER
  BAXTER HLTHCARE
    2,000 UNITS/100ML .... N018814 002   JUL 09, 1985

HEPARIN SODIUM 10,000 UNITS IN SODIUM CHLORIDE 0.9%
  ABBOTT
    10,000 UNITS/100ML .... N018911 003   JAN 30, 1985
    10,000 UNITS/100ML .... N018916 002   JAN 31, 1984

HEPARIN SODIUM (continued)
Injectable; Injection

HEPARIN SODIUM 10,000 UNITS IN SODIUM CHLORIDE 0.45%
  ABBOTT
    10,000 UNITS/100ML .... N018911 001   JAN 30, 1985
    10,000 UNITS/100ML .... N018916 005   JAN 31, 1984

HEPARIN SODIUM 12,500 UNITS IN DEXTROSE 5%
  ABBOTT
    5,000 UNITS/100ML .... N018911 007   JAN 30, 1985

HEPARIN SODIUM 12,500 UNITS IN SODIUM CHLORIDE 0.9%
  ABBOTT
    5,000 UNITS/100ML .... N018911 005   JAN 30, 1985
    5,000 UNITS/100ML .... N018916 003   JAN 31, 1984

HEPARIN SODIUM 12,500 UNITS IN SODIUM CHLORIDE 0.45% IN PLASTIC CONTAINER
  B BRAUN
    5,000 UNITS/100ML .... N019802 001   JUL 20, 1992

HEPARIN SODIUM 25,000 UNITS IN DEXTROSE 5%
  ABBOTT
    10,000 UNITS/100ML .... N018911 008   JAN 30, 1985
    5,000 UNITS/100ML .... N018911 009   JAN 30, 1985

HEPARIN SODIUM 25,000 UNITS IN DEXTROSE 5% IN PLASTIC CONTAINER
  B BRAUN
    5,000 UNITS/100ML .... N019134 001   MAR 29, 1985

HEPARIN SODIUM 25,000 UNITS IN SODIUM CHLORIDE 0.9%
  ABBOTT
    5,000 UNITS/100ML .... N018911 004   JAN 30, 1985

HEPARIN SODIUM 25,000 UNITS IN SODIUM CHLORIDE 0.9% IN PLASTIC CONTAINER
  ABBOTT
    5,000 UNITS/100ML .... N018916 009   JAN 31, 1984
                               N019135 001   MAR 29, 1985
  B BRAUN
    5,000 UNITS/100ML .... N019802 003   JUL 20, 1992

HEPARIN SODIUM 25,000 UNITS IN SODIUM CHLORIDE 0.45% IN PLASTIC CONTAINER
  B BRAUN
    10,000 UNITS/100ML .... N019802 002   JUL 20, 1992
    5,000 UNITS/100ML .... N019802 005   JUL 20, 1992

HEPARIN SODIUM PRESERVATIVE FREE
  PHARMA SERVE NY
    1,000 UNITS/ML N086129 001

LIPO-HEPIN
  3M
    1,000 UNITS/0.5ML N017027 001
    1,000 UNITS/ML N017027 006
    5,000 UNITS/0.5ML N017027 002
    5,000 UNITS/ML N017027 008
    7,500 UNITS/0.5ML N017027 010
    10,000 UNITS/0.5ML N017027 003
    10,000 UNITS/ML N017027 009

Discontinued Drug Products (continued)

HEPARIN SODIUM (continued)
Injectable; Injection
LIPO-HEPIN
  3M
  - 15,000 UNITS/0.5ML — N017027 011
  - 20,000 UNITS/0.5ML — N017027 004
  - 20,000 UNITS/ML — N017027 007
  - 40,000 UNITS/ML — N017027 005
LIQUAEMIN LOCK FLUSH
  ORGANON USA INC
  - 100 UNITS/ML — N000552 007
LIQUAEMIN SODIUM
  ORGANON USA INC
  - 1,000 UNITS/ML — N000552 004
  - 5,000 UNITS/ML — N000552 003
  - 10,000 UNITS/ML — N000552 005
  - 20,000 UNITS/ML — N000552 001
  - 40,000 UNITS/ML — N000552 002
LIQUAEMIN SODIUM PRESERVATIVE FREE
  ORGANON USA INC
  - 1,000 UNITS/ML — N000552 011 — APR 11, 1986
  - 5,000 UNITS/ML — N000552 012 — APR 11, 1986
  - 10,000 UNITS/ML — N000552 013 — APR 11, 1986
PANHEPRIN
  ABBOTT
  - 1,000 UNITS/ML — N005264 004
  - 5,000 UNITS/ML — N005264 006
  - 10,000 UNITS/ML — N005264 007
  - 20,000 UNITS/ML — N005264 008
  - 40,000 UNITS/ML — N005264 009
SODIUM HEPARIN
  AM PHARM PARTNERS
  - 5,000 UNITS/ML — N017033 002
  - 10,000 UNITS/ML — N017033 003
  - 20,000 UNITS/ML — N017033 004

HEPARIN SODIUM *MULTIPLE*
SEE DIHYDROERGOTAMINE MESYLATE; HEPARIN SODIUM; LIDOCAINE HYDROCHLORIDE

HETACILLIN
For Suspension; Oral
VERSAPEN
  BRISTOL
  - EQ 112.5MG AMPICIL/5ML — N050060 001
  - EQ 112.5MG AMPICIL/ML — N050060 003
  - EQ 112.5MG AMPICIL/ML — N061398 001
  - EQ 225MG AMPICIL/5ML — N061398 002

HETACILLIN POTASSIUM
Capsule; Oral
VERSAPEN-K
  BRISTOL
  - EQ 225MG AMPICIL — N061396 001
  - EQ 450MG AMPICIL — N061396 002

HEXACHLOROPHENE
Aerosol; Topical
SEPTISOL
  VESTAL LABS — 0.23% — N017424 001

HEXACHLOROPHENE (continued)
Aerosol; Topical
TURGEX
  XTTRIUM — 3% — N018375 001
Emulsion; Topical
HEXA-GERM
  HUNTINGTON LABS — 3% — N017411 001
PHISOHEX
  SANOFI SYNTHELABO — 3% — N008402 001
SOY-DOME
  BAYER PHARMS — 3% — N017405 001
TURGEX
  XTTRIUM — 3% — N019055 001 — NOV 30, 1984
Soap; Topical
GAMOPHEN
  ARBROOK — 2% — N006270 003
Solution; Topical
DIAL
  DIAL — 0.25% — N017421 002
GERMA-MEDICA
  HUNTINGTON LABS — 1% — N017412 001
GERMA-MEDICA "MG"
  HUNTINGTON LABS — 0.25% — N017412 002
SEPTI-SOFT
  CALGON — 0.25% — N017460 001
SEPTISOL
  VESTAL LABS — 0.25% — N017423 001
Sponge; Topical
E-Z SCRUB
  BECTON DICKINSON — 450MG — N017452 001
HEXASCRUB
  PROF DSPLS — 3% — N018363 001
PHISO-SCRUB
  SANOFI SYNTHELABO — 3% — N017446 001
SCRUBTEAM SURGICAL SPONGEBRUSH
  3M — 330MG — N017413 001

HEXAFLUORENIUM BROMIDE
Injectable; Injection
MYLAXEN
  MEDPOINTE PHARM HLC — 20MG/ML — N009789 003

HEXOCYCLIUM METHYLSULFATE
Tablet; Oral
TRAL
  ABBOTT — 25MG — N010599 001

HEXYLCAINE HYDROCHLORIDE
Solution; Topical
CYCLAINE
  MERCK — 5% — N008472 001

Discontinued Drug Products *(continued)*

HISTAMINE PHOSPHATE
Injectable; Injection
HISTAMINE PHOSPHATE

LILLY	EQ 0.1MG BASE/ML	N000734 003
	EQ 0.2MG BASE/ML	N000734 002
	EQ 1MG BASE/ML	N000734 001

HISTRELIN ACETATE
Injectable; Injection
SUPPRELIN

SHIRE LABS	EQ 0.2MG BASE/ML	N019836 001	DEC 24, 1991
	EQ 0.5MG BASE/ML	N019836 002	DEC 24, 1991
	EQ 1MG BASE/ML	N019836 003	DEC 24, 1991

HOMATROPINE METHYLBROMIDE
Tablet, Chewable; Oral
EQUIPIN

MISSION PHARMA	3MG	N086310 001

Tablet; Oral
HOMAPIN-5

MISSION PHARMA	5MG	N086309 001

HOMAPIN-10

MISSION PHARMA	10MG	N086308 001

HOMATROPINE METHYLBROMIDE; HYDROCODONE BITARTRATE
Syrup; Oral
HYDROPANE

HALSEY	1.5MG/5ML;5MG/5ML	N088066 001	JUN 28, 1985

HYALURONIDASE
Injectable; Injection
WYDASE

WYETH AYERST	1,500 UNITS/VIAL	N006343 005
	150 UNITS/ML	N006343 002
	150 UNITS/VIAL	N006343 006

HYDRALAZINE HYDROCHLORIDE
Injectable; Injection
APRESOLINE

NOVARTIS	20MG/ML	N008303 003

HYDRALAZINE HCL

AM PHARM PARTNERS	20MG/ML	N089532 001	AUG 11, 1987
		N088518 001	
SMITH AND NEPHEW	20MG/ML	N088517 001	APR 20, 1984
SOLOPAK	20MG/ML		AUG 22, 1985

Tablet; Oral
DRALZINE

TEVA	25MG	N084301 001

HYDRALAZINE HYDROCHLORIDE *(continued)*
Tablet; Oral
HYDRALAZINE HCL

AMIDE PHARM	25MG	N088560 001	OCT 04, 1984
	50MG	N088649 001	OCT 18, 1984
ASCOT	25MG	N088310 001	DEC 19, 1984
	50MG	N088311 001	DEC 19, 1984
EON	50MG	N085088 001	
HALSEY	10MG	N088728 001	APR 11, 1985
	10MG	N089218 001	
	25MG	N084106 002	JAN 22, 1986
	25MG	N089130 001	
	50MG	N084107 002	JAN 15, 1986
	50MG	N089222 001	
	100MG	N088729 001	JAN 22, 1986
	100MG	N089178 001	APR 11, 1985
IMPAX LABS	25MG	N084922 001	JAN 15, 1986
IVAX PHARMS	10MG	N084443 001	
	25MG	N084437 001	
	50MG	N084469 002	
	100MG	N084581 001	
PUREPAC PHARM	25MG	N088177 001	JUL 29, 1983
	50MG	N088178 001	AUG 15, 1983
QUANTUM PHARMICS	10MG	N088671 001	MAY 01, 1984
	25MG	N088657 001	JUN 15, 1984
	50MG	N088652 001	MAY 08, 1984
	100MG	N088686 001	MAY 01, 1984
SUPERPHARM	10MG	N088787 001	AUG 28, 1984
	25MG	N088788 001	AUG 28, 1984
	50MG	N088789 001	AUG 28, 1984
USL PHARMA	25MG	N087780 001	MAR 29, 1982
	50MG	N087751 001	MAR 29, 1982
VANGARD	25MG	N087712 001	
	50MG	N087908 001	MAY 07, 1982
VITARINE	25MG	N086088 001	

Discontinued Drug Products (continued)

HYDRALAZINE HYDROCHLORIDE (continued)
Tablet; Oral

HYDRALAZINE HCL

Manufacturer	Strength	Appl. No.	Date
WATSON LABS	25MG	N085532 002	MAY 24, 1982
	50MG	N085533 002	MAY 25, 1982
WEST WARD	25MG	N088240 001	MAY 27, 1983
	50MG	N088241 001	MAY 27, 1983

HYDRALAZINE HYDROCHLORIDE; HYDROCHLOROTHIAZIDE
Capsule; Oral

APRESAZIDE

Manufacturer	Strength	Appl. No.	Date
NOVARTIS	100MG;50MG	N084811 001	

HYDRALAZINE HCL AND HYDROCHLOROTHIAZIDE

Manufacturer	Strength	Appl. No.	Date
SOLVAY	50MG;50MG	N087213 001	FEB 08, 1982
	25MG;25MG	N087608 001	FEB 08, 1982
	100MG;50MG	N087609 001	FEB 08, 1982
SUPERPHARM	25MG;25MG	N089200 001	FEB 09, 1987
WATSON LAB	100MG;50MG	N085440 001	MAR 04, 1982
	50MG;50MG	N085446 001	MAR 04, 1982
	25MG;25MG	N085457 001	MAR 04, 1982

HYDRALAZINE HCL W/ HYDROCHLOROTHIAZIDE 25/25

Manufacturer	Strength	Appl. No.	Date
IVAX PHARMS	25MG;25MG	N088356 001	APR 10, 1984

HYDRALAZINE HCL W/ HYDROCHLOROTHIAZIDE 50/50

Manufacturer	Strength	Appl. No.	Date
IVAX PHARMS	50MG;50MG	N088357 001	APR 10, 1984

HYDRALAZINE HCL W/ HYDROCHLOROTHIAZIDE 100/50

Manufacturer	Strength	Appl. No.	Date
IVAX PHARMS	100MG;50MG	N088358 001	APR 10, 1984

Tablet; Oral

APRESOLINE-ESIDRIX

Manufacturer	Strength	Appl. No.
NOVARTIS	25MG;15MG	N012026 002

HYDRALAZINE AND HYDROCHLORTHIAZIDE

Manufacturer	Strength	Appl. No.
WATSON LABS	25MG;15MG	N085827 001

HYDROCHLOROTHIAZIDE W/ HYDRALAZINE

Manufacturer	Strength	Appl. No.
WATSON LAB	25MG;15MG	N085373 001

HYDRALAZINE HYDROCHLORIDE; HYDROCHLOROTHIAZIDE; RESERPINE
Tablet; Oral

CAM-AP-ES

Manufacturer	Strength	Appl. No.
ABC HOLDING	25MG;15MG;0.1MG	N084897 001

HYDRALAZINE HCL, HYDROCHLOROTHIAZIDE AND RESERPINE

Manufacturer	Strength	Appl. No.
IVAX PHARMS	25MG;15MG;0.1MG	N084291 001

HYDRALAZINE HYDROCHLORIDE; HYDROCHLOROTHIAZIDE; RESERPINE (continued)
Tablet; Oral

HYDRALAZINE HCL-HYDROCHLOROTHIAZIDE-RESERPINE

Manufacturer	Strength	Appl. No.
MYLAN	25MG;15MG;0.1MG	N087085 001

HYDRALAZINE, HYDROCHLOROTHIAZIDE W/ RESERPINE

Manufacturer	Strength	Appl. No.
WATSON LABS	25MG;15MG;0.1MG	N085771 001

HYDRAP-ES

Manufacturer	Strength	Appl. No.
EON	25MG;15MG;0.1MG	N084876 001

HYDROCHLOROTHIAZIDE W/ RESERPINE AND HYDRALAZINE

Manufacturer	Strength	Appl. No.
WATSON LAB	25MG;15MG;0.1MG	N083770 001

HYDROSERPINE PLUS (R-H-H)

Manufacturer	Strength	Appl. No.
IVAX PHARMS	25MG;15MG;0.1MG	N083877 001

RESERPINE, HYDRALAZINE HCL AND HYDROCHLOROTHIAZIDE

Manufacturer	Strength	Appl. No.	Date
WATSON LABS	25MG;15MG;0.1MG	N085549 001	
	25MG;15MG;0.1MG	N087556 001	
	25MG;15MG;0.1MG	N088376 001	OCT 28, 1983
SOLVAY	25MG;15MG;0.1MG	N088570 001	APR 10, 1984
HALSEY	25MG;15MG;0.1MG	N087709 001	MAY 13, 1982

RESERPINE, HYDROCHLOROTHIAZIDE, AND HYDRALAZINE HCL

Manufacturer	Strength	Appl. No.
LEDERLE	25MG;15MG;0.1MG	N087210 001

SER-A-GEN

Manufacturer	Strength	Appl. No.
SOLVAY	25MG;15MG;0.1MG	N012193 005

SER-AP-ES

Manufacturer	Strength	Appl. No.
NOVARTIS	25MG;15MG;0.1MG	N085893 001
UNIPRES	25MG;15MG;0.1MG	N086298 001
SOLVAY		

HYDRALAZINE HYDROCHLORIDE; RESERPINE
Tablet; Oral

DRALSERP

Manufacturer	Strength	Appl. No.
EON	25MG;0.1MG	N084617 001

SERPASIL-APRESOLINE

Manufacturer	Strength	Appl. No.
NOVARTIS	25MG;0.1MG	N009296 004
	50MG;0.2MG	N009296 002

HYDROCHLOROTHIAZIDE
Solution; Oral

HYDROCHLOROTHIAZIDE

Manufacturer	Strength	Appl. No.	Date
MORTON GROVE	50MG/5ML	N089661 001	JUN 20, 1988

HYDROCHLOROTHIAZIDE INTENSOL

Manufacturer	Strength	Appl. No.	Date
ROXANE	100MG/ML	N088588 001	JUL 02, 1984

Tablet; Oral

ESIDRIX

Manufacturer	Strength	Appl. No.
NOVARTIS	100MG	N011793 009

HYDRO-D

Manufacturer	Strength	Appl. No.
HALSEY	25MG	N086504 001
	50MG	N083891 002

Discontinued Drug Products *(continued)*

HYDROCHLOROTHIAZIDE *(continued)*
Tablet; Oral

HYDROCHLOROTHIAZIDE

Firm	Strength	Number
ALRA	25MG	N086369 001
	50MG	N083554 001
ASCOT	25MG	N087539 001 FEB 03, 1982
	50MG	N087540 001 FEB 03, 1982
BARR	50MG	N084771 001
CLONMEL HLTHCARE	100MG	N087060 001
ELKINS SINN	50MG	N085152 002
EON	25MG	N083899 001
HALSEY	25MG	N083972 002
	50MG	N083972 003
	100MG	N084135 001
HEATHER	50MG	N084029 001
IMPAX LABS	25MG	N083607 002
	50MG	N085098 001
	100MG	N084776 001
INWOOD LABS	25MG	N085067 001
	25MG	N084776 002
IVAX PHARMS	50MG	N084658 001
MAST MM	50MG	N086192 001
	50MG	N086192 002
MYLAN	25MG	N084880 001
	50MG	N085112 001
PHARMERAL	25MG	N084325 001
	50MG	N084324 001
PVT FORM	50MG	N086597 001
ROXANE	25MG	N085004 001
	50MG	N085005 001
SOLVAY	25MG	N085323 001
SUPERPHARM	25MG	N088827 001 DEC 28, 1984
	50MG	N088828 001 DEC 28, 1984
	100MG	N088829 001 DEC 28, 1984
TEVA	25MG	N088924 001 FEB 07, 1985
	50MG	N088923 001 FEB 07, 1985
USL PHARMA	25MG	N087827 001 APR 19, 1982
	50MG	N087752 001 APR 19, 1982
VANGARD	25MG	N087638 001
	50MG	N087610 001
WARNER CHILCOTT	25MG	N087586 001 MAY 03, 1982
	50MG	N087587 001 MAY 03, 1982
WATSON LAB	25MG	N083458 001
	50MG	N083456 001
	100MG	N085099 001

HYDROCHLOROTHIAZIDE *(continued)*
Tablet; Oral

HYDROCHLOROTHIAZIDE

Firm	Strength	Number
WATSON LABS	25MG	N085232 002
	50MG	N083232 001
	50MG	N085233 001
	50MG	N086087 001
	50MG	N086594 001
	100MG	N081190 001 JAN 24, 1992
WEST WARD	100MG	N087002 001
	25MG	N084899 001
	50MG	N084878 001
WHITEWORTH TOWN PLSN	25MG	N083809 002
	50MG	N083809 001
	100MG	N085347 001

HYDRODIURIL

Firm	Strength	Number
MERCK	25MG	N011835 003
	50MG	N011835 006
	100MG	N011835 007

ORETIC

Firm	Strength	Number
ABBOTT	25MG	N011971 001

ZIDE

Firm	Strength	Number
SOLVAY	50MG	N083925 001

HYDROCHLOROTHIAZIDE; IRBESARTAN
Tablet; Oral

AVALIDE

Firm	Strength	Number
SANOFI SYNTHELABO	12.5MG;75MG	N020758 001 SEP 30, 1997

HYDROCHLOROTHIAZIDE; LABETALOL HYDROCHLORIDE
Tablet; Oral

NORMOZIDE

Firm	Strength	Number
SCHERING	25MG;100MG	N019046 001 APR 06, 1987
	25MG;200MG	N019046 002 APR 06, 1987
	25MG;300MG	N019046 003 APR 06, 1987
	25MG;400MG	N019046 004 APR 06, 1987

TRANDATE HCT

Firm	Strength	Number
GLAXOSMITHKLINE	25MG;100MG	N019174 001 APR 10, 1987
	25MG;200MG	N019174 002 APR 10, 1987
	25MG;300MG	N019174 003 APR 10, 1987
	25MG;400MG	N019174 004 APR 10, 1987

Discontinued Drug Products *(continued)*

HYDROCHLOROTHIAZIDE; METHYLDOPA
Tablet; Oral

METHYLDOPA AND HYDROCHLOROTHIAZIDE

Manufacturer	Strength	NDC	Date
INVAMED	15MG;250MG	N070829 001	MAR 09, 1987
	25MG;250MG	N070830 001	MAR 09, 1987
IVAX PHARMS	15MG;250MG	N071458 001	MAR 08, 1988
	25MG;250MG	N071459 001	MAR 08, 1988
	30MG;500MG	N071460 001	MAR 08, 1988
	50MG;500MG	N071461 001	MAR 08, 1988
PARKE DAVIS	15MG;250MG	N071897 001	NOV 23, 1987
	25MG;250MG	N071898 001	NOV 23, 1987
	30MG;500MG	N071899 001	NOV 23, 1987
	50MG;500MG	N071900 001	NOV 23, 1987
PUREPAC PHARM	25MG;250MG	N070688 001	APR 24, 1986
	50MG;500MG	N070689 001	APR 24, 1986
	15MG;250MG	N070853 001	OCT 08, 1986
	30MG;500MG	N070854 001	OCT 08, 1986
TEVA	15MG;250MG	N071819 001	APR 08, 1988
	25MG;250MG	N071820 001	APR 08, 1988
	30MG;500MG	N071821 001	APR 08, 1988
	50MG;500MG	N071822 001	APR 08, 1988
WATSON LAB	15MG;250MG	N070365 001	MAR 19, 1986
	25MG;250MG	N070366 001	APR 16, 1986
	30MG;500MG	N070367 001	MAR 19, 1986
	50MG;500MG	N070368 001	APR 16, 1986
WATSON LABS	15MG;250MG	N071920 001	AUG 29, 1988
	25MG;250MG	N071921 001	AUG 29, 1988
	30MG;500MG	N071922 001	AUG 29, 1988
	50MG;500MG	N071923 001	AUG 29, 1988

HYDROCHLOROTHIAZIDE; PINDOLOL
Tablet; Oral

VISKAZIDE

Manufacturer	Strength	NDC	Date
NOVARTIS	25MG;5MG	N018872 001	JUL 22, 1987
	25MG;10MG	N018872 002	JUL 22, 1987

HYDROCHLOROTHIAZIDE; PROPRANOLOL HYDROCHLORIDE
Capsule, Extended Release; Oral

INDERIDE LA 80/50

Manufacturer	Strength	NDC	Date
WYETH AYERST	50MG;80MG	N019059 001	JUL 03, 1985

INDERIDE LA 120/50

Manufacturer	Strength	NDC	Date
WYETH AYERST	50MG;120MG	N019059 002	JUL 03, 1985

INDERIDE LA 160/50

Manufacturer	Strength	NDC	Date
WYETH AYERST	50MG;160MG	N019059 003	JUL 03, 1985

Tablet; Oral

PROPRANOLOL HCL HYDROCHLOROTHIAZIDE

Manufacturer	Strength	NDC	Date
DURAMED PHARM BARR	25MG;40MG	N071126 001	MAR 02, 1987
	25MG;80MG	N071127 001	MAR 02, 1987

PROPRANOLOL HCL AND HYDROCHLOROTHIAZIDE

Manufacturer	Strength	NDC	Date
IVAX PHARMS	25MG;40MG	N071552 001	DEC 01, 1988
	25MG;80MG	N071553 001	DEC 01, 1988
WARNER CHILCOTT	25MG;40MG	N071771 001	JAN 26, 1988
	25MG;80MG	N071772 001	JAN 26, 1988
WATSON LABS	25MG;40MG	N071498 001	DEC 18, 1991
	25MG;80MG	N071501 001	DEC 18, 1991

HYDROCHLOROTHIAZIDE; RESERPINE
Tablet; Oral

H.R.-50

Manufacturer	Strength	NDC	Date
WHITEWORTH TOWN PLSN	50MG;0.125MG	N085338 001	

HYDRO-RESERP

Manufacturer	Strength	NDC	Date
ABC HOLDING	50MG;0.125MG	N084714 002	JUN 29, 1982

HYDRO-SERP "25"

Manufacturer	Strength	NDC	Date
EON	25MG;0.125MG	N084827 001	

HYDRO-SERP "50"

Manufacturer	Strength	NDC	Date
EON	50MG;0.125MG	N085213 001	

HYDROCHLOROTHIAZIDE W/ RESERPINE

Manufacturer	Strength	NDC	Date
IVAX PHARMS	25MG;0.1MG	N083571 001	
	50MG;0.1MG	N083572 001	
		N083568 001	

Discontinued Drug Products (continued)

HYDROCHLOROTHIAZIDE; RESERPINE (continued)
Tablet; Oral
HYDROCHLOROTHIAZIDE W/ RESERPINE

IVAX PHARMS	50MG;0.125MG	N083573 001
PHARMERAL	25MG;0.125MG	N085421 001
	50MG;0.125MG	N085420 001
ROXANE	50MG;0.125MG	N084603 001
WATSON LAB	25MG;0.125MG	N085317 001
	50MG;0.125MG	N083666 001
WATSON LABS	25MG;0.125MG	N084466 001
	50MG;0.125MG	N086330 002
	25MG;0.125MG	N084467 001
	50MG;0.125MG	N086331 001

HYDROPRES 25
MERCK   25MG;0.125MG   N011958 002

HYDROPRES 50
MERCK   50MG;0.125MG   N011958 003

RESERPINE AND HYDROCHLOROTHIAZIDE

BARR	25MG;0.125MG	N084580 001
	50MG;0.125MG	N084579 001
	50MG;0.125MG	N088200 001
GENEVA PHARMS		JAN 31, 1984

RESERPINE AND HYDROCHLOROTHIAZIDE-50
WEST WARD   50MG;0.125MG   N088189 001
MAY 10, 1984

SERPASIL-ESIDRIX #1
NOVARTIS   25MG;0.1MG   N011878 003

SERPASIL-ESIDRIX #2
NOVARTIS   50MG;0.1MG   N011878 005

HYDROCHLOROTHIAZIDE; SPIRONOLACTONE
Tablet; Oral
SPIRONOLACTONE + HYDROCHLOROTHIAZIDE
ASCOT   25MG;25MG   N088025 001
NOV 23, 1984

SPIRONOLACTONE AND HYDROCHLOROTHIAZIDE
PUREPAC PHARM   25MG;25MG   N087999 001
NOV 06, 1985
SUPERPHARM   25MG;25MG   N089137 001
AUG 26, 1985

SPIRONOLACTONE W/ HYDROCHLOROTHIAZIDE

IVAX PHARMS	25MG;25MG	N087004 002 MAY 24, 1982
LEDERLE	25MG;25MG	N080054 001
PUREPAC PHARM	25MG;25MG	AUG 18, 1983
UPSHER SMITH	25MG;25MG	N087553 001
USL PHARMA	25MG;25MG	N087651 001
VANGARD	25MG;25MG	N087655 001
WATSON LAB	25MG;25MG	N085974 001
WATSON LABS	25MG;25MG	N086026 001

HYDROCHLOROTHIAZIDE; TRIAMTERENE
Capsule; Oral
DYAZIDE
GLAXOSMITHKLINE   25MG;50MG   N016042 002
TRIAMTERENE AND HYDROCHLOROTHIAZIDE
NOVARTIS   25MG;37.5MG   N074857 001   SEP 09, 1997
VITARINE   25MG;50MG   N071737 001   FEB 12, 1988
Tablet; Oral
TRIAMTERENE AND HYDROCHLOROTHIAZIDE
AM THERAP   50MG;75MG   N072022 001   APR 17, 1988
QUANTUM PHARMICS   50MG;75MG   N071980 001   APR 17, 1988

HYDROCHLOROTHIAZIDE *MULTIPLE*
SEE   BISOPROLOL FUMARATE; HYDROCHLOROTHIAZIDE
SEE   CAPTOPRIL; HYDROCHLOROTHIAZIDE
SEE   DESERPIDINE; HYDROCHLOROTHIAZIDE
SEE   GUANETHIDINE MONOSULFATE; HYDROCHLOROTHIAZIDE
SEE   HYDRALAZINE HYDROCHLORIDE; HYDROCHLOROTHIAZIDE
SEE   HYDRALAZINE HYDROCHLORIDE; HYDROCHLOROTHIAZIDE; RESERPINE

HYDROCODONE BITARTRATE; PHENYLPROPANOLAMINE HYDROCHLORIDE
Syrup; Oral
CODAMINE
ALPHARMA   5MG/5ML;25MG/5ML   N075103 001   SEP 29, 2000
HYCOMINE
ENDO PHARMS   5MG/5ML;25MG/5ML   N019410 001   AUG 17, 1990
HYCOMINE PEDIATRIC
ENDO PHARMS   2.5MG/5ML;12.5MG/5ML   N019411 001   AUG 17, 1990

HYDROCODONE BITARTRATE *MULTIPLE*
SEE   ACETAMINOPHEN; HYDROCODONE BITARTRATE
SEE   ASPIRIN; HYDROCODONE BITARTRATE
SEE   HOMATROPINE METHYLBROMIDE; HYDROCODONE BITARTRATE

HYDROCORTAMATE HYDROCHLORIDE
Ointment; Topical
MAGNACORT
PFIZER   0.5%   N010554 001

HYDROCORTISONE
Aerosol; Topical
AEROSEB-HC
ALLERGAN HERBERT   0.5%   N085805 001
Cream; Topical
CORT-DOME
BAYER PHARMS   0.5%   N009585 003

Discontinued Drug Products (continued)

HYDROCORTISONE (continued)

Cream; Topical

Product	Company	Strength	Number	Date
CORT-DOME	BAYER PHARMS	1%	N009585 001	
DERMACORT				
MONARCH PHARMS		1%	N083011 002	
ELDECORT	ICN	1%	N080459 001	
		2.5%	N084055 001	
FLEXICORT	WESTWOOD SQUIBB	0.5%	N087136 003	APR 08, 1982
		1%	N087136 002	APR 08, 1982
		2.5%	N087136 001	APR 08, 1982
H-CORT	PHARM ASSOC	0.5%	N086823 001	
HC #1	BAYER PHARMS	0.5%	N080438 001	
HC #4	BAYER PHARMS	1%	N080438 002	
HC (HYDROCORTISONE)	C AND M PHARMA	0.5%	N080482 003	
		1%	N080482 004	
HYDROCORTISONE	ALPHARMA	2.5%	N089754 001	FEB 01, 1989
	AMBIX	1%	N086080 001	
		2.5%	N086271 001	
	CLAY PARK	0.5%	N084970 002	
		1%	N085026 001	
	EVERYLIFE	0.5%	N080452 001	
	G AND W LABS	1%	N084059 001	
	IVAX PHARMS	1%	N085733 001	
	NASKA	1%	N089706 001	MAR 10, 1988
	PHARMADERM	1%	N088845 001	FEB 27, 1986
	PHARMAFAIR	1%	N087838 001	JUL 28, 1982
	STIEFEL	1%	N086170 001	
	TARO	0.5%	N086154 001	
	TEVA	0.5%	N080400 002	
		1%	N080400 003	
		1%	N085191 001	
		2.5%	N080400 004	
TOPIDERM		1%	N089273 001	FEB 17, 1989
USL PHARMA		1%	N088027 001	SEP 27, 1983
		2.5%	N088029 001	SEP 27, 1983
WHITEWORTH TOWN				
PLSN		1%	N080496 002	

HYDROCORTISONE (continued)

Cream; Topical

Product	Company	Strength	Number	Date
NOGENIC HC	IVAX PHARMS	1%	N087427 001	APR 04, 1988
NUTRACORT	HEALTHPOINT	0.5%	N080442 002	
		1%	N080442 003	
PROCTOCORT	MONARCH PHARMS	1%	N083011 001	
SYNACORT	MEDICIS	0.5%	N087459 001	

Gel; Topical

Product	Company	Strength	Number	Date
NUTRACORT	HEALTHPOINT	1%	N084698 001	
PENECORT	ALLERGAN HERBERT	1%	N088215 001	JUN 06, 1984

Injectable; Injection

Product	Company	Strength	Number
CORTEF	PHARMACIA AND UPJOHN	50MG/ML	N009864 001

Lotion; Topical

Product	Company	Strength	Number	Date
ACTICORT	BAKER NORTON	1%	N086535 001	
BALNEOL-HC	SOLVAY	1%	N088041 001	DEC 03, 1982
BETA-HC	BETA DERMAC	1%	N089495 001	JAN 25, 1988
CORT-DOME	BAYER PHARMS	0.5%	N009895 003	
		1%	N009895 001	
DERMACORT	SOLVAY	0.5%	N084573 002	
		1%	N086462 001	
GLYCORT	HERAN	1%	N087489 001	OCT 03, 1983
H-CORT	PHARM ASSOC	0.5%	N086824 001	
HYDROCORTISONE	ALPHARMA	0.5%	N087317 001	JUN 07, 1982
		1%	N087315 001	JUN 07, 1982
	CLAY PARK	0.5%	N085662 001	
		1%	N085663 001	
	MERICON	0.5%	N085282 001	
		1%	N085282 002	FEB 26, 1987
	NASKA	1%	N089705 001	APR 25, 1988
	TARO	1%	N089024 001	

Discontinued Drug Products (continued)

HYDROCORTISONE (continued)

Lotion; Topical

HYDROCORTISONE
- TARO — FEB 12, 1986

NUTRACORT
- HEALTHPOINT — 0.5% — N080443 002

Ointment; Topical

HC (HYDROCORTISONE)
- C AND M PHARMA — 0.5% — N080481 001
- 1% — N080481 002

HYDROCORTISONE
- ALTANA — 0.5% — N080489 002
- AMBIX — 1% — N086079 001
- 2.5% — N086272 001
- CLAY PARK — 0.5% — N084969 003
- 1% — N085028 001
- NASKA — 1% — N089704 001, MAR 10, 1988
- N088842 001
- FEB 09, 1987
- PHARMADERM — 1% — N086256 001
- TARO — 0.5% — N088061 001, SEP 27, 1983
- USL PHARMA — 1% — N088039 001, SEP 27, 1983
- 2.5%

HYTONE
- DERMIK LABS — 1% — N080474 003
- 2.5% — N080474 004

PENECORT
- ALLERGAN HERBERT — 2.5% — N088217 001, JUN 06, 1984

Powder; For Rx Compounding

H-CORT
- TORCH — 100% — N087834 001, MAR 29, 1982

Tablet; Oral

CORTRIL
- PFIZER — 10MG — N009127 005
- 20MG — N009127 003

HYDROCORTISONE
- ANABOLIC — 20MG — N083140 001
- BARR — 20MG — N083999 001
- ELKINS SINN — 20MG — N080624 001
- EON — 20MG — N080642 002
- FERRANTE — 10MG — N080568 001
- 20MG — N080568 002
- IMPAX LABS — 20MG — N080781 001
- INWOOD LABS — 20MG — N080732 001
- LANNETT — 20MG — N085070 001
- PANRAY — 10MG — N009659 001
- 20MG — N009659 002
- PARKE DAVIS — 20MG — N084243 001
- 20MG — N084247 003, AUG 31, 1982
- PUREPAC PHARM — 10MG — N080395 001
- 20MG — N084247 002

HYDROCORTISONE (continued)

Tablet; Oral

HYDROCORTISONE
- ROXANE — 10MG — N088539 001, MAR 21, 1984
- 20MG — N080355 001
- WATSON LABS
- WHITEWORTH TOWN
- PLSN — 10MG — N080344 001
- 20MG — N080344 002

Tablet; Vaginal

CORTRIL
- PFIPHARMECS — 10MG — N009796 001

HYDROCORTISONE; NEOMYCIN SULFATE

Cream; Topical

NEO-CCRT-DOME
- BAYER PHARMS — 0.5%;EQ 3.5MG BASE/GM — N050237 006, JUN 05, 1984
- 1%;EQ 3.5MG BASE/GM — N050237 005, JUN 05, 1984

HYDROCORTISONE; NEOMYCIN SULFATE; POLYMYXIN B SULFATE

Solution/Drops; Otic

NEOMYCIN SULFATE-POLYMYXIN B SULFATE-HYDROCORTISONE
- PHARMAFAIR — 1%;EQ 3.5MG BASE/ML;10,000 UNITS/ML — N062394 001, SEP 29, 1982

OTOCORT
- STERIS — 1%;EQ 3.5MG BASE/ML;10,000 UNITS/ML — N060730 002

Suspension;Drops; Ophthalmic

NEOMYCIN SULFATE-POLYMYXIN B SULFATE-HYDROCORTISONE
- PHARMAFAIR — 1%;EQ 3.5MG BASE/ML;10,000 UNITS/ML — N062623 001, SEP 24, 1985

Suspension;Drops; Otic

NEOMYCIN SULFATE, POLYMYXIN B SULFATE HYDROCORTISONE
- PHARMAFAIR — 1%;EQ 3.5MG BASE/ML;10,000 UNITS/ML — N062617 001, SEP 18, 1985

OTICAIR
- PHARMAFAIR — 1%;EQ 3.5MG BASE/ML;10,000 UNITS/ML — N062399 001, NOV 18, 1982

OTOBIONE
- SCHERING — 1%;EQ 3.5MG BASE/ML;10,000 UNITS/ML — N061816 001

OTOCORT
- STERIS — 1%;EQ 3.5MG BASE/ML;10,000 UNITS/ML — N062521 001, JUL 11, 1985

HYDROCORTISONE ACETATE (continued)

Ointment; Ophthalmic, Otic

HYDROCORTONE			
MERCK	1.5%		N009018 003

Ointment; Topical

CORTEF ACETATE			
PHARMACIA AND UPJOHN	2.5%	*SEE ANNUAL PREFACE INTRODUCTION DISCONTINUED SECTION*	N008917 002
	1%		N008917 001

HYDROCORTISONE ACETATE; NEOMYCIN SULFATE

Cream; Topical

NEO-CORTEF		
PHARMACIA AND UPJOHN	1%;EQ 3.5MG BASE/GM	N061049 001
	2.5%;EQ 3.5MG BASE/GM	N061049 002

Ointment; Ophthalmic

NEO-CORTEF		
PHARMACIA AND UPJOHN	0.5%;EQ 3.5MG BASE/GM	N060610 001
	1.5%;EQ 3.5MG BASE/GM	N060610 002

Ointment; Topical

NEO-CORTEF		
PHARMACIA AND UPJOHN	0.5%;EQ 3.5MG BASE/GM	N060751 001
	1%;EQ 3.5MG BASE/GM	N060751 002
	2.5%;EQ 3.5MG BASE/GM	N060751 003

Suspension/Drops; Ophthalmic

COR-OTICIN		
AKORN	1.5%;EQ 3.5MG BASE/ML	N060188 001
NEO-CORTEF		
PHARMACIA AND UPJOHN	0.5%;EQ 3.5MG BASE/ML	N060612 002
	1.5%;EQ 3.5MG BASE/ML	N060612 001

HYDROCORTISONE ACETATE; PRAMOXINE HYDROCHLORIDE

Lotion; Topical

PRAMOSONE		
FERNDALE LABS	0.5%;1%	N083213 002

HYDROCORTISONE ACETATE *MULTIPLE*

SEE BACITRACIN; HYDROCORTISONE ACETATE; NEOMYCIN SULFATE; POLYMYXIN B SULFATE

SEE CHLORAMPHENICOL; HYDROCORTISONE ACETATE

SEE CHLORAMPHENICOL; HYDROCORTISONE ACETATE; POLYMYXIN B SULFATE

HYDROCORTISONE BUTYRATE

Cream; Topical

LOCOID			
YAMANOUCHI	0.1%	N018795 001	JAN 07, 1983

Discontinued Drug Products (continued)

HYDROCORTISONE; POLYMYXIN B SULFATE

Solution/Drops; Otic

PYOCIDIN		
FORREST LABS	5MG/ML;EQ 10,000 UNITS BASE/ML	N061606 001

HYDROCORTISONE; TETRACYCLINE HYDROCHLORIDE

Ointment; Ophthalmic

ACHROMYCIN		
LEDERLE	1.5%;1%	N050272 001

HYDROCORTISONE; UREA

Cream; Topical

ALPHADERM		
BIOGLAN	1%;10%	N086008 001
CALMURID HC		
PHARMACIA AND UPJOHN	1%;10%	N083947 001

HYDROCORTISONE *MULTIPLE*

SEE ACETIC ACID, GLACIAL; HYDROCORTISONE

SEE ACETIC ACID, GLACIAL; HYDROCORTISONE; NEOMYCIN SULFATE

SEE BACITRACIN ZINC; HYDROCORTISONE; NEOMYCIN SULFATE; POLYMYXIN B SULFATE

HYDROCORTISONE ACETATE

Cream; Topical

HEMSOL-HC			
ABLE	1%	N081274 001	JUN 19, 1992

HYDROCORTISONE ACETATE

CENCI	1%	N080419 001	JAN 25, 1982
PARKE DAVIS	1%	N089914 001	JAN 03, 1989
PUREPAC PHARM	0.5%	N086050 001	
	1%	N086052 001	

Injectable; Injection

CORTEF ACETATE		
PHARMACIA AND UPJOHN	50MG/ML	N009378 002
CORTRIL		
PFIZER	25MG/ML	N009164 001

HYDROCORTISONE ACETATE

AKORN	25MG/ML	N009637 001
	50MG/ML	N009637 002
BEL MAR	25MG/ML	N083739 001
	50MG/ML	N083739 002
STERIS	25MG/ML	N083128 001
	25MG/ML	N083759 001
	50MG/ML	N083759 002
	50MG/ML	N085214 001

HYDROCORTONE		
MERCK	25MG/ML	N008228 001
	50MG/ML	N008228 004

HYDROFLUMETHIAZIDE (continued)

Tablet; Oral

HYDROFLUMETHIAZIDE
WATSON LAB	50MG	N088031 001	APR 06, 1983
WATSON LABS	50MG	N088528 001	AUG 15, 1984

HYDROFLUMETHIAZIDE; RESERPINE

Tablet; Oral

HYDROFLUMETHIAZIDE AND RESERPINE
USL PHARMA	50MG;0.125MG	N088195 001	OCT 26, 1983
WATSON LAB	25MG;0.125MG	N088127 001	MAR 22, 1983
	50MG;0.125MG	N088110 001	MAR 22, 1983

RESERPINE AND HYDROFLUMETHIAZIDE
IVAX PHARMS	50MG;0.125MG	N088932 001	JAN 11, 1985
PAR PHARM	50MG;0.125MG	N088907 001	SEP 20, 1985

SALUTENSIN-DEMI
SHIRE LABS	25MG;0.125MG	N012359 004	

HYDROXOCOBALAMIN

Injectable; Injection

ALPHAREDISOL
MERCK	1MG/ML	N080778 001

HYDROXOCOBALAMIN
AM P-IARM PARTNERS	1MG/ML	N084921 001
STERIS	1MG/ML	N085528 001

HYDROXOMIN
BEL MAR	1MG/ML	N084629 001

HYDROXYAMPHETAMINE HYDROBROMIDE

Solution/Drops; Ophthalmic

PAREDRINE
AKORN	1%	N000004 004

HYDROXYPROGESTERONE CAPROATE

Injectable; Injection

DELALUTIN
BRISTOL MYERS SQUIBB	125MG/ML	N010347 004
	125MG/ML	N016911 001
	250MG/ML	N010347 002
	250MG/ML	N016911 002

HYDROXYPROGESTERONE CAPROATE
AKORN	125MG/ML	N018004 001	
QUAD PHARMS	125MG/ML	N089330 001	JAN 02, 1987
	250MG/ML	N089331 001	
STERIS	125MG/ML	N017439 001	JAN 02, 1987

Discontinued Drug Products (continued)

HYDROCORTISONE BUTYRATE (continued)

Ointment; Topical

LOCOID
YAMANOUCHI	0.1%	N019106 001	JUL 03, 1984

Solution; Topical

LOCOID
YAMANOUCHI	0.1%	N019819 001	SEP 15, 1988

HYDROCORTISONE SODIUM PHOSPHATE

Injectable; Injection

HYDROCORTISONE SODIUM PHOSPHATE
QUAD PHARMS	EQ 50MG BASE/ML	N089581 001	MAY 28, 1987

HYDROCORTONE
MERCK	EQ 50MG BASE/ML	N012052 001

HYDROCORTISONE SODIUM SUCCINATE

Injectable; Injection

A-HYDROCORT
ABBOTT	EQ 1GM BASE/VIAL	N089580 001	APR 11, 1989
	EQ 100MG BASE/VIAL	N085928 001	
	EQ 100MG BASE/VIAL	N089577 001	APR 11, 1989
	EQ 250MG BASE/VIAL	N089578 001	APR 11, 1989
	EQ 500MG BASE/VIAL	N089579 001	APR 11, 1989

HYDROCORTISONE SODIUM SUCCINATE
AM PHARM PARTNERS	EQ 100MG BASE/VIAL	N088667 001	JUN 08, 1984
	EQ 250MG BASE/VIAL	N088668 001	JUN 08, 1984
	EQ 500MG BASE/VIAL	N088669 001	JUN 08, 1984
	EQ 1GM BASE/VIAL	N088670 001	JUN 08, 1984
	EQ 100MG BASE/VIAL	N088712 001	JUN 08, 1984
ELKINS SINN	EQ 100MG BASE/VIAL	N086619 001	
	EQ 250MG BASE/VIAL	N087567 001	
	EQ 500MG BASE/VIAL	N087568 001	
	EQ 1GM BASE/VIAL	N087569 001	
STERIS	EQ 250MG BASE/VIAL	N084737 001	
	EQ 100MG BASE/VIAL	N084737 002	
	EQ 100MG BASE/VIAL	N084738 001	
	EQ 500MG BASE/VIAL	N084747 001	
	EQ 1GM BASE/VIAL	N084748 001	

HYDROFLUMETHIAZIDE

Tablet; Oral

DIUCARDIN
WYETH AYERST	50MG	N083383 001

Discontinued Drug Products (continued)

HYDROXYPROGESTERONE CAPROATE (continued)
Injectable; Injection

HYDROXYPROGESTERONE CAPROATE

Company	Strength	Appl. No.	Date
STERIS	250MG/ML	N017439 002	

HYDROXYSTILBAMIDINE ISETHIONATE
Injectable; Injection

HYDROXYSTILBAMIDINE ISETHIONATE

Company	Strength	Appl. No.	Date
AVENTIS PHARMS	225MG/AMP	N009166 001	

HYDROXYZINE HYDROCHLORIDE
Injectable; Injection

HYDROXYZINE

Company	Strength	Appl. No.	Date
ELKINS SINN	50MG/ML	N085551 002	

HYDROXYZINE HCL

Company	Strength	Appl. No.	Date
ABBOTT	50MG/ML	N086821 001	
ALTANA	25MG/ML	N087273 001	APR 20, 1982
	50MG/ML	N087273 002	APR 20, 1982
AM PHARM PARTNERS	25MG/ML	N088184 001	MAR 31, 1983
	50MG/ML	N088185 001	MAR 31, 1983
ELKINS SINN	25MG/ML	N085551 001	
PHARMAFAIR	25MG/ML	N088862 001	FEB 14, 1986
	25MG/ML	N089106 001	FEB 14, 1986
	50MG/ML	N088881 001	FEB 14, 1986
	50MG/ML	N089107 001	FEB 14, 1986
SMITH AND NEPHEW SOLOPAK	25MG/ML	N087592 001	
	25MG/ML	N086822 001	
	25MG/ML	N087591 001	
	50MG/ML	N087310 001	
	50MG/ML	N087593 001	
	50MG/ML	N087595 001	
	50MG/ML	N087596 001	
STERIS	25MG/ML	N085778 001	
	25MG/ML	N087274 001	
	50MG/ML	N087274 002	
WYETH AYERST	25MG/ML	N086258 001	
	50MG/ML	N086258 002	

ORGATRAX

Company	Strength	Appl. No.	Date
ORGANON USA INC	25MG/ML	N087014 001	
	50MG/ML	N087014 002	

Syrup; Oral

HYDROXYZINE HCL

Company	Strength	Appl. No.	Date
ALPHARMA	10MG/5ML	N088785 001	FEB 03, 1988
KV PHARM	10MG/5ML	N087730 001	JUL 01, 1982

HYDROXYZINE HYDROCHLORIDE (continued)
Tablet; Oral

ATARAX

Company	Strength	Appl. No.	Date
PFIZER	10MG	N010392 001	
	25MG	N010392 004	
	50MG	N010392 006	
	100MG	N010392 005	

HYDROXYZINE HCL

Company	Strength	Appl. No.	Date
AMIDE PHARM	10MG	N089071 001	
	10MG	N089072 001	JUL 22, 1986
	25MG	N089073 001	JUL 22, 1986
	50MG	N087246 002	JUL 22, 1986
EON	10MG	N085247 001	
	25MG	N087245 001	
	50MG	N088409 001	NOV 15, 1983
HALSEY	10MG	N089366 001	
	25MG	N087857 001	MAY 02, 1988
	25MG	N089117 001	APR 18, 1983
	50MG	N087860 001	MAY 02, 1988
	50MG	N089396 001	APR 18, 1983
	100MG	N087862 001	MAY 02, 1988
	100MG	N087216 001	APR 18, 1983
IVAX PHARMS	10MG	N087410 001	
	25MG	N087411 001	
	50MG	N087819 001	
KV PHARM	10MG	N087820 001	JUN 23, 1982
	25MG	N087821 001	JUN 23, 1982
	50MG	N087822 001	JUN 23, 1982
	100MG	N087602 001	JUN 23, 1982
PAR PHARM	10MG	N087603 001	JAN 22, 1982
	25MG	N087604 001	JAN 22, 1982
PLIVA	50MG	N081054 001	JAN 22, 1982
	100MG	N088120 001	SEP 25, 1995
PUREPAC PHARM	10MG	N088121 001	SEP 25, 1984
	25MG	N088122 001	SEP 25, 1984
QUANTUM PHARMICS	10MG	N088540 001	SEP 25, 1984

Discontinued Drug Products (continued)

HYDROXYZINE HYDROCHLORIDE (continued)

Syrup; Oral

HYDROXYZINE HCL

Applicant	Strength	Appl. No.	Date
QUANTUM PHARMICS	25MG	N088551 001	OCT 22, 1985
	50MG	N088529 001	OCT 22, 1985
SUPERPHARM	10MG	N088794 001	DEC 05, 1984
		N087795 001	DEC 05, 1984
	25MG	N088796 001	DEC 05, 1984
	50MG	N089121 001	MAR 20, 1986
USL PHARMA	10MG	N089122 001	MAR 20, 1986
	25MG	N089123 001	MAR 20, 1986
	50MG		
WATSON LABS	10MG	N086827 001	
	25MG	N086829 001	
	50MG	N086836 001	

HYDROXYZINE PAMOATE

Capsule; Oral

HY-PAM "25"

Applicant	Strength	Appl. No.	Date
TEVA	EQ 25MG HCL	N088713 001	MAR 04, 1985

HYDROXYZINE PAMOATE

Applicant	Strength	Appl. No.	Date
DURAMED PHARM BARR	EQ 25MG HCL	N088593 001	FEB 29, 1984
	EQ 50MG HCL	N088594 001	FEB 29, 1984
	EQ 100MG HCL	N088595 001	FEB 29, 1984
GENEVA PHARMS	EQ 50MG HCL	N081128 001	JUN 28, 1991
	EQ 100MG HCL	N081129 001	JUN 28, 1991
PAR PHARM	EQ 25MG HCL	N087656 001	JUN 11, 1982
	EQ 25MG HCL	N089145 001	MAR 17, 1986
	EQ 50MG HCL	N087657 001	JUN 11, 1982
	EQ 50MG HCL	N089146 001	MAR 17, 1986
	EQ 100MG HCL	N087658 001	JUN 11, 1982
SUPERPHARM	EQ 25MG HCL	N089031 001	JAN 02, 1987
	EQ 50MG HCL	N089032 001	JAN 02, 1987
	EQ 100MG HCL	N089033 001	JAN 02, 1987
VANGARD	EQ 25MG HCL	N088392 001	

HYDROXYZINE PAMOATE (continued)

Capsule; Oral

HYDROXYZINE PAMOATE

Applicant	Strength	Appl. No.	Date
VANGARD	EQ 50MG HCL	N088393 001	SEP 19, 1983
WATSON LAB	EQ 25MG HCL	N086698 001	SEP 19, 1983
	EQ 50MG HCL	N086695 001	
	EQ 100MG HCL	N086697 001	
	EQ 25MG HCL	N086840 001	JUL 01, 1982
WATSON LABS	EQ 50MG HCL	N086705 001	JUL 01, 1982
	EQ 50MG HCL	N087767 001	AUG 16, 1982
	EQ 100MG HCL	N086728 001	OCT 05, 1982
	EQ 100MG HCL	N087790 001	AUG 16, 1982

IBUPROFEN

Capsule; Oral

MIDOL

Applicant	Strength	Appl. No.	Date
BAYER	200MG *SEE ANNUAL PREFACE INTRODUCTION DISCONTINUED SECTION*	N070626 001	SEP 02, 1987
	200MG *SEE ANNUAL PREFACE INTRODUCTION DISCONTINUED SECTION*	N071002 001	SEP 02, 1987

Suspension/Drops; Oral

MOTRIN

Applicant	Strength	Appl. No.	Date
MCNEIL	40MG/ML	N020476 001	MAY 25, 1995

Suspension; Oral

IBU

Applicant	Strength	Appl. No.	Date
ABBOTT	100MG/5ML	N019784 001	DEC 18, 1989

Tablet, Chewable; Oral

MOTRIN

Applicant	Strength	Appl. No.	Date
MCNEIL CONS SPECLT	50MG	N020135 001	NOV 16, 1994
	100MG	N020135 002	NOV 16, 1994

Tablet; Oral

ACHES-N-PAIN

Applicant	Strength	Appl. No.	Date
LEDERLE	200MG	N071065 001	MAY 28, 1987

IBU-TAB

Applicant	Strength	Appl. No.	Date
ALRA	800MG	N071965 001	AUG 11, 1988

IBUPRIN

Applicant	Strength	Appl. No.	Date
PLIVA	200MG	N071773 001	JUL 16, 1987

Discontinued Drug Products *(continued)*

IBUPROFEN *(continued)*
Tablet; Oral

IBUPROFEN

Manufacturer	Strength	Appl. No.	Date
ABBOTT	600MG	N070556 001	JUN 14, 1985
	800MG	N071264 001	JUL 25, 1986
BARR	200MG	N070493 001	DEC 24, 1985
	200MG	N070908 001	SEP 26, 1986
	200MG	N071462 001	OCT 02, 1986
	400MG	N070079 001	JUL 24, 1985
	600MG	N070080 001	JUL 24, 1985
	800MG	N071448 001	FEB 18, 1987
HALSEY	200MG	N071027 001	SEP 29, 1987
	300MG	N071028 001	MAR 23, 1987
	400MG	N071029 001	MAR 23, 1987
	600MG	N071030 001	MAR 23, 1987
	800MG	N072137 001	FEB 05, 1988
INVAMED	400MG	N072064 001	JAN 14, 1988
	600MG	N072065 001	JAN 14, 1988
	800MG	N071938 001	JAN 14, 1988
IVAX PHARMS	200MG	N071154 001	OCT 27, 1987
	200MG	N072040 001	APR 29, 1988
LEDERLE	400MG	N070629 001	SEP 19, 1986
	600MG	N070630 001	SEP 19, 1986
MCNEIL	400MG	N070081 001	JUN 16, 1986
	600MG	N070476 001	JUN 16, 1986
PAR PHARM	300MG	N070328 001	AUG 06, 1985
PUREPAC PHARM	200MG	N071122 001	OCT 03, 1986
	200MG	N071664 001	FEB 03, 1987
	300MG	N071123 001	SEP 19, 1986
	400MG	N071124 001	SEP 19, 1986

IBUPROFEN *(continued)*
Tablet; Oral

IBUPROFEN

Manufacturer	Strength	Appl. No.	Date
PUREPAC PHARM	600MG	N071125 001	SEP 19, 1986
	800MG	N071964 001	FEB 01, 1988
SUPERPHARM	600MG	N070709 001	APR 25, 1986
TEVA	200MG	N073141 001	MAY 29, 1992
	400MG	N073343 001	JUN 30, 1992
	600MG	N073344 001	JUN 30, 1992
	800MG	N073345 001	JUN 30, 1992
WATSON LABS	200MG	N071765 001	SEP 04, 1987
	200MG	N071905 001	MAR 08, 1988
	300MG	N071338 001	DEC 01, 1986
	400MG	N070038 001	SEP 06, 1985
	600MG	N070041 001	SEP 06, 1985
	800MG	N071911 001	OCT 13, 1987

MIDOL

Manufacturer	Strength	Appl. No.	Date
BAYER	200MG	N070591 001	SEP 02, 1987
	200MG	N071001 001	SEP 02, 1987

MOTRIN

Manufacturer	Strength	Appl. No.	Date
MCNEIL CONS SPECLT	100MG	N020418 001	NOV 16, 1994

NUPRIN

Manufacturer	Strength	Appl. No.	Date
BRISTOL MYERS	200MG	N072035 001	FEB 16, 1988
	200MG	N072036 001	FEB 16, 1988
MCNEIL	200MG	N019012 001	MAY 18, 1984
	200MG	N019012 002	JUL 29, 1987

RUFEN

Manufacturer	Strength	Appl. No.	Date
BASF	600MG	N018197 002	MAR 05, 1984

IDARUBICIN HYDROCHLORIDE
Injectable; Injection

IDAMYCIN

Manufacturer	Strength	Appl. No.	Date
PHARMACIA AND UPJOHN	5MG/VIAL	N050661 002	SEP 27, 1990

Discontinued Drug Products (continued)

IDARUBICIN HYDROCHLORIDE (continued)
Injectable; Injection

IDAMYCIN

Company	Strength	NDA	Date
PHARMACIA AND UPJOHN	10MG/VIAL	N050661 001	SEP 27, 1990
	20MG/VIAL	N050661 003	APR 25, 1995

IDOXURIDINE
Ointment; Ophthalmic

STOXIL

Company	Strength	NDA
GLAXOSMITHKLINE	0.5%	N015868 001

Solution/Drops; Ophthalmic

STOXIL

Company	Strength	NDA
GLAXOSMITHKLINE	0.1%	N013934 001

IFOSFAMIDE
Injectable; Injection

IFEX

Company	Strength	NDA	Date	Note
BRISTOL MYERS SQUIBB	1GM/VIAL	N019763 001	DEC 30, 1988	*SEE ANNUAL PREFACE INTRODUCTION DISCONTINUED SECTION*
	3GM/VIAL	N019763 002	DEC 30, 1988	*SEE ANNUAL PREFACE INTRODUCTION DISCONTINUED SECTION*

IMATINIB MESYLATE
Capsule; Oral

GLEEVEC

Company	Strength	NDA	Date
NOVARTIS	50MG	N021335 001	MAY 10, 2001

IMIPRAMINE HYDROCHLORIDE
Injectable; Injection

TOFRANIL

Company	Strength	NDA
NOVARTIS	12.5MG/ML	N011838 002

Tablet; Oral

IMIPRAMINE HCL

Company	Strength	NDA	Date
EON	10MG	N085200 001	
	25MG	N084869 002	
	50MG	N085133 001	
LEDERLE	10MG	N086269 001	
	25MG	N086267 001	
	50MG	N086268 001	
ROXANE	25MG	N083799 002	
	50MG	N083799 003	
USL PHARMA	25MG	N087776 001	FEB 10, 1982
	10MG	N088036 001	NOV 03, 1982
VANGARD	10MG	N087619 001	FEB 09, 1982
	25MG		

IMIPRAMINE HYDROCHLORIDE (continued)
Tablet; Oral

IMIPRAMINE HCL

Company	Strength	NDA	Date
VANGARD	50MG	N087631 001	JAN 04, 1982
WATSON LAB	10MG	N085220 001	
	25MG	N084252 002	
	50MG	N085221 001	
WATSON LABS	10MG	N085875 001	
	25MG	N085878 001	
	50MG	N085877 001	
WEST WARD	25MG	N088222 001	MAY 26, 1983
	50MG	N088223 001	MAY 26, 1983

JANIMINE

Company	Strength	NDA
ABBOTT	10MG	N017895 001
	25MG	N017895 002
	50MG	N017895 003

PRAMINE

Company	Strength	NDA
ALRA	10MG	N083827 001
	25MG	N083827 002
	50MG	N083827 003

PRESAMINE

Company	Strength	NDA
AVENTIS	10MG	N011836 006
	25MG	N011836 003
	50MG	N011836 007

INAMRINONE LACTATE
Injectable; Injection

INOCOR

Company	Strength	NDA	Date
SANOFI SYNTHELABO	EQ 5MG BASE/ML	N018700 001	JUL 31, 1984

INDAPAMIDE
Tablet; Oral

INDAPAMIDE

Company	Strength	NDA	Date
TEVA	1.25MG	N074665 001	APR 04, 1997
	2.5MG	N074665 002	APR 04, 1997

INDECAINIDE HYDROCHLORIDE
Tablet, Extended Release; Oral

DECABID

Company	Strength	NDA	Date
LILLY	EQ 50MG BASE	N019693 001	DEC 29, 1989
	EQ 75MG BASE	N019693 002	DEC 29, 1989
	EQ 100MG BASE	N019693 003	DEC 29, 1989

Discontinued Drug Products (continued)

INDOCYANINE GREEN
Injectable; Injection
CARDIO-GREEN
AKORN
- 10MG/VIAL — N011525 003
- 40MG/VIAL — N011525 004
- 50MG/VIAL — N011525 002

INDOMETHACIN
Capsule, Extended Release; Oral
INDOCIN SR
MERCK
- 75MG — N018185 001 — FEB 23, 1982

Capsule; Oral
INDOMETHACIN
DURAMED PHARM BARR
- 25MG — N070326 001 — OCT 18, 1985
- 50MG — N070327 001 — OCT 18, 1985

HALSEY
- 25MG — N070067 001 — OCT 03, 1986
- 25MG — N070782 001 — JUN 03, 1987
- 50MG — N070068 001 — OCT 03, 1986
- 50MG — N070635 001 — JUN 03, 1987

IVAX PHARMS
- 25MG — N018730 001 — MAY 04, 1984
- 50MG — N018730 002 — MAY 04, 1984

PARKE DAVIS
- 25MG — N018806 001 — NOV 23, 1984
- 50MG — N018806 002 — NOV 23, 1984

PIONEER PHARMS
- 25MG — N070813 001 — AUG 11, 1986
- 50MG — N070592 001 — AUG 11, 1986

ROXANE
- 25MG — N070353 001 — JUN 18, 1985
- 50MG — N070354 001 — JUN 18, 1985

SUPERPHARM
- 25MG — N070487 001 — OCT 10, 1986
- 50MG — N070488 001 — OCT 10, 1986

WATSON LAB
- 25MG — N070784 001 — OCT 10, 1986
- 50MG — N070785 001 — AUG 20, 1986

WATSON LABS
- 25MG — N018690 001 — JUL 31, 1984
- 25MG — N070529 001 — OCT 18, 1985
- 25MG — N072996 001 — JUL 31, 1991

INDOMETHACIN (continued)
Capsule; Oral
INDOMETHACIN
WATSON LABS
- 50MG — N018690 002 — JUL 31, 1984
- 50MG — N070530 001 — OCT 18, 1985
- 50MG — N071635 001 — MAY 18, 1987
- 50MG — N072997 001 — JUL 31, 1991

Suppository; Rectal
INDOCIN
MERCK
- 50MG — N017814 001 — AUG 13, 1984

INSULIN PORK
Injectable; Injection
ILETIN I
LILLY
- 500 UNITS/ML — N017931 001

INSULIN
NOVO NORDISK
- 40 UNITS/ML — N017926 001

REGULAR INSULIN
NOVO NORDISK
- 100 UNITS/ML — N017926 003

INSULIN PURIFIED BEEF
Injectable; Injection
REGULAR ILETIN II
LILLY
- 100 UNITS/ML — N018478 001

INSULIN PURIFIED PORK
Injectable; Injection
REGULAR PURIFIED PORK INSULIN
NOVO NORDISK
- 100 UNITS/ML — N018381 001

VELOSULIN
NOVO NORDISK
- 100 UNITS/ML — N018193 001

INSULIN PURIFIED PORK; INSULIN SUSP ISOPHANE PURIFIED PORK
Injectable; Injection
INSULIN NORDISK MIXTARD (PORK)
NOVO NORDISK
- 30 UNITS/ML;70 UNITS/ML — N018195 001

INSULIN RECOMBINANT HUMAN
Injectable; Injection
HUMULIN BR
LILLY
- 100 UNITS/ML — N019529 001 — APR 28, 1986

INSULIN RECOMBINANT PURIFIED HUMAN
Injectable; Injection
NOVOLIN R
NOVO NORDISK
- 100 UNITS/ML — N018778 001 — AUG 30, 1983

Discontinued Drug Products (continued)

INSULIN RECOMBINANT PURIFIED HUMAN (continued)
Injectable; Injection
VELOSULIN BR HUMAN
NOVO NORDISK — 100 UNITS/ML — N019450 001 — MAY 30, 1986

INSULIN RECOMBINANT PURIFIED HUMAN; INSULIN SUSP ISOPHANE SEMISYNTHETIC PURIFIED HUMAN
Injectable; Injection
MIXTARD HUMAN 70/30
BAYER PHARMS — 30 UNITS/ML;70 UNITS/ML — N019585 001 — MAR 11, 1988
NOVOLIN 70/30
NOVO NORDISK — 30 UNITS/ML;70 UNITS/ML — N019441 001 — JUL 11, 1986

INSULIN SUSP ISOPHANE BEEF
Injectable; Injection
NPH INSULIN
NOVO NORDISK — 40 UNITS/ML — N017929 001

INSULIN SUSP ISOPHANE BEEF/PORK
Injectable; Injection
NPH ILETIN I (BEEF-PORK)
LILLY — 40 UNITS/ML — N017936 001

INSULIN SUSP ISOPHANE PURIFIED BEEF
Injectable; Injection
NPH ILETIN II
LILLY — 100 UNITS/ML — N018479 001

INSULIN SUSP ISOPHANE PURIFIED PORK
Injectable; Injection
INSULIN INSULATARD NPH NORDISK
NOVO NORDISK — 100 UNITS/ML — N018194 001
NPH PURIFIED PORK ISOPHANE INSULIN
NOVO NORDISK — 100 UNITS/ML — N018623 001

INSULIN SUSP ISOPHANE PURIFIED PORK *MULTIPLE*
SEE INSULIN PURIFIED PORK; INSULIN SUSP ISOPHANE PURIFIED PORK

INSULIN SUSP ISOPHANE SEMISYNTHETIC PURIFIED HUMAN
Injectable; Injection
INSULATARD NPH HUMAN
NOVO NORDISK — 100 UNITS/ML — N019449 001 — MAY 30, 1986
NOVOLIN N
NOVO NORDISK — 100 UNITS/ML — N019065 001 — JAN 23, 1985

INSULIN SUSP ISOPHANE SEMISYNTHETIC PURIFIED HUMAN *MULTIPLE*
SEE INSULIN RECOMBINANT PURIFIED HUMAN; INSULIN SUSP ISOPHANE SEMISYNTHETIC PURIFIED HUMAN

INSULIN SUSP PROTAMINE ZINC BEEF/PORK
Injectable; Injection
PROTAMINE, ZINC ILETIN I (BEEF-PORK)
LILLY — 40 UNITS/ML — N017932 001
LILLY — 100 UNITS/ML — N017932 002

INSULIN SUSP PROTAMINE ZINC PURIFIED BEEF
Injectable; Injection
PROTAMINE ZINC AND ILETIN II
LILLY — 100 UNITS/ML — N018476 001
PROTAMINE ZINC INSULIN
BRISTOL MYERS SQUIBB — 40 UNITS/ML — N017928 001
BRISTOL MYERS SQUIBB — 100 UNITS/ML — N017928 003

INSULIN SUSP PROTAMINE ZINC PURIFIED PORK
Injectable; Injection
PROTAMINE ZINC AND ILETIN II (PORK)
LILLY — 100 UNITS/ML — N018346 001

INSULIN ZINC SUSP BEEF
Injectable; Injection
LENTE INSULIN
NOVO NORDISK — 40 UNITS/ML — N017998 001
NOVO NORDISK — 100 UNITS/ML — N017998 003

INSULIN ZINC SUSP EXTENDED BEEF
Injectable; Injection
ULTRALENTE INSULIN
NOVO NORDISK — 100 UNITS/ML — N017997 003

INSULIN ZINC SUSP EXTENDED PURIFIED BEEF
Injectable; Injection
ULTRALENTE
NOVO NORDISK — 100 UNITS/ML — N018385 001

INSULIN ZINC SUSP EXTENDED RECOMBINANT HUMAN
Injectable; Injection
HUMULIN U
LILLY — 40 UNITS/ML — N019571 001 — JUN 10, 1987

INSULIN ZINC SUSP PROMPT BEEF
Injectable; Injection
SEMILENTE INSULIN
NOVO NORDISK — 100 UNITS/ML — N017996 003

Discontinued Drug Products (continued)

INSULIN ZINC SUSP PROMPT PURIFIED PORK
Injectable; Injection
SEMILENTE
NOVO NORDISK   100 UNITS/ML   N018382 001

INSULIN ZINC SUSP PURIFIED BEEF
Injectable; Injection
LENTE ILETIN II
LILLY   100 UNITS/ML   N018477 001

INSULIN ZINC SUSP PURIFIED BEEF/PORK
Injectable; Injection
LENTARD
NOVO NORDISK   100 UNITS/ML   N018384 001

INSULIN ZINC SUSP PURIFIED PORK
Injectable; Injection
LENTE
NOVO NORDISK   100 UNITS/ML   N018383 001

INSULIN ZINC SUSP SEMISYNTHETIC PURIFIED HUMAN
Injectable; Injection
NOVOLIN L
NOVO NORDISK   100 UNITS/ML   N018777 001 AUG 30, 1983

INTRINSIC FACTOR *MULTIPLE*
SEE   COBALT CHLORIDE, CO-60; CYANOCOBALAMIN; CYANOCOBALAMIN, CO-60;
       INTRINSIC FACTOR
SEE   CYANOCOBALAMIN; CYANOCOBALAMIN, CO-57; INTRINSIC FACTOR

INVERT SUGAR
Injectable; Injection
TRAVERT 10% IN PLASTIC CONTAINER
BAXTER HLTHCARE   10GM/100ML   N016717 001

IOCETAMIC ACID
Tablet; Oral
CHOLEBRINE
MALLINCKRODT   750MG   N017129 001

IODAMIDE MEGLUMINE
Injectable; Injection
RENOVUE-65
BRACCO   65%   N017902 001
RENOVUE-DIP
BRACCO   24%   N017903 001

IODIPAMIDE MEGLUMINE
Injectable; Injection
CHOLOGRAFIN MEGLUMINE
BRACCO   10.3%   N009321 007

IODIPAMIDE SODIUM
Injectable; Injection
CHOLOGRAFIN SODIUM
BRACCO   20%   N009321 001

IODIXANOL
Injectable; Injection
VISIPAQUE 270
AMERSHAM HLTH   55%   N020808 001 AUG 29, 1997
VISIPAQUE 320
AMERSHAM HLTH   65.2%   N020808 002 AUG 29, 1997

IODOHIPPURATE SODIUM, I-123
Injectable; Injection
NEPHROFLOW
AMERSHAM HLTH   1mCi/ML   N018289 001 DEC 28, 1984

IODOHIPPURATE SODIUM, I-131
Injectable; Injection
HIPPURAN I 131
MALLINCKRODT   0.25mCi/ML   N016666 001
HIPPUTOPE
BRACCO   1-2mCi/VIAL   N015419 002
IODOHIPPURATE SODIUM I 131
CIS   0.2mCi/ML   N017313 001

IODOXAMATE MEGLUMINE
Injectable; Injection
CHOLOVUE
BRACCO   9.9%   N018077 001
          40.3%   N018076 001

IOFETAMINE HYDROCHLORIDE I-123
Injectable; Injection
SPECTAMINE
IMP   1mCi/ML   N019432 001 DEC 24, 1987

IOHEXOL
Injectable; Injection
OMNIPAQUE 210
AMERSHAM HLTH   45.3%   N018956 006 JUN 30, 1989
Solution; Urethral
OMNIPAQUE 70
AMERSHAM HLTH   15.1%   N018956 007 JUN 01, 1994

Discontinued Drug Products (continued)

IOPAMIDOL
Injectable; Injection

Product / Firm	Strength	Appl. No.	Date
IOPAMIDOL			
ELKINS SINN PHARM	41%	N074629 001	NOV 06, 1996
	51%	N074629 004	MAR 31, 1998
	61%	N074629 002	NOV 06, 1996
	76%	N074629 003	NOV 06, 1996
FAULDING	61%	N074734 001	DEC 10, 1996
	76%	N074734 002	DEC 10, 1996
IOPAMIDOL-300			
ABBOTT	61%	N074638 001	APR 30, 1997
ISOVUE-128			
BRACCO	26%	N018735 005	OCT 21, 1986
ISOVUE-200			
BRACCO	41%	N020327 001	OCT 12, 1994

IOPHENDYLATE
Injectable; Injection

Product / Firm	Strength	Appl. No.	Date
PANTOPAQUE			
ALCON	100%	N005319 001	

IOTHALAMATE SODIUM
Injectable; Injection

Product / Firm	Strength	Appl. No.	Date
ANGIO-CONRAY			
MALLINCKRODT	80%	N013319 001	
CONRAY 325			
MALLINCKRODT	54.3%	N017685 001	

IOTROLAN
Injectable; Intrathecal

Product / Firm	Strength	Appl. No.	Date
OSMOVIST 190			
BERLEX LABS	40.6%	N019580 001	DEC 07, 1989
OSMOVIST 240			
BERLEX LABS	51.3%	N019580 002	DEC 07, 1989

IOVERSOL
Injectable; Injection

Product / Firm	Strength	Appl. No.	Date
OPTIRAY 240			
MALLINCKRODT	51%	N020923 001	MAY 28, 1998
OPTIRAY 320			
MALLINCKRODT	68%	N020923 002	MAY 29, 1998

IPODATE CALCIUM
Granule; Oral

Product / Firm	Strength	Appl. No.	Date
ORAGRAFIN CALCIUM			
BRACCO	3GM/PACKET	N012968 001	

IPODATE SODIUM
Capsule; Oral

Product / Firm	Strength	Appl. No.	Date
BILIVIST			
BERLEX	500MG	N087768 001	AUG 11, 1982
ORAGRAFIN SODIUM			
BRACCO	500MG	N012967 001	

IRBESARTAN *MULTIPLE*
SEE HYDROCHLOROTHIAZIDE; IRBESARTAN

IRON DEXTRAN
Injectable; Injection

Product / Firm	Strength	Appl. No.	Date
IRON DEXTRAN			
FISONs	EQ 50MG IRON/ML	N010787 002	

ISOETHARINE HYDROCHLORIDE
Solution; Inhalation

Product / Firm	Strength	Appl. No.	Date
BRONKCSOL			
SANOFI SYNTHELABO	0.25%	N012339 009	
	1%	N012339 008	
ISOETHARINE HCL			
ALPHARMA	1%	N087101 001	
ASTRAZENECA	0.2%	N088471 001	MAR 14, 1984
	0.2%	N089617 001	JUN 13, 1991
	0.25%	N088472 001	MAR 14, 1984
	0.25%	N089618 001	JUN 13, 1991
	0.062%	N087937 001	NOV 15, 1982
	0.062%	N089614 001	JUN 13, 1991
	0.125%	N087938 001	NOV 15, 1982
	0.125%	N089615 001	JUN 13, 1991
	0.167%	N088470 001	MAR 14, 1984
	0.167%	N089616 001	JUN 13, 1991
BAXTER HLTHCARE	0.08%	N088144 001	JUL 29, 1983
	0.14%	N088145 001	MAR 26, 1984
DEY	0.25%	N088146 001	AUG 01, 1983
	0.08%	N088187 001	

Discontinued Drug Products (continued)

ISOETHARINE HYDROCHLORIDE (continued)

Solution; Inhalation

ISOETHARINE HCL

Firm	Strength	Appl. No.	Date
DEY	0.17%	N087390 001	DEC 03, 1982
	0.25%	N088188 001	DEC 03, 1982
INTL MEDICATION	1%	N086763 001	
	0.1%	N086651 003	
	0.2%	N086651 006	
	0.25%	N086651 007	
	0.077%	N086651 001	
	0.167%	N086651 005	
	1%	N086651 008	
PARKE DAVIS	0.5%	N085997 001	
	1%	N085889 001	
ROXANE	0.1%	N087396 001	
	0.25%	N088275 001	JUN 03, 1983

ISOETHARINE HCL S/F

Firm	Strength	Appl. No.	Date
DEY	0.125%	N087025 001	
	0.1%	N089818 001	NOV 22, 1988
	0.08%	N089817 001	NOV 22, 1988
	0.17%	N089819 001	NOV 22, 1988
	0.25%	N089820 001	NOV 22, 1988
	1%	N089252 001	SEP 15, 1986

ISOETHARINE MESYLATE

Aerosol, Metered; Inhalation

Firm	Strength	Appl. No.	Date
BRONKOMETER			
SANOFI SYNTHELABO	0.34MG/INH	N012339 007	
ISOETHARINE MESYLATE			
ALPHARMA	0.34MG/INH	N087858 001	AUG 21, 1984

ISOFLUROPHATE

Ointment; Ophthalmic

Firm	Strength	Appl. No.	Date
FLOROPRYL			
MERCK	0.025%	N010656 001	

ISONIAZID

Injectable; Injection

Firm	Strength	Appl. No.	Date
ISONIAZID			
QUAD PHARMS	100MG/ML	N089816 001	OCT 28, 1988
RIMIFON			
ROCHE	25MG/ML	N008420 002	
	100MG/ML	N008420 003	

ISONIAZID (continued)

Syrup; Oral

Firm	Strength	Appl. No.	Date
ISONIAZID			
MIKART	50MG/5ML	N081118 001	JUL 21, 1997
LANIAZID			
LANNETT	50MG/5ML	N089243 001	FEB 03, 1986
RIMIFON			
ROCHE	50MG/5ML	N008420 001	

Tablet; Oral

Firm	Strength	Appl. No.	Date
DOW-ISONIAZID			
DOW PHARM	300MG	N080330 002	
HYZYD			
MEDPOINTE PHARM HLC	100MG	N080134 003	
	300MG	N080134 004	
INH			
NOVARTIS	300MG	N080935 001	
ISONIAZID			
ANABOLIC	100MG	N084050 001	
AXIOM PHARM	100MG	N080136 001	
DURAMED PHARM BARR	100MG	N088231 001	MAR 17, 1983
HALSEY	50MG	N083632 001	
IMPAX LABS	100MG	N080153 001	
IVAX PHARMS	100MG	N080270 001	
	300MG	N083610 001	
LILLY	100MG	N008499 002	
	300MG	N008499 003	
MK LABS	50MG	N080941 001	
PANRAY	100MG	N008428 002	
	300MG	N008428 003	
PERRIGO	100MG	N083060 001	
PHARMAVITE	100MG	N085091 001	
PHOENIX LABS NY	50MG	N080368 001	
	100MG	N080368 002	
PUREPAC PHARM	50MG	N080132 003	JUL 14, 1982
	100MG	N080132 004	JUL 14, 1982
WATSON LAB	100MG	N080401 001	
	300MG	N083178 001	
WATSON LABS	50MG	N080522 001	
	100MG	N080523 001	
WHITEWORTH TOWN PLSN	100MG	N085790 001	
	300MG	N085784 001	
NYDRAZID			
BRISTOL MYERS SQUIBB	100MG	N080120 002	
	300MG	N008392 003	
STANOZIDE			
EVERYLIFE	100MG	N080126 001	
	300MG	N080126 002	

Discontinued Drug Products (continued)

ISOPROPAMIDE IODIDE
Tablet; Oral

Brand	Manufacturer	Strength	Number	Date
DARBID	GLAXOSMITHKLINE	EQ 5MG BASE	N010744 001	

ISOPROTERENOL HYDROCHLORIDE
Aerosol, Metered; Inhalation

Brand	Manufacturer	Strength	Number	Date
ISOPROTERENOL HCL	3M	0.12MG/INH	N010375 004	
ALPHARMA		0.12MG/INH	N085904 001	
ISUPREL	SANOFI SYNTHELABO	0.103MG/INH	N011178 001	

Disc; Inhalation

Brand	Manufacturer	Strength	Number	Date
NORISODRINE AEROTROL	ABBOTT	0.25%	N016814 001	

Injectable; Injection

Brand	Manufacturer	Strength	Number	Date
ISOPROTERENOL HCL	AM PHARM PARTNERS	0.2MG/ML	N083431 001	
	BAXTER HLTHCARE	0.2MG/ML	N083486 001	

Solution; Inhalation

Brand	Manufacturer	Strength	Number	Date
AEROLONE	LILLY	0.25%	N007245 001	
ISOPROTERENOL HCL	ARMOUR PHARM	0.031%	N087935 001	NOV 18, 1982
		0.062%	N087936 001	NOV 18, 1982
	DEY	0.5%	N086764 001	JAN 04, 1982
	PARKE DAVIS	0.5%	N085540 001	
		0.25%	N085994 001	
ISUPREL	SANOFI SYNTHELABO	0.5%	N006327 002	
		1%	N006327 003	
VAPO-ISO	FISONS	0.5%	N016813 001	

Tablet; Rectal, Sublingual

Brand	Manufacturer	Strength	Number	Date
ISUPREL	SANOFI SYNTHELABO	10MG	N006328 001	
		15MG	N006328 002	

ISOPROTERENOL HYDROCHLORIDE; PHENYLEPHRINE BITARTRATE
Aerosol, Metered; Inhalation

Brand	Manufacturer	Strength	Number	Date
DUO-MEDIHALER	3M	0.16MG/INH;0.24MG/INH	N013296 001	

ISOPROTERENOL HYDROCHLORIDE *MULTIPLE*
SEE   ACETYLCYSTEINE; ISOPROTERENOL HYDROCHLORIDE

ISOPROTERENOL SULFATE
Aerosol, Metered; Inhalation

Brand	Manufacturer	Strength	Number	Date
MEDIHALER-ISO	3M	0.08MG/INH	N010375 003	

ISOPROTERENOL SULFATE (continued)
Powder; Inhalation

Brand	Manufacturer	Strength	Number	Date
NORISODRINE	ABBOTT	10%	N006905 003	
		25%	N006905 002	

ISOSORBIDE
Solution; Oral

Brand	Manufacturer	Strength	Number	Date
ISMOTIC	ALCON	100GM/220ML	N017063 001	

ISOSORBIDE DINITRATE
Capsule, Extended Release; Oral

Brand	Manufacturer	Strength	Number	Date
ISORDIL	WYETH AYERST	40MG	N012882 002	JUL 29, 1988

Tablet, Chewable; Oral

Brand	Manufacturer	Strength	Number	Date
SORBITRATE	ASTRAZENECA	5MG	N016776 002	APR 01, 1996

Tablet, Extended Release; Oral

Brand	Manufacturer	Strength	Number	Date
ISORDIL	WYETH AYERST	40MG	N012882 001	JUL 29, 1988

Tablet; Oral

Brand	Manufacturer	Strength	Number	Date
ISOSORBIDE DINITRATE	HALSEY	5MG	N086166 002	SEP 19, 1986
		10MG	N086169 001	SEP 19, 1986
		20MG	N086167 001	SEP 19, 1986
		30MG	N087564 001	SEP 18, 1986
	SUPERPHARM	5MG	N089190 001	FEB 17, 1987
		10MG	N089191 001	FEB 17, 1987
		20MG	N089192 001	FEB 17, 1987
SORBITRATE	ASTRAZENECA	5MG	N016192 001	APR 01, 1996
		10MG	N016192 002	APR 01, 1996
		30MG	N088124 001	AUG 21, 1990

Tablet; Sublingual

Brand	Manufacturer	Strength	Number	Date
ISOSORBIDE DINITRATE	HALSEY	2.5MG	N084204 001	SEP 18, 1986
		5MG	N086168 001	SEP 18, 1986
		10MG	N087545 001	SEP 18, 1986

Discontinued Drug Products (continued)

ISOSORBIDE DINITRATE (continued)
Tablet; Sublingual
SORBITRATE

ASTRAZENECA	2.5MG	N016191 002	APR 01, 1996
	5MG	N016191 001	APR 01, 1996

KANAMYCIN SULFATE
Capsule; Oral
KANTREX

APOTHECON	EQ 500MG BASE	N060516 001
	EQ 500MG BASE	N061911 001

Injectable; Injection
KANAMYCIN

ELKINS SINN	EQ 1GM BASE/3ML	N062324 003
	EQ 75MG BASE/2ML	N062324 001
	EQ 500MG BASE/2ML	N062324 002

KANAMYCIN SULFATE

AM PHARM PARTNERS	EQ 1GM BASE/3ML	N062504 003	APR 05, 1984
	EQ 75MG BASE/2ML	N062504 001	APR 05, 1984
	EQ 500MG BASE/2ML	N062504 002	APR 05, 1984
INTL MEDICATION	EQ 1GM BASE/3ML	N062466 002	SEP 30, 1983
	EQ 500MG BASE/2ML	N062466 001	SEP 30, 1983
LOCH	EQ 1GM BASE/3ML	N063025 001	JUL 31, 1992
	EQ 75MG BASE/2ML	N063021 001	JUL 31, 1992
	EQ 500MG BASE/2ML	N063022 001	JUL 31, 1992
PHARMAFAIR	EQ 1GM BASE/3ML	N062669 001	MAY 07, 1987
	EQ 75MG BASE/2ML	N062668 001	MAY 07, 1987
	EQ 500MG BASE/2ML	N062672 001	MAY 07, 1987
QUAD PHARMS	EQ 1GM BASE/3ML	N062642 003	FEB 03, 1986
	EQ 75MG BASE/2ML	N062642 001	FEB 03, 1986
	EQ 500MG BASE/2ML	N062642 002	FEB 03, 1986
SOLOPAK	EQ 1GM BASE/3ML	N062605 002	FEB 26, 1986
	EQ 75MG BASE/2ML	N062605 003	FEB 26, 1986
	EQ 500MG BASE/2ML	N062605 001	FEB 26, 1986
STERIS	EQ 1GM BASE/3ML	N062520 003	MAY 09, 1985
WARNER CHILCOTT	EQ 1GM BASE/3ML	N063092 001	

KANAMYCIN SULFATE (continued)
Injectable; Injection
KANAMYCIN SULFATE
WARNER CHILCOTT
KANTREX

APOTHECON	EQ 1GM BASE/3ML	N061655 002	OCT 11, 1989
	EQ 1GM BASE/3ML	N062564 003	SEP 21, 1984
	EQ 75MG BASE/2ML	N061655 003	
	EQ 75MG BASE/2ML	N062564 001	SEP 21, 1984
	EQ 500MG BASE/2ML	N061655 001	
	EQ 500MG BASE/2ML	N062564 002	SEP 21, 1984

KLEBCIL

KING PHARMS	EQ 1GM BASE/3ML	N062170 003
	EQ 75MG BASE/2ML	N062170 001
	EQ 500MG BASE/2ML	N062170 002

KETAMINE HYDROCHLORIDE
Injectable; Injection
KETAMINE HCL

QUAD PHARMS	EQ 10MG BASE/ML	N071949 001	APR 11, 1988
	EQ 50MG BASE/ML	N071950 001	APR 11, 1988
	EQ 100MG BASE/ML	N071951 001	APR 11, 1988

KETOCONAZOLE
Suspension; Oral
NIZORAL

JANSSEN	100MG/5ML	N070767 001	NOV 07, 1986

KETOPROFEN
Capsule; Oral
ORUDIS

WYETH AYERST	25MG	N018754 001	JUL 31, 1987
	50MG	N018754 002	JAN 09, 1986
	75MG	N018754 003	JAN 09, 1986

KETOROLAC TROMETHAMINE
Injectable; Injection
KETOROLAC TROMETHAMINE

APOTHECON	15MG/ML	N075348 001	NOV 28, 2000
	30MG/ML	N075348 002	NOV 28, 2000
BEDFORD	15MG/ML	N075230 002	OCT 25, 1999
	30MG/ML	N075230 001	

Discontinued Drug Products (continued)

KETOROLAC TROMETHAMINE (continued)
Injectable; Injection
- KETOROLAC TROMETHAMINE
  - BEDFORD — OCT 25, 1999

Tablet; Oral
- KETOROLAC TROMETHAMINE
  - ROXANE — 10MG — N074790 001 JUN 26, 1997

KRYPTON, KR-81M
Gas; Inhalation
- MPI KRYPTON 81M GAS GENERATOR
  - AMERSHAM HLTH — N/A — N018088 001

LABETALOL HYDROCHLORIDE
Injectable; Injection
- LABETALOL HCL
  - APOTHECON — 5MG/ML — N075355 001 NOV 29, 1999

Tablet; Oral
- NORMODYNE
  - SCHERING — 400MG — N018687 004 AUG 01, 1984
- TRANDATE
  - PROMETHEUS LABS — 400MG — N018716 004 AUG 01, 1984

LABETALOL HYDROCHLORIDE *MULTIPLE*
SEE HYDROCHLOROTHIAZIDE; LABETALOL HYDROCHLORIDE

LACTULOSE
Solution; Oral
- DUPHALAC
  - SOLVAY — 10GM/15ML — N072372 001 MAR 22, 1989
- LACTULOSE
  - MORTON GROVE — 10GM/15ML — N071841 001 SEP 22, 1988
  - PACO — 10GM/15ML — N073160 001 AUG 25, 1992

Solution; Oral, Rectal
- CEPHULAC
  - AVENTIS PHARMS — 10GM/15ML — N017657 001
- GENERLAC
  - MORTON GROVE — 10GM/15ML — N071842 001 SEP 27, 1988
- LACTULOSE
  - PACO — 10GM/15ML — N072029 001 AUG 25, 1992
  - ROXANE — 10GM/15ML — N073590 001 MAY 29, 1992
  - SOLVAY — 10GM/15ML — N017906 001
- PORTALAC
  - SOLVAY — 10GM/15ML — N072374 001 MAR 22, 1989

LAMOTRIGINE
Tablet, Chewable; Oral
- LAMICTAL CD
  - GLAXOSMITHKLINE — 100MG — N020764 003 AUG 24, 1998

Tablet; Oral
- LAMICTAL
  - GLAXOSMITHKLINE — 50MG — N020241 006 DEC 27, 1994
  - GLAXOSMITHKLINE — 250MG — N020241 004 DEC 27, 1994

LEFLUNOMIDE
Tablet; Oral
- ARAVA
  - AVENTIS PHARMS — 100MG — N020905 003 SEP 10, 1998

LEUCOVORIN CALCIUM
For Solution; Oral
- LEUCOVORIN CALCIUM
  - XANODYNE PHARM — EQ 60MG BASE/VIAL — N008107 003 JAN 30, 1987

Injectable; Injection
- LEUCOVORIN CALCIUM
  - ABIC — EQ 3MG BASE/VIAL — N089352 001 JUN 01, 1988
  - ABIC — EQ 50MG BASE/VIAL — N089353 001 JUN 01, 1988
  - AM PHARM PARTNERS — EQ 50MG BASE/VIAL — N088939 001 DEC 01, 1986
  - ELKINS SINN — EQ 50MG BASE/VIAL — N070480 001 JAN 02, 1987
  - ELKINS SINN — EQ 100MG BASE/VIAL — N081224 001 JUN 03, 1994
  - QUAD PHARMS — EQ 5MG BASE/ML — N089503 001 OCT 05, 1987
  - QUAD PHARMS — EQ 5MG BASE/ML — N089504 001 DEC 22, 1987
  - QUAD PHARMS — EQ 50MG BASE/VIAL — N089496 001 MAR 05, 1987
  - QUAD PHARMS — EQ 100MG BASE/VIAL — N089636 001 DEC 24, 1987
  - XANODYNE PHARM — EQ 3MG BASE/ML — N008107 001
- WELLCOVORIN
  - GLAXOSMITHKLINE — EQ 25MG BASE/VIAL — N089833 001 JAN 23, 1989
  - GLAXOSMITHKLINE — EQ 50MG BASE/VIAL — N089465 001 JAN 23, 1989
  - GLAXOSMITHKLINE — EQ 100MG BASE/VIAL — N089834 001 JAN 23, 1989

Tablet; Oral
- LEUCOVORIN CALCIUM
  - PAR PHARM — EQ 5MG BASE — N071600 001 OCT 14, 1987
  - PAR PHARM — EQ 25MG BASE — N071598 001

Discontinued Drug Products *(continued)*

LEUCOVORIN CALCIUM *(continued)*
Tablet; Oral
  LEUCOVORIN CALCIUM
    PAR PHARM   OCT 14, 1987
  LEUCOVORIN
  WELLCOVORIN
    GLAXOSMITHKLINE   EQ 5MG BASE   N018342 001   JUL 08, 1983
        EQ 25MG BASE   N018342 002   JUL 08, 1983

LEUPROLIDE ACETATE
Injectable; Injection
  LUPRON DEPOT-PED
    TAP PHARM   3.75MG/VIAL;7.5MG/VIAL   N020263 003   APR 16, 1993
        7.5MG/VIAL;7.5MG/VIAL   N020263 004   APR 16, 1993

LEVALLORPHAN TARTRATE
Injectable; Injection
  LORFAN
    ROCHE   1MG/ML   N010423 001

LEVOCARNITINE
Solution; Oral
  CARNITOR
    SIGMA TAU   1GM/10ML   N018948 002   APR 27, 1988

LEVODOPA
Capsule; Oral
  BENDOPA
    ICN   100MG   N016948 003
        250MG   N016948 001
        500MG   N016948 002
  DOPAR
    SHIRE LABS   100MG   N016913 003
        250MG   N016913 001
        500MG   N016913 002
  LARODOPA
    ROCHE   100MG   N016912 002
        250MG   N016912 001
        500MG   N016912 006
Tablet; Oral
  DOPAR
    SHIRE LABS   250MG   N016913 004
        500MG   N016913 005
  LARODOPA
    ROCHE   100MG   N016912 005
        250MG   N016912 003
        500MG   N016912 004

LEVODOPA *MULTIPLE*
  SEE   CARBIDOPA; LEVODOPA

LEVONORDEFRIN; MEPIVACAINE HYDROCHLORIDE
Injectable; Injection
  ARESTOCAINE HCL W/ LEVONORDEFRIN
    SOLVAY   0.05MG/ML;2%   N085010 001

LEVONORDEFRIN; PROCAINE HYDROCHLORIDE; PROPOXYCAINE HYDROCHLORIDE
Injectable; Injection
  RAVOCAINE AND NOVOCAIN W/ NEO-COBEFRIN
    EASTMAN KODAK   0.05MG/ML;2%;0.4%   N008592 007

LEVONORGESTREL
Implant; Implantation
  LEVONORGESTREL
    WYETH PHARMS INC   75MG/IMPLANT   N020627 001   AUG 15, 1996
  NORPLANT
    POPULATION COUNCIL   36MG/IMPLANT   N019897 001   DEC 10, 1990
  NORPLANT SYSTEM IN PLASTIC CONTAINER
    WYETH PHARMS INC   36MG/IMPLANT   N020088 001   DEC 10, 1990

LEVOPROPOXYPHENE NAPSYLATE, ANHYDROUS
Capsule; Oral
  NOVRAD
    LILLY   EQ 50MG BASE   N012928 006
        EQ 100MG BASE   N012928 004
Suspension; Oral
  NOVRAD
    LILLY   EQ 50MG BASE/5ML   N012928 002

LEVORPHANOL TARTRATE
Tablet; Oral
  LEVO-DROMORAN
    ICN   2MG   N008720 001   DEC 19, 1991

LIDOCAINE
Aerosol; Oral
  XYLOCAINE
    ASTRAZENECA   10%   N014394 001
Film, Extended Release; Buccal
  LIDOCAINE
    NOVEN   23MG/PATCH   N020575 001   MAY 21, 1996
Ointment; Topical
  ALPHACAINE
    CARLISLE   5%   N084944 001
        5%   N084946 001
  XYLOCAINE
    ASTRAZENECA   5%   N008048 001

Discontinued Drug Products (continued)

LIDOCAINE (continued)

Suppository; Rectal

Product	Applicant	Strength	Appl No
XYLOCAINE	ASTRAZENECA	100MG	N013077 001

LIDOCAINE *MULTIPLE*

SEE BACITRACIN ZINC; LIDOCAINE; NEOMYCIN SULFATE; POLYMYXIN B SULFATE
SEE CEFTRIAXONE SODIUM; LIDOCAINE

LIDOCAINE HYDROCHLORIDE

Injectable; Injection

Product	Applicant	Strength	Appl No	Date
ALPHACAINE HCL	CARLISLE	2%	N084721 001	
LIDOCAINE HCL	ABBOTT	1.5%	N088330 001	
		10%	N087980 001	MAY 17, 1984
		20%	N089362 001	FEB 02, 1983
				MAY 25, 1988
	AKORN	1%	N085037 001	
		2%	N085037 002	
	AM PHARM PARTNERS	1%	N080390 001	
		1%	N080420 001	
		1.5%	N086761 001	
		1%	N080420 005	
		2%	N017508 001	
		2%	N080390 002	
		2%	N080420 002	
		2%	N080420 004	
		4%	N086761 002	
		20%	N017508 002	
			N017508 004	
	BEL MAR	1%	N080710 001	
		2%	N080760 001	
	DELL LABS	1%	N083387 001	
		2%	N083388 001	
	ELKINS SINN	0.5%	N085131 001	
		1%	N080407 001	
		2%	N080407 002	
		4%	N084626 001	
	GD SEARLE LLC	1%	N083135 001	
		2%	N083135 002	
	INTL MEDICATION	1%	N017701 002	
		1GM/VIAL	N018543 001	
		2%	N017701 001	
		2GM/VIAL	N018543 002	
	MILES	1%	N080414 001	
		2%	N080414 002	
	STERIS	1%	N080377 001	
		2%	N083627 001	
		1%	N080377 002	
		2%	N083627 002	
	WYETH AYERST	1%	N083083 001	
		2%	N083083 002	

LIDOCAINE HYDROCHLORIDE (continued)

Injectable; Injection

Product	Applicant	Strength	Appl No	Date
LIDOCAINE HCL 0.1% AND DEXTROSE 5% IN PLASTIC CONTAINER	BAXTER HLTHCARE	100MG/100ML	N018461 001	
LIDOCAINE HCL 0.2% IN DEXTROSE 5% IN PLASTIC CONTAINER	ABBOTT	200MG/100ML	N018954 001	JUL 09, 1985
LIDOCAINE HCL PRESERVATIVE FREE	ELKINS SINN	1%	N084625 001	
		2%	N084625 002	
	INTL MEDICATION	4%	N017702 002	
LIDOCATON	PHARMATON	2%	N084727 001	AUG 17, 1983
XYLOCAINE	ASTRAZENECA	1%	N010418 005	
		1.5%	N010418 009	
		2%	N006488 002	
		2%	N010418 007	

Injectable; Spinal

Product	Applicant	Strength	Appl No	Date
XYLOCAINE 5% W/ GLUCOSE 7.5%	ASTRAZENECA	5%	N010496 002	JUL 07, 1982

Solution; Oral

Product	Applicant	Strength	Appl No	Date
LIDOCAINE HCL VISCOUS	INTL MEDICATION	2%	N086389 001	FEB 02, 1982

Solution; Topical

Product	Applicant	Strength	Appl No	Date
LARYNGOTRACHEAL ANESTHESIA KIT	KENDALL IL	4%	N087931 001	JUN 10, 1983
LIDOCAINE HCL	PACO	4%	N089688 001	JUN 30, 1989
PEDIATRIC LTA KIT	ABBOTT	2%	N088572 001	JUL 31, 1984

LIDOCAINE HYDROCHLORIDE *MULTIPLE*

SEE DEXAMETHASONE SODIUM PHOSPHATE; LIDOCAINE HYDROCHLORIDE
SEE DIHYDROERGOTAMINE MESYLATE; HEPARIN SODIUM; LIDOCAINE HYDROCHLORIDE
SEE EPINEPHRINE; LIDOCAINE HYDROCHLORIDE

LINCOMYCIN HYDROCHLORIDE

Capsule; Oral

Product	Applicant	Strength	Appl No
LINCOCIN	PHARMACIA AND UPJOHN	EQ 250MG BASE	N050316 001
		EQ 500MG BASE	N050316 002

Injectable; Injection

Product	Applicant	Strength	Appl No	Date
LINCOMYCIN HCL	QUAD PHARMS	EQ 300MG BASE/ML	N062784 001	MAR 14, 1988
	STERIS	EQ 300MG BASE/ML	N063180 001	

Discontinued Drug Products (continued)

LINCOMYCIN HYDROCHLORIDE (continued)
Injectable; Injection

LINCOMYCIN HCL			
STERIS			APR 16, 1991

LINDANE
Cream; Topical

KWELL			
REED AND CARNRICK	1%	N006309 001	
	1%	N084218 001	

Lotion; Topical

GAMENE			
SOLA BARNES HIND	1%	N084989 001	
KWELL			
REED AND CARNRICK	1%	N006309 003	
	1%	N084218 002	
SCABENE			
STIEFEL	1%	N086769 001	

Shampoo; Topical

GAMENE			
SOLA BARNES HIND	1%	N084988 001	
KWELL			
REED AND CARNRICK	1%	N010718 001	
	1%	N084219 001	
SCABENE			
STIEFEL	1%	N087940 001	APR 08, 1983

LINEZOLID
Tablet; Oral

ZYVOX			
PHARMACIA AND UPJOHN	400MG	N021130 001	APR 18, 2000

LIOTHYRONINE SODIUM
Tablet; Oral

LIOTHYRONINE SODIUM			
WATSON LAB	EQ 0.05MG BASE	N085753 001	FEB 03, 1982
	EQ 0.025MG BASE	N085755 001	JAN 25, 1982

LIOTRIX (T4;T3)
Tablet; Oral

EUTHROID-0.5		
PARKE DAVIS	0.03MG;0.0075MG	N016680 001
EUTHROID-1		
PARKE DAVIS	0.06MG;0.015MG	N016680 002
EUTHROID-2		
PARKE DAVIS	0.12MG;0.03MG	N016680 003
EUTHROID-3		
PARKE DAVIS	0.18MG;0.045MG	N016680 004

LIOTRIX (T4;T3) (continued)
Tablet; Oral

THYROLAR-5		
FORREST LABS	0.25MG;0.0625MG	N016807 006

LIPASE *MULTIPLE*
SEE PANCRELIPASE (AMYLASE;LIPASE;PROTEASE)

LITHIUM CARBONATE
Capsule; Oral

LITHIUM CARBONATE			
USL PHARMA	300MG	N072542 001	FEB 01, 1989
WATSON LAB	300MG	N070407 001	MAR 19, 1987
LITHONATE			
SOLVAY	300MG	N016782 001	

Tablet; Oral

ESKALITH			
GLAXOSMITHKLINE	300MG	N017971 001	
LITHANE			
BAYER PHARMS	300MG	N018833 001	JUL 18, 1985
LITHOTABS			
SOLVAY	300MG	N016980 001	

LITHIUM CITRATE
Syrup; Oral

LITHONATE		
SOLVAY	EQ 300MG CARBONATE/5ML	N017672 001

LOPERAMIDE HYDROCHLORIDE
Capsule; Oral

IMODIUM			
MCNEIL CONS SPECLT	2MG	N017690 001	
LOPERAMIDE HCL			
ROXANE	2MG	N073080 001	NOV 27, 1991

Solution; Oral

IMODIUM			
JANSSEN	1MG/5ML	N019037 001	JUL 31, 1984
LOPERAMIDE HCL			
ALPHARMA	1MG/5ML	N073187 001	SEP 15, 1992
WATSON LABS	1MG/5ML	N073062 001	MAY 28, 1993

Tablet; Oral

LOPERAMIDE HCL			
ABLE	2MG	N073528 001	NOV 30, 1993

Discontinued Drug Products (continued)

LORATADINE
Syrup; Oral

CLARITIN

Firm	Strength	NDA	Date
SCHERING	1MG/ML	N020641 001	OCT 10, 1996

Tablet, Orally Disintegrating; Oral

CLARITIN REDITABS

Firm	Strength	NDA	Date
SCHERING	10MG	N020704 001	DEC 23, 1996

Tablet; Oral

CLARITIN

Firm	Strength	NDA	Date
SCHERING	10MG	N019658 001	APR 12, 1993

LORAZEPAM
Tablet; Oral

LORAZ

Firm	Strength	NDA	Date
QUANTUM PHARMICS	0.5MG	N070200 001	AUG 09, 1985
	1MG	N070201 001	AUG 09, 1985
	2MG	N070202 001	AUG 09, 1985

LORAZEPAM

Firm	Strength	NDA	Date
AM THERAP	0.5MG	N070727 001	MAR 07, 1986
	1MG	N070728 001	MAR 07, 1986
	2MG	N070729 001	MAR 07, 1986
HALSEY	0.5MG	N070472 001	MAR 07, 1986
	0.5MG	N071434 001	DEC 10, 1985
	1MG	N070473 001	SEP 01, 1987
	1MG	N071435 001	DEC 10, 1985
	2MG	N070474 001	SEP 01, 1987
	2MG	N071436 001	DEC 10, 1985
PAR PHARM	0.5MG	N070675 001	SEP 01, 1987
	1MG	N070676 001	DEC 01, 1986
	2MG	N070677 001	DEC 01, 1986
SUPERPHARM	0.5MG	N071245 001	DEC 01, 1986
	1MG	N071246 001	FEB 09, 1987
	2MG	N071247 001	FEB 09, 1987
USL PHARMA	1MG	N070539 001	DEC 22, 1986

LORAZEPAM (continued)
Tablet; Oral

LORAZEPAM

Firm	Strength	NDA	Date
USL PHARMA	2MG	N070540 001	DEC 22, 1986
WARNER CHILCOTT	1MG	N071038 001	JAN 12, 1988
	2MG	N071039 001	JAN 12, 1988
WATSON LABS	0.5MG	N071086 001	MAR 23, 1987

LOTEPREDNOL ETABONATE
Suspension/Drops; Ophthalmic

LOTEMAX

Firm	Strength	NDA	Date
PHARMOS	0.5%	N020841 001	MAR 09, 1998

LOXAPINE HYDROCHLORIDE
Concentrate; Oral

LOXITANE C

Firm	Strength	NDA
WATSON LABS	EQ 25MG BASE/ML	N017658 001

Injectable; Injection

LOXITANE IM

Firm	Strength	NDA
WATSON LABS	EQ 50MG BASE/ML	N018039 001

LOXAPINE SUCCINATE
Tablet; Oral

LOXITANE

Firm	Strength	NDA
WATSON LABS	EQ 10MG BASE	N017525 006
	EQ 25MG BASE	N017525 007
	EQ 50MG BASE	N017525 008

LYPRESSIN
Solution; Nasal

DIAPID

Firm	Strength	NDA
NOVARTIS	0.185MG/ML	N016755 001

MAGNESIUM ACETATE *MULTIPLE*

SEE AMINO ACIDS; MAGNESIUM ACETATE; PHOSPHORIC ACID; POTASSIUM ACETATE; SODIUM CHLORIDE

SEE AMINO ACIDS; MAGNESIUM ACETATE; POTASSIUM ACETATE; SODIUM CHLORIDE

SEE AMINO ACIDS; MAGNESIUM ACETATE; POTASSIUM ACETATE; SODIUM CHLORIDE; SODIUM PHOSPHATE, DIBASIC, HEPTAHYDRATE

Discontinued Drug Products *(continued)*

MAGNESIUM CHLORIDE; POTASSIUM CHLORIDE; POTASSIUM PHOSPHATE, MONOBASIC; SODIUM ACETATE; SODIUM CHLORIDE; SODIUM GLUCONATE; SODIUM PHOSPHATE, DIBASIC, HEPTAHYDRATE
Injectable; Injection
ISOLYTE S PH 7.4 IN PLASTIC CONTAINER
  B BRAUN   30MG/100ML;37MG/100ML;0.82MG/100ML;370MG/100ML;530MG/100ML;500MG/100ML;12MG/100ML   N019006 001   APR 04, 1984

MAGNESIUM CHLORIDE; POTASSIUM CHLORIDE; SODIUM ACETATE; SODIUM CHLORIDE; SODIUM GLUCONATE
Solution; Irrigation
PHYSIOSOL IN PLASTIC CONTAINER
  ABBOTT   14MG/100ML;37MG/100ML;222MG/100ML;526MG/100ML;502MG/100ML   N018406 001

SYNOVALYTE IN PLASTIC CONTAINER
  BAXTER HLTHCARE   30MG/100ML;37MG/100ML;368MG/100ML;526MG/100ML;502MG/100ML   N019326 001   JAN 25, 1985

MAGNESIUM CHLORIDE *MULTIPLE*
SEE   AMINO ACIDS; CALCIUM CHLORIDE; DEXTROSE; MAGNESIUM CHLORIDE; POTASSIUM CHLORIDE; POTASSIUM PHOSPHATE, DIBASIC; SODIUM CHLORIDE
SEE   AMINO ACIDS; DEXTROSE; MAGNESIUM CHLORIDE; POTASSIUM ACETATE; POTASSIUM CHLORIDE; POTASSIUM PHOSPHATE, DIBASIC; SODIUM CHLORIDE
SEE   AMINO ACIDS; DEXTROSE; MAGNESIUM CHLORIDE; POTASSIUM CHLORIDE; POTASSIUM PHOSPHATE, DIBASIC; SODIUM CHLORIDE
SEE   AMINO ACIDS; DEXTROSE; MAGNESIUM CHLORIDE; SODIUM CHLORIDE
SEE   SODIUM CHLORIDE; MAGNESIUM CHLORIDE; SODIUM PHOSPHATE, DIBASIC, HEPTAHYDRATE
SEE   AMINO ACIDS; MAGNESIUM CHLORIDE; POTASSIUM ACETATE; POTASSIUM CHLORIDE; SODIUM ACETATE
SEE   AMINO ACIDS; MAGNESIUM CHLORIDE; POTASSIUM CHLORIDE; POTASSIUM PHOSPHATE, DIBASIC; SODIUM CHLORIDE
SEE   AMINO ACIDS; MAGNESIUM CHLORIDE; POTASSIUM CHLORIDE; SODIUM PHOSPHATE, DIBASIC; SODIUM CHLORIDE
SEE   CALCIUM CHLORIDE; DEXTROSE; MAGNESIUM CHLORIDE; POTASSIUM CHLORIDE; SODIUM ACETATE; SODIUM CHLORIDE
SEE   CALCIUM CHLORIDE; DEXTROSE; MAGNESIUM CHLORIDE; POTASSIUM CHLORIDE; SODIUM CITRATE
SEE   CALCIUM CHLORIDE; DEXTROSE; MAGNESIUM CHLORIDE; SODIUM CHLORIDE; SODIUM ACETATE; SODIUM CHLORIDE
SEE   CALCIUM CHLORIDE; DEXTROSE; MAGNESIUM CHLORIDE; SODIUM CHLORIDE; SODIUM LACTATE
SEE   CALCIUM CHLORIDE; MAGNESIUM CHLORIDE; POTASSIUM CHLORIDE; SODIUM ACETATE; SODIUM CHLORIDE
SEE   CALCIUM CHLORIDE; MAGNESIUM CHLORIDE; POTASSIUM CHLORIDE; SODIUM ACETATE; SODIUM CHLORIDE; SODIUM CITRATE

MAGNESIUM TRISILICATE *MULTIPLE*
SEE   ALUMINUM HYDROXIDE; MAGNESIUM TRISILICATE

MANGANESE CHLORIDE TETRAHYDRATE
For Solution; Oral
LUMENHANCE
  BRACCO   3.49MG/GM   N020686 001   DEC 19, 1997

MANGANESE SULFATE
Injectable; Injection
MANGANESE SULFATE
  AM PHARM PARTNERS   EQ 0.1MG MANGANESE/ML   N019228 001   MAY 05, 1987

MANNITOL
Injectable; Injection
MANNITOL 5%
  ABBOTT   5GM/100ML   N016269 001
MANNITOL 10%
  ABBOTT   10GM/100ML   N016269 002
  MILES   10GM/100ML   N016472 002
MANNITOL 15%
  ABBOTT   15GM/100ML   N016269 003
  MILES   15GM/100ML   N016472 005
MANNITOL 20%
  ABBOTT   20GM/100ML   N016269 004
  MILES   20GM/100ML   N016472 004
MANNITOL 25%
  ABBOTT   12.5GM/50ML   N016269 005
  AM PHARM PARTNERS   12.5GM/50ML   N086754 001
  ASTRAZENECA   12.5GM/50ML   N089239 001   MAY 06, 1987
     12.5GM/50ML   N089240 001   MAY 06, 1987
  MERCK   12.5GM/50ML   N005620 001
  STERIS   12.5GM/50ML   N087460 001   JUN 27, 1983

Solution; Irrigation
RESECTISOL
  B BRAUN   5GM/100ML   N016704 002

MANNITOL; SORBITOL
Solution; Irrigation
SORBITOL-MANNITOL
  ABBOTT   540MG/100ML;2.7GM/100ML   N080224 001

MAPROTILINE HYDROCHLORIDE
Tablet; Oral
MAPROTILINE HCL
  AM THERAP   25MG   N072129 001   JAN 14, 1988
     50MG   N072130 001   JAN 14, 1988

Discontinued Drug Products (continued)

MAPROTILINE HYDROCHLORIDE (continued)

Tablet; Oral

MAPROTILINE HCL

Manufacturer	Strength	Appl. No.	Date
AM THERAP	75MG	N072131 001	JAN 14, 1988
		N071943 001	
WATSON LAB	25MG		DEC 30, 1987
		N071944 001	DEC 30, 1987
	50MG	N071945 001	DEC 30, 1987
	75MG		DEC 30, 1987

MASOPROCOL

Cream; Topical

ACTINEX

Manufacturer	Strength	Appl. No.	Date
UNIV AZ CANCER CTR	10%	N019940 001	SEP 04, 1992

MAZINDOL

Tablet; Oral

MAZANOR

Manufacturer	Strength	Appl. No.
WYETH AYERST	1MG	N017980 002
	2MG	N017980 001

SANOREX

Manufacturer	Strength	Appl. No.
NOVARTIS	1MG	N017247 001
	2MG	N017247 002

MEBUTAMATE

Tablet; Oral

DORMATE

Manufacturer	Strength	Appl. No.
MEDPOINTE PHARM HLC	600MG	N017374 001

MECLIZINE HYDROCHLORIDE

Tablet; Chewable; Oral

MECLIZINE HCL

Manufacturer	Strength	Appl. No.
ANABOLIC	25MG	N086392 001
IVAX PHARMS	25MG	N084976 001

Tablet; Oral

MECLIZINE HCL

Manufacturer	Strength	Appl. No.	Date
ANABOLIC	25MG	N085891 001	
IVAX PHARMS	12.5MG	N083784 001	
KV PHARM	12.5MG	N085524 001	
	25MG	N085523 001	
SUPERPHARM	12.5MG	N089113 001	AUG 20, 1985
		N089114 001	AUG 20, 1985
	25MG	N088256 001	AUG 20, 1985
UDL	12.5MG	N088257 001	JUN 13, 1983
	25MG		JUN 13, 1983
		N087877 001	APR 20, 1982
VANGARD	12.5MG	N087620 001	JAN 04, 1982
	25MG		

MECLIZINE HYDROCHLORIDE (continued)

Tablet; Oral

MECLIZINE HCL

Manufacturer	Strength	Appl. No.
WATSON LAB	12.5MG	N085195 001
WATSON LABS	12.5MG	N085269 001

MECLOCYCLINE SULFOSALICYLATE

Cream; Topical

MECLAN

Manufacturer	Strength	Appl. No.
JOHNSON AND JOHNSON	1%	N050518 001

MECLOFENAMATE SODIUM

Capsule; Oral

MECLODIUM

Manufacturer	Strength	Appl. No.	Date
QUANTUM PHARMICS	EQ 50MG BASE	N071380 001	JUL 14, 1987
		N071381 001	JUL 14, 1987
	EQ 100MG BASE		JUL 14, 1987

MECLOFENAMATE SODIUM

Manufacturer	Strength	Appl. No.	Date
AM THERAP	EQ 50MG BASE	N071362 001	FEB 10, 1987
		N071363 001	FEB 10, 1987
	EQ 100MG BASE		FEB 10, 1987
BARR	EQ 50MG BASE	N072848 001	MAR 20, 1989
	EQ 100MG BASE	N072809 001	MAR 20, 1989
PAR PHARM	EQ 50MG BASE	N072077 001	MAR 10, 1988
	EQ 100MG BASE	N072078 001	MAR 10, 1988
USL PHARMA	EQ 50MG BASE	N071007 001	MAR 25, 1988
	EQ 100MG BASE	N071008 001	MAR 25, 1988
VITARINE	EQ 50MG BASE	N071710 001	JUN 15, 1988
	EQ 100MG BASE	N071684 001	JUN 15, 1988
WATSON LAB	EQ 50MG BASE	N070400 001	NOV 25, 1986
	EQ 100MG BASE	N070401 001	NOV 25, 1986
WATSON LABS	EQ 50MG BASE	N071640 001	AUG 11, 1987
	EQ 100MG BASE	N071641 001	AUG 11, 1987

MECLOMEN

Manufacturer	Strength	Appl. No.
PARKE DAVIS	EQ 50MG BASE	N018006 001
	EQ 100MG BASE	N018006 002

Discontinued Drug Products (continued)

MEDROXYPROGESTERONE ACETATE

Injectable; Injection

Product / Firm	Strength	Application No.	Date
DEPO-PROVERA			
PHARMACIA AND UPJOHN	100MG/ML *SEE ANNUAL PREFACE INTRODUCTION DISCONTINUED SECTION*	N012541 002	

Tablet; Oral

Product / Firm	Strength	Application No.	Date
AMEN			
AMARIN PHARMS	10MG	N083242 001	
CURRETAB			
SOLVAY	10MG	N085686 001	
CYCRIN			
ESI	2.5MG	N081239 001	OCT 30, 1992
	5MG	N081240 001	OCT 30, 1992
	10MG	N089386 001	SEP 09, 1987

MEDROXYPROGESTERONE ACETATE *MULTIPLE*
SEE   ESTROGENS, CONJUGATED; MEDROXYPROGESTERONE ACETATE

MEFLOQUINE HYDROCHLORIDE

Tablet; Oral

Product / Firm	Strength	Application No.	Date
MEFLOQUINE HCL			
US ARMY WALTER REED	250MG	N019578 001	MAY 02, 1989

MEGESTROL ACETATE

Tablet; Oral

Product / Firm	Strength	Application No.	Date
MEGESTROL ACETATE			
USL PHARMA	20MG	N070646 001	OCT 02, 1987
	40MG	N070647 001	OCT 02, 1987

MEGLUMINE *MULTIPLE*
SEE   CALCIUM; MEGLUMINE; METRIZOIC ACID

MEGLUMINE METRIZOATE *MULTIPLE*
SEE   CALCIUM METRIZOATE; MEGLUMINE METRIZOATE; METRIZOATE MAGNESIUM; METRIZOATE SODIUM

MENADIOL SODIUM DIPHOSPHATE

Injectable; Injection

Product / Firm	Strength	Application No.	Date
KAPPADIONE			
LILLY	10MG/ML	N005725 001	
SYNKAYVITE			
ROCHE	5MG/ML	N003718 004	
	10MG/ML	N003718 006	
	37.5MG/ML	N003718 008	

Tablet; Oral

Product / Firm	Strength	Application No.	Date
SYNKAYVITE			
ROCHE	5MG	N003718 010	

MENADIONE

Tablet; Oral

Product / Firm	Strength	Application No.	Date
MENADIONE			
LILLY	5MG	N002139 003	

MENOTROPINS (FSH;LH)

Injectable; Injection

Product / Firm	Strength	Application No.	Date
HUMEGON			
ORGANON USA INC	75 IU/VIAL;75 IU/VIAL	N020328 001	SEP 01, 1994
	150 IU/VIAL;150 IU/VIAL	N020328 002	SEP 01, 1994
MENOTROPINS			
FERRING	75 IU/VIAL;75 IU/VIAL	N073598 001	JAN 30, 1997
	150 IU/VIAL;150 IU/VIAL	N073599 001	JAN 30, 1997
PERGONAL			
SERONO	150 IU/AMP;150 IU/AMP	N017646 002	MAY 20, 1985
REPRONEX			
FERRING	150 IU/VIAL;150 IU/VIAL	N021047 002	AUG 27, 1999

MEPENZOLATE BROMIDE

Solution; Oral

Product / Firm	Strength	Application No.	Date
CANTIL			
AVENTIS PHARMS	25MG/5ML	N010679 004	

MEPERIDINE HYDROCHLORIDE

Injectable; Injection

Product / Firm	Strength	Application No.	Date
DEMEROL			
SANOFI SYNTHELABO	25MG/ML	N005010 007	
	50MG/ML	N005010 002	
	75MG/ML	N005010 009	
	100MG/ML	N005010 003	
MEPERIDINE HCL			
ABBOTT	25MG/ML	N080388 001	
	50MG/ML	N080385 001	
	50MG/ML	N080387 001	
	75MG/ML	N080389 001	
	100MG/ML	N080386 001	
	25MG/ML	N089781 001	MAR 31, 1989
ASTRAZENECA	50MG/ML	N089782 001	MAR 31, 1989
	50MG/ML	N089783 001	MAR 31, 1989
	50MG/ML	N089784 001	MAR 31, 1989
	75MG/ML	N089785 001	MAR 31, 1989
	100MG/ML	N089786 001	MAR 31, 1989
	100MG/ML	N089787 001	MAR 31, 1989

MEPREDNISONE

Tablet; Oral

Product / Applicant	Strength	Appl. No.
BETAPAR		
SCHERING	4MG	N016053 002

MEPROBAMATE

Capsule, Extended Release; Oral

Product / Applicant	Strength	Appl. No.
MEPROSPAN		
MEDPOINTE PHARM HLC	200MG	N011284 001
	400MG	N011284 002

Capsule; Oral

Product / Applicant	Strength	Appl. No.
EQUANIL		
WYETH-AYERST	400MG	N012455 002

Tablet; Oral

Product / Applicant	Strength	Appl. No.
AMOSENE		
FERNDALE LABS	400MG	N084030 001
BAMATE		
ALRA	200MG	N080380 001
	400MG	N080380 002
EQUANIL		
WYETH AYERST	200MG	N010028 005
	400MG	N010028 004
MEPRIAM		
TEVA	400MG	N016069 001
MEPROBAMATE		
ANABOLIC	200MG	N084220 001
	400MG	N084589 001
	600MG	N084230 001
BARR	200MG	N015426 002
	400MG	N015426 001
ELKINS SINN	200MG	N080699 001
	400MG	N080699 002
HALSEY	400MG	N016928 003
HEATHER	600MG	N084329 001
ICN	200MG	N015139 006
	400MG	N015139 005
IMPAX LABS	200MG	N014322 002
	400MG	N014322 001
IVAX PHARMS	200MG	N015438 001
	400MG	N015438 002
LANNETT	600MG	N084181 001
	200MG	N014882 002
	400MG	N014882 001
LEDERLE	400MG	N086299 001
LEE KM	400MG	N089538 001 (NOV 25, 1987)
MALLARD	400MG	N015072 002
MK LABS	200MG	N014368 004
	400MG	N014368 002
PARKE DAVIS	200MG	N084744 001
	400MG	N084744 002
PERRIGO	200MG	N084546 001
	400MG	N084547 001
PHARMAVITE	400MG	N084438 001
PHARMERAL	400MG	N084153 001
PUREPAC PHARM	200MG	N084804 001

Discontinued Drug Products *(continued)*

MEPERIDINE HYDROCHLORIDE *(continued)*

Injectable; Injection

Product / Applicant	Strength	Appl. No.	Date
MEPERIDINE HCL			
ASTRAZENECA	100MG/ML	N089788 001	MAR 31, 1989
ELKINS SINN	25MG/ML	N088279 001	MAR 31, 1989
	50MG/ML	N088280 001	JUN 15, 1984
	75MG/ML	N088281 001	JUN 15, 1984
	100MG/ML	N088282 001	JUN 15, 1984
INTL MEDICATION	10MG/ML	N086332 001	JUN 15, 1984
PARKE DAVIS	50MG/ML	N080364 002	
	75MG/ML	N080364 003	
	100MG/ML	N080364 001	

Tablet; Oral

Product / Applicant	Strength	Appl. No.
MEPERIDINE HCL		
WYETH AYERST	50MG	N080454 001

MEPERIDINE HYDROCHLORIDE; PROMETHAZINE HYDROCHLORIDE

Injectable; Injection

Product / Applicant	Strength	Appl. No.
MEPERGAN		
BAXTER HLTHCARE CORP	25MG/ML;25MG/ML	N011730 001

MEPERIDINE HYDROCHLORIDE *MULTIPLE*

SEE ATROPINE SULFATE: MEPERIDINE HYDROCHLORIDE

MEPHENTERMINE SULFATE

Injectable; Injection

Product / Applicant	Strength	Appl. No.
WYAMINE SULFATE		
BAXTER HLTHCARE CORP	EQ 15MG BASE/ML	N008248 002
	EQ 30MG BASE/ML	N008248 001

MEPHENYTOIN

Tablet; Oral

Product / Applicant	Strength	Appl. No.
MESANTOIN		
NOVARTIS	100MG	N006008 001

MEPIVACAINE HYDROCHLORIDE

Injectable; Injection

Product / Applicant	Strength	Appl. No.	Date
ARESTOCAINE HCL			
SOLVAY	3%	N084777 002	APR 18, 1982
MEPIVACAINE HCL			
INTL MEDICATION	1%	N087509 001	OCT 05, 1982

MEPIVACAINE HYDROCHLORIDE *MULTIPLE*

SEE LEVONORDEFRIN: MEPIVACAINE HYDROCHLORIDE

Discontinued Drug Products *(continued)*

MEPROBAMATE *(continued)*
Tablet; Oral

MEPROBAMATE			
PUREPAC PHARM	400MG		N084804 002
PVT FORM	400MG		N014601 001
SOLVAY	200MG		N084435 001
STANLABS PHARM	200MG		N014474 002
	400MG		N014474 004
USL PHARMA	200MG		N087825 001 MAR 18, 1982
	400MG		N087826 001 MAR 18, 1982
VANGARD	400MG		N088011 001 JUL 14, 1982
WATSON LABS	600MG		N084274 001
	600MG		N085719 001

MILTOWN			
WHITEWORTH TOWN	200MG		N083830 001
PLSN	400MG		N083442 001

MEDPOINTE PHARM HLC	600MG		N083919 001

NEURAMATE			
HALSEY	200MG		N014359 002
	400MG		N014359 001

TRANMEP			
SOLVAY	400MG		N084369 001

MEPROBAMATE *MULTIPLE*
SEE ASPIRIN; MEPROBAMATE
SEE ESTROGENS, CONJUGATED; MEPROBAMATE

MERSALYL SODIUM; THEOPHYLLINE
Injectable; Injection

MERSALYL-THEOPHYLLINE		
STERIS	100MG/ML;50MG/ML	N084875 001

MESALAMINE
Suppository; Rectal

ROWASA		
SOLVAY	500MG *SEE ANNUAL PREFACE INTRODUCTION DISCONTINUED SECTION*	N019919 001 DEC 18, 1990

MESORIDAZINE BESYLATE
Injectable; Injection

SERENTIL		
NOVARTIS	EQ 25MG BASE/ML	N016775 001

Tablet; Oral

SERENTIL		
NOVARTIS	EQ 10MG BASE	N016774 001
	EQ 50MG BASE	N016774 003

MESTRANOL; NORETHINDRONE
Tablet; Oral-20

NORINYL		
WATSON LABS	0.1MG;2MG	N013625 004

Tablet; Oral-21

NORINYL 1+80 21-DAY		
GD SEARLE LLC	0.08MG;1MG	N016724 001
ORTHO-NOVUM 1/80 21		
ORTHO MCNEIL PHARM	0.08MG;1MG	N016715 001
ORTHO-NOVUM 2-21		
ORTHO MCNEIL PHARM	0.1MG;2MG	N012728 005
ORTHO-NOVUM 10-21		
ORTHO MCNEIL PHARM	0.06MG;10MG	N012728 001

Tablet; Oral-28

NORINYL 1+80 28-DAY		
GD SEARLE LLC	0.08MG;1MG	N016725 001
ORTHO-NOVUM 1/80 28		
ORTHO MCNEIL PHARM	0.08MG;1MG	N016715 002

MESTRANOL; NORETHYNODREL
Tablet; Oral

ENOVID		
GD SEARLE LLC	0.15MG;9.85MG	N010976 005
	0.075MG;5MG	N010976 008

Tablet; Oral-20

ENOVID		
GD SEARLE LLC	0.075MG;5MG	N010976 004
ENOVID-E		
GD SEARLE LLC	0.1MG;2.5MG	N010976 006

Tablet; Oral-21

ENOVID-E 21		
GD SEARLE LLC	0.1MG;2.5MG	N010976 007

MESTRANOL *MULTIPLE*
SEE ETHYNODIOL DIACETATE; MESTRANOL

METAPROTERENOL SULFATE
Solution; Inhalation

ALUPENT		
BOEHRINGER INGELHEIM	5%	N017659 001

METAPROTERENOL SULFATE			
ASTRAZENECA	0.4%	JUL 27, 1988	N071275 001
	0.6%	JUL 27, 1988	N071018 001
DEY	0.5%	AUG 05, 1988	N071805 001
	0.33%	AUG 05, 1988	N071806 001
	5%	AUG 17, 1987	N070805 001
MORTON GROVE	5%	JUN 07, 1988	N072190 001

Discontinued Drug Products (continued)

METAPROTERENOL SULFATE (continued)

Solution; Inhalation

PROMETA			
MURO	5%	N073340 001	MAR 30, 1992

Syrup; Oral

ALUPENT			
BOEHRINGER INGELHEIM	10MG/5ML	N017571 001	
METAPROTERENOL SULFATE			
COPLEY PHARM	10MG/5ML	N073034 001	AUG 30, 1991
MORTON GROVE	10MG/5ML	N071656 001	OCT 13, 1987
TEVA	10MG/5ML	N072761 001	FEB 27, 1992
PROMETA			
MURO	10MG/5ML	N072023 001	SEP 15, 1988

Tablet; Oral

ALUPENT			
BOEHRINGER INGELHEIM	10MG	N015874 002	
	20MG	N015874 001	
METAPROTERENOL SULFATE			
AM THERAP	10MG	N072054 001	JUN 23, 1988
	20MG	N072055 001	JUN 23, 1988
USL PHARMA	10MG	N071013 001	JAN 25, 1988
	20MG	N071014 001	JAN 25, 1988

METARAMINOL BITARTRATE

Injectable; Injection

METARAMINOL BITARTRATE		
AM PHARM PARTNERS	EQ 10MG BASE/ML	N080431 001
ELKINS SINN	EQ 10MG BASE/ML	N083363 001
GD SEARLE LLC	EQ 10MG BASE/ML	N086418 001
	EQ 20MG BASE/ML	N086418 002

METFORMIN HYDROCHLORIDE

Tablet; Oral

GLUCOPHAGE			
BRISTOL MYERS SQUIBB	625MG *SEE ANNUAL PREFACE INTRODUCTION DISCONTINUED SECTION*	N020357 003	NOV 05, 1998
	750MG *SEE ANNUAL PREFACE INTRODUCTION DISCONTINUED SECTION*	N020357 004	NOV 05, 1998

METHACYCLINE HYDROCHLORIDE

Capsule; Oral

RONDOMYCIN		
MEDPOINTE PHARM HLC	EQ 140MG BASE	N060641 001
	EQ 280MG BASE	N060641 002

Syrup; Oral

RONDOMYCIN		
MEDPOINTE PHARM HLC	EQ 70MG BASE/5ML	N060641 003

METHADONE HYDROCHLORIDE

Syrup; Oral

DOLOPHINE HCL		
ROXANE	10MG/30ML	N006134 004

Tablet, Dispersible; Oral

WESTADONE		
EON	2.5MG	N017108 001

Tablet, Effervescent; Oral

WESTADONE		
EON	5MG	N017108 002
	10MG	N017108 003
	40MG	N017108 004

METHAMPHETAMINE HYDROCHLORIDE

Tablet, Extended Release; Oral

DESOXYN		
OVATION PHARMS	5MG	N005378 004
	10MG	N005378 003
	15MG	N005378 005

Tablet; Oral

METHAMPEX		
TEVA	10MG	N083889 001
METHAMPHETAMINE HCL		
REXAR	5MG	N084931 001
	10MG	N084931 002
TEVA	5MG	N086359 001

METHANTHELINE BROMIDE

Tablet; Oral

BANTHINE		
SHIRE LABS	50MG	N007390 001

METHARBITAL

Tablet; Oral

GEMONIL		
ABBOTT	100MG	N008322 001

METHAZOLAMIDE

Tablet; Oral

METHAZOLAMIDE			
APPLIED ANAL	25MG	N040011 001	JUL 17, 1997
	50MG	N040011 002	JUL 17, 1997

METHOCARBAMOL (continued)

Tablet; Oral
METHOCARBAMOL

Firm	Strength	Appl. No.	Date
ASCOT	750MG	N087661 001	OCT 27, 1982
		N084488 001	
HALSEY	500MG	N084486 001	
	750MG	N084675 001	
HEATHER	500MG	N084924 001	
	750MG	N085137 001	
INWOOD LABS	500MG	N084648 001	
IVAX PHARMS	500MG	N084649 001	
	750MG		
KV PHARM	500MG	N085658 001	
	750MG	N085660 001	
LEDERLE	500MG	N085961 001	
	750MG	N085963 001	
MYLAN	500MG	N084259 001	
	750MG	N084323 001	
PHARMERAL	500MG	N084231 002	
	750MG	N084471 001	
PIONEER PHARMS	500MG	N088731 001	DEC 13, 1985
	750MG	N089082 001	DEC 13, 1985
PUREPAC PHARM	500MG	N085718 001	
	750MG	N085718 002	
ROXANE	500MG	N088646 001	
	750MG	N088647 001	FEB 29, 1984
SOLVAY	500MG	N084448 001	FEB 29, 1984
	750MG	N084449 001	
UPSHER SMITH	500MG	N087453 001	
WATSON LAB	500MG	N087454 001	
	750MG	N083605 001	
	750MG	N083605 002	

METHOCARBAMOL *MULTIPLE*

SEE ASPIRIN; METHOCARBAMOL

METHOTREXATE SODIUM

Injectable; Injection
ABITREXATE

Firm	Strength	Appl. No.	Date
ABIC	EQ 25MG BASE/ML	N089161 001	MAR 10, 1987
	EQ 50MG BASE/VIAL	N089354 001	JUL 17, 1987
	EQ 100MG BASE/VIAL	N089355 001	JUL 17, 1987
	EQ 250MG BASE/VIAL	N089356 001	JUL 17, 1987
FOLEX PFS			
PHARMACIA AND UPJOHN	EQ 25MG BASE/ML	N081242 001	AUG 23, 1991
	EQ 25MG BASE/ML	N089180 001	

Discontinued Drug Products (continued)

METHAZOLAMIDE (continued)

Tablet; Oral
NEPTAZANE

Firm	Strength	Appl. No.	Date
LEDERLE	25MG	N011721 002	NOV 25, 1991
	50MG	N011721 001	

METHDILAZINE

Tablet, Chewable; Oral
TACARYL

Firm	Strength	Appl. No.
WESTWOOD SQUIBB	3.6MG	N011950 009

METHDILAZINE HYDROCHLORIDE

Syrup; Oral
METHDILAZINE HCL

Firm	Strength	Appl. No.
ALPHARMA	4MG/5ML	N087122 001

TACARYL

Firm	Strength	Appl. No.
WESTWOOD SQUIBB	4MG/5ML	N011950 007

Tablet; Oral
TACARYL

Firm	Strength	Appl. No.
WESTWOOD SQUIBB	8MG	N011950 006

METHICILLIN SODIUM

Injectable; Injection
STAPHCILLIN

Firm	Strength	Appl. No.
APOTHECON	EQ 3.6GM BASE/VIAL	N050117 002
	EQ 3.6GM BASE/VIAL	N061449 002
	EQ 5.4GM BASE/VIAL	N050117 003
	EQ 5.4GM BASE/VIAL	N061449 003
	EQ 900MG BASE/VIAL	N050117 001
	EQ 900MG BASE/VIAL	N061449 001

METHIXENE HYDROCHLORIDE

Tablet; Oral
TREST

Firm	Strength	Appl. No.
NOVARTIS	1MG	N013420 001

METHOCARBAMOL

Injectable; Injection
METHOCARBAMOL

Firm	Strength	Appl. No.	Date
MARSAM PHARMS LLC	100MG/ML	N089849 001	DEC 27, 1991

Tablet; Oral
METHOCARBAMOL
DELAXIN

Firm	Strength	Appl. No.	Date
FERNDALE LABS	500MG	N085454 001	

FORBAXIN

Firm	Strength	Appl. No.
FORREST LABS	750MG	N085136 001

METHOCARBAMOL

Firm	Strength	Appl. No.	Date
AM THERAP	500MG	N089417 001	FEB 11, 1987
	750MG	N089418 001	FEB 11, 1987
ASCOT	500MG	N087660 001	OCT 27, 1982

Discontinued Drug Products (continued)

METHOTREXATE SODIUM (continued)

Injectable; Injection

Product / Applicant	Strength	Appl. No.	Date
FOLEX PFS			JAN 03, 1986
PHARMACIA AND UPJOHN			
METHOTREXATE SODIUM			
AM PHARM PARTNERS			
	EQ 2.5MG BASE/ML	N089323 001	JUN 13, 1986
	EQ 20MG BASE/VIAL	N088935 001	OCT 11, 1985
	EQ 25MG BASE/ML	N089263 001	JUN 13, 1986
	EQ 25MG BASE/ML	N089322 001	JUN 13, 1986
	EQ 50MG BASE/VIAL	N088936 001	OCT 11, 1985
	EQ 100MG BASE/VIAL	N088937 001	OCT 11, 1985
QUAD PHARMS			
	EQ 20MG BASE/VIAL	N089293 001	JUL 10, 1986
	EQ 25MG BASE/ML	N089308 001	JUL 10, 1986
	EQ 25MG BASE/ML	N089309 001	JUL 10, 1986
	EQ 50MG BASE/VIAL	N089294 001	JUL 10, 1986
	EQ 100MG BASE/VIAL	N089295 001	JUL 10, 1986
	EQ 250MG BASE/VIAL	N089296 001	JUL 10, 1986
WYETH PHARMS INC			
	EQ 2.5MG BASE/ML	N011719 004	
	EQ 50MG BASE/VIAL	N011719 003	
	EQ 100MG BASE/VIAL	N011719 006	
MEXATE			
BRISTOL			
	EQ 20MG BASE/VIAL	N086358 001	
	EQ 50MG BASE/VIAL	N086358 002	
	EQ 100MG BASE/VIAL	N086358 003	
	EQ 250MG BASE/VIAL	N086358 004	
MEXATE-AQ PRESERVED			
BRISTOL MYERS SQUIBB			
	EQ 25MG BASE/ML	N089887 001	APR 14, 1989

METHOTRIMEPRAZINE

Injectable; Injection

Product / Applicant	Strength	Appl. No.
LEVOPROME		
IMMUNEX	20MG/ML	N015865 001

METHOXAMINE HYDROCHLORIDE

Injectable; Injection

Product / Applicant	Strength	Appl. No.
VASOXYL		
GLAXOSMITHKLINE	10MG/ML	N006772 002
	20MG/ML	N006772 001

METHOXSALEN

Capsule; Oral

Product / Applicant	Strength	Appl. No.	Date
METHOXSALEN			
GENEVA PHARMS	10MG	N087781 001	JUN 08, 1982

METHOXYFLURANE

Liquid; Inhalation

Product / Applicant	Strength	Appl. No.
PENTHRANE		
ABBOTT	99.9%	N013056 001

METHSCOPOLAMINE BROMIDE

Tablet; Oral

Product / Applicant	Strength	Appl. No.
METHSCOPOLAMINE BROMIDE		
PVT FORM	2.5MG	N080970 001

METHYCLOTHIAZIDE

Tablet; Oral

Product / Applicant	Strength	Appl. No.	Date
AQUATENSEN			
MEDPOINTE PHARM HLC	5MG	N017364 001	
METHYCLOTHIAZIDE			
IVAX PHARMS	5MG	N087786 001	MAY 18, 1982
	2.5MG	N087671 001	AUG 17, 1982
MYLAN	2.5MG	N089135 001	FEB 12, 1986
PAR PHARM	2.5MG	N089136 001	FEB 12, 1986
	5MG	N088745 001	MAR 21, 1985
USL PHARMA	5MG	N085487 001	MAR 11, 1982
WATSON LAB	2.5MG	N085476 001	MAR 11, 1982
	5MG	N088750 001	SEP 06, 1984
WATSON LABS	2.5MG		

METHYCLOTHIAZIDE; PARGYLINE HYDROCHLORIDE

Tablet; Oral

Product / Applicant	Strength	Appl. No.
EUTRON		
ABBOTT	5MG;25MG	N016047 001

METHYCLOTHIAZIDE; RESERPINE

Tablet; Oral

Product / Applicant	Strength	Appl. No.
DIUTENSEN-R		
MEDPOINTE PHARM HLC	2.5MG;0.1MG	N012708 005

METHYCLOTHIAZIDE *MULTIPLE*

SEE DESERPIDINE; METHYCLOTHIAZIDE

Discontinued Drug Products (continued)

METHYLDOPA
Suspension; Oral
ALDOMET
- MERCK — 250MG/5ML — N018389 001

Tablet; Oral
ALDOMET
- MERCK — 125MG — N013400 003
- MERCK — 250MG — N013400 001

METHYLDOPA
- DURAMED PHARM BARR — 250MG — N071006 001 — DEC 16, 1986
- DURAMED PHARM BARR — 500MG — N071009 001 — DEC 16, 1986
- HALSEY — 125MG — N070073 001 — OCT 09, 1986
- HALSEY — 125MG — N071751 001 — MAR 28, 1988
- HALSEY — 250MG — N070060 001 — OCT 09, 1986
- HALSEY — 250MG — N071752 001 — MAR 28, 1988
- HALSEY — 500MG — N070074 001 — OCT 09, 1986
- HALSEY — 500MG — N071753 001 — MAR 28, 1988
- LEDERLE — 125MG — N070070 003 — OCT 15, 1985
- PARKE DAVIS — 125MG — N070331 001 — APR 15, 1986
- PARKE DAVIS — 250MG — N070332 001 — APR 15, 1986
- PARKE DAVIS — 500MG — N070333 001 — APR 15, 1986
- PUREPAC PHARM — 125MG — N070749 001 — FEB 07, 1986
- PUREPAC PHARM — 250MG — N070750 001 — FEB 07, 1986
- PUREPAC PHARM — 500MG — N070452 001 — FEB 07, 1986
- ROXANE — 125MG — N070192 001 — APR 25, 1986
- ROXANE — 250MG — N070193 001 — APR 25, 1986
- ROXANE — 500MG — N070194 001 — APR 25, 1986
- TEVA — 125MG — N071105 001 — DEC 05, 1986
- TEVA — 250MG — N071106 001 — DEC 05, 1986
- TEVA — 500MG — N071067 001 — DEC 05, 1986
- WATSON LAB — 125MG — N070245 001 — FEB 25, 1986
- WATSON LAB — 250MG — N070246 001 — FEB 25, 1986
- WATSON LAB — 500MG — N070247 001 — FEB 25, 1986

METHYLDOPA (continued)
Tablet; Oral
METHYLDOPA
- WATSON LABS — 125MG — N070260 001 — JUN 24, 1985
- WATSON LABS — 250MG — N070261 001 — JUN 24, 1985
- WATSON LABS — 500MG — N070262 001 — JUN 24, 1985

METHYLDOPA *MULTIPLE*
SEE CHLOROTHIAZIDE; METHYLDOPA
SEE HYDROCHLOROTHIAZIDE; METHYLDOPA

METHYLDOPATE HYDROCHLORIDE
Injectable; Injection
METHYLDOPATE HCL
- AM PHARM PARTNERS — 50MG/ML — N070652 001 — JUN 03, 1986
- ELKINS SINN — 50MG/ML — N070291 001 — JUL 01, 1986
- FAULDING — 50MG/ML — N070691 001 — JUN 19, 1987
- FAULDING — 50MG/ML — N070849 001 — JUN 19, 1987
- MARSAM PHARMS LLC — 50MG/ML — N071812 001 — DEC 22, 1987
- QUAD PHARMS — 50MG/ML — N071024 001 — SEP 18, 1986
- SMITH AND NEPHEW — 50MG/ML — N070841 001 — JAN 02, 1987

METHYLPREDNISOLONE
Tablet; Oral
METHYLPREDNISOLONE
- EON — 4MG — N087341 001
- HEATHER — 4MG — N085650 001
- WATSON LABS — 4MG — N086161 001 — FEB 09, 1982
- WATSON LABS — 16MG — N086159 001 — FEB 09, 1982

METHYLPREDNISOLONE; NEOMYCIN SULFATE
Ointment; Ophthalmic
NEO-MEDROL
- PHARMACIA AND UPJOHN — 0.1%;EQ 3.5MG BASE/GM — N060645 001

METHYLPREDNISOLONE ACETATE
Enema; Rectal
MEDROL
- PHARMACIA AND UPJOHN — 40MG/BOT — N018102 001

Discontinued Drug Products (continued)

METHYLPREDNISOLONE ACETATE (continued)
Injectable; Injection

Product / Firm	Strength	Appl No	Date
M-PREDROL			
BEL MAR	40MG/ML	N086666 001	
	80MG/ML	N087135 001	
METHYLPREDNISOLONE ACETATE			
AKORN	40MG/ML	N086903 001	OCT 20, 1982
	80MG/ML	N086903 002	OCT 20, 1982
STERIS	20MG/ML	N085597 001	
	20MG/ML	N087248 001	
	40MG/ML	N085374 001	
	40MG/ML	N085600 001	
	80MG/ML	N085595 001	
	80MG/ML	N086507 001	

Ointment; Topical

Product / Firm	Strength	Appl No
MEDROL ACETATE		
PHARMACIA AND	0.25%	N012421 001
UPJOHN	1%	N012421 002

METHYLPREDNISOLONE ACETATE; NEOMYCIN SULFATE
Cream; Topical

Product / Firm	Strength	Appl No
NEO-MEDROL ACETATE		
PHARMACIA AND	0.25%;EQ 3.5MG BASE/GM	N060611 002
UPJOHN	1%;EQ 3.5MG BASE/GM	N060611 001

METHYLPREDNISOLONE SODIUM SUCCINATE
Injectable; Injection

Firm	Strength	Appl No	Date
A-METHAPRED			
ABBOTT	EQ 1GM BASE/VIAL	N089576 001	FEB 22, 1991
	EQ 40MG BASE/VIAL	N089573 001	FEB 22, 1991
	EQ 125MG BASE/VIAL	N089574 001	FEB 22, 1991
	EQ 500MG BASE/VIAL	N089575 001	FEB 22, 1991
METHYLPREDNISOLONE			
ELKINS SINN	EQ 1GM BASE/VIAL	N086906 004	
	EQ 125MG BASE/VIAL	N086906 002	
	EQ 500MG BASE/VIAL	N086906 003	
ORGANON USA INC	EQ 1GM BASE/VIAL	N087535 002	JUN 25, 1982
	EQ 500MG BASE/VIAL	N087535 001	JUN 25, 1982
METHYLPREDNISOLONE SODIUM SUCCINATE			
AM PHARM PARTNERS	EQ 40MG BASE/VIAL	N088676 001	JUN 08, 1984
	EQ 125MG BASE/VIAL	N088677 001	JUN 08, 1984
	EQ 500MG BASE/VIAL	N088678 001	JUN 08, 1984
	EQ 1GM BASE/VIAL	N088679 001	JUN 08, 1984

METHYLPREDNISOLONE SODIUM SUCCINATE (continued)
Injectable; Injection
METHYLPREDNISOLONE SODIUM SUCCINATE

Firm	Strength	Appl No	Date
AM PHARM PARTNERS	EQ 40MG BASE/VIAL	N089143 001	MAR 28, 1986
	EQ 125MG BASE/VIAL	N089144 001	MAR 28, 1986
	EQ 500MG BASE/VIAL	N089186 001	MAR 28, 1986
	EQ 500MG BASE/VIAL	N089187 001	MAR 28, 1986
	EQ 1GM BASE/VIAL	N089188 001	MAR 28, 1986
	EQ 1GM BASE/VIAL	N089189 001	MAR 28, 1986
ELKINS SINN	EQ 40MG BASE/VIAL	N086906 001	
	EQ 500MG BASE/VIAL	N081267 001	NOV 30, 1992
GENS A SICOR PHARMS	EQ 1GM BASE/VIAL	N081268 001	NOV 30, 1992
INTL MEDICATION	EQ 40MG BASE/VIAL	N087812 001	FEB 09, 1983
	EQ 125MG BASE/VIAL	N087813 001	FEB 09, 1983
	EQ 500MG BASE/VIAL	N087851 001	FEB 09, 1983
	EQ 1GM BASE/VIAL	N087852 001	FEB 09, 1983
QUAD PHARMS	EQ 40MG BASE/VIAL	N089264 001	JAN 22, 1986
	EQ 125MG BASE/VIAL	N089265 001	JAN 22, 1986
	EQ 500MG BASE/VIAL	N089266 001	JAN 22, 1986
	EQ 1GM BASE/VIAL	N089267 001	JAN 22, 1986
STERIS	EQ 40MG BASE/VIAL	N086953 001	JUL 22, 1982
	EQ 125MG BASE/VIAL	N087030 001	JUL 22, 1982
	EQ 500MG BASE/VIAL	N088523 001	JUL 24, 1984
	EQ 1GM BASE/VIAL	N088524 001	JUL 24, 1984

METHYLTESTOSTERONE
Capsule; Oral

Product / Firm	Strength	Appl No
METHYLTESTOSTERONE		
HEATHER	10MG	N084967 001

Tablet; Buccal

Product / Firm	Strength	Appl No
ANDRO ID 5		
ICN	5MG	N087222 001
ORETON		
SCHERING	10MG	N080281 001

Discontinued Drug Products (continued)

METHYLTESTOSTERONE (continued)

Tablet; Buccal/Sublingual

Product / Firm	Strength	Appl. No.
METANDREN		
NOVARTIS	5MG	N003240 004
	10MG	N003240 005
METHYLTESTOSTERONE		
IMPAX LABS	10MG	N084287 001
LILLY	10MG	N080256 001
PUREPAC PHARM	10MG	N080308 001
	10MG	N080475 001
PVT FORM	5MG	N083836 001
TABLICAPS	10MG	N085125 001
USL PHARMA	10MG	N080271 001

Tablet; Oral

Product / Firm	Strength	Appl. No.
METANDREN		
NOVARTIS	10MG	N003240 001
	25MG	N003240 003
METHYLTESTOSTERONE		
INWOOD LABS	10MG	N080839 001
	25MG	N080973 001
KV PHARM	10MG	N084312 001
LANNETT	10MG	N087092 001 NOV 05, 1982
	25MG	N087111 001 JAN 27, 1983
LILLY	25MG	N080256 002
PARKE DAVIS	10MG	N084244 001
	25MG	N084241 001
PUREPAC PHARM	10MG	N080309 001
	25MG	N080475 002
	25MG	N080310 001
	5MG	N080475 003
PVT FORM	10MG	N080214 001
	10MG	N080214 002
	25MG	N080214 003
TABLICAPS	10MG	N080313 001
	25MG	N085270 001
WATSON LABS	10MG	N080933 001
WEST WARD	10MG	N080931 001
	10MG	N084331 001
	25MG	N084331 002
	25MG	N084642 001
ORETON METHYL		
SCHERING	10MG	N003158 001
	25MG	N003158 002

METHYPRYLON

Capsule; Oral

Product / Firm	Strength	Appl. No.
NOLUDAR		
ROCHE	300MG	N009660 008

Elixir; Oral

Product / Firm	Strength	Appl. No.
NOLUDAR		
ROCHE	50MG/5ML	N009660 007

Tablet; Oral

Product / Firm	Strength	Appl. No.
NOLUDAR		
ROCHE	50MG	N009660 002

METHYPRYLON (continued)

Tablet; Oral

Product / Firm	Strength	Appl. No.
NOLUDAR		
ROCHE	200MG	N009660 004

METHYSERGIDE MALEATE

Tablet; Oral

Product / Firm	Strength	Appl. No.
SANSERT		
NOVARTIS	2MG	N012516 001

METOCLOPRAMIDE HYDROCHLORIDE

Injectable; Injection

Product / Firm	Strength	Appl. No.	Date
METOCLOPRAMIDE HCL			
ABBOTT	EQ 5MG BASE/ML	N070506 001	JUN 22, 1989
	EQ 10MG BASE/2ML	N070293 001	JAN 24, 1986
AM PHARM PARTNERS	EQ 5MG BASE/ML	N072155 001	MAR 30, 1992
BEDFORD	EQ 5MG BASE/ML	N072244 001	MAR 30, 1992
	EQ 5MG BASE/ML	N072247 001	MAY 18, 1992
FAULDING	EQ 5MG BASE/ML	N071990 001	JAN 18, 1989
NORBROOK	EQ 10MG BASE/2ML	N070892 001	AUG 26, 1988
QUAD PHARMS	EQ 10MG BASE/2ML	N070671 001	MAY 27, 1986
SMITH AND NEPHEW	EQ 5MG BASE/ML	N070623 001	MAR 02, 1987
	EQ 10MG BASE/2ML	N070622 001	MAR 02, 1987
REGLAN			
ROBINS AH	EQ 10MG BASE/ML	N017862 004	MAY 28, 1987

Solution; Oral

Product / Firm	Strength	Appl. No.	Date
METOCLOPRAMIDE HCL			
MORTON GROVE	EQ 5MG BASE/5ML	N070949 001	MAR 06, 1987
PACO	EQ 5MG BASE/5ML	N071665 001	DEC 05, 1988
REGLAN			
ROBINS AH	EQ 5MG BASE/5ML	N018821 001	MAR 25, 1983

Tablet; Oral

Product / Firm	Strength	Appl. No.	Date
CLOPRA			
QUANTUM PHARMICS	EQ 5MG BASE	N072384 001	JUN 02, 1988
	EQ 10MG BASE	N070294 001	JUL 29, 1985
CLOPRA-"YELLOW"			
QUANTUM PHARMICS	EQ 10MG BASE	N070632 001	OCT 28, 1985
MAXOLON			
KING PHARMS	EQ 10MG BASE	N070106 001	

Discontinued Drug Products *(continued)*

METOCLOPRAMIDE HYDROCHLORIDE *(continued)*
Tablet; Oral

MAXOLON			
KING PHARMS			MAR 04, 1986
METOCLOPRAMIDE HCL			
HALSEY	EQ 10MG BASE		N070660 001
			FEB 10, 1987
	EQ 10MG BASE		N070906 001
			OCT 28, 1986
INTERPHARM	EQ 10MG BASE		N071213 001
			SEP 24, 1986
INVAMED	EQ 5MG BASE		N072436 001
			JUN 22, 1989
	EQ 10MG BASE		N070850 001
			FEB 03, 1987
LEDERLE	EQ 10MG BASE		N072639 001
			MAY 09, 1991
MUTUAL PHARM	EQ 5MG BASE		N071536 002
			JAN 16, 1997
	EQ 10MG BASE		N071536 001
			APR 28, 1993
PAR PHARM	EQ 10MG BASE		N070342 001
			MAR 25, 1986
SCHERING	EQ 10MG BASE		N070598 001
			FEB 02, 1987
SUPERPHARM	EQ 10MG BASE		N070926 001
			JUN 26, 1987
USL PHARMA	EQ 10MG BASE		N070339 001
			JUL 29, 1985
WATSON LAB	EQ 10MG BASE		N070363 001
			MAR 02, 1987
WATSON LABS	EQ 10MG BASE		N070453 001
			JUN 06, 1986
	EQ 10MG BASE		N070645 001
			MAY 11, 1987

METOCURINE IODIDE
Injectable; Injection

METOCURINE IODIDE		
QUAD PHARMS	2MG/ML	N089443 001
		JUN 01, 1988
METUBINE IODIDE		
LILLY	2MG/ML	N006632 003

METOLAZONE
Tablet; Oral

DIULO		
GD SEARLE LLC	2.5MG	N018535 001
	5MG	N018535 002
	10MG	N018535 003

METOPROLOL FUMARATE
Tablet, Extended Release; Oral

LOPRESSOR		
NOVARTIS	EQ 100MG TARTRATE	N019786 001
		DEC 27, 1989

METOPROLOL FUMARATE *(continued)*
Tablet, Extended Release; Oral

LOPRESSOR		
NOVARTIS	EQ 200MG TARTRATE	N019786 002
		DEC 27, 1989
	EQ 300MG TARTRATE	N019786 003
		DEC 27, 1989
	EQ 400MG TARTRATE	N019786 004
		DEC 27, 1989

METOPROLOL TARTRATE
Tablet; Oral

METOPROLOL TARTRATE		
PUREPAC PHARM	50MG	N074380 001
		JUL 29, 1994
	100MG	N074380 002
		JUL 29, 1994

METOPROLOL TARTRATE *MULTIPLE*
SEE   CHLORTHALIDONE; METOPROLOL TARTRATE

METRIZAMIDE
Injectable; Injection

AMIPAQUE		
AMERSHAM HLTH	2.5GM/VIAL	N017982 003
		SEP 12, 1983
	3.75GM/VIAL	N017982 001
		JUN 26, 1987
	6.75GM/VIAL	N017982 002
	13.5GM/VIAL	N017982 004
		SEP 12, 1983

METRIZOATE MAGNESIUM *MULTIPLE*
SEE   CALCIUM METRIZOATE; MEGLUMINE METRIZOATE; METRIZOATE MAGNESIUM; METRIZOATE SODIUM

METRIZOATE SODIUM *MULTIPLE*
SEE   CALCIUM METRIZOATE; MEGLUMINE METRIZOATE; METRIZOATE MAGNESIUM; METRIZOATE SODIUM

METRIZOIC ACID *MULTIPLE*
SEE   CALCIUM; MEGLUMINE; METRIZOIC ACID

METRONIDAZOLE
Injectable; Injection

METRO I.V.		
B BRAUN	500MG/100ML	N018674 001
		AUG 31, 1982
METRONIDAZOLE		
ABBOTT	500MG/100ML	N018889 001
		NOV 18, 1983
AM PHARM PARTNERS	500MG/100ML	N070071 001
		DEC 03, 1984
ELKINS SINN	500MG/100ML	N018907 001
		MAR 30, 1984

Discontinued Drug Products (continued)

METRONIDAZOLE (continued)

Injectable; Injection

METRONIDAZOLE

INTL MEDICATION	500MG/100ML	N070004 001	MAY 08, 1985
STERIS	500MG/100ML	N070042 001	DEC 20, 1984
	500MG/100ML	N070170 001	APR 01, 1986

Tablet; Oral

METRONIDAZOLE

HALSEY	250MG	N018818 001	FEB 16, 1983
	250MG	N070021 001	APR 02, 1985
	500MG	N018818 002	FEB 16, 1983
	500MG	N070593 001	FEB 27, 1986
SUPERPHARM	250MG	N070008 001	DEC 11, 1984
	500MG	N070009 001	DEC 11, 1984
WATSON LABS	250MG	N018599 001	SEP 17, 1982
	500MG	N018599 002	FEB 13, 1984

PROTOSTAT

ORTHO MCNEIL PHARM	250MG	N018871 001	MAR 02, 1983
	500MG	N018871 002	MAR 02, 1983

SATRIC

SAVAGE LABS	250MG	N070029 001	MAR 19, 1985
	500MG	N070731 001	JUN 08, 1987

METRONIDAZOLE HYDROCHLORIDE

Injectable; Injection

METRONIDAZOLE HCL

AM PHARM PARTNERS	EQ 500MG BASE/VIAL	N070295 001	OCT 15, 1985

METYRAPONE

Tablet; Oral

METOPIRONE

NOVARTIS	250MG	N012911 001

MEZLOCILLIN SODIUM MONOHYDRATE

Injectable; Injection

MEZLIN

BAYER PHARMS	EQ 1GM BASE/VIAL	N050549 001
	EQ 1GM BASE/VIAL	N062333 001
	EQ 1GM BASE/VIAL	N062372 005

MEZLOCILLIN SODIUM MONOHYDRATE (continued)

Injectable; Injection

MEZLIN

BAYER PHARMS	EQ 2GM BASE/VIAL	N050549 002	JAN 13, 1983
	EQ 2GM BASE/VIAL	N062333 002	
	EQ 2GM BASE/VIAL	N062372 001	
	EQ 3GM BASE/VIAL	N050549 003	MAY 13, 1982
	EQ 3GM BASE/VIAL	N062333 003	
	EQ 3GM BASE/VIAL	N062372 002	MAY 13, 1982
	EQ 4GM BASE/VIAL	N062697 001	JAN 22, 1987
	EQ 4GM BASE/VIAL	N050549 004	
	EQ 4GM BASE/VIAL	N062333 004	
	EQ 4GM BASE/VIAL	N062372 003	
	EQ 4GM BASE/VIAL	N062697 002	MAY 13, 1982
	EQ 20GM BASE/VIAL	N050549 005	JAN 22, 1987
	EQ 20GM BASE/VIAL	N062372 004	MAR 02, 1988
			MAR 02, 1988

MICONAZOLE

Injectable; Injection

MONISTAT

JANSSEN	10MG/ML	N018040 001

MICONAZOLE NITRATE

Cream, Insert; Topical, Vaginal

MONISTAT DUAL- PAK

PERSONAL PRODS	1.2GM;2%	N020968 001	JUN 30, 1999

Lotion; Topical

MONISTAT-DERM

JOHNSON AND JOHNSON	2%	N017739 001

Tampon; Vaginal

MONISTAT 5

PERSONAL PRODS	100MG	N018592 001	OCT 27, 1989

MIDAZOLAM HYDROCHLORIDE

Injectable; Injection

MIDAZOLAM HCL

APOTHECON	EQ 1MG BASE/ML	N075620 001	NOV 01, 2000
	EQ 5MG BASE/ML	N075620 002	NOV 01, 2000
	EQ 5MG BASE/ML	N075641 001	OCT 19, 2000
ASTRAZENECA	EQ 5MG BASE/ML	N075263 001	JUN 26, 2000
BEDFORD	EQ 5MG BASE/ML	N075249 001	

MINOXIDIL (continued)

Tablet; Oral

MINODYL			
QUANTUM PHARMICS	10MG		JUL 13, 1988
		N071534 001	MAR 19, 1987

MINOXIDIL			
ROYCE LABS	2.5MG	N071799 001	NOV 10, 1987
	10MG	N071796 001	NOV 10, 1987
USL PHARMA	2.5MG	N071537 001	DEC 16, 1988

MITOMYCIN

Injectable; Injection

MUTAMYCIN		
BRISTOL	5MG/VIAL	N050450 001
	20MG/VIAL	N050450 002

MIVACURIUM CHLORIDE

Injectable; Injection

MIVACRON IN DEXTROSE 5% IN PLASTIC CONTAINER			
ABBOTT	EQ 0.5MG BASE/ML	N020098 002	JAN 22, 1992

MOLINDONE HYDROCHLORIDE

Capsule; Oral

MOBAN		
ENDO PHARMS	5MG	N017111 001
	10MG	N017111 002
	25MG	N017111 003

MONOCTANOIN

Liquid; Perfusion, Biliary

MOCTANIN			
ETHITEK	100%	N019368 001	OCT 29, 1985

MOXALACTAM DISODIUM

Injectable; Injection

MOXAM		
LILLY	EQ 1GM BASE/VIAL	N050550 003
	EQ 2GM BASE/VIAL	N050550 004
	EQ 10GM BASE/VIAL	N050550 008
	EQ 250MG BASE/VIAL	N050550 001
	EQ 500MG BASE/VIAL	N050550 002

NABILONE

Capsule; Oral

CESAMET			
LILLY	1MG	N018677 001	DEC 26, 1985

Discontinued Drug Products (continued)

MIDAZOLAM HYDROCHLORIDE (continued)

Injectable; Injection

MIDAZOLAM HCL			
BEDFORD	EQ 5MG BASE/ML		JUN 23, 2000
BEN VENUE		N075455 001	JUN 20, 2000

VERSED			
HLR	EQ 1MG BASE/ML	N018654 002	MAY 26, 1987
	EQ 5MG BASE/ML	N018654 001	DEC 20, 1985

Syrup; Oral

VERSED			
ROCHE	EQ 2MG BASE/ML	N020942 001	OCT 15, 1998

MILRINONE LACTATE

Injectable; Injection

PRIMACOR IN DEXTROSE 5% IN PLASTIC CONTAINER			
SANOFI SYNTHELABO	EQ 10MG BASE/100ML	N020343 001	AUG 09, 1994
	EQ 15MG BASE/100ML	N020343 002	AUG 09, 1994

MINOCYCLINE HYDROCHLORIDE

Capsule; Oral

MINOCIN		
LEDERLE	EQ 50MG BASE	N050315 002
	EQ 100MG BASE	N050315 001

VECTRIN			
MEDICIS	EQ 75MG BASE	N063067 002	SEP 15, 1999
	EQ 100MG BASE	N063067 001	JUL 31, 1990

Injectable; Injection

MINOCIN		
LEDERLE	EQ 100MG BASE/VIAL	N062139 001

Suspension; Oral

MINOCIN		
LEDERLE	EQ 50MG BASE/5ML	N050445 001

Tablet; Oral

MINOCYCLINE HCL			
LEDERLE	EQ 50MG BASE *SEE ANNUAL PREFACE INTRODUCTION DISCONTINUED SECTION*	N050451 003	AUG 10, 1982
	EQ 100MG BASE *SEE ANNUAL PREFACE INTRODUCTION DISCONTINUED SECTION*	N050451 002	AUG 10, 1982

MINOXIDIL

Tablet; Oral

MINODYL		
QUANTUM PHARMICS	2.5MG	N072153 001

Discontinued Drug Products (continued)

NAFCILLIN SODIUM

Capsule; Oral

UNIPEN			
WYETH AYERST	EQ 250MG BASE	N050111 001	

For Solution; Oral

UNIPEN			
WYETH AYERST	EQ 250MG BASE/5ML	N050199 001	

Injectable; Injection

NAFCILLIN SODIUM			
APOTHECON	EQ 1GM BASE/VIAL	N061984 002	
	EQ 2GM BASE/VIAL	N061984 003	
	EQ 4GM BASE/VIAL	N061984 005	
	EQ 500MG BASE/VIAL	N061984 001	
MARSAM PHARMS LLC	EQ 1.5GM BASE/VIAL	N062844 003	OCT 26, 1988
	EQ 1GM BASE/VIAL	N062844 002	OCT 26, 1988
	EQ 2GM BASE/VIAL	N062844 004	OCT 26, 1988
	EQ 4GM BASE/VIAL	N062844 005	OCT 26, 1988
	EQ 10GM BASE/VIAL	N063008 001	SEP 29, 1988
	EQ 500MG BASE/VIAL	N062844 001	OCT 26, 1988
NALLPEN			
GLAXOSMITHKLINE	EQ 1GM BASE/VIAL	N061999 002	
	EQ 1GM BASE/VIAL	N062755 001	DEC 19, 1986
	EQ 2GM BASE/VIAL	N061999 003	
	EQ 2GM BASE/VIAL	N062755 002	DEC 19, 1986
	EQ 10GM BASE/VIAL	N061999 004	
	EQ 500MG BASE/VIAL	N061999 001	
UNIPEN			
WYETH AYERST	EQ 1GM BASE/VIAL	N062717 002	DEC 16, 1986
	EQ 2GM BASE/VIAL	N050320 003	
	EQ 2GM BASE/VIAL	N062717 004	DEC 16, 1986
	EQ 4GM BASE/VIAL	N050320 004	
	EQ 10GM BASE/VIAL	N050320 005	
	EQ 20GM BASE/VIAL	N050320 006	
	EQ 500MG BASE/VIAL	N050320 001	
	EQ 500MG BASE/VIAL	N062717 001	DEC 16, 1986
UNIPEN IN PLASTIC CONTAINER			
WYETH AYERST	EQ 1GM BASE/VIAL	N050320 002	
UNIPEN			
WYETH AYERST	EQ 500MG BASE	N050462 001	

NAFTIFINE HYDROCHLORIDE

Cream; Topical

NAFTIN			
ALLERGAN HERBERT	1%	N019599 001	

NAFTIFINE HYDROCHLORIDE (continued)

Cream; Topical

NAFTIN			
ALLERGAN HERBERT			FEB 29, 1988

Gel; Topical

NAFTIN			
ALLERGAN HERBERT	1%	N019356 001	JUN 18, 1990

NALBUPHINE HYDROCHLORIDE

Injectable; Injection

NALBUPHINE			
AM PHARM PARTNERS	10MG/ML	N070751 001	JUL 02, 1986
	20MG/ML	N070752 001	SEP 24, 1986
QUAD PHARMS	10MG/ML	N070692 001	MAR 25, 1986
	20MG/ML	N070693 001	SEP 24, 1986
NALBUPHINE HCL			
ABBOTT	1.5MG/ML	N020200 001	MAR 12, 1993
ASTRAZENECA	10MG/ML	N072070 001	APR 10, 1989
	10MG/ML	N072071 001	APR 10, 1989
	10MG/ML	N072072 001	APR 10, 1989
	20MG/ML	N072073 001	APR 10, 1989
	20MG/ML	N072074 001	APR 10, 1989
	20MG/ML	N072075 001	APR 10, 1989
KING PHARMS	10MG/ML	N074471 001	MAR 19, 1998
	20MG/ML	N074471 002	MAR 19, 1998

NALIDIXIC ACID

Suspension; Oral

NEGGRAM			
SANOFI SYNTHELABO	250MG/5ML	N017430 001	

Tablet; Oral

NALIDIXIC ACID			
HALSEY	1GM	N070272 001	JUN 29, 1988
	250MG	N070270 001	JUN 29, 1988
	500MG	N070271 001	JUN 29, 1988

Discontinued Drug Products *(continued)*

NALOXONE HYDROCHLORIDE

Injectable; Injection

NALOXONE

Manufacturer	Strength	Number	Date
ELKINS SINN	0.4MG/ML	N070299 001	SEP 24, 1986
	0.4MG/ML	N070496 001	SEP 24, 1986
ELKINS SINN PHARM	0.4MG/ML	N070298 001	SEP 24, 1986
WYETH AYERST	0.02MG/ML	N070188 001	SEP 24, 1986
	0.02MG/ML	N070189 001	SEP 24, 1986
	0.4MG/ML	N070190 001	SEP 24, 1986
	0.4MG/ML	N070191 001	SEP 24, 1986

NALOXONE HCL

Manufacturer	Strength	Number	Date
ABBOTT	0.4MG/ML	N070172 001	SEP 24, 1986
AM PHARM PARTNERS	0.02MG/ML	N070648 001	NOV 17, 1986
	0.02MG/ML	N070661 001	NOV 17, 1986
	0.4MG/ML	N070649 001	NOV 17, 1986
	1MG/ML	N071604 001	DEC 16, 1988
ASTRAZENECA	0.02MG/ML	N072081 001	APR 11, 1989
	0.02MG/ML	N072082 001	APR 11, 1989
	0.02MG/ML	N072083 001	APR 11, 1989
	0.02MG/ML	N072084 001	APR 11, 1989
	0.02MG/ML	N072085 001	APR 11, 1989
	0.02MG/ML	N072086 001	APR 11, 1989
	0.4MG/ML	N072087 001	APR 11, 1989
	0.4MG/ML	N072088 001	APR 11, 1989
	0.4MG/ML	N072089 001	APR 11, 1989
	0.4MG/ML	N072090 001	APR 11, 1989
	1MG/ML	N072091 001	APR 11, 1989
	1MG/ML	N072092 001	APR 11, 1989
	1MG/ML	N072093 001	APR 11, 1989
ELKINS SINN	0.02MG/ML	N071272 001	MAY 24, 1988
	1MG/ML	N071273 001	

NALOXONE HYDROCHLORIDE *(continued)*

Injectable; Injection

NALOXONE HCL

Manufacturer	Strength	Number	Date
ELKINS SINN	1MG/ML	N071274 001	MAY 24, 1988
	1MG/ML	N071287 001	MAY 24, 1988
INTL MEDICATION	0.4MG/ML	N070417 001	MAY 24, 1988
	1MG/ML	N072115 001	SEP 24, 1986
MARSAM PHARMS LLC	0.4MG/ML	N071811 001	APR 27, 1988
QUAD PHARMS	0.02MG/ML	N070678 001	JUL 19, 1988
	0.4MG/ML	N070679 001	DEC 18, 1986
	1MG/ML	N070680 001	DEC 18, 1986
SMITH AND NEPHEW	0.02MG/ML	N071671 001	DEC 18, 1986
	0.4MG/ML	N071681 001	NOV 17, 1987
	0.4MG/ML	N071682 001	NOV 17, 1987
SOLOPAK	0.02MG/ML	N071672 001	NOV 17, 1987
STERIS	0.4MG/ML	N071683 001	NOV 17, 1987
	0.4MG/ML	N071339 001	NOV 17, 1987
NARCAN BRISTOL MYERS SQUIBB	0.4MG/ML	N071083 001	NOV 18, 1987
	1MG/ML	N071084 001	JUL 28, 1988
	1MG/ML	N071311 001	JUL 28, 1988

NANDROLONE DECANOATE

Injectable; Injection

DECA-DURABOLIN

Manufacturer	Strength	Number	Date
ORGANON USA INC	50MG/ML	N013132 001	JUN 12, 1986
	100MG/ML	N013132 002	JUN 12, 1986
	200MG/ML	N013132 003	JUN 12, 1986

NANDROLONE DECANOATE

Manufacturer	Strength	Number	Date
AKORN	100MG/ML	N087519 001	SEP 28, 1983
AM PHARM PARTNERS	100MG/ML	N088290 001	OCT 03, 1983
	200MG/ML	N088317 001	

Discontinued Drug Products (continued)

NANDROLONE DECANOATE (continued)

Injectable; Injection

NANDROLONE DECANOATE
  AM PHARM PARTNERS

Manufacturer	Strength	NDA Number	Date
QUAD PHARMS	50MG/ML	N089248 001	OCT 14, 1983
	100MG/ML	N089249 001	JUN 25, 1986
	200MG/ML	N089250 001	JUN 25, 1986
STERIS	50MG/ML	N087598 001	JUN 25, 1986
	50MG/ML	N088554 001	OCT 06, 1983
	100MG/ML	N087599 001	FEB 10, 1986
			OCT 06, 1983

NANDROLONE PHENPROPIONATE

Injectable; Injection

DURABOLIN

Manufacturer	Strength	NDA Number	Date
ORGANON USA INC	25MG/ML	N011891 001	
	50MG/ML	N011891 002	

NANDROLONE PHENPROPIONATE

Manufacturer	Strength	NDA Number	Date
QUAD PHARMS	25MG/ML	N089297 001	OCT 01, 1986
	50MG/ML	N089298 001	OCT 01, 1986
STERIS	25MG/ML	N086386 001	JUN 17, 1983
	50MG/ML	N087488 001	JUN 17, 1983

NAPHAZOLINE HYDROCHLORIDE

Solution/Drops; Ophthalmic

NAFAZAIR

Manufacturer	Strength	NDA Number	Date
PHARMAFAIR	0.1%	N088101 001	APR 15, 1983

NAPHCON FORTE

Manufacturer	Strength	NDA Number	Date
ALCON	0.1%	N080229 001	

OPCON

Manufacturer	Strength	NDA Number	Date
BAUSCH AND LOMB	0.1%	N087506 001	

NAPROXEN

Tablet; Oral

NAPROXEN

Manufacturer	Strength	NDA Number	Date
HAMILTON PHARMS	250MG	N074110 001	OCT 30, 1992
	375MG	N074110 002	OCT 30, 1992
	500MG	N074110 003	OCT 30, 1992

NAPROXEN SODIUM

Tablet, Extended Release; Oral

NAPRELAN

Manufacturer	Strength	NDA Number	Date
ELAN PHARMA	EQ 750MG BASE	N020353 003	JAN 05, 1996

Tablet; Oral

NAPROXEN SODIUM

Manufacturer	Strength	NDA Number	Date
HAMILTON PHARMS	EQ 250MG BASE	N074106 001	AUG 31, 1993
	EQ 500MG BASE	N074106 002	AUG 31, 1993
PUREPAC PHARM	EQ 250MG BASE	N074319 001	MAR 20, 1995
	EQ 500MG BASE	N074319 002	MAR 20, 1995

NEDOCROMIL SODIUM

Solution; Inhalation

TILADE

Manufacturer	Strength	NDA Number	Date
AVENTIS	0.5%	N020750 001	OCT 01, 1997

NEFAZODONE HYDROCHLORIDE

Tablet; Oral

SERZONE

Manufacturer	Strength	NDA Number	Date
BRISTOL MYERS SQUIBB	300MG	N020152 006	DEC 22, 1994

NEOMYCIN SULFATE

Solution; Oral

MYCIFRADIN

Manufacturer	Strength	NDA Number	Date
PHARMACIA AND UPJOHN	EQ 87.5MG BASE/5ML	N050285 001	

Tablet; Oral

MYCIFRADIN

Manufacturer	Strength	NDA Number	Date
PHARMACIA AND UPJOHN	EQ 350MG BASE	N060520 001	

NEOBIOTIC

Manufacturer	Strength	NDA Number	Date
PFIZER	EQ 350MG BASE	N060475 001	

NEOMYCIN SULFATE

Manufacturer	Strength	NDA Number	Date
BRISTOL MYERS SQUIBB	EQ 350MG BASE	N060365 001	
EON	EQ 350MG BASE	N061586 001	
LANNETT	EQ 350MG BASE	N060607 001	
LILLY	EQ 350MG BASE	N060385 001	
ROXANE	EQ 350MG BASE	N062173 001	

NEOMYCIN SULFATE; POLYMYXIN B SULFATE

Cream; Topical

NEOSPORIN

Manufacturer	Strength	NDA Number	Date
GLAXOSMITHKLINE	EQ 3.5MG BASE/GM;10,000 UNITS/GM	N050176 002	JAN 14, 1985

NEOMYCIN SULFATE *MULTIPLE*

SEE ACETIC ACID, GLACIAL; HYDROCORTISONE; NEOMYCIN SULFATE
SEE BACITRACIN; HYDROCORTISONE ACETATE; NEOMYCIN SULFATE; POLYMYXIN B SULFATE
SEE BACITRACIN; NEOMYCIN SULFATE; POLYMYXIN B SULFATE
SEE BACITRACIN ZINC; HYDROCORTISONE; NEOMYCIN SULFATE; POLYMYXIN B SULFATE
SEE BACITRACIN ZINC; LIDOCAINE; NEOMYCIN SULFATE; POLYMYXIN B SULFATE
SEE BACITRACIN ZINC; NEOMYCIN SULFATE; POLYMYXIN B SULFATE
SEE DEXAMETHASONE; NEOMYCIN SULFATE; POLYMYXIN B SULFATE
SEE DEXAMETHASONE SODIUM PHOSPHATE; NEOMYCIN SULFATE
SEE FLUOCINOLONE ACETONIDE; NEOMYCIN SULFATE
SEE FLURANDRENOLIDE; NEOMYCIN SULFATE
SEE GRAMICIDIN; NEOMYCIN SULFATE; POLYMYXIN B SULFATE
SEE HYDROCORTISONE; NEOMYCIN SULFATE
SEE HYDROCORTISONE; NEOMYCIN SULFATE; POLYMYXIN B SULFATE
SEE HYDROCORTISONE ACETATE; NEOMYCIN SULFATE
SEE METHYLPREDNISOLONE; NEOMYCIN SULFATE
SEE METHYLPREDNISOLONE ACETATE; NEOMYCIN SULFATE

NETILMICIN SULFATE

Injectable; Injection

NETROMYCIN

SCHERING	EQ 10MG BASE/ML	N050544 001	FEB 28, 1983
	EQ 25MG BASE/ML	N050544 002	FEB 28, 1983
	EQ 100MG BASE/ML	N050544 003	FEB 28, 1983

NIACIN

Capsule; Oral

WAMPOCAP

MEDPOINTE PHARM HLC	500MG	N011073 003

Tablet, Extended Release; Oral

NIASPAN

KOS	375MG	N020381 001	JUL 28, 1997

NIASPAN TITRATION STARTER PACK

KOS	375MG;500MG;750MG	N020381 005	JUL 28, 1997

Tablet; Oral

NIACIN

EVERYLIFE	500MG	N083203 001
GENEVA PHARMS	500MG	N083306 001
HALSEY	500MG	N083453 001
IMPAX LABS	500MG	N083115 001
IVAX PHARMS	500MG	N083180 001
PUREPAC PHARM	500MG	N083271 001
WATSON LAB	500MG	N083136 001
WATSON LABS	500MG	N083305 001
	500MG	N085172 001
WEST WARD	500MG	N083718 001

Discontinued Drug Products (continued)

NEOMYCIN SULFATE; POLYMYXIN B SULFATE (continued)

Ointment; Ophthalmic

STATROL

ALCON	EQ 3.5MG BASE/GM;10,000 UNITS/GM	N050344 002

Solution/Drops; Ophthalmic

STATROL

ALCON	EQ 3.5MG BASE/ML;16,250 UNITS/ML	N050456 001	
	EQ 3.5MG BASE/ML;16,250 UNITS/ML	N062339 001	NOV 30, 1984

Solution; Irrigation

NEOMYCIN AND POLYMYXIN B SULFATES

STERIS	EQ 40MG BASE/ML;200,000 UNITS/ML	N062664 001	APR 08, 1986

NEOMYCIN SULFATE; PREDNISOLONE ACETATE

Ointment; Ophthalmic

NEO-DELTA-CORTEF

PHARMACIA AND UPJOHN	EQ 3.5MG BASE/GM;0.5%	N061039 001
	EQ 3.5MG BASE/GM;0.25%	N061039 002

Suspension/Drops; Ophthalmic

NEO-DELTA-CORTEF

PHARMACIA AND UPJOHN	EQ 3.5MG BASE/ML;0.25%	N061037 001

NEOMYCIN SULFATE; PREDNISOLONE SODIUM PHOSPHATE

Ointment; Ophthalmic

NEO-HYDELTRASOL

MERCK	EQ 3.5MG BASE/GM;EQ 0.25% PHOSPHATE	N050378 001

NEOMYCIN SULFATE; TRIAMCINOLONE ACETONIDE

Cream; Topical

MYTREX A

SAVAGE LABS	EQ 3.5MG BASE/GM;0.1%	N062598 001	JUL 21, 1986

NEOMYCIN SULFATE-TRIAMCINOLONE ACETONIDE

FOUGERA	EQ 3.5MG BASE/GM;0.1%	N062600 001	JUL 21, 1986
PHARMADERM	EQ 3.5MG BASE/GM;0.1%	N062595 001	JUL 21, 1986

Ointment; Topical

MYTREX A

SAVAGE LABS	EQ 3.5MG BASE/GM;0.1%	N062609 001	MAY 23, 1986

NEOMYCIN SULFATE-TRIAMCINOLONE ACETONIDE

FOUGERA	EQ 3.5MG BASE/GM;0.1%	N062608 001	MAY 23, 1986
PHARMADERM	EQ 3.5MG BASE/GM;0.1%	N062607 001	MAY 23, 1986

Discontinued Drug Products (continued)

NIACINAMIDE; PYRIDOXINE HYDROCHLORIDE; TYROSINE
Suspension; Oral
TPN SUSPENSION
INTL MINERALS   15MG/5ML;3.75MG/5ML;600MG/5ML   N008378 003

NIACINAMIDE *MULTIPLE*
SEE   ALPHA-TOCOPHEROL; ASCORBIC ACID; BIOTIN; CHOLECALCIFEROL; CYANOCOBALAMIN; FOLIC ACID; NIACINAMIDE; PANTOTHENIC ACID; PYRIDOXINE; RIBOFLAVIN; THIAMINE; VITAMIN A

SEE   ASCORBIC ACID; BIOTIN; CYANOCOBALAMIN; DEXPANTHENOL; ERGOCALCIFEROL; FOLIC ACID; NIACINAMIDE; PYRIDOXINE PHOSPHATE SODIUM; THIAMINE; VITAMIN A; VITAMIN E

SEE   ASCORBIC ACID; BIOTIN; CYANOCOBALAMIN; DEXPANTHENOL; ERGOCALCIFEROL; FOLIC ACID; NIACINAMIDE; PYRIDOXINE HYDROCHLORIDE; RIBOFLAVIN PHOSPHATE SODIUM; THIAMINE; VITAMIN A PALMITATE; VITAMIN E

SEE   ASCORBIC ACID; BIOTIN; CYANOCOBALAMIN; DEXPANTHENOL; ERGOCALCIFEROL; FOLIC ACID; NIACINAMIDE; PYRIDOXINE HYDROCHLORIDE; RIBOFLAVIN PHOSPHATE SODIUM; THIAMINE; VITAMIN A; VITAMIN E

SEE   ASCORBIC ACID; BIOTIN; CYANOCOBALAMIN; ERGOCALCIFEROL; FOLIC ACID; NIACINAMIDE; PANTOTHENIC ACID; PHYTONADIONE; PYRIDOXINE; RIBOFLAVIN; THIAMINE; VITAMIN A PALMITATE; VITAMIN E

NICLOSAMIDE
Tablet, Chewable; Oral
NICLOCIDE
BAYER PHARMS   500MG   N018669 001   MAY 14, 1982

NICOTINE
Inhalant; Inhalation
NICOTROL
PHARMACIA AND UPJOHN   4MG/CARTRIDGE   N020714 001   MAY 02, 1997

NIFEDIPINE
Capsule; Oral
ADALAT
BAYER PHARMS   10MG   N019478 001   NOV 27, 1985
                20MG   N019478 002   SEP 17, 1986
NIFEDIPINE
CHASE LABS NJ   10MG   N072409 001   JUL 04, 1990
                 20MG   N073421 001   JUN 19, 1991
Tablet, Extended Release; Oral
NIFEDIPINE
MYLAN   30MG   N075108 001   DEC 17, 1999

NILUTAMIDE
Tablet; Oral
NILANDRON
AVENTIS PHARMS   50MG   N020169 001   SEP 19, 1996

NITROFURANTOIN
Capsule; Oral
NITROFURANTOIN
WATSON LAB   50MG   N084326 001
              100MG   N084326 002
Tablet; Oral
FURADANTIN
PROCTER AND GAMBLE   50MG   N008693 001
                      100MG   N008693 002
FURALAN
LANNETT   50MG   N080017 001
           100MG   N080017 002
NITROFURANTOIN
ELKINS SINN   50MG   N080003 001
               100MG   N080003 002
EON   50MG   N080043 001
       100MG   N080043 002
IVAX PHARMS   50MG   N080078 002
               100MG   N080078 001
WATSON LAB   50MG   N080447 001
              100MG   N080447 002
WATSON LABS   50MG   N085797 001
               100MG   N085796 001
WHITEWORTH TOWN PLSN   100MG   N084085 002

NITROFURANTOIN SODIUM
Injectable; Injection
IVADANTIN
PROCTER AND GAMBLE   EQ 180MG BASE/VIAL   N012402 001

NITROFURANTOIN, MACROCRYSTALLINE
Capsule; Oral
NITROFURANTOIN MACROCRYSTALLINE
WATSON LAB   50MG   N070248 001   JUN 24, 1988
              100MG   N070249 001   JUN 24, 1988

NITROFURAZONE
Cream; Topical
FURACIN
SHIRE LABS   0.2%   N083789 001
Dressing; Topical
ACTIN-N
SHERWOOD MEDCL   0.2%   N017343 001
Ointment; Topical
FURACIN
SHIRE PHARM   0.2%   N005795 001

Discontinued Drug Products (continued)

NITROFURAZONE (continued)

Ointment; Topical
NITROFURAZONE
AMBIX 0.2% N086077 001
CLAY PARK 0.2% N084968 001
LANNETT 0.2% N084393 001

Powder; Topical
FURACIN
SHIRE PHARM 0.2% N083791 001

Solution; Topical
NITROFURAZONE
CLAY PARK 0.2% N085130 001

NITROGLYCERIN

Aerosol; Sublingual
NITROLINGUAL
POHL BOSKAMP 0.4MG/SPRAY N018705 001 OCT 31, 1985

Injectable; Injection
NITRO IV
POHL BOSKAMP 5MG/ML N018672 002 AUG 30, 1983
NITRO-BID
AVENTIS PHARMS 10MG/ML N071159 001 FEB 28, 1990
NITROGLYCERIN
AM PHARM PARTNERS 5MG/ML N070077 001 DEC 13, 1985
5MG/ML N071203 001 MAY 08, 1987
INTL MEDICATION 5MG/ML N070026 001 SEP 10, 1985
LUITPOLD 5MG/ML N071492 001 MAY 24, 1988
QUAD PHARMS 5MG/ML N071094 001 JUL 31, 1987
10MG/ML N071095 001 JUL 31, 1987
SMITH AND NEPHEW 5MG/ML N070633 001 JUN 19, 1986
5MG/ML N070634 001 JUN 19, 1986
NITROL
RORER 0.8MG/ML N018774 001 JAN 19, 1983
NITRONAL
POHL BOSKAMP 1MG/ML N018672 001 AUG 30, 1983
NITROSTAT
PARKE DAVIS 0.8MG/ML N018588 001
5MG/ML N018588 002 DEC 23, 1983
5MG/ML N070863 001 JAN 08, 1987
5MG/ML N070871 001 JAN 08, 1987
10MG/ML JAN 08, 1987

NITROGLYCERIN (continued)

Injectable; Injection
NITROSTAT
PARKE DAVIS 10MG/ML N070872 001 JAN 08, 1987
TRIDIL
FAULDING 0.5MG/ML N018537 002 JUN 16, 1983
5MG/ML N018537 001

NONOXYNOL-9

Aerosol; Vaginal
DELFEN
PERSONAL PRODS 12.5% N014349 002

Sponge; Vaginal
TODAY
ALLENDALE PHARMS 1GM N018683 001 APR 01, 1983

NOREPINEPHRINE BITARTRATE; PROCAINE HYDROCHLORIDE; PROPOXYCAINE HYDROCHLORIDE

Injectable; Injection
RAVOCAINE AND NOVOCAIN W/ LEVOPHED
EASTMAN KODAK EQ 0.033MG BASE/ML;2%;0.4% N008592 003

NORETHINDRONE

Tablet; Oral
NORLUTIN
PARKE DAVIS 5MG N010895 002

NORETHINDRONE *MULTIPLE*

SEE ETHINYL ESTRADIOL; FERROUS FUMARATE; NORETHINDRONE
SEE ETHINYL ESTRADIOL; NORETHINDRONE
SEE MESTRANOL; NORETHINDRONE

NORETHINDRONE ACETATE

Tablet; Oral
NORLUTATE
PARKE DAVIS 5MG N012184 002

NORETHINDRONE ACETATE *MULTIPLE*

SEE ETHINYL ESTRADIOL; FERROUS FUMARATE; NORETHINDRONE ACETATE
SEE ETHINYL ESTRADIOL; NORETHINDRONE ACETATE

NORETHYNODREL *MULTIPLE*

SEE MESTRANOL; NORETHYNODREL

NORFLOXACIN

Solution/Drops; Ophthalmic
CHIBROXIN
MERCK 0.3% N019757 001 JUN 17, 1991

Discontinued Drug Products (continued)

NORGESTIMATE *MULTIPLE*
SEE ETHINYL ESTRADIOL; NORGESTIMATE

NOVOBIOCIN SODIUM
Capsule; Oral
- ALBAMYCIN
  - PHARMACIA AND UPJOHN — EQ 250MG BASE — N050339 001 — DEC 17, 1987

NYSTATIN

Cream; Topical
- CANDEX
  - BAYER PHARMS — 100,000 UNITS/GM — N061810 001
- MYKINAC
  - ALPHARMA — 100,000 UNITS/GM — N062387 001 — JUL 29, 1982
- NILSTAT
  - LEDERLE — 100,000 UNITS/GM — N061445 001
- NYSTATIN
  - TEVA — 100,000 UNITS/GM — N061966 001

Lotion; Topical
- CANDEX
  - BAYER PHARMS — 100,000 UNITS/ML — N050233 001

Ointment; Topical
- MYCOSTATIN
  - WESTWOOD SQUIBB — 100,000 UNITS/GM — N060571 001
- MYKINAC
  - ALPHARMA — 100,000 UNITS/GM — N062731 001 — SEP 22, 1986
- NILSTAT
  - LEDERLE — 100,000 UNITS/GM — N061444 001

Powder; Oral
- BARSTATIN 100
  - BARLAN — 100% — N062489 001 — APR 27, 1988

Suppository; Vaginal
- NYSERT
  - PROCTER AND GAMBLE — 100,000 UNITS — N050478 001

Suspension; Oral
- NYSTATIN
  - ALPHARMA — 100,000 UNITS/ML — N062571 001 — OCT 29, 1985
  - MORTON GROVE — 100,000 UNITS/ML — N062835 001 — NOV 19, 1987
  - PHARMADERM — 100,000 UNITS/ML — N062518 001 — JUL 06, 1984
  - PHARMAFAIR — 100,000 UNITS/ML — N062541 001 — JAN 16, 1985
  - PHARMAFAIR — N062832 001 — DEC 27, 1991
  - ROXANE — 100,000 UNITS/ML — N062876 001
  - TARO — 100,000 UNITS/ML — N062670 001 — FEB 29, 1988
  - TEVA — 100,000 UNITS/ML — N062776 001 — JUN 18, 1987

NYSTATIN (continued)

Suspension; Oral
- NYSTATIN
  - TEVA — N061151 001 — DEC 17, 1987

Tablet; Oral
- NILSTAT
  - LEDERLE — 500,000 UNITS — N062065 001
- NYSTATIN
  - EON — 500,000 UNITS — N062524 001 — OCT 29, 1984
  - QUANTUM PHARMICS — 500,000 UNITS — N062525 001 — NOV 26, 1985
  - USL PHARMA — 500,000 UNITS — N062402 001
  - WATSON LABS — 500,000 UNITS — N061718 001 — DEC 16, 1982

Tablet; Vaginal
- KOROSTATIN
  - HOLLAND RANTOS — 100,000 UNITS — N060577 001
- MYCOSTATIN
  - BRISTOL MYERS SQUIBB — 100,000 UNITS — N061325 001
- NILSTAT
  - LEDERLE — 100,000 UNITS — N061965 001
- NYSTATIN
  - EON — 100,000 UNITS — N062509 001 — APR 03, 1984
  - QUANTUM PHARMICS — 100,000 UNITS — N062502 001 — DEC 23, 1983
  - TEVA — 100,000 UNITS — N062176 001
  - WATSON LABS — 100,000 UNITS

NYSTATIN; TRIAMCINOLONE ACETONIDE

Cream; Topical
- MYCOLOG-II
  - APOTHECON — 100,000 UNITS/GM;0.1% — N060576 002 — MAY 01, 1985
- NYSTATIN AND TRIAMCINOLONE ACETONIDE
  - ALPHARMA — 100,000 UNITS/GM;0.1% — N063010 001 — DEC 20, 1988
  - CLAY PARK — 100,000 UNITS/GM;0.1% — N062186 002 — JUN 06, 1985
  - PHARMAFAIR — 100,000 UNITS/GM;0.1% — N062657 001 — JUL 30, 1986
- NYSTATIN-TRIAMCINOLONE ACETONIDE
  - PHARMADERM — 100,000 UNITS/GM;0.1% — N062596 001 — OCT 08, 1985

Ointment; Topical
- MYCO-TRIACET II
  - TEVA — 100,000 UNITS/GM;0.1% — N062045 002 — NOV 26, 1985
- NYSTATIN AND TRIAMCINOLONE ACETONIDE
  - CLAY PARK — 100,000 UNITS/GM;0.1% — N062280 002 — OCT 10, 1985
  - PHARMAFAIR — 100,000 UNITS/GM;0.1% — N062656 001 — JUL 30, 1986

Discontinued Drug Products (continued)

NYSTATIN; TRIAMCINOLONE ACETONIDE (continued)
Ointment; Topical
NYSTATIN-TRIAMCINOLONE ACETONIDE

Labeler	Strength	Appl. No.	Date
PHARMADERM	100,000 UNITS/GM;0.1%	N062603 001	OCT 09, 1985

NYSTATIN *MULTIPLE*
SEE   CLIOQUINOL; NYSTATIN

OFLOXACIN
Injectable; Injection
FLOXIN

Labeler	Strength	Appl. No.	Date
ORTHO MCNEIL PHARM	20MG/ML	N020087 002	MAR 31, 1992

FLOXIN IN DEXTROSE 5% IN PLASTIC CONTAINER

Labeler	Strength	Appl. No.	Date
ORTHO MCNEIL PHARM	4MG/ML	N020087 004	MAR 31, 1992

ORPHENADRINE CITRATE
Tablet, Extended Release; Oral
ORPHENADRINE CITRATE

Labeler	Strength	Appl. No.	Date
ASCOT	100MG	N088067 001	APR 06, 1983
GENEVA PHARMS	100MG	N085046 001	
WATSON LAB	100MG	N084303 001	

ORPHENADRINE HYDROCHLORIDE
Tablet; Oral
DISIPAL

Labeler	Strength	Appl. No.	Date
3M	50MG	N010653 001	

OXACILLIN SODIUM
Capsule; Oral
OXACILLIN SODIUM

Labeler	Strength	Appl. No.	Date
APOTHECON	EQ 250MG BASE	N061450 002	
	EQ 500MG BASE	N061450 001	

PROSTAPHLIN

Labeler	Strength	Appl. No.	Date
APOTHECON	EQ 500MG BASE	N050118 002	

For Solution; Oral
PROSTAPHLIN

Labeler	Strength	Appl. No.	Date
APOTHECON	EQ 250MG BASE/5ML	N050194 001	

Injectable; Injection
BACTOCILL

Labeler	Strength	Appl. No.	Date
GLAXOSMITHKLINE	EQ 1GM BASE/VIAL	N061334 006	MAR 26, 1982
	EQ 1GM BASE/VIAL	N062736 001	DEC 19, 1986
	EQ 2GM BASE/VIAL	N061334 007	MAR 26, 1982
	EQ 2GM BASE/VIAL	N062736 002	DEC 19, 1986
	EQ 4GM BASE/VIAL	N061334 008	MAR 26, 1982
	EQ 10GM BASE/VIAL	N061334 010	

OXACILLIN SODIUM (continued)
Injectable; Injection
BACTOCILL

Labeler	Strength	Appl. No.	Date
GLAXOSMITHKLINE	EQ 500MG BASE/VIAL	N061334 009	MAR 26, 1982

OXACILLIN SODIUM

Labeler	Strength	Appl. No.	Date
APOTHECON	EQ 1GM BASE/VIAL	N050195 003	
	EQ 2GM BASE/VIAL	N050195 004	
	EQ 4GM BASE/VIAL	N050195 005	
	EQ 250MG BASE/VIAL	N050195 001	
	EQ 500MG BASE/VIAL	N050195 002	
ELKINS SINN	EQ 1GM BASE/VIAL	N062711 003	FEB 03, 1989
	EQ 2GM BASE/VIAL	N062711 004	FEB 03, 1989
	EQ 4GM BASE/VIAL	N062711 005	FEB 03, 1989
	EQ 10GM BASE/VIAL	N062711 006	FEB 03, 1989
	EQ 250MG BASE/VIAL	N062711 001	FEB 03, 1989
	EQ 500MG BASE/VIAL	N062711 002	FEB 03, 1989
IBI	EQ 1GM BASE/VIAL	N062798 001	FEB 03, 1989
	EQ 2GM BASE/VIAL	N062798 002	DEC 11, 1995
	EQ 125MG BASE/VIAL	N062798 003	DEC 11, 1995
	EQ 250MG BASE/VIAL	N062798 004	DEC 11, 1995
	EQ 500MG BASE/VIAL	N062798 005	DEC 11, 1995

OXAZEPAM
Capsule; Oral
OXAZEPAM

Labeler	Strength	Appl. No.	Date
AM THERAP	10MG	N071955 001	
	15MG	N071956 001	MAR 03, 1988
	30MG	N071957 001	MAR 03, 1988
HALSEY	10MG	N070957 001	AUG 10, 1987
	15MG	N071025 001	AUG 10, 1987
	30MG	N071026 001	AUG 10, 1987
MYLAN	10MG	N071713 001	OCT 20, 1987
	15MG	N071714 001	OCT 20, 1987
	30MG	N071715 001	OCT 20, 1987

Discontinued Drug Products (continued)

OXAZEPAM (continued)
Capsule; Oral

ZAXOPAM				
QUANTUM PHARMICS	10MG	N070650 001	MAR 01, 1988	
	15MG	N070640 001	MAR 01, 1988	
	30MG	N070641 001	MAR 01, 1988	

Tablet; Oral

OXAZEPAM				
HALSEY	15MG	N070683 001	JAN 16, 1987	
PARKE DAVIS	15MG	N071508 001	FEB 02, 1987	
WATSON LABS	15MG	N071494 001	APR 21, 1987	

OXPRENOLOL HYDROCHLORIDE
Capsule; Oral

TRASICOR			
NOVARTIS	20MG	N018166 001	DEC 28, 1983
	40MG	N018166 002	DEC 28, 1983
	80MG	N018166 003	DEC 28, 1983
	160MG	N018166 004	DEC 28, 1983

OXTRIPHYLLINE
Solution; Oral

CHOLEDYL			
PARKE DAVIS	100MG/5ML	N009268 012	NOV 27, 1984
OXTRIPHYLLINE			
MORTON GROVE	100MG/5ML	N088243 001	DEC 05, 1983

Syrup; Oral

CHOLEDYL			
PARKE DAVIS	50MG/5ML	N009268 011	
OXTRIPHYLLINE PEDIATRIC			
MORTON GROVE	50MG/5ML	N088242 001	DEC 05, 1983

Tablet, Delayed Release; Oral

CHOLEDYL			
PARKE DAVIS	100MG	N009268 003	
	200MG	N009268 007	
OXTRIPHYLLINE			
WATSON LAB	100MG	N087866 001	AUG 25, 1983
	200MG	N087835 001	AUG 25, 1983

OXYBUTYNIN CHLORIDE
Tablet; Oral

OXYBUTYNIN CHLORIDE			
QUANTUM PHARMICS	5MG	N072296 001	DEC 08, 1988
USL PHARMA	5MG	N070746 001	MAR 10, 1988
WATSON LAB	5MG	N072485 001	APR 19, 1989

OXYCODONE HYDROCHLORIDE
Tablet, Extended Release; Oral

OXYCONTIN			
PURDUE PHARMA LP	160MG	N020553 005	MAR 15, 2000
ROXICODONE			
ROXANE	10MG	N020932 001	OCT 26, 1998
	30MG	N020932 002	OCT 26, 1998

OXYCODONE HYDROCHLORIDE *MULTIPLE*
SEE ACETAMINOPHEN; OXYCODONE HYDROCHLORIDE
SEE ACETAMINOPHEN; OXYCODONE HYDROCHLORIDE; OXYCODONE TEREPHTHALATE
SEE ASPIRIN; OXYCODONE HYDROCHLORIDE; OXYCODONE TEREPHTHALATE

OXYCODONE TEREPHTHALATE *MULTIPLE*
SEE ACETAMINOPHEN; OXYCODONE HYDROCHLORIDE; OXYCODONE TEREPHTHALATE
SEE ASPIRIN; OXYCODONE HYDROCHLORIDE; OXYCODONE TEREPHTHALATE

OXYPHENBUTAZONE
Tablet; Oral

OXYPHENBUTAZONE			
WATSON LAB	100MG	N088399 001	SEP 17, 1984
TANDEARIL			
NOVARTIS	100MG	N012542 004	SEP 03, 1982

OXYPHENCYCLIMINE HYDROCHLORIDE
Tablet; Oral

DARICON			
PFIZER	10MG	N011612 001	

OXYPHENONIUM BROMIDE
Tablet; Oral

ANTRENYL			
NOVARTIS	5MG	N008492 002	

Discontinued Drug Products (continued)

OXYTETRACYCLINE
Tablet; Oral
TERRAMYCIN
| PFIZER | 250MG | N050287 001 |

OXYTETRACYCLINE CALCIUM
Syrup; Oral
TERRAMYCIN
| PFIZER | EQ 125MG BASE/5ML | N060595 001 |

OXYTETRACYCLINE HYDROCHLORIDE
Capsule; Oral
OXY-KESSO-TETRA
| FERRANTE | EQ 250MG BASE | N060179 001 |

OXYTETRACYCLINE HCL
IMPAX LABS	EQ 250MG BASE	N060760 001
PROTER	EQ 250MG BASE	N060869 001
PUREPAC PHARM	EQ 250MG BASE	N060634 001
WEST WARD	EQ 250MG BASE	N060770 001

TERRAMYCIN
| PFIZER | EQ 125MG BASE | N050286 001 |

Injectable; Injection
TERRAMYCIN
| PFIZER | EQ 250MG BASE/VIAL | N060586 001 |
| | EQ 500MG BASE/VIAL | N060586 002 |

OXYTETRACYCLINE HYDROCHLORIDE; POLYMYXIN B SULFATE
Ointment; Otic
TERRAMYCIN W/ POLYMYXIN
| PFIZER | EQ 5MG BASE/GM;10,000 UNITS/GM | N061841 001 |

Tablet; Vaginal
TERRAMYCIN-POLYMYXIN
| PFIZER | EQ 100MG BASE;100,000 UNITS | N061009 001 |

OXYTOCIN
Injectable; Injection
OXYTOCIN
| BAXTER HLTHCARE CORP | 10USP UNITS/ML | N018243 001 |

OXYTOCIN 5 USP UNITS IN DEXTROSE 5%
| ABBOTT | 1USP UNITS/100ML | N019185 001 | MAR 29, 1985 |

OXYTOCIN 10 USP UNITS IN DEXTROSE 5%
| ABBOTT | 1USP UNITS/100ML | N019185 004 | MAR 29, 1985 |
| | 2USP UNITS/100ML | N019185 003 | MAR 29, 1985 |

OXYTOCIN 20 USP UNITS IN DEXTROSE 5%
| ABBOTT | 2USP UNITS/100ML | N019185 002 | MAR 29, 1985 |

Solution; Nasal
SYNTOCINON
| NOVARTIS | 40USP UNITS/ML | N012285 001 |

PANCRELIPASE (AMYLASE;LIPASE;PROTEASE)
Capsule; Oral
COTAZYM
| ORGANON USA INC | 30,000USP UNITS;8,000USP UNITS;30,000USP UNITS | N020580 001 | DEC 09, 1996 |

PANCURONIUM BROMIDE
Injectable; Injection
PANCURONIUM BROMIDE
ASTRAZENECA	1MG/ML	N072210 001	MAR 31, 1988
	2MG/ML	N072211 001	MAR 31, 1988
	2MG/ML	N072212 001	MAR 31, 1988
	2MG/ML	N072213 001	MAR 31, 1988
QUAD PHARMS	1MG/ML	N072209 001	JUN 03, 1988
	2MG/ML	N072208 001	JUN 03, 1988

PAVULON
| ORGANON USA INC | 1MG/ML | N017015 002 |
| | 2MG/ML | N017015 001 |

PANTOTHENIC ACID *MULTIPLE*
SEE ALPHA-TOCOPHEROL; ASCORBIC ACID; BIOTIN; CHOLECALCIFEROL; CYANOCOBALAMIN; FOLIC ACID; NIACINAMIDE; PANTOTHENIC ACID; PYRIDOXINE; RIBOFLAVIN; THIAMINE; VITAMIN A

SEE ASCORBIC ACID; BIOTIN; CYANOCOBALAMIN; ERGOCALCIFEROL; FOLIC ACID; NIACINAMIDE; PANTOTHENIC ACID; PHYTONADIONE; PYRIDOXINE; RIBOFLAVIN; THIAMINE; VITAMIN A PALMITATE; VITAMIN E

PARAMETHADIONE
Capsule; Oral
PARADIONE
| ABBOTT | 150MG | N006800 003 |
| | 300MG | N006800 001 |

Solution; Oral
PARADIONE
| ABBOTT | 300MG/ML | N006800 002 |

PARAMETHASONE ACETATE
Tablet; Oral
HALDRONE
| LILLY | 1MG | N012772 005 |
| | 2MG | N012772 006 |

PARGYLINE HYDROCHLORIDE
Tablet; Oral
EUTONYL
ABBOTT	10MG	N013448 002
	25MG	N013448 003
	50MG	N013448 004

Discontinued Drug Products (continued)

PARGYLINE HYDROCHLORIDE *MULTIPLE*
SEE METHYCLOTHIAZIDE; PARGYLINE HYDROCHLORIDE

PAROMOMYCIN SULFATE
Capsule; Oral
- HUMATIN
  - PARKEDALE — EQ 250MG BASE — N060521 001

Syrup; Oral
- HUMATIN
  - PARKE DAVIS — EQ 125MG BASE/5ML — N060522 001

PAROXETINE HYDROCHLORIDE
Capsule; Oral
- PAXIL
  - GLAXOSMITHKLINE — EQ 10MG BASE — N020885 001 — OCT 09, 1998
  - EQ 20MG BASE — N020885 002 — OCT 09, 1998
  - EQ 30MG BASE — N020885 003 — OCT 09, 1998
  - EQ 40MG BASE — N020885 004 — OCT 09, 1998

Tablet; Oral
- PAXIL
  - GLAXOSMITHKLINE — EQ 50MG BASE — N020031 004 — DEC 29, 1992

PENBUTOLOL SULFATE
Tablet; Oral
- LEVATOL
  - SCHWARZ PHARMA — 10MG — N018976 001 — DEC 30, 1987

PENICILLIN G BENZATHINE
Injectable; Injection
- BICILLIN L-A
  - WYETH AYERST — 300,000 UNITS/ML — N050131 001

Suspension; Oral
- BICILLIN
  - WYETH AYERST — 300,000 UNITS/5ML — N050126 002

Tablet; Oral
- BICILLIN
  - WYETH AYERST — 200,000 UNITS — N050128 001

PENICILLIN G POTASSIUM
For Solution; Oral
- PENICILLIN
  - TEVA — 200,000 UNITS/5ML — N060307 002
  - 400,000 UNITS/5ML — N060307 004
- PENICILLIN G POTASSIUM
  - MYLAN — 200,000 UNITS/5ML — N060752 003
  - 250,000 UNITS/5ML — N060752 002
  - 400,000 UNITS/5ML — N060752 001
  - PUREPAC PHARM — 250,000 UNITS/5ML — N061740 001

PENICILLIN G POTASSIUM (continued)
For Solution; Oral
- PENICILLIN G POTASSIUM
  - PUREPAC PHARM — 400,000 UNITS/5ML — N061740 002
- PENICILLIN-2
  - TEVA — 250,000 UNITS/5ML — N060307 003
- PENTIDS '200'
  - APOTHECON — 200,000 UNITS/5ML — N062149 001
- PENTIDS '400'
  - APOTHECON — 400,000 UNITS/5ML — N062149 002
- PFIZERPEN G
  - PFIZER — 400,000 UNITS/5ML — N060587 001

Injectable; Injection
- PENICILLIN G POTASSIUM
  - APOTHECON — 1,000,000 UNITS/VIAL — N060362 001
  - 5,000,000 UNITS/VIAL — N060362 003
  - 10,000,000 UNITS/VIAL — N060362 004
  - 20,000,000 UNITS/VIAL — N060362 002
  - CONSOLIDATED PHARM — 1,000,000 UNITS/VIAL — N060806 002
  - 5,000,000 UNITS/VIAL — N060806 003
  - 10,000,000 UNITS/VIAL — N060806 004
  - 500,000 UNITS/VIAL — N060806 001
  - LILLY — 1,000,000 UNITS/VIAL — N060384 002
  - 5,000,000 UNITS/VIAL — N060384 001
  - 20,000,000 UNITS/VIAL — N060384 005
  - 20,000,000 UNITS/VIAL — N060601 001
  - 200,000 UNITS/VIAL — N060384 004
  - PARKE DAVIS — 500,000 UNITS/VIAL — N060384 003
  - 1,000,000 UNITS/VIAL — N062003 001
  - 5,000,000 UNITS/VIAL — N062003 002

Tablet; Oral
- PENICILLIN G POTASSIUM
  - APOTHECON — 250,000 UNITS — N060392 003
  - 400,000 UNITS — N060073 004
  - IVAX PHARMS — 250,000 UNITS — N060403 001
  - LILLY — 200,000 UNITS — N060781 001
  - 250,000 UNITS — N060781 002
  - MYLAN — 400,000 UNITS — N060781 003
  - 500,000 UNITS — N060781 005
  - 800,000 UNITS — N060781 004
  - PUREPAC PHARM — 200,000 UNITS — N061588 001
  - 250,000 UNITS — N061588 002
  - 400,000 UNITS — N061588 003
  - TEVA — 200,000 UNITS — N060306 001
  - 250,000 UNITS — N060306 003
  - 400,000 UNITS — N060306 004
  - WYETH AYERST — 500,000 UNITS — N060413 001
  - 200,000 UNITS — N060413 002
  - 400,000 UNITS — N060413 003
- PENTIDS '200'
  - APOTHECON — 200,000 UNITS — N062155 001
- PENTIDS '250'
  - APOTHECON — 250,000 UNITS — N062155 002
- PENTIDS '400'
  - APOTHECON — 400,000 UNITS — N060392 004

PENICILLIN V POTASSIUM (continued)

For Solution; Oral

Product / Firm	Strength	Application No.
PEN-VEE K — WYETH AYERST	EQ 125MG BASE/5ML	N060007 001
	EQ 250MG BASE/5ML	N060007 002
PENAPAR-VK — PARKE DAVIS	EQ 125MG BASE/5ML	N062002 001
	EQ 250MG BASE/5ML	N062002 002
PENICILLIN V POTASSIUM — MYLAN	EQ 125MG BASE/5ML	N061624 002
	EQ 250MG BASE/5ML	N061624 001
PUREPAC PHARM	EQ 125MG BASE/5ML	N061758 001
	EQ 250MG BASE/5ML	N061758 002
PFIZERPEN VK — PFIZER	EQ 125MG BASE/5ML	N061815 001
	EQ 250MG BASE/5ML	N061815 002
V-CILLIN K — LILLY	EQ 125MG BASE/5ML	N060004 001
	EQ 250MG BASE/5ML	N060004 002
VEETIDS '125' — APOTHECON	EQ 125MG BASE/5ML	N061206 001
	EQ 125MG BASE/5ML	N062153 001
VEETIDS '250' — APOTHECON	EQ 250MG BASE/5ML	N061206 002
	EQ 250MG BASE/5ML	N062153 002

Tablet; Oral

Product / Firm	Strength	Application No.
LEDERCILLIN VK — LEDERLE	EQ 250MG BASE	N060134 001
	EQ 500MG BASE	N060134 002
PEN-VEE K — WYETH AYERST	EQ 125MG BASE	N060006 001
	EQ 250MG BASE	N060006 002
	EQ 500MG BASE	N060006 003
PENAPAR-VK — PARKE DAVIS	EQ 250MG BASE	N062001 001
	EQ 500MG BASE	N062001 002
PENICILLIN V POTASSIUM — IVAX PHARMS	EQ 125MG BASE	N060518 001
	EQ 250MG BASE	N060518 002
	EQ 500MG BASE	N060518 003
MYLAN	EQ 250MG BASE	N061530 001
	EQ 500MG BASE	N061530 002
PUREPAC PHARM	EQ 125MG BASE	N061571 001
	EQ 250MG BASE	N061571 002
	EQ 500MG BASE	N061571 003
PFIZERPEN VK — PFIZER	EQ 250MG BASE	N061836 001
	EQ 500MG BASE	N061836 002
UTICILLIN VK — PHARMACIA AND UPJOHN	EQ 500MG BASE	N061651 002
V-CILLIN K — LILLY	EQ 125MG BASE	N060003 001
	EQ 250MG BASE	N060003 002
	EQ 500MG BASE	N060003 003

Discontinued Drug Products (continued)

PENICILLIN G POTASSIUM (continued)

Tablet; Oral

Product / Firm	Strength	Application No.
PENTIDS '400' — APOTHECON	400,000 UNITS	N062155 003
PENTIDS '800' — APOTHECON	800,000 UNITS	N060392 005
	800,000 UNITS	N062155 004
PFIZERPEN G — PFIZER	50,000 UNITS	N060075 001
	100,000 UNITS	N060075 002
	200,000 UNITS	N060075 003
	250,000 UNITS	N060075 004
	400,000 UNITS	N060075 005
	800,000 UNITS	N060075 006

PENICILLIN G PROCAINE

Injectable; Injection

Product / Firm	Strength	Application No.
DURACILLIN A.S. — LILLY	300,000 UNITS/ML	N060093 001
PENICILLIN G PROCAINE — CONSOLIDATED PHARM	300,000 UNITS/ML	N060800 001
	600,000 UNITS/1.2ML	N060800 002
PARKE DAVIS	300,000 UNITS/ML	N062029 001
	1,500,000 UNITS/VIAL	N060099 002
PFIZERPEN-AS — PFIZER	300,000 UNITS/VIAL	N060099 001
	300,000 UNITS/ML	N060286 001
	600,000 UNITS/ML	N060286 002

PENICILLIN G SODIUM

Injectable; Im-Iv

Product / Firm	Strength	Application No.
PENICILLIN G SODIUM — MARSAM PHARMS LLC	5,000,000 UNITS/VIAL	N063014 001 SEP 13, 1988

Injectable; Injection

Product / Firm	Strength	Application No.
PENICILLIN G SODIUM — BRISTOL MYERS SQUIBB	5,000,000 UNITS/VIAL	N061935 001
COPANOS	5,000,000 UNITS/VIAL	N061051 001
PHARMACIA AND UPJOHN	1,000,000 UNITS/VIAL	N061046 001

PENICILLIN V

For Suspension; Oral

Product / Firm	Strength	Application No.
V-CILLIN — LILLY	125MG/0.6ML	N060002 001

PENICILLIN V POTASSIUM

For Solution; Oral

Product / Firm	Strength	Application No.
BETAPEN-VK — APOTHECON	EQ 125MG BASE/5ML	N061149 001
	EQ 250MG BASE/5ML	N061149 002
LEDERCILLIN VK — LEDERLE	EQ 125MG BASE/5ML	N060136 001
	EQ 250MG BASE/5ML	N060136 002

Discontinued Drug Products (continued)

PENICILLIN V POTASSIUM (continued)
Tablet; Oral
VEETIDS '250'
   APOTHECON   EQ 250MG BASE   N061164 001
                  EQ 250MG BASE   N062156 002
VEETIDS '500'
   APOTHECON   EQ 500MG BASE   N061164 002
                  EQ 500MG BASE   N062156 001

PENTAGASTRIN
Injectable; Injection
PEPTAVLON
   WYETH AYERST   0.25MG/ML   N017048 001

PENTAMIDINE ISETHIONATE
Injectable; Injection
PENTACARINAT
   ARMOUR PHARM   300MG/VIAL   N073447 001   APR 28, 1994
PENTAMIDINE ISETHIONATE
   ELKINS SINN   300MG/VIAL   N073617 001   DEC 18, 1995

PENTAZOCINE HYDROCHLORIDE
Tablet; Oral
TALWIN 50
   SANOFI SYNTHELABO   EQ 50MG BASE   N016732 001

PENTAZOCINE HYDROCHLORIDE *MULTIPLE*
SEE ASPIRIN; PENTAZOCINE HYDROCHLORIDE

PENTETATE CALCIUM TRISODIUM YB-169
Injectable; Injection
YTTERBIUM YB 169 DTPA
   3M   2mCi/ML   N017518 001

PENTOBARBITAL
Elixir; Oral
NEMBUTAL
   ABBOTT   18.2MG/5ML   N083244 001

PENTOBARBITAL SODIUM
Capsule; Oral
NEMBUTAL SODIUM
   ABBOTT   50MG   N084093 001
PENTOBARBITAL SODIUM
   LANNETT   50MG   N085937 001
              100MG   N085915 001
              100MG   N083284 001
   VITARINE
   WHITEWORTH TOWN
   PLSN   100MG   N083338 001
SODIUM PENTOBARBITAL
   ANABOLIC   100MG   N084590 001
   ELKINS SINN   100MG   N083368 001

PENTOBARBITAL SODIUM (continued)
Capsule; Oral
SODIUM PENTOBARBITAL
   EVERYLIFE   100MG   N083259 001
   HALSEY   100MG   N084677 001
   IVAX PHARMS   50MG   N083461 001
                 100MG   N083461 002
   PARKE DAVIS   100MG   N084156 001
   PERRIGO   100MG   N084560 001
   PUREPAC PHARM   100MG   N083301 001
   WATSON LABS   100MG   N085791 001
   WYETH AYERST   100MG   N083239 001
Injectable; Injection
PENTOBARBITAL SODIUM
   ELKINS SINN   50MG/ML   N083270 001
SODIUM PENTOBARBITAL
   WYETH AYERST   50MG/ML   N083261 001
Suppository; Rectal
NEMBUTAL
   ABBOTT   30MG   N083247 001   JAN 25, 1982
              60MG   N083247 002   JAN 25, 1982
              120MG   N083247 003   JAN 25, 1982
              200MG   N083247 004   JAN 25, 1982
Tablet; Oral
PENTOBARBITAL SODIUM
   VITARINE   100MG   N083285 001
SODIUM PENTOBARBITAL
   ANABOLIC   100MG   N084238 001

PENTOLINIUM TARTRATE
Injectable; Injection
ANSOLYSEN
   WYETH AYERST   10MG/ML   N009372 001

PERFLUBRON
Liquid; Oral
IMAGENT
   ALLIANCE PHARM   100%   N020091 001   AUG 13, 1993

PERMETHRIN
Lotion; Topical
NIX
   GLAXOSMITHKLINE   1%   N019435 001   MAR 31, 1986

PERPHENAZINE
Concentrate; Oral
TRILAFON
   SCHERING   16MG/5ML   N011557 001

Discontinued Drug Products (continued)

PERPHENAZINE (continued)

Syrup; Oral
TRILAFON

SCHERING	2MG/5ML	N011294 002	

Tablet, Extended Release; Oral
TRILAFON

SCHERING	8MG	N011361 002	

Tablet; Oral
TRILAFON

SCHERING	2MG	N010775 001	
	4MG	N010775 002	
	8MG	N010775 003	
	16MG	N010775 004	

PERPHENAZINE *MULTIPLE*
SEE AMITRIPTYLINE HYDROCHLORIDE; PERPHENAZINE

PHENACEMIDE

Tablet; Oral
PHENURONE

ABBOTT	500MG	N007707 001	

PHENAZOPYRIDINE HYDROCHLORIDE; SULFAMETHOXAZOLE

Tablet; Oral
AZO GANTANOL

ROCHE	100MG;500MG	N013294 001	SEP 10, 1987

PHENAZOPYRIDINE HYDROCHLORIDE; SULFAMETHOXAZOLE; TRIMETHOPRIM

SULFAMETHOXAZOLE AND TRIMETHOPRIM AND PENAZOPYRIDINE HCL

ABLE	200MG;800MG;160MG	N021105 001	JUN 26, 2001

PHENAZOPYRIDINE HYDROCHLORIDE; SULFISOXAZOLE

Tablet; Oral
AZO GANTRISIN

ROCHE	50MG;500MG	N019358 001	AUG 31, 1990

PHENDIMETRAZINE TARTRATE

Capsule, Extended Release; Oral
MELFIAT-105

NUMARK	105MG	N087487 001	OCT 13, 1982

PHENDIMETRAZINE TARTRATE

GENEVA PHARMS	105MG	N087378 001	
GRAHAM DM	105MG	N087214 001	MAY 26, 1982
	105MG	N088020 001	
	105MG	N088028 001	AUG 16, 1982
	105MG		AUG 16, 1982

PHENDIMETRAZINE TARTRATE (continued)

Capsule, Extended Release; Oral
PHENDIMETRAZINE TARTRATE

GRAHAM DM	105MG	N088062 001	SEP 13, 1982
		N088063 001	SEP 10, 1982
	105MG	N088111 001	OCT 18, 1982
	105MG		

SPRX-105

NUMARK	105MG	N088024 001	DEC 22, 1982

Capsule; Oral
PHENAZINE

MAST MM	35MG	N086523 001	
	35MG	N086524 001	
	35MG	N086525 001	

PHENDIMETRAZINE TARTRATE

EON	35MG	N085633 001	
	35MG	N085694 001	
	35MG	N085702 001	
	35MG	N085634 001	
VITARINE	35MG	N085645 001	
	35MG	N085670 001	
	35MG	N086403 001	
	35MG	N086408 001	
	35MG	N086410 001	
	35MG	N087424 001	

SPRX-3

SOLVAY	35MG	N085897 001	

STATOBEX

TEVA	35MG	N085507 001	

Tablet; Oral
ADPHEN

FERNDALE LABS	35MG	N083655 001	

ALPHAZINE

EON	35MG	N085034 001	

DI-METREX

PVT FORM	35MG	N085698 001	

MELFIAT

NUMARK	35MG	N083790 002	

METRA

FOREST PHARMS	35MG	N083754 001	

PHENAZINE

MAST MM	35MG	N087305 001	

PHENAZINE-35

ABC HOLDING	35MG	N085512 001	

PHENDIMETRAZINE TARTRATE

ANABOLIC	35MG	N086020 001	
BARR	35MG	N083644 001	
	35MG	N083684 001	
	35MG	N083686 001	
	35MG	N083687 001	
	35MG	N084831 001	
	35MG	N084834 001	
	35MG	N084835 001	

Discontinued Drug Products *(continued)*

PHENDIMETRAZINE TARTRATE *(continued)*
Tablet; Oral

Product / Firm	Strength	Appl. No.
PHENDIMETRAZINE TARTRATE		
EON	35MG	N085402 001
	35MG	N085497 001
FERNDALE LABS	35MG	N086834 001
		SEP 15, 1983
GENEVA PHARMS	35MG	N086365 001
	35MG	N086370 001
INWOOD LABS	35MG	N084740 001
	35MG	N084741 001
	35MG	N084742 001
	35MG	N084743 001
IVAX PHARMS	35MG	N083682 001
	35MG	N085611 001
KV PHARM	35MG	N085612 001
	35MG	N084138 001
	35MG	N084141 001
MFG CHEMISTS	35MG	N085525 001
	35MG	N085914 001
NUMARK	35MG	N083790 001
PVT FORM	35MG	N085199 001
	35MG	N085697 001
SOLVAY	35MG	N083993 001
USL PHARMA	35MG	N083805 001
	35MG	N084398 001
	35MG	N084399 001
VITARINE	35MG	N085519 001
	35MG	N086005 001
	35MG	N086106 001
WATSON LABS	35MG	N085767 001
	35MG	N085768 001
	35MG	N085770 001
	35MG	N085773 001
PLEGINE		
WYETH AYERST	35MG	N012248 001
STATOBEX		
TEVA	35MG	N086013 001
STATOBEX-G		
TEVA	35MG	N085095 001
X-TROZINE		
SHIRE RICHWOOD	35MG	N086550 001
	35MG	N086551 001
	35MG	N086552 001

PHENINDIONE
Tablet; Oral

Product / Firm	Strength	Appl. No.
HEDULIN		
AVENTIS PHARMS	50MG	N008767 002

PHENMETRAZINE HYDROCHLORIDE
Tablet, Extended Release; Oral

Product / Firm	Strength	Appl. No.
PRELUDIN		
BOEHRINGER INGELHEIM	50MG	N011752 004
	75MG	N011752 003

PHENMETRAZINE HYDROCHLORIDE *(continued)*
Tablet; Oral

Product / Firm	Strength	Appl. No.
PRELUDIN		
BOEHRINGER INGELHEIM	25MG	N010460 005

PHENPROCOUMON
Tablet; Oral

Product / Firm	Strength	Appl. No.
LIQUAMAR		
ORGANON	3MG	N011228 001

PHENSUXIMIDE
Capsule; Oral

Product / Firm	Strength	Appl. No.
MILONTIN		
PARKE DAVIS	500MG	N008855 004

PHENTERMINE HYDROCHLORIDE
Capsule; Oral

Product / Firm	Strength	Appl. No.
FASTIN		
GLAXOSMITHKLINE	30MG	N017352 001
OBESTIN-30		
FERNDALE LABS	30MG	N087144 001
OBY-TRIM		
SHIRE RICHWOOD	30MG	N087764 001
		MAR 18, 1982
PHENTERMINE HCL		
ABC HOLDING	30MG	N085411 001
DURAMED PHARM BARR	30MG	N088948 001
		APR 25, 1986
EON	37.5MG	N088414 001
		OCT 19, 1983
		N086329 001
		N087022 001
		FEB 03, 1983
IVAX PHARMS	30MG	N086911 001
LANNETT	30MG	N087126 001
		N087777 001
		NOV 01, 1985
TEVA	30MG	N088612 001
		APR 04, 1984
		N088613 001
		APR 09, 1984
		N088614 001
		APR 09, 1984
USL PHARMA	30MG	N084487 001
		APR 09, 1982
		N088430 001
		MAR 27, 1984
VITARINE	30MG	N087202 001
		N087235 001
		N086740 001
		MAR 21, 1985
WATSON LABS	30MG	

Tablet; Oral

Product / Firm	Strength	Appl. No.
PHENTERMINE HCL		
EON	8MG	N085671 001

Discontinued Drug Products (continued)

PHENTERMINE HYDROCHLORIDE (continued)
Tablet; Oral

PHENTERMINE HCL
EON	8MG	N085689 001
IVAX PHARMS	8MG	N085553 001
VITARINE	8MG	N086453 001
	8MG	N086456 001
	8MG	N085739 001
WATSON LABS	8MG	
TORA		
SOLVAY	8MG	N084035 001

PHENTERMINE RESIN COMPLEX
Capsule, Extended Release; Oral

PHENTERMINE RESIN 30
QUANTUM PHARMICS	EQ 30MG BASE	N089120 001
		FEB 04, 1988

PHENYL AMINOSALICYLATE
Powder; Oral

PHENY-PAS-TEBAMIN
PURDUE FREDERICK	50%	N011695 002

Tablet; Oral

PHENY-PAS-TEBAMIN
PURDUE FREDERICK	500MG	N011695 003

PHENYLBUTAZONE
Capsule; Oral

AZOLID
AVENTIS	100MG	N087260 001

BUTAZOLIDIN
NOVARTIS	100MG	N008319 009

PHENYLBUTAZONE
GENEVA PHARMS	100MG	N087774 001
		JUN 16, 1982
	100MG	N088994 001
		DEC 04, 1985
HALSEY	100MG	N088218 001
IVAX PHARMS	100MG	N087674 001
		JUN 24, 1983
WATSON LABS	100MG	N087756 001
		DEC 17, 1982

Tablet; Oral

AZOLID
AVENTIS	100MG	N087091 001

BUTAZOLIDIN
NOVARTIS	100MG	N008319 008

PHENYLBUTAZONE
GENEVA PHARMS	100MG	N084339 001
HALSEY	100MG	N088863 001
		DEC 04, 1985
WATSON LABS	100MG	N086151 001
	100MG	N087674 001
		APR 21, 1982

PHENYLEPHRINE BITARTRATE *MULTIPLE*
SEE   ISOPROTERENOL HYDROCHLORIDE; PHENYLEPHRINE BITARTRATE

PHENYLEPHRINE HYDROCHLORIDE; PROMETHAZINE HYDROCHLORIDE
Syrup; Oral

PHENERGAN VC
WYETH AYERST	5MG/5ML;6.25MG/5ML	N008604 003
		APR 02, 1984

PHERAZINE VC
HALSEY	5MG/5ML;6.25MG/5ML	N088868 001
		MAR 02, 1987

PROMETHAZINE VC PLAIN
CENCI	5MG/5ML;6.25MG/5ML	N088815 001
		NOV 22, 1985

PHENYLEPHRINE HYDROCHLORIDE; PYRILAMINE MALEATE
Solution/Drops; Ophthalmic

PREFRIN-A
ALLERGAN	0.12%;0.1%	N007953 001

PHENYLEPHRINE HYDROCHLORIDE *MULTIPLE*
SEE   CODEINE PHOSPHATE; PHENYLEPHRINE HYDROCHLORIDE; PROMETHAZINE HYDROCHLORIDE

PHENYLPROPANOLAMINE HYDROCHLORIDE *MULTIPLE*
SEE   BROMPHENIRAMINE MALEATE; CODEINE PHOSPHATE; PHENYLPROPANOLAMINE HYDROCHLORIDE
SEE   BROMPHENIRAMINE MALEATE; PHENYLPROPANOLAMINE HYDROCHLORIDE
SEE   CHLORPHENIRAMINE MALEATE; PHENYLPROPANOLAMINE HYDROCHLORIDE
SEE   CLEMASTINE FUMARATE; PHENYLPROPANOLAMINE HYDROCHLORIDE
SEE   HYDROCODONE BITARTRATE; PHENYLPROPANOLAMINE HYDROCHLORIDE

PHENYLPROPANOLAMINE POLISTIREX *MULTIPLE*
SEE   CHLORPHENIRAMINE POLISTIREX; PHENYLPROPANOLAMINE POLISTIREX

PHENYTOIN
Suspension; Oral

DILANTIN-30
PARKE DAVIS	30MG/5ML	N008762 002

PHENYTOIN SODIUM
Injectable; Injection

DILANTIN
PARKE DAVIS	50MG/ML	N010151 001

PHENYTOIN SODIUM
ABBOTT	50MG/ML	N089521 001
		MAR 17, 1987
	50MG/ML	N089744 001
		DEC 18, 1987
AM PHARM PARTNERS	50MG/ML	N089003 001
		MAY 31, 1985
MARSAM PHARMS LLC	50MG/ML	N089501 001
		OCT 13, 1987
	50MG/ML	N089779 001
		NOV 27, 1992
SMITH AND NEPHEW	50MG/ML	N088519 001

Discontinued Drug Products *(continued)*

PHENYTOIN SODIUM *(continued)*
Injectable; Injection
  PHENYTOIN SODIUM
    SMITH AND NEPHEW   50MG/ML   DEC 19, 1984 N088521 001
                                DEC 18, 1984 N088520 001
    SOLOPAK   50MG/ML   DEC 17, 1984 N085434 001
    STERIS   50MG/ML   N089900 001
    WARNER CHILCOTT   50MG/ML   MAR 30, 1990

PHENYTOIN SODIUM, EXTENDED
Capsule; Oral
  EXTENDED PHENYTOIN SODIUM
    PLIVA   100MG   N089441 001 DEC 18, 1986
  PHENYTEX
    WATSON LAB   100MG   N088711 001 DEC 21, 1984

PHENYTOIN SODIUM, PROMPT
Capsule; Oral
  DIPHENYLAN SODIUM
    LANNETT   30MG   N080857 001
                  100MG   N080857 002
  PHENYTOIN SODIUM
    PHARMERAL   100MG   N085435 001
    WATSON LABS   100MG   N085894 001
  PROMPT PHENYTOIN SODIUM
    WATSON LABS   100MG   N080905 001

PHOSPHORIC ACID *MULTIPLE*
  SEE AMINO ACIDS; MAGNESIUM ACETATE; PHOSPHORIC ACID; POTASSIUM ACETATE; SODIUM CHLORIDE

PHYTONADIONE
Injectable; Injection
  KONAKION
    ROCHE   1MG/0.5ML   N011745 001
              10MG/ML   N011745 003
  PHYTONADIONE
    GLAXOSMITHKLINE   1MG/0.5ML   N084060 001
                       10MG/ML   N084060 002
  VITAMIN K1
    ABBOTT   10MG/ML   N087956 001 JUL 25, 1983

PHYTONADIONE *MULTIPLE*
  SEE ASCORBIC ACID; BIOTIN; CYANOCOBALAMIN; ERGOCALCIFEROL; FOLIC ACID; NIACINAMIDE; PANTOTHENIC ACID; PHYTONADIONE; PYRIDOXINE; RIBOFLAVIN; THIAMINE; VITAMIN A PALMITATE; VITAMIN E

PILOCARPINE
Drug Delivery System; Ophthalmic
  OCUSERT PILO-40
    AKORN   11MG   N017548 001
Insert, Extended Release; Ophthalmic
  OCUSERT PILO-20
    AKORN   5MG   N017431 001

PILOCARPINE HYDROCHLORIDE *MULTIPLE*
  SEE BETAXOLOL HYDROCHLORIDE; PILOCARPINE HYDROCHLORIDE

PINACIDIL
Capsule, Extended Release; Oral
  PINDAC
    LEO PHARM   12.5MG   N019456 001 DEC 28, 1989
                  25MG   N019456 002 DEC 28, 1989

PINDOLOL
Tablet; Oral
  PINDOLOL
    PUREPAC PHARM   5MG   N074125 001 APR 28, 1993
                      10MG   N074125 002 APR 28, 1993

PINDOLOL *MULTIPLE*
  SEE HYDROCHLOROTHIAZIDE; PINDOLOL

PIPECURONIUM BROMIDE
Injectable; Injection
  ARDUAN
    ORGANON USA INC   10MG/VIAL   N019638 001 JUN 26, 1990

PIPERACETAZINE
Tablet; Oral
  QUIDE
    DOW PHARM   10MG   N013615 001
                  25MG   N013615 002

PIPERACILLIN SODIUM
Injectable; Injection
  PIPRACIL
    WYETH PHARMS INC   EQ 2GM BASE/VIAL   N050545 002 OCT 13, 1987
                       EQ 2GM BASE/VIAL   N062750 001
                       EQ 3GM BASE/VIAL   N050545 003 OCT 13, 1987
                       EQ 3GM BASE/VIAL   N062750 002 OCT 13, 1987
                       EQ 4GM BASE/VIAL   N050545 004
                       EQ 4GM BASE/VIAL   N062750 003 OCT 13, 1987

Discontinued Drug Products *(continued)*

PIPERACILLIN SODIUM *(continued)*
Injectable; Injection
PIPRACIL
- WYETH PHARMS INC — EQ 40GM BASE/VIAL *SEE ANNUAL PREFACE INTRODUCTION DISCONTINUED SECTION* — N050545 006 — SEP 30, 1985

PIPERAZINE CITRATE
Syrup; Oral
ANTEPAR
- GLAXOSMITHKLINE — EQ 500MG BASE/5ML — N009102 001
BRYREL
- SANOFI SYNTHELABO — EQ 500MG BASE/5ML — N017796 001
PIPERAZINE CITRATE
- ALPHARMA — EQ 500MG BASE/5ML — N080774 001
- LANNETT — EQ 500MG BASE/5ML — N080963 001
VERMIDOL
- SOLVAY — EQ 500MG BASE/5ML — N080992 001
Tablet; Oral
ANTEPAR
- GLAXOSMITHKLINE — EQ 500MG BASE — N009102 003
PIPERAZINE CITRATE
- IMPAX LABS — EQ 250MG BASE — N080874 001

PIPOBROMAN
Tablet; Oral
VERCYTE
- ABBOTT — 10MG — N016245 001
- — 25MG — N016245 002

PIRBUTEROL ACETATE
Aerosol, Metered; Inhalation
MAXAIR
- 3M — EQ 0.2MG BASE/INH — N019009 001 — DEC 30, 1986

PIROXICAM
Capsule; Oral
PIROXICAM
- ROXANE — 10MG — N073651 001 — FEB 26, 1993
- — 20MG — N073651 002 — FEB 26, 1993

POLYESTRADIOL PHOSPHATE
Injectable; Injection
ESTRADURIN
- WYETH AYERST — 40MG/AMP — N010753 001

POLYETHYLENE GLYCOL 3350; POTASSIUM CHLORIDE; SODIUM BICARBONATE; SODIUM CHLORIDE; SODIUM SULFATE, ANHYDROUS
For Solution; Oral
COLYTE
- SCHWARZ PHARMA — 227.1GM/PACKET;2.82GM/PACKET;6.36GM/PACKET;5.53GM/PACKET:21.5GM/PACKET — N018983 004 — OCT 26, 1984
- — 120GM/PACKET;1.49GM/PACKET;3.36GM/PACKET;2.92GM/PACKET;11.36GM/PACKET — N018983 005 — OCT 26, 1984
- — 360GM/PACKET;4.47GM/PACKET;10.08GM/PACKET;8.76GM/PACKET;34.08GM/PACKET — N018983 006 — OCT 26, 1984

For Suspension; Oral
PEG-LYTE
- INVAMED — 236GM/BOT;2.97GM/BOT;6.74GM/BOT;5.86GM/BOT;22.74GM/BOT — N073098 001 — AUG 31, 1993

POLYMYXIN B SULFATE
Injectable; Injection
AEROSPORIN
- GLAXOSMITHKLINE — EQ 500,000 U BASE/VIAL — N062036 001
Powder; For Rx Compounding
POLYMYXIN B SULFATE
- PADDOCK — 100,000,000 UNITS/BOT — N062455 001 — JUL 27, 1983

POLYMYXIN B SULFATE *MULTIPLE*
- SEE BACITRACIN;HYDROCORTISONE ACETATE; NEOMYCIN SULFATE; POLYMYXIN B SULFATE
- SEE BACITRACIN; NEOMYCIN SULFATE; POLYMYXIN B SULFATE
- SEE BACITRACIN; POLYMYXIN B SULFATE
- SEE BACITRACIN ZINC; HYDROCORTISONE; NEOMYCIN SULFATE; POLYMYXIN B SULFATE
- SEE BACITRACIN ZINC; LIDOCAINE; NEOMYCIN SULFATE; POLYMYXIN B SULFATE
- SEE BACITRACIN ZINC; NEOMYCIN SULFATE; POLYMYXIN B SULFATE
- SEE BACITRACIN ZINC; POLYMYXIN B SULFATE
- SEE CHLORAMPHENICOL; HYDROCORTISONE ACETATE; POLYMYXIN B SULFATE
- SEE CHLORAMPHENICOL; POLYMYXIN B SULFATE
- SEE DEXAMETHASONE; NEOMYCIN SULFATE; POLYMYXIN B SULFATE
- SEE GRAMICIDIN; NEOMYCIN SULFATE; POLYMYXIN B SULFATE
- SEE HYDROCORTISONE; NEOMYCIN SULFATE; POLYMYXIN B SULFATE
- SEE HYDROCORTISONE; POLYMYXIN B SULFATE
- SEE NEOMYCIN SULFATE; POLYMYXIN B SULFATE
- SEE OXYTETRACYCLINE HYDROCHLORIDE; POLYMYXIN B SULFATE

Discontinued Drug Products (continued)

POTASSIUM ACETATE *MULTIPLE*

SEE   AMINO ACIDS; DEXTROSE; MAGNESIUM CHLORIDE; POTASSIUM ACETATE; POTASSIUM ACETATE; POTASSIUM CHLORIDE; POTASSIUM PHOSPHATE, DIBASIC; SODIUM CHLORIDE

SEE   AMINO ACIDS; MAGNESIUM ACETATE; PHOSPHORIC ACID; POTASSIUM ACETATE; SODIUM CHLORIDE

SEE   AMINO ACIDS; MAGNESIUM ACETATE; POTASSIUM ACETATE; SODIUM CHLORIDE

SEE   AMINO ACIDS; MAGNESIUM ACETATE; POTASSIUM ACETATE; SODIUM CHLORIDE; SODIUM PHOSPHATE, DIBASIC, HEPTAHYDRATE

SEE   AMINO ACIDS; MAGNESIUM CHLORIDE; POTASSIUM ACETATE; POTASSIUM CHLORIDE; SODIUM ACETATE

POTASSIUM AMINOSALICYLATE

Powder; Oral

POTASSIUM AMINOSALICYLATE			
HEXCEL	100%		N080098 001

POTASSIUM CHLORIDE

Capsule, Extended Release; Oral

K-LEASE			
SAVAGE LABS	8MEQ		N073398 001
			JAN 28, 1992
	10MEQ		N072427 001
			MAR 28, 1990

For Suspension, Extended Release; Oral

MICRO-K LS			
KV PHARM	20MEQ/PACKET		N019561 003
			AUG 26, 1988

Injectable; Injection

POTASSIUM CHLORIDE			
ABBOTT	1MEQ/ML		N080205 003
	1MEQ/ML		N083345 003
	2.4MEQ/ML		N080205 004
	3.2MEQ/ML		N080205 005
	2MEQ/ML		N088286 001
			SEP 05, 1985
AM PHARM PARTNERS	2MEQ/ML		N080204 001
	2MEQ/ML		N084290 001
	2MEQ/ML		N086713 001
	2MEQ/ML		N086714 001
	2MEQ/ML		N087787 001
			APR 20, 1982
	2MEQ/ML		N087885 001
			FEB 03, 1983
	2MEQ/ML		N080203 001
ELKINS SINN	2MEQ/ML		N086219 001
GD SEARLE LLC	1MEQ/ML		N086219 002
	2MEQ/ML		N086220 002
	3MEQ/ML		N086219 003
	3MEQ/ML		N086220 001
	4MEQ/ML		N086219 004
LILLY	2MEQ/ML		N007865 002
LUITPOLD	2MEQ/ML		N080221 001
	2MEQ/ML		N080736 001
MILES	1MEQ/ML		N080195 002

POTASSIUM CHLORIDE (continued)

Injectable; Injection

POTASSIUM CHLORIDE			
MILES	2MEQ/ML		N080195 001
	3MEQ/ML		N080195 003
	4MEQ/ML		N080195 004
	2MEQ/ML		N086208 001
	2MEQ/ML		N089163 001
			MAR 10, 1988
STERIS	2MEQ/ML		N089421 001
			JAN 02, 1987
	3MEQ/ML		N086210 001

POTASSIUM CHLORIDE 10MEQ IN PLASTIC CONTAINER			
ABBOTT	745MG/100ML		N020161 001
			NOV 30, 1992
	14.9MG/ML		N020161 005
			NOV 30, 1992

POTASSIUM CHLORIDE 20MEQ IN PLASTIC CONTAINER			
ABBOTT	1.49GM/100ML		N020161 002
			NOV 30, 1992

Tablet, Extended Release; Oral

KAON CL			
SAVAGE LABS	6.7MEQ		N017046 001
KAON CL-10			
SAVAGE LABS	10MEQ		N017046 002
TEN-K			
NOVARTIS	10MEQ		N019381 001
			APR 16, 1986

POTASSIUM CHLORIDE; SODIUM CHLORIDE

Injectable; Injection

POTASSIUM CHLORIDE 0.3% IN SODIUM CHLORIDE 0.9% IN PLASTIC CONTAINER			
B BRAUN	300MG/100ML;900MG/100ML		N019708 006
			SEP 29, 1989

POTASSIUM CHLORIDE 0.11% IN SODIUM CHLORIDE 0.9% IN PLASTIC CONTAINER			
B BRAUN	110MG/100ML;900MG/100ML		N019708 003
			SEP 29, 1989

POTASSIUM CHLORIDE 0.22% IN SODIUM CHLORIDE 0.9% IN PLASTIC CONTAINER			
B BRAUN	220MG/100ML;900MG/100ML		N019708 005
			SEP 29, 1989

POTASSIUM CHLORIDE 0.037% IN SODIUM CHLORIDE 0.9% IN PLASTIC CONTAINER			
B BRAUN	37MG/100ML;900MG/100ML		N019708 001
			SEP 29, 1989

POTASSIUM CHLORIDE 0.075% IN SODIUM CHLORIDE 0.9% IN PLASTIC CONTAINER			
B BRAUN	75MG/100ML;900MG/100ML		N019708 002
			SEP 29, 1989

SODIUM CHLORIDE 0.9% AND POTASSIUM CHLORIDE 0.075% IN PLASTIC CONTAINER			
BAXTER HLTHCARE	75MG/100ML;900MG/100ML		N017648 004
B BRAUN	75MG/100ML;900MG/100ML		N018722 001

POTASSIUM CHLORIDE *MULTIPLE* (continued)

SEE DEXTROSE; POTASSIUM CHLORIDE
SEE DEXTROSE; POTASSIUM CHLORIDE; SODIUM CHLORIDE
SEE MAGNESIUM CHLORIDE; POTASSIUM CHLORIDE; POTASSIUM PHOSPHATE, MONOBASIC; SODIUM ACETATE; SODIUM CHLORIDE; SODIUM GLUCONATE; SODIUM PHOSPHATE, DIBASIC, HEPTAHYDRATE
SEE MAGNESIUM CHLORIDE; POTASSIUM CHLORIDE; SODIUM ACETATE; SODIUM CHLORIDE; SODIUM GLUCONATE
SEE POLYETHYLENE GLYCOL 3350; POTASSIUM CHLORIDE; SODIUM BICARBONATE; SODIUM CHLORIDE; SODIUM SULFATE, ANHYDROUS

POTASSIUM CITRATE
For Solution; Oral

POTASSIUM CITRATE			
MISSION PHARMA	10MEQ/PACKET	N019647 002	OCT 13, 1988
	20MEQ/PACKET	N019647 001	OCT 13, 1988

POTASSIUM IODIDE
Solution; Oral

POTASSIUM IODIDE			
ROXANE	1GM/ML	N018551 001	FEB 19, 1982

POTASSIUM PHOSPHATE, DIBASIC *MULTIPLE*

SEE AMINO ACIDS; CALCIUM CHLORIDE; DEXTROSE; MAGNESIUM CHLORIDE; POTASSIUM CHLORIDE; POTASSIUM PHOSPHATE, DIBASIC; SODIUM CHLORIDE
SEE AMINO ACIDS; DEXTROSE; MAGNESIUM CHLORIDE; POTASSIUM ACETATE; POTASSIUM CHLORIDE; POTASSIUM PHOSPHATE, DIBASIC; SODIUM CHLORIDE
SEE AMINO ACIDS; DEXTROSE; MAGNESIUM CHLORIDE; POTASSIUM CHLORIDE; POTASSIUM PHOSPHATE, DIBASIC; SODIUM CHLORIDE
SEE AMINO ACIDS; MAGNESIUM CHLORIDE; POTASSIUM CHLORIDE; POTASSIUM PHOSPHATE, DIBASIC, HEPTAHYDRATE

POTASSIUM PHOSPHATE, MONOBASIC *MULTIPLE*

SEE MAGNESIUM CHLORIDE; POTASSIUM CHLORIDE; POTASSIUM PHOSPHATE, MONOBASIC; SODIUM ACETATE; SODIUM CHLORIDE; SODIUM GLUCONATE; SODIUM PHOSPHATE, DIBASIC, HEPTAHYDRATE

PRALIDOXIME CHLORIDE
Injectable; Injection

PRALIDOXIME CHLORIDE			
BAXTER HLTHCARE CORP	300MG/ML	N018799 001	DEC 13, 1982
QUAD PHARMS	1GM/VIAL	N072224 001	NOV 23, 1988

Tablet; Oral

PROTOPAM CHLORIDE			
WYETH AYERST	500MG	N014122 002	

Discontinued Drug Products (continued)

POTASSIUM CHLORIDE; SODIUM CHLORIDE (continued)
Injectable; Injection

SODIUM CHLORIDE 0.9% AND POTASSIUM CHLORIDE 0.075% IN PLASTIC CONTAINER

B BRAUN			NOV 09, 1982

SODIUM CHLORIDE 0.9% AND POTASSIUM CHLORIDE 0.15% IN PLASTIC CONTAINER

B BRAUN	150MG/100ML;900MG/100ML	N018722 002	NOV 09, 1982

SODIUM CHLORIDE 0.9% AND POTASSIUM CHLORIDE 0.22% IN PLASTIC CONTAINER

B BRAUN	220MG/100ML;900MG/100ML	N018722 003	NOV 09, 1982

SODIUM CHLORIDE 0.9% AND POTASSIUM CHLORIDE 0.3% IN PLASTIC CONTAINER

B BRAUN	300MG/100ML;900MG/100ML	N018722 004	NOV 09, 1982

POTASSIUM CHLORIDE; SODIUM CHLORIDE; TROMETHAMINE
Injectable; Injection

THAM-E			
ABBOTT	370MG/VIAL;1.75GM/VIAL;.36GM/VIAL	N013025 001	

POTASSIUM CHLORIDE *MULTIPLE*

SEE AMINO ACIDS; CALCIUM CHLORIDE; DEXTROSE; MAGNESIUM CHLORIDE; POTASSIUM CHLORIDE; POTASSIUM PHOSPHATE, DIBASIC; SODIUM CHLORIDE
SEE AMINO ACIDS; DEXTROSE; MAGNESIUM CHLORIDE; POTASSIUM CHLORIDE; POTASSIUM ACETATE; POTASSIUM PHOSPHATE, DIBASIC; SODIUM CHLORIDE
SEE AMINO ACIDS; DEXTROSE; MAGNESIUM CHLORIDE; POTASSIUM CHLORIDE; POTASSIUM PHOSPHATE, DIBASIC; SODIUM CHLORIDE
SEE AMINO ACIDS; DEXTROSE; POTASSIUM PHOSPHATE, DIBASIC; SODIUM CHLORIDE
SEE AMINO ACIDS; DEXTROSE; MAGNESIUM CHLORIDE; POTASSIUM CHLORIDE; SODIUM PHOSPHATE, DIBASIC, HEPTAHYDRATE
SEE AMINO ACIDS; MAGNESIUM CHLORIDE; POTASSIUM ACETATE; POTASSIUM CHLORIDE; SODIUM ACETATE
SEE AMINO ACIDS; MAGNESIUM CHLORIDE; POTASSIUM CHLORIDE; POTASSIUM PHOSPHATE, DIBASIC; SODIUM CHLORIDE
SEE AMINO ACIDS; MAGNESIUM CHLORIDE; POTASSIUM CHLORIDE; SODIUM PHOSPHATE, DIBASIC, HEPTAHYDRATE
SEE CALCIUM CHLORIDE; DEXTROSE; MAGNESIUM CHLORIDE; POTASSIUM CHLORIDE; SODIUM ACETATE; SODIUM CHLORIDE
SEE CALCIUM CHLORIDE; DEXTROSE; MAGNESIUM CHLORIDE; POTASSIUM CHLORIDE; SODIUM CITRATE
SEE CALCIUM CHLORIDE; DEXTROSE; POTASSIUM CHLORIDE; SODIUM CHLORIDE; SODIUM LACTATE
SEE CALCIUM CHLORIDE; MAGNESIUM CHLORIDE; POTASSIUM CHLORIDE; SODIUM ACETATE; SODIUM CHLORIDE
SEE CALCIUM CHLORIDE; MAGNESIUM CHLORIDE; POTASSIUM CHLORIDE; SODIUM ACETATE; SODIUM CHLORIDE; SODIUM CITRATE
SEE CALCIUM CHLORIDE; POTASSIUM CHLORIDE; SODIUM ACETATE; SODIUM CHLORIDE; SODIUM CITRATE
SEE CALCIUM CHLORIDE; POTASSIUM CHLORIDE; SODIUM CHLORIDE
SEE CALCIUM CHLORIDE; POTASSIUM CHLORIDE; SODIUM CHLORIDE; SODIUM LACTATE

Discontinued Drug Products (continued)

PRALIDOXIME CHLORIDE *MULTIPLE*
  SEE ATROPINE; PRALIDOXIME CHLORIDE

PRAMIPEXOLE DIHYDROCHLORIDE
  Tablet; Oral
    MIRAPEX
      PHARMACIA AND
      UPJOHN   1.25MG   N020667 004
                                 JUL 01, 1997

PRAMOXINE HYDROCHLORIDE *MULTIPLE*
  SEE HYDROCORTISONE ACETATE; PRAMOXINE HYDROCHLORIDE

PRAZEPAM
  Capsule; Oral
    CENTRAX
    PARKE DAVIS   5MG   N018144 001
                  10MG   N018144 002
                  20MG   N018144 003
                           MAY 10, 1982
    PRAZEPAM
    USL PHARMA   5MG   N070427 001
                           NOV 06, 1987
                  10MG   N070428 001
                           NOV 06, 1987
  Tablet; Oral
    CENTRAX
    PARKE DAVIS   10MG   N017415 001

PRAZOSIN HYDROCHLORIDE
  Capsule; Oral
    PRAZOSIN HCL
    AM THERAP   EQ 1MG BASE   N072782 001
                                     MAY 16, 1989
              EQ 2MG BASE   N072783 001
                                     MAY 16, 1989
              EQ 5MG BASE   N072784 001
                                     MAY 16, 1989
    PUREPAC PHARM EQ 1MG BASE   N072991 001
                                     MAY 16, 1989
              EQ 2MG BASE   N072921 001
                                     MAY 16, 1989
              EQ 5MG BASE   N072992 001
                                     MAY 16, 1989

PREDNISOLONE
  Cream; Topical
    METI-DERM
    SCHERING   0.5%   N010209 002
  Tablet; Oral
    CORTALONE
    HALSEY   1MG   N080304 003
               2.5MG   N080304 002
               5MG   N080304 001

PREDNISOLONE (continued)
  Tablet; Oral
    DELTA-CORTEF
      PHARMACIA AND
      UPJOHN   5MG   N009987 004
    FERNISOLONE-P
    FERNDALE LABS 5MG   N083941 001
    PREDNISOLONE
    BARR   5MG   N084426 002
    BUNDY   5MG   N083675 001
    ELKINS SINN   5MG   N080625 001
    EON   5MG   N084773 001
    EVERYLIFE   1MG   N084439 001
    FERRANTE   2.5MG   N080562 001
               5MG   N080562 002
    GENEVA PHARMS 5MG   N080339 001
    HEATHER   5MG   N080326 001
    ICN   5MG   N080236 001
    IMPAX LABS   5MG   N080780 001
    INWOOD LABS   5MG   N080748 001
    IVAX PHARMS   5MG   N080378 001
    PANRAY   1MG   N080351 001
               5MG   N080351 002
    PERRIGO   5MG   N084542 001
    PHOENIX LABS NY 5MG   N080322 001
    PUREPAC PHARM 5MG   N080325 001
    PVT FORM   5MG   N080211 001
    ROXANE   5MG   N080327 002
    SUPERPHARM   5MG   N088892 001
                                 FEB 26, 1985
    TABLICAPS   5MG   N085170 001
    TEVA   5MG   N080398 001
    UDL   5MG   N087987 001
                                  JAN 18, 1983
               5MG   N080534 001
    VITARINE   5MG   N085085 002
    WATSON LABS   5MG   N085415 001
               5MG   N085416 001
    WEST WARD   5MG   N080324 001
    WHITEWORTH TOWN
    PLSN   5MG   N080342 001
    STERANE
    PFIZER   5MG   N009996 001

PREDNISOLONE *MULTIPLE*
  SEE CHLORAMPHENICOL; PREDNISOLONE

PREDNISOLONE ACETATE
  Injectable; Injection
    METICORTELONE
    SCHERING   25MG/ML   N010255 002
    PREDNISOLONE ACETATE
    AKORN   25MG/ML   N083032 001
               50MG/ML   N084492 001
    BEL MAR   25MG/ML   N083738 001
               50MG/ML   N083738 002

PREDNISOLONE SODIUM PHOSPHATE *(continued)*

Ointment; Ophthalmic, Otic

HYDELTRASOL			
MERCK	EQ 0.25% PHOSPHATE	N011028 001	

Solution/Drops; Ophthalmic

METRETON			
SCHERING	EQ 0.5% PHOSPHATE	N083834 001	
PREDAIR			
PHARMAFAIR	EQ 0.11% PHOSPHATE	N088415 001	FEB 29, 1984
PREDAIR FORTE			
PHARMAFAIR	EQ 0.9% PHOSPHATE	N088165 001	MAR 28, 1983

PREDNISOLONE SODIUM PHOSPHATE

AKORN	EQ 0.11% PHOSPHATE	N083358 001	
	EQ 0.9% PHOSPHATE	N083358 002	
	EQ 0.11% PHOSPHATE	N081043 001	OCT 24, 1991
ALCON UNIVERSAL	EQ 0.9% PHOSPHATE	N081044 001	OCT 24, 1991
	EQ 0.9% PHOSPHATE	N084168 001	
SOLA BARNES HIND	EQ 0.9% PHOSPHATE	N084169 001	
	EQ 0.11% PHOSPHATE	N084171 001	
	EQ 0.9% PHOSPHATE	N084172 001	

PREDNISOLONE SODIUM PHOSPHATE; SULFACETAMIDE SODIUM

Solution/Drops; Ophthalmic

SULSTER			
AKORN	EQ 0.23% PHOSPHATE;10%	N074511 001	JUL 30, 1996

PREDNISOLONE SODIUM PHOSPHATE *MULTIPLE*
SEE NEOMYCIN SULFATE; PREDNISOLONE SODIUM PHOSPHATE

PREDNISOLONE TEBUTATE

Injectable; Injection

HYDELTRA-TBA			
MERCK	20MG/ML	N010562 001	
PREDNISOLONE TEBUTATE			
STERIS	20MG/ML	N083362 001	FEB 17, 1984

PREDNISONE

Solution; Oral

PREDNISONE			
MORTON GROVE	5MG/5ML	N089726 001	AUG 02, 1988

Syrup; Oral

LIQUID PRED			
MURO	5MG/5ML	N087611 002	SEP 07, 1982

Tablet; Oral

CORTAN			
HALSEY	20MG	N087480 001	

Discontinued Drug Products *(continued)*

PREDNISOLONE ACETATE *(continued)*

Injectable; Injection

PREDNISOLONE ACETATE		
CENT PHARMS	25MG/ML	N084717 001
	50MG/ML	N084717 002
	25MG/ML	N083654 001
	40MG/ML	N083767 001
STERANE		
PFIZER	25MG/ML	N011446 001

Suspension/Drops; Ophthalmic

ECONOPRED		
ALCON	0.125%	N017468 001

PREDNISOLONE ACETATE; SULFACETAMIDE SODIUM

Ointment; Ophthalmic

CETAPRED			
ALCON	0.25%;10%	N087771 001	AUG 06, 1993
METIMYD			
SCHERING	0.5%;10%	N010210 002	SEP 09, 1984
PREDSULFAIR			
PHARMAFAIR	0.5%;10%	N088032 001	APR 15, 1983

Suspension/Drops; Ophthalmic

METIMYD			
SCHERING	0.5%;10%	N010210 001	
PREDAMIDE			
AKORN	0.5%;10%	N088059 001	JUL 29, 1983
PREDSULFAIR			
PHARMAFAIR	0.5%;10%	N088007 001	APR 19, 1983
PREDSULFAIR II			
PHARMAFAIR	0.2%;10%	N088837 001	DEC 24, 1985
SULPHRIN			
BAUSCH AND LOMB	0.5%;10%	N088089 001	DEC 28, 1982

Suspension; Ophthalmic

ISOPTO CETAPRED			
ALCON	0.25%;10%	N087547 001	

PREDNISOLONE ACETATE *MULTIPLE*
SEE NEOMYCIN SULFATE; PREDNISOLONE ACETATE

PREDNISOLONE SODIUM PHOSPHATE

Injectable; Injection

HYDELTRASOL		
MERCK	EQ 20MG PHOSPHATE/ML	N011583 002
PREDNISOLONE SODIUM PHOSPHATE		
STERIS	EQ 20MG PHOSPHATE/ML	N080517 001

Discontinued Drug Products *(continued)*

PREDNISONE *(continued)*
Tablet; Oral

Trade Name / Applicant	Strength	Appl. No.	Date
DELTA-DOME			
BAYER PHARMS	5MG	N080293 001	
FERNISONE			
FERNDALE LABS	5MG	N083364 001	
METICORTEN			
SCHERING	1MG	N009766 002	
	5MG	N009766 001	
ORASONE			
SOLVAY	1MG	N083009 001	
	5MG	N083009 002	
	10MG	N083009 003	
	20MG	N083009 004	
	50MG	N085999 001	
PARACORT			
PARKE DAVIS	5MG	N010962 002	
PREDNICEN-M			
SCHWARZ PHARMA	5MG	N084655 001	
PREDNISONE			
AM THERAP	5MG	N089387 001	NOV 06, 1986
	5MG	N089388 001	NOV 06, 1986
	10MG	N089389 001	NOV 06, 1986
	20MG	N083676 001	NOV 06, 1986
BUNDY	5MG	N088394 001	OCT 04, 1983
DURAMED PHARM BARR	5MG	N088395 001	OCT 04, 1983
	10MG	N088396 001	OCT 04, 1983
	20MG	N080491 001	
ELKINS SINN	5MG	N085811 001	
	20MG	N084774 001	
EON	5MG	N084440 001	
EVERYLIFE	1MG	N084440 002	
	2.5MG	N084440 003	
	5MG	N080563 001	
FERRANTE	2.5MG	N080563 002	
	5MG	N080336 002	
GENEVA PHARMS	5MG	N080300 001	
HALSEY	5MG	N080701 001	
	5MG	N086595 001	
	10MG	N084634 001	
	20MG	N086596 001	
	50MG	N080320 001	
HEATHER	5MG	N084341 001	
	10MG	N084417 001	
	20MG	N085543 001	
ICN	20MG	N086946 001	
	50MG	N080237 001	
IMPAX LABS	5MG	N080782 001	
INTERPHARM	5MG	N089597 001	OCT 05, 1987

PREDNISONE *(continued)*
Tablet; Oral

Trade Name / Applicant	Strength	Appl. No.	Date
PREDNISONE			
INTERPHARM	10MG	N089598 001	OCT 05, 1987
	20MG	N089599 001	OCT 05, 1987
INWOOD LABS	1MG	N080328 001	
	2.5MG	N080306 001	
	5MG	N080279 001	
IVAX PHARMS	5MG	N080283 001	
	10MG	N084133 001	
	20MG	N084134 001	
KV PHARM	5MG	N084236 001	
LANNETT	5MG	N080514 001	
	20MG	N084275 001	
LEDERLE	5MG	N086968 001	
NYLOS	5MG	N085115 001	
PANRAY	1MG	N080350 001	
	2.5MG	N080350 002	
	5MG	N080350 003	
PERRIGO	5MG	N083059 001	
PHARMAVITE	5MG	N084662 002	
PHOENIX LABS NY	5MG	N080321 001	
	20MG	N083807 001	
PUREPAC PHARM	5MG	N080353 001	
	10MG	N086062 001	
	20MG	N086061 001	
PVT FORM	20MG	N085151 001	
REXALL	5MG	N080232 001	
ROXANE	20MG	N017109 001	
	25MG	N087833 001	MAY 04, 1982
SCHERER LABS	5MG	N080371 001	
SPERTI	1MG	N080359 001	
	2.5MG	N080359 002	
	5MG	N080359 003	
SUPERPHARM	5MG	N088865 001	OCT 25, 1984
	10MG	N088866 001	OCT 25, 1984
	20MG	N088867 001	OCT 25, 1984
TEVA	5MG	N080397 001	
UDL	5MG	N087984 001	JAN 18, 1983
	10MG	N087985 001	JAN 18, 1983
	20MG	N087986 001	JAN 18, 1983
UPSHER SMITH	5MG	N087471 001	
	20MG	N087470 001	
VANGARD	5MG	N087682 001	JAN 15, 1982
	20MG	N087701 001	JAN 15, 1982
VITARINE	5MG	N080334 001	

Discontinued Drug Products (continued)

PREDNISONE (continued)
Tablet; Oral
PREDNISONE

VITARINE	5MG	N080506 001
WATSON LABS	5MG	N085084 002
	50MG	N086867 001
WHITEWORTH TOWN		
PLSN	2.5MG	N084913 001
	5MG	N080343 001
	10MG	N089028 001
		JUL 24, 1986
	20MG	N084913 002

SERVISONE

LEDERLE	5MG	N080223 001

PRILOCAINE HYDROCHLORIDE
Injectable; Injection
CITANEST

ASTRAZENECA	1%	N014763 004
	2%	N014763 005
	3%	N014763 003

CITANEST PLAIN

ASTRAZENECA	4%	N014763 007

PRILOCAINE HYDROCHLORIDE *MULTIPLE*
SEE   EPINEPHRINE BITARTRATE; PRILOCAINE HYDROCHLORIDE

PRIMAQUINE PHOSPHATE *MULTIPLE*
SEE   CHLOROQUINE PHOSPHATE; PRIMAQUINE PHOSPHATE

PRIMIDONE
Suspension; Oral
MYSOLINE

XCEL PHARMS	250MG/5ML	N010401 001

Tablet; Oral
PRIMIDONE

WATSON LAB	250MG	N085052 001

PROBENECID
Tablet; Oral
BENEMID

MERCK	500MG	N007898 004

PROBENECID

LEDERLE	500MG	N086917 001
WATSON LABS	500MG	N086150 002
		APR 23, 1982

PROBENECID *MULTIPLE*
SEE   AMPICILLIN/AMPICILLIN TRIHYDRATE; PROBENECID
SEE   COLCHICINE; PROBENECID

PROBUCOL
Tablet; Oral
LORELCO

AVENTIS PHARMS	250MG	N017535 001
	500MG	N017535 002
		JUL 06, 1988

PROCAINAMIDE HYDROCHLORIDE
Capsule; Oral
PROCAINAMIDE HCL

ASCOT	250MG	N087542 001
		JAN 08, 1982
	375MG	N087697 001
		MAR 01, 1983
	500MG	N087543 001
		JAN 08, 1982
LANNETT	500MG	N084696 001
LEDERLE	250MG	N086942 001
	375MG	N086952 001
	500MG	N086943 001
ROXANE	250MG	N088989 001
		APR 26, 1985
	500MG	N088990 001
		APR 26, 1985
VANGARD	250MG	N087643 001
		JUN 01, 1982
	500MG	N087875 001
		JUN 01, 1982
WATSON LAB	250MG	N083795 001
	500MG	N084357 001
WATSON LABS	250MG	N085167 001
	375MG	N087020 001
	500MG	N087021 001

PROCAN

PARKE DAVIS	250MG	N085804 001
	375MG	N087502 001
	500MG	N085079 001

PROCAPAN

PANRAY	250MG	N083553 002

Injectable; Injection
PROCAINAMIDE HCL

AM PHARM PARTNERS	100MG/ML	N089415 001
		NOV 17, 1986
	500MG/ML	N089416 001
		NOV 17, 1986
ELKINS SINN	100MG/ML	N089029 001
		APR 17, 1986
	500MG/ML	N089030 001
		APR 17, 1986
PHARMAFAIR	100MG/ML	N088824 001
		NOV 20, 1985
	500MG/ML	N088830 001
		NOV 20, 1985
QUAD PHARMS	100MG/ML	N089256 001
		MAY 30, 1986
	500MG/ML	N089257 001

Discontinued Drug Products (continued)

PROCAINAMIDE HYDROCHLORIDE (continued)

Injectable; Injection

PROCAINAMIDE HCL

Firm	Strength	Number	Date
QUAD PHARMS			
SMITH AND NEPHEW	100MG/ML	N088530 001	MAY 30, 1986
SOLOPAK	500MG/ML	N088531 001	MAR 04, 1985
STERIS	500MG/ML	N088532 001	MAR 04, 1985
WARNER CHILCOTT	100MG/ML	N087079 001	MAR 04, 1985
	100MG/ML	N087080 001	
	100MG/ML	N089528 001	MAY 03, 1988
	500MG/ML	N089529 001	MAY 03, 1988

Tablet, Extended Release; Oral

PROCAINAMIDE HCL

Firm	Strength	Number	Date
INVAMED	500MG	N089284 001	JUN 23, 1986
INWOOD LABS	500MG	N089840 001	MAR 06, 1989
PLIVA	250MG	N088958 001	DEC 02, 1985
WATSON LAB	1GM	N089520 001	JAN 15, 1987
	250MG	N088533 001	DEC 03, 1984
	500MG	N088534 001	DEC 03, 1984
	750MG	N088535 001	DEC 03, 1984

PROCAN SR

Firm	Strength	Number	Date
PARKE DAVIS	250MG	N086468 001	NOV 03, 1984
PARKEDALE	1GM	N088489 001	JAN 16, 1985
	500MG	N086065 001	
	750MG	N087510 001	APR 01, 1982

PROCAINE HYDROCHLORIDE

Injectable; Injection

PROCAINE HCL

Firm	Strength	Number
AM PHARM PARTNERS	1%	N080384 002
	2%	N080384 003
BEL MAR	1%	N080711 001
	2%	N080756 001
GD SEARLE LLC	1%	N086202 001
	2%	N086202 002
MILES	1%	N080415 001
	2%	N080415 002
STERIS	1%	N083535 001
	2%	N083535 002

PROCAINE HYDROCHLORIDE; TETRACYCLINE HYDROCHLORIDE

Injectable; Injection

ACHROMYCIN

Firm	Strength	Number
LEDERLE	40MG/VIAL;100MG/VIAL	N050276 001
	40MG/VIAL;250MG/VIAL	N050276 003

TETRACYN

Firm	Strength	Number
PFIZER	40MG/VIAL;100MG/VIAL	N060285 002
	40MG/VIAL;250MG/VIAL	N060285 003

PROCAINE HYDROCHLORIDE *MULTIPLE*

SEE   EPINEPHRINE; PROCAINE HYDROCHLORIDE
SEE   LEVONORDEFRIN; PROCAINE HYDROCHLORIDE; PROPOXYCAINE HYDROCHLORIDE
SEE   NOREPINEPHRINE BITARTRATE; PROCAINE HYDROCHLORIDE; PROPOXYCAINE HYDROCHLORIDE

PROCAINE MERETHOXYLLINE; THEOPHYLLINE

Injectable; Injection

DICURIN PROCAINE

Firm	Strength	Number
LILLY	100MG/ML;50MG/ML	N008869 001

PROCHLORPERAZINE EDISYLATE

Concentrate; Oral

COMPAZINE

Firm	Strength	Number	Date
GLAXOSMITHKLINE	EQ 10MG BASE/ML	N011276 001	

PROCHLORPERAZINE

Firm	Strength	Number	Date
ALPHARMA	EQ 10MG BASE/ML	N087153 001	JUN 08, 1982

PROCHLORPERAZINE EDISYLATE

Firm	Strength	Number	Date
MORTON GROVE	EQ 10MG BASE/ML	N088598 001	OCT 25, 1984

Injectable; Injection

PROCHLORPERAZINE EDISYLATE

Firm	Strength	Number	Date
ELKINS SINN	EQ 5MG BASE/ML	N089523 001	MAY 03, 1988
		N089675 001	DEC 05, 1988
MARSAM PHARMS LLC	EQ 5MG BASE/ML	N089637 001	FEB 01, 1988
QUAD PHARMS	EQ 5MG BASE/ML	N089638 001	FEB 01, 1988
SMITH AND NEPHEW	EQ 5MG BASE/ML	N089251 001	DEC 04, 1986
STERIS	EQ 5MG BASE/ML	N089605 001	JUL 08, 1987
	EQ 5MG BASE/ML	N089606 001	JUL 08, 1987
WYETH AYERST	EQ 5MG BASE/ML	N086348 001	

Syrup; Oral

PROCHLORPERAZINE EDISYLATE

Firm	Strength	Number	Date
ALPHARMA	EQ 5MG BASE/5ML	N087154 001	SEP 01, 1982
MORTON GROVE	EQ 5MG BASE/5ML	N088597 001	OCT 25, 1984

Discontinued Drug Products (continued)

PROCHLORPERAZINE MALEATE

Capsule, Extended Release; Oral

COMPAZINE		
GLAXOSMITHKLINE	EQ 10MG BASE	N011000 001
	EQ 15MG BASE	N011000 002
	EQ 30MG BASE	N011000 003
	EQ 75MG BASE	N011000 004

Tablet; Oral

PROCHLORPERAZINE		
WATSON LAB	EQ 5MG BASE	N085580 001
	EQ 10MG BASE	N085178 001
	EQ 25MG BASE	N085579 001
PROCHLORPERAZINE MALEATE		
DURAMED PHARM BARR	EQ 5MG BASE	N089484 001 JAN 20, 1987
		N089485 001 JAN 20, 1987
	EQ 10MG BASE	N089486 001 JAN 20, 1987
	EQ 25MG BASE	

PROCYCLIDINE HYDROCHLORIDE

Tablet; Oral

KEMADRIN		
MONARCH PHARMS	2MG	N009818 005

PROGESTERONE

Capsule; Oral

PROMETRIUM		
UNIMED PHARMS	300MG	N019781 003 OCT 15, 1999

Injectable; Injection

PROGESTERONE		
LILLY	25MG/ML	N009238 002
	50MG/ML	N009238 001

Insert, Extended Release; Intrauterine

PROGESTASERT		
ALZA	38MG	N017553 001

PROMAZINE HYDROCHLORIDE

Concentrate; Oral

SPARINE		
WYETH AYERST	30MG/ML	N010942 001
	100MG/ML	N010942 004

Injectable; Injection

PROMAZINE HCL		
STERIS	25MG/ML	N084510 001
	50MG/ML	N084517 001
SPARINE		
WYETH AYERST	25MG/ML	N010349 008
	50MG/ML	N010349 006

Syrup; Oral

SPARINE		
WYETH AYERST	10MG/5ML	N010942 003

PROMAZINE HYDROCHLORIDE (continued)

Tablet; Oral

SPARINE		
WYETH AYERST	10MG	N010348 006
	25MG	N010348 001
	50MG	N010348 002
	100MG	N010348 003
	200MG	N010348 004

PROMETHAZINE HYDROCHLORIDE

Injectable; Injection

PHENERGAN		
WYETH AYERST	25MG/ML	N008857 002
	50MG/ML	N008857 003
PROMETHAZINE HCL		
ABBOTT	25MG/ML	N084223 001
	50MG/ML	N084222 001
	25MG/ML	N083955 002
	50MG/ML	N083955 001
AKORN	25MG/ML	N089463 001 MAY 02, 1988
MARSAM PHARMS LLC	50MG/ML	N089477 001 MAY 02, 1988
STERIS	25MG/ML	N083532 001
	50MG/ML	N083532 002
ZIPAN-25		
ALTANA	25MG/ML	N083997 001
ZIPAN-50		
ALTANA	50MG/ML	N083997 002

Suppository; Rectal

PROMETHACON		
POLYMEDICA	50MG	N084902 001

Syrup; Oral

MYMETHAZINE FORTIS		
USL PHARMA	25MG/5ML	N087996 001 JAN 18, 1983
PHENERGAN FORTIS		
WYETH AYERST	25MG/5ML	N008381 003
PHENERGAN PLAIN		
WYETH AYERST	6.25MG/5ML	N008381 004 APR 18, 1984
PROMETH FORTIS		
ALPHARMA	25MG/5ML	N084772 001
PROMETHAZINE		
CENCI	6.25MG/5ML	N089013 001 SEP 20, 1985
PROMETHAZINE HCL		
KV PHARM	6.25MG/5ML	N085388 001
	25MG/5ML	N085385 001
PHARM ASSOC	6.25MG/5ML	N087518 001

Tablet; Oral

PROMETHAZINE HCL		
ABBOTT	12.5MG	N084160 001
	25MG	N084166 001
	50MG	N084539 001

Discontinued Drug Products *(continued)*

PROMETHAZINE HYDROCHLORIDE *(continued)*
Tablet; Oral
PROMETHAZINE HCL

EON	25MG	N085146 001
	50MG	N085146 002
GENEVA PHARMS	12.5MG	N084233 001
HALSEY	12.5MG	N084555 001
	25MG	N084554 001
	50MG	N084557 001
	25MG	N084214 002 JUL 07, 1982
IMPAX LABS	25MG	N083604 001
	50MG	N083603 001
IVAX PHARMS	12.5MG	N083613 001
	25MG	N080949 001
	50MG	N080949 002
LANNETT	12.5MG	N080949 003
	25MG	N083214 001
	50MG	N083658 001
PVT FORM	12.5MG	N084080 001
	25MG	N084027 001
TABLICAPS	12.5MG	N089109 001
	25MG	SEP 10, 1985
TEVA	25MG	N083401 001
WATSON LAB	12.5MG	N083204 001
	25MG	N083403 001
	50MG	N083712 001
WATSON LABS	12.5MG	N085986 001
	25MG	N085684 001
	50MG	N085664 001
REMSED		
BRISTOL MYERS		
SQUIBB	25MG	N083176 002
	50MG	N083176 001

PROMETHAZINE HYDROCHLORIDE *MULTIPLE*
SEE   CODEINE PHOSPHATE; PHENYLEPHRINE HYDROCHLORIDE; PROMETHAZINE HYDROCHLORIDE
SEE   CODEINE PHOSPHATE; PROMETHAZINE HYDROCHLORIDE
SEE   DEXTROMETHORPHAN HYDROBROMIDE; PROMETHAZINE HYDROCHLORIDE
SEE   MEPERIDINE HYDROCHLORIDE; PROMETHAZINE HYDROCHLORIDE
SEE   PHENYLEPHRINE HYDROCHLORIDE; PROMETHAZINE HYDROCHLORIDE

PROPANTHELINE BROMIDE
Injectable; Injection
PRO-BANTHINE

GD SEARLE LLC	30MG/VIAL	N008843 001

Tablet; Oral
PROPANTHELINE BROMIDE

ASCOT	15MG	N087663 001 OCT 25, 1982
GENEVA PHARMS	15MG	N080928 001
HEATHER	15MG	N085780 001
IMPAX LABS	15MG	N084541 002
MYLAN	15MG	N083706 001
PAR PHARM	15MG	N088377 001

PROPANTHELINE BROMIDE *(continued)*
Tablet; Oral
PROPANTHELINE BROMIDE

PAR PHARM	15MG	DEC 08, 1983
PVT FORM	15MG	N080977 001
TABLICAPS	15MG	N084428 001
WATSON LAB	15MG	N083151 001
WATSON LABS	15MG	N083029 002

PROPARACAINE HYDROCHLORIDE
Solution/Drops; Ophthalmic
KAINAIR

PHARMAFAIR	0.5%	N088087 001 JUN 07, 1983

PROPARACAINE HCL

SOLA BARNES HIND	0.5%	N084144 001
	0.5%	N084151 001

PROPIOLACTONE
Solution; Irrigation
BETAPRONE

FORREST LABS	N/A	N011657 001

PROPIOMAZINE HYDROCHLORIDE
Injectable; Injection
LARGON

BAXTER HLTHCARE		
CORP	20MG/ML	N012382 002

PROPOFOL
Injectable; Injection
DIPRIVAN

ASTRAZENECA	10MG/ML	N019627 001 OCT 02, 1989

PROPOXYCAINE HYDROCHLORIDE *MULTIPLE*
SEE   LEVONORDEFRIN; PROCAINE HYDROCHLORIDE; PROPOXYCAINE HYDROCHLORIDE
SEE   NOREPINEPHRINE BITARTRATE; PROCAINE HYDROCHLORIDE; PROPOXYCAINE HYDROCHLORIDE

PROPOXYPHENE HYDROCHLORIDE
Capsule; Oral
PROPHENE 65

HALSEY	65MG	N083538 002

PROPOXYPHENE HCL

ALRA	65MG	N083184 001
ANABOLIC	65MG	N083185 001
EON	32MG	N084014 001
	65MG	N083688 001
	65MG	N083870 002
GENEVA PHARMS	65MG	N086495 001
	65MG	N083125 002
HALSEY	65MG	N083186 001

Discontinued Drug Products (continued)

PROPOXYPHENE HYDROCHLORIDE (continued)

Capsule; Oral

PROPOXYPHENE HCL

Firm	Strength	Application	Date
IMPAX LABS	65MG	N083317 001	
IVAX PHARMS	32MG	N083597 001	
MYLAN	65MG	N083299 001	
PUREPAC PHARM	65MG	N083278 001	
PVT FORM	32MG	N083464 001	
	65MG	N083113 001	
ROXANE	32MG	N083089 001	
	65MG	N083089 002	
WATSON LABS	65MG	N080908 002	
	65MG	N085190 001	

PROPOXYPHENE HCL 65

Firm	Strength	Application	Date
WARNER CHILCOTT	65MG	N083786 001	

PROPOXYPHENE HYDROCHLORIDE *MULTIPLE*
SEE ACETAMINOPHEN; PROPOXYPHENE HYDROCHLORIDE
SEE ASPIRIN; CAFFEINE; PROPOXYPHENE HYDROCHLORIDE

PROPOXYPHENE NAPSYLATE *MULTIPLE*
SEE ACETAMINOPHEN; PROPOXYPHENE NAPSYLATE
SEE ASPIRIN; PROPOXYPHENE NAPSYLATE

PROPRANOLOL HYDROCHLORIDE

Capsule, Extended Release; Oral

PROPRANOLOL HCL

Firm	Strength	Application	Date
INWOOD LABS	60MG	N072499 001	APR 11, 1989
	80MG	N072500 001	APR 11, 1989
	120MG	N072501 001	APR 11, 1989
	160MG	N072502 001	APR 11, 1989

Injectable; Injection

PROPRANOLOL HCL

Firm	Strength	Application	Date
SMITH AND NEPHEW	1MG/ML	N070135 001	APR 15, 1986
	1MG/ML	N070137 001	APR 15, 1986
SOLOPAK	1MG/ML	N070136 001	APR 15, 1986

Solution; Oral

PROPRANOLOL HCL

Firm	Strength	Application	Date
MORTON GROVE	20MG/5ML	N071984 001	MAR 03, 1989
	40MG/5ML	N071985 001	MAR 03, 1989

Suspension; Oral

INDERAL

Firm	Strength	Application	Date
WYETH AYERST	10MG/ML	N019536 001	DEC 12, 1986

PROPRANOLOL HYDROCHLORIDE (continued)

Tablet; Oral

INDERAL

Firm	Strength	Application	Date
WYETH PHARMS INC	90MG	N016418 010	OCT 18, 1982

PROPRANOLOL HCL

Firm	Strength	Application	Date
DURAMED PHARM BARR	10MG	N070306 001	SEP 09, 1985
	20MG	N070307 001	SEP 09, 1985
	40MG	N070308 001	SEP 09, 1985
	60MG	N070309 001	OCT 01, 1986
	80MG	N070310 001	SEP 09, 1985
	90MG	N071327 001	OCT 01, 1986
HALSEY	10MG	N070319 001	OCT 22, 1985
	20MG	N070320 001	OCT 22, 1985
	40MG	N070103 001	OCT 22, 1985
	60MG	N070321 001	SEP 24, 1986
	80MG	N070322 001	AUG 04, 1986
INTERPHARM	10MG	N071368 001	MAY 05, 1987
	20MG	N071369 001	MAY 05, 1987
	40MG	N071370 001	MAY 05, 1987
	80MG	N071371 001	MAY 05, 1987
INVAMED	10MG	N071658 001	JUL 05, 1988
	20MG	N071687 001	JUL 05, 1988
	40MG	N071688 001	JUL 05, 1988
	60MG	N072197 001	JUL 05, 1988
	80MG	N071689 001	JUL 05, 1988
	90MG	N072198 001	JUL 05, 1988
IVAX PHARMS	10MG	N072063 001	JUL 29, 1988
	20MG	N072066 001	JUL 29, 1988
	40MG	N072067 001	JUL 29, 1988
	60MG	N072068 001	JUL 29, 1988
	80MG	N072069 001	

Discontinued Drug Products (continued)

PROPRANOLOL HYDROCHLORIDE (continued)

Suspension; Oral
PROPRANOLOL HCL

Firm	Strength	Date	Appl. No.
IVAX PHARMS			
LEDERLE	10MG	JUL 29, 1988	N070125 001
	10MG	JUL 30, 1985	N072117 001
	20MG	JUN 23, 1988	N070126 001
	20MG	JUL 30, 1985	N072118 001
	40MG	JUN 23, 1988	N070127 001
	40MG	JUL 30, 1985	N072119 001
	60MG	JUN 23, 1988	N071495 001
	80MG	DEC 31, 1987	N070128 001
	80MG	JUL 30, 1985	N072120 001
	90MG	JUN 23, 1988	N071496 001
MYLAN	60MG	DEC 31, 1987	N072275 001
PUREPAC PHARM	10MG	JUN 09, 1989	N070814 001
	20MG	NOV 03, 1986	N070815 001
	40MG	NOV 03, 1986	N070816 001
	60MG	NOV 03, 1986	N070817 001
	80MG	NOV 03, 1986	N070757 001
ROXANE	10MG	NOV 03, 1986	N070516 001
	20MG	JUL 07, 1986	N070517 001
	40MG	JUL 07, 1986	N070518 001
	60MG	JUL 07, 1986	N070519 001
	80MG	SEP 24, 1986	N070520 001
	90MG	JUL 07, 1986	N070521 001
SCHERING	10MG	SEP 24, 1986	N070120 001
	20MG	AUG 06, 1985	N070121 001
	40MG	AUG 06, 1985	N070122 001
	60MG	AUG 06, 1985	N070123 001
	80MG	OCT 29, 1986	N070124 001

PROPRANOLOL HYDROCHLORIDE (continued)

Suspension; Oral
PROPRANOLOL HCL

Firm	Strength	Date	Appl. No.
SCHERING			
SUPERPHARM	10MG	AUG 06, 1985	N071515 001
	20MG	JUN 08, 1988	N071516 001
	40MG	JUN 08, 1988	N071517 001
	80MG	JUN 08, 1988	N071518 001
TEVA	10MG	JUN 08, 1988	N070232 001
	20MG	OCT 07, 1987	N070233 001
WARNER CHILCOTT	10MG	JUN 23, 1986	N070438 001
	20MG	SEP 15, 1986	N070439 001
	40MG	SEP 15, 1986	N070440 001
	60MG	SEP 15, 1986	N070441 001
	80MG	SEP 24, 1986	N070442 001
WATSON LAB	10MG	SEP 15, 1986	N070378 001
	20MG	MAR 19, 1987	N070379 001
	40MG	MAR 19, 1987	N070380 001
	60MG	MAR 19, 1987	N070381 001
	80MG	MAR 19, 1987	N070382 001
WATSON LABS	10MG	MAR 19, 1987	N070140 001
	20MG	JUL 30, 1985	N070141 001
	20MG	JUL 30, 1985	N070549 001
	40MG	APR 11, 1986	N070142 001
	60MG	JUL 30, 1985	N070143 001
	60MG	JAN 15, 1987	N071098 001
	80MG	OCT 06, 1986	N070144 001
	90MG	JUL 30, 1985	N071183 001
		OCT 06, 1986	

PROPRANOLOL HYDROCHLORIDE *MULTIPLE*
SEE   HYDROCHLOROTHIAZIDE; PROPRANOLOL HYDROCHLORIDE

Discontinued Drug Products *(continued)*

PROPYLIODONE

Suspension; Intratracheal

Brand	Manufacturer	Strength	Number
DIONOSIL AQUEOUS	GLAXOSMITHKLINE	50%	N009309 001
DIONOSIL OILY	GLAXOSMITHKLINE	60%	N009309 002

PROPYLTHIOURACIL

Tablet; Oral

PROPYLTHIOURACIL

Manufacturer	Strength	Number
ABBOTT	50MG	N084075 001
ANABOLIC	50MG	N080285 001
HALSEY	50MG	N080015 001
	50MG	N083982 001
IVAX PHARMS	50MG	N080215 001
LANNETT	50MG	N080016 001
LILLY	50MG	N006213 001
PERRIGO	50MG	N084543 001
TABLICAPS	50MG	N080840 001
WATSON LABS	50MG	N080932 001
	50MG	N085201 001

PROTAMINE SULFATE

Injectable; Injection

PROTAMINE SULFATE

Manufacturer	Strength	Number	Date
ELKINS SINN	10MG/ML	N089474 001	NOV 05, 1986
	10MG/ML	N089475 001	NOV 05, 1986
PHARMACIA AND UPJOHN	50MG/VIAL	N007413 001	
	250MG/VIAL	N007413 002	AUG 02, 1984
QUAD PHARMS	10MG/ML	N089306 001	MAY 30, 1986
	50MG/VIAL	N089307 001	MAY 30, 1986

PROTEIN HYDROLYSATE

Injectable; Injection

Brand	Manufacturer	Strength	Number	Date
AMINOSOL 5%	ABBOTT	5%	N005932 012	JAN 31, 1985
HYPROTIGEN 5%	B BRAUN	5%	N006170 003	JAN 10, 1984

PROTIRELIN

Injectable; Injection

Brand	Manufacturer	Strength	Number
THYPINONE	ABBOTT	0.5MG/ML	N017638 001

PROTOKYLOL HYDROCHLORIDE

Tablet; Oral

Brand	Manufacturer	Strength	Number
VENTAIRE	AVENTIS PHARMS	2MG	N083459 001

PROTRIPTYLINE HYDROCHLORIDE

Tablet; Oral

Brand	Manufacturer	Strength	Number
VIVACTIL	PLIVA	5MG	N016012 001
		10MG	N016012 002

PSEUDOEPHEDRINE HYDROCHLORIDE

Capsule, Extended Release; Oral

Brand	Manufacturer	Strength	Number
NOVAFED	AVENTIS PHARMS	120MG	N017603 001
SUDAFED 12 HOUR	GLAXOSMITHKLINE	120MG *SEE ANNUAL PREFACE INTRODUCTION DISCONTINUED SECTION*	N017941 002

PSEUDOEPHEDRINE HYDROCHLORIDE; TRIPROLIDINE HYDROCHLORIDE

Capsule, Extended Release; Oral

Brand	Manufacturer	Strength	Number	Date
ACTIFED	GLAXOSMITHKLINE	120MG;5MG	N018996 001	JUN 17, 1985
TRIPROLIDINE AND PSEUDOEPHEDRINE HYDROCHLORIDES	KV PHARM	120MG;5MG	N071798 001	MAR 16, 1989

Syrup; Oral

Brand	Manufacturer	Strength	Number	Date
ACTAHIST	CENCI	30MG/5ML;1.25MG/5ML	N088344 001	FEB 09, 1984
HISTAFED	CENCI	30MG/5ML;1.25MG/5ML	N088283 001	APR 20, 1984
MYFED	USL PHARMA	30MG/5ML;1.25MG/5ML	N088116 001	MAR 04, 1983
TRILITRON	NEWTRON PHARMS	30MG/5ML;1.25MG/5ML	N088474 001	FEB 12, 1985

Tablet; Oral

Brand	Manufacturer	Strength	Number	Date
ALLERFED	PVT FORM	60MG;2.5MG	N088860 001	JAN 31, 1985
TRIPHED	TEVA	60MG;2.5MG	N088630 001	MAY 17, 1984
TRIPROLIDINE AND PSEUDOEPHEDRINE	WEST WARD	60MG;2.5MG	N088117 001	APR 19, 1983
		60MG;2.5MG	N088318 002	JAN 13, 1984
	WATSON LAB	60MG;2.5MG		

Discontinued Drug Products (continued)

PSEUDOEPHEDRINE HYDROCHLORIDE; TRIPROLIDINE HYDROCHLORIDE (continued)
Tablet; Oral
TRIPROLIDINE HCL AND PSEUDOEPHEDRINE HCL
  60MG;2.5MG
IVAX PHARMS   N085273 001   DEC 12, 1984

PSEUDOEPHEDRINE HYDROCHLORIDE *MULTIPLE*
SEE BROMPHENIRAMINE MALEATE: DEXTROMETHORPHAN HYDROBROMIDE: PSEUDOEPHEDRINE HYDROCHLORIDE
SEE CHLORPHENIRAMINE MALEATE: PSEUDOEPHEDRINE HYDROCHLORIDE
SEE CODEINE PHOSPHATE: PSEUDOEPHEDRINE HYDROCHLORIDE: TRIPROLIDINE HYDROCHLORIDE
SEE DIPHENHYDRAMINE HYDROCHLORIDE: PSEUDOEPHEDRINE HYDROCHLORIDE

PSEUDOEPHEDRINE POLISTIREX
Suspension, Extended Release; Oral
PSEUDO-12   EQ 60MG HCL/5ML
CELLTECH PHARMS   N019401 001   JUN 19, 1987

PSEUDOEPHEDRINE SULFATE *MULTIPLE*
SEE DEXBROMPHENIRAMINE MALEATE: PSEUDOEPHEDRINE SULFATE

PYRIDOSTIGMINE BROMIDE
Injectable; Injection
REGONOL   5MG/ML
SABEX 2002   N017398 001
Tablet; Oral
PYRIDOSTIGMINE BROMIDE
SOLVAY   30MG   N089572 001   NOV 27, 1990
US ARMY   30MG   N020414 001   FEB 05, 2003

PYRIDOXINE *MULTIPLE*
SEE ALPHA-TOCOPHEROL: ASCORBIC ACID: BIOTIN: CHOLECALCIFEROL: CYANOCOBALAMIN: FOLIC ACID: NIACINAMIDE: PANTOTHENIC ACID: PYRIDOXINE: RIBOFLAVIN: THIAMINE: VITAMIN A
SEE ASCORBIC ACID: BIOTIN: CYANOCOBALAMIN: DEXPANTHENOL: ERGOCALCIFEROL: FOLIC ACID: NIACINAMIDE: PYRIDOXINE: RIBOFLAVIN PHOSPHATE SODIUM: THIAMINE: VITAMIN A: VITAMIN E
SEE ASCORBIC ACID: BIOTIN: CYANOCOBALAMIN: ERGOCALCIFEROL: FOLIC ACID: NIACINAMIDE: PANTOTHENIC ACID: PHYTONADIONE: PYRIDOXINE: RIBOFLAVIN: THIAMINE: VITAMIN A PALMITATE: VITAMIN E

PYRIDOXINE HYDROCHLORIDE
Injectable; Injection
HEXA-BETALIN   100MG/ML
LILLY   N080854 001
PYRIDOXINE HCL   100MG/ML
AKORN   N087967 001   OCT 01, 1982

PYRIDOXINE HYDROCHLORIDE (continued)
Injectable; Injection
PYRIDOXINE HCL
BEL MAR   100MG/ML   N080761 001
DELL LABS   50MG/ML   N083771 001
   100MG/ML   N083772 001
ELKINS SINN   100MG/ML   N080581 001
LUITPOLD   100MG/ML   N080669 001
STERIS   100MG/ML   N083760 001

PYRIDOXINE HYDROCHLORIDE *MULTIPLE*
SEE ASCORBIC ACID: BIOTIN: CYANOCOBALAMIN: DEXPANTHENOL: ERGOCALCIFEROL: FOLIC ACID: NIACINAMIDE: PYRIDOXINE HYDROCHLORIDE: RIBOFLAVIN PHOSPHATE SODIUM: THIAMINE HYDROCHLORIDE: VITAMIN A PALMITATE: VITAMIN E
SEE ASCORBIC ACID: BIOTIN: CYANOCOBALAMIN: DEXPANTHENOL: ERGOCALCIFEROL: FOLIC ACID: NIACINAMIDE: PYRIDOXINE HYDROCHLORIDE: RIBOFLAVIN PHOSPHATE SODIUM: THIAMINE HYDROCHLORIDE: VITAMIN A: VITAMIN E
SEE DOXYLAMINE SUCCINATE: PYRIDOXINE HYDROCHLORIDE
SEE NIACINAMIDE: PYRIDOXINE HYDROCHLORIDE: TYROSINE

PYRILAMINE MALEATE
Tablet; Oral
PYRILAMINE MALEATE   25MG   N085231 001
WATSON LABS

PYRILAMINE MALEATE *MULTIPLE*
SEE PHENYLEPHRINE HYDROCHLORIDE: PYRILAMINE MALEATE

PYRITHIONE ZINC
Lotion; Topical
HEAD SHOULDERS CONDITIONER   0.3%
PROCTER AND GAMBLE   N019412 002   MAR 10, 1986

PYRVINIUM PAMOATE
Suspension; Oral
POVAN   EQ 50MG BASE/5ML   N011964 001
PARKE DAVIS
Tablet; Oral
POVAN   EQ 50MG BASE   N012485 002
PARKE DAVIS

QUINESTROL
Tablet; Oral
ESTROVIS   0.1MG   N016768 002
PARKE DAVIS   0.2MG   N016768 003

QUINETHAZONE
Tablet; Oral
HYDROMOX   50MG   N013264 001
LEDERLE

Discontinued Drug Products *(continued)*

QUINETHAZONE; RESERPINE
Tablet; Oral
  HYDROMOX R
    LEDERLE   50MG;0.125MG   N013927 001

QUINIDINE GLUCONATE
Tablet, Extended Release; Oral
  DURAQUIN
    WARNER CHILCOTT   330MG   N017917 001
  QUINAGLUTE
    BERLEX LABS   324MG   N016647 001
  QUINALAN
    LANNETT   324MG   N088081 001 FEB 10, 1986
  QUINATIME
    WATSON LAB   324MG   N087448 001
QUINIDINE GLUCONATE
  ASCOT   324MG   N088582 001 JUN 17, 1985
  GENEVA PHARMS   324MG   N089894 001 DEC 15, 1988
  HALSEY   324MG   N089476 001 APR 10, 1987
  ROXANE   324MG   N088431 001 JAN 06, 1984
  SUPERPHARM   324MG   N089164 001 NOV 21, 1985
  WATSON LABS   324MG   N087785 001 JAN 24, 1983
       324MG   N087810 001 SEP 29, 1982
Tablet; Oral
  QUINACT
    BERLEX   266MG   N085978 001
         400MG   N086099 001

QUINIDINE POLYGALACTURONATE
Tablet; Oral
  CARDIOQUIN
    PURDUE FREDERICK   275MG   N011642 002

QUINIDINE SULFATE
Capsule; Oral
  CIN-QUIN
    SOLVAY   200MG   N085296 001
        300MG   N085297 001
  QUINIDINE SULFATE
    LILLY   200MG   N085103 001
Tablet, Extended Release; Oral
  QUINIDEX
    WYETH PHARMS INC   300MG   N012796 002
Tablet; Oral
  CIN-QUIN
    SOLVAY   100MG   N085299 001
        200MG   N084932 001

QUINIDINE SULFATE *(continued)*
Tablet; Oral
  CIN-QUIN
    SOLVAY   300MG   N085298 001
  QUINIDINE SULFATE
    BARR   200MG   N084177 001
    ELKINS SINN   200MG   N083622 001
    EVERYLIFE   200MG   N083439 001
    HALSEY   200MG   N083583 001
    ICN   200MG   N083393 001
    IMPAX LABS   200MG   N083347 001
    IVAX PHARMS   200MG   N084549 001
    KING PHARMS   200MG   N085175 001
    KV PHARM   200MG   N085276 001
    LEDERLE   200MG   N086176 001
    LILLY   200MG   N085038 001
    MUTUAL PHARM   300MG   N081031 001 APR 14, 1989
    PERRIGO   200MG   N085322 001
    PHARMAVITE   200MG   N084627 001
    PUREPAC PHARM   200MG   N084003 001
    SCHERER LABS   200MG   N085068 001
    USL PHARMA   200MG   N087837 001 APR 14, 1982
    VANGARD   200MG   N087909 001 JUL 13, 1982
    VINTAGE PHARMS   200MG   N083963 001
    WARNER CHILCOTT   200MG   N083879 001
    WATSON LABS   100MG   N085584 001
    WEST WARD   200MG   N083362 001
    WHITEWORTH TOWN
    PLSN   200MG   N085444 001
  QUINORA
    KEY PHARMS   200MG   N083576 001
    SCHERING   300MG   N085222 001

QUINUPRISTIN *MULTIPLE*
  SEE DALFOPRISTIN; QUINUPRISTIN

RABEPRAZOLE SODIUM
Tablet, Delayed Release; Oral
  ACIPHEX
    EISAI MEDCL RES   10MG   N020973 001 MAY 29, 2002

RANITIDINE BISMUTH CITRATE
Tablet; Oral
  TRITEC
    GLAXOSMITHKLINE   400MG   N020559 001 AUG 08, 1996

RANITIDINE HYDROCHLORIDE
Capsule; Oral
  ZANTAC 150
    GLAXOSMITHKLINE   EQ 150MG BASE   N020095 001

Discontinued Drug Products (continued)

RANITIDINE HYDROCHLORIDE (continued)

Capsule; Oral

ZANTAC 150	GLAXOSMITHKLINE			MAR 08, 1994
ZANTAC 300	GLAXOSMITHKLINE	EQ 300MG BASE	N020095 002	MAR 08, 1994

Injectable; Injection

ZANTAC IN PLASTIC CONTAINER	GLAXOSMITHKLINE	EQ 50MG BASE/100ML	N019593 001	DEC 17, 1986

Tablet, Effervescent; Oral

ZANTAC 75	WARNER LAMBERT	EQ 75MG BASE	N020745 001	FEB 26, 1998

Tablet; Oral

RANITIDINE HCL	BOEHRINGER INGELHEIM	EQ 150MG BASE	N074662 001	AUG 29, 1997
		EQ 300MG BASE	N074662 002	AUG 29, 1997

RAPACURONIUM BROMIDE

Injectable; Injection

RAPLON	ORGANON USA INC	100MG/VIAL	N020984 001	AUG 18, 1999
		200MG/VIAL	N020984 002	AUG 18, 1999

RAUWOLFIA SERPENTINA

Tablet; Oral

Product	Firm	Strength	Code
HIWOLFIA	BOWMAN PHARMS	50MG	N009276 003
		50MG	N009276 005
		100MG	N009276 004
HYSERPIN	PHYS PRODS VA	50MG	N010581 001
KOGLUCOID	PANRAY	50MG	N009278 001
		100MG	N009278 002
RAUDIXIN	APOTHECON	50MG	N008842 001
		100MG	N008842 002
RAUSERPIN	FERNDALE LABS	50MG	N009926 002
		100MG	N009926 004
RAUVAL	PAL PAK	50MG	N009108 002
		100MG	N009108 004
RAUWOLFIA SERPENTINA	BUNDY	50MG	N009477 001
		100MG	N009477 002
	HALSEY	50MG	N080498 001

RAUWOLFIA SERPENTINA (continued)

Tablet; Oral
RAUWOLFIA SERPENTINA

Product	Firm	Strength	Code
	HALSEY	100MG	N080498 002
	ICN	50MG	N009668 001
		100MG	N009668 002
	IMPAX LABS	50MG	N009273 001
		100MG	N009273 002
	IVAX PHARMS	50MG	N011521 001
		100MG	N011521 002
	PUREPAC PHARM	50MG	N080842 001
		100MG	N080842 002
	PVT FORM	50MG	N080583 001
		100MG	N080583 002
	SOLVAY	50MG	N080500 001
		100MG	N080500 002
	TABLICAPS	50MG	N083867 001
		100MG	N083444 001
	WATSON LABS	50MG	N080907 001
		100MG	N080914 001
WOLFINA	FOREST PHARMS	50MG	N009255 008
		100MG	N009255 006

RESCINNAMINE

Capsule; Oral

Product	Firm	Strength	Code
CINNASIL	PANRAY	0.5MG	N084736 001

RESERPINE

Elixir; Oral

Product	Firm	Strength	Code
SERPASIL	NOVARTIS	0.2MG/4ML	N009115 005

Injectable; Injection

Product	Firm	Strength	Code
SANDRIL	LILLY	2.5MG/ML	N010012 001
SERPASIL	NOVARTIS	2.5MG/ML	N009434 002

Tablet; Oral

Product	Firm	Strength	Code
HISERPIA	BOWMAN PHARMS	0.1MG	N009631 002
		0.25MG	N009631 004
RAU-SED	BRISTOL MYERS SQUIBB	0.1MG	N009357 001
		0.5MG	N009357 006
		0.25MG	N009357 004
		1MG	N009357 008
RESERPINE	BARR	0.25MG	N080721 002
	BELL PHARMA	0.1MG	N083058 001
		0.25MG	N083058 002
	BUNDY	0.1MG	N009663 001
		0.25MG	N009663 003
	ELKINS SINN	0.1MG	N083145 001
		0.25MG	N083145 002

Discontinued Drug Products (continued)

RESERPINE (continued)
Tablet; Oral

RESERPINE

EVERYLIFE	0.1MG	N010441 001
	0.5MG	N010441 003
	0.25MG	N010441 002
	1MG	N010441 004
HALSEY	0.1MG	N080457 002
	0.25MG	N080457 001
	1MG	N080457 003
ICN	0.1MG	N009667 001
	0.25MG	N009667 002
IMPAX LABS	0.1MG	N009627 001
	0.25MG	N009627 002
IVAX PHARMS	0.1MG	N011185 001
	0.25MG	N011185 002
MARSHALL PHARMA	0.1MG	N080492 001
	0.25MG	N080492 002
MK LABS	0.1MG	N080525 002
	0.25MG	N080525 001
MYLAN	1MG	N084974 001
PHARMAVITE	0.25MG	N084663 001
PUREPAC PHARM	0.1MG	N080753 002
PVT FORM	0.1MG	N080753 001
	0.25MG	N086117 001
	0.25MG	N080582 001
	0.25MG	N085775 001
	1MG	N080582 002
REXALL	0.25MG	N080637 001
ROXANE	0.1MG	N009859 001
	0.25MG	N009859 002
SOLVAY	0.25MG	N080446 001
TABLICAPS	0.25MG	N085207 001
TEVA	0.1MG	N089020 001
	0.25MG	MAR 07, 1985 N089019 001
	0.25MG	MAR 07, 1985 N080679 001
WATSON LABS	0.1MG	N080393 001
	0.25MG	N085401 001
	0.25MG	N080749 001
	1MG	N080975 001
WEST WARD	0.1MG	N080975 002
	0.25MG	N080975 003
WHITEWORTH TOWN PLSN	0.1MG	N080723 001
	0.25MG	N080723 002
	1MG	N080723 003

SANDRIL

LILLY	0.1MG	N009376 004
	0.25MG	N009376 001

SERPANRAY

PANRAY	0.1MG	N009391 001
	0.25MG	N009391 002
	1MG	N009391 004

SERPASIL

NOVARTIS	0.1MG	N009115 001

RESERPINE (continued)
Tablet; Oral

SERPASIL

NOVARTIS	0.25MG	N009115 003
	1MG	N009115 004

SERPATE

VALE	0.1MG	N009453 001
	0.25MG	N009453 002

SERPIVITE

VITARINE	0.25MG	N009645 002

RESERPINE; TRICHLORMETHIAZIDE
Tablet; Oral

METATENSIN #2

AVENTIS PHARMS	0.1MG;2MG	N012972 001

METATENSIN #4

AVENTIS PHARMS	0.1MG;4MG	N012972 002

NAQUIVAL

SCHERING	0.1MG;4MG	N012265 003

TRICHLORMETHIAZIDE W/ RESERPINE

WATSON LAB	0.1MG;4MG	N085248 001

RESERPINE *MULTIPLE*

- SEE CHLOROTHIAZIDE; RESERPINE
- SEE CHLORTHALIDONE; RESERPINE
- SEE HYDRALAZINE HYDROCHLORIDE; HYDROCHLOROTHIAZIDE; RESERPINE
- SEE HYDRALAZINE HYDROCHLORIDE; RESERPINE
- SEE HYDROCHLOROTHIAZIDE; RESERPINE
- SEE HYDROFLUMETHIAZIDE; RESERPINE
- SEE METHYCLOTHIAZIDE; RESERPINE
- SEE QUINETHAZONE; RESERPINE

RIBOFLAVIN *MULTIPLE*

- SEE ALPHA-TOCOPHEROL; ASCORBIC ACID; BIOTIN; CHOLECALCIFEROL; CYANOCOBALAMIN; FOLIC ACID; NIACINAMIDE; PANTOTHENIC ACID; PYRIDOXINE; RIBOFLAVIN; THIAMINE; VITAMIN A
- SEE ASCORBIC ACID; BIOTIN; CYANOCOBALAMIN; ERGOCALCIFEROL; FOLIC ACID; NIACINAMIDE; PANTOTHENIC ACID; PHYTONADIONE; PYRIDOXINE; RIBOFLAVIN; THIAMINE; VITAMIN A PALMITATE; VITAMIN E

RIBOFLAVIN PHOSPHATE SODIUM *MULTIPLE*

- SEE ASCORBIC ACID; BIOTIN; CYANOCOBALAMIN; DEXPANTHENOL; ERGOCALCIFEROL; FOLIC ACID; NIACINAMIDE; PYRIDOXINE; RIBOFLAVIN PHOSPHATE SODIUM; THIAMINE; VITAMIN A; VITAMIN E
- SEE ASCORBIC ACID; BIOTIN; CYANOCOBALAMIN; DEXPANTHENOL; ERGOCALCIFEROL; FOLIC ACID; NIACINAMIDE; PYRIDOXINE; RIBOFLAVIN PHOSPHATE SODIUM; THIAMINE; VITAMIN A PALMITATE; VITAMIN E
- SEE ASCORBIC ACID; BIOTIN; CYANOCOBALAMIN; DEXPANTHENOL; ERGOCALCIFEROL; FOLIC ACID; NIACINAMIDE; PYRIDOXINE; RIBOFLAVIN PHOSPHATE SODIUM; THIAMINE; VITAMIN A; VITAMIN E

Discontinued Drug Products *(continued)*

RISPERIDONE
Tablet; Oral
RISPERDAL
JANSSEN PHARMA   5MG   N020272 005   DEC 29, 1993

RITODRINE HYDROCHLORIDE
Injectable; Injection
RITODRINE HCL
AM PHARM PARTNERS   10MG/ML   N071188 001   JUL 23, 1987
15MG/ML   N071189 001   JUL 23, 1987
QUAD PHARMS   10MG/ML   N070700 001   OCT 06, 1986
15MG/ML   N070701 001   OCT 06, 1986
YUTOPAR
ASTRAZENECA   10MG/ML   N018580 001
15MG/ML   N018580 002
Tablet; Oral
YUTOPAR
ASTRAZENECA   10MG   N018555 001

RITONAVIR
Capsule; Oral
NORVIR
ABBOTT   100MG   N020680 001   MAR 01, 1996

ROCURONIUM BROMIDE
Injectable; Injection
ZEMURON
ORGANON USA INC   10MG/ML   N020214 002   MAR 17, 1994

ROSE BENGAL SODIUM, I-131
Injectable; Injection
ROBENGATOPE
BRACCO   0.5mCi/VIAL   N016224 001
1mCi/VIAL   N016224 002
2mCi/VIAL   N016224 003
SODIUM ROSE BENGAL I 131
SORIN   0.5mCi/ML   N017318 001

SAFFLOWER OIL
Injectable; Injection
LIPOSYN 10%
ABBOTT   10% (10GM/100ML)   N018203 001
LIPOSYN 20%
ABBOTT   20% (20GM/100ML)   N018614 001

SARALASIN ACETATE
Injectable; Injection
SARENIN
PROCTER AND GAMBLE   EQ 0.6MG BASE/ML   N018009 001

SECOBARBITAL SODIUM
Capsule; Oral
SECOBARBITAL SODIUM
ICN   100MG   N085477 001
IVAX PHARMS   100MG   N085869 001
LANNETT   50MG   N085909 001
100MG   N085903 001
PARKE DAVIS   100MG   N084762 001
PUREPAC PHARM   100MG   N085867 001
VITARINE   100MG   N085898 001
WHITEWORTH TOWN   100MG   N086273 001
PLSN   100MG   N085798 001
WYETH AYERST   100MG   N086390 001
SODIUM SECOBARBITAL
ANABOLIC   100MG   N084422 001
BARR   100MG   N084225 001
HALSEY   100MG   N084676 001
KV PHARM   100MG   N085285 001
PERRIGO   100MG   N084561 001
WATSON LABS   100MG   N085792 001
Injectable; Injection
SECONAL SODIUM
LILLY   50MG/ML   N007392 002
SODIUM SECOBARBITAL
WYETH AYERST   50MG/ML   N083262 001
Suppository; Rectal
SECONAL SODIUM
LILLY   30MG   N086530 001
60MG   N086530 002
120MG   N086530 003
200MG   N086530 004

SECRETIN
Injectable; Injection
SECRETIN-FERRING
FERRING   75CU/VIAL   N018290 001

SELENIUM SULFIDE
Lotion/Shampoo; Topical
SELENIUM SULFIDE
IVAX PHARMS   2.5%   N085777 001
TARO   2.5%   N086209 001

SELENOMETHIONINE, SE-75
Injectable; Injection
SELENOMETHIONINE SE 75
AMERSHAM HLTH   250uCi/ML   N017257 001
CIS   500uCi/ML   N017322 001
MALLINCKRODT   100uCi/ML   N017098 001

SODIUM ACETATE *MULTIPLE* (continued)
SEE   MAGNESIUM CHLORIDE; POTASSIUM CHLORIDE; POTASSIUM PHOSPHATE, MONOBASIC; SODIUM ACETATE; SODIUM CHLORIDE; SODIUM GLUCONATE; SODIUM PHOSPHATE, DIBASIC, HEPTAHYDRATE
SEE   MAGNESIUM CHLORIDE; POTASSIUM CHLORIDE; SODIUM ACETATE; SODIUM CHLORIDE; SODIUM GLUCONATE

SODIUM BENZOATE; SODIUM PHENYLACETATE
Solution; Oral
UCEPHAN
B BRAUN   100MG/ML;100MG/ML   N019530 001   DEC 23, 1987

SODIUM BICARBONATE
Injectable; Injection
SODIUM BICARBONATE IN PLASTIC CONTAINER
ABBOTT   0.9MEQ/ML   N019443 001   JUN 03, 1986
               1MEQ/ML   N019443 002   JUN 03, 1986

SODIUM BICARBONATE *MULTIPLE*
SEE   POLYETHYLENE GLYCOL 3350; POTASSIUM CHLORIDE; SODIUM BICARBONATE; SODIUM CHLORIDE; SODIUM SULFATE, ANHYDROUS

SODIUM CHLORIDE
Injectable; Injection
BACTERIOSTATIC SODIUM CHLORIDE 0.9% IN PLASTIC CONTAINER
AM P-IARM PARTNERS   9MG/ML   N088909 001   FEB 07, 1985
SODIUM CHLORIDE
ABBOTT   20GM/100ML   N017013 001
B BRAUN   20GM/100ML   N017038 001
SODIUM CHLORIDE 0.9% IN PLASTIC CONTAINER
ABBOTT   9MG/ML   N019218 001   JUL 13, 1984
MILES   900MG/100ML   N018502 001
SODIUM CHLORIDE 0.45% IN PLASTIC CONTAINER
B BRAUN   450MG/100ML   N018184 001
MILES   450MG/100ML   N018503 001
SODIUM CHLORIDE 3% IN PLASTIC CONTAINER
B BRAUN   3GM/100ML   N019635 003   MAR 09, 1988
SODIUM CHLORIDE 5% IN PLASTIC CONTAINER
B BRAUN   5GM/100ML   N019635 004   MAR 09, 1988
SODIUM CHLORIDE 23.4% IN PLASTIC CONTAINER
AM PHARM PARTNERS   234MG/ML   N019329 001   APR 22, 1987

Solution; Irrigation
SODIUM CHLORIDE 0.45% IN PLASTIC CONTAINER
ABBOTT   450MG/100ML   N018380 001
BAXTER HLTHCARE 450MG/100ML   N018497 001   FEB 19, 1982

Discontinued Drug Products (continued)

SELENOMETHIONINE, SE-75 (continued)
Injectable; Injection
SETHOTOPE
BRACCO   85-550uCi/ML   N017047 001

SERACTIDE ACETATE
Injectable; Injection
ACTHAR GEL-SYNTHETIC
ARMOUR PHARM   40 UNITS/ML   N017861 001
                80 UNITS/ML   N017861 002

SERMORELIN ACETATE
Injectable; Injection
GEREF
SERONO   EQ 0.5MG BASE/VIAL   N020443 001   SEP 26, 1997
                EQ 1MG BASE/VIAL   N020443 002   SEP 26, 1997

SERTRALINE HYDROCHLORIDE
Tablet; Oral
ZOLOFT
PFIZER   EQ 150MG BASE   N019839 003   DEC 30, 1991
                EQ 200MG BASE   N019839 004   DEC 30, 1991

SILVER SULFADIAZINE
Dressing; Topical
SILDAFLO
FRANKLIN PHARMS   1%   N019608 001   NOV 30, 1989

SIMETHICONE-CELLULOSE
Suspension; Oral
SONORX
BRACCO   7.5MG/ML   N020773 001   OCT 29, 1998

SODIUM ACETATE *MULTIPLE*
SEE   AMINO ACIDS; MAGNESIUM CHLORIDE; POTASSIUM ACETATE; POTASSIUM CHLORIDE; SODIUM ACETATE
SEE   CALCIUM CHLORIDE; DEXTROSE; MAGNESIUM CHLORIDE; POTASSIUM CHLORIDE; SODIUM CHLORIDE
SEE   CALCIUM CHLORIDE; DEXTROSE; MAGNESIUM CHLORIDE; POTASSIUM CHLORIDE; SODIUM CHLORIDE; SODIUM CITRATE
SEE   CALCIUM CHLORIDE; DEXTROSE; MAGNESIUM CHLORIDE; POTASSIUM CHLORIDE; SODIUM ACETATE; SODIUM CHLORIDE
SEE   CALCIUM CHLORIDE; MAGNESIUM CHLORIDE; POTASSIUM CHLORIDE; SODIUM ACETATE; SODIUM CHLORIDE
SEE   CALCIUM CHLORIDE; MAGNESIUM CHLORIDE; POTASSIUM CHLORIDE; SODIUM ACETATE; SODIUM CHLORIDE; SODIUM CITRATE
SEE   CALCIUM CHLORIDE; POTASSIUM CHLORIDE; SODIUM ACETATE; SODIUM CHLORIDE

Discontinued Drug Products *(continued)*

SODIUM CHLORIDE *(continued)*
Solution; Irrigation
SODIUM CHLORIDE IN PLASTIC CONTAINER
    MILES   900MG/100ML   N018247 001

SODIUM CHLORIDE *MULTIPLE*
SEE   AMINO ACIDS; CALCIUM CHLORIDE; DEXTROSE; MAGNESIUM CHLORIDE; POTASSIUM CHLORIDE; POTASSIUM PHOSPHATE, DIBASIC; SODIUM CHLORIDE
SEE   AMINO ACIDS; DEXTROSE; MAGNESIUM CHLORIDE; POTASSIUM ACETATE; POTASSIUM CHLORIDE; POTASSIUM PHOSPHATE, DIBASIC; SODIUM CHLORIDE
SEE   AMINO ACIDS; DEXTROSE; MAGNESIUM CHLORIDE; POTASSIUM CHLORIDE; POTASSIUM PHOSPHATE, DIBASIC; SODIUM CHLORIDE
SEE   AMINO ACIDS; DEXTROSE; MAGNESIUM CHLORIDE; POTASSIUM CHLORIDE; SODIUM CHLORIDE; SODIUM PHOSPHATE, DIBASIC, HEPTAHYDRATE
SEE   AMINO ACIDS; MAGNESIUM ACETATE; PHOSPHORIC ACID; POTASSIUM ACETATE; SODIUM CHLORIDE
SEE   AMINO ACIDS; MAGNESIUM ACETATE; POTASSIUM ACETATE; SODIUM CHLORIDE
SEE   AMINO ACIDS; MAGNESIUM CHLORIDE; POTASSIUM ACETATE; SODIUM CHLORIDE; SODIUM PHOSPHATE, DIBASIC, HEPTAHYDRATE
SEE   AMINO ACIDS; MAGNESIUM CHLORIDE; POTASSIUM CHLORIDE; POTASSIUM PHOSPHATE, DIBASIC; SODIUM CHLORIDE
SEE   AMINO ACIDS; MAGNESIUM CHLORIDE; POTASSIUM CHLORIDE; SODIUM CHLORIDE; SODIUM PHOSPHATE, DIBASIC, HEPTAHYDRATE
SEE   CALCIUM CHLORIDE; DEXTROSE; MAGNESIUM CHLORIDE; POTASSIUM CHLORIDE; SODIUM ACETATE; SODIUM CHLORIDE
SEE   CALCIUM CHLORIDE; DEXTROSE; MAGNESIUM CHLORIDE; SODIUM CHLORIDE; SODIUM CITRATE
SEE   CALCIUM CHLORIDE; DEXTROSE; MAGNESIUM CHLORIDE; SODIUM ACETATE; SODIUM CHLORIDE
SEE   CALCIUM CHLORIDE; DEXTROSE; MAGNESIUM CHLORIDE; SODIUM CHLORIDE
SEE   CALCIUM CHLORIDE; DEXTROSE; POTASSIUM CHLORIDE; SODIUM CHLORIDE; SODIUM LACTATE
SEE   CALCIUM CHLORIDE; DEXTROSE; SODIUM CHLORIDE; SODIUM LACTATE
SEE   CALCIUM CHLORIDE; DEXTROSE; SODIUM CHLORIDE; SODIUM LACTATE
SEE   CALCIUM CHLORIDE; MAGNESIUM CHLORIDE; POTASSIUM CHLORIDE; SODIUM ACETATE; SODIUM CHLORIDE
SEE   CALCIUM CHLORIDE; MAGNESIUM CHLORIDE; POTASSIUM CHLORIDE; SODIUM ACETATE; SODIUM CHLORIDE; SODIUM CITRATE
SEE   CALCIUM CHLORIDE; POTASSIUM CHLORIDE; SODIUM CHLORIDE
SEE   CALCIUM CHLORIDE; POTASSIUM CHLORIDE; SODIUM CHLORIDE; SODIUM LACTATE
SEE   DEXTROSE; POTASSIUM CHLORIDE; SODIUM CHLORIDE
SEE   DEXTROSE; SODIUM CHLORIDE
SEE   MAGNESIUM CHLORIDE; POTASSIUM CHLORIDE; POTASSIUM PHOSPHATE, MONOBASIC; SODIUM ACETATE; SODIUM CHLORIDE; SODIUM GLUCONATE; SODIUM PHOSPHATE, DIBASIC, HEPTAHYDRATE
SEE   MAGNESIUM CHLORIDE; POTASSIUM CHLORIDE; SODIUM ACETATE; SODIUM CHLORIDE; SODIUM GLUCONATE
SEE   POLYETHYLENE GLYCOL 3350; POTASSIUM CHLORIDE; SODIUM BICARBONATE; SODIUM CHLORIDE; SODIUM SULFATE, ANHYDROUS
SEE   POTASSIUM CHLORIDE; SODIUM CHLORIDE
SEE   POTASSIUM CHLORIDE; SODIUM CHLORIDE; TROMETHAMINE

SODIUM CHROMATE, CR-51
Injectable; Injection
CHROMITOPE SODIUM
    BRACCO   2mCi/VIAL   N013993 002

SODIUM CITRATE *MULTIPLE*
SEE   CALCIUM CHLORIDE; DEXTROSE; MAGNESIUM CHLORIDE; POTASSIUM CHLORIDE; SODIUM ACETATE; SODIUM CHLORIDE; SODIUM CITRATE
SEE   CALCIUM CHLORIDE; MAGNESIUM CHLORIDE; POTASSIUM CHLORIDE; SODIUM ACETATE; SODIUM CHLORIDE; SODIUM CITRATE

SODIUM FLUORIDE, F-18
Injectable; Intravenous
FLUORINE F-18
    AMERSHAM HLTH   2mCi/ML   N017042 001

SODIUM GLUCONATE *MULTIPLE*
SEE   MAGNESIUM CHLORIDE; POTASSIUM CHLORIDE; POTASSIUM PHOSPHATE, MONOBASIC; SODIUM ACETATE; SODIUM CHLORIDE; SODIUM GLUCONATE; SODIUM PHOSPHATE, DIBASIC, HEPTAHYDRATE
SEE   MAGNESIUM CHLORIDE; POTASSIUM CHLORIDE; SODIUM ACETATE; SODIUM CHLORIDE; SODIUM GLUCONATE

SODIUM IODIDE, I-123
Capsule; Oral
SODIUM IODIDE I 123
    SYNCOR PHARMS   400uCi   N018671 003   MAY 27, 1982

SODIUM IODIDE, I-131
Capsule; Oral
IODOTOPE
    BRACCO   1-150mCi   N010929 003
SODIUM IODIDE I 131
    CIS   50uCi   N017316 001
        100uCi   N017316 002
    MALLINCKRODT   0.8-100mCi   N016515 002
Solution; Oral
IODOTOPE
    BRACCO   7-106mCi/BOT   N010929 002

SODIUM LACTATE
Injectable; Injection
SODIUM LACTATE 0.167 MOLAR IN PLASTIC CONTAINER
    B BRAUN   1.87GM/100ML   N018186 001

SODIUM LACTATE *MULTIPLE*
SEE   CALCIUM CHLORIDE; DEXTROSE; MAGNESIUM CHLORIDE; SODIUM CHLORIDE; SODIUM LACTATE
SEE   CALCIUM CHLORIDE; DEXTROSE; POTASSIUM CHLORIDE; SODIUM CHLORIDE; SODIUM LACTATE
SEE   CALCIUM CHLORIDE; DEXTROSE; SODIUM CHLORIDE; SODIUM LACTATE
SEE   CALCIUM CHLORIDE; POTASSIUM CHLORIDE; SODIUM CHLORIDE; SODIUM LACTATE

Discontinued Drug Products (continued)

SODIUM NITROPRUSSIDE
Injectable; Injection
NIPRIDE
  ROCHE   50MG/VIAL   N017546 001
NITROPRESS
  ABBOTT   50MG/VIAL   N018450 001
     50MG/VIAL   N071555 001   NOV 16, 1987
SODIUM NITROPRUSSIDE
  AM PHARM PARTNERS   50MG/VIAL   N070031 001   JAN 17, 1985
  ELKINS SINN   50MG/VIAL   N018581 001   JUL 28, 1982

SODIUM PHENYLACETATE *MULTIPLE*
SEE   SODIUM BENZOATE; SODIUM PHENYLACETATE

SODIUM PHOSPHATE, DIBASIC, HEPTAHYDRATE *MULTIPLE*
SEE   AMINO ACIDS; DEXTROSE; MAGNESIUM CHLORIDE; POTASSIUM CHLORIDE; SODIUM CHLORIDE; SODIUM PHOSPHATE, DIBASIC, HEPTAHYDRATE
SEE   AMINO ACIDS; MAGNESIUM ACETATE; POTASSIUM ACETATE; SODIUM CHLORIDE; SODIUM PHOSPHATE, DIBASIC, HEPTAHYDRATE
SEE   AMINO ACIDS; MAGNESIUM CHLORIDE; POTASSIUM CHLORIDE; SODIUM CHLORIDE; SODIUM PHOSPHATE, DIBASIC, HEPTAHYDRATE
SEE   MAGNESIUM CHLORIDE; POTASSIUM CHLORIDE; POTASSIUM PHOSPHATE, MONOBASIC; SODIUM ACETATE; SODIUM CHLORIDE; SODIUM GLUCONATE; SODIUM PHOSPHATE, DIBASIC, HEPTAHYDRATE

SODIUM PHOSPHATE, P-32
Solution; Injection, Oral
PHOSPHOTOPE
  BRACCO   1-8mCi/VIAL   N010927 001
SODIUM PHOSPHATE P 32
  MALLINCKRODT   1.5mCi/VIAL   N011777 002

SODIUM POLYSTYRENE SULFONATE
Powder; Oral, Rectal
SODIUM POLYSTYRENE SULFONATE
  MORTON GROVE   453.6GM/BOT   N088786 001   SEP 11, 1984
Suspension; Oral, Rectal
SODIUM POLYSTYRENE SULFONATE
  MORTON GROVE   15GM/60ML   N088717 001   SEP 11, 1984
  ROXANE   15GM/60ML   N088453 001   NOV 17, 1983

SODIUM SUCCINATE
Injectable; Injection
SODIUM SUCCINATE
  ELKINS SINN   30%   N080516 001

SODIUM SULFATE, ANHYDROUS *MULTIPLE*
SEE   POLYETHYLENE GLYCOL 3350; POTASSIUM CHLORIDE; SODIUM BICARBONATE; SODIUM CHLORIDE; SODIUM SULFATE, ANHYDROUS

SODIUM TETRADECYL SULFATE
Injectable; Injection
SOTRADECOL
  ELKINS SINN   1% *SEE ANNUAL PREFACE INTRODUCTION DISCONTINUED SECTION*   N005970 004
     3% *SEE ANNUAL PREFACE INTRODUCTION DISCONTINUED SECTION*   N005970 005

SOMATROPIN
Injectable; Injection
ASELLACRIN 2
  SERONO   2 IU/VIAL   N017726 002   JUL 21, 1983
ASELLACRIN 10
  SERONO   10 IU/VIAL   N017726 001
CRESCORMON
  GENENTECH   4 IU/VIAL   N017992 001

SOMATROPIN RECOMBINANT
Injectable; Injection
BIO-TROPIN
  BIO TECH GEN   4.8MG/VIAL   N019774 001   MAY 25, 1995
HUMATROPE
  LILLY   2MG/VIAL   N019640 001   JUN 23, 1987
NORDITROPIN
  NOVO NORDISK   4MG/VIAL   N019721 001   MAY 08, 1995
     8MG/VIAL   N019721 002   MAY 08, 1995

SORBITOL
Solution; Irrigation
SORBITOL 3% IN PLASTIC CONTAINER
  BAXTER HLTHCARE   3GM/100ML   N018512 001   MAY 27, 1982

SORBITOL *MULTIPLE*
SEE   MANNITOL; SORBITOL

SOTALOL HYDROCHLORIDE
Tablet; Oral
BETAPACE
  BERLEX LABS   320MG   N019865 004   OCT 30, 1992
BETAPACE AF
  BERLEX LABS   40MG   N021151 006

SPIRONOLACTONE *MULTIPLE*
SEE HYDROCHLOROTHIAZIDE; SPIRONOLACTONE

STAVUDINE
Tablet; Oral
ZERIT
BRISTOL MYERS SQUIBB — 5MG — N020412 001 — JUN 24, 1994

STREPTOMYCIN SULFATE
Injectable; Injection
STREPTOMYCIN SULFATE

COPANOS	EQ 500MG BASE/ML	N060684 001
LILLY	EQ 1GM BASE/2ML	N060404 001
	EQ 1GM BASE/VIAL	N060107 001
	EQ 5GM BASE/VIAL	N060107 002
PFIZER	EQ 1GM BASE/VIAL	N060076 001
	EQ 5GM BASE/VIAL	N060076 002

SUCCINYLCHOLINE CHLORIDE
Injectable; Injection
ANECTINE
GLAXOSMITHKLINE — 50MG/ML — N008453 003
QUELICIN PRESERVATIVE FREE
ABBOTT — 50MG/ML — N008845 002
SUCCINYLCHOLINE CHLORIDE
INTL MEDICATION — 100MG/VIAL — N085400 001 — FEB 04, 1982
SUCOSTRIN
APOTHECON — 20MG/ML — N008847 001
— 100MG/ML — N008847 003

SUFENTANIL CITRATE
Injectable; Injection
SUFENTANIL CITRATE
STERIS — EQ 0.05MG BASE/ML — N074406 001 — DEC 15, 1995

SULBACTAM SODIUM *MULTIPLE*
SEE AMPICILLIN SODIUM; SULBACTAM SODIUM

SULCONAZOLE NITRATE
Solution; Topical
EXELDERM
WESTWOOD SQUIBB — 1% — N018738 001 — AUG 30, 1985

SULFACETAMIDE *MULTIPLE*
SEE TRIPLE SULFA (SULFABENZAMIDE;SULFACETAMIDE;SULFATHIAZOLE)

Discontinued Drug Products (continued)

SOTALOL HYDROCHLORIDE (continued)
Tablet; Oral
BETAPACE AF
BERLEX LABS — 60MG — N021151 007 — APR 02, 2003
— 100MG — N021151 005 — MAR 14, 2003

SOYBEAN OIL
Injectable; Injection
TRAVAMULSION 10%
BAXTER HLTHCARE — 10% — N018660 001 — FEB 26, 1982
TRAVAMULSION 20%
BAXTER HLTHCARE — 20% — N018758 001 — FEB 15, 1983

SPECTINOMYCIN HYDROCHLORIDE
Injectable; Injection
TROBICIN
PHARMACIA AND UPJOHN — EQ 4GM BASE/VIAL — N050347 002

SPIRAPRIL HYDROCHLORIDE
Tablet; Oral
RENORMAX
SCHERING — 3MG — N020240 001 — DEC 29, 1994
— 6MG — N020240 002 — DEC 29, 1994
— 12MG — N020240 003 — DEC 29, 1994
— 24MG — N020240 004 — DEC 29, 1994

SPIRONOLACTONE
Tablet; Oral
SPIRONOLACTONE

Company	Strength	Appl No	Date
ASCOT	25MG	N087687 001	OCT 20, 1982
IVAX PHARMS	25MG	N087108 001	
LEDERLE	25MG	N087634 001	
PUREPAC PHARM	25MG	N087998 001	OCT 14, 1983
	25MG	N088053 001	AUG 25, 1983
UPSHER SMITH	25MG	N087554 001	
VANGARD	25MG	N087648 001	FEB 01, 1982
WARNER CHILCOTT	25MG	N087952 001	NOV 18, 1982
WATSON LAB	25MG	N086898 002	MAR 02, 1982
WATSON LABS	25MG	N087078 001	

Discontinued Drug Products (continued)

SULFACETAMIDE SODIUM

Ointment; Ophthalmic

- BLEPH-10
  - ALLERGAN — 10% — N084015 001
- SODIUM SULAMYD
  - SCHERING — 10% — N005963 002
- SULFAIR 10
  - PHARMAFAIR — 10% — N088000 001 DEC 22, 1982

Solution/Drops; Ophthalmic

- OCUSULF-30
  - MIZA PHARMS USA — 30% — N080660 002
- SODIUM SULAMYD
  - SCHERING — 10% — N005963 001
  - — 30% — N005963 003
- SODIUM SULFACETAMIDE
  - AKORN — 10% — N083021 001
  - — 15% — N083021 002
  - — 30% — N083021 003
  - SOLA BARNES HIND — 10% — N084143 001
  - — 10% — N084145 001
  - — 30% — N084146 001
  - — 30% — N084147 001
- SULFACETAMIDE SODIUM
  - PHARMAFAIR — 10% — N088947 001 MAY 17, 1985
- SULFAIR 10
  - PHARMAFAIR — 10% — N087949 001 DEC 13, 1982
- SULFAIR FORTE
  - PHARMAFAIR — 30% — N088385 001 OCT 13, 1983
- SULFAIR-15
  - PHARMAFAIR — 15% — N088186 001 MAY 25, 1983
- SULTEN-10
  - BAUSCH AND LOMB — 10% — N087818 001 FEB 03, 1983

SULFACETAMIDE SODIUM *MULTIPLE*

SEE PREDNISOLONE ACETATE; SULFACETAMIDE SODIUM
SEE PREDNISOLONE SODIUM PHOSPHATE; SULFACETAMIDE SODIUM

SULFADIAZINE

Tablet; Oral

- SULFADIAZINE
  - ABBOTT — 300MG — N004125 005
  - EVERYLIFE — 500MG — N080088 001
  - IMPAX LABS — 500MG — N080081 001
  - LANNETT — 500MG — N080084 001
  - LEDERLE — 500MG — N004054 001
  - LILLY — 500MG — N004122 002

SULFADIAZINE; SULFAMERAZINE

Suspension; Oral

- SULFONAMIDES DUPLEX
  - LILLY — 250MG/5ML;250MG/5ML — N006317 007

SULFADIAZINE SODIUM

Injectable; Injection

- SULFADIAZINE SODIUM
  - LEDERLE — 250MG/ML — N004054 002

SULFAMERAZINE *MULTIPLE*

SEE SULFADIAZINE; SULFAMERAZINE
SEE TRISULFAPYRIMIDINES (SULFADIAZINE;SULFAMERAZINE;SULFAMETHAZINE)

SULFAMETER

Tablet; Oral

- SULLA
  - BERLEX — 500MG — N016000 002

SULFAMETHIZOLE

Tablet; Oral

- MICROSUL
  - FOREST PHARMS — 1GM — N086012 001
- PROKLAR
  - FOREST PHARMS — 500MG — N080273 001
- THIOSULFIL
  - WYETH AYERST — 250MG — N008565 001
  - — 500MG — N008565 004

SULFAMETHOXAZOLE

Suspension; Oral

- GANTANOL
  - ROCHE — 500MG/5ML — N013664 002

Tablet; Oral

- GANTANOL
  - ROCHE — 500MG — N012715 002
- GANTANOL-DS
  - ROCHE — 1GM — N012715 003
- SULFAMETHOXAZOLE
  - ASCOT — 500MG — N087662 001 OCT 20, 1982
  - — 500MG — N087189 001 JUL. 25, 1983
  - BARR — 500MG — N085844 001
  - GENEVA PHARMS — 500MG — N086163 001
  - HEATHER — 1GM — N086000 001
  - WATSON LAB — 500MG — N085053 001
- UROBAK
  - SHIONOGI — 500MG — N087307 001

SULFAMETHOXAZOLE; TRIMETHOPRIM

Injectable; Injection

- SEPTRA
  - MONARCH PHARMS — 80MG/ML;16MG/ML — N018452 001

SULFAMETHOXAZOLE; TRIMETHOPRIM *(continued)*

Tablet; Oral

SULFAMETHOXAZOLE AND TRIMETHOPRIM

Firm	Strength	Appl. No.	Date
USL PHARMA			
WATSON LABS	400MG;80MG	N070002 001	NOV 08, 1985
	800MG;160MG	N070000 001	NOV 07, 1984

SULFAMETHOXAZOLE AND TRIMETHOPRIM DOUBLE STRENGTH

Firm	Strength	Appl. No.	Date
HALSEY	800MG;160MG	N070007 001	NOV 07, 1984
MARTEC	800MG;160MG	N072417 001	NOV 14, 1984
ROXANE	800MG;160MG	N072769 001	DEC 07, 1988
SULFATRIM-DS SUPERPHARM	800MG;160MG	N070066 001	AUG 30, 1991
SULFATRIM-SS SUPERPHARM	400MG;80MG	N070065 002	JUN 24, 1985
UROPLUS DS SHIONOGI	800MG;160MG	N071816 001	JUN 24, 1985
UROPLUS SS SHIONOGI	400MG;80MG	N071815 001	SEP 28, 1987

SULFAMETHOXAZOLE *MULTIPLE*

SEE   PHENAZOPYRIDINE HYDROCHLORIDE; SULFAMETHOXAZOLE

SEE   PHENAZOPYRIDINE HYDROCHLORIDE; SULFAMETHOXAZOLE; TRIMETHOPRIM

SULFAPHENAZOLE

Suspension; Oral

SULFABID

Firm	Strength	Appl. No.
PURDUE FREDERICK	500MG/5ML	N013093 001

Tablet; Oral

SULFABID

Firm	Strength	Appl. No.
PURDUE FREDERICK	500MG	N013092 002

SULFAPYRIDINE

Tablet; Oral

SULFAPYRIDINE

Firm	Strength	Appl. No.
LILLY	500MG	N000159 001

SULFASALAZINE

Suspension; Oral

AZULFIDINE

Firm	Strength	Appl. No.
PHARMACIA AND UPJOHN	250MG/5ML	N018605 001

Tablet, Delayed Release; Oral

SULFASALAZINE

Firm	Strength	Appl. No.	Date
WATSON LAB	500MG	N088052 001	MAY 24, 1983

Discontinued Drug Products *(continued)*

SULFAMETHOXAZOLE; TRIMETHOPRIM *(continued)*

Injectable; Injection

SULFAMETHOXAZOLE TRIMETHOPRIM

Firm	Strength	Appl. No.	Date
QUAD PHARMS	80MG/ML;16MG/ML	N071341 001	AUG 07, 1987

SULFAMETHOXAZOLE AND TRIMETHOPRIM

Firm	Strength	Appl. No.	Date
AM PHARM PARTNERS	80MG/ML;16MG/ML	N070223 001	DEC 29, 1987
BEDFORD	80MG/ML;16MG/ML	N072383 001	APR 29, 1992
STERIS	80MG/ML;16MG/ML	N071556 001	DEC 29, 1987

Suspension; Oral

BACTRIM

Firm	Strength	Appl. No.
WOMEN FIRST HLTHCARE	200MG/5ML;40MG/5ML	N017560 001

BACTRIM PEDIATRIC

Firm	Strength	Appl. No.
WOMEN FIRST HLTHCARE	200MG/5ML;40MG/5ML	N017560 002

SULMEPRIM

Firm	Strength	Appl. No.	Date
USL PHARMA	200MG/5ML;40MG/5ML	N070063 001	AUG 01, 1986

SULMEPRIM PEDIATRIC

Firm	Strength	Appl. No.	Date
USL PHARMA	200MG/5ML;40MG/5ML	N070064 001	AUG 01, 1986

TRIMETH/SULFA

Firm	Strength	Appl. No.	Date
ALPHARMA	200MG/5ML;40MG/5ML	N072289 001	MAY 23, 1988
	200MG/5ML;40MG/5ML	N072398 001	MAY 23, 1988
NASKA	200MG/5ML;40MG/5ML	N072399 001	MAY 23, 1988

Tablet; Oral

SULFAMETHOXAZOLE TRIMETHOPRIM

Firm	Strength	Appl. No.	Date
HEATHER	400MG;80MG	N018946 001	AUG 10, 1984
	800MG;160MG	N018946 002	AUG 10, 1984

SULFAMETHOXAZOLE AND TRIMETHOPRIM

Firm	Strength	Appl. No.	Date
EON	400MG;80MG	N018598 003	MAY 19, 1982
HALSEY	400MG;80MG	N070006 001	NOV 14, 1984
INTERPHARM	400MG;80MG	N071299 001	OCT 27, 1987
	800MG;160MG	N071300 001	OCT 27, 1987
MARTEC	400MG;80MG	N072408 001	DEC 07, 1988
ROXANE	400MG;80MG	N072768 001	AUG 30, 1991
TEVA	400MG;80MG	N018242 001	
	800MG;160MG	N018242 002	
USL PHARMA	400MG;80MG	N070203 001	NOV 08, 1985
	800MG;160MG	N070204 001	

Discontinued Drug Products (continued)

SULFASALAZINE (continued)
Tablet; Oral

S.A.S.-500			
	SOLVAY	500MG	N083450 001
SULFASALAZINE			
	EON	500MG	N086184 001
	LEDERLE	500MG	N080197 001
	SUPERPHARM	500MG	N089339 001
			OCT 26, 1987
	WATSON LAB	500MG	N084964 001

SULFINPYRAZONE
Capsule; Oral

SULFINPYRAZONE			
	VANGARD	200MG	N088666 001
			FEB 17, 1984

Tablet; Oral

SULFINPYRAZONE			
	IVAX PHARMS	100MG	N087769 001
			JUN 01, 1982
	WATSON LABS	100MG	N087667 001
			MAY 26, 1982

SULFISOXAZOLE
Tablet; Oral

GANTRISIN			
	ROCHE	500MG	N006525 001
SOXAZOLE			
	ALRA	500MG	N080366 001
SULFALAR			
	PARKE DAVIS	500MG	N084955 001
SULFISOXAZOLE			
	BARR	500MG	N084031 001
	GENEVA PHARMS	500MG	N085628 001
	HEATHER	500MG	N080189 001
	IMPAX LABS	500MG	N080109 001
	LANNETT	500MG	N080085 001
	LEDERLE	500MG	N087649 001
	PHARMERAL	500MG	N084385 001
	PUREPAC PHARM	500MG	N080087 001
	VITARINE	500MG	N087332 001
	WATSON LABS	500MG	N085534 001
	WEST WARD	500MG	N080379 001
SULSOXIN			
	SOLVAY	500MG	N080040 001

SULFISOXAZOLE *MULTIPLE*
SEE   PHENAZOPYRIDINE HYDROCHLORIDE; SULFISOXAZOLE

SULFISOXAZOLE ACETYL
Emulsion; Oral

LIPO GANTRISIN			
	ROCHE	EQ 1GM BASE/5ML	N009182 009

SULFISOXAZOLE ACETYL (continued)
Syrup; Oral

GANTRISIN			
	ROCHE	EQ 500MG BASE/5ML	N009182 002

SULFISOXAZOLE ACETYL *MULTIPLE*
SEE   ERYTHROMYCIN ESTOLATE; SULFISOXAZOLE ACETYL

SULFISOXAZOLE DIOLAMINE
Injectable; Injection

GANTRISIN			
	ROCHE	EQ 400MG BASE/ML	N006917 001

Ointment; Ophthalmic

GANTRISIN			
	ROCHE	EQ 4% BASE	N008414 002

Solution/Drops; Ophthalmic

GANTRISIN			
	ROCHE	EQ 4% BASE	N007757 002
SULFISOXAZOLE DIOLAMINE			
	SOLA BARNES HIND	EQ 4% BASE	N084148 001

SULFOXONE SODIUM
Tablet, Delayed Release; Oral

DIASONE SODIUM			
	ABBOTT	165MG	N006044 003

SULFUR
Powder; Topical

BENSULFOID			
	POYTHRESS	33.32%	N002918 001

SUPROFEN
Solution/Drops; Ophthalmic

PROFENAL			
	ALCON	1%	N019387 001
			DEC 23, 1988

SUTILAINS
Ointment; Topical

TRAVASE			
	ABBOTT	82,000 UNITS/GM *SEE ANNUAL PREFACE INTRODUCTION DISCONTINUED SECTION*	N012828 001

TALBUTAL
Tablet; Oral

LOTUSATE			
	SANOFI SYNTHELABO	120MG	N009410 005

TANNIC ACID *MULTIPLE*
SEE   CYANOCOBALAMIN; TANNIC ACID; ZINC ACETATE

Discontinued Drug Products (*continued*)

TECHNETIUM TC-99M ALBUMIN AGGREGATED
Injectable; Injection
  TC 99M-LUNGAGGREGATE   5mCi/ML
    AMERSHAM HLTH   N017848 001

TECHNETIUM TC-99M ALBUMIN AGGREGATED KIT
Injectable; Injection
  A-N STANNOUS AGGREGATED ALBUMIN N/A
    SYNCOR PHARMS   N017916 001
  AN-MAA N/A
    CIS   N017792 001
  LUNGAGGREGATE REAGENT N/A
    AMERSHAM HLTH   N017838 001
  TECHNETIUM TC 99M MAA N/A
    AMERSHAM HLTH   N017773 001

TECHNETIUM TC-99M ALBUMIN COLLOID KIT
Injectable; Injection
  MICROLITE N/A
    CIS   N018263 001
      MAR 25, 1983

TECHNETIUM TC-99M ALBUMIN KIT
Injectable; Injection
  TECHNETIUM TC 99M HSA N/A
    AMERSHAM HLTH   N017775 001

TECHNETIUM TC-99M ALBUMIN MICROSPHERES KIT
Injectable; Injection
  INSTANT MICROSPHERES N/A
    3M   N017832 001

TECHNETIUM TC-99M ETIDRONATE KIT
Injectable; Injection
  CINTICHEM TECHNETIUM 99M HEDSPA N/A
    AMERSHAM HLTH   N017653 001
  MPI STANNOUS DIPHOSPHONATE N/A
    AMERSHAM HLTH   N017667 001
  OSTEOSCAN N/A
    MALLINCKRODT   N017454 001
  TECHNETIUM TC 99M DIPHOSPHONATE-TIN KIT N/A
    AMERSHAM HLTH   N017562 001

TECHNETIUM TC-99M FERPENTETATE KIT
Injectable; Injection
  RENOTEC N/A
    BRACCO   N017045 001

TECHNETIUM TC-99M GLUCEPTATE KIT
Injectable; Injection
  GLUCOSCAN N/A
    BRISTOL MYERS SQUIBB   N017907 001

TECHNETIUM TC-99M LIDOFENIN KIT
Injectable; Injection
  TECHNESCAN HIDA N/A
    DRAXIMAGE   N018489 001
      OCT 31, 1986

TECHNETIUM TC-99M MEDRONATE KIT
Injectable; Injection
  AMERSCAN MDP KIT N/A
    AMERSHAM HLTH   N018335 001
      AUG 05, 1982

TECHNETIUM TC-99M PENTETATE KIT
Injectable; Injection
  MPI DTPA KIT - CHELATE N/A
    AMERSHAM HLTH   N017255 001

TECHNETIUM TC-99M POLYPHOSPHATE KIT
Injectable; Injection
  SODIUM POLYPHOSPHATE-TIN KIT N/A
    AMERSHAM HLTH   N017664 001

TECHNETIUM TC-99M PYRO/TRIMETA PHOSPHATES KIT
Injectable; Injection
  PYROLITE N/A
    CIS   N017684 001

TECHNETIUM TC-99M RED BLOOD CELL KIT
Injectable; Injection
  RBC-SCAN N/A
    CADEMA   N020063 001
      JUN 11, 1992

TECHNETIUM TC-99M SODIUM PERTECHNETATE
Solution; Injection, Oral
  SODIUM PERTECHNETATE TC 99M
    AMERSHAM HLTH 2-100mCi/ML N017471 001
    CIS 12mCi/ML N017321 001
      24mCi/ML N017321 002
      48mCi/ML N017321 003
    MALLINCKRODT 10-60mCi/ML N017725 001

TECHNETIUM TC-99M SODIUM PERTECHNETATE GENERATOR
Solution; Injection, Oral
  MINITEC 0.22-2.22 CI/GENERATOR
    BRACCO   N017339 001
  TECHNETIUM TC 99M GENERATOR 830-16600mCi/GENERATOR
    AMERSHAM HLTH   N017693 001

TECHNETIUM TC-99M SULFUR COLLOID
Solution; Injection, Oral
  TECHNETIUM TC 99M SULFUR COLLOID 4mCi/ML
    AMERSHAM HLTH   N017456 001

Discontinued Drug Products *(continued)*

TECHNETIUM TC-99M SULFUR COLLOID *(continued)*
Solution; Oral
TECHNETIUM TC 99M SULFUR COLLOID
MALLINCKRODT — 3mCi/ML — N017724 001

TECHNETIUM TC-99M SULFUR COLLOID KIT
Solution; Injection, Oral
TECHNETIUM TC 99M TSC
AMERSHAM HLTH — N/A — N017784 001
TESULOID
BRACCO — N/A — N016923 001

TEMAZEPAM
Capsule; Oral
TEMAZ
QUANTUM PHARMICS — 15MG — N070564 001 — OCT 15, 1985
— 30MG — N070547 001 — OCT 15, 1985
TEMAZEPAM
DURAMED PHARM BARR — 15MG — N071708 001 — SEP 29, 1988
— 30MG — N071709 001 — SEP 29, 1988
HALSEY — 15MG — N071174 001 — JUL 10, 1986
— 30MG — N071175 001 — JUL 10, 1986
USL PHARMA — 15MG — N070489 001 — JUL 07, 1986
— 30MG — N070490 001 — JUL 07, 1986
WATSON LAB — 15MG — N070383 001 — MAR 23, 1987
— 30MG — N070384 001 — MAR 23, 1987

TERBINAFINE
Gel; Topical
LAMISIL
NOVARTIS — 1% — N020846 001 — APR 29, 1998

TERBUTALINE SULFATE
Aerosol, Metered; Inhalation
BRETHAIRE
NOVARTIS — 0.2MG/INH — N018762 001 — AUG 17, 1984
BRICANYL
AVENTIS PHARMS — 0.2MG/INH — N018000 001 — MAR 19, 1985
Injectable; Injection
BRICANYL
AVENTIS PHARMS — 1MG/ML — N017466 001

TERBUTALINE SULFATE *(continued)*
Tablet; Oral
BRICANYL
AVENTIS PHARMS — 2.5MG — N017618 001
— 5MG — N017618 002

TERIPARATIDE ACETATE
Injectable; Injection
PARATHAR
AVENTIS — 200 UNITS/VIAL — N019498 001 — DEC 23, 1987

TESTOLACTONE
Injectable; Irjection
TESLAC
BRISTOL MYERS SQUIBB — 100MG/ML — N016119 001
Tablet; Oral
TESLAC
BRISTOL MYERS SQUIBB — 250MG — N016118 002

TESTOSTERONE
Injectable; Injection
TESTOSTERONE
STERIS — 25MG/ML — N086420 001 — MAY 10, 1983
— 50MG/ML — N086419 001 — AUG 23, 1983

TESTOSTERONE CYPIONATE
Injectable; Injection
DEPO-TESTOSTERONE
PHARMACIA AND UPJOHN — 50MG/ML — N085635 001
TESTOSTERONE CYPIONATE
QUAD PHARMS — 100MG/ML — N089326 001 — OCT 28, 1988
— 200MG/ML — N089327 001 — OCT 28, 1988
STERIS — 100MG/ML — N084401 001
— 200MG/ML — N084401 002

TESTOSTERONE CYPIONATE *MULTIPLE*
SEE ESTRADIOL CYPIONATE; TESTOSTERONE CYPIONATE

TESTOSTERONE ENANTHATE
Injectable; Injection
DELATESTRYL
BTG — 200MG/ML — N009165 001
TESTOSTERONE ENANTHATE
QUAD PHARMS — 100MG/ML — N089324 001 — SEP 16, 1986
— 200MG/ML — N089325 001

TETRACYCLINE HYDROCHLORIDE (continued)

Capsule; Oral

TETRACYCLINE HCL

Firm	Strength	Appl. No.	Date
EON	250MG	N061471 001	
FERRANTE	125MG	N060173 001	
	250MG	N060173 002	
HEATHER	250MG	N061148 001	
	500MG	N061148 002	
ICN	250MG	N060471 001	
	500MG	N060471 002	
PUREPAC PHARM	250MG	N060290 001	
	500MG	N060290 002	
PVT FORM	250MG	N062686 001	JUL 24, 1986
	500MG	N062686 002	JUL 24, 1986
SUPERPHARM	250MG	N062540 001	MAR 21, 1985
	500MG	N062540 002	MAR 21, 1985
WARNER CHILCOTT	250MG	N062300 001	
	500MG	N062300 002	
WATSON LABS	250MG	N062103 001	
	500MG	N062103 002	
	250MG	N062343 001	
	500MG	N062343 002	
WEST WARD	500MG	N060768 001	
	500MG	N060768 002	
WYETH AYERST	250MG	N061685 001	
	500MG	N061685 002	
TETRACYN			
PFIPHARMECS	250MG	N060082 003	
	500MG	N060082 004	

Fiber, Extended Release; Periodontal

Firm	Strength	Appl. No.	Date
ACTISITE			
ALZA	12.7MG/FIBER	N050653 001	MAR 25, 1994

For Solution; Topical

Firm	Strength	Appl. No.	Date
TOPICYCLINE			
SHIRE LABS	2.2MG/ML	N050493 001	

Injectable; Injection

Firm	Strength	Appl. No.	Date
ACHROMYCIN			
LEDERLE	250MG/VIAL	N050273 002	
	500MG/VIAL	N050273 003	
TETRACYN			
PFIZER	250MG/VIAL	N060096 001	
	500MG/VIAL	N060096 002	

Ointment; Ophthalmic

Firm	Strength	Appl. No.	Date
ACHROMYCIN			
STORZ	10MG/GM	N050266 001	

Suspension/Drops; Ophthalmic

Firm	Strength	Appl. No.	Date
ACHROMYCIN			
STORZ	1%	N050268 001	

Suspension; Oral

Firm	Strength	Appl. No.	Date
ACHROMYCIN V			
LEDERLE	125MG/5ML	N050263 002	

Discontinued Drug Products (continued)

TESTOSTERONE ENANTHATE (continued)

Injectable; Injection

TESTOSTERONE ENANTHATE

Firm	Strength	Appl. No.	Date
QUAD PHARMS	100MG/ML	N085599 001	SEP 16, 1986
STERIS	100MG/ML	N083667 001	
	200MG/ML	N083667 002	

TESTOSTERONE ENANTHATE *MULTIPLE*

SEE ESTRADIOL VALERATE; TESTOSTERONE ENANTHATE

TESTOSTERONE PROPIONATE

Injectable; Injection

TESTOSTERONE PROPIONATE

Firm	Strength	Appl. No.	Date
BEL MAR	25MG/ML	N080741 001	
	50MG/ML	N080742 001	
	100MG/ML	N080743 001	
ELKINS SINN	25MG/ML	N080276 001	
LILLY	50MG/ML	N080254 002	
QUAD PHARMS	100MG/ML	N089283 001	
STERIS	25MG/ML	N085490 001	NOV 03, 1986
	50MG/ML	N085490 002	
	100MG/ML	N083595 003	

TETRACYCLINE HYDROCHLORIDE

Capsule; Oral

Firm	Strength	Appl. No.
ACHROMYCIN V		
CLONMEL HLTHCARE	250MG	N050278 003
	500MG	N050278 001
CYCLOPAR		
WARNER CHILCOTT	250MG	N061725 001
	250MG	N062175 001
	250MG	N062332 001
	500MG	N061725 002
	500MG	N062332 002
PANMYCIN		
PHARMACIA AND UPJOHN	250MG	N060347 001
RETET		
SOLVAY	250MG	N061443 001
	500MG	N061443 002
ROBITET		
WYETH AYERST	250MG	N061734 001
	500MG	N061734 002
SUMYCIN		
APOTHECON	100MG	N060429 002
	125MG	N060429 004
TETRACHEL		
ANGUS	250MG	N060343 001
	500MG	N060343 003
TETRACYCLINE HCL		
ABBOTT	250MG	N061802 001
	500MG	N061802 002
ELKINS SINN	250MG	N060059 001

Discontinued Drug Products (continued)

TETRACYCLINE HYDROCHLORIDE (continued)
Suspension; Oral

TETRACYCLINE HCL			
ALPHARMA	125MG/5ML	N060633 001	
FERRANTE	125MG/5ML	N060174 001	
PROTER	125MG/5ML	N060446 001	
PUREPAC PHARM	125MG/5ML	N060291 001	
TETRACYN			
PFIPHARMECS	125MG/5ML	N060095 001	
TETRAMED			
IVAX PHARMS	125MG/5ML	N061468 001	

Tablet; Oral

PANMYCIN			
PHARMACIA AND	250MG	N061705 001	
UPJOHN	500MG	N061705 002	
SUMYCIN			
PAR PHARM	50MG	N061147 003	
	100MG	N061147 002	

TETRACYCLINE HYDROCHLORIDE *MULTIPLE*
SEE   HYDROCORTISONE; TETRACYCLINE HYDROCHLORIDE
SEE   PROCAINE HYDROCHLORIDE; TETRACYCLINE HYDROCHLORIDE

TETRACYCLINE PHOSPHATE COMPLEX
Capsule; Oral

TETREX			
BRISTOL	EQ 250MG HCL	N050212 002	
	EQ 500MG HCL	N050212 003	

THALLOUS CHLORIDE, TL-201
Injectable; Injection

THALLOUS CHLORIDE TL 201			
BRACCO	1mCi/ML	N018548 001	DEC 30, 1982

THEOPHYLLINE
Capsule, Extended Release; Oral

ELIXOPHYLLIN SR			
FORREST LABS	125MG	N086826 001	JAN 29, 1985
	250MG	N086826 002	JAN 29, 1985
SLO-PHYLLIN			
AVENTIS	60MG	N085206 001	MAY 24, 1982
	125MG	N085203 001	MAY 24, 1982
	250MG	N085205 001	MAY 24, 1982
SOMOPHYLLIN-CRT			
GRAHAM DM	50MG	N087763 001	FEB 27, 1985
	100MG	N087194 001	
	200MG	N088382 001	

THEOPHYLLINE (continued)
Capsule, Extended Release; Oral

SOMOPHYLLIN-CRT			
GRAHAM DM	250MG	N087193 001	FEB 27, 1985
	300MG	N088383 001	FEB 27, 1985
THEO-DUR			
SCHERING	50MG	N088022 001	SEP 10, 1985
	75MG	N088015 001	SEP 10, 1985
	125MG	N088016 001	SEP 10, 1985
	200MG	N087995 001	SEP 10, 1985
THEOBID			
WHITBY	260MG	N085983 001	MAR 20, 1985
THEOBID JR.			
WHITBY	130MG	N087854 001	MAR 20, 1985
THEOCLEAR L.A.-130			
SCHWARZ PHARMA	130MG	N086569 001	MAY 27, 1982
THEOCLEAR L.A.-260			
SCHWARZ PHARMA	260MG	N086569 002	MAY 27, 1982
THEOPHYL-SR			
ORTHO MCNEIL PHARM	125MG	N086480 001	FEB 08, 1985
	250MG	N086471 001	FEB 08, 1985
THEOPHYLLINE			
CENT PHARMS	125MG	N088654 001	FEB 12, 1985
	250MG	N088689 001	FEB 12, 1985
EON	260MG	N087462 001	MAY 11, 1982
FAULDING	100MG	N089976 001	JAN 04, 1995
	200MG	N089977 001	JAN 04, 1995
	300MG	N089932 001	JAN 04, 1995
THEOPHYLLINE-SR			
SCHERER RP	300MG	N088255 001	JUN 12, 1986
THEOVENT			
SCHERING	125MG	N087010 001	JAN 31, 1985
	250MG	N087910 001	JAN 31, 1985

Discontinued Drug Products *(continued)*

THEOPHYLLINE *(continued)*

Capsule: Oral

	Strength	Appl. No.	Date
BRONKODYL			
SANOFI SYNTHELABO	100MG	N085264 001	
	200MG	N085264 002	
ELIXOPHYLLIN			
FORREST LABS	100MG	N085545 001	JUL 31, 1984
	200MG	N083921 001	JUL 31, 1984
SOMOPHYLLIN-T			
FISONS	100MG	N087155 001	FEB 25, 1985
	200MG	N087155 002	FEB 25, 1985
	250MG	N087155 003	FEB 25, 1985
THEOPHYLLINE			
KV PHARM	100MG	N085263 001	
	200MG	N085263 002	
SCHERER RP	100MG	N084731 002	NOV 07, 1986
	200MG	N084731 001	NOV 07, 1986
	250MG	N084731 003	NOV 07, 1986

Elixir; Oral

	Strength	Appl. No.	Date
ELIXOMIN			
CENCI	80MG/15ML	N088303 001	JAN 25, 1984
LANOPHYLLIN			
LANNETT	80MG/15ML	N084578 001	
THEOLIXIR			
PANRAY	80MG/15ML	N084559 001	
THEOPHYL-225			
ORTHO MCNEIL PHARM	112.5MG/15ML	N086485 001	
THEOPHYLLINE			
ALPHARMA	80MG/15ML	N089223 001	MAY 27, 1988
	80MG/15ML	N087679 001	APR 15, 1982
CENCI	80MG/15ML	N085169 001	
HALSEY	80MG/15ML	N085952 001	
PERRIGO	80MG/15ML	N084739 001	
ROXANE			

Injectable: Injection

	Strength	Appl. No.	Date
THEOPHYLLINE 0.2% AND DEXTROSE 5% IN PLASTIC CONTAINER			
B BRAUN	200MG/100ML	N019212 001	NOV 07, 1984
	200MG/100ML	N019826 004	AUG 14, 1992
THEOPHYLLINE 0.04% AND DEXTROSE 5% IN PLASTIC CONTAINER			
B BRAUN	40MG/100ML	N019083 001	NOV 07, 1984
THEOPHYLLINE 0.4% AND DEXTROSE 5% IN PLASTIC CONTAINER			
B BRAUN	400MG/100ML	N019212 002	NOV 07, 1984

THEOPHYLLINE *(continued)*

Injectable: Injection

	Strength	Appl. No.	Date
THEOPHYLLINE 0.4% AND DEXTROSE 5% IN PLASTIC CONTAINER			
B BRAUN	4MG/ML	N019212 003	NOV 07, 1984
	400MG/100ML	N019826 005	AUG 14, 1992
THEOPHYLLINE 0.08% AND DEXTROSE 5% IN PLASTIC CONTAINER			
B BRAUN	80MG/100ML	N019083 002	NOV 07, 1984
THEOPHYLLINE 0.16% AND DEXTROSE 5% IN PLASTIC CONTAINER			
B BRAUN	160MG/100ML	N019083 003	NOV 07, 1984

Suspension; Oral

	Strength	Appl. No.	Date
ELIXICON			
FORREST LABS	100MG/5ML	N085502 001	

Syrup; Oral

	Strength	Appl. No.	Date
ACCURBRON			
AVENTIS PHARMS	150MG/15ML	N088746 001	NOV 22, 1985
AQUAPHYLLIN			
FERNDALE LABS	80MG/15ML	N087917 001	JAN 18, 1983
THEOCLEAR-80			
CENT PHARMS	80MG/15ML	N087095 001	MAR 01, 1982
THEOPHYLLINE			
ALPHARMA	80MG/15ML	N086001 001	
	150MG/15ML	N086545 001	

Tablet, Chewable; Oral

	Strength	Appl. No.	Date
THEOPHYL			
ORTHO MCNEIL PHARM	100MG	N086506 001	SEP 12, 1985

Tablet, Extended Release; Oral

	Strength	Appl. No.	Date
DURAPHYL			
FORREST LABS	100MG	N088503 001	APR 03, 1985
	200MG	N088504 001	APR 03, 1985
	300MG	N088505 001	APR 03, 1985
LABID			
PROCTER AND GAMBLE	250MG	N087225 001	
SUSTAIRE			
ROERIG	100MG	N085665 001	
	300MG	N085665 002	

Tablet; Oral

	Strength	Appl. No.	Date
THEOCLEAR-100			
CENT PHARMS	100MG	N085353 002	
THEOCLEAR-200			
CENT PHARMS	200MG	N085353 001	
THEOPHYL-225			
ORTHO MCNEIL PHARM	225MG	N084726 001	

THIAMYLAL SODIUM *(continued)*
Injectable; Injection
  SURITAL
    PARKEDALE   10GM/VIAL   N007600 009

THIETHYLPERAZINE MALATE
Injectable; Injection
  TORECAN
    NOVARTIS   5MG/ML   N012754 002

THIETHYLPERAZINE MALEATE
Suppository; Rectal
  TORECAN
    NOVARTIS   10MG   N013247 001

THIOPENTAL SODIUM
Suspension; Rectal
  PENTOTHAL
    ABBOTT   400MG/GM   N011679 001

THIORIDAZINE
Suspension; Oral
  MELLARIL-S
    NOVARTIS   EQ 25MG HCL/5ML   N017923 001
                EQ 100MG HCL/5ML   N017923 002

THIORIDAZINE HYDROCHLORIDE
Concentrate; Oral
  MELLARIL
    NOVARTIS   30MG/ML   N011808 012
                100MG/ML   N011808 018
  THIORIDAZINE HCL
    ALPHARMA   30MG/ML   N087766 001   APR 26, 1983
    GENEVA PHARMS   30MG/ML   N088307 001   NOV 23, 1983
                100MG/ML   N088308 001   NOV 23, 1983
    MORTON GROVE   30MG/ML   N088258 001   JUL 25, 1983
                100MG/ML   N088227 001   JUL 05, 1983
Tablet; Oral
  MELLARIL
    NOVARTIS   10MG   N011808 003
                15MG   N011808 016
                25MG   N011808 006
                50MG   N011808 011
                100MG   N011808 009
                150MG   N011808 017
                200MG   N011808 015
  THIORIDAZINE HCL
    HALSEY   10MG   N088375 001   NOV 18, 1983
            15MG   N088461 001

Discontinued Drug Products *(continued)*

THEOPHYLLINE *MULTIPLE*
SEE MERSALYL SODIUM; THEOPHYLLINE
SEE PROCAINE MERETHOXYLLINE; THEOPHYLLINE

THEOPHYLLINE SODIUM GLYCINATE
Elixir; Oral
  SYNOPHYLATE
    CENT PHARMS   EQ 165MG BASE/15ML   N006333 008
Tablet; Oral
  ASBRON
    NOVARTIS   EQ 150MG BASE   N085148 001

THIAMINE *MULTIPLE*
SEE ALPHA-TOCOPHEROL; ASCORBIC ACID; BIOTIN; CHOLECALCIFEROL; CYANOCOBALAMIN; FOLIC ACID; NIACINAMIDE; PANTOTHENIC ACID; PYRIDOXINE; RIBOFLAVIN; THIAMINE; VITAMIN A
SEE ASCORBIC ACID; BIOTIN; CYANOCOBALAMIN; DEXPANTHENOL; ERGOCALCIFEROL; FOLIC ACID; NIACINAMIDE; PYRIDOXINE; RIBOFLAVIN PHOSPHATE SODIUM; THIAMINE; VITAMIN A; VITAMIN E
SEE ASCORBIC ACID; BIOTIN; CYANOCOBALAMIN; ERGOCALCIFEROL; FOLIC ACID; NIACINAMIDE; PANTOTHENIC ACID; PHYTONADIONE; PYRIDOXINE; RIBOFLAVIN; THIAMINE; VITAMIN A PALMITATE; VITAMIN E

THIAMINE HYDROCHLORIDE
Injectable; Injection
  BETALIN S
    LILLY   100MG/ML   N080853 001
  THIAMINE HCL
    AKORN   100MG/ML   N087968 001   OCT 01, 1982
                          N080509 001
    AM PHARM PARTNERS   100MG/ML   N080718 001
    BEL MAR   100MG/ML   N080712 001
             200MG/ML   N083775 001
    DELL LABS   100MG/ML   N080667 001
    LUITPOLD   100MG/ML   N080770 001
    PARKE DAVIS   100MG/ML   N083534 001
    STERIS   200MG/ML   N083534 002
    WYETH AYERST   100MG/ML   N080553 001

THIAMINE HYDROCHLORIDE *MULTIPLE*
SEE ASCORBIC ACID; BIOTIN; CYANOCOBALAMIN; DEXPANTHENOL; ERGOCALCIFEROL; FOLIC ACID; NIACINAMIDE; PYRIDOXINE HYDROCHLORIDE; RIBOFLAVIN PHOSPHATE SODIUM; THIAMINE HYDROCHLORIDE; VITAMIN A PALMITATE; VITAMIN E
SEE ASCORBIC ACID; BIOTIN; CYANOCOBALAMIN; DEXPANTHENOL; ERGOCALCIFEROL; FOLIC ACID; NIACINAMIDE; PYRIDOXINE HYDROCHLORIDE; RIBOFLAVIN PHOSPHATE SODIUM; THIAMINE HYDROCHLORIDE; VITAMIN A; VITAMIN E

THIAMYLAL SODIUM
Injectable; Injection
  SURITAL
    PARKEDALE   1GM/VIAL   N007600 003
                5GM/VIAL   N007600 005

Discontinued Drug Products (continued)

THIORIDAZINE HYDROCHLORIDE (continued)
Tablet; Oral
THIORIDAZINE HCL

	Strength	Date	Appl No.
HALSEY	25MG	NOV 18, 1983	N087264 001
	100MG	NOV 18, 1983	N088379 001
	150MG	NOV 16, 1983	N088737 001
	200MG	SEP 26, 1984	N088738 001
IVAX PHARMS	50MG	OCT 16, 1984	N088194 001
	100MG	APR 14, 1983	N088273 001
MYLAN	10MG	OCT 03, 1983	N088332 001
	25MG	JUN 27, 1983	N088333 001
	50MG	JUN 27, 1983	N088334 001
	100MG	JUN 27, 1983	N088335 001
PAR PHARM	10MG	NOV 18, 1983	N088351 001
	15MG	DEC 05, 1983	N088352 001
	25MG	DEC 05, 1983	N088336 001
	50MG	DEC 05, 1983	N088322 001
	100MG	DEC 05, 1983	N088480 001
	150MG	DEC 29, 1983	N089764 001
	200MG	FEB 09, 1988	N089765 001
ROXANE	10MG	FEB 09, 1988	N088663 001
	25MG	MAR 15, 1984	N088664 001
	50MG	MAR 15, 1984	N088665 001
	100MG	MAR 15, 1984	N089048 001
SUPERPHARM	10MG	FEB 26, 1985	N089103 001
	25MG	JUL 02, 1985	N089104 001
	50MG	JUL 02, 1985	N089105 001
TEVA	10MG	JUL 02, 1985	N088493 001
WATSON LAB	10MG	MAY 17, 1985	N088412 001
	15MG	SEP 12, 1983	N088345 001

THIORIDAZINE HYDROCHLORIDE (continued)
Tablet; Oral
THIORIDAZINE HCL

	Strength	Date	Appl No.
WATSON LAB	25MG	JUL 28, 1983	N088296 001
	50MG	JUL 28, 1983	N088323 001
	100MG	JUL 28, 1983	N088284 001
	150MG	AUG 25, 1983	N088410 001
	200MG	MAR 05, 1984	N088381 001
WATSON LABS	10MG	MAR 14, 1984	N088561 001
	15MG	MAY 11, 1984	N088562 001
	25MG	MAY 11, 1984	N088755 001
WEST WARD	10MG	JUL 24, 1984	N088658 001
	15MG	MAR 26, 1984	N088659 001
	25MG	MAR 26, 1984	N088660 001
	50MG	MAR 26, 1984	N088661 001

THIOTEPA
Injectable; Injection
THIOTEPA

IMMUNEX	15MG/VIAL		N011683 001

THIOTHIXENE
Capsule; Oral
THIOTHIXENE

	Strength	Date	Appl No.
AM THERAP	1MG	AUG 12, 1987	N071884 001
	2MG	AUG 12, 1987	N071885 001
	5MG	AUG 12, 1987	N071886 001
	10MG	AUG 12, 1987	N071887 001
	20MG	DEC 17, 1987	N072200 001
WATSON LABS	2MG	JUN 25, 1987	N071626 001
	5MG	JUN 25, 1987	N071627 001
	10MG	JUN 25, 1987	N071628 001

Discontinued Drug Products *(continued)*

THIOTHIXENE HYDROCHLORIDE
Concentrate; Oral
THIOTHIXENE HCL
Firm	Strength	Appl. No.	Date
ALPHARMA	EQ 5MG BASE/ML	N070969 001	OCT 16, 1987
PACO	EQ 1MG BASE/ML	N071917 001	SEP 20, 1989
	EQ 5MG BASE/ML	N071939 001	DEC 16, 1988
TEVA	EQ 5MG BASE/ML	N071184 001	JUN 22, 1987

THIOTHIXENE HCL INTENSOL
Firm	Strength	Appl. No.	Date
ROXANE	EQ 5MG BASE/ML	N073494 001	JUN 30, 1992

Injectable; Injection
NAVANE
Firm	Strength	Appl. No.
PFIZER	EQ 2MG BASE/ML	N016904 001

THYROGLOBULIN
Tablet; Oral
PROLOID
Firm	Strength	Appl. No.
PARKE DAVIS	16MG	N002245 009
	32MG	N002245 005
	65MG	N002245 002
	100MG	N002245 008
	130MG	N002245 010
	200MG	N002245 007
	325MG	N002245 004

THYROGLOBULIN
Firm	Strength	Appl. No.
IMPAX LABS	64.8MG	N080151 001

THYROTROPIN
Injectable; Injection
THYTROPAR
Firm	Strength	Appl. No.
AVENTIS	10 IU/VIAL	N008682 001

TIAGABINE HYDROCHLORIDE
Tablet; Oral
GABITRIL
Firm	Strength	Appl. No.	Date
CEPHALON	20MG	N020646 004	SEP 30, 1997

TICARCILLIN DISODIUM
Injectable; Injection
TICAR
Firm	Strength	Appl. No.	Date
GLAXOSMITHKLINE	EQ 3GM BASE/VIAL	N062690 001	DEC 19, 1986
	EQ 6GM BASE/VIAL	N050497 003	

TICLOPIDINE HYDROCHLORIDE
Tablet; Oral
TICLID
Firm	Strength	Appl. No.	Date
ROCHE PALO	125MG	N019979 001	MAR 24, 1993

TIMOLOL MALEATE
Solution/Drops; Ophthalmic
TIMOLOL MALEATE
Firm	Strength	Appl. No.	Date
FALCON PHARMS	EQ 0.5% BASE	N074262 001	APR 28, 1995
	EQ 0.25% BASE	N074261 001	APR 28, 1995

Tablet; Oral
TIMOLOL MALEATE
Firm	Strength	Appl. No.	Date
QUANTUM PHARMCS	5MG	N072466 001	MAY 19, 1989
	10MG	N072467 001	MAY 19, 1989
	20MG	N072468 001	MAY 19, 1989
TEVA	5MG	N072648 001	JUN 16, 1993
	10MG	N072649 001	JUN 16, 1993
	20MG	N072650 001	JUN 16, 1993
USL PHARMA	5MG	N072001 001	APR 11, 1989
	10MG	N072002 001	APR 11, 1989
	20MG	N072003 001	APR 11, 1989
WATSON LAB	5MG	N072269 001	APR 11, 1989
	10MG	N072270 001	APR 11, 1989
	20MG	N072271 001	APR 11, 1989

TIOCONAZOLE
Cream; Topical
TZ-3
Firm	Strength	Appl. No.	Date
PFIZER	1%	N018682 001	FEB 18, 1983

TOBRAMYCIN
Solution/Drops; Ophthalmic
TOBRAMYCIN
Firm	Strength	Appl. No.	Date
ALCON UNIVERSAL	0.3%	N063176 001	MAY 25, 1994

TOBRAMYCIN SULFATE
Injectable; Injection
TOBRAMYCIN SULFATE
Firm	Strength	Appl. No.	Date
APOTHECON	EQ 40MG BASE/ML	N064026 001	MAY 31, 1994
ASTRAZENECA	EQ 10MG BASE/ML	N063119 001	OCT 31, 1994
	EQ 40MG BASE/ML	N063120 001	OCT 31, 1994
	EQ 40MG BASE/ML	N063121 001	OCT 31, 1994

TOLBUTAMIDE

Tablet; Oral

Applicant	Strength	Appl. No.	Approval
ORINASE			
PHARMACIA AND UPJOHN	250MG	N010670 002	
	500MG	N010670 001	
TOLBUTAMIDE			
ALRA	500MG	N086141 001	
ASCOT	500MG	N087541 001	MAR 01, 1983
BARR	500MG	N087121 001	
EON	500MG	N012678 001	
PARKE DAVIS	500MG	N086047 001	
PUREPAC PHARM	500MG	N088950 001	JUN 17, 1985
SUPERPHARM	500MG	N088893 001	NOV 19, 1984
VANGARD	500MG	N087876 001	APR 20, 1982
WATSON LAB	250MG	N089110 001	MAY 29, 1987
	500MG	N089111 001	MAY 29, 1987

TOLBUTAMIDE SODIUM

Injectable; Injection

Applicant	Strength	Appl. No.	Approval
ORINASE DIAGNOSTIC			
PHARMACIA AND UPJOHN	EQ 1GM BASE/VIAL	N012095 001	

TOLMETIN SODIUM

Capsule; Oral

Applicant	Strength	Appl. No.	Approval
TOLMETIN SODIUM			
GENEVA PHARMS	EQ 400MG BASE	N073462 001	APR 30, 1992

Tablet; Oral

Applicant	Strength	Appl. No.	Approval
TOLMETIN SODIUM			
TEVA	EQ 600MG BASE	N074729 001	FEB 27, 1997

TOPIRAMATE

Capsule; Oral

Applicant	Strength	Appl. No.	Approval
TOPAMAX SPRINKLE			
ORTHO MCNEIL	50MG	N020844 003	OCT 26, 1998

Tablet; Oral

Applicant	Strength	Appl. No.	Approval
TOPAMAX			
ORTHO MCNEIL PHARM	50MG	N020505 005	DEC 24, 1996
	300MG	N020505 003	DEC 24, 1996
	400MG	N020505 006	DEC 24, 1996

Discontinued Drug Products (continued)

TOBRAMYCIN SULFATE (continued)

Injectable; Injection

Applicant	Strength	Appl. No.	Approval
TOBRAMYCIN SULFATE			
ASTRAZENECA	EQ 40MG BASE/ML	N063122 001	OCT 31, 1994
	EQ 10MG BASE/ML	N063128 001	OCT 31, 1994
ELKINS SINN	EQ 40MG BASE/ML	N063127 001	NOV 27, 1991
	EQ 10MG BASE/ML	N063113 001	NOV 27, 1991
LEDERLE	EQ 10MG BASE/ML		APR 26, 1991

TOLAZAMIDE

Tablet; Oral

Applicant	Strength	Appl. No.	Approval
TOLAZAMIDE			
BARR	100MG	N070162 001	JAN 14, 1986
	250MG	N070163 001	JAN 14, 1986
	500MG	N070164 001	JAN 14, 1986
DURAMED PHARM BARR	100MG	N070165 001	JAN 10, 1986
	250MG	N070166 001	JAN 10, 1986
	500MG	N070167 001	JAN 10, 1986
INTERPHARM	250MG	N071270 001	SEP 23, 1986
	500MG	N071271 001	SEP 23, 1986
SUPERPHARM	250MG	N070763 001	JUN 16, 1986
	500MG	N070764 001	JUN 16, 1986
USL PHARMA	100MG	N071355 001	JAN 11, 1988
	250MG	N070168 001	APR 02, 1986
	500MG	N070169 001	APR 02, 1986
WATSON LAB	100MG	N070242 001	AUG 01, 1986
	250MG	N070243 001	AUG 01, 1986
	500MG	N070244 001	AUG 01, 1986

TOLAZOLINE HYDROCHLORIDE

Injectable; Injection

Applicant	Strength	Appl. No.	Approval
PRISCOLINE			
NOVARTIS	25MG/ML	N006403 005	FEB 22, 1985

Discontinued Drug Products (continued)

TRAMADOL HYDROCHLORIDE
Tablet; Oral

Trade / Firm	Strength	Appl. No.	Date
ULTRAM			
ORTHO MCNEIL PHARM	100MG	N020281 001	MAR 03, 1995

TRANEXAMIC ACID
Tablet; Oral

Trade / Firm	Strength	Appl. No.	Date
CYKLOKAPRON			
PHARMACIA AND UPJOHN	500MG	N019280 001	DEC 30, 1986

TRAZODONE HYDROCHLORIDE
Tablet; Oral

Trade / Firm	Strength	Appl. No.	Date
TRAZODONE HCL			
AM THERAP	50MG	N071139 001	OCT 29, 1986
	100MG	N071140 001	OCT 29, 1986
QUANTUM PHARMICS	100MG	N070921 001	DEC 01, 1986
USL PHARMA	50MG	N070491 001	APR 29, 1987
	100MG	N070492 001	APR 29, 1987
WATSON LAB	50MG	N071112 001	NOV 17, 1986
	100MG	N071113 001	NOV 17, 1986
TRIALODINE			
QUANTUM PHARMICS	50MG	N070942 001	DEC 01, 1986

TRETINOIN
Swab; Topical

Trade / Firm	Strength	Appl. No.	Date
RETIN-A			
JOHNSON AND JOHNSON	0.05%	N016921 002	

TRIAMCINOLONE
Tablet; Oral

Trade / Firm	Strength	Appl. No.	Date
ARISTOCORT			
FUJISAWA HLTHCARE	1MG	N011161 009	
	2MG	N011161 004	
	8MG	N011161 011	
	16MG	N011161 010	
KENACORT			
BRISTOL MYERS SQUIBB	1MG	N011283 003	
	2MG	N011283 008	
TRIAMCINOLONE			
BARR	2MG	N084286 001	
	2MG	N084318 001	
	4MG	N084267 001	

TRIAMCINOLONE (continued)
Tablet; Oral

Trade / Firm	Strength	Appl. No.	Date
TRIAMCINOLONE			
BARR	4MG	N084319 001	
	8MG	N084268 001	
	8MG	N084320 001	
GENEVA PHARMS	4MG	N085601 001	
IMPAX LABS	4MG	N084340 001	
IVAX PHARMS	4MG	N083750 001	
MYLAN	2MG	N084406 001	
PUREPAC PHARM	2MG	N084020 002	
	4MG	N084020 003	
ROXANE	2MG	N084708 001	
	4MG	N084709 001	
	8MG	N084707 001	
TEVA	4MG	N084775 001	
WATSON LABS	4MG	N085834 001	

TRIAMCINOLONE ACETONIDE
Cream; Topical

Trade / Firm	Strength	Appl. No.	Date
FLUTEX			
IVAX PHARMS	0.1%	N085539 002	
	0.5%	N085539 003	
	0.025%	N085539 001	
KENALOG-H			
APOTHECON	0.1%	N086240 001	
TRIACORT			
SOLVAY	0.1%	N087113 001	
TRIAMCINOLONE ACETONIDE			
ALPHARMA	0.025%	N087797 001	JUN 07, 1982
MORTON GROVE	0.1%	N088095 001	SEP 01, 1983
	0.5%	N088096 001	SEP 01, 1983
	0.025%	N088094 001	SEP 01, 1983
PHARMADERM	0.1%	N087991 001	JUL 07, 1983
	0.5%	N087992 001	JUL 07, 1983
PHARMAFAIR	0.025%	N087990 001	JUL 07, 1983
	0.1%	N087912 001	JUL 07, 1983
	0.5%	N087922 001	AUG 10, 1982
	0.025%	N087921 001	AUG 10, 1982
TARO	0.025%	N040038 001	OCT 26, 1994
TOPIDERM	0.1%	N089275 001	FEB 21, 1989
	0.5%	N089276 001	FEB 21, 1989
	0.025%	N089274 001	

TRIAMCINOLONE ACETONIDE (continued)

Ointment; Topical
TRIAMCINOLONE ACETONIDE

MORTON GROVE	0.5%	SEP 01, 1983	N088092 001
	0.025%	SEP 01, 1983	N088090 001
PHARMADERM	0.1%	SEP 01, 1983	N088690 001
	0.025%	AUG 02, 1984	N088692 001
		AUG 02, 1984	

Spray, Metered; Nasal
TRI-NASAL

MURO	0.05MG/SPRAY	N020120 001	FEB 04, 2000

TRIAMCINOLONE ACETONIDE *MULTIPLE*

SEE NEOMYCIN SULFATE; TRIAMCINOLONE ACETONIDE
SEE NYSTATIN; TRIAMCINOLONE ACETONIDE

TRIAMCINOLONE DIACETATE

Injectable; Injection
TRIAMCINOLONE DIACETATE

AKORN	25MG/ML	N085122 001
	40MG/ML	N086394 001
STERIS	40MG/ML	N084072 001
	40MG/ML	N085529 001

Syrup; Oral
ARISTOCORT

FUJISAWA HLTHCARE	2MG/5ML	N011960 004
KENACORT		
BRISTOL MYERS SQUIBB	EQ 4MG BASE/5ML	N012515 001

TRIAMTERENE *MULTIPLE*

SEE HYDROCHLOROTHIAZIDE; TRIAMTERENE

TRIAZOLAM

Tablet; Oral
HALCION

PHARMACIA AND UPJOHN	0.5MG	N017892 002	NOV 15, 1982

TRICHLORMETHIAZIDE

Tablet; Oral
METAHYDRIN

AVENTIS PHARMS	2MG	N012594 001	JUN 16, 1988
	4MG	N012594 002	JUN 16, 1988
NAQUA			
SCHERING	2MG	N012265 001	

Discontinued Drug Products (continued)

TRIAMCINOLONE ACETONIDE (continued)

Cream; Topical
TRIAMCINOLONE ACETONIDE

TOPIDERM			FEB 21, 1989
TRIATEX			
IVAX PHARMS	0.1%	N087429 001	NOV 01, 1988
	0.5%	N087428 001	NOV 01, 1988
	0.025%	N087430 001	NOV 01, 1988
TRYMEX			
SAVAGE LABS	0.5%	N088198 001	MAR 25, 1983

Gel; Topical
ARISTOGEL

FUJISAWA HLTHCARE	0.1%	N083380 001

Injectable; Injection
TRIAMCINOLONE ACETONIDE

PARNELL	3MG/ML	N019503 001	OCT 16, 1987
STERIS	40MG/ML	N085825 001	

Lotion; Topical
KENALOG

BRISTOL MYERS SQUIBB	0.1%	N011602 001
	0.025%	N011602 003

TRIAMCINOLONE ACETONIDE

ALPHARMA	0.1%	N087192 001	SEP 08, 1982
	0.025%	N087191 001	SEP 08, 1982

Ointment; Topical
ARISTOCORT

FUJISAWA HLTHCARE	0.5%	N080745 002	
ARISTOCORT A			
FUJISAWA HLTHCARE	0.5%	N080745 003	
	0.5%	N088781 001	OCT 05, 1984
FLUTEX			
IVAX PHARMS	0.1%	N087377 001	NOV 01, 1988
	0.5%	N087376 001	NOV 01, 1988
	0.025%	N087375 001	NOV 01, 1988
KENALOG			
APOTHECON	0.5%	N083944 001	

TRIAMCINOLONE ACETONIDE

ALPHARMA	0.5%	N089913 001	DEC 23, 1988
G AND W LABS	0.1%	N089796 001	DEC 23, 1988
	0.025%	N089795 001	DEC 23, 1988
MORTON GROVE	0.1%	N088091 001	

TRIFLUOPERAZINE HYDROCHLORIDE (continued)

Tablet; Oral

TRIFLUOPERAZINE HCL

Firm	Strength	NDA	Date
DURAMED PHARM BARR			
IVAX PHARMS	EQ 1MG BASE	N087612 001	APR 23, 1985
	EQ 2MG BASE	N087613 001	NOV 19, 1982
	EQ 5MG BASE	N087328 001	NOV 19, 1982
	EQ 10MG BASE	N087614 001	NOV 19, 1982
WATSON LAB	EQ 1MG BASE	N085975 001	NOV 19, 1982
	EQ 2MG BASE	N085976 001	JUN 23, 1988
	EQ 5MG BASE	N085973 001	JUN 23, 1988
	EQ 10MG BASE	N088710 001	JUN 23, 1988
			JUN 23, 1988

TRIFLUPROMAZINE

Suspension; Oral

VESPRIN

Firm	Strength	NDA
APOTHECON	EQ 50MG HCL/5ML	N011491 004

TRIFLUPROMAZINE HYDROCHLORIDE

Injectable; Injection

VESPRIN

Firm	Strength	NDA
APOTHECON	3MG/ML	N011325 005
	10MG/ML	N011325 004
	20MG/ML	N011325 001

Tablet; Oral

VESPRIN

Firm	Strength	NDA
BRISTOL MYERS SQUIBB	10MG	N011123 001
	25MG	N011123 002
	50MG	N011123 003

TRIHEXYPHENIDYL HYDROCHLORIDE

Capsule, Extended Release; Oral

ARTANE

Firm	Strength	NDA
LEDERLE	5MG	N006773 010
	5MG	N012947 001

Elixir; Oral

ARTANE

Firm	Strength	NDA
LEDERLE	2MG/5ML	N006773 009

Tablet; Oral

ARTANE

Firm	Strength	NDA
LEDERLE	2MG	N006773 005
	5MG	N006773 003

TREMIN

Firm	Strength	NDA
SCHERING	2MG	N080381 001
	5MG	N080381 003

Discontinued Drug Products (continued)

TRICHLORMETHIAZIDE (continued)

Tablet; Oral

TRICHLOREX

Firm	Strength	NDA
LANNETT	4MG	N083436 001
	4MG	N085630 001

TRICHLORMAS

Firm	Strength	NDA
MAST MM	4MG	N086259 001

TRICHLORMETHIAZIDE

Firm	Strength	NDA
EON	4MG	N086171 001
IMPAX LABS	4MG	N083967 001
WATSON LAB	4MG	N083462 001
WATSON LABS	2MG	N083847 001
	2MG	N086458 001
	4MG	N083855 001
	4MG	N085962 001

TRICHLORMETHIAZIDE *MULTIPLE*

SEE RESERPINE; TRICHLORMETHIAZIDE

TRICLOFOS SODIUM

Solution; Oral

TRICLOS

Firm	Strength	NDA
AVENTIS PHARMS	1.5GM/15ML	N016830 001

Tablet; Oral

TRICLOS

Firm	Strength	NDA
AVENTIS PHARMS	750MG	N016809 002

TRIDIHEXETHYL CHLORIDE

Injectable; Injection

PATHILON

Firm	Strength	NDA
LEDERLE	10MG/ML	N009729 001

Tablet; Oral

PATHILON

Firm	Strength	NDA
LEDERLE	25MG	N009489 005

TRIFLUOPERAZINE HYDROCHLORIDE

Concentrate; Oral

TRIFLUOPERAZINE HCL

Firm	Strength	NDA	Date
GENEVA PHARMS	EQ 10MG BASE/ML	N085787 001	APR 15, 1982
MORTON GROVE	EQ 10MG BASE/ML	N088143 001	JUL 26, 1983

Injectable; Injection

TRIFLUOPERAZINE HCL

Firm	Strength	NDA	Date
QUAD PHARMS	EQ 2MG BASE/ML	N089893 001	OCT 17, 1988

Tablet; Oral

TRIFLUOPERAZINE HCL

Firm	Strength	NDA	Date
DURAMED PHARM BARR	EQ 1MG BASE	N088967 001	APR 23, 1985
	EQ 2MG BASE	N088968 001	APR 23, 1985
	EQ 5MG BASE	N088969 001	APR 23, 1985
	EQ 10MG BASE	N088970 001	APR 23, 1985

TRIMETHOBENZAMIDE HYDROCHLORIDE (continued)

Injectable; Injection

TRIMETHOBENZAMIDE HCL

STERIS	100MG/ML	N086577 001	OCT 19, 1982
	100MG/ML	N087939 001	DEC 28, 1982

TRIMETHOPRIM

Tablet; Oral

PROLOPRIM			
MONARCH PHARMS	200MG	N017943 003	JUL 14, 1982
TRIMETHOPRIM			
HALSEY	100MG	N070494 001	JAN 22, 1986
	200MG	N070495 001	SEP 24, 1986
TRIMPEX			
ROCHE	100MG	N017952 001	
TRIMPEX 200			
ROCHE	200MG	N017952 002	NOV 09, 1982

TRIMETHOPRIM *MULTIPLE*

SEE PHENAZOPYRIDINE HYDROCHLORIDE; SULFAMETHOXAZOLE;
    TRIMETHOPRIM
SEE SULFAMETHOXAZOLE; TRIMETHOPRIM

TRIMETHOPRIM HYDROCHLORIDE

Solution; Oral

PRIMSOL			
ASCENT PEDS	EQ 25MG BASE/5ML	N074374 001	JUN 23, 1995

TRIMIPRAMINE MALEATE

Capsule; Oral

TRIMIPRAMINE MALEATE			
USL PHARMA	EQ 25MG BASE	N071283 001	DEC 08, 1987
	EQ 50MG BASE	N071284 001	DEC 08, 1987
	EQ 100MG BASE	N071285 001	DEC 08, 1987

TRIOXSALEN

Tablet; Oral

TRISORALEN			
ICN	5MG	N012697 001	

TRIPELENNAMINE CITRATE

Elixir; Oral

PBZ			
NOVARTIS	EQ 25MG HCL/5ML	N005914 004	

Discontinued Drug Products (continued)

TRIHEXYPHENIDYL HYDROCHLORIDE (continued)

Tablet; Oral

TRIHEXYPHENIDYL HCL			
VANGARD	2MG	N088035 001	JUL 30, 1982
WATSON LAB	2MG	N085117 001	
	5MG	N085105 001	

TRILOSTANE

Capsule; Oral

MODRASTANE			
BIOENVISION	30MG	N018719 002	DEC 31, 1984
	60MG	N018719 001	DEC 31, 1984

TRIMEPRAZINE TARTRATE

Capsule, Extended Release; Oral

TEMARIL			
ALLERGAN HERBERT	EQ 5MG BASE	N011316 004	

Syrup; Oral

TEMARIL			
ALLERGAN HERBERT	EQ 2.5MG BASE/5ML	N011316 003	
TRIMEPRAZINE TARTRATE			
ALPHARMA	EQ 2.5MG BASE/5ML	N085015 001	FEB 18, 1982
MORTON GROVE	EQ 2.5MG BASE/5ML	N088285 001	APR 11, 1985

Tablet; Oral

TEMARIL			
ALLERGAN HERBERT	EQ 2.5MG BASE	N011316 001	

TRIMETHADIONE

Capsule; Oral

TRIDIONE			
ABBOTT	300MG	N005856 005	

Solution; Oral

TRIDIONE			
ABBOTT	200MG/5ML	N005856 002	

TRIMETHAPHAN CAMSYLATE

Injectable; Injection

ARFONAD			
ROCHE	50MG/ML	N008983 001	

TRIMETHOBENZAMIDE HYDROCHLORIDE

Injectable; Injection

TRIMETHOBENZAMIDE HCL			
SMITH AND NEPHEW	100MG/ML	N088960 001	APR 04, 1986
	100MG/ML	N089043 001	APR 04, 1986
SOLOPAK	100MG/ML	N089094 001	APR 04, 1986

Discontinued Drug Products *(continued)*

TRIPELENNAMINE HYDROCHLORIDE

Tablet, Extended Release; Oral

PBZ-SR		
NOVARTIS	50MG	N010533 002
	100MG	N010533 001

Tablet; Oral

TRIPELENNAMINE HCL		
ANABOLIC	50MG	N083037 001
BARR	50MG	N080744 001
HEATHER	50MG	N083989 001
IMPAX LABS	50MG	N080785 001
PARKE DAVIS	25MG	N083625 001
	50MG	N083626 001
WATSON LAB	50MG	N080790 001
WATSON LABS	50MG	N085188 001

TRIPLE SULFA (SULFABENZAMIDE;SULFACETAMIDE;SULFATHIAZOLE)

Cream; Vaginal

TRIPLE SULFA			
FOUGERA	3.7%;2.86%;3.42%	N086424 001	
VAGILIA			
TEVA	3.7%;2.86%;3.42%	N088821 001	NOV 09, 1987

Tablet; Vaginal

SULTRIN			
ORTHO MCNEIL PHARM	184MG;143.75MG;172.5MG	N005794 002	
TRIPLE SULFA			
FOUGERA	184MG;143.75MG;172.5MG	N088463 001	JAN 03, 1985
PHARMADERM	184MG;143.75MG;172.5MG	N088462 001	JAN 03, 1985

TRIPROLIDINE HYDROCHLORIDE

Syrup; Oral

ACTIDIL			
GLAXOSMITHKLINE	1.25MG/5ML	N011496 002	JUL 01, 1983
MYIDYL			
USL PHARMA	1.25MG/5ML	N087963 001	JAN 18, 1983
TRIPROLIDINE HCL			
ALPHARMA	1.25MG/5ML	N085940 001	
HALSEY	1.25MG/5ML	N088735 001	JAN 17, 1985
PHARM ASSOC	1.25MG/5ML	N087514 001	FEB 10, 1982

Tablet; Oral

ACTIDIL			
GLAXOSMITHKLINE	2.5MG	N011110 002	JUL 01, 1983
TRIPROLIDINE HCL			
VITARINE	2.5MG	N085610 001	
WATSON LABS	2.5MG	N085094 001	

TRIPROLIDINE HYDROCHLORIDE *MULTIPLE*

SEE CODEINE PHOSPHATE; PSEUDOEPHEDRINE HYDROCHLORIDE; TRIPROLIDINE HYDROCHLORIDE;

SEE PSEUDOEPHEDRINE HYDROCHLORIDE; TRIPROLIDINE HYDROCHLORIDE

TRISULFAPYRIMIDINES (SULFADIAZINE;SULFAMERAZINE;SULFAMETHAZINE)

Suspension; Oral

LANTRISUL		
LANNETT	167MG/5ML;167MG/5ML;167MG/5ML	N080123 002
NEOTRIZINE		
LILLY	167MG/5ML;167MG/5ML;167MG/5ML	N006317 012
SULFALOID		
FOREST PHARMS	167MG/5ML;167MG/5ML;167MG/5ML	N080100 001
SULFOSE		
WYETH AYERST	167MG/5ML;167MG/5ML;167MG/5ML	N080013 002
TERFONYL		
BRISTOL MYERS SQUIBB	167MG/5ML;167MG/5ML;167MG/5ML	N006904 002
TRIPLE SULFA		
ALPHARMA	167MG/5ML;167MG/5ML;167MG/5ML	N080280 001
TRIPLE SULFAS		
LEDERLE	167MG/5ML;167MG/5ML;167MG/5ML	N006920 003

Tablet; Oral

NEOTRIZINE		
LILLY	167MG;167MG;167MG	N006317 011
SULFA-TRIPLE #2		
IMPAX LABS	167MG;167MG;167MG	N080079 001
SULFALOID		
FOREST PHARMS	167MG;167MG;167MG	N080099 001
SULFOSE		
WYETH AYERST	167MG;167MG;167MG	N080013 001
TERFONYL		
BRISTOL MYERS SQUIBB	167MG;167MG;167MG	N006904 001
TRIPLE SULFA		
PUREPAC PHARM	167MG;167MG;167MG	N080086 001
TRIPLE SULFAS		
LEDERLE	167MG;167MG;167MG	N006920 002

TROGLITAZONE

Tablet; Oral

PRELAY			
SANKYO	200MG	N020719 001	JAN 29, 1997
	300MG	N020719 003	AUG 04, 1997
	400MG	N020719 002	

Discontinued Drug Products (continued)

TROGLITAZONE (continued)
Tablet; Oral
PRELAY
  SANKYO   JAN 29, 1997
REZULIN
  PFIZER PHARMS   200MG   N020720 001   JAN 29, 1997
                   300MG   N020720 003   JAN 29, 1997
                                           AUG 04, 1997
                   400MG   N020720 002   JAN 29, 1997

TROLEANDOMYCIN
Suspension; Oral
TAO
  PFIZER   EQ 125MG BASE/5ML   N050332 001

TROMETHAMINE *MULTIPLE*
SEE POTASSIUM CHLORIDE; SODIUM CHLORIDE; TROMETHAMINE

TROPICAMIDE
Solution/Drops; Ophthalmic
MYDRIACYL
  ALCON   0.5%   N012111 002
               1%   N012111 004
MYDRIAFAIR
  PHARMAFAIR   0.5%   N088274 001   SEP 16, 1983
               1%   N088230 001   SEP 16, 1983
TROPICAMIDE
  AKORN   1%   N088447 001   AUG 28, 1985
  STERIS   0.5%   N089171 001   DEC 28, 1990

TROVAFLOXACIN MESYLATE *MULTIPLE*
SEE AZITHROMYCIN DIHYDRATE; TROVAFLOXACIN MESYLATE

TUBOCURARINE CHLORIDE
Injectable; Injection
TUBOCURARINE CHLORIDE
  LILLY   3MG/ML   N006325 001
  QUAD PHARMS   3MG/ML   N089442 001   AUG 12, 1988

TYROPANOATE SODIUM
Capsule; Oral
BILOPAQUE
  AMERSHAM HLTH   750MG   N013731 001

TYROSINE *MULTIPLE*
SEE NIACINAMIDE; PYRIDOXINE HYDROCHLORIDE; TYROSINE

UNDECOYLIUM CHLORIDE; UNDECOYLIUM CHLORIDE IODINE COMPLEX
Solution; Topical
VIRAC REX
  CHESEBROUGH PONDS   0.5%;1.8%   N011914 001

UNDECOYLIUM CHLORIDE IODINE COMPLEX *MULTIPLE*
SEE UNDECOYLIUM CHLORIDE; UNDECOYLIUM CHLORIDE IODINE COMPLEX

URACIL MUSTARD
Capsule; Oral
URACIL MUSTARD
  SHIRE PHARM   1MG   N012892 001

UREA
Injectable; Injection
STERILE UREA
  ABBOTT   40GM/VIAL   N017698 001

UREA *MULTIPLE*
SEE HYDROCORTISONE; UREA

UREA, C-13
For Solution; Oral
HELICOSOL
  METABOLIC SOLUTIONS   125MG/VIAL   N021092 001   DEC 17, 1999
MERETEK UBT KIT (W/ PRANACTIN)
  MERETEK   125MG/VIAL   N020586 001   SEP 17, 1996
PYLORI-CHEK BREATH TEST
  DEVICES   100MG/VIAL   N020900 001   FEB 04, 1999

UROFOLLITROPIN
Injectable; Intramuscular
METRODIN
  SERONO   75 IU/AMP   N019415 002   SEP 18, 1986
            150 IU/AMP   N019415 003   SEP 18, 1986
Injectable; Subcutaneous
FERTINEX
  SERONO   150 IU/AMP   N019415 004   AUG 23, 1996

URSODIOL
Capsule; Oral
ACTIGALL
  WATSON PHARMS   150MG   N019594 001   DEC 31, 1987

Discontinued Drug Products (continued)

VALACYCLOVIR HYDROCHLORIDE
Tablet; Oral

VALTREX

GLAXOSMITHKLINE	EQ 1GM BASE	N020487 002	JUN 23, 1995
	EQ 500MG BASE	N020487 001	JUN 23, 1995

VALPROIC ACID
Capsule; Oral

VALPROIC ACID

PAR PHARM	250MG	N070431 001	FEB 28, 1986
SCHERER RP	250MG	N070195 001	JUL 02, 1987

VALSARTAN
Capsule; Oral

DIOVAN

NOVARTIS	80MG	N020665 001	DEC 23, 1996
	160MG	N020665 002	DEC 23, 1996

VANCOMYCIN HYDROCHLORIDE
For Solution; Oral

VANCOLED

LEDERLE	EQ 250MG BASE/5ML	N063321 002	OCT 15, 1993
	EQ 500MG BASE/6ML	N063321 003	OCT 15, 1993

Injectable; Injection

VANCOMYCIN HCL

ELKINS SINN	EQ 1GM BASE/VIAL	N062879 002	AUG 02, 1988
	EQ 500MG BASE/VIAL	N062879 001	AUG 02, 1988
QUAD PHARMS	EQ 1GM BASE/VIAL	N062845 002	JUL 15, 1988
	EQ 500MG BASE/VIAL	N062845 001	JUL 15, 1988

VANCOR

PHARMACIA AND UPJOHN	EQ 1GM BASE/VIAL	N062956 002	AUG 01, 1988
	EQ 500MG BASE/VIAL	N062956 001	AUG 01, 1988

VASOPRESSIN TANNATE
Injectable; Injection

PITRESSIN TANNATE

PARKE DAVIS	5PRESSOR UNITS/ML	N003402 001	

VECURONIUM BROMIDE
Injectable; Injection

NORCURON

ORGANON USA INC	10MG/VIAL	N018776 002	APR 30, 1984
	20MG/VIAL	N018776 003	JAN 03, 1992

VENLAFAXINE HYDROCHLORIDE
Capsule, Extended Release; Oral

EFFEXOR XR

WYETH PHARMS INC	EQ 100MG BASE	N020699 003	OCT 20, 1997

Tablet; Oral

EFFEXOR

WYETH PHARMS INC	EQ 12.5MG BASE	N020151 001	DEC 28, 1993

VERAPAMIL HYDROCHLORIDE
Injectable; Injection

CALAN

GD SEARLE LLC	2.5MG/ML	N018925 001	MAR 30, 1984
	2.5MG/ML	N019038 001	MAR 30, 1984

VERAPAMIL HCL

AM PHARM PARTNERS	2.5MG/ML	N070348 001	MAY 01, 1986
MARSAM PHARMS LLC	2.5MG/ML	N072233 001	FEB 26, 1993
	2.5MG/ML	N073485 001	SEP 27, 1993
QUAD PHARMS	2.5MG/ML	N070672 001	MAR 07, 1986
SMITH AND NEPHEW	2.5MG/ML	N070696 001	JUL 31, 1987
	2.5MG/ML	N070697 001	JUL 31, 1987
SOLOPAK	2.5MG/ML	N070695 001	JUL 31, 1987

Tablet, Extended Release; Oral

VERAPAMIL HCL

BARR	120MG	N075072 001	MAY 25, 1999
	240MG	N075072 003	MAY 25, 1999

Tablet; Oral

CALAN

GD SEARLE LLC	160MG	N018817 004	FEB 23, 1988

VERAPAMIL HCL

HALSEY	80MG	N070482 001	SEP 24, 1986
	120MG	N070483 001	SEP 24, 1986
WARNER CHILCOTT	80MG	N070340 001	

Discontinued Drug Products (continued)

VERAPAMIL HYDROCHLORIDE (continued)
Tablet; Oral
VERAPAMIL HCL
WARNER CHILCOTT   120MG   SEP 24, 1986   N070341 001
                                         SEP 24, 1986
WATSON LABS   40MG   N072799 001
                     APR 28, 1989

VERATRUM VIRIDE
Tablet; Oral
VERTAVIS
MEDPOINTE PHARM HLC   130CSR UNIT   N005691 002

VIDARABINE
Injectable; Injection
VIRA-A
PARKEDALE   EQ 187.4MG BASE/ML   N050523 001
Ointment; Ophthalmic
VIRA-A
PARKEDALE   3%   N050486 001

VINBLASTINE SULFATE
Injectable; Injection
VELBAN
LILLY   10MG/VIAL   N012665 001
VINBLASTINE SULFATE
AM PHARM PARTNERS   10MG/VIAL   N089011 001
                                NOV 18, 1985
QUAD PHARMS   1MG/ML   N089311 001
                       MAR 23, 1987
              10MG/VIAL   N089365 001
                          AUG 07, 1986

VINCRISTINE SULFATE
Injectable; Injection
ONCOVIN
LILLY   1MG/VIAL   N014103 001
        5MG/VIAL   N014103 002
VINCREX
BRISTOL MYERS SQUIBB   5MG/VIAL   N070867 001
                                  JUL 12, 1988
VINCRISTINE SULFATE
ABIC   1MG/ML   N070873 001
                FEB 19, 1987
AM PHARM PARTNERS   1MG/ML   N070411 001
                             SEP 10, 1986
FAULDING   1MG/VIAL   N071559 001
                      APR 11, 1988
           2MG/VIAL   N071560 001
                      APR 11, 1988
           5MG/VIAL   N071561 001
                      APR 11, 1988
QUAD PHARMS   1MG/ML   N070777 001

VINCRISTINE SULFATE (continued)
Injectable; Injection
VINCRISTINE SULFATE
QUAD PHARMS   1MG/ML   APR 29, 1986   N070778 001
                      MAY 01, 1986   N071222 001
              1MG/VIAL   MAR 07, 1988   N071223 001
              2MG/VIAL   MAR 07, 1988   N071937 001
              5MG/VIAL   MAR 07, 1988

VIOMYCIN SULFATE
Injectable; Injection
VIOCIN SULFATE
PFIZER   EQ 1GM BASE/VIAL   N061086 001
         EQ 5GM BASE/VIAL   N061086 002

VITAMIN A
Capsule; Oral
AQUASOL A
ASTRAZENECA   25,000USP UNITS   N083080 002
              50,000USP UNITS   N083080 001
VITAMIN A
BANNER PHARMACAPS   50,000USP UNITS   N083973 001
CHASE CHEM   50,000 IU   N083351 001
EVERYLIFE   50,000 IU   N083134 001
IMPAX LABS   50,000USP UNITS   N080952 001

VITAMIN A *MULTIPLE*
SEE   ALPHA-TOCOPHEROL; ASCORBIC ACID; BIOTIN; CHOLECALCIFEROL; CYANOCOBALAMIN; FOLIC ACID; NIACINAMIDE; PANTOTHENIC ACID; PYRIDOXINE; RIBOFLAVIN; THIAMINE; VITAMIN A
SEE   ASCORBIC ACID; BIOTIN; CYANOCOBALAMIN; DEXPANTHENOL; ERGOCALCIFEROL; FOLIC ACID; NIACINAMIDE; PYRIDOXINE; RIBOFLAVIN PHOSPHATE SODIUM; THIAMINE; VITAMIN A; VITAMIN E
SEE   ASCORBIC ACID; BIOTIN; CYANOCOBALAMIN; DEXPANTHENOL; ERGOCALCIFEROL; FOLIC ACID; NIACINAMIDE; PYRIDOXINE HYDROCHLORIDE; RIBOFLAVIN; VITAMIN A; VITAMIN E

VITAMIN A PALMITATE
Capsule; Oral
AFAXIN
STERLING WINTHROP   EQ 50,000 UNITS BASE   N083187 001
ALPHALIN
LILLY   EQ 50,000 UNITS BASE   N080883 001
DEL-VI-A
DEL RAY LABS   EQ 50,000 UNITS BASE   N080830 001
VI-DOM-A
BAYER PHARMS   EQ 50,000 UNITS BASE   N080972 001
VITAMIN A
BANNER PHARMACAPS   EQ 50,000 UNITS BASE   N080702 001

Discontinued Drug Products (continued)

VITAMIN A PALMITATE (continued)

Capsule; Oral

VITAMIN A

Firm	Strength	Number
BRISTOL MYERS SQUIBB	EQ 50,000 UNITS BASE	N080860 001
CHASE CHEM	EQ 50,000 UNITS BASE	N080746 001
	EQ 50,000 UNITS BASE	N083207 001
	EQ 50,000 UNITS BASE	N085479 001
ELKINS SINN	EQ 50,000 UNITS BASE	N080943 001
EVERYLIFE	EQ 50,000 UNITS BASE	N083114 001
IMPAX LABS	EQ 50,000 UNITS BASE	N080953 001
	EQ 50,000 UNITS BASE	N080955 001
IVAX PHARMS	EQ 50,000 UNITS BASE	N083035 001
	EQ 50,000 UNITS BASE	N083190 001
WEST WARD	EQ 50,000 UNITS BASE	N080967 001
WHARTON LABS	EQ 50,000 UNITS BASE	N083665 001

VITAMIN A PALMITATE

Firm	Strength	Number
BANNER PHARMACAPS	EQ 50,000 UNITS BASE	N083948 001
	EQ 50,000 UNITS BASE	N083981 001

VITAMIN A SOLUBILIZED

Firm	Strength	Number
TEVA	EQ 50,000 UNITS BASE	N080921 001

Injectable; Injection

VITAMIN A PALMITATE

Firm	Strength	Number
BEL MAR	EQ 50,000 UNITS BASE/ML	N080819 001

VITAMIN A PALMITATE *MULTIPLE*

SEE ASCORBIC ACID; BIOTIN; CYANOCOBALAMIN; DEXPANTHENOL; ERGOCALCIFEROL; FOLIC ACID; NIACINAMIDE; PYRIDOXINE HYDROCHLORIDE; RIBOFLAVIN PHOSPHATE SODIUM; THIAMINE HYDROCHLORIDE; VITAMIN A PALMITATE; VITAMIN E

SEE ASCORBIC ACID; BIOTIN; CYANOCOBALAMIN; ERGOCALCIFEROL; FOLIC ACID; NIACINAMIDE; PANTOTHENIC ACID; PHYTONADIONE; PYRIDOXINE; RIBOFLAVIN; THIAMINE; VITAMIN A PALMITATE; VITAMIN E

VITAMIN E *MULTIPLE*

SEE ASCORBIC ACID; BIOTIN; CYANOCOBALAMIN; DEXPANTHENOL; ERGOCALCIFEROL; FOLIC ACID; NIACINAMIDE; PYRIDOXINE; RIBOFLAVIN PHOSPHATE SODIUM; THIAMINE; VITAMIN A; VITAMIN E

SEE ASCORBIC ACID; BIOTIN; CYANOCOBALAMIN; DEXPANTHENOL; ERGOCALCIFEROL; FOLIC ACID; NIACINAMIDE; PYRIDOXINE HYDROCHLORIDE; RIBOFLAVIN PHOSPHATE SODIUM; THIAMINE HYDROCHLORIDE; VITAMIN A PALMITATE; VITAMIN E

SEE ASCORBIC ACID; BIOTIN; CYANOCOBALAMIN; DEXPANTHENOL; ERGOCALCIFEROL; FOLIC ACID; NIACINAMIDE; PYRIDOXINE HYDROCHLORIDE; RIBOFLAVIN PHOSPHATE SODIUM; THIAMINE; VITAMIN A; VITAMIN E

SEE ASCORBIC ACID; BIOTIN; CYANOCOBALAMIN; ERGOCALCIFEROL; FOLIC ACID; NIACINAMIDE; PANTOTHENIC ACID; PHYTONADIONE; PYRIDOXINE; RIBOFLAVIN; THIAMINE; VITAMIN A PALMITATE; VITAMIN E

WARFARIN POTASSIUM

Tablet; Oral

ATHROMBIN-K

Firm	Strength	Number
PURDUE FREDERICK	2MG	N011771 007
	5MG	N011771 004
	10MG	N011771 005

WARFARIN POTASSIUM (continued)

Tablet; Oral

ATHROMBIN-K

Firm	Strength	Number
PURDUE FREDERICK	25MG	N011771 006

WARFARIN SODIUM

Injectable; Injection

COUMADIN

Firm	Strength	Number
BRISTOL MYERS SQUIBB	50MG/VIAL	N009218 020
	75MG/VIAL	N009218 012

Tablet; Oral

ATHROMBIN

Firm	Strength	Number
PURDUE FREDERICK	5MG	N011771 003
	10MG	N011771 002
	25MG	N011771 001

PANWARFIN

Firm	Strength	Number
ABBOTT	2.5MG	N017020 002
	2MG	N017020 001
	5MG	N017020 003
	7.5MG	N017020 004
	10MG	N017020 005

WARFARIN SODIUM

Firm	Strength	Number	Date
USL PHARMA	2.5MG	N088720 001	AUG 06, 1985
	2MG	N088719 001	JUN 27, 1985
	5MG	N088721 001	JUL 02, 1985
WATSON LAB	2.5MG	N086120 001	AUG 17, 1982
	2MG	N086123 001	AUG 17, 1982
	5MG	N086119 001	AUG 17, 1982
	7.5MG	N086118 001	AUG 17, 1982
	10MG	N086122 001	AUG 17, 1982

WATER FOR INJECTION, STERILE

Liquid; N/A

BACTERIOSTATIC WATER FOR INJECTION IN PLASTIC CONTAINER

Firm	Strength	Number	Date
AM PHARM PARTNERS	100%	N089099 001	DEC 29, 1987
	100%	N089100 001	DEC 29, 1987

WATER FOR IRRIGATION, STERILE

Liquid; Irrigation

STERILE WATER IN PLASTIC CONTAINER

Firm	Strength	Number
MILES	100%	N018246 001

Discontinued Drug Products *(continued)*

XENON, XE-127
Gas; Inhalation
XENON XE 127
MALLINCKRODT 5mCi/VIAL N018536 001
OCT 01, 1982
10mCi/VIAL N018536 002
OCT 01, 1982

XENON, XE-133
Gas; Inhalation
XENON XE 133
AMERSHAM HLTH 1 Ci/AMP N017256 002
10mCi/VIAL N017687 002
20mCi/VIAL N017687 003
XENON XE 133-V.S.S.
AMERSHAM HLTH 10mCi/VIAL N017687 001
Injectable; Injection
XENON XE 133
AMERSHAM HLTH 1.3-1.7 Ci/AMP N017256 001
BRISTOL MYERS
SQUIBB 6.3mCi/ML N017283 001
Solution; Inhalation, Injection
XENEISOL
MALLINCKRODT 18-25mCi/AMP N017262 002

XYLOSE
Powder; Oral
XYLO-PFAN
SAVAGE LABS 25GM/BOT N017605 001
XYLOSE
LYNE 25GM/BOT N018856 001
MAR 26, 1987

ZIDOVUDINE
Tablet; Oral
RETROVIR
GLAXOSMITHKLINE 200MG N020518 001
DEC 19, 1995

ZILEUTON
Tablet; Oral
ZYFLO
ABBOTT 300MG N020471 001
DEC 09, 1996

ZINC ACETATE *MULTIPLE*
SEE CYANOCOBALAMIN; TANNIC ACID; ZINC ACETATE

ZINC SULFATE
Injectable
ZINC SULFATE EQ 1MG ZINC/ML N019229 001

CUMULATIVE LIST OF ORPHAN PRODUCT DESIGNATIONS AND APPROVALS

NAME *Generic/Chemical* *TN=Trade Name*	INDICATION DESIGNATED	SPONSOR AND ADDRESS *DD=Date Designated* *MA=Marketing Approval*
(+/-)-7-[3-(4-ACETYL-3-METHOXY-2-PROPYLPHENOXY)PROPOXY]-3,4-DIHYDRO-8-PROPYL-2H-1-BENZOPYRAN-2-CARBOXYLIC ACID	PREVENTION OF SERIOUS ADVERSE EVENTS ASSOCIATED WITH VASCULAR LEAK SYNDROME CAUSED BY INTERLEUKIN-2 THERAPY	BIOMEDICINES, INC. 2000 POWELL STREET SUITE 1640 EMERYVILLE CA 94608 DD 3/31/2003
(4S)-4-ETHYL-4-HYDROXY-3,14-DIOXO-3,4,12,14-TETRAHYDRO-1-H-PYRANO[3 ,4 :6,7]-INDOLIZINO-[1,2-B]-QUINOLINE-11-CARBALDEHYDE O-(TERT-BUTYL)-(E)-OXIME TN=GIMATECAN	TREATMENT MALIGNANT GLIOMA	SIGMA-TAU RESEARCH, INC. 800 SOUTH FREDERICK AVENUE SUITE 103 GAITHERSBURG MD 20877-4150 DD 11/29/2002
(R)-N-[2-(6-CHLORO-5-METHOXY-1H-INDOL-3-YL)PROPYL]ACETAMIDE	TREATMENT OF CIRCADIAN RHYTHM SLEEP DISORDERS IN BLIND PEOPLE WITH NO LIGHT PERCEPTION	PHASE 2 DISCOVERY, INC. 3130 HIGHLAND AVENUE, THIRD FLOOR CINCINNATI OH 45219-2374 DD 10/3/2001
1,5-(BUTYLIMINO)-1,5 DIDEOX-Y,D-GLUCITOL	TREATMENT OF FABRY'S DISEASE.	OXFORD GLYCOSCIENCES 10, THE QUADRANT ABINGTON SCIENCE PARK, ABINGTON OXFORDSHIRE OX14 3YS UK DD 5/12/1998
1,5-(BUTYLIMINO)-1,5 DIDEOX-Y,D-GLUCITOL	TREATMENT OF GAUCHER DISEASE.	OXFORD GLYCOSCIENCES 10, THE QUADRANT ABINGTON SCIENCE PARK, ABINGTON OXFORDSHIRE OX14 3YS UK DD 5/29/1998
1-(11-DODECYLAMINO-10-HYDROXYUNDECYL)-3,7-DIMETHYL-XANTHINE HYDROGEN METHANESULFONATE	TREATMENT OF HORMONE REFRACTORY PROSTATE CARCINOMA.	CELL THERAPEUTICS, INC. 201 ELLIOTT AVENUE WEST SUITE 400 SEATTLE WA 98119 DD 1/18/2000
111INDIUM PENTETREOTIDE TN=SOMATOTHER	TREATMENT OF SOMATOSTATIN RECEPTOR POSITIVE NEUROENDOCRINE TUMORS.	LOUISIANA STATE UNIVERSITY MEDICAL CENTER FOUNDATION 1600 CANAL ST. 10TH FLOOR NEW ORLEANS LA 70112 DD 6/10/1999
166HO-DOTMP	TREATMENT OF MULTIPLE MYELOMA.	NEORX CORPORATION 410 W. HARRISON STREET SEATTLE WA 98119-4007 DD 2/10/1999
2',3',5'-TRI-O-ACETYLURIDINE	TREATMENT OF MITOCHONDRIAL DISEASE	REPLIGEN CORPORATION 41 SEYON STREET BUILDING 1, SUITE 100 WALTHAM MA 02453 DD 1/13/2003
2'-3'-DIDEOXYADENOSINE	TREATMENT OF AQUIRED IMMUNODEFICIENCY SYNDROME.	NATIONAL CANCER INSTITUTE, DCT NIH, EXEC. PLAZA N., ROOM 7-18 BETHESDA MD 20892 DD 7/21/1987

NAME *Generic/Chemical* *TN=Trade Name*	INDICATION DESIGNATED	SPONSOR AND ADDRESS *DD=Date Designated* *MA=Marketing Approval*
2'-DEOXYCYTIDINE	AS A HOST-PROTECTIVE AGENT IN THE TREATMENT OF ACUTE MYELOGENOUS LEUKEMIA.	GRANT, STEVEN M.D. MASSEY CANCER CENTER, VCU P.O. BOX 980230 RICHMOND VA 23298-0230 DD 9/9/1996
2-0-DESULFATED HEPARIN TN=AEROPIN	TREATMENT OF CYSTIC FIBROSIS.	KENNEDY & HOIDAL, M.D.'S UNIVERSITY OF UTAH HEALTH SCIENCES CENTER 50 NORTH MEDICAL DRIVE, ROOM 4R240 SALT LAKE CITY UT 84132 DD 9/17/1993
2-CHLOROETHYL-3-SARCOSINA-MIDE-1-NITROSOUREA	TREATMENT FOR MALIGNANT GLIOMAS	LAWRENCE PANASCI, MD PROFESSOR OF MEDICINE, MCGILL UNIVERSITY 3755 COTE STE CATHERINE MONTREAL, QUEBEC H3T 1E2 DD 8/3/2001
2-CHLOROETHYL-3-SARCOSINA-MIDE-1-NITROSOUREA TN=SARMUSTINE	TREATMENT FOR MALIGNANT GLIOMA	PANGENE CORPORATION 5500 STEWART AVENUE FREMONT CA 94538 DD 11/15/2001
2-METHOXYESTRADIOL TN=PANZEM	TREATMENT OF MULTIPLE MYELOMA	ENTREMED, INC. 9640 MEDICAL CENTER DRIVE ROCKVILLE MD 20850 DD 7/10/2001
24,25 DIHYDROXYCHOLECALCI-FEROL	TREATMENT OF UREMIC OSTEODYSTROPHY.	LEMMON COMPANY 1510 DELP DRIVE KULPSVILLE PA 19443 DD 2/27/1987
3'-AZIDO-2',3'DIDEOXYURIDINE TN=AZDU	TREATMENT OF ACQUIRED IMMUNODEFICIENCY SYNDROME.	BERLEX LABORATORIES, INC. 1401 HARBOR BAY PARKWAY ALAMEDA CA 94501 DD 11/20/1989
3,4-DIAMINOPYRIDINE	TREATMENT OF LAMBERT-EATON MYASTHENIC SYNDROME.	JACOBUS PHARMACEUTICAL COMPANY 37 CLEVELAND AVENUE P.O. BOX 5290 PRINCETON NJ 08540 DD 12/18/1990
3,5,3'-TRIIODOTHYROACETATE	TREATMENT OF WELL-DIFFERENTIATED PAPILLARY, FOLLICULAR OR COMBINED PAPILLARY/FOLLICULAR CARCINOMAS OF THE THYROID GLAND.	ELLIOT DANFORTH, JR., M.D. UNIVERSITY OF VERMONT 84 BEARTOWN ROAD UNDERHILL VT 05489 DD 9/20/2000
3-(3,5-DIMETHYL-1H-2YLMETHY-LENE)-1,3-DIHYDRO-INDOL-2-ONE	TREATMENT OF VON HIPPEL-LINDAU DISEASE.	SUGEN, INC. 230 EAST GRAND AVE. SOUTH SAN FRANCISCO CA 94080 DD 3/23/2000
3-(3,5-DIMETHYL-1H-2YLMETHY-LENE)-1,3-DIHYDRO-INDOL-2-ONE	TREATMENT OF KAPOSI'S SARCOMA.	SUGEN, INC. 230 EAST GRAND AVE. SOUTH SAN FRANCISCO CA 94080-4811 DD 9/11/1998

NAME *Generic/Chemical* *TN=Trade Name*	INDICATION DESIGNATED	SPONSOR AND ADDRESS *DD=Date Designated* *MA=Marketing Approval*
3-(4'AMINOISOINDOLINE-1'-ONE)- 1-PIPERIDINE-2,6-DIONE TN=REVIMID (PROPOSED)	TREATMENT FOR MULTIPLE MYELOMA	CELEGENE CORPORATION 7 POWDER HORN DRIVE WARREN NJ 07059 DD 9/20/2001
4-AMINOSALICYLIC ACID TN=PAMISYL (P-D), REZIPAS (SQUIBB)	TREATMENT OF MILD TO MODERATE ULCERATIVE COLITIS IN PATIENTS INTOLERANT TO SULFASALA-ZINE.	BEEKEN, WARREN M.D. UNIVERSITY OF VERMONT GIVEN C-317 BURLINGTON VT 05405 DD 12/13/1989
4,5-DIBROMORHODAMINE 123 TN=THERALUX IRRADIATION DE-VICE	TREATMENT OF CHRONIC MYELOGENOUS LEUKE-MIA.	CELMED BIOSCIENCES, INC. 2310 BOUL ALFRED-NOBEL SAINT-LAURENT, QUEBEC CANADA H4S 2A4 DD 04/10/2003
40SD02	TREATMENT OF CHRONIC IRON OVERLOAD RESULT-ING FROM CONVENTIONAL TRANSFUSIONAL TREAT-MENT OF BETA-THALASSEMIA MAJOR AND SICKLE CELL ANEMIA.	BIOMEDICAL FRONTIERS, INC. 1095 10TH AVE., S.E. MINNEAPOLIS MN 55414 DD 12/21/1998
5,6-DIHYDRO-5-AZACYTIDINE	TREATMENT OF MALIGNANT MESOTHELIOMA.	ILEX ONCOLOGY, INC. 4545 HORIZON HILL BLVD. SAN ANTONIO TX 78229-2263 DD 5/11/1992
5-AZA-2'-DEOXYCYTIDINE	TREATMENT OF ACUTE LEUKEMIA.	SUPERGEN, INC. 4140 DUBLIN BLVD. SUITE 200 DUBLIN CA 94568 DD 8/3/1987
506U78	TREATMENT OF CHRONIC LYMPHOCYTIC LEUKEMIA.	GLAXOSMITHKLINE FIVE MOORE DR. P.O. BOX 13398 RESEARCH TRIANGLE PARK NC 27709-3398 DD 9/2/1999
5A8, MONOCLONAL ANTIBODY TO CD4	FOR USE IN POST-EXPOSURE PROPHYLAXIS FOR OC-CUPATIONAL EXPOSURE TO HUMAN IMMUNODEFI-CIENCY VIRUS.	BIOGEN, INC. 14 CAMBRIDGE CENTER CAMBRIDGE MA 02142 DD 12/20/1993
6-HYDROXYMETHYLACYLFUL-VENE	TREATMENT OF HISTOLOGICALLY CONFIRMED AD-VANCED OR METASTATIC PANCREATIC CANCER.	MGI PHARMA, INC. 6300 WEST OLD SHAKOPPE RD. SUITE 110 BLOOMINGTON MN 55438-2318 DD 4/6/1999
6-HYDROXYMETHYLACYLFUL-VENE	TREATMENT OF RENAL CELL CARCINOMA.	MGI PHARMA, INC. 6300 WEST OLD SHAKOPPE RD. SUITE 110 BLOOMINGTON MN 55438-2318 DD 7/27/1999
6-HYDROXYMETHYLACYLFUL-VENE	TREATMENT OF OVARIAN CANCER.	MGI PHARMA, INC. 5775 WEST OLD SHAKOPPE RD. SUITE 100 BLOOMINGTON MN 55437-3107 DD 7/6/1999

NAME *Generic/Chemical* *TN=Trade Name*	INDICATION DESIGNATED	SPONSOR AND ADDRESS *DD=Date Designated* *MA=Marketing Approval*
8 CYCLOPENTYL 1,3-DIPROPYL-XANTHINE	TREATMENT OF CYSTIC FIBROSIS.	SCICLONE PHARMACEU-TICALS, INC. 901 MARINER'S ISLAND BOULE-VARD SAN MATEO CA 94404-1593 DD 3/24/1997
8-METHOXSALEN TN=UVADEX	FOR USE IN CONJUNCTION WITH THE UVAR PHOTO-PHERESIS TO TREAT DIFFUSE SYSTEMIC SCLERO-SIS.	THERAKOS, INC. OAKLANDS CORPORATE CENTER 437 CREAMERY WAY EXTON PA 19341 DD 6/22/1993
8-METHOXSALEN TN=UVADEX	FOR THE PREVENTION OF ACUTE REJECTION OF CARDIAC ALLOGRAFTS.	THERAKOS, INC. OAKLANDS CORPORATE CENTER 437 CREAMERY WAY EXTON PA 19341 DD 5/12/1994
9-CIS RETINOIC ACID TN=PANRETIN	TREATMENT OF ACUTE PROMYELOCYTIC LEUKEMIA.	LIGAND PHARMACEUTICALS, INC. 10275 SCIENCE CENTER DR. SAN DIEGO CA 92121-1117 DD 4/10/1992
9-CIS-RETINOIC ACID	PREVENTION OF RETINAL DETACHMENT DUE TO PROLIFERATIVE VITREORETINOPATHY.	ALLERGAN, INC. 2525 DUPONT DRIVE P.O. BOX 19534 IRVINE CA 92623-9534 DD 1/2/1997
9-NITRO-20-(S)-CAMPTOTHECIN	TREATMENT OF PANCREATIC CANCER.	SUPERGEN, INC. 4140 DUBLIN BLVD. SUITE 200 DUBLIN CA 94568 DD 9/16/1996
9-NITRO-20-(S)-CAMPTOTHECIN TN=CAMVIREX	TREATMENT OF PEDIATRIC HIV INFECTION/AIDS	NOVOMED PHARMACEU-TICALS, INC. P.O. BOX 900 GERMANTOWN MD 20875-0900 DD 5/15/2001
AI-RSA	TREATMENT OF AUTOIMMUNE UVEITIS.	AUTOIMMUNE, INC. 128 SPRING STREET LEXINGTON MA 02173 DD 10/8/1992
AMG 531	TREATMENT OF IMMUNE THROMBOCYTOPENIC PUR-PURA.	AMGEN, INC. ONE AMGEN CENTER DRIVE THOUSAND OAKS CA 91320-1799 DD 3/27/2003
AP1903	TREATMENT OF ACUTE GRAFT-VERSUS-HOST DIS-EASE IN PATIENTS UNDERGOING BONE MARROW TRANSPLANTATION.	ARIAD GENE THERAPEUTICS, INC. 26 LANDSDOWNE ST. CAMBRIDGE MA 02139-4234 DD 11/24/1999
APL 400-020 V-BETA DNA VAC-CINE	TREATMENT OF CUTANEOUS T CELL LYMPHOMA.	WYETH-LEDERLE VACCINES AND PEDIATRICS 211 BAILEY RD. WEST HENRIETTA NY 14586-9728 DD 3/8/1995

NAME *Generic/Chemical* *TN=Trade Name*	**INDICATION DESIGNATED**	SPONSOR AND ADDRESS *DD=Date Designated* *MA=Marketing Approval*
ABETIMUS	TREATMENT OF LUPUS NEPHRITIS.	LA JOLLA PHARMACEUTICAL CO. 6455 NANCY RIDGE DR. SAN DIEGO CA 92121 DD 7/28/2000
ACETYLCYSTEINE TN=MUCOMYST/MUCOMYST 10 IV	INTRAVENOUS TREATMENT OF PATIENTS PRESENT- ING WITH MODERATE TO SEVERE ACETAMINOPHEN OVERDOSE.	BRISTOL-MYERS SQUIBB COMPANY P.O. BOX 4500 PRINCETON NJ 08543-4500 DD 8/13/1987
ACONIAZIDE	TREATMENT OF TUBERCULOSIS.	LINCOLN DIAGNOSTICS P.O. BOX 1128 DECATUR IL 62525 DD 6/20/1988
ADENO-ASSOCIATED VIRAL VEC- TOR CONTAINING THE GENE FOR HUMAN COAGULATION FAC- TOR IX TN=COAGULIN-B	INTRAMUSCULAR TREATMENT OF PATIENTS WITH MODERATE TO SEVERE HEMOPHILIA	AVIGEN, INC. 1301 HARBOR BAY PARKWAY ALAMEDA CA 94502 DD 6/13/2001
ADENO-ASSOCIATED VIRAL VEC- TOR CONTAINING THE GENE FOR HUMAN COAGULATION FAC- TOR IX TN=COAGULIN-B	INTRAHEPATIC TREATMENT OF PATIENTS WITH MOD- ERATE TO SEVERE HEMOPHILIA	AVIGEN, INC. 1301 HARBOR BAY PARKWAY ALAMEDA CA 94502 DD 6/13/2001
ADENO-ASSOCIATED VIRAL- BASED VECTOR CYSTIC FIBRO- SIS GENE THERAPY	TREATMENT OF CYSTIC FIBROSIS.	TARGETED GENETICS CORPORATION 1100 OLIVE WAY, SUITE 100 SEATTLE WA 98101 DD 2/15/1995
ADENOSINE	FOR USE IN CONJUNCTION WITH BCNU IN THE TREAT- MENT OF BRAIN TUMORS.	MEDCO RESEARCH, INC. 8455 BEVERLY BOULEVARD SUITE 308 LOS ANGELES CA 90048 DD 8/1/1989
ADENOVIRUS-BASED VECTOR FACTOR VIII COMPLEMENTARY DNA TO SOMATIC CELLS TN=MINIADFVIII	TREATMENT OF HEMOPHILIA A.	GENSTAR THERAPEUTICS CORPORATION 10835 ALTMAN ROW SUITE 150 SAN DIEGO CA 92121 DD 12/15/1999
AEROSOLIZED POOLED IMMUNE GLOBULIN	TREATMENT OF RESPIRATORY SYNCYTIAL VIRUS LOWER RESPIRATORY TRACT DISEASE.	PEDIATRIC PHARMACEU- TICALS, INC. 718 BRADFORD AVENUE WESTFIELD NJ 07090 DD 1/3/1989
ALBENDAZOLE TN=ALBENZA	TREATMENT OF NEUROCYSTICERCOSIS DUE TO TAENIA SOLIUM AS: 1) CHEMOTHERAPY OF PAR- ENCHYMAL, SUBARACHNOIDAL AND RACEMOSE (CYSTS IN SPINAL FLUID) NEUROCYSTICERCOSIS IN SYMPTOMATIC CASES AND 2) PROPHYLAXIS OF EPI- LEPSY AND OTHER SEQUELAE IN ASYMPTOMATIC NEUROCYS	SMITHKLINE BEECHAM PHARMACEUTICALS ONE FRANKLIN PLAZA P.O. BOX 7929 PHILADELPHIA PA 19101 DD 1/18/1996 MA 6/11/1996
ALBENDAZOLE TN=ALBENZA	TREATMENT OF HYDATID DISEASE (CYSTIC ECHINO- COCCOSIS DUE TO E. GRANULOSUS LARVAE OR AL- VEOLAR ECHINOCOCCOSIS DUE TO E. MULTILOCULARIS LARVAE).	SMITHKLINE BEECHAM PHARMACEUTICALS ONE FRANKLIN PLAZA P.O. BOX 7929 PHILADELPHIA PA 19101 DD 1/17/1996 MA 6/11/1996

NAME *Generic/Chemical* *TN=Trade Name*	INDICATION DESIGNATED	SPONSOR AND ADDRESS *DD=Date Designated* *MA=Marketing Approval*
ALDESLEUKIN TN=PROLEUKIN	TREATMENT OF METASTATIC MELANOMA.	CHIRON CORPORATION 4560 HORTON STREET EMERYVILLE CA 94608-2916 DD 9/10/1996 MA 1/9/1998
ALDESLEUKIN TN=PROLEUKIN	FOR THE TREATMENT NON-HODGKIN'S LYMPHOMA.	CHIRON CORPORATION 4560 HORTON ST. EMERYVILLE CA 94608-2916 DD 11/24/1998
ALDESLEUKIN TN=PROLEUKIN	TREATMENT OF METASTATIC RENAL CELL CARCINO-MA.	CHIRON CORPORATION 4560 HORTON STREET EMERYVILLE CA 94608-2916 DD 9/14/1988 MA 5/5/1992
ALDESLEUKIN TN=PROLEUKIN	TREATMENT OF ACUTE MYELOGENOUS LEUKEMIA.	CHIRON CORPORATION 4560 HORTON ST. EMERYVILLE CA 94608-2916 DD 7/31/1998
ALDESLEUKIN TN=PROLEUKIN	TREATMENT OF PRIMARY IMMUNODEFICIENCY DIS-EASE ASSOCIATED WITH T-CELL DEFECTS.	CHIRON CORPORATION 4560 HORTON STREET EMERYVILLE CA 94608-2916 DD 3/22/1989
ALENDRONATE DISODIUM TN=FOSAMAX	TREATMENT OF THE BONE MANIFESTATIONS OF GAUCHER DISEASE	RICHARD J. WENSTRUP, M.D. DIVISION OF HUMAN GENETICS CHILDREN'S HOSPITAL RESEARCH FOUNDATION CINCINNATI OH 45229-3039 DD 2/13/2001
ALGLUCERASE INJECTION TN=CEREDASE	FOR REPLACEMENT THERAPY IN PATIENTS WITH GAUCHER'S DISEASE TYPE I.	GENZYME CORPORATION ONE KENDALL SQUARE CAMBRIDGE MA 02139-1562 DD 3/11/1985 MA 4/5/1991
ALGLUCERASE INJECTION TN=CEREDASE	REPLACEMENT THERAPY IN PATIENTS WITH TYPE II AND III GAUCHER'S DISEASE.	GENZYME CORPORATION ONE KENDALL SQUARE CAMBRIDGE MA 02139-1562 DD 7/21/1995
ALITRETINOIN TN=PANRETIN	TOPICAL TREATMENT OF CUTANEOUS LESIONS IN PATIENTS WITH AIDS-RELATED KAPOSI'S SARCOMA.	LIGAND PHARMACEUTICALS INC. 10275 SCIENCE CENTER DRIVE SAN DIEGO CA 92121-1117 DD 3/24/1998 MA 2/2/1999
ALLOGENEIC HUMAN RETINAL PIGMENT EPITHELIAL CELLS ON GELATIN MICROCARRIERS TN=SPHERAMINE	TREATMENT OF HOEHN AND YAHR STAGE 3 AND 4 PARKINSON'S DISEASE.	TITAN PHARMACEUTICALS, INC. POST OFFICE PLAZA 50 DIVISION STREET, SUITE 503 SOMERVILLE NJ 08876 DD 7/18/1997
ALLOGENEIC PERIPHERAL BLOOD MONONUCLEAR CELLS SENSITIZED AGAINST PATIENT ALLOANTIGENS BY MIXED LYM-PHOCYTE CULTURE TN=CYTOIMPLANT	TREATMENT OF PANCREATIC CANCER.	APPLIED IMMUNOTHERA-PEUTICS, LLC 14132 E. FIRESTONE BOULEVARD SANTA FE SPRINGS CA 90670 DD 6/13/1997

NAME *Generic/Chemical* *TN=Trade Name*	INDICATION DESIGNATED	SPONSOR AND ADDRESS *DD=Date Designated* *MA=Marketing Approval*
ALLOPURINOL RIBOSIDE	TREATMENT OF CHAGAS' DISEASE.	BURROUGHS WELLCOME COMPANY 3030 CORNWALLIS ROAD P.O. BOX 12700 RESEARCH TRIANGLE PARK NC 27709 DD 12/4/1985
ALLOPURINOL RIBOSIDE	TREATMENT OF CUTANEOUS AND VISCERAL LEISH-MANIASIS.	BURROUGHS WELLCOME COMPANY 3030 CORNWALLIS ROAD P.O. BOX 12700 RESEARCH TRIANGLE PARK NC 27709 DD 12/4/1985
ALLOPURINOL SODIUM	EX-VIVO PRESERVATION OF CADAVERIC KIDNEYS FOR TRANSPLANTATION	BURROUGHS WELLCOME COMPANY 3030 CORNWALLIS ROAD RESEARCH TRIANGLE PK NC 27709 DD 11/9/1987
ALLOPURINOL SODIUM TN=ALOPRIM FOR INJECTION	MANAGEMENT OF PATIENTS WITH LEUKEMIA, LYM-PHOMA, AND SOLID TUMOR MALIGNANCIES WHO ARE RECEIVING CANCER THERAPY WHICH CAUSES ELEVATIONS OF SERUM AND URINARY URIC ACID LE-VELS AND WHO CANNOT TOLERATE ORAL THERAPY.	CATALYTICA PHARMACEU-TICALS, INC PO BOX 1887 GREENVILLE NC 27835-1887 DD 10/16/1992 MA 5/17/1996
ALPHA-1-ANTITRYPSIN (RECOM-BINANT DNA ORIGIN)	AS SUPPLEMENTATION THERAPY FOR ALPHA-1-ANTI-TRYPSIN DEFICIENCY IN THE ZZ PHENOTYPE POPU-LATION.	CHIRON CORPORATION 4560 HORTON STREET EMERYVILLE CA 94608-2916 DD 1/1/1984
ALPHA-GALACTOSIDASE A TN=REPLAGAL	LONG-TERM ENZYME REPLACEMENT THERAPY FOR THE TREATMENT OF FABRY DISEASE.	TRANSKARYOTIC THERAPIES INC. 195 ALBANY ST. CAMBRIDGE MA 02139 DD 6/22/1998
ALPHA-GALACTOSIDASE A TN=CC-GALACTOSIDASE	TREATMENT OF ALPHA-GALACTOSIDASE A DEFI-CIENCY (FABRY'S DISEASE).	ORPHAN MEDICAL, INC. 13911 RIDGEDALE DRIVE SUITE 475 MINNETONKA MN 55305 DD 6/17/1991
ALPHA-GALACTOSIDASE A TN=FABRASE	TREATMENT OF FABRY'S DISEASE.	DESNICK, ROBERT J. M.D. THE MOUNT SINAI SCHOOL OF MEDICINE FIFTH AVENUE AT 100TH STREET, BOX 1203 NEW YORK NY 10029 DD 7/20/1990
ALPHA-MELANOCYTE STIMULAT-ING HORMONE	PREVENTION AND TREATMENT OF INTRINSIC ACUTE RENAL FAILURE DUE TO ISCHEMIA.	NATIONAL INSTITUTE OF DIABETES, AND DIGESTIVE AND KIDNEY DISEASES NATIONAL INSTITUTES OF HEALTH, 31 CENTER DRIVE MSC 2560 BUILDING 31, ROOM 9N-222 BETHESDA MD 20892-2560 DD 8/19/1997

NAME *Generic/Chemical* *TN=Trade Name*	INDICATION DESIGNATED	SPONSOR AND ADDRESS *DD=Date Designated* *MA=Marketing Approval*
ALPHA1-PROTEINASE INHIBITOR (HUMAN)	FOR SLOWING THE PROGRESSION OF EMPHYSEMA IN ALPHA1-ANTITRYPSIN DEFICIENT PATIENTS.	AVENTIS BEHRING L.L.C. 1020 FIRST AVE. PO BOX 61501 KING OF PRUSSIA PA 19406-0901 DD 11/24/1999
ALPHA1-PROTEINASE INHIBITOR (HUMAN) TN=PROLASTIN	FOR REPLACEMENT THERAPY IN THE ALPHA-1-PROTEINASE INHIBITOR CONGENITAL DEFICIENCY STATE.	BAYER CORPORATION PHARMACEUTICAL DIVISION, BIOLOGICAL PRODUCTS 400 MORGAN LANE NEW HAVEN CT 06516 DD 12/7/1984 MA 12/2/1987
ALPROSTADIL	TREATMENT OF SEVERE PERIPHERAL ARTERIAL OCCLUSIVE DISEASE (CRITICAL LIMB ISCHEMIA) IN PATIENTS WHERE OTHER PROCEDURES, GRAFTS OR ANGIOPLASTY, ARE NOT INDICATED.	SCHWARZ PHARMA, INC. P.O. BOX 2038 MILWAUKEE WI 53201 DD 10/20/1993
ALRONIDASE TN=ALDURAZYME	TREATMENT OF PATIENTS WITH MUCOPOLYSACCHARIDOSIS-I.	BIOMARIN PHARMACEUTICAL, INC. 371 BEL MARIN KEYS BOULEVARD, SUITE 210 NOVATO CA 94949-5608 DD 9/24/1997
ALTRETAMINE TN=HEXALEN	TREATMENT OF ADVANCED ADENOCARCINOMA OF THE OVARY.	MEDIMMUNE ONCOLOGY, INC. ONE TOWER BRIDGE 100 FRONT STREET, SUITE 400 CONSHOHOCKEN PA 19428 DD 2/9/1984 MA 12/26/1990
AMIFOSTINE TN=ETHYOL	REDUCTION OF THE INCIDENCE OF MODERATE TO SEVERE XEROSTOMIA IN PATIENTS UNDERGOING POST-OPERATIVE RADIATION TREATMENT FOR HEAD AND NECK CANCER.	MEDIMMUNE ONCOLOGY, INC. ONE TOWER BRIDGE 100 FRONT STREET, SUITE 400 CONSHOHOCKEN PA 19428 DD 5/12/1998 MA 6/24/1999
AMIFOSTINE TN=ETHYOL	FOR USE AS A CHEMOPROTECTIVE AGENT FOR CISPLATIN IN THE TREATMENT OF METASTATIC MELANOMA.	MEDIMMUNE ONCOLOGY, INC. 35 WEST WATKINS MILLS RD. GAITHERSBURG MD 20878 DD 5/30/1990
AMIFOSTINE TN=ETHYOL	TREATMENT OF MYELODYSPLASTIC SYNDROMES.	MEDIMMUNE ONCOLOGY, INC. 35 WEST WATKINS MILL RD. GAITHERSBURG MD 20878 DD 10/4/1999
AMIFOSTINE TN=ETHYOL	FOR THE REDUCTION OF THE INCIDENCE AND SEVERITY OF TOXICITIES ASSOCIATED WITH CISPLATIN ADMINISTRATION.	MEDIMMUNE ONCOLOGY, INC. 35 WEST WATKINS MILL RD. GAITHERSBURG MD 20878 DD 11/24/1998
AMIFOSTINE TN=ETHYOL	FOR USE AS A CHEMOPROTECTIVE AGENT FOR CISPLATIN IN THE TREATMENT OF ADVANCED OVARIAN CARCINOMA.	MEDIMMUNE ONCOLOGY, INC. ONE TOWER BRIDGE 100 FRONT STREET, SUITE 400 WEST CONSHOHOCKEN PA 19428 DD 5/30/1990 MA 12/8/1995
AMIFOSTINE TN=ETHYOL	FOR USE AS A CHEMOPROTECTIVE AGENT FOR CYCLOPHOSPHAMIDE IN THE TREATMENT OF ADVANCED OVARIAN CARCINOMA.	MEDIMMUNE ONCOLOGY, INC. 35 WEST WATKINS MILL RD. GAITHERSBURG MD 20878 DD 5/30/1990

NAME *Generic/Chemical* *TN=Trade Name*	INDICATION DESIGNATED	SPONSOR AND ADDRESS *DD=Date Designated* *MA=Marketing Approval*
AMILORIDE HCL SOLUTION FOR INHALATION	TREATMENT OF CYSTIC FIBROSIS.	GLAXO WELLCOME RESEARCH AND DEVELOPMENT 5 MOORE DRIVE PO BOX 13398 RESEARCH TRIANGLE PARK NC 27709 DD 7/18/1990
AMINOCAPROIC ACID TN=CAPROGEL	FOR THE TOPICAL TREATMENT OF TRAUMATIC HYPHEMA OF THE EYE.	EASTERN VIRGINIA MEDICAL SCHOOL DEPARTMENT OF OPHTHALOMOLOGY 880 KEMPSVILLE ROAD, SUITE 2500 NORFOLK VA 23502-3990 DD 1/6/1995
AMINOSALICYLATE SODIUM	TREATMENT OF CROHN'S DISEASE.	SYNCOM PHARMACEUTICALS, INC. 66 HANOVER ROAD FLORHAM PARK NJ 07932 DD 4/6/1993
AMINOSALICYLIC ACID TN=PASER GRANULES	TREATMENT OF TUBERCULOSIS INFECTIONS.	JACOBUS PHARMACEUTICAL COMPANY 37 CLEVELAND LANE P.O. BOX 5290 PRINCETON NJ 08540 DD 2/19/1992 MA 6/30/1994
AMINOSIDINE TN=GABBROMICINA	TREATMENT OF TUBERCULOSIS.	KANYOK, THOMAS P. PHARM.D. UNIVERSITY OF ILLINOIS AT CHICAGO COLLEGE OF PHARMACY 833 SOUTH WOOD STREET (M/C886) RM. 176 CHICAGO IL 60612 DD 5/14/1993
AMINOSIDINE TN=GABBROMICINA	TREATMENT OF MYCOBACTERIUM AVIUM COMPLEX.	KANYOK, THOMAS P. PHARM.D. UNIVERSITY OF ILLINOIS AT CHICAGO COLLEGE OF PHARMACY 833 SOUTH WOOD STREET (M/C886) RM. 176 CHICAGO IL 60612 DD 11/15/1993
AMINOSIDINE TN=PAROMOMYCIN	TREATMENT OF VISCERAL LEISHMANIASIS (KALA-AZAR).	KANYOK, THOMAS P. PHARM.D. UNIVERSITY OF ILLINOIS AT CHICAGO COLLEGE OF PHARMACY 833 SOUTH WOOD STREET (M/C886) RM. 176 CHICAGO IL 60612 DD 9/9/1994
AMIODARONE TN=AMIO-AQUEOUS	TREATMENT OF INCESSANT VENTRICULAR TACHYCARDIA.	WYETH-AYERST RESEARCH PO BOX 8299 PHILADELPHIA PA 19101-8299 DD 8/17/1993
AMIODARONE HCL TN=CORDARONE	FOR THE ACUTE TREATMENT AND PROPHYLAXIS OF LIFE-THREATENING VENTRICULAR TACHYCARDIA OR VENTRICULAR FIBRILLATION.	WYETH-AYERST LABORATORIES P.O. BOX 8299 PHILADELPHIA PA 19101 DD 3/16/1994 MA 8/3/1995

NAME *Generic/Chemical* *TN=Trade Name*	INDICATION DESIGNATED	SPONSOR AND ADDRESS *DD=Date Designated* *MA=Marketing Approval*
AMMONIUM TETRATHIOMOLYB-DATE	TREATMENT OF WILSON'S DISEASE.	BREWER, GEORGE J. M.D. UNIVERSITY OF MICHIGAN MEDICAL SCHOOL 4708 MEDICAL SCIENCE BUILDING II 0618 ANN ARBOR MI 48109 DD 1/31/1994
AMPHOTERICIN B LIPID COMPLEX TN=ABELCET	TREATMENT OF INVASIVE PROTOTHECOSIS.	THE LIPOSOME COMPANY, INC. ONE RESEARCH WAY PRINCETON NJ 08540 DD 8/21/1996
AMPHOTERICIN B LIPID COMPLEX TN=ABELCET	TREATMENT OF INVASIVE FUNGAL INFECTIONS.	LIPOSOME COMPANY, INC. ONE RESEARCH WAY PRINCETON NJ 08540 DD 12/3/1996 MA 10/18/1996
AMPHOTERICIN B LIPID COMPLEX TN=ABELCET	TREATMENT OF INVASIVE ZYGOMYCOSIS.	THE LIPOSOME COMPANY, INC. ONE RESEARCH WAY PRINCETON NJ 08540 DD 5/6/1996
AMPHOTERICIN B LIPID COMPLEX TN=ABELCET	TREATMENT OF INVASIVE CANDIDIASIS.	THE LIPOSOME COMPANY, INC. ONE RESEARCH WAY PRINCETON NJ 08540 DD 6/27/1996
AMPHOTERICIN B LIPID COMPLEX TN=ABELCET	TREATMENT OF INVASIVE COCCIDIOIDOMYCOSIS.	THE LIPOSOME COMPANY, INC. ONE RESEARCH WAY PRINCETON NJ 08540 DD 5/6/1996
AMPHOTERICIN B LIPID COMPLEX TN=ABELCET	TREATMENT OF INVASIVE SPOROTRICHOSIS.	THE LIPOSOME COMPANY, INC. ONE RESEARCH WAY PRINCETON NJ 08540 DD 9/23/1996
AMSACRINE TN=AMSIDYL	TREATMENT OF ACUTE ADULT LEUKEMIA.	WARNER-LAMBERT COMPANY PARKE-DAVIS PHARMACEUTICAL RESEARCH DIVISION 2800 PLYMOUTH ROAD ANN ARBOR MI 48106 DD 12/7/1984
ANAGRELIDE TN=AGRYLIN	TREATMENT OF POLYCYTHEMIA VERA.	ROBERTS PHARMACEUTICAL CORP. MERIDIAN CENTER II 4 INDUSTRIAL WAY WEST EATONTOWN NJ 07724-2274 DD 6/11/1985
ANAGRELIDE TN=AGRYLIN	TREATMENT OF THROMBOCYTOSIS IN CHRONIC MYELOGENOUS LEUKEMIA.	ROBERTS PHARMACEUTICAL CORP. MERIDIAN CENTER II 4 INDUSTRIAL WAY WEST EATONTOWN NJ 07724-2274 DD 7/14/1986
ANAGRELIDE TN=AGRYLIN	TREATMENT OF ESSENTIAL THROMBOCYTHEMIA.	ROBERTS PHARMACEUTICAL CORP. MERIDIAN CENTER III 6 INDUSTRIAL WAY WEST EATONTOWN NJ 07724 DD 1/27/1988 MA 3/14/1997

NAME *Generic/Chemical* *TN=Trade Name*	INDICATION DESIGNATED	SPONSOR AND ADDRESS *DD=Date Designated* *MA=Marketing Approval*
ANANAIN, COMOSAIN TN=VIANAIN	FOR THE ENZYMATIC DEBRIDEMENT OF SEVERE BURNS.	GENZYME CORPORATION ONE KENDALL SQUARE CAMBRIDGE MA 02139 DD 1/21/1992
ANARITIDE ACETATE TN=AURICULIN	TREATMENT OF PATIENTS WITH ACUTE RENAL FAILURE.	SCIOS, INC. 2450 BAYSHORE PARKWAY MOUNTAIN VIEW CA 94043 DD 8/27/1992
ANARITIDE ACETATE TN=AURICULIN	IMPROVEMENT OF EARLY RENAL ALLOGRAFT FUNCTION FOLLOWING RENAL TRANSPLANTATION.	SCIOS, INC. 2450 BAYSHORE PARKWAY MOUNTAIN VIEW CA 94043 DD 4/10/1992
ANCESTIM TN=STEMGEN	FOR USE IN COMBINATION WITH FILGRASTIM TO DECREASE THE NUMBER OF PHERESES REQUIRED TO COLLECT PERIPHERAL BLOOD PROGENITOR CELLS CAPABLE OF PROVIDING RAPID MULTI-LINEAGE HEMATOPOIETIC RECONSTITUTION FOLLOWING MYELOSUPPRESSIVE OR MYELOABLATIVE THERAPY.	AMGEN, INC. ONE AMGEN CENTER DRIVE THOUSAND OAKS CA 91320-1799 DD 7/5/1995
ANCROD TN=VIPRINEX	TO ESTABLISH AND MAINTAIN ANTICOAGULATION IN HEPARIN-INTOLERANT PATIENTS UNDERGOING CARDIOPULMONARY BYPASS.	KNOLL PHARMACEUTICAL COMPANY 3000 CONTINENTAL DR., NORTH MT. OLIVE NJ 07828 DD 10/20/1989
ANGIOTENSIN 1-7	TREATMENT OF NEUTROPENIA ASSOCIATED WITH AUTOLOGOUS BONE MARROW TRANSPLANTATION.	MARET PHARMACEUTICALS 4041 MACARTHUR BLVD. SUITE 375 NEWPORT BEACH CA 92660 DD 2/16/2000
ANGIOTENSIN 1-7 TN=MARSTEM	TREATMENT OF MYELODYSPLASTIC SYNDROME	MARET PHARMACEUTICAL CORPORATION 4041 MACARTHUR BOULEVARD, SUITE 375 NEWPORT BEACH CA 92660 DD 8/3/2001
ANTI PAN T LYMPHOCYTE MONOCLONAL ANTIBODY TN=ANTI-T LYMPHOCYTE IMMUNOTOXIN XMMLY-H65-RTA	FOR IN-VIVO TREATMENT OF BONE MARROW RECIPIENTS TO PREVENT GRAFT REJECTION AND GRAFT VERSUS HOST DISEASE.	XOMA CORPORATION 2910 SEVENTH STREET BERKELEY CA 94710 DD 1/29/1986
ANTI PAN T LYMPHOCYTE MONOCLONAL ANTIBODY TN=ANTI-T LYMPHOCYTE IMMUNOTOXIN XMMLY-H65-RTA	FOR EX-VIVO TREATMENT TO ELIMINATE MATURE T CELLS FROM POTENTIAL BONE MARROW GRAFTS.	XOMA CORPORATION 2910 SEVENTH STREET BERKELEY CA 94710 DD 1/29/1986
ANTI-CD45 MONOCLONAL ANTIBODIES	PREVENTION OF ACUTE GRAFT REJECTION OF HUMAN ORGAN TRANSPLANTS.	BAXTER HEALTHCARE CORPORATION 1620 WAUKEGAN ROAD MCGAW PARK IL 60085 DD 9/10/1990
ANTI-CEA SHEEP-HUMAN CHIMERIC MONOCLONAL ANTIBODY LABELED W/IODINE-131 (KAb620I)	TREATMENT OF PANCREATIC CANCER.	KS BIOMEDIX, LTD. 1 OCCAM COURT GROUND FLOOR SURVEY RESEARCH PARK GULFORD, SURREY UNITED KINGDOM GU2 7HJ DD 5/21/2003

NAME Generic/Chemical TN=Trade Name	INDICATION DESIGNATED	SPONSOR AND ADDRESS DD=Date Designated MA=Marketing Approval
ANTI-CYTOMEGALOVIRUS MONOCLONAL ANTIBODIES	PREVENTION OF HUMAN CYTOMEGALOVIRUS INFECTION IN PATIENTS DIAGNOSED WITH AIDS.	BIOMEDICAL RESEARCH INSTITUTE 345 NORTH SMITH AVENUE ST. PAUL MN 55102 DD 5/3/1990
ANTI-CYTOMEGALOVIRUS MONOCLONAL ANTIBODIES	TREATMENT OF HUMAN CYTOMEGALOVIRUS INFECTION IN PATIENTS DIAGNOSED WITH AIDS.	BIOMEDICAL RESEARCH INSTITUTE 345 NORTH SMITH AVENUE ST. PAUL MN 55102 DD 5/3/1990
ANTI-CYTOMEGALOVIRUS MONOCLONAL ANTIBODIES	PREVENTION OF HUMAN CYTOMEGALOVIRUS INFECTION IN BONE MARROW AND ORGAN TRANSPLANT PATIENTS.	BIOMEDICAL RESEARCH INSTITUTE 345 NORTH SMITH AVENUE ST. PAUL MN 55102 DD 5/2/1990
ANTI-CYTOMEGALOVIRUS MONOCLONAL ANTIBODIES	TREATMENT OF HUMAN CYTOMEGALOVIRUS INFECTION IN BONE MARROW AND ORGAN TRANSPLANT PATIENTS.	BIOMEDICAL RESEARCH INSTITUTE 345 NORTH SMITH AVENUE ST. PAUL MN 55102 DD 5/2/1990
ANTI-TAP-72 IMMUNOTOXIN TN=XOMAZYME-791	TREATMENT OF METASTATIC COLORECTAL ADENOCARCINOMA.	XOMA CORPORATION 2910 SEVENTH STREET BERKELEY CA 94710 DD 3/6/1987
ANTI-THYMOCYTE GLOBULIN (RABBITT) TN=THYMOGLOBULIN	TREATMENT OF MYELODYSPLASTIC SYNDROME (MDS)	SANGSTAT MEDICAL CORPORATION 6300 DUMBARTON CIRCLE FREEMONT CA 94555 DD 9/6/2000
ANTI-THYMOCYTE SERUM TN=NASHVILLE RABBIT ANTI-THYMOCYTE SERUM	TREATMENT OF ALLOGRAFT REJECTION, INCLUDING SOLID ORGAN (KIDNEY, LIVER, HEART, LUNG, AND PANCREAS) AND BONE MARROW TRANSPLANTATION.	APPLIED MEDICAL RESEARCH 1600 HAYES STREET NASHVILLE TN 37203 DD 6/2/1993
ANTIEPILEPSIRINE	TREATMENT OF DRUG RESISTANT GENERALIZED TONIC-CLONIC EPILEPSY IN CHILDREN AND ADULTS.	CHILDREN'S HOSPITAL 700 CHILDREN'S DRIVE COLUMBUS OH 43205 DD 3/23/1989
ANTIHEMOPHILIC FACTOR (HUMAN) TN=ALPHANATE	TREATMENT OF VON WILLEBRAND'S DISEASE.	ALPHA THERAPEUTIC CORPORATION 5555 VALLEY BOULEVARD LOS ANGELES CA 90032-3520 DD 1/5/1996
ANTIHEMOPHILIC FACTOR (RECOMBINANT) TN=REFACTO	FOR THE CONTROL AND PREVENTION OF HEMORRHAGIC EPISODES AND FOR SURGICAL PROPHYLAXIS IN PATIENTS WITH HEMOPHILIA A (CONGENITAL FACTOR VIII DEFICIENCY OR CLASSIC HEMOPHILIA).	GENETICS INSTITUTE, INC. 87 CAMBRIDGEPARK DRIVE CAMBRIDGE MA 02140 DD 2/8/1996
ANTIHEMOPHILIC FACTOR (RECOMBINANT) TN=KOGENATE	PROPHYLAXIS AND TREATMENT OF BLEEDING IN INDIVIDUALS WITH HEMOPHILIA A OR FOR PROPHYLAXIS WHEN SURGERY IS REQUIRED IN INDIVIDUALS WITH HEMOPHILIA A.	BAYER CORPORATION 1884 MILES AVENUE ELKHART IN 46515 DD 9/25/1989 MA 2/25/1993

NAME *Generic/Chemical* *TN=Trade Name*	INDICATION DESIGNATED	SPONSOR AND ADDRESS *DD=Date Designated* *MA=Marketing Approval*
ANTIHEMOPHILIC FACTOR/VON WILLEBRAND FACTOR COMPLEX (HUMAN), DRIED, PASTEURIZED TN=HUMATE-P	TREATMENT AND PREVENTION OF BLEEDING IN HEMOPHILIA A (CLASSICAL HEMOPHILIA) IN ADULT PATIENTS; AND TREATMENT OF SPONTANEOUS AND TRAUMA-INDUCED BLEEDING EPISODES IN SEVERE VON WILLEBRAND DISEASE, AND IN MILD AND MODERATE VON WILLEBRAND DISEASE WHERE USE OF	AVENTIS BEHRING L.L.C. 1020 FIRST AVENUE PO BOX 61501 KING OF PRUSSIA PA 19406-0901 DD 10/16/1992 MA 4/1/1999
ANTIMELANOMA ANTIBODY XMMME-001-DTPA 111 INDIUM TN=ANTIMELANOMA ANTIBODY XMMME-001-DTPA 111 INDIUM	DIAGNOSTIC USE IN IMAGING SYSTEMIC AND NODAL MELANOMA METASTASIS.	XOMA CORPORATION 2910 SEVENTH STREET BERKELEY CA 94710 DD 11/14/1984
ANTIMELANOMA ANTIBODY XMMME-001-RTA TN=ANTIMELANOMA ANTIBODY XMMME-001-RTA	TREATMENT OF STAGE III MELANOMA NOT AMENABLE TO SURGICAL RESECTION.	XOMA CORPORATION 2910 SEVENTH STREET BERKELEY CA 94710 DD 11/14/1984
ANTIPYRINE TEST	FOR USE AS AN INDEX OF HEPATIC DRUG-METABOLIZING CAPACITY.	UPSHER-SMITH LABORATORIES, INC 4905 23RD AVENUE NORTH MINNEAPOLIS MN 55447 DD 2/21/1985
ANTISENSE 20-MER PHOSPHOROTHIOATE OLEGONUCLEOTIDE [COMPLEMENTARY TO THE CODING REGION OF R2 COMPONENT OF THE HUMAN RIBUNUCLEOTIDE REDUCTASE mRNA] TN=GTI-2040	TREATMENT FOR RENAL CELL CARCINOMA.	LORUS THERAPEUTICS, INC. 2 MERIDAN ROAD TORONTO, ONTARIO CANADA M9W427 DD 3/12/2003
ANTITHROMBIN III (HUMAN) TN=ATNATIV	FOR THE TREATMENT OF PATIENTS WITH HEREDITARY ANTITHROMBIN III DEFICIENCY IN CONNECTION WITH SURGICAL OR OBSTETRICAL PROCE-DURES OR WHEN THEY SUFFER FROM THROMBOEMBOLISM.	PHARMACIA & UPJOHN AB LINDHAGENSGATAN 133 SE-112 87 STOCKHOLM SWEDEN SE DD 2/8/1985 MA 12/13/1989
ANTITHROMBIN III (HUMAN) TN=THROMBATE III	FOR REPLACEMENT THERAPY IN CONGENITAL DEFICIENCY OF AT-III FOR PREVENTION AND TREATMENT OF THROMBOSIS AND PULMONARY EMBOLI.	BAYER CORPORATION PHARMACEUTICAL DIVISION, BIOLOGICAL PRODUCTS 400 MORGAN LANE NEW HAVEN CT 06516 DD 11/26/1984 MA 12/30/1991
ANTITHROMBIN III (HUMAN) CONCENTRATE IV TN=KYBERNIN P	FOR PROPHYLAXIS AND TREATMENT OF THROMBOEMBOLIC EPISODES IN PATIENTS WITH GENETIC AT-III DEFICIENCY.	AVENTIS BEHRING L.L.C. 1020 FIRST AVE. PO BOX 61501 KING OF PRUSSIA PA 19406-0901 DD 7/2/1985
ANTITHROMBIN III HUMAN TN=ANTITHROMBIN III HUMAN	PREVENTING OR ARRESTING EPISODES OF THROMBOSIS IN PATIENTS WITH CONGENITAL AT-III DEFICIENCY AND/OR TO PREVENT THE OCCURRENCE OF THROMBOSIS IN PATIENTS WITH AT-III DEFICIENCY WHO HAVE UNDERGONE TRAUMA OR WHO ARE ABOUT TO UNDERGO SURGERY OR PARTURITION.	AMERICAN NATIONAL RED CROSS 9312 OLD GEORGETOWN ROAD BETHESDA MD 20814 DD 1/2/1986
ANTIVENIN, CROTALIDAE POLYVALENT IMMUNE FAB (OVINE) TN=CROFAB	TREATMENT OF ENVENOMATIONS INFLICTED BY NORTH AMERICAN CROTALID SNAKES.	PROTHERICS, INC. 1207 17TH AVE. S., SUITE 103 NASHVILLE TN 37212 DD 1/12/1994 MA 10/2/2000

NAME *Generic/Chemical* *TN=Trade Name*	INDICATION DESIGNATED	SPONSOR AND ADDRESS *DD=Date Designated* *MA=Marketing Approval*
ANTIVENOM (CROTALIDAE) PURIFIED (AVIAN)	TREATMENT OF ENVENOMATION BY POISONOUS SNAKES BELONGING TO THE CROTALIDAE FAMILY.	OPHIDIAN PHARMACEUTICALS, INC. 5445 EAST CHERYL PARKWAY MADISON WI 53711 DD 2/12/1991
APOMORPHINE	TREATMENT OF THE ON-OFF FLUCTUATIONS ASSOCIATED WITH LATE-STAGE PARKINSON'S DISEASE.	PENTECH PHARMACEUTICALS, INC. 1110 LAKE COOK RD. SUITE 257 BUFFALO GROVE IL 60089 DD 7/17/1995
APOMORPHINE	FOR USE AS RESCUE TREATMENT FOR EARLY MORNING MOTOR DYSFUNCTION IN LATE-STAGE PARKINSON'S DISEASE.	SCHERER DDS FRANKLAND ROAD SWINDON SN5 8RU WILTSHIRE UK DD 10/20/1997
APOMORPHINE HCL	TREATMENT OF THE ON-OFF FLUCTUATIONS ASSOCIATED WITH LATE-STAGE PARKINSON'S DISEASE.	MYLAN PHARMACEUTICALS, INC. 781 CHESTNUT RIDGE RD. PO BOX 4310 MORGANTOWN WV 26505-4310 DD 4/22/1993
APROTININ TN=TRASYLOL	FOR PROPHYLACTIC USE TO REDUCE PERIOPERATIVE BLOOD LOSS AND THE HOMOLOGOUS BLOOD TRANSFUSION REQUIREMENT IN PATIENTS UNDERGOING CARDIOPULMONARY BYPASS SURGERY IN THE COURSE OF REPEAT CORONARY ARTERY BYPASS GRAFT SURGERY, AND IN SELECTED CASES OF PRIMARY C	BAYER CORPORATION PHARMACEUTICAL DIVISION 400 MORGAN LANE WEST HAVEN CT 06516 DD 11/17/1993 MA 12/29/1993
ARCITUMOMAB TN=99M TC-LABELED CEA-SCAN	DIAGNOSIS AND LOCALIZATION OF PRIMARY, RESIDUAL, RECURRENT AND METASTATIC MEDULLARY THYROID CARCINOMA.	IMMUNOMEDICS, INC. 300 AMERICAN ROAD MORRIS PLAINS NJ 07950 DD 5/10/1996
ARGININE BUTYRATE	TREATMENT OF BETA-HEMOGLOBINOPATHIES AND BETA-THALASSEMIA.	PERRINE, SUSAN P., M.D. BOSTON UNIVERSITY CANCER RESEARCH CENTER BOSTON MA 02118 DD 4/7/1992
ARGININE BUTYRATE	TREATMENT OF SICKLE CELL DISEASE AND BETA THALASSEMIA.	VERTEX PHARMACEUTICALS INC. 130 WAVERLY STREET CAMBRIDGE MA 02139-4242 DD 5/25/1994
ARSENIC TRIOXIDE TN=TRISENOX	TREATMENT OF ACUTE PROMYELOCYTIC LEUKEMIA.	CELL THERAPEUTICS, INC. 201 ELLIOTT AVE. WEST SUITE 400 SEATTLE WA 98119 DD 3/3/1998 MA 9/25/2000
ARSENIC TRIOXIDE TN=TRISENOX	TREATMENT OF MULTIPLE MYELOMA.	CELL THERAPEUTICS, INC. 201 ELLIOTT AVE. WEST, SUITE 400 SEATTLE WA 98119 DD 4/28/2000

NAME *Generic/Chemical* *TN=Trade Name*	INDICATION DESIGNATED	SPONSOR AND ADDRESS *DD=Date Designated* *MA=Marketing Approval*
ARSENIC TRIOXIDE TN=TRISENOX	TREATMENT OF MYELODYSPLASTIC SYNDROME.	CELL THERAPEUTICS, INC. 201 ELLIOTT AVENUE WEST SUITE 400 SEATTLE, WA 98119 DD 7/17/2000
ARSENIC TRIOXIDE TN=TRISENOX	TREATMENT OF CHRONIC LYMPHOCYTIC LEUKEMIA.	CELL THERAPEUTICS, INC. 501 ELLIOTT AVENUE WEST SUITE 400 SEATTLE, WA 98119 DD 5/13/2003
ARSENIC TRIOXIDE TN=TRISENOX	TREATMENT OF LIVER CANCER.	CELL THERAPEUTICS, INC. 501 ELLIOTT AVENUE WEST SUITE 400 SEATTLE, WA 98119 DD 6/13/2003
ARTESUNATE	TREATMENT OF MALARIA.	WORLD HEALTH ORGANISATION SPECIAL PROGRAMME FOR RE- SEARCH AND TRAINING IN TRO- PICAL DISEASES VIA APPIA , GENEVA 27 SWITZERLAND CH DD 7/19/1999
AS-101	TREATMENT OF ACQUIRED IMMUNODEFICIENCY SYNDROME.	NPDC-AS101, INC. 783 JERSEY AVENUE NEW BRUNSWICK NJ 08901 DD 11/9/1987
ATOVAQUONE TN=MEPRON	PREVENTION OF PNEUMOCYSTIS CARINII PNEUMO- NIA (PCP) IN HIGH-RISK, HIV-INFECTED PATIENTS DE- FINED BY A HISTORY OF ONE OR MORE EPISODES OF PCP AND/OR A PERIPHERAL CD4+ (T4 HELPER/INDU- CER) LYMPHOCYTE COUNT LESS THAN OR EQUAL TO 200/MM3.	GLAXO WELLCOME RESEARCH AND DEVELOPMENT 5 MOORE DRIVE PO BOX 13398 RESEARCH TRIANGLE PARK NC 27709 DD 8/14/1991 MA 1/5/1999
ATOVAQUONE TN=MEPRON	PRIMARY PROPHYLAXIS OF HIV-INFECTED PERSONS AT HIGH RISK FOR DEVELOPING TOXOPLASMA GON- DII ENCEPHALITIS.	GLAXO WELLCOME INC. 5 MOORE DRIVE PO BOX 13398 RESEARCH TRIANGLE PARK NC 27709 DD 3/16/1993
ATOVAQUONE TN=MEPRON	TREATMENT AND SUPPRESSION OF TOXOPLASMA GONDII ENCEPHALITIS.	GLAXO WELLCOME INC. 5 MOORE DRIVE PO BOX 13398 RESEARCH TRIANGLE PARK NC 27709-3398 DD 3/16/1993
ATOVAQUONE TN=MEPRON	TREATMENT OF AIDS ASSOCIATED PNEUMOCYSTIS CARINII PNEUMONIA.	GLAXO WELLCOME INC. 5 MOORE DRIVE RESEARCH TRIANGLE PARK NC 27709 DD 9/10/1990 MA 11/25/1992
AUTOLOGOUS DNP-CONJU- GATED TUMOR VACCINE TN=M-VAX	FOR ADJUVANT THERAPY IN MELANOMA PATIENTS WITH SURGICALLY RESECTABLE LYMPH NODE ME- TASTASIS (STAGE III AND LIMITED STAGE IV DIS- EASE).	AVAX TECHNOLOGIES, INC. 9200 INDIAN CREEK PARKWAY BUILDING 9, SUITE 200 OVERLAND PARK KS 66210 DD 2/23/1999

NAME *Generic/Chemical* *TN=Trade Name*	INDICATION DESIGNATED	SPONSOR AND ADDRESS *DD=Date Designated* *MA=Marketing Approval*
AUTOLOGOUS DENDRITIC CELLS PULSED WITH AUTOLOGOUS GLIOBLASTOMA MULTIFORME ACID-ELUTED TUMOR ANTIGENS TN=DCVAX-BRAIN	TREATMENT OF GLIOBLASTOMA MULTIFORME	NORTHWEST BIOTHERA-PEUTICS, INC. 21720 23RD DRIVE, SE SUITE 100 BOTHELL WA 98021 DD 11/29/2002
AUTOLYMPHOCYTE THERAPY	TREATMENT OF RENAL CELL CARCINOMA.	CYTOGEN CORPORATION 600 COLLEGE ROAD EAST CN 5308 PRINCETON NJ 08540-5308 DD 7/12/1994
AZATHIOPRINE TN=IMURAN	TREATMENT OF ORAL MANIFESTATIONS OF GRAFT-VERSUS-HOST DISEASE.	ORAL SOLUTIONS, INC. 787 SEVENTH AVE., 48TH FLOOR NEW YORK NY 10019 DD 9/14/1999
B LYMPHOCYTE STIMULATOR TN=BLYS	TREATMENT OF COMMON VARIABLE IMMUNODEFI-CIENCY (CVID)	HUMAN GENOME SCIENCES, INC. 9410 KEY WEST AVENUE ROCKVILLE MD 20850 DD 2/21/2001
BMY-45622	TREATMENT OF OVARIAN CANCER.	BRISTOL-MYERS SQUIBB 5 RESEARCH PARKWAY WALLINGFORD CT 06492 DD 10/15/1990
BW 12C	TREATMENT OF SICKLE CELL DISEASE.	BURROUGHS WELLCOME COMPANY 3030 CORNWALLIS ROAD P.O. BOX 12700 RESEARCH TRIANGLE PK NC 27709 DD 10/23/1987
BACITRACIN TN=ALTRACIN	TREATMENT OF ANTIBIOTIC-ASSOCIATED PSEUDO-MEMBRANOUS ENTEROCOLITIS CAUSED BY TOXINS A AND B ELABORATED BY CLOSTRIDIUM DIFFICILE.	A. L. LABORATORIES, INC. ONE EXECUTIVE DRIVE P.O. BOX 1399 FORT LEE NJ 07024 DD 3/13/1984
BACLOFEN TN=LIORESAL INTRATHECAL	TREATMENT OF SPASTICITY ASSOCIATED WITH CER-EBRAL PALSY.	MEDTRONIC, INC. 800 53RD AVENUE N.E. P.O. 1250 MINNEAPOLIS MN 55440-9087 DD 9/26/1994
BACLOFEN	TREATMENT OF INTRACTABLE SPASTICITY DUE TO MULTIPLE SCLEROSIS OR SPINAL CORD INJURY.	INFUSAID, INC. 1400 PROVIDENCE HIGHWAY NORWOOD MA 02062 DD 12/16/1991
BACLOFEN TN=LIORESAL INTRATHECAL	TREATMENT OF INTRACTABLE SPASTICITY CAUSED BY SPINAL CORD INJURY, MULTIPLE SCLEROSIS, AND OTHER SPINAL DISEASES (INCLUDING SPINAL ISCHEMIA, SPINAL TUMOR, TRANSVERSE MYELITIS, CERVICAL SPONDYLOSIS, AND DEGENERATIVE MYE-LOPATHY).	MEDTRONIC, INC. 800 53RD AVENUE N.E. MINNEAPOLIS MN 55432 DD 11/10/1987 MA 6/25/1992
BASILIXIMAB TN=SIMULECT	PROPHYLAXIS OF SOLID ORGAN REJECTION.	NOVARTIS PHARMACEUTICALS CORPORATION 59 ROUTE 10 EAST HANOVER NJ 07936-1080 DD 12/12/1997 MA 5/12/1998

NAME *Generic/Chemical* *TN=Trade Name*	INDICATION DESIGNATED	SPONSOR AND ADDRESS *DD=Date Designated* *MA=Marketing Approval*
BECLOMETHASONE DIPROPIO-NATE	FOR ORAL ADMINISTRATION IN THE TREATMENT OF INTESTINAL GRAFT-VERSUS-HOST DISEASE.	GEORGE B. MCDONALD, M.D. FRED HUTCHINSON CANCER RE-SEARCH CENTER 1100 FAIRVIEW AVENUE NORTH (SC-113); PO BOX 19024 SEATTLE WA 98109 DD 3/27/1998
BENZOATE AND PHENYLACE-TATE TN=UCEPHAN	FOR ADJUNCTIVE THERAPY IN THE PREVENTION AND TREATMENT OF HYPERAMMONEMIA IN PATIENTS WITH UREA CYCLE ENZYMOPATHY DUE TO CARBA-MYLPHOSPHATE SYNTHETASE, ORNITHINE, TRANS-CARBAMYLASE, OR ARGININOSUCCINATE SYNTHETASE DEFICIENCY.	IMMUNEXIMMUNEX 2525 MCGAW AVENUE P.O. BOX 19791 IRVINE CA 92623 DD 1/21/1986 MA 12/23/1987
BENZOPHENONE-3, OCTYL-METHOXYCINNAMATE, AVOBEN-ZONE, TITANIUM DIOXIDE, ZINC OXIDE TN=TOTAL BLOCK VL SPF 75	FOR THE PREVENTION OF VISIBLE LIGHT INDUCED SKIN PHOTOSENSITIVITY AS A RESULT OF PORFIMER SODIUM PHOTODYNAMIC THERAPY	FALLIEN COSMECEUTICALS LTD. 677 W. DEKALB PIKE KING OF PRUSSIA PA 19406 DD 8/13/2001
BENZYDAMINE HYDROCHLOR-IDE TN=TANTUM	PROPHYLACTIC TREATMENT OF ORAL MUCOSITIS RESULTING FROM RADIATION THERAPY FOR HEAD AND NECK CANCER.	ANGELINI PHARMACEUTICALS, INC. 70 GRAND AVENUE RIVER EDGE NJ 07661 DD 5/18/1998
BENZYLPENICILLIN, BENZYLPE-NICILLOIC, BENZYLPENILLOIC ACID TN=PRE-PEN/MDM	ASSESSING THE RISK OF ADMINISTRATING PENICIL-LIN WHEN IT IS THE PREFERRED DRUG OF CHOICE IN ADULT PATIENTS WHO HAVE PREVIOUSLY RE-CEIVED PENICILLIN AND HAVE A HISTORY OF CLINI-CAL SENSITIVITY.	HOLLISTER-STIER LABORA-TORIES LLC PO BOX 3145 SPOKANE WA 99220-3145 DD 9/29/1987
BERACTANT TN=SURVANTA INTRATRACHEAL SUSPENSION	TREATMENT OF FULL-TERM NEWBORN INFANTS WITH RESPIRATORY FAILURE CAUSED BY MECONIUM ASPIRATION SYNDROME, PERSISTENT PULMONARY HYPERTENSION OF THE NEWBORN, OR PNEUMONIA AND SEPSIS.	ROSS LABORATORIES 625 CLEVELAND AVENUE COLUMBUS OH 43215 DD 12/20/1993
BERACTANT TN=SURVANTA INTRATRACHEAL SUSPENSION	PREVENTION OF NEONATAL RESPIRATORY DIS-TRESS SYNDROME.	ROSS LABORATORIES 625 CLEVELAND AVENUE COLUMBUS OH 43215 DD 2/5/1986 MA 7/1/1991
BERACTANT TN=SURVANTA INTRATRACHEAL SUSPENSION	TREATMENT OF NEONATAL RESPIRATORY DISTRESS SYNDROME.	ROSS LABORATORIES 625 CLEVELAND AVENUE COLUMBUS OH 43215 DD 2/5/1986 MA 7/1/1991
BERAPROST	TREATMENT OF PULMONARY ARTERIAL HYPERTEN-SION ASSOCIATED WITH ANY NEW YORK HEART AS-SOCIATION CLASSIFICATION (CLASS I, II, III, OR IV).	UNITED THERAPEUTICS CORPORATION 68 T.W. ALEXANDER DRIVE, PO BOX 14186 RESEARCH TRIANGLE PARK NC 27709 DD 4/29/1999
BETA ALETHINE TN=BETATHINE	TREATMENT OF METASTATIC MELANOMA.	DOVETAIL TECHNOLOGIES, INC. BLDG. 337, PAINT BRANCH DRIVE COLLEGE PARK MD 20742 DD 3/24/1997

NAME *Generic/Chemical* *TN=Trade Name*	INDICATION DESIGNATED	SPONSOR AND ADDRESS *DD=Date Designated* *MA=Marketing Approval*
BETA ALETHINE TN=BETATHINE	TREATMENT OF MULTIPLE MYELOMA.	DOVETAIL TECHNOLOGIES, INC. BLDG. 337, PAINT BRANCH DRIVE COLLEGE PARK MD 20742 DD 3/24/1997
BETAINE TN=CYSTADANE	TREATMENT OF HOMOCYSTINURIA.	ORPHAN MEDICAL, INC. 13911 RIDGEDALE DRIVE SUITE 475 MINNETONKA MN 55305 DD 5/16/1994 MA 10/25/1996
BETHANIDINE SULFATE	TREATMENT OF PRIMARY VENTRICULAR FIBRILLATION.	MEDCO RESEARCH, INC. 8455 BEVERLY BLVD. SUITE 308 LOS ANGELES CA 90048 DD 9/20/1988
BETHANIDINE SULFATE	PREVENTION OF RECURRENCE OF PRIMARY VENTRICULAR FIBRILLATION.	MEDCO RESEARCH, INC. 8455 BEVERLY BLVD. SUITE 308 LOS ANGELES CA 90048 DD 11/24/1989
BEXAROTENE TN=TARGRETIN	TREATMENT OF CUTANEOUS MANIFESTATIONS OF CUTANEOUS T-CELL LYMPHOMA IN PATIENTS WHO ARE REFRACTORY TO AT LEAST ONE PRIOR SYSTEMIC THERAPY.	LIGAND PHARMACEUTICALS, INC. 10275 SCIENCE CENTER DR. SAN DIEGO CA 92121 DD 6/18/1999 MA 12/29/1999
BINDARIT	TREATMENT OF LUPUS NEPHRITIS.	ANGELINI PHARMACEUTICALS, INC. 70 GRAND AVENUE RIVER EDGE NJ 07661 DD 2/3/1998
BIOARTIFICIAL LIVER SYSTEM UTILIZING XENOGENIC HEPATOCYTES IN A HOLLOW FIBER BIOREACTOR CARTRIDGE (BAL)	TREATMENT OF PATIENTS WITH ACUTE LIVER FAILURE PRESENTING WITH ENCEPHALOPATHY DETERIORATING BEYOND PARSON'S GRADE 2	EXCORP MEDICAL, INC. SUITE 235 7200 HUDSON BLVD. OAKDALE MN 55128 DD 2/11/2002
BIS(4-FLUOROPHENYL)PHENYLACETAMIDE	TREATMENT OF SICKLE CELL DISEASE.	ICAGEN INC. ION CHANNEL ADVANCES PO BOX 14487 DURHAM NC 27709 DD 3/2/2000
BISPECIFIC ANTIBODY 520C9X22	FOR IN VIVO SEROTHERAPY OF PATIENTS WITH OVARIAN CANCER.	MEDAREX, INC. 67 BEAVER AVENUE ANNANDALE NJ 08801-0953 DD 10/5/1993
BLEOMYCIN TN=BLENOXANE	TREATMENT OF PANCREATIC CANCER.	GENETRONICS, INC. 11199 SORRENTO VALLEY RD. SAN DIEGO CA 92121-1334 DD 2/9/1999
BLEOMYCIN SULFATE TN=BLENOXANE	TREATMENT OF MALIGNANT PLEURAL EFFUSION.	BRISTOL-MYERS SQUIBB PHARMACEUTICAL RESEARCH INSTITUTE P.O. BOX 4000 PRINCETON NJ 08543 DD 9/17/1993 MA 2/20/1996

NAME *Generic/Chemical* *TN=Trade Name*	INDICATION DESIGNATED	SPONSOR AND ADDRESS *DD=Date Designated* *MA=Marketing Approval*
BOSENTAN TN=TRACLEER	TREATMENT OF PULMONARY ARTERIAL HYPERTEN-SION.	ACTELION LIFE SCIENCES LTD. 1840 GATEWAY DR. 2ND FLOOR SAN MATEO CA 94404 DD 10/6/2000 MA 11/20/2001
BOTULINUM TOXIN TYPE A TN=DYSPORT	TREATMENT OF ESSENTIAL BLEPHAROSPASM.	PORTON INTERNATIONAL, INC. 1155 15TH STREET, N.W., #315 WASHINGTON DC 20005 DD 3/23/1989
BOTULINUM TOXIN TYPE A TN=BOTOX	TREATMENT OF DYNAMIC MUSCLE CONTRACTURE IN PEDIATRIC CEREBRAL PALSY PATIENTS.	ALLERGAN, INC. 2525 DUPONT DRIVE P.O. BOX 19534 IRVINE CA 92623-9534 DD 12/6/1991
BOTULINUM TOXIN TYPE A TN=DYSPORT	TREATMENT OF SPASMODIC TORTICOLLIS (CERVI-CAL DYSTONIA).	IPSEN LIMITED 1 BATH ROAD MAIDENHEAD, BERKSHIRE U.K. SL6 4UH GB DD 8/12/1998
BOTULINUM TOXIN TYPE A TN=BOTOX	TREATMENT OF STRABISMUS ASSOCIATED WITH DYSTONIA IN ADULTS (PATIENTS 12 YEARS OF AGE AND ABOVE).	ALLERGAN, INC. 2525 DUPONT DRIVE P.O. BOX 19534 IRVINE CA 92713 DD 3/22/1984 MA 12/29/1989
BOTULINUM TOXIN TYPE A TN=DYSPORT	TREATMENT OF DYNAMIC MUSCLE CONTRACTURES IN PEDIATRIC CEREBRAL PALSY PATIENTS.	IPSEN LIMITED 1 BATH RD., MAIDENHEAD BERKSHIRE SL6 4UH ENGLAND GB DD 10/20/1999
BOTULINUM TOXIN TYPE A TN=BOTOX	TREATMENT OF BLEPHAROSPASM ASSOCIATED WITH DYSTONIA IN ADULTS (PATIENTS 12 YEARS OF AGE AND ABOVE).	ALLERGAN, INC. 2525 DUPONT DRIVE P.O. BOX 19534 IRVINE CA 92713 DD 3/22/1984 MA 12/29/1989
BOTULINUM TOXIN TYPE A	TREATMENT OF SYNKINETIC CLOSURE OF THE EYE-LID ASSOCIATED WITH VII CRANIAL NERVE ABER-RANT REGENERATION.	BOTULINUM TOXIN RESEARCH ASSOCIATES, INC. 1261 FURNACE BROOK PARKWAY QUINCY MA 02169 DD 9/15/1992
BOTULINUM TOXIN TYPE A TN=BOTOX	TREATMENT OF CERVICAL DYSTONIA.	ALLERGAN, INC. 2525 DUPONT DRIVE P.O. BOX 19534 IRVINE CA 92623-9534 DD 8/20/1986 MA 12/21/2000
BOTULINUM TOXIN TYPE B TN=NEUROBLOC	TREATMENT OF CERVICAL DYSTONIA.	ELAN PHARMACEUTICALS, INC. 800 GATEWAY BLVD. SOUTH SAN FRANCISCO CA 94080 DD 1/16/1992 MA 12/8/2000

NAME *Generic/Chemical* *TN=Trade Name*	INDICATION DESIGNATED	SPONSOR AND ADDRESS *DD=Date Designated* *MA=Marketing Approval*
BOTULINUM TOXIN TYPE F	TREATMENT OF ESSENTIAL BLEPHAROSPASM.	IPSEN LIMITED (NAME CHANGED FROM PORTON INTERNATIONAL INC) MILFORD MA DD 12/5/1991
BOTULINUM TOXIN TYPE F	TREATMENT OF SPASMODIC TORTICOLLIS (CERVI-CAL DYSTONIA).	IPSEN LIMITED (NAME CHANGED FROM PORTON INTERNATIONAL INC.) MILFORD MA DD 10/24/1991
BOTULISM IMMUNE GLOBULIN	TREATMENT OF INFANT BOTULISM.	CALIFORNIA DEPARTMENT OF HEALTH SERVICES 2151 BERKELEY WAY BERKELEY CA 94704-1011 DD 1/31/1989
BOVINE COLOSTRUM	TREATMENT OF AIDS-RELATED DIARRHEA.	HASTINGS, DONALD DVM 1030 NORTH PARKVIEW DRIVE BISMARCK ND 58501 DD 11/19/1990
BOVINE IMMUNOGLOBULIN CON-CENTRATE, CRYPTOSPORIDIUM PARVUM TN=SPORIDIN-G	TREATMENT AND SYMPTOMATIC RELIEF OF CRYP-TOSPORIDIUM PARVUM INFECTION OF THE GASTRO-INTESTINAL TRACT IN IMMUNOCOM-PROMISED PATIENTS.	GALAGEN, INC. 4001 LEXINGTON AVENUE NORTH ARDEN HILLS MN 55126 DD 3/1/1994
BOVINE WHEY PROTEIN CON-CENTRATE TN=IMMUNO-C	TREATMENT OF CRYPTOSPORIDIOSIS CAUSED BY THE PRESENCE OF CRYPTOSPORIDIUM PARVUM IN THE GASTROINTESTINAL TRACT OF PATIENTS WHO ARE IMMUNODEFICIENT/IMMUNOCOMPROMISED OR IMMUNOCOMPETENT.	BIOMUNE SYSTEMS, INC. 540 ARAPEEN DRIVE, SUITE 202 SALT LAKE CITY UT 84108 DD 9/30/1993
BRANCHED CHAIN AMINO ACIDS	TREATMENT OF AMYOTROPHIC LATERAL SCLERO-SIS.	MOUNT SINAI MEDICAL CENTER ONE GUSTAVE L. LEVY PLACE NEW YORK NY 10029 DD 12/23/1988
BRIMONIDINE TN=ALPHAGAN	TREATMENT OF ANTERIOR ISCHEMIC OPTIC NEURO-PATHY.	ALLERGAN, INC. 2525 DUPONT DR. P.O. BOX 19534 IRVINE CA 92623-9534 DD 2/7/2000
BROMHEXINE TN=BISOLVON	TREATMENT OF MILD TO MODERATE KERATOCON-JUNCTIVITIS SICCA IN PATIENTS WITH SJOGREN'S SYNDROME.	BOEHRINGER INGELHEIM PHAR-MACEUTICALS, INC. 900 RIDGEBURY ROAD, BOX 368 RIDGEFIELD CT 06877-0368 DD 5/15/1989
BROXURIDINE TN=BROXINE/NEOMARK	RADIATION SENSITIZER IN THE TREATMENT OF PRI-MARY BRAIN TUMORS.	NEOPHARM, INC. 225 EAST DEERPATH, SUITE 250 LAKE FOREST IL 60045 DD 9/18/1995
BUFFERED INTRATHECAL ELEC-TROLYTE/DEXTROSE INJECTION TN=ELLIOTTS B SOLUTION	FOR USE AS A DILUENT IN THE INTRATHECAL ADMIN-ISTRATION OF METHOTREXATE AND CYTARABINE FOR THE PREVENTION OR TREATMENT MENINGEAL LEUKEMIA AND LYMPHOCYTIC LYMPHOMA.	ORPHAN MEDICAL, INC. 13911 RIDGEDALE DRIVE SUITE 475 MINNETONKA MN 55305 DD 8/24/1994 MA 9/27/1996

NAME Generic/Chemical TN=Trade Name	INDICATION DESIGNATED	SPONSOR AND ADDRESS DD=Date Designated MA=Marketing Approval
BUPRENORPHINE HYDRO-CHLORIDE TN=SUBUTEX	TREATMENT OF OPIATE ADDICTION IN OPIATE USERS.	RECKITT BENCKISER PHARMA-CEUTICALS, INC. 1901 HUGUENOT ROAD RICHMOND VA 23235 DD 6/15/1994 MA 10/8/2002
BUPRENORPHINE IN COMBINA-TION WITH NALOXONE TN=SUBOXONE	TREATMENT OF OPIATE ADDICTION IN OPIATE USERS.	RECKITT BENCKISER PHARMA-CEUTICALS, INC. 1901 HUGUENOT ROAD RICHMOND VA 23235 DD 10/27/1994 MA 10/8/2002
BUSULFAN TN=SPARTAJECT	FOR USE AS PREPARATIVE THERAPY FOR MALIG-NANCIES TREATED WITH BONE MARROW TRANS-PLANTATION.	SPARTA PHARMACEUTICALS, INC. 111 ROCK ROAD HORSHAM PA 19044-2310 DD 4/21/1994
BUSULFAN TN=BUSULFEX	AS PREPARATIVE THERAPY IN THE TREATMENT OF MALIGNANCIES WITH BONE MARROW TRANSPLANTA-TION.	ORPHAN MEDICAL, INC. 13911 RIDGEDALE DRIVE SUITE 250 MINNETONKA MN 55305 DD 7/28/1994 MA 2/4/1999
BUSULFAN TN=SPARTAJECT	TREATMENT OF PRIMARY BRAIN MALIGNANCIES.	SUPERGEN, INC. TWO ANNABEL LANE, SUITE 220 SAN RAMON CA 94583 DD 7/7/1997
BUSULFAN TN=SPARTAJET-BUSULFAN	INTRATHECAL THERAPY FOR NEOPLASTIC MENINGI-TIS	SUPERGEN, INC. 4140 DUBLIN BOULEVARD DUBLIN CA 94568 DD 3/5/2001
BUTYRYLCHOLINESTERASE	TREATMENT OF POST-SURGICAL APNEA.	SHIRE LABORATORIES INC. 1550 EAST GUDE DRIVE ROCKVILLE MD 20850 DD 9/30/1992
BUTYRYLCHOLINESTERASE	FOR THE REDUCTION AND CLEARANCE OF TOXIC BLOOD LEVELS OF COCAINE ENCOUNTERED DURING A DRUG OVERDOSE.	SHIRE LABORATORIES INC. 1550 EAST GUDE DRIVE ROCKVILLE MD 20850 DD 3/25/1992
C1 ESTERASE INHIBITOR (HU-MAN)	TREATMENT AND PREVENTION OF ANGIOEDEMA CAUSED BY C1-ESTERASE INHIBITOR DEFICIENCY.	ALPHA THERAPEUTIC CORPORATION 5555 VALLEY BOULEVARD LOS ANGELES CA 90032 DD 8/21/1996
C1-ESTERASE-INHIBITOR, HU-MAN, PASTEURIZED TN=BERINERT P	PREVENTION AND/OR TREATMENT OF ACUTE AT-TACKS OF HEREDITARY ANGIOEDEMA.	AVENTIS BEHRING L.L.C. 1020 FIRST AVE. PO BOX 61501 KING OF PRUSSIA PA 19406-0901 DD 10/16/1992
C1-INHIBITOR TN=C1-INHIBITOR (HUMAN) VA-POR HEATED, IMMUNO	TREATMENT OF ACUTE ATTACKS OF ANGIOEDEMA.	BAXTER HEALTHCARE CORP. HYLAND DIVISION (BAXTER HYLAND) 550 NORTH BRAND BLVD. GLENDALE CA 91203 DD 8/30/1990

NAME *Generic/Chemical* *TN=Trade Name*	INDICATION DESIGNATED	SPONSOR AND ADDRESS *DD=Date Designated* *MA=Marketing Approval*
C1-INHIBITOR TN=C1-INHIBITOR (HUMAN) VA-POR HEATED, IMMUNO	PREVENTION OF ACUTE ATTACKS OF ANGIOEDEMA, INCLUDING SHORT-TERM PROPHYLAXIS FOR PATIENTS REQUIRING DENTAL OR OTHER SURGICAL PROCEDURES.	BAXTER HEALTHCARE CORP. HYLAND DIVISION (BAXTER HYLAND) 550 NORTH BRAND BLVD. GLENDALE CA 91203 DD 8/30/1990
CD4 HUMAN TRUNCATED 369 AA POLYPEPTIDE TN=SOLUBLE T4	TREATMENT OF ACQUIRED IMMUNODEFICIENCY SYNDROME.	SMITHKLINE BEECHAM ROUTE 23 & WOODMONT AVE., P.O. BOX 1510 KING OF PRUSSIA PA 19406 DD 11/21/1989
CD5-T LYMPHOCYTE IMMUNO-TOXIN TN=XOMAZYME-H65	TREATMENT OF GRAFT VERSUS HOST DISEASE AND/OR REJECTION IN PATIENTS WHO HAVE RECEIVED BONE MARROW TRANSPLANTS.	XOMA CORPORATION 2910 SEVENTH STREET BERKELEY CA 94710 DD 8/27/1987
CDP571	TREATMENT OF CROHN'S DISEASE.	CELLTECH CHIROSCIENCE LIMITED 216 BATH ROAD SLOUGH SL1 4EN BERKSHIRE UK DD 12/11/1997
CT-2584 MESYLATE	TREATMENT OF MALIGNANT MESOTHELIOMA.	CELL THERAPEUTICS, INC. 201 ELLIOTT AVE. WEST SEATTLE WA 98119 DD 4/16/1999
CT-2584 MESYLATE	TREATMENT OF ADULT SOFT TISSUE SARCOMA.	CELL THERAPEUTICS, INC. 201 ELLIOTT AVE. WEST SUITE 400 SEATTLE WA 98119 DD 4/16/1999
CY-1503 TN=CYLEXIN	TREATMENT OF POST-ISCHEMIC PULMONARY RE-PERFUSION EDEMA FOLLOWING SURGICAL TREATMENT FOR CHRONIC THROMBOEMBOLIC PULMONARY HYPERTENSION.	CYTEL CORPORATION 3525 JOHN HOPKINS COURT SAN DIEGO CA 92121 DD 12/22/1993
CY-1503 TN=CYLEXIN	TREATMENT OF NEONATES AND INFANTS UNDER-GOING CARDIOPULMONARY BYPASS DURING SURGI-CAL REPAIR OF CONGENITAL HEART LESIONS.	CYTEL CORPORATION 3525 JOHN HOPKINS COURT SAN DIEGO CA 92121 DD 7/18/1997
CY-1899	TREATMENT OF CHRONIC ACTIVE HEPATITIS B IN-FECTION IN HLA-A2 POSITIVE PATIENTS.	CYTEL CORPORATION 3525 JOHN HOPKINS COURT SAN DIEGO CA 92121 DD 3/16/1994
CAFFEINE TN=CAFCIT	TREATMENT OF APNEA OF PREMATURITY.	O.P.R. DEVELOPMENT, L.P. 1501 WAKARUSA DRIVE LAWRENCE KS 66047 DD 9/20/1988 MA 9/21/1999
CALCITONIN SALMON NASAL SPRAY TN=MIACALCIN NASAL SPRAY	TREATMENT OF SYMPTOMATIC PAGET'S DISEASE (OSTEITIS DEFORMANS).	SANDOZ PHARMACEUTICALS CORP. 59 ROUTE 10 EAST HANOVER NJ 07936 DD 10/29/1990
CALCITONIN-HUMAN FOR INJEC-TION TN=CIBACALCIN	TREATMENT OF SYMPTOMATIC PAGET'S DISEASE (OSTEITIS DEFORMANS).	NOVARTIS PHARMACEUTICAL CORPORATION 59 ROUTE 10 EAST HANOVER NJ 07936 DD 1/20/1987 MA 10/31/1986

NAME Generic/Chemical TN=Trade Name	INDICATION DESIGNATED	SPONSOR AND ADDRESS DD=Date Designated MA=Marketing Approval
CALCIUM ACETATE TN=PHOS-LO	TREATMENT OF HYPERPHOSPHATEMIA IN END STAGE RENAL FAILURE.	BRAINTREE LABORATORIES 60 COLUMBIAN STREET P.O. BOX 361 BRAINTREE MA 02184 DD 12/22/1988 MA 12/10/1990
CALCIUM ACETATE	TREATMENT OF HYPERPHOSPHATEMIA IN END STAGE RENAL DISEASE.	PHARMEDIC COMPANY 28101 BALLARD ROAD, SUITE F LAKE FOREST IL 60045 DD 6/27/1989
CALCIUM CARBONATE TN=R & D CALCIUM CARBONATE/ 600	TREATMENT OF HYPERPHOSPHATEMIA IN PATIENTS WITH END STAGE RENAL DISEASE.	R & D LABORATORIES, INC. 4204 GLENCOE AVENUE MARINA DEL REY CA 90292 DD 6/6/1990
CALCIUM GLUCONATE TN=CALGONATE	FOR USE AS A WASH FOR HYDROFLUORIC ACID SPILLS ON HUMAN SKIN.	CALGONATE CORP. 190 COMMERCE DRIVE WARWICK RI 02886 DD 11/20/1997
CALCIUM GLUCONATE GEL TN=H-F GEL	FOR USE IN THE EMERGENCY TOPICAL TREATMENT OF HYDROGEN FLUORIDE (HYDROFLUORIC ACID) BURNS.	LTR PHARMACEUTICALS, INC. 145 SAKONNET BLVD. NARRAGANSETT RI 02882 DD 5/21/1991
CALCIUM GLUCONATE GEL 2.5%	EMERGENCY TOPICAL TREATMENT OF HYDROGEN FLUORIDE (HYDROFLUORIC ACID) BURNS.	PADDOCK LABORATORIES, INC. 3940 QUEBEC AVENUE NORTH MINNEAPOLIS MN 55427 DD 9/10/1990
CALFACTANT TN=INFASURF	ACUTE RESPIRATORY DISTRESS SYNDROME (ARDS)	ONY, INC. BAIRD RESEARCH PARK 1576 SWEET HOME ROAD AMHERST NY 14228 DD 9/5/2000
CAPSAICIN	TREATMENT OF PAINFUL HIV-ASSOCIATED NEURO-PATHY.	NEUROGESX, INC. SAN CARLOS BUSINESS PARK 981F INDUSTRIAL ROAD SAN CAROLS, CA 94070-4117 DD 5/2/2003
CARBAMYLGLUTAMIC ACID	TREATMENT OF N-ACETYLGLUTAMATE SYNTHETASE DEFICIENCY.	ORPHAN EUROPE IMMEUBLE ""LE GUILLAUMET"" 60, AVENUE DU GENERAL DE GAULLE - CEDEX 70 92046 PARIS LA DEFENSE FR DD 1/20/1998
CARBOVIR	TREATMENT OF PERSONS WITH AIDS AND IN PA-TIENTS WITH SYMPTOMATIC HIV INFECTION AND A CD4 COUNT LESS THAN 200/MM3.	GLAXO WELLCOME INC. 5 MOORE DRIVE RESEARCH TRIANGLE PARK NC 27709 DD 12/13/1989
CARMUSTINE	TREATMENT OF INTRACRANIAL MALIGNANCIES.	DIRECT THERAPEUTICS, INC. 460 SEAPORT COURT SUITE 220 REDWOOD CA 94063 DD 7/3/2000
CASCARA SAGRADA FLUID EX-TRACT	TREATMENT OF ORAL DRUG OVERDOSAGE TO SPEED LOWER BOWEL EVACUATION.	INTRAMED CORPORATION 102 TREMONT WAY AUGUSTA GA 30907 DD 3/21/1989

NAME *Generic/Chemical* *TN=Trade Name*	INDICATION DESIGNATED	SPONSOR AND ADDRESS *DD=Date Designated* *MA=Marketing Approval*
CENTRUROIDES IMMUNE F(AB)2 TN=ALACRAMYN	TREATMENT OF SCORPION ENVENOMATIONS RE-QUIRING MEDICAL ATTENTION.	SILANES LABORATORIES S.A. DE C.V. AMORES #1034 COL DEL VALLE C.P. 03100 MEXICO D.F. DD 6/12/2000
CERAMIDE TRIHEXOSIDASE/AL-PHA-GALACTOSIDASE A TN=FABRAZYME	TREATMENT OF FABRY'S DISEASE.	GENZYME CORPORATION ONE KENDALL SQUARE CAMBRIDGE MA 02139-1562 DD 1/19/1988
CETIEDIL CITRATE INJECTION	TREATMENT OF SICKLE CELL DISEASE CRISIS.	BAKER CUMMINS PHARMACEUTICALS, INC. DD 12/22/1988
CETUXIMAB	TREATMENT OF SQUAMOUS CELL CANCER OF THE HEAD AND NECK IN PATIENTS WHO EXPRESS EPI-DERMAL GROWTH FACTOR RECEPTOR.	IMCLONE SYSTEMS I NCORPORATED BRANCHBURG CORPORATE CENTER 22 CHUBB WAY SOMERVILLE NJ 08876 DD 7/3/2000
CHENODIOL TN=CHENIX	FOR PATIENTS WITH RADIOLUCENT STONES IN WELL OPACIFYING GALLBLADDERS, IN WHOM ELECTIVE SURGERY WOULD BE UNDERTAKEN EXCEPT FOR THE PRESENCE OF INCREASED SURGICAL RISK DUE TO SYSTEMIC DISEASE OR AGE.	SOLVAY 901 SAWYER ROAD MARIETTA GA 30062 DD 9/21/1984 MA 7/28/1983
CHIMERIC (HUMAN-MURINE) G250 IGG MONOCLONAL ANTI-BODY	TREATMENT OF RENAL CELL CARCINOMA.	WILEX BIOTECHNOLOGY GMBH GRILLPARZERSTRASSE 10B 81675 MUNICH GERMANY DE DD 7/24/2000
CHIMERIC M-T412 (HUMAN-MUR-INE) IGG MONOCLONAL ANTI-CD4	TREATMENT OF MULTIPLE SCLEROSIS.	CENTOCOR, INC. 244 GREAT VALLEY PARKWAY MALVERN PA 19355 DD 6/5/1991
CHIMERIC, HUMANIZED MONO-CLONAL ANTIBODY TO STAPHY-LOCOCCUS	PROPHYLAXIS OF STAPHYLOCOCCUS EPIDERMIDIS SEPSIS IN LOW BIRTH WEIGHT (1500 GRAMS OR LESS) INFANTS.	BIOSYNEXUS, INC. 9610 MEDICAL CENTER DRIVE SUITE 100 ROCKVILLE MD 20850 DD 8/3/2000
CHLORHEXIDINE GLUCONATE MOUTHRINSE TN=PERIDEX	FOR USE IN THE AMELIORATION OF ORAL MUCOSITIS ASSOCIATED WITH CYTOREDUCTIVE THERAPY USED IN CONDITIONING PATIENTS FOR BONE MARROW TRANSPLANTATION THERAPY.	PROCTER & GAMBLE COMPANY SHARON WOOD TECHNICAL CENTER 11370 REED HARTMAN HIGHWAY CINCINNATI OH 45241 DD 8/18/1986
CHOLINE CHLORIDE TN=INTRACHOL	TREATMENT OF CHOLINE DEFICIENCY, SPECIFI-CALLY THE CHOLINE DEFICIENCY, HEPATIC STEATO-SIS, AND CHOLESTASIS, ASSOCIATED WITH LONG-TERM PARENTERAL NUTRITION.	ORPHAN MEDICAL, INC. 13911 RIDGEDALE DRIVE SUITE 250 MINNETONKA MN 55305 DD 2/10/1994
CHONDROCYTE-ALGINATE GEL SUSPENSION	FOR USE IN CORRECTING VESICOURETERAL REFLUX IN THE PEDIATRIC POPULATION.	CURIS, INC. 61 MOULTON STREET CAMBRIDGE MA 02138 DD 12/1/1997

NAME *Generic/Chemical* *TN=Trade Name*	INDICATION DESIGNATED	SPONSOR AND ADDRESS *DD=Date Designated* *MA=Marketing Approval*
CHONDROITINASE	TREATMENT OF PATIENTS UNDERGOING VITRECT-OMY.	BAUSCH & LOMB PHARMACEUTI-CALS, INC. 8500 HIDDEN RIVER PKWY. TAMPA FL 33637 DD 2/9/1995
CILIARY NEUROTROPHIC FAC-TOR	TREATMENT OF AMYOTROPHIC LATERAL SCLERO-SIS.	REGENERON PHARMACEU-TICALS INC 777 OLD SAW MILL RIVER ROAD TARRYTOWN NY 10591 DD 1/30/1992
CILIARY NEUROTROPHIC FAC-TOR, RECOMBINANT HUMAN	TREATMENT OF MOTOR NEURON DISEASE (INCLUD-ING AMYOTROPHIC LATERAL SCLEROSIS, PROGRES-SIVE MUSCULAR ATROPHY, PROGRESSIVE BULBAR PALSY, AND PRIMARY LATERAL SCLEROSIS).	SYNTEX-SYNERGEN NEUROSCIENCE 3200 WALNUT STREET BOULDER CO 80301 DD 5/8/1992
CILIARY NEUROTROPHIC FAC-TOR, RECOMBINANT HUMAN	TREATMENT OF SPINAL MUSCULAR ATROPHIES.	SYNTEX-SYNERGEN NEUROSCIENCE 3200 WALNUT STREET BOULDER CO 80301 DD 4/2/1992
CINACALCET	TREATMENT OF HYPERCALCEMIA IN PATIENTS WITH PARATHYROID CARCINOMA.	AMGEN, INC. ONE AMGEN CENTER DRIVE THOUSAND OAKS, CA 91320-1799 DD 5/12/2003
CISPLATIN/EPINEPHRINE TN=INTRADOSE	TREATMENT OF METASTATIC MALIGNANT MELANO-MA.	MATRIX PHARMACEUTICAL, INC. 34700 CAMPUS DRIVE FREMONT CA 94555-3612 DD 9/7/2000
CISPLATIN/EPINEPHRINE TN=INTRADOSE	TREATMENT OF SQUAMOUS CELL CARCINOMA OF THE HEAD AND NECK.	MATRIX PHARMACEUTICAL, INC. 34700 CAMPUS DRIVE FREMONT CA 94555-3612 DD 4/3/2000
CITRIC ACID, GLUCONO-DELTA-LACTONE AND MAGNESIUM CAR-BONATE TN=RENACIDIN IRRIGATION	TREATMENT OF RENAL AND BLADDER CALCULI OF THE APATITE OR STRUVITE VARIETY.	UNITED-GUARDIAN, INC. P.O. BOX 2500 SMITHTOWN NY 11787 DD 8/28/1989 MA 10/2/1990
CLADRIBINE TN=LEUSTATIN INJECTION	TREATMENT OF HAIRY CELL LEUKEMIA.	R. W. JOHNSON PHARMACEUTI-CAL RESEARCH INSTITUTE ROUTE 202, P.O. BOX 300 RARITAN NJ 08869 DD 11/15/1990 MA 2/26/1993
CLADRIBINE TN=MYLINAX	TREATMENT OF THE CHRONIC PROGRESSIVE FORM OF MULTIPLE SCLEROSIS.	R. W. JOHNSON PHARMACEUTI-CAL RESEARCH INSTITUTE ROUTE 202 PO BOX 300 RARITAN NJ 08869-0602 DD 4/19/1994
CLADRIBINE TN=LEUSTATIN	TREATMENT OF ACUTE MYELOID LEUKEMIA.	R. W. JOHNSON PHARMACEUTI-CAL RESEARCH INSTITUTE ROUTE 202 P.O. BOX 300 RARITAN NJ 08869 DD 7/20/1990

NAME Generic/Chemical TN=Trade Name	INDICATION DESIGNATED	SPONSOR AND ADDRESS DD=Date Designated MA=Marketing Approval
CLADRIBINE TN=LEUSTATIN INJECTION	TREATMENT OF CHRONIC LYMPHOCYTIC LEUKEMIA.	R. W. JOHNSON PHARMACEUTICAL RESEARCH INSTITUTE ROUTE 202, P.O. BOX 300 RARITAN NJ 08869-0602 DD 12/31/1990
CLADRIBINE TN=LEUSTATIN INJECTION	TREATMENT OF NON-HODGKIN'S LYMPHOMA.	R. W. JOHNSON PHARMACEUTICAL RESEARCH INSTITUTE ROUTE 202 SOUTH, P.O. BOX 300 RARITAN NJ 08869-0602 DD 4/19/1993
CLINDAMYCIN TN=CLEOCIN	PREVENTION OF PNEUMOCYSTIS CARINII PNEUMONIA IN AIDS PATIENTS.	PHARMACIA & UPJOHN 7000 PORTAGE ROAD UNIT 0633-298-113 KALAMAZOO MI 49001-0199 DD 10/28/1988
CLINDAMYCIN TN=CLEOCIN	TREATMENT OF PNEUMOCYSTIS CARINII PNEUMONIA ASSOCIATED WITH AIDS PATIENTS.	PHARMACIA & UPJOHN 7000 PORTAGE ROAD UNIT 0633-298-113 KALAMAZOO MI 49001-0199 DD 10/28/1988
CLOFAZIMINE TN=LAMPRENE	TREATMENT OF LEPROMATOUS LEPROSY, INCLUDING DAPSONE-RESISTANT LEPROMATOUS LEPROSY AND LEPROMATOUS LEPROSY COMPLICATED BY ERYTHEMA NODOSUM LEPROSUM.	NOVARTIS PHARMACEUTICAL CORPORATION 59 ROUTE 10 EAST HANOVER NJ 07936 DD 6/11/1984 MA 12/15/1986
CLONAZEPAM TN=KLONOPIN	TREATMENT OF HYPEREKPLEXIA (STARTLE DISEASE).	HOFFMANN-LA ROCHE, INC. 340 KINGSLAND STREET NUTLEY NJ 07110 DD 8/4/1994
CLONIDINE TN=DURACLON	FOR CONTINOUS EPIDURAL ADMINISTRATION AS ADJUNCTIVE THERAPY WITH INTRASPINAL OPIATES FOR THE TREATMENT OF PAIN IN CANCER PATIENTS TOLERANT TO, OR UNRESPONSIVE TO, INTRASPINAL OPIATES.	ROXANE LABORATORIES, INC. PO BOX 16532 COLUMBUS OH 43216-6532 DD 1/24/1989 MA 10/2/1996
CLOSTRIDIAL COLLAGENASE	TREATMENT OF ADVANCED (INVOLUTIONAL OR RESIDUAL STAGE) DUPUYTREN'S DISEASE.	HURST, L. M.D. & BADALAMENTE, M. PH.D. STATE UNIVERSITY OF NEW YORK AT STONY BROOK SCHOOL OF MEDICINE, HEALTH SCIENCES CENTER T18-020 STONY BROOK NY 11794-8181 DD 5/23/1996
CLOTRIMAZOLE	TREATMENT OF SICKLE CELL DISEASE.	BRUGNARA, CARLO M.D. THE CHILDREN'S HOSPITAL 300 LONGWOOD AVENUE, BADER 760 BOSTON MA 02115 DD 4/24/1995
COAGULATION FACTOR IX (HUMAN) TN=ALPHANINE	FOR USE AS REPLACEMENT THERAPY IN PATIENTS WITH HEMOPHILIA B FOR THE PREVENTION AND CONTROL OF BLEEDING EPISODES, AND DURING SURGERY TO CORRECT DEFECTIVE HEMOSTASIS.	ALPHA THERAPEUTIC CORPORATION 5555 VALLEY BOULEVARD LOS ANGELES CA 90032 DD 7/5/1990 MA 12/31/1990

NAME *Generic/Chemical* *TN=Trade Name*	INDICATION DESIGNATED	SPONSOR AND ADDRESS *DD=Date Designated* *MA=Marketing Approval*
COAGULATION FACTOR IX (RE-COMBINANT) TN=BENEFIX	TREATMENT OF HEMOPHILIA B.	GENETICS INSTITUTE, INC. 87 CAMBRIDGE PARK DRIVE CAMBRIDGE MA 02140 DD 10/3/1994 MA 2/11/1997
COAGULATION FACTOR IX TN=MONONINE	REPLACEMENT TREATMENT AND PROPHYLAXIS OF THE HEMORRHAGIC COMPLICATIONS OF HEMOPHILIA B.	ARMOUR PHARMACEUTICAL COMPANY 500 ARCOLA ROAD, P.O. BOX 1200 COLLEGEVILLE PA 19426 DD 6/27/1989 MA 8/20/1992
COAGULATION FACTOR VIIA (RE-COMBINANT) TN=NOVOSEVEN	TREATMENT OF BLEEDING EPISODES IN HEMOPHILIA A OR B PATIENTS WITH INHIBITORS TO FACTOR VIII OR FACTOR IX.	NOVO NORDISK PHARMACEUTI-CALS, INC. 100 OVERLOOK CENTER SUITE 200 PRINCETON NJ 08540-7810 DD 6/6/1988 MA 3/25/1999
COENZYME Q10	FOR THE TREATRMENT OF HUNTINGTON'S DISEASE	VITALINE CORPORATION 385 WILLIAMSON WAY ASHLAND OR 97520 DD 3/5/2001
COLCHICINE	FOR ARRESTING THE PROGRESSION OF NEUROLO-GIC DISABILITY CAUSED BY CHRONIC PROGRESSIVE MULTIPLE SCLEROSIS.	PHARMACONTROL CORPORATION 661 PALISADE AVE., P.O. BOX 931 ENGLEWOOD CLIFFS NJ 07632 DD 12/9/1985
COLFOSCERIL PALMITATE, CE-TYL ALCOHOL, TYLOXAPOL TN=EXOSURF	TREATMENT OF ADULT RESPIRATORY DISTRESS SYNDROME.	GLAXOSMITHKLINE 5 MOORE DRIVE P.O. BOX 13398 RESEARCH TRIANGLE PARK NC 27709 DD 1/11/1993
COLFOSCERIL PALMITATE, CE-TYL ALCOHOL, TYLOXAPOL TN=EXOSURF NEONATAL FOR INTRATRACHEAL SUSPENSION	TREATMENT OF ESTABLISHED HYALINE MEMBRANE DISEASE AT ALL GESTATIONAL AGES.	GLAXO WELLCOME INC. 5 MOORE DRIVE RESEARCH TRIANGLE PARK NC 27709 DD 10/20/1989 MA 8/2/1990
COLFOSCERIL PALMITATE, CE-TYL ALCOHOL, TYLOXAPOL TN=EXOSURF NEONATAL FOR INTRATRACHEAL SUSPENSION	PREVENTION OF HYALINE MEMBRANE DISEASE, ALSO KNOWN AS RESPIRATORY DISTRESS SYN-DROME, IN INFANTS BORN AT 32 WEEKS GESTATION OR LESS.	GLAXO WELLCOME INC. 5 MOORE DRIVE RESEARCH TRIANGLE PARK NC 27709 DD 10/20/1989 MA 8/2/1990
COLLAGENASE (LYOPHILIZED) FOR INJECTION TN=PLAQUASE	TREATMENT OF PEYRONIE'S DISEASE.	ADVANCE BIOFACTURES CORPORATION 35 WILBUR STREET LYNBROOK NY 11563-2358 DD 3/12/1996
CORTICORELIN OVINE TRIFLU-TATE TN=ACTHREL	FOR USE IN DIFFERENTIATING PITUITARY AND ECTO-PIC PRODUCTION OF ACTH IN PATIENTS WITH ACTH-DEPENDENT CUSHINGS SYNDROME.	FERRING LABORATORIES, INC. 400 RELLA BOULEVARD, SUITE 201 SUFFERN NY 10901 DD 11/24/1989 MA 5/23/1996

NAME *Generic/Chemical* *TN=Trade Name*	INDICATION DESIGNATED	SPONSOR AND ADDRESS *DD=Date Designated* *MA=Marketing Approval*
CORTICOTROPIN-RELEASING FACTOR, HUMAN TN=XERECEPT	TREATMENT OF PERITUMORAL BRAIN EDEMA.	NEUROBIOLOGICAL TECHNOLOGIES, INC. 1387 MARINA WAY SOUTH RICHMOND CA 94804 DD 4/6/1998
COUMARIN TN=ONKOLOX	TREATMENT OF RENAL CELL CARCINOMA.	DROSSAPHARM LTD 4002 BASEL SWITZERLAND CH DD 12/22/1994
CROMOLYN SODIUM TN=GASTROCROM	TREATMENT OF MASTOCYTOSIS.	FISONS CORPORATION 755 JEFFERSON RD P.O. BOX 1710 ROCHESTER NY 14603 DD 3/8/1984 MA 12/22/1989
CROMOLYN SODIUM 4% OPHTHALMIC SOLUTION TN=OPTICROM 4% OPHTHALMIC SOLUTION	TREATMENT OF VERNAL KERATOCONJUNCTIVITIS.	FISONS CORPORATION 755 JEFFERSON RD. P.O. BOX 1710 ROCHESTER NY 14603 DD 7/24/1985 MA 10/3/1984
CRYPTOSPORIDIUM HYPERIM-MUNE BOVINE COLOSTRUM IGG CONCENTRATE	TREATMENT OF DIARRHEA IN AIDS PATIENTS CAUSED BY INFECTION WITH CRYPTOSPORIDIUM PARVUM.	IMMUCELL CORPORATION 56 EVERGREEN DRIVE PORTLAND ME 04103 DD 12/30/1991
CYCLOSPORINE 2% OPHTHAL-MIC OINTMENT	FOR USE IN CORNEAL MELTING SYNDROMES OF KNOWN OR PRESUMED IMMUNOLOGIC ETIOPATHO-GENESIS, INCLUDING MOOREN'S ULCER.	ALLERGAN, INC. 2525 DUPONT DRIVE P.O. BOX 19534 IRVINE CA 92623-9534 DD 8/1/1991
CYCLOSPORINE 2% OPHTHAL-MIC OINTMENT	TREATMENT OF PATIENTS AT HIGH RISK OF GRAFT REJECTION FOLLOWING PENETRATING KERATO-PLASTY.	ALLERGAN, INC. 2525 DUPONT DRIVE P.O. BOX 19534 IRVINE CA 92623-9534 DD 8/1/1991
CYCLOSPORINE IN COMBINA-TION WITH OMEGA-3 POLYUNSA-TURATED FATTY ACIDS	PREVENTION OF SOLID ORGAN GRAFT REJECTION.	RTP PHARMA CORPORATION 200 WESTPARK CORPORATE CENTER 4364 SOUTH ALSTON AVENUE DURHAM NC 27713-2280 DD 12/6/2000
CYCLOSPORINE OPHTHALMIC TN=OPTIMMUNE	TREATMENT OF SEVERE KERATOCONJUNCTIVITIS SICCA ASSOCIATED WITH SJOGREN'S SYNDROME.	UNIVERSITY OF GEORGIA COLLEGE OF VETERINARY MEDI-CINE DEPARTMENT OF SMALL ANIMAL MEDICINE ATHENS GA 30602 DD 11/9/1988
CYPROTERONE ACETATE TN=ANDROCUR	TREATMENT OF SEVERE HIRSUTISM.	BERLEX LABORATORIES, INC. 300 FAIRFIELD ROAD WAYNE NJ 07470 DD 10/26/1984
CYSTEAMINE	TREATMENT OF NEPHROPATHIC CYSTINOSIS.	THOENE, JESS G., M.D. UNIVERSITY OF MICHIGAN MEDICAL SCHOOL 300 NIB, 1192 SE ANN ARBOR MI 48109-0408 DD 5/1/1986

NAME *Generic/Chemical* *TN=Trade Name*	INDICATION DESIGNATED	SPONSOR AND ADDRESS *DD=Date Designated* *MA=Marketing Approval*
CYSTEAMINE TN=CYSTAGON	TREATMENT OF NEPHROPATHIC CYSTINOSIS.	MYLAN LABORATORIES, INC. 781 CHESTNUT RIDGE ROAD P.O. BOX 4310 MORGANTOWN WV 26504 DD 1/25/1991 MA 8/15/1994
CYSTEAMINE HYDROCHLORIDE	TREATMENT OF CORNEAL CYSTINE CRYSTAL ACCU-MULATION IN CYSTINOSIS PATIENTS.	SIGMA-TAU PHARMACEU-TICALS, INC. 800 SOUTH FREDERICK AVENUE GAITHERSBURG MD 20877 DD 8/19/1997
CYSTIC FIBROSIS TR GENE THERAPY (RECOMBINANT ADE-NOVIRUS) TN=ADGVCFTR.10	TREATMENT OF CYSTIC FIBROSIS.	GENVEC, INC. 12111 PARKLAWN DRIVE ROCKVILLE MD 20852 DD 3/9/1995
CYSTIC FIBROSIS GENE THER-APY	TREATMENT OF CYSTIC FIBROSIS.	GENZYME CORPORATION ONE MOUNTAIN RD. P.O. BOX 9322 FRAMINGHAM MA 01701-9322 DD 6/30/1992
CYSTIC FIBROSIS TRANSMEM-BRANE CONDUCTANCE REGULA-TOR	FOR CYSTIC FIBROSIS TRANSMEMBRANE CONDUC-TANCE REGULATOR PROTEIN REPLACEMENT THER-APY IN CYSTIC FIBROSIS PATIENTS.	GENZYME CORPORATION ONE MOUNTAIN ROAD P.O. BOX 9322 FRAMINGHAM MA 01701-9322 DD 1/14/1992
CYSTIC FIBROSIS TRANSMEM-BRANE CONDUCTANCE REGULA-TOR GENE	TREATMENT OF CYSTIC FIBROSIS.	GENETIC THERAPY, INC. 938 CLOPPER ROAD GAITHERSBURG MD 20878 DD 1/8/1993
CYTARABINE LIPOSOMAL TN=DEPOCYT	TREATMENT OF NEOPLASTIC MENINGITIS.	DEPOTECH CORPORATION 10450 SCIENCE CENTER DRIVE SAN DIEGO CA 92121 DD 6/2/1993 MA 4/1/1999
CYTOMEGALOVIRUS IMMUNE GLOBULIN (HUMAN) TN=CYTOGAM	PREVENTION OR ATTENUATION OF PRIMARY CYTO-MEGALOVIRUS DISEASE IN IMMUNOSUPPRESSED RECIPIENTS OF ORGAN TRANSPLANTS.	MASSACHUSSETTS PUBLIC HEALTH BIOLOGIC LABORATORIES 305 SOUTH STREET BOSTON MA 02130-3597 DD 8/3/1987 MA 12/4/1998
CYTOMEGALOVIRUS IMMUNE GLOBULIN INTRAVENOUS (HU-MAN)	FOR USE IN CONJUNCTION WITH GANCICLOVIR SO-DIUM FOR THE TREATMENT OF CYTOMEGALOVIRUS PNEUMONIA IN BONE MARROW TRANSPLANT PA-TIENTS.	BAYER CORPORATION PHARMACEUTICAL DIVISION, BI-OLOGICAL PRODUCTS 400 MORGAN LANE NEW HAVEN CT 06516 DD 1/28/1991
D-PEPTIDE OF THE SEQUENCE AKRHHGYKRKFH - NH2 TN=PULMADEX	TREATMENT OF CYSTIC FIBROSIS	DEMEGEN, INC. 1051 BRINTON ROAD PITTSBURGH PA 15221 DD 10/23/2002
DHA-PACLITAXEL TN=TAXOPREXIN	TREATMENT OF METASTATIC MALIGNANT MELANO-MA	PROTARGA, INC. 2200 RENAISSANCE BOULEVARD SUITE 450 KING OF PRUSSIA PA 19406 DD 10/10/2002

NAME *Generic/Chemical* *TN=Trade Name*	INDICATION DESIGNATED	SPONSOR AND ADDRESS *DD=Date Designated* *MA=Marketing Approval*
DHA-PACLITAXEL TN=TAXOPREXIN	TREATMENT OF PANCREATIC CANCER	PROTARGA, INC. 2200 RENAISSANCE BLVD. SUITE 450 KING OF PRUSSIA PA 19406 DD 9/25/2001
DMP 777	THERAPEUTIC MANAGEMENT OF PATIENTS WITH LUNG DISEASE ATTRIBUTABLE TO CYSTIC FIBROSIS.	DUPONT PHARMACEUTICALS COMPANY CHESTNUT RUN, MAPLE RUN CENTRE RD. WILMINGTON DE 19805 DD 6/4/1996
DNA-LIPID COMPLEX (DMRIE/ DOPE)/PLASMID VECTOR (VCL-1102, VICAL) EXPRESSING HUMAN INTERLEUKIN-2 TN=LEUVECTIN	TREATMENT OF RENAL CELL CARCINOMA.	VICAL INCORPORATED 9373 TOWNE CENTER DR. SUITE 100 SAN DIEGO CA 92121-3088 DD 4/28/2000
DNP-MODIFIED AUTOLOGOUS TUMOR VACCINE TN=O-VAX	ADJUVANT THERAPY FOR THE TREATMENT OF OVARIAN CANCER	AVAX TECHNOLOGIES, INC. 9200 INDIAN CREEK PARKWAY BUILDING 9, SUITE 200 OVERLAND PARK KS 66210 DD 9/21/2000
DACLIZUMAB TN=ZENAPAX	PREVENTION OF ACUTE RENAL ALLOGRAFT REJECTION.	HOFFMANN-LA ROCHE, INC. 340 KINGSLAND STREET NUTLEY NJ 07110 DD 3/5/1993 MA 12/10/1997
DANTROLENE SODIUM TN=DANTRIUM	TREATMENT OF THE NEUROLEPTIC MALIGNANT SYNDROME.	NORWICH EATON PHARMACEUTICALS P.O. BOX 191 NORWICH NY 13815 DD 12/14/1987
DAPSONE	PROPHYLAXIS OF TOXOPLASMOSIS IN SEVERELY IMMUNOCOMPROMISED PATIENTS WITH CD4 COUNTS BELOW 100.	JACOBUS PHARMACEUTICAL COMPANY, INC. 37 CLEVELAND LANE P.O. BOX 5290 PRINCETON NJ 08540 DD 11/7/1994
DAPSONE USP TN=DAPSONE	FOR THE COMBINATION TREATMENT OF PNEUMOCYSTIS CARINII PNEUMONIA IN CONJUNCTION WITH TRIMETHOPRIM.	JACOBUS PHARMACEUTICAL COMPANY 37 CLEVELAND LANE P.O. BOX 5290 PRINCETON NJ 08540 DD 1/8/1992
DAPSONE USP TN=DAPSONE	PROPHYLAXIS FOR PNEUMOCYSTIS CARINII PNEUMONIA.	JACOBUS PHARMACEUTICAL COMPANY 37 CLEVELAND LANE P.O. BOX 5290 PRINCETON NJ 08540 DD 12/24/1991
DAUNORUBICIN CITRATE LIPOSOME INJECTION TN=DAUNOXOME	TREATMENT OF PATIENTS WITH ADVANCED HIV-ASSOCIATED KAPOSI'S SARCOMA.	NEXSTAR PHARMACEUTICALS, INC. 650 CLIFFSIDE DRIVE SAN DIMAS CA 91773 DD 5/14/1993 MA 4/8/1996

NAME *Generic/Chemical* *TN=Trade Name*	INDICATION DESIGNATED	SPONSOR AND ADDRESS *DD=Date Designated* *MA=Marketing Approval*
DECITABINE	TREATMENT OF CHRONIC MYELOGENOUS LEUKEMIA.	SUPERGEN, INC. 4140 DUBLIN BLVD. SUITE 200 DUBLIN CA 94568 DD 3/8/1999
DECITABINE	TREATMENT OF MYELODYSPLASTIC SYNDROMES.	SUPERGEN, INC. 4140 DUBLIN BLVD.4140 DUBLIN BLVD. SUITE 200 DUBLIN CA 94568 DD 3/8/1999
DEFERASIROX	TREATMENT OF CHRONIC IRON OVERLOAD IN PATIENTS WITH TRANSFUSION-DEPENDENT ANEMIAS	NOVARTIS PHARMACEUTICALS CORPORATION 59 ROUTE 10 EAST HANOVER NJ 07936-1080 DD 11/21/2002
DEFIBROTIDE	TREATMENT OF THROMBOTIC THROMBOCYTOPENIC PURPURA.	CRINOS INTERNATIONAL VIA BELVEDERE 1 VILLA GUARDIA, ITALY 22079 DD 7/5/1985
DEFIBROTIDE	FOR THE TREATMENT OF HEPATIC VENO-OCCLUSIVE DISEASE.	GENTIUM SPA PIAZZA XX VILLA SETTEMBRE, 2 GUARDIA (CO) ITALY 22079 DD 5/21/2003
DEHYDROEPIANDROSTERONE	TREATMENT OF SYSTEMIC LUPUS ERYTHEMATOSUS (SLE) AND THE REDUCTION IN THE USE OF STEROIDS IN STEROID-DEPENDENT SLE PATIENTS.	GENELABS TECHNOLOGIES, INC. 505 PENOBSCOT DRIVE REDWOOD CITY CA 94063 DD 7/13/1994
DEHYDROEPIANDROSTERONE SULFATE SODIUM	TREATMENT OF SERIOUS BURNS REQUIRING HOSPITALIZATION.	PHARMADIGM, INC. 2401 FOOTHILL DRIVE SALT LAKE CITY UT 84109-1405 DD 1/29/1997
DEHYDROEPIANDROSTERONE SULFATE SODIUM	TO ACCELERATE THE RE-EPITHELIALIZATION OF DONOR SITES IN THOSE HOSPITALIZED BURN PATIENTS WHO MUST UNDERGO AUTOLOGOUS SKIN GRAFTING.	PHARMADIGM, INC. 2401 FOOTHILL DRIVE SALT LAKE CITY UT 84109-1405 DD 1/28/1997
DENILEUKIN DIFTITOX TN=ONTAK	TREATMENT OF PATIENTS WITH PERSISTENT OR RECURRENT CUTANEOUS T-CELL LYMPHOMA WHOSE MALIGNANT CELLS EXPRESS THE CD25 COMPONENT OF THE IL-2 RECEPTOR.	LIGAND PHARMACEUTICALS INC. 10275 SCIENCE CENTER DRIVE SAN DIEGO CA 92121 DD 8/21/1996 MA 2/5/1999
DEOXYRIBOSE, PHOSPHOROTHIOATE	TREATMENT OF ADVANCED MALIGNANT MELANOMA (STAGES II,III, IV).	GENTA, INC. 99 HAYDEN AVE., SUITE 200 LEXINGTON MA 02421-7966 DD 7/31/2000
DESLORELIN TN=SOMAGARD		ROBERTS PHARMACEUTICAL CORP. MERIDIAN CENTER II FOUR INDUSTRIAL WAY WEST EATONTOWN NJ 07724-2274 DD 11/5/1987

NAME Generic/Chemical TN=Trade Name	INDICATION DESIGNATED	SPONSOR AND ADDRESS DD=Date Designated MA=Marketing Approval
DESMOPRESSIN ACETATE	TREATMENT OF MILD HEMOPHILIA A AND VON WILL-EBRAND'S DISEASE.	AVENTIS BEHRING L.L.C. 1020 FIRST AVENUE PO BOX 61501 KING OF PRUSSIA PA 19406-0901 DD 1/22/1991 MA 3/7/1994
DEXAMETHASONE	FOR USE IN POSTERIOR SEGMENT DRUG DELIVERY SYSTEM IN THE TREATMENT OF IDIOPATHIC INTER-MEDIATE UVEITIS.	OCULEX PHARMACEUTICALS, INC. 639 N. PASTORIA AVENUE SUNNYVALE CA 94086-2917 DD 9/11/1998
DEXRAZOXANE TN=ZINECARD	FOR THE PREVENTION OF CARDIOMYOPATHY ASSO-CIATED WITH DOXORUBICIN ADMINISTRATION.	PHARMACIA & UPJOHN 7000 PORTAGE ROAD KALAMAZOO MI 49001-0199 DD 12/17/1991 MA 5/26/1995
DEXTRAN 70 TN=DEHYDREX	TREATMENT OF RECURRENT CORNEAL EROSION UN-RESPONSIVE TO CONVENTIONAL THERAPY.	HOLLES LABORATORIES, INC. 30 FOREST NOTCH COHASSET MA 02025 DD 3/5/1990
DEXTRAN AND DEFEROXAMINE TN=BIO-RESCUE	TREATMENT OF ACUTE IRON POISONING.	BIOMEDICAL FRONTIERS, INC. 1095 10TH AVENUE S.E. MINNEAPOLIS MN 55414 DD 3/8/1991
DEXTRAN SULFATE (INHALED, AEROSOLIZED) TN=UENDEX	FOR USE AS AN ADJUNCT TO THE TREATMENT OF CYSTIC FIBROSIS.	KENNEDY & HOIDAL, M.D.'S UNIVERSITY OF UTAH MEDICAL CENTER 50 NORTH MEDICAL DRIVE, ROOM 4R240 SALT LAKE CITY UT 84132 DD 10/5/1990
DEXTRAN SULFATE SODIUM	TREATMENT OF AQUIRED IMMUNODEFICIENCY SYN-DROME.	UENO FINE CHEMICALS INDUSTRY, LTD. 2-31 KORAIBASHI, HIGASHI-KU OSAKA 541, JAPAN DD 11/19/1987
DHA-PACLITAXEL TN=TAXOPREXIN	TREATMENT OF ADENOCARCINOMA OF THE STO-MACH OR LOWER ESOPHAGUS.	PROTARGA, INC. 2200 RENAISSANCE BOULEVARD SUITE 450 KING OF PRUSSIA, PA 19406 DD 5/1/2003
DIANEAL PERITONEAL DIALYSIS SOLUTION WITH 1.1% AMINO ACIDS TN=NUTRINEAL (PERITONEAL DIALYSIS SOLUTION WITH 1.1% AMINO ACID	FOR USE AS A NUTRITIONAL SUPPLEMENT FOR THE TREATMENT OF MALNOURISHMENT IN PATIENTS UN-DERGOING CONTINUOUS AMBULATORY PERITONEAL DIALYSIS.	BAXTER HEALTHCARE CORPORATION 1620 WAUKEGAN ROAD MCGAW PARK IL 60085 DD 6/11/1992
DIAZEPAM VISCOUS SOLUTION FOR RECTAL ADMINISTRATION	FOR THE MANAGEMENT OF SELECTED, REFRAC-TORY, PATIENTS WITH EPILEPSY, ON STABLE REGI-MENS OF ANTIEPILEPTIC DRUGS (AEDS), WHO REQUIRE INTERMITTENT USE OF DIAZEPAM TO CON-TROL BOUTS OF INCREASED SEIZURE ACTIVITY.	ATHENA NEUROSCIENCES, INC. 800F GATEWAY BOULEVARD SOUTH SAN FRANCISCO CA 94080 DD 2/25/1992 MA 7/29/1997
DIAZIQUONE	TREATMENT OF PRIMARY BRAIN MALIGNANCIES (GRADE III AND IV ASTROCYTOMAS).	WARNER-LAMBERT COMPANY 2800 PLYMOUTH RD., P.O. BOX 1047 ANN ARBOR MI 48106 DD 11/10/1983

NAME *Generic/Chemical* *TN=Trade Name*	INDICATION DESIGNATED	SPONSOR AND ADDRESS *DD=Date Designated* *MA=Marketing Approval*
DIDEOXYINOSINE	TREATMENT OF ACQUIRED IMMUNODEFICIENCY SYNDROME.	BRISTOL-MYERS SQUIBB DD 6/22/1988
DIETHYLDITHIOCARBAMATE TN=IMUTHIOL	TREATMENT OF AIDS.	CONNAUGHT LABORATORIES ROUTE 611, P.O. BOX 187 SWIFTWATER PA 18370 DD 4/3/1986
DIFERULOYLMETHANE	TREATMENT OF CYSTIC FIBROSIS.	SEER PHARMACEUTICALS, LLC P.O. BOX 138 SOUTHPORT, CT 06890 DD 6/13/2003
DIGOXIN IMMUNE FAB (OVINE) TN=DIGIBIND	TREATMENT OF POTENTIALLY LIFE THREATENING DIGITALIS INTOXICATION IN PATIENTS WHO ARE REFRACTORY TO MANAGEMENT BY CONVENTIONAL THERAPY.	GLAXO WELLCOME INC. 5 MOORE DRIVE RESEARCH TRIANGLE PARK NC 27709 DD 11/1/1984 MA 4/22/1986
DIGOXIN IMMUNE FAB(OVINE) TN=DIGIDOTE	TREATMENT OF LIFE-THREATENING ACUTE CARDIAC GLYCOSIDE INTOXICATION MANIFESTED BY CONDUCTION DISORDERS, ECTOPIC VENTRICULAR ACTIVITY AND (IN SOME CASES) HYPERKALEMIA.	BOEHRINGER MANNHEIM CORP. 1301 PICCARD DRIVE ROCKVILLE MD 20850 DD 3/11/1985
DIHYDROTESTOSTERONE TN=ANDROGEL -DHT	TREATMENT OF WEIGHT LOSS IN AIDS PATIENTS WITH HIV-ASSOCIATED WASTING.	UNIMED PHARMACEUTICALS, INC. FOUR PARKWAY NORTH DEERFIELD IL 60015-2544 DD 2/5/1996
DIMETHYL SULFOXIDE	TREATMENT OF INCREASED INTRACRANIAL PRESSURE IN PATIENTS WITH SEVERE, CLOSED-HEAD INJURY, ALSO KNOWN AS TRAUMATIC BRAIN COMA, FOR WHOM NO OTHER EFFECTIVE TREATMENT IS AVAILABLE.	PHARMA 21 C/O UNIV. OF CALIF., SAN DIEGO 9500 GILMAN DR. LA JOLLA CA 92093-0624 DD 11/22/1994
DIMETHYL SULFOXIDE	TREATMENT OF CUTANEOUS MANIFESTATIONS OF SCLERODERMA.	RESEARCH INDUSTRIES CORP. DD 6/6/1986
DIMETHYLSULFOXIDE	TOPICAL TREATMENT FOR THE PREVENTION OF SOFT TISSUE INJURY FOLLOWING EXTRAVASTION OF CYTOTOXIC DRUGS.	CANCER TECHNOLOGIES, INC. 7301 EAST 22ND STREET SUITE 10E TUCSON AZ 85710 DD 4/15/1997
DIMETHYLSULFOXIDE	TREATMENT OF PALMAR-PLANTAR ERYTHRODYSETHESIA SYNDROME.	CANCER TECHNOLOGIES, INC. 7301 EAST 22ND STREET SUITE 10E TUCSON AZ 85710 DD 4/6/1998
DIPALMITOYLPHOSPHATIDYL-CHOLINE /PHOSPHATIDYLGLY-CEROL TN=ALEC	PREVENTION AND TREATMENT OF NEONATAL RESPIRATORY DISTRESS SYNDROME.	FORUM PRODUCTS, INC. 33 FLYING POINT ROAD SOUTHAMPTON NY 11968 DD 7/28/1988
DIPHENYLCYCLOPENONE	TREATMENT OF CHRONIC SEVERE FORMS OF ALOPECIA AREATA (ALOPECIA TOTALIS [AT]/ALOPECIA UNIVERSALIS [AU]).	LLOYD E. KING, JR. 1900 PATTERSON STREET SUITE 104 NASHVILLE, TN 37203 DD 6/13/2003

NAME *Generic/Chemical* *TN=Trade Name*	INDICATION DESIGNATED	SPONSOR AND ADDRESS *DD=Date Designated* *MA=Marketing Approval*
DISACCHARIDE TRIPEPTIDE GLYCEROL DIPALMITOYL TN=IMMTHER	TREATMENT OF PULMONARY AND HEPATIC METAS-TASES IN PATIENTS WITH COLORECTAL ADENOCAR-CINOMA.	IMMUNOTHERAPEUTICS, INC. 3505 RIVERVIEW CIRCLE MOORHEAD MN 56560 DD 3/1/1990
DISODIUM CLODRONATE	TREATMENT OF HYPERCALCEMIA OF MALIGNANCY.	DISCOVERY EXPERIMENTAL & DEVELOPMENT, INC. 29949 S.R. 54 WEST WESLEY CHAPEL FL 33543 DD 6/16/1993
DISODIUM CLODRONATE TETRA-HYDRATE TN=BONEFOS	TREATMENT OF INCREASED BONE RESORPTION DUE TO MALIGNANCY.	ANTHRA PHARMACEUTICALS, INC. 103 CARNEGIE CENTER, SUITE 102 PRINCETON NJ 08540 DD 3/5/1990
DISODIUM SILIBININ DIHEMISUC-CINATE TN=LEGALON	TREATMENT OF HEPATIC INTOXICATION BY AMANITA PHALLOIDES (MUSHROOM POISONING).	PHARMAQUEST CORPORATION 4470 REDWOOD HIGHWAY SAN RAFAEL CA 94903 DD 7/10/1986
DORNASE ALFA TN=PULMOZYME	TO REDUCE MUCOUS VISCOSITY AND ENABLE THE CLEARANCE OF AIRWAY SECRETIONS IN PATIENTS WITH CYSTIC FIBROSIS.	GENENTECH, INC. 460 POINT SAN BRUNO BOULEVARD SOUTH SAN FRANCISCO CA 94080 DD 1/16/1991 MA 12/30/1993
DOXORUBICIN LIPOSOME TN=DOXIL	TREATMENT OF OVARIAN CANCER.	ALZA CORPORATION 1550 PLYMOUTH ST. PO BOX 7210 MOUNTAIN VIEW CA 94039-7210 DD 11/4/1998 MA 6/28/1999
DRONABINOL TN=MARINOL	FOR THE STIMULATION OF APPETITE AND PREVEN-TION OF WEIGHT LOSS IN PATIENTS WITH A CON-FIRMED DIAGNOSIS OF AIDS.	UNIMED PHARMACEUTICALS, INC. 2150 EAST LAKE COOK ROAD, SUITE 210 BUFFALO GROVE IL 60089-1862 DD 1/15/1991 MA 12/22/1992
DURAMYCIN	TREATMENT OF CYSTIC FIBROSIS.	MOLICHEM MEDICINES INC. 207 SOUTH ELLIOTT ROAD PMB#231 CHAPEL HILL NC 27514 DD 12/11/1997
DYNAMINE	TREATMENT OF LAMBERT EATON MYASTHENIC SYN-DROME.	MAYO FOUNDATION 200 FIRST STREET SOUTHWEST ROCHESTER MN 55905 DD 2/5/1990
DYNAMINE	TREATMENT OF HEREDITARY MOTOR AND SENSORY NEUROPATHY TYPE I (CHARCOT-MARIE-TOOTH DIS-EASE).	MAYO FOUNDATION 200 FIRST STREET SOUTHWEST ROCHESTER MN 55905 DD 10/16/1991

NAME *Generic/Chemical* *TN=Trade Name*	INDICATION DESIGNATED	SPONSOR AND ADDRESS *DD=Date Designated* *MA=Marketing Approval*
EFLORNITHINE HCL TN=ORNIDYL	TREATMENT OF PNEUMOCYSTIS CARINII PNEUMONIA IN AIDS PATIENTS.	MARION MERRELL DOW, INC. P.O. BOX 9627 KANSAS CITY MO 64134 DD 4/18/1986
EFLORNITHINE HCL TN=ORNIDYL	TREATMENT OF TRYPANOSOMA BRUCEI GAMBIENSE INFECTION (SLEEPING SICKNESS).	HOECHST MARION ROUSSEL P.O. BOX 9627 KANSAS CITY MO 64134 DD 4/23/1986 MA 11/28/1990
ELCATONIN	INTRATHECAL TREATMENT OF INTRACTABLE PAIN.	INNAPHARMA, INC. 10 MOUNTAINVIEW ROAD UPPER SADDLE RIVER NJ 07458 DD 9/25/1995
ENADOLINE HYDROCHLORIDE	TREATMENT OF SEVERE HEAD INJURY.	WARNER-LAMBERT COMPANY PARKE-DAVIS PHARMACEUTI-CAL RESEARCH DIVISION 2800 PLYMOUTH ROAD ANN ARBOR MI 48105 DD 1/28/1997
ENCAPSULATED PORCINE ISLET PREPARATION TN=BETARX	TREATMENT OF TYPE I DIABETIC PATIENTS WHO ARE ALREADY ON IMMUNOSUPPRESSION.	VIVORX 2825 SANTA MONICA BLVD. 2ND FLOOR SANTA MONICA CA 90404-2429 DD 7/5/1995
ENISOPROST	FOR USE WITH CYCLOSPORINE IN ORGAN TRANS-PLANT RECIPIENTS TO REDUCE ACUTE TRANSPLANT REJECTION.	G.D. SEARLE & COMPANY 4901 SEARLE PARKWAY SKOKIE IL 60077 DD 10/20/1989
ENISOPROST	FOR USE IN ORGAN TRANSPLANT PATIENTS TO DI-MINISH THE NEPHROTOXICITY INDUCED BY CYCLOS-PORINE.	G.D. SEARLE & COMPANY 4901 SEARLE PARKWAY SKOKIE IL 60077 DD 10/20/1989
EPIDERMAL GROWTH FACTOR (HUMAN)	FOR ACCELERATION OF CORNEAL EPITHELIAL RE-GENERATION AND THE HEALING OF STROMAL TIS-SUE IN THE CONDITION OF NON-HEALING CORNEAL DEFECTS.	CHIRON VISION 500 IOLAB DRIVE CLAREMONT CA 91711 DD 10/5/1987
EPIDERMAL GROWTH FACTOR (HUMAN)	FOR PROMOTION OF CUTANEOUS WOUND HEALING IN EXTREME BURN TREATMENT PROTOCOLS.	ETHICON, INC. P.O. BOX 151 SOMERVILLE NJ 08876 DD 3/6/1985
EPIRUBICIN TN=ELLENCE	TREATMENT OF BREAST CANCER.	PHARMACIA & UPJOHN COMPANY 0634-298-113 7000 PORTAGE RD. KALAMAZOO MI 49001-0199 DD 9/14/1999 MA 9/15/1999
EPOETIN ALFA TN=EPOGEN	TREATMENT OF ANEMIA ASSOCIATED WITH HIV IN-FECTION OR HIV TREATMENT.	AMGEN, INC. 1840 DEHAVILLAND DRIVE THOUSAND OAKS CA 91320 DD 7/1/1991 MA 12/31/1990

NAME Generic/Chemical TN=Trade Name	INDICATION DESIGNATED	SPONSOR AND ADDRESS DD=Date Designated MA=Marketing Approval
EPOETIN ALFA TN=EPOGEN	TREATMENT OF ANEMIA ASSOCIATED WITH END STAGE RENAL DISEASE.	AMGEN, INC. 1840 DEHAVILLAND DRIVE THOUSAND OAKS CA 91320 DD 4/10/1986 MA 6/1/1989
EPOETIN ALFA	TREATMENT OF MYELODYSPLASTIC SYNDROME.	R. W. JOHNSON PHARMACEUTI-CAL RESEARCH INSTITUTE ROUTE 202, P.O. BOX 300 RARITAN NJ 08869-0602 DD 12/20/1993
EPOETIN ALPHA TN=PROCRIT	TREATMENT OF ANEMIA ASSOCIATED WITH END STAGE RENAL DISEASE.	R. W. JOHNSON PHARMACEUTI-CAL RESEARCH INSTITUTE ROUTE 202 SOUTH P.O. BOX 300 RARITAN NJ 08869 DD 8/27/1987
EPOETIN ALPHA TN=PROCRIT	TREATMENT OF HIV ASSOCIATED ANEMIA RELATED TO HIV INFECTION OR HIV TREATMENT.	R. W. JOHNSON PHARMACEUTI-CAL RESEARCH INSTITUTE ROUTE 202, P.O. BOX 300 RARITAN NJ 08869 DD 3/7/1989
EPOETIN ALPHA TN=PROCRIT	TREATMENT OF ANEMIA OF PREMATURITY IN PRE-TERM INFANTS.	R. W. JOHNSON PHARMACEUTI-CAL RESEARCH INSTITUTE ROUTE 202, P.O. BOX 300 RARITAN NJ 08869-0602 DD 7/21/1988
EPOETIN BETA TN=MAROGEN	TREATMENT OF ANEMIA ASSOCIATED WITH END STAGE RENAL DISEASE.	CHUGAI-USA, INC. 3780 HAWTHORN COURT WAUKEGAN IL 60087 DD 10/22/1987
EPOPROSTENOL TN=FLOLAN	TREATMENT OF PRIMARY PULMONARY HYPERTEN-SION.	GLAXO WELLCOME INC. 5 MOORE DRIVE RESEARCH TRIANGLE PARK NC 27709 DD 9/25/1985 MA 9/20/1995
EPOPROSTENOL TN=FLOLAN	REPLACEMENT OF HEPARIN IN PATIENTS REQUIRING HEMODIALYSIS AND WHO ARE AT INCREASED RISK OF HEMORRHAGE.	GLAXO WELLCOME INC. 5 MOORE DRIVE RESEARCH TRIANGLE PARK NC 27709 DD 3/29/1984
EPOPROSTENOL TN=FLOLAN	TREATMENT OF SECONDARY PULMONARY HYPER-TENSION DUE TO INTRINSIC PRECAPILLARY PUL-MONARY VASCULAR DISEASE.	GLAXOSMITHKLINE FIVE MOORE DR. PO BOX 13398 RESEARCH TRIANGLE PARK NC 27709-3398 DD 3/22/1999 MA 4/14/2000
EPOPROSTENOL TN=CYCLOPROSTIN	REPLACEMENT OF HEPARIN IN PATIENTS REQUIRING HEMODIALYSIS AND WHO ARE AT INCREASED RISK OF HEMORRHAGE.	UPJOHN COMPANY 301 HENRIETTA STREET KALAMAZOO MI 49001 DD 10/29/1984
ERWINIA L-ASPARAGINASE TN=ERWINASE	TREATMENT OF ACUTE LYMPHOCYTIC LEUKEMIA.	PORTON INTERNATIONAL, INC. 7114 SPRINGBROOK TERRACE, #200 SPOTSYLVANIA VA 22553 DD 7/30/1986

NAME *Generic/Chemical* *TN=Trade Name*	INDICATION DESIGNATED	SPONSOR AND ADDRESS *DD=Date Designated* *MA=Marketing Approval*
ERWINIA L-ASPARAGINASE	FOR USE AS AN ALTERNATIVE TO E. COLI ASPARAGI-NASE IN THOSE SITUATIONS WHERE REPEAT COURSES OF ASPARAGINASE THERAPY FOR ACUTE LYMPHOBLASTIC LEUKEMIA ARE REQUIRED OR WHERE ALLERGIC REACTIONS FORCE THE DISCON-TINUANCE OF THE E. COLI PREPARATION.	LYPHOMED, INC. DD 1/25/1985
ERYTHROPOIETIN (HUMAN, RE-COMBINANT)	TREATMENT OF ANEMIA ASSOCIATED WITH END STAGE RENAL DISEASE.	ORGANON TEKNIKA CORPORATION DD 11/19/1987
ERYTHROPOIETIN (RECOMBI-NANT HUMAN)	TREATMENT OF ANEMIA ASSOCIATED WITH END STAGE RENAL DISEASE.	MCDONNELL DOUGLAS CORP P.O. BOX 516, 107/2 MS10 ST. LOUIS MO 63166 DD 8/19/1987
ETANERCEPT TN=ENBREL	TREATMENT OF WEGENER'S GRANULOMATOSIS.	IMMUNEX CORPORATION 51 UNIVERSITY STREET SEATTLE WA 98101-2936 DD 4/6/1999
ETANERCEPT TN=ENBREL	REDUCTION IN SIGNS AND SYMPTOMS OF MODER-ATELY TO SEVERELY ACTIVE POLYARTICULAR-COURSE JUVENILE RHEUMATOID ARTHRITIS IN PA-TIENTS WHO HAVE HAD AN INADEQUATE RESPONSE TO ONE OR MORE DISEASE-MODIFYING ANTI-RHEU-MATIC DRUGS.	IMMUNEX CORPORATION 51 UNIVERSITY ST. SEATTLE WA 98101-2936 DD 10/27/1998 MA 5/27/1999
ETHANOLAMINE OLEATE TN=ETHAMOLIN	TREATMENT OF PATIENTS WITH ESOPHAGEAL VARICES THAT HAVE RECENTLY BLED, TO PREVENT REBLEEDING.	BLOCK DRUG COMPANY, INC. 257 CORNELISON AVENUE JERSEY CITY NJ 07302 DD 3/22/1984 MA 12/22/1988
ETHINYL ESTRADIOL, USP	TREATMENT OF TURNER'S SYNDROME.	BIO-TECHNOLOGY GENERAL CORP. 70 WOOD AVENUE, SOUTH ISELIN NJ 08830 DD 6/22/1988
ETHIOFOS	USE AS A CHEMOPROTECTIVE AGENT FOR CISPLA-TIN AND CYCLOPHOSPHAMIDE IN THE TREATMENT OF OVARIAN CANCER.	U.S. BIOSCIENCE DD 8/1/1989
ETHYL EICOSAPENTAENOATE	TREATMENT OF HUNTINGTON'S DISEASE.	LAXDALE LTD. KINGS PARK HOUSE, LAURELHILL BUSINESS PARK POLMAISE ROAD, STIRLING FK7 9JQ UNITED KINGDOM UK DD 4/6/2000
ETIDRONATE DISODIUM TN=DIDRONEL IV INFUSION	PREVENTION OF DEGENERATIVE METABOLIC BONE DISEASE OCCURRING IN PATIENTS WHO REQUIRE LONG TERM (6 MONTHS OR GREATER) TOTAL PAR-ENTERAL NUTRITION.	MGI PHARMA, INC. 6300 WEST OLD SHAKOPPE RD. SUITE 110 BLOOMINGTON MN 55438-2318 DD 5/2/1991
ETIDRONATE DISODIUM TN=DIDRONEL	TREATMENT OF HYPERCALCEMIA OF MALIGNANCY INADEQUATELY MANAGED BY DIETARY MODIFICA-TION AND/OR ORAL HYDRATION.	MGI PHARMA, INC. 6300 WEST OLD SHAKOPPE RD. SUITE 110 BLOOMINGTON MN 55438-2318 DD 3/21/1986 MA 4/21/1987

NAME *Generic/Chemical* *TN=Trade Name*	INDICATION DESIGNATED	SPONSOR AND ADDRESS *DD=Date Designated* *MA=Marketing Approval*
ETIDRONATE DISODIUM TN=DIDRONEL IV INFUSION	TREATMENT OF DEGENERATIVE METABOLIC BONE DISEASE OCCURRING IN PATIENTS WHO REQUIRE LONG TERM (6 MONTHS OR GREATER) TOTAL PARENTERAL NUTRITION.	MGI PHARMA, INC. 6300 WEST OLD SHAKOPPE RD. SUITE 110 BLOOMINGTON MN 55438-2318 DD 5/2/1991
ETIOCHOLANEDIONE	TREATMENT OF PRADER-WILLI SYNDROME.	SUPERGEN, INC. TWO ANNABEL LANE, SUITE 220 SAN RAMON CA 94583 DD 5/7/1996
ETIOCHOLANEDIONE	TREATMENT OF APLASTIC ANEMIA.	SUPERGEN, INC. TWO ANNABEL LANE, SUITE 220 SUITE 10 SAN RAMON CA 94583 DD 11/3/1995
EXEMESTANE TN=AROMASIN	TREATMENT OF ADVANCED BREAST CANCER IN POSTMENOPAUSAL WOMEN WHOSE DISEASE HAS PROGRESSED FOLLOWING TAMOXIFEN THERAPY.	PHARMACIA & UPJOHN 7000 PORTAGE ROAD MAIL STOP: 0636-298-113 KALAMAZOO MI 49001-0199 DD 9/19/1991 MA 10/21/1999
EXISULIND	FOR THE SUPPRESSION AND CONTROL OF COLONIC ADENOMATOUS POLYPS IN THE INHERITED DISEASE ADENOMATOUS POLYPOSIS COLI.	CELL PATHWAYS, INC. 702 ELECTRONIC DRIVE HORSHAM PA 19044 DD 2/14/1994
FIAU	ADJUNCTIVE TREATMENT OF CHRONIC ACTIVE HEPATITIS B.	OCLASSEN PHARMACEUTICALS, INC. 100 PELICAN WAY SAN RAFAEL CA 94901 DD 7/24/1992
FACTOR XIII, RECOMBINANT	TREATMENT OF CONGENITAL FACTOR XIII DEFICIENCY.	ZYMOGENETICS, INC. 4225 ROOSEVELT WAY SEATTLE WA 98105 DD 4/22/1993
FACTOR XIII [A2] HOMODIMER, RECOMBINANT DNA ORIGIN	TREATMENT OF CONGENITAL FXIII DEFICIENCY.	ZYMOGENETICS, INC. 1201 EASTLAKE AVENUE EAST SEATTLE WA 98102 DD 5/21/2003
FAMPRIDINE TN=NEURELAN	RELIEF OF SYMPTOMS OF MULTIPLE SCLEROSIS.	ACORDA THERAPEUTICS 15 SKYLINE DR. HAWTHORNE NY 10532 DD 6/2/1987
FAMPRIDINE TN=NEURELAN	TREATMENT OF CHRONIC, INCOMPLETE SPINAL CORD INJURY.	ACORDA THERAPEUTICS, INC. 15 SKYLINE DR. HAWTHORNE NY 10532 DD 6/2/1997
FELBAMATE TN=FELBATOL	TREATMENT OF LENNOX-GASTAUT SYNDROME.	WALLACE LABORATORIES 301B COLLEGE ROAD EAST PRINCETON NJ 08540 DD 1/24/1989 MA 7/29/1993
FERRIC HEXACYANOFERRATE (II) "PRUSSIAN BLUE"	TREATMENT OF PATIENTS WITH KNOWN OR SUSPECTED INTERNAL CONTAMINATION WITH RADIOACTIVE OR NON-RADIOACTIVE CESIUM OR THALLIUM.	DEGUSSA AG WEISSFRAUENSTR.9 FRANKFURT GERMANY D-60287 DD 6/26/2003

NAME *Generic/Chemical* *TN=Trade Name*	**INDICATION DESIGNATED**	SPONSOR AND ADDRESS *DD=Date Designated* *MA=Marketing Approval*
FIBRINOGEN (HUMAN)	FOR THE CONTROL OF BLEEDING AND PROPHYLACTIC TREATMENT OF PATIENTS DEFICIENT IN FIBRINOGEN.	ALPHA THERAPEUTIC CORPORATION 5555 VALLEY BOULEVARD LOS ANGELES CA 90032 DD 8/23/1995
FIBRONECTIN (HUMAN PLASMA DERIVED)	TREATMENT OF NON-HEALING CORNEAL ULCERS OR EPITHELIAL DEFECTS WHICH HAVE BEEN UNRESPONSIVE TO CONVENTIONAL THERAPY AND THE UNDERLYING CAUSE HAS BEEN ELIMINATED.	MELVILLE BIOLOGICS, INC. 310 EAST 67TH STREET NEW YORK NY 10021 DD 9/5/1988
FIBRONECTIN (PLASMA DERIVED)	TREATMENT OF NON-HEALING CORNEAL ULCERS OR EPITHELIAL DEFECTS WHICH ARE UNRESPONSIVE TO CONVENTIONAL THERAPY AND FOR WHICH ANY INFECTIOUS CAUSE OF THE DEFECT HAS BEEN ELIMINATED.	CHIRON VISION 9342 JERONIMO ROAD IRVINE CA 92718 DD 12/5/1988
FILGRASTIM TN=NEUPOGEN	FOR USE IN THE MOBILIZATION OF PERIPHERAL BLOOD PROGENITOR CELLS FOR COLLECTION IN PATIENTS WHO WILL RECEIVE MYELOABLATIVE OR MYELOSUPPRESSIVE CHEMOTHERAPY.	AMGEN, INC. 1840 DEHAVILLAND DRIVE THOUSAND OAKS CA 91320 DD 7/17/1995 MA 12/28/1995
FILGRASTIM TN=NEUPOGEN	TREATMENT OF PATIENTS WITH SEVERE CHRONIC NEUTROPENIA (ABSOLUTE NEUTROPHIL COUNT LESS THAN 500/MM3).	AMGEN, INC. 1840 DEHAVILLAND DRIVE THOUSAND OAKS CA 91320 DD 11/7/1990 MA 12/19/1994
FILGRASTIM TN=NEUPOGEN	TREATMENT OF MYELODYSPLASTIC SYNDROME.	AMGEN, INC. 1840 DEHAVILLAND DRIVE THOUSAND OAKS CA 91320 DD 8/30/1990
FILGRASTIM TN=NEUPOGEN	REDUCTION IN THE DURATION OF NEUTROPENIA, FEVER, ANTIBIOTIC USE, AND HOSPITALIZATION, FOLLOWING INDUCTION AND CONSOLIDATION TREATMENT FOR ACUTE MYELOID LEUKEMIA.	AMGEN, INC. ONE AMGEN CENTER DR. THOUSAND OAKS CA 91320-1799 DD 11/7/1996 MA 4/2/1998
FILGRASTIM TN=NEUPOGEN	TREATMENT OF NEUTROPENIA ASSOCIATED WITH BONE MARROW TRANSPLANTS.	AMGEN, INC. 1840 DEHAVILLAND DRIVE THOUSAND OAKS CA 91320 DD 10/1/1990 MA 6/15/1994
FILGRASTIM TN=NEUPOGEN	TREATMENT OF PATIENTS WITH AIDS WHO, IN ADDITION, ARE AFFLICTED WITH CYTOMEGALOVIRUS RETINITIS AND ARE BEING TREATED WITH GANCICLOVIR.	AMGEN, INC. ONE AMGEN CENTER DR. THOUSAND OAKS CA 91320-1799 DD 9/3/1991
FLUCINOLONE	TREATMENT UVEITIS INVOLVING THE POSTERIOR SEGMENT OF THE EYE.	BAUSCH & LOMB PHARMACEUTICALS, INC. 8500 HIDDEN RIVER PARKWAY TAMPA FL 33637 DD 7/31/2000
FLUDARABINE PHOSPHATE TN=FLUDARA	TREATMENT AND MANAGEMENT OF PATIENTS WITH NON-HODGKINS LYMPHOMA.	BERLEX LABORATORIES, INC. 15049 SAN PABLO AVENUE P.O. BOX 4099 RICHMOND CA 94804-0099 DD 4/18/1989

NAME *Generic/Chemical* *TN=Trade Name*	INDICATION DESIGNATED	SPONSOR AND ADDRESS *DD=Date Designated* *MA=Marketing Approval*
FLUDARABINE PHOSPHATE TN=FLUDARA	TREATMENT OF CHRONIC LYMPHOCYTIC LEUKEMIA (CLL), INCLUDING REFRACTORY CLL.	BERLEX LABORATORIES, INC. 15049 SAN PABLO AVENUE, P.O. BOX 4099 RICHMOND CA 94804 DD 4/18/1989 MA 4/18/1991
FLUMECINOL TN=ZIXORYN	TREATMENT OF HYPERBILIRUBINEMIA IN NEWBORN INFANTS UNRESPONSIVE TO PHOTOTHERAPY.	FARMACON, INC. POST HOUSE, SUITE 213 1720 POST ROAD EAST WESTPORT CT 06880-5643 DD 1/15/1985
FLUNARIZINE TN=SIBELIUM	TREATMENT OF ALTERNATING HEMIPLEGIA.	JANSSEN RESEARCH FOUNDATION P.O. BOX 200 TITUSVILLE NJ 08560 DD 1/6/1986
FLUOROURACIL	FOR USE IN COMBINATION WITH INTERFERON ALPHA-2A, RECOMBINANT, FOR THE TREATMENT OF ESOPHAGEAL CARCINOMA.	HOFFMANN-LA ROCHE, INC. 340 KINGSLAND STREET NUTLEY NJ 07110-1199 DD 10/27/1989
FLUOROURACIL TN=ADRUCIL	FOR USE IN COMBINATION WITH LEUCOVORIN FOR THERAPY OF METASTATIC ADENOCARCINOMA OF THE COLON AND RECTUM.	LEDERLE LABORATORIES DIVISION OF AMERICAN CYANAMID COMPANY 401 N. MIDDLETOWN ROAD PEARL RIVER NY 10965 DD 2/6/1989
FLUOROURACIL	FOR USE IN COMBINATION WITH INTERFERON ALPHA-2A, RECOMBINANT, FOR THE TREATMENT OF ADVANCED COLORECTAL CARCINOMA.	HOFFMANN-LA ROCHE, INC. 340 KINGSLAND STREET NUTLEY NJ 07110-1199 DD 4/18/1990
FLUOROURACIL	TREATMENT OF GLIOBLASTOMA MULTIFORME.	ETHYPHARM SA 194 BUREAUX DE LA COLLINE - BATIMENT D 92213 SAINT-CLOUD CEDEX FRANCE FR DD 6/29/2000
FLUOXETINE TN=PROZAC	TREATMENT OF AUTISM.	HOLLANDER, MD, ERIC MT. SINAI SCHOOL OF MEDICINE, DEPT. OF PSYCHIATRY BOX 1230, ONE GUSTAVE L. LEVY PLACE NEW YORK NY 10029-6574 DD 4/30/1999
FOLLITROPIN ALFA, RECOMBINANT TN=GONAL-F	FOR THE INITIATION AND RE-INITIATION OF SPERMATOGENESIS IN ADULT MALES WITH REPRODUCTIVE FAILURE DUE TO HYPOTHALAMIC OR PITUITARY DYSFUNCTION, HYPOGONADOTROPIC HYPOGONADISM. AMENDED INDICATION 6/27/00: FOR THE INDUCTION OF SPERMATOGENESIS IN MEN WITH PR	SERONO LABORATORIES, INC. 100 LONGWATER CIRCLE NORWELL MA 02061 DD 12/21/1998 MA 5/24/2000
FOMEPIZOLE TN=ANTIZOLE	TREATMENT OF METHANOL OR ETHYLENE GLYCOL POISONING.	ORPHAN MEDICAL, INC. 13911 RIDGEDALE DRIVE SUITE 250 MINNETONKA MN 55305 DD 12/22/1988 MA 12/8/2000

NAME *Generic/Chemical* *TN=Trade Name*	INDICATION DESIGNATED	SPONSOR AND ADDRESS *DD=Date Designated* *MA=Marketing Approval*
FOMEPIZOLE TN=ANTIZOLE	TREATMENT OF METHANOL OR ETHYLENE GLYCOL POISONING.	ORPHAN MEDICAL, INC. 13911 RIDGEDALE DRIVE SUITE 250 MINNETONKA MN 55305 DD 12/22/1988 MA 12/4/1997
FOSPHENYTOIN TN=CEREBYX	FOR THE ACUTE TREATMENT OF PATIENTS WITH STATUS EPILEPTICUS OF THE GRAND MAL TYPE.	WARNER-LAMBERT COMPANY 2800 PLYMOUTH ROAD ANN ARBOR MI 48106 DD 6/4/1991 MA 8/5/1996
FRUCTOSE-1,6-DIPHOSPHATE TN=CORDOX	TREATMENT OF PAINFUL VASO-OCCLUSIVE EPISODES ASSOCIATED WITH SICKLE CELL DISEASE.	QUESTCOR PHARMACEUTICALS, INC. 3260 WHIPPLE ROAD UNION CITY CA 94587-1217 DD 5/29/1998
G17DT IMMUNOGEN	TREATMENT OF GASTRIC CANCER	APHTON CORPORATION 26 HARTER AVENUE SUITE 14 WOODLAND CA 95776 DD 7/18/2002
G17DT IMMUNOGEN	TREATMENT OF ADENOCARCINOMA OF THE PANCREAS	APHTON CORPORATION 26 HARTER AVENUE SUITE 14 WOODLAND CA 95776 DD 7/10/2002
GABAPENTIN TN=NEURONTIN	TREATMENT OF AMYOTROPHIC LATERAL SCLEROSIS.	WARNER-LAMBERT COMPANY PARKE-DAVIS PHARMACEUTICAL RESEARCH DIVISION 2800 PLYMOUTH ROAD ANN ARBOR MI 48105 DD 7/5/1995
GALLIUM NITRATE INJECTION TN=GANITE	TREATMENT OF HYPERCALCEMIA OF MALIGNANCY.	SOLOPAK PHARMACEUTICAL CO. 1845 TONNE ROAD ELK GROVE VILLAGE IL 60007 DD 12/5/1988 MA 1/17/1991
GAMMA HYDROXYBUTYRATE	TREATMENT OF NARCOLEPSY AND THE AUXILIARY SYMPTOMS OF CATAPLEXY, SLEEP PARALYSIS, HYPNAGOGIC HALLUCINATIONS AND AUTOMATIC BEHAVIOR.	BIOCRAFT LABORATORIES, INC. 18-01 RIVER ROAD FAIR LAWN NJ 07410 DD 12/3/1987
GAMMA-HYDROXYBUTYRIC ACID	TREATMENT OF NARCOLEPSY AND THE AUXILIARY SYMPTOMS OF CATAPLEXY, SLEEP PARALYSIS, HYPNAGOGIC HALLUCINATIONS, AND AUTOMATIC BEHAVIOR.	SIGMA CHEMICAL COMPANY DD 1/22/1985
GAMMALINOLENIC ACID	TREATMENT OF JUVENILE RHEUMATOID ARTHRITIS.	ZURIER, ROBERT B. M.D. UNIVERSITY OF MASSACHUSETTS MEDICAL CENTER 55 LAKE AVENUE WORCESTER MA 01655 DD 7/27/1994
GANAXOLONE	TREATMENT OF INFANTILE SPASMS.	PURDUE PHARMA L.P.PURDUE PHARMA L.P. ONE STAMFORD FORUM STAMFORD CT 06901-3431 DD 5/25/1994

NAME *Generic/Chemical* *TN=Trade Name*	INDICATION DESIGNATED	SPONSOR AND ADDRESS *DD=Date Designated* *MA=Marketing Approval*
GANCICLOVIR INTRAVITREAL IMPLANT TN=VITRASERT IMPLANT	TREATMENT OF CYTOMEGALOVIRUS RETINITIS.	BAUSCH & LOMB SURGICAL, CHIRON VISION PRODUCTS 9342 JERONIMO ROAD IRVINE CA 92718-1903 DD 6/7/1995 MA 3/4/1996
GANCICLOVIR SODIUM TN=CYTOVENE	TREATMENT OF CYTOMEGALOVIRUS RETINITIS IN IMMUNOCOMPROMISED PATIENTS WITH AIDS.	SYNTEX (USA), INC. 3401 HILLVIEW AVENUE PALO ALTO CA 94304 DD 10/31/1985 MA 6/23/1989
GANCYCLOVIR	TREATMENT OF SEVERE HUMAN CYTOMEGALOVIRUS INFECTIONS IN SPECIFIC IMMUNOSUPPRESSED PATIENT POPULATIONS.	BURROUGHS WELLCOME COMPANY 3030 CORNWALLIS ROAD DD 6/7/1985
GANGLIOSIDES AS SODIUM SALTS TN=CRONASSIAL	TREATMENT OF RETINITIS PIGMENTOSA.	FIDIA PHARMACEUTICAL CORP. 1401 EYE STREET, N.W. SUITE 900 WASHINGTON DC 20005 DD 11/17/1988
GAVILIMOMAB	ACUTE GRAFT-VERSUS-HOST DISEASE (AGVHD)	ABGENIX, INC. 7601 DUMBARTON CIRCLE FREMONT CA 94555 DD 11/20/2000
GEMTUZUMAB ZOGAMICIN TN=MYLOTARG	TREATMENT OF CD33-POSITIVE ACUTE MYELOID LEUKEMIA.	WYETH-AYERST LABORATORIES PO BOX 8299 PHILADELPHIA PA 19101-8299 DD 11/24/1999 MA 5/17/2000
GENE PLASMID HVEGF165 DRIVEN BY HUMAN CYTOMEGALOVIRUS, AND [2,3-BIS(OLEOYL)-PROPYL]TRIMETHYL AMMONIUM AND DIOLEOYL PHOSPHATIDYL ETHANOLAMINE TN=TRINAM	PREVENTION OF COMPLICATIONS DUE TO NEOINTIMAL HYPERPLASIA DISEASE IN CERTAIN VASCULAR ANASTOMOSES.	ARK THERAPEUTICS LTD. 1 FITZROY MEWS LONDON W1T6DE UK DD 10/24/2000
GENTAMICIN IMPREGNATED PMMA BEADS ON SURGICAL WIRE TN=SEPTOPAL	TREATMENT OF CHRONIC OSTEOMYELITIS OF POST-TRAUMATIC, POSTOPERATIVE, OR HEMATOGENOUS ORIGIN.	LIPHA PHARMACEUTICALS, INC. 9 WEST 57TH STREET SUITE 3825 NEW YORK NY 10019-2701 DD 1/31/1991
GENTAMICIN LIPOSOME INJECTION TN=MAITEC	TREATMENT OF DISSEMINATED MYCOBACTERIUM AVIUM-INTRACELLULARE INFECTION.	LIPOSOME COMPANY, INC. ONE RESEARCH WAY PRINCETON NJ 08540 DD 7/10/1990
GLATIRAMER ACETATE TN=COPAXONE	TREATMENT OF MULTIPLE SCLEROSIS.	TEVA PHARMACEUTICALS USA 1510 DELP DRIVE KULPSVILLE PA 19443 DD 11/9/1987 MA 12/20/1996
GLATIRAMER ACETATE FOR INJECTION TN=COPAXONE	TREATMENT OF PRIMARY-PROGRESSIVE MULTIPLE SCLEROSIS	TEVA PHARMACEUTICALS, USA 1090 HORSHAM ROAD NORTH WALES PA 19454 DD 6/5/2001

NAME *Generic/Chemical* *TN=Trade Name*	INDICATION DESIGNATED	SPONSOR AND ADDRESS *DD=Date Designated* *MA=Marketing Approval*
GLUTAMINE	FOR USE WITH HUMAN GROWTH HORMONE IN THE TREATMENT OF SHORT BOWEL SYNDROME (NUTRIENT MALABSORPTION FROM THE GASTROINTESTINAL TRACT RESULTING FROM AN INADEQUATE ABSORPTIVE SURFACE).	NUTRITIONAL RESTART PHARMACEUTICAL, L.P. 4364 SOUTH ALSTON AVENUE DURHAM NC 27713 DD 3/6/1995
GLYCEOL	TO DECREASE INTRACRANIAL HYPERTENSION AND/OR ALLEVIATE CEREBRAL EDEMA IN PATIENTS WHO MAY BENEFIT FROM OSMOTHERAPY.	CHUGAI PHARMACEUTICAL CO., LTD. DD 2/22/1990
GLYCERYL TRIOLEATE AND GLYCERYL TRIERUCATE	TREATMENT OF ADRENOLEUKODYSTROPHY.	MOSER, HUGO W. M.D. JOHNS HOPKINS UNIVERSITY KENNEDY KRIEGER INSTITUTE, 707 NORTH BROADWAY BALTIMORE MD 21205 DD 2/14/1995
GONADORELIN ACETATE TN=LUTREPULSE	FOR INDUCTION OF OVULATION IN WOMEN WITH HYPOTHALAMIC AMENORRHEA DUE TO A DEFICIENCY OR ABSENCE IN THE QUANTITY OR PULSE PATTERN OF ENDOGENOUS GNRH SECRETION.	FERRING LABORATORIES, INC. 400 RELLA BOULEVARD, SUITE 201 SUFFERN NY 10901 DD 4/22/1987 MA 10/10/1989
GOSSYPOL	TREATMENT OF CANCER OF THE ADRENAL CORTEX.	REIDENBERG, MARCUS M. M.D. THE NEW YORK HOSPITAL - CORNELL MEDICAL CENTER 525 EAST 68TH STREET, BOX 70 NEW YORK NY 10021 DD 10/22/1990
GP100 ADENOVIRAL GENE THERAPY	TREATMENT OF METASTATIC MELANOMA.	GENZYME CORPORATION ONE MOUNTAIN RD. P.O. BOX 9322 FRAMINGHAM MA 01701-9322 DD 3/25/1997
GRANULOCYTE MACROPHAGE-COLONY STIMULATING FACTOR TN=LEUCOMAX	TREATMENT OF NEUTROPENIA ASSOCIATED WITH BONE MARROW TRANSPLANTS.	SCHERING CORPORATION 2000 GALLOPING HILL ROAD KENILWORTH NJ 07033 DD 12/12/1989
GRANULOCYTE MACROPHAGE-COLONY STIMULATING FACTOR TN=LEUCOMAX	TREATMENT OF NEUTROPENIA DUE TO HAIRY CELL LEUKEMIA.	SCHERING CORPORATION 2000 GALLOPING HILL ROAD KENILWORTH NJ 07033 DD 5/3/1990
GRANULOCYTE MACROPHAGE-COLONY STIMULATING FACTOR TN=LEUCOMAX	TREATMENT OF CHRONIC LYMPHOCYTIC LEUKEMIA TO INCREASE GRANULOCYTE COUNT.	SCHERING CORPORATION 2000 GALLOPING HILL ROAD KENILWORTH NJ 07033 DD 5/4/1990
GRANULOCYTE MACROPHAGE-COLONY STIMULATING FACTOR TN=LEUCOMAX	TREATMENT OF MYELODYSPLASTIC SYNDROME.	SCHERING CORPORATION 2000 GALLOPING HILL ROAD KENILWORTH NJ 07033 DD 8/7/1989
GRANULOCYTE MACROPHAGE-COLONY STIMULATING FACTOR TN=LEUCOMAX	TREATMENT OF SEVERE THERMAL INJURIES IN PATIENTS WITH GREATER THAN 40% FULL OR PARTIAL THICKNESS BURNS.	SCHERING CORPORATION 2000 GALLOPING HILL ROAD KENILWORTH NJ 07033 DD 6/6/1989
GROUP B STREPTOCOCCUS IMMUNE GLOBULIN	TREATMENT OF NEONATES FOR DISSEMINATED GROUP B STREPTOCOCCAL INFECTION.	NORTH AMERICAN BIOLOGICALS, INC. 12280 WILKINS AVENUE ROCKVILLE MD 20852 DD 5/8/1990

NAME *Generic/Chemical* *TN=Trade Name*	INDICATION DESIGNATED	SPONSOR AND ADDRESS *DD=Date Designated* *MA=Marketing Approval*
GROWTH HORMONE RELEASING FACTOR	FOR THE LONG-TERM TREATMENT OF CHILDREN WHO HAVE GROWTH FAILURE DUE TO A LACK OF ADEQUATE ENDOGENOUS GROWTH HORMONE SECRETION.	ICN PHARMACEUTICALS, INC. ICN PLAZA 3300 HYLAND AVENUE COSTA MESA CA 92626 DD 8/7/1989
GUANETHIDINE MONOSULFATE TN=ISMELIN	TREATMENT OF MODERATE TO SEVERE REFLEX SYMPATHETIC DYSTROPHY AND CAUSALGIA.	NOVARTIS PHARMACEUTICALS CORPORATION 59 ROUTE 10 EAST HANOVER NJ 07936-1080 DD 1/6/1986
GUANFACINE TN=TENEX	TREATMENT OF FRAGILE X SYNDROME.	WATSON LABORATORIES, INC. 311 BONNIE CIRCLE PO BOX 1900 CORONA CA 91718-1900 DD 8/5/1999
GUSPERIMUS TN=SPANIDIN	TREATMENT OF ACUTE RENAL GRAFT REJECTION EPISODES.	BRISTOL-MYERS SQUIBB PHARMACEUTICAL RESEARCH INSTITUTE 5 RESEARCH PARKWAY P.O. BOX 5100 WALLINGFORD CT 06492-7660 DD 6/27/1996
HIV NEUTRALIZING ANTIBODIES TN=IMMUPATH	TREATMENT OF ACQUIRED IMMUNODEFICIENCY SYNDROME.	HEMACARE CORPORATION 4954 VAN NUYS BOULEVARD SHERMAN OAKS CA 91403 DD 3/24/1992
HLA-B7/BETA2M DNA LIPID (DMRIE/DOPE) COMPLEX TN=ALLOVECTIN-7	TREATMENT OF INVASIVE AND METASTATIC MELANOMA (STAGES II, III, AND IV).	VICAL INCORPORATED 9373 TOWNE CENTRE DR., SUITE 100 SAN DIEGO CA 92121 DD 9/30/1999
HPA-23	TREATMENT OF ACQUIRED IMMUNODEFICIENCY SYNDROME.	RHONE-POULENC RORER PHARM. 500 ARCOLA ROAD COLLEGEVILLE PA 19426 DD 7/17/1985
HALOFANTRINE TN=HALFAN	TREATMENT OF MILD TO MODERATE ACUTE MALARIA CAUSED BY SUSCEPTIBLE STRAINS OF P. FALCIPARUM AND P. VIVAX.	SMITHKLINE BEECHAM PHARMACEUTICALS ONE FRANKLIN PLAZA P.O. BOX 7929 PHILADELPHIA PA 19101 DD 11/4/1991 MA 7/24/1992
HALOFUGINONE TN=STENOROL	TREATMENT OF SYSTEMIC SCLEROSIS.	COLLGARD BIOPHARMACEUTICALS LTD. TEXTILE HOUSE, 2 KOIFMAN ST. TEL-AVIV 68012 ISRAEL IL DD 2/7/2000
HEME ARGINATE TN=NORMOSANG	TREATMENT OF SYMPTOMATIC STAGE OF ACUTE PORPHYRIA.	BERLEX LABORATORIES, INC. 15049 SAN PABLO AVENUE RICHMOND CA 94804-0099 DD 3/10/1988
HEME ARGINATE TN=NORMOSANG	TREATMENT OF MYELODYSPLASTIC SYNDROMES.	BERLEX LABORATORIES, INC. 15049 SAN PABLO AVENUE RICHMOND CA 94804-0099 DD 3/1/1994

NAME *Generic/Chemical* *TN=Trade Name*	INDICATION DESIGNATED	SPONSOR AND ADDRESS *DD=Date Designated* *MA=Marketing Approval*
HEMIN TN=PANHEMATIN	AMELIORATION OF RECURRENT ATTACKS OF ACUTE INTERMITTENT PORPHYRIA (AIP) TEMPORARILY RELATED TO THE MENSTRUAL CYCLE IN SUSCEPTIBLE WOMEN AND SIMILAR SYMPTOMS WHICH OCCUR IN OTHER PATIENTS WITH AIP, PORPHYRIA VARIEGATA AND HEREDITARY COPROPORPHYRIA.	ABBOTT LABORATORIES DIAGNOSTICS DIVISION ABBOTT PARK IL 60064 DD 3/16/1984 MA 7/20/1983
HEMIN AND ZINC MESOPOR-PHYRIN TN=HEMEX	TREATMENT OF ACUTE PORPHYRIC SYNDROMES.	BONKOVSKY, HERBERT L. M.D. UNIVERSITY OF MASSACHU-SETTS MEDICAL CENTER 55 LAKE AVENUE NORTH WORCESTER MA 01655 DD 12/20/1993
HEPATITIS B IMMUNE GLOBULIN INTRAVENOUS (HUMAN) TN=NABI-HB	PROPHYLAXIS AGAINST HEPATITIS B VIRUS REINFECTION IN LIVER TRANSPLANT PATIENTS.	NABI 12280 WILKINS AVENUE ROCKVILLE MD 20852 DD 3/8/1995
HEPATITIS C VIRUS IMMUNE GLOBULIN (HUMAN)	PROPHYLAXIS OF HEPATITIS C INFECTION IN LIVER TRANSPLANT RECIPIENTS.	NABI 5800 PARK OF COMMERCE BLVD., N.W. BOCA RATON FL 33487 DD 11/14/2002
HERPES SIMPLEX VIRUS GENE	TREATMENT OF PRIMARY AND METASTATIC BRAIN TUMORS.	GENETIC THERAPY, INC. 938 CLOPPER ROAD GAITHERSBURG MD 20878 DD 10/16/1992
HISTAMINE TN=MAXAMINE	ADJUNCT TO CYTOKINE THERAPY IN THE TREATMENT OF ACUTE MYELOID LEUKEMIA.	MAXIM PHARMACEUTICALS, INC. 8899 UNIVERSITY CENTER LANE SUITE 400 SAN DIEGO CA 92122 DD 12/15/1999
HISTAMINE TN=MAXAMINE	FOR USE AS AN ADJUNCT TO CYTOKINE THERAPY IN THE TREATMENT OF MALIGNANT MELANOMA.	MAXIM PHARMACEUTICALS, INC. 8899 UNIVERSITY CENTER LANE SUITE 400 SAN DIEGO CA 92122 DD 2/1/2000
HISTRELIN	TREATMENT OF ACUTE INTERMITTENT PORPHYRIA, HEREDITARY COPROPORPHYRIA, AND VARIEGATE PORPHYRIA.	ANDERSON, KARL E., M.D. UNIVERSITY OF TEXAS MEDICAL BRANCH AT GALVESTON ROUTE J-09, 700 THE STRAND GALVESTON TX 77550 DD 5/3/1991
HISTRELIN ACETATE TN=SUPPRELIN INJECTION	TREATMENT OF CENTRAL PRECOCIOUS PUBERTY.	ROBERTS PHARMACEUTICAL CORP. MERIDIAN CENTER III 6 INDUSTRIAL WAY WEST EATONTOWN NJ 07724 DD 8/10/1988 MA 12/24/1991
HSP E7	TREATMENT OF RECURRENT RESPIRATORY PAPIL-LOMATOSIS (RRP)	STRESSGEN BIOTECHNOLO-GIES, INC. 409 2ND AVENUE SUITE 201 COLLEGEVILLE PA 19426-2655 DD 3/19/2001

NAME *Generic/Chemical* *TN=Trade Name*	INDICATION DESIGNATED	SPONSOR AND ADDRESS *DD=Date Designated* *MA=Marketing Approval*
HU1D10, HUMANIZED MONOCLO-NAL ANTIBODY TN=REMITOGEN	FOR USE IN THE TREATMENT OF 1D10+ B CELL NON-HODGKIN S LYMPHOMA	PROTEIN DESIGN LABS, INC. 34801 CAMPUS DRIVE FREMONT CA 94555 DD 11/28/2001
HUMAN ANTI-TUMOR NECROSIS FACTOR ALPHA MONOCLONAL ANTIBODY	TREATMENT OF UVEITIS OF THE POSTERIOR SEG-MENT OF NON-INFECTIOUS ETIOLOGY, AND UVEITIS OF THE ANTERIOR SEGMENT OF NON-INFECTIOUS ETIOLOGY AND REFRACTORY TO CONVENTIONAL THERAPY	CENTOCOR, INC. 200 GREAT VALLEY PARKWAY MALVERN PA 19355-1307 DD 1/16/2003
HUMAN IGM MONOCLONAL ANTI-BODY (C-58) TO CMV TN=CENTOVIR	TREATMENT OF CYTOMEGALOVIRUS INFECTIONS IN ALLOGENIC BONE MARROW TRANSPLANT PATIENTS.	CENTOCOR, INC. 244 GREAT VALLEY PARKWAY MALVERN PA 19355 DD 8/7/1989
HUMAN IGM MONOCLONAL ANTI-BODY (C-58) TO CMV TN=CENTOVIR	PROPHYLAXIS OF CYTOMEGALOVIRUS INFECTIONS IN BONE MARROW TRANSPLANT PATIENTS.	CENTOCOR, INC. 244 GREAT VALLEY PARKWAY MALVERN PA 19355 DD 8/7/1989
HUMAN T-LYMPHOTROPIC VIRUS TYPE III GP160 ANTIGENS TN=VAXSYN HIV-1	TREATMENT OF AIDS.	MICROGENESYS, INC. 1000 RESEARCH PARKWAY MERIDEN CT 06450 DD 11/20/1989
HUMAN ACID PRECURSOR AL-PHA-GLUCOSIDASE, RECOMBI-NANT	TREATMENT OF GLYCOGEN STORAGE DISEASE TYPE II.	PHARMING/GENZYME LLC C/O GENZYME CORPORATION 1 MOUNTAIN RD. FRAMINGHAM MA 01701-9322 DD 9/10/1996
HUMAN IMMUNODEFICIENCY VIRUS IMMUNE GLOBULIN TN=HIVIG	TREATMENT OF HIV-INFECTED PEDIATRIC PATIENTS.	NABI 5800 PARK OF COMMERCE BLVD., NW BOCA RATON FL 33487 DD 1/4/1995
HUMAN IMMUNODEFICIENCY VIRUS IMMUNE GLOBULIN	TREATMENT OF AIDS.	NABI 5800 PARK OF COMMERCE BLVD., NW BOCA RATON FL 33487 DD 11/21/1989
HUMAN IMMUNODEFICIENCY VIRUS IMMUNE GLOBULIN	TREATMENT OF HIV-INFECTED PREGNANT WOMEN AND INFANTS OF HIV-INFECTED MOTHERS.	NABI 5800 PARK OF COMMERCE BLVD., N.W. BOCA RATON FL 33487 DD 3/25/1992
HUMANIZED MAB (IDEC-131) TO CD40L	TREATMENT OF SYSTEMIC LUPUS ERYTHEMATOSUS.	IDEC PHARMACEUTICALS CORPORATION 3030 CALLAN RD. SAN DIEGO CA 92121 DD 2/9/1999
HUMANIZED ANTI-CD2 MONO-CLONAL ANTIBODY	TREATMENT OF GRAFT-VERSUS-HOST DISEASE.	MEDIMMUNE, INC. 35 WEST WATKINS MILL RD. GAITHERSBURG MD 20878 DD 11/13/1998
HUMANIZED ANTI-HUMAN CD2 MAB TN=MEDI-507	FOR THE INDUCTION OF DONOR-SPECIFIC IMMUNO-LOGIC UNRESPONSIVENESS RESULTING IN PROPHY-LAXIS OF ORGAN REJECTION WITHOUT THE NEED FOR CHRONIC IMMUNOSUPPRESSIVE THERAPY, IN PATIENTS RECEIVING ALLOGENEIC RENAL TRANS-PLANTS.	BIOTRANSPLANT, INC. BUILDING 75, 3RD. AVE. CHARLESTOWN NAVY YARD CHARLESTOWN MA 02129 DD 9/17/1998

NAME *Generic/Chemical* *TN=Trade Name*	INDICATION DESIGNATED	SPONSOR AND ADDRESS *DD=Date Designated* *MA=Marketing Approval*
HUMANIZED ANTI-TAC TN=ZENAPAX	PREVENTION OF ACUTE GRAFT-VS-HOST DISEASE FOLLOWING BONE MARROW TRANSPLANTATION.	HOFFMANN-LA ROCHE, INC. 340 KINGSLAND STREET NUTLEY NJ 07110-1199 DD 3/5/1993
HYDROXOCOBALAMIN TN=CYANOKIT	TREATMENT OF ACUTE CYANIDE POISONING	ORPHAN MEDICAL, INC. 13911 RIDGEDALE DRIVE SUITE 250 MINNETONKA MN 55305 DD 9/22/2000
HYDROXYCOBALAMIN/SODIUM THIOSULFATE	TREATMENT OF SEVERE ACUTE CYANIDE POISON-ING.	HALL, ALAN H., M.D. MILE 5.0 PASS CREEK ROAD PO BOX 24 ELK MOUNTAIN WY 82324 DD 10/4/1985
HYDROXYUREA TN=DROXIA	TREATMENT OF PATIENTS WITH SICKLE CELL ANEMIA AS SHOWN BY THE PRESENCE OF HEMOGLOBIN S.	BRISTOL-MYERS SQUIBB PHARMACEUTICAL RESEARCH INSTITUTE P.O. BOX 4000 PRINCETON NJ 08543 DD 10/1/1990 MA 2/25/1998
HYPERICIN	TREATMENT OF CUTANEOUS T-CELL LYMPHOMA.	NEXELL THERAPEUTICS, INC. 2751 CENTERVILLE RD., SUITE 210 WILMINGTON DE 19808 DD 2/7/2000
HYPERICIN	TREATMENT OF GLIOBLASTOMA MULTIFORME.	NEXELL THERAPEUTICS 2751 CENTERVILLE RD., SUITE 210 WILMINGTON DE 19808 DD 8/3/2000
I(131)-TM-601 (CHLOROTOXIN)	TREATMENT OF MALIGNANT GLIOMA	TRANSMOLECULAR, INC. 3800 COLONNADE PARKWAY SUITE 240 BIRMINGHAM AL 35243 DD 2/14/2002
IL-4 PSEUDOMONAS TOXIN FU-SION PROTEIN (IL-4(38-37)-PE38KDEL)	TREATMENT OF ASTROCYTIC GLIOMA.	NEUROCRINE BIOSCIENCES, INC. 10555 SCIENCE CENTER DR. SAN DIEGO CA 92121 DD 4/6/2000
IL13-PE38QQR	TREATMENT OF MALIGNANT GLIOMA	NEOPHARM, INC. 150 FIELD DRIVE SUITE 195 LAKE FOREST IL 60045 DD 11/2/2001
INGN 201 TN=ADVEXIN	TREATMENT OF HEAD AND NECK CANCER	INTROGEN THERAPEUTICS, INC. 2250 HOLCOMBE BLVD HOUSTON TX 77030 DD 1/27/2003
INH-A00021 TN=VERONATE	REDUCTION (PREVENTION) OF NOSOCOMIAL BAC-TEREMIA CAUSED BY STAPHYLOCOCCI IN VERY LOW BIRTH WEIGHT INFANTS.	INHIBITEX, INC. 8995 WESTSIDE PARKWAY SUITE 150 ALPHARETTA GA 30004 DD 6/13/2001

NAME *Generic/Chemical* *TN=Trade Name*	INDICATION DESIGNATED	SPONSOR AND ADDRESS *DD=Date Designated* *MA=Marketing Approval*
IBUPROFEN I.V. SOLUTION	TREATMENT OF PATENT DUCTUS ARTERIOSUS.	FARMACON-IL-LLC 1720 POST ROAD EAST SUITE 213 WESTPORT CT 06880-5643 DD 10/29/1996
IBUPROFEN I.V. SOLUTION TN=SALPROFEN	PREVENTION OF PATENT DUCTUS ARTERIOSUS.	FARMACON-IL, LLC 1720 POST ROAD EAST SUITE 213 WESTPORT CT 06880-5643 DD 10/29/1996
ICODEXTRIN 7.5% WITH ELEC- TROLYTES PERITONEAL DIALY- SIS SOLUTION TN=EXTRANEAL (WITH 7.5% ICO- DEXTRIN) PERITONEAL DIALYSIS SOLUTIO	TREATMENT OF THOSE PATIENTS HAVING END STAGE RENAL DISEASE AND REQUIRING PERITO- NEAL DIALYSIS TREATMENT.	BAXTER HEALTHCARE CORPORATION RENAL DIVISION 1620 WAUKEGAN ROAD MCGAW PARK IL 60085 DD 7/18/1997
IDARUBICIN TN=IDAMYCIN	TREATMENT OF CHRONIC MYELOGENOUS LEUKE- MIA.	PHARMACIA & UPJOHN 7000 PORTAGE ROAD UNIT 0633-298-113 KALAMAZOO MI 49001-0199 DD 12/2/1992
IDARUBICIN TN=IDAMYCIN	TREATMENT OF MYELODYSPLASTIC SYNDROMES.	PHARMACIA & UPJOHN 7000 PORTAGE ROAD UNIT 0633-298-113 KALAMAZOO MI 49001-0199 DD 12/1/1992
IDARUBICIN HCL FOR INJECTION TN=IDAMYCIN	TREATMENT OF ACUTE LYMPHOBLASTIC LEUKEMIA IN PEDIATRIC PATIENTS.	PHARMACIA & UPJOHN 7000 PORTAGE ROAD UNIT 0633-298-113 KALAMAZOO MI 49001-0199 DD 2/12/1991
IDARUBICIN HCL FOR INJECTION TN=IDAMYCIN	TREATMENT OF ACUTE MYELOGENOUS LEUKEMIA, ALSO REFERRED TO AS ACUTE NONLYMPHOCYTIC LEUKEMIA.	ADRIA LABORATORIES, INC. P.O. BOX 16529 COLUMBUS OH 43216 DD 7/25/1988 MA 9/27/1990
IDOXURIDINE	TREATMENT OF NONPARENCHYMATOUS SARCO- MAS.	NEOPHARM, INC. 225 EAST DEERPATH, SUITE 250 LAKE FOREST IL 60045 DD 4/8/1996
IFOSFAMIDE TN=IFEX	TREATMENT OF SOFT TISSUE SARCOMAS.	BRISTOL-MYERS SQUIBB PHARMACEUTICAL RESEARCH INSTITUTE P.O. BOX 4000 PRINCETON NJ 08543 DD 8/7/1985
IFOSFAMIDE TN=IFEX	TREATMENT OF TESTICULAR CANCER.	BRISTOL-MYERS SQUIBB PHARMACEUTICAL RESEARCH INSTITUTE 5 RESEARCH PARKWAY, P.O. BOX 5100 WALLINGFORD CT 06492 DD 1/20/1987 MA 12/30/1988

NAME *Generic/Chemical* *TN=Trade Name*	INDICATION DESIGNATED	SPONSOR AND ADDRESS *DD=Date Designated* *MA=Marketing Approval*
IFOSFAMIDE TN=IFEX	TREATMENT OF BONE SARCOMAS.	BRISTOL-MYERS SQUIBB PHARMACEUTICAL RESEARCH INSTITUTE P.O. BOX 4000 PRINCETON NJ 08543-4000 DD 8/7/1985
ILOPROST SOLUTION FOR INFU- SION	TREATMENT OF RAYNAUD'S PHENOMENON SECOND- ARY TO SYSTEMIC SCLEROSIS.	BERLEX LABORATORIES, INC. 300 FAIRFIELD ROAD WAYNE NJ 07470 DD 9/21/1989
ILOPROST SOLUTION FOR INFU- SION	TREATMENT OF HEPARIN-ASSOCIATED THROMBO- CYTOPENIA.	BERLEX LABORATORIES, INC. 300 FAIRFIELD ROAD WAYNE NJ 07470 DD 5/14/1990
IMATINIB TN=GLEEVEC	TREATMENT OF CHRONIC MYELOGENOUS LEUKEMIA	NOVARTIS PHARMACEUTICALS CORPORATION 59 ROUTE 10 EAST HANOVER NJ 07936-1080 DD 1/31/2001 MA 5/10/2001
IMCIROMAB PENTETATE TN=MYOSCINT	DETECTING EARLY NECROSIS AS AN INDICATION OF REJECTION OF ORTHOTOPIC CARDIAC TRANS- PLANTS.	CENTOCOR, INC. 244 GREAT VALLEY PARKWAY MALVERN PA 19355 DD 1/25/1989
IMEXON TN=N/A	TREATMENT OF METASTATIC MALIGNANT MELANO- MA	AMPLIMED CORPORATION 2321 CAMINO LA ZORRELA TUCSON AZ 85718 DD 8/3/2001
IMEXON	TREATMENT OF MULTIPLE MYELOMA.	AMPLIMED CORPORATION 2321 CAMINO LA ZORRELA TUCSON AZ 85718 DD 11/8/1996
IMIGLUCERASE TN=CEREZYME	REPLACEMENT THERAPY IN PATIENTS WITH TYPES I, II, AND III GAUCHER'S DISEASE.	GENZYME CORPORATION ONE KENDALL SQUARE CAMBRIDGE MA 02139-1562 DD 11/5/1991 MA 5/23/1994
IMMUNE GLOBULIN INTRAVE- NOUS (HUMAN) TN=IVEEGAM, IMMUNO	TREATMENT OF POLYMYOSITIS/DERMATOMYOSITIS.	IMMUNO CLINICAL RESEARCH CORP. 155 EAST 56TH STREET NEW YORK NY 10022 DD 10/13/1992
IMMUNE GLOBULIN INTRAVE- NOUS (HUMAN) TN=IVEEGAM, IMMUNO	TREATMENT OF JUVENILE RHEUMATOID ARTHRITIS.	IMMUNO CLINICAL RESEARCH CORP. 750 LEXINGTON AVENUE, 19TH FLOOR NEW YORK NY 10022 DD 12/16/1992
IMMUNE GLOBULIN INTRAVE- NOUS (HUMAN) TN=IMMUNE GLOBULIN INTRAVE- NOUS (HUMAN) IMMUNO, IVEE- GAM	TREATMENT OF PATIENTS WITH ACUTE MYOCARDI- TIS.	IMMUNO CLINICAL RESEARCH CORP. 750 LEXINGTON AVENUE NEW YORK NY 10022 DD 11/22/1993

NAME Generic/Chemical TN=Trade Name	INDICATION DESIGNATED	SPONSOR AND ADDRESS DD=Date Designated MA=Marketing Approval
IMMUNE GLOBULIN INTRAVE-NOUS, HUMAN TN=GAMIMUNE N	INFECTION PROPHYLAXIS IN PEDIATRIC PATIENTS AFFECTED WITH THE HUMAN IMMUNODEFICIENCY VIRUS.	BAYER CORPORATION PHARMACEUTICAL DIVISION, BI-OLOGICAL PRODUCTS 400 MORGAN LANE NEW HAVEN CT 06516 DD 2/18/1993 MA 12/27/1993
IMPORTED FIRE ANT VENOM, AL-LERGENIC EXTRACT	FOR SKIN TESTING OF VICTIMS OF FIRE ANT STINGS TO CONFIRM FIRE ANT SENSITIVITY AND IF POSITIVE, FOR USE AS IMMUNOTHERAPY FOR THE PREVEN-TION OF IGE-MEDIATED ANAPHYLACTIC REACTIONS.	ALK LABORATORIES, INC. RESEARCH CENTER 27 VILLAGE LANE WALLINGFORD CT 06492 DD 5/12/1992
INDIUM IN 111 MURINE MONO-CLONAL ANTIBODY FAB TO MYO-SIN TN=MYOSCINT	TO AID IN THE DIAGNOSIS OF MYOCARDITIS.	CENTOCOR, INC. 244 GREAT VALLEY PARKWAY MALVERN PA 19355 DD 8/7/1989
INDIUM IN-111 ALTUMOMAB PEN-TETATE TN=HYBRI-CEAKER	DETECTION OF SUSPECTED AND PREVIOUSLY UNI-DENTIFIED TUMOR FOCI OF RECURRENT COLOREC-TAL CARCINOMA.	HYBRITECH, INC. 11095 TORREYANNA ROAD SAN DIEGO CA 92196 DD 2/6/1990
INFLIXIMAB TN=REMICADE	TREATMENT OF MODERATELY TO SEVERELY ACTIVE CROHN'S DISEASE FOR THE REDUCTION OF THE SIGNS AND SYMPTOMS, IN PATIENTS WHO HAVE AN INADEQUATE RESPONSE TO CONVENTIONAL THER-APY; AND TREATMENT OF PATIENTS WITH FISTULIZ-ING CROHN'S DISEASE FOR THE REDUCTION IN TH	CENTOCOR, INC. 200 GREAT VALLEY PARKWAY MALVERN PA 19355-1307 DD 11/14/1995 MA 8/24/1998
INFLIXIMAB TN=REMICADE	TREATMENT OF CHRONIC SARCOIDOSIS.	CENTOCOR, INC. 200 GREAT VALLEY PARKWAY MALVERN PA 19355-1307 DD 5/21/2003
INFLIXIMAB TN=REMICADE	TREATMENT OF GIANT CELL ARTERITIS.	CENTOCOR, INC. 200 GREAT VALLEY PARKWAY MALVERN PA 19355-1307 DD 5/6/2003
INOSINE PRANOBEX TN=ISOPRINOSINE	TREATMENT OF SUBACUTE SCLEROSING PANENCE-PHALITIS.	NEWPORT PHARMACEUTICALS 897 WEST SIXTEENTH STREET NEWPORT BEACH CA 92663 DD 9/20/1988
INTERFERON BETA-1A TN=AVONEX	TREATMENT OF JUVENILE RHEUMATOID ARTHRITIS.	BIOGEN, INC. 14 CAMBRIDGE CENTER CAMBRIDGE MA 02142 DD 10/14/1998
INTERFERON ALFA-2A TN=ROFERON A	TREATMENT OF CHRONIC MYELOGENOUS LEUKE-MIA.	HOFFMANN-LA ROCHE, INC. 340 KINGSLAND STREET NUTLEY NJ 07110 DD 6/6/1989 MA 10/19/1995
INTERFERON ALFA-2A (RECOM-BINANT) TN=ROFERON-A	FOR THE CONCOMITANT ADMINISTRATION WITH TE-CELEUKIN FOR THE TREATMENT OF METASTATIC RE-NAL CELL CARCINOMA.	HOFFMANN-LA ROCHE, INC. 340 KINGSLAND STREET NUTLEY NJ 07119 DD 5/2/1990
INTERFERON ALFA-2A (RECOM-BINANT) TN=ROFERON-A	FOR THE TREATMENT OF METASTATIC MALIGNANT MELANOMA IN COMBINATION WITH TECELEUKIN.	HOFFMANN-LA ROCHE, INC. 340 KINGSLAND STREET NUTLEY NJ 07110 DD 5/11/1990

NAME *Generic/Chemical* *TN=Trade Name*	**INDICATION DESIGNATED**	SPONSOR AND ADDRESS *DD=Date Designated* *MA=Marketing Approval*
INTERFERON ALFA-2A (RECOMBINANT) TN=ROFERON-A	FOR THE CONCOMITANT ADMINISTRATION WITH FLUOROURACIL FOR THE TREATMENT OF ADVANCED COLORECTAL CANCER.	HOFFMANN-LA ROCHE, INC. 340 KINGSLAND STREET NUTLEY NJ 07110-1199 DD 5/14/1990
INTERFERON ALFA-2A (RECOMBINANT) TN=ROFERON-A	FOR USE IN COMBINATION WITH FLUOROURACIL FOR THE TREATMENT OF ESOPHAGEAL CARCINOMA.	HOFFMANN-LA ROCHE, INC. 340 KINGSLAND STREET NUTLEY NJ 07110-1199 DD 10/27/1989
INTERFERON ALFA-2A (RECOMBINANT) TN=ROFERON-A	TREATMENT OF AIDS RELATED KAPOSI'S SARCOMA.	HOFFMANN-LA ROCHE, INC. 340 KINGSLAND STREET NUTLEY NJ 07110 DD 12/14/1987 MA 11/21/1988
INTERFERON ALFA-2A (RECOMBINANT) TN=ROFERON-A	TREATMENT OF RENAL CELL CARCINOMA.	HOFFMANN-LA ROCHE, INC. 340 KINGSLAND STREET NUTLEY NJ 07110-1199 DD 4/18/1988
INTERFERON ALFA-2B (RECOMBINANT) TN=INTRON A	TREATMENT OF METASTATIC RENAL CELL CARCINOMA.	SCHERING CORPORATION 2000 GALLOPING HILL ROAD KENILWORTH NJ 07033 DD 6/22/1987
INTERFERON ALFA-2B (RECOMBINANT) TN=INTRON A	TREATMENT OF PRIMARY MALIGNANT BRAIN TUMORS.	SCHERING CORPORATION 2000 GALLOPING HILL ROAD KENILWORTH NJ 07033 DD 5/13/1988
INTERFERON ALFA-2B (RECOMBINANT) TN=INTRON A	TREATMENT OF ACUTE HEPATITIS B.	SCHERING CORPORATION 2000 GALLOPING HILL ROAD KENILWORTH NJ 07033 DD 11/17/1988
INTERFERON ALFA-2B (RECOMBINANT) TN=INTRON A	TREATMENT OF AIDS-RELATED KAPOSI'S SARCOMA.	SCHERING CORPORATION 2000 GALLOPING HILL ROAD KENILWORTH NJ 07033 DD 6/24/1987 MA 11/21/1988
INTERFERON ALFA-2B (RECOMBINANT) TN=INTRON A	TREATMENT OF CHRONIC MYELOGENOUS LEUKEMIA.	SCHERING CORPORATION 2000 GALLOPING HILL ROAD KENILWORTH NJ 07033 DD 6/22/1987
INTERFERON ALFA-2B (RECOMBINANT) TN=INTRON A	TREATMENT OF OVARIAN CARCINOMA.	SCHERING CORPORATION 2000 GALLOPING HILL ROAD KENILWORTH NJ 07033 DD 8/3/1987
INTERFERON ALFA-2B (RECOMBINANT) TN=INTRON A	TREATMENT OF INVASIVE CARCINOMA OF THE CERVIX.	SCHERING CORPORATION 2000 GALLOPING HILL ROAD KENILWORTH NJ 07033 DD 4/18/1988
INTERFERON ALFA-2B (RECOMBINANT) TN=INTRON A	TREATMENT OF CHRONIC DELTA HEPATITIS.	SCHERING CORPORATION 2000 GALLOPING HILL ROAD KENILWORTH NJ 07033 DD 5/4/1990
INTERFERON ALFA-2B (RECOMBINANT) TN=INTRON A	TREATMENT OF LARYNGEAL (RESPIRATORY) PAPILLOMATOSIS.	SCHERING CORPORATION 2000 GALLOPING HILL ROAD KENILWORTH NJ 07033 DD 8/17/1988

NAME *Generic/Chemical* *TN=Trade Name*	INDICATION DESIGNATED	SPONSOR AND ADDRESS *DD=Date Designated* *MA=Marketing Approval*
INTERFERON ALFA-2B (RECOMBINANT) TN=INTRON A	TREATMENT OF CARCINOMA IN SITU OF THE URINARY BLADDER.	SCHERING CORPORATION 2000 GALLOPING HILL ROAD KENILWORTH NJ 07033 DD 8/10/1988
INTERFERON ALFA-NL TN=WELLFERON	TREATMENT OF HUMAN PAPILLOMAVIRUS IN PATIENTS WITH SEVERE RESISTANT/RECURRENT RESPIRATORY (LARYNGEAL) PAPILLOMATOSIS.	GLAXO WELLCOME INC. 5 MOORE DRIVE RESEARCH TRIANGLE PARK NC 27709 DD 10/16/1987
INTERFERON ALFA-NL TN=WELLFERON	TREATMENT OF AIDS RELATED KAPOSI'S SARCOMA.	BURROUGHS WELLCOME COMPANY 3030 CORNWALLIS ROAD RESEARCH TRIANGLE PK NC 27709 DD 8/25/1986
INTERFERON BETA (RECOMBINANT HUMAN) TN=AVONEX	TREATMENT OF PRIMARY BRAIN TUMORS.	BIOGEN, INC. 14 CAMBRIDGE CENTER CAMBRIDGE MA 02142 DD 1/13/1993
INTERFERON BETA (RECOMBINANT) TN=R-HUIFN-BETA	FOR THE INTRALESIONAL AND/OR SYSTEMIC TREATMENT OF AIDS-RELATED KAPOSI'S SARCOMA.	BIOGEN, INC. 14 CAMBRIDGE CENTER CAMBRIDGE MA 02142 DD 5/9/1991
INTERFERON BETA (RECOMBINANT) TN=R-HUIFN-BETA	FOR THE SYSTEMIC TREATMENT OF CUTANEOUS T-CELL LYMPHOMA.	BIOGEN, INC. 14 CAMBRIDGE CENTER CAMBRIDGE MA 02142 DD 4/18/1991
INTERFERON BETA (RECOMBINANT) TN=R-IFN-BETA	FOR THE SYSTEMIC TREATMENT OF METASTATIC RENAL CELL CARCINOMA.	BIOGEN, INC. 14 CAMBRIDGE CENTER CAMBRIDGE MA 02142 DD 2/12/1991
INTERFERON BETA, RECOMBINANT HUMAN TN=BETASERON	TREATMENT OF ACQUIRED IMMUNODEFICIENCY SYNDROME.	BERLEX LABORATORIES, INC. 15049 SAN PABLO AVENUE, P.O. BOX 4099 RICHMOND CA 94804 DD 11/15/1988
INTERFERON BETA-1A TN=REBIF	TREATMENT OF PATIENTS WITH SECONDARY PROGRESSIVE MULTIPLE SCLEROSIS.	SERONO LABORATORIES, INC. 100 LONGWATER CIRCLE NORWELL MA 02061 DD 3/11/1996
INTERFERON BETA-1A TN=AVONEX	TREATMENT OF MULTIPLE SCLEROSIS.	BIOGEN, INC. 14 CAMBRIDGE CENTER CAMBRIDGE MA 02142 DD 12/16/1991 MA 5/17/1996
INTERFERON BETA-1A (RECOMBINANT HUMAN) TN=AVONEX	TREATMENT OF PULMONARY FIBROSIS.	BIOGEN, INC. 14 CAMBRIDGE CENTER CAMBRIDGE MA 02142 DD 1/7/1999
INTERFERON BETA-1A (RECOMBINANT HUMAN)	TREATMENT OF ACUTE NON-A, NON-B HEPATITIS.	BIOGEN, INC. 14 CAMBRIDGE CENTER CAMBRIDGE MA 02142 DD 7/24/1992

NAME *Generic/Chemical* *TN=Trade Name*	INDICATION DESIGNATED	SPONSOR AND ADDRESS *DD=Date Designated* *MA=Marketing Approval*
INTERFERON BETA-1A (RECOMBINANT) TN=REBIF	TREATMENT OF SYMPTOMATIC PATIENTS WITH AIDS INCLUDING ALL PATIENTS WITH CD4 T-CELL COUNTS LESS THAN 200 CELLS PER MM3.	SERONO LABORATORIES, INC. 100 LONGWATER CIRCLE NORWELL MA 02061 DD 12/2/1992
INTERFERON BETA-1A (RECOMBINANT) TN=R-HUIFN-BETA	FOR THE SYSTEMIC TREATMENT OF CUTANEOUS MALIGNANT MELANOMA.	BIOGEN, INC. 14 CAMBRIDGE CENTER CAMBRIDGE MA 02142 DD 4/3/1991
INTERFERON BETA-1B TN=BETASERON	TREATMENT OF MULTIPLE SCLEROSIS.	CHIRON CORP. & BERLEX LABORATORIES 4560 HORTON STREET EMERYVILLE CA 94608 DD 11/17/1988 MA 7/23/1993
INTERFERON GAMMA 1-B TN=ACTIMMUNE	TREATMENT OF CHRONIC GRANULOMATOUS DISEASE.	GENENTECH, INC. 460 POINT SAN BRUNO BOULEVARD SOUTH SAN FRANCISCO CA 94080 DD 9/30/1988 MA 12/20/1990
INTERFERON GAMMA-1B TN=ACTIMMUNE	TREATMENT OF RENAL CELL CARCINOMA.	GENENTECH, INC. 1 DNA WAY SOUTH SAN FRANCISCO CA 94080-4990 DD 12/4/1995
INTERFERON GAMMA-1B TN=ACTIMMUNE	DELAYING TIME TO DISEASE PROGRESSION IN PATIENTS WITH SEVERE, MALIGNANT OSTEOPETROSIS.	INTERMUNE , INC. 3280 BAYSHORE BOULEVARD BRISBANE CA 94005 DD 9/30/1996 MA 2/10/2000
INTERFERON-ALFA-1B	TREATMENT OF MULTIPLE MYELOMA	ERNEST C.BORDEN CENTER FOR CANCER DRUD DISCOVERY AND DEVELOPMENT 9500 EUCLID AVENUE CLEVLAND OH 44195 DD 4/17/2001
INTERLEUKIN-1 ALPHA, HUMAN RECOMBINANT	FOR THE PROMOTION OF EARLY ENGRAFTMENT IN BONE MARROW TRANSPLANTATION.	IMMUNEX CORPORATION 51 UNIVERSITY STREET SEATTLE WA 98101 DD 6/17/1991
INTERLEUKIN-1 ALPHA, HUMAN RECOMBINANT	FOR HEMATOPOIETIC POTENTIATION IN APLASTIC ANEMIA.	IMMUNEX CORPORATION 51 UNIVERSITY STREET SEATTLE WA 98101 DD 6/17/1991
INTERLEUKIN-1 RECEPTOR ANTAGONIST, HUMAN RECOMBINANT TN=ANTRIL	PREVENTION AND TREATMENT OF GRAFT VERSUS HOST DISEASE IN TRANSPLANT RECIPIENTS.	AMGEN, INC. ONE AMGEN CENTER DRIVE THOUSAND OAKS CA 91320-1799 DD 10/16/1992
INTERLEUKIN-1 RECEPTOR ANTAGONIST, HUMAN RECOMBINANT TN=ANTRIL	TREATMENT OF JUVENILE RHEUMATOID ARTHRITIS.	AMGEN, INC. ONE AMGEN CENTER DRIVE THOUSAND OAKS CA 91320-1799 DD 9/23/1991

NAME *Generic/Chemical* *TN=Trade Name*	INDICATION DESIGNATED	SPONSOR AND ADDRESS *DD=Date Designated* *MA=Marketing Approval*
INTERLEUKIN-2 TN=TECELEUKIN	TREATMENT OF METASTATIC RENAL CELL CARCINO-MA.	HOFFMANN-LA ROCHE, INC. 340 KINGSLAND STREET NUTLEY NJ 07110 DD 2/5/1990
INTERLEUKIN-2 TN=TECELEUKIN	IN COMBINATION WITH INTERFERON ALFA-2A FOR THE TREATMENT OF METASTATIC MALIGNANT MELANOMA.	HOFFMANN-LA ROCHE, INC. 340 KINGSLAND STREET NUTLEY NJ 07110 DD 5/11/1990
INTERLEUKIN-2 TN=TELELEUKIN	TREATMENT OF METASTATIC MALIGNANT MELANO-MA.	HOFFMANN-LA ROCHE, INC. 340 KINGSLAND STREET NUTLEY NJ 07110 DD 2/6/1990
INTERLEUKIN-2 TN=TECELEUKIN	IN COMBINATION WITH INTERFERON ALFA-2A FOR THE TREATMENT OF METASTATIC RENAL CELL CARCINOMA.	HOFFMANN-LA ROCHE, INC. 340 KINGSLAND STREET NUTLEY NJ 07110 DD 5/3/1990
INTERLEUKIN-3 HUMAN (RECOMBINANT)	PROMOTION OF ERYTHROPOIESIS IN DIAMOND-BLACKFAN ANEMIA (CONGENITAL PURE RED CELL APLASIA).	IMMUNEX CORPORATION 51 UNIVERSITY STREET SEATTLE WA 98101 DD 5/20/1991
INTERLEUKIN-3, HUMAN, RE-COMBINANT	FOR SEQUENTIAL ADMINISTRATION WITH SARGRA-MOSTIM TO ACCELERATE NEUTROPHIL AND PLATE-LET RECOVERY IN PATIENTS UNDERGOING AUTOLOGOUS BONE MARROW TRANSPLANTATION FOR THE TREATMENT OF HODGKIN'S DISEASE OR NON-HODGKIN'S LYMPHOMA.	SANDOZ PHARMACEUTICALS CORP. 59 ROUTE 10 EAST HANOVER NJ 07936 DD 9/30/1993
INTRAORAL FLUORIDE RELEASING SYSTEM TN=IFRS	PREVENTION OF DENTAL CARIES DUE TO RADIATION-INDUCED XEROSTOMIA IN PATIENTS WITH HEAD AND NECK CANCER	DIGESTIVE CARE, INC. 1120 WIN DRIVE BETHLEHEM PA 18017 DD 7/31/2001
IOBENGUANE SULFATE I 131	FOR USE AS A DIAGNOSTIC ADJUNCT IN PATIENTS WITH PHEOCHROMOCYTOMA.	UNIVERSITY OF MICHIGAN UH B1 H410/0028 1500 E. MEDICAL CENTER DRIVE ANN ARBOR MI 48109-0028 DD 11/14/1984 MA 3/21/1990
IODINE 131 6B-IODOMETHYL-19-NORCHOLESTEROL	FOR USE IN ADRENAL CORTICAL IMAGING.	DAVID E. KUHL, M.D. UNIVERSITY OF MICHIGAN MEDI-CAL CENTER/1500 E. MED. CTR. DRIVE B1G412 /0028 UNIVERSITY HOS-PITAL ANN ARBOR MI 48109-0028 DD 8/1/1984
IODINE I 123 MURINE MONOCLO-NAL ANTIBODY TO ALPHA-FETO-PROTEIN	DETECTION OF ALPHA-FETOPROTEIN PRODUCING GERM CELL TUMORS.	IMMUNOMEDICS, INC. 300 AMERICAN ROAD MORRIS PLAINS NJ 07950 DD 9/30/1988
IODINE I 123 MURINE MONOCLO-NAL ANTIBODY TO ALPHA-FETO-PROTEIN	DETECTION OF HEPATOCELLULAR CARCINOMA AND HEPATOBLASTOMA.	IMMUNOMEDICS, INC. 300 AMERICAN ROAD MORRIS PLAINS NJ 07950 DD 9/30/1988
IODINE I 123 MURINE MONOCLO-NAL ANTIBODY TO HCG	DETECTION OF HCG PRODUCING TUMORS SUCH AS GERM CELL AND TROPHOBLASTIC CELL TUMORS.	IMMUNOMEDICS, INC. 300 AMERICAN ROAD MORRIS PLAINS NJ 07950 DD 11/7/1988

NAME *Generic/Chemical* *TN=Trade Name*	INDICATION DESIGNATED	SPONSOR AND ADDRESS *DD=Date Designated* *MA=Marketing Approval*
IODINE I 131 LYM-1 MONOCLO-NAL ANTIBODY	TREATMENT OF B-CELL LYMPHOMA.	LEDERLE LABORATORIES DIVISION AMERICAN CYANAMIDE COMPANY PEARL RIVER NY 10965 DD 11/2/1987
IODINE I 131 BIS(INDIUM-DIETHY-LENETRIAMINEPENTAACETIC ACID)TYROSYLLYSINE/HMN-14 X M734 F(AB')2 BISPECIFIC MONO-CLONAL ANTIBODY TN=PENTACEA	TREATMENT OF SMALL-CELL LUNG CANCER.	IBC PHARMACEUTICALS, L.L.C. 300 AMERICAN RD. MORRIS PLAINS NJ 07950 DD 2/22/2000
IODINE I 131 MURINE MONOCLO-NAL ANTIBODY IGG2A TO B CELL TN=IMMURAIT, LL-2-I-131	TREATMENT OF B-CELL LEUKEMIA AND B-CELL LYM-PHOMA.	IMMUNOMEDICS, INC. 300 AMERICAN ROAD MORRIS PLAINS NJ 07950 DD 9/18/1989
IODINE I 131 MURINE MONOCLO-NAL ANTIBODY TO ALPHA-FETO-PROTEIN	TREATMENT OF HEPATOCELLULAR CARCINOMA AND HEPATOBLASTOMA.	IMMUNOMEDICS, INC. 300 AMERICAN ROAD MORRIS PLAINS NJ 07950 DD 9/30/1988
IODINE I 131 MURINE MONOCLO-NAL ANTIBODY TO ALPHA-FETO-PROTEIN	TREATMENT OF ALPHA-FETOPROTEIN PRODUCING GERM CELL TUMORS.	IMMUNOMEDICS, INC. 300 AMERICAN ROAD MORRIS PLAINS NJ 07950 DD 9/30/1988
IODINE I 131 MURINE MONOCLO-NAL ANTIBODY TO HCG	TREATMENT OF HCG PRODUCING TUMORS SUCH AS GERM CELL AND TROPHOBLASTIC CELL TUMORS.	IMMUNOMEDICS, INC. 300 AMERICAN ROAD MORRIS PLAINS NJ 07950 DD 11/7/1988
IODINE I-131 RADIOLABELED CHI-MERIC MAB TUMOR NECROSIS TREATMENT (TNT-1B) TN=131ICHTNT-1	TREATMENT OF GLIOBLASTOMA MULTIFORME AND ANAPLASTIC ASTROCYTOMA.	PEREGRINE PHARMACEUTI-CALS, INC. 14282 FRANKLIN AVE. TUSTIN CA 92780-7017 DD 2/12/1999
IRON(III)-HEXACYANOFERRA-TE(II) TN=RADIOGARDASE-CS/ANTIDOTUM	TREATMENT OF PATIENTS WITH KNOWN OR SUS-PECTED INTERNAL CONTAMINATION WITH RADIOAC-TIVE OR NON-RADIOACTIVE CESIUM OR THALLIUM.	HEYL CHEMISCH-PHARMZEU-TISCHE FABRIK GMBH 7 CO, KG GOERZALLE 253 BERLIN, FEDERAL REPUBLIC OF GERMANY D-14167 DD 5/1/2003
ISOBUTYRAMIDE	TREATMENT OF SICKLE CELL DISEASE AND BETA THALASSEMIA.	ALPHA THERAPEUTIC COR-PORATION 5555 VALLEY BOULEVARD LOS ANGELES CA 90032 DD 5/25/1994
ISOBUTYRAMIDE TN=ISOBUTYRAMIDE ORAL SO-LUTION	TREATMENT OF BETA-HEMOGLOBINOPATHIES AND BETA-THALASSEMIA SYNDROMES.	PERRINE, SUSAN P., M.D. BOSTON UNIVERSITY CANCER RESEARCH CENTER BOSTON MA 02118 DD 12/18/1992
JAPANESE ENCEPHALITIS VAC-CINE (LIVE, ATTENUATED)	PREVENTION OF JAPANESE ENCEPHALITIS.	BORAN PHARMACEUTICALS 3F, KORYO ACADEMYTEL, 437-3 AHYUN-DONG, MAPO-GU, SEOUL 121-010 SOUTH KOREA KR DD 5/19/1999

NAME *Generic/Chemical* *TN=Trade Name*	INDICATION DESIGNATED	SPONSOR AND ADDRESS *DD=Date Designated* *MA=Marketing Approval*
KETOCONAZOLE TN=NIZORAL	FOR USE WITH CYCLOSPORINE A TO DIMINISH THE NEPHROTOXICITY INDUCED BY CYCLOSPORINE IN ORGAN TRANSPLANTATION.	PHARMEDIC COMPANY 28101 BALLARD ROAD LAKE FOREST IL 60045 DD 3/27/1991
L-2-OXOTHIAZOLIDINE-4-CAR-BOXYLIC ACID TN=PROCYSTEINE	TREATMENT OF ADULT RESPIRATORY DISTRESS SYNDROME.	TRANSCEND THERAPEUTICS, INC. 640 MEMORIAL DRIVE, 3RD FLOOR WEST CAMBRIDGE MA 02139 DD 6/14/1994
L-2-OXOTHIAZOLIDINE-4-CAR-BOXYLIC ACID TN=PROCYSTEINE	TREATMENT OF AMYOTROPHIC LATERAL SCLERO-SIS.	TRANSCEND THERAPEUTICS, INC. 640 MEMORIAL DRIVE, 3RD FLOOR WEST CAMBRIDGE MA 02139 DD 7/30/1996
L-5-HYDROXYTRYPTOPHAN	TREATMENT OF TETRAHYDROBIOPTERIN DEFI-CIENCY.	WATSON LABORATORIES, INC. 311 BONNIE CIRCLE P.O. BOX 1900 CORONA CA 91718-1900 DD 1/20/1999
L-BACLOFEN	TREATMENT OF TRIGEMINAL NEURALGIA.	FROMM, GERHARD M.D. UNIVERSITY OF PITTSBURGH SCHOOL OF MEDICINE PITTSBURGH PA 15261 DD 7/13/1990
L-BACLOFEN TN=NEURALGON	TREATMENT OF INTRACTABLE SPASTICITY ASSO-CIATED WITH SPINAL CORD INJURY OR MULTIPLE SCLEROSIS.	PHARMASCIENCE INC. 6111 ROYALMOUNT, SUITE 100 MONTREAL, QUEBEC H4P 2T4 CANADA CA DD 12/17/1991
L-BACLOFEN TN=NEURALGON	TREATMENT OF INTRACTABLE SPASTICITY IN CHIL-DREN WITH CEREBRAL PALSY.	PHARMASCIENCE INC. 6111 ROYALMOUNT, SUITE 100 MONTREAL, QUEBEC H4P 2T4 CANADA CA DD 1/30/1992
L-BACLOFEN	TREATMENT OF TRIGEMINAL NEURALGIA.	PHARMASCIENCE INC. 6111 ROYALMOUNT, #100 MONTREAL, QUEBEC CANADA H4P 2T4 CA DD 1/6/1998
L-CYCLOSERINE	TREATMENT OF GAUCHER'S DISEASE.	LEV, MEIR M.D. THE CITY COLLEGE, CITY UNI-VERSITY OF NY MEDICAL SCHOOL CONVENT AVENUE AT 138 STREET NEW YORK NY 10031 DD 8/1/1989
L-CYSTEINE	FOR THE PREVENTION AND LESSENING OF PHOTO-SENSITIVITY IN ERYTHROPOIETIC PROTOPORPHYR-IA.	ORPHAN PHARMACEUTICALS, U.S.A., INC. 1101 KERMIT DR.1101 KERMIT DR. SUITE 608 NASHVILLE TN 37217 DD 5/16/1994

NAME *Generic/Chemical* *TN=Trade Name*	INDICATION DESIGNATED	SPONSOR AND ADDRESS *DD=Date Designated* *MA=Marketing Approval*
L-GLUTAMINE	TREATMENT OF SICKLE CELL DISEASE	ORPHAN DRUGS INTERNA-TIONAL, LLC (D.B.A. HOPE THER-APEUTICS) PO BOX 0401 MONTROSE CA 91021-0401 DD 8/1/2001
L-GLUTAMYL-L-TRYPTOPHAN	TREATMENT OF AIDS-RELATED KAPOSI'S SARCOMA.	CYTRAN INCORPORATED 10230 N.E. POINTS DR. SUITE 530 KIRKLAND WA 98033-7869 DD 10/20/1999
L-LEUCOVORIN TN=ISOVORIN	FOR USE IN COMBINATION CHEMOTHERAPY WITH THE APPROVED AGENT 5-FLUOROURACIL IN THE PALLIATIVE TREATMENT OF METASTATIC ADENO-CARCINOMA OF THE COLON AND RECTUM.	LEDERLE LABORATORIES DIVISION OF AMERICAN CYANA-MID COMPANY 401 N. MIDDLETOWN ROAD PEARL RIVER NY 10965 DD 12/18/1990
L-LEUCOVORIN TN=ISOVORIN	FOR USE IN CONJUNCTION WITH HIGH-DOSE METHO-TREXATE IN THE TREATMENT OF OSTEOSARCOMA.	LEDERLE LABORATORIES DIVISION OF AMERICAN CYANA-MID COMPANY 401 N. MIDDLETOWN ROAD PEARL RIVER NY 10965 DD 8/1/1991
L-THREONINE TN=THREOSTAT	TREATMENT OF AMYOTROPHIC LATERAL SCLERO-SIS.	TYSON AND ASSOCIATES 12832 CHADRON AVENUE HAWTHORNE CA 90250 DD 2/6/1989
L-THREONINE	TREATMENT OF SPASTICITY ASSOCIATED WITH FA-MILIAL SPASTIC PARAPARESIS.	INTERNEURON PHARMACEUTI-CALS, INC. 99 HAYDEN AVE., SUITE 200 LEXINGTON MA 02421-7966 DD 7/24/1992
LACTIC ACID TN=APHTHAID	TREATMENT OF SEVERE APHTHOUS STOMATITIS IN SEVERELY, TERMINALLY IMMUNOCOMPROMISED PA-TIENTS.	FRONTIER PHARMACEUTICAL, INC. SUNY FARMINGDALE CONKLIN HALL FARMINGDALE NY 11735 DD 6/29/1999
LACTOBIN TN=LACTOBIN	TREATMENT OF AIDS-ASSOCIATED DIARRHEA UNRE-SPONSIVE TO INITIAL ANTIDIARRHEAL THERAPY.	ROXANE LABORATORIES, INC. P.O. BOX 16532 COLUMBUS OH 43216-6532 DD 9/12/1990
LAMOTRIGINE TN=LAMICTAL	TREATMENT OF LENNOX-GASTAUT SYNDROME.	GLAXO WELLCOME RESEARCH AND DEVELOPMENT 5 MOORE DRIVE P.O. BOX 13398 RESEARCH TRIANGLE PARK NC 27709 DD 8/23/1995 MA 8/24/1998
LANREOTIDE, SOMATOSTATIN TN=IPSTYL	TREATMENT FOR ACROMEGLY	IPSEN, INC. 27 MAPLE STREET MILFORD MA 01757 DD 9/11/2000

NAME *Generic/Chemical* *TN=Trade Name*	**INDICATION DESIGNATED**	**SPONSOR AND ADDRESS** *DD=Date Designated* *MA=Marketing Approval*
LATRODECTUS IMMUNE F(AB)2 TN=ARACMYN	TREATMENT OF BLACK WIDOW SPIDER ENVENOMA-TIONS	RARE DISEASE THERAPEUTICS, INC. 1101 KERMIT DRIVE, SUITE 608 NASHVILLE TN 37217 DD 6/18/2001
LEFLUNOMIDE	PREVENTION OF ACUTE AND CHRONIC REJECTION IN PATIENTS WHO HAVE RECEIVED SOLID ORGAN TRANSPLANTS.	WILLIAMS, MD, JAMES W. RUSH-PRESBYTERIAN-ST. LUKE'S MEDICAL CTR., DEPT. OF GENERAL SURGERY 1653 WEST CONGRESS PARK-WAY CHICAGO IL 60612-3833 DD 10/18/1996
LEPIRUDIN TN=REFLUDEN	TREATMENT OF HEPARIN-ASSOCIATED THROMBO-CYTOPENIA TYPE II.	HOECHST MARION ROUSSEL FRANKFURT AM MAIN GERMANY DE DD 2/13/1997 MA 3/6/1998
LEUCOVORIN TN=LEUCOVORIN CALCIUM	FOR RESCUE USE AFTER HIGH DOSE METHOTREX-ATE THERAPY IN THE TREATMENT OF OSTEOSARCO-MA.	IMMUNEX CORPORATION 51 UNIVERSITY STREET SEATTLE WA 98101 DD 8/17/1988 MA 8/31/1988
LEUCOVORIN TN=LEUCOVORIN CALCIUM	FOR USE IN COMBINATION WITH 5-FLUOROURACIL FOR THE TREATMENT OF METASTATIC COLORECTAL CANCER.	IMMUNEX CORPORATION 51 UNIVERSITY STREET SEATTLE WA 98101 DD 12/8/1986 MA 12/12/1991
LEUCOVORIN CALCIUM TN=WELLCOVORIN	FOR USE IN COMBINATION WITH 5-FLUOROURACIL FOR THE TREATMENT OF METASTATIC COLORECTAL CANCER.	GLAXO WELLCOME RESEARCH AND DEVELOPMENT 5 MOORE DRIVE PO BOX 13398 RESEARCH TRIANGLE PARK NC 27709 DD 6/23/1988
LEUPEPTIN	FOR USE AS AN ADJUNCT TO MICROSURGICAL PE-RIPHERAL NERVE REPAIR.	NEUROMUSCULAR ADJUNCTS, INC. S.U.N.Y. AT STONY BROOK H.S.C. T18-020 STONY BROOK NY 11794-8181 DD 9/18/1990
LEUPROLIDE ACETATE TN=LUPRON INJECTION	TREATMENT OF CENTRAL PRECOCIOUS PUBERTY.	TAP PHARMACEUTICALS, INC. 2355 WAUKEGAN ROAD DEERFIELD IL 60015 DD 7/25/1988 MA 4/16/1993
LEVOCABASTINE HCL OPH-THALMIC SUSPENSION 0.05%	TREATMENT OF VERNAL KERATOCONJUNCTIVITIS.	IOLAB PHARMACEUTICALS 500 IOLAB DRIVE CLAREMONT CA 94608 DD 2/29/1988
LEVOCARNITINE TN=CARNITOR	TREATMENT OF PRIMARY AND SECONDARY CARNI-TINE DEFICIENCY OF GENETIC ORIGIN.	SIGMA-TAU PHARMACEUTICALS, INC. 800 SOUTH FREDERICK AVENUE GAITHERSBURG MD 20877 DD 7/26/1984 MA 12/16/1992

NAME *Generic/Chemical* *TN=Trade Name*	INDICATION DESIGNATED	SPONSOR AND ADDRESS *DD=Date Designated* *MA=Marketing Approval*
LEVOCARNITINE TN=CARNITOR	TREATMENT OF GENETIC CARNITINE DEFICIENCY.	SIGMA-TAU PHARMACEUTICALS, INC. 800 SOUTH FREDERICK AVENUE GAITHERSBURG MD 20877 DD 2/28/1984 MA 4/10/1986
LEVOCARNITINE TN=CARNITOR	FOR THE TREATMENT OF SECONDARY CARNITINE DEFICIENCY IN VALPROIC ACID TOXICITY.	SIGMA-TAU PHARMACEUTICALS, INC. 800 SOUTH FREDERICK AVENUE GAITHERSBURG MD 20877 DD 11/15/1989
LEVOCARNITINE TN=CARNITOR	TREATMENT OF ZIDOVUDINE-INDUCED MITOCHONDRIAL MYOPATHY.	SIGMA-TAU PHARMACEUTICALS, INC. 800 S. FREDERICK AVENUE, SUITE 300 GAITHERSBURG MD 20877 DD 4/7/1997
LEVOCARNITINE TN=CARNITOR	TREATMENT OF MANIFESTATIONS OF CARNITINE DEFICIENCY IN PATIENTS WITH END STAGE RENAL DISEASE WHO REQUIRE DIALYSIS.	SIGMA-TAU PHARMACEUTICALS, INC. 800 SOUTH FREDERICK AVENUE GAITHERSBURG MD 20877 DD 11/24/1986
LEVOCARNITINE TN=CARNITOR	TREATMENT OF MANIFESTATIONS OF CARNITINE DEFICIENCY IN PATIENTS WITH END STAGE RENAL DISEASE WHO REQUIRE DIALYSIS.	SIGMA-TAU PHARMACEUTICALS, INC. 800 SOUTH FREDERICK AVENUE, SUITE 300 GAITHERSBURG MD 20877 DD 9/6/1988 MA 12/15/1999
LEVOCARNITINE TN=CARNITOR	TREATMENT OF PEDIATRIC CARDIOMYOPATHY.	SIGMA-TAU PHARMACEUTICALS, INC. 800 SOUTH FREDERICK AVENUE GAITHERSBURG MD 20877 DD 11/22/1993
LEVOCARNITINE TN=CARNITOR	FOR THE PREVENTION OF SECONDARY CARNITINE DEFICIENCY IN VALPROIC ACID TOXICITY.	SIGMA-TAU PHARMACEUTICALS, INC. 800 SOUTH FREDERICK AVENUE GAITHERSBURG MD 20877 DD 11/15/1989
LEVODOPA AND CARBIDOPA TN=DUODOPA	TREATMENT OF LATE STAGE PARKINSON'S DISEASE.	NOUVEL PHARMA, INC. 11384 STRANG LINE ROAD LENEXA KS 66215 DD 1/18/2000
LEVOMETHADYL ACETATE HYDROCHLORIDE TN=ORLAAM	TREATMENT OF HEROIN ADDICTS SUITABLE FOR MAINTENANCE ON OPIATE AGONISTS.	BIODEVELOPMENT CORPORATION 8180 GREENSBORO DRIVE, SUITE 1000 MCLEAN VA 22102 DD 1/24/1985 MA 7/9/1993
LIDOCAINE PATCH 5% TN=LIDODERM PATCH	FOR RELIEF OF ALLODYNIA (PAINFUL HYPERSENSITIVITY), AND CHRONIC PAIN IN POST-HERPETIC NEURALGIA.	TEIKOKU PHARMA USA, INC. 745-D CAMDEN AVE. CAMPBELL CA 95008-4146 DD 10/24/1995 MA 3/19/1999

NAME *Generic/Chemical* *TN=Trade Name*	INDICATION DESIGNATED	SPONSOR AND ADDRESS *DD=Date Designated* *MA=Marketing Approval*
LIOTHYRONINE SODIUM INJECTION TN=TRIOSTAT	TREATMENT OF MYXEDEMA COMA/PRECOMA.	SMITHKLINE BEECHAM PHARMACEUTICALS ONE FRANKLIN PLAZA P.O. BOX 7929 PHILADELPHIA PA 19101 DD 7/30/1990 MA 12/31/1991
LIPID/DNA HUMAN CYSTIC FIBROSIS GENE	TREATMENT OF CYSTIC FIBROSIS.	GENZYME CORPORATION ONE MOUNTAIN ROAD P.O. BOX 9322 FRAMINGHAM MA 01701-9322 DD 4/8/1996
LIPOSOMAL N-ACETYLGLUCOS-MINYL-N-ACETYLMURAMLY-L-ALA-D-ISOGLN-L-ALA -GYLCERO-LIDPALMITOYL TN=IMMTHER	TREATMENT OF OSTEOSARCOMA.	ENDOREX CORP. 900 NORTH SHORE DRIVE LAKE BLUFF IL 60044 DD 6/10/1998
LIPOSOMAL N-ACETYLGLUCOS-MINYL-N-ACETYLMURAMLY-L-ALA-D-ISOGLN-L-ALA -GYLCERO-LIDPALMITOYL TN=IMMTHER	TREATMENT OF EWING'S SARCOMA.	ENDOREX CORP. 900 NORTH SHORE DRIVE LAKE BLUFF IL 60044 DD 6/10/1998
LIPOSOMAL AMPHOTERICIN B TN=AMBISOME	TREATMENT OF HISTOPLASMOSIS.	FUJISAWA USA, INC. 3 PARKWAY NORTH CENTER DEERFIELD IL 60015 DD 12/10/1996
LIPOSOMAL AMPHOTERICIN B TN=AMBISOME	TREATMENT OF CRYPTOCOCCAL MENINGITIS.	FUJISAWA USA, INC. 3 PARKWAY NORTH CENTER DEERFIELD IL 60015 DD 12/10/1996 MA 8/11/1997
LIPOSOMAL AMPHOTERICIN B TN=AMBISOME	TREATMENT OF VISCERAL LEISHMANIASIS.	FUJISAWA USA, INC. 3 PARKWAY NORTH CENTER DEERFIELD IL 60015 DD 12/6/1996 MA 8/11/1997
LIPOSOMAL CYCLOSPORIN A TN=CYCLOSPIRE	FOR AEROSOLIZED ADMINISTRATION IN THE PREVENTION AND TREATMENT OF LUNG ALLOGRAFT REJECTION AND PULMONARY REJECTION EVENTS ASSOCIATED WITH BONE MARROW TRANSPLANTATION.	VERNON KNIGHT, M.D. BAYLOR COLLEGE OF MEDICINE, DEPT. OF MOLECULAR PHYSIOLOGY ONE BAYLOR PLAZA HOUSTON TX 77030 DD 4/30/1998
LIPOSOMAL NYSTATIN TN=NYOTRAN	TREATMENT OF INVASIVE FUNGAL INFECTIONS.	ANTIGENICS, INC. 34 COMMERCE WAY WOBURN MA 01801 DD 6/13/2000
LIPOSOMAL PROSTAGLANDIN E1 INJECTION	TREATMENT OF ACUTE RESPIRATORY DISTRESS SYNDROME.	LIPOSOME COMPANY, INC. ONE RESEARCH WAY PRINCETON NJ 08540 DD 4/25/1996
LIPOSOMAL-CIS-BIS-NEODECA-NOATO-TRANS-R,R-1,2-DIAMINO-CYCLOHEXANE-PT (II)	TREATMENT OF MALIGNANT MESOTHELIOMA.	ANTIGENICS INCORPORATED 34 COMMERCE WAY WOBURN MA 01801 DD 9/1/1999

NAME Generic/Chemical TN=Trade Name	INDICATION DESIGNATED	SPONSOR AND ADDRESS DD=Date Designated MA=Marketing Approval
LIPOSOME ENCAPSULATED RECOMBINANT INTERLEUKIN-2	TREATMENT OF CANCERS OF THE KIDNEY AND RENAL PELVIS.	BIOMIRA USA, INC. 1002 EASTPARK BOULEVARD CRANBURY NJ 08512 DD 6/20/1994
LIPOSOME ENCAPSULATED RECOMBINANT INTERLEUKIN-2	TREATMENT OF BRAIN AND CNS TUMORS.	BIOMIRA USA, INC. 1002 EASTPARK BOULEVARD CRANBURY NJ 08512 DD 11/25/1991
LISOFYLLINE	TREATMENT OF PATIENTS UNDERGOING INDUCTION THERAPY FOR ACUTE MYELOID LEUKEMIA.	CELL THERAPEUTICS, INC. 201 ELLIOT AVENUE WEST201 ELLIOTT AVENUE WEST201 ELLIOTT AVENUE WEST SUITE 400 SEATTLE WA 98119 DD 6/10/1999
LODOXAMIDE TROMETHAMINE TN=ALOMIDE OPHTHALMIC SOLUTION	TREATMENT OF VERNAL KERATOCONJUNCTIVITIS.	ALCON LABORATORIES, INC. 6201 SOUTH FREEWAY FORT WORTH TX 76134 DD 10/16/1991 MA 9/23/1993
LOXORIBINE	TREATMENT OF COMMON VARIABLE IMMUNODEFICIENCY.	R. W. JOHNSON PHARMACEUTICAL RESEARCH INSTITUTE ROUTE 202, P.O. BOX 300 RARITAN NJ 08869 DD 2/24/1992
LUCINACTANT TN=SURFAXIN	TREATMENT OF MECONIUM ASPIRATION SYNDROME IN NEWBORN INFANTS.	DISCOVERY LABORATORIES, INC. 350 SOUTH MAIN STREET SUITE 307 DOYLESTOWN PA 18901 DD 7/30/1996
LUCINACTANT TN=SURFAXIN	TREATMENT OF ACUTE RESPIRATORY DISTRESS SYNDROME IN ADULTS.	DISCOVERY LABORATORIES, INC. 350 SOUTH MAIN STREET SUITE 307 DOYLESTOWN PA 18901 DD 7/17/1995
LUCINACTANT TN=SURFAXIN	TREATMENT OF RESPIRATORY DISTRESS SYNDROME IN PREMATURE INFANTS.	DISCOVERY LABORATORIES, INC. 350 SOUTH MAIN STREET SUITE 307 DOYLESTOWN PA 18901 DD 10/18/1995
LYSINE ACETYLSALICYLATE INJECTABLE	TREATMENT OF PAIN AND FEVER SECONDARY TO SICKLE CELL DISEASE CRISIS.	G.D. SEARLE & COMPANY DD 8/1/1989
MART-1 ADENOVIRAL GENE THERAPY FOR MALIGNANT MELANOMA	TREATMENT OF METASTATIC MELANOMA.	GENZYME CORPORATION ONE MOUNTAIN ROAD P.O. BOX 9322 FRAMINGHAM MA 01701-9322 DD 3/28/1997
MN14 MONOCLONAL ANTIBODY TO CARCINOEMBRYONIC ANTIGEN TN=CEA-CIDE	TREATMENT OF PANCREATIC CANCER.	IMMUNOMEDICS, INC. 300 AMERICAN ROAD MORRIS PLAINS NJ 07950 DD 11/24/1998
MN14 MONOCLONAL ANTIBODY TO CARCINOEMBRYONIC ANTIGEN TN=CEA-CIDE	FOR THE TREATMENT OF SMALL CELL LUNG CANCER.	IMMUNOMEDICS, INC. 300 AMERICAN RD. MORRIS PLAINS NJ 07950 DD 9/18/1998

NAME *Generic/Chemical* *TN=Trade Name*	INDICATION DESIGNATED	SPONSOR AND ADDRESS *DD=Date Designated* *MA=Marketing Approval*
MTC-DOX FOR INJECTION	TREATMENT OF HEPATOCELLULAR CARCINOMA	FERX INCORPORATED 4330 LA JOLLA VILLAGE DRIVE SUITE #250 SAN DIEGO CA 92122 DD 1/3/2001
MAFENIDE ACETATE SOLUTION TN=SULFAMYLON SOLUTION	FOR USE AS AN ADJUNCTIVE TOPICAL ANTIMICRO-BIAL AGENT TO CONTROL BACTERIAL INFECTION WHEN USED UNDER MOIST DRESSINGS OVER MESHED AUTOGRAFTS ON EXCISED BURN WOUNDS.	MYLAN LABORATORIES, INC. 781 CHESTNUT RIDGE ROAD P.O. BOX 4310 MORGANTOWN WV 26504-4310 DD 7/18/1990 MA 6/5/1998
MAFOSFAMIDE	TREATMENT OF NEOPLASTIC MENINGITIS	BAXTER ONCOLOGY GMBH (FORMERLY ASTA MEDICA ONCOLOGY) DAIMLERSTRASSE 40 60314 FRANFURT/MAIN GERMANY DD 1/21/2003
MARIJUANA	TREATMENT OF HIV-ASSOCIATED WASTING SYN-DROME.	MULTIDISCIPLINARY ASSOCIA-TION FOR PSYCHEDELIC STUDIES, INC. 3 FRANCIS ST. BELMONT MA 02478 DD 5/25/1999
MATRIX METALLOPROTEINASE INHIBITOR TN=GALARDIN	TREATMENT OF CORNEAL ULCERS.	GLYCOMED, INC 860 ATLANTIC AVENUE ALAMEDA CA 94501 DD 12/5/1991
MAXADFVIII	TREATMENT OF HEMOPHILIA A	GENSTAR THERAEUTICS CORPORATION 10865 ALTMAN ROW SUITE 200 SAN DIEGO CA 92121-1113 DD 3/3/2003
MAZINDOL TN=SANOREX	TREATMENT OF DUCHENNE MUSCULAR DYSTRO-PHY.	COLLIPP, PLATON J. M.D. 176 MEMORIAL DRIVE JESUP GA 31545 DD 12/8/1986
MECAMYLAMINE TN=INVERSINE	TREATMENT OF TOURETTE'S SYNDROME.	TARGACEPT, INC. 200 EAST FIRST ST. SUITE 300 WINSTON-SALEM NC 27101-4165 DD 10/14/1998
MECASERMIN TN=MYOTROPHIN	TREATMENT OF AMYOTROPHIC LATERAL SCLERO-SIS.	CEPHALON, INC. 145 BRANDYWINE PARKWAY WEST CHESTER PA 19380-4245 DD 8/5/1991
MECASERMIN	TREATMENT OF GROWTH HORMONE INSUFFICENCY SYNDROME.	GENENTECH, INC. 460 POINT SAN BRUNO BOULE-VARD SOUTH SAN FRANCISCO CA 94080 DD 12/12/1995

NAME *Generic/Chemical* *TN=Trade Name*	INDICATION DESIGNATED	SPONSOR AND ADDRESS *DD=Date Designated* *MA=Marketing Approval*
MEDROXYPROGESTERONE ACE- TATE TN=HEMATROL	TREATMENT OF IMMUNE THROMBOCYTOPENIC PUR- PURA.	INKINE PHARMACEUTICAL COM- PANY, INC. 1787 SENTRY PARKWAY WEST BUILDING 18, SUITE 440 BLUE BELL PA 19422 DD 2/22/2001
MEFLOQUINE HCL TN=MEPHAQUIN	PREVENTION OF CHLOROQUINE-RESISTANT FALCI- PARUM MALARIA.	MEPHA AG 4143 DORNACH POSTFASH 137 AESCH BASEL, SWITZERLAND CH DD 7/22/1987
MEFLOQUINE HCL TN=LARIAM	TREATMENT OF ACUTE MALARIA DUE TO PLASMO- DIUM FALCIPARUM AND PLASMODIUM VIVAX.	HOFFMANN-LA ROCHE, INC. 340 KINGSLAND STREET NUTLEY NJ 07110 DD 4/13/1988 MA 5/2/1989
MEFLOQUINE HCL TN=MEPHAQUIN	TREATMENT OF CHLOROQUINE-RESISTANT FALCI- PARUMMALARIA.	MEPHA AG 4143 DORNACH POSTFASH 137 AESCH BASEL, SWITZERLAND CH DD 7/22/1987
MEFLOQUINE HCL TN=LARIAM	PROPHYLAXIS OF PLASMODIUM FALCIPARUM MA- LARIA WHICH IS RESISTANT TO OTHER AVAILABLE DRUGS.	HOFFMANN-LA ROCHE, INC. 340 KINGSLAND STREET NUTLEY NJ 07110 DD 4/13/1988 MA 5/2/1989
MEGESTROL ACETATE TN=MEGACE	TREATMENT OF PATIENTS WITH ANOREXIA, CACHEX- IA, OR SIGNIFICANT WEIGHT LOSS (=/>10% OF BASE- LINE BODY WEIGHT) AND CONFIRMED DIAGNOSIS OF AIDS.	BRISTOL-MYERS SQUIBB PHARMACEUTICAL RESEARCH INSTITUTE 2400 WEST LLOYD EXPRESSWAY EVANSVILLE IN 47721 DD 4/13/1988 MA 9/10/1993
MELANOMA CELL VACCINE	TREATMENT OF INVASIVE MELANOMA.	MORTON, DONALD L. M.D. JOHN WAYNE CANCER INSTI- TUTE 2200 SANTA MONICA BOULE- VARD SANTA MONICA CA 90404 DD 10/13/1994
MELANOMA VACCINE TN=MELACINE	TREATMENT OF STAGE III - IV MELANOMA.	RIBI IMMUNOCHEM RESEARCH, INC. 533 OLD CORVALLIS ROAD HAMILTON MT 59840 DD 12/20/1989
MELATONIN	TREATMENT OF CIRCADIAN RHYTHM SLEEP DISOR- DERS IN BLIND PEOPLE WITH NO LIGHT PERCEPTION.	SACK, ROBERT, M.D. OREGON HEALTH SCIENCES UNIVERSITY 3181 S.W. SAM JACKSON PARK ROAD PORTLAND OR 97201 DD 11/15/1993

NAME Generic/Chemical TN=Trade Name	INDICATION DESIGNATED	SPONSOR AND ADDRESS DD=Date Designated MA=Marketing Approval
MELPHALAN TN=ALKERAN FOR INJECTION	FOR USE IN HYPERTHERMIC REGIONAL LIMB PERFUSION TO TREAT METASTATIC MELANOMA OF THE EXTREMITY.	GLAXO WELLCOME RESEARCH AND DEVELOPMENT 5 MOORE DRIVE PO BOX 13398 RESEARCH TRIANGLE PARK NC 27709 DD 3/3/1992
MELPHALAN TN=ALKERAN FOR INJECTION	TREATMENT OF PATIENTS WITH MULTIPLE MYELOMA FOR WHOM ORAL THERAPY IS INAPPROPRIATE.	GLAXO WELLCOME INC. 5 MOORE DRIVE RESEARCH TRIANGLE PARK NC 27709 DD 2/24/1992 MA 11/18/1992
MEROPENEM TN=MERREM IV	MANAGEMENT OF ACUTE PULMONARY EXACERBATIONS, IN CYSTIC FIBROSIS PATIENTS, DUE TO RESPIRATORY TRACT INFECTION WITH SUSCEPTIBLE ORGANISMS.	ZENECA PHARMACEUTICALS 1800 CONCORD PIKE PO BOX 15437 WILMINGTON DE 19850-5437 DD 4/27/2000
MESNA	INHIBITION OF THE UROTOXIC EFFECTS INDUCED BY OXAZAPHOSPHORINE COMPOUNDS SUCH AS CYCLOPHOSPHAMIDE.	ASTA MEDICA , INC. 890 EAST ST. TEWKSBURY MA 01876-1496 DD 12/16/1987
MESNA TN=MESNEX	FOR USE AS A PROPHYLACTIC AGENT IN REDUCING THE INCIDENCE OF IFOSFAMIDE-INDUCED HEMORRHAGIC CYSTITIS.	DEGUSSA CORPORATION 65 CHALLENGER ROAD RIDGEFIELD PARK NJ 07660 DD 11/14/1985 MA 12/30/1988
METHIONINE/L-METHIONINE	TREATMENT OF AIDS MYELOPATHY.	DI ROCCO, ALESSANDRO M.D. BETH ISRAEL MEDICAL CENTER, PHILLIPS AMBULATORY CARE CTR. PHILIPS BUILDING, SUITE 2R; 10 UNION SQUARE EAST NEW YORK NY 10003 DD 8/21/1996
METHOTREXATE TN=RHEUMATREX	TREATMENT OF JUVENILE RHEUMATOID ARTHRITIS.	WYETH-AYERST LABORATORIES P.O. BOX 8299 PHILADELPHIA PA 19101-8299 DD 8/23/1993
METHOTREXATE SODIUM TN=METHOTREXATE	TREATMENT OF OSTEOGENIC SARCOMA.	LEDERLE LABORATORIES DIVISION OF AMERICAN CYANAMID COMPANY 401 N. MIDDLETOWN ROAD PEARL RIVER NY 10965 DD 10/21/1985 MA 4/7/1988
METHOTREXATE WITH LAUROCAPRAM TN=METHOTREXATE/AZONE	TOPICAL TREATMENT OF MYCOSIS FUNGOIDES.	DURHAM PHARMACEUTICALS LLC 200 WESTPARK CORPORATE CENTER 4364 SOUTH ALSTON AVENUE DURHAM NC 27713-2280 DD 10/15/1990
METHOXSALEN TN=UVADEX	FOR USE IN CONJUNCTION WITH THE UVAR PHOTOPHERESIS SYSTEM TO TREAT GRAFT VERSUS HOST DISEASE.	THERAKOS, INC. 437 CREAMERY WAY EXTON PA 19431 DD 10/14/1998

NAME *Generic/Chemical* *TN=Trade Name*	INDICATION DESIGNATED	SPONSOR AND ADDRESS *DD=Date Designated* *MA=Marketing Approval*
METHYLNALTREXONE	TREATMENT OF CHRONIC OPIOID-INDUCED CONSTIPATION UNRESPONSIVE TO CONVENTIONAL THERAPY.	UNIVERSITY OF CHICAGO 5841 SOUTH MARYLAND AVENUE MC 4028 CHICAGO IL 60637 DD 6/17/1996
METRONIDAZOLE TN=METROGEL	TREATMENT OF PERIORAL DERMATITIS.	GALDERMA LABORATORIES, INC. P.O. BOX 331329 FORT WORTH TX 76163 DD 10/24/1991
METRONIDAZOLE (TOPICAL) TN=FLAGYL	TREATMENT OF GRADE III AND IV, ANAEROBICALLY INFECTED, DECUBITUS ULCERS.	SEARLE 4901 SEARLE PARKWAY SKOKIE IL 60077 DD 11/24/1987
METRONIDAZOLE (TOPICAL) TN=METROGEL	TREATMENT OF ACNE ROSACEA.	GALDERMA LABORATORIES, INC. P.O. BOX 331329 FORT WORTH TX 76163 DD 10/22/1987 MA 11/22/1988
MICROBUBBLE CONTRAST AGENT TN=FILMIX NEUROSONO-GRAPHIC CONTRAST AGENT	INTRAOPERATIVE AID IN THE IDENTIFICATION AND LOCALIZATION OF INTRACRANIAL TUMORS.	CAV-CON, INC. 55 KNOLLWOOD ROAD FARMINGTON CT 06032 DD 11/16/1990
MIDODRINE HCL TN=AMATINE	TREATMENT OF PATIENTS WITH SYMPTOMATIC ORTHOSTATIC HYPOTENSION.	SCHIER RIDGEWOOD F.K.A. (ROBERTS PHARMACEUTICAL CORP.) MERIDIAN CENTER III 6 INDUSTRIAL WAY WEST EATONTOWN NJ 07724 DD 12/5/1996 MA 9/6/1996
MINOCYCLINE HCL TN=MINOCIN INTRAVENOUS	TREATMENT OF CHRONIC MALIGNANT PLEURAL EFFUSION.	LEDERLE LABORATORIES DIVISION PEARL RIVER NY 10965 DD 6/19/1992
MITOGUAZONE TN=APEP	TREATMENT OF DIFFUSE NON-HODGKIN'S LYMPHOMA, INCLUDING AIDS-RELATED DIFFUSE NON-HODGKIN'S LYMPHOMA.	ILEX ONCOLOGY, INC. 4545 HORIZON HILL BLVD. SAN ANTONIO TX 78229-2263 DD 3/18/1994
MITOLACTOL	AS ADJUVANT THERAPY IN THE TREATMENT OF PRIMARY BRAIN TUMORS.	BIOPHARMACEUTICS, INC. 990 STATION ROAD BELLPORT NY 11713 DD 7/12/1995
MITOLACTOL	TREATMENT OF RECURRENT INVASIVE OR METASTATIC SQUAMOUS CARCINOMA OF THE CERVIX.	BIOPHARMACEUTICS, INC. 990 STATION ROAD BELLPORT NY 11713 DD 1/23/1989
MITOMYCIN-C	TREATMENT OF REFRACTORY GLAUCOMA AS AN ADJUNCT TO AB EXTERNO GLAUCOMA SURGERY.	IOP INC. 3100 AIRWAY AVENUE, SUITE 106 COSTA MESA CA 92626 DD 8/20/1993

NAME *Generic/Chemical* *TN=Trade Name*	INDICATION DESIGNATED	SPONSOR AND ADDRESS *DD=Date Designated* *MA=Marketing Approval*
MITOXANTRONE TN=NOVANTRONE	TREATMENT OF HORMONE REFRACTORY PROSTATE CANCER.	SERONO ONE TECHNOLOGY PLACE ROCKLAND MA 02370 DD 8/21/1996 MA 11/13/1996
MITOXANTRONE TN=NOVANTRONE	TREATMENT OF SECONDARY-PROGRESSIVE MULTI-PLE SCLEROSIS.	IMMUNEX CORPORATION 51 UNIVERSITY ST. SEATTLE WA 98101 DD 8/13/1999 MA 10/13/2000
MITOXANTRONE TN=NOVANTRONE	TREATMENT OF PROGRESSIVE-RELAPSING MULTI-PLE SCLEROSIS.	IMMUNEX CORPORATION 51 UNIVERSITY ST. SEATTLE WA 98101 DD 8/13/1999 MA 10/13/2000
MITOXANTRONE HCL TN=NOVANTRONE	TREATMENT OF ACUTE MYELOGENOUS LEUKEMIA, ALSO REFERRED TO AS ACUTE NONLYMPHOCYTIC LEUKEMIA.	LEDERLE LABORATORIES DIVISION OF AMERICAN CYANAMID COMPANY 401 N. MIDDLETOWN ROAD PEARL RIVER NY 10965 DD 7/13/1987 MA 12/23/1987
MODAFINIL TN=PROVIGIL	TREATMENT OF EXCESSIVE DAYTIME SLEEPINESS IN NARCOLEPSY.	CEPHALON, INC. 145 BRANDYWINE PARKWAY WEST CHESTER PA 19380 DD 3/15/1993 MA 12/24/1998
MOLGRAMOSTIM TN=LEUCOMAX	TREATMENT OF AIDS PATIENTS WITH NEUTROPENIA DUE TO THE DISEASE, AZTOR GANCICLOVIR.	SCHERING CORPORATION 2000 GALLOPING HILL ROAD KENILWORTH NJ 07033 DD 1/24/1989
MOLGRAMOSTIM TN=LEUCOMAX	TREATMENT OF APLASTIC ANEMIA.	SCHERING CORPORATION 2000 GALLOPING HILL ROAD KENILWORTH NJ 07033 DD 9/25/1989
MONOCLONAL AB(MURINE) ANTI-IDIOTYPE MELANOMA-ASSO-CIATED ANTIGEN TN=MELIMMUNE	TREATMENT OF INVASIVE CUTANEOUS MELANOMA.	IDEC PHARMACEUTICALS CORPORATION 3030 CALLAN ROAD SAN DIEGO CA 92121 DD 9/19/1994
MONOCLONAL ANTIBODIES (MURINE OR HUMAN) TO B-CELL LYMPHOMA	TREATMENT OF B-CELL LYMPHOMA.	IDEC PHARMACEUTICALS CORPORATION 11011 TORREYANA ROAD SAN DIEGO CA 92121 DD 5/6/1986
MONOCLONAL ANTIBODIES PM-81 AND AML-2-23	FOR THE EXOGENOUS DEPLETION OF CD14 AND CD15 POSITIVE ACUTE MYELOID LEUKEMIC BONE MARROW CELLS FROM PATIENTS UNDERGOING BONE MARROW TRANSPLANTATION.	MEDAREX, INC. 67 BEAVER AVENUE ANNANDALE NJ 08801-0953 DD 3/12/1990
MONOCLONAL ANTIBODY 17-1A TN=PANOREX	TREATMENT OF PANCREATIC CANCER.	CENTOCOR, INC. 244 GREAT VALLEY PARKWAY MALVERN PA 19355 DD 4/4/1988

NAME *Generic/Chemical* *TN=Trade Name*	INDICATION DESIGNATED	SPONSOR AND ADDRESS *DD=Date Designated* *MA=Marketing Approval*
MONOCLONAL ANTIBODY PM-81	ADJUNCTIVE TREATMENT OF ACUTE MYELOGENOUS LEUKEMIA.	MEDAREX, INC. 519 ROUTE 173 WEST BLOOMSBURY NJ 08804 DD 6/27/1991
MONOCLONAL ANTIBODY FOR IMMUNIZATION AGAINST LUPUS NEPHRITIS	TREATMENT OF LUPUS NEPHRITIS.	VIVORX AUTOIMMUNE, INC. 2825 SANTA MONICA BLVD., SUITE 200 SANTA MONICA CA 90404 DD 1/7/1993
MONOCLONAL ANTIBODY TO CYTOMEGALOVIRUS (HUMAN)	TREATMENT OF CYTOMEGALOVIRUS RETINITIS IN PATIENTS WITH AIDS.	PROTEIN DESIGN LABS, INC. 2375 GARCIA AVENUE MOUNTAIN VIEW CA 94043 DD 11/15/1991
MONOCLONAL ANTIBODY TO CYTOMEGALOVIRUS (HUMAN)	PROPHYLAXIS OF CYTOMEGALOVIRUS DISEASE IN PATIENTS UNDERGOING SOLID ORGAN TRANSPLANTATION.	PROTEIN DESIGN LABS, INC. 2375 GARCIA AVENUE MOUNTAIN VIEW CA 94043 DD 9/13/1991
MONOCLONAL ANTIBODY TO HEPATITIS B VIRUS (HUMAN)	PROPHYLAXIS OF HEPATITIS B REINFECTION IN PATIENTS UNDERGOING LIVER TRANSPLANTATION SECONDARY TO END-STAGE CHRONIC HEPATITIS B INFECTION.	PROTEIN DESIGN LABS, INC. 34801 CAMPUS DR. FREMONT CA 94555 DD 6/17/1991
MONOCLONAL ANTIBODY-B43.13 TN=OVAREX MAB-B43.13	TREATMENT OF EPITHELIAL OVARIAN CANCER.	ALTAREX US CORP. 610 LINCOLN STREET WALTHAM MA 02451 DD 11/25/1996
MONOCLONAL ANTIENDOTOXIN ANTIBODY XMMEN-0E5	TREATMENT OF PATIENTS WITH GRAM-NEGATIVE SEPSIS WHICH HAS PROGRESSED TO SHOCK.	PFIZER, INC. 235 EAST 42ND STREET NEW YORK NY 10017 DD 11/4/1985
MONOLAURIN TN=GLYLORIN	TREATMENT OF CONGENITAL PRIMARY ICHTHYOSIS.	GLAXO WELLCOME INC. 5 MOORE DRIVE PO BOX 13398 RESEARCH TRIANGLE PARK NC 27709 DD 4/29/1993
MONOOCTANOIN TN=MOCTANIN	FOR DISSOLUTION OF CHOLESTEROL GALLSTONES RETAINED IN THE COMMON BILE DUCT.	ETHITEK PHARMACEUTICALS, INC. 7855 GROSS POINT ROAD, UNIT L SKOKIE IL 60077 DD 5/30/1984 MA 10/31/1985
MORPHINE SULFATE CONCENTRATE (PRESERVATIVE FREE) TN=INFUMORPH	FOR USE IN MICROINFUSION DEVICES FOR INTRASPINAL ADMINISTRATION IN THE TREATMENT OF INTRACTABLE CHRONIC PAIN.	ELKINS-SINN, INC. 2 ESTERBROOK LANE CHERRY HILL NJ 08003 DD 7/12/1990 MA 7/19/1991
MUCOID EXOPOLYSACCHARIDE PSEUDOMONAS HYPERIMMUNE GLOBULIN TN=MEP IGIV	PREVENTION OF PULMONARY INFECTIONS DUE TO PSEUDOMONAS AERUGINOSA IN PATIENTS WITH CYSTIC FIBROSIS.	NORTH AMERICAN BIOLOGICALS, INC. 12280 WILKINS AVENUE ROCKVILLE MD 20852 DD 11/7/1990

NAME *Generic/Chemical* *TN=Trade Name*	INDICATION DESIGNATED	SPONSOR AND ADDRESS *DD=Date Designated* *MA=Marketing Approval*
MUCOID EXOPOLYSACCHARIDE PSEUDOMONAS HYPERIMMUNE GLOBULIN TN=MEP IGIV	TREATMENT OF PULMONARY INFECTIONS DUE TO PSEUDOMONAS AERUGINOSA IN PATIENTS WITH CYSTIC FIBROSIS.	NORTH AMERICAN BIOLOGICALS, INC. 12280 WILKINS AVENUE ROCKVILLE MD 20852 DD 1/9/1991
MULTI-VITAMIN INFUSION (NEO-NATAL FORMULA)	FOR ESTABLISHMENT AND MAINTENANCE OF TOTAL PARENTERAL NUTRITION IN VERY LOW BIRTH WEIGHT INFANTS.	ASTRA PHARMACEUTICALS, L.P. 725 CHESTERBROOK BLVD. WAYNE PA 19087-5677 DD 12/12/1989
MURINE MAB (LYM-1) AND IODINE 131-I RADIOLABELED MURINE MAB (LYM-1) TO HUMAN B-CELL LYMPHOMA TN=ONCOLYM	TREATMENT OF B-CELL NON-HODGKIN'S LYMPHOMA.	PEREGRINE PHARMACEUTI-CALS, INC. 14272 FRANKLIN AVE. SUITE 100 TUSTIN CA 92780 DD 11/27/1998
MURINE MAB TO POLYMORPHIC EPITHELIAL MUCIN, HUMAN MILK FAT GLOBULE 1 TN=THERAGYN	ADJUVANT TREATMENT OF OVARIAN CANCER.	ANTISOMA PLC WEST AFRICA HOUSE HANGER LANE EALING LONDON W5 3QR UK DD 3/22/1999
MYCOBACTERIUM AVIUM SENSI-TIN RS-10	FOR USE IN THE DIAGNOSIS OF INVASIVE MYCOBAC-TERIUM AVIUM DISEASE IN IMMUNOCOMPETENT IN-DIVIDUALS.	STATENS SERUMINSTITUT 5 ARTILLERIVEJ DK-2300 COPENHAGEN S DENMARK DD 10/11/1995
MYELIN	TREATMENT OF MULTIPLE SCLEROSIS.	AUTOIMMUNE, INC. 128 SPRING STREET LEXINGTON MA 02173 DD 6/27/1991
MYRISTOYLATED RECOMBINANT SCR1-3 OF HUMAN COMPLE-MENT RESEPTOR TYPE 1 TN=APT070	PREVENTION OF DELAYED GRAFT FUNCTION IN SO-LID ORGAN TRANSPLANT.	ADPROTECH, LTD. CHESTERFORD RESEARCH PARK, LITTLE CHESTERFORD, SAFFRON WALDEN, ESSEX, CB10 1XK UK DD 5/21/2003
N-[4-BROMO-2-(1H-1,2,3,4-TETRA-ZOL-5-YL)PHENYL]-N'-[3,5-BIS(-TRIFLUOROMETHYL)PHENY-L]UREA	TREATMENT OF SICKLE CELL DISEASE	NEUROSEARCH A/S 93 PEDERSTRUPVEJ DK-2750 BALLERUP DENMARK DD 5/13/2002
N-ACETYL-PROCAINAMIDE	PREVENTION OF LIFE-THREATENING VENTRICULAR ARRHYTHMIAS IN PATIENTS WITH DOCUMENTED PROCAINAMIDE-INDUCED LUPUS.	NAPA OF THE BAHAMAS 3560 PENNSYLVANIA AVENUE, SUITE 7 DUBUQUE IA 52002 DD 12/10/1996
N-ACETYLCYSTEINATE LYSINE TN=NACYSTELYN DRY POWDER INHALER	FOR THE MANAGEMENT OF CYSTIC FIBROSIS	GALEPHAR PHARMACEUTICAL RESEARCH, INC. ROAD 198, NO. 100 KM. 14.7 JUNCOS INDUSTRIAL PARK JUNCOS PR 00777-3873 DD 12/27/2000

NAME *Generic/Chemical* *TN=Trade Name*	INDICATION DESIGNATED	SPONSOR AND ADDRESS *DD=Date Designated* *MA=Marketing Approval*
N-ACETYLCYSTEINE	TREATMENT OF ACUTE LIVER FAILURE	WILLIAM M. LEE, MD, FACP UNIVERSITY OF TEXAS SOUTH- WESTERN MEDICAL CENTER AT DALLAS 5323 HARRY HINES BLVD DALLAS TX 75390-9151 DD 9/9/2002
N-ACETYLGALACTOSAMINE-4- SULFATASE, RECOMBINANT HU- MAN	TREATMENT OF MUCOPOLYSACCHARIDOSIS TYPE VI (MAROTEAUX-LAMY SYNDROME).	BIOMARIN PHARMACEUTICAL, INC. 11 PIMENTAL COURT NOVATO CA 94949-5608 DD 2/17/1999
N-ACETYLPROCAINAMIDE TN=NAPA	TO LOWER THE DEFIBRILLATION ENERGY REQUIRE- MENT SUFFICIENTLY TO ALLOW AUTOMATIC IMPLAN- TABLE CARDIOVERTER DEFIBRILLATOR THERAPY IN THOSE PATIENTS WHO COULD OTHERWISE NOT USE THE DEVICE.	MEDCO RESEARCH, INC. 8455 BEVERLY BLVD. SUITE 308 LOS ANGELES CA 90048 DD 3/23/1990
NDROGE	TREATMENT OF POSTANOXIC INTENTION MYOCLO- NUS.	WATSON LABORATORIES, INC. 33 RALPH AVENUE P.O. BOX 30 COPIAQUE NY 11726-0030 DD 11/1/1984
NG-29 TN=SOMATREL	DIAGNOSTIC MEASURE OF THE CAPACITY OF THE PI- TUITARY GLAND TO RELEASE GROWTH HORMONE.	FERRING LABORATORIES, INC. 400 RELLA BOULEVARD, SUITE 201 SUFFERN NY 10901 DD 8/8/1989
NZ-1002	ENZYME REPLACEMENT THERAPY IN PATIENTS WITH ALL SUBTYPES OF MUCOPOLYSACCHARIDOSIS I.	NOVAZYME PHARMACEUTICALS, INC. 800 RESEARCH PARKWAY SUITE 200 OKLAHOMA CITY OK 73104 DD 4/11/2001
NAFARELIN ACETATE TN=SYNAREL NASAL SOLUTION	TREATMENT OF CENTRAL PRECOCIOUS PUBERTY.	SYNTEX (USA), INC. 3401 HILLVIEW AVENUE PALO ALTO CA 94303 DD 7/20/1988 MA 2/26/1992
NALTREXONE HCL TN=TREXAN	FOR BLOCKADE OF THE PHARMACOLOGICAL EF- FECTS OF EXOGENOUSLY ADMINISTERED OPIOIDS AS AN ADJUNCT TO THE MAINTENANCE OF THE OPIOID-FREE STATE IN DETOXIFIED FORMERLY OPIOID-DEPENDENT INDIVIDUALS.	DUPONT PHARMACEUTICALS E.I. DU PONT DE NEMOURS & CO. WILMINGTON DE 19880 DD 3/11/1985 MA 11/30/1984
NATURAL HUMAN LYMPHOBLAS- TOID INTERFERON-ALPHA	TREATMENT OF PAPILLOMAVIRUS WARTS IN THE ORAL CAVITY OF HIV POSITIVE PATIENTS.	ATRIX LABORATORIES, INC. 2579 MIDPOINT DRIVE FORT COLLINS CO 80525-4417 DD 8/10/2000
NATURAL HUMAN LYMPHOBLAS- TOID INTERFERON-ALPHA	TREATMENT OF BEHCET'S DISEASE.	AMARILLO BIOSCIENCES, INC. 800 WEST NINTH AVENUE AMARILLO TX 79101-3206 DD 1/18/2000
NATURAL HUMAN LYMPHOBLAS- TOID INTERFERON-ALPHA	TREATMENT OF POLYCYTHEMIA VERA	AMARILLO BIOSCIENCES, INC. 800 WEST 9TH AVENUE AMARILLO TX 79101 DD 11/18/2002

NAME *Generic/Chemical* *TN=Trade Name*	INDICATION DESIGNATED	SPONSOR AND ADDRESS *DD=Date Designated* *MA=Marketing Approval*
NEBACUMAB TN=CENTOXIN	TREATMENT OF PATIENTS WITH GRAM-NEGATIVE BACTEREMIA WHICH HAS PROGRESSED TO ENDO-TOXIN SHOCK.	CENTOCOR, INC. 200 GREAT VALLEY PARKWAY MALVERN PA 19355 DD 10/1/1986
NEUROTROPHIN-1	TREATMENT OF MOTOR NEURON DISEASE/AMYO-TROPHIC LATERAL SCLEROSIS.	ERICSSON, ARTHUR DALE, M.D. 6560 FANNIN, SCURLOCK TOWER, SUITE 720 HOUSTON TX 77303 DD 9/13/1994
NIFEDIPINE	TREATMENT OF INTERSTITIAL CYSTITIS.	FLEISCHMANN, JONATHAN M.D. METROHEALTH MEDICAL CEN-TER 3395 SCRANTON ROAD CLEVELAND OH 44109 DD 6/13/1991
NITAZOXANIDE TN=ALINIA	TREATMENT OF CRYPTOSPORIDIOSIS.	ROMARK LABORATORIES, L.C. 6200 COURTNEY CAMPBELL CAUSEWAY SUITE 880 TAMPA FL 33607 DD 12/12/1996 MA 11/22/2002
NITISINONE TN=ORFADIN	TREATMENT OF ALKAPTONURIA	SWEDISH ORPHAN AB KUNGSGATAN 37, 7TH FLOOR SE-111 56 STOCKHOLM, SWEDEN DD 10/19/2001
NITISINONE TN=ORFADIN	TREATMENT OF TYROSINEMIA TYPE 1.	SWEDISH ORPHAN AB DROTTNINGGATAN 98 SE-111 60 STOCKHOLM SWEDEN SE DD 5/16/1995 MA 1/18/2002
NITRIC OXIDE	TREATMENT OF ACUTE RESPIRATORY DISTRESS SYNDROME IN ADULTS.	INO THERAPEUTICS, INC. 54 OLD HIGHWAY 22 CLINTON NJ 08809 DD 7/10/1995
NITRIC OXIDE TN=INOMAX	TREATMENT OF PERSISTENT PULMONARY HYPER-TENSION IN THE NEWBORN.	INO THERAPEUTICS, INC. 54 OLD HIGHWAY 22 CLINTON NJ 08809 DD 6/22/1993 MA 12/23/1999
NITROPRUSSIDE	TREATMENT AND PREVENTION OF CEREBRAL VA-SOSPASM FOLLOWING SUBARACHNOID HEMOR-RHAGE.	THOMAS, MD, JEFFREY EVAN THOMAS JEFFERSON UNIVER-SITY AND WILLS NEUROSEN-SORY INSTITUTE 834 WALNUT STREET, SUITE 650 PHILADELPHIA PA 19107-5102 DD 2/21/2001
NOVEL ACTING THROMBOLYTIC (NAT)	TREATMENT OF PERIPHERAL ARTERIAL OCCLUSION (PAO)	AMGEN, INC. ONE AMGEN CENTER DRIVE THOUSAND OAKS CA 91320-1799 DD 1/26/2001
OM 401 TN=DREPANOL	PROPHYLACTIC TREATMENT OF SICKLE CELL DIS-EASE.	OMEX INTERNATIONAL, INC. 6001 SAVOY, SUITE 110 HOUSTON TX 77036 DD 10/24/1991

NAME *Generic/Chemical* *TN=Trade Name*	INDICATION DESIGNATED	SPONSOR AND ADDRESS *DD=Date Designated* *MA=Marketing Approval*
OCTREOTIDE TN=SANDOSTATIN LAR	TREATMENT OF ACROMEGALY.	NOVARTIS PHARMACEUTICALS CORPORATION 59 ROUTE 10 EAST HANOVER NJ 07936-1080 DD 8/24/1998 MA 11/25/1998
OCTREOTIDE TN=SANDOSTATIN LAR	TREATMENT OF SEVERE DIARRHEA AND FLUSHING ASSOCIATED WITH MALIGNANT CARCINOID TUMORS.	NOVARTIS PHARMACEUTICALS CORPORATION 59 ROUTE 10 EAST HANOVER NJ 07936-1080 DD 8/24/1998 MA 11/25/1998
OCTREOTIDE TN=SANDOSTATIN LAR	TREATMENT OF DIARRHEA ASSOCIATED WITH VA-SOACTIVE INTESTINAL PEPTIDE TUMORS (VIPOMA).	NOVARTIS PHARMACEUTICALS CORPORATION 59 ROUTE 10 EAST HANOVER NJ 07936-1080 DD 8/24/1998 MA 11/25/1998
OFLOXACIN TN=OCUFLOX OPHTHALMIC SO-LUTION	TREATMENT OF BACTERIAL CORNEAL ULCERS.	ALLERGAN, INC. 2525 DUPONT DRIVE P.O. BOX 19534 IRVINE CA 92713 DD 4/18/1991 MA 5/22/1996
OMEGA-3 (N-3) POLYUNSATU-RATED FATTY ACID WITH ALL DOUBLE BONDS IN THE CIS CON-FIGURATION	PREVENTION OF ORGAN GRAFT REJECTION.	RESEARCH TRIANGLE PHARMACEUTICALS 4364 SOUTH ALSTON AVENUE DURHAM NC 27713 DD 11/22/1995
OMEGA-3 (N-3) POLYUNSATU-RATED FATTY ACIDS TN=OMACOR	TREATMENT OF IGA NEPHROPATHY.	PRONOVA BIOCARE, AS PO BOX 420 1327 LYSAKER NORWAY DD 5/4/2000
ONCORAD OV103	TREATMENT OF OVARIAN CANCER.	CYTOGEN CORPORATION 600 COLLEGE ROAD EAST PRINCETON NJ 08540 DD 4/24/1990
OPRELVEKIN TN=NEUMEGA	PREVENTION OF SEVERE CHEMOTHERAPY-INDUCED THROMBOCYTOPENIA.	GENETICS INSTITUTE, INC. 87 CAMBRIDGE PARK DRIVE CAMBRIDGE MA 02140 DD 12/17/1996 MA 11/25/1997
ORGOTEIN FOR INJECTION	TREATMENT OF FAMILIAL AMYOTROPHIC LATERAL SCLEROSIS ASSOCIATED WITH A MUTATION OF THE GENE (ON CHROMOSOME 21Q) FOR COPPER, ZINC SUPEROXIDE DISMUTASE.	OXIS INTERNATIONAL, INC. 6040 N. CUTTER CIRCLE, SUITE 317 PORTLAND OR 97217-3935 DD 12/22/1994
OXALIPLATIN	TREATMENT OF OVARIAN CANCER.	DEBIO PHARM S.A. RUE DES TERREAUX 17 CH-1000 LAUSANNE 9 SWITZERLAND CH DD 10/6/1992

NAME *Generic/Chemical* *TN=Trade Name*	INDICATION DESIGNATED	SPONSOR AND ADDRESS *DD=Date Designated* *MA=Marketing Approval*
OXANDROLONE TN=OXANDRIN	ADJUNCTIVE THERAPY FOR AIDS PATIENTS SUFFERING FROM HIV-WASTING SYNDROME.	BIO-TECHNOLOGY GENERAL CORP. ONE TOWER CENTER BOULEVARD, 12 TH FLOOR EAST BRUNSWICK NJ 08816 DD 9/6/1991
OXANDROLONE	TREATMENT OF CONSTITUTIONAL DELAY OF GROWTH AND PUBERTY.	BIO-TECHNOLOGY GENERAL CORP. 70 WOOD AVENUE, SOUTH ISELIN NJ 08830 DD 10/5/1990
OXANDROLONE TN=OXANDRIN	TREATMENT OF SHORT STATURE ASSOCIATED WITH TURNER'S SYNDROME.	BIO-TECHNOLOGY GENERAL CORP. 70 WOOD AVENUE, SOUTH ISELIN NJ 08830 DD 7/5/1990
OXANDROLONE TN=OXANDRIN	TREATMENT OF PATIENTS WITH DUCHENNE'S MUSCULAR DYSTROPHY AND BECKER'S MUSCULAR DYSTROPHY.	BIO-TECHNOLOGY GENERAL CORP. ONE TOWER CENTER BOULEVARD, 12TH FLOOR EAST BRUNSWICK NJ 08816 DD 4/22/1997
OXANDROLONE TN=HEPANDRIN	TREATMENT OF MODERATE/SEVERE ACUTE ALCOHOLIC HEPATITIS IN THE PRESENCE OF MODERATE PROTEIN CALORIE MALNUTRITION.	BIO-TECHNOLOGY GENERAL CORP. 70 WOOD AVENUE SOUTH ISELIN NJ 08830 DD 3/18/1994
OXYBATE TN=XYREM	TREATMENT OF NARCOLEPSY.	ORPHAN MEDICAL, INC. 13911 RIDGEDALE DRIVE SUITE 250 MINNETONKA MN 55305 DD 11/7/1994 MA 7/17/2002
OXYMORPHONE TN=NUMORPHAN H.P.	FOR RELIEF OF SEVERE INTRACTABLE PAIN IN NARCOTIC-TOLERANT PATIENTS.	DUPONT MERCK PHARMACEUTICAL COMPANY P.O. BOX 80027 WILMINGTON DE 19880 DD 3/19/1985
OXYPURINOL	TREATMENT OF HYPERURICEMIA IN PATIENTS INTOLERANT TO ALLOPURINOL.	CARDIOME PHARMA CORP. 3650 WESTBROOK MALL VANCOUVER, B.C. CANADA V65 2L2 DD 11/9/1998
P1, P4-DI(URIDINE 5'-TETRAPHOSPHATE), TETRASODIUM SALT	TREATMENT OF CYSTIC FIBROSIS.	INSPIRE PHARMACEUTICALS, INC. 4222 EMPEROR BLVD., SUITE 470 DURHAM NC 27703 DD 10/27/1998
PEG-GLUCOCEREBROSIDASE TN=LYSODASE	FOR USE AS CHRONIC ENZYME REPLACEMENT THERAPY IN PATIENTS WITH GAUCHER'S DISEASE WHO ARE DEFICIENT IN GLUCOCEREBROSIDASE.	NATIONAL INSTITUTE OF MENTAL HEALTH, NIH 49 CONVENT DR. MSC4405 BLDG. 49, ROOM B1EE16 BETHESDA MD 20892-4405 DD 12/9/1992
PEG-INTERLEUKIN-2	TREATMENT OF PRIMARY IMMUNODEFICIENCIES ASSOCIATED WITH T-CELL DEFECTS.	CHIRON CORPORATION 4560 HORTON STREET EMERYVILLE CA 94608 DD 2/1/1990

NAME Generic/Chemical TN=Trade Name	INDICATION DESIGNATED	SPONSOR AND ADDRESS DD=Date Designated MA=Marketing Approval
PR-225 (REDOX-ACYCLOVIR)	TREATMENT OF HERPES SIMPLEX ENCEPHALITIS IN INDIVIDUALS AFFLICTED WITH AIDS.	PHARMOS 2 INNOVATION DRIVE ALACHUA FL 32615 DD 5/29/1990
PR-239 (REDOX PENICILLIN G)	TREATMENT OF AIDS ASSOCIATED NEUROSYPHILIS.	PHARMOS 2 INNOVATION DRIVE ALACHUA FL 32615 DD 5/23/1990
PACLITAXEL TN=PAXENE	TREATMENT OF AIDS-RELATED KAPOSI'S SARCOMA.	BAKER NORTON PHARMACEUTI-CALS, INC. 4400 BISCAYNE BOULEVARD MIAMI FL 33137 DD 4/15/1997
PACLITAXEL TN=TAXOL	TREATMENT OF AIDS-RELATED KAPOSI'S SARCOMA.	BRISTOL-MYERS SQUIBB PHARMACEUTICAL RESEARCH INSTITUTE 5 RESEARCH PARKWAY P.O. BOX 5100 WALLINGFORD CT 06492-7660 DD 3/25/1997 MA 8/4/1997
PAPAIN, TRYPSIN, AND CHYMO-TRYPSIN TN=WOBE-MUGOS	TREATMENT OF MULTIPLE MYELOMA.	MARLYN NUTRACEUTICALS, INC. 14851 N. SCOTTSDALE RD. SCOTTSDALE AZ 85254 DD 12/21/1998
PAPAVERINE TOPICAL GEL	TREATMENT OF SEXUAL DYSFUNCTION IN SPINAL CORD INJURY PATIENTS.	PHARMEDIC COMPANY 417 HARVESTER COURT WHEELING IL 60090 DD 2/6/1992
PAROVIRUS B19 (RECOMBINANT VP1 AND VP2; S.FRUGIPERDA CELLS) VACCINE TN=MEDI-491	PREVENTION OF TRANSIENT APLASTIC CRISIS IN PA-TIENTS WITH SICKLE CELL ANEMIA.	MEDIMMUNE, INC. 35 WEST WATKINS MILL RD. GAITHERSBURG MD 20878 DD 5/7/1999
PATUL-END	TREATMENT OF PATULOUS EUSTACHIAN TUBE.	EAR FOUNDATION 2420 CASTILLO STREET, SUITE 100 SANTA BARBARA CA 93105 DD 2/18/1997
PEGADEMASE BOVINE TN=ADAGEN	FOR ENZYME REPLACEMENT THERAPY FOR ADA DE-FICIENCY IN PATIENTS WITH SEVERE COMBINED IM-MUNODEFICIENCY.	ENZON, INC. 20 KINGSBRIDGE ROAD PISCATAWAY NJ 08854 DD 5/29/1984 MA 3/21/1990
PEGASPARGASE TN=ONCASPAR	TREATMENT OF ACUTE LYMPHOCYTIC LEUKEMIA.	ENZON, INC. 20 KINGSBRIDGE ROAD PISCATAWAY NJ 08854 DD 10/20/1989 MA 2/1/1994
PEGINTERFERON ALFA-2A TN=PEGASYS	TREATMENT OF RENAL CELL CARCINOMA.	HOFFMAN-LA ROCHE INC. 340 KINGSLAND ST. NUTLEY NJ 07110-1199 DD 7/13/1998
PEGINTERFERON ALFA-2A TN=PEGASYS	TREATMENT OF CHRONIC MYELOGENOUS LEUKE-MIA.	HOFFMAN-LA ROCHE INC. 340 KINGSLAND ST. NUTLEY NJ 07110-1199 DD 9/30/1999

NAME *Generic/Chemical* *TN=Trade Name*	INDICATION DESIGNATED	SPONSOR AND ADDRESS *DD=Date Designated* *MA=Marketing Approval*
PEGVISOMANT TN=SOMAVERT	TREATMENT OF ACROMEGALY.	SENSUS CORPORATION SUITE 430, 98 SAN JACINTO BOULEVARD AUSTIN TX 78701 DD 6/24/1997
PEGYLATED ARGININE DEIMI- NASE TN=HEPACID	TREATMENT OF HEPATOCELLULAR CARCINOMA.	PHOENIX PHARMACOLOGICS, INC. 115 JOHN ROBERT THOMAS DR. EXTON PA 19341 DD 3/26/1999
PEGYLATED ARGININE DEIMI- NASE TN=MELANOCID	TREATMENT OF INVASIVE MALIGNANT MELANOMA.	PHOENIX PHARMACOLOGICS, INC. 115 JOHN ROBERT THOMAS DR. EXTON PA 19341 DD 4/12/1999
PEGYLATED RECOMBINANT HU- MAN MEGAKARYOCYTE GROWTH AND DEVELOPMENT FACTOR TN=MEGAGEN	FOR REDUCING THE PERIOD OF THROMBOCYTOPE- NIA IN PATIENTS UNDERGOING HEMATOPOIETIC STEM CELL TRANSPLANTATION.	AMGEN, INC. ONE AMGEN CENTER DR. THOUSAND OAKS CA 91320-1789 DD 10/20/1997
PELDESINE	TREATMENT OF CUTANEOUS T-CELL LYMPHOMA.	BIOCRYST PHARMACEUTICALS, INC. 2190 PARKWAY LAKE DRIVE BIRMINGHAM AL 35244 DD 10/5/1993
PENTAMIDINE ISETHIONATE TN=NEBUPENT	PREVENTION OF PNEUMOCYSTIS CARINII PNEUMO- NIA IN PATIENTS AT HIGH RISK OF DEVELOPING THIS DISEASE.	FUJISAWA USA, INC. 3 PARKWAY NORTH CENTER DEERFIELD IL 60015 DD 1/12/1988 MA 6/15/1989
PENTAMIDINE ISETHIONATE TN=PENTAM 300	TREATMENT OF PNEUMOCYSTIS CARINII PNEUMO- NIA.	FUJISAWA USA, INC. 3 PARKWAY NORTH CENTER DEERFIELD IL 60015 DD 2/28/1984 MA 10/16/1984
PENTAMIDINE ISETHIONATE	TREATMENT OF PNEUMOCYSTIS CARINII PNEUMO- NIA.	AVENTIS BEHRING L.L.C. 1020 FIRST AVENUE PO BOX 61501 KING OF PRUSSIA PA 19406-0901 DD 10/29/1984
PENTAMIDINE ISETHIONATE (IN- HALATION) TN=PNEUMOPENT	PREVENTION OF PNEUMOCYSTIS CARINII PNEUMO- NIA IN PATIENTS AT HIGH RISK OF DEVELOPING THIS DISEASE.	FISONS CORPORATION 755 JEFFERSON RD., P.O. BOX 1710 ROCHESTER NY 14603 DD 10/5/1987
PENTASTARCH TN=PENTASPAN	AS AN ADJUNCT IN LEUKAPHERESIS TO IMPROVE THE HARVESTING AND INCREASE THE YIELD OF LEU- KOCYTES BY CENTRIFUGAL MEANS.	DU PONT PHARMACEUTICALS E.I. DU PONT DE NEMOURS & CO. WILMINGTON DE 19898 DD 8/28/1985 MA 5/19/1987
PENTOSAN POLYSULFATE SO- DIUM TN=ELMIRON	TREATMENT OF INTERSTITIAL CYSTITIS.	ALZA CORPORATION 950 PAGE MILL RD. PO BOX 10950 PALO ALTO CA 94303-0802 DD 8/7/1985 MA 9/26/1996

NAME *Generic/Chemical* *TN=Trade Name*	INDICATION DESIGNATED	SPONSOR AND ADDRESS *DD=Date Designated* *MA=Marketing Approval*
PENTOSTATIN TN=NIPENT	TREATMENT OF PATIENTS WITH CHRONIC LYMPHO-CYTIC LEUKEMIA.	SUPERGEN, INC. 4140 DUBLIN BLVD. SUITE 200 DUBLIN CA 94568 DD 1/29/1991
PENTOSTATIN TN=NIPENT	TREATMENT OF CUTANEOUS T-CELL LYMPHOMA.	SUPERGEN, INC. 4140 DUBLIN BLVD. SUITE 200 DUBLIN CA 94568 DD 3/27/1998
PENTOSTATIN TN=NIPENT	TREATMENT OF PERIPHERAL T-CELL LYMPHOMAS.	SUPERGEN, INC. 4140 DUBLIN BLVD. SUITE 200 DUBLIN CA 94568 DD 11/24/1999
PENTOSTATIN FOR INJECTION TN=NIPENT	TREATMENT OF HAIRY CELL LEUKEMIA.	SUPERGEN, INC. 4140 DUBLIN BLVD. SUITE 200 DUBLIN CA 94568 DD 9/10/1987 MA 10/11/1991
PERFLUBRON TN=LIQUIVENT	TREATMENT OF ACUTE RESPIRATORY DISTRESS DISEASE (ARDS) IN ADULTS	ALLIANCE PHARMACEUTICAL CORP. 3040 SCIENCE PARK ROAD SAN DIEGO CA 92191 DD 4/26/2001
PERFOSFAMIDE TN=PERGAMID	FOR USE IN THE EX-VIVO TREATMENT OF AUTOLO-GOUS BONE MARROW AND SUBSEQUENT REINFU-SION IN PATIENTS WITH ACUTE MYELOGENOUS LEUKEMIA, ALSO REFERRED TO AS ACUTE NONLYM-PHOCYTIC LEUKEMIA.	SCIOS NOVA, INC. 2450 BAYSHORE PARKWAY MOUNTAIN VIEW CA 94043 DD 12/4/1989
PERGOLIDE TN=PERMAX	TREATMENT OF TOURETTE'S SYNDROME.	SALLEE, FLOYD R. M.D., PH.D. CINCINNATI CHILDREN'S HOSPI-TAL MEDICAL CENTER 3333 BURNET AVE. CINCINNATI OH 45229-3039 DD 11/20/1997
PHENYLACETATE	FOR USE AS AN ADJUNCT TO SURGERY, RADIATION THERAPY AND CHEMOTHERAPY FOR THE TREAT-MENT OF PATIENTS WITH PRIMARY OR RECURRENT MALIGNANT GLIOMA.	ELAN DRUG DELIVERY, INC. 1300 GOULD DR. GAINESVILLE GA 30504 DD 3/6/1998
PHENYLALANINE AMMONIA-LYASE TN=PHENYLASE	TREATMENT OF HYPERPHENYLALANINEMIA.	IBEX TECHNOLOGIES, INC. 5485 PARE MONTREAL, QUEBEC CANADA H4P 1P7 CA DD 3/8/1995
PHENYLBUTYRATE	TREATMENT OF ACUTE PROMYELOCYTIC LEUKEMIA.	ELAN DRUG DELIVERY, INC. 1300 GOULD DR. GAINESVILLE GA 30504 DD 1/19/2000
PHOSPHOCYSTEAMINE	TREATMENT OF CYSTINOSIS.	MEDEA RESEARCH LABORA-TORIES PORT JEFFERSON BUSINESS CENTER 200 WILSON STREET, BUILDING D-6 PORT JEFFERSON NY 11776 DD 9/12/1988

NAME *Generic/Chemical* *TN=Trade Name*	INDICATION DESIGNATED	SPONSOR AND ADDRESS *DD=Date Designated* *MA=Marketing Approval*
PILOCARPINE TN=SALAGEN	TREATMENT OF XEROSTOMIA INDUCED BY RADIATION THERAPY FOR HEAD AND NECK CANCER.	MGI PHARMA, INC. 6300 WEST OLD SHAKOPEE RD. SUITE 110 BLOOMINGTON MN 55438-2318 DD 9/24/1990 MA 3/22/1994
PILOCARPINE HCL TN=SALAGEN	TREATMENT OF XEROSTOMIA AND KERATOCONJUNCTIVITIS SICCA IN SJOGREN'S SYNDROME PATIENTS.	MGI PHARMA, INC. 6300 WEST OLD SHAKOPEE RD. SUITE 110 BLOOMINGTON MN 55438-2318 DD 2/28/1992 MA 2/11/1998
PIRACETAM TN=NOOTROPIL	TREATMENT OF MYOCLONUS.	UCB PHARMA, INC. 1950 LAKE PARK DRIVE SMYRNA GA 30080 DD 10/2/1987
PIRITREXIM ISETHIONATE	TREATMENT OF INFECTIONS CAUSED BY PNEUMOCYSTIS CARINII, TOXOPLASMA GONDII, AND MYCOBACTERIUM AVIUM-INTRACELLULARE.	BURROUGHS WELLCOME COMPANY 3030 CORNWALLIS ROAD P.O. BOX 12700 RESEARCH TRIANGLE PARK NC 27709 DD 6/13/1988
POLIFEPROSAN 20 WITH CARMUSTINE TN=GLIADEL	TREATMENT OF MALIGNANT GLIOMA.	GUILFORD PHARMACEUTICALS, INC. 6611 TRIBUTARY STREET BALTIMORE MD 21224 DD 12/13/1989 MA 9/23/1996
POLOXAMER 188	TREATMENT OF VASOSPASM IN SUBARACHNOID HEMORRHAGE PATIENTS FOLLOWING SURGICAL REPAIR OF A RUPTURED CEREBRAL ANEURYSM.	CYTRX CORPORATION 154 TECHNOLOGY PARKWAY NORCROSS GA 30092 DD 8/5/1997
POLOXAMER 188 TN=FLOCOR	TREATMENT OF SICKLE CELL CRISIS.	CYTRX CORPORATION 154 TECHNOLOGY PARKWAY NORCROSS GA 30092 DD 6/27/1989
POLOXAMER 188 TN=FLORCOR	TREATMENT OF SEVERE BURNS REQUIRING HOSPITALIZATION.	CYTRX CORPORATION 154 TECHNOLOGY PARKWAY NORCROSS GA 30092 DD 2/22/1990
POLOXAMER 331 TN=PROTOX	INITIAL THERAPY OF TOXOPLASMOSIS IN PATIENTS WITH AIDS.	CYTRX CORPORATION 154 TECHNOLOGY PARKWAY NORCROSS GA 30092 DD 3/21/1991
POLY I: POLY C12U TN=AMPLIGEN	TREATMENT OF RENAL CELL CARCINOMA.	HEMISPHERX BIOPHARMA, INC. ONE PENN CENTER 1617 JFK BOULEVARD PHILADELPHIA PA 19103 DD 5/20/1991
POLY I: POLY C12U TN=AMPLIGEN	TREATMENT OF AIDS.	HEMISPHERX BIOPHARMA, INC. ONE PENN CENTER 1617 JFK BOULEVARD PHILADELPHIA PA 19103 DD 7/19/1988

NAME *Generic/Chemical* *TN=Trade Name*	INDICATION DESIGNATED	SPONSOR AND ADDRESS *DD=Date Designated* *MA=Marketing Approval*
POLY I: POLY C12U TN=AMPLIGEN	TREATMENT OF CHRONIC FATIGUE SYNDROME.	HEMISPHERX BIOPHARMA, INC. ONE PENN CENTER 1617 JFK BOULEVARD PHILADELPHIA PA 19103 DD 12/9/1993
POLY I: POLY C12U TN=AMPLIGEN	TREATMENT OF INVASIVE METASTATIC MELANOMA (STAGE IIB, III, IV).	HEMISPHERX BIOPHARMA, INC. ONE PENN CENTER 1617 JFK BOULEVARD PHILADELPHIA PA 19103 DD 12/9/1993
POLY-ICLC	TREATMENT OF PRIMARY BRAIN TUMORS.	SALAZAR, ANDRES M. M.D. AND LEVY, HILTON B. PH.D. 3202 CLEVELAND AVENUE N.W. WASHINGTON DC 20008 DD 3/17/1997
POLYETHYLENE GLYCOL (PEG)-URICASE	TO CONTROL THE CLINICAL CONSEQUENCES OF HYPERURICEMIA IN PATIENTS WITH SEVERE GOUT IN WHOM CONVENTIONAL THERAPY IS CONTRAINDICATED OR HAS BEEN INEFFECTIVE.	BIO-TECHNOLOGY GENERAL CORPORATION ONE TOWER CENTER BOULEVARD, 12TH FLOOR EAST BRUNSWICK NJ 08816 DD 2/21/2001
POLYETHYLENE GLYCOL-MODIFIED URICASE TN=ZURASE	PROPHYLAXIS OF HYPERURICEMIA IN CANCER PATIENTS PRONE TO DEVELOP TUMOR LYSIS SYNDROME DURING CHEMOTHERAPY.	PHOENIX PHARMACOLOGICS, INC. 115 JOHN ROBERT THOMAS DR. EXTON PA 19341 DD 9/14/1999
POLYETHYLENE GLYCOL-MODIFIED URICASE TN=ZURASE	TREATMENT OF TUMOR LYSIS SYNDROME IN CANCER PATIENTS UNDERGOING CHEMOTHERAPY.	PHOENIX PHARMACOLOGICS, INC. 115 JOHN ROBERT THOMAS DR. EXTON PA 19341 DD 12/21/1998
POLYMERIC OXYGEN	TREATMENT OF SICKLE CELL ANEMIA.	CAPMED USA P.O. BOX 14 BRYN MAWR PA 19010 DD 3/25/1992
PORCINE SERTOLI CELLS ASEPTICALLY PREPARED FOR INTRACEREBRAL CO-IMPLANTATION WITH FETAL NEURAL TISSUE TN=N-GRAFT	TREATMENT OF HOEHN AND YAHR STAGE FOUR AND FIVE PARKINSON'S DISEASE.	TITAN PHARMACEUTICALS, INC. POST OFFICE PLAZA 50 DIVISION STREET, SUITE 503 SOMERVILLE NJ 08876 DD 6/24/1997
PORCINE FETAL NEURAL DOPAMINERGIC CELLS AND/OR PRECURSORS ASEPTICALLY PREPARED AND COATED WITH ANTI-MHC-1 AB FOR INTRACEREBRAL IMPLANTATION TN=NEUROCELL-PD	TREATMENT OF HOEHN AND YAHR STAGE 4 AND 5 PARKINSON'S DISEASE.	DIACRIN/GENZYME LLC ONE KENDALL SQUARE CAMBRIDGE MA 02139-1562 DD 12/17/1996
PORCINE FETAL NEURAL DOPAMINERGIC CELLS AND/OR PRECURSORS ASEPTICALLY PREPARED FOR INTRACEREBRAL IMPLANTATION. TN=NEUROCELL-PD	TREATMENT OF HOEHN AND YAHR STAGE 4 AND 5 PARKINSON'S DISEASE.	DIACRIN/GENZYME LLC ONE KENDALL SQUARE CAMBRIDGE MA 02139-1562 DD 12/17/1996

NAME *Generic/Chemical* *TN=Trade Name*	INDICATION DESIGNATED	SPONSOR AND ADDRESS *DD=Date Designated* *MA=Marketing Approval*
PORCINE FETAL NEURAL GA-BAERGIC CELLS AND/OR PRE-CURSORS ASEPTICALLY PREPARED AND COATED WITH ANTI-MHC-1 AB FOR INTRACEREBRAL IMPLANTATION TN=NEUROCELL-HD	TREATMENT OF HUNTINGTON'S DISEASE.	DIACRIN/GENZYME LLC ONE KENDALL SQUARE CAMBRIDGE MA 02129-1562 DD 12/10/1996
PORCINE FETAL NEURAL GA-BAERGIC CELLS AND/OR PRE-CURSORS ASEPTICALLY PREPARED FOR INTRACEREBRAL IMPLANTATION FOR HUNTINGTON'S DISEASE. TN=NEUROCELL-HD	TREATMENT OF HUNTINGTON'S DISEASE.	DIACRIN/GENZYME LLC ONE KENDALL SQUARE CAMBRIDGE MA 02139-1562 DD 12/10/1996
PORFIMER SODIUM TN=PHOTOFRIN	FOR THE PHOTODYNAMIC THERAPY OF PATIENTS WITH PRIMARY OR RECURRENT OBSTRUCTING (EITHER PARTIALLY OR COMPLETELY) ESOPHAGEAL CARCINOMA.	QLT PHOTOTHERAPEUTICS, INC. LEDERLE LABORATORIES 401 NORTH MIDDLETOWN ROAD PEARL RIVER NY 10965 DD 6/6/1989 MA 12/27/1995
PORFIMER SODIUM TN=PHOTOFRIN	FOR THE PHOTODYNAMIC THERAPY OF PATIENTS WITH TRANSITIONAL CELL CARCINOMA IN SITU OF THE URINARY BLADDER.	QLT PHOTOTHERAPEUTICS, INC. LEDERLE LABORATORIES 401 NORTH MIDDLETOWN ROAD PEARL RIVER NY 10965 DD 11/15/1989
PORFIROMYCIN TN=PROMYCIN	TREATMENT OF HEAD AND NECK CANCER.	BOEHRINGER INGELHEIM PHAR-MACEUTICALS, INC. 900 RIDGEBURY ROAD PO BOX 368 RIDGEFIELD CT 06877 DD 9/19/1995
PORFIROMYCIN TN=PROMYCIN	TREATMENT OF CERVICAL CANCER.	BOEHRINGER INGELHEIM PHAR-MACEUTICALS, INC. 900 RIDGEBURY ROAD PO BOX 368 RIDGEFIELD CT 06877 DD 3/13/1997
POTASSIUM CITRATE TN=UROCIT-K	PREVENTION OF CALCIUM RENAL STONES IN PATIENTS WITH HYPOCITRATURIA.	UNIVERSITY OF TEXAS HEALTH SCIENCE CENTER AT DALLAS 5323 HARRY HINES BLVD DALLAS TX 75235 DD 9/16/1985 MA 8/30/1985
POTASSIUM CITRATE TN=UROCIT-K	PREVENTION OF URIC ACID NEPHROLITHIASIS.	UNIVERSITY OF TEXAS HEALTH SCIENCE CENTER AT DALLAS 5323 HARRY HINES BOULEVARD DALLAS TX 75235 DD 11/1/1984 MA 8/30/1985
POTASSIUM CITRATE TN=UROCIT-K	FOR AVOIDANCE OF THE COMPLICATION OF CALCIUM STONE FORMATION IN PATIENTS WITH URIC LITHIASIS.	UNIVERSITY OF TEXAS HEALTH SCIENCE CENTER AT DALLAS 5323 HARRY HINES BLVD DALLAS TX 75235 DD 9/12/1985 MA 8/30/1985

NAME *Generic/Chemical* *TN=Trade Name*	INDICATION DESIGNATED	SPONSOR AND ADDRESS *DD=Date Designated* *MA=Marketing Approval*
POTASSIUM CITRATE AND CITRIC ACID	FOR THE DISSOLUTION AND CONTROL OF URIC ACID AND CYSTEINE CALCULI IN THE URINARY TRACT.	WILLEN DRUG COMPANY DD 2/14/1986
PR-122 (REDOX-PHENYTOIN)	FOR THE EMERGENCY RESCUE TREATMENT OF STATUS EPILEPTICUS, GRAND MAL TYPE.	PHARMOS 2 INNOVATION DRIVE ALACHUA FL 32615 DD 7/5/1990
PR-320 (MOLECUSOL-CARBAMAZEPINE)	FOR THE EMERGENCY RESCUE TREATMENT OF STATUS EPILEPTICUS, GRAND MAL TYPE.	PHARMOS 2 INNOVATION DRIVE ALACHUA FL 32615 DD 7/20/1990
PRAMIRACETAM SULFATE	FOR THE MANAGEMENT OF COGNITIVE DYSFUNCTION AND ENHANCEMENT OF ANTIDEPRESSANT ACTIVITY ASSOCIATED WITH ELECTROCONVULSIVE THERAPY.	CAMBRIDGE NEUROSCIENCE, INC. 1 KENDALL SQUARE, BLDG. 700 CAMBRIDGE MA 02139 DD 11/4/1991
PRAZIQUANTEL	TREATMENT OF NEUROCYSTICERCOSIS.	EM PHARMEUTICALS, INC. DD 4/18/1988
PREDNIMUSTINE TN=STERECYT	TREATMENT OF MALIGNANT NON-HODGKIN'S LYMPHOMAS.	PHARMACIA INC. P.O. BOX 16529 COLUMBUS OH 43216-6529 DD 6/17/1985
PRIMAQUINE PHOSPHATE	FOR USE IN COMBINATION WITH CLINDAMYCIN HYDROCHLORIDE IN THE TREATMENT OF PNEUMOCYSTIS CARINII PNEUMONIA ASSOCIATED WITH AIDS.	SANOFI WINTHROP, INC. 90 PARK AVENUE NEW YORK NY 10016 DD 7/23/1993
PROGESTERONE	ESTABLISHMENT AND MAINTENANCE OF PREGNANCY IN WOMEN UNDERGOING IN VITRO FERTILIZATION OR EMBRYO TRANSFER PROCEDURES.	WATSON LABORATORIES, INC. 311 BONNIE CIRCLE CORONA CA 91720 DD 12/22/1994
PROPAMIDINE ISETHIONATE 0.1% OPHTHALMIC SOLUTION TN=BROLENE	TREATMENT OF ACANTHAMOEBA KERATITIS.	BAUSCH & LOMB PHARMACEUTICALS DIVISION 8500 HIDDEN RIVER PARKWAY TAMPA FL 33637 DD 3/10/1988
PROSTAGLANDIN E1 ENOL ESTER (AS-013)	TREATMENT OF FONTAINE STAGE IV CHRONIC CRITICAL LIMB ISCHEMIA.	WELFIDE INTERNATIONAL CORPORATION 5555 VALLEY BOULEVARD LOS ANGELES CA 90032 DD 6/12/1998
PROSTAGLANDIN E1 IN LIPID EMULSION TN=LIPO-PGE1	TREATMENT OF ISCHEMIC ULCERATION OF THE LOWER LIMBS DUE TO PERIPHERAL ARTERIAL DISEASE.	ALPHA THERAPEUTIC CORPORATION 5555 VALLEY BOULEVARD LOS ANGELES CA 90032 DD 9/10/1996
PROTAXEL	TREATMENT OF OVARIAN CANCER.	BIOPHYSICA, INC. 3333 NORTH TORREY PINES COURT SUITE 100 LA JOLLA CA 92037 DD 5/21/2003
PROTEIN C CONCENTRATE TN=PROTEIN C CONCENTRATE (HUMAN) VAPOR HEATED, IMMUNO	FOR REPLACEMENT THERAPY IN PATIENTS WITH CONGENITAL OR ACQUIRED PROTEIN C DEFICIENCY FOR THE PREVENTION AND TREATMENT OF WARFARIN-INDUCED SKIN NECROSIS DURING ORAL ANTICOAGULATION.	IMMUNO CLINICAL RESEARCH CORP. 750 LEXINGTON AVENUE, 19TH FLOOR NEW YORK NY 10022 DD 6/19/1992

NAME *Generic/Chemical* *TN=Trade Name*	INDICATION DESIGNATED	SPONSOR AND ADDRESS *DD=Date Designated* *MA=Marketing Approval*
PROTEIN C CONCENTRATE TN=PROTEIN C CONCENTRATE (HUMAN) VAPOR HEATED, IMMU- NO	FOR USE IN THE PREVENTION AND TREATMENT OF PURPURA FULMINANS IN MENINGOCOCCEMIA.	IMMUNO CLINICAL RESEARCH CORP. 750 LEXINGTON AVENUE, 19TH FLOOR NEW YORK NY 10022 DD 4/22/1993
PROTEIN C CONCENTRATE TN=PROTEIN C CONCENTRATE (HUMAN) VAPOR HEATED, IMMU- NO	FOR REPLACEMENT THERAPY IN CONGENITAL PRO- TEIN C DEFICIENCY FOR THE PREVENTION AND TREATMENT OF THROMBOSIS, PULMONARY EMBOLI, AND PURPURA FULMINANS.	BAXTER HEALTHCARE CORPORATION HYLAND DIVISION (BAXTER HYLAND) 550 NORTH BRAND BLVD. GLENDALE CA 91203 DD 6/23/1992
PROTIRELIN	PREVENTION OF INFANT RESPIRATORY DISTRESS SYNDROME ASSOCIATED WITH PREMATURITY.	UCB PHARMA, INC. 1950 LAKE PARK DRIVE SMYRNA GA 30080 DD 8/24/1993
PROTIRELIN INJECTION	TREATMENT OF AMYOTHROPHIC LATERAL SCLERO- SIS.	ABBOTT LABORATORIES DD 1/10/1985
PULMONARY SURFACTANT RE- PLACEMENT	PREVENTION AND TREATMENT OF INFANT RESPIRA- TORY DISTRESS SYNDROME.	SCIOS NOVA, INC. 2450 BAYSHORE PARKWAY MOUNTAIN VIEW CA 94043 DD 12/5/1988
PULMONARY SURFACTANT RE- PLACEMENT, PORCINE TN=CUROSURF	FOR THE TREATMENT AND PREVENTION OF RE- SPIRATORY DISTRESS SYNDROME IN PREMATURE INFANTS.	DEY LABORATORIES 2751 NAPA VALLEY CORPORATE DRIVE NAPA CA 94558 DD 8/2/1993
PURIFIED EXTRACT OF PSEUDO- MONAS AERUGINOSA TN=IMMUDYN	TREATMENT OF IMMUNE THROMBOCYTOPENIA PUR- PURA WHERE IT IS REQUIRED TO INCREASE PLATE- LET COUNTS.	DYNAGEN, INC. 99 ERIE STREET CAMBRIDGE MA 02139 DD 9/22/1997
PURIFIED TYPE II COLLAGEN TN=COLLORAL	TREATMENT OF JUVENILE RHEUMATOID ARTHRITIS.	AUTOIMMUNE, INC. 128 SPRING STREET LEXINGTON MA 02421 DD 2/9/1995
PYRUVATE	TREATMENT OF INTERSTITIAL LUNG DISEASE.	CELLULAR SCIENCES, INC 84 PARK AVENUE P.O. BOX 968 FLEMINGTON NJ 08822 DD 2/21/2001
QUINACRINE HYDROCHLORIDE	FOR PREVENTION OF RECURRENCE OF PNEU- MOTHORAX IN PATIENTS AT HIGH RISK OF RECUR- RENCE.	LYPHOMED, INC. DD 10/17/1984
R-ETODOLAC	THE TREATMENT OF CHRONIC LYMPHOCYTIC LEUKE- MIA	SALMEDIX, INC. 4330 LA JOLLA VILLAGE DRIVE SUITE 250 SAN DIEGO CA 92122 DD 12/9/2002
RGG0853, E1A LIPID COMPLEX	TREATMENT OF OVARIAN CANCER.	TARGETED GENETICS CORPORATION 1100 OLIVE WAY, SUITE 100 SEATTLE WA 98101 DD 9/15/1995

NAME *Generic/Chemical* *TN=Trade Name*	INDICATION DESIGNATED	SPONSOR AND ADDRESS *DD=Date Designated* *MA=Marketing Approval*
RII RETINAMIDE	TREATMENT OF MYELODYSPLASTIC SYNDROMES.	SPARTA PHARMACEUTICALS, INC. 111 ROCK ROAD HORSHAM PA 19044-2310 DD 5/6/1993
RECOMBINANT HUMAN ALPHA-FETOPROTEIN (RHAFP)	TREATMENT OF MYASTHENIA GRAVIS	MERRIMACK PHARMACEUTICALS, INC. 101 BINNEY STREET CAMBRIDGE MA 02142 DD 2/22/2001
RECOMBINANT BACTERICIDAL/PERMEABILITY-INCREASING PROTEIN TN=NEUPREX	TREATMENT OF SEVERE MENINGOCOCCAL DISEASE.	XOMA CORPORATION 2910 SEVENTH STREET BERKELEY CA 94710 DD 6/22/1998
RECOMBINANT GLYCINE2-HUMAN GLUCAGON-LIKE PEPTIDE-2	TREATMENT OF SHORT BOWEL SYNDROME.	NPS ALLELIX CORP. 6850 GOREWAY DR. MISSISSAUGA, ONTARIO L4V 1V7 CANADA CA DD 6/29/2000
RECOMBINANT HUMAN C1-ESTERASE INHIBITOR	PROPHYLACTIC TREATMENT OF ANGIOEDEMA CAUSED BY HEREDITARY OR ACQUIRED C1-ESTERASE INHIBITOR DEFICIENCY.	PHARMING N.V. CIPALSTREET 3 B-2440 GEEL BELGIUM BE DD 2/23/1999
RECOMBINANT HUMAN C1-ESTERASE INHIBITOR	TREATMENT OF (ACUTE ATTACKS OF) ANGIOEDEMA CAUSED BY HEREDITARY OR ACQUIRED C1-ESTERASE INHIBITOR DEFICIENCY.	PHARMING N.V. CIPALSTREET 3 B-2440 GEEL BELGIUM BE DD 2/23/1999
RECOMBINANT HUMAN CD4 IMMUNOGLOBULIN G	TREATMENT OF AIDS RESULTING FROM INFECTION WITH HIV-1.	GENENTECH, INC. 460 POINT SAN BRUNO BOULEVARD SOUTH SAN FRANCISCO CA 94080 DD 8/30/1990
RECOMBINANT HUMAN CLARA CELL 10KDA PROTEIN	PREVENTION OF NEONATAL BRONCHOPULMONARY DYSPLASIA IN PREMATURE NEONATES WITH RESPIRATORY DISTRESS SYNDROME.	CLARAGEN, INC. 335 PAINT BRANCH DRIVE COLLEGE PARK MD 20742 DD 7/13/1998
RECOMBINANT HUMAN ACID ALPHA-GLUCOSIDASE	TREATMENT OF GLYCOGEN STORAGE DISEASE TYPE II.	GENZYME CORPORATION ONE KENDALL SQUARE CAMBRIDGE MA 02139 DD 8/19/1997
RECOMBINANT HUMAN ANTITHROMBIN III	TREATMENT OF ANTITHROMBIN III DEPENDENT HEPARIN RESISTANCE REQUIRING ANTICOAGULATION.	AT III LLC C/O GENZYME CORPORATION 15 PLEASANT ST. CONNECTOR, P.O. BOX 9322 FRAMINGHAM MA 01701 DD 4/6/2000
RECOMBINANT HUMAN GELSOLIN	TREATMENT OF ACUTE AND CHRONIC RESPIRATORY SYMPTOMS OF BRONCHIECTASIS.	BIOGEN, INC. 14 CAMBRIDGE CENTER CAMBRIDGE MA 02142 DD 3/6/1995

NAME Generic/Chemical TN=Trade Name	INDICATION DESIGNATED	SPONSOR AND ADDRESS DD=Date Designated MA=Marketing Approval
RECOMBINANT HUMAN GELSO-LIN	TREATMENT OF THE RESPIRATORY SYMPTOMS OF CYSTIC FIBROSIS.	BIOGEN, INC. 14 CAMBRIDGE CENTER CAMBRIDGE MA 02124 DD 1/12/1994
RECOMBINANT HUMAN HIGHLY PHOSPHORYLATED ACID AL-PHA-GLUCOSIDASE TN=TBD	FOR ENZYME REPLACEMENT THERAPY IN PATIENTS WITH ALL SUBTYPES OF GLYCOGEN STORAGE DIS-EASE TYPE II (GSDII, POMPE DISEASE)	NOVAZYME PHARMACEUTICALS, INC. 800 RESEARCH PARKWAY SUITE 200 OKLAHOMA CITY OK 73104 DD 9/20/2000
RECOMBINANT HUMAN INSULIN-LIKE GROWTH FACTOR 1 TN=IGF-1	TREATMENT OF ANTIBODY-MEDIATED GROWTH HOR-MONE RESISTANCE IN PATIENTS WITH ISOLATED GROWTH HORMONE DEFICIENCY IA.	PHARMACIA & UPJOHN 7000 PORTAGE ROAD KALAMAZOO MI 49001-0199 DD 6/7/1995
RECOMBINANT HUMAN INSULIN-LIKE GROWTH FACTOR 1 TN=IGF-1	TREATMENT OF GROWTH HORMONE RECEPTOR DE-FICIENCY.	PHARMACIA & UPJOHN 7000 PORTAGE ROAD KALAMAZOO MI 49001-0199 DD 6/7/1995
RECOMBINANT HUMAN INSULIN-LIKE GROWTH FACTOR-I TN=PV802	TREATMENT OF SHORT-BOWEL SYNDROME AS A RE-SULT OF RESECTION OF THE SMALL BOWEL OR AS A RESULT OF CONGENITAL DYSFUNCTION OF THE IN-TESTINES.	GROPEP PTY LTD. GATE 11, VICTORIA DR. ADELAIDE SA 5000 AUSTRALIA AU DD 2/16/2000
RECOMBINANT HUMAN INSULIN-LIKE GROWTH FACTOR-I	TREATMENT OF POST-POLIOMYELITIS SYNDROME.	CEPHALON, INC. 145 BRANDYWINE PARKWAY WEST CHESTER PA 19380-4245 DD 10/13/1995
RECOMBINANT HUMAN INSULIN-LIKE GROWTH FACTOR-I/INSU-LIN-LIKE GROWTH FACTOR BIND-ING PROTEIN-3	TREATMENT OF MAJOR BURNS THAT REQUIRE HOS-PITALIZATION.	CELTRIX PHARMACEUTICALS, INC. P.O. BOX 2400 GLEN ALLEN VA 23058-2400 DD 6/15/1999
RECOMBINANT HUMAN INTER-LEUKIN-12	TREATMENT OF RENAL CELL CARCINOMA.	GENETICS INSTITUTE, INC. 87 CAMBRIDGEPARK DRIVE CAMBRIDGE MA 02140 DD 10/20/1997
RECOMBINANT HUMAN KERATI-NOCYTE GROWTH FACTOR	REDUCING THE INCIDENCE AND SEVERITY OF RADIA-TION-INDUCED XEROSTOMIA.	AMGEN INC. ONE AMGEN CENTER DR. THOUSAND OAKS CA 91320-1799 DD 12/20/1999
RECOMBINANT HUMAN LUTEI-NIZING HORMONE TN=LHADI	FOR USE IN ASSOCIATION WITH RECOMBINANT HU-MAN FOLLICLE STIMULATING HORMONE FOR THE TREATMENT OF WOMEN WITH CHRONIC ANOVULA-TION DUE TO HYPOGONADOTROPIC HYPOGONAD-ISM.	SERONO LABORATORIES, INC. 100 LONGWATER CIRCLE NORWELL MA 02061 DD 10/7/1994
RECOMBINANT HUMAN NERVE GROWTH FACTOR	TREATMENT OF HIV-ASSOCIATED SENSORY NEURO-PATHY.	GENENTECH, INC. 1 DNA WAY SOUTH SAN FRANCISCO CA 94080 DD 4/16/1999
RECOMBINANT HUMAN RELAXIN	TREATMENT OF PROGRESSIVE SYSTEMIC SCLERO-SIS.	CONNETICS CORPORATION 3400 WEST BAYSHORE ROAD PALO ALTO CA 94303 DD 11/3/1995

NAME *Generic/Chemical* *TN=Trade Name*	INDICATION DESIGNATED	SPONSOR AND ADDRESS *DD=Date Designated* *MA=Marketing Approval*
RECOMBINANT HUMAN SUPER- OXIDE DISMUTASE TN=OXSODROL	PREVENTION OF BRONCHOPULMONARY DYSPLASIA IN PREMATURE NEONATES WEIGHING LESS THAN 1500 GRAMS.	BIO-TECHNOLOGY GENERAL CORP. ONE TOWER CENTER BOULEVARD, 12TH FLOOR EAST BRUNSWICK NJ 08816 DD 4/18/1991
RECOMBINANT HUMAN THROM- BOPOIETIN	FOR USE IN ACCELERATING PLATELET RECOVERY IN PATIENTS UNDERGOING HEMATOPOIETIC STEM CELL TRANSPLANTATION.	GENENTECH, INC. 1 DNA WAY SOUTH SAN FRANCISCO CA 94080-4990 DD 9/29/1997
RECOMBINANT HUMANIZED MAB 5C8	PREVENTION AND TREATMENT OF FACTOR VIII/FAC-TOR IX INHIBITORS IN PATIENTS WITH HEMOPHILIA A OR B.	BIOGEN, INC. 14 CAMBRIDGE CENTER CAMBRIDGE MA 02142 DD 10/14/1998
RECOMBINANT HUMANIZED MAB 5C8	PREVENTION OF REJECTION OF PANCREATIC ISLET CELL TRANSPLANTS.	BIOGEN, INC. 14 CAMBRIDGE CENTER CAMBRIDGE MA 02142 DD 3/22/1999
RECOMBINANT HUMANIZED MAB 5C8	PREVENTION OF REJECTION OF SOLID ORGAN TRANSPLANTS.	BIOGEN, INC. 14 CAMBRIDGE CENTER CAMBRIDGE MA 02142 DD 3/22/1999
RECOMBINANT HUMANIZED MONCLONAL ANTIBODY 5C8	TREATMENT OF IMMUNE THROMBOCYTOPENIC PUR-PURA.	BIOGEN, INC. 14 CAMBRIDGE CENTER CAMBRIDGE MA 02142 DD 2/3/1998
RECOMBINANT HUMANIZED MONOCLONAL ANTIBODY 5C8	TREATMENT OF SYSTEMIC LUPUS ERYTHEMATOSUS.	BIOGEN, INC. 14 CAMBRIDGE CENTER CAMBRIDGE MA 02142 DD 2/18/1998
RECOMBINANT METHIONYL BRAIN-DERIVED NEURO-TROPHIC FACTOR	TREATMENT OF AMYOTROPHIC LATERAL SCLERO-SIS.	AMGEN, INC. ONE AMGEN CENTER DR. THOUSAND OAKS CA 91320-1799 DD 11/28/1994
RECOMBINANT METHIONYL HU-MAN STEM CELL FACTOR	TREATMENT OF PRIMARY BONE MARROW FAILURE.	AMGEN, INC. ONE AMGEN CENTER DRIVE THOUSAND OAKS CA 91320-1799 DD 11/22/1995
RECOMBINANT RETROVIRAL VECTOR - GLUCOCEREBROSI-DASE	FOR USE AS ENZYME REPLACEMENT THERAPY FOR PATIENTS WITH TYPES I, II, OR III GAUCHER DISEASE.	GENETIC THERAPY, INC. 938 CLOPPER ROAD GAITHERSBURG MD 20878 DD 11/15/1993
RECOMBINANT SECRETORY LEUCOCYTE PROTEASE INHIBI-TOR	TREATMENT OF CYSTIC FIBROSIS.	AMGEN, INC. 3200 WALNUT STREET BOULDER CO 80301 DD 3/29/1991
RECOMBINANT SECRETORY LEUCOCYTE PROTEASE INHIBI-TOR	TREATMENT OF CONGENITAL ALPHA-1 ANTITRYPSIN DEFICIENCY.	AMGEN INC. 3200 WALNUT STREET BOULDER CO 80301 DD 3/29/1991

NAME *Generic/Chemical* *TN=Trade Name*	INDICATION DESIGNATED	SPONSOR AND ADDRESS *DD=Date Designated* *MA=Marketing Approval*
RECOMBINANT SOLUBLE HUMAN CD4 TN=RECEPTIN	TREATMENT OF ACQUIRED IMMUNODEFICIENCY SYNDROME.	BIOGEN, INC. 14 CAMBRIDGE CENTER CAMBRIDGE MA 02142 DD 11/20/1989
RECOMBINANT SOLUBLE HUMAN CD4 (RCD4)	TREATMENT OF AIDS IN PATIENTS INFECTED WITH HIV VIRUS.	GENENTECH, INC. 460 POINT SAN BRUNO BOULEVARD SOUTH SAN FRANCISCO CA 94080 DD 3/23/1989
RECOMBINANT T-CELL RECEPTOR	TREATMENT OF MULTIPLE SCLEROSIS PATIENTS WHO ARE BOTH HLA-DR2 POSITIVE AND GLYCOPROTEIN RESIDUES 35-55 AUTOREACTIVE TO MYELIN OLIGODENDROCYTE.	VIROGENOMICS, INC. 9020 SW WASHINGTON SQUARE ROAD SUITE 380 TIGARD OR 97223-4332 DD 5/2/2003
RECOMBINANT URATE OXIDASE	PROPHYLAXIS OF CHEMOTHERAPY-INDUCED HYPERURICEMIA.	SANOFI-SYNTHELABO RESEARCH 9 GREAT VALLEY PARKWAY MALVERN PA 19355 DD 10/11/2000
RECOMBINANT VACCINIA (HUMAN PAPILLOMAVIRUS) TN=TA-HPV	TREATMENT OF CERVICAL CANCER.	XENOVA RESEARCH LIMITED 310 CAMBRIDGE SCIENCE PARK CAMBRIDGE CB4 0WG GREAT BRITAIN GB DD 8/24/1994
REDUCED L-GLUTATHIONE TN=CACHEXON	TREATMENT OF AIDS-ASSOCIATED CACHEXIA.	TELLURIDE PHARMACEUTICAL CORPORATION 146 FLANDERS DRIVE HILLSBOROUGH NJ 08876 DD 2/14/1994
REMACEMIDE TN=ECOVIA	TREATMENT OF HUNTINGTON'S DISEASE.	ASTRAZENECA LP 725 CHESTERBROOK BLVD. WAYNE PA 19087-5677 DD 3/6/2000
REPOSITORY CORTICOTROPIN OR ADRENOCORTICOTROPIC HORMONE TN=H.P. ACTHAR GEL	TREATMENT OF INFANTILE SPASMS.	QUESTCOR PHARMACEUTICALS, INC. 3260 WHIPPLE ROAD UNION CITY CA 94587-1217 DD 5/21/2003
RESINIFERATOXIN	TREATMENT OF INTRACTABLE PAIN AT END-STAGE DISEASE.	ANDREW J. MANNES, MD BLDG 10/RM 2N236-DASS/PPCS/NIDCR/NIH 10 CONVENT DRIVE BETHESDA MD 20892 DD 5/13/2003
RESPIRATORY SYNCYTIAL VIRUS IMMUNE GLOBULIN (HUMAN) TN=HYPERMUNE RSV	TREATMENT OF RESPIRATORY SYNCYTIAL VIRUS LOWER RESPIRATORY TRACT INFECTIONS IN HOSPITALIZED INFANTS AND YOUNG CHILDREN.	MEDIMMUNE, INC. 35 WEST WATKINS MILL ROAD GAITHERSBURG MD 20878 DD 9/27/1990
RESPIRATORY SYNCYTIAL VIRUS IMMUNE GLOBULIN (HUMAN) TN=RESPIGAM	PROPHYLAXIS OF RESPIRATORY SYNCYTIAL VIRUS LOWER RESPIRATORY TRACT INFECTIONS IN INFANTS AND YOUNG CHILDREN AT HIGH RISK OF RSV DISEASE.	MEDIMMUNE & MASSACHUSETTS PUBLIC HEALTH BIOLOGICS LABS. 35 WEST WATKINS MILL ROAD GAITHERSBURG MD 20878 DD 9/27/1990 MA 1/18/1996

NAME Generic/Chemical TN=Trade Name	INDICATION DESIGNATED	SPONSOR AND ADDRESS DD=Date Designated MA=Marketing Approval
RETROVIRAL VECTOR, R-GC AND GC GENE 1750	TREATMENT OF GAUCHER DISEASE.	GENZYME CORPORATION ONE MOUNTAIN ROAD P.O. BOX 9322 FRAMINGHAM MA 01701-9322 DD 5/6/1997
REVIPARIN SODIUM TN=CLIVARINE	TREATMENT OF DEEP VEIN THROMBOSIS WHICH MAY LEAD TO PULMONARY EMBOLISM IN PEDIATRIC PATIENTS	KNOLL AG LUDWIGSHAFEN, GERMANY DD 6/18/2001
REVIPARIN SODIUM TN=CLIVARINE	LONG-TERM TREATMENT OF ACUTE DEEP VEIN TROMBOSIS WITH OR WITHOUT PULMONARY EMBOLISM IN PREGNANT PATIENTS	KNOLL AG LUDWIGSHAFEN, GERMANY DD 6/18/2001
RHO (D) IMMUNE GLOBULIN INTRAVENOUS (HUMAN) TN=WINRHO SD	TREATMENT OF IMMUNE THROMBOCYTOPENIC PURPURA.	RH PHARMACEUTICALS, INC. 104 CHANCELLOR MATHESON ROAD WINNIPEG, MANITOBA CANADA R3T 2N2 CA DD 11/9/1993 MA 3/24/1995
RIBAVIRIN TN=REBETOL	TREATMENT OF CHRONIC HEPATITIS C IN PEDIATRIC PATIENTS.	SCHERING CORPORATION 2000 GALLOPING HILL ROAD KENILWORTH NJ 07033 DD 4/4/2003 MA 7/29/2003
RIBAVIRIN TN=VIRAZOLE	TREATMENT OF HEMORRHAGIC FEVER WITH RENAL SYNDROME.	ICN PHARMACEUTICALS, INC. ICN PLAZA 3300 HYLAND AVENUE COSTA MESA CA 92626 DD 4/12/1991
RICIN (BLOCKED) CONJUGATED MURINE MCA (ANTI-B4)	TREATMENT OF B-CELL LEUKEMIA AND B-CELL LYMPHOMA.	IMMUNOGEN, INC. 148 SIDNEY STREET CAMBRIDGE MA 02139 DD 11/17/1988
RICIN (BLOCKED) CONJUGATED MURINE MCA (ANTI-MY9)	TREATMENT OF MYELOID LEUKEMIA, INCLUDING AML, AND BLAST CRISIS OF CML.	IMMUNOGEN, INC. 148 SIDNEY STREET CAMBRIDGE MA 02139 DD 8/3/1989
RICIN (BLOCKED) CONJUGATED MURINE MCA (ANTI-MY9)	FOR USE IN THE EX-VIVO TREATMENT OF AUTOLOGOUS BONE MARROW AND SUBSEQUENT REINFUSION IN PATIENTS WITH ACUTE MYELOGENOUS LEUKEMIA.	IMMUNOGEN, INC. 148 SIDNEY STREET CAMBRIDGE MA 02139 DD 2/1/1990
RICIN (BLOCKED) CONJUGATED MURINE MCA (N901)	TREATMENT OF SMALL CELL LUNG CANCER.	IMMUNOGEN, INC. 148 SIDNEY STREET CAMBRIDGE MA 02139 DD 1/25/1991
RICIN (BLOCKED) CONJUGATED MURINE MCA (ANTI-B4)	FOR THE EX-VIVO PURGING OF LEUKEMIC CELLS FROM THE BONE MARROW OF NON-T CELL ACUTE LYMPHOCYTIC LEUKEMIA PATIENTS WHO ARE IN COMPLETE REMISSION.	IMMUNOGEN, INC. 148 SIDNEY STREET CAMBRIDGE MA 02139 DD 1/24/1991
RICIN (BLOCKED) CONJUGATED MURINE MONOCLONAL ANTIBODY (CD6)	TREATMENT OF CUTANEOUS T-CELL LYMPHOMAS, ACUTE T-CELL LEUKEMIA-LYMPHOMA, AND RELATED MATURE T-CELL MALIGNANCIES.	IMMUNOGEN, INC. 148 SIDNEY STREET CAMBRIDGE MA 02139 DD 9/6/1994

NAME *Generic/Chemical* *TN=Trade Name*	INDICATION DESIGNATED	SPONSOR AND ADDRESS *DD=Date Designated* *MA=Marketing Approval*
RIFABUTIN	TREATMENT OF DISSEMINATED MYCOBACTERIUM AVIUM COMPLEX DISEASE.	PHARMACIA & UPJOHN 7000 PORTAGE ROAD UNIT 0633-298-113 KALAMAZOO MI 49001-0199 DD 12/18/1989
RIFABUTIN TN=MYCOBUTIN	PREVENTION OF DISSEMINATED MYCOBACTERIUM AVIUM COMPLEX DISEASE IN PATIENTS WITH ADVANCED HIV INFECTION.	ADRIA LABORATORIES, INC. P.O. BOX 16529 COLUMBUS OH 43216 DD 12/18/1989 MA 12/23/1992
RIFALAZIL	TREATMENT OF PULMONARY TUBERCULOSIS.	PATHOGENESIS CORPORATION 201 ELLIOTT AVENUE WEST SUITE 150 SEATTLE WA 98119 DD 4/13/1999
RIFAMPIN TN=RIFADIN I.V.	FOR ANTITUBERCULOSIS TREATMENT WHERE USE OF THE ORAL FORM OF THE DRUG IS NOT FEASIBLE.	HOECHST MARION ROUSSEL P.O. BOX 9627 KANSAS CITY MO 64134 DD 12/9/1985 MA 5/25/1989
RIFAMPIN, ISONIAZID, PYRAZINAMIDE TN=RIFATER	FOR THE SHORT-COURSE TREATMENT OF TUBERCULOSIS.	HOECHST MARION ROUSSEL P.O. BOX 9627 KANSAS CITY MO 64134 DD 9/12/1985 MA 5/31/1994
RIFAPENTINE TN=PRIFTIN	PROPHYLACTIC TREATMENT OF MYCOBACTERIUM AVIUM COMPLEX IN PATIENTS WITH AIDS AND A CD4+ COUNT LESS THAN OR EQUAL TO 75/MM3.	HOECHST MARION ROUSSEL, INC. P.O. BOX 9627 MAIL STATION: H3-M2516 KANSAS CITY MO 64134-0627 DD 3/12/1996
RIFAPENTINE TN=PRIFTIN	TREATMENT OF MYCOBACTERIUM AVIUM COMPLEX IN PATIENTS WITH AIDS.	HOECHST MARION ROUSSEL, INC. P.O. BOX 9627 MAIL STATION: H3-M2516 KANSAS CITY MO 64134-0627 DD 6/9/1995
RIFAPENTINE TN=PRIFTIN	TREATMENT OF PULMONARY TUBERCULOSIS.	HOECHST MARION ROUSSEL P.O. BOX 9627 MAIL STATION: H3-M2516 KANSAS CITY MO 64134-0627 DD 6/9/1995 MA 6/22/1998
RIFAXIMIN TN=NORMIX	TREATMENT OF HEPATIC ENCEPHALOPATHY.	SALIX PHARMACEUTICALS, INC. 3600 W. BAYSHORE ROAD, SUITE 205 PALO ALTO CA 94303 DD 2/10/1998
RILUZOLE TN=RILUTEK	TREATMENT OF HUNTINGTON'S DISEASE.	RHONE-POULENC RORER PHARMACEUTICALS, INC. 500 ARCOLA ROAD PO BOX 5096 COLLEGEVILLE PA 19426-0800 DD 10/15/1996

NAME *Generic/Chemical* *TN=Trade Name*	INDICATION DESIGNATED	SPONSOR AND ADDRESS *DD=Date Designated* *MA=Marketing Approval*
RILUZOLE TN=RILUTEK	TREATMENT OF AMYOTROPHIC LATERAL SCLEROSIS.	RHONE-POULENC RORER PHARMACEUTICALS, INC. 500 ARCOLA ROAD, P.O. BOX 1200 COLLEGEVILLE PA 19426 DD 3/16/1993 MA 12/12/1995
RITUXIMAB TN=RITUXAN	TREATMENT OF NON-HODGKIN'S B-CELL LYMPHOMA.	IDEC PHARMACEUTICALS CORPORATION 3030 CALLAN ROAD SAN DIEGO CA 92121 DD 6/13/1994 MA 11/26/1997
ROQUINIMEX TN=LINOMIDE	TO PROLONG TIME TO RELAPSE IN LEUKEMIA PATIENTS WHO HAVE UNDERGONE AUTOLOGOUS BONE MARROW TRANSPLANTATION.	PHARMACIA & UPJOHN 7000 PORTAGE ROAD KALAMAZOO MI 49001-0199 DD 7/1/1993
S(-)-3-[3-AMINO-PHTHALIMIDO]-GLUTARAMIDE	TREATMENT OF MULTIPLE MYELOMA	ENTREMED INCORPORATED 9640 MEDICAL CENTER DR. ROCKVILLE MD 20850 DD 3/14/2002
S-ADENOSYLMETHIONINE	TREATMENT OF AIDS-MYELOPATHY.	DI ROCCO, ALESSANDRO M.D. BETH ISRAEL MEDICAL CENTER, PHILLIPS AMBULATORY CARE CENTER PHILIPS BUILDING, SUITE 2Q; 10 UNION SQUARE EAST NEW YORK NY 10003 DD 4/30/1998
SB-408075	FOR PANCREATIC CANCER	SMITHKLINE BEECHAM PHARMACEUTICALS 1250 S. COLLEGEVILLE ROAD COLLEGEVILLE PA 19426-0989 DD 12/7/2000
SCH 58500	TREATMENT OF PRIMARY OVARIAN CANCER.	SCHERING CORPORATION 2000 GALLOPING HILL RD. KENILWORTH NJ 07033 DD 4/12/1999
SK&F 110679	FOR THE LONG TERM TREATMENT OF CHILDREN WHO HAVE GROWTH FAILURE DUE TO A LACK OF ADEQUATE ENDOGENOUS GROWTH HORMONE SECRETION.	SMITHKLINE BEECHAM PHARMACEUTICALS ONE FRANKLIN PLAZA PHILADELPHIA PA 19101 DD 5/23/1990
SS1(DSFV)-PE38	TREATMENT OF MALIGNANT MESOTHELIOMA	NEOPHARM INCORPORATED 150 FIELD DRIVE SUITE 195 LAKE FOREST IL 60045 DD 2/11/2002
SS1(DSFV)-PE38	TREATMENT OF EPITHELIAL OVARIAN CANCER	NEOPHARM, INC. 150 FIELD DRIVE SUITE 195 LAKE FOREST IL 60045 DD 2/11/2002
ST1-RTA IMMUNOTOXIN (SR 44163)	PREVENTION OF ACUTE GRAFT VERSUS HOST DISEASE IN ALLOGENIC BONE MARROW TRANSPLANTATION.	SANOFI WINTHROP, INC. 9 GREAT VALLEY PARKWAY MALVERN PA 19355 DD 8/12/1987

NAME *Generic/Chemical* *TN=Trade Name*	INDICATION DESIGNATED	SPONSOR AND ADDRESS *DD=Date Designated* *MA=Marketing Approval*
ST1-RTA IMMUNOTOXIN (SR 44163)	TREATMENT OF PATIENTS WITH B-CHRONIC LYM-PHOCYTIC LEUKEMIA.	SANOFI WINTHROP, INC. 9 GREAT VALLEY PARKWAY MALVERN PA 19355 DD 8/12/1987
SU101	TREATMENT OF MALIGNANT GLIOMA.	SUGEN, INC. 230 EAST GRAND AVE. SOUTH SAN FRANCISCO CA 94080-4811 DD 5/25/1995
SU101	TREATMENT OF OVARIAN CANCER.	SUGEN, INC. 230 EAST GRAND AVE. SOUTH SAN FRANCISCO CA 94080-4811 DD 3/12/1996
SACROSIDASE TN=SUCRAID	TREATMENT OF CONGENITAL SUCRASE-ISOMAL-TASE DEFICIENCY.	ORPHAN MEDICAL, INC. 13911 RIDGEDALE DRIVE SUITE 475 MINNETONKA MN 55305 DD 12/10/1993 MA 4/9/1998
SARGRAMOSTIM TN=LEUKINE	TO REDUCE NEUTROPENIA AND LEUKOPENIA AND DECREASE THE INCIDENCE OF DEATH DUE TO INFEC-TION IN PATIENTS WITH ACUTE MYELOGENOUS LEU-KEMIA.	IMMUNEX CORPORATION 51 UNIVERSITY STREET SEATTLE WA 98101 DD 3/6/1995 MA 9/15/1995
SARGRAMOSTIM TN=LEUKINE	TREATMENT OF NEUTROPENIA ASSOCIATED WITH BONE MARROW TRANSPLANT, FOR THE TREATMENT OF GRAFT FAILURE AND DELAY OF ENGRAFTMENT, AND FOR THE PROMOTION OF EARLY ENGRAFT-MENT.	IMMUNEX CORPORATION 51 UNIVERSITY STREET SEATTLE WA 98101 DD 5/3/1990 MA 3/5/1991
SATUMOMAB PENDETIDE TN=ONCOSCINT CR/OV	DETECTION OF OVARIAN CARCINOMA.	CYTOGEN CORPORATION 600 COLLEGE ROAD EAST PRINCETON NJ 08540 DD 9/25/1989 MA 12/29/1992
SECALCIFEROL TN=OSTEO-D	TREATMENT OF FAMILIAL HYPOPHOSPHATEMIC RICKETS.	TEVA PHARMACEUTICALS USA 650 CATHILL RD. SELLERSVILLE PA 18960 DD 7/26/1993
SECRETORY LEUKOCYTE PRO-TEASE INHIBITOR	TREATMENT OF BRONCHOPULMONARY DYSPLASIA.	SYNERGEN, INC. 1885 33RD STREET BOULDER CO 80301 DD 6/30/1992
SELEGILINE HCL TN=ELDEPRYL	AS AN ADJUVANT TO LEVODOPA AND CARBIDOPA TREATMENT OF IDIOPATHIC PARKINSON'S DISEASE (PARALYSIS AGITANS), POSTENCEPHALITIC PARKIN-SONISM, AND SYMPTOMATIC PARKINSONISM.	SOMERSET PHARMACEUTICALS, INC. 777 SOUTH HARBOR ISLAND BOULEVARD TAMPA FL 33602 DD 11/7/1984 MA 6/5/1989
SERMORELIN ACETATE TN=GEREF	TREATMENT OF AIDS-ASSOCIATED CATABOLISM/WEIGHT LOSS.	SERONO LABORATORIES, INC. ONE TECHNOLOGY PLACE ROCKLAND MA 02370 DD 12/5/1991

NAME *Generic/Chemical* *TN=Trade Name*	**INDICATION DESIGNATED**	**SPONSOR AND ADDRESS** *DD=Date Designated* *MA=Marketing Approval*
SERMORELIN ACETATE TN=GEREF	ADJUNCT TO GONADOTROPIN THERAPY IN THE IN-DUCTION OF OVULATION IN WOMEN WITH ANOVULA-TORY OR OLIGO-OVULATORY INFERTILITY WHO FAIL TO OVULATE IN RESPONSE TO ADEQUATE TREAT-MENT WITH CLOMIPHENE CITRATE ALONE AND GO-NADOTROPIN THERAPY ALONE.	SERONO LABORATORIES, INC. ONE TECHNOLOGY PLACE ROCKLAND MA 02370 DD 2/13/1990
SERMORELIN ACETATE TN=GEREF	TREATMENT OF IDIOPATHIC OR ORGANIC GROWTH HORMONE DEFICIENCY IN CHILDREN WITH GROWTH FAILURE.	SERONO LABORATORIES, INC. 100 LONGWATER CIRCLE NORWELL MA 02061 DD 9/14/1988 MA 9/26/1997
SERRATIA MARCESCENS EX-TRACT (POLYRIBOSOMES) TN=IMUVERT	TREATMENT OF PRIMARY BRAIN MALIGNANCIES.	CELL TECHNOLOGY, INC. 1668 VALTEC LANE BOULDER CO 80306 DD 9/7/1988
SHORT CHAIN FATTY ACID ENE-MA TN=COLOMED	TREATMENT OF CHRONIC RADIATION PROCTITIS.	RICHARD I. BREUER, M.D. 1000 CENTRAL STREET, SUITE 615 EVANSTON IL 60201 DD 8/19/1997
SHORT CHAIN FATTY ACID SOLU-TION TN=COLOMED	TREATMENT OF THE ACTIVE PHASE OF ULCERATIVE COLITIS WITH INVOLVEMENT RESTRICTED TO THE LEFT SIDE OF THE COLON.	RICHARD I. BREUER 1000 CENTRAL STREET, SUITE 615 EVANSTON IL 60201 DD 5/29/1990
SILVER SULFADIAZINE AND CER-IUM NITRATE TN=FLAMMACERIUM	PREVENTION OF MORTALITY IN SEVERELY BURNED PATIENTS.	SYNTHES (USA) 1690 RUSSELL ROAD PO BOX 1766 PAOLI PA 19301 DD 11/17/1999
SODIUM 1,3-PROPANEDISULFO-NATE	TREATMENT OF SECONDARY AMYLOIDOSIS.	NEUROCHEM, INC. 7220 FREDERICK BANTING, SUITE 100 SAINT-LAURENT, QUEBEC CANADA H4S 2A1 CA DD 4/6/1999
SODIUM MONOMERCAPTOUN-DECAHYDRO-CLOSO-DODECA-BORATE TN=BOROCELL	FOR USE IN BORON NEUTRON CAPTURE THERAPY (BNCT) IN THE TREATMENT OF GLIOBLASTOMA MUL-TIFORME.	NEUTRON TECHNOLOGY CORP. & NEUTRON R&D PARTNER 877 MAIN STREET, SUITE 402 BOISE ID 83702 DD 4/15/1992
SODIUM DICHLOROACETATE	TREATMENT OF CONGENITAL LACTIC ACIDOSIS.	STACPOOLE, PETER W. M.D., PH.D. UNIVERSITY OF FLORIDA P.O. BOX 100277 GAINESVILLE FL 32610 DD 6/11/1990
SODIUM DICHLOROACETATE	TREATMENT OF CONGENITAL LACTIC ACIDOSIS.	QUESTCOR PHARMACEUTICALS, INC. 3260 WHIPPLE RD. UNION CITY CA 94587-1217 DD 12/31/1997
SODIUM DICHLOROACETATE TN=CERESINE	TREATMENT OF SEVERE HEAD INJURY.	QUESTCOR PHARMACEUTICALS, INC. 26118 RESEARCH ROAD HAYWARD CA 94545 DD 6/14/1999

NAME *Generic/Chemical* *TN=Trade Name*	INDICATION DESIGNATED	SPONSOR AND ADDRESS *DD=Date Designated* *MA=Marketing Approval*
SODIUM DICHLOROACETATE	TREATMENT OF LACTIC ACIDOSIS IN PATIENTS WITH SEVERE MALARIA.	STACPOOLE, PETER W. M.D., PH.D. UNIVERSITY OF FLORIDA P.O. BOX 100277 GAINESVILLE FL 32610 DD 11/10/1994
SODIUM DICHLOROACETATE	TREATMENT OF HOMOZYGOUS FAMILIAL HYPERCH-OLESTEROLEMIA.	STACPOOLE, PETER W. M.D., PH.D. UNIVERSITY OF FLORIDA P.O. BOX 100277 GAINESVILLE FL 32610 DD 6/11/1990
SODIUM MONOMERCAPTOUN-DECAHYDRO-CLOSO-DODECA-BORATE	FOR USE IN CONJUNCTION WITH A THERMAL OR EPITHERMAL NEUTRON BEAM IN BORON NUCLEAR CAPTURE THERAPY OF GLIOBLASTOMA MULTI-FORME.	THERAGENICS CORPORATION DD 12/18/1984
SODIUM PHENYLBUTYRATE	FOR USE AS AN ADJUCT TO SURGERY, RADIATION THERAPY AND CHEMOTHERAPY FOR THE TREAT-MENT OF PATIENTS WITH PRIMARY OR RECURRENT MALIGNANT GLIOMA.	ELAN DRUG DELIVERY, INC. 1300 GOULD DR. GAINESVILLE GA 30504 DD 4/24/1998
SODIUM PYRUVATE	TREATMENT OF CYSTIC FIBROSIS	CELLULAR SCIENCES, INC. 84 PARK AVENUE P. O. BOX 968 FLEMINGTON NJ 08822 DD 3/31/2003
SODIUM TETRADECYL SULFATE TN=SOTRADECOL	TREATMENT OF BLEEDING ESOPHAGEAL VARICES.	ELKINS-SINN, INC. 2 ESTERBROOK LANE CHERRY HILL NJ 08003 DD 6/10/1986
SOLUBLE COMPLEMENT RECEP-TOR TYPE 1	PREVENTION OF POST-CARDIOPULMONARY BYPASS SYNDROME IN CHILDREN UNDERGOING CARDIOPUL-MONARY BYPASS.	AVANT IMMUNOTHERAPEUTICS, INC. 119 FOURTH AVE. NEEDHAM MA 02494-2725 DD 3/6/2000
SOLUBLE RECOMBINANT HUMAN COMPLEMENT RECEPTOR TYPE 1	PREVENTION OR REDUCTION OF ADULT RESPIRA-TORY DISTRESS SYNDROME.	T CELL SCIENCES, INC. 119 FOURTH AVENUE NEEDHAM HEIGHTS MA 02194 DD 11/21/1994
SOMATOSTATIN	TREATMENT OF BLEEDING ESOPHAGEAL VARICES.	UCB PHARMACEUTICALS, INC. 1950 LAKE PARK DRIVE SMYRNA GA 30080 DD 12/22/1994
SOMATOSTATIN TN=ZECNIL	ADJUNCT TO THE NON-OPERATIVE MANAGEMENT OF SECRETING CUTANEOUS FISTULAS OF THE STO-MACH, DUODENUM, SMALL INTESTINE (JEJUNUM AND ILEUM), OR PANCREAS.	FERRING LABORATORIES, INC. 400 RELLA BOULEVARD, SUITE 201 SUFFERN NY 10901 DD 6/20/1988
SOMATREM FOR INJECTION TN=PROTROPIN	FOR LONG-TERM TREATMENT OF CHILDREN WHO HAVE GROWTH FAILURE DUE TO A LACK OF ADE-QUATE ENDOGENOUS GROWTH HORMONE SECRE-TION.	GENENTECH, INC. 460 POINT SAN BRUNO BOULEVARD SOUTH SAN FRANCISCO CA 94080 DD 12/9/1985 MA 10/17/1985

NAME *Generic/Chemical* *TN=Trade Name*	INDICATION DESIGNATED	SPONSOR AND ADDRESS *DD=Date Designated* *MA=Marketing Approval*
SOMATREM FOR INJECTION TN=PROTROPIN	TREATMENT OF SHORT STATURE ASSOCIATED WITH TURNER'S SYNDROME.	GENENTECH, INC. 460 POINT SAN BRUNO BOULEVARD SOUTH SAN FRANCISCO CA 94080 DD 12/9/1985
SOMATROPIN TN=NORDITROPIN	ADJUNCT FOR THE INDUCTION OF OVULATION IN WOMEN WITH INFERTILITY DUE TO HYPOGONADOTROPIC HYPOGONADISM OR BILATERAL TUBAL OCCLUSION OR UNEXPLAINED INFERTILITY, WHO ARE UNDERGOING IN VIVO OR IN VITRO FERTILIZATION PROCEDURES.	NOVO NORDISK PHARMACEUTICALS 100 OVERLOOK CENTER SUITE 200 PRINCETON NJ 08540 DD 9/1/1987
SOMATROPIN TN=NORDITROPIN	TREATMENT OF SHORT STATURE ASSOCIATED WITH TURNER'S SYNDROME.	NOVO NORDISK PHARMACEUTICALS 100 OVERLOOK CENTER SUITE 200 PRINCETON NJ 08540 DD 11/5/1987
SOMATROPIN TN=BIOTROPIN	TREATMENT OF CACHEXIA ASSOCIATED WITH AIDS.	BIO-TECHNOLOGY GENERAL CORP. 70 WOOD AVENUE, SOUTH ISELIN NJ 08830 DD 2/12/1993
SOMATROPIN TN=NUTROPIN	FOR USE IN THE LONG-TERM TREATMENT OF CHILDREN WHO HAVE GROWTH FAILURE DUE TO A LACK OF ADEQUATE ENDOGENOUS GROWTH HORMONE SECRETION.	GENENTECH, INC. 460 POINT SAN BRUNO BOULEVARD SOUTH SAN FRANCISCO CA 94080 DD 3/6/1987 MA 10/17/1985
SOMATROPIN TN=GENOTROPIN	TREATMENT OF ADULTS WITH GROWTH HORMONE DEFICIENCY.	PHARMACIA & UPJOHN 7000 PORTAGE ROAD KALAMAZOO MI 49001-0199 DD 9/6/1994 MA 10/31/1997
SOMATROPIN TN=HUMATROPE	TREATMENT OF SHORT STATURE ASSOCIATED WITH TURNER SYNDROME.	ELI LILLY AND COMPANY LILLY CORPORATE CENTER INDIANAPOLIS IN 46285 DD 5/8/1990 MA 12/30/1996
SOMATROPIN (RDNA) TN=SAIZEN	FOR THE ENHANCEMENT OF NITROGEN RETENTION IN HOSPITALIZED PATIENTS SUFFERING FROM SEVERE BURNS.	SERONO LABORATORIES, INC. ONE TECHNOLOGY PLACE ROCKLAND MA 02370 DD 5/3/1989
SOMATROPIN (R-DNA) TN=SEROSTIM	FOR USE ALONE OR IN COMBINATION WITH GLUTAMINE IN THE TREATMENT OF SHORT BOWEL SYNDROME.	SERONO LABORATORIES, INC. ONE TECHNOLOGY PLACE ROACKLAND MA 02370 DD 3/6/1995
SOMATROPIN (R-DNA) FOR INJECTION TN=SEROSTIM	TREATMENT OF CHILDREN WITH AIDS-ASSOCIATED FAILURE-TO-THRIVE INCLUDING AIDS-ASSOCIATED WASTING.	SERONO LABORATORIES, INC. ONE TECHNOLOGY PLACE ROCKLAND MA 02370 DD 3/26/1996
SOMATROPIN (RDNA ORIGIN) TN=SAIZEN	TREATMENT OF IDIOPATHIC OR ORGANIC GROWTH HORMONE DEFICIENCY IN CHILDREN WITH GROWTH FAILURE.	SERONO LABORATORIES, INC. 100 LONGWATER CIRCLE NORWELL MA 02061 DD 3/6/1987

NAME *Generic/Chemical* *TN=Trade Name*	INDICATION DESIGNATED	SPONSOR AND ADDRESS *DD=Date Designated* *MA=Marketing Approval*
SOMATROPIN (RDNA ORIGIN) TN=NUTROPIN DEPOT	LONG-TERM TREATMENT OF CHILDREN WHO HAVE GROWTH FAILURE DUE TO A LACK OF ADEQUATE ENDOGENOUS GROWTH HORMONE SECRETION.	GENENTECH, INC. 1 DNA WAY SOUTH SAN FRANCISCO CA 94080-4990 DD 10/28/1999
SOMATROPIN (RDNA ORIGIN) INJECTION TN=NORDITROPIN	TREATMENT OF GROWTH FAILURE IN CHILDREN DUE TO INADEQUATE GROWTH HORMONE SECRETION.	NOVO NORDISK PHARMACEUTICALS 100 OVERLOOK CENTER SUITE 200 PRINCETON NJ 08540 DD 7/10/1987
SOMATROPIN [RDNA] TN=GENOTROPIN	TREATMENT OF SHORT STATURE IN PATIENTS WITH PRADER-WILLI SYNDROME.	PHARMACIA & UPJOHN 7000 PORTAGE RD. 0633-298-113 KALAMAZOO MI 49001-0199 DD 7/6/1999 MA 6/20/2000
SOMATROPIN FOR INJECTION TN=NUTROPIN	AS REPLACEMENT THERAPY FOR GROWTH HORMONE DEFICIENCY IN ADULTS AFTER EPIPHYSEAL CLOSURE.	GENENTECH, INC. 460 POINT SAN BRUNO BOULEVARD SOUTH SAN FRANCISCO CA 94080 DD 11/18/1996 MA 12/15/1997
SOMATROPIN FOR INJECTION TN=HUMATROPE	FOR THE LONG-TERM TREATMENT OF CHILDREN WHO HAVE GROWTH FAILURE DUE TO INADEQUATE SECRETION OF NORMAL ENDOGENOUS GROWTH HORMONE.	ELI LILLY AND COMPANY LILLY CORPORATE CENTER INDIANAPOLIS IN 46285 DD 6/12/1986 MA 3/8/1987
SOMATROPIN FOR INJECTION TN=NUTROPIN	TREATMENT OF SHORT STATURE ASSOCIATED WITH TURNER'S SYNDROME.	GENENTECH, INC. 460 POINT SAN BRUNO BOULEVARD SOUTH SAN FRANCISCO CA 94080 DD 3/23/1989 MA 12/30/1996
SOMATROPIN FOR INJECTION TN=SEROSTIM	TREATMENT OF AIDS-ASSOCIATED CATABOLISM/WEIGHT LOSS.	SERONO LABORATORIES, INC. 100 LONGWATER CIRCLE NORWELL MA 02061 DD 11/15/1991 MA 8/23/1996
SOMATROPIN FOR INJECTION TN=NUTROPIN	TREATMENT OF GROWTH RETARDATION ASSOCIATED WITH CHRONIC RENAL FAILURE.	GENENTECH, INC. 460 POINT SAN BRUNO BOULEVARD SOUTH SAN FRANCISCO CA 94080 DD 8/4/1989 MA 11/17/1993
SORIVUDINE TN=BRAVAVIR	TREATMENT OF HERPES ZOSTER (SHINGLES) IN IMMUNOCOMPROMISED PATIENTS.	BRISTOL-MYERS SQUIBB 5 RESEARCH PARKWAY P.O. BOX 5100 WALLINGFORD CT 06492 DD 11/9/1995
SOTALOL HCL TN=BETAPACE	PREVENTION OF LIFE THREATENING VENTRICULAR TACHYARRHYTHMIAS.	BERLEX LABORATORIES, INC. 300 FAIRFIELD ROAD WAYNE NJ 07470 DD 9/23/1988

NAME *Generic/Chemical* *TN=Trade Name*	INDICATION DESIGNATED	SPONSOR AND ADDRESS *DD=Date Designated* *MA=Marketing Approval*
SOTALOL HCL TN=BETAPACE	TREATMENT OF LIFE-THREATENING VENTRICULAR TACHYARRHYTHMIAS.	BERLEX LABORATORIES, INC. 300 FAIRFIELD ROAD WAYNE NJ 07470 DD 9/23/1988 MA 10/30/1992
SPIRAMYCIN TN=ROVAMYCINE	FOR SYMPTOMATIC RELIEF AND PARASITIC CURE OF CHRONIC CRYPTOSPORIDIOSIS IN PATIENTS WITH IMMUNODEFICIENCY.	RHONE-POULENC RORER PHARMACEUTICALS 500 ARCOLA ROAD COLLEGEVILLE PA 19426 DD 10/17/1984
STERILE TALC TN=STERITALC	TREATMENT OF PNEUMOTHORAX.	NOVATECH SA AVENUE DU VENT DES DAMES - Z.L. LES PALUDS 13685 AUBAGNE FRANCE DD 12/8/1997
STERILE TALC TN=STERITALC	TREATMENT OF MALIGNANT PLEURAL EFFUSION.	NOVATECH SA AVENUE DU VENT DES DAMES - Z.L. LES PALUDS 13685 AUBAGNE FRANCE DD 12/8/1997
STERILE TALC POWDER TN=SCLEROSOL INTRAPLEURAL AEROSOL	TREATMENT OF MALIGNANT PLEURAL EFFUSION.	BRYAN CORPORATION 4 PLYMPTON STREET WOBURN MA 01801 DD 9/18/1995 MA 12/24/1997
SUBEROYLANILIDE HYDROXA-MIC ACID	TREATMENT OF MULTIPLE MYELOMA.	ATON PHARMA, INC. 777 OLD SAW MILL RIVER ROAD TARRYTOWN NY 10591-6717 DD 6/12/2003
SUCCIMER TN=CHEMET CAPSULES	TREATMENT OF LEAD POISONING IN CHILDREN.	BOCK PHARMACAL COMPANY P.O. BOX 419056 SAINT LOUIS MO 63141-9056 DD 5/9/1984 MA 12/22/1988
SUCCIMER TN=CHEMET	PREVENTION OF CYSTINE KIDNEY STONE FORMA-TION IN PATIENTS WITH HOMOZYGOUS CYSTINURIA WHO ARE PRONE TO STONE DEVELOPMENT.	SANOFI WINTHROP, INC. 90 PARK AVENUE NEW YORK NY 10016-1389 DD 11/5/1990
SUCCIMER TN=CHEMET	TREATMENT OF MERCURY INTOXICATION.	SANOFI WINTHROP, INC. 90 PARK AVENUE NEW YORK NY 10016-1389 DD 3/22/1991
SUCRALFATE	TREATMENT OF ORAL MUCOSITIS AND STOMATITIS FOLLOWING RADIATION THERAPY FOR HEAD AND NECK CANCER.	FUISZ TECHNOLOGIES, LTD. 14555 AVION AT LAKESIDE CHANTILLY VA 20151 DD 7/15/1993
SUCRALFATE SUSPENSION	TREATMENT OF ORAL COMPLICATIONS OF CHE-MOTHERAPY IN BONE MARROW TRANSPLANT PA-TIENTS.	DARBY PHARMACEUTICALS, INC. 100 BANKS AVENUE ROCKVILLE CENTRE NY 11570 DD 3/12/1990
SUCRALFATE SUSPENSION	TREATMENT OF ORAL ULCERATIONS AND DYSPHA-GIA IN PATIENTS WITH EPIDERMOLYSIS BULLOSA.	DARBY PHARMACEUTICALS, INC. 100 BANKS AVENUE ROCKVILLE CENTRE NY 11570 DD 3/4/1991

NAME Generic/Chemical TN=Trade Name	INDICATION DESIGNATED	SPONSOR AND ADDRESS DD=Date Designated MA=Marketing Approval
SULFADIAZINE	FOR USE IN COMBINATION WITH PYRIMETHAMINE FOR THE TREATMENT OF TOXOPLASMA GONDIIENCEPHALITIS IN PATIENTS WITH AND WITHOUT AIDS.	EON LABS MANUFACTURING, INC. 227-15 NORTH CONDUIT AVENUE LAURELTON NY 11413 DD 3/14/1994 MA 7/29/1994
SULFAPYRIDINE	TREATMENT OF DERMATITIS HERPETIFORMIS.	JACOBUS PHARMACEUTICAL COMPANY 37 CLEVELAND LANE P.O. BOX 5290 PRINCETON NJ 08540 DD 9/10/1990
SUPEROXIDE DISMUTASE (HUMAN)	FOR PROTECTION OF DONOR ORGAN TISSUE FROM DAMAGE OR INJURY MEDIATED BY OXYGEN-DERIVED FREE RADICALS THAT ARE GENERATED DURING THE NECESSARY PERIODS OF ISCHEMIA (HYPOXIA, ANOXIA), AND ESPECIALLY REPERFUSION, ASSOCIATED WITH THE OPERATIVE PROCEDURE.	PHARMACIA-CHIRON PARTNERSHIP 4560 HORTON STREET EMERYVILLE CA 94608 DD 3/6/1985
SUPEROXIDE DISMUTASE (RECOMBINANT HUMAN) TN=OXSODROL	PREVENTION OF REPERFUSION INJURY TO DONOR ORGAN TISSUE.	BIO-TECHNOLOGY GENERAL CORP. 70 WOOD AVENUE, SOUTH ISELIN NJ 08830 DD 5/17/1988
SURAMIN TN=METARET	TREATMENT OF HORMONE-REFRACTORY PROSTATE CANCER.	WARNER-LAMBERT COMPANY PARKE-DAVIS PHARMACEUTICAL RESEARCH DIVISION 2800 PLYMOUTH ROAD ANN ARBOR MI 48105-2430 DD 5/6/1997
SURFACE ACTIVE EXTRACT OF SALINE LAVAGE OF BOVINE LUNGS TN=INFASURF	TREATMENT AND PREVENTION OF RESPIRATORY FAILURE DUE TO PULMONARY SURFACTANT DEFICIENCY IN PRETERM INFANTS.	ONY, INC. 1576 SWEET HOME ROAD AMHERST NY 14228 DD 6/7/1985
SURFACTANT (HUMAN) (AMNIOTIC FLUID DERIVED) TN=HUMAN SURF	PREVENTION AND TREATMENT OF NEONATAL RESPIRATORY DISTRESS SYNDROME.	MERRITT, T. ALLEN M.D. 2516 STOCKTON BOULEVARD SACRAMENTO CA 95817 DD 3/25/1987
SYNSORB PK	TREATMENT OF VEROCYTOTOXOGENIC E. COLI INFECTIONS.	SYNSORB BIOTECH INC. 201, 1204 KENSINGTON ROAD, N.W. CALGARY, ALBERTA CANADA T2N 3P5 CA DD 7/17/1995
SYNTHETIC HUMAN PARATHYROID HORMONE 1-34	TREATMENT OF HYPOPARATHYROIDISM	ORPHAN PHARMACEUTICALS, U.S., INC. 1101 KERMIT DRIVE, SUITE 608 NASHVILLE TN 37217 DD 1/26/2001
SYNTHETIC HUMAN SECRETIN	FOR USE IN OBTAINING DESQUAMATED PANCREATIC CELLS FOR CYTOPATHOLOGIC EXAMINATION IN PANCREATIC CARCINOMA.	CHIRHOCLIN, INC. 15500 GALLAUDET AVE. SILVER SPRING MD 20905-4176 DD 6/16/1999
SYNTHETIC HUMAN SECRETIN	FOR USE IN THE EVALUATION OF EXOCRINE PANCREAS FUNCTION.	CHIRHOCLIN, INC. 1550 GALLAUDET AVE. SILVER SPRING MD 20905-4176 DD 6/16/1999

NAME Generic/Chemical TN=Trade Name	INDICATION DESIGNATED	SPONSOR AND ADDRESS DD=Date Designated MA=Marketing Approval
SYNTHETIC HUMAN SECRETIN	FOR USE IN THE DIAGNOSIS OF GASTRINOMA ASSOCIATED WITH ZOLLINGER-ELLISON SYNDROME.	CHIRHOCLIN, INC. 15500 GALLAUDET AVE. SILVER SPRING MD 20905-4176 DD 6/16/1999
SYNTHETIC HUMAN SECRETIN	FOR USE IN CONJUNCTION WITH DIAGNOSTIC PROCEDURES FOR PANCREATIC DISORDERS TO INCREASE PANCREATIC FLUID SECRETION.	CHIRHOCLIN, INC. 15500 GALLAUDET AVE. SILVER SPRING MD 20905-4176 DD 3/7/2000
SYNTHETIC PORCINE SECRETIN	FOR USE IN OBTAINING DESQUAMATED PANCREATIC CELLS FOR CYTOPATHOLOGIC EXAMINATION IN PANCREATIC CARCINOMA.	CHIRHOCLIN, INC. 15500 GALLAUDET AVE. SILVER SPRING MD 20905-4176 DD 6/18/1999
SYNTHETIC PORCINE SECRETIN	FOR USE IN THE EVALUATION OF EXOCRINE PANCREAS FUNCTION.	CHIRHOCLIN, INC. 15500 GALLAUDET AVE. SILVER SPRING MD 20905-4176 DD 6/18/1999 MA 11/1/2002
SYNTHETIC PORCINE SECRETIN	FOR USE IN THE DIAGNOSIS OF GASTRINOMA ASSOCIATED WITH ZOLLINGER-ELLISON SYNDROME.	CHIRHOCLIN, INC. 15500 GALLAUDET AVE. SILVER SPRING MD 20905-4176 DD 6/18/1999 MA 4/4/2002
SYNTHETIC PORCINE SECRETIN	FOR USE IN CONJUNCTION WITH DIAGNOSTIC PROCEDURES FOR PANCREATIC DISORDERS TO INCREASE PANCREATIC FLUID SECRETION.	CHIRHOCLIN, INC. 15500 GALLAUDET AVE. SILVER SPRING MD 20905-4176 DD 3/7/2000 MA 4/4/2002
T-CELL DEPLETED STEM CELL ENRICHED CELLULAR PRODUCT FROM PERIPHEAL BLOOD STEM CELLS	TREATMENT OF CHRONIC GRANULOMATOUS DISEASE	NEXELL THERAPEUTICS INC. 9 PARKER IRVINE CA 92618-1605 DD 11/1/2001
T4 ENDONUCLEASE V, LIPOSOME ENCAPSULATED	TO PREVENT CUTANEOUS NEOPLASMS AND OTHER SKIN ABNORMALITIES IN XERODERMA PIGMENTOSUM.	AGI DERMATICS 205 BUFFALO AVENUE FREEPORT NY 11520 DD 6/27/1989
TAK-603	TREATMENT OF CROHN'S DISEASE.	TAP HOLDINGS INC. 2355 WAUKEGAN ROAD DEERFIELD IL 60015 DD 5/13/1998
TGF(BETA)2-SPECIFIC PHOSPHOROTHIOATE ANTISENSE OLIGODEOXYNUCLEOTIDE TN=ONCOMUN	TREATMENT OF MALIGNANT GLIOMA	ANTISENSE PHARMA GMBH JOSEF-ENGERT-STR. 9 93053 REGENSBERG GERMANY DD 6/5/2002
TACROLIMUS TN=PROGRAF	PROPHYLAXIS OF GRAFT-VERSUS-HOST-DISEASE.	FUJISAWA USA, INC. 3 PARKWAY NORTH CENTER DEERFIELD IL 60015 DD 4/6/1998
TECHNETIUM TC 99M PTEROTETRAMIDE	FOR THE IDENTIFICATION OF OVARIAN CARCINOMAS.	ENDOCYTE, INC. 1205 KENT AVE. LAFAYETTE IN 47906 DD 2/16/2000

NAME *Generic/Chemical* *TN=Trade Name*	INDICATION DESIGNATED	SPONSOR AND ADDRESS *DD=Date Designated* *MA=Marketing Approval*
TECHNETIUM TC99M ANTI-MELA-NOMA MURINE MONOCLONAL ANTIBODY TN=ONCOTRAC MELANOMA IMAGING KIT	FOR USE IN DETECTING, BY IMAGING, METASTASES OF MALIGNANT MELANOMA.	NEORX CORPORATION 410 WEST HARRISON SEATTLE WA 98119-4007 DD 6/2/1987
TECHNETIUM TC99M MURINE MONOCLONAL ANTIBODY (IGG2A) TO B CELL TN=LYMPHOSCAN	DIAGNOSTIC IMAGING IN THE EVALUATION OF THE EXTENT OF DISEASE IN PATIENTS WITH HISTOLOGI-CALLY CONFIRMED DIAGNOSIS OF NON-HODGKIN'S B-CELL LYMPHOMA, ACUTE B-CELL LYMPHOBLASTIC LEUKEMIA (IN CHILDREN AND ADULTS), AND CHRONIC B-CELL LYMPHOCYTIC LEUKEMIA.	IMMUNOMEDICS, INC. 300 AMERICAN ROAD MORRIS PLAINS NJ 07950 DD 4/7/1992
TECHNETIUM TC99M MURINE MONOCLONAL ANTIBODY TO HCG TN=IMMURAID, HCG-TC-99M	DETECTION OF HCG PRODUCING TUMORS SUCH AS GERM CELL AND TROPHOBLASTIC CELL TUMORS.	IMMUNOMEDICS, INC. 300 AMERICAN ROAD MORRIS PLAINS NJ 07950 DD 8/7/1989
TECHNETIUM TC99M MURINE MONOCLONAL ANTIBODY TO HU-MAN AFP TN=AFP-SCAN	DETECTION OF ALPHA-FETOPROTEIN PRODUCING GERM CELL TUMORS.	IMMUNOMEDICS, INC. 300 AMERICAN ROAD MORRIS PLAINS NJ 07950 DD 8/1/1989
TECHNETIUM TC99M MURINE MONOCLONAL ANTIBODY TO HU-MAN ALPHA-FETOPROTEIN TN=IMMURAID, AFP-SCAN	DETECTION OF HEPATOCELLULAR CARCINOMA AND HEPATOBLASTOMA.	IMMUNOMEDICS, INC. 300 AMERICAN ROAD MORRIS PLAINS NJ 07950 DD 8/1/1989
TECHNETIUM TC99M RH-ANNEX-IN V TN=APOMATE	DIAGNOSIS OR ASSESSMENT OF REJECTION STATUS IN HEART, HEART-LUNG, SINGLE LUNG, OR BILAT-ERAL LUNG TRANSPLANTS.	THESEUS IMAGING CORPORA-TION 124 MOUNT AUBURN STREET SUITE 200 NORTH CAMBRIDGE MA 02138 DD 11/3/2000
TEMOPORFIN TN=FOSCAN	PALLIATIVE TREATMENT OF RECURRENT, REFRAC-TORY OR SECOND PRIMARY SQUAMOUS CELL CAR-CINOMAS OF THE HEAD AND NECK IN PATIENTS CONSIDERED TO BE INCURABLE WITH SURGERY OR RADIOTHERAPY.	SCOTIA PHARMACEUTICALS LTD. SCOTIA HOUSE, CASTLE BUSINESS PARK STIRLING SCOTLAND FK9 4TZ GB DD 10/28/1999
TEMOZOLOMIDE TN=TEMODAR	TREATMENT OF RECURRENT MALIGNANT GLIOMA.	SCHERING-PLOUGH RESEARCH INSTITUTE 2000 GALLOPING HILL RD. KENILWORTH NJ 07033 DD 10/5/1998 MA 8/11/1999
TEMOZOLOMIDE TN=TEMODAL	TREATMENT OF ADVANCED METASTATIC MELANO-MA.	SCHERING-PLOUGH RESEARCH INSTITUTE 2000 GALLOPING HILL RD. KENILWORTH NJ 07033 DD 10/14/1998
TENIPOSIDE TN=VUMON FOR INJECTION	TREATMENT OF REFRACTORY CHILDHOOD ACUTE LYMPHOCYTIC LEUKEMIA.	BRISTOL-MYERS SQUIBB PHARMACEUTICAL RESEARCH INSTITUTE 5 RESEARCH PARKWAY P.O. BOX 5100 WALLINGFORD CT 06492 DD 11/1/1984 MA 7/14/1992

NAME *Generic/Chemical* *TN=Trade Name*	INDICATION DESIGNATED	SPONSOR AND ADDRESS *DD=Date Designated* *MA=Marketing Approval*
TERIPARATIDE TN=PARATHAR	TREATMENT OF IDIOPATHIC OSTEOPOROSIS.	HENRI BEAUFOUR INSTITUTE USA, INC. 27 MAPLE ST. MILFORD MA 01757 DD 10/28/1999
TERIPARATIDE TN=PARATHAR	DIAGNOSTIC AGENT TO ASSIST IN ESTABLISHING THE DIAGNOSIS IN PATIENTS PRESENTING WITH CLINICAL AND LABORATORY EVIDENCE OF HYPO-CALCEMIA DUE TO EITHER HYPOPARATHYROIDISM OR PSEUDOHYPOPARATHYROIDISM.	RHONE-POULENC RORER PHARMACEUTICALS, INC. 500 ARCOLA ROAD COLLEGEVILLE PA 19426 DD 1/9/1987 MA 12/23/1987
TERLIPRESSIN TN=GLYPRESSIN	TREATMENT OF BLEEDING ESOPHAGEAL VARICES.	FERRING LABORATORIES, INC. 400 RELLA BOULEVARD, SUITE 201 SUFFERN NY 10901 DD 3/6/1986
TESTOSTERONE TN=THERADERM TESTOSTER-ONE TRANSDERMAL SYSTEM	FOR USE AS PHYSIOLOGIC TESTOSTERONE REPLA-CEMENT IN ANDROGEN DEFICIENT HIV+ PATIENTS WITH AN ASSOCIATED WEIGHT LOSS.	WATSON LABORATORIES RESEARCH PARK 417 WAKARA WAY SALT LAKE CITY UT 84108 DD 9/22/1997
TESTOSTERONE TN=ANDROGEL	TREATMENT OF WEIGHT LOSS IN AIDS PATIENTS WITH HIV-ASSOCIATED WASTING.	UNIMED PHARMACEUTICALS, INC. FOUR PARKWAY NORTH DEERFIELD IL 60015-2544 DD 2/5/1996
TESTOSTERONE PROPIONATE OINTMENT 2%	TREATMENT OF VULVAR DYSTROPHIES.	STAR PHARMACEUTICALS, INC. 1990 N.W. 44TH STREET POMPANO BEACH FL 33064 DD 7/31/1991
TESTOSTERONE SUBLINGUAL	TREATMENT OF CONSTITUTIONAL DELAY OF GROWTH AND PUBERTY IN BOYS.	BIO-TECHNOLOGY GENERAL CORP. 70 WOOD AVENUE SOUTH ISELIN NJ 08830 DD 1/16/1991
TETRABENAZINE	TREATMENT OF HUNTINGTON'S DISEASE.	LIFEHEALTH LIMITED 23 WINKFIELD ROADDOLTIC HOUSE KINGFISHER WA WINDOR, BERKSHIRE SL4 4BA UK DD 12/11/1997
TETRABENAZINE	TREATMENT OF MODERATE/SEVERE TARDIVE DYSKI-NESIA.	LIFEHEALTH LIMITED 23 WINKFIELD ROAD WINDSOR, BERKSHIRE SL4 4BA UK DD 5/12/1998
TETRAIODOTHYROACETIC ACID	SUPPRESSION OF THYROID STIMULATING HORMONE IN PATIENTS WITH WELL-DIFFERENTIATED CANCER OF THE THYROID GLAND.	DANFORTH, JR., MD, ELLIOT UNIVERSITY OF VERMONT 84 BEARTOWN RD. UNDERHILL VT 05489 DD 5/1/2000
TEZACITABINE	TREATMENT OF ADENOCARCINOMA OF THE ESO-PHAGUS AND STOMACH	CHIRON CORPORATION 4560 HORTON STREET EMERYVILLE CA 94608-2916 DD 1/27/2003

NAME Generic/Chemical TN=Trade Name	INDICATION DESIGNATED	SPONSOR AND ADDRESS DD=Date Designated MA=Marketing Approval
THALIDOMIDE TN=THALOMID	TREATMENT OF MULTIPLE MYELOMA.	CELGENE CORPORATION 7 POWDER HORN DR. WARREN NJ 07059 DD 10/14/1998
THALIDOMIDE	TREATMENT AND PREVENTION OF RECURRENT APHTHOUS ULCERS IN SEVERELY, TERMINALLY IMMUNOCOMPROMISED PATIENTS.	ANDRULIS RESEARCH CORPORATION 11800 BALTIMORE AVENUE, SUITE 113 BELTSVILLE MD 20705 DD 5/15/1995
THALIDOMIDE TN=THALOMID	TREATMENT OF CROHN'S DISEASE.	CELGENE CORPORATION 7 POWDER HORN DR. WARREN NJ 07059 DD 4/6/1999
THALIDOMIDE	TREATMENT AND MAINTENANCE OF REACTIONAL LEPROMATOUS LEPROSY.	PEDIATRIC PHARMACEUTICALS, INC. 718 BRADFORD AVENUE WESTFIELD NJ 07090 DD 11/15/1988
THALIDOMIDE	TREATMENT OF GRAFT VERSUS HOST DISEASE.	ANDRULIS RESEARCH CORPORATION 11800 BALTIMORE AVENUE, SUITE 113 BELTSVILLE MD 20705 DD 3/5/1990
THALIDOMIDE	TREATMENT OF KAPOSI'S SARCOMA.	CELGENE CORPORATION 7 POWDER HORN DR. WARREN NJ 07059 DD 7/29/1998
THALIDOMIDE	TREATMENT OF PRIMARY BRAIN MALIGNANCIES.	CELGENE CORPORATION 7 POWDER HORN DR. WARREN NJ 07059 DD 2/27/1998
THALIDOMIDE	PREVENTION OF GRAFT VERSUS HOST DISEASE.	ANDRULIS RESEARCH CORPORATION 11800 BALTIMORE AVENUE, SUITE 113 BELTSVILLE MD 20705 DD 3/5/1990
THALIDOMIDE	TREATMENT OF GRAFT VERSUS HOST DISEASE IN PATIENTS RECEIVING BONE MARROW TRANSPLANTATION.	PEDIATRIC PHARMACEUTICALS, INC. 718 BRADFORD AVENUE WESTFIELD NJ 07090 DD 9/19/1988
THALIDOMIDE TN=THALOMID	TREATMENT OF ERYTHEMA NODOSUM LEPROSUM.	CELGENE CORPORATION P.O. BOX 4914 7 POWDER HORN DRIVE WARREN NJ 07059 DD 7/26/1995 MA 7/16/1998
THALIDOMIDE	TREATMENT OF SEVERE RECURRENT APHTHOUS STOMATITIS IN SEVERELY, TERMINALLY IMMUNOCOMPROMISED PATIENTS.	CELGENE CORPORATION P.O. BOX 4914 7 POWDER HORN SRIVE WARREN NJ 07059 DD 5/1/1995

NAME *Generic/Chemical* *TN=Trade Name*	INDICATION DESIGNATED	SPONSOR AND ADDRESS *DD=Date Designated* *MA=Marketing Approval*
THALIDOMIDE TN=SYNOVIR	TREATMENT OF HIV-ASSOCIATED WASTING SYNDROME.	CELGENE CORPORATION P.O. BOX 4914 7 POWDER HORN DRIVE WARREN NJ 07059 DD 3/11/1996
THALIDOMIDE	TREATMENT OF THE CLINICAL MANIFESTATIONS OF MYCOBACTERIAL INFECTION CAUSED BY MYCOBACTERIUM TUBERCULOSIS AND NON-TUBERCULOUS MYCOBACTERIA.	CELGENE CORPORATION P.O. BOX 4914 7 POWDER HORN DRIVE WARREN NJ 07059 DD 1/12/1993
THALIDOMIDE	PREVENTION OF GRAFT VERSUS HOST DISEASE IN PATIENTS RECEIVING BONE MARROW TRANSPLANTATION.	PEDIATRIC PHARMACEUTICALS, INC. 718 BRADFORD AVENUE WESTFIELD NJ 07090 DD 9/19/1988
THYMALFASIN TN=ZADAXIN	TREATMENT OF HEPATOCELLULAR CARCINOMA.	SCICLONE PHARMACEUTICALS, INC. 901 MARINER'S BLVD., SUITE 205 SAN MATEO CA 94404 DD 3/6/2000
THYMALFASIN TN=ZADAXIN	TREATMENT OF CHRONIC ACTIVE HEPATITIS B.	SCICLONE PHARMACEUTICALS, INC. 901 MARINER'S ISLAND BLVD. SAN MATEO CA 94404-1593 DD 5/3/1991
THYMALFASIN TN=ZADAXIN	TREATMENT OF DIGEORGE ANOMALY WITH IMMUNE DEFECTS.	SCICLONE PHARMACEUTICALS, INC. 901 MARINER'S ISLAND BLVD. SAN MATEO CA 94404-1593 DD 1/8/1998
THYMOXAMINE HCL	REVERSAL OF PHENYLEPHRINE-INDUCED MYDRIASIS IN PATIENTS WHO HAVE NARROW ANTERIOR ANGLES AND ARE AT RISK OF DEVELOPING AN ACUTE ATTACK OF ANGLE-CLOSURE GLAUCOMA FOLLOWING MYDRIASIS.	IOLAB PHARMACEUTICALS 500 IOLAB DRIVE CLAREMONT CA 91711 DD 11/16/1987
THYROTROPIN ALFA TN=THYROGEN	TREATMENT OF WELL-DIFFERENTIATED PAPILLARY, FOLLICULAR OR COMBINED PAPILLARY/FOLLICULAR CARCINOMAS OF THE THYROID	GENZYME CORPORATION ONE KENDALL SQUARE CAMBRIDGE MA 02139-1562 DD 8/3/2001
THYROTROPIN ALPHA TN=THYROGEN	AS AN ADJUNCT IN THE DIAGNOSIS OF THYROID CANCER.	GENZYME CORPORATION ONE KENDALL SQUARE CAMBRIDGE MA 02139 DD 2/24/1992 MA 11/30/1998
TIAPRIDE	TREATMENT OF TOURETTE'S SYNDROME.	SANOFI-SYNTHELABO, INC. 9 GREAT VALLEY PARKWAY PO BOX 3026 MALVERN PA 19355 DD 4/21/1998
TIAZOFURIN (2-BETA-D-RIBO-FURANOSYL-4-THIAZOLECARBOXAMIDE)	CHRONIC MYELOGENOUS LEUKEMIA (CML)	RIBAPHARM 3300 HYLAND AVENUE COSTA MESA CA 92626 DD 12/27/2000

NAME *Generic/Chemical* *TN=Trade Name*	INDICATION DESIGNATED	SPONSOR AND ADDRESS *DD=Date Designated* *MA=Marketing Approval*
TIOPRONIN TN=THIOLA	PREVENTION OF CYSTINE NEPHROLITHIASIS IN PATIENTS WITH HOMOZYGOUS CYSTINURIA.	PAK, CHARLES Y.C. M.D. THE UNIVERSITY OF TEXAS HEALTH SCIENC CENTER AT DALLAS 5323 HARRY HINES BOULEVARD DALLAS TX 75235 DD 1/17/1986 MA 8/11/1988
TIRATRICOL TN=TRIACANA	FOR USE IN COMBINATION WITH LEVO-THYROXINE TO SUPPRESS THYROID STIMULATING HORMONE IN PATIENTS WITH WELL-DIFFERENTIATED THYROID CANCER WHO ARE INTOLERANT TO ADEQUATE DOSES OF LEVO-THYROXINE ALONE.	LAPHAL LABORATOIRES 48 BIS, RUE DES BELLES-FEUILLES 75116 PARIS FRANCE FR DD 8/13/1991
TIZANIDINE HCL TN=ZANAFLEX	TREATMENT OF SPASTICITY ASSOCIATED WITH MULTIPLE SCLEROSIS AND SPINAL CORD INJURY.	ATHENA NEUROSCIENCES, INC. 800 GATEWAY BOULEVARD SOUTH SAN FRANCISCO CA 94080 DD 1/31/1994
TOBRAMYCIN TN=TOBI	TREATMENT OF BRONCHIECTASIS PATIENTS INFECTED WITH PSEUDOMONAS AERUGINOSA.	CHIRON CORPORATION 201 ELLIOTT AVENUE WEST SUITE 150 SEATTLE WA 98119 DD 6/18/1999
TOBRAMYCIN FOR INHALATION TN=TOBI	TREATMENT OF BRONCHOPULMONARY INFECTIONS OF PSEUDOMONAS AERUGINOSA IN CYSTIC FIBROSIS PATIENTS.	PATHOGENESIS CORPORATION 201 ELLIOTT AVENUE WEST, SUITE 150 SEATTLE WA 98119 DD 10/13/1994 MA 12/22/1997
TOCOPHERSOLAN ORAL SOLUTION (VITAMIN E-TPGS)	TREATMENT OF VITAMIN E DEFICIENCY RESULTING FROM MALABSORPTION DUE TO PROLONGED CHOLESTATIC HEPATOBILIARY DISEASE.	STERLING WINTHROP 9 GREAT VALLEY PARKWAY MALVERN PA 19355 DD 4/15/1988
TOPIRAMATE TN=TOPAMAX	TREATMENT OF LENNOX-GASTAUT SYNDROME.	R. W. JOHNSON PHARMACEUTICAL RESEARCH INSTITUTE ROUTE 202, P.O. BOX 300 RARITAN NJ 08869-0602 DD 11/25/1992 MA 8/28/2001
TOREMIFENE	TREATMENT OF DESMOID TUMORS.	ORION CORPORATION P.O. BOX 65 02101 ESPOO FINLAND DD 8/17/1993
TOREMIFENE TN=FARESTON	HORMONAL THERAPY OF METASTATIC CARCINOMA OF THE BREAST.	ORION CORPORATION P.O. BOX 65 02101 ESPOO FINLAND DD 9/19/1991 MA 5/29/1997
TOSITUMOMAB AND IODINE I 131 TOSITUMOMAB TN=BEXXAR	TREATMENT OF NON-HODGKIN'S B-CELL LYMPHOMA.	COULTER PHARMACEUTICAL, INC. 550 CALIFORNIA AVENUE SUITE 200 PALO ALTO CA 94306 DD 5/16/1994

NAME *Generic/Chemical* *TN=Trade Name*	INDICATION DESIGNATED	SPONSOR AND ADDRESS *DD=Date Designated* *MA=Marketing Approval*
TRANEXAMIC ACID TN=CYKLOKAPRON	TREATMENT OF PATIENTS WITH CONGENITAL COAGULOPATHIES WHO ARE UNDERGOING SURGICAL PROCEDURES (E.G. DENTAL EXTRACTIONS).	PHARMACIA INC. P.O. BOX 16529 COLUMBUS OH 43216 DD 10/29/1985 MA 12/30/1986
TRANEXAMIC ACID TN=CYKLOKAPRON	TREATMENT OF HEREDITARY ANGIONEUROTIC EDEMA.	PHARMACIA INC. P.O. BOX 16529 COLUMBUS OH 43216 DD 9/9/1985
TRANEXAMIC ACID TN=CYKLOKAPRON	TREATMENT OF PATIENTS UNDERGOING PROSTATECTOMY WHERE THERE IS HEMORRHAGE OR RISK OF HEMORRHAGE AS A RESULT OF INCREASED FIBRINOLYSIS OR FIBRINOGENOLYSIS.	PHARMACIA INC. P.O. BOX 16529 COLUMBUS OH 43216 DD 7/23/1987
TRANSFORMING GROWTH FACTOR-BETA 2	TREATMENT OF FULL THICKNESS MACULAR HOLES.	CELTRIX PHARMACEUTICALS, INC. 3055 PATRICK HENRY DRIVE SANTA CLARA CA 95054 DD 12/18/1992
TRANSGENIC HUMAN ALPHA 1 ANTITRYPSIN	TREATMENT OF EMPHYSEMA SECONDARY TO ALPHA 1 ANTITRYPSIN DEFICIENCY.	PPL THERAPEUTICS (SCOTLAND) LIMITED ROSLIN, EDINBURGH EH25 9PP SCOTLAND GB DD 5/19/1999
TRASTUZUMAB TN=HERCEPTIN	TREATMENT OF PATIENTS WITH PANCREATIC CANCER THAT OVEREXPRESS P185HER2.	GENENTECH, INC. 1 DNA WAY SOUTH SAN FRANCISCO CA 94080-4990 DD 12/14/1999
TREOSULFAN TN=OVASTAT	TREATMENT OF OVARIAN CANCER.	MEDAC GMBH FEHLANDTSTRASSE 3 D-20354 HAMBURG GERMANY DE DD 5/16/1994
TRETINOIN	TREATMENT OF SQUAMOUS METAPLASIA OF THE OCULAR SURFACE EPITHELIA (CONJUNCTIVA AND/OR CORNEA) WITH MUCOUS DEFICIENCY AND KERATINIZATION.	HANNAN OPHTHALMIC MARKETING SERVICES, INC 34 SHERRILL RD. MARSHFIELD MA 02050 DD 4/15/1985
TRETINOIN TN=VESANOID	TREATMENT OF ACUTE PROMYELOCYTIC LEUKEMIA.	HOFFMANN-LA ROCHE, INC. 340 KINGSLAND STREET NUTLEY NJ 07110 DD 10/24/1990 MA 11/22/1995
TRETINOIN TN=ATRA-IV	TREATMENT OF T-CELL NON-HODGKIN'S LYMPHOMA.	ANTIGENICS, INC. 34 COMMERCE WAY WOBURN MA 01801 DD 4/11/2003
TRETINOIN TN=ATRA-IV	TREATMENT OF ACUTE AND CHRONIC LEUKEMIA.	ANTIGENICS, INC. 34 COMMERCE WAY WOBURN MA 01801 DD 1/14/1993

NAME *Generic/Chemical* *TN=Trade Name*	INDICATION DESIGNATED	SPONSOR AND ADDRESS *DD=Date Designated* *MA=Marketing Approval*
TRIENTINE HCL TN=SYPRINE	TREATMENT OF PATIENTS WITH WILSON'S DISEASE WHO ARE INTOLERANT, OR INADEQUATELY RESPONSIVE TO PENICILLAMINE.	MERCK SHARP & DOHME RESEARCH DIVISION OF MERCK AND COMPANY WEST POINT PA 19486 DD 12/24/1984 MA 11/8/1985
TRIMETREXATE TN=NEUTREXIN	TREATMENT OF METASTATIC OSTEOGENIC SARCOMA.	MEDIMMUNE ONCOLOGY, INC. ONE TOWER BRIDGE 100 FRONT ST., SUITE 400 WEST CONSHOHOCKEN PA 19428 DD 8/10/2000
TRIMETREXATE GLUCURONATE	TREATMENT OF METASTATIC CARCINOMA OF THE HEAD AND NECK (I.E. BUCCAL CAVITY, PHARYNX, AND LARYNX).	MEDIMMUNE ONCOLOGY, INC. 35 WEST WATKINS MILLS ROAD GAITHERSBURG MD 20878 DD 7/25/1985
TRIMETREXATE GLUCURONATE TN=NEUTREXIN	TREATMENT OF PNEUMOCYSTIS CARINII PNEUMONIA IN AIDS PATIENTS.	MEDIMMUNE ONCOLOGY, INC. ONE TOWER BRIDGE 100 FRONT STREET, SUITE 400 WEST CONSHOHOCKEN PA 19428 DD 5/15/1986 MA 12/17/1993
TRIMETREXATE GLUCURONATE	TREATMENT OF METASTATIC COLORECTAL ADENOCARCINOMA.	MEDIMMUNE ONCOLOGY, INC. ONE TOWER BRIDGE 100 FRONT STREET, SUITE 400 WEST CONSHOHOCKEN PA 19428 DD 7/25/1985
TRIMETREXATE GLUCURONATE	TREATMENT OF PANCREATIC ADENOCARCINOMA.	MEDIMMUNE ONCOLOGY, INC. ONE TOWER BRIDGE 100 FRONT STREET, SUITE 400 WEST CONSHOHOCKEN PA 19428 DD 7/25/1985
TRIMETREXATE GLUCURONATE	TREATMENT OF PATIENTS WITH ADVANCED NON-SMALL CELL CARCINOMA OF THE LUNG.	MEDIMMUNE ONCOLOGY, INC. ONE TOWER BRIDGE 100 FRONT STREET, SUITE 400 WEST CONSHOHOCKEN PA 19428 DD 1/13/1988
TRIPTORELIN PAMOATE TN=DECAPEPTYL INJECTION	FOR USE IN THE PALLIATIVE TREATMENT OF ADVANCED OVARIAN CARCINOMA OF EPITHELIAL ORIGIN.	DEBIO R.A. INC. 7929 WESTPARK DRIVE, SUITE 400 MCLEAN VA 22102 DD 8/10/1990
TRISACCHARIDES A AND B TN=BIOSYNJECT	FOR USE IN ABO-INCOMPATIBLE SOLID ORGAN TRANSPLANTATION, INCLUDING KIDNEY, HEART, LIVER AND PANCREAS.	CHEMBIOMED, LTD. P.O. BOX 8050, STATION F EDMONTON, ALBERTA CANADA T6H 4NP CA DD 4/20/1987
TRISACCHARIDES A AND B TN=BIOSYNJECT	PREVENTION OF ABO MEDICAL HEMOLYTIC REACTIONS ARISING FROM ABO-INCOMPATIBLE BONE MARROW TRANSPLANTATION.	CHEMBIOMED, LTD. P.O. BOX 8050, STATION F EDMONTON, ALBERTA CANADA T6H 4NP CA DD 4/15/1988

NAME *Generic/Chemical* *TN=Trade Name*	INDICATION DESIGNATED	SPONSOR AND ADDRESS *DD=Date Designated* *MA=Marketing Approval*
TRISACCHARIDES A AND B TN=BIOSYNJECT	TREATMENT OF MODERATE TO SEVERE CLINICAL FORMS OF HEMOLYTIC DISEASE OF THE NEWBORN ARISING FROM PLACENTAL TRANSFER OF ANTIBODIES AGAINST BLOOD GROUP SUBSTANCES A AND B.	CHEMBIOMED, LTD. P.O. BOX 8050, STATION F EDMONTON, ALBERTA CANADA T6H 4NP CA DD 4/12/1987
TRISACCHARIDES A AND B	TREATMENT OF MODERATE TO VERY SEVERE CLINICAL FORMS OF TRANSFUSION REACTIONS ARISING FROM ABO INCOMPATIBLE TRANSFUSIONS OF BLOOD, BLOOD PRODUCTS, AND BLOOD DERIVATIVES.	CHEMBIOMED, LTD. P.O. BOX 8050, EDMONTON, ALBERTA CA DD 8/3/1987
TRISODIUM CITRATE CONCENTRATION TN=HEMOCITRATE	FOR USE IN LEUKAPHERESIS PROCEDURES.	HEMOTEC MEDICAL PRODUCTS, INC. BOX 19255 JOHNSTON RI 02919 DD 6/15/1995
TROLEANDOMYCIN	TREATMENT OF SEVERE STEROID-REQUIRING ASTHMA.	SZEFLER, STANLEY M. M.D. NATIONAL JEWISH CENTER FOR IMMUNOLOGY AND RESPIRATORY MEDICINE 1400 JACKSON STREET DENVER CO 80206 DD 9/21/1989
TUMOR NECROSIS FACTOR-BINDING PROTEIN 1	TREATMENT OF SYMPTOMATIC PATIENTS WITH AIDS INCLUDING ALL PATIENTS WITH CD4 COUNTS LESS THAN 200 CELLS PER MM3.	SERONO LABORATORIES, INC. 100 LONGWATER CIRCLE NORWELL MA 02061 DD 1/6/1993
TUMOR NECROSIS FACTOR-BINDING PROTEIN II	TREATMENT OF SYMPTOMATIC PATIENTS WITH THE AIDS INCLUDING ALL PATIENTS WITH CD4 T-CELL COUNTS LESS THAN 200 CELLS PER MM3.	SERONO LABORATORIES, INC. 100 LONGWATER CIRCLE NORWELL MA 02061 DD 1/6/1993
TYLOXAPOL TN=SUPERVENT	TREATMENT OF CYSTIC FIBROSIS.	KENNEDY & HOIDAL, M.D.'S UNIVERSITY OF UTAH HEALTH SCIENCES CENTER 50 NORTH MEDICAL DRIVE, ROOM 4R240 SALT LAKE CITY UT 84132-0001 DD 3/8/1995
UBIQUINONE TN=UBIQGEL	TREATMENT OF MITOCHONDRIAL CYTOPATHIES.	GEL-TEC, DIVISION OF TISHCON CORP. 30 NEW YORK AVE. PO BOX 331 WESTBURY NY 11590 DD 12/14/1999
UNCONJUGATED CHIMERIC (HUMAN-MURINE) G250 IGG MONOCLONAL ANTIBODY	TREATMENT OF RENAL CELL CARCINOMA.	WILEX BIOTECHNOLOGY GMBH GRILLPARZERSTRASSE 10B 81675 MUNICH GERMANY DE DD 3/22/2001
URIDINE 5'-TRIPHOSPHATE	TO FACILITATE THE REMOVAL OF LUNG SECRETIONS IN THE TREATMENT OF PATIENTS WITH PRIMARY CILIARY DYSKINESIA.	INSPIRE PHARMACEUTICALS, INC. 4222 EMPEROR BOULEVARD, SUITE 470 DURHAM NC 27703 DD 6/26/1996

NAME *Generic/Chemical* *TN=Trade Name*	INDICATION DESIGNATED	SPONSOR AND ADDRESS *DD=Date Designated* *MA=Marketing Approval*
URIDINE 5'-TRIPHOSPHATE	TREATMENT OF CYSTIC FIBROSIS.	INSPIRE PHARMACEUTICALS, INC. 4222 EMPEROR BOULEVARD, SUITE 470 DURHAM NC 27703 DD 12/4/1995
UROFOLLITROPIN TN=METRODIN	FOR INDUCTION OF OVULATION IN PATIENTS WITH POLYCYSTIC OVARIAN DISEASE WHO HAVE AN ELEVATED LH/FSH RATIO AND WHO HAVE FAILED TO RESPOND TO ADEQUATE CLOMIPHENE CITRATE THERAPY.	SERONO LABORATORIES, INC. 100 LONGWATER CIRCLE NORWELL MA 02061 DD 11/25/1987 MA 9/18/1986
UROFOLLITROPIN TN=FERTINEX	FOR THE INITIATION AND RE-INITIATION OF SPERMATOGENESIS IN ADULT MALES WITH REPRODUCTIVE FAILURE DUE TO HYPOTHALAMIC OR PITUITARY DYSFUNCTION, HYPOGONADOTROPIC HYPOGONADISM.	SERONO LABORATORIES, INC. 100 LONGWATER CIRCLE NORWELL MA 02061 DD 12/5/1997
UROGASTRONE	FOR ACCELERATION OF CORNEAL EPITHELIAL REGENERATION AND HEALING OF STROMAL INCISIONS FROM CORNEAL TRANSPLANT SURGERY.	CHIRON VISION 500 IOLAB DRIVE CLAREMONT CA 91711 DD 11/1/1984
URSODIOL TN=URSO	TREATMENT OF PATIENTS WITH PRIMARY BILIARY CIRRHOSIS.	AXCAN PHARMA INC. 597 LAURIER BLVD MOUNT ST. HILAIRE QUEBEC H7L 4S3 CANADA CA DD 6/20/1991 MA 12/10/1997
URSODIOL TN=ACTIGALL	MANAGEMENT OF THE CLINICAL SIGNS AND SYMPTOMS ASSOCIATED WITH PRIMARY BILIARY CIRRHOSIS.	NOVARTIS PHARMACEUTICALS CORPORATION 59 ROUTE 10 EAST HANOVER NJ 07936-1080 DD 2/19/1991
VALINE, ISOLEUCINE AND LEUCINE TN=VIL	TREATMENT OF HYPERPHENYLALANINEMIA.	LEAS RESEARCH PRODUCTS 78 FALLON DRIVE NORTH HAVEN CT 06473 DD 1/5/1996
VALRUBICIN TN=VALSTAR	TREATMENT OF CARCINOMA IN SITU OF THE URINARY BLADDER.	ANTHRA PHARMACEUTICALS, INC. 103 CARNEGIE CENTER, SUITE 102 PRINCETON NJ 08540 DD 5/23/1994 MA 9/25/1998
VAPREOTIDE TN=OCTASTATIN	TREATMENT OF GASTROINTESTINAL AND PANCREATIC FISTULAS.	DEBIOPHARM S.A. 17 RUE DES TERREAUX CH-1000 LAUSANNE 9 SWITZERLAND CH DD 1/10/2000
VAPREOTIDE TN=OCTASTATIN	PREVENTION OF EARLY POSTOPERATIVE COMPLICATIONS FOLLOWING PANCREATIC RESECTION.	DEBIOPHARM S.A. 17 RUE DES TERREAUX CH-1000 LAUSANNE 9 SWITZERLAND CH DD 3/6/2000
VAPREOTIDE TN=OCTASTATIN	TREATMENT OF ESOPHAGEAL VARICEAL HEMORRHAGE PATIENTS WITH PORTAL HYPERTENSION.	DEBIOPHARM S.A. 17 RUE DES TERREAUX CH-1000 LAUSANNE 9 SWITZERLAND CH DD 1/10/2000

NAME *Generic/Chemical* *TN=Trade Name*	INDICATION DESIGNATED	SPONSOR AND ADDRESS *DD=Date Designated* *MA=Marketing Approval*
VASOACTIVE INTESTINAL PEP-TIDE	TREATMENT OF ACUTE RESPIRATORY DISTRESS SYNDROME.	SAMI I. SAID, M.D. STATE UNIVERSITY OF NEW YORK AT STONY BROOKHEALTH SCIENCES CENTER T17, 040 HEALTH SCIENCES CENTER T17, 040 STONY BROOK NY 11794-8172 DD 3/9/2001
VASOACTIVE INTESTINAL POLY-PEPTIDE	TREATMENT OF ACUTE ESOPHAGEAL FOOD IMPAC-TION.	RESEARCH TRIANGLE PHARMACEUTICALS 200 WESTPARK CORPORATE CENTER 4364 SOUTH ALSTON AVENUE DURHAM NC 27713-2280 DD 6/23/1993
VILOXAZINE HCL TN=CATATROL	TREATMENT OF CATAPLEXY.	STUART PHARMACEUTICALS DIVISION OF ICI AMERICAS WILMINGTON DE 19897 DD 6/11/1984
VILOXAZINE HCL TN=CATATROL	TREATMENT OF NARCOLEPSY.	STUART PHARMACEUTICALS DIVISION OF ICI AMERICAS WILMINGTON DE 19897 DD 6/11/1984
VIRULIZIN TN=VIRULIZIN	TREATMENT OF PANCREATIC CANCER.	LORUS THERAPEUTICS INC. 7100 WOODBINE AVENUE, SUITE 215 MARKHAM, ON L3R 5J2 CANADA DD 2/1/2001
XENOGENEIC HEPATOCYTES TN=HEPATASSIST LIVER ASSIST SYSTEM	TREATMENT OF SEVERE LIVER FAILURE.	CIRCE BIOMEDICAL, INC. 99 HAYDEN AVE. LEXINGTON MA 02421-7995 DD 11/27/1998
YTTRIUM-90 RADIOLABELED HU-MANIZED MONOCLONAL ANTI-CARCINOEMBROYONIC ANTIGEN IGG ANTIBODY TN=CEA-CIDE	TREATMENT OF OVARIAN CARCINOMA.	IMMUNOMEDICS, INC. 300 AMERICAN RD. MORRIS PLAINS NJ 07950 DD 8/3/1999
ZALCITABINE	TREATMENT OF AIDS.	NATIONAL CANCER INSTITUTE, DCT NIH, EXECUTIVE PLAZA NORTH, ROOM 7-18 BETHESDA MD 20892 DD 12/9/1986
ZALCITABINE TN=HIVID	TREATMENT OF AIDS.	HOFFMANN-LA ROCHE, INC. 340 KINGSLAND STREET NUTLEY NJ 07110 DD 6/28/1988 MA 6/19/1992
ZIDOVUDINE TN=RETROVIR	TREATMENT OF AIDS.	GLAXO WELLCOME INC. 5 MOORE DRIVE RESEARCH TRIANGLE PARK NC 27709 DD 7/17/1985 MA 3/19/1987

NAME *Generic/Chemical* *TN=Trade Name*	INDICATION DESIGNATED	SPONSOR AND ADDRESS *DD=Date Designated* *MA=Marketing Approval*
ZIDOVUDINE TN=RETROVIR	TREATMENT OF AIDS RELATED COMPLEX.	GLAXO WELLCOME INC. 5 MOORE DRIVE RESEARCH TRIANGLE PARK NC 27709 DD 5/12/1987 MA 3/19/1987
ZINC ACETATE TN=GALZIN	TREATMENT OF WILSON'S DISEASE.	LEMMON COMPANY 1510 DELP DRIVE KULPSVILLE PA 19443 DD 11/6/1985 MA 1/28/1997
ZOLEDRONATE TN=ZOMETA, ZABEL	TREATMENT OF TUMOR INDUCED HYPERCALCEMIA.	NOVARTIS PHARMACEUTICALS CORP. 59 ROUTE 10 EAST HANOVER NJ 07936-1080 DD 8/18/2000 MA 8/20/2001
A-(3-AMINOPHTHALIMIDO) GLU-TARAMIDE TN=ACTIMID	TREATMENT OF MULTIPLE MYELOMA	CELGENE CORPORATION 7 POWDER HORN DRIVE WARREN NJ 07059 DD 1/15/2003
A-GALACTOSIDASE A TN=PLANT-PRODUCED HUMAN A-GLACTOSIDASE A	TREATMENT OF FABRY'S DISEASE	LARGE SCALE BIOLOGY COR-PORATION 3333 VACAVILLE PARKWAY SUITE 1000 VACAVILLE CA 95688 DD 1/21/2003
ACETYLCYSTEINE TN=ACETADOTE	FOR THE INTRAVENOUS TREATMENT OF MODERATE TO SEVERE ACETAMINOPHEN OVERDOSE	LIGAND 209 10TH STREET SOUTH SUITE 332 NASHVILLE TN 37203 DD 10/19/2001
ADENOVIRUS-MEDIATED HERPES SIMPLEX VIRUS-THYMI-DINE KINASE GENE	USE WITH GANCYCLOVIR IN THE TREATMENT OF MA-LIGNANT GLIOMA	ARK THERAPEUTICS LTD 6 WARREN MEWS LONDON W1T6AR UK DD 7/31/2001
ALBUTEROL	PREVENTION OF PARALYSIS DUE TO SPINAL CORD INJURY	MOTOGEN, INC. 3 PINE VIEW ROAD MOUNT KISCO NY 10549 DD 3/12/2002
ALEMTUZUMAB TN=CAMPATH	TREATMENT OF CHRONIC LYMPHOCYTIC LEUKEMIA.	MILLENNIUM AND ILEX PART-NERS, LP 75 SIDNEY STREET CAMBRIDGE MA 02138 DD 10/20/1997 MA 5/7/2001
ALENDRONATE TN=FOSAMAX	TREATMENT OF OSTEOGENESIS IMPERFECTA IN PE-DIATRIC PATIENTS 4 YEARS OF AGE AND OLDER	MERCK & CO., INC. 126 EAST LINCOLN AVE. RAHWAY NJ 07065-0900 DD 3/31/2003
ALLANTOIN TN=ALWEXTIN	TREATMENT OF SKIN BLISTERING AND EROSIONS AS-SOCIATED WITH INHERITED EPIDERMOLYSIS BULLO-SA	ALWYN COMPANY, INC. 2301 HIGHWAY 60 EAST LAKE CRYSTAL MN 56055 DD 11/21/2002

NAME *Generic/Chemical* *TN=Trade Name*	INDICATION DESIGNATED	SPONSOR AND ADDRESS *DD=Date Designated* *MA=Marketing Approval*
ALTEPLASE TN=ACTIVASE	TREATMENT OF INTRAVENTRICULAR HEMMORAGE ASSOCIATED WITH INTRACEREBRAL HEMMOR-RHAGE	DANIEL F. HANLEY, MD JOHNS HOPKINS UNIVERSITY 600 N. WOLFE ST., JEFFERSON 1-109 BALTIMORE MD 21287 DD 1/27/2003
ANTI-CD23 IGG1, KAPPA MONO-CLONAL ANTIBODY	TREATMENT OF CHRONIC LYMPHOCYTIC LEUKEMIA	IDEC PHARMACEUTICALS, INC. 3030 CALLAN ROAD SAN DIEGO CA 92121 DD 2/12/2003
ANTIANGIOGENIC COMPONENTS EXTRACTED FROM MARINE CAR-TILAGE TN=NEOVASTAT (AE-941)	TREATMENT OF RENAL CELL CARCINOMA	AETERNA LABORATORIES, INC. DR. CLAUDE HARITON, CHIEF MEDICAL OFFICER, VP, CLINICAL & REGULATORY AFFAIRS 1405 BOUL. DU PARC - TECHNO-LOGIQUE QUEBEC G1P 4P5 CANADA DD 10/16/2002
ARSENIC TN=TRISENOX	TREATMENT OF ACUTE MYELOCYTIC LEUKEMIA SUB-TYPES M0, M1, M2, M4, M5, M6 AND M7	CELL THERAPEUTICS, INC. 201 ELLIOTT AVENUE WEST SUITE 400 SEATTLE WA 98119 DD 11/2/2001
ARSENIC TRIOXIDE TN=TRISENOX	TREATMENT OF CHRONIC MYELOID LEUKEMIA	CELL THERAPEUTICS, INC. 201 ELLIOTT AVENUE WEST SUITE 400 SEATTLE WA 98119 DD 10/18/2001
ARSENIC TRIOXIDE TN=TRISENOX	TREATMENT OF MYELODYSPLASTIC SYNDROME.	CELL THERAPEUTICS, INC. 201 ELLIOTT AVENUE WEST SUITE 400 SEATTLE WA 98119 DD 7/17/2000
AUGMEROSEN TN=GENASENSE	TREATMENT OF CHRONIC LYMPHOCYTIC LEUKEMIA	GENTA INCORPORATED TWO OAK WAY BERKELEY HEIGHTS NJ 07922 DD 8/28/2001
AUGMEROSEN TN=GENASENSE	TREATMENT OF MULTIPLE MYELOMA	GENTA INCORPORATED TWO OAK WAY BERKELEY HEIGHTS NJ 07922 DD 8/28/2001
AUGMEROSEN TN=GENASENSE	TREATMENT OF ACUTE MYELOCYTIC LEUKEMIA	GENTA INCORPORATED TWO OAK WAY BERKELEY HEIGHTS NJ 07922 DD 8/28/2001
AUTOLOGOUS ANTIGEN PRE-SENTING CELLS PULSED WITH AUTOLOGOUS TUMOR IG IDIO-TYPE TN=MYLOVENGE	TREATMENT OF MULTIPLE MYELOMA	DENDREON CORPORATION 3005 FIRST AVENUE SEATTLE WA 98121 DD 4/18/2002
AUTOLOGOUS TUMOR-DERIVED GP96 HEAT SHOCK PROTEIN-PEPTIDE COMPLEX TN=ONCOPHAGE	TREATMENT OF METASTATIC MELANOMA	ANTIGENICS, INC. 34 COMMERCE WAY WOBURN MA 01702 DD 7/11/2002

NAME *Generic/Chemical* *TN=Trade Name*	INDICATION DESIGNATED	SPONSOR AND ADDRESS *DD=Date Designated* *MA=Marketing Approval*
AUTOLOGOUS TUMOR-DERIVED GP96 HEAT SHOCK PROTEIN-PEPTIDE COMPLEX TN=ONCOPHAGE	TREATMENT OF RENAL CELL CARCINOMA	ANTIGENICS, INC. 34 COMMERCE WAY WOBURN MA 01702 DD 5/10/2002
AZACITIDINE	TREATAMENT OF MYELODYSPLASTIC SYNDROMES	PHARMION CORPORATION 4865 RIVERBEND ROAD BOULDER CO 80301 DD 12/3/2001
AZTREONAM	INHALATION THERAPY FOR CONTROL OF GRAM-NEGATIVE BACTERIA IN THE RESPIRATORY TRACT OF PATIENTS WITH CYSTIC FIBROSIS	CORUS PHARMA 2025 FIRST AVE., SUITE 800 SEATTLE WA 98121 DD 3/12/2002
BECLOMETHASONE 17,21-DI-PROPIONATE	PREVENTION OF GASTROINTESTINAL GRAFT-VERSUS-HOST DISEASE	ENTERON PHARMACEUTICALS, INC. 1680 MICHIGAN AVE. SUITE 700 MIAMI FL 33139 DD 8/28/2001
BENZOATE/PHENYLACETATE TN=AMMONUL	FOR THE TREATMENT OF ACUTE HYPERAMMONEMIA AND ASSOCIATED ENCEPHALOPATHY IN PATIENTS WITH DEFICIENCIES IN ENZYMES OF THE UREA CYCLE.	MEDICIS PHARMACEUTICAL CORP. 8125 N. HAYDEN ROAD SCOTTSDALE AZ 85258 DD 11/22/1993
BIFIDOBACTERIUM LONGUM INFANTIS 35624	TREATMENT OF PEDIATRIC CROHN'S DISEASE	ALIMENTARY HEALTH LIMITED GUARDWELL, KINSALE COUNTY CORK, IRELAND DD 1/16/2003
BORTEZOMIB TN=VELCADE	TO TREAT MULTIPLE MYELOMA	MILLENNIUM PHARMACEUTICALS, INC. 75 SIDNEY STREET CAMBRIDGE MA 02139 DD 1/15/2003
BRYOSTATIN-1	FOR USE IN COMBINATION WITH PACLITAXEL IN THE TREATMENT OF ESOPHAGEAL CANCER	GPC BIOTECH, INC. 610 LINCOLN STREET WALTHAM MA 02451 DD 12/3/2001
BUSULFAN TN=PARTAJECT	PREPARATIVE THERAPY FOR PEDIATRIC PATIENTS UNDERGOING BONE MARROW TRANSPLANTATION	SUPERGEN, INC. 4140 DUBLIN BLVD SUITE 200 DUBLIN CA 94568 DD 11/25/2002
CAPSAICIN	TREATMENT OF ERYTHROMELALGIA	NEUROGESX, INC. 981F INDUSTRIAL ROAD SAN CARLOS CA 94070 DD 10/23/2002
CARBAMIC ACID, [[4-[[3-[[4-[1-(4-HYDROXYPHENYL)-1-METHYL-ETHYL]PHENOXY]METHYL]PHE-NYL]METHOXY]-PHENYL]IMINO-METHYL]-,ETHYL ESTER	MANAGEMENT OF CYSTIC FIBROSIS	BOEHRINGER INGELHEIM PHARMACEUTICALS, INC 900 RIDGEBURY ROAD P.O. BOX 368 RIDGEFIELD CT 06877 DD 1/15/2002

NAME *Generic/Chemical* *TN=Trade Name*	INDICATION DESIGNATED	SPONSOR AND ADDRESS *DD=Date Designated* *MA=Marketing Approval*
CELLS PRODUCED USING THE AASTROMREPLICELLE SYSTEM AND SC-I THERAPY KIT	FOR USE IN PATIENTS RECEIVING HIGH DOSE CHEMOTHERAPY WHO ARE UNABLE TO GENERATE AN ACCEPTABLE DOSE OF PERIPHERAL BLOOD STEM CELLS AND WHO HAVE A SUFFICIENT BONE MARROW ASPIRATE WITHOUT MORPHOLOGICAL EVIDENCE OF TUMOR	AASTROM BIOSCIENCES INCORPORATED P.O. BOX 376 ANN ARBOR MI 48106 DD 7/10/2002
CIVAMIDE TN=ZUCAPSAICIN	TREATMENT OF POSTHERPETIC NEURALGIA OF THE TRIGEMINAL NERVE	WINSTON LABORATORIES, INC. 100 FAIRWAY DRIVE, SUITE 134 VERNON HILLS IL 60061 DD 12/9/2002
CLOFARABINE TN=CLOFAREX	TREATMENT OF ACUTE LYMPHOBLASTIC LEUKEMIA	ILEX PRODUCTS, INC. 4545 HORIZON HILL BLVD. SAN ANTONIO TX 78229-2263 DD 2/7/2002
CLOFARABINE TN=CLOFAREX	TREATMENT OF ACUTE MYELOGENOUS LEUKEMIA	ILEX PRODUCTS, INC. 4545 HORIZON HILL BLVD. SAN ANTONIO TX 78229-2263 DD 3/14/2002
CONJUGATE OF HUMAN TRANSFERRIN AND A MUTANT DIPHTHERIA TOXIN (CRM 107) TN=TRANSMID	TREATMENT OF MALIGNANT TUMORS OF THE CENTRAL NERVOUS SYSTEM	INTELLIGENE EXPRESSIONS INC. 1938-94 ST. EDMONTON, AB T6N 1J3 DD 12/3/2001
CREATINE TN=CREAPURE	TREATMENT OF AMYOTROPHIC LATERAL SCLEROSIS	AVICENA GROUP, INC. 580 CALIFORNIA ST. SUITE 1600 SAN FRANCISCO CA 94104 DD 2/12/2002
DECITABINE	TREATMENT OF SICKLE CELL ANEMIA	SUPERGEN, INC. 4140 DUBLIN BLVD., SUITE 200 DUBLIN CA 94568 DD 9/9/2002
DEFERIPRONE TN=FERRIPROX	TREATMENT OF IRON OVERLOAD IN PATIENTS WITH HEMATOLOGIC DISORDERS REQUIRING CHRONIC TRANSFUSION THERAPY	APOTEX RESEARCH INC. 150 SIGNET DRIVE TORONTO, CANADA M9L 1T9 DD 12/12/2001
DEXTRAN 1	TREATMENT OF CYSTIC FIBROSIS	BCY LIFESCIENCES INC. 160 EGLINTON AVE. EAST SUITE 600 TORONTO, ONTARIO M4P 3B5 DD 3/21/2003
DIGITOXIN	TREATMENT OF OVARIAN CANCER	PRIMECYTE, INC. 130 FIFTH AVE., N. SEATTLE WA 98109-4933 DD 11/2/2001
DIGITOXIN	TREATMENT OF SOFT TISSUE SARCOMAS	PRIMECYTE, INC. 130 FIFTH AVE., N. SEATTLE WA 98109-4933 DD 10/18/2001
DOCOSAHEXANOIC ACID-PACLITAXEL TN=TAXOPREXIN	TREATMENT OF HORMONE-REFRACTORY PROSTATE CANCER.	PROTARGA, INC. 1100 EAST HECTOR STREET SUITE 450 CONSHOHOCKEN PA 19428-2377 DD 3/5/2001

NAME Generic/Chemical TN=Trade Name	INDICATION DESIGNATED	SPONSOR AND ADDRESS DD=Date Designated MA=Marketing Approval
ECULIZUMAB	IDIOPATHIC MEMBRANOUS GLOMERULAR NEPHRO-PATHY	ALEXION PHARMACEUTICALS, INC. 352 KNOTTER DRIVE CHESHIRE CT 06410 DD 3/5/2001
EPRATUZUMAB TN=LYMPHOCIDE	TREATMENT OF NON-HODGKIN'S LYMPHOMA.	AMGEN ONE AMGEN CENTER DRIVE THOUSAND OAKS CA 20857 DD 7/13/1998
FACTOR XIII CONCENTRATE (HU-MAN), PASTEURIZED TN=FIBROGAMMIN P	TREATMENT OF CONGENITAL FACTOR XIII DEFI-CIENCY.	AVENTIS BEHRING L.L.C. 1020 FIRST AVE. PO BOX 61501 KING OF PRUSSIA PA 19406-0901 DD 1/16/1985
GENETICALLY ENGINEERED HERPES SIMPLEX VIRUS (G207)	TRETAMENT OF MALIGNANT GLIOMA	MEDIGENE, INC. 9880 CAMPUS POINT DRIVE, SUITE A SAN DIEGO CA 92121 DD 4/29/2002
H5G1.1-MAB	TREATMENT OF DERMATOMYOSITIS	ALEXION PHARMACEUTICALS, INC.ALEXION PHARMACEUTI-CALS, INC. 352 KNOTTER DRIVE25 SCIENCE PARK CHESHIRE CT 06410 DD 9/21/2000
HEAT KILLED MYCOBACTERIUM WITH IMMUNOMODULATOR TN=CADI MW	ADJUVANT TO MULTI-DRUG THERAPY IN THE MAN-AGEMENT OF MULTIBACILLARY LEPROSY	CPL, INC. 16020 SWINGLEY RIDGE ROAD SUITE 145 CHESTERFIELD MO 63017 DD 11/21/2002
HOMOHARRINGTONINE	TREATMENT FOR CHRONIC MYELOGENOUS LEUKE-MIA	AMERICAN BIOSCIENCE, INC. 2730 WILSHIRE BLVD. #110 SANTA MONICA CA 90403 DD 2/8/2002
HUMAN ANTI-TRANSFORMING GROWTH FACTOR BETA 1 MONO-CLONAL ANTIBODY	TREATMENT OF SYSTEMIC SCLEROSIS	GENZYME CORPORATION ONE KENDALL SQUARE CAMBRIDGE MA 02139 DD 1/11/2002
HUMAN GAMMAGLOBULIN	TREATMENT OF GASTROINTESTINAL DISTURBANCES (TO INCLUDE CONSTIPATION, DIARRHEA, AND AB-DOMINAL PAIN) ASSOCIATED WITH REGRESSION-ON-SET AUTISM IN PEDIATRIC PATIENTS.	PROTEIN THERAPEUTICS, INC. 9040 S. RITA ROAD SUITE 1100 TUCSON AZ 85747 DD 9/16/2002
HUMAN GAMMAGLOBULIN	TREATMENT FOR JUVENILE RHEUMATOID ARTHRITIS	PROTEIN THERAPEUTICS, INC 9040 S. RITA RD., SUITE 1100 TUCSON AZ 84747 DD 5/25/2001
HUMANIZED MONOCLONAL ANTI-BODY AGAINST SHIGA-LIKE TOX-IN II	TO PREVENT THE DEVELOPMENT OF OR TO DE-CREASE THE INCIDENCE AND SEVERITY OF HEMOLY-TIC UREMIC SYNDROME AND ASSOCIATED SEQUELAE OF SHIGA-LIKE TOXIN-PRODUCING E. COLI.	TEIJIN AMERICA, INC. 600 ALEXANDER PARK SUITE 304 PRINCETON NJ 08540 DD 9/12/2001
HYALURONIC ACID	TREATMENT OF EMPHYSEMA IN PATIENTS DUE TO ALPHA-1 ANTITRYPSIN DEFICIENCY	EXHALE THERAPEUTICS, INC. 1301 SHOREWAY ROAD SUITE 320 BELMONT CA 94002 DD 3/19/2002

NAME *Generic/Chemical* *TN=Trade Name*	INDICATION DESIGNATED	SPONSOR AND ADDRESS *DD=Date Designated* *MA=Marketing Approval*
IBRITUMOMAB TIUXETAN TN=ZEVALIN	TREATMENT OF B-CELL NON-HODGKIN'S LYMPHOMA.	IDEC PHARMACEUTICALS COR- PORATION 3030 CALLAN ROAD SAN DIEGO CA 92121 DD 9/6/1994 MA 2/19/2002
IDURONATE-2-SULFATASE	LONG TERM ENZYME REPLACEMENT THERAPY FOR PATIENTS WITH MPS II (HUNTER SYNDROME)	TRANSKARYOTIC THERAPIES INC. 195 ALBANY STREET CAMBRIDGE MA 02139 DD 11/28/2001
IMATINIB MESYLATE TN=GLEEVEC	TREATMENT OF GASTROINTESTINAL STROMAL TU-MORS	NOVARTIS PHARMACEUTICALS CORP. ONE HEALTH PLAZA EAST HANOVER NJ 07936-1080 DD 11/1/2001 MA 2/1/2002
INFLIXIMAB TN=REMICADE	TREATMENT OF JUVENILE RHEUMATOID ARTHRITIS	CENTOCOR, INC. 200 GREAT VALLEY PARKWAY MALVERN PA 19355-1307 DD 10/23/2002
INOLIMOMAB TN=LEUKOTAC	TREATMENT OF GRAFT VERSUS HOST DISEASE	OPI 6, CHEMIN DE L'INDUSTRIE 69570 DARDILLY - FRANCE DD 10/23/2002
INTERFERON GAMMA-1B TN=ACTIMMUNE	TREATMENT OF IDIOPATHIC PULMONARY FIBROSIS	INTERMUNE, INC. 3280 BAYSHORE BOULEVARD BRISBANE CA 94005 DD 9/12/2002
LACTIC ACID BACTERIA (LACTO-BACILLI, BIFIDOBACTERIA, AND STEPTOCOCCI)	TREATMENT OF ACTIVE CHRONIC POUCHITIS	VSL PHARMACEUTICALS, INC. 800 S. FREDERICK AVENUE GAITHERSBURG MD 20877 DD 1/15/2002
LACTIC ACID BACTERIA (LACTO-BACILLI, BIFIDOBACTERIA, AND STREPTOCOCCUS SPECIES)	PREVENTION OF DISEASE RELAPSE IN PATIENTS WITH CHRONIC POUCHITIS	VSL PHARMACEUTICALS, INC. 800 S. FREDERICK AVE. GAITHERSBURG MD 20877 DD 1/15/2002
LINTUZUMAB TN=ZAMYL	TREATMENT OF ACUTE MYELOGENOUS LEUKEMIA	PROTEIN DESIGN LABS, INC. 34801 CAMPUS DRIVE FREMONT CA 94555 DD 9/9/2002
LIPASE, AMYLASE, AND PRO-TEASE TN=THERACLEC-TOTAL	TREATMENT OF PANCREATIC INSUFFICIENCY	ALTUS BIOLOGICS INC. 625 PUTNAM AVENUE CAMBRIDGE MA 02139 DD 1/23/2002
MELOXICAM TN=MOBIC	TREATMENT OF JUVENILE RHEUMATOID ARTHRITIS	BOEHRINGER INGELHEIM PHAR-MACEUTICALS, INC. 900 RIDGEBURY ROAD P. O. BOX 368 RIDGEFIELD CT 06877-0368 DD 11/22/2002

NAME Generic/Chemical TN=Trade Name	INDICATION DESIGNATED	SPONSOR AND ADDRESS DD=Date Designated MA=Marketing Approval
METHYLBICYCLONE	TREATMENT OF CYSTIC FIBROSIS	SUCAMPO PHARMACEUTICALS, INC. 4733 BETHESDA AVE. SUITE 450 BETHESDA MD 20814 DD 11/14/2002
METRELEPTIN	TREATMENT OF METABOLIC DISORDERS SECONDARY TO LIPODYSTROPHY	AMGEN, INC., ONE AMGEN CENTER DRIVE THOUSAND OAKS CA 91320-1799 DD 8/22/2001
METRELEPTIN	TREATMENT OF LEPTIN DEFICIENCY SECONDARY TO GENERALIZEDLIPODYSTROPHY AND PARTIAL FAMILIAL LIPODYSTROPHY	AMGEN, INC. ONE AMGEN CENTER DRIVE THOUSAND OAKS CA 91320-1799 DD 8/22/2001
MOTEXAFIN GADOLINIUM TN=XCYTRIN	FOR USE IN CONJUNCTION WITH WHOLE BRAIN RADIATION FOR THE TREATMENT OF BRAIN METASTASES ARISING FROM SOLID TUMORS	PHARMACYCLICS, INC. 999 EAST ARQUES AVENUE SUNNYVALE CA 94085-4521 DD 1/27/2003
MURAMYLTRIPEPTIDE, PHOSPHATIDYL-ETHANOLAMINE ENCASED IN MULTI-LAMELLAR LIPOSOMES	TREATMENT OF CHILDREN AND ADOLESCENT OSTEOSARCOMA	JENNER BIOTHERAPIES, INC. 541 KENOSA STREET WALWORTH WI 53184 DD 6/5/2001
NITAZOXANIDE TN=ALINIA	TREATMENT OF INTESTINAL GIARDIASIS	ROMARK LABORATORIES, L.C. 6200 COURTNEY CAMPBELL CAUSEWAY SUITE 880 TAMPA FL 33607 DD 2/14/2002 MA 11/22/2002
NITAZOXANIDE TN=CRYPTAZ	TREATMENT FOR INTESTINAL AMEBIASIS	ROMARK LABORATORIES, L.C. 6200 COURTNEY CAMPBELL CAUSEWAY SUITE 880 TAMPA FL 33607 DD 10/23/2001
NOLATREXED TN=THYMITAQ	TREATMENT OF HEPATOCELLULAR CARCINOMA	ZARIX, INC. 1055 WESTLAKES DRIVE SUITE 200 BERWYN PA 19312 DD 10/18/2001
OCTAVALENT PSUEDOMONAS AERUGINOSA O-POLYSACCAHARIDE-TOXIN A CONJUGATE TN=AERUGEN	PREVENTION OF PSUEDOMONAS AERUGINOSA INFECTIONS IN PATIENTS WITH CYSTIC FIBROSIS	ORPHAN EUROPE IMMEUBLE ""LE WILSON"" 70 AVENUE DU GENERAL DE GAULLE, 92046 PARIS LA DEFENSE FRANCE DD 5/16/2002
OGLUFANIDE DISODIUM	TREATMENT OF OVARIAN CANCER	CYTRAN, INC. 10230 NE POINTS DR., NE SUITE 530 KIRKLAND WA 98033-7869 DD 9/24/2001
P1-(URIDINE 5'-)-P4-(2'-DEOXYCYTIDINE 5'-) TETRAPHOSPHATE, TETRASODIUM SALT	FOR THE TREATMENT OF CYSTIC FIBROSIS	INSPIRE PHARMACEUTICALS, INC. 4222 EMPEROR BLVD. SUITE 470 DURHAM NC 27703 DD 3/7/2001

NAME *Generic/Chemical* *TN=Trade Name*	INDICATION DESIGNATED	SPONSOR AND ADDRESS *DD=Date Designated* *MA=Marketing Approval*
PVGI.1(VEGF2)	TREATMENT OF THROMBOANGIITIS OBLITERANS.	VASCULAR GENETICS, INC. 200 WESTPARK CORPORATE CENTER 4364 SOUTH ALSTON AVE. DURHAM NC 27713-2280 DD 11/9/1999
PEMETREXED DISODIUM TN=ALIMTA	TREATMENT OF MALIGNANT PLEURAL MESOTHELIO-MA	ELI LILLY AND COMPANY LILLY CORPORATE CENTER INDIANAPOLIS IN 46285 DD 8/28/2001
PHENYLEPHRINE	TREATMENT OF ILEAL POUCH ANAL ANASTOMOSIS RELATED FECAL INCONTINENCE	S.L.A. PHARMA UNIT 3, HILL FARM INDUSTRIAL ESTATE LEAVESDEN, WATFORD UNITED KINGDOM WD25 7SA DD 2/14/2002
PHYSOSTIGMINE SALICYLATE-PHYSOSTIGMINE SALICYLATE	TREATMENT OF FRIEDREICH'S AND OTHER INHER-ITED ATAXIAS.	FOREST PHARMACEUTICALS.3-.3-.30 6 150 EAST 58TH STREET NEW YORK NY 10155 DD 1/16/1985
POLYINOSINIC-POLYCYTIDILIC ACID TN=POLY-ICLC	TREATMENT OF FLAVIVIRUS INFECTIONS INCLUDING THOSE DUE TO WEST NILE, JAPANESE ENCEPHALI-TIS, DENGUE, ST. LOUIS ENCEPHALITIS, YELLOW FE-VER, MURRAY VALLEY, AND BANZAI VIRUSES	RIBOPHARM, INC. 3203 CLEVELAND AVE., NW WASHINGTON DC 20008-3450 DD 3/3/2003
POLYINOSINIC-POLYCYTIDILIC ACID TN=POLY-ICLC	TREATMENT FOR ORTHOPOX VIRUS INFECTIONS	RIBOPHARM, INC. 3203 CLEVELAND AVE., NW WASHINGTON DC 20008-3450 DD 11/19/2002
POLYINOSINIC-POLYCYTIDILIC ACID TN=POLY-ICLC	AS AN ADJUVANT TO SMALLPOX VACCINATION	RIBOPHARM, INC. 3203 CLEVELAND AVE., NW WASHINGTON DC 20008-3450 DD 8/2/2002
PORFIMER TN=PHOTOFRIN	FOR THE ABLATION OF HIGH-GRADE DYSPLASIA IN BARRETT'S ESOPHAGUS IN PATIENTS WHO ARE NOT CONSIDERED TO BE CANDIDATES FOR ESOPHA-GECTOMY	AXCAN SCANDIPHARM INC. 22 INVERNESS PARKWAY SUITE 310 BIRMINGHAM AL 35242 DD 10/19/2001
RSP-C LUNG SURFACTANT TN=VENTICUTE	TREATMENT OF ADULT RESPIRATORY DISTRESS SYNDROME.	BYK GULDEN PHARMACEUTI-CALS BYK-GULDEN STRABE 2 78467 KONSTANZ GERMANY DE DD 4/3/2000
RASBURICASE TN=ELITEK	TREATMENT OF MALIGNANCY-ASSOCIATED OR CHE-MOTHERAPY-INDUCED HYPERURICEMIA.	SANOFI-SYNTHELABO RE-SEARCH 9 GREAT VALLEY PARKWAY MALVERN PA 19355 DD 10/11/2000 MA 7/12/2002
RECOMBINANT ADENO-ASSO-CIATED VIRUS ALPHA 1-ANTI-TRYPSIN VECTOR TN=RAAV-AAT	TREATMENT OF ALPHA1-ANTITRYPSIN DEFICIENCY	APPLIED GENETIC TECHNOLO-GIES CORP. 12085 RESEARCH DRIVE SUITE 110 ALACHUA FL 32615 DD 1/27/2003

NAME *Generic/Chemical* *TN=Trade Name*	INDICATION DESIGNATED	SPONSOR AND ADDRESS *DD=Date Designated* *MA=Marketing Approval*
RECOMBINANT HUMAN ALPHA 1-ANTITRYPSIN (RAAT)	TREATMENT OF CYSTIC FIBROSIS	ARRIVA PHARMACEUTICALS, INC. 2020 CHALLENGER DRIVE ALAMEDA CA 94501 DD 11/20/2001
RECOMBINANT HUMAN ALPHA-1 ANTITRYPSIN	TREATMENT OF CYSTIC FIBROSIS.	PPL THERAPEUTICS (SCOTLAND) LIMITED ROSLIN, EDINBURGH EH25 9PP SCOTLAND GB DD 3/6/1998
RECOMBINANT HUMAN ALPHA-1 ANTITRYPSIN (RAAT)	TO DELAY PROGRESSION OF CHRONIC OBSTRUCTIVE PULMONARY DISEASE RESULTING FROM AAT DEFICIENCY-MEDIATED EMPHYSEMA AND BRONCHIECTASIS	BAXTER HEALTHCARE CORPORATION 550 N. BRAND BLVD. GLENDALE CA 91203 DD 8/28/2001
RECOMBINANT HUMAN ENDOSTATIN PROTEIN	TREATMENT OF METASTATIC MELANOMA	ENTREMED, INC. 9640 MEDICAL CENTER DRIVE ROCKVILLE MD 20850 DD 2/21/2002
RECOMBINANT HUMAN ENDOSTATIN PROTEIN	TREATMENT OF NEUROENDOCRINE TUMORS.	ENTREMED, INC. 9640 MEDICAL CENTER DRIVE ROCKVILLE MD 20850 DD 8/13/2001
RECOMBINANT HUMAN INSULIN-LIKE GROWTH FACTOR-I/INSULIN-LIKE GROWTH FACTOR BINDING PROTEIN-3 TN=SOMATOKINE	TREATMENT OF GROWTH HORMONE INSENSITIVITY SYNDROME	CELTRIX PHARMACEUTICALS, INC. A SUBSIDIARY OF INSMED, INC. 4851 LAKE BROOK DRIVE GLEN ALLEN VA 23060 DD 5/17/2002
RECOMBINANT HUMAN MONOCLONAL ANTIBODY TO HSP90 TN=MYCOGRAB	TREATMENT OF INVASIVE CANDIDIASIS	NEUTEC PHARMA PLC 2DN FLOOR, CLINICAL SCIENCES BLDG. CENTRAL MANCHESTER HEALTHCARE TRUST, OXFORD RD., MANCHESTER M139WL, UK DD 9/16/2002
RECOMBINANT HUMAN PORPHOBILINOGEN DEAMINASE	TREATMENT OF ACUTE INTERMITTENT PORPHYRIA ATTACKS	HEMEBIOTECH A/S ROSKILDEVEJ 12C 3400 HILLEROD DENMARK DD 9/9/2002
RECOMBINANT HUMAN PORPHOBILINOGEN DEAMINASE, ERYTHROPOETIC FORM	TREATMENT OF ACUTE INTERMITTENT PORPHYRIA PREVENTING ATTACKS	HEMEBIOTECH A/S ROSKILDEVEJ 12C 3400 HILLEROD DENMARK DD 7/11/2002
RECOMBINANT INHIBITOR OF HUMAN PLASMA KALLIKREIN	TREATMENT OF ANGIOEDEMA	DYAX CORP 300 TECHNOLOGY SQUARE CAMBRIDGE MA 02139 DD 2/4/2003
REPERTAXIN	PREVENTION OF DELAYED GRAFT FUNCTION IN SOLID ORGAN TRANSPLANT	DOMPE S.P.A. VIA CAMPO DI PILE 67100 - L'AQUILA ITALY DD 1/27/2003

NAME *Generic/Chemical* *TN=Trade Name*	INDICATION DESIGNATED	SPONSOR AND ADDRESS *DD=Date Designated* *MA=Marketing Approval*
RETROVIRAL GAMMA-C CDNA CONTAINING VECTOR	TREATMENT OF X LINKED SEVERE COMBINED IMMUNE DEFICIENCY DISEASE	AVAX TECHNOLOGIES, INC. 9200 INDIAN CREEK PARKWAY BUILDING 9, SUITE 200 OVERLAND PARK KS 66210 DD 4/29/2002
RITUXIMAB TN=RITUXAN	TREATMENT OF IMMUNE THROMBOCYTOPENIC PURPURA	GENENTECH, INC. 1 DNA WAY SOUTH SAN FRANCISCO CA 94080-4990 DD 3/12/2002
RUBITECAN	TREATMENT OF PEDIATRIC PATIENTS INFECTED WITH HUMAN IMMUNODEFICIENCY VIRUS AND ACQUIRED IMMUNODEFICIENCY SYNDROME	SUPERGEN, INC. 4140 DUBLIN BLVD. SUITE 200 DUBLIN CA 94568 DD 7/17/2002
SODIUM PHENYLBUTYRATE	TREATMENT FOR SICKLING DISORDERS, WHICH INCLUDE S-S HEMOGLOBINOPATHY, S-C HEMOGLOBINOPATHY, AND S-THALASSEMIA HEMOGLOBINOPATHY.	MEDICIS PHARMACEUTICAL CORP. 8125 N. HAYDEN ROAD SCOTTSDALE AZ 85258 DD 7/2/1992
SODIUM PHENYLBUTYRATE TN=BUPHENYL	TREATMENT OF UREA CYCLE DISORDERS: CARBAMYLPHOSPHATE SYNTHETASE DEFICIENCY, ORNITHINE TRANSCARBAMYLASE DEFICIENCY, AND ARGINIOSUCCINIC ACID SYNTHETASE DEFICIENCY.	MEDICIS PHARMACEUTICAL CORP. 8125 N. HAYDEN ROAD SCOTTSDALE AZ 85258 DD 11/22/1993 MA 4/30/1996
SOMATROPIN [RDNA] TN=GENOTROPIN	TREATMENT OF GROWTH FAILURE IN CHILDREN WHO WERE BORN SMALL FOR GESTATIONAL AGE.	PHARMACIA AND UPJOHN COMPANY 7000 PORTAGE ROAD KALAMAZOO MI 49001 DD 12/27/2000 MA 7/25/2001
SQUALAMINE LACTATE	TREATMENT OF OVARIAN CANCER REFRACTORY OR RESISTANT TO STANDARD CHEMOTHERAPY	GENAERA CORPORATION 5110 CAMPUS DRIVE PLYMOUTH MEETING PA 19462 DD 5/11/2001
TINIDAZOLE	TREATMENT OF GIARDIASIS	PRESUTTI LABORATORIES, INC. 1607 N. DOUGLAS AVE. ARLINGTON HEIGHTS IL 60004 DD 4/18/2002
TIRAPAZAMINE	FOR THE TREATMENT OF HEAD AND NECK CANCER	SANOFI-SYNTHELABO RESEARCH 9 GREAT VALLEY PARKWAY MALVERN PA 19355 DD 10/23/2002
TORALIZUMAB	TREATMENT OF IMMUNE THROMBOCYTOPENIC PURPURA	IDEC PHARMACEUTICALS CORPORATION 3030 CALLAN ROAD SAN DIEGO CA 92121 DD 3/14/2002
TREPROSTINIL TN=REMODULIN	TREATMENT OF PULMONARY ARTERIAL HYPERTENSION.	UNITED THERAPEUTICS CORP. 68 T.W. ALEXANDER DR. P.O. BOX 14186 RESEARCH TRIANGLE PARK NC 27709 DD 6/4/1997 MA 5/21/2002

NAME *Generic/Chemical* *TN=Trade Name*	INDICATION DESIGNATED	SPONSOR AND ADDRESS *DD=Date Designated* *MA=Marketing Approval*
TRI-ANTENNARY GLYCOTRIPEP- TIDE DERIVATIVE OF 5-FLUORO- DEOXYURIDINE MONOPHO- SPHATE	TREATMENT FOR HEPATOCELLULAR CARCINOMA	CELL WORKS INC. 6200 SEAFORTH STREET BALTIMORE MD 21224-6506 DD 11/23/2001
VIGABATRIN TN=SABRIL	TREATMENT OF INFANTILE SPASMS.	AVENTIS PHARMACEUTICALS INC. P.O. BOX 9627 KANSAS CITY MO 64137 DD 6/12/2000

DRUG PRODUCTS WHICH MUST DEMONSTRATE *IN VIVO* BIOAVAILABILITY ONLY IF PRODUCT FAILS TO ACHIEVE ADEQUATE DISSOLUTION

ACETAMINOPHEN; ASPIRIN; BUTALBITAL
CAPSULE OR TABLET; ORAL
160-165MG; 160-165MG; 50MG

ACETAMINOPHEN; ASPIRIN; BUTALBITAL
CAPSULE OR TABLET; ORAL
325MG; 325MG; 50MG

ACETAMINOPHEN; ASPIRIN; BUTALBITAL; CAFFEINE
CAPSULE OR TABLET; ORAL
160-165MG; 160-165MG; 50MG; 40MG

ACETAMINOPHEN; ASPIRIN; BUTALBITAL; CAFFEINE
CAPSULE OR TABLET; ORAL
325MG; 325MG; 50MG; 40MG

ACETAMINOPHEN; BUTALBITAL
CAPSULE OR TABLET; ORAL
325MG; 50MG
650MG; 50MG

ACETAMINOPHEN; BUTALBITAL; CAFFEINE
CAPSULE OR TABLET; ORAL
325MG; 50MG; 40MG
650MG; 50MG; 40MG
500MG; 50MG; 40MG

AMINOPHYLLINE
TABLET; ORAL
100MG
200MG

ASPIRIN; BUTALBITAL
CAPSULE OR TABLET; ORAL
325MG; 50MG
650MG; 50MG

ASPIRIN; BUTALBITAL; CAFFEINE
CAPSULE OR TABLET; ORAL
325MG; 50MG; 40MG
650MG; 50MG; 40MG

ASPIRIN; CAFFEINE; CARISOPRODOL
TABLET; ORAL
160MG; 32MG; 200MG

ASPIRIN; CAFFEINE; CARISOPRODOL; CODEINE PHOS-
PHATE
TABLET; ORAL
160MG; 32MG; 200MG; 16MG

ASPIRIN; CARISOPRODOL
TABLET; ORAL
325MG; 200MG

ASPIRIN; CARISOPRODOL; CODEINE PHOSPHATE
TABLET; ORAL
325MG; 200MG; 16MG

ASPIRIN; MEPROBAMATE
TABLET; ORAL
325MG; 200MG

ASPIRIN; METHOCARBAMOL
TABLET; ORAL
325MG; 400MG

CHLOROTHIAZIDE
TABLET; ORAL
250MG

HYDROXYZINE HYDROCHLORIDE
TABLET; ORAL
10MG; 25MG;
50MG; 100MG

PREDNISONE
TABLET; ORAL
1MG; 2.5MG; 5MG; 10MG; 20MG; 25MG; 50MG

APPENDIX A
PRODUCT NAME INDEX

8

8-HOUR BAYER, ASPIRIN (OTC)
8-MOP, METHOXSALEN

A

A-HYDROCORT, HYDROCORTISONE SODIUM
    SUCCINATE
A-METHAPRED, METHYLPREDNISOLONE SODIUM
    SUCCINATE
A-N STANNOUS AGGREGATED ALBUMIN, TECHNETIUM
    TC-99M ALBUMIN AGGREGATED KIT
A-POXIDE, CHLORDIAZEPOXIDE HYDROCHLORIDE
A.P.L., GONADOTROPIN, CHORIONIC
A/T/S, ERYTHROMYCIN
ABELCET, AMPHOTERICIN B
ABILIFY, ARIPIPRAZOLE
ABITREXATE, METHOTREXATE SODIUM
ABREVA, DOCOSANOL (OTC)
ACCOLATE, ZAFIRLUKAST
ACCUNEB, ALBUTEROL SULFATE
ACCUPRIL, QUINAPRIL HYDROCHLORIDE
ACCURBRON, THEOPHYLLINE
ACCURETIC, HYDROCHLOROTHIAZIDE
ACCUTANE, ISOTRETINOIN
ACEBUTOLOL HCL, ACEBUTOLOL HYDROCHLORIDE
ACEON, PERINDOPRIL ERBUMINE
ACEPHEN, ACETAMINOPHEN (OTC)
ACETAMINOPHEN AND BUTALBITAL AND CAFFEINE,
    ACETAMINOPHEN
ACETAMINOPHEN AND CODEINE PHOSPAHTE,
    ACETAMINOPHEN
ACETAMINOPHEN AND CODEINE PHOSPHATE #2,
    ACETAMINOPHEN
ACETAMINOPHEN AND CODEINE PHOSPHATE #3,
    ACETAMINOPHEN
ACETAMINOPHEN AND CODEINE PHOSPHATE #4,
    ACETAMINOPHEN
ACETAMINOPHEN AND CODEINE PHOSPHATE NO. 2,
    ACETAMINOPHEN
ACETAMINOPHEN AND CODEINE PHOSPHATE NO. 3,
    ACETAMINOPHEN
ACETAMINOPHEN AND CODEINE PHOSPHATE NO. 4,
    ACETAMINOPHEN
ACETAMINOPHEN AND CODEINE PHOSPHATE,
    ACETAMINOPHEN
ACETAMINOPHEN AND HYDROCODONE BITARTRATE,
    ACETAMINOPHEN
ACETAMINOPHEN AND PENTAZOCINE HCL,
    ACETAMINOPHEN
ACETAMINOPHEN W/ CODEINE #2, ACETAMINOPHEN
ACETAMINOPHEN W/ CODEINE #4, ACETAMINOPHEN
ACETAMINOPHEN W/ CODEINE NO. 2, ACETAMINOPHEN
ACETAMINOPHEN W/ CODEINE NO. 3, ACETAMINOPHEN
ACETAMINOPHEN W/ CODEINE PHOSPHATE #3,
    ACETAMINOPHEN
ACETAMINOPHEN W/ CODEINE PHOSPHATE,
    ACETAMINOPHEN
ACETAMINOPHEN W/ CODEINE, ACETAMINOPHEN
ACETAMINOPHEN, ACETAMINOPHEN (OTC)
ACETAMINOPHEN, ASPIRIN AND CAFFEINE,
    ACETAMINOPHEN (OTC)
ACETAMINOPHEN, ASPIRIN, AND CODEINE
    PHOSPHATE, ACETAMINOPHEN

ACETAMINOPHEN, BUTALBITAL AND CAFFEINE,
    ACETAMINOPHEN
ACETAMINOPHEN, BUTALBITAL, AND CAFFEINE,
    ACETAMINOPHEN
ACETAMINOPHEN, BUTALBITAL, CAFFEINE, AND
    CODEINE PHOSPHATE, ACETAMINOPHEN
ACETAMINOPHEN, CAFFEINE, AND DIHYDROCODEINE
    BITARTRATE, ACETAMINOPHEN
ACETASOL HC, ACETIC ACID, GLACIAL
ACETASOL, ACETIC ACID, GLACIAL
ACETATED RINGER'S IN PLASTIC CONTAINER, CALCIUM
    CHLORIDE
ACETAZOLAMIDE SODIUM, ACETAZOLAMIDE SODIUM
ACETAZOLAMIDE, ACETAZOLAMIDE
ACETIC ACID 0.25% IN PLASTIC CONTAINER, ACETIC
    ACID, GLACIAL
ACETIC ACID 2% IN AQUEOUS ALUMINUM ACETATE,
    ACETIC ACID, GLACIAL
ACETIC ACID W/ HYDROCORTISONE, ACETIC ACID,
    GLACIAL
ACETIC ACID, ACETIC ACID, GLACIAL
ACETOHEXAMIDE, ACETOHEXAMIDE
ACETYLCYSTEINE, ACETYLCYSTEINE
ACHES-N-PAIN, IBUPROFEN (OTC)
ACHROMYCIN V, TETRACYCLINE HYDROCHLORIDE
ACHROMYCIN, HYDROCORTISONE
ACHROMYCIN, PROCAINE HYDROCHLORIDE
ACHROMYCIN, TETRACYCLINE HYDROCHLORIDE
ACILAC, LACTULOSE
ACIPHEX, RABEPRAZOLE SODIUM
ACLOVATE, ALCLOMETASONE DIPROPIONATE
ACTAHIST, PSEUDOEPHEDRINE HYDROCHLORIDE
ACTH, CORTICOTROPIN
ACTHAR GEL-SYNTHETIC, SERACTIDE ACETATE
ACTHAR, CORTICOTROPIN
ACTHREL, CORTICORELIN OVINE TRIFLUTATE
ACTICORT, HYDROCORTISONE
ACTIDIL, TRIPROLIDINE HYDROCHLORIDE (OTC)
ACTIFED W/ CODEINE, CODEINE PHOSPHATE
ACTIFED, PSEUDOEPHEDRINE HYDROCHLORIDE (OTC)
ACTIGALL, URSODIOL
ACTIN-N, NITROFURAZONE
ACTINEX, MASOPROCOL
ACTIQ, FENTANYL CITRATE
ACTISITE, TETRACYCLINE HYDROCHLORIDE
ACTIVELLA, ESTRADIOL
ACTONEL, RISEDRONATE SODIUM
ACTOS, PIOGLITAZONE HYDROCHLORIDE
ACTRON, KETOPROFEN (OTC)
ACULAR LS, KETOROLAC TROMETHAMINE
ACULAR PRESERVATIVE FREE, KETOROLAC
    TROMETHAMINE
ACULAR, KETOROLAC TROMETHAMINE
ACUTECT, TECHNETIUM TC-99M APCITIDE
ACYCLOVIR IN SODIUM CHLORIDE 0.9% PRESERVATIVE
    FREE, ACYCLOVIR SODIUM
ACYCLOVIR SODIUM, ACYCLOVIR SODIUM
ACYCLOVIR, ACYCLOVIR
ACYCLOVIR, ACYCLOVIR SODIUM
ACYLANID, ACETYLDIGITOXIN
ADAGEN, PEGADEMASE BOVINE
ADALAT CC, NIFEDIPINE
ADALAT, NIFEDIPINE
ADDERALL 5, AMPHETAMINE ASPARTATE
ADDERALL 7.5, AMPHETAMINE ASPARTATE
ADDERALL 10, AMPHETAMINE ASPARTATE
ADDERALL 12.5, AMPHETAMINE ASPARTATE

APPENDIX A
PRODUCT NAME INDEX (*continued*)

ADDERALL 15, AMPHETAMINE ASPARTATE
ADDERALL 20, AMPHETAMINE ASPARTATE
ADDERALL 30, AMPHETAMINE ASPARTATE
ADDERALL XR 5, AMPHETAMINE ASPARTATE
ADDERALL XR 10, AMPHETAMINE ASPARTATE
ADDERALL XR 15, AMPHETAMINE ASPARTATE
ADDERALL XR 20, AMPHETAMINE ASPARTATE
ADDERALL XR 25, AMPHETAMINE ASPARTATE
ADDERALL XR 30, AMPHETAMINE ASPARTATE
ADENOCARD, ADENOSINE
ADENOSCAN, ADENOSINE
ADIPEX-P, PHENTERMINE HYDROCHLORIDE
ADPHEN, PHENDIMETRAZINE TARTRATE
ADRIAMYCIN PFS, DOXORUBICIN HYDROCHLORIDE
ADRIAMYCIN RDF, DOXORUBICIN HYDROCHLORIDE
ADRUCIL, FLUOROURACIL
ADVAIR DISKUS 100/50, FLUTICASONE PROPIONATE
ADVAIR DISKUS 250/50, FLUTICASONE PROPIONATE
ADVAIR DISKUS 500/50, FLUTICASONE PROPIONATE
ADVICOR, LOVASTATIN
ADVIL ALLERGY SINUS, CHLORPHENIRAMINE MALEATE
    (OTC)
ADVIL COLD AND SINUS, IBUPROFEN (OTC)
ADVIL LIQUI-GELS, IBUPROFEN POTASSIUM (OTC)
ADVIL MIGRAINE LIQUI-GELS, IBUPROFEN POTASSIUM
    (OTC)
ADVIL, IBUPROFEN (OTC)
AEROBID, FLUNISOLIDE
AEROLATE III, THEOPHYLLINE
AEROLATE JR, THEOPHYLLINE
AEROLATE SR, THEOPHYLLINE
AEROLATE, THEOPHYLLINE
AEROLONE, ISOPROTERENOL HYDROCHLORIDE
AEROSEB-DEX, DEXAMETHASONE
AEROSEB-HC, HYDROCORTISONE
AEROSPORIN, POLYMYXIN B SULFATE
AFAXIN, VITAMIN A PALMITATE
AFRINOL, PSEUDOEPHEDRINE SULFATE (OTC)
AGENERASE, AMPRENAVIR
AGGRASTAT, TIROFIBAN HYDROCHLORIDE
AGGRENOX, ASPIRIN
AGRYLIN, ANAGRELIDE HYDROCHLORIDE
AK-PENTOLATE, CYCLOPENTOLATE HYDROCHLORIDE
AKBETA, LEVOBUNOLOL HYDROCHLORIDE
AKINETON, BIPERIDEN HYDROCHLORIDE
AKINETON, BIPERIDEN LACTATE
AKNE-MYCIN, ERYTHROMYCIN
AKPENTOLATE, CYCLOPENTOLATE HYDROCHLORIDE
AKPRO, DIPIVEFRIN HYDROCHLORIDE
AKRINOL, ACRISORCIN
AKTOB, TOBRAMYCIN
ALA-CORT, HYDROCORTISONE
ALA-SCALP, HYDROCORTISONE
ALAMAST, PEMIROLAST POTASSIUM
ALAVERT, LORATADINE (OTC)
ALBALON, NAPHAZOLINE HYDROCHLORIDE
ALBAMYCIN, NOVOBIOCIN SODIUM
ALBENZA, ALBENDAZOLE
ALBUMOTOPE 125 I, ALBUMIN IODINATED I-125 SERUM
ALBUTEROL SULFATE, ALBUTEROL SULFATE
ALBUTEROL, ALBUTEROL
ALCAINE, PROPARACAINE HYDROCHLORIDE
ALCOHOL 5% AND DEXTROSE 5%, ALCOHOL
ALCOHOL 10% AND DEXTROSE 5%, ALCOHOL
ALCOHOL 5% IN D5-W, ALCOHOL
ALCOHOL 5% IN DEXTROSE 5% IN WATER, ALCOHOL
ALCOHOL 5% IN DEXTROSE 5%, ALCOHOL
ALDACTAZIDE, HYDROCHLOROTHIAZIDE
ALDACTONE, SPIRONOLACTONE

ALDARA, IMIQUIMOD
ALDOCLOR-150, CHLOROTHIAZIDE
ALDOCLOR-250, CHLOROTHIAZIDE
ALDOMET, METHYLDOPA
ALDOMET, METHYLDOPATE HYDROCHLORIDE
ALDORIL 15, HYDROCHLOROTHIAZIDE
ALDORIL 25, HYDROCHLOROTHIAZIDE
ALDORIL D30, HYDROCHLOROTHIAZIDE
ALDORIL D50, HYDROCHLOROTHIAZIDE
ALESSE, ETHINYL ESTRADIOL
ALEVE COLD AND SINUS, NAPROXEN SODIUM (OTC)
ALEVE, NAPROXEN SODIUM (OTC)
ALFENTA, ALFENTANIL HYDROCHLORIDE
ALFENTANIL, ALFENTANIL HYDROCHLORIDE
ALINIA, NITAZOXANIDE
ALKERAN, MELPHALAN
ALKERAN, MELPHALAN HYDROCHLORIDE
ALKERGOT, ERGOLOID MESYLATES
ALLAY, ACETAMINOPHEN
ALLEGRA, FEXOFENADINE HYDROCHLORIDE
ALLEGRA-D, FEXOFENADINE HYDROCHLORIDE
ALLERFED, PSEUDOEPHEDRINE HYDROCHLORIDE
ALLOPURINOL, ALLOPURINOL
ALOCRIL, NEDOCROMIL SODIUM
ALOMIDE, LODOXAMIDE TROMETHAMINE
ALOPRIM, ALLOPURINOL SODIUM
ALORA, ESTRADIOL
ALPHA CHYMAR, CHYMOTRYPSIN
ALPHACAINE HCL W/ EPINEPHRINE, EPINEPHRINE
ALPHACAINE HCL, LIDOCAINE HYDROCHLORIDE
ALPHACAINE, LIDOCAINE
ALPHADERM, HYDROCORTISONE
ALPHADROL, FLUPREDNISOLONE
ALPHAGAN P, BRIMONIDINE TARTRATE
ALPHAGAN, BRIMONIDINE TARTRATE
ALPHALIN, VITAMIN A PALMITATE
ALPHAREDISOL, HYDROXOCOBALAMIN
ALPHATREX, BETAMETHASONE DIPROPIONATE
ALPHAZINE, PHENDIMETRAZINE TARTRATE
ALPRAZOLAM, ALPRAZOLAM
ALPROSTADIL, ALPROSTADIL
ALREX, LOTEPREDNOL ETABONATE
ALTACE, RAMIPRIL
ALTOCOR, LOVASTATIN
ALUMINUM HYDROXIDE AND MAGNESIUM TRISILICATE,
    ALUMINUM HYDROXIDE (OTC)
ALUPENT, METAPROTERENOL SULFATE
AMANTADINE HCL, AMANTADINE HYDROCHLORIDE
AMARYL, GLIMEPIRIDE
AMBENYL, BROMODIPHENHYDRAMINE
    HYDROCHLORIDE
AMBIEN, ZOLPIDEM TARTRATE
AMBISOME, AMPHOTERICIN B
AMBODRYL, BROMODIPHENHYDRAMINE
    HYDROCHLORIDE
AMCILL, AMPICILLIN/AMPICILLIN TRIHYDRATE
AMCINONIDE, AMCINONIDE
AMEN, MEDROXYPROGESTERONE ACETATE
AMERGE, NARATRIPTAN HYDROCHLORIDE
AMERSCAN MDP KIT, TECHNETIUM TC-99M
    MEDRONATE KIT
AMICAR, AMINOCAPROIC ACID
AMIDATE, ETOMIDATE
AMIKACIN SULFATE IN SODIUM CHLORIDE 0.9% IN
    PLASTIC CONTAINER, AMIKACIN SULFATE
AMIKACIN SULFATE, AMIKACIN SULFATE
AMIKIN IN SODIUM CHLORIDE 0.9% IN PLASTIC
    CONTAINER, AMIKACIN SULFATE
AMIKIN, AMIKACIN SULFATE

APPENDIX A
PRODUCT NAME INDEX (*continued*)

AMILORIDE HCL AND HYDROCHLOROTHIAZIDE, AMILORIDE HYDROCHLORIDE

AMILORIDE HCL, AMILORIDE HYDROCHLORIDE

AMINESS 5.2% ESSENTIAL AMINO ACIDS W/ HISTADINE, AMINO ACIDS

AMINOACETIC ACID 1.5% IN PLASTIC CONTAINER, GLYCINE

AMINOCAPROIC ACID IN PLASTIC CONTAINER, AMINOCAPROIC ACID

AMINOCAPROIC ACID, AMINOCAPROIC ACID

AMINOCAPROIC, AMINOCAPROIC ACID

AMINOHIPPURATE SODIUM, AMINOHIPPURATE SODIUM

AMINOPHYLLIN, AMINOPHYLLINE

AMINOPHYLLINE DYE FREE, AMINOPHYLLINE

AMINOPHYLLINE IN SODIUM CHLORIDE 0.45% IN PLASTIC CONTAINER, AMINOPHYLLINE

AMINOPHYLLINE IN SODIUM CHLORIDE 0.45%, AMINOPHYLLINE

AMINOPHYLLINE, AMINOPHYLLINE

AMINOSOL 5%, PROTEIN HYDROLYSATE

AMINOSYN 10% (PH6), AMINO ACIDS

AMINOSYN 10%, AMINO ACIDS

AMINOSYN 3.5% IN PLASTIC CONTAINER, AMINO ACIDS

AMINOSYN 3.5% M IN PLASTIC CONTAINER, AMINO ACIDS

AMINOSYN 3.5% M, AMINO ACIDS

AMINOSYN 3.5% W/ DEXTROSE 25% IN PLASTIC CONTAINER, AMINO ACIDS

AMINOSYN 3.5% W/ DEXTROSE 5% IN PLASTIC CONTAINER, AMINO ACIDS

AMINOSYN 3.5%, AMINO ACIDS

AMINOSYN 4.25% W/ DEXTROSE 25% IN PLASTIC CONTAINER, AMINO ACIDS

AMINOSYN 5%, AMINO ACIDS

AMINOSYN 7% (PH6), AMINO ACIDS

AMINOSYN 7% W/ ELECTROLYTES, AMINO ACIDS

AMINOSYN 7%, AMINO ACIDS

AMINOSYN 8.5% (PH6), AMINO ACIDS

AMINOSYN 8.5% W/ ELECTROLYTES, AMINO ACIDS

AMINOSYN 8.5%, AMINO ACIDS

AMINOSYN II 10% IN PLASTIC CONTAINER, AMINO ACIDS

AMINOSYN II 10% W/ ELECTROLYTES, AMINO ACIDS

AMINOSYN II 10%, AMINO ACIDS

AMINOSYN II 15% IN PLASTIC CONTAINER, AMINO ACIDS

AMINOSYN II 3.5% IN DEXTROSE 25% IN PLASTIC CONTAINER, AMINO ACIDS

AMINOSYN II 3.5% IN DEXTROSE 5% IN PLASTIC CONTAINER, AMINO ACIDS

AMINOSYN II 3.5% IN PLASTIC CONTAINER, AMINO ACIDS

AMINOSYN II 3.5% M IN DEXTROSE 5% IN PLASTIC CONTAINER, AMINO ACIDS

AMINOSYN II 3.5% M IN PLASTIC CONTAINER, AMINO ACIDS

AMINOSYN II 3.5% M, AMINO ACIDS

AMINOSYN II 3.5% W/ ELECTROLYTES IN DEXTROSE 25% IN PLASTIC CONTAINER, AMINO ACIDS

AMINOSYN II 3.5% W/ ELECTROLYTES IN DEXTROSE 25% W/ CALCIUM IN PLASTIC CONTAINER, AMINO ACIDS

AMINOSYN II 3.5%, AMINO ACIDS

AMINOSYN II 4.25% IN DEXTROSE 10% IN PLASTIC CONTAINER, AMINO ACIDS

AMINOSYN II 4.25% IN DEXTROSE 20% IN PLASTIC CONTAINER, AMINO ACIDS

AMINOSYN II 4.25% IN DEXTROSE 25% IN PLASTIC CONTAINER, AMINO ACIDS

AMINOSYN II 4.25% M IN DEXTROSE 10% IN PLASTIC CONTAINER, AMINO ACIDS

AMINOSYN II 4.25% W/ ELECT AND ADJUSTED PHOSPHATE IN DEXTROSE 10% IN PLASTIC CONTAINER, AMINO ACIDS

AMINOSYN II 4.25% W/ ELECTROLYTES IN DEXTROSE 20% W/ CALCIUM IN PLASTIC CONTAINER, AMINO ACIDS

AMINOSYN II 4.25% W/ ELECTROLYTES IN DEXTROSE 25% IN PLASTIC CONTAINER, AMINO ACIDS

AMINOSYN II 4.25% W/ ELECTROLYTES IN DEXTROSE 25% W/ CALCIUM IN PLASTIC CONTAINER, AMINO ACIDS

AMINOSYN II 5% IN DEXTROSE 25% IN PLASTIC CONTAINER, AMINO ACIDS

AMINOSYN II 5% W/ ELECTROLYTES IN DEXTROSE 25% W/ CALCIUM IN PLASTIC CONTAINER, AMINO ACIDS

AMINOSYN II 5%, AMINO ACIDS

AMINOSYN II 7% W/ ELECTROLYTES, AMINO ACIDS

AMINOSYN II 7%, AMINO ACIDS

AMINOSYN II 8.5% W/ ELECTROLYTES, AMINO ACIDS

AMINOSYN II 8.5%, AMINO ACIDS

AMINOSYN-HBC 7% IN PLASTIC CONTAINER, AMINO ACIDS

AMINOSYN-HBC 7%, AMINO ACIDS

AMINOSYN-HF 8%, AMINO ACIDS

AMINOSYN-PF 7%, AMINO ACIDS

AMINOSYN-PF 10%, AMINO ACIDS

AMINOSYN-RF 5.2%, AMINO ACIDS

AMIODARONE HCL, AMIODARONE HYDROCHLORIDE

AMIPAQUE, METRIZAMIDE

AMITID, AMITRIPTYLINE HYDROCHLORIDE

AMITRIL, AMITRIPTYLINE HYDROCHLORIDE

AMITRIPTYLINE HCL, AMITRIPTYLINE HYDROCHLORIDE

AMITRIPTYLINE HYDROCHLORIDE, AMITRIPTYLINE HYDROCHLORIDE

AMMONIUM CHLORIDE 0.9% IN NORMAL SALINE, AMMONIUM CHLORIDE

AMMONIUM CHLORIDE 2.14%, AMMONIUM CHLORIDE

AMMONIUM CHLORIDE IN PLASTIC CONTAINER, AMMONIUM CHLORIDE

AMMONIUM CHLORIDE, AMMONIUM CHLORIDE

AMMONIUM LACTATE, AMMONIUM LACTATE

AMNESTEEM, ISOTRETINOIN

AMNESTROGEN, ESTROGENS, ESTERIFIED

AMOSENE, MEPROBAMATE

AMOXAPINE, AMOXAPINE

AMOXICILLIN

AMOXICILLIN AND CLAVULANATE POTASSIUM, AMOXICILLIN

AMOXICILLIN AND CLAVULANATE POTSSSIUM, AMOXICILLIN

AMOXICILLIN PEDIATRIC, AMOXICILLIN

AMOXICILLIN, AMOXICILLIN

AMOXIL, AMOXICILLIN

AMPHETAMINE SULFATE, AMPHETAMINE SULFATE

AMPHICOL, CHLORAMPHENICOL

AMPHOTEC, AMPHOTERICIN B

AMPHOTERICIN B, AMPHOTERICIN B

AMPICILLIN AND SULBACTAM, AMPICILLIN SODIUM

AMPICILLIN SODIUM, AMPICILLIN SODIUM

AMPICILLIN TRIHYDRATE, AMPICILLIN/AMPICILLIN TRIHYDRATE

AMPICILLIN, AMPICILLIN/AMPICILLIN TRIHYDRATE

AMRINONE LACTATE, INAMRINONE LACTATE

AMRINONE, INAMRINONE LACTATE

AN-DTPA, TECHNETIUM TC-99M PENTETATE KIT

AN-MAA, TECHNETIUM TC-99M ALBUMIN AGGREGATED KIT

AN-SULFUR COLLOID, TECHNETIUM TC-99M SULFUR COLLOID KIT

APPENDIX A
PRODUCT NAME INDEX (*continued*)

ANADROL-50, OXYMETHOLONE
ANAFRANIL, CLOMIPRAMINE HYDROCHLORIDE
ANAPROX DS, NAPROXEN SODIUM
ANAPROX, NAPROXEN SODIUM
ANCEF IN DEXTROSE 5% IN PLASTIC CONTAINER,
    CEFAZOLIN SODIUM
ANCEF IN PLASTIC CONTAINER, CEFAZOLIN SODIUM
ANCEF IN SODIUM CHLORIDE 0.9% IN PLASTIC
    CONTAINER, CEFAZOLIN SODIUM
ANCEF, CEFAZOLIN SODIUM
ANCOBON, FLUCYTOSINE
ANDRODERM, TESTOSTERONE
ANDROGEL, TESTOSTERONE
ANDROID 5, METHYLTESTOSTERONE
ANDROID 10, METHYLTESTOSTERONE
ANDROID 25, METHYLTESTOSTERONE
ANDROID-F, FLUOXYMESTERONE
ANECTINE, SUCCINYLCHOLINE CHLORIDE
ANESTACON, LIDOCAINE HYDROCHLORIDE
ANEXSIA 5/325, ACETAMINOPHEN
ANEXSIA 7.5/325, ACETAMINOPHEN
ANEXSIA 7.5/650, ACETAMINOPHEN
ANEXSIA, ACETAMINOPHEN
ANGIO-CONRAY, IOTHALAMATE SODIUM
ANGIOMAX, BIVALIRUDIN
ANGIOVIST 282, DIATRIZOATE MEGLUMINE
ANGIOVIST 292, DIATRIZOATE MEGLUMINE
ANGIOVIST 370, DIATRIZOATE MEGLUMINE
ANHYDRON, CYCLOTHIAZIDE
ANISOTROPINE METHYLBROMIDE, ANISOTROPINE
    METHYLBROMIDE
ANOQUAN, ACETAMINOPHEN
ANSAID, FLURBIPROFEN
ANSOLYSEN, PENTOLINIUM TARTRATE
ANSPOR, CEPHRADINE
ANTABUSE, DISULFIRAM
ANTAGON, GANIRELIX ACETATE
ANTAGONATE, CHLORPHENIRAMINE MALEATE
ANTEPAR, PIPERAZINE CITRATE
ANTITUSSIVE, DIPHENHYDRAMINE HYDROCHLORIDE
    (OTC)
ANTIVERT, MECLIZINE HYDROCHLORIDE
ANTIZOL, FOMEPIZOLE
ANTRENYL, OXYPHENONIUM BROMIDE
ANTURANE, SULFINPYRAZONE
ANUSOL HC, HYDROCORTISONE
ANZEMET, DOLASETRON MESYLATE MONOHYDRATE
APAP W/ CODEINE PHOSPHATE, ACETAMINOPHEN
APHTHASOL, AMLEXANOX
APOGEN, GENTAMICIN SULFATE
APRESAZIDE, HYDRALAZINE HYDROCHLORIDE
APRESOLINE, HYDRALAZINE HYDROCHLORIDE
APRESOLINE-ESIDRIX, HYDRALAZINE
    HYDROCHLORIDE
AQUAMEPHYTON, PHYTONADIONE
AQUAPHYLLIN, THEOPHYLLINE
AQUASOL A, VITAMIN A
AQUASOL A, VITAMIN A PALMITATE
AQUATAG, BENZTHIAZIDE
AQUATENSEN, METHYCLOTHIAZIDE
ARALEN HCL, CHLOROQUINE HYDROCHLORIDE
ARALEN PHOSPHATE W/ PRIMAQUINE PHOSPHATE,
    CHLOROQUINE PHOSPHATE
ARALEN, CHLOROQUINE PHOSPHATE
ARAMINE, METARAMINOL BITARTRATE
ARAVA, LEFLUNOMIDE
ARDUAN, PIPECURONIUM BROMIDE
AREDIA, PAMIDRONATE DISODIUM
ARESTIN, MINOCYCLINE HYDROCHLORIDE

ARESTOCAINE HCL W/ LEVONORDEFRIN,
    LEVONORDEFRIN
ARESTOCAINE HCL, MEPIVACAINE HYDROCHLORIDE
ARFONAD, TRIMETHAPHAN CAMSYLATE
ARGATROBAN, ARGATROBAN
ARICEPT, DONEPEZIL HYDROCHLORIDE
ARIMIDEX, ANASTROZOLE
ARISTOCORT A, TRIAMCINOLONE ACETONIDE
ARISTOCORT, TRIAMCINOLONE
ARISTOCORT, TRIAMCINOLONE ACETONIDE
ARISTOCORT, TRIAMCINOLONE DIACETATE
ARISTOGEL, TRIAMCINOLONE ACETONIDE
ARISTOSPAN, TRIAMCINOLONE HEXACETONIDE
ARIXTRA, FONDAPARINUX SODIUM
AROMASIN, EXEMESTANE
ARTANE, TRIHEXYPHENIDYL HYDROCHLORIDE
ARTHROTEC, DICLOFENAC SODIUM
ASACOL, MESALAMINE
ASBRON, THEOPHYLLINE SODIUM GLYCINATE
ASELLACRIN 2, SOMATROPIN
ASELLACRIN 10, SOMATROPIN
ASENDIN, AMOXAPINE
ASPIRIN AND CAFFEINE W/ BUTALBITAL, ASPIRIN
ASTELIN, AZELASTINE HYDROCHLORIDE
ASTRAMORPH PF, MORPHINE SULFATE
ATACAND HCT, CANDESARTAN CILEXETIL
ATACAND, CANDESARTAN CILEXETIL
ATARAX, HYDROXYZINE HYDROCHLORIDE
ATENOLOL AND CHLORTHALIDONE, ATENOLOL
ATENOLOL, ATENOLOL
ATHROMBIN, WARFARIN SODIUM
ATHROMBIN-K, WARFARIN POTASSIUM
ATIVAN, LORAZEPAM
ATNAA, ATROPINE
ATRACURIUM BESYLATE PRESERVATIVE FREE,
    ATRACURIUM BESYLATE
ATRACURIUM BESYLATE, ATRACURIUM BESYLATE
ATRIDOX, DOXYCYCLINE HYCLATE
ATROMID-S, CLOFIBRATE
ATROPEN, ATROPINE
ATROPINE AND DEMEROL, ATROPINE SULFATE
ATROPINE SULFATE ANSYR PLASTIC SYRINGE,
    ATROPINE SULFATE
ATROPINE SULFATE, ATROPINE SULFATE
ATROPINE, ATROPINE
ATROVENT, IPRATROPIUM BROMIDE
AUGMENTIN '125', AMOXICILLIN
AUGMENTIN '200', AMOXICILLIN
AUGMENTIN '250', AMOXICILLIN
AUGMENTIN '400', AMOXICILLIN
AUGMENTIN '500', AMOXICILLIN
AUGMENTIN '875', AMOXICILLIN
AUGMENTIN ES-600, AMOXICILLIN
AUGMENTIN XR, AMOXICILLIN
AUREOMYCIN, CHLORTETRACYCLINE
    HYDROCHLORIDE
AVAGARD, ALCOHOL (OTC)
AVAGE, TAZAROTENE
AVALIDE, HYDROCHLOROTHIAZIDE
AVANDAMET, METFORMIN HYDROCHLORIDE
AVANDIA, ROSIGLITAZONE MALEATE
AVAPRO, IRBESARTAN
AVC, SULFANILAMIDE
AVELOX IN SODIUM CHLORIDE 0.8% IN PLASTIC
    CONTAINER, MOXIFLOXACIN HYDROCHLORIDE
AVELOX, MOXIFLOXACIN HYDROCHLORIDE
AVENTYL HCL, NORTRIPTYLINE HYDROCHLORIDE
AVIANE-21, ETHINYL ESTRADIOL
AVIANE-28, ETHINYL ESTRADIOL

APPENDIX A
PRODUCT NAME INDEX (*continued*)

AVINZA, MORPHINE SULFATE
AVITA, TRETINOIN
AVODART, DUTASTERIDE
AXERT, ALMOTRIPTAN MALATE
AXID AR, NIZATIDINE (OTC)
AXID, NIZATIDINE
AXOTAL, ASPIRIN
AYGESTIN, NORETHINDRONE ACETATE
AZACTAM IN PLASTIC CONTAINER, AZTREONAM
AZACTAM, AZTREONAM
AZASAN, AZATHIOPRINE
AZATHIOPRINE SODIUM, AZATHIOPRINE SODIUM
AZATHIOPRINE, AZATHIOPRINE
AZATHIOPRINE, AZATHIOPRINE SODIUM
AZDONE, ASPIRIN
AZELEX, AZELAIC ACID
AZLIN, AZLOCILLIN SODIUM
AZMACORT, TRIAMCINOLONE ACETONIDE
AZO GANTANOL, PHENAZOPYRIDINE HYDROCHLORIDE
AZO GANTRISIN, PHENAZOPYRIDINE HYDROCHLORIDE
AZOLID, PHENYLBUTAZONE
AZOPT, BRINZOLAMIDE
AZULFIDINE EN-TABS, SULFASALAZINE
AZULFIDINE, SULFASALAZINE

B

BACI-RX, BACITRACIN
BACIGUENT, BACITRACIN
BACIIM, BACITRACIN
BACITRACIN ZINC AND POLYMYXIN B SULFATE, BACITRACIN ZINC
BACITRACIN ZINC-NEOMYCIN SULFATE-POLYMYXIN B SULFATE, BACITRACIN ZINC
BACITRACIN ZINC-NEOMYCIN SULFATE-POLYMYXIN B SULFATE, BACITRACIN ZINC (OTC)
BACITRACIN ZINC-POLYMYXIN B SULFATE, BACITRACIN ZINC (OTC)
BACITRACIN, BACITRACIN
BACITRACIN, BACITRACIN (OTC)
BACITRACIN-NEOMYCIN-POLYMYXIN W/ HYDROCORTISONE ACETATE, BACITRACIN
BACITRACIN-NEOMYCIN-POLYMYXIN, BACITRACIN ZINC
BACLOFEN, BACLOFEN
BACTERIOSTATIC SODIUM CHLORIDE 0.9% IN PLASTIC CONTAINER, SODIUM CHLORIDE
BACTERIOSTATIC WATER FOR INJECTION IN PLASTIC CONTAINER, WATER FOR INJECTION, STERILE
BACTOCILL IN PLASTIC CONTAINER, OXACILLIN SODIUM
BACTOCILL, OXACILLIN SODIUM
BACTRIM DS, SULFAMETHOXAZOLE
BACTRIM PEDIATRIC, SULFAMETHOXAZOLE
BACTRIM, SULFAMETHOXAZOLE
BACTROBAN, MUPIROCIN
BACTROBAN, MUPIROCIN CALCIUM
BAL, DIMERCAPROL
BALNEOL-HC, HYDROCORTISONE
BAMATE, MEPROBAMATE
BANAN, CEFPODOXIME PROXETIL
BANCAP HC, ACETAMINOPHEN
BANCAP, ACETAMINOPHEN
BANTHINE, METHANTHELINE BROMIDE
BAROS, SODIUM BICARBONATE
BARSTATIN 100, NYSTATIN
BAYCOL, CERIVASTATIN SODIUM
BAYER EXTRA STRENGTH ASPIRIN FOR MIGRAINE PAIN, ASPIRIN (OTC)

BECLOVENT, BECLOMETHASONE DIPROPIONATE
BECONASE AQ, BECLOMETHASONE DIPROPIONATE MONOHYDRATE
BECONASE, BECLOMETHASONE DIPROPIONATE
BEEPEN-VK, PENICILLIN V POTASSIUM
BELDIN, DIPHENHYDRAMINE HYDROCHLORIDE (OTC)
BELIX, DIPHENHYDRAMINE HYDROCHLORIDE
BENADRYL PRESERVATIVE FREE, DIPHENHYDRAMINE HYDROCHLORIDE
BENADRYL, DIPHENHYDRAMINE HYDROCHLORIDE
BENDECTIN, DOXYLAMINE SUCCINATE
BENDOPA, LEVODOPA
BENEMID, PROBENECID
BENICAR HCT, HYDROCHLOROTHIAZIDE
BENICAR, OLMESARTAN MEDOXOMIL
BENOQUIN, MONOBENZONE
BENOXINATE HCL, BENOXINATE HYDROCHLORIDE
BENSULFOID, SULFUR
BENTYL PRESERVATIVE FREE, DICYCLOMINE HYDROCHLORIDE
BENTYL, DICYCLOMINE HYDROCHLORIDE
BENYLIN, DIPHENHYDRAMINE HYDROCHLORIDE (OTC)
BENZACLIN, BENZOYL PEROXIDE
BENZAMYCIN PAK, BENZOYL PEROXIDE
BENZAMYCIN, BENZOYL PEROXIDE
BENZONATATE, BENZONATATE
BENZTHIAZIDE, BENZTHIAZIDE
BENZTROPINE MESYLATE, BENZTROPINE MESYLATE
BENZYL BENZOATE, BENZYL BENZOATE
BEPADIN, BEPRIDIL HYDROCHLORIDE
BEROCCA PN, ASCORBIC ACID
BERUBIGEN, CYANOCOBALAMIN
BETA-2, ISOETHARINE HYDROCHLORIDE
BETA-HC, HYDROCORTISONE
BETA-VAL, BETAMETHASONE VALERATE
BETADERM, BETAMETHASONE VALERATE
BETADINE, POVIDONE-IODINE
BETAGAN, LEVOBUNOLOL HYDROCHLORIDE
BETALIN 12, CYANOCOBALAMIN
BETALIN S, THIAMINE HYDROCHLORIDE
BETAMETHASONE DIPROPIONATE, BETAMETHASONE DIPROPIONATE
BETAMETHASONE SODIUM PHOSPHATE, BETAMETHASONE SODIUM PHOSPHATE
BETAMETHASONE VALERATE, BETAMETHASONE VALERATE
BETAPACE AF, SOTALOL HYDROCHLORIDE
BETAPACE, SOTALOL HYDROCHLORIDE
BETAPAR, MEPREDNISONE
BETAPEN-VK, PENICILLIN V POTASSIUM
BETAPRONE, PROPIOLACTONE
BETATREX, BETAMETHASONE VALERATE
BETAXOLOL HCL, BETAXOLOL HYDROCHLORIDE
BETAXOLOL, BETAXOLOL HYDROCHLORIDE
BETAXON, LEVOBETAXOLOL HYDROCHLORIDE
BETHANECHOL CHLORIDE, BETHANECHOL CHLORIDE
BETIMOL, TIMOLOL
BETOPTIC PILO, BETAXOLOL HYDROCHLORIDE
BETOPTIC S, BETAXOLOL HYDROCHLORIDE
BETOPTIC, BETAXOLOL HYDROCHLORIDE
BEXTRA, VALDECOXIB
BIAXIN XL, CLARITHROMYCIN
BIAXIN, CLARITHROMYCIN
BICILLIN C-R 900/300, PENICILLIN G BENZATHINE
BICILLIN C-R, PENICILLIN G BENZATHINE
BICILLIN L-A, PENICILLIN G BENZATHINE
BICILLIN, PENICILLIN G BENZATHINE
BICNU, CARMUSTINE
BILIVIST, IPODATE SODIUM

APPENDIX A
PRODUCT NAME INDEX (*continued*)

BILOPAQUE, TYROPANOATE SODIUM
BILTRICIDE, PRAZIQUANTEL
BIO-TROPIN, SOMATROPIN RECOMBINANT
BIOSCRUB, CHLORHEXIDINE GLUCONATE (OTC)
BIPHETAMINE 7.5, AMPHETAMINE RESIN COMPLEX
BIPHETAMINE 12.5, AMPHETAMINE RESIN COMPLEX
BIPHETAMINE 20, AMPHETAMINE RESIN COMPLEX
BIPHETAP, BROMPHENIRAMINE MALEATE
BISOPROLOL FUMARATE AND
    HYDROCHLOROTHIAZIDE, BISOPROLOL FUMARATE
BISOPROLOL FUMARATE, BISOPROLOL FUMARATE
BLENOXANE, BLEOMYCIN SULFATE
BLEOMYCIN SULFATE, BLEOMYCIN SULFATE
BLEOMYCIN, BLEOMYCIN SULFATE
BLEPH-10, SULFACETAMIDE SODIUM
BLEPH-30, SULFACETAMIDE SODIUM
BLEPHAMIDE S.O.P., PREDNISOLONE ACETATE
BLEPHAMIDE, PREDNISOLONE ACETATE
BLOCADREN, TIMOLOL MALEATE
BONIVA, IBANDRONATE SODIUM
BONTRIL PDM, PHENDIMETRAZINE TARTRATE
BONTRIL, PHENDIMETRAZINE TARTRATE
BOROFAIR, ACETIC ACID, GLACIAL
BRANCHAMIN 4% IN PLASTIC CONTAINER, AMINO
    ACIDS
BRANCHAMIN 4%, AMINO ACIDS
BRAVELLE, UROFOLLITROPIN
BREATHTEK UBT FOR H-PYLORI, UREA, C-13
BRETHAIRE, TERBUTALINE SULFATE
BRETHINE, TERBUTALINE SULFATE
BRETYLIUM TOSYLATE IN DEXTROSE 5% IN PLASTIC
    CONTAINER, BRETYLIUM TOSYLATE
BRETYLIUM TOSYLATE IN DEXTROSE 5%, BRETYLIUM
    TOSYLATE
BRETYLIUM TOSYLATE IN PLASTIC CONTAINER,
    BRETYLIUM TOSYLATE
BRETYLIUM TOSYLATE, BRETYLIUM TOSYLATE
BRETYLOL, BRETYLIUM TOSYLATE
BREVIBLOC DOUBLE STRENGTH IN PLASTIC
    CONTAINER, ESMOLOL HYDROCHLORIDE
BREVIBLOC IN PLASTIC CONTAINER, ESMOLOL
    HYDROCHLORIDE
BREVIBLOC, ESMOLOL HYDROCHLORIDE
BREVICON 21-DAY, ETHINYL ESTRADIOL
BREVICON 28-DAY, ETHINYL ESTRADIOL
BREVITAL SODIUM, METHOHEXITAL SODIUM
BRIAN CARE, CHLORHEXIDINE GLUCONATE (OTC)
BRICANYL, TERBUTALINE SULFATE
BRIMONIDINE TARTRATE, BRIMONIDINE TARTRATE
BRISTACYCLINE, TETRACYCLINE HYDROCHLORIDE
BRISTAGEN, GENTAMICIN SULFATE
BRISTAMYCIN, ERYTHROMYCIN STEARATE
BROMANATE DC, BROMPHENIRAMINE MALEATE
BROMANATE DM, BROMPHENIRAMINE MALEATE
BROMANATE, BROMPHENIRAMINE MALEATE
BROMANYL, BROMODIPHENHYDRAMINE
    HYDROCHLORIDE
BROMATAPP, BROMPHENIRAMINE MALEATE (OTC)
BROMFED-DM, BROMPHENIRAMINE MALEATE
BROMOCRIPTINE MESYLATE, BROMOCRIPTINE
    MESYLATE
BROMPHENIRAMINE MALEATE, BROMPHENIRAMINE
    MALEATE
BROMPHERIL, DEXBROMPHENIRAMINE MALEATE (OTC)
BRONCHO SALINE, SODIUM CHLORIDE (OTC)
BRONITIN MIST, EPINEPHRINE BITARTRATE (OTC)
BRONKAID MIST, EPINEPHRINE (OTC)
BRONKODYL, THEOPHYLLINE
BRONKOMETER, ISOETHARINE MESYLATE

BRONKOSOL, ISOETHARINE HYDROCHLORIDE
BRYREL, PIPERAZINE CITRATE
BSS PLUS, CALCIUM CHLORIDE
BSS, CALCIUM CHLORIDE
BUCET, ACETAMINOPHEN
BUCLADIN-S, BUCLIZINE HYDROCHLORIDE
BUMETANIDE, BUMETANIDE
BUMEX, BUMETANIDE
BUPHENYL, SODIUM PHENYLBUTYRATE
BUPIVACAINE HCL AND EPINEPHRINE, BUPIVACAINE
    HYDROCHLORIDE
BUPIVACAINE HCL KIT, BUPIVACAINE HYDROCHLORIDE
BUPIVACAINE HCL, BUPIVACAINE HYDROCHLORIDE
BUPIVACAINE, BUPIVACAINE HYDROCHLORIDE
BUPIVACINE HCL PRESERVATIVE FREE, BUPIVACAINE
    HYDROCHLORIDE
BUPRENEX, BUPRENORPHINE HYDROCHLORIDE
BUPRENORPHINE HCL, BUPRENORPHINE
    HYDROCHLORIDE
BUPROPION HCL, BUPROPION HYDROCHLORIDE
BUSPAR, BUSPIRONE HYDROCHLORIDE
BUSPIRONE HCL, BUSPIRONE HYDROCHLORIDE
BUSULFEX, BUSULFAN
BUTABARB, BUTABARBITAL SODIUM
BUTABARBITAL SODIUM, BUTABARBITAL SODIUM
BUTARARBITAL, BUTABARBITAL SODIUM
BUTAL COMPOUND, ASPIRIN
BUTALAN, BUTABARBITAL SODIUM
BUTALBITAL AND ACETAMINOPHEN, ACETAMINOPHEN
BUTALBITAL ASPIRIN AND CAFFEINE, ASPIRIN
BUTALBITAL COMPOUND, ASPIRIN
BUTALBITAL W/ ASPIRIN ACETAMINOPHEN; AND
    CAFFEINE WITH CODEINE PHOSPHATE,
    ACETAMINOPHEN
BUTAPAP, ACETAMINOPHEN
BUTAZOLIDIN, PHENYLBUTAZONE
BUTICAPS, BUTABARBITAL SODIUM
BUTISOL SODIUM, BUTABARBITAL SODIUM
BUTORPHANOL TARTRATE PRESERVATIVE FREE,
    BUTORPHANOL TARTRATE
BUTORPHANOL TARTRATE, BUTORPHANOL TARTRATE

C

C-SOLVE-2, ERYTHROMYCIN
CAFCIT, CAFFEINE CITRATE
CAFERGOT, CAFFEINE
CALAN, VERAPAMIL HYDROCHLORIDE
CALCIBIND, CELLULOSE SODIUM PHOSPHATE
CALCIJEX, CALCITRIOL
CALCIMAR, CALCITONIN, SALMON
CALCIPARINE, HEPARIN CALCIUM
CALCITONIN-SALMON, CALCITONIN, SALMON
CALCITRIOL, CALCITRIOL
CALCIUM CHLORIDE 10% IN PLASTIC CONTAINER,
    CALCIUM CHLORIDE
CALCIUM DISODIUM VERSENATE, EDETATE CALCIUM
    DISODIUM
CALCIUM GLUCEPTATE, CALCIUM GLUCEPTATE
CALDEROL, CALCIFEDIOL
CALMURID HC, HYDROCORTISONE
CAM-AP-ES, HYDRALAZINE HYDROCHLORIDE
CAM-METRAZINE, PHENDIMETRAZINE TARTRATE
CAMILA, NORETHINDRONE
CAMOQUIN HCL, AMODIAQUINE HYDROCHLORIDE
CAMPTOSAR, IRINOTECAN HYDROCHLORIDE
CANASA, MESALAMINE
CANCIDAS, CASPOFUNGIN ACETATE
CANDEX, NYSTATIN

APPENDIX A
PRODUCT NAME INDEX (*continued*)

CANTIL, MEPENZOLATE BROMIDE
CAP-PROFEN, IBUPROFEN (OTC)
CAPASTAT SULFATE, CAPREOMYCIN SULFATE
CAPITAL AND CODEINE, ACETAMINOPHEN
CAPITAL WITH CODEINE, ACETAMINOPHEN
CAPITROL, CHLOROXINE
CAPOTEN, CAPTOPRIL
CAPOZIDE 25/15, CAPTOPRIL
CAPOZIDE 25/25, CAPTOPRIL
CAPOZIDE 50/15, CAPTOPRIL
CAPOZIDE 50/25, CAPTOPRIL
CAPTOPRIL AND HYDROCHLOROTHIAZIDE, CAPTOPRIL
CAPTOPRIL, CAPTOPRIL
CARAC, FLUOROURACIL
CARAFATE, SUCRALFATE
CARBACHOL, CARBACHOL
CARBAMAZEPINE, CARBAMAZEPINE
CARBASTAT, CARBACHOL
CARBATROL, CARBAMAZEPINE
CARBIDOPA AND LEVODOPA, CARBIDOPA
CARBINOXAMINE MALEATE, CARBINOXAMINE
    MALEATE
CARBOCAINE W/ NEO-COBEFRIN, LEVONORDEFRIN
CARBOCAINE, MEPIVACAINE HYDROCHLORIDE
CARDENE SR, NICARDIPINE HYDROCHLORIDE
CARDENE, NICARDIPINE HYDROCHLORIDE
CARDIO-GREEN, INDOCYANINE GREEN
CARDIOGEN-82, RUBIDIUM CHLORIDE RB-82
CARDIOGRAFIN, DIATRIZOATE MEGLUMINE
CARDIOLITE, TECHNETIUM TC-99M SESTAMIBI KIT
CARDIOPLEGIC IN PLASTIC CONTAINER, CALCIUM
    CHLORIDE
CARDIOQUIN, QUINIDINE POLYGALACTURONATE
CARDIOTEC, TECHNETIUM TC-99M TEBOROXIME KIT
CARDIZEM CD, DILTIAZEM HYDROCHLORIDE
CARDIZEM LA, DILTIAZEM HYDROCHLORIDE
CARDIZEM SR, DILTIAZEM HYDROCHLORIDE
CARDIZEM, DILTIAZEM HYDROCHLORIDE
CARDRASE, ETHOXZOLAMIDE
CARDURA, DOXAZOSIN MESYLATE
CARISOPRODOL AND ASPIRIN, ASPIRIN
CARISOPRODOL COMPOUND, ASPIRIN
CARISOPRODOL, ASPIRIN AND CODEINE PHOSPHATE,
    ASPIRIN
CARISOPRODOL, CARISOPRODOL
CARMOL HC, HYDROCORTISONE ACETATE
CARNITOR, LEVOCARNITINE
CARTEOLOL HCL, CARTEOLOL HYDROCHLORIDE
CARTIA XT, DILTIAZEM HYDROCHLORIDE
CARTROL, CARTEOLOL HYDROCHLORIDE
CASODEX, BICALUTAMIDE
CATAFLAM, DICLOFENAC POTASSIUM
CATAPRES, CLONIDINE HYDROCHLORIDE
CATAPRES-TTS-1, CLONIDINE
CATAPRES-TTS-2, CLONIDINE
CATAPRES-TTS-3, CLONIDINE
CATARASE, CHYMOTRYPSIN
CAVERJECT, ALPROSTADIL
CECLOR CD, CEFACLOR
CECLOR, CEFACLOR
CEDAX, CEFTIBUTEN DIHYDRATE
CEDILANID-D, DESLANOSIDE
CEENU, LOMUSTINE
CEFACLOR, CEFACLOR
CEFADROXIL, CEFADROXIL/CEFADROXIL
    HEMIHYDRATE
CEFADYL, CEPHAPIRIN SODIUM
CEFAZOLIN AND DEXTROSE, CEFAZOLIN SODIUM
CEFAZOLIN SODIUM, CEFAZOLIN SODIUM

CEFIZOX IN DEXTROSE 5% IN PLASTIC CONTAINER,
    CEFTIZOXIME SODIUM
CEFIZOX IN PLASTIC CONTAINER, CEFTIZOXIME
    SODIUM
CEFIZOX, CEFTIZOXIME SODIUM
CEFMAX, CEFMENOXIME HYDROCHLORIDE
CEFOBID IN PLASTIC CONTAINER, CEFOPERAZONE
    SODIUM
CEFOBID, CEFOPERAZONE SODIUM
CEFOTAN IN PLASTIC CONTAINER, CEFOTETAN
    DISODIUM
CEFOTAN, CEFOTETAN DISODIUM
CEFOTAXIME, CEFOTAXIME SODIUM
CEFOXITIN, CEFOXITIN SODIUM
CEFPIRAMIDE SODIUM, CEFPIRAMIDE SODIUM
CEFPODOXIME PROXETIL, CEFPODOXIME PROXETIL
CEFTAZIDIME SODIUM IN PLASTIC CONTAINER,
    CEFTAZIDIME SODIUM
CEFTIN, CEFUROXIME AXETIL
CEFUROXIME AND DEXTROSE IN DUPLEX CONTAINER,
    CEFUROXIME SODIUM
CEFUROXIME AXETIL, CEFUROXIME AXETIL
CEFUROXIME SODIUM, CEFUROXIME SODIUM
CEFUROXIME, CEFUROXIME SODIUM
CEFZIL, CEFPROZIL
CELEBREX, CELECOXIB
CELESTONE SOLUSPAN, BETAMETHASONE ACETATE
CELESTONE, BETAMETHASONE
CELESTONE, BETAMETHASONE SODIUM PHOSPHATE
CELEXA, CITALOPRAM HYDROBROMIDE
CELLCEPT, MYCOPHENOLATE MOFETIL
CELLCEPT, MYCOPHENOLATE MOFETIL
    HYDROCHLORIDE
CELONTIN, METHSUXIMIDE
CENESTIN, ESTROGENS, CONJUGATED SYNTHETIC A
CENTRAX, PRAZEPAM
CEPHALEXIN, CEPHALEXIN
CEPHALOTHIN SODIUM W/ DEXTROSE IN PLASTIC
    CONTAINER, CEPHALOTHIN SODIUM
CEPHALOTHIN SODIUM W/ SODIUM CHLORIDE IN
    PLASTIC CONTAINER, CEPHALOTHIN SODIUM
CEPHALOTHIN SODIUM, CEPHALOTHIN SODIUM
CEPHALOTHIN, CEPHALOTHIN SODIUM
CEPHAPIRIN SODIUM, CEPHAPIRIN SODIUM
CEPHRADINE, CEPHRADINE
CEPHULAC, LACTULOSE
CEPTAZ, CEFTAZIDIME (ARGININE FORMULATION)
CERADON, CEFOTIAM HYDROCHLORIDE
CEREBYX, FOSPHENYTOIN SODIUM
CEREDASE, ALGLUCERASE
CERETEC, TECHNETIUM TC-99M EXAMETAZIME KIT
CEREZYME, IMIGLUCERASE
CERNEVIT-12, ALPHA-TOCOPHEROL
CERUBIDINE, DAUNORUBICIN HYDROCHLORIDE
CERUMENEX, TROLAMINE POLYPEPTIDE OLEATE
    CONDENSATE
CERVIDIL, DINOPROSTONE
CESAMET, NABILONE
CETACORT, HYDROCORTISONE
CETAMIDE, SULFACETAMIDE SODIUM
CETAPRED, PREDNISOLONE ACETATE
CETROTIDE, CETRORELIX
CHEMET, SUCCIMER
CHENIX, CHENODIOL
CHG SCRUB, CHLORHEXIDINE GLUCONATE (OTC)
CHIBROXIN, NORFLOXACIN
CHILDREN'S ADVIL COLD, IBUPROFEN (OTC)
CHILDREN'S ADVIL, IBUPROFEN
CHILDREN'S ADVIL, IBUPROFEN (OTC)

APPENDIX A
PRODUCT NAME INDEX (*continued*)

CHILDREN'S ADVIL-FLAVORED, IBUPROFEN (OTC)
CHILDREN'S IBUPROFEN, IBUPROFEN (OTC)
CHILDREN'S MOTRIN COLD, IBUPROFEN (OTC)
CHILDREN'S MOTRIN, IBUPROFEN (OTC)
CHIROCAINE, LEVOBUPIVACAINE HYDROCHLORIDE
CHLOR-TRIMETON, CHLORPHENIRAMINE MALEATE
CHLOR-TRIMETON, CHLORPHENIRAMINE MALEATE
    (OTC)
CHLORAMPHENICOL SODIUM SUCCINATE,
    CHLORAMPHENICOL SODIUM SUCCINATE
CHLORAMPHENICOL, CHLORAMPHENICOL
CHLORAMPHENICOL, CHLORAMPHENICOL SODIUM
    SUCCINATE
CHLORAPREP ONE-STEP SEPP, CHLORHEXIDINE
    GLUCONATE (OTC)
CHLORAPREP, CHLORHEXIDINE GLUCONATE (OTC)
CHLORDIAZACHEL, CHLORDIAZEPOXIDE
    HYDROCHLORIDE
CHLORDIAZEPOXIDE AND AMITRIPTYLINE HCL,
    AMITRIPTYLINE HYDROCHLORIDE
CHLORDIAZEPOXIDE HCL, CHLORDIAZEPOXIDE
    HYDROCHLORIDE
CHLORHEXIDINE GLUCONATE, CHLORHEXIDINE
    GLUCONATE
CHLORHEXIDINE GLUCONATE, CHLORHEXIDINE
    GLUCONATE (OTC)
CHLORMERODRIN HG 197, CHLORMERODRIN, HG-197
CHLOROFAIR, CHLORAMPHENICOL
CHLOROHENIRAMINE MALEATE AND
    PHENYLPROPANOLAMINE HCL,
    CHLORPHENIRAMINE MALEATE
CHLOROMYCETIN HYDROCORTISONE,
    CHLORAMPHENICOL
CHLOROMYCETIN PALMITATE, CHLORAMPHENICOL
    PALMITATE
CHLOROMYCETIN, CHLORAMPHENICOL
CHLOROMYCETIN, CHLORAMPHENICOL SODIUM
    SUCCINATE
CHLOROMYXIN, CHLORAMPHENICOL
CHLOROPROCAINE HCL, CHLOROPROCAINE
    HYDROCHLORIDE
CHLOROPTIC S.O.P., CHLORAMPHENICOL
CHLOROPTIC, CHLORAMPHENICOL
CHLOROPTIC-P S.O.P., CHLORAMPHENICOL
CHLOROQUINE PHOSPHATE, CHLOROQUINE
    PHOSPHATE
CHLOROTHIAZIDE AND RESERPINE, CHLOROTHIAZIDE
CHLOROTHIAZIDE W/ RESERPINE, CHLOROTHIAZIDE
CHLOROTHIAZIDE, CHLOROTHIAZIDE
CHLOROTHIAZIDE-RESERPINE, CHLOROTHIAZIDE
CHLOROTRIANISENE, CHLOROTRIANISENE
CHLORPHENIRAMINE MALEATE AND
    PHENYLPROPANOLAMINE HCL,
    CHLORPHENIRAMINE MALEATE
CHLORPHENIRAMINE MALEATE, CHLORPHENIRAMINE
    MALEATE
CHLORPHENIRAMINE MALEATE, CHLORPHENIRAMINE
    MALEATE (OTC)
CHLORPROMAZINE HCL INTENSOL, CHLORPROMAZINE
    HYDROCHLORIDE
CHLORPROMAZINE HCL, CHLORPROMAZINE
    HYDROCHLORIDE
CHLORPROPAMIDE, CHLORPROPAMIDE
CHLORTHALIDONE, CHLORTHALIDONE
CHLORZOXAZONE, CHLORZOXAZONE
CHOLAC, LACTULOSE
CHOLEBRINE, IOCETAMIC ACID
CHOLEDYL SA, OXTRIPHYLLINE
CHOLEDYL, OXTRIPHYLLINE

CHOLESTYRAMINE LIGHT, CHOLESTYRAMINE
CHOLESTYRAMINE, CHOLESTYRAMINE
CHOLETEC, TECHNETIUM TC-99M MEBROFENIN KIT
CHOLOGRAFIN MEGLUMINE, IODIPAMIDE MEGLUMINE
CHOLOGRAFIN SODIUM, IODIPAMIDE SODIUM
CHOLOVUE, IODOXAMATE MEGLUMINE
CHOLOXIN, DEXTROTHYROXINE SODIUM
CHOLYBAR, CHOLESTYRAMINE
CHORIONIC GONADOTROPIN, GONADOTROPIN,
    CHORIONIC
CHROMALBIN, ALBUMIN CHROMATED CR-51 SERUM
CHROMIC CHLORIDE IN PLASTIC CONTAINER,
    CHROMIC CHLORIDE
CHROMIC CHLORIDE, CHROMIC CHLORIDE
CHROMITOPE SODIUM, SODIUM CHROMATE, CR-51
CHRONULAC, LACTULOSE
CHYMEX, BENTIROMIDE
CHYMODIACTIN, CHYMOPAPAIN
CIBACALCIN, CALCITONIN HUMAN
CIDA-STAT, CHLORHEXIDINE GLUCONATE (OTC)
CILOXAN, CIPROFLOXACIN HYDROCHLORIDE
CIMETIDINE HCL IN SODIUM CHLORIDE 0.9% IN PLASTIC
    CONTAINER, CIMETIDINE HYDROCHLORIDE
CIMETIDINE HCL, CIMETIDINE
CIMETIDINE HCL, CIMETIDINE HYDROCHLORIDE
CIMETIDINE, CIMETIDINE
CIMETIDINE, CIMETIDINE (OTC)
CIN-QUIN, QUINIDINE SULFATE
CINNASIL, RESCINNAMINE
CINOBAC, CINOXACIN
CINOXACIN, CINOXACIN
CINTICHEM TECHNETIUM 99M HEDSPA, TECHNETIUM
    TC-99M ETIDRONATE KIT
CIPRO HC, CIPROFLOXACIN HYDROCHLORIDE
CIPRO IN DEXTROSE 5% IN PLASTIC CONTAINER,
    CIPROFLOXACIN
CIPRO IN SODIUM CHLORIDE 0.9% IN PLASTIC
    CONTAINER, CIPROFLOXACIN
CIPRO XR, CIPROFLOXACIN
CIPRO, CIPROFLOXACIN
CIPRO, CIPROFLOXACIN HYDROCHLORIDE
CIRCANOL, ERGOLOID MESYLATES
CIS-MDP, TECHNETIUM TC-99M MEDRONATE KIT
CIS-PYRO, TECHNETIUM TC-99M PYROPHOSPHATE KIT
CISPLATIN, CISPLATIN
CITANEST FORTE, EPINEPHRINE BITARTRATE
CITANEST PLAIN, PRILOCAINE HYDROCHLORIDE
CITANEST, PRILOCAINE HYDROCHLORIDE
CLADRIBINE, CLADRIBINE
CLAFORAN IN DEXTROSE 5% IN PLASTIC CONTAINER,
    CEFOTAXIME SODIUM
CLAFORAN IN SODIUM CHLORIDE 0.9% IN PLASTIC
    CONTAINER, CEFOTAXIME SODIUM
CLAFORAN, CEFOTAXIME SODIUM
CLARAVIS, ISOTRETINOIN
CLARINEX, DESLORATADINE
CLARITIN REDITABS, LORATADINE
CLARITIN REDITABS, LORATADINE (OTC)
CLARITIN, LORATADINE
CLARITIN, LORATADINE (OTC)
CLARITIN-D 24 HOUR, LORATADINE (OTC)
CLARITIN-D, LORATADINE (OTC)
CLEMASTINE FUMARATE, CLEMASTINE FUMARATE
CLEMASTINE FUMARATE, CLEMASTINE FUMARATE
    (OTC)
CLEOCIN HCL, CLINDAMYCIN HYDROCHLORIDE
CLEOCIN PHOSPHATE IN DEXTROSE 5% IN PLASTIC
    CONTAINER, CLINDAMYCIN PHOSPHATE
CLEOCIN PHOSPHATE, CLINDAMYCIN PHOSPHATE

APPENDIX A
PRODUCT NAME INDEX (*continued*)

CLEOCIN T, CLINDAMYCIN PHOSPHATE
CLEOCIN, CLINDAMYCIN HYDROCHLORIDE
CLEOCIN, CLINDAMYCIN PALMITATE HYDROCHLORIDE
CLEOCIN, CLINDAMYCIN PHOSPHATE
CLIMARA, ESTRADIOL
CLINDA-DERM, CLINDAMYCIN PHOSPHATE
CLINDAGEL, CLINDAMYCIN PHOSPHATE
CLINDAMYCIN HCL, CLINDAMYCIN HYDROCHLORIDE
CLINDAMYCIN PHOSPHATE IN DEXTROSE 5% IN
　　PLASTIC CONTAINER, CLINDAMYCIN PHOSPHATE
CLINDAMYCIN PHOSPHATE IN DEXTROSE 5%,
　　CLINDAMYCIN PHOSPHATE
CLINDAMYCIN PHOSPHATE, CLINDAMYCIN
　　PHOSPHATE
CLINDETS, CLINDAMYCIN PHOSPHATE
CLINIMIX 2.75/10 SULFITE FREE IN DEXTROSE 10% IN
　　PLASTIC CONTAINER, AMINO ACIDS
CLINIMIX 2.75/25 SULFITE FREE IN DEXTROSE 25% IN
　　PLASTIC CONTAINER, AMINO ACIDS
CLINIMIX 2.75/5 SULFITE FREE IN DEXTROSE 5% IN
　　PLASTIC CONTAINER, AMINO ACIDS
CLINIMIX 4.25/10 SULFITE FREE IN DEXTROSE 10% IN
　　PLASTIC CONTAINER, AMINO ACIDS
CLINIMIX 4.25/20 SULFITE FREE IN DEXTROSE 20% IN
　　PLASTIC CONTAINER, AMINO ACIDS
CLINIMIX 4.25/25 SULFITE FREE IN DEXTROSE 25% IN
　　PLASTIC CONTAINER, AMINO ACIDS
CLINIMIX 4.25/5 SULFITE FREE IN DEXTROSE 5% IN
　　PLASTIC CONTAINER, AMINO ACIDS
CLINIMIX 5/10 SULFITE FREE IN DEXTROSE 10% IN
　　PLASTIC CONTAINER, AMINO ACIDS
CLINIMIX 5/15 SULFITE FREE IN DEXTROSE 15% IN
　　PLASTIC CONTAINER, AMINO ACIDS
CLINIMIX 5/20 SULFITE FREE IN DEXTROSE 20% IN
　　PLASTIC CONTAINER, AMINO ACIDS
CLINIMIX 5/25 SULFITE FREE IN DEXTROSE 25% IN
　　PLASTIC CONTAINER, AMINO ACIDS
CLINIMIX 5/35 SULFITE FREE IN DEXTROSE 35% IN
　　PLASTIC CONTAINER, AMINO ACIDS
CLINIMIX E 2.75/10 SULFITE-FREE W/ ELECT IN
　　DEXTROSE 10% W/ CALCIUM IN PLASTIC
　　CONTAINER, AMINO ACIDS
CLINIMIX E 2.75/25 SULFITE-FREE W/ ELECT IN
　　DEXTROSE 25% W/ CALCIUM IN PLASTIC
　　CONTAINER, AMINO ACIDS
CLINIMIX E 2.75/5 SULFITE-FREE W/ ELECT IN
　　DEXTROSE 5% W/ CALCIUM IN PLASTIC CONTAINER,
　　AMINO ACIDS
CLINIMIX E 4.25/10 SULFITE-FREE W/ ELECT IN
　　DEXTROSE 10% W/ CALCIUM IN PLASTIC
　　CONTAINER, AMINO ACIDS
CLINIMIX E 4.25/20 SULFITE-FREE W/ ELECT IN
　　DEXTROSE 20% W/ CALCIUM IN PLASTIC
　　CONTAINER, AMINO ACIDS
CLINIMIX E 4.25/25 SULFITE-FREE W/ ELECT IN
　　DEXTROSE 25% W/ CALCIUM IN PLASTIC
　　CONTAINER, AMINO ACIDS
CLINIMIX E 4.25/5 SULFITE-FREE W/ ELECT IN
　　DEXTROSE 5% W/ CALCIUM IN PLASTIC CONTAINER,
　　AMINO ACIDS
CLINIMIX E 5/10 SULFITE-FREE W/ ELECT IN DEXTROSE
　　10% W/ CALCIUM IN PLASTIC CONTAINER, AMINO
　　ACIDS
CLINIMIX E 5/15 SULFITE-FREE W/ ELECT IN DEXTROSE
　　15% W/ CALCIUM IN PLASTIC CONTAINER, AMINO
　　ACIDS
CLINIMIX E 5/20 SULFITE-FREE W/ ELECT IN 20%
　　DEXTROSE W/ CALCIUM IN PLASTIC CONTAINER,
　　AMINO ACIDS

CLINIMIX E 5/25 SULFITE-FREE W/ ELECT IN DEXTROSE
　　25% W/ CALCIUM IN PLASTIC CONTAINER, AMINO
　　ACIDS
CLINIMIX E 5/35 SULFITE FREE W/ ELECT IN DEXTROSE
　　35% W/ CALCIUM IN PLASTIC CONTAINER, AMINO
　　ACIDS
CLINISOL 15% SULFITE FREE IN PLASTIC CONTAINER,
　　AMINO ACIDS
CLINORIL, SULINDAC
CLISTIN, CARBINOXAMINE MALEATE
CLOBETASOL PROPIONATE (EMOLLIENT),
　　CLOBETASOL PROPIONATE
CLOBETASOL PROPIONATE, CLOBETASOL
　　PROPIONATE
CLODERM, CLOCORTOLONE PIVALATE
CLOFIBRATE, CLOFIBRATE
CLOMID, CLOMIPHENE CITRATE
CLOMIPHENE CITRATE, CLOMIPHENE CITRATE
CLOMIPRAMINE HCL, CLOMIPRAMINE
　　HYDROCHLORIDE
CLONAZEPAM, CLONAZEPAM
CLONIDINE HCL AND CHLORTHALIDONE,
　　CHLORTHALIDONE
CLONIDINE HCL, CLONIDINE HYDROCHLORIDE
CLOPRA, METOCLOPRAMIDE HYDROCHLORIDE
CLOPRA-"YELLOW", METOCLOPRAMIDE
　　HYDROCHLORIDE
CLORAZEPATE DIPOTASSIUM, CLORAZEPATE
　　DIPOTASSIUM
CLORPRES, CHLORTHALIDONE
CLOTRIMAZOLE AND BETAMETHASONE
　　DIPROPIONATE, BETAMETHASONE DIPROPIONATE
CLOTRIMAZOLE, CLOTRIMAZOLE
CLOTRIMAZOLE, CLOTRIMAZOLE (OTC)
CLOXACILLIN SODIUM, CLOXACILLIN SODIUM
CLOXAPEN, CLOXACILLIN SODIUM
CLOZAPINE, CLOZAPINE
CLOZARIL, CLOZAPINE
CO-GESIC, ACETAMINOPHEN
CO-LAV, POLYETHYLENE GLYCOL 3350
COACTIN, AMDINOCILLIN
COBAVITE, CYANOCOBALAMIN
CODAMINE, HYDROCODONE BITARTRATE
CODEINE PHOSPHATE AND ACETAMINOPHEN,
　　ACETAMINOPHEN
CODEINE, ASPIRIN, APAP FORMULA NO. 2,
　　ACETAMINOPHEN
CODEINE, ASPIRIN, APAP FORMULA NO. 3,
　　ACETAMINOPHEN
CODEINE, ASPIRIN, APAP FORMULA NO. 4,
　　ACETAMINOPHEN
CODIMAL-L.A. 12, CHLORPHENIRAMINE MALEATE (OTC)
CODOXY, ASPIRIN
CODRIX, ACETAMINOPHEN
COGENTIN, BENZTROPINE MESYLATE
COGNEX, TACRINE HYDROCHLORIDE
COL-PROBENECID, COLCHICINE
COLAZAL, BALSALAZIDE DISODIUM
COLBENEMID, COLCHICINE
COLD CAPSULE IV, CHLORPHENIRAMINE MALEATE
　　(OTC)
COLD CAPSULE V, CHLORPHENIRAMINE MALEATE
　　(OTC)
COLESTID, COLESTIPOL HYDROCHLORIDE
COLGATE TOTAL, SODIUM FLUORIDE (OTC)
COLISTIMETHATE, COLISTIMETHATE SODIUM
COLOCORT, HYDROCORTISONE
COLONAID, ATROPINE SULFATE
COLOVAGE, POLYETHYLENE GLYCOL 3350

APPENDIX A
PRODUCT NAME INDEX (*continued*)

COLY-MYCIN M, COLISTIMETHATE SODIUM
COLY-MYCIN S, COLISTIN SULFATE
COLYTE WITH FLAVOR PACKS, POLYETHYLENE
  GLYCOL 3350
COLYTE, POLYETHYLENE GLYCOL 3350
COLYTE-FLAVORED, POLYETHYLENE GLYCOL 3350
COMBIPATCH, ESTRADIOL
COMBIPRES, CHLORTHALIDONE
COMBIVENT, ALBUTEROL SULFATE
COMBIVIR, LAMIVUDINE
COMMIT, NICOTINE POLACRILEX (OTC)
COMPAZINE, PROCHLORPERAZINE
COMPAZINE, PROCHLORPERAZINE EDISYLATE
COMPAZINE, PROCHLORPERAZINE MALEATE
COMPOUND 65, ASPIRIN
COMPRO, PROCHLORPERAZINE
COMTAN, ENTACAPONE
CONCENTRAID, DESMOPRESSIN ACETATE
CONCERTA, METHYLPHENIDATE HYDROCHLORIDE
CONDYLOX, PODOFILOX
CONRAY 30, IOTHALAMATE MEGLUMINE
CONRAY 43, IOTHALAMATE MEGLUMINE
CONRAY 325, IOTHALAMATE SODIUM
CONRAY 400, IOTHALAMATE SODIUM
CONRAY, IOTHALAMATE MEGLUMINE
CONSTILAC, LACTULOSE
CONSTULOSE, LACTULOSE
CONTAC 12 HOUR, CHLORPHENIRAMINE MALEATE
  (OTC)
CONTAC, CHLORPHENIRAMINE MALEATE (OTC)
COPAXONE, GLATIRAMER ACETATE
COPEGUS, RIBAVIRIN
COPPER T MODEL TCU 380A, COPPER
COR-OTICIN, HYDROCORTISONE ACETATE
CORDARONE, AMIODARONE HYDROCHLORIDE
CORDRAN SP, FLURANDRENOLIDE
CORDRAN, FLURANDRENOLIDE
CORDRAN-N, FLURANDRENOLIDE
COREG, CARVEDILOL
CORGARD, NADOLOL
CORLOPAM, FENOLDOPAM MESYLATE
CORMAX, CLOBETASOL PROPIONATE
CORPHED, PSEUDOEPHEDRINE HYDROCHLORIDE
CORSYM, CHLORPHENIRAMINE POLISTIREX (OTC)
CORT-DOME, HYDROCORTISONE
CORTALONE, PREDNISOLONE
CORTAN, PREDNISONE
CORTEF ACETATE, HYDROCORTISONE ACETATE
CORTEF, HYDROCORTISONE
CORTEF, HYDROCORTISONE CYPIONATE
CORTENEMA, HYDROCORTISONE
CORTICOTROPIN, CORTICOTROPIN
CORTIFOAM, HYDROCORTISONE ACETATE
CORTISONE ACETATE, CORTISONE ACETATE
CORTISPORIN, BACITRACIN ZINC
CORTISPORIN, HYDROCORTISONE
CORTISPORIN, HYDROCORTISONE ACETATE
CORTONE, CORTISONE ACETATE
CORTRIL, HYDROCORTISONE
CORTRIL, HYDROCORTISONE ACETATE
CORTROPHIN-ZINC, CORTICOTROPIN-ZINC
  HYDROXIDE
CORTROSYN, COSYNTROPIN
CORVERT, IBUTILIDE FUMARATE
CORZIDE, BENDROFLUMETHIAZIDE
COSMEGEN, DACTINOMYCIN
COSOPT, DORZOLAMIDE HYDROCHLORIDE
COTAZYM, LIPASE
COTRIM D.S., SULFAMETHOXAZOLE

COTRIM, SULFAMETHOXAZOLE
COUMADIN, WARFARIN SODIUM
COVERA-HS, VERAPAMIL HYDROCHLORIDE
COZAAR, LOSARTAN POTASSIUM
CRESCORMON, SOMATROPIN
CRINONE, PROGESTERONE
CRIXIVAN, INDINAVIR SULFATE
CROLOM, CROMOLYN SODIUM
CROMOLYN SODIUM, CROMOLYN SODIUM
CROMOLYN SODIUM, CROMOLYN SODIUM (OTC)
CROMOPTIC, CROMOLYN SODIUM
CROTAN, CROTAMITON
CRYSELLE, ETHINYL ESTRADIOL
CRYSTODIGIN, DIGITOXIN
CU-7, COPPER
CUPRIC CHLORIDE IN PLASTIC CONTAINER, CUPRIC
  CHLORIDE
CUPRIC SULFATE, CUPRIC SULFATE
CUPRIMINE, PENICILLAMINE
CUROSURF, PORACTANT ALFA
CURRETAB, MEDROXYPROGESTERONE ACETATE
CUTIVATE, FLUTICASONE PROPIONATE
CYANOCOBALAMIN CO 57 SCHILLING TEST KIT,
  CYANOCOBALAMIN
CYANOCOBALAMIN, CYANOCOBALAMIN
CYCLACILLIN, CYCLACILLIN
CYCLAINE, HEXYLCAINE HYDROCHLORIDE
CYCLAPEN-W, CYCLACILLIN
CYCLESSA, DESOGESTREL
CYCLOBENZAPRINE HCL, CYCLOBENZAPRINE
  HYDROCHLORIDE
CYCLOCORT, AMCINONIDE
CYCLOGYL, CYCLOPENTOLATE HYDROCHLORIDE
CYCLOMYDRIL, CYCLOPENTOLATE HYDROCHLORIDE
CYCLOPAR, TETRACYCLINE HYDROCHLORIDE
CYCLOPENTOLATE HCL, CYCLOPENTOLATE
  HYDROCHLORIDE
CYCLOPHOSPHAMIDE, CYCLOPHOSPHAMIDE
CYCLOSPORINE, CYCLOSPORINE
CYCRIN, MEDROXYPROGESTERONE ACETATE
CYKLOKAPRON, TRANEXAMIC ACID
CYLERT, PEMOLINE
CYPROHEPTADINE HCL, CYPROHEPTADINE
  HYDROCHLORIDE
CYSTADANE, BETAINE, ANHYDROUS
CYSTAGON, CYSTEAMINE BITARTRATE
CYSTEINE HCL, CYSTEINE HYDROCHLORIDE
CYSTO-CONRAY II, IOTHALAMATE MEGLUMINE
CYSTOGRAFIN DILUTE, DIATRIZOATE MEGLUMINE
CYSTOGRAFIN, DIATRIZOATE MEGLUMINE
CYTADREN, AMINOGLUTETHIMIDE
CYTARABINE, CYTARABINE
CYTOMEL, LIOTRIX (T4;T3)
CYTOSAR-U, CYTARABINE
CYTOTEC, MISOPROSTOL
CYTOVENE IV, GANCICLOVIR SODIUM
CYTOVENE, GANCICLOVIR
CYTOXAN, CYCLOPHOSPHAMIDE

D

D.H.E. 45, DIHYDROERGOTAMINE MESYLATE
DACARBAZINE, DACARBAZINE
DALGAN, DEZOCINE
DALMANE, FLURAZEPAM HYDROCHLORIDE
DANAZOL, DANAZOL
DANOCRINE, DANAZOL
DANTRIUM, DANTROLENE SODIUM
DAPSONE, DAPSONE

APPENDIX A
PRODUCT NAME INDEX (*continued*)

DARANIDE, DICHLORPHENAMIDE
DARAPRIM, PYRIMETHAMINE
DARBID, ISOPROPAMIDE IODIDE
DARICON, OXYPHENCYCLIMINE HYDROCHLORIDE
DARVOCET, ACETAMINOPHEN
DARVOCET-N 50, ACETAMINOPHEN
DARVOCET-N 100, ACETAMINOPHEN
DARVON COMPOUND, ASPIRIN
DARVON COMPOUND-65, ASPIRIN
DARVON W/ ASA, ASPIRIN
DARVON, PROPOXYPHENE HYDROCHLORIDE
DARVON-N W/ ASA, ASPIRIN
DARVON-N, PROPOXYPHENE NAPSYLATE
DAUNORUBICIN HCL, DAUNORUBICIN
  HYDROCHLORIDE
DAUNOXOME, DAUNORUBICIN CITRATE
DAYPRO ALTA, OXAPROZIN POTASSIUM
DAYPRO, OXAPROZIN
DDAVP (NEEDS NO REFRIGERATION), DESMOPRESSIN
  ACETATE
DDAVP, DESMOPRESSIN ACETATE
DEAPRIL-ST, ERGOLOID MESYLATES
DECA-DURABOLIN, NANDROLONE DECANOATE
DECABID, INDECAINIDE HYDROCHLORIDE
DECADERM, DEXAMETHASONE
DECADRON W/ XYLOCAINE, DEXAMETHASONE SODIUM
  PHOSPHATE
DECADRON, DEXAMETHASONE
DECADRON, DEXAMETHASONE SODIUM PHOSPHATE
DECADRON-LA, DEXAMETHASONE ACETATE
DECAPRYN, DOXYLAMINE SUCCINATE
DECASPRAY, DEXAMETHASONE
DECLOMYCIN, DEMECLOCYCLINE HYDROCHLORIDE
DEFINITY, PERFLUTREN
DEL-VI-A, VITAMIN A PALMITATE
DELALUTIN, HYDROXYPROGESTERONE CAPROATE
DELATESTRYL, TESTOSTERONE ENANTHATE
DELAXIN, METHOCARBAMOL
DELCOBESE, AMPHETAMINE ADIPATE
DELESTROGEN, ESTRADIOL VALERATE
DELFEN, NONOXYNOL-9 (OTC)
DELFLEX W/ DEXTROSE 1.5% IN PLASTIC CONTAINER,
  CALCIUM CHLORIDE
DELFLEX W/ DEXTROSE 1.5% LOW MAGNESIUM IN
  PLASTIC CONTAINER, CALCIUM CHLORIDE
DELFLEX W/ DEXTROSE 1.5% LOW MAGNESIUM LOW
  CALCIUM IN PLASTIC CONTAINER, CALCIUM
  CHLORIDE
DELFLEX W/ DEXTROSE 2.5% IN PLASTIC CONTAINER,
  CALCIUM CHLORIDE
DELFLEX W/ DEXTROSE 2.5% LOW MAGNESIUM IN
  PLASTIC CONTAINER, CALCIUM CHLORIDE
DELFLEX W/ DEXTROSE 2.5% LOW MAGNESIUM LOW
  CALCIUM IN PLASTIC CONTAINER, CALCIUM
  CHLORIDE
DELFLEX W/ DEXTROSE 3.5% IN PLASTIC CONTAINER,
  CALCIUM CHLORIDE
DELFLEX W/ DEXTROSE 4.25% IN PLASTIC CONTAINER,
  CALCIUM CHLORIDE
DELFLEX W/ DEXTROSE 4.25% LOW MAGNESIUM IN
  PLASTIC CONTAINER, CALCIUM CHLORIDE
DELFLEX W/ DEXTROSE 4.25% LOW MAGNESIUM LOW
  CALCIUM IN PLASTIC CONTAINER, CALCIUM
  CHLORIDE
DELFLEX-LM W/ DEXTROSE 1.5% IN PLASTIC
  CONTAINER, CALCIUM CHLORIDE
DELFLEX-LM W/ DEXTROSE 2.5% IN PLASTIC
  CONTAINER, CALCIUM CHLORIDE

DELFLEX-LM W/ DEXTROSE 3.5% IN PLASTIC
  CONTAINER, CALCIUM CHLORIDE
DELFLEX-LM W/ DEXTROSE 4.25% IN PLASTIC
  CONTAINER, CALCIUM CHLORIDE
DELSYM, DEXTROMETHORPHAN POLISTIREX (OTC)
DELTA-CORTEF, PREDNISOLONE
DELTA-DOME, PREDNISONE
DELTALIN, ERGOCALCIFEROL
DELTASONE, PREDNISONE
DEMADEX, TORSEMIDE
DEMAZIN, CHLORPHENIRAMINE MALEATE (OTC)
DEMEROL, MEPERIDINE HYDROCHLORIDE
DEMI-REGROTON, CHLORTHALIDONE
DEMSER, METYROSINE
DEMULEN 1/35-21, ETHINYL ESTRADIOL
DEMULEN 1/35-28, ETHINYL ESTRADIOL
DEMULEN 1/50-21, ETHINYL ESTRADIOL
DEMULEN 1/50-28, ETHINYL ESTRADIOL
DENAVIR, PENCICLOVIR SODIUM
DENDRID, IDOXURIDINE
DEPACON, VALPROATE SODIUM
DEPAKENE, VALPROIC ACID
DEPAKOTE CP, DIVALPROEX SODIUM
DEPAKOTE ER, DIVALPROEX SODIUM
DEPAKOTE, DIVALPROEX SODIUM
DEPEN, PENICILLAMINE
DEPINAR, CYANOCOBALAMIN
DEPO-ESTRADIOL, ESTRADIOL CYPIONATE
DEPO-MEDROL, METHYLPREDNISOLONE ACETATE
DEPO-PROVERA, MEDROXYPROGESTERONE ACETATE
DEPO-TESTADIOL, ESTRADIOL CYPIONATE
DEPO-TESTOSTERONE, TESTOSTERONE CYPIONATE
DEPOCYT, CYTARABINE
DERMA-SMOOTHE/FS, FLUOCINOLONE ACETONIDE
DERMABET, BETAMETHASONE VALERATE
DERMACORT, HYDROCORTISONE
DERMATOP E EMOLLIENT, PREDNICARBATE
DERMATOP, PREDNICARBATE
DESFERAL, DEFEROXAMINE MESYLATE
DESIPRAMINE HCL, DESIPRAMINE HYDROCHLORIDE
DESMOPRESSIN ACETATE PRESERVATIVE FREE,
  DESMOPRESSIN ACETATE
DESMOPRESSIN ACETATE, DESMOPRESSIN ACETATE
DESOGEN, DESOGESTREL
DESOGESTREL AND ETHINYL ESTRADIOL,
  DESOGESTREL
DESONIDE, DESONIDE
DESOWEN, DESONIDE
DESOXIMETASONE, DESOXIMETASONE
DESOXYN, METHAMPHETAMINE HYDROCHLORIDE
DESYREL, TRAZODONE HYDROCHLORIDE
DETROL LA, TOLTERODINE TARTRATE
DETROL, TOLTERODINE TARTRATE
DEXACEN-4, DEXAMETHASONE SODIUM PHOSPHATE
DEXACIDIN, DEXAMETHASONE
DEXACORT, DEXAMETHASONE SODIUM PHOSPHATE
DEXAIR, DEXAMETHASONE SODIUM PHOSPHATE
DEXAMETHASONE ACETATE, DEXAMETHASONE
  ACETATE
DEXAMETHASONE INTENSOL, DEXAMETHASONE
DEXAMETHASONE SODIUM PHOSPHATE,
  DEXAMETHASONE SODIUM PHOSPHATE
DEXAMETHASONE, DEXAMETHASONE
DEXAMETHASONE, DEXAMETHASONE SODIUM
  PHOSPHATE
DEXAMPEX, DEXTROAMPHETAMINE SULFATE
DEXASPORIN, DEXAMETHASONE
DEXCHLORPHENIRAMINE MALEATE,
  DEXCHLORPHENIRAMINE MALEATE

APPENDIX A
PRODUCT NAME INDEX (*continued*)

APPENDIX A
PRODUCT NAME INDEX (*continued*)

DEXTROSE 5%, SODIUM CHLORIDE 0.33% AND POTASSIUM CHLORIDE 15MEQ IN PLASTIC CONTAINER, DEXTROSE

DEXTROSE 5%, SODIUM CHLORIDE 0.33% AND POTASSIUM CHLORIDE 20MEQ IN PLASTIC CONTAINER, DEXTROSE

DEXTROSE 5%, SODIUM CHLORIDE 0.33% AND POTASSIUM CHLORIDE 30MEQ IN PLASTIC CONTAINER, DEXTROSE

DEXTROSE 5%, SODIUM CHLORIDE 0.33% AND POTASSIUM CHLORIDE 40MEQ IN PLASTIC CONTAINER, DEXTROSE

DEXTROSE 5%, SODIUM CHLORIDE 0.33% AND POTASSIUM CHLORIDE 5MEQ IN PLASTIC CONTAINER, DEXTROSE

DEXTROSE 5%, SODIUM CHLORIDE 0.45% AND POTASSIUM CHLORIDE 0.075%, DEXTROSE

DEXTROSE 5%, SODIUM CHLORIDE 0.45% AND POTASSIUM CHLORIDE 0.15% IN PLASTIC CONTAINER, DEXTROSE

DEXTROSE 5%, SODIUM CHLORIDE 0.45% AND POTASSIUM CHLORIDE 0.22% IN PLASTIC CONTAINER, DEXTROSE

DEXTROSE 5%, SODIUM CHLORIDE 0.45% AND POTASSIUM CHLORIDE 0.3% IN PLASTIC CONTAINER, DEXTROSE

DEXTROSE 5%, SODIUM CHLORIDE 0.45% AND POTASSIUM CHLORIDE 15MEQ IN PLASTIC CONTAINER, DEXTROSE

DEXTROSE 5%, SODIUM CHLORIDE 0.45% AND POTASSIUM CHLORIDE 20MEQ (K) IN PLASTIC CONTAINER, DEXTROSE

DEXTROSE 5%, SODIUM CHLORIDE 0.45% AND POTASSIUM CHLORIDE 5MEQ IN PLASTIC CONTAINER, DEXTROSE

DEXTROSE 50% IN PLASTIC CONTAINER, DEXTROSE

DEXTROSE 60% IN PLASTIC CONTAINER, DEXTROSE

DEXTROSE 60%, DEXTROSE

DEXTROSE 7.7% IN PLASTIC CONTAINER, DEXTROSE

DEXTROSE 70% IN PLASTIC CONTAINER, DEXTROSE

DEXTROSTAT, DEXTROAMPHETAMINE SULFATE

DHC PLUS, ACETAMINOPHEN

DI-ATRO, ATROPINE SULFATE

DI-METREX, PHENDIMETRAZINE TARTRATE

DIABETA, GLYBURIDE

DIABINESE, CHLORPROPAMIDE

DIAL, HEXACHLOROPHENE

DIALYTE CONCENTRATE W/ DEXTROSE 30% IN PLASTIC CONTAINER, CALCIUM CHLORIDE

DIALYTE CONCENTRATE W/ DEXTROSE 50% IN PLASTIC CONTAINER, CALCIUM CHLORIDE

DIALYTE LM/ DEXTROSE 1.5% IN PLASTIC CONTAINER, CALCIUM CHLORIDE

DIALYTE LM/ DEXTROSE 2.5% IN PLASTIC CONTAINER, CALCIUM CHLORIDE

DIALYTE LM/ DEXTROSE 4.25% IN PLASTIC CONTAINER, CALCIUM CHLORIDE

DIALYTE W/ DEXTROSE 1.5% IN PLASTIC CONTAINER, CALCIUM CHLORIDE

DIALYTE W/ DEXTROSE 4.25% IN PLASTIC CONTAINER, CALCIUM CHLORIDE

DIAMOX, ACETAZOLAMIDE

DIAMOX, ACETAZOLAMIDE SODIUM

DIANEAL 137 W/ DEXTROSE 1.5% IN PLASTIC CONTAINER, CALCIUM CHLORIDE

DIANEAL 137 W/ DEXTROSE 2.5% IN PLASTIC CONTAINER, CALCIUM CHLORIDE

DIANEAL 137 W/ DEXTROSE 4.25% IN PLASTIC CONTAINER, CALCIUM CHLORIDE

DIANEAL LOW CALCIUM W/ DEXTROSE 1.5% IN PLASTIC CONTAINER, CALCIUM CHLORIDE

DIANEAL LOW CALCIUM W/ DEXTROSE 2.5% IN PLASTIC CONTAINER, CALCIUM CHLORIDE

DIANEAL LOW CALCIUM W/ DEXTROSE 3.5% IN PLASTIC CONTAINER, CALCIUM CHLORIDE

DIANEAL LOW CALCIUM W/ DEXTROSE 4.25% IN PLASTIC CONTAINER, CALCIUM CHLORIDE

DIANEAL PD-1 W/ DEXTROSE 1.5% IN PLASTIC CONTAINER, CALCIUM CHLORIDE

DIANEAL PD-1 W/ DEXTROSE 2.5% IN PLASTIC CONTAINER, CALCIUM CHLORIDE

DIANEAL PD-1 W/ DEXTROSE 3.5% IN PLASTIC CONTAINER, CALCIUM CHLORIDE

DIANEAL PD-1 W/ DEXTROSE 4.25% IN PLASTIC CONTAINER, CALCIUM CHLORIDE

DIANEAL PD-2 W/ DEXTROSE 1.5% IN PLASTIC CONTAINER, CALCIUM CHLORIDE

DIANEAL PD-2 W/ DEXTROSE 2.5% IN PLASTIC CONTAINER, CALCIUM CHLORIDE

DIANEAL PD-2 W/ DEXTROSE 3.5% IN PLASTIC CONTAINER, CALCIUM CHLORIDE

DIANEAL PD-2 W/ DEXTROSE 4.25% IN PLASTIC CONTAINER, CALCIUM CHLORIDE

DIAPID, LYPRESSIN

DIASONE SODIUM, SULFOXONE SODIUM

DIASTAT, DIAZEPAM

DIATRIZOATE MEGLUMINE, DIATRIZOATE MEGLUMINE

DIATRIZOATE-60, DIATRIZOATE MEGLUMINE

DIAZEPAM INTENSOL, DIAZEPAM

DIAZEPAM, DIAZEPAM

DIAZOXIDE, DIAZOXIDE

DIBENIL, DIPHENHYDRAMINE HYDROCHLORIDE

DIBENZYLINE, PHENOXYBENZAMINE HYDROCHLORIDE

DICLOFENAC POTASSIUM, DICLOFENAC POTASSIUM

DICLOFENAC SODIUM, DICLOFENAC SODIUM

DICLOXACILLIN SODIUM, DICLOXACILLIN SODIUM

DICOPAC KIT, CYANOCOBALAMIN

DICUMAROL, DICUMAROL

DICURIN PROCAINE, PROCAINE MERETHOXYLLINE

DICYCLOMINE HCL (PRESERVATIVE-FREE), DICYCLOMINE HYDROCHLORIDE

DICYCLOMINE HCL, DICYCLOMINE HYDROCHLORIDE

DIDREX, BENZPHETAMINE HYDROCHLORIDE

DIDRONEL, ETIDRONATE DISODIUM

DIENESTROL, DIENESTROL

DIETHYLPROPION HCL, DIETHYLPROPION HYDROCHLORIDE

DIETHYLSTILBESTROL, DIETHYLSTILBESTROL

DIFFERIN, ADAPALENE

DIFLORASONE DIACETATE, DIFLORASONE DIACETATE

DIFLUCAN IN DEXTROSE 5% IN PLASTIC CONTAINER, FLUCONAZOLE

DIFLUCAN IN SODIUM CHLORIDE 0.9% IN PLASTIC CONTAINER, FLUCONAZOLE

DIFLUCAN IN SODIUM CHLORIDE 0.9%, FLUCONAZOLE

DIFLUCAN, FLUCONAZOLE

DIFLUNISAL, DIFLUNISAL

DIGOXIN PEDIATRIC, DIGOXIN

DIGOXIN, DIGOXIN

DIHYDROERGOTAMINE MESYLATE, DIHYDROERGOTAMINE MESYLATE

DIHYDROEROGTAMINE MESYLATE, DIHYDROERGOTAMINE MESYLATE

DILACOR XR, DILTIAZEM HYDROCHLORIDE

DILANTIN, PHENYTOIN

DILANTIN, PHENYTOIN SODIUM

DILANTIN, PHENYTOIN SODIUM, EXTENDED

DILANTIN-125, PHENYTOIN

APPENDIX A
PRODUCT NAME INDEX (*continued*)

DILANTIN-30, PHENYTOIN
DILATRATE-SR, ISOSORBIDE DINITRATE
DILAUDID, HYDROMORPHONE HYDROCHLORIDE
DILAUDID-HP, HYDROMORPHONE HYDROCHLORIDE
DILOR, DYPHYLLINE
DILOR-400, DYPHYLLINE
DILTIAZEM HCL, DILTIAZEM HYDROCHLORIDE
DIMENHYDRINATE, DIMENHYDRINATE
DIMETANE, BROMPHENIRAMINE MALEATE
DIMETANE, BROMPHENIRAMINE MALEATE (OTC)
DIMETANE-DC, BROMPHENIRAMINE MALEATE
DIMETANE-DX, BROMPHENIRAMINE MALEATE
DIMETANE-TEN, BROMPHENIRAMINE MALEATE
DIMETAPP, BROMPHENIRAMINE MALEATE (OTC)
DIMETHYL SULFOXIDE, DIMETHYL SULFOXIDE
DIONOSIL AQUEOUS, PROPYLIODONE
DIONOSIL OILY, PROPYLIODONE
DIOVAN HCT, HYDROCHLOROTHIAZIDE
DIOVAN, VALSARTAN
DIPENTUM, OLSALAZINE SODIUM
DIPHEN, DIPHENHYDRAMINE HYDROCHLORIDE
DIPHEN, DIPHENHYDRAMINE HYDROCHLORIDE (OTC)
DIPHENHYDRAMINE HCL PRESERVATIVE FREE, DIPHENHYDRAMINE HYDROCHLORIDE
DIPHENHYDRAMINE HCL, DIPHENHYDRAMINE HYDROCHLORIDE
DIPHENHYDRAMINE HCL, DIPHENHYDRAMINE HYDROCHLORIDE (OTC)
DIPHENOXYLATE HCL AND ATROPINE SULFATE, ATROPINE SULFATE
DIPHENOXYLATE HCL W/ ATROPINE SULFATE, ATROPINE SULFATE
DIPHENYLAN SODIUM, PHENYTOIN SODIUM, PROMPT
DIPIVEFRIN HCL, DIPIVEFRIN HYDROCHLORIDE
DIPRIVAN, PROPOFOL
DIPROLENE AF, BETAMETHASONE DIPROPIONATE
DIPROLENE, BETAMETHASONE DIPROPIONATE
DIPROSONE, BETAMETHASONE DIPROPIONATE
DIPYRIDAMOLE, DIPYRIDAMOLE
DISCASE, CHYMOPAPAIN
DISIPAL, ORPHENADRINE HYDROCHLORIDE
DISOBROM, DEXBROMPHENIRAMINE MALEATE (OTC)
DISODIUM EDETATE, EDETATE DISODIUM
DISOMER, DEXBROMPHENIRAMINE MALEATE
DISOPHROL, DEXBROMPHENIRAMINE MALEATE (OTC)
DISOPYRAMIDE PHOSPHATE, DISOPYRAMIDE PHOSPHATE
DISULFIRAM, DISULFIRAM
DITATE-DS, ESTRADIOL VALERATE
DITROPAN XL, OXYBUTYNIN CHLORIDE
DITROPAN, OXYBUTYNIN CHLORIDE
DIUCARDIN, HYDROFLUMETHIAZIDE
DIULO, METOLAZONE
DIUPRES-250, CHLOROTHIAZIDE
DIUPRES-500, CHLOROTHIAZIDE
DIURIL, CHLOROTHIAZIDE
DIURIL, CHLOROTHIAZIDE SODIUM
DIUTENSEN-R, METHYCLOTHIAZIDE
DIZAC, DIAZEPAM
DOBUTAMINE HCL IN DEXTROSE 5% IN PLASTIC CONTAINER, DOBUTAMINE HYDROCHLORIDE
DOBUTAMINE HCL IN DEXTROSE 5%, DOBUTAMINE HYDROCHLORIDE
DOBUTAMINE HCL, DOBUTAMINE HYDROCHLORIDE
DOBUTREX, DOBUTAMINE HYDROCHLORIDE
DOCA, DESOXYCORTICOSTERONE ACETATE
DOLENE AP-65, ACETAMINOPHEN
DOLENE, PROPOXYPHENE HYDROCHLORIDE
DOLOBID, DIFLUNISAL
DOLOPHINE HCL, METHADONE HYDROCHLORIDE
DOMEBORO, ACETIC ACID, GLACIAL
DOPAMINE HCL AND DEXTROSE 5% IN PLASTIC CONTAINER, DOPAMINE HYDROCHLORIDE
DOPAMINE HCL AND DEXTROSE 5%, DOPAMINE HYDROCHLORIDE
DOPAMINE HCL IN DEXTROSE 5% IN PLASTIC CONTAINER, DOPAMINE HYDROCHLORIDE
DOPAMINE HCL IN DEXTROSE 5%, DOPAMINE HYDROCHLORIDE
DOPAMINE HCL, DOPAMINE HYDROCHLORIDE
DOPAR, LEVODOPA
DOPRAM, DOXAPRAM HYDROCHLORIDE
DORAL, QUAZEPAM
DORIDEN, GLUTETHIMIDE
DORMATE, MEBUTAMATE
DORYX, DOXYCYCLINE HYCLATE
DOSTINEX, CABERGOLINE
DOVONEX, CALCIPOTRIENE
DOW-ISONIAZID, ISONIAZID
DOXAPRAM HCL, DOXAPRAM HYDROCHLORIDE
DOXAZOSIN MESYLATE, DOXAZOSIN MESYLATE
DOXEPIN HCL, DOXEPIN HYDROCHLORIDE
DOXIL, DOXORUBICIN HYDROCHLORIDE
DOXORUBICIN HCL, DOXORUBICIN HYDROCHLORIDE
DOXY 100, DOXYCYCLINE HYCLATE
DOXY 200, DOXYCYCLINE HYCLATE
DOXY-LEMMON, DOXYCYCLINE HYCLATE
DOXY-SLEEP-AID, DOXYLAMINE SUCCINATE (OTC)
DOXYCHEL HYCLATE, DOXYCYCLINE HYCLATE
DOXYCHEL, DOXYCYCLINE
DOXYCYCLINE HYCLATE, DOXYCYCLINE HYCLATE
DOXYCYCLINE HYLATE, DOXYCYCLINE HYCLATE
DOXYCYCLINE, DOXYCYCLINE
DOXYCYCLINE, DOXYCYCLINE HYCLATE
DOXYLAMINE SUCCINATE, DOXYLAMINE SUCCINATE
DOXYLAMINE SUCCINATE, DOXYLAMINE SUCCINATE (OTC)
DRALSERP, HYDRALAZINE HYDROCHLORIDE
DRALZINE, HYDRALAZINE HYDROCHLORIDE
DRICORT, HYDROCORTISONE ACETATE
DRISDOL, ERGOCALCIFEROL
DRIXORAL PLUS, ACETAMINOPHEN (OTC)
DRIXORAL, DEXBROMPHENIRAMINE MALEATE (OTC)
DRIZE, CHLORPHENIRAMINE MALEATE
DROLBAN, DROMOSTANOLONE PROPIONATE
DROPERIDOL, DROPERIDOL
DROXIA, HYDROXYUREA
DTIC-DOME, DACARBAZINE
DTPA, TECHNETIUM TC-99M PENTETATE KIT
DUAC, BENZOYL PEROXIDE
DUO-MEDIHALER, ISOPROTERENOL HYDROCHLORIDE
DUOCAINE, BUPIVACAINE HYDROCHLORIDE
DUONEB, ALBUTEROL SULFATE
DUPHALAC, LACTULOSE
DURABOLIN, NANDROLONE PHENPROPIONATE
DURACILLIN A.S., PENICILLIN G PROCAINE
DURACLON, CLONIDINE HYDROCHLORIDE
DURADYNE DHC, ACETAMINOPHEN
DURAGESIC, FENTANYL
DURAMORPH PF, MORPHINE SULFATE
DURANEST, EPINEPHRINE
DURANEST, EPINEPHRINE BITARTRATE
DURANEST, ETIDOCAINE HYDROCHLORIDE
DURAPHYL, THEOPHYLLINE
DURAQUIN, QUINIDINE GLUCONATE
DURICEF, CEFADROXIL/CEFADROXIL HEMIHYDRATE
DUVOID, BETHANECHOL CHLORIDE
DV, DIENESTROL

APPENDIX A
PRODUCT NAME INDEX (*continued*)

DYAZIDE, HYDROCHLOROTHIAZIDE
DYCILL, DICLOXACILLIN SODIUM
DYCLONE, DYCLONINE HYDROCHLORIDE
DYMELOR, ACETOHEXAMIDE
DYNA-HEX, CHLORHEXIDINE GLUCONATE (OTC)
DYNABAC, DIRITHROMYCIN
DYNACIRC CR, ISRADIPINE
DYNACIRC, ISRADIPINE
DYNAPEN, DICLOXACILLIN SODIUM
DYRENIUM, TRIAMTERENE

E

E-BASE, ERYTHROMYCIN
E-GLADES, ERYTHROMYCIN
E-MYCIN E, ERYTHROMYCIN ETHYLSUCCINATE
E-MYCIN, ERYTHROMYCIN
E-SOLVE 2, ERYTHROMYCIN
E-Z PREP 220, POVIDONE-IODINE (OTC)
E-Z PREP, POVIDONE-IODINE (OTC)
E-Z SCRUB 201, POVIDONE-IODINE (OTC)
E-Z SCRUB 241, POVIDONE-IODINE (OTC)
E-Z SCRUB, CHLORHEXIDINE GLUCONATE (OTC)
E-Z SCRUB, HEXACHLOROPHENE
E-Z-EM PREP LYTE, POLYETHYLENE GLYCOL 3350
E.E.S. 200, ERYTHROMYCIN ETHYLSUCCINATE
E.E.S. 400, ERYTHROMYCIN ETHYLSUCCINATE
E.E.S., ERYTHROMYCIN ETHYLSUCCINATE
EC-NAPROSYN, NAPROXEN
ECONAZOLE NITRATE, ECONAZOLE NITRATE
ECONOCHLOR, CHLORAMPHENICOL
ECONOPRED PLUS, PREDNISOLONE ACETATE
ECONOPRED, PREDNISOLONE ACETATE
EDECRIN, ETHACRYNATE SODIUM
EDECRIN, ETHACRYNIC ACID
EDETATE DISODIUM, EDETATE DISODIUM
EDEX, ALPROSTADIL
EDROPHONIUM CHLORIDE PRESERVATIVE FREE,
    EDROPHONIUM CHLORIDE
EDROPHONIUM CHLORIDE, EDROPHONIUM CHLORIDE
EFFEXOR XR, VENLAFAXINE HYDROCHLORIDE
EFFEXOR, VENLAFAXINE HYDROCHLORIDE
EFIDAC 24 CHLORPHENIRAMINE MALEATE,
    CHLORPHENIRAMINE MALEATE (OTC)
EFIDAC 24 PSEUDOEPHEDRINE HCL,
    PSEUDOEPHEDRINE HYDROCHLORIDE (OTC)
EFIDAC 24 PSEUDOEPHEDRINE HCL/
    BROMPHENIRAMINE MALEATE, BROMPHENIRAMINE
    MALEATE (OTC)
EFUDEX, FLUOROURACIL
ELASE-CHLOROMYCETIN, CHLORAMPHENICOL
ELAVIL, AMITRIPTYLINE HYDROCHLORIDE
ELDECORT, HYDROCORTISONE
ELDEPRYL, SELEGILINE HYDROCHLORIDE
ELIDEL, PIMECROLIMUS
ELIGARD, LEUPROLIDE ACETATE
ELIMITE, PERMETHRIN
ELIXICON, THEOPHYLLINE
ELIXOMIN, THEOPHYLLINE
ELIXOPHYLLIN SR, THEOPHYLLINE
ELIXOPHYLLIN, THEOPHYLLINE
ELLENCE, EPIRUBICIN HYDROCHLORIDE
ELLIOTTS B SOLUTION, CALCIUM CHLORIDE
ELMIRON, PENTOSAN POLYSULFATE SODIUM
ELOCON, MOMETASONE FUROATE
ELOXATIN, OXALIPLATIN
EMADINE, EMEDASTINE DIFUMARATE
EMBELINE E, CLOBETASOL PROPIONATE
EMBELINE, CLOBETASOL PROPIONATE

EMBOLEX, DIHYDROERGOTAMINE MESYLATE
EMCYT, ESTRAMUSTINE PHOSPHATE SODIUM
EMEND, APREPITANT
EMETE-CON, BENZQUINAMIDE HYDROCHLORIDE
EMGEL, ERYTHROMYCIN
EMLA, LIDOCAINE
EMPRACET W/ CODEINE PHOSPHATE #3,
    ACETAMINOPHEN
EMPRACET W/ CODEINE PHOSPHATE #4,
    ACETAMINOPHEN
ENALAPRIL MALEATE AND HYDROCHLOROTHIAZIDE,
    ENALAPRIL MALEATE
ENALAPRIL MALEATE, ENALAPRIL MALEATE
ENALAPRILAT, ENALAPRILAT
ENDEP, AMITRIPTYLINE HYDROCHLORIDE
ENDOSOL EXTRA, CALCIUM CHLORIDE
ENDRATE, EDETATE DISODIUM
ENDURON, METHYCLOTHIAZIDE
ENDURONYL FORTE, DESERPIDINE
ENDURONYL, DESERPIDINE
ENFLURANE, ENFLURANE
ENLON, EDROPHONIUM CHLORIDE
ENLON-PLUS, ATROPINE SULFATE
ENOVID, MESTRANOL
ENOVID-E 21, MESTRANOL
ENOVID-E, MESTRANOL
ENPRESSE-21, ETHINYL ESTRADIOL
ENPRESSE-28, ETHINYL ESTRADIOL
ENTOCORT EC, BUDESONIDE
ENULOSE, LACTULOSE
EPI E Z PEN JR, EPINEPHRINE
EPICORT, HYDROCORTISONE
EPIFOAM, HYDROCORTISONE ACETATE
EPINEPHRINE, EPINEPHRINE (OTC)
EPIPEN E Z PEN, EPINEPHRINE
EPIPEN JR., EPINEPHRINE
EPIPEN, EPINEPHRINE
EPITOL, CARBAMAZEPINE
EPIVIR, LAMIVUDINE
EPIVIR-HBV, LAMIVUDINE
EQUAGESIC, ASPIRIN
EQUANIL, MEPROBAMATE
EQUIPIN, HOMATROPINE METHYLBROMIDE
ERCATAB, CAFFEINE
ERGAMISOL, LEVAMISOLE HYDROCHLORIDE
ERGOLOID MESYLATES, ERGOLOID MESYLATES
ERGOMAR, ERGOTAMINE TARTRATE
ERGOSTAT, ERGOTAMINE TARTRATE
ERRIN, NORETHINDRONE
ERY-TAB, ERYTHROMYCIN
ERYC 125, ERYTHROMYCIN
ERYC SPRINKLES, ERYTHROMYCIN
ERYC, ERYTHROMYCIN
ERYCETTE, ERYTHROMYCIN
ERYDERM, ERYTHROMYCIN
ERYGEL, ERYTHROMYCIN
ERYMAX, ERYTHROMYCIN
ERYPAR, ERYTHROMYCIN STEARATE
ERYPED, ERYTHROMYCIN ETHYLSUCCINATE
ERYTHRA-DERM, ERYTHROMYCIN
ERYTHRO-STATIN, ERYTHROMYCIN
ERYTHROCIN STEARATE, ERYTHROMYCIN STEARATE
ERYTHROCIN, ERYTHROMYCIN LACTOBIONATE
ERYTHROMYCIN ESTOLATE, ERYTHROMYCIN
    ESTOLATE
ERYTHROMYCIN ETHYLSUCCINATE AND
    SULFISOXAZOLE ACETYL, ERYTHROMYCIN
    ETHYLSUCCINATE

APPENDIX A
PRODUCT NAME INDEX (*continued*)

ERYTHROMYCIN ETHYLSUCCINATE, ERYTHROMYCIN
    ETHYLSUCCINATE
ERYTHROMYCIN LACTOBIONATE, ERYTHROMYCIN
    LACTOBIONATE
ERYTHROMYCIN STEARATE, ERYTHROMYCIN
    STEARATE
ERYTHROMYCIN, ERYTHROMYCIN
ERYTHROMYCIN, ERYTHROMYCIN LACTOBIONATE
ERYZOLE, ERYTHROMYCIN ETHYLSUCCINATE
ESCLIM, ESTRADIOL
ESGIC, ACETAMINOPHEN
ESGIC-PLUS, ACETAMINOPHEN
ESIDRIX, HYDROCHLOROTHIAZIDE
ESIMIL, GUANETHIDINE MONOSULFATE
ESKALITH CR, LITHIUM CARBONATE
ESKALITH, LITHIUM CARBONATE
ESTAZOLAM, ESTAZOLAM
ESTERIFIED ESTROGENS, ESTROGENS, ESTERIFIED
ESTINYL, ETHINYL ESTRADIOL
ESTRACE, ESTRADIOL
ESTRADERM, ESTRADIOL
ESTRADIOL CYPIONATE, ESTRADIOL CYPIONATE
ESTRADIOL VALERATE, ESTRADIOL VALERATE
ESTRADIOL, ESTRADIOL
ESTRADURIN, POLYESTRADIOL PHOSPHATE
ESTRAGUARD, DIENESTROL
ESTRATAB, ESTROGENS, ESTERIFIED
ESTRING, ESTRADIOL
ESTROGENIC SUBSTANCE, ESTRONE
ESTRONE, ESTRONE
ESTROPIPATE, ESTROPIPATE
ESTROSTEP 21, ETHINYL ESTRADIOL
ESTROSTEP FE, ETHINYL ESTRADIOL
ESTROVIS, QUINESTROL
ETHAMBUTOL HCL, ETHAMBUTOL HYDROCHLORIDE
ETHAMIDE, ETHOXZOLAMIDE
ETHAMOLIN, ETHANOLAMINE OLEATE
ETHCHLORVYNOL, ETHCHLORVYNOL
ETHIODOL, ETHIODIZED OIL
ETHMOZINE, MORICIZINE HYDROCHLORIDE
ETHOSUXIMIDE, ETHOSUXIMIDE
ETHRANE, ENFLURANE
ETHRIL 250, ERYTHROMYCIN STEARATE
ETHRIL 500, ERYTHROMYCIN STEARATE
ETHYOL, AMIFOSTINE
ETIDRONATE DISODIUM, ETIDRONATE DISODIUM
ETODOLAC, ETODOLAC
ETOMIDATE, ETOMIDATE
ETOPOPHOS PRESERVATIVE FREE, ETOPOSIDE
    PHOSPHATE
ETOPOSIDE, ETOPOSIDE
ETRAFON 2-10, AMITRIPTYLINE HYDROCHLORIDE
ETRAFON 2-25, AMITRIPTYLINE HYDROCHLORIDE
ETRAFON-A, AMITRIPTYLINE HYDROCHLORIDE
ETRAFON-FORTE, AMITRIPTYLINE HYDROCHLORIDE
EULEXIN, FLUTAMIDE
EURAX, CROTAMITON
EUTHROID-0.5, LIOTRIX (T4;T3)
EUTHROID-1, LIOTRIX (T4;T3)
EUTHROID-2, LIOTRIX (T4;T3)
EUTHROID-3, LIOTRIX (T4;T3)
EUTONYL, PARGYLINE HYDROCHLORIDE
EUTRON, METHYCLOTHIAZIDE
EVALOSE, LACTULOSE
EVANS BLUE, EVANS BLUE
EVEX, ESTROGENS, ESTERIFIED
EVISTA, RALOXIFENE HYDROCHLORIDE
EVOXAC, CEVIMELINE HYDROCHLORIDE
EXCEDRIN (MIGRAINE), ACETAMINOPHEN (OTC)

EXELDERM, SULCONAZOLE NITRATE
EXELON, RIVASTIGMINE TARTRATE
EXIDINE, CHLORHEXIDINE GLUCONATE (OTC)
EXNA, BENZTHIAZIDE
EXOSURF NEONATAL, CETYL ALCOHOL
EXSEL, SELENIUM SULFIDE
EXTENDED PHENYTOIN SODIUM, PHENYTOIN SODIUM,
    EXTENDED
EXTRA-STRENGTH AIM, SODIUM
    MONOFLUOROPHOSPHATE (OTC)
EXTRANEAL, ICODEXTRIN

F

FACTIVE, GEMIFLOXACIN MESYLATE
FACTREL, GONADORELIN HYDROCHLORIDE
FAMOTIDINE PRESERVATIVE FREE (PHARMACY BULK),
    FAMOTIDINE
FAMOTIDINE PRESERVATIVE FREE IN PLASTIC
    CONTAINER, FAMOTIDINE
FAMOTIDINE PRESERVATIVE FREE, FAMOTIDINE
FAMOTIDINE, FAMOTIDINE
FAMOTIDINE, FAMOTIDINE (OTC)
FAMVIR, FAMCICLOVIR
FANSIDAR, PYRIMETHAMINE
FARESTON, TOREMIFENE CITRATE
FASLODEX, FULVESTRANT
FASTIN, PHENTERMINE HYDROCHLORIDE
FELBATOL, FELBAMATE
FELDENE, PIROXICAM
FEMARA, LETROZOLE
FEMCET, ACETAMINOPHEN
FEMHRT, ETHINYL ESTRADIOL
FEMINONE, ETHINYL ESTRADIOL
FEMOGEN, ESTROGENS, ESTERIFIED
FEMPATCH, ESTRADIOL
FEMRING, ESTRADIOL ACETATE
FEMSTAT 3, BUTOCONAZOLE NITRATE (OTC)
FEMSTAT, BUTOCONAZOLE NITRATE
FENOFIBRATE (MICRONIZED), FENOFIBRATE
FENOPROFEN CALCIUM, FENOPROFEN CALCIUM
FENTANYL CITRATE AND DROPERIDOL, DROPERIDOL
FENTANYL CITRATE PRESERVATIVE FREE, FENTANYL
    CITRATE
FENTANYL CITRATE, FENTANYL CITRATE
FENTANYL, FENTANYL CITRATE
FERIDEX I.V., FERUMOXIDES
FERNDEX, DEXTROAMPHETAMINE SULFATE
FERNISOLONE-P, PREDNISOLONE
FERNISONE, PREDNISONE
FERRISELTZ, FERRIC AMMONIUM CITRATE
FERRLECIT, SODIUM FERRIC GLUCONATE COMPLEX
FERROUS CITRATE FE 59, FERROUS CITRATE, FE-59
FERTINEX, UROFOLLITROPIN
FINACEA, AZELAIC ACID
FIORICET W/ CODEINE, ACETAMINOPHEN
FIORICET, ACETAMINOPHEN
FIORINAL W/CODEINE NO 3, ASPIRIN
FIORINAL, ASPIRIN
FLAGYL ER, METRONIDAZOLE
FLAGYL I.V. RTU IN PLASTIC CONTAINER,
    METRONIDAZOLE
FLAGYL I.V., METRONIDAZOLE HYDROCHLORIDE
FLAGYL, METRONIDAZOLE
FLAREX, FLUOROMETHOLONE ACETATE
FLAVORED COLESTID, COLESTIPOL HYDROCHLORIDE
FLAXEDIL, GALLAMINE TRIETHIODIDE
FLECAINIDE ACETATE, FLECAINIDE ACETATE
FLEXERIL, CYCLOBENZAPRINE HYDROCHLORIDE

APPENDIX A
PRODUCT NAME INDEX (*continued*)

APPENDIX A
PRODUCT NAME INDEX (*continued*)

GENTAFAIR, GENTAMICIN SULFATE
GENTAK, GENTAMICIN SULFATE
GENTAMICIN SULFATE IN SODIUM CHLORIDE 0.9% IN
    PLASTIC CONTAINER, GENTAMICIN SULFATE
GENTAMICIN SULFATE, GENTAMICIN SULFATE
GENTAMICIN, GENTAMICIN SULFATE
GEOCILLIN, CARBENICILLIN INDANYL SODIUM
GEODON, ZIPRASIDONE HYDROCHLORIDE
GEODON, ZIPRASIDONE MESYLATE
GEOPEN, CARBENICILLIN DISODIUM
GEREF, SERMORELIN ACETATE
GERIMAL, ERGOLOID MESYLATES
GERMA-MEDICA "MG", HEXACHLOROPHENE
GERMA-MEDICA, HEXACHLOROPHENE
GLEEVEC, IMATINIB MESYLATE
GLIADEL, CARMUSTINE
GLIPIZIDE, GLIPIZIDE
GLOFIL-125, IOTHALAMATE SODIUM, I-125
GLUCAGEN, GLUCAGON HYDROCHLORIDE
    RECOMBINANT
GLUCAGON, GLUCAGON HYDROCHLORIDE
GLUCAGON, GLUCAGON RECOMBINANT
GLUCAMIDE, CHLORPROPAMIDE
GLUCOPHAGE XR, METFORMIN HYDROCHLORIDE
GLUCOPHAGE, METFORMIN HYDROCHLORIDE
GLUCOSCAN, TECHNETIUM TC-99M GLUCEPTATE KIT
GLUCOTROL XL, GLIPIZIDE
GLUCOTROL, GLIPIZIDE
GLUCOVANCE, GLYBURIDE
GLUTETHIMIDE, GLUTETHIMIDE
GLYBURIDE (MICRONIZED), GLYBURIDE
GLYBURIDE, GLYBURIDE
GLYCINE 1.5% IN PLASTIC CONTAINER, GLYCINE
GLYCOPREP, POLYETHYLENE GLYCOL 3350
GLYCOPYRROLATE, GLYCOPYRROLATE
GLYCORT, HYDROCORTISONE
GLYNASE, GLYBURIDE
GLYSET, MIGLITOL
GO-EVAC, POLYETHYLENE GLYCOL 3350
GOLYTELY, POLYETHYLENE GLYCOL 3350
GONAL-F, FOLLITROPIN ALFA
GONAL-F, FOLLITROPIN ALFA/BETA
GRIFULVIN V, GRISEOFULVIN, MICROCRYSTALLINE
GRIS-PEG, GRISEOFULVIN, ULTRAMICROCRYSTALLINE
GRISACTIN ULTRA, GRISEOFULVIN,
    ULTRAMICROCRYSTALLINE
GRISACTIN, GRISEOFULVIN, MICROCRYSTALLINE
GUANABENZ ACETATE, GUANABENZ ACETATE
GUANETHIDINE MONOSULFATE, GUANETHIDINE
    MONOSULFATE
GUANFACINE HCL, GUANFACINE HYDROCHLORIDE
GUANIDINE HCL, GUANIDINE HYDROCHLORIDE
GVS, GENTIAN VIOLET
GYNAZOLE-1, BUTOCONAZOLE NITRATE
GYNE-LOTRIMIN 3 COMBINATION PACK,
    CLOTRIMAZOLE (OTC)
GYNE-LOTRIMIN 3, CLOTRIMAZOLE (OTC)
GYNE-LOTRIMIN COMBINATION PACK, CLOTRIMAZOLE
    (OTC)
GYNE-LOTRIMIN, CLOTRIMAZOLE (OTC)
GYNE-SULF, TRIPLE SULFA
    (SULFABENZAMIDE;SULFACETAMIDE;
    SULFATHIAZOLE)
GYNIX, CLOTRIMAZOLE (OTC)
GYNODIOL, ESTRADIOL
GYNOREST, DYDROGESTERONE

H

H-CORT, HYDROCORTISONE
H.P. ACTHAR GEL, CORTICOTROPIN
H.R.-50, HYDROCHLOROTHIAZIDE
HABITROL, NICOTINE (OTC)
HALCION, TRIAZOLAM
HALDOL SOLUTAB, HALOPERIDOL
HALDOL, HALOPERIDOL
HALDOL, HALOPERIDOL DECANOATE
HALDOL, HALOPERIDOL LACTATE
HALDRONE, PARAMETHASONE ACETATE
HALFAN, HALOFANTRINE HYDROCHLORIDE
HALOG, HALCINONIDE
HALOG-E, HALCINONIDE
HALOPERIDOL DECANOATE, HALOPERIDOL
    DECANOATE
HALOPERIDOL INTENSOL, HALOPERIDOL LACTATE
HALOPERIDOL LACTATE, HALOPERIDOL LACTATE
HALOPERIDOL, HALOPERIDOL
HALOPERIDOL, HALOPERIDOL LACTATE
HALOTESTIN, FLUOXYMESTERONE
HALOTEX, HALOPROGIN
HALOTHANE, HALOTHANE
HARMONYL, DESERPIDINE
HC #1, HYDROCORTISONE
HC #4, HYDROCORTISONE
HC (HYDROCORTISONE), HYDROCORTISONE
HC (HYDROCORTISONE), HYDROCORTISONE (OTC)
HEAD IN PLASTIC CONTAINER, HEPARIN SODIUM
HEPARIN SODIUM 1,000 UNITS IN DEXTROSE 5% IN
    PLASTIC CONTAINER, HEPARIN SODIUM
HEPARIN SODIUM 1,000 UNITS IN SODIUM CHLORIDE
    0.9% IN PLASTIC CONTAINER, HEPARIN SODIUM
HEPARIN SODIUM 10,000 UNITS IN DEXTROSE 5% IN
    PLASTIC CONTAINER, HEPARIN SODIUM
HEPARIN SODIUM 10,000 UNITS IN DEXTROSE 5%,
    HEPARIN SODIUM
HEPARIN SODIUM 10,000 UNITS IN SODIUM CHLORIDE
    0.45%, HEPARIN SODIUM
HEPARIN SODIUM 10,000 UNITS IN SODIUM CHLORIDE
    0.9%, HEPARIN SODIUM
HEPARIN SODIUM 12,500 UNITS IN DEXTROSE 5% IN
    PLASTIC CONTAINER, HEPARIN SODIUM
HEPARIN SODIUM 12,500 UNITS IN DEXTROSE 5%,
    HEPARIN SODIUM
HEPARIN SODIUM 12,500 UNITS IN SODIUM CHLORIDE
    0.45% IN PLASTIC CONTAINER, HEPARIN SODIUM
HEPARIN SODIUM 12,500 UNITS IN SODIUM CHLORIDE
    0.9%, HEPARIN SODIUM
HEPARIN SODIUM 2,000 UNITS AND SODIUM CHLORIDE
    0.9% IN PLASTIC CONTAINER, HEPARIN SODIUM
HEPARIN SODIUM 2,000 UNITS IN DEXTROSE 5% IN
    PLASTIC CONTAINER, HEPARIN SODIUM
HEPARIN SODIUM 2,000 UNITS IN SODIUM CHLORIDE
    0.9% IN PLASTIC CONTAINER, HEPARIN SODIUM
HEPARIN SODIUM 20,000 UNITS AND DEXTROSE 5% IN
    PLASTIC CONTAINER, HEPARIN SODIUM
HEPARIN SODIUM 20,000 UNITS IN DEXTROSE 5% IN
    PLASTIC CONTAINER, HEPARIN SODIUM
HEPARIN SODIUM 25,000 UNITS AND DEXTROSE 5% IN
    PLASTIC CONTAINER, HEPARIN SODIUM
HEPARIN SODIUM 25,000 UNITS IN DEXTROSE 5% IN
    PLASTIC CONTAINER, HEPARIN SODIUM
HEPARIN SODIUM 25,000 UNITS IN DEXTROSE 5%,
    HEPARIN SODIUM
HEPARIN SODIUM 25,000 UNITS IN SODIUM CHLORIDE
    0.45% IN PLASTIC CONTAINER, HEPARIN SODIUM

APPENDIX A
PRODUCT NAME INDEX (*continued*)

HEPARIN SODIUM 25,000 UNITS IN SODIUM CHLORIDE 0.9% IN PLASTIC CONTAINER, HEPARIN SODIUM
HEPARIN SODIUM 25,000 UNITS IN SODIUM CHLORIDE 0.9%, HEPARIN SODIUM
HEPARIN SODIUM 5,000 UNITS AND SODIUM CHLORIDE 0.9% IN PLASTIC CONTAINER, HEPARIN SODIUM
HEPARIN SODIUM 5,000 UNITS IN DEXTROSE 5% IN PLASTIC CONTAINER, HEPARIN SODIUM
HEPARIN SODIUM 5,000 UNITS IN SODIUM CHLORIDE 0.45%, HEPARIN SODIUM
HEPARIN SODIUM 5,000 UNITS IN SODIUM CHLORIDE 0.9% IN PLASTIC CONTAINER, HEPARIN SODIUM
HEPARIN SODIUM 5,000 UNITS IN SODIUM CHLORIDE 0.9%, HEPARIN SODIUM
HEPARIN SODIUM IN PLASTIC CONTAINER, HEPARIN SODIUM
HEPARIN SODIUM PRESERVATIVE FREE, HEPARIN SODIUM
HEPARIN SODIUM, HEPARIN SODIUM
HEPATAMINE 8%, AMINO ACIDS
HEPATASOL 8%, AMINO ACIDS
HEPATOLITE, TECHNETIUM TC-99M DISOFENIN KIT
HEPFLUSH-10, HEPARIN SODIUM
HEPSERA, ADEFOVIR DIPIVOXIL
HEPTALAC, LACTULOSE
HERPLEX, IDOXURIDINE
HETRAZAN, DIETHYLCARBAMAZINE CITRATE
HEXA-BETALIN, PYRIDOXINE HYDROCHLORIDE
HEXA-GERM, HEXACHLOROPHENE
HEXABRIX, IOXAGLATE MEGLUMINE
HEXADROL, DEXAMETHASONE
HEXADROL, DEXAMETHASONE SODIUM PHOSPHATE
HEXALEN, ALTRETAMINE
HEXASCRUB, HEXACHLOROPHENE
HI-COR, HYDROCORTISONE
HIBICLENS, CHLORHEXIDINE GLUCONATE (OTC)
HIBISTAT, CHLORHEXIDINE GLUCONATE (OTC)
HIPPURAN I 131, IODOHIPPURATE SODIUM, I-131
HIPPUTOPE, IODOHIPPURATE SODIUM, I-131
HIPREX, METHENAMINE HIPPURATE
HISERPIA, RESERPINE
HISPRIL, DIPHENYLPYRALINE HYDROCHLORIDE
HISTAFED, PSEUDOEPHEDRINE HYDROCHLORIDE
HISTALOG, BETAZOLE HYDROCHLORIDE
HISTAMINE PHOSPHATE, HISTAMINE PHOSPHATE
HIVID, ZALCITABINE
HIWOLFIA, RAUWOLFIA SERPENTINA
HMS, MEDRYSONE
HOMAPIN-5, HOMATROPINE METHYLBROMIDE
HOMAPIN-10, HOMATROPINE METHYLBROMIDE
HOMATROPRINE METHYLBROMIDE AND HYDROCODONE BITARTRATE, HOMATROPINE METHYLBROMIDE
HUMALOG MIX 50/50, INSULIN LISPRO
HUMALOG MIX 75/25, INSULIN LISPRO
HUMALOG PEN, INSULIN LISPRO
HUMALOG, INSULIN LISPRO
HUMATIN, PAROMOMYCIN SULFATE
HUMATROPE, SOMATROPIN RECOMBINANT
HUMEGON, MENOTROPINS (FSH;LH)
HUMORSOL, DEMECARIUM BROMIDE
HUMULIN 50/50, INSULIN RECOMBINANT HUMAN (OTC)
HUMULIN 70/30 PEN, INSULIN RECOMBINANT HUMAN (OTC)
HUMULIN 70/30, INSULIN RECOMBINANT HUMAN (OTC)
HUMULIN BR, INSULIN RECOMBINANT HUMAN (OTC)
HUMULIN L, INSULIN ZINC SUSP RECOMBINANT HUMAN (OTC)

HUMULIN N, INSULIN SUSP ISOPHANE RECOMBINANT HUMAN (OTC)
HUMULIN R PEN, INSULIN RECOMBINANT HUMAN (OTC)
HUMULIN R, INSULIN RECOMBINANT HUMAN
HUMULIN R, INSULIN RECOMBINANT HUMAN (OTC)
HUMULIN U, INSULIN ZINC SUSP EXTENDED RECOMBINANT HUMAN (OTC)
HY-PAM "25", HYDROXYZINE PAMOATE
HY-PHEN, ACETAMINOPHEN
HYCAMTIN, TOPOTECAN HYDROCHLORIDE
HYCODAN, HOMATROPINE METHYLBROMIDE
HYCOMINE PEDIATRIC, HYDROCODONE BITARTRATE
HYCOMINE, HYDROCODONE BITARTRATE
HYDELTRA-TBA, PREDNISOLONE TEBUTATE
HYDELTRASOL, PREDNISOLONE SODIUM PHOSPHATE
HYDERGINE LC, ERGOLOID MESYLATES
HYDERGINE, ERGOLOID MESYLATES
HYDRA-ZIDE, HYDRALAZINE HYDROCHLORIDE
HYDRALAZINE AND HYDROCHLORTHIAZIDE, HYDRALAZINE HYDROCHLORIDE
HYDRALAZINE HCL AND HYDROCHLOROTHIAZIDE, HYDRALAZINE HYDROCHLORIDE
HYDRALAZINE HCL W/ HYDROCHLOROTHIAZIDE 100/50, HYDRALAZINE HYDROCHLORIDE
HYDRALAZINE HCL W/ HYDROCHLOROTHIAZIDE 25/25, HYDRALAZINE HYDROCHLORIDE
HYDRALAZINE HCL W/ HYDROCHLOROTHIAZIDE 50/50, HYDRALAZINE HYDROCHLORIDE
HYDRALAZINE HCL, HYDRALAZINE HYDROCHLORIDE
HYDRALAZINE HCL, HYDROCHLOROTHIAZIDE AND RESERPINE, HYDRALAZINE HYDROCHLORIDE
HYDRALAZINE HCL-HYDROCHLOROTHIAZIDE-RESERPINE, HYDRALAZINE HYDROCHLORIDE
HYDRALAZINE, HYDROCHLOROTHIAZIDE W/ RESERPINE, HYDRALAZINE HYDROCHLORIDE
HYDRAMINE, DIPHENHYDRAMINE HYDROCHLORIDE
HYDRAMINE, DIPHENHYDRAMINE HYDROCHLORIDE (OTC)
HYDRAP-ES, HYDRALAZINE HYDROCHLORIDE
HYDREA, HYDROXYUREA
HYDRO-D, HYDROCHLOROTHIAZIDE
HYDRO-RESERP, HYDROCHLOROTHIAZIDE
HYDRO-RIDE, AMILORIDE HYDROCHLORIDE
HYDRO-SERP "25", HYDROCHLOROTHIAZIDE
HYDRO-SERP "50", HYDROCHLOROTHIAZIDE
HYDROCET, ACETAMINOPHEN
HYDROCHLOROTHIAZIDE INTENSOL, HYDROCHLOROTHIAZIDE
HYDROCHLOROTHIAZIDE W/ HYDRALAZINE, HYDRALAZINE HYDROCHLORIDE
HYDROCHLOROTHIAZIDE W/ RESERPINE AND HYDRALAZINE, HYDRALAZINE HYDROCHLORIDE
HYDROCHLOROTHIAZIDE W/ RESERPINE, HYDROCHLOROTHIAZIDE
HYDROCHLOROTHIAZIDE, HYDROCHLOROTHIAZIDE
HYDROCODONE BITARTRATE AND ACETAMINOPHEN, ACETAMINOPHEN
HYDROCODONE BITARTRATE AND HOMATROPINE METHYLBROMIDE, HOMATROPINE METHYLBROMIDE
HYDROCODONE BITARTRATE AND IBUPROFEN, HYDROCODONE BITARTRATE
HYDROCODONE COMPOUND, HOMATROPINE METHYLBROMIDE
HYDROCORTISONE ACETATE 1% AND PRAMOXINE HCL 1%, HYDROCORTISONE ACETATE
HYDROCORTISONE ACETATE, HYDROCORTISONE ACETATE

APPENDIX A
PRODUCT NAME INDEX (*continued*)

HYDROCORTISONE AND ACETIC ACID, ACETIC ACID, GLACIAL
HYDROCORTISONE IN ABSORBASE, HYDROCORTISONE
HYDROCORTISONE SODIUM PHOSPHATE, HYDROCORTISONE SODIUM PHOSPHATE
HYDROCORTISONE SODIUM SUCCINATE, HYDROCORTISONE SODIUM SUCCINATE
HYDROCORTISONE VALERATE, HYDROCORTISONE VALERATE
HYDROCORTISONE, HYDROCORTISONE
HYDROCORTONE, HYDROCORTISONE
HYDROCORTONE, HYDROCORTISONE ACETATE
HYDROCORTONE, HYDROCORTISONE SODIUM PHOSPHATE
HYDRODIURIL, HYDROCHLOROTHIAZIDE
HYDROFLUMETHIAZIDE AND RESERPINE, HYDROFLUMETHIAZIDE
HYDROFLUMETHIAZIDE, HYDROFLUMETHIAZIDE
HYDROGENATED ERGOT ALKALOIDS, ERGOLOID MESYLATES
HYDROMORPHONE HCL, HYDROMORPHONE HYDROCHLORIDE
HYDROMOX R, QUINETHAZONE
HYDROMOX, QUINETHAZONE
HYDROPANE, HOMATROPINE METHYLBROMIDE
HYDROPRES 25, HYDROCHLOROTHIAZIDE
HYDROPRES 50, HYDROCHLOROTHIAZIDE
HYDROSERPINE PLUS (R-H-H), HYDRALAZINE HYDROCHLORIDE
HYDROXOCOBALAMIN, HYDROXOCOBALAMIN
HYDROXOMIN, HYDROXOCOBALAMIN
HYDROXYCHLOROQINE SULFATE, HYDROXYCHLOROQUINE SULFATE
HYDROXYCHLOROQUINE SULFATE, HYDROXYCHLOROQUINE SULFATE
HYDROXYPROGESTERONE CAPROATE, HYDROXYPROGESTERONE CAPROATE
HYDROXYSTILBAMIDINE ISETHIONATE, HYDROXYSTILBAMIDINE ISETHIONATE
HYDROXYUREA, HYDROXYUREA
HYDROXYZINE HCL, HYDROXYZINE HYDROCHLORIDE
HYDROXYZINE PAMOATE, HYDROXYZINE PAMOATE
HYDROXYZINE, HYDROXYZINE HYDROCHLORIDE
HYGROTON, CHLORTHALIDONE
HYLOREL, GUANADREL SULFATE
HYPAQUE SODIUM 20%, DIATRIZOATE SODIUM
HYPAQUE, DIATRIZOATE MEGLUMINE
HYPAQUE, DIATRIZOATE SODIUM
HYPAQUE-76, DIATRIZOATE MEGLUMINE
HYPAQUE-CYSTO, DIATRIZOATE MEGLUMINE
HYPAQUE-M,75%, DIATRIZOATE MEGLUMINE
HYPAQUE-M,90%, DIATRIZOATE MEGLUMINE
HYPERSTAT, DIAZOXIDE
HYPROTIGEN 5%, PROTEIN HYDROLYSATE
HYSERPIN, RAUWOLFIA SERPENTINA
HYTONE, HYDROCORTISONE
HYTRIN, TERAZOSIN HYDROCHLORIDE
HYZAAR, HYDROCHLOROTHIAZIDE
HYZYD, ISONIAZID

I

IBRIN, FIBRINOGEN, I-125
IBU, IBUPROFEN
IBU-TAB 200, IBUPROFEN (OTC)
IBU-TAB, IBUPROFEN
IBUPRIN, IBUPROFEN (OTC)
IBUPROFEN AND PSEUDOEPHEDRINE HCL, IBUPROFEN (OTC)
IBUPROFEN, IBUPROFEN
IBUPROFEN, IBUPROFEN (OTC)
IBUPROHM COLD AND SINUS, IBUPROFEN (OTC)
IBUPROHM, IBUPROFEN
IBUPROHM, IBUPROFEN (OTC)
IDAMYCIN PFS, IDARUBICIN HYDROCHLORIDE
IDAMYCIN, IDARUBICIN HYDROCHLORIDE
IDARUBICIN HCL PFS, IDARUBICIN HYDROCHLORIDE
IDARUBICIN HCL, IDARUBICIN HYDROCHLORIDE
IDKIT:HP, CITRIC ACID
IFEX, IFOSFAMIDE
IFEX/MESNEX KIT, IFOSFAMIDE
IFOSFAMIDE/MESNA KIT, IFOSFAMIDE
IFSOFAMIDE, IFOSFAMIDE
ILETIN I, INSULIN PORK
ILETIN II, INSULIN PURIFIED PORK
ILOSONE SULFA, ERYTHROMYCIN ESTOLATE
ILOSONE, ERYTHROMYCIN ESTOLATE
ILOTYCIN GLUCEPTATE, ERYTHROMYCIN GLUCEPTATE
ILOTYCIN, ERYTHROMYCIN
IMAGENT, DIMYRISTOYL LECITHIN
IMAGENT, PERFLUBRON
IMDUR, ISOSORBIDE MONONITRATE
IMIPRAMINE HCL, IMIPRAMINE HYDROCHLORIDE
IMITREX, SUMATRIPTAN
IMITREX, SUMATRIPTAN SUCCINATE
IMODIUM A-D, LOPERAMIDE HYDROCHLORIDE (OTC)
IMODIUM ADVANCED, LOPERAMIDE HYDROCHLORIDE (OTC)
IMODIUM, LOPERAMIDE HYDROCHLORIDE
IMURAN, AZATHIOPRINE
IMURAN, AZATHIOPRINE SODIUM
INAPSINE, DROPERIDOL
INDAPAMIDE, INDAPAMIDE
INDERAL LA, PROPRANOLOL HYDROCHLORIDE
INDERAL, PROPRANOLOL HYDROCHLORIDE
INDERIDE LA 80/50, HYDROCHLOROTHIAZIDE
INDERIDE LA 120/50, HYDROCHLOROTHIAZIDE
INDERIDE LA 160/50, HYDROCHLOROTHIAZIDE
INDERIDE-40/25, HYDROCHLOROTHIAZIDE
INDERIDE-80/25, HYDROCHLOROTHIAZIDE
INDIUM IN-111 OXYQUINOLINE, INDIUM IN-111 OXYQUINOLINE
INDO-LEMMON, INDOMETHACIN
INDOCIN I.V., INDOMETHACIN SODIUM
INDOCIN SR, INDOMETHACIN
INDOCIN, INDOMETHACIN
INDOMETHACIN, INDOMETHACIN
INDOMETHEGAN, INDOMETHACIN
INFANTS' FEVERALL, ACETAMINOPHEN (OTC)
INFASURF PRESERVATIVE FREE, CALFACTANT
INFED, IRON DEXTRAN
INFLAMASE FORTE, PREDNISOLONE SODIUM PHOSPHATE
INFLAMASE MILD, PREDNISOLONE SODIUM PHOSPHATE
INFUMORPH, MORPHINE SULFATE
INFUVITE ADULT, ALPHA-TOCOPHEROL ACETATE
INFUVITE PEDIATRIC, ASCORBIC ACID
INH, ISONIAZID
INJECTAPAP, ACETAMINOPHEN
INNOFEM, ESTRADIOL
INNOHEP, TINZAPARIN SODIUM
INNOPRAN XL, PROPRANOLOL HYDROCHLORIDE
INNOVAR, DROPERIDOL
INOCOR, INAMRINONE LACTATE
INOMAX, NITRIC OXIDE

APPENDIX A
PRODUCT NAME INDEX (*continued*)

INPERSOL-LC/LM W/ DEXTROSE 1.5% IN PLASTIC
    CONTAINER, CALCIUM CHLORIDE
INPERSOL-LC/LM W/ DEXTROSE 2.5% IN PLASTIC
    CONTAINER, CALCIUM CHLORIDE
INPERSOL-LC/LM W/ DEXTROSE 3.5% IN PLASTIC
    CONTAINER, CALCIUM CHLORIDE
INPERSOL-LC/LM W/ DEXTROSE 4.25% IN PLASTIC
    CONTAINER, CALCIUM CHLORIDE
INPERSOL-ZM W/ DEXTROSE 1.5% IN PLASTIC
    CONTAINER, CALCIUM CHLORIDE
INPERSOL-ZM W/ DEXTROSE 2.5% IN PLASTIC
    CONTAINER, CALCIUM CHLORIDE
INPERSOL-ZM W/ DEXTROSE 4.25% IN PLASTIC
    CONTAINER, CALCIUM CHLORIDE
INSPRA, EPLERENONE
INSTANT MICROSPHERES, TECHNETIUM TC-99M
    ALBUMIN MICROSPHERES KIT
INSULATARD NPH HUMAN, INSULIN SUSP ISOPHANE
    SEMISYNTHETIC PURIFIED HUMAN (OTC)
INSULIN INSULATARD NPH NORDISK, INSULIN SUSP
    ISOPHANE PURIFIED PORK (OTC)
INSULIN NORDISK MIXTARD (PORK), INSULIN PURIFIED
    PORK (OTC)
INSULIN, INSULIN PORK (OTC)
INTAL, CROMOLYN SODIUM
INTEGRILIN, EPTIFIBATIDE
INTRALIPID 10%, SOYBEAN OIL
INTRALIPID 20%, SOYBEAN OIL
INTRALIPID 30%, SOYBEAN OIL
INTROPIN, DOPAMINE HYDROCHLORIDE
INULIN AND SODIUM CHLORIDE, INULIN
INVAGESIC FORTE, ASPIRIN
INVAGESIC, ASPIRIN
INVANZ, ERTAPENEM SODIUM
INVERSINE, MECAMYLAMINE HYDROCHLORIDE
INVIRASE, SAQUINAVIR MESYLATE
IOBENGUANE SULFATE I 131, IOBENGUANE SULFATE
    I-131
IODOHIPPURATE SODIUM I 131, IODOHIPPURATE
    SODIUM, I-131
IODOTOPE, SODIUM IODIDE, I-131
IONAMIN, PHENTERMINE RESIN COMPLEX
IONOSOL B AND DEXTROSE 5% IN PLASTIC
    CONTAINER, DEXTROSE
IONOSOL MB AND DEXTROSE 5% IN PLASTIC
    CONTAINER, DEXTROSE
IONOSOL T AND DEXTROSE 5% IN PLASTIC CONTAINER,
    DEXTROSE
IONTOCAINE, EPINEPHRINE
IOPAMIDOL, IOPAMIDOL
IOPAMIDOL-200 IN PLASTIC CONTAINER, IOPAMIDOL
IOPAMIDOL-200, IOPAMIDOL
IOPAMIDOL-250 IN PLASTIC CONTAINER, IOPAMIDOL
IOPAMIDOL-250, IOPAMIDOL
IOPAMIDOL-300 IN PLASTIC CONTAINER, IOPAMIDOL
IOPAMIDOL-300, IOPAMIDOL
IOPAMIDOL-370 IN PLASTIC CONTAINER, IOPAMIDOL
IOPAMIDOL-370, IOPAMIDOL
IOPIDINE, APRACLONIDINE HYDROCHLORIDE
IOSAT, POTASSIUM IODIDE (OTC)
IPATROPIUM BROMIDE, IPRATROPIUM BROMIDE
IPRATROPIUM BROMIDE, IPRATROPIUM BROMIDE
IPRIVASK, DESIRUDIN
IRESSA, GEFITINIB
IRON DEXTRAN, IRON DEXTRAN
IRRIGATING SOLUTION G IN PLASTIC CONTAINER,
    CITRIC ACID

ISMELIN, GUANETHIDINE MONOSULFATE
ISMO, ISOSORBIDE MONONITRATE
ISMOTIC, ISOSORBIDE
ISOCAINE HCL W/ LEVONORDEFRIN, LEVONORDEFRIN
ISOCAINE HCL, MEPIVACAINE HYDROCHLORIDE
ISOCLOR, CHLORPHENIRAMINE MALEATE (OTC)
ISOETHARINE HCL S/F, ISOETHARINE HYDROCHLORIDE
ISOETHARINE HCL, ISOETHARINE HYDROCHLORIDE
ISOETHARINE MESYLATE, ISOETHARINE MESYLATE
ISOFLURANE, ISOFLURANE
ISOLYTE E IN DEXTROSE 5% IN PLASTIC CONTAINER,
    CALCIUM CHLORIDE
ISOLYTE E IN PLASTIC CONTAINER, CALCIUM
    CHLORIDE
ISOLYTE E W/ DEXTROSE 5% IN PLASTIC CONTAINER,
    CALCIUM CHLORIDE
ISOLYTE H IN DEXTROSE 5% IN PLASTIC CONTAINER,
    DEXTROSE
ISOLYTE H W/ DEXTROSE 5% IN PLASTIC CONTAINER,
    DEXTROSE
ISOLYTE M IN DEXTROSE 5% IN PLASTIC CONTAINER,
    DEXTROSE
ISOLYTE M W/ DEXTROSE 5% IN PLASTIC CONTAINER,
    DEXTROSE
ISOLYTE P IN DEXTROSE 5% IN PLASTIC CONTAINER,
    DEXTROSE
ISOLYTE P W/ DEXTROSE 5% IN PLASTIC CONTAINER,
    DEXTROSE
ISOLYTE R IN DEXTROSE 5% IN PLASTIC CONTAINER,
    CALCIUM CHLORIDE
ISOLYTE R W/ DEXTROSE 5% IN PLASTIC CONTAINER,
    CALCIUM CHLORIDE
ISOLYTE S IN DEXTROSE 5% IN PLASTIC CONTAINER,
    DEXTROSE
ISOLYTE S IN PLASTIC CONTAINER, MAGNESIUM
    CHLORIDE
ISOLYTE S PH 7.4 IN PLASTIC CONTAINER, MAGNESIUM
    CHLORIDE
ISOLYTE S W/ DEXTROSE 5% IN PLASTIC CONTAINER,
    DEXTROSE
ISONIAZID, ISONIAZID
ISOPAQUE 280, CALCIUM
ISOPAQUE 440, CALCIUM METRIZOATE
ISOPROTERENOL HCL, ISOPROTERENOL
    HYDROCHLORIDE
ISOPTIN SR, VERAPAMIL HYDROCHLORIDE
ISOPTIN, VERAPAMIL HYDROCHLORIDE
ISOPTO CETAMIDE, SULFACETAMIDE SODIUM
ISOPTO CETAPRED, PREDNISOLONE ACETATE
ISORDIL, ISOSORBIDE DINITRATE
ISOSORBIDE DINITRATE, ISOSORBIDE DINITRATE
ISOSORBIDE MONONITRATE, ISOSORBIDE
    MONONITRATE
ISOTONIC GENTAMICIN SULFATE IN PLASTIC
    CONTAINER, GENTAMICIN SULFATE
ISOTRETINOIN, ISOTRETINOIN
ISOVUE-128, IOPAMIDOL
ISOVUE-200, IOPAMIDOL
ISOVUE-250, IOPAMIDOL
ISOVUE-300, IOPAMIDOL
ISOVUE-370, IOPAMIDOL
ISOVUE-M 200, IOPAMIDOL
ISOVUE-M 300, IOPAMIDOL
ISUPREL, ISOPROTERENOL HYDROCHLORIDE
IV PERSANTINE, DIPYRIDAMOLE
IVADANTIN, NITROFURANTOIN SODIUM
IVY BLOCK, BENTOQUATAM (OTC)

APPENDIX A
PRODUCT NAME INDEX (*continued*)

J

JANIMINE, IMIPRAMINE HYDROCHLORIDE
JUNEL 1.5/30, ETHINYL ESTRADIOL
JUNEL 1/20, ETHINYL ESTRADIOL
JUNIOR STRENGTH ADVIL, IBUPROFEN (OTC)
JUNIOR STRENGTH IBUPROFEN, IBUPROFEN (OTC)
JUNIOR STRENGTH MOTRIN, IBUPROFEN (OTC)

K

K+8, POTASSIUM CHLORIDE
K+10, POTASSIUM CHLORIDE
K-DUR 10, POTASSIUM CHLORIDE
K-DUR 20, POTASSIUM CHLORIDE
K-LEASE, POTASSIUM CHLORIDE
K-TAB, POTASSIUM CHLORIDE
KADIAN, MORPHINE SULFATE
KAFOCIN, CEPHALOGLYCIN
KAINAIR, PROPARACAINE HYDROCHLORIDE
KALETRA, LOPINAVIR
KANAMYCIN SULFATE, KANAMYCIN SULFATE
KANAMYCIN, KANAMYCIN SULFATE
KANTREX, KANAMYCIN SULFATE
KAON CL, POTASSIUM CHLORIDE
KAON CL-10, POTASSIUM CHLORIDE
KAPPADIONE, MENADIOL SODIUM DIPHOSPHATE
KARIVA, DESOGESTREL
KAYEXALATE, SODIUM POLYSTYRENE SULFONATE
KEFLET, CEPHALEXIN
KEFLEX, CEPHALEXIN
KEFLIN IN PLASTIC CONTAINER, CEPHALOTHIN SODIUM
KEFLIN, CEPHALOTHIN SODIUM
KEFTAB, CEPHALEXIN HYDROCHLORIDE
KEFUROX IN PLASTIC CONTAINER, CEFUROXIME
    SODIUM
KEFUROX, CEFUROXIME SODIUM
KEFZOL, CEFAZOLIN SODIUM
KEMADRIN, PROCYCLIDINE HYDROCHLORIDE
KENACORT, TRIAMCINOLONE
KENACORT, TRIAMCINOLONE DIACETATE
KENALOG IN ORABASE, TRIAMCINOLONE ACETONIDE
KENALOG, TRIAMCINOLONE ACETONIDE
KENALOG-10, TRIAMCINOLONE ACETONIDE
KENALOG-40, TRIAMCINOLONE ACETONIDE
KENALOG-H, TRIAMCINOLONE ACETONIDE
KEPPRA, LEVETIRACETAM
KERLEDEX, BETAXOLOL HYDROCHLORIDE
KERLONE, BETAXOLOL HYDROCHLORIDE
KESSO-GESIC, PROPOXYPHENE HYDROCHLORIDE
KETALAR, KETAMINE HYDROCHLORIDE
KETAMINE HCL, KETAMINE HYDROCHLORIDE
KETOCONAZOLE, KETOCONAZOLE
KETOPROFEN, KETOPROFEN
KETOPROFEN, KETOPROFEN (OTC)
KETOROLAC TROMETHAMINE, KETOROLAC
    TROMETHAMINE
KETOZOLE, KETOCONAZOLE
KINEVAC, SINCALIDE
KIONEX, SODIUM POLYSTYRENE SULFONATE
KLARON, SULFACETAMIDE SODIUM
KLEBCIL, KANAMYCIN SULFATE
KLONOPIN RAPIDLY DISINTEGRATING, CLONAZEPAM
KLONOPIN, CLONAZEPAM
KLOR-CON M10, POTASSIUM CHLORIDE
KLOR-CON M15, POTASSIUM CHLORIDE
KLOR-CON M20, POTASSIUM CHLORIDE
KLOR-CON, POTASSIUM CHLORIDE

KLOROMIN, CHLORPHENIRAMINE MALEATE
KLOTRIX, POTASSIUM CHLORIDE
KOGLUCOID, RAUWOLFIA SERPENTINA
KONAKION, PHYTONADIONE
KOROSTATIN, NYSTATIN
KWELL, LINDANE
KYTRIL, GRANISETRON HYDROCHLORIDE

L

LABETALOL HCL, LABETALOL HYDROCHLORIDE
LABID, THEOPHYLLINE
LAC-HYDRIN, AMMONIUM LACTATE
LACRISERT, HYDROXYPROPYL CELLULOSE
LACTATED RINGER'S AND DEXTROSE 5% IN PLASTIC
    CONTAINER, CALCIUM CHLORIDE
LACTATED RINGER'S IN PLASTIC CONTAINER, CALCIUM
    CHLORIDE
LACTULOSE, LACTULOSE
LAMICTAL CD, LAMOTRIGINE
LAMICTAL, LAMOTRIGINE
LAMISIL AT, TERBINAFINE HYDROCHLORIDE (OTC)
LAMISIL, TERBINAFINE
LAMISIL, TERBINAFINE HYDROCHLORIDE
I AMISIL, TERBINAFINE HYDROCHLORIDE (OTC)
LAMPRENE, CLOFAZIMINE
LANABIOTIC, BACITRACIN (OTC)
LANABIOTIC, BACITRACIN ZINC (OTC)
LANIAZID, ISONIAZID
LANOPHYLLIN, THEOPHYLLINE
LANORINAL, ASPIRIN
LANOXICAPS, DIGOXIN
LANOXIN PEDIATRIC, DIGOXIN
LANOXIN, DIGOXIN
LANTRISUL, TRISULFAPYRIMIDINES (SULFADIAZINE;
    SULFAMERAZINE; SULFAMETHAZINE)
LANTUS, INSULIN GLARGINE
LARGON, PROPIOMAZINE HYDROCHLORIDE
LARIAM, MEFLOQUINE HYDROCHLORIDE
LARODOPA, LEVODOPA
LAROTID, AMOXICILLIN
LARYNG-O-JET KIT, LIDOCAINE HYDROCHLORIDE
LARYNGOTRACHEAL ANESTHESIA KIT, LIDOCAINE
    HYDROCHLORIDE
LASIX, FUROSEMIDE
LAXILOSE, LACTULOSE
LEDERCILLIN VK, PENICILLIN V POTASSIUM
LENTARD, INSULIN ZINC SUSP PURIFIED BEEF/PORK
    (OTC)
LENTE ILETIN II (PORK), INSULIN ZINC SUSP PURIFIED
    PORK (OTC)
LENTE ILETIN II, INSULIN ZINC SUSP PURIFIED BEEF
    (OTC)
LENTE INSULIN, INSULIN ZINC SUSP BEEF (OTC)
LENTE, INSULIN ZINC SUSP PURIFIED PORK (OTC)
LERITINE, ANILERIDINE HYDROCHLORIDE
LERITINE, ANILERIDINE PHOSPHATE
LESCOL XL, FLUVASTATIN SODIUM
LESCOL, FLUVASTATIN SODIUM
LESSINA-21, ETHINYL ESTRADIOL
LESSINA-28, ETHINYL ESTRADIOL
LEUCOVORIN CALCIUM PRESERVATIVE FREE,
    LEUCOVORIN CALCIUM
LEUCOVORIN CALCIUM, LEUCOVORIN CALCIUM
LEUKERAN, CHLORAMBUCIL
LEUPROLIDE ACETATE, LEUPROLIDE ACETATE
LEUSTATIN, CLADRIBINE
LEVAQUIN IN DEXTROSE 5% IN PLASTIC CONTAINER,
    LEVOFLOXACIN

APPENDIX A
PRODUCT NAME INDEX (*continued*)

LEVAQUIN, LEVOFLOXACIN
LEVATOL, PENBUTOLOL SULFATE
LEVLITE, ETHINYL ESTRADIOL
LEVO-DROMORAN, LEVORPHANOL TARTRATE
LEVO-T, LIOTRIX (T4;T3)
LEVOBUNOLOL HCL, LEVOBUNOLOL HYDROCHLORIDE
LEVOCARNITINE, LEVOCARNITINE
LEVOLET, LIOTRIX (T4;T3)
LEVONORGESTREL AND ETHINYL ESTRADIOL, ETHINYL
    ESTRADIOL
LEVONORGESTREL, LEVONORGESTREL
LEVOPHED, NOREPINEPHRINE BITARTRATE
LEVOPROME, LEVOMEPROMAZINE
LEVORA 0.15/30-21, ETHINYL ESTRADIOL
LEVORA 0.15/30-28, ETHINYL ESTRADIOL
LEVORPHANOL TARTRATE, LEVORPHANOL TARTRATE
LEVOTHYROXINE SODIUM, LIOTRIX (T4;T3)
LEVOXYL, LIOTRIX (T4;T3)
LEVULAN, AMINOLEVULINIC ACID HYDROCHLORIDE
LEXAPRO, ESCITALOPRAM OXALATE
LEXXEL, ENALAPRIL MALEATE
LIBRELEASE, CHLORDIAZEPOXIDE
LIBRITABS, CHLORDIAZEPOXIDE
LIBRIUM, CHLORDIAZEPOXIDE HYDROCHLORIDE
LIDEX, FLUOCINONIDE
LIDEX-E, FLUOCINONIDE
LIDOCAINE HCL 0.1% AND DEXTROSE 5% IN PLASTIC
    CONTAINER, LIDOCAINE HYDROCHLORIDE
LIDOCAINE HCL 0.2% AND DEXTROSE 5% IN PLASTIC
    CONTAINER, LIDOCAINE HYDROCHLORIDE
LIDOCAINE HCL 0.2% IN DEXTROSE 5% IN PLASTIC
    CONTAINER, LIDOCAINE HYDROCHLORIDE
LIDOCAINE HCL 0.2% IN DEXTROSE 5%, LIDOCAINE
    HYDROCHLORIDE
LIDOCAINE HCL 0.4% AND DEXTROSE 5% IN PLASTIC
    CONTAINER, LIDOCAINE HYDROCHLORIDE
LIDOCAINE HCL 0.4% IN DEXTROSE 5% IN PLASTIC
    CONTAINER, LIDOCAINE HYDROCHLORIDE
LIDOCAINE HCL 0.4% IN DEXTROSE 5%, LIDOCAINE
    HYDROCHLORIDE
LIDOCAINE HCL 0.8% AND DEXTROSE 5% IN PLASTIC
    CONTAINER, LIDOCAINE HYDROCHLORIDE
LIDOCAINE HCL 0.8% IN DEXTROSE 5% IN PLASTIC
    CONTAINER, LIDOCAINE HYDROCHLORIDE
LIDOCAINE HCL 5% AND DEXTROSE 7.5%, LIDOCAINE
    HYDROCHLORIDE
LIDOCAINE HCL AND EPINEPHRINE, EPINEPHRINE
LIDOCAINE HCL IN PLASTIC CONTAINER, LIDOCAINE
    HYDROCHLORIDE
LIDOCAINE HCL PRESERVATIVE FREE IN PLASTIC
    CONTAINER, LIDOCAINE HYDROCHLORIDE
LIDOCAINE HCL PRESERVATIVE FREE, LIDOCAINE
    HYDROCHLORIDE
LIDOCAINE HCL VISCOUS, LIDOCAINE
    HYDROCHLORIDE
LIDOCAINE HCL W/ EPINEPHRINE, EPINEPHRINE
LIDOCAINE HCL, LIDOCAINE HYDROCHLORIDE
LIDOCAINE VISCOUS, LIDOCAINE HYDROCHLORIDE
LIDOCAINE, LIDOCAINE
LIDOCATON, EPINEPHRINE
LIDOCATON, LIDOCAINE HYDROCHLORIDE
LIDODERM, LIDOCAINE
LIDOPEN, LIDOCAINE HYDROCHLORIDE
LIGNOSPAN FORTE, EPINEPHRINE BITARTRATE
LIGNOSPAN STANDARD, EPINEPHRINE BITARTRATE
LIMBITROL DS, AMITRIPTYLINE HYDROCHLORIDE
LIMBITROL, AMITRIPTYLINE HYDROCHLORIDE
LINCOCIN, LINCOMYCIN HYDROCHLORIDE
LINCOMYCIN HCL, LINCOMYCIN HYDROCHLORIDE

LINDANE, LINDANE
LIORESAL, BACLOFEN
LIOTHYRONINE SODIUM, LIOTRIX (T4;T3)
LIPIDIL, FENOFIBRATE
LIPITOR, ATORVASTATIN CALCIUM
LIPO GANTRISIN, SULFISOXAZOLE ACETYL
LIPO-HEPIN, HEPARIN SODIUM
LIPOSYN 10%, SAFFLOWER OIL
LIPOSYN 20%, SAFFLOWER OIL
LIPOSYN II 10%, SAFFLOWER OIL
LIPOSYN II 20%, SAFFLOWER OIL
LIPOSYN III 10%, SOYBEAN OIL
LIPOSYN III 20%, SOYBEAN OIL
LIPOSYN III 30%, SOYBEAN OIL
LIQUAEMIN LOCK FLUSH, HEPARIN SODIUM
LIQUAEMIN SODIUM PRESERVATIVE FREE, HEPARIN
    SODIUM
LIQUAEMIN SODIUM, HEPARIN SODIUM
LIQUAMAR, PHENPROCOUMON
LIQUID PRED, PREDNISONE
LISINOPRIL AND HYDROCHLOROTHIAZIDE,
    HYDROCHLOROTHIAZIDE
LISINOPRIL, LISINOPRIL
LITHANE, LITHIUM CARBONATE
LITHIUM CARBONATE, LITHIUM CARBONATE
LITHIUM CITRATE, LITHIUM CITRATE
LITHOBID, LITHIUM CARBONATE
LITHONATE, LITHIUM CARBONATE
LITHONATE, LITHIUM CITRATE
LITHOSTAT, ACETOHYDROXAMIC ACID
LITHOTABS, LITHIUM CARBONATE
LIVOSTIN, LEVOCABASTINE HYDROCHLORIDE
LO-TROL, ATROPINE SULFATE
LO/OVRAL, ETHINYL ESTRADIOL
LO/OVRAL-28, ETHINYL ESTRADIOL
LOCHOLEST LIGHT, CHOLESTYRAMINE
LOCHOLEST, CHOLESTYRAMINE
LOCOID LIPOCREAM, HYDROCORTISONE BUTYRATE
LOCOID, HYDROCORTISONE BUTYRATE
LOCORTEN, FLUMETHASONE PIVALATE
LODINE XL, ETODOLAC
LODINE, ETODOLAC
LODOSYN, CARBIDOPA
LOESTRIN 21 1/20, ETHINYL ESTRADIOL
LOESTRIN 21 1.5/30, ETHINYL ESTRADIOL
LOESTRIN FE 1/20, ETHINYL ESTRADIOL
LOESTRIN FE 1.5/30, ETHINYL ESTRADIOL
LOGEN, ATROPINE SULFATE
LOMANATE, ATROPINE SULFATE
LOMOTIL, ATROPINE SULFATE
LONITEN, MINOXIDIL
LONOX, ATROPINE SULFATE
LOPERAMIDE HCL AND SIMETHICONE, LOPERAMIDE
    HYDROCHLORIDE (OTC)
LOPERAMIDE HCL, LOPERAMIDE HYDROCHLORIDE
LOPERAMIDE HCL, LOPERAMIDE HYDROCHLORIDE
    (OTC)
LOPID, GEMFIBROZIL
LOPRESSIDONE, CHLORTHALIDONE
LOPRESSOR HCT, HYDROCHLOROTHIAZIDE
LOPRESSOR, METOPROLOL FUMARATE
LOPRESSOR, METOPROLOL TARTRATE
LOPROX, CICLOPIROX
LOPURIN, ALLOPURINOL
LORABID, LORACARBEF
LORATADINE AND PSEUDOEPHEDRINE HCL,
    LORATADINE (OTC)
LORATADINE AND PSEUDOEPHEDRINE SULFATE,
    LORATADINE (OTC)

APPENDIX A
PRODUCT NAME INDEX (*continued*)

LORATADINE, LORATADINE (OTC)
LORAZ, LORAZEPAM
LORAZEPAM INTENSOL, LORAZEPAM
LORAZEPAM, LORAZEPAM
LORCET-HD, ACETAMINOPHEN
LORELCO, PROBUCOL
LORFAN, LEVALLORPHAN TARTRATE
LORTAB, ACETAMINOPHEN
LOTEMAX, LOTEPREDNOL ETABONATE
LOTENSIN HCT, BENAZEPRIL HYDROCHLORIDE
LOTENSIN, BENAZEPRIL HYDROCHLORIDE
LOTREL, AMLODIPINE BESYLATE
LOTRIMIN ULTRA, BUTENAFINE HYDROCHLORIDE
   (OTC)
LOTRIMIN, CLOTRIMAZOLE
LOTRISONE, BETAMETHASONE DIPROPIONATE
LOTRONEX, ALOSETRON HYDROCHLORIDE
LOTUSATE, TALBUTAL
LOVASTATIN, LOVASTATIN
LOVENOX, ENOXAPARIN SODIUM
LOW-OGESTREL-21, ETHINYL ESTRADIOL
LOW-OGESTREL-28, ETHINYL ESTRADIOL
LOW-QUEL, ATROPINE SULFATE
LOXAPINE SUCCINATE, LOXAPINE SUCCINATE
LOXITANE C, LOXAPINE HYDROCHLORIDE
LOXITANE IM, LOXAPINE HYDROCHLORIDE
LOXITANE, LOXAPINE SUCCINATE
LOZOL, INDAPAMIDE
LTA II KIT, LIDOCAINE HYDROCHLORIDE
LUDIOMIL, MAPROTILINE HYDROCHLORIDE
LUFYLLIN, DYPHYLLINE
LUMENHANCE, MANGANESE CHLORIDE
   TETRAHYDRATE
LUMIGAN, BIMATOPROST
LUNELLE, ESTRADIOL CYPIONATE
LUNGAGGREGATE REAGENT, TECHNETIUM TC-99M
   ALBUMIN AGGREGATED KIT
LUPRON DEPOT, LEUPROLIDE ACETATE
LUPRON DEPOT-3, LEUPROLIDE ACETATE
LUPRON DEPOT-4, LEUPROLIDE ACETATE
LUPRON DEPOT-PED, LEUPROLIDE ACETATE
LUPRON, LEUPROLIDE ACETATE
LUTREPULSE KIT, GONADORELIN ACETATE
LUVOX, FLUVOXAMINE MALEATE
LUXIQ, BETAMETHASONE VALERATE
LYGEN, CHLORDIAZEPOXIDE HYDROCHLORIDE
LYMPHAZURIN, ISOSULFAN BLUE
LYNORAL, ETHINYL ESTRADIOL
LYOPHILIZED CYTOXAN, CYCLOPHOSPHAMIDE
LYSODREN, MITOTANE

M

M-PREDROL, METHYLPREDNISOLONE ACETATE
M-ZOLE 3 COMBINATION PACK, MICONAZOLE NITRATE
   (OTC)
M-ZOLE 7 DUAL PACK, MICONAZOLE NITRATE (OTC)
M.V.C. 9+3, ASCORBIC ACID
M.V.I. PEDIATRIC, ASCORBIC ACID
M.V.I.-12 LYOPHILIZED, ASCORBIC ACID
M.V.I.-12, ASCORBIC ACID
MACROBID, NITROFURANTOIN
MACRODANTIN, NITROFURANTOIN,
   MACROCRYSTALLINE
MACROTEC, TECHNETIUM TC-99M ALBUMIN
   AGGREGATED KIT
MAGNACORT, HYDROCORTAMATE HYDROCHLORIDE
MAGNESIUM SULFATE IN DEXTROSE 5% IN PLASTIC
   CONTAINER, MAGNESIUM SULFATE

MAGNESIUM SULFATE IN PLASTIC CONTAINER,
   MAGNESIUM SULFATE
MAGNESIUM SULFATE, MAGNESIUM SULFATE
MAGNEVIST, GADOPENTETATE DIMEGLUMINE
MALARONE PEDIATRIC, ATOVAQUONE
MALARONE, ATOVAQUONE
MANDOL, CEFAMANDOLE NAFATE
MANGANESE CHLORIDE IN PLASTIC CONTAINER,
   MANGANESE CHLORIDE
MANGANESE SULFATE, MANGANESE SULFATE
MANNITOL 10% IN PLASTIC CONTAINER, MANNITOL
MANNITOL 10% W/ DEXTROSE 5% IN DISTILLED WATER,
   MANNITOL
MANNITOL 10%, MANNITOL
MANNITOL 15% IN PLASTIC CONTAINER, MANNITOL
MANNITOL 15% W/ DEXTROSE 5% IN SODIUM CHLORIDE
   0.45%, MANNITOL
MANNITOL 15%, MANNITOL
MANNITOL 20% IN PLASTIC CONTAINER, MANNITOL
MANNITOL 20%, MANNITOL
MANNITOL 25%, MANNITOL
MANNITOL 5% IN PLASTIC CONTAINER, MANNITOL
MANNITOL 5% W/ DEXTROSE 5% IN SODIUM CHLORIDE
   0.12%, MANNITOL
MANNITOL 5%, MANNITOL
MAOLATE, CHLORPHENESIN CARBAMATE
MAPROTILINE HCL, MAPROTILINE HYDROCHLORIDE
MARCAINE HCL PRESERVATIVE FREE, BUPIVACAINE
   HYDROCHLORIDE
MARCAINE HCL W/ EPINEPHRINE PRESERVATIVE FREE,
   BUPIVACAINE HYDROCHLORIDE
MARCAINE HCL W/ EPINEPHRINE, BUPIVACAINE
   HYDROCHLORIDE
MARCAINE HCL, BUPIVACAINE HYDROCHLORIDE
MARCAINE, BUPIVACAINE HYDROCHLORIDE
MAREZINE, CYCLIZINE LACTATE
MARINOL, DRONABINOL
MARPLAN, ISOCARBOXAZID
MATULANE, PROCARBAZINE HYDROCHLORIDE
MAVIK, TRANDOLAPRIL
MAXAIR, PIRBUTEROL ACETATE
MAXALT, RIZATRIPTAN BENZOATE
MAXALT-MLT, RIZATRIPTAN BENZOATE
MAXAQUIN, LOMEFLOXACIN HYDROCHLORIDE
MAXIBOLIN, ETHYLESTRENOL
MAXIDEX, DEXAMETHASONE
MAXIDEX, DEXAMETHASONE SODIUM PHOSPHATE
MAXIPIME, CEFEPIME HYDROCHLORIDE (ARGININE
   FORMULATION)
MAXITROL, DEXAMETHASONE
MAXOLON, METOCLOPRAMIDE HYDROCHLORIDE
MAXZIDE, HYDROCHLOROTHIAZIDE
MAXZIDE-25, HYDROCHLOROTHIAZIDE
MAZANOR, MAZINDOL
MD-50, DIATRIZOATE SODIUM
MD-60, DIATRIZOATE MEGLUMINE
MD-76, DIATRIZOATE MEGLUMINE
MD-76R, DIATRIZOATE MEGLUMINE
MD-GASTROVIEW, DIATRIZOATE MEGLUMINE
MDP-BRACCO, TECHNETIUM TC-99M MEDRONATE KIT
MEASURIN, ASPIRIN (OTC)
MEBENDAZOLE, MEBENDAZOLE
MECLAN, MECLOCYCLINE SULFOSALICYLATE
MECLIZINE HCL, MECLIZINE HYDROCHLORIDE
MECLODIUM, MECLOFENAMATE SODIUM
MECLOFENAMATE SODIUM, MECLOFENAMATE SODIUM
MECLOMEN, MECLOFENAMATE SODIUM
MEDIGESIC PLUS, ACETAMINOPHEN
MEDIHALER ERGOTAMINE, ERGOTAMINE TARTRATE

APPENDIX A
PRODUCT NAME INDEX (*continued*)

MEDIHALER-EPI, EPINEPHRINE BITARTRATE (OTC)
MEDIHALER-ISO, ISOPROTERENOL SULFATE
MEDIPREN, IBUPROFEN (OTC)
MEDROL ACETATE, METHYLPREDNISOLONE ACETATE
MEDROL, METHYLPREDNISOLONE
MEDROL, METHYLPREDNISOLONE ACETATE
MEDROXYPROGESTERONE ACETATE,
    MEDROXYPROGESTERONE ACETATE
MEFLOQUINE HCL, MEFLOQUINE HYDROCHLORIDE
MEFOXIN IN DEXTROSE 5% IN PLASTIC CONTAINER,
    CEFOXITIN SODIUM
MEFOXIN IN PLASTIC CONTAINER, CEFOXITIN SODIUM
MEFOXIN IN SODIUM CHLORIDE 0.9% IN PLASTIC
    CONTAINER, CEFOXITIN SODIUM
MEFOXIN, CEFOXITIN SODIUM
MEGACE, MEGESTROL ACETATE
MEGATOPE, ALBUMIN IODINATED I-131 SERUM
MEGESTROL ACETATE, MEGESTROL ACETATE
MELFIAT, PHENDIMETRAZINE TARTRATE
MELFIAT-105, PHENDIMETRAZINE TARTRATE
MELLARIL, THIORIDAZINE HYDROCHLORIDE
MELLARIL-S, THIORIDAZINE
MENADIONE, MENADIONE
MENEST, ESTROGENS, ESTERIFIED
MENOTROPINS, MENOTROPINS (FSH;LH)
MENRIUM 5-2, CHLORDIAZEPOXIDE
MENRIUM 5-4, CHLORDIAZEPOXIDE
MENRIUM 10-4, CHLORDIAZEPOXIDE
MENTAX, BUTENAFINE HYDROCHLORIDE
MENTAX-TC, BUTENAFINE HYDROCHLORIDE
MEPERGAN, MEPERIDINE HYDROCHLORIDE
MEPERIDINE AND ATROPINE SULFATE, ATROPINE
    SULFATE
MEPERIDINE HCL PRESERVATIVE FREE, MEPERIDINE
    HYDROCHLORIDE
MEPERIDINE HCL, MEPERIDINE HYDROCHLORIDE
MEPHYTON, PHYTONADIONE
MEPIVACAINE HCL W/ LEVONORDEFRIN,
    LEVONORDEFRIN
MEPIVACAINE HCL, MEPIVACAINE HYDROCHLORIDE
MEPRIAM, MEPROBAMATE
MEPRO-ASPIRIN, ASPIRIN
MEPROBAMATE AND ASPIRIN, ASPIRIN
MEPROBAMATE, MEPROBAMATE
MEPRON, ATOVAQUONE
MEPROSPAN, MEPROBAMATE
MERETEK UBT KIT (W/ PRANACTIN), UREA, C-13
MERIDIA, SIBUTRAMINE HYDROCHLORIDE
MERREM I.V., MEROPENEM
MERSALYL-THEOPHYLLINE, MERSALYL SODIUM
MESANTOIN, MEPHENYTOIN
MESNA, MESNA
MESNEX, MESNA
MESTINON, PYRIDOSTIGMINE BROMIDE
METADATE CD, METHYLPHENIDATE HYDROCHLORIDE
METADATE ER, METHYLPHENIDATE HYDROCHLORIDE
METAGLIP, GLIPIZIDE
METAHYDRIN, TRICHLORMETHIAZIDE
METANDREN, METHYLTESTOSTERONE
METAPROTERENOL SULFATE, METAPROTERENOL
    SULFATE
METARAMINOL BITARTRATE, METARAMINOL
    BITARTRATE
METASTRON, STRONTIUM CHLORIDE, SR-89
METATENSIN #2, RESERPINE
METATENSIN #4, RESERPINE
METFORMIN HCL, METFORMIN HYDROCHLORIDE
METHADONE HCL INTENSOL, METHADONE
    HYDROCHLORIDE

METHADONE HCL, METHADONE HYDROCHLORIDE
METHADOSE, METHADONE HYDROCHLORIDE
METHAMPEX, METHAMPHETAMINE HYDROCHLORIDE
METHAMPHETAMINE HCL, METHAMPHETAMINE
    HYDROCHLORIDE
METHAZOLAMIDE, METHAZOLAMIDE
METHDILAZINE HCL, METHDILAZINE HYDROCHLORIDE
METHENAMINE HIPPURATE, METHENAMINE
    HIPPURATE
METHERGINE, METHYLERGONOVINE MALEATE
METHIMAZOLE, METHIMAZOLE
METHOCARBAMOL AND ASPIRIN, ASPIRIN
METHOCARBAMOL, METHOCARBAMOL
METHOTREXATE LPF, METHOTREXATE SODIUM
METHOTREXATE PRESERVATIVE FREE,
    METHOTREXATE SODIUM
METHOTREXATE SODIUM PRESERVATIVE FREE,
    METHOTREXATE SODIUM
METHOTREXATE SODIUM, METHOTREXATE SODIUM
METHOTREXATE, METHOTREXATE SODIUM
METHOXSALEN, METHOXSALEN
METHSCOPOLAMINE BROMIDE, METHSCOPOLAMINE
    BROMIDE
METHYCLOTHIAZIDE AND DESERPIDINE, DESERPIDINE
METHYCLOTHIAZIDE, METHYCLOTHIAZIDE
METHYLDOPA AND CHLOROTHIAZIDE,
    CHLOROTHIAZIDE
METHYLDOPA AND HYDROCHLOROTHIAZIDE,
    HYDROCHLOROTHIAZIDE
METHYLDOPA, METHYLDOPA
METHYLDOPATE HCL, METHYLDOPATE
    HYDROCHLORIDE
METHYLIN ER, METHYLPHENIDATE HYDROCHLORIDE
METHYLIN, METHYLPHENIDATE HYDROCHLORIDE
METHYLPHENIDATE HCL, METHYLPHENIDATE
    HYDROCHLORIDE
METHYLPREDNISOLONE ACETATE,
    METHYLPREDNISOLONE ACETATE
METHYLPREDNISOLONE SODIUM SUCCINATE,
    METHYLPREDNISOLONE SODIUM SUCCINATE
METHYLPREDNISOLONE, METHYLPREDNISOLONE
METHYLPREDNISOLONE, METHYLPREDNISOLONE
    SODIUM SUCCINATE
METHYLTESTOSTERONE, METHYLTESTOSTERONE
METI-DERM, PREDNISOLONE
METICORTELONE, PREDNISOLONE ACETATE
METICORTEN, PREDNISONE
METIMYD, PREDNISOLONE ACETATE
METIPRANOLOL, METIPRANOLOL HYDROCHLORIDE
METOCLOPRAMIDE HCL, METOCLOPRAMIDE
    HYDROCHLORIDE
METOCLOPRAMIDE INTENSOL, METOCLOPRAMIDE
    HYDROCHLORIDE
METOCLOPRAMIDE, METOCLOPRAMIDE
    HYDROCHLORIDE
METOCURINE IODIDE, METOCURINE IODIDE
METOPIRONE, METYRAPONE
METOPROLOL TARTRATE, METOPROLOL TARTRATE
METRA, PHENDIMETRAZINE TARTRATE
METRETON, PREDNISOLONE SODIUM PHOSPHATE
METRO I.V. IN PLASTIC CONTAINER, METRONIDAZOLE
METRO I.V., METRONIDAZOLE
METROCREAM, METRONIDAZOLE
METRODIN, UROFOLLITROPIN
METROGEL, METRONIDAZOLE
METROGEL-VAGINAL, METRONIDAZOLE
METROLOTION, METRONIDAZOLE
METROMIDOL, METRONIDAZOLE

APPENDIX A
PRODUCT NAME INDEX (*continued*)

METRONIDAZOLE HCL, METRONIDAZOLE
    HYDROCHLORIDE
METRONIDAZOLE IN PLASTIC CONTAINER,
    METRONIDAZOLE
METRONIDAZOLE, METRONIDAZOLE
METUBINE IODIDE, METOCURINE IODIDE
MEVACOR, LOVASTATIN
MEXATE, METHOTREXATE SODIUM
MEXATE-AQ PRESERVED, METHOTREXATE SODIUM
MEXATE-AQ, METHOTREXATE SODIUM
MEXILETINE HCL, MEXILETINE HYDROCHLORIDE
MEXITIL, MEXILETINE HYDROCHLORIDE
MEZLIN, MEZLOCILLIN SODIUM MONOHYDRATE
MIACALCIN, CALCITONIN, SALMON
MICARDIS HCT, HYDROCHLOROTHIAZIDE
MICARDIS, TELMISARTAN
MICONAZOLE 7, MICONAZOLE NITRATE (OTC)
MICONAZOLE NITRATE COMBINATION PACK,
    MICONAZOLE NITRATE (OTC)
MICONAZOLE NITRATE, MICONAZOLE NITRATE
MICONAZOLE NITRATE, MICONAZOLE NITRATE (OTC)
MICORT-HC, HYDROCORTISONE ACETATE
MICRAININ, ASPIRIN
MICRO-K 10, POTASSIUM CHLORIDE
MICRO-K LS, POTASSIUM CHLORIDE
MICRO-K, POTASSIUM CHLORIDE
MICRODERM, CHLORHEXIDINE GLUCONATE (OTC)
MICROGESTIN FE 1/20, ETHINYL ESTRADIOL
MICROGESTIN FE 1.5/30, ETHINYL ESTRADIOL
MICROLITE, TECHNETIUM TC-99M ALBUMIN COLLOID
    KIT
MICRONASE, GLYBURIDE
MICRONOR, NORETHINDRONE
MICROSUL, SULFAMETHIZOLE
MICROZIDE, HYDROCHLOROTHIAZIDE
MIDAMOR, AMILORIDE HYDROCHLORIDE
MIDAZOLAM HCL, MIDAZOLAM HYDROCHLORIDE
MIDOL, IBUPROFEN (OTC)
MIFEPREX, MIFEPRISTONE
MIGERGOT, CAFFEINE
MIGRANAL, DIHYDROERGOTAMINE MESYLATE
MILONTIN, PHENSUXIMIDE
MILOPHENE, CLOMIPHENE CITRATE
MILPREM-200, ESTROGENS, CONJUGATED
MILPREM-400, ESTROGENS, CONJUGATED
MILRINONE LACTATE IN DEXTROSE 5% IN PLASTIC
    CONTAINER, MILRINONE LACTATE
MILRINONE LACTATE, MILRINONE LACTATE
MILRINONE LACTOSE IN 5% DEXTROSE, MILRINONE
    LACTATE
MILTOWN, MEPROBAMATE
MINIPRESS XL, PRAZOSIN HYDROCHLORIDE
MINIPRESS, PRAZOSIN HYDROCHLORIDE
MINIRIN, DESMOPRESSIN ACETATE
MINITEC, TECHNETIUM TC-99M SODIUM
    PERTECHNETATE GENERATOR
MINITRAN, NITROGLYCERIN
MINIZIDE, POLYTHIAZIDE
MINOCIN, MINOCYCLINE HYDROCHLORIDE
MINOCYCLINE HCL, MINOCYCLINE HYDROCHLORIDE
MINODYL, MINOXIDIL
MINOXIDIL (FOR MEN), MINOXIDIL (OTC)
MINOXIDIL (FOR WOMEN), MINOXIDIL (OTC)
MINOXIDIL EXTRA STRENGTH (FOR MEN), MINOXIDIL
    (OTC)
MINOXIDIL, MINOXIDIL
MINTEZOL, THIABENDAZOLE
MIOCHOL, ACETYLCHOLINE CHLORIDE
MIOCHOL-E, ACETYLCHOLINE CHLORIDE

MIOSTAT, CARBACHOL
MIRADON, ANISINDIONE
MIRALAX, POLYETHYLENE GLYCOL 3350
MIRALUMA, TECHNETIUM TC-99M SESTAMIBI KIT
MIRAPEX, PRAMIPEXOLE DIHYDROCHLORIDE
MIRCETTE, DESOGESTREL
MIRENA, LEVONORGESTREL
MIRTAZAPINE, MIRTAZAPINE
MISOPROSTOL, MISOPROSTOL
MITHRACIN, PLICAMYCIN
MITOMYCIN, MITOMYCIN
MIVACRON IN DEXTROSE 5% IN PLASTIC CONTAINER,
    MIVACURIUM CHLORIDE
MIVACRON, MIVACURIUM CHLORIDE
MIXTARD HUMAN 70/30, INSULIN RECOMBINANT
    PURIFIED HUMAN (OTC)
MOBAN, MOLINDONE HYDROCHLORIDE
MOBIC, MELOXICAM
MOCTANIN, MONOCTANOIN
MODERIL, RESCINNAMINE
MODICON 21, ETHINYL ESTRADIOL
MODICON 28, ETHINYL ESTRADIOL
MODRASTANE, TRILOSTANE
MODURETIC 5-50, AMILORIDE HYDROCHLORIDE
MOEXIPRIL HCL, MOEXIPRIL HYDROCHLORIDE
MOMETASONE FUROATE, MOMETASONE FUROATE
MONISTAT 3 COMBINATION PACK (PREFILLED),
    MICONAZOLE NITRATE (OTC)
MONISTAT 3 COMBINATION PACK, MICONAZOLE
    NITRATE (OTC)
MONISTAT 3, MICONAZOLE NITRATE
MONISTAT 3, MICONAZOLE NITRATE (OTC)
MONISTAT 5, MICONAZOLE NITRATE
MONISTAT 7 COMBINATION PACK, MICONAZOLE
    NITRATE (OTC)
MONISTAT 7, MICONAZOLE NITRATE (OTC)
MONISTAT DUAL- PAK, MICONAZOLE NITRATE
MONISTAT, MICONAZOLE
MONISTAT-3 COMBINATION PACK, MICONAZOLE
    NITRATE (OTC)
MONISTAT-DERM, MICONAZOLE NITRATE
MONOCID, CEFONICID SODIUM
MONODOX, DOXYCYCLINE
MONOKET, ISOSORBIDE MONONITRATE
MONOPRIL, FOSINOPRIL SODIUM
MONOPRIL-HCT, FOSINOPRIL SODIUM
MONUROL, FOSFOMYCIN TROMETHAMINE
MORPHINE SULFATE, MORPHINE SULFATE
MOTOFEN HALF-STRENGTH, ATROPINE SULFATE
MOTOFEN, ATROPINE SULFATE
MOTRIN IB, IBUPROFEN (OTC)
MOTRIN MIGRAINE PAIN, IBUPROFEN (OTC)
MOTRIN, IBUPROFEN
MOXAM, MOXALACTAM DISODIUM
MPI DMSA KIDNEY REAGENT, TECHNETIUM TC-99M
    SUCCIMER KIT
MPI DTPA KIT - CHELATE, TECHNETIUM TC-99M
    PENTETATE KIT
MPI INDIUM DTPA IN 111, INDIUM IN-111 PENTETATE
    DISODIUM
MPI KRYPTON 81M GAS GENERATOR, KRYPTON, KR-
    81M
MPI STANNOUS DIPHOSPHONATE, TECHNETIUM TC-
    99M ETIDRONATE KIT
MS CONTIN, MORPHINE SULFATE
MUCINEX, GUAIFENESIN (OTC)
MUCOMYST W/ ISOPROTERENOL, ACETYLCYSTEINE
MUCOMYST, ACETYLCYSTEINE
MUCOSIL-10, ACETYLCYSTEINE

APPENDIX A
PRODUCT NAME INDEX (*continued*)

MUCOSIL-20, ACETYLCYSTEINE
MULTIFUGE, PIPERAZINE CITRATE
MUPIROCIN, MUPIROCIN
MUSE, ALPROSTADIL
MUSTARGEN, MECHLORETHAMINE HYDROCHLORIDE
MUTAMYCIN, MITOMYCIN
MVC PLUS, ASCORBIC ACID
MYAMBUTOL, ETHAMBUTOL HYDROCHLORIDE
MYBANIL, BROMODIPHENHYDRAMINE
    HYDROCHLORIDE
MYCELEX, CLOTRIMAZOLE
MYCELEX-7 COMBINATION PACK, CLOTRIMAZOLE
    (OTC)
MYCELEX-7, CLOTRIMAZOLE (OTC)
MYCELEX-G, CLOTRIMAZOLE
MYCHEL, CHLORAMPHENICOL
MYCHEL-S, CHLORAMPHENICOL SODIUM SUCCINATE
MYCIFRADIN, NEOMYCIN SULFATE
MYCITRACIN, BACITRACIN
MYCO-TRIACET II, NYSTATIN
MYCOBUTIN, RIFABUTIN
MYCODONE, HOMATROPINE METHYLBROMIDE
MYCOLOG-II, NYSTATIN
MYCOSTATIN, NYSTATIN
MYDRIACYL, TROPICAMIDE
MYDRIAFAIR, TROPICAMIDE
MYFED, PSEUDOEPHEDRINE HYDROCHLORIDE (OTC)
MYIDYL, TRIPROLIDINE HYDROCHLORIDE
MYKACET, NYSTATIN
MYKINAC, NYSTATIN
MYKROX, METOLAZONE
MYLARAMINE, DEXCHLORPHENIRAMINE MALEATE
MYLAXEN, HEXAFLUORENIUM BROMIDE
MYLERAN, BUSULFAN
MYLOTARG, GEMTUZUMAB OZOGAMICIN
MYMETHASONE, DEXAMETHASONE
MYMETHAZINE FORTIS, PROMETHAZINE
    HYDROCHLORIDE
MYOTONACHOL, BETHANECHOL CHLORIDE
MYOVIEW, TECHNETIUM TC-99M TETROFOSMIN KIT
MYPHETANE DC, BROMPHENIRAMINE MALEATE
MYPHETANE DX, BROMPHENIRAMINE MALEATE
MYPROIC ACID, VALPROIC ACID
MYSOLINE, PRIMIDONE
MYTELASE, AMBENONIUM CHLORIDE
MYTOZYTREX, MITOMYCIN
MYTREX A, NEOMYCIN SULFATE
MYTREX F, NYSTATIN

N

N.E.E. 1/35 21, ETHINYL ESTRADIOL
N.E.E. 1/35 28, ETHINYL ESTRADIOL
NABUMETONE, NABUMETONE
NADOLOL, NADOLOL
NAFAZAIR, NAPHAZOLINE HYDROCHLORIDE
NAFCILLIN SODIUM, NAFCILLIN SODIUM
NAFTIN, NAFTIFINE HYDROCHLORIDE
NALBUPHINE HCL, NALBUPHINE HYDROCHLORIDE
NALBUPHINE, NALBUPHINE HYDROCHLORIDE
NALFON 200, FENOPROFEN CALCIUM
NALFON, FENOPROFEN CALCIUM
NALIDIXIC ACID, NALIDIXIC ACID
NALLPEN IN PLASTIC CONTAINER, NAFCILLIN SODIUM
NALLPEN, NAFCILLIN SODIUM
NALOXONE HCL AND PENTAZOCAINE, NALOXONE
    HYDROCHLORIDE
NALOXONE HCL, NALOXONE HYDROCHLORIDE
NALOXONE, NALOXONE HYDROCHLORIDE

NALTREXONE HCL, NALTREXONE HYDROCHLORIDE
NANDROLONE DECANOATE, NANDROLONE
    DECANOATE
NANDROLONE PHENPROPIONATE, NANDROLONE
    PHENPROPIONATE
NAPHAZOLINE HCL, NAPHAZOLINE HYDROCHLORIDE
NAPHCON FORTE, NAPHAZOLINE HYDROCHLORIDE
NAPHCON-A, NAPHAZOLINE HYDROCHLORIDE (OTC)
NAPRELAN, NAPROXEN SODIUM
NAPROSYN, NAPROXEN
NAPROXEN SODIUM, NAPROXEN SODIUM
NAPROXEN SODIUM, NAPROXEN SODIUM (OTC)
NAPROXEN, NAPROXEN
NAQUA, TRICHLORMETHIAZIDE
NAQUIVAL, RESERPINE
NARCAN, NALOXONE HYDROCHLORIDE
NARDIL, PHENELZINE SULFATE
NAROPIN, ROPIVACAINE HYDROCHLORIDE
    MONOHYDRATE
NASACORT AQ, TRIAMCINOLONE ACETONIDE
NASACORT, TRIAMCINOLONE ACETONIDE
NASALCROM, CROMOLYN SODIUM (OTC)
NASALIDE, FLUNISOLIDE
NASAREL, FLUNISOLIDE
NASCOBAL, CYANOCOBALAMIN
NASONEX, MOMETASONE FUROATE MONOHYDRATE
NATACYN, NATAMYCIN
NATRECOR, NESIRITIDE
NATURAL ESTROGENIC SUBSTANCE-ESTRONE,
    ESTRONE
NATURETIN-10, BENDROFLUMETHIAZIDE
NATURETIN-2.5, BENDROFLUMETHIAZIDE
NATURETIN-5, BENDROFLUMETHIAZIDE
NAVANE, THIOTHIXENE
NAVANE, THIOTHIXENE HYDROCHLORIDE
NAVELBINE, VINORELBINE TARTRATE
NEBCIN, TOBRAMYCIN SULFATE
NEBUPENT, PENTAMIDINE ISETHIONATE
NEGGRAM, NALIDIXIC ACID
NEMBUTAL SODIUM, PENTOBARBITAL SODIUM
NEMBUTAL, PENTOBARBITAL
NEMBUTAL, PENTOBARBITAL SODIUM
NEO TECT KIT, TECHNETIUM TC-99M DEPREOTIDE
NEO-CORT-DOME, ACETIC ACID, GLACIAL
NEO-CORT-DOME, HYDROCORTISONE
NEO-CORTEF, HYDROCORTISONE ACETATE
NEO-DELTA-CORTEF, NEOMYCIN SULFATE
NEO-FRADIN, NEOMYCIN SULFATE
NEO-HYDELTRASOL, NEOMYCIN SULFATE
NEO-MEDROL ACETATE, METHYLPREDNISOLONE
    ACETATE
NEO-MEDROL, METHYLPREDNISOLONE
NEO-POLYCIN, BACITRACIN ZINC
NEO-POLYCIN, GRAMICIDIN
NEO-RX, NEOMYCIN SULFATE
NEO-SYNALAR, FLUOCINOLONE ACETONIDE
NEOBIOTIC, NEOMYCIN SULFATE
NEODECADRON, DEXAMETHASONE SODIUM
    PHOSPHATE
NEOMYCIN , AMINO ACIDS
NEORAL, CYCLOSPORINE
NEOSAR, CYCLOPHOSPHAMIDE
NEOSCAN, GALLIUM CITRATE, GA-67
NEOSPORIN G.U. IRRIGANT, NEOMYCIN SULFATE
NEOSPORIN, BACITRACIN ZINC
NEOSPORIN, GRAMICIDIN
NEOSPORIN, NEOMYCIN SULFATE (OTC)
NEOTHYLLINE, DYPHYLLINE

APPENDIX A
PRODUCT NAME INDEX (*continued*)

NEOTRIZINE, TRISULFAPYRIMIDINES
(SULFADIAZINE;SULFAMERAZINE;
SULFAMETHAZINE)
NEPHRAMINE 5.4%, AMINO ACIDS
NEPHROFLOW, IODOHIPPURATE SODIUM, I-123
NEPTAZANE, METHAZOLAMIDE
NESACAINE, CHLOROPROCAINE HYDROCHLORIDE
NESACAINE-MPF, CHLOROPROCAINE
HYDROCHLORIDE
NETROMYCIN, NETILMICIN SULFATE
NEURAMATE, MEPROBAMATE
NEUROLITE, TECHNETIUM TC-99M BICISATE KIT
NEURONTIN, GABAPENTIN
NEUTREXIN, TRIMETREXATE GLUCURONATE
NEXIUM, ESOMEPRAZOLE MAGNESIUM
NIACIN, NIACIN
NIACOR, NIACIN
NIASPAN TITRATION STARTER PACK, NIACIN
NIASPAN, NIACIN
NICARDIPINE HCL, NICARDIPINE HYDROCHLORIDE
NICLOCIDE, NICLOSAMIDE
NICODERM CQ, NICOTINE (OTC)
NICOLAR, NIACIN
NICORETTE (0RANGE), NICOTINE POLACRILEX (OTC)
NICORETTE (MINT), NICOTINE POLACRILEX (OTC)
NICORETTE (ORANGE), NICOTINE POLACRILEX (OTC)
NICORETTE, NICOTINE POLACRILEX (OTC)
NICOTINE POLACRILEX, NICOTINE POLACRILEX (OTC)
NICOTINE, NICOTINE
NICOTROL, NICOTINE
NICOTROL, NICOTINE (OTC)
NIFEDIPINE, NIFEDIPINE
NILANDRON, NILUTAMIDE
NILSTAT, NYSTATIN
NIMBEX PRESERVATIVE FREE, CISATRACURIUM
BESYLATE
NIMBEX, CISATRACURIUM BESYLATE
NIMOTOP, NIMODIPINE
NIPENT, PENTOSTATIN
NIPRIDE, SODIUM NITROPRUSSIDE
NITRO IV, NITROGLYCERIN
NITRO-BID, NITROGLYCERIN
NITRO-DUR, NITROGLYCERIN
NITROFURANTION, NITROFURANTOIN,
MACROCRYSTALLINE
NITROFURANTOIN MACROCRYSTALLINE,
NITROFURANTOIN, MACROCRYSTALLINE
NITROFURANTOIN, NITROFURANTOIN
NITROFURANTOIN, NITROFURANTOIN,
MACROCRYSTALLINE
NITROFURAZONE, NITROFURAZONE
NITROGLYCERIN IN DEXTROSE 5%, NITROGLYCERIN
NITROGLYCERIN, NITROGLYCERIN
NITROL, NITROGLYCERIN
NITROLINGUAL PUMPSPRAY, NITROGLYCERIN
NITROLINGUAL, NITROGLYCERIN
NITRONAL, NITROGLYCERIN
NITROPRESS, SODIUM NITROPRUSSIDE
NITROSTAT, NITROGLYCERIN
NIX, PERMETHRIN
NIX, PERMETHRIN (OTC)
NIZATIDINE, NIZATIDINE
NIZORAL A-D, KETOCONAZOLE (OTC)
NIZORAL, KETOCONAZOLE
NOGENIC HC, HYDROCORTISONE
NOLUDAR, METHYPRYLON
NOLVADEX, TAMOXIFEN CITRATE
NOR-QD, NORETHINDRONE
NORCEPT-E 1/35 21, ETHINYL ESTRADIOL

NORCEPT-E 1/35 28, ETHINYL ESTRADIOL
NORCET, ACETAMINOPHEN
NORCO, ACETAMINOPHEN
NORCURON, VECURONIUM BROMIDE
NORDETTE-21, ETHINYL ESTRADIOL
NORDETTE-28, ETHINYL ESTRADIOL
NORDITROPIN, SOMATROPIN RECOMBINANT
NOREPINEPHRINE BITARTRATE, NOREPINEPHRINE
BITARTRATE
NORETHIN 1/35E-21, ETHINYL ESTRADIOL
NORETHIN 1/35E-28, ETHINYL ESTRADIOL
NORETHIN 1/50M-21, MESTRANOL
NORETHIN 1/50M-28, MESTRANOL
NORETHINDRONE ACETATE, NORETHINDRONE
ACETATE
NORETHINDRONE AND ETHINYL ESTRADIOL (10/11),
ETHINYL ESTRADIOL
NORETHINDRONE AND ETHINYL ESTRADIOL (7/14),
ETHINYL ESTRADIOL
NORETHINDRONE AND ETHINYL ESTRADIOL, ETHINYL
ESTRADIOL
NORETHINDRONE AND MESTRANOL, MESTRANOL
NORFLEX, ORPHENADRINE CITRATE
NORGESIC FORTE, ASPIRIN
NORGESIC, ASPIRIN
NORINYL 1+35 21-DAY, ETHINYL ESTRADIOL
NORINYL 1+35 28-DAY, ETHINYL ESTRADIOL
NORINYL 1+50 21-DAY, MESTRANOL
NORINYL 1+50 28-DAY, MESTRANOL
NORINYL 1+80 21-DAY, MESTRANOL
NORINYL 1+80 28-DAY, MESTRANOL
NORINYL, MESTRANOL
NORISODRINE AEROTROL, ISOPROTERENOL
HYDROCHLORIDE
NORISODRINE, ISOPROTERENOL SULFATE
NORITATE, METRONIDAZOLE
NORLESTRIN 21 1/50, ETHINYL ESTRADIOL
NORLESTRIN 21 2.5/50, ETHINYL ESTRADIOL
NORLESTRIN 28 1/50, ETHINYL ESTRADIOL
NORLESTRIN FE 1/50, ETHINYL ESTRADIOL
NORLESTRIN FE 2.5/50, ETHINYL ESTRADIOL
NORLUTATE, NORETHINDRONE ACETATE
NORLUTIN, NORETHINDRONE
NORMIFLO, ARDEPARIN SODIUM
NORMODYNE, LABETALOL HYDROCHLORIDE
NORMOSOL-M AND DEXTROSE 5% IN PLASTIC
CONTAINER, DEXTROSE
NORMOSOL-R AND DEXTROSE 5% IN PLASTIC
CONTAINER, DEXTROSE
NORMOSOL-R IN PLASTIC CONTAINER, MAGNESIUM
CHLORIDE
NORMOZIDE, HYDROCHLOROTHIAZIDE
NOROXIN, NORFLOXACIN
NORPACE CR, DISOPYRAMIDE PHOSPHATE
NORPACE, DISOPYRAMIDE PHOSPHATE
NORPLANT II, LEVONORGESTREL
NORPLANT SYSTEM IN PLASTIC CONTAINER,
LEVONORGESTREL
NORPLANT, LEVONORGESTREL
NORPRAMIN, DESIPRAMINE HYDROCHLORIDE
NORQUEST FE, ETHINYL ESTRADIOL
NORTREL 0.5/35-21, ETHINYL ESTRADIOL
NORTREL 0.5/35-28, ETHINYL ESTRADIOL
NORTREL 1/35-21, ETHINYL ESTRADIOL
NORTREL 1/35-28, ETHINYL ESTRADIOL
NORTREL 7/7/7, ETHINYL ESTRADIOL
NORTRIPTYLINE HCL, NORTRIPTYLINE
HYDROCHLORIDE
NORVASC, AMLODIPINE BESYLATE

APPENDIX A
PRODUCT NAME INDEX (*continued*)

NORVIR, RITONAVIR
NOVAFED, PSEUDOEPHEDRINE HYDROCHLORIDE
NOVAMINE 11.4%, AMINO ACIDS
NOVAMINE 15% SULFITE FREE IN PLASTIC CONTAINER,
    AMINO ACIDS
NOVAMINE 15%, AMINO ACIDS
NOVAMINE 8.5%, AMINO ACIDS
NOVANTRONE, MITOXANTRONE HYDROCHLORIDE
NOVOCAIN, PROCAINE HYDROCHLORIDE
NOVOLIN 70/30, INSULIN RECOMBINANT HUMAN (OTC)
NOVOLIN 70/30, INSULIN RECOMBINANT PURIFIED
    HUMAN (OTC)
NOVOLIN L, INSULIN ZINC SUSP RECOMBINANT HUMAN
    (OTC)
NOVOLIN L, INSULIN ZINC SUSP SEMISYNTHETIC
    PURIFIED HUMAN (OTC)
NOVOLIN N, INSULIN SUSP ISOPHANE RECOMBINANT
    HUMAN (OTC)
NOVOLIN N, INSULIN SUSP ISOPHANE SEMISYNTHETIC
    PURIFIED HUMAN (OTC)
NOVOLIN R, INSULIN RECOMBINANT HUMAN (OTC)
NOVOLIN R, INSULIN RECOMBINANT PURIFIED HUMAN
    (OTC)
NOVOLOG MIX 70/30, INSULIN ASPART
NOVOLOG, INSULIN ASPART
NOVOTHYROX, LIOTRIX (T4;T3)
NOVRAD, LEVOPROPOXYPHENE NAPSYLATE,
    ANHYDROUS
NPH ILETIN I (BEEF-PORK), INSULIN SUSP ISOPHANE
    BEEF/PORK (OTC)
NPH ILETIN II (PORK), INSULIN SUSP ISOPHANE
    PURIFIED PORK (OTC)
NPH ILETIN II, INSULIN SUSP ISOPHANE PURIFIED BEEF
    (OTC)
NPH INSULIN, INSULIN SUSP ISOPHANE BEEF (OTC)
NPH PURIFIED PORK ISOPHANE INSULIN, INSULIN SUSP
    ISOPHANE PURIFIED PORK (OTC)
NUBAIN, NALBUPHINE HYDROCHLORIDE
NULYTELY, POLYETHYLENE GLYCOL 3350
NULYTELY-FLAVORED, POLYETHYLENE GLYCOL 3350
NUMORPHAN, OXYMORPHONE HYDROCHLORIDE
NUPRIN, IBUPROFEN (OTC)
NUROMAX, DOXACURIUM CHLORIDE
NUTRACORT, HYDROCORTISONE
NUTRILIPID 10%, SOYBEAN OIL
NUTRILIPID 20%, SOYBEAN OIL
NUTROPIN AQ PEN, SOMATROPIN RECOMBINANT
NUTROPIN AQ, SOMATROPIN RECOMBINANT
NUTROPIN DEPOT, SOMATROPIN RECOMBINANT
NUTROPIN, SOMATROPIN RECOMBINANT
NUVARING, ETHINYL ESTRADIOL
NYDRAZID, ISONIAZID
NYSERT, NYSTATIN
NYSTAFORM, CLIOQUINOL
NYSTATIN AND TRIAMCINOLONE ACETONIDE,
    NYSTATIN
NYSTATIN, NYSTATIN
NYSTATIN-TRIAMCINOLONE ACETONIDE, NYSTATIN
NYSTEX, NYSTATIN
NYSTOP, NYSTATIN

O

OBESTIN-30, PHENTERMINE HYDROCHLORIDE
OBY-TRIM, PHENTERMINE HYDROCHLORIDE
OCL, POLYETHYLENE GLYCOL 3350
OCTOCAINE, EPINEPHRINE
OCTREOSCAN, INDIUM IN-111 PENTETREOTIDE KIT
OCUCLEAR, OXYMETAZOLINE HYDROCHLORIDE (OTC)

OCUFEN, FLURBIPROFEN SODIUM
OCUFLOX, OFLOXACIN
OCUMYCIN, BACITRACIN ZINC
OCUPRESS, CARTEOLOL HYDROCHLORIDE
OCUSERT PILO-20, PILOCARPINE
OCUSERT PILO-40, PILOCARPINE
OCUSULF-10, SULFACETAMIDE SODIUM
OCUSULF-30, SULFACETAMIDE SODIUM
OFLOXACIN, OFLOXACIN
OGEN .625, ESTROPIPATE
OGEN 1.25, ESTROPIPATE
OGEN 2.5, ESTROPIPATE
OGEN 5, ESTROPIPATE
OGEN, ESTROPIPATE
OGESTREL 0.5/50-21, ETHINYL ESTRADIOL
OGESTREL 0.5/50-28, ETHINYL ESTRADIOL
OLUX FOAM, CLOBETASOL PROPIONATE
OMEPRAZOLE, OMEPRAZOLE
OMNICEF, CEFDINIR
OMNIPAQUE 70, IOHEXOL
OMNIPAQUE 140, IOHEXOL
OMNIPAQUE 180, IOHEXOL
OMNIPAQUE 210, IOHEXOL
OMNIPAQUE 240, IOHEXOL
OMNIPAQUE 300, IOHEXOL
OMNIPAQUE 350, IOHEXOL
OMNIPEN (AMPICILLIN), AMPICILLIN/AMPICILLIN
    TRIHYDRATE
OMNIPEN-N, AMPICILLIN SODIUM
OMNISCAN, GADODIAMIDE
ONA MAST, PHENTERMINE HYDROCHLORIDE
ONA-MAST, PHENTERMINE HYDROCHLORIDE
ONCOVIN, VINCRISTINE SULFATE
OPCON, NAPHAZOLINE HYDROCHLORIDE
OPCON-A, NAPHAZOLINE HYDROCHLORIDE (OTC)
OPHTHAINE, PROPARACAINE HYDROCHLORIDE
OPHTHETIC, PROPARACAINE HYDROCHLORIDE
OPHTHOCHLOR, CHLORAMPHENICOL
OPHTHOCORT, CHLORAMPHENICOL
OPTICROM, CROMOLYN SODIUM
OPTIMARK IN PLASTIC CONTAINER,
    GADOVERSETAMIDE
OPTIMARK, GADOVERSETAMIDE
OPTIMINE, AZATADINE MALEATE
OPTIPRANOLOL, METIPRANOLOL HYDROCHLORIDE
OPTIRAY 160, IOVERSOL
OPTIRAY 240, IOVERSOL
OPTIRAY 300, IOVERSOL
OPTIRAY 320, IOVERSOL
OPTIRAY 350, IOVERSOL
OPTISON, ALBUMIN HUMAN
OPTIVAR, AZELASTINE HYDROCHLORIDE
OPTOMYCIN, CHLORAMPHENICOL
ORA-TESTRYL, FLUOXYMESTERONE
ORABASE HCA, HYDROCORTISONE ACETATE
ORACORT, TRIAMCINOLONE ACETONIDE
ORAGRAFIN CALCIUM, IPODATE CALCIUM
ORAGRAFIN SODIUM, IPODATE SODIUM
ORALONE, TRIAMCINOLONE ACETONIDE
ORAMORPH SR, MORPHINE SULFATE
ORAP, PIMOZIDE
ORAPRED, PREDNISOLONE SODIUM PHOSPHATE
ORASONE, PREDNISONE
ORETIC, HYDROCHLOROTHIAZIDE
ORETICYL 25, DESERPIDINE
ORETICYL 50, DESERPIDINE
ORETICYL FORTE, DESERPIDINE
ORETON METHYL, METHYLTESTOSTERONE
ORETON, METHYLTESTOSTERONE

APPENDIX A
PRODUCT NAME INDEX (*continued*)

ORFADIN, NITISINONE
ORGARAN, DANAPAROID SODIUM
ORGATRAX, HYDROXYZINE HYDROCHLORIDE
ORINASE DIAGNOSTIC, TOLBUTAMIDE SODIUM
ORINASE, TOLBUTAMIDE
ORLAAM, LEVOMETHADYL ACETATE HYDROCHLORIDE
ORLEX HC, ACETIC ACID, GLACIAL
ORLEX, ACETIC ACID, GLACIAL
ORNADE, CHLORPHENIRAMINE MALEATE
ORNIDYL, EFLORNITHINE HYDROCHLORIDE
ORPHENADRINE CITRATE, ASPIRIN, AND CAFFEINE,
     ASPIRIN
ORPHENADRINE CITRATE, ORPHENADRINE CITRATE
ORPHENGESIC FORTE, ASPIRIN
ORPHENGESIC, ASPIRIN
ORTHO CYCLEN-21, ETHINYL ESTRADIOL
ORTHO CYCLEN-28, ETHINYL ESTRADIOL
ORTHO EVRA, ETHINYL ESTRADIOL
ORTHO TRI-CYCLEN LO, ETHINYL ESTRADIOL
ORTHO TRI-CYCLEN, ETHINYL ESTRADIOL
ORTHO-CEPT, DESOGESTREL
ORTHO-EST, ESTROPIPATE
ORTHO-NOVUM 1/35-21, ETHINYL ESTRADIOL
ORTHO-NOVUM 1/35-28, ETHINYL ESTRADIOL
ORTHO-NOVUM 1/50 21, MESTRANOL
ORTHO-NOVUM 1/50 28, MESTRANOL
ORTHO-NOVUM 1/80 21, MESTRANOL
ORTHO-NOVUM 1/80 28, MESTRANOL
ORTHO-NOVUM 10-21, MESTRANOL
ORTHO-NOVUM 10/11-21, ETHINYL ESTRADIOL
ORTHO-NOVUM 10/11-28 IN PLASTIC CONTAINER,
     ETHINYL ESTRADIOL
ORTHO-NOVUM 2-21, MESTRANOL
ORTHO-NOVUM 7/14-21, ETHINYL ESTRADIOL
ORTHO-NOVUM 7/14-28, ETHINYL ESTRADIOL
ORTHO-NOVUM 7/7/7-21, ETHINYL ESTRADIOL
ORTHO-NOVUM 7/7/7-28, ETHINYL ESTRADIOL
ORUDIS KT, KETOPROFEN (OTC)
ORUDIS, KETOPROFEN
ORUVAIL, KETOPROFEN
OSMITROL 10% IN WATER IN PLASTIC CONTAINER,
     MANNITOL
OSMITROL 10% IN WATER, MANNITOL
OSMITROL 15% IN WATER IN PLASTIC CONTAINER,
     MANNITOL
OSMITROL 15% IN WATER, MANNITOL
OSMITROL 20% IN WATER IN PLASTIC CONTAINER,
     MANNITOL
OSMITROL 20% IN WATER, MANNITOL
OSMITROL 5% IN WATER IN PLASTIC CONTAINER,
     MANNITOL
OSMITROL 5% IN WATER, MANNITOL
OSMOVIST 190, IOTROLAN
OSMOVIST 240, IOTROLAN
OSTEOLITE, TECHNETIUM TC-99M MEDRONATE KIT
OSTEOSCAN, TECHNETIUM TC-99M ETIDRONATE KIT
OTICAIR, HYDROCORTISONE
OTOBIONE, HYDROCORTISONE
OTOBIOTIC, HYDROCORTISONE
OTOCORT, HYDROCORTISONE
OVCON-35, ETHINYL ESTRADIOL
OVCON-50, ETHINYL ESTRADIOL
OVIDE, MALATHION
OVIDREL, CHORIOGONADOTROPIN ALFA
OVRAL, ETHINYL ESTRADIOL
OVRAL-28, ETHINYL ESTRADIOL
OVRETTE, NORGESTREL
OVULEN, ETHYNODIOL DIACETATE
OVULEN-21, ETHYNODIOL DIACETATE

OVULEN-28, ETHYNODIOL DIACETATE
OXACILLIN SODIUM, OXACILLIN SODIUM
OXANDRIN, OXANDROLONE
OXAPROZIN, OXAPROZIN
OXAZEPAM, OXAZEPAM
OXILAN-300, IOXILAN
OXILAN-350, IOXILAN
OXISTAT, OXICONAZOLE NITRATE
OXSORALEN, METHOXSALEN
OXSORALEN-ULTRA, METHOXSALEN
OXTRIPHYLLINE PEDIATRIC, OXTRIPHYLLINE
OXTRIPHYLLINE, OXTRIPHYLLINE
OXY-KESSO-TETRA, OXYTETRACYCLINE
     HYDROCHLORIDE
OXYBUTYNIN CHLORIDE, OXYBUTYNIN CHLORIDE
OXYCET, ACETAMINOPHEN
OXYCODONE 2.5/APAP 500, ACETAMINOPHEN
OXYCODONE 5/APAP 500, ACETAMINOPHEN
OXYCODONE AND ACETAMINOPHEN, ACETAMINOPHEN
OXYCODONE AND ASPIRIN (HALF-STRENGTH), ASPIRIN
OXYCODONE AND ASPIRIN, ASPIRIN
OXYCONTIN, OXYCODONE HYDROCHLORIDE
OXYLONE, FLUOROMETHOLONE
OXYPHENBUTAZONE, OXYPHENBUTAZONE
OXYTETRACYCLINE HCL, OXYTETRACYCLINE
     HYDROCHLORIDE
OXYTOCIN 5 USP UNITS IN DEXTROSE 5%, OXYTOCIN
OXYTOCIN 10 USP UNITS IN DEXTROSE 5%, OXYTOCIN
OXYTOCIN 20 USP UNITS IN DEXTROSE 5%, OXYTOCIN
OXYTOCIN, OXYTOCIN
OXYTROL, OXYBUTYNIN

P

P.A.S. SODIUM, AMINOSALICYLATE SODIUM
PACERONE, AMIODARONE HYDROCHLORIDE
PACLITAXEL, PACLITAXEL
PAGITANE, CYCRIMINE HYDROCHLORIDE
PAMELOR, NORTRIPTYLINE HYDROCHLORIDE
PAMIDRONATE DISODIUM, PAMIDRONATE DISODIUM
PAMINE FORTE, METHSCOPOLAMINE BROMIDE
PAMINE, METHSCOPOLAMINE BROMIDE
PANCURONIUM BROMIDE, PANCURONIUM BROMIDE
PANCURONIUM, PANCURONIUM BROMIDE
PANDEL, HYDROCORTISONE PROBUTATE
PANHEPRIN, HEPARIN SODIUM
PANMYCIN, TETRACYCLINE HYDROCHLORIDE
PANRETIN, ALITRETINOIN
PANTOPAQUE, IOPHENDYLATE
PANWARFIN, WARFARIN SODIUM
PAPA-DEINE #3, ACETAMINOPHEN
PAPA-DEINE #4, ACETAMINOPHEN
PARACAINE, PROPARACAINE HYDROCHLORIDE
PARACORT, PREDNISONE
PARADIONE, PARAMETHADIONE
PARAFLEX, CHLORZOXAZONE
PARAFON FORTE DSC, CHLORZOXAZONE
PARAPLATIN, CARBOPLATIN
PARASAL SODIUM, AMINOSALICYLATE SODIUM
PARASAL, AMINOSALICYLIC ACID
PARATHAR, TERIPARATIDE ACETATE
PAREDRINE, HYDROXYAMPHETAMINE
     HYDROBROMIDE
PAREMYD, HYDROXYAMPHETAMINE HYDROBROMIDE
PARLODEL, BROMOCRIPTINE MESYLATE
PARNATE, TRANYLCYPROMINE SULFATE
PAROMOMYCIN SULFATE, PAROMOMYCIN SULFATE
PARSIDOL, ETHOPROPAZINE HYDROCHLORIDE
PASER, AMINOSALICYLIC ACID

APPENDIX A
PRODUCT NAME INDEX (*continued*)

PASKALIUM, POTASSIUM AMINOSALICYLATE
PATANOL, OLOPATADINE HYDROCHLORIDE
PATHILON, TRIDIHEXETHYL CHLORIDE
PATHOCIL, DICLOXACILLIN SODIUM
PAVULON, PANCURONIUM BROMIDE
PAXIL CR, PAROXETINE HYDROCHLORIDE
PAXIL, PAROXETINE HYDROCHLORIDE
PAXIPAM, HALAZEPAM
PBZ, TRIPELENNAMINE CITRATE
PBZ, TRIPELENNAMINE HYDROCHLORIDE
PBZ-SR, TRIPELENNAMINE HYDROCHLORIDE
PCE, ERYTHROMYCIN
PEDIAMYCIN 400, ERYTHROMYCIN ETHYLSUCCINATE
PEDIAMYCIN, ERYTHROMYCIN ETHYLSUCCINATE
PEDIAPRED, PREDNISOLONE SODIUM PHOSPHATE
PEDIATRIC ADVIL, IBUPROFEN (OTC)
PEDIATRIC LTA KIT, LIDOCAINE HYDROCHLORIDE
PEDIAZOLE, ERYTHROMYCIN ETHYLSUCCINATE
PEDIOTIC, HYDROCORTISONE
PEG-LYTE, POLYETHYLENE GLYCOL 3350
PEGANONE, ETHOTOIN
PEMOLINE, PEMOLINE
PEN-VEE K, PENICILLIN V POTASSIUM
PENAPAR-VK, PENICILLIN V POTASSIUM
PENBRITIN, AMPICILLIN/AMPICILLIN TRIHYDRATE
PENBRITIN-S, AMPICILLIN SODIUM
PENECORT, HYDROCORTISONE
PENETREX, ENOXACIN
PENICILLIN G POTASSIUM IN PLASTIC CONTAINER,
    PENICILLIN G POTASSIUM
PENICILLIN G POTASSIUM, PENICILLIN G POTASSIUM
PENICILLIN G PROCAINE, PENICILLIN G PROCAINE
PENICILLIN G SODIUM, PENICILLIN G SODIUM
PENICILLIN V POTASSIUM, PENICILLIN V POTASSIUM
PENICILLIN, PENICILLIN G POTASSIUM
PENICILLIN-2, PENICILLIN G POTASSIUM
PENICILLIN-VK, PENICILLIN V POTASSIUM
PENLAC, CICLOPIROX
PENNTUSS, CHLORPHENIRAMINE POLISTIREX (OTC)
PENTACARINAT, PENTAMIDINE ISETHIONATE
PENTACEF, CEFTAZIDIME (ARGININE FORMULATION)
PENTAM, PENTAMIDINE ISETHIONATE
PENTAMIDINE ISETHIONATE, PENTAMIDINE
    ISETHIONATE
PENTASA, MESALAMINE
PENTAZOCINE AND NALOXONE HYDROCHLORIDES,
    NALOXONE HYDROCHLORIDE
PENTAZOCINE HCL AND ACETAMINOPHEN,
    ACETAMINOPHEN
PENTHRANE, METHOXYFLURANE
PENTIDS '200', PENICILLIN G POTASSIUM
PENTIDS '250', PENICILLIN G POTASSIUM
PENTIDS '400', PENICILLIN G POTASSIUM
PENTIDS '800', PENICILLIN G POTASSIUM
PENTOBARBITAL SODIUM, PENTOBARBITAL SODIUM
PENTOLAIR, CYCLOPENTOLATE HYDROCHLORIDE
PENTOTHAL, THIOPENTAL SODIUM
PENTOXIFYLLINE, PENTOXIFYLLINE
PENTOXIL, PENTOXIFYLLINE
PEPCID AC, FAMOTIDINE (OTC)
PEPCID COMPLETE, CALCIUM CARBONATE,
    PRECIPITATED (OTC)
PEPCID PRESERVATIVE FREE IN PLASTIC CONTAINER,
    FAMOTIDINE
PEPCID PRESERVATIVE FREE, FAMOTIDINE
PEPCID RPD, FAMOTIDINE
PEPCID, FAMOTIDINE
PEPTAVLON, PENTAGASTRIN
PERCHLORACAP, POTASSIUM PERCHLORATE

PERCOCET, ACETAMINOPHEN
PERCODAN, ASPIRIN
PERCODAN-DEMI, ASPIRIN
PERCORTEN, DESOXYCORTICOSTERONE ACETATE
PERCORTEN, DESOXYCORTICOSTERONE PIVALATE
PERGOLIDE MESYLATE, PERGOLIDE MESYLATE
PERGONAL, MENOTROPINS (FSH;LH)
PERIACTIN, CYPROHEPTADINE HYDROCHLORIDE
PERIDEX, CHLORHEXIDINE GLUCONATE
PERIOCHIP, CHLORHEXIDINE GLUCONATE
PERIOGARD, CHLORHEXIDINE GLUCONATE
PERIOSTAT, DOXYCYCLINE HYCLATE
PERMAPEN, PENICILLIN G BENZATHINE
PERMAX, PERGOLIDE MESYLATE
PERMETHRIN, PERMETHRIN
PERMETHRIN, PERMETHRIN (OTC)
PERMITIL, FLUPHENAZINE HYDROCHLORIDE
PERPHENAZINE AND AMITRIPTYLINE HCL,
    AMITRIPTYLINE HYDROCHLORIDE
PERPHENAZINE, PERPHENAZINE
PERSANTINE, DIPYRIDAMOLE
PERTOFRANE, DESIPRAMINE HYDROCHLORIDE
PFIZER-E, ERYTHROMYCIN STEARATE
PFIZERPEN G, PENICILLIN G POTASSIUM
PFIZERPEN VK, PENICILLIN V POTASSIUM
PFIZERPEN, PENICILLIN G POTASSIUM
PFIZERPEN-A, AMPICILLIN/AMPICILLIN TRIHYDRATE
PFIZERPEN-AS, PENICILLIN G PROCAINE
PHARMASEAL SCRUB CARE, CHLORHEXIDINE
    GLUCONATE (OTC)
PHENAPHEN W/ CODEINE NO. 2, ACETAMINOPHEN
PHENAPHEN W/ CODEINE NO. 3, ACETAMINOPHEN
PHENAPHEN W/ CODEINE NO. 4, ACETAMINOPHEN
PHENAPHEN-650 W/ CODEINE, ACETAMINOPHEN
PHENAZINE, PHENDIMETRAZINE TARTRATE
PHENAZINE-35, PHENDIMETRAZINE TARTRATE
PHENDIMETRAZINE TARTRATE, PHENDIMETRAZINE
    TARTRATE
PHENERGAN FORTIS, PROMETHAZINE
    HYDROCHLORIDE
PHENERGAN PLAIN, PROMETHAZINE HYDROCHLORIDE
PHENERGAN VC W/ CODEINE, CODEINE PHOSPHATE
PHENERGAN VC, PHENYLEPHRINE HYDROCHLORIDE
PHENERGAN W/ CODEINE, CODEINE PHOSPHATE
PHENERGAN W/ DEXTROMETHORPHAN,
    DEXTROMETHORPHAN HYDROBROMIDE
PHENERGAN, PROMETHAZINE HYDROCHLORIDE
PHENETRON, CHLORPHENIRAMINE MALEATE
PHENTERMINE HCL, PHENTERMINE HYDROCHLORIDE
PHENTERMINE RESIN 30, PHENTERMINE RESIN
    COMPLEX
PHENTOLAMINE MESYLATE, PHENTOLAMINE
    MESYLATE
PHENTYTOIN, PHENYTOIN
PHENURONE, PHENACEMIDE
PHENY-PAS-TEBAMIN, PHENYL AMINOSALICYLATE
PHENYLBUTAZONE, PHENYLBUTAZONE
PHENYLPROPANOLAMINE HCL W/
    CHLORPHENIRAMINE MALEATE,
    CHLORPHENIRAMINE MALEATE (OTC)
PHENYTEK, PHENYTOIN SODIUM, EXTENDED
PHENYTEX, PHENYTOIN SODIUM, EXTENDED
PHENYTOIN SODIUM, PHENYTOIN SODIUM
PHENYTOIN SODIUM, PHENYTOIN SODIUM, PROMPT
PHENYTOIN, PHENYTOIN
PHENYTOIN, PHENYTOIN SODIUM
PHERAZINE DM, DEXTROMETHORPHAN
    HYDROBROMIDE
PHERAZINE VC W/ CODEINE, CODEINE PHOSPHATE

APPENDIX A
PRODUCT NAME INDEX (*continued*)

PHERAZINE VC, PHENYLEPHRINE HYDROCHLORIDE
PHERAZINE W/ CODEINE, CODEINE PHOSPHATE
PHISO-SCRUB, HEXACHLOROPHENE
PHISOHEX, HEXACHLOROPHENE
PHOSLO GELCAPS, CALCIUM ACETATE
PHOSLO, CALCIUM ACETATE
PHOSPHOCOL P32, CHROMIC PHOSPHATE, P-32
PHOSPHOLINE IODIDE, ECHOTHIOPHATE IODIDE
PHOSPHOTEC, TECHNETIUM TC-99M
    PYROPHOSPHATE KIT
PHOSPHOTOPE, SODIUM PHOSPHATE, P-32
PHOTOFRIN, PORFIMER SODIUM
PHRENILIN FORTE, ACETAMINOPHEN
PHRENILIN WITH CAFFEINE AND CODEINE,
    ACETAMINOPHEN
PHRENILIN, ACETAMINOPHEN
PHYLLOCONTIN, AMINOPHYLLINE
PHYSIOLYTE IN PLASTIC CONTAINER, MAGNESIUM
    CHLORIDE
PHYSIOSOL IN PLASTIC CONTAINER, MAGNESIUM
    CHLORIDE
PHYSIOSOL PH 7.4 IN PLASTIC CONTAINER,
    MAGNESIUM CHLORIDE
PHYTONADIONE, PHYTONADIONE
PILOPINE HS, PILOCARPINE HYDROCHLORIDE
PINDAC, PINACIDIL
PINDOLOL, PINDOLOL
PIPERAZINE CITRATE, PIPERAZINE CITRATE
PIPRACIL, PIPERACILLIN SODIUM
PIROXICAM, PIROXICAM
PITOCIN, OXYTOCIN
PITRESSIN TANNATE, VASOPRESSIN TANNATE
PLACIDYL, ETHCHLORVYNOL
PLAN B, LEVONORGESTREL
PLAQUENIL, HYDROXYCHLOROQUINE SULFATE
PLASMA-LYTE 56 AND DEXTROSE 5% IN PLASTIC
    CONTAINER, DEXTROSE
PLASMA-LYTE 148 AND DEXTROSE 5% IN PLASTIC
    CONTAINER, DEXTROSE
PLASMA-LYTE 148 IN WATER IN PLASTIC CONTAINER,
    MAGNESIUM CHLORIDE
PLASMA-LYTE 56 IN PLASTIC CONTAINER, MAGNESIUM
    ACETATE TETRAHYDRATE
PLASMA-LYTE A IN PLASTIC CONTAINER, MAGNESIUM
    CHLORIDE
PLASMA-LYTE M AND DEXTROSE 5% IN PLASTIC
    CONTAINER, CALCIUM CHLORIDE
PLASMA-LYTE R IN PLASTIC CONTAINER, CALCIUM
    CHLORIDE
PLATINOL, CISPLATIN
PLATINOL-AQ, CISPLATIN
PLAVIX, CLOPIDOGREL BISULFATE
PLEGINE, PHENDIMETRAZINE TARTRATE
PLEGISOL IN PLASTIC CONTAINER, CALCIUM CHLORIDE
PLENDIL, FELODIPINE
PLETAL, CILOSTAZOL
PMB 200, ESTROGENS, CONJUGATED
PMB 400, ESTROGENS, CONJUGATED
PODOFILOX, PODOFILOX
POLARAMINE, DEXCHLORPHENIRAMINE MALEATE
POLOCAINE W/ LEVONORDEFRIN, LEVONORDEFRIN
POLOCAINE, MEPIVACAINE HYDROCHLORIDE
POLOCAINE-MPF, MEPIVACAINE HYDROCHLORIDE
POLY-PRED, NEOMYCIN SULFATE
POLY-RX, POLYMYXIN B SULFATE
POLYCILLIN, AMPICILLIN/AMPICILLIN TRIHYDRATE
POLYCILLIN-N, AMPICILLIN SODIUM
POLYCILLIN-PRB, AMPICILLIN/AMPICILLIN TRIHYDRATE
POLYMOX, AMOXICILLIN

POLYMYXIN B SULFATE, POLYMYXIN B SULFATE
POLYSPORIN, BACITRACIN ZINC
POLYSPORIN, BACITRACIN ZINC (OTC)
POLYTRIM, POLYMYXIN B SULFATE
PONSTEL, MEFENAMIC ACID
PORTALAC, LACTULOSE
PORTIA-21, ETHINYL ESTRADIOL
PORTIA-28, ETHINYL ESTRADIOL
POTASSIUM ACETATE IN PLASTIC CONTAINER,
    POTASSIUM ACETATE
POTASSIUM AMINOSALICYLATE, POTASSIUM
    AMINOSALICYLATE
POTASSIUM CHLORIDE 0.037% IN DEXTROSE 10% AND
    SODIUM CHLORIDE 0.2% IN PLASTIC CONTAINER,
    DEXTROSE
POTASSIUM CHLORIDE 0.037% IN DEXTROSE 10% AND
    SODIUM CHLORIDE 0.45% IN PLASTIC CONTAINER,
    DEXTROSE
POTASSIUM CHLORIDE 0.037% IN DEXTROSE 10% AND
    SODIUM CHLORIDE 0.9% IN PLASTIC CONTAINER,
    DEXTROSE
POTASSIUM CHLORIDE 0.037% IN DEXTROSE 5% AND
    SODIUM CHLORIDE 0.11% IN PLASTIC CONTAINER,
    DEXTROSE
POTASSIUM CHLORIDE 0.037% IN DEXTROSE 5% AND
    SODIUM CHLORIDE 0.2% IN PLASTIC CONTAINER,
    DEXTROSE
POTASSIUM CHLORIDE 0.037% IN DEXTROSE 5% AND
    SODIUM CHLORIDE 0.33% IN PLASTIC CONTAINER,
    DEXTROSE
POTASSIUM CHLORIDE 0.037% IN DEXTROSE 5% AND
    SODIUM CHLORIDE 0.45% IN PLASTIC CONTAINER,
    DEXTROSE
POTASSIUM CHLORIDE 0.037% IN DEXTROSE 5% AND
    SODIUM CHLORIDE 0.9% IN PLASTIC CONTAINER,
    DEXTROSE
POTASSIUM CHLORIDE 0.037% IN DEXTROSE 5% IN
    PLASTIC CONTAINER, DEXTROSE
POTASSIUM CHLORIDE 0.037% IN SODIUM CHLORIDE
    0.9% IN PLASTIC CONTAINER, POTASSIUM
    CHLORIDE
POTASSIUM CHLORIDE 0.075% IN DEXTROSE 10% AND
    SODIUM CHLORIDE 0.2% IN PLASTIC CONTAINER,
    DEXTROSE
POTASSIUM CHLORIDE 0.075% IN DEXTROSE 10% AND
    SODIUM CHLORIDE 0.45% IN PLASTIC CONTAINER,
    DEXTROSE
POTASSIUM CHLORIDE 0.075% IN DEXTROSE 10% AND
    SODIUM CHLORIDE 0.9% IN PLASTIC CONTAINER,
    DEXTROSE
POTASSIUM CHLORIDE 0.075% IN DEXTROSE 3.3% AND
    SODIUM CHLORIDE 0.3% IN PLASTIC CONTAINER,
    DEXTROSE
POTASSIUM CHLORIDE 0.075% IN DEXTROSE 5% AND
    SODIUM CHLORIDE 0.11% IN PLASTIC CONTAINER,
    DEXTROSE
POTASSIUM CHLORIDE 0.075% IN DEXTROSE 5% AND
    SODIUM CHLORIDE 0.2% IN PLASTIC CONTAINER,
    DEXTROSE
POTASSIUM CHLORIDE 0.075% IN DEXTROSE 5% AND
    SODIUM CHLORIDE 0.33% IN PLASTIC CONTAINER,
    DEXTROSE
POTASSIUM CHLORIDE 0.075% IN DEXTROSE 5% AND
    SODIUM CHLORIDE 0.45% IN PLASTIC CONTAINER,
    DEXTROSE
POTASSIUM CHLORIDE 0.075% IN DEXTROSE 5% AND
    SODIUM CHLORIDE 0.9% IN PLASTIC CONTAINER,
    DEXTROSE

APPENDIX A
PRODUCT NAME INDEX (*continued*)

POTASSIUM CHLORIDE 0.075% IN DEXTROSE 5% IN PLASTIC CONTAINER, DEXTROSE

POTASSIUM CHLORIDE 0.075% IN SODIUM CHLORIDE 0.9% IN PLASTIC CONTAINER, POTASSIUM CHLORIDE

POTASSIUM CHLORIDE 0.11% IN DEXTROSE 10% AND SODIUM CHLORIDE 0.2% IN PLASTIC CONTAINER, DEXTROSE

POTASSIUM CHLORIDE 0.11% IN DEXTROSE 10% AND SODIUM CHLORIDE 0.45% IN PLASTIC CONTAINER, DEXTROSE

POTASSIUM CHLORIDE 0.11% IN DEXTROSE 10% AND SODIUM CHLORIDE 0.9% IN PLASTIC CONTAINER, DEXTROSE

POTASSIUM CHLORIDE 0.11% IN DEXTROSE 3.3% AND SODIUM CHLORIDE 0.3% IN PLASTIC CONTAINER, DEXTROSE

POTASSIUM CHLORIDE 0.11% IN DEXTROSE 5% AND SODIUM CHLORIDE 0.11% IN PLASTIC CONTAINER, DEXTROSE

POTASSIUM CHLORIDE 0.11% IN DEXTROSE 5% AND SODIUM CHLORIDE 0.2% IN PLASTIC CONTAINER, DEXTROSE

POTASSIUM CHLORIDE 0.11% IN DEXTROSE 5% AND SODIUM CHLORIDE 0.33% IN PLASTIC CONTAINER, DEXTROSE

POTASSIUM CHLORIDE 0.11% IN DEXTROSE 5% AND SODIUM CHLORIDE 0.45% IN PLASTIC CONTAINER, DEXTROSE

POTASSIUM CHLORIDE 0.11% IN DEXTROSE 5% AND SODIUM CHLORIDE 0.9% IN PLASTIC CONTAINER, DEXTROSE

POTASSIUM CHLORIDE 0.11% IN DEXTROSE 5% IN PLASTIC CONTAINER, DEXTROSE

POTASSIUM CHLORIDE 0.11% IN SODIUM CHLORIDE 0.9% IN PLASTIC CONTAINER, POTASSIUM CHLORIDE

POTASSIUM CHLORIDE 0.15% IN DEXTROSE 10% AND SODIUM CHLORIDE 0.2% IN PLASTIC CONTAINER, DEXTROSE

POTASSIUM CHLORIDE 0.15% IN DEXTROSE 10% AND SODIUM CHLORIDE 0.45% IN PLASTIC CONTAINER, DEXTROSE

POTASSIUM CHLORIDE 0.15% IN DEXTROSE 10% AND SODIUM CHLORIDE 0.9% IN PLASTIC CONTAINER, DEXTROSE

POTASSIUM CHLORIDE 0.15% IN DEXTROSE 3.3% AND SODIUM CHLORIDE 0.3% IN PLASTIC CONTAINER, DEXTROSE

POTASSIUM CHLORIDE 0.15% IN DEXTROSE 5% AND SODIUM CHLORIDE 0.11% IN PLASTIC CONTAINER, DEXTROSE

POTASSIUM CHLORIDE 0.15% IN DEXTROSE 5% AND SODIUM CHLORIDE 0.2% IN PLASTIC CONTAINER, DEXTROSE

POTASSIUM CHLORIDE 0.15% IN DEXTROSE 5% AND SODIUM CHLORIDE 0.33% IN PLASTIC CONTAINER, DEXTROSE

POTASSIUM CHLORIDE 0.15% IN DEXTROSE 5% AND SODIUM CHLORIDE 0.45% IN PLASTIC CONTAINER, DEXTROSE

POTASSIUM CHLORIDE 0.15% IN DEXTROSE 5% AND SODIUM CHLORIDE 0.9% IN PLASTIC CONTAINER, DEXTROSE

POTASSIUM CHLORIDE 0.15% IN DEXTROSE 5% IN PLASTIC CONTAINER, DEXTROSE

POTASSIUM CHLORIDE 0.15% IN SODIUM CHLORIDE 0.9% IN PLASTIC CONTAINER, POTASSIUM CHLORIDE

POTASSIUM CHLORIDE 0.22% IN DEXTROSE 10% AND SODIUM CHLORIDE 0.2% IN PLASTIC CONTAINER, DEXTROSE

POTASSIUM CHLORIDE 0.22% IN DEXTROSE 10% AND SODIUM CHLORIDE 0.45% IN PLASTIC CONTAINER, DEXTROSE

POTASSIUM CHLORIDE 0.22% IN DEXTROSE 10% AND SODIUM CHLORIDE 0.9% IN PLASTIC CONTAINER, DEXTROSE

POTASSIUM CHLORIDE 0.22% IN DEXTROSE 3.3% AND SODIUM CHLORIDE 0.3% IN PLASTIC CONTAINER, DEXTROSE

POTASSIUM CHLORIDE 0.22% IN DEXTROSE 5% AND SODIUM CHLORIDE 0.11% IN PLASTIC CONTAINER, DEXTROSE

POTASSIUM CHLORIDE 0.22% IN DEXTROSE 5% AND SODIUM CHLORIDE 0.2% IN PLASTIC CONTAINER, DEXTROSE

POTASSIUM CHLORIDE 0.22% IN DEXTROSE 5% AND SODIUM CHLORIDE 0.33% IN PLASTIC CONTAINER, DEXTROSE

POTASSIUM CHLORIDE 0.22% IN DEXTROSE 5% AND SODIUM CHLORIDE 0.45% IN PLASTIC CONTAINER, DEXTROSE

POTASSIUM CHLORIDE 0.22% IN DEXTROSE 5% AND SODIUM CHLORIDE 0.9% IN PLASTIC CONTAINER, DEXTROSE

POTASSIUM CHLORIDE 0.22% IN DEXTROSE 5% IN PLASTIC CONTAINER, DEXTROSE

POTASSIUM CHLORIDE 0.22% IN SODIUM CHLORIDE 0.9% IN PLASTIC CONTAINER, POTASSIUM CHLORIDE

POTASSIUM CHLORIDE 0.3% IN DEXTROSE 10% AND SODIUM CHLORIDE 0.2% IN PLASTIC CONTAINER, DEXTROSE

POTASSIUM CHLORIDE 0.3% IN DEXTROSE 10% AND SODIUM CHLORIDE 0.45% IN PLASTIC CONTAINER, DEXTROSE

POTASSIUM CHLORIDE 0.3% IN DEXTROSE 10% AND SODIUM CHLORIDE 0.9% IN PLASTIC CONTAINER, DEXTROSE

POTASSIUM CHLORIDE 0.3% IN DEXTROSE 3.3% AND SODIUM CHLORIDE 0.3% IN PLASTIC CONTAINER, DEXTROSE

POTASSIUM CHLORIDE 0.3% IN DEXTROSE 5% AND SODIUM CHLORIDE 0.11% IN PLASTIC CONTAINER, DEXTROSE

POTASSIUM CHLORIDE 0.3% IN DEXTROSE 5% AND SODIUM CHLORIDE 0.2% IN PLASTIC CONTAINER, DEXTROSE

POTASSIUM CHLORIDE 0.3% IN DEXTROSE 5% AND SODIUM CHLORIDE 0.33% IN PLASTIC CONTAINER, DEXTROSE

POTASSIUM CHLORIDE 0.3% IN DEXTROSE 5% AND SODIUM CHLORIDE 0.45% IN PLASTIC CONTAINER, DEXTROSE

POTASSIUM CHLORIDE 0.3% IN DEXTROSE 5% AND SODIUM CHLORIDE 0.9% IN PLASTIC CONTAINER, DEXTROSE

POTASSIUM CHLORIDE 0.3% IN DEXTROSE 5% IN PLASTIC CONTAINER, DEXTROSE

POTASSIUM CHLORIDE 0.3% IN SODIUM CHLORIDE 0.9% IN PLASTIC CONTAINER, POTASSIUM CHLORIDE

POTASSIUM CHLORIDE 10MEQ IN DEXTROSE 5% AND LACTATED RINGER'S IN PLASTIC CONTAINER, CALCIUM CHLORIDE

POTASSIUM CHLORIDE 10MEQ IN DEXTROSE 5% AND SODIUM CHLORIDE 0.225% IN PLASTIC CONTAINER, DEXTROSE

APPENDIX A
PRODUCT NAME INDEX (*continued*)

POTASSIUM CHLORIDE 10MEQ IN DEXTROSE 5% AND SODIUM CHLORIDE 0.3% IN PLASTIC CONTAINER, DEXTROSE

POTASSIUM CHLORIDE 10MEQ IN DEXTROSE 5% AND SODIUM CHLORIDE 0.45% IN PLASTIC CONTAINER, DEXTROSE

POTASSIUM CHLORIDE 10MEQ IN DEXTROSE 5% AND SODIUM CHLORIDE 0.9% IN PLASTIC CONTAINER, DEXTROSE

POTASSIUM CHLORIDE 10MEQ IN PLASTIC CONTAINER, POTASSIUM CHLORIDE

POTASSIUM CHLORIDE 15MEQ IN DEXTROSE 5% AND LACTATED RINGER'S IN PLASTIC CONTAINER, CALCIUM CHLORIDE

POTASSIUM CHLORIDE 15MEQ IN DEXTROSE 5% AND SODIUM CHLORIDE 0.225% IN PLASTIC CONTAINER, DEXTROSE

POTASSIUM CHLORIDE 15MEQ IN DEXTROSE 5% AND SODIUM CHLORIDE 0.3% IN PLASTIC CONTAINER, DEXTROSE

POTASSIUM CHLORIDE 15MEQ IN DEXTROSE 5% AND SODIUM CHLORIDE 0.45% IN PLASTIC CONTAINER, DEXTROSE

POTASSIUM CHLORIDE 15MEQ IN DEXTROSE 5% AND SODIUM CHLORIDE 0.9% IN PLASTIC CONTAINER, DEXTROSE

POTASSIUM CHLORIDE 20MEQ IN DEXTROSE 5% AND LACTATED RINGER'S IN PLASTIC CONTAINER, CALCIUM CHLORIDE

POTASSIUM CHLORIDE 20MEQ IN DEXTROSE 5% AND SODIUM CHLORIDE 0.225% IN PLASTIC CONTAINER, DEXTROSE

POTASSIUM CHLORIDE 20MEQ IN DEXTROSE 5% AND SODIUM CHLORIDE 0.3% IN PLASTIC CONTAINER, DEXTROSE

POTASSIUM CHLORIDE 20MEQ IN DEXTROSE 5% AND SODIUM CHLORIDE 0.45% IN PLASTIC CONTAINER, DEXTROSE

POTASSIUM CHLORIDE 20MEQ IN DEXTROSE 5% AND SODIUM CHLORIDE 0.9% IN PLASTIC CONTAINER, DEXTROSE

POTASSIUM CHLORIDE 20MEQ IN DEXTROSE 5% IN PLASTIC CONTAINER, DEXTROSE

POTASSIUM CHLORIDE 20MEQ IN DEXTROSE 5% IN SODIUM CHLORIDE 0.3% IN PLASTIC CONTAINER, DEXTROSE

POTASSIUM CHLORIDE 20MEQ IN PLASTIC CONTAINER, POTASSIUM CHLORIDE

POTASSIUM CHLORIDE 20MEQ IN SODIUM CHLORIDE 0.9% IN PLASTIC CONTAINER, POTASSIUM CHLORIDE

POTASSIUM CHLORIDE 30MEQ IN DEXTROSE 5% AND LACTATED RINGER'S IN PLASTIC CONTAINER, CALCIUM CHLORIDE

POTASSIUM CHLORIDE 30MEQ IN DEXTROSE 5% AND SODIUM CHLORIDE 0.225% IN PLASTIC CONTAINER, DEXTROSE

POTASSIUM CHLORIDE 30MEQ IN DEXTROSE 5% AND SODIUM CHLORIDE 0.3% IN PLASTIC CONTAINER, DEXTROSE

POTASSIUM CHLORIDE 30MEQ IN DEXTROSE 5% AND SODIUM CHLORIDE 0.45% IN PLASTIC CONTAINER, DEXTROSE

POTASSIUM CHLORIDE 30MEQ IN DEXTROSE 5% AND SODIUM CHLORIDE 0.9% IN PLASTIC CONTAINER, DEXTROSE

POTASSIUM CHLORIDE 30MEQ IN DEXTROSE 5% IN PLASTIC CONTAINER, DEXTROSE

POTASSIUM CHLORIDE 30MEQ IN PLASTIC CONTAINER, POTASSIUM CHLORIDE

POTASSIUM CHLORIDE 40MEQ IN DEXTROSE 5% AND LACTATED RINGER'S IN PLASTIC CONTAINER, CALCIUM CHLORIDE

POTASSIUM CHLORIDE 40MEQ IN DEXTROSE 5% AND SODIUM CHLORIDE 0.225% IN PLASTIC CONTAINER, DEXTROSE

POTASSIUM CHLORIDE 40MEQ IN DEXTROSE 5% AND SODIUM CHLORIDE 0.3% IN PLASTIC CONTAINER, DEXTROSE

POTASSIUM CHLORIDE 40MEQ IN DEXTROSE 5% AND SODIUM CHLORIDE 0.45% IN PLASTIC CONTAINER, DEXTROSE

POTASSIUM CHLORIDE 40MEQ IN DEXTROSE 5% AND SODIUM CHLORIDE 0.9% IN PLASTIC CONTAINER, DEXTROSE

POTASSIUM CHLORIDE 40MEQ IN DEXTROSE 5% IN PLASTIC CONTAINER, DEXTROSE

POTASSIUM CHLORIDE 40MEQ IN PLASTIC CONTAINER, POTASSIUM CHLORIDE

POTASSIUM CHLORIDE 40MEQ IN SODIUM CHLORIDE 0.9% IN PLASTIC CONTAINER, POTASSIUM CHLORIDE

POTASSIUM CHLORIDE 5MEQ IN DEXTROSE 5% AND LACTATED RINGER'S IN PLASTIC CONTAINER, CALCIUM CHLORIDE

POTASSIUM CHLORIDE 5MEQ IN DEXTROSE 5% AND SODIUM CHLORIDE 0.225% IN PLASTIC CONTAINER, DEXTROSE

POTASSIUM CHLORIDE 5MEQ IN DEXTROSE 5% AND SODIUM CHLORIDE 0.3% IN PLASTIC CONTAINER, DEXTROSE

POTASSIUM CHLORIDE 5MEQ IN DEXTROSE 5% AND SODIUM CHLORIDE 0.45% IN PLASTIC CONTAINER, DEXTROSE

POTASSIUM CHLORIDE 5MEQ IN DEXTROSE 5% AND SODIUM CHLORIDE 0.9% IN PLASTIC CONTAINER, DEXTROSE

POTASSIUM CHLORIDE IN PLASTIC CONTAINER, POTASSIUM CHLORIDE

POTASSIUM CHLORIDE, POTASSIUM CHLORIDE

POTASSIUM CITRATE, POTASSIUM CITRATE

POTASSIUM IODIDE, POTASSIUM IODIDE (OTC)

POVAN, PYRVINIUM PAMOATE

POVIDONE IODINE, POVIDONE-IODINE (OTC)

PRALIDOXIME CHLORIDE, PRALIDOXIME CHLORIDE

PRAMINE, IMIPRAMINE HYDROCHLORIDE

PRAMOSONE, HYDROCORTISONE ACETATE

PRANDIN, REPAGLINIDE

PRANTAL, DIPHEMANIL METHYLSULFATE

PRAVACHOL, PRAVASTATIN SODIUM

PRAVIGARD PAC (COPACKAGED), ASPIRIN

PRAZEPAM, PRAZEPAM

PRAZOSIN HCL, PRAZOSIN HYDROCHLORIDE

PRE-OP II, HEXACHLOROPHENE

PRE-OP, HEXACHLOROPHENE

PRE-PEN, BENZYL PENICILLOYL-POLYLYSINE

PRE-SATE, CHLORPHENTERMINE HYDROCHLORIDE

PRECEDEX, DEXMEDETOMIDINE

PRECEF, CEFORANIDE

PRECOSE, ACARBOSE

PRED FORTE, PREDNISOLONE ACETATE

PRED MILD, PREDNISOLONE ACETATE

PRED-G, GENTAMICIN SULFATE

PREDAIR FORTE, PREDNISOLONE SODIUM PHOSPHATE

PREDAIR, PREDNISOLONE SODIUM PHOSPHATE

PREDAMIDE, PREDNISOLONE ACETATE

APPENDIX A
PRODUCT NAME INDEX (*continued*)

PREDNICEN-M, PREDNISONE
PREDNISOLONE ACETATE, PREDNISOLONE ACETATE
PREDNISOLONE SODIUM PHOSPHATE, PREDNISOLONE SODIUM PHOSPHATE
PREDNISOLONE TEBUTATE, PREDNISOLONE TEBUTATE
PREDNISOLONE, PREDNISOLONE
PREDNISONE INTENSOL, PREDNISONE
PREDNISONE, PREDNISONE
PREDSULFAIR II, PREDNISOLONE ACETATE
PREDSULFAIR, PREDNISOLONE ACETATE
PREFEST, ESTRADIOL
PREFRIN-A, PHENYLEPHRINE HYDROCHLORIDE
PREGNYL, GONADOTROPIN, CHORIONIC
PRELAY, TROGLITAZONE
PRELONE, PREDNISOLONE
PRELUDIN, PHENMETRAZINE HYDROCHLORIDE
PREMARIN, ESTROGENS, CONJUGATED
PREMASOL 10% IN PLASTIC CONTAINER, AMINO ACIDS
PREMASOL 6% IN PLASTIC CONTAINER, AMINO ACIDS
PREMPHASE (PREMARIN;CYCRIN 14/14), ESTROGENS, CONJUGATED
PREMPHASE 14/14, ESTROGENS, CONJUGATED
PREMPRO (PREMARIN;CYCRIN), ESTROGENS, CONJUGATED
PREMPRO, ESTROGENS, CONJUGATED
PREPIDIL, DINOPROSTONE
PRESAMINE, IMIPRAMINE HYDROCHLORIDE
PREVACARE R, CHLORHEXIDINE GLUCONATE (OTC)
PREVACID, LANSOPRAZOLE
PREVALITE, CHOLESTYRAMINE
PREVEN EMERGENCY CONTRACEPTIVE KIT, ETHINYL ESTRADIOL
PREVPAC, AMOXICILLIN
PRIFTIN, RIFAPENTINE
PRILOSEC, OMEPRAZOLE
PRILOSEC, OMEPRAZOLE MAGNESIUM (OTC)
PRIMACOR IN DEXTROSE 5% IN PLASTIC CONTAINER, MILRINONE LACTATE
PRIMACOR, MILRINONE LACTATE
PRIMAQUINE, PRIMAQUINE PHOSPHATE
PRIMATENE MIST, EPINEPHRINE (OTC)
PRIMAXIN, CILASTATIN SODIUM
PRIMIDONE, PRIMIDONE
PRIMSOL, TRIMETHOPRIM HYDROCHLORIDE
PRINCIPEN '125', AMPICILLIN/AMPICILLIN TRIHYDRATE
PRINCIPEN '250', AMPICILLIN/AMPICILLIN TRIHYDRATE
PRINCIPEN '500', AMPICILLIN/AMPICILLIN TRIHYDRATE
PRINCIPEN W/ PROBENECID, AMPICILLIN/AMPICILLIN TRIHYDRATE
PRINCIPEN, AMPICILLIN/AMPICILLIN TRIHYDRATE
PRINIVIL, LISINOPRIL
PRINZIDE, HYDROCHLOROTHIAZIDE
PRISCOLINE, TOLAZOLINE HYDROCHLORIDE
PRO-BANTHINE, PROPANTHELINE BROMIDE
PROAMATINE, MIDODRINE HYDROCHLORIDE
PROBALAN, PROBENECID
PROBAMPACIN, AMPICILLIN/AMPICILLIN TRIHYDRATE
PROBEN-C, COLCHICINE
PROBENECID AND COLCHICINE, COLCHICINE
PROBENECID W/ COLCHICINE, COLCHICINE
PROBENECID, PROBENECID
PROCAINAMIDE HCL, PROCAINAMIDE HYDROCHLORIDE
PROCAINE HCL W/ EPINEPHRINE, EPINEPHRINE
PROCAINE HCL, PROCAINE HYDROCHLORIDE
PROCALAMINE, AMINO ACIDS
PROCAN SR, PROCAINAMIDE HYDROCHLORIDE
PROCAN, PROCAINAMIDE HYDROCHLORIDE

PROCANBID, PROCAINAMIDE HYDROCHLORIDE
PROCAPAN, PROCAINAMIDE HYDROCHLORIDE
PROCARDIA XL, NIFEDIPINE
PROCARDIA, NIFEDIPINE
PROCHLORPERAZINE EDISYLATE, PROCHLORPERAZINE EDISYLATE
PROCHLORPERAZINE MALEATE, PROCHLORPERAZINE MALEATE
PROCHLORPERAZINE, PROCHLORPERAZINE
PROCHLORPERAZINE, PROCHLORPERAZINE EDISYLATE
PROCHLORPERAZINE, PROCHLORPERAZINE MALEATE
PROCTOCORT, HYDROCORTISONE
PROCTOFOAM HC, HYDROCORTISONE ACETATE
PROFEN, IBUPROFEN (OTC)
PROFENAL, SUPROFEN
PROFERDEX, IRON DEXTRAN
PROGESTASERT, PROGESTERONE
PROGESTERONE, PROGESTERONE
PROGLYCEM, DIAZOXIDE
PROGRAF, TACROLIMUS
PROHANCE, GADOTERIDOL
PROKETAZINE, CARPHENAZINE MALEATE
PROKLAR, SULFAMETHIZOLE
PROLIXIN DECANOATE, FLUPHENAZINE DECANOATE
PROLIXIN ENANTHATE, FLUPHENAZINE ENANTHATE
PROLIXIN, FLUPHENAZINE HYDROCHLORIDE
PROLOID, THYROGLOBULIN
PROLOPRIM, TRIMETHOPRIM
PROMAPAR, CHLORPROMAZINE HYDROCHLORIDE
PROMAZINE HCL, PROMAZINE HYDROCHLORIDE
PROMETA, METAPROTERENOL SULFATE
PROMETH FORTIS, PROMETHAZINE HYDROCHLORIDE
PROMETH PLAIN, PROMETHAZINE HYDROCHLORIDE
PROMETH VC PLAIN, PHENYLEPHRINE HYDROCHLORIDE
PROMETH VC W/ CODEINE, CODEINE PHOSPHATE
PROMETH W/ CODEINE, CODEINE PHOSPHATE
PROMETH W/ DEXTROMETHORPHAN, DEXTROMETHORPHAN HYDROBROMIDE
PROMETHACON, PROMETHAZINE HYDROCHLORIDE
PROMETHAZINE HCL AND CODEINE PHOSPHATE, CODEINE PHOSPHATE
PROMETHAZINE HCL AND DEXTROMETHORPHAN HYDROBROMIDE, DEXTROMETHORPHAN HYDROBROMIDE
PROMETHAZINE HCL, PROMETHAZINE HYDROCHLORIDE
PROMETHAZINE PLAIN, PROMETHAZINE HYDROCHLORIDE
PROMETHAZINE VC PLAIN, PHENYLEPHRINE HYDROCHLORIDE
PROMETHAZINE VC W/ CODEINE, CODEINE PHOSPHATE
PROMETHAZINE W/ CODEINE, CODEINE PHOSPHATE
PROMETHAZINE W/ DEXTROMETHORPHAN, DEXTROMETHORPHAN HYDROBROMIDE
PROMETHAZINE, PROMETHAZINE HYDROCHLORIDE
PROMETHEGAN, PROMETHAZINE HYDROCHLORIDE
PROMETRIUM, PROGESTERONE
PROMPT PHENYTOIN SODIUM, PHENYTOIN SODIUM, PROMPT
PRONESTYL, PROCAINAMIDE HYDROCHLORIDE
PRONESTYL-SR, PROCAINAMIDE HYDROCHLORIDE
PROPACET 100, ACETAMINOPHEN
PROPAFENONE HCL, PROPAFENONE HYDROCHLORIDE
PROPANTHELINE BROMIDE, PROPANTHELINE BROMIDE

APPENDIX A
PRODUCT NAME INDEX (*continued*)

PROPARACAINE HCL, PROPARACAINE
    HYDROCHLORIDE
PROPECIA, FINASTERIDE
PROPHENE 65, PROPOXYPHENE HYDROCHLORIDE
PROPINE, DIPIVEFRIN HYDROCHLORIDE
PROPOFOL, PROPOFOL
PROPOXYPHENE COMPOUND 65, ASPIRIN
PROPOXYPHENE COMPOUND-65, ASPIRIN
PROPOXYPHENE HCL 65, PROPOXYPHENE
    HYDROCHLORIDE
PROPOXYPHENE HCL AND ACETAMINOPHEN,
    ACETAMINOPHEN
PROPOXYPHENE HCL W/ ASPIRIN AND CAFFEINE,
    ASPIRIN
PROPOXYPHENE HCL, PROPOXYPHENE
    HYDROCHLORIDE
PROPOXYPHENE NAPSYLATE AND ACETAMINOPHEN,
    ACETAMINOPHEN
PROPRANOLOL HCL SULFITE FREE IN PLASTIC
    CONTAINER, AMINO ACIDS
PROSOM, ESTAZOLAM
PROSTAPHLIN, OXACILLIN SODIUM
PROSTEP, NICOTINE (OTC)
PROSTIN E2, DINOPROSTONE
PROSTIN F2 AI PHA, DINOPROST TROMETHAMINE
PROSTIN VR PEDIATRIC, ALPROSTADIL
PROTAMINE SULFATE, PROTAMINE SULFATE
PROTAMINE ZINC AND ILETIN II (PORK), INSULIN SUSP
    PROTAMINE ZINC PURIFIED PORK (OTC)
PROTAMINE ZINC AND ILETIN II, INSULIN SUSP
    PROTAMINE ZINC PURIFIED BEEF (OTC)
PROTAMINE ZINC INSULIN, INSULIN SUSP PROTAMINE
    ZINC PURIFIED BEEF (OTC)
PROTAMINE, ZINC 3, ACETAMINOPHEN
PROVENTIL, ALBUTEROL
PROVENTIL, ALBUTEROL SULFATE
PROVENTIL-HFA, ALBUTEROL SULFATE
PROVERA, MEDROXYPROGESTERONE ACETATE
PROVIGIL, MODAFINIL
PROVOCHOLINE, METHACHOLINE CHLORIDE
PROZAC WEEKLY, FLUOXETINE HYDROCHLORIDE
PROZAC, FLUOXETINE HYDROCHLORIDE
PSEUDO-12, PSEUDOEPHEDRINE POLISTIREX (OTC)
PSEUDOEPHEDRINE HCL AND CHLORPHENIRAMINE
    MALEATE, CHLORPHENIRAMINE MALEATE (OTC)
PSEUDOEPHEDRINE HCL AND TRIPROLIDINE HCL,
    PSEUDOEPHEDRINE HYDROCHLORIDE
PSEUDOEPHEDRINE HCL, PSEUDOEPHEDRINE
    HYDROCHLORIDE (OTC)
PSEUDOEPHEDRINE HCL/CHLORPHENIRAMINE
    MALEATE, CHLORPHENIRAMINE MALEATE (OTC)
PSORCON, DIFLORASONE DIACETATE
PULMICORT RESPULES, BUDESONIDE
PULMICORT, BUDESONIDE
PULMOLITE, TECHNETIUM TC-99M ALBUMIN
    AGGREGATED KIT
PURIFIED CORTROPHIN GEL, CORTICOTROPIN
PURINETHOL, MERCAPTOPURINE
PYLORI-CHEK BREATH TEST, UREA, C-13
PYOCIDIN, HYDROCORTISONE
PYOPEN, CARBENICILLIN DISODIUM
PYRAZINAMIDE, PYRAZINAMIDE
PYRIDAMAL 100, CHLORPHENIRAMINE MALEATE
PYRIDOSTIGMINE BROMIDE, PYRIDOSTIGMINE
    BROMIDE
PYRIDOXINE HCL, PYRIDOXINE HYDROCHLORIDE
PYRILAMINE MALEATE, PYRILAMINE MALEATE
PYROLITE, TECHNETIUM TC-99M PYRO/TRIMETA
    PHOSPHATES KIT

PYTEST KIT, UREA, C-14
PYTEST, UREA, C-14

Q

Q-GESIC, ASPIRIN
Q-PAM, DIAZEPAM
QUADRAMET, SAMARIUM SM 153 LEXIDRONAM
    PENTASODIUM
QUARZAN, CLIDINIUM BROMIDE
QUELICIN PRESERVATIVE FREE, SUCCINYLCHOLINE
    CHLORIDE
QUELICIN, SUCCINYLCHOLINE CHLORIDE
QUESTRAN LIGHT, CHOLESTYRAMINE
QUESTRAN, CHOLESTYRAMINE
QUIBRON-T, THEOPHYLLINE
QUIBRON-T/SR, THEOPHYLLINE
QUIDE, PIPERACETAZINE
QUINACT, QUINIDINE GLUCONATE
QUINAGLUTE, QUINIDINE GLUCONATE
QUINALAN, QUINIDINE GLUCONATE
QUINAPRIL HCL, QUINAPRIL HYDROCHLORIDE
QUINATIME, QUINIDINE GLUCONATE
QUINIDEX, QUINIDINE SULFATE
QUINIDINE GLUCONATE, QUINIDINE GLUCONATE
QUINIDINE SULFATE, QUINIDINE SULFATE
QUINORA, QUINIDINE SULFATE
QUIXIN, LEVOFLOXACIN
QVAR 40, BECLOMETHASONE DIPROPIONATE
QVAR 80, BECLOMETHASONE DIPROPIONATE

R

R-GENE 10, ARGININE HYDROCHLORIDE
R-P MYCIN, ERYTHROMYCIN
RADIO-IODINATED (I 125) SERUM ALBUMIN (HUMAN),
    ALBUMIN IODINATED I-125 SERUM
RADIOIODINATED SERUM ALBUMIN (HUMAN) IHSA I 125,
    ALBUMIN IODINATED I-125 SERUM
RADIONUCLIDE-LABELED (125 I) FIBRINOGEN (HUMAN)
    SENSOR, FIBRINOGEN, I-125
RANITIDINE HCL, RANITIDINE HYDROCHLORIDE
RANITIDINE, RANITIDINE HYDROCHLORIDE
RANITIDINE, RANITIDINE HYDROCHLORIDE (OTC)
RAPAMUNE, SIROLIMUS
RAPLON, RAPACURONIUM BROMIDE
RAU-SED, RESERPINE
RAUDIXIN, RAUWOLFIA SERPENTINA
RAUSERPIN, RAUWOLFIA SERPENTINA
RAUTENSIN, ALSEROXYLON
RAUVAL, RAUWOLFIA SERPENTINA
RAUWILOID, ALSEROXYLON
RAUWOLFIA SERPENTINA, RAUWOLFIA SERPENTINA
RAVOCAINE AND NOVOCAIN W/ LEVOPHED,
    NOREPINEPHRINE BITARTRATE
RAVOCAINE AND NOVOCAIN W/ NEO-COBEFRIN,
    LEVONORDEFRIN
RAXAR, GREPAFLOXACIN HYDROCHLORIDE
RBC-SCAN, TECHNETIUM TC-99M RED BLOOD CELL KIT
REBETOL, RIBAVIRIN
REDISOL, CYANOCOBALAMIN
REFLUDAN, LEPIRUDIN
REGITINE, PHENTOLAMINE MESYLATE
REGLAN, METOCLOPRAMIDE HYDROCHLORIDE
REGONOL, PYRIDOSTIGMINE BROMIDE
REGROTON, CHLORTHALIDONE
REGULAR ILETIN II (PORK), INSULIN PURIFIED PORK
    (OTC)

APPENDIX A
PRODUCT NAME INDEX (*continued*)

REGULAR ILETIN II, INSULIN PURIFIED BEEF (OTC)
REGULAR INSULIN, INSULIN PORK (OTC)
REGULAR PURIFIED PORK INSULIN, INSULIN PURIFIED
    PORK (OTC)
RELA, CARISOPRODOL
RELAFEN, NABUMETONE
RELENZA, ZANAMIVIR
RELPAX, ELETRIPTAN HYDROBROMIDE
REMERON SOLTAB, MIRTAZAPINE
REMERON, MIRTAZAPINE
REMINYL, GALANTAMINE HYDROBROMIDE
REMODULIN, TREPROSTINIL SODIUM
REMSED, PROMETHAZINE HYDROCHLORIDE
RENACIDIN, CITRIC ACID
RENAGEL, SEVELAMER HYDROCHLORIDE
RENAMIN W/O ELECTROLYTES, AMINO ACIDS
RENESE, POLYTHIAZIDE
RENESE-R, POLYTHIAZIDE
RENO-30, DIATRIZOATE MEGLUMINE
RENO-60, DIATRIZOATE MEGLUMINE
RENO-DIP, DIATRIZOATE MEGLUMINE
RENOCAL-76, DIATRIZOATE MEGLUMINE
RENOGRAFIN-60, DIATRIZOATE MEGLUMINE
RENOGRAFIN-76, DIATRIZOATE MEGLUMINE
RENOQUID, SULFACYTINE
RENORMAX, SPIRAPRIL HYDROCHLORIDE
RENOTEC, TECHNETIUM TC-99M FERPENTETATE KIT
RENOVA, TRETINOIN
RENOVIST II, DIATRIZOATE MEGLUMINE
RENOVIST, DIATRIZOATE MEGLUMINE
RENOVUE-65, IODAMIDE MEGLUMINE
RENOVUE-DIP, IODAMIDE MEGLUMINE
REPRONEX, MENOTROPINS (FSH;LH)
REQUIP, ROPINIROLE HYDROCHLORIDE
RESCRIPTOR, DELAVIRDINE MESYLATE
RESCULA, UNOPROSTONE ISOPROPYL
RESECTISOL IN PLASTIC CONTAINER, MANNITOL
RESECTISOL, MANNITOL
RESERPINE AND HYDROCHLOROTHIAZIDE,
    HYDROCHLOROTHIAZIDE
RESERPINE AND HYDROCHLOROTHIAZIDE-50,
    HYDROCHLOROTHIAZIDE
RESERPINE AND HYDROFLUMETHIAZIDE,
    HYDROFLUMETHIAZIDE
RESERPINE, HYDRALAZINE HCL AND
    HYDROCHLOROTHIAZIDE, HYDRALAZINE
    HYDROCHLORIDE
RESERPINE, HYDROCHLOROTHIAZIDE, AND
    HYDRALAZINE HCL, HYDRALAZINE
    HYDROCHLORIDE
RESERPINE, RESERPINE
RESPORAL, DEXBROMPHENIRAMINE MALEATE (OTC)
RESTASIS, CYCLOSPORINE
RESTORIL, TEMAZEPAM
RETET, TETRACYCLINE HYDROCHLORIDE
RETIN-A MICRO, TRETINOIN
RETIN-A, TRETINOIN
RETROVIR, ZIDOVUDINE
REV-EYES, DAPIPRAZOLE HYDROCHLORIDE
REVERSOL, EDROPHONIUM CHLORIDE
REVEX, NALMEFENE HYDROCHLORIDE
REVIA, NALTREXONE HYDROCHLORIDE
REYATAZ, ATAZANAVIR SULFATE
REZIPAS, AMINOSALICYLIC ACID RESIN COMPLEX
REZULIN, TROGLITAZONE
RHINOCORT, BUDESONIDE
RID MOUSSE, PIPERONYL BUTOXIDE (OTC)
RIDAURA, AURANOFIN
RIFADIN, RIFAMPIN

RIFAMATE, ISONIAZID
RIFAMPIN, RIFAMPIN
RIFATER, ISONIAZID
RILUTEK, RILUZOLE
RILUZOLE, RILUZOLE
RIMACTANE, RIFAMPIN
RIMADYL, CARPROFEN
RIMANTADINE HCL, RIMANTADINE HYDROCHLORIDE
RIMIFON, ISONIAZID
RIMSO-50, DIMETHYL SULFOXIDE
RINGER'S IN PLASTIC CONTAINER, CALCIUM CHLORIDE
RISPERDAL, RISPERIDONE
RITALIN LA, METHYLPHENIDATE HYDROCHLORIDE
RITALIN, METHYLPHENIDATE HYDROCHLORIDE
RITALIN-SR, METHYLPHENIDATE HYDROCHLORIDE
RITODRINE HCL IN DEXTROSE 5% IN PLASTIC
    CONTAINER, RITODRINE HYDROCHLORIDE
RITODRINE HCL, RITODRINE HYDROCHLORIDE
ROBAXIN, METHOCARBAMOL
ROBAXIN-750, METHOCARBAMOL
ROBAXISAL, ASPIRIN
ROBENGATOPE, ROSE BENGAL SODIUM, I-131
ROBIMYCIN, ERYTHROMYCIN
ROBINUL FORTE, GLYCOPYRROLATE
ROBINUL, GLYCOPYRROLATE
ROBITET, TETRACYCLINE HYDROCHLORIDE
ROCALTROL, CALCITRIOL
ROCEPHIN KIT, CEFTRIAXONE SODIUM
ROCEPHIN W/ DEXTROSE IN PLASTIC CONTAINER,
    CEFTRIAXONE SODIUM
ROCEPHIN, CEFTRIAXONE SODIUM
ROGAINE (FOR MEN), MINOXIDIL (OTC)
ROGAINE (FOR WOMEN), MINOXIDIL (OTC)
ROGAINE EXTRA STRENGTH (FOR MEN), MINOXIDIL
    (OTC)
ROMAZICON, FLUMAZENIL
RONDOMYCIN, METHACYCLINE HYDROCHLORIDE
ROWASA, MESALAMINE
ROXICET 5/500, ACETAMINOPHEN
ROXICET, ACETAMINOPHEN
ROXICODONE, OXYCODONE HYDROCHLORIDE
ROXILOX, ACETAMINOPHEN
ROXIPRIN, ASPIRIN
RUBEX, DOXORUBICIN HYDROCHLORIDE
RUBIVITE, CYANOCOBALAMIN
RUBRAMIN PC, CYANOCOBALAMIN
RUBRATOPE-57 KIT, COBALT CHLORIDE, CO-57
RUBRATOPE-57, CYANOCOBALAMIN, CO-57
RUBRATOPE-60 KIT, COBALT CHLORIDE, CO-60
RUBRATOPE-60, CYANOCOBALAMIN, CO-60
RUFEN, IBUPROFEN
RUVITE, CYANOCOBALAMIN
RYTHMOL, PROPAFENONE HYDROCHLORIDE

S

S.A.S.-500, SULFASALAZINE
SAIZEN, SOMATROPIN RECOMBINANT
SALAGEN, PILOCARPINE HYDROCHLORIDE
SALPIX, ACETRIZOATE SODIUM
SALURON, HYDROFLUMETHIAZIDE
SALUTENSIN, HYDROFLUMETHIAZIDE
SALUTENSIN-DEMI, HYDROFLUMETHIAZIDE
SANDIMMUNE, CYCLOSPORINE
SANDOSTATIN LAR, OCTREOTIDE ACETATE
SANDOSTATIN, OCTREOTIDE ACETATE
SANDRIL, RESERPINE
SANOREX, MAZINDOL
SANSAC, ERYTHROMYCIN

APPENDIX A
PRODUCT NAME INDEX (*continued*)

SANSERT, METHYSERGIDE MALEATE
SARAFEM, FLUOXETINE HYDROCHLORIDE
SARENIN, SARALASIN ACETATE
SARISOL NO. 1, BUTABARBITAL SODIUM
SARISOL NO. 2, BUTABARBITAL SODIUM
SARISOL, BUTABARBITAL SODIUM
SATRIC, METRONIDAZOLE
SCABENE, LINDANE
SCANDONEST L, LEVONORDEFRIN
SCANDONEST PLAIN, MEPIVACAINE HYDROCHLORIDE
SCLEROSOL, TALC
SCRUBTEAM SURGICAL SPONGEBRUSH,
    HEXACHLOROPHENE
SECOBARBITAL SODIUM, SECOBARBITAL SODIUM
SECONAL SODIUM, SECOBARBITAL SODIUM
SECREFLO, SECRETIN
SECRETIN-FERRING, SECRETIN
SECTRAL, ACEBUTOLOL HYDROCHLORIDE
SEDAPAP, ACETAMINOPHEN
SEFFIN, CEPHALOTHIN SODIUM
SELEGILINE HCL, SELEGILINE HYDROCHLORIDE
SELENIUM SULFIDE, SELENIUM SULFIDE
SELENOMETHIONINE SE 75, SELENOMETHIONINE, SE-
    75
SELSUN, SELENIUM SULFIDE
SEMILENTE INSULIN, INSULIN ZINC SUSP PROMPT
    BEEF (OTC)
SEMILENTE, INSULIN ZINC SUSP PROMPT PURIFIED
    PORK (OTC)
SEMPREX-D, ACRIVASTINE
SENSORCAINE, BUPIVACAINE HYDROCHLORIDE
SEPTI-SOFT, HEXACHLOROPHENE
SEPTISOL, HEXACHLOROPHENE
SEPTOCAINE, ARTICAINE HYDROCHLORIDE
SEPTRA DS, SULFAMETHOXAZOLE
SEPTRA GRAPE, SULFAMETHOXAZOLE
SEPTRA, SULFAMETHOXAZOLE
SER-A-GEN, HYDRALAZINE HYDROCHLORIDE
SER-AP-ES, HYDRALAZINE HYDROCHLORIDE
SERAX, OXAZEPAM
SERENTIL, MESORIDAZINE BESYLATE
SEREVENT, SALMETEROL XINAFOATE
SEROMYCIN, CYCLOSERINE
SEROPHENE, CLOMIPHENE CITRATE
SEROQUEL, QUETIAPINE FUMARATE
SEROSTIM, SOMATROPIN RECOMBINANT
SERPALAN, RESERPINE
SERPANRAY, RESERPINE
SERPASIL, RESERPINE
SERPASIL-APRESOLINE, HYDRALAZINE
    HYDROCHLORIDE
SERPASIL-ESIDRIX #1, HYDROCHLOROTHIAZIDE
SERPASIL-ESIDRIX #2, HYDROCHLOROTHIAZIDE
SERPATE, RESERPINE
SERPIVITE, RESERPINE
SERVISONE, PREDNISONE
SERZONE, NEFAZODONE HYDROCHLORIDE
SETHOTOPE, SELENOMETHIONINE, SE-75
SEVOFLURANE, SEVOFLURANE
SHADE UVAGUARD, AVOBENZONE (OTC)
SILDAFLO, SILVER SULFADIAZINE
SILPHEN, DIPHENHYDRAMINE HYDROCHLORIDE (OTC)
SILVADENE, SILVER SULFADIAZINE
SINE-AID IB, IBUPROFEN (OTC)
SINEMET CR, CARBIDOPA
SINEMET, CARBIDOPA
SINEQUAN, DOXEPIN HYDROCHLORIDE
SINGULAIR, MONTELUKAST SODIUM
SINOGRAFIN, DIATRIZOATE MEGLUMINE

SKELAXIN, METAXALONE
SKELID, TILUDRONATE DISODIUM
SKIN EXPOSURE REDUCTION PASTE AGAINST
    CHEMICAL WARFARE AGENTS,
    PERFLUOROPOLYMETHYLISOPROPYL ETHER
SLO-BID, THEOPHYLLINE
SLO-PHYLLIN, THEOPHYLLINE
SLOW-K, POTASSIUM CHLORIDE
SODIUM ACETATE IN PLASTIC CONTAINER, SODIUM
    ACETATE, ANHYDROUS
SODIUM AMINOSALICYLATE, AMINOSALICYLATE
    SODIUM
SODIUM BICARBONATE IN PLASTIC CONTAINER,
    SODIUM BICARBONATE
SODIUM BUTABARBITAL, BUTABARBITAL SODIUM
SODIUM CHLORIDE 0.45% IN PLASTIC CONTAINER,
    SODIUM CHLORIDE
SODIUM CHLORIDE 0.9% AND POTASSIUM CHLORIDE
    0.075% IN PLASTIC CONTAINER, POTASSIUM
    CHLORIDE
SODIUM CHLORIDE 0.9% AND POTASSIUM CHLORIDE
    0.15% IN PLASTIC CONTAINER, POTASSIUM
    CHLORIDE
SODIUM CHLORIDE 0.9% AND POTASSIUM CHLORIDE
    0.22% IN PLASTIC CONTAINER, POTASSIUM
    CHLORIDE
SODIUM CHLORIDE 0.9% AND POTASSIUM CHLORIDE
    0.224%, POTASSIUM CHLORIDE
SODIUM CHLORIDE 0.9% AND POTASSIUM CHLORIDE
    0.3% IN PLASTIC CONTAINER, POTASSIUM
    CHLORIDE
SODIUM CHLORIDE 0.9% IN PLASTIC CONTAINER,
    SODIUM CHLORIDE
SODIUM CHLORIDE 0.9% IN STERILE PLASTIC
    CONTAINER, SODIUM CHLORIDE
SODIUM CHLORIDE 23.4% IN PLASTIC CONTAINER,
    SODIUM CHLORIDE
SODIUM CHLORIDE 3% IN PLASTIC CONTAINER,
    SODIUM CHLORIDE
SODIUM CHLORIDE 5% IN PLASTIC CONTAINER,
    SODIUM CHLORIDE
SODIUM CHLORIDE IN PLASTIC CONTAINER, SODIUM
    CHLORIDE
SODIUM CHLORIDE, SODIUM CHLORIDE
SODIUM CHROMATE CR 51, SODIUM CHROMATE, CR-51
SODIUM HEPARIN, HEPARIN SODIUM
SODIUM IODIDE I 123, SODIUM IODIDE, I-123
SODIUM IODIDE I 131, KIT, SODIUM IODIDE, I-131
SODIUM IODIDE I 131, SODIUM IODIDE, I-131
SODIUM LACTATE 0.167 MOLAR IN PLASTIC
    CONTAINER, SODIUM LACTATE
SODIUM LACTATE 1/6 MOLAR IN PLASTIC CONTAINER,
    SODIUM LACTATE
SODIUM LACTATE IN PLASTIC CONTAINER, SODIUM
    LACTATE
SODIUM NITROPRUSSIDE, SODIUM NITROPRUSSIDE
SODIUM P.A.S., AMINOSALICYLATE SODIUM
SODIUM PENTOBARBITAL, PENTOBARBITAL SODIUM
SODIUM PERTECHNETATE TC 99M, TECHNETIUM TC-
    99M SODIUM PERTECHNETATE
SODIUM PHOSPHATE P 32, SODIUM PHOSPHATE, P-32
SODIUM PHOSPHATES IN PLASTIC CONTAINER,
    SODIUM PHOSPHATE, DIBASIC, HEPTAHYDRATE
SODIUM POLYPHOSPHATE-TIN KIT, TECHNETIUM TC-
    99M POLYPHOSPHATE KIT
SODIUM POLYSTYRENE SULFONATE, SODIUM
    POLYSTYRENE SULFONATE
SODIUM ROSE BENGAL I 131, ROSE BENGAL SODIUM, I-
    131

APPENDIX A
PRODUCT NAME INDEX (continued)

SODIUM SECOBARBITAL, SECOBARBITAL SODIUM
SODIUM SUCCINATE, SODIUM SUCCINATE
SODIUM SULAMYD, SULFACETAMIDE SODIUM
SODIUM SULFACETAMIDE, SULFACETAMIDE SODIUM
SODIUM THIOSULFATE, SODIUM THIOSULFATE
SODIUM VERSENATE, EDETATE DISODIUM
SOLAGE, MEQUINOL
SOLARAZE, DICLOFENAC SODIUM
SOLATENE, BETA-CAROTENE
SOLU-CORTEF, HYDROCORTISONE SODIUM
    SUCCINATE
SOLU-MEDROL, METHYLPREDNISOLONE SODIUM
    SUCCINATE
SOMA COMPOUND W/ CODEINE, ASPIRIN
SOMA COMPOUND, ASPIRIN
SOMA, CARISOPRODOL
SOMAVERT, PEGVISOMANT
SOMOPHYLLIN, AMINOPHYLLINE
SOMOPHYLLIN-CRT, THEOPHYLLINE
SOMOPHYLLIN-DF, AMINOPHYLLINE
SOMOPHYLLIN-T, THEOPHYLLINE
SONATA, ZALEPLON
SONAZINE, CHLORPROMAZINE HYDROCHLORIDE
SONORX, SIMETHICONE-CELLULOSE
SORBITOL 3% IN PLASTIC CONTAINER, SORBITOL
SORBITOL 3.3% IN PLASTIC CONTAINER, SORBITOL
SORBITOL-MANNITOL IN PLASTIC CONTAINER,
    MANNITOL
SORBITOL-MANNITOL, MANNITOL
SORBITRATE, ISOSORBIDE DINITRATE
SORIATANE, ACITRETIN
SORINE, SOTALOL HYDROCHLORIDE
SOSOL, SULFISOXAZOLE
SOTALOL HCL, SOTALOL HYDROCHLORIDE
SOTRADECOL, SODIUM TETRADECYL SULFATE
SOTRET, ISOTRETINOIN
SOXAZOLE, SULFISOXAZOLE
SOY-DOME, HEXACHLOROPHENE
SOYACAL 10%, SOYBEAN OIL
SOYACAL 20%, SOYBEAN OIL
SPARINE, PROMAZINE HYDROCHLORIDE
SPECTAMINE, IOFETAMINE HYDROCHLORIDE I-123
SPECTAZOLE, ECONAZOLE NITRATE
SPECTRACEF, CEFDITOREN PIVOXIL
SPECTROBID, BACAMPICILLIN HYDROCHLORIDE
SPIRONOLACTONE + HYDROCHLOROTHIAZIDE,
    HYDROCHLOROTHIAZIDE
SPIRONOLACTONE AND HYDROCHLOROTHIAZIDE,
    HYDROCHLOROTHIAZIDE
SPIRONOLACTONE W/ HYDROCHLOROTHIAZIDE,
    HYDROCHLOROTHIAZIDE
SPIRONOLACTONE, SPIRONOLACTONE
SPIRONOLACTONE/HYDROCHLOROTHIAZIDE,
    HYDROCHLOROTHIAZIDE
SPORANOX, ITRACONAZOLE
SPRINTEC, ETHINYL ESTRADIOL
SPRX-3, PHENDIMETRAZINE TARTRATE
SPRX-105, PHENDIMETRAZINE TARTRATE
SPS, SODIUM POLYSTYRENE SULFONATE
SSD AF, SILVER SULFADIAZINE
SSD, SILVER SULFADIAZINE
STADOL PRESERVATIVE FREE, BUTORPHANOL
    TARTRATE
STADOL, BUTORPHANOL TARTRATE
STALEVO 50, CARBIDOPA
STALEVO 100, CARBIDOPA
STALEVO 150, CARBIDOPA
STANOZIDE, ISONIAZID
STAPHCILLIN, METHICILLIN SODIUM

STARLIX, NATEGLINIDE
STATICIN, ERYTHROMYCIN
STATOBEX, PHENDIMETRAZINE TARTRATE
STATOBEX-G, PHENDIMETRAZINE TARTRATE
STATROL, NEOMYCIN SULFATE
STELAZINE, TRIFLUOPERAZINE HYDROCHLORIDE
STERANE, PREDNISOLONE
STERANE, PREDNISOLONE ACETATE
STERI-STAT, CHLORHEXIDINE GLUCONATE (OTC)
STERILE UREA, UREA
STERILE WATER FOR INJECTION IN PLASTIC
    CONTAINER, WATER FOR INJECTION, STERILE
STERILE WATER IN PLASTIC CONTAINER, WATER FOR
    IRRIGATION, STERILE
STERILE WATER, WATER FOR IRRIGATION, STERILE
STIE-CORT, HYDROCORTISONE
STILBESTROL, DIETHYLSTILBESTROL
STILBETIN, DIETHYLSTILBESTROL
STILPHOSTROL, DIETHYLSTILBESTROL DIPHOSPHATE
STIMATE, DESMOPRESSIN ACETATE
STOXIL, IDOXURIDINE
STRATTERA, ATOMOXETINE HYDROCHLORIDE
STREPTOMYCIN SULFATE, STREPTOMYCIN SULFATE
STRIANT, TESTOSTERONE
STRIFON FORTE DSC, CHLORZOXAZONE
STROMECTOL, IVERMECTIN
STRONTIUM CHLORIDE SR-89, STRONTIUM CHLORIDE,
    SR-89
SUBLIMAZE PRESERVATIVE FREE, FENTANYL CITRATE
SUBOXONE, BUPRENORPHINE HYDROCHLORIDE
SUBUTEX, BUPRENORPHINE HYDROCHLORIDE
SUCCINYLCHOLINE CHLORIDE, SUCCINYLCHOLINE
    CHLORIDE
SUCOSTRIN, SUCCINYLCHOLINE CHLORIDE
SUCRAID, SACROSIDASE
SUCRALFATE, SUCRALFATE
SUDAFED 12 HOUR, PSEUDOEPHEDRINE
    HYDROCHLORIDE (OTC)
SUFENTA, SUFENTANIL CITRATE
SUFENTANIL CITRATE, SUFENTANIL CITRATE
SULAR, NISOLDIPINE
SULF-10, SULFACETAMIDE SODIUM
SULF-15, SULFACETAMIDE SODIUM
SULFA-TRIPLE #2, TRISULFAPYRIMIDINES
    (SULFADIAZINE; SULFAMERAZINE;
    SULFAMETHAZINE)
SULFABID, SULFAPHENAZOLE
SULFACEL-15, SULFACETAMIDE SODIUM
SULFACETAMIDE SODIUM AND PREDNISOLONE
    SODIUM PHOSPHATE, PREDNISOLONE SODIUM
    PHOSPHATE
SULFACETAMIDE SODIUM, SULFACETAMIDE SODIUM
SULFADIAZINE SODIUM, SULFADIAZINE SODIUM
SULFADIAZINE, TRISULFAPYRIMIDINES (SULFADIAZINE;
    SULFAMERAZINE; SULFAMETHAZINE)
SULFAIR 10, SULFACETAMIDE SODIUM
SULFAIR FORTE, SULFACETAMIDE SODIUM
SULFAIR-15, SULFACETAMIDE SODIUM
SULFALAR, SULFISOXAZOLE
SULFALOID, TRISULFAPYRIMIDINES (SULFADIAZINE;
    SULFAMERAZINE; SULFAMETHAZINE)
SULFAMETHOPRIM, SULFAMETHOXAZOLE
SULFAMETHOPRIM-DS, SULFAMETHOXAZOLE
SULFAMETHOXAZOLE AND TRIMETHOPRIM AND
    PENAZOPYRIDINE HCL, PHENAZOPYRIDINE
    HYDROCHLORIDE
SULFAMETHOXAZOLE AND TRIMETHOPRIM DOUBLE
    STRENGTH, SULFAMETHOXAZOLE

APPENDIX A
PRODUCT NAME INDEX (*continued*)

SULFAMETHOXAZOLE AND TRIMETHOPRIM SINGLE STRENGTH, SULFAMETHOXAZOLE
SULFAMETHOXAZOLE AND TRIMETHOPRIM, SULFAMETHOXAZOLE
SULFAMETHOXAZOLE, SULFAMETHOXAZOLE
SULFAMYLON, MAFENIDE ACETATE
SULFANILAMIDE, SULFANILAMIDE
SULFAPYRIDINE, SULFAPYRIDINE
SULFASALAZINE, SULFASALAZINE
SULFATRIM PEDIATRIC, SULFAMETHOXAZOLE
SULFATRIM, SULFAMETHOXAZOLE
SULFATRIM-DS, SULFAMETHOXAZOLE
SULFATRIM-SS, SULFAMETHOXAZOLE
SULFENTANIL CITRATE, SUFENTANIL CITRATE
SULFINPYRAZONE, SULFINPYRAZONE
SULFISOXAZOLE DIOLAMINE, SULFISOXAZOLE DIOLAMINE
SULFISOXAZOLE, SULFISOXAZOLE
SULFONAMIDES DUPLEX, TRISULFAPYRIMIDINES (SULFADIAZINE; SULFAMERAZINE; SULFAMETHAZINE)
SULFOSE, TRISULFAPYRIMIDINES (SULFADIAZINE; SULFAMERAZINE; SULFAMETHAZINE)
SULINDAC, SULINDAC
SULLA, SULFAMETER
SULMEPRIM PEDIATRIC, SULFAMETHOXAZOLE
SULMEPRIM, SULFAMETHOXAZOLE
SULPHRIN, PREDNISOLONE ACETATE
SULSOXIN, SULFISOXAZOLE
SULSTER, PREDNISOLONE SODIUM PHOSPHATE
SULTEN-10, SULFACETAMIDE SODIUM
SULTRIN, TRIPLE SULFA (SULFABENZAMIDE; SULFACETAMIDE; SULFATHIAZOLE)
SUMYCIN, TETRACYCLINE HYDROCHLORIDE
SUPPRELIN, HISTRELIN ACETATE
SUPRANE, DESFLURANE
SUPRAX, CEFIXIME
SURITAL, THIAMYLAL SODIUM
SURMONTIL, TRIMIPRAMINE MALEATE
SURVANTA, BERACTANT
SUS-PHRINE SULFITE-FREE, EPINEPHRINE
SUSTAIRE, THEOPHYLLINE
SUSTIVA, EFAVIRENZ
SYMADINE, AMANTADINE HYDROCHLORIDE
SYMMETREL, AMANTADINE HYDROCHLORIDE
SYNACORT, HYDROCORTISONE
SYNALAR, FLUOCINOLONE ACETONIDE
SYNALAR-HP, FLUOCINOLONE ACETONIDE
SYNALGOS-DC, ASPIRIN
SYNALGOS-DC-A, ACETAMINOPHEN
SYNAREL, NAFARELIN ACETATE
SYNCURINE, DECAMETHONIUM BROMIDE
SYNERCID, DALFOPRISTIN
SYNKAYVITE, MENADIOL SODIUM DIPHOSPHATE
SYNOPHYLATE, THEOPHYLLINE SODIUM GLYCINATE
SYNOVALYTE IN PLASTIC CONTAINER, MAGNESIUM CHLORIDE
SYNTHROID, LIOTRIX (T4;T3)
SYNTOCINON, OXYTOCIN
SYPRINE, TRIENTINE HYDROCHLORIDE

T

T-PHYL, THEOPHYLLINE
T-STAT, ERYTHROMYCIN
TAB-PROFEN, IBUPROFEN (OTC)
TACARYL, METHDILAZINE
TACARYL, METHDILAZINE HYDROCHLORIDE
TACE, CHLOROTRIANISENE

TAGAMET HB 200, CIMETIDINE (OTC)
TAGAMET HB, CIMETIDINE (OTC)
TAGAMET HCL IN SODIUM CHLORIDE 0.9% IN PLASTIC CONTAINER, CIMETIDINE HYDROCHLORIDE
TAGAMET, CIMETIDINE
TAGAMET, CIMETIDINE HYDROCHLORIDE
TALACEN, ACETAMINOPHEN
TALWIN 50, PENTAZOCINE HYDROCHLORIDE
TALWIN COMPOUND, ASPIRIN
TALWIN NX, NALOXONE HYDROCHLORIDE
TALWIN, PENTAZOCINE LACTATE
TAMBOCOR, FLECAINIDE ACETATE
TAMIFLU, OSELTAMIVIR PHOSPHATE
TAMOXIFEN CITRATE, TAMOXIFEN CITRATE
TANDEARIL, OXYPHENBUTAZONE
TAO, TROLEANDOMYCIN
TAPAZOLE, METHIMAZOLE
TARACTAN, CHLORPROTHIXENE
TARGRETIN, BEXAROTENE
TARKA, TRANDOLAPRIL
TASMAR, TOLCAPONE
TATUM-T, COPPER
TAVIST ALLERGY/SINUS/HEADACHE, ACETAMINOPHEN (OTC)
TAVIST D, CLEMASTINE FUMARATE
TAVIST, CLEMASTINE FUMARATE
TAVIST-1, CLEMASTINE FUMARATE
TAVIST-1, CLEMASTINE FUMARATE (OTC)
TAVIST-D, CLEMASTINE FUMARATE (OTC)
TAXOL, PACLITAXEL
TAXOTERE, DOCETAXEL
TAZICEF, CEFTAZIDIME
TAZIDIME IN PLASTIC CONTAINER, CEFTAZIDIME
TAZIDIME, CEFTAZIDIME
TAZORAC, TAZAROTENE
TAZTIA XT, DILTIAZEM HYDROCHLORIDE
TC 99M-LUNGAGGREGATE, TECHNETIUM TC-99M ALBUMIN AGGREGATED
TECHNECOLL, TECHNETIUM TC-99M SULFUR COLLOID KIT
TECHNELITE, TECHNETIUM TC-99M SODIUM PERTECHNETATE GENERATOR
TECHNESCAN GLUCEPTATE, TECHNETIUM TC-99M GLUCEPTATE KIT
TECHNESCAN HDP, TECHNETIUM TC-99M OXIDRONATE KIT
TECHNESCAN HIDA, TECHNETIUM TC-99M LIDOFENIN KIT
TECHNESCAN MAA, TECHNETIUM TC-99M ALBUMIN AGGREGATED KIT
TECHNESCAN MAG3, TECHNETIUM TC-99M MERTIATIDE KIT
TECHNESCAN MDP KIT, TECHNETIUM TC-99M MEDRONATE KIT
TECHNESCAN PYP KIT, TECHNETIUM TC-99M PYROPHOSPHATE KIT
TECHNETIUM TC 99M ALBUMIN AGGREGATED KIT, TECHNETIUM TC-99M ALBUMIN AGGREGATED KIT
TECHNETIUM TC 99M DIPHOSPHONATE-TIN KIT, TECHNETIUM TC-99M ETIDRONATE KIT
TECHNETIUM TC 99M GENERATOR, TECHNETIUM TC-99M SODIUM PERTECHNETATE GENERATOR
TECHNETIUM TC 99M HSA, TECHNETIUM TC-99M ALBUMIN KIT
TECHNETIUM TC 99M MAA, TECHNETIUM TC-99M ALBUMIN AGGREGATED KIT
TECHNETIUM TC 99M MPI MDP, TECHNETIUM TC-99M MEDRONATE KIT

APPENDIX A
PRODUCT NAME INDEX (continued)

TECHNETIUM TC 99M SULFUR COLLOID, TECHNETIUM TC-99M SULFUR COLLOID
TECHNETIUM TC 99M TSC, TECHNETIUM TC-99M SULFUR COLLOID KIT
TECHNETIUM TC-99M PENTETATE KIT, TECHNETIUM TC-99M PENTETATE KIT
TECZEM, DILTIAZEM MALATE
TEEBACIN, AMINOSALICYLATE SODIUM
TEGISON, ETRETINATE
TEGOPEN, CLOXACILLIN SODIUM
TEGRETOL, CARBAMAZEPINE
TEGRETOL-XR, CARBAMAZEPINE
TELDRIN, CHLORPHENIRAMINE MALEATE (OTC)
TELEPAQUE, IOPANOIC ACID
TEMARIL, TRIMEPRAZINE TARTRATE
TEMAZ, TEMAZEPAM
TEMAZEPAM, TEMAZEPAM
TEMODAR, TEMOZOLOMIDE
TEMOVATE E, CLOBETASOL PROPIONATE
TEMOVATE, CLOBETASOL PROPIONATE
TEN-K, POTASSIUM CHLORIDE
TENATHAN, BETHANIDINE SULFATE
TENCON, ACETAMINOPHEN
TENEX, GUANFACINE HYDROCHLORIDE
TENORETIC 50, ATENOLOL
TENORETIC 100, ATENOLOL
TENORMIN, ATENOLOL
TENSILON PRESERVATIVE FREE, EDROPHONIUM CHLORIDE
TENSILON, EDROPHONIUM CHLORIDE
TENUATE DOSPAN, DIETHYLPROPION HYDROCHLORIDE
TENUATE, DIETHYLPROPION HYDROCHLORIDE
TEPANIL TEN-TAB, DIETHYLPROPION HYDROCHLORIDE
TEPANIL, DIETHYLPROPION HYDROCHLORIDE
TEQUIN, GATIFLOXACIN
TERAZOL 3, TERCONAZOLE
TERAZOL 7, TERCONAZOLE
TERAZOSIN HCL, TERAZOSIN HYDROCHLORIDE
TERBUTALINE SULFATE, TERBUTALINE SULFATE
TERFONYL, TRISULFAPYRIMIDINES (SULFADIAZINE; SULFAMERAZINE; SULFAMETHAZINE)
TERRA-CORTRIL, HYDROCORTISONE ACETATE
TERRAMYCIN W/ POLYMYXIN B SULFATE, OXYTETRACYCLINE HYDROCHLORIDE
TERRAMYCIN W/ POLYMYXIN, OXYTETRACYCLINE HYDROCHLORIDE
TERRAMYCIN, LIDOCAINE HYDROCHLORIDE
TERRAMYCIN, OXYTETRACYCLINE
TERRAMYCIN, OXYTETRACYCLINE CALCIUM
TERRAMYCIN, OXYTETRACYCLINE HYDROCHLORIDE
TERRAMYCIN-POLYMYXIN, OXYTETRACYCLINE HYDROCHLORIDE
TESLAC, TESTOLACTONE
TESLASCAN, MANGAFODIPIR TRISODIUM
TESSALON, BENZONATATE
TESTIM, TESTOSTERONE
TESTODERM TTS, TESTOSTERONE
TESTODERM, TESTOSTERONE
TESTOSTERONE CYPIONATE, TESTOSTERONE CYPIONATE
TESTOSTERONE CYPIONATE-ESTRADIOL CYPIONATE, ESTRADIOL CYPIONATE
TESTOSTERONE ENANTHATE AND ESTRADIOL VALERATE, ESTRADIOL VALERATE
TESTOSTERONE ENANTHATE, TESTOSTERONE ENANTHATE
TESTOSTERONE PROPIONATE, TESTOSTERONE PROPIONATE

TESTOSTERONE, TESTOSTERONE
TESTRED, METHYLTESTOSTERONE
TESULOID, TECHNETIUM TC-99M SULFUR COLLOID KIT
TETRACHEL, TETRACYCLINE HYDROCHLORIDE
TETRACYCLINE HCL, TETRACYCLINE HYDROCHLORIDE
TETRACYN, PROCAINE HYDROCHLORIDE
TETRACYN, TETRACYCLINE HYDROCHLORIDE
TETRAMED, TETRACYCLINE HYDROCHLORIDE
TETREX, TETRACYCLINE PHOSPHATE COMPLEX
TEV-TROPIN, SOMATROPIN RECOMBINANT
TEVETEN HCT, EPROSARTAN MESYLATE
TEVETEN, EPROSARTAN MESYLATE
TEXACORT, HYDROCORTISONE
THALITONE, CHLORTHALIDONE
THALLOUS CHLORIDE TL 201, THALLOUS CHLORIDE, TL-201
THALOMID, THALIDOMIDE
THAM, TROMETHAMINE
THAM-E, POTASSIUM CHLORIDE
THEELIN, ESTRONE
THEO-24, THEOPHYLLINE
THEO-DUR, THEOPHYLLINE
THEOBID JR., THEOPHYLLINE
THEOBID, THEOPHYLLINE
THEOCHRON, THEOPHYLLINE
THEOCLEAR L.A.-130, THEOPHYLLINE
THEOCLEAR L.A.-260, THEOPHYLLINE
THEOCLEAR-80, THEOPHYLLINE
THEOCLEAR-100, THEOPHYLLINE
THEOCLEAR-200, THEOPHYLLINE
THEOLAIR, THEOPHYLLINE
THEOLAIR-SR, THEOPHYLLINE
THEOLIXIR, THEOPHYLLINE
THEOPHYL, THEOPHYLLINE
THEOPHYL-225, THEOPHYLLINE
THEOPHYL-SR, THEOPHYLLINE
THEOPHYLLINE 0.04% AND DEXTROSE 5% IN PLASTIC CONTAINER, THEOPHYLLINE
THEOPHYLLINE 0.08% AND DEXTROSE 5% IN PLASTIC CONTAINER, THEOPHYLLINE
THEOPHYLLINE 0.16% AND DEXTROSE 5% IN PLASTIC CONTAINER, THEOPHYLLINE
THEOPHYLLINE 0.2% AND DEXTROSE 5% IN PLASTIC CONTAINER, THEOPHYLLINE
THEOPHYLLINE 0.32% AND DEXTROSE 5% IN PLASTIC CONTAINER, THEOPHYLLINE
THEOPHYLLINE 0.4% AND DEXTROSE 5% IN PLASTIC CONTAINER, THEOPHYLLINE
THEOPHYLLINE AND DEXTROSE 5% IN PLASTIC CONTAINER, THEOPHYLLINE
THEOPHYLLINE IN DEXTROSE 5% IN PLASTIC CONTAINER, THEOPHYLLINE
THEOPHYLLINE, THEOPHYLLINE
THEOPHYLLINE-SR, THEOPHYLLINE
THEOVENT, THEOPHYLLINE
THERMAZENE, SILVER SULFADIAZINE
THIAMINE HCL, THIAMINE HYDROCHLORIDE
THIOGUANINE, THIOGUANINE
THIOPLEX, THIOTEPA
THIORIDAZINE HCL INTENSOL, THIORIDAZINE HYDROCHLORIDE
THIORIDAZINE HCL, THIORIDAZINE HYDROCHLORIDE
THIOSULFIL, SULFAMETHIZOLE
THIOTEPA, THIOTEPA
THIOTHIXENE HCL INTENSOL, THIOTHIXENE HYDROCHLORIDE
THIOTHIXENE HCL, THIOTHIXENE HYDROCHLORIDE
THIOTHIXENE, THIOTHIXENE
THORAZINE, CHLORPROMAZINE

APPENDIX A
PRODUCT NAME INDEX (*continued*)

THORAZINE, CHLORPROMAZINE HYDROCHLORIDE
THYPINONE, PROTIRELIN
THYREL TRH, PROTIRELIN
THYRO-BLOCK, POTASSIUM IODIDE (OTC)
THYRO-TABS, LIOTRIX (T4;T3)
THYROGEN, THYROTROPIN ALFA
THYROGLOBULIN, THYROGLOBULIN
THYROLAR-0.25, LIOTRIX (T4;T3)
THYROLAR-0.5, LIOTRIX (T4;T3)
THYROLAR-1, LIOTRIX (T4;T3)
THYROLAR-2, LIOTRIX (T4;T3)
THYROLAR-3, LIOTRIX (T4;T3)
THYROLAR-5, LIOTRIX (T4;T3)
THYROSAFE, POTASSIUM IODIDE (OTC)
THYTROPAR, THYROTROPIN
TIAMATE, DILTIAZEM MALATE
TIAZAC, DILTIAZEM HYDROCHLORIDE
TICAR, TICARCILLIN DISODIUM
TICLID, TICLOPIDINE HYDROCHLORIDE
TICLOPIDINE HCL, TICLOPIDINE HYDROCHLORIDE
TIGAN, TRIMETHOBENZAMIDE HYDROCHLORIDE
TIKOSYN, DOFETILIDE
TILADE, NEDOCROMIL SODIUM
TIMENTIN IN PLASTIC CONTAINER, CLAVULANATE
    POTASSIUM
TIMENTIN, CLAVULANATE POTASSIUM
TIMOLIDE 10-25, HYDROCHLOROTHIAZIDE
TIMOLOL MALEATE, TIMOLOL MALEATE
TIMOPTIC IN OCUDOSE, TIMOLOL MALEATE
TIMOPTIC, TIMOLOL MALEATE
TIMOPTIC-XE, TIMOLOL MALEATE
TINDAL, ACETOPHENAZINE MALEATE
TIOCONAZOLE, TIOCONAZOLE (OTC)
TIOPRONIN, TIOPRONIN
TIS-U-SOL IN PLASTIC CONTAINER, MAGNESIUM
    SULFATE
TIS-U-SOL, MAGNESIUM SULFATE
TIZANIDINE HCL, TIZANIDINE HYDROCHLORIDE
TOBI, TOBRAMYCIN
TOBRADEX, DEXAMETHASONE
TOBRAMYCIN (PHARMACY BULK), TOBRAMYCIN
    SULFATE
TOBRAMYCIN AND DEXAMETHASONE,
    DEXAMETHASONE
TOBRAMYCIN SULFATE IN SODIUM CHLORIDE 0.9% IN
    PLASTIC CONTAINER, TOBRAMYCIN SULFATE
TOBRAMYCIN SULFATE, TOBRAMYCIN SULFATE
TOBRAMYCIN, TOBRAMYCIN
TOBRAMYCIN, TOBRAMYCIN SULFATE
TOBRASONE, FLUOROMETHOLONE ACETATE
TOBREX, TOBRAMYCIN
TODAY, NONOXYNOL-9 (OTC)
TOFRANIL, IMIPRAMINE HYDROCHLORIDE
TOFRANIL-PM, IMIPRAMINE PAMOATE
TOLAZAMIDE, TOLAZAMIDE
TOLBUTAMIDE, TOLBUTAMIDE
TOLECTIN 600, TOLMETIN SODIUM
TOLECTIN DS, TOLMETIN SODIUM
TOLECTIN, TOLMETIN SODIUM
TOLINASE, TOLAZAMIDE
TOLMETIN SODIUM, TOLMETIN SODIUM
TONOCARD, TOCAINIDE HYDROCHLORIDE
TOPAMAX SPRINKLE, TOPIRAMATE
TOPAMAX, TOPIRAMATE
TOPICORT LP, DESOXIMETASONE
TOPICORT, DESOXIMETASONE
TOPICYCLINE, TETRACYCLINE HYDROCHLORIDE
TOPOSAR, ETOPOSIDE
TOPROL-XL, METOPROLOL SUCCINATE

TORA, PHENTERMINE HYDROCHLORIDE
TORADOL, KETOROLAC TROMETHAMINE
TORECAN, THIETHYLPERAZINE MALATE
TORECAN, THIETHYLPERAZINE MALEATE
TORNALATE, BITOLTEROL MESYLATE
TORSEMIDE, TORSEMIDE
TOTACILLIN, AMPICILLIN/AMPICILLIN TRIHYDRATE
TOTACILLIN-N, AMPICILLIN SODIUM
TPN ELECTROLYTES IN PLASTIC CONTAINER, CALCIUM
    CHLORIDE
TPN SUSPENSION, NIACINAMIDE
TRACLEER, BOSENTAN
TRACRIUM PRESERVATIVE FREE, ATRACURIUM
    BESYLATE
TRACRIUM, ATRACURIUM BESYLATE
TRAL, HEXOCYCLIUM METHYLSULFATE
TRAMADOL HCL, TRAMADOL HYDROCHLORIDE
TRANCOPAL, CHLORMEZANONE
TRANDATE HCT, HYDROCHLOROTHIAZIDE
TRANDATE, LABETALOL HYDROCHLORIDE
TRANMEP, MEPROBAMATE
TRANSDERM SCOP, SCOPOLAMINE
TRANSDERM-NITRO, NITROGLYCERIN
TRANXENE SD, CLORAZEPATE DIPOTASSIUM
TRANXENE, CLORAZEPATE DIPOTASSIUM
TRASICOR, OXPRENOLOL HYDROCHLORIDE
TRASYLOL, APROTININ BOVINE
TRAVAMULSION 10%, SOYBEAN OIL
TRAVAMULSION 20%, SOYBEAN OIL
TRAVASE, SUTILAINS
TRAVASOL 10% IN PLASTIC CONTAINER, AMINO ACIDS
TRAVASOL 10% W/O ELECTROLYTES, AMINO ACIDS
TRAVASOL 2.75% IN DEXTROSE 10% IN PLASTIC
    CONTAINER, AMINO ACIDS
TRAVASOL 2.75% IN DEXTROSE 15% IN PLASTIC
    CONTAINER, AMINO ACIDS
TRAVASOL 2.75% IN DEXTROSE 20% IN PLASTIC
    CONTAINER, AMINO ACIDS
TRAVASOL 2.75% IN DEXTROSE 25% IN PLASTIC
    CONTAINER, AMINO ACIDS
TRAVASOL 2.75% IN DEXTROSE 5% IN PLASTIC
    CONTAINER, AMINO ACIDS
TRAVASOL 2.75% SULFITE FREE W/ ELECTROLYTES IN
    DEXTROSE 10% IN PLASTIC CONTAINER, AMINO
    ACIDS
TRAVASOL 2.75% SULFITE FREE W/ ELECTROLYTES IN
    DEXTROSE 15% IN PLASTIC CONTAINER, AMINO
    ACIDS
TRAVASOL 2.75% SULFITE FREE W/ ELECTROLYTES IN
    DEXTROSE 20% IN PLASTIC CONTAINER, AMINO
    ACIDS
TRAVASOL 2.75% SULFITE FREE W/ ELECTROLYTES IN
    DEXTROSE 25% IN PLASTIC CONTAINER, AMINO
    ACIDS
TRAVASOL 2.75% SULFITE FREE W/ ELECTROLYTES IN
    DEXTROSE 5% IN PLASTIC CONTAINER, AMINO
    ACIDS
TRAVASOL 3.5% SULFITE FREE W/ ELECTROLYTES IN
    PLASTIC CONTAINER, AMINO ACIDS
TRAVASOL 3.5% W/ ELECTROLYTES, AMINO ACIDS
TRAVASOL 4.25% IN DEXTROSE 10% IN PLASTIC
    CONTAINER, AMINO ACIDS
TRAVASOL 4.25% IN DEXTROSE 15% IN PLASTIC
    CONTAINER, AMINO ACIDS
TRAVASOL 4.25% IN DEXTROSE 20% IN PLASTIC
    CONTAINER, AMINO ACIDS
TRAVASOL 4.25% IN DEXTROSE 25% IN PLASTIC
    CONTAINER, AMINO ACIDS

APPENDIX A
PRODUCT NAME INDEX (*continued*)

TRAVASOL 4.25% IN DEXTROSE 5% IN PLASTIC CONTAINER, AMINO ACIDS
TRAVASOL 4.25% SULFITE FREE W/ ELECTROLYTES IN DEXTROSE 10% IN PLASTIC CONTAINER, AMINO ACIDS
TRAVASOL 4.25% SULFITE FREE W/ ELECTROLYTES IN DEXTROSE 15% IN PLASTIC CONTAINER, AMINO ACIDS
TRAVASOL 4.25% SULFITE FREE W/ ELECTROLYTES IN DEXTROSE 20% IN PLASTIC CONTAINER, AMINO ACIDS
TRAVASOL 4.25% SULFITE FREE W/ ELECTROLYTES IN DEXTROSE 25% IN PLASTIC CONTAINER, AMINO ACIDS
TRAVASOL 4.25% SULFITE FREE W/ ELECTROLYTES IN DEXTROSE 5% IN PLASTIC CONTAINER, AMINO ACIDS
TRAVASOL 5.5% IN PLASTIC CONTAINER, AMINO ACIDS
TRAVASOL 5.5% SULFITE FREE W/ ELECTROLYTES IN PLASTIC CONTAINER, AMINO ACIDS
TRAVASOL 5.5% W/ ELECTROLYTES, AMINO ACIDS
TRAVASOL 5.5% W/O ELECTROLYTES, AMINO ACIDS
TRAVASOL 8.5% IN PLASTIC CONTAINER, AMINO ACIDS
TRAVASOL 8.5% SULFITE FREE W/ ELECTROLYTES IN PLASTIC CONTAINER, AMINO ACIDS
TRAVASOL 8.5% W/ ELECTROLYTES, AMINO ACIDS
TRAVASOL 8.5% W/O ELECTROLYTES, AMINO ACIDS
TRAVATAN, TRAVOPROST
TRAVERT 10% IN PLASTIC CONTAINER, INVERT SUGAR
TRAZODONE HCL, TRAZODONE HYDROCHLORIDE
TRECATOR-SC, ETHIONAMIDE
TRELSTAR DEPOT, TRIPTORELIN PAMOATE
TRELSTAR, TRIPTORELIN PAMOATE
TREMIN, TRIHEXYPHENIDYL HYDROCHLORIDE
TRENTAL, PENTOXIFYLLINE
TREST, METHIXENE HYDROCHLORIDE
TRETINOIN, TRETINOIN
TREXALL, METHOTREXATE SODIUM
TRI-LUMA, FLUOCINOLONE ACETONIDE
TRI-NASAL, TRIAMCINOLONE ACETONIDE
TRI-NORINYL 21-DAY, ETHINYL ESTRADIOL
TRI-NORINYL 28-DAY, ETHINYL ESTRADIOL
TRI-SPRINTEC, ETHINYL ESTRADIOL
TRIACET, TRIAMCINOLONE ACETONIDE
TRIACIN-C, CODEINE PHOSPHATE
TRIACORT, TRIAMCINOLONE ACETONIDE
TRIAD, ACETAMINOPHEN
TRIALODINE, TRAZODONE HYDROCHLORIDE
TRIAMCINOLONE ACETONIDE IN ABSORBASE, TRIAMCINOLONE ACETONIDE
TRIAMCINOLONE ACETONIDE, TRIAMCINOLONE ACETONIDE
TRIAMCINOLONE DIACETATE, TRIAMCINOLONE DIACETATE
TRIAMCINOLONE, TRIAMCINOLONE
TRIAMINIC-12, CHLORPHENIRAMINE MALEATE (OTC)
TRIAMTERENE AND HYDROCHLOROTHIAZIDE, HYDROCHLOROTHIAZIDE
TRIAPRIN, ACETAMINOPHEN
TRIATEX, TRIAMCINOLONE ACETONIDE
TRIAVIL 2-10, AMITRIPTYLINE HYDROCHLORIDE
TRIAVIL 2-25, AMITRIPTYLINE HYDROCHLORIDE
TRIAVIL 4-10, AMITRIPTYLINE HYDROCHLORIDE
TRIAVIL 4-25, AMITRIPTYLINE HYDROCHLORIDE
TRIAVIL 4-50, AMITRIPTYLINE HYDROCHLORIDE
TRIAZOLAM, TRIAZOLAM
TRICHLOREX, TRICHLORMETHIAZIDE
TRICHLORMAS, TRICHLORMETHIAZIDE
TRICHLORMETHIAZIDE W/ RESERPINE, RESERPINE

TRICHLORMETHIAZIDE, TRICHLORMETHIAZIDE
TRICLOS, TRICLOFOS SODIUM
TRICOR (MICRONIZED), FENOFIBRATE
TRICOR, FENOFIBRATE
TRIDERM, TRIAMCINOLONE ACETONIDE
TRIDESILON, ACETIC ACID, GLACIAL
TRIDESILON, DESONIDE
TRIDIL, NITROGLYCERIN
TRIDIONE, TRIMETHADIONE
TRIFLUOPERAZINE HCL, TRIFLUOPERAZINE HYDROCHLORIDE
TRIFLURIDINE, TRIFLURIDINE
TRIHEXYPHENIDYL HCL, TRIHEXYPHENIDYL HYDROCHLORIDE
TRILAFON, PERPHENAZINE
TRILEPTAL, OXCARBAZEPINE
TRILITRON, PSEUDOEPHEDRINE HYDROCHLORIDE
TRIMEPRAZINE TARTRATE, TRIMEPRAZINE TARTRATE
TRIMETH/SULFA, SULFAMETHOXAZOLE
TRIMETHOBENZAMIDE HCL, TRIMETHOBENZAMIDE HYDROCHLORIDE
TRIMETHOPRIM SULFATE AND POLYMYXIN B SULFATE, POLYMYXIN B SULFATE
TRIMETHOPRIM, TRIMETHOPRIM
TRIMIPRAMINE MALEATE, TRIMIPRAMINE MALEATE
TRIMOX, AMOXICILLIN
TRIMPEX 200, TRIMETHOPRIM
TRIMPEX, TRIMETHOPRIM
TRINALIN, AZATADINE MALEATE
TRIOSTAT, LIOTRIX (T4;T3)
TRIPELENNAMINE HCL, TRIPELENNAMINE HYDROCHLORIDE
TRIPHASIL-21, ETHINYL ESTRADIOL
TRIPHASIL-28, ETHINYL ESTRADIOL
TRIPHED, PSEUDOEPHEDRINE HYDROCHLORIDE
TRIPLE SULFA, TRIPLE SULFA (SULFABENZAMIDE; SULFACETAMIDE; SULFATHIAZOLE)
TRIPLE SULFA, TRISULFAPYRIMIDINES (SULFADIAZINE; SULFAMERAZINE; SULFAMETHAZINE)
TRIPLE SULFAS, TRISULFAPYRIMIDINES (SULFADIAZINE; SULFAMERAZINE; SULFAMETHAZINE)
TRIPLE SULFOID, TRISULFAPYRIMIDINES (SULFADIAZINE; SULFAMERAZINE; SULFAMETHAZINE)
TRIPROLIDINE AND PSEUDOEPHEDRINE HYDROCHLORIDES W/ CODEINE, CODEINE PHOSPHATE
TRIPROLIDINE AND PSEUDOEPHEDRINE HYDROCHLORIDES, PSEUDOEPHEDRINE HYDROCHLORIDE (OTC)
TRIPROLIDINE AND PSEUDOEPHEDRINE, PSEUDOEPHEDRINE HYDROCHLORIDE
TRIPROLIDINE AND PSEUDOEPHEDRINE, PSEUDOEPHEDRINE HYDROCHLORIDE (OTC)
TRIPROLIDINE HCL AND PSEUDOEPHEDRINE HCL, PSEUDOEPHEDRINE HYDROCHLORIDE
TRIPROLIDINE HCL, PSEUDOEPHEDRINE HCL AND CODEINE PHOSPHATE, CODEINE PHOSPHATE
TRIPROLIDINE HCL, TRIPROLIDINE HYDROCHLORIDE
TRISENOX, ARSENIC TRIOXIDE
TRISORALEN, TRIOXSALEN
TRITEC, RANITIDINE BISMUTH CITRATE
TRIVAGIZOLE 3, CLOTRIMAZOLE (OTC)
TRIVORA-21, ETHINYL ESTRADIOL
TRIVORA-28, ETHINYL ESTRADIOL
TRIZIVIR, ABACAVIR SULFATE
TROBICIN, SPECTINOMYCIN HYDROCHLORIDE
TROPHAMINE 10%, AMINO ACIDS

APPENDIX A
PRODUCT NAME INDEX (*continued*)

TROPHAMINE, AMINO ACIDS
TROPICACYL, TROPICAMIDE
TROPICAMIDE, TROPICAMIDE
TROVAN PRESERVATIVE FREE, ALATROFLOXACIN
    MESYLATE
TROVAN, TROVAFLOXACIN MESYLATE
TROVAN/ZITHROMAX COMPLIANCE PAK,
    AZITHROMYCIN DIHYDRATE
TRUPHYLLINE, AMINOPHYLLINE
TRUSOPT, DORZOLAMIDE HYDROCHLORIDE
TRYMEX, TRIAMCINOLONE ACETONIDE
TRYSUL, TRIPLE SULFA (SULFABENZAMIDE;
    SULFACETAMIDE; SULFATHIAZOLE)
TUBOCURARINE CHLORIDE, TUBOCURARINE
    CHLORIDE
TURGEX, HEXACHLOROPHENE
TUSSIGON, HOMATROPINE METHYLBROMIDE
TUSSIONEX, CHLORPHENIRAMINE POLISTIREX
TWINJECT, EPINEPHRINE
TYCOLET, ACETAMINOPHEN
TYLENOL (CAPLET), ACETAMINOPHEN (OTC)
TYLENOL (GELTAB), ACETAMINOPHEN (OTC)
TYLENOL W/ CODEINE NO. 1, ACETAMINOPHEN
TYLENOL W/ CODEINE NO. 2, ACETAMINOPHEN
TYLENOL W/ CODEINE NO. 3, ACETAMINOPHEN
TYLENOL W/ CODEINE NO. 4, ACETAMINOPHEN
TYLENOL W/ CODEINE, ACETAMINOPHEN
TYLENOL, ACETAMINOPHEN (OTC)
TYLOX, ACETAMINOPHEN
TYLOX-325, ACETAMINOPHEN
TYMTRAN, CERULETIDE DIETHYLAMINE
TYZINE, TETRAHYDROZOLINE HYDROCHLORIDE
TZ-3, TIOCONAZOLE (OTC)

U

U-CORT, HYDROCORTISONE ACETATE
U-GENCIN, GENTAMICIN SULFATE
UCEPHAN, SODIUM BENZOATE
ULO, CHLOPHEDIANOL HYDROCHLORIDE
ULTANE, SEVOFLURANE
ULTIVA, REMIFENTANIL HYDROCHLORIDE
ULTRA-TECHNEKOW FM, TECHNETIUM TC-99M SODIUM
    PERTECHNETATE GENERATOR
ULTRACEF, CEFADROXIL/CEFADROXIL HEMIHYDRATE
ULTRACET, ACETAMINOPHEN
ULTRAGRIS-165, GRISEOFULVIN,
    ULTRAMICROCRYSTALLINE
ULTRAGRIS-330, GRISEOFULVIN,
    ULTRAMICROCRYSTALLINE
ULTRALENTE INSULIN, INSULIN ZINC SUSP EXTENDED
    BEEF (OTC)
ULTRALENTE, INSULIN ZINC SUSP EXTENDED PURIFIED
    BEEF (OTC)
ULTRAM, TRAMADOL HYDROCHLORIDE
ULTRATAG, TECHNETIUM TC-99M RED BLOOD CELL KIT
ULTRAVATE, HALOBETASOL PROPIONATE
ULTRAVIST (PHARMACY BULK), IOPROMIDE
ULTRAVIST 150, IOPROMIDE
ULTRAVIST 240, IOPROMIDE
ULTRAVIST 300, IOPROMIDE
ULTRAVIST 370, IOPROMIDE
UNASYN, AMPICILLIN SODIUM
UNI-DUR, THEOPHYLLINE
UNIPEN IN PLASTIC CONTAINER, NAFCILLIN SODIUM
UNIPEN, NAFCILLIN SODIUM
UNIPHYL, THEOPHYLLINE
UNIPRES, HYDRALAZINE HYDROCHLORIDE
UNIRETIC, HYDROCHLOROTHIAZIDE

UNISOM, DOXYLAMINE SUCCINATE (OTC)
UNITENSEN, CRYPTENAMINE ACETATES
UNITENSEN, CRYPTENAMINE TANNATES
UNITHROID, LIOTRIX (T4;T3)
UNIVASC, MOEXIPRIL HYDROCHLORIDE
URACIL MUSTARD, URACIL MUSTARD
UREAPHIL, UREA
URECHOLINE, BETHANECHOL CHLORIDE
URESE, BENZTHIAZIDE
UREX, METHENAMINE HIPPURATE
URISPAS, FLAVOXATE HYDROCHLORIDE
UROBAK, SULFAMETHOXAZOLE
UROLOGIC G IN PLASTIC CONTAINER, CITRIC ACID
UROPLUS DS, SULFAMETHOXAZOLE
UROPLUS SS, SULFAMETHOXAZOLE
UROVIST CYSTO PEDIATRIC, DIATRIZOATE MEGLUMINE
UROVIST CYSTO, DIATRIZOATE MEGLUMINE
UROVIST MEGLUMINE DIU/CT, DIATRIZOATE
    MEGLUMINE
UROVIST SODIUM 300, DIATRIZOATE SODIUM
UROXATRAL, ALFUZOSIN HYDROCHLORIDE
URSO, URSODIOL
URSODIOL, URSODIOL
UTICILLIN VK, PENICILLIN V POTASSIUM
UTICORT, BETAMETHASONE BENZOATE
UTIMOX, AMOXICILLIN
UVADEX, METHOXSALEN

V

V-CILLIN K, PENICILLIN V POTASSIUM
V-CILLIN, PENICILLIN V
VAGIFEM, ESTRADIOL
VAGILIA, TRIPLE SULFA
    (SULFABENZAMIDE;SULFACETAMIDE;
    SULFATHIAZOLE)
VAGISTAT-1, TIOCONAZOLE (OTC)
VALCYTE, VALGANCICLOVIR HYDROCHLORIDE
VALISONE, BETAMETHASONE VALERATE
VALIUM, DIAZEPAM
VALMID, ETHINAMATE
VALNAC, BETAMETHASONE VALERATE
VALPIN 50, ANISOTROPINE METHYLBROMIDE
VALPROATE SODIUM, VALPROATE SODIUM
VALPROIC ACID, VALPROIC ACID
VALRELEASE, DIAZEPAM
VALSTAR PRESERVATIVE FREE, VALRUBICIN
VALTREX, VALACYCLOVIR HYDROCHLORIDE
VANCENASE AQ, BECLOMETHASONE DIPROPIONATE
    MONOHYDRATE
VANCENASE, BECLOMETHASONE DIPROPIONATE
VANCERIL DOUBLE STRENGTH, BECLOMETHASONE
    DIPROPIONATE
VANCERIL, BECLOMETHASONE DIPROPIONATE
VANCOCIN HCL IN PLASTIC CONTAINER, VANCOMYCIN
    HYDROCHLORIDE
VANCOCIN HCL, VANCOMYCIN HYDROCHLORIDE
VANCOLED, VANCOMYCIN HYDROCHLORIDE
VANCOMYCIN HCL, VANCOMYCIN HYDROCHLORIDE
VANCOR, VANCOMYCIN HYDROCHLORIDE
VANIQA, EFLORNITHINE HYDROCHLORIDE
VANOBID, CANDICIDIN
VANSIL, OXAMNIQUINE
VANTIN, CEFPODOXIME PROXETIL
VAPO-ISO, ISOPROTERENOL HYDROCHLORIDE
VASCOR, BEPRIDIL HYDROCHLORIDE
VASCORAY, IOTHALAMATE MEGLUMINE
VASERETIC, ENALAPRIL MALEATE
VASOCIDIN, PREDNISOLONE ACETATE

APPENDIX A
PRODUCT NAME INDEX (*continued*)

VASOCIDIN, PREDNISOLONE SODIUM PHOSPHATE
VASOCON, NAPHAZOLINE HYDROCHLORIDE
VASOCON-A, ANTAZOLINE PHOSPHATE (OTC)
VASOTEC, ENALAPRIL MALEATE
VASOTEC, ENALAPRILAT
VASOXYL, METHOXAMINE HYDROCHLORIDE
VECTRIN, MINOCYCLINE HYDROCHLORIDE
VECURONIUM BROMIDE, VECURONIUM BROMIDE
VEETIDS '125', PENICILLIN V POTASSIUM
VEETIDS '250', PENICILLIN V POTASSIUM
VEETIDS '500', PENICILLIN V POTASSIUM
VEETIDS, PENICILLIN V POTASSIUM
VEINAMINE 8%, AMINO ACIDS
VELBAN, VINBLASTINE SULFATE
VELCADE, BORTEZOMIB
VELOSEF '125', CEPHRADINE
VELOSEF '250', CEPHRADINE
VELOSEF '500', CEPHRADINE
VELOSEF, CEPHRADINE
VELOSULIN BR HUMAN, INSULIN RECOMBINANT
    PURIFIED HUMAN (OTC)
VELOSULIN BR, INSULIN RECOMBINANT HUMAN (OTC)
VELOSULIN, INSULIN PURIFIED PORK (OTC)
VENOFER, IRON SUCROSE
VENTAIRE, PROTOKYLOL HYDROCHLORIDE
VENTOLIN HFA, ALBUTEROL SULFATE
VENTOLIN ROTACAPS, ALBUTEROL SULFATE
VENTOLIN, ALBUTEROL
VENTOLIN, ALBUTEROL SULFATE
VEPESID, ETOPOSIDE
VERAPAMIL HCL, VERAPAMIL HYDROCHLORIDE
VERCYTE, PIPOBROMAN
VERELAN PM, VERAPAMIL HYDROCHLORIDE
VERELAN, VERAPAMIL HYDROCHLORIDE
VERILOID, ALKAVERVIR
VERMIDOL, PIPERAZINE CITRATE
VERMOX, MEBENDAZOLE
VERSAPEN, HETACILLIN
VERSAPEN-K, HETACILLIN POTASSIUM
VERSED, MIDAZOLAM HYDROCHLORIDE
VERTAVIS, VERATRUM VIRIDE
VESANOID, TRETINOIN
VESPRIN, TRIFLUPROMAZINE
VESPRIN, TRIFLUPROMAZINE HYDROCHLORIDE
VEXOL, RIMEXOLONE
VFEND, VORICONAZOLE
VI-DOM-A, VITAMIN A PALMITATE
VI-TWEL, CYANOCOBALAMIN
VIADUR, LEUPROLIDE ACETATE
VIAGRA, SILDENAFIL CITRATE
VIBISONE, CYANOCOBALAMIN
VIBRA-TABS, DOXYCYCLINE HYCLATE
VIBRAMYCIN, DOXYCYCLINE
VIBRAMYCIN, DOXYCYCLINE CALCIUM
VIBRAMYCIN, DOXYCYCLINE HYCLATE
VICKS FORMULA 44, DIPHENHYDRAMINE
    HYDROCHLORIDE (OTC)
VICODIN ES, ACETAMINOPHEN
VICODIN HP, ACETAMINOPHEN
VICODIN, ACETAMINOPHEN
VICOPRIN, ASPIRIN
VICOPROFEN, HYDROCODONE BITARTRATE
VIDEX EC, DIDANOSINE
VIDEX, DIDANOSINE
VIGAMOX, MOXIFLOXACIN HYDROCHLORIDE
VINBLASTINE SULFATE, VINBLASTINE SULFATE
VINCASAR PFS, VINCRISTINE SULFATE
VINCREX, VINCRISTINE SULFATE
VINCRISTINE SULFATE PFS, VINCRISTINE SULFATE

VINCRISTINE SULFATE, VINCRISTINE SULFATE
VINORELBINE TARTRATE, VINORELBINE TARTRATE
VIOCIN SULFATE, VIOMYCIN SULFATE
VIOXX, ROFECOXIB
VIRA-A, VIDARABINE
VIRAC REX, UNDECOYLIUM CHLORIDE
VIRACEPT, NELFINAVIR MESYLATE
VIRAMUNE, NEVIRAPINE
VIRAZOLE, RIBAVIRIN
VIREAD, TENOFOVIR DISOPROXIL FUMARATE
VIRILON, METHYLTESTOSTERONE
VIROPTIC, TRIFLURIDINE
VISICOL, SODIUM PHOSPHATE, DIBASIC, ANHYDROUS
VISINE L.R., OXYMETAZOLINE HYDROCHLORIDE (OTC)
VISINE-A, NAPHAZOLINE HYDROCHLORIDE (OTC)
VISIPAQUE 270, IODIXANOL
VISIPAQUE 320, IODIXANOL
VISKAZIDE, HYDROCHLOROTHIAZIDE
VISKEN, PINDOLOL
VISTARIL, HYDROXYZINE HYDROCHLORIDE
VISTARIL, HYDROXYZINE PAMOATE
VISTIDE, CIDOFOVIR
VISUDYNE, VERTEPORFIN
VITAMIN A PALMITATE, VITAMIN A PALMITATE
VITAMIN A SOLUBILIZED, VITAMIN A PALMITATE
VITAMIN A, VITAMIN A
VITAMIN A, VITAMIN A PALMITATE
VITAMIN D, ERGOCALCIFEROL
VITAMIN K1, PHYTONADIONE
VITAPED, ASCORBIC ACID
VITRASERT, GANCICLOVIR
VITRAVENE PRESERVATIVE FREE, FOMIVIRSEN
    SODIUM
VIVACTIL, PROTRIPTYLINE HYDROCHLORIDE
VIVELLE, ESTRADIOL
VIVELLE-DOT, ESTRADIOL
VOLMAX, ALBUTEROL SULFATE
VOLTAREN, DICLOFENAC SODIUM
VOLTAREN-XR, DICLOFENAC SODIUM
VONTROL, DIPHENIDOL HYDROCHLORIDE
VOSOL HC, ACETIC ACID, GLACIAL
VOSOL, ACETIC ACID, GLACIAL
VUMON, TENIPOSIDE

W

WAMPOCAP, NIACIN
WARFARIN SODIUM, WARFARIN SODIUM
WELCHOL, COLESEVELAM HYDROCHLORIDE
WELLBUTRIN SR, BUPROPION HYDROCHLORIDE
WELLBUTRIN, BUPROPION HYDROCHLORIDE
WELLCOVORIN, LEUCOVORIN CALCIUM
WESTADONE, METHADONE HYDROCHLORIDE
WESTCORT, HYDROCORTISONE VALERATE
WIGRAINE, CAFFEINE
WIGRETTES, ERGOTAMINE TARTRATE
WINSTROL, STANOZOLOL
WOLFINA, RAUWOLFIA SERPENTINA
WYAMINE SULFATE, MEPHENTERMINE SULFATE
WYAMYCIN E, ERYTHROMYCIN ETHYLSUCCINATE
WYAMYCIN S, ERYTHROMYCIN STEARATE
WYCILLIN, PENICILLIN G PROCAINE
WYDASE, HYALURONIDASE
WYGESIC, ACETAMINOPHEN
WYMOX, AMOXICILLIN
WYTENSIN, GUANABENZ ACETATE

APPENDIX A
PRODUCT NAME INDEX (*continued*)

X

X-TROZINE L.A., PHENDIMETRAZINE TARTRATE
X-TROZINE, PHENDIMETRAZINE TARTRATE
XALATAN, LATANOPROST
XANAX XR, ALPRAZOLAM
XANAX, ALPRAZOLAM
XELODA, CAPECITABINE
XENEISOL, XENON, XE-133
XENICAL, ORLISTAT
XENON XE 127, XENON, XE-127
XENON XE 133, XENON, XE-133
XENON XE 133-V.S.S., XENON, XE-133
XOPENEX, LEVALBUTEROL HYDROCHLORIDE
XYLO-PFAN, XYLOSE
XYLOCAINE 1.5% W/ DEXTROSE 7.5%, LIDOCAINE
    HYDROCHLORIDE
XYLOCAINE 4% PRESERVATIVE FREE, LIDOCAINE
    HYDROCHLORIDE
XYLOCAINE 5% W/ GLUCOSE 7.5%, LIDOCAINE
    HYDROCHLORIDE
XYLOCAINE PRESERVATIVE FREE, LIDOCAINE
    HYDROCHLORIDE
XYLOCAINE VISCOUS, LIDOCAINE HYDROCHLORIDE
XYLOCAINE W/ EPINEPHRINE, EPINEPHRINE
XYLOCAINE, LIDOCAINE
XYLOCAINE, LIDOCAINE HYDROCHLORIDE
XYLOSE, XYLOSE
XYREM, SODIUM OXYBATE

Y

YASMIN, DROSPIRENONE
YTTERBIUM YB 169 DTPA, PENTETATE CALCIUM
    TRISODIUM YB-169
YUTOPAR, RITODRINE HYDROCHLORIDE

Z

ZADITOR, KETOTIFEN FUMARATE
ZAGAM, SPARFLOXACIN
ZANAFLEX, TIZANIDINE HYDROCHLORIDE
ZANOSAR, STREPTOZOCIN
ZANTAC 150, RANITIDINE HYDROCHLORIDE
ZANTAC 300, RANITIDINE HYDROCHLORIDE
ZANTAC 75, RANITIDINE HYDROCHLORIDE (OTC)
ZANTAC IN PLASTIC CONTAINER, RANITIDINE
    HYDROCHLORIDE
ZANTAC, RANITIDINE HYDROCHLORIDE
ZARONTIN, ETHOSUXIMIDE
ZAROXOLYN, METOLAZONE
ZAXOPAM, OXAZEPAM
ZEBETA, BISOPROLOL FUMARATE
ZEFAZONE IN PLASTIC CONTAINER, CEFMETAZOLE
    SODIUM
ZEFAZONE, CEFMETAZOLE SODIUM

ZELNORM, TEGASEROD MALEATE
ZEMPLAR, PARICALCITOL
ZEMURON (P/F), ROCURONIUM BROMIDE
ZEMURON, ROCURONIUM BROMIDE
ZERIT XR, STAVUDINE
ZERIT, STAVUDINE
ZESTORETIC, HYDROCHLOROTHIAZIDE
ZESTRIL, LISINOPRIL
ZETIA, EZETIMIBE
ZIAC, BISOPROLOL FUMARATE
ZIAGEN, ABACAVIR SULFATE
ZIBA-RX, BACITRACIN ZINC
ZIDE, HYDROCHLOROTHIAZIDE
ZINACEF IN PLASTIC CONTAINER, CEFUROXIME
    SODIUM
ZINACEF, CEFUROXIME SODIUM
ZINC BACITRACIN,NEOMYCIN SULFATE,POLYMYXIN B
    SULFATE & HYDROCORTISONE, BACITRACIN ZINC
ZINC CHLORIDE IN PLASTIC CONTAINER, ZINC
    CHLORIDE
ZINC SULFATE, ZINC SULFATE
ZINECARD, DEXRAZOXANE HYDROCHLORIDE
ZIPAN-25, PROMETHAZINE HYDROCHLORIDE
ZIPAN-50, PROMETHAZINE HYDROCHLORIDE
ZITHROMAX, AZITHROMYCIN DIHYDRATE
ZOCOR, SIMVASTATIN
ZOFRAN IN PLASTIC CONTAINER, ONDANSETRON
    HYDROCHLORIDE
ZOFRAN ODT, ONDANSETRON
ZOFRAN PRESERVATIVE FREE, ONDANSETRON
    HYDROCHLORIDE
ZOFRAN, ONDANSETRON HYDROCHLORIDE
ZOLADEX, GOSERELIN ACETATE
ZOLOFT, SERTRALINE HYDROCHLORIDE
ZOLYSE, CHYMOTRYPSIN
ZOMETA, ZOLEDRONIC ACID
ZOMIG, ZOLMITRIPTAN
ZOMIG-ZMT, ZOLMITRIPTAN
ZONALON, DOXEPIN HYDROCHLORIDE
ZONEGRAN, ZONISAMIDE
ZOSYN IN PLASTIC CONTAINER, PIPERACILLIN SODIUM
ZOSYN, PIPERACILLIN SODIUM
ZOVIA 1/35E-21, ETHINYL ESTRADIOL
ZOVIA 1/35E-28, ETHINYL ESTRADIOL
ZOVIA 1/50E-21, ETHINYL ESTRADIOL
ZOVIA 1/50E-28, ETHINYL ESTRADIOL
ZOVIRAX, ACYCLOVIR
ZOVIRAX, ACYCLOVIR SODIUM
ZYBAN, BUPROPION HYDROCHLORIDE
ZYFLO, ZILEUTON
ZYLOPRIM, ALLOPURINOL
ZYMAR, GATIFLOXACIN
ZYPREXA ZYDIS, OLANZAPINE
ZYPREXA, OLANZAPINE
ZYRTEC, CETIRIZINE HYDROCHLORIDE
ZYRTEC-D 12 HOUR, CETIRIZINE HYDROCHLORIDE
ZYVOX, LINEZOLID

APPENDIX B
PRODUCT NAME INDEX
LISTED BY APPLICANT

3

3M
3M CO
   SCRUBTEAM SURGICAL SPONGEBRUSH,
      HEXACHLOROPHENE
3M HEALTH CARE INC
   AVAGARD, ALCOHOL (OTC)
3M MEDICAL PRODUCTS DIV
   INSTANT MICROSPHERES, TECHNETIUM TC-99M
      ALBUMIN MICROSPHERES KIT
   YTTERBIUM YB 169 DTPA, PENTETATE CALCIUM
      TRISODIUM YB-169
3M PHARMACEUTICALS INC
   ALDARA, IMIQUIMOD
   CALCIUM DISODIUM VERSENATE, EDETATE CALCIUM
      DISODIUM
   CIRCANOL, ERGOLOID MESYLATES
   DISIPAL, ORPHENADRINE HYDROCHLORIDE
   DUO-MEDIHALER, ISOPROTERENOL HYDROCHLORIDE
   ISOPROTERENOL HCL, ISOPROTERENOL
      HYDROCHLORIDE
   LIPO-HEPIN, HEPARIN SODIUM
   MAXAIR, PIRBUTEROL ACETATE
   MEDIHALER ERGOTAMINE, ERGOTAMINE TARTRATE
   MEDIHALER-EPI, EPINEPHRINE BITARTRATE (OTC)
   MEDIHALER-ISO, ISOPROTERENOL SULFATE
   METROGEL-VAGINAL, METRONIDAZOLE
   MINITRAN, NITROGLYCERIN
   NORFLEX, ORPHENADRINE CITRATE
   NORGESIC FORTE, ASPIRIN
   NORGESIC, ASPIRIN
   PROVENTIL-HFA, ALBUTEROL SULFATE
   QVAR 40, BECLOMETHASONE DIPROPIONATE
   QVAR 80, BECLOMETHASONE DIPROPIONATE
   RAUWILOID, ALSEROXYLON
   SODIUM VERSENATE, EDETATE DISODIUM
   TAMBOCOR, FLECAINIDE ACETATE
   TEPANIL TEN-TAB, DIETHYLPROPION HYDROCHLORIDE
   TEPANIL, DIETHYLPROPION HYDROCHLORIDE
   THEOLAIR, THEOPHYLLINE
   THEOLAIR-SR, THEOPHYLLINE
   ULO, CHLOPHEDIANOL HYDROCHLORIDE
   UREX, METHENAMINE HIPPURATE
   VERILOID, ALKAVERVIR

A

AAI PHARMA
AAI PHARMA LLC
   DARVON, PROPOXYPHENE HYDROCHLORIDE
AAIPHARMA
AAIPHARMA INC
   ACYCLOVIR, ACYCLOVIR
   AQUASOL A, VITAMIN A PALMITATE
   BRETHINE, TERBUTALINE SULFATE
   CALCITRIOL, CALCITRIOL
   DOLOPHINE HCL, METHADONE HYDROCHLORIDE
   M.V.I. PEDIATRIC, ASCORBIC ACID
   M.V.I.-12, ASCORBIC ACID
AAIPHARMA LLC
AAIPHARMA LLC
   AZASAN, AZATHIOPRINE
   DARVOCET, ACETAMINOPHEN

   DARVOCET-N 100, ACETAMINOPHEN
   DARVOCET-N 50, ACETAMINOPHEN
   DARVON COMPOUND, ASPIRIN
   DARVON COMPOUND-65, ASPIRIN
   DARVON W/ ASA, ASPIRIN
   DARVON-N W/ ASA, ASPIRIN
   DARVON-N, PROPOXYPHENE NAPSYLATE
AB GENERICS
AB GENERICS LP
   MORPHINE SULFATE, MORPHINE SULFATE
ABANA
ABANA PHARMACEUTICALS INC
   NORCET, ACETAMINOPHEN
ABBOTT
ABBOTT LABORATORIES
   A-METHAPRED, METHYLPREDNISOLONE SODIUM
      SUCCINATE
   ACETAZOLAMIDE SODIUM, ACETAZOLAMIDE SODIUM
   ACETYLCYSTEINE, ACETYLCYSTEINE
   ACYCLOVIR SODIUM, ACYCLOVIR SODIUM
   ACYCLOVIR, ACYCLOVIR SODIUM
   AKINETON, BIPERIDEN HYDROCHLORIDE
   AKINETON, BIPERIDEN LACTATE
   ALCOHOL 5% IN D5-W, ALCOHOL
   ALFENTANIL, ALFENTANIL HYDROCHLORIDE
   AMIDATE, ETOMIDATE
   AMIKACIN SULFATE IN SODIUM CHLORIDE 0.9% IN
      PLASTIC CONTAINER, AMIKACIN SULFATE
   AMIKACIN SULFATE, AMIKACIN SULFATE
   AMINOCAPROIC ACID IN PLASTIC CONTAINER,
      AMINOCAPROIC ACID
   AMINOPHYLLINE, AMINOPHYLLINE
   AMINOSYN 10% (PH6), AMINO ACIDS
   AMINOSYN 10%, AMINO ACIDS
   AMINOSYN 3.5% M, AMINO ACIDS
   AMINOSYN 3.5%, AMINO ACIDS
   AMINOSYN 5%, AMINO ACIDS
   AMINOSYN 7% (PH6), AMINO ACIDS
   AMINOSYN 7% W/ ELECTROLYTES, AMINO ACIDS
   AMINOSYN 7%, AMINO ACIDS
   AMINOSYN 8.5% (PH6), AMINO ACIDS
   AMINOSYN 8.5% W/ ELECTROLYTES, AMINO ACIDS
   AMINOSYN 8.5%, AMINO ACIDS
   AMINOSYN II 10%, AMINO ACIDS
   AMINOSYN II 3.5% IN DEXTROSE 25% IN PLASTIC
      CONTAINER, AMINO ACIDS
   AMINOSYN II 3.5% IN DEXTROSE 5% IN PLASTIC
      CONTAINER, AMINO ACIDS
   AMINOSYN II 3.5% M IN DEXTROSE 5% IN PLASTIC
      CONTAINER, AMINO ACIDS
   AMINOSYN II 3.5% W/ ELECTROLYTES IN DEXTROSE
      25% W/ CALCIUM IN PLASTIC CONTAINER, AMINO
      ACIDS
   AMINOSYN II 3.5%, AMINO ACIDS
   AMINOSYN II 4.25% IN DEXTROSE 10% IN PLASTIC
      CONTAINER, AMINO ACIDS
   AMINOSYN II 4.25% IN DEXTROSE 20% IN PLASTIC
      CONTAINER, AMINO ACIDS
   AMINOSYN II 4.25% IN DEXTROSE 25% IN PLASTIC
      CONTAINER, AMINO ACIDS
   AMINOSYN II 4.25% M IN DEXTROSE 10% IN PLASTIC
      CONTAINER, AMINO ACIDS
   AMINOSYN II 4.25% W/ ELECT AND ADJUSTED
      PHOSPHATE IN DEXTROSE 10% IN PLASTIC
      CONTAINER, AMINO ACIDS

APPENDIX B
PRODUCT NAME INDEX
LISTED BY APPLICANT (*continued*)

AMINOSYN II 4.25% W/ ELECTROLYTES IN DEXTROSE 20% W/ CALCIUM IN PLASTIC CONTAINER, AMINO ACIDS

AMINOSYN II 4.25% W/ ELECTROLYTES IN DEXTROSE 25% W/ CALCIUM IN PLASTIC CONTAINER, AMINO ACIDS

AMINOSYN II 5% IN DEXTROSE 25% IN PLASTIC CONTAINER, AMINO ACIDS

AMINOSYN II 5% W/ ELECTROLYTES IN DEXTROSE 25% W/ CALCIUM IN PLASTIC CONTAINER, AMINO ACIDS

AMINOSYN II 5%, AMINO ACIDS

AMINOSYN II 7%, AMINO ACIDS

AMINOSYN II 8.5%, AMINO ACIDS

AMINOSYN-HF 8%, AMINO ACIDS

AMINOSYN-PF 7%, AMINO ACIDS

AMINOSYN-RF 5.2%, AMINO ACIDS

AMMONIUM CHLORIDE IN PLASTIC CONTAINER, AMMONIUM CHLORIDE

AMPHOTERICIN B, AMPHOTERICIN B

ATRACURIUM BESYLATE PRESERVATIVE FREE, ATRACURIUM BESYLATE

ATRACURIUM BESYLATE, ATRACURIUM BESYLATE

ATROPINE AND DEMEROL, ATROPINE SULFATE

BACTERIOSTATIC WATER FOR INJECTION IN PLASTIC CONTAINER, WATER FOR INJECTION, STERILE

BIAXIN XL, CLARITHROMYCIN

BIAXIN, CLARITHROMYCIN

BRETYLIUM TOSYLATE IN DEXTROSE 5% IN PLASTIC CONTAINER, BRETYLIUM TOSYLATE

BUMETANIDE, BUMETANIDE

BUPIVACAINE HCL KIT, BUPIVACAINE HYDROCHLORIDE

BUPIVACAINE HCL, BUPIVACAINE HYDROCHLORIDE

BUPIVACAINE, BUPIVACAINE HYDROCHLORIDE

BUPRENORPHINE HCL, BUPRENORPHINE HYDROCHLORIDE

BUTORPHANOL TARTRATE PRESERVATIVE FREE, BUTORPHANOL TARTRATE

BUTORPHANOL TARTRATE, BUTORPHANOL TARTRATE

CALCIUM CHLORIDE 10% IN PLASTIC CONTAINER, CALCIUM CHLORIDE

CARTROL, CARTEOLOL HYDROCHLORIDE

CIMETIDINE HCL IN SODIUM CHLORIDE 0.9% IN PLASTIC CONTAINER, CIMETIDINE HYDROCHLORIDE

CIMETIDINE HCL, CIMETIDINE HYDROCHLORIDE

CLINDAMYCIN PHOSPHATE IN DEXTROSE 5% IN PLASTIC CONTAINER, CLINDAMYCIN PHOSPHATE

CYCLOSPORINE, CYCLOSPORINE

DEMEROL, MEPERIDINE HYDROCHLORIDE

DEPAKOTE ER, DIVALPROEX SODIUM

DEPAKOTE, DIVALPROEX SODIUM

DESMOPRESSIN ACETATE, DESMOPRESSIN ACETATE

DEXTROSE 50% IN PLASTIC CONTAINER, DEXTROSE

DEXTROSE 70% IN PLASTIC CONTAINER, DEXTROSE

DIAZEPAM, DIAZEPAM

DIGOXIN PEDIATRIC, DIGOXIN

DIGOXIN, DIGOXIN

DILTIAZEM HCL, DILTIAZEM HYDROCHLORIDE

DIPHENHYDRAMINE HCL, DIPHENHYDRAMINE HYDROCHLORIDE

DIPYRIDAMOLE, DIPYRIDAMOLE

DOBUTAMINE HCL IN DEXTROSE 5% IN PLASTIC CONTAINER, DOBUTAMINE HYDROCHLORIDE

DOBUTAMINE HCL IN DEXTROSE 5%, DOBUTAMINE HYDROCHLORIDE

DOBUTAMINE HCL, DOBUTAMINE HYDROCHLORIDE

DOPAMINE HCL IN DEXTROSE 5%, DOPAMINE HYDROCHLORIDE

DOPAMINE HCL, DOPAMINE HYDROCHLORIDE

DROPERIDOL, DROPERIDOL

EDROPHONIUM CHLORIDE, EDROPHONIUM CHLORIDE

ENALAPRILAT, ENALAPRILAT

ERYTHROCIN, ERYTHROMYCIN LACTOBIONATE

ETOPOSIDE, ETOPOSIDE

FAMOTIDINE PRESERVATIVE FREE IN PLASTIC CONTAINER, FAMOTIDINE

FAMOTIDINE, FAMOTIDINE

FENTANYL CITRATE PRESERVATIVE FREE, FENTANYL CITRATE

FUROSEMIDE, FUROSEMIDE

GENGRAF, CYCLOSPORINE

GENTAMICIN SULFATE IN SODIUM CHLORIDE 0.9% IN PLASTIC CONTAINER, GENTAMICIN SULFATE

GENTAMICIN SULFATE, GENTAMICIN SULFATE

GLYCINE 1.5% IN PLASTIC CONTAINER, GLYCINE

HEPARIN LOCK FLUSH, HEPARIN SODIUM

HEPARIN SODIUM PRESERVATIVE FREE, HEPARIN SODIUM

HEPARIN SODIUM, HEPARIN SODIUM

HYDROMORPHONE HCL, HYDROMORPHONE HYDROCHLORIDE

HYDROXYZINE HCL, HYDROXYZINE HYDROCHLORIDE

IONOSOL B AND DEXTROSE 5% IN PLASTIC CONTAINER, DEXTROSE

IONOSOL MB AND DEXTROSE 5% IN PLASTIC CONTAINER, DEXTROSE

IONOSOL T AND DEXTROSE 5% IN PLASTIC CONTAINER, DEXTROSE

IOPAMIDOL-200 IN PLASTIC CONTAINER, IOPAMIDOL

IOPAMIDOL-200, IOPAMIDOL

IOPAMIDOL-250 IN PLASTIC CONTAINER, IOPAMIDOL

IOPAMIDOL-250, IOPAMIDOL

IOPAMIDOL-300 IN PLASTIC CONTAINER, IOPAMIDOL

IOPAMIDOL-300, IOPAMIDOL

IOPAMIDOL-370 IN PLASTIC CONTAINER, IOPAMIDOL

IOPAMIDOL-370, IOPAMIDOL

ISOFLURANE, ISOFLURANE

ISUPREL, ISOPROTERENOL HYDROCHLORIDE

KALETRA, LOPINAVIR

KETAMINE HCL, KETAMINE HYDROCHLORIDE

KETOROLAC TROMETHAMINE, KETOROLAC TROMETHAMINE

LABETALOL HCL, LABETALOL HYDROCHLORIDE

LEUCOVORIN CALCIUM PRESERVATIVE FREE, LEUCOVORIN CALCIUM

LEVOPHED, NOREPINEPHRINE BITARTRATE

LIDOCAINE HCL PRESERVATIVE FREE IN PLASTIC CONTAINER, LIDOCAINE HYDROCHLORIDE

LIDOCAINE HCL, LIDOCAINE HYDROCHLORIDE

LIPOSYN II 20%, SAFFLOWER OIL

LIPOSYN III 10%, SOYBEAN OIL

LIPOSYN III 20%, SOYBEAN OIL

LORAZEPAM, LORAZEPAM

MAGNESIUM SULFATE, MAGNESIUM SULFATE

MARCAINE HCL PRESERVATIVE FREE, BUPIVACAINE HYDROCHLORIDE

MARCAINE HCL W/ EPINEPHRINE PRESERVATIVE FREE, BUPIVACAINE HYDROCHLORIDE

MARCAINE HCL W/ EPINEPHRINE, BUPIVACAINE HYDROCHLORIDE

MARCAINE HCL, BUPIVACAINE HYDROCHLORIDE

MARCAINE, BUPIVACAINE HYDROCHLORIDE

METHYLDOPATE HCL, METHYLDOPATE HYDROCHLORIDE

METOCLOPRAMIDE HCL, METOCLOPRAMIDE HYDROCHLORIDE

METOPROLOL TARTRATE, METOPROLOL TARTRATE

APPENDIX B
PRODUCT NAME INDEX
LISTED BY APPLICANT (*continued*)

MIDAZOLAM HCL, MIDAZOLAM HYDROCHLORIDE
MILRINONE LACTATE IN DEXTROSE 5% IN PLASTIC
  CONTAINER, MILRINONE LACTATE
MILRINONE LACTATE, MILRINONE LACTATE
MIVACRON IN DEXTROSE 5% IN PLASTIC CONTAINER,
  MIVACURIUM CHLORIDE
MIVACRON, MIVACURIUM CHLORIDE
NALBUPHINE HCL, NALBUPHINE HYDROCHLORIDE
NALOXONE HCL, NALOXONE HYDROCHLORIDE
NIMBEX PRESERVATIVE FREE, CISATRACURIUM
  BESYLATE
NIMBEX, CISATRACURIUM BESYLATE
NITROGLYCERIN IN DEXTROSE 5%, NITROGLYCERIN
NITROGLYCERIN, NITROGLYCERIN
NITROPRESS, SODIUM NITROPRUSSIDE
NORVIR, RITONAVIR
NOVOCAIN, PROCAINE HYDROCHLORIDE
NUROMAX, DOXACURIUM CHLORIDE
OMNICEF, CEFDINIR
PACLITAXEL, PACLITAXEL
PANCURONIUM BROMIDE, PANCURONIUM BROMIDE
PENTAMIDINE ISETHIONATE, PENTAMIDINE
  ISETHIONATE
POTASSIUM CHLORIDE 10MEQ IN PLASTIC CONTAINER,
  POTASSIUM CHLORIDE
POTASSIUM CHLORIDE 20MEQ IN DEXTROSE 5% IN
  PLASTIC CONTAINER, DEXTROSE
POTASSIUM CHLORIDE 20MEQ IN PLASTIC CONTAINER,
  POTASSIUM CHLORIDE
POTASSIUM CHLORIDE 30MEQ IN DEXTROSE 5% IN
  PLASTIC CONTAINER, DEXTROSE
POTASSIUM CHLORIDE 30MEQ IN PLASTIC CONTAINER,
  POTASSIUM CHLORIDE
POTASSIUM CHLORIDE 40MEQ IN DEXTROSE 5% IN
  PLASTIC CONTAINER, DEXTROSE
POTASSIUM CHLORIDE 40MEQ IN PLASTIC CONTAINER,
  POTASSIUM CHLORIDE
PRECEDEX, DEXMEDETOMIDINE
PROCAINAMIDE HCL, PROCAINAMIDE
  HYDROCHLORIDE
PROCHLORPERAZINE EDISYLATE,
  PROCHLORPERAZINE EDISYLATE
PROMETHAZINE HCL, PROMETHAZINE
  HYDROCHLORIDE
QUELICIN PRESERVATIVE FREE, SUCCINYLCHOLINE
  CHLORIDE
QUELICIN, SUCCINYLCHOLINE CHLORIDE
RINGER'S IN PLASTIC CONTAINER, CALCIUM CHLORIDE
RITODRINE HCL IN DEXTROSE 5% IN PLASTIC
  CONTAINER, RITODRINE HYDROCHLORIDE
SODIUM ACETATE IN PLASTIC CONTAINER, SODIUM
  ACETATE, ANHYDROUS
SODIUM PHOSPHATES IN PLASTIC CONTAINER,
  SODIUM PHOSPHATE, DIBASIC, HEPTAHYDRATE
SORBITOL-MANNITOL IN PLASTIC CONTAINER,
  MANNITOL
STERILE WATER FOR INJECTION IN PLASTIC
  CONTAINER, WATER FOR INJECTION, STERILE
SULFAMETHOXAZOLE AND TRIMETHOPRIM,
  SULFAMETHOXAZOLE
SULFENTANIL CITRATE, SUFENTANIL CITRATE
SYNTHROID, LIOTRIX (T4;T3)
TALWIN, PENTAZOCINE LACTATE
TAZICEF, CEFTAZIDIME
THIAMINE HCL, THIAMINE HYDROCHLORIDE
TOBRAMYCIN SULFATE, TOBRAMYCIN SULFATE
TRACRIUM PRESERVATIVE FREE, ATRACURIUM
  BESYLATE

TRACRIUM, ATRACURIUM BESYLATE
TRICOR, FENOFIBRATE
TRIMETHOBENZAMIDE HCL, TRIMETHOBENZAMIDE
  HYDROCHLORIDE
ULTANE, SEVOFLURANE
ULTIVA, REMIFENTANIL HYDROCHLORIDE
VANCOMYCIN HCL, VANCOMYCIN HYDROCHLORIDE
VECURONIUM BROMIDE, VECURONIUM BROMIDE
VERAPAMIL HCL, VERAPAMIL HYDROCHLORIDE
ZEMPLAR, PARICALCITOL
ZYFLO, ZILEUTON
ABBOTT LABORATORIES HOSP PRODUCTS DIV
A-HYDROCORT, HYDROCORTISONE SODIUM
  SUCCINATE
A-METHAPRED, METHYLPREDNISOLONE SODIUM
  SUCCINATE
ACYCLOVIR SODIUM, ACYCLOVIR SODIUM
AMIKACIN SULFATE, AMIKACIN SULFATE
AMINOCAPROIC ACID, AMINOCAPROIC ACID
AMINOPHYLLINE, AMINOPHYLLINE
AMINOSYN II 10% IN PLASTIC CONTAINER, AMINO ACIDS
AMINOSYN II 15% IN PLASTIC CONTAINER, AMINO ACIDS
AMINOSYN II 3.5% IN DEXTROSE 25% IN PLASTIC
  CONTAINER, AMINO ACIDS
AMINOSYN II 3.5% IN DEXTROSE 5% IN PLASTIC
  CONTAINER, AMINO ACIDS
AMINOSYN II 3.5% M IN DEXTROSE 5% IN PLASTIC
  CONTAINER, AMINO ACIDS
AMINOSYN II 3.5% W/ ELECTROLYTES IN DEXTROSE
  25% W/ CALCIUM IN PLASTIC CONTAINER, AMINO
  ACIDS
AMINOSYN II 4.25% IN DEXTROSE 10% IN PLASTIC
  CONTAINER, AMINO ACIDS
AMINOSYN II 4.25% IN DEXTROSE 20% IN PLASTIC
  CONTAINER, AMINO ACIDS
AMINOSYN II 4.25% IN DEXTROSE 25% IN PLASTIC
  CONTAINER, AMINO ACIDS
AMINOSYN II 4.25% W/ ELECT AND ADJUSTED
  PHOSPHATE IN DEXTROSE 10% IN PLASTIC
  CONTAINER, AMINO ACIDS
AMINOSYN II 4.25% W/ ELECTROLYTES IN DEXTROSE
  20% W/ CALCIUM IN PLASTIC CONTAINER, AMINO
  ACIDS
AMINOSYN II 4.25% W/ ELECTROLYTES IN DEXTROSE
  25% W/ CALCIUM IN PLASTIC CONTAINER, AMINO
  ACIDS
AMINOSYN II 5% IN DEXTROSE 25% IN PLASTIC
  CONTAINER, AMINO ACIDS
AMINOSYN II 5% W/ ELECTROLYTES IN DEXTROSE 25%
  W/ CALCIUM IN PLASTIC CONTAINER, AMINO ACIDS
AMINOSYN-HBC 7%, AMINO ACIDS
AMIODARONE HCL, AMIODARONE HYDROCHLORIDE
AMRINONE, INAMRINONE LACTATE
ATROPINE SULFATE ANSYR PLASTIC SYRINGE,
  ATROPINE SULFATE
BRETYLIUM TOSYLATE IN PLASTIC CONTAINER,
  BRETYLIUM TOSYLATE
BRETYLIUM TOSYLATE, BRETYLIUM TOSYLATE
BUPIVACAINE HCL AND EPINEPHRINE, BUPIVACAINE
  HYDROCHLORIDE
CALCIJEX, CALCITRIOL
CHROMIC CHLORIDE IN PLASTIC CONTAINER,
  CHROMIC CHLORIDE
CLINDAMYCIN PHOSPHATE, CLINDAMYCIN
  PHOSPHATE
CORLOPAM, FENOLDOPAM MESYLATE
CUPRIC CHLORIDE IN PLASTIC CONTAINER, CUPRIC
  CHLORIDE

APPENDIX B
PRODUCT NAME INDEX
LISTED BY APPLICANT (*continued*)

DEXTROSE 25%, DEXTROSE
DEXTROSE 5% IN PLASTIC CONTAINER, DEXTROSE
DEXTROSE 50% IN PLASTIC CONTAINER, DEXTROSE
DIAZEPAM, DIAZEPAM
DOBUTAMINE HCL, DOBUTAMINE HYDROCHLORIDE
DOPAMINE HCL IN DEXTROSE 5% IN PLASTIC
    CONTAINER, DOPAMINE HYDROCHLORIDE
DOPAMINE HCL, DOPAMINE HYDROCHLORIDE
ENFLURANE, ENFLURANE
ERYTHROCIN, ERYTHROMYCIN LACTOBIONATE
FENTANYL CITRATE AND DROPERIDOL, DROPERIDOL
FENTANYL CITRATE, FENTANYL CITRATE
HEPARIN LOCK FLUSH IN PLASTIC CONTAINER,
    HEPARIN SODIUM
HEPARIN LOCK FLUSH, HEPARIN SODIUM
HEPARIN SODIUM 20,000 UNITS IN DEXTROSE 5% IN
    PLASTIC CONTAINER, HEPARIN SODIUM
HEPARIN SODIUM 25,000 UNITS IN DEXTROSE 5% IN
    PLASTIC CONTAINER, HEPARIN SODIUM
HEPARIN SODIUM PRESERVATIVE FREE, HEPARIN
    SODIUM
ISOPROTERENOL HCL, ISOPROTERENOL
    HYDROCHLORIDE
LIDOCAINE HCL 0.2% IN DEXTROSE 5% IN PLASTIC
    CONTAINER, LIDOCAINE HYDROCHLORIDE
LIDOCAINE HCL 0.4% IN DEXTROSE 5% IN PLASTIC
    CONTAINER, LIDOCAINE HYDROCHLORIDE
LIDOCAINE HCL 0.8% IN DEXTROSE 5% IN PLASTIC
    CONTAINER, LIDOCAINE HYDROCHLORIDE
LIDOCAINE HCL 5% AND DEXTROSE 7.5%, LIDOCAINE
    HYDROCHLORIDE
LIDOCAINE HCL AND EPINEPHRINE, EPINEPHRINE
LIDOCAINE HCL, LIDOCAINE HYDROCHLORIDE
LIPOSYN III 30%, SOYBEAN OIL
MAGNESIUM SULFATE IN DEXTROSE 5% IN PLASTIC
    CONTAINER, MAGNESIUM SULFATE
MAGNESIUM SULFATE IN PLASTIC CONTAINER,
    MAGNESIUM SULFATE
MANGANESE CHLORIDE IN PLASTIC CONTAINER,
    MANGANESE CHLORIDE
METOCLOPRAMIDE HCL, METOCLOPRAMIDE
    HYDROCHLORIDE
MIDAZOLAM HCL, MIDAZOLAM HYDROCHLORIDE
MORPHINE SULFATE, MORPHINE SULFATE
NALBUPHINE HCL, NALBUPHINE HYDROCHLORIDE
NALOXONE HCL, NALOXONE HYDROCHLORIDE
NITROGLYCERIN IN DEXTROSE 5%, NITROGLYCERIN
NITROPRESS, SODIUM NITROPRUSSIDE
PANCURONIUM BROMIDE, PANCURONIUM BROMIDE
PANHEPRIN, HEPARIN SODIUM
PENTHRANE, METHOXYFLURANE
PENTOTHAL, THIOPENTAL SODIUM
PHENYTOIN SODIUM, PHENYTOIN SODIUM
POTASSIUM ACETATE IN PLASTIC CONTAINER,
    POTASSIUM ACETATE
POTASSIUM CHLORIDE 10MEQ IN DEXTROSE 5% AND
    LACTATED RINGER'S IN PLASTIC CONTAINER,
    CALCIUM CHLORIDE
POTASSIUM CHLORIDE 15MEQ IN DEXTROSE 5% AND
    LACTATED RINGER'S IN PLASTIC CONTAINER,
    CALCIUM CHLORIDE
POTASSIUM CHLORIDE 20MEQ IN DEXTROSE 5% AND
    LACTATED RINGER'S IN PLASTIC CONTAINER,
    CALCIUM CHLORIDE
POTASSIUM CHLORIDE 20MEQ IN SODIUM CHLORIDE
    0.9% IN PLASTIC CONTAINER, POTASSIUM
    CHLORIDE

POTASSIUM CHLORIDE 30MEQ IN DEXTROSE 5% AND
    LACTATED RINGER'S IN PLASTIC CONTAINER,
    CALCIUM CHLORIDE
POTASSIUM CHLORIDE 40MEQ IN DEXTROSE 5% AND
    LACTATED RINGER'S IN PLASTIC CONTAINER,
    CALCIUM CHLORIDE
POTASSIUM CHLORIDE 40MEQ IN SODIUM CHLORIDE
    0.9% IN PLASTIC CONTAINER, POTASSIUM
    CHLORIDE
POTASSIUM CHLORIDE 5MEQ IN DEXTROSE 5% AND
    LACTATED RINGER'S IN PLASTIC CONTAINER,
    CALCIUM CHLORIDE
PROMETHAZINE HCL, PROMETHAZINE
    HYDROCHLORIDE
RITODRINE HCL, RITODRINE HYDROCHLORIDE
SODIUM CHLORIDE 0.45% IN PLASTIC CONTAINER,
    SODIUM CHLORIDE
SODIUM CHLORIDE 0.9% IN PLASTIC CONTAINER,
    SODIUM CHLORIDE
SODIUM CHLORIDE IN PLASTIC CONTAINER, SODIUM
    CHLORIDE
SODIUM LACTATE IN PLASTIC CONTAINER, SODIUM
    LACTATE
STERILE WATER FOR INJECTION IN PLASTIC
    CONTAINER, WATER FOR INJECTION, STERILE
THAM, TROMETHAMINE
THAM-E, POTASSIUM CHLORIDE
TOBRAMYCIN SULFATE IN SODIUM CHLORIDE 0.9% IN
    PLASTIC CONTAINER, TOBRAMYCIN SULFATE
TOBRAMYCIN SULFATE, TOBRAMYCIN SULFATE
TPN ELECTROLYTES IN PLASTIC CONTAINER, CALCIUM
    CHLORIDE
TUBOCURARINE CHLORIDE, TUBOCURARINE
    CHLORIDE
UREAPHIL, UREA
VANCOMYCIN HCL, VANCOMYCIN HYDROCHLORIDE
ZINC CHLORIDE IN PLASTIC CONTAINER, ZINC
    CHLORIDE
ABBOTT LABORATORIES PHARMACEUTICAL PRODUCTS
DIV
    A-HYDROCORT, HYDROCORTISONE SODIUM
        SUCCINATE
    A-METHAPRED, METHYLPREDNISOLONE SODIUM
        SUCCINATE
    A-POXIDE, CHLORDIAZEPOXIDE HYDROCHLORIDE
    ACETIC ACID 0.25% IN PLASTIC CONTAINER, ACETIC
        ACID, GLACIAL
    AMINOPHYLLINE IN SODIUM CHLORIDE 0.45% IN
        PLASTIC CONTAINER, AMINOPHYLLINE
    AMINOPHYLLINE IN SODIUM CHLORIDE 0.45%,
        AMINOPHYLLINE
    AMINOSOL 5%, PROTEIN HYDROLYSATE
    AMINOSYN 3.5% IN PLASTIC CONTAINER, AMINO ACIDS
    AMINOSYN 3.5% M IN PLASTIC CONTAINER, AMINO
        ACIDS
    AMINOSYN 3.5% W/ DEXTROSE 25% IN PLASTIC
        CONTAINER, AMINO ACIDS
    AMINOSYN 3.5% W/ DEXTROSE 5% IN PLASTIC
        CONTAINER, AMINO ACIDS
    AMINOSYN 4.25% W/ DEXTROSE 25% IN PLASTIC
        CONTAINER, AMINO ACIDS
    AMINOSYN II 10% W/ ELECTROLYTES, AMINO ACIDS
    AMINOSYN II 3.5% IN DEXTROSE 25% IN PLASTIC
        CONTAINER, AMINO ACIDS
    AMINOSYN II 3.5% IN DEXTROSE 5% IN PLASTIC
        CONTAINER, AMINO ACIDS
    AMINOSYN II 3.5% IN PLASTIC CONTAINER, AMINO
        ACIDS

APPENDIX B
PRODUCT NAME INDEX
LISTED BY APPLICANT (*continued*)

AMINOSYN II 3.5% M IN DEXTROSE 5% IN PLASTIC
CONTAINER, AMINO ACIDS
AMINOSYN II 3.5% M IN PLASTIC CONTAINER, AMINO
ACIDS
AMINOSYN II 3.5% M, AMINO ACIDS
AMINOSYN II 3.5% W/ ELECTROLYTES IN DEXTROSE
25% IN PLASTIC CONTAINER, AMINO ACIDS
AMINOSYN II 4.25% IN DEXTROSE 25% IN PLASTIC
CONTAINER, AMINO ACIDS
AMINOSYN II 4.25% M IN DEXTROSE 10% IN PLASTIC
CONTAINER, AMINO ACIDS
AMINOSYN II 4.25% W/ ELECTROLYTES IN DEXTROSE
25% IN PLASTIC CONTAINER, AMINO ACIDS
AMINOSYN II 5% IN DEXTROSE 25% IN PLASTIC
CONTAINER, AMINO ACIDS
AMINOSYN II 7% W/ ELECTROLYTES, AMINO ACIDS
AMINOSYN II 8.5% W/ ELECTROLYTES, AMINO ACIDS
AMINOSYN-HBC 7% IN PLASTIC CONTAINER, AMINO
ACIDS
AMINOSYN-PF 10%, AMINO ACIDS
AMMONIUM CHLORIDE, AMMONIUM CHLORIDE
BACTERIOSTATIC SODIUM CHLORIDE 0.9% IN PLASTIC
CONTAINER, SODIUM CHLORIDE
BIAXIN, CLARITHROMYCIN
BRETYLIUM TOSYLATE IN DEXTROSE 5%, BRETYLIUM
TOSYLATE
BUPIVACAINE HCL, BUPIVACAINE HYDROCHLORIDE
CALCIUM GLUCEPTATE, CALCIUM GLUCEPTATE
CEPHALOTHIN SODIUM, CEPHALOTHIN SODIUM
CHLOROPROCAINE HCL, CHLOROPROCAINE
HYDROCHLORIDE
CHLORPROMAZINE HCL, CHLORPROMAZINE
HYDROCHLORIDE
CHLORTHALIDONE, CHLORTHALIDONE
CHOLOXIN, DEXTROTHYROXINE SODIUM
CHYMODIACTIN, CHYMOPAPAIN
CLINDAMYCIN PHOSPHATE, CLINDAMYCIN
PHOSPHATE
CYLERT, PEMOLINE
DEPACON, VALPROATE SODIUM
DEPAKENE, VALPROIC ACID
DEPAKOTE CP, DIVALPROEX SODIUM
DEPAKOTE, DIVALPROEX SODIUM
DEXTROSE 10% IN PLASTIC CONTAINER, DEXTROSE
DEXTROSE 2.5% AND SODIUM CHLORIDE 0.45% IN
PLASTIC CONTAINER, DEXTROSE
DEXTROSE 20% IN PLASTIC CONTAINER, DEXTROSE
DEXTROSE 3.3% AND SODIUM CHLORIDE 0.3% IN
PLASTIC CONTAINER, DEXTROSE
DEXTROSE 30% IN PLASTIC CONTAINER, DEXTROSE
DEXTROSE 38.5% IN PLASTIC CONTAINER, DEXTROSE
DEXTROSE 40% IN PLASTIC CONTAINER, DEXTROSE
DEXTROSE 5% AND LACTATED RINGER'S IN PLASTIC
CONTAINER, CALCIUM CHLORIDE
DEXTROSE 5% AND RINGER'S IN PLASTIC CONTAINER,
CALCIUM CHLORIDE
DEXTROSE 5% AND SODIUM CHLORIDE 0.225% IN
PLASTIC CONTAINER, DEXTROSE
DEXTROSE 5% AND SODIUM CHLORIDE 0.3% IN
PLASTIC CONTAINER, DEXTROSE
DEXTROSE 5% AND SODIUM CHLORIDE 0.45% IN
PLASTIC CONTAINER, DEXTROSE
DEXTROSE 5% AND SODIUM CHLORIDE 0.9% IN
PLASTIC CONTAINER, DEXTROSE
DEXTROSE 5% IN PLASTIC CONTAINER, DEXTROSE
DEXTROSE 50% IN PLASTIC CONTAINER, DEXTROSE
DEXTROSE 60% IN PLASTIC CONTAINER, DEXTROSE
DEXTROSE 70% IN PLASTIC CONTAINER, DEXTROSE

DIASONE SODIUM, SULFOXONE SODIUM
DICUMAROL, DICUMAROL
DILAUDID, HYDROMORPHONE HYDROCHLORIDE
DILAUDID-HP, HYDROMORPHONE HYDROCHLORIDE
DISCASE, CHYMOPAPAIN
DROPERIDOL, DROPERIDOL
E-MYCIN, ERYTHROMYCIN
E.E.S. 200, ERYTHROMYCIN ETHYLSUCCINATE
E.E.S. 400, ERYTHROMYCIN ETHYLSUCCINATE
E.E.S., ERYTHROMYCIN ETHYLSUCCINATE
ENDRATE, EDETATE DISODIUM
ENDURON, METHYCLOTHIAZIDE
ENDURONYL FORTE, DESERPIDINE
ENDURONYL, DESERPIDINE
ERY-TAB, ERYTHROMYCIN
ERYDERM, ERYTHROMYCIN
ERYPED, ERYTHROMYCIN ETHYLSUCCINATE
ERYTHROCIN STEARATE, ERYTHROMYCIN STEARATE
ERYTHROCIN, ERYTHROMYCIN LACTOBIONATE
ERYTHROMYCIN, ERYTHROMYCIN
EUTONYL, PARGYLINE HYDROCHLORIDE
EUTRON, METHYCLOTHIAZIDE
FENTANYL CITRATE, FENTANYL CITRATE
GEMONIL, METHARBITAL
GENTAMICIN SULFATE IN SODIUM CHLORIDE 0.9% IN
PLASTIC CONTAINER, GENTAMICIN SULFATE
GENTAMICIN SULFATE, GENTAMICIN SULFATE
GLYCOPYRROLATE, GLYCOPYRROLATE
HALOTHANE, HALOTHANE
HARMONYL, DESERPIDINE
HEPARIN SODIUM 1,000 UNITS IN SODIUM CHLORIDE
0.9% IN PLASTIC CONTAINER, HEPARIN SODIUM
HEPARIN SODIUM 10,000 UNITS IN DEXTROSE 5% IN
PLASTIC CONTAINER, HEPARIN SODIUM
HEPARIN SODIUM 10,000 UNITS IN DEXTROSE 5%,
HEPARIN SODIUM
HEPARIN SODIUM 10,000 UNITS IN SODIUM CHLORIDE
0.45%, HEPARIN SODIUM
HEPARIN SODIUM 10,000 UNITS IN SODIUM CHLORIDE
0.9%, HEPARIN SODIUM
HEPARIN SODIUM 12,500 UNITS IN DEXTROSE 5% IN
PLASTIC CONTAINER, HEPARIN SODIUM
HEPARIN SODIUM 12,500 UNITS IN DEXTROSE 5%,
HEPARIN SODIUM
HEPARIN SODIUM 12,500 UNITS IN SODIUM CHLORIDE
0.45% IN PLASTIC CONTAINER, HEPARIN SODIUM
HEPARIN SODIUM 12,500 UNITS IN SODIUM CHLORIDE
0.9%, HEPARIN SODIUM
HEPARIN SODIUM 2,000 UNITS IN SODIUM CHLORIDE
0.9% IN PLASTIC CONTAINER, HEPARIN SODIUM
HEPARIN SODIUM 25,000 UNITS IN DEXTROSE 5% IN
PLASTIC CONTAINER, HEPARIN SODIUM
HEPARIN SODIUM 25,000 UNITS IN DEXTROSE 5%,
HEPARIN SODIUM
HEPARIN SODIUM 25,000 UNITS IN SODIUM CHLORIDE
0.45% IN PLASTIC CONTAINER, HEPARIN SODIUM
HEPARIN SODIUM 25,000 UNITS IN SODIUM CHLORIDE
0.9% IN PLASTIC CONTAINER, HEPARIN SODIUM
HEPARIN SODIUM 25,000 UNITS IN SODIUM CHLORIDE
0.9%, HEPARIN SODIUM
HEPARIN SODIUM 5,000 UNITS IN SODIUM CHLORIDE
0.45%, HEPARIN SODIUM
HEPARIN SODIUM 5,000 UNITS IN SODIUM CHLORIDE
0.9%, HEPARIN SODIUM
HYDROXYZINE HCL, HYDROXYZINE HYDROCHLORIDE
HYTRIN, TERAZOSIN HYDROCHLORIDE
IBU, IBUPROFEN
IBUPROFEN, IBUPROFEN

APPENDIX B
PRODUCT NAME INDEX
LISTED BY APPLICANT (*continued*)

ISOPROTERENOL HCL, ISOPROTERENOL HYDROCHLORIDE
ISOPTIN SR, VERAPAMIL HYDROCHLORIDE
ISOPTIN, VERAPAMIL HYDROCHLORIDE
JANIMINE, IMIPRAMINE HYDROCHLORIDE
K-TAB, POTASSIUM CHLORIDE
LACTATED RINGER'S IN PLASTIC CONTAINER, CALCIUM CHLORIDE
LIDOCAINE HCL 0.2% IN DEXTROSE 5% IN PLASTIC CONTAINER, LIDOCAINE HYDROCHLORIDE
LIDOCAINE HCL 0.2% IN DEXTROSE 5%, LIDOCAINE HYDROCHLORIDE
LIDOCAINE HCL 0.4% IN DEXTROSE 5%, LIDOCAINE HYDROCHLORIDE
LIDOCAINE HCL AND EPINEPHRINE, EPINEPHRINE
LIDOCAINE HCL IN PLASTIC CONTAINER, LIDOCAINE HYDROCHLORIDE
LIDOCAINE HCL PRESERVATIVE FREE, LIDOCAINE HYDROCHLORIDE
LIDOCAINE HCL W/ EPINEPHRINE, EPINEPHRINE
LIDOCAINE HCL, LIDOCAINE HYDROCHLORIDE
LIPIDIL, FENOFIBRATE
LIPOSYN 10%, SAFFLOWER OIL
LIPOSYN 20%, SAFFLOWER OIL
LIPOSYN II 10%, SAFFLOWER OIL
LOPURIN, ALLOPURINOL
LTA II KIT, LIDOCAINE HYDROCHLORIDE
MANNITOL 10% IN PLASTIC CONTAINER, MANNITOL
MANNITOL 10%, MANNITOL
MANNITOL 15% IN PLASTIC CONTAINER, MANNITOL
MANNITOL 15%, MANNITOL
MANNITOL 20% IN PLASTIC CONTAINER, MANNITOL
MANNITOL 20%, MANNITOL
MANNITOL 25%, MANNITOL
MANNITOL 5% IN PLASTIC CONTAINER, MANNITOL
MANNITOL 5%, MANNITOL
MAVIK, TRANDOLAPRIL
MEPERIDINE HCL PRESERVATIVE FREE, MEPERIDINE HYDROCHLORIDE
MEPERIDINE HCL, MEPERIDINE HYDROCHLORIDE
MERIDIA, SIBUTRAMINE HYDROCHLORIDE
METRONIDAZOLE IN PLASTIC CONTAINER, METRONIDAZOLE
METRONIDAZOLE, METRONIDAZOLE
MORPHINE SULFATE, MORPHINE SULFATE
NALOXONE HCL, NALOXONE HYDROCHLORIDE
NEMBUTAL SODIUM, PENTOBARBITAL SODIUM
NEMBUTAL, PENTOBARBITAL
NEMBUTAL, PENTOBARBITAL SODIUM
NITROPRESS, SODIUM NITROPRUSSIDE
NORISODRINE AEROTROL, ISOPROTERENOL HYDROCHLORIDE
NORISODRINE, ISOPROTERENOL SULFATE
NORMOSOL-M AND DEXTROSE 5% IN PLASTIC CONTAINER, DEXTROSE
NORMOSOL-R AND DEXTROSE 5% IN PLASTIC CONTAINER, DEXTROSE
NORMOSOL-R IN PLASTIC CONTAINER, MAGNESIUM CHLORIDE
NORVIR, RITONAVIR
OCL, POLYETHYLENE GLYCOL 3350
ORETIC, HYDROCHLOROTHIAZIDE
ORETICYL 25, DESERPIDINE
ORETICYL 50, DESERPIDINE
ORETICYL FORTE, DESERPIDINE
OXYTOCIN 10 USP UNITS IN DEXTROSE 5%, OXYTOCIN
OXYTOCIN 20 USP UNITS IN DEXTROSE 5%, OXYTOCIN
OXYTOCIN 5 USP UNITS IN DEXTROSE 5%, OXYTOCIN

PANWARFIN, WARFARIN SODIUM
PARADIONE, PARAMETHADIONE
PCE, ERYTHROMYCIN
PEDIATRIC LTA KIT, LIDOCAINE HYDROCHLORIDE
PHENURONE, PHENACEMIDE
PHENYTOIN SODIUM, PHENYTOIN SODIUM
PHYSIOSOL IN PLASTIC CONTAINER, MAGNESIUM CHLORIDE
PHYSIOSOL PH 7.4 IN PLASTIC CONTAINER, MAGNESIUM CHLORIDE
PLACIDYL, ETHCHLORVYNOL
PLEGISOL IN PLASTIC CONTAINER, CALCIUM CHLORIDE
POTASSIUM CHLORIDE 10MEQ IN DEXTROSE 5% AND SODIUM CHLORIDE 0.225% IN PLASTIC CONTAINER, DEXTROSE
POTASSIUM CHLORIDE 10MEQ IN DEXTROSE 5% AND SODIUM CHLORIDE 0.3% IN PLASTIC CONTAINER, DEXTROSE
POTASSIUM CHLORIDE 10MEQ IN DEXTROSE 5% AND SODIUM CHLORIDE 0.45% IN PLASTIC CONTAINER, DEXTROSE
POTASSIUM CHLORIDE 10MEQ IN DEXTROSE 5% AND SODIUM CHLORIDE 0.9% IN PLASTIC CONTAINER, DEXTROSE
POTASSIUM CHLORIDE 15MEQ IN DEXTROSE 5% AND SODIUM CHLORIDE 0.225% IN PLASTIC CONTAINER, DEXTROSE
POTASSIUM CHLORIDE 15MEQ IN DEXTROSE 5% AND SODIUM CHLORIDE 0.3% IN PLASTIC CONTAINER, DEXTROSE
POTASSIUM CHLORIDE 15MEQ IN DEXTROSE 5% AND SODIUM CHLORIDE 0.45% IN PLASTIC CONTAINER, DEXTROSE
POTASSIUM CHLORIDE 15MEQ IN DEXTROSE 5% AND SODIUM CHLORIDE 0.9% IN PLASTIC CONTAINER, DEXTROSE
POTASSIUM CHLORIDE 20MEQ IN DEXTROSE 5% AND SODIUM CHLORIDE 0.225% IN PLASTIC CONTAINER, DEXTROSE
POTASSIUM CHLORIDE 20MEQ IN DEXTROSE 5% AND SODIUM CHLORIDE 0.3% IN PLASTIC CONTAINER, DEXTROSE
POTASSIUM CHLORIDE 20MEQ IN DEXTROSE 5% AND SODIUM CHLORIDE 0.45% IN PLASTIC CONTAINER, DEXTROSE
POTASSIUM CHLORIDE 20MEQ IN DEXTROSE 5% AND SODIUM CHLORIDE 0.9% IN PLASTIC CONTAINER, DEXTROSE
POTASSIUM CHLORIDE 20MEQ IN DEXTROSE 5% IN SODIUM CHLORIDE 0.3% IN PLASTIC CONTAINER, DEXTROSE
POTASSIUM CHLORIDE 30MEQ IN DEXTROSE 5% AND SODIUM CHLORIDE 0.225% IN PLASTIC CONTAINER, DEXTROSE
POTASSIUM CHLORIDE 30MEQ IN DEXTROSE 5% AND SODIUM CHLORIDE 0.3% IN PLASTIC CONTAINER, DEXTROSE
POTASSIUM CHLORIDE 30MEQ IN DEXTROSE 5% AND SODIUM CHLORIDE 0.45% IN PLASTIC CONTAINER, DEXTROSE
POTASSIUM CHLORIDE 30MEQ IN DEXTROSE 5% AND SODIUM CHLORIDE 0.9% IN PLASTIC CONTAINER, DEXTROSE
POTASSIUM CHLORIDE 40MEQ IN DEXTROSE 5% AND SODIUM CHLORIDE 0.225% IN PLASTIC CONTAINER, DEXTROSE

APPENDIX B
PRODUCT NAME INDEX
LISTED BY APPLICANT (*continued*)

POTASSIUM CHLORIDE 40MEQ IN DEXTROSE 5% AND SODIUM CHLORIDE 0.3% IN PLASTIC CONTAINER, DEXTROSE
POTASSIUM CHLORIDE 40MEQ IN DEXTROSE 5% AND SODIUM CHLORIDE 0.45% IN PLASTIC CONTAINER, DEXTROSE
POTASSIUM CHLORIDE 40MEQ IN DEXTROSE 5% AND SODIUM CHLORIDE 0.9% IN PLASTIC CONTAINER, DEXTROSE
POTASSIUM CHLORIDE 5MEQ IN DEXTROSE 5% AND SODIUM CHLORIDE 0.225% IN PLASTIC CONTAINER, DEXTROSE
POTASSIUM CHLORIDE 5MEQ IN DEXTROSE 5% AND SODIUM CHLORIDE 0.3% IN PLASTIC CONTAINER, DEXTROSE
POTASSIUM CHLORIDE 5MEQ IN DEXTROSE 5% AND SODIUM CHLORIDE 0.45% IN PLASTIC CONTAINER, DEXTROSE
POTASSIUM CHLORIDE 5MEQ IN DEXTROSE 5% AND SODIUM CHLORIDE 0.9% IN PLASTIC CONTAINER, DEXTROSE
POTASSIUM CHLORIDE, POTASSIUM CHLORIDE
PROCAINE HCL, PROCAINE HYDROCHLORIDE
PROMETHAZINE HCL, PROMETHAZINE HYDROCHLORIDE
PROPYLTHIOURACIL, PROPYLTHIOURACIL
PROSOM, ESTAZOLAM
RADIONUCLIDE-LABELED (125 I) FIBRINOGEN (HUMAN) SENSOR, FIBRINOGEN, I-125
RINGER'S IN PLASTIC CONTAINER, CALCIUM CHLORIDE
RYTHMOL, PROPAFENONE HYDROCHLORIDE
SODIUM BICARBONATE IN PLASTIC CONTAINER, SODIUM BICARBONATE
SODIUM CHLORIDE 0.45% IN PLASTIC CONTAINER, SODIUM CHLORIDE
SODIUM CHLORIDE 0.9% IN PLASTIC CONTAINER, SODIUM CHLORIDE
SODIUM CHLORIDE, SODIUM CHLORIDE
SODIUM LACTATE 0.167 MOLAR IN PLASTIC CONTAINER, SODIUM LACTATE
SORBITOL-MANNITOL IN PLASTIC CONTAINER, MANNITOL
SORBITOL-MANNITOL, MANNITOL
STERILE UREA, UREA
STERILE WATER FOR INJECTION IN PLASTIC CONTAINER, WATER FOR INJECTION, STERILE
STERILE WATER IN PLASTIC CONTAINER, WATER FOR IRRIGATION, STERILE
SULFADIAZINE, TRISULFAPYRIMIDINES (SULFADIAZINE; SULFAMERAZINE; SULFAMETHAZINE)
TARKA, TRANDOLAPRIL
TETRACYCLINE HCL, TETRACYCLINE HYDROCHLORIDE
THEOPHYLLINE IN DEXTROSE 5% IN PLASTIC CONTAINER, THEOPHYLLINE
THYPINONE, PROTIRELIN
TPN ELECTROLYTES IN PLASTIC CONTAINER, CALCIUM CHLORIDE
TRAL, HEXOCYCLIUM METHYLSULFATE
TRAVASE, SUTILAINS
TRICOR (MICRONIZED), FENOFIBRATE
TRIDIONE, TRIMETHADIONE
UROLOGIC G IN PLASTIC CONTAINER, CITRIC ACID
VERAPAMIL HCL, VERAPAMIL HYDROCHLORIDE
VERCYTE, PIPOBROMAN
VICODIN ES, ACETAMINOPHEN
VICODIN HP, ACETAMINOPHEN
VICODIN, ACETAMINOPHEN
VICOPRIN, ASPIRIN
VICOPROFEN, HYDROCODONE BITARTRATE
VITAMIN K1, PHYTONADIONE

ABC HOLDING
ABC HOLDING CORP
CAM-AP-ES, HYDRALAZINE HYDROCHLORIDE
CAM-METRAZINE, PHENDIMETRAZINE TARTRATE
CHLOROTHIAZIDE, CHLOROTHIAZIDE
CYPROHEPTADINE HCL, CYPROHEPTADINE HYDROCHLORIDE
DIETHYLPROPION HCL, DIETHYLPROPION HYDROCHLORIDE
HYDRALAZINE HCL, HYDRALAZINE HYDROCHLORIDE
HYDRO-RESERP, HYDROCHLOROTHIAZIDE
HYDROCHLOROTHIAZIDE, HYDROCHLOROTHIAZIDE
MECLIZINE HCL, MECLIZINE HYDROCHLORIDE
PHENAZINE-35, PHENDIMETRAZINE TARTRATE
PHENDIMETRAZINE TARTRATE, PHENDIMETRAZINE TARTRATE
PHENTERMINE HCL, PHENTERMINE HYDROCHLORIDE
TRICHLORMETHIAZIDE, TRICHLORMETHIAZIDE

ABIC
ABIC LTD
ABITREXATE, METHOTREXATE SODIUM
FLUOROURACIL, FLUOROURACIL
LEUCOVORIN CALCIUM, LEUCOVORIN CALCIUM
VINCRISTINE SULFATE, VINCRISTINE SULFATE

ABLE
ABLE LABORATORIES INC
ACETAMINOPHEN AND CODEINE PHOSPHATE, ACETAMINOPHEN
ACETAMINOPHEN AND HYDROCODONE BITARTRATE, ACETAMINOPHEN
ACETAMINOPHEN, ACETAMINOPHEN (OTC)
BUTALBITAL, ACETAMINOPHEN AND CAFFEINE, ACETAMINOPHEN
CARISOPRODOL, CARISOPRODOL
CLORAZEPATE DIPOTASSIUM, CLORAZEPATE DIPOTASSIUM
DIPHENOXYLATE HCL AND ATROPINE SULFATE, ATROPINE SULFATE
HEMSOL-HC, HYDROCORTISONE ACETATE
HYDROCODONE BITARTRATE AND ACETAMINOPHEN, ACETAMINOPHEN
INDOMETHACIN, INDOMETHACIN
LITHIUM CARBONATE, LITHIUM CARBONATE
LOPERAMIDE HCL, LOPERAMIDE HYDROCHLORIDE (OTC)
METHOCARBAMOL, METHOCARBAMOL
METHYLPHENIDATE HCL, METHYLPHENIDATE HYDROCHLORIDE
METRONIDAZOLE, METRONIDAZOLE
PHENTERMINE HCL, PHENTERMINE HYDROCHLORIDE
PROCHLORPERAZINE, PROCHLORPERAZINE
PROMETHAZINE HCL, PROMETHAZINE HYDROCHLORIDE
PROPOXYPHENE NAPSYLATE AND ACETAMINOPHEN, ACETAMINOPHEN
SULFAMETHOXAZOLE AND TRIMETHOPRIM AND PENAZOPYRIDINE HCL, PHENAZOPYRIDINE HYDROCHLORIDE

ACTELION
ACTELION LTD
TRACLEER, BOSENTAN

ADAMS LABS
ADAMS LABORATORIES INC
MUCINEX, GUAIFENESIN (OTC)

APPENDIX B
PRODUCT NAME INDEX
LISTED BY APPLICANT (*continued*)

ADV CARE
ADVANCED CARE PRODUCTS DIV ORTHO PHARMACEUTI-
CAL CORP
    MONISTAT 7 COMBINATION PACK, MICONAZOLE
      NITRATE (OTC)
    MONISTAT 7, MICONAZOLE NITRATE (OTC)
    MONISTAT-3 COMBINATION PACK, MICONAZOLE
      NITRATE (OTC)
ADV MAGNETICS
ADVANCED MAGNETICS INC
    FERIDEX I.V., FERUMOXIDES
    GASTROMARK, FERUMOXSIL
ADVANCED CARE PRODS
ADVANCED CARE PRODUCTS
    MONISTAT 3, MICONAZOLE NITRATE (OTC)
    MONISTAT 7, MICONAZOLE NITRATE (OTC)
AEGIS PHARMS
AEGIS PHARMACEUTICALS INC
    TAMOXIFEN CITRATE, TAMOXIFEN CITRATE
AESGEN
AESGEN INC
    PAMIDRONATE DISODIUM, PAMIDRONATE DISODIUM
AGOURON
AGOURON PHARMACEUTICALS INC
    RESCRIPTOR, DELAVIRDINE MESYLATE
    VIRACEPT, NELFINAVIR MESYLATE
AH ROBINS INC
AH ROBINS INC
    EXNA, BENZTHIAZIDE
AKORN
AKORN INC
    AK-PENTOLATE, CYCLOPENTOLATE HYDROCHLORIDE
    AKBETA, LEVOBUNOLOL HYDROCHLORIDE
    AKPENTOLATE, CYCLOPENTOLATE HYDROCHLORIDE
    AKPRO, DIPIVEFRIN HYDROCHLORIDE
    AKTOB, TOBRAMYCIN
    ALFENTA, ALFENTANIL HYDROCHLORIDE
    BACITRACIN ZINC AND POLYMYXIN B SULFATE,
      BACITRACIN ZINC
    BAL, DIMERCAPROL
    BETAXOLOL, BETAXOLOL HYDROCHLORIDE
    CARDIO-GREEN, INDOCYANINE GREEN
    CHLORAMPHENICOL, CHLORAMPHENICOL
    COR-OTICIN, HYDROCORTISONE ACETATE
    CROMOLYN SODIUM, CROMOLYN SODIUM
    CYANOCOBALAMIN, CYANOCOBALAMIN
    DEXAMETHASONE SODIUM PHOSPHATE,
      DEXAMETHASONE SODIUM PHOSPHATE
    ENDOSOL EXTRA, CALCIUM CHLORIDE
    ERYTHROMYCIN, ERYTHROMYCIN
    GENTAK, GENTAMICIN SULFATE
    GENTAMICIN SULFATE, GENTAMICIN SULFATE
    HEPARIN SODIUM, HEPARIN SODIUM
    HYDROCORTISONE ACETATE, HYDROCORTISONE
      ACETATE
    HYDROXYPROGESTERONE CAPROATE,
      HYDROXYPROGESTERONE CAPROATE
    INAPSINE, DROPERIDOL
    LIDOCAINE HCL, LIDOCAINE HYDROCHLORIDE
    LORAZEPAM, LORAZEPAM
    METHYLPREDNISOLONE ACETATE,
      METHYLPREDNISOLONE ACETATE
    NANDROLONE DECANOATE, NANDROLONE
      DECANOATE
    OCUSERT PILO-20, PILOCARPINE
    OCUSERT PILO-40, PILOCARPINE
    PAREDRINE, HYDROXYAMPHETAMINE
      HYDROBROMIDE

    PAREMYD, HYDROXYAMPHETAMINE HYDROBROMIDE
    POTASSIUM CHLORIDE, POTASSIUM CHLORIDE
    PREDAMIDE, PREDNISOLONE ACETATE
    PREDNISOLONE ACETATE, PREDNISOLONE ACETATE
    PREDNISOLONE SODIUM PHOSPHATE, PREDNISOLONE
      SODIUM PHOSPHATE
    PROMETHAZINE HCL, PROMETHAZINE
      HYDROCHLORIDE
    PYRIDOXINE HCL, PYRIDOXINE HYDROCHLORIDE
    SODIUM SULFACETAMIDE, SULFACETAMIDE SODIUM
    SUFENTA, SUFENTANIL CITRATE
    SULFACETAMIDE SODIUM, SULFACETAMIDE SODIUM
    SULSTER, PREDNISOLONE SODIUM PHOSPHATE
    THIAMINE HCL, THIAMINE HYDROCHLORIDE
    TIMOLOL MALEATE, TIMOLOL MALEATE
    TRIAMCINOLONE DIACETATE, TRIAMCINOLONE
      DIACETATE
    TROPICACYL, TROPICAMIDE
    TROPICAMIDE, TROPICAMIDE
AKORN MFG
AKORN MANUFACTURING INC
    INNOVAR, DROPERIDOL
    SUBLIMAZE PRESERVATIVE FREE, FENTANYL CITRATE
AL HIKMA
AL HIKMA PHARMACEUTICALS
    NAPROXEN SODIUM, NAPROXEN SODIUM
ALARA PHARM
ALARA PHARMACEUTICAL CORPORATION
    LEVO-T, LIOTRIX (T4;T3)
ALCON
ALCON INC
    SULFACETAMIDE SODIUM AND PREDNISOLONE
      SODIUM PHOSPHATE, PREDNISOLONE SODIUM
      PHOSPHATE
    VIGAMOX, MOXIFLOXACIN HYDROCHLORIDE
ALCON LABORATORIES INC
    ALCAINE, PROPARACAINE HYDROCHLORIDE
    ALOMIDE, LODOXAMIDE TROMETHAMINE
    AZOPT, BRINZOLAMIDE
    BETADINE, POVIDONE-IODINE
    BETAXON, LEVOBETAXOLOL HYDROCHLORIDE
    BETOPTIC PILO, BETAXOLOL HYDROCHLORIDE
    BETOPTIC S, BETAXOLOL HYDROCHLORIDE
    BETOPTIC, BETAXOLOL HYDROCHLORIDE
    BSS PLUS, CALCIUM CHLORIDE
    BSS, CALCIUM CHLORIDE
    CARTEOLOL HCL, CARTEOLOL HYDROCHLORIDE
    CETAMIDE, SULFACETAMIDE SODIUM
    CETAPRED, PREDNISOLONE ACETATE
    CHLORAMPHENICOL, CHLORAMPHENICOL
    CILOXAN, CIPROFLOXACIN HYDROCHLORIDE
    CIPRO HC, CIPROFLOXACIN HYDROCHLORIDE
    CROMOLYN SODIUM, CROMOLYN SODIUM
    CYCLOGYL, CYCLOPENTOLATE HYDROCHLORIDE
    CYCLOMYDRIL, CYCLOPENTOLATE HYDROCHLORIDE
    DENDRID, IDOXURIDINE
    ECONOCHLOR, CHLORAMPHENICOL
    ECONOPRED, PREDNISOLONE ACETATE
    EMADINE, EMEDASTINE DIFUMARATE
    FLAREX, FLUOROMETHOLONE ACETATE
    IOPIDINE, APRACLONIDINE HYDROCHLORIDE
    ISMOTIC, ISOSORBIDE
    ISOPTO CETAMIDE, SULFACETAMIDE SODIUM
    ISOPTO CETAPRED, PREDNISOLONE ACETATE
    MAXIDEX, DEXAMETHASONE
    MAXIDEX, DEXAMETHASONE SODIUM PHOSPHATE
    MAXITROL, DEXAMETHASONE
    MIOSTAT, CARBACHOL

APPENDIX B
PRODUCT NAME INDEX
LISTED BY APPLICANT (*continued*)

MYDRIACYL, TROPICAMIDE
NAPHCON FORTE, NAPHAZOLINE HYDROCHLORIDE
NAPHCON-A, NAPHAZOLINE HYDROCHLORIDE (OTC)
NATACYN, NATAMYCIN
NEOMYCIN AND POLYMYXIN B SULFATES AND
    HYDROCORTISONE, HYDROCORTISONE
PANTOPAQUE, IOPHENDYLATE
PATANOL, OLOPATADINE HYDROCHLORIDE
PILOPINE HS, PILOCARPINE HYDROCHLORIDE
PROFENAL, SUPROFEN
STATROL, NEOMYCIN SULFATE
TOBRADEX, DEXAMETHASONE
TOBRASONE, FLUOROMETHOLONE ACETATE
TOBREX, TOBRAMYCIN
TRIFLURIDINE, TRIFLURIDINE
VEXOL, RIMEXOLONE
ZOLYSE, CHYMOTRYPSIN
ALCON UNIVERSAL
ALCON UNIVERSAL LTD
    CYCLOPENTOLATE HCL, CYCLOPENTOLATE
        HYDROCHLORIDE
    DEXAMETHASONE SODIUM PHOSPHATE,
        DEXAMETHASONE SODIUM PHOSPHATE
    GENTAMICIN SULFATE, GENTAMICIN SULFATE
    NEOMYCIN AND POLYMYXIN B SULFATES AND
        DEXAMETHASONE, DEXAMETHASONE
    NEOMYCIN AND POLYMYXIN B SULFATES AND
        HYDROCORTISONE, HYDROCORTISONE
    NEOMYCIN SULFATE-DEXAMETHASONE SODIUM
        PHOSPHATE, DEXAMETHASONE SODIUM
        PHOSPHATE
    PREDNISOLONE SODIUM PHOSPHATE, PREDNISOLONE
        SODIUM PHOSPHATE
    SULFACETAMIDE SODIUM, SULFACETAMIDE SODIUM
    TOBRAMYCIN, TOBRAMYCIN
    TRAVATAN, TRAVOPROST
    TROPICAMIDE, TROPICAMIDE
ALLEGIANCE HLTHCARE
ALLEGIANCE HEALTHCARE CORP
    POVIDONE IODINE, POVIDONE-IODINE (OTC)
ALLENDALE PHARMS
ALLENDALE PHARMACEUTICALS
    TODAY, NONOXYNOL-9 (OTC)
ALLERGAN
ALLERGAN
    ACULAR LS, KETOROLAC TROMETHAMINE
    BLEPH-10, SULFACETAMIDE SODIUM
    BLEPH-30, SULFACETAMIDE SODIUM
    GENOPTIC, GENTAMICIN SULFATE
ALLERGAN INC
    ACULAR PRESERVATIVE FREE, KETOROLAC
        TROMETHAMINE
    ACULAR, KETOROLAC TROMETHAMINE
    ALBALON, NAPHAZOLINE HYDROCHLORIDE
    ALOCRIL, NEDOCROMIL SODIUM
    ALPHAGAN P, BRIMONIDINE TARTRATE
    ALPHAGAN, BRIMONIDINE TARTRATE
    AVAGE, TAZAROTENE
    AZELEX, AZELAIC ACID
    ELIMITE, PERMETHRIN
    LUMIGAN, BIMATOPROST
    OCUFLOX, OFLOXACIN
    OPTICROM, CROMOLYN SODIUM
    POLYTRIM, POLYMYXIN B SULFATE
    RESTASIS, CYCLOSPORINE
    TAZORAC, TAZAROTENE
    ZYMAR, GATIFLOXACIN

ALLERGAN PHARMACEUTICAL
    BETAGAN, LEVOBUNOLOL HYDROCHLORIDE
    BLEPH-10, SULFACETAMIDE SODIUM
    BLEPHAMIDE S.O.P., PREDNISOLONE ACETATE
    BLEPHAMIDE, PREDNISOLONE ACETATE
    CHLOROPTIC S.O.P., CHLORAMPHENICOL
    CHLOROPTIC, CHLORAMPHENICOL
    CHLOROPTIC-P S.O.P., CHLORAMPHENICOL
    ETHAMIDE, ETHOXZOLAMIDE
    FML FORTE, FLUOROMETHOLONE
    FML, FLUOROMETHOLONE
    FML-S, FLUOROMETHOLONE
    HERPLEX, IDOXURIDINE
    HMS, MEDRYSONE
    OCUFEN, FLURBIPROFEN SODIUM
    OPHTHETIC, PROPARACAINE HYDROCHLORIDE
    POLY-PRED, NEOMYCIN SULFATE
    PRED FORTE, PREDNISOLONE ACETATE
    PRED MILD, PREDNISOLONE ACETATE
    PRED-G, GENTAMICIN SULFATE
    PREFRIN-A, PHENYLEPHRINE HYDROCHLORIDE
    PROPINE, DIPIVEFRIN HYDROCHLORIDE
ALLERGAN HERBERT
ALLERGAN HERBERT DIV ALLERGAN INC
    AEROSEB-DEX, DEXAMETHASONE
    AEROSEB-HC, HYDROCORTISONE
    ERYGEL, ERYTHROMYCIN
    ERYMAX, ERYTHROMYCIN
    EXSEL, SELENIUM SULFIDE
    FLUONID, FLUOCINOLONE ACETONIDE
    FLUOROPLEX, FLUOROURACIL
    PENECORT, HYDROCORTISONE
ALLERGAN HERBERT SKIN CARE DIV ALLERGAN INC
    FLUOROPLEX, FLUOROURACIL
    NAFTIN, NAFTIFINE HYDROCHLORIDE
    PENECORT, HYDROCORTISONE
    TEMARIL, TRIMEPRAZINE TARTRATE
ALLIANCE PHARM
ALLIANCE PHARMACEUTICAL CORP
    IMAGENT, DIMYRISTOYL LECITHIN
    IMAGENT, PERFLUBRON
ALPHA THERA
ALPHA THERAPEUTIC CORP
    SOYACAL 10%, SOYBEAN OIL
    SOYACAL 20%, SOYBEAN OIL
ALPHAPHARM
ALPHAPHARM PARTY LTD
    ALPRAZOLAM, ALPRAZOLAM
    AMIODARONE HCL, AMIODARONE HYDROCHLORIDE
    CLONAZEPAM, CLONAZEPAM
    DICLOFENAC SODIUM, DICLOFENAC SODIUM
    FLECAINIDE ACETATE, FLECAINIDE ACETATE
    FLUOXETINE HCL, FLUOXETINE HYDROCHLORIDE
    FLUOXETINE, FLUOXETINE HYDROCHLORIDE
    GLIPIZIDE, GLIPIZIDE
    INDAPAMIDE, INDAPAMIDE
    METFORMIN HCL, METFORMIN HYDROCHLORIDE
    MIRTAZAPINE, MIRTAZAPINE
    NAPROXEN, NAPROXEN
    SELEGILINE HCL, SELEGILINE HYDROCHLORIDE
    TRAMADOL HCL, TRAMADOL HYDROCHLORIDE
    TRIAZOLAM, TRIAZOLAM
ALPHARMA
ALPHARMA INC
    SULFATRIM PEDIATRIC, SULFAMETHOXAZOLE
    SULFATRIM, SULFAMETHOXAZOLE

APPENDIX B
PRODUCT NAME INDEX
LISTED BY APPLICANT (*continued*)

ALPHARMA USPD INC
ACETAMINOPHEN AND CODEINE PHOSPHATE, ACETAMINOPHEN
ACETASOL HC, ACETIC ACID, GLACIAL
ACETASOL, ACETIC ACID, GLACIAL
ACYCLOVIR, ACYCLOVIR
ALBUTEROL SULFATE, ALBUTEROL SULFATE
AMANTADINE HCL, AMANTADINE HYDROCHLORIDE
AMINOPHYLLINE DYE FREE, AMINOPHYLLINE
BETAMETHASONE DIPROPIONATE, BETAMETHASONE DIPROPIONATE
BETAMETHASONE VALERATE, BETAMETHASONE VALERATE
BROMANATE DC, BROMPHENIRAMINE MALEATE
BROMANATE DM, BROMPHENIRAMINE MALEATE
BROMANATE, BROMPHENIRAMINE MALEATE
BROMANYL, BROMODIPHENHYDRAMINE HYDROCHLORIDE
BROMPHENIRAMINE MALEATE, BROMPHENIRAMINE MALEATE
BUTABARB, BUTABARBITAL SODIUM
CAPITAL AND CODEINE, ACETAMINOPHEN
CHLORHEXIDINE GLUCONATE, CHLORHEXIDINE GLUCONATE
CHLORPROMAZINE HCL, CHLORPROMAZINE HYDROCHLORIDE
CIMETIDINE HCL, CIMETIDINE HYDROCHLORIDE
CLEMASTINE FUMARATE, CLEMASTINE FUMARATE
CLINDAMYCIN PHOSPHATE, CLINDAMYCIN PHOSPHATE
CODAMINE, HYDROCODONE BITARTRATE
CONSTULOSE, LACTULOSE
CROMOLYN SODIUM, CROMOLYN SODIUM
CROMOLYN SODIUM, CROMOLYN SODIUM (OTC)
CYPROHEPTADINE HCL, CYPROHEPTADINE HYDROCHLORIDE
DEXAMETHASONE, DEXAMETHASONE
DICYCLOMINE HCL, DICYCLOMINE HYDROCHLORIDE
DIPHENHYDRAMINE HCL, DIPHENHYDRAMINE HYDROCHLORIDE (OTC)
ENULOSE, LACTULOSE
EPINEPHRINE, EPINEPHRINE (OTC)
ERYTHROMYCIN ESTOLATE, ERYTHROMYCIN ESTOLATE
ERYTHROMYCIN ETHYLSUCCINATE, ERYTHROMYCIN ETHYLSUCCINATE
ERYTHROMYCIN, ERYTHROMYCIN
FLUOCET, FLUOCINOLONE ACETONIDE
FLUOCINOLONE ACETONIDE, FLUOCINOLONE ACETONIDE
FLUOCINONIDE, FLUOCINONIDE
FLUOXETINE, FLUOXETINE HYDROCHLORIDE
FLURANDRENOLIDE, FLURANDRENOLIDE
GENTAMICIN SULFATE, GENTAMICIN SULFATE
HALOPERIDOL, HALOPERIDOL LACTATE
HYDRAMINE, DIPHENHYDRAMINE HYDROCHLORIDE
HYDRAMINE, DIPHENHYDRAMINE HYDROCHLORIDE (OTC)
HYDROCODONE COMPOUND, HOMATROPINE METHYLBROMIDE
HYDROCORTISONE, HYDROCORTISONE
HYDROXYZINE HCL, HYDROXYZINE HYDROCHLORIDE
IBUPROFEN, IBUPROFEN
IBUPROFEN, IBUPROFEN (OTC)
IPRATROPIUM BROMIDE, IPRATROPIUM BROMIDE
ISOETHARINE HCL, ISOETHARINE HYDROCHLORIDE
ISOETHARINE MESYLATE, ISOETHARINE MESYLATE

ISOPROTERENOL HCL, ISOPROTERENOL HYDROCHLORIDE
LIDOCAINE HCL VISCOUS, LIDOCAINE HYDROCHLORIDE
LINDANE, LINDANE
LOMANATE, ATROPINE SULFATE
LOPERAMIDE HCL, LOPERAMIDE HYDROCHLORIDE (OTC)
M-ZOLE 7 DUAL PACK, MICONAZOLE NITRATE (OTC)
METHDILAZINE HCL, METHDILAZINE HYDROCHLORIDE
METOCLOPRAMIDE HCL, METOCLOPRAMIDE HYDROCHLORIDE
MINOXIDIL (FOR MEN), MINOXIDIL (OTC)
MINOXIDIL EXTRA STRENGTH (FOR MEN), MINOXIDIL (OTC)
MYKINAC, NYSTATIN
NYSTATIN AND TRIAMCINOLONE ACETONIDE, NYSTATIN
NYSTATIN, NYSTATIN
PERMETHRIN, PERMETHRIN
PERMETHRIN, PERMETHRIN (OTC)
PHENYTOIN, PHENYTOIN
PIPERAZINE CITRATE, PIPERAZINE CITRATE
PROCHLORPERAZINE EDISYLATE, PROCHLORPERAZINE EDISYLATE
PROCHLORPERAZINE, PROCHLORPERAZINE EDISYLATE
PROMETH FORTIS, PROMETHAZINE HYDROCHLORIDE
PROMETH PLAIN, PROMETHAZINE HYDROCHLORIDE
PROMETH VC PLAIN, PHENYLEPHRINE HYDROCHLORIDE
PROMETH VC W/ CODEINE, CODEINE PHOSPHATE
PROMETH W/ CODEINE, CODEINE PHOSPHATE
PROMETH W/ DEXTROMETHORPHAN, DEXTROMETHORPHAN HYDROBROMIDE
SELENIUM SULFIDE, SELENIUM SULFIDE
TETRACYCLINE HCL, TETRACYCLINE HYDROCHLORIDE
THEOPHYLLINE, THEOPHYLLINE
THIORIDAZINE HCL, THIORIDAZINE HYDROCHLORIDE
THIOTHIXENE HCL, THIOTHIXENE HYDROCHLORIDE
TRIACIN-C, CODEINE PHOSPHATE
TRIAMCINOLONE ACETONIDE, TRIAMCINOLONE ACETONIDE
TRIMEPRAZINE TARTRATE, TRIMEPRAZINE TARTRATE
TRIMETH/SULFA, SULFAMETHOXAZOLE
TRIPLE SULFA, TRIPLE SULFA (SULFABENZAMIDE; SULFACETAMIDE; SULFATHIAZOLE)
TRIPLE SULFA, TRISULFAPYRIMIDINES (SULFADIAZINE; SULFAMERAZINE; SULFAMETHAZINE)
TRIPROLIDINE HCL, TRIPROLIDINE HYDROCHLORIDE
ALPHARMA US PHARM
ALPHARMA US PHARMACEUTICAL DIV
ACETAMINOPHEN, ACETAMINOPHEN (OTC)
BETAMETHASONE DIPROPIONATE, BETAMETHASONE DIPROPIONATE
BETAMETHASONE VALERATE, BETAMETHASONE VALERATE
CLOBETASOL PROPIONATE, CLOBETASOL PROPIONATE
CLOTRIMAZOLE AND BETAMETHASONE DIPROPIONATE, BETAMETHASONE DIPROPIONATE
CLOTRIMAZOLE, CLOTRIMAZOLE (OTC)
FLUOCINONIDE EMULSIFIED BASE, FLUOCINONIDE
FLUOCINONIDE, FLUOCINONIDE
HYDROCORTISONE, HYDROCORTISONE
INFANTS' FEVERALL, ACETAMINOPHEN (OTC)
M-ZOLE 3 COMBINATION PACK, MICONAZOLE NITRATE (OTC)

I/678 **Approved Drug Products with Therapeutic Equivalence Evaluations**

USP DI

APPENDIX B
PRODUCT NAME INDEX
LISTED BY APPLICANT (*continued*)

MICONAZOLE 7, MICONAZOLE NITRATE (OTC)
MICONAZOLE NITRATE, MICONAZOLE NITRATE
MICONAZOLE NITRATE, MICONAZOLE NITRATE (OTC)
MYKACET, NYSTATIN
TRIAMCINOLONE ACETONIDE, TRIAMCINOLONE
ACETONIDE
VALNAC, BETAMETHASONE VALERATE

ALRA
ALRA LABORATORIES INC
ACETAZOLAMIDE, ACETAZOLAMIDE
BAMATE, MEPROBAMATE
CHOLAC, LACTULOSE
COMPOUND 65, ASPIRIN
CONSTILAC, LACTULOSE
DIMENHYDRINATE, DIMENHYDRINATE
DIPHENHYDRAMINE HCL, DIPHENHYDRAMINE
HYDROCHLORIDE
ERYZOLE, ERYTHROMYCIN ETHYLSUCCINATE
GEN-XENE, CLORAZEPATE DIPOTASSIUM
HYDROCHLOROTHIAZIDE, HYDROCHLOROTHIAZIDE
IBU-TAB 200, IBUPROFEN (OTC)
IBU-TAB, IBUPROFEN
K+10, POTASSIUM CHLORIDE
K+8, POTASSIUM CHLORIDE
LYGEN, CHLORDIAZEPOXIDE HYDROCHLORIDE
PRAMINE, IMIPRAMINE HYDROCHLORIDE
PROPOXYPHENE HCL, PROPOXYPHENE
HYDROCHLORIDE
SOXAZOLE, SULFISOXAZOLE
TOLBUTAMIDE, TOLBUTAMIDE

ALTANA
ALTANA INC
AMCINONIDE, AMCINONIDE
BACITRACIN ZINC AND POLYMYXIN B SULFATE,
BACITRACIN ZINC
BACITRACIN, BACITRACIN
BACITRACIN-NEOMYCIN-POLYMYXIN W/
HYDROCORTISONE ACETATE, BACITRACIN
BACITRACIN-NEOMYCIN-POLYMYXIN, BACITRACIN
ZINC
BETAMETHASONE DIPROPIONATE, BETAMETHASONE
DIPROPIONATE
CHLORAMPHENICOL, CHLORAMPHENICOL
CLINDAMYCIN PHOSPHATE, CLINDAMYCIN
PHOSPHATE
CLOBETASOL PROPIONATE (EMOLLIENT),
CLOBETASOL PROPIONATE
CLOBETASOL PROPIONATE, CLOBETASOL
PROPIONATE
CLOTRIMAZOLE AND BETAMETHASONE
DIPROPIONATE, BETAMETHASONE DIPROPIONATE
DESONIDE, DESONIDE
DESOXIMETASONE, DESOXIMETASONE
DIFLORASONE DIACETATE, DIFLORASONE DIACETATE
ECONAZOLE NITRATE, ECONAZOLE NITRATE
ERYTHROMYCIN, ERYTHROMYCIN
FLUOCINONIDE, FLUOCINONIDE
HYDROCORTISONE ACETATE, HYDROCORTISONE
ACETATE
HYDROCORTISONE VALERATE, HYDROCORTISONE
VALERATE
HYDROCORTISONE, HYDROCORTISONE
HYDROXYZINE HCL, HYDROXYZINE HYDROCHLORIDE
NYSTATIN, NYSTATIN
SULFACETAMIDE SODIUM, SULFACETAMIDE SODIUM
TOBRAMYCIN, TOBRAMYCIN
TRIAMCINOLONE ACETONIDE, TRIAMCINOLONE
ACETONIDE

ZIPAN-25, PROMETHAZINE HYDROCHLORIDE
ZIPAN-50, PROMETHAZINE HYDROCHLORIDE
ALZA
ALZA CORP
ACTISITE, TETRACYCLINE HYDROCHLORIDE
DITROPAN XL, OXYBUTYNIN CHLORIDE
DITROPAN, OXYBUTYNIN CHLORIDE
DOXIL, DOXORUBICIN HYDROCHLORIDE
DURAGESIC, FENTANYL
EFIDAC 24 CHLORPHENIRAMINE MALEATE,
CHLORPHENIRAMINE MALEATE (OTC)
EFIDAC 24 PSEUDOEPHEDRINE HCL,
PSEUDOEPHEDRINE HYDROCHLORIDE (OTC)
EFIDAC 24 PSEUDOEPHEDRINE HCL/
BROMPHENIRAMINE MALEATE, BROMPHENIRAMINE
MALEATE (OTC)
PROGESTASERT, PROGESTERONE
TESTODERM TTS, TESTOSTERONE
TESTODERM, TESTOSTERONE
VIADUR, LEUPROLIDE ACETATE
AM PHARM
AMERICAN PHARMACEUTICAL PARTNERS INC
DEXAMETHASONE SODIUM PHOSPHATE,
DEXAMETHASONE SODIUM PHOSPHATE
VALPROATE SODIUM, VALPROATE SODIUM
AM PHARM PARTNERS
ACYCLOVIR SODIUM, ACYCLOVIR SODIUM
AMINOCAPROIC ACID, AMINOCAPROIC ACID
AMINOPHYLLINE, AMINOPHYLLINE
AMIODARONE HCL, AMIODARONE HYDROCHLORIDE
AMPHOTERICIN B, AMPHOTERICIN B
BACITRACIN, BACITRACIN
BACTERIOSTATIC SODIUM CHLORIDE 0.9% IN PLASTIC
CONTAINER, SODIUM CHLORIDE
BACTERIOSTATIC WATER FOR INJECTION IN PLASTIC
CONTAINER, WATER FOR INJECTION, STERILE
BRETYLIUM TOSYLATE, BRETYLIUM TOSYLATE
CALCITRIOL, CALCITRIOL
CALCIUM GLUCEPTATE, CALCIUM GLUCEPTATE
CEFAZOLIN SODIUM, CEFAZOLIN SODIUM
CEFIZOX, CEFTIZOXIME SODIUM
CEFOTAXIME, CEFOTAXIME SODIUM
CEFOXITIN, CEFOXITIN SODIUM
CEFUROXIME SODIUM, CEFUROXIME SODIUM
CEFUROXIME, CEFUROXIME SODIUM
CEPHALOTHIN SODIUM, CEPHALOTHIN SODIUM
CEPHAPIRIN SODIUM, CEPHAPIRIN SODIUM
CHLORAMPHENICOL SODIUM SUCCINATE,
CHLORAMPHENICOL SODIUM SUCCINATE
CHLORPROMAZINE HCL, CHLORPROMAZINE
HYDROCHLORIDE
CHORIONIC GONADOTROPIN, GONADOTROPIN,
CHORIONIC
CHROMIC CHLORIDE, CHROMIC CHLORIDE
CISPLATIN, CISPLATIN
CLINDAMYCIN PHOSPHATE IN DEXTROSE 5%,
CLINDAMYCIN PHOSPHATE
CLINDAMYCIN PHOSPHATE, CLINDAMYCIN
PHOSPHATE
CUPRIC SULFATE, CUPRIC SULFATE
CYANOCOBALAMIN, CYANOCOBALAMIN
DACARBAZINE, DACARBAZINE
DEXAMETHASONE SODIUM PHOSPHATE,
DEXAMETHASONE SODIUM PHOSPHATE
DEXAMETHASONE, DEXAMETHASONE SODIUM
PHOSPHATE
DIAZEPAM, DIAZEPAM
DIAZOXIDE, DIAZOXIDE

APPENDIX B
PRODUCT NAME INDEX
LISTED BY APPLICANT (*continued*)

DIGOXIN, DIGOXIN
DIPHENHYDRAMINE HCL PRESERVATIVE FREE,
    DIPHENHYDRAMINE HYDROCHLORIDE
DIPHENHYDRAMINE HCL, DIPHENHYDRAMINE
    HYDROCHLORIDE
DIPYRIDAMOLE, DIPYRIDAMOLE
DOPAMINE HCL, DOPAMINE HYDROCHLORIDE
DOXORUBICIN HCL, DOXORUBICIN HYDROCHLORIDE
DOXY 100, DOXYCYCLINE HYCLATE
DOXY 200, DOXYCYCLINE HYCLATE
DROPERIDOL, DROPERIDOL
ERYTHROMYCIN LACTOBIONATE, ERYTHROMYCIN
    LACTOBIONATE
ETOPOSIDE, ETOPOSIDE
FAMOTIDINE PRESERVATIVE FREE, FAMOTIDINE
FAMOTIDINE, FAMOTIDINE
FLOXURIDINE, FLOXURIDINE
FLUOROURACIL, FLUOROURACIL
FLUPHENAZINE DECANOATE, FLUPHENAZINE
    DECANOATE
FLUPHENAZINE HCL, FLUPHENAZINE HYDROCHLORIDE
FOLIC ACID, FOLIC ACID
FUROSEMIDE, FUROSEMIDE
GENTAMICIN SULFATE, GENTAMICIN SULFATE
GLYCOPYRROLATE, GLYCOPYRROLATE
HALOPERIDOL DECANOATE, HALOPERIDOL
    DECANOATE
HALOPERIDOL, HALOPERIDOL LACTATE
HEP FLUSH KIT IN PLASTIC CONTAINER, HEPARIN
    SODIUM
HEPARIN LOCK FLUSH PRESERVATIVE FREE IN
    PLASTIC CONTAINER, HEPARIN SODIUM
HEPARIN LOCK FLUSH PRESERVATIVE FREE, HEPARIN
    SODIUM
HEPARIN LOCK FLUSH, HEPARIN SODIUM
HEPARIN SODIUM IN PLASTIC CONTAINER, HEPARIN
    SODIUM
HEPARIN SODIUM PRESERVATIVE FREE, HEPARIN
    SODIUM
HEPARIN SODIUM, HEPARIN SODIUM
HEPFLUSH-10, HEPARIN SODIUM
HYDRALAZINE HCL, HYDRALAZINE HYDROCHLORIDE
HYDROCORTISONE SODIUM SUCCINATE,
    HYDROCORTISONE SODIUM SUCCINATE
HYDROXOCOBALAMIN, HYDROXOCOBALAMIN
HYDROXYZINE HCL, HYDROXYZINE HYDROCHLORIDE
IFSOFAMIDE, IFOSFAMIDE
IOPAMIDOL-250, IOPAMIDOL
IOPAMIDOL-300, IOPAMIDOL
IOPAMIDOL-370, IOPAMIDOL
ISOPROTERENOL HCL, ISOPROTERENOL
    HYDROCHLORIDE
KANAMYCIN SULFATE, KANAMYCIN SULFATE
KANAMYCIN, KANAMYCIN SULFATE
KETOROLAC TROMETHAMINE, KETOROLAC
    TROMETHAMINE
LEUCOVORIN CALCIUM, LEUCOVORIN CALCIUM
LIDOCAINE HCL IN PLASTIC CONTAINER, LIDOCAINE
    HYDROCHLORIDE
LIDOCAINE HCL PRESERVATIVE FREE, LIDOCAINE
    HYDROCHLORIDE
LIDOCAINE HCL, LIDOCAINE HYDROCHLORIDE
M.V.C. 9+3, ASCORBIC ACID
MAGNESIUM SULFATE, MAGNESIUM SULFATE
MANGANESE SULFATE, MANGANESE SULFATE
MANNITOL 25%, MANNITOL
MESNA, MESNA

METARAMINOL BITARTRATE, METARAMINOL
    BITARTRATE
METHOTREXATE SODIUM, METHOTREXATE SODIUM
METHYLDOPATE HCL, METHYLDOPATE
    HYDROCHLORIDE
METHYLPREDNISOLONE SODIUM SUCCINATE,
    METHYLPREDNISOLONE SODIUM SUCCINATE
METOCLOPRAMIDE HCL, METOCLOPRAMIDE
    HYDROCHLORIDE
METRONIDAZOLE HCL, METRONIDAZOLE
    HYDROCHLORIDE
METRONIDAZOLE, METRONIDAZOLE
MIDAZOLAM HCL, MIDAZOLAM HYDROCHLORIDE
MILRINONE LACTATE, MILRINONE LACTATE
NALBUPHINE, NALBUPHINE HYDROCHLORIDE
NALOXONE HCL, NALOXONE HYDROCHLORIDE
NANDROLONE DECANOATE, NANDROLONE
    DECANOATE
NEBUPENT, PENTAMIDINE ISETHIONATE
NITROGLYCERIN, NITROGLYCERIN
OXYTOCIN, OXYTOCIN
PAMIDRONATE DISODIUM, PAMIDRONATE DISODIUM
PENTAM, PENTAMIDINE ISETHIONATE
PHENYTOIN SODIUM, PHENYTOIN SODIUM
POTASSIUM CHLORIDE IN PLASTIC CONTAINER,
    POTASSIUM CHLORIDE
POTASSIUM CHLORIDE, POTASSIUM CHLORIDE
PROCAINAMIDE HCL, PROCAINAMIDE
    HYDROCHLORIDE
PROCAINE HCL, PROCAINE HYDROCHLORIDE
PROGESTERONE, PROGESTERONE
PROTAMINE SULFATE, PROTAMINE SULFATE
PYRIDOXINE HCL, PYRIDOXINE HYDROCHLORIDE
RITODRINE HCL, RITODRINE HYDROCHLORIDE
SODIUM CHLORIDE 0.9% IN PLASTIC CONTAINER,
    SODIUM CHLORIDE
SODIUM CHLORIDE 23.4% IN PLASTIC CONTAINER,
    SODIUM CHLORIDE
SODIUM HEPARIN, HEPARIN SODIUM
SODIUM NITROPRUSSIDE, SODIUM NITROPRUSSIDE
STERILE WATER FOR INJECTION IN PLASTIC
    CONTAINER, WATER FOR INJECTION, STERILE
SULFAMETHOXAZOLE AND TRIMETHOPRIM,
    SULFAMETHOXAZOLE
THIAMINE HCL, THIAMINE HYDROCHLORIDE
THIOTEPA, THIOTEPA
TOBRAMYCIN (PHARMACY BULK), TOBRAMYCIN
    SULFATE
TOBRAMYCIN, TOBRAMYCIN SULFATE
VANCOMYCIN HCL, VANCOMYCIN HYDROCHLORIDE
VERAPAMIL HCL, VERAPAMIL HYDROCHLORIDE
VIBISONE, CYANOCOBALAMIN
VINBLASTINE SULFATE, VINBLASTINE SULFATE
VINCRISTINE SULFATE, VINCRISTINE SULFATE
ZINC SULFATE, ZINC SULFATE
AM THERAP
AMERICAN THERAPEUTICS INC
    ACETAMINOPHEN AND CODEINE PHOSPHATE NO. 2,
        ACETAMINOPHEN
    ACETAMINOPHEN AND CODEINE PHOSPHATE NO. 3,
        ACETAMINOPHEN
    ACETAMINOPHEN AND CODEINE PHOSPHATE NO. 4,
        ACETAMINOPHEN
    ALBUTEROL SULFATE, ALBUTEROL SULFATE
    AMITRIPTYLINE HCL, AMITRIPTYLINE HYDROCHLORIDE
    CLONIDINE HCL, CLONIDINE HYDROCHLORIDE
    CLORAZEPATE DIPOTASSIUM, CLORAZEPATE
        DIPOTASSIUM

APPENDIX B
PRODUCT NAME INDEX
LISTED BY APPLICANT (*continued*)

CYPROHEPTADINE HCL, CYPROHEPTADINE
   HYDROCHLORIDE
DANAZOL, DANAZOL
FENOPROFEN CALCIUM, FENOPROFEN CALCIUM
LORAZEPAM, LORAZEPAM
MAPROTILINE HCL, MAPROTILINE HYDROCHLORIDE
MECLOFENAMATE SODIUM, MECLOFENAMATE SODIUM
METAPROTERENOL SULFATE, METAPROTERENOL
   SULFATE
METHOCARBAMOL, METHOCARBAMOL
OXAZEPAM, OXAZEPAM
PRAZOSIN HCL, PRAZOSIN HYDROCHLORIDE
PREDNISONE, PREDNISONE
THIOTHIXENE, THIOTHIXENE
TRAZODONE HCL, TRAZODONE HYDROCHLORIDE
TRIAMTERENE AND HYDROCHLOROTHIAZIDE,
   HYDROCHLOROTHIAZIDE

AMARIN PHARMS
AMARIN PHARMACEUTICALS INC
   ACETAMINOPHEN AND CODEINE PHOSPHATE,
     ACETAMINOPHEN
   AMEN, MEDROXYPROGESTERONE ACETATE
   BONTRIL PDM, PHENDIMETRAZINE TARTRATE
   MOTOFEN HALF-STRENGTH, ATROPINE SULFATE
   MOTOFEN, ATROPINE SULFATE
   PHRENILIN FORTE, ACETAMINOPHEN
   PHRENILIN WITH CAFFEINE AND CODEINE,
     ACETAMINOPHEN
   PHRENILIN, ACETAMINOPHEN

AMBI PHARMS
AMBI PHARMACEUTICALS INC
   PHENTERMINE HCL, PHENTERMINE HYDROCHLORIDE

AMBIX
AMBIX LABORATORIES DIV ORGANICS CORP AMERICA
   HYDROCORTISONE, HYDROCORTISONE
   NITROFURAZONE, NITROFURAZONE
   TRIAMCINOLONE ACETONIDE, TRIAMCINOLONE
     ACETONIDE

AMERSHAM HLTH
AMERSHAM HEALTH
   AMERSCAN MDP KIT, TECHNETIUM TC-99M
     MEDRONATE KIT
   AMIPAQUE, METRIZAMIDE
   BILOPAQUE, TYROPANOATE SODIUM
   CERETEC, TECHNETIUM TC-99M EXAMETAZIME KIT
   CINTICHEM TECHNETIUM 99M HEDSPA, TECHNETIUM
     TC-99M ETIDRONATE KIT
   DICOPAC KIT, CYANOCOBALAMIN
   FLUORINE F-18, SODIUM FLUORIDE, F-18
   GALLIUM CITRATE GA 67, GALLIUM CITRATE, GA-67
   HYPAQUE SODIUM 20%, DIATRIZOATE SODIUM
   HYPAQUE, DIATRIZOATE MEGLUMINE
   HYPAQUE, DIATRIZOATE SODIUM
   HYPAQUE-76, DIATRIZOATE MEGLUMINE
   HYPAQUE-CYSTO, DIATRIZOATE MEGLUMINE
   HYPAQUE-M,75%, DIATRIZOATE MEGLUMINE
   HYPAQUE-M,90%, DIATRIZOATE MEGLUMINE
   IBRIN, FIBRINOGEN, I-125
   INDIUM IN-111 OXYQUINOLINE, INDIUM IN-111
     OXYQUINOLINE
   ISOPAQUE 280, CALCIUM
   ISOPAQUE 440, CALCIUM METRIZOATE
   LUNGAGGREGATE REAGENT, TECHNETIUM TC-99M
     ALBUMIN AGGREGATED KIT
   METASTRON, STRONTIUM CHLORIDE, SR-89
   MPI DMSA KIDNEY REAGENT, TECHNETIUM TC-99M
     SUCCIMER KIT

MPI DTPA KIT - CHELATE, TECHNETIUM TC-99M
   PENTETATE KIT
MPI INDIUM DTPA IN 111, INDIUM IN-111 PENTETATE
   DISODIUM
MPI KRYPTON 81M GAS GENERATOR, KRYPTON, KR-
   81M
MPI STANNOUS DIPHOSPHONATE, TECHNETIUM TC-
   99M ETIDRONATE KIT
MYOVIEW, TECHNETIUM TC-99M TETROFOSMIN KIT
NEOSCAN, GALLIUM CITRATE, GA-67
NEPHROFLOW, IODOHIPPURATE SODIUM, I-123
OMNIPAQUE 140, IOHEXOL
OMNIPAQUE 180, IOHEXOL
OMNIPAQUE 210, IOHEXOL
OMNIPAQUE 240, IOHEXOL
OMNIPAQUE 300, IOHEXOL
OMNIPAQUE 350, IOHEXOL
OMNIPAQUE 70, IOHEXOL
OMNISCAN, GADODIAMIDE
OPTISON, ALBUMIN HUMAN
SELENOMETHIONINE SE 75, SELENOMETHIONINE, SE-
   75
SODIUM IODIDE I 123, SODIUM IODIDE, I-123
SODIUM PERTECHNETATE TC 99M, TECHNETIUM TC-
   99M SODIUM PERTECHNETATE
SODIUM POLYPHOSPHATE-TIN KIT, TECHNETIUM TC-
   99M POLYPHOSPHATE KIT
TC 99M-LUNGAGGREGATE, TECHNETIUM TC-99M
   ALBUMIN AGGREGATED
TECHNETIUM TC 99M DIPHOSPHONATE-TIN KIT,
   TECHNETIUM TC-99M ETIDRONATE KIT
TECHNETIUM TC 99M GENERATOR, TECHNETIUM TC-
   99M SODIUM PERTECHNETATE GENERATOR
TECHNETIUM TC 99M HSA, TECHNETIUM TC-99M
   ALBUMIN KIT
TECHNETIUM TC 99M MAA, TECHNETIUM TC-99M
   ALBUMIN AGGREGATED KIT
TECHNETIUM TC 99M MPI MDP, TECHNETIUM TC-99M
   MEDRONATE KIT
TECHNETIUM TC 99M SULFUR COLLOID, TECHNETIUM
   TC-99M SULFUR COLLOID
TECHNETIUM TC 99M TSC, TECHNETIUM TC-99M
   SULFUR COLLOID KIT
TECHNETIUM TC-99M PENTETATE KIT, TECHNETIUM
   TC-99M PENTETATE KIT
TELEPAQUE, IOPANOIC ACID
TESLASCAN, MANGAFODIPIR TRISODIUM
THALLOUS CHLORIDE TL 201, THALLOUS CHLORIDE, TL-
   201
VISIPAQUE 270, IODIXANOL
VISIPAQUE 320, IODIXANOL
XENON XE 133, XENON, XE-133
XENON XE 133-V.S.S., XENON, XE-133

AMIDE PHARM
AMIDE PHARMACEUTICAL INC
   ACETAMINOPHEN AND PENTAZOCINE HCL,
     ACETAMINOPHEN
   BETAXOLOL HCL, BETAXOLOL HYDROCHLORIDE
   CARISOPRODOL AND ASPIRIN, ASPIRIN
   CARISOPRODOL, ASPIRIN AND CODEINE PHOSPHATE,
     ASPIRIN
   CARISOPRODOL, CARISOPRODOL
   CHLORZOXAZONE, CHLORZOXAZONE
   DIGOXIN, DIGOXIN
   GLYBURIDE, GLYBURIDE
   GUANFACINE HCL, GUANFACINE HYDROCHLORIDE

APPENDIX B
PRODUCT NAME INDEX
LISTED BY APPLICANT (*continued*)

HOMATROPRINE METHYLBROMIDE AND
    HYDROCODONE BITARTRATE, HOMATROPINE
    METHYLBROMIDE
HYDRALAZINE HCL, HYDRALAZINE HYDROCHLORIDE
HYDROXYZINE HCL, HYDROXYZINE HYDROCHLORIDE
MEPERIDINE HCL, MEPERIDINE HYDROCHLORIDE
MIRTAZAPINE, MIRTAZAPINE
NALOXONE HCL AND PENTAZOCAINE, NALOXONE
    HYDROCHLORIDE
NALTREXONE HCL, NALTREXONE HYDROCHLORIDE
OXYCODONE AND ACETAMINOPHEN, ACETAMINOPHEN
PEMOLINE, PEMOLINE
PHENTERMINE HCL, PHENTERMINE HYDROCHLORIDE
RIMANTADINE HCL, RIMANTADINE HYDROCHLORIDE
URSODIOL, URSODIOL

AMPAHSTAR
AMPAHSTAR PHARMACEUTICALS INC
    CORTROSYN, COSYNTROPIN
    DUOCAINE, BUPIVACAINE HYDROCHLORIDE

ANABOLIC
ANABOLIC INC
    BROMPHENIRAMINE MALEATE, BROMPHENIRAMINE
        MALEATE
    BUTALBITAL, ASPIRIN, CAFFEINE, AND CODEINE
        PHOSPHATE, ASPIRIN
    CHLORPHENIRAMINE MALEATE, CHLORPHENIRAMINE
        MALEATE
    DIMENHYDRINATE, DIMENHYDRINATE
    DIPHENHYDRAMINE HCL, DIPHENHYDRAMINE
        HYDROCHLORIDE
    FOLIC ACID, FOLIC ACID
    HYDROCORTISONE, HYDROCORTISONE
    ISONIAZID, ISONIAZID
    MECLIZINE HCL, MECLIZINE HYDROCHLORIDE
    MEPROBAMATE, MEPROBAMATE
    PHENDIMETRAZINE TARTRATE, PHENDIMETRAZINE
        TARTRATE
    PROPOXYPHENE HCL, PROPOXYPHENE
        HYDROCHLORIDE
    PROPYLTHIOURACIL, PROPYLTHIOURACIL
    SODIUM PENTOBARBITAL, PENTOBARBITAL SODIUM
    SODIUM SECOBARBITAL, SECOBARBITAL SODIUM
    TRIPELENNAMINE HCL, TRIPELENNAMINE
        HYDROCHLORIDE

ANBEX
ANBEX INC
    IOSAT, POTASSIUM IODIDE (OTC)

ANDRX
ANDRX CORP
    ALTOCOR, LOVASTATIN
    DILTIAZEM HCL, DILTIAZEM HYDROCHLORIDE

ANDRX PHARMS
ANDRX PHARMACEUTICALS INC
    ACETAMINOPHEN AND CODEINE PHOSPAHTE,
        ACETAMINOPHEN
    CARTIA XT, DILTIAZEM HYDROCHLORIDE
    CODRIX, ACETAMINOPHEN
    HYDROCODONE BITARTRATE AND ACETAMINOPHEN,
        ACETAMINOPHEN
    KETOPROFEN, KETOPROFEN
    LORATADINE AND PSEUDOEPHEDRINE HCL,
        LORATADINE (OTC)
    METFORMIN HCL, METFORMIN HYDROCHLORIDE
    MIRTAZAPINE, MIRTAZAPINE
    NAPROXEN SODIUM, NAPROXEN SODIUM
    OMEPRAZOLE, OMEPRAZOLE
    POTASSIUM CHLORIDE, POTASSIUM CHLORIDE
    TAMOXIFEN CITRATE, TAMOXIFEN CITRATE

TAZTIA XT, DILTIAZEM HYDROCHLORIDE
ANDRX PHARMACEUTICALS LLC
    CODRIX, ACETAMINOPHEN
    ETODOLAC, ETODOLAC

ANESTA
ANESTA CORP
    ACTIQ, FENTANYL CITRATE
    FENTANYL, FENTANYL CITRATE

ANGELINI
ANGELINI PHARMACEUTICALS INC
    REV-EYES, DAPIPRAZOLE HYDROCHLORIDE

ANGUS
ANGUS CHEMICAL CO
    MYCHEL-S, CHLORAMPHENICOL SODIUM SUCCINATE
    TETRACHEL, TETRACYCLINE HYDROCHLORIDE

ANTHRA
ANTHRA PHARMACEUTICALS INC
    VALSTAR PRESERVATIVE FREE, VALRUBICIN

APOTEX
APOTEX CORP
    AMIODARONE HCL, AMIODARONE HYDROCHLORIDE
    BUTORPHANOL TARTRATE PRESERVATIVE FREE,
        BUTORPHANOL TARTRATE
    BUTORPHANOL TARTRATE, BUTORPHANOL TARTRATE
    CARBAMAZEPINE, CARBAMAZEPINE
    CEFUROXIME AXETIL, CEFUROXIME AXETIL
    DILTIAZEM HCL, DILTIAZEM HYDROCHLORIDE
    DIPYRIDAMOLE, DIPYRIDAMOLE
    EDETATE DISODIUM, EDETATE DISODIUM
    ETODOLAC, ETODOLAC
    FAMOTIDINE PRESERVATIVE FREE (PHARMACY BULK),
        FAMOTIDINE
    FAMOTIDINE PRESERVATIVE FREE, FAMOTIDINE
    FAMOTIDINE, FAMOTIDINE
    FLUPHENAZINE DECANOATE, FLUPHENAZINE
        DECANOATE
    HALOPERIDOL DECANOATE, HALOPERIDOL
        DECANOATE
    KETOROLAC TROMETHAMINE, KETOROLAC
        TROMETHAMINE
    LABETALOL HCL, LABETALOL HYDROCHLORIDE
    LISINOPRIL, LISINOPRIL
    MIDAZOLAM HCL, MIDAZOLAM HYDROCHLORIDE
    SELEGILINE HCL, SELEGILINE HYDROCHLORIDE
    SOTALOL HCL, SOTALOL HYDROCHLORIDE

APOTHECON
APOTHECON INC DIV BRISTOL MYERS SQUIBB
    ACYCLOVIR SODIUM, ACYCLOVIR SODIUM
    ACYCLOVIR, ACYCLOVIR
    AMIKIN IN SODIUM CHLORIDE 0.9% IN PLASTIC
        CONTAINER, AMIKACIN SULFATE
    AMIKIN, AMIKACIN SULFATE
    AMOXICILLIN, AMOXICILLIN
    AMPICILLIN SODIUM, AMPICILLIN SODIUM
    BETAPEN-VK, PENICILLIN V POTASSIUM
    BISOPROLOL FUMARATE AND
        HYDROCHLOROTHIAZIDE, BISOPROLOL FUMARATE
    CAPOZIDE 25/15, CAPTOPRIL
    CAPOZIDE 25/25, CAPTOPRIL
    CAPOZIDE 50/15, CAPTOPRIL
    CAPOZIDE 50/25, CAPTOPRIL
    CAPTOPRIL, CAPTOPRIL
    CEFADROXIL, CEFADROXIL/CEFADROXIL
        HEMIHYDRATE
    CEFADYL, CEPHAPIRIN SODIUM
    CEFAZOLIN SODIUM, CEFAZOLIN SODIUM
    CEPHALEXIN, CEPHALEXIN
    CLOXACILLIN SODIUM, CLOXACILLIN SODIUM

APPENDIX B
PRODUCT NAME INDEX
LISTED BY APPLICANT (*continued*)

CORGARD, NADOLOL
DESYREL, TRAZODONE HYDROCHLORIDE
DICLOXACILLIN SODIUM, DICLOXACILLIN SODIUM
DILTIAZEM HCL, DILTIAZEM HYDROCHLORIDE
DYNAPEN, DICLOXACILLIN SODIUM
ENALAPRIL MALEATE, ENALAPRIL MALEATE
FAMOTIDINE PRESERVATIVE FREE, FAMOTIDINE
FAMOTIDINE, FAMOTIDINE
FUNGIZONE, AMPHOTERICIN B
KANTREX, KANAMYCIN SULFATE
KENALOG IN ORABASE, TRIAMCINOLONE ACETONIDE
KENALOG, TRIAMCINOLONE ACETONIDE
KENALOG-10, TRIAMCINOLONE ACETONIDE
KENALOG-40, TRIAMCINOLONE ACETONIDE
KENALOG-H, TRIAMCINOLONE ACETONIDE
KETOROLAC TROMETHAMINE, KETOROLAC
    TROMETHAMINE
KLOTRIX, POTASSIUM CHLORIDE
LABETALOL HCL, LABETALOL HYDROCHLORIDE
METOPROLOL TARTRATE, METOPROLOL TARTRATE
MIDAZOLAM HCL, MIDAZOLAM HYDROCHLORIDE
MUCOMYST, ACETYLCYSTEINE
MYCOLOG-II, NYSTATIN
MYCOSTATIN, NYSTATIN
NAFCILLIN SODIUM, NAFCILLIN SODIUM
NATURETIN-10, BENDROFLUMETHIAZIDE
NATURETIN-2.5, BENDROFLUMETHIAZIDE
NATURETIN-5, BENDROFLUMETHIAZIDE
NYDRAZID, ISONIAZID
OPHTHAINE, PROPARACAINE HYDROCHLORIDE
OXACILLIN SODIUM, OXACILLIN SODIUM
PENICILLIN G POTASSIUM, PENICILLIN G POTASSIUM
POLYCILLIN, AMPICILLIN/AMPICILLIN TRIHYDRATE
POLYCILLIN-PRB, AMPICILLIN/AMPICILLIN TRIHYDRATE
POLYMOX, AMOXICILLIN
PRECEF, CEFORANIDE
PRINCIPEN, AMPICILLIN/AMPICILLIN TRIHYDRATE
PROLIXIN ENANTHATE, FLUPHENAZINE ENANTHATE
PROLIXIN, FLUPHENAZINE HYDROCHLORIDE
PRONESTYL, PROCAINAMIDE HYDROCHLORIDE
PRONESTYL-SR, PROCAINAMIDE HYDROCHLORIDE
PROSTAPHLIN, OXACILLIN SODIUM
QUESTRAN, CHOLESTYRAMINE
RAUDIXIN, RAUWOLFIA SERPENTINA
STADOL PRESERVATIVE FREE, BUTORPHANOL
    TARTRATE
STADOL, BUTORPHANOL TARTRATE
STAPHCILLIN, METHICILLIN SODIUM
SUCOSTRIN, SUCCINYLCHOLINE CHLORIDE
SUMYCIN, TETRACYCLINE HYDROCHLORIDE
TEGOPEN, CLOXACILLIN SODIUM
TOBRAMYCIN SULFATE, TOBRAMYCIN SULFATE
TRIMOX, AMOXICILLIN
ULTRACEF, CEFADROXIL/CEFADROXIL HEMIHYDRATE
VEETIDS, PENICILLIN V POTASSIUM
VELOSEF ',125', CEPHRADINE
VELOSEF ',250', CEPHRADINE
VELOSEF, CEPHRADINE
VESPRIN, TRIFLUPROMAZINE HYDROCHLORIDE
APOTHECON SUB BRISTOL MYERS SQUIBB CO
ATENOLOL, ATENOLOL
OXACILLIN SODIUM, OXACILLIN SODIUM
PENICILLIN G POTASSIUM, PENICILLIN G POTASSIUM
PENTIDS ',200', PENICILLIN G POTASSIUM
PENTIDS ',250', PENICILLIN G POTASSIUM
PENTIDS ',400', PENICILLIN G POTASSIUM
PENTIDS ',800', PENICILLIN G POTASSIUM
PRINCIPEN ',125', AMPICILLIN/AMPICILLIN TRIHYDRATE

PRINCIPEN ',250', AMPICILLIN/AMPICILLIN TRIHYDRATE
PRINCIPEN ',500', AMPICILLIN/AMPICILLIN TRIHYDRATE
PRINCIPEN W/ PROBENECID, AMPICILLIN/AMPICILLIN
    TRIHYDRATE
TRIMOX, AMOXICILLIN
VEETIDS ',125', PENICILLIN V POTASSIUM
VEETIDS ',250', PENICILLIN V POTASSIUM
VEETIDS ',500', PENICILLIN V POTASSIUM
VESPRIN, TRIFLUPROMAZINE
APOTHEKERNES
APOTHEKERNES LABORATORIUM A/S
BACITRACIN, BACITRACIN
APPLIED ANAL
APPLIED ANALYTICAL INDUSTRIES
    METHAZOLAMIDE, METHAZOLAMIDE
APPLIED ANALYTICAL INDUSTRIES INC
    ESTRADIOL, ESTRADIOL
ARBROOK
ARBROOK INC
    GAMOPHEN, HEXACHLOROPHENE
ARCUM
ARCUM PHARMACEUTICAL CORP
    VITAMIN A PALMITATE, VITAMIN A PALMITATE
ARMENPHARM
ARMENPHARM LTD
    MYCHEL, CHLORAMPHENICOL
ARMOUR PHARM
ARMOUR PHARMACEUTICAL CO
    ACTHAR GEL-SYNTHETIC, SERACTIDE ACETATE
    DEPINAR, CYANOCOBALAMIN
    ISOPROTERENOL HCL, ISOPROTERENOL
        HYDROCHLORIDE
    PENTACARINAT, PENTAMIDINE ISETHIONATE
ARMSTRONG PHARMS
ARMSTRONG PHARMACEUTICALS INC
    ALBUTEROL, ALBUTEROL
ASCENT PEDS
ASCENT PEDIATRICS INC
    ORAPRED, PREDNISOLONE SODIUM PHOSPHATE
    PRIMSOL, TRIMETHOPRIM HYDROCHLORIDE
ASCHER
BF ASCHER AND CO INC
    DRIZE, CHLORPHENIRAMINE MALEATE
    HY-PHEN, ACETAMINOPHEN
ASCOT
ASCOT HOSP PHARMACEUTICALS INC DIV TRAVENOL LA-
BORATORIES INC
    ACETAZOLAMIDE, ACETAZOLAMIDE
    AMINOPHYLLINE, AMINOPHYLLINE
    BETHANECHOL CHLORIDE, BETHANECHOL CHLORIDE
    CHLORDIAZEPOXIDE HCL, CHLORDIAZEPOXIDE
        HYDROCHLORIDE
    CHLORTHALIDONE, CHLORTHALIDONE
    CYPROHEPTADINE HCL, CYPROHEPTADINE
        HYDROCHLORIDE
    DIPHENOXYLATE HCL AND ATROPINE SULFATE,
        ATROPINE SULFATE
    HYDRALAZINE HCL, HYDRALAZINE HYDROCHLORIDE
    HYDROCHLOROTHIAZIDE, HYDROCHLOROTHIAZIDE
    METHOCARBAMOL, METHOCARBAMOL
    ORPHENADRINE CITRATE, ORPHENADRINE CITRATE
    PROCAINAMIDE HCL, PROCAINAMIDE
        HYDROCHLORIDE
    PROPANTHELINE BROMIDE, PROPANTHELINE
        BROMIDE
    QUINIDINE GLUCONATE, QUINIDINE GLUCONATE
    SPIRONOLACTONE + HYDROCHLOROTHIAZIDE,
        HYDROCHLOROTHIAZIDE

APPENDIX B
PRODUCT NAME INDEX
LISTED BY APPLICANT (*continued*)

SPIRONOLACTONE, SPIRONOLACTONE
SULFAMETHOXAZOLE, SULFAMETHOXAZOLE
TOLBUTAMIDE, TOLBUTAMIDE

ASLUNG PHARM
ASLUNG PHARMACEUTICAL LP
  IPRATROPIUM BROMIDE, IPRATROPIUM BROMIDE

ASTA
ASTA MEDICA INC
  TRAMADOL HCL, TRAMADOL HYDROCHLORIDE

ASTRAZENECA
ASTRAZENECA LP
  AMIKACIN SULFATE, AMIKACIN SULFATE
  AQUASOL A, VITAMIN A
  ASTRAMORPH PF, MORPHINE SULFATE
  BRETYLIUM TOSYLATE, BRETYLIUM TOSYLATE
  CALCITONIN-SALMON, CALCITONIN, SALMON
  CITANEST FORTE, EPINEPHRINE BITARTRATE
  CITANEST PLAIN, PRILOCAINE HYDROCHLORIDE
  CITANEST, PRILOCAINE HYDROCHLORIDE
  CLINDAMYCIN PHOSPHATE, CLINDAMYCIN
    PHOSPHATE
  DALGAN, DEZOCINE
  DOBUTAMINE HCL, DOBUTAMINE HYDROCHLORIDE
  DOPAMINE HCL, DOPAMINE HYDROCHLORIDE
  DROPERIDOL, DROPERIDOL
  DURANEST, EPINEPHRINE
  DURANEST, EPINEPHRINE BITARTRATE
  DURANEST, ETIDOCAINE HYDROCHLORIDE
  DYCLONE, DYCLONINE HYDROCHLORIDE
  EMLA, LIDOCAINE
  ENTOCORT EC, BUDESONIDE
  FENTANYL CITRATE AND DROPERIDOL, DROPERIDOL
  FOSCAVIR, FOSCARNET SODIUM
  FUROSEMIDE, FUROSEMIDE
  ISOETHARINE HCL, ISOETHARINE HYDROCHLORIDE
  M.V.I.-12 LYOPHILIZED, ASCORBIC ACID
  MANNITOL 25%, MANNITOL
  MEPERIDINE HCL PRESERVATIVE FREE, MEPERIDINE
    HYDROCHLORIDE
  MEPERIDINE HCL, MEPERIDINE HYDROCHLORIDE
  METAPROTERENOL SULFATE, METAPROTERENOL
    SULFATE
  NALBUPHINE HCL, NALBUPHINE HYDROCHLORIDE
  NALOXONE HCL, NALOXONE HYDROCHLORIDE
  NAROPIN, ROPIVACAINE HYDROCHLORIDE
    MONOHYDRATE
  NESACAINE, CHLOROPROCAINE HYDROCHLORIDE
  NESACAINE-MPF, CHLOROPROCAINE
    HYDROCHLORIDE
  NEXIUM, ESOMEPRAZOLE MAGNESIUM
  PANCURONIUM BROMIDE, PANCURONIUM BROMIDE
  POLOCAINE, MEPIVACAINE HYDROCHLORIDE
  POLOCAINE-MPF, MEPIVACAINE HYDROCHLORIDE
  PRILOSEC, OMEPRAZOLE
  PRILOSEC, OMEPRAZOLE MAGNESIUM (OTC)
  PULMICORT RESPULES, BUDESONIDE
  RHINOCORT, BUDESONIDE
  SENSORCAINE, BUPIVACAINE HYDROCHLORIDE
  SEROQUEL, QUETIAPINE FUMARATE
  TENORMIN, ATENOLOL
  TOBRAMYCIN SULFATE, TOBRAMYCIN SULFATE
  TOPROL-XL, METOPROLOL SUCCINATE
  XYLOCAINE 1.5% W/ DEXTROSE 7.5%, LIDOCAINE
    HYDROCHLORIDE
  XYLOCAINE 4% PRESERVATIVE FREE, LIDOCAINE
    HYDROCHLORIDE
  XYLOCAINE 5% W/ GLUCOSE 7.5%, LIDOCAINE
    HYDROCHLORIDE
  XYLOCAINE PRESERVATIVE FREE, LIDOCAINE
    HYDROCHLORIDE
  XYLOCAINE VISCOUS, LIDOCAINE HYDROCHLORIDE
  XYLOCAINE W/ EPINEPHRINE, EPINEPHRINE
  XYLOCAINE, LIDOCAINE
  XYLOCAINE, LIDOCAINE HYDROCHLORIDE
  YUTOPAR, RITODRINE HYDROCHLORIDE
ASTRAZENECA PHARMACEUTICALS LP
  ATACAND HCT, CANDESARTAN CILEXETIL
  ATACAND, CANDESARTAN CILEXETIL
  CEFOTAN IN PLASTIC CONTAINER, CEFOTETAN
    DISODIUM
  CEFOTAN, CEFOTETAN DISODIUM
  ELAVIL, AMITRIPTYLINE HYDROCHLORIDE
  FASLODEX, FULVESTRANT
  LEXXEL, ENALAPRIL MALEATE
  MIDAZOLAM HCL, MIDAZOLAM HYDROCHLORIDE
  NOLVADEX, TAMOXIFEN CITRATE
  PLENDIL, FELODIPINE
  PULMICORT, BUDESONIDE
  SORBITRATE, ISOSORBIDE DINITRATE
  TENORETIC 100, ATENOLOL
  TENORETIC 50, ATENOLOL
  TENORMIN, ATENOLOL
  TONOCARD, TOCAINIDE HYDROCHLORIDE
  ZOMIG-ZMT, ZOLMITRIPTAN
ASTRAZENECA UK LTD
  ACCOLATE, ZAFIRLUKAST
  ARIMIDEX, ANASTROZOLE
  CASODEX, BICALUTAMIDE
  DIPRIVAN, PROPOFOL
  IRESSA, GEFITINIB
  MERREM I.V., MEROPENEM
  ZESTORETIC, HYDROCHLOROTHIAZIDE
  ZESTRIL, LISINOPRIL
  ZOLADEX, GOSERELIN ACETATE

ATRIX
ATRIX LABORATORIES INC
  ATRIDOX, DOXYCYCLINE HYCLATE
  ELIGARD, LEUPROLIDE ACETATE

AUXILIUM A2
AUXILIUM A2 INC
  TESTIM, TESTOSTERONE

AVENTIS
AVENTIS PHARMACEUTICAL PRODUCTS INC
  ACTHAR, CORTICOTROPIN
  AZMACORT, TRIAMCINOLONE ACETONIDE
  AZOLID, PHENYLBUTAZONE
  CALCIMAR, CALCITONIN, SALMON
  CERUBIDINE, DAUNORUBICIN HYDROCHLORIDE
  DDAVP (NEEDS NO REFRIGERATION), DESMOPRESSIN
    ACETATE
  DDAVP, DESMOPRESSIN ACETATE
  DORIDEN, GLUTETHIMIDE
  INTAL, CROMOLYN SODIUM
  LOVENOX, ENOXAPARIN SODIUM
  LOZOL, INDAPAMIDE
  NASACORT AQ, TRIAMCINOLONE ACETONIDE
  NASACORT, TRIAMCINOLONE ACETONIDE
  NICOLAR, NIACIN
  PARATHAR, TERIPARATIDE ACETATE
  PENETREX, ENOXACIN
  PERTOFRANE, DESIPRAMINE HYDROCHLORIDE
  PRESAMINE, IMIPRAMINE HYDROCHLORIDE
  RILUTEK, RILUZOLE
  SLO-BID, THEOPHYLLINE
  SLO-PHYLLIN, THEOPHYLLINE
  THYTROPAR, THYROTROPIN

APPENDIX B
PRODUCT NAME INDEX
LISTED BY APPLICANT (*continued*)

TILADE, NEDOCROMIL SODIUM

AVENTIS BEHRING
AVENTIS BEHRING LLC
   FLURBIPROFEN SODIUM, FLURBIPROFEN SODIUM
   STIMATE, DESMOPRESSIN ACETATE

AVENTIS PHARMS
AVENTIS PHARMACEUTICALS INC
   A/T/S, ERYTHROMYCIN
   ACCURBRON, THEOPHYLLINE
   ALLEGRA, FEXOFENADINE HYDROCHLORIDE
   ALLEGRA-D, FEXOFENADINE HYDROCHLORIDE
   AMARYL, GLIMEPIRIDE
   ANZEMET, DOLASETRON MESYLATE MONOHYDRATE
   ARAVA, LEFLUNOMIDE
   BENDECTIN, DOXYLAMINE SUCCINATE
   BENTYL PRESERVATIVE FREE, DICYCLOMINE
      HYDROCHLORIDE
   BENTYL, DICYCLOMINE HYDROCHLORIDE
   BRICANYL, TERBUTALINE SULFATE
   CANTIL, MEPENZOLATE BROMIDE
   CARAFATE, SUCRALFATE
   CARDIZEM CD, DILTIAZEM HYDROCHLORIDE
   CARDIZEM SR, DILTIAZEM HYDROCHLORIDE
   CARDIZEM, DILTIAZEM HYDROCHLORIDE
   CEPHULAC, LACTULOSE
   CHRONULAC, LACTULOSE
   CLAFORAN IN DEXTROSE 5% IN PLASTIC CONTAINER,
      CEFOTAXIME SODIUM
   CLAFORAN IN SODIUM CHLORIDE 0.9% IN PLASTIC
      CONTAINER, CEFOTAXIME SODIUM
   CLAFORAN, CEFOTAXIME SODIUM
   CLOMID, CLOMIPHENE CITRATE
   CYANOCOBALAMIN, CYANOCOBALAMIN
   DECAPRYN, DOXYLAMINE SUCCINATE
   DEMI-REGROTON, CHLORTHALIDONE
   DIABETA, GLYBURIDE
   DV, DIENESTROL
   GAVISCON, ALUMINUM HYDROXIDE (OTC)
   GLYBURIDE (MICRONIZED), GLYBURIDE
   HEDULIN, PHENINDIONE
   HIPREX, METHENAMINE HIPPURATE
   HYDROXYSTILBAMIDINE ISETHIONATE,
      HYDROXYSTILBAMIDINE ISETHIONATE
   HYGROTON, CHLORTHALIDONE
   INTAL, CROMOLYN SODIUM
   IPRIVASK, DESIRUDIN
   LANTUS, INSULIN GLARGINE
   LASIX, FUROSEMIDE
   LORELCO, PROBUCOL
   METAHYDRIN, TRICHLORMETHIAZIDE
   METATENSIN #2, RESERPINE
   METATENSIN #4, RESERPINE
   NICODERM CQ, NICOTINE (OTC)
   NILANDRON, NILUTAMIDE
   NITRO-BID, NITROGLYCERIN
   NORPRAMIN, DESIPRAMINE HYDROCHLORIDE
   NOVAFED, PSEUDOEPHEDRINE HYDROCHLORIDE
   ORNIDYL, EFLORNITHINE HYDROCHLORIDE
   PRIFTIN, RIFAPENTINE
   REGROTON, CHLORTHALIDONE
   RIFADIN, RIFAMPIN
   RIFAMATE, ISONIAZID
   RIFATER, ISONIAZID
   TACE, CHLOROTRIANISENE
   TAXOTERE, DOCETAXEL
   TENUATE DOSPAN, DIETHYLPROPION
      HYDROCHLORIDE
   TENUATE, DIETHYLPROPION HYDROCHLORIDE

   TRENTAL, PENTOXIFYLLINE
   TRICLOS, TRICLOFOS SODIUM
   VANOBID, CANDICIDIN
   VENTAIRE, PROTOKYLOL HYDROCHLORIDE

AXCAN SCANDIPHARM
AXCAN SCANDIPHARM INC
   CANASA, MESALAMINE
   CHENIX, CHENODIOL
   PHOTOFRIN, PORFIMER SODIUM
   URSO, URSODIOL

AXIOM PHARM
AXIOM PHARMACEUTICAL CORP
   BUTALBITAL, APAP, AND CAFFEINE, ACETAMINOPHEN
   DOXYCYCLINE HYCLATE, DOXYCYCLINE HYCLATE
   DOXYCYCLINE HYLATE, DOXYCYCLINE HYCLATE
   DOXYCYCLINE, DOXYCYCLINE
   HYDROCODONE BITARTRATE AND ACETAMINOPHEN,
      ACETAMINOPHEN
   HYDROCODONE BITARTRATE AND HOMATROPINE
      METHYLBROMIDE, HOMATROPINE
      METHYLBROMIDE
   ISONIAZID, ISONIAZID
   MEPERIDINE HCL, MEPERIDINE HYDROCHLORIDE
   OXYCODONE AND ACETAMINOPHEN, ACETAMINOPHEN
   OXYCODONE AND ASPIRIN, ASPIRIN
   PREDNISOLONE, PREDNISOLONE
   TETRACYCLINE HCL, TETRACYCLINE HYDROCHLORIDE

AYERST
AYERST LABORATORIES INC
   PHOSPHOLINE IODIDE, ECHOTHIOPHATE IODIDE

B

B BRAUN
B BRAUN MEDICAL INC
   ACETATED RINGER'S IN PLASTIC CONTAINER, CALCIUM
      CHLORIDE
   ACETIC ACID 0.25% IN PLASTIC CONTAINER, ACETIC
      ACID, GLACIAL
   ALCOHOL 10% AND DEXTROSE 5%, ALCOHOL
   ALCOHOL 5% AND DEXTROSE 5%, ALCOHOL
   AMMONIUM CHLORIDE 2.14%, AMMONIUM CHLORIDE
   BRETYLIUM TOSYLATE IN DEXTROSE 5% IN PLASTIC
      CONTAINER, BRETYLIUM TOSYLATE
   CEFAZOLIN AND DEXTROSE, CEFAZOLIN SODIUM
   CEFUROXIME AND DEXTROSE IN DUPLEX CONTAINER,
      CEFUROXIME SODIUM
   DEXTROSE 10% AND SODIUM CHLORIDE 0.11% IN
      PLASTIC CONTAINER, DEXTROSE
   DEXTROSE 10% AND SODIUM CHLORIDE 0.2% IN
      PLASTIC CONTAINER, DEXTROSE
   DEXTROSE 10% AND SODIUM CHLORIDE 0.33% IN
      PLASTIC CONTAINER, DEXTROSE
   DEXTROSE 10% AND SODIUM CHLORIDE 0.45% IN
      PLASTIC CONTAINER, DEXTROSE
   DEXTROSE 10% AND SODIUM CHLORIDE 0.9% IN
      PLASTIC CONTAINER, DEXTROSE
   DEXTROSE 10% IN PLASTIC CONTAINER, DEXTROSE
   DEXTROSE 2.5% AND SODIUM CHLORIDE 0.11% IN
      PLASTIC CONTAINER, DEXTROSE
   DEXTROSE 2.5% AND SODIUM CHLORIDE 0.2% IN
      PLASTIC CONTAINER, DEXTROSE
   DEXTROSE 2.5% AND SODIUM CHLORIDE 0.33% IN
      PLASTIC CONTAINER, DEXTROSE
   DEXTROSE 2.5% AND SODIUM CHLORIDE 0.45% IN
      PLASTIC CONTAINER, DEXTROSE

APPENDIX B
PRODUCT NAME INDEX
LISTED BY APPLICANT (*continued*)

DEXTROSE 2.5% AND SODIUM CHLORIDE 0.9% IN PLASTIC CONTAINER, DEXTROSE

DEXTROSE 2.5% IN HALF-STRENGTH LACTATED RINGER'S IN PLASTIC CONTAINER, CALCIUM CHLORIDE

DEXTROSE 2.5% IN PLASTIC CONTAINER, DEXTROSE

DEXTROSE 3.3% AND SODIUM CHLORIDE 0.3% IN PLASTIC CONTAINER, DEXTROSE

DEXTROSE 4% IN MODIFIED LACTATED RINGER'S IN PLASTIC CONTAINER, CALCIUM CHLORIDE

DEXTROSE 5% AND SODIUM CHLORIDE 0.11% IN PLASTIC CONTAINER, DEXTROSE

DEXTROSE 5% AND SODIUM CHLORIDE 0.2% IN PLASTIC CONTAINER, DEXTROSE

DEXTROSE 5% AND SODIUM CHLORIDE 0.33% IN PLASTIC CONTAINER, DEXTROSE

DEXTROSE 5% AND SODIUM CHLORIDE 0.45% IN PLASTIC CONTAINER, DEXTROSE

DEXTROSE 5% AND SODIUM CHLORIDE 0.9% IN PLASTIC CONTAINER, DEXTROSE

DEXTROSE 5% IN ACETATED RINGER'S IN PLASTIC CONTAINER, CALCIUM CHLORIDE

DEXTROSE 5% IN LACTATED RINGER'S IN PLASTIC CONTAINER, CALCIUM CHLORIDE

DEXTROSE 5% IN PLASTIC CONTAINER, DEXTROSE

DEXTROSE 5% IN RINGER'S IN PLASTIC CONTAINER, CALCIUM CHLORIDE

DEXTROSE 5%, SODIUM CHLORIDE 0.2% AND POTASSIUM CHLORIDE 0.075%, DEXTROSE

DEXTROSE 5%, SODIUM CHLORIDE 0.2% AND POTASSIUM CHLORIDE 0.15% IN PLASTIC CONTAINER, DEXTROSE

DEXTROSE 5%, SODIUM CHLORIDE 0.2% AND POTASSIUM CHLORIDE 0.224% IN PLASTIC CONTAINER, DEXTROSE

DEXTROSE 5%, SODIUM CHLORIDE 0.2% AND POTASSIUM CHLORIDE 0.3% IN PLASTIC CONTAINER, DEXTROSE

DEXTROSE 5%, SODIUM CHLORIDE 0.33% AND POTASSIUM CHLORIDE 0.075% IN PLASTIC CONTAINER, DEXTROSE

DEXTROSE 5%, SODIUM CHLORIDE 0.33% AND POTASSIUM CHLORIDE 0.15% IN PLASTIC CONTAINER, DEXTROSE

DEXTROSE 5%, SODIUM CHLORIDE 0.33% AND POTASSIUM CHLORIDE 0.22% IN PLASTIC CONTAINER, DEXTROSE

DEXTROSE 5%, SODIUM CHLORIDE 0.33% AND POTASSIUM CHLORIDE 0.30% IN PLASTIC CONTAINER, DEXTROSE

DEXTROSE 5%, SODIUM CHLORIDE 0.45% AND POTASSIUM CHLORIDE 0.075%, DEXTROSE

DEXTROSE 5%, SODIUM CHLORIDE 0.45% AND POTASSIUM CHLORIDE 0.15% IN PLASTIC CONTAINER, DEXTROSE

DEXTROSE 5%, SODIUM CHLORIDE 0.45% AND POTASSIUM CHLORIDE 0.22% IN PLASTIC CONTAINER, DEXTROSE

DEXTROSE 5%, SODIUM CHLORIDE 0.45% AND POTASSIUM CHLORIDE 0.3% IN PLASTIC CONTAINER, DEXTROSE

DEXTROSE 60% IN PLASTIC CONTAINER, DEXTROSE

DEXTROSE 60%, DEXTROSE

DEXTROSE 7.7% IN PLASTIC CONTAINER, DEXTROSE

DIALYTE CONCENTRATE W/ DEXTROSE 30% IN PLASTIC CONTAINER, CALCIUM CHLORIDE

DIALYTE CONCENTRATE W/ DEXTROSE 50% IN PLASTIC CONTAINER, CALCIUM CHLORIDE

DIALYTE LM/ DEXTROSE 1.5% IN PLASTIC CONTAINER, CALCIUM CHLORIDE

DIALYTE LM/ DEXTROSE 2.5% IN PLASTIC CONTAINER, CALCIUM CHLORIDE

DIALYTE LM/ DEXTROSE 4.25% IN PLASTIC CONTAINER, CALCIUM CHLORIDE

DIALYTE W/ DEXTROSE 1.5% IN PLASTIC CONTAINER, CALCIUM CHLORIDE

DIALYTE W/ DEXTROSE 4.25% IN PLASTIC CONTAINER, CALCIUM CHLORIDE

DOPAMINE HCL AND DEXTROSE 5% IN PLASTIC CONTAINER, DOPAMINE HYDROCHLORIDE

DOPAMINE HCL AND DEXTROSE 5%, DOPAMINE HYDROCHLORIDE

FREAMINE 8.5%, AMINO ACIDS

FREAMINE HBC 6.9%, AMINO ACIDS

FREAMINE II 8.5%, AMINO ACIDS

FREAMINE III 10%, AMINO ACIDS

FREAMINE III 3% W/ ELECTROLYTES, AMINO ACIDS

FREAMINE III 8.5% W/ ELECTROLYTES, AMINO ACIDS

FREAMINE III 8.5%, AMINO ACIDS

GENTAMICIN SULFATE IN SODIUM CHLORIDE 0.9% IN PLASTIC CONTAINER, GENTAMICIN SULFATE

GLYCINE 1.5% IN PLASTIC CONTAINER, GLYCINE

HEPARIN SODIUM 1,000 UNITS IN SODIUM CHLORIDE 0.9% IN PLASTIC CONTAINER, HEPARIN SODIUM

HEPARIN SODIUM 12,500 UNITS IN SODIUM CHLORIDE 0.45% IN PLASTIC CONTAINER, HEPARIN SODIUM

HEPARIN SODIUM 2,000 UNITS IN SODIUM CHLORIDE 0.9% IN PLASTIC CONTAINER, HEPARIN SODIUM

HEPARIN SODIUM 20,000 UNITS IN DEXTROSE 5% IN PLASTIC CONTAINER, HEPARIN SODIUM

HEPARIN SODIUM 25,000 UNITS IN DEXTROSE 5% IN PLASTIC CONTAINER, HEPARIN SODIUM

HEPARIN SODIUM 25,000 UNITS IN SODIUM CHLORIDE 0.45% IN PLASTIC CONTAINER, HEPARIN SODIUM

HEPARIN SODIUM 25,000 UNITS IN SODIUM CHLORIDE 0.9% IN PLASTIC CONTAINER, HEPARIN SODIUM

HEPARIN SODIUM 5,000 UNITS IN SODIUM CHLORIDE 0.9% IN PLASTIC CONTAINER, HEPARIN SODIUM

HEPATAMINE 8%, AMINO ACIDS

HYPROTIGEN 5%, PROTEIN HYDROLYSATE

ISOLYTE E IN DEXTROSE 5% IN PLASTIC CONTAINER, CALCIUM CHLORIDE

ISOLYTE E IN PLASTIC CONTAINER, CALCIUM CHLORIDE

ISOLYTE E W/ DEXTROSE 5% IN PLASTIC CONTAINER, CALCIUM CHLORIDE

ISOLYTE H IN DEXTROSE 5% IN PLASTIC CONTAINER, DEXTROSE

ISOLYTE H W/ DEXTROSE 5% IN PLASTIC CONTAINER, DEXTROSE

ISOLYTE M IN DEXTROSE 5% IN PLASTIC CONTAINER, DEXTROSE

ISOLYTE M W/ DEXTROSE 5% IN PLASTIC CONTAINER, DEXTROSE

ISOLYTE P IN DEXTROSE 5% IN PLASTIC CONTAINER, DEXTROSE

ISOLYTE P W/ DEXTROSE 5% IN PLASTIC CONTAINER, DEXTROSE

ISOLYTE R IN DEXTROSE 5% IN PLASTIC CONTAINER, CALCIUM CHLORIDE

ISOLYTE R W/ DEXTROSE 5% IN PLASTIC CONTAINER, CALCIUM CHLORIDE

ISOLYTE S IN DEXTROSE 5% IN PLASTIC CONTAINER, DEXTROSE

ISOLYTE S IN PLASTIC CONTAINER, MAGNESIUM CHLORIDE

APPENDIX B
PRODUCT NAME INDEX
LISTED BY APPLICANT (*continued*)

ISOLYTE S PH 7.4 IN PLASTIC CONTAINER, MAGNESIUM CHLORIDE
ISOLYTE S W/ DEXTROSE 5% IN PLASTIC CONTAINER, DEXTROSE
LACTATED RINGER'S IN PLASTIC CONTAINER, CALCIUM CHLORIDE
LIDOCAINE HCL 0.2% AND DEXTROSE 5% IN PLASTIC CONTAINER, LIDOCAINE HYDROCHLORIDE
LIDOCAINE HCL 0.4% AND DEXTROSE 5% IN PLASTIC CONTAINER, LIDOCAINE HYDROCHLORIDE
LIDOCAINE HCL 0.8% AND DEXTROSE 5% IN PLASTIC CONTAINER, LIDOCAINE HYDROCHLORIDE
MANNITOL 10% IN PLASTIC CONTAINER, MANNITOL
MANNITOL 10% W/ DEXTROSE 5% IN DISTILLED WATER, MANNITOL
MANNITOL 10%, MANNITOL
MANNITOL 15% IN PLASTIC CONTAINER, MANNITOL
MANNITOL 15% W/ DEXTROSE 5% IN SODIUM CHLORIDE 0.45%, MANNITOL
MANNITOL 15%, MANNITOL
MANNITOL 20% IN PLASTIC CONTAINER, MANNITOL
MANNITOL 20%, MANNITOL
MANNITOL 5% IN PLASTIC CONTAINER, MANNITOL
MANNITOL 5% W/ DEXTROSE 5% IN SODIUM CHLORIDE 0.12%, MANNITOL
MANNITOL 5%, MANNITOL
METRO I.V. IN PLASTIC CONTAINER, METRONIDAZOLE
METRO I.V., METRONIDAZOLE
NEPHRAMINE 5.4%, AMINO ACIDS
NUTRILIPID 10%, SOYBEAN OIL
NUTRILIPID 20%, SOYBEAN OIL
PHYSIOLYTE IN PLASTIC CONTAINER, MAGNESIUM CHLORIDE
POTASSIUM CHLORIDE 0.037% IN DEXTROSE 10% AND SODIUM CHLORIDE 0.2% IN PLASTIC CONTAINER, DEXTROSE
POTASSIUM CHLORIDE 0.037% IN DEXTROSE 10% AND SODIUM CHLORIDE 0.45% IN PLASTIC CONTAINER, DEXTROSE
POTASSIUM CHLORIDE 0.037% IN DEXTROSE 10% AND SODIUM CHLORIDE 0.9% IN PLASTIC CONTAINER, DEXTROSE
POTASSIUM CHLORIDE 0.037% IN DEXTROSE 5% AND SODIUM CHLORIDE 0.11% IN PLASTIC CONTAINER, DEXTROSE
POTASSIUM CHLORIDE 0.037% IN DEXTROSE 5% AND SODIUM CHLORIDE 0.2% IN PLASTIC CONTAINER, DEXTROSE
POTASSIUM CHLORIDE 0.037% IN DEXTROSE 5% AND SODIUM CHLORIDE 0.33% IN PLASTIC CONTAINER, DEXTROSE
POTASSIUM CHLORIDE 0.037% IN DEXTROSE 5% AND SODIUM CHLORIDE 0.45% IN PLASTIC CONTAINER, DEXTROSE
POTASSIUM CHLORIDE 0.037% IN DEXTROSE 5% AND SODIUM CHLORIDE 0.9% IN PLASTIC CONTAINER, DEXTROSE
POTASSIUM CHLORIDE 0.037% IN DEXTROSE 5% IN PLASTIC CONTAINER, DEXTROSE
POTASSIUM CHLORIDE 0.037% IN SODIUM CHLORIDE 0.9% IN PLASTIC CONTAINER, POTASSIUM CHLORIDE
POTASSIUM CHLORIDE 0.075% IN DEXTROSE 10% AND SODIUM CHLORIDE 0.2% IN PLASTIC CONTAINER, DEXTROSE
POTASSIUM CHLORIDE 0.075% IN DEXTROSE 10% AND SODIUM CHLORIDE 0.45% IN PLASTIC CONTAINER, DEXTROSE

POTASSIUM CHLORIDE 0.075% IN DEXTROSE 10% AND SODIUM CHLORIDE 0.9% IN PLASTIC CONTAINER, DEXTROSE
POTASSIUM CHLORIDE 0.075% IN DEXTROSE 3.3% AND SODIUM CHLORIDE 0.3% IN PLASTIC CONTAINER, DEXTROSE
POTASSIUM CHLORIDE 0.075% IN DEXTROSE 5% AND SODIUM CHLORIDE 0.11% IN PLASTIC CONTAINER, DEXTROSE
POTASSIUM CHLORIDE 0.075% IN DEXTROSE 5% AND SODIUM CHLORIDE 0.2% IN PLASTIC CONTAINER, DEXTROSE
POTASSIUM CHLORIDE 0.075% IN DEXTROSE 5% AND SODIUM CHLORIDE 0.33% IN PLASTIC CONTAINER, DEXTROSE
POTASSIUM CHLORIDE 0.075% IN DEXTROSE 5% AND SODIUM CHLORIDE 0.45% IN PLASTIC CONTAINER, DEXTROSE
POTASSIUM CHLORIDE 0.075% IN DEXTROSE 5% AND SODIUM CHLORIDE 0.9% IN PLASTIC CONTAINER, DEXTROSE
POTASSIUM CHLORIDE 0.075% IN DEXTROSE 5% IN PLASTIC CONTAINER, DEXTROSE
POTASSIUM CHLORIDE 0.075% IN SODIUM CHLORIDE 0.9% IN PLASTIC CONTAINER, POTASSIUM CHLORIDE
POTASSIUM CHLORIDE 0.11% IN DEXTROSE 10% AND SODIUM CHLORIDE 0.2% IN PLASTIC CONTAINER, DEXTROSE
POTASSIUM CHLORIDE 0.11% IN DEXTROSE 10% AND SODIUM CHLORIDE 0.45% IN PLASTIC CONTAINER, DEXTROSE
POTASSIUM CHLORIDE 0.11% IN DEXTROSE 10% AND SODIUM CHLORIDE 0.9% IN PLASTIC CONTAINER, DEXTROSE
POTASSIUM CHLORIDE 0.11% IN DEXTROSE 3.3% AND SODIUM CHLORIDE 0.3% IN PLASTIC CONTAINER, DEXTROSE
POTASSIUM CHLORIDE 0.11% IN DEXTROSE 5% AND SODIUM CHLORIDE 0.11% IN PLASTIC CONTAINER, DEXTROSE
POTASSIUM CHLORIDE 0.11% IN DEXTROSE 5% AND SODIUM CHLORIDE 0.2% IN PLASTIC CONTAINER, DEXTROSE
POTASSIUM CHLORIDE 0.11% IN DEXTROSE 5% AND SODIUM CHLORIDE 0.33% IN PLASTIC CONTAINER, DEXTROSE
POTASSIUM CHLORIDE 0.11% IN DEXTROSE 5% AND SODIUM CHLORIDE 0.45% IN PLASTIC CONTAINER, DEXTROSE
POTASSIUM CHLORIDE 0.11% IN DEXTROSE 5% AND SODIUM CHLORIDE 0.9% IN PLASTIC CONTAINER, DEXTROSE
POTASSIUM CHLORIDE 0.11% IN DEXTROSE 5% IN PLASTIC CONTAINER, DEXTROSE
POTASSIUM CHLORIDE 0.11% IN SODIUM CHLORIDE 0.9% IN PLASTIC CONTAINER, POTASSIUM CHLORIDE
POTASSIUM CHLORIDE 0.15% IN DEXTROSE 10% AND SODIUM CHLORIDE 0.2% IN PLASTIC CONTAINER, DEXTROSE
POTASSIUM CHLORIDE 0.15% IN DEXTROSE 10% AND SODIUM CHLORIDE 0.45% IN PLASTIC CONTAINER, DEXTROSE
POTASSIUM CHLORIDE 0.15% IN DEXTROSE 10% AND SODIUM CHLORIDE 0.9% IN PLASTIC CONTAINER, DEXTROSE

APPENDIX B
PRODUCT NAME INDEX
LISTED BY APPLICANT (*continued*)

POTASSIUM CHLORIDE 0.15% IN DEXTROSE 3.3% AND SODIUM CHLORIDE 0.3% IN PLASTIC CONTAINER, DEXTROSE

POTASSIUM CHLORIDE 0.15% IN DEXTROSE 5% AND SODIUM CHLORIDE 0.11% IN PLASTIC CONTAINER, DEXTROSE

POTASSIUM CHLORIDE 0.15% IN DEXTROSE 5% AND SODIUM CHLORIDE 0.2% IN PLASTIC CONTAINER, DEXTROSE

POTASSIUM CHLORIDE 0.15% IN DEXTROSE 5% AND SODIUM CHLORIDE 0.33% IN PLASTIC CONTAINER, DEXTROSE

POTASSIUM CHLORIDE 0.15% IN DEXTROSE 5% AND SODIUM CHLORIDE 0.45% IN PLASTIC CONTAINER, DEXTROSE

POTASSIUM CHLORIDE 0.15% IN DEXTROSE 5% AND SODIUM CHLORIDE 0.9% IN PLASTIC CONTAINER, DEXTROSE

POTASSIUM CHLORIDE 0.15% IN DEXTROSE 5% IN PLASTIC CONTAINER, DEXTROSE

POTASSIUM CHLORIDE 0.15% IN SODIUM CHLORIDE 0.9% IN PLASTIC CONTAINER, POTASSIUM CHLORIDE

POTASSIUM CHLORIDE 0.22% IN DEXTROSE 10% AND SODIUM CHLORIDE 0.2% IN PLASTIC CONTAINER, DEXTROSE

POTASSIUM CHLORIDE 0.22% IN DEXTROSE 10% AND SODIUM CHLORIDE 0.45% IN PLASTIC CONTAINER, DEXTROSE

POTASSIUM CHLORIDE 0.22% IN DEXTROSE 10% AND SODIUM CHLORIDE 0.9% IN PLASTIC CONTAINER, DEXTROSE

POTASSIUM CHLORIDE 0.22% IN DEXTROSE 3.3% AND SODIUM CHLORIDE 0.3% IN PLASTIC CONTAINER, DEXTROSE

POTASSIUM CHLORIDE 0.22% IN DEXTROSE 5% AND SODIUM CHLORIDE 0.11% IN PLASTIC CONTAINER, DEXTROSE

POTASSIUM CHLORIDE 0.22% IN DEXTROSE 5% AND SODIUM CHLORIDE 0.2% IN PLASTIC CONTAINER, DEXTROSE

POTASSIUM CHLORIDE 0.22% IN DEXTROSE 5% AND SODIUM CHLORIDE 0.33% IN PLASTIC CONTAINER, DEXTROSE

POTASSIUM CHLORIDE 0.22% IN DEXTROSE 5% AND SODIUM CHLORIDE 0.45% IN PLASTIC CONTAINER, DEXTROSE

POTASSIUM CHLORIDE 0.22% IN DEXTROSE 5% AND SODIUM CHLORIDE 0.9% IN PLASTIC CONTAINER, DEXTROSE

POTASSIUM CHLORIDE 0.22% IN DEXTROSE 5% IN PLASTIC CONTAINER, DEXTROSE

POTASSIUM CHLORIDE 0.22% IN SODIUM CHLORIDE 0.9% IN PLASTIC CONTAINER, POTASSIUM CHLORIDE

POTASSIUM CHLORIDE 0.3% IN DEXTROSE 10% AND SODIUM CHLORIDE 0.2% IN PLASTIC CONTAINER, DEXTROSE

POTASSIUM CHLORIDE 0.3% IN DEXTROSE 10% AND SODIUM CHLORIDE 0.45% IN PLASTIC CONTAINER, DEXTROSE

POTASSIUM CHLORIDE 0.3% IN DEXTROSE 10% AND SODIUM CHLORIDE 0.9% IN PLASTIC CONTAINER, DEXTROSE

POTASSIUM CHLORIDE 0.3% IN DEXTROSE 3.3% AND SODIUM CHLORIDE 0.3% IN PLASTIC CONTAINER, DEXTROSE

POTASSIUM CHLORIDE 0.3% IN DEXTROSE 5% AND SODIUM CHLORIDE 0.11% IN PLASTIC CONTAINER, DEXTROSE

POTASSIUM CHLORIDE 0.3% IN DEXTROSE 5% AND SODIUM CHLORIDE 0.2% IN PLASTIC CONTAINER, DEXTROSE

POTASSIUM CHLORIDE 0.3% IN DEXTROSE 5% AND SODIUM CHLORIDE 0.33% IN PLASTIC CONTAINER, DEXTROSE

POTASSIUM CHLORIDE 0.3% IN DEXTROSE 5% AND SODIUM CHLORIDE 0.45% IN PLASTIC CONTAINER, DEXTROSE

POTASSIUM CHLORIDE 0.3% IN DEXTROSE 5% AND SODIUM CHLORIDE 0.9% IN PLASTIC CONTAINER, DEXTROSE

POTASSIUM CHLORIDE 0.3% IN DEXTROSE 5% IN PLASTIC CONTAINER, DEXTROSE

POTASSIUM CHLORIDE 0.3% IN SODIUM CHLORIDE 0.9% IN PLASTIC CONTAINER, POTASSIUM CHLORIDE

POTASSIUM CHLORIDE, POTASSIUM CHLORIDE

PROCALAMINE, AMINO ACIDS

RESECTISOL IN PLASTIC CONTAINER, MANNITOL

RESECTISOL, MANNITOL

RINGER'S IN PLASTIC CONTAINER, CALCIUM CHLORIDE

SODIUM CHLORIDE 0.45% IN PLASTIC CONTAINER, SODIUM CHLORIDE

SODIUM CHLORIDE 0.9% AND POTASSIUM CHLORIDE 0.075% IN PLASTIC CONTAINER, POTASSIUM CHLORIDE

SODIUM CHLORIDE 0.9% AND POTASSIUM CHLORIDE 0.15% IN PLASTIC CONTAINER, POTASSIUM CHLORIDE

SODIUM CHLORIDE 0.9% AND POTASSIUM CHLORIDE 0.22% IN PLASTIC CONTAINER, POTASSIUM CHLORIDE

SODIUM CHLORIDE 0.9% AND POTASSIUM CHLORIDE 0.3% IN PLASTIC CONTAINER, POTASSIUM CHLORIDE

SODIUM CHLORIDE 0.9% IN PLASTIC CONTAINER, SODIUM CHLORIDE

SODIUM CHLORIDE 3% IN PLASTIC CONTAINER, SODIUM CHLORIDE

SODIUM CHLORIDE 5% IN PLASTIC CONTAINER, SODIUM CHLORIDE

SODIUM CHLORIDE, SODIUM CHLORIDE

SODIUM LACTATE 0.167 MOLAR IN PLASTIC CONTAINER, SODIUM LACTATE

SODIUM LACTATE 1/6 MOLAR IN PLASTIC CONTAINER, SODIUM LACTATE

SORBITOL 3.3% IN PLASTIC CONTAINER, SORBITOL

STERILE WATER FOR INJECTION IN PLASTIC CONTAINER, WATER FOR INJECTION, STERILE

STERILE WATER IN PLASTIC CONTAINER, WATER FOR IRRIGATION, STERILE

THEOPHYLLINE 0.04% AND DEXTROSE 5% IN PLASTIC CONTAINER, THEOPHYLLINE

THEOPHYLLINE 0.08% AND DEXTROSE 5% IN PLASTIC CONTAINER, THEOPHYLLINE

THEOPHYLLINE 0.16% AND DEXTROSE 5% IN PLASTIC CONTAINER, THEOPHYLLINE

THEOPHYLLINE 0.2% AND DEXTROSE 5% IN PLASTIC CONTAINER, THEOPHYLLINE

THEOPHYLLINE 0.32% AND DEXTROSE 5% IN PLASTIC CONTAINER, THEOPHYLLINE

THEOPHYLLINE 0.4% AND DEXTROSE 5% IN PLASTIC CONTAINER, THEOPHYLLINE

TROPHAMINE 10%, AMINO ACIDS

APPENDIX B
PRODUCT NAME INDEX
LISTED BY APPLICANT (*continued*)

TROPHAMINE, AMINO ACIDS
UCEPHAN, SODIUM BENZOATE

BAKER NORTON

BAKER NORTON
  PROGLYCEM, DIAZOXIDE
BAKER NORTON PHARMACEUTICALS INC
  ACTICORT, HYDROCORTISONE
  PACLITAXEL, PACLITAXEL
  PROGLYCEM, DIAZOXIDE

BALLARD MEDCL

BALLARD MEDICAL PRODUCTS INC
  PYTEST KIT, UREA, C-14
  PYTEST, UREA, C-14

BANNER PHARMACAPS

BANNER PHARMACAPS INC
  BENZONATATE, BENZONATATE
  CHLOROTRIANISENE, CHLOROTRIANISENE
  CLOFIBRATE, CLOFIBRATE
  ETHCHLORVYNOL, ETHCHLORVYNOL
  ETHOSUXIMIDE, ETHOSUXIMIDE
  IBUPROFEN, IBUPROFEN (OTC)
  VALPROIC ACID, VALPROIC ACID
  VITAMIN A PALMITATE, VITAMIN A PALMITATE
  VITAMIN A, VITAMIN A
  VITAMIN A, VITAMIN A PALMITATE
  VITAMIN D, ERGOCALCIFEROL

BARLAN

BARLAN PHARMACAL CO INC
  BARSTATIN 100, NYSTATIN

BARR

BARR LABORATORIES INC
  ACETOHEXAMIDE, ACETOHEXAMIDE
  AMILORIDE HCL AND HYDROCHLOROTHIAZIDE,
    AMILORIDE HYDROCHLORIDE
  AMINOPHYLLINE, AMINOPHYLLINE
  AMIODARONE HCL, AMIODARONE HYDROCHLORIDE
  BROMPHENIRAMINE MALEATE, BROMPHENIRAMINE
    MALEATE
  CAMILA, NORETHINDRONE
  CEFADROXIL, CEFADROXIL/CEFADROXIL
    HEMIHYDRATE
  CEPHALEXIN, CEPHALEXIN
  CEPHRADINE, CEPHRADINE
  CHLORDIAZEPOXIDE HCL, CHLORDIAZEPOXIDE
    HYDROCHLORIDE
  CHLORPROPAMIDE, CHLORPROPAMIDE
  CHLORZOXAZONE, CHLORZOXAZONE
  CLARAVIS, ISOTRETINOIN
  CORTISONE ACETATE, CORTISONE ACETATE
  DANAZOL, DANAZOL
  DEXTROAMP SACCHARATE, AMP ASPARTATE,
    DEXTROAMP SULFATE AND AMP SULFATE,
    AMPHETAMINE ASPARTATE
  DEXTROAMPHETAMINE SULFATE,
    DEXTROAMPHETAMINE SULFATE
  DIAZEPAM, DIAZEPAM
  DIPHENHYDRAMINE HCL, DIPHENHYDRAMINE
    HYDROCHLORIDE
  DIPYRIDAMOLE, DIPYRIDAMOLE
  E-BASE, ERYTHROMYCIN
  ERRIN, NORETHINDRONE
  ERYTHROMYCIN ESTOLATE, ERYTHROMYCIN
    ESTOLATE
  ERYTHROMYCIN ETHYLSUCCINATE AND
    SULFISOXAZOLE ACETYL, ERYTHROMYCIN
    ETHYLSUCCINATE
  ERYTHROMYCIN ETHYLSUCCINATE, ERYTHROMYCIN
    ETHYLSUCCINATE

ERYTHROMYCIN STEARATE, ERYTHROMYCIN
  STEARATE
ERYTHROMYCIN, ERYTHROMYCIN
ESTRADIOL, ESTRADIOL
ESTROPIPATE, ESTROPIPATE
ETHAMBUTOL HCL, ETHAMBUTOL HYDROCHLORIDE
EXTENDED PHENYTOIN SODIUM, PHENYTOIN SODIUM,
  EXTENDED
FLECAINIDE ACETATE, FLECAINIDE ACETATE
FLUDROCORTISONE ACETATE, FLUDROCORTISONE
  ACETATE
FLUOXETINE HCL, FLUOXETINE HYDROCHLORIDE
FLUOXETINE, FLUOXETINE HYDROCHLORIDE
FLUTAMIDE, FLUTAMIDE
FLUVOXAMINE MALEATE, FLUVOXAMINE MALEATE
FOLIC ACID, FOLIC ACID
GENCEPT 10/11-21, ETHINYL ESTRADIOL
GENCEPT 10/11-28, ETHINYL ESTRADIOL
HYDROCHLOROTHIAZIDE, HYDROCHLOROTHIAZIDE
HYDROCODONE BITARTRATE AND ACETAMINOPHEN,
  ACETAMINOPHEN
HYDROCORTISONE, HYDROCORTISONE
HYDROXYUREA, HYDROXYUREA
HYDROXYZINE PAMOATE, HYDROXYZINE PAMOATE
IBUPROFEN, IBUPROFEN
IBUPROFEN, IBUPROFEN (OTC)
ISONIAZID, ISONIAZID
JUNEL 1.5/30, ETHINYL ESTRADIOL
JUNEL 1/20, ETHINYL ESTRADIOL
KARIVA, DESOGESTREL
LESSINA-21, ETHINYL ESTRADIOL
LESSINA-28, ETHINYL ESTRADIOL
LEVONORGESTREL AND ETHINYL ESTRADIOL, ETHINYL
  ESTRADIOL
LITHIUM CARBONATE, LITHIUM CARBONATE
MECLOFENAMATE SODIUM, MECLOFENAMATE SODIUM
MEDROXYPROGESTERONE ACETATE,
  MEDROXYPROGESTERONE ACETATE
MEGESTROL ACETATE, MEGESTROL ACETATE
MEPERIDINE HCL, MEPERIDINE HYDROCHLORIDE
MEPROBAMATE, MEPROBAMATE
METFORMIN HCL, METFORMIN HYDROCHLORIDE
METHOTREXATE SODIUM, METHOTREXATE SODIUM
NALTREXONE HCL, NALTREXONE HYDROCHLORIDE
NORETHINDRONE ACETATE, NORETHINDRONE
  ACETATE
NORTREL 0.5/35-21, ETHINYL ESTRADIOL
NORTREL 0.5/35-28, ETHINYL ESTRADIOL
NORTREL 1/35-21, ETHINYL ESTRADIOL
NORTREL 1/35-28, ETHINYL ESTRADIOL
NORTREL 7/7/7, ETHINYL ESTRADIOL
OXYCODONE AND ACETAMINOPHEN, ACETAMINOPHEN
PHENDIMETRAZINE TARTRATE, PHENDIMETRAZINE
  TARTRATE
PORTIA-21, ETHINYL ESTRADIOL
PORTIA-28, ETHINYL ESTRADIOL
PREDNISOLONE, PREDNISOLONE
PROPRANOLOL HCL AND HYDROCHLOROTHIAZIDE,
  HYDROCHLOROTHIAZIDE
QUINIDINE SULFATE, QUINIDINE SULFATE
RESERPINE AND HYDROCHLOROTHIAZIDE,
  HYDROCHLOROTHIAZIDE
RESERPINE, RESERPINE
SODIUM SECOBARBITAL, SECOBARBITAL SODIUM
SPRINTEC, ETHINYL ESTRADIOL
SULFAMETHOXAZOLE, SULFAMETHOXAZOLE
SULFINPYRAZONE, SULFINPYRAZONE
SULFISOXAZOLE, SULFISOXAZOLE

APPENDIX B
PRODUCT NAME INDEX
LISTED BY APPLICANT (*continued*)

TAMOXIFEN CITRATE, TAMOXIFEN CITRATE
TETRACYCLINE HCL, TETRACYCLINE HYDROCHLORIDE
TIZANIDINE HCL, TIZANIDINE HYDROCHLORIDE
TOLAZAMIDE, TOLAZAMIDE
TOLBUTAMIDE, TOLBUTAMIDE
TRAZODONE HCL, TRAZODONE HYDROCHLORIDE
TREXALL, METHOTREXATE SODIUM
TRI-SPRINTEC, ETHINYL ESTRADIOL
TRIAMCINOLONE, TRIAMCINOLONE
TRIAMTERENE AND HYDROCHLOROTHIAZIDE,
   HYDROCHLOROTHIAZIDE
TRIPELENNAMINE HCL, TRIPELENNAMINE
   HYDROCHLORIDE
VERAPAMIL HCL, VERAPAMIL HYDROCHLORIDE
WARFARIN SODIUM, WARFARIN SODIUM
BARR PHARMACEUTICALS
   LEUCOVORIN CALCIUM, LEUCOVORIN CALCIUM
BARR PHARMS
BARR PHARMACEUTICALS INC
   REVIA, NALTREXONE HYDROCHLORIDE
BARTOR
BARTOR PHARMACAL CO
   TESTOSTERONE, TESTOSTERONE
BASF
BASF CORP
   IBU, IBUPROFEN
   IBUPROFEN, IBUPROFEN
   IBUPROFEN, IBUPROFEN (OTC)
   LOPURIN, ALLOPURINOL
   RUFEN, IBUPROFEN
   SSD AF, SILVER SULFADIAZINE
   SSD, SILVER SULFADIAZINE
BAUSCH AND LOMB
BAUSCH AND LOMB INC
   ALBUTEROL SULFATE, ALBUTEROL SULFATE
   ALREX, LOTEPREDNOL ETABONATE
   CARTEOLOL HCL, CARTEOLOL HYDROCHLORIDE
   IPRATROPIUM BROMIDE, IPRATROPIUM BROMIDE
   LOTEMAX, LOTEPREDNOL ETABONATE
   OPCON-A, NAPHAZOLINE HYDROCHLORIDE (OTC)
   SULPHRIN, PREDNISOLONE ACETATE
   SULTEN-10, SULFACETAMIDE SODIUM
   TIMOLOL MALEATE, TIMOLOL MALEATE
BAUSCH AND LOMB PHARMACEUTICALS INC
   ACETIC ACID 2% IN AQUEOUS ALUMINUM ACETATE,
     ACETIC ACID, GLACIAL
   BACITRACIN ZINC AND POLYMYXIN B SULFATE,
     BACITRACIN ZINC
   BETAXOLOL HCL, BETAXOLOL HYDROCHLORIDE
   BRIMONIDINE TARTRATE, BRIMONIDINE TARTRATE
   CROLOM, CROMOLYN SODIUM
   CROMOLYN SODIUM, CROMOLYN SODIUM
   CROMOLYN SODIUM, CROMOLYN SODIUM (OTC)
   DESMOPRESSIN ACETATE, DESMOPRESSIN ACETATE
   DEXAMETHASONE SODIUM PHOSPHATE,
     DEXAMETHASONE SODIUM PHOSPHATE
   DEXASPORIN, DEXAMETHASONE
   DIPIVEFRIN HCL, DIPIVEFRIN HYDROCHLORIDE
   ERYTHROMYCIN, ERYTHROMYCIN
   FLUNISOLIDE, FLUNISOLIDE
   FLUOCINOLONE ACETONIDE, FLUOCINOLONE
     ACETONIDE
   GENTAMICIN SULFATE, GENTAMICIN SULFATE
   HYDROCORTISONE AND ACETIC ACID, ACETIC ACID,
     GLACIAL
   IPRATROPIUM BROMIDE, IPRATROPIUM BROMIDE
   LEVOBUNOLOL HCL, LEVOBUNOLOL HYDROCHLORIDE
   MINOXIDIL (FOR MEN), MINOXIDIL (OTC)

NAFAZAIR, NAPHAZOLINE HYDROCHLORIDE
NEOMYCIN AND POLYMYXIN B SULFATES AND
   BACITRACIN ZINC, BACITRACIN ZINC
NEOMYCIN AND POLYMYXIN B SULFATES AND
   DEXAMETHASONE, DEXAMETHASONE
NEOMYCIN AND POLYMYXIN B SULFATES AND
   GRAMICIDIN, GRAMICIDIN
NEOMYCIN AND POLYMYXIN B SULFATES AND
   HYDROCORTISONE, HYDROCORTISONE
NEOMYCIN AND POLYMYXIN B SULFATES, BACITRACIN
   ZINC AND HYDROCORTISONE, BACITRACIN ZINC
NEOMYCIN SULFATE AND DEXAMETHASONE SODIUM
   PHOSPHATE, DEXAMETHASONE SODIUM
   PHOSPHATE
NYSTATIN, NYSTATIN
OPCON, NAPHAZOLINE HYDROCHLORIDE
OPTIPRANOLOL, METIPRANOLOL HYDROCHLORIDE
OTICAIR, HYDROCORTISONE
PENTOLAIR, CYCLOPENTOLATE HYDROCHLORIDE
PREDNISOLONE SODIUM PHOSPHATE, PREDNISOLONE
   SODIUM PHOSPHATE
PROPARACAINE HCL, PROPARACAINE
   HYDROCHLORIDE
SULFACETAMIDE SODIUM AND PREDNISOLONE
   SODIUM PHOSPHATE, PREDNISOLONE SODIUM
   PHOSPHATE
SULFACETAMIDE SODIUM, SULFACETAMIDE SODIUM
TIMOLOL MALEATE, TIMOLOL MALEATE
TOBRAMYCIN AND DEXAMETHASONE,
   DEXAMETHASONE
TOBRAMYCIN, TOBRAMYCIN
TRIMETHOPRIM SULFATE AND POLYMYXIN B SULFATE,
   POLYMYXIN B SULFATE
TROPICAMIDE, TROPICAMIDE
BAUSCH AND LOMB SURGICAL INC
   VITRASERT, GANCICLOVIR
BAXTER HLTHCARE
BAXTER HEALTHCARE CORP
   ACETIC ACID 0.25% IN PLASTIC CONTAINER, ACETIC
     ACID, GLACIAL
   ALCOHOL 5% IN DEXTROSE 5% IN WATER, ALCOHOL
   AMINOACETIC ACID 1.5% IN PLASTIC CONTAINER,
     GLYCINE
   ANCEF IN DEXTROSE 5% IN PLASTIC CONTAINER,
     CEFAZOLIN SODIUM
   ANCEF IN PLASTIC CONTAINER, CEFAZOLIN SODIUM
   ANCEF IN SODIUM CHLORIDE 0.9% IN PLASTIC
     CONTAINER, CEFAZOLIN SODIUM
   BACTOCILL IN PLASTIC CONTAINER, OXACILLIN
     SODIUM
   BRANCHAMIN 4% IN PLASTIC CONTAINER, AMINO
     ACIDS
   BRANCHAMIN 4%, AMINO ACIDS
   BRETYLIUM TOSYLATE IN DEXTROSE 5% IN PLASTIC
     CONTAINER, BRETYLIUM TOSYLATE
   CARDIOPLEGIC IN PLASTIC CONTAINER, CALCIUM
     CHLORIDE
   CEFTAZIDIME SODIUM IN PLASTIC CONTAINER,
     CEFTAZIDIME SODIUM
   CEPHALOTHIN SODIUM W/ DEXTROSE IN PLASTIC
     CONTAINER, CEPHALOTHIN SODIUM
   CEPHALOTHIN SODIUM W/ SODIUM CHLORIDE IN
     PLASTIC CONTAINER, CEPHALOTHIN SODIUM
   CERNEVIT-12, ALPHA-TOCOPHEROL
   CLINDAMYCIN PHOSPHATE IN DEXTROSE 5% IN
     PLASTIC CONTAINER, CLINDAMYCIN PHOSPHATE
   CLINIMIX 2.75/10 SULFITE FREE IN DEXTROSE 10% IN
     PLASTIC CONTAINER, AMINO ACIDS

APPENDIX B
PRODUCT NAME INDEX
LISTED BY APPLICANT (*continued*)

CLINIMIX 2.75/25 SULFITE FREE IN DEXTROSE 25% IN PLASTIC CONTAINER, AMINO ACIDS
CLINIMIX 2.75/5 SULFITE FREE IN DEXTROSE 5% IN PLASTIC CONTAINER, AMINO ACIDS
CLINIMIX 4.25/10 SULFITE FREE IN DEXTROSE 10% IN PLASTIC CONTAINER, AMINO ACIDS
CLINIMIX 4.25/20 SULFITE FREE IN DEXTROSE 20% IN PLASTIC CONTAINER, AMINO ACIDS
CLINIMIX 4.25/25 SULFITE FREE IN DEXTROSE 25% IN PLASTIC CONTAINER, AMINO ACIDS
CLINIMIX 4.25/5 SULFITE FREE IN DEXTROSE 5% IN PLASTIC CONTAINER, AMINO ACIDS
CLINIMIX 5/10 SULFITE FREE IN DEXTROSE 10% IN PLASTIC CONTAINER, AMINO ACIDS
CLINIMIX 5/15 SULFITE FREE IN DEXTROSE 15% IN PLASTIC CONTAINER, AMINO ACIDS
CLINIMIX 5/20 SULFITE FREE IN DEXTROSE 20% IN PLASTIC CONTAINER, AMINO ACIDS
CLINIMIX 5/25 SULFITE FREE IN DEXTROSE 25% IN PLASTIC CONTAINER, AMINO ACIDS
CLINIMIX 5/35 SULFITE FREE IN DEXTROSE 35% IN PLASTIC CONTAINER, AMINO ACIDS
CLINIMIX E 2.75/10 SULFITE-FREE W/ ELECT IN DEXTROSE 10% W/ CALCIUM IN PLASTIC CONTAINER, AMINO ACIDS
CLINIMIX E 2.75/25 SULFITE-FREE W/ ELECT IN DEXTROSE 25% W/ CALCIUM IN PLASTIC CONTAINER, AMINO ACIDS
CLINIMIX E 2.75/5 SULFITE-FREE W/ ELECT IN DEXTROSE 5% W/ CALCIUM IN PLASTIC CONTAINER, AMINO ACIDS
CLINIMIX E 4.25/10 SULFITE-FREE W/ ELECT IN DEXTROSE 10% W/ CALCIUM IN PLASTIC CONTAINER, AMINO ACIDS
CLINIMIX E 4.25/20 SULFITE-FREE W/ ELECT IN DEXTROSE 20% W/ CALCIUM IN PLASTIC CONTAINER, AMINO ACIDS
CLINIMIX E 4.25/25 SULFITE-FREE W/ ELECT IN DEXTROSE 25% W/ CALCIUM IN PLASTIC CONTAINER, AMINO ACIDS
CLINIMIX E 4.25/5 SULFITE-FREE W/ ELECT IN DEXTROSE 5% W/ CALCIUM IN PLASTIC CONTAINER, AMINO ACIDS
CLINIMIX E 5/10 SULFITE-FREE W/ ELECT IN DEXTROSE 10% W/ CALCIUM IN PLASTIC CONTAINER, AMINO ACIDS
CLINIMIX E 5/15 SULFITE-FREE W/ ELECT IN DEXTROSE 15% W/ CALCIUM IN PLASTIC CONTAINER, AMINO ACIDS
CLINIMIX E 5/20 SULFITE-FREE W/ ELECT IN 20% DEXTROSE W/ CALCIUM IN PLASTIC CONTAINER, AMINO ACIDS
CLINIMIX E 5/25 SULFITE-FREE W/ ELECT IN DEXTROSE 25% W/ CALCIUM IN PLASTIC CONTAINER, AMINO ACIDS
CLINIMIX E 5/35 SULFITE FREE W/ ELECT IN DEXTROSE 35% W/ CALCIUM IN PLASTIC CONTAINER, AMINO ACIDS
CYCLOPHOSPHAMIDE, CYCLOPHOSPHAMIDE
DEXTROSE 10% AND SODIUM CHLORIDE 0.9% IN PLASTIC CONTAINER, DEXTROSE
DEXTROSE 10% IN PLASTIC CONTAINER, DEXTROSE
DEXTROSE 2.5% AND SODIUM CHLORIDE 0.45% IN PLASTIC CONTAINER, DEXTROSE
DEXTROSE 20% IN PLASTIC CONTAINER, DEXTROSE
DEXTROSE 30% IN PLASTIC CONTAINER, DEXTROSE
DEXTROSE 40% IN PLASTIC CONTAINER, DEXTROSE

DEXTROSE 5% AND ELECTROLYTE NO 75 IN PLASTIC CONTAINER, DEXTROSE
DEXTROSE 5% AND ELECTROLYTE NO.48 IN PLASTIC CONTAINER, DEXTROSE
DEXTROSE 5% IN PLASTIC CONTAINER, DEXTROSE
DEXTROSE 5% IN RINGER'S IN PLASTIC CONTAINER, CALCIUM CHLORIDE
DEXTROSE 5% IN SODIUM CHLORIDE 0.2% IN PLASTIC CONTAINER, DEXTROSE
DEXTROSE 5% IN SODIUM CHLORIDE 0.33% IN PLASTIC CONTAINER, DEXTROSE
DEXTROSE 5% IN SODIUM CHLORIDE 0.45% IN PLASTIC CONTAINER, DEXTROSE
DEXTROSE 5% IN SODIUM CHLORIDE 0.9% IN PLASTIC CONTAINER, DEXTROSE
DEXTROSE 5%, SODIUM CHLORIDE 0.2% AND POTASSIUM CHLORIDE 10MEQ, DEXTROSE
DEXTROSE 5%, SODIUM CHLORIDE 0.2% AND POTASSIUM CHLORIDE 15MEQ (K), DEXTROSE
DEXTROSE 5%, SODIUM CHLORIDE 0.2% AND POTASSIUM CHLORIDE 20MEQ (K), DEXTROSE
DEXTROSE 5%, SODIUM CHLORIDE 0.2% AND POTASSIUM CHLORIDE 20MEQ, DEXTROSE
DEXTROSE 5%, SODIUM CHLORIDE 0.2% AND POTASSIUM CHLORIDE 30MEQ, DEXTROSE
DEXTROSE 5%, SODIUM CHLORIDE 0.2% AND POTASSIUM CHLORIDE 40MEQ, DEXTROSE
DEXTROSE 5%, SODIUM CHLORIDE 0.2% AND POTASSIUM CHLORIDE 5MEQ (K), DEXTROSE
DEXTROSE 5%, SODIUM CHLORIDE 0.2% AND POTASSIUM CHLORIDE 5MEQ, DEXTROSE
DEXTROSE 5%, SODIUM CHLORIDE 0.33% AND POTASSIUM CHLORIDE 10MEQ IN PLASTIC CONTAINER, DEXTROSE
DEXTROSE 5%, SODIUM CHLORIDE 0.33% AND POTASSIUM CHLORIDE 15MEQ IN PLASTIC CONTAINER, DEXTROSE
DEXTROSE 5%, SODIUM CHLORIDE 0.33% AND POTASSIUM CHLORIDE 20MEQ IN PLASTIC CONTAINER, DEXTROSE
DEXTROSE 5%, SODIUM CHLORIDE 0.33% AND POTASSIUM CHLORIDE 30MEQ IN PLASTIC CONTAINER, DEXTROSE
DEXTROSE 5%, SODIUM CHLORIDE 0.33% AND POTASSIUM CHLORIDE 40MEQ IN PLASTIC CONTAINER, DEXTROSE
DEXTROSE 5%, SODIUM CHLORIDE 0.33% AND POTASSIUM CHLORIDE 5MEQ IN PLASTIC CONTAINER, DEXTROSE
DEXTROSE 5%, SODIUM CHLORIDE 0.45% AND POTASSIUM CHLORIDE 15MEQ IN PLASTIC CONTAINER, DEXTROSE
DEXTROSE 5%, SODIUM CHLORIDE 0.45% AND POTASSIUM CHLORIDE 20MEQ (K) IN PLASTIC CONTAINER, DEXTROSE
DEXTROSE 5%, SODIUM CHLORIDE 0.45% AND POTASSIUM CHLORIDE 5MEQ IN PLASTIC CONTAINER, DEXTROSE
DEXTROSE 50% IN PLASTIC CONTAINER, DEXTROSE
DEXTROSE 60% IN PLASTIC CONTAINER, DEXTROSE
DEXTROSE 70% IN PLASTIC CONTAINER, DEXTROSE
DIANEAL 137 W/ DEXTROSE 1.5% IN PLASTIC CONTAINER, CALCIUM CHLORIDE
DIANEAL 137 W/ DEXTROSE 2.5% IN PLASTIC CONTAINER, CALCIUM CHLORIDE
DIANEAL 137 W/ DEXTROSE 4.25% IN PLASTIC CONTAINER, CALCIUM CHLORIDE

APPENDIX B
PRODUCT NAME INDEX
LISTED BY APPLICANT (*continued*)

DIANEAL LOW CALCIUM W/ DEXTROSE 1.5% IN PLASTIC
    CONTAINER, CALCIUM CHLORIDE
DIANEAL LOW CALCIUM W/ DEXTROSE 2.5% IN PLASTIC
    CONTAINER, CALCIUM CHLORIDE
DIANEAL LOW CALCIUM W/ DEXTROSE 3.5% IN PLASTIC
    CONTAINER, CALCIUM CHLORIDE
DIANEAL LOW CALCIUM W/ DEXTROSE 4.25% IN
    PLASTIC CONTAINER, CALCIUM CHLORIDE
DIANEAL PD-1 W/ DEXTROSE 1.5% IN PLASTIC
    CONTAINER, CALCIUM CHLORIDE
DIANEAL PD-1 W/ DEXTROSE 2.5% IN PLASTIC
    CONTAINER, CALCIUM CHLORIDE
DIANEAL PD-1 W/ DEXTROSE 3.5% IN PLASTIC
    CONTAINER, CALCIUM CHLORIDE
DIANEAL PD-1 W/ DEXTROSE 4.25% IN PLASTIC
    CONTAINER, CALCIUM CHLORIDE
DIANEAL PD-2 W/ DEXTROSE 1.5% IN PLASTIC
    CONTAINER, CALCIUM CHLORIDE
DIANEAL PD-2 W/ DEXTROSE 2.5% IN PLASTIC
    CONTAINER, CALCIUM CHLORIDE
DIANEAL PD-2 W/ DEXTROSE 3.5% IN PLASTIC
    CONTAINER, CALCIUM CHLORIDE
DIANEAL PD-2 W/ DEXTROSE 4.25% IN PLASTIC
    CONTAINER, CALCIUM CHLORIDE
DOBUTAMINE HCL IN DEXTROSE 5% IN PLASTIC
    CONTAINER, DOBUTAMINE HYDROCHLORIDE
DOPAMINE HCL IN DEXTROSE 5% IN PLASTIC
    CONTAINER, DOPAMINE HYDROCHLORIDE
EXTRANEAL, ICODEXTRIN
FAMOTIDINE PRESERVATIVE FREE, FAMOTIDINE
FAMOTIDINE, FAMOTIDINE
FLAGYL I.V. RTU IN PLASTIC CONTAINER,
    METRONIDAZOLE
GLYCINE 1.5% IN PLASTIC CONTAINER, GLYCINE
HEPARIN SODIUM 1,000 UNITS AND SODIUM CHLORIDE
    0.9% IN PLASTIC CONTAINER, HEPARIN SODIUM
HEPARIN SODIUM 10,000 UNITS IN DEXTROSE 5% IN
    PLASTIC CONTAINER, HEPARIN SODIUM
HEPARIN SODIUM 2,000 UNITS AND SODIUM CHLORIDE
    0.9% IN PLASTIC CONTAINER, HEPARIN SODIUM
HEPARIN SODIUM 20,000 UNITS AND DEXTROSE 5% IN
    PLASTIC CONTAINER, HEPARIN SODIUM
HEPARIN SODIUM 25,000 UNITS AND DEXTROSE 5% IN
    PLASTIC CONTAINER, HEPARIN SODIUM
HEPARIN SODIUM 5,000 UNITS AND SODIUM CHLORIDE
    0.9% IN PLASTIC CONTAINER, HEPARIN SODIUM
HEPATASOL 8%, AMINO ACIDS
IRRIGATING SOLUTION G IN PLASTIC CONTAINER,
    CITRIC ACID
ISOETHARINE HCL, ISOETHARINE HYDROCHLORIDE
ISOTONIC GENTAMICIN SULFATE IN PLASTIC
    CONTAINER, GENTAMICIN SULFATE
LACTATED RINGER'S AND DEXTROSE 5% IN PLASTIC
    CONTAINER, CALCIUM CHLORIDE
LACTATED RINGER'S IN PLASTIC CONTAINER, CALCIUM
    CHLORIDE
LIDOCAINE HCL 0.1% AND DEXTROSE 5% IN PLASTIC
    CONTAINER, LIDOCAINE HYDROCHLORIDE
LIDOCAINE HCL 0.2% AND DEXTROSE 5% IN PLASTIC
    CONTAINER, LIDOCAINE HYDROCHLORIDE
LIDOCAINE HCL 0.4% AND DEXTROSE 5% IN PLASTIC
    CONTAINER, LIDOCAINE HYDROCHLORIDE
LIDOCAINE HCL 0.8% AND DEXTROSE 5% IN PLASTIC
    CONTAINER, LIDOCAINE HYDROCHLORIDE
MESNEX, MESNA
MILRINONE LACTATE IN DEXTROSE 5% IN PLASTIC
    CONTAINER, MILRINONE LACTATE
NALLPEN IN PLASTIC CONTAINER, NAFCILLIN SODIUM

NITROGLYCERIN IN DEXTROSE 5%, NITROGLYCERIN
NOVAMINE 15% SULFITE FREE IN PLASTIC CONTAINER,
    AMINO ACIDS
OSMITROL 10% IN WATER IN PLASTIC CONTAINER,
    MANNITOL
OSMITROL 10% IN WATER, MANNITOL
OSMITROL 15% IN WATER IN PLASTIC CONTAINER,
    MANNITOL
OSMITROL 15% IN WATER, MANNITOL
OSMITROL 20% IN WATER IN PLASTIC CONTAINER,
    MANNITOL
OSMITROL 20% IN WATER, MANNITOL
OSMITROL 5% IN WATER IN PLASTIC CONTAINER,
    MANNITOL
OSMITROL 5% IN WATER, MANNITOL
PENICILLIN G POTASSIUM IN PLASTIC CONTAINER,
    PENICILLIN G POTASSIUM
PLASMA-LYTE 148 AND DEXTROSE 5% IN PLASTIC
    CONTAINER, DEXTROSE
PLASMA-LYTE 148 IN WATER IN PLASTIC CONTAINER,
    MAGNESIUM CHLORIDE
PLASMA-LYTE 56 AND DEXTROSE 5% IN PLASTIC
    CONTAINER, DEXTROSE
PLASMA-LYTE 56 IN PLASTIC CONTAINER, MAGNESIUM
    ACETATE TETRAHYDRATE
PLASMA-LYTE A IN PLASTIC CONTAINER, MAGNESIUM
    CHLORIDE
PLASMA-LYTE M AND DEXTROSE 5% IN PLASTIC
    CONTAINER, CALCIUM CHLORIDE
PLASMA-LYTE R IN PLASTIC CONTAINER, CALCIUM
    CHLORIDE
POTASSIUM CHLORIDE 10MEQ IN DEXTROSE 5% AND
    LACTATED RINGER'S IN PLASTIC CONTAINER,
    CALCIUM CHLORIDE
POTASSIUM CHLORIDE 10MEQ IN DEXTROSE 5% AND
    SODIUM CHLORIDE 0.45% IN PLASTIC CONTAINER,
    DEXTROSE
POTASSIUM CHLORIDE 10MEQ IN DEXTROSE 5% AND
    SODIUM CHLORIDE 0.9% IN PLASTIC CONTAINER,
    DEXTROSE
POTASSIUM CHLORIDE 10MEQ IN PLASTIC CONTAINER,
    POTASSIUM CHLORIDE
POTASSIUM CHLORIDE 15MEQ IN DEXTROSE 5% AND
    LACTATED RINGER'S IN PLASTIC CONTAINER,
    CALCIUM CHLORIDE
POTASSIUM CHLORIDE 20MEQ IN DEXTROSE 5% AND
    LACTATED RINGER'S IN PLASTIC CONTAINER,
    CALCIUM CHLORIDE
POTASSIUM CHLORIDE 20MEQ IN DEXTROSE 5% AND
    SODIUM CHLORIDE 0.45% IN PLASTIC CONTAINER,
    DEXTROSE
POTASSIUM CHLORIDE 20MEQ IN DEXTROSE 5% AND
    SODIUM CHLORIDE 0.9% IN PLASTIC CONTAINER,
    DEXTROSE
POTASSIUM CHLORIDE 20MEQ IN PLASTIC CONTAINER,
    POTASSIUM CHLORIDE
POTASSIUM CHLORIDE 30MEQ IN DEXTROSE 5% AND
    LACTATED RINGER'S IN PLASTIC CONTAINER,
    CALCIUM CHLORIDE
POTASSIUM CHLORIDE 30MEQ IN DEXTROSE 5% AND
    SODIUM CHLORIDE 0.45% IN PLASTIC CONTAINER,
    DEXTROSE
POTASSIUM CHLORIDE 30MEQ IN DEXTROSE 5% AND
    SODIUM CHLORIDE 0.9% IN PLASTIC CONTAINER,
    DEXTROSE
POTASSIUM CHLORIDE 30MEQ IN PLASTIC CONTAINER,
    POTASSIUM CHLORIDE

APPENDIX B
PRODUCT NAME INDEX
LISTED BY APPLICANT (*continued*)

POTASSIUM CHLORIDE 40MEQ IN DEXTROSE 5% AND LACTATED RINGER'S IN PLASTIC CONTAINER, CALCIUM CHLORIDE
POTASSIUM CHLORIDE 40MEQ IN DEXTROSE 5% AND SODIUM CHLORIDE 0.45% IN PLASTIC CONTAINER, DEXTROSE
POTASSIUM CHLORIDE 40MEQ IN DEXTROSE 5% AND SODIUM CHLORIDE 0.9% IN PLASTIC CONTAINER, DEXTROSE
POTASSIUM CHLORIDE 40MEQ IN PLASTIC CONTAINER, POTASSIUM CHLORIDE
POTASSIUM CHLORIDE 5MEQ IN DEXTROSE 5% AND LACTATED RINGER'S IN PLASTIC CONTAINER, CALCIUM CHLORIDE
POTASSIUM CHLORIDE 5MEQ IN DEXTROSE 5% AND SODIUM CHLORIDE 0.45% IN PLASTIC CONTAINER, DEXTROSE
POTASSIUM CHLORIDE 5MEQ IN DEXTROSE 5% AND SODIUM CHLORIDE 0.9% IN PLASTIC CONTAINER, DEXTROSE
POTASSIUM CHLORIDE, POTASSIUM CHLORIDE
PREMASOL 10% IN PLASTIC CONTAINER, AMINO ACIDS
PREMASOL 6% IN PLASTIC CONTAINER, AMINO ACIDS
RENAMIN W/O ELECTROLYTES, AMINO ACIDS
RINGER'S IN PLASTIC CONTAINER, CALCIUM CHLORIDE
SEVOFLURANE, SEVOFLURANE
SODIUM CHLORIDE 0.45% IN PLASTIC CONTAINER, SODIUM CHLORIDE
SODIUM CHLORIDE 0.9% AND POTASSIUM CHLORIDE 0.075% IN PLASTIC CONTAINER, POTASSIUM CHLORIDE
SODIUM CHLORIDE 0.9% AND POTASSIUM CHLORIDE 0.15% IN PLASTIC CONTAINER, POTASSIUM CHLORIDE
SODIUM CHLORIDE 0.9% AND POTASSIUM CHLORIDE 0.224%, POTASSIUM CHLORIDE
SODIUM CHLORIDE 0.9% AND POTASSIUM CHLORIDE 0.3% IN PLASTIC CONTAINER, POTASSIUM CHLORIDE
SODIUM CHLORIDE 0.9% IN PLASTIC CONTAINER, SODIUM CHLORIDE
SODIUM CHLORIDE 0.9% IN STERILE PLASTIC CONTAINER, SODIUM CHLORIDE
SODIUM CHLORIDE 3% IN PLASTIC CONTAINER, SODIUM CHLORIDE
SODIUM CHLORIDE 5% IN PLASTIC CONTAINER, SODIUM CHLORIDE
SODIUM HEPARIN, HEPARIN SODIUM
SODIUM LACTATE 0.167 MOLAR IN PLASTIC CONTAINER, SODIUM LACTATE
SORBITOL 3% IN PLASTIC CONTAINER, SORBITOL
STERILE WATER FOR INJECTION IN PLASTIC CONTAINER, WATER FOR INJECTION, STERILE
STERILE WATER IN PLASTIC CONTAINER, WATER FOR IRRIGATION, STERILE
STERILE WATER, WATER FOR IRRIGATION, STERILE
SYNOVALYTE IN PLASTIC CONTAINER, MAGNESIUM CHLORIDE
THEOPHYLLINE AND DEXTROSE 5% IN PLASTIC CONTAINER, THEOPHYLLINE
TIS-U-SOL IN PLASTIC CONTAINER, MAGNESIUM SULFATE
TIS-U-SOL, MAGNESIUM SULFATE
TRAVAMULSION 10%, SOYBEAN OIL
TRAVAMULSION 20%, SOYBEAN OIL
TRAVASOL 10% IN PLASTIC CONTAINER, AMINO ACIDS
TRAVASOL 10% W/O ELECTROLYTES, AMINO ACIDS

TRAVASOL 2.75% IN DEXTROSE 10% IN PLASTIC CONTAINER, AMINO ACIDS
TRAVASOL 2.75% IN DEXTROSE 15% IN PLASTIC CONTAINER, AMINO ACIDS
TRAVASOL 2.75% IN DEXTROSE 20% IN PLASTIC CONTAINER, AMINO ACIDS
TRAVASOL 2.75% IN DEXTROSE 25% IN PLASTIC CONTAINER, AMINO ACIDS
TRAVASOL 2.75% IN DEXTROSE 5% IN PLASTIC CONTAINER, AMINO ACIDS
TRAVASOL 2.75% SULFITE FREE W/ ELECTROLYTES IN DEXTROSE 10% IN PLASTIC CONTAINER, AMINO ACIDS
TRAVASOL 2.75% SULFITE FREE W/ ELECTROLYTES IN DEXTROSE 15% IN PLASTIC CONTAINER, AMINO ACIDS
TRAVASOL 2.75% SULFITE FREE W/ ELECTROLYTES IN DEXTROSE 20% IN PLASTIC CONTAINER, AMINO ACIDS
TRAVASOL 2.75% SULFITE FREE W/ ELECTROLYTES IN DEXTROSE 25% IN PLASTIC CONTAINER, AMINO ACIDS
TRAVASOL 2.75% SULFITE FREE W/ ELECTROLYTES IN DEXTROSE 5% IN PLASTIC CONTAINER, AMINO ACIDS
TRAVASOL 3.5% SULFITE FREE W/ ELECTROLYTES IN PLASTIC CONTAINER, AMINO ACIDS
TRAVASOL 3.5% W/ ELECTROLYTES, AMINO ACIDS
TRAVASOL 4.25% IN DEXTROSE 10% IN PLASTIC CONTAINER, AMINO ACIDS
TRAVASOL 4.25% IN DEXTROSE 15% IN PLASTIC CONTAINER, AMINO ACIDS
TRAVASOL 4.25% IN DEXTROSE 20% IN PLASTIC CONTAINER, AMINO ACIDS
TRAVASOL 4.25% IN DEXTROSE 25% IN PLASTIC CONTAINER, AMINO ACIDS
TRAVASOL 4.25% IN DEXTROSE 5% IN PLASTIC CONTAINER, AMINO ACIDS
TRAVASOL 4.25% SULFITE FREE W/ ELECTROLYTES IN DEXTROSE 10% IN PLASTIC CONTAINER, AMINO ACIDS
TRAVASOL 4.25% SULFITE FREE W/ ELECTROLYTES IN DEXTROSE 15% IN PLASTIC CONTAINER, AMINO ACIDS
TRAVASOL 4.25% SULFITE FREE W/ ELECTROLYTES IN DEXTROSE 20% IN PLASTIC CONTAINER, AMINO ACIDS
TRAVASOL 4.25% SULFITE FREE W/ ELECTROLYTES IN DEXTROSE 25% IN PLASTIC CONTAINER, AMINO ACIDS
TRAVASOL 4.25% SULFITE FREE W/ ELECTROLYTES IN DEXTROSE 5% IN PLASTIC CONTAINER, AMINO ACIDS
TRAVASOL 5.5% IN PLASTIC CONTAINER, AMINO ACIDS
TRAVASOL 5.5% SULFITE FREE W/ ELECTROLYTES IN PLASTIC CONTAINER, AMINO ACIDS
TRAVASOL 5.5% W/ ELECTROLYTES, AMINO ACIDS
TRAVASOL 5.5% W/O ELECTROLYTES, AMINO ACIDS
TRAVASOL 8.5% IN PLASTIC CONTAINER, AMINO ACIDS
TRAVASOL 8.5% SULFITE FREE W/ ELECTROLYTES IN PLASTIC CONTAINER, AMINO ACIDS
TRAVASOL 8.5% W/ ELECTROLYTES, AMINO ACIDS
TRAVASOL 8.5% W/O ELECTROLYTES, AMINO ACIDS
TRAVERT 10% IN PLASTIC CONTAINER, INVERT SUGAR
VANCOCIN HCL IN PLASTIC CONTAINER, VANCOMYCIN HYDROCHLORIDE

APPENDIX B
PRODUCT NAME INDEX
LISTED BY APPLICANT (*continued*)

BAXTER HEALTHCARE CORP ANESTHESIA AND CRITICAL CARE
- CHLORPROMAZINE HCL, CHLORPROMAZINE HYDROCHLORIDE
- DIPHENHYDRAMINE HCL, DIPHENHYDRAMINE HYDROCHLORIDE
- DOPAMINE HCL, DOPAMINE HYDROCHLORIDE
- DURAMORPH PF, MORPHINE SULFATE
- FAMOTIDINE PRESERVATIVE FREE, FAMOTIDINE
- FAMOTIDINE, FAMOTIDINE
- FUROSEMIDE, FUROSEMIDE
- GENTAMICIN SULFATE, GENTAMICIN SULFATE
- HEP-LOCK U/P, HEPARIN SODIUM
- HEP-LOCK, HEPARIN SODIUM
- HEPARIN SODIUM, HEPARIN SODIUM
- INFUMORPH, MORPHINE SULFATE
- ISOPROTERENOL HCL, ISOPROTERENOL HYDROCHLORIDE
- MIDAZOLAM HCL, MIDAZOLAM HYDROCHLORIDE
- MILRINONE LACTATE IN DEXTROSE 5% IN PLASTIC CONTAINER, MILRINONE LACTATE
- MILRINONE LACTATE, MILRINONE LACTATE
- PROMETHAZINE HCL, PROMETHAZINE HYDROCHLORIDE
- WYDASE, HYALURONIDASE

BAXTER HEALTHCARE INTERNATIONAL SPECIALTY THERAPIES DIV
- FAMOTIDINE PRESERVATIVE FREE IN PLASTIC CONTAINER, FAMOTIDINE
- PROSOL 20% SULFITE FREE IN PLASTIC CONTAINER, AMINO ACIDS

BAXTER HLTHCARE CORP
BAXTER HEALTHCARE CORP ANESTHESIA CRITICAL CARE
- AMRINONE LACTATE, INAMRINONE LACTATE
- ATIVAN, LORAZEPAM
- ATRACURIUM BESYLATE PRESERVATIVE FREE, ATRACURIUM BESYLATE
- ATRACURIUM BESYLATE, ATRACURIUM BESYLATE
- BREVIBLOC DOUBLE STRENGTH IN PLASTIC CONTAINER, ESMOLOL HYDROCHLORIDE
- BREVIBLOC IN PLASTIC CONTAINER, ESMOLOL HYDROCHLORIDE
- BREVIBLOC, ESMOLOL HYDROCHLORIDE
- DOPRAM, DOXAPRAM HYDROCHLORIDE
- ENLON, EDROPHONIUM CHLORIDE
- ENLON-PLUS, ATROPINE SULFATE
- ETHRANE, ENFLURANE
- FACTREL, GONADORELIN HYDROCHLORIDE
- FORANE, ISOFLURANE
- HEPARIN LOCK FLUSH, HEPARIN SODIUM
- HEPARIN SODIUM, HEPARIN SODIUM
- INDERAL, PROPRANOLOL HYDROCHLORIDE
- KETOROLAC TROMETHAMINE, KETOROLAC TROMETHAMINE
- LARGON, PROPIOMAZINE HYDROCHLORIDE
- MEPERGAN, MEPERIDINE HYDROCHLORIDE
- MEPERIDINE HCL, MEPERIDINE HYDROCHLORIDE
- MIDAZOLAM HCL, MIDAZOLAM HYDROCHLORIDE
- MILRINONE LACTATE, MILRINONE LACTATE
- OXYTOCIN, OXYTOCIN
- PRALIDOXIME CHLORIDE, PRALIDOXIME CHLORIDE
- REVEX, NALMEFENE HYDROCHLORIDE
- SUPRANE, DESFLURANE
- WYAMINE SULFATE, MEPHENTERMINE SULFATE

BAYER
BAYER HEALTHCARE LLC
- 8-HOUR BAYER, ASPIRIN (OTC)
- ACTRON, KETOPROFEN (OTC)
- ALEVE COLD AND SINUS, NAPROXEN SODIUM (OTC)
- ALEVE, NAPROXEN SODIUM (OTC)
- BAYER EXTRA STRENGTH ASPIRIN FOR MIGRAINE PAIN, ASPIRIN (OTC)
- MEASURIN, ASPIRIN (OTC)
- MIDOL, IBUPROFEN (OTC)

BAYER PHARMS
BAYER PHARMACEUTICALS CORP
- ADALAT CC, NIFEDIPINE
- ADALAT, NIFEDIPINE
- ANTAGONATE, CHLORPHENIRAMINE MALEATE
- AVELOX IN SODIUM CHLORIDE 0.8% IN PLASTIC CONTAINER, MOXIFLOXACIN HYDROCHLORIDE
- AVELOX, MOXIFLOXACIN HYDROCHLORIDE
- AZLIN, AZLOCILLIN SODIUM
- BAYCOL, CERIVASTATIN SODIUM
- BILTRICIDE, PRAZIQUANTEL
- CANDEX, NYSTATIN
- CIPRO IN DEXTROSE 5% IN PLASTIC CONTAINER, CIPROFLOXACIN
- CIPRO IN SODIUM CHLORIDE 0.9% IN PLASTIC CONTAINER, CIPROFLOXACIN
- CIPRO XR, CIPROFLOXACIN
- CIPRO, CIPROFLOXACIN
- CIPRO, CIPROFLOXACIN HYDROCHLORIDE
- CORT-DOME, HYDROCORTISONE
- DELTA-DOME, PREDNISONE
- DOMEBORO, ACETIC ACID, GLACIAL
- DTIC-DOME, DACARBAZINE
- HC #1, HYDROCORTISONE
- HC #4, HYDROCORTISONE
- LITHANE, LITHIUM CARBONATE
- MEZLIN, MEZLOCILLIN SODIUM MONOHYDRATE
- MIXTARD HUMAN 70/30, INSULIN RECOMBINANT PURIFIED HUMAN (OTC)
- MYCELEX, CLOTRIMAZOLE
- MYCELEX-7 COMBINATION PACK, CLOTRIMAZOLE (OTC)
- MYCELEX-7, CLOTRIMAZOLE (OTC)
- MYCELEX-G, CLOTRIMAZOLE
- NEO-CORT-DOME, ACETIC ACID, GLACIAL
- NEO-CORT-DOME, HYDROCORTISONE
- NICLOCIDE, NICLOSAMIDE
- NIMOTOP, NIMODIPINE
- NYSTAFORM, CLIOQUINOL
- PRECOSE, ACARBOSE
- RADIO-IODINATED (I 125) SERUM ALBUMIN (HUMAN), ALBUMIN IODINATED I-125 SERUM
- SOY-DOME, HEXACHLOROPHENE
- STILPHOSTROL, DIETHYLSTILBESTROL DIPHOSPHATE
- TRASYLOL, APROTININ BOVINE
- TRIDESILON, ACETIC ACID, GLACIAL
- VI-DOM-A, VITAMIN A PALMITATE

BECKLOFF
BECKLOFF ASSOC INC
- CHLORAPREP ONE-STEP SEPP, CHLORHEXIDINE GLUCONATE (OTC)

BECTON DICKINSON
BECTON DICKINSON AND CO
- E-Z PREP 220, POVIDONE-IODINE (OTC)
- E-Z PREP, POVIDONE-IODINE (OTC)
- E-Z SCRUB 201, POVIDONE-IODINE (OTC)
- E-Z SCRUB 241, POVIDONE-IODINE (OTC)
- E-Z SCRUB, HEXACHLOROPHENE

BECTON DICKINSON SURGICAL SYSTEM
- E-Z SCRUB, CHLORHEXIDINE GLUCONATE (OTC)

APPENDIX B
PRODUCT NAME INDEX
LISTED BY APPLICANT (*continued*)

BEDFORD
BEDFORD LABORATORIES DIV BEN VENUE LABORA-
TORIES INC
  ACETAZOLAMIDE SODIUM, ACETAZOLAMIDE SODIUM
  ACETYLCYSTEINE, ACETYLCYSTEINE
  ACYCLOVIR SODIUM, ACYCLOVIR SODIUM
  ALPROSTADIL, ALPROSTADIL
  AMIKACIN SULFATE, AMIKACIN SULFATE
  AMIODARONE HCL, AMIODARONE HYDROCHLORIDE
  AMRINONE, INAMRINONE LACTATE
  ATRACURIUM BESYLATE PRESERVATIVE FREE,
    ATRACURIUM BESYLATE
  ATRACURIUM BESYLATE, ATRACURIUM BESYLATE
  AZATHIOPRINE SODIUM, AZATHIOPRINE SODIUM
  BLEOMYCIN, BLEOMYCIN SULFATE
  BUMETANIDE, BUMETANIDE
  BUTORPHANOL TARTRATE PRESERVATIVE FREE,
    BUTORPHANOL TARTRATE
  BUTORPHANOL TARTRATE, BUTORPHANOL TARTRATE
  CEFAZOLIN SODIUM, CEFAZOLIN SODIUM
  CERUBIDINE, DAUNORUBICIN HYDROCHLORIDE
  CHLOROPROCAINE HCL, CHLOROPROCAINE
    HYDROCHLORIDE
  CISPLATIN, CISPLATIN
  CLADRIBINE, CLADRIBINE
  CLINDAMYCIN PHOSPHATE, CLINDAMYCIN
    PHOSPHATE
  CYCLOSPORINE, CYCLOSPORINE
  CYTARABINE, CYTARABINE
  DACARBAZINE, DACARBAZINE
  DAUNORUBICIN HCL, DAUNORUBICIN
    HYDROCHLORIDE
  DESMOPRESSIN ACETATE PRESERVATIVE FREE,
    DESMOPRESSIN ACETATE
  DESMOPRESSIN ACETATE, DESMOPRESSIN ACETATE
  DICYCLOMINE HCL (PRESERVATIVE-FREE),
    DICYCLOMINE HYDROCHLORIDE
  DIHYDROERGOTAMINE MESYLATE,
    DIHYDROERGOTAMINE MESYLATE
  DILTIAZEM HCL, DILTIAZEM HYDROCHLORIDE
  DIPYRIDAMOLE, DIPYRIDAMOLE
  DOBUTAMINE HCL, DOBUTAMINE HYDROCHLORIDE
  DOXAPRAM HCL, DOXAPRAM HYDROCHLORIDE
  DOXORUBICIN HCL, DOXORUBICIN HYDROCHLORIDE
  DOXYCYCLINE, DOXYCYCLINE HYCLATE
  ENALAPRILAT, ENALAPRILAT
  ETOMIDATE, ETOMIDATE
  ETOPOSIDE, ETOPOSIDE
  FAMOTIDINE PRESERVATIVE FREE, FAMOTIDINE
  FAMOTIDINE, FAMOTIDINE
  FLOXURIDINE, FLOXURIDINE
  FLUOROURACIL, FLUOROURACIL
  FLUPHENAZINE DECANOATE, FLUPHENAZINE
    DECANOATE
  HALOPERIDOL DECANOATE, HALOPERIDOL
    DECANOATE
  HALOPERIDOL, HALOPERIDOL LACTATE
  KETAMINE HCL, KETAMINE HYDROCHLORIDE
  KETOROLAC TROMETHAMINE, KETOROLAC
    TROMETHAMINE
  LABETALOL HCL, LABETALOL HYDROCHLORIDE
  LEUCOVORIN CALCIUM PRESERVATIVE FREE,
    LEUCOVORIN CALCIUM
  LEUCOVORIN CALCIUM, LEUCOVORIN CALCIUM
  LEVOCARNITINE, LEVOCARNITINE
  METHOTREXATE SODIUM, METHOTREXATE SODIUM
  METOCLOPRAMIDE HCL, METOCLOPRAMIDE
    HYDROCHLORIDE

  MIDAZOLAM HCL, MIDAZOLAM HYDROCHLORIDE
  MILRINONE LACTATE, MILRINONE LACTATE
  MITOMYCIN, MITOMYCIN
  OFLOXACIN, OFLOXACIN
  PACLITAXEL, PACLITAXEL
  PAMIDRONATE DISODIUM, PAMIDRONATE DISODIUM
  PHENTOLAMINE MESYLATE, PHENTOLAMINE
    MESYLATE
  POLYMYXIN B SULFATE, POLYMYXIN B SULFATE
  PROPRANOLOL HCL, PROPRANOLOL HYDROCHLORIDE
  RIFAMPIN, RIFAMPIN
  SULFAMETHOXAZOLE AND TRIMETHOPRIM,
    SULFAMETHOXAZOLE
  THIOTEPA, THIOTEPA
  VALPROATE SODIUM, VALPROATE SODIUM
  VECURONIUM BROMIDE, VECURONIUM BROMIDE
  VERAPAMIL HCL, VERAPAMIL HYDROCHLORIDE
  VINBLASTINE SULFATE, VINBLASTINE SULFATE
BEDFORD LABS
BEDFORD LABORATORIES
  AMIODARONE HCL, AMIODARONE HYDROCHLORIDE
  ORPHENADRINE CITRATE, ORPHENADRINE CITRATE
BEDFORD LABORATORIES INC
  LEUPROLIDE ACETATE, LEUPROLIDE ACETATE
BEECHAM
BEECHAM LABORATORIES DIV BEECHAM INC
  PROBENECID AND COLCHICINE, COLCHICINE
BEL MAR
BEL MAR LABORATORIES INC
  CHLORPHENIRAMINE MALEATE, CHLORPHENIRAMINE
    MALEATE
  CHORIONIC GONADOTROPIN, GONADOTROPIN,
    CHORIONIC
  DEXAMETHASONE SODIUM PHOSPHATE,
    DEXAMETHASONE SODIUM PHOSPHATE
  DIPHENHYDRAMINE HCL, DIPHENHYDRAMINE
    HYDROCHLORIDE
  HYDROCORTISONE ACETATE, HYDROCORTISONE
    ACETATE
  HYDROXOMIN, HYDROXOCOBALAMIN
  LIDOCAINE HCL W/ EPINEPHRINE, EPINEPHRINE
  LIDOCAINE HCL, LIDOCAINE HYDROCHLORIDE
  M-PREDROL, METHYLPREDNISOLONE ACETATE
  PREDNISOLONE ACETATE, PREDNISOLONE ACETATE
  PROCAINE HCL W/ EPINEPHRINE, EPINEPHRINE
  PROCAINE HCL, PROCAINE HYDROCHLORIDE
  PYRIDAMAL 100, CHLORPHENIRAMINE MALEATE
  PYRIDOXINE HCL, PYRIDOXINE HYDROCHLORIDE
  RUBIVITE, CYANOCOBALAMIN
  TESTOSTERONE PROPIONATE, TESTOSTERONE
    PROPIONATE
  THIAMINE HCL, THIAMINE HYDROCHLORIDE
  VITAMIN A PALMITATE, VITAMIN A PALMITATE
BELL PHARMA
BELL PHARMACAL CORP
  CHLORPHENIRAMINE MALEATE, CHLORPHENIRAMINE
    MALEATE
  RESERPINE, RESERPINE
BEN VENUE
BEN VENUE LABORATORIES INC
  AMIODARONE HCL, AMIODARONE HYDROCHLORIDE
  FAMOTIDINE PRESERVATIVE FREE, FAMOTIDINE
  MIDAZOLAM HCL, MIDAZOLAM HYDROCHLORIDE
BERLEX
BERLEX
  FINACEA, AZELAIC ACID
BERLEX LABORATORIES INC SUB SCHERING AG
  ANGIOVIST 282, DIATRIZOATE MEGLUMINE

APPENDIX B
PRODUCT NAME INDEX
LISTED BY APPLICANT (*continued*)

ANGIOVIST 292, DIATRIZOATE MEGLUMINE
ANGIOVIST 370, DIATRIZOATE MEGLUMINE
BILIVIST, IPODATE SODIUM
FLUDARA, FLUDARABINE PHOSPHATE
GASTROVIST, DIATRIZOATE MEGLUMINE
MAGNEVIST, GADOPENTETATE DIMEGLUMINE
QUINACT, QUINIDINE GLUCONATE
SULLA, SULFAMETER
UROVIST CYSTO PEDIATRIC, DIATRIZOATE MEGLUMINE
UROVIST CYSTO, DIATRIZOATE MEGLUMINE
UROVIST MEGLUMINE DIU/CT, DIATRIZOATE
    MEGLUMINE
UROVIST SODIUM 300, DIATRIZOATE SODIUM
VI-TWEL, CYANOCOBALAMIN
BERLEX LABS
BERLEX LABORATORIES INC
    BETAPACE AF, SOTALOL HYDROCHLORIDE
    BETAPACE, SOTALOL HYDROCHLORIDE
    CLIMARA, ESTRADIOL
    LEVLITE, ETHINYL ESTRADIOL
    MAGNEVIST, GADOPENTETATE DIMEGLUMINE
    MIRENA, LEVONORGESTREL
    OSMOVIST 190, IOTROLAN
    OSMOVIST 240, IOTROLAN
    QUINAGLUTE, QUINIDINE GLUCONATE
    REFLUDAN, LEPIRUDIN
    ULTRAVIST (PHARMACY BULK), IOPROMIDE
    ULTRAVIST 150, IOPROMIDE
    ULTRAVIST 240, IOPROMIDE
    ULTRAVIST 300, IOPROMIDE
    ULTRAVIST 370, IOPROMIDE
    YASMIN, DROSPIRENONE
BERTEK
BERTEK PHARMACEUTICALS INC
    MENTAX-TC, BUTENAFINE HYDROCHLORIDE
BERTEK PHARMS

    AVITA, TRETINOIN
    MENTAX, BUTENAFINE HYDROCHLORIDE
    SULFAMYLON, MAFENIDE ACETATE
BETA DERMAC
BETA DERMACEUTICALS INC
    BETA-HC, HYDROCORTISONE
BH
BH CHEMICALS INC
    HALOTHANE, HALOTHANE
BIGMAR
BIGMAR INC
    DAUNORUBICIN HCL, DAUNORUBICIN
        HYDROCHLORIDE
    FLUOROURACIL, FLUOROURACIL
    LEUCOVORIN CALCIUM PRESERVATIVE FREE,
        LEUCOVORIN CALCIUM
    METHOTREXATE PRESERVATIVE FREE,
        METHOTREXATE SODIUM
    METHOTREXATE, METHOTREXATE SODIUM
BIO NUCLEONICS
BIO NUCLEONICS INC
    STRONTIUM CHLORIDE SR-89, STRONTIUM CHLORIDE,
        SR-89
BIO TECH GEN
BIO TECHNOLOGY GENERAL CORP
    BIO-TROPIN, SOMATROPIN RECOMBINANT
    OXANDRIN, OXANDROLONE
    TEV-TROPIN, SOMATROPIN RECOMBINANT
BIOCHEMIE
BIOCHEMIE GMBH
    AMOXICILLIN, AMOXICILLIN

AMPICILLIN TRIHYDRATE, AMPICILLIN/AMPICILLIN
    TRIHYDRATE
PENICILLIN G SODIUM, PENICILLIN G SODIUM
PENICILLIN V POTASSIUM, PENICILLIN V POTASSIUM
BIOENVISION
BIOENVISION INC
    MODRASTANE, TRILOSTANE
BIOGLAN
BIOGLAN LABORATORIES LTD
    ALPHADERM, HYDROCORTISONE
BIOGLAN PHARMA
BIOGLAN PHARMA INC
    C-SOLVE-2, ERYTHROMYCIN
    SOLARAZE, DICLOFENAC SODIUM
BIOGLAN PHARMS
BIOGLAN PHARMACEUTICALS CO
    ZONALON, DOXEPIN HYDROCHLORIDE
BIONICHE (CANADA)
BIONICHE PHARMA (CANADA) LTD
    AMIODARONE HCL, AMIODARONE HYDROCHLORIDE
    DIMETHYL SULFOXIDE, DIMETHYL SULFOXIDE
    EDETATE DISODIUM, EDETATE DISODIUM
    KETAMINE HCL, KETAMINE HYDROCHLORIDE
    MILRINONE LACTATE, MILRINONE LACTATE
BIOVAIL
BIOVAIL CORP INTERNATIONAL
    TIAZAC, DILTIAZEM HYDROCHLORIDE
BIOVAIL LABORATORIES INC
    ATIVAN, LORAZEPAM
    CARDIZEM LA, DILTIAZEM HYDROCHLORIDE
    CARDIZEM, DILTIAZEM HYDROCHLORIDE
    DICLOFENAC SODIUM, DICLOFENAC SODIUM
    DILTIAZEM HCL, DILTIAZEM HYDROCHLORIDE
    ISORDIL, ISOSORBIDE DINITRATE
    NIFEDIPINE, NIFEDIPINE
    PENTOXIFYLLINE, PENTOXIFYLLINE
    TECZEM, DILTIAZEM MALATE
    VASERETIC, ENALAPRIL MALEATE
    VASOTEC, ENALAPRIL MALEATE
    VASOTEC, ENALAPRILAT
BIOVAIL TECHNOLOGIES
    CEDAX, CEFTIBUTEN DIHYDRATE
BIOVAIL PHARMS
BIOVAIL PHARMACEUTICALS INC
    TEVETEN HCT, EPROSARTAN MESYLATE
    TEVETEN, EPROSARTAN MESYLATE
BLAIREX
BLAIREX LABORATORIES INC
    BRONCHO SALINE, SODIUM CHLORIDE (OTC)
BLUE RIDGE
BLUE RIDGE LABORATORIES INC
    CARAFATE, SUCRALFATE
BLULINE
BLULINE LABORATORIES INC
    EPICORT, HYDROCORTISONE
    MULTIFUGE, PIPERAZINE CITRATE
BOEHRINGER INGELHEIM
BOEHRINGER INGELHEIM
    ALUPENT, METAPROTERENOL SULFATE
    CATAPRES, CLONIDINE HYDROCHLORIDE
    CATAPRES-TTS-1, CLONIDINE
    CATAPRES-TTS-2, CLONIDINE
    CATAPRES-TTS-3, CLONIDINE
    MEXITIL, MEXILETINE HYDROCHLORIDE
    MICARDIS HCT, HYDROCHLOROTHIAZIDE
    MICARDIS, TELMISARTAN
BOEHRINGER INGELHEIM CORP
    RANITIDINE HCL, RANITIDINE HYDROCHLORIDE

APPENDIX B
PRODUCT NAME INDEX
LISTED BY APPLICANT (*continued*)

BOEHRINGER INGELHEIM PHARMACEUTICALS INC
  AGGRENOX, ASPIRIN
  ALUPENT, METAPROTERENOL SULFATE
  ATROVENT, IPRATROPIUM BROMIDE
  COMBIPRES, CHLORTHALIDONE
  COMBIVENT, ALBUTEROL SULFATE
  FLOMAX, TAMSULOSIN HYDROCHLORIDE
  IV PERSANTINE, DIPYRIDAMOLE
  MOBIC, MELOXICAM
  PERSANTINE, DIPYRIDAMOLE
  PRELUDIN, PHENMETRAZINE HYDROCHLORIDE
  VIRAMUNE, NEVIRAPINE
BONE CARE
BONE CARE INTERNATIONAL INC
  HECTOROL, DOXERCALCIFEROL
BOWMAN PHARMS
BOWMAN PHARMACEUTICALS INC
  HISERPIA, RESERPINE
  HIWOLFIA, RAUWOLFIA SERPENTINA
BRACCO
BRACCO DIAGNOSTICS INC
  CARDIOGEN-82, RUBIDIUM CHLORIDE RB-82
  CARDIOGRAFIN, DIATRIZOATE MEGLUMINE
  CARDIOTEC, TECHNETIUM TC-99M TEBOROXIME KIT
  CHLORMERODRIN HG 197, CHLORMERODRIN, HG-197
  CHOLETEC, TECHNETIUM TC-99M MEBROFENIN KIT
  CHOLOGRAFIN MEGLUMINE, IODIPAMIDE MEGLUMINE
  CHOLOGRAFIN SODIUM, IODIPAMIDE SODIUM
  CHOLOVUE, IODOXAMATE MEGLUMINE
  CHROMITOPE SODIUM, SODIUM CHROMATE, CR-51
  CYSTOGRAFIN DILUTE, DIATRIZOATE MEGLUMINE
  CYSTOGRAFIN, DIATRIZOATE MEGLUMINE
  DIATRIZOATE MEGLUMINE, DIATRIZOATE MEGLUMINE
  GASTROGRAFIN, DIATRIZOATE MEGLUMINE
  HIPPUTOPE, IODOHIPPURATE SODIUM, I-131
  IODOTOPE, SODIUM IODIDE, I-131
  ISOVUE-128, IOPAMIDOL
  ISOVUE-200, IOPAMIDOL
  ISOVUE-250, IOPAMIDOL
  ISOVUE-300, IOPAMIDOL
  ISOVUE-370, IOPAMIDOL
  ISOVUE-M 200, IOPAMIDOL
  ISOVUE-M 300, IOPAMIDOL
  KINEVAC, SINCALIDE
  LUMENHANCE, MANGANESE CHLORIDE
    TETRAHYDRATE
  MACROTEC, TECHNETIUM TC-99M ALBUMIN
    AGGREGATED KIT
  MDP-BRACCO, TECHNETIUM TC-99M MEDRONATE KIT
  MINITEC, TECHNETIUM TC-99M SODIUM
    PERTECHNETATE GENERATOR
  ORAGRAFIN CALCIUM, IPODATE CALCIUM
  ORAGRAFIN SODIUM, IPODATE SODIUM
  PHOSPHOTEC, TECHNETIUM TC-99M
    PYROPHOSPHATE KIT
  PHOSPHOTOPE, SODIUM PHOSPHATE, P-32
  PROHANCE, GADOTERIDOL
  RENO-30, DIATRIZOATE MEGLUMINE
  RENO-60, DIATRIZOATE MEGLUMINE
  RENO-DIP, DIATRIZOATE MEGLUMINE
  RENOCAL-76, DIATRIZOATE MEGLUMINE
  RENOGRAFIN-60, DIATRIZOATE MEGLUMINE
  RENOGRAFIN-76, DIATRIZOATE MEGLUMINE
  RENOTEC, TECHNETIUM TC-99M FERPENTETATE KIT
  RENOVIST II, DIATRIZOATE MEGLUMINE
  RENOVIST, DIATRIZOATE MEGLUMINE
  RENOVUE-65, IODAMIDE MEGLUMINE
  RENOVUE-DIP, IODAMIDE MEGLUMINE

  ROBENGATOPE, ROSE BENGAL SODIUM, I-131
  RUBRATOPE-57 KIT, COBALT CHLORIDE, CO-57
  RUBRATOPE-57, CYANOCOBALAMIN, CO-57
  RUBRATOPE-60 KIT, COBALT CHLORIDE, CO-60
  RUBRATOPE-60, CYANOCOBALAMIN, CO-60
  SETHOTOPE, SELENOMETHIONINE, SE-75
  SINOGRAFIN, DIATRIZOATE MEGLUMINE
  SONORX, SIMETHICONE-CELLULOSE
  TESULOID, TECHNETIUM TC-99M SULFUR COLLOID KIT
  THALLOUS CHLORIDE TL 201, THALLOUS CHLORIDE, TL-
  201
BRADLEY PHARMS
BRADLEY PHARMACEUTICALS INC
  PAMINE FORTE, METHSCOPOLAMINE BROMIDE
  PAMINE, METHSCOPOLAMINE BROMIDE
BRAINTREE
BRAINTREE LABORATORIES INC
  GOLYTELY, POLYETHYLENE GLYCOL 3350
  MIRALAX, POLYETHYLENE GLYCOL 3350
  NULYTELY, POLYETHYLENE GLYCOL 3350
  NULYTELY-FLAVORED, POLYETHYLENE GLYCOL 3350
  PHOSLO GELCAPS, CALCIUM ACETATE
  PHOSLO, CALCIUM ACETATE
BRIGHTSTONE
BRIGHTSTONE PHARMA INC
  ISOSORBIDE MONONITRATE, ISOSORBIDE
    MONONITRATE
BRISTOL
BRISTOL LABORATORIES INC DIV BRISTOL MYERS CO
  BETAPEN-VK, PENICILLIN V POTASSIUM
  BICNU, CARMUSTINE
  BRISTACYCLINE, TETRACYCLINE HYDROCHLORIDE
  BRISTAGEN, GENTAMICIN SULFATE
  BRISTAMYCIN, ERYTHROMYCIN STEARATE
  CEPHALOTHIN SODIUM, CEPHALOTHIN SODIUM
  LYSODREN, MITOTANE
  MEXATE, METHOTREXATE SODIUM
  MUTAMYCIN, MITOMYCIN
  POLYCILLIN, AMPICILLIN/AMPICILLIN TRIHYDRATE
  POLYCILLIN-N, AMPICILLIN SODIUM
  POLYCILLIN-PRB, AMPICILLIN/AMPICILLIN TRIHYDRATE
  PRECEF, CEFORANIDE
  TETREX, TETRACYCLINE PHOSPHATE COMPLEX
  ULTRACEF, CEFADROXIL/CEFADROXIL HEMIHYDRATE
  VEPESID, ETOPOSIDE
  VERSAPEN, HETACILLIN
  VERSAPEN-K, HETACILLIN POTASSIUM
BRISTOL MYERS
BRISTOL MYERS CO
  MEXATE-AQ, METHOTREXATE SODIUM
  MUTAMYCIN, MITOMYCIN
  PLATINOL, CISPLATIN
  PLATINOL-AQ, CISPLATIN
  QUESTRAN LIGHT, CHOLESTYRAMINE
  QUESTRAN, CHOLESTYRAMINE
BRISTOL MYERS PRODUCTS INC
  EXCEDRIN (MIGRAINE), ACETAMINOPHEN (OTC)
  NUPRIN, IBUPROFEN (OTC)
BRISTOL MYERS SQUIBB
BRISTOL MYERS SQUIBB
  AZACTAM, AZTREONAM
  DELALUTIN, HYDROXYPROGESTERONE CAPROATE
  DEXTROSE 5% AND POTASSIUM CHLORIDE 0.075% IN
    PLASTIC CONTAINER, DEXTROSE
  DEXTROSE 5% AND POTASSIUM CHLORIDE 0.15% IN
    PLASTIC CONTAINER, DEXTROSE
  DEXTROSE 5% AND POTASSIUM CHLORIDE 0.224% IN
    PLASTIC CONTAINER, DEXTROSE

APPENDIX B
PRODUCT NAME INDEX
LISTED BY APPLICANT (*continued*)

DEXTROSE 5% AND POTASSIUM CHLORIDE 0.3% IN
    PLASTIC CONTAINER, DEXTROSE
FOLLUTEIN, GONADOTROPIN, CHORIONIC
GLUCOVANCE, GLYBURIDE
HALOG, HALCINONIDE
MEGACE, MEGESTROL ACETATE
MEXATE-AQ PRESERVED, METHOTREXATE SODIUM
MONOPRIL-HCT, FOSINOPRIL SODIUM
MYCOSTATIN, NYSTATIN
ORA-TESTRYL, FLUOXYMESTERONE
PRAVACHOL, PRAVASTATIN SODIUM
STILBESTROL, DIETHYLSTILBESTROL
STILBETIN, DIETHYLSTILBESTROL
TESLAC, TESTOLACTONE
VINCREX, VINCRISTINE SULFATE
BRISTOL MYERS SQUIBB CO
    AMITID, AMITRIPTYLINE HYDROCHLORIDE
    AMNESTROGEN, ESTROGENS, ESTERIFIED
    AZACTAM IN PLASTIC CONTAINER, AZTREONAM
    CEENU, LOMUSTINE
    DROXIA, HYDROXYUREA
    ESTRACE, ESTRADIOL
    ETHRIL 250, ERYTHROMYCIN STEARATE
    ETHRIL 500, ERYTHROMYCIN STEARATE
    ETOPOPHOS PRESERVATIVE FREE, ETOPOSIDE
        PHOSPHATE
    FUNGIZONE, AMPHOTERICIN B
    GLUCOPHAGE XR, METFORMIN HYDROCHLORIDE
    HYDREA, HYDROXYUREA
    KENACORT, TRIAMCINOLONE
    KENACORT, TRIAMCINOLONE DIACETATE
    METAGLIP, GLIPIZIDE
    MYCOSTATIN, NYSTATIN
    NEOMYCIN SULFATE, NEOMYCIN SULFATE
    NYDRAZID, ISONIAZID
    PRAVIGARD PAC (COPACKAGED), ASPIRIN
    PROLIXIN DECANOATE, FLUPHENAZINE DECANOATE
    PROTAMINE ZINC INSULIN, INSULIN SUSP PROTAMINE
        ZINC PURIFIED BEEF (OTC)
    RAU-SED, RESERPINE
    REYATAZ, ATAZANAVIR SULFATE
    REZIPAS, AMINOSALICYLIC ACID RESIN COMPLEX
    RUBEX, DOXORUBICIN HYDROCHLORIDE
    RUBRAMIN PC, CYANOCOBALAMIN
    SUSTIVA, EFAVIRENZ
    TERFONYL, TRISULFAPYRIMIDINES (SULFADIAZINE;
        SULFAMERAZINE; SULFAMETHAZINE)
    TESLAC, TESTOLACTONE
    TUBOCURARINE CHLORIDE, TUBOCURARINE
        CHLORIDE
    VAGISTAT-1, TIOCONAZOLE (OTC)
    VELOSEF, CEPHRADINE
    VEPESID, ETOPOSIDE
    VESPRIN, TRIFLUPROMAZINE HYDROCHLORIDE
    VIDEX EC, DIDANOSINE
    VITAMIN A, VITAMIN A PALMITATE
    ZERIT XR, STAVUDINE
BRISTOL MYERS SQUIBB CO PHARMACEUTICAL RE-
SEARCH INSTITUTE
    BLENOXANE, BLEOMYCIN SULFATE
    BUSPAR, BUSPIRONE HYDROCHLORIDE
    CEFZIL, CEFPROZIL
    CYTOXAN, CYCLOPHOSPHAMIDE
    DEAPRIL-ST, ERGOLOID MESYLATES
    DOVONEX, CALCIPOTRIENE
    ESTRACE, ESTRADIOL
    ETOPOPHOS PRESERVATIVE FREE, ETOPOSIDE
        PHOSPHATE

GLUCOPHAGE, METFORMIN HYDROCHLORIDE
IFEX, IFOSFAMIDE
IFEX/MESNEX KIT, IFOSFAMIDE
KENALOG, TRIAMCINOLONE ACETONIDE
LYOPHILIZED CYTOXAN, CYCLOPHOSPHAMIDE
MAXIPIME, CEFEPIME HYDROCHLORIDE (ARGININE
    FORMULATION)
MONOPRIL, FOSINOPRIL SODIUM
PARAPLATIN, CARBOPLATIN
SERZONE, NEFAZODONE HYDROCHLORIDE
STADOL, BUTORPHANOL TARTRATE
TAXOL, PACLITAXEL
TEQUIN, GATIFLOXACIN
VIDEX, DIDANOSINE
VUMON, TENIPOSIDE
ZERIT, STAVUDINE
BRISTOL MYERS SQUIBB MEDICAL IMAGING
    DEFINITY, PERFLUTREN
    GALLIUM CITRATE GA 67, GALLIUM CITRATE, GA-67
    NEUROLITE, TECHNETIUM TC-99M BICISATE KIT
    TECHNELITE, TECHNETIUM TC-99M SODIUM
        PERTECHNETATE GENERATOR
    THALLOUS CHLORIDE TL 201, THALLOUS CHLORIDE, TL-
        201
    XENON XE 133, XENON, XE-133
BRISTOL MYERS SQUIBB PHARMA CO
    CARDIOLITE, TECHNETIUM TC-99M SESTAMIBI KIT
    CLINDAMYCIN PHOSPHATE, CLINDAMYCIN
        PHOSPHATE
    COUMADIN, WARFARIN SODIUM
    GLUCOSCAN, TECHNETIUM TC-99M GLUCEPTATE KIT
    LODOSYN, CARBIDOPA
    MIRALUMA, TECHNETIUM TC-99M SESTAMIBI KIT
    NARCAN, NALOXONE HYDROCHLORIDE
    OXYCODONE 2.5/APAP 500, ACETAMINOPHEN
    OXYCODONE 5/APAP 500, ACETAMINOPHEN
    REMSED, PROMETHAZINE HYDROCHLORIDE
    SINEMET CR, CARBIDOPA
    SINEMET, CARBIDOPA
    SUSTIVA, EFAVIRENZ
BRISTOL MYERS SQUIBB SPA
    PENICILLIN G SODIUM, PENICILLIN G SODIUM
BRYAN
BRYAN CORP
    SCLEROSOL, TALC
BUNDY
CM BUNDY CO
    BUTABARBITAL, BUTABARBITAL SODIUM
    DIPHENHYDRAMINE HCL, DIPHENHYDRAMINE
        HYDROCHLORIDE
    MECLIZINE HCL, MECLIZINE HYDROCHLORIDE
    PREDNISOLONE, PREDNISOLONE
    PREDNISONE, PREDNISONE
    RAUWOLFIA SERPENTINA, RAUWOLFIA SERPENTINA
    RESERPINE, RESERPINE

C

C AND M PHARMA
C AND M PHARMACAL INC
    HC (HYDROCORTISONE), HYDROCORTISONE
    HC (HYDROCORTISONE), HYDROCORTISONE (OTC)
    HI-COR, HYDROCORTISONE
CADEMA
CADEMA MEDICAL PRODUCTS INC
    RBC-SCAN, TECHNETIUM TC-99M RED BLOOD CELL KIT

APPENDIX B
PRODUCT NAME INDEX
LISTED BY APPLICANT (*continued*)

CALGON
CALGON CORP DIV MERCK AND CO INC
  SEPTI-SOFT, HEXACHLOROPHENE
CAMALL
CAMALL CO INC
  CAM-METRAZINE, PHENDIMETRAZINE TARTRATE
  PHENTERMINE HCL, PHENTERMINE HYDROCHLORIDE
CARACO
CARACO PHARMACEUTICAL LABORATORIES LTD
  CARBAMAZEPINE, CARBAMAZEPINE
  CLONAZEPAM, CLONAZEPAM
  CLOZAPINE, CLOZAPINE
  DIGOXIN, DIGOXIN
  FLURBIPROFEN, FLURBIPROFEN
  MEPERIDINE HCL, MEPERIDINE HYDROCHLORIDE
  METFORMIN HCL, METFORMIN HYDROCHLORIDE
  METOPROLOL TARTRATE, METOPROLOL TARTRATE
  OXAPROZIN, OXAPROZIN
  PAROMOMYCIN SULFATE, PAROMOMYCIN SULFATE
  TICLOPIDINE HCL, TICLOPIDINE HYDROCHLORIDE
  TRAMADOL HCL, TRAMADOL HYDROCHLORIDE
CARLISLE
CARLISLE LABORATORIES INC
  ALPHACAINE HCL W/ EPINEPHRINE, EPINEPHRINE
  ALPHACAINE HCL, LIDOCAINE HYDROCHLORIDE
  ALPHACAINE, LIDOCAINE
CARLSBAD
CARLSBAD TECHNOLOGY INC
  ACYCLOVIR, ACYCLOVIR
  DICLOFENAC SODIUM, DICLOFENAC SODIUM
  FAMOTIDINE, FAMOTIDINE
  FLUOXETINE, FLUOXETINE HYDROCHLORIDE
  LOVASTATIN, LOVASTATIN
CARNRICK
CARNRICK LABORATORIES INC DIV GW CARNRICK CO
  CAPITAL WITH CODEINE, ACETAMINOPHEN
CAROLINA MEDCL
CAROLINA MEDICAL PRODUCTS CO
  AMANTADINE HCL, AMANTADINE HYDROCHLORIDE
  HYDROCORTISONE IN ABSORBASE,
    HYDROCORTISONE
  ISONIAZID, ISONIAZID
  SODIUM POLYSTYRENE SULFONATE, SODIUM
    POLYSTYRENE SULFONATE
  SPS, SODIUM POLYSTYRENE SULFONATE
  TRIAMCINOLONE ACETONIDE IN ABSORBASE,
    TRIAMCINOLONE ACETONIDE
CELGENE
CELGENE CORP
  THALOMID, THALIDOMIDE
CELL THERAP
CELL THERAPEUTICS INC
  TRISENOX, ARSENIC TRIOXIDE
CELLTECH MFG
CELLTECH MANUFACTURING INC
  METADATE ER, METHYLPHENIDATE HYDROCHLORIDE
  METHYLPHENIDATE HCL, METHYLPHENIDATE
    HYDROCHLORIDE
CELLTECH PHARMS
CELLTECH PHARMACEUTICALS INC
  ALBUTEROL SULFATE, ALBUTEROL SULFATE
  AMITRIPTYLINE HCL, AMITRIPTYLINE HYDROCHLORIDE
  BIPHETAMINE 12.5, AMPHETAMINE RESIN COMPLEX
  BIPHETAMINE 20, AMPHETAMINE RESIN COMPLEX
  BIPHETAMINE 7.5, AMPHETAMINE RESIN COMPLEX
  CORSYM, CHLORPHENIRAMINE POLISTIREX (OTC)
  DELSYM, DEXTROMETHORPHAN POLISTIREX (OTC)
  DEXACORT, DEXAMETHASONE SODIUM PHOSPHATE

  DIETHYLPROPION HCL, DIETHYLPROPION
    HYDROCHLORIDE
  GASTROCROM, CROMOLYN SODIUM
  GLUTETHIMIDE, GLUTETHIMIDE
  IONAMIN, PHENTERMINE RESIN COMPLEX
  METADATE CD, METHYLPHENIDATE HYDROCHLORIDE
  METADATE ER, METHYLPHENIDATE HYDROCHLORIDE
  MYKROX, METOLAZONE
  PEDIAPRED, PREDNISOLONE SODIUM PHOSPHATE
  PSEUDO-12, PSEUDOEPHEDRINE POLISTIREX (OTC)
  SEMPREX-D, ACRIVASTINE
  TUSSIONEX, CHLORPHENIRAMINE POLISTIREX
  ZAROXOLYN, METOLAZONE
CENCI
CENCI POWDER PRODUCTS INC
  THEOPHYLLINE, THEOPHYLLINE
HR CENCI LABORATORIES INC
  ACTAHIST, PSEUDOEPHEDRINE HYDROCHLORIDE
  DIBENIL, DIPHENHYDRAMINE HYDROCHLORIDE
  DIPHENHYDRAMINE HCL, DIPHENHYDRAMINE
    HYDROCHLORIDE
  ELIXOMIN, THEOPHYLLINE
  HISTAFED, PSEUDOEPHEDRINE HYDROCHLORIDE
  HYDROCORTISONE ACETATE, HYDROCORTISONE
    ACETATE
  PROMETHAZINE VC PLAIN, PHENYLEPHRINE
    HYDROCHLORIDE
  PROMETHAZINE VC W/ CODEINE, CODEINE
    PHOSPHATE
  PROMETHAZINE W/ CODEINE, CODEINE PHOSPHATE
  PROMETHAZINE, PROMETHAZINE HYDROCHLORIDE
  TRIPROLIDINE AND PSEUDOEPHEDRINE
    HYDROCHLORIDES W/ CODEINE, CODEINE
    PHOSPHATE
CENT PHARMS
CENTRAL PHARMACEUTICALS INC
  ACETAMINOPHEN AND HYDROCODONE BITARTRATE,
    ACETAMINOPHEN
  AZDONE, ASPIRIN
  CO-GESIC, ACETAMINOPHEN
  DEXACEN-4, DEXAMETHASONE SODIUM PHOSPHATE
  PHENYLPROPANOLAMINE HCL W/
    CHLORPHENIRAMINE MALEATE,
    CHLORPHENIRAMINE MALEATE (OTC)
  PREDNISOLONE ACETATE, PREDNISOLONE ACETATE
  PSEUDOEPHEDRINE HCL AND CHLORPHENIRAMINE
    MALEATE, CHLORPHENIRAMINE MALEATE (OTC)
  SYNOPHYLATE, THEOPHYLLINE SODIUM GLYCINATE
  THEOCLEAR-100, THEOPHYLLINE
  THEOCLEAR-200, THEOPHYLLINE
  THEOCLEAR-80, THEOPHYLLINE
  THEOPHYLLINE, THEOPHYLLINE
CENTURY PHARMS
CENTURY PHARMACEUTICALS INC
  P.A.S. SODIUM, AMINOSALICYLATE SODIUM
CEPH INTL
CEPH INTERNATIONAL CORP
  CECLOR, CEFACLOR
  KEFLEX, CEPHALEXIN
CEPHALON
CEPHALON INC
  GABITRIL, TIAGABINE HYDROCHLORIDE
  PROVIGIL, MODAFINIL
CHAMBERLIN PARENTERL
CHAMBERLIN PARENTERAL CORP
  HEPARIN SODIUM, HEPARIN SODIUM

APPENDIX B
PRODUCT NAME INDEX
LISTED BY APPLICANT (*continued*)

CHASE CHEM
CHASE CHEMICAL CO LP
    VITAMIN A, VITAMIN A
    VITAMIN A, VITAMIN A PALMITATE
    VITAMIN D, ERGOCALCIFEROL
CHASE LABS NJ
CHASE LABORATORIES INC
    NIFEDIPINE, NIFEDIPINE
CHATTEM
CHATTEM INC
    SELSUN, SELENIUM SULFIDE
CHESEBROUGH PONDS
CHESEBROUGH PONDS INC
    EXTRA-STRENGTH AIM, SODIUM
        MONOFLUOROPHOSPHATE (OTC)
    VIRAC REX, UNDECOYLIUM CHLORIDE
CHIRHOCLIN
CHIRHOCLIN INC
    SECREFLO, SECRETIN
CHIRON
CHIRON CORP
    TOBI, TOBRAMYCIN
CIBA
CIBA VISION CORP DIV NOVARTIS CO
    CATARASE, CHYMOTRYPSIN
CIS
CIS BIOINDUSTRIES COMPAGNIE
    SODIUM IODIDE I 131, SODIUM IODIDE, I-131
CIS US INC
    AN-DTPA, TECHNETIUM TC-99M PENTETATE KIT
    AN-MAA, TECHNETIUM TC-99M ALBUMIN AGGREGATED
        KIT
    AN-SULFUR COLLOID, TECHNETIUM TC-99M SULFUR
        COLLOID KIT
    CIS-MDP, TECHNETIUM TC-99M MEDRONATE KIT
    CIS-PYRO, TECHNETIUM TC-99M PYROPHOSPHATE KIT
    HEPATOLITE, TECHNETIUM TC-99M DISOFENIN KIT
    IOBENGUANE SULFATE I 131, IOBENGUANE SULFATE I
        131
    IODOHIPPURATE SODIUM I 131, IODOHIPPURATE
        SODIUM, I-131
    MICROLITE, TECHNETIUM TC-99M ALBUMIN COLLOID
        KIT
    OSTEOLITE, TECHNETIUM TC-99M MEDRONATE KIT
    PULMOLITE, TECHNETIUM TC-99M ALBUMIN
        AGGREGATED KIT
    PYROLITE, TECHNETIUM TC-99M PYRO/TRIMETA
        PHOSPHATES KIT
    SELENOMETHIONINE SE 75, SELENOMETHIONINE, SE-
        75
    SODIUM PERTECHNETATE TC 99M, TECHNETIUM TC-
        99M SODIUM PERTECHNETATE
CLAY PARK
CLAY PARK LABORATORIES INC
    AMMONIUM LACTATE, AMMONIUM LACTATE
    BETAMETHASONE DIPROPIONATE, BETAMETHASONE
        DIPROPIONATE
    BETAMETHASONE VALERATE, BETAMETHASONE
        VALERATE
    CLINDAMYCIN PHOSPHATE, CLINDAMYCIN
        PHOSPHATE
    ERYTHROMYCIN, ERYTHROMYCIN
    FLUOCINOLONE ACETONIDE, FLUOCINOLONE
        ACETONIDE
    FLUOCINONIDE, FLUOCINONIDE
    GENTAMICIN, GENTAMICIN SULFATE
    HYDROCORTISONE VALERATE, HYDROCORTISONE
        VALERATE

    HYDROCORTISONE, HYDROCORTISONE
    MINOXIDIL EXTRA STRENGTH (FOR MEN), MINOXIDIL
        (OTC)
    MOMETASONE FUROATE, MOMETASONE FUROATE
    NITROFURAZONE, NITROFURAZONE
    NYSTATIN AND TRIAMCINOLONE ACETONIDE,
        NYSTATIN
    NYSTATIN, NYSTATIN
    PERMETHRIN, PERMETHRIN
    PERMETHRIN, PERMETHRIN (OTC)
    PROMETHAZINE HCL, PROMETHAZINE
        HYDROCHLORIDE
    SELENIUM SULFIDE, SELENIUM SULFIDE
    TRIAMCINOLONE ACETONIDE, TRIAMCINOLONE
        ACETONIDE
    TRIDESILON, DESONIDE
    TRIPLE SULFA, TRIPLE SULFA (SULFABENZAMIDE;
        SULFACETAMIDE; SULFATHIAZOLE)
CLINTEC NUTR
CLINTEC NUTRITION CO SUB CLINIQUE
    CLINISOL 15% SULFITE FREE IN PLASTIC CONTAINER,
        AMINO ACIDS
CLONMEL
CLONMEL HEALTHCARE
    ACETAMINOPHEN AND CODEINE PHOSPHATE,
        ACETAMINOPHEN
    AMOXICILLIN, AMOXICILLIN
    AMPICILLIN TRIHYDRATE, AMPICILLIN/AMPICILLIN
        TRIHYDRATE
    PENICILLIN V POTASSIUM, PENICILLIN V POTASSIUM
    PYRAZINAMIDE, PYRAZINAMIDE
CLONMEL HLTHCARE
CLONMEL HEALTHCARE LTD
    ACHROMYCIN V, TETRACYCLINE HYDROCHLORIDE
    ACYCLOVIR, ACYCLOVIR
    ALBUTEROL SULFATE, ALBUTEROL SULFATE
    ALPRAZOLAM, ALPRAZOLAM
    ATENOLOL, ATENOLOL
    CAPTOPRIL, CAPTOPRIL
    CEFACLOR, CEFACLOR
    CHLORPROPAMIDE, CHLORPROPAMIDE
    CHLORTHALIDONE, CHLORTHALIDONE
    CIMETIDINE HCL, CIMETIDINE HYDROCHLORIDE
    CIMETIDINE, CIMETIDINE
    CLONIDINE HCL, CLONIDINE HYDROCHLORIDE
    CLORAZEPATE DIPOTASSIUM, CLORAZEPATE
        DIPOTASSIUM
    DIAZEPAM, DIAZEPAM
    DILTIAZEM HCL, DILTIAZEM HYDROCHLORIDE
    DIPYRIDAMOLE, DIPYRIDAMOLE
    DOLENE, PROPOXYPHENE HYDROCHLORIDE
    DOXEPIN HCL, DOXEPIN HYDROCHLORIDE
    ESTRADIOL, ESTRADIOL
    FENOPROFEN CALCIUM, FENOPROFEN CALCIUM
    FUROSEMIDE, FUROSEMIDE
    GEMFIBROZIL, GEMFIBROZIL
    GLYBURIDE (MICRONIZED), GLYBURIDE
    HYDRALAZINE HCL, HYDRALAZINE HYDROCHLORIDE
    HYDROCHLOROTHIAZIDE, HYDROCHLOROTHIAZIDE
    LORAZEPAM, LORAZEPAM
    METHOTREXATE SODIUM, METHOTREXATE SODIUM
    NAPROXEN, NAPROXEN
    SELEGILINE HCL, SELEGILINE HYDROCHLORIDE
COLGATE
COLGATE ORAL PHARMACEUTICALS INC
    ORABASE HCA, HYDROCORTISONE ACETATE
    PERIOGARD, CHLORHEXIDINE GLUCONATE

APPENDIX B
PRODUCT NAME INDEX
LISTED BY APPLICANT (*continued*)

COLGATE PALMOLIVE
COLGATE PALMOLIVE
  COLGATE TOTAL, SODIUM FLUORIDE (OTC)
COLLAGENEX
COLLAGENEX INC
  PERIOSTAT, DOXYCYCLINE HYCLATE
COLLAGENEX PHARMS
COLLAGENEX PHARMACEUTICALS INC
  PERIOSTAT, DOXYCYCLINE HYCLATE
COLUMBIA LABS
COLUMBIA LABORATORIES INC
  STRIANT, TESTOSTERONE
COLUMBIA RES LABS
COLUMBIA RESEARCH LABORATORIES INC
  CRINONE, PROGESTERONE
COMBE
COMBE INC
  BACITRACIN, BACITRACIN (OTC)
  LANABIOTIC, BACITRACIN (OTC)
  LANABIOTIC, BACITRACIN ZINC (OTC)
CONNETICS
CONNETICS CORP
  LUXIQ, BETAMETHASONE VALERATE
  OLUX FOAM, CLOBETASOL PROPIONATE
CONSOLIDATED MIDLAND
CONSOLIDATED MIDLAND CORP
  TEEBACIN, AMINOSALICYLATE SODIUM
CONSOLIDATED PHARM
CONSOLIDATED PHARMACEUTICAL GROUP INC
  AMOXICILLIN, AMOXICILLIN
  AMPICILLIN SODIUM, AMPICILLIN SODIUM
  AMPICILLIN TRIHYDRATE, AMPICILLIN/AMPICILLIN
    TRIHYDRATE
  PENICILLIN G POTASSIUM, PENICILLIN G POTASSIUM
  PENICILLIN G PROCAINE, PENICILLIN G PROCAINE
  PENICILLIN V POTASSIUM, PENICILLIN V POTASSIUM
CONTROLLED THERAP
CONTROLLED THERAPEUTICS (SCOTLAND) LTD
  CERVIDIL, DINOPROSTONE
COOK IMAGING
COOK IMAGING CORP
  IOPAMIDOL-200, IOPAMIDOL
  IOPAMIDOL-250, IOPAMIDOL
  IOPAMIDOL-300, IOPAMIDOL
  IOPAMIDOL-370, IOPAMIDOL
COPANOS
JOHN D COPANOS AND CO INC
  PENICILLIN G SODIUM, PENICILLIN G SODIUM
  STREPTOMYCIN SULFATE, STREPTOMYCIN SULFATE
COPLEY PHARM
COPLEY PHARMACEUTICAL INC
  ACYCLOVIR, ACYCLOVIR
  ALBUTEROL SULFATE, ALBUTEROL SULFATE
  AMANTADINE HCL, AMANTADINE HYDROCHLORIDE
  AMIODARONE HCL, AMIODARONE HYDROCHLORIDE
  AMITRIPTYLINE HCL, AMITRIPTYLINE HYDROCHLORIDE
  ATENOLOL, ATENOLOL
  BETAMETHASONE DIPROPIONATE, BETAMETHASONE
    DIPROPIONATE
  BETAMETHASONE VALERATE, BETAMETHASONE
    VALERATE
  BISOPROLOL FUMARATE, BISOPROLOL FUMARATE
  BROMATAPP, BROMPHENIRAMINE MALEATE (OTC)
  BROMPHERIL, DEXBROMPHENIRAMINE MALEATE (OTC)
  CAPTOPRIL, CAPTOPRIL
  CHOLESTYRAMINE LIGHT, CHOLESTYRAMINE
  CHOLESTYRAMINE, CHOLESTYRAMINE
  CIMETIDINE HCL, CIMETIDINE HYDROCHLORIDE

  CLEMASTINE FUMARATE, CLEMASTINE FUMARATE
  CLINDAMYCIN PHOSPHATE, CLINDAMYCIN
    PHOSPHATE
  CLOBETASOL PROPIONATE, CLOBETASOL
    PROPIONATE
  CO-LAV, POLYETHYLENE GLYCOL 3350
  DESONIDE, DESONIDE
  DICLOFENAC SODIUM, DICLOFENAC SODIUM
  DILTIAZEM HCL, DILTIAZEM HYDROCHLORIDE
  DOXEPIN HCL, DOXEPIN HYDROCHLORIDE
  DOXYLAMINE SUCCINATE, DOXYLAMINE SUCCINATE
    (OTC)
  ETHOSUXIMIDE, ETHOSUXIMIDE
  EVALOSE, LACTULOSE
  FLUOCINONIDE, FLUOCINONIDE
  FLUPHENAZINE HCL, FLUPHENAZINE HYDROCHLORIDE
  GO-EVAC, POLYETHYLENE GLYCOL 3350
  GUANABENZ ACETATE, GUANABENZ ACETATE
  GYNIX, CLOTRIMAZOLE (OTC)
  HALOPERIDOL, HALOPERIDOL LACTATE
  HEPTALAC, LACTULOSE
  HYDROCORTISONE ACETATE 1% AND PRAMOXINE HCL
    1%, HYDROCORTISONE ACETATE
  HYDROCORTISONE VALERATE, HYDROCORTISONE
    VALERATE
  HYDROCORTISONE, HYDROCORTISONE
  HYDROXYCHLOROQUINE SULFATE,
    HYDROXYCHLOROQUINE SULFATE
  LIDOCAINE HCL, LIDOCAINE HYDROCHLORIDE
  MEBENDAZOLE, MEBENDAZOLE
  MEGESTROL ACETATE, MEGESTROL ACETATE
  METAPROTERENOL SULFATE, METAPROTERENOL
    SULFATE
  METHAZOLAMIDE, METHAZOLAMIDE
  METOPROLOL TARTRATE, METOPROLOL TARTRATE
  MICONAZOLE NITRATE, MICONAZOLE NITRATE (OTC)
  MINOXIDIL (FOR MEN), MINOXIDIL (OTC)
  NABUMETONE, NABUMETONE
  NADOLOL, NADOLOL
  NAPROXEN SODIUM, NAPROXEN SODIUM
  NAPROXEN, NAPROXEN
  PEMOLINE, PEMOLINE
  PIROXICAM, PIROXICAM
  POTASSIUM CHLORIDE, POTASSIUM CHLORIDE
  PREDNISOLONE, PREDNISOLONE
  PROCAINAMIDE HCL, PROCAINAMIDE
    HYDROCHLORIDE
  PROCHLORPERAZINE MALEATE, PROCHLORPERAZINE
    MALEATE
  QUINIDINE SULFATE, QUINIDINE SULFATE
  THIORIDAZINE HCL, THIORIDAZINE HYDROCHLORIDE
  THIOTHIXENE HCL, THIOTHIXENE HYDROCHLORIDE
  TRETINOIN, TRETINOIN
  URSODIOL, URSODIOL
  VALPROIC ACID, VALPROIC ACID
COREPHARMA
COREPHARMA LLC
  ACETAMINOPHEN, ACETAMINOPHEN (OTC)
  BENZTROPINE MESYLATE, BENZTROPINE MESYLATE
  CARISOPRODOL, CARISOPRODOL
  DEXTROAMP SACCHARATE, AMP ASPARTATE,
    DEXTROAMP SULFATE AND AMP SULFATE,
    AMPHETAMINE ASPARTATE
  GLYBURIDE, GLYBURIDE
  METHENAMINE HIPPURATE, METHENAMINE
    HIPPURATE
  PYRIDOSTIGMINE BROMIDE, PYRIDOSTIGMINE
    BROMIDE

APPENDIX B
PRODUCT NAME INDEX
LISTED BY APPLICANT (*continued*)

RIMANTADINE HCL, RIMANTADINE HYDROCHLORIDE
TIZANIDINE HCL, TIZANIDINE HYDROCHLORIDE
TRAMADOL HCL, TRAMADOL HYDROCHLORIDE
CUMBERLAND SWAN
CUMBERLAND SWAN INC
   DIPHENHYDRAMINE HCL, DIPHENHYDRAMINE
     HYDROCHLORIDE (OTC)
CYTOGEN
CYTOGEN CORP
   QUADRAMET, SAMARIUM SM 153 LEXIDRONAM
     PENTASODIUM

D

DAIICHI
DAIICHI PHARMACEUTICAL CO LTD
   FLOXIN, OFLOXACIN
DAIICHI PHARMACEUTICAL CORP
   EVOXAC, CEVIMELINE HYDROCHLORIDE
DAINIPPON
DAINIPPON PHARMACEUTICAL USA CORP
   ZONEGRAN, ZONISAMIDE
DANCO LABS LLC
DANCO LABORATORIES LLC
   MIFEPREX, MIFEPRISTONE
DAVIS AND GECK
DAVIS AND GECK DIV AMERICAN CYANAMID CO
   FLAXEDIL, GALLAMINE TRIETHIODIDE
   PRE-OP II, HEXACHLOROPHENE
   PRE-OP, HEXACHLOROPHENE
DEL RAY LABS
DEL RAY LABORATORIES INC
   ALA-CORT, HYDROCORTISONE
   ALA-SCALP, HYDROCORTISONE
   DEL-VI-A, VITAMIN A PALMITATE
   TRIDERM, TRIAMCINOLONE ACETONIDE
DELL LABS
DELL LABORATORIES INC
   CYANOCOBALAMIN, CYANOCOBALAMIN
   DEXAMETHASONE SODIUM PHOSPHATE,
     DEXAMETHASONE SODIUM PHOSPHATE
   HEPARIN SODIUM, HEPARIN SODIUM
   LIDOCAINE HCL W/ EPINEPHRINE, EPINEPHRINE
   LIDOCAINE HCL, LIDOCAINE HYDROCHLORIDE
   PYRIDOXINE HCL, PYRIDOXINE HYDROCHLORIDE
   THIAMINE HCL, THIAMINE HYDROCHLORIDE
DENTSPLY PHARM
DENTSPLY PHARMACEUTICAL
   CITANEST FORTE, EPINEPHRINE BITARTRATE
   CITANEST PLAIN, PRILOCAINE HYDROCHLORIDE
   DURANEST, EPINEPHRINE BITARTRATE
   POLOCAINE W/ LEVONORDEFRIN, LEVONORDEFRIN
   POLOCAINE, MEPIVACAINE HYDROCHLORIDE
   XYLOCAINE W/ EPINEPHRINE, EPINEPHRINE
   XYLOCAINE, LIDOCAINE HYDROCHLORIDE
DEPROCO
DEPROCO INC
   LIGNOSPAN FORTE, EPINEPHRINE BITARTRATE
   LIGNOSPAN STANDARD, EPINEPHRINE BITARTRATE
   SCANDONEST L, LEVONORDEFRIN
   SCANDONEST PLAIN, MEPIVACAINE HYDROCHLORIDE
   SEPTOCAINE, ARTICAINE HYDROCHLORIDE
DERMIK LABS
DERMIK LABORATORIES DIV AVENTIS PHARMACEUTICALS
INC
   BENZACLIN, BENZOYL PEROXIDE
   BENZAMYCIN PAK, BENZOYL PEROXIDE

   BENZAMYCIN, BENZOYL PEROXIDE
   CARAC, FLUOROURACIL
   DERMATOP, PREDNICARBATE
   HYTONE, HYDROCORTISONE
   KLARON, SULFACETAMIDE SODIUM
   NORITATE, METRONIDAZOLE
   PSORCON, DIFLORASONE DIACETATE
DERMIK LABORATORIES INC
   DERMATOP E EMOLLIENT, PREDNICARBATE
   PENLAC, CICLOPIROX
DERMIK LABORATORIES INC SUB RORER
   HYTONE, HYDROCORTISONE
DESERET
DESERET MEDICAL INC DIV BECTON DICKINSON AND CO
   CHLORHEXIDINE GLUCONATE, CHLORHEXIDINE
     GLUCONATE (OTC)
DEXCEL LTD
DEXCEL LTD
   DICLOFENAC SODIUM, DICLOFENAC SODIUM
   ISOSORBIDE MONONITRATE, ISOSORBIDE
     MONONITRATE
DEXCEL PHARMA
DEXCEL PHARMA TECHNOLOGIES LTD
   PERIOCHIP, CHLORHEXIDINE GLUCONATE
DEY
DEY LP
   ACCUNEB, ALBUTEROL SULFATE
   ALBUTEROL SULFATE, ALBUTEROL SULFATE
   CROMOLYN SODIUM, CROMOLYN SODIUM
   CUROSURF, PORACTANT ALFA
   DUONEB, ALBUTEROL SULFATE
   IPRATROPIUM BROMIDE, IPRATROPIUM BROMIDE
   ISOETHARINE HCL S/F, ISOETHARINE HYDROCHLORIDE
   ISOETHARINE HCL, ISOETHARINE HYDROCHLORIDE
   ISOPROTERENOL HCL, ISOPROTERENOL
     HYDROCHLORIDE
   METAPROTERENOL SULFATE, METAPROTERENOL
     SULFATE
   MUCOSIL-10, ACETYLCYSTEINE
   MUCOSIL-20, ACETYLCYSTEINE
DHL
DHL LABORATORIES INC
   DEXTROSE 5% IN PLASTIC CONTAINER, DEXTROSE
DIAL
DIAL CORP DIV GREYHOUND CO
   DIAL, HEXACHLOROPHENE
DIATIDE RES LABS
DIATIDE RESEARCH LABORATORIES DIV BERLEX LABS
INC
   ACUTECT, TECHNETIUM TC-99M APCITIDE
   NEO TECT KIT, TECHNETIUM TC-99M DEPREOTIDE
DISTA
DISTA PRODUCTS CO DIV ELI LILLY AND CO
   ERYTHROMYCIN ETHYLSUCCINATE, ERYTHROMYCIN
     ETHYLSUCCINATE
   ILOSONE, ERYTHROMYCIN ESTOLATE
   ILOTYCIN GLUCEPTATE, ERYTHROMYCIN GLUCEPTATE
   ILOTYCIN, ERYTHROMYCIN
   NALFON, FENOPROFEN CALCIUM
   VALMID, ETHINAMATE
DOW PHARM
DOW PHARMACEUTICAL CORP SUB DOW CHEMICAL CO
   DOW-ISONIAZID, ISONIAZID
   NEO-POLYCIN, BACITRACIN ZINC
   NEO-POLYCIN, GRAMICIDIN
   QUIDE, PIPERACETAZINE

APPENDIX B
PRODUCT NAME INDEX
LISTED BY APPLICANT (*continued*)

DOWNSTATE CLINCL
DOWNSTATE CLINICAL PET CENTER
    FLUDEOXYGLUCOSE F 18, FLUDEOXYGLUCOSE, F-18
DPT
DPT LABORATORIES INC
    EMBELINE, CLOBETASOL PROPIONATE
DR REDDYS LABS INC
DR REDDYS LABORATORIES INC
    FLUOXETINE HCL, FLUOXETINE HYDROCHLORIDE
    FLUOXETINE, FLUOXETINE HYDROCHLORIDE
    IBUPROFEN, IBUPROFEN
    IBUPROFEN, IBUPROFEN (OTC)
    NAPROXEN SODIUM, NAPROXEN SODIUM (OTC)
    TIZANIDINE HCL, TIZANIDINE HYDROCHLORIDE
DR REDDYS LABS LTD
DR REDDYS LABORATORIES LTD
    ENALAPRIL MALEATE AND HYDROCHLOROTHIAZIDE,
        ENALAPRIL MALEATE
    FAMOTIDINE, FAMOTIDINE
    FAMOTIDINE, FAMOTIDINE (OTC)
    OXAPROZIN, OXAPROZIN
    RANITIDINE HCL, RANITIDINE HYDROCHLORIDE
    RANITIDINE, RANITIDINE HYDROCHLORIDE (OTC)
DRAXIMAGE
DRAXIMAGE INC
    DTPA, TECHNETIUM TC-99M PENTETATE KIT
    SODIUM IODIDE I 131, KIT, SODIUM IODIDE, I-131
    TECHNESCAN GLUCEPTATE, TECHNETIUM TC-99M
        GLUCEPTATE KIT
    TECHNESCAN HIDA, TECHNETIUM TC-99M LIDOFENIN
        KIT
    TECHNESCAN MDP KIT, TECHNETIUM TC-99M
        MEDRONATE KIT
    TECHNETIUM TC 99M ALBUMIN AGGREGATED KIT,
        TECHNETIUM TC-99M ALBUMIN AGGREGATED KIT
DSM PHARMS
DSM PHARMACEUTICALS INC
    ALOPRIM, ALLOPURINOL SODIUM
DUNHALL
DUNHALL PHARMACEUTICALS INC
    TRIAPRIN, ACETAMINOPHEN
DURAMED
DURAMED PHARMACEUTICALS INC
    CENESTIN, ESTROGENS, CONJUGATED SYNTHETIC A
DURAMED PHARM BARR
DURAMED PHARMACEUTICALS INC SUB BARR LABORA-
TORIES INC
    ACETAMINOPHEN AND CODEINE PHOSPHATE,
        ACETAMINOPHEN
    AMINOPHYLLINE, AMINOPHYLLINE
    AVIANE-21, ETHINYL ESTRADIOL
    AVIANE-28, ETHINYL ESTRADIOL
    AYGESTIN, NORETHINDRONE ACETATE
    CHLORPROPAMIDE, CHLORPROPAMIDE
    CIMETIDINE HCL, CIMETIDINE
    CLONIDINE HCL, CLONIDINE HYDROCHLORIDE
    CRYSELLE, ETHINYL ESTRADIOL
    CYPROHEPTADINE HCL, CYPROHEPTADINE
        HYDROCHLORIDE
    DESOGESTREL AND ETHINYL ESTRADIOL,
        DESOGESTREL
    DIAMOX, ACETAZOLAMIDE
    DIAMOX, ACETAZOLAMIDE SODIUM
    DIAZEPAM, DIAZEPAM
    ENPRESSE-21, ETHINYL ESTRADIOL
    ENPRESSE-28, ETHINYL ESTRADIOL
    ESTROPIPATE, ESTROPIPATE
    GLIPIZIDE, GLIPIZIDE

    GYNODIOL, ESTRADIOL
    HALOPERIDOL, HALOPERIDOL
    HYDROXYUREA, HYDROXYUREA
    HYDROXYZINE PAMOATE, HYDROXYZINE PAMOATE
    INDOMETHACIN, INDOMETHACIN
    ISONIAZID, ISONIAZID
    LOPERAMIDE HCL, LOPERAMIDE HYDROCHLORIDE
        (OTC)
    MEDROXYPROGESTERONE ACETATE,
        MEDROXYPROGESTERONE ACETATE
    MEPERIDINE HCL, MEPERIDINE HYDROCHLORIDE
    METHOTREXATE SODIUM, METHOTREXATE SODIUM
    METHYLDOPA, METHYLDOPA
    METHYLPREDNISOLONE, METHYLPREDNISOLONE
    OXYCODONE AND ACETAMINOPHEN, ACETAMINOPHEN
    PHENTERMINE HCL, PHENTERMINE HYDROCHLORIDE
    PREDNISONE, PREDNISONE
    PROCHLORPERAZINE MALEATE, PROCHLORPERAZINE
        MALEATE
    PROPRANOLOL HCL & HYDROCHLOROTHIAZIDE,
        HYDROCHLOROTHIAZIDE
    PROPRANOLOL HCL, PROPRANOLOL HYDROCHLORIDE
    TEMAZEPAM, TEMAZEPAM
    TOLAZAMIDE, TOLAZAMIDE
    TRIAMTERENE AND HYDROCHLOROTHIAZIDE,
        HYDROCHLOROTHIAZIDE
    TRIFLUOPERAZINE HCL, TRIFLUOPERAZINE
        HYDROCHLORIDE
    ZEBETA, BISOPROLOL FUMARATE
    ZIAC, BISOPROLOL FUMARATE
DUSA
DUSA PHARMACEUTICALS INC
    LEVULAN, AMINOLEVULINIC ACID HYDROCHLORIDE
DXS DEVICES
DIAGNOSTICS AND DEVICES INC
    PYLORI-CHEK BREATH TEST, UREA, C-13
DYNAPHARM
DYNAPHARM INC
    COLOVAGE, POLYETHYLENE GLYCOL 3350

E

E Z EM
E Z EM CO INC
    E-Z-EM PREP LYTE, POLYETHYLENE GLYCOL 3350
EASTMAN KODAK
EASTMAN KODAK CO
    CARBOCAINE W/ NEO-COBEFRIN, LEVONORDEFRIN
    CARBOCAINE, MEPIVACAINE HYDROCHLORIDE
    LIDOCAINE HCL AND EPINEPHRINE, EPINEPHRINE
    RAVOCAINE AND NOVOCAIN W/ LEVOPHED,
        NOREPINEPHRINE BITARTRATE
    RAVOCAINE AND NOVOCAIN W/ NEO-COBEFRIN,
        LEVONORDEFRIN
ECOLAB
ECOLAB INC
    CHG SCRUB, CHLORHEXIDINE GLUCONATE (OTC)
    CIDA-STAT, CHLORHEXIDINE GLUCONATE (OTC)
EGIS
EGIS PHARMACEUTICALS
    BUSPIRONE HCL, BUSPIRONE HYDROCHLORIDE
    PIROXICAM, PIROXICAM
EGIS PHARMS
EGIS PHARMACEUTICALS LTD
    CAPTOPRIL, CAPTOPRIL

APPENDIX B
PRODUCT NAME INDEX
LISTED BY APPLICANT (*continued*)

ELAN DRUG
ELAN DRUG DELIVERY INC
  VERELAN, VERAPAMIL HYDROCHLORIDE
ELAN PHARM
ELAN PHARMACEUTICAL RESEARCH CORP
  ISOSORBIDE MONONITRATE, ISOSORBIDE
    MONONITRATE
  KETOPROFEN, KETOPROFEN
  NIFEDIPINE, NIFEDIPINE
  PROSTEP, NICOTINE (OTC)
  VERELAN PM, VERAPAMIL HYDROCHLORIDE
ELAN PHARMA
ELAN PHARMACEUTICALS INC
  NAPRELAN, NAPROXEN SODIUM
ELAN PHARMS
ELAN PHARMACEUTICALS
  FROVA, FROVATRIPTAN SUCCINATE
  ORAMORPH SR, MORPHINE SULFATE
  ZANAFLEX, TIZANIDINE HYDROCHLORIDE
ELAN PHARMACEUTICALS INC
  DURACLON, CLONIDINE HYDROCHLORIDE
  ROXICODONE, OXYCODONE HYDROCHLORIDE
  ZANAFLEX, TIZANIDINE HYDROCHLORIDE
ELKINS SINN
ELKINS SINN DIV AH ROBINS CO INC
  AMIKACIN SULFATE, AMIKACIN SULFATE
  AMINOCAPROIC ACID, AMINOCAPROIC ACID
  AMINOPHYLLINE, AMINOPHYLLINE
  AMPICILLIN SODIUM, AMPICILLIN SODIUM
  BRETYLIUM TOSYLATE, BRETYLIUM TOSYLATE
  CEFAZOLIN SODIUM, CEFAZOLIN SODIUM
  CEPHAPIRIN SODIUM, CEPHAPIRIN SODIUM
  CHLORAMPHENICOL, CHLORAMPHENICOL SODIUM
    SUCCINATE
  CHLORPHENIRAMINE MALEATE, CHLORPHENIRAMINE
    MALEATE
  CLINDAMYCIN PHOSPHATE, CLINDAMYCIN
    PHOSPHATE
  CORTISONE ACETATE, CORTISONE ACETATE
  CYANOCOBALAMIN, CYANOCOBALAMIN
  DEXAMETHASONE, DEXAMETHASONE SODIUM
    PHOSPHATE
  DIAZEPAM, DIAZEPAM
  DIGOXIN, DIGOXIN
  DIMENHYDRINATE, DIMENHYDRINATE
  DIPHENHYDRAMINE HCL, DIPHENHYDRAMINE
    HYDROCHLORIDE
  DIPYRIDAMOLE, DIPYRIDAMOLE
  DOBUTAMINE HCL, DOBUTAMINE HYDROCHLORIDE
  DOXYCYCLINE, DOXYCYCLINE HYCLATE
  ERYTHROMYCIN, ERYTHROMYCIN LACTOBIONATE
  FENTANYL CITRATE PRESERVATIVE FREE, FENTANYL
    CITRATE
  HYDROCHLOROTHIAZIDE, HYDROCHLOROTHIAZIDE
  HYDROCORTISONE SODIUM SUCCINATE,
    HYDROCORTISONE SODIUM SUCCINATE
  HYDROCORTISONE, HYDROCORTISONE
  HYDROXYZINE HCL, HYDROXYZINE HYDROCHLORIDE
  HYDROXYZINE, HYDROXYZINE HYDROCHLORIDE
  KANAMYCIN, KANAMYCIN SULFATE
  LEUCOVORIN CALCIUM, LEUCOVORIN CALCIUM
  LIDOCAINE HCL AND EPINEPHRINE, EPINEPHRINE
  LIDOCAINE HCL PRESERVATIVE FREE, LIDOCAINE
    HYDROCHLORIDE
  LIDOCAINE HCL, LIDOCAINE HYDROCHLORIDE
  LORAZEPAM, LORAZEPAM
  MEPERIDINE HCL, MEPERIDINE HYDROCHLORIDE
  MEPROBAMATE, MEPROBAMATE

METARAMINOL BITARTRATE, METARAMINOL
  BITARTRATE
METHYLDOPATE HCL, METHYLDOPATE
  HYDROCHLORIDE
METHYLPREDNISOLONE SODIUM SUCCINATE,
  METHYLPREDNISOLONE SODIUM SUCCINATE
METHYLPREDNISOLONE, METHYLPREDNISOLONE
  SODIUM SUCCINATE
METRONIDAZOLE, METRONIDAZOLE
NALOXONE HCL, NALOXONE HYDROCHLORIDE
NALOXONE, NALOXONE HYDROCHLORIDE
NITROFURANTOIN, NITROFURANTOIN
OXACILLIN SODIUM, OXACILLIN SODIUM
PANCURONIUM, PANCURONIUM BROMIDE
PENTAMIDINE ISETHIONATE, PENTAMIDINE
  ISETHIONATE
PENTOBARBITAL SODIUM, PENTOBARBITAL SODIUM
PHENYTOIN, PHENYTOIN SODIUM
POTASSIUM CHLORIDE, POTASSIUM CHLORIDE
PREDNISOLONE, PREDNISOLONE
PREDNISONE, PREDNISONE
PROCAINAMIDE HCL, PROCAINAMIDE
  HYDROCHLORIDE
PROCAINE HCL, PROCAINE HYDROCHLORIDE
PROCI ILORPERAZINE EDISYLATE,
  PROCHLORPERAZINE EDISYLATE
PROCHLORPERAZINE, PROCHLORPERAZINE
  EDISYLATE
PROTAMINE SULFATE, PROTAMINE SULFATE
PYRIDOXINE HCL, PYRIDOXINE HYDROCHLORIDE
QUINIDINE SULFATE, QUINIDINE SULFATE
RESERPINE, RESERPINE
SECOBARBITAL SODIUM, SECOBARBITAL SODIUM
SODIUM NITROPRUSSIDE, SODIUM NITROPRUSSIDE
SODIUM PENTOBARBITAL, PENTOBARBITAL SODIUM
SODIUM SUCCINATE, SODIUM SUCCINATE
SOTRADECOL, SODIUM TETRADECYL SULFATE
SUFENTANIL CITRATE, SUFENTANIL CITRATE
SULFAMETHOXAZOLE AND TRIMETHOPRIM,
  SULFAMETHOXAZOLE
TESTOSTERONE PROPIONATE, TESTOSTERONE
  PROPIONATE
TETRACYCLINE HCL, TETRACYCLINE HYDROCHLORIDE
THIAMINE HCL, THIAMINE HYDROCHLORIDE
TOBRAMYCIN SULFATE, TOBRAMYCIN SULFATE
VANCOMYCIN HCL, VANCOMYCIN HYDROCHLORIDE
VITAMIN A, VITAMIN A PALMITATE
ELKINS SINN PHARM
ELKINS SINN PHARMACEUTICAL CO
  IOPAMIDOL, IOPAMIDOL
  NALOXONE, NALOXONE HYDROCHLORIDE
ENCYSIVE
ENCYSIVE PHARMACEUTICALS INC
  ARGATROBAN, ARGATROBAN
ENDO LABS
ENDO LABORATORIES INC DIV DUPONT MERCK PHARMA-
CEUTICAL CO
  CAPTOPRIL, CAPTOPRIL
ENDO LABORATORIES LLC
  CAPTOPRIL AND HYDROCHLOROTHIAZIDE, CAPTOPRIL
ENDO PHARMS
ENDO PHARMACEUTICALS INC
  BUTALBITAL, ASPIRIN, CAFFEINE, AND CODEINE
    PHOSPHATE, ASPIRIN
  CIMETIDINE HCL, CIMETIDINE HYDROCHLORIDE
  CIMETIDINE, CIMETIDINE
  DEXTROAMPHETAMINE SULFATE,
    DEXTROAMPHETAMINE SULFATE

APPENDIX B
PRODUCT NAME INDEX
LISTED BY APPLICANT (*continued*)

ETODOLAC, ETODOLAC
GLIPIZIDE, GLIPIZIDE
HYCODAN, HOMATROPINE METHYLBROMIDE
HYCOMINE PEDIATRIC, HYDROCODONE BITARTRATE
HYCOMINE, HYDROCODONE BITARTRATE
HYDROCODONE BITARTRATE AND ACETAMINOPHEN,
    ACETAMINOPHEN
MOBAN, MOLINDONE HYDROCHLORIDE
MORPHINE SULFATE, MORPHINE SULFATE
NARCAN, NALOXONE HYDROCHLORIDE
NUBAIN, NALBUPHINE HYDROCHLORIDE
NUMORPHAN, OXYMORPHONE HYDROCHLORIDE
OXYCODONE AND ACETAMINOPHEN, ACETAMINOPHEN
PERCOCET, ACETAMINOPHEN
PERCODAN, ASPIRIN
PERCODAN-DEMI, ASPIRIN
SELEGILINE HCL, SELEGILINE HYDROCHLORIDE
SYMMETREL, AMANTADINE HYDROCHLORIDE
VALPIN 50, ANISOTROPINE METHYLBROMIDE

ENVIRODERM
ENVIRODERM PHARMACEUTICALS INC
    IVY BLOCK, BENTOQUATAM (OTC)

ENZON
ENZON INC
    ABELCET, AMPHOTERICIN B
    ADAGEN, PEGADEMASE BOVINE

EON
EON LABORATORIES MANUFACTURING INC
    ACETAMINOPHEN AND CODEINE PHOSPHATE,
        ACETAMINOPHEN
    ALKERGOT, ERGOLOID MESYLATES
    ALPHAZINE, PHENDIMETRAZINE TARTRATE
    AMIODARONE HCL, AMIODARONE HYDROCHLORIDE
    BETHANECHOL CHLORIDE, BETHANECHOL CHLORIDE
    BISOPROLOL FUMARATE AND
        HYDROCHLOROTHIAZIDE, BISOPROLOL FUMARATE
    BISOPROLOL FUMARATE, BISOPROLOL FUMARATE
    BUMETANIDE, BUMETANIDE
    BUPROPION HCL, BUPROPION HYDROCHLORIDE
    BUTABARBITAL SODIUM, BUTABARBITAL SODIUM
    CAPTOPRIL, CAPTOPRIL
    CARISOPRODOL AND ASPIRIN, ASPIRIN
    CARISOPRODOL, ASPIRIN AND CODEINE PHOSPHATE,
        ASPIRIN
    CARISOPRODOL, CARISOPRODOL
    CHLORDIAZEPOXIDE HCL, CHLORDIAZEPOXIDE
        HYDROCHLORIDE
    CHLOROTHIAZIDE, CHLOROTHIAZIDE
    CHLORPROPAMIDE, CHLORPROPAMIDE
    CHLORTHALIDONE, CHLORTHALIDONE
    CHOLESTYRAMINE LIGHT, CHOLESTYRAMINE
    CHOLESTYRAMINE, CHOLESTYRAMINE
    CLONAZEPAM, CLONAZEPAM
    CYCLOSPORINE, CYCLOSPORINE
    DESIPRAMINE HCL, DESIPRAMINE HYDROCHLORIDE
    DEXTROAMP SACCHARATE, AMP ASPARTATE,
        DEXTROAMP SULFATE AND AMP SULFATE,
        AMPHETAMINE ASPARTATE
    DICLOFENAC POTASSIUM, DICLOFENAC POTASSIUM
    DIETHYLPROPION HCL, DIETHYLPROPION
        HYDROCHLORIDE
    DIPHENHYDRAMINE HCL, DIPHENHYDRAMINE
        HYDROCHLORIDE
    DIPHENOXYLATE HCL W/ ATROPINE SULFATE,
        ATROPINE SULFATE
    DOXAZOSIN MESYLATE, DOXAZOSIN MESYLATE
    DOXYCYCLINE, DOXYCYCLINE
    DRALSERP, HYDRALAZINE HYDROCHLORIDE

ENALAPRIL MALEATE AND HYDROCHLOROTHIAZIDE,
    ENALAPRIL MALEATE
ENALAPRIL MALEATE, ENALAPRIL MALEATE
ETODOLAC, ETODOLAC
FAMOTIDINE, FAMOTIDINE
FAMOTIDINE, FAMOTIDINE (OTC)
FLUOXETINE HCL, FLUOXETINE HYDROCHLORIDE
FLUOXETINE, FLUOXETINE HYDROCHLORIDE
FLUTAMIDE, FLUTAMIDE
FLUVOXAMINE MALEATE, FLUVOXAMINE MALEATE
FOLIC ACID, FOLIC ACID
FUROSEMIDE, FUROSEMIDE
GUANABENZ ACETATE, GUANABENZ ACETATE
HYDRALAZINE HCL, HYDRALAZINE HYDROCHLORIDE
HYDRAP-ES, HYDRALAZINE HYDROCHLORIDE
HYDRO-SERP "25", HYDROCHLOROTHIAZIDE
HYDRO-SERP "50", HYDROCHLOROTHIAZIDE
HYDROCHLOROTHIAZIDE, HYDROCHLOROTHIAZIDE
HYDROCODONE BITARTRATE AND ACETAMINOPHEN,
    ACETAMINOPHEN
HYDROCORTISONE, HYDROCORTISONE
HYDROXYZINE HCL, HYDROXYZINE HYDROCHLORIDE
HYDROXYZINE PAMOATE, HYDROXYZINE PAMOATE
IMIPRAMINE HCL, IMIPRAMINE HYDROCHLORIDE
INDOCIN SR, INDOMETHACIN
ISONIAZID, ISONIAZID
LABETALOL HCL, LABETALOL HYDROCHLORIDE
LISINOPRIL AND HYDROCHLOROTHIAZIDE,
    HYDROCHLOROTHIAZIDE
LISINOPRIL, LISINOPRIL
LOCHOLEST LIGHT, CHOLESTYRAMINE
LOCHOLEST, CHOLESTYRAMINE
LOVASTATIN, LOVASTATIN
MEPRO-ASPIRIN, ASPIRIN
MEPROBAMATE, MEPROBAMATE
METFORMIN HCL, METFORMIN HYDROCHLORIDE
METHADONE HCL, METHADONE HYDROCHLORIDE
METHIMAZOLE, METHIMAZOLE
METHOCARBAMOL, METHOCARBAMOL
METHYLPREDNISOLONE, METHYLPREDNISOLONE
METRONIDAZOLE, METRONIDAZOLE
MIRTAZAPINE, MIRTAZAPINE
NABUMETONE, NABUMETONE
NALTREXONE HCL, NALTREXONE HYDROCHLORIDE
NEOMYCIN SULFATE, NEOMYCIN SULFATE
NITROFURANTOIN, NITROFURANTOIN
NIZATIDINE, NIZATIDINE
NYSTATIN, NYSTATIN
OMEPRAZOLE, OMEPRAZOLE
ORPHENADRINE CITRATE, ASPIRIN, AND CAFFEINE,
    ASPIRIN
ORPHENADRINE CITRATE, ORPHENADRINE CITRATE
OXAPROZIN, OXAPROZIN
PHENDIMETRAZINE TARTRATE, PHENDIMETRAZINE
    TARTRATE
PHENTERMINE HCL, PHENTERMINE HYDROCHLORIDE
PREDNISOLONE, PREDNISOLONE
PREDNISONE, PREDNISONE
PROBENECID AND COLCHICINE, COLCHICINE
PROMETHAZINE HCL, PROMETHAZINE
    HYDROCHLORIDE
PROPOXYPHENE COMPOUND 65, ASPIRIN
PROPOXYPHENE HCL, PROPOXYPHENE
    HYDROCHLORIDE
PSEUDOEPHEDRINE HCL AND TRIPROLIDINE HCL,
    PSEUDOEPHEDRINE HYDROCHLORIDE
QUINIDINE SULFATE, QUINIDINE SULFATE
RESERPINE, RESERPINE

APPENDIX B
PRODUCT NAME INDEX
LISTED BY APPLICANT (*continued*)

RIFAMPIN, RIFAMPIN
SOTALOL HCL, SOTALOL HYDROCHLORIDE
SULFADIAZINE, TRISULFAPYRIMIDINES (SULFADIAZINE;
    SULFAMERAZINE; SULFAMETHAZINE)
SULFAMETHOXAZOLE AND TRIMETHOPRIM DOUBLE
    STRENGTH, SULFAMETHOXAZOLE
SULFAMETHOXAZOLE AND TRIMETHOPRIM,
    SULFAMETHOXAZOLE
SULFASALAZINE, SULFASALAZINE
TETRACYCLINE HCL, TETRACYCLINE HYDROCHLORIDE
THEOPHYLLINE, THEOPHYLLINE
TICLOPIDINE HCL, TICLOPIDINE HYDROCHLORIDE
TIZANIDINE HCL, TIZANIDINE HYDROCHLORIDE
TOLBUTAMIDE, TOLBUTAMIDE
TRAMADOL HCL, TRAMADOL HYDROCHLORIDE
TRICHLORMETHIAZIDE, TRICHLORMETHIAZIDE
WESTADONE, METHADONE HYDROCHLORIDE

ERSANA
ERSANA INC SUB ER SQUIBB AND SONS
    VELOSEF ',250', CEPHRADINE
    VELOSEF ',500', CEPHRADINE

ESI
ESI PHARMACAL
    CYCRIN, MEDROXYPROGESTERONE ACETATE

ESI LEDERLE
ESI LEDERLE GENERICS
    VECURONIUM BROMIDE, VECURONIUM BROMIDE
ESI LEDERLE INC
    ACYCLOVIR IN SODIUM CHLORIDE 0.9% PRESERVATIVE
        FREE, ACYCLOVIR SODIUM
    ACYCLOVIR SODIUM, ACYCLOVIR SODIUM
    AMPICILLIN AND SULBACTAM, AMPICILLIN SODIUM
    ATRACURIUM BESYLATE PRESERVATIVE FREE,
        ATRACURIUM BESYLATE
    ATRACURIUM BESYLATE, ATRACURIUM BESYLATE
    CEFOXITIN, CEFOXITIN SODIUM
    MILRINONE LACTOSE IN 5% DEXTROSE, MILRINONE
        LACTATE
    MITOMYCIN, MITOMYCIN
    MORPHINE SULFATE, MORPHINE SULFATE
    PENTOXIFYLLINE, PENTOXIFYLLINE
    VINORELBINE TARTRATE, VINORELBINE TARTRATE

ESP PHARMA
ESP PHARMA INC
    BUSULFEX, BUSULFAN
    ISMO, ISOSORBIDE MONONITRATE
    SECTRAL, ACEBUTOLOL HYDROCHLORIDE
    TENEX, GUANFACINE HYDROCHLORIDE

ETHITEK
ETHITEK PHARMACEUTICALS CO
    MOCTANIN, MONOCTANOIN

EVERYLIFE
EVERYLIFE
    APAP W/ CODEINE PHOSPHATE, ACETAMINOPHEN
    CORTISONE ACETATE, CORTISONE ACETATE
    FOLIC ACID, FOLIC ACID
    HYDROCORTISONE, HYDROCORTISONE
    NIACIN, NIACIN
    PREDNISOLONE, PREDNISOLONE
    PREDNISONE, PREDNISONE
    QUINIDINE SULFATE, QUINIDINE SULFATE
    RESERPINE, RESERPINE
    SECOBARBITAL SODIUM, SECOBARBITAL SODIUM
    SODIUM PENTOBARBITAL, PENTOBARBITAL SODIUM
    STANOZIDE, ISONIAZID
    SULFADIAZINE, TRISULFAPYRIMIDINES (SULFADIAZINE;
        SULFAMERAZINE; SULFAMETHAZINE)
    VITAMIN A, VITAMIN A

VITAMIN A, VITAMIN A PALMITATE
VITAMIN D, ERGOCALCIFEROL

F

FALCON PHARMS
FALCON PHARMACEUTICALS INC
    TIMOLOL MALEATE, TIMOLOL MALEATE
FALCON PHARMACEUTICALS LTD
    DICLOFENAC SODIUM, DICLOFENAC SODIUM
    DIPIVEFRIN HCL, DIPIVEFRIN HYDROCHLORIDE
    ECONOPRED PLUS, PREDNISOLONE ACETATE
    GENTAMICIN SULFATE, GENTAMICIN SULFATE
    LEVOBUNOLOL HCL, LEVOBUNOLOL HYDROCHLORIDE
    MAXITROL, DEXAMETHASONE
    METIPRANOLOL, METIPRANOLOL HYDROCHLORIDE
    TIMOLOL MALEATE, TIMOLOL MALEATE
    TOBREX, TOBRAMYCIN
    TRIMETHOPRIM SULFATE AND POLYMYXIN B SULFATE,
        POLYMYXIN B SULFATE

FAULDING
FAULDING PHARMACEUTICAL CO
    ACETYLCYSTEINE, ACETYLCYSTEINE
    ACYCLOVIR SODIUM, ACYCLOVIR SODIUM
    AMIKACIN SULFATE, AMIKACIN SULFATE
    AMIODARONE HCL, AMIODARONE HYDROCHLORIDE
    ATRACURIUM BESYLATE PRESERVATIVE FREE,
        ATRACURIUM BESYLATE
    ATRACURIUM BESYLATE, ATRACURIUM BESYLATE
    BLEOMYCIN, BLEOMYCIN SULFATE
    BRETYLOL, BRETYLIUM TOSYLATE
    BUTORPHANOL TARTRATE PRESERVATIVE FREE,
        BUTORPHANOL TARTRATE
    CYTARABINE, CYTARABINE
    DACARBAZINE, DACARBAZINE
    DROPERIDOL, DROPERIDOL
    ENALAPRILAT, ENALAPRILAT
    FAMOTIDINE PRESERVATIVE FREE, FAMOTIDINE
    FAMOTIDINE, FAMOTIDINE
    FUDR, FLOXURIDINE
    HYDROMORPHONE HCL, HYDROMORPHONE
        HYDROCHLORIDE
    INTROPIN, DOPAMINE HYDROCHLORIDE
    IOPAMIDOL, IOPAMIDOL
    LABETALOL HCL, LABETALOL HYDROCHLORIDE
    MEPERIDINE HCL PRESERVATIVE FREE, MEPERIDINE
        HYDROCHLORIDE
    METHYLDOPATE HCL, METHYLDOPATE
        HYDROCHLORIDE
    METOCLOPRAMIDE HCL, METOCLOPRAMIDE
        HYDROCHLORIDE
    MIDAZOLAM HCL, MIDAZOLAM HYDROCHLORIDE
    MILRINONE LACTATE, MILRINONE LACTATE
    MITOMYCIN, MITOMYCIN
    PAMIDRONATE DISODIUM, PAMIDRONATE DISODIUM
    TRIDIL, NITROGLYCERIN
    VINBLASTINE SULFATE, VINBLASTINE SULFATE
    VINCRISTINE SULFATE PFS, VINCRISTINE SULFATE
    VINCRISTINE SULFATE, VINCRISTINE SULFATE
FH FAULDING AND CO LTD
    DORYX, DOXYCYCLINE HYCLATE
    ERYC SPRINKLES, ERYTHROMYCIN
    ERYC, ERYTHROMYCIN
    THEOPHYLLINE, THEOPHYLLINE

APPENDIX B
PRODUCT NAME INDEX
LISTED BY APPLICANT (*continued*)

FAULDING PHARMS
FAULDING PHARMACEUTICALS INC
  KADIAN, MORPHINE SULFATE
  SERAX, OXAZEPAM
FEI
FEI ACQUISITION LLC
  COPPER T MODEL TCU 380A, COPPER
FERNDALE LABS
FERNDALE LABORATORIES INC
  ADPHEN, PHENDIMETRAZINE TARTRATE
  AMOSENE, MEPROBAMATE
  AQUAPHYLLIN, THEOPHYLLINE
  DELAXIN, METHOCARBAMOL
  DIAZEPAM, DIAZEPAM
  FERNDEX, DEXTROAMPHETAMINE SULFATE
  FERNISOLONE-P, PREDNISOLONE
  FERNISONE, PREDNISONE
  HYDROCORTISONE ACETATE, HYDROCORTISONE
    ACETATE
  LOCOID LIPOCREAM, HYDROCORTISONE BUTYRATE
  LOCOID, HYDROCORTISONE BUTYRATE
  MICORT-HC, HYDROCORTISONE ACETATE
  OBESTIN-30, PHENTERMINE HYDROCHLORIDE
  PHENDIMETRAZINE TARTRATE, PHENDIMETRAZINE
    TARTRATE
  PRAMOSONE, HYDROCORTISONE ACETATE
  RAUSERPIN, RAUWOLFIA SERPENTINA
  STRIFON FORTE DSC, CHLORZOXAZONE
FERRANTE
JOHN J FERRANTE
  AMPHICOL, CHLORAMPHENICOL
  CHLORDIAZEPOXIDE HCL, CHLORDIAZEPOXIDE
    HYDROCHLORIDE
  HYDROCORTISONE, HYDROCORTISONE
  OXY-KESSO-TETRA, OXYTETRACYCLINE
    HYDROCHLORIDE
  PREDNISOLONE, PREDNISOLONE
  PREDNISONE, PREDNISONE
  TETRACYCLINE HCL, TETRACYCLINE HYDROCHLORIDE
FERRING
FERRING PHARMACEUTICALS INC
  ACTHREL, CORTICORELIN OVINE TRIFLUTATE
  BRAVELLE, UROFOLLITROPIN
  CONCENTRAID, DESMOPRESSIN ACETATE
  LUTREPULSE KIT, GONADORELIN ACETATE
  MENOTROPINS, MENOTROPINS (FSH;LH)
  MINIRIN, DESMOPRESSIN ACETATE
  REPRONEX, MENOTROPINS (FSH;LH)
  SECRETIN-FERRING, SECRETIN
  THYREL TRH, PROTIRELIN
FIRST HORIZON
FIRST HORIZON PHARMACEUTICAL CORP
  COGNEX, TACRINE HYDROCHLORIDE
  FURADANTIN, NITROFURANTOIN
  PONSTEL, MEFENAMIC ACID
  ROBINUL FORTE, GLYCOPYRROLATE
  ROBINUL, GLYCOPYRROLATE
  SULAR, NISOLDIPINE
FISAI MEDCL RES
EISAI MEDICAL RESEARCH INC
  ACIPHEX, RABEPRAZOLE SODIUM
  ARICEPT, DONEPEZIL HYDROCHLORIDE
FISONS
FISONS CORP
  IRON DEXTRAN, IRON DEXTRAN
  ISOCLOR, CHLORPHENIRAMINE MALEATE (OTC)
  PENNTUSS, CHLORPHENIRAMINE POLISTIREX (OTC)
  SOMOPHYLLIN, AMINOPHYLLINE

  SOMOPHYLLIN-DF, AMINOPHYLLINE
  SOMOPHYLLIN-T, THEOPHYLLINE
  VAPO-ISO, ISOPROTERENOL HYDROCHLORIDE
FLEMING PHARMS
FLEMING AND CO PHARMACEUTICALS INC
  AEROLATE III, THEOPHYLLINE
  AEROLATE JR, THEOPHYLLINE
  AEROLATE SR, THEOPHYLLINE
  AEROLATE, THEOPHYLLINE
FLEMINGTON PHARM
FLEMINGTON PHARMACEUTICAL CORP
  NIFEDIPINE, NIFEDIPINE
FONDA BV
FONDA BV
  ARIXTRA, FONDAPARINUX SODIUM
FOREST LABS
FOREST LABORATORIES INC
  CELEXA, CITALOPRAM HYDROBROMIDE
  FLUMADINE, RIMANTADINE HYDROCHLORIDE
  LEXAPRO, ESCITALOPRAM OXALATE
  TESSALON, BENZONATATE
FOREST PHARMS
FOREST PHARMACEUTICALS INC
  BANCAP HC, ACETAMINOPHEN
  BANCAP, ACETAMINOPHEN
  DURADYNE DHC, ACETAMINOPHEN
  ESGIC, ACETAMINOPHEN
  METRA, PHENDIMETRAZINE TARTRATE
  MICROSUL, SULFAMETHIZOLE
  PROKLAR, SULFAMETHIZOLE
  SULFALOID, TRISULFAPYRIMIDINES (SULFADIAZINE;
    SULFAMERAZINE; SULFAMETHAZINE)
  WOLFINA, RAUWOLFIA SERPENTINA
FORREST LABS
FORREST LABORATORIES INC
  AMBENYL, BROMODIPHENHYDRAMINE
    HYDROCHLORIDE
  BETAPRONE, PROPIOLACTONE
  DURAPHYL, THEOPHYLLINE
  ELIXICON, THEOPHYLLINE
  ELIXOPHYLLIN SR, THEOPHYLLINE
  ELIXOPHYLLIN, THEOPHYLLINE
  FORBAXIN, METHOCARBAMOL
  PYOCIDIN, HYDROCORTISONE
  SUS-PHRINE SULFITE-FREE, EPINEPHRINE
  THYROLAR-0.25, LIOTRIX (T4;T3)
  THYROLAR-0.5, LIOTRIX (T4;T3)
  THYROLAR-1, LIOTRIX (T4;T3)
  THYROLAR-2, LIOTRIX (T4;T3)
  THYROLAR-3, LIOTRIX (T4;T3)
  THYROLAR-5, LIOTRIX (T4;T3)
FOUGERA
E FOUGERA DIV ALTANA INC
  BETAMETHASONE DIPROPIONATE, BETAMETHASONE
    DIPROPIONATE
  BETAMETHASONE VALERATE, BETAMETHASONE
    VALERATE
  CLINDAMYCIN PHOSPHATE, CLINDAMYCIN
    PHOSPHATE
  CLOBETASOL PROPIONATE, CLOBETASOL
    PROPIONATE
  ERYTHROMYCIN, ERYTHROMYCIN
  FLUOCINOLONE ACETONIDE, FLUOCINOLONE
    ACETONIDE
  FLUOCINONIDE, FLUOCINONIDE
  GENTAMICIN SULFATE, GENTAMICIN SULFATE
  HYDROCORTISONE, HYDROCORTISONE
  LIDOCAINE, LIDOCAINE

APPENDIX B
PRODUCT NAME INDEX
LISTED BY APPLICANT (*continued*)

NEOMYCIN AND POLYMYXIN B SULFATES AND
    DEXAMETHASONE, DEXAMETHASONE
NEOMYCIN SULFATE-TRIAMCINOLONE ACETONIDE,
    NEOMYCIN SULFATE
NITROGLYCERIN, NITROGLYCERIN
NYSTATIN, NYSTATIN
NYSTATIN-TRIAMCINOLONE ACETONIDE, NYSTATIN
TIMOLOL MALEATE, TIMOLOL MALEATE
TRIPLE SULFA, TRIPLE SULFA (SULFABENZAMIDE;
    SULFACETAMIDE; SULFATHIAZOLE)

FRANKLIN PHARMS
FRANKLIN PHARMACEUTICALS INC
    SILDAFLO, SILVER SULFADIAZINE

FRESENIUS
FRESENIUS USA INC
    INPERSOL-LC/LM W/ DEXTROSE 1.5% IN PLASTIC
        CONTAINER, CALCIUM CHLORIDE
    INPERSOL-LC/LM W/ DEXTROSE 2.5% IN PLASTIC
        CONTAINER, CALCIUM CHLORIDE
    INPERSOL-LC/LM W/ DEXTROSE 3.5% IN PLASTIC
        CONTAINER, CALCIUM CHLORIDE
    INPERSOL-LC/LM W/ DEXTROSE 4.25% IN PLASTIC
        CONTAINER, CALCIUM CHLORIDE

FRESENIUS KABI
FRESENIUS KABI CLAYTON L P
    AMINESS 5.2% ESSENTIAL AMINO ACIDS W/ HISTADINE,
        AMINO ACIDS
    CYSTEINE HCL, CYSTEINE HYDROCHLORIDE
    INTRALIPID 10%, SOYBEAN OIL
    INTRALIPID 20%, SOYBEAN OIL
    INTRALIPID 30%, SOYBEAN OIL
    NEOPHAM 6.4%, AMINO ACIDS
    VITAPED, ASCORBIC ACID
FRESENIUS KABI CLAYTON R&D INC
    NOVAMINE 11.4%, AMINO ACIDS
    NOVAMINE 15%, AMINO ACIDS
    NOVAMINE 8.5%, AMINO ACIDS
    VEINAMINE 8%, AMINO ACIDS

FRESENIUS MEDCL
FRESENIUS MEDICAL CARE NORTH AMERICA
    DELFLEX W/ DEXTROSE 1.5% IN PLASTIC CONTAINER,
        CALCIUM CHLORIDE
    DELFLEX W/ DEXTROSE 1.5% LOW MAGNESIUM IN
        PLASTIC CONTAINER, CALCIUM CHLORIDE
    DELFLEX W/ DEXTROSE 1.5% LOW MAGNESIUM LOW
        CALCIUM IN PLASTIC CONTAINER, CALCIUM
        CHLORIDE
    DELFLEX W/ DEXTROSE 2.5% IN PLASTIC CONTAINER,
        CALCIUM CHLORIDE
    DELFLEX W/ DEXTROSE 2.5% LOW MAGNESIUM IN
        PLASTIC CONTAINER, CALCIUM CHLORIDE
    DELFLEX W/ DEXTROSE 2.5% LOW MAGNESIUM LOW
        CALCIUM IN PLASTIC CONTAINER, CALCIUM
        CHLORIDE
    DELFLEX W/ DEXTROSE 3.5% IN PLASTIC CONTAINER,
        CALCIUM CHLORIDE
    DELFLEX W/ DEXTROSE 4.25% IN PLASTIC CONTAINER,
        CALCIUM CHLORIDE
    DELFLEX W/ DEXTROSE 4.25% LOW MAGNESIUM IN
        PLASTIC CONTAINER, CALCIUM CHLORIDE
    DELFLEX W/ DEXTROSE 4.25% LOW MAGNESIUM LOW
        CALCIUM IN PLASTIC CONTAINER, CALCIUM
        CHLORIDE
    DELFLEX-LM W/ DEXTROSE 1.5% IN PLASTIC
        CONTAINER, CALCIUM CHLORIDE
    DELFLEX-LM W/ DEXTROSE 2.5% IN PLASTIC
        CONTAINER, CALCIUM CHLORIDE

DELFLEX-LM W/ DEXTROSE 3.5% IN PLASTIC
    CONTAINER, CALCIUM CHLORIDE
DELFLEX-LM W/ DEXTROSE 4.25% IN PLASTIC
    CONTAINER, CALCIUM CHLORIDE
INPERSOL-ZM W/ DEXTROSE 1.5% IN PLASTIC
    CONTAINER, CALCIUM CHLORIDE
INPERSOL-ZM W/ DEXTROSE 2.5% IN PLASTIC
    CONTAINER, CALCIUM CHLORIDE
INPERSOL-ZM W/ DEXTROSE 4.25% IN PLASTIC
    CONTAINER, CALCIUM CHLORIDE

FUJISAWA HLTHCARE
FUJISAWA HEALTHCARE INC
    ADENOCARD, ADENOSINE
    ADENOSCAN, ADENOSINE
    AMBISOME, AMPHOTERICIN B
    ARISTOCORT A, TRIAMCINOLONE ACETONIDE
    ARISTOCORT, TRIAMCINOLONE
    ARISTOCORT, TRIAMCINOLONE ACETONIDE
    ARISTOCORT, TRIAMCINOLONE DIACETATE
    ARISTOGEL, TRIAMCINOLONE ACETONIDE
    ARISTOSPAN, TRIAMCINOLONE HEXACETONIDE
    CEFIZOX IN DEXTROSE 5% IN PLASTIC CONTAINER,
        CEFTIZOXIME SODIUM
    CEFIZOX IN PLASTIC CONTAINER, CEFTIZOXIME
        SODIUM
    CEFIZOX, CEFTIZOXIME SODIUM
    CYCLOCORT, AMCINONIDE
    PROGRAF, TACROLIMUS
    PROTOPIC, TACROLIMUS

G

G AND W LABS
G AND W LABORATORIES INC
    ACEPHEN, ACETAMINOPHEN (OTC)
    FLUOCINOLONE ACETONIDE, FLUOCINOLONE
        ACETONIDE
    GYNE-SULF, TRIPLE SULFA (SULFABENZAMIDE;
        SULFACETAMIDE; SULFATHIAZOLE)
    HYDROCORTISONE, HYDROCORTISONE
    INDOMETHEGAN, INDOMETHACIN
    MICONAZOLE NITRATE, MICONAZOLE NITRATE (OTC)
    MIGERGOT, CAFFEINE
    PROCHLORPERAZINE, PROCHLORPERAZINE
    PROMETHAZINE HCL, PROMETHAZINE
        HYDROCHLORIDE
    PROMETHEGAN, PROMETHAZINE HYDROCHLORIDE
    TRIAMCINOLONE ACETONIDE, TRIAMCINOLONE
        ACETONIDE
    TRUPHYLLINE, AMINOPHYLLINE

GALDERMA LABS
GALDERMA LABORATORIES INC
    SOLAGE, MEQUINOL

GALDERMA LABS LP
GALDERMA LABORATORIES LP
    CLINDAGEL, CLINDAMYCIN PHOSPHATE
    DESOWEN, DESONIDE
    DIFFERIN, ADAPALENE
    FS SHAMPOO, FLUOCINOLONE ACETONIDE
    METROCREAM, METRONIDAZOLE
    METROGEL, METRONIDAZOLE
    METROLOTION, METRONIDAZOLE

GALEN CHEM
GALEN CHEMICAL LTD
    ESTROSTEP 21, ETHINYL ESTRADIOL
    ESTROSTEP FE, ETHINYL ESTRADIOL
    FEMHRT, ETHINYL ESTRADIOL

APPENDIX B
PRODUCT NAME INDEX
LISTED BY APPLICANT (*continued*)

LOESTRIN 21 1.5/30, ETHINYL ESTRADIOL
LOESTRIN 21 1/20, ETHINYL ESTRADIOL
LOESTRIN FE 1.5/30, ETHINYL ESTRADIOL
LOESTRIN FE 1/20, ETHINYL ESTRADIOL

GALEN LTD
GALEN LTD
FEMRING, ESTRADIOL ACETATE

GD SEARLE LLC
GD SEARLE LLC
ALDACTAZIDE, HYDROCHLOROTHIAZIDE
ALDACTONE, SPIRONOLACTONE
AMINOPHYLLIN, AMINOPHYLLINE
AMMONIUM CHLORIDE, AMMONIUM CHLORIDE
ARTHROTEC, DICLOFENAC SODIUM
BEXTRA, VALDECOXIB
CALAN, VERAPAMIL HYDROCHLORIDE
CELEBREX, CELECOXIB
CLORAZEPATE DIPOTASSIUM, CLORAZEPATE
    DIPOTASSIUM
COVERA-HS, VERAPAMIL HYDROCHLORIDE
CU-7, COPPER
CYTOTEC, MISOPROSTOL
DAYPRO, OXAPROZIN
DEMULEN 1/35-21, ETHINYL ESTRADIOL
DEMULEN 1/35-28, ETHINYL ESTRADIOL
DEMULEN 1/50-21, ETHINYL ESTRADIOL
DEMULEN 1/50-28, ETHINYL ESTRADIOL
DIULO, METOLAZONE
ENOVID, MESTRANOL
ENOVID-E 21, MESTRANOL
ENOVID-E, MESTRANOL
FLAGYL ER, METRONIDAZOLE
FLAGYL I.V. RTU IN PLASTIC CONTAINER,
    METRONIDAZOLE
FLAGYL I.V., METRONIDAZOLE HYDROCHLORIDE
FLAGYL, METRONIDAZOLE
INSPRA, EPLERENONE
LIDOCAINE HCL, LIDOCAINE HYDROCHLORIDE
LOMOTIL, ATROPINE SULFATE
METARAMINOL BITARTRATE, METARAMINOL
    BITARTRATE
NORINYL 1+80 21-DAY, MESTRANOL
NORINYL 1+80 28-DAY, MESTRANOL
NORPACE CR, DISOPYRAMIDE PHOSPHATE
NORPACE, DISOPYRAMIDE PHOSPHATE
NORQUEST FE, ETHINYL ESTRADIOL
OVULEN, ETHYNODIOL DIACETATE
OVULEN-21, ETHYNODIOL DIACETATE
OVULEN-28, ETHYNODIOL DIACETATE
POTASSIUM CHLORIDE, POTASSIUM CHLORIDE
PRO-BANTHINE, PROPANTHELINE BROMIDE
PROCAINE HCL, PROCAINE HYDROCHLORIDE
SYNAREL, NAFARELIN ACETATE
TATUM-T, COPPER

GEN ELECTRIC
GENERAL ELECTRIC CO
XENON XE 133, XENON, XE-133

GENENTECH
GENENTECH INC
CRESCORMON, SOMATROPIN
NUTROPIN AQ PEN, SOMATROPIN RECOMBINANT
NUTROPIN AQ, SOMATROPIN RECOMBINANT
NUTROPIN DEPOT, SOMATROPIN RECOMBINANT
NUTROPIN, SOMATROPIN RECOMBINANT
PROTROPIN, SOMATREM

GENESOFT PHARMS
GENESOFT PHARMACEUTICALS INC
FACTIVE, GEMIFLOXACIN MESYLATE

GENEVA PHARMS
GENEVA PHARMACEUTICALS INC
ACETAMINOPHEN AND CODEINE PHOSPHATE,
    ACETAMINOPHEN
ALBUTEROL SULFATE, ALBUTEROL SULFATE
ALLOPURINOL, ALLOPURINOL
ALPRAZOLAM, ALPRAZOLAM
AMANTADINE HCL, AMANTADINE HYDROCHLORIDE
AMILORIDE HCL AND HYDROCHLOROTHIAZIDE,
    AMILORIDE HYDROCHLORIDE
AMINOPHYLLINE, AMINOPHYLLINE
AMITRIPTYLINE HCL, AMITRIPTYLINE HYDROCHLORIDE
AMOXAPINE, AMOXAPINE
AMOXICILLIN AND CLAVULANATE POTASSIUM,
    AMOXICILLIN
ATENOLOL, ATENOLOL
BROMPHENIRAMINE MALEATE, BROMPHENIRAMINE
    MALEATE
BUSPIRONE HCL, BUSPIRONE HYDROCHLORIDE
BUTABARBITAL SODIUM, BUTABARBITAL SODIUM
BUTAL COMPOUND, ASPIRIN
CAPTOPRIL, CAPTOPRIL
CARBIDOPA AND LEVODOPA, CARBIDOPA
CARISOPRODOL, CARISOPRODOL
CHLORDIAZEPOXIDE HCL, CHLORDIAZEPOXIDE
    HYDROCHLORIDE
CHLORPHENIRAMINE MALEATE AND
    PHENYLPROPANOLAMINE HCL,
    CHLORPHENIRAMINE MALEATE
CHLORPHENIRAMINE MALEATE, CHLORPHENIRAMINE
    MALEATE
CHLORPHENIRAMINE MALEATE, CHLORPHENIRAMINE
    MALEATE (OTC)
CHLORPROMAZINE HCL, CHLORPROMAZINE
    HYDROCHLORIDE
CHLORPROPAMIDE, CHLORPROPAMIDE
CHLORTHALIDONE, CHLORTHALIDONE
CHLORZOXAZONE, CHLORZOXAZONE
CIMETIDINE, CIMETIDINE
CLEMASTINE FUMARATE, CLEMASTINE FUMARATE
CLEMASTINE FUMARATE, CLEMASTINE FUMARATE
    (OTC)
CLOFIBRATE, CLOFIBRATE
CLOMIPRAMINE HCL, CLOMIPRAMINE
    HYDROCHLORIDE
CLONIDINE HCL, CLONIDINE HYDROCHLORIDE
CLORAZEPATE DIPOTASSIUM, CLORAZEPATE
    DIPOTASSIUM
CLOZAPINE, CLOZAPINE
CORPHED, PSEUDOEPHEDRINE HYDROCHLORIDE
CYCLOBENZAPRINE HCL, CYCLOBENZAPRINE
    HYDROCHLORIDE
CYPROHEPTADINE HCL, CYPROHEPTADINE
    HYDROCHLORIDE
DESIPRAMINE HCL, DESIPRAMINE HYDROCHLORIDE
DEXAMETHASONE, DEXAMETHASONE
DEXTROAMPHETAMINE SULFATE,
    DEXTROAMPHETAMINE SULFATE
DIAZEPAM, DIAZEPAM
DICLOFENAC SODIUM, DICLOFENAC SODIUM
DIFLUNISAL, DIFLUNISAL
DIPHENHYDRAMINE HCL, DIPHENHYDRAMINE
    HYDROCHLORIDE
DIPYRIDAMOLE, DIPYRIDAMOLE
DISOBROM, DEXBROMPHENIRAMINE MALEATE (OTC)
DISOPYRAMIDE PHOSPHATE, DISOPYRAMIDE
    PHOSPHATE
DOXEPIN HCL, DOXEPIN HYDROCHLORIDE

APPENDIX B
PRODUCT NAME INDEX
LISTED BY APPLICANT (*continued*)

ENALAPRIL MALEATE, ENALAPRIL MALEATE
ERCATAB, CAFFEINE
ESTERIFIED ESTROGENS, ESTROGENS, ESTERIFIED
ETODOLAC, ETODOLAC
FAMOTIDINE, FAMOTIDINE
FENOPROFEN CALCIUM, FENOPROFEN CALCIUM
FLECAINIDE ACETATE, FLECAINIDE ACETATE
FLUOXETINE HCL, FLUOXETINE HYDROCHLORIDE
FLUOXETINE, FLUOXETINE HYDROCHLORIDE
FLUPHENAZINE HCL, FLUPHENAZINE HYDROCHLORIDE
FLURAZEPAM HCL, FLURAZEPAM HYDROCHLORIDE
FLURBIPROFEN, FLURBIPROFEN
FLUVOXAMINE MALEATE, FLUVOXAMINE MALEATE
FUROSEMIDE, FUROSEMIDE
GLIPIZIDE, GLIPIZIDE
GLUTETHIMIDE, GLUTETHIMIDE
HALOPERIDOL, HALOPERIDOL
HYDRALAZINE HCL, HYDRALAZINE HYDROCHLORIDE
HYDROCHLOROTHIAZIDE, HYDROCHLOROTHIAZIDE
HYDROXYCHLOROQUINE SULFATE,
    HYDROXYCHLOROQUINE SULFATE
HYDROXYZINE HCL, HYDROXYZINE HYDROCHLORIDE
HYDROXYZINE PAMOATE, HYDROXYZINE PAMOATE
IBUPROFEN, IBUPROFEN
IBUPROFEN, IBUPROFEN (OTC)
IMIPRAMINE HCL, IMIPRAMINE HYDROCHLORIDE
INDOMETHACIN, INDOMETHACIN
ISOSORBIDE DINITRATE, ISOSORBIDE DINITRATE
KETOPROFEN, KETOPROFEN
LONOX, ATROPINE SULFATE
LOPERAMIDE HCL, LOPERAMIDE HYDROCHLORIDE
LORATADINE, LORATADINE (OTC)
LORAZEPAM, LORAZEPAM
LOVASTATIN, LOVASTATIN
MECLIZINE HCL, MECLIZINE HYDROCHLORIDE
MECLOFENAMATE SODIUM, MECLOFENAMATE SODIUM
MEFLOQUINE HCL, MEFLOQUINE HYDROCHLORIDE
MEPROBAMATE, MEPROBAMATE
METFORMIN HCL, METFORMIN HYDROCHLORIDE
METHAZOLAMIDE, METHAZOLAMIDE
METHOCARBAMOL, METHOCARBAMOL
METHOXSALEN, METHOXSALEN
METHYCLOTHIAZIDE, METHYCLOTHIAZIDE
METHYLDOPA AND HYDROCHLOROTHIAZIDE,
    HYDROCHLOROTHIAZIDE
METHYLDOPA, METHYLDOPA
METHYLPREDNISOLONE, METHYLPREDNISOLONE
METOCLOPRAMIDE HCL, METOCLOPRAMIDE
    HYDROCHLORIDE
METOPROLOL TARTRATE, METOPROLOL TARTRATE
METRONIDAZOLE, METRONIDAZOLE
MEXILETINE HCL, MEXILETINE HYDROCHLORIDE
MIRTAZAPINE, MIRTAZAPINE
NAPROXEN SODIUM, NAPROXEN SODIUM
NAPROXEN, NAPROXEN
NIACIN, NIACIN
NITROFURANTOIN, NITROFURANTOIN,
    MACROCRYSTALLINE
NORTRIPTYLINE HCL, NORTRIPTYLINE
    HYDROCHLORIDE
ORPHENADRINE CITRATE, ORPHENADRINE CITRATE
OXAPROZIN, OXAPROZIN
OXAZEPAM, OXAZEPAM
PENICILLIN G POTASSIUM, PENICILLIN G POTASSIUM
PERPHENAZINE AND AMITRIPTYLINE HCL,
    AMITRIPTYLINE HYDROCHLORIDE
PERPHENAZINE, PERPHENAZINE

PHENDIMETRAZINE TARTRATE, PHENDIMETRAZINE
    TARTRATE
PHENYLBUTAZONE, PHENYLBUTAZONE
PINDOLOL, PINDOLOL
PRAZOSIN HCL, PRAZOSIN HYDROCHLORIDE
PREDNISOLONE, PREDNISOLONE
PREDNISONE, PREDNISONE
PROCAINAMIDE HCL, PROCAINAMIDE
    HYDROCHLORIDE
PROMETHAZINE HCL, PROMETHAZINE
    HYDROCHLORIDE
PROPANTHELINE BROMIDE, PROPANTHELINE
    BROMIDE
PROPOXYPHENE COMPOUND-65, ASPIRIN
PROPOXYPHENE HCL AND ACETAMINOPHEN,
    ACETAMINOPHEN
PROPOXYPHENE HCL, PROPOXYPHENE
    HYDROCHLORIDE
PROPOXYPHENE NAPSYLATE AND ACETAMINOPHEN,
    ACETAMINOPHEN
PROPRANOLOL HCL AND HYDROCHLOROTHIAZIDE,
    HYDROCHLOROTHIAZIDE
PROPRANOLOL HCL, PROPRANOLOL HYDROCHLORIDE
QUINIDINE GLUCONATE, QUINIDINE GLUCONATE
QUINIDINE SULFATE, QUINIDINE SULFATE
RANITIDINE HCL, RANITIDINE HYDROCHLORIDE
RANITIDINE, RANITIDINE HYDROCHLORIDE (OTC)
RESERPINE AND HYDROCHLOROTHIAZIDE,
    HYDROCHLOROTHIAZIDE
RIMACTANE, RIFAMPIN
SONAZINE, CHLORPROMAZINE HYDROCHLORIDE
SPIRONOLACTONE AND HYDROCHLOROTHIAZIDE,
    HYDROCHLOROTHIAZIDE
SPIRONOLACTONE, SPIRONOLACTONE
SULFAMETHOXAZOLE AND TRIMETHOPRIM,
    SULFAMETHOXAZOLE
SULFAMETHOXAZOLE, SULFAMETHOXAZOLE
SULFISOXAZOLE, SULFISOXAZOLE
SULINDAC, SULINDAC
TEMAZEPAM, TEMAZEPAM
TERAZOSIN HCL, TERAZOSIN HYDROCHLORIDE
THIORIDAZINE HCL, THIORIDAZINE HYDROCHLORIDE
THIOTHIXENE, THIOTHIXENE
TIMOLOL MALEATE, TIMOLOL MALEATE
TOLAZAMIDE, TOLAZAMIDE
TOLBUTAMIDE, TOLBUTAMIDE
TOLMETIN SODIUM, TOLMETIN SODIUM
TRAZODONE HCL, TRAZODONE HYDROCHLORIDE
TRIAMCINOLONE, TRIAMCINOLONE
TRIAMTERENE AND HYDROCHLOROTHIAZIDE,
    HYDROCHLOROTHIAZIDE
TRIFLUOPERAZINE HCL, TRIFLUOPERAZINE
    HYDROCHLORIDE
VERAPAMIL HCL, VERAPAMIL HYDROCHLORIDE
GENEVA PHARMS TECH
GENEVA PHARMACEUTICALS TECHNOLOGY CORP
    ATENOLOL, ATENOLOL
    BISOPROLOL FUMARATE AND
        HYDROCHLOROTHIAZIDE, BISOPROLOL FUMARATE
    BUPROPION HCL, BUPROPION HYDROCHLORIDE
    CAPTOPRIL, CAPTOPRIL
    CIMETIDINE, CIMETIDINE
    CLOMIPRAMINE HCL, CLOMIPRAMINE
        HYDROCHLORIDE
    CLONAZEPAM, CLONAZEPAM
    CYCLOBENZAPRINE HCL, CYCLOBENZAPRINE
        HYDROCHLORIDE
    DICLOFENAC POTASSIUM, DICLOFENAC POTASSIUM

APPENDIX B
PRODUCT NAME INDEX
LISTED BY APPLICANT (*continued*)

DOXAZOSIN MESYLATE, DOXAZOSIN MESYLATE
ETODOLAC, ETODOLAC
GEMFIBROZIL, GEMFIBROZIL
GLIPIZIDE, GLIPIZIDE
GLYBURIDE (MICRONIZED), GLYBURIDE
HYDROXYCHLOROQUINE SULFATE,
    HYDROXYCHLOROQUINE SULFATE
INDAPAMIDE, INDAPAMIDE
INVAGESIC FORTE, ASPIRIN
INVAGESIC, ASPIRIN
LEUCOVORIN CALCIUM, LEUCOVORIN CALCIUM
LISINOPRIL AND HYDROCHLOROTHIAZIDE,
    HYDROCHLOROTHIAZIDE
LISINOPRIL, LISINOPRIL
METOCLOPRAMIDE HCL, METOCLOPRAMIDE
    HYDROCHLORIDE
NADOLOL, NADOLOL
NAPROXEN SODIUM, NAPROXEN SODIUM
NAPROXEN, NAPROXEN
NORTRIPTYLINE HCL, NORTRIPTYLINE
    HYDROCHLORIDE
ORPHENADRINE CITRATE, ORPHENADRINE CITRATE
PEMOLINE, PEMOLINE
PROCHLORPERAZINE MALEATE, PROCHLORPERAZINE
    MALEATE
TICLOPIDINE HCL, TICLOPIDINE HYDROCHLORIDE
TRIFLUOPERAZINE HCL, TRIFLUOPERAZINE
    HYDROCHLORIDE
WARFARIN SODIUM, WARFARIN SODIUM
GENPHARM
GENPHARM INC
  ACYCLOVIR, ACYCLOVIR
  ALBUTEROL, ALBUTEROL
  AMNESTEEM, ISOTRETINOIN
  AZATHIOPRINE, AZATHIOPRINE
  DOXAZOSIN MESYLATE, DOXAZOSIN MESYLATE
  ENALAPRIL MALEATE, ENALAPRIL MALEATE
  ETIDRONATE DISODIUM, ETIDRONATE DISODIUM
  ETODOLAC, ETODOLAC
  ETOPOSIDE, ETOPOSIDE
  FAMOTIDINE, FAMOTIDINE
  FAMOTIDINE, FAMOTIDINE (OTC)
  FLUTAMIDE, FLUTAMIDE
  FLUVOXAMINE MALEATE, FLUVOXAMINE MALEATE
  GUANFACINE HCL, GUANFACINE HYDROCHLORIDE
  LOVASTATIN, LOVASTATIN
  METFORMIN HCL, METFORMIN HYDROCHLORIDE
  METHIMAZOLE, METHIMAZOLE
  NICARDIPINE HCL, NICARDIPINE HYDROCHLORIDE
  NIZATIDINE, NIZATIDINE
  NOVOTHYROX, LIOTRIX (T4;T3)
  OXAPROZIN, OXAPROZIN
  RANITIDINE HCL, RANITIDINE HYDROCHLORIDE
  RANITIDINE, RANITIDINE HYDROCHLORIDE (OTC)
  SOTALOL HCL, SOTALOL HYDROCHLORIDE
  TICLOPIDINE HCL, TICLOPIDINE HYDROCHLORIDE
GENPHARM PHARMACEUTICALS INC
  ATENOLOL, ATENOLOL
  PINDOLOL, PINDOLOL
  PIROXICAM, PIROXICAM
GENSIA
GENSIA LABORATORIES LTD
  VECURONIUM BROMIDE, VECURONIUM BROMIDE
GENSIA AUTOMEDICS
GENSIA AUTOMEDICS INC
  GENESA, ARBUTAMINE HYDROCHLORIDE
GENSIA SICOR PHARMS
GENSIA SICOR PHARMACEUTICALS INC

ACYCLOVIR SODIUM, ACYCLOVIR SODIUM
ACYCLOVIR, ACYCLOVIR SODIUM
ALPROSTADIL, ALPROSTADIL
AMIKACIN SULFATE, AMIKACIN SULFATE
AMINOPHYLLINE, AMINOPHYLLINE
AMPHOTERICIN B, AMPHOTERICIN B
ATRACURIUM BESYLATE, ATRACURIUM BESYLATE
BLEOMYCIN, BLEOMYCIN SULFATE
BUMETANIDE, BUMETANIDE
CALCITRIOL, CALCITRIOL
CIMETIDINE HCL, CIMETIDINE HYDROCHLORIDE
CISPLATIN, CISPLATIN
CLINDAMYCIN PHOSPHATE, CLINDAMYCIN
    PHOSPHATE
CYTARABINE, CYTARABINE
CYTOSAR-U, CYTARABINE
DACARBAZINE, DACARBAZINE
DAUNORUBICIN HCL, DAUNORUBICIN
    HYDROCHLORIDE
DESMOPRESSIN ACETATE, DESMOPRESSIN ACETATE
DEXAMETHASONE SODIUM PHOSPHATE,
    DEXAMETHASONE SODIUM PHOSPHATE
DILTIAZEM HCL, DILTIAZEM HYDROCHLORIDE
DIPYRIDAMOLE, DIPYRIDAMOLE
DOBUTAMINE HCL, DOBUTAMINE HYDROCHLORIDE
DOPAMINE HCL, DOPAMINE HYDROCHLORIDE
DOXORUBICIN HCL, DOXORUBICIN HYDROCHLORIDE
ENALAPRILAT, ENALAPRILAT
ERYTHROMYCIN LACTOBIONATE, ERYTHROMYCIN
    LACTOBIONATE
ETOPOSIDE, ETOPOSIDE
FLUOROURACIL, FLUOROURACIL
FLUPHENAZINE DECANOATE, FLUPHENAZINE
    DECANOATE
GENTAMICIN SULFATE, GENTAMICIN SULFATE
GLYCOPYRROLATE, GLYCOPYRROLATE
HALOPERIDOL DECANOATE, HALOPERIDOL
    DECANOATE
HALOPERIDOL, HALOPERIDOL LACTATE
HYDRALAZINE HCL, HYDRALAZINE HYDROCHLORIDE
IDARUBICIN HCL PFS, IDARUBICIN HYDROCHLORIDE
IDARUBICIN HCL, IDARUBICIN HYDROCHLORIDE
IFOSFAMIDE/MESNA KIT, IFOSFAMIDE
LEUCOVORIN CALCIUM PRESERVATIVE FREE,
    LEUCOVORIN CALCIUM
LEUCOVORIN CALCIUM, LEUCOVORIN CALCIUM
LEUPROLIDE ACETATE, LEUPROLIDE ACETATE
LEVOCARNITINE, LEVOCARNITINE
MESNA, MESNA
METHYLDOPATE HCL, METHYLDOPATE
    HYDROCHLORIDE
METHYLPREDNISOLONE SODIUM SUCCINATE,
    METHYLPREDNISOLONE SODIUM SUCCINATE
METOCLOPRAMIDE HCL, METOCLOPRAMIDE
    HYDROCHLORIDE
NOREPINEPHRINE BITARTRATE, NOREPINEPHRINE
    BITARTRATE
PAMIDRONATE DISODIUM, PAMIDRONATE DISODIUM
PANCURONIUM BROMIDE, PANCURONIUM BROMIDE
PROCHLORPERAZINE EDISYLATE,
    PROCHLORPERAZINE EDISYLATE
PROMETHAZINE HCL, PROMETHAZINE
    HYDROCHLORIDE
PROPOFOL, PROPOFOL
SODIUM NITROPRUSSIDE, SODIUM NITROPRUSSIDE
SULFAMETHOXAZOLE AND TRIMETHOPRIM,
    SULFAMETHOXAZOLE
THIOTEPA, THIOTEPA

APPENDIX B
PRODUCT NAME INDEX
LISTED BY APPLICANT (*continued*)

TOBRAMYCIN SULFATE, TOBRAMYCIN SULFATE
VINCRISTINE SULFATE PFS, VINCRISTINE SULFATE
VINORELBINE TARTRATE, VINORELBINE TARTRATE
ZANOSAR, STREPTOZOCIN
GENTA
GENTA INC
  GANITE, GALLIUM NITRATE
GENZYME
GENZYME CORP
  CEREDASE, ALGLUCERASE
  CEREZYME, IMIGLUCERASE
  LEUPROLIDE ACETATE, LEUPROLIDE ACETATE
  RENAGEL, SEVELAMER HYDROCHLORIDE
  THYROGEN, THYROTROPIN ALFA
GILBERT LABS
GILBERT LABORATORIES
  ACETAMINOPHEN, BUTALBITAL AND CAFFEINE,
    ACETAMINOPHEN
GILEAD
GILEAD SCIENCES INC
  DAUNOXOME, DAUNORUBICIN CITRATE
  HEPSERA, ADEFOVIR DIPIVOXIL
  VIREAD, TENOFOVIR DISOPROXIL FUMARATE
  VISTIDE, CIDOFOVIR
GLADES PHARMS
GLADES PHARMACEUTICALS INC
  E-GLADES, ERYTHROMYCIN
GLAXO WELLCOME
GLAXO WELLCOME INC
  LANOXICAPS, DIGOXIN
  LANOXIN, DIGOXIN
GLAXOSMITHKLINE
GLAXOSMITHKLINE
  ABREVA, DOCOSANOL (OTC)
  ACLOVATE, ALCLOMETASONE DIPROPIONATE
  ACTIDIL, TRIPROLIDINE HYDROCHLORIDE (OTC)
  ACTIFED W/ CODEINE, CODEINE PHOSPHATE
  ACTIFED, PSEUDOEPHEDRINE HYDROCHLORIDE (OTC)
  ADVAIR DISKUS 100/50, FLUTICASONE PROPIONATE
  ADVAIR DISKUS 250/50, FLUTICASONE PROPIONATE
  ADVAIR DISKUS 500/50, FLUTICASONE PROPIONATE
  AEROSPORIN, POLYMYXIN B SULFATE
  AGENERASE, AMPRENAVIR
  ALBENZA, ALBENDAZOLE
  ALKERAN, MELPHALAN
  ALKERAN, MELPHALAN HYDROCHLORIDE
  AMERGE, NARATRIPTAN HYDROCHLORIDE
  AMOXIL, AMOXICILLIN
  ANCEF, CEFAZOLIN SODIUM
  ANECTINE, SUCCINYLCHOLINE CHLORIDE
  ANSPOR, CEPHRADINE
  ANTEPAR, PIPERAZINE CITRATE
  AUGMENTIN ',125', AMOXICILLIN
  AUGMENTIN ',200', AMOXICILLIN
  AUGMENTIN ',250', AMOXICILLIN
  AUGMENTIN ',400', AMOXICILLIN
  AUGMENTIN ',500', AMOXICILLIN
  AUGMENTIN ',875', AMOXICILLIN
  AUGMENTIN ES-600, AMOXICILLIN
  AUGMENTIN XR, AMOXICILLIN
  AVODART, DUTASTERIDE
  BACTOCILL, OXACILLIN SODIUM
  BACTROBAN, MUPIROCIN
  BACTROBAN, MUPIROCIN CALCIUM
  BECLOVENT, BECLOMETHASONE DIPROPIONATE
  BECONASE AQ, BECLOMETHASONE DIPROPIONATE
    MONOHYDRATE
  BECONASE, BECLOMETHASONE DIPROPIONATE

BEEPEN-VK, PENICILLIN V POTASSIUM
CEFAZOLIN SODIUM, CEFAZOLIN SODIUM
CEFTIN, CEFUROXIME AXETIL
CEPTAZ, CEFTAZIDIME (ARGININE FORMULATION)
CLOXAPEN, CLOXACILLIN SODIUM
COMBIVIR, LAMIVUDINE
COMPAZINE, PROCHLORPERAZINE
COMPAZINE, PROCHLORPERAZINE EDISYLATE
COMPAZINE, PROCHLORPERAZINE MALEATE
CONTAC 12 HOUR, CHLORPHENIRAMINE MALEATE
  (OTC)
COREG, CARVEDILOL
CUTIVATE, FLUTICASONE PROPIONATE
DARAPRIM, PYRIMETHAMINE
DARBID, ISOPROPAMIDE IODIDE
DEXEDRINE, DEXTROAMPHETAMINE SULFATE
DIONOSIL AQUEOUS, PROPYLIODONE
DIONOSIL OILY, PROPYLIODONE
DYAZIDE, HYDROCHLOROTHIAZIDE
DYCILL, DICLOXACILLIN SODIUM
EMGEL, ERYTHROMYCIN
EMPRACET W/ CODEINE PHOSPHATE #3,
  ACETAMINOPHEN
EMPRACET W/ CODEINE PHOSPHATE #4,
  ACETAMINOPHEN
EPIVIR, LAMIVUDINE
EPIVIR-HBV, LAMIVUDINE
ESKALITH CR, LITHIUM CARBONATE
ESKALITH, LITHIUM CARBONATE
EXOSURF NEONATAL, CETYL ALCOHOL
FASTIN, PHENTERMINE HYDROCHLORIDE
FLOLAN, EPOPROSTENOL SODIUM
FLONASE, FLUTICASONE PROPIONATE
FLOVENT DISKUS 100, FLUTICASONE PROPIONATE
FLOVENT DISKUS 250, FLUTICASONE PROPIONATE
FLOVENT DISKUS 50, FLUTICASONE PROPIONATE
FLOVENT, FLUTICASONE PROPIONATE
FORTAZ IN PLASTIC CONTAINER, CEFTAZIDIME SODIUM
FORTAZ, CEFTAZIDIME
HALFAN, HALOFANTRINE HYDROCHLORIDE
HISPRIL, DIPHENYLPYRALINE HYDROCHLORIDE
HYCAMTIN, TOPOTECAN HYDROCHLORIDE
IMITREX, SUMATRIPTAN
IMITREX, SUMATRIPTAN SUCCINATE
LAMICTAL CD, LAMOTRIGINE
LAMICTAL, LAMOTRIGINE
LANOXIN PEDIATRIC, DIGOXIN
LANOXIN, DIGOXIN
LAROTID, AMOXICILLIN
LEUKERAN, CHLORAMBUCIL
LOTRONEX, ALOSETRON HYDROCHLORIDE
MALARONE PEDIATRIC, ATOVAQUONE
MALARONE, ATOVAQUONE
MAREZINE, CYCLIZINE LACTATE
MEPRON, ATOVAQUONE
MONOCID, CEFONICID SODIUM
MYLERAN, BUSULFAN
NALLPEN, NAFCILLIN SODIUM
NAVELBINE, VINORELBINE TARTRATE
NEOSPORIN, NEOMYCIN SULFATE (OTC)
NICORETTE (0RANGE), NICOTINE POLACRILEX (OTC)
NICORETTE (MINT), NICOTINE POLACRILEX (OTC)
NICORETTE (ORANGE), NICOTINE POLACRILEX (OTC)
NICORETTE, NICOTINE POLACRILEX (OTC)
NIX, PERMETHRIN
ORNADE, CHLORPHENIRAMINE MALEATE
OXISTAT, OXICONAZOLE NITRATE
PARNATE, TRANYLCYPROMINE SULFATE

APPENDIX B
PRODUCT NAME INDEX
LISTED BY APPLICANT (*continued*)

PAXIL CR, PAROXETINE HYDROCHLORIDE
PAXIL, PAROXETINE HYDROCHLORIDE
PENTACEF, CEFTAZIDIME (ARGININE FORMULATION)
PHYTONADIONE, PHYTONADIONE
POLYSPORIN, BACITRACIN ZINC (OTC)
PURINETHOL, MERCAPTOPURINE
PYOPEN, CARBENICILLIN DISODIUM
RELAFEN, NABUMETONE
RELENZA, ZANAMIVIR
REQUIP, ROPINIROLE HYDROCHLORIDE
RETROVIR, ZIDOVUDINE
SEFFIN, CEPHALOTHIN SODIUM
SEREVENT, SALMETEROL XINAFOATE
STELAZINE, TRIFLUOPERAZINE HYDROCHLORIDE
STOXIL, IDOXURIDINE
SUDAFED 12 HOUR, PSEUDOEPHEDRINE
    HYDROCHLORIDE (OTC)
SYNCURINE, DECAMETHONIUM BROMIDE
TAGAMET HB 200, CIMETIDINE (OTC)
TAGAMET HB, CIMETIDINE (OTC)
TAGAMET HCL IN SODIUM CHLORIDE 0.9% IN PLASTIC
    CONTAINER, CIMETIDINE HYDROCHLORIDE
TAGAMET, CIMETIDINE
TAGAMET, CIMETIDINE HYDROCHLORIDE
TELDRIN, CHLORPHENIRAMINE MALEATE (OTC)
TEMOVATE E, CLOBETASOL PROPIONATE
TEMOVATE, CLOBETASOL PROPIONATE
THIOGUANINE, THIOGUANINE
THORAZINE, CHLORPROMAZINE
THORAZINE, CHLORPROMAZINE HYDROCHLORIDE
TICAR, TICARCILLIN DISODIUM
TIMENTIN IN PLASTIC CONTAINER, CLAVULANATE
    POTASSIUM
TIMENTIN, CLAVULANATE POTASSIUM
TOTACILLIN, AMPICILLIN/AMPICILLIN TRIHYDRATE
TOTACILLIN-N, AMPICILLIN SODIUM
TRANDATE HCT, HYDROCHLOROTHIAZIDE
TRITEC, RANITIDINE BISMUTH CITRATE
TRIZIVIR, ABACAVIR SULFATE
VALTREX, VALACYCLOVIR HYDROCHLORIDE
VASOXYL, METHOXAMINE HYDROCHLORIDE
VENTOLIN HFA, ALBUTEROL SULFATE
VENTOLIN ROTACAPS, ALBUTEROL SULFATE
VENTOLIN, ALBUTEROL
VENTOLIN, ALBUTEROL SULFATE
VONTROL, DIPHENIDOL HYDROCHLORIDE
WELLBUTRIN SR, BUPROPION HYDROCHLORIDE
WELLBUTRIN, BUPROPION HYDROCHLORIDE
WELLCOVORIN, LEUCOVORIN CALCIUM
ZANTAC 150, RANITIDINE HYDROCHLORIDE
ZANTAC 300, RANITIDINE HYDROCHLORIDE
ZANTAC IN PLASTIC CONTAINER, RANITIDINE
    HYDROCHLORIDE
ZANTAC, RANITIDINE HYDROCHLORIDE
ZIAGEN, ABACAVIR SULFATE
ZINACEF IN PLASTIC CONTAINER, CEFUROXIME
    SODIUM
ZINACEF, CEFUROXIME SODIUM
ZOFRAN IN PLASTIC CONTAINER, ONDANSETRON
    HYDROCHLORIDE
ZOFRAN ODT, ONDANSETRON
ZOFRAN PRESERVATIVE FREE, ONDANSETRON
    HYDROCHLORIDE
ZOFRAN, ONDANSETRON HYDROCHLORIDE
ZOVIRAX, ACYCLOVIR
ZOVIRAX, ACYCLOVIR SODIUM
ZYBAN, BUPROPION HYDROCHLORIDE

GLAXOSMITHKLINE CONS
GLAXOSMITHKLINE CONSUMER HEALTHCARE
    APHTHASOL, AMLEXANOX
    COMMIT, NICOTINE POLACRILEX (OTC)
GLENWOOD
GLENWOOD INC
    MYOTONACHOL, BETHANECHOL CHLORIDE
    PASKALIUM, POTASSIUM AMINOSALICYLATE
    RENOQUID, SULFACYTINE
GOLDLINE
GOLDLINE LABORATORIES INC
    GLYCOPREP, POLYETHYLENE GLYCOL 3350
    METFORMIN HCL, METFORMIN HYDROCHLORIDE
GRAHAM CHEM
GRAHAM CHEMICAL CO
    LIDOCAINE HCL AND EPINEPHRINE, EPINEPHRINE
    LIDOCAINE HCL, LIDOCAINE HYDROCHLORIDE
    LIDOCAINE, LIDOCAINE
    MEPIVACAINE HCL W/ LEVONORDEFRIN,
        LEVONORDEFRIN
    MEPIVACAINE HCL, MEPIVACAINE HYDROCHLORIDE
GRAHAM DM
DM GRAHAM LABORATORIES INC
    BUTALBITAL, ACETAMINOPHEN, CAFFEINE,
        ACETAMINOPHEN
    COLD CAPSULE IV, CHLORPHENIRAMINE MALEATE
        (OTC)
    COLD CAPSULE V, CHLORPHENIRAMINE MALEATE
        (OTC)
    PHENDIMETRAZINE TARTRATE, PHENDIMETRAZINE
        TARTRATE
    PSEUDOEPHEDRINE HCL/CHLORPHENIRAMINE
        MALEATE, CHLORPHENIRAMINE MALEATE (OTC)
    SOMOPHYLLIN-CRT, THEOPHYLLINE
GRIFFEN
KW GRIFFEN CO
    BIOSCRUB, CHLORHEXIDINE GLUCONATE (OTC)
GRUPPO LEPETIT
GRUPPO LEPETIT SPA SUB MERRELL DOW PHARMACEU-
TICALS INC
    CHLORAMPHENICOL SODIUM SUCCINATE,
        CHLORAMPHENICOL SODIUM SUCCINATE
GUARDIAN DRUG
GUARDIAN DRUG CO INC
    FOAMCOAT, ALUMINUM HYDROXIDE (OTC)
GUERBET
GUERBET LLC
    OXILAN-300, IOXILAN
    OXILAN-350, IOXILAN
GUILFORD PHARMS
GUILFORD PHARMACEUTICALS INC
    GLIADEL, CARMUSTINE
GYNETICS
GYNETICS INC
    PREVEN EMERGENCY CONTRACEPTIVE KIT, ETHINYL
        ESTRADIOL
GYNOPHARMA
GYNOPHARMA INC
    NORCEPT-E 1/35 21, ETHINYL ESTRADIOL
    NORCEPT-E 1/35 28, ETHINYL ESTRADIOL

H

HALLMARK PHARMS
HALLMARK PHARMACEUTICALS
    CAPTOPRIL, CAPTOPRIL

APPENDIX B
PRODUCT NAME INDEX
LISTED BY APPLICANT (*continued*)

HALOCARBON
HALOCARBON LABORATORIES DIV HALOCARBON PRO-
DUCTS CORP
   HALOTHANE, HALOTHANE
HALOCARBON PRODS
HALOCARBON PRODUCTS CORP
   ISOFLURANE, ISOFLURANE
HALSEY
HALSEY DRUG CO INC
   ACETAMINOPHEN AND CODEINE PHOSPHATE,
      ACETAMINOPHEN
   ACETAMINOPHEN W/ CODEINE PHOSPHATE,
      ACETAMINOPHEN
   ACETAMINOPHEN W/ CODEINE, ACETAMINOPHEN
   ALLOPURINOL, ALLOPURINOL
   AMINOPHYLLINE, AMINOPHYLLINE
   AMITRIPTYLINE HCL, AMITRIPTYLINE HYDROCHLORIDE
   BELDIN, DIPHENHYDRAMINE HYDROCHLORIDE (OTC)
   BELIX, DIPHENHYDRAMINE HYDROCHLORIDE
   BUTALBITAL AND ACETAMINOPHEN, ACETAMINOPHEN
   BUTALBITAL, ASPIRIN & CAFFEINE, ASPIRIN
   CHLORDIAZEPOXIDE AND AMITRIPTYLINE HCL,
      AMITRIPTYLINE HYDROCHLORIDE
   CHLORDIAZEPOXIDE HCL, CHLORDIAZEPOXIDE
      HYDROCHLORIDE
   CHLORPHENIRAMINE MALEATE, CHLORPHENIRAMINE
      MALEATE
   CHLORPROPAMIDE, CHLORPROPAMIDE
   CHLORTHALIDONE, CHLORTHALIDONE
   CLONIDINE HCL, CLONIDINE HYDROCHLORIDE
   CODOXY, ASPIRIN
   CORTALONE, PREDNISOLONE
   CORTAN, PREDNISONE
   CYCLOBENZAPRINE HCL, CYCLOBENZAPRINE
      HYDROCHLORIDE
   CYPROHEPTADINE HCL, CYPROHEPTADINE
      HYDROCHLORIDE
   DEXAMETHASONE, DEXAMETHASONE
   DEXTROAMPHETAMINE SULFATE,
      DEXTROAMPHETAMINE SULFATE
   DIAZEPAM, DIAZEPAM
   DICYCLOMINE HCL, DICYCLOMINE HYDROCHLORIDE
   DIPHENHYDRAMINE HCL, DIPHENHYDRAMINE
      HYDROCHLORIDE
   DIPHENOXYLATE HCL AND ATROPINE SULFATE,
      ATROPINE SULFATE
   DISOPYRAMIDE PHOSPHATE, DISOPYRAMIDE
      PHOSPHATE
   DOXEPIN HCL, DOXEPIN HYDROCHLORIDE
   DOXYCYCLINE HYCLATE, DOXYCYCLINE HYCLATE
   ERGOLOID MESYLATES, ERGOLOID MESYLATES
   FENOPROFEN CALCIUM, FENOPROFEN CALCIUM
   FLURAZEPAM HCL, FLURAZEPAM HYDROCHLORIDE
   FOLIC ACID, FOLIC ACID
   FUROSEMIDE, FUROSEMIDE
   GLUTETHIMIDE, GLUTETHIMIDE
   HALOPERIDOL, HALOPERIDOL
   HYDRALAZINE HCL, HYDRALAZINE HYDROCHLORIDE
   HYDRO-D, HYDROCHLOROTHIAZIDE
   HYDROCHLOROTHIAZIDE, HYDROCHLOROTHIAZIDE
   HYDROCODONE BITARTRATE AND ACETAMINOPHEN,
      ACETAMINOPHEN
   HYDROPANE, HOMATROPINE METHYLBROMIDE
   HYDROXYZINE HCL, HYDROXYZINE HYDROCHLORIDE
   IBUPROFEN, IBUPROFEN
   IBUPROFEN, IBUPROFEN (OTC)
   INDOMETHACIN, INDOMETHACIN
   ISONIAZID, ISONIAZID

   ISOSORBIDE DINITRATE, ISOSORBIDE DINITRATE
   KLOROMIN, CHLORPHENIRAMINE MALEATE
   LORAZEPAM, LORAZEPAM
   LOW-QUEL, ATROPINE SULFATE
   MEPROBAMATE, MEPROBAMATE
   METHOCARBAMOL, METHOCARBAMOL
   METHYLDOPA, METHYLDOPA
   METOCLOPRAMIDE HCL, METOCLOPRAMIDE
      HYDROCHLORIDE
   METRONIDAZOLE, METRONIDAZOLE
   NALIDIXIC ACID, NALIDIXIC ACID
   NEURAMATE, MEPROBAMATE
   NIACIN, NIACIN
   OXAZEPAM, OXAZEPAM
   OXYCODONE AND ACETAMINOPHEN, ACETAMINOPHEN
   OXYCODONE AND ASPIRIN, ASPIRIN
   PERPHENAZINE AND AMITRIPTYLINE HCL,
      AMITRIPTYLINE HYDROCHLORIDE
   PHENYLBUTAZONE, PHENYLBUTAZONE
   PHERAZINE DM, DEXTROMETHORPHAN
      HYDROBROMIDE
   PHERAZINE VC W/ CODEINE, CODEINE PHOSPHATE
   PHERAZINE VC, PHENYLEPHRINE HYDROCHLORIDE
   PHERAZINE W/ CODEINE, CODEINE PHOSPHATE
   PREDNISONE, PREDNISONE
   PROMETHAZINE HCL, PROMETHAZINE
      HYDROCHLORIDE
   PROPHENE 65, PROPOXYPHENE HYDROCHLORIDE
   PROPOXYPHENE HCL, PROPOXYPHENE
      HYDROCHLORIDE
   PROPOXYPHENE NAPSYLATE AND ACETAMINOPHEN,
      ACETAMINOPHEN
   PROPRANOLOL HCL, PROPRANOLOL HYDROCHLORIDE
   PROPYLTHIOURACIL, PROPYLTHIOURACIL
   QUINIDINE GLUCONATE, QUINIDINE GLUCONATE
   QUINIDINE SULFATE, QUINIDINE SULFATE
   RAUWOLFIA SERPENTINA, RAUWOLFIA SERPENTINA
   RESERPINE, HYDRALAZINE HCL AND
      HYDROCHLOROTHIAZIDE, HYDRALAZINE
      HYDROCHLORIDE
   RESERPINE, RESERPINE
   SARISOL NO. 1, BUTABARBITAL SODIUM
   SARISOL NO. 2, BUTABARBITAL SODIUM
   SARISOL, BUTABARBITAL SODIUM
   SODIUM PENTOBARBITAL, PENTOBARBITAL SODIUM
   SODIUM SECOBARBITAL, SECOBARBITAL SODIUM
   SPIRONOLACTONE AND HYDROCHLOROTHIAZIDE,
      HYDROCHLOROTHIAZIDE
   SPIRONOLACTONE, SPIRONOLACTONE
   SULFAMETHOXAZOLE AND TRIMETHOPRIM DOUBLE
      STRENGTH, SULFAMETHOXAZOLE
   SULFAMETHOXAZOLE AND TRIMETHOPRIM,
      SULFAMETHOXAZOLE
   TEMAZEPAM, TEMAZEPAM
   THEOPHYLLINE, THEOPHYLLINE
   THIORIDAZINE HCL, THIORIDAZINE HYDROCHLORIDE
   TRIMETHOPRIM, TRIMETHOPRIM
   TRIPROLIDINE HCL, TRIPROLIDINE HYDROCHLORIDE
   VERAPAMIL HCL, VERAPAMIL HYDROCHLORIDE
HAMILTON PHARMS
HAMILTON PHARMACEUTICALS LTD
   NAPROXEN SODIUM, NAPROXEN SODIUM
   NAPROXEN, NAPROXEN
HANFORD GC
GC HANFORD MANUFACTURING CO
   AMPICILLIN SODIUM, AMPICILLIN SODIUM
   CEFAZOLIN SODIUM, CEFAZOLIN SODIUM
   CEFUROXIME SODIUM, CEFUROXIME SODIUM

APPENDIX B
PRODUCT NAME INDEX
LISTED BY APPLICANT (*continued*)

HARVEST PHARMS
HARVEST PHARMACEUTICALS INC
   ERGOMAR, ERGOTAMINE TARTRATE
HEALTHPOINT
HEALTHPOINT LTD
   AKNE-MYCIN, ERYTHROMYCIN
   CETACORT, HYDROCORTISONE
   CLODERM, CLOCORTOLONE PIVALATE
   CORMAX, CLOBETASOL PROPIONATE
   EMBELINE E, CLOBETASOL PROPIONATE
   EMBELINE, CLOBETASOL PROPIONATE
   NUTRACORT, HYDROCORTISONE
   SANSAC, ERYTHROMYCIN
HEATHER
HEATHER DRUG CO INC
   CORTISONE ACETATE, CORTISONE ACETATE
   DIMENHYDRINATE, DIMENHYDRINATE
   DIPHENHYDRAMINE HCL, DIPHENHYDRAMINE
     HYDROCHLORIDE
   DIPHENOXYLATE HCL AND ATROPINE SULFATE,
     ATROPINE SULFATE
   DOXYCYCLINE HYCLATE, DOXYCYCLINE HYCLATE
   HYDROCHLOROTHIAZIDE, HYDROCHLOROTHIAZIDE
   MEPROBAMATE, MEPROBAMATE
   METHOCARBAMOL, METHOCARBAMOL
   METHYLPREDNISOLONE, METHYLPREDNISOLONE
   METHYLTESTOSTERONE, METHYLTESTOSTERONE
   PREDNISOLONE, PREDNISOLONE
   PREDNISONE, PREDNISONE
   PROPANTHELINE BROMIDE, PROPANTHELINE
     BROMIDE
   SULFAMETHOXAZOLE & TRIMETHOPRIM,
     SULFAMETHOXAZOLE
   SULFAMETHOXAZOLE, SULFAMETHOXAZOLE
   SULFISOXAZOLE, SULFISOXAZOLE
   TETRACYCLINE HCL, TETRACYCLINE HYDROCHLORIDE
   TRIPELENNAMINE HCL, TRIPELENNAMINE
     HYDROCHLORIDE
HERAN
HERAN PHARMACEUTICAL INC
   GLYCORT, HYDROCORTISONE
HERCON LABS
HERCON LABORATORIES CORP
   NITROGLYCERIN, NITROGLYCERIN
HEXCEL
HEXCEL CHEMICAL PRODUCTS
   POTASSIUM AMINOSALICYLATE, POTASSIUM
     AMINOSALICYLATE
   SODIUM AMINOSALICYLATE, AMINOSALICYLATE
     SODIUM
HI TECH PHARMA
HI TECH PHARMACAL CO INC
   ACETAMINOPHEN AND CODEINE PHOSPHATE,
     ACETAMINOPHEN
   ALBUTEROL SULFATE, ALBUTEROL SULFATE
   AMANTADINE HCL, AMANTADINE HYDROCHLORIDE
   CHLORHEXIDINE GLUCONATE, CHLORHEXIDINE
     GLUCONATE
   CIMETIDINE HCL, CIMETIDINE HYDROCHLORIDE
   DIPHENHYDRAMINE HCL, DIPHENHYDRAMINE
     HYDROCHLORIDE (OTC)
   ERYTHRO-STATIN, ERYTHROMYCIN
   FLUOXETINE HCL, FLUOXETINE HYDROCHLORIDE
   HYDROXYZINE HCL, HYDROXYZINE HYDROCHLORIDE
   LACTULOSE, LACTULOSE
   LIDOCAINE HCL, LIDOCAINE HYDROCHLORIDE
   LOPERAMIDE HCL, LOPERAMIDE HYDROCHLORIDE
     (OTC)

   MINOXIDIL (FOR MEN), MINOXIDIL (OTC)
   PREDNISOLONE SODIUM PHOSPHATE, PREDNISOLONE
     SODIUM PHOSPHATE
   PREDNISOLONE, PREDNISOLONE
   PROMETHAZINE HCL AND CODEINE PHOSPHATE,
     CODEINE PHOSPHATE
   PROMETHAZINE HCL AND DEXTROMETHORPHAN
     HYDROBROMIDE, DEXTROMETHORPHAN
     HYDROBROMIDE
   PROMETHAZINE HCL, PROMETHAZINE
     HYDROCHLORIDE
   SULFAMETHOXAZOLE AND TRIMETHOPRIM,
     SULFAMETHOXAZOLE
   THIORIDAZINE HCL, THIORIDAZINE HYDROCHLORIDE
   TIMOLOL MALEATE, TIMOLOL MALEATE
HIGH TECH PHARMA
HIGH TECHNOLOGY PHARMACAL CO INC
   VALPROIC ACID, VALPROIC ACID
HIKMA
HIKMA FARMACEUTICA LDA
   CEFOTAXIME, CEFOTAXIME SODIUM
HILL DERMAC
HILL DERMACEUTICALS INC
   DERMA-SMOOTHE/FS, FLUOCINOLONE ACETONIDE
   TRI-LUMA, FLUOCINOLONE ACETONIDE
HLR
HLR TECHNOLOGY
   ACCUTANE, ISOTRETINOIN
   FORTOVASE, SAQUINAVIR
   INVIRASE, SAQUINAVIR MESYLATE
   ROCEPHIN KIT, CEFTRIAXONE SODIUM
   ROCEPHIN W/ DEXTROSE IN PLASTIC CONTAINER,
     CEFTRIAXONE SODIUM
   ROCEPHIN, CEFTRIAXONE SODIUM
   ROMAZICON, FLUMAZENIL
   SORIATANE, ACITRETIN
   VERSED, MIDAZOLAM HYDROCHLORIDE
   XELODA, CAPECITABINE
   XENICAL, ORLISTAT
HOLLAND RANTOS
HOLLAND RANTOS CO INC
   KOROSTATIN, NYSTATIN
HOLLISTER STIER LABS
HOLLISTER STIER LABORATORIES LLC
   TWINJECT, EPINEPHRINE
HUNTINGTON LABS
HUNTINGTON LABORATORIES INC
   GERMA-MEDICA "MG", HEXACHLOROPHENE
   GERMA-MEDICA, HEXACHLOROPHENE
   HEXA-GERM, HEXACHLOROPHENE

I

IBI
ISTITUTO BIOCHIMICO ITALIANO SPA
   AMPICILLIN SODIUM, AMPICILLIN SODIUM
   OXACILLIN SODIUM, OXACILLIN SODIUM
ICN
ICN PHARMACEUTICALS INC
   8-MOP, METHOXSALEN
   AMINOPHYLLINE, AMINOPHYLLINE
   ANCOBON, FLUCYTOSINE
   ANDROID 10, METHYLTESTOSTERONE
   ANDROID 25, METHYLTESTOSTERONE
   ANDROID 5, METHYLTESTOSTERONE
   ANDROID-F, FLUOXYMESTERONE
   BENDOPA, LEVODOPA

APPENDIX B
PRODUCT NAME INDEX
LISTED BY APPLICANT (*continued*)

BENOQUIN, MONOBENZONE
CHLORPHENIRAMINE MALEATE, CHLORPHENIRAMINE
  MALEATE
CODEINE PHOSPHATE AND ACETAMINOPHEN,
  ACETAMINOPHEN
DALMANE, FLURAZEPAM HYDROCHLORIDE
DIPHENHYDRAMINE HCL, DIPHENHYDRAMINE
  HYDROCHLORIDE
DIPHENOXYLATE HCL W/ ATROPINE SULFATE,
  ATROPINE SULFATE
EFUDEX, FLUOROURACIL
ELDECORT, HYDROCORTISONE
FLUOXYMESTERONE, FLUOXYMESTERONE
FOLIC ACID, FOLIC ACID
LEVO-DROMORAN, LEVORPHANOL TARTRATE
LIBRELEASE, CHLORDIAZEPOXIDE
LIBRITABS, CHLORDIAZEPOXIDE
LIBRIUM, CHLORDIAZEPOXIDE HYDROCHLORIDE
LIMBITROL DS, AMITRIPTYLINE HYDROCHLORIDE
LIMBITROL, AMITRIPTYLINE HYDROCHLORIDE
MEPROBAMATE, MEPROBAMATE
MESTINON, PYRIDOSTIGMINE BROMIDE
OXSORALEN, METHOXSALEN
OXSORALEN ULTRA, METHOXSALEN
PREDNISOLONE, PREDNISOLONE
PREDNISONE, PREDNISONE
PROPOXYPHENE HCL, PROPOXYPHENE
  HYDROCHLORIDE
QUINIDINE SULFATE, QUINIDINE SULFATE
RAUWOLFIA SERPENTINA, RAUWOLFIA SERPENTINA
RESERPINE, RESERPINE
SECOBARBITAL SODIUM, SECOBARBITAL SODIUM
SODIUM PENTOBARBITAL, PENTOBARBITAL SODIUM
SULFISOXAZOLE, SULFISOXAZOLE
TENSILON PRESERVATIVE FREE, EDROPHONIUM
  CHLORIDE
TENSILON, EDROPHONIUM CHLORIDE
TESTRED, METHYLTESTOSTERONE
TETRACYCLINE HCL, TETRACYCLINE HYDROCHLORIDE
TRISORALEN, TRIOXSALEN
VIRAZOLE, RIBAVIRIN
ICN PUERTO RICO
ICN PUERTO RICO INC
  FLUOROURACIL, FLUOROURACIL
IMMUNEX
IMMUNEX CORP
  LEVOPROME, LEVOMEPROMAZINE
  THIOPLEX, THIOTEPA
  THIOTEPA, THIOTEPA
IMP
IMP INC
  SPECTAMINE, IOFETAMINE HYDROCHLORIDE I-123
IMPAX LABS
IMPAX LABORATORIES INC
  AMINOPHYLLINE, AMINOPHYLLINE
  CHLORDIAZEPOXIDE HCL, CHLORDIAZEPOXIDE
    HYDROCHLORIDE
  CHLOROQUINE PHOSPHATE, CHLOROQUINE
    PHOSPHATE
  CHLORPHENIRAMINE MALEATE, CHLORPHENIRAMINE
    MALEATE
  CORTISONE ACETATE, CORTISONE ACETATE
  DEXAMETHASONE, DEXAMETHASONE
  DIPHENHYDRAMINE HCL, DIPHENHYDRAMINE
    HYDROCHLORIDE
  FLUDROCORTISONE ACETATE, FLUDROCORTISONE
    ACETATE
  FOLIC ACID, FOLIC ACID

HYDRALAZINE HCL, HYDRALAZINE HYDROCHLORIDE
HYDROCHLOROTHIAZIDE, HYDROCHLOROTHIAZIDE
HYDROCORTISONE, HYDROCORTISONE
ISONIAZID, ISONIAZID
LORATADINE AND PSEUDOEPHEDRINE SULFATE,
  LORATADINE (OTC)
MEPROBAMATE, MEPROBAMATE
METHOCARBAMOL, METHOCARBAMOL
METHYLTESTOSTERONE, METHYLTESTOSTERONE
MINOCYCLINE HCL, MINOCYCLINE HYDROCHLORIDE
NIACIN, NIACIN
OMEPRAZOLE, OMEPRAZOLE
OXYTETRACYCLINE HCL, OXYTETRACYCLINE
  HYDROCHLORIDE
PENTOXIFYLLINE, PENTOXIFYLLINE
PIPERAZINE CITRATE, PIPERAZINE CITRATE
PREDNISOLONE, PREDNISOLONE
PREDNISONE, PREDNISONE
PROBENECID AND COLCHICINE, COLCHICINE
PROMETHAZINE HCL, PROMETHAZINE
  HYDROCHLORIDE
PROPANTHELINE BROMIDE, PROPANTHELINE
  BROMIDE
PROPOXYPHENE HCL, PROPOXYPHENE
  HYDROCHLORIDE
PROPYLTHIOURACIL, PROPYLTHIOURACIL
PYRIDOSTIGMINE BROMIDE, PYRIDOSTIGMINE
  BROMIDE
PYRILAMINE MALEATE, PYRILAMINE MALEATE
QUINIDINE SULFATE, QUINIDINE SULFATE
RAUWOLFIA SERPENTINA, RAUWOLFIA SERPENTINA
RESERPINE, RESERPINE
RILUZOLE, RILUZOLE
RIMANTADINE HCL, RIMANTADINE HYDROCHLORIDE
SULFA-TRIPLE #2, TRISULFAPYRIMIDINES
  (SULFADIAZINE; SULFAMERAZINE;
  SULFAMETHAZINE)
SULFADIAZINE, TRISULFAPYRIMIDINES (SULFADIAZINE;
  SULFAMERAZINE; SULFAMETHAZINE)
SULFISOXAZOLE, SULFISOXAZOLE
TERBUTALINE SULFATE, TERBUTALINE SULFATE
TETRACYCLINE HCL, TETRACYCLINE HYDROCHLORIDE
THYROGLOBULIN, THYROGLOBULIN
TRIAMCINOLONE, TRIAMCINOLONE
TRICHLORMETHIAZIDE, TRICHLORMETHIAZIDE
TRIPELENNAMINE HCL, TRIPELENNAMINE
  HYDROCHLORIDE
VITAMIN A, VITAMIN A
VITAMIN A, VITAMIN A PALMITATE
VITAMIN D, ERGOCALCIFEROL
IMPAX PHARM
IMPAX PHARMACEUTICALS
  ORPHENADRINE CITRATE, ORPHENADRINE CITRATE
  SOTALOL HCL, SOTALOL HYDROCHLORIDE
INALCO
INALCO SPA
  LACTULOSE, LACTULOSE
INGRAM PHARM
INGRAM PHARMACEUTICAL CO
  DRICORT, HYDROCORTISONE ACETATE
  HYDROCORTISONE, HYDROCORTISONE
INKINE
INKINE PHARMACEUTICAL CO INC
  VISICOL, SODIUM PHOSPHATE, DIBASIC, ANHYDROUS
INO
INO THERAPEUTICS INC
  INOMAX, NITRIC OXIDE

APPENDIX B
PRODUCT NAME INDEX
LISTED BY APPLICANT (*continued*)

INSIGHT PHARMS
INSIGHT PHARMACEUTICALS CORP
  NIX, PERMETHRIN (OTC)
INTERMUNE PHARMS
INTERMUNE PHARMACEUTICALS INC
  AMPHOTEC, AMPHOTERICIN B
INTERPHARM
INTERPHARM INC
  CLONIDINE HCL, CLONIDINE HYDROCHLORIDE
  DISOPYRAMIDE PHOSPHATE, DISOPYRAMIDE
    PHOSPHATE
  DOXYCYCLINE HYCLATE, DOXYCYCLINE HYCLATE
  IBUPROFEN, IBUPROFEN
  IBUPROFEN, IBUPROFEN (OTC)
  METOCLOPRAMIDE HCL, METOCLOPRAMIDE
    HYDROCHLORIDE
  NAPROXEN, NAPROXEN
  PREDNISONE, PREDNISONE
  PROPRANOLOL HCL, PROPRANOLOL HYDROCHLORIDE
  SULFAMETHOXAZOLE AND TRIMETHOPRIM,
    SULFAMETHOXAZOLE
  TOLAZAMIDE, TOLAZAMIDE
INTL MEDICATED
INTERNATIONAL MEDICATED SYSTEMS LTD
  BUPIVACINE HCL PRESERVATIVE FREE, BUPIVACAINE
    HYDROCHLORIDE
  MILRINONE LACTATE, MILRINONE LACTATE
INTL MEDICATION
INTERNATIONAL MEDICATION SYSTEM
  AMINOPHYLLINE, AMINOPHYLLINE
  BRETYLIUM TOSYLATE, BRETYLIUM TOSYLATE
  DIPHENHYDRAMINE HCL PRESERVATIVE FREE,
    DIPHENHYDRAMINE HYDROCHLORIDE
  DOPAMINE HCL, DOPAMINE HYDROCHLORIDE
  FUROSEMIDE, FUROSEMIDE
  ISOPROTERENOL HCL, ISOPROTERENOL
    HYDROCHLORIDE
  LARYNG-O-JET KIT, LIDOCAINE HYDROCHLORIDE
  LIDOCAINE HCL PRESERVATIVE FREE, LIDOCAINE
    HYDROCHLORIDE
  LIDOCAINE HCL W/ EPINEPHRINE, EPINEPHRINE
  LIDOCAINE HCL, LIDOCAINE HYDROCHLORIDE
  MANNITOL 25%, MANNITOL
  MEPERIDINE HCL PRESERVATIVE FREE, MEPERIDINE
    HYDROCHLORIDE
  MEPIVACAINE HCL, MEPIVACAINE HYDROCHLORIDE
  NALOXONE HCL, NALOXONE HYDROCHLORIDE
  PHYTONADIONE, PHYTONADIONE
  POTASSIUM CHLORIDE, POTASSIUM CHLORIDE
  PROCAINAMIDE HCL, PROCAINAMIDE
    HYDROCHLORIDE
  VERAPAMIL HCL, VERAPAMIL HYDROCHLORIDE
INTERNATIONAL MEDICATION SYSTEMS LTD
  AMINOPHYLLINE, AMINOPHYLLINE
  AMPICILLIN SODIUM, AMPICILLIN SODIUM
  CEPHALOTHIN, CEPHALOTHIN SODIUM
  DEXAMETHASONE SODIUM PHOSPHATE,
    DEXAMETHASONE SODIUM PHOSPHATE
  DIATRIZOATE-60, DIATRIZOATE MEGLUMINE
  DILTIAZEM HCL, DILTIAZEM HYDROCHLORIDE
  FUROSEMIDE, FUROSEMIDE
  GENTAMICIN, GENTAMICIN SULFATE
  HEPARIN LOCK FLUSH, HEPARIN SODIUM
  HYDROCORTISONE SODIUM SUCCINATE,
    HYDROCORTISONE SODIUM SUCCINATE
  ISOETHARINE HCL, ISOETHARINE HYDROCHLORIDE
  KANAMYCIN SULFATE, KANAMYCIN SULFATE

  LIDOCAINE HCL VISCOUS, LIDOCAINE
    HYDROCHLORIDE
  LIDOCAINE HCL, LIDOCAINE HYDROCHLORIDE
  MEPERIDINE HCL, MEPERIDINE HYDROCHLORIDE
  METHYLPREDNISOLONE SODIUM SUCCINATE,
    METHYLPREDNISOLONE SODIUM SUCCINATE
  METRONIDAZOLE, METRONIDAZOLE
  NALOXONE HCL, NALOXONE HYDROCHLORIDE
  NITROGLYCERIN, NITROGLYCERIN
  SUCCINYLCHOLINE CHLORIDE, SUCCINYLCHOLINE
    CHLORIDE
INTL MINERALS
INTERNATIONAL MINERALS CHEMICAL CORP
  TPN SUSPENSION, NIACINAMIDE
INVAMED
INVAMED INC
  FAMOTIDINE, FAMOTIDINE
  IBUPROFEN, IBUPROFEN
  IBUPROFEN, IBUPROFEN (OTC)
  METHAZOLAMIDE, METHAZOLAMIDE
  METHYLDOPA AND HYDROCHLOROTHIAZIDE,
    HYDROCHLOROTHIAZIDE
  METOCLOPRAMIDE HCL, METOCLOPRAMIDE
    HYDROCHLORIDE
  NABUMETONE, NABUMETONE
  NAPROXEN SODIUM, NAPROXEN SODIUM (OTC)
  OXAPROZIN, OXAPROZIN
  PEG-LYTE, POLYETHYLENE GLYCOL 3350
  PROCAINAMIDE HCL, PROCAINAMIDE
    HYDROCHLORIDE
  PROPRANOLOL HCL, PROPRANOLOL HYDROCHLORIDE
  TERAZOSIN HCL, TERAZOSIN HYDROCHLORIDE
INWOOD LABS
INWOOD LABORATORIES INC SUB FOREST LABORA-
TORIES INC
  CARBAMAZEPINE, CARBAMAZEPINE
  CORTISONE ACETATE, CORTISONE ACETATE
  DIPHENOXYLATE HCL AND ATROPINE SULFATE,
    ATROPINE SULFATE
  HYDROCHLOROTHIAZIDE, HYDROCHLOROTHIAZIDE
  HYDROCORTISONE, HYDROCORTISONE
  INDOMETHACIN, INDOMETHACIN
  ISOSORBIDE DINITRATE, ISOSORBIDE DINITRATE
  METHOCARBAMOL, METHOCARBAMOL
  METHYLTESTOSTERONE, METHYLTESTOSTERONE
  PHENDIMETRAZINE TARTRATE, PHENDIMETRAZINE
    TARTRATE
  PREDNISOLONE, PREDNISOLONE
  PREDNISONE, PREDNISONE
  PROCAINAMIDE HCL, PROCAINAMIDE
    HYDROCHLORIDE
  PROPRANOLOL HCL, PROPRANOLOL HYDROCHLORIDE
  THEOCHRON, THEOPHYLLINE
  THEOPHYLLINE, THEOPHYLLINE
IOMED
IOMED INC
  IONTOCAINE, EPINEPHRINE
IPHARM
IPHARM DIV LYPHOMED INC
  NEOMYCIN AND POLYMYXIN B SULFATES AND
    GRAMICIDIN, GRAMICIDIN
IPR
IPR PHARMACEUTICALS INC
  ATENOLOL AND CHLORTHALIDONE, ATENOLOL
  ATENOLOL, ATENOLOL
  ZOMIG, ZOLMITRIPTAN

APPENDIX B
PRODUCT NAME INDEX
LISTED BY APPLICANT (*continued*)

ISO TEX
ISO TEX DIAGNOSTICS INC
  ALBUMOTOPE 125 I, ALBUMIN IODINATED I-125 SERUM
  CHROMALBIN, ALBUMIN CHROMATED CR-51 SERUM
  MEGATOPE, ALBUMIN IODINATED I-131 SERUM
IVAX PHARMS
IVAX PHARMACEUTICALS INC
  ACYCLOVIR, ACYCLOVIR
  ALBUTEROL SULFATE, ALBUTEROL SULFATE
  ALBUTEROL, ALBUTEROL
  ALLAY, ACETAMINOPHEN
  ALPRAZOLAM, ALPRAZOLAM
  AMPICILLIN TRIHYDRATE, AMPICILLIN/AMPICILLIN
    TRIHYDRATE
  BACLOFEN, BACLOFEN
  BETHANECHOL CHLORIDE, BETHANECHOL CHLORIDE
  BISOPROLOL FUMARATE AND
    HYDROCHLOROTHIAZIDE, BISOPROLOL FUMARATE
  BROMPHENIRAMINE MALEATE, BROMPHENIRAMINE
    MALEATE
  BUMETANIDE, BUMETANIDE
  BUTALBITAL COMPOUND, ASPIRIN
  C-SOLVE-2, ERYTHROMYCIN
  CAPTOPRIL AND HYDROCHLOROTHIAZIDE, CAPTOPRIL
  CAPTOPRIL, CAPTOPRIL
  CEFACLOR, CEFACLOR
  CEFADROXIL, CEFADROXIL/CEFADROXIL
    HEMIHYDRATE
  CEPHALEXIN, CEPHALEXIN
  CEPHRADINE, CEPHRADINE
  CHLORAMPHENICOL, CHLORAMPHENICOL
  CHLORDIAZEPOXIDE HCL, CHLORDIAZEPOXIDE
    HYDROCHLORIDE
  CHLORPHENIRAMINE MALEATE, CHLORPHENIRAMINE
    MALEATE
  CHLORPROMAZINE HCL, CHLORPROMAZINE
    HYDROCHLORIDE
  CHLORPROPAMIDE, CHLORPROPAMIDE
  CHLORTHALIDONE, CHLORTHALIDONE
  CHOLESTYRAMINE, CHOLESTYRAMINE
  CIMETIDINE, CIMETIDINE
  CIMETIDINE, CIMETIDINE (OTC)
  CLOZAPINE, CLOZAPINE
  CORTISONE ACETATE, CORTISONE ACETATE
  CROMOLYN SODIUM, CROMOLYN SODIUM
  CYPROHEPTADINE HCL, CYPROHEPTADINE
    HYDROCHLORIDE
  DIAZEPAM, DIAZEPAM
  DILTIAZEM HCL, DILTIAZEM HYDROCHLORIDE
  DIPHENHYDRAMINE HCL, DIPHENHYDRAMINE
    HYDROCHLORIDE
  DIPHENOXYLATE HCL W/ ATROPINE SULFATE,
    ATROPINE SULFATE
  DISOPYRAMIDE PHOSPHATE, DISOPYRAMIDE
    PHOSPHATE
  DOXAZOSIN MESYLATE, DOXAZOSIN MESYLATE
  DOXYCYCLINE HYCLATE, DOXYCYCLINE HYCLATE
  ENALAPRIL MALEATE AND HYDROCHLOROTHIAZIDE,
    ENALAPRIL MALEATE
  ENALAPRIL MALEATE, ENALAPRIL MALEATE
  ERYTHROMYCIN ESTOLATE, ERYTHROMYCIN
    ESTOLATE
  ERYTHROMYCIN STEARATE, ERYTHROMYCIN
    STEARATE
  ESTAZOLAM, ESTAZOLAM
  ETODOLAC, ETODOLAC
  FAMOTIDINE, FAMOTIDINE
  FAMOTIDINE, FAMOTIDINE (OTC)

FENOPROFEN CALCIUM, FENOPROFEN CALCIUM
FLUOXETINE, FLUOXETINE HYDROCHLORIDE
FLURBIPROFEN, FLURBIPROFEN
FLUTAMIDE, FLUTAMIDE
FLUTEX, TRIAMCINOLONE ACETONIDE
FLUVOXAMINE MALEATE, FLUVOXAMINE MALEATE
FOLIC ACID, FOLIC ACID
FUROSEMIDE, FUROSEMIDE
GLIPIZIDE, GLIPIZIDE
GUANABENZ ACETATE, GUANABENZ ACETATE
HYDRALAZINE HCL W/ HYDROCHLOROTHIAZIDE 100/50,
  HYDRALAZINE HYDROCHLORIDE
HYDRALAZINE HCL W/ HYDROCHLOROTHIAZIDE 25/25,
  HYDRALAZINE HYDROCHLORIDE
HYDRALAZINE HCL W/ HYDROCHLOROTHIAZIDE 50/50,
  HYDRALAZINE HYDROCHLORIDE
HYDRALAZINE HCL, HYDRALAZINE HYDROCHLORIDE
HYDRALAZINE HCL, HYDROCHLOROTHIAZIDE AND
  RESERPINE, HYDRALAZINE HYDROCHLORIDE
HYDROCHLOROTHIAZIDE W/ RESERPINE,
  HYDROCHLOROTHIAZIDE
HYDROCHLOROTHIAZIDE, HYDROCHLOROTHIAZIDE
HYDROCODONE BITARTRATE AND ACETAMINOPHEN,
  ACETAMINOPHEN
HYDROCORTISONE, HYDROCORTISONE
HYDROGENATED ERGOT ALKALOIDS, ERGOLOID
  MESYLATES
HYDROSERPINE PLUS (R-H-H), HYDRALAZINE
  HYDROCHLORIDE
HYDROXYZINE HCL, HYDROXYZINE HYDROCHLORIDE
HYDROXYZINE PAMOATE, HYDROXYZINE PAMOATE
IBUPROFEN, IBUPROFEN
IBUPROFEN, IBUPROFEN (OTC)
INDAPAMIDE, INDAPAMIDE
INDOMETHACIN, INDOMETHACIN
IPRATROPIUM BROMIDE, IPRATROPIUM BROMIDE
ISONIAZID, ISONIAZID
ISOSORBIDE MONONITRATE, ISOSORBIDE
  MONONITRATE
LABETALOL HCL, LABETALOL HYDROCHLORIDE
LISINOPRIL AND HYDROCHLOROTHIAZIDE,
  HYDROCHLOROTHIAZIDE
LISINOPRIL, LISINOPRIL
MECLIZINE HCL, MECLIZINE HYDROCHLORIDE
MEPROBAMATE, MEPROBAMATE
METHOCARBAMOL AND ASPIRIN, ASPIRIN
METHOCARBAMOL, METHOCARBAMOL
METHYCLOTHIAZIDE, METHYCLOTHIAZIDE
METHYLDOPA AND HYDROCHLOROTHIAZIDE,
  HYDROCHLOROTHIAZIDE
METHYLDOPA, METHYLDOPA
METRONIDAZOLE, METRONIDAZOLE
MISOPROSTOL, MISOPROSTOL
NABUMETONE, NABUMETONE
NADOLOL, NADOLOL
NAPROXEN SODIUM, NAPROXEN SODIUM
NAPROXEN, NAPROXEN
NIACIN, NIACIN
NICARDIPINE HCL, NICARDIPINE HYDROCHLORIDE
NITROFURANTOIN, NITROFURANTOIN
NITROFURANTOIN, NITROFURANTOIN,
  MACROCRYSTALLINE
NOGENIC HC, HYDROCORTISONE
OXAPROZIN, OXAPROZIN
OXAZEPAM, OXAZEPAM
PACLITAXEL, PACLITAXEL
PENICILLIN G POTASSIUM, PENICILLIN G POTASSIUM
PENICILLIN V POTASSIUM, PENICILLIN V POTASSIUM

APPENDIX B
PRODUCT NAME INDEX
LISTED BY APPLICANT (continued)

PERPHENAZINE AND AMITRIPTYLINE HCL,
    AMITRIPTYLINE HYDROCHLORIDE
PERPHENAZINE, PERPHENAZINE
PHENDIMETRAZINE TARTRATE, PHENDIMETRAZINE
    TARTRATE
PHENTERMINE HCL, PHENTERMINE HYDROCHLORIDE
PHENYLBUTAZONE, PHENYLBUTAZONE
PINDOLOL, PINDOLOL
PIROXICAM, PIROXICAM
PRAZOSIN HCL, PRAZOSIN HYDROCHLORIDE
PREDNISOLONE, PREDNISOLONE
PREDNISONE, PREDNISONE
PROBENECID AND COLCHICINE, COLCHICINE
PROBENECID, PROBENECID
PROCAINAMIDE HCL, PROCAINAMIDE
    HYDROCHLORIDE
PROCHLORPERAZINE MALEATE, PROCHLORPERAZINE
    MALEATE
PROMETHAZINE HCL, PROMETHAZINE
    HYDROCHLORIDE
PROMPT PHENYTOIN SODIUM, PHENYTOIN SODIUM,
    PROMPT
PROPOXYPHENE COMPOUND 65, ASPIRIN
PROPOXYPHENE HCL, PROPOXYPHENE
    HYDROCHLORIDE
PROPOXYPHENE NAPSYLATE AND ACETAMINOPHEN,
    ACETAMINOPHEN
PROPRANOLOL HCL AND HYDROCHLOROTHIAZIDE,
    HYDROCHLOROTHIAZIDE
PROPRANOLOL HCL, PROPRANOLOL HYDROCHLORIDE
PROPYLTHIOURACIL, PROPYLTHIOURACIL
QUINIDINE SULFATE, QUINIDINE SULFATE
RANITIDINE HCL, RANITIDINE HYDROCHLORIDE
RANITIDINE, RANITIDINE HYDROCHLORIDE (OTC)
RAUWOLFIA SERPENTINA, RAUWOLFIA SERPENTINA
RESERPINE AND HYDROFLUMETHIAZIDE,
    HYDROFLUMETHIAZIDE
RESERPINE, RESERPINE
SECOBARBITAL SODIUM, SECOBARBITAL SODIUM
SELEGILINE HCL, SELEGILINE HYDROCHLORIDE
SELENIUM SULFIDE, SELENIUM SULFIDE
SODIUM BUTABARBITAL, BUTABARBITAL SODIUM
SODIUM PENTOBARBITAL, PENTOBARBITAL SODIUM
SPIRONOLACTONE W/ HYDROCHLOROTHIAZIDE,
    HYDROCHLOROTHIAZIDE
SPIRONOLACTONE, SPIRONOLACTONE
SULFINPYRAZONE, SULFINPYRAZONE
SULFISOXAZOLE, SULFISOXAZOLE
TAMOXIFEN CITRATE, TAMOXIFEN CITRATE
TERAZOSIN HCL, TERAZOSIN HYDROCHLORIDE
TETRACYCLINE HCL, TETRACYCLINE HYDROCHLORIDE
TETRAMED, TETRACYCLINE HYDROCHLORIDE
THIORIDAZINE HCL, THIORIDAZINE HYDROCHLORIDE
TOLAZAMIDE, TOLAZAMIDE
TOLBUTAMIDE, TOLBUTAMIDE
TOLMETIN SODIUM, TOLMETIN SODIUM
TRAMADOL HCL, TRAMADOL HYDROCHLORIDE
TRIAMCINOLONE, TRIAMCINOLONE
TRIAMTERENE AND HYDROCHLOROTHIAZIDE,
    HYDROCHLOROTHIAZIDE
TRIATEX, TRIAMCINOLONE ACETONIDE
TRIFLUOPERAZINE HCL, TRIFLUOPERAZINE
    HYDROCHLORIDE
TRIPROLIDINE HCL AND PSEUDOEPHEDRINE HCL,
    PSEUDOEPHEDRINE HYDROCHLORIDE
VERAPAMIL HCL, VERAPAMIL HYDROCHLORIDE
VITAMIN A, VITAMIN A PALMITATE

IVAX RES
IVAX RESEARCH INC
    NASALIDE, FLUNISOLIDE
    NASAREL, FLUNISOLIDE

J

J AND J
JOHNSON AND JOHNSON CONSUMER PRODUCTS INC
    ERYCETTE, ERYTHROMYCIN
    GRIFULVIN V, GRISEOFULVIN, MICROCRYSTALLINE
JOHNSON AND JOHNSON MEDICAL INC
    MICRODERM, CHLORHEXIDINE GLUCONATE (OTC)
    PREVACARE R, CHLORHEXIDINE GLUCONATE (OTC)
JACOBUS
JACOBUS PHARMACEUTICAL CO
    DAPSONE, DAPSONE
    PASER, AMINOSALICYLIC ACID
JANSSEN
JANSSEN PHARMACEUTICA INC
    IMODIUM, LOPERAMIDE HYDROCHLORIDE
    MONISTAT, MICONAZOLE
    NIZORAL, KETOCONAZOLE
JANSSEN ORTHO
JANSSEN ORTHO LLC
    AXERT, ALMOTRIPTAN MALATE
JANSSEN PHARM
JANSSEN PHARMACEUTICAL
    RISPERDAL, RISPERIDONE
JANSSEN PHARMA
JANSSEN PHARMACEUTICA PRODUCTS LP
    ERGAMISOL, LEVAMISOLE HYDROCHLORIDE
    NIZORAL, KETOCONAZOLE
    PROPULSID QUICKSOLV, CISAPRIDE MONOHYDRATE
    PROPULSID, CISAPRIDE MONOHYDRATE
    REMINYL, GALANTAMINE HYDROBROMIDE
    RISPERDAL, RISPERIDONE
    SPORANOX, ITRACONAZOLE
JOHNSON AND JOHNSON
JOHNSON AND JOHNSON CONSUMER COMPANIES INC
    GRIFULVIN V, GRISEOFULVIN, MICROCRYSTALLINE
    MECLAN, MECLOCYCLINE SULFOSALICYLATE
    MONISTAT-DERM, MICONAZOLE NITRATE
    MUPIROCIN, MUPIROCIN
    RENOVA, TRETINOIN
    RETIN-A MICRO, TRETINOIN
    RETIN-A, TRETINOIN
    SPECTAZOLE, ECONAZOLE NITRATE
JOHNSON AND JOHNSON PHARMACEUTICAL RESEARCH
AND DEVELOPMENT
    ELMIRON, PENTOSAN POLYSULFATE SODIUM
    ORTHO TRI-CYCLEN LO, ETHINYL ESTRADIOL
    RISPERDAL, RISPERIDONE
JONES PHARMA
JONES PHARMA INC SUB KING PHARMACEUTICALS INC
    CYTOMEL, LIOTRIX (T4;T3)
    LEVOXYL, LIOTRIX (T4;T3)
    METHIMAZOLE, METHIMAZOLE
    SONATA, ZALEPLON
    TRIOSTAT, LIOTRIX (T4;T3)
    TUSSIGON, HOMATROPINE METHYLBROMIDE
JONES PHARMA INC
JONES PHARMA INC
    SKELAXIN, METAXALONE

APPENDIX B
PRODUCT NAME INDEX
LISTED BY APPLICANT (*continued*)

JVL
JVL CORP
   METOCLOPRAMIDE, METOCLOPRAMIDE
      HYDROCHLORIDE

K

KALAPHARM
KALAPHARM INC
   FUROSEMIDE, FUROSEMIDE
   GENTAMICIN SULFATE, GENTAMICIN SULFATE
KENDALL IL
KENDALL CO
   CHLORHEXIDINE GLUCONATE, CHLORHEXIDINE
      GLUCONATE (OTC)
   LARYNGOTRACHEAL ANESTHESIA KIT, LIDOCAINE
      HYDROCHLORIDE
KENDALL LP
KENDALL CO LP
   THERMAZENE, SILVER SULFADIAZINE
KENWOOD LABS
KENWOOD LABORATORIES DIV BRADLEY PHARMACEUTI-
CALS
   CARMOL HC, HYDROCORTISONE ACETATE
   TYZINE, TETRAHYDROZOLINE HYDROCHLORIDE
KEY PHARMS
KEY PHARMACEUTICALS INC SUB SCHERING PLOUGH
CORP
   GENAPAX, GENTIAN VIOLET
   K-DUR 10, POTASSIUM CHLORIDE
   K-DUR 20, POTASSIUM CHLORIDE
   NITRO-DUR, NITROGLYCERIN
   QUINORA, QUINIDINE SULFATE
KIEL
KIEL LABORATORIES INC
   ORPHENADRINE CITRATE, ORPHENADRINE CITRATE
KING PHARMS
KING PHARMACEUTICALS INC
   ALTACE, RAMIPRIL
   AMINOPHYLLINE, AMINOPHYLLINE
   APOGEN, GENTAMICIN SULFATE
   BICILLIN C-R 900/300, PENICILLIN G BENZATHINE
   BICILLIN C-R, PENICILLIN G BENZATHINE
   BICILLIN L-A, PENICILLIN G BENZATHINE
   BREVITAL SODIUM, METHOHEXITAL SODIUM
   CORZIDE, BENDROFLUMETHIAZIDE
   CROMOPTIC, CROMOLYN SODIUM
   DELESTROGEN, ESTRADIOL VALERATE
   FLORINEF, FLUDROCORTISONE ACETATE
   FLUPHENAZINE DECANOATE, FLUPHENAZINE
      DECANOATE
   HALOPERIDOL DECANOATE, HALOPERIDOL
      DECANOATE
   HUMATIN, PAROMOMYCIN SULFATE
   KLEBCIL, KANAMYCIN SULFATE
   LORABID, LORACARBEF
   MAXOLON, METOCLOPRAMIDE HYDROCHLORIDE
   NALBUPHINE HCL, NALBUPHINE HYDROCHLORIDE
   PREFEST, ESTRADIOL
   PROCANBID, PROCAINAMIDE HYDROCHLORIDE
   QUINIDINE SULFATE, QUINIDINE SULFATE
   SILVADENE, SILVER SULFADIAZINE
   SYNERCID, DALFOPRISTIN
   TIGAN, TRIMETHOBENZAMIDE HYDROCHLORIDE
   WYCILLIN, PENICILLIN G PROCAINE
KOS
KOS PHARMACEUTICALS INC
   ADVICOR, LOVASTATIN

   NIASPAN TITRATION STARTER PACK, NIACIN
   NIASPAN, NIACIN
KREMERS URBAN
KREMERS URBAN CO
   ISOSORBIDE MONONITRATE, ISOSORBIDE
      MONONITRATE
KREMERS URBAN DEV
KREMERS URBAN DEVELOPMENT CO
   OMEPRAZOLE, OMEPRAZOLE
KRKA DD NOVO MESTO
KRKA DD NOVO MESTO
   ENALAPRIL MALEATE, ENALAPRIL MALEATE
KV PHARM
KV PHARMACEUTICAL CO
   ACETAMINOPHEN AND CODEINE PHOSPHATE,
      ACETAMINOPHEN
   ACETIC ACID W/ HYDROCORTISONE, ACETIC ACID,
      GLACIAL
   ACETIC ACID, ACETIC ACID, GLACIAL
   AMINOPHYLLINE, AMINOPHYLLINE
   BROMPHENIRAMINE MALEATE, BROMPHENIRAMINE
      MALEATE
   BUSPIRONE HCL, BUSPIRONE HYDROCHLORIDE
   CHLORPHENIRAMINE MALEATE, CHLORPHENIRAMINE
      MALEATE
   CHLORPROMAZINE HCL, CHLORPROMAZINE
      HYDROCHLORIDE
   CHLORTHALIDONE, CHLORTHALIDONE
   CYPROHEPTADINE HCL, CYPROHEPTADINE
      HYDROCHLORIDE
   DEXTROAMPHETAMINE SULFATE,
      DEXTROAMPHETAMINE SULFATE
   DIPHENHYDRAMINE HCL, DIPHENHYDRAMINE
      HYDROCHLORIDE
   DIPHENOXYLATE HCL W/ ATROPINE SULFATE,
      ATROPINE SULFATE
   DISOPYRAMIDE PHOSPHATE, DISOPYRAMIDE
      PHOSPHATE
   DOXAZOSIN MESYLATE, DOXAZOSIN MESYLATE
   ERGOLOID MESYLATES, ERGOLOID MESYLATES
   GYNAZOLE-1, BUTOCONAZOLE NITRATE
   HYDROCODONE BITARTRATE AND ACETAMINOPHEN,
      ACETAMINOPHEN
   HYDROXYZINE HCL, HYDROXYZINE HYDROCHLORIDE
   ISOSORBIDE MONONITRATE, ISOSORBIDE
      MONONITRATE
   MECLIZINE HCL, MECLIZINE HYDROCHLORIDE
   METHOCARBAMOL, METHOCARBAMOL
   METHYLTESTOSTERONE, METHYLTESTOSTERONE
   MICRO-K 10, POTASSIUM CHLORIDE
   MICRO-K LS, POTASSIUM CHLORIDE
   MICRO-K, POTASSIUM CHLORIDE
   PHENDIMETRAZINE TARTRATE, PHENDIMETRAZINE
      TARTRATE
   POTASSIUM CHLORIDE, POTASSIUM CHLORIDE
   PREDNISOLONE, PREDNISOLONE
   PREDNISONE, PREDNISONE
   PROMETHAZINE HCL, PROMETHAZINE
      HYDROCHLORIDE
   PROPAFENONE HCL, PROPAFENONE
      HYDROCHLORIDE
   PSEUDOEPHEDRINE HCL AND CHLORPHENIRAMINE
      MALEATE, CHLORPHENIRAMINE MALEATE (OTC)
   QUINIDINE SULFATE, QUINIDINE SULFATE
   SODIUM SECOBARBITAL, SECOBARBITAL SODIUM
   THEOPHYLLINE, THEOPHYLLINE

APPENDIX B
PRODUCT NAME INDEX
LISTED BY APPLICANT (*continued*)

TRIPROLIDINE AND PSEUDOEPHEDRINE
   HYDROCHLORIDES, PSEUDOEPHEDRINE
   HYDROCHLORIDE (OTC)

L

LABS AF
LABORATORIOS APLICACIONES FARMACEUTICAS SA DE
CV
   METROMIDOL, METRONIDAZOLE
LABS ATRAL
LABORATORIOS ATRAL SARL
   AMOXICILLIN, AMOXICILLIN
   CEPHALEXIN, CEPHALEXIN
   TETRACYCLINE HCL, TETRACYCLINE HYDROCHLORIDE
LAFAYETTE PHARMS
LAFAYETTE PHARMACEUTICALS INC
   BAROS, SODIUM BICARBONATE
LANNETT
LANNETT CO INC
   ACETAZOLAMIDE, ACETAZOLAMIDE
   AMINOPHYLLINE, AMINOPHYLLINE
   AMPHETAMINE SULFATE, AMPHETAMINE SULFATE
   BENZYL BENZOATE, BENZYL BENZOATE
   BETHANECHOL CHLORIDE, BETHANECHOL CHLORIDE
   BUTALAN, BUTABARBITAL SODIUM
   CORTISONE ACETATE, CORTISONE ACETATE
   DEXTROAMPHETAMINE SULFATE,
      DEXTROAMPHETAMINE SULFATE
   DICYCLOMINE HCL, DICYCLOMINE HYDROCHLORIDE
   DIPHENHYDRAMINE HCL, DIPHENHYDRAMINE
      HYDROCHLORIDE
   DIPHENOXYLATE HCL AND ATROPINE SULFATE,
      ATROPINE SULFATE
   DIPHENYLAN SODIUM, PHENYTOIN SODIUM, PROMPT
   FOLIC ACID, FOLIC ACID
   FURALAN, NITROFURANTOIN
   GLUTETHIMIDE, GLUTETHIMIDE
   HYDROCORTISONE, HYDROCORTISONE
   LANIAZID, ISONIAZID
   LANOPHYLLIN, THEOPHYLLINE
   LANORINAL, ASPIRIN
   LANTRISUL, TRISULFAPYRIMIDINES (SULFADIAZINE;
      SULFAMERAZINE; SULFAMETHAZINE)
   MEPROBAMATE, MEPROBAMATE
   METHOCARBAMOL, METHOCARBAMOL
   METHYLTESTOSTERONE, METHYLTESTOSTERONE
   NEOMYCIN SULFATE, NEOMYCIN SULFATE
   NITROFURAZONE, NITROFURAZONE
   PENTOBARBITAL SODIUM, PENTOBARBITAL SODIUM
   PHENETRON, CHLORPHENIRAMINE MALEATE
   PHENTERMINE HCL, PHENTERMINE HYDROCHLORIDE
   PIPERAZINE CITRATE, PIPERAZINE CITRATE
   PREDNISOLONE, PREDNISOLONE
   PREDNISONE, PREDNISONE
   PRIMIDONE, PRIMIDONE
   PROBALAN, PROBENECID
   PROCAINAMIDE HCL, PROCAINAMIDE
      HYDROCHLORIDE
   PROMETHAZINE HCL, PROMETHAZINE
      HYDROCHLORIDE
   PROPYLTHIOURACIL, PROPYLTHIOURACIL
   QUINALAN, QUINIDINE GLUCONATE
   QUINIDINE SULFATE, QUINIDINE SULFATE
   SECOBARBITAL SODIUM, SECOBARBITAL SODIUM
   SERPALAN, RESERPINE
   SODIUM BUTABARBITAL, BUTABARBITAL SODIUM

SODIUM P.A.S., AMINOSALICYLATE SODIUM
   SULFADIAZINE, TRISULFAPYRIMIDINES (SULFADIAZINE;
      SULFAMERAZINE; SULFAMETHAZINE)
   SULFISOXAZOLE, SULFISOXAZOLE
   TRICHLOREX, TRICHLORMETHIAZIDE
   TRIPELENNAMINE HCL, TRIPELENNAMINE
      HYDROCHLORIDE
   VITAMIN D, ERGOCALCIFEROL
LEDERLE
LEDERLE LABORATORIES DIV AMERICAN CYANAMID CO
   ACETAMINOPHEN W/ CODEINE, ACETAMINOPHEN
   ACHES-N-PAIN, IBUPROFEN (OTC)
   ACHROMYCIN V, TETRACYCLINE HYDROCHLORIDE
   ACHROMYCIN, HYDROCORTISONE
   ACHROMYCIN, PROCAINE HYDROCHLORIDE
   ACHROMYCIN, TETRACYCLINE HYDROCHLORIDE
   AMITRIPTYLINE HCL, AMITRIPTYLINE HYDROCHLORIDE
   AMPICILLIN, AMPICILLIN/AMPICILLIN TRIHYDRATE
   ARTANE, TRIHEXYPHENIDYL HYDROCHLORIDE
   ASENDIN, AMOXAPINE
   AUREOMYCIN, CHLORTETRACYCLINE
      HYDROCHLORIDE
   CHLORDIAZEPOXIDE HCL, CHLORDIAZEPOXIDE
      HYDROCHLORIDE
   CHLOROTHIAZIDE, CHLOROTHIAZIDE
   CHLORPHENIRAMINE MALEATE, CHLORPHENIRAMINE
      MALEATE
   CHLORPROMAZINE HCL, CHLORPROMAZINE
      HYDROCHLORIDE
   CLORAZEPATE DIPOTASSIUM, CLORAZEPATE
      DIPOTASSIUM
   DECLOMYCIN, DEMECLOCYCLINE HYDROCHLORIDE
   DIAZEPAM, DIAZEPAM
   DIPHENHYDRAMINE HCL, DIPHENHYDRAMINE
      HYDROCHLORIDE
   DIPHENOXYLATE HCL AND ATROPINE SULFATE,
      ATROPINE SULFATE
   DOLENE AP-65, ACETAMINOPHEN
   ERGOLOID MESYLATES, ERGOLOID MESYLATES
   ERYTHROMYCIN STEARATE, ERYTHROMYCIN
      STEARATE
   FOLVRON, FERROUS SULFATE
   HALOPERIDOL, HALOPERIDOL
   HETRAZAN, DIETHYLCARBAMAZINE CITRATE
   HYDROMOX R, QUINETHAZONE
   HYDROMOX, QUINETHAZONE
   IBUPROFEN, IBUPROFEN
   IMIPRAMINE HCL, IMIPRAMINE HYDROCHLORIDE
   INDOMETHACIN, INDOMETHACIN
   KETOPROFEN, KETOPROFEN
   LEDERCILLIN VK, PENICILLIN V POTASSIUM
   MEPROBAMATE, MEPROBAMATE
   METHOCARBAMOL, METHOCARBAMOL
   METHYLDOPA AND HYDROCHLOROTHIAZIDE,
      HYDROCHLOROTHIAZIDE
   METHYLDOPA, METHYLDOPA
   METOCLOPRAMIDE HCL, METOCLOPRAMIDE
      HYDROCHLORIDE
   MINOCIN, MINOCYCLINE HYDROCHLORIDE
   MINOCYCLINE HCL, MINOCYCLINE HYDROCHLORIDE
   MYAMBUTOL, ETHAMBUTOL HYDROCHLORIDE
   NAPROXEN, NAPROXEN
   NEPTAZANE, METHAZOLAMIDE
   NILSTAT, NYSTATIN
   PATHILON, TRIDIHEXETHYL CHLORIDE
   PRAZOSIN HCL, PRAZOSIN HYDROCHLORIDE
   PREDNISONE, PREDNISONE
   PROBENECID W/ COLCHICINE, COLCHICINE

APPENDIX B
PRODUCT NAME INDEX
LISTED BY APPLICANT (*continued*)

PROBENECID, PROBENECID
PROCAINAMIDE HCL, PROCAINAMIDE
    HYDROCHLORIDE
PROPRANOLOL HCL, PROPRANOLOL HYDROCHLORIDE
PROPYLTHIOURACIL, PROPYLTHIOURACIL
QUINIDINE SULFATE, QUINIDINE SULFATE
RESERPINE, HYDROCHLOROTHIAZIDE, AND
    HYDRALAZINE HCL, HYDRALAZINE
    HYDROCHLORIDE
SERVISONE, PREDNISONE
SPIRONOLACTONE W/ HYDROCHLOROTHIAZIDE,
    HYDROCHLOROTHIAZIDE
SPIRONOLACTONE, SPIRONOLACTONE
SULFADIAZINE SODIUM, SULFADIAZINE SODIUM
SULFADIAZINE, TRISULFAPYRIMIDINES (SULFADIAZINE;
    SULFAMERAZINE; SULFAMETHAZINE)
SULFASALAZINE, SULFASALAZINE
SULFISOXAZOLE, SULFISOXAZOLE
SULINDAC, SULINDAC
SUPRAX, CEFIXIME
TOLBUTAMIDE, TOLBUTAMIDE
TRIPLE SULFAS, TRISULFAPYRIMIDINES
    (SULFADIAZINE; SULFAMERAZINE;
    SULFAMETHAZINE)
VANCOLED, VANCOMYCIN HYDROCHLORIDE
VERAPAMIL HCL, VERAPAMIL HYDROCHLORIDE
LEDERLE PARENTERALS INC
    CLINDAMYCIN PHOSPHATE, CLINDAMYCIN
        PHOSPHATE
    DOXYCYCLINE HYCLATE, DOXYCYCLINE HYCLATE
    ERYTHROMYCIN LACTOBIONATE, ERYTHROMYCIN
        LACTOBIONATE
    FUROSEMIDE, FUROSEMIDE
    TOBRAMYCIN SULFATE, TOBRAMYCIN SULFATE
    VANCOLED, VANCOMYCIN HYDROCHLORIDE
LEE KM
KM LEE LABORATORIES INC
    MEPROBAMATE, MEPROBAMATE
LEINER
LEINER HEALTH PRODUCTS INC
    CIMETIDINE, CIMETIDINE (OTC)
    IBUPROFEN, IBUPROFEN (OTC)
    LOPERAMIDE HCL, LOPERAMIDE HYDROCHLORIDE
        (OTC)
    NAPROXEN SODIUM, NAPROXEN SODIUM (OTC)
    RANITIDINE, RANITIDINE HYDROCHLORIDE (OTC)
LEK PHARM
LEK PHARMACEUTICAL AND CHEMICAL CO DD
    ACYCLOVIR, ACYCLOVIR
    BROMOCRIPTINE MESYLATE, BROMOCRIPTINE
        MESYLATE
LEK PHARMS
LEK PHARMACEUTICALS D D
    0, AMOXICILLIN
    AMOXICILLIN AND CLAVULANATE POTASSIUM,
        AMOXICILLIN
    AMOXICILLIN AND CLAVULANATE POTSSSIUM,
        AMOXICILLIN
    BROMOCRIPTINE MESYLATE, BROMOCRIPTINE
        MESYLATE
    CIMETIDINE, CIMETIDINE
    CIMETIDINE, CIMETIDINE (OTC)
    ENALAPRIL MALEATE, ENALAPRIL MALEATE
    LISINOPRIL, LISINOPRIL
    OMEPRAZOLE, OMEPRAZOLE
LEO PHARM
LEO PHARMACEUTICAL PRODUCTS LTD
    PINDAC, PINACIDIL

LIFE LABS
LIFE LABORATORIES INC
    ERYTHROMYCIN ESTOLATE, ERYTHROMYCIN
        ESTOLATE
LIGAND
LIGAND PHARMACEUTICALS INC
    AVINZA, MORPHINE SULFATE
    PANRETIN, ALITRETINOIN
    TARGRETIN, BEXAROTENE
LILLY
ELI LILLY AND CO
    AEROLONE, ISOPROTERENOL HYDROCHLORIDE
    ALPHALIN, VITAMIN A PALMITATE
    AMPICILLIN SODIUM, AMPICILLIN SODIUM
    ANHYDRON, CYCLOTHIAZIDE
    AVENTYL HCL, NORTRIPTYLINE HYDROCHLORIDE
    BACITRACIN, BACITRACIN
    BETALIN 12, CYANOCOBALAMIN
    BETALIN S, THIAMINE HYDROCHLORIDE
    CALCIUM GLUCEPTATE, CALCIUM GLUCEPTATE
    CAPASTAT SULFATE, CAPREOMYCIN SULFATE
    CECLOR CD, CEFACLOR
    CECLOR, CEFACLOR
    CESAMET, NABILONE
    CINOBAC, CINOXACIN
    CORDRAN-N, FLURANDRENOLIDE
    CRYSTODIGIN, DIGITOXIN
    DECABID, INDECAINIDE HYDROCHLORIDE
    DELTALIN, ERGOCALCIFEROL
    DICUMAROL, DICUMAROL
    DICURIN PROCAINE, PROCAINE MERETHOXYLLINE
    DIETHYLSTILBESTROL, DIETHYLSTILBESTROL
    DOBUTREX, DOBUTAMINE HYDROCHLORIDE
    DROLBAN, DROMOSTANOLONE PROPIONATE
    DURACILLIN A.S., PENICILLIN G PROCAINE
    ERYTHROMYCIN, ERYTHROMYCIN
    EVISTA, RALOXIFENE HYDROCHLORIDE
    FOLIC ACID, FOLIC ACID
    FORTEO, TERIPARATIDE ACETATE
    GEMZAR, GEMCITABINE HYDROCHLORIDE
    GLUCAGON, GLUCAGON HYDROCHLORIDE
    GLUCAGON, GLUCAGON RECOMBINANT
    HALDRONE, PARAMETHASONE ACETATE
    HEPARIN SODIUM, HEPARIN SODIUM
    HEXA-BETALIN, PYRIDOXINE HYDROCHLORIDE
    HISTALOG, BETAZOLE HYDROCHLORIDE
    HISTAMINE PHOSPHATE, HISTAMINE PHOSPHATE
    HUMALOG MIX 50/50, INSULIN LISPRO
    HUMALOG MIX 75/25, INSULIN LISPRO
    HUMALOG PEN, INSULIN LISPRO
    HUMALOG, INSULIN LISPRO
    HUMATROPE, SOMATROPIN RECOMBINANT
    HUMULIN 50/50, INSULIN RECOMBINANT HUMAN (OTC)
    HUMULIN 70/30 PEN, INSULIN RECOMBINANT HUMAN
        (OTC)
    HUMULIN 70/30, INSULIN RECOMBINANT HUMAN (OTC)
    HUMULIN BR, INSULIN RECOMBINANT HUMAN (OTC)
    HUMULIN L, INSULIN ZINC SUSP RECOMBINANT HUMAN
        (OTC)
    HUMULIN N, INSULIN SUSP ISOPHANE RECOMBINANT
        HUMAN (OTC)
    HUMULIN R PEN, INSULIN RECOMBINANT HUMAN (OTC)
    HUMULIN R, INSULIN RECOMBINANT HUMAN
    HUMULIN R, INSULIN RECOMBINANT HUMAN (OTC)
    HUMULIN U, INSULIN ZINC SUSP EXTENDED
        RECOMBINANT HUMAN (OTC)
    ILETIN I, INSULIN PORK
    ILETIN II, INSULIN PURIFIED PORK

APPENDIX B
PRODUCT NAME INDEX
LISTED BY APPLICANT (*continued*)

ILOSONE SULFA, ERYTHROMYCIN ESTOLATE
ILOSONE, ERYTHROMYCIN ESTOLATE
ISONIAZID, ISONIAZID
KAFOCIN, CEPHALOGLYCIN
KAPPADIONE, MENADIOL SODIUM DIPHOSPHATE
KEFLET, CEPHALEXIN
KEFLEX, CEPHALEXIN
KEFLIN IN PLASTIC CONTAINER, CEPHALOTHIN SODIUM
KEFLIN, CEPHALOTHIN SODIUM
KEFTAB, CEPHALEXIN HYDROCHLORIDE
KEFUROX IN PLASTIC CONTAINER, CEFUROXIME
    SODIUM
KEFUROX, CEFUROXIME SODIUM
KEFZOL, CEFAZOLIN SODIUM
LENTE ILETIN II (PORK), INSULIN ZINC SUSP PURIFIED
    PORK (OTC)
LENTE ILETIN II, INSULIN ZINC SUSP PURIFIED BEEF
    (OTC)
MANDOL, CEFAMANDOLE NAFATE
MENADIONE, MENADIONE
METHYLTESTOSTERONE, METHYLTESTOSTERONE
METUBINE IODIDE, METOCURINE IODIDE
MOXAM, MOXALACTAM DISODIUM
NEBCIN, TOBRAMYCIN SULFATE
NEOMYCIN SULFATE, NEOMYCIN SULFATE
NEOTRIZINE, TRISULFAPYRIMIDINES (SULFADIAZINE;
    SULFAMERAZINE; SULFAMETHAZINE)
NPH ILETIN I (BEEF-PORK), INSULIN SUSP ISOPHANE
    BEEF/PORK (OTC)
NPH ILETIN II (PORK), INSULIN SUSP ISOPHANE
    PURIFIED PORK (OTC)
NPH ILETIN II, INSULIN SUSP ISOPHANE PURIFIED BEEF
    (OTC)
ONCOVIN, VINCRISTINE SULFATE
PAGITANE, CYCRIMINE HYDROCHLORIDE
PENICILLIN G POTASSIUM, PENICILLIN G POTASSIUM
PERMAX, PERGOLIDE MESYLATE
POTASSIUM CHLORIDE, POTASSIUM CHLORIDE
PROGESTERONE, PROGESTERONE
PROPYLTHIOURACIL, PROPYLTHIOURACIL
PROTAMINE SULFATE, PROTAMINE SULFATE
PROTAMINE ZINC AND ILETIN II (PORK), INSULIN SUSP
    PROTAMINE ZINC PURIFIED PORK (OTC)
PROTAMINE ZINC AND ILETIN II, INSULIN SUSP
    PROTAMINE ZINC PURIFIED BEEF (OTC)
PROTAMINE, ZINC & ILETIN I (BEEF-PORK), INSULIN
    SUSP PROTAMINE ZINC BEEF/PORK (OTC)
PROZAC WEEKLY, FLUOXETINE HYDROCHLORIDE
PROZAC, FLUOXETINE HYDROCHLORIDE
QUINIDINE GLUCONATE, QUINIDINE GLUCONATE
QUINIDINE SULFATE, QUINIDINE SULFATE
REGULAR ILETIN II (PORK), INSULIN PURIFIED PORK
    (OTC)
REGULAR ILETIN II, INSULIN PURIFIED BEEF (OTC)
SANDRIL, RESERPINE
SECONAL SODIUM, SECOBARBITAL SODIUM
SEROMYCIN, CYCLOSERINE
STRATTERA, ATOMOXETINE HYDROCHLORIDE
STREPTOMYCIN SULFATE, STREPTOMYCIN SULFATE
SULFADIAZINE, TRISULFAPYRIMIDINES (SULFADIAZINE;
    SULFAMERAZINE; SULFAMETHAZINE)
SULFAPYRIDINE, SULFAPYRIDINE
SULFONAMIDES DUPLEX, TRISULFAPYRIMIDINES
    (SULFADIAZINE; SULFAMERAZINE;
    SULFAMETHAZINE)
TAPAZOLE, METHIMAZOLE
TAZIDIME IN PLASTIC CONTAINER, CEFTAZIDIME
TAZIDIME, CEFTAZIDIME

TESTOSTERONE PROPIONATE, TESTOSTERONE
    PROPIONATE
TUBOCURARINE CHLORIDE, TUBOCURARINE
    CHLORIDE
V-CILLIN K, PENICILLIN V POTASSIUM
V-CILLIN, PENICILLIN V
VANCOCIN HCL, VANCOMYCIN HYDROCHLORIDE
VELBAN, VINBLASTINE SULFATE
ZYPREXA ZYDIS, OLANZAPINE
ZYPREXA, OLANZAPINE
ELI LILLY INDUSTRIES INC
    DYMELOR, ACETOHEXAMIDE
    NOVRAD, LEVOPROPOXYPHENE NAPSYLATE,
        ANHYDROUS
LILLY RESEARCH LABORATORIES DIV ELI LILLY AND CO
    CECLOR, CEFACLOR
    ILOSONE, ERYTHROMYCIN ESTOLATE
    PROZAC, FLUOXETINE HYDROCHLORIDE
    SARAFEM, FLUOXETINE HYDROCHLORIDE
LILLY RES LABS
LILLY RESEARCH LABORATORIES
    DYNABAC, DIRITHROMYCIN
LLOYD
LLOYD INC
    THYRO-TABS, LIOTRIX (T4;T3)
LNK
LNK INTERNATIONAL INC
    DIPHENHYDRAMINE HCL, DIPHENHYDRAMINE
        HYDROCHLORIDE
    IBUPROFEN, IBUPROFEN (OTC)
    LOPERAMIDE HCL, LOPERAMIDE HYDROCHLORIDE
        (OTC)
    METRONIDAZOLE, METRONIDAZOLE
LOCH
LOCH PHARMACEUTICALS INC
    CLINDAMYCIN PHOSPHATE, CLINDAMYCIN
        PHOSPHATE
    FOLIC ACID, FOLIC ACID
    KANAMYCIN SULFATE, KANAMYCIN SULFATE
LOREX
LOREX PHARMACEUTICALS
    AMBIEN, ZOLPIDEM TARTRATE
    KERLEDEX, BETAXOLOL HYDROCHLORIDE
    KERLONE, BETAXOLOL HYDROCHLORIDE
LPI
LPI HOLDINGS INC
    N.E.E. 1/35 21, ETHINYL ESTRADIOL
    N.E.E. 1/35 28, ETHINYL ESTRADIOL
LUITPOLD
LUITPOLD PHARMACEUTICALS INC
    ACETYLCYSTEINE, ACETYLCYSTEINE
    AMINOCAPROIC ACID, AMINOCAPROIC ACID
    AMINOPHYLLINE, AMINOPHYLLINE
    BRETYLIUM TOSYLATE, BRETYLIUM TOSYLATE
    CIMETIDINE HCL, CIMETIDINE HYDROCHLORIDE
    CYANOCOBALAMIN, CYANOCOBALAMIN
    DEXAMETHASONE SODIUM PHOSPHATE,
        DEXAMETHASONE SODIUM PHOSPHATE
    DEXFERRUM, IRON DEXTRAN
    DOBUTAMINE HCL, DOBUTAMINE HYDROCHLORIDE
    DOPAMINE HCL, DOPAMINE HYDROCHLORIDE
    DROPERIDOL, DROPERIDOL
    FUROSEMIDE, FUROSEMIDE
    GLYCOPYRROLATE, GLYCOPYRROLATE
    HEPARIN LOCK FLUSH, HEPARIN SODIUM
    HEPARIN SODIUM, HEPARIN SODIUM
    HYDRALAZINE HCL, HYDRALAZINE HYDROCHLORIDE
    HYDROXYZINE HCL, HYDROXYZINE HYDROCHLORIDE

APPENDIX B
PRODUCT NAME INDEX
LISTED BY APPLICANT (*continued*)

LEUCOVORIN CALCIUM PRESERVATIVE FREE,
 LEUCOVORIN CALCIUM
LEVOCARNITINE, LEVOCARNITINE
LIDOCAINE HCL, LIDOCAINE HYDROCHLORIDE
MANNITOL 25%, MANNITOL
METHYLDOPATE HCL, METHYLDOPATE
 HYDROCHLORIDE
NITROGLYCERIN, NITROGLYCERIN
PIPERAZINE CITRATE, PIPERAZINE CITRATE
POTASSIUM CHLORIDE, POTASSIUM CHLORIDE
PYRIDOXINE HCL, PYRIDOXINE HYDROCHLORIDE
THIAMINE HCL, THIAMINE HYDROCHLORIDE
VENOFER, IRON SUCROSE
VERAPAMIL HCL, VERAPAMIL HYDROCHLORIDE

LYNE
LYNE LABORATORIES INC
 XYLOSE, XYLOSE

M

MALLARD
MALLARD INC
 MEPROBAMATE, MEPROBAMATE
MALLINCKRODT
MALLINCKRODT CHEMICAL INC
 ANEXSIA 7.5/650, ACETAMINOPHEN
 ANEXSIA, ACETAMINOPHEN
 BONTRIL, PHENDIMETRAZINE TARTRATE
 BUCET, ACETAMINOPHEN
 BUTALBITAL, ACETAMINOPHEN AND CAFFEINE,
  ACETAMINOPHEN
 BUTALBITAL, ACETAMINOPHEN, CAFFEINE,
  ACETAMINOPHEN
 FEMCET, ACETAMINOPHEN
 HYDROCET, ACETAMINOPHEN
 HYDROCODONE BITARTRATE AND ACETAMINOPHEN,
  ACETAMINOPHEN
 LORCET-HD, ACETAMINOPHEN
 LORTAB, ACETAMINOPHEN
 MEPERIDINE HCL PRESERVATIVE FREE, MEPERIDINE
  HYDROCHLORIDE
 METHADONE HCL, METHADONE HYDROCHLORIDE
 METHADOSE, METHADONE HYDROCHLORIDE
 MORPHINE SULFATE, MORPHINE SULFATE
 OXYCODONE AND ACETAMINOPHEN, ACETAMINOPHEN
 TENCON, ACETAMINOPHEN
 TRIAD, ACETAMINOPHEN
MALLINCKRODT INC
 ACETAMINOPHEN AND CODEINE PHOSPHATE,
  ACETAMINOPHEN
 ANEXSIA 5/325, ACETAMINOPHEN
 ANEXSIA 7.5/325, ACETAMINOPHEN
 DEXTROAMPHETAMINE SULFATE,
  DEXTROAMPHETAMINE SULFATE
 FERROUS CITRATE FE 59, FERROUS CITRATE, FE-59
 FLUOXETINE, FLUOXETINE HYDROCHLORIDE
 HYDROCODONE BITARTRATE AND ACETAMINOPHEN,
  ACETAMINOPHEN
 MD-50, DIATRIZOATE SODIUM
 MEPERIDINE HCL, MEPERIDINE HYDROCHLORIDE
 METHYLIN ER, METHYLPHENIDATE HYDROCHLORIDE
 METHYLIN, METHYLPHENIDATE HYDROCHLORIDE
 METHYLPHENIDATE HCL, METHYLPHENIDATE
  HYDROCHLORIDE
 NALTREXONE HCL, NALTREXONE HYDROCHLORIDE
 OPTIMARK IN PLASTIC CONTAINER,
  GADOVERSETAMIDE

OPTIMARK, GADOVERSETAMIDE
OSTEOSCAN, TECHNETIUM TC-99M ETIDRONATE KIT
OXYCET, ACETAMINOPHEN
PEMOLINE, PEMOLINE
PROPOXYPHENE NAPSYLATE AND ACETAMINOPHEN,
 ACETAMINOPHEN
SELENOMETHIONINE SE 75, SELENOMETHIONINE, SE-
 75
TRAMADOL HCL, TRAMADOL HYDROCHLORIDE
XENEISOL, XENON, XE-133
MALLINCKRODT MEDICAL INC
 ANGIO-CONRAY, IOTHALAMATE SODIUM
 CHOLEBRINE, IOCETAMIC ACID
 CONRAY 30, IOTHALAMATE MEGLUMINE
 CONRAY 325, IOTHALAMATE SODIUM
 CONRAY 400, IOTHALAMATE SODIUM
 CONRAY 43, IOTHALAMATE MEGLUMINE
 CONRAY, IOTHALAMATE MEGLUMINE
 CYANOCOBALAMIN CO 57 SCHILLING TEST KIT,
  CYANOCOBALAMIN
 CYSTO-CONRAY II, IOTHALAMATE MEGLUMINE
 GALLIUM CITRATE GA 67, GALLIUM CITRATE, GA-67
 HEXABRIX, IOXAGLATE MEGLUMINE
 HIPPURAN I 131, IODOHIPPURATE SODIUM, I-131
 MD-60, DIATRIZOATE MEGLUMINE
 MD-76, DIATRIZOATE MEGLUMINE
 MD-76R, DIATRIZOATE MEGLUMINE
 MD-GASTROVIEW, DIATRIZOATE MEGLUMINE
 OCTREOSCAN, INDIUM IN-111 PENTETREOTIDE KIT
 OPTIRAY 160, IOVERSOL
 OPTIRAY 240, IOVERSOL
 OPTIRAY 300, IOVERSOL
 OPTIRAY 320, IOVERSOL
 OPTIRAY 350, IOVERSOL
 PERCHLORACAP, POTASSIUM PERCHLORATE
 PHOSPHOCOL P32, CHROMIC PHOSPHATE, P-32
 RADIOIODINATED SERUM ALBUMIN (HUMAN) IHSA I 125,
  ALBUMIN IODINATED I-125 SERUM
 SODIUM CHROMATE CR 51, SODIUM CHROMATE, CR-51
 SODIUM IODIDE I 123, SODIUM IODIDE, I-123
 SODIUM IODIDE I 131, SODIUM IODIDE, I-131
 SODIUM PERTECHNETATE TC 99M, TECHNETIUM TC-
  99M SODIUM PERTECHNETATE
 SODIUM PHOSPHATE P 32, SODIUM PHOSPHATE, P-32
 TECHNECOLL, TECHNETIUM TC-99M SULFUR COLLOID
  KIT
 TECHNESCAN HDP, TECHNETIUM TC-99M OXIDRONATE
  KIT
 TECHNESCAN MAA, TECHNETIUM TC-99M ALBUMIN
  AGGREGATED KIT
 TECHNESCAN MAG3, TECHNETIUM TC-99M
  MERTIATIDE KIT
 TECHNESCAN PYP KIT, TECHNETIUM TC-99M
  PYROPHOSPHATE KIT
 TECHNETIUM TC 99M SULFUR COLLOID, TECHNETIUM
  TC-99M SULFUR COLLOID
 THALLOUS CHLORIDE TL 201, THALLOUS CHLORIDE, TL-
  201
 ULTRA-TECHNEKOW FM, TECHNETIUM TC-99M SODIUM
  PERTECHNETATE GENERATOR
 ULTRATAG, TECHNETIUM TC-99M RED BLOOD CELL KIT
 VASCORAY, IOTHALAMATE MEGLUMINE
 XENON XE 127, XENON, XE-127
 XENON XE 133, XENON, XE-133
MALLINCKRODT BAKER
MALLINCKRODT BAKER INC
 METHYLIN, METHYLPHENIDATE HYDROCHLORIDE

APPENDIX B
PRODUCT NAME INDEX
LISTED BY APPLICANT (*continued*)

MARCHAR
MARCHAR LABORATORIES INC LTD
　FLUOROURACIL, FLUOROURACIL
MARSAM PHARMS LLC
MARSAM PHARMACEUTICALS LLC
　AMPICILLIN SODIUM, AMPICILLIN SODIUM
　ATRACURIUM BESYLATE PRESERVATIVE FREE,
　　ATRACURIUM BESYLATE
　ATRACURIUM BESYLATE, ATRACURIUM BESYLATE
　CEFACLOR, CEFACLOR
　CEFAZOLIN SODIUM, CEFAZOLIN SODIUM
　CEFUROXIME SODIUM, CEFUROXIME SODIUM
　CHLORPROMAZINE HCL, CHLORPROMAZINE
　　HYDROCHLORIDE
　CLINDAMYCIN PHOSPHATE, CLINDAMYCIN
　　PHOSPHATE
　DIAZEPAM, DIAZEPAM
　DOBUTAMINE HCL, DOBUTAMINE HYDROCHLORIDE
　ETOPOSIDE, ETOPOSIDE
　FENTANYL CITRATE PRESERVATIVE FREE, FENTANYL
　　CITRATE
　FUROSEMIDE, FUROSEMIDE
　HALOPERIDOL, HALOPERIDOL LACTATE
　HEPARIN SODIUM PRESERVATIVE FREE, HEPARIN
　　SODIUM
　HEPARIN SODIUM, HEPARIN SODIUM
　ISOFLURANE, ISOFLURANE
　LORAZEPAM, LORAZEPAM
　METHOCARBAMOL, METHOCARBAMOL
　METHYLDOPATE HCL, METHYLDOPATE
　　HYDROCHLORIDE
　NAFCILLIN SODIUM, NAFCILLIN SODIUM
　NALOXONE HCL, NALOXONE HYDROCHLORIDE
　OXACILLIN SODIUM, OXACILLIN SODIUM
　PENICILLIN G POTASSIUM, PENICILLIN G POTASSIUM
　PENICILLIN G SODIUM, PENICILLIN G SODIUM
　PHENYTOIN SODIUM, PHENYTOIN SODIUM
　PROCHLORPERAZINE EDISYLATE,
　　PROCHLORPERAZINE EDISYLATE
　PROMETHAZINE HCL, PROMETHAZINE
　　HYDROCHLORIDE
　TOBRAMYCIN SULFATE, TOBRAMYCIN SULFATE
　VERAPAMIL HCL, VERAPAMIL HYDROCHLORIDE
MARSHALL PHARMA
MARSHALL PHARMACAL CORP
　CHLORPHENIRAMINE MALEATE, CHLORPHENIRAMINE
　　MALEATE
　PREDNISOLONE, PREDNISOLONE
　PREDNISONE, PREDNISONE
　RESERPINE, RESERPINE
　SODIUM BUTABARBITAL, BUTABARBITAL SODIUM
MARTEC
MARTEC PHARMACEUTICALS INC
　ATENOLOL AND CHLORTHALIDONE, ATENOLOL
　ATENOLOL, ATENOLOL
　DIAZEPAM, DIAZEPAM
　PINDOLOL, PINDOLOL
　SULFAMETHOXAZOLE AND TRIMETHOPRIM DOUBLE
　　STRENGTH, SULFAMETHOXAZOLE
　SULFAMETHOXAZOLE AND TRIMETHOPRIM,
　　SULFAMETHOXAZOLE
MARTEC SCIENTIFIC INC
　DICLOFENAC SODIUM, DICLOFENAC SODIUM
MAST MM
MM MAST AND CO
　CHLORDIAZEPOXIDE HCL, CHLORDIAZEPOXIDE
　　HYDROCHLORIDE

DEXTROAMPHETAMINE SULFATE,
　DEXTROAMPHETAMINE SULFATE
HYDROCHLOROTHIAZIDE, HYDROCHLOROTHIAZIDE
ONA MAST, PHENTERMINE HYDROCHLORIDE
ONA-MAST, PHENTERMINE HYDROCHLORIDE
PHENAZINE, PHENDIMETRAZINE TARTRATE
TETRACYCLINE HCL, TETRACYCLINE HYDROCHLORIDE
TRICHLORMAS, TRICHLORMETHIAZIDE
MATRIX MEDCL
MATRIX MEDICAL CORP
　STERI-STAT, CHLORHEXIDINE GLUCONATE (OTC)
MAYRAND
MAYRAND INC
　SEDAPAP, ACETAMINOPHEN
MCGAW
MCGAW INC
　AMMONIUM CHLORIDE 0.9% IN NORMAL SALINE,
　　AMMONIUM CHLORIDE
　HEPARIN SODIUM 1,000 UNITS IN DEXTROSE 5% IN
　　PLASTIC CONTAINER, HEPARIN SODIUM
　HEPARIN SODIUM 2,000 UNITS IN DEXTROSE 5% IN
　　PLASTIC CONTAINER, HEPARIN SODIUM
　HEPARIN SODIUM 5,000 UNITS IN DEXTROSE 5% IN
　　PLASTIC CONTAINER, HEPARIN SODIUM
MCNEIL
MCNEIL CONSUMER PRODUCTS CO DIV MCNEILAB INC
　CHILDREN'S MOTRIN, IBUPROFEN (OTC)
　IBUPROFEN, IBUPROFEN
　IBUPROFEN, IBUPROFEN (OTC)
　IMODIUM A-D, LOPERAMIDE HYDROCHLORIDE (OTC)
　IMODIUM ADVANCED, LOPERAMIDE HYDROCHLORIDE
　　(OTC)
　JUNIOR STRENGTH MOTRIN, IBUPROFEN (OTC)
　MEDIPREN, IBUPROFEN (OTC)
　METHOCARBAMOL AND ASPIRIN, ASPIRIN
　MOTRIN IB, IBUPROFEN (OTC)
　MOTRIN MIGRAINE PAIN, IBUPROFEN (OTC)
　MOTRIN, IBUPROFEN
　NUPRIN, IBUPROFEN (OTC)
MCNEIL PHARMACEUTICAL CO DIV MCNEILAB INC
　CLISTIN, CARBINOXAMINE MALEATE
MCNEIL CONS SPECLT
MCNEIL CONSUMER AND SPECIALTY PHARMACEUTICALS
　CONCERTA, METHYLPHENIDATE HYDROCHLORIDE
MCNEIL CONSUMER AND SPECIALTY PHARMACEUTICALS
DIV MCNEIL PCC
　CHILDREN'S MOTRIN COLD, IBUPROFEN (OTC)
　FLEXERIL, CYCLOBENZAPRINE HYDROCHLORIDE
　IMODIUM ADVANCED, LOPERAMIDE HYDROCHLORIDE
　　(OTC)
　IMODIUM, LOPERAMIDE HYDROCHLORIDE
　MOTRIN, IBUPROFEN
　NIZORAL A-D, KETOCONAZOLE (OTC)
　NIZORAL, KETOCONAZOLE
　SINE-AID IB, IBUPROFEN (OTC)
　TYLENOL (CAPLET), ACETAMINOPHEN (OTC)
　TYLENOL (GELTAB), ACETAMINOPHEN (OTC)
　TYLENOL, ACETAMINOPHEN (OTC)
　VERMOX, MEBENDAZOLE
MD PHARM
MD PHARMACEUTICAL INC
　CHLOROQUINE PHOSPHATE, CHLOROQUINE
　　PHOSPHATE
　CYPROHEPTADINE HCL, CYPROHEPTADINE
　　HYDROCHLORIDE
　DI-ATRO, ATROPINE SULFATE

APPENDIX B
PRODUCT NAME INDEX
LISTED BY APPLICANT (*continued*)

MEAD JOHNSON
MEAD JOHNSON AND CO
    CAFCIT, CAFFEINE CITRATE
MEAD JOHNSON AND CO SUB BRISTOL MYERS CO
    MUCOMYST W/ ISOPROTERENOL, ACETYLCYSTEINE
MEDI FLEX HOSP
MEDI FLEX HOSP PRODUCTS INC
    CHLORAPREP, CHLORHEXIDINE GLUCONATE (OTC)
MEDICIS
MEDICIS PHARMACEUTICAL CORP
    BUPHENYL, SODIUM PHENYLBUTYRATE
    LIDEX, FLUOCINONIDE
    LIDEX-E, FLUOCINONIDE
    LOPROX, CICLOPIROX
    NEO-SYNALAR, FLUOCINOLONE ACETONIDE
    OVIDE, MALATHION
    SYNACORT, HYDROCORTISONE
    SYNALAR, FLUOCINOLONE ACETONIDE
    SYNALAR-HP, FLUOCINOLONE ACETONIDE
    TOPICORT LP, DESOXIMETASONE
    TOPICORT, DESOXIMETASONE
    VECTRIN, MINOCYCLINE HYDROCHLORIDE
MEDIMMUNE ONCOLOGY
MEDIMMUNE ONCOLOGY INC
    ETHYOL, AMIFOSTINE
    NEUTREXIN, TRIMETREXATE GLUCURONATE
MEDPOINTE
MEDPOINTE HEALTHCARE INC
    FELBATOL, FELBAMATE
MEDPOINTE PHARM HLC
MEDPOINTE PHARMACEUTICALS MEDPOINTE HEALTH-
CARE INC
    AQUATENSEN, METHYCLOTHIAZIDE
    ASTELIN, AZELASTINE HYDROCHLORIDE
    BEPADIN, BEPRIDIL HYDROCHLORIDE
    BUTICAPS, BUTABARBITAL SODIUM
    BUTISOL SODIUM, BUTABARBITAL SODIUM
    COLONAID, ATROPINE SULFATE
    DEPEN, PENICILLAMINE
    DIUTENSEN-R, METHYCLOTHIAZIDE
    DORAL, QUAZEPAM
    DORMATE, MEBUTAMATE
    HYZYD, ISONIAZID
    LUFYLLIN, DYPHYLLINE
    MEPROSPAN, MEPROBAMATE
    MICRAININ, ASPIRIN
    MILPREM-200, ESTROGENS, CONJUGATED
    MILPREM-400, ESTROGENS, CONJUGATED
    MILTOWN, MEPROBAMATE
    MYLAXEN, HEXAFLUORENIUM BROMIDE
    NEOPASALATE, AMINOSALICYLATE SODIUM
    OPTIVAR, AZELASTINE HYDROCHLORIDE
    RONDOMYCIN, METHACYCLINE HYDROCHLORIDE
    SOMA COMPOUND W/ CODEINE, ASPIRIN
    SOMA COMPOUND, ASPIRIN
    SOMA, CARISOPRODOL
    THYRO-BLOCK, POTASSIUM IODIDE (OTC)
    UNITENSEN, CRYPTENAMINE ACETATES
    UNITENSEN, CRYPTENAMINE TANNATES
    VERTAVIS, VERATRUM VIRIDE
    VOSOL HC, ACETIC ACID, GLACIAL
    VOSOL, ACETIC ACID, GLACIAL
    WAMPOCAP, NIACIN
MEDS (TMC)
MEDICINES CO (TMC)
    ANGIOMAX, BIVALIRUDIN

MEDTRONIC
MEDTRONIC INC
    LIORESAL, BACLOFEN
MEPHA
MEPHA AG
    PIROXICAM, PIROXICAM
MERCK
MERCK AND CO INC
    ALDOCLOR-150, CHLOROTHIAZIDE
    ALDOCLOR-250, CHLOROTHIAZIDE
    ALDOMET, METHYLDOPA
    ALDOMET, METHYLDOPATE HYDROCHLORIDE
    ALDORIL 15, HYDROCHLOROTHIAZIDE
    ALDORIL 25, HYDROCHLOROTHIAZIDE
    ALDORIL D30, HYDROCHLOROTHIAZIDE
    ALDORIL D50, HYDROCHLOROTHIAZIDE
    ALPHAREDISOL, HYDROXOCOBALAMIN
    AMINOHIPPURATE SODIUM, AMINOHIPPURATE SODIUM
    AQUAMEPHYTON, PHYTONADIONE
    ARAMINE, METARAMINOL BITARTRATE
    BENEMID, PROBENECID
    COGENTIN, BENZTROPINE MESYLATE
    COLBENEMID, COLCHICINE
    CORTONE, CORTISONE ACETATE
    CUPRIMINE, PENICILLAMINE
    CYCLAINE, HEXYLCAINE HYDROCHLORIDE
    DARANIDE, DICHLORPHENAMIDE
    DECADERM, DEXAMETHASONE
    DECADRON W/ XYLOCAINE, DEXAMETHASONE SODIUM
       PHOSPHATE
    DECADRON, DEXAMETHASONE
    DECADRON, DEXAMETHASONE SODIUM PHOSPHATE
    DECASPRAY, DEXAMETHASONE
    DEMSER, METYROSINE
    DIUPRES-250, CHLOROTHIAZIDE
    DIUPRES-500, CHLOROTHIAZIDE
    DIURIL, CHLOROTHIAZIDE
    DIURIL, CHLOROTHIAZIDE SODIUM
    DOLOBID, DIFLUNISAL
    EDECRIN, ETHACRYNATE SODIUM
    EDECRIN, ETHACRYNIC ACID
    EMEND, APREPITANT
    FLOROPRYL, ISOFLUROPHATE
    FOSAMAX, ALENDRONATE SODIUM
    HUMORSOL, DEMECARIUM BROMIDE
    HYDELTRA-TBA, PREDNISOLONE TEBUTATE
    HYDELTRASOL, PREDNISOLONE SODIUM PHOSPHATE
    HYDROCORTONE, HYDROCORTISONE
    HYDROCORTONE, HYDROCORTISONE ACETATE
    HYDROCORTONE, HYDROCORTISONE SODIUM
       PHOSPHATE
    HYDRODIURIL, HYDROCHLOROTHIAZIDE
    HYDROPRES 25, HYDROCHLOROTHIAZIDE
    HYDROPRES 50, HYDROCHLOROTHIAZIDE
    HYZAAR, HYDROCHLOROTHIAZIDE
    INVANZ, ERTAPENEM SODIUM
    LERITINE, ANILERIDINE HYDROCHLORIDE
    LERITINE, ANILERIDINE PHOSPHATE
    MANNITOL 25%, MANNITOL
    MAXALT, RIZATRIPTAN BENZOATE
    MAXALT-MLT, RIZATRIPTAN BENZOATE
    MEFOXIN IN DEXTROSE 5% IN PLASTIC CONTAINER,
       CEFOXITIN SODIUM
    MEFOXIN IN SODIUM CHLORIDE 0.9% IN PLASTIC
       CONTAINER, CEFOXITIN SODIUM
    MEFOXIN, CEFOXITIN SODIUM
    MEPHYTON, PHYTONADIONE
    MIDAMOR, AMILORIDE HYDROCHLORIDE

APPENDIX B
PRODUCT NAME INDEX
LISTED BY APPLICANT (*continued*)

MINTEZOL, THIABENDAZOLE
MUSTARGEN, MECHLORETHAMINE HYDROCHLORIDE
NEO-HYDELTRASOL, NEOMYCIN SULFATE
NEODECADRON, DEXAMETHASONE SODIUM
    PHOSPHATE
PERIACTIN, CYPROHEPTADINE HYDROCHLORIDE
PRIMAXIN, CILASTATIN SODIUM
PROSCAR, FINASTERIDE
REDISOL, CYANOCOBALAMIN
SINGULAIR, MONTELUKAST SODIUM
SYPRINE, TRIENTINE HYDROCHLORIDE
TIAMATE, DILTIAZEM MALATE
TIMOLIDE 10-25, HYDROCHLOROTHIAZIDE
MERCK RESEARCH LABORATORIES DIV MERCK CO INC
    AGGRASTAT, TIROFIBAN HYDROCHLORIDE
    ALDOMET, METHYLDOPA
    BLOCADREN, TIMOLOL MALEATE
    CHIBROXIN, NORFLOXACIN
    CLINORIL, SULINDAC
    COSMEGEN, DACTINOMYCIN
    COSOPT, DORZOLAMIDE HYDROCHLORIDE
    COZAAR, LOSARTAN POTASSIUM
    CRIXIVAN, INDINAVIR SULFATE
    DECADRON-LA, DEXAMETHASONE ACETATE
    INDOCIN I.V., INDOMETHACIN SODIUM
    INDOCIN SR, INDOMETHACIN
    INDOCIN, INDOMETHACIN
    LACRISERT, HYDROXYPROPYL CELLULOSE
    MEFOXIN IN PLASTIC CONTAINER, CEFOXITIN SODIUM
    MEVACOR, LOVASTATIN
    MODURETIC 5-50, AMILORIDE HYDROCHLORIDE
    NOROXIN, NORFLOXACIN
    PEPCID AC, FAMOTIDINE (OTC)
    PEPCID COMPLETE, CALCIUM CARBONATE,
        PRECIPITATED (OTC)
    PEPCID PRESERVATIVE FREE IN PLASTIC CONTAINER,
        FAMOTIDINE
    PEPCID PRESERVATIVE FREE, FAMOTIDINE
    PEPCID RPD, FAMOTIDINE
    PEPCID, FAMOTIDINE
    PRINIVIL, LISINOPRIL
    PRINZIDE, HYDROCHLOROTHIAZIDE
    PROPECIA, FINASTERIDE
    SINGULAIR, MONTELUKAST SODIUM
    STROMECTOL, IVERMECTIN
    TIMOPTIC IN OCUDOSE, TIMOLOL MALEATE
    TIMOPTIC, TIMOLOL MALEATE
    TIMOPTIC-XE, TIMOLOL MALEATE
    TRUSOPT, DORZOLAMIDE HYDROCHLORIDE
    VIOXX, ROFECOXIB
    ZOCOR, SIMVASTATIN
MERCK RES
MERCK RESEARCH LABORATORIES
    CANCIDAS, CASPOFUNGIN ACETATE
MERETEK
MERETEK DIAGNOSTICS INC
    BREATHTEK UBT FOR H-PYLORI, UREA, C-13
    MERETEK UBT KIT (W/ PRANACTIN), UREA, C-13
MERICON
MERICON INDUSTRIES INC
    HYDROCORTISONE, HYDROCORTISONE
MERIDIAN MEDCL TECHN
MERIDIAN MEDICAL TECHNOLOGIES INC
    ACYCLOVIR SODIUM, ACYCLOVIR SODIUM
    ATROPEN, ATROPINE
    BUTORPHANOL TARTRATE, BUTORPHANOL TARTRATE
    DILTIAZEM HCL, DILTIAZEM HYDROCHLORIDE
    EPI E Z PEN JR, EPINEPHRINE

    EPIPEN E Z PEN, EPINEPHRINE
    EPIPEN JR., EPINEPHRINE
    EPIPEN, EPINEPHRINE
    LIDOPEN, LIDOCAINE HYDROCHLORIDE
    MORPHINE SULFATE, MORPHINE SULFATE
    PRALIDOXIME CHLORIDE, PRALIDOXIME CHLORIDE
METABOLIC SOLUTIONS
METABOLIC SOLUTIONS INC
    HELICOSOL, UREA, C-13
METHAPHARM
METHAPHARM INC
    PROVOCHOLINE, METHACHOLINE CHLORIDE
MFG CHEMISTS
MANUFACTURING CHEMISTS INC
    PHENDIMETRAZINE TARTRATE, PHENDIMETRAZINE
        TARTRATE
MGI PHARMA INC
MGI PHARMA INC
    DIDRONEL, ETIDRONATE DISODIUM
    HEXALEN, ALTRETAMINE
    SALAGEN, PILOCARPINE HYDROCHLORIDE
MIKART
MIKART INC
    ACETAMINOPHEN AND BUTALBITAL AND CAFFEINE,
        ACETAMINOPHEN
    ACETAMINOPHEN AND CODEINE PHOSPHATE,
        ACETAMINOPHEN
    ACETAMINOPHEN, ASPIRIN, AND CODEINE
        PHOSPHATE, ACETAMINOPHEN
    ACETAMINOPHEN, BUTALBITAL, AND CAFFEINE,
        ACETAMINOPHEN
    ACETAMINOPHEN, CAFFEINE, AND DIHYDROCODEINE
        BITARTRATE, ACETAMINOPHEN
    AMANTADINE HCL, AMANTADINE HYDROCHLORIDE
    AMINOCAPROIC ACID, AMINOCAPROIC ACID
    AMINOCAPROIC, AMINOCAPROIC ACID
    BUTALBITAL, ACETAMINOPHEN AND CAFFEINE,
        ACETAMINOPHEN
    BUTAPAP, ACETAMINOPHEN
    CARBINOXAMINE MALEATE, CARBINOXAMINE
        MALEATE
    ESGIC-PLUS, ACETAMINOPHEN
    HYDROCODONE BITARTRATE AND ACETAMINOPHEN,
        ACETAMINOPHEN
    ISONIAZID, ISONIAZID
    METHAZOLAMIDE, METHAZOLAMIDE
    OXYBUTYNIN CHLORIDE, OXYBUTYNIN CHLORIDE
    PHENDIMETRAZINE TARTRATE, PHENDIMETRAZINE
        TARTRATE
    PYRAZINAMIDE, PYRAZINAMIDE
    TRIHEXYPHENIDYL HCL, TRIHEXYPHENIDYL
        HYDROCHLORIDE
MILES
MILES LABORATORIES INC
    ALCOHOL 5% IN DEXTROSE 5%, ALCOHOL
    DEXTROSE 10% IN PLASTIC CONTAINER, DEXTROSE
    DEXTROSE 5% AND SODIUM CHLORIDE 0.2% IN
        PLASTIC CONTAINER, DEXTROSE
    DEXTROSE 5% AND SODIUM CHLORIDE 0.3% IN
        PLASTIC CONTAINER, DEXTROSE
    DEXTROSE 5% AND SODIUM CHLORIDE 0.45% IN
        PLASTIC CONTAINER, DEXTROSE
    DEXTROSE 5% AND SODIUM CHLORIDE 0.9% IN
        PLASTIC CONTAINER, DEXTROSE
    DEXTROSE 5% IN LACTATED RINGER'S IN PLASTIC
        CONTAINER, CALCIUM CHLORIDE
    LACTATED RINGER'S IN PLASTIC CONTAINER, CALCIUM
        CHLORIDE

APPENDIX B
PRODUCT NAME INDEX
LISTED BY APPLICANT (*continued*)

LIDOCAINE HCL, LIDOCAINE HYDROCHLORIDE
MANNITOL 10%, MANNITOL
MANNITOL 15%, MANNITOL
MANNITOL 20%, MANNITOL
POTASSIUM CHLORIDE, POTASSIUM CHLORIDE
PROCAINE HCL, PROCAINE HYDROCHLORIDE
SODIUM CHLORIDE 0.45% IN PLASTIC CONTAINER,
SODIUM CHLORIDE
SODIUM CHLORIDE 0.9% IN PLASTIC CONTAINER,
SODIUM CHLORIDE
SODIUM CHLORIDE IN PLASTIC CONTAINER, SODIUM
CHLORIDE
STERILE WATER IN PLASTIC CONTAINER, WATER FOR
IRRIGATION, STERILE
MILEX
MILEX PRODUCTS INC
MILOPHENE, CLOMIPHENE CITRATE
MILLENNIUM PHARMS
MILLENNIUM PHARMACEUTICALS INC
INTEGRILIN, EPTIFIBATIDE
VELCADE, BORTEZOMIB
MINRAD
MINRAD INC
ENFLURANE, ENFLURANE
ISOFLURANE, ISOFLURANE
MISSION PHARMA
MISSION PHARMACAL CO
CALCIBIND, CELLULOSE SODIUM PHOSPHATE
EQUIPIN, HOMATROPINE METHYLBROMIDE
FOLICET, FOLIC ACID
HOMAPIN-10, HOMATROPINE METHYLBROMIDE
HOMAPIN-5, HOMATROPINE METHYLBROMIDE
LITHOSTAT, ACETOHYDROXAMIC ACID
POTASSIUM CITRATE, POTASSIUM CITRATE
TIOPRONIN, TIOPRONIN
MIZA PHARMS USA
MIZA PHARMACEUTICALS USA INC
OCUSULF-10, SULFACETAMIDE SODIUM
OCUSULF-30, SULFACETAMIDE SODIUM
TROPICAMIDE, TROPICAMIDE
MJ PHARMS
MJ PHARMACEUTICALS LTD
CEPHALEXIN, CEPHALEXIN
MK LABS
MK LABORATORIES INC
DIPHENHYDRAMINE HCL, DIPHENHYDRAMINE
HYDROCHLORIDE
FOLIC ACID, FOLIC ACID
ISONIAZID, ISONIAZID
KESSO-GESIC, PROPOXYPHENE HYDROCHLORIDE
MEPROBAMATE, MEPROBAMATE
NIACIN, NIACIN
RESERPINE, RESERPINE
SOSOL, SULFISOXAZOLE
VITAMIN A, VITAMIN A PALMITATE
MONARCH PHARMS
MONARCH PHARMACEUTICALS INC
CORTISPORIN, BACITRACIN ZINC
CORTISPORIN, HYDROCORTISONE
CORTISPORIN, HYDROCORTISONE ACETATE
DERMACORT, HYDROCORTISONE
KEMADRIN, PROCYCLIDINE HYDROCHLORIDE
MENEST, ESTROGENS, ESTERIFIED
NEOSPORIN G.U. IRRIGANT, NEOMYCIN SULFATE
NEOSPORIN, BACITRACIN ZINC
NEOSPORIN, GRAMICIDIN
PEDIOTIC, HYDROCORTISONE
POLYSPORIN, BACITRACIN ZINC

PROCTOCORT, HYDROCORTISONE
PROLOPRIM, TRIMETHOPRIM
QUIBRON-T, THEOPHYLLINE
QUIBRON-T/SR, THEOPHYLLINE
SEPTRA DS, SULFAMETHOXAZOLE
SEPTRA GRAPE, SULFAMETHOXAZOLE
SEPTRA, SULFAMETHOXAZOLE
THALITONE, CHLORTHALIDONE
VIROPTIC, TRIFLURIDINE
MORTON GROVE
MORTON GROVE ACQUISITION CORP
CLEMASTINE FUMARATE, CLEMASTINE FUMARATE
FLUOXETINE HCL, FLUOXETINE HYDROCHLORIDE
MINOXIDIL EXTRA STRENGTH (FOR MEN), MINOXIDIL
(OTC)
OXYBUTYNIN CHLORIDE, OXYBUTYNIN CHLORIDE
PREDNISOLONE SODIUM PHOSPHATE, PREDNISOLONE
SODIUM PHOSPHATE
MORTON GROVE PHARMACEUTICALS INC
ACETAMINOPHEN AND CODEINE PHOSPHATE,
ACETAMINOPHEN
ACETIC ACID, ACETIC ACID, GLACIAL
ALBUTEROL SULFATE, ALBUTEROL SULFATE
AMANTADINE HCL, AMANTADINE HYDROCHLORIDE
AMINOPHYLLINE, AMINOPHYLLINE
BIPHETAP, BROMPHENIRAMINE MALEATE
BUTABARBITAL SODIUM, BUTABARBITAL SODIUM
CARBAMAZEPINE, CARBAMAZEPINE
CHLORPROMAZINE HCL, CHLORPROMAZINE
HYDROCHLORIDE
CIMETIDINE HCL, CIMETIDINE HYDROCHLORIDE
CLINDAMYCIN PHOSPHATE, CLINDAMYCIN
PHOSPHATE
CLOBETASOL PROPIONATE, CLOBETASOL
PROPIONATE
CROMOLYN SODIUM, CROMOLYN SODIUM
CYPROHEPTADINE HCL, CYPROHEPTADINE
HYDROCHLORIDE
DIPHEN, DIPHENHYDRAMINE HYDROCHLORIDE (OTC)
DOXEPIN HCL, DOXEPIN HYDROCHLORIDE
ERYTHROMYCIN, ERYTHROMYCIN
FLUOCINOLONE ACETONIDE, FLUOCINOLONE
ACETONIDE
FUROSEMIDE, FUROSEMIDE
GENERLAC, LACTULOSE
HALOPERIDOL, HALOPERIDOL LACTATE
HYDROCHLOROTHIAZIDE, HYDROCHLOROTHIAZIDE
HYDROCORTISONE AND ACETIC ACID, ACETIC ACID,
GLACIAL
HYDROXYZINE HCL, HYDROXYZINE HYDROCHLORIDE
LACTULOSE, LACTULOSE
LIDOCAINE HCL, LIDOCAINE HYDROCHLORIDE
LINDANE, LINDANE
LITHIUM CITRATE, LITHIUM CITRATE
LOPERAMIDE HCL, LOPERAMIDE HYDROCHLORIDE
(OTC)
METAPROTERENOL SULFATE, METAPROTERENOL
SULFATE
METOCLOPRAMIDE HCL, METOCLOPRAMIDE
HYDROCHLORIDE
MINOXIDIL (FOR MEN), MINOXIDIL (OTC)
MYBANIL, BROMODIPHENHYDRAMINE
HYDROCHLORIDE
MYCODONE, HOMATROPINE METHYLBROMIDE
MYLARAMINE, DEXCHLORPHENIRAMINE MALEATE
MYMETHASONE, DEXAMETHASONE
MYPHETANE DC, BROMPHENIRAMINE MALEATE
MYPHETANE DX, BROMPHENIRAMINE MALEATE

APPENDIX B
PRODUCT NAME INDEX
LISTED BY APPLICANT (*continued*)

MYPROIC ACID, VALPROIC ACID
NYSTATIN, NYSTATIN
OXTRIPHYLLINE PEDIATRIC, OXTRIPHYLLINE
OXTRIPHYLLINE, OXTRIPHYLLINE
PHENYTOIN, PHENYTOIN
PREDNISONE, PREDNISONE
PROCHLORPERAZINE EDISYLATE,
    PROCHLORPERAZINE EDISYLATE
PROMETHAZINE PLAIN, PROMETHAZINE
    HYDROCHLORIDE
PROMETHAZINE VC PLAIN, PHENYLEPHRINE
    HYDROCHLORIDE
PROMETHAZINE VC W/ CODEINE, CODEINE
    PHOSPHATE
PROMETHAZINE W/ CODEINE, CODEINE PHOSPHATE
PROMETHAZINE W/ DEXTROMETHORPHAN,
    DEXTROMETHORPHAN HYDROBROMIDE
PROPRANOLOL HCL, PROPRANOLOL HYDROCHLORIDE
SELENIUM SULFIDE, SELENIUM SULFIDE
SODIUM POLYSTYRENE SULFONATE, SODIUM
    POLYSTYRENE SULFONATE
THEOPHYLLINE, THEOPHYLLINE
THIORIDAZINE HCL, THIORIDAZINE HYDROCHLORIDE
TRETINOIN, TRETINOIN
TRIAMCINOLONE ACETONIDE, TRIAMCINOLONE
    ACETONIDE
TRIFLUOPERAZINE HCL, TRIFLUOPERAZINE
    HYDROCHLORIDE
TRIMEPRAZINE TARTRATE, TRIMEPRAZINE TARTRATE
TRIPROLIDINE HCL, PSEUDOEPHEDRINE HCL AND
    CODEINE PHOSPHATE, CODEINE PHOSPHATE
MOUNT SINAI MEDCTR
MOUNT SINAI MEDCTR
    THALLOUS CHLORIDE TL 201, THALLOUS CHLORIDE, TL-
    201
MOVA
MOVA PHARMACEUTICALS CORP
    ALBUTEROL SULFATE, ALBUTEROL SULFATE
MSP SINGAPORE
MSP SINGAPORE CO LLC
    ZETIA, EZETIMIBE
MURO
MURO PHARMACEUTICAL INC
    LIQUID PRED, PREDNISONE
    PRELONE, PREDNISOLONE
    PROMETA, METAPROTERENOL SULFATE
    TRI-NASAL, TRIAMCINOLONE ACETONIDE
    VOLMAX, ALBUTEROL SULFATE
MUTUAL PHARM
MUTUAL PHARMACEUTICAL CO INC
    ACETAMINOPHEN AND CODEINE PHOSPHATE,
        ACETAMINOPHEN
    ACETAZOLAMIDE, ACETAZOLAMIDE
    ALBUTEROL SULFATE, ALBUTEROL SULFATE
    ALLOPURINOL, ALLOPURINOL
    AMITRIPTYLINE HCL, AMITRIPTYLINE HYDROCHLORIDE
    ATENOLOL AND CHLORTHALIDONE, ATENOLOL
    ATENOLOL, ATENOLOL
    BENZTROPINE MESYLATE, BENZTROPINE MESYLATE
    BISOPROLOL FUMARATE, BISOPROLOL FUMARATE
    CARISOPRODOL, CARISOPRODOL
    CHLORTHALIDONE, CHLORTHALIDONE
    CHLORZOXAZONE, CHLORZOXAZONE
    DICLOFENAC POTASSIUM, DICLOFENAC POTASSIUM
    DIPHENHYDRAMINE HCL, DIPHENHYDRAMINE
        HYDROCHLORIDE
    DOXYCYCLINE HYCLATE, DOXYCYCLINE HYCLATE
    ERGOLOID MESYLATES, ERGOLOID MESYLATES

FAMOTIDINE, FAMOTIDINE
FENOPROFEN CALCIUM, FENOPROFEN CALCIUM
FLUVOXAMINE MALEATE, FLUVOXAMINE MALEATE
HYDRALAZINE HCL, HYDRALAZINE HYDROCHLORIDE
HYDROXYZINE HCL, HYDROXYZINE HYDROCHLORIDE
IBUPROFEN, IBUPROFEN
IBUPROFEN, IBUPROFEN (OTC)
IMIPRAMINE HCL, IMIPRAMINE HYDROCHLORIDE
INDOMETHACIN, INDOMETHACIN
LABETALOL HCL, LABETALOL HYDROCHLORIDE
LORAZEPAM, LORAZEPAM
METOCLOPRAMIDE HCL, METOCLOPRAMIDE
    HYDROCHLORIDE
METOPROLOL TARTRATE, METOPROLOL TARTRATE
METRONIDAZOLE, METRONIDAZOLE
MINOXIDIL, MINOXIDIL
NYSTATIN, NYSTATIN
PINDOLOL, PINDOLOL
PIROXICAM, PIROXICAM
PREDNISONE, PREDNISONE
PROPAFENONE HCL, PROPAFENONE
    HYDROCHLORIDE
QUINIDINE GLUCONATE, QUINIDINE GLUCONATE
QUINIDINE SULFATE, QUINIDINE SULFATE
SOTALOL HCL, SOTALOL HYDROCHLORIDE
SPIRONOLACTONE AND HYDROCHLOROTHIAZIDE,
    HYDROCHLOROTHIAZIDE
SPIRONOLACTONE, SPIRONOLACTONE
SULFAMETHOXAZOLE AND TRIMETHOPRIM,
    SULFAMETHOXAZOLE
SULFASALAZINE, SULFASALAZINE
SULINDAC, SULINDAC
THIORIDAZINE HCL, THIORIDAZINE HYDROCHLORIDE
TOLAZAMIDE, TOLAZAMIDE
TOLMETIN SODIUM, TOLMETIN SODIUM
TRAMADOL HCL, TRAMADOL HYDROCHLORIDE
TRAZODONE HCL, TRAZODONE HYDROCHLORIDE
VERAPAMIL HCL, VERAPAMIL HYDROCHLORIDE
MUTUAL PHARMA
MUTUAL PHARMACAL CO
    FLUOXETINE, FLUOXETINE HYDROCHLORIDE
    KETOCONAZOLE, KETOCONAZOLE
    METFORMIN HCL, METFORMIN HYDROCHLORIDE
MYLAN
MYLAN LABORATORIES INC
    ACYCLOVIR, ACYCLOVIR
    CAPTOPRIL, CAPTOPRIL
    ETODOLAC, ETODOLAC
    IBUPROFEN, IBUPROFEN
    TERAZOSIN HCL, TERAZOSIN HYDROCHLORIDE
MYLAN PHARMACEUTICALS INC
    ACEBUTOLOL HCL, ACEBUTOLOL HYDROCHLORIDE
    ACYCLOVIR, ACYCLOVIR
    ALBUTEROL SULFATE, ALBUTEROL SULFATE
    ALLOPURINOL, ALLOPURINOL
    ALPRAZOLAM, ALPRAZOLAM
    AMILORIDE HCL AND HYDROCHLOROTHIAZIDE,
        AMILORIDE HYDROCHLORIDE
    AMITRIPTYLINE HCL, AMITRIPTYLINE HYDROCHLORIDE
    AMOXICILLIN, AMOXICILLIN
    AMPICILLIN TRIHYDRATE, AMPICILLIN/AMPICILLIN
        TRIHYDRATE
    ATENOLOL AND CHLORTHALIDONE, ATENOLOL
    ATENOLOL, ATENOLOL
    BISOPROLOL FUMARATE AND
        HYDROCHLOROTHIAZIDE, BISOPROLOL FUMARATE
    BUPROPION HCL, BUPROPION HYDROCHLORIDE
    BUSPIRONE HCL, BUSPIRONE HYDROCHLORIDE

APPENDIX B
PRODUCT NAME INDEX
LISTED BY APPLICANT (*continued*)

BUTORPHANOL TARTRATE, BUTORPHANOL TARTRATE
CAPTOPRIL AND HYDROCHLOROTHIAZIDE, CAPTOPRIL
CARBIDOPA AND LEVODOPA, CARBIDOPA
CHLORDIAZEPOXIDE AND AMITRIPTYLINE HCL, AMITRIPTYLINE HYDROCHLORIDE
CHLORDIAZEPOXIDE HCL, CHLORDIAZEPOXIDE HYDROCHLORIDE
CHLOROTHIAZIDE, CHLOROTHIAZIDE
CHLOROTHIAZIDE-RESERPINE, CHLOROTHIAZIDE
CHLORPROPAMIDE, CHLORPROPAMIDE
CHLORTHALIDONE, CHLORTHALIDONE
CIMETIDINE, CIMETIDINE
CLOMIPRAMINE HCL, CLOMIPRAMINE HYDROCHLORIDE
CLONAZEPAM, CLONAZEPAM
CLONIDINE HCL, CLONIDINE HYDROCHLORIDE
CLORAZEPATE DIPOTASSIUM, CLORAZEPATE DIPOTASSIUM
CLORPRES, CHLORTHALIDONE
CLOZAPINE, CLOZAPINE
CYCLOBENZAPRINE HCL, CYCLOBENZAPRINE HYDROCHLORIDE
CYPROHEPTADINE HCL, CYPROHEPTADINE HYDROCHLORIDE
CYSTAGON, CYSTEAMINE BITARTRATE
DIAZEPAM, DIAZEPAM
DICLOFENAC POTASSIUM, DICLOFENAC POTASSIUM
DICLOFENAC SODIUM, DICLOFENAC SODIUM
DICYCLOMINE HCL, DICYCLOMINE HYDROCHLORIDE
DILTIAZEM HCL, DILTIAZEM HYDROCHLORIDE
DIPHENOXYLATE HCL AND ATROPINE SULFATE, ATROPINE SULFATE
DISOPYRAMIDE PHOSPHATE, DISOPYRAMIDE PHOSPHATE
DOXAZOSIN MESYLATE, DOXAZOSIN MESYLATE
DOXEPIN HCL, DOXEPIN HYDROCHLORIDE
DOXYCYCLINE HYCLATE, DOXYCYCLINE HYCLATE
ENALAPRIL MALEATE AND HYDROCHLOROTHIAZIDE, ENALAPRIL MALEATE
ENALAPRIL MALEATE, ENALAPRIL MALEATE
ERYTHROMYCIN ETHYLSUCCINATE, ERYTHROMYCIN ETHYLSUCCINATE
ERYTHROMYCIN STEARATE, ERYTHROMYCIN STEARATE
ESTRADIOL, ESTRADIOL
ESTROPIPATE, ESTROPIPATE
ETODOLAC, ETODOLAC
EXTENDED PHENYTOIN SODIUM, PHENYTOIN SODIUM, EXTENDED
FAMOTIDINE, FAMOTIDINE
FENOPROFEN CALCIUM, FENOPROFEN CALCIUM
FLUOXETINE, FLUOXETINE HYDROCHLORIDE
FLUPHENAZINE HCL, FLUPHENAZINE HYDROCHLORIDE
FLURAZEPAM HCL, FLURAZEPAM HYDROCHLORIDE
FLURBIPROFEN, FLURBIPROFEN
FLUVOXAMINE MALEATE, FLUVOXAMINE MALEATE
FUROSEMIDE, FUROSEMIDE
GEMFIBROZIL, GEMFIBROZIL
GLIPIZIDE, GLIPIZIDE
GLYBURIDE (MICRONIZED), GLYBURIDE
GUANFACINE HCL, GUANFACINE HYDROCHLORIDE
HALOPERIDOL, HALOPERIDOL
HYDRALAZINE HCL-HYDROCHLOROTHIAZIDE-RESERPINE, HYDRALAZINE HYDROCHLORIDE
HYDROCHLOROTHIAZIDE, HYDROCHLOROTHIAZIDE
HYDROXYCHLOROQINE SULFATE, HYDROXYCHLOROQUINE SULFATE
IBUPROFEN, IBUPROFEN

IBUPROFEN, IBUPROFEN (OTC)
INDAPAMIDE, INDAPAMIDE
INDOMETHACIN, INDOMETHACIN
KETOCONAZOLE, KETOCONAZOLE
KETOPROFEN, KETOPROFEN
KETOROLAC TROMETHAMINE, KETOROLAC TROMETHAMINE
LEVOTHYROXINE SODIUM, LIOTRIX (T4;T3)
LISINOPRIL AND HYDROCHLOROTHIAZIDE, HYDROCHLOROTHIAZIDE
LISINOPRIL, LISINOPRIL
LOPERAMIDE HCL, LOPERAMIDE HYDROCHLORIDE
LORAZEPAM, LORAZEPAM
LOVASTATIN, LOVASTATIN
MAPROTILINE HCL, MAPROTILINE HYDROCHLORIDE
MAXZIDE, HYDROCHLOROTHIAZIDE
MAXZIDE-25, HYDROCHLOROTHIAZIDE
MECLOFENAMATE SODIUM, MECLOFENAMATE SODIUM
MEPROBAMATE, MEPROBAMATE
METFORMIN HCL, METFORMIN HYDROCHLORIDE
METHOCARBAMOL, METHOCARBAMOL
METHOTREXATE SODIUM, METHOTREXATE SODIUM
METHYCLOTHIAZIDE, METHYCLOTHIAZIDE
METHYLDOPA AND HYDROCHLOROTHIAZIDE, HYDROCHLOROTHIAZIDE
METHYLDOPA, METHYLDOPA
METOPROLOL TARTRATE, METOPROLOL TARTRATE
MIRTAZAPINE, MIRTAZAPINE
NADOLOL, NADOLOL
NAPROXEN SODIUM, NAPROXEN SODIUM
NAPROXEN, NAPROXEN
NICARDIPINE HCL, NICARDIPINE HYDROCHLORIDE
NIFEDIPINE, NIFEDIPINE
NITROFURANTION, NITROFURANTOIN, MACROCRYSTALLINE
NITROFURANTOIN, NITROFURANTOIN, MACROCRYSTALLINE
NIZATIDINE, NIZATIDINE
NORTRIPTYLINE HCL, NORTRIPTYLINE HYDROCHLORIDE
OMEPRAZOLE, OMEPRAZOLE
OXAPROZIN, OXAPROZIN
OXAZEPAM, OXAZEPAM
PACLITAXEL, PACLITAXEL
PENICILLIN G POTASSIUM, PENICILLIN G POTASSIUM
PENICILLIN V POTASSIUM, PENICILLIN V POTASSIUM
PENTOXIFYLLINE, PENTOXIFYLLINE
PERPHENAZINE AND AMITRIPTYLINE HCL, AMITRIPTYLINE HYDROCHLORIDE
PHENYTEK, PHENYTOIN SODIUM, EXTENDED
PINDOLOL, PINDOLOL
PIROXICAM, PIROXICAM
PRAZOSIN HCL, PRAZOSIN HYDROCHLORIDE
PROBENECID, PROBENECID
PROCHLORPERAZINE MALEATE, PROCHLORPERAZINE MALEATE
PROPANTHELINE BROMIDE, PROPANTHELINE BROMIDE
PROPOXYPHENE HCL AND ACETAMINOPHEN, ACETAMINOPHEN
PROPOXYPHENE HCL, PROPOXYPHENE HYDROCHLORIDE
PROPOXYPHENE NAPSYLATE AND ACETAMINOPHEN, ACETAMINOPHEN
PROPRANOLOL HCL AND HYDROCHLOROTHIAZIDE, HYDROCHLOROTHIAZIDE
PROPRANOLOL HCL, PROPRANOLOL HYDROCHLORIDE
RANITIDINE HCL, RANITIDINE HYDROCHLORIDE

APPENDIX B
PRODUCT NAME INDEX
LISTED BY APPLICANT (continued)

RESERPINE, RESERPINE
SOTALOL HCL, SOTALOL HYDROCHLORIDE
SPIRONOLACTONE AND HYDROCHLOROTHIAZIDE,
  HYDROCHLOROTHIAZIDE
SPIRONOLACTONE, SPIRONOLACTONE
SULFAMYLON, MAFENIDE ACETATE
SULINDAC, SULINDAC
TAMOXIFEN CITRATE, TAMOXIFEN CITRATE
TEMAZEPAM, TEMAZEPAM
TETRACYCLINE HCL, TETRACYCLINE HYDROCHLORIDE
THIORIDAZINE HCL, THIORIDAZINE HYDROCHLORIDE
THIOTHIXENE, THIOTHIXENE
TICLOPIDINE HCL, TICLOPIDINE HYDROCHLORIDE
TIMOLOL MALEATE, TIMOLOL MALEATE
TIZANIDINE HCL, TIZANIDINE HYDROCHLORIDE
TOLAZAMIDE, TOLAZAMIDE
TOLBUTAMIDE, TOLBUTAMIDE
TOLMETIN SODIUM, TOLMETIN SODIUM
TRAMADOL HCL, TRAMADOL HYDROCHLORIDE
TRAZODONE HCL, TRAZODONE HYDROCHLORIDE
TRIAMCINOLONE, TRIAMCINOLONE
TRIAMTERENE AND HYDROCHLOROTHIAZIDE,
  HYDROCHLOROTHIAZIDE
TRIFLUOPERAZINE HCL, TRIFLUOPERAZINE
  HYDROCHLORIDE
VERAPAMIL HCL, VERAPAMIL HYDROCHLORIDE
ZAGAM, SPARFLOXACIN
MYLAN TECHNOLOGIES
MYLAN TECHNOLOGIES INC
  ESTRADIOL, ESTRADIOL
  NITROGLYCERIN, NITROGLYCERIN
  TERAZOSIN HCL, TERAZOSIN HYDROCHLORIDE

N

NAPRO
NAPRO BIOTHERAPEUTICS INC
  PACLITAXEL, PACLITAXEL
NASKA
NASKA PHARMACAL CO INC DIV RUGBY DARBY GROUP
COSMETICS
  BACITRACIN ZINC-NEOMYCIN SULFATE-POLYMYXIN B
    SULFATE, BACITRACIN ZINC (OTC)
  BACITRACIN ZINC-POLYMYXIN B SULFATE, BACITRACIN
    ZINC (OTC)
  BACITRACIN, BACITRACIN (OTC)
  CYPROHEPTADINE HCL, CYPROHEPTADINE
    HYDROCHLORIDE
  DIPHENHYDRAMINE HCL, DIPHENHYDRAMINE
    HYDROCHLORIDE
  ERYTHROMYCIN ETHYLSUCCINATE, ERYTHROMYCIN
    ETHYLSUCCINATE
  HYDROCORTISONE, HYDROCORTISONE
  TRIMETH/SULFA, SULFAMETHOXAZOLE
NEOSAN PHARMS
NEOSAN PHARMACEUTICALS
  ACYCLOVIR, ACYCLOVIR
  DARVON-N, PROPOXYPHENE NAPSYLATE
  ETODOLAC, ETODOLAC
  KETOCONAZOLE, KETOCONAZOLE
NEPHRON
NEPHRON CORP
  ALBUTEROL SULFATE, ALBUTEROL SULFATE
  BETA-2, ISOETHARINE HYDROCHLORIDE
  IPRATROPIUM BROMIDE, IPRATROPIUM BROMIDE
NEPHRON PHARMACEUTICALS CORP

METAPROTERENOL SULFATE, METAPROTERENOL
  SULFATE
NEW RIVER
NEW RIVER PHARMACEUTICALS INC
  DOXEPIN HCL, DOXEPIN HYDROCHLORIDE
  PROFERDEX, IRON DEXTRAN
  TRIAVIL 2-10, AMITRIPTYLINE HYDROCHLORIDE
  TRIAVIL 2-25, AMITRIPTYLINE HYDROCHLORIDE
  TRIAVIL 4-10, AMITRIPTYLINE HYDROCHLORIDE
  TRIAVIL 4-25, AMITRIPTYLINE HYDROCHLORIDE
  TRIAVIL 4-50, AMITRIPTYLINE HYDROCHLORIDE
NEWTRON PHARMS
NEWTRON PHARMACEUTICALS INC
  BROMPHENIRAMINE MALEATE, BROMPHENIRAMINE
    MALEATE
  CHLORPHENIRAMINE MALEATE, CHLORPHENIRAMINE
    MALEATE
  DIPHENHYDRAMINE HCL, DIPHENHYDRAMINE
    HYDROCHLORIDE
  TRILITRON, PSEUDOEPHEDRINE HYDROCHLORIDE
NORBROOK
NORBROOK LABORATORIES LTD
  METHOTREXATE SODIUM, METHOTREXATE SODIUM
  METOCLOPRAMIDE HCL, METOCLOPRAMIDE
    HYDROCHLORIDE
NOVARTIS
NOVARTIS CONSUMER HEALTH INC
  ASBRON, THEOPHYLLINE SODIUM GLYCINATE
  CONTAC, CHLORPHENIRAMINE MALEATE (OTC)
  DENAVIR, PENCICLOVIR SODIUM
  FOAMICON, ALUMINUM HYDROXIDE (OTC)
  HABITROL, NICOTINE (OTC)
  LAMISIL AT, TERBINAFINE HYDROCHLORIDE (OTC)
  LAMISIL, TERBINAFINE
  LAMISIL, TERBINAFINE HYDROCHLORIDE
  LAMISIL, TERBINAFINE HYDROCHLORIDE (OTC)
  RAUTENSIN, ALSEROXYLON
  TAVIST ALLERGY/SINUS/HEADACHE, ACETAMINOPHEN
    (OTC)
  TRANSDERM SCOP, SCOPOLAMINE
NOVARTIS OPHTHALMICS INC
  CARBASTAT, CARBACHOL
  CATARASE, CHYMOTRYPSIN
  DEXACIDIN, DEXAMETHASONE
  FLUOR-OP, FLUOROMETHOLONE
  FUNDUSCEIN-25, FLUORESCEIN SODIUM
  GENTACIDIN, GENTAMICIN SULFATE
  INFLAMASE FORTE, PREDNISOLONE SODIUM
    PHOSPHATE
  INFLAMASE MILD, PREDNISOLONE SODIUM
    PHOSPHATE
  LIVOSTIN, LEVOCABASTINE HYDROCHLORIDE
  MIOCHOL, ACETYLCHOLINE CHLORIDE
  MIOCHOL-E, ACETYLCHOLINE CHLORIDE
  OCUPRESS, CARTEOLOL HYDROCHLORIDE
  RESCULA, UNOPROSTONE ISOPROPYL
  SULF-10, SULFACETAMIDE SODIUM
  SULF-15, SULFACETAMIDE SODIUM
  VASOCIDIN, PREDNISOLONE ACETATE
  VASOCIDIN, PREDNISOLONE SODIUM PHOSPHATE
  VASOCON, NAPHAZOLINE HYDROCHLORIDE
  VASOCON-A, ANTAZOLINE PHOSPHATE (OTC)
  VITRAVENE PRESERVATIVE FREE, FOMIVIRSEN
    SODIUM
  VOLTAREN, DICLOFENAC SODIUM
  ZADITOR, KETOTIFEN FUMARATE
NOVARTIS PHARMACEUTICALS CORP
  ACYLANID, ACETYLDIGITOXIN

APPENDIX B
PRODUCT NAME INDEX
LISTED BY APPLICANT (*continued*)

ANTRENYL, OXYPHENONIUM BROMIDE
ANTURANE, SULFINPYRAZONE
APRESAZIDE, HYDRALAZINE HYDROCHLORIDE
APRESOLINE, HYDRALAZINE HYDROCHLORIDE
APRESOLINE-ESIDRIX, HYDRALAZINE
    HYDROCHLORIDE
AREDIA, PAMIDRONATE DISODIUM
BRETHAIRE, TERBUTALINE SULFATE
BUTAZOLIDIN, PHENYLBUTAZONE
CAFERGOT, CAFFEINE
CATAFLAM, DICLOFENAC POTASSIUM
CEDILANID-D, DESLANOSIDE
CIBACALCIN, CALCITONIN HUMAN
CLOZARIL, CLOZAPINE
COMBIPATCH, ESTRADIOL
CYTADREN, AMINOGLUTETHIMIDE
DESFERAL, DEFEROXAMINE MESYLATE
DIAPID, LYPRESSIN
DIOVAN HCT, HYDROCHLOROTHIAZIDE
DIOVAN, VALSARTAN
ELIDEL, PIMECROLIMUS
EMBOLEX, DIHYDROERGOTAMINE MESYLATE
ESIDRIX, HYDROCHLOROTHIAZIDE
ESIMIL, GUANETHIDINE MONOSULFATE
ESTRADERM, ESTRADIOL
EXELON, RIVASTIGMINE TARTRATE
FAMVIR, FAMCICLOVIR
FEMARA, LETROZOLE
FOCALIN, DEXMETHYLPHENIDATE HYDROCHLORIDE
FORADIL, FORMOTEROL FUMARATE
GLEEVEC, IMATINIB MESYLATE
HEAVY SOLUTION NUPERCAINE, DIBUCAINE
    HYDROCHLORIDE
HYDERGINE LC, ERGOLOID MESYLATES
HYDERGINE, ERGOLOID MESYLATES
IMIPRAMINE HCL, IMIPRAMINE HYDROCHLORIDE
INH, ISONIAZID
ISMELIN, GUANETHIDINE MONOSULFATE
LAMISIL, TERBINAFINE HYDROCHLORIDE
LAMPRENE, CLOFAZIMINE
LESCOL XL, FLUVASTATIN SODIUM
LESCOL, FLUVASTATIN SODIUM
LIORESAL, BACLOFEN
LOCORTEN, FLUMETHASONE PIVALATE
LOPRESSIDONE, CHLORTHALIDONE
LOPRESSOR HCT, HYDROCHLOROTHIAZIDE
LOPRESSOR, METOPROLOL FUMARATE
LOPRESSOR, METOPROLOL TARTRATE
LOTENSIN HCT, BENAZEPRIL HYDROCHLORIDE
LOTENSIN, BENAZEPRIL HYDROCHLORIDE
LOTREL, AMLODIPINE BESYLATE
LUDIOMIL, MAPROTILINE HYDROCHLORIDE
MELLARIL, THIORIDAZINE HYDROCHLORIDE
MELLARIL-S, THIORIDAZINE
MESANTOIN, MEPHENYTOIN
METANDREN, METHYLTESTOSTERONE
METHERGINE, METHYLERGONOVINE MALEATE
METOPIRONE, METYRAPONE
MIACALCIN, CALCITONIN, SALMON
NEORAL, CYCLOSPORINE
PARLODEL, BROMOCRIPTINE MESYLATE
PBZ, TRIPELENNAMINE CITRATE
PBZ, TRIPELENNAMINE HYDROCHLORIDE
PBZ-SR, TRIPELENNAMINE HYDROCHLORIDE
PERCORTEN, DESOXYCORTICOSTERONE ACETATE
PERCORTEN, DESOXYCORTICOSTERONE PIVALATE
PRISCOLINE, TOLAZOLINE HYDROCHLORIDE
REGITINE, PHENTOLAMINE MESYLATE

RITALIN LA, METHYLPHENIDATE HYDROCHLORIDE
RITALIN, METHYLPHENIDATE HYDROCHLORIDE
RITALIN-SR, METHYLPHENIDATE HYDROCHLORIDE
SANDIMMUNE, CYCLOSPORINE
SANDOSTATIN LAR, OCTREOTIDE ACETATE
SANDOSTATIN, OCTREOTIDE ACETATE
SANOREX, MAZINDOL
SANSERT, METHYSERGIDE MALEATE
SER-AP-ES, HYDRALAZINE HYDROCHLORIDE
SERENTIL, MESORIDAZINE BESYLATE
SERPASIL, RESERPINE
SERPASIL-APRESOLINE, HYDRALAZINE
    HYDROCHLORIDE
SERPASIL-ESIDRIX #1, HYDROCHLOROTHIAZIDE
SERPASIL-ESIDRIX #2, HYDROCHLOROTHIAZIDE
SLOW-K, POTASSIUM CHLORIDE
STARLIX, NATEGLINIDE
SYNTOCINON, OXYTOCIN
TANDEARIL, OXYPHENBUTAZONE
TAVIST D, CLEMASTINE FUMARATE
TAVIST, CLEMASTINE FUMARATE
TAVIST-1, CLEMASTINE FUMARATE
TAVIST-1, CLEMASTINE FUMARATE (OTC)
TAVIST-D, CLEMASTINE FUMARATE (OTC)
TEGRETOL, CARBAMAZEPINE
TEGRETOL-XR, CARBAMAZEPINE
TEN-K, POTASSIUM CHLORIDE
TOFRANIL, IMIPRAMINE HYDROCHLORIDE
TORECAN, THIETHYLPERAZINE MALATE
TORECAN, THIETHYLPERAZINE MALEATE
TRANSDERM-NITRO, NITROGLYCERIN
TRASICOR, OXPRENOLOL HYDROCHLORIDE
TREST, METHIXENE HYDROCHLORIDE
TRIAMINIC-12, CHLORPHENIRAMINE MALEATE (OTC)
TRIAMTERENE AND HYDROCHLOROTHIAZIDE,
    HYDROCHLOROTHIAZIDE
TRILEPTAL, OXCARBAZEPINE
VISKAZIDE, HYDROCHLOROTHIAZIDE
VISKEN, PINDOLOL
VIVELLE, ESTRADIOL
VIVELLE-DOT, ESTRADIOL
VOLTAREN, DICLOFENAC SODIUM
VOLTAREN-XR, DICLOFENAC SODIUM
ZELNORM, TEGASEROD MALEATE
ZOMETA, ZOLEDRONIC ACID
NOVAVAX
NOVAVAX INC
    AVC, SULFANILAMIDE
NOVEN
NOVEN PHARMACEUTICALS INC
    LIDOCAINE, LIDOCAINE
NOVEX
NOVEX PHARMA
    ALBUTEROL SULFATE, ALBUTEROL SULFATE
    BETAXOLOL, BETAXOLOL HYDROCHLORIDE
    BUTORPHANOL TARTRATE, BUTORPHANOL TARTRATE
    CARTEOLOL HCL, CARTEOLOL HYDROCHLORIDE
    CHLORHEXIDINE GLUCONATE, CHLORHEXIDINE
        GLUCONATE
    CIMETIDINE HCL, CIMETIDINE HYDROCHLORIDE
    CLEMASTINE FUMARATE, CLEMASTINE FUMARATE
    CROMOLYN SODIUM, CROMOLYN SODIUM
    FLUOXETINE, FLUOXETINE HYDROCHLORIDE
    IPRATROPIUM BROMIDE, IPRATROPIUM BROMIDE
    LACTULOSE, LACTULOSE
    LEVOBUNOLOL HCL, LEVOBUNOLOL HYDROCHLORIDE
    METAPROTERENOL SULFATE, METAPROTERENOL
        SULFATE

APPENDIX B
PRODUCT NAME INDEX
LISTED BY APPLICANT (*continued*)

MINOXIDIL (FOR MEN), MINOXIDIL (OTC)
MINOXIDIL (FOR WOMEN), MINOXIDIL (OTC)
MINOXIDIL EXTRA STRENGTH (FOR MEN), MINOXIDIL
  (OTC)
OXYBUTYNIN CHLORIDE, OXYBUTYNIN CHLORIDE
TIMOLOL MALEATE, TIMOLOL MALEATE
TOBRAMYCIN, TOBRAMYCIN
NOVO NORDISK
NOVO NORDISK PHARMACEUTICALS INC
  ACTIVELLA, ESTRADIOL
  GLUCAGEN, GLUCAGON HYDROCHLORIDE
    RECOMBINANT
  INNOFEM, ESTRADIOL
  INSULATARD NPH HUMAN, INSULIN SUSP ISOPHANE
    SEMISYNTHETIC PURIFIED HUMAN (OTC)
  INSULIN INSULATARD NPH NORDISK, INSULIN SUSP
    ISOPHANE PURIFIED PORK (OTC)
  INSULIN NORDISK MIXTARD (PORK), INSULIN PURIFIED
    PORK (OTC)
  INSULIN, INSULIN PORK (OTC)
  LENTARD, INSULIN ZINC SUSP PURIFIED BEEF/PORK
    (OTC)
  LENTE INSULIN, INSULIN ZINC SUSP BEEF (OTC)
  LENTE, INSULIN ZINC SUSP PURIFIED PORK (OTC)
  NORDITROPIN, SOMATROPIN RECOMBINANT
  NOVOLIN 70/30, INSULIN RECOMBINANT HUMAN (OTC)
  NOVOLIN 70/30, INSULIN RECOMBINANT PURIFIED
    HUMAN (OTC)
  NOVOLIN L, INSULIN ZINC SUSP RECOMBINANT HUMAN
    (OTC)
  NOVOLIN L, INSULIN ZINC SUSP SEMISYNTHETIC
    PURIFIED HUMAN (OTC)
  NOVOLIN N, INSULIN SUSP ISOPHANE RECOMBINANT
    HUMAN (OTC)
  NOVOLIN N, INSULIN SUSP ISOPHANE SEMISYNTHETIC
    PURIFIED HUMAN (OTC)
  NOVOLIN R, INSULIN RECOMBINANT HUMAN (OTC)
  NOVOLIN R, INSULIN RECOMBINANT PURIFIED HUMAN
    (OTC)
  NOVOLOG MIX 70/30, INSULIN ASPART
  NOVOLOG, INSULIN ASPART
  NPH INSULIN, INSULIN SUSP ISOPHANE BEEF (OTC)
  NPH PURIFIED PORK ISOPHANE INSULIN, INSULIN SUSP
    ISOPHANE PURIFIED PORK (OTC)
  PRANDIN, REPAGLINIDE
  REGULAR INSULIN, INSULIN PORK (OTC)
  REGULAR PURIFIED PORK INSULIN, INSULIN PURIFIED
    PORK (OTC)
  SEMILENTE INSULIN, INSULIN ZINC SUSP PROMPT
    BEEF (OTC)
  SEMILENTE, INSULIN ZINC SUSP PROMPT PURIFIED
    PORK (OTC)
  ULTRALENTE INSULIN, INSULIN ZINC SUSP EXTENDED
    BEEF (OTC)
  ULTRALENTE, INSULIN ZINC SUSP EXTENDED PURIFIED
    BEEF (OTC)
  VAGIFEM, ESTRADIOL
  VELOSULIN BR HUMAN, INSULIN RECOMBINANT
    PURIFIED HUMAN (OTC)
  VELOSULIN BR, INSULIN RECOMBINANT HUMAN (OTC)
  VELOSULIN, INSULIN PURIFIED PORK (OTC)
NOVOCOL
NOVOCOL PHARMACEUTICAL INC
  ISOCAINE HCL W/ LEVONORDEFRIN, LEVONORDEFRIN
  ISOCAINE HCL, MEPIVACAINE HYDROCHLORIDE
NUMARK
NUMARK LABORATORIES INC
  MELFIAT, PHENDIMETRAZINE TARTRATE

MELFIAT-105, PHENDIMETRAZINE TARTRATE
PHENDIMETRAZINE TARTRATE, PHENDIMETRAZINE
  TARTRATE
SPRX-105, PHENDIMETRAZINE TARTRATE
NYLOS
NYLOS TRADING CO INC
  METHOCARBAMOL, METHOCARBAMOL
  PREDNISONE, PREDNISONE
  TRIHEXYPHENIDYL HCL, TRIHEXYPHENIDYL
    HYDROCHLORIDE
  TRIPELENNAMINE HCL, TRIPELENNAMINE
    HYDROCHLORIDE

O

OCLASSEN
OCLASSEN PHARMACEUTICALS INC
  CONDYLOX, PODOFILOX
  CORDRAN SP, FLURANDRENOLIDE
  CORDRAN, FLURANDRENOLIDE
  MONODOX, DOXYCYCLINE
ODYSSEY PHARMS
ODYSSEY PHARMACEUTICALS INC
  ANTABUSE, DISULFIRAM
  NYSTATIN, NYSTATIN
  URECHOLINE, BETHANECHOL CHLORIDE
  VIVACTIL, PROTRIPTYLINE HYDROCHLORIDE
OHM
OHM CORP
  IBUPROFEN, IBUPROFEN (OTC)
OHM LABS
OHM LABORATORIES INC
  CHLORZOXAZONE, CHLORZOXAZONE
  IBUPROFEN, IBUPROFEN
  IBUPROHM COLD AND SINUS, IBUPROFEN (OTC)
  IBUPROHM, IBUPROFEN
  IBUPROHM, IBUPROFEN (OTC)
  LOPERAMIDE HCL, LOPERAMIDE HYDROCHLORIDE
    (OTC)
ONY
ONY INC
  INFASURF PRESERVATIVE FREE, CALFACTANT
OPTOPICS
OPTOPICS LABORATORIES CORP
  OPTOMYCIN, CHLORAMPHENICOL
  PARACAINE, PROPARACAINE HYDROCHLORIDE
  SULFACEL-15, SULFACETAMIDE SODIUM
ORAPHARMA
ORAPHARMA INC
  ARESTIN, MINOCYCLINE HYDROCHLORIDE
ORGANICS LAGRANGE
ORGANICS LAGRANGE INC
  CORTICOTROPIN, CORTICOTROPIN
ORGANON
ORGANON INC SUB AKZONA INC
  LIQUAMAR, PHENPROCOUMON
ORGANON USA
ORGANON USA INC
  HEXADROL, DEXAMETHASONE
ORGANON USA INC

  ANTAGON, GANIRELIX ACETATE
  ARDUAN, PIPECURONIUM BROMIDE
  CALDEROL, CALCIFEDIOL
  CORTROPHIN-ZINC, CORTICOTROPIN-ZINC
    HYDROXIDE
  COTAZYM, LIPASE

APPENDIX B
PRODUCT NAME INDEX
LISTED BY APPLICANT (*continued*)

CYCLESSA, DESOGESTREL
DECA-DURABOLIN, NANDROLONE DECANOATE
DESOGEN, DESOGESTREL
DOCA, DESOXYCORTICOSTERONE ACETATE
DURABOLIN, NANDROLONE PHENPROPIONATE
FOLLISTIM, FOLLITROPIN ALFA/BETA
FUROSEMIDE, FUROSEMIDE
HEPARIN SODIUM, HEPARIN SODIUM
HEXADROL, DEXAMETHASONE
HEXADROL, DEXAMETHASONE SODIUM PHOSPHATE
HUMEGON, MENOTROPINS (FSH;LH)
LIQUAEMIN LOCK FLUSH, HEPARIN SODIUM
LIQUAEMIN SODIUM PRESERVATIVE FREE, HEPARIN
    SODIUM
LIQUAEMIN SODIUM, HEPARIN SODIUM
LYNORAL, ETHINYL ESTRADIOL
MAXIBOLIN, ETHYLESTRENOL
METHYLPREDNISOLONE, METHYLPREDNISOLONE
    SODIUM SUCCINATE
MIRCETTE, DESOGESTREL
NORCURON, VECURONIUM BROMIDE
NUVARING, ETHINYL ESTRADIOL
ORGARAN, DANAPAROID SODIUM
ORGATRAX, HYDROXYZINE HYDROCHLORIDE
PAVULON, PANCURONIUM BROMIDE
PREGNYL, GONADOTROPIN, CHORIONIC
PURIFIED CORTROPHIN GEL, CORTICOTROPIN
RAPLON, RAPACURONIUM BROMIDE
REMERON SOLTAB, MIRTAZAPINE
REMERON, MIRTAZAPINE
REVERSOL, EDROPHONIUM CHLORIDE
SUCCINYLCHOLINE CHLORIDE, SUCCINYLCHOLINE
    CHLORIDE
WIGRAINE, CAFFEINE
WIGRETTES, ERGOTAMINE TARTRATE
ZEMURON (P/F), ROCURONIUM BROMIDE
ZEMURON, ROCURONIUM BROMIDE
ORIDION
ORIDION BREATHID INC
    IDKIT:HP, CITRIC ACID
ORION
ORION CORP
    COMTAN, ENTACAPONE
    FARESTON, TOREMIFENE CITRATE
ORION PHARMA INC
ORION PHARMACEUTICALS INC
    STALEVO 100, CARBIDOPA
    STALEVO 150, CARBIDOPA
    STALEVO 50, CARBIDOPA
ORPHAN MEDCL
ORPHAN MEDICAL INC
    ANTIZOL, FOMEPIZOLE
    CYSTADANE, BETAINE, ANHYDROUS
    XYREM, SODIUM OXYBATE
ORTHO BIOTECH
ORTHO BIOTECH PRODUCTS LP
    LEUSTATIN, CLADRIBINE
ORTHO MCNEIL
ORTHO MCNEIL PHARMACEUTICAL
    DIENESTROL, DIENESTROL
    HALDOL, HALOPERIDOL
    HALDOL, HALOPERIDOL DECANOATE
    HALDOL, HALOPERIDOL LACTATE
    TOPAMAX SPRINKLE, TOPIRAMATE
ORTHO MCNEIL PHARM
ORTHO MCNEIL PHARMACEUTICAL INC
    CLISTIN, CARBINOXAMINE MALEATE
    ESTRADIOL, ESTRADIOL

FLOXIN IN DEXTROSE 5% IN PLASTIC CONTAINER,
    OFLOXACIN
FLOXIN IN DEXTROSE 5%, OFLOXACIN
FLOXIN, OFLOXACIN
HALDOL SOLUTAB, HALOPERIDOL
INJECTAPAP, ACETAMINOPHEN
LEVAQUIN IN DEXTROSE 5% IN PLASTIC CONTAINER,
    LEVOFLOXACIN
LEVAQUIN, LEVOFLOXACIN
MICRONOR, NORETHINDRONE
MODICON 21, ETHINYL ESTRADIOL
MODICON 28, ETHINYL ESTRADIOL
MONISTAT 3, MICONAZOLE NITRATE
ORTHO CYCLEN-21, ETHINYL ESTRADIOL
ORTHO CYCLEN-28, ETHINYL ESTRADIOL
ORTHO EVRA, ETHINYL ESTRADIOL
ORTHO TRI-CYCLEN, ETHINYL ESTRADIOL
ORTHO-CEPT, DESOGESTREL
ORTHO-N0VUM 1/80 28, MESTRANOL
ORTHO-NOVUM 1/35-21, ETHINYL ESTRADIOL
ORTHO-NOVUM 1/35-28, ETHINYL ESTRADIOL
ORTHO-NOVUM 1/50 21, MESTRANOL
ORTHO-NOVUM 1/50 28, MESTRANOL
ORTHO-NOVUM 1/80 21, MESTRANOL
ORTHO-NOVUM 10-21, MESTRANOL
ORTHO-NOVUM 10/11-21, ETHINYL ESTRADIOL
ORTHO-NOVUM 10/11-28 IN PLASTIC CONTAINER,
    ETHINYL ESTRADIOL
ORTHO-NOVUM 2-21, MESTRANOL
ORTHO-NOVUM 7/14-21, ETHINYL ESTRADIOL
ORTHO-NOVUM 7/14-28, ETHINYL ESTRADIOL
ORTHO-NOVUM 7/7/7-21, ETHINYL ESTRADIOL
ORTHO-NOVUM 7/7/7-28, ETHINYL ESTRADIOL
PARAFLEX, CHLORZOXAZONE
PARAFON FORTE DSC, CHLORZOXAZONE
PROTOSTAT, METRONIDAZOLE
SALPIX, ACETRIZOATE SODIUM
SULTRIN, TRIPLE SULFA (SULFABENZAMIDE;
    SULFACETAMIDE; SULFATHIAZOLE)
TERAZOL 3, TERCONAZOLE
TERAZOL 7, TERCONAZOLE
THEOPHYL, THEOPHYLLINE
THEOPHYL-225, THEOPHYLLINE
THEOPHYL-SR, THEOPHYLLINE
TOLECTIN 600, TOLMETIN SODIUM
TOLECTIN DS, TOLMETIN SODIUM
TOLECTIN, TOLMETIN SODIUM
TOPAMAX, TOPIRAMATE
TYCOLET, ACETAMINOPHEN
TYLENOL W/ CODEINE NO. 1, ACETAMINOPHEN
TYLENOL W/ CODEINE NO. 2, ACETAMINOPHEN
TYLENOL W/ CODEINE NO. 3, ACETAMINOPHEN
TYLENOL W/ CODEINE NO. 4, ACETAMINOPHEN
TYLENOL W/ CODEINE, ACETAMINOPHEN
TYLOX, ACETAMINOPHEN
TYLOX-325, ACETAMINOPHEN
ULTRACET, ACETAMINOPHEN
ULTRAM, TRAMADOL HYDROCHLORIDE
URISPAS, FLAVOXATE HYDROCHLORIDE
VASCOR, BEPRIDIL HYDROCHLORIDE
OTSUKA
OTSUKA PHARMACEUTICAL CO LTD
    ABILIFY, ARIPIPRAZOLE
    FERRISELTZ, FERRIC AMMONIUM CITRATE
    PLETAL, CILOSTAZOL
    RAXAR, GREPAFLOXACIN HYDROCHLORIDE
OVATION PHARMS
OVATION PHARMACEUTICALS INC

APPENDIX B
PRODUCT NAME INDEX
LISTED BY APPLICANT (*continued*)

DESOXYN, METHAMPHETAMINE HYDROCHLORIDE
PEGANONE, ETHOTOIN
TRANXENE SD, CLORAZEPATE DIPOTASSIUM
TRANXENE, CLORAZEPATE DIPOTASSIUM
OXFORD PHARM
OXFORD PHARMACEUTICAL SERVICES INC
   MARPLAN, ISOCARBOXAZID

P

PACIFIC PHARMA
PACIFIC PHARMA
   TIMOLOL MALEATE, TIMOLOL MALEATE
PACIFIC PHARMA INC
   TIMOLOL MALEATE, TIMOLOL MALEATE
PACO
PACO PHARMACEUTICAL SERVICES INC
   LACTULOSE, LACTULOSE
PACO RESEARCH CORP
   GENTAMICIN SULFATE, GENTAMICIN SULFATE
   LIDOCAINE HCL, LIDOCAINE HYDROCHLORIDE
   METOCLOPRAMIDE HCL, METOCLOPRAMIDE
     HYDROCHLORIDE
   THIOTHIXENE HCL, THIOTHIXENE HYDROCHLORIDE
PADDOCK
PADDOCK LABORATORIES INC
   AMMONIUM LACTATE, AMMONIUM LACTATE
   BACITRACIN, BACITRACIN
   CLINDA-DERM, CLINDAMYCIN PHOSPHATE
   COLOCORT, HYDROCORTISONE
   COMPRO, PROCHLORPERAZINE
   CONDYLOX, PODOFILOX
   DIHYDROEROGTAMINE MESYLATE,
     DIHYDROERGOTAMINE MESYLATE
   ERYTHRA-DERM, ERYTHROMYCIN
   ERYTHROMYCIN, ERYTHROMYCIN
   HYDROCORTISONE, HYDROCORTISONE
   KIONEX, SODIUM POLYSTYRENE SULFONATE
   NYSTATIN, NYSTATIN
   NYSTOP, NYSTATIN
   PODOFILOX, PODOFILOX
   POLYMYXIN B SULFATE, POLYMYXIN B SULFATE
   PROMETHAZINE HCL, PROMETHAZINE
     HYDROCHLORIDE
PAL PAK
PAL PAK INC
   AMINOPHYLLINE, AMINOPHYLLINE
   RAUVAL, RAUWOLFIA SERPENTINA
   TRIPLE SULFOID, TRISULFAPYRIMIDINES
     (SULFADIAZINE; SULFAMERAZINE;
     SULFAMETHAZINE)
PANRAY
PANRAY CORP SUB ORMONT DRUG AND CHEMICAL CO
INC
   AMINOPHYLLINE, AMINOPHYLLINE
   CHLORPHENIRAMINE MALEATE, CHLORPHENIRAMINE
     MALEATE
   CINNASIL, RESCINNAMINE
   CORTISONE ACETATE, CORTISONE ACETATE
   HYDROCORTISONE, HYDROCORTISONE
   ISONIAZID, ISONIAZID
   KOGLUCOID, RAUWOLFIA SERPENTINA
   PARASAL SODIUM, AMINOSALICYLATE SODIUM
   PARASAL, AMINOSALICYLIC ACID
   PREDNISOLONE, PREDNISOLONE
   PREDNISONE, PREDNISONE
   PROCAPAN, PROCAINAMIDE HYDROCHLORIDE

   SERPANRAY, RESERPINE
   THEOLIXIR, THEOPHYLLINE
PAR PHARM
PAR PHARMACEUTICAL INC
   ACEBUTOLOL HCL, ACEBUTOLOL HYDROCHLORIDE
   ALLOPURINOL, ALLOPURINOL
   AMILORIDE HCL, AMILORIDE HYDROCHLORIDE
   AMITRIPTYLINE HCL, AMITRIPTYLINE HYDROCHLORIDE
   BENZTROPINE MESYLATE, BENZTROPINE MESYLATE
   BROMPHENIRAMINE MALEATE, BROMPHENIRAMINE
     MALEATE
   BUSPIRONE HCL, BUSPIRONE HYDROCHLORIDE
   CAPOTEN, CAPTOPRIL
   CAPTOPRIL, CAPTOPRIL
   CARISOPRODOL AND ASPIRIN, ASPIRIN
   CHLORDIAZEPOXIDE AND AMITRIPTYLINE HCL,
     AMITRIPTYLINE HYDROCHLORIDE
   CHLORPROPAMIDE, CHLORPROPAMIDE
   CHLORZOXAZONE, CHLORZOXAZONE
   CLOMIPHENE CITRATE, CLOMIPHENE CITRATE
   CLONIDINE HCL AND CHLORTHALIDONE,
     CHLORTHALIDONE
   CLONIDINE HCL, CLONIDINE HYDROCHLORIDE
   CYPROHEPTADINE HCL, CYPROHEPTADINE
     HYDROCHLORIDE
   DEXAMETHASONE, DEXAMETHASONE
   DIAZEPAM, DIAZEPAM
   DIPHENOXYLATE HCL AND ATROPINE SULFATE,
     ATROPINE SULFATE
   DISULFIRAM, DISULFIRAM
   DOXEPIN HCL, DOXEPIN HYDROCHLORIDE
   DOXY-SLEEP-AID, DOXYLAMINE SUCCINATE (OTC)
   DOXYCYCLINE HYCLATE, DOXYCYCLINE HYCLATE
   DOXYCYCLINE, DOXYCYCLINE
   FENOPROFEN CALCIUM, FENOPROFEN CALCIUM
   FLUPHENAZINE HCL, FLUPHENAZINE HYDROCHLORIDE
   FLURAZEPAM HCL, FLURAZEPAM HYDROCHLORIDE
   HALOPERIDOL, HALOPERIDOL
   HYDRA-ZIDE, HYDRALAZINE HYDROCHLORIDE
   HYDRALAZINE HCL, HYDRALAZINE HYDROCHLORIDE
   HYDRO-RIDE, AMILORIDE HYDROCHLORIDE
   HYDROFLUMETHIAZIDE, HYDROFLUMETHIAZIDE
   HYDROXYUREA, HYDROXYUREA
   HYDROXYZINE HCL, HYDROXYZINE HYDROCHLORIDE
   HYDROXYZINE PAMOATE, HYDROXYZINE PAMOATE
   IBUPROFEN, IBUPROFEN
   IBUPROFEN, IBUPROFEN (OTC)
   IMIPRAMINE HCL, IMIPRAMINE HYDROCHLORIDE
   INDOMETHACIN, INDOMETHACIN
   ISOSORBIDE DINITRATE, ISOSORBIDE DINITRATE
   LEUCOVORIN CALCIUM, LEUCOVORIN CALCIUM
   LISINOPRIL, LISINOPRIL
   LORAZEPAM, LORAZEPAM
   MECLIZINE HCL, MECLIZINE HYDROCHLORIDE
   MECLOFENAMATE SODIUM, MECLOFENAMATE SODIUM
   MEGESTROL ACETATE, MEGESTROL ACETATE
   MEPROBAMATE AND ASPIRIN, ASPIRIN
   METAPROTERENOL SULFATE, METAPROTERENOL
     SULFATE
   METHOCARBAMOL AND ASPIRIN, ASPIRIN
   METHOCARBAMOL, METHOCARBAMOL
   METHYCLOTHIAZIDE, METHYCLOTHIAZIDE
   METHYLDOPA AND CHLOROTHIAZIDE,
     CHLOROTHIAZIDE
   METHYLDOPA AND HYDROCHLOROTHIAZIDE,
     HYDROCHLOROTHIAZIDE
   METHYLDOPA, METHYLDOPA
   METHYLPREDNISOLONE, METHYLPREDNISOLONE

APPENDIX B
PRODUCT NAME INDEX
LISTED BY APPLICANT (*continued*)

METOCLOPRAMIDE HCL, METOCLOPRAMIDE
    HYDROCHLORIDE
METOPROLOL TARTRATE, METOPROLOL TARTRATE
METRONIDAZOLE, METRONIDAZOLE
MINOCYCLINE HCL, MINOCYCLINE HYDROCHLORIDE
MINOXIDIL, MINOXIDIL
NYSTATIN, NYSTATIN
ORPHENGESIC FORTE, ASPIRIN
ORPHENGESIC, ASPIRIN
PERPHENAZINE AND AMITRIPTYLINE HCL,
    AMITRIPTYLINE HYDROCHLORIDE
PROPANTHELINE BROMIDE, PROPANTHELINE
    BROMIDE
PROPRANOLOL HCL, PROPRANOLOL HYDROCHLORIDE
RANITIDINE HCL, RANITIDINE HYDROCHLORIDE
RESERPINE AND HYDROFLUMETHIAZIDE,
    HYDROFLUMETHIAZIDE
SULFAMETHOPRIM, SULFAMETHOXAZOLE
SULFAMETHOPRIM-DS, SULFAMETHOXAZOLE
SULFINPYRAZONE, SULFINPYRAZONE
SUMYCIN, TETRACYCLINE HYDROCHLORIDE
TEMAZEPAM, TEMAZEPAM
THIORIDAZINE HCL, THIORIDAZINE HYDROCHLORIDE
TOLAZAMIDE, TOLAZAMIDE
TORSEMIDE, TORSEMIDE
TRICHLORMETHIAZIDE, TRICHLORMETHIAZIDE
VALPROIC ACID, VALPROIC ACID
PARKE DAVIS
PARKE DAVIS DIV WARNER LAMBERT CO
    AMBODRYL, BROMODIPHENHYDRAMINE
        HYDROCHLORIDE
    AMCILL, AMPICILLIN/AMPICILLIN TRIHYDRATE
    BENADRYL PRESERVATIVE FREE, DIPHENHYDRAMINE
        HYDROCHLORIDE
    BENADRYL, DIPHENHYDRAMINE HYDROCHLORIDE
    BENYLIN, DIPHENHYDRAMINE HYDROCHLORIDE (OTC)
    CAMOQUIN HCL, AMODIAQUINE HYDROCHLORIDE
    CELONTIN, METHSUXIMIDE
    CENTRAX, PRAZEPAM
    CEREBYX, FOSPHENYTOIN SODIUM
    CHLORDIAZEPOXIDE HCL, CHLORDIAZEPOXIDE
        HYDROCHLORIDE
    CHOLEDYL SA, OXTRIPHYLLINE
    CHOLEDYL, OXTRIPHYLLINE
    CHOLYBAR, CHOLESTYRAMINE
    COLY-MYCIN S, COLISTIN SULFATE
    DILANTIN, PHENYTOIN SODIUM, EXTENDED
    DILANTIN-125, PHENYTOIN
    DILANTIN-30, PHENYTOIN
    DIPHENOXYLATE HCL AND ATROPINE SULFATE,
        ATROPINE SULFATE
    ERGOSTAT, ERGOTAMINE TARTRATE
    ERYC 125, ERYTHROMYCIN
    ERYC, ERYTHROMYCIN
    ERYPAR, ERYTHROMYCIN STEARATE
    ERYTHROMYCIN ETHYLSUCCINATE, ERYTHROMYCIN
        ETHYLSUCCINATE
    ESTROVIS, QUINESTROL
    EUTHROID-0.5, LIOTRIX (T4;T3)
    EUTHROID-1, LIOTRIX (T4;T3)
    EUTHROID-2, LIOTRIX (T4;T3)
    EUTHROID-3, LIOTRIX (T4;T3)
    EVANS BLUE, EVANS BLUE
    HEPARIN LOCK FLUSH, HEPARIN SODIUM
    HEPARIN SODIUM, HEPARIN SODIUM
    HUMATIN, PAROMOMYCIN SULFATE
    HYDROCORTISONE ACETATE, HYDROCORTISONE
        ACETATE

    HYDROCORTISONE, HYDROCORTISONE
    INDOMETHACIN, INDOMETHACIN
    ISOPROTERENOL HCL, ISOPROTERENOL
        HYDROCHLORIDE
    MECLOMEN, MECLOFENAMATE SODIUM
    MEPERIDINE HCL, MEPERIDINE HYDROCHLORIDE
    MEPROBAMATE, MEPROBAMATE
    METHYLDOPA AND HYDROCHLOROTHIAZIDE,
        HYDROCHLOROTHIAZIDE
    METHYLDOPA, METHYLDOPA
    METHYLTESTOSTERONE, METHYLTESTOSTERONE
    MILONTIN, PHENSUXIMIDE
    NARDIL, PHENELZINE SULFATE
    NEURONTIN, GABAPENTIN
    NITROSTAT, NITROGLYCERIN
    NORLUTATE, NORETHINDRONE ACETATE
    NORLUTIN, NORETHINDRONE
    OXAZEPAM, OXAZEPAM
    PARACORT, PREDNISONE
    PARSIDOL, ETHOPROPAZINE HYDROCHLORIDE
    PENAPAR-VK, PENICILLIN V POTASSIUM
    PENICILLIN G POTASSIUM, PENICILLIN G POTASSIUM
    PENICILLIN G PROCAINE, PENICILLIN G PROCAINE
    PITRESSIN TANNATE, VASOPRESSIN TANNATE
    POVAN, PYRVINIUM PAMOATE
    PRE-SATE, CHLORPHENTERMINE HYDROCHLORIDE
    PROCAN SR, PROCAINAMIDE HYDROCHLORIDE
    PROCAN, PROCAINAMIDE HYDROCHLORIDE
    PROLOID, THYROGLOBULIN
    PROMAPAR, CHLORPROMAZINE HYDROCHLORIDE
    SECOBARBITAL SODIUM, SECOBARBITAL SODIUM
    SODIUM PENTOBARBITAL, PENTOBARBITAL SODIUM
    SPIRONOLACTONE W/ HYDROCHLOROTHIAZIDE,
        HYDROCHLOROTHIAZIDE
    SULFALAR, SULFISOXAZOLE
    THIAMINE HCL, THIAMINE HYDROCHLORIDE
    TOLBUTAMIDE, TOLBUTAMIDE
    TRIPELENNAMINE HCL, TRIPELENNAMINE
        HYDROCHLORIDE
    UTICORT, BETAMETHASONE BENZOATE
    UTIMOX, AMOXICILLIN
    ZARONTIN, ETHOSUXIMIDE
PARKE DAVIS LABORATORIES DIV WARNER LAMBERT CO
    NORLESTRIN 21 1/50, ETHINYL ESTRADIOL
    NORLESTRIN 21 2.5/50, ETHINYL ESTRADIOL
    NORLESTRIN 28 1/50, ETHINYL ESTRADIOL
    NORLESTRIN FE 1/50, ETHINYL ESTRADIOL
    NORLESTRIN FE 2.5/50, ETHINYL ESTRADIOL
PARKE DAVIS PHARMACEUTICAL RESEARCH DIV WARNER
LAMBERT CO
    CHLOROMYCETIN PALMITATE, CHLORAMPHENICOL
        PALMITATE
    CHLOROMYCETIN, CHLORAMPHENICOL
    CHLOROMYXIN, CHLORAMPHENICOL
    DILANTIN, PHENYTOIN SODIUM
    ELASE-CHLOROMYCETIN, CHLORAMPHENICOL
    FEMPATCH, ESTRADIOL
    ISOETHARINE HCL, ISOETHARINE HYDROCHLORIDE
    UTICORT, BETAMETHASONE BENZOATE
    ZARONTIN, ETHOSUXIMIDE
PARKEDALE
PARKEDALE PHARMACEUTICALS INC
    ACTH, CORTICOTROPIN
    ANUSOL HC, HYDROCORTISONE
    CHLOROMYCETIN HYDROCORTISONE,
        CHLORAMPHENICOL
    CHLOROMYCETIN, CHLORAMPHENICOL

APPENDIX B
PRODUCT NAME INDEX
LISTED BY APPLICANT (*continued*)

CHLOROMYCETIN, CHLORAMPHENICOL SODIUM
    SUCCINATE
COLY-MYCIN M, COLISTIMETHATE SODIUM
COLY-MYCIN S, COLISTIN SULFATE
HUMATIN, PAROMOMYCIN SULFATE
KETALAR, KETAMINE HYDROCHLORIDE
OPHTHOCHLOR, CHLORAMPHENICOL
OPHTHOCORT, CHLORAMPHENICOL
PITOCIN, OXYTOCIN
PROCAN SR, PROCAINAMIDE HYDROCHLORIDE
SURITAL, THIAMYLAL SODIUM
THEELIN, ESTRONE
VIRA-A, VIDARABINE
PARNELL
PARNELL PHARMACEUTICALS INC
    TRIAMCINOLONE ACETONIDE, TRIAMCINOLONE
      ACETONIDE
PEDINOL
PEDINOL PHARMACAL INC
    GRIS-PEG, GRISEOFULVIN, ULTRAMICROCRYSTALLINE
PENNEX
PENNEX PRODUCTS CO INC
    ALUMINUM HYDROXIDE AND MAGNESIUM TRISILICATE,
      ALUMINUM HYDROXIDE (OTC)
PERRIGO
L PERRIGO CO
    ACETAMINOPHEN, ACETAMINOPHEN (OTC)
    ACETAMINOPHEN, ASPIRIN AND CAFFEINE,
      ACETAMINOPHEN (OTC)
    ANTITUSSIVE, DIPHENHYDRAMINE HYDROCHLORIDE
      (OTC)
    CAP-PROFEN, IBUPROFEN (OTC)
    CHILDREN'S IBUPROFEN, IBUPROFEN (OTC)
    CIMETIDINE, CIMETIDINE (OTC)
    CROMOLYN SODIUM, CROMOLYN SODIUM (OTC)
    DIPHENHYDRAMINE HCL, DIPHENHYDRAMINE
      HYDROCHLORIDE
    DOXYLAMINE SUCCINATE, DOXYLAMINE SUCCINATE
      (OTC)
    IBUPROFEN, IBUPROFEN (OTC)
    ISONIAZID, ISONIAZID
    KETOPROFEN, KETOPROFEN (OTC)
    LOPERAMIDE HCL AND SIMETHICONE, LOPERAMIDE
      HYDROCHLORIDE (OTC)
    LOPERAMIDE HCL, LOPERAMIDE HYDROCHLORIDE
      (OTC)
    MEPROBAMATE, MEPROBAMATE
    MICONAZOLE NITRATE, MICONAZOLE NITRATE (OTC)
    MINOXIDIL EXTRA STRENGTH (FOR MEN), MINOXIDIL
      (OTC)
    NAPROXEN SODIUM, NAPROXEN SODIUM (OTC)
    PREDNISOLONE, PREDNISOLONE
    PREDNISONE, PREDNISONE
    PROPYLTHIOURACIL, PROPYLTHIOURACIL
    QUINIDINE SULFATE, QUINIDINE SULFATE
    RANITIDINE, RANITIDINE HYDROCHLORIDE (OTC)
    SODIUM PENTOBARBITAL, PENTOBARBITAL SODIUM
    SODIUM SECOBARBITAL, SECOBARBITAL SODIUM
    TAB-PROFEN, IBUPROFEN (OTC)
    THEOPHYLLINE, THEOPHYLLINE
    TIOCONAZOLE, TIOCONAZOLE (OTC)
PERRIGO CO
    CIMETIDINE, CIMETIDINE (OTC)
    CLEMASTINE FUMARATE, CLEMASTINE FUMARATE
      (OTC)
    IBUPROFEN, IBUPROFEN (OTC)
    JUNIOR STRENGTH IBUPROFEN, IBUPROFEN (OTC)

LOPERAMIDE HCL, LOPERAMIDE HYDROCHLORIDE
    (OTC)
MICONAZOLE NITRATE COMBINATION PACK,
    MICONAZOLE NITRATE (OTC)
MINOXIDIL (FOR MEN), MINOXIDIL (OTC)
MINOXIDIL (FOR WOMEN), MINOXIDIL (OTC)
PSEUDOEPHEDRINE HCL, PSEUDOEPHEDRINE
    HYDROCHLORIDE (OTC)
PERSONAL PRODS
PERSONAL PRODUCTS CO
    DELFEN, NONOXYNOL-9 (OTC)
    MONISTAT 3 COMBINATION PACK (PREFILLED),
      MICONAZOLE NITRATE (OTC)
    MONISTAT 3 COMBINATION PACK, MICONAZOLE
      NITRATE (OTC)
    MONISTAT 5, MICONAZOLE NITRATE
    MONISTAT DUAL- PAK, MICONAZOLE NITRATE
PFIPHARMECS
PFIPHARMECS DIV PFIZER INC
    CORTRIL, HYDROCORTISONE
    TETRACYN, TETRACYCLINE HYDROCHLORIDE
PFIZER
PFIZER AGRICULTURAL DIV
    ANTIVERT, MECLIZINE HYDROCHLORIDE
    NORVASC, AMLODIPINE BESYLATE
    VIAGRA, SILDENAFIL CITRATE
PFIZER CENTRAL RESEARCH
    DIFLUCAN, FLUCONAZOLE
    TROVAN, TROVAFLOXACIN MESYLATE
    ZITHROMAX, AZITHROMYCIN DIHYDRATE
PFIZER CHEMICALS DIV PFIZER INC
    DIFLUCAN, FLUCONAZOLE
    TROVAN PRESERVATIVE FREE, ALATROFLOXACIN
      MESYLATE
    ZITHROMAX, AZITHROMYCIN DIHYDRATE
PFIZER INC
    ATARAX, HYDROXYZINE HYDROCHLORIDE
    CEFOBID, CEFOPERAZONE SODIUM
    DIFLUCAN IN DEXTROSE 5% IN PLASTIC CONTAINER,
      FLUCONAZOLE
    DIFLUCAN IN SODIUM CHLORIDE 0.9% IN PLASTIC
      CONTAINER, FLUCONAZOLE
    DIFLUCAN IN SODIUM CHLORIDE 0.9%, FLUCONAZOLE
    EMETE-CON, BENZQUINAMIDE HYDROCHLORIDE
    GEODON, ZIPRASIDONE HYDROCHLORIDE
    GEODON, ZIPRASIDONE MESYLATE
    GLUCOTROL XL, GLIPIZIDE
    GLUCOTROL, GLIPIZIDE
    LIPITOR, ATORVASTATIN CALCIUM
    LITHIUM CARBONATE, LITHIUM CARBONATE
    MINIPRESS XL, PRAZOSIN HYDROCHLORIDE
    MINIZIDE, POLYTHIAZIDE
    NAVANE, THIOTHIXENE
    NAVANE, THIOTHIXENE HYDROCHLORIDE
    PROCARDIA, NIFEDIPINE
    RENESE, POLYTHIAZIDE
    RID MOUSSE, PIPERONYL BUTOXIDE (OTC)
    UNASYN, AMPICILLIN SODIUM
    VFEND, VORICONAZOLE
    VISINE-A, NAPHAZOLINE HYDROCHLORIDE (OTC)
    ZITHROMAX, AZITHROMYCIN DIHYDRATE
    ZYRTEC, CETIRIZINE HYDROCHLORIDE
    ZYRTEC-D 12 HOUR, CETIRIZINE HYDROCHLORIDE
PFIZER LABORATORIES DIV PFIZER INC
    BACITRACIN, BACITRACIN
    CARDURA, DOXAZOSIN MESYLATE
    CEFOBID IN PLASTIC CONTAINER, CEFOPERAZONE
      SODIUM

APPENDIX B
PRODUCT NAME INDEX
LISTED BY APPLICANT (*continued*)

CEFOBID, CEFOPERAZONE SODIUM
CORTRIL, HYDROCORTISONE
CORTRIL, HYDROCORTISONE ACETATE
DARICON, OXYPHENCYCLIMINE HYDROCHLORIDE
DIABINESE, CHLORPROPAMIDE
FELDENE, PIROXICAM
FOVANE, BENZTHIAZIDE
GEOCILLIN, CARBENICILLIN INDANYL SODIUM
MAGNACORT, HYDROCORTAMATE HYDROCHLORIDE
MINIPRESS, PRAZOSIN HYDROCHLORIDE
MITHRACIN, PLICAMYCIN
MODERIL, RESCINNAMINE
NEOBIOTIC, NEOMYCIN SULFATE
PENICILLIN G POTASSIUM, PENICILLIN G POTASSIUM
PENICILLIN G PROCAINE, PENICILLIN G PROCAINE
PERMAPEN, PENICILLIN G BENZATHINE
PFIZER-E, ERYTHROMYCIN STEARATE
PFIZERPEN G, PENICILLIN G POTASSIUM
PFIZERPEN VK, PENICILLIN V POTASSIUM
PFIZERPEN, PENICILLIN G POTASSIUM
PFIZERPEN-A, AMPICILLIN/AMPICILLIN TRIHYDRATE
PFIZERPEN-AS, PENICILLIN G PROCAINE
PROCARDIA XL, NIFEDIPINE
RENESE-R, POLYTHIAZIDE
SINEQUAN, DOXEPIN HYDROCHLORIDE
SPECTROBID, BACAMPICILLIN HYDROCHLORIDE
STERANE, PREDNISOLONE
STERANE, PREDNISOLONE ACETATE
STREPTOMYCIN SULFATE, STREPTOMYCIN SULFATE
TAO, TROLEANDOMYCIN
TERRA-CORTRIL, HYDROCORTISONE ACETATE
TERRAMYCIN W/ POLYMYXIN B SULFATE,
    OXYTETRACYCLINE HYDROCHLORIDE
TERRAMYCIN W/ POLYMYXIN, OXYTETRACYCLINE
    HYDROCHLORIDE
TERRAMYCIN, LIDOCAINE HYDROCHLORIDE
TERRAMYCIN, OXYTETRACYCLINE
TERRAMYCIN, OXYTETRACYCLINE CALCIUM
TERRAMYCIN, OXYTETRACYCLINE HYDROCHLORIDE
TERRAMYCIN-POLYMYXIN, OXYTETRACYCLINE
    HYDROCHLORIDE
TETRACYN, PROCAINE HYDROCHLORIDE
TETRACYN, TETRACYCLINE HYDROCHLORIDE
TZ-3, TIOCONAZOLE (OTC)
UNASYN, AMPICILLIN SODIUM
UNISOM, DOXYLAMINE SUCCINATE (OTC)
URESE, BENZTHIAZIDE
VANSIL, OXAMNIQUINE
VIBRA-TABS, DOXYCYCLINE HYCLATE
VIBRAMYCIN, DOXYCYCLINE
VIBRAMYCIN, DOXYCYCLINE CALCIUM
VIBRAMYCIN, DOXYCYCLINE HYCLATE
VIOCIN SULFATE, VIOMYCIN SULFATE
VISINE L.R., OXYMETAZOLINE HYDROCHLORIDE (OTC)
VISTARIL, HYDROXYZINE HYDROCHLORIDE
VISTARIL, HYDROXYZINE PAMOATE
PFIZER PHARMACEUTICALS INC
    TAO, TROLEANDOMYCIN
    TROVAN/ZITHROMAX COMPLIANCE PAK,
        AZITHROMYCIN DIHYDRATE
    ZOLOFT, SERTRALINE HYDROCHLORIDE
PFIZER PHARMACEUTICALS PRODUCTION CORP LTD
    TIKOSYN, DOFETILIDE
PFIZER IRELAND
PFIZER IRELAND PHARMACEUTICALS
    RELPAX, ELETRIPTAN HYDROBROMIDE
PFIZER PHARMS
PFIZER PHARMACEUTICALS LTD

ACCUPRIL, QUINAPRIL HYDROCHLORIDE
ACCURETIC, HYDROCHLOROTHIAZIDE
DILANTIN, PHENYTOIN
LOPID, GEMFIBROZIL
NEURONTIN, GABAPENTIN
NITROSTAT, NITROGLYCERIN
REZULIN, TROGLITAZONE
PHARM ASSOC
PHARMACEUTICAL ASSOC INC
    NORTRIPTYLINE HCL, NORTRIPTYLINE
        HYDROCHLORIDE
    PERPHENAZINE, PERPHENAZINE
    PREDNISOLONE SODIUM PHOSPHATE, PREDNISOLONE
        SODIUM PHOSPHATE
PHARMACEUTICAL ASSOC INC DIV BEACH PRODUCTS
    ACETAMINOPHEN AND CODEINE PHOSPHATE,
        ACETAMINOPHEN
    AMANTADINE HCL, AMANTADINE HYDROCHLORIDE
    BROMPHENIRAMINE MALEATE, BROMPHENIRAMINE
        MALEATE
    CHLORPHENIRAMINE MALEATE, CHLORPHENIRAMINE
        MALEATE
    CHLORPROMAZINE HCL, CHLORPROMAZINE
        HYDROCHLORIDE
    CIMETIDINE HCL, CIMETIDINE HYDROCHLORIDE
    DIPHENHYDRAMINE HCL, DIPHENHYDRAMINE
        HYDROCHLORIDE
    ETHOSUXIMIDE, ETHOSUXIMIDE
    FLUOXETINE, FLUOXETINE HYDROCHLORIDE
    FLUPHENAZINE HCL, FLUPHENAZINE HYDROCHLORIDE
    H-CORT, HYDROCORTISONE
    HALOPERIDOL, HALOPERIDOL LACTATE
    HYDROCODONE BITARTRATE AND ACETAMINOPHEN,
        ACETAMINOPHEN
    LACTULOSE, LACTULOSE
    METOCLOPRAMIDE HCL, METOCLOPRAMIDE
        HYDROCHLORIDE
    OXYBUTYNIN CHLORIDE, OXYBUTYNIN CHLORIDE
    PREDNISOLONE, PREDNISOLONE
    PROMETHAZINE HCL AND CODEINE PHOSPHATE,
        CODEINE PHOSPHATE
    PROMETHAZINE HCL, PROMETHAZINE
        HYDROCHLORIDE
    THEOPHYLLINE, THEOPHYLLINE
    THIORIDAZINE HCL, THIORIDAZINE HYDROCHLORIDE
    TRIHEXYPHENIDYL HCL, TRIHEXYPHENIDYL
        HYDROCHLORIDE
    TRIPROLIDINE HCL, TRIPROLIDINE HYDROCHLORIDE
    VALPROIC ACID, VALPROIC ACID
PHARM FORM
PHARMACEUTICAL FORMULATIONS INC
    CIMETIDINE, CIMETIDINE (OTC)
    IBUPROFEN AND PSEUDOEPHEDRINE HCL, IBUPROFEN
        (OTC)
    IBUPROFEN, IBUPROFEN (OTC)
PHARM SPEC
PHARMACEUTICAL SPECIALIST ASSOC
    GENTAMICIN SULFATE, GENTAMICIN SULFATE
    HEPARIN SODIUM, HEPARIN SODIUM
PHARM VENTURES
PHARMACEUTICAL VENTURES LTD
    METOCLOPRAMIDE HCL, METOCLOPRAMIDE
        HYDROCHLORIDE
    TRIHEXYPHENIDYL HCL, TRIHEXYPHENIDYL
        HYDROCHLORIDE
PHARMA SERVE NY
PHARMA SERVE INC SUB TORIGIAN LABORATORIES
    AMINOPHYLLINE, AMINOPHYLLINE

APPENDIX B
PRODUCT NAME INDEX
LISTED BY APPLICANT (*continued*)

HEPARIN SODIUM PRESERVATIVE FREE, HEPARIN
    SODIUM
POTASSIUM CHLORIDE, POTASSIUM CHLORIDE
PHARMA TEK
PHARMA TEK INC
    AMPHOTERICIN B, AMPHOTERICIN B
    BACI-RX, BACITRACIN
    BACIIM, BACITRACIN
    COLISTIMETHATE, COLISTIMETHATE SODIUM
    HYDROCORTISONE ACETATE, HYDROCORTISONE
        ACETATE
    HYDROCORTISONE, HYDROCORTISONE
    NEO-RX, NEOMYCIN SULFATE
    POLY-RX, POLYMYXIN B SULFATE
    POLYMYXIN B SULFATE, POLYMYXIN B SULFATE
    STREPTOMYCIN SULFATE, STREPTOMYCIN SULFATE
    TOBRAMYCIN, TOBRAMYCIN SULFATE
    ZIBA-RX, BACITRACIN ZINC
PHARMACHEMIE
PHARMACHEMIE BV
    CISPLATIN, CISPLATIN
    DOXORUBICIN HCL, DOXORUBICIN HYDROCHLORIDE
    ETOPOSIDE, ETOPOSIDE
    LEUCOVORIN CALCIUM, LEUCOVORIN CALCIUM
    TAMOXIFEN CITRATE, TAMOXIFEN CITRATE
PHARMACHEMIE USA
PHARMACHEMIE USA INC
    LEUCOVORIN CALCIUM, LEUCOVORIN CALCIUM
    METHOTREXATE SODIUM, METHOTREXATE SODIUM
PHARMACIA
PHARMACIA CORP
    DAYPRO ALTA, OXAPROZIN POTASSIUM
    MAXAQUIN, LOMEFLOXACIN HYDROCHLORIDE
PHARMACIA AND UPJOHN
PHARMACIA AND UPJOHN
    XANAX XR, ALPRAZOLAM
PHARMACIA AND UPJOHN CO
    ADRIAMYCIN PFS, DOXORUBICIN HYDROCHLORIDE
    ADRIAMYCIN RDF, DOXORUBICIN HYDROCHLORIDE
    ADRUCIL, FLUOROURACIL
    ALBAMYCIN, NOVOBIOCIN SODIUM
    ALPHADROL, FLUPREDNISOLONE
    ANSAID, FLURBIPROFEN
    AROMASIN, EXEMESTANE
    AZULFIDINE EN-TABS, SULFASALAZINE
    AZULFIDINE, SULFASALAZINE
    BACIGUENT, BACITRACIN
    BACITRACIN, BACITRACIN
    BERUBIGEN, CYANOCOBALAMIN
    BLEOMYCIN SULFATE, BLEOMYCIN SULFATE
    CALMURID HC, HYDROCORTISONE
    CAMPTOSAR, IRINOTECAN HYDROCHLORIDE
    CARDRASE, ETHOXZOLAMIDE
    CAVERJECT, ALPROSTADIL
    CLEOCIN HCL, CLINDAMYCIN HYDROCHLORIDE
    CLEOCIN PHOSPHATE IN DEXTROSE 5% IN PLASTIC
        CONTAINER, CLINDAMYCIN PHOSPHATE
    CLEOCIN PHOSPHATE, CLINDAMYCIN PHOSPHATE
    CLEOCIN T, CLINDAMYCIN PHOSPHATE
    CLEOCIN, CLINDAMYCIN HYDROCHLORIDE
    CLEOCIN, CLINDAMYCIN PALMITATE HYDROCHLORIDE
    CLEOCIN, CLINDAMYCIN PHOSPHATE
    COLESTID, COLESTIPOL HYDROCHLORIDE
    CORTEF ACETATE, HYDROCORTISONE ACETATE
    CORTEF, HYDROCORTISONE
    CORTEF, HYDROCORTISONE CYPIONATE
    CORTISONE ACETATE, CORTISONE ACETATE
    CORVERT, IBUTILIDE FUMARATE

CYKLOKAPRON, TRANEXAMIC ACID
DELTA-CORTEF, PREDNISOLONE
DELTASONE, PREDNISONE
DEPO-ESTRADIOL, ESTRADIOL CYPIONATE
DEPO-MEDROL, METHYLPREDNISOLONE ACETATE
DEPO-PROVERA, MEDROXYPROGESTERONE ACETATE
DEPO-TESTADIOL, ESTRADIOL CYPIONATE
DEPO-TESTOSTERONE, TESTOSTERONE CYPIONATE
DETROL LA, TOLTERODINE TARTRATE
DETROL, TOLTERODINE TARTRATE
DIDREX, BENZPHETAMINE HYDROCHLORIDE
DIPENTUM, OLSALAZINE SODIUM
DIZAC, DIAZEPAM
DOSTINEX, CABERGOLINE
E-MYCIN E, ERYTHROMYCIN ETHYLSUCCINATE
EMCYT, ESTRAMUSTINE PHOSPHATE SODIUM
ESTRING, ESTRADIOL
FEMINONE, ETHINYL ESTRADIOL
FLAVORED COLESTID, COLESTIPOL HYDROCHLORIDE
FLORONE E, DIFLORASONE DIACETATE
FLORONE, DIFLORASONE DIACETATE
FLUIDIL, CYCLOTHIAZIDE
FOLEX PFS, METHOTREXATE SODIUM
FOLEX, METHOTREXATE SODIUM
FRAGMIN, DALTEPARIN SODIUM
GENOTROPIN PRESERVATIVE FREE, SOMATROPIN
    RECOMBINANT
GENOTROPIN, SOMATROPIN RECOMBINANT
GLYNASE, GLYBURIDE
GLYSET, MIGLITOL
HALCION, TRIAZOLAM
HALOTESTIN, FLUOXYMESTERONE
HEMABATE, CARBOPROST TROMETHAMINE
HEPARIN SODIUM, HEPARIN SODIUM
HYLOREL, GUANADREL SULFATE
IDAMYCIN PFS, IDARUBICIN HYDROCHLORIDE
IDAMYCIN, IDARUBICIN HYDROCHLORIDE
LINCOCIN, LINCOMYCIN HYDROCHLORIDE
LONITEN, MINOXIDIL
LUNELLE, ESTRADIOL CYPIONATE
MAOLATE, CHLORPHENESIN CARBAMATE
MEDROL ACETATE, METHYLPREDNISOLONE ACETATE
MEDROL, METHYLPREDNISOLONE
MEDROL, METHYLPREDNISOLONE ACETATE
MICRONASE, GLYBURIDE
MIRAPEX, PRAMIPEXOLE DIHYDROCHLORIDE
MYCIFRADIN, NEOMYCIN SULFATE
MYCITRACIN, BACITRACIN
MYCOBUTIN, RIFABUTIN
NEO-CORTEF, HYDROCORTISONE ACETATE
NEO-DELTA-CORTEF, NEOMYCIN SULFATE
NEO-MEDROL ACETATE, METHYLPREDNISOLONE
    ACETATE
NEO-MEDROL, METHYLPREDNISOLONE
NEOSAR, CYCLOPHOSPHAMIDE
NICOTROL, NICOTINE
NICOTROL, NICOTINE (OTC)
NORMIFLO, ARDEPARIN SODIUM
OGEN .625, ESTROPIPATE
OGEN 1.25, ESTROPIPATE
OGEN 2.5, ESTROPIPATE
OGEN 5, ESTROPIPATE
OGEN, ESTROPIPATE
ORINASE DIAGNOSTIC, TOLBUTAMIDE SODIUM
ORINASE, TOLBUTAMIDE
OXYLONE, FLUOROMETHOLONE
PANMYCIN, TETRACYCLINE HYDROCHLORIDE
PENICILLIN G SODIUM, PENICILLIN G SODIUM

APPENDIX B
PRODUCT NAME INDEX
LISTED BY APPLICANT (*continued*)

PREPIDIL, DINOPROSTONE
PROSTIN E2, DINOPROSTONE
PROSTIN F2 ALPHA, DINOPROST TROMETHAMINE
PROSTIN VR PEDIATRIC, ALPROSTADIL
PROTAMINE SULFATE, PROTAMINE SULFATE
PROVERA, MEDROXYPROGESTERONE ACETATE
PSORCON, DIFLORASONE DIACETATE
R-GENE 10, ARGININE HYDROCHLORIDE
ROGAINE (FOR MEN), MINOXIDIL (OTC)
ROGAINE (FOR WOMEN), MINOXIDIL (OTC)
ROGAINE EXTRA STRENGTH (FOR MEN), MINOXIDIL
    (OTC)
SOLU-CORTEF, HYDROCORTISONE SODIUM
    SUCCINATE
SOLU-MEDROL, METHYLPREDNISOLONE SODIUM
    SUCCINATE
SOMAVERT, PEGVISOMANT
TOLINASE, TOLAZAMIDE
TOPOSAR, ETOPOSIDE
TRELSTAR DEPOT, TRIPTORELIN PAMOATE
TRELSTAR, TRIPTORELIN PAMOATE
TROBICIN, SPECTINOMYCIN HYDROCHLORIDE
TYMTRAN, CERULETIDE DIETHYLAMINE
U-GENCIN, GENTAMICIN SULFATE
UTICILLIN VK, PENICILLIN V POTASSIUM
VANCOR, VANCOMYCIN HYDROCHLORIDE
VANTIN, CEFPODOXIME PROXETIL
VINCASAR PFS, VINCRISTINE SULFATE
XALATAN, LATANOPROST
XANAX, ALPRAZOLAM
ZEFAZONE IN PLASTIC CONTAINER, CEFMETAZOLE
    SODIUM
ZEFAZONE, CEFMETAZOLE SODIUM
ZINECARD, DEXRAZOXANE HYDROCHLORIDE
ZYVOX, LINEZOLID
PHARMACIA AND UPJOHN CO NUTRITION DIV
  ELLENCE, EPIRUBICIN HYDROCHLORIDE
PHARMACIA UPJOHN
PHARMACIA AND UPJOHN CONSUMER HEALTHCARE
  NASALCROM, CROMOLYN SODIUM (OTC)
PHARMADERM
PHARMADERM DIV ALTANA INC
  BACITRACIN, BACITRACIN
  BACITRACIN-NEOMYCIN-POLYMYXIN W/
    HYDROCORTISONE ACETATE, BACITRACIN
  BACITRACIN-NEOMYCIN-POLYMYXIN, BACITRACIN
    ZINC
  BETAMETHASONE DIPROPIONATE, BETAMETHASONE
    DIPROPIONATE
  BETAMETHASONE VALERATE, BETAMETHASONE
    VALERATE
  ERYTHROMYCIN, ERYTHROMYCIN
  FLUOCINOLONE ACETONIDE, FLUOCINOLONE
    ACETONIDE
  GENTAMICIN SULFATE, GENTAMICIN SULFATE
  HYDROCORTISONE, HYDROCORTISONE
  NEOMYCIN SULFATE-TRIAMCINOLONE ACETONIDE,
    NEOMYCIN SULFATE
  NYSTATIN, NYSTATIN
  NYSTATIN-TRIAMCINOLONE ACETONIDE, NYSTATIN
  TRIAMCINOLONE ACETONIDE, TRIAMCINOLONE
    ACETONIDE
  TRIPLE SULFA, TRIPLE SULFA (SULFABENZAMIDE;
    SULFACETAMIDE; SULFATHIAZOLE)
PHARMAFAIR
PHARMAFAIR INC
  BACITRACIN ZINC-NEOMYCIN SULFATE-POLYMYXIN B
    SULFATE, BACITRACIN ZINC

BACITRACIN, BACITRACIN
BETAMETHASONE VALERATE, BETAMETHASONE
    VALERATE
BOROFAIR, ACETIC ACID, GLACIAL
CARBACHOL, CARBACHOL
CHLOROFAIR, CHLORAMPHENICOL
DEXAIR, DEXAMETHASONE SODIUM PHOSPHATE
DEXASPORIN, DEXAMETHASONE
ERYTHROMYCIN ETHYLSUCCINATE, ERYTHROMYCIN
    ETHYLSUCCINATE
ERYTHROMYCIN, ERYTHROMYCIN
FLUOCINOLONE ACETONIDE, FLUOCINOLONE
    ACETONIDE
GENTAFAIR, GENTAMICIN SULFATE
HYDROCORTISONE, HYDROCORTISONE
HYDROXYZINE HCL, HYDROXYZINE HYDROCHLORIDE
KAINAIR, PROPARACAINE HYDROCHLORIDE
KANAMYCIN SULFATE, KANAMYCIN SULFATE
MYDRIAFAIR, TROPICAMIDE
NAFAZAIR, NAPHAZOLINE HYDROCHLORIDE
NEOMYCIN & POLYMYXIN B SULFATES & BACITRACIN
    ZINC & HYDROCORTISONE, BACITRACIN ZINC
NEOMYCIN SULFATE AND POLYMYXIN B SULFATE
    GRAMICIDIN, GRAMICIDIN
NEOMYCIN SULFATE, POLYMYXIN B SULFATE &
    HYDROCORTISONE, HYDROCORTISONE
NEOMYCIN SULFATE-DEXAMETHASONE SODIUM
    PHOSPHATE, DEXAMETHASONE SODIUM
    PHOSPHATE
NEOMYCIN SULFATE-POLYMYXIN B SULFATE-
    HYDROCORTISONE, HYDROCORTISONE
NYSTATIN AND TRIAMCINOLONE ACETONIDE,
    NYSTATIN
NYSTATIN, NYSTATIN
OCUMYCIN, BACITRACIN ZINC
OTICAIR, HYDROCORTISONE
PENTOLAIR, CYCLOPENTOLATE HYDROCHLORIDE
PREDAIR FORTE, PREDNISOLONE SODIUM
    PHOSPHATE
PREDAIR, PREDNISOLONE SODIUM PHOSPHATE
PREDSULFAIR II, PREDNISOLONE ACETATE
PREDSULFAIR, PREDNISOLONE ACETATE
PROCAINAMIDE HCL, PROCAINAMIDE
    HYDROCHLORIDE
SULFACETAMIDE SODIUM, SULFACETAMIDE SODIUM
SULFAIR 10, SULFACETAMIDE SODIUM
SULFAIR FORTE, SULFACETAMIDE SODIUM
SULFAIR-15, SULFACETAMIDE SODIUM
TRIAMCINOLONE ACETONIDE, TRIAMCINOLONE
    ACETONIDE
ZINC BACITRACIN,NEOMYCIN SULFATE,POLYMYXIN B
    SULFATE & HYDROCORTISONE, BACITRACIN ZINC
PHARMAFORCE
PHARMAFORCE INC
  PROMETHAZINE HCL, PROMETHAZINE
    HYDROCHLORIDE
PHARMASEAL
PHARMASEAL DIV BAXTER HEALTHCARE CORP
  PHARMASEAL SCRUB CARE, CHLORHEXIDINE
    GLUCONATE (OTC)
PHARMATEK
PHARMATEK INC
  NEO-FRADIN, NEOMYCIN SULFATE
PHARMATON
PHARMATON LTD
  LIDOCATON, EPINEPHRINE
  LIDOCATON, LIDOCAINE HYDROCHLORIDE

APPENDIX B
PRODUCT NAME INDEX
LISTED BY APPLICANT (*continued*)

PHARMAVITE
PHARMAVITE PHARMACEUTICALS
    CHLORPHENIRAMINE MALEATE, CHLORPHENIRAMINE
        MALEATE
    ISONIAZID, ISONIAZID
    MEPROBAMATE, MEPROBAMATE
    PREDNISONE, PREDNISONE
    QUINIDINE SULFATE, QUINIDINE SULFATE
    RESERPINE, RESERPINE
PHARMERAL
PHARMERAL INC
    ACETAMINOPHEN AND CODEINE PHOSPHATE,
        ACETAMINOPHEN
    BUTALBITAL W/ ASPIRIN & CAFFEINE, ASPIRIN
    CHLORPHENIRAMINE MALEATE, CHLORPHENIRAMINE
        MALEATE
    FOLIC ACID, FOLIC ACID
    HYDROCHLOROTHIAZIDE W/ RESERPINE,
        HYDROCHLOROTHIAZIDE
    HYDROCHLOROTHIAZIDE, HYDROCHLOROTHIAZIDE
    MEPROBAMATE, MEPROBAMATE
    METHOCARBAMOL, METHOCARBAMOL
    PHENYTOIN SODIUM, PHENYTOIN SODIUM, PROMPT
    SULFISOXAZOLE, SULFISOXAZOLE
PHARMEX PRODS
PHARMEX PRODUCTS INC
    BUSPIRONE HCL, BUSPIRONE HYDROCHLORIDE
PHARMION
PHARMION CORP
    INNOHEP, TINZAPARIN SODIUM
PHARMOS
PHARMOS CORP
    LOTEMAX, LOTEPREDNOL ETABONATE
PHOENIX LABS NY
PHOENIX LABORATORIES INC
    CHLORPHENIRAMINE MALEATE, CHLORPHENIRAMINE
        MALEATE
    DEXAMETHASONE, DEXAMETHASONE
    ISONIAZID, ISONIAZID
    PREDNISOLONE, PREDNISOLONE
    PREDNISONE, PREDNISONE
PHYS PRODS VA
PHYSICIANS PRODUCTS CO INC DIV INTERNATIONAL LA-
TEX CORP
    HYSERPIN, RAUWOLFIA SERPENTINA
PIERRE FABRE
PIERRE FABRE MEDICAMENT
    ETOPOSIDE, ETOPOSIDE
PIONEER PHARMS
PIONEER PHARMACEUTICALS INC
    BROMPHENIRAMINE MALEATE, BROMPHENIRAMINE
        MALEATE
    CARISOPRODOL, CARISOPRODOL
    CHLORDIAZEPOXIDE HCL, CHLORDIAZEPOXIDE
        HYDROCHLORIDE
    CHLORPHENIRAMINE MALEATE, CHLORPHENIRAMINE
        MALEATE
    CHLORTHALIDONE, CHLORTHALIDONE
    CHLORZOXAZONE, CHLORZOXAZONE
    CYPROHEPTADINE HCL, CYPROHEPTADINE
        HYDROCHLORIDE
    DIAZEPAM, DIAZEPAM
    DICYCLOMINE HCL, DICYCLOMINE HYDROCHLORIDE
    DIPHENHYDRAMINE HCL, DIPHENHYDRAMINE
        HYDROCHLORIDE
    FOLIC ACID, FOLIC ACID
    INDOMETHACIN, INDOMETHACIN
    METHOCARBAMOL, METHOCARBAMOL

RESPORAL, DEXBROMPHENIRAMINE MALEATE (OTC)
PLANTEX
PLANTEX USA INC DIV IKAPHARM INC
    SULFAMETHOXAZOLE AND TRIMETHOPRIM SINGLE
        STRENGTH, SULFAMETHOXAZOLE
PLIVA
PLIVA INC
    ALBUTEROL SULFATE, ALBUTEROL SULFATE
    ALBUTEROL, ALBUTEROL
    AMITRIPTYLINE HCL, AMITRIPTYLINE HYDROCHLORIDE
    ANTABUSE, DISULFIRAM
    ATENOLOL AND CHLORTHALIDONE, ATENOLOL
    ATENOLOL, ATENOLOL
    BENZTROPINE MESYLATE, BENZTROPINE MESYLATE
    CARBAMAZEPINE, CARBAMAZEPINE
    CHLORPROPAMIDE, CHLORPROPAMIDE
    CHLORTHALIDONE, CHLORTHALIDONE
    CIMETIDINE, CIMETIDINE
    CYCLOBENZAPRINE HCL, CYCLOBENZAPRINE
        HYDROCHLORIDE
    CYCLOSPORINE, CYCLOSPORINE
    CYPROHEPTADINE HCL, CYPROHEPTADINE
        HYDROCHLORIDE
    DESIPRAMINE HCL, DESIPRAMINE HYDROCHLORIDE
    DEXCHLORPHENIRAMINE MALEATE,
        DEXCHLORPHENIRAMINE MALEATE
    DICLOFENAC SODIUM, DICLOFENAC SODIUM
    DOXAZOSIN MESYLATE, DOXAZOSIN MESYLATE
    DOXYCYCLINE HYCLATE, DOXYCYCLINE HYCLATE
    EXTENDED PHENYTOIN SODIUM, PHENYTOIN SODIUM,
        EXTENDED
    FLUOXETINE, FLUOXETINE HYDROCHLORIDE
    FLURBIPROFEN, FLURBIPROFEN
    GLIPIZIDE, GLIPIZIDE
    HYDRALAZINE HCL, HYDRALAZINE HYDROCHLORIDE
    HYDROXYZINE HCL, HYDROXYZINE HYDROCHLORIDE
    IBUPRIN, IBUPROFEN (OTC)
    IBUPROFEN, IBUPROFEN
    INDOMETHACIN, INDOMETHACIN
    KETOCONAZOLE, KETOCONAZOLE
    KETOROLAC TROMETHAMINE, KETOROLAC
        TROMETHAMINE
    MECLIZINE HCL, MECLIZINE HYDROCHLORIDE
    METHYLDOPA, METHYLDOPA
    METOCLOPRAMIDE HCL, METOCLOPRAMIDE
        HYDROCHLORIDE
    METRONIDAZOLE, METRONIDAZOLE
    NAPROXEN SODIUM, NAPROXEN SODIUM
    NAPROXEN, NAPROXEN
    OXYBUTYNIN CHLORIDE, OXYBUTYNIN CHLORIDE
    PENTOXIFYLLINE, PENTOXIFYLLINE
    PROCAINAMIDE HCL, PROCAINAMIDE
        HYDROCHLORIDE
    PROPRANOLOL HCL AND HYDROCHLOROTHIAZIDE,
        HYDROCHLOROTHIAZIDE
    PROPRANOLOL HCL, PROPRANOLOL HYDROCHLORIDE
    SULFAMETHOXAZOLE AND TRIMETHOPRIM,
        SULFAMETHOXAZOLE
    SURMONTIL, TRIMIPRAMINE MALEATE
    THEOPHYLLINE, THEOPHYLLINE
    TRAMADOL HCL, TRAMADOL HYDROCHLORIDE
    TRAZODONE HCL, TRAZODONE HYDROCHLORIDE
    TRIAMTERENE AND HYDROCHLOROTHIAZIDE,
        HYDROCHLOROTHIAZIDE
    ULTRAGRIS-165, GRISEOFULVIN,
        ULTRAMICROCRYSTALLINE
    ULTRAGRIS-330, GRISEOFULVIN,
        ULTRAMICROCRYSTALLINE

APPENDIX B
PRODUCT NAME INDEX
LISTED BY APPLICANT (*continued*)

URECHOLINE, BETHANECHOL CHLORIDE
VERAPAMIL HCL, VERAPAMIL HYDROCHLORIDE
VIVACTIL, PROTRIPTYLINE HYDROCHLORIDE

PLIVA PHARM IND
PLIVA PHARMACEUTICAL INDUSTRY INC
TORSEMIDE, TORSEMIDE

POHL BOSKAMP
G POHL BOSKAMP GMBH AND CO
NITRO IV, NITROGLYCERIN
NITROLINGUAL PUMPSPRAY, NITROGLYCERIN
NITROLINGUAL, NITROGLYCERIN
NITRONAL, NITROGLYCERIN

POINT HOLDINGS
POINT HOLDINGS INC
ETODOLAC, ETODOLAC

POLYMEDICA
POLYMEDICA INDUSTRIES INC
ANESTACON, LIDOCAINE HYDROCHLORIDE
NEOPAP, ACETAMINOPHEN (OTC)
PROMETHACON, PROMETHAZINE HYDROCHLORIDE

POPULATION COUNCIL
POPULATION COUNCIL
NORPLANT, LEVONORGESTREL
POPULATION COUNCIL CENTER FOR BIOMEDICAL RE-
SEARCH
NORPLANT II, LEVONORGESTREL

POYTHRESS
WILLIAM P POYTHRESS AND CO INC
BENSULFOID, SULFUR

PROCTER AND GAMBLE
PROCTER AND GAMBLE CO
DANTRIUM, DANTROLENE SODIUM
HEAD & SHOULDERS CONDITIONER, PYRITHIONE ZINC
(OTC)
MACRODANTIN, NITROFURANTOIN,
MACROCRYSTALLINE
VICKS FORMULA 44, DIPHENHYDRAMINE
HYDROCHLORIDE (OTC)
PROCTER AND GAMBLE PHARMACEUTICALS INC SUB
PROCTER AND GAMBL
ACTONEL, RISEDRONATE SODIUM
ASACOL, MESALAMINE
DANTRIUM, DANTROLENE SODIUM
DIDRONEL, ETIDRONATE DISODIUM
FURADANTIN, NITROFURANTOIN
IVADANTIN, NITROFURANTOIN SODIUM
LABID, THEOPHYLLINE
MACROBID, NITROFURANTOIN
NYSERT, NYSTATIN
ORLEX HC, ACETIC ACID, GLACIAL
ORLEX, ACETIC ACID, GLACIAL
SARENIN, SARALASIN ACETATE

PROF DSPLS
PROFESSIONAL DISPOSABLES INC
HEXASCRUB, HEXACHLOROPHENE

PROMETHEUS LABS
PROMETHEUS LABORATORIES INC
HELIDAC, BISMUTH SUBSALICYLATE
IMURAN, AZATHIOPRINE
IMURAN, AZATHIOPRINE SODIUM
RIDAURA, AURANOFIN
TRANDATE, LABETALOL HYDROCHLORIDE
ZYLOPRIM, ALLOPURINOL

PROTER
PROTER LABORATORY SPA
OXYTETRACYCLINE HCL, OXYTETRACYCLINE
HYDROCHLORIDE
TETRACYCLINE HCL, TETRACYCLINE HYDROCHLORIDE

PURDUE FREDERICK
PURDUE FREDERICK CO
ATHROMBIN, WARFARIN SODIUM
ATHROMBIN-K, WARFARIN POTASSIUM
CARDIOQUIN, QUINIDINE POLYGALACTURONATE
CERUMENEX, TROLAMINE POLYPEPTIDE OLEATE
CONDENSATE
DHC PLUS, ACETAMINOPHEN
MS CONTIN, MORPHINE SULFATE
PHENY-PAS-TEBAMIN, PHENYL AMINOSALICYLATE
PHYLLOCONTIN, AMINOPHYLLINE
SULFABID, SULFAPHENAZOLE
T-PHYL, THEOPHYLLINE
UNIPHYL, THEOPHYLLINE

PURDUE PHARMA LP
PURDUE PHARMA LP
CHIROCAINE, LEVOBUPIVACAINE HYDROCHLORIDE
OXYCONTIN, OXYCODONE HYDROCHLORIDE
SPECTRACEF, CEFDITOREN PIVOXIL

PUREPAC PHARM
PUREPAC PHARMACEUTICAL CO DIV PUREPAC INC
ACETAMINOPHEN AND CODEINE PHOSPHATE #3,
ACETAMINOPHEN
ACETAMINOPHEN AND CODEINE PHOSPHATE,
ACETAMINOPHEN
ACYCLOVIR, ACYCLOVIR
ALLOPURINOL, ALLOPURINOL
ALPRAZOLAM, ALPRAZOLAM
AMINOPHYLLINE, AMINOPHYLLINE
AMITRIPTYLINE HCL, AMITRIPTYLINE HYDROCHLORIDE
AMPICILLIN TRIHYDRATE, AMPICILLIN/AMPICILLIN
TRIHYDRATE
ASPIRIN AND CAFFEINE W/ BUTALBITAL, ASPIRIN
BISOPROLOL FUMARATE AND
HYDROCHLOROTHIAZIDE, BISOPROLOL FUMARATE
CAPTOPRIL, CAPTOPRIL
CARBAMAZEPINE, CARBAMAZEPINE
CARBIDOPA AND LEVODOPA, CARBIDOPA
CEFADROXIL, CEFADROXIL/CEFADROXIL
HEMIHYDRATE
CEPHALEXIN, CEPHALEXIN
CHLORDIAZEPOXIDE HCL, CHLORDIAZEPOXIDE
HYDROCHLORIDE
CHLOROQUINE PHOSPHATE, CHLOROQUINE
PHOSPHATE
CHLORPHENIRAMINE MALEATE, CHLORPHENIRAMINE
MALEATE
CHLORPROMAZINE HCL, CHLORPROMAZINE
HYDROCHLORIDE
CHLORTHALIDONE, CHLORTHALIDONE
CLONAZEPAM, CLONAZEPAM
CLONIDINE HCL, CLONIDINE HYDROCHLORIDE
CLORAZEPATE DIPOTASSIUM, CLORAZEPATE
DIPOTASSIUM
CORTISONE ACETATE, CORTISONE ACETATE
DEXTROAMPHETAMINE SULFATE,
DEXTROAMPHETAMINE SULFATE
DIAZEPAM, DIAZEPAM
DICLOFENAC SODIUM, DICLOFENAC SODIUM
DIFLUNISAL, DIFLUNISAL
DILTIAZEM HCL, DILTIAZEM HYDROCHLORIDE
DIPHENHYDRAMINE HCL, DIPHENHYDRAMINE
HYDROCHLORIDE
DIPYRIDAMOLE, DIPYRIDAMOLE
DOXAZOSIN MESYLATE, DOXAZOSIN MESYLATE
DOXEPIN HCL, DOXEPIN HYDROCHLORIDE
ERYTHROMYCIN STEARATE, ERYTHROMYCIN
STEARATE

APPENDIX B
PRODUCT NAME INDEX
LISTED BY APPLICANT (*continued*)

ETODOLAC, ETODOLAC
FAMOTIDINE, FAMOTIDINE
FENOPROFEN CALCIUM, FENOPROFEN CALCIUM
FLURAZEPAM HCL, FLURAZEPAM HYDROCHLORIDE
FLUVOXAMINE MALEATE, FLUVOXAMINE MALEATE
FOLIC ACID, FOLIC ACID
GEMFIBROZIL, GEMFIBROZIL
HALOPERIDOL, HALOPERIDOL
HYDRALAZINE HCL, HYDRALAZINE HYDROCHLORIDE
HYDROCHLOROTHIAZIDE, HYDROCHLOROTHIAZIDE
HYDROCORTISONE ACETATE, HYDROCORTISONE
    ACETATE
HYDROCORTISONE, HYDROCORTISONE
HYDROXYZINE HCL, HYDROXYZINE HYDROCHLORIDE
IBUPROFEN, IBUPROFEN
IBUPROFEN, IBUPROFEN (OTC)
INDAPAMIDE, INDAPAMIDE
ISONIAZID, ISONIAZID
ISOSORBIDE MONONITRATE, ISOSORBIDE
    MONONITRATE
LISINOPRIL AND HYDROCHLOROTHIAZIDE,
    HYDROCHLOROTHIAZIDE
LISINOPRIL, LISINOPRIL
LORAZEPAM, LORAZEPAM
LOVASTATIN, LOVASTATIN
MEPROBAMATE, MEPROBAMATE
METFORMIN HCL, METFORMIN HYDROCHLORIDE
METHOCARBAMOL, METHOCARBAMOL
METHYLDOPA AND HYDROCHLOROTHIAZIDE,
    HYDROCHLOROTHIAZIDE
METHYLDOPA, METHYLDOPA
METHYLPHENIDATE HCL, METHYLPHENIDATE
    HYDROCHLORIDE
METHYLTESTOSTERONE, METHYLTESTOSTERONE
METOCLOPRAMIDE HCL, METOCLOPRAMIDE
    HYDROCHLORIDE
METOPROLOL TARTRATE, METOPROLOL TARTRATE
MIRTAZAPINE, MIRTAZAPINE
NAPROXEN SODIUM, NAPROXEN SODIUM
NAPROXEN, NAPROXEN
NIACIN, NIACIN
NIFEDIPINE, NIFEDIPINE
OXAPROZIN, OXAPROZIN
OXAZEPAM, OXAZEPAM
OXYTETRACYCLINE HCL, OXYTETRACYCLINE
    HYDROCHLORIDE
PENICILLIN G POTASSIUM, PENICILLIN G POTASSIUM
PENICILLIN V POTASSIUM, PENICILLIN V POTASSIUM
PENTOXIFYLLINE, PENTOXIFYLLINE
PHENTERMINE HCL, PHENTERMINE HYDROCHLORIDE
PINDOLOL, PINDOLOL
PRAZOSIN HCL, PRAZOSIN HYDROCHLORIDE
PREDNISOLONE, PREDNISOLONE
PREDNISONE, PREDNISONE
PROPOXYPHENE HCL, PROPOXYPHENE
    HYDROCHLORIDE
PROPOXYPHENE NAPSYLATE AND ACETAMINOPHEN,
    ACETAMINOPHEN
PROPRANOLOL HCL AND HYDROCHLOROTHIAZIDE,
    HYDROCHLOROTHIAZIDE
PROPRANOLOL HCL, PROPRANOLOL HYDROCHLORIDE
PROPYLTHIOURACIL, PROPYLTHIOURACIL
QUINIDINE SULFATE, QUINIDINE SULFATE
RAUWOLFIA SERPENTINA, RAUWOLFIA SERPENTINA
RESERPINE, RESERPINE
SECOBARBITAL SODIUM, SECOBARBITAL SODIUM
SODIUM PENTOBARBITAL, PENTOBARBITAL SODIUM

SPIRONOLACTONE AND HYDROCHLOROTHIAZIDE,
    HYDROCHLOROTHIAZIDE
SPIRONOLACTONE W/ HYDROCHLOROTHIAZIDE,
    HYDROCHLOROTHIAZIDE
SPIRONOLACTONE, SPIRONOLACTONE
SULFISOXAZOLE, SULFISOXAZOLE
TEMAZEPAM, TEMAZEPAM
TETRACYCLINE HCL, TETRACYCLINE HYDROCHLORIDE
TICLOPIDINE HCL, TICLOPIDINE HYDROCHLORIDE
TIZANIDINE HCL, TIZANIDINE HYDROCHLORIDE
TOLBUTAMIDE, TOLBUTAMIDE
TOLMETIN SODIUM, TOLMETIN SODIUM
TRAMADOL HCL, TRAMADOL HYDROCHLORIDE
TRAZODONE HCL, TRAZODONE HYDROCHLORIDE
TRIAMCINOLONE, TRIAMCINOLONE
TRIPLE SULFA, TRISULFAPYRIMIDINES (SULFADIAZINE;
    SULFAMERAZINE; SULFAMETHAZINE)
VERAPAMIL HCL, VERAPAMIL HYDROCHLORIDE
PVT FORM
PRIVATE FORMULATIONS INC
    ALLERFED, PSEUDOEPHEDRINE HYDROCHLORIDE
    BENZTHIAZIDE, BENZTHIAZIDE
    CHLORPHENIRAMINE MALEATE, CHLORPHENIRAMINE
        MALEATE
    CHLORPROMAZINE HCL, CHLORPROMAZINE
        HYDROCHLORIDE
    DEXAMETHASONE, DEXAMETHASONE
    DI-METREX, PHENDIMETRAZINE TARTRATE
    DIPHENHYDRAMINE HCL, DIPHENHYDRAMINE
        HYDROCHLORIDE
    DIPHENOXYLATE HCL W/ ATROPINE SULFATE,
        ATROPINE SULFATE
    DOXYCYCLINE HYCLATE, DOXYCYCLINE HYCLATE
    ESTERIFIED ESTROGENS, ESTROGENS, ESTERIFIED
    FEMOGEN, ESTROGENS, ESTERIFIED
    FOLIC ACID, FOLIC ACID
    HYDROCHLOROTHIAZIDE, HYDROCHLOROTHIAZIDE
    IBUPROFEN, IBUPROFEN
    IBUPROFEN, IBUPROFEN (OTC)
    MEPROBAMATE, MEPROBAMATE
    METHSCOPOLAMINE BROMIDE, METHSCOPOLAMINE
        BROMIDE
    METHYLTESTOSTERONE, METHYLTESTOSTERONE
    NAPROXEN SODIUM, NAPROXEN SODIUM (OTC)
    PHENDIMETRAZINE TARTRATE, PHENDIMETRAZINE
        TARTRATE
    PREDNISOLONE, PREDNISOLONE
    PREDNISONE, PREDNISONE
    PROFEN, IBUPROFEN (OTC)
    PROMETHAZINE HCL, PROMETHAZINE
        HYDROCHLORIDE
    PROPANTHELINE BROMIDE, PROPANTHELINE
        BROMIDE
    PROPOXYPHENE HCL, PROPOXYPHENE
        HYDROCHLORIDE
    QUINIDINE SULFATE, QUINIDINE SULFATE
    RAUWOLFIA SERPENTINA, RAUWOLFIA SERPENTINA
    RESERPINE, RESERPINE
    TETRACYCLINE HCL, TETRACYCLINE HYDROCHLORIDE

Q

QLT
QLT INC
    VISUDYNE, VERTEPORFIN
QOL MEDCL
QOL MEDICAL LLC

APPENDIX B
PRODUCT NAME INDEX
LISTED BY APPLICANT (*continued*)

ELLIOTTS B SOLUTION, CALCIUM CHLORIDE
SUCRAID, SACROSIDASE
QUAD PHARMS
QUAD PHARMACEUTICALS INC
ACETAZOLAMIDE SODIUM, ACETAZOLAMIDE SODIUM
ACETYLCYSTEINE, ACETYLCYSTEINE
AMINOCAPROIC ACID, AMINOCAPROIC ACID
AMINOHIPPURATE SODIUM, AMINOHIPPURATE SODIUM
AZATHIOPRINE, AZATHIOPRINE SODIUM
BACITRACIN, BACITRACIN
BETHANECHOL CHLORIDE, BETHANECHOL CHLORIDE
BRETYLIUM TOSYLATE, BRETYLIUM TOSYLATE
CHORIONIC GONADOTROPIN, GONADOTROPIN,
    CHORIONIC
CLINDAMYCIN PHOSPHATE, CLINDAMYCIN
    PHOSPHATE
CYTARABINE, CYTARABINE
DACARBAZINE, DACARBAZINE
DEXAMETHASONE SODIUM PHOSPHATE,
    DEXAMETHASONE SODIUM PHOSPHATE
DIAZOXIDE, DIAZOXIDE
DOXYCYCLINE HYCLATE, DOXYCYCLINE HYCLATE
DROPERIDOL, DROPERIDOL
ERYTHROMYCIN LACTOBIONATE, ERYTHROMYCIN
    LACTOBIONATE
ESTRADIOL CYPIONATE, ESTRADIOL CYPIONATE
FLOXURIDINE, FLOXURIDINE
FLUOROURACIL, FLUOROURACIL
FLUPHENAZINE HCL, FLUPHENAZINE HYDROCHLORIDE
FLUPHENAZINE, FLUPHENAZINE DECANOATE
GLUCAGON, GLUCAGON HYDROCHLORIDE
GLYCOPYRROLATE, GLYCOPYRROLATE
HALOPERIDOL, HALOPERIDOL LACTATE
HYDROCORTISONE SODIUM PHOSPHATE,
    HYDROCORTISONE SODIUM PHOSPHATE
HYDROXYPROGESTERONE CAPROATE,
    HYDROXYPROGESTERONE CAPROATE
ISONIAZID, ISONIAZID
KANAMYCIN SULFATE, KANAMYCIN SULFATE
KETAMINE HCL, KETAMINE HYDROCHLORIDE
LEUCOVORIN CALCIUM, LEUCOVORIN CALCIUM
LINCOMYCIN HCL, LINCOMYCIN HYDROCHLORIDE
METHOTREXATE SODIUM, METHOTREXATE SODIUM
METHYLDOPATE HCL, METHYLDOPATE
    HYDROCHLORIDE
METHYLPREDNISOLONE SODIUM SUCCINATE,
    METHYLPREDNISOLONE SODIUM SUCCINATE
METOCLOPRAMIDE HCL, METOCLOPRAMIDE
    HYDROCHLORIDE
METOCURINE IODIDE, METOCURINE IODIDE
NALBUPHINE, NALBUPHINE HYDROCHLORIDE
NALOXONE HCL, NALOXONE HYDROCHLORIDE
NANDROLONE DECANOATE, NANDROLONE
    DECANOATE
NANDROLONE PHENPROPIONATE, NANDROLONE
    PHENPROPIONATE
NITROGLYCERIN, NITROGLYCERIN
PANCURONIUM BROMIDE, PANCURONIUM BROMIDE
PRALIDOXIME CHLORIDE, PRALIDOXIME CHLORIDE
PROCAINAMIDE HCL, PROCAINAMIDE
    HYDROCHLORIDE
PROCHLORPERAZINE EDISYLATE,
    PROCHLORPERAZINE EDISYLATE
PROTAMINE SULFATE, PROTAMINE SULFATE
RITODRINE HCL, RITODRINE HYDROCHLORIDE
SULFAMETHOPRIM, SULFAMETHOXAZOLE
TESTOSTERONE CYPIONATE, TESTOSTERONE
    CYPIONATE

TESTOSTERONE ENANTHATE, TESTOSTERONE
    ENANTHATE
TESTOSTERONE PROPIONATE, TESTOSTERONE
    PROPIONATE
TRIFLUOPERAZINE HCL, TRIFLUOPERAZINE
    HYDROCHLORIDE
TUBOCURARINE CHLORIDE, TUBOCURARINE
    CHLORIDE
VANCOMYCIN HCL, VANCOMYCIN HYDROCHLORIDE
VERAPAMIL HCL, VERAPAMIL HYDROCHLORIDE
VINBLASTINE SULFATE, VINBLASTINE SULFATE
VINCRISTINE SULFATE, VINCRISTINE SULFATE
QUANTUM PHARMICS
QUANTUM PHARMICS LTD
BENZTROPINE MESYLATE, BENZTROPINE MESYLATE
BUTALBITAL ASPIRIN AND CAFFEINE, ASPIRIN
CLOPRA, METOCLOPRAMIDE HYDROCHLORIDE
CLOPRA-"YELLOW", METOCLOPRAMIDE
    HYDROCHLORIDE
CLORAZEPATE DIPOTASSIUM, CLORAZEPATE
    DIPOTASSIUM
DOXEPIN HCL, DOXEPIN HYDROCHLORIDE
DOXYLAMINE SUCCINATE, DOXYLAMINE SUCCINATE
FENOPROFEN CALCIUM, FENOPROFEN CALCIUM
HALOPERIDOL, HALOPERIDOL
HYDRALAZINE HCL, HYDRALAZINE HYDROCHLORIDE
HYDROXYZINE HCL, HYDROXYZINE HYDROCHLORIDE
LORAZ, LORAZEPAM
MECLODIUM, MECLOFENAMATE SODIUM
MINODYL, MINOXIDIL
NYSTATIN, NYSTATIN
OXYBUTYNIN CHLORIDE, OXYBUTYNIN CHLORIDE
PHENTERMINE RESIN 30, PHENTERMINE RESIN
    COMPLEX
Q-GESIC, ASPIRIN
Q-PAM, DIAZEPAM
TEMAZ, TEMAZEPAM
TIMOLOL MALEATE, TIMOLOL MALEATE
TRAZODONE HCL, TRAZODONE HYDROCHLORIDE
TRIALODINE, TRAZODONE HYDROCHLORIDE
TRIAMTERENE AND HYDROCHLOROTHIAZIDE,
    HYDROCHLOROTHIAZIDE
ZAXOPAM, OXAZEPAM
QUESTCOR PHARMS
QUESTCOR PHARMACEUTICALS INC
ETHAMOLIN, ETHANOLAMINE OLEATE
GLOFIL-125, IOTHALAMATE SODIUM, I-125
H.P. ACTHAR GEL, CORTICOTROPIN
INULIN AND SODIUM CHLORIDE, INULIN
NASCOBAL, CYANOCOBALAMIN

R

R AND D LABS
R AND D LABORATORIES INC
FERRLECIT, SODIUM FERRIC GLUCONATE COMPLEX
R AND S PHARMA
R AND S PHARMA INC
DIPHENOXYLATE HCL AND ATROPINE SULFATE,
    ATROPINE SULFATE
R R REGISTRATIONS
R AND R REGISTRATIONS
THYROSAFE, POTASSIUM IODIDE (OTC)
RACHELLE
RACHELLE LABORATORIES INC
CHLORDIAZACHEL, CHLORDIAZEPOXIDE
    HYDROCHLORIDE

APPENDIX B
PRODUCT NAME INDEX
LISTED BY APPLICANT (*continued*)

DOXYCHEL HYCLATE, DOXYCYCLINE HYCLATE
DOXYCHEL, DOXYCYCLINE
RANBAXY
RANBAXY LABORATORIES LTD
  ACYCLOVIR, ACYCLOVIR
  AMOXICILLIN AND CLAVULANATE POTASSIUM,
    AMOXICILLIN
  AMOXICILLIN, AMOXICILLIN
  CEFADROXIL, CEFADROXIL/CEFADROXIL
    HEMIHYDRATE
  CEFPODOXIME PROXETIL, CEFPODOXIME PROXETIL
  CEFUROXIME AXETIL, CEFUROXIME AXETIL
  CEPHALEXIN, CEPHALEXIN
  CLINDAMYCIN HCL, CLINDAMYCIN HYDROCHLORIDE
  DOXYCYCLINE, DOXYCYCLINE
  ENALAPRIL MALEATE, ENALAPRIL MALEATE
  ETODOLAC, ETODOLAC
  FLECAINIDE ACETATE, FLECAINIDE ACETATE
  FLUOXETINE, FLUOXETINE HYDROCHLORIDE
  GANCICLOVIR, GANCICLOVIR
  LORAZEPAM, LORAZEPAM
  MIDAZOLAM HCL, MIDAZOLAM HYDROCHLORIDE
  MINOCYCLINE HCL, MINOCYCLINE HYDROCHLORIDE
  RANITIDINE, RANITIDINE HYDROCHLORIDE
  RANITIDINE, RANITIDINE HYDROCHLORIDE (OTC)
  SOTRET, ISOTRETINOIN
  TERAZOSIN HCL, TERAZOSIN HYDROCHLORIDE
RANBAXY PHARMACEUTICALS INC
  ACETAMINOPHEN AND CODEINE PHOSPHATE,
    ACETAMINOPHEN
  ACETAMINOPHEN W/ CODEINE PHOSPHATE #3,
    ACETAMINOPHEN
  AMOXICILLIN AND CLAVULANATE POTASSIUM,
    AMOXICILLIN
  AMOXICILLIN, AMOXICILLIN
  AVENTYL HCL, NORTRIPTYLINE HYDROCHLORIDE
  CEFACLOR, CEFACLOR
  CEFADROXIL, CEFADROXIL/CEFADROXIL
    HEMIHYDRATE
  DOXYCYCLINE HYCLATE, DOXYCYCLINE HYCLATE
  ISOTRETINOIN, ISOTRETINOIN
  LISINOPRIL AND HYDROCHLOROTHIAZIDE,
    HYDROCHLOROTHIAZIDE
  LISINOPRIL, LISINOPRIL
  NALFON 200, FENOPROFEN CALCIUM
  NALFON, FENOPROFEN CALCIUM
  PENTAZOCINE AND NALOXONE HYDROCHLORIDES,
    NALOXONE HYDROCHLORIDE
  RANITIDINE HCL, RANITIDINE HYDROCHLORIDE
  RANITIDINE, RANITIDINE HYDROCHLORIDE (OTC)
  SECONAL SODIUM, SECOBARBITAL SODIUM
RATIOPHARM
RATIOPHARM GMBH AND CO ARZNEIMITTEL
  SUCRALFATE, SUCRALFATE
RECKITT BENCKISER
RECKITT BENCKISER PHARMACEUTICALS INC
  BUPRENEX, BUPRENORPHINE HYDROCHLORIDE
  SUBOXONE, BUPRENORPHINE HYDROCHLORIDE
  SUBUTEX, BUPRENORPHINE HYDROCHLORIDE
REED AND CARNRICK
REED AND CARNRICK PHARMACEUTICALS DIV BLOCK
DRUG CO INC
  KWELL, LINDANE
RELIANT PHARMS
RELIANT PHARMACEUTICALS LLC
  AXID, NIZATIDINE
  DYNACIRC CR, ISRADIPINE
  DYNACIRC, ISRADIPINE

  INNOPRAN XL, PROPRANOLOL HYDROCHLORIDE
RES INDS
RESEARCH INDUSTRIES CORP
  RIMSO-50, DIMETHYL SULFOXIDE
REXALL
REXALL DRUG CO
  PREDNISONE, PREDNISONE
  RESERPINE, RESERPINE
REXAR
REXAR PHARMACAL
  METHAMPHETAMINE HCL, METHAMPHETAMINE
    HYDROCHLORIDE
RHODIA
RHODIA LTD
  ISOFLURANE, ISOFLURANE
ROACO
TJ ROACO LTD
  BETADERM, BETAMETHASONE VALERATE
ROBINS AH
AH ROBINS CO
  DIMETANE-DC, BROMPHENIRAMINE MALEATE
  DIMETANE-DX, BROMPHENIRAMINE MALEATE
  PHENAPHEN W/ CODEINE NO. 2, ACETAMINOPHEN
  PHENAPHEN W/ CODEINE NO. 3, ACETAMINOPHEN
  PHENAPHEN W/ CODEINE NO. 4, ACETAMINOPHEN
  PHENAPHEN-650 W/ CODEINE, ACETAMINOPHEN
  REGLAN, METOCLOPRAMIDE HYDROCHLORIDE
  ROBAXIN, METHOCARBAMOL
  ROBAXISAL, ASPIRIN
  ROBIMYCIN, ERYTHROMYCIN
  ROBINUL, GLYCOPYRROLATE
  TENATHAN, BETHANIDINE SULFATE
ROCHE
HOFFMANN LA ROCHE INC
  ARFONAD, TRIMETHAPHAN CAMSYLATE
  AZO GANTANOL, PHENAZOPYRIDINE HYDROCHLORIDE
  AZO GANTRISIN, PHENAZOPYRIDINE HYDROCHLORIDE
  BEROCCA PN, ASCORBIC ACID
  BONIVA, IBANDRONATE SODIUM
  BUMEX, BUMETANIDE
  COACTIN, AMDINOCILLIN
  COPEGUS, RIBAVIRIN
  DEMADEX, TORSEMIDE
  ENDEP, AMITRIPTYLINE HYDROCHLORIDE
  FANSIDAR, PYRIMETHAMINE
  FUZEON, ENFUVIRTIDE
  GANTANOL, SULFAMETHOXAZOLE
  GANTANOL-DS, SULFAMETHOXAZOLE
  GANTRISIN PEDIATRIC, SULFISOXAZOLE ACETYL
  GANTRISIN, SULFISOXAZOLE
  GANTRISIN, SULFISOXAZOLE ACETYL
  GANTRISIN, SULFISOXAZOLE DIOLAMINE
  HIVID, ZALCITABINE
  KLONOPIN RAPIDLY DISINTEGRATING, CLONAZEPAM
  KLONOPIN, CLONAZEPAM
  KONAKION, PHYTONADIONE
  KYTRIL, GRANISETRON HYDROCHLORIDE
  LARIAM, MEFLOQUINE HYDROCHLORIDE
  LARODOPA, LEVODOPA
  LIPO GANTRISIN, SULFISOXAZOLE ACETYL
  LORFAN, LEVALLORPHAN TARTRATE
  MENRIUM 10-4, CHLORDIAZEPOXIDE
  MENRIUM 5-2, CHLORDIAZEPOXIDE
  MENRIUM 5-4, CHLORDIAZEPOXIDE
  NIPRIDE, SODIUM NITROPRUSSIDE
  NOLUDAR, METHYPRYLON
  QUARZAN, CLIDINIUM BROMIDE
  RIMADYL, CARPROFEN

APPENDIX B
PRODUCT NAME INDEX
LISTED BY APPLICANT (*continued*)

RIMIFON, ISONIAZID
ROCALTROL, CALCITRIOL
ROCEPHIN, CEFTRIAXONE SODIUM
SOLATENE, BETA-CAROTENE
SYNKAYVITE, MENADIOL SODIUM DIPHOSPHATE
TAMIFLU, OSELTAMIVIR PHOSPHATE
TARACTAN, CHLORPROTHIXENE
TASMAR, TOLCAPONE
TEGISON, ETRETINATE
TRIMPEX 200, TRIMETHOPRIM
TRIMPEX, TRIMETHOPRIM
VALIUM, DIAZEPAM
VALRELEASE, DIAZEPAM
VERSED, MIDAZOLAM HYDROCHLORIDE
VESANOID, TRETINOIN
ROCHE PALO
ROCHE PALO ALTO LLC
    AEROBID, FLUNISOLIDE
    ANAPROX DS, NAPROXEN SODIUM
    ANAPROX, NAPROXEN SODIUM
    CARDENE SR, NICARDIPINE HYDROCHLORIDE
    CARDENE, NICARDIPINE HYDROCHLORIDE
    CELLCEPT, MYCOPHENOLATE MOFETIL
    CELLCEPT, MYCOPHENOLATE MOFETIL
        HYDROCHLORIDE
    CYTOVENE IV, GANCICLOVIR SODIUM
    CYTOVENE, GANCICLOVIR
    EC-NAPROSYN, NAPROXEN
    EVEX, ESTROGENS, ESTERIFIED
    FEMSTAT 3, BUTOCONAZOLE NITRATE (OTC)
    FEMSTAT, BUTOCONAZOLE NITRATE
    NAPROSYN, NAPROXEN
    TICLID, TICLOPIDINE HYDROCHLORIDE
    TORADOL, KETOROLAC TROMETHAMINE
    VALCYTE, VALGANCICLOVIR HYDROCHLORIDE
ROERIG
ROERIG DIV PFIZER INC
    ATARAX, HYDROXYZINE HYDROCHLORIDE
    EMETE-CON, BENZQUINAMIDE HYDROCHLORIDE
    GEOPEN, CARBENICILLIN DISODIUM
    SUSTAIRE, THEOPHYLLINE
ROMARK
ROMARK LABORATORIES
    ALINIA, NITAZOXANIDE
RORER
RORER PHARMACEUTICAL CORP SUB RORER GROUP
    NITROL, NITROGLYCERIN
ROSS LABS
ROSS LABORATORIES DIV ABBOTT LABORATORIES
    MIDAZOLAM HCL, MIDAZOLAM HYDROCHLORIDE
ROSS LABORATORIES DIV ABBOTT LABORATORIES INC
    PEDIAMYCIN 400, ERYTHROMYCIN ETHYLSUCCINATE
    PEDIAMYCIN, ERYTHROMYCIN ETHYLSUCCINATE
    PEDIAZOLE, ERYTHROMYCIN ETHYLSUCCINATE
    SURVANTA, BERACTANT
ROXANE
ROXANE LABORATORIES INC
    ACETAMINOPHEN AND CODEINE PHOSPHATE NO. 4,
        ACETAMINOPHEN
    ACETAMINOPHEN AND CODEINE PHOSPHATE,
        ACETAMINOPHEN
    ACETAMINOPHEN W/ CODEINE NO. 2, ACETAMINOPHEN
    ACETAMINOPHEN W/ CODEINE NO. 3, ACETAMINOPHEN
    ACETAMINOPHEN W/ CODEINE, ACETAMINOPHEN
    ACETAMINOPHEN, ACETAMINOPHEN (OTC)
    ACETYLCYSTEINE, ACETYLCYSTEINE
    ACYCLOVIR, ACYCLOVIR
    ALBUTEROL SULFATE, ALBUTEROL SULFATE

ALPRAZOLAM, ALPRAZOLAM
AMINOPHYLLINE, AMINOPHYLLINE
AMITRIPTYLINE HCL, AMITRIPTYLINE HYDROCHLORIDE
AZATHIOPRINE, AZATHIOPRINE
BUTORPHANOL TARTRATE, BUTORPHANOL TARTRATE
CHLORDIAZEPOXIDE HCL, CHLORDIAZEPOXIDE
    HYDROCHLORIDE
CHLORPHENIRAMINE MALEATE, CHLORPHENIRAMINE
    MALEATE
CHLORPROMAZINE HCL INTENSOL, CHLORPROMAZINE
    HYDROCHLORIDE
CHLORPROMAZINE HCL, CHLORPROMAZINE
    HYDROCHLORIDE
CIMETIDINE HCL, CIMETIDINE HYDROCHLORIDE
CIMETIDINE, CIMETIDINE
CROMOLYN SODIUM, CROMOLYN SODIUM
CYCLOPHOSPHAMIDE, CYCLOPHOSPHAMIDE
DEXAMETHASONE INTENSOL, DEXAMETHASONE
DEXAMETHASONE, DEXAMETHASONE
DIAZEPAM INTENSOL, DIAZEPAM
DIAZEPAM, DIAZEPAM
DICLOFENAC SODIUM, DICLOFENAC SODIUM
DIFLUNISAL, DIFLUNISAL
DIPHENHYDRAMINE HCL, DIPHENHYDRAMINE
    HYDROCHLORIDE
DIPHENOXYLATE HCL AND ATROPINE SULFATE,
    ATROPINE SULFATE
DOLOPHINE HCL, METHADONE HYDROCHLORIDE
FLECAINIDE ACETATE, FLECAINIDE ACETATE
FUROSEMIDE, FUROSEMIDE
HALOPERIDOL INTENSOL, HALOPERIDOL LACTATE
HALOPERIDOL, HALOPERIDOL
HYDROCHLOROTHIAZIDE INTENSOL,
    HYDROCHLOROTHIAZIDE
HYDROCHLOROTHIAZIDE W/ RESERPINE,
    HYDROCHLOROTHIAZIDE
HYDROCHLOROTHIAZIDE, HYDROCHLOROTHIAZIDE
HYDROCORTISONE, HYDROCORTISONE
HYDROMORPHONE HCL, HYDROMORPHONE
    HYDROCHLORIDE
HYDROXYUREA, HYDROXYUREA
IMIPRAMINE HCL, IMIPRAMINE HYDROCHLORIDE
INDOMETHACIN, INDOMETHACIN
IPATROPIUM BROMIDE, IPRATROPIUM BROMIDE
ISOETHARINE HCL, ISOETHARINE HYDROCHLORIDE
KETOROLAC TROMETHAMINE, KETOROLAC
    TROMETHAMINE
LACTULOSE, LACTULOSE
LEUCOVORIN CALCIUM, LEUCOVORIN CALCIUM
LEVORPHANOL TARTRATE, LEVORPHANOL TARTRATE
LIDOCAINE HCL, LIDOCAINE HYDROCHLORIDE
LIDOCAINE VISCOUS, LIDOCAINE HYDROCHLORIDE
LITHIUM CARBONATE, LITHIUM CARBONATE
LITHIUM CITRATE, LITHIUM CITRATE
LOPERAMIDE HCL, LOPERAMIDE HYDROCHLORIDE
LOPERAMIDE HCL, LOPERAMIDE HYDROCHLORIDE
    (OTC)
LORAZEPAM INTENSOL, LORAZEPAM
LORAZEPAM, LORAZEPAM
MEGESTROL ACETATE, MEGESTROL ACETATE
MEPERIDINE HCL, MEPERIDINE HYDROCHLORIDE
MEPROBAMATE, MEPROBAMATE
METHADONE HCL INTENSOL, METHADONE
    HYDROCHLORIDE
METHADONE HCL, METHADONE HYDROCHLORIDE
METHOCARBAMOL, METHOCARBAMOL
METHOTREXATE SODIUM, METHOTREXATE SODIUM
METHYLDOPA, METHYLDOPA

APPENDIX B
PRODUCT NAME INDEX
LISTED BY APPLICANT (*continued*)

METOCLOPRAMIDE HCL, METOCLOPRAMIDE
   HYDROCHLORIDE
METOCLOPRAMIDE INTENSOL, METOCLOPRAMIDE
   HYDROCHLORIDE
MIDAZOLAM HCL, MIDAZOLAM HYDROCHLORIDE
MIRTAZAPINE, MIRTAZAPINE
NAPROXEN SODIUM, NAPROXEN SODIUM
NAPROXEN, NAPROXEN
NEOMYCIN SULFATE, NEOMYCIN SULFATE
NYSTATIN, NYSTATIN
ORLAAM, LEVOMETHADYL ACETATE HYDROCHLORIDE
OXYCODONE AND ASPIRIN (HALF-STRENGTH), ASPIRIN
PIROXICAM, PIROXICAM
POTASSIUM IODIDE, POTASSIUM IODIDE (OTC)
PREDNISOLONE, PREDNISOLONE
PREDNISONE INTENSOL, PREDNISONE
PREDNISONE, PREDNISONE
PROCAINAMIDE HCL, PROCAINAMIDE
   HYDROCHLORIDE
PROPANTHELINE BROMIDE, PROPANTHELINE
   BROMIDE
PROPOXYPHENE HCL, PROPOXYPHENE
   HYDROCHLORIDE
PROPRANOLOL HCL INTENSOL, PROPRANOLOL
   HYDROCHLORIDE
PROPRANOLOL HCL, PROPRANOLOL HYDROCHLORIDE
QUINIDINE GLUCONATE, QUINIDINE GLUCONATE
QUINIDINE SULFATE, QUINIDINE SULFATE
RESERPINE, RESERPINE
ROXICET 5/500, ACETAMINOPHEN
ROXICET, ACETAMINOPHEN
ROXICODONE, OXYCODONE HYDROCHLORIDE
ROXILOX, ACETAMINOPHEN
ROXIPRIN, ASPIRIN
SODIUM POLYSTYRENE SULFONATE, SODIUM
   POLYSTYRENE SULFONATE
SULFAMETHOXAZOLE AND TRIMETHOPRIM DOUBLE
   STRENGTH, SULFAMETHOXAZOLE
SULFAMETHOXAZOLE AND TRIMETHOPRIM,
   SULFAMETHOXAZOLE
SULFISOXAZOLE, SULFISOXAZOLE
TAMOXIFEN CITRATE, TAMOXIFEN CITRATE
TETRACYCLINE HCL, TETRACYCLINE HYDROCHLORIDE
THEOPHYLLINE, THEOPHYLLINE
THIORIDAZINE HCL INTENSOL, THIORIDAZINE
   HYDROCHLORIDE
THIORIDAZINE HCL, THIORIDAZINE HYDROCHLORIDE
THIOTHIXENE HCL INTENSOL, THIOTHIXENE
   HYDROCHLORIDE
TRIAMCINOLONE, TRIAMCINOLONE
TRIAZOLAM, TRIAZOLAM
ROYCE LABS
ROYCE LABORATORIES INC
   HALOPERIDOL, HALOPERIDOL
   MINOXIDIL, MINOXIDIL

S

SABEX 2002
SABEX 2002 INC
   INFUVITE ADULT, ALPHA-TOCOPHEROL ACETATE
   INFUVITE PEDIATRIC, ASCORBIC ACID
   PROPRANOLOL HCL, PROPRANOLOL HYDROCHLORIDE
   REGONOL, PYRIDOSTIGMINE BROMIDE
SALIX PHARMS
SALIX PHARMACEUTICALS INC
   COLAZAL, BALSALAZIDE DISODIUM

SANKYO
SANKYO PHARMA INC
   BENICAR HCT, HYDROCHLOROTHIAZIDE
   BENICAR, OLMESARTAN MEDOXOMIL
   WELCHOL, COLESEVELAM HYDROCHLORIDE
SANKYO USA CORP
   BANAN, CEFPODOXIME PROXETIL
   PRELAY, TROGLITAZONE
SANO
SANO CORP
   NICOTINE, NICOTINE
SANOFI
SANOFI RESEARCH DIV SANOFI INC
   ELOXATIN, OXALIPLATIN
SANOFI SYN RES
SANOFI SYNTHELABO RESEARCH DIV SANOFI SYNTHELA-
BO INC
   UROXATRAL, ALFUZOSIN HYDROCHLORIDE
SANOFI SYNTHELABO
SANOFI SYNTHELABO INC
   ARALEN HCL, CHLOROQUINE HYDROCHLORIDE
   ARALEN PHOSPHATE W/ PRIMAQUINE PHOSPHATE,
     CHLOROQUINE PHOSPHATE
   ARALEN, CHLOROQUINE PHOSPHATE
   AVALIDE, HYDROCHLOROTHIAZIDE
   AVAPRO, IRBESARTAN
   BRONKODYL, THEOPHYLLINE
   BRONKOMETER, ISOETHARINE MESYLATE
   BRONKOSOL, ISOETHARINE HYDROCHLORIDE
   BRYREL, PIPERAZINE CITRATE
   CALCIPARINE, HEPARIN CALCIUM
   CHEMET, SUCCIMER
   DANOCRINE, DANAZOL
   DEMEROL, MEPERIDINE HYDROCHLORIDE
   DRISDOL, ERGOCALCIFEROL
   INOCOR, INAMRINONE LACTATE
   ISUPREL, ISOPROTERENOL HYDROCHLORIDE
   KAYEXALATE, SODIUM POLYSTYRENE SULFONATE
   LOTUSATE, TALBUTAL
   MYTELASE, AMBENONIUM CHLORIDE
   NEGGRAM, NALIDIXIC ACID
   PHISO-SCRUB, HEXACHLOROPHENE
   PHISOHEX, HEXACHLOROPHENE
   PLAQUENIL, HYDROXYCHLOROQUINE SULFATE
   PLAVIX, CLOPIDOGREL BISULFATE
   PRIMACOR IN DEXTROSE 5% IN PLASTIC CONTAINER,
     MILRINONE LACTATE
   PRIMACOR, MILRINONE LACTATE
   PRIMAQUINE, PRIMAQUINE PHOSPHATE
   SKELID, TILUDRONATE DISODIUM
   TALACEN, ACETAMINOPHEN
   TALWIN 50, PENTAZOCINE HYDROCHLORIDE
   TALWIN COMPOUND, ASPIRIN
   TALWIN NX, NALOXONE HYDROCHLORIDE
   TORNALATE, BITOLTEROL MESYLATE
   TRANCOPAL, CHLORMEZANONE
   WINSTROL, STANOZOLOL
SANTEN
SANTEN INC
   ALAMAST, PEMIROLAST POTASSIUM
   QUIXIN, LEVOFLOXACIN
SANTEN OY
SANTEN OY
   BETIMOL, TIMOLOL
SAVAGE LABS
SAVAGE LABORATORIES INC DIV ALTANA INC
   ALPHATREX, BETAMETHASONE DIPROPIONATE
   AXOTAL, ASPIRIN

APPENDIX B
PRODUCT NAME INDEX
LISTED BY APPLICANT (*continued*)

BETATREX, BETAMETHASONE VALERATE
CHYMEX, BENTIROMIDE
DILOR, DYPHYLLINE
DILOR-400, DYPHYLLINE
DITATE-DS, ESTRADIOL VALERATE
ETHIODOL, ETHIODIZED OIL
FLUOTREX, FLUOCINOLONE ACETONIDE
GVS, GENTIAN VIOLET
K-LEASE, POTASSIUM CHLORIDE
KAON CL, POTASSIUM CHLORIDE
KAON CL-10, POTASSIUM CHLORIDE
MYTREX A, NEOMYCIN SULFATE
MYTREX F, NYSTATIN
NYSTEX, NYSTATIN
PANDEL, HYDROCORTISONE PROBUTATE
RUVITE, CYANOCOBALAMIN
SATRIC, METRONIDAZOLE
TRYMEX, TRIAMCINOLONE ACETONIDE
TRYSUL, TRIPLE SULFA (SULFABENZAMIDE;
　　SULFACETAMIDE; SULFATHIAZOLE)
XYLO-PFAN, XYLOSE
SAVIENT PHARMS
SAVIENT PHARMACEUTICALS INC
　DELATESTRYL, TESTOSTERONE ENANTHATE
SB PHARMCO
SB PHARMCO PUERTO RICO INC
　AVANDAMET, METFORMIN HYDROCHLORIDE
　AVANDIA, ROSIGLITAZONE MALEATE
SCHEIN
SCHEIN PHARMACEUTICAL INC
　INFED, IRON DEXTRAN
　PROGESTERONE, PROGESTERONE
SCHERER LABS
SCHERER LABORATORIES INC
　CODEINE, ASPIRIN, APAP FORMULA NO. 2,
　　ACETAMINOPHEN
　CODEINE, ASPIRIN, APAP FORMULA NO. 3,
　　ACETAMINOPHEN
　CODEINE, ASPIRIN, APAP FORMULA NO. 4,
　　ACETAMINOPHEN
　MEPROBAMATE, MEPROBAMATE
　PREDNISONE, PREDNISONE
　QUINIDINE SULFATE, QUINIDINE SULFATE
SCHERER RP
RP SCHERER CORP
　NIFEDIPINE, NIFEDIPINE
RP SCHERER NORTH AMERICA
　NIFEDIPINE, NIFEDIPINE
　THEOPHYLLINE, THEOPHYLLINE
　VALPROIC ACID, VALPROIC ACID
RP SCHERER NORTH AMERICA DIV RP SCHERER CORP
　DIPHENOXYLATE HCL W/ ATROPINE SULFATE,
　　ATROPINE SULFATE
　THEOPHYLLINE-SR, THEOPHYLLINE
　VALPROIC ACID, VALPROIC ACID
SCHERING
SCHERING CORP
　CLARINEX, DESLORATADINE
　CLARITIN REDITABS, LORATADINE
　CLARITIN REDITABS, LORATADINE (OTC)
　CLARITIN, LORATADINE
　CLARITIN, LORATADINE (OTC)
　CLARITIN-D 24 HOUR, LORATADINE (OTC)
　DIPROLENE AF, BETAMETHASONE DIPROPIONATE
　GUANIDINE HCL, GUANIDINE HYDROCHLORIDE
　IMDUR, ISOSORBIDE MONONITRATE
　LOTRISONE, BETAMETHASONE DIPROPIONATE
　QUINORA, QUINIDINE SULFATE

RENORMAX, SPIRAPRIL HYDROCHLORIDE
TEMODAR, TEMOZOLOMIDE
THEO-DUR, THEOPHYLLINE
UNI-DUR, THEOPHYLLINE
VALISONE, BETAMETHASONE VALERATE
VANCENASE AQ, BECLOMETHASONE DIPROPIONATE
　MONOHYDRATE
VANCERIL DOUBLE STRENGTH, BECLOMETHASONE
　DIPROPIONATE
SCHERING CORP SUB SCHERING PLOUGH CORP
　AKRINOL, ACRISORCIN
　BETAPAR, MEPREDNISONE
　CELESTONE SOLUSPAN, BETAMETHASONE ACETATE
　CELESTONE, BETAMETHASONE
　CELESTONE, BETAMETHASONE SODIUM PHOSPHATE
　CHLOR-TRIMETON, CHLORPHENIRAMINE MALEATE
　CLARITIN, LORATADINE
　CLARITIN, LORATADINE (OTC)
　CLARITIN-D, LORATADINE (OTC)
　DIPROLENE, BETAMETHASONE DIPROPIONATE
　DIPROSONE, BETAMETHASONE DIPROPIONATE
　DISOMER, DEXBROMPHENIRAMINE MALEATE
　DISOPHROL, DEXBROMPHENIRAMINE MALEATE (OTC)
　FLOCON, MOMETASONE FUROATE
　ESTINYL, ETHINYL ESTRADIOL
　ETRAFON 2-10, AMITRIPTYLINE HYDROCHLORIDE
　ETRAFON 2-25, AMITRIPTYLINE HYDROCHLORIDE
　ETRAFON-A, AMITRIPTYLINE HYDROCHLORIDE
　ETRAFON-FORTE, AMITRIPTYLINE HYDROCHLORIDE
　EULEXIN, FLUTAMIDE
　FULVICIN P/G 165, GRISEOFULVIN,
　　ULTRAMICROCRYSTALLINE
　FULVICIN P/G 330, GRISEOFULVIN,
　　ULTRAMICROCRYSTALLINE
　FULVICIN P/G, GRISEOFULVIN,
　　ULTRAMICROCRYSTALLINE
　FULVICIN-U/F, GRISEOFULVIN, MICROCRYSTALLINE
　GARAMYCIN, GENTAMICIN SULFATE
　HYPERSTAT, DIAZOXIDE
　LOTRIMIN, CLOTRIMAZOLE
　METI-DERM, PREDNISOLONE
　METICORTELONE, PREDNISOLONE ACETATE
　METICORTEN, PREDNISONE
　METIMYD, PREDNISOLONE ACETATE
　METOCLOPRAMIDE HCL, METOCLOPRAMIDE
　　HYDROCHLORIDE
　METRETON, PREDNISOLONE SODIUM PHOSPHATE
　MIRADON, ANISINDIONE
　NAQUA, TRICHLORMETHIAZIDE
　NAQUIVAL, RESERPINE
　NETROMYCIN, NETILMICIN SULFATE
　NORMODYNE, LABETALOL HYDROCHLORIDE
　NORMOZIDE, HYDROCHLOROTHIAZIDE
　OPTIMINE, AZATADINE MALEATE
　ORETON METHYL, METHYLTESTOSTERONE
　ORETON, METHYLTESTOSTERONE
　OTOBIONE, HYDROCORTISONE
　OTOBIOTIC, HYDROCORTISONE
　PAXIPAM, HALAZEPAM
　PERMITIL, FLUPHENAZINE HYDROCHLORIDE
　POLARAMINE, DEXCHLORPHENIRAMINE MALEATE
　PRANTAL, DIPHEMANIL METHYLSULFATE
　PROPRANOLOL HCL, PROPRANOLOL HYDROCHLORIDE
　PROVENTIL, ALBUTEROL
　PROVENTIL, ALBUTEROL SULFATE
　RELA, CARISOPRODOL
　SODIUM SULAMYD, SULFACETAMIDE SODIUM
　THEOVENT, THEOPHYLLINE

APPENDIX B
PRODUCT NAME INDEX
LISTED BY APPLICANT (*continued*)

TINDAL, ACETOPHENAZINE MALEATE
TREMIN, TRIHEXYPHENIDYL HYDROCHLORIDE
TRILAFON, PERPHENAZINE
TRINALIN, AZATADINE MALEATE
UNI-DUR, THEOPHYLLINE
VALISONE, BETAMETHASONE VALERATE
VANCENASE AQ, BECLOMETHASONE DIPROPIONATE
    MONOHYDRATE
VANCENASE, BECLOMETHASONE DIPROPIONATE
VANCERIL, BECLOMETHASONE DIPROPIONATE
SCHERING PLOUGH
SCHERING PLOUGH CORP
    CLARINEX, DESLORATADINE
    NASONEX, MOMETASONE FUROATE MONOHYDRATE
SCHERING PLOUGH HEALTHCARE PRODUCTS INC
    AFRINOL, PSEUDOEPHEDRINE SULFATE (OTC)
    CHLOR-TRIMETON, CHLORPHENIRAMINE MALEATE
    CHLOR-TRIMETON, CHLORPHENIRAMINE MALEATE
        (OTC)
    DEMAZIN, CHLORPHENIRAMINE MALEATE (OTC)
    DISOPHROL, DEXBROMPHENIRAMINE MALEATE (OTC)
    DRIXORAL PLUS, ACETAMINOPHEN (OTC)
    DRIXORAL, DEXBROMPHENIRAMINE MALEATE (OTC)
    GYNE-LOTRIMIN 3 COMBINATION PACK,
        CLOTRIMAZOLE (OTC)
    GYNE-LOTRIMIN 3, CLOTRIMAZOLE (OTC)
    GYNE-LOTRIMIN COMBINATION PACK, CLOTRIMAZOLE
        (OTC)
    GYNE-LOTRIMIN, CLOTRIMAZOLE (OTC)
    LOTRIMIN ULTRA, BUTENAFINE HYDROCHLORIDE
        (OTC)
    LOTRIMIN, CLOTRIMAZOLE
    OCUCLEAR, OXYMETAZOLINE HYDROCHLORIDE (OTC)
    SHADE UVAGUARD, AVOBENZONE (OTC)
SCHERING PLOUGH RES
SCHERING PLOUGH RESEARCH INSTITUTE
    LOTRISONE, BETAMETHASONE DIPROPIONATE
    REBETOL, RIBAVIRIN
SCHWARZ
SCHWARZ GMBH
    MONOKET, ISOSORBIDE MONONITRATE
SCHWARZ PHARMA
SCHWARZ PHARMA AG
    EDEX, ALPROSTADIL
    PRE-PEN, BENZYL PENICILLOYL-POLYLYSINE
SCHWARZ PHARMA INC
    CO-GESIC, ACETAMINOPHEN
    CODIMAL-L.A. 12, CHLORPHENIRAMINE MALEATE (OTC)
    COLYTE WITH FLAVOR PACKS, POLYETHYLENE
        GLYCOL 3350
    COLYTE, POLYETHYLENE GLYCOL 3350
    COLYTE-FLAVORED, POLYETHYLENE GLYCOL 3350
    CORTIFOAM, HYDROCORTISONE ACETATE
    DILATRATE-SR, ISOSORBIDE DINITRATE
    EPIFOAM, HYDROCORTISONE ACETATE
    LEVATOL, PENBUTOLOL SULFATE
    PREDNICEN-M, PREDNISONE
    PROCTOFOAM HC, HYDROCORTISONE ACETATE
    REGLAN, METOCLOPRAMIDE HYDROCHLORIDE
    ROBAXIN, METHOCARBAMOL
    ROBAXIN-750, METHOCARBAMOL
    THEOCLEAR L.A.-130, THEOPHYLLINE
    THEOCLEAR L.A.-260, THEOPHYLLINE
    UNIRETIC, HYDROCHLOROTHIAZIDE
    UNIVASC, MOEXIPRIL HYDROCHLORIDE
SCIOS
SCIOS INC
    NATRECOR, NESIRITIDE

SCS
SCS PHARMACEUTICALS
    ATENOLOL, ATENOLOL
    CARBIDOPA AND LEVODOPA, CARBIDOPA
    HALOPERIDOL, HALOPERIDOL
    HALOPERIDOL, HALOPERIDOL LACTATE
    PIROXICAM, PIROXICAM
SEPRACOR
SEPRACOR INC
    XOPENEX, LEVALBUTEROL HYDROCHLORIDE
SEPTODONT
SEPTODONT INC
    OCTOCAINE, EPINEPHRINE
SERONO
SERONO LABORATORIES INC
    ASELLACRIN 10, SOMATROPIN
    ASELLACRIN 2, SOMATROPIN
    FERTINEX, UROFOLLITROPIN
    GEREF, SERMORELIN ACETATE
    GONAL-F, FOLLITROPIN ALFA
    GONAL-F, FOLLITROPIN ALFA/BETA
    METRODIN, UROFOLLITROPIN
    PERGONAL, MENOTROPINS (FSH;LH)
    SAIZEN, SOMATROPIN RECOMBINANT
    SEROPHENE, CLOMIPHENE CITRATE
    SEROSTIM, SOMATROPIN RECOMBINANT
SERONO INC
SERONO INC
    CETROTIDE, CETRORELIX
    NOVANTRONE, MITOXANTRONE HYDROCHLORIDE
    OVIDREL, CHORIOGONADOTROPIN ALFA
SHERWOOD MEDCL
SHERWOOD MEDICAL CO
    ACTIN-N, NITROFURAZONE
SHIONOGI
SHIONOGI USA INC
    UROBAK, SULFAMETHOXAZOLE
    UROPLUS DS, SULFAMETHOXAZOLE
    UROPLUS SS, SULFAMETHOXAZOLE
SHIRE LABS
SHIRE LABORATORIES INC
    ADDERALL 10, AMPHETAMINE ASPARTATE
    ADDERALL 12.5, AMPHETAMINE ASPARTATE
    ADDERALL 15, AMPHETAMINE ASPARTATE
    ADDERALL 20, AMPHETAMINE ASPARTATE
    ADDERALL 30, AMPHETAMINE ASPARTATE
    ADDERALL 5, AMPHETAMINE ASPARTATE
    ADDERALL 7.5, AMPHETAMINE ASPARTATE
    ADDERALL XR 10, AMPHETAMINE ASPARTATE
    ADDERALL XR 15, AMPHETAMINE ASPARTATE
    ADDERALL XR 20, AMPHETAMINE ASPARTATE
    ADDERALL XR 25, AMPHETAMINE ASPARTATE
    ADDERALL XR 30, AMPHETAMINE ASPARTATE
    ADDERALL XR 5, AMPHETAMINE ASPARTATE
    AGRYLIN, ANAGRELIDE HYDROCHLORIDE
    BANTHINE, METHANTHELINE BROMIDE
    DOPAR, LEVODOPA
    ETHMOZINE, MORICIZINE HYDROCHLORIDE
    FURACIN, NITROFURAZONE
    FUROXONE, FURAZOLIDONE
    PENTASA, MESALAMINE
    PRO-BANTHINE, PROPANTHELINE BROMIDE
    SALURON, HYDROFLUMETHIAZIDE
    SALUTENSIN, HYDROFLUMETHIAZIDE
    SALUTENSIN-DEMI, HYDROFLUMETHIAZIDE
    SUPPRELIN, HISTRELIN ACETATE
    TOPICYCLINE, TETRACYCLINE HYDROCHLORIDE

APPENDIX B
PRODUCT NAME INDEX
LISTED BY APPLICANT (*continued*)

SHIRE PHARM
SHIRE PHARMACEUTICAL DEVELOPMENT INC
  ANOQUAN, ACETAMINOPHEN
  CARBATROL, CARBAMAZEPINE
  FURACIN, NITROFURAZONE
  PROAMATINE, MIDODRINE HYDROCHLORIDE
  URACIL MUSTARD, URACIL MUSTARD
SHIRE RICHWOOD
SHIRE RICHWOOD INC
  DEXTROSTAT, DEXTROAMPHETAMINE SULFATE
  OBY-TRIM, PHENTERMINE HYDROCHLORIDE
  X-TROZINE L.A., PHENDIMETRAZINE TARTRATE
  X-TROZINE, PHENDIMETRAZINE TARTRATE
SIEGFRIED
SIEGFRIED LTD
  FLUOXETINE, FLUOXETINE HYDROCHLORIDE
  SELEGILINE HCL, SELEGILINE HYDROCHLORIDE
SIGHT PHARMS
SIGHT PHARMACEUTICALS INC
  MINOXIDIL (FOR MEN), MINOXIDIL (OTC)
  MINOXIDIL (FOR WOMEN), MINOXIDIL (OTC)
SIGMA TAU
SIGMA TAU PHARMACEUTICALS INC
  CARNITOR, LEVOCARNITINE
  MATULANE, PROCARBAZINE HYDROCHLORIDE
SILARX
SILARX PHARMACEUTICALS INC
  CLEMASTINE FUMARATE, CLEMASTINE FUMARATE
  DOXEPIN HCL, DOXEPIN HYDROCHLORIDE
  HALOPERIDOL, HALOPERIDOL LACTATE
  METAPROTERENOL SULFATE, METAPROTERENOL
    SULFATE
  METOCLOPRAMIDE HCL, METOCLOPRAMIDE
    HYDROCHLORIDE
  OXYBUTYNIN CHLORIDE, OXYBUTYNIN CHLORIDE
  SILPHEN, DIPHENHYDRAMINE HYDROCHLORIDE (OTC)
SIRIUS LABS
SIRIUS LABORATORIES INC
  TEXACORT, HYDROCORTISONE
SKYEPHARMA
SKYEPHARMA INC
  DEPOCYT, CYTARABINE
SMITH AND NEPHEW
SMITH AND NEPHEW SOLOPAK DIV SMITH AND NEPHEW
  AMINOPHYLLINE, AMINOPHYLLINE
  DOPAMINE HCL, DOPAMINE HYDROCHLORIDE
  DROPERIDOL, DROPERIDOL
  FLUOROURACIL, FLUOROURACIL
  FUROSEMIDE, FUROSEMIDE
  HALOPERIDOL, HALOPERIDOL LACTATE
  HEPARIN LOCK FLUSH, HEPARIN SODIUM
  HEPARIN SODIUM, HEPARIN SODIUM
  HYDRALAZINE HCL, HYDRALAZINE HYDROCHLORIDE
  HYDROXYZINE HCL, HYDROXYZINE HYDROCHLORIDE
  METHYLDOPATE HCL, METHYLDOPATE
    HYDROCHLORIDE
  METOCLOPRAMIDE HCL, METOCLOPRAMIDE
    HYDROCHLORIDE
  NALOXONE HCL, NALOXONE HYDROCHLORIDE
  NITROGLYCERIN, NITROGLYCERIN
  PHENYTOIN SODIUM, PHENYTOIN SODIUM
  PROCAINAMIDE HCL, PROCAINAMIDE
    HYDROCHLORIDE
  PROCHLORPERAZINE EDISYLATE,
    PROCHLORPERAZINE EDISYLATE
  PROPRANOLOL HCL, PROPRANOLOL HYDROCHLORIDE
  TRIMETHOBENZAMIDE HCL, TRIMETHOBENZAMIDE
    HYDROCHLORIDE

  VERAPAMIL HCL, VERAPAMIL HYDROCHLORIDE
SOAPCO
SOAPCO INC
  BRIAN CARE, CHLORHEXIDINE GLUCONATE (OTC)
SOLA BARNES HIND
SOLA BARNES HIND
  ALPHA CHYMAR, CHYMOTRYPSIN
  BENOXINATE HCL, BENOXINATE HYDROCHLORIDE
  CYCLOPENTOLATE HCL, CYCLOPENTOLATE
    HYDROCHLORIDE
  DEXAMETHASONE SODIUM PHOSPHATE,
    DEXAMETHASONE SODIUM PHOSPHATE
  GAMENE, LINDANE
  PREDNISOLONE SODIUM PHOSPHATE, PREDNISOLONE
    SODIUM PHOSPHATE
  PROPARACAINE HCL, PROPARACAINE
    HYDROCHLORIDE
  SODIUM SULFACETAMIDE, SULFACETAMIDE SODIUM
  SULFISOXAZOLE DIOLAMINE, SULFISOXAZOLE
    DIOLAMINE
SOLOPAK
SOLOPAK LABORATORIES INC
  CLINDAMYCIN PHOSPHATE, CLINDAMYCIN
    PHOSPHATE
  DROPERIDOL, DROPERIDOL
  GENTAMICIN SULFATE, GENTAMICIN SULFATE
  HALOPERIDOL, HALOPERIDOL LACTATE
  HYDRALAZINE HCL, HYDRALAZINE HYDROCHLORIDE
  HYDROXYZINE HCL, HYDROXYZINE HYDROCHLORIDE
  KANAMYCIN SULFATE, KANAMYCIN SULFATE
SOLOPAK MEDICAL PRODUCTS INC
  CYANOCOBALAMIN, CYANOCOBALAMIN
  HALOPERIDOL, HALOPERIDOL LACTATE
  HEPARIN LOCK FLUSH, HEPARIN SODIUM
  HEPARIN SODIUM, HEPARIN SODIUM
  HYDROXYZINE HCL, HYDROXYZINE HYDROCHLORIDE
  NALOXONE HCL, NALOXONE HYDROCHLORIDE
  PHENYTOIN SODIUM, PHENYTOIN SODIUM
  PROCAINAMIDE HCL, PROCAINAMIDE
    HYDROCHLORIDE
  PROPRANOLOL HCL, PROPRANOLOL HYDROCHLORIDE
  TRIMETHOBENZAMIDE HCL, TRIMETHOBENZAMIDE
    HYDROCHLORIDE
  VERAPAMIL HCL, VERAPAMIL HYDROCHLORIDE
SOLVAY
SOLVAY PHARMACEUTICALS
  AQUATAG, BENZTHIAZIDE
  ARESTOCAINE HCL W/ LEVONORDEFRIN,
    LEVONORDEFRIN
  ARESTOCAINE HCL, MEPIVACAINE HYDROCHLORIDE
  ATROPINE, ATROPINE
  BALNEOL-HC, HYDROCORTISONE
  BUTABARBITAL SODIUM, BUTABARBITAL SODIUM
  CIN-QUIN, QUINIDINE SULFATE
  CORTENEMA, HYDROCORTISONE
  CURRETAB, MEDROXYPROGESTERONE ACETATE
  DERMACORT, HYDROCORTISONE
  DEXONE 0.5, DEXAMETHASONE
  DEXONE 0.75, DEXAMETHASONE
  DEXONE 1.5, DEXAMETHASONE
  DEXONE 4, DEXAMETHASONE
  DUPHALAC, LACTULOSE
  ESTRAGUARD, DIENESTROL
  ESTRATAB, ESTROGENS, ESTERIFIED
  GYNOREST, DYDROGESTERONE
  HYDRALAZINE HCL AND HYDROCHLOROTHIAZIDE,
    HYDRALAZINE HYDROCHLORIDE
  HYDROCHLOROTHIAZIDE, HYDROCHLOROTHIAZIDE

APPENDIX B
PRODUCT NAME INDEX
LISTED BY APPLICANT (*continued*)

LACTULOSE, LACTULOSE
LITHOBID, LITHIUM CARBONATE
LITHONATE, LITHIUM CARBONATE
LITHONATE, LITHIUM CITRATE
LITHOTABS, LITHIUM CARBONATE
LUVOX, FLUVOXAMINE MALEATE
MEPROBAMATE, MEPROBAMATE
METHOCARBAMOL, METHOCARBAMOL
ORASONE, PREDNISONE
PHENDIMETRAZINE TARTRATE, PHENDIMETRAZINE
   TARTRATE
PORTALAC, LACTULOSE
PROVAL #3, ACETAMINOPHEN
PYRIDOSTIGMINE BROMIDE, PYRIDOSTIGMINE
   BROMIDE
R-P MYCIN, ERYTHROMYCIN
RAUWOLFIA SERPENTINA, RAUWOLFIA SERPENTINA
RESERPINE, HYDRALAZINE HCL AND
   HYDROCHLOROTHIAZIDE, HYDRALAZINE
   HYDROCHLORIDE
RESERPINE, RESERPINE
RETET, TETRACYCLINE HYDROCHLORIDE
ROWASA, MESALAMINE
S.A.S.-500, SULFASALAZINE
SER-A-GEN, HYDRALAZINE HYDROCHLORIDE
SPRX-3, PHENDIMETRAZINE TARTRATE
SULSOXIN, SULFISOXAZOLE
SYMADINE, AMANTADINE HYDROCHLORIDE
TORA, PHENTERMINE HYDROCHLORIDE
TRANMEP, MEPROBAMATE
TRIACORT, TRIAMCINOLONE ACETONIDE
UNIPRES, HYDRALAZINE HYDROCHLORIDE
VERMIDOL, PIPERAZINE CITRATE
ZIDE, HYDROCHLOROTHIAZIDE
SOLVAY PHARMA
SOLVAY PHARMA INC
ACEON, PERINDOPRIL ERBUMINE
SOMERSET
SOMERSET PHARMACEUTICALS INC
ELDEPRYL, SELEGILINE HYDROCHLORIDE
SELEGILINE HCL, SELEGILINE HYDROCHLORIDE
SORIN
SORIN BIOMEDICA SPA
SODIUM ROSE BENGAL I 131, ROSE BENGAL SODIUM, I-
   131
SPEAR PHARMS
SPEAR PHARMACEUTICALS INC
TRETINOIN, TRETINOIN
SPERTI
SPERTI DRUG PRODUCTS INC
PREDNISOLONE, PREDNISOLONE
PREDNISONE, PREDNISONE
SSL INTL
SSL INTERNATIONAL
HIBICLENS, CHLORHEXIDINE GLUCONATE (OTC)
HIBISTAT, CHLORHEXIDINE GLUCONATE (OTC)
STANLABS PHARM
STANLABS PHARMACEUTICAL CO SUB SIMPAK CORP
MEPROBAMATE, MEPROBAMATE
STAR PHARMS FL
STAR PHARMACEUTICALS INC
VIRILON, METHYLTESTOSTERONE
STASON
STASON INDUSTRIAL CORP
ACYCLOVIR, ACYCLOVIR
CAPTOPRIL, CAPTOPRIL
SELEGILINE HCL, SELEGILINE HYDROCHLORIDE

STERIS
STERIS LABORATORIES INC
AMITRIPTYLINE HCL, AMITRIPTYLINE HYDROCHLORIDE
BETAMETHASONE SODIUM PHOSPHATE,
   BETAMETHASONE SODIUM PHOSPHATE
BROMPHENIRAMINE MALEATE, BROMPHENIRAMINE
   MALEATE
CHLORPHENIRAMINE MALEATE, CHLORPHENIRAMINE
   MALEATE
CHLORPROMAZINE HCL, CHLORPROMAZINE
   HYDROCHLORIDE
CHORIONIC GONADOTROPIN, GONADOTROPIN,
   CHORIONIC
CLINDAMYCIN PHOSPHATE, CLINDAMYCIN
   PHOSPHATE
COBAVITE, CYANOCOBALAMIN
CORTICOTROPIN, CORTICOTROPIN
CORTISONE ACETATE, CORTISONE ACETATE
CYANOCOBALAMIN, CYANOCOBALAMIN
DEXAMETHASONE ACETATE, DEXAMETHASONE
   ACETATE
DEXAMETHASONE SODIUM PHOSPHATE,
   DEXAMETHASONE SODIUM PHOSPHATE
DEXAMETHASONE, DEXAMETHASONE
DIAZEPAM, DIAZEPAM
DICYCLOMINE HCL, DICYCLOMINE HYDROCHLORIDE
DIMENHYDRINATE, DIMENHYDRINATE
DIPHENHYDRAMINE HCL PRESERVATIVE FREE,
   DIPHENHYDRAMINE HYDROCHLORIDE
DIPHENHYDRAMINE HCL, DIPHENHYDRAMINE
   HYDROCHLORIDE
DISODIUM EDETATE, EDETATE DISODIUM
DOBUTAMINE HCL, DOBUTAMINE HYDROCHLORIDE
DOXAPRAM HCL, DOXAPRAM HYDROCHLORIDE
DROPERIDOL, DROPERIDOL
EDETATE DISODIUM, EDETATE DISODIUM
EDROPHONIUM CHLORIDE PRESERVATIVE FREE,
   EDROPHONIUM CHLORIDE
EDROPHONIUM CHLORIDE, EDROPHONIUM CHLORIDE
ESTRADIOL CYPIONATE, ESTRADIOL CYPIONATE
ESTRADIOL VALERATE, ESTRADIOL VALERATE
ESTRONE, ESTRONE
ETOPOSIDE, ETOPOSIDE
FENTANYL CITRATE, FENTANYL CITRATE
FLUOROURACIL, FLUOROURACIL
FUROSEMIDE, FUROSEMIDE
GENTAMICIN SULFATE, GENTAMICIN SULFATE
GLYCOPYRROLATE, GLYCOPYRROLATE
HALOPERIDOL, HALOPERIDOL LACTATE
HEPARIN LOCK FLUSH, HEPARIN SODIUM
HEPARIN SODIUM, HEPARIN SODIUM
HYDROCORTISONE ACETATE, HYDROCORTISONE
   ACETATE
HYDROCORTISONE SODIUM SUCCINATE,
   HYDROCORTISONE SODIUM SUCCINATE
HYDROMORPHONE HCL, HYDROMORPHONE
   HYDROCHLORIDE
HYDROXOCOBALAMIN, HYDROXOCOBALAMIN
HYDROXYPROGESTERONE CAPROATE,
   HYDROXYPROGESTERONE CAPROATE
HYDROXYZINE HCL, HYDROXYZINE HYDROCHLORIDE
KANAMYCIN SULFATE, KANAMYCIN SULFATE
LIDOCAINE HCL W/ EPINEPHRINE, EPINEPHRINE
LIDOCAINE HCL, LIDOCAINE HYDROCHLORIDE
LINCOMYCIN HCL, LINCOMYCIN HYDROCHLORIDE
LORAZEPAM, LORAZEPAM
MANNITOL 25%, MANNITOL

APPENDIX B
PRODUCT NAME INDEX
LISTED BY APPLICANT (*continued*)

MEPERIDINE HCL PRESERVATIVE FREE, MEPERIDINE
    HYDROCHLORIDE
MEPERIDINE HCL, MEPERIDINE HYDROCHLORIDE
MEPIVACAINE HCL, MEPIVACAINE HYDROCHLORIDE
MERSALYL-THEOPHYLLINE, MERSALYL SODIUM
METHOCARBAMOL, METHOCARBAMOL
METHYLPREDNISOLONE ACETATE,
    METHYLPREDNISOLONE ACETATE
METHYLPREDNISOLONE SODIUM SUCCINATE,
    METHYLPREDNISOLONE SODIUM SUCCINATE
METOPROLOL TARTRATE, METOPROLOL TARTRATE
METRONIDAZOLE, METRONIDAZOLE
MORPHINE SULFATE, MORPHINE SULFATE
MVC PLUS, ASCORBIC ACID
NALOXONE HCL, NALOXONE HYDROCHLORIDE
NANDROLONE DECANOATE, NANDROLONE
    DECANOATE
NANDROLONE PHENPROPIONATE, NANDROLONE
    PHENPROPIONATE
NATURAL ESTROGENIC SUBSTANCE-ESTRONE,
    ESTRONE
NEOMYCIN AND POLYMYXIN B SULFATES AND
    GRAMICIDIN, GRAMICIDIN
NEOMYCIN AND POLYMYXIN B SULFATES, NEOMYCIN
    SULFATE
ORPHENADRINE CITRATE, ORPHENADRINE CITRATE
OTOCORT, HYDROCORTISONE
PENTAMIDINE ISETHIONATE, PENTAMIDINE
    ISETHIONATE
PHENYTOIN SODIUM, PHENYTOIN SODIUM
POTASSIUM CHLORIDE, POTASSIUM CHLORIDE
PREDNISOLONE ACETATE, PREDNISOLONE ACETATE
PREDNISOLONE SODIUM PHOSPHATE, PREDNISOLONE
    SODIUM PHOSPHATE
PREDNISOLONE TEBUTATE, PREDNISOLONE
    TEBUTATE
PROCAINAMIDE HCL, PROCAINAMIDE
    HYDROCHLORIDE
PROCAINE HCL, PROCAINE HYDROCHLORIDE
PROCHLORPERAZINE EDISYLATE,
    PROCHLORPERAZINE EDISYLATE
PROMAZINE HCL, PROMAZINE HYDROCHLORIDE
PROMETHAZINE HCL, PROMETHAZINE
    HYDROCHLORIDE
PYRIDOXINE HCL, PYRIDOXINE HYDROCHLORIDE
SUFENTANIL CITRATE, SUFENTANIL CITRATE
SULFACETAMIDE SODIUM, SULFACETAMIDE SODIUM
SULFAMETHOXAZOLE AND TRIMETHOPRIM,
    SULFAMETHOXAZOLE
TESTOSTERONE CYPIONATE, TESTOSTERONE
    CYPIONATE
TESTOSTERONE CYPIONATE-ESTRADIOL CYPIONATE,
    ESTRADIOL CYPIONATE
TESTOSTERONE ENANTHATE AND ESTRADIOL
    VALERATE, ESTRADIOL VALERATE
TESTOSTERONE ENANTHATE, TESTOSTERONE
    ENANTHATE
TESTOSTERONE PROPIONATE, TESTOSTERONE
    PROPIONATE
TESTOSTERONE, TESTOSTERONE
THIAMINE HCL, THIAMINE HYDROCHLORIDE
TRIAMCINOLONE ACETONIDE, TRIAMCINOLONE
    ACETONIDE
TRIAMCINOLONE DIACETATE, TRIAMCINOLONE
    DIACETATE
TRIMETHOBENZAMIDE HCL, TRIMETHOBENZAMIDE
    HYDROCHLORIDE
TROPICAMIDE, TROPICAMIDE

VECURONIUM BROMIDE, VECURONIUM BROMIDE
STERLING
STERLING HEALTH DIV STERLING WINTHROP INC
    BRONKAID MIST, EPINEPHRINE (OTC)
STERLING WINTHROP
STERLING WINTHROP INC
    AFAXIN, VITAMIN A PALMITATE
    CARBOCAINE, MEPIVACAINE HYDROCHLORIDE
STEVENS J
JEROME STEVENS PHARMACEUTICALS INC
    BUTALBITAL, ASPIRIN, CAFFEINE, AND CODEINE
        PHOSPHATE, ASPIRIN
    CEPHALEXIN, CEPHALEXIN
    DIGOXIN, DIGOXIN
    METHOCARBAMOL AND ASPIRIN, ASPIRIN
    ORPHENADRINE CITRATE, ASPIRIN, AND CAFFEINE,
        ASPIRIN
    UNITHROID, LIOTRIX (T4;T3)
STIEFEL
STIEFEL LABORATORIES INC
    CLINDAMYCIN PHOSPHATE, CLINDAMYCIN
        PHOSPHATE
    CLINDETS, CLINDAMYCIN PHOSPHATE
    CLOBETASOL PROPIONATE, CLOBETASOL
        PROPIONATE
    DUAC, BENZOYL PEROXIDE
    ERYTHROMYCIN, ERYTHROMYCIN
    HYDROCORTISONE, HYDROCORTISONE
    SCABENE, LINDANE
    STIE-CORT, HYDROCORTISONE
STORZ
STORZ OPHTHALMICS INC SUB AMERICAN CYANAMID CO
    ACHROMYCIN, TETRACYCLINE HYDROCHLORIDE
STUART PHARMS
STUART PHARMACEUTICALS DIV ICI AMERICAS
    BUCLADIN-S, BUCLIZINE HYDROCHLORIDE
SUMMERS
SUMMERS LABORATORIES INC
    CROTAN, CROTAMITON
SUPERGEN
SUPERGEN INC
    DAUNORUBICIN HCL, DAUNORUBICIN
        HYDROCHLORIDE
    ETOPOSIDE, ETOPOSIDE
    MITOMYCIN, MITOMYCIN
    MYTOZYTREX, MITOMYCIN
    NIPENT, PENTOSTATIN
SUPERPHARM
SUPERPHARM CORP
    ACETAMINOPHEN AND CODEINE PHOSPHATE #2,
        ACETAMINOPHEN
    ACETAMINOPHEN AND CODEINE PHOSPHATE #3,
        ACETAMINOPHEN
    ACETAMINOPHEN AND CODEINE PHOSPHATE #4,
        ACETAMINOPHEN
    ALLOPURINOL, ALLOPURINOL
    AMITRIPTYLINE HCL, AMITRIPTYLINE HYDROCHLORIDE
    CHLORDIAZEPOXIDE HCL, CHLORDIAZEPOXIDE
        HYDROCHLORIDE
    CHLORPHENIRAMINE MALEATE, CHLORPHENIRAMINE
        MALEATE
    CHLORPROPAMIDE, CHLORPROPAMIDE
    CHLORTHALIDONE, CHLORTHALIDONE
    CYPROHEPTADINE HCL, CYPROHEPTADINE
        HYDROCHLORIDE
    DIPHENHYDRAMINE HCL, DIPHENHYDRAMINE
        HYDROCHLORIDE

APPENDIX B
PRODUCT NAME INDEX
LISTED BY APPLICANT (*continued*)

DISOPYRAMIDE PHOSPHATE, DISOPYRAMIDE
   PHOSPHATE
DOXYCYCLINE HYCLATE, DOXYCYCLINE HYCLATE
ERGOLOID MESYLATES, ERGOLOID MESYLATES
FLURAZEPAM HCL, FLURAZEPAM HYDROCHLORIDE
FUROSEMIDE, FUROSEMIDE
HYDRALAZINE HCL AND HYDROCHLOROTHIAZIDE,
   HYDRALAZINE HYDROCHLORIDE
HYDRALAZINE HCL, HYDRALAZINE HYDROCHLORIDE
HYDROCHLOROTHIAZIDE, HYDROCHLOROTHIAZIDE
HYDROXYZINE HCL, HYDROXYZINE HYDROCHLORIDE
HYDROXYZINE PAMOATE, HYDROXYZINE PAMOATE
IBUPROFEN, IBUPROFEN
INDOMETHACIN, INDOMETHACIN
ISOSORBIDE DINITRATE, ISOSORBIDE DINITRATE
LOGEN, ATROPINE SULFATE
LORAZEPAM, LORAZEPAM
MECLIZINE HCL, MECLIZINE HYDROCHLORIDE
METHOCARBAMOL, METHOCARBAMOL
METHYLDOPA, METHYLDOPA
METOCLOPRAMIDE HCL, METOCLOPRAMIDE
   HYDROCHLORIDE
METRONIDAZOLE, METRONIDAZOLE
PREDNISOLONE, PREDNISOLONE
PREDNISONE, PREDNISONE
PROPOXYPHENE NAPSYLATE AND ACETAMINOPHEN,
   ACETAMINOPHEN
PROPRANOLOL HCL, PROPRANOLOL HYDROCHLORIDE
QUINIDINE GLUCONATE, QUINIDINE GLUCONATE
QUINIDINE SULFATE, QUINIDINE SULFATE
SPIRONOLACTONE AND HYDROCHLOROTHIAZIDE,
   HYDROCHLOROTHIAZIDE
SPIRONOLACTONE, SPIRONOLACTONE
SULFASALAZINE, SULFASALAZINE
SULFATRIM-DS, SULFAMETHOXAZOLE
SULFATRIM-SS, SULFAMETHOXAZOLE
TETRACYCLINE HCL, TETRACYCLINE HYDROCHLORIDE
THIORIDAZINE HCL, THIORIDAZINE HYDROCHLORIDE
TOLAZAMIDE, TOLAZAMIDE
TOLBUTAMIDE, TOLBUTAMIDE
TRIPROLIDINE HCL AND PSEUDOEPHEDRINE HCL,
   PSEUDOEPHEDRINE HYDROCHLORIDE

SUPPOSITORIA
SUPPOSITORIA LABORATORIES INC
   ACETAMINOPHEN, ACETAMINOPHEN (OTC)
SWEDISH ORPHAN
SWEDISH ORPHAN AB
   ORFADIN, NITISINONE
SYNCOR PHARMS
SYNCOR PHARMACEUTICALS INC
   A-N STANNOUS AGGREGATED ALBUMIN, TECHNETIUM
      TC-99M ALBUMIN AGGREGATED KIT
   SODIUM IODIDE I 123, SODIUM IODIDE, I-123
SYNTHON PHARMS
SYNTHON PHARMACEUTICALS LTD
   FLUVOXAMINE MALEATE, FLUVOXAMINE MALEATE
SYOSSET
SYOSSET LABORATORIES INC
   E-SOLVE 2, ERYTHROMYCIN
   HYDROCORTISONE, HYDROCORTISONE

T

TABLICAPS
TABLICAPS INC
   AMINOPHYLLINE, AMINOPHYLLINE

CHLORPHENIRAMINE MALEATE, CHLORPHENIRAMINE
   MALEATE
FOLIC ACID, FOLIC ACID
MEPROBAMATE, MEPROBAMATE
METHOCARBAMOL, METHOCARBAMOL
METHYLTESTOSTERONE, METHYLTESTOSTERONE
NIACIN, NIACIN
PREDNISOLONE, PREDNISOLONE
PROMETHAZINE HCL, PROMETHAZINE
   HYDROCHLORIDE
PROPANTHELINE BROMIDE, PROPANTHELINE
   BROMIDE
PROPYLTHIOURACIL, PROPYLTHIOURACIL
RAUWOLFIA SERPENTINA, RAUWOLFIA SERPENTINA
RESERPINE, RESERPINE
STILBESTROL, DIETHYLSTILBESTROL
TAKEDA
TAKEDA CHEMICAL INDUSTRIES LTD
   CERADON, CEFOTIAM HYDROCHLORIDE
TAKEDA PHARMS NA
TAKEDA PHARMACEUTICALS NORTH AMERICA INC
   ACTOS, PIOGLITAZONE HYDROCHLORIDE
TAP PHARM
TAP PHARMACEUTICAL PRODUCTS INC
   CEFMAX, CEFMENOXIME HYDROCHLORIDE
   LUPRON DEPOT, LEUPROLIDE ACETATE
   LUPRON DEPOT-3, LEUPROLIDE ACETATE
   LUPRON DEPOT-4, LEUPROLIDE ACETATE
   LUPRON DEPOT-PED, LEUPROLIDE ACETATE
   LUPRON, LEUPROLIDE ACETATE
   PREVACID, LANSOPRAZOLE
   PREVPAC, AMOXICILLIN
TARGACEPT
TARGACEPT INC
   INVERSINE, MECAMYLAMINE HYDROCHLORIDE
TARO
TARO PHARMACEUTICAL INDUSTRIES LTD
   ACETAZOLAMIDE, ACETAZOLAMIDE
   CARBAMAZEPINE, CARBAMAZEPINE
   CLOMIPRAMINE HCL, CLOMIPRAMINE
      HYDROCHLORIDE
   ENALAPRIL MALEATE, ENALAPRIL MALEATE
   ETODOLAC, ETODOLAC
   KETOCONAZOLE, KETOCONAZOLE
TARO PHARMACEUTICALS INC
   BETAMETHASONE DIPROPIONATE, BETAMETHASONE
      DIPROPIONATE
   CLOBETASOL PROPIONATE, CLOBETASOL
      PROPIONATE
   CLOTRIMAZOLE, CLOTRIMAZOLE
   CLOTRIMAZOLE, CLOTRIMAZOLE (OTC)
   DESOXIMETASONE, DESOXIMETASONE
   DIFLORASONE DIACETATE, DIFLORASONE DIACETATE
   FLUOCINOLONE ACETONIDE, FLUOCINOLONE
      ACETONIDE
   FLUOCINONIDE, FLUOCINONIDE
   HYDROCORTISONE VALERATE, HYDROCORTISONE
      VALERATE
   MICONAZOLE NITRATE, MICONAZOLE NITRATE (OTC)
   NORTRIPTYLINE HCL, NORTRIPTYLINE
      HYDROCHLORIDE
   TRIAMCINOLONE ACETONIDE, TRIAMCINOLONE
      ACETONIDE
   WARFARIN SODIUM, WARFARIN SODIUM
TARO PHARMACEUTICALS USA INC
   ACETIC ACID, ACETIC ACID, GLACIAL
   AMIODARONE HCL, AMIODARONE HYDROCHLORIDE
   AMMONIUM LACTATE, AMMONIUM LACTATE

APPENDIX B
PRODUCT NAME INDEX
LISTED BY APPLICANT (*continued*)

BETAMETHASONE DIPROPIONATE, BETAMETHASONE
  DIPROPIONATE
BETAMETHASONE VALERATE, BETAMETHASONE
  VALERATE
CLOBETASOL PROPIONATE (EMOLLIENT),
  CLOBETASOL PROPIONATE
CLOBETASOL PROPIONATE, CLOBETASOL
  PROPIONATE
CLORAZEPATE DIPOTASSIUM, CLORAZEPATE
  DIPOTASSIUM
CLOTRIMAZOLE AND BETAMETHASONE
  DIPROPIONATE, BETAMETHASONE DIPROPIONATE
CLOTRIMAZOLE, CLOTRIMAZOLE
DERMABET, BETAMETHASONE VALERATE
DESONIDE, DESONIDE
DIFLORASONE DIACETATE, DIFLORASONE DIACETATE
ECONAZOLE NITRATE, ECONAZOLE NITRATE
FLUOCINOLONE ACETONIDE, FLUOCINOLONE
  ACETONIDE
FLUOCINONIDE EMULSIFIED BASE, FLUOCINONIDE
FLUOCINONIDE, FLUOCINONIDE
GENTAMICIN SULFATE, GENTAMICIN SULFATE
HYDROCORTISONE AND ACETIC ACID, ACETIC ACID,
  GLACIAL
HYDROCORTISONE, HYDROCORTISONE
KETOZOLE, KETOCONAZOLE
LIDOCAINE, LIDOCAINE
NITROFURAZONE, NITROFURAZONE
NYSTATIN AND TRIAMCINOLONE ACETONIDE,
  NYSTATIN
NYSTATIN, NYSTATIN
ORACORT, TRIAMCINOLONE ACETONIDE
ORALONE, TRIAMCINOLONE ACETONIDE
SELENIUM SULFIDE, SELENIUM SULFIDE
THEOPHYLLINE, THEOPHYLLINE
TRIAMCINOLONE ACETONIDE, TRIAMCINOLONE
  ACETONIDE
TRIVAGIZOLE 3, CLOTRIMAZOLE (OTC)
U-CORT, HYDROCORTISONE ACETATE
TARO PHARM INDS
TARO PHARMACEUTICAL INDUSTRIES LTD
  AMCINONIDE, AMCINONIDE
  CARBAMAZEPINE, CARBAMAZEPINE
  ENALAPRIL MALEATE AND HYDROCHLOROTHIAZIDE,
    ENALAPRIL MALEATE
  ETODOLAC, ETODOLAC
TAYLOR
TAYLOR PHARMACEUTICALS
  LABETALOL HCL, LABETALOL HYDROCHLORIDE
  LORAZEPAM, LORAZEPAM
  MIDAZOLAM HCL, MIDAZOLAM HYDROCHLORIDE
  NAPHAZOLINE HCL, NAPHAZOLINE HYDROCHLORIDE
TAYLOR PHARMA
TAYLOR PHARMACAL CO
  DILTIAZEM HCL, DILTIAZEM HYDROCHLORIDE
  MIDAZOLAM HCL, MIDAZOLAM HYDROCHLORIDE
  PROPARACAINE HCL, PROPARACAINE
    HYDROCHLORIDE
  TRIMETHOPRIM SULFATE AND POLYMYXIN B SULFATE,
    POLYMYXIN B SULFATE
TECHNILAB
TECHNILAB INC
  ACILAC, LACTULOSE
  LAXILOSE, LACTULOSE
TEIKOKU PHARMA USA
TEIKOKU PHARMA USA INC
  LIDODERM, LIDOCAINE

TEVA
TEVA PHARMACEUTICALS USA INC
  ACETAMINOPHEN AND CODEINE PHOSPHATE,
    ACETAMINOPHEN
  ACETAMINOPHEN W/ CODEINE #2, ACETAMINOPHEN
  ACETAMINOPHEN W/ CODEINE #4, ACETAMINOPHEN
  ACYCLOVIR, ACYCLOVIR
  ADIPEX-P, PHENTERMINE HYDROCHLORIDE
  ALBUTEROL SULFATE, ALBUTEROL SULFATE
  ALPRAZOLAM, ALPRAZOLAM
  AMILORIDE HCL AND HYDROCHLOROTHIAZIDE,
    AMILORIDE HYDROCHLORIDE
  AMIODARONE HCL, AMIODARONE HYDROCHLORIDE
  AMITRIPTYLINE HCL, AMITRIPTYLINE HYDROCHLORIDE
  AMOXICILLIN AND CLAVULANATE POTASSIUM,
    AMOXICILLIN
  AMOXICILLIN PEDIATRIC, AMOXICILLIN
  AMOXICILLIN, AMOXICILLIN
  AMPICILLIN TRIHYDRATE, AMPICILLIN/AMPICILLIN
    TRIHYDRATE
  ATENOLOL, ATENOLOL
  BACLOFEN, BACLOFEN
  BETA-VAL, BETAMETHASONE VALERATE
  BETAMETHASONE DIPROPIONATE, BETAMETHASONE
    DIPROPIONATE
  BISOPROLOL FUMARATE AND
    HYDROCHLOROTHIAZIDE, BISOPROLOL FUMARATE
  BUPROPION HCL, BUPROPION HYDROCHLORIDE
  BUSPIRONE HCL, BUSPIRONE HYDROCHLORIDE
  BUTABARBITAL SODIUM, BUTABARBITAL SODIUM
  CALCITRIOL, CALCITRIOL
  CAPTOPRIL AND HYDROCHLOROTHIAZIDE, CAPTOPRIL
  CAPTOPRIL, CAPTOPRIL
  CARBIDOPA AND LEVODOPA, CARBIDOPA
  CEFACLOR, CEFACLOR
  CEFADROXIL, CEFADROXIL/CEFADROXIL
    HEMIHYDRATE
  CEFAZOLIN SODIUM, CEFAZOLIN SODIUM
  CEFUROXIME, CEFUROXIME SODIUM
  CEPHALEXIN, CEPHALEXIN
  CEPHRADINE, CEPHRADINE
  CHLORDIAZEPOXIDE HCL, CHLORDIAZEPOXIDE
    HYDROCHLORIDE
  CHLORHEXIDINE GLUCONATE, CHLORHEXIDINE
    GLUCONATE
  CHLOROQUINE PHOSPHATE, CHLOROQUINE
    PHOSPHATE
  CHLORPROPAMIDE, CHLORPROPAMIDE
  CHLORTHALIDONE, CHLORTHALIDONE
  CHLORZOXAZONE, CHLORZOXAZONE
  CHOLESTYRAMINE LIGHT, CHOLESTYRAMINE
  CHOLESTYRAMINE, CHOLESTYRAMINE
  CIMETIDINE HCL, CIMETIDINE HYDROCHLORIDE
  CIMETIDINE, CIMETIDINE
  CINOXACIN, CINOXACIN
  CLEMASTINE FUMARATE, CLEMASTINE FUMARATE
  CLEMASTINE FUMARATE, CLEMASTINE FUMARATE
    (OTC)
  CLINDAMYCIN HCL, CLINDAMYCIN HYDROCHLORIDE
  CLINDAMYCIN PHOSPHATE, CLINDAMYCIN
    PHOSPHATE
  CLOFIBRATE, CLOFIBRATE
  CLOMIPRAMINE HCL, CLOMIPRAMINE
    HYDROCHLORIDE
  CLONAZEPAM, CLONAZEPAM
  CLONIDINE HCL, CLONIDINE HYDROCHLORIDE
  CLOTRIMAZOLE, CLOTRIMAZOLE
  CLOXACILLIN SODIUM, CLOXACILLIN SODIUM

APPENDIX B
PRODUCT NAME INDEX
LISTED BY APPLICANT (*continued*)

COPAXONE, GLATIRAMER ACETATE
COTRIM D.S., SULFAMETHOXAZOLE
COTRIM, SULFAMETHOXAZOLE
CYCLACILLIN, CYCLACILLIN
DELCOBESE, AMPHETAMINE ADIPATE
DEXAMPEX, DEXTROAMPHETAMINE SULFATE
DICLOFENAC POTASSIUM, DICLOFENAC POTASSIUM
DICLOFENAC SODIUM, DICLOFENAC SODIUM
DICLOXACILLIN SODIUM, DICLOXACILLIN SODIUM
DIETHYLPROPION HCL, DIETHYLPROPION
    HYDROCHLORIDE
DIFLUNISAL, DIFLUNISAL
DILTIAZEM HCL, DILTIAZEM HYDROCHLORIDE
DIPHENHYDRAMINE HCL, DIPHENHYDRAMINE
    HYDROCHLORIDE
DISOPYRAMIDE PHOSPHATE, DISOPYRAMIDE
    PHOSPHATE
DOXAZOSIN MESYLATE, DOXAZOSIN MESYLATE
DOXY-LEMMON, DOXYCYCLINE HYCLATE
DRALZINE, HYDRALAZINE HYDROCHLORIDE
ENALAPRIL MALEATE AND HYDROCHLOROTHIAZIDE,
    ENALAPRIL MALEATE
ENALAPRIL MALEATE, ENALAPRIL MALEATE
EPITOL, CARBAMAZEPINE
ESTAZOLAM, ESTAZOLAM
ETODOLAC, ETODOLAC
FAMOTIDINE, FAMOTIDINE
FAMOTIDINE, FAMOTIDINE (OTC)
FENOFIBRATE (MICRONIZED), FENOFIBRATE
FLUOCINONIDE EMULSIFIED BASE, FLUOCINONIDE
FLUOCINONIDE, FLUOCINONIDE
FLUOXETINE HCL, FLUOXETINE HYDROCHLORIDE
FLUOXETINE, FLUOXETINE HYDROCHLORIDE
FLURBIPROFEN, FLURBIPROFEN
FLUTAMIDE, FLUTAMIDE
FLUVOXAMINE MALEATE, FLUVOXAMINE MALEATE
GALZIN, ZINC ACETATE
GEMFIBROZIL, GEMFIBROZIL
GLIPIZIDE, GLIPIZIDE
GLUCAMIDE, CHLORPROPAMIDE
GLYBURIDE (MICRONIZED), GLYBURIDE
GLYBURIDE, GLYBURIDE
HALOPERIDOL, HALOPERIDOL LACTATE
HY-PAM "25", HYDROXYZINE PAMOATE
HYDROCHLOROTHIAZIDE, HYDROCHLOROTHIAZIDE
HYDROCODONE BITARTRATE AND IBUPROFEN,
    HYDROCODONE BITARTRATE
HYDROCORTISONE, HYDROCORTISONE
IBUPROFEN, IBUPROFEN
IBUPROFEN, IBUPROFEN (OTC)
IMIPRAMINE HCL, IMIPRAMINE HYDROCHLORIDE
INDAPAMIDE, INDAPAMIDE
INDO-LEMMON, INDOMETHACIN
INDOMETHACIN, INDOMETHACIN
ISOSORBIDE MONONITRATE, ISOSORBIDE
    MONONITRATE
KETOCONAZOLE, KETOCONAZOLE
KETOPROFEN, KETOPROFEN
KETOROLAC TROMETHAMINE, KETOROLAC
    TROMETHAMINE
LABETALOL HCL, LABETALOL HYDROCHLORIDE
LISINOPRIL AND HYDROCHLOROTHIAZIDE,
    HYDROCHLOROTHIAZIDE
LISINOPRIL, LISINOPRIL
LOPERAMIDE HCL, LOPERAMIDE HYDROCHLORIDE
LOPERAMIDE HCL, LOPERAMIDE HYDROCHLORIDE
    (OTC)
LOVASTATIN, LOVASTATIN

MEGESTROL ACETATE, MEGESTROL ACETATE
MEPRIAM, MEPROBAMATE
METAPROTERENOL SULFATE, METAPROTERENOL
    SULFATE
METFORMIN HCL, METFORMIN HYDROCHLORIDE
METHAMPEX, METHAMPHETAMINE HYDROCHLORIDE
METHAMPHETAMINE HCL, METHAMPHETAMINE
    HYDROCHLORIDE
METHYLDOPA AND HYDROCHLOROTHIAZIDE,
    HYDROCHLOROTHIAZIDE
METHYLDOPA, METHYLDOPA
METOCLOPRAMIDE HCL, METOCLOPRAMIDE
    HYDROCHLORIDE
METOPROLOL TARTRATE, METOPROLOL TARTRATE
METRONIDAZOLE, METRONIDAZOLE
MEXILETINE HCL, MEXILETINE HYDROCHLORIDE
MICONAZOLE NITRATE, MICONAZOLE NITRATE (OTC)
MINOCYCLINE HCL, MINOCYCLINE HYDROCHLORIDE
MINOXIDIL (FOR MEN), MINOXIDIL (OTC)
MINOXIDIL EXTRA STRENGTH (FOR MEN), MINOXIDIL
    (OTC)
MIRTAZAPINE, MIRTAZAPINE
MOEXIPRIL HCL, MOEXIPRIL HYDROCHLORIDE
MYCO-TRIACET II, NYSTATIN
NABUMETONE, NABUMETONE
NAPROXEN SODIUM, NAPROXEN SODIUM
NAPROXEN, NAPROXEN
NEOMYCIN SULFATE, NEOMYCIN SULFATE
NEOTHYLLINE, DYPHYLLINE
NICARDIPINE HCL, NICARDIPINE HYDROCHLORIDE
NIFEDIPINE, NIFEDIPINE
NIZATIDINE, NIZATIDINE
NORTRIPTYLINE HCL, NORTRIPTYLINE
    HYDROCHLORIDE
NYSTATIN, NYSTATIN
ORAP, PIMOZIDE
OXACILLIN SODIUM, OXACILLIN SODIUM
OXAPROZIN, OXAPROZIN
PENICILLIN G POTASSIUM, PENICILLIN G POTASSIUM
PENICILLIN, PENICILLIN G POTASSIUM
PENICILLIN-2, PENICILLIN G POTASSIUM
PENICILLIN-VK, PENICILLIN V POTASSIUM
PENTOXIFYLLINE, PENTOXIFYLLINE
PERGOLIDE MESYLATE, PERGOLIDE MESYLATE
PHENTERMINE HCL, PHENTERMINE HYDROCHLORIDE
PINDOLOL, PINDOLOL
PIROXICAM, PIROXICAM
POTASSIUM CHLORIDE, POTASSIUM CHLORIDE
PREDNISOLONE, PREDNISOLONE
PREDNISONE, PREDNISONE
PRELONE, PREDNISOLONE
PROBAMPACIN, AMPICILLIN/AMPICILLIN TRIHYDRATE
PROMETHAZINE HCL, PROMETHAZINE
    HYDROCHLORIDE
PROPACET 100, ACETAMINOPHEN
PROPOXYPHENE COMPOUND 65, ASPIRIN
PROPOXYPHENE HCL, PROPOXYPHENE
    HYDROCHLORIDE
PROPOXYPHENE NAPSYLATE AND ACETAMINOPHEN,
    ACETAMINOPHEN
PROPRANOLOL HCL, PROPRANOLOL HYDROCHLORIDE
QUINAPRIL HCL, QUINAPRIL HYDROCHLORIDE
RANITIDINE HCL, RANITIDINE HYDROCHLORIDE
RESERPINE, RESERPINE
SELEGILINE HCL, SELEGILINE HYDROCHLORIDE
SOTALOL HCL, SOTALOL HYDROCHLORIDE
STATOBEX, PHENDIMETRAZINE TARTRATE
STATOBEX-G, PHENDIMETRAZINE TARTRATE

APPENDIX B
PRODUCT NAME INDEX
LISTED BY APPLICANT (*continued*)

SUCRALFATE, SUCRALFATE
SULFAMETHOXAZOLE AND TRIMETHOPRIM DOUBLE
    STRENGTH, SULFAMETHOXAZOLE
SULFAMETHOXAZOLE AND TRIMETHOPRIM,
    SULFAMETHOXAZOLE
SULFANILAMIDE, SULFANILAMIDE
SULINDAC, SULINDAC
TAMOXIFEN CITRATE, TAMOXIFEN CITRATE
TERAZOSIN HCL, TERAZOSIN HYDROCHLORIDE
THIORIDAZINE HCL, THIORIDAZINE HYDROCHLORIDE
THIOTHIXENE HCL, THIOTHIXENE HYDROCHLORIDE
TICLOPIDINE HCL, TICLOPIDINE HYDROCHLORIDE
TIMOLOL MALEATE, TIMOLOL MALEATE
TIZANIDINE HCL, TIZANIDINE HYDROCHLORIDE
TOLMETIN SODIUM, TOLMETIN SODIUM
TORSEMIDE, TORSEMIDE
TRAMADOL HCL, TRAMADOL HYDROCHLORIDE
TRAZODONE HCL, TRAZODONE HYDROCHLORIDE
TRIACET, TRIAMCINOLONE ACETONIDE
TRIAMCINOLONE, TRIAMCINOLONE
TRIMETHOPRIM, TRIMETHOPRIM
TRIPHED, PSEUDOEPHEDRINE HYDROCHLORIDE
VAGILIA, TRIPLE SULFA (SULFABENZAMIDE;
    SULFACETAMIDE; SULFATHIAZOLE)
VITAMIN A SOLUBILIZED, VITAMIN A PALMITATE
THERAKOS
THERAKOS INC
    UVADEX, METHOXSALEN
TOPIDERM
TOPIDERM INC
    HYDROCORTISONE, HYDROCORTISONE
    TRIAMCINOLONE ACETONIDE, TRIAMCINOLONE
      ACETONIDE
TORCH
TORCH LABORATORIES INC
    H-CORT, HYDROCORTISONE
TORPHARM
TORPHARM INC
    BUSPIRONE HCL, BUSPIRONE HYDROCHLORIDE
    CAPTOPRIL, CAPTOPRIL
    CIMETIDINE, CIMETIDINE
    CIMETIDINE, CIMETIDINE (OTC)
    CLONAZEPAM, CLONAZEPAM
    CYCLOSPORINE, CYCLOSPORINE
    DILTIAZEM HCL, DILTIAZEM HYDROCHLORIDE
    DOXAZOSIN MESYLATE, DOXAZOSIN MESYLATE
    ENALAPRIL MALEATE, ENALAPRIL MALEATE
    ETODOLAC, ETODOLAC
    FAMOTIDINE, FAMOTIDINE
    FAMOTIDINE, FAMOTIDINE (OTC)
    FLUVOXAMINE MALEATE, FLUVOXAMINE MALEATE
    GEMFIBROZIL, GEMFIBROZIL
    GLIPIZIDE, GLIPIZIDE
    KETOCONAZOLE, KETOCONAZOLE
    METFORMIN HCL, METFORMIN HYDROCHLORIDE
    NIZATIDINE, NIZATIDINE
    PENTOXIFYLLINE, PENTOXIFYLLINE
    RANITIDINE HCL, RANITIDINE HYDROCHLORIDE
    RANITIDINE, RANITIDINE HYDROCHLORIDE (OTC)
    SELEGILINE HCL, SELEGILINE HYDROCHLORIDE
    TERAZOSIN HCL, TERAZOSIN HYDROCHLORIDE
    TICLOPIDINE HCL, TICLOPIDINE HYDROCHLORIDE
    TRAMADOL HCL, TRAMADOL HYDROCHLORIDE
TRIGEN
TRIGEN LABORATORIES INC
    INDAPAMIDE, INDAPAMIDE
    METHYLPREDNISOLONE, METHYLPREDNISOLONE
    PREDNISONE, PREDNISONE

PROCHLORPERAZINE MALEATE, PROCHLORPERAZINE
    MALEATE
TYCO HLTHCARE
TYCO HEALTHCARE GROUP LP
    ANAFRANIL, CLOMIPRAMINE HYDROCHLORIDE
    PAMELOR, NORTRIPTYLINE HYDROCHLORIDE
    RESTORIL, TEMAZEPAM
    TOFRANIL, IMIPRAMINE HYDROCHLORIDE
    TOFRANIL-PM, IMIPRAMINE PAMOATE

U

UCB
UCB PHARMA INC
    HYDROCODONE BITARTRATE AND ACETAMINOPHEN,
      ACETAMINOPHEN
    KEPPRA, LEVETIRACETAM
    LORTAB, ACETAMINOPHEN
    THEO-24, THEOPHYLLINE
UDL
UDL LABORATORIES INC
    ALBUTEROL SULFATE, ALBUTEROL SULFATE
    FOLIC ACID, FOLIC ACID
    HALOPERIDOL LACTATE, HALOPERIDOL LACTATE
    MECLIZINE HCL, MECLIZINE HYDROCHLORIDE
    METHADONE HCL, METHADONE HYDROCHLORIDE
    NYSTATIN, NYSTATIN
    PREDNISOLONE, PREDNISOLONE
    PREDNISONE, PREDNISONE
    VALPROIC ACID, VALPROIC ACID
UNIMED
UNIMED INC
    MARINOL, DRONABINOL
UNIMED PHARMS
UNIMED PHARMACEUTICALS INC
    ANADROL-50, OXYMETHOLONE
    ANDROGEL, TESTOSTERONE
    PROMETRIUM, PROGESTERONE
UNITED GUARDIAN
UNITED GUARDIAN INC
    RENACIDIN, CITRIC ACID
UNITED THERAP
UNITED THERAPEUTICS CORP
    REMODULIN, TREPROSTINIL SODIUM
UNIV AZ CANCER CTR
UNIV ARIZONA CANCER CENTER
    ACTINEX, MASOPROCOL
UPSHER SMITH
UPSHER SMITH LABORATORIES INC
    DEXAMETHASONE, DEXAMETHASONE
    KLOR-CON M10, POTASSIUM CHLORIDE
    KLOR-CON M15, POTASSIUM CHLORIDE
    KLOR-CON M20, POTASSIUM CHLORIDE
    KLOR-CON, POTASSIUM CHLORIDE
    METHOCARBAMOL, METHOCARBAMOL
    NIACOR, NIACIN
    PACERONE, AMIODARONE HYDROCHLORIDE
    PENTOXIL, PENTOXIFYLLINE
    PREDNISONE, PREDNISONE
    PREVALITE, CHOLESTYRAMINE
    SORINE, SOTALOL HYDROCHLORIDE
    SPIRONOLACTONE W/ HYDROCHLOROTHIAZIDE,
      HYDROCHLOROTHIAZIDE
    SPIRONOLACTONE, SPIRONOLACTONE
US ARMY
UNITED STATES ARMY OFFICE SURGEON GENERAL
    ATROPINE SULFATE, ATROPINE SULFATE

APPENDIX B
PRODUCT NAME INDEX
LISTED BY APPLICANT (*continued*)

PYRIDOSTIGMINE BROMIDE, PYRIDOSTIGMINE
    BROMIDE
SODIUM THIOSULFATE, SODIUM THIOSULFATE
US ARMY MEDICAL RESEARCH MATERIEL COMMAND
    ATNAA, ATROPINE
    DIAZEPAM, DIAZEPAM
    SKIN EXPOSURE REDUCTION PASTE AGAINST
        CHEMICAL WARFARE AGENTS,
        PERFLUOROPOLYMETHYLISOPROPYL ETHER
US ARMY WALTER REED
UNITED STATES ARMY WALTER REED ARMY INSTITUTE
RESEARCH
    MEFLOQUINE HCL, MEFLOQUINE HYDROCHLORIDE
US CHEM
US CHEMICAL MARKETING GROUP INC
    MEDIGESIC PLUS, ACETAMINOPHEN
US SURGCL
UNITED STATES SURGICAL DIV TYCO HEALTHCARE
GROUP LP
    LYMPHAZURIN, ISOSULFAN BLUE
USL PHARMA
USL PHARMA INC
    ACETAMINOPHEN W/ CODEINE PHOSPHATE,
        ACETAMINOPHEN
    ACETOHEXAMIDE, ACETOHEXAMIDE
    AMANTADINE HCL, AMANTADINE HYDROCHLORIDE
    AMITRIPTYLINE HCL, AMITRIPTYLINE HYDROCHLORIDE
    BACLOFEN, BACLOFEN
    BENZTROPINE MESYLATE, BENZTROPINE MESYLATE
    BROMPHENIRAMINE MALEATE, BROMPHENIRAMINE
        MALEATE
    CARBAMAZEPINE, CARBAMAZEPINE
    CHLORDIAZEPOXIDE AND AMITRIPTYLINE HCL,
        AMITRIPTYLINE HYDROCHLORIDE
    CHLORDIAZEPOXIDE HCL, CHLORDIAZEPOXIDE
        HYDROCHLORIDE
    CHLORPROMAZINE HCL, CHLORPROMAZINE
        HYDROCHLORIDE
    CHLORPROPAMIDE, CHLORPROPAMIDE
    CHLORTHALIDONE, CHLORTHALIDONE
    CLOFIBRATE, CLOFIBRATE
    CLORAZEPATE DIPOTASSIUM, CLORAZEPATE
        DIPOTASSIUM
    DESIPRAMINE HCL, DESIPRAMINE HYDROCHLORIDE
    DIPHEN, DIPHENHYDRAMINE HYDROCHLORIDE
    DIPHENOXYLATE HCL W/ ATROPINE SULFATE,
        ATROPINE SULFATE
    ESTRADIOL, ESTRADIOL
    FENOPROFEN CALCIUM, FENOPROFEN CALCIUM
    FLUOCINOLONE ACETONIDE, FLUOCINOLONE
        ACETONIDE
    FLUOXYMESTERONE, FLUOXYMESTERONE
    FLURAZEPAM HCL, FLURAZEPAM HYDROCHLORIDE
    FOLIC ACID, FOLIC ACID
    HYDRALAZINE HCL, HYDRALAZINE HYDROCHLORIDE
    HYDROCHLOROTHIAZIDE, HYDROCHLOROTHIAZIDE
    HYDROCODONE BITARTRATE AND ACETAMINOPHEN,
        ACETAMINOPHEN
    HYDROCORTISONE, HYDROCORTISONE
    HYDROFLUMETHIAZIDE AND RESERPINE,
        HYDROFLUMETHIAZIDE
    HYDROXYZINE HCL, HYDROXYZINE HYDROCHLORIDE
    IMIPRAMINE HCL, IMIPRAMINE HYDROCHLORIDE
    LITHIUM CARBONATE, LITHIUM CARBONATE
    LORAZEPAM, LORAZEPAM
    MECLOFENAMATE SODIUM, MECLOFENAMATE SODIUM
    MEDROXYPROGESTERONE ACETATE,
        MEDROXYPROGESTERONE ACETATE

MEGESTROL ACETATE, MEGESTROL ACETATE
MEPROBAMATE, MEPROBAMATE
METAPROTERENOL SULFATE, METAPROTERENOL
    SULFATE
METHYCLOTHIAZIDE, METHYCLOTHIAZIDE
METHYLTESTOSTERONE, METHYLTESTOSTERONE
METOCLOPRAMIDE HCL, METOCLOPRAMIDE
    HYDROCHLORIDE
MINOXIDIL, MINOXIDIL
MYFED, PSEUDOEPHEDRINE HYDROCHLORIDE (OTC)
MYIDYL, TRIPROLIDINE HYDROCHLORIDE
MYMETHAZINE FORTIS, PROMETHAZINE
    HYDROCHLORIDE
NYSTATIN, NYSTATIN
OXYBUTYNIN CHLORIDE, OXYBUTYNIN CHLORIDE
PHENDIMETRAZINE TARTRATE, PHENDIMETRAZINE
    TARTRATE
PHENTERMINE HCL, PHENTERMINE HYDROCHLORIDE
PRAZEPAM, PRAZEPAM
QUINIDINE SULFATE, QUINIDINE SULFATE
SPIRONOLACTONE W/ HYDROCHLOROTHIAZIDE,
    HYDROCHLOROTHIAZIDE
SULFAMETHOXAZOLE AND TRIMETHOPRIM,
    SULFAMETHOXAZOLE
SULMEPRIM PEDIATRIC, SULFAMETHOXAZOLE
SULMEPRIM, SULFAMETHOXAZOLE
TEMAZEPAM, TEMAZEPAM
TIMOLOL MALEATE, TIMOLOL MALEATE
TOLAZAMIDE, TOLAZAMIDE
TRAZODONE HCL, TRAZODONE HYDROCHLORIDE
TRIMIPRAMINE MALEATE, TRIMIPRAMINE MALEATE
VALPROIC ACID, VALPROIC ACID
WARFARIN SODIUM, WARFARIN SODIUM

V

VALE
VALE CHEMICAL CO INC
    AMINOPHYLLINE, AMINOPHYLLINE
    SERPATE, RESERPINE
VANGARD
VANGARD LABORATORIES INC DIV MIDWAY MEDICAL CO
    ACETAZOLAMIDE, ACETAZOLAMIDE
    AMINOPHYLLINE, AMINOPHYLLINE
    AMITRIPTYLINE HCL, AMITRIPTYLINE HYDROCHLORIDE
    CHLORDIAZEPOXIDE HCL, CHLORDIAZEPOXIDE
        HYDROCHLORIDE
    CHLORPROMAZINE HCL, CHLORPROMAZINE
        HYDROCHLORIDE
    CHLORTHALIDONE, CHLORTHALIDONE
    DIPHENHYDRAMINE HCL, DIPHENHYDRAMINE
        HYDROCHLORIDE
    ERGOLOID MESYLATES, ERGOLOID MESYLATES
    FOLIC ACID, FOLIC ACID
    HYDRALAZINE HCL, HYDRALAZINE HYDROCHLORIDE
    HYDROCHLOROTHIAZIDE, HYDROCHLOROTHIAZIDE
    HYDROXYZINE PAMOATE, HYDROXYZINE PAMOATE
    IMIPRAMINE HCL, IMIPRAMINE HYDROCHLORIDE
    LO-TROL, ATROPINE SULFATE
    MECLIZINE HCL, MECLIZINE HYDROCHLORIDE
    MEPROBAMATE, MEPROBAMATE
    PAPA-DEINE #3, ACETAMINOPHEN
    PAPA-DEINE #4, ACETAMINOPHEN
    PREDNISONE, PREDNISONE
    PROCAINAMIDE HCL, PROCAINAMIDE
        HYDROCHLORIDE
    QUINIDINE SULFATE, QUINIDINE SULFATE

APPENDIX B
PRODUCT NAME INDEX
LISTED BY APPLICANT (*continued*)

SPIRONOLACTONE W/ HYDROCHLOROTHIAZIDE,
    HYDROCHLOROTHIAZIDE
SPIRONOLACTONE, SPIRONOLACTONE
SULFINPYRAZONE, SULFINPYRAZONE
TOLBUTAMIDE, TOLBUTAMIDE
TRIHEXYPHENIDYL HCL, TRIHEXYPHENIDYL
    HYDROCHLORIDE

VERSAPHARM
VERSAPHARM INC
    RIFAMPIN, RIFAMPIN

VERUM PHARMS
VERUM PHARMACEUTICALS INC
    BROMFED-DM, BROMPHENIRAMINE MALEATE

VESTAL LABS
VESTAL LABORATORIES DIV CHEMED CORP
    SEPTISOL, HEXACHLOROPHENE

VINTAGE PHARMS
VINTAGE PHARMACEUTICALS INC
    ACETAMINOPHEN AND CODEINE PHOSPHATE,
      ACETAMINOPHEN
    ACETAMINOPHEN, BUTALBITAL, CAFFEINE, AND
      CODEINE PHOSPHATE, ACETAMINOPHEN
    ALLOPURINOL, ALLOPURINOL
    AMINOPHYLLINE, AMINOPHYLLINE
    AMITRIPTYLINE HYDROCHLORIDE, AMITRIPTYLINE
      HYDROCHLORIDE
    CARISOPRODOL, CARISOPRODOL
    DOXYCYCLINE HYCLATE, DOXYCYCLINE HYCLATE
    FOLIC ACID, FOLIC ACID
    HYDROCHLOROTHIAZIDE, HYDROCHLOROTHIAZIDE
    HYDROCODONE BITARTRATE AND ACETAMINOPHEN,
      ACETAMINOPHEN
    HYDROXYZINE HCL, HYDROXYZINE HYDROCHLORIDE
    IBUPROFEN, IBUPROFEN
    IBUPROFEN, IBUPROFEN (OTC)
    LACTULOSE, LACTULOSE
    LEVOLET, LIOTRIX (T4;T3)
    MECLIZINE HCL, MECLIZINE HYDROCHLORIDE
    MEPERIDINE HCL, MEPERIDINE HYDROCHLORIDE
    METHOCARBAMOL, METHOCARBAMOL
    METHYLPREDNISOLONE, METHYLPREDNISOLONE
    OXYBUTYNIN CHLORIDE, OXYBUTYNIN CHLORIDE
    OXYCODONE AND ACETAMINOPHEN, ACETAMINOPHEN
    PEMOLINE, PEMOLINE
    PERPHENAZINE, PERPHENAZINE
    PHENTERMINE HCL, PHENTERMINE HYDROCHLORIDE
    PREDNISONE, PREDNISONE
    PROPAFENONE HCL, PROPAFENONE
      HYDROCHLORIDE
    PROPOXYPHENE NAPSYLATE AND ACETAMINOPHEN,
      ACETAMINOPHEN
    QUINIDINE SULFATE, QUINIDINE SULFATE
    SULFASALAZINE, SULFASALAZINE
    TRIHEXYPHENIDYL HCL, TRIHEXYPHENIDYL
      HYDROCHLORIDE

VISTAPHARM
VISTAPHARM INC
    LACTULOSE, LACTULOSE
    METOCLOPRAMIDE, METOCLOPRAMIDE
      HYDROCHLORIDE
    PHENYTOIN, PHENYTOIN

VITARINE
VITARINE PHARMACEUTICALS INC
    ACETAMINOPHEN W/ CODEINE PHOSPHATE,
      ACETAMINOPHEN
    AMPICILLIN, AMPICILLIN/AMPICILLIN TRIHYDRATE
    BROMPHENIRAMINE MALEATE, BROMPHENIRAMINE
      MALEATE

CEPHALEXIN, CEPHALEXIN
CEPHRADINE, CEPHRADINE
CHLORPHENIRAMINE MALEATE, CHLORPHENIRAMINE
    MALEATE
CORTISONE ACETATE, CORTISONE ACETATE
CYPROHEPTADINE HCL, CYPROHEPTADINE
    HYDROCHLORIDE
DEXTROAMPHETAMINE SULFATE,
    DEXTROAMPHETAMINE SULFATE
GLUTETHIMIDE, GLUTETHIMIDE
HYDRALAZINE HCL, HYDRALAZINE HYDROCHLORIDE
MECLOFENAMATE SODIUM, MECLOFENAMATE SODIUM
PENTOBARBITAL SODIUM, PENTOBARBITAL SODIUM
PHENDIMETRAZINE TARTRATE, PHENDIMETRAZINE
    TARTRATE
PHENTERMINE HCL, PHENTERMINE HYDROCHLORIDE
PREDNISOLONE, PREDNISOLONE
PREDNISONE, PREDNISONE
SECOBARBITAL SODIUM, SECOBARBITAL SODIUM
SERPIVITE, RESERPINE
SULFISOXAZOLE, SULFISOXAZOLE
TRIAMTERENE AND HYDROCHLOROTHIAZIDE,
    HYDROCHLOROTHIAZIDE
TRIPROLIDINE HCL, TRIPROLIDINE HYDROCHLORIDE
VITAMIN D, ERGOCALCIFEROL

VIVUS
VIVUS INC
    MUSE, ALPROSTADIL

W

WARNER CHILCOTT
WARNER CHILCOTT BERMUDA LTD
    CHOLEDYL SA, OXTRIPHYLLINE
    DORYX, DOXYCYCLINE HYCLATE
WARNER CHILCOTT DIV WARNER LAMBERT CO
    ACETAMINOPHEN AND CODEINE PHOSPHATE,
      ACETAMINOPHEN
    ACETAMINOPHEN W/ CODEINE PHOSPHATE,
      ACETAMINOPHEN
    ALBUTEROL SULFATE, ALBUTEROL SULFATE
    AMITRIL, AMITRIPTYLINE HYDROCHLORIDE
    CARBAMAZEPINE, CARBAMAZEPINE
    CHLORTHALIDONE, CHLORTHALIDONE
    CLONIDINE HCL, CLONIDINE HYDROCHLORIDE
    CLORAZEPATE DIPOTASSIUM, CLORAZEPATE
      DIPOTASSIUM
    CYCLOPAR, TETRACYCLINE HYDROCHLORIDE
    DIAZEPAM, DIAZEPAM
    DOPAMINE HCL, DOPAMINE HYDROCHLORIDE
    DOXYCYCLINE HYCLATE, DOXYCYCLINE HYCLATE
    DURAQUIN, QUINIDINE GLUCONATE
    ERYPAR, ERYTHROMYCIN STEARATE
    FENOPROFEN CALCIUM, FENOPROFEN CALCIUM
    FLURAZEPAM HCL, FLURAZEPAM HYDROCHLORIDE
    FUROSEMIDE, FUROSEMIDE
    HYDROCHLOROTHIAZIDE, HYDROCHLOROTHIAZIDE
    KANAMYCIN SULFATE, KANAMYCIN SULFATE
    LORAZEPAM, LORAZEPAM
    PHENYTOIN SODIUM, PHENYTOIN SODIUM
    PROCAINAMIDE HCL, PROCAINAMIDE
      HYDROCHLORIDE
    PROPOXYPHENE HCL 65, PROPOXYPHENE
      HYDROCHLORIDE
    PROPRANOLOL HCL AND HYDROCHLOROTHIAZIDE,
      HYDROCHLOROTHIAZIDE
    PROPRANOLOL HCL, PROPRANOLOL HYDROCHLORIDE

APPENDIX B
PRODUCT NAME INDEX
LISTED BY APPLICANT (*continued*)

QUINIDINE SULFATE, QUINIDINE SULFATE
SPIRONOLACTONE, SPIRONOLACTONE
VERAPAMIL HCL, VERAPAMIL HYDROCHLORIDE
WARNER CHILCOTT INC
  CARBAMAZEPINE, CARBAMAZEPINE
  CYANOCOBALAMIN, CYANOCOBALAMIN
  DURICEF, CEFADROXIL/CEFADROXIL HEMIHYDRATE
  ERYC, ERYTHROMYCIN
  ESTRACE, ESTRADIOL
  FLURAZEPAM HCL, FLURAZEPAM HYDROCHLORIDE
  FLURBIPROFEN, FLURBIPROFEN
  OVCON-35, ETHINYL ESTRADIOL
  OVCON-50, ETHINYL ESTRADIOL
  PROPRANOLOL HCL, PROPRANOLOL HYDROCHLORIDE
  SULINDAC, SULINDAC
  TETRACYCLINE HCL, TETRACYCLINE HYDROCHLORIDE
WARNER LAMBERT
WARNER LAMBERT CO
  SUDAFED 12 HOUR, PSEUDOEPHEDRINE
    HYDROCHLORIDE (OTC)
  ZANTAC 75, RANITIDINE HYDROCHLORIDE (OTC)
WARRICK PHARMS
WARRICK PHARMACEUTICALS
  CROMOLYN SODIUM, CROMOLYN SODIUM
  IPRATROPIUM BROMIDE, IPRATROPIUM BROMIDE
WATSON LAB
WATSON LABORATORIES INC
  ACETAZOLAMIDE, ACETAZOLAMIDE
  ALLOPURINOL, ALLOPURINOL
  AMANTADINE HCL, AMANTADINE HYDROCHLORIDE
  ANISOTROPINE METHYLBROMIDE, ANISOTROPINE
    METHYLBROMIDE
  BETHANECHOL CHLORIDE, BETHANECHOL CHLORIDE
  CARISOPRODOL COMPOUND, ASPIRIN
  CARISOPRODOL, CARISOPRODOL
  CHLOROTHIAZIDE W/ RESERPINE, CHLOROTHIAZIDE
  CHLOROTHIAZIDE, CHLOROTHIAZIDE
  CHLORPHENIRAMINE MALEATE, CHLORPHENIRAMINE
    MALEATE
  CHLORPROPAMIDE, CHLORPROPAMIDE
  CHLORTHALIDONE, CHLORTHALIDONE
  CLOMIPRAMINE HCL, CLOMIPRAMINE
    HYDROCHLORIDE
  CLONIDINE HCL, CLONIDINE HYDROCHLORIDE
  CYPROHEPTADINE HCL, CYPROHEPTADINE
    HYDROCHLORIDE
  DEXAMETHASONE, DEXAMETHASONE
  DICYCLOMINE HCL, DICYCLOMINE HYDROCHLORIDE
  DIPHENHYDRAMINE HCL, DIPHENHYDRAMINE
    HYDROCHLORIDE
  DISOPYRAMIDE PHOSPHATE, DISOPYRAMIDE
    PHOSPHATE
  ERGOLOID MESYLATES, ERGOLOID MESYLATES
  FLUOXYMESTERONE, FLUOXYMESTERONE
  FLUPHENAZINE HCL, FLUPHENAZINE HYDROCHLORIDE
  FOLIC ACID, FOLIC ACID
  GLIPIZIDE, GLIPIZIDE
  GLYCOPYRROLATE, GLYCOPYRROLATE
  GUANETHIDINE MONOSULFATE, GUANETHIDINE
    MONOSULFATE
  HALOPERIDOL, HALOPERIDOL
  HYDRALAZINE HCL AND HYDROCHLOROTHIAZIDE,
    HYDRALAZINE HYDROCHLORIDE
  HYDROCHLOROTHIAZIDE W/ HYDRALAZINE,
    HYDRALAZINE HYDROCHLORIDE
  HYDROCHLOROTHIAZIDE W/ RESERPINE AND
    HYDRALAZINE, HYDRALAZINE HYDROCHLORIDE

HYDROCHLOROTHIAZIDE W/ RESERPINE,
  HYDROCHLOROTHIAZIDE
HYDROCHLOROTHIAZIDE, HYDROCHLOROTHIAZIDE
HYDROFLUMETHIAZIDE AND RESERPINE,
  HYDROFLUMETHIAZIDE
HYDROFLUMETHIAZIDE, HYDROFLUMETHIAZIDE
HYDROXYZINE PAMOATE, HYDROXYZINE PAMOATE
IMIPRAMINE HCL, IMIPRAMINE HYDROCHLORIDE
INDOMETHACIN, INDOMETHACIN
ISONIAZID, ISONIAZID
LIOTHYRONINE SODIUM, LIOTRIX (T4;T3)
LITHIUM CARBONATE, LITHIUM CARBONATE
MAPROTILINE HCL, MAPROTILINE HYDROCHLORIDE
MECLIZINE HCL, MECLIZINE HYDROCHLORIDE
MECLOFENAMATE SODIUM, MECLOFENAMATE SODIUM
METHOCARBAMOL, METHOCARBAMOL
METHYCLOTHIAZIDE AND DESERPIDINE, DESERPIDINE
METHYCLOTHIAZIDE, METHYCLOTHIAZIDE
METHYLDOPA AND HYDROCHLOROTHIAZIDE,
  HYDROCHLOROTHIAZIDE
METHYLDOPA, METHYLDOPA
METOCLOPRAMIDE HCL, METOCLOPRAMIDE
  HYDROCHLORIDE
NIACIN, NIACIN
NICOTINE POLACRILEX, NICOTINE POLACRILEX (OTC)
NITROFURANTOIN MACROCRYSTALLINE,
  NITROFURANTOIN, MACROCRYSTALLINE
NITROFURANTOIN, NITROFURANTOIN
ORPHENADRINE CITRATE, ORPHENADRINE CITRATE
OXTRIPHYLLINE, OXTRIPHYLLINE
OXYBUTYNIN CHLORIDE, OXYBUTYNIN CHLORIDE
OXYPHENBUTAZONE, OXYPHENBUTAZONE
PERPHENAZINE AND AMITRIPTYLINE HCL,
  AMITRIPTYLINE HYDROCHLORIDE
PHENYTEX, PHENYTOIN SODIUM, EXTENDED
PRIMIDONE, PRIMIDONE
PROBENECID W/ COLCHICINE, COLCHICINE
PROCAINAMIDE HCL, PROCAINAMIDE
  HYDROCHLORIDE
PROCHLORPERAZINE, PROCHLORPERAZINE MALEATE
PROMETHAZINE HCL, PROMETHAZINE
  HYDROCHLORIDE
PROPANTHELINE BROMIDE, PROPANTHELINE
  BROMIDE
PROPOXYPHENE NAPSYLATE AND ACETAMINOPHEN,
  ACETAMINOPHEN
PROPRANOLOL HCL, PROPRANOLOL HYDROCHLORIDE
QUINATIME, QUINIDINE GLUCONATE
SPIRONOLACTONE W/ HYDROCHLOROTHIAZIDE,
  HYDROCHLOROTHIAZIDE
SPIRONOLACTONE, SPIRONOLACTONE
SULFAMETHOXAZOLE, SULFAMETHOXAZOLE
SULFASALAZINE, SULFASALAZINE
TEMAZEPAM, TEMAZEPAM
THIORIDAZINE HCL, THIORIDAZINE HYDROCHLORIDE
TIMOLOL MALEATE, TIMOLOL MALEATE
TOLAZAMIDE, TOLAZAMIDE
TOLBUTAMIDE, TOLBUTAMIDE
TRAZODONE HCL, TRAZODONE HYDROCHLORIDE
TRICHLORMETHIAZIDE W/ RESERPINE, RESERPINE
TRICHLORMETHIAZIDE, TRICHLORMETHIAZIDE
TRIFLUOPERAZINE HCL, TRIFLUOPERAZINE
  HYDROCHLORIDE
TRIHEXYPHENIDYL HCL, TRIHEXYPHENIDYL
  HYDROCHLORIDE
TRIPELENNAMINE HCL, TRIPELENNAMINE
  HYDROCHLORIDE

APPENDIX B
PRODUCT NAME INDEX
LISTED BY APPLICANT (*continued*)

TRIPROLIDINE AND PSEUDOEPHEDRINE,
    PSEUDOEPHEDRINE HYDROCHLORIDE (OTC)
WARFARIN SODIUM, WARFARIN SODIUM
WATSON LABS
WATSON LABORATORIES
  FOLIC ACID, FOLIC ACID
  METFORMIN HCL, METFORMIN HYDROCHLORIDE
  MICROGESTIN FE 1.5/30, ETHINYL ESTRADIOL
  MICROGESTIN FE 1/20, ETHINYL ESTRADIOL
  NORCO, ACETAMINOPHEN
  OXAPROZIN, OXAPROZIN
  OXYCODONE AND ACETAMINOPHEN, ACETAMINOPHEN
  PENTAZOCINE HCL AND ACETAMINOPHEN,
    ACETAMINOPHEN
  PROPAFENONE HCL, PROPAFENONE
    HYDROCHLORIDE
  TRAMADOL HCL, TRAMADOL HYDROCHLORIDE
WATSON LABORATORIES INC
  ACEBUTOLOL HCL, ACEBUTOLOL HYDROCHLORIDE
  ACETAMINOPHEN AND CODEINE PHOSPHATE,
    ACETAMINOPHEN
  ACETAMINOPHEN W/ CODEINE PHOSPHATE,
    ACETAMINOPHEN
  ACETAZOLAMIDE, ACETAZOLAMIDE
  ACETOHEXAMIDE, ACETOHEXAMIDE
  ACYCLOVIR, ACYCLOVIR
  ALBUTEROL SULFATE, ALBUTEROL SULFATE
  ALLOPURINOL, ALLOPURINOL
  ALORA, ESTRADIOL
  ALPRAZOLAM, ALPRAZOLAM
  AMILORIDE HCL AND HYDROCHLOROTHIAZIDE,
    AMILORIDE HYDROCHLORIDE
  AMINOPHYLLINE, AMINOPHYLLINE
  AMITRIPTYLINE HCL, AMITRIPTYLINE HYDROCHLORIDE
  AMOXAPINE, AMOXAPINE
  ANDRODERM, TESTOSTERONE
  ATENOLOL AND CHLORTHALIDONE, ATENOLOL
  ATENOLOL, ATENOLOL
  BACLOFEN, BACLOFEN
  BETHANECHOL CHLORIDE, BETHANECHOL CHLORIDE
  BISOPROLOL FUMARATE AND
    HYDROCHLOROTHIAZIDE, BISOPROLOL FUMARATE
  BREVICON 21-DAY, ETHINYL ESTRADIOL
  BREVICON 28-DAY, ETHINYL ESTRADIOL
  BROMPHENIRAMINE MALEATE, BROMPHENIRAMINE
    MALEATE
  BUSPIRONE HCL, BUSPIRONE HYDROCHLORIDE
  BUTABARBITAL SODIUM, BUTABARBITAL SODIUM
  BUTALBITAL AND ACETAMINOPHEN, ACETAMINOPHEN
  BUTALBITAL, ACETAMINOPHEN AND CAFFEINE,
    ACETAMINOPHEN
  BUTALBITAL, ASPIRIN AND CAFFEINE, ASPIRIN
  BUTALBITAL, ASPIRIN, CAFFEINE, AND CODEINE
    PHOSPHATE, ASPIRIN
  CAPTOPRIL AND HYDROCHLOROTHIAZIDE, CAPTOPRIL
  CAPTOPRIL, CAPTOPRIL
  CARBIDOPA AND LEVODOPA, CARBIDOPA
  CARISOPRODOL, CARISOPRODOL
  CHLORDIAZEPOXIDE AND AMITRIPTYLINE HCL,
    AMITRIPTYLINE HYDROCHLORIDE
  CHLORDIAZEPOXIDE HCL, CHLORDIAZEPOXIDE
    HYDROCHLORIDE
  CHLOROHENIRAMINE MALEATE AND
    PHENYLPROPANOLAMINE HCL,
    CHLORPHENIRAMINE MALEATE
  CHLOROQUINE PHOSPHATE, CHLOROQUINE
    PHOSPHATE
  CHLOROTHIAZIDE, CHLOROTHIAZIDE

  CHLORPHENIRAMINE MALEATE, CHLORPHENIRAMINE
    MALEATE
  CHLORPROMAZINE HCL, CHLORPROMAZINE
    HYDROCHLORIDE
  CHLORPROPAMIDE, CHLORPROPAMIDE
  CHLORTHALIDONE, CHLORTHALIDONE
  CHLORZOXAZONE, CHLORZOXAZONE
  CIMETIDINE, CIMETIDINE
  CIMETIDINE, CIMETIDINE (OTC)
  CLINDAMYCIN HCL, CLINDAMYCIN HYDROCHLORIDE
  CLOFIBRATE, CLOFIBRATE
  CLOMIPRAMINE HCL, CLOMIPRAMINE
    HYDROCHLORIDE
  CLONAZEPAM, CLONAZEPAM
  CLONIDINE HCL, CLONIDINE HYDROCHLORIDE
  CLORAZEPATE DIPOTASSIUM, CLORAZEPATE
    DIPOTASSIUM
  COL-PROBENECID, COLCHICINE
  CORTISONE ACETATE, CORTISONE ACETATE
  CYCLOBENZAPRINE HCL, CYCLOBENZAPRINE
    HYDROCHLORIDE
  CYPROHEPTADINE HCL, CYPROHEPTADINE
    HYDROCHLORIDE
  DEXAMETHASONE, DEXAMETHASONE
  DEXTROAMP SACCHARATE, AMP ASPARATE,
    DEXTROAMP SULFATE AND AMP SULFATE,
    AMPHETAMINE ASPARTATE
  DIAZEPAM, DIAZEPAM
  DICLOFENAC POTASSIUM, DICLOFENAC POTASSIUM
  DICYCLOMINE HCL, DICYCLOMINE HYDROCHLORIDE
  DIETHYLPROPION HCL, DIETHYLPROPION
    HYDROCHLORIDE
  DIFLUNISAL, DIFLUNISAL
  DILACOR XR, DILTIAZEM HYDROCHLORIDE
  DIMENHYDRINATE, DIMENHYDRINATE
  DIPHENHYDRAMINE HCL, DIPHENHYDRAMINE
    HYDROCHLORIDE
  DIPHENOXYLATE HCL AND ATROPINE SULFATE,
    ATROPINE SULFATE
  DIPYRIDAMOLE, DIPYRIDAMOLE
  DISOPYRAMIDE PHOSPHATE, DISOPYRAMIDE
    PHOSPHATE
  DISULFIRAM, DISULFIRAM
  DOXAZOSIN MESYLATE, DOXAZOSIN MESYLATE
  DOXEPIN HCL, DOXEPIN HYDROCHLORIDE
  DOXYCYCLINE HYCLATE, DOXYCYCLINE HYCLATE
  ENALAPRIL MALEATE, ENALAPRIL MALEATE
  ERGOLOID MESYLATES, ERGOLOID MESYLATES
  ERYTHROMYCIN ESTOLATE, ERYTHROMYCIN
    ESTOLATE
  ERYTHROMYCIN STEARATE, ERYTHROMYCIN
    STEARATE
  ESTAZOLAM, ESTAZOLAM
  ESTRADIOL, ESTRADIOL
  ESTROPIPATE, ESTROPIPATE
  ETODOLAC, ETODOLAC
  FAMOTIDINE, FAMOTIDINE
  FAMOTIDINE, FAMOTIDINE (OTC)
  FENOPROFEN CALCIUM, FENOPROFEN CALCIUM
  FLUOXETINE, FLUOXETINE HYDROCHLORIDE
  FLURAZEPAM HCL, FLURAZEPAM HYDROCHLORIDE
  FLUVOXAMINE MALEATE, FLUVOXAMINE MALEATE
  FOLIC ACID, FOLIC ACID
  FUROSEMIDE, FUROSEMIDE
  GEMFIBROZIL, GEMFIBROZIL
  GERIMAL, ERGOLOID MESYLATES
  GLIPIZIDE, GLIPIZIDE
  GLUTETHIMIDE, GLUTETHIMIDE

APPENDIX B
PRODUCT NAME INDEX
LISTED BY APPLICANT (*continued*)

GLYCOPYRROLATE, GLYCOPYRROLATE
GUANABENZ ACETATE, GUANABENZ ACETATE
GUANFACINE HCL, GUANFACINE HYDROCHLORIDE
HALOPERIDOL, HALOPERIDOL
HYDRALAZINE AND HYDROCHLORTHIAZIDE,
   HYDRALAZINE HYDROCHLORIDE
HYDRALAZINE HCL, HYDRALAZINE HYDROCHLORIDE
HYDRALAZINE, HYDROCHLOROTHIAZIDE W/
   RESERPINE, HYDRALAZINE HYDROCHLORIDE
HYDROCHLOROTHIAZIDE W/ RESERPINE,
   HYDROCHLOROTHIAZIDE
HYDROCHLOROTHIAZIDE, HYDROCHLOROTHIAZIDE
HYDROCODONE BITARTRATE AND ACETAMINOPHEN,
   ACETAMINOPHEN
HYDROCORTISONE, HYDROCORTISONE
HYDROFLUMETHIAZIDE, HYDROFLUMETHIAZIDE
HYDROXYCHLOROQUINE SULFATE,
   HYDROXYCHLOROQUINE SULFATE
HYDROXYZINE HCL, HYDROXYZINE HYDROCHLORIDE
HYDROXYZINE PAMOATE, HYDROXYZINE PAMOATE
IBUPROFEN, IBUPROFEN
IBUPROFEN, IBUPROFEN (OTC)
IMIPRAMINE HCL, IMIPRAMINE HYDROCHLORIDE
INDAPAMIDE, INDAPAMIDE
INDOMETHACIN, INDOMETHACIN
ISONIAZID, ISONIAZID
ISOSORBIDE DINITRATE, ISOSORBIDE DINITRATE
KETOROLAC TROMETHAMINE, KETOROLAC
   TROMETHAMINE
LABETALOL HCL, LABETALOL HYDROCHLORIDE
LEVORA 0.15/30-21, ETHINYL ESTRADIOL
LEVORA 0.15/30-28, ETHINYL ESTRADIOL
LISINOPRIL, LISINOPRIL
LOPERAMIDE HCL, LOPERAMIDE HYDROCHLORIDE
   (OTC)
LORAZEPAM, LORAZEPAM
LOW-OGESTREL-21, ETHINYL ESTRADIOL
LOW-OGESTREL-28, ETHINYL ESTRADIOL
LOXAPINE SUCCINATE, LOXAPINE SUCCINATE
LOXITANE C, LOXAPINE HYDROCHLORIDE
LOXITANE IM, LOXAPINE HYDROCHLORIDE
LOXITANE, LOXAPINE SUCCINATE
MAPROTILINE HCL, MAPROTILINE HYDROCHLORIDE
MECLIZINE HCL, MECLIZINE HYDROCHLORIDE
MECLOFENAMATE SODIUM, MECLOFENAMATE SODIUM
MEPERIDINE HCL, MEPERIDINE HYDROCHLORIDE
MEPROBAMATE, MEPROBAMATE
METAPROTERENOL SULFATE, METAPROTERENOL
   SULFATE
METHOCARBAMOL, METHOCARBAMOL
METHYCLOTHIAZIDE, METHYCLOTHIAZIDE
METHYLDOPA AND HYDROCHLOROTHIAZIDE,
   HYDROCHLOROTHIAZIDE
METHYLDOPA, METHYLDOPA
METHYLPHENIDATE HCL, METHYLPHENIDATE
   HYDROCHLORIDE
METHYLPREDNISOLONE, METHYLPREDNISOLONE
METHYLTESTOSTERONE, METHYLTESTOSTERONE
METOCLOPRAMIDE HCL, METOCLOPRAMIDE
   HYDROCHLORIDE
METOPROLOL TARTRATE, METOPROLOL TARTRATE
METRONIDAZOLE, METRONIDAZOLE
MEXILETINE HCL, MEXILETINE HYDROCHLORIDE
MICROZIDE, HYDROCHLOROTHIAZIDE
MINOCYCLINE HCL, MINOCYCLINE HYDROCHLORIDE
MINOXIDIL, MINOXIDIL
MIRTAZAPINE, MIRTAZAPINE
MORPHINE SULFATE, MORPHINE SULFATE

NALIDIXIC ACID, NALIDIXIC ACID
NAPROXEN SODIUM, NAPROXEN SODIUM
NAPROXEN, NAPROXEN
NIACIN, NIACIN
NICARDIPINE HCL, NICARDIPINE HYDROCHLORIDE
NITROFURANTOIN, NITROFURANTOIN
NITROFURANTOIN, NITROFURANTOIN,
   MACROCRYSTALLINE
NIZATIDINE, NIZATIDINE
NORCO, ACETAMINOPHEN
NORETHIN 1/35E-21, ETHINYL ESTRADIOL
NORETHIN 1/35E-28, ETHINYL ESTRADIOL
NORETHIN 1/50M-21, MESTRANOL
NORETHIN 1/50M-28, MESTRANOL
NORETHINDRONE AND ETHINYL ESTRADIOL (10/11),
   ETHINYL ESTRADIOL
NORETHINDRONE AND ETHINYL ESTRADIOL (7/14),
   ETHINYL ESTRADIOL
NORETHINDRONE AND ETHINYL ESTRADIOL, ETHINYL
   ESTRADIOL
NORETHINDRONE AND MESTRANOL, MESTRANOL
NORINYL 1+35 21-DAY, ETHINYL ESTRADIOL
NORINYL 1+35 28-DAY, ETHINYL ESTRADIOL
NORINYL 1+50 21-DAY, MESTRANOL
NORINYL 1+50 28-DAY, MESTRANOL
NORINYL, MESTRANOL
NORTRIPTYLINE HCL, NORTRIPTYLINE
   HYDROCHLORIDE
NYSTATIN, NYSTATIN
OGESTREL 0.5/50-21, ETHINYL ESTRADIOL
OGESTREL 0.5/50-28, ETHINYL ESTRADIOL
OXAZEPAM, OXAZEPAM
OXYCODONE AND ACETAMINOPHEN, ACETAMINOPHEN
OXYCODONE AND ASPIRIN, ASPIRIN
PEMOLINE, PEMOLINE
PENTAZOCINE AND NALOXONE HYDROCHLORIDES,
   NALOXONE HYDROCHLORIDE
PENTOXIFYLLINE, PENTOXIFYLLINE
PERPHENAZINE AND AMITRIPTYLINE HCL,
   AMITRIPTYLINE HYDROCHLORIDE
PHENDIMETRAZINE TARTRATE, PHENDIMETRAZINE
   TARTRATE
PHENTERMINE HCL, PHENTERMINE HYDROCHLORIDE
PHENYLBUTAZONE, PHENYLBUTAZONE
PHENYTOIN SODIUM, PHENYTOIN SODIUM, PROMPT
PINDOLOL, PINDOLOL
PIROXICAM, PIROXICAM
PRAZOSIN HCL, PRAZOSIN HYDROCHLORIDE
PREDNISOLONE, PREDNISOLONE
PREDNISONE, PREDNISONE
PRIMIDONE, PRIMIDONE
PROBEN-C, COLCHICINE
PROBENECID, PROBENECID
PROCAINAMIDE HCL, PROCAINAMIDE
   HYDROCHLORIDE
PROMETHAZINE HCL, PROMETHAZINE
   HYDROCHLORIDE
PROMPT PHENYTOIN SODIUM, PHENYTOIN SODIUM,
   PROMPT
PROPANTHELINE BROMIDE, PROPANTHELINE
   BROMIDE
PROPOXYPHENE HCL AND ACETAMINOPHEN,
   ACETAMINOPHEN
PROPOXYPHENE HCL W/ ASPIRIN AND CAFFEINE,
   ASPIRIN
PROPOXYPHENE HCL, PROPOXYPHENE
   HYDROCHLORIDE

APPENDIX B
PRODUCT NAME INDEX
LISTED BY APPLICANT (*continued*)

PROPRANOLOL HCL AND HYDROCHLOROTHIAZIDE,
   HYDROCHLOROTHIAZIDE
PROPRANOLOL HCL, PROPRANOLOL HYDROCHLORIDE
PROPYLTHIOURACIL, PROPYLTHIOURACIL
PYRILAMINE MALEATE, PYRILAMINE MALEATE
QUINIDINE GLUCONATE, QUINIDINE GLUCONATE
QUINIDINE SULFATE, QUINIDINE SULFATE
RANITIDINE HCL, RANITIDINE HYDROCHLORIDE
RANITIDINE, RANITIDINE HYDROCHLORIDE (OTC)
RAUWOLFIA SERPENTINA, RAUWOLFIA SERPENTINA
RESERPINE, HYDRALAZINE HCL AND
   HYDROCHLOROTHIAZIDE, HYDRALAZINE
   HYDROCHLORIDE
RESERPINE, RESERPINE
SODIUM PENTOBARBITAL, PENTOBARBITAL SODIUM
SODIUM SECOBARBITAL, SECOBARBITAL SODIUM
SOTALOL HCL, SOTALOL HYDROCHLORIDE
SPIRONOLACTONE W/ HYDROCHLOROTHIAZIDE,
   HYDROCHLOROTHIAZIDE
SPIRONOLACTONE, SPIRONOLACTONE
SPIRONOLACTONE/HYDROCHLOROTHIAZIDE,
   HYDROCHLOROTHIAZIDE
SULFAMETHOXAZOLE AND TRIMETHOPRIM DOUBLE
   STRENGTH, SULFAMETHOXAZOLE
SULFAMETHOXAZOLE AND TRIMETHOPRIM,
   SULFAMETHOXAZOLE
SULFASALAZINE, SULFASALAZINE
SULFINPYRAZONE, SULFINPYRAZONE
SULFISOXAZOLE, SULFISOXAZOLE
SULINDAC, SULINDAC
TEMAZEPAM, TEMAZEPAM
TETRACYCLINE HCL, TETRACYCLINE HYDROCHLORIDE
THIORIDAZINE HCL, THIORIDAZINE HYDROCHLORIDE
THIOTHIXENE, THIOTHIXENE
TICLOPIDINE HCL, TICLOPIDINE HYDROCHLORIDE
TIMOLOL MALEATE, TIMOLOL MALEATE
TOLAZAMIDE, TOLAZAMIDE
TOLBUTAMIDE, TOLBUTAMIDE
TRAZODONE HCL, TRAZODONE HYDROCHLORIDE
TRI-NORINYL 21-DAY, ETHINYL ESTRADIOL
TRI-NORINYL 28-DAY, ETHINYL ESTRADIOL
TRIAMCINOLONE, TRIAMCINOLONE
TRIAMTERENE AND HYDROCHLOROTHIAZIDE,
   HYDROCHLOROTHIAZIDE
TRIAZOLAM, TRIAZOLAM
TRICHLORMETHIAZIDE, TRICHLORMETHIAZIDE
TRIHEXYPHENIDYL HCL, TRIHEXYPHENIDYL
   HYDROCHLORIDE
TRIMETHOPRIM, TRIMETHOPRIM
TRIPELENNAMINE HCL, TRIPELENNAMINE
   HYDROCHLORIDE
TRIPROLIDINE HCL, TRIPROLIDINE HYDROCHLORIDE
TRIVORA-21, ETHINYL ESTRADIOL
TRIVORA-28, ETHINYL ESTRADIOL
VERAPAMIL HCL, VERAPAMIL HYDROCHLORIDE
ZOVIA 1/35E-21, ETHINYL ESTRADIOL
ZOVIA 1/35E-28, ETHINYL ESTRADIOL
ZOVIA 1/50E-21, ETHINYL ESTRADIOL
ZOVIA 1/50E-28, ETHINYL ESTRADIOL
WATSON LABS INC
  LISINOPRIL AND HYDROCHLOROTHIAZIDE,
    HYDROCHLOROTHIAZIDE
WATSON LABS (UTAH)
WATSON LABORATORIES INC
  NOR-QD, NORETHINDRONE
  OXYTROL, OXYBUTYNIN
WATSON PHARMS
WATSON PHARMACEUTICALS INC

ACTIGALL, URSODIOL
FIORICET W/ CODEINE, ACETAMINOPHEN
FIORICET, ACETAMINOPHEN
FIORINAL W/CODEINE NO 3, ASPIRIN
FIORINAL, ASPIRIN
WE PHARMS
WE PHARMACEUTICALS INC
  PREDNISOLONE SODIUM PHOSPHATE, PREDNISOLONE
    SODIUM PHOSPHATE
  PREDNISOLONE, PREDNISOLONE
WELLSPRING PHARM
WELLSPRING PHARMACEUTICAL CORP
  DIBENZYLINE, PHENOXYBENZAMINE HYDROCHLORIDE
  DUVOID, BETHANECHOL CHLORIDE
  DYRENIUM, TRIAMTERENE
WENDT
WENDT LABORATORIES INC
  NITROFURAZONE, NITROFURAZONE
WEST WARD
WEST WARD PHARMACEUTICAL CORP
  AMINOPHYLLINE, AMINOPHYLLINE
  AMITRIPTYLINE HCL, AMITRIPTYLINE HYDROCHLORIDE
  BUTALBITAL, ACETAMINOPHEN AND CAFFEINE,
    ACETAMINOPHEN
  BUTALBITAL, ACETAMINOPHEN, AND CAFFEINE,
    ACETAMINOPHEN
  BUTALBITAL, ASPIRIN AND CAFFEINE, ASPIRIN
  BUTALBITAL; ACETAMINOPHEN; AND CAFFEINE WITH
    CODEINE PHOSPHATE, ACETAMINOPHEN
  CAPTOPRIL, CAPTOPRIL
  CARISOPRODOL, CARISOPRODOL
  CHLORDIAZEPOXIDE HCL, CHLORDIAZEPOXIDE
    HYDROCHLORIDE
  CHLOROQUINE PHOSPHATE, CHLOROQUINE
    PHOSPHATE
  CHLOROTHIAZIDE AND RESERPINE, CHLOROTHIAZIDE
  CHLOROTHIAZIDE, CHLOROTHIAZIDE
  CHLORPHENIRAMINE MALEATE, CHLORPHENIRAMINE
    MALEATE
  CHLORPROMAZINE HCL, CHLORPROMAZINE
    HYDROCHLORIDE
  CORTISONE ACETATE, CORTISONE ACETATE
  CYANOCOBALAMIN, CYANOCOBALAMIN
  DICYCLOMINE HCL, DICYCLOMINE HYDROCHLORIDE
  DIPHENHYDRAMINE HCL, DIPHENHYDRAMINE
    HYDROCHLORIDE
  DIPHENOXYLATE HCL AND ATROPINE SULFATE,
    ATROPINE SULFATE
  DOXYCYCLINE HYCLATE, DOXYCYCLINE HYCLATE
  ETHAMBUTOL HCL, ETHAMBUTOL HYDROCHLORIDE
  FLURAZEPAM HCL, FLURAZEPAM HYDROCHLORIDE
  FOLIC ACID, FOLIC ACID
  HYDRALAZINE HCL, HYDRALAZINE HYDROCHLORIDE
  HYDROCHLOROTHIAZIDE, HYDROCHLOROTHIAZIDE
  HYDROCORTISONE, HYDROCORTISONE
  IMIPRAMINE HCL, IMIPRAMINE HYDROCHLORIDE
  ISONIAZID, ISONIAZID
  ISOSORBIDE DINITRATE, ISOSORBIDE DINITRATE
  ISOSORBIDE MONONITRATE, ISOSORBIDE
    MONONITRATE
  LISINOPRIL AND HYDROCHLOROTHIAZIDE,
    HYDROCHLOROTHIAZIDE
  LISINOPRIL, LISINOPRIL
  LITHIUM CARBONATE, LITHIUM CARBONATE
  MEPROBAMATE, MEPROBAMATE
  METHOCARBAMOL, METHOCARBAMOL
  METHYLTESTOSTERONE, METHYLTESTOSTERONE
  NIACIN, NIACIN

APPENDIX B
PRODUCT NAME INDEX
LISTED BY APPLICANT (*continued*)

OXYTETRACYCLINE HCL, OXYTETRACYCLINE
   HYDROCHLORIDE
PREDNISOLONE, PREDNISOLONE
PREDNISONE, PREDNISONE
PROPOXYPHENE HCL, PROPOXYPHENE
   HYDROCHLORIDE
PROPYLTHIOURACIL, PROPYLTHIOURACIL
QUINIDINE SULFATE, QUINIDINE SULFATE
RESERPINE AND HYDROCHLOROTHIAZIDE-50,
   HYDROCHLOROTHIAZIDE
RESERPINE, RESERPINE
SODIUM BUTABARBITAL, BUTABARBITAL SODIUM
SODIUM SECOBARBITAL, SECOBARBITAL SODIUM
SULFISOXAZOLE, SULFISOXAZOLE
TETRACYCLINE HCL, TETRACYCLINE HYDROCHLORIDE
THIORIDAZINE HCL, THIORIDAZINE HYDROCHLORIDE
TRIHEXYPHENIDYL HCL, TRIHEXYPHENIDYL
   HYDROCHLORIDE
TRIPROLIDINE AND PSEUDOEPHEDRINE,
   PSEUDOEPHEDRINE HYDROCHLORIDE
VITAMIN A, VITAMIN A
VITAMIN A, VITAMIN A PALMITATE
VITAMIN D, ERGOCALCIFEROL
WESTWARD
WESTWARD PHARMACEUTICAL CORP
   CEFAZOLIN SODIUM, CEFAZOLIN SODIUM
WESTWOOD SQUIBB
WESTWOOD SQUIBB PHARMACEUTICALS INC
   CAPITROL, CHLOROXINE
   EURAX, CROTAMITON
   EXELDERM, SULCONAZOLE NITRATE
   FLEXICORT, HYDROCORTISONE
   HALOG, HALCINONIDE
   HALOG-E, HALCINONIDE
   HALOTEX, HALOPROGIN
   LAC-HYDRIN, AMMONIUM LACTATE
   MYCOSTATIN, NYSTATIN
   STATICIN, ERYTHROMYCIN
   T-STAT, ERYTHROMYCIN
   TACARYL, METHDILAZINE
   TACARYL, METHDILAZINE HYDROCHLORIDE
   ULTRAVATE, HALOBETASOL PROPIONATE
   WESTCORT, HYDROCORTISONE VALERATE
WHARTON LABS
WHARTON LABORATORIES INC DIV US ETHICALS
   VITAMIN A, VITAMIN A PALMITATE
WHITBY
WHITBY PHARMACEUTICALS INC
   THEOBID JR., THEOPHYLLINE
   THEOBID, THEOPHYLLINE
WHITEHALL ROBINS
WHITEHALL ROBINS HEALTHCARE DIV AMERICAN HOME
PRODUCTS CORP
   BRONITIN MIST, EPINEPHRINE BITARTRATE (OTC)
   PRIMATENE MIST, EPINEPHRINE (OTC)
WHITEWORTH TOWN PLSN
WHITEWORTH TOWNE PAULSEN INC
   ACETAMINOPHEN W/ CODEINE PHOSPHATE,
     ACETAMINOPHEN
   BUTABARBITAL SODIUM, BUTABARBITAL SODIUM
   CORTISONE ACETATE, CORTISONE ACETATE
   DEXAMETHASONE, DEXAMETHASONE
   DIPHENHYDRAMINE HCL, DIPHENHYDRAMINE
     HYDROCHLORIDE
   FOLIC ACID, FOLIC ACID
   H.R.-50, HYDROCHLOROTHIAZIDE
   HYDROCHLOROTHIAZIDE, HYDROCHLOROTHIAZIDE
   HYDROCORTISONE, HYDROCORTISONE

ISONIAZID, ISONIAZID
MEPROBAMATE, MEPROBAMATE
NITROFURANTOIN, NITROFURANTOIN
PENTOBARBITAL SODIUM, PENTOBARBITAL SODIUM
PREDNISOLONE, PREDNISOLONE
PREDNISONE, PREDNISONE
PROMETHAZINE HCL, PROMETHAZINE
   HYDROCHLORIDE
PROPOXYPHENE HCL, PROPOXYPHENE
   HYDROCHLORIDE
QUINIDINE SULFATE, QUINIDINE SULFATE
RESERPINE, RESERPINE
SECOBARBITAL SODIUM, SECOBARBITAL SODIUM
WOCKHARDT
WOCKHARDT AMERICAS INC
   CAPTOPRIL, CAPTOPRIL
   ENALAPRIL MALEATE, ENALAPRIL MALEATE
   FAMOTIDINE, FAMOTIDINE
   RANITIDINE HCL, RANITIDINE HYDROCHLORIDE
WOCKHARDT LTD
   NIACIN, NIACIN
WOMEN FIRST HLTHCARE
WOMEN FIRST HEALTHCARE INC
   BACTRIM DS, SULFAMETHOXAZOLE
   BACTRIM PEDIATRIC, SULFAMETHOXAZOLE
   BACTRIM, SULFAMETHOXAZOLE
   EQUAGESIC, ASPIRIN
   ESCLIM, ESTRADIOL
   ORTHO-EST, ESTROPIPATE
   SYNALGOS-DC, ASPIRIN
   SYNALGOS-DC-A, ACETAMINOPHEN
   VANIQA, EFLORNITHINE HYDROCHLORIDE
   WYGESIC, ACETAMINOPHEN
WOMENS CAPITAL
WOMENS CAPITAL CORP
   PLAN B, LEVONORGESTREL
WYETH AYERST
WYETH AYERST LABORATORIES
   A.P.L., GONADOTROPIN, CHORIONIC
   ANSOLYSEN, PENTOLINIUM TARTRATE
   ATROMID-S, CLOFIBRATE
   BICILLIN L-A, PENICILLIN G BENZATHINE
   BICILLIN, PENICILLIN G BENZATHINE
   CEFPIRAMIDE SODIUM, CEFPIRAMIDE SODIUM
   CHLORPROMAZINE HCL, CHLORPROMAZINE
     HYDROCHLORIDE
   CYANOCOBALAMIN, CYANOCOBALAMIN
   CYCLAPEN-W, CYCLACILLIN
   DEXAMETHASONE SODIUM PHOSPHATE,
     DEXAMETHASONE SODIUM PHOSPHATE
   DIGOXIN, DIGOXIN
   DIMENHYDRINATE, DIMENHYDRINATE
   DIMETANE-TEN, BROMPHENIRAMINE MALEATE
   DIPHENHYDRAMINE HCL, DIPHENHYDRAMINE
     HYDROCHLORIDE
   DIUCARDIN, HYDROFLUMETHIAZIDE
   EQUANIL, MEPROBAMATE
   ESTRADURIN, POLYESTRADIOL PHOSPHATE
   ESTROGENIC SUBSTANCE, ESTRONE
   FLUOTHANE, HALOTHANE
   FUROSEMIDE, FUROSEMIDE
   GENTAMICIN SULFATE, GENTAMICIN SULFATE
   GRISACTIN ULTRA, GRISEOFULVIN,
     ULTRAMICROCRYSTALLINE
   GRISACTIN, GRISEOFULVIN, MICROCRYSTALLINE
   HYDROXYZINE HCL, HYDROXYZINE HYDROCHLORIDE
   INDERAL, PROPRANOLOL HYDROCHLORIDE
   INDERIDE LA 120/50, HYDROCHLOROTHIAZIDE

APPENDIX B
PRODUCT NAME INDEX
LISTED BY APPLICANT (*continued*)

INDERIDE LA 160/50, HYDROCHLOROTHIAZIDE
INDERIDE LA 80/50, HYDROCHLOROTHIAZIDE
ISORDIL, ISOSORBIDE DINITRATE
LIDOCAINE HCL, LIDOCAINE HYDROCHLORIDE
MAZANOR, MAZINDOL
MEPERIDINE AND ATROPINE SULFATE, ATROPINE
    SULFATE
MEPERIDINE HCL, MEPERIDINE HYDROCHLORIDE
NALOXONE, NALOXONE HYDROCHLORIDE
OMNIPEN (AMPICILLIN), AMPICILLIN/AMPICILLIN
    TRIHYDRATE
OMNIPEN-N, AMPICILLIN SODIUM
ORUDIS, KETOPROFEN
PATHOCIL, DICLOXACILLIN SODIUM
PEN-VEE K, PENICILLIN V POTASSIUM
PENBRITIN, AMPICILLIN/AMPICILLIN TRIHYDRATE
PENBRITIN-S, AMPICILLIN SODIUM
PENICILLIN G POTASSIUM, PENICILLIN G POTASSIUM
PEPTAVLON, PENTAGASTRIN
PHENERGAN FORTIS, PROMETHAZINE
    HYDROCHLORIDE
PHENERGAN PLAIN, PROMETHAZINE HYDROCHLORIDE
PHENERGAN VC W/ CODEINE, CODEINE PHOSPHATE
PHENERGAN VC, PHENYLEPHRINE HYDROCHLORIDE
PHENERGAN W/ CODEINE, CODEINE PHOSPHATE
PHENERGAN W/ DEXTROMETHORPHAN,
    DEXTROMETHORPHAN HYDROBROMIDE
PHENERGAN, PROMETHAZINE HYDROCHLORIDE
PLEGINE, PHENDIMETRAZINE TARTRATE
PMB 200, ESTROGENS, CONJUGATED
PMB 400, ESTROGENS, CONJUGATED
PROCHLORPERAZINE EDISYLATE,
    PROCHLORPERAZINE EDISYLATE
PROKETAZINE, CARPHENAZINE MALEATE
PROTOPAM CHLORIDE, PRALIDOXIME CHLORIDE
ROBITET, TETRACYCLINE HYDROCHLORIDE
SECOBARBITAL SODIUM, SECOBARBITAL SODIUM
SODIUM PENTOBARBITAL, PENTOBARBITAL SODIUM
SODIUM SECOBARBITAL, SECOBARBITAL SODIUM
SPARINE, PROMAZINE HYDROCHLORIDE
SULFOSE, TRISULFAPYRIMIDINES (SULFADIAZINE;
    SULFAMERAZINE; SULFAMETHAZINE)
TETRACYCLINE HCL, TETRACYCLINE HYDROCHLORIDE
THIAMINE HCL, THIAMINE HYDROCHLORIDE
THIOSULFIL, SULFAMETHIZOLE
UNIPEN IN PLASTIC CONTAINER, NAFCILLIN SODIUM
UNIPEN, NAFCILLIN SODIUM
WYAMYCIN E, ERYTHROMYCIN ETHYLSUCCINATE
WYAMYCIN S, ERYTHROMYCIN STEARATE
WYMOX, AMOXICILLIN
WYTENSIN, GUANABENZ ACETATE
WYETH AYERST RESEARCH
    CERUBIDINE, DAUNORUBICIN HYDROCHLORIDE
WYETH CONS
WYETH CONSUMER HEALTHCARE
    ADVIL ALLERGY SINUS, CHLORPHENIRAMINE MALEATE
      (OTC)
    ADVIL COLD AND SINUS, IBUPROFEN (OTC)
    ADVIL LIQUI-GELS, IBUPROFEN POTASSIUM (OTC)
    ADVIL MIGRAINE LIQUI-GELS, IBUPROFEN POTASSIUM
      (OTC)
    ADVIL, IBUPROFEN (OTC)
    ALAVERT, LORATADINE (OTC)
    AXID AR, NIZATIDINE (OTC)
    CHILDREN'S ADVIL COLD, IBUPROFEN (OTC)
    CHILDREN'S ADVIL, IBUPROFEN
    CHILDREN'S ADVIL, IBUPROFEN (OTC)
    CHILDREN'S ADVIL-FLAVORED, IBUPROFEN (OTC)

DIMETANE, BROMPHENIRAMINE MALEATE
DIMETANE, BROMPHENIRAMINE MALEATE (OTC)
DIMETAPP, BROMPHENIRAMINE MALEATE (OTC)
JUNIOR STRENGTH ADVIL, IBUPROFEN (OTC)
LORATADINE, LORATADINE (OTC)
ORUDIS KT, KETOPROFEN (OTC)
PEDIATRIC ADVIL, IBUPROFEN (OTC)
WYETH PHARMS INC
WYETH PHARMACEUTICALS INC
    ALESSE, ETHINYL ESTRADIOL
    CORDARONE, AMIODARONE HYDROCHLORIDE
    DECLOMYCIN, DEMECLOCYCLINE HYDROCHLORIDE
    EFFEXOR XR, VENLAFAXINE HYDROCHLORIDE
    EFFEXOR, VENLAFAXINE HYDROCHLORIDE
    FOLVITE, FOLIC ACID
    INDERAL LA, PROPRANOLOL HYDROCHLORIDE
    INDERAL, PROPRANOLOL HYDROCHLORIDE
    INDERIDE-40/25, HYDROCHLOROTHIAZIDE
    INDERIDE-80/25, HYDROCHLOROTHIAZIDE
    LEVONORGESTREL, LEVONORGESTREL
    LO/OVRAL, ETHINYL ESTRADIOL
    LO/OVRAL-28, ETHINYL ESTRADIOL
    LODINE XL, ETODOLAC
    LODINE, ETODOLAC
    METHOTREXATE LPF, METHOTREXATE SODIUM
    METHOTREXATE SODIUM PRESERVATIVE FREE,
      METHOTREXATE SODIUM
    METHOTREXATE SODIUM, METHOTREXATE SODIUM
    MINOCIN, MINOCYCLINE HYDROCHLORIDE
    MYLOTARG, GEMTUZUMAB OZOGAMICIN
    NORDETTE-21, ETHINYL ESTRADIOL
    NORDETTE-28, ETHINYL ESTRADIOL
    NORPLANT SYSTEM IN PLASTIC CONTAINER,
      LEVONORGESTREL
    ORUVAIL, KETOPROFEN
    OVRAL, ETHINYL ESTRADIOL
    OVRAL-28, ETHINYL ESTRADIOL
    OVRETTE, NORGESTREL
    PHENERGAN, PROMETHAZINE HYDROCHLORIDE
    PIPRACIL, PIPERACILLIN SODIUM
    PREMARIN, ESTROGENS, CONJUGATED
    PREMPHASE (PREMARIN;CYCRIN 14/14), ESTROGENS,
      CONJUGATED
    PREMPHASE 14/14, ESTROGENS, CONJUGATED
    PREMPRO (PREMARIN;CYCRIN), ESTROGENS,
      CONJUGATED
    PREMPRO, ESTROGENS, CONJUGATED
    PROTONIX IV, PANTOPRAZOLE SODIUM
    PROTONIX, PANTOPRAZOLE SODIUM
    QUINIDEX, QUINIDINE SULFATE
    RAPAMUNE, SIROLIMUS
    TRECATOR-SC, ETHIONAMIDE
    TRIPHASIL-21, ETHINYL ESTRADIOL
    TRIPHASIL-28, ETHINYL ESTRADIOL
    ZOSYN IN PLASTIC CONTAINER, PIPERACILLIN SODIUM
    ZOSYN, PIPERACILLIN SODIUM

X

XANODYNE PHARM
XANODYNE PHARMACAL INC
    AMICAR, AMINOCAPROIC ACID
    LEUCOVORIN CALCIUM, LEUCOVORIN CALCIUM
XCEL PHARM
XCEL PHARMACEUTICALS INC
    MIGRANAL, DIHYDROERGOTAMINE MESYLATE

APPENDIX B
PRODUCT NAME INDEX
LISTED BY APPLICANT (*continued*)

XCEL PHARMS
XCEL PHARMACEUTICALS
    D.H.E. 45, DIHYDROERGOTAMINE MESYLATE
    DIASTAT, DIAZEPAM
    MYSOLINE, PRIMIDONE

XTTRIUM
XTTRIUM LABORATORIES INC
    DYNA-HEX, CHLORHEXIDINE GLUCONATE (OTC)
    EXIDINE, CHLORHEXIDINE GLUCONATE (OTC)
    TURGEX, HEXACHLOROPHENE

Y

YAMANOUCHI
YAMANOUCHI EUROPE BV
    LOCOID, HYDROCORTISONE BUTYRATE

YOSHITOMI
YOSHITOMI PHARMACEUTICAL INDUSTRIES LTD
    CEPHALEXIN, CEPHALEXIN

Z

ZAMBON
ZAMBON CORP
    MONUROL, FOSFOMYCIN TROMETHAMINE

ZENITH GOLDLINE
ZENITH GOLDLINE LABORATORIES INC
    METFORMIN HCL, METFORMIN HYDROCHLORIDE
ZENITH GOLDLINE PHARMACEUTICALS
    BUSPIRONE HCL, BUSPIRONE HYDROCHLORIDE
    FLUOXETINE HCL, FLUOXETINE HYDROCHLORIDE
ZENITH GOLDLINE PHARMACEUTICALS INC
    NIZATIDINE, NIZATIDINE

ZILA
ZILA PHARMACEUTICALS INC
    PERIDEX, CHLORHEXIDINE GLUCONATE

APPENDIX C
UNIFORM TERMS

DOSAGE FORMS
AEROSOL
AEROSOL, METERED
BAR, CHEWABLE
CAPSULE
CAPSULE, COATED PELLETS
CAPSULE, DELAYED REL PELLETS
CAPSULE, EXTENDED RELEASE
CONCENTRATE
CREAM
CREAM, AUGMENTED
CREAM, SUPPOSITORY
DISC
DRESSING
DRUG DELIVERY SYSTEM
ELIXIR
EMULSION
ENEMA
FIBER, EXTENDED RELEASE
FILM, EXTENDED RELEASE
FOR SOLUTION
FOR SUSPENSION
FOR SUSPENSION, EXTENDED RELEASE
GAS
GEL
GEL, METERED
GRANULE
GRANULE, DELAYED RELEASE
GRANULE, EFFERVESCENT
GUM, CHEWING
IMPLANT
INHALANT
INJECTABLE
INJECTABLE, LIPID COMPLEX
INJECTABLE, LIPOSOMAL
INSERT
INSERT, EXTENDED RELEASE
INTRAUTERINE DEVICE
JELLY
LIQUID
LIQUID, EXTENDED RELEASE
LOTION
LOTION, AUGMENTED
LOTION, SHAMPOO
N/A
OIL
OINTMENT
OINTMENT, AUGMENTED
PASTE
PASTILLE
PELLET
POWDER
POWDER, EXTENDED RELEASE
POWDER, METERED
RING
SHAMPOO
SOAP
SOLUTION
SOLUTION FOR SLUSH
SOLUTION/DROPS
SOLUTION, CONCENTRATE
SOLUTION, GEL FORMING/DROPS
SPONGE
SPRAY
SPRAY, METERED
SUPPOSITORY

SUSPENSION
SUSPENSION/DROPS
SUSPENSION, EXTENDED RELEASE
SWAB
SYRUP
TABLET
TABLET, CHEWABLE
TABLET, CHEWABLE, TABLET, CAPSULE
TABLET, COATED PARTICLES
TABLET, DELAYED RELEASE
TABLET, DISPERSIBLE
TABLET, EFFERVESCENT
TABLET, EXTENDED RELEASE
TABLET, ORALLY DISINTEGRATING
TAMPON
TAPE
TROCHE/LOZENGE

ROUTES OF ADMINISTRATION
BUCCAL
BUCCAL/SUBLINGUAL
DENTAL
ENDOCERVICAL
FOR RX COMPOUNDING
IMPLANTATION
IM-IV
IM-IV-SC
IM-SCI
INHALATION
INJECTION
INTRACRANIAL
INTRALYMPHATIC
INTRAMUSCULAR
INTRAOCULAR
INTRAPERITONEAL
INTRAPLEURAL
INTRATHECAL
INTRATRACHEAL
INTRAUTERINE
INTRAVASCULAR
INTRAVENOUS
INTRAVESICAL
IONTOPHORESIS
IRRIGATION
IV (INFUSION)
N/A
NASAL
OPHTHALMIC
ORAL
ORAL-20
ORAL-21
ORAL-28
OTIC
PERFUSION, BILIARY
PERFUSION, CARDIAC
PERIODONTAL
RECTAL
SPINAL
SUBCUTANEOUS
SUBLINGUAL
TOPICAL
TOPICAL, VAGINAL
TRANSDERMAL
URETERAL
URETHRAL
VAGINAL

APPENDIX C
UNIFORM TERMS (*continued*)

ABBREVIATIONS

AMP	AMPULE	INH	INHALATION
AMPICIL	AMPICILLIN	IU	INTERNATIONAL UNITS
APPROX	APPROXIMATELY	KIU	KALLIKREIN INHIBITOR UNITS
BOT	BOTTLE	MCI	MILLICURIE
CI	CURIE	MEQ	MILLIEQUIVALENT
CSR	CAROTID SINUS REFLEX	MG	MILLIGRAM
CU	CLINICAL UNITS	ML	MILLILITER
DIPROP	DIPROPIONATE	N/A	NOT APPLICABLE
EQ	EQUIVALENT TO	PPM	PARTS PER MILLION
ELECT	ELECTROLYTE	REL	RELEASE
ER	EXTENDED RELEASE	SQ CM	SQUARE CENTIMETER
GM	GRAM	U	UNITS
HBR	HYDROBROMIDE	UCI	MICROCURIE
HCL	HYDROCHLORIDE	UGM	MICROGRAM
HR	HOUR	UMOLAR	MICROMOLAR
		USP	UNITED STATES PHARMACOPEIA

PATENT AND EXCLUSIVITY INFORMATION ADDENDUM

This *Addendum* identifies drugs that qualify under the Drug Price Competition and Patent Term Restoration Act (1984 Amendments) for periods of exclusivity, during which abbreviated new drug applications (ANDAs) and applications described in Section 505(b)(2) of the Federal Food, Drug, and Cosmetic Act (the Act) for those drug products may, in some instances, not be submitted or made effective as described below, and provides patent information concerning the listed drug products. Those drugs that have qualified for Orphan Drug Exclusivity pursuant to Section 527 of the Act and those drugs that have qualified for Pediatric Exclusivity pursuant to Section 505A are also included in this *Addendum*. This section is arranged in alphabetical order by active ingredient name. For those drug products with multiple active ingredients, only the first active ingredient (in alphabetical order) will appear. For an explanation of the codes used in the *Addendum*, see the *Patent and Exclusivity Terms* page. Exclusivity prevents the submission or effective approval of ANDAs or applications described in Section 505(b)(2) of the Act. It does not prevent the submission or approval of a second full NDA. Applications qualifying for periods of exclusivity are:

(1) A new drug application approved after September 24, 1984, for a drug product all active ingredients (including any ester or salt of the active ingredient) of which had never been approved in any other new drug application under Section 505(b) of the Act. No subsequent ANDA or application described in Section 505(b)(2) of the Act for the same drug may be submitted for a period of five years from the date of approval of the original application, except that such an application may be *submitted* after four years if it contains a certification that a patent claiming the drug is invalid or will not be infringed by the product for which approval is sought.

(2) A new drug application approved after September 24, 1984, for a drug product containing an active ingredient (including any ester or salt of that active ingredient) that has been approved in an earlier new drug application and that includes reports of new clinical investigations (other than bioavailability studies). Such investigations must have been conducted or sponsored by the applicant and must have been essential to approval of the application. If these requirements are met, the approval of a subsequent ANDA or an application described in Section 505(b)(2) of the Act may not be made effective for the same drug or use, if for a new indication,

before the expiration of *three years* from the date of approval of the original application. If an applicant has exclusivity for a new use or indication, this does not preclude the approval of an ANDA application or 505(b)(2) application for the drug product with indications not covered by the exclusivity.

(3) A supplement to a new drug application for a drug containing a previously approved active ingredient (including any ester or salt of the active ingredient) approved after September 24, 1984, that contains reports of new clinical investigations (other than bioavailability studies) essential to the approval of the supplement and conducted or sponsored by the applicant. The approval of a subsequent application for a change approved in the supplement may not be *made effective* for *three years* from the date of approval of the original supplement.

The Act requires that patent information must now be filed with all newly submitted Section 505 drug applications, and that no NDA may be approved after September 24, 1984, without the submission of pertinent patent information to the Agency. The patent numbers and the expiration dates of appropriate patents claiming drug products that are the subject of approved applications will be published in this *Addendum* or in the monthly Cumulative Supplement to this publication. Patent information on unapproved applications or on patents beyond the scope of the Act (i.e., process or manufacturing patents) will not be published.

The patents that FDA regards as covered by the statutory provisions for submission of patent information are: patents that claim the active ingredient or ingredients; drug product patents, which include formulation/composition patents; and use patents for a particular approved indication or method of using the product. NDA holders or applicants amending or supplementing applications with formulation/ composition patent information are asked to declare that the patent(s) is appropriate for publication and refers to an approved product or one for which approval is being sought. The Agency asks all applicants or application holders with use patents to provide information as to the approved indications or uses covered by such patents. This information will be included in the Cumulative Supplement to the List as it becomes available.

Since all parts of this publication are subject to changes, additions, or deletions, the *Addendum* must be used in conjunction with the most current Cumulative Supplement.

PATENT AND EXCLUSIVITY TERMS

DUE TO SPACE LIMITATIONS IN THE EXCLUSIVITY COLUMN, THE FOLLOWING ABBREVIATIONS HAVE BEEN DEVELOPED. PLEASE REFER TO THIS PAGE FOR AN EXPLANATION OF THE PATENT AND EXCLUSIVITY ABBREVIATIONS FOUND IN THE ADDENDUM.

ABBREVIATIONS

D	NEW DOSING SCHEDULE (SEE REFERENCES, BELOW)
I	NEW INDICATION (SEE REFERENCES, BELOW)
NC	NEW COMBINATION
NCE	NEW CHEMICAL ENTITY
NDF	NEW DOSAGE FORM
NE	NEW ESTER OR SALT OF AN ACTIVE INGREDIENT
NP	NEW PRODUCT
NP*	NEW PRODUCT (MINT FLAVORED)
NPP	NEW PATIENT POPULATION
NR	NEW ROUTE
NS	NEW STRENGTH
ODE	ORPHAN DRUG EXCLUSIVITY
PC	PATENT CHALLENGE
PED	PEDIATRIC EXCLUSIVITY
RTO	RX TO OTC SWITCH OR OTC USE
U	PATENT USE CODE (SEE REFERENCES, BELOW)
W	EXCLUSIVITY ON THIS APPLICATION EXPIRING ON THIS DATE HAS BEEN WAIVED BY SPONSOR - SEE SECTION 1.3 OF SUPPLEMENT WAIVED EXCLUSIVITY

REFERENCES

EXCLUSIVITY DOSING SCHEDULE

D-1	ONCE A DAY APPLICATION
D-2	ONCE DAILY DOSING
D-3	SEVEN DAYS/SEVEN DAYS/SEVEN DAYS DOSING SCHEDULE
D-4	SEVEN DAYS/FOURTEEN DAYS DOSING SCHEDULE
D-5	TEN DAYS/ELEVEN DAYS DOSING SCHEDULE
D-6	SEVEN DAYS/NINE DAYS/FIVE DAYS DOSING SCHEDULE
D-7	BID DOSING
D-8	INTRAVENOUS, EPIDURAL AND INTRATHECAL DOSING
D-9	NARCOTIC OVERDOSE IN ADULTS
D-10	NARCOTIC OVERDOSE IN CHILDREN
D-11	POSTOPERATIVE NARCOTIC DEPRESSION IN CHILDREN
D-12	BEDTIME DOSING OF 800MG FOR TREATMENT OF ACTIVE DUODENAL ULCER
D-13	INCREASED MAXIMUM DAILY DOSAGE RECOMMENDATION
D-14	BEDTIME DOSING OF 800MG FOR TREATMENT OF ACTIVE BENIGN GASTRIC ULCER
D-15	SINGLE DAILY DOSE OF 25MG/37.5MG
D-16	CONTINUOUS INTRAVENOUS INFUSION
D-17	400MG EVERY 12 HOURS FOR THREE DAYS FOR UNCOMPLICATED URINARY TRACT INFECTIONS
D-18	LOWER RECOMMENDED STARTING DOSE GUIDELINES
D-19	BOLUS DOSING GUIDELINES
D-20	SINGLE 32MG DOSE
D-21	ALTERNATIVE DOSAGE OF 300MG ONCE DAILY AFTER THE EVENING MEAL
D-22	REDUCTION IN INFUSION TIME FROM 24 TO 4 HOURS FOR THE 60MG DOSE
D-23	INCREASE MAXIMUM DOSE AND VARIATIONS IN THE DOSING REGIMEN
D-24	FOR OVARIAN CANCER THE RECOMMENDED REGIMEN IS 135MG/M^2 OR 175MG/M^2 INTRAVENOUSLY OVER THREE HOURS EVERY THREE WEEKS
D-25	ADDITIONAL DOSAGE REGIMEN EQUAL TO HALF OF THE ORIGINAL DOSING REGIMEN
D-26	ONCE WEEKLY APPLICATION
D-27	BID DOSING IN PATIENTS 12 YEARS OF AGE AND OLDER FOR PREVENTION OF NAUSEA AND VOMITING ASSOCIATED WITH MODERATELY EMETOGENIC CANCER CHEMOTHERAPY
D-28	USE OF ISOVUE-370 IN EXCRETORY UROGRAPHY AT EQUIVALENT GRAMS OF IODINE TO THE CURRENTLY APPROVED ISOVUE-250 AND ISOVUE-300
D-29	INCREASE OF CUMULATIVE DOSE TO 0.3MMOL/KG FOR MRI OF THE CNS IN ADULTS
D-30	5000 IU DOSE FOR PHOPHYLAXIS AGAINST DEEP VEIN THROMBOSIS
D-31	CHANGE IN RECOMMENDED TOTAL DAILY DOSE TO 80MG (40MG BID)
D-32	REMOVAL OF THE RESTRICTIONS LIMITING TREATMENT TO TWO CONSECUTIVE WEEKS AND TO SMALL AREAS
D-33	ONCE DAILY DOSING FOR PLAQUE PSORIASIS
D-34	EVERY FOUR MONTHS DOSAGE REGIMEN

EXCLUSIVITY TERMS

EXCLUSIVITY DOSING SCHEDULE (continued)

D-35	FOR A ONE WEEK DOSING PERIOD FOR INTERDIGITAL TINEA PEDIS
D-36	FOR A SINGLE 2MG DOSE AS AN ALTERNATIVE TO THE 1MG DOSE GIVE TWICE DAILY
D-37	DOSING REGIMEN FOR ADMINISTRATION EITHER ONCE DAILY (QD) OR TWICE DAILY (BID)
D-38	CONTINUOUS INFUSION AS AN ALTERNATE METHOD OF ADMINISTRATION
D-39	CHANGE IN TIME TO TAKE THE DRUG PRIOR TO A MEAL TO PREVENT MEAL-INDUCED HEARTBURN SYMPTOMS FROM ". . 1/2-1 HOUR BEFORE EATING . ." TO " . . RIGHT BEFORE EATING OR UP TO 60 MIN BEFORE CONSUMING . ."
D-40	ONCE-A-DAY DOSING REGIMEN
D-41	DRUG MAY BE DOSED RIGHT BEFORE A MEAL OR ANY TIME UP TO 30 MIN BEFORE EATING OR DRINKING FOOD AND BEVERAGES THAT WOULD BE EXPECTED TO CAUSE SYMPTOMS
D-42	TEN DAY DOSING REGIMEN FOR TRIPLE THERAPY, PREVACID IN COMBINATION WITH CLARITHROMYCIN AND AMOXICCLIN, FOR THE ERADICATION OF H. PYLORI IN PATIENTS WITH DUODENAL ULCER DISEASE
D-43	INITIATION OF TREATMENT WITH 900MG/DAY BY DELETION OF THE REQUIREMENT TO TITRATE TO 900MG/DAY OVER A 3-DAY PERIOD
D-44	IN A CLINICAL TRIAL, FEWER DISCONTINUATIONS DUE TO ADVERSE EVENTS, ESPECIALLY DIZZINESS AND VERTIGO, WERE OBSERVED WHEN TITRATING THE DOSE IN INCREMENTS OF 50MG/DAY EVERY THREE DAYS UNTIL AN EFFECTIVE DOSE (NOT EXCEEDING 400MG/DAY) WAS REACHED
D-45	ONCE DAILY DOSING FOR MAINTENANCE ONLY
D-46	NEW DOSING REGIMEN OF 80MG DAILY
D-47	PREVENTION OF HEARTBURN SYMPTOMS WHEN ADMINISTERED FROM 15 MINUTES UP TO, BUT NOT INCLUDING, 1 HOUR PRIOR TO A PROVOCATIVE MEAL
D-48	ADMINISTRATION OF CISATRICURIUM, A NEUROMUSCULAR BLOCKING AGENT AT DOSES OF 3 AND 4X THE ED95 OF CISATRICUNIUM FOLLOWING INDUCTION WITH THIOPENTAL
D-49	PEDIATRIC DOSING GUIDELINES
D-50	INFORMATION FOR USE OF CORVERT IN POST-CARDIAC SURGERY PATIENTS
D-51	OPTIONAL STARTING DOSE OF 40MG/DAY
D-52	ALTERNATE DOSING REGIMEN OF 1250MG TWICE DAILY
D-53	USE IN PEDIATRIC PATIENTS FROM 1 MONTH TO 16 YEARS OF AGE
D-54	USE OF ZYBAN FOR MAINTENANCE THERAPY. TREATMENT UP TO 6 MONTHS WAS SHOWN EFFICACIOUS
D-55	ADDITION OF A HIGHER DOSE OF NUTROPIN FOR PUBERTAL PATIENTS (PUBERTAL DOSE LESS THAN OR EQUAL TO 0.7MG/KG/WEEK)
D-56	ADDITION OF POSTPRANDIAL DOSING
D-57	3-HOUR INFUSION OF TAXOL GIVEN EVERY THREE WEEKS AT A DOSE OF 175MG/M2 FOLLOWED BY CISPLATIN AT A DOSE OF 75MG/M2 FOR THE FIRST-LINE TREATMENT OF ADVANCED OVARIAN CANCER
D-58	CHANGE IN DOSING INTERVAL TO ONCE-DAILY ADMINISTRATION
D-59	REDUCTION OF ELEVATED LDL-C IN A NEW, HIGHER STRENGTH TABLET, 0.8MG, AND FOR EXTENSION OF THE DOSAGE RANGE TO 0.8MG DAILY
D-60	ADDITION OF A POST-OPERATIVE DOSING REGIMEN
D-61	ONCE WEEKLY DOSING FOR THE TREATMENT OF POSTMENOPAUSAL OSTEOPOROSIS
D-62	ONCE WEEKLY DOSING FOR THE PREVENTION OF POSTMENOPAUSAL OSTEOPOROSIS
D-63	TO ALLOW A TITRATION DOSING REGIMEN USING A 25MG DOSE
D-64	INCREASING DOSAGE FOR NERVE BLOCK ANESTHESIA USING NAROPIN 7.5MG/ML AND FOR EXTENDING THE DURATION OF TREATMENT FOR POSTOPERATIVE ANALGESIA USING NAROPIN 2MG/ML
D-65	CHANGE DOSING AND ADMINISTRATION TO INDICATE MAINTENANCE OF WEIGHT LOSS OVER AN 18 MONTH PERIOD THUS EXTENDING THE USE OF THIS DRUG FROM ONE TO TWO YEARS
D-66	DOSING RECOMMENDATIONS FOR PATIENTS UNDERGOING PCI
D-67	SHORTER TREATMENT COURSE OF THREE DAYS IN THE TREATMENT OF RECURRENT EPISODES OF GENITAL HERPES
D-68	CHANGE OF ADMIN RATE FOR INFUSION OF AREDIA FOR TREATMENT OF MODERATE AND SEVERE HYPERCALCEMIA OF MALIGNANCY FROM 24 HOURS TO 2 HOURS UP TO BUT NOT INCLUDING 24 HOURS
D-69	SHORTENED DOSING REGIMEN TO 5 DAYS FOR THE TREATMENT OF ACUTE EXACERBATION OF CHRONIC BRONCHITIS
D-70	80MG ONCE DAILY DOSING REGIMEN
D-71	EIGHT WEEK DOSING REGIMEN
D-72	INFORMATION REGARDING INCREASED RATE OF INFUSION FOR DEPACON
D-73	ONCE A WEEK DOSING FOR THE TREATMENT OF POSTMENOPAUSAL OSTEOPOROSIS
D-74	ONCE A WEEK DOSING FOR THE PREVENTION OF POSTMENOPAUSAL OSTEOPOROSIS
D-75	INTERMITTENT DOSING REGIMEN, STARTING DAILY DOSE 14 DAYS PRIOR TO THE ANTICIPATED ONSET OF MENSTRUATION THROUGH THE FIRST FULL DAY OF MENSES AND REPEATING WITH EACH NEW CYCLE
D-76	FOR USE ON AN "AS NEEDED" OR PRN BASIS FOR THE MANAGEMENT OF NASAL SYMPTOMS IN PATIENTS FOR WHOM THE DRUG IS INDICATED
D-77	ADDITION OF 20MG AND 40MG DAILY AS OPTIONAL STARTING DOSES WITH 40MG INTENDED FOR PATIENTS WHO REQUIRE A LARGE REDUCTION IN LDL-C (MORE THAN 45%)
D-78	USE OF FLEXERIL 5MG FOR THE RELIEF OF MUSCLE SPASM ASSOCIATED WITH ACUTE, PAINFUL, MUSCULOSKELETAL CONDITIONS
D-79	NEW LOWER STARTING DOSE FOR TREATMENT OF MODERATE TO SEVERE VASOMOTOR SYMPTOMS AND/OR MODERATE TO SEVERE SYMPTOMS OF VULVAR AND VAGINAL ATROPHY ASSOCIATED W/THE MENOPAUSE

EXCLUSIVITY TERMS
EXCLUSIVITY DOSING SCHEDULE (continued)

D-80   CHANGE OF DOSING SCHEDULE FOR LANTUS FROM ONCE DAILY AT BEDTIME TO FLEXIBLE DAILY DOSING
D-81   NEW LOWER STARTING DOES FOR THE PREVENTION OF POSTMENOPAUSAL OSTEOPORSIS

EXCLUSIVITY INDICATION

I-1   DYSMENORRHEA
I-2   CHOLANGIOPANCREATOGRAPHY
I-3   INTRAVENOUS DIGITAL SUBTRACTION ANGIOGRAPHY
I-4   PERIPHERAL VENOGRAPHY (PHLEBOGRAPHY)
I-5   HYSTEROSALPINGOGRAPHY
I-6   TREATMENT OF JUVENILE ARTHRITIS
I-7   BIOPSY PROVEN MINIMAL CHANGE NEPHROTIC SYNDROME IN CHILDREN
I-8   ADULT INTRAVENOUS CONTRAST-ENHANCED COMPUTED TOMOGRAPHY OF THE HEAD AND BODY
I-9   PREVENTION OF POSTOPERATIVE NAUSEA AND VOMITING
I-10   PREVENTION OF POSTOPERATIVE DEEP VENOUS THROMBOSIS AND PULMONARY EMBOLISM IN TOTAL
        HIP REPLACEMENT SURGERY
I-11   RELIEF OF MILD TO MODERATE PAIN
I-12   TREATMENT OF CUTANEOUS CANDIDIASIS
I-13   URINARY TRACT INFECTION (UTI) PREVENTION FOR PERIODS UP TO FIVE MONTHS IN WOMEN WITH A
        HISTORY OF RECURRENT UTI
I-14   SEBORRHEIC DERMATITIS
I-15   PHOTOPHERESIS IN THE PALLIATIVE TREATMENT OF SKIN MANIFESTATIONS OF CUTANEOUS T-CELL
        LYMPHOMA IN PERSONS NOT RESPONSIVE TO OTHER TREATMENT
I-16   STIMULATE THE DEVELOPMENT OF MULTIPLE FOLLICLES/OOCYTES IN OVULATORY PATIENTS PARTICI-
        PATING IN AN IN VITRO FERTILIZATION PROGRAM
I-17   MANAGEMENT OF CONGESTIVE HEART FAILURE
I-18   ENDOSCOPIC RETROGRADE PANCREATOGRAPHY
I-19   HERNIOGRAPHY
I-20   KNEE ARTHROGRAPHY
I-21   HIGH DOSE METHOTREXATE WITH LEUCOVORIN RESCUE IN COMBINATION WITH OTHER CHEMOTHERA-
        PEUTIC AGENTS TO DELAY RECURRENCE IN PATIENTS WITH NONMETASTATIC OSTEOSARCOMA WHO
        HAVE UNDERGONE SURGICAL RESECTION OR AMPUTATION FOR THE PRIMARY TUMOR
I-22   RESCUE AFTER HIGH-DOSE METHOTREXATE THERAPY IN OSTEOSARCOMA
I-23   SHORT-TERM TREATMENT OF ACTIVE BENIGN GASTRIC ULCER
I-24   TREATMENT OF RHEUMATOID ARTHRITIS
I-25   ADULT INTRA-ARTERIAL DIGITAL SUBTRACTION ANGIOGRAPHY OF THE HEAD, NECK, ABDOMINAL, RENAL
        AND PERIPHERAL VESSELS
I-26   TREATMENT OF LIVER FLUKES
I-27   ADJUNCTIVE THERAPY TO DIET TO REDUCE THE RISK OF CORONARY ARTERY DISEASE
I-28   SELECTIVE ADULT VISCERAL ARTERIOGRAPHY
I-29   METASTATIC BREAST CANCER IN PREMENOPAUSAL WOMEN AS AN ALTERNATIVE TO OOPHORECTOMY
        OR OVARIAN IRRADIATION
I-30   TREATMENT OF TINEA PEDIS
I-31   CONTRAST ENHANCEMENT AGENT TO FACILITATE VISUALIZATION OF LESIONS IN THE SPINE AND ASSO-
        CIATED TISSUES
I-32   PEDIATRIC MYELOGRAPHY
I-33   ORAL USE OF DILUTED OMNIPAQUE INJECTION IN ADULTS FOR CONTRAST ENHANCED COMPUTED TO-
        MOGRAPHY OF THE ABDOMEN
I-34   ORAL USE IN ADULTS FOR PASS-THROUGH EXAMINATION OF THE GASTROINTESTINAL TRACT
I-35   PEDIATRIC CONTRAST ENHANCEMENT OF COMPUTED TOMOGRAPHIC HEAD IMAGING
I-36   ARTHROGRAPHY OF THE SHOULDER JOINTS IN ADULTS
I-37   RADIOGRAPHY OF THE TEMPOROMANDIBULAR JOINT IN ADULTS
I-38   CONTRAST ENHANCEMENT AGENT TO FACILITATE VISUALIZATION OF LESIONS OF THE CENTRAL NER-
        VOUS SYSTEM IN CHILDREN (2 YEARS OF AGE AND OLDER)
I-39   TREATMENT OF ACUTE MYOCARDIAL INFARCTION
I-40   PRIMARY NOCTURNAL ENURESIS
I-41   MIGRAINE HEADACHE PROPHYLAXIS
I-42   HERPES ZOSTER
I-43   HERPES SIMPLEX ENCEPHALITIS
I-44   MAINTENANCE THERAPY IN HEALED DUODENAL ULCER PATIENTS AT DOSE OF 1 GRAM TWICE DAILY
I-45   ACUTE TREATMENT OF VARICELLA ZOSTER VIRUS
I-46   USE IN PEDIATRIC COMPUTED TOMOGRAPHIC HEAD AND BODY IMAGING
I-47   TREATMENT OF PEDIATRIC PATIENTS WITH SYMPTOMATIC HUMAN IMMUNODEFICIENCY VIRUS (HIV) DIS-
        EASE
I-48   PEDIATRIC ANGIOCARDIOGRAPHY

EXCLUSIVITY TERMS

EXCLUSIVITY INDICATION (continued)

I-49	TREATMENT OF TRAVELERS' DIARRHEA DUE TO SUSCEPTIBLE STRAINS OF ENTEROTOXIGENIC ESCHERICHIA COLI
I-50	FOR USE IN WOMEN WITH AXILLARY NODE-NEGATIVE BREAST CANCER
I-51	TREATMENT OF PRIMARY DYSMENORRHEA AND FOR THE TREATMENT OF IDIOPATHIC HEAVY MENSTRUAL BLOOD LOSS
I-52	PEDIATRIC EXCRETORY UROGRAPHY
I-53	TREATMENT OF PANIC DISORDER, WITH OR WITHOUT AGORAPHOBIA
I-54	RENAL CONCENTRATION CAPACITY TEST
I-55	HYPERTENSION
I-56	EROSIVE GASTROESOPHAGEAL REFLUX DISEASE
I-57	SHORT-TERM TREATMENT OF ACTIVE DUODENAL ULCER
I-58	INITIAL TREATMENT OF ADVANCED OVARIAN CARCINOMA IN COMBINATION WITH OTHER APPROVED CHEMOTHERAPEUTIC AGENTS
I-59	ENDOSCOPICALLY DIAGNOSED ESOPHAGITIS, INCLUDING EROSIVE AND ULCERATIVE ESOPHAGITIS, AND ASSOCIATED HEARTBURN DUE TO GASTROESOPHAGEAL REFLUX DISEASE
I-60	SINGLE APPLICATION TREATMENT OF HEAD LICE IN CHILDREN TWO MONTHS TO TWO YEARS IN AGE
I-61	FEMALE ANDROGENETIC ALOPECIA
I-62	PREVENTION AND TREATMENT OF POSTMENOPAUSAL OSTEOPOROSIS
I-63	ONCE DAILY TREATMENT AS INITIAL THERAPY IN THE TREATMENT OF HYPERTENSION
I-64	PREVENTION OF SUPRAVENTRICULAR TACHYCARDIAS
I-65	PREVENTION OF UPPER GASTROINTESTINAL BLEEDING IN CRITICALLY ILL PATIENTS
I-66	UNCOMPLICATED GONORRHEA
I-67	TREATMENT OF ACUTE ASTHMATIC ATTACKS IN CHILDREN SIX YEARS OF AGE AND OLDER
I-68	CENTRAL PRECOCIOUS PUBERTY
I-69	SHORT TERM TREATMENT OF PATIENTS WITH SYMPTOMS OF GASTROESOPHAGEAL REFLUX DISEASE (GERD), AND FOR THE SHORT TERM TREATMENT OF ESOPHAGITIS DUE TO GERD INCLUDING ULCERATIVE DISEASE DIAGNOSED BY ENDOSCOPY
I-70	USE IN COMBINATION WITH 5-FLUOROURACIL TO PROLONG SURVIVAL IN THE PALLIATIVE TREATMENT OF PATIENTS WITH ADVANCED COLORECTAL CANCER
I-71	VARICELLA INFECTIONS (CHICKENPOX)
I-72	PREVENTION OF CMV DISEASE IN TRANSPLANT PATIENTS AT RISK FOR CMV DISEASE
I-73	INITIATE AND MAINTAIN MONITORED ANESTHESIA CARE (MAC) SEDATION DURING DIAGNOSTIC PROCEDURES
I-74	INTRAVENOUS DIGITAL SUBTRACTION ANGIOGRAPHY
I-75	TREATMENT OF ENDOSCOPICALLY DIAGNOSED EROSIVE ESOPHAGITIS
I-76	PREVENTION OF OSTEOPOROSIS
I-77	DERMAL INFECTIONS-TINEA PEDIS, TINEA CORPORIS, TINEA CRURIS DUE TO EPIDERMOPHYTON FLOCCOSUM
I-78	CONTRAST ENHANCED COMPUTED TOMOGRAPHIC IMAGING OF THE HEAD AND BODY AND INTRAVENOUS EXCRETORY UROGRAPHY
I-79	MANAGEMENT OF CHRONIC STABLE ANGINA AND ANGINA DUE TO CORONARY ARTERY SPASM
I-80	DIAGNOSIS AND LOCALIZATION OF ISCHEMIA AND CORONARY HEART DISEASE
I-81	PROPHYLAXIS IN DESIGNATED IMMUNOCOMPROMISED CONDITIONS TO REDUCE THE INCIDENCE OF OROPHARYNGEAL CANDIDIASIS
I-82	TREATMENT OF TRAVELERS' DIARRHEA
I-83	ANGIOCARDIOGRAPHY, CONTRAST ENHANCED COMPUTED TOMOGRAPHIC IMAGING OF THE HEAD AND BODY, AND INTRAVENOUS EXCRETORY UROGRAPHY IN CHILDREN
I-84	INTRAOPERATIVE AND POSTOPERATIVE TACHYCARDIA AND/OR HYPERTENSION
I-85	TREATMENT OF ANOREXIA ASSOCIATED WITH WEIGHT LOSS IN PATIENTS WITH AIDS
I-86	TREATMENT OF SECONDARY CARNITINE DEFICIENCY
I-87	RENAL IMAGING AGENT FOR USE IN CHILDREN
I-88	MANAGEMENT OF ENDOMETRIOSIS
I-89	EPIDURAL USE IN LABOR AND DELIVERY AS AN ANALGESIC ADJUNCT TO BUPIVACAINE
I-90	INTENSIVE CARE UNIT SEDATION
I-91	MONOTHERAPY USE FOR HYPERTENSION
I-92	ADJUNCTIVE THERAPY IN THE MANAGEMENT OF HEART FAILURE
I-93	PREVENTION OF EXERCISE-INDUCED BRONCHOSPASM IN CHILDREN AGES 4-11 YEARS
I-94	USE WITH MRI IN ADULTS TO PROVIDE CONTRAST ENHANCEMENT AND FACILITATE VISUALIZATION OF LESIONS IN THE BODY [EXCLUDING THE HEART]
I-95	TREATMENT OF LEFT VENTRICULAR DYSFUNCTION FOLLOWING MYOCARDIAL INFARCTION
I-96	TREATMENT OF SYMPTOMATIC BENIGN PROSTATIC HYPERPLASIA
I-97	ORAL OR RECTAL USE IN CHILDREN FOR THE EXAMINATION OF THE GASTROINTESTINAL TRACT
I-98	TREATMENT OF CHILDREN WHO HAVE GROWTH FAILURE ASSOCIATED WITH CHRONIC RENAL INSUFFICIENCY
I-99	PEDIATRIC ANESTHESIA IN CHILDREN 3 YEARS AND OLDER
I-100	TO DECREASE THE INCIDENCE OF CANDIDIASIS IN PATIENTS UNDERGOING BONE MARROW TRANSPLANTATION WHO RECEIVE CYTOTOXIC CHEMOTHERAPY AND/OR RADIATION THERAPY

EXCLUSIVITY TERMS

EXCLUSIVITY INDICATION (continued)

I-101	TREATMENT OF DIABETIC NEPHROPATHY IN PATIENTS WITH TYPE I INSULIN-DEPENDENT DIABETES MELLITUS AND RETINOPATHY
I-102	TREATMENT OF OBSESSIVE-COMPULSIVE DISORDER
I-103	PROPHYLAXIS AGAINST PNEUMOCYSTIS CARINII PNEUMONIA IN INDIVIDUALS WHO ARE IMMUNOCOMPROMISED AND CONSIDERED TO BE AT RISK OF DEVELOPING PNEUMOCYSTIS CARINII PNEUMONIA
I-104	TREATMENT OF PULMONARY AND EXTRAPULMONARY ASPERGILLOSIS IN PATIENTS WHO ARE INTOLERANT OF OR WHO ARE REFRACTORY TO AMPHOTERICIN B THERAPY
I-105	TREATMENT OF METASTATIC CARCINOMA OF THE BREAST AFTER FAILURE OF FIRST-LINE OR SUBSEQUENT CHEMOTHERAPY
I-106	TREATMENT OF ACROMEGALY
I-107	VAGINAL CANDIDIASIS
I-108	EXPANDED USE-FOR ICU PATIENTS UNDERGOING LONG-TERM INFUSION DURING MECHANICAL VENTILATION
I-109	TYPHOID FEVER
I-110	PREVENTION OF NAUSEA AND VOMITING ASSOCIATED WITH RADIOTHERAPY
I-111	TREATMENT OF PAGET'S DISEASE OF BONE
I-112	MANAGEMENT OF MODERATE TO SEVERE PAIN
I-113	TREATMENT OF PROSTATITIS
I-114	USE IN CHILDREN TO VISUALIZE LESIONS WITH ABNORMAL VASCULARITY IN THE BRAIN (INTRACRANIAL LESIONS), SPINE AND ASSOCIATED TISSUE
I-115	USE IN MRI IN ADULTS TO VISUALIZE LESIONS IN THE HEAD AND NECK
I-116	MAINTENANCE OF HEALING OF EROSIVE ESOPHAGITIS
I-117	TO SLOW THE PROGRESSION OF CORONARY ATHEROSCLEROSIS IN PATIENTS WITH CORONARY HEART DISEASE
I-118	PREVENTION OF DEEP VEIN THROMBOSIS, WHICH MAY LEAD TO PULMONARY EMBOLISM, FOLLOWING KNEE REPLACEMENT SURGERY
I-119	TREATMENT OF ANEMIA CAUSED BY UTERINE LEIOMYOMATA IN WOMEN WHO FAIL IRON THERAPY
I-120	MAINTENANCE THERAPY FOR GASTRIC ULCER PATIENTS AT REDUCED DOSAGE AFTER HEALING ACUTE ULCERS
I-121	EXPANDED PATIENT POPULATION - USE IN ICU PATIENTS
I-122	PSORIASIS OF THE SCALP
I-123	RELIEF OF MILD TO MODERATE PAIN IN PATIENTS AGED 6 MONTHS AND OLDER
I-124	LEUCOCYTE LABELED SCINTIGRAPHY AS AN ADJUNCT IN THE LOCALIZATION OF INTRA-ABDOMINAL INFECTION AND INFLAMMATORY BOWEL DISEASE
I-125	EXPANSION OF CONSCIOUS SEDATION INDICATION TO INCLUDE SHORT THERAPEUTIC PROCEDURES
I-126	ADJUNCT TO THALLIUM-201 MYOCARDIAL PERFUSION IN PATIENTS UNABLE TO EXERCISE ADEQUATELY
I-127	TREATMENT OF ACYCLOVIR-RESISTANT HERPES IN IMMUNOCOMPROMISED PATIENTS
I-128	IN PATIENTS WITH CORONARY HEART DISEASE AND HYPERCHOLESTEROLEMIA: TO REDUCE THE RISK OF TOTAL MORTALITY BY REDUCING CORONARY DEATH; REDUCE THE RISK OF NON-FATAL MYOCARDIAL INFARCTION; REDUCE THE RISK FOR UNDERGOING MYOCARDIAL REVASCULARIZATION PROCEDURES; REDUCTION OF ELEVATED TOTAL AND LDL CHOLESTEROL LEVELS IN PATIENTS WITH PRIMARY HYPERCHOLESTEROLEMIA (TYPES IIA AND IIB)
I-129	TREATMENT OF ALCOHOL DEPENDENCE
I-130	MAINTENANCE OF HEALING OF EROSIVE ESOPHAGITIS
I-131	PERIPHERAL ARTERIOGRAPHY
I-132	TREATMENT OF MANIC PHASE OF BIPOLAR DISORDER
I-133	MANAGEMENT OF CHRONIC STABLE ANGINA
I-134	HEART FAILURE POST MYOCARDIAL INFARCTION
I-135	BONE METASTASES ASSOCIATED WITH MULTIPLE MYELOMA
I-136	IDIOPATHIC CHRONIC URTICARIA
I-137	PREVENTION OF MEAL-INDUCED HEARTBURN, ACID INDIGESTION, AND SOUR STOMACH WHEN TAKEN 30 MINUTES PRIOR TO CONSUMING FOOD OR BEVERAGES
I-138	TREATMENT OF ACUTE RECURRENT GENITAL HERPES
I-139	PALLIATIVE TREATMENT OF ADVANCED BREAST CANCER IN PRE- AND PERIMENOPAUSAL WOMEN
I-140	PREVENTION OF CYTOMEGALOVIRUS (CMV) DISEASE IN INDIVIDUALS WITH HIV INFECTION AT RISK FOR DEVELOPING CMV DISEASE
I-141	TREATMENT OF HEMODYNAMICALLY STABLE PATIENTS WITHIN 24 HOURS OF ACUTE MYOCARDIAL INFRACTION TO IMPROVE SURVIVAL
I-142	LOCALIZE MYOCARDIAL ISCHEMIA (REVERSIBLE DEFECT) AND INFARCTION (NON-REVERSIBLE DEFECTS) IN EVALUATING MYOCARDIAL FUNCTION
I-143	EPISODIC TREATMENT OF RECURRENT GENITAL HERPES IN IMMUNOCOMPETENT ADULTS
I-144	ENHANCEMENT OF MRI OF THE ADULT BODY INTERNAL ORGANS
I-145	0.1MMOL/KG AS A SINGLE INTRAVENOUS BOLUS FOR MRI OF THE CNS IN CHILDREN
I-146	CONTRAST ENHANCEMENT AND FACILITATION OF VISUALIZATION OF EXTRACRANIAL HEAD AND NECK LESIONS
I-147	PREVENTION OF GALLSTONE FORMATION IN OBESE PATIENTS EXPERIENCING RAPID WEIGHT LOSS
I-148	TREATMENT OF ACUTE PNEUMOCYSTIC CARINII PNEUMONIA (PCP) IN HIV-INFECTED PATIENTS WHOSE ALVEOLAR-ARTERIAL OXYGEN DIFFERENCE (AaDO$_2$) IS LESS THAN OR EQUAL TO 55 TORR

EXCLUSIVITY TERMS

EXCLUSIVITY INDICATION (continued)

I-149	TREATMENT OF PATIENTS WITH NON-SMALL CELL LUNG CANCER
I-150	TREATMENT OF OBSESSIVE COMPULSIVE DISORDER AND PANIC DISORDER
I-151	PREVENTION OF AND PREVENTION OF FURTHER POSTOPERATIVE NAUSEA AND VOMITING IN PEDIATRIC PATIENTS RECEIVING GENERAL ANESTHESIA
I-152	SLOWING THE PROGRESSION OF CORONARY ATHEROSCLEROSIS AND REDUCING THE RISK OF ACUTE CORONARY EVENTS
I-153	MANAGEMENT OF SEVERE SPASTICITY [ENCOMPASSES SPINAL AND CEREBRAL ORIGIN]
I-154	PATIENT POPULATION ALTERED TO INCLUDE PEDIATRIC USE
I-155	TREATMENT OF ONCHOMYCOSIS DUE TO DERMATOPHYTES (TINEA UNGUIUM) OF THE TOENAIL WITH OR WITHOUT FINGERNAIL INVOLVEMENT
I-156	ADDITIONAL DATA REGARDING THE SAFE USE OF NORVASC IN PATIENTS WITH HEART FAILURE
I-157	TREATMENT OF ACUTE UNCOMPLICATED CYSTITIS IN FEMALES
I-158	TREATMENT OF OSTEOLYTIC BONE METASTASES OF BREAST CANCER
I-159	FOR HYPERCHOLESTEROLEMIC PATIENTS WITHOUT CLINICALLY EVIDENT HEART DISEASE REDUCE THE RISK OF MYOCARDIAL INFARCTION, REVASCULARIZATION, AND DEATH DUE TO CARDIOVASCULAR CAUSES WITH NO INCREASE IN DEATH FROM NON-CARDIOVASCULAR CAUSES
I-160	TREATMENT OF BACTERIAL CORNEAL ULCERS
I-161	TREATMENT OF ADULT-ONSET OR CHILDHOOD-ONSET ADULT GROWTH HORMONE DEFICIENCY
I-162	FOR USE IN PATIENTS 6-11 YEARS OF AGE
I-163	TREATMENT OF PHOTOPHOBIA
I-164	CHRONIC BACTERIAL PROSTATITIS
I-165	MANAGEMENT OF ADULTS WITH ACTIVE, CLASSIC AND DEFINITIVE RHEUMATOID ARTHRITIS WHO HAVE HAD AN INSUFFICIENT THERAPEUTIC RESPONSE TO OR ARE INTOLERANT OF AN ADEQUATE TRIAL OF FULL DOSES OF ONE OR MORE NON-STEROIDAL ANTI-INFLAMMATORY DRUGS
I-166	TREATMENT OF BULIMIA
I-167	COMPLICATED INTRA-ABDOMINAL INFECTIONS (USED IN COMBINATION WITH METRONIDAZOLE) CAUSED BY MIXED AEROBIC/ANAEROBIC PATHOGENS
I-168	MANAGEMENT OF LOCALLY CONFINED STAGE B2-C METASTATIC CARCINOMA OF THE PROSTATE (IN COMBINATION WITH LHRH AGONISTS)
I-169	USE IN COMBINATION WITH CORTICOSTEROIDS AS INITIAL CHEMOTHERAPY FOR THE TREATMENT OF PATIENTS WITH PAIN RELATED TO ADVANCED HORMONE-REFRACTORY PROSTATE CANCER
I-170	PROPHYLACTIC USE DURING HEAD LICE EPIDEMICS
I-171	RELIEF OF SYMPTOMS OF THE COMMON COLD
I-172	TREATMENT OF INITIAL EPISODE OF GENITAL HERPES
I-173	PREOPERATIVELY FOR THE PREVENTION OF INFECTION IN TRANSRECTAL PROSTATE BIOPSY
I-174	PELVIC INFLAMMATORY DISEASE
I-175	TREATMENT OF TINEA CORPORIS AND TINEA CRURIS
I-176	TREATMENT OF POSTOPERATIVE INFLAMMATION IN PATIENTS WHO HAVE UNDERGONE CATARACT EX-TRACTION
I-177	TREATMENT OF MODERATE ACNE VULGARIS IN FEMALES, GREATER OR EQUAL TO 15 YEARS OF AGE, WHO HAVE NO KNOWN CONTRAINDICATIONS TO ORAL CONTRACEPTIVE THERAPY, DESIRE CONTRACEP-TION, HAVE ACHIEVED MENARCHE AND ARE UNRESPONSIVE TO TOPICAL ANTI-ACNE MEDICATIONS
I-178	TREATMENT OF ONCHOMYCOSIS OF THE FINGERNAIL WITHOUT CONCOMITANT ONCHOMYCOSIS OF THE TOENAIL WITH A PULSE DOSING REGIMEN
I-179	NOSOCOMIAL PNEUMONIA-MILD TO MODERATE AND SEVERE CAUSED BY HAEMOPHILUS INFLUENZAE OR KLEBSIELLA PNEUMONIAE
I-180	TREATMENT OF PLANTAR TINEA PEDIS (MOCCASIN TYPE)
I-181	TREATMENT OF PATIENTS WITH COMPLEX PARTIAL SEIZURES WITH AND WITHOUT SECONDARY GENER-ALIZATION
I-182	TREATMENT OF GROWTH FAILURE ASSOCIATED WITH TURNER SYNDROME
I-183	MAINTENANCE THERAPY IN THE MANAGEMENT OF MILD TO MODERATE ASTHMA IN PEDIATRIC PATIENTS AGES 6-11
I-184	TREATMENT OF PANIC DISORDER AT A RECOMMENDED DOSE RANGE OF 1 TO 2 MG/DAY (MAXIMUM OF 4MG)
I-185	PREVENTION OF OSTEOPOROSIS IN POSTMENOPAUSAL WOMEN
I-186	TREATMENT OF TINEA (PITYRIASIS) VERSICOLOR CAUSED BY OR PRESUMED TO BE CAUSED BY PITYR-OSPORUM ORBICULARE (ALSO KNOWN AS MALASSEZIA FURFUR OR M. ORBICULARE)
I-187	PREVENTION OF FRACTURES IN THE TREATMENT OF POSTMENOPAUSAL OSTEOPOROSIS
I-188	TREATMENT OF ACUTE SINUSITIS AND ACUTE EXACERBATION OF CHRONIC SINUSITIS
I-189	TREATMENT OF ACUTE OTITIS MEDIA IN PEDIATRIC PATIENTS
I-190	PLANAR IMAGING AS A SECOND LINE DIAGNOSTIC DRUG AFTER MAMMOGRAPHY TO ASSIST IN THE EVA-LUATION OF BREAST LESIONS IN PATIENTS WITH AN ABNORMAL MAMMOGRAM OR A PALPABLE BREAST MASS
I-191	ENDOMETRIAL THINNING AGENT PRIOR TO ENDOMETRIAL ABLATION FOR DYSFUNCTIONAL UTERINE BLEEDING
I-192	THE PREVENTION OF DEEP VEIN THROMBOSIS, WHICH MAY LEAD TO PULMONARY EMBOLISM, IN PA-TIENTS UNDERGOING ABDOMINAL SURGERY WHO ARE AT RISK FOR THROMBOEMBOLIC COMPLICA-TIONS AND A NEW DOSAGE REGIMEN, 40MG ONCE DAILY, FOR THIS INDICATION

EXCLUSIVITY TERMS

EXCLUSIVITY INDICATION (continued)

I-193	TREATMENT OF PANIC DISORDER IN A RECOMMENDED DOSE RANGE OF 50 TO 200MG/DAY
I-194	CONGESTIVE HEART FAILURE
I-195	USE OF LANSOPRAZOLE IN COMBINATION WITH CLARITHROMYCIN AND AMOXICILLIN FOR THE ERADICATION OF HELICOBACTER PYLORI IN PATIENTS WITH ACTIVE DUODENAL ULCER DISEASE OR A ONE-YEAR HISTORY OF DUODENAL ULCER
I-196	ACUTE TREATMENT OF ACTIVE BENIGN GASTRIC ULCER
I-197	MAINTENANCE OF HEALING OF DUODENAL ULCER
I-198	USE OF LANSOPRAZOLE IN COMBINATION WITH AMOXICILLIN FOR THE ERADICATION OF HELICOBACTER PYLORI IN PATIENTS WITH ACTIVE DUODENAL ULCER DISEASE OR A ONE-YEAR HISTORY OF A DUODENAL ULCER
I-199	MONOTHERAPY AND COMBINATION THERAPY WITH SULFONYLUREAS IN THE TREATMENT OF TYPE II DIABETES
I-200	TREATMENT OF TINEA (PITYRIASIS) VERSICOLOR
I-201	EMPIRICAL THERAPY FOR FEBRILE NEUTROPENIC PATIENTS
I-202	SECOND-LINE TREATMENT OF AIDS-RELATED KAPOSI'S SARCOMA
I-203	MAINTENANCE OF REMISSION OF ULCERATIVE COLITIS
I-204	USE IN PEDIATRIC PATIENTS BETWEEN THE AGES OF 6 AND 11 FOR THE TREATMENT OF THE NASAL SYMPTOMS OF SEASONAL AND PERENNIAL ALLERGIC RHINITIS
I-205	INITIAL ANTICONVULSANT TREATMENT OF STATUS EPILEPTICUS
I-206	TREATMENT OF EDEMA ASSOCIATED WITH CHRONIC RENAL FAILURE
I-207	FOR THE SUPPRESSION OF RECURRENT EPISODES OF GENITAL HERPES IN IMMUNOCOMPETENT ADULTS
I-208	TREATMENT OF OBSESSIVE COMPULSIVE DISORDER IN THE PEDIATRIC POPULATION
I-209	PAROXYSMAL SUPRAVENTRICULAR TACHYCARDIA (PSVT)
I-210	TO SLOW THE PROGRESSION OF CORONARY ATHEROSCLEROSIS IN PATIENTS WITH CORONARY HEART DISEASE AS PART OF A TREATENT STRATEGY TO LOWER TOTAL AND LDL CHOLESTEROL TO TARGET LEVELS
I-211	FOR USE IN THE PEDIATRIC POPULATION
I-212	TREATMENT OF SYMPTOMS OF DRY MOUTH IN PATIENTS WITH SJOGREN?S SYNDROME
I-213	TEMPORARY RELIEF OF PAIN AND PHOTOPHOBIA IN PATIENTS UNDERGOING CORNEAL REFRACTIVE SURGERY
I-214	TREATMENT OF OSTEOPOROSIS
I-215	PRE-PROCEDURAL APPLICATION TO ADULT MALE GENITAL SKIN PRIOR TO SITE-SPECIFIC SUBCUTANEOUS INFILTRATION WITH LIDOCAINE FOR THE REMOVAL OF GENITAL WARTS
I-216	FOR THE LONG-TERM TWICE-DAILY (MORNING AND EVENING) ADMINISTRATION IN THE MAINTENANCE TREATMENT OF BRONCHOSPASM ASSOCIATED WITH COPD, INCLUDING CHRONIC BRONCHITIS AND EMPHYSEMA
I-217	PREVENTION (DURING AND FOLLOWING HOSPITALIZATION) OF DEEP VEIN THROMBOSIS, WHICH MAY LEAD TO PULMONARY EMBOLISM, IN PATIENTS UNDERGOING HIP REPLACEMENT SURGERY
I-218	USE OF LIPITOR AS AN ADJUNCTIVE THERAPY TO DIET FOR THE TREATMENT OF PATIENTS WITH ELEVATED SERUM TRIGLYCERIDE LEVELS (FREDERICKSON TYPE IV)
I-219	USE OF LIPITOR BY PATIENTS WITH PRIMARY DYSBETALIPOPROTEINEMIA (FREDERICKSON TYPE III) WHO DO NOT RESPOND ADEQUATELY TO DIET
I-220	TREATMENT OF EPISODIC HEARTBURN, ACID INDIGESTION AND SOUR STOMACH
I-221	TREATMENT OF BENIGN PROSTATIC HYPERPLASIA (BPH) IN MEN WITH AN ENLARGED PROSTATE TO IMPROVE SYMPTOMS, REDUCE THE RISK OF ACUTE URINARY RETENTION AND REDUCE THE RISK OF THE NEED OF SURGERY
I-222	PREVENTION OF ISCHEMIC COMPLICATIONS OF UNSTABLE ANGINA AND NON-Q-WAVE MYOCARDIAL INFARCTION, WHEN CONCURRENTLY ADMINISTERED WITH ASPIRIN
I-223	USE IN THE SYMPTOMATIC RELIEF OF RHINORRHEA ASSOICATED WITH ALLERGIC AND NONALLERGIC PERENNIAL RHINITIS IN CHILDREN AGE 6-11 YEARS
I-224	FOR THE USE IN PEDIATRIC PATIENTS 4 TO 11 YEARS OF AGE FOR THE MANAGEMENT OF THE NASAL SYMPTOMS OF SEASONAL AND PERENNIAL ALLERGIC RHINITIS
I-225	USE IN PATIENTS WITH PREVIOUS MI AND NORMAL CHOLESTEROL LEVELS, TO REDUCE RISK OF RECURRENT MI, MYOCARDIAL REVASCULARIZATION, AND CEREBROVASCULAR DISEASE EVENTS
I-226	FIRST-LINE THERAPY FOR THE TREATMENT OF ADVANCED CARCINOMA OF THE OVARY IN COMBINATION WITH CISPLATIN
I-227	SHORT-TERM TREATMENT OF SYMPTOMATIC GASTROESOPHAGEAL REFLUX DISEASE (GERD)
I-228	PREVENTION OF MEAL INDUCED HEARTBURN AT A DOSE OF 75MG TAKEN 30-60 MIN PRIOR TO A MEAL
I-229	PRILOSEC (OMEPRAZOLE), AMOXICILLIN AND CLARITHROMYCIN FOR THE ERADICATION OF H. PYLORI IN PATIENTS WITH DUODENAL ULCER DISEASE
I-230	IN COMBINATION WITH CISPLATIN, FOR THE FIRST-LINE TREATMENT OF NON-SMALL CELL LUNG CANCER IN PATIENTS WHO ARE NOT CANDIDATES FOR POTENTIALLY CURATIVE SURGERY AND/OR RADIATION
I-231	TREATMENT OF PATIENTS WITH LOCALLY ADVANCED OR METASTATIC BREAST CANCER AFTER FAILURE OF PRIOR CHEMOTHERAPY
I-232	TREATMENT OF RECURRENT MUCOCUTANEOUS HERPES SIMPLEX INFECTIONS IN HIV-AFFECTED PATIENTS AT A DOSE OF 500MG TWICE DAILY

EXCLUSIVITY TERMS

EXCLUSIVITY INDICATION (continued)

I-233	PROPHYLACTIC USE TO REDUCE PERIOPERATIVE BLOOD LOSS AND THE NEED FOR BLOOD TRANSFUSION IN PATIENTS UNDERGOING CARDIOPULMONARY BYPASS IN THE COURSE OF CORONARY ARTERY BYPASS GRAFT SURGERY
I-234	FOR USE IN COMBINATION WITH CISPLATIN FOR THE FIRST-LINE TREATMENT OF PATIENTS WITH INOPERABLE LOCALLY ADVANCED (STAGE IIIA OR IIIB) OR METASTATIC (STAGE IV) NON-SMALL CELL LUNG CANCER
I-235	PREVENTION OF EXERCISE-INDUCED BRONCHOSPASM IN PATIENTS 12 YEARS OF AGE AND OLDER
I-236	PREVENTION OF EXERCISE-INDUCED BRONCHOSPASM IN PATIENTS 4 YEARS OF AGE AND OLDER
I-237	MAINTENANCE TREATMENT OF ASTHMA AND PREVENTION OF BRONCHOSPASM IN PATIENTS 4 YEARS OF AGE AND OLDER
I-238	ADJUNCTIVE TREATMENT OF LENNOX-GASTAUT SYNDROME IN PEDIATRIC AND ADULT PATIENTS
I-239	TREATMENT OF PATIENTS WITH HOMOZYGOUS FAMILIAL HYPERCHOLESTEROLEMIA
I-240	MANAGEMENT OF SECONDARY HYPERPARATHYROIDISM AND RESULTANT METABOLIC BONE DISEASE IN PATIENTS WITH MODERATE TO SEVERE CHRONIC RENAL FAILURE (Ccr 15 TO 55ML MIN) NOT YET ON DIALYSIS
I-241	USE IN PHOTODYNAMIC THERAPY (PDT) FOR REDUCTION OF OBSTRUCTION AND PALLIATION OF SYMPTOMS IN PATIENTS WITH COMPLETELY OR PARTIALLY OBSTRUCTING ENDOBRONCHIAL NONSMALL CELL LUNG CANCER
I-242	TREATMENT OF MODERATE TO SEVERE VASOMOTOR SYMPTOMS ASSOCIATED WITH THE MENOPAUSE AND IN THE TREATMENT OF VULVAR AND VAGINAL ATROPHY IN WOMEN WITH AN INTACT UTERUS
I-243	USE IN THE SYMPTOMATIC RELIEF OF RHINORRHEA ASSOCIATED WITH THE COMMON COLD IN CHILDREN AGE 5 TO 11 YEARS
I-244	REDUCE THE INCIDENCE OF BREAST CANCER IN WOMEN AT HIGH RISK FOR BREAST CANCER
I-245	TREATMENT OF ACUTE SINUSITIS
I-246	TREATMENT OF UNCOMPLICATED URINARY TRACT INFECTIONS
I-247	USE IN CONVERSION TO MONOTHERAPY IN ADULTS WITH PARTIAL SEIZURES WHO ARE RECEIVING TREATMENT WITH A SINGLE ENZYME-INDUCING ANTIEPILEPTIC DRUG
I-248	INPATIENT TREATMENT OF ACUTE DEEP VEIN THROMBOSIS WITH/WITHOUT PULMONARY EMBOLISM WHEN ADMIN IN CONJUNCTION WITH WARFARIN SODIUM AND OUTPATIENT TREATMENT OF ACUTE DEEP VEIN THROMBOSIS WITHOUT PULMONARY EMBOLISM WHEN ADMINISTERED IN CONJUNCITON WITH WARFARIN SODIUM
I-249	TREATMENT OF CHRONIC HEPATITIS C IN PATIENTS WITH COMPENSATED LIVER DISEASE PREVIOUSLY UNTREATED WITH ALPHA INTERFERON THERAPY
I-250	PRIMARY PREVENTION OF CORONARY HEART DISEASE IN PATIENTS WITHOUT SYMPTOMATIC CARDIOVASCULAR DISEASE WHO HAVE AVERAGE TO MODERATELY ELEVATED TOTAL-C AND LDL-C AND BELOW AVERAGE HDL-C
I-251	TREATMENT OF GENERALIZED ANXIETY DISORDER
I-252	NEW COMBINATION USE OF PRECOSE FOR PATIENTS WITH TYPE 2 DIABETES TREATED WITH DIET PLUS METFORMIN
I-253	COMBINATION USE OF PRECOSE FOR PATIENTS WITH TYPE 2 DIABETES TREATED WITH DIET PLUS INSULIN
I-254	PREVENTION OF POSTMENOPAUSAL OSTEOPOROSIS (LOSS OF BONE MASS)
I-255	PREVENTION OF PNEUMOCYSTIS CARINII PNEUMONIA (PCP)
I-256	USE IN TREATMENT OF SMALL CELL LUNG CANCER SENSITIVE DISEASE AFTER FAILURE OF FIRST-LINE CHEMOTHERAPY
I-257	TREATMENT OF CHRONIC HEPATITIS B ASSOCIATED WITH EVIDENCE OF HEPATITIS B VIRAL REPLICATION AND ACTIVE LIVER INFLAMMATION
I-258	FOR PERENNIAL NONALLERGIC RHINITIS FOR AGES FOUR AND ABOVE
I-259	PROPHYLAXIS OF DEEP VEIN THROMBOSIS (DVT), WHICH MAY LEAD TO PULMONARY EMBOLISM, IN PATIENTS UNDERGOING HIP REPLACEMENT SURGERY
I-260	EXPANDED PEDIATRIC USE IN CHILDREN YOUNGER THAN ONE MONTH OF AGE TO BIRTH (WITH A GESTATIONAL AGE OF 37 WEEKS OR GREATER)
I-261	TREATMENT OF SOCIAL ANXIETY DISORDER
I-262	TREATMENT OR PREVENTION OF BRONCHOSPASM WITH REVERSIBLE OBSTRUCTIVE AIRWAY DISEASE AND FOR THE PREVENTION OF EXERCISE INDUCED BRONCHOSPASM IN CHILDREN AGES 4-12
I-263	TREATMENT OF UNSTABLE ANGINA AND NON-Q-WAVE MYOCARDIAL INFARCTION FOR THE PREVENTION OF ISCHEMIC COMPLICATIONS IN PATIENTS ON CONCURRENT ASPIRIN THERAPY
I-264	PREVENTION OF NAUSEA AND VOMITING ASSOCIATED WITH RADIATION, INCLUDING TOTAL BODY IRRADIATION (TBI) AND FRACTIONATED ABDOMINAL RADIATION
I-265	TREATMENT OF ATOPIC DERMATITIS IN PEDIATRIC PATIENTS 6 YEARS AND OLDER
I-266	USE OF TOPAMAX AS ADJUNCTIVE THERAPY IN PEDIATRIC PATIENTS AGES 2-16 YEARS WITH PARTIAL ONSET SEIZURES
I-267	USE IN PEDIATRIC PATIENTS 3 MONTHS OLD AND OLDER-FOR CORTICOSTEROID-RESPONSIVE DERMATOSES
I-268	PROPHYLAXIS AND CHRONIC TREATMENT OF ASTHMA IN PATIENTS 7-11 YEARS OF AGE
I-269	PREVENTION OF NAUSEA AND VOMITING ASSOCIATED WITH HIGHLY EMETOGENIC CANCER CHEMOTHERAPY, INCLUDING CISPLATIN

EXCLUSIVITY TERMS
EXCLUSIVITY INDICATION (continued)

I-270   ADJUVANT TREATMENT OF NODE-POSITIVE BREAST CANCER ADMINISTERED SEQUENTIALLY TO STAN-
         DARD DOXORUBICIN-CONTAINING COMBINATION CHEMOTHERAPY

I-271   TREATMENT OF OSTEOPOROSIS IN POSTMENOPAUSAL WOMEN

I-272   TREATMENT OF GLUCOCORTICOID-INDUCED OSTEOPOROSIS IN MEN AND WOMEN RECEIVING GLUCO-
         CORTICOIDS IN A DAILY DOSE EQUIVALENT TO 7.5MG OR GREATER OF PREDNISONE AND WHO HAVE
         LOW BONE MINERAL DENSITY

I-273   ADJUNCT TO DIET TO INCREASE HDL-C IN PATIENTS WITH PRIMARY HYPERCHOLESTEROLEMIA (HETERO-
         ZYGOUS FAMILIAL AND NONFAMILIAL) AND MIXED DYSLIPIDEMIA (FREDERICKSON TYPES IIA AND IIB)

I-274   USE OF TOPAMAX AS ADJUNCTIVE THERAPY IN THE TREATMENT OF PRIMARY GENERALIZED TONIC-CLO-
         NIC SEIZURES

I-275   USE IN COMBINATION WITH METFORMIN AND SULFONYLUREAS IN PATIENTS WITH TYPE 2 DIABETES

I-276   USE OF REZULIN IN COMBINATION WITH METFORMIN AND SULFONYLUREAS IN PATIENTS WITH TYPE 2
         DIABETES

I-277   TREATMENT OF TYPE III HYPERLIPOPROTEINEMIA

I-278   TREATMENT OF PATIENTS WITH ISOLATED HYPERTRIGLYCERIDEMIA (FREDERICKSON TYPE IV)

I-279   TREATMENT OF POST-TRAUMATIC STRESS DISORDER

I-280   USE OF CARNITOR INJECTION FOR THE PREVENTION AND TREATMENT OF CARNITINE DEFICIENCY IN PA-
         TIENTS WITH END STAGE RENAL DISEASE WHO ARE UNDERGOING DIALYSIS

I-281   INCREASING HDL-C IN PATIENTS WITH PRIMARY HYPERCHOLESTEROLEMIA (HETEROZYGOUS FAMILIAL
         AND NON-FAMILIAL) AND MIXED DYSLIPIDEMIA (FREDERICKSON TYPES IIa and IIb)

I-282   TREATMENT OF PATIENTS WITH LOCALLY ADVANCED OR METASTATIC NON-SMALL CELL LUNG CANCER
         AFTER FAILURE OF PRIOR PLATINUM-BASED CHEMOTHERAPY

I-283   TO REDUCE THE INCIDENCE OF MODERATE TO SEVERE XEROSTOMIA IN PATIENTS UNDERGOING POST-
         OPERATIVE RADIATION TREATMENT FOR HEAD AND NECK CANCER, WHERE THE RADIATION PORT IN-
         CLUDES A SUBSTANTIAL PORTION OF THE PAROTID GLANDS

I-284   TO REDUCE THE NUMBER OF ADENOMATOUS COLORECTAL POLYPS IN FAMILIAL ADENOMATOUS POLY-
         POSIS PATIENTS AS AN ADJUNCT TO USUAL CARE

I-285   TREATMENT OF NASAL SYMPTOMS OF SEASONAL AND PERENNIAL RHINITIS IN ADULTS AND CHILDREN 3
         YEARS OF AGE AND OLDER

I-286   TREATMENT OF PATIENTS WITH FREDERICKSON TYPE III

I-287   USE OF PRAVASTATIN IN PATIENTS WITH EVIDENT CORONARY HEART DISEASE TO REDUCE THE RISK OF
         TOTAL MORTALITY BY REDUCING CORONARY DEATH

I-288   CHANGES SEVERAL SECTIONS OF THE PACKAGE INSERT TO INCORPORATE STATEMENTS CONCERNING
         THE USE OF HIGH DOSES OF LISINOPRIL TO REDUCE THE RISK OF THE COMBINED OUTCOMES OF MOR-
         TALITY AND HOSPITALIZATION IN PATIENTS WITH CONGESTIVE HEART FAILURE

I-289   USE OF AVANDIA IN COMBINATION WITH A SULFONYLUREA IN PATIENTS WITH TYPE 2 DIABETES MELLLI-
         TUS WHEN DIET AND EXERCISE WITH EITHER SINGLE AGENT DOES NOT ACHIEVE ADEQUATE GLYCEMIC
         CONTROL

I-290   TREATMENT OF CORTICOSTEOID-INDUCED OSTEOPOROSIS

I-291   PREVENTION OF POSTMENOPAUSAL OSTEOPOROSIS

I-292   TREATMENT OF POSTMENOPAUSAL OSTEOPOROSIS

I-293   TREATMENT OF CORTICOSTEOID-INDUCED OSTEOPOROSIS

I-294   TREATMENT OF UNCOMPLICATED ACUTE ILLNESS DUE TO INFLUENZA A AND B IN PEDIATRIC PATIENTS 7
         YEARS AND OLDER WHO HAVE BEEN SYMPTOMATIC FOR NO MORE THAN 2 DAYS

I-295   PREVENTION OF POSTMENOPAUSAL OSTEOPOROSIS FOR WOMEN WITH AN INTACT UTERUS

I-296   LONG-TERM INTRAVENOUS TREATMENT OF PULMONARY HYPERTENSION ASSOCIATED WITH THE
         SCLERODERMA SPECTRUM OF DISEASE IN NYHA CLASS III AND CLASS IV PATIENTS WHO DO NOT RE-
         SPOND TO CONVENTIONAL THERAPY

I-297   SHORT-TERM TREATMENT OF ACUTE MANIC EPISODES ASSOCIATED WITH BIPOLAR I DISORDER

I-298   TREATMENT OF PATIENTS WITH FREDERICKSON TYPE IIA AND IIB HYPERLIPOPROTEINEMIA

I-299   USE OF CAMPTOSAR AS A COMPONENT OF FIRST-LINE THERAPY IN COMBINATION WITH 5-FLUROURACIL
         AND LEUCOVARIN FOR PATIENTS WITH METASTATIC CARCINOMA OF THE COLON OR RECTUM

I-300   PROPHYLAXIS FOR ASTHMA IN CHILDREN 2-5 YEARS OF AGE

I-301   TREATMENT OF SIGNS AND SYMPTOMS OF ALLERGIC CONJUNCTIVITIS

I-302   TREATMENT OF PEDIATRIC PATIENTS WITH PRADER-WILLI SYNDROME

I-303   INCREASING HDL-CHOLESTEROL IN PATIENTS WITH PRIMARY HYPERCHOLESTEROLEMIA AND MIXED
         DYSLIPIDEMIAS

I-304   TREATMENT OF PATIENTS WITH FREDERICKSON TYPE IV

I-305   TREATMENT OF LEVOFLOXACIN SUSCEPTIBLE STRAINS OF PENICILLIN-RESISTANT STREPTOCOCCUS
         PNEUMONIAE IN PATIENTS WITH COMMUNITY ACQUIRED PNEUMONIA

I-306   INDUCTION OF SPERMATOGENESIS IN MEN WITH PRIMARY AND SECONDARY HYPOGONADOTROPIC HY-
         POGONADISM IN WHOM THE CAUSE OF INFERTILITY IS NOT DUE TO PRIMARY TESTICULAR FAILURE

I-307   NEW COMBINATION USE OF METFORMIN AND INSULIN IN TYPE 2 DIABETES

I-308   TREATMENT OF PEDIATRIC PATIENTS WITH POLYARTICULAR COURSE JUVENILE RHEUMOTOID ARTHRI-
         TIS WHO RESPONDED INADEQUATELY TO SALICYLATES OR OTHER NSAIDS

I-309   INCREASE BONE MASS IN MEN WITH OSTEOPOROSIS

I-310   REDUCTION IN RISK OF MYOCARDIAL INFARCTION, STROKE, AND DEATH FROM CARDIOVASCULAR
         CAUSES

EXCLUSIVITY TERMS

EXCLUSIVITY INDICATION (continued)

I-311	ADJUNCTIVE THERAPY IN THE TREATMENT OF PARTIAL SEIZURES IN PEDIATRIC PATIENTS AGE 3 TO 12 YEARS
I-312	FIRST LINE TREATMENT OF POSTMENOPAUSAL WOMEN WITH HORMONE RECEPTOR POSITIVE OR HORMONE RECEPTOR UNKNOWN LOCALLY ADVANCED OR METASTATIC BREAST CANCER
I-313	EXTENSION OF INDICATION TO PROVIDE FOR MAINTENANCE OF RESPONSE
I-314	TOPICAL ANESTHETIC FOR SUPERFICIAL MINOR SURGERY OF GENITAL MUCOUS MEMBRANES AND AS AN ADJUNCT FOR LOCAL INFILTRATION ANESTHESIA IN GENITAL MUCOUS MEMBRANES
I-315	THROMBOPROPHYLAXIS OF DEEP VEIN THROMBOSIS, WHICH MAY LEAD TO PULMONARY EMBOLISM, IN MEDICAL PATIENTS WHO ARE AT RISK FOR THROMBOEMBOLIC COMPLICATIONS DUE TO SEVERELY RESTRICTED MOBILITY DURING ACUTE ILLNESS
I-316	TREATMENT OF NSAID-ASSOCIATED GASTRIC ULCER PATIENTS WHO CONTINUE NSAID USE AND REDUCING RISK OF NSAID-ASSOCIATED GASTRIC ULCERS IN PATIENTS WITH HISTORY OF DOCUMENTED GASTRIC ULCER WHO REQUIRE USE OF AN NSAID
I-317	PROPHYLAXIS OF INFLUENZA IN ADULTS AND ADOLESCENTS 13 YEARS AND OLDER
I-318	FIRSTLINE TREATMENT OF POSTMENOPAUSAL WOMEN WITH HORMONE RECEPTOR POSITIVE OR HORMONE RECEPTOR UNKNOWN LOCALLY ADVANCED OR METASTATIC BREAST CANCER
I-319	USE FOR SUSPECTED OR CONFIRMED METHANOL POISONING, EITHER ALONE OR IN COMBINATION WITH HEMODIALYSIS
I-320	TREATMENT OF TYPE 2 DIABETES IN PEDIATRIC PATIENTS (AGES 10-16 YEARS)
I-321	JUVENILE RHEUMATOID ARTHRITIS
I-322	USE OF DIPRIVAN IN PATIENTS 3 MONTHS TO 16 YEARS
I-323	COLORECTAL CANCER
I-324	REDUCING NEUROLOGIC DISABILITY AND/OR FREQUENCY OF CLINICAL RELAPSES IN PATIENTS WITH SECONDARY (CHRONIC) PROGRESSIVE, PROGRESSIVE RELAPSING, OR WORSENING RELAPSING-REMITTING MULTIPLE SCLEROSIS
I-325	PREVENTION OF RELAPSE AND RECURRENCE OF DEPRESSION
I-326	GENERALIZED ANXIETY DISORDER
I-327	SYMPTOMATIC RELIEF OF RHINOORRHEA ASSOCIATED WITH SEASONAL ALLERGIC RHINITIS IN PATIENTS 5 YEARS AND OLDER
I-328	PROPHYLAXIS AND CHRONIC TREATMENT OF ASTHMA IN PATIENTS 5-6 YEARS OF AGE
I-329	UNCOMPLICATED SKIN AND SKIN STRUCTURE INFECTIONS
I-330	MAINTENANCE OF HEALING OF EROSIVE ESOPHAGITIS AND CONTROL OF DAYTIME AND NIGHTTIME HEARTBURN SYSTOMS IN PATIENTS WITH GERD
I-331	TREATMENT OF MODERATE ACNE VULGARIS
I-332	EMPIRIC THERAPY IN FEBRILE NEUTROPENIC PATIENTS WITH SUSPECTED FUNGAL INFECTIONS (ETFN)
I-333	TOPICAL TREATMENT OF TINEA (PITYRIASIS) VERSICOLOR DUE TO MALASSEZIA FURFUR (FORMERLY PITYROSPORUM ORBICULARE)
I-334	LONG-TERM TREATMENT OF GROWTH FAILURE IN CHILDREN BORN SMALL FOR GESTATIONAL AGE WHO FAIL TO MANIFEST CATCH-UP GROWTH BY TWO YEARS OF AGE
I-335	ADJUNCTIVE THERAPY IN PATIENTS TWO YEARS AND OLDER WITH SEIZURES ASSOCIATED WITH LENNOX-GASTAUT SYNDROME
I-336	EXPANSION OF INDICATION TO INCLUDE THE TREATMENT OF PATIENTS WITH PREDOMINATELY CLASSIC SUBFOVEAL CHOROIDAL NEOVASCULARIZATION DUE TO PATHOLOGIC MYOPIA OR PRESUMED OCULAR HISTOPLASMOSIS
I-337	PATHOLOGICAL HYPERSECRETION ASSOCIATED WITH ZOLLINGER-ELLISON SNYDROME
I-338	MANAGEMENT OF ACUTE PAIN IN ADULTS AND TREATMENT OF PRIMARY DYSMENORRHEA
I-339	TREATMENT OF HEPATITIS B IN PEDIATRIC PATIENTS AGES 2-17 YEARS
I-340	ATOPIC DERMATITIS IN PEDIATRIC PATIENTS AGES 2-5
I-341	BREAST CANCER COMBINATION THERAPY
I-342	USE OF FORADIL FOR LONG-TERM, TWICE DAILY (MORNING AND EVENING) ADMINISTRATION IN THE MAINTENANCE TREATMENT OF BRONCHO-CONSTRICTION IN PATIENTS WITH COPD INCLUDING CHRONIC BRONCHITIS AND EMPHYSEMA
I-343	USE OF COREG FOR SEVERE HEART FAILURE
I-344	ACNE VULGARIS
I-345	TREATMENT OF POSTTRAUMATIC STRESS DISORDER
I-346	TREATMENT OF SYMPTOMATIC GASTRO ESOPHAGEAL REFLUX DISEASE (GERD)
I-347	TREATMENT OR PREVENTION OF BRONCHOSPASM IN CHILDREN 6 YEARS OF AGE AND OLDER WITH OBSTRUCTIVE AIRWAY DISEASE
I-348	LONG-TERM, TWICE-DAILY (MORNING AND EVENING) ADMINISTRATION IN THE MAINTENANCE TREATMENT OF BRONCHOSPASM ASSOCIATED WITH COPD (INCLUDING EMPHYSEMA AND CHRONIC BRONCHITIS)
I-349	ACUTE CORONARY SYNDROME
I-350	TREATMENT OF HETEROZYGOUS FAMILIAL HYPERCHOLESTEROLEMIA IN ADOLESCENT BOYS AND GIRLS AT LEAST ONE YEAR POSTMENARCHAL, AGES 10 TO 17 YEARS, WITH A RECOMMENDED DOSING RANGE OF 10 TO 40MG ONCE DAILY
I-351	PREVENTION OF POSTMENOPAUSAL OSTEOPOROSIS FOR ALL STRENGTHS
I-352	ANTICOAGULANT IN PATIENTS WITH OR AT RISK FOR HEPARIN-INDUCED THROMBOCYTOPENIA UNDERGOING PERCUTANEOUS CORONARY INTERVENTIONS (PCI)

EXCLUSIVITY TERMS
EXCLUSIVITY INDICATION (continued)

I-353	TREATMENT OF SIGNS AND SYMPTOMS OF RHEUMATOID ARTHRITIS
I-354	MANAGEMENT OF POST HERPETIC NEURALGIA
I-355	PREMENSTRUAL DYSPHORIC DISORDER
I-356	TREATMENT OF PATHOLOGICAL HYPERSECRETORY CONDITIONS, INCLUDING ZOLLINGER-ELLISON SYNDROME
I-357	TREATMENT OF COMPLICATED SKIN AND SKIN STRUCTURE INFECTIONS
I-358	TREATMENT OF PANIC DISORDER
I-359	TREATMENT OF VULVAR AND VAGINAL ATROPHY ASSOCIATED WITH THE MENOPAUSE
I-360	TREATMENT OF NASAL SYMPTOMS OF SEASONAL AND PERENNIAL RHINITIS IN CHILDREN AGES TWO UP TO AGE THREE
I-361	TREATMENT OF MULTIPLE MYELOMA AND DOCUMENTED BONE METASTASES FROM SOLID TUMORS, IN CONJUNCTION WITH STANDARD ANTINEOPLASTIC THERAPY. PROSTATE CANCER SHOULD HAVE PROGRESSED AFTER TREATMENT WITH AT LEAST ONE HORMONAL THERAPY
I-362	TREATMENT OF PANIC DISORDER, WITH OR WITHOUT AGORAPHOBIA
I-363	ADJUVANT TREATMENT OF POST MENOPAUSAL WOMEN WITH HORMONE RECEPTOR POSITIVE EARLY BREAST CANCER
I-364	TREATMENT OF COMMUNITY-ACQUIRED PNEUMONIA IN ADULTS
I-365	TREATMENT OF HEART FAILURE (NYHA CLASS II-IV) IN PATIENTS WHO ARE INTOLERANT TO AN ACE INHIBITOR
I-366	PREVENTION OF RELAPSE FOLLOWING LONG-TERM TREATMENT OF MAJOR DEPRESSIVE DISORDER
I-367	COMBINATION THERAPY WITH THIAZOLIDINEDIONE TO LOWER BLOOD GLUCOSE IN PTS WHOSE HYPERGLYCEMIA CANNOT BE CONTROLLED BY DIET/EXERCISE PLUS MONOTHERAPY WITH ANY OF THE FOLLOWING AGENTS:METFORMIN,SULFONYLUREAS,REPAGLINIDE,OR THIAZOLIDINEDIONES
I-368	USE OF GLUCOVANCE WITH A THIAZOLIDINEDIONE WHEN GLYCEMIC CONTROL IS NOT OBTAINED WITH GLUCOVANCE ALONE
I-369	PREVENTION AND TREATMENT OF POSTOPERATIVE NAUSEA AND VOMITING
I-370	TREATMENT OF HETEROZYGOUS FAMILIAL HYPERCHOLESTEROLEMIA IN CHILDREN, AGES 8-13 YEARS, WITH RECOMMENDED DOSE OF 20MG ONCE DAILY AND IN ADOLESCENTS, AGES 14-18 WITH A RECOMMENDED DOSE OF 40ONCE DAILY MG
I-371	HELICOBACTER PYLORI ERADICATION TO REDUCE THE RISK OF DUODENAL ULCER RECURRENCE
I-372	NOSOCOMIAL PNEUMONIA
I-373	TREATMENT OF TYPE 2 DIABETIC NEPHROPATHY
I-374	SHORT TERM TOPICAL TREATMENT OF MILD TO MODERATE PLAQUE-TYPE PSORIASIS OF NON SCALP REGIONS
I-375	FIRST LINE THERAPY FOR THE REDUCTION OF INTRAOCULAR PRESSURE IN PATIENTS WITH OPEN-ANGLE GLAUCOMA OR OCULAR HYPERTENSION
I-376	TREATMENT OF NEWLY DIAGNOSED ADULT PATIENTS WITH PHILADELPHIA CHROMOSOME POSITIVE CHRONIC MYELOID LEUKEMIA (CML)
1-377	USE OF BRAVELLE FOR MULTIPLE FOLLICULAR DEVELOPMENT (CONTROLLED OVARIAN STIMULATION) DURING ASSISTED REPRODUCTIVE TECHNOLOGY CYCLES IN PATIENTS WHO HAVE PREVIOUSLY RECEIVED PITUITARY SUPPRESSION
I-378	RELIEF OF SYMPTOMS OF SEASONAL ALLERGIC RHINITIS IN ADULTS AND PEDIATRIC PATIENTS 2 YEARS OF AGE AND OLDER
I-379	USE TAXOTERE IN COMBINATION WITH CISPLATIN FOR THE TREATMENT OF PATIENTS WITH UNRESECTABLE, LOCALLY ADVANCED OR METASTATIC NON-SMALL CELL LUNG CANCER WHO HAVE NOT PREVIOUSLY RECEIVED CHEMOTHERAPY FOR THIS CONDITION
I-380	TO TREAT PATIENTS WITH SCHIZOPHRENIA OR SCHIZOAFFECTIVE DISORDER AT RISK FOR EMERGENT SUICIDAL BEHAVIOR
I-381	TREATMENT OF COLD SORES (HERPES LABIALIS) IN ADULT AND ADOLESCENT PATIENTS 12 YEARS OF AGE AND OLDER
I-382	FOR NEWLY-DIAGNOSED HIGH GRADE MALIGNANT GLIOMA PATIENTS AS AN ADJUNCT TO SURGERY AND RADIATION
I-383	TREATMENT OF TYPE 2 DIABETIC NEPHROPATHY
I-384	USE IN COMBINATION WITH INSULIN FOR THE TREATMENT OF PATIENTS WITH TYPE 2 DIABETES
I-385	MODIFICATION OF THE INDICATION FOR COMMUNITY ACQUIRED PNEUMONIA TO ADD "INCLUDING PENICILLIN-RESISTANT STRAINS, MIC PENICILLIN>=2MCG/ML TO STREPTOCOCCUS PNEUMONIAE
I-386	RAPAMUNE (SIROLIMUS) WITHIN AN IMMUNOSUPPRESSIVE REGIMEN THAT WOULD ALLOW FOR THE WITHDRAWAL OF CYCLOSPORINE 2 TO 4 MONTHS AFTER RENAL TRANSPLANTATION IN PATIENTS CONSIDERED AT LOW TO MODERATE IMMUNOLOGIC RISK FOR RENAL TRANSPLANT REJECTION
I-387	ADJUNCTIVE THERAPY OF PARTIAL SEIZURES IN PEDIATRIC PATIENTS GREATER THAT OR EQUAL TO 2 YEARS OF AGE
I-388	TREATMENT OF PATIENTS WITH LEFT VENTRICULAR DYSFUNCTION FOLLOWING MYOCARDIAL INFARCTION
I-389	SUPPRESSION OF RECURRENT GENITAL HERPES IN HIV-INFECTED INDIVIDUALS
I-390	USE IN PTS AT HIGH RISK CORONARY EVENTS DUE TO EXISTING CORONARY HEART DISEASE, DIABETES, PERIPHERAL VESSEL DISEASE, STROKE HISTORY, OTHER CV DISEASE TO REDUCE RISK TOTAL MORTALITY BY REDUCING CORONARY DEATH, REDUCE NONFATAL MI & STROKE.....

EXCLUSIVITY TERMS

EXCLUSIVITY INDICATION (continued)

I-391   USE IN PTS AT HIGH RISK CORONARY EVENTS DUE TO EXISTING CORONARY HEART DISEASE,DIABETE-S,PERIPHERAL VESSEL DISEASE,STROKE HISTORY,OTHER CV DISEASE TO REDUCE RISK TOTAL MORTALITY BY REDUCING CORONARY DEATH,REDUCE NONFATAL MI & STROKE.....

I-392   TX OF PED PATIENTS W/PH+ CHRONIC PHASE CML DISEASE RECUR AFTER STEM CELL TRNSPLT OR RESIST TO INTERFERON ALPHA THERAPY.NO CONTROLLED TRIALS DEMONSTRATING A CLINICAL BENEFIT SUCH AS IMPROVE IN DISEASE RELATED SX OR INCREASED SURVIVAL

I-393   CHRONIC BACTERIAL PROSTATITIS

I-394   USE IN PATIENTS WITH CORONARY HEART DISEASE TO REDUCE THE RISK OF UNDERGOING CORONARY REVASCULARIZATION PROCEDURES

I-395   TO IMPROVE PHYSICAL FUNCTION

EXCLUSIVITY TERMS

MISCELLANEOUS EXCLUSIVITY CODES

M-1   INFORMATION REGARDING SUPERIORITY CLAIM OVER RANITIDINE FOR DAY AND NIGHT HEARTBURN ADDED TO CLINICAL STUDIES SECTION

M-2   APPROVAL FOR ADDTION TO CLINICAL PHARMACOLOGY SECTION OF THE LABEL REGARDING (1) IMPROVEMENT IN BONE MINERAL DENSITY IN CHILDHOOD-ONSET ADULT GROWTH HORMONE DEFICIENT PATIENTS AND (2) INCREASES IN SERUM ALKALINE PHOSPHATASE

M-3   ADDITION OF EFFICACY AND SAFETY INFORMATION IN WHICH FOSAMAX WAS USED CONCOMITANTLY WITH ESTROGEN ALONE OR WITH ESTROGEN PLUS PROGESTIN

M-4   CHANGES TO PEDIATRIC USE SECTION TO PROVIDE INFORMATION REGARDING SAFETY AND EFFICACY IN PEDIATRIC PATIENTS AS YOUNG AS 2 YEARS OLD

M-5   INFORMATION REGARDING EFFECTS IN PATIENTS WITH ASTHMA ON CONCOMITANT INHALED CORTICOSTEROIDS IN CLINICAL PHARMACOLOGY SECTION

M-6   ADDITIONAL INFORMATION REGARDING CLINICAL STUDIES DONE WITH GLUCOPHAGE/GLYBURIDE COMBINATION ADDED TO CLIN PHARM AND DOSING AND ADMIN

M-7   CLINICAL PHARMACOLOGY IN PEDIATRIC PATIENTS; DOSAGE AND ADMINISTRATION INFORMATION

M-8   ADDITIONAL INFORMATION FOR THE USE OF SONATA CAPSULES FOR UP TO 5 WEEKS (35 NIGHTS) OF TREATMENT IN A CONTROLLED TRIAL SETTING

M-9   ADDITION TO THE CLINICAL STUDIES SECTION OF THE LABELING OF TEXT AND TWO TABLES CONTAINING INFORMATION FOR THE PRESCRIBING PHYSICIAN ON BLOOD PRESSURE, HEART RATE, AND HEART RATE VARIABILITY

M-10   INFORMATION REGARDING MAINTENANCE OF AN ANTIDEPRESSANT EFFECT UP TO 1 YEAR OF DOSING

M-11   USE FOR LONG-TERM TREATMENT OF POSTTRAUMATIC STRESS DISORDER

M-12   NEW LANGUAGE FOR PEDIATRIC USE

M-13   INFORMATION FROM PEDIATRIC STUDIES ADDED TO CLINICAL PHARMACOLOGY, PRECAUTIONS, AND DOSAGE AND ADMINISTRATION

M-14   ADDITIONAL CLINICAL TRIAL INFORMATION ADDED TO PEDIATRIC USE SUBSECTION

M-15   LONGER TERM EFFICACY INFORMATION FOR RISPERIDONE IN THE TREATMENT OF SCHIZOPHRENIA

M-16   CHANGE IN WORDING OF THE PEDIATRIC SECTION OF THE PACKAGE INSERT

M-17   INFORMATION REGARDING USE OF ULTANE IN PEDIATRIC PATIENTS WITH CONGENITAL HEART DISEASE

M-18   INFORMATION DENOTING THE EFFICACY OF REMERON IN MAINTAINING A RESPONSE IN PATIENTS WITH MAJOR DEPRESSIVE DISORDER (MDD)

M-19   INFORMATION REGARDING USE IN PEDIATRIC PATIENTS TWO YEARS OF AGE AND OLDER

M-20   LABELING REVISIONS RELATED TO MCCUNE ALBRIGHT SYNDROME

M-21   COMPARSION DATA ON THE ANTIHYPERTENSIVE EFFECTS OF ATACAND AND COZAAR

M-22   CHANGE I TIME TO ONSET OF ACTION

M-23   INFORMATION REGARDING ELIMINATION ADDED TO CLINICAL PHARMACOLOGY, STUDY RESULTS IN PATIENTS WITH HEPATIC AND RENAL IMPAIRMENT

M-24   INFORMATION ON RESULTS OF A LONG TERM LONGITUDINAL GROWTH STUDY AND PEDIATRIC SAFETY INFORMATION

M-25   ADDITIONAL SAFETY & PK INFORMATION IN CHILDREN 6 MONTHS TO LESS THAN 6 YEARS OF AGE ADDED TO PKG INSERT

M-26   INCORPORATION OF INFORMATION CONTAINED IN THE PEG-INTRON PACKAGE INSERT INTO THE REBETOL PACKAGE INSERT AND MEDGUIDE-PEG-INTRON WAS APPROVED FOR USE IN COMBINATION WITH REBETOL FOR TREATMENT OF CHRONIC HEPATITIS C VIRUS INFECTION ON 8/7/01

PATENT USE

U-1   PREVENTION OF PREGNANCY

U-2   TREATMENT OR PROPHYLAXIS OF ANGINA PECTORIS AND ARRHYTHMIA

U-3   TREATMENT OF HYPERTENSION

EXCLUSIVITY TERMS

PATENT USE (continued)

U-4　PROVIDING PREVENTION AND TREATMENT OF EMESIS AND NAUSEA IN MAMMALS
U-5　METHOD OF PRODUCING BRONCHODILATION
U-6　METHOD OF PRODUCING SYMPATHOMIMETIC EFFECTS
U-7　INCREASING CARDIAC CONTRACTILITY
U-8　ACUTE MYOCARDIAL INFARCTION
U-9　CONTROL OF EMESIS ASSOCIATED WITH ANY CANCER CHEMOTHERAPY AGENT
U-10　DIAGNOSTIC METHOD FOR DISTINGUISHING BETWEEN HYPOTHALAMIC MALFUNCTIONS OR LESIONS IN HUMANS
U-11　TREATMENT OR PROPHYLAXIS OF CARDIAC DISORDERS
U-12　METHOD OF TREATING [A] HUMAN SUFFERING FROM DEPRESSION
U-13　A METHOD FOR TREATING ANXIETY IN A HUMAN SUBJECT IN NEED OF SUCH TREATMENT
U-14　ADJUNCTIVE THERAPY FOR THE PREVENTION AND TREATMENT OF HYPERAMMONEMIA IN THE CHRONIC MANAGEMENT OF PATIENTS WITH UREA CYCLE ENZYMOPATHIES
U-15　METHOD OF LOWERING INTRAOCULAR PRESSURE
U-16　USE IN LUNG SCANNING PROCEDURES
U-17　TREATMENT OF VENTRICULAR AND SUPRAVENTRICULAR ARRHYTHMIAS
U-18　METHOD FOR INHIBITING GASTRIC SECRETION IN MAMMALS
U-19　TREATMENT OF INFLAMMATION
U-20　A PROCESS FOR TREATING A PATIENT SUFFERING FROM PARKINSON'S SYNDROME AND IN NEED OF TREATMENT
U-21　TREATMENT OF HUMANS SUFFERING UNDESIRED UROTOXIC SIDE EFFECTS CAUSED BY CYTOSTATICALLY ACTIVE ALKYLATING AGENTS
U-22　METHOD OF COMBATTING PATHOLOGICALLY REDUCED CEREBRAL FUNCTIONS AND PERFORMANCE WEAKNESSES, CEREBRAL INSUFFICIENCY AND DISORDERS IN CEREBRAL CIRCULATION AND METABOLISM IN WARM-BLOODED ANIMALS
U-23　METHOD FOR TREATING PROSTATIC CARCINOMA COMPRISING ADMINISTERING FLUTAMIDE
U-24　METHOD FOR TREATING PROSTATE ADENOCARCINOMA COMPRISING ADMINISTERING AN ANTIANDROGEN INCLUDING FLUTAMIDE AND AN LHRH AGONIST
U-25　REDUCING CHOLESTEROL IN CHOLELITHIASIS PATIENTS
U-26　REDUCING CHOLESTEROL GALLSTONES AND/OR FRAGMENTS THEREOF
U-27　DISSOLVING CHOLESTEROL GALLSTONES AND/OR FRAGMENTS THEREOF
U-28　CEREBRAL, CORONARY, PERIPHERAL, VISCERAL AND RENAL ARTERIOGRAPHY, AORTOGRAPHY AND LEFT VENTRICULOGRAPHY
U-29　CT IMAGING OF THE HEAD AND BODY, AND INTRAVENOUS EXCRETORY UROGRAPHY
U-30　CEREBRAL ANGIOGRAPHY, AND VENOGRAPHY
U-31　INTRA-ARTERIAL DIGITAL SUBTRACTION ANGIOGRAPHY
U-32　PALLIATIVE TREATMENT OF PATIENTS WITH OVARIAN CARCINOMA RECURRENT AFTER PRIOR CHEMOTHERAPY, INCLUDING PATIENTS WHO HAVE BEEN PREVIOUSLY TREATED WITH CISPLATIN
U-33　TREATING VIRAL INFECTIONS IN A MAMMAL
U-34　TREATING VIRAL INFECTIONS IN A WARM-BLOODED ANIMAL
U-35　TREATING CYTOMEGALOVIRUS IN A HUMAN WITH AN INJECTABLE COMPOSITION
U-36　METHODS OF TREATING BACTERIAL ILLNESSES
U-37　METHOD OF TREATING GASTROINTESTINAL DISEASE
U-38　TREATMENT OF PAROXYSMAL SUPRAVENTRICULAR TACHYCARDIA
U-39　ANGINA PECTORIS
U-40　METHOD OF TREATMENT OF BURNS
U-41　METHOD OF TREATING CARDIAC ARRHYTHMIAS
U-42　ADJUVANT TREATMENT IN COMBINATION WITH FLUOROURACIL AFTER SURGICAL RESECTION IN PATIENTS WITH DUKES' STAGE C COLON CANCER
U-43　MANAGEMENT OF CHRONIC PAIN IN PATIENTS REQUIRING OPIOID ANALGESIA
U-44　RELIEF OF NAUSEA AND VOMITING
U-45　TREATMENT OF INFLAMMATION AND ANALGESIA
U-46　TREATMENT OF PANIC DISORDER
U-47　STIMULATION OF THE RELEASE OF GROWTH HORMONE
U-48　ANALGESIA
U-49　SYMPTOMATIC CANCER-RELATED HYPERCALCEMIA
U-50　USE IN TREATING INFLAMMATORY DERMATOSES
U-51　BLOOD POOL IMAGING, INCLUDING CARDIAC FIRST PASS AND GATED EQUILIBRIUM IMAGING AND FOR DETECTION OF SITES OF GASTROINTESTINAL BLEEDING
U-52　TREATMENT OF ADULT AND PEDIATRIC PATIENTS (OVER SIX MONTHS OF AGE) WITH ADVANCED HIV INFECTION
U-53　HYPERCALCEMIA OF MALIGNANCY
U-54　REVERSAL AGENT OR ANTAGONIST OF NONDEPOLARIZING NEUROMUSCULAR BLOCKING AGENTS
U-55　TREATMENT OF PAIN
U-56　AID TO SMOKING CESSATION
U-57　OPHTHALMIC USE OF NORFLOXACIN
U-58　METHOD OF TREATING INFLAMMATORY INTESTINAL DISEASES
U-59　METHOD OF TREATING HYPERCHOLESTEROLEMIA

EXCLUSIVITY TERMS
PATENT USE (continued)

U-60	NASAL ADMINISTRATION OF BUTORPHANOL
U-61	CEREBRAL AND PERIPHERAL ARTERIOGRAPHY AND CT IMAGING OF THE HEAD
U-62	CORONARY ARTERIOGRAPHY, LEFT VENTRICULOGRAPHY, CT IMAGING OF THE BODY, INTRAVENOUS EXCRETORY UROGRAPHY, INTRAVENOUS DIGITAL SUBTRACTION ANGIOGRAPHY AND VENOGRAPHY
U-63	ISOPRENALINE ANTAGONISM ON THE HEART RATE OR BLOOD PRESSURE
U-64	TREATMENT OF VIRAL INFECTIONS
U-65	METHOD OF TREATMENT OF A PATIENT INFECTED WITH HIV
U-66	TRIPHASIC REGIMEN
U-67	METHOD OF INDUCING ANESTHESIA IN A WARM BLOODED ANIMAL
U-68	TREATMENT OF ACTINIC KERATOSIS
U-69	TREATMENT OF PNEUMOCYSTIS CARINII INFECTIONS
U-70	TREATMENT OF TRANSIENT INSOMNIA
U-71	METHOD OF TREATMENT OF HEART FAILURE
U-72	TREATMENT OF MIGRAINE
U-73	METHOD OF TREATING DISEASES OR INFECTIONS CAUSED BY MYCETES
U-74	METHOD OF PROVIDING HYPNOTIC EFFECT
U-75	RELIEF OF OCULAR ITCHING DUE TO SEASONAL ALLERGIC CONJUNCTIVITIS
U-76	USE TO IMAGE A SUBJECT WITH A MAGNETIC RESONANCE IMAGING SYSTEM
U-77	TREATMENT OF SYMPTOMS OF SEASONAL ALLERGIC RHINITIS
U-78	ULCERATIVE COLITIS
U-79	SYMPTOMATIC TREATMENT OF PATIENTS WITH NOCTURNAL HEARTBURN DUE TO GERD
U-80	METHOD OF TREATING OCULAR BACTERIAL INFECTIONS
U-81	RELIEF OF SYMPTOMS ASSOCIATED WITH SEASONAL ALLERGIC RHINITIS
U-82	TREATMENT FOR DEMENTIA IN PATIENTS WITH ALZHEIMER'S DISEASE
U-83	TREATMENT OF SEIZURES
U-84	A METHOD OF BLOCKING THE UPTAKE OF MONOAMINES BY BRAIN NEURONS IN ANIMALS
U-85	NASAL TREATMENT OF SEASONAL AND PERENNIAL ALLERGIC RHINITIS SYMPTOMS
U-86	METHOD OF TREATING CERTAIN FORMS OF EPILEPSY
U-87	METHOD FOR NONINVASIVE ADMINISTRATION OF SEDATIVES, ANALGESICS, AND ANESTHETICS
U-88	TREATMENT OF MODERATE PLAQUE PSORIASIS
U-89	TREATMENT OR PROPHYLAXIS OF EMESIS
U-90	TREATMENT OF PSYCHOTIC DISORDERS
U-91	ALTERNATIVE THERAPY TO TRIMETHOPRIM-SULFAMETHOXAZOLE FOR TREATMENT OF MODERATE-TO-SEVERE PNEUMOCYSTIS CARINII PNEUMONIA IN IMMUNOCOMPROMISED AND AIDS PATIENTS
U-92	TREATMENT OF DIABETIC NEPHROPATHY IN PATIENTS WITH TYPE I INSULIN DEPENDENT DIABETES MELLITUS AND RETINOPATHY
U-93	USE AS AN ANTIHISTAMINE/ DECONGESTANT
U-94	TREATMENT OF ADULTS WITH ADVANCED HIV INFECTION WHO ARE INTOLERANT OF APPROVED THERAPIES WITH PROVEN CLINICAL BENEFIT OR WHO HAVE EXPERIENCED SIGNIFICANT CLINICAL OR IMMUNOLOGIC DETERIORATION WHILE RECEIVING THESE THERAPIES OR FOR WHOM SUCH THERAPIES ARE CONTRAINDICATED
U-95	SHORT TERM MANAGEMENT OF MODERATE PRURITUS IN ADULTS WITH ATOPIC DERMATITIS AND LICHEN SIMPLEX CHRONICUS
U-96	METHOD OF TREATING VARICELLA ZOSTER (SHINGLES) INFECTIONS
U-97	A METHOD OF TREATING A PATIENT IN NEED OF MEMORY ENHANCEMENT
U-98	A METHOD OF INDUCING REGRESSION OF LEUKEMIA CELL GROWTH IN A MAMMAL
U-99	METHOD OF PROVIDING POTASSIUM TO A SUBJECT IN NEED OF POTASSIUM
U-100	METHOD OF TREATING OCULAR INFLAMMATION
U-101	ADJUNCT TO CONVENTIONAL CT OR MRI IMAGING IN THE LOCALIZATION OF STROKE IN PATIENTS IN WHOM STROKE HAS ALREADY BEEN DIAGNOSED
U-102	METHOD OF HORMONALLY TREATING MENOPAUSAL OR POST-MENOPAUSAL DISORDERS IN WOMEN
U-103	TREATMENT OF OCULAR HYPERTENSION
U-104	TREATMENT OF AQUEOUS HUMOR FORMATION AND INTRAOCULAR PRESSURE
U-105	EMESIS
U-106	TREATMENT OF EPILEPSY
U-107	TREATMENT OF HYPERTENSION AND ANGINA PECTORIS
U-108	SHORT-TERM TREATMENT OF ACTIVE DUODENAL ULCER, GASTROESOPHAGEAL REFLUX DISEASE (GERD), SEVERE EROSIVE ESOPHAGITIS, POORLY RESPONSIVE SYMPTOMATIC GERD, PATHOLOGICAL HYPERSECRETORY CONDITIONS AND MAINTENANCE OF HEALING OF EROSIVE ESOPHAGITIS
U-109	USE AS AN ADJUNCT TO DIET IN THE TREATMENT OF ELEVATED TOTAL CHOLESTEROL AND LDL-C LEVELS IN PATIENTS WITH PRIMARY HYPERCHOLESTEROLEMIA WHOSE RESPONSE TO DIETARY RESTRICTION OF SATURATED FAT AND CHOLESTEROL AND OTHER NONPHARMACOLOGICAL MEASURES HAS NOT BEEN ADEQUATE
U-110	USE AS A RETRIEVABLE PESSARY
U-111	DIABETES
U-112	CONTRACEPTION
U-113	METHOD OF CONDUCTING A RADIOLOGICAL EXAMINATION OF A PATIENT BY ADMINISTERING TO SAID PATIENT A RADIOPAQUE AMOUNT OF IOPROMIDE

EXCLUSIVITY TERMS

PATENT USE (continued)

U-114	USE FOR INHIBITING BONE RESORPTION
U-115	USE OF VASODILATORS TO EFFECT AND ENHANCE AN ERECTION (AND THUS TREAT ERECTILE DYSFUNCTION), BY INJECTION INTO THE PENIS
U-116	METHOD OF MYOCARDIAL IMAGING
U-117	TREATMENT OF OCULAR ALLERGIC RESPONSE IN HUMAN EYES
U-118	METHOD OF LOWERING BLOOD SUGAR LEVEL
U-119	TREATMENT OF NASAL HYPERSECRETION
U-120	CONTROLLING OR PREVENTING POST-OPERATIVE INTRAOCULAR PRESSURE RISES ASSOCIATED WITH OPHTHALMIC LASER SURGICAL PROCEDURES
U-121	METHOD OF TREATING CONDITIONS MEDIATED THROUGH HISTAMINE H2-RECEPTORS
U-122	A THERAPEUTIC METHOD FOR CONTROLLING THROMBOSIS
U-123	METHOD FOR CONTROLLING THROMBOSIS AND DECREASING BLOOD HYPERCOAGULATION AND HEMORRHAGING RISKS
U-124	TREATMENT OF ACNE
U-125	TREATING NEUROGENERATIVE DISEASES
U-126	TREATMENT OF GASTRITIS
U-127	METHOD OF PRODUCING NEUROMUSCULAR BLOCKADE
U-128	METHODS FOR TREATMENT OF TUMORS
U-129	METHOD TO DESTROY OR IMPAIR TARGET CELLS
U-130	MANAGEMENT OF PATIENTS WITH MASTOCYTOSIS
U-131	PHOTODAMAGED SKIN
U-132	INHIBITING HIV PROTEASE
U-133	MANAGEMENT OF OBESITY INCLUDING WEIGHT LOSS AND MAINTENANCE IN PATIENTS ON A REDUCED-CALORIE DIET
U-134	TREATMENT OF ACNE VULGARIS
U-135	ANTITUMOR AGENT
U-136	PROCESS FOR WASTE NITROGEN REMOVAL
U-137	METHOD OF TREATING BACTERIAL VAGINOSIS
U-138	TREATMENT OF ALLERGIC RHINITIS
U-139	TREATMENT OF ALLERGIC REACTIONS
U-140	USE OF NORVIR TO INHIBIT HIV PROTESASE OR TO INHIBIT AN HIV INFECTION
U-141	TREATMENT OF ULCERATIVE COLITIS
U-142	METHOD OF TREATING ALLERGIC REACTIONS IN A MAMMAL BY USING THIS ACTIVE METABOLITE
U-143	BIODEGRADABLE SUPERPARAMAGNETIC METAL OXIDES AS CONTRAST AGENTS FOR MR IMAGING
U-144	BIOLOGICALLY DEGRADABLE SUPERPARAMAGNETIC MATERIALS FOR USE IN CLINICAL APPLICATIONS
U-145	BIOLOGICALLY DEGRADABLE SUPERPARAMAGNETIC PARTICLES FOR USE AS NUCLEAR MAGNETIC RESONANCE IMAGING AGENTS
U-146	METHOD OF TREATING SUSCEPTIBLE NEOPLASMS IN MAMMALS
U-147	DETECTION OF GASTROINTESTINAL DISORDERS AND THE SUBSEQUENT BREATH COLLECTION AND MEASUREMENT OF $^{13}CO_2$
U-148	DEVICE FOR COLLECTING A BREATH SAMPLE
U-149	METHOD OF TREATING AN ANIMAL, INCLUDING A HUMAN SUFFERING FROM OR SUSCEPTIBLE TO PSYCHOSIS, ACUTE MANIA OR MILD ANXIETY STATES
U-150	METHOD OF USE FOR CONTROLLING HYPERGLYCEMIA BY ADMINISTRATION OF THIS SUSTAINED RELEASE DOSAGE FORM OF GLIPIZIDE
U-151	RELIEF OF SYMPTOMS OF THE COMMON COLD
U-152	METHOD OF TREATING ANXIETY RELATED DISORDERS INCLUDING OBSESSIVE COMPULSIVE DISORDER
U-153	TREATMENT OF INITIAL EPISODE GENITAL HERPES
U-154	METHOD OF TREATING ANIMALS SUFFERING FROM AN APPETITE DISORDER
U-155	TREATMENT OF ERECTILE DYSFUNCTION
U-156	METHOD OF PROVIDING ANESTHESIA
U-157	TREATMENT OF A HUMAN SUFFERING FROM VITAMIN B12 DEFICIENCY
U-158	ANGINA
U-159	TREATMENT OF INTERSTITIAL CYSTITIS
U-160	TREATMENT OF BACTERIAL INFECTIOUS DISEASE
U-161	METHOD OF INHIBITING CHOLESTEROL BIOSYNTHESIS IN A PATIENT
U-162	METHOD OF USE TO INHIBIT CHOLESTEROL SYNTHESIS IN A HUMAN SUFFERING FROM HYPERCHOLESTEROLEMIA
U-163	METHOD OF USING TROGLITAZONE TO TREAT IMPAIRED GLUCOSE TOLERANCE TO PREVENT OR DELAY THE ONSET OF NONINSULIN-DEPENDENT DIABETES MELLITUS
U-164	METHOD OF USING TROGLITAZONE TO PREVENT OR DELAY THE ONSET OF NONINSULIN-DEPENDENT DIABETES MELLITUS IN A DEFINED POPULATION OF PATIENTS
U-165	TREATMENT OF SYMPTOMATIC BENIGN PROSTATIC HYPERPLASIA
U-166	TREATMENT OF H. PYLORI ASSOCIATED DUODENAL ULCER
U-167	METHOD FOR TREATING HIV-1 INFECTION
U-168	METHOD OF INHIBITING LIPOXYGENASE ACTIVITY IN A MAMMAL WHICH IS THE MODE OF ACTION IN THE TREATMENT OF ASTHMA

EXCLUSIVITY TERMS

PATENT USE (continued)

U-169	METHODS OF USING THE COMPOUND/DRUG PRODUCT AS A CONTRAST AGENT IN MAGNETIC RESONANCE IMAGING
U-170	METHOD OF OBTAINING AN MR IMAGE USING THE COMPOSITION/DRUG PRODUCT AS A CONTRAST AGENT
U-171	METHODS OF USING THE COMPOUND/DRUG PRODUCT AS AN ORAL CONTRAST AGENT IN MAGNETIC RESONANCE IMAGING OF THE GASTROINTESTINAL TRACT
U-172	TREATMENT OF GENITAL WARTS
U-173	ADMINISTRATION TO A HOST SUFFERING FROM GESTATIONAL DIABETES
U-174	USE AS AN ANTIHISTAMINE AGENT
U-175	METHOD OF TREATING MALIGNANT TUMORS
U-176	METHOD OF TREATING A PATIENT SUFFERING FROM LISTED CONDITIONS, INCLUDING SPECIFIC PSYCHOSIS
U-177	FUNGICIDE
U-178	FACILITATED ADHERENCE OF AGENTS TO SKIN
U-179	ENHANCED CUTANEOUS PENETRATION OF A DERMALLY-APPLIED PHARMACOLOGICALLY ACTIVE AGENT
U-180	TREATMENT OF ADULT AND PEDIATRIC PATIENTS (OVER SIX MONTHS OF AGE) WITH ADVANCED HIV INFECTION
U-181	PRODUCING ALPHA ADRENERGIC ANTAGONISTIC ACTION IN A HOST
U-182	USE OF SALMETEROL IN PATIENTS WITH REVERSIBLE AIRWAY OBSTRUCTION
U-183	TREATMENT OF CONDITIONS CAUSED BY DISTURBANCE OF NEURONAL 5HT FUNCTION
U-184	TREATING ALLERGIC EYE DISEASES IN HUMANS
U-185	METHOD OF TREATING HYPERTENSION
U-186	METHOD FOR TREATING GI DISORDERS CAUSED BY H. PYLORI WHICH COMPRISES ADMINISTRATION OF RANITIDINE BISMUTH CITRATE AND CLARITHROMYCIN FOR A GREATER THAN ADDITIVE EFFECT
U-187	THERAPEUTIC TREATMENT OF CALCIFIC TUMORS
U-188	TREATMENT OF H. PYLORI ASSOCIATED DUODENAL ULCER
U-189	ENHANCEMENT OF THE BIOAVAILABILITY OF THE DRUG SUBSTANCE
U-190	USE OF RITONAVIR IN COMBINATION WITH ANY REVERSE TRANSCRIPTASE INHIBITOR
U-191	METHOD OF TREATMENT FOR CONTROLLING AND LOWERING INTRAOCULAR PRESSURE IN A HUMAN
U-192	USE IN TREATING ALLERGIC REACTIONS
U-193	PSORIASIS
U-194	TREATING AGINA PECTORIS AND HIGH BLOOD PRESSURE
U-195	METHOD FOR THE DIAGNOSIS OF GASTROINTESTINAL DISORDERS BY UREA ISOTOAC OR NITROGEN LABELED CARBON
U-196	TREATMENT OF METASTIC BREAST CANCER IN POSTMENOPAUSAL WOMEN WITH ESTROGEN RECEPTOR POSITIVE TUMORS
U-197	USE IN COMBINATION WITH CERTAIN LHRH ANALOGUES FOR THE TREATMENT OF ADVANCED PROSTATE CANCER
U-198	TREATMENT METASTATIC CARCINOMA OF OVARY AFTER FIRST-LINE FAILURE OR SUBSEQUENT CHEMOTHERAPY, TREATMENT OF BREAST CANCER AFTER FAILURE OF COMBINATION CHEMOTHERAPY FOR METASTATIC DISEASE AND SECOND-LINE TREATMENT OF AIDS-RELATED KAPOSI'S SARCOMA
U-199	METHOD OF TREATING INFECTIOUS UPPER GI TRACT DISORDERS CAUSED BY CAMPYLOBACTER PYLORDIS INFECTION COMPRISING ADMINISTRATION OF A BISMUTH AGENT AND AN ANTIMICROBIAL AGENT
U-200	METHOD OF TREATING GI DISORDERS COMPRISING ADMINISTRATION OF A BISMUTH-CONTAINING AGENT AND H2 RECEPTOR BLOCKING ANTI-SECRETORY AGENT
U-201	METHOD OF TREATING GI DISORDERS COMPRISING ADMINISTRATION OF CAMPYLOBACTER-INHIBITING ANTIMICROBIAL AGENT AND H2 RECEPTOR BLOCKING ANTI-SECRETORY AGENT
U-202	METHOD OF TREATING PEPTIC ULCER DISEASE CAUSED BY CAMPYLOBACTER PYLORIDIS COMPRISING ORAL ADMINISTRATION OF 50 TO 5,000MG BISMUTH DAILY FOR 3-56 DAYS
U-203	TREATMENT OF ADVANCED BREAST CANCER IN POSTMENOPAUSAL WOMEN WITH DISEASE PROGRESSION FOLLOWING ANTIESTROGEN THERAPY
U-204	USE OF TAXOL IN COMBINATION WITH G-CSF FOR TREATMENT OF PATIENTS WITH AIDS-RELATED KAPOSI?S SARCOMA
U-205	METHOD FOR TREATING HEARTBURN
U-206	METHOD OF USING FSH ALONE, WITHOUT THE PRESENCE OF EXOGENOUS LH, IN IN VITRO FERTILIZATION
U-207	USE AS NASAL SPRAY
U-208	VAGINAL ADMINISTRATION USING SPECIFIED FORMULATION
U-209	VAGINAL ADMINISTRATION OF PROGESTERONE USING SPECIFIED FORMULATION
U-210	METHOD OF TREATING CONGESTIVE HEART FAILURE
U-211	USE IN PATIENTS WITH REVERSIBLE AIRWAY OBSTRUCTION
U-212	METHOD OF TREATMENT OF PARKINSON'S DISEASE
U-213	METHOD OF INHIBITING CHOLESTEROL BIOSYNTHESIS AND TREATING HYPERCHOLESTEROLEMIA AND METHOD FOR TREATING HYPERLIPIDEMIA
U-214	USE AS A BLOOD GLUCOSE-LOWERING AGENT
U-215	TREATMENT OF EPILEPSY TWICE DAILY. TREATING A PATIENT BY ADMINISTERING CARBAMAZEPINE IN A DOSAGE FORM CAPABLE OF MAINTAINING BLOOD CONCENTRATION FROM 4-12MCG/ML OVER 12 HOURS

EXCLUSIVITY TERMS

PATENT USE (continued)

U-216	TREATMENT OF ADENOCARCINOMA, INCLUDING STAGE B2-C, BY ADMINISTERING AN AGONIST OF LR-RH AND FLUTAMIDE
U-217	METHOD OF PRODUCING ANESTHESIA
U-218	METHOD FOR LIMITING THE POTENTIAL FOR MICROBIAL GROWTH IN THE DRUG PRODUCT
U-219	TREATMENT OF PARKISON'S DISEASE
U-220	METHOD OF DIAGNOSIS
U-221	SELECTIVE VASODILATION BY CONTINUOUS ADENOSINE INFUSION
U-222	METHOD OF TREATING PAGET'S DISEASE USING ACTONEL
U-223	TREATMENT OF BACTERIAL CONJUNCTIVITIS CAUSED BY SUSCEPTIBLE STRAINS OF MICROORGANISMS
U-224	CONTROLLING INTRAOCULAR PRESSURE
U-225	METHOD FOR DELIVERY
U-226	METHOD OF ENHANCING THE DISSOLUTION PROFILE OF A PHARMACEUTICAL FROM A SOLID DOSAGE FORM CONTAINING THE PHARMACEUTICAL AND SIMETHICONE
U-227	NASAL ADMINISTRATION
U-228	ASTHMA
U-229	CARDIAC INSUFFICIENCY (CONGESTIVE HEART FAILURE)
U-230	PREVENTION OF ACUTE CARDIAC ISCHEMIC EVENTS
U-231	USE IN PARKINSON'S DISEASE
U-232	METHOD OF TREATING MIGRAINE
U-233	DECREASING MORTALITY CAUSED BY CONGESTIVE HEART FAILURE
U-234	METHOD OF USING RIBAVIRIN TO TREAT VIRAL INFECTIONS IN MAMMALS
U-235	METHOD OF MODULATING TH1 AND TH2 RESPONSE IN ACTIVATED T CELLS OF A HUMAN COMPRISING ADMINISTERING RIBAVIRIN TO THE T CELLS IN A DOSAGE WHICH PROMOTES THE TH1 RESPONSE AND SUPPRESSES THE TH2 RESPONSE
U-236	TREATING MALE PATTERN BALDNESS WITH 0.05 TO 3 MG/DAY
U-237	METHOD OF PERFORMING NMR IMAGING WITH A PATIENT COMPRISING ADMINISTERING TO THE PATIENT AN EFFECTIVE AMOUNT OF CONTRAST AGENT DISCLOSED IN THE CLAIMS
U-238	IMAGING A BODY TISSUE AND SUBJECTING TO NMR TOMOGRAPHY, ADMINISTERING AN AMOUNT OF PHARMACEUTICAL AGENT FOR AFFECTING THE RELAXATION TIMES OF ATOMS IN BODY TISSUES UNDER-GOING NMR DIAGNOSIS, WHEREBY THE IMAGE CONTRAST IN ENHANCED....
U-239	TREATING OR CONTROLLING OCULAR INFLAMMATION WHICH COMPRISES TOPICALLY ADMINISTERING TO THE AFFECTED EYE A COMPOSITION COMPRISING AN NSAID, A POLYMERIC QUATERNARY AMMONIUM COMPOUND AND BORIC ACID
U-240	TREATMENT OF ACUTE MIGRAINE ATTACKS
U-241	FOR SHORT-TERM TREATMENT ACTIVE DUODENAL ULCER, MAINTENANCE THERAPY FOR DUODENAL UL-CER PATIENTS AT REDUCED DOSAGE AFTER HEALING OF ACTIVE ULCER, SHORT-TERM TREATMENT AC-TIVE BENIGN GASTRIC ULCER & GERD, PATHOLOGICAL HYPERSECRETORY CONDITIONS
U-242	USE OF FOLLITROPIN ALPHA ALONE IN IN-VITRO FERTILIZATION
U-243	TOPICAL ADMINISTRATION
U-244	PLATELET AGGREGATION INHIBITORS
U-245	TREATMENT OF SEBORRHEA DERMATITIS IN HUMANS
U-246	PHOSPHATE BINDING
U-247	TREATMENT OF RHEUMATOID ARTHRITIS
U-248	TREATMENT OF HIV
U-249	METHOD OF TREATING ALLERGIC OR NON-ALLERGIC RHINITIS IN PATIENTS BY ADMINISTERING AEROSO-LIZED PARTICLES OF MOMETASONE FUROATE
U-250	TREATMENT OF HEPATITIS B INFECTION
U-251	USE OF TROGLITAZONE IN COMBINATION WITH SULFONYLUREAS IN THE TREATMENT OF TYPE II DIA-BETES
U-252	METHOD OF TREATING A HUMAN SUBJECT HAVING GAUCHER?S DISEASE
U-253	ORAL TRANSMUCOSAL USE
U-254	USE OF AGGRASTAT IN COMBINATION WITH HEPARIN
U-255	IMPROVED WAKEFULNESS IN PATIENTS WITH EXCESSIVE DAYTIME SLEEPINESS ASSOCIATED WITH NAR-COLEPSY
U-256	TREATMENT OF HIV INFECITON IN COMBINATION WITH ONE OR MORE ADDITIONAL HIV ANTIVIRAL AGENTS
U-257	TREATMENT OF HIV INFECTION
U-258	TREATMENT OF NEURODEGENERATIVE DISEASES
U-259	TREATMENT OF ANDROGENIC ALOPECIA BY ORAL ADMINISTRATION OF DRUG SUBSTANCE
U-260	REDUCTION OF INTRAOCULAR PRESSURE IN PATIENTS WITH OPEN ANGLE GLAUCOMA AND OCULAR HY-PERTENSION WHO ARE INTOLERANT OF OTHER IOP LOWERING MEDICATIONS OR INSUFFICIENTLY RE-SPONSIVE TO ANOTHER IOP LOWERING MEDICATION
U-261	TREATING BENIGN PROSTATIC HYPERPLASIA WITH A GENUS OF COMPOUNDS, INCLUDING FINASTERIDE
U-262	TREATING BENIGN PROSTATIC HYPERTROPHY WITH FINASTERIDE
U-263	METHOD OF TREATING A MALIGNANT CONDITION THROUGH INTRAVASCULAR ADMINISTRATION OF BU-SULFAN. METHOD FOR TREATING LEUKEMIA OR LYMPHOMA IN A PATIENT UNDERGOING A BONE MAR-ROW TRANSPLANT THROUGH INTRAVENOUS ADMINISTRATION OF BUSULFAN.

EXCLUSIVITY TERMS

PATENT USE (continued)

U-264	METHOD OF TREATING A MALIGNANT DISEASE THROUGH PARENTERAL ADMINISTRATION OF BUSULFAN. METHOD FOR TREATING A PATIENT UNDERGOING A BONE MARROW TRANSPLANT THROUGH INTRAVASCULAR ADMINISTRATION OF BUSULFAN
U-265	USE AS A LAXATIVE
U-266	RELIEF OF THE SIGNS AND SYMPTOMS OF OSTEOARTHRITIS; MANAGEMENT OF ACUTE PAIN IN ADULTS; TREATMENT OF PRIMARY DYSMENORRHEA
U-267	PREVENTING HEARTBURN EPISODES FOLLOWING INGESTION OF HEARTBURN-INDUCING FOOD/BEVERAGE, COMPRISING ADMIN TO PT, 30 MIN PRIOR TO CONSUMPTION BY THE PT THE FOOD/BEVERAGE, A COMPOSITION COMPRISING 10MG FAMOTIDINE
U-268	ACROMEGALY
U-269	EXCESS GH-SECRETION OR GASTRO-INTESTINAL DISORDERS
U-270	METHOD FOR IMPROVING THE TIME FOR ADMINISTRATION OR THE TIME BETWEEN CHANGES OF GIVING SETS FOR THE DRUG PRODUCT
U-271	METHOD OF TREATING TUMORS
U-272	METHOD OF TREATING CARCINOMA
U-273	CUTANEOUS T-CELL LYMPHOMA
U-274	ZANAMIVIR FOR INHALATION
U-275	METHOD OF USE OF THE DRUG SUBSTANCE
U-276	METHOD OF USE OF LEVOBUPIVACAINE
U-277	NEUROLOGICAL AND OTHER DISORDERS (TREATMENT OF EPILEPSY, BID ORAL DOSING)
U-278	METHOD OF USE OF THE INDICATION OF THE DRUG PRODUCT
U-279	METHOD OF USE OF THE APPROVED PRODUCT
U-280	TREATING PRECIPITATED ACUTE URINARY RETENTION WITH FINASTERIDE
U-281	ANTIMYCOTIC USES, SPECIFICALLY, TREATMENT OF ONYCHOMYCOSIS
U-282	METHOD OF TREATING BACTERIAL INFECTIONS
U-283	METHOD FOR TREATING MENOPAUSAL SYMPTOMS IN A POSTMENOPAUSAL FEMALE
U-284	MENOPAUSAL AND POSTMENOPAUSAL DISORDERS (INCLUDING VASOMOTOR SYMPTOMS ASSOCIATED WITH MENOPAUSE, AND VULVAR AND VAGINAL ATROPHY) AND OSTEOPOROSIS
U-285	DEPRESSION AND SOCIAL ANXIETY DISORDER/SOCIAL PHOBIA
U-286	DEPRESSION
U-287	TREATMENT OR PREVENTION OF OSTEOPOROSIS
U-288	THERAPY OF INFLUENZA
U-289	TREATMENT OF NON-HYPERKERATOTIC ACTINIC KERATOSES OF FACE AND SCALP
U-290	INHIBITING TRANSPLANT REJECTION USING RAPAMYCIN (SIROLIMUS)
U-291	INHIBITING TRANSPLANT REJECTION USING RAPAMYCIN (SIROLIMUS) IN COMBINATION WITH CYCLOSPORIN
U-292	INHIBITING TRANSPLANT REJECTION USING RAPAMYCIN (SIROLIMUS) IN COMBINATION WITH AZATHIOPRINE
U-293	INHIBITING TRANSPLANT REJECTION USING RAPAMYCIN (SIROLIMUS) IN COMBINATION WITH A CORTICOSTEROID
U-294	TREATMENT OF HYPERPIGMENTARY DISORDERS
U-295	TREATMENT OF SEASONAL AND PERENNIAL ALLERGIC RHINITIS SYMPTOMS
U-296	TREATING MIGRAINE PAIN AND ONE OR MORE OF A CLUSTER OF SYMPTOMS CHARACTERISTIC OF A MIGRAINE ATTACK SYMPTOMS BEING SELECTED FROM PHOTOPHOBIA, PHONOPHOBIA, NAUSEA AND FUNCTIONAL DISABILITY
U-297	PREVENTION OR TREATMENT OF REVERSIBLE VASOCONSTRICTION BY THE INHALATION OF NITRIC OXIDE WITH AN OXYGEN CONTAINING GAS
U-298	METHOD OF COMBATING BACTERIA IN A PATIENT
U-299	TREATMENT OF ADENOMATOUS POLYPS
U-300	INDICATED FOR THE REDUCTION OF ELEVATED TOTAL AND LDL CHOLESTEROL LEVELS IN PATIENTS WITH PRIMARY HYPERCHOLESTEROLEMIA
U-301	USE OF TROGLITAZONE IN COMBINATION WITH SULFONYLUREAS AND BIGUANIDES IN THE TREATMENT OF TYPE II DIABETES
U-302	TO REDUCE THE RISK OF STROKE IN PATIENTS WHO HAVE HAD TRANSIENT ISCHEMIA OF THE BRAIN OR COMPLETED ISCHEMIC STROKE DUE TO THROMBOSIS
U-303	METHOD OF USE PATENT-PRODUCT APPROVED FOR TREATMENT OF OSTEOPORISIS, PAGET'S DISEASE, PREVENTION AND TREATMENT OF GLUCOCORTICOID-INDUCED OSTEOPOROSIS
U-304	A METHOD OF TREATMENT OF A CONDITION INVOLVING AN ANTIBODY ANTIGEN REACTION
U-305	METHODS FOR USING THE DRUG PRODUCT
U-306	TREATMENT OF POST-MENOPAUSAL UROGENITAL SYMPTOMS ASSOCIATED WITH ESTROGEN DEFICIENCY
U-307	CLAIMS AN OLANZAPINE POLYMORPH USEFUL FOR TREATING ANY NUMBER OF LISTED CONDITIONS, INCLUDING SPECIFIC PSYCHOSES, EMPLOYING OLANZAPINE AS PER THE INDICATION OF THIS NDA
U-308	CLAIMS A SOLID ORAL FORMULATION INCLUDING TABLETS AND GRANULES OF OLANZAPINE USEFUL FOR TREATING ANY NUMBER OF LISTED CONDITIONS, INCLUDING SPECIFIC PSYCHOSES, EMPLOYING OLANZAPINE AS PER THE INDICATION OF THIS NDA
U-309	TREATING SJOEGREN SYNDROME
U-310	TREATMENT OF XEROSTOMIA

EXCLUSIVITY TERMS

PATENT USE (continued)

U-311	HORMONE REPLACEMENT
U-312	PANIC DISORDER OBSESSIVE-COMPULSIVE DISORDER POSTTRAUMATIC STRESS DISORDER
U-313	TREATMENT OF CONGESTIVE HEART FAILURE
U-314	METHOD FOR TREATING HYPERPARATHYROIDISM WHICH COMPRISES SUPPRESSING PARATHYROID AC-TIVITY
U-315	METHOD FOR ADMINISTERING DRUG TO GASTROINTESTINAL TRACT
U-316	METHOD OF TREATING A SUBJECT SUFFERING FROM PROSTATE CANCER
U-317	METHOD OF USING TROGLITAZONE TO TREAT PATIENTS HAVING INSULIN RESISTANCE
U-318	TREATMENT OF PATIENTS WITH AN OVERACTIVE BLADDER WITH SYMPTOMS OF URINARY FREQUENCY, URGENCY, OR URGE INCONTINENCE
U-319	TREATMENT OF MICROBIAL INFECTIONS
U-320	INHIBITING OR ELIMINATING ACUTE MYELOID LEUKEMIA
U-321	REDUCTION OF ELEVATED IPTH LEVELS IN THE MGT OF SECONDARY HYPERPARATHYROIDISM IN PA-TIENTS UNDERGONG CHRONIC RENAL DIALYSIS
U-322	TREATMENT OF ALZHEIMER?S DEMENTIA
U-323	USE AS A BILE ACID SEQUESTRANT
U-324	METHOD OF TREATING AN ANIMAL, INCLUDING A HUMAN, SUFFERING FROM OR SUSCEPTIBLE TO PSY-CHOSIS OR ACUTE MANIA EMPLOYING OLANZAPINE
U-325	METHOD OF TREATING A PATIENT SUFFERING FROM ANY OF A NUMBER OF LISTED CONDITIONS, INCLUD-ING "BIPOLAR DISORDER NOS" EMPLOYING OLANZAPINE
U-326	METHOD OF TREATING SCHIZOPHRENIA AND BIPOLAR DISORDER
U-327	METHOD OF TREATING A PATIENT SUFFERING FROM ANY OF A NUMBER OF LISTED PSYCHOTIC CONDI-TIONS EMPLOYING OLANZAPINE
U-328	METHOD OF TREATING A PATIENT SUFFERING FROM ANY OF A NUMBER OF LISTED CONDITIONS INCLUD-ING "A PSYCHOTIC CONDITION" EMPLOYING AN OLANZAPINE POLYMORPH
U-329	USE OF AVANDIA AS MONOTHERAPY, IN COMBINATION WITH METFORMIN, AND IN COMBINATION WITH SULFONYLUREAS TO IMPROVE GLYCEMIC CONTROL IN PATIENTS WITH TYPE 2 DIABETES MELLITUS
U-330	TREATMENT OF NAUSEA AND VOMITING
U-331	METHOD OF TREATING HYPERLIPIDEMIA WITH NICOTINIC ACID BY DOSING ONCE PER DAY IN THE EVE-NING OR AT NIGHT
U-332	TREATMENT OR PREVENTION OF BRONCHOSPASM
U-333	METHOD OF TREATING OCULAR HYPERTENSION
U-334	TREATMENT OF EXCESSIVE FEMALE FACIAL HAIR
U-335	USE OF PRAVASTATIN SODIUM FOR SECONDARY PREVENTION OF CORONARY EVENTS IN MEN AND WO-MEN WHO HAVE HAD A MYOCARDIAL INFARCTION AND HAVE NORMAL CHOLESTEROL LEVELS
U-336	DIAGNOSTIC RADIOIMAGING
U-337	USE OF CARDIOLITE/MIRALUMA KIT FOR THE PREPARATION OF TC99M SESTAMIBI
U-338	METHODS FOR TREATING DISTURBANCES OF MOOD, DISTURBANCES OF APPETITE, DEPRESSED MOOD, OR CARBOHYDRATE CRAVING ALL ASSOCIATED WITH PREMENSTRUAL SYNDROME
U-339	PREVENTION OF CARDIO-TOXICITY CAUSED BY THE ADMINISTRATION OF DOXORUBICIN
U-340	THE LONG TERM TREATMENT OF GROWTH FAILURE DUE TO LACK OF ADEQUATE ENDOGENOUS GROWTH HORMONE SECRETION IN CHILDREN
U-341	METHOD FOR ENHANCING THE TREATMENT OF ... LATE LUTEAL PHASE DYSPHORIC DISORDER
U-342	METHOD FOR TREATMENT OF LATE LUTEAL PHASE DYSPHORIC DISORDER
U-343	REDUCTION OF INTESTINAL GAS, CRAMPING AND ANORECTAL IRRITATION
U-344	METHOD FOR INHIBITING HIV INFECTION BY ADMINISTERING RITONAVIR IN COMBINATION WITH ANOTHER HIV PROTEASE INHIBITOR
U-345	RITONAVIR AND ANOTHER HIV PROTEASE INHIBITOR FOR CONCOMITANT ADMINISTRATION FOR THE TREATMENT OF AN HIV INFECTION
U-346	METHOD FOR INHIBITING CYTOCHROME P450 MONOOXYGENASE WITH RITONAVIR AND A METHOD FOR IMPROVING THE PHARMCOKINETICS OF A DRUG THAT IS METABOLIZED BY CYTOCHROME P450 MONO-OXYGENASE BY ADMIN THE DRUG AND RITONAVIR
U-347	METHOD OF USE IN COMBINATION WITH REVERSE TRANSCRIPTASE INHIBITORS
U-348	METHOD OF USE FOR INHIBITING HIV INFECTION
U-349	METHOD OF USE WHICH IS SUBJECT OF THE APPLICATION
U-350	PREPARATION OF A PHARMACEUTICAL COMPOSITION FOR CONCOMITANT ADMIN WITH A REVERSE TRANSCRIPTASE INHIBITOR
U-351	INHIBITING PROTEASE WITH LOPINAVIR AND INHIBITING AN HIV INFECTION WITH LOPINAVIR
U-352	INHIBITING HIV INFECTION BY ADMINISTERING RITONAVIR IN COMBINATION WITH A REVERSE TRAN-SCRIPTASE INHIBITOR
U-353	PREVENTION AND TREATMENT OF OSTEOPOROSIS
U-354	METHOD OF TREATING HYPERLIPIDEMIA WITH NICOTINIC ACID WITHOUT CAUSING TREATMENT-LIMITING ELEVATIONS IN URIC ACID OR GLUCOSE LEVELS OR CAUSING LIVER DAMAGE, BY DOSING ONCE PER DAY IN THE EVENING OR AT NIGHT
U-355	METHOD OF ASSISTING PERSON TO QUIT SMOKING...TRANSDERMALLY ADMIN NICOTINE VIA...PATCH AD-HERED TO SKIN AT DOSING RATE APPROX SAME AS ABSORBED FROM SMOKING
U-356	DELIVERING A MEDICINAL AEROSOL FORMULATION USING CFC-FREE PROPELLANT 134A

EXCLUSIVITY TERMS

PATENT USE (continued)

U-357	USE OF THE DRUG PRODUCT IN PHOTODYNAMIC THERAPEUTIC PROTOCOLS FOR THE TREATMENT OF AGE-RELATED MACULAR DEGENERATION AND RELATED CONDITIONS INVOLVING UNWANTED NEOVASCULATURE IN THE EYE
U-358	DEPRESSION, OBSESSIVE COMPULSIVE DISORDER, PANIC DISORDER AND SOCIAL ANXIETY DISORDER
U-359	METHOD OF USE OF VISICOL
U-360	METHOD OF TREATING A PATIENT SUFFERING FROM ANY OF A NUMBER OF PATHOLOGICAL PSYCHOLOGICAL CONDITIONS INCLUDING MENTAL DISORDERS EMPLOYING OLANZAPINE AS PER THE INDICATION WHICH IS THE SUBJECT MATTER OF THIS SNDA-011
U-361	MANAGEMENT OF ANXIETY DISORDERS AND THE SHORT-TERM RELIEF OF THE SYMPTOMS OF ANXIETY
U-362	USE OF APPROVED FORMULATIONS TO TREAT ALL APPROVED DISEASE INDICATIONS
U-363	METHOD OF TREATING A PATIENT SUFFERING FROM ANY OF A NUMBER OF PATHOLOGICAL PSYCHOLOGICAL CONDITIONS THAT RELATE TO THE USE OF A PSYCHOACTIVE SUBSTANCE EMPLOYING OLANZAPINE AS PER THE INDICATION WHICH IS THE SUBJECT MATER OF THIS SNDA-011
U-364	TREATING A PATIENT SUFFERING FROM OR SUSCEPTIBLE TO ANY NUMBER OF LISTED CONDITIONS INCLUDING PSYCHOSIS, EMPLOYING OLANZAPINE AS PER THE INDICATION WHICH IS THE SUBJECT MATTER OF THIS SNDA-011
U-365	METHOD FOR THE TREATMENT OF CARDIOVASCULAR DISEASE THROUGH THE ADMINISTRATION OF A CALCIUM BLOCKING VASODILATOR IN OUR EXTENDED, CONTROLLED RELEASE FORMULATION
U-366	METHOD FOR THE TREATMENT OF CARDIOVASCULAR DISEASE THROUGH THE ADMINISTRATION OF A CALCIUM BLOCKING VASODILATOR IN A DELAYED RELEASE FORMULATION
U-367	TREATMENT OF CARDIOVASCULAR DISORDERS
U-368	HEARTBURN
U-369	METHOD OF CONTROLLING AND LOWERING INTRAOCULAR PRESSURE
U-370	INTRAVAGINAL TREATMENT OF VAGINAL INFECTIONS WITH BUFFERED METRONIDAZOLE COMPOSITIONS
U-371	APPROVAL FOR MARKETING ONLY UNDER A SPECIAL RESTRICTION PROGRAM APPROVED BY FDA CALLED "SYSTEM FOR THALIDOMIDE EDUCATION AND PRESCRIBING SAFETY" (S.T.E.P.S.)
U-372	METHOD FOR ADMINISTERING A BENEFICIAL DRUG TO THE GI TRACT OF AN ANIMAL, WHICH METHOD COMPRISES ADMITTING AN OSMOTIC DEVICE ORALLY INTO THE ANIMAL...
U-373	GENERAL USE CLAIM SUBMITTED FOR 12 NEXIUM PATIENTS STATING "PERTINENT TO THE CAPSULE FORMULATION FOR NEXIUM AND ITS INDICATIONS FOR THE TREATMENT OFGERD AND ERADICATION OF H.PYLORI TO REDUCE THE RISK OF DUODENAL ULCER RECURRENCE
U-374	KIT ADAPTED AND DESIGNED TO PROVIDE BOTH DATA ON THE CURRENT REPRODUCTIVE STATUS OF A PATIENT AND CONTRACEPTION FOR THOSE WHO ARE NOT PREGNANT, BUT RECENTLY ENGAGED IN UNPROTECTED SEX
U-375	METHOD OF USING RIBAVIRIN FOR TREATING A DISEASE RESPONSIVE TO RIBAVIRIN, E.G. HEPATITIS C
U-376	TREATMENT OF INFLUENZA
U-377	METHOD OF TREATING PT WITH CHRONIC HEPATITIS C HAVING HCV GENOTYPE 1 AND VIRAL LOAD GREATER THAN 2 MILLION COPIES/ML TO ERADICATE DETECTABLE HCV-RNA BY ADMIN COMBINATION OF RIBAVIRIN AND INTERFERON ALFA-2B FOR A LEAST 24 WEEKS
U-378	METHOD FOR TREATING INCONTINENCE
U-379	METHOD OF TREATING ONYCHROMYCOSIS
U-380	COMBINATIONS OF TAXOL (PACLITAXEL) AND CISPLATIN WHICH ARE SUITABLE FOR THE TREATMENT OF OVARIAN AND NON-SMALL CELL LUNG CARCINOMAS
U-381	TREATMENT OF HYPERPHOSPHATEMIA
U-382	METHOD OF STABLIZING PROSTAGLANDIN
U-383	METHOD FOR TREATING GLAUCOMA AND OCULAR HYPERTENSION
U-384	TREATMENT OF CMV RETINITIS
U-385	TREATMENT OF PEPTIC ULCERS
U-386	TREATMENT OF PATIENTS SUFFERING FROM A LATE ASTHMATIC REACTION OR LATE PHASE ASTHMA
U-387	TREATMENT OF PATIENTS WITH RESPIRATORY DISORDERS
U-388	SMOKING CESSATION AID APPLIED TO THE SKIN
U-389	SMOKING CESSATION AID APPLIED TO THE SKIN ON WAKING AND REMOVED PRIOR TO SLEEP AFTER ABOUT 16 HOURS
U-390	METHOD OF USING THE DRUG TO TREAT NEUROIMMUNOLOGIC DISEASES (INCLUDING MULTIPLE SCLEROSIS)
U-391	USE OF CASODEX IN COMBINATION WITH LHRH AGONISTS FOR THE TREATMENT OF PROSTATE CANCER
U-392	TREATMENT OF PATIENTS FOR INFLAMMATION
U-393	MANAGEMENT OF INCONTINENCE, MGT OF HORMONE REPLACEMENT THERAPY, TREATMENT OF INVOLUNTARY INCONTINENCE, MGT OVERACTIVE BLADDER AND INCREASING COMPLIANCE IN SUCH PT
U-394	METHOD OF USE OF ALPHAGAN
U-395	METHOD OF USE OF ALPHAGAN P
U-396	METHOD OF TREATING PEOPLE SUFFERING FROM DEPRESSION
U-397	METHOD OF TREATING PEOPLE SUFFERING FROM DEPRESSION WITHOUT AN INCREASE IN NAUSEA
U-398	TREATMENT OF GENERALIZED ANXIETY DISORDER
U-399	IN-THE-EYE USE OF CHLORINE DIOXIDE CONTAINING COMPOSITIONS
U-400	USE OF RIBAVIRIN TO INCREASE TYPE 1 CYTOKINE RESPONSE AND SUPPRESS TYPE 2 CYTOKINE RESPONSE TO LYMPHOCYTES, INCLUDING METHODS THAT TAKE ADVANTAGE OF SUCH MODULATION TO TREAT INFECTIONS AND INFESTATIONS

EXCLUSIVITY TERMS

PATENT USE (continued)

U-401	USE OF LOPINAVIR IN COMBINATION WITH REVERSE TRANSCRIPTASE INHIBITORS FOR TREATING HIV INFECTION AND IN COMBO WITH OTHER HIV PROTEASE INHIBITORS
U-402	TREATMENT OF ACTINIC KERATOSES
U-403	ANTI-ALLERGIC FOR VARIOUS ALLERGIC DISEASES
U-404	TREATMENT OF ALLERGIC CONJUNCTIVITIS
U-405	METHOD OF USE OF LOTRONEX
U-406	METHOD OF USE OF ATOVAQUONE AND PROGUANIL
U-407	METHOD OF TREATING OTOPATHY
U-408	FOR INDUCING OVULATION IN CONJUNCTION WITH A GONADOTROPIN RELEASING FACTOR ANTAGONIST AND RECRUITING OOCYTES FOR IN-VITRO FERTILIZATION
U-409	METHOD OF TREATING INFLAMMATION USING DRUG SUBSTANCE
U-410	METHOD OF REDUCING AMOUNT OF RESPECTIVE ACTIVE COMPONENTS ADMINISTERED TO A DIABETIC PATIENT BY ADMINISTERING A CHEMICAL COMPOUND HAVING A PARTICULAR FORMULA (INCLUDING PIOGLITAZONE) IN COMBINATION WITH AN INSULIN SECRETION ENHANCER
U-411	METHOD OF REDUCING THE SIDE EFFECTS OF ACTIVE COMPONENTS ADMINISTERED TO A DIABETIC PATIENT BY ADMINISTERING A CHEMICAL COMPOUND HAVING A PARTICULAR FORMULA(WHICH INCLUDES PIOGLITAZONE) IN COMBINATION WITH AN INSULIN PREPARATION
U-412	TREATMENT OF TYPE 2 DIABETES
U-413	USE OF THE ACTIVE INGREDIENT FOR INHIBITING THE BIOSYNTHESIS OF CHOLESTEROL AND TREATMENT OF ATHEROSCLEROSIS
U-414	A METHOD OF TREATING GLYCOMETABOLISM DISORDERS BY ADMINISTERING AN INSULIN SENSITIVITY ENHANCER (INCLUDING PIOGLITAZONE) IN COMBINATION WITH A BIGUANIDE
U-415	A METHOD FOR REDUCING THE AMOUNT OF ACTIVE COMPONENTS ADMINISTERED TO A DIABETIC PATIENT BY ADMINISTERING AN INSULIN SENSITIVITY ENHANCER (INCLUDING PIOGLITAZONE) IN COMBINATION WITH A BIGUANIDE AS SAID ACTIVE COMPONENTS
U-416	A METHOD FOR REDUCING SIDE EFFECTS OF ACTIVE COMPONENTS ADMINISTERED TO A DIABETIC PATIENT BY ADMINISTERING AN INSULIN SENSITIVITY ENHANCER (INCLUDING PIOGLITAZONE) IN COMBINATION WITH A BIGUANIDE AS SAID ACTIVE COMPONENTS
U-417	COMBINATION USE OF AD-4833 WITH A BIGUANIDE
U-418	A METHOD OF TREATING LIPID METABOLISM DISORDERS BY ADMINISTERING A CHEMICAL COMPOUND HAVING A PARTICULAR FORMULA (WHICH INCLUDES PIOGLITAZONE) IN COMBINATION WITH AN INSULIN SECRETION ENHANCER
U-419	A METHOD OF TREATING LIPID METABOLISM DISORDERS BY ADMINISTERING AN INSULIN SENSITIVITY ENHANCER (INCLUDING PIOGLITAZONE) IN COMBINATION WITH A BIGUANIDE
U-420	METHOD OF TREATMENT OF TYPE II DIABETES
U-421	USE FOR SEDATION
U-422	METHOD OF TREATING AT LEAST ONE OF ATTENTION DEFICIT DISORDER AND ATTENTION DEFICIT HYPERACTIVITY DISORDER
U-423	METHOD OF TREATING AT LEAST ONE OF ATTENTION DEFICIT DISORDER, ATTENTION DEFICIT HYPERACTIVITY DISORDER, OR AIDS RELATED DEMENTIA
U-424	FOR ONCE DAILY, BOLUS ADMINISTRATION TO A PATIENT IN ORDER TO ENGENDER TREATMENT FOR A NERVOUS DISORDER FOR SUBSTANTIALLY AN ENTIRE DAY ON A CHRONIC BASIS
U-425	METHOD OF REDUCING SIDE EFFECTS OF ACTIVE COMPONENTS ADMIN TO A DIABETIC BY ADMIN A CHEMICAL COMPOUND HAVING FORMULA (INCL PIOGLITAZONE) IN COMBINATION WITH AN INSULIN SECRETION ENHANCER
U-426	PREVENTION OF PREMATURE LH SURGES IN WOMEN UNDERGOING CONTROLLED OVARIAN STIMULATION
U-427	METHOD OF TREATING ALLERGIC REACTIONS IN MAMMALS
U-428	METHOD OF TREATING ALLERGY IN A MAMMAL USING THIS ACTIVE METABOLITE
U-429	METHOD OF USING DESLORATADINE TO TREAT ALLERGIC RHINITIS
U-430	METHOD OF TREATING A DIABETIC BY ADMINISTERING AN INSULIN SENSITIZER IN COMBINATION WITH AN INSULIN SECRETION ENHANCER, AND A DRUG PRODUCT COMPRISING AN INSULIN SENSITIZER AND AN INSULIN SECRETION ENHANCER
U-431	POSTTRAUMATIC STRESS DISORDER
U-432	REDUCTION OF ATHEROSCLEROTIC EVENTS (MYOCARDIAL INFARCTION, STROKE, AND VASCULAR DEATH) IN PATIENTS WITH ATHEROSCLEROSIS DOCUMENTED BY RECENT STROKE, RECENT MYOCARDIAL INFARCTION, OR ESTABLISHED PERIPHERAL ARTERIAL DISEASE
U-433	USE OF LEVOCARITINE IN PREVENTION AND TREATMENT OF CARNITINE DEFICIENCY IN PATIENTS WITH END STAGE RENAL DISEASE WHO ARE UNDERGOING DIALYSIS
U-434	CONTROLLED SYMPTOMS OF DIARRHEA, BLOATING PRESSURE AND CRAMPS, COMMONLY REFERRED TO AS GAS
U-435	A TITRATION DOSING REGIMEN FOR THE TREATMENT OF PAIN USING AN INITIAL DOSE OF ABOUT 25MG
U-436	ACUTE TREATMENT OF MIGRAINE ATTACKS WITH OR WITHOUT AURA IN ADULTS
U-437	METHOD OF USE EQUAL TO PROCESS OF PREPARATION
U-438	TREATMENT/PREVENTION OF NEURODEGENERATIVE DISEASE
U-439	TREATMENT OF OBESITY
U-440	METHOD FOR TRANSDERMAL ADMINISTRATION OF A DRUG THROUGH NON-SCROTAL SKIN USING A TRANSDERMAL DRUG DELIVERY DEVICE CONTAINING THE DRUG AND HAVING AN ADHESIVE SURFACE

EXCLUSIVITY TERMS

PATENT USE (continued)

U-441	METHOD OF TREATING MS BY ADMINISTERING COPAXONE
U-442	METHOD FOR DELIVERING A DRUG TO A PATIENT IN NEED OF THE DRUG, WHILE AVOIDING THE OCCURENCE OF AN ADVERSE SIDE EFFECT KNOWN OR SUSPECTED OF BEING CAUSED BY SAID DRUG
U-443	MANAGEMENT OF MODERATE TO SEVERE PAIN WHEN A CONTINUOUS, AROUND-THE-CLOCK ANALGESIC IS NEEDED FOR AN EXTENDED PERIOD OF TIME
U-444	METHOD OF TREATING
U-445	USE AS AN ANTIMYCOTIC AGENT
U-446	TOPICAL TREATMENT OF OCULAR HYPERTENSION AND GLAUCOMA
U-447	METHOD OF TREATING HYPERLIPIDEMIA WITH NICOTINIC ACID BY DOSING ONCE PER DAY IN THE EVENING OR AT NIGHT
U-448	METHOD OF TREATING HYPERLIPIDEMIA WITH NICOTINIC ACID WITHOUT CAUSING TREATMENT- LIMITING ELEVATIONS IN URIC ACID OR GLUCOSE LEVELS OR CAUSING LIVER DAMAGE, BY DOSING ONCE PER DAY IN THE EVENING OR AT NIGHT
U-449	USE IN COMBINATION WITH 5-FLUOROURACIL AND LEUCOVORIN FOR THE TREATMENT OF METASTATIC COLORECTAL CANCER WHERE THE DOSE OF LEUCOVORIN IS AT LEAST 200MG PER SQUARE METER
U-450	INTERMEDIATE REL NICOTINIC ACID FORMULATIONS HAVING UNIQUE URINARY METAB PROFILES RESULTING FROM ABSORPTION PROFILES OF NICOTINIC ACID FROM THE INTERMEDIATE NICOTINIC ACID FORMULATIONS, SUITABLE FOR TX HYPERLIPIDEMIA FOLLOWING QD DOSING
U-451	TREATMENT OF DEPRESSION AND GENERALIZED ANXIETY DISORDER
U-452	USE OF LANSOPRAZOLE FOR COMBATTING DISEASES CAUSED BY THE GENUS CAMPYLOBACTER (C.PYLORI=H.PYLORI)
U-453	TREATMENT OF PLATELET ASSOCIATED ISCHEMIC DISORDERS
U-454	METHOD OF TX A PT SUSPECTED OF HAVING HEPATITIS C BY ADMIN, IN COMBINATION, A CONJUGATE COMPRISING PEG 12000 & INTERFERON ALFA-2B IN AN AMT OF FROM 0.5MCG/KG TO 2MCG/KG, ONCE WEEKLY, AND RIBAVIRIN
U-455	TREATMENT OF PULMONARY HYPERTENSION WITH UT-15
U-456	METHOD OF DECREASING THE PRODUCTION OF A-BETA USING A COMPOSITION WHICH DECREASES BLOOD CHOLESTEROL IN PATIENTS AT RISK OF OR EXHIBITING SYMPTOMS OF ALZHEIMER'S DISEASE
U-457	METHOD OF TREATING A VAGINAL FUNGAL INFECTION IN A FEMALE HUMAN
U-458	METHOD OF USE OF IMAGENT
U-459	TREATMENT OF DEPRESSION AND GENERALIZED ANXIETY DISORDER
U-460	METHOD OF TREATING PSYCHIATRIC SYMPTOMS ASSOCIATED WITH PREMENSTRUAL DISORDERS USING SERTRALINE
U-461	METHOD OF TREATMENT OF LATE LUTEAL PHASE DYSPHORIC DISORDER (PMDD) USING SERTRALINE
U-462	SIGNS AND SYMPTOMS OF OSTEOARTHRITIS AND ADULT RHEUMATOID ARTHRITIS AND TREATMENT OF PRIMARY DYSMENORRHEA
U-463	VENOGRAPHY
U-464	PERIPHERAL ARTERIOGRAPHY
U-465	CT IMAGING OF THE HEAD
U-466	TREATMENT OF IRRITABLE BOWEL SYNDROME
U-467	USE OF EPLERENONE IN COMBINATION WITH AN ANGIOTENSIN CONVERTING ENZYME (ACE) INHIBITOR FOR TREATING HYPERTENSION
U-468	METHOD OF USING FEXOFENADINE HCL IN TREATING ALLERGIC RHINITIS
U-469	TREATMENT OF GASTROESOPHAGEAL REFLEX DISEASE (GERD) AND ERADICATION OF H.PYLORI TO REDUCE RISK OF DUODENAL ULCER RECURRENCE
U-470	THERAPY IN CHRONIC HEPATITIS B VIRUS INFECTION
U-471	METHOD OF TREATING A PATIENT SUFFERING FROM DIABETES MELLITUS
U-472	TREATMENT OF ATTENTION DEFICIT HYPERACTIVITY DISORDER USING METHYLPHENIDATE BI-MODAL RELEASE PROFILE EXTENDED-RELEASE CAPSULES
U-473	TO REDUCE PLASMA CHOLESTEROL LEVELS IN A MAMMAL
U-474	TO REDUCE PLASMA CHOLESTEROL LEVELS BY ADMIN EZETIMIBE IN COMBO WITH CHOLESTERO BIOSYNTHESIS INHIB SELECTED FROM GROUP CONSISTING OF HMG COA REDUCTASE INHIBITORS INCL SIMVASTATIN
U-475	TREATMENT OF CUTANEOUS MANIFESTATIONS OF CUTANEOUS T-CELL LYMPHOMA IN PATIENTS WHO ARE REFRACTORY TO AT LEAST ONE PRIOR SYSTEMIC THERAPY
U-476	METHOD OF TREATING ANDROGEN RESPONSIVE/MEDIATED CONDITION IN MAMMAL BY ADMIN A SAFE, EFFECTIVE AMOUNT OF DUTASTERIDE OR PHARMACEUTICALLY ACCEPTABLE DERIVATIVE THEREOF..- CONDITIONS INCLUDE BENIGN PROSTATIC HYPERTROPHY
U-477	METHOD OF INHIBITING 5 ALPHA TESTOSTERONE REDUCTASE ENZYME WITH DUTASTERIDE OR ITS DERIVATIVE AND TREATING ANDROGEN RESPONSIVE/MEDIATED DISEASE INCLUDING BENIGN PROSTATIC HYPERPLASIA
U-478	METHOD OF TREATING HEPATITIS C VIRAL INFECTION BY CONTINUOUS PARENTERAL ADMIN INTERFERON ALPHA 2-10 MILLION IU WEEKLY, SUBCUTANEOUSLY, INJECTION OF POLYMER-INTERFERONALPHA CONJUGATE-POLYMER IS PEG-INTERFERON IS ALPHA 2B
U-479	METHOD OF USING PEG-INTRON/REBETOL COMBINATION THERAPY AND INTRON/REBETOL COMBINATION THERAPY
U-480	CONTRAST AGENT FOR MRI

EXCLUSIVITY TERMS

PATENT USE (continued)

U-481	DISUBSTITUTED ACETYLENES BEARING HETEROAROMATIC AND HETEROBICYCLIC GROUPS HAVING RETINOID-LIKE ACTIVITY
U-482	METHOD OF IN VITRO FERTILIZATION THERAPY INCLUDING MEANS FOR INDUCING OVULATION....
U-483	METHOD FOR THE ADMINISTRATION OF DRUGS USING THAT COMPOUND
U-484	METHOD OF TREATING A SKIN DISEASE WITH A CORTICOSTEROID-CONTAINING PHARMACEUTICAL COMPOSITION
U-485	METHOD AND COMPOSITION FOR REDUCING NERVE INJURY PAIN ASSOCIATED WITH SHINGLES (HERPES ZOSTER AND POST-HERPETIC NEURALGIA)
U-486	EXTERNAL PREPARATION FOR APPLICATION TO THE SKIN CONTAINING LIDOCAINE-DRUG RETAINING LAYER PLACED ON SUPPORT AND COMPRISES ADHESIVE GEL BASE 1-10% BY WEIGHT OF LIDOCAINE
U-487	METHOD AND COMPOSITION FOR REDUCING NERVE INJURY PAIN ASSOCIATED WITH SHINGLES (HERPES ZOSTER AND POST-HERPETIC NEURALGIA)
U-488	METHOD FOR REDUCING THE PAIN ASSOCIATED WITH HERPES-ZOSTER AND POST-HERPETIC NEURALGIA
U-489	EXPECTORANT
U-490	TESTOSTERONE REPLACEMENT THERAPY IN MALES FOR CONDITIONS ASSOCIATED WITH A DEFICIENCY OR ABSENCE OF ENDOGENOUS TESTOSTERONE
U-491	METHOD OF DELIVERING A DRUG TO THE LUNG
U-492	METHOD FOR THE TREATMENT OF SKIN, SUFFERING FROM A CONDITION SELECTED FROM A GROUP CONSISTING OF NONACNE INFLAMMATORY DERMATOSES... COMPRISING APPLYING TO AFFECTED AREA. A THERAPEUTICALLY EFFECTIVE AMT AZELAIC ACID
U-493	TREATMENT OF TYPE 2 DIABETES MELLITUS
U-494	TREATMENT OF ATTENTION-DEFICIT HYPERACTIVITY DISORDER
U-495	PERITONEAL DIALYSIS SOLUTION
U-496	METHOD FOR TREATING CHRONIC RENAL FAILURE
U-497	RELIEF OF THE SIGNS AND SYMPTOMS OF OSTEOARTHRITIS AND RHEUMATOID ARTHRITIS
U-498	INTRA-ARTERIAL AND INTRAVENOUS USES OF ULTRAVIST
U-499	METHOD OF USING REBETOL CAPSULES IN COMBINATION WITH A CONJUGATE COMPRISING POLYETHYLENE GLYCOL(PEG) AND AN ALPHA INTERFERON, INCLUDING, FOR EXAMPLE, PEG-INTRON POWDER FOR INJECTION
U-500	USE AS AN ANTIHYPERTENSIVE AGENT
U-501	TREATMENT OF RECURRENT HERPES LABIALIS (COLD SORES) IN ADULTS
U-502	PITYRIASIS VERSICOLOR
U-503	GENERATOR MUST BE USED WITH INFUSION SYSTEM SPECIFICALLY LABELED FOR USE WITH GENERATOR
U-504	TINEA PEDIS, TINEA CRURIS, TINEA CORPORIS
U-505	ULTRASOUND CONTRAST AGENT
U-506	PHARM PRODUCT CONTAINER 1ST CHAMBER IS DISPOSED AQUEOUS DILUENT SOL 2ND CHAMBER PHARM ACTIVE AGENT COMPRISING ACETYLCHOLINE,BUFFER IN 1ST CHAM IS SUFFICIENT TO BUFFER PH OF MIXED SOL RESULTING MIXTURE OF AQUEOUS DILUENT SOL & PHARM ACTIVE.
U-507	ACROMEGALY IN PATIENTS W/INADEQUATE RESPONSE TO SURGERY AND/OR RADIATION THERAPY AND/OR MEDICAL THERAPIES, OR FOR WHOM THESE THERAPIES ARE NOT APPROPRIATE
U-508	METHOD OF RELEASING 17-BETA OESTRADIOL PRECURSOR IN A SUBSTANTIALLY ZERO ORDER PATTERN FOR AT LEAST THREE WEEKS
U-509	TREATMENT OF CUTANEOUS MANIFESTATIONS OF CUTANEIOUS T-CELL LYMPHOMA IN PATIENTS WHO ARE REFRACTORY TO AT LEAST ONE PRIOR SYSTEMIC THERAPY
U-510	TOPICAL TREATMENT OF CUTANEOUS LESIONS IN PATIENTS WITH CUTANEOUS T-CELL LYMPHOMA (STAGE IA AND IB) WHO HAVE REFRACTORY OR PERSISTENT DISEASE AFTER OTHER THERAPIES OR WHO HAVE NOT TOLERATED OTHER THERAPIES
U-511	USE OF QUINOLONE COMPOUNDS AGAINST ANAEROBIC PATHOGENIC BACTERIA
U-512	USE OF QUINOLONE COMPOUNDS AGAINST ATYPICAL UPPER RESPIRATORY PATHOGENIC BACTERIA
U-513	METHODS OF USE OF ANTIMICROBIAL COMPOUNDS AGAINST PATHOGENIC AMYCOPLASMA BACTERIA
U-514	PREVENTION OF OVULATION IN A WOMAN
U-515	TREATMENT OF MULTIPLE MYELOMA PATIENTS WHO HAVE RECEIVED AT LEAST TWO PRIOR THERAPIES AND HAVE DEMONSTRATED DISEASE PROGRESSION ON THE LAST THERAPY
U-516	METHOD OF TREATING A PSYCHOTIC DISEASE
U-517	STABLE GEL FORMULATION FOR TOPICAL TREATMENT OF SKIN CONDITIONS

PRESCRIPTION AND OTC PRODUCT
PATENT AND EXCLUSIVITY DATA
*PED and PED represent Pediatric Exclusivity

APPL/PROD NUMBER	INGREDIENT NAME; TRADE NAME	PATENT NUMBER	PATENT EXPIRES	USE CODE	EX-CLUS CODE	EXCLUS EXPIRES
021205 001	ABACAVIR SULFATE; TRIZIVIR	4724232	SEP 17,2005		PED	JUN 17,2004
		4818538	SEP 17,2005		PED	JUN 17,2004
		4828838	SEP 17,2005		PED	JUN 17,2004
		4833130	SEP 17,2005		PED	JUN 17,2004
		4837208	SEP 17,2005		PED	JUN 17,2004
		5034394	JUN 26,2009		PED	JUN 17,2004
		5034394*PED	DEC 26,2009		PED	JUN 17,2004
		5047407	NOV 17,2009		PED	JUN 17,2004
		5047407*PED	MAY 17,2010		PED	JUN 17,2004
		5089500	JUN 26,2009	U-248	PED	JUN 17,2004
		5089500*PED	DEC 26,2009	U-248	PED	JUN 17,2004
		5905082	MAY 18,2016		PED	JUN 17,2004
		5905082*PED	NOV 18,2016		PED	JUN 17,2004
		6180639	JAN 30,2018	U-248	PED	JUN 17,2004
		6180639*PED	JUL 30,2018	U-248	PED	JUN 17,2004
		6294540	MAY 14,2018	U-65	PED	JUN 17,2004
		6294540*PED	NOV 14,2018	U-65	PED	JUN 17,2004
		6417191	MAR 28,2016	U-248	PED	JUN 17,2004
020977 001	ABACAVIR SULFATE; ZIAGEN	5034394	DEC 18,2011		NCE	DEC 17,2003
		5034394*PED	JUN 18,2012		NCE	DEC 17,2003
		5089500	JUN 26,2009	U-248	NCE	DEC 17,2003
		5089500*PED	DEC 26,2009		NCE	DEC 17,2003
		6294540	MAY 14,2018	U-65	NCE	DEC 17,2003
		6294540*PED	NOV 14,2018	U-65	NCE	DEC 17,2003
020978 001	ABACAVIR SULFATE; ZIAGEN	5034394	DEC 18,2011		NCE	DEC 17,2003
		5034394*PED	JUN 18,2012		NCE	DEC 17,2003
		5089500	JUN 26,2009	U-248	NCE	DEC 17,2003
		5089500*PED	DEC 26,2009		NCE	DEC 17,2003
		6294540	MAY 14,2018	U-65	NCE	DEC 17,2003
		6294540*PED	NOV 14,2018	U-65	NCE	DEC 17,2003
020482 001	ACARBOSE; PRECOSE	4904769	FEB 27,2007			
020482 002	ACARBOSE; PRECOSE	4904769	FEB 27,2007			
020482 004	ACARBOSE; PRECOSE	4904769	FEB 27,2007			
020802 001	ACETAMINOPHEN; EXCEDRIN (MIGRAINE)	4943565	JUL 24,2007			
		5972916	JUL 14,2017	U-296		
021082 001	ACETAMINOPHEN; TAVIST ALLERGY/SINUS/ HEADACHE				NC	MAR 01,2004
019872 001	ACETAMINOPHEN; TYLENOL (CAPLET)	4820522	JUL 27,2007			
		4968509	NOV 06,2007			
		5004613	JUL 27,2007			
021123 001	ACETAMINOPHEN; ULTRACET	5336691	AUG 09,2011		NC	AUG 15,2004
020213 001	ACETYLCHOLINE CHLORIDE; MIOCHOL-E	6261546	APR 29,2019	U-506		
019806 001	ACRIVASTINE; SEMPREX-D	4501893	FEB 01,2003			
		4650807	MAR 26,2008	U-93		
021478 001	ACYCLOVIR; ZOVIRAX				NDF	DEC 30,2005
020338 001	ADAPALENE; DIFFERIN	4717720	MAY 31,2010			
		RE34440	MAR 31,2010	U-275		
020380 001	ADAPALENE; DIFFERIN	4717720	MAY 31,2010			
		RE34440	MAY 31,2010	U-275		
020748 001	ADAPALENE; DIFFERIN	4717720	MAY 31,2010		NDF	MAY 26,2003
		RE34440	MAY 31,2010	U-275	NDF	MAY 26,2003
021449 001	ADEFOVIR DIPIVOXIL; HEPSERA	4724233	APR 21,2006	U-470	NCE	SEP 20,2007
		4808716	APR 25,2006		NCE	SEP 20,2007
		5663159	SEP 02,2014	U-470	NCE	SEP 20,2007
		6451340	JUL 23,2018	U-470	NCE	SEP 20,2007
019937 002	ADENOSINE; ADENOCARD	4673563	JUN 16,2004	U-38		
020059 001	ADENOSINE; ADENOSCAN	5070877	MAY 18,2009	U-116		
		5731296	MAR 24,2015	U-221		
020760 001	ALATROFLOXACIN MESYLATE; TROVAN PRESERVATIVE FREE	5164402	NOV 17,2009	U-282	NCE	DEC 18,2002
		5763454	JUN 15,2015	U-282	NCE	DEC 18,2002
		6080756	JUL 05,2016		NCE	DEC 18,2002
		6194429	JUL 23,2018		NCE	DEC 18,2002
020760 002	ALATROFLOXACIN MESYLATE; TROVAN PRESERVATIVE FREE	5164402	NOV 17,2009	U-282	NCE	DEC 18,2002
		5763454	JUN 15,2015	U-282	NCE	DEC 18,2002
		6080756	JUL 05,2016		NCE	DEC 18,2002
		6194429	JUL 23,2018		NCE	DEC 18,2002

PRESCRIPTION AND OTC PRODUCT
PATENT AND EXCLUSIVITY DATA
*PED and PED represent Pediatric Exclusivity (*continued*)

APPL/PROD NUMBER	INGREDIENT NAME; TRADE NAME	PATENT NUMBER	PATENT EXPIRES	USE CODE	EX-CLUS CODE	EXCLUS EXPIRES
020666 001	ALBENDAZOLE; ALBENZA				ODE	JUN 11,2003
020899 001	ALBUMIN HUMAN; OPTISON	5529766	JUN 25,2013	U-505		
		5558094	FEB 28,2012	U-505		
		5573751	APR 25,2012			
020949 001	ALBUTEROL SULFATE; ACCUNEB				NP	APR 30,2004
020949 002	ALBUTEROL SULFATE; ACCUNEB				NP	APR 30,2004
020291 001	ALBUTEROL SULFATE; COMBIVENT	5603918	JUN 09,2015			
020950 001	ALBUTEROL SULFATE; DUONEB				NP	MAR 21,2004
018062 001	ALBUTEROL SULFATE; PROVENTIL	4499108	JUN 08,2003			
020503 001	ALBUTEROL SULFATE; PROVENTIL-HFA	5225183	JUL 06,2010			
		5439670	JUL 06,2010			
		5605674	FEB 25,2014			
		5695743	JUL 06,2010	U-491		
		5766573	JUN 16,2015			
		6352684	NOV 28,2009			
019621 001	ALBUTEROL SULFATE; VENTOLIN	4594359	JUN 10,2003			
020983 001	ALBUTEROL SULFATE; VENTOLIN HFA	6251368	DEC 04,2012			
019604 001	ALBUTEROL SULFATE; VOLMAX	4751071	JUN 14,2005			
		4777049	OCT 11,2005			
		4851229	JUN 14,2005			
019604 002	ALBUTEROL SULFATE; VOLMAX	4751071	JUN 14,2005			
		4777049	OCT 11,2005			
		4851229	JUN 14,2005			
021074 001	ALCOHOL; AVAGARD	5897031	JUN 21,2016		NC	JUN 07,2004
020560 001	ALENDRONATE SODIUM; FOSAMAX	4621077	AUG 06,2007	U-114	I-309	SEP 29,2003
		4621077*PED	FEB 06,2008	U-114	I-309	SEP 29,2003
		5358941	DEC 02,2012		I-309	SEP 29,2003
		5358941*PED	JUN 02,2013		I-309	SEP 29,2003
		5681590	DEC 02,2012		I-309	SEP 29,2003
		5681590*PED	JUN 02,2013		I-309	SEP 29,2003
		5849726	JUN 06,2015		I-309	SEP 29,2003
		5849726*PED	DEC 06,2015		I-309	SEP 29,2003
		6008207	JUN 06,2015	U-303	I-309	SEP 29,2003
		6008207*PED	DEC 06,2015	U-303	I-309	SEP 29,2003
		6090410	DEC 02,2012		I-309	SEP 29,2003
		6090410*PED	JUN 02,2013		I-309	SEP 29,2003
		6194004	DEC 02,2012		I-309	SEP 29,2003
		6194004*PED	JUN 02,2013		I-309	SEP 29,2003
020560 002	ALENDRONATE SODIUM; FOSAMAX	4621077	AUG 06,2007	U-114	M-3	NOV 24,2002
		4621077*PED	FEB 06,2008	U-114	M-3	NOV 24,2002
		5358941	DEC 02,2012		M-3	NOV 24,2002
		5358941*PED	JUN 02,2013		M-3	NOV 24,2002
		5681590	DEC 02,2012		M-3	NOV 24,2002
		5681590*PED	JUN 02,2013		M-3	NOV 24,2002
		5849726	JUN 06,2015		M-3	NOV 24,2002
		5849726*PED	DEC 06,2015		M-3	NOV 24,2002
		6008207	JUN 06,2015	U-303	M-3	NOV 24,2002
		6008207*PED	JUN 06,2015	U-303	M-3	NOV 24,2002
		6090410	DEC 02,2012		M-3	NOV 24,2002
		6090410*PED	JUN 02,2013		M-3	NOV 24,2002
020560 003	ALENDRONATE SODIUM; FOSAMAX	4621077	AUG 06,2007	U-114	M-3	NOV 24,2002
		4621077*PED	FEB 06,2008	U-114	M-3	NOV 24,2002
		5358941	DEC 02,2012		M-3	NOV 24,2002
		5358941*PED	JUN 02,2013		M-3	NOV 24,2002
		5681590	DEC 02,2012		M-3	NOV 24,2002
		5681590*PED	JUN 02,2013		M-3	NOV 24,2002
		5849726	JUN 06,2015		M-3	NOV 24,2002
		5849726*PED	DEC 06,2015		M-3	NOV 24,2002
		6008207	JUN 06,2015	U-303	M-3	NOV 24,2002
		6008207*PED	DEC 06,2015	U-303	M-3	NOV 24,2002
		6090410	DEC 02,2012		M-3	NOV 24,2002
		6090410*PED	JUN 02,2013		M-3	NOV 24,2002
020560 004	ALENDRONATE SODIUM; FOSAMAX	4621077	AUG 06,2007	U-114	PED	APR 20,2004
		4621077*PED	FEB 06,2008	U-114	PED	APR 20,2004
		5358941	DEC 02,2012		PED	APR 20,2004
		5358941*PED	JUN 02,2013		PED	APR 20,2004
		5681590	DEC 02,2012		PED	APR 20,2004
		5681590*PED	JUN 02,2013		PED	APR 20,2004
		5849726	JUN 06,2015		PED	APR 20,2004
		5849726*PED	DEC 16,2015		PED	APR 20,2004
		5994329	JUL 17,2018		PED	APR 20,2004

PRESCRIPTION AND OTC PRODUCT
PATENT AND EXCLUSIVITY DATA
PED and PED represent Pediatric Exclusivity (continued)

APPL/PROD NUMBER	INGREDIENT NAME; TRADE NAME	PATENT NUMBER	PATENT EXPIRES	USE CODE	EX- CLUS CODE	EXCLUS EXPIRES
		5994329*PED	JAN 17,2019		PED	APR 20,2004
		6008207	JUN 06,2015		PED	APR 20,2004
		6008207*PED	DEC 06,2015		PED	APR 20,2004
		6015801	JUL 17,2018	U-353	PED	APR 20,2004
		6015801*PED	JAN 17,2019	U-353	PED	APR 20,2004
		6090410	DEC 02,2012		PED	APR 20,2004
		6090410*PED	JUN 02,2013		PED	APR 20,2004
		6225294	JUL 17,2018		PED	APR 20,2004
		6225294*PED	JAN 17,2019		PED	APR 20,2004
020560 005	ALENDRONATE SODIUM; FOSAMAX	4621077	AUG 06,2007	U-114	D-62	OCT 20,2003
		4621077*PED	FEB 06,2008	U-114	D-62	OCT 20,2003
		5358941	DEC 02,2012		D-62	OCT 20,2003
		5358941*PED	JUN 02,2013		D-62	OCT 20,2003
		5681590	DEC 02,2012		D-62	OCT 20,2003
		5681590*PED	JUN 02,2013		D-62	OCT 20,2003
		5849726	JUN 06,2015		D-62	OCT 20,2003
		5849726*PED	DEC 06,2015		D-62	OCT 20,2003
		5994329	JUL 17,2018		D-62	OCT 20,2003
		5994329*PED	JAN 17,2019		D-62	OCT 20,2003
		6008207	JUN 06,2015		D-62	OCT 20,2003
		6008207*PED	DEC 06,2015		D-62	OCT 20,2003
		6015801	JUL 17,2018	U-353	D-62	OCT 20,2003
		6015801*PED	JAN 17,2019	U-353	D-62	OCT 20,2003
		6090410	DEC 02,2012		D-62	OCT 20,2003
		6090410*PED	JUN 02,2013		D-62	OCT 20,2003
		6225294	JUL 17,2018		D-62	OCT 20,2003
		6225294*PED	JAN 17,2019		D-62	OCT 20,2003
021287 001	ALFUZOSIN HYDROCHLORIDE; UROXATRAL	4661491	MAY 27,2006		NCE	JUN 12,2008
		6149940	AUG 22,2017		NCE	JUN 12,2008
020886 001	ALITRETINOIN; PANRETIN				NCE	FEB 02,2004
020298 001	ALLOPURINOL SODIUM; ALOPRIM				ODE	MAY 17,2003
021001 001	ALMOTRIPTAN MALATE; AXERT	5565447	OCT 15,2013		NCE	MAY 07,2006
021001 002	ALMOTRIPTAN MALATE; AXERT	5565447	OCT 15,2013		NCE	MAY 07,2006
021107 001	ALOSETRON HYDROCHLORIDE; LOTRONEX	5360800	FEB 02,2010		NCE	FEB 09,2005
		6284770	OCT 05,2018	U-405	NCE	FEB 09,2005
018276 001	ALPRAZOLAM; XANAX	4508726	SEP 16,2002	U-46		
018276 002	ALPRAZOLAM; XANAX	4508726	SEP 16,2002	U-46		
018276 003	ALPRAZOLAM; XANAX	4508726	SEP 16,2002	U-46		
018276 004	ALPRAZOLAM; XANAX	4508726	SEP 16,2002	U-46		
		5061494	OCT 29,2008			
021434 001	ALPRAZOLAM; XANAX XR				NDF	JAN 17,2006
021434 002	ALPRAZOLAM; XANAX XR				NDF	JAN 17,2006
021434 003	ALPRAZOLAM; XANAX XR				NDF	JAN 17,2006
021434 004	ALPRAZOLAM; XANAX XR				NDF	JAN 17,2006
020379 001	ALPROSTADIL; CAVERJECT	5741523	APR 21,2015			
020379 002	ALPROSTADIL; CAVERJECT	5741523	APR 21,2015			
020379 003	ALPROSTADIL; CAVERJECT	5741523	APR 21,2015			
020379 004	ALPROSTADIL; CAVERJECT	5741523	APR 21,2015			
021212 001	ALPROSTADIL; CAVERJECT				NP	JUN 11,2005
021212 002	ALPROSTADIL; CAVERJECT				NP	JUN 11,2005
020700 001	ALPROSTADIL; MUSE	4801587	JAN 31,2007	U-155		
		5242391	SEP 07,2010	U-155		
		5474535	DEC 12,2012	U-155		
020700 002	ALPROSTADIL; MUSE	4801587	JAN 31,2007	U-155		
		5242391	SEP 07,2010	U-155		
		5474535	DEC 12,2012	U-155		
020700 003	ALPROSTADIL; MUSE	4801587	JAN 31,2007	U-155		
		5242391	SEP 07,2010	U-155		
		5474535	DEC 12,2012	U-155		
020700 004	ALPROSTADIL; MUSE	4801587	JAN 31,2007	U-155		
		5242391	SEP 07,2010	U-155		
		5474535	DEC 12,2012	U-155		
020221 001	AMIFOSTINE; ETHYOL	5424471	JUL 31,2012		ODE	DEC 08,2002
		5591731	JUL 31,2012		ODE	DEC 08,2002
		5994409	DEC 08,2017	U-305	ODE	DEC 08,2002
020221 002	AMIFOSTINE; ETHYOL	5424471	JUL 31,2012		ODE	DEC 08,2002
		5591731	JUL 31,2012		ODE	DEC 08,2002
		5994409	DEC 08,2017	U-305	ODE	DEC 08,2002
020965 001	AMINOLEVULINIC ACID HYDROCHLORIDE; LEVULAN	5079262	JUL 28,2009	U-289	NCE	DEC 03,2004
		5211938	MAY 18,2010	U-289	NCE	DEC 03,2004

PRESCRIPTION AND OTC PRODUCT
PATENT AND EXCLUSIVITY DATA
*PED and PED represent Pediatric Exclusivity (continued)

APPL/PROD NUMBER	INGREDIENT NAME; TRADE NAME	PATENT NUMBER	PATENT EXPIRES	USE CODE	EX-CLUS CODE	EXCLUS EXPIRES
		5422093	JUL 28,2009	U-289	NCE	DEC 03,2004
		5954703	OCT 31,2017	U-289	NCE	DEC 03,2004
020377 001	AMIODARONE HYDROCHLORIDE; CORDARONE				ODE	AUG 03,2002
020511 001	AMLEXANOX; APHTHASOL	5362737	NOV 08,2011	U-243		
020364 002	AMLODIPINE BESYLATE; LOTREL	4410520	AUG 11,2003			
		4410520*PED	FEB 11,2004			
		4572909	JUL 31,2006			
		4879303	MAR 25,2007			
		6162802	DEC 19,2017	U-367		
020364 003	AMLODIPINE BESYLATE; LOTREL	4410520	AUG 11,2003			
		4410520*PED	FEB 11,2004			
		4572909	JUL 31,2006			
		4879303	MAR 25,2007			
		6162802	DEC 19,2017	U-367		
020364 004	AMLODIPINE BESYLATE; LOTREL	4410520	AUG 11,2003			
		4410520*PED	FEB 11,2004			
		4572909	JUL 31,2006			
		4879303	MAR 25,2007			
		6162802	DEC 19,2017	U-367		
020364 005	AMLODIPINE BESYLATE; LOTREL	4410520	AUG 11,2003		PED	DEC 20,2005
		4410520*PED	FEB 11,2004		PED	DEC 20,2005
		4572909	JUL 31,2006		PED	DEC 20,2005
		4879303	MAR 25,2007		PED	DEC 20,2005
		6162802	DEC 19,2017	U-367	PED	DEC 20,2005
019787 001	AMLODIPINE BESYLATE; NORVASC	4572909	JUL 31,2006			
		4572909*PED	JAN 31,2007			
		4879303	MAR 25,2007			
		4879303*PED	SEP 25,2007			
019787 002	AMLODIPINE BESYLATE; NORVASC	4572909	JUL 31,2006			
		4572909*PED	JAN 31,2007			
		4879303	MAR 25,2007			
		4879303*PED	SEP 25,2007			
019787 003	AMLODIPINE BESYLATE; NORVASC	4572909	JUL 31,2006			
		4572909*PED	JAN 31,2007			
		4879303	MAR 25,2007			
		4879303*PED	SEP 25,2007			
020508 001	AMMONIUM LACTATE; LAC-HYDRIN				PED	FEB 25,2004
011522 007	AMPHETAMINE ASPARTATE; ADDERALL 10	6384020	JUL 06,2020			
011522 012	AMPHETAMINE ASPARTATE; ADDERALL 12.5	6384020	JUL 06,2020			
011522 013	AMPHETAMINE ASPARTATE; ADDERALL 15	6384020	JUL 06,2020			
011522 008	AMPHETAMINE ASPARTATE; ADDERALL 20	6384020	JUL 06,2020			
011522 010	AMPHETAMINE ASPARTATE; ADDERALL 30	6384020	JUL 06,2020			
011522 009	AMPHETAMINE ASPARTATE; ADDERALL 5	6384020	JUL 06,2020			
011522 011	AMPHETAMINE ASPARTATE; ADDERALL 7.5	6384020	JUL 06,2020			
021303 001	AMPHETAMINE ASPARTATE; ADDERALL XR 10	6322819	OCT 21,2018		NDF	OCT 11,2004
021303 006	AMPHETAMINE ASPARTATE; ADDERALL XR 15	6322819	OCT 21,2018		NDF	OCT 11,2004
021303 002	AMPHETAMINE ASPARTATE; ADDERALL XR 20	6322819	OCT 21,2018		NDF	OCT 11,2004
021303 004	AMPHETAMINE ASPARTATE; ADDERALL XR 25	6322819	OCT 21,2018		NDF	OCT 11,2004
021303 003	AMPHETAMINE ASPARTATE; ADDERALL XR 30	6322819	OCT 21,2018		NDF	OCT 11,2004
021303 005	AMPHETAMINE ASPARTATE; ADDERALL XR 5	6322819	OCT 21,2018		NDF	OCT 11,2004
040422 005	AMPHETAMINE ASPARTATE; DEXTROAMP SACCHARATE, AMP ASPARTATE, DEXTROAMP SULFATE AND AMP SULFATE				PC	SEP 15,2003
040422 006	AMPHETAMINE ASPARTATE; DEXTROAMP SACCHARATE, AMP ASPARTATE, DEXTROAMP SULFATE AND AMP SULFATE				PC	SEP 15,2003
040422 007	AMPHETAMINE ASPARTATE; DEXTROAMP SACCHARATE, AMP ASPARTATE, DEXTROAMP SULFATE AND AMP SULFATE				PC	SEP 15,2003
050724 001	AMPHOTERICIN B; ABELCET				ODE	OCT 18,2003
050740 001	AMPHOTERICIN B; AMBISOME				ODE	AUG 11,2004
021007 001	AMPRENAVIR; AGENERASE	5585397	DEC 17,2013		NCE	APR 15,2004
		5646180	JUL 08,2014	U-257	NCE	APR 15,2004
		5723490	MAR 03,2013	U-257	NCE	APR 15,2004
021007 002	AMPRENAVIR; AGENERASE	5585397	DEC 17,2013		NCE	APR 15,2004
		5646180	JUL 08,2014	U-257	NCE	APR 15,2004
		5723490	MAR 03,2015	U-257	NCE	APR 15,2004
021039 001	AMPRENAVIR; AGENERASE	5585397	DEC 17,2013		NCE	APR 15,2004
		5646180	JUL 08,2014	U-257	NCE	APR 15,2004
		5723490	MAR 03,2015	U-257	NCE	APR 15,2004
020333 001	ANAGRELIDE HYDROCHLORIDE; AGRYLIN				ODE	MAR 14,2004

PRESCRIPTION AND OTC PRODUCT
PATENT AND EXCLUSIVITY DATA
*PED and PED represent Pediatric Exclusivity (*continued*)

APPL/PROD NUMBER	INGREDIENT NAME; TRADE NAME	PATENT NUMBER	PATENT EXPIRES	USE CODE	EX-CLUS CODE	EXCLUS EXPIRES
020333 002	ANAGRELIDE HYDROCHLORIDE; AGRYLIN				ODE	MAR 14,2004
020541 001	ANASTROZOLE; ARIMIDEX	RE36617	DEC 27,2009		I-363	SEP 05,2005
019779 001	APRACLONIDINE HYDROCHLORIDE; IOPIDINE	5212196	MAY 18,2010	U-120		
021549 001	APREPITANT; EMEND	5538982	JUL 23,2013		NCE	MAR 26,2008
		5719147	JUN 29,2012		NCE	MAR 26,2008
		6048859	JUN 29,2012		NCE	MAR 26,2008
		6096742	JUL 01,2018		NCE	MAR 26,2008
		6235735	JUN 29,2012		NCE	MAR 26,2008
021549 002	APREPITANT; EMEND	5538982	JUL 23,2013		NCE	MAR 26,2008
		5719147	JUN 29,2012		NCE	MAR 26,2008
		6048859	JUN 29,2012		NCE	MAR 26,2008
		6096742	JUL 01,2018		NCE	MAR 26,2008
		6235735	JUN 29,2012		NCE	MAR 26,2008
020420 001	ARBUTAMINE HYDROCHLORIDE; GENESA	5108363	APR 28,2009	U-220	NCE	SEP 12,2002
		5234404	AUG 10,2010	U-220	NCE	SEP 12,2002
		5395970	MAR 07,2012		NCE	SEP 12,2002
020883 001	ARGATROBAN; ARGATROBAN	5214052	MAR 13,2012		I-352	APR 03,2005
		5925760	AUG 04,2017		I-352	APR 03,2005
021436 001	ARIPIPRAZOLE; ABILIFY	4734416	MAR 29,2005		NCE	NOV 15,2007
		5006528	OCT 20,2009		NCE	NOV 15,2007
021436 002	ARIPIPRAZOLE; ABILIFY	4734416	MAR 29,2005		NCE	NOV 15,2007
		5006528	OCT 20,2009		NCE	NOV 15,2007
021436 003	ARIPIPRAZOLE; ABILIFY	4734416	MAR 29,2005		NCE	NOV 15,2007
		5006528	OCT 20,2009		NCE	NOV 15,2007
021436 004	ARIPIPRAZOLE; ABILIFY	4734416	MAR 29,2005		NCE	NOV 15,2007
		5006528	OCT 20,2009		NCE	NOV 15,2007
021436 005	ARIPIPRAZOLE; ABILIFY	4734416	MAR 29,2005		NCE	NOV 15,2007
		5006528	OCT 20,2009		NCE	NOV 15,2007
021436 006	ARIPIPRAZOLE; ABILIFY	4734416	MAR 29,2005		NCE	NOV 15,2007
		5006528	OCT 20,2009		NCE	NOV 15,2007
021248 001	ARSENIC TRIOXIDE; TRISENOX				NCE	SEP 25,2005
020971 001	ARTICAINE HYDROCHLORIDE; SEPTOCAINE				NC	APR 03,2003
020884 001	ASPIRIN; AGGRENOX	6015577	JAN 18,2017	U-302	NC	NOV 22,2002
021317 001	ASPIRIN; BAYER EXTRA STRENGTH ASPIRIN FOR MIGRAINE PAIN				NP	OCT 18,2004
021387 001	ASPIRIN; PRAVIGARD PAC (COPACKAGED)	4346227	OCT 20,2005			
		4346227*PED	APR 20,2006			
		5030447	JUL 09,2008			
		5030447*PED	JAN 09,2009			
		5180589	JUL 09,2208			
		5180589*PED	JAN 09,2009			
		5622985	APR 22,2014	U-335		
		5622985*PED	OCT 22,2014	U-335		
021387 002	ASPIRIN; PRAVIGARD PAC (COPACKAGED)	4346227	OCT 20,2005			
		4346227*PED	APR 20,2006			
		5030447	JUL 09,2008			
		5030447*PED	JAN 09,2009			
		5180589	JUL 09,2008			
		5180589*PED	JAN 09,2009			
		5622985	APR 22,2014	U-335		
		5622985*PED	OCT 22,2014	U-335		
021387 003	ASPIRIN; PRAVIGARD PAC (COPACKAGED)	4346227	OCT 20,2005			
		4346227*PED	APR 20,2006			
		5030447	JUL 09,2008			
		5030447*PED	JAN 09,2009			
		5180589	JUL 09,2008			
		5180589*PED	JAN 09,2009			
		5622985	APR 22,2014	U-335		
		5622985*PED	OCT 22,2014	U-335		
021387 004	ASPIRIN; PRAVIGARD PAC (COPACKAGED)	4346227	OCT 20,2005			
		4346227*PED	APR 20,2006			
		5030447	JUL 09,2008			
		5030447*PED	JAN 09,2009			
		5180589	JUL 09,2008			
		5180589*PED	JAN 09,2009			
		5622985	APR 22,2014	U-335		
		5622985*PED	OCT 22,2014	U-335		
021387 005	ASPIRIN; PRAVIGARD PAC (COPACKAGED)	4346227	OCT 20,2005			
		4346227*PED	APR 20,2006			
		5030447	JUL 09,2008			
		5030447*PED	JAN 09,2009			

PRESCRIPTION AND OTC PRODUCT
PATENT AND EXCLUSIVITY DATA
*PED and PED represent Pediatric Exclusivity (*continued*)

APPL/PROD NUMBER	INGREDIENT NAME; TRADE NAME	PATENT NUMBER	PATENT EXPIRES	USE CODE	EX-CLUS CODE	EXCLUS EXPIRES
		5180589	JUL 09,2008			
		5180589*PED	JAN 09,2009			
		5622985	APR 22,2014	U-335		
		5622985*PED	OCT 22,2014	U-335		
021387 006	ASPIRIN; PRAVIGARD PAC (COPACKAGED)	4346227	OCT 20,2005			
		4346227*PED	APR 20,2006			
		5030447	JUL 09,2008			
		5030447*PED	JAN 09,2009			
		5180589	JUL 09,2008			
		5180589*PED	JAN 09,2009			
		5622985	APR 22,2014	U-335		
		5622985*PED	OCT 22,2014	U-335		
012365 005	ASPIRIN; SOMA COMPOUND	4534973	AUG 13,2002			
012366 002	ASPIRIN; SOMA COMPOUND W/ CODEINE	4534974	AUG 13,2002			
021411 001	ATOMOXETINE HYDROCHLORIDE; STRATTERA	5658590	JAN 11,2015	U-494	PED	MAY 26,2008
		5658590*PED	JUL 11,2015	U-494	PED	MAY 26,2008
021411 002	ATOMOXETINE HYDROCHLORIDE; STRATTERA	5658590	JAN 11,2015	U-494	PED	MAY 26,2008
		5658590*PED	JUL 11,2015	U-494	PED	MAY 26,2008
021411 003	ATOMOXETINE HYDROCHLORIDE; STRATTERA	5658590	JAN 11,2015	U-494	PED	MAY 26,2008
		5658590*PED	JUL 11,2015	U-494	PED	MAY 26,2008
021411 004	ATOMOXETINE HYDROCHLORIDE; STRATTERA	5658590	JAN 11,2015	U-494	PED	MAY 26,2008
		5658590*PED	JUL 11,2015	U-494	PED	MAY 26,2008
021411 005	ATOMOXETINE HYDROCHLORIDE; STRATTERA	5658590	JAN 11,2015	U-494	PED	MAY 26,2008
		5658590*PED	JUL 11,2015	U-494	PED	MAY 26,2008
021411 006	ATOMOXETINE HYDROCHLORIDE; STRATTERA	5658590	JAN 11,2015	U-494	PED	MAY 26,2008
		5658590*PED	JUL 11,2015	U-494	PED	MAY 26,2008
020702 001	ATORVASTATIN CALCIUM; LIPITOR	4681893	SEP 24,2009	U-161	PED	JUN 02,2003
		4681893*PED	MAR 24,2010	U-161	PED	JUN 02,2003
		5273995	DEC 28,2010	U-162	PED	JUN 02,2003
		5273995*PED	JUN 28,2011	U-162	PED	JUN 02,2003
		5686104	NOV 11,2014	U-213	PED	JUN 02,2003
		5686104*PED	MAY 11,2015	U-213	PED	JUN 02,2003
		5969156	JUL 08,2016		PED	JUN 02,2003
		5969156*PED	JAN 08,2017		PED	JUN 02,2003
		6126971	JAN 19,2013		PED	JUN 02,2003
		6126971*PED	JUL 19,2013		PED	JUN 02,2003
020702 002	ATORVASTATIN CALCIUM; LIPITOR	4681893	SEP 24,2009	U-161	I-281	DEC 02,2002
		4681893*PED	MAR 24,2010	U-161	I-281	DEC 02,2002
		5273995	DEC 28,2010	U-162	I-281	DEC 02,2002
		5273995*PED	JUN 28,2011	U-162	I-281	DEC 02,2002
		5686104	NOV 11,2014	U-213	I-281	DEC 02,2002
		5686104*PED	MAY 11,2015	U-213	I-281	DEC 02,2002
		5969156	JUL 08,2016		I-281	DEC 02,2002
		5969156*PED	JAN 18,2017		I-281	DEC 02,2002
		6126971	JAN 19,2013		I-281	DEC 02,2002
		6126971*PED	JUL 19,2013		I-281	DEC 02,2002
020702 003	ATORVASTATIN CALCIUM; LIPITOR	4681893	SEP 24,2009	U-161	I-281	DEC 02,2002
		4681893*PED	MAR 24,2010	U-161	I-281	DEC 02,2002
		5273995	DEC 28,2010	U-162	I-281	DEC 02,2002
		5273995*PED	JUN 28,2011	U-162	I-281	DEC 02,2002
		5686104	NOV 11,2014	U-213	I-281	DEC 02,2002
		5686104*PED	MAY 11,2015	U-213	I-281	DEC 02,2002
		5969156	JUL 08,2016		I-281	DEC 02,2002
		5969156*PED	JAN 08,2017		I-281	DEC 02,2002
		6126971	JAN 19,2013		I-281	DEC 02,2002
		6126971*PED	JUL 19,2013		I-281	DEC 02,2002
020702 004	ATORVASTATIN CALCIUM; LIPITOR	4681893	SEP 24,2009	U-161	I-281	DEC 02,2002
		4681893*PED	MAR 24,2010	U-161	I-281	DEC 02,2002
		5273995	DEC 28,2010	U-162	I-281	DEC 02,2002
		5273995*PED	JUN 28,2011	U-162	I-281	DEC 02,2002
		5686104	NOV 11,2014	U-213	I-281	DEC 02,2002
		5686104*PED	MAY 11,2015	U-213	I-281	DEC 02,2002
		5969156	JUL 08,2016		I-281	DEC 02,2002
		5969156*PED	JAN 08,2017		I-281	DEC 02,2002
		6126971	JAN 19,2013		I-281	DEC 02,2002
		6126971*PED	JUL 19,2013		I-281	DEC 02,2002
021078 001	ATOVAQUONE; MALARONE	5053432	OCT 01,2008		NC	JUL 14,2003
		6166046	NOV 25,2013	U-406	NC	JUL 14,2003
		6291488	NOV 25,2013		NC	JUL 14,2003
021078 002	ATOVAQUONE; MALARONE PEDIATRIC	5053432	OCT 01,2008		NC	JUL 14,2003
		6166046	NOV 25,2013		NC	JUL 14,2003

PRESCRIPTION AND OTC PRODUCT
PATENT AND EXCLUSIVITY DATA
*PED and PED represent Pediatric Exclusivity (*continued*)

APPL/PROD NUMBER	INGREDIENT NAME; TRADE NAME	PATENT NUMBER	PATENT EXPIRES	USE CODE	EX-CLUS CODE	EXCLUS EXPIRES
		6291488	NOV 25,2013	U-406	NC	JUL 14,2003
020259 001	ATOVAQUONE; MEPRON	4981874	AUG 15,2009	U-69		
		5053432	OCT 01,2008			
020500 001	ATOVAQUONE; MEPRON	4981874	AUG 15,2009	U-69	ODE	JAN 05,2006
		5053432	OCT 01,2008		ODE	JAN 05,2006
019677 001	ATROPINE SULFATE; ENLON-PLUS	4952586	AUG 28,2007	U-54		
019678 001	ATROPINE SULFATE; ENLON-PLUS	4952586	AUG 28,2007	U-54		
021470 001	AZELAIC ACID; FINACEA	4713394	JAN 17,2006	U-492	NDF	DEC 24,2005
		6534070	NOV 18,2018		NDF	DEC 24,2005
020114 001	AZELASTINE HYDROCHLORIDE; ASTELIN	5164194	OCT 16,2011	U-207		
021127 001	AZELASTINE HYDROCHLORIDE; OPTIVAR	5164194	NOV 01,2010		PED	NOV 22,2003
		5164194*PED	MAY 01,2011		PED	NOV 22,2003
020610 001	BALSALAZIDE DISODIUM; COLAZAL				NCE	JUL 18,2005
020911 002	BECLOMETHASONE DIPROPIONATE; QVAR 40	5605674	FEB 25,2014		NPP	MAY 10,2005
		5683677	NOV 04,2014		NPP	MAY 10,2005
		5695743	JUL 06,2010		NPP	MAY 10,2005
		5766573	NOV 28,2009	U-356	NPP	MAY 10,2005
		5776432	JUL 07,2015		NPP	MAY 10,2005
		6352684	NOV 28,2009		NPP	MAY 10,2005
020911 001	BECLOMETHASONE DIPROPIONATE; QVAR 80	5605674	FEB 25,2014		NPP	MAY 10,2005
		5683677	NOV 04,2014		NPP	MAY 10,2005
		5695743	JUL 06,2010		NPP	MAY 10,2005
		5766573	NOV 28,2009	U-356	NPP	MAY 10,2005
		5776432	JUL 07,2015		NPP	MAY 10,2005
		6352684	NOV 28,2009		NPP	MAY 10,2005
019851 001	BENAZEPRIL HYDROCHLORIDE; LOTENSIN	4410520	AUG 11,2003			
		4410520*PED	FEB 11,2004			
019851 002	BENAZEPRIL HYDROCHLORIDE; LOTENSIN	4410520	AUG 11,2003			
		4410520*PED	FEB 11,2004			
019851 003	BENAZEPRIL HYDROCHLORIDE; LOTENSIN	4410520	AUG 11,2003			
		4410520*PED	FEB 11,2004			
019851 004	BENAZEPRIL HYDROCHLORIDE; LOTENSIN	4410520	AUG 11,2003			
		4410520*PED	FEB 11,2004			
020033 001	BENAZEPRIL HYDROCHLORIDE; LOTENSIN HCT	4410520	AUG 11,2003			
		4410520*PED	FEB 11,2004			
020033 002	BENAZEPRIL HYDROCHLORIDE; LOTENSIN HCT	4410520	AUG 11,2003			
		4410520*PED	FEB 11,2004			
020033 003	BENAZEPRIL HYDROCHLORIDE; LOTENSIN HCT	4410520	AUG 11,2003			
		4410520*PED	FEB 11,2004			
020033 004	BENAZEPRIL HYDROCHLORIDE; LOTENSIN HCT	4410520	AUG 11,2003			
		4410520*PED	FEB 11,2004			
020032 001	BERACTANT; SURVANTA	4397839	JUL 01,2005			
020576 001	BETAINE, ANHYDROUS; CYSTADANE				ODE	OCT 25,2003
019408 001	BETAMETHASONE DIPROPIONATE; DIPROLENE	4489070	MAY 13,2003			
019408 002	BETAMETHASONE DIPROPIONATE; DIPROLENE	4489070	MAY 13,2003			
019716 001	BETAMETHASONE DIPROPIONATE; DIPROLENE	4775529	MAY 21,2007			
019555 001	BETAMETHASONE DIPROPIONATE; DIPROLENE AF	4489071	DEC 09,2003			
020010 001	BETAMETHASONE DIPROPIONATE; LOTRISONE				NP	DEC 08,2003
020934 001	BETAMETHASONE VALERATE; LUXIQ	6126920	MAR 01,2016	U-484		
020619 001	BETAXOLOL HYDROCHLORIDE; BETOPTIC PILO	5635172	JUN 03,2014	U-191		
019845 001	BETAXOLOL HYDROCHLORIDE; BETOPTIC S	4911920	MAR 27,2007			
021055 001	BEXAROTENE; TARGRETIN	5466861	NOV 14,2012		ODE	DEC 29,2006
		5780676	JUL 14,2015	U-509	ODE	DEC 29,2006
		5962731	OCT 05,2016	U-475	ODE	DEC 29,2006
021056 001	BEXAROTENE; TARGRETIN	5466861	NOV 14,2012		ODE	DEC 29,2006
		5780676	JUL 14,2015	U-510	ODE	DEC 29,2006
		5962731	OCT 05,2016		ODE	DEC 29,2006
020498 001	BICALUTAMIDE; CASODEX	4636505	OCT 01,2008			
021275 001	BIMATOPROST; LUMIGAN	5688819	SEP 21,2012		NCE	MAR 16,2006
		6403649	SEP 21,2012	U-446	NCE	MAR 16,2006
020873 001	BIVALIRUDIN; ANGIOMAX	5196404	MAR 23,2010		NCE	DEC 15,2005
050443 001	BLEOMYCIN SULFATE; BLENOXANE				ODE	FEB 20,2003
050443 002	BLEOMYCIN SULFATE; BLENOXANE				ODE	FEB 20,2003
021602 001	BORTEZOMIB; VELCADE	5780454	OCT 28,2014		NCE	MAY 13,2008
		6083903	OCT 28,2014	U-515	NCE	MAY 13,2008
		6297217	OCT 28,2014	U-515	NCE	MAY 13,2008
021290 001	BOSENTAN; TRACLEER				NCE	NOV 20,2006
021290 002	BOSENTAN; TRACLEER				NCE	NOV 20,2006
020490 001	BRIMONIDINE TARTRATE; ALPHAGAN				PED	JUN 20,2005
020613 001	BRIMONIDINE TARTRATE; ALPHAGAN	6194415	JUN 28,2015	U-394	PED	JUN 20,2005
		6194415*PED	DEC 28,2015	U-394	PED	JUN 20,2005

PRESCRIPTION AND OTC PRODUCT
PATENT AND EXCLUSIVITY DATA
*PED and PED represent Pediatric Exclusivity (*continued*)

APPL/PROD NUMBER	INGREDIENT NAME; TRADE NAME	PATENT NUMBER	PATENT EXPIRES	USE CODE	EX-CLUS CODE	EXCLUS EXPIRES
		6248741	JUN 28,2015	U-394	PED	JUN 20,2005
		6248741*PED	DEC 28,2015	U-394	PED	JUN 20,2005
		6465464	JUN 28,2015	U-394	PED	JUN 20,2005
		6465464*PED	DEC 28,2015	U-394	PED	JUN 20,2005
021262 001	BRIMONIDINE TARTRATE; ALPHAGAN P	5424078	JUN 13,2012		PED	SEP 16,2004
		5424078*PED	DEC 13,2012		PED	SEP 16,2004
		5736165	APR 07,2015	U-399	PED	SEP 16,2004
		5736165*PED	OCT 07,2015	U-399	PED	SEP 16,2004
		6194415	JUN 28,2015	U-395	PED	SEP 16,2004
		6194415*PED	DEC 28,2015	U-395	PED	SEP 16,2004
		6248741	JUN 28,2015	U-395	PED	SEP 16,2004
		6248741*PED	DEC 28,2015	U-395	PED	SEP 16,2004
		6465464	JUN 28,2015	U-395	PED	SEP 16,2004
		6465464*PED	DEC 28,2015	U-395	PED	SEP 16,2004
		6562873	JUL 10,2021		PED	SEP 16,2004
		6562873*PED	JAN 10,2022		PED	SEP 16,2004
076260 001	BRIMONIDINE TARTRATE; BRIMONIDINE TARTRATE				PC	SEP 16,2003
020816 001	BRINZOLAMIDE; AZOPT	5240923	AUG 31,2010	U-224	NCE	APR 01,2003
		5378703	APR 01,2012	U-224	NCE	APR 01,2003
		5461081	OCT 24,2012	U-225	NCE	APR 01,2003
019672 001	BROMPHENIRAMINE MALEATE; EFIDAC 24 PSEUDOEPHEDRINE HCL/BROMPHENIRAMINE MALEATE	4662880	MAR 14,2006			
		4673405	MAR 18,2003			
		4801461	MAR 14,2006			
		4810502	MAR 14,2006			
021324 001	BUDESONIDE; ENTOCORT EC	5643602	JUL 01,2014		PED	APR 02,2005
		5643602*PED	JAN 01,2015		PED	APR 02,2005
020441 002	BUDESONIDE; PULMICORT	4668218	APR 11,2006			
		4668218*PED	OCT 11,2006			
		4907583	MAR 13,2007			
		4907583*PED	SEP 13,2007			
020441 003	BUDESONIDE; PULMICORT	4668218	APR 11,2006			
		4668218*PED	OCT 11,2006			
		4907583	MAR 13,2007			
		4907583*PED	SEP 13,2007			
020929 001	BUDESONIDE; PULMICORT RESPULES	4787536	FEB 27,2006		PED	FEB 08,2004
		4787536*PED	AUG 27,2006		PED	FEB 08,2004
020929 002	BUDESONIDE; PULMICORT RESPULES	4787536	FEB 27,2006		NDF	AUG 08,2003
		4787536*PED	AUG 27,2006		NDF	AUG 08,2003
020929 003	BUDESONIDE; PULMICORT RESPULES	4787536	FEB 27,2006		PED	FEB 08,2004
		4787536*PED	AUG 27,2006		PED	FEB 08,2004
020746 001	BUDESONIDE; RHINOCORT	6291445	APR 29,2017		M-22	OCT 26,2004
		6291445*PED	OCT 29,2017		M-22	OCT 26,2004
020746 002	BUDESONIDE; RHINOCORT	6291445	APR 29,2017		M-22	OCT 26,2004
		6291445*PED	OCT 29,2017		M-22	OCT 26,2004
020733 001	BUPRENORPHINE HYDROCHLORIDE; SUBOXONE				ODE	OCT 08,2009
020733 002	BUPRENORPHINE HYDROCHLORIDE; SUBOXONE				ODE	OCT 08,2009
020732 002	BUPRENORPHINE HYDROCHLORIDE; SUBUTEX				ODE	OCT 08,2009
020732 003	BUPRENORPHINE HYDROCHLORIDE; SUBUTEX				ODE	OCT 08,2009
020358 001	BUPROPION HYDROCHLORIDE; WELLBUTRIN SR	5358970	AUG 12,2013		M-10	JUN 11,2004
		5427798	AUG 12,2013		M-10	JUN 11,2004
		5731000	AUG 12,2013		M-10	JUN 11,2004
		5763493	AUG 12,2013		M-10	JUN 11,2004
020358 002	BUPROPION HYDROCHLORIDE; WELLBUTRIN SR	5358970	AUG 12,2013		M-10	JUN 11,2004
		5427798	AUG 12,2013		M-10	JUN 11,2004
		5731000	AUG 12,2013		M-10	JUN 11,2004
		5763493	AUG 12,2013		M-10	JUN 11,2004
020358 003	BUPROPION HYDROCHLORIDE; WELLBUTRIN SR	5358970	AUG 12,2013		M-10	JUN 11,2004
		5427798	AUG 12,2013		M-10	JUN 11,2004
		5731000	AUG 12,2013		M-10	JUN 11,2004
		5763493	AUG 12,2013		M-10	JUN 11,2004
020358 004	BUPROPION HYDROCHLORIDE; WELLBUTRIN SR	5358970	AUG 12,2013		M-10	JUN 11,2004
		5427798	AUG 12,2013		M-10	JUN 11,2004
		5731000	AUG 12,2013		M-10	JUN 11,2004
		5763493	AUG 12,2013		M-10	JUN 11,2004
020711 002	BUPROPION HYDROCHLORIDE; ZYBAN	5358970	AUG 12,2013		D-54	SEP 10,2002
		5427798	AUG 12,2013		D-54	SEP 10,2002
		5731000	AUG 12,2013		D-54	SEP 10,2002
		5763493	AUG 12,2013		D-54	SEP 10,2002

PRESCRIPTION AND OTC PRODUCT
PATENT AND EXCLUSIVITY DATA
PED and PED represent Pediatric Exclusivity (continued)

APPL/PROD NUMBER	INGREDIENT NAME; TRADE NAME	PATENT NUMBER	PATENT EXPIRES	USE CODE	EX-CLUS CODE	EXCLUS EXPIRES
020711 003	BUPROPION HYDROCHLORIDE; ZYBAN	5358970	AUG 12,2013		D-54	SEP 10,2002
		5427798	AUG 12,2013		D-54	SEP 10,2002
		5731000	AUG 12,2013		D-54	SEP 10,2002
		5763493	AUG 12,2013		D-54	SEP 10,2002
018731 001	BUSPIRONE HYDROCHLORIDE; BUSPAR				PED	JAN 19,2005
018731 002	BUSPIRONE HYDROCHLORIDE; BUSPAR				PED	JAN 19,2005
018731 003	BUSPIRONE HYDROCHLORIDE; BUSPAR				W	JUL 19,2004
018731 004	BUSPIRONE HYDROCHLORIDE; BUSPAR				M-12	JUL 19,2004
021190 001	BUSPIRONE HYDROCHLORIDE; BUSPAR	5015646	MAY 14,2008			
		5015646*PED	NOV 14,2008			
021190 002	BUSPIRONE HYDROCHLORIDE; BUSPAR	5015646	MAY 14,2008			
		5015646*PED	NOV 14,2008			
021190 003	BUSPIRONE HYDROCHLORIDE; BUSPAR	5015646	MAY 14,2008			
		5015646*PED	NOV 14,2008			
021190 004	BUSPIRONE HYDROCHLORIDE; BUSPAR	5015646	MAY 14,2008			
		5015646*PED	NOV 14,2008			
020954 001	BUSULFAN; BUSULFEX	5430057	SEP 30,2013	U-263	PED	AUG 04,2006
		5430057*PED	MAR 30,2014	U-263	PED	AUG 04,2006
		5559148	MAY 24,2015	U-264	PED	AUG 04,2006
		5559148*PED	NOV 24,2015	U-264	PED	AUG 04,2006
020524 001	BUTENAFINE HYDROCHLORIDE; MENTAX	5021458	OCT 18,2010	U-177	I-333	JUN 06,2004
021408 001	BUTENAFINE HYDROCHLORIDE; MENTAX-TC				NP	OCT 17,2005
019881 001	BUTOCONAZOLE NITRATE; GYNAZOLE-1	4551148	NOV 05,2002			
		5266329	NOV 30,2010	U-457		
020664 001	CABERGOLINE; DOSTINEX	4526892	DEC 29,2005			
020793 001	CAFFEINE CITRATE; CAFCIT				NE	SEP 21,2002
020273 001	CALCIPOTRIENE; DOVONEX	4866048	DEC 29,2007			
020554 001	CALCIPOTRIENE; DOVONEX	4866048	DEC 29,2007			
020611 001	CALCIPOTRIENE; DOVONEX	4866048	DEC 29,2007			
020313 002	CALCITONIN, SALMON; MIACALCIN	5733569	MAR 31,2015	U-227		
		5759565	MAR 31,2015			
018874 001	CALCITRIOL; CALCIJEX	6051567	AUG 02,2019		M-14	NOV 16,2004
		6051567*PED	FEB 02,2020		M-14	NOV 16,2004
		6265392	AUG 02,2019		M-14	NOV 16,2004
		6265392*PED	FEB 02,2020		M-14	NOV 16,2004
		6274169	AUG 02,2019		M-14	NOV 16,2004
		6274169*PED	FEB 02,2020		M-14	NOV 16,2004
018874 002	CALCITRIOL; CALCIJEX	6051567	AUG 02,2019		PED	MAY 16,2005
		6051567*PED	FEB 02,2020		PED	MAY 16,2005
		6265392	AUG 02,2019		PED	MAY 16,2005
		6265392*PED	FEB 02,2020		PED	MAY 16,2005
		6274169	AUG 02,2019		PED	MAY 16,2005
		6274169*PED	FEB 02,2020		PED	MAY 16,2005
075766 001	CALCITRIOL; CALCITRIOL				PC	SEP 17,2003
075766 002	CALCITRIOL; CALCITRIOL				PC	SEP 17,2003
075823 001	CALCITRIOL; CALCITRIOL				PC	SEP 17,2003
075823 002	CALCITRIOL; CALCITRIOL				PC	SEP 17,2003
075836 001	CALCITRIOL; CALCITRIOL				PC	SEP 17,2003
075836 002	CALCITRIOL; CALCITRIOL				PC	SEP 17,2003
019976 001	CALCIUM ACETATE; PHOSLO	4870105	APR 07,2007	U-381		
021160 001	CALCIUM ACETATE; PHOSLO	4870105	APR 07,2007	U-381		
021160 002	CALCIUM ACETATE; PHOSLO	4870105	APR 07,2007	U-381		
		6576665	APR 03,2021			
021160 003	CALCIUM ACETATE; PHOSLO GELCAPS	4870105	APR 07,2007	U-381		
		6576665	APR 03,2021			
020958 001	CALCIUM CARBONATE, PRECIPITATED; PEPCID COMPLETE	5229137	MAY 16,2012	U-349	PED	APR 15,2004
		5229137*PED	NOV 16,2012		PED	APR 15,2004
		5817340	DEC 01,2012		PED	APR 15,2004
		5817340*PED	JUN 01,2013		PED	APR 15,2004
		5989588	SEP 30,2015	U-349	PED	APR 15,2004
		5989588*PED	MAR 30,2018	U-349	PED	APR 15,2004
018469 001	CALCIUM CHLORIDE; BSS PLUS	4550022	OCT 29,2002			
020577 001	CALCIUM CHLORIDE; ELLIOTTS B SOLUTION				ODE	SEP 27,2003
021321 001	CALCIUM CHLORIDE; EXTRANEAL	4761237	AUG 02,2005	U-495		
		4886789	DEC 12,2006	U-495		
		6077836	JUN 20,2017	U-495		
		6248726	JUN 19,2018	U-495		
020521 001	CALFACTANT; INFASURF PRESERVATIVE FREE				NCE	JUL 01,2003
020838 001	CANDESARTAN CILEXETIL; ATACAND	5196444	JUN 04,2012	U-3	M-21	SEP 13,2005
		5534534	JUL 09,2013		M-21	SEP 13,2005

PRESCRIPTION AND OTC PRODUCT
PATENT AND EXCLUSIVITY DATA
*PED and PED represent Pediatric Exclusivity (*continued*)

APPL/PROD NUMBER	INGREDIENT NAME; TRADE NAME	PATENT NUMBER	PATENT EXPIRES	USE CODE	EX-CLUS CODE	EXCLUS EXPIRES
		5703110	APR 18,2011		M-21	SEP 13,2005
		5705517	APR 18,2011		M-21	SEP 13,2005
020838 002	CANDESARTAN CILEXETIL; ATACAND	5196444	JUN 04,2012	U-3	NCE	JUN 04,2003
		5534534	JUL 09,2013		NCE	JUN 04,2003
		5703110	APR 18,2011		NCE	JUN 04,2003
		5705517	APR 18,2011		NCE	JUN 04,2003
020838 003	CANDESARTAN CILEXETIL; ATACAND	5196444	JUN 04,2012	U-3	NCE	JUN 04,2003
		5534534	JUL 09,2013		NCE	JUN 04,2003
		5703110	APR 18,2011		NCE	JUN 04,2003
		5705517	APR 18,2011		NCE	JUN 04,2003
020838 004	CANDESARTAN CILEXETIL; ATACAND	5196444	JUN 04,2012	U-3	NCE	JUN 04,2003
		5534534	JUL 09,2013		NCE	JUN 04,2003
		5703110	APR 18,2011		NCE	JUN 04,2003
		5705517	APR 18,2011		NCE	JUN 04,2003
021093 001	CANDESARTAN CILEXETIL; ATACAND HCT	5196444	JUN 04,2012	U-3	NC	SEP 05,2003
		5534534	JUL 09,2013		NC	SEP 05,2003
		5703110	APR 18,2011	U-3	NC	SEP 05,2003
		5705517	APR 18,2011	U-3	NC	SEP 05,2003
		5721263	FEB 24,2015	U-3	NC	SEP 05,2003
		5958961	JUN 06,2014	U-3	NC	SEP 05,2003
021093 002	CANDESARTAN CILEXETIL; ATACAND HCT	5196444	JUN 04,2012	U-3	NCE	JUN 04,2003
		5534534	JUL 09,2013		NCE	JUN 04,2003
		5703110	APR 18,2011	U-3	NCE	JUN 04,2003
		5705517	APR 18,2011	U-3	NCE	JUN 04,2003
		5721263	FEB 24,2015	U-3	NCE	JUN 04,2003
		5958961	JUN 06,2014	U-3	NCE	JUN 04,2003
020896 001	CAPECITABINE; XELODA	4966891	JAN 13,2011	U-272	I-323	APR 30,2004
		5472949	DEC 14,2013	U-271	I-323	APR 30,2004
020896 002	CAPECITABINE; XELODA	4966891	JAN 13,2011	U-272	I-341	SEP 07,2004
		5472949	DEC 14,2013	U-271	I-341	SEP 07,2004
018343 001	CAPTOPRIL; CAPOTEN	5238924	AUG 24,2010	U-92		
018343 002	CAPTOPRIL; CAPOTEN	5238924	AUG 24,2010	U-92		
018343 003	CAPTOPRIL; CAPOTEN	5238924	AUG 24,2010	U-92		
018343 004	CAPTOPRIL; CAPOTEN	5238924	AUG 24,2010	U-92		
018343 005	CAPTOPRIL; CAPOTEN	5238924	AUG 24,2010	U-92		
018343 006	CAPTOPRIL; CAPOTEN	5238924	AUG 24,2010	U-92		
018343 007	CAPTOPRIL; CAPOTEN	5238924	AUG 24,2010	U-92		
020712 001	CARBAMAZEPINE; CARBATROL	5326570	JUL 05,2011	U-215		
		5912013	JUN 15,2016	U-277		
020712 002	CARBAMAZEPINE; CARBATROL	5326570	JUL 05,2011	U-215		
		5912013	JUN 15,2016	U-277		
020234 001	CARBAMAZEPINE; TEGRETOL-XR	5284662	FEB 08,2011			
		RE34990	JUL 29,2007			
020234 002	CARBAMAZEPINE; TEGRETOL-XR	5284662	FEB 08,2011			
		RE34990	JUL 29,2007			
020234 003	CARBAMAZEPINE; TEGRETOL-XR	5284662	FEB 08,2011			
		RE34990	JUL 29,2007			
019856 001	CARBIDOPA; SINEMET CR	4832957	JUN 16,2006			
		4900755	JUN 16,2006			
019856 002	CARBIDOPA; SINEMET CR	4832957	JUN 16,2006			
		4900755	JUN 16,2006			
021485 002	CARBIDOPA; STALEVO 100	4963590	NOV 27,2007		NCE	OCT 19,2004
		5112861	MAY 12,2009		NCE	OCT 19,2004
		5135950	OCT 31,2010		NCE	OCT 19,2004
		5446194	AUG 29,2012		NCE	OCT 19,2004
		6500867	JUN 29,2020		NCE	OCT 19,2004
021485 003	CARBIDOPA; STALEVO 150	4963590	NOV 27,2007		NCE	OCT 19,2004
		5112861	MAY 12,2009		NCE	OCT 19,2004
		5135950	OCT 31,2010		NCE	OCT 19,2004
		5446194	AUG 29,2012		NCE	OCT 19,2004
		6500867	JUN 29,2020		NCE	OCT 19,2004
021485 001	CARBIDOPA; STALEVO 50	4963590	NOV 27,2007		NCE	OCT 19,2004
		5112861	MAY 12,2009		NCE	OCT 19,2004
		5135950	OCT 31,2010		NCE	OCT 19,2004
		5446194	AUG 29,2012		NCE	OCT 19,2004
		6500867	JUN 29,2020		NCE	OCT 19,2004
019880 001	CARBOPLATIN; PARAPLATIN	4657927	APR 14,2004	U-175		
019880 002	CARBOPLATIN; PARAPLATIN	4657927	APR 14,2004	U-175		
019880 003	CARBOPLATIN; PARAPLATIN	4657927	APR 14,2004	U-175		
020637 001	CARMUSTINE; GLIADEL	4757128	AUG 01,2006		I-382	FEB 25,2006
		4789724	AUG 01,2006		I-382	FEB 25,2006

PRESCRIPTION AND OTC PRODUCT
PATENT AND EXCLUSIVITY DATA
*PED and PED represent Pediatric Exclusivity (*continued*)

APPL/PROD NUMBER	INGREDIENT NAME; TRADE NAME	PATENT NUMBER	PATENT EXPIRES	USE CODE	EX-CLUS CODE	EXCLUS EXPIRES
020297 001	CARVEDILOL; COREG	4503067	MAR 05,2007	U-3	I-388	MAR 27,2006
		5760069	JUN 07,2015	U-233	I-388	MAR 27,2006
		5902821	FEB 07,2016	U-313	I-388	MAR 27,2006
020297 002	CARVEDILOL; COREG	4503067	MAR 05,2007	U-3	I-343	NOV 01,2004
		5760069	JUN 07,2015	U-233	I-343	NOV 01,2004
		5902821	FEB 07,2016	U-313	I-343	NOV 01,2004
020297 003	CARVEDILOL; COREG	4503067	MAR 05,2007	U-3	I-343	NOV 01,2004
		5760069	JUN 07,2015	U-233	I-343	NOV 01,2004
		5902821	FEB 07,2016	U-313	I-343	NOV 01,2004
020297 004	CARVEDILOL; COREG	4503067	MAR 05,2007	U-3	I-343	NOV 01,2004
		5760069	JUN 07,2015	U-233	I-343	NOV 01,2004
		5902821	FEB 07,2016	U-313	I-343	NOV 01,2004
021227 001	CASPOFUNGIN ACETATE; CANCIDAS	5378804	MAR 16,2013		NCE	JAN 26,2006
		5514650	MAR 16,2013		NCE	JAN 26,2006
		5792746	MAR 16,2013		NCE	JAN 26,2006
		5952300	MAR 28,2017		NCE	JAN 26,2006
		6136783	MAR 28,2017		NCE	JAN 26,2006
021227 002	CASPOFUNGIN ACETATE; CANCIDAS	5378804	MAR 16,2013		NCE	JAN 26,2006
		5514650	MAR 16,2013		NCE	JAN 26,2006
		5792746	MAR 16,2013		NCE	JAN 26,2006
		5952300	MAR 28,2017		NCE	JAN 26,2006
		6136783	MAR 28,2017		NCE	JAN 26,2006
021222 001	CEFDITOREN PIVOXIL; SPECTRACEF	4839350	JUN 13,2006		I-364	AUG 21,2005
		4918068	JUN 13,2006		I-364	AUG 21,2005
		5958915	OCT 14,2016		I-364	AUG 21,2005
020998 001	CELECOXIB; CELEBREX	5466823	NOV 30,2013		I-338	OCT 17,2004
		5563165	NOV 30,2013		I-338	OCT 17,2004
		5760068	JUN 02,2015	U-19	I-338	OCT 17,2004
		5760068	JUN 02,2015	U-299	I-338	OCT 17,2004
		5972986	OCT 14,2017	U-299	I-338	OCT 17,2004
020998 002	CELECOXIB; CELEBREX	5466823	NOV 30,2013		NCE	DEC 31,2003
		5563165	NOV 30,2013		NCE	DEC 31,2003
		5760068	JUN 02,2015	U-19	NCE	DEC 31,2003
		5760068	JUN 02,2015	U-299	NCE	DEC 31,2003
		5972986	OCT 14,2017	U-299	NCE	DEC 31,2003
020998 003	CELECOXIB; CELEBREX	5466823	NOV 30,2013		I-284	DEC 23,2002
		5563165	NOV 30,2013		I-284	DEC 23,2002
		5760068	JUN 02,2015	U-19	I-284	DEC 23,2002
		5760068	JUN 02,2015	U-299	I-284	DEC 23,2002
		5972986	OCT 14,2017	U-299	I-284	DEC 23,2002
020740 001	CERIVASTATIN SODIUM; BAYCOL	5006530	JUN 26,2011		D-59	JUL 21,2003
		5177080	NOV 26,2011		D-59	JUL 21,2003
020740 002	CERIVASTATIN SODIUM; BAYCOL	5006530	JUN 26,2011		D-59	JUL 21,2003
		5177080	NOV 26,2011		D-59	JUL 21,2003
020740 003	CERIVASTATIN SODIUM; BAYCOL	5006530	JUN 26,2011		I-303	JUL 21,2003
		5177080	NOV 26,2011		I-303	JUL 21,2003
020740 004	CERIVASTATIN SODIUM; BAYCOL	5006530	JUN 26,2011		D-59	JUL 21,2003
		5177080	NOV 26,2011		D-59	JUL 21,2003
020740 005	CERIVASTATIN SODIUM; BAYCOL	5006530	JUN 26,2011		D-59	JUL 21,2003
		5177080	NOV 26,2011		D-59	JUL 21,2003
020740 006	CERIVASTATIN SODIUM; BAYCOL	5006530	JUN 26,2011		D-59	JUL 21,2003
		5177080	JAN 26,2011		D-59	JUL 21,2003
019835 001	CETIRIZINE HYDROCHLORIDE; ZYRTEC	4525358	JUN 25,2007		PED	APR 21,2006
		4525358*PED	DEC 25,2007		PED	APR 21,2006
019835 002	CETIRIZINE HYDROCHLORIDE; ZYRTEC	4525358	JUN 25,2007		NPP	OCT 21,2005
		4525358*PED	DEC 25,2007		NPP	OCT 21,2005
020346 001	CETIRIZINE HYDROCHLORIDE; ZYRTEC	4525358	JUN 25,2007		PED	APR 21,2006
		4525358*PED	DEC 25,2007		PED	APR 21,2006
021150 001	CETIRIZINE HYDROCHLORIDE; ZYRTEC-D 12 HOUR	4525358	JUN 25,2007	U-295		
		4525358*PED	DEC 25,2007	U-295		
		6469009	JUL 13,2019	U-295		
		6489329	APR 08,2016			
021197 001	CETRORELIX; CETROTIDE	4800191	JUL 17,2007		NCE	AUG 11,2005
		5198533	JUL 17,2007		NCE	AUG 11,2005
		6319192	APR 23,2018	U-426	NCE	AUG 11,2005
021197 002	CETRORELIX; CETROTIDE	4800191	JUL 17,2007		NCE	AUG 11,2005
		5198533	JUL 17,2007		NCE	AUG 11,2005
		6319192	APR 23,2018	U-426	NCE	AUG 11,2005
020044 001	CETYL ALCOHOL; EXOSURF NEONATAL	4312860	AUG 20,2003			
		4826821	MAY 02,2006			
		5110806	MAY 02,2006			

PRESCRIPTION AND OTC PRODUCT
PATENT AND EXCLUSIVITY DATA
*PED and PED represent Pediatric Exclusivity (continued)

APPL/PROD NUMBER	INGREDIENT NAME; TRADE NAME	PATENT NUMBER	PATENT EXPIRES	USE CODE	EX-CLUS CODE	EXCLUS EXPIRES
020989 002	CEVIMELINE HYDROCHLORIDE; EVOXAC	4855290	AUG 08,2006		NCE	JAN 11,2005
		5340821	AUG 23,2011	U-309	NCE	JAN 11,2005
		5580880	JUN 06,2015	U-310	NCE	JAN 11,2005
020832 001	CHLORHEXIDINE GLUCONATE; CHLORAPREP				NC	JUL 14,2003
021555 001	CHLORHEXIDINE GLUCONATE; CHLORAPREP ONE-STEP SEPP				NP	OCT 07,2005
021441 001	CHLORPHENIRAMINE MALEATE; ADVIL ALLERGY SINUS				NP	DEC 19,2005
019746 002	CHLORPHENIRAMINE MALEATE; EFIDAC 24 CHLORPHENIRAMINE MALEATE	4576604	MAR 18,2003			
		4673405	MAR 18,2003			
		4857330	AUG 15,2006			
019111 001	CHLORPHENIRAMINE POLISTIREX; TUSSIONEX	4762709	AUG 09,2005			
019574 001	CHLORTHALIDONE; THALITONE	4933360	JUN 12,2007			
021149 001	CHORIOGONADOTROPIN ALFA; OVIDREL	5767251	JUN 16,2015		NP	SEP 20,2003
021159 001	CICLOPIROX; LOPROX				NDF	FEB 28,2006
021022 001	CICLOPIROX; PENLAC	4957730	SEP 18,2007	U-379	NDF	DEC 17,2002
020638 001	CIDOFOVIR; VISTIDE	5142051	JUN 26,2010			
020863 001	CILOSTAZOL; PLETAL				NCE	JAN 15,2004
020863 002	CILOSTAZOL; PLETAL				NCE	JAN 15,2004
019992 001	CIPROFLOXACIN HYDROCHLORIDE; CILOXAN	4670444	DEC 09,2003			
		4670444*PED	JUN 09,2004			
020369 001	CIPROFLOXACIN HYDROCHLORIDE; CILOXAN	4670444	DEC 09,2003	U-223		
		4670444*PED	JUN 09,2004	U-223		
019537 001	CIPROFLOXACIN HYDROCHLORIDE; CIPRO	4670444	DEC 09,2003	U-36		
		5286754	FEB 15,2011			
019537 002	CIPROFLOXACIN HYDROCHLORIDE; CIPRO	4670444	DEC 09,2003	U-36		
		5286754	FEB 15,2011			
019537 003	CIPROFLOXACIN HYDROCHLORIDE; CIPRO	4670444	DEC 09,2003	U-36		
		5286754	FEB 15,2011			
019537 004	CIPROFLOXACIN HYDROCHLORIDE; CIPRO	4670444	DEC 09,2003	U-36		
		5286754	FEB 15,2011			
020805 001	CIPROFLOXACIN HYDROCHLORIDE; CIPRO HC	4670444	DEC 09,2003			
		4670444*PED	JUN 09,2004			
		4844902	FEB 11,2008			
019847 001	CIPROFLOXACIN; CIPRO	4670444	DEC 09,2003			
		4705789	NOV 10,2004			
		4808583	FEB 28,2006			
020780 001	CIPROFLOXACIN; CIPRO	4670444	DEC 09,2003			
		5695784	DEC 09,2014			
		6136347	JAN 06,2013	U-362		
020780 002	CIPROFLOXACIN; CIPRO	4670444	DEC 09,2003			
		5695784	DEC 09,2014			
		6136347	JAN 06,2013	U-362		
019857 001	CIPROFLOXACIN; CIPRO IN DEXTROSE 5% IN PLASTIC CONTAINER	4670444	DEC 09,2003			
		4705789	NOV 10,2004			
		4808583	FEB 28,2006			
		4957922	SEP 18,2007			
019858 001	CIPROFLOXACIN; CIPRO IN SODIUM CHLORIDE 0.9% IN PLASTIC CONTAINER	4670444	DEC 09,2003			
		4705789	NOV 10,2004			
		4808583	FEB 28,2006			
		4957922	SEP 18,2007			
021473 001	CIPROFLOXACIN; CIPRO XR	4670444	DEC 09,2003		NDF	DEC 13,2005
020210 001	CISAPRIDE MONOHYDRATE; PROPULSID	4962115	OCT 09,2007	U-79		
020210 002	CISAPRIDE MONOHYDRATE; PROPULSID	4962115	OCT 09,2007	U-79		
020398 001	CISAPRIDE MONOHYDRATE; PROPULSID	4962115	OCT 09,2007	U-79		
020767 001	CISAPRIDE MONOHYDRATE; PROPULSID QUICKSOLV	4962115	OCT 09,2007	U-79		
		5648093	JUL 15,2014			
020551 001	CISATRACURIUM BESYLATE; NIMBEX	5453510	SEP 26,2012	U-127		
020551 002	CISATRACURIUM BESYLATE; NIMBEX PRESERVATIVE FREE	5453510	SEP 26,2012	U-127		
020551 003	CISATRACURIUM BESYLATE; NIMBEX PRESERVATIVE FREE	5453510	SEP 26,2012	U-127		
020822 001	CITALOPRAM HYDROBROMIDE; CELEXA				NCE	JUL 17,2003
020822 002	CITALOPRAM HYDROBROMIDE; CELEXA				PED	JAN 17,2004
020822 003	CITALOPRAM HYDROBROMIDE; CELEXA				NCE	JUL 17,2003
020822 004	CITALOPRAM HYDROBROMIDE; CELEXA				NCE	JUL 17,2003
021046 001	CITALOPRAM HYDROBROMIDE; CELEXA				PED	JAN 17,2004

PRESCRIPTION AND OTC PRODUCT
PATENT AND EXCLUSIVITY DATA
*PED and PED represent Pediatric Exclusivity (*continued*)

APPL/PROD NUMBER	INGREDIENT NAME; TRADE NAME	PATENT NUMBER	PATENT EXPIRES	USE CODE	EX-CLUS CODE	EXCLUS EXPIRES
021142 001	CLOBETASOL PROPIONATE; OLUX FOAM	6126920	MAR 01,2016	U-484	I-374	DEC 20,2005
020615 001	CLONIDINE HYDROCHLORIDE; DURACLON				ODE	OCT 02,2003
018891 001	CLONIDINE; CATAPRES-TTS-1	4559222	MAY 04,2003			
018891 002	CLONIDINE; CATAPRES-TTS-2	4559222	MAY 04,2003			
018891 003	CLONIDINE; CATAPRES-TTS-3	4559222	MAY 04,2003			
020839 001	CLOPIDOGREL BISULFATE; PLAVIX	4529596	JUL 05,2003		I-349	FEB 27,2005
		4847265	NOV 17,2011		I-349	FEB 27,2005
		5576328	JAN 31,2014	U-432	I-349	FEB 27,2005
		6429210	JUN 10,2019		I-349	FEB 27,2005
		6504030	JUN 10,2019		I-349	FEB 27,2005
019758 001	CLOZAPINE; CLOZARIL				I-380	DEC 18,2005
019758 002	CLOZAPINE; CLOZARIL				I-380	DEC 18,2005
021141 001	COLESEVELAM HYDROCHLORIDE; WELCHOL	5607669	JUN 10,2014	U-323	NCE	MAY 26,2005
		5679717	APR 29,2014	U-323	NCE	MAY 26,2005
		5693675	DEC 02,2014		NCE	MAY 26,2005
		5917007	APR 29,2014	U-323	NCE	MAY 26,2005
		5919832	JUN 10,2014		NCE	MAY 26,2005
		6066678	JUN 10,2014	U-323	NCE	MAY 26,2005
		6433026	JUN 10,2014		NCE	MAY 26,2005
021176 001	COLESEVELAM HYDROCHLORIDE; WELCHOL	5607669	JUN 10,2014	U-323	NCE	MAY 26,2005
		5679717	APR 29,2014	U-323	NCE	MAY 26,2005
		5693675	DEC 02,2014		NCE	MAY 26,2005
		5917007	APR 29,2014	U-323	NCE	MAY 26,2005
		5919832	JUN 10,2014		NCE	MAY 26,2005
		6066678	JUN 10,2014	U-323	NCE	MAY 26,2005
		6433026	JUN 10,2014		NCE	MAY 26,2005
019722 001	CYANOCOBALAMIN; NASCOBAL	4724231	APR 16,2005	U-157		
017821 001	CYCLOBENZAPRINE HYDROCHLORIDE; FLEXERIL				D-78	FEB 03,2006
021041 001	CYTARABINE; DEPOCYT				ODE	APR 01,2006
020287 001	DALTEPARIN SODIUM; FRAGMIN	4303651	JAN 04,2005		D-60	AUG 03,2003
020287 003	DALTEPARIN SODIUM; FRAGMIN	4303651	JAN 04,2005		D-60	AUG 03,2003
020287 004	DALTEPARIN SODIUM; FRAGMIN	4303651	JAN 04,2005		D-60	AUG 03,2003
020430 001	DANAPAROID SODIUM; ORGARAN	5164377	OCT 03,2010			
019849 001	DAPIPRAZOLE HYDROCHLORIDE; REV-EYES	4252721	FEB 07,2003			
050704 002	DAUNORUBICIN CITRATE; DAUNOXOME				ODE	APR 08,2003
020705 001	DELAVIRDINE MESYLATE; RESCRIPTOR	5563142	OCT 08,2013			
		6177101	JUN 11,2018			
020118 001	DESFLURANE; SUPRANE	4762856	FEB 02,2007	U-67		
021165 001	DESLORATADINE; CLARINEX	4659716	APR 21,2004	U-427	PED	JUN 21,2007
		4659716*PED	OCT 21,2004	U-427	PED	JUN 21,2007
		4804666	FEB 14,2006	U-428	PED	JUN 21,2007
		4804666*PED	AUG 14,2006	U-428	PED	JUN 21,2007
		4863931	SEP 15,2008		PED	JUN 21,2007
		4863931*PED	MAR 15,2009		PED	JUN 21,2007
		5595997	DEC 30,2014	U-429	PED	JUN 21,2007
		5595997*PED	JUN 30,2015	U-429	PED	JUN 21,2007
		6100274	JUL 07,2019		PED	JUN 21,2007
		6100274*PED	JAN 07,2020		PED	JUN 21,2007
021312 001	DESLORATADINE; CLARINEX				PED	JUN 21,2007
017922 001	DESMOPRESSIN ACETATE; DDAVP	5500413	JUN 29,2013			
		5674850	DEC 23,2013			
		5763407	JUN 29,2013			
017922 002	DESMOPRESSIN ACETATE; DDAVP	5500413	JUN 29,2013			
		5674850	DEC 23,2013			
		5763407	JUN 29,2013			
018938 001	DESMOPRESSIN ACETATE; DDAVP	5500413	JUN 29,2013			
		5763407	JUN 29,2013			
018938 002	DESMOPRESSIN ACETATE; DDAVP	5500413	JUN 29,2013			
		5763407	JUN 29,2013			
019955 001	DESMOPRESSIN ACETATE; DDAVP	5047398	SEP 10,2008			
		5500413	JUN 29,2013			
		5674850	DEC 23,2013			
		5763407	JUN 29,2013			
019955 002	DESMOPRESSIN ACETATE; DDAVP	5047398	SEP 10,2008			
		5500413	JUN 29,2013			
		5674850	DEC 23,2013			
		5763407	JUN 29,2013			
017922 003	DESMOPRESSIN ACETATE; DDAVP (NEEDS NO REFRIGERATION)	5482931	JUN 29,2013			
		5500413	JUN 29,2013			
		5674850	DEC 23,2013			

PRESCRIPTION AND OTC PRODUCT
PATENT AND EXCLUSIVITY DATA
*PED and PED represent Pediatric Exclusivity (*continued*)

APPL/PROD NUMBER	INGREDIENT NAME; TRADE NAME	PATENT NUMBER	PATENT EXPIRES	USE CODE	EX-CLUS CODE	EXCLUS EXPIRES
		5763407	JUN 29,2013			
021090 001	DESOGESTREL; CYCLESSA	4544554	SEP 26,2003		NP	DEC 20,2003
		4616006	OCT 07,2003		NP	DEC 20,2003
		4628051	SEP 26,2003		NP	DEC 20,2003
020713 001	DESOGESTREL; MIRCETTE	RE35724	OCT 20,2008			
021038 001	DEXMEDETOMIDINE; PRECEDEX	4910214	JUL 15,2008	U-421	NCE	DEC 17,2004
021278 001	DEXMETHYLPHENIDATE HYDROCHLORIDE; FOCALIN	5908850	DEC 04,2015	U-422	NP	NOV 13,2004
		6355656	DEC 04,2015		NP	NOV 13,2004
021278 002	DEXMETHYLPHENIDATE HYDROCHLORIDE; FOCALIN	5908850	DEC 04,2015	U-422	NP	NOV 13,2004
		6355656	DEC 04,2015		NP	NOV 13,2004
021278 003	DEXMETHYLPHENIDATE HYDROCHLORIDE; FOCALIN	5908850	DEC 04,2015	U-422	NP	NOV 13,2004
		6355656	DEC 04,2015		NP	NOV 13,2004
020212 001	DEXRAZOXANE HYDROCHLORIDE; ZINECARD	4275063	JUN 23,2003			
		4963551	DEC 21,2007			
		5242901	SEP 07,2010	U-339		
020212 002	DEXRAZOXANE HYDROCHLORIDE; ZINECARD	4275063	JUN 23,2003			
		4963551	DEC 21,2007			
		5242901	SEP 07,2010	U-339		
019082 001	DEZOCINE; DALGAN	4605671	AUG 12,2003			
019082 002	DEZOCINE; DALGAN	4605671	AUG 12,2003			
019082 003	DEZOCINE; DALGAN	4605671	AUG 12,2003			
020648 001	DIAZEPAM; DIASTAT	5462740	OCT 31,2012		ODE	JUL 29,2004
020648 002	DIAZEPAM; DIASTAT	5462740	OCT 31,2012		ODE	JUL 29,2004
020648 003	DIAZEPAM; DIASTAT	5462740	OCT 31,2012		ODE	JUL 29,2004
020648 004	DIAZEPAM; DIASTAT	5462740	OCT 31,2012		ODE	JUL 29,2004
020648 005	DIAZEPAM; DIASTAT	5462740	OCT 31,2012		ODE	JUL 29,2004
020607 001	DICLOFENAC SODIUM; ARTHROTEC	5601843	FEB 11,2014			
		5698225	FEB 03,2017	U-392		
020607 002	DICLOFENAC SODIUM; ARTHROTEC	5601843	FEB 11,2014			
		5698225	FEB 03,2017	U-392		
020809 001	DICLOFENAC SODIUM; DICLOFENAC SODIUM	5603929	NOV 16,2014	U-239		
		5653972	NOV 16,2014	U-239		
021005 001	DICLOFENAC SODIUM; SOLARAZE	5639738	JUN 17,2014	U-402	NP	OCT 16,2003
		5792753	AUG 11,2015		NP	OCT 16,2003
		5852002	JUN 17,2014	U-402	NP	OCT 16,2003
		5914322	AUG 11,2015		NP	OCT 16,2003
		5929048	JUL 27,2016	U-402	NP	OCT 16,2003
		5985850	NOV 16,2016		NP	OCT 16,2003
020037 001	DICLOFENAC SODIUM; VOLTAREN	4829088	APR 14,2007			
		4960799	OCT 03,2007			
020154 002	DIDANOSINE; VIDEX	4861759	AUG 29,2006	U-248	PED	APR 28,2003
		4861759*PED	MAR 01,2007	U-248	PED	APR 28,2003
		5254539	AUG 29,2006	U-248	PED	APR 28,2003
		5254539*PED	MAR 01,2007	U-248	PED	APR 28,2003
		5616566	AUG 29,2006	U-180	PED	APR 28,2003
		5616566*PED	MAR 01,2007	U-180	PED	APR 28,2003
		5880106	JUL 22,2011		PED	APR 28,2003
		5880106*PED	JAN 22,2012		PED	APR 28,2003
020154 003	DIDANOSINE; VIDEX	4861759	AUG 29,2006	U-248	PED	APR 28,2003
		4861759*PED	MAR 01,2007	U-248	PED	APR 28,2003
		5254539	AUG 29,2006	U-248	PED	APR 28,2003
		5254539*PED	MAR 01,2007	U-248	PED	APR 28,2003
		5616566	AUG 29,2006	U-180	PED	APR 28,2003
		5616566*PED	MAR 01,2007	U-180	PED	APR 28,2003
		5880106	JUL 22,2011		PED	APR 28,2003
		5880106*PED	JAN 22,2012		PED	APR 28,2003
020154 004	DIDANOSINE; VIDEX	4861759	AUG 29,2006	U-248	PED	APR 28,2003
		4861759*PED	MAR 01,2007	U-248	PED	APR 28,2003
		5254539	AUG 29,2006	U-248	PED	APR 28,2003
		5254539*PED	MAR 01,2007	U-248	PED	APR 28,2003
		5616566	AUG 29,2006	U-180	PED	APR 28,2003
		5616566*PED	MAR 01,2007	U-180	PED	APR 28,2003
		5880106	JUL 22,2011		PED	APR 28,2003
		5880106*PED	JAN 22,2012		PED	APR 28,2003
020154 005	DIDANOSINE; VIDEX	4861759	AUG 29,2006	U-248	D-58	OCT 28,2002
		4861759*PED	MAR 01,2007	U-248	D-58	OCT 28,2002
		5254539	AUG 29,2006	U-248	D-58	OCT 28,2002
		5254539*PED	MAR 01,2007	U-248	D-58	OCT 28,2002

PRESCRIPTION AND OTC PRODUCT
PATENT AND EXCLUSIVITY DATA
*PED and PED represent Pediatric Exclusivity (*continued*)

APPL/PROD NUMBER	INGREDIENT NAME; TRADE NAME	PATENT NUMBER	PATENT EXPIRES	USE CODE	EX-CLUS CODE	EXCLUS EXPIRES
		5616566	AUG 29,2006	U-180	D-58	OCT 28,2002
		5616566*PED	MAR 01,2007	U-180	D-58	OCT 28,2002
		5880106	JUL 22,2011		D-58	OCT 28,2002
		5880106*PED	JAN 22,2012		D-58	OCT 28,2002
020154 006	DIDANOSINE; VIDEX	4861759	AUG 29,2006	U-248	NS	OCT 28,2002
		4861759*PED	MAR 01,2007	U-248	NS	OCT 28,2002
		5254539	AUG 29,2006	U-248	NS	OCT 28,2002
		5254539*PED	MAR 01,2007	U-248	NS	OCT 28,2002
		5616566	AUG 29,2006	U-180	NS	OCT 28,2002
		5616566*PED	MAR 01,2007	U-180	NS	OCT 28,2002
		5880106	JUL 22,2011		NS	OCT 28,2002
		5880106*PED	JAN 22,2012		NS	OCT 28,2002
020155 003	DIDANOSINE; VIDEX	4861759	AUG 29,2006	U-248		
		4861759*PED	MAR 01,2007	U-248		
		5254539	AUG 29,2006	U-248		
		5254539*PED	MAR 01,2007	U-248		
		5616566	AUG 29,2006	U-180		
		5616566*PED	MAR 01,2007	U-180		
020155 004	DIDANOSINE; VIDEX	4861759	AUG 29,2006	U-248		
		4861759*PED	MAR 01,2007	U-248		
		5254539	AUG 29,2006	U-248		
		5254539*PED	MAR 01,2007	U-248		
		5616566	AUG 29,2006	U-180		
		5616566*PED	MAR 01,2007	U-180		
020155 005	DIDANOSINE; VIDEX	4861759	AUG 29,2006	U-248		
		4861759*PED	MAR 01,2007	U-248		
		5254539	AUG 29,2006	U-248		
		5254539*PED	MAR 01,2007	U-248		
		5616566	AUG 29,2006	U-180		
		5616566*PED	MAR 01,2007	U-180		
020155 006	DIDANOSINE; VIDEX	4861759	AUG 29,2006	U-52		
		4861759*PED	MAR 01,2007	U-248		
		5254539	AUG 29,2006	U-248		
		5254539*PED	MAR 01,2007	U-248		
		5616566	AUG 29,2006	U-180		
		5616566*PED	MAR 01,2007	U-180		
020156 001	DIDANOSINE; VIDEX	4861759	AUG 29,2006	U-248		
		4861759*PED	MAR 01,2007	U-248		
		5254539	AUG 29,2006	U-248		
		5254539*PED	MAR 01,2007	U-248		
		5616566	AUG 29,2006	U-180		
		5616566*PED	MAR 01,2007	U-180		
021183 001	DIDANOSINE; VIDEX EC	4861759	AUG 29,2006	U-248	PED	MAY 01,2004
		4861759*PED	MAR 01,2007	U-248	PED	MAY 01,2004
		5254539	AUG 29,2006	U-248	PED	MAY 01,2004
		5254539*PED	MAR 01,2007	U-248	PED	MAY 01,2004
021183 002	DIDANOSINE; VIDEX EC	4861759	AUG 29,2006	U-248	PED	MAY 01,2004
		4861759*PED	MAR 01,2007	U-248	PED	MAY 01,2004
		5254539	AUG 29,2006	U-248	PED	MAY 01,2004
		5254539*PED	MAR 01,2007	U-248	PED	MAY 01,2004
021183 003	DIDANOSINE; VIDEX EC	4861759	AUG 29,2006	U-248	PED	MAY 01,2004
		4861759*PED	MAR 01,2007	U-248	PED	MAY 01,2004
		5254539	AUG 29,2006	U-248	PED	MAY 01,2004
		5254539*PED	MAR 01,2007	U-248	PED	MAY 01,2004
021183 004	DIDANOSINE; VIDEX EC	4861759	AUG 29,2006	U-248	PED	MAY 01,2004
		4861759*PED	MAR 01,2007	U-248	PED	MAY 01,2004
		5254539	AUG 29,2006	U-248	PED	MAY 01,2004
		5254539*PED	MAR 01,2007	U-248	PED	MAY 01,2004
020148 001	DIHYDROERGOTAMINE MESYLATE; MIGRANAL	5169849	DEC 08,2009	U-227		
020062 001	DILTIAZEM HYDROCHLORIDE; CARDIZEM CD	4894240	JAN 16,2007			
		5002776	MAR 26,2008			
		5286497	MAY 20,2011			
		5364620	NOV 14,2011	U-3		
		5439689	AUG 08,2012	U-107		
		5470584	MAY 20,2011			
020062 002	DILTIAZEM HYDROCHLORIDE; CARDIZEM CD	4894240	JAN 16,2007			
		5002776	MAR 26,2008			
		5286497	MAY 20,2011			
		5364620	NOV 14,2011	U-3		
		5439689	AUG 08,2012	U-107		
		5470584	MAY 20,2011			

PRESCRIPTION AND OTC PRODUCT
PATENT AND EXCLUSIVITY DATA
*PED and PED represent Pediatric Exclusivity (*continued*)

APPL/PROD NUMBER	INGREDIENT NAME; TRADE NAME	PATENT NUMBER	PATENT EXPIRES	USE CODE	EX-CLUS CODE	EXCLUS EXPIRES
020062 003	DILTIAZEM HYDROCHLORIDE; CARDIZEM CD	4894240	JAN 16,2007			
		5002776	MAR 26,2008			
		5286497	MAY 20,2011			
		5364620	NOV 14,2011	U-3		
		5439689	AUG 08,2012	U-107		
		5470584	MAY 20,2011			
020062 004	DILTIAZEM HYDROCHLORIDE; CARDIZEM CD	4894240	JAN 16,2007			
		5002776	MAR 26,2008			
		5286497	MAY 20,2011			
		5364620	NOV 14,2011	U-3		
		5439689	AUG 08,2012	U-107		
		5470584	MAY 20,2011			
021392 001	DILTIAZEM HYDROCHLORIDE; CARDIZEM LA	5288505	JUN 26,2011		NDF	FEB 06,2006
		5529791	JUN 25,2013		NDF	FEB 06,2006
021392 002	DILTIAZEM HYDROCHLORIDE; CARDIZEM LA	5288505	JUN 26,2011		NDF	FEB 06,2006
		5529791	JUN 25,2013		NDF	FEB 06,2006
021392 003	DILTIAZEM HYDROCHLORIDE; CARDIZEM LA	5288505	JUN 26,2011		NDF	FEB 06,2006
		5529791	JUN 25,2013		NDF	FEB 06,2006
021392 004	DILTIAZEM HYDROCHLORIDE; CARDIZEM LA	5288505	JUN 26,2011		NDF	FEB 06,2006
		5529791	JUN 25,2013		NDF	FEB 06,2006
021392 005	DILTIAZEM HYDROCHLORIDE; CARDIZEM LA	5288505	JUN 26,2011		NDF	FEB 06,2006
		5529791	JUN 25,2013		NDF	FEB 06,2006
021392 006	DILTIAZEM HYDROCHLORIDE; CARDIZEM LA	5288505	JUN 26,2011		NDF	FEB 06,2006
		5529791	JUN 25,2013		NDF	FEB 06,2006
019471 001	DILTIAZEM HYDROCHLORIDE; CARDIZEM SR	4721619	JAN 26,2005			
019471 002	DILTIAZEM HYDROCHLORIDE; CARDIZEM SR	4721619	JAN 26,2005			
019471 003	DILTIAZEM HYDROCHLORIDE; CARDIZEM SR	4721619	JAN 26,2005			
019471 004	DILTIAZEM HYDROCHLORIDE; CARDIZEM SR	4721619	JAN 26,2005			
020092 001	DILTIAZEM HYDROCHLORIDE; DILACOR XR	4839177	DEC 09,2006			
		5422123	JUN 06,2012			
020092 002	DILTIAZEM HYDROCHLORIDE; DILACOR XR	4839177	DEC 09,2006			
		5422123	JUN 06,2012			
020092 003	DILTIAZEM HYDROCHLORIDE; DILACOR XR	4839177	DEC 09,2006			
		5422123	JUN 06,2012			
020939 001	DILTIAZEM HYDROCHLORIDE; DILTIAZEM HCL	5288505	JUN 26,2011			
		5529791	JUN 25,2013			
020939 002	DILTIAZEM HYDROCHLORIDE; DILTIAZEM HCL	5288505	JUN 26,2011			
		5529791	JUN 25,2013			
020939 003	DILTIAZEM HYDROCHLORIDE; DILTIAZEM HCL	5288505	JUN 26,2011			
		5529791	JUN 25,2013			
020939 004	DILTIAZEM HYDROCHLORIDE; DILTIAZEM HCL	5288505	JUN 26,2011			
		5529791	JUN 25,2013			
020401 001	DILTIAZEM HYDROCHLORIDE; TIAZAC	5529791	JUN 25,2013			
020401 002	DILTIAZEM HYDROCHLORIDE; TIAZAC	5529791	JUN 25,2013			
020401 003	DILTIAZEM HYDROCHLORIDE; TIAZAC	5529791	JUN 25,2013			
020401 004	DILTIAZEM HYDROCHLORIDE; TIAZAC	5529791	JUN 25,2013			
020401 005	DILTIAZEM HYDROCHLORIDE; TIAZAC	5529791	JUN 25,2013			
020401 006	DILTIAZEM HYDROCHLORIDE; TIAZAC	5529791	JUN 25,2013			
020507 001	DILTIAZEM MALATE; TECZEM	4880631	SEP 24,2007			
		4968507	JUL 25,2006			
		4983598	JAN 08,2008			
020506 001	DILTIAZEM MALATE; TIAMATE	4880631	SEP 24,2007			
		4968507	JUL 25,2006			
020506 002	DILTIAZEM MALATE; TIAMATE	4880631	SEP 24,2007			
		4968507	JUL 25,2006			
020506 003	DILTIAZEM MALATE; TIAMATE	4880631	SEP 24,2007			
		4968507	JUL 25,2006			
021191 001	DIMYRISTOYL LECITHIN; IMAGENT	5605673	FEB 25,2014		NCE	MAY 31,2007
		5626833	MAY 16,2014	U-458	NCE	MAY 31,2007
		5639443	JUN 17,2014		NCE	MAY 31,2007
		5695741	DEC 09,2014	U-458	NCE	MAY 31,2007
		5720938	FEB 24,2015		NCE	MAY 31,2007
		5798091	AUG 25,2015	U-458	NCE	MAY 31,2007
		6280704	JUL 30,2013		NCE	MAY 31,2007
		6280705	JUL 30,2013		NCE	MAY 31,2007
		6287539	JUL 30,2013		NCE	MAY 31,2007
020411 001	DINOPROSTONE; CERVIDIL	4931288	JAN 16,2007			
		5269321	DEC 14,2010	U-110		
019617 001	DINOPROSTONE; PREPIDIL	4680312	JUL 14,2004			
018723 001	DIVALPROEX SODIUM; DEPAKOTE	4988731	JAN 29,2008			
		5212326	JAN 29,2008			

PRESCRIPTION AND OTC PRODUCT
PATENT AND EXCLUSIVITY DATA
*PED and PED represent Pediatric Exclusivity (continued)

APPL/PROD NUMBER	INGREDIENT NAME; TRADE NAME	PATENT NUMBER	PATENT EXPIRES	USE CODE	EX-CLUS CODE	EXCLUS EXPIRES
018723 002	DIVALPROEX SODIUM; DEPAKOTE	4988731	JAN 29,2008			
		5212326	JAN 29,2008			
018723 003	DIVALPROEX SODIUM; DEPAKOTE	4988731	JAN 29,2008			
		5212326	JAN 29,2008			
019680 001	DIVALPROEX SODIUM; DEPAKOTE	4988731	JAN 29,2008			
		5212326	JAN 29,2008			
019794 001	DIVALPROEX SODIUM; DEPAKOTE CP	4988731	JAN 29,2008			
		5212326	JAN 29,2008			
019794 002	DIVALPROEX SODIUM; DEPAKOTE CP	4988731	JAN 29,2008			
		5212326	JAN 29,2008			
021168 001	DIVALPROEX SODIUM; DEPAKOTE ER	4913906	APR 03,2007		NP	AUG 04,2003
		4988731	JAN 29,2008		NP	AUG 04,2003
		6419953	DEC 18,2018		NP	AUG 04,2003
		6511678	DEC 18,2018		NP	AUG 04,2003
021168 002	DIVALPROEX SODIUM; DEPAKOTE ER	4913906	APR 03,2007		NP	AUG 04,2003
		4988731	JAN 29,2008		NP	AUG 04,2003
		6511678	DEC 18,2018		NP	AUG 04,2003
020449 001	DOCETAXEL; TAXOTERE	4814470	MAY 14,2010	I-379		NOV 27,2005
		5438072	NOV 22,2013	I-379		NOV 27,2005
		5698582	JUL 03,2012	I-379		NOV 27,2005
		5714512	JUL 03,2012	I-379		NOV 27,2005
020941 001	DOCOSANOL; ABREVA	4874794	APR 28,2014		NCE	JUL 25,2005
020931 001	DOFETILIDE; TIKOSYN	6124363	OCT 09,2018		NCE	OCT 01,2004
020931 002	DOFETILIDE; TIKOSYN	6124363	OCT 09,2018		NCE	OCT 01,2004
020931 003	DOFETILIDE; TIKOSYN	6124363	OCT 09,2018		NCE	OCT 01,2004
020623 001	DOLASETRON MESYLATE MONOHYDRATE; ANZEMET	4906755	JUL 02,2011		NCE	SEP 11,2002
020623 002	DOLASETRON MESYLATE MONOHYDRATE; ANZEMET	4906755	JUL 02,2011		NCE	SEP 11,2002
020624 001	DOLASETRON MESYLATE MONOHYDRATE; ANZEMET	4906755	JUL 02,2011		NCE	SEP 11,2002
020690 001	DONEPEZIL HYDROCHLORIDE; ARICEPT	4895841	NOV 25,2010			
		5985864	DEC 30,2016			
		6140321	DEC 30,2016			
		6245911	DEC 01,2018			
		6372760	MAR 31,2019			
020690 002	DONEPEZIL HYDROCHLORIDE; ARICEPT	4895841	NOV 25,2010			
		5985864	DEC 30,2016			
		6140321	DEC 30,2016			
		6245911	DEC 01,2018			
		6372760	MAR 31,2019			
020869 001	DORZOLAMIDE HYDROCHLORIDE; COSOPT	4619939	OCT 28,2003	U-104		
		4797413	APR 28,2008	U-103		
		6248735	APR 17,2011			
020408 001	DORZOLAMIDE HYDROCHLORIDE; TRUSOPT	4619939	OCT 28,2003	U-104		
		4797413	APR 28,2008	U-103		
019946 001	DOXACURIUM CHLORIDE; NUROMAX	4701460	MAR 06,2005			
020862 001	DOXERCALCIFEROL; HECTOROL	5602116	FEB 11,2014	U-278	NCE	JUN 09,2004
		5707980	AUG 17,2010	U-278	NCE	JUN 09,2004
		5861386	AUG 02,2008	U-278	NCE	JUN 09,2004
		5869473	AUG 02,2008	U-278	NCE	JUN 09,2004
021027 001	DOXERCALCIFEROL; HECTOROL	5602116	FEB 11,2014	U-321	NCE	JUN 09,2004
		5707980	AUG 17,2010	U-321	NCE	JUN 09,2004
050718 001	DOXORUBICIN HYDROCHLORIDE; DOXIL				ODE	JUN 28,2006
021098 001	DROSPIRENONE; YASMIN	5569652	OCT 29,2013	U-1	NC	MAY 11,2004
021319 001	DUTASTERIDE; AVODART	5565467	OCT 15,2013		NCE	NOV 20,2006
		5846976	DEC 08,2015	U-476	NCE	NOV 20,2006
		5998427	OCT 15,2013	U-477	NCE	NOV 20,2006
020972 001	EFAVIRENZ; SUSTIVA	5519021	MAY 21,2013		NCE	SEP 17,2003
		5663169	SEP 02,2014	U-257	NCE	SEP 17,2003
		5811423	AUG 07,2012	U-256	NCE	SEP 17,2003
		6238695	APR 06,2019		NCE	SEP 17,2003
		6555133	APR 06,2019	U-248	NCE	SEP 17,2003
020972 002	EFAVIRENZ; SUSTIVA	5519021	MAY 21,2013		NCE	SEP 17,2003
		5663169	SEP 02,2014	U-257	NCE	SEP 17,2003
		5811423	AUG 07,2012	U-256	NCE	SEP 17,2003
		6238695	APR 06,2019		NCE	SEP 17,2003
		6555133	APR 06,2019	U-248	NCE	SEP 17,2003
020972 003	EFAVIRENZ; SUSTIVA	5519021	MAY 21,2013		NCE	SEP 17,2003
		5663169	SEP 02,2014	U-257	NCE	SEP 17,2003
		5811423	AUG 07,2012	U-256	NCE	SEP 17,2003

PRESCRIPTION AND OTC PRODUCT
PATENT AND EXCLUSIVITY DATA
*PED and PED represent Pediatric Exclusivity (*continued*)

APPL/PROD NUMBER	INGREDIENT NAME; TRADE NAME	PATENT NUMBER	PATENT EXPIRES	USE CODE	EX-CLUS CODE	EXCLUS EXPIRES
		6238695	APR 06,2019		NCE	SEP 17,2003
021360 001	EFAVIRENZ; SUSTIVA	6555133	APR 06,2019	U-248	NCE	SEP 17,2003
		5519021	MAY 21,2013		NCE	SEP 17,2003
		5663169	SEP 02,2014		NCE	SEP 17,2003
		5811423	AUG 07,2012	U-256	NCE	SEP 17,2003
021360 002	EFAVIRENZ; SUSTIVA	5519021	MAY 21,2013		NCE	SEP 17,2003
		5663169	SEP 02,2014	U-248	NCE	SEP 17,2003
		5811423	AUG 07,2012	U-256	NCE	SEP 17,2003
021145 001	EFLORNITHINE HYDROCHLORIDE; VANIQA	4720489	JAN 19,2005	U-334	NP	JUL 27,2003
		5648394	JUL 15,2014	U-334	NP	JUL 27,2003
021016 001	ELETRIPTAN HYDROBROMIDE; RELPAX	5545644	AUG 13,2013		NCE	DEC 26,2007
021016 002	ELETRIPTAN HYDROBROMIDE; RELPAX	5545644	AUG 13,2013		NCE	DEC 26,2007
020706 001	EMEDASTINE DIFUMARATE; EMADINE	4430343	AUG 14,2005	U-403	NCE	DEC 29,2002
		5441958	DEC 08,2013	U-404	NCE	DEC 29,2002
020668 001	ENALAPRIL MALEATE; LEXXEL	4703038	OCT 07,2005	U-3		
		4803081	APR 03,2007			
		4803081*PED	OCT 03,2007			
020668 002	ENALAPRIL MALEATE; LEXXEL	4703038	OCT 07,2005	U-3		
		4803081	APR 03,2007			
		4803081*PED	OCT 03,2007			
018998 001	ENALAPRIL MALEATE; VASOTEC				PED	AUG 13,2004
018998 002	ENALAPRIL MALEATE; VASOTEC				M-7	FEB 13,2004
018998 003	ENALAPRIL MALEATE; VASOTEC				PED	AUG 13,2004
018998 005	ENALAPRIL MALEATE; VASOTEC				M-7	FEB 13,2004
021481 001	ENFUVIRTIDE; FUZEON	5112861	MAY 12,2009		NCE	MAR 13,2008
		5464933	JUN 07,2013		NCE	MAR 13,2008
		6133418	JUN 07,2013		NCE	MAR 13,2008
		6475491	JUN 07,2015	U-248	NCE	MAR 13,2008
		6500867	JUN 29,2020		NCE	MAR 13,2008
020164 001	ENOXAPARIN SODIUM; LOVENOX	4692435	DEC 24,2004	U-123	I-315	NOV 17,2003
		5389618	FEB 14,2012		I-315	NOV 17,2003
020164 002	ENOXAPARIN SODIUM; LOVENOX	4692435	DEC 24,2004	U-123	I-315	NOV 17,2003
		5389618	FEB 14,2012		I-315	NOV 17,2003
020164 003	ENOXAPARIN SODIUM; LOVENOX	4692435	DEC 24,2004	U-123	I-315	NOV 17,2003
		5389618	FEB 14,2012		I-315	NOV 17,2003
020164 004	ENOXAPARIN SODIUM; LOVENOX	4692435	DEC 24,2004	U-123	I-315	NOV 17,2003
		5389618	FEB 14,2012		I-315	NOV 17,2003
020164 005	ENOXAPARIN SODIUM; LOVENOX	4692435	DEC 24,2004	U-123	I-315	NOV 17,2003
		5389618	FEB 14,2012		I-315	NOV 17,2003
020164 006	ENOXAPARIN SODIUM; LOVENOX	4692435	DEC 24,2004	U-123		
		5389618	FEB 14,2012			
020164 007	ENOXAPARIN SODIUM; LOVENOX	4692435	DEC 24,2004	U-123		
		5389618	FEB 14,2012			
020164 008	ENOXAPARIN SODIUM; LOVENOX	4692435	DEC 24,2004	U-123		
		5389618	FEB 14,2012			
020796 001	ENTACAPONE; COMTAN	4963590	NOV 27,2007		NCE	OCT 19,2004
		5112861	MAY 12,2009		NCE	OCT 19,2004
		5135950	OCT 31,2010		NCE	OCT 19,2004
		5446194	AUG 29,2012		NCE	OCT 19,2004
050778 001	EPIRUBICIN HYDROCHLORIDE; ELLENCE				ODE	SEP 15,2006
021437 001	EPLERENONE; INSPRA	4559332	APR 09,2004		NCE	SEP 27,2007
		6410054	DEC 08,2019	U-3	NCE	SEP 27,2007
		6410524	NOV 05,2019	U-467	NCE	SEP 27,2007
		6495165	DEC 08,2019	U-3	NCE	SEP 27,2007
		6534093	DEC 08,2019	U-3	NCE	SEP 27,2007
021437 002	EPLERENONE; INSPRA	4559332	APR 09,2004		NCE	SEP 27,2007
		6410054	DEC 08,2019	U-3	NCE	SEP 27,2007
		6410524	NOV 05,2019	U-467	NCE	SEP 27,2007
		6495165	DEC 08,2019	U-3	NCE	SEP 27,2007
		6534093	DEC 08,2019	U-3	NCE	SEP 27,2007
021437 003	EPLERENONE; INSPRA	4559332	APR 09,2004		NCE	SEP 27,2007
		6410054	DEC 08,2019	U-3	NCE	SEP 27,2007
		6410524	NOV 05,2019	U-467	NCE	SEP 27,2007
		6495165	DEC 08,2019	U-3	NCE	SEP 27,2007
		6534093	DEC 08,2019	U-3	NCE	SEP 27,2007
020444 001	EPOPROSTENOL SODIUM; FLOLAN	4539333	SEP 03,2002		I-296	APR 14,2003
		4883812	MAY 12,2006	U-185	I-296	APR 14,2003
020444 002	EPOPROSTENOL SODIUM; FLOLAN	4539333	SEP 03,2002		I-296	APR 14,2003
		4883812	MAY 12,2006	U-185	I-296	APR 14,2003
020738 004	EPROSARTAN MESYLATE; TEVETEN	5185351	FEB 09,2010	U-3	NCE	DEC 22,2002
		5656650	AUG 12,2014	U-3	NCE	DEC 22,2002

PRESCRIPTION AND OTC PRODUCT
PATENT AND EXCLUSIVITY DATA
*PED and PED represent Pediatric Exclusivity (*continued*)

APPL/PROD NUMBER	INGREDIENT NAME; TRADE NAME	PATENT NUMBER	PATENT EXPIRES	USE CODE	EX-CLUS CODE	EXCLUS EXPIRES
020738 005	EPROSARTAN MESYLATE; TEVETEN	5185351	FEB 09,2010	U-3	NCE	DEC 22,2002
		5656650	AUG 12,2014	U-3	NCE	DEC 22,2002
020738 006	EPROSARTAN MESYLATE; TEVETEN	5185351	FEB 09,2010	U-3	NCE	DEC 22,2002
		5656650	AUG 12,2014	U-3	NCE	DEC 22,2002
021268 001	EPROSARTAN MESYLATE; TEVETEN HCT	5185351	FEB 09,2010	U-3	NCE	DEC 22,2002
		5656650	AUG 12,2014	U-3	NCE	DEC 22,2002
021268 002	EPROSARTAN MESYLATE; TEVETEN HCT	5185351	FEB 09,2010	U-3	NC	NOV 01,2004
		5656650	AUG 12,2014	U-3	NC	NOV 01,2004
020718 001	EPTIFIBATIDE; INTEGRILIN	5686570	NOV 11,2014		D-66	JUN 08,2004
		5747447	MAY 05,2015		D-66	JUN 08,2004
		5756451	NOV 11,2014		D-66	JUN 08,2004
		5807825	SEP 15,2015	U-244	D-66	JUN 08,2004
		5968902	JUN 02,2015	U-453	D-66	JUN 08,2004
020718 002	EPTIFIBATIDE; INTEGRILIN	5686570	NOV 11,2014		D-66	JUN 08,2004
		5747447	MAY 05,2015		D-66	JUN 08,2004
		5756451	NOV 11,2014		D-66	JUN 08,2004
		5807825	SEP 15,2015	U-244	D-66	JUN 08,2004
		5968902	JUN 02,2015	U-453	D-66	JUN 08,2004
021337 001	ERTAPENEM SODIUM; INVANZ	5478820	FEB 02,2013		NCE	NOV 21,2006
		5652233	FEB 02,2013		NCE	NOV 21,2006
		5952323	MAY 15,2017		NCE	NOV 21,2006
021323 001	ESCITALOPRAM OXALATE; LEXAPRO	RE34712	JUN 08,2009		PED	FEB 14,2006
		RE34712*PED	DEC 08,2009		PED	FEB 14,2006
021323 002	ESCITALOPRAM OXALATE; LEXAPRO	RE34712	JUN 08,2009		PED	FEB 14,2006
		RE34712*PED	DEC 08,2009		PED	FEB 14,2006
021323 003	ESCITALOPRAM OXALATE; LEXAPRO	RE34712	JUN 08,2009		PED	MAR 01,2006
		RE34712*PED	DEC 08,2009		PED	MAR 01,2006
021365 001	ESCITALOPRAM OXALATE; LEXAPRO				PED	FEB 14,2006
019386 002	ESMOLOL HYDROCHLORIDE; BREVIBLOC	4593119	JUN 03,2003			
		5017609	MAY 21,2008			
019386 003	ESMOLOL HYDROCHLORIDE; BREVIBLOC	4593119	JUN 03,2003			
		5017609	MAY 21,2008			
019386 006	ESMOLOL HYDROCHLORIDE; BREVIBLOC	4593119	JUN 03,2003			
		6310094	JAN 12,2021			
		6528540	JAN 12,2021			
019386 005	ESMOLOL HYDROCHLORIDE; BREVIBLOC DOUBLE STRENGTH IN PLASTIC CONTAINER	4593119	JUN 03,2003			
		6310094	JAN 12,2021			
		6528540	JAN 12,2021			
019386 004	ESMOLOL HYDROCHLORIDE; BREVIBLOC IN PLASTIC CONTAINER	4593119	JUN 03,2003			
		6310094	JAN 12,2021			
		6528540	JAN 12,2021			
021153 001	ESOMEPRAZOLE MAGNESIUM; NEXIUM	4738974	APR 19,2005	U-373	PED	AUG 20,2004
		4738974*PED	OCT 19,2005	U-373	PED	AUG 20,2004
		4786505	APR 20,2007	U-373	PED	AUG 20,2004
		4786505*PED	OCT 20,2007	U-373	PED	AUG 20,2004
		4853230	APR 20,2007	U-373	PED	AUG 20,2004
		4853230*PED	OCT 20,2007	U-373	PED	AUG 20,2004
		5690960	NOV 25,2014	U-373	PED	AUG 20,2004
		5690960*PED	MAY 25,2015	U-373	PED	AUG 20,2004
		5714504	FEB 03,2015	U-373	PED	AUG 20,2004
		5714504*PED	AUG 03,2015	U-373	PED	AUG 20,2004
		5877192	MAY 27,2014	U-373	PED	AUG 20,2004
		5877192*PED	NOV 27,2014	U-373	PED	AUG 20,2004
		5900424	MAY 04,2016	U-373	PED	AUG 20,2004
		5900424*PED	NOV 04,2016	U-373	PED	AUG 20,2004
		6147103	OCT 09,2018		PED	AUG 20,2004
		6147103*PED	APR 09,2019		PED	AUG 20,2004
		6166213	OCT 09,2018		PED	AUG 20,2004
		6166213*PED	APR 09,2019		PED	AUG 20,2004
		6191148	OCT 09,2018		PED	AUG 20,2004
		6191148*PED	APR 09,2019		PED	AUG 20,2004
		6369085	MAY 25,2018		PED	AUG 20,2004
		6369085*PED	NOV 25,2018		PED	AUG 20,2004
		6428810	NOV 03,2018	U-469	PED	AUG 20,2004
		6428810*PED	MAY 03,2020	U-469	PED	AUG 20,2004
021153 002	ESOMEPRAZOLE MAGNESIUM; NEXIUM	4738974	APR 19,2005	U-373	PED	AUG 20,2004
		4738974*PED	OCT 19,2005	U-373	PED	AUG 20,2004
		4786505	APR 20,2007	U-373	PED	AUG 20,2004
		4786505*PED	OCT 20,2007	U-373	PED	AUG 20,2004

PRESCRIPTION AND OTC PRODUCT
PATENT AND EXCLUSIVITY DATA
*PED and PED represent Pediatric Exclusivity (*continued*)

APPL/PROD NUMBER	INGREDIENT NAME; TRADE NAME	PATENT NUMBER	PATENT EXPIRES	USE CODE	EX-CLUS CODE	EXCLUS EXPIRES
		4853230	APR 20,2007	U-373	PED	AUG 20,2004
		4853230*PED	OCT 20,2007	U-373	PED	AUG 20,2004
		5690960	NOV 25,2014	U-373	PED	AUG 20,2004
		5690960*PED	MAY 25,2015	U-373	PED	AUG 20,2004
		5714504	FEB 03,2015	U-373	PED	AUG 20,2004
		5714504*PED	AUG 03,2015	U-373	PED	AUG 20,2004
		5877192	MAY 27,2014	U-373	PED	AUG 20,2004
		5877192*PED	NOV 27,2014	U-373	PED	AUG 20,2004
		5900424	MAY 04,2016	U-373	PED	AUG 20,2004
		5900424*PED	NOV 04,2016	U-373	PED	AUG 20,2004
		6147103	OCT 09,2018		PED	AUG 20,2004
		6147103*PED	APR 09,2019		PED	AUG 20,2004
		6166213	OCT 09,2018		PED	AUG 20,2004
		6166213*PED	APR 09,2019		PED	AUG 20,2004
		6191148	OCT 09,2018		PED	AUG 20,2004
		6191148*PED	APR 09,2019		PED	AUG 20,2004
		6369085	MAY 25,2018		PED	AUG 20,2004
		6369085*PED	NOV 25,2018		PED	AUG 20,2004
		6428810	NOV 03,2019	U-469	PED	AUG 20,2004
		6428810*PED	MAY 03,2020	U-469	PED	AUG 20,2004
021367 001	ESTRADIOL ACETATE; FEMRING	5855906	DEC 19,2015	U-508	NP	MAR 20,2006
021367 002	ESTRADIOL ACETATE; FEMRING	5855906	DEC 19,2015	U-508	NP	MAR 20,2006
020874 001	ESTRADIOL CYPIONATE; LUNELLE				NP	OCT 05,2003
020907 001	ESTRADIOL; ACTIVELLA	RE36247	MAY 02,2006		I-295	APR 11,2003
020655 001	ESTRADIOL; ALORA	5122383	MAY 17,2011		I-351	APR 05,2005
		5164190	DEC 11,2010		I-351	APR 05,2005
		5212199	MAY 17,2011		I-351	APR 05,2005
		5227169	MAY 17,2011		I-351	APR 05,2005
020655 002	ESTRADIOL; ALORA	5122383	MAY 17,2011		I-351	APR 05,2005
		5164190	DEC 11,2010		I-351	APR 05,2005
		5212199	MAY 17,2011		I-351	APR 05,2005
		5227169	MAY 17,2011		I-351	APR 05,2005
020655 003	ESTRADIOL; ALORA	5122383	MAY 17,2011		I-351	APR 05,2005
		5164190	DEC 11,2010		I-351	APR 05,2005
		5212199	MAY 17,2011		I-351	APR 05,2005
		5227169	MAY 17,2011		I-351	APR 05,2005
020655 004	ESTRADIOL; ALORA	5122383	MAY 17,2011		I-351	APR 05,2005
		5164190	DEC 11,2010		I-351	APR 05,2005
		5212199	MAY 17,2011		I-351	APR 05,2005
		5227169	MAY 17,2011		I-351	APR 05,2005
020375 001	ESTRADIOL; CLIMARA	5223261	JUN 29,2010			
020375 002	ESTRADIOL; CLIMARA	5223261	JUN 29,2010			
020375 003	ESTRADIOL; CLIMARA	5223261	JUN 29,2010			
020375 004	ESTRADIOL; CLIMARA	5223261	JUN 29,2010			
020870 001	ESTRADIOL; COMBIPATCH	5474783	DEC 12,2012			
		5656286	AUG 12,2014			
		5958446	DEC 12,2012			
		6024976	JAN 07,2014			
020870 002	ESTRADIOL; COMBIPATCH	5474783	DEC 12,2012			
		5656286	AUG 12,2014			
		5958446	DEC 12,2012			
		6024976	JAN 07,2014			
020847 001	ESTRADIOL; ESCLIM	4842864	MAR 25,2008			
020847 002	ESTRADIOL; ESCLIM	4842864	MAR 25,2008			
020847 003	ESTRADIOL; ESCLIM	4842864	MAR 25,2008			
020847 004	ESTRADIOL; ESCLIM	4842864	MAR 25,2008			
020847 005	ESTRADIOL; ESCLIM	4842864	MAR 25,2008			
020472 001	ESTRADIOL; ESTRING	4871543	JUN 12,2007	U-306		
		5188835	JUN 12,2007	U-306		
020417 001	ESTRADIOL; FEMPATCH	4906463	MAR 06,2007			
		5006342	APR 09,2008			
021040 001	ESTRADIOL; PREFEST	5108995	APR 28,2009	U-311		
		5382573	JAN 17,2012			
020323 001	ESTRADIOL; VIVELLE	4814168	MAR 04,2008		I-254	AUG 16,2003
		4994267	MAR 04,2008		I-254	AUG 16,2003
		4994278	MAR 04,2008		I-254	AUG 16,2003
		5300291	APR 05,2011		I-254	AUG 16,2003
020323 002	ESTRADIOL; VIVELLE	4814168	MAR 04,2008		I-254	AUG 16,2003
		4994267	MAR 04,2008		I-254	AUG 16,2003
		4994278	MAR 04,2008		I-254	AUG 16,2003
		5300291	APR 05,2011		I-254	AUG 16,2003

PRESCRIPTION AND OTC PRODUCT
PATENT AND EXCLUSIVITY DATA
*PED and PED represent Pediatric Exclusivity (*continued*)

APPL/PROD NUMBER	INGREDIENT NAME; TRADE NAME	PATENT NUMBER	PATENT EXPIRES	USE CODE	EX- CLUS CODE	EXCLUS EXPIRES
020323 003	ESTRADIOL; VIVELLE	4814168	MAR 04,2008		I-254	AUG 16,2003
		4994267	MAR 04,2008		I-254	AUG 16,2003
		4994278	MAR 04,2008		I-254	AUG 16,2003
		5300291	APR 05,2011		I-254	AUG 16,2003
020323 004	ESTRADIOL; VIVELLE	4814168	MAR 04,2008		I-254	AUG 16,2003
		4994267	MAR 04,2008		I-254	AUG 16,2003
		4994278	MAR 04,2008		I-254	AUG 16,2003
		5300291	APR 05,2011		I-254	AUG 16,2003
020323 005	ESTRADIOL; VIVELLE	4814168	MAR 04,2008		I-254	AUG 16,2003
		4994267	MAR 04,2008		I-254	AUG 16,2003
		4994278	MAR 04,2008		I-254	AUG 16,2003
		5300291	APR 05,2011		I-254	AUG 16,2003
020538 005	ESTRADIOL; VIVELLE-DOT	5474783	DEC 12,2012		I-254	AUG 16,2003
		5656286	AUG 12,2014		I-254	AUG 16,2003
		5958446	DEC 12,2012		I-254	AUG 16,2003
		6024976	JAN 07,2014		I-254	AUG 16,2003
020538 006	ESTRADIOL; VIVELLE-DOT	5474783	DEC 12,2012		I-254	AUG 16,2003
		5656286	AUG 12,2014		I-254	AUG 16,2003
		5958446	DEC 12,2012		I-254	AUG 16,2003
		6024976	JAN 07,2014		I-254	AUG 16,2003
020538 007	ESTRADIOL; VIVELLE-DOT	5474783	DEC 12,2012		I-254	AUG 16,2003
		5656286	AUG 12,2014		I-254	AUG 16,2003
		5958446	DEC 12,2012		I-254	AUG 16,2003
		6024976	JAN 07,2014		I-254	AUG 16,2003
020538 008	ESTRADIOL; VIVELLE-DOT	5474783	DEC 12,2012		I-254	AUG 16,2003
		5656286	AUG 12,2014		I-254	AUG 16,2003
		5958446	DEC 12,2012		I-254	AUG 16,2003
		6024976	JAN 07,2014		I-254	AUG 16,2003
020992 001	ESTROGENS, CONJUGATED SYNTHETIC A; CENESTIN	5908638	JUL 26,2015		I-359	JUN 21,2005
020992 002	ESTROGENS, CONJUGATED SYNTHETIC A; CENESTIN	5908638	JUL 26,2015			
020992 003	ESTROGENS, CONJUGATED SYNTHETIC A; CENESTIN	5908638	JUL 26,2015			
020992 004	ESTROGENS, CONJUGATED SYNTHETIC A; CENESTIN	5908638	JUL 26,2015			
010971 005	ESTROGENS, CONJUGATED; PMB 200	5210081	FEB 26,2012			
010971 003	ESTROGENS, CONJUGATED; PMB 400	5210081	FEB 26,2012			
004782 001	ESTROGENS, CONJUGATED; PREMARIN	5210081	FEB 26,2012			
004782 002	ESTROGENS, CONJUGATED; PREMARIN	5210081	FEB 26,2012			
004782 003	ESTROGENS, CONJUGATED; PREMARIN	5210081	FEB 26,2012			
004782 004	ESTROGENS, CONJUGATED; PREMARIN	5210081	FEB 26,2012			
004782 005	ESTROGENS, CONJUGATED; PREMARIN	5210081	FEB 26,2012			
010402 001	ESTROGENS, CONJUGATED; PREMARIN	5210081	FEB 26,2012			
020216 001	ESTROGENS, CONJUGATED; PREMARIN	5210081	FEB 26,2012			
020303 002	ESTROGENS, CONJUGATED; PREMPHASE (PREMARIN;CYCRIN 14/14)	5210081	FEB 26,2012			
020527 002	ESTROGENS, CONJUGATED; PREMPHASE 14/14	5210081	FEB 26,2012			
		5547948	JAN 17,2015			
020527 001	ESTROGENS, CONJUGATED; PREMPRO	5210081	FEB 26,2012		D-79	MAR 12,2006
		5547948	JAN 17,2015		D-79	MAR 12,2006
		RE36247	MAY 02,2006	U-284	D-79	MAR 12,2006
020527 003	ESTROGENS, CONJUGATED; PREMPRO	5210081	FEB 26,2012		D-79	MAR 12,2006
		5547948	JAN 17,2015		D-79	MAR 12,2006
		RE36247	MAY 02,2006	U-284	D-79	MAR 12,2006
020527 004	ESTROGENS, CONJUGATED; PREMPRO	5210081	FEB 26,2012		D-81	JUN 04,2006
		5547948	JAN 17,2015		D-79	MAR 12,2006
		RE36247	MAY 02,2006		NP	MAR 12,2006
020527 005	ESTROGENS, CONJUGATED; PREMPRO	5210081	FEB 26, 2012		NS	JUN 04,2006
					D-81	JUN 04,2006
020303 001	ESTROGENS, CONJUGATED; PREMPRO (PREMARIN;CYCRIN)	5210081	FEB 26,2012			
		RE36247	MAY 02,2006	U-284		
020130 001	ETHINYL ESTRADIOL; ESTROSTEP 21	4962098	OCT 09,2007	U-112	I-331	JUL 01,2004
		5010070	APR 23,2008		I-331	JUL 01,2004
020130 002	ETHINYL ESTRADIOL; ESTROSTEP FE	4962098	OCT 09,2007	U-112	I-331	JUL 01,2004
		5010070	APR 23,2008		I-331	JUL 01,2004
021065 002	ETHINYL ESTRADIOL; FEMHRT	5208225	MAY 04,2010	U-283	NP	OCT 15,2002
021187 001	ETHINYL ESTRADIOL; NUVARING	5989581	APR 08,2018		NP	OCT 03,2004
021180 001	ETHINYL ESTRADIOL; ORTHO EVRA	5876746	JUN 07,2015	U-514	NP	NOV 20,2004
		5972377	JUN 07,2015	U-514	NP	NOV 20,2004

PRESCRIPTION AND OTC PRODUCT
PATENT AND EXCLUSIVITY DATA
*PED and PED represent Pediatric Exclusivity (continued)

APPL/PROD NUMBER	INGREDIENT NAME; TRADE NAME	PATENT NUMBER	PATENT EXPIRES	USE CODE	EX-CLUS CODE	EXCLUS EXPIRES
019697 001	ETHINYL ESTRADIOL; ORTHO TRI-CYCLEN	4530839	SEP 26,2003	U-112		
		4544554	SEP 26,2003	U-66		
		4616006	SEP 26,2003	U-66		
		4628051	SEP 26,2003	U-66		
019697 002	ETHINYL ESTRADIOL; ORTHO TRI-CYCLEN	4530839	SEP 26,2003	U-112		
		4544554	SEP 26,2003	U-66		
		4616006	SEP 26,2003	U-66		
		4628051	SEP 26,2003	U-66		
021241 001	ETHINYL ESTRADIOL; ORTHO TRI-CYCLEN LO	4530839	SEP 26,2003	U-112	NP	AUG 22,2005
		4544554	SEP 26,2003	U-112	NP	AUG 22,2005
		4616006	SEP 26,2003	U-112	NP	AUG 22,2005
		4628051	SEP 26,2003	U-112	NP	AUG 22,2005
		6214815	JUN 09,2019	U-112	NP	AUG 22,2005
018985 001	ETHINYL ESTRADIOL; ORTHO-NOVUM 7/7/7-21	4530839	SEP 26,2003			
		4544554	SEP 26,2003			
		4616006	SEP 26,2003			
		4628051	SEP 26,2003			
018985 002	ETHINYL ESTRADIOL; ORTHO-NOVUM 7/7/7-28	4530839	SEP 26,2003			
		4544554	SEP 26,2003			
		4616006	SEP 26,2003			
		4628051	SEP 26,2003			
020946 001	ETHINYL ESTRADIOL; PREVEN EMERGENCY CONTRACEPTIVE KIT	6156742	DEC 05,2020	U-374		
020584 001	ETODOLAC; LODINE XL	4966768	OCT 30,2007		PED	FEB 11,2004
		4966768*PED	APR 30,2008		PED	FEB 11,2004
020584 002	ETODOLAC; LODINE XL	4966768	OCT 30,2007		PED	FEB 11,2004
		4966768*PED	APR 30,2008		PED	FEB 11,2004
020584 003	ETODOLAC; LODINE XL	4966768	OCT 30,2007		PED	FEB 11,2004
		4966768*PED	APR 30,2008		PED	FEB 11,2004
020457 001	ETOPOSIDE PHOSPHATE; ETOPOPHOS PRESERVATIVE FREE	5041424	AUG 20,2008	U-135		
		RE35524	MAY 17,2010			
020906 001	ETOPOSIDE PHOSPHATE; ETOPOPHOS PRESERVATIVE FREE	5041424	AUG 20,2008	U-135		
		RE35524	MAY 17,2010			
020906 002	ETOPOSIDE PHOSPHATE; ETOPOPHOS PRESERVATIVE FREE	5041424	AUG 20,2008	U-135		
		RE35524	MAY 17,2010			
020753 001	EXEMESTANE; AROMASIN	4808616	JUL 07,2006		ODE	OCT 21,2006
		4904650	JUL 07,2006		ODE	OCT 21,2006
021445 001	EZETIMIBE; ZETIA	5846966	SEP 21,2013	U-474	NCE	OCT 25,2007
		RE37721	JUN 16,2015	U-473	NCE	OCT 25,2007
020363 001	FAMCICLOVIR; FAMVIR	5246937	SEP 21,2010	U-96		
020363 002	FAMCICLOVIR; FAMVIR	5246937	SEP 21,2010	U-96		
020363 003	FAMCICLOVIR; FAMVIR	5246937	SEP 21,2010	U-96		
020325 001	FAMOTIDINE; PEPCID AC	5667794	MAY 02,2015	U-205		
		5667794*PED	NOV 02,2015	U-205		
		5854267	DEC 29,2015	U-267		
		5854267*PED	JUN 29,2016	U-267		
020801 001	FAMOTIDINE; PEPCID AC	5075114	DEC 24,2008			
		5075114*PED	JUN 24,2009			
		5667794	MAY 02,2015			
		5667794*PED	NOV 02,2015			
		5854267	DEC 29,2015	U-267		
		5854267*PED	JUN 29,2016			
020902 001	FAMOTIDINE; PEPCID AC	4820524	FEB 20,2007			
		4820524*PED	AUG 20,2007			
		5667794	MAY 02,2015			
		5667794*PED	NOV 02,2015	U-368		
		5854267	DEC 29,2015	U-368		
		5854267*PED	JUN 29,2016	U-368		
020189 001	FELBAMATE; FELBATOL	4978680	SEP 26,2009	U-83		
		5082861	SEP 26,2009	U-83		
020189 002	FELBAMATE; FELBATOL	4978680	SEP 26,2009	U-83		
		5082861	SEP 26,2009	U-83		
020189 003	FELBAMATE; FELBATOL	4978680	SEP 26,2009	U-83		
		5082861	SEP 26,2009	U-83		

PRESCRIPTION AND OTC PRODUCT
PATENT AND EXCLUSIVITY DATA
*PED and PED represent Pediatric Exclusivity (*continued*)

APPL/PROD NUMBER	INGREDIENT NAME; TRADE NAME	PATENT NUMBER	PATENT EXPIRES	USE CODE	EX-CLUS CODE	EXCLUS EXPIRES
019834 001	FELODIPINE; PLENDIL	4803081	APR 03,2007			
		4803081*PED	OCT 03,2007			
019834 002	FELODIPINE; PLENDIL	4803081	APR 03,2007			
		4803081*PED	OCT 03,2007			
019834 004	FELODIPINE; PLENDIL	4803081	APR 03,2007			
		4803081*PED	OCT 03,2007			
075753 002	FENOFIBRATE; FENOFIBRATE (MICRONIZED)				PC	SEP 15,2002
075753 003	FENOFIBRATE; FENOFIBRATE (MICRONIZED)				PC	SEP 15,2002
021203 001	FENOFIBRATE; TRICOR	4895726	JAN 19,2009		I-298	APR 24,2003
		6074670	JAN 09,2018		I-298	APR 24,2003
		6277405	JAN 09,2018		I-298	APR 24,2003
021203 003	FENOFIBRATE; TRICOR	4895726	JAN 19,2009		I-298	APR 24,2003
		6074670	JAN 09,2018		I-298	APR 24,2003
		6277405	JAN 09,2018		I-298	APR 24,2003
019304 002	FENOFIBRATE; TRICOR (MICRONIZED)	4895726	JAN 19,2009		I-298	APR 24,2003
019304 003	FENOFIBRATE; TRICOR (MICRONIZED)	4895726	JAN 19,2009		I-298	APR 24,2003
019304 004	FENOFIBRATE; TRICOR (MICRONIZED)	4895726	JAN 19,2009		I-298	APR 24,2003
019922 001	FENOLDOPAM MESYLATE; CORLOPAM				NCE	SEP 23,2002
020747 001	FENTANYL CITRATE; ACTIQ	4671953	MAY 01,2005	U-253		
		4863737	SEP 05,2006			
		5785989	SEP 05,2006			
020747 002	FENTANYL CITRATE; ACTIQ	4671953	MAY 01,2005	U-253		
		4863737	SEP 05,2006			
		5785989	SEP 05,2006			
020747 003	FENTANYL CITRATE; ACTIQ	4671953	MAY 01,2005	U-253		
		4863737	SEP 05,2006			
		5785989	SEP 05,2006			
020747 004	FENTANYL CITRATE; ACTIQ	4671953	MAY 01,2005	U-253		
		4863737	SEP 05,2006			
		5785989	SEP 05,2006			
020747 005	FENTANYL CITRATE; ACTIQ	4671953	MAY 01,2005	U-253		
		4863737	SEP 05,2006			
		5785989	SEP 05,2006			
020747 006	FENTANYL CITRATE; ACTIQ	4671953	MAY 01,2005	U-253		
		4863737	SEP 05,2006			
		5785989	SEP 05,2006			
020195 001	FENTANYL CITRATE; FENTANYL	4671953	MAY 01,2005	U-87		
020195 002	FENTANYL CITRATE; FENTANYL	4671953	MAY 01,2005	U-87		
020195 003	FENTANYL CITRATE; FENTANYL	4671953	MAY 01,2005	U-87		
020195 007	FENTANYL CITRATE; FENTANYL	4671953	MAY 01,2005	U-87		
019813 001	FENTANYL; DURAGESIC	4588580	JUL 23,2004	U-43	NPP	MAY 20,2006
		4588580*PED	JAN 23,2005	U-43	PED	NOV 20,2006
019813 002	FENTANYL; DURAGESIC	4588580	JUL 23,2004	U-43	NPP	MAY 20,2006
		4588580*PED	JAN 23,2005	U-43	PED	NOV 20,2006
019813 003	FENTANYL; DURAGESIC	4588580	JUL 23,2004	U-43	NPP	MAY 20,2006
		4588580*PED	JAN 23,2005	U-43	PED	NOV 20,2006
019813 004	FENTANYL; DURAGESIC	4588580	JUL 23,2004	U-43	NPP	MAY 20,2006
		4588580*PED	JAN 23,2005	U-43	PED	NOV 20,2006
020416 001	FERUMOXIDES; FERIDEX I.V.	4770183	SEP 13,2005	U-145		
		4827945	MAY 09,2006	U-144		
		4951675	AUG 28,2007	U-143		
		5055288	OCT 08,2008			
		5102652	FEB 06,2009			
		5219554	JUN 15,2010			
		5248492	SEP 28,2010			
020410 001	FERUMOXSIL; GASTROMARK	4695392	SEP 22,2004			
		4695393	SEP 22,2004			
		4770183	SEP 13,2005	U-169		
		4827945	MAY 09,2006	U-170		
		4951675	SEP 13,2005	U-169		
		5055288	OCT 08,2008			
		5069216	MAY 09,2006	U-171		
		5219554	JUN 15,2010			
020625 001	FEXOFENADINE HYDROCHLORIDE; ALLEGRA	5578610	NOV 26,2013	U-192	M-25	MAY 12,2006
		5578610*PED	MAY 26,2014	U-192	PED	NOV 12,2006
		5738872	FEB 28,2015		PED	NOV 12,2006
		5738872*PED	AUG 28,2015		PED	NOV 12,2006
		5855912	FEB 28,2015		PED	NOV 12,2006
		5855912*PED	AUG 28,2015		PED	NOV 12,2006
		5932247	FEB 28,2015		PED	NOV 12,2006
		5932247*PED	AUG 28,2015		PED	NOV 12,2006

PRESCRIPTION AND OTC PRODUCT
PATENT AND EXCLUSIVITY DATA
*PED and PED represent Pediatric Exclusivity (continued)

APPL/PROD NUMBER	INGREDIENT NAME; TRADE NAME	PATENT NUMBER	PATENT EXPIRES	USE CODE	EX-CLUS CODE	EXCLUS EXPIRES
		6037353	MAR 14,2017	U-138	PED	NOV 12,2006
		6037353*PED	SEP 14,2017	U-138	PED	NOV 12,2006
		6113942	FEB 28,2015		PED	NOV 12,2006
		6113942*PED	AUG 28,2015		PED	NOV 12,2006
		6187791	MAY 11,2012	U-138	PED	NOV 12,2006
		6187791*PED	NOV 11,2012	U-138	PED	NOV 12,2006
		6399632	MAY 11,2012	U-468	PED	NOV 12,2006
		6399632*PED	NOV 11,2012	U-468	PED	NOV 12,2006
020872 001	FEXOFENADINE HYDROCHLORIDE; ALLEGRA	5578610	NOV 26,2013	U-139	PED	AUG 25,2003
		5578610*PED	MAY 26,2014	U-139	PED	AUG 25,2003
		5855912	FEB 28,2015		M-25	MAY 12,2006
		5855912*PED	AUG 28,2015		PED	AUG 25,2003
		5932247	FEB 28,2015		PED	AUG 25,2003
		5932247*PED	AUG 28,2015		PED	AUG 25,2003
		6037353	MAR 14,2017	U-138	PED	NOV 12,2006
		6037353*PED	SEP 14,2017	U-138	PED	AUG 25,2003
		6113942	FEB 28,2015		PED	AUG 25,2003
		6113942*PED	AUG 28,2015		PED	AUG 25,2003
		6187791	MAY 11,2012	U-138	PED	AUG 25,2003
		6187791*PED	NOV 11,2012	U-138	PED	AUG 25,2003
		6399632	MAY 11,2012	U-468	PED	AUG 25,2003
		6399632*PED	NOV 11,2012	U-468	PED	AUG 25,2003
020872 002	FEXOFENADINE HYDROCHLORIDE; ALLEGRA	5578610	NOV 26,2013	U-139	NDF	FEB 25,2003
		5578610*PED	MAY 26,2014	U-139	PED	AUG 25,2003
		5855912	FEB 28,2015		M-25	MAY 12,2006
		5855912*PED	AUG 28,2015		PED	AUG 25,2003
		5932247	FEB 28,2015		PED	AUG 25,2003
		5932247*PED	AUG 28,2015		PED	AUG 25,2003
		6037353	MAR 14,2017	U-138	PED	NOV 12,2006
		6037353*PED	SEP 14,2017	U-138	PED	AUG 25,2003
		6113942	FEB 28,2015		PED	AUG 25,2003
		6113942*PED	AUG 28,2015		PED	AUG 25,2003
		6187791	MAY 11,2012	U-138	PED	AUG 25,2003
		6187791*PED	NOV 11,2012	U-138	PED	AUG 25,2003
		6399632	MAY 11,2012	U-468	PED	AUG 25,2003
		6399632*PED	NOV 11,2012	U-468	PED	AUG 25,2003
020872 004	FEXOFENADINE HYDROCHLORIDE; ALLEGRA	5578610	NOV 26,2013	U-139	NDF	FEB 25,2003
		5578610*PED	MAY 26,2014	U-139	NDF	FEB 25,2003
		5855912	FEB 28,2015		M-25	MAY 12,2006
		5855912*PED	AUG 28,2015		NDF	FEB 25,2003
		5932247	FEB 28,2015		NDF	FEB 25,2003
		5932247*PED	AUG 28,2015		NDF	FEB 25,2003
		6037353	MAR 14,2017	U-138	PED	NOV 12,2006
		6037353*PED	SEP 14,2017	U-138	NDF	FEB 25,2003
		6113942	FEB 28,2015		NDF	FEB 25,2003
		6113942*PED	AUG 28,2015		NDF	FEB 25,2003
		6187791	MAY 11,2012	U-138	NDF	FEB 25,2003
		6187791*PED	NOV 11,2012	U-138	NDF	FEB 25,2003
		6399632	MAY 11,2012	U-468	NDF	FEB 25,2003
		6399632*PED	NOV 11,2012	U-468	NDF	FEB 25,2003
020786 001	FEXOFENADINE HYDROCHLORIDE; ALLEGRA-D	5578610	NOV 26,2013		M-25	MAY 12,2006
		5578610*PED	MAY 26,2014		PED	NOV 12,2006
		5855912	FEB 28,2015		PED	NOV 12,2006
		5855912*PED	AUG 28,2015		PED	NOV 12,2006
		6037353	MAR 14,2017	U-138	PED	NOV 12,2006
		6037353*PED	SEP 14,2017	U-138	PED	NOV 12,2006
		6039974	JUL 31,2018		PED	NOV 12,2006
		6113942	FEB 28,2015		PED	NOV 12,2006
		6113942*PED	AUG 28,2015		PED	NOV 12,2006
		6187791	MAY 11,2012	U-138	PED	NOV 12,2006
		6187791*PED	NOV 11,2012	U-138	PED	NOV 12,2006
		6399632	MAY 11,2012	U-468	PED	NOV 12,2006
		6399632*PED	NOV 11,2012	U-468	PED	NOV 12,2006
020788 001	FINASTERIDE; PROPECIA	4760071	JUN 19,2006			
		5547957	OCT 15,2013	U-236		
		5571817	NOV 05,2013	U-259		
		5886184	NOV 19,2012			
020180 001	FINASTERIDE; PROSCAR	4760071	JUN 19,2006	U-262		
		5886184	NOV 19,2012			
		5942519	OCT 23,2018	U-280		
		6046183	MAR 20,2011			

PRESCRIPTION AND OTC PRODUCT
PATENT AND EXCLUSIVITY DATA
*PED and PED represent Pediatric Exclusivity (*continued*)

APPL/PROD NUMBER	INGREDIENT NAME; TRADE NAME	PATENT NUMBER	PATENT EXPIRES	USE CODE	EX-CLUS CODE	EXCLUS EXPIRES
075442 001	FLECAINIDE ACETATE; FLECAINIDE ACETATE				PC	OCT 28,2002
075442 002	FLECAINIDE ACETATE; FLECAINIDE ACETATE				PC	OCT 28,2002
075442 003	FLECAINIDE ACETATE; FLECAINIDE ACETATE				PC	OCT 28,2002
018830 001	FLECAINIDE ACETATE; TAMBOCOR	4642384	FEB 10,2004			
018830 002	FLECAINIDE ACETATE; TAMBOCOR	4642384	FEB 10,2004			
018830 003	FLECAINIDE ACETATE; TAMBOCOR	4642384	FEB 10,2004			
018830 004	FLECAINIDE ACETATE; TAMBOCOR	4642384	FEB 10,2004			
019949 001	FLUCONAZOLE; DIFLUCAN	4404216	JAN 29,2004			
019949 002	FLUCONAZOLE; DIFLUCAN	4404216	JAN 29,2004			
019949 003	FLUCONAZOLE; DIFLUCAN	4404216	JAN 29,2004			
019949 004	FLUCONAZOLE; DIFLUCAN	4404216	JAN 29,2004			
020090 001	FLUCONAZOLE; DIFLUCAN	4404216	JAN 29,2004			
020090 002	FLUCONAZOLE; DIFLUCAN	4404216	JAN 29,2004			
019950 003	FLUCONAZOLE; DIFLUCAN IN DEXTROSE 5% IN PLASTIC CONTAINER	4404216	JAN 29,2004			
019950 005	FLUCONAZOLE; DIFLUCAN IN DEXTROSE 5% IN PLASTIC CONTAINER	4404216	JAN 29,2004			
019950 001	FLUCONAZOLE; DIFLUCAN IN SODIUM CHLORIDE 0.9%	4404216	JAN 29,2004			
019950 002	FLUCONAZOLE; DIFLUCAN IN SODIUM CHLORIDE 0.9% IN PLASTIC CONTAINER	4404216	JAN 29,2004			
019950 004	FLUCONAZOLE; DIFLUCAN IN SODIUM CHLORIDE 0.9% IN PLASTIC CONTAINER	4404216	JAN 29,2004			
020038 001	FLUDARABINE PHOSPHATE; FLUDARA	4357324	FEB 24,2003			
		4357324*PED	AUG 24,2003			
020073 001	FLUMAZENIL; ROMAZICON	4316839	OCT 10,2004			
018340 001	FLUNISOLIDE; AEROBID	4933168	JUN 12,2007			
018148 001	FLUNISOLIDE; NASALIDE	4933168	JUN 12,2007			
020409 001	FLUNISOLIDE; NASAREL	4782047	MAY 22,2006			
		4933168	JUN 12,2007			
		4983595	MAY 22,2006			
019452 001	FLUOCINOLONE ACETONIDE; DERMA-SMOOTHE/FS				I-340	OCT 10,2004
021112 001	FLUOCINOLONE ACETONIDE; TRI-LUMA				NC	JAN 18,2005
020985 001	FLUOROURACIL; CARAC	4690825	OCT 04,2005		NP	OCT 27,2003
018936 001	FLUOXETINE HYDROCHLORIDE; PROZAC	4626549	DEC 02,2003	U-154	I-362	JUL 29,2005
		4626549*PED	JUN 02,2004	U-154	I-362	JUL 29,2005
018936 003	FLUOXETINE HYDROCHLORIDE; PROZAC	4626549	DEC 02,2003	U-154	I-362	JUL 29,2005
		4626549*PED	JUN 02,2004	U-154	I-362	JUL 29,2005
018936 004	FLUOXETINE HYDROCHLORIDE; PROZAC	4626549	DEC 02,2003	U-154	I-362	JUL 29,2005
		4626549*PED	JUN 02,2004	U-154	I-362	JUL 29,2005
018936 006	FLUOXETINE HYDROCHLORIDE; PROZAC	4626549	DEC 02,2003	U-154	I-362	JUL 29,2005
		4626549*PED	JUN 02,2004	U-154	I-362	JUL 29,2005
020101 001	FLUOXETINE HYDROCHLORIDE; PROZAC	4626549	DEC 02,2003	U-154	PED	JUL 03,2006
		4626549*PED	JUN 02,2004	U-154	PED	JUL 03,2006
020974 001	FLUOXETINE HYDROCHLORIDE; PROZAC	4626549	DEC 02,2003	U-154	NPP	JAN 03,2006
		4626549*PED	JUN 02,2004	U-154	NPP	JAN 03,2006
020974 002	FLUOXETINE HYDROCHLORIDE; PROZAC	4626549	DEC 02,2003	U-154	I-362	JUL 29,2005
		4626549*PED	JUN 02,2004	U-154	I-362	JUL 29,2005
021235 001	FLUOXETINE HYDROCHLORIDE; PROZAC WEEKLY				NDF	FEB 26,2004
018936 007	FLUOXETINE HYDROCHLORIDE; SARAFEM	4971998	NOV 20,2007	U-338	D-75	JUN 12,2005
		4971998*PED	MAY 20,2008	U-338	D-75	JUN 12,2005
018936 008	FLUOXETINE HYDROCHLORIDE; SARAFEM	4971998	NOV 20,2007	U-338	NP	JUL 06,2003
		4971998*PED	MAY 20,2008	U-338	NP	JUL 06,2003
021077 001	FLUTICASONE PROPIONATE; ADVAIR DISKUS 100/50	4335121	NOV 14,2003		NC	AUG 24,2003
		4335121*PED	MAY 14,2004		NC	AUG 24,2003
		4992474	FEB 12,2008	U-211	NC	AUG 24,2003
		5126375	FEB 12,2008		NC	AUG 24,2003
		5225445	FEB 12,2008	U-211	NC	AUG 24,2003
		5270305	SEP 07,2010	U-387	NC	AUG 24,2003
		5290815	MAR 01,2011	U-386	NC	AUG 24,2003
021077 002	FLUTICASONE PROPIONATE; ADVAIR DISKUS 250/50	4335121	NOV 14,2003		NC	AUG 24,2003
		4335121*PED	MAY 14,2004		NC	AUG 24,2003
		4992474	FEB 12,2008	U-211	NC	AUG 24,2003
		5126375	FEB 12,2008		NC	AUG 24,2003
		5225445	FEB 12,2008	U-211	NC	AUG 24,2003
		5270305	SEP 07,2010	U-387	NC	AUG 24,2003
		5290815	MAR 01,2011	U-386	NC	AUG 24,2003

PRESCRIPTION AND OTC PRODUCT
PATENT AND EXCLUSIVITY DATA
*PED and PED represent Pediatric Exclusivity (*continued*)

APPL/PROD NUMBER	INGREDIENT NAME; TRADE NAME	PATENT NUMBER	PATENT EXPIRES	USE CODE	EX-CLUS CODE	EXCLUS EXPIRES
021077 003	FLUTICASONE PROPIONATE; ADVAIR DISKUS 500/50	4335121	NOV 14,2003		NC	AUG 24,2003
		4335121*PED	MAY 14,2004		NC	AUG 24,2003
		4992474	FEB 12,2008	U-211	NC	AUG 24,2003
		5126375	FEB 12,2008		NC	AUG 24,2003
		5225445	FEB 12,2008	U-211	NC	AUG 24,2003
		5270305	SEP 07,2010	U-387	NC	AUG 24,2003
		5290815	MAR 01,2011	U-386	NC	AUG 24,2003
019957 001	FLUTICASONE PROPIONATE; CUTIVATE	4335121	NOV 14,2003			
		4335121*PED	MAY 14,2004			
019958 001	FLUTICASONE PROPIONATE; CUTIVATE	4335121	NOV 14,2003			
		4335121*PED	MAY 14,2004			
020121 001	FLUTICASONE PROPIONATE; FLONASE	4335121	NOV 14,2003		D-76	MAY 23,2005
		4335121*PED	MAY 14,2004		PED	NOV 23,2005
					M-24	MAY 01,2006
					PED	NOV 01,2006
020548 001	FLUTICASONE PROPIONATE; FLOVENT	4335121	NOV 14,2003			
		4335121*PED	MAY 14,2004			
020548 002	FLUTICASONE PROPIONATE; FLOVENT	4335121	NOV 14,2003			
		4335121*PED	MAY 14,2004			
020548 003	FLUTICASONE PROPIONATE; FLOVENT	4335121	NOV 14,2003			
		4335121*PED	MAY 14,2004			
020549 001	FLUTICASONE PROPIONATE; FLOVENT	4335121	NOV 14,2003	U-409		
		4335121*PED	MAY 14,2004	U-409		
020549 002	FLUTICASONE PROPIONATE; FLOVENT	4335121	NOV 14,2003	U-409		
		4335121*PED	MAY 14,2004	U-409		
020549 003	FLUTICASONE PROPIONATE; FLOVENT	4335121	NOV 14,2003	U-409		
		4335121*PED	MAY 14,2004	U-409		
020833 002	FLUTICASONE PROPIONATE; FLOVENT DISKUS 100	4335121	NOV 14,2003	U-409		
		4335121*PED	MAY 14,2004	U-409		
020833 003	FLUTICASONE PROPIONATE; FLOVENT DISKUS 250	4335121	NOV 14,2003	U-409		
		4335121*PED	MAY 14,2004	U-409		
020833 001	FLUTICASONE PROPIONATE; FLOVENT DISKUS 50	4335121	NOV 14,2003	U-409		
		4335121*PED	MAY 14,2004	U-409		
020261 001	FLUVASTATIN SODIUM; LESCOL	5354772	OCT 11,2011	U-413	I-394	MAY 27,2006
		5354772	OCT 11,2011	U-109	I-394	MAY 27,2006
		5356896	DEC 12,2011		I-394	MAY 27,2006
020261 002	FLUVASTATIN SODIUM; LESCOL	5354772	OCT 11,2011	U-413	I-394	MAY 27,2006
		5354772	OCT 11,2011	U-109	I-394	MAY 27,2006
		5356896	DEC 12,2011		I-394	MAY 27,2006
021192 001	FLUVASTATIN SODIUM; LESCOL XL	5354772	OCT 11,2011	U-413	I-394	MAY 27,2006
		5354772	OCT 11,2011	U-109	I-394	MAY 27,2006
		5356896	DEC 12,2011		I-394	MAY 27,2006
		6242003	APR 13,2020		I-394	MAY 27,2006
020582 001	FOLLITROPIN ALFA/BETA; FOLLISTIM	4589402	JUL 26,2004	U-206	I-306	FEB 07,2005
		5270057	MAR 20,2011		I-306	FEB 07,2005
		5767251	JUN 16,2015		I-306	FEB 07,2005
020582 002	FOLLITROPIN ALFA/BETA; FOLLISTIM	4589402	JUL 26,2004	U-206	I-306	FEB 07,2005
		5270057	MAR 20,2011		I-306	FEB 07,2005
		5767251	JUN 16,2015		I-306	FEB 07,2005
020378 001	FOLLITROPIN ALFA/BETA; GONAL-F	4589402	JUL 26,2004	U-242	I-306	MAY 24,2003
		5767251	JUN 16,2015		I-306	MAY 24,2003
020378 002	FOLLITROPIN ALFA/BETA; GONAL-F	4589402	JUL 26,2004	U-242	I-306	MAY 24,2003
		5767251	JUN 16,2015		I-306	MAY 24,2003
020378 003	FOLLITROPIN ALFA/BETA; GONAL-F	4589402	JUL 26,2004	U-242	I-306	MAY 24,2003
		5767251	JUN 16,2015		I-306	MAY 24,2003
020696 001	FOMEPIZOLE; ANTIZOL				I-319	DEC 08,2003
020961 001	FOMIVIRSEN SODIUM; VITRAVENE PRESERVATIVE FREE				NCE	AUG 26,2003
021345 001	FONDAPARINUX SODIUM; ARIXTRA	4818816	AUG 19,2003		NCE	DEC 07,2006
020831 001	FORMOTEROL FUMARATE; FORADIL	6488027	MAR 08,2019		I-342	SEP 25,2004
					NPP	JUN 27,2006
019915 002	FOSINOPRIL SODIUM; MONOPRIL	4337201	DEC 04,2002			
		4337201*PED	JUN 04,2003			
		5006344	JUL 10,2009			
		5006344*PED	JAN 10,2010			
019915 003	FOSINOPRIL SODIUM; MONOPRIL	4337201	DEC 04,2002			
		4337201*PED	JUN 04,2003			
		5006344	JUL 10,2009			

PRESCRIPTION AND OTC PRODUCT
PATENT AND EXCLUSIVITY DATA
*PED and PED represent Pediatric Exclusivity (*continued*)

APPL/PROD NUMBER	INGREDIENT NAME; TRADE NAME	PATENT NUMBER	PATENT EXPIRES	USE CODE	EX-CLUS CODE	EXCLUS EXPIRES
019915 004	FOSINOPRIL SODIUM; MONOPRIL	5006344*PED	JAN 10,2010			
		4337201	DEC 04,2002			
		4337201*PED	JUN 04,2003			
		5006344	JUL 10,2009			
020286 001	FOSINOPRIL SODIUM; MONOPRIL-HCT	5006344*PED	JAN 10,2010			
		4337201	DEC 04,2002			
		4337201*PED	JUN 04,2003			
		5006344	JUL 10,2009			
020286 002	FOSINOPRIL SODIUM; MONOPRIL-HCT	5006344*PED	JAN 10,2010			
		4337201	DEC 04,2002			
		4337201*PED	JUN 04,2003			
		5006344	JUL 10,2009			
020450 001	FOSPHENYTOIN SODIUM; CEREBYX	5006344*PED	JAN 10,2010			
		4260769	APR 07,2003		ODE	AUG 05,2003
		4925860	AUG 05,2007		ODE	AUG 05,2003
021006 001	FROVATRIPTAN SUCCINATE; FROVA	5464864	NOV 07,2012	U-436	NCE	NOV 08,2006
		5616603	APR 01,2014	U-436	NCE	NOV 08,2006
		5637611	JUN 10,2014	U-436	NCE	NOV 08,2006
		5827871	OCT 27,2015	U-436	NCE	NOV 08,2006
		5962501	DEC 16,2013	U-436	NCE	NOV 08,2006
021344 001	FULVESTRANT; FASLODEX	4659516	OCT 01,2004		NCE	APR 25,2007
020235 001	GABAPENTIN; NEURONTIN	4894476	MAY 02,2008		PED	APR 12,2004
		4894476*PED	NOV 02,2008		PED	APR 12,2004
		6054482	APR 25,2017		PED	APR 12,2004
		6054482*PED	OCT 25,2017		PED	APR 12,2004
020235 002	GABAPENTIN; NEURONTIN	4894476	MAY 02,2008		I-311	OCT 12,2003
		4894476*PED	NOV 02,2008		I-311	OCT 12,2003
		6054482	APR 25,2017		I-311	OCT 12,2003
		6054482*PED	OCT 25,2017		I-311	OCT 12,2003
020235 003	GABAPENTIN; NEURONTIN	4894476	MAY 02,2008		I-311	OCT 12,2003
		4894476*PED	NOV 02,2008		I-311	OCT 12,2003
		6054482	APR 25,2017		I-311	OCT 12,2003
		6054482*PED	OCT 25,2017		I-311	OCT 12,2003
020882 001	GABAPENTIN; NEURONTIN	4894476	MAY 02,2008		I-354	MAY 24,2005
		4894476*PED	NOV 02,2008		I-354	MAY 24,2005
		6054482	APR 25,2017		I-354	MAY 24,2005
		6054482*PED	OCT 25,2017		I-354	MAY 24,2005
020882 002	GABAPENTIN; NEURONTIN	4894476	MAY 02,2008		I-311	OCT 12,2003
		4894476*PED	NOV 02,2008		I-311	OCT 12,2003
		6054482	APR 25,2017		I-311	OCT 12,2003
		6054482*PED	OCT 25,2017		I-311	OCT 12,2003
021129 001	GABAPENTIN; NEURONTIN	4894476	MAY 02,2008		PED	APR 12,2004
		4894476*PED	NOV 02,2008		PED	APR 12,2004
		6054482	APR 25,2017		PED	APR 12,2004
		6054482*PED	OCT 25,2017		PED	APR 12,2004
020123 001	GADODIAMIDE; OMNISCAN	4687659	MAY 04,2007	U-76		
019596 001	GADOPENTETATE DIMEGLUMINE; MAGNEVIST	4647447	MAR 03,2004			
		4957939	MAR 03,2004			
		4963344	MAR 03,2004			
		5362475	NOV 08,2011			
		5560903	OCT 01,2013			
021037 001	GADOPENTETATE DIMEGLUMINE; MAGNEVIST	4647447	MAR 03,2004			
		4957939	MAR 03,2004			
		4963344	MAR 03,2004			
		5362475	NOV 08,2011			
		5560903	OCT 01,2013			
020131 001	GADOTERIDOL; PROHANCE	4885363	DEC 05,2006			
		5474756	DEC 12,2012	U-480		
		5846519	DEC 08,2015			
		6143274	DEC 12,2012	U-480		
020937 001	GADOVERSETAMIDE; OPTIMARK	5130120	JUL 14,2009		NCE	DEC 08,2004
		5137711	JUL 14,2009		NCE	DEC 08,2004
020975 001	GADOVERSETAMIDE; OPTIMARK	5130120	JUL 14,2009		NCE	DEC 08,2004
		5137711	JUL 14,2009		NCE	DEC 08,2004
020976 001	GADOVERSETAMIDE; OPTIMARK IN PLASTIC CONTAINER	5130120	JUL 14,2009		NCE	DEC 08,2004
		5137711	JUL 14,2009		NCE	DEC 08,2004
021169 001	GALANTAMINE HYDROBROMIDE; REMINYL	4663318	JAN 15,2006		NCE	FEB 28,2006
		6099863	JUN 06,2017		NCE	FEB 28,2006
021169 002	GALANTAMINE HYDROBROMIDE; REMINYL	4663318	JAN 15,2006		NCE	FEB 28,2006
		6099863	JUN 06,2017		NCE	FEB 28,2006

PRESCRIPTION AND OTC PRODUCT
PATENT AND EXCLUSIVITY DATA
*PED and PED represent Pediatric Exclusivity (*continued*)

APPL/PROD NUMBER	INGREDIENT NAME; TRADE NAME	PATENT NUMBER	PATENT EXPIRES	USE CODE	EX-CLUS CODE	EXCLUS EXPIRES
021169 003	GALANTAMINE HYDROBROMIDE; REMINYL	4663318	JAN 15,2006		NCE	FEB 28,2006
		6099863	JUN 06,2017		NCE	FEB 28,2006
021224 001	GALANTAMINE HYDROBROMIDE; REMINYL	4663318	JAN 15,2006		NCE	FEB 28,2006
019961 002	GALLIUM NITRATE; GANITE	4529593	JAN 17,2005	U-49		
019661 001	GANCICLOVIR SODIUM; CYTOVENE IV	4355032	JUN 23,2003	U-64		
020460 001	GANCICLOVIR; CYTOVENE	4355032	JUN 23,2003	U-64		
		4642346	JUN 24,2005			
020460 002	GANCICLOVIR; CYTOVENE	4355032	JUN 23,2003	U-64		
		4642346	JUN 24,2005			
020569 001	GANCICLOVIR; VITRASERT	5378475	JAN 03,2012		ODE	MAR 04,2003
021057 001	GANIRELIX ACETATE; ANTAGON	4801577	FEB 05,2007		NCE	JUL 29,2004
		5767082	JUN 16,2015		NCE	JUL 29,2004
021061 001	GATIFLOXACIN; TEQUIN	4980470	DEC 25,2007		D-69	OCT 12,2004
		5880283	DEC 05,2015		D-69	OCT 12,2004
021061 002	GATIFLOXACIN; TEQUIN	4980470	DEC 25,2007		NCE	DEC 17,2004
		5880283	DEC 05,2015		NCE	DEC 17,2004
021062 001	GATIFLOXACIN; TEQUIN	4980470	DEC 25,2007		D-69	OCT 12,2004
		5880283	DEC 05,2015		D-69	OCT 12,2004
021062 002	GATIFLOXACIN; TEQUIN	4980470	DEC 25,2007		D-69	OCT 12,2004
		5880283	DEC 05,2015		D-69	OCT 12,2004
021062 003	GATIFLOXACIN; TEQUIN	4980470	DEC 25,2007		NCE	DEC 17,2004
		5880283	DEC 05,2015		NCE	DEC 17,2004
021062 004	GATIFLOXACIN; TEQUIN	4980470	DEC 25,2007		NCE	DEC 17,2004
		5880283	DEC 05,2015		NCE	DEC 17,2004
021493 001	GATIFLOXACIN; ZYMAR	4980470	DEC 15,2009		NCE	DEC 17,2004
		5880283	DEC 05,2015		NDF	MAR 28,2006
021399 001	GEFITINIB; IRESSA				NCE	DEC 17,2004
020509 001	GEMCITABINE HYDROCHLORIDE; GEMZAR	4808614	MAY 15,2010			
		5464826	NOV 07,2012	U-146		
020509 002	GEMCITABINE HYDROCHLORIDE; GEMZAR	4808614	MAY 15,2010			
		5464826	NOV 07,2012	U-146		
021158 001	GEMIFLOXACIN MESYLATE; FACTIVE	5633262	JUN 15,2015		NCE	APR 04,2008
		5776944	JUN 15,2015		NCE	APR 04,2008
		5962468	JUN 15,2015	U-282	NCE	APR 04,2008
		6262071	SEP 21,2019	U-513	NCE	APR 04,2008
		6331550	SEP 21,2019	U-511	NCE	APR 04,2008
		6340689	SEP 14,2019	U-512	NCE	APR 04,2008
		6455540	SEP 21,2019	U-511	NCE	APR 04,2008
021174 001	GEMTUZUMAB OZOGAMICIN; MYLOTARG	4970198	NOV 30,2007		NCE	MAY 17,2005
		5079233	JAN 07,2009		NCE	MAY 17,2005
		5585089	DEC 17,2013		NCE	MAY 17,2005
		5606040	FEB 25,2014		NCE	MAY 17,2005
		5693762	DEC 02,2014		NCE	MAY 17,2005
		5739116	APR 14,2015		NCE	MAY 17,2005
		5767285	JUN 16,2015		NCE	MAY 17,2005
		5773001	JUN 30,2015	U-320	NCE	MAY 17,2005
020622 001	GLATIRAMER ACETATE; COPAXONE	5981589	MAY 24,2014		ODE	DEC 20,2003
		6054430	MAY 24,2014		ODE	DEC 20,2003
		6342476	MAY 24,2014	U-441	ODE	DEC 20,2003
		6362161	MAY 24,2014	U-441	ODE	DEC 20,2003
020496 001	GLIMEPIRIDE; AMARYL	4379785	APR 06,2005	U-118		
020496 002	GLIMEPIRIDE; AMARYL	4379785	APR 06,2005	U-118		
020496 003	GLIMEPIRIDE; AMARYL	4379785	APR 06,2005	U-118		
020329 001	GLIPIZIDE; GLUCOTROL XL	4612008	SEP 16,2003			
		5024843	SEP 05,2009			
		5082668	SEP 16,2003			
		5091190	SEP 05,2009	U-111		
		5545413	JUL 21,2008	U-111		
		5591454	JAN 07,2014	U-150		
020329 002	GLIPIZIDE; GLUCOTROL XL	4612008	SEP 16,2003			
		5024843	SEP 05,2009			
		5082668	SEP 16,2003			
		5091190	SEP 05,2009	U-111		
		5545413	JUL 21,2008	U-111		
		5591454	JAN 07,2014	U-150		
020329 003	GLIPIZIDE; GLUCOTROL XL	4612008	SEP 16,2003			
		5024843	SEP 05,2009			
		5082668	SEP 16,2003			
		5091190	SEP 05,2009	U-111		
		5545413	JUL 21,2008	U-111		
		5591454	JAN 07,2014	U-111		

PRESCRIPTION AND OTC PRODUCT
PATENT AND EXCLUSIVITY DATA
*PED and PED represent Pediatric Exclusivity (*continued*)

APPL/PROD NUMBER	INGREDIENT NAME; TRADE NAME	PATENT NUMBER	PATENT EXPIRES	USE CODE	EX-CLUS CODE	EXCLUS EXPIRES
021460 001	GLIPIZIDE; METAGLIP				NC	OCT 21,2005
021460 002	GLIPIZIDE; METAGLIP				NC	OCT 21,2005
021460 003	GLIPIZIDE; METAGLIP				NC	OCT 21,2005
021178 001	GLYBURIDE; GLUCOVANCE	6303146	JUL 14,2019	U-412	I-368	SEP 30,2005
021178 002	GLYBURIDE; GLUCOVANCE	6303146	JUL 14,2019	U-412	NC	JUL 31,2003
021178 003	GLYBURIDE; GLUCOVANCE	6303146	JUL 14,2019	U-412	NC	JUL 31,2003
020051 001	GLYBURIDE; GLYNASE	4735805	APR 05,2005			
		4916163	APR 10,2007			
020051 002	GLYBURIDE; GLYNASE	4735805	APR 05,2005			
		4916163	APR 10,2007			
020051 003	GLYBURIDE; GLYNASE	4735805	APR 05,2005			
		4916163	APR 10,2007			
020051 004	GLYBURIDE; GLYNASE	4735805	APR 05,2005			
		4916163	APR 10,2007			
019726 001	GOSERELIN ACETATE; ZOLADEX	4767628	AUG 30,2005			
		5366734	NOV 22,2011			
020578 001	GOSERELIN ACETATE; ZOLADEX	4767628	AUG 30,2005			
		5366734	NOV 22,2011			
020239 001	GRANISETRON HYDROCHLORIDE; KYTRIL	4886808	DEC 29,2007	U-89	I-369	AUG 16,2005
		6294548	MAY 04,2019		I-369	AUG 16,2005
020239 002	GRANISETRON HYDROCHLORIDE; KYTRIL	4886808	DEC 29,2007	U-89	I-369	AUG 16,2005
		6294548	MAY 04,2019		I-369	AUG 16,2005
020305 001	GRANISETRON HYDROCHLORIDE; KYTRIL	4886808	DEC 29,2007	U-105	I-264	JUL 27,2002
020305 002	GRANISETRON HYDROCHLORIDE; KYTRIL	4886808	DEC 20,2007	U-105	I-264	JUL 27,2002
021238 001	GRANISETRON HYDROCHLORIDE; KYTRIL	4886808	DEC 29,2007	U-105	I-264	JUL 27,2002
020695 001	GREPAFLOXACIN HYDROCHLORIDE; RAXAR	5563138	OCT 08,2013		NCE	NOV 06,2002
021282 001	GUAIFENESIN; MUCINEX	6372252	APR 28,2020	U-489		
021282 002	GUAIFENESIN; MUCINEX	6372252	APR 28,2020	U-489		
019967 001	HALOBETASOL PROPIONATE; ULTRAVATE	4619921	DEC 17,2004			
019968 001	HALOBETASOL PROPIONATE; ULTRAVATE	4619921	DEC 17,2004			
020125 001	HYDROCHLOROTHIAZIDE; ACCURETIC	4344949	OCT 03,2002	U-3	PED	JUN 28,2003
		4344949*PED	APR 03,2003	U-3	PED	JUN 28,2003
		4743450	FEB 24,2007		PED	JUN 28,2003
		4743450*PED	AUG 24,2007		PED	JUN 28,2003
020125 002	HYDROCHLOROTHIAZIDE; ACCURETIC	4344949	OCT 03,2002	U-3	NC	DEC 28,2002
		4344949*PED	APR 03,2003	U-3	NC	DEC 28,2002
		4743450	FEB 24,2007		NC	DEC 28,2002
		4743450*PED	AUG 24,2007		NC	DEC 28,2002
020125 003	HYDROCHLOROTHIAZIDE; ACCURETIC	4344949	OCT 03,2002	U-3	NC	DEC 28,2002
		4344949*PED	APR 03,2003	U-3	NC	DEC 28,2002
		4743450	FEB 24,2007		NC	DEC 28,2002
		4743450*PED	AUG 24,2007		NC	DEC 28,2002
020758 001	HYDROCHLOROTHIAZIDE; AVALIDE	5270317	SEP 30,2011		NCE	SEP 30,2002
		5994348	JUN 07,2015		NCE	SEP 30,2002
020758 002	HYDROCHLOROTHIAZIDE; AVALIDE	5270317	SEP 30,2011		NCE	SEP 30,2002
		5994348	JUN 07,2015		NCE	SEP 30,2002
020758 003	HYDROCHLOROTHIAZIDE; AVALIDE	5270317	SEP 30,2011		NCE	SEP 30,2002
		5994348	JUN 07,2015		NCE	SEP 30,2002
021532 002	HYDROCHLOROTHIAZIDE; BENICAR HCT	5616599	APR 01,2014	U-500	NC	JUN 05,2006
					NCE	APR 25,2007
021532 003	HYDROCHLOROTHIAZIDE; BENICAR HCT	5616599	APR 01,2014	U-500	NC	JUN 05,2006
					NCE	APR 25,2007
021532 005	HYDROCHLOROTHIAZIDE; BENICAR HCT	5616599	APR 01,2014	U-500	NC	JUN 25,2007
					NCE	APR 25,2007
020818 001	HYDROCHLOROTHIAZIDE; DIOVAN HCT	5399578	MAR 21,2012	U-3		
		6294197	JUN 18,2017	U-3		
020818 002	HYDROCHLOROTHIAZIDE; DIOVAN HCT	5399578	MAR 21,2012	U-3		
		6294197	JUN 18,2017	U-3		
020387 001	HYDROCHLOROTHIAZIDE; HYZAAR	5138069	AUG 11,2009			
		5138069*PED	FEB 11,2010			
		5153197	OCT 06,2009	U-3		
		5153197*PED	APR 06,2010	U-3		
		5608075	MAR 04,2014			
		5608075*PED	SEP 04,2014			
020387 002	HYDROCHLOROTHIAZIDE; HYZAAR	5138069	AUG 11,2009			
		5138069*PED	FEB 11,2010			
		5153197	OCT 06,2009	U-3		
		5153197*PED	APR 06,2010	U-3		
		5608075	MAR 04,2014			
		5608075*PED	SEP 04,2014			
019129 001	HYDROCHLOROTHIAZIDE; MAXZIDE	4444769	JUL 27,2002			

PRESCRIPTION AND OTC PRODUCT
PATENT AND EXCLUSIVITY DATA
*PED and PED represent Pediatric Exclusivity (*continued*)

APPL/PROD NUMBER	INGREDIENT NAME; TRADE NAME	PATENT NUMBER	PATENT EXPIRES	USE CODE	EX-CLUS CODE	EXCLUS EXPIRES
019129 003	HYDROCHLOROTHIAZIDE; MAXZIDE-25	4444769	JUL 27,2002			
021162 001	HYDROCHLOROTHIAZIDE; MICARDIS HCT	5591762	JAN 07,2014	U-3	NC	NOV 17,2003
021162 002	HYDROCHLOROTHIAZIDE; MICARDIS HCT	5591762	JAN 07,2014	U-3	NC	NOV 17,2003
020729 001	HYDROCHLOROTHIAZIDE; UNIRETIC	4743450	FEB 24,2007			
020729 002	HYDROCHLOROTHIAZIDE; UNIRETIC	4743450	FEB 24,2007			
020729 003	HYDROCHLOROTHIAZIDE; UNIRETIC	4743450	FEB 24,2007			
020716 001	HYDROCODONE BITARTRATE; VICOPROFEN	4587252	DEC 18,2004	U-55		
		6348216	JUN 10,2017			
020769 001	HYDROCORTISONE BUTYRATE; LOCOID LIPOCREAM	5635497	JUN 03,2014			
020453 001	HYDROCORTISONE PROBUTATE; PANDEL	4794106	AUG 28,2006			
016295 002	HYDROXYUREA; DROXIA				ODE	FEB 25,2005
016295 003	HYDROXYUREA; DROXIA				ODE	FEB 25,2005
016295 004	HYDROXYUREA; DROXIA				ODE	FEB 25,2005
021455 001	IBANDRONATE SODIUM; BONIVA				NCE	MAY 16,2008
020402 002	IBUPROFEN POTASSIUM; ADVIL MIGRAINE LIQUI-GELS				NP	MAR 16,2003
019771 001	IBUPROFEN; ADVIL COLD AND SINUS	4552899	APR 09,2004			
		4552899*PED	OCT 09,2004			
021374 001	IBUPROFEN; ADVIL COLD AND SINUS	5071643	DEC 10,2008			
		5071643*PED	JUN 10,2009			
		5360615	DEC 10,2008			
		5360615*PED	JUN 10,2009			
019833 002	IBUPROFEN; CHILDREN'S ADVIL	4788220	NOV 29,2005			
		4788220*PED	MAY 29,2006			
020589 001	IBUPROFEN; CHILDREN'S ADVIL	4788220	JUL 08,2007			
		4788220*PED	JAN 08,2008			
021373 001	IBUPROFEN; CHILDREN'S ADVIL COLD				PED	FEB 01,2004
020516 001	IBUPROFEN; CHILDREN'S MOTRIN	5374659	DEC 20,2011			
		5374659*PED	JUN 20,2012			
020601 001	IBUPROFEN; CHILDREN'S MOTRIN	5215755	JUN 01,2010			
		5215755*PED	DEC 01,2010			
020603 001	IBUPROFEN; CHILDREN'S MOTRIN	5374659	DEC 20,2011			
		5374659*PED	JUN 20,2012			
021128 001	IBUPROFEN; CHILDREN'S MOTRIN COLD	6211246	JUN 10,2019		NP	AUG 01,2003
020601 003	IBUPROFEN; JUNIOR STRENGTH MOTRIN	5215755	JUN 01,2010			
		5215755*PED	DEC 01,2010			
019842 001	IBUPROFEN; MOTRIN	5374659	DEC 20,2011			
		5374659*PED	JUN 20,2012			
020135 001	IBUPROFEN; MOTRIN	5215755	JUN 01,2010			
		5215755*PED	DEC 01,2010			
		5320855	JUN 14,2011			
		5320855*PED	DEC 14,2011			
020135 002	IBUPROFEN; MOTRIN	5215755	JUN 01,2010			
		5215755*PED	DEC 01,2010			
		5320855	JUN 14,2011			
		5320855*PED	DEC 14,2011			
019012 004	IBUPROFEN; MOTRIN MIGRAINE PAIN				NP	FEB 26,2003
020491 001	IBUTILIDE FUMARATE; CORVERT	5155268	DEC 28,2009			
019763 001	IFOSFAMIDE; IFEX	4882452	MAR 03,2008			
019763 002	IFOSFAMIDE; IFEX	4882452	MAR 03,2008			
019763 003	IFOSFAMIDE; IFEX/MESNEX KIT	4882452	MAR 03,2008			
		5696172	OCT 06,2013			
019763 004	IFOSFAMIDE; IFEX/MESNEX KIT	4882452	MAR 03,2008			
		5696172	OCT 06,2013			
075874 001	IFOSFAMIDE; IFOSFAMIDE/MESNA KIT				PC	OCT 05,2002
075874 002	IFOSFAMIDE; IFOSFAMIDE/MESNA KIT				PC	OCT 05,2002
021335 001	IMATINIB MESYLATE; GLEEVEC	5521184	MAY 28,2013		ODE	MAY 10,2008
					I-392	MAY 20,2006
021335 002	IMATINIB MESYLATE; GLEEVEC	5521184	MAY 28,2013		ODE	MAY 10,2008
					I-392	MAY 20,2006
021588 001	IMATINIB MESYLATE; GLEEVEC	5521184	MAY 28,2013		NCE	MAY 10,2006
					I-376	DEC 20,2005
					ODE	FEB 01,2009
					ODE	MAY 10,2008
					I-392	MAY 20,2006
021588 002	IMATINIB MESYLATE; GLEEVEC	5521184	MAY 28,2013		NCE	MAY 10,2006
					I-376	DEC 20,2005
					ODE	FEB 01,2009
					ODE	MAY 10,2008
					I-392	MAY 20,2006

PRESCRIPTION AND OTC PRODUCT
PATENT AND EXCLUSIVITY DATA
*PED and PED represent Pediatric Exclusivity (*continued*)

APPL/PROD NUMBER	INGREDIENT NAME; TRADE NAME	PATENT NUMBER	PATENT EXPIRES	USE CODE	EX- CLUS CODE	EXCLUS EXPIRES
020367 001	IMIGLUCERASE; CEREZYME	5236838	AUG 17,2010			
		5549892	AUG 27,2013	U-252		
020723 001	IMIQUIMOD; ALDARA	4689338	AUG 25,2009	U-172		
		5238944	AUG 24,2010			
019693 001	INDECAINIDE HYDROCHLORIDE; DECABID	4452745	JUN 05,2003			
019693 002	INDECAINIDE HYDROCHLORIDE; DECABID	4452745	JUN 05,2003			
019693 003	INDECAINIDE HYDROCHLORIDE; DECABID	4452745	JUN 05,2003			
020685 001	INDINAVIR SULFATE; CRIXIVAN	5413999	MAY 09,2012	U-132		
020685 003	INDINAVIR SULFATE; CRIXIVAN	5413999	MAY 09,2012	U-132		
020685 005	INDINAVIR SULFATE; CRIXIVAN	5413999	MAY 09,2012	U-132		
020685 006	INDINAVIR SULFATE; CRIXIVAN	5413999	MAY 09,2012	U-132		
020986 001	INSULIN ASPART; NOVOLOG	5618913	APR 08,2014		NR	DEC 21,2004
		5866538	JUN 20,2017		NR	DEC 21,2004
021172 001	INSULIN ASPART; NOVOLOG MIX 70/30	5547930	SEP 28,2013		NC	NOV 01,2004
		5618913	APR 08,2014		NC	NOV 01,2004
		5834422	SEP 28,2013	U-471	NC	NOV 01,2004
		5840680	SEP 28,2013	U-471	NC	NOV 01,2004
		5948751	JUN 19,2017		NC	NOV 01,2004
021081 001	INSULIN GLARGINE; LANTUS	5656722	SEP 12,2014		D-80	MAY 01,2006
		5656722*PED	MAR 12,2015		D-80	MAY 01,2006
020563 001	INSULIN LISPRO; HUMALOG	5474978	JUN 16,2014		D-56	APR 04,2003
		5514646	MAY 07,2013	U-111	D-56	APR 04,2003
021018 001	INSULIN LISPRO; HUMALOG MIX 50/50	5461031	JUN 26,2014		NC	DEC 22,2002
		5474978	JUN 16,2014		NC	DEC 22,2002
		5514646	MAY 07,2013		NC	DEC 22,2002
		5747642	JUN 16,2014		NC	DEC 22,2002
021017 001	INSULIN LISPRO; HUMALOG MIX 75/25	5461031	JUN 16,2014		NC	DEC 22,2002
		5474978	JUN 16,2014		NC	DEC 22,2002
		5514646	MAY 07,2013		NC	DEC 22,2002
		5747642	JUN 16,2014		NC	DEC 22,2002
020563 002	INSULIN LISPRO; HUMALOG PEN	5474978	JUN 16,2014		D-56	APR 04,2003
		5514646	MAY 07,2013	U-111	D-56	APR 04,2003
021028 001	INSULIN RECOMBINANT HUMAN; VELOSULIN BR				NP	JUL 19,2002
020084 001	IOBENGUANE SULFATE I 131; IOBENGUANE SULFATE I 131	4584187	APR 22,2003			
020351 001	IODIXANOL; VISIPAQUE 270	5349085	SEP 20,2011			
020808 001	IODIXANOL; VISIPAQUE 270	5349085	SEP 20,2011			
020351 002	IODIXANOL; VISIPAQUE 320	5349085	SEP 20,2011			
020808 002	IODIXANOL; VISIPAQUE 320	5349085	SEP 20,2011			
021425 001	IOPROMIDE; ULTRAVIST (PHARMACY BULK)	4364921	MAR 06,2005	U-498		
021425 002	IOPROMIDE; ULTRAVIST (PHARMACY BULK)	4364921	MAR 06,2005	U-498		
020220 004	IOPROMIDE; ULTRAVIST 150	4364921	MAR 06,2005	U-113		
020220 003	IOPROMIDE; ULTRAVIST 240	4364921	MAR 06,2005	U-113		
020220 002	IOPROMIDE; ULTRAVIST 300	4364921	MAR 06,2005	U-113		
020220 001	IOPROMIDE; ULTRAVIST 370	4364921	MAR 06,2005	U-113		
019710 003	IOVERSOL; OPTIRAY 160	4396598	DEC 30,2002	U-31		
019710 002	IOVERSOL; OPTIRAY 240	4396598	DEC 30,2002	U-29		
		4396598	DEC 30,2002	U-30		
020923 001	IOVERSOL; OPTIRAY 240	4396598	DEC 30,2002			
019710 004	IOVERSOL; OPTIRAY 300	4396598	DEC 30,2002	U-29		
		4396598	DEC 30,2002	U-30		
		4396598	DEC 30,2002	U-464		
019710 001	IOVERSOL; OPTIRAY 320	4396598	DEC 30,2002	U-29		
		4396598	DEC 30,2002	U-463		
		4396598	DEC 30,2002	U-28		
020923 002	IOVERSOL; OPTIRAY 320	4396598	DEC 30,2002			
019710 005	IOVERSOL; OPTIRAY 350	4396598	DEC 30,2002	U-464		
		4396598	DEC 30,2002	U-465		
		4396598	DEC 30,2002	U-62		
020923 003	IOVERSOL; OPTIRAY 350	4396598	DEC 30,2002			
020316 001	IOXILAN; OXILAN-300	4954348	DEC 21,2009			
020316 002	IOXILAN; OXILAN-350	4954348	DEC 21,2009			
020394 001	IPRATROPIUM BROMIDE; ATROVENT				I-327	OCT 27,2003
020757 001	IRBESARTAN; AVAPRO	5270317	SEP 30,2011		I-373	SEP 17,2005
		6342247	JUN 07,2015		I-373	SEP 17,2005
020757 002	IRBESARTAN; AVAPRO	5270317	SEP 30,2011		NCE	SEP 30,2002
		6342247	JUN 07,2015		NCE	SEP 30,2002
020757 003	IRBESARTAN; AVAPRO	5270317	SEP 30,2011		NCE	SEP 30,2002
		6342247	JUN 07,2015		NCE	SEP 30,2002
020571 001	IRINOTECAN HYDROCHLORIDE; CAMPTOSAR	4604463	AUG 20,2007		I-299	APR 20,2003
		6403569	APR 28,2020	U-449	I-299	APR 20,2003

PRESCRIPTION AND OTC PRODUCT
PATENT AND EXCLUSIVITY DATA
*PED and PED represent Pediatric Exclusivity (continued)

APPL/PROD NUMBER	INGREDIENT NAME; TRADE NAME	PATENT NUMBER	PATENT EXPIRES	USE CODE	EX-CLUS CODE	EXCLUS EXPIRES
040024 001	IRON DEXTRAN; DEXFERRUM	5624668	SEP 29,2015			
021135 001	IRON SUCROSE; VENOFER				NP	NOV 07,2003
018662 002	ISOTRETINOIN; ACCUTANE				PED	NOV 02,2005
018662 003	ISOTRETINOIN; ACCUTANE				PED	NOV 02,2005
018662 004	ISOTRETINOIN; ACCUTANE				M-12	MAY 02,2005
019546 001	ISRADIPINE; DYNACIRC	4466972	AUG 21,2003	U-3		
019546 002	ISRADIPINE; DYNACIRC	4466972	AUG 21,2003	U-3		
020336 001	ISRADIPINE; DYNACIRC CR	4466972	AUG 21,2003	U-3		
		4783337	SEP 16,2003	U-3		
		4816263	OCT 02,2007	U-3		
		4946687	AUG 07,2007			
		4950486	AUG 21,2007			
		5030456	JUL 09,2008			
020336 002	ISRADIPINE; DYNACIRC CR	4466972	AUG 21,2003	U-3		
		4783337	SEP 16,2003	U-3		
		4816263	OCT 02,2007	U-3		
		4946687	AUG 07,2007			
		4950486	AUG 21,2007			
		5030456	JUL 09,2008			
020083 001	ITRACONAZOLE; SPORANOX	5633015	MAY 27,2014			
020657 001	ITRACONAZOLE; SPORANOX	4727064	FEB 23,2005		I-332	MAY 09,2004
		5707975	JAN 13,2015		I-332	MAY 09,2004
		6407079	JUN 18,2019		I-332	MAY 09,2004
020966 001	ITRACONAZOLE; SPORANOX	4727064	FEB 23,2005		I-332	MAY 09,2004
		4791111	DEC 23,2005		I-332	MAY 09,2004
		6407079	JUN 18,2019		I-332	MAY 09,2004
019084 001	KETOCONAZOLE; NIZORAL	4942162	FEB 11,2003			
019927 001	KETOCONAZOLE; NIZORAL	4942162	FEB 11,2003			
020310 001	KETOCONAZOLE; NIZORAL A-D	4942162	FEB 11,2003	U-245		
		5456851	APR 07,2014			
019700 001	KETOROLAC TROMETHAMINE; ACULAR	4454151*PED	SEP 22,2002	U-75	M-16	FEB 08,2005
		5110493	MAY 05,2009	U-75	M-16	FEB 08,2005
		5110493*PED	NOV 05,2009	U-75	M-16	FEB 08,2005
021528 001	KETOROLAC TROMETHAMINE; ACULAR LS	5110493	MAY 05,2009		NP	MAY 30,2006
		5110493*PED	NOV 05,2009		NP	MAY 30,2006
020811 001	KETOROLAC TROMETHAMINE; ACULAR PRESERVATIVE FREE	4454151*PED	SEP 22,2002		M-16	FEB 08,2005
021066 001	KETOTIFEN FUMARATE; ZADITOR				NCE	JUL 02,2004
020857 001	LAMIVUDINE; COMBIVIR	4724232	SEP 17,2005			
		4818538	SEP 17,2005			
		4828838	SEP 17,2005			
		4833130	SEP 17,2005			
		4837208	SEP 17,2005			
		5047407	NOV 17,2009			
		5047407*PED	MAY 17,2010			
		5859021	MAY 15,2012	U-248		
		5859021*PED	NOV 15,2012	U-248		
		5905082	MAY 18,2016	U-248		
		5905082*PED	NOV 18,2016	U-248		
		6113920	OCT 23,2017	U-257		
		6113920*PED	APR 23,2018	U-257		
		6180639	JAN 30,2018	U-248		
		6180639*PED	JUL 30,2018	U-248		
020564 001	LAMIVUDINE; EPIVIR	5047407	NOV 17,2009		D-2	JUN 24,2005
		5047407*PED	MAY 17,2010		D-2	JUN 24,2005
		5905082	MAY 18,2016		D-2	JUN 24,2005
		5905082*PED	NOV 18,2016		D-2	JUN 24,2005
		6180639	JAN 30,2018	U-248	D-2	JUN 24,2005
		6180639*PED	JUL 30,2018	U-248	D-2	JUN 24,2005
020596 001	LAMIVUDINE; EPIVIR	5047407	NOV 17,2009		D-2	JUN 24,2005
		5047407*PED	MAY 17,2010		D-2	JUN 24,2005
		6004968	MAR 20,2018		D-2	JUN 24,2005
		6004968*PED	SEP 20,2018		D-2	JUN 24,2005
		6180639	JAN 30,2018	U-248	D-2	JUN 24,2005
		6180639*PED	JUL 30,2018	U-248	D-2	JUN 24,2005
021003 001	LAMIVUDINE; EPIVIR-HBV	5047407	NOV 17,2009		PED	FEB 16,2005
		5047407*PED	MAY 17,2010		PED	FEB 16,2005
		5532246	JUL 02,2013	U-250	PED	FEB 16,2005
		5532246*PED	JAN 02,2014	U-250	PED	FEB 16,2005
		5905082	MAY 18,2016		PED	FEB 16,2005
		5905082*PED	NOV 18,2016		PED	FEB 16,2005

PRESCRIPTION AND OTC PRODUCT
PATENT AND EXCLUSIVITY DATA
*PED and PED represent Pediatric Exclusivity (*continued*)

APPL/PROD NUMBER	INGREDIENT NAME; TRADE NAME	PATENT NUMBER	PATENT EXPIRES	USE CODE	EX-CLUS CODE	EXCLUS EXPIRES
021004 001	LAMIVUDINE; EPIVIR-HBV	5047407	NOV 17,2009		I-339	AUG 16,2004
		5047407*PED	MAY 17,2010		I-339	AUG 16,2004
		5532246	JUL 02,2013	U-250	I-339	AUG 16,2004
		5532246*PED	JAN 02,2014	U-250	I-339	AUG 16,2004
		6004968	MAR 20,2018		I-339	AUG 16,2004
		6004968*PED	SEP 20,2018		I-339	AUG 16,2004
020241 001	LAMOTRIGINE; LAMICTAL	4602017	JUL 22,2008	U-106	I-387	JAN 17,2006
020241 002	LAMOTRIGINE; LAMICTAL	4602017	JUL 22,2008	U-106	ODE	AUG 24,2005
020241 003	LAMOTRIGINE; LAMICTAL	4602017	JUL 22,2008	U-106	ODE	AUG 24,2005
020241 004	LAMOTRIGINE; LAMICTAL	4602017	JUL 22,2008	U-106	ODE	AUG 24,2005
020241 005	LAMOTRIGINE; LAMICTAL	4602017	JUL 22,2008	U-106	I-387	JAN 17,2006
020241 006	LAMOTRIGINE; LAMICTAL	4602017	JUL 22,2008	U-106	I-387	JAN 17,2006
020764 001	LAMOTRIGINE; LAMICTAL CD	4602017	JUL 22,2008	U-106	I-387	JAN 17,2006
		5698226	JAN 29,2012		I-387	JAN 17,2006
020764 002	LAMOTRIGINE; LAMICTAL CD	4602017	JUL 22,2008	U-106	ODE	AUG 24,2005
		5698226	JAN 29,2012		ODE	AUG 24,2005
020764 003	LAMOTRIGINE; LAMICTAL CD	4602017	JUL 22,2008	U-106	ODE	AUG 24,2005
		5698226	JAN 29,2012		ODE	AUG 24,2005
020764 004	LAMOTRIGINE; LAMICTAL CD				I-387	JAN 17,2006
020406 001	LANSOPRAZOLE; PREVACID	4628098	MAY 10,2009		I-316	NOV 30,2003
		4689333	JUL 29,2005	U-126	I-316	NOV 30,2003
		5013743	FEB 12,2010	U-452	I-316	NOV 30,2003
		5026560	JUN 25,2008		I-316	NOV 30,2003
		5045321	SEP 03,2008		I-316	NOV 30,2003
		5093132	SEP 03,2008		I-316	NOV 30,2003
		5433959	SEP 03,2008		I-316	NOV 30,2003
020406 002	LANSOPRAZOLE; PREVACID	4628098	MAY 10,2009		I-316	NOV 30,2003
		4689333	JUL 29,2005	U-126	I-316	NOV 30,2003
		5013743	FEB 12,2010	U-452	I-316	NOV 30,2003
		5026560	JUN 25,2008		I-316	NOV 30,2003
		5045321	SEP 03,2008		I-316	NOV 30,2003
		5093132	SEP 03,2008		I-316	NOV 30,2003
		5433959	SEP 03,2008		I-316	NOV 30,2003
021281 001	LANSOPRAZOLE; PREVACID				M-1	JUL 06,2002
021281 002	LANSOPRAZOLE; PREVACID				I-316	NOV 30,2003
021428 001	LANSOPRAZOLE; PREVACID	4628098	MAY 10,2009			
		4689333	JUL 29,2005	U-126		
		5013743	FEB 12,2010	U-452		
		5026560	JUN 25,2008			
		5045321	SEP 03,2008			
		5093132	SEP 03,2008			
		5433959	SEP 03,2008			
		5464632	NOV 07,2012			
		6123962	FEB 13,2007			
		6328994	MAY 17,2009			
021428 002	LANSOPRAZOLE; PREVACID	4628098	MAY 10,2009			
		4689333	JUL 29,2005	U-126		
		5013743	FEB 12,2010	U-452		
		5026560	JUN 25,2008			
		5045321	SEP 03,2008			
		5093132	SEP 03,2008			
		5433959	SEP 03,2008			
		5464632	NOV 07,2012			
		6123962	FEB 13,2007			
		6328994	MAY 17,2009			
020597 001	LATANOPROST; XALATAN	4599353	JUL 28,2006	U-260	I-375	DEC 20,2005
		5296504	MAR 22,2011	U-260	I-375	DEC 20,2005
		5422368	MAR 22,2011	U-260	I-375	DEC 20,2005
		6429226	SEP 06,2009	U-260	I-375	DEC 20,2005
020905 001	LEFLUNOMIDE; ARAVA				I-395	JUN 13,2006
020905 002	LEFLUNOMIDE; ARAVA				I-395	JUN 13,2006
020905 003	LEFLUNOMIDE; ARAVA				I-395	JUN 13,2006
020807 001	LEPIRUDIN; REFLUDAN	5180668	JAN 19,2010		NCE	MAR 06,2003
020726 001	LETROZOLE; FEMARA	4978672	JUN 03,2011	U-203	I-318	JAN 10,2004
021343 001	LEUPROLIDE ACETATE; ELIGARD	4938763	OCT 03,2008		NP	JAN 23,2005
		5278201	JAN 11,2011		NP	JAN 23,2005
		5324519	OCT 20,2011		NP	JAN 23,2005
		5599552	FEB 04,2014		NP	JAN 23,2005
		5733950	OCT 03,2008		NP	JAN 23,2005
		5739176	OCT 03,2008		NP	JAN 23,2005
021379 001	LEUPROLIDE ACETATE; ELIGARD	4938763	OCT 03,2008		NP	JUL 24,2005

PRESCRIPTION AND OTC PRODUCT
PATENT AND EXCLUSIVITY DATA
*PED and PED represent Pediatric Exclusivity (*continued*)

APPL/PROD NUMBER	INGREDIENT NAME; TRADE NAME	PATENT NUMBER	PATENT EXPIRES	USE CODE	EX-CLUS CODE	EXCLUS EXPIRES
		5278201	JAN 11,2011		NP	JUL 24,2005
		5324519	OCT 20,2011		NP	JUL 24,2005
		5599552	FEB 04,2014		NP	JUL 24,2005
		5733950	OCT 03,2008		NP	JUL 24,2005
		5739176	OCT 03,2008		NP	JUL 24,2005
021488 001	LEUPROLIDE ACETATE; ELIGARD				NP	FEB 13,2006
019732 001	LEUPROLIDE ACETATE; LUPRON DEPOT	4652441	NOV 01,2004			
		4677191	JUL 03,2005			
		4728721	MAY 01,2006			
		4849228	JUL 18,2006			
		4917893	NOV 01,2004			
		5330767	NOV 01,2004			
		5476663	NOV 01,2004			
		5575987	SEP 02,2013			
		5631020	MAY 20,2014			
		5631020	NOV 01,2004			
		5716640	SEP 02,2013			
		6036976	DEC 13,2013			
020011 001	LEUPROLIDE ACETATE; LUPRON DEPOT	4652441	NOV 01,2004			
		4677191	JUL 03,2005			
		4728721	MAY 01,2006			
		4849228	JUL 18,2006			
		4917893	NOV 01,2004			
		5330767	NOV 01,2004			
		5476663	NOV 01,2004			
		5575987	SEP 02,2013			
		5631020	NOV 01,2004			
		5631021	MAY 20,2014			
		5716640	SEP 02,2013			
020517 001	LEUPROLIDE ACETATE; LUPRON DEPOT	4728721	MAY 01,2006			
		4849228	JUL 18,2006			
		5330767	NOV 01,2004			
		5476663	NOV 01,2004			
		5480656	JAN 02,2013			
		5575987	NOV 19,2013			
		5631020	MAY 20,2014			
		5631021	NOV 01,2004			
		5643607	JAN 02,2013			
		5716640	SEP 02,2013			
		5814342	FEB 01,2011			
		6036976	DEC 13,2016			
020708 001	LEUPROLIDE ACETATE; LUPRON DEPOT-3	4728721	MAY 01,2006			
		4849228	JUL 18,2006			
		4954298	NOV 01,2004			
		5330767	NOV 01,2004			
		5476663	NOV 01,2004			
		5480656	JAN 02,2013			
		5575987	NOV 19,2013			
		5631020	MAY 20,2014			
		5631021	NOV 01,2004			
		5643607	JAN 02,2013			
		5716640	SEP 02,2013			
		5814342	FEB 01,2011			
		6036976	DEC 13,2016			
020517 002	LEUPROLIDE ACETATE; LUPRON DEPOT-4	4728721	MAY 01,2006			
		4849228	JUL 18,2006			
		5330767	NOV 01,2004			
		5476663	NOV 01,2004			
		5480656	JAN 02,2013			
		5575987	NOV 19,2013			
		5631020	MAY 20,2014			
		5631021	NOV 01,2004			
		5643607	JAN 02,2013			
		5716640	SEP 02,2013			
		5814342	FEB 01,2011			
		6036976	DEC 13,2016			
020263 002	LEUPROLIDE ACETATE; LUPRON DEPOT-PED	4652441	NOV 01,2004			
		4677191	JUL 03,2005			
		4728721	MAY 01,2006			
		4849228	JUL 18,2006			
		4917893	NOV 01,2004			

PRESCRIPTION AND OTC PRODUCT
PATENT AND EXCLUSIVITY DATA
*PED and PED represent Pediatric Exclusivity (*continued*)

APPL/PROD NUMBER	INGREDIENT NAME; TRADE NAME	PATENT NUMBER	PATENT EXPIRES	USE CODE	EX-CLUS CODE	EXCLUS EXPIRES
		5330767	NOV 01,2004			
		5476663	NOV 01,2004			
		5575987	SEP 02,2013			
		5631020	MAY 20,2014			
		5631021	NOV 01,2004			
		5716640	SEP 02,2013			
		6036976	DEC 13,2013			
020263 003	LEUPROLIDE ACETATE; LUPRON DEPOT-PED	4652441	NOV 01,2004			
		4677191	JUL 03,2005			
		4728721	MAY 01,2006			
		4849228	JUL 18,2006			
		4917893	NOV 01,2004			
		5330767	NOV 01,2004			
		5476663	NOV 01,2004			
		5575987	SEP 02,2013			
		5631020	MAY 20,2014			
		5631021	NOV 01,2004			
		5716640	SEP 02,2013			
		6036976	DEC 13,2013			
020263 004	LEUPROLIDE ACETATE; LUPRON DEPOT-PED	4652441	NOV 01,2004			
		4677191	JUL 03,2005			
		4728721	MAY 01,2006			
		4049228	JUL 18,2006			
		4917893	NOV 01,2004			
		5330767	NOV 01,2004			
		5476663	NOV 01,2004			
		5575987	SEP 02,2013			
		5631020	MAY 20,2014			
		5631021	NOV 01,2004			
		5716640	SEP 02,2013			
		6036976	DEC 13,2013			
020263 005	LEUPROLIDE ACETATE; LUPRON DEPOT-PED	4652441	NOV 01,2004			
		4677191	JUL 03,2005			
		4728721	MAY 01,2006			
		4849228	JUL 18,2006			
		4917893	NOV 01,2004			
		5330767	NOV 01,2004			
		5476663	NOV 01,2004			
		5575987	SEP 02,2013			
		5631020	MAY 20,2014			
		5631021	NOV 01,2004			
		5716640	SEP 02,2013			
		6036976	DEC 13,2013			
020263 006	LEUPROLIDE ACETATE; LUPRON DEPOT-PED	4652441	NOV 01,2004			
		4677191	JUL 03,2005			
		4728721	MAY 01,2006			
		4849228	JUL 18,2006			
		4917893	NOV 01,2004			
		5330767	NOV 01,2004			
		5476663	NOV 01,2004			
		5575987	SEP 02,2013			
		5631020	MAY 20,2014			
		5631021	NOV 01,2004			
		5716640	SEP 02,2013			
		6036976	DEC 13,2013			
021088 001	LEUPROLIDE ACETATE; VIADUR	5728396	JAN 30,2017	U-316	NP	MAR 03,2003
		5932547	JUN 13,2017		NP	MAR 03,2003
		5985305	JAN 30,2017		NP	MAR 03,2003
		6113938	JUL 24,2018		NP	MAR 03,2003
		6124261	JUN 13,2017		NP	MAR 03,2003
		6132420	JAN 30,2017		NP	MAR 03,2003
		6156331	JAN 30,2017		NP	MAR 03,2003
		6235712	JUN 13,2017		NP	MAR 03,2003
		6375978	DEC 17,2018		NP	MAR 03,2003
		6395292	JAN 30,2017		NP	MAR 03,2003
020837 001	LEVALBUTEROL HYDROCHLORIDE; XOPENEX	5362755	NOV 08,2011	U-332	I-347	JAN 30,2005
		5547994	AUG 20,2013	U-332	I-347	JAN 30,2005
		5760090	JAN 05,2010	U-332	I-347	JAN 30,2005
		5844002	JAN 05,2010	U-332	I-347	JAN 30,2005
		6083993	JAN 05,2010	U-332	I-347	JAN 30,2005
		6451289	MAR 21,2021		I-347	JAN 30,2005

PRESCRIPTION AND OTC PRODUCT
PATENT AND EXCLUSIVITY DATA
*PED and PED represent Pediatric Exclusivity (*continued*)

APPL/PROD NUMBER	INGREDIENT NAME; TRADE NAME	PATENT NUMBER	PATENT EXPIRES	USE CODE	EX-CLUS CODE	EXCLUS EXPIRES
020837 002	LEVALBUTEROL HYDROCHLORIDE; XOPENEX	5362755	NOV 08,2011	U-332	I-347	JAN 30,2005
		5547994	AUG 20,2013	U-332	I-347	JAN 30,2005
		5760090	JAN 05,2010	U-332	I-347	JAN 30,2005
		5844002	JAN 05,2010	U-332	I-347	JAN 30,2005
		6083993	JAN 05,2010	U-332	I-347	JAN 30,2005
		6451289	MAR 21,2021		I-347	JAN 30,2005
020837 003	LEVALBUTEROL HYDROCHLORIDE; XOPENEX	5362755	NOV 08,2011	U-332	I-347	JAN 30,2005
		5547994	AUG 20,2013	U-332	I-347	JAN 30,2005
		5760090	JAN 05,2010	U-332	I-347	JAN 30,2005
		5844002	JAN 05,2010	U-332	I-347	JAN 30,2005
		6083993	JAN 05,2010	U-332	I-347	JAN 30,2005
		6451289	MAR 21,2021		I-347	JAN 30,2005
020035 001	LEVAMISOLE HYDROCHLORIDE; ERGAMISOL	4584305	JUN 18,2004	U-42		
021035 001	LEVETIRACETAM; KEPPRA	4837223	JUN 06,2006		NCE	NOV 30,2004
		4943639	JUL 06,2006		NCE	NOV 30,2004
021035 002	LEVETIRACETAM; KEPPRA	4837223	JUN 06,2006		NCE	NOV 30,2004
		4943639	JUL 06,2006		NCE	NOV 30,2004
021035 003	LEVETIRACETAM; KEPPRA	4837223	JUN 06,2006		NCE	NOV 30,2004
		4943639	JUL 06,2006		NCE	NOV 30,2004
021114 001	LEVOBETAXOLOL HYDROCHLORIDE; BETAXON	4911920	MAR 27,2007	U-369	NP	FEB 23,2003
		5540918	JUL 30,2013		NP	FEB 23,2003
020997 001	LEVOBUPIVACAINE HYDROCHLORIDE; CHIROCAINE	5708011	OCT 13,2014	U-276	NP	AUG 05,2002
020997 002	LEVOBUPIVACAINE HYDROCHLORIDE; CHIROCAINE	5708011	OCT 13,2014	U-276	NP	AUG 05,2002
020997 003	LEVOBUPIVACAINE HYDROCHLORIDE; CHIROCAINE	5708011	OCT 13,2014	U-276	NP	AUG 05,2002
020219 001	LEVOCABASTINE HYDROCHLORIDE; LIVOSTIN	4369184	DEC 02,2004			
020182 001	LEVOCARNITINE; CARNITOR	6335369	JAN 18,2021	U-433	ODE	DEC 15,2006
		6429230	JAN 18,2021	U-433	ODE	DEC 15,2006
020634 001	LEVOFLOXACIN; LEVAQUIN	5053407	DEC 20,2010		I-357	APR 08,2003
					I-393	MAY 23,2006
020634 002	LEVOFLOXACIN; LEVAQUIN	5053407	DEC 20,2010		I-357	APR 08,2003
					I-393	MAY 23,2006
020634 003	LEVOFLOXACIN; LEVAQUIN	5053407	DEC 20,2010		I-357	APR 08,2003
					I-393	MAY 23,2006
020635 001	LEVOFLOXACIN; LEVAQUIN	5053407	DEC 20,2010		I-357	APR 08,2003
					I-393	MAY 23,2006
020635 002	LEVOFLOXACIN; LEVAQUIN IN DEXTROSE 5% IN PLASTIC CONTAINER	5053407	DEC 20,2010		I-305	FEB 02,2003
					I-393	MAY 23,2006
020635 003	LEVOFLOXACIN; LEVAQUIN IN DEXTROSE 5% IN PLASTIC CONTAINER	5053407	DEC 20,2010		I-357	APR 08,2003
					I-393	MAY 23,2006
021199 001	LEVOFLOXACIN; QUIXIN	4382892	SEP 02,2003		NDF	AUG 18,2003
		4551456	NOV 14,2003		NDF	AUG 18,2003
		5503407	DEC 20,2010		NDF	AUG 18,2003
021225 001	LEVONORGESTREL; MIRENA				NP	DEC 06,2003
021045 001	LEVONORGESTREL; PLAN B				NP	JUL 28,2002
021342 001	LEVOTHYROXINE SODIUM; LEVO-T	6399101	MAR 30,2020			
021342 002	LEVOTHYROXINE SODIUM; LEVO-T	6399101	MAR 30,2020			
021342 003	LEVOTHYROXINE SODIUM; LEVO-T	6399101	MAR 30,2020			
021342 004	LEVOTHYROXINE SODIUM; LEVO-T	6399101	MAR 30,2020			
021342 005	LEVOTHYROXINE SODIUM; LEVO-T	6399101	MAR 30,2020			
021342 006	LEVOTHYROXINE SODIUM; LEVO-T	6399101	MAR 30,2020			
021342 007	LEVOTHYROXINE SODIUM; LEVO-T	6399101	MAR 30,2020			
021342 008	LEVOTHYROXINE SODIUM; LEVO-T	6399101	MAR 30,2020			
021342 009	LEVOTHYROXINE SODIUM; LEVO-T	6399101	MAR 30,2020			
021342 010	LEVOTHYROXINE SODIUM; LEVO-T	6399101	MAR 30,2020			
021342 011	LEVOTHYROXINE SODIUM; LEVO-T	6399101	MAR 30,2020			
021301 001	LEVOTHYROXINE SODIUM; LEVOXYL	6555581	FEB 15,2022			
021301 002	LEVOTHYROXINE SODIUM; LEVOXYL	6555581	FEB 15,2022			
021301 003	LEVOTHYROXINE SODIUM; LEVOXYL	6555581	FEB 15,2022			
021301 004	LEVOTHYROXINE SODIUM; LEVOXYL	6555581	FEB 15,2022			
021301 005	LEVOTHYROXINE SODIUM; LEVOXYL	6555581	FEB 15,2022			
021301 006	LEVOTHYROXINE SODIUM; LEVOXYL	6555581	FEB 15,2022			
021301 007	LEVOTHYROXINE SODIUM; LEVOXYL	6555581	FEB 15,2022			
021301 008	LEVOTHYROXINE SODIUM; LEVOXYL	6555581	FEB 15,2022			
021301 009	LEVOTHYROXINE SODIUM; LEVOXYL	6555581	FEB 15,2022			
021301 010	LEVOTHYROXINE SODIUM; LEVOXYL	6555581	FEB 15,2022			
021301 011	LEVOTHYROXINE SODIUM; LEVOXYL	6555581	FEB 15,2022			

PRESCRIPTION AND OTC PRODUCT
PATENT AND EXCLUSIVITY DATA
*PED and PED represent Pediatric Exclusivity (*continued*)

APPL/PROD NUMBER	INGREDIENT NAME; TRADE NAME	PATENT NUMBER	PATENT EXPIRES	USE CODE	EX-CLUS CODE	EXCLUS EXPIRES
021301 012	LEVOTHYROXINE SODIUM; LEVOXYL	6555581	FEB 15,2022			
019941 001	LIDOCAINE; EMLA	4529601	JUL 16,2002		I-314	JAN 28,2003
		4562060	DEC 31,2002		I-314	JAN 28,2003
020575 001	LIDOCAINE; LIDOCAINE	5234957	FEB 27,2011			
		5332576	JUL 26,2011			
		5446070	FEB 27,2011			
020575 002	LIDOCAINE; LIDOCAINE	5234957	FEB 27,2011			
		5332576	JUL 26,2011			
		5446070	FEB 27,2011			
020612 001	LIDOCAINE; LIDODERM	5411738	MAY 02,2012		ODE	MAR 19,2006
		5589180	MAR 17,2009	U-485	ODE	MAR 19,2006
		5601838	MAY 02,2012	U-488	ODE	MAR 19,2006
		5709869	MAR 17,2009	U-485	ODE	MAR 19,2006
		5827529	OCT 27,2015	U-486	ODE	MAR 19,2006
021130 001	LINEZOLID; ZYVOX	5688792	NOV 18,2014	U-319	NPP	DEC 19,2005
021130 002	LINEZOLID; ZYVOX	5688792	NOV 18,2014	U-319	NPP	DEC 19,2005
021131 001	LINEZOLID; ZYVOX	5688792	NOV 18,2014	U-319	NPP	DEC 19,2005
021132 001	LINEZOLID; ZYVOX	5688792	NOV 18,2014	U-319	NPP	DEC 19,2005
019777 001	LISINOPRIL; ZESTRIL				PED	AUG 07,2003
019777 002	LISINOPRIL; ZESTRIL				I-288	FEB 07,2003
019777 003	LISINOPRIL; ZESTRIL				I-288	FEB 07,2003
019777 004	LISINOPRIL; ZESTRIL				I-288	FEB 07,2003
019777 005	LISINOPRIL; ZESTRIL				I-288	FEB 07,2003
019777 006	LISINOPRIL; ZESTRIL				PED	AUG 07,2003
020191 001	LODOXAMIDE TROMETHAMINE; ALOMIDE	5457126	OCT 10,2012	U-117		
020013 001	LOMEFLOXACIN HYDROCHLORIDE; MAXAQUIN	4528287	FEB 21,2006	U-36		
020448 001	LOPERAMIDE HYDROCHLORIDE; IMODIUM A-D	5489436	FEB 06,2013			
020606 001	LOPERAMIDE HYDROCHLORIDE; IMODIUM ADVANCED	5248505	JUL 28,2010			
		5489436	FEB 06,2013			
		5612054	SEP 28,2010			
		5679376	OCT 21,2014			
		5716641	MAY 21,2012	U-226		
021140 001	LOPERAMIDE HYDROCHLORIDE; IMODIUM ADVANCED	5248505	SEP 28,2010	U-434		
		5612054	SEP 28,2010			
		6103260	JUL 17,2017			
021226 001	LOPINAVIR; KALETRA	5541206	JUL 30,2013	U-348	NC	SEP 15,2003
		5635523	JUN 30,2014	U-352	NC	SEP 15,2003
		5648497	JUL 15,2014		NC	SEP 15,2003
		5674882	OCT 07,2014	U-344	NC	SEP 15,2003
		5846987	DEC 29,2012	U-350	NC	SEP 15,2003
		5886036	DEC 29,2012	U-345	NC	SEP 15,2003
		5914332	DEC 13,2015	U-351	NC	SEP 15,2003
		6037157	JUN 26,2016	U-346	NC	SEP 15,2003
		6232333	NOV 07,2017		NC	SEP 15,2003
		6284767	FEB 14,2016	U-401	NC	SEP 15,2003
		6458818	NOV 07,2017		NC	SEP 15,2003
		6521651	NOV 01,2017		NC	SEP 15,2003
021251 001	LOPINAVIR; KALETRA	5541206	JUL 30,2013	U-348	NC	SEP 15,2003
		5635523	JUN 03,2014	U-352	NC	SEP 15,2003
		5648497	JUL 15,2014		NC	SEP 15,2003
		5674882	OCT 07,2014	U-344	NC	SEP 15,2003
		5846987	DEC 29,2012	U-350	NC	SEP 15,2003
		5886036	DEC 29,2012	U-345	NC	SEP 15,2003
		5914332	DEC 13,2005	U-351	NC	SEP 15,2003
		6037157	JUN 26,2016	U-346	NC	SEP 15,2003
		6284767	FEB 14,2016	U-401	NC	SEP 15,2003
019658 001	LORATADINE; CLARITIN	4282233*PED	DEC 19,2002	U-77		
		4659716	APR 21,2004	U-142		
		4659716*PED	OCT 21,2004	U-142		
		4863931	SEP 15,2008			
		4863931*PED	MAR 15,2009			
019658 002	LORATADINE; CLARITIN	4659716	APR 21,2004	U-142		
		4659716*PED	OCT 21,2004	U-142		
		4863931	SEP 15,2008			
		4863931*PED	MAR 15,2009			
020641 001	LORATADINE; CLARITIN	4282233*PED	DEC 19,2002	U-77		
		4659716	APR 21,2004	U-142		
		4659716*PED	OCT 21,2004	U-142		
		4863931	SEP 15,2008			

PRESCRIPTION AND OTC PRODUCT
PATENT AND EXCLUSIVITY DATA
*PED and PED represent Pediatric Exclusivity (*continued*)

APPL/PROD NUMBER	INGREDIENT NAME; TRADE NAME	PATENT NUMBER	PATENT EXPIRES	USE CODE	EX-CLUS CODE	EXCLUS EXPIRES
		4863931*PED	MAR 15,2009			
		6132758	JUN 01,2018			
020641 002	LORATADINE; CLARITIN	4659716	APR 21,2004	U-142		
		4659716*PED	OCT 21,2004	U-142		
		4863931	SEP 15,2008			
		4863931*PED	MAR 15,2009			
		6132758	JUN 01,2018			
020704 001	LORATADINE; CLARITIN REDITABS	4282233*PED	DEC 19,2002	U-77		
		4659716	APR 21,2004	U-142		
		4659716*PED	OCT 21,2004	U-142		
		4863931	SEP 15,2008			
		4863931*PED	MAR 15,2009			
020704 002	LORATADINE; CLARITIN REDITABS	4659716	APR 21,2004	U-142		
		4659716*PED	OCT 21,2004	U-142		
		4863931	SEP 15,2008			
		4863931*PED	MAR 15,2009			
019670 002	LORATADINE; CLARITIN-D	4659716	APR 21,2004	U-142		
		4659716*PED	OCT 21,2004	U-142		
		4863931	SEP 15,2008			
		4863931*PED	MAR 15,2009			
020470 002	LORATADINE; CLARITIN-D 24 HOUR	4659716	APR 21,2004	U-142		
		4659716*PED	OCT 21,2004	U-142		
		4863931	SEP 15,2008			
		4863931*PED	MAR 15,2009			
		5314697	OCT 23,2012			
		5314697*PED	APR 23,2013			
075209 001	LORATADINE; LORATADINE				PC	JUL 21,2003
075822 001	LORATADINE; LORATADINE				PC	AUG 09,2003
075706 001	LORATADINE; LORATADINE AND PSEUDOEPHEDRINE HCL				PC	NOV 29,2003
076050 001	LORATADINE; LORATADINE AND PSEUDOEPHEDRINE SULFATE				PC	JUL 30,2003
020386 001	LOSARTAN POTASSIUM; COZAAR	5138069	AUG 11,2009		I-383	SEP 17,2005
		5138069*PED	FEB 11,2010		I-383	SEP 17,2005
		5153197	OCT 06,2009	U-3	I-383	SEP 17,2005
		5153197*PED	APR 06,2010	U-3	I-383	SEP 17,2005
		5210079	MAY 11,2010	U-496	I-383	SEP 17,2005
		5210079*PED	NOV 11,2010	U-496	I-383	SEP 17,2005
		5608075	MAR 04,2014		I-383	SEP 17,2005
		5608075*PED	SEP 04,2014		I-383	SEP 17,2005
020386 002	LOSARTAN POTASSIUM; COZAAR	5138069	AUG 11,2009		I-383	SEP 17,2005
		5138069*PED	FEB 11,2010		I-383	SEP 17,2005
		5153197	OCT 06,2009	U-3	I-383	SEP 17,2005
		5153197*PED	APR 06,2010	U-3	I-383	SEP 17,2005
		5210079	MAY 11,2010	U-496	I-383	SEP 17,2005
		5210079*PED	NOV 11,2010	U-496	I-383	SEP 17,2005
		5608075	MAR 04,2014		I-383	SEP 17,2005
		5608075*PED	SEP 04,2014		I-383	SEP 17,2005
020386 003	LOSARTAN POTASSIUM; COZAAR	5138069	AUG 11,2009		I-383	SEP 17,2005
		5138069*PED	FEB 11,2010		I-383	SEP 17,2005
		5153197	OCT 06,2009	U-3	I-383	SEP 17,2005
		5153197*PED	APR 06,2010	U-3	I-383	SEP 17,2005
		5210079	MAY 11,2010	U-496	I-383	SEP 17,2005
		5210079*PED	NOV 11,2010	U-496	I-383	SEP 17,2005
		5608075	MAR 04,2014		I-383	SEP 17,2005
		5608075*PED	SEP 04,2014		I-383	SEP 17,2005
020803 001	LOTEPREDNOL ETABONATE; ALREX	4996335	MAR 09,2012		NCE	MAR 09,2003
		5540930	OCT 25,2013		NCE	MAR 09,2003
020583 001	LOTEPREDNOL ETABONATE; LOTEMAX	4996335	MAR 09,2012		NCE	MAR 09,2003
		5540930	OCT 25,2013		NCE	MAR 09,2003
020841 001	LOTEPREDNOL ETABONATE; LOTEMAX	4996335	FEB 26,2008		NCE	MAR 09,2003
		5540930	OCT 25,2013		NCE	MAR 09,2003
021249 001	LOVASTATIN; ADVICOR	6080428	MAY 27,2017	U-447	NC	DEC 17,2004
		6129930	SEP 20,2013	U-448	NC	DEC 17,2004
		6406715	OCT 31,2017	U-450	NC	DEC 17,2004
021249 002	LOVASTATIN; ADVICOR	6080428	MAY 27,2017	U-447	NC	DEC 17,2004
		6129930	SEP 20,2013	U-448	NC	DEC 17,2004
		6406715	OCT 31,2017	U-450	NC	DEC 17,2004
021249 003	LOVASTATIN; ADVICOR	6080428	MAY 27,2017	U-447	NC	DEC 17,2004
		6129930	SEP 20,2013	U-448	NC	DEC 17,2004
		6406715	OCT 31,2017	U-450	NC	DEC 17,2004

PRESCRIPTION AND OTC PRODUCT
PATENT AND EXCLUSIVITY DATA
*PED and PED represent Pediatric Exclusivity (*continued*)

APPL/PROD NUMBER	INGREDIENT NAME; TRADE NAME	PATENT NUMBER	PATENT EXPIRES	USE CODE	EX-CLUS CODE	EXCLUS EXPIRES
021316 001	LOVASTATIN; ALTOCOR	5916595	DEC 12,2017		NDF	JUN 26,2005
		6080778	MAR 23,2018	U-456	NDF	JUN 26,2005
021316 002	LOVASTATIN; ALTOCOR	5916595	DEC 12,2017		NDF	JUN 26,2005
		6080778	MAR 23,2018	U-456	NDF	JUN 26,2005
021316 003	LOVASTATIN; ALTOCOR	5916595	DEC 12,2017		NDF	JUN 26,2005
		6080778	MAR 23,2018	U-456	NDF	JUN 26,2005
021316 004	LOVASTATIN; ALTOCOR	5916595	DEC 12,2017		NDF	JUN 26,2005
		6080778	MAR 23,2018	U-456	NDF	JUN 26,2005
019643 002	LOVASTATIN; MEVACOR				PED	AUG 14,2005
019643 003	LOVASTATIN; MEVACOR				PED	AUG 14,2005
019643 004	LOVASTATIN; MEVACOR				PED	SEP 11,2002
019832 003	MAFENIDE ACETATE; SULFAMYLON				ODE	JUN 05,2005
020652 001	MANGAFODIPIR TRISODIUM; TESLASCAN	4647447	MAR 03,2004	U-238	NCE	NOV 26,2002
		4933456	NOV 27,2011		NCE	NOV 26,2002
		4992554	FEB 12,2008		NCE	NOV 26,2002
		5091169	FEB 25,2009		NCE	NOV 26,2002
		5223243	JUN 29,2010	U-237	NCE	NOV 26,2002
019940 001	MASOPROCOL; ACTINEX	4695590	APR 17,2008			
		5008294	APR 15,2008	U-68		
019591 001	MEFLOQUINE HYDROCHLORIDE; LARIAM	4579855	OCT 01,2004			
076175 001	MEFLOQUINE HYDROCHLORIDE; MEFLOQUINE HCL				PC	NOV 03,2002
020264 001	MEGESTROL ACETATE; MEGACE	5338732	AUG 16,2011			
020938 001	MELOXICAM; MOBIC				NCE	APR 13,2005
020938 002	MELOXICAM; MOBIC				NCE	APR 13,2005
020207 001	MELPHALAN HYDROCHLORIDE; ALKERAN	4997651	NOV 18,2008			
021047 001	MENOTROPINS (FSH; REPRONEX				NP	AUG 27,2002
021047 002	MENOTROPINS (FSH; REPRONEX				NP	AUG 27,2002
020922 001	MEQUINOL; SOLAGE	5194247	MAR 16,2010	U-294	NC	DEC 10,2004
		5470567	MAR 19,2010	U-294	NC	DEC 10,2004
		6353029	AUG 24,2020		NC	DEC 10,2004
019651 001	MESALAMINE; ASACOL	5541170	JUL 30,2013	U-141		
		5541171	JUL 30,2013	U-141		
019618 001	MESALAMINE; ROWASA	4657900	APR 14,2004			
		RE33239	MAY 12,2004			
019884 001	MESNA; MESNEX	5696172	OCT 06,2013			
020855 001	MESNA; MESNEX	5252341	JUL 16,2011		NDF	MAR 21,2005
		5262169	JUL 16,2011		NDF	MAR 21,2005
013217 001	METAXALONE; SKELAXIN	6407128	DEC 03,2021	U-189		
013217 003	METAXALONE; SKELAXIN	6407128	DEC 03,2021	U-189		
021410 001	METFORMIN HYDROCHLORIDE; AVANDAMET	5002953	AUG 30,2008	U-493	NCE	MAY 25,2004
		5741803	APR 21,2015	U-493	NCE	MAY 25,2004
		5965584	JUN 19,2016	U-493	NCE	MAY 25,2004
		6166042	JUN 19,2016	U-493	NCE	MAY 25,2004
		6288095	FEB 11,2017	U-493	NCE	MAY 25,2004
021410 002	METFORMIN HYDROCHLORIDE; AVANDAMET	5002953	AUG 30,2008	U-493	NCE	MAY 25,2004
		5741803	APR 21,2015	U-493	NCE	MAY 25,2004
		5965584	JUN 19,2016	U-493	NCE	MAY 25,2004
		6166042	JUN 19,2016	U-493	NCE	MAY 25,2004
		6288095	FEB 11,2017	U-493	NCE	MAY 25,2004
021410 003	METFORMIN HYDROCHLORIDE; AVANDAMET	5002953	AUG 30,2008	U-493	NCE	MAY 25,2004
		5741803	APR 21,2015	U-493	NCE	MAY 25,2004
		5965584	JUN 19,2016	U-493	NCE	MAY 25,2004
		6166042	JUN 19,2016	U-493	NCE	MAY 25,2004
		6288095	FEB 11,2017	U-493	NCE	MAY 25,2004
020357 001	METFORMIN HYDROCHLORIDE; GLUCOPHAGE				I-320	DEC 15,2003
020357 002	METFORMIN HYDROCHLORIDE; GLUCOPHAGE				I-320	DEC 15,2003
020357 003	METFORMIN HYDROCHLORIDE; GLUCOPHAGE				I-320	DEC 15,2003
020357 004	METFORMIN HYDROCHLORIDE; GLUCOPHAGE				I-320	DEC 15,2003
020357 005	METFORMIN HYDROCHLORIDE; GLUCOPHAGE				M-6	APR 19,2004
021202 001	METFORMIN HYDROCHLORIDE; GLUCOPHAGE XR	6475521	MAR 19,2018		NDF	OCT 13,2003
021202 004	METFORMIN HYDROCHLORIDE; GLUCOPHAGE XR	6475521	MAR 19,2018		NDF	OCT 13,2003
020969 001	METHOXSALEN; UVADEX	4845075	APR 11,2009			
		4999375	MAR 12,2008			
		5036102	JUL 30,2008	U-273		
021121 001	METHYLPHENIDATE HYDROCHLORIDE; CONCERTA	4519801	JUL 12,2002		NP	AUG 01,2003
		4612008	SEP 16,2003		NP	AUG 01,2003
		4783337	SEP 16,2003	U-372	NP	AUG 01,2003
		5082668	SEP 16,2003		NP	AUG 01,2003

PRESCRIPTION AND OTC PRODUCT
PATENT AND EXCLUSIVITY DATA
*PED and PED represent Pediatric Exclusivity (*continued*)

APPL/PROD NUMBER	INGREDIENT NAME; TRADE NAME	PATENT NUMBER	PATENT EXPIRES	USE CODE	EX-CLUS CODE	EXCLUS EXPIRES
021121 002	METHYLPHENIDATE HYDROCHLORIDE; CONCERTA	4519801	JUL 12,2002		NP	AUG 01,2003
		4612008	SEP 16,2003		NP	AUG 01,2003
		4783337	SEP 16,2003	U-372	NP	AUG 01,2003
		5082668	SEP 16,2003		NP	AUG 01,2003
021121 003	METHYLPHENIDATE HYDROCHLORIDE; CONCERTA	4519801	JUL 12,2002		NP	AUG 01,2003
		4612008	SEP 16,2003		NP	AUG 01,2003
		4783337	SEP 16,2003	U-372	NP	AUG 01,2003
		5082668	SEP 16,2003		NP	AUG 01,2003
021121 004	METHYLPHENIDATE HYDROCHLORIDE; CONCERTA	4519801	JUL 12,2002		NP	AUG 01,2003
		4612008	SEP 16,2003		NP	AUG 01,2003
		4783337	SEP 16,2003	U-372	NP	AUG 01,2003
		5082668	SEP 16,2003		NP	AUG 01,2003
021259 001	METHYLPHENIDATE HYDROCHLORIDE; METADATE CD	6344215	OCT 27,2020		NDF	APR 03,2004
021259 002	METHYLPHENIDATE HYDROCHLORIDE; METADATE CD	6344215	OCT 27,2020		NDF	APR 03,2004
021284 001	METHYLPHENIDATE HYDROCHLORIDE; RITALIN LA	5837284	MAY 15,2016		NP	JUN 07,2005
		6228398	MAY 01,2019	U-472	NP	JUN 07,2005
021284 002	METHYLPHENIDATE HYDROCHLORIDE; RITALIN LA	5837284	MAY 15,2016		NP	JUN 07,2005
		6228398	MAY 01,2019	U-472	NP	JUN 07,2005
021284 003	METHYLPHENIDATE HYDROCHLORIDE; RITALIN LA	5837284	MAY 15,2016		NP	JUN 07,2005
		6228398	NOV 01,2019	U-472	NP	JUN 07,2005
017862 001	METOCLOPRAMIDE HYDROCHLORIDE; REGLAN	4536386	AUG 20,2002	U-9		
017862 004	METOCLOPRAMIDE HYDROCHLORIDE; REGLAN	4536386	AUG 20,2002	U-9		
019532 001	METOLAZONE; MYKROX	4517179	APR 29,2003			
019786 003	METOPROLOL FUMARATE; LOPRESSOR	4892739	JAN 09,2007			
019786 004	METOPROLOL FUMARATE; LOPRESSOR	4892739	JAN 09,2007			
019962 001	METOPROLOL SUCCINATE; TOPROL-XL	4927640	MAY 22,2007		I-194	FEB 05,2004
		4957745	SEP 18,2007	U-107	I-194	FEB 05,2004
		5001161	MAR 19,2008		I-194	FEB 05,2004
		5081154	JAN 14,2009		I-194	FEB 05,2004
019962 002	METOPROLOL SUCCINATE; TOPROL-XL	4927640	MAY 22,2007		I-194	FEB 05,2004
		4957745	SEP 18,2007	U-107	I-194	FEB 05,2004
		5001161	MAR 19,2008		I-194	FEB 05,2004
		5081154	JAN 14,2009		I-194	FEB 05,2004
019962 003	METOPROLOL SUCCINATE; TOPROL-XL	4927640	MAY 22,2007		I-194	FEB 05,2004
		4957745	SEP 18,2007	U-107	I-194	FEB 05,2004
		5001161	MAR 19,2008		I-194	FEB 05,2004
		5081154	JAN 14,2009		I-194	FEB 05,2004
019962 004	METOPROLOL SUCCINATE; TOPROL-XL	4927640	MAY 22,2007		NS	FEB 05,2004
		4957745	SEP 18,2007	U-107	NS	FEB 05,2004
		5001161	MAR 19,2008	U-107	NS	FEB 05,2004
		5081154	JAN 14,2009	U-107	NS	FEB 05,2004
019737 001	METRONIDAZOLE; METROGEL	4837378	JUN 06,2006			
020208 001	METRONIDAZOLE; METROGEL-VAGINAL	4837378	JUN 06,2006			
		5536743	JUL 16,2013	U-137		
		5840744	JAN 15,2008	U-370		
020968 001	MICONAZOLE NITRATE; MONISTAT DUAL- PAK	5514698	MAR 21,2014			
019815 001	MIDODRINE HYDROCHLORIDE; PROAMATINE				ODE	SEP 06,2003
019815 002	MIDODRINE HYDROCHLORIDE; PROAMATINE				ODE	SEP 06,2003
019815 003	MIDODRINE HYDROCHLORIDE; PROAMATINE				ODE	SEP 06,2003
020687 001	MIFEPRISTONE; MIFEPREX	4626531	OCT 12,2004		NCE	SEP 28,2005
020682 001	MIGLITOL; GLYSET	4639436	JAN 27,2009	U-111		
020682 002	MIGLITOL; GLYSET	4639436	JAN 27,2009	U-111		
020682 003	MIGLITOL; GLYSET	4639436	JAN 27,2009	U-111		
076119 001	MIRTAZAPINE; MIRTAZAPINE				PC	JUN 16,2003
076119 002	MIRTAZAPINE; MIRTAZAPINE				PC	JUN 16,2003
020415 001	MIRTAZAPINE; REMERON				M-18	APR 09,2005
020415 002	MIRTAZAPINE; REMERON				M-18	APR 09,2005
020415 003	MIRTAZAPINE; REMERON				M-18	APR 09,2005
021208 001	MIRTAZAPINE; REMERON SOLTAB	5178878	JAN 12,2010		M-18	APR 09,2005
021208 002	MIRTAZAPINE; REMERON SOLTAB	5178878	JAN 12,2010		M-18	APR 09,2005
021208 003	MIRTAZAPINE; REMERON SOLTAB	5178878	JAN 12,2010		M-18	APR 09,2005
019297 001	MITOXANTRONE HYDROCHLORIDE; NOVANTRONE	4617319	JUN 13,2005	U-390	ODE	OCT 13,2007
		4820738	APR 11,2006	U-98	ODE	OCT 13,2007
020098 001	MIVACURIUM CHLORIDE; MIVACRON	4761418	JAN 22,2006			
020098 002	MIVACURIUM CHLORIDE; MIVACRON IN DEXTROSE 5% IN PLASTIC CONTAINER	4761418	JAN 22,2006			

PRESCRIPTION AND OTC PRODUCT
PATENT AND EXCLUSIVITY DATA
*PED and PED represent Pediatric Exclusivity (*continued*)

APPL/PROD NUMBER	INGREDIENT NAME; TRADE NAME	PATENT NUMBER	PATENT EXPIRES	USE CODE	EX-CLUS CODE	EXCLUS EXPIRES
020717 001	MODAFINIL; PROVIGIL	4927855	MAY 22,2007	U-255	NCE	DEC 24,2003
		RE37516	OCT 06,2014	U-255	NCE	DEC 24,2003
020717 002	MODAFINIL; PROVIGIL	4927855	MAY 22,2007	U-255	ODE	DEC 24,2005
		RE37516	OCT 06,2014	U-255	ODE	DEC 24,2005
076204 001	MOEXIPRIL HYDROCHLORIDE; MOEXIPRIL HCL				PC	SEP 21,2003
076204 002	MOEXIPRIL HYDROCHLORIDE; MOEXIPRIL HCL				PC	SEP 21,2003
020312 001	MOEXIPRIL HYDROCHLORIDE; UNIVASC	4743450	FEB 24,2007			
020312 002	MOEXIPRIL HYDROCHLORIDE; UNIVASC	4743450	FEB 24,2007			
020762 001	MOMETASONE FUROATE MONOHYDRATE; NASONEX	5837699	JAN 27,2014	U-249	I-360	JUL 17,2005
		5837699*PED	JUL 27,2014	U-249	I-360	JUL 17,2005
		6127353	OCT 03,2017		I-360	JUL 17,2005
		6127353*PED	APR 03,2018		I-360	JUL 17,2005
019625 001	MOMETASONE FUROATE; ELOCON	4808610	OCT 02,2006			
		4808610*PED	APR 02,2007			
019796 001	MOMETASONE FUROATE; ELOCON	4775529	MAY 21,2007			
		4775529*PED	NOV 21,2007			
020829 002	MONTELUKAST SODIUM; SINGULAIR	5565473	FEB 03,2012	U-228	I-378	DEC 31,2005
		5565473*PED	AUG 03,2012	U-228	I-378	DEC 31,2005
020830 001	MONTELUKAST SODIUM; SINGULAIR	5565473	FEB 03,2012	U-228	PED	AUG 20,2003
		5565473*PED	AUG 03,2012	U-228	PED	AUG 20,2003
020830 002	MONTELUKAST SODIUM; SINGULAIR	5565473	FEB 03,2012	U-228	NCE	FEB 20,2003
		5565473*PED	AUG 03,2012	U-228	NCE	FEB 20,2003
021409 001	MONTELUKAST SODIUM; SINGULAIR	5565473	FEB 03,2012		NCE	FEB 20,2003
		5565473*PED	AUG 03,2012		NCE	FEB 20,2003
021260 001	MORPHINE SULFATE; AVINZA	6066339	NOV 25,2017		NP	MAR 20,2005
021260 002	MORPHINE SULFATE; AVINZA	6066339	NOV 25,2017		NP	MAR 20,2005
021260 003	MORPHINE SULFATE; AVINZA	6066339	NOV 25,2017		NP	MAR 20,2005
021260 004	MORPHINE SULFATE; AVINZA	6066339	NOV 25,2017		NP	MAR 20,2005
020616 001	MORPHINE SULFATE; KADIAN	5202128	APR 13,2010			
		5378474	MAR 23,2010			
020616 002	MORPHINE SULFATE; KADIAN	5202128	APR 13,2010			
		5378474	MAR 23,2010			
020616 003	MORPHINE SULFATE; KADIAN	5202128	APR 13,2010			
		5378474	MAR 23,2010			
021085 001	MOXIFLOXACIN HYDROCHLORIDE; AVELOX	4990517	JUN 30,2009	U-298	I-385	FEB 28,2006
		5607942	MAR 04,2014	U-298	I-385	FEB 28,2006
		5849752	DEC 05,2016	U-298	I-385	FEB 28,2006
021277 001	MOXIFLOXACIN HYDROCHLORIDE; AVELOX IN SODIUM CHLORIDE 0.8% IN PLASTIC CONTAINER	4990517	JUN 30,2009	U-298	I-329	APR 27,2004
		5607942	MAR 04,2014	U-298	I-329	APR 27,2004
		5849752	DEC 05,2016	U-298	I-329	APR 27,2004
021598 001	MOXIFLOXACIN HYDROCHLORIDE; VIGAMOX	4990517	JUN 30,2009		PED	OCT 15,2006
		4990517*PED	DEC 30,2009		PED	OCT 15,2006
		5607942	MAR 04,2014		PED	OCT 15,2006
		5607942*PED	SEP 04,2014		PED	OCT 15,2006
		5849752	DEC 05,2016		PED	OCT 15,2006
		5849752*PED	JUN 05,2017		PED	OCT 15,2006
021076 001	NAPROXEN SODIUM; ALEVE COLD AND SINUS				NC	NOV 29,2002
020353 001	NAPROXEN SODIUM; NAPRELAN	5637320	JUN 10,2014			
020353 002	NAPROXEN SODIUM; NAPRELAN	5637320	JUN 10,2014			
020353 003	NAPROXEN SODIUM; NAPRELAN	5637320	JUN 10,2014			
020763 001	NARATRIPTAN HYDROCHLORIDE; AMERGE	4997841	JUL 07,2010	U-232	NCE	FEB 10,2003
020763 002	NARATRIPTAN HYDROCHLORIDE; AMERGE	4997841	JUL 07,2010	U-232	NCE	FEB 10,2003
021204 001	NATEGLINIDE; STARLIX	5463116	OCT 21,2012		NCE	DEC 22,2005
		5488150	JAN 30,2013		NCE	DEC 22,2005
		6559188	SEP 17,2019		NCE	DEC 22,2005
		RE34878	MAR 28,2006		NCE	DEC 22,2005
021204 002	NATEGLINIDE; STARLIX	5463116	OCT 21,2012		NCE	DEC 22,2005
		5488150	JAN 30,2013		NCE	DEC 22,2005
		6559188	SEP 17,2019		NCE	DEC 22,2005
		RE34878	MAR 28,2006		NCE	DEC 22,2005
021009 001	NEDOCROMIL SODIUM; ALOCRIL	4474787	OCT 02,2006	U-304	NP	DEC 08,2002
		4760072	JUL 26,2005		NP	DEC 08,2002
019660 001	NEDOCROMIL SODIUM; TILADE	4474787	OCT 02,2006			
		4760072	JUL 26,2005			
020152 001	NEFAZODONE HYDROCHLORIDE; SERZONE	4338317	MAR 16,2003			
		4338317*PED	SEP 16,2003			
		5256664	APR 28,2012			
		5256664*PED	OCT 28,2012			

PRESCRIPTION AND OTC PRODUCT
PATENT AND EXCLUSIVITY DATA
*PED and PED represent Pediatric Exclusivity (*continued*)

APPL/PROD NUMBER	INGREDIENT NAME; TRADE NAME	PATENT NUMBER	PATENT EXPIRES	USE CODE	EX-CLUS CODE	EXCLUS EXPIRES
020152 002	NEFAZODONE HYDROCHLORIDE; SERZONE	4338317	MAR 16,2003			
		4338317*PED	SEP 16,2003			
		5256664	APR 28,2012			
		5256664*PED	OCT 28,2012			
020152 003	NEFAZODONE HYDROCHLORIDE; SERZONE	4338317	MAR 16,2003			
		4338317*PED	SEP 16,2003			
		5256664	APR 28,2012			
		5256664*PED	OCT 28,2012			
020152 004	NEFAZODONE HYDROCHLORIDE; SERZONE	4338317	MAR 16,2003			
		4338317*PED	SEP 16,2003			
		5256664	APR 28,2012			
		5256664*PED	OCT 28,2012			
020152 005	NEFAZODONE HYDROCHLORIDE; SERZONE	4338317	MAR 16,2003			
		4338317*PED	SEP 16,2003			
		5256664	APR 28,2012			
		5256664*PED	OCT 28,2012			
020152 006	NEFAZODONE HYDROCHLORIDE; SERZONE	4338317	MAR 16,2003			
		4338317*PED	SEP 16,2003			
		5256664	APR 28,2012			
		5256664*PED	OCT 28,2012			
020778 001	NELFINAVIR MESYLATE; VIRACEPT	5484926	OCT 07,2013		D-52	NOV 24,2002
		5952343	OCT 07,2013	U-257	D-52	NOV 24,2002
		6162812	OCT 07,2013	U-248	D-52	NOV 24,2002
020779 001	NELFINAVIR MESYLATE; VIRACEPT	5484926	OCT 07,2013		D-52	NOV 24,2002
		5952343	OCT 07,2013	U-257	D-52	NOV 24,2002
		6162812	OCT 07,2013	U-248	D-52	NOV 24,2002
020920 001	NESIRITIDE; NATRECOR	5114923	MAY 19,2009		NCE	AUG 10,2006
		5674710	OCT 07,2014		NCE	AUG 10,2006
020636 001	NEVIRAPINE; VIRAMUNE	5366972	NOV 22,2011	U-167		
		5366972*PED	MAY 22,2012			
020933 001	NEVIRAPINE; VIRAMUNE	5366972	NOV 22,2011			
		5366972*PED	MAY 22,2012			
020381 001	NIACIN; NIASPAN	6080428	MAY 27,2017	U-331		
		6129930	SEP 20,2013	U-354		
		6406715	OCT 31,2017	U-450		
020381 002	NIACIN; NIASPAN	6080428	MAY 27,2017	U-331		
		6129930	SEP 20,2013	U-354		
		6406715	OCT 31,2017	U-450		
020381 003	NIACIN; NIASPAN	6080428	MAY 27,2017	U-331		
		6129930	SEP 20,2013	U-354		
		6406715	OCT 31,2017	U-450		
020381 004	NIACIN; NIASPAN	6080428	MAY 27,2017	U-331		
		6129930	SEP 20,2013	U-354		
		6406715	OCT 31,2017	U-450		
020381 005	NIACIN; NIASPAN TITRATION STARTER PACK	6080428	MAY 27,2017	U-331		
		6129930	SEP 20,2013	U-354		
		6406715	OCT 31,2017	U-450		
019734 001	NICARDIPINE HYDROCHLORIDE; CARDENE	4880823	NOV 14,2006			
		5164405	NOV 17,2009			
020005 001	NICARDIPINE HYDROCHLORIDE; CARDENE SR	5198226	MAR 30,2010			
020005 002	NICARDIPINE HYDROCHLORIDE; CARDENE SR	5198226	MAR 30,2010			
020005 003	NICARDIPINE HYDROCHLORIDE; CARDENE SR	5198226	MAR 30,2010			
021330 001	NICOTINE POLACRILEX; COMMIT	5110605	AUG 21,2010		NDF	OCT 31,2005
021330 002	NICOTINE POLACRILEX; COMMIT	5110605	AUG 21,2010		NDF	OCT 31,2005
020076 004	NICOTINE; HABITROL	4597961	JAN 23,2005	U-56	D-71	NOV 12,2002
		5016652	MAY 21,2008		D-71	NOV 12,2002
		5834011	MAY 01,2007	U-355	D-71	NOV 12,2002
020076 005	NICOTINE; HABITROL	4597961	JAN 23,2005	U-56	D-71	NOV 12,2002
		5016652	MAY 21,2008		D-71	NOV 12,2002
		5834011	MAY 01,2007	U-355	D-71	NOV 12,2002
020076 006	NICOTINE; HABITROL	4597961	JAN 23,2005	U-56	D-71	NOV 12,2002
		5016652	MAY 21,2008		D-71	NOV 12,2002
		5834011	MAY 01,2007	U-355	D-71	NOV 12,2002
020165 004	NICOTINE; NICODERM CQ	5004610	JUN 14,2008			
		5342623	JUN 14,2008			
		5344656	JUN 14,2008			
		5364630	JUN 14,2008			
		5462745	JUN 14,2008			
		5508038	APR 16,2013			
		5633008	JUN 14,2008	U-389		
		6165497	JUN 14,2008	U-388		

PRESCRIPTION AND OTC PRODUCT
PATENT AND EXCLUSIVITY DATA
*PED and PED represent Pediatric Exclusivity (*continued*)

APPL/PROD NUMBER	INGREDIENT NAME; TRADE NAME	PATENT NUMBER	PATENT EXPIRES	USE CODE	EX-CLUS CODE	EXCLUS EXPIRES
020165 005	NICOTINE; NICODERM CQ	5004610	JUN 14,2008			
		5342623	JUN 14,2008			
		5344656	JUN 14,2008			
		5364630	JUN 14,2008			
		5462745	JUN 14,2008			
		5508038	APR 16,2013			
		5633008	JUN 14,2008	U-389		
		6165497	JUN 14,2008	U-388		
020165 006	NICOTINE; NICODERM CQ	5004610	JUN 14,2008			
		5342623	JUN 14,2008			
		5344656	JUN 14,2008			
		5364630	JUN 14,2008			
		5462745	JUN 14,2008			
		5508038	APR 16,2013			
		5633008	JUN 14,2008	U-389		
		6165497	JUN 14,2008	U-388		
020385 001	NICOTINE; NICOTROL	5656255	AUG 12,2014			
020536 001	NICOTINE; NICOTROL	5501236	JUN 08,2010			
		6098632	JUN 08,2010			
020714 001	NICOTINE; NICOTROL	4793366	DEC 27,2005			
		4800903	JAN 31,2006			
		4917120	APR 17,2007			
		5167242	JUN 08,2010			
		5400808	JUN 08,2010			
		5501236	JUN 08,2010			
		6098632	JUN 08,2010			
019983 003	NICOTINE; PROSTEP	4946853	AUG 07,2007	U-56		
019983 004	NICOTINE; PROSTEP	4946853	AUG 07,2007	U-56		
020198 001	NIFEDIPINE; ADALAT CC	4892741	JUN 08,2008			
		5264446	NOV 23,2010			
020198 002	NIFEDIPINE; ADALAT CC	4892741	JUN 08,2008			
		5264446	NOV 23,2010			
020198 003	NIFEDIPINE; ADALAT CC	4892741	JUN 08,2008			
		5264446	NOV 23,2010			
019684 001	NIFEDIPINE; PROCARDIA XL	4612008	SEP 16,2003			
		4765989	SEP 16,2003			
		4783337	SEP 16,2003			
		5264446	NOV 23,2010			
019684 002	NIFEDIPINE; PROCARDIA XL	4612008	SEP 16,2003			
		4765989	SEP 16,2003			
		4783337	SEP 16,2003			
		5264446	NOV 23,2010			
019684 003	NIFEDIPINE; PROCARDIA XL	4612008	SEP 16,2003			
		4765989	SEP 16,2003			
		4783337	SEP 16,2003			
		5264446	NOV 23,2010			
018869 001	NIMODIPINE; NIMOTOP	4406906	SEP 27,2002	U-22		
020356 001	NISOLDIPINE; SULAR	4703038	OCT 07,2005	U-3		
		4892741	JUN 08,2008			
020356 002	NISOLDIPINE; SULAR	4703038	OCT 07,2005	U-3		
		4892741	JUN 08,2008			
020356 003	NISOLDIPINE; SULAR	4703038	OCT 07,2005	U-3		
		4892741	JUN 08,2008			
020356 004	NISOLDIPINE; SULAR	4703038	OCT 07,2005	U-3		
		4892741	JUN 08,2008			
021498 001	NITAZOXANIDE; ALINIA				ODE	NOV 22,2009
021232 001	NITISINONE; ORFADIN				ODE	JAN 18,2009
021232 002	NITISINONE; ORFADIN				NCE	JAN 18,2007
021232 003	NITISINONE; ORFADIN				NCE	JAN 18,2007
020845 002	NITRIC OXIDE; INOMAX	5485827	JAN 23,2013	U-297	NCE	DEC 23,2004
		5873359	JAN 23,2013	U-297	NCE	DEC 23,2004
020845 003	NITRIC OXIDE; INOMAX	5485827	JAN 23,2013	U-297	ODE	DEC 23,2006
		5873359	JAN 23,2013	U-297	ODE	DEC 23,2006
020064 001	NITROFURANTOIN; MACROBID	4772473	JUN 16,2006			
		4798725	JUN 16,2006			
020145 001	NITROGLYCERIN; NITRO-DUR	5186938	FEB 16,2010			
020145 002	NITROGLYCERIN; NITRO-DUR	5186938	FEB 16,2010			
020145 003	NITROGLYCERIN; NITRO-DUR	5186938	FEB 16,2010			
020145 004	NITROGLYCERIN; NITRO-DUR	5186938	FEB 16,2010			
020145 005	NITROGLYCERIN; NITRO-DUR	5186938	FEB 16,2010			
020145 006	NITROGLYCERIN; NITRO-DUR	5186938	FEB 16,2010			

PRESCRIPTION AND OTC PRODUCT
PATENT AND EXCLUSIVITY DATA
PED and PED represent Pediatric Exclusivity (continued)

APPL/PROD NUMBER	INGREDIENT NAME; TRADE NAME	PATENT NUMBER	PATENT EXPIRES	USE CODE	EX-CLUS CODE	EXCLUS EXPIRES
018705 002	NITROGLYCERIN; NITROLINGUAL PUMPSPRAY	5186925	FEB 16,2010			
021134 001	NITROGLYCERIN; NITROSTAT	6500456	SEP 16,2018		NDF	MAY 01,2003
021134 002	NITROGLYCERIN; NITROSTAT	6500456	SEP 16,2018		NDF	MAY 01,2003
021134 003	NITROGLYCERIN; NITROSTAT	6500456	SEP 16,2018		NDF	MAY 01,2003
019757 001	NORFLOXACIN; CHIBROXIN	4551456	NOV 14,2003	U-57		
019384 002	NORFLOXACIN; NOROXIN	4639458	JAN 22,2005			
019667 001	OCTREOTIDE ACETATE; SANDOSTATIN	4395403	OCT 21,2002			
		5753618	MAY 19,2015			
019667 002	OCTREOTIDE ACETATE; SANDOSTATIN	4395403	OCT 21,2002			
		5753618	MAY 19,2015			
019667 003	OCTREOTIDE ACETATE; SANDOSTATIN	4395403	OCT 21,2002			
		5753618	MAY 19,2015			
019667 004	OCTREOTIDE ACETATE; SANDOSTATIN	4395403	OCT 21,2002			
		5753618	MAY 19,2015			
019667 005	OCTREOTIDE ACETATE; SANDOSTATIN	4395403	OCT 21,2002			
021008 001	OCTREOTIDE ACETATE; SANDOSTATIN LAR	4395403	NOV 21,2002	U-269	ODE	NOV 25,2005
		5538739	JUL 23,2013		ODE	NOV 25,2005
		5639480	JUN 17,2014		ODE	NOV 25,2005
		5688530	NOV 18,2014	U-268	ODE	NOV 25,2005
		5922338	JUL 13,2016		ODE	NOV 25,2005
		5922682	JUL 13,2016		ODE	NOV 25,2005
		6395292	JAN 30,2017		ODE	NOV 25,2005
021008 002	OCTREOTIDE ACETATE; SANDOSTATIN LAR	4395403	NOV 21,2002	U-269	ODE	NOV 25,2005
		5538739	JUL 23,2013		ODE	NOV 25,2005
		5639480	JUN 17,2014		ODE	NOV 25,2005
		5688530	NOV 18,2014	U-268	ODE	NOV 25,2005
		5922338	JUL 13,2016		ODE	NOV 25,2005
		5922682	JUL 13,2016		ODE	NOV 25,2005
021008 003	OCTREOTIDE ACETATE; SANDOSTATIN LAR	4395403	NOV 21,2002	U-269	ODE	NOV 25,2005
		5538739	JUL 23,2013		ODE	NOV 25,2005
		5639480	JUN 17,2014		ODE	NOV 25,2005
		5688530	NOV 18,2014	U-268	ODE	NOV 25,2005
		5922338	JUL 13,2016		ODE	NOV 25,2005
		5922682	JUL 13,2016		ODE	NOV 25,2005
019735 001	OFLOXACIN; FLOXIN	4382892	SEP 02,2003			
019735 002	OFLOXACIN; FLOXIN	4382892	SEP 02,2003			
019735 003	OFLOXACIN; FLOXIN	4382892	SEP 02,2003			
020799 001	OFLOXACIN; FLOXIN	5401741	MAR 27,2012	U-407		
019921 001	OFLOXACIN; OCUFLOX	4382892	SEP 02,2003		PED	NOV 22,2003
		4382892*PED	MAR 02,2004		PED	NOV 22,2003
		4551456	NOV 14,2003	U-80	PED	NOV 22,2003
		4551456*PED	MAY 14,2004	U-80	PED	NOV 22,2003
020592 001	OLANZAPINE; ZYPREXA	5229382	APR 23,2011	U-149	I-313	NOV 09,2003
020592 002	OLANZAPINE; ZYPREXA	5229382	APR 23,2011	U-149	I-313	NOV 09,2003
020592 003	OLANZAPINE; ZYPREXA	5229382	APR 23,2011	U-149	I-297	MAR 17,2003
020592 004	OLANZAPINE; ZYPREXA	5229382	APR 23,2011	U-149	I-313	NOV 09,2003
020592 005	OLANZAPINE; ZYPREXA	5229382	APR 23,2011	U-149	I-313	NOV 09,2003
020592 006	OLANZAPINE; ZYPREXA	5229382	APR 23,2011	U-149	I-313	NOV 09,2003
021086 001	OLANZAPINE; ZYPREXA ZYDIS	5229382	APR 23,2011	U-324		
021086 002	OLANZAPINE; ZYPREXA ZYDIS	5229382	APR 23,2011	U-324		
021086 003	OLANZAPINE; ZYPREXA ZYDIS	5229382	APR 23,2011	U-324		
021086 004	OLANZAPINE; ZYPREXA ZYDIS	5229382	APR 23,2011	U-324		
021286 001	OLMESARTAN MEDOXOMIL; BENICAR	5616599	APR 01,2014	U-500	NCE	APR 25,2007
021286 003	OLMESARTAN MEDOXOMIL; BENICAR	5616599	APR 01,2014	U-500	NCE	APR 25,2007
021286 004	OLMESARTAN MEDOXOMIL; BENICAR				NCE	APR 25,2007
020688 001	OLOPATADINE HYDROCHLORIDE; PATANOL	4871865	OCT 03,2006		I-301	MAR 20,2003
		4923892	MAY 08,2007	U-174	I-301	MAR 20,2003
		5116863	DEC 18,2010		I-301	MAR 20,2003
		5641805	JUN 06,2015	U-184	I-301	MAR 20,2003
019715 001	OLSALAZINE SODIUM; DIPENTUM	4559330	JUL 31,2004	U-58		
021229 001	OMEPRAZOLE MAGNESIUM; PRILOSEC	4738974	APR 19,2005		RTO	JUN 20,2006
		4786505	APR 20,2007		RTO	JUN 20,2006
		4786505*PED	OCT 20,2007		RTO	JUN 20,2006
		4853230	APR 20,2007		RTO	JUN 20,2006
		4853230*PED	OCT 20,2007		RTO	JUN 20,2006
		5690960	NOV 25,2014		RTO	JUN 20,2006
		5753265	JUN 07,2015		RTO	JUN 20,2006
		5817338	OCT 06,2015		RTO	JUN 20,2006
		5900424	MAY 04,2016		RTO	JUN 20,2006
		6403616	NOV 15,2019		RTO	JUN 20,2006
		6428810	NOV 03,2019		RTO	JUN 20,2006

PRESCRIPTION AND OTC PRODUCT
PATENT AND EXCLUSIVITY DATA
*PED and PED represent Pediatric Exclusivity (*continued*)

APPL/PROD NUMBER	INGREDIENT NAME; TRADE NAME	PATENT NUMBER	PATENT EXPIRES	USE CODE	EX-CLUS CODE	EXCLUS EXPIRES
019810 001	OMEPRAZOLE; PRILOSEC	4508905*PED	OCT 02,2002		PED	JAN 12,2006
		4786505	APR 20,2007	U-108	PED	JAN 12,2006
		4786505*PED	OCT 20,2007	U-108	PED	JAN 12,2006
		4853230	APR 20,2007	U-108	PED	JAN 12,2006
		4853230*PED	OCT 20,2007	U-108	PED	JAN 12,2006
		6147103	OCT 09,2018		PED	JAN 12,2006
		6147103*PED	APR 09,2019		PED	JAN 12,2006
		6150380	NOV 10,2018		PED	JAN 12,2006
		6150380*PED	MAY 10,2019		PED	JAN 12,2006
		6166213	OCT 09,2018		PED	JAN 12,2006
		6166213*PED	APR 09,2019		PED	JAN 12,2006
		6191148	OCT 09,2018		PED	JAN 12,2006
		6191148*PED	APR 09,2019		PED	JAN 12,2006
019810 002	OMEPRAZOLE; PRILOSEC	4508905*PED	OCT 02,2002		M-19	JUL 12,2005
		4786505	APR 20,2007	U-108	M-19	JUL 12,2005
		4786505*PED	OCT 20,2007	U-108	M-19	JUL 12,2005
		4853230	APR 20,2007	U-108	M-19	JUL 12,2005
		4853230*PED	OCT 20,2007	U-108	M-19	JUL 12,2005
		6147103	OCT 09,2018		M-19	JUL 12,2005
		6147103*PED	APR 09,2019		M-19	JUL 12,2005
		6150380	NOV 10,2018		M-19	JUL 12,2005
		6150380*PED	MAY 10,2019		M-19	JUL 12,2005
		6166213	OCT 09,2018		M-19	JUL 12,2005
		6166213*PED	APR 09,2019		M-19	JUL 12,2005
		6191148	OCT 09,2018		M-19	JUL 12,2005
		6191148*PED	APR 09,2019		M-19	JUL 12,2005
019810 003	OMEPRAZOLE; PRILOSEC	4508905*PED	OCT 02,2002		M-19	JUL 12,2005
		4786505	APR 20,2007	U-108	M-19	JUL 12,2005
		4786505*PED	OCT 20,2007	U-108	M-19	JUL 12,2005
		4853230	APR 20,2007	U-108	M-19	JUL 12,2005
		4853230*PED	OCT 20,2007	U-108	M-19	JUL 12,2005
		6147103	OCT 09,2018		M-19	JUL 12,2005
		6147103*PED	APR 09,2019		M-19	JUL 12,2005
		6150380	NOV 10,2018		M-19	JUL 12,2005
		6150380*PED	MAY 10,2019		M-19	JUL 12,2005
		6166213	OCT 09,2018		M-19	JUL 12,2005
		6166213*PED	APR 09,2019		M-19	JUL 12,2005
		6191148	OCT 09,2018		M-19	JUL 12,2005
		6191148*PED	APR 09,2019		M-19	JUL 12,2005
020007 001	ONDANSETRON HYDROCHLORIDE; ZOFRAN	4695578	JAN 25,2005			
		4753789	JUN 24,2006	U-44		
		5578628	FEB 16,2005	U-44		
020103 001	ONDANSETRON HYDROCHLORIDE; ZOFRAN	4695578	JAN 25,2005		I-269	AUG 27,2002
		4753789	JUN 24,2006	U-44	I-269	AUG 27,2002
		5344658	SEP 06,2011		I-269	AUG 27,2002
		5578628	FEB 16,2005	U-44	I-269	AUG 27,2002
020103 002	ONDANSETRON HYDROCHLORIDE; ZOFRAN	4695578	JAN 25,2005		I-269	AUG 27,2002
		4753789	JUN 24,2006	U-44	I-269	AUG 27,2002
		5344658	SEP 06,2011		I-269	AUG 27,2002
		5578628	FEB 16,2005	U-44	I-269	AUG 27,2002
020103 003	ONDANSETRON HYDROCHLORIDE; ZOFRAN	4695578	JAN 25,2005		I-269	AUG 27,2002
		4753789	JUN 24,2006	U-44	I-269	AUG 27,2002
		5344658	SEP 06,2011		I-269	AUG 27,2002
		5578628	FEB 16,2005	U-44	I-269	AUG 27,2002
020605 001	ONDANSETRON HYDROCHLORIDE; ZOFRAN	4695578	JAN 25,2005	U-183		
		4753789	JUN 24,2006	U-44		
		5578628	FEB 16,2005	U-44		
020403 001	ONDANSETRON HYDROCHLORIDE; ZOFRAN IN PLASTIC CONTAINER	4695578	JAN 25,2005			
		4753789	JUN 24,2006	U-44		
		5578628	FEB 16,2005	U-44		
020007 003	ONDANSETRON HYDROCHLORIDE; ZOFRAN PRESERVATIVE FREE	4695578	JAN 25,2005			
		4753789	JUN 24,2006	U-44		
		5578628	FEB 16,2005	U-44		
020781 001	ONDANSETRON; ZOFRAN ODT	4695578	JAN 25,2005	U-330		
		4753789	JUN 24,2006	U-330		
		5578628	FEB 16,2005	U-330		
		5955488	NOV 14,2015			
		6063802	NOV 14,2015			
020781 002	ONDANSETRON; ZOFRAN ODT	4695578	JAN 25,2005	U-330		

PRESCRIPTION AND OTC PRODUCT
PATENT AND EXCLUSIVITY DATA
*PED and PED represent Pediatric Exclusivity (*continued*)

APPL/PROD NUMBER	INGREDIENT NAME; TRADE NAME	PATENT NUMBER	PATENT EXPIRES	USE CODE	EX-CLUS CODE	EXCLUS EXPIRES
		4753789	JUN 24,2006	U-330		
		5578628	FEB 16,2005	U-330		
		5955488	NOV 14,2015			
		6063802	NOV 14,2015			
020766 001	ORLISTAT; XENICAL	4598089	JUN 18,2009		NCE	APR 23,2004
		6004996	JAN 06,2018		NCE	APR 23,2004
021087 001	OSELTAMIVIR PHOSPHATE; TAMIFLU	5763483	DEC 27,2016		I-317	NOV 17,2003
		5866601	FEB 02,2016		I-317	NOV 17,2003
		5952375	FEB 02,2016		I-317	NOV 17,2003
021246 001	OSELTAMIVIR PHOSPHATE; TAMIFLU	5763483	DEC 27,2016	U-376	NDF	DEC 14,2003
		5866601	FEB 02,2016		NDF	DEC 14,2003
		5952375	FEB 02,2016		NDF	DEC 14,2003
021492 001	OXALIPLATIN; ELOXATIN	5290961	JAN 12,2013		NCE	AUG 09,2007
		5338874	APR 07,2013		NCE	AUG 09,2007
		5420319	APR 07,2013		NCE	AUG 09,2007
021492 002	OXALIPLATIN; ELOXATIN	5290961	JAN 12,2013		NCE	AUG 09,2007
		5338874	APR 07,2013		NCE	AUG 09,2007
		5420319	APR 07,2013		NCE	AUG 09,2007
020776 001	OXAPROZIN POTASSIUM; DAYPRO ALTA	6030643	MAY 16,2017	U-497	NE	OCT 17,2005
015539 002	OXAZEPAM; SERAX	4620974	NOV 04,2003			
015539 004	OXAZEPAM; SERAX	4620974	NOV 04,2003			
015539 006	OXAZEPAM; SERAX	4620974	NOV 04,2003			
021014 001	OXCARBAZEPINE; TRILEPTAL				NCE	JAN 14,2005
021014 002	OXCARBAZEPINE; TRILEPTAL				NCE	JAN 14,2005
021014 003	OXCARBAZEPINE; TRILEPTAL				NCE	JAN 14,2005
021285 001	OXCARBAZEPINE; TRILEPTAL				NCE	JAN 14,2005
017577 001	OXYBUTYNIN CHLORIDE; DITROPAN				PED	OCT 15,2006
					NPP	APR 15,2006
018211 001	OXYBUTYNIN CHLORIDE; DITROPAN				PED	OCT 15,2006
					NPP	APR 15,2006
020897 001	OXYBUTYNIN CHLORIDE; DITROPAN XL	4519801	JUL 12,2002		PED	OCT 15,2006
		4519801*PED	JAN 12,2003		PED	OCT 15,2006
		4612008	SEP 16,2003		PED	OCT 15,2006
		4612008*PED	MAR 16,2004		PED	OCT 15,2006
		4783337	SEP 16,2003		PED	OCT 15,2006
		4783337*PED	MAR 16,2004		PED	OCT 15,2006
		5082668	SEP 16,2003		PED	OCT 15,2006
		5082668*PED	MAR 16,2004		PED	OCT 15,2006
		5674895	MAY 22,2015		PED	OCT 15,2006
		5674895*PED	NOV 22,2015		PED	OCT 15,2006
		5840754	MAY 22,2015		PED	OCT 15,2006
		5840754*PED	NOV 22,2015		PED	OCT 15,2006
		5912268	MAY 22,2015		PED	OCT 15,2006
		5912268*PED	NOV 22,2015		PED	OCT 15,2006
		6124355	MAY 22,2015	U-378	PED	OCT 15,2006
		6124355*PED	NOV 22,2015	U-378	PED	OCT 15,2006
		6262115	MAY 22,2015	U-393	PED	OCT 15,2006
		6262115*PED	NOV 22,2015	U-393	PED	OCT 15,2006
					NPP	APR 15,2006
020897 002	OXYBUTYNIN CHLORIDE; DITROPAN XL	4519801	JUL 12,2002		NPP	APR 15,2006
		4519801*PED	JAN 12,2003		NPP	APR 15,2006
		4612008	SEP 16,2003		NPP	APR 15,2006
		4612008*PED	MAR 16,2004		NPP	APR 15,2006
		4783337	SEP 16,2003		NPP	APR 15,2006
		4783337*PED	MAR 16,2004		NPP	APR 15,2006
		5082668	SEP 16,2003		NPP	APR 15,2006
		5082668*PED	MAR 16,2004		NPP	APR 15,2006
		5674895	MAY 22,2015		NPP	APR 15,2006
		5674895*PED	NOV 22,2015		NPP	APR 15,2006
		5840754	MAY 22,2015		NPP	APR 15,2006
		5840754*PED	NOV 22,2015		NPP	APR 15,2006
		5912268	MAY 22,2015		NPP	APR 15,2006
		5912268*PED	NOV 22,2015		NPP	APR 15,2006
		6124355	MAY 22,2015	U-378	NPP	APR 15,2006
		6124355*PED	NOV 22,2015	U-378	NPP	APR 15,2006
		6262115	MAY 22,2015	U-393	NPP	APR 15,2006
		6262115*PED	NOV 22,2015	U-393	NPP	APR 15,2006
					PED	OCT 15,2006
020897 003	OXYBUTYNIN CHLORIDE; DITROPAN XL	4519801	JUL 12,2002		NPP	APR 15,2006
		4519801*PED	JAN 12,2003		NPP	APR 15,2006
		4612008	SEP 16,2003		NPP	APR 15,2006

PRESCRIPTION AND OTC PRODUCT
PATENT AND EXCLUSIVITY DATA
*PED and PED represent Pediatric Exclusivity (*continued*)

APPL/PROD NUMBER	INGREDIENT NAME; TRADE NAME	PATENT NUMBER	PATENT EXPIRES	USE CODE	EX-CLUS CODE	EXCLUS EXPIRES
		4612008*PED	MAR 16,2004		NPP	APR 15,2006
		4783337	SEP 16,2003		NPP	APR 15,2006
		4783337*PED	MAR 16,2004		NPP	APR 15,2006
		5082668	SEP 16,2003		NPP	APR 15,2006
		5082668*PED	MAR 16,2004		NPP	APR 15,2006
		5674895	MAY 22,2015		NPP	APR 15,2006
		5674895*PED	NOV 22,2015		NPP	APR 15,2006
		5840754	MAY 22,2015		NPP	APR 15,2006
		5840754*PED	NOV 22,2015		NPP	APR 15,2006
		5912268	MAY 22,2015		NPP	APR 15,2006
		5912268*PED	NOV 22,2015		NPP	APR 15,2006
		6124355	MAY 22,2015	U-378	NPP	APR 15,2006
		6124355*PED	NOV 22,2015	U-378	NPP	APR 15,2006
		6262115	MAY 22,2015	U-393	NPP	APR 15,2006
		6262115*PED	NOV 22,2015	U-393	NPP	APR 15,2006
					PED	OCT 15,2006
021351 002	OXYBUTYNIN; OXYTROL				NDF	FEB 26,2006
020553 001	OXYCODONE HYDROCHLORIDE; OXYCONTIN	4861598	AUG 29,2006			
		4970075	AUG 29,2006			
		5266331	OCT 26,2007			
		5508042	APR 16,2013	U-443		
		5549912	OCT 26,2007			
		5656295	OCT 26,2007	U-443		
020553 002	OXYCODONE HYDROCHLORIDE; OXYCONTIN	4861598	AUG 29,2006			
		4970075	AUG 29,2006			
		5266331	OCT 26,2007			
		5508042	APR 16,2013	U-443		
		5549912	OCT 26,2007			
		5656295	OCT 26,2007	U-443		
020553 003	OXYCODONE HYDROCHLORIDE; OXYCONTIN	4861598	AUG 29,2006			
		4970075	AUG 29,2006			
		5266331	OCT 26,2007			
		5508042	APR 16,2013	U-443		
		5549912	OCT 26,2007			
		5656295	OCT 26,2007	U-443		
020553 004	OXYCODONE HYDROCHLORIDE; OXYCONTIN	4861598	AUG 29,2006			
		4970075	AUG 29,2006			
		5266331	OCT 26,2007			
		5508042	APR 16,2013	U-443		
		5549912	OCT 26,2007			
		5656295	OCT 26,2007	U-443		
020553 005	OXYCODONE HYDROCHLORIDE; OXYCONTIN	4861598	AUG 29,2006			
		4970075	AUG 29,2006			
		5266331	OCT 26,2007			
		5508042	APR 16,2013	U-443		
		5549912	OCT 26,2007			
		5656295	OCT 26,2007	U-443		
020262 001	PACLITAXEL; TAXOL				ODE	AUG 04,2004
020036 001	PAMIDRONATE DISODIUM; AREDIA	4711880	JUL 29,2005		D-68	AUG 20,2004
020036 003	PAMIDRONATE DISODIUM; AREDIA	4711880	JUL 29,2005		D-68	AUG 20,2004
020036 004	PAMIDRONATE DISODIUM; AREDIA	4711880	JUL 29,2005		D-68	AUG 20,2004
020987 001	PANTOPRAZOLE SODIUM; PROTONIX	4758579	JUL 19,2005		I-356	APR 19,2005
		5997903	DEC 07,2016		I-356	APR 19,2005
020987 002	PANTOPRAZOLE SODIUM; PROTONIX	4758579	JUL 19,2005		I-356	APR 19,2005
		5997903	DEC 07,2016		I-356	APR 19,2005
020988 001	PANTOPRAZOLE SODIUM; PROTONIX IV	4758579	JUL 19,2005		I-337	OCT 19,2004
020819 001	PARICALCITOL; ZEMPLAR	5246925	APR 17,2012	U-314	NCE	APR 17,2003
		5587497	DEC 24,2013		NCE	APR 17,2003
		6136799	APR 08,2018		NCE	APR 17,2003
020031 001	PAROXETINE HYDROCHLORIDE; PAXIL	4721723	DEC 29,2006	U-12	PED	OCT 13,2004
		4721723*PED	JUN 29,2007	U-12	PED	OCT 13,2004
		5789449	JAN 06,2009	U-285	PED	OCT 13,2004
		5789449*PED	JUL 06,2009	U-285	PED	OCT 13,2004
		5872132	MAY 19,2015		PED	OCT 13,2004
		5872132*PED	NOV 19,2015		PED	OCT 13,2004
		5900423	MAY 19,2015		PED	OCT 13,2004
		5900423*PED	NOV 19,2015		PED	OCT 13,2004
		6063927	APR 23,2019		PED	OCT 13,2004
		6063927*PED	OCT 23,2019		PED	OCT 13,2004
		6080759	MAY 19,2015		PED	OCT 13,2004
		6080759*PED	NOV 19,2015		PED	OCT 13,2004

PRESCRIPTION AND OTC PRODUCT
PATENT AND EXCLUSIVITY DATA
*PED and PED represent Pediatric Exclusivity (continued)

APPL/PROD NUMBER	INGREDIENT NAME; TRADE NAME	PATENT NUMBER	PATENT EXPIRES	USE CODE	EX- CLUS CODE	EXCLUS EXPIRES
		6113944	DEC 14,2014		PED	OCT 13,2004
		6113944*PED	JUN 14,2015		PED	OCT 13,2004
		6121291	MAR 17,2017	U-286	PED	OCT 13,2004
		6121291	MAR 17,2017	U-431	PED	OCT 13,2004
		6121291*PED	SEP 17,2017	U-286	PED	OCT 13,2004
		6121291*PED	SEP 17,2017	U-431	PED	OCT 13,2004
		6133289	MAY 19,2015	U-358	PED	OCT 13,2004
		6133289*PED	NOV 19,2015	U-358	PED	OCT 13,2004
		6172233	JAN 15,2018		PED	OCT 13,2004
		6172233*PED	JUL 15,2018		PED	OCT 13,2004
020031 002	PAROXETINE HYDROCHLORIDE; PAXIL	4721723	DEC 29,2006	U-12	I-326	APR 13,2004
		4721723*PED	JUN 29,2007	U-12	I-326	APR 13,2004
		5789449	JAN 06,2009	U-285	I-326	APR 13,2004
		5789449*PED	JUL 06,2009	U-285	I-326	APR 13,2004
		5872132	MAY 19,2015		I-326	APR 13,2004
		5872132*PED	NOV 19,2015		I-326	APR 13,2004
		5900423	MAY 19,2015		I-326	APR 13,2004
		5900423*PED	NOV 19,2015		I-326	APR 13,2004
		6063927	APR 23,2019		I-326	APR 13,2004
		6063927*PED	OCT 23,2019		I-326	APR 13,2004
		6080759	MAY 19,2015		I-326	APR 13,2004
		6080759*PED	NOV 19,2015		I-326	APR 13,2004
		6113944	DEC 14,2014		I-326	APR 13,2004
		6113944*PED	JUN 14,2015		I-326	APR 13,2004
		6121291	MAR 17,2017	U-286	I-326	APR 13,2004
		6121291	MAR 17,2017	U-431	I-326	APR 13,2004
		6121291*PED	SEP 17,2017	U-286	I-326	APR 13,2004
		6121291*PED	SEP 17,2017	U-431	I-326	APR 13,2004
		6133289	MAY 19,2015	U-358	I-326	APR 13,2004
		6133289*PED	NOV 19,2015	U-358	I-326	APR 13,2004
		6172233	JAN 15,2018		I-326	APR 13,2004
		6172233*PED	JUL 15,2018		I-326	APR 13,2004
020031 003	PAROXETINE HYDROCHLORIDE; PAXIL	4721723	DEC 29,2006		I-326	APR 13,2004
		4721723*PED	JUN 29,2007	U-12	I-326	APR 13,2004
		5789449	JAN 06,2009	U-285	I-326	APR 13,2004
		5789449*PED	JUL 06,2009	U-285	I-326	APR 13,2004
		5872132	MAY 19,2015		I-326	APR 13,2004
		5872132*PED	NOV 19,2015		I-326	APR 13,2004
		5900423	MAY 19,2015		I-326	APR 13,2004
		5900423*PED	NOV 19,2015		I-326	APR 13,2004
		6063927	APR 23,2019		I-326	APR 13,2004
		6063927*PED	OCT 23,2019		I-326	APR 13,2004
		6080759	MAY 19,2015		I-326	APR 13,2004
		6080759*PED	NOV 19,2015		I-326	APR 13,2004
		6113944	DEC 14,2014		I-326	APR 13,2004
		6113944*PED	JUN 14,2015		I-326	APR 13,2004
		6121291	MAR 17,2017	U-286	I-326	APR 13,2004
		6121291	MAR 17,2017	U-431	I-326	APR 13,2004
		6121291*PED	SEP 17,2017	U-286	I-326	APR 13,2004
		6121291*PED	SEP 17,2017	U-431	I-326	APR 13,2004
		6133289	MAY 19,2015	U-358	I-326	APR 13,2004
		6133289*PED	NOV 19,2015	U-358	I-326	APR 13,2004
		6172233	JAN 15,2018		I-326	APR 13,2004
		6172233*PED	JUL 15,2018		I-326	APR 13,2004
020031 004	PAROXETINE HYDROCHLORIDE; PAXIL	4721723	DEC 29,2006		I-345	DEC 14,2004
		4721723*PED	JUN 29,2007	U-12	I-345	DEC 14,2004
		5789449	JAN 06,2009	U-285	I-345	DEC 14,2004
		5789449*PED	JUL 06,2009	U-285	I-345	DEC 14,2004
		5872132	MAY 19,2015		I-345	DEC 14,2004
		5872132*PED	NOV 19,2015		I-345	DEC 14,2004
		5900423	MAY 19,2015		I-345	DEC 14,2004
		5900423*PED	NOV 19,2015		I-345	DEC 14,2004
		6063927	APR 23,2019		I-345	DEC 14,2004
		6063927*PED	OCT 23,2019		I-345	DEC 14,2004
		6080759	MAY 19,2015		I-345	DEC 14,2004
		6080759*PED	NOV 19,2015		I-345	DEC 14,2004
		6113944	DEC 14,2014		I-345	DEC 14,2004
		6113944*PED	JUN 14,2015		I-345	DEC 14,2004
		6121291	MAR 17,2017	U-286	I-345	DEC 14,2004
		6121291	MAR 17,2017	U-431	I-345	DEC 14,2004
		6121291*PED	SEP 17,2017	U-286	I-345	DEC 14,2004

PRESCRIPTION AND OTC PRODUCT
PATENT AND EXCLUSIVITY DATA
*PED and PED represent Pediatric Exclusivity (*continued*)

APPL/PROD NUMBER	INGREDIENT NAME; TRADE NAME	PATENT NUMBER	PATENT EXPIRES	USE CODE	EX-CLUS CODE	EXCLUS EXPIRES
		6121291*PED	SEP 17,2017	U-431	I-345	DEC 14,2004
		6133289	MAY 15,2015	U-358	I-345	DEC 14,2004
		6133289*PED	NOV 19,2015	U-358	I-345	DEC 14,2004
		6172233	JAN 15,2018		I-345	DEC 14,2004
		6172233*PED	JUL 15,2018		I-345	DEC 14,2004
020031 005	PAROXETINE HYDROCHLORIDE; PAXIL	4721723	DEC 29,2006	U-12	I-345	DEC 14,2004
		4721723*PED	JUN 29,2007	U-12	I-345	DEC 14,2004
		5789449	JAN 06,2009	U-285	I-345	DEC 14,2004
		5789449*PED	JUL 06,2009	U-285	I-345	DEC 14,2004
		5872132	MAY 19,2015		I-345	DEC 14,2004
		5872132*PED	NOV 19,2015		I-345	DEC 14,2004
		5900423	MAY 19,2015		I-345	DEC 14,2004
		5900423*PED	NOV 19,2015		I-345	DEC 14,2004
		6063927	APR 23,2019		I-345	DEC 14,2004
		6063927*PED	OCT 23,2019		I-345	DEC 14,2004
		6080759	MAY 19,2015		I-345	DEC 14,2004
		6080759*PED	NOV 19,2015		I-345	DEC 14,2004
		6113944	DEC 14,2014		I-345	DEC 14,2004
		6113944*PED	JUN 14,2015		I-345	DEC 14,2004
		6121291	MAR 17,2017	U-286	I-345	DEC 14,2004
		6121291	MAR 17,2017	U-431	I-345	DEC 14,2004
		6121291*PED	SEP 17,2017	U-286	I-345	DEC 14,2004
		6121291*PED	SEP 17,2017	U-431	I-345	DEC 14,2004
		6133289	MAY 15,2015	U-358	I-345	DEC 14,2004
		6133289*PED	NOV 19,2015	U-358	I-345	DEC 14,2004
		6172233	JAN 15,2018		I-345	DEC 14,2004
		6172233*PED	JUL 15,2018		I-345	DEC 14,2004
020710 001	PAROXETINE HYDROCHLORIDE; PAXIL	4721723	DEC 29,2006		I-326	APR 13,2004
		4721723*PED	JUN 29,2007		I-326	APR 13,2004
		5789449	JAN 06,2009	U-285	I-326	APR 13,2004
		5789449*PED	JUL 06,2009	U-285	I-326	APR 13,2004
		5811436	SEP 22,2015		I-326	APR 13,2004
		5811436*PED	MAR 22,2016		I-326	APR 13,2004
		5872132	MAY 19,2015		I-326	APR 13,2004
		5872132*PED	NOV 19,2015		I-326	APR 13,2004
		5900423	MAY 19,2015		I-326	APR 13,2004
		5900423*PED	NOV 19,2015		I-326	APR 13,2004
		6063927	APR 23,2019		I-326	APR 13,2004
		6063927*PED	OCT 23,2019		I-326	APR 13,2004
		6080759	MAY 19,2015		I-326	APR 13,2004
		6080759*PED	NOV 19,2015		I-326	APR 13,2004
		6121291	MAR 17,2017	U-286	I-326	APR 13,2004
		6121291	MAR 17,2017	U-431	I-326	APR 13,2004
		6121291*PED	SEP 17,2017	U-286	I-326	APR 13,2004
		6121291*PED	SEP 17,2017	U-431	I-326	APR 13,2004
		6133289	MAY 19,2015	U-358	I-326	APR 13,2004
		6133289*PED	NOV 19,2015	U-358	I-326	APR 13,2004
		6172233	JAN 15,2018		I-326	APR 13,2004
		6172233*PED	JUL 15,2018		I-326	APR 13,2004
020885 001	PAROXETINE HYDROCHLORIDE; PAXIL	4721723	DEC 29,2006	U-12	PED	OCT 13,2004
		4721723*PED	JUN 29,2007	U-12	PED	OCT 13,2004
		5789449	JAN 06,2009	U-285	PED	OCT 13,2004
		5789449*PED	JUL 06,2009	U-285	PED	OCT 13,2004
		5872132	MAY 19,2015		PED	OCT 13,2004
		5872132*PED	NOV 19,2015		PED	OCT 13,2004
		5900423	MAY 19,2015		PED	OCT 13,2004
		5900423*PED	NOV 19,2015		PED	OCT 13,2004
		6063927	APR 23,2019		PED	OCT 13,2004
		6063927*PED	OCT 23,2019		PED	OCT 13,2004
		6080759	MAY 19,2015		PED	OCT 13,2004
		6080759*PED	NOV 19,2015		PED	OCT 13,2004
		6121291	MAR 17,2017	U-286	PED	OCT 13,2004
		6121291	MAR 17,2017	U-431	PED	OCT 13,2004
		6121291*PED	SEP 17,2017	U-286	PED	OCT 13,2004
		6121291*PED	SEP 17,2017	U-431	PED	OCT 13,2004
		6133289	MAY 19,2015	U-358	PED	OCT 13,2004
		6133289*PED	NOV 19,2015	U-358	PED	OCT 13,2004
		6172233	JAN 15,2018		PED	OCT 13,2004
		6172233*PED	JUL 15,2018		PED	OCT 13,2004
020885 002	PAROXETINE HYDROCHLORIDE; PAXIL	4721723	DEC 29,2006	U-12	I-326	APR 13,2004
		4721723*PED	JUN 29,2007	U-12	I-326	APR 13,2004

PRESCRIPTION AND OTC PRODUCT
PATENT AND EXCLUSIVITY DATA
*PED and PED represent Pediatric Exclusivity (*continued*)

APPL/PROD NUMBER	INGREDIENT NAME; TRADE NAME	PATENT NUMBER	PATENT EXPIRES	USE CODE	EX-CLUS CODE	EXCLUS EXPIRES
		5789449	JAN 06,2009	U-285	I-326	APR 13,2004
		5789449*PED	JUL 06,2009	U-285	I-326	APR 13,2004
		5872132	MAY 19,2015		I-326	APR 13,2004
		5872132*PED	NOV 19,2015		I-326	APR 13,2004
		5900423	MAY 19,2015		I-326	APR 13,2004
		5900423*PED	NOV 19,2015		I-326	APR 13,2004
		6063927	APR 23,2019		I-326	APR 13,2004
		6063927*PED	OCT 23,2019		I-326	APR 13,2004
		6080759	MAY 19,2015		I-326	APR 13,2004
		6080759*PED	NOV 19,2015		I-326	APR 13,2004
		6121291	MAR 17,2017	U-286	I-326	APR 13,2004
		6121291	MAR 17,2017	U-431	I-326	APR 13,2004
		6121291*PED	SEP 17,2017	U-286	I-326	APR 13,2004
		6121291*PED	SEP 17,2017	U-431	I-326	APR 13,2004
		6133289	MAY 19,2015	U-358	I-326	APR 13,2004
		6133289*PED	NOV 19,2015	U-358	I-326	APR 13,2004
		6172233	JAN 15,2018		I-326	APR 13,2004
		6172233*PED	JUL 15,2018		I-326	APR 13,2004
020885 003	PAROXETINE HYDROCHLORIDE; PAXIL	4721723	DEC 29,2006	U-12	PED	NOV 17,2002
		4721723*PED	JUN 29,2007	U-12	PED	NOV 17,2002
		5789449	JAN 06,2009	U-285	PED	NOV 17,2002
		5789449*PED	JUL 06,2009	U-285	PED	NOV 17,2002
		5872132	MAY 19,2015		PED	NOV 17,2002
		5872132*PED	NOV 19,2015		PED	NOV 17,2002
		5900423	MAY 19,2015		PED	NOV 17,2002
		5900423*PED	NOV 19,2015		PED	NOV 17,2002
		6063927	APR 23,2019		PED	NOV 17,2002
		6063927*PED	OCT 23,2019		PED	NOV 17,2002
		6080759	MAY 19,2015		PED	NOV 17,2002
		6080759*PED	NOV 19,2015		PED	NOV 17,2002
		6121291	MAR 17,2017	U-286	PED	NOV 17,2002
		6121291	MAR 17,2017	U-431	PED	NOV 17,2002
		6121291*PED	SEP 17,2017	U-286	PED	NOV 17,2002
		6121291*PED	SEP 17,2017	U-431	PED	NOV 17,2002
		6133289	MAY 19,2015	U-358	PED	NOV 17,2002
		6133289*PED	NOV 19,2015	U-358	PED	NOV 17,2002
		6172233	JAN 15,2018		PED	NOV 17,2002
		6172233*PED	JUL 15,2018		PED	NOV 17,2002
020885 004	PAROXETINE HYDROCHLORIDE; PAXIL	4721723	DEC 29,2006	U-12	I-345	DEC 14,2004
		4721723*PED	JUN 29,2007	U-12	I-345	DEC 14,2004
		5789449	JAN 06,2009	U-285	I-345	DEC 14,2004
		5789449*PED	JUL 06,2009	U-285	I-345	DEC 14,2004
		5872132	MAY 19,2015		I-345	DEC 14,2004
		5872132*PED	NOV 19,2015		I-345	DEC 14,2004
		5900423	MAY 19,2015		I-345	DEC 14,2004
		5900423*PED	NOV 19,2015		I-345	DEC 14,2004
		6062927	APR 23,2019		I-345	DEC 14,2004
		6063927*PED	OCT 23,2019		I-345	DEC 14,2004
		6080759	MAY 19,2015		I-345	DEC 14,2004
		6080759*PED	NOV 19,2015		I-345	DEC 14,2004
		6121291	MAR 17,2017	U-286	I-345	DEC 14,2004
		6121291	MAR 17,2017	U-431	I-345	DEC 14,2004
		6121291*PED	SEP 17,2017	U-286	I-345	DEC 14,2004
		6121291*PED	SEP 17,2017	U-431	I-345	DEC 14,2004
		6133289	MAY 19,2015	U-358	I-345	DEC 14,2004
		6133289*PED	NOV 19,2015	U-358	I-345	DEC 14,2004
		6172233	JAN 15,2018		I-345	DEC 14,2004
		6172233*PED	JUL 15,2018		I-345	DEC 14,2004
020936 001	PAROXETINE HYDROCHLORIDE; PAXIL CR	4721723	DEC 29,2006		PED	AUG 12,2005
		4721723*PED	JUN 29,2007		PED	AUG 12,2005
		4839177	JUN 13,2006		PED	AUG 12,2005
		4839177*PED	DEC 13,2006		PED	AUG 12,2005
		5422123	JUN 06,2012		PED	AUG 12,2005
		5422123*PED	DEC 06,2012		PED	AUG 12,2005
		5789449	JAN 06,2009	U-286	PED	AUG 12,2005
		5789449*PED	JUL 06,2009	U-286	PED	AUG 12,2005
		5872132	MAY 19,2015		PED	AUG 12,2005
		5872132*PED	NOV 19,2015		PED	AUG 12,2005
		5900423	MAY 19,2015		PED	AUG 12,2005
		5900423*PED	NOV 19,2015		PED	AUG 12,2005
		6063927	APR 23,2019		PED	AUG 12,2005

PRESCRIPTION AND OTC PRODUCT
PATENT AND EXCLUSIVITY DATA
*PED and PED represent Pediatric Exclusivity (*continued*)

APPL/PROD NUMBER	INGREDIENT NAME; TRADE NAME	PATENT NUMBER	PATENT EXPIRES	USE CODE	EX-CLUS CODE	EXCLUS EXPIRES
		6063927*PED	OCT 23,2019		PED	AUG 12,2005
		6080759	MAY 19,2015		PED	AUG 12,2005
		6080759*PED	NOV 19,2015		PED	AUG 12,2005
		6121291	MAR 17,2017	U-286	PED	AUG 12,2005
		6121291*PED	SEP 17,2017	U-286	PED	AUG 12,2005
		6133289	MAY 19,2015	U-286	PED	AUG 12,2005
		6133289*PED	NOV 19,2015	U-286	PED	AUG 12,2005
		6172233	JAN 15,2018		PED	AUG 12,2005
		6172233*PED	JUL 15,2018		PED	AUG 12,2005
		6548084	JUL 19,2016		PED	AUG 12,2005
		6548084*PED	JAN 19,2017		PED	AUG 12,2005
020936 002	PAROXETINE HYDROCHLORIDE; PAXIL CR	4721723	DEC 29,2006		PED	AUG 12,2005
		4721723*PED	JUN 29,2007		PED	AUG 12,2005
		4839177	JUN 13,2006		PED	AUG 12,2005
		4839177*PED	DEC 13,2006		PED	AUG 12,2005
		5422123	JUN 06,2012		PED	AUG 12,2005
		5422123*PED	DEC 06,2012		PED	AUG 12,2005
		5789449	JAN 06,2009	U-286	PED	AUG 12,2005
		5789449*PED	JUL 06,2009	U-286	PED	AUG 12,2005
		5872132	MAY 19,2015		PED	AUG 12,2005
		5872132*PED	NOV 19,2015		PED	AUG 12,2005
		5900423	MAY 19,2015		PED	AUG 12,2005
		5900423*PED	NOV 19,2015		PED	AUG 12,2005
		6063927	APR 23,2019		PED	AUG 12,2005
		6063927*PED	OCT 23,2019		PED	AUG 12,2005
		6080759	MAY 19,2015		PED	AUG 12,2005
		6080759*PED	NOV 19,2015		PED	AUG 12,2005
		6121291	MAR 17,2017	U-286	PED	AUG 12,2005
		6121291*PED	SEP 17,2017	U-286	PED	AUG 12,2005
		6133289	MAY 19,2015	U-286	PED	AUG 12,2005
		6133289*PED	NOV 19,2015	U-286	PED	AUG 12,2005
		6172233	JAN 15,2018		PED	AUG 12,2005
		6172233*PED	JUL 15,2018		PED	AUG 12,2005
		6548084	JUL 19,2016		PED	AUG 12,2005
		6548084*PED	JAN 19,2017		PED	AUG 12,2005
020936 003	PAROXETINE HYDROCHLORIDE; PAXIL CR	4721723	DEC 29,2006		PED	AUG 12,2005
		4721723*PED	JUN 29,2007		PED	AUG 12,2005
		4839177	JUN 13,2006		PED	AUG 12,2005
		4839177*PED	DEC 13,2006		PED	AUG 12,2005
		5422123	JUN 06,2012		PED	AUG 12,2005
		5422123*PED	DEC 06,2012		PED	AUG 12,2005
		5789449	JAN 06,2009	U-286	PED	AUG 12,2005
		5789449*PED	JUL 06,2009	U-286	PED	AUG 12,2005
		5872132	MAY 19,2015		PED	AUG 12,2005
		5872132*PED	NOV 19,2015		PED	AUG 12,2005
		5900423	MAY 19,2015		PED	AUG 12,2005
		5900423*PED	NOV 19,2015		PED	AUG 12,2005
		6063927	APR 23,2019		PED	AUG 12,2005
		6063927*PED	OCT 23,2019		PED	AUG 12,2005
		6080759	MAY 19,2015		PED	AUG 12,2005
		6080759*PED	NOV 19,2015		PED	AUG 12,2005
		6121291	MAR 17,2017	U-286	PED	AUG 12,2005
		6121291*PED	SEP 17,2017	U-286	PED	AUG 12,2005
		6133289	MAY 19,2015	U-286	PED	AUG 12,2005
		6133289*PED	NOV 19,2015	U-286	PED	AUG 12,2005
		6172233	JAN 15,2018		PED	AUG 12,2005
		6172233*PED	JUL 15,2018		PED	AUG 12,2005
		6548084	JUL 19,2016		PED	AUG 12,2005
		6548084*PED	JAN 19,2017		PED	AUG 12,2005
021106 001	PEGVISOMANT; SOMAVERT	5350836	SEP 27,2011	U-507	NCE	MAR 25,2008
		5681809	SEP 27,2011	U-507	NCE	MAR 25,2008
		5849535	SEP 21,2015		NCE	MAR 25,2008
		5958879	SEP 27,2011	U-507	NCE	MAR 25,2008
		6057292	SEP 21,2015	U-507	NCE	MAR 25,2008
021106 002	PEGVISOMANT; SOMAVERT	5350836	SEP 27,2011	U-507	NCE	MAR 25,2008
		5681809	SEP 27,2011	U-507	NCE	MAR 25,2008
		5849535	SEP 21,2015		NCE	MAR 25,2008
		5958879	SEP 27,2011	U-507	NCE	MAR 25,2008
		6057292	SEP 21,2015	U-507	NCE	MAR 25,2008
021106 003	PEGVISOMANT; SOMAVERT	5350836	SEP 27,2011	U-507	NCE	MAR 25,2008
		5681809	SEP 27,2011	U-507	NCE	MAR 25,2008

PRESCRIPTION AND OTC PRODUCT
PATENT AND EXCLUSIVITY DATA
PED and PED represent Pediatric Exclusivity (continued)

APPL/PROD NUMBER	INGREDIENT NAME; TRADE NAME	PATENT NUMBER	PATENT EXPIRES	USE CODE	EX-CLUS CODE	EXCLUS EXPIRES
		5849535	SEP 21,2015		NCE	MAR 25,2008
		5958879	SEP 27,2011	U-507	NCE	MAR 25,2008
		6057292	SEP 21,2015	U-507	NCE	MAR 25,2008
021079 001	PEMIROLAST POTASSIUM; ALAMAST	5034230	DEC 23,2008	U-184	NCE	SEP 24,2004
		5034230*PED	JUN 23,2009	U-184	NCE	SEP 24,2004
020629 001	PENCICLOVIR SODIUM; DENAVIR	5075445	SEP 24,2010			
		6469015	OCT 22,2019	U-501		
		6573378	SEP 24,2010			
		6579981	JUN 17,2020	U-501		
020193 001	PENTOSAN POLYSULFATE SODIUM; ELMIRON	5180715	JAN 19,2010	U-159	ODE	SEP 26,2003
021084 001	PERFLUOROPOLYMETHYLISOPROPYL ETHER; SKIN EXPOSURE REDUCTION PASTE AGAINST CHEMICAL WARFARE AGENTS	5607979	MAY 30,2015		NCE	FEB 17,2005
021064 001	PERFLUTREN; DEFINITY	5527521	APR 05,2011		NCE	JUL 31,2006
		5547656	APR 05,2011		NCE	JUL 31,2006
		5769080	JUL 20,2010		NCE	JUL 31,2006
076061 001	PERGOLIDE MESYLATE; PERGOLIDE MESYLATE				PC	MAY 31,2003
076061 002	PERGOLIDE MESYLATE; PERGOLIDE MESYLATE				PC	MAY 31,2003
076061 003	PERGOLIDE MESYLATE; PERGOLIDE MESYLATE				PC	MAY 31,2003
019385 001	PERGOLIDE MESYLATE; PERMAX	4797405	OCT 26,2007			
		5114948	OCT 19,2009			
019385 002	PERGOLIDE MESYLATE; PERMAX	4797405	OCT 26,2007			
		5114948	OCT 19,2009			
019385 003	PERGOLIDE MESYLATE; PERMAX	4797405	OCT 26,2007			
		5114948	OCT 19,2009			
020184 001	PERINDOPRIL ERBUMINE; ACEON	4508729	AUG 21,2006			
020184 002	PERINDOPRIL ERBUMINE; ACEON	4508729	AUG 21,2006			
020184 003	PERINDOPRIL ERBUMINE; ACEON	4508729	AUG 21,2006			
020237 001	PILOCARPINE HYDROCHLORIDE; SALAGEN				ODE	FEB 11,2005
021302 001	PIMECROLIMUS; ELIDEL	5912238	JUN 15,2016		PED	JUN 13,2007
		5912238*PED	DEC 15,2016		PED	JUN 13,2007
		6352998	OCT 26,2015		PED	JUN 13,2007
		6352998*PED	APR 26,2016		PED	JUN 13,2007
		6423722	JUN 26,2018		PED	JUN 13,2007
		6423722*PED	DEC 26,2018		PED	JUN 13,2007
021073 001	PIOGLITAZONE HYDROCHLORIDE; ACTOS	4687777	JAN 17,2011		NCE	JUL 15,2004
		5965584	JUN 19,2016	U-417	NCE	JUL 15,2004
		6150383	JUN 19,2016	U-418	NCE	JUL 15,2004
		6150384	JUN 19,2016	U-419	NCE	JUL 15,2004
		6166042	JUN 19,2016	U-414	NCE	JUL 15,2004
		6166043	JUN 19,2016	U-415	NCE	JUL 15,2004
		6172090	JUN 19,2016	U-416	NCE	JUL 15,2004
		6211205	JUN 19,2016	U-410	NCE	JUL 15,2004
		6271243	JUN 19,2016	U-411	NCE	JUL 15,2004
		6303640	AUG 09,2016	U-425	NCE	JUL 15,2004
		6329404	JUN 19,2016	U-430	NCE	JUL 15,2004
021073 002	PIOGLITAZONE HYDROCHLORIDE; ACTOS	4687777	JAN 17,2011		NCE	JUL 15,2004
		5965584	JUN 19,2016	U-417	NCE	JUL 15,2004
		6150383	JUN 19,2016	U-418	NCE	JUL 15,2004
		6150384	JUN 19,2016	U-419	NCE	JUL 15,2004
		6166042	JUN 19,2016	U-414	NCE	JUL 15,2004
		6166043	JUN 19,2016	U-415	NCE	JUL 15,2004
		6172090	JUN 19,2016	U-416	NCE	JUL 15,2004
		6211205	JUN 19,2016	U-410	NCE	JUL 15,2004
		6271243	JUN 19,2016	U-411	NCE	JUL 15,2004
		6303640	AUG 09,2016	U-425	NCE	JUL 15,2004
		6329404	JUN 19,2016	U-430	NCE	JUL 15,2004
021073 003	PIOGLITAZONE HYDROCHLORIDE; ACTOS	4687777	JAN 17,2011		NCE	JUL 15,2004
		5965584	JUN 19,2016	U-417	NCE	JUL 15,2004
		6150383	JUN 19,2016	U-418	NCE	JUL 15,2004
		6150384	JUN 19,2016		NCE	JUL 15,2004
		6166042	JUN 19,2016	U-414	NCE	JUL 15,2004
		6166043	JUN 19,2016	U-415	NCE	JUL 15,2004
		6172090	JUN 19,2016	U-416	NCE	JUL 15,2004
		6211205	JUN 19,2016	U-410	NCE	JUL 15,2004
		6271243	JUN 19,2016	U-411	NCE	JUL 15,2004
		6303640	AUG 09,2016	U-425	NCE	JUL 15,2004
		6329404	JUN 19,2016	U-430	NCE	JUL 15,2004
020014 001	PIRBUTEROL ACETATE; MAXAIR	4664107	MAY 12,2004			
020529 001	PODOFILOX; CONDYLOX	4680399	JUL 14,2004			
		5057616	OCT 15,2008			

PRESCRIPTION AND OTC PRODUCT
PATENT AND EXCLUSIVITY DATA
*PED and PED represent Pediatric Exclusivity (*continued*)

APPL/PROD NUMBER	INGREDIENT NAME; TRADE NAME	PATENT NUMBER	PATENT EXPIRES	USE CODE	EX- CLUS CODE	EXCLUS EXPIRES
020698 001	POLYETHYLENE GLYCOL 3350; MIRALAX	5710183	JUL 14,2015	U-265		
		6048901	APR 20,2019	U-343		
020744 001	PORACTANT ALFA; CUROSURF				NCE	NOV 18,2004
020451 001	PORFIMER SODIUM; PHOTOFRIN	4649151	MAR 10,2004		ODE	DEC 27,2002
		4866168	MAR 10,2004		ODE	DEC 27,2002
		4932934	JUN 12,2007	U-128	ODE	DEC 27,2002
		5028621	MAR 10,2004		ODE	DEC 27,2002
		5145863	DEC 15,2009	U-129	ODE	DEC 27,2002
		5438071	AUG 01,2012		ODE	DEC 27,2002
019439 002	POTASSIUM CHLORIDE; K-DUR 10	4863743	SEP 05,2006	U-99		
019439 001	POTASSIUM CHLORIDE; K-DUR 20	4863743	SEP 05,2006	U-99		
074726 003	POTASSIUM CHLORIDE; KLOR-CON M15				PC	DEC 24,2003
020667 001	PRAMIPEXOLE DIHYDROCHLORIDE; MIRAPEX	4843086	NOV 23,2007	U-231	NCE	JUL 01,2002
		4886812	MAR 25,2011		NCE	JUL 01,2002
020667 002	PRAMIPEXOLE DIHYDROCHLORIDE; MIRAPEX	4843086	NOV 23,2007	U-231	NCE	JUL 01,2002
		4886812	MAR 25,2011		NCE	JUL 01,2002
020667 003	PRAMIPEXOLE DIHYDROCHLORIDE; MIRAPEX	4843086	NOV 23,2007	U-231	NCE	JUL 01,2002
		4886812	MAR 25,2011		NCE	JUL 01,2002
020667 004	PRAMIPEXOLE DIHYDROCHLORIDE; MIRAPEX	4843086	NOV 23,2007	U-231	NCE	JUL 01,2002
		4886812	MAR 25,2011		NCE	JUL 01,2002
020667 005	PRAMIPEXOLE DIHYDROCHLORIDE; MIRAPEX	4843086	NOV 23,2007	U-231	NCE	JUL 01,2002
		4886812	MAR 25,2011		NCE	JUL 01,2002
020667 006	PRAMIPEXOLE DIHYDROCHLORIDE; MIRAPEX	4843086	NOV 23,2007	U-231		
		4886812	MAR 25,2011			
019898 002	PRAVASTATIN SODIUM; PRAVACHOL	4346227	OCT 20,2005		I-304	JAN 18,2003
		4346227*PED	APR 20,2006		I-304	JAN 18,2003
		5030447	JUL 09,2008		I-304	JAN 18,2003
		5030447*PED	JAN 09,2009		I-304	JAN 18,2003
		5180589	JUL 09,2008		I-304	JAN 18,2003
		5180589*PED	JAN 09,2009		I-304	JAN 18,2003
		5622985	APR 22,2014	U-335	I-304	JAN 18,2003
		5622985*PED	OCT 22,2014	U-335	I-304	JAN 18,2003
019898 003	PRAVASTATIN SODIUM; PRAVACHOL	4346227	OCT 20,2005		I-304	JAN 18,2003
		4346227*PED	APR 20,2006		I-304	JAN 18,2003
		5030447	JUL 09,2008		I-304	JAN 18,2003
		5030447*PED	JAN 09,2009		I-304	JAN 18,2003
		5180589	JUL 09,2008		I-304	JAN 18,2003
		5180589*PED	JAN 09,2009		I-304	JAN 18,2003
		5622985	APR 22,2014	U-335	I-304	JAN 18,2003
		5622985*PED	OCT 22,2014	U-335	I-304	JAN 18,2003
019898 004	PRAVASTATIN SODIUM; PRAVACHOL	4346227	OCT 20,2005		I-281	JUN 09,2003
		4346227*PED	APR 20,2006		I-281	JUN 09,2003
		5030447	JUL 09,2008		I-281	JUN 09,2003
		5030447*PED	JAN 09,2009		I-281	JUN 09,2003
		5180589	JUL 09,2008		I-281	JUN 09,2003
		5180589*PED	JAN 09,2009		I-281	JUN 09,2003
		5622985	APR 22,2014	U-335	I-281	JUN 09,2003
		5622985*PED	OCT 22,2014	U-335	I-281	JUN 09,2003
019898 008	PRAVASTATIN SODIUM; PRAVACHOL	4346227	OCT 20,2005		NS	DEC 18,2004
		4346227*PED	APR 20,2006		NS	DEC 18,2004
		5030447	JUL 09,2008		NS	DEC 18,2004
		5030447*PED	JAN 09,2009		NS	DEC 18,2004
		5180589	JUL 09,2008		NS	DEC 18,2004
		5180589*PED	JAN 09,2009		NS	DEC 18,2004
		5622985	APR 22,2014	U-335	NS	DEC 18,2004
		5622985*PED	OCT 22,2014	U-335	NS	DEC 18,2004
019775 001	PRAZOSIN HYDROCHLORIDE; MINIPRESS XL	4612008	SEP 16,2003			
		4765989	SEP 16,2003			
		4783337	SEP 16,2003			
		5082668	SEP 16,2003			
019775 002	PRAZOSIN HYDROCHLORIDE; MINIPRESS XL	4612008	SEP 16,2003			
		4765989	SEP 16,2003			
		4783337	SEP 16,2003			
		5082668	SEP 16,2003			
019157 001	PREDNISOLONE SODIUM PHOSPHATE; PEDIAPRED	4448774	DEC 22,2002			
020545 001	PROCAINAMIDE HYDROCHLORIDE; PROCANBID	5656296	AUG 12,2014			
020545 002	PROCAINAMIDE HYDROCHLORIDE; PROCANBID	5656296	AUG 12,2014			
020701 001	PROGESTERONE; CRINONE	4615697	OCT 07,2003	U-208		
		5543150	SEP 15,2013	U-209		
020701 002	PROGESTERONE; CRINONE	4615697	OCT 07,2003	U-208		

PRESCRIPTION AND OTC PRODUCT
PATENT AND EXCLUSIVITY DATA
*PED and PED represent Pediatric Exclusivity (*continued*)

APPL/PROD NUMBER	INGREDIENT NAME; TRADE NAME	PATENT NUMBER	PATENT EXPIRES	USE CODE	EX-CLUS CODE	EXCLUS EXPIRES
		5543150	SEP 15,2013	U-209		
019627 002	PROPOFOL; DIPRIVAN	5714520	MAR 22,2015		PED	AUG 20,2004
		5714520*PED	SEP 22,2015		PED	AUG 20,2004
		5731355	MAR 22,2015	U-217	PED	AUG 20,2004
		5731355*PED	SEP 22,2015	U-217	PED	AUG 20,2004
		5731356	MAR 22,2015	U-218	PED	AUG 20,2004
		5731356*PED	SEP 22,2015	U-218	PED	AUG 20,2004
		5908869	MAR 22,2015	U-270	PED	AUG 20,2004
		5908869*PED	SEP 22,2015	U-270	PED	AUG 20,2004
019536 001	PROPRANOLOL HYDROCHLORIDE; INDERAL	4600708	JUL 19,2005			
021438 001	PROPRANOLOL HYDROCHLORIDE; INNOPRAN XL	6500454	DEC 31,2022		NP	MAR 12,2006
021438 002	PROPRANOLOL HYDROCHLORIDE; INNOPRAN XL	6500454	DEC 31,2022		NP	MAR 12,2006
020021 002	PSEUDOEPHEDRINE HYDROCHLORIDE; EFIDAC 24 PSEUDOEPHEDRINE HCL	4576604	MAR 18,2003			
		4801461	MAR 14,2006			
020639 001	QUETIAPINE FUMARATE; SEROQUEL	4879288	SEP 26,2011		NCE	SEP 26,2002
020639 002	QUETIAPINE FUMARATE; SEROQUEL	4879288	SEP 26,2011		NCE	SEP 26,2002
020639 003	QUETIAPINE FUMARATE; SEROQUEL	4879288	SEP 26,2011		NCE	SEP 26,2002
020639 004	QUETIAPINE FUMARATE; SEROQUEL	4879288	SEP 26,2011		NCE	SEP 26,2002
020639 005	QUETIAPINE FUMARATE; SEROQUEL	4879288	SEP 26,2011		NCE	SEP 26,2002
019885 001	QUINAPRIL HYDROCHLORIDE; ACCUPRIL	4344949	OCT 03,2002	U-3		
		4344949*PED	APR 03,2003	U-3		
		4743450	FEB 24,2007			
		4743450*PED	AUG 24,2007			
		5684016	NOV 04,2014	U-210		
		5684016*PED	MAY 04,2015	U-210		
		5747504	APR 10,2005	U-210		
		5747504*PED	OCT 10,2005	U-210		
019885 002	QUINAPRIL HYDROCHLORIDE; ACCUPRIL	4344949	OCT 03,2002	U-3		
		4344949*PED	APR 03,2003	U-3		
		4743450	FEB 24,2007			
		4743450*PED	AUG 24,2007			
		5684016	NOV 04,2014	U-210		
		5684016*PED	MAY 04,2015	U-210		
		5747504	APR 10,2005	U-210		
		5747504*PED	OCT 10,2005	U-210		
019885 003	QUINAPRIL HYDROCHLORIDE; ACCUPRIL	4344949	OCT 03,2002	U-3		
		4344949*PED	APR 03,2003	U-3		
		4743450	FEB 24,2007			
		4743450*PED	AUG 24,2007			
		5684016	NOV 04,2014	U-210		
		5684016*PED	MAY 04,2015	U-210		
		5747504	APR 10,2005	U-210		
		5747504*PED	OCT 10,2005	U-210		
019885 004	QUINAPRIL HYDROCHLORIDE; ACCUPRIL	4344949	OCT 03,2002	U-3		
		4344949*PED	APR 03,2003	U-3		
		4743450	FEB 24,2007			
		4743450*PED	AUG 24,2007			
		5684016	NOV 04,2014	U-210		
		5684016*PED	MAY 04,2015	U-210		
		5747504	APR 10,2005	U-210		
		5747504*PED	OCT 10,2005	U-210		
020973 001	RABEPRAZOLE SODIUM; ACIPHEX	5035899	APR 04,2009	U-385	I-346	FEB 12,2005
		5045552	SEP 03,2008	U-385	I-346	FEB 12,2005
020973 002	RABEPRAZOLE SODIUM; ACIPHEX	5035899	APR 04,2009	U-385	I-346	FEB 12,2005
		5045552	SEP 03,2008	U-385	I-346	FEB 12,2005
020815 001	RALOXIFENE HYDROCHLORIDE; EVISTA	4418068	APR 03,2003		NCE	DEC 09,2002
		5393763	JUL 28,2012	U-114	NCE	DEC 09,2002
		5457117	JUL 28,2012	U-114	NCE	DEC 09,2002
		5478847	MAR 02,2014	U-114	NCE	DEC 09,2002
		5811120	MAR 02,2014		NCE	DEC 09,2002
		5972383	MAR 02,2014	U-287	NCE	DEC 09,2002
		6458811	MAR 10,2017		NCE	DEC 09,2002
019901 001	RAMIPRIL; ALTACE	4587258	JAN 27,2005		I-310	OCT 04,2003
		5061722	OCT 19,2008		I-310	OCT 04,2003
		5403856	APR 04,2012	U-71	I-310	OCT 04,2003
019901 002	RAMIPRIL; ALTACE	4587258	JAN 27,2005		I-310	OCT 04,2003
		5061722	OCT 19,2008		I-310	OCT 04,2003
		5403856	APR 01,2012	U-71	I-310	OCT 04,2003
019901 003	RAMIPRIL; ALTACE	4587258	JAN 27,2005		I-310	OCT 04,2003
		5061722	OCT 19,2008		I-310	OCT 04,2003

PRESCRIPTION AND OTC PRODUCT
PATENT AND EXCLUSIVITY DATA
*PED and PED represent Pediatric Exclusivity (continued)

APPL/PROD NUMBER	INGREDIENT NAME; TRADE NAME	PATENT NUMBER	PATENT EXPIRES	USE CODE	EX-CLUS CODE	EXCLUS EXPIRES
019901 004	RAMIPRIL; ALTACE	5403856	APR 01,2012	U-71	I-310	OCT 04,2003
		4587258	JAN 27,2005		I-310	OCT 04,2003
		5061722	OCT 19,2008		I-310	OCT 04,2003
		5403856	APR 04,2012	U-71	I-310	OCT 04,2003
020559 001	RANITIDINE BISMUTH CITRATE; TRITEC	5008256	JUL 17,2009			
		5256684	OCT 26,2010	U-199		
		5403830	APR 04,2012	U-200		
		5407688	APR 04,2012	U-201		
		5456925	OCT 10,2012			
		5601848	FEB 11,2014	U-202		
		5629297	MAY 13,2014	U-186		
019090 001	RANITIDINE HYDROCHLORIDE; ZANTAC	4521431*PED	DEC 04,2002		PED	APR 29,2003
		4585790	MAY 11,2004		PED	APR 29,2003
		4585790*PED	NOV 11,2004		PED	APR 29,2003
019675 001	RANITIDINE HYDROCHLORIDE; ZANTAC	4521431*PED	DEC 04,2002		PED	APR 29,2003
		4585790	MAY 11,2004		PED	APR 29,2003
		4585790*PED	NOV 11,2004		PED	APR 29,2003
		5068249	NOV 26,2008		PED	APR 29,2003
		5068249*PED	MAY 26,2009		PED	APR 29,2003
018703 001	RANITIDINE HYDROCHLORIDE; ZANTAC 150	4521431*PED	DEC 04,2002		PED	APR 29,2003
		4880636	MAY 13,2008		PED	APR 29,2003
		4880636*PED	NOV 13,2008		PED	APR 29,2003
020095 001	RANITIDINE HYDROCHLORIDE; ZANTAC 150	4521431*PED	DEC 04,2002		PED	APR 29,2003
		5028432	FEB 22,2010		PED	APR 29,2003
		5028432*PED	AUG 22,2010		PED	APR 29,2003
020251 001	RANITIDINE HYDROCHLORIDE; ZANTAC 150	4521431*PED	DEC 04,2002		PED	APR 29,2003
		5102665	JUN 23,2009		PED	APR 29,2003
		5102665*PED	DEC 23,2009		PED	APR 29,2003
020251 002	RANITIDINE HYDROCHLORIDE; ZANTAC 150	4521431*PED	DEC 04,2002		PED	APR 29,2003
		5102665	JUN 23,2009		PED	APR 29,2003
		5102665*PED	DEC 23,2009		PED	APR 29,2003
018703 002	RANITIDINE HYDROCHLORIDE; ZANTAC 300	4521431*PED	DEC 04,2002		D-53	OCT 29,2002
		4880636	MAY 13,2008		D-53	OCT 29,2002
		4880636*PED	NOV 13,2008		D-53	OCT 29,2002
020095 002	RANITIDINE HYDROCHLORIDE; ZANTAC 300	4521431*PED	DEC 04,2002		PED	APR 29,2003
		5028432	FEB 22,2010		PED	APR 29,2003
		5028432*PED	AUG 22,2010		PED	APR 29,2003
020520 001	RANITIDINE HYDROCHLORIDE; ZANTAC 75	4521431*PED	DEC 04,2002			
		4880636	MAY 13,2008			
		4880636*PED	NOV 13,2008			
019593 001	RANITIDINE HYDROCHLORIDE; ZANTAC IN PLASTIC CONTAINER	4521431*PED	DEC 04,2002		PED	APR 29,2003
		4585790	MAY 11,2004		PED	APR 29,2003
019593 002	RANITIDINE HYDROCHLORIDE; ZANTAC IN PLASTIC CONTAINER	4521431*PED	DEC 04,2002		PED	APR 29,2003
		4585790	MAY 11,2004		PED	APR 29,2003
		4585790*PED	NOV 11,2004		PED	APR 29,2003
020984 001	RAPACURONIUM BROMIDE; RAPLON	5418226	APR 14,2013		NCE	AUG 18,2004
020984 002	RAPACURONIUM BROMIDE; RAPLON	5418226	APR 14,2013		NCE	AUG 18,2004
020630 001	REMIFENTANIL HYDROCHLORIDE; ULTIVA	5019583	FEB 15,2009		PED	APR 15,2003
		5019583*PED	AUG 15,2009		PED	APR 15,2003
		5466700	AUG 30,2013	U-156	PED	APR 15,2003
		5466700*PED	MAR 01,2014	U-156	PED	APR 15,2003
020630 002	REMIFENTANIL HYDROCHLORIDE; ULTIVA	5019583	FEB 15,2009		NPP	OCT 15,2002
		5019583*PED	AUG 15,2009		NPP	OCT 15,2002
		5466700	AUG 30,2013	U-156	NPP	OCT 15,2002
		5466700*PED	MAR 01,2014		NPP	OCT 15,2002
020630 003	REMIFENTANIL HYDROCHLORIDE; ULTIVA	5019583	FEB 15,2009		NPP	OCT 15,2002
		5019583*PED	AUG 15,2009		NPP	OCT 15,2002
		5466700	AUG 30,2013	U-156	NPP	OCT 15,2002
		5466700*PED	MAR 01,2014	U-156	NPP	OCT 15,2002
020741 001	REPAGLINIDE; PRANDIN	5312924	SEP 05,2006		I-367	OCT 21,2005
		6143769	SEP 05,2006		I-367	OCT 21,2005
		RE37035	MAR 14,2009		I-367	OCT 21,2005
020741 002	REPAGLINIDE; PRANDIN	5312924	SEP 05,2006	U-214	I-367	OCT 21,2005
		6143769	SEP 05,2006		I-367	OCT 21,2005
		RE37035	MAR 14,2009		I-367	OCT 21,2005
020741 003	REPAGLINIDE; PRANDIN	5312924	SEP 05,2006	U-214	I-367	OCT 21,2005
		6143769	SEP 05,2006		I-367	OCT 21,2005
		RE37035	MAR 14,2009		I-367	OCT 21,2005
021511 001	RIBAVIRIN; COPEGUS				NP	DEC 03,2005

PRESCRIPTION AND OTC PRODUCT
PATENT AND EXCLUSIVITY DATA
*PED and PED represent Pediatric Exclusivity (*continued*)

APPL/PROD NUMBER	INGREDIENT NAME; TRADE NAME	PATENT NUMBER	PATENT EXPIRES	USE CODE	EX-CLUS CODE	EXCLUS EXPIRES
020903 001	RIBAVIRIN; REBETOL	5767097	JAN 23,2016	U-235	M-26	MAR 06,2005
		5767097*PED	JUL 23,2016	U-235	M-26	MAR 06,2005
		5914128	DEC 22,2017		M-26	MAR 06,2005
		5914128*PED	JUN 22,2018		M-26	MAR 06,2005
		6051252	DEC 22,2017		M-26	MAR 06,2005
		6051252*PED	JUN 22,2018		M-26	MAR 06,2005
		6063772	JAN 23,2016	U-375	M-26	MAR 06,2005
		6063772*PED	JUL 23,2016	U-375	M-26	MAR 06,2005
		6172046	SEP 21,2017	U-377	M-26	MAR 06,2005
		6172046*PED	MAR 21,2018	U-377	M-26	MAR 06,2005
		6177074	NOV 01,2016	U-454	M-26	MAR 06,2005
		6177074*PED	MAY 01,2017	U-454	M-26	MAR 06,2005
		6335032	DEC 22,2017		M-26	MAR 06,2005
		6335032*PED	JUN 22,2018		M-26	MAR 06,2005
		6337090	DEC 22,2017		M-26	MAR 06,2005
		6337090*PED	JUN 22,2018		M-26	MAR 06,2005
		6461605	NOV 01,2016	U-478	M-26	MAR 06,2005
		6461605*PED	MAY 01,2017	U-478	M-26	MAR 06,2005
		6472373	SEP 21,2017	U-479	M-26	MAR 06,2005
		6472373*PED	MAR 21,2018	U-479	M-26	MAR 06,2005
		6524570	NOV 01,2016	U-499	M-26	MAR 06,2005
		6524570*PED	MAY 01,2017	U-499	M-26	MAR 06,2005
020903 002	RIBAVIRIN; REBETOL	5767097	JAN 23,2016	U-235	M-26	MAR 06,2005
		5767097*PED	JUL 23,2016	U-235	M-26	MAR 06,2005
		5914128	DEC 22,2017		M-26	MAR 06,2005
		5914128*PED	JUN 22,2018		M-26	MAR 06,2005
		6051252	DEC 22,2017		M-26	MAR 06,2005
		6051252*PED	JUN 22,2018		M-26	MAR 06,2005
		6063772	JAN 23,2016	U-375	M-26	MAR 06,2005
		6063772*PED	JUL 23,2016	U-375	M-26	MAR 06,2005
		6172046	SEP 21,2017	U-377	M-26	MAR 06,2005
		6172046*PED	MAR 21,2018	U-377	M-26	MAR 06,2005
		6335032	DEC 22,2017		M-26	MAR 06,2005
		6335032*PED	JUN 22,2018		M-26	MAR 06,2005
		6337090	DEC 22,2017		M-26	MAR 06,2005
		6337090*PED	JUN 22,2018		M-26	MAR 06,2005
018859 001	RIBAVIRIN; VIRAZOLE	6150337	NOV 21,2017	U-400		
021024 001	RIFAPENTINE; PRIFTIN				ODE	JUN 22,2005
020599 001	RILUZOLE; RILUTEK	5527814	JUN 18,2013		ODE	DEC 12,2002
020474 001	RIMEXOLONE; VEXOL	4686214	JUL 22,2008	U-100		
020835 001	RISEDRONATE SODIUM; ACTONEL	5583122	DEC 10,2013	U-222	I-290	APR 14,2003
		6096342	MAR 12,2017		I-290	APR 14,2003
		6165513	JUN 10,2018		I-290	APR 14,2003
020835 002	RISEDRONATE SODIUM; ACTONEL	5583122	DEC 10,2013	U-222	I-292	APR 14,2003
		6096342	MAR 12,2017		I-292	APR 14,2003
		6165513	JUN 10,2018		I-292	APR 14,2003
020835 003	RISEDRONATE SODIUM; ACTONEL	5994329	JUL 17,2018	U-353	NCE	MAR 27,2003
		6015801	JUL 17,2018	U-353	NCE	MAR 27,2003
020272 001	RISPERIDONE; RISPERDAL	4804663	DEC 29,2007	U-90	M-15	MAR 03,2005
020272 002	RISPERIDONE; RISPERDAL	4804663	DEC 29,2007	U-90	M-15	MAR 03,2005
020272 003	RISPERIDONE; RISPERDAL	4804663	DEC 29,2007	U-90	M-15	MAR 03,2005
020272 004	RISPERIDONE; RISPERDAL	4804663	DEC 29,2007	U-90	M-15	MAR 03,2005
020272 005	RISPERIDONE; RISPERDAL	4804663	DEC 29,2007	U-90	M-15	MAR 03,2005
020272 007	RISPERIDONE; RISPERDAL	4804663	DEC 29,2007	U-90	M-15	MAR 03,2005
020272 008	RISPERIDONE; RISPERDAL	4804663	DEC 29,2007	U-90	M-15	MAR 03,2005
020588 001	RISPERIDONE; RISPERDAL	4804663	DEC 29,2007	U-90	M-15	MAR 03,2005
		5453425	JUL 11,2014		M-15	MAR 03,2005
		5616587	JUL 11,2014		M-15	MAR 03,2005
021444 001	RISPERIDONE; RISPERDAL	4804663	DEC 29,2007	U-516	M-15	MAR 03,2005
		5648093	JUL 15,2004		M-15	MAR 03,2005
		6224905	JUN 10,2017	U-516	M-15	MAR 03,2005
021444 002	RISPERIDONE; RISPERDAL	4804663	DEC 29,2007	U-516	M-15	MAR 03,2005
		5648093	JUL 15,2004		M-15	MAR 03,2005
		6224905	JUN 10,2017	U-516	M-15	MAR 03,2005
021444 003	RISPERIDONE; RISPERDAL	4804663	DEC 29,2007	U-516	M-15	MAR 03,2005
		5648093	JUL 15,2004		M-15	MAR 03,2005
		6224905	JUN 10,2017	U-516	M-15	MAR 03,2005
		6224905	JUN 10,2017	U-516	M-15	MAR 03,2005
020659 001	RITONAVIR; NORVIR	5484801	JAN 28,2014			
		5541206	JUL 30,2013	U-140		
		5635523	JUN 03,2014	U-190		

PRESCRIPTION AND OTC PRODUCT
PATENT AND EXCLUSIVITY DATA
*PED and PED represent Pediatric Exclusivity (*continued*)

APPL/PROD NUMBER	INGREDIENT NAME; TRADE NAME	PATENT NUMBER	PATENT EXPIRES	USE CODE	EX-CLUS CODE	EXCLUS EXPIRES
		5648497	JUL 15,2014			
		5674882	OCT 07,2014			
		5846987	DEC 29,2012	U-190		
		5886036	DEC 29,2012			
		6037157	JUN 26,2016			
020680 001	RITONAVIR; NORVIR	5541206	JUL 30,2013	U-140		
		5635523	JUN 03,2014	U-190		
		5648497	JUL 15,2014			
		5846987	DEC 29,2012	U-190		
		5948436	SEP 13,2013			
020945 001	RITONAVIR; NORVIR	5541206	JUL 30,2013	U-348		
		5635523	JUN 03,2014	U-347		
		5648497	JUL 15,2014			
		5846987	DEC 29,2012	U-347		
		6232333	NOV 07,2017			
020823 003	RIVASTIGMINE TARTRATE; EXELON	4948807	AUG 14,2007	U-322	NCE	APR 21,2005
		5602176	FEB 11,2014	U-322	NCE	APR 21,2005
020823 004	RIVASTIGMINE TARTRATE; EXELON	4948807	AUG 14,2007	U-322	NCE	APR 21,2005
		5602176	FEB 11,2014	U-322	NCE	APR 21,2005
020823 005	RIVASTIGMINE TARTRATE; EXELON	4948807	AUG 14,2007	U-322	NCE	APR 21,2005
		5602176	FEB 11,2014	U-322	NCE	APR 21,2005
020823 006	RIVASTIGMINE TARTRATE; EXELON	4948807	AUG 14,2007	U-322	NCE	APR 21,2005
		5602176	FEB 11,2014	U-322	NCE	APR 21,2005
021025 001	RIVASTIGMINE TARTRATE; EXELON	4948807	AUG 14,2007	U-322	NCE	APR 21,2005
		5602176	FEB 11,2014	U-322	NCE	APR 21,2005
020864 001	RIZATRIPTAN BENZOATE; MAXALT	5298520	JUN 29,2012	U-240	NCE	JUN 29,2003
		5602162	FEB 11,2014		NCE	JUN 29,2003
020864 002	RIZATRIPTAN BENZOATE; MAXALT	5298520	JUN 29,2012	U-240	NCE	JUN 29,2003
		5602162	FEB 11,2014		NCE	JUN 29,2003
020865 001	RIZATRIPTAN BENZOATE; MAXALT-MLT	5298520	JUN 29,2012	U-240	NCE	JUN 29,2003
		5457895	OCT 01,2013		NCE	JUN 29,2003
		5602162	FEB 11,2014	U-240	NCE	JUN 29,2003
020865 002	RIZATRIPTAN BENZOATE; MAXALT-MLT	5298520	JUN 29,2012	U-240	NCE	JUN 29,2003
		5457895	OCT 01,2013		NCE	JUN 29,2003
		5602162	FEB 11,2014	U-240	NCE	JUN 29,2003
020214 002	ROCURONIUM BROMIDE; ZEMURON	4894369	APR 13,2008			
020214 001	ROCURONIUM BROMIDE; ZEMURON (P/F)	4894369	APR 13,2008			
021042 001	ROFECOXIB; VIOXX	5474995	JUN 24,2013	U-266	I-353	APR 11,2005
		5691374	MAY 18,2015		I-353	APR 11,2005
		6063811	MAY 06,2017	U-266	I-353	APR 11,2005
		6239173	JUN 24,2013		I-353	APR 11,2005
021042 002	ROFECOXIB; VIOXX	5474995	JUN 24,2013	U-266	NCE	MAY 20,2004
		5691374	MAY 18,2015		NCE	MAY 20,2004
		6063811	MAY 06,2017	U-266	NCE	MAY 20,2004
		6239173	JUN 24,2013		NCE	MAY 20,2004
021042 003	ROFECOXIB; VIOXX	5474995	JUN 24,2013	U-266	NCE	MAY 20,2004
		5691374	MAY 18,2015		NCE	MAY 20,2004
		6063811	MAY 06,2017		NCE	MAY 20,2004
		6239173	JUN 24,2013		NCE	MAY 20,2004
021052 001	ROFECOXIB; VIOXX	5474995	JUN 24,2013	U-266	I-353	APR 11,2005
		5691374	MAY 18,2015		I-353	APR 11,2005
		6063811	MAY 06,2017	U-266	I-353	APR 11,2005
		6239173	JUN 24,2013		I-353	APR 11,2005
021052 002	ROFECOXIB; VIOXX	5474995	JUN 24,2013	U-266	NCE	MAY 20,2004
		5691374	MAY 18,2015		NCE	MAY 20,2004
		6063811	MAY 06,2017	U-266	NCE	MAY 20,2004
		6239173	JUN 24,2013		NCE	MAY 20,2004
020658 001	ROPINIROLE HYDROCHLORIDE; REQUIP	4452808	DEC 07,2007		NCE	SEP 19,2002
		4824860	MAY 19,2008	U-212	NCE	SEP 19,2002
020658 002	ROPINIROLE HYDROCHLORIDE; REQUIP	4452808	DEC 07,2007		NCE	SEP 19,2002
		4824860	MAY 19,2008	U-212	NCE	SEP 19,2002
020658 003	ROPINIROLE HYDROCHLORIDE; REQUIP	4452808	DEC 07,2007		NCE	SEP 19,2002
		4824860	MAY 19,2008	U-212	NCE	SEP 19,2002
020658 004	ROPINIROLE HYDROCHLORIDE; REQUIP	4452808	DEC 07,2007		NCE	SEP 19,2002
		4824860	MAY 19,2008	U-212	NCE	SEP 19,2002
020658 005	ROPINIROLE HYDROCHLORIDE; REQUIP	4452808	DEC 07,2007		NCE	SEP 19,2002
		4824860	MAY 19,2008	U-212	NCE	SEP 19,2002
020658 006	ROPINIROLE HYDROCHLORIDE; REQUIP	4452808	DEC 07,2007			
020658 007	ROPINIROLE HYDROCHLORIDE; REQUIP	4452808	DEC 07,2007			
020533 001	ROPIVACAINE HYDROCHLORIDE MONOHYDRATE; NAROPIN	4695576	SEP 22,2004		D-64	NOV 02,2003

PRESCRIPTION AND OTC PRODUCT
PATENT AND EXCLUSIVITY DATA
*PED and PED represent Pediatric Exclusivity (*continued*)

APPL/PROD NUMBER	INGREDIENT NAME; TRADE NAME	PATENT NUMBER	PATENT EXPIRES	USE CODE	EX-CLUS CODE	EXCLUS EXPIRES
		4870086	JUL 28,2010		D-64	NOV 02,2003
020533 003	ROPIVACAINE HYDROCHLORIDE MONOHYDRATE; NAROPIN	4695576	SEP 22,2004		D-64	NOV 02,2003
		4870086	JUL 28,2010		D-64	NOV 02,2003
020533 004	ROPIVACAINE HYDROCHLORIDE MONOHYDRATE; NAROPIN	4695576	SEP 22,2004		D-64	NOV 02,2003
		4870086	JUL 28,2010		D-64	NOV 02,2003
020533 005	ROPIVACAINE HYDROCHLORIDE MONOHYDRATE; NAROPIN	4695576	SEP 22,2004		D-64	NOV 02,2003
		4870086	JUL 28,2010		D-64	NOV 02,2003
021071 002	ROSIGLITAZONE MALEATE; AVANDIA	5002953	AUG 30,2008	U-329	I-289	APR 03,2003
		5741803	APR 21,2015	U-329	I-289	APR 03,2003
		6288095	FEB 11,2017	U-420	I-289	APR 03,2003
021071 003	ROSIGLITAZONE MALEATE; AVANDIA	5002953	AUG 30,2008	U-329	NCE	MAY 25,2004
		5741803	APR 21,2015	U-329	NCE	MAY 25,2004
		6288095	FEB 11,2017	U-420	NCE	MAY 25,2004
021071 004	ROSIGLITAZONE MALEATE; AVANDIA	5002953	AUG 30,2008	U-329	NCE	MAY 25,2004
		5741803	APR 21,2015	U-329	NCE	MAY 25,2004
		6288095	FEB 11,2017	U-420	NCE	MAY 25,2004
019414 001	RUBIDIUM CHLORIDE RB-82; CARDIOGEN-82	4400358	AUG 23,2002			
		4562829	MAY 01,2004	U-503		
020772 001	SACROSIDASE; SUCRAID				NCE	APR 09,2003
020236 001	SALMETEROL XINAFOATE; SEREVENT	4992474	FEB 12,2008		M-5	JUN 30,2003
		5126375	FEB 12,2008		M-5	JUN 30,2003
		5225445	FEB 12,2008	U-182	M-5	JUN 30,2003
020692 001	SALMETEROL XINAFOATE; SEREVENT	4992474	FEB 12,2008		I-348	MAR 22,2005
		5126375	FEB 12,2008		I-348	MAR 22,2005
		5225445	FEB 12,2008	U-211	I-348	MAR 22,2005
		5290815	MAR 01,2011	U-386	I-348	MAR 22,2005
020570 001	SAMARIUM SM 153 LEXIDRONAM PENTASODIUM; QUADRAMET	4898724	FEB 06,2007	U-187		
020628 001	SAQUINAVIR MESYLATE; INVIRASE	5196438	NOV 19,2010			
020828 001	SAQUINAVIR; FORTOVASE	5196438	NOV 19,2010			
		6008228	JUN 06,2015			
		6352717	NOV 16,2019			
021209 001	SECRETIN; SECREFLO				ODE	APR 04,2009
019863 001	SERMORELIN ACETATE; GEREF	4703035	DEC 28,2004	U-47		
020443 001	SERMORELIN ACETATE; GEREF	4703035	DEC 28,2004		ODE	SEP 26,2004
020443 002	SERMORELIN ACETATE; GEREF	4703035	DEC 28,2004		ODE	SEP 26,2004
019839 001	SERTRALINE HYDROCHLORIDE; ZOLOFT	4536518	DEC 30,2005	U-12	M-11	AUG 06,2004
		4536518*PED	JUN 30,2006	U-12	M-11	AUG 06,2004
		4962128	NOV 02,2009	U-152	M-11	AUG 06,2004
		4962128*PED	MAY 02,2010	U-152	M-11	AUG 06,2004
		5248699	AUG 13,2012		M-11	AUG 06,2004
		5248699*PED	FEB 13,2013		M-11	AUG 06,2004
		5744501	JAN 06,2009	U-461	M-11	AUG 06,2004
		5789449	JAN 06,2009	U-460	M-11	AUG 06,2004
019839 002	SERTRALINE HYDROCHLORIDE; ZOLOFT	4536518	DEC 30,2005	U-12	I-279	DEC 07,2002
		4536518*PED	JUN 30,2006	U-12	I-279	DEC 07,2002
		4962128	NOV 02,2009	U-152	I-279	DEC 07,2002
		4962128*PED	MAY 02,2010	U-152	I-279	DEC 07,2002
		5248699	AUG 13,2012		I-279	DEC 07,2002
		5248699*PED	FEB 13,2013		I-279	DEC 07,2002
		5744501	JAN 06,2009	U-461	I-279	DEC 07,2002
		5789449	JAN 06,2009	U-460	I-279	DEC 07,2002
019839 003	SERTRALINE HYDROCHLORIDE; ZOLOFT	4536518	DEC 30,2005	U-12	I-279	DEC 07,2002
		4536518*PED	JUN 30,2006	U-12	I-279	DEC 07,2002
		4962128	NOV 02,2009	U-152	I-279	DEC 07,2002
		4962128*PED	MAY 02,2010	U-152	I-279	DEC 07,2002
		5248699	AUG 13,2012		I-279	DEC 07,2002
		5248699*PED	FEB 13,2013		I-279	DEC 07,2002
		5744501	JAN 06,2009	U-461	I-279	DEC 07,2002
		5789449	JAN 06,2009	U-460	I-279	DEC 07,2002
019839 004	SERTRALINE HYDROCHLORIDE; ZOLOFT	4536518	DEC 30,2005	U-12	I-279	DEC 07,2002
		4536518*PED	JUN 30,2006	U-12	I-279	DEC 07,2002
		4962128	NOV 02,2009	U-152	I-279	DEC 07,2002
		4962128*PED	MAY 02,2010	U-152	I-279	DEC 07,2002
		5248699	AUG 13,2012		I-279	DEC 07,2002
		5248699*PED	FEB 13,2013		I-279	DEC 07,2002
		5744501	JAN 06,2009	U-461	I-279	DEC 07,2002
		5789449	JAN 06,2009	U-460	I-279	DEC 07,2002

PRESCRIPTION AND OTC PRODUCT
PATENT AND EXCLUSIVITY DATA
*PED and PED represent Pediatric Exclusivity (*continued*)

APPL/PROD NUMBER	INGREDIENT NAME; TRADE NAME	PATENT NUMBER	PATENT EXPIRES	USE CODE	EX-CLUS CODE	EXCLUS EXPIRES
019839 005	SERTRALINE HYDROCHLORIDE; ZOLOFT	4536518	DEC 30,2005	U-12	M-11	AUG 06,2004
		4536518*PED	JUN 30,2006	U-12	M-11	AUG 06,2004
		4962128	NOV 02,2009	U-152	M-11	AUG 06,2004
		4962128*PED	MAY 02,2010	U-152	M-11	AUG 06,2004
		5248699	AUG 13,2012		M-11	AUG 06,2004
		5248699*PED	FEB 13,2013		M-11	AUG 06,2004
		5744501	JAN 06,2009	U-461	M-11	AUG 06,2004
		5789449	JAN 06,2009	U-460	M-11	AUG 06,2004
020990 001	SERTRALINE HYDROCHLORIDE; ZOLOFT	4536518	DEC 30,2005	U-286	PED	FEB 06,2005
		4536518*PED	JUN 30,2006	U-286	PED	FEB 06,2005
		5248699	AUG 13,2012		PED	FEB 06,2005
		5248699*PED	FEB 13,2013		PED	FEB 06,2005
		5744501	JAN 06,2009	U-461	PED	FEB 06,2005
		5789449	JAN 06,2009	U-460	PED	FEB 06,2005
020926 001	SEVELAMER HYDROCHLORIDE; RENAGEL	5496545	AUG 11,2013	U-246	NCE	OCT 30,2003
		5667775	SEP 16,2014	U-246	NCE	OCT 30,2003
		6509013	AUG 13,2013		NCE	OCT 30,2003
021179 001	SEVELAMER HYDROCHLORIDE; RENAGEL	5496545	AUG 11,2013	U-246	NCE	OCT 30,2003
		5667775	SEP 16,2014	U-246	NCE	OCT 30,2003
		6509013	AUG 13,2013		NCE	OCT 30,2003
021179 002	SEVELAMER HYDROCHLORIDE; RENAGEL	5496545	AUG 11,2013	U-246	NCE	OCT 30,2003
		5667775	SEP 16,2014	U-246	NCE	OCT 30,2003
		6509013	AUG 13,2013		NCE	OCT 30,2003
020478 001	SEVOFLURANE; ULTANE	5990176	JAN 27,2017		PED	SEP 30,2004
		5990176*PED	JUL 27,2017		PED	SEP 30,2004
		6074668	JAN 09,2018		PED	SEP 30,2004
		6074668*PED	JUL 09,2018		PED	SEP 30,2004
		6288127	JAN 27,2017		PED	SEP 30,2004
		6288127*PED	JUL 27,2017		PED	SEP 30,2004
		6444859	JAN 27,2017		PED	SEP 30,2004
		6444859*PED	JUL 27,2017		PED	SEP 30,2004
020632 001	SIBUTRAMINE HYDROCHLORIDE; MERIDIA	4746680	JUN 11,2007		M-9	FEB 16,2004
		4929629	MAY 29,2007		M-9	FEB 16,2004
		5436272	JUL 25,2012	U-439	M-9	FEB 16,2004
020632 002	SIBUTRAMINE HYDROCHLORIDE; MERIDIA	4746680	JUN 11,2007		D-65	FEB 16,2004
		4929629	MAY 29,2007		D-65	FEB 16,2004
		5436272	JUL 25,2012	U-439	D-65	FEB 16,2004
020632 003	SIBUTRAMINE HYDROCHLORIDE; MERIDIA	4746680	JUN 11,2007		D-65	FEB 16,2004
		4929629	MAY 29,2007		D-65	FEB 16,2004
		5436272	JUL 25,2012	U-439	D-65	FEB 16,2004
020895 001	SILDENAFIL CITRATE; VIAGRA	5250534	MAR 27,2012		NCE	MAR 27,2003
		6469012	OCT 22,2019	U-155	NCE	MAR 27,2003
020895 002	SILDENAFIL CITRATE; VIAGRA	5250534	MAR 27,2012		NCE	MAR 27,2003
		6469012	OCT 22,2019	U-155	NCE	MAR 27,2003
020895 003	SILDENAFIL CITRATE; VIAGRA	5250534	MAR 27,2012		NCE	MAR 27,2003
		6469012	OCT 22,2019	U-155	NCE	MAR 27,2003
019608 001	SILVER SULFADIAZINE; SILDAFLO	4563184	JAN 07,2003			
019766 001	SIMVASTATIN; ZOCOR	4444784	DEC 23,2005	U-59	I-273	AUG 05,2002
		4444784*PED	JUN 23,2006	U-59	I-273	AUG 05,2002
		RE36481	JUL 10,2007	U-300	I-273	AUG 05,2002
		RE36481*PED	JAN 10,2008	U-300	I-273	AUG 05,2002
		RE36520	MAY 26,2009	U-300	I-273	AUG 05,2002
		RE36520*PED	NOV 26,2009	U-300	I-273	AUG 05,2002
019766 002	SIMVASTATIN; ZOCOR	4444784	DEC 23,2005	U-59	I-277	NOV 22,2002
		4444784*PED	JUN 23,2006	U-59	I-277	NOV 22,2002
		RE36481	JUL 10,2007	U-300	I-277	NOV 22,2002
		RE36481*PED	JAN 10,2008	U-300	I-277	NOV 22,2002
		RE36520	MAY 26,2009	U-300	I-277	NOV 22,2002
		RE36520*PED	NOV 26,2009	U-300	I-277	NOV 22,2002
019766 003	SIMVASTATIN; ZOCOR	4444784	DEC 23,2005	U-59	I-277	NOV 22,2002
		4444784*PED	JUN 23,2006	U-59	I-277	NOV 22,2002
		RE36481	JUL 10,2007	U-300	I-277	NOV 22,2002
		RE36481*PED	JAN 10,2008	U-300	I-277	NOV 22,2002
		RE36520	MAY 26,2009	U-300	I-277	NOV 22,2002
		RE36520*PED	NOV 26,2009	U-300	I-277	NOV 22,2002
019766 004	SIMVASTATIN; ZOCOR	4444784	DEC 23,2005	U-59	I-277	NOV 22,2002
		4444784*PED	JUN 23,2006	U-59	I-277	NOV 22,2002
		RE36481	JUL 10,2007	U-300	I-277	NOV 22,2002
		RE36481*PED	JAN 10,2008	U-300	I-277	NOV 22,2002
		RE36520	MAY 26,2009	U-300	I-277	NOV 22,2002
		RE36520*PED	NOV 26,2009	U-300	I-277	NOV 22,2002

PRESCRIPTION AND OTC PRODUCT
PATENT AND EXCLUSIVITY DATA
*PED and PED represent Pediatric Exclusivity (*continued*)

APPL/PROD NUMBER	INGREDIENT NAME; TRADE NAME	PATENT NUMBER	PATENT EXPIRES	USE CODE	EX- CLUS CODE	EXCLUS EXPIRES
019766 005	SIMVASTATIN; ZOCOR	4444784	DEC 23,2005	U-59	I-277	NOV 22,2002
		4444784*PED	JUN 23,2006	U-59	I-277	NOV 22,2002
		RE36481	JUL 10,2007	U-300	I-277	NOV 22,2002
		RE36481*PED	JAN 10,2008	U-300	I-277	NOV 22,2002
		RE36520	MAY 26,2009	U-300	I-277	NOV 22,2002
		RE36520*PED	NOV 26,2009	U-300	I-277	NOV 22,2002
021083 001	SIROLIMUS; RAPAMUNE	5100899	JUN 06,2009	U-290	I-386	APR 11,2006
		5212155	MAY 18,2010	U-291	I-386	APR 11,2006
		5308847	MAY 03,2011	U-292	I-386	APR 11,2006
		5403833	APR 04,2012	U-293	I-386	APR 11,2006
		5536729	SEP 30,2013		I-386	APR 11,2006
021110 001	SIROLIMUS; RAPAMUNE	5100899	JUN 06,2009	U-290	I-386	APR 11,2006
		5212155	MAY 18,2010	U-291	I-386	APR 11,2006
		5308847	MAY 03,2011	U-292	I-386	APR 11,2006
		5403833	APR 04,2012	U-293	I-386	APR 11,2006
		5989591	MAR 11,2018		I-386	APR 11,2006
021110 002	SIROLIMUS; RAPAMUNE	5100899	JUN 06,2009	U-290	NCE	SEP 15,2004
		5212155	MAY 18,2010	U-291	NCE	SEP 15,2004
		5308847	MAY 03,2011	U-292	NCE	SEP 15,2004
		5403833	APR 04,2012	U-293	NCE	SEP 15,2004
		5989591	MAR 11,2018		NCE	SEP 15,2004
020955 001	SODIUM FERRIC GLUCONATE COMPLEX; FERRLECIT				NCE	FEB 18,2004
020231 001	SODIUM FLUORIDE; COLGATE TOTAL	5288480	JUL 16,2008			
021196 001	SODIUM OXYBATE; XYREM				NCE	JUL 17,2007
020572 001	SODIUM PHENYLBUTYRATE; BUPHENYL	4457942	AUG 20,2004	U-136		
020573 001	SODIUM PHENYLBUTYRATE; BUPHENYL	4457942	AUG 20,2004	U-136	ODE	APR 30,2003
021097 001	SODIUM PHOSPHATE, DIBASIC, ANHYDROUS; VISICOL	5616346	MAY 18,2013	U-359	NP	SEP 21,2003
019107 001	SOMATREM; PROTROPIN	4658021	APR 14,2004			
020280 006	SOMATROPIN RECOMBINANT; GENOTROPIN	4968299	JUN 28,2008		ODE	JUL 25,2008
		5633352	MAR 10,2015		ODE	JUL 25,2008
020280 007	SOMATROPIN RECOMBINANT; GENOTROPIN	4968299	JUN 28,2008		ODE	JUL 25,2008
		5633352	MAR 10,2015		ODE	JUL 25,2008
020280 001	SOMATROPIN RECOMBINANT; GENOTROPIN PRESERVATIVE FREE	5435076	APR 16,2013		ODE	JUN 20,2007
		5633352	MAR 10,2015		ODE	JUN 20,2007
		5716338	FEB 10,2015		ODE	JUN 20,2007
		6152897	JUN 11,2018		ODE	JUN 20,2007
020280 002	SOMATROPIN RECOMBINANT; GENOTROPIN PRESERVATIVE FREE	5435076	APR 16,2013		ODE	JUN 20,2007
		5633352	MAR 10,2015		ODE	JUN 20,2007
		5716338	FEB 10,2015		ODE	JUN 20,2007
		6152897	JUN 11,2018		ODE	JUN 20,2007
020280 003	SOMATROPIN RECOMBINANT; GENOTROPIN PRESERVATIVE FREE	5435076	APR 16,2013		ODE	JUN 20,2007
		5633352	MAR 10,2015		ODE	JUN 20,2007
		5716338	FEB 10,2015		ODE	JUN 20,2007
		6152897	JUN 11,2018		ODE	JUN 20,2007
020280 004	SOMATROPIN RECOMBINANT; GENOTROPIN PRESERVATIVE FREE	5633352	MAR 10,2015		ODE	JUL 25,2008
020280 005	SOMATROPIN RECOMBINANT; GENOTROPIN PRESERVATIVE FREE	5435076	APR 16,2013		ODE	JUL 25,2008
		5633352	MAR 10,2015		ODE	JUL 25,2008
		5716338	FEB 10,2015		ODE	JUL 25,2008
		6152897	JUN 11,2018		ODE	JUL 25,2008
020280 008	SOMATROPIN RECOMBINANT; GENOTROPIN PRESERVATIVE FREE	5435076	APR 16,2013		ODE	JUL 25,2008
		5633352	MAR 10,2015		ODE	JUL 25,2008
		5716338	FEB 10,2015		ODE	JUL 25,2008
		6152897	JUN 11,2018		ODE	JUL 25,2008
020280 009	SOMATROPIN RECOMBINANT; GENOTROPIN PRESERVATIVE FREE	5435076	APR 16,2013		ODE	JUN 20,2007
		5633352	MAR 10,2015		ODE	JUN 20,2007
		5716338	FEB 10,2015		ODE	JUN 20,2007
		6152897	JUN 11,2018		ODE	JUN 20,2007
020280 010	SOMATROPIN RECOMBINANT; GENOTROPIN PRESERVATIVE FREE	5435076	APR 16,2013		ODE	JUN 20,2007
		5633352	MAR 10,2015		ODE	JUN 20,2007
		5716338	FEB 10,2015		ODE	JUN 20,2007

PRESCRIPTION AND OTC PRODUCT
PATENT AND EXCLUSIVITY DATA
*PED and PED represent Pediatric Exclusivity (*continued*)

APPL/PROD NUMBER	INGREDIENT NAME; TRADE NAME	PATENT NUMBER	PATENT EXPIRES	USE CODE	EX-CLUS CODE	EXCLUS EXPIRES
020280 011	SOMATROPIN RECOMBINANT; GENOTROPIN PRESERVATIVE FREE	5435076	APR 16,2013		ODE	JUL 25,2008
		5633352	MAR 10,2015		ODE	JUL 25,2008
		5716338	FEB 10,2015		ODE	JUL 25,2008
020280 012	SOMATROPIN RECOMBINANT; GENOTROPIN PRESERVATIVE FREE	5435076	APR 16,2013		ODE	JUL 25,2008
		5633352	MAR 10,2015		ODE	JUL 25,2008
		5716338	FEB 10,2015		ODE	JUL 25,2008
020280 013	SOMATROPIN RECOMBINANT; GENOTROPIN PRESERVATIVE FREE	5435076	APR 16,2013		ODE	JUL 25,2008
		5633352	MAR 10,2015		ODE	JUL 25,2008
		5716338	FEB 10,2015		ODE	JUL 25,2008
019640 001	SOMATROPIN RECOMBINANT; HUMATROPE				ODE	DEC 30,2003
019640 004	SOMATROPIN RECOMBINANT; HUMATROPE				ODE	DEC 30,2003
019640 005	SOMATROPIN RECOMBINANT; HUMATROPE				ODE	DEC 30,2003
019640 006	SOMATROPIN RECOMBINANT; HUMATROPE				ODE	DEC 30,2003
019640 007	SOMATROPIN RECOMBINANT; HUMATROPE				ODE	DEC 30,2003
019721 001	SOMATROPIN RECOMBINANT; NORDITROPIN	5633352	MAY 27,2014			
019721 002	SOMATROPIN RECOMBINANT; NORDITROPIN	5633352	MAY 27,2014			
021148 001	SOMATROPIN RECOMBINANT; NORDITROPIN	5633352	MAY 27,2014			
		5849700	DEC 15,2015	U-340		
		5849704	DEC 15,2015			
021148 002	SOMATROPIN RECOMBINANT; NORDITROPIN	5633352	MAY 27,2014			
		5849700	DEC 15,2015	U-340		
		5849704	DEC 15,2015			
021148 003	SOMATROPIN RECOMBINANT; NORDITROPIN	5633352	MAY 27,2014			
		5849700	DEC 15,2015	U-340		
		5849704	DEC 15,2015			
020168 001	SOMATROPIN RECOMBINANT; NUTROPIN				ODE	DEC 30,2003
020168 002	SOMATROPIN RECOMBINANT; NUTROPIN				ODE	DEC 30,2003
020522 001	SOMATROPIN RECOMBINANT; NUTROPIN AQ				M-2	DEC 01,2002
021075 001	SOMATROPIN RECOMBINANT; NUTROPIN DEPOT	5654010	AUG 05,2014		NP	DEC 22,2002
		5656297	JUL 25,2014		NP	DEC 22,2002
		5912015	MAR 12,2012		NP	DEC 22,2002
		6051259	DEC 02,2012	U-340	NP	DEC 22,2002
021075 002	SOMATROPIN RECOMBINANT; NUTROPIN DEPOT	5654010	AUG 05,2014		NP	DEC 22,2002
		5656297	JUL 25,2014		NP	DEC 22,2002
		5912015	MAR 12,2012		NP	DEC 22,2002
		6051259	DEC 02,2012	U-340	NP	DEC 22,2002
021075 003	SOMATROPIN RECOMBINANT; NUTROPIN DEPOT	5654010	AUG 05,2014		NP	DEC 22,2002
		5656297	JUL 25,2014		NP	DEC 22,2002
		5912015	MAR 12,2012		NP	DEC 22,2002
		6051259	DEC 02,2012	U-340	NP	DEC 22,2002
020604 001	SOMATROPIN RECOMBINANT; SEROSTIM				ODE	AUG 23,2003
020604 002	SOMATROPIN RECOMBINANT; SEROSTIM				ODE	AUG 23,2003
020604 004	SOMATROPIN RECOMBINANT; SEROSTIM				ODE	AUG 23,2003
019865 001	SOTALOL HYDROCHLORIDE; BETAPACE				M-13	OCT 01,2004
019865 002	SOTALOL HYDROCHLORIDE; BETAPACE				PED	APR 01,2005
019865 003	SOTALOL HYDROCHLORIDE; BETAPACE				M-13	OCT 01,2004
019865 004	SOTALOL HYDROCHLORIDE; BETAPACE				PED	APR 01,2005
019865 005	SOTALOL HYDROCHLORIDE; BETAPACE				PED	APR 01,2005
021151 001	SOTALOL HYDROCHLORIDE; BETAPACE AF				PED	AUG 22,2003
021151 002	SOTALOL HYDROCHLORIDE; BETAPACE AF				PED	AUG 22,2003
021151 003	SOTALOL HYDROCHLORIDE; BETAPACE AF				PED	AUG 22,2003
021151 005	SOTALOL HYDROCHLORIDE; BETAPACE AF				NP	FEB 22,2003
					PED	AUG 22,2003
021151 006	SOTALOL HYDROCHLORIDE; BETAPACE AF				NP	FEB 22,2003
					PED	AUG 22,2003
021151 007	SOTALOL HYDROCHLORIDE; BETAPACE AF				NP	FEB 22,2003
					PED	AUG 22,2003
020677 001	SPARFLOXACIN; ZAGAM	4795751	FEB 04,2010	U-160		
020240 001	SPIRAPRIL HYDROCHLORIDE; RENORMAX	4470972	SEP 11,2003	U-3		
020240 002	SPIRAPRIL HYDROCHLORIDE; RENORMAX	4470972	SEP 11,2003	U-3		
020240 003	SPIRAPRIL HYDROCHLORIDE; RENORMAX	4470972	SEP 11,2003	U-3		
020240 004	SPIRAPRIL HYDROCHLORIDE; RENORMAX	4470972	SEP 11,2003	U-3		
020412 001	STAVUDINE; ZERIT	4978655	JUN 24,2008	U-94		
		4978655*PED	DEC 24,2008	U-94		
020412 002	STAVUDINE; ZERIT	4978655	JUN 24,2008	U-94		
		4978655*PED	DEC 24,2008	U-94		
020412 003	STAVUDINE; ZERIT	4978655	JUN 24,2008	U-94		
		4978655*PED	DEC 24,2008	U-94		

PRESCRIPTION AND OTC PRODUCT
PATENT AND EXCLUSIVITY DATA
*PED and PED represent Pediatric Exclusivity (continued)

APPL/PROD NUMBER	INGREDIENT NAME; TRADE NAME	PATENT NUMBER	PATENT EXPIRES	USE CODE	EX-CLUS CODE	EXCLUS EXPIRES
020412 004	STAVUDINE; ZERIT	4978655	JUN 24,2008	U-94		
		4978655*PED	DEC 24,2008	U-94		
020412 005	STAVUDINE; ZERIT	4978655	JUN 24,2008	U-94		
		4978655*PED	DEC 24,2008	U-94		
020413 001	STAVUDINE; ZERIT	4978655	JUN 24,2008			
		4978655*PED	DEC 24,2008			
021453 001	STAVUDINE; ZERIT XR	4978655	JUN 24,2008	U-248	NDF	DEC 31,2005
		4978655*PED	DEC 24,2008	U-248	PED	JUL 01,2006
021453 002	STAVUDINE; ZERIT XR	4978655	JUN 24,2008	U-248	NDF	DEC 31,2005
		4978655*PED	DEC 24,2008	U-248	PED	JUL 01,2006
021453 003	STAVUDINE; ZERIT XR	4978655	JUN 24,2008	U-248	NDF	DEC 31,2005
		4978655*PED	DEC 24,2008	U-248	PED	JUL 01,2006
021453 004	STAVUDINE; ZERIT XR	4978655	JUN 24,2008	U-248	NDF	DEC 31,2005
		4978655*PED	DEC 24,2008	U-248	PED	JUL 01,2006
007073 002	SULFASALAZINE; AZULFIDINE EN-TABS				I-308	AUG 18,2003
020080 001	SUMATRIPTAN SUCCINATE; IMITREX	4816470	DEC 28,2006	U-72		
		5037845	AUG 06,2008	U-72		
020132 001	SUMATRIPTAN SUCCINATE; IMITREX	4816470	DEC 28,2006	U-72		
		5037845	AUG 06,2008	U-72		
		5863559	JAN 26,2016	U-72		
		6020001	MAR 02,2012	U-444		
		6368627	MAR 02,2012	U-444		
020132 002	SUMATRIPTAN SUCCINATE; IMITREX	4816470	DEC 28,2006	U-72		
		5037845	AUG 06,2008	U-72		
		5863559	JAN 26,2016	U-72		
		6020001	MAR 02,2012	U-444		
		6368627	MAR 02,2012	U-444		
020132 003	SUMATRIPTAN SUCCINATE; IMITREX	4816470	DEC 28,2006	U-72		
		5037845	AUG 06,2008	U-72		
		5863559	JAN 26,2016	U-72		
		6020001	MAR 02,2012	U-444		
		6368627	MAR 02,2012	U-444		
020626 001	SUMATRIPTAN; IMITREX	4816470	DEC 28,2006	U-72		
		5037845	AUG 06,2008			
		5307953	DEC 02,2012			
		5554639	SEP 10,2013	U-232		
		5705520	DEC 10,2011	U-232		
020626 002	SUMATRIPTAN; IMITREX	4816470	DEC 28,2006	U-72		
		5037845	AUG 06,2008			
		5307953	DEC 02,2012			
		5554639	SEP 10,2013	U-232		
		5705520	DEC 10,2011	U-232		
020626 003	SUMATRIPTAN; IMITREX	4816470	DEC 28,2006	U-72		
		5037845	AUG 06,2008			
		5307953	DEC 02,2012			
		5554639	SEP 10,2013	U-232		
		5705520	DEC 10,2011	U-232		
019387 001	SUPROFEN; PROFENAL	4559343	DEC 17,2002			
020070 001	TACRINE HYDROCHLORIDE; COGNEX	4631286	OCT 25,2004	U-97		
		4816456	SEP 09,2007			
020070 002	TACRINE HYDROCHLORIDE; COGNEX	4631286	OCT 25,2004	U-97		
		4816456	SEP 09,2007			
020070 003	TACRINE HYDROCHLORIDE; COGNEX	4631286	OCT 25,2004	U-97		
		4816456	SEP 09,2007			
020070 004	TACRINE HYDROCHLORIDE; COGNEX	4631286	OCT 25,2004	U-97		
		4816456	SEP 09,2007			
020587 001	TALC; SCLEROSOL				ODE	DEC 24,2004
017970 001	TAMOXIFEN CITRATE; NOLVADEX	4536516	AUG 20,2002		PED	MAR 01,2006
		4536516*PED	FEB 20,2003		PED	MAR 01,2006
017970 002	TAMOXIFEN CITRATE; NOLVADEX	4536516	AUG 20,2002			
		4536516*PED	FEB 20,2003			
020579 001	TAMSULOSIN HYDROCHLORIDE; FLOMAX	4703063	OCT 27,2009			
		4731478	OCT 27,2004			
		4772475	FEB 27,2006			
		4868216	SEP 19,2006	U-181		
021184 003	TAZAROTENE; AVAGE	5089509	JUN 13,2011	U-481	NP	SEP 30,2005
020600 001	TAZAROTENE; TAZORAC	5089509	JUN 13,2011	U-481		
		5089509	JUN 13,2011	U-193		
		5914334	JUN 07,2014	U-517		
		6258830	JUN 07,2014	U-517		
020600 002	TAZAROTENE; TAZORAC	5089509	JUN 13,2011	U-481		

PRESCRIPTION AND OTC PRODUCT
PATENT AND EXCLUSIVITY DATA
*PED and PED represent Pediatric Exclusivity (*continued*)

APPL/PROD NUMBER	INGREDIENT NAME; TRADE NAME	PATENT NUMBER	PATENT EXPIRES	USE CODE	EX-CLUS CODE	EXCLUS EXPIRES
		5089509	JUN 13,2011	U-193		
		5914334	JUN 07,2014	U-517		
		6258830	JUN 07,2014	U-517		
021184 001	TAZAROTENE; TAZORAC	5089509	JUN 13,2011	U-481	NDF	SEP 29,2003
021184 002	TAZAROTENE; TAZORAC	5089509	JUN 13,2011	U-481	I-344	OCT 11,2004
020887 001	TECHNETIUM TC-99M APCITIDE; ACUTECT	5443815	AUG 22,2012		NCE	SEP 14,2003
		5508020	APR 16,2013		NCE	SEP 14,2003
		5645815	JUL 08,2014		NCE	SEP 14,2003
020256 001	TECHNETIUM TC-99M BICISATE KIT; NEUROLITE	5279811	NOV 23,2008	U-101		
		5431900	JUL 11,2012	U-336		
021012 001	TECHNETIUM TC-99M DEPREOTIDE; NEO TECT KIT				NCE	AUG 03,2004
019829 001	TECHNETIUM TC-99M EXAMETAZIME KIT; CERETEC	4615876	OCT 07,2003			
		4789736	DEC 06,2005			
019981 001	TECHNETIUM TC-99M RED BLOOD CELL KIT; ULTRATAG	4755375	JUL 05,2005	U-51		
019785 001	TECHNETIUM TC-99M SESTAMIBI KIT; CARDIOLITE	4452774	DEC 21,2004			
		4885100	SEP 11,2007			
		4894445	JAN 16,2007	U-337		
		4988827	JAN 29,2008			
		5324824	JAN 16,2007			
019785 003	TECHNETIUM TC-99M SESTAMIBI KIT; MIRALUMA	4452774	DEC 21,2004			
		4885100	SEP 11,2007			
		4894445	JAN 16,2007	U-337		
		4988827	JAN 29,2008			
		5324824	JAN 16,2007			
019928 001	TECHNETIUM TC-99M TEBOROXIME KIT; CARDIOTEC	4705849	NOV 10,2004			
020372 001	TECHNETIUM TC-99M TETROFOSMIN KIT; MYOVIEW	5045302	AUG 14,2008			
021200 001	TEGASEROD MALEATE; ZELNORM	5510353	APR 26,2013	U-466	NCE	JUL 24,2007
021200 002	TEGASEROD MALEATE; ZELNORM	5510353	APR 26,2013	U-466	NCE	JUL 24,2007
020850 001	TELMISARTAN; MICARDIS	5591762	JAN 07,2014	U-3	NCE	NOV 10,2003
020850 002	TELMISARTAN; MICARDIS	5591762	JAN 07,2014	U-3	NCE	NOV 10,2003
018163 003	TEMAZEPAM; RESTORIL	5030632	JUL 09,2008	U-70		
		5211954	MAY 18,2010			
		5326758	JUL 09,2008	U-70		
021029 001	TEMOZOLOMIDE; TEMODAR	5260291	NOV 09,2010		PED	FEB 11,2005
		5260291*PED	MAY 09,2011		PED	FEB 11,2005
021029 002	TEMOZOLOMIDE; TEMODAR	5260291	NOV 09,2010		NCE	AUG 11,2004
		5260291*PED	MAY 09,2011		NCE	AUG 11,2004
021029 003	TEMOZOLOMIDE; TEMODAR	5260291	NOV 09,2010		ODE	AUG 11,2006
		5260291*PED	MAY 09,2011		ODE	AUG 11,2006
021029 004	TEMOZOLOMIDE; TEMODAR	5260291	NOV 09,2010		PED	FEB 11,2005
		5260291*PED	MAY 09,2011		PED	FEB 11,2005
021356 001	TENOFOVIR DISOPROXIL FUMARATE; VIREAD	4808716	APR 25,2006	U-248	NCE	OCT 26,2006
		5922695	JUL 25,2017	U-248	NCE	OCT 26,2006
		5935946	JUL 25,2017	U-248	NCE	OCT 26,2006
		5977089	JUL 25,2017	U-248	NCE	OCT 26,2006
		6043230	JUL 25,2017	U-248	NCE	OCT 26,2006
		6057305	MAY 02,2017	U-248	NCE	OCT 26,2006
019057 001	TERAZOSIN HYDROCHLORIDE; HYTRIN	5212176	JUN 29,2010			
		5294615	APR 29,2013	U-165		
		5294615	APR 29,2013	U-3		
		5412095	APR 29,2013			
019057 002	TERAZOSIN HYDROCHLORIDE; HYTRIN	5212176	JUN 29,2010			
		5294615	APR 29,2013	U-165		
		5294615	APR 29,2013	U-3		
		5412095	APR 29,2013			
019057 003	TERAZOSIN HYDROCHLORIDE; HYTRIN	5212176	JUN 29,2010			
		5294615	APR 29,2013	U-165		
		5294615	APR 29,2013	U-3		
		5412095	APR 29,2013			
019057 004	TERAZOSIN HYDROCHLORIDE; HYTRIN	5212176	JUN 29,2010			
		5294615	APR 29,2013	U-165		
		5294615	APR 29,2013	U-3		
		5412095	APR 29,2013			
020347 001	TERAZOSIN HYDROCHLORIDE; HYTRIN	5212176	JUN 29,2010			
		5294615	APR 29,2013	U-165		
		5294615	APR 29,2013	U-3		

PRESCRIPTION AND OTC PRODUCT
PATENT AND EXCLUSIVITY DATA
*PED and PED represent Pediatric Exclusivity (*continued*)

APPL/PROD NUMBER	INGREDIENT NAME; TRADE NAME	PATENT NUMBER	PATENT EXPIRES	USE CODE	EX-CLUS CODE	EXCLUS EXPIRES
		5412095	APR 29,2013			
020347 002	TERAZOSIN HYDROCHLORIDE; HYTRIN	5212176	JUN 29,2010			
		5294615	APR 29,2013	U-165		
		5294615	APR 29,2013	U-3		
		5412095	APR 29,2013			
020347 003	TERAZOSIN HYDROCHLORIDE; HYTRIN	5212176	JUN 29,2010			
		5294615	APR 29,2013	U-165		
		5294615	APR 29,2013	U-3		
		5412095	APR 29,2013			
020347 004	TERAZOSIN HYDROCHLORIDE; HYTRIN	5212176	JUN 29,2010			
		5294615	APR 29,2013	U-165		
		5294615	APR 29,2013	U-3		
		5412095	APR 29,2013			
020192 001	TERBINAFINE HYDROCHLORIDE; LAMISIL	4755534	DEC 30,2006	U-73		
020539 001	TERBINAFINE HYDROCHLORIDE; LAMISIL	4680291	JUL 14,2004	U-281		
		4755534	DEC 30,2006	U-73		
020749 001	TERBINAFINE HYDROCHLORIDE; LAMISIL	4755534	DEC 30,2006			
		6121314	MAY 18,2012	U-502		
020980 001	TERBINAFINE HYDROCHLORIDE; LAMISIL	4680291	JUL 14,2004	U-73		
		4755534	DEC 30,2006	U-73		
021124 001	TERBINAFINE HYDROCHLORIDE; LAMISIL AT	4680291	JUL 14,2004	U-73		
		4755534	DEC 30,2006	U-73		
		5681849	OCT 28,2014			
		6121314	MAY 18,2012	U-504		
020846 001	TERBINAFINE; LAMISIL	4680291	JUL 14,2004	U-445		
		4755534	DEC 30,2006	U-445		
021318 001	TERIPARATIDE ACETATE; FORTEO				NP	NOV 26,2005
020489 001	TESTOSTERONE; ANDRODERM	4849224	NOV 12,2007			
		4855294	SEP 06,2008			
		4863970	NOV 14,2006			
		4983395	NOV 12,2007			
		5152997	DEC 11,2010	U-490		
		5164190	DEC 11,2010			
020489 002	TESTOSTERONE; ANDRODERM	4849224	NOV 12,2007			
		4855294	SEP 06,2008			
		4863970	NOV 14,2006			
		4983395	NOV 12,2007			
		5152997	DEC 11,2010	U-490		
		5164190	DEC 11,2010			
021015 001	TESTOSTERONE; ANDROGEL	6503894	AUG 30,2020	U-490	NDF	FEB 28,2003
021543 001	TESTOSTERONE; STRIANT				NP	JUN 19,2006
021454 001	TESTOSTERONE; TESTIM	5023252	JUN 11,2008	U-483	NP	OCT 31,2005
019762 001	TESTOSTERONE; TESTODERM	4704282	NOV 03,2004			
		4725439	FEB 16,2005			
		4867982	FEB 16,2005			
		5840327	AUG 15,2016			
019762 002	TESTOSTERONE; TESTODERM	4704282	NOV 03,2004			
		4725439	FEB 16,2005			
		4867982	FEB 16,2005			
		5840327	AUG 15,2016			
020791 001	TESTOSTERONE; TESTODERM TTS	6348210	NOV 10,2019	U-440		
020785 001	THALIDOMIDE; THALOMID	6045501	AUG 28,2018	U-371	ODE	JUL 16,2005
		6315720	OCT 23,2020	U-442	ODE	JUL 16,2005
		6561976	AUG 28,2018	U-371	ODE	JUL 16,2005
		6561977	OCT 23,2020	U-371	ODE	JUL 16,2005
020785 002	THALIDOMIDE; THALOMID	6045501	AUG 28,2018	U-371	ODE	JUL 16,2005
		6315720	OCT 23,2020	U-442	ODE	JUL 16,2005
		6561976	AUG 28,2018	U-371	NCE	JUL 16,2003
		6561977	OCT 23,2020	U-371	ODE	JUL 16,2005
020785 003	THALIDOMIDE; THALOMID	6045501	AUG 28,2018	U-371	ODE	JUL 16,2005
		6315720	OCT 23,2020	U-442	ODE	JUL 16,2005
		6561976	AUG 28,2018	U-371	NCE	JUL 16,2003
		6561977	OCT 23,2020	U-371	ODE	JUL 16,2005
020898 001	THYROTROPIN ALFA; THYROGEN	5240832	AUG 31,2010		NCE	NOV 30,2003
		5602006	FEB 11,2014		NCE	NOV 30,2003
		5658760	AUG 19,2014		NCE	NOV 30,2003
		5674711	AUG 31,2010		NCE	NOV 30,2003
		5840566	NOV 24,2015		NCE	NOV 30,2003
		6114144	NOV 24,2015		NCE	NOV 30,2003
020646 001	TIAGABINE HYDROCHLORIDE; GABITRIL	5010090	SEP 30,2011		NCE	SEP 30,2002
		5354760	MAR 24,2012		NCE	SEP 30,2002

PRESCRIPTION AND OTC PRODUCT
PATENT AND EXCLUSIVITY DATA
*PED and PED represent Pediatric Exclusivity (*continued*)

APPL/PROD NUMBER	INGREDIENT NAME; TRADE NAME	PATENT NUMBER	PATENT EXPIRES	USE CODE	EX-CLUS CODE	EXCLUS EXPIRES
		5866590	APR 29,2016		NCE	SEP 30,2002
		5958951	JUN 10,2017		NCE	SEP 30,2002
020646 002	TIAGABINE HYDROCHLORIDE; GABITRIL	5010090	SEP 30,2011		NCE	SEP 30,2002
		5354760	MAR 24,2012		NCE	SEP 30,2002
		5866590	APR 29,2016		NCE	SEP 30,2002
		5958951	JUN 10,2017		NCE	SEP 30,2002
020646 003	TIAGABINE HYDROCHLORIDE; GABITRIL	5010090	SEP 30,2011		NCE	SEP 30,2002
		5354760	MAR 24,2012		NCE	SEP 30,2002
		5866590	APR 29,2016		NCE	SEP 30,2002
		5958951	JUN 10,2017		NCE	SEP 30,2002
020646 004	TIAGABINE HYDROCHLORIDE; GABITRIL	5010090	SEP 30,2011		NCE	SEP 30,2002
		5354760	MAR 24,2012		NCE	SEP 30,2002
		5866590	APR 29,2016		NCE	SEP 30,2002
		5958951	JUN 10,2017		NCE	SEP 30,2002
020646 005	TIAGABINE HYDROCHLORIDE; GABITRIL	5010090	SEP 30,2011		NCE	SEP 30,2002
		5354760	MAR 24,2012		NCE	SEP 30,2002
		5866590	APR 29,2016		NCE	SEP 30,2002
		5958951	JUN 10,2017		NCE	SEP 30,2002
019979 001	TICLOPIDINE HYDROCHLORIDE; TICLID	4591592	MAY 27,2003			
019979 002	TICLOPIDINE HYDROCHLORIDE; TICLID	4591592	MAY 27,2003			
020707 001	TILUDRONATE DISODIUM; SKELID	4876248	JAN 30,2010			
		4980171	APR 06,2009			
020963 001	TIMOLOL MALEATE; TIMOLOL MALEATE	6174524	MAR 26,2019			
020963 002	TIMOLOL MALEATE; TIMOLOL MALEATE	6174524	MAR 26,2019			
020330 001	TIMOLOL MALEATE; TIMOPTIC-XE	4861760	AUG 29,2006			
		4861760	SEP 25,2006			
020330 002	TIMOLOL MALEATE; TIMOPTIC-XE	4861760	SEP 25,2006			
		4861760	AUG 29,2006			
020439 001	TIMOLOL; BETIMOL	5231095	JUL 27,2010			
020439 002	TIMOLOL; BETIMOL	5231095	JUL 27,2010			
020484 001	TINZAPARIN SODIUM; INNOHEP				NCE	JUL 14,2005
020912 001	TIROFIBAN HYDROCHLORIDE; AGGRASTAT	5292756	MAY 14,2012	U-230	NCE	MAY 14,2003
		5658929	MAR 08,2011		NCE	MAY 14,2003
		5733919	OCT 23,2016		NCE	MAY 14,2003
		5880136	SEP 27,2010	U-254	NCE	MAY 14,2003
		5965581	OCT 23,2016		NCE	MAY 14,2003
		5972967	OCT 23,2016		NCE	MAY 14,2003
		5978698	OCT 08,2017		NCE	MAY 14,2003
		6136794	JAN 29,2019		NCE	MAY 14,2003
020913 001	TIROFIBAN HYDROCHLORIDE; AGGRASTAT	5292756	MAY 14,2012	U-230	NCE	MAY 14,2003
		5658929	MAR 08,2011		NCE	MAY 14,2003
		5733919	OCT 23,2016		NCE	MAY 14,2003
		5880136	SEP 27,2010	U-254	NCE	MAY 14,2003
		5965581	OCT 23,2016		NCE	MAY 14,2003
		5972967	OCT 23,2016		NCE	MAY 14,2003
		5978698	OCT 08,2017		NCE	MAY 14,2003
		6136794	JAN 29,2019		NCE	MAY 14,2003
021447 001	TIZANIDINE HYDROCHLORIDE; ZANAFLEX	6455557	NOV 28,2021			
021447 002	TIZANIDINE HYDROCHLORIDE; ZANAFLEX	6455557	NOV 28,2021			
021447 003	TIZANIDINE HYDROCHLORIDE; ZANAFLEX	6455557	NOV 28,2021			
050753 001	TOBRAMYCIN; TOBI				ODE	DEC 22,2004
020697 001	TOLCAPONE; TASMAR	5236952	JAN 29,2012		NCE	JAN 29,2003
		5476875	DEC 19,2012	U-219	NCE	JAN 29,2003
020697 002	TOLCAPONE; TASMAR	5236952	JAN 29,2012		NCE	JAN 29,2003
		5476875	DEC 19,2012	U-219	NCE	JAN 29,2003
020771 001	TOLTERODINE TARTRATE; DETROL	5382600	JAN 17,2012		NCE	MAR 25,2003
		5559269	NOV 05,2013	U-318	NCE	MAR 25,2003
020771 002	TOLTERODINE TARTRATE; DETROL	5382600	JAN 17,2012		NCE	MAR 25,2003
		5559269	NOV 05,2013	U-318	NCE	MAR 25,2003
021228 001	TOLTERODINE TARTRATE; DETROL LA	5382600	JAN 17,2012		NCE	MAR 25,2003
		5559269	NOV 05,2013	U-318	NCE	MAR 25,2003
021228 002	TOLTERODINE TARTRATE; DETROL LA	5382600	JAN 17,2012		NCE	MAR 25,2003
		5559269	NOV 05,2013	U-318	NCE	MAR 25,2003
020505 001	TOPIRAMATE; TOPAMAX	4513006	SEP 26,2004		I-266	JUL 23,2002
020505 002	TOPIRAMATE; TOPAMAX	4513006	SEP 26,2004		I-266	JUL 23,2002
020505 003	TOPIRAMATE; TOPAMAX	4513006	SEP 26,2004		I-266	JUL 23,2002
020505 004	TOPIRAMATE; TOPAMAX	4513006	SEP 26,2004		ODE	AUG 28,2008
020505 005	TOPIRAMATE; TOPAMAX	4513006	SEP 26,2004		ODE	AUG 28,2008
020505 006	TOPIRAMATE; TOPAMAX	4513006	SEP 26,2004		I-274	OCT 01,2002
020844 001	TOPIRAMATE; TOPAMAX SPRINKLE	4513006	SEP 26,2004		I-266	JUL 23,2002
020844 002	TOPIRAMATE; TOPAMAX SPRINKLE	4513006	SEP 26,2004		I-274	OCT 01,2002

PRESCRIPTION AND OTC PRODUCT
PATENT AND EXCLUSIVITY DATA
*PED and PED represent Pediatric Exclusivity (*continued*)

APPL/PROD NUMBER	INGREDIENT NAME; TRADE NAME	PATENT NUMBER	PATENT EXPIRES	USE CODE	EX-CLUS CODE	EXCLUS EXPIRES
020844 003	TOPIRAMATE; TOPAMAX SPRINKLE	4513006	SEP 26,2004		ODE	AUG 28,2008
020671 001	TOPOTECAN HYDROCHLORIDE; HYCAMTIN	5004758	MAY 28,2010			
		5004758*PED	NOV 28,2010			
020497 001	TOREMIFENE CITRATE; FARESTON	4696949	SEP 29,2009	U-196	ODE	MAY 29,2004
020136 001	TORSEMIDE; DEMADEX	RE34672	AUG 11,2006			
020136 002	TORSEMIDE; DEMADEX	RE34672	AUG 11,2006			
020136 003	TORSEMIDE; DEMADEX	RE34672	AUG 11,2006			
020136 004	TORSEMIDE; DEMADEX	RE34672	AUG 11,2006			
020137 002	TORSEMIDE; DEMADEX	4861786	JUL 08,2007			
		RE34672	AUG 11,2006			
076110 001	TORSEMIDE; TORSEMIDE				PC	FEB 17,2003
076110 002	TORSEMIDE; TORSEMIDE				PC	DEC 10,2002
076110 003	TORSEMIDE; TORSEMIDE				PC	DEC 07,2002
076110 004	TORSEMIDE; TORSEMIDE				PC	DEC 10,2002
020281 001	TRAMADOL HYDROCHLORIDE; ULTRAM	6339105	OCT 12,2019	U-435		
		6339105*PED	APR 12,2020	U-435		
020281 002	TRAMADOL HYDROCHLORIDE; ULTRAM	6339105	OCT 12,2019	U-435	PED	JUN 23,2003
		6339105*PED	APR 12,2020	U-435	PED	JUN 23,2003
020528 001	TRANDOLAPRIL; MAVIK	4933361	JUN 12,2007			
		5744496	APR 28,2015	U-229		
020528 002	TRANDOLAPRIL; MAVIK	4933361	JUN 12,2007			
		5744496	APR 28,2015	U-229		
020528 003	TRANDOLAPRIL; MAVIK	4933361	JUN 12,2007			
		5744496	APR 28,2015	U-229		
020591 001	TRANDOLAPRIL; TARKA	4933361	JUN 12,2007			
		5721244	FEB 24,2015			
020591 002	TRANDOLAPRIL; TARKA	4933361	JUN 12,2007			
		5721244	FEB 24,2015			
020591 003	TRANDOLAPRIL; TARKA	4933361	JUN 12,2007			
		5721244	FEB 24,2015			
020591 004	TRANDOLAPRIL; TARKA	4933361	JUN 12,2007			
		5721244	FEB 24,2015			
021257 001	TRAVOPROST; TRAVATAN	5631287	DEC 22,2014	U-382	M-23	FEB 13,2006
		5849792	DEC 22,2014	U-383	M-23	FEB 13,2006
		5889052	AUG 03,2013	U-383	M-23	FEB 13,2006
		6011062	DEC 22,2014	U-382	M-23	FEB 13,2006
		6235781	JUN 15,2019	U-382	M-23	FEB 13,2006
021272 001	TREPROSTINIL SODIUM; REMODULIN	5153222	OCT 06,2009	U-455	ODE	MAY 21,2009
021272 002	TREPROSTINIL SODIUM; REMODULIN	5153222	OCT 06,2009	U-455	NCE	MAY 21,2007
021272 003	TREPROSTINIL SODIUM; REMODULIN	5153222	OCT 06,2009	U-455	NCE	MAY 21,2007
021272 004	TREPROSTINIL SODIUM; REMODULIN	5153222	OCT 06,2009	U-455	ODE	MAY 21,2009
020404 003	TRETINOIN; AVITA	4971800	NOV 20,2007	U-178		
		5045317	SEP 03,2008	U-179		
019963 001	TRETINOIN; RENOVA	4603146	JUL 29,2003	U-131		
		RE36068	JUL 29,2003	U-131		
021108 001	TRETINOIN; RENOVA	4603146	JUL 29,2003	U-131	NP	AUG 31,2003
		6531141	MAR 07,2020		NP	AUG 31,2003
		RE36068	JUL 29,2003	U-131	NP	AUG 31,2003
020475 001	TRETINOIN; RETIN-A MICRO	4690825	OCT 04,2005	U-134		
		5955109	SEP 21,2016	U-134		
020475 002	TRETINOIN; RETIN-A MICRO	4690825	OCT 04,2005	U-134	NS	MAY 10,2005
		5955109	SEP 21,2016	U-134	NS	MAY 10,2005
020438 001	TRETINOIN; VESANOID				ODE	NOV 22,2002
019798 001	TRIAMCINOLONE ACETONIDE; NASACORT	4767612	JAN 23,2007	U-85		
020468 001	TRIAMCINOLONE ACETONIDE; NASACORT AQ	5976573	JUL 03,2016	U-295		
		6143329	JUL 03,2016			
074973 001	TRIMETHOPRIM HYDROCHLORIDE; PRIMSOL	5763449	AUG 07,2016			
		5962461	AUG 07,2016			
020326 001	TRIMETREXATE GLUCURONATE; NEUTREXIN	4376858	MAY 09,2004			
		4694007	MAY 20,2006	U-91		
		6017922	MAY 18,2018			
020326 002	TRIMETREXATE GLUCURONATE; NEUTREXIN	6017922	MAY 18,2018			
021288 001	TRIPTORELIN PAMOATE; TRELSTAR	5225205	JUL 20,2010		NCE	JUN 15,2005
020715 001	TRIPTORELIN PAMOATE; TRELSTAR DEPOT	5225205	JUL 20,2010		NCE	JUN 15,2005
		5776885	JUL 07,2015		NCE	JUN 15,2005
020719 001	TROGLITAZONE; PRELAY	4572912	NOV 09,2008			
		5602133	SEP 15,2013	U-173		
		5859037	NOV 13,2017	U-251		
		6011049	NOV 13,2017	U-301		
		6046202	SEP 15,2013	U-317		
020719 002	TROGLITAZONE; PRELAY	4572912	NOV 09,2008			

PRESCRIPTION AND OTC PRODUCT
PATENT AND EXCLUSIVITY DATA
PED and PED represent Pediatric Exclusivity (continued)

APPL/PROD NUMBER	INGREDIENT NAME; TRADE NAME	PATENT NUMBER	PATENT EXPIRES	USE CODE	EX- CLUS CODE	EXCLUS EXPIRES
		5602133	SEP 15,2013	U-173		
		5859037	NOV 13,2017	U-251		
		6011049	NOV 13,2017	U-301		
		6046202	SEP 15,2013	U-317		
020719 003	TROGLITAZONE; PRELAY	4572912	NOV 09,2008			
		5602133	SEP 15,2013	U-173		
		5859037	NOV 13,2017	U-251		
		6011049	NOV 13,2017	U-301		
		6046202	SEP 15,2013	U-317		
020720 001	TROGLITAZONE; REZULIN	4572912	NOV 09,2008			
		5602133	SEP 15,2013	U-173		
		5859037	NOV 13,2017	U-251		
		6011049	NOV 13,2017	U-301		
		6046202	SEP 15,2013	U-317		
020720 002	TROGLITAZONE; REZULIN	4572912	NOV 09,2008			
		5602133	SEP 15,2013	U-173		
		5859037	NOV 13,2017	U-251		
		6011049	NOV 13,2017	U-301		
		6046202	SEP 15,2013	U-317		
020720 003	TROGLITAZONE; REZULIN	4572912	NOV 09,2008			
		5602133	SEP 15,2013	U-173		
		5859037	NOV 13,2017	U-251		
		6011049	NOV 13,2017	U-301		
		6046202	SEP 15,2013	U-317		
020759 001	TROVAFLOXACIN MESYLATE; TROVAN	5164402	DEC 18,2011	U-282	NCE	DEC 18,2002
		5763454	JUN 15,2015	U-282	NCE	DEC 18,2002
		6187341	JAN 20,2019		NCE	DEC 18,2002
020759 002	TROVAFLOXACIN MESYLATE; TROVAN	5164402	DEC 18,2011	U-282	NCE	DEC 18,2002
		5763454	JUN 15,2015	U-282	NCE	DEC 18,2002
		6187341	JAN 20,2019		NCE	DEC 18,2002
021214 001	UNOPROSTONE ISOPROPYL; RESCULA	5001153	SEP 19,2008		NCE	AUG 03,2005
		5151444	MAR 19,2008	U-333	NCE	AUG 03,2005
		5166178	NOV 24,2009	U-333	NCE	AUG 03,2005
		5208256	MAY 21,2011	U-333	NCE	AUG 03,2005
		5212200	MAY 18,2010	U-333	NCE	AUG 03,2005
		5221763	JUN 22,2010		NCE	AUG 03,2005
020586 002	UREA, C-13; BREATHTEK UBT FOR H-PYLORI	4830010	OCT 27,2009	U-147		
		5140993	AUG 24,2009	U-148		
021092 001	UREA, C-13; HELICOSOL				NP	DEC 17,2002
020586 001	UREA, C-13; MERETEK UBT KIT (W/ PRANACTIN)	4830010	OCT 27,2009	U-147		
		5140993	AUG 24,2009	U-148		
020617 001	UREA, C-14; PYTEST	4830010	MAY 15,2006	U-195		
020617 002	UREA, C-14; PYTEST KIT	4830010	MAY 15,2006	U-195		
021289 001	UROFOLLITROPIN; BRAVELLE				I-377	DEC 19,2005
019415 004	UROFOLLITROPIN; FERTINEX	4589402	JUL 26,2004	U-482		
		4725579	FEB 21,2005	U-408		
		4845077	JUL 04,2006	U-408		
		5767067	JUN 16,2015			
019415 005	UROFOLLITROPIN; FERTINEX	4589402	JUL 26,2004	U-482		
		4725579	FEB 21,2005	U-408		
		4845077	JUL 04,2006	U-408		
		5767067	JUN 16,2015			
020675 001	URSODIOL; URSO	4859660	AUG 22,2006		ODE	DEC 10,2004
020487 001	VALACYCLOVIR HYDROCHLORIDE; VALTREX	4957924	JUN 23,2009			
		5879706	JAN 19,2016			
		6107302	JAN 19,2016			
020487 002	VALACYCLOVIR HYDROCHLORIDE; VALTREX	4957924	JUN 23,2009			
		5879706	JAN 19,2016			
		6107302	JAN 19,2016			
020550 001	VALACYCLOVIR HYDROCHLORIDE; VALTREX	4957924	JUN 23,2009		I-389	APR 01,2006
		5879706	JAN 19,2016		I-389	APR 01,2006
		6107302	JAN 19,2016		I-389	APR 01,2006
020550 002	VALACYCLOVIR HYDROCHLORIDE; VALTREX	4957924	JUN 23,2009		I-389	APR 01,2006
		5879706	JAN 19,2016		I-389	APR 01,2006
		6107302	JAN 19,2016		I-389	APR 01,2006
021341 002	VALDECOXIB; BEXTRA	5633272	FEB 13,2015	U-462	NCE	NOV 16,2006
021341 003	VALDECOXIB; BEXTRA	5633272	FEB 13,2015	U-462	NCE	NOV 16,2006
021304 001	VALGANCICLOVIR HYDROCHLORIDE; VALCYTE	6083953	JUL 28,2014	U-384	NE	MAR 29,2004
020593 001	VALPROATE SODIUM; DEPACON				D-72	JAN 24,2005
020892 001	VALRUBICIN; VALSTAR PRESERVATIVE FREE				ODE	SEP 25,2005
020665 001	VALSARTAN; DIOVAN	5399578	MAR 21,2012	U-3	I-365	AUG 14,2005

PRESCRIPTION AND OTC PRODUCT
PATENT AND EXCLUSIVITY DATA
*PED and PED represent Pediatric Exclusivity (*continued*)

APPL/PROD NUMBER	INGREDIENT NAME; TRADE NAME	PATENT NUMBER	PATENT EXPIRES	USE CODE	EX-CLUS CODE	EXCLUS EXPIRES
020665 002	VALSARTAN; DIOVAN	5399578	MAR 21,2012	U-3	I-365	AUG 14,2005
021283 001	VALSARTAN; DIOVAN	5399578	MAR 21,2012		I-365	AUG 14,2005
021283 002	VALSARTAN; DIOVAN	6294197	JUN 18,2017	U-3	I-365	AUG 14,2005
		5399578	MAR 21,2012		I-365	AUG 14,2005
021283 003	VALSARTAN; DIOVAN	6294197	JUN 18,2017	U-3	I-365	AUG 14,2005
		5399578	MAR 21,2012		I-365	AUG 14,2005
		6294197	JUN 18,2017	U-3	I-365	AUG 14,2005
020151 001	VENLAFAXINE HYDROCHLORIDE; EFFEXOR	4535186	DEC 13,2007		PED	NOV 02,2004
		4535186*PED	JUN 13,2008		PED	NOV 02,2004
020151 002	VENLAFAXINE HYDROCHLORIDE; EFFEXOR	4535186	DEC 13,2007		I-325	MAY 02,2004
		4535186*PED	JUN 13,2008		I-325	MAY 02,2004
020151 003	VENLAFAXINE HYDROCHLORIDE; EFFEXOR	4535186	DEC 13,2007		I-325	MAY 02,2004
		4535186*PED	JUN 13,2008		I-325	MAY 02,2004
020151 004	VENLAFAXINE HYDROCHLORIDE; EFFEXOR	4535186	DEC 13,2007		I-325	MAY 02,2004
		4535186*PED	JUN 13,2008		I-325	MAY 02,2004
020151 005	VENLAFAXINE HYDROCHLORIDE; EFFEXOR	4535186	DEC 13,2007		I-325	MAY 02,2004
		4535186*PED	JUN 13,2008		I-325	MAY 02,2004
020151 006	VENLAFAXINE HYDROCHLORIDE; EFFEXOR	4535186	DEC 13,2007		I-325	MAY 02,2004
		4535186*PED	JUN 13,2008		I-325	MAY 02,2004
020699 001	VENLAFAXINE HYDROCHLORIDE; EFFEXOR XR	4535186	DEC 13,2007		PED	NOV 02,2004
		4535186*PED	JUN 13,2008		PED	NOV 02,2004
		5916923	JUN 28,2013	U-398	PED	NOV 02,2004
		5916923*PED	DEC 28,2013	U-398	PED	NOV 02,2004
		6274171	MAR 20,2017		PED	NOV 02,2004
		6274171*PED	SEP 20,2017		PED	NOV 02,2004
		6403120	MAR 20,2017	U-451	PED	NOV 02,2004
		6403120*PED	SEP 20,2017	U-451	PED	NOV 02,2004
		6419958	MAR 20,2017	U-459	PED	NOV 02,2004
		6419958*PED	SEP 20,2017	U-459	PED	NOV 02,2004
		6444708	JUN 28,2013		PED	NOV 02,2004
		6444708*PED	DEC 28,2013		PED	NOV 02,2004
020699 002	VENLAFAXINE HYDROCHLORIDE; EFFEXOR XR	4535186	DEC 13,2007		I-261	FEB 11,2006
		4535186*PED	JUN 13,2008		I-261	FEB 11,2006
		5916923	JUN 28,2013	U-398	I-261	FEB 11,2006
		5916923*PED	DEC 28,2013	U-398	I-261	FEB 11,2006
		6274171	MAR 20,2017		I-261	FEB 11,2006
		6274171*PED	SEP 20,2017		I-261	FEB 11,2006
		6403120	MAR 20,2017	U-451	I-261	FEB 11,2006
		6403120*PED	SEP 20,2017	U-451	I-261	FEB 11,2006
		6419958	MAR 20,2017	U-459	I-261	FEB 11,2006
		6419958*PED	SEP 20,2017	U-459	I-261	FEB 11,2006
		6444708	JUN 28,2013		I-261	FEB 11,2006
		6444708*PED	DEC 28,2013		I-261	FEB 11,2006
020699 003	VENLAFAXINE HYDROCHLORIDE; EFFEXOR XR	4535186	DEC 13,2007		PED	NOV 02,2004
		4535186*PED	JUN 13,2008		PED	NOV 02,2004
		5916923	JUN 28,2013	U-398	PED	NOV 02,2004
		5916923*PED	DEC 28,2013	U-398	PED	NOV 02,2004
		6274171	MAR 20,2017		PED	NOV 02,2004
		6274171*PED	SEP 20,2017		PED	NOV 02,2004
		6403120	MAR 20,2017	U-451	PED	NOV 02,2004
		6403120*PED	SEP 20,2017	U-451	PED	NOV 02,2004
		6419958	MAR 20,2017	U-459	PED	NOV 02,2004
		6419958*PED	SEP 20,2017	U-459	PED	NOV 02,2004
		6444708	JUN 28,2013		PED	NOV 02,2004
		6444708*PED	DEC 28,2013		PED	NOV 02,2004
020699 004	VENLAFAXINE HYDROCHLORIDE; EFFEXOR XR	4535186	DEC 13,2007		I-261	FEB 11,2006
		4535186*PED	JUN 13,2008		I-261	FEB 11,2006
		5916923	JUN 28,2013	U-398	I-261	FEB 11,2006
		5916923*PED	DEC 28,2013	U-398	I-261	FEB 11,2006
		6274171	MAR 20,2017		I-261	FEB 11,2006
		6274171*PED	SEP 20,2017		I-261	FEB 11,2006
		6403120	MAR 20,2017	U-451	I-261	FEB 11,2006
		6403120*PED	SEP 20,2017	U-451	I-261	FEB 11,2006
		6419958	MAR 20,2017	U-459	I-261	FEB 11,2006
		6419958*PED	SEP 20,2017	U-459	I-261	FEB 11,2006
		6444708	JUN 28,2013		I-261	FEB 11,2006
		6444708*PED	DEC 28,2013		I-261	FEB 11,2006
020552 001	VERAPAMIL HYDROCHLORIDE; COVERA-HS	4612008	SEP 16,2003			
		4783337	SEP 16,2003			
		4946687	OCT 02,2007			
		5030456	NOV 07,2008			

PRESCRIPTION AND OTC PRODUCT
PATENT AND EXCLUSIVITY DATA
*PED and PED represent Pediatric Exclusivity (*continued*)

APPL/PROD NUMBER	INGREDIENT NAME; TRADE NAME	PATENT NUMBER	PATENT EXPIRES	USE CODE	EX-CLUS CODE	EXCLUS EXPIRES
		5082668	JAN 21,2009			
		5141752	JUN 27,2006			
		5160744	JUN 27,2011			
		5190765	AUG 14,2007			
		5200196	JAN 22,2008			
		5232705	AUG 31,2010			
		5252338	JUN 27,2011			
		5785994	OCT 22,2009	U-315		
		6096339	APR 04,2017	U-365		
		6146662	AUG 14,2007	U-366		
020552 002	VERAPAMIL HYDROCHLORIDE; COVERA-HS	4612008	SEP 16,2003			
		4783337	SEP 16,2003			
		4946687	OCT 02,2007			
		5030456	NOV 07,2008			
		5082668	JAN 21,2009			
		5141752	JUN 27,2006			
		5160744	JUN 27,2011			
		5190765	AUG 14,2007			
		5200196	JAN 22,2008			
		5232705	AUG 31,2010			
		5252338	JUN 27,2011			
		5785994	OCT 22,2009	U-315		
		6096339	APR 04,2017	U-365		
		6146662	AUG 14,2007	U-366		
019614 001	VERAPAMIL HYDROCHLORIDE; VERELAN	4863742	JUN 19,2007	U-3		
019614 002	VERAPAMIL HYDROCHLORIDE; VERELAN	4863742	JUN 19,2007	U-3		
019614 003	VERAPAMIL HYDROCHLORIDE; VERELAN	4863742	JUN 19,2007	U-3		
019614 004	VERAPAMIL HYDROCHLORIDE; VERELAN	4863742	JUN 19,2007			
020943 001	VERAPAMIL HYDROCHLORIDE; VERELAN PM	4863742	JUN 19,2007			
020943 002	VERAPAMIL HYDROCHLORIDE; VERELAN PM	4863742	JUN 19,2007			
020943 003	VERAPAMIL HYDROCHLORIDE; VERELAN PM	4863742	JUN 19,2007			
021119 001	VERTEPORFIN; VISUDYNE	4883790	JAN 20,2007		I-336	AUG 22,2004
		4920143	APR 24,2007		I-336	AUG 22,2004
		5095030	APR 24,2007		I-336	AUG 22,2004
		5214036	MAY 25,2010		I-336	AUG 22,2004
		5283255	JAN 20,2007	U-357	I-336	AUG 22,2004
		5707608	AUG 02,2015		I-336	AUG 22,2004
		5756541	MAR 11,2016	U-357	I-336	AUG 22,2004
		5770619	JAN 06,2015	U-357	I-336	AUG 22,2004
		5798349	AUG 25,2015	U-357	I-336	AUG 22,2004
		6074666	FEB 05,2012		I-336	AUG 22,2004
014103 003	VINCRISTINE SULFATE; ONCOVIN	4619935	OCT 28,2003			
020388 001	VINORELBINE TARTRATE; NAVELBINE	4307100	JUL 08,2002			
		4307100*PED	JAN 08,2003			
021266 001	VORICONAZOLE; VFEND				NCE	MAY 24,2007
021266 002	VORICONAZOLE; VFEND				NCE	MAY 24,2007
021267 001	VORICONAZOLE; VFEND				NCE	MAY 24,2007
020547 001	ZAFIRLUKAST; ACCOLATE	4859692	SEP 26,2010		I-328	SEP 17,2002
		5294636	DEC 11,2011		I-328	SEP 17,2002
		5319097	DEC 11,2011		I-328	SEP 17,2002
		5482963	JAN 09,2013		I-328	SEP 17,2002
		5583152	SEP 26,2010		I-328	SEP 17,2002
		5612367	MAR 18,2014	U-189	I-328	SEP 17,2002
		6143775	DEC 11,2011		I-328	SEP 17,2002
020547 003	ZAFIRLUKAST; ACCOLATE	4859692	SEP 26,2010		I-328	SEP 17,2002
		5294636	DEC 11,2011		I-328	SEP 17,2002
		5319097	DEC 11,2011		I-328	SEP 17,2002
		5482963	JAN 09,2013		I-328	SEP 17,2002
		5583152	SEP 26,2010		I-328	SEP 17,2002
		5612367	MAR 18,2014	U-189	I-328	SEP 17,2002
		6143775	DEC 11,2011		I-328	SEP 17,2002
020199 001	ZALCITABINE; HIVID	4879277	NOV 07,2006	U-65		
		5028595	JUL 02,2008	U-65		
020199 002	ZALCITABINE; HIVID	4879277	NOV 07,2006	U-65		
		5028595	JUL 02,2008	U-65		
020859 001	ZALEPLON; SONATA	4626538	JUN 06,2008		M-8	FEB 22,2004
020859 002	ZALEPLON; SONATA	4626538	JUN 06,2008		M-8	FEB 22,2004
021036 001	ZANAMIVIR; RELENZA	5360817	NOV 01,2011		NCE	JUL 26,2004
		5648379	JUL 15,2014	U-274	NCE	JUL 26,2004
		6294572	DEC 15,2014		NCE	JUL 26,2004
019655 001	ZIDOVUDINE; RETROVIR	4724232	SEP 17,2005			

PRESCRIPTION AND OTC PRODUCT
PATENT AND EXCLUSIVITY DATA
*PED and PED represent Pediatric Exclusivity (*continued*)

APPL/PROD NUMBER	INGREDIENT NAME; TRADE NAME	PATENT NUMBER	PATENT EXPIRES	USE CODE	EX-CLUS CODE	EXCLUS EXPIRES
		4818538	SEP 17,2005			
		4828838	SEP 17,2005			
		4833130	SEP 17,2005			
		4837208	SEP 17,2005			
019910 001	ZIDOVUDINE; RETROVIR	4724232	SEP 17,2005			
		4818538	SEP 17,2005			
		4833130	SEP 17,2005			
		4837208	SEP 17,2005			
019951 001	ZIDOVUDINE; RETROVIR	4724232	SEP 17,2005			
		4818538	SEP 17,2005			
		4833130	SEP 17,2005			
		4837208	SEP 17,2005			
020518 001	ZIDOVUDINE; RETROVIR	4724232	SEP 17,2005			
		4818538	SEP 17,2005			
		4828838	SEP 17,2005			
		4833130	SEP 17,2005			
		4837208	SEP 17,2005			
020518 002	ZIDOVUDINE; RETROVIR	4724232	SEP 17,2005			
		4818538	SEP 17,2005			
		4828838	SEP 17,2005			
		4833130	SEP 17,2005			
		4837208	SEP 17,2005			
020471 001	ZILEUTON; ZYFLO	4873259	DEC 10,2010	U-168		
020471 003	ZILEUTON; ZYFLO	4873259	DEC 10,2010	U-168		
020458 001	ZINC ACETATE; GALZIN				ODE	JAN 28,2004
020458 002	ZINC ACETATE; GALZIN				ODE	JAN 28,2004
020825 001	ZIPRASIDONE HYDROCHLORIDE; GEODON	4831031	MAR 02,2007		NCE	FEB 05,2006
		5312925	SEP 01,2012		NCE	FEB 05,2006
		6150366	MAY 27,2019		NCE	FEB 05,2006
020825 002	ZIPRASIDONE HYDROCHLORIDE; GEODON	4831031	MAR 02,2007		NCE	FEB 05,2006
		5312925	SEP 01,2012		NCE	FEB 05,2006
		6150366	MAY 27,2019		NCE	FEB 05,2006
020825 003	ZIPRASIDONE HYDROCHLORIDE; GEODON	4831031	MAR 02,2007		NCE	FEB 05,2006
		5312925	SEP 01,2012		NCE	FEB 05,2006
		6150366	MAY 27,2019		NCE	FEB 05,2006
020825 004	ZIPRASIDONE HYDROCHLORIDE; GEODON	4831031	MAR 02,2007		NCE	FEB 05,2006
		5312925	SEP 01,2012		NCE	FEB 05,2006
		6150366	MAY 27,2019		NCE	FEB 05,2006
020919 001	ZIPRASIDONE MESYLATE; GEODON	4831031	MAR 02,2007		NDF	JUN 21,2005
		6110918	MAR 26,2017		NDF	JUN 21,2005
		6232304	APR 01,2017		NDF	JUN 21,2005
		6399777	APR 01,2017		NDF	JUN 21,2005
021223 001	ZOLEDRONIC ACID; ZOMETA	4777163	JUL 24,2007		ODE	AUG 20,2008
		4939130	NOV 13,2007	U-53	ODE	AUG 20,2008
020768 001	ZOLMITRIPTAN; ZOMIG	5466699	NOV 14,2012		NCE	NOV 25,2002
		5863935	NOV 14,2012		NCE	NOV 25,2002
020768 002	ZOLMITRIPTAN; ZOMIG	5466699	NOV 14,2012		NCE	NOV 25,2002
		5863935	NOV 14,2012		NCE	NOV 25,2002
021231 001	ZOLMITRIPTAN; ZOMIG-ZMT	5466699	NOV 14,2012		NCE	NOV 25,2002
019908 001	ZOLPIDEM TARTRATE; AMBIEN	4382938	OCT 21,2006	U-74		
019908 002	ZOLPIDEM TARTRATE; AMBIEN	4382938	OCT 21,2006	U-74		
020789 001	ZONISAMIDE; ZONEGRAN	6342515	DEC 21,2018	U-438	NCE	MAR 27,2005

Section II

LISTING OF B-RATED DRUGS

*Cumulative through the June Supplement to the 2003
"Orange Book"*

The listing of "B-rated" drugs that follows has been extracted by the USPC from the "Orange Book" (*Approved Drug Products with Therapeutic Equivalence Evaluations*) listings. It is intended to provide a concise listing of drug products that the Food and Drug Administration (FDA) has approved but does not list as therapeutically equivalent. For each product with a "B" rating, the "Orange Book" entry for the entire dosage form of that particular drug substance is included so that practitioners will be able to readily determine whether there are other products available containing the same substance and in the same dosage form that are considered by FDA to be therapeutically equivalent.

The fact that a drug product is not listed in the "B listing" does not necessarily mean FDA considers it therapeutically equivalent to other products containing the same drug substance. For example, this listing is derived from the list of FDA-approved products and does not cover "grandfathered" (pre-1938) products that have not gone through the NDA process. Similarly, other products not specifically approved by FDA do not have therapeutic equivalency ratings assigned and do not appear in the "Orange Book."

The two-letter coding system for therapeutic equivalence evaluations used in the "Orange Book" is constructed to allow users to determine quickly whether FDA has evaluated a particular approved product as therapeutically equivalent to other pharmaceutically equivalent products (first letter) and to provide additional information on the basis of FDA's evaluations (second letter). The application and product numbers and final approval date have been omitted (because of space constraints). Please see the "Orange Book" section of this volume for the complete listings.

The two basic categories into which multisource drugs have been placed are indicated by the first letter as follows:

A—Drug products that FDA considers to be therapeutically equivalent to other pharmaceutically equivalent products, i.e., drug products for which:

(1) there are no known or suspected bioequivalence problems. These are designated **AA, AN, AO, AP,** or **AT,** depending on the dosage form; or

(2) actual or potential bioequivalence problems have been resolved with adequate *in vivo* and/or *in vitro* evidence supporting bioequivalence. These are designated AB.

B—Drug products that FDA at this time considers not to be therapeutically equivalent to other pharmaceutically equivalent products, i.e., drug products for which actual or potential bioequivalence problems have not been resolved by adequate evidence of bioequiv-alence. Often the problem is with specific dosage forms rather than with the active ingredients. These are designated BC, BD, BE, BN, BP, BR, BS, BT, BX, or B*.

Drug products designated with a **"B"** code fall under one of three main policies:

(1) the drug products contain active ingredients or are manufactured in dosage forms that have been identified by the Agency as having documented bioequivalence problems or a significant potential for such problems and for which no adequate studies demonstrating bioequivalence have been submitted to FDA; or

(2) the quality standards are inadequate or FDA has an insufficient basis to determine therapeutic equivalence; or

(3) the drug products are under regulatory review.

The specific coding definitions and policies for the "**B**" subcodes are as follows:

B*

Drug products requiring further FDA investigation and review to determine therapeutic equivalence

The code **B*** is assigned to products that were previously assigned an **A** or **B** code if FDA receives new information that raises a significant question regarding therapeutic equivalence that can be resolved only through further Agency investigation and/or review of data and information submitted by the applicant. The **B*** code signifies that the Agency will take no position regarding the therapeutic equivalence of the product until the Agency completes its investigation and review.

BC

Extended-release tablets, extended-release capsules, and extended-release injectables

An extended-release dosage form is defined by the official compendia as one that allows at least a twofold reduction in dosing frequency as compared to that drug presented as a conventional dosage form (e.g., as a solution or a prompt drug-releasing, conventional solid dosage form).

Although bioavailability studies have been conducted on these dosage forms, they are subject to bioavailability differences, primarily because firms developing extended-release products for the same active ingredient rarely employ the same formulation approach. FDA, therefore, does not consider different extended-release dosage forms containing the same active ingredient in equal strength to be therapeutically equivalent unless equivalence between individual products in both rate and extent has been specifically demonstrated through appropriate bioequivalence studies. Extended-release products for which such bioequivalence data have not been submitted are coded **BC**, while those for which such data are available have been coded **AB**.

BD

Active ingredients and dosage forms with documented bioequivalence problems

The **BD** code denotes products containing active ingredients with known bioequivalence problems and for which adequate studies have not been submitted to FDA demonstrating bioequivalence. Where studies showing bioequivalence have been submitted, the product has been coded **AB**.

BE

Delayed-release oral dosage forms

A delayed-release dosage form is defined by the official compendia as one that releases a drug (or drugs) at a time other than promptly after administration. Enteric-coated articles are delayed-release dosage forms.

Drug products in delayed-release dosage forms containing the same active ingredients are subject to significant differences in absorption. Unless otherwise specifically noted, the Agency considers different delayed-release products containing the same active ingredients as presenting a potential bioequivalence problem and codes these products **BE** in the absence of *in vivo* studies showing bioequivalence. If adequate *in vivo* studies have demonstrated the bioequivalence of specific delayed-release products, such products are coded **AB**.

BN

Products in aerosol-nebulizer drug delivery systems

This code applies to drug solutions or powders that are marketed only as a component of, or as compatible with, a specific drug delivery system. There may, for example, be significant differences in the dose of drug and particle size delivered by different products of this type. Therefore, the Agency does not consider different metered aerosol dosage forms containing the same active ingredient(s) in equal strengths to be therapeutically equivalent unless the drug products meet an appropriate bioequivalence standard.

BP

Active ingredients and dosage forms with potential bioequivalence problems

FDA's bioequivalence regulations (21 CFR 320.33) contain criteria and procedures for determining whether a specific active ingredient in a specific dosage form has a potential for causing a bioequivalence problem. It is FDA's policy to consider an ingredient meeting these criteria as having a potential bioequivalence problem even in the absence of positive data demonstrating inequivalence. Pharmaceutically equivalent products containing these ingredients in oral dosage forms are coded **BP** until adequate in vivo bioequivalence data are submitted.

Injectable suspensions containing an active ingredient suspended in an aqueous or oleaginous vehicle have also been coded **BP**. Injectable suspensions are subject to bioequivalence problems because differences in particle size, polymorphic structure of the suspended active ingredient, or the suspension formulation can significantly affect the rate of release and absorption. FDA does not consider pharmaceutical equivalents of these products bioequivalent without adequate evidence of bioequivalence.

BR

Suppositories or enemas that deliver drugs for systemic absorption

The absorption of active ingredients from suppositories or enemas that are intended to have a systemic effect (as distinct from suppositories administered for local effect) can vary significantly from product to product. Therefore, FDA considers pharmaceutically equivalent systemic suppositories or enemas bioequivalent only if *in vivo* evidence of bioequivalence is available. In those cases where *in vivo* evidence is available, the product is coded **AB**. If such evidence is not available, the products are coded **BR**.

BS

Products having drug standard deficiencies

If the drug standards for an active ingredient in a particular dosage form are found by FDA to be deficient so as to prevent an FDA evaluation of either pharmaceutical or therapeutic equivalence, all drug products containing that active ingredient in that dosage form are coded **BS**. For example, if the standards permit a wide variation in pharmacologically active components of the active ingredient such that pharmaceutical equivalence is in question, all products containing that active ingredient in that dosage form are coded **BS**.

BT

Topical products with bioequivalence issues

This code applies mainly to post-1962 dermatologic, ophthalmic, otic, rectal, and vaginal products for topical administration, including creams, ointments, gels, lotions, pastes, and sprays, as well as suppositories not intended for systemic drug absorption. Topical products evaluated as having acceptable performance, but that are not bioequivalent to other pharmaceutically equivalent products or that lack sufficient evidence of bioequivalence will be coded **BT**.

BX

Insufficient data

The code **BX** is assigned to specific drug products for which the data that has been reviewed by the Agency are insufficient to determine therapeutic equivalence under the policies stated in this document. In these situations, the drug products are presumed to be therapeutically inequivalent until the Agency has determined that there is adequate information to make a full evaluation of therapeutic equivalence.

LISTING OF B-RATED DRUGS

ALBUTEROL
Aerosol, Metered; Inhalation
ALBUTEROL
AB	ARMSTRONG PHARMS	0.09MG/INH
AB	GENPHARM	0.09MG/INH
AB	IVAX PHARMS	0.09MG/INH
AB	PLIVA	0.09MG/INH

PROVENTIL
| BN | + SCHERING | 0.09MG/INH |

VENTOLIN
| AB | + GLAXOSMITHKLINE | 0.09MG/INH |

ALBUTEROL SULFATE
Aerosol, Metered; Inhalation
PROVENTIL-HFA
| BX | + 3M | EQ 0.09MG BASE/INH |

VENTOLIN HFA
| BX | + GLAXOSMITHKLINE | EQ 0.09MG BASE/INH |

Tablet, Extended Release; Oral
ALBUTEROL SULFATE
| AB | PLIVA | EQ 4MG BASE |
| AB | PLIVA | EQ 8MG BASE |

PROVENTIL
| BC | SCHERING | EQ 4MG BASE |

VOLMAX
| AB | + MURO | EQ 4MG BASE |
| AB | + | EQ 8MG BASE |

BECLOMETHASONE DIPROPIONATE
Aerosol, Metered; Inhalation
QVAR 40
| | + 3M | 0.04MG/INH |
QVAR 80
| | + 3M | 0.08MG/INH |
VANCERIL
| BN | + SCHERING | 0.042MG/INH |
VANCERIL DOUBLE STRENGTH
| | + SCHERING | 0.084MG/INH |

BECLOMETHASONE DIPROPIONATE MONOHYDRATE
Spray, Metered; Nasal
BECONASE AQ
| BN | + GLAXOSMITHKLINE | EQ 0.042MG DIPROP/SPRAY |
VANCENASE AQ
| BN | + SCHERING | EQ 0.042MG DIPROP/SPRAY |

CHLOROTHIAZIDE; RESERPINE
Tablet; Oral
DIUPRES-250
| BP | MERCK | 250MG;0.125MG |

CHLOROTHIAZIDE; RESERPINE
(continued)
Tablet; Oral
DIUPRES-500
| BP | + MERCK | 500MG;0.125MG |

CHLORPROMAZINE HYDROCHLORIDE
Tablet; Oral
CHLORPROMAZINE HCL
GENEVA PHARMS
BP		10MG
BP		25MG
BP		50MG
BP		100MG
BP		200MG

USL PHARMA
BP		10MG
BP		25MG
BP		50MG
BP		100MG
BP		200MG

THORAZINE
	+ GLAXOSMITHKLINE	
BP		10MG
BP		25MG
BP		50MG
BP	+	100MG
BP	+	200MG

CLINDAMYCIN PHOSPHATE
Gel; Topical
CLEOCIN T
| AB | + PHARMACIA AND UPJOHN | EQ 1% BASE |
CLINDAGEL
| BT | GALDERMA LABS LP | EQ 1% BASE |
CLINDAMYCIN PHOSPHATE
| AB | ALTANA | EQ 1% BASE |

CLOTRIMAZOLE
Cream; Topical
CLOTRIMAZOLE
| AB | TARO | 1% |
LOTRIMIN
| AB | + SCHERING PLOUGH | 1% |
MYCELEX
| BT | BAYER PHARMS | 1% |

COLCHICINE; PROBENECID
Tablet; Oral
COL-PROBENECID
| BP | + WATSON LABS | 0.5MG;500MG |
PROBENECID AND COLCHICINE
| BP | IVAX PHARMS | 0.5MG;500MG |

CORTICOTROPIN
Injectable; Injection
CORTICOTROPIN
	+ ORGANICS LAGRANGE	40 UNITS/ML
		80 UNITS/ML
BC	H.P. ACTHAR GEL	
BC	+ QUESTCOR PHARMS	80 UNITS/ML

CORTISONE ACETATE
Tablet; Oral
CORTISONE ACETATE
PHARMACIA AND UPJOHN
		5MG
		10MG
BP	+	25MG
BP	+ WEST WARD	25MG

CYCLOSPORINE
Capsule; Oral
CYCLOSPORINE
AB1	EON	25MG
AB1		100MG
AB1	PLIVA	25MG
AB1		100MG
AB2	TORPHARM	25MG
AB2		100MG

GENGRAF
ABBOTT
AB1		25MG
BX		50MG
AB1		100MG

NEORAL
NOVARTIS
| AB1 | | 25MG |
| AB1 | | 100MG |

SANDIMMUNE
+ NOVARTIS
AB2		25MG
BX		50MG
AB2	+	100MG

Solution; Oral
CYCLOSPORINE
| AB | ABBOTT | 100MG/ML |
| AB | PLIVA | 100MG/ML |

NEORAL
| AB | + NOVARTIS | 100MG/ML |

SANDIMMUNE
| BX | + NOVARTIS | 100MG/ML |

DEXAMETHASONE
Tablet; Oral
DECADRON
MERCK
AB		0.5MG
BP	+	0.25MG
AB	+	0.75MG
AB		1.5MG
AB		4MG
BP	+	6MG

Listing of B-rated Drugs (continued)

DEXAMETHASONE (continued)
Tablet; Oral

DEXAMETHASONE
BP	PAR PHARM	0.5MG
BP		0.25MG
BP		0.75MG
BP		1.5MG
BP		4MG
BP		6MG
AB	ROXANE	0.5MG
AB		0.75MG
AB		1.5MG
		1MG
		2MG
AB		4MG
BP		6MG

HEXADROL
BP	ORGANON USA	4MG

DIFLORASONE DIACETATE
Cream; Topical

DIFLORASONE DIACETATE
AB1	ALTANA	0.05%
AB2		0.05%
AB1	TARO	0.05%

FLORONE
BX +	PHARMACIA AND UPJOHN	0.05%

FLORONE E
AB2 +	PHARMACIA AND UPJOHN	0.05%

PSORCON
AB1 +	DERMIK LABS	0.05%

DYPHYLLINE
Tablet; Oral

DILOR
BP	SAVAGE LABS	200MG

DILOR-400
BP	SAVAGE LABS	400MG

LUFYLLIN
BP	MEDPOINTE PHARM HLC	200MG
BP		400MG

EPIRUBICIN HYDROCHLORIDE
Injectable; Injection

ELLENCE
BX +	PHARMACIA AND UPJOHN	2MG/ML

ESTRADIOL
Film, Extended Release; Transdermal

ALORA
BX	WATSON LABS	0.1MG/24HR

ESTRADIOL (continued)
Film, Extended Release; Transdermal

ALORA
BX		0.05MG/24HR
BX		0.025MG/24HR
BX		0.075MG/24HR

CLIMARA
AB2 +	BERLEX LABS	0.1MG/24HR
AB2 +		0.05MG/24HR
+		0.06MG/24HR
BX +		0.025MG/24HR
BX +		0.075MG/24HR
BX +		0.0375MG/24HR

ESCLIM
BX	WOMEN FIRST HLTHCARE	0.1MG/24HR
BX		0.05MG/24HR
BX		0.025MG/24HR
BX		0.075MG/24HR
BX		0.0375MG/24HR

ESTRADERM
BX +	NOVARTIS	0.1MG/24HR
BX		0.05MG/24HR

ESTRADIOL
AB2	MYLAN TECHNOLOGIES	0.1MG/24HR
AB2		0.05MG/24HR

VIVELLE
AB1 +	NOVARTIS	0.1MG/24HR
+		0.05MG/24HR
+		0.025MG/24HR
+		0.075MG/24HR
AB1 +		0.0375MG/24HR

VIVELLE-DOT
AB1	NOVARTIS	0.1MG/24HR
AB1		0.05MG/24HR
AB1		0.075MG/24HR
AB1		0.0375MG/24HR

FLUNISOLIDE
Spray, Metered; Nasal

FLUNISOLIDE
AB	BAUSCH AND LOMB	0.025MG/SPRAY

NASALIDE
AB +	IVAX RES	0.025MG/SPRAY

NASAREL
BX +	IVAX RES	0.025MG/SPRAY

FLUOXYMESTERONE
Tablet; Oral

FLUOXYMESTERONE
BP	USL PHARMA	10MG

HALOTESTIN
	PHARMACIA AND UPJOHN	2MG
		5MG

FLUOXYMESTERONE (continued)
Tablet; Oral

HALOTESTIN
BP +		10MG

FOLLITROPIN ALFA/BETA
Injectable; Injection

FOLLISTIM
BX	ORGANON USA INC	75 IU/VIAL
BX		150 IU/VIAL

GONAL-F
BX	SERONO	75 IU/VIAL
BX		150 IU/VIAL

GALLIUM CITRATE, GA-67
Injectable; Injection

GALLIUM CITRATE GA 67
BS	BRISTOL MYERS SQUIBB	2mCi/ML
BS	MALLINCKRODT	2mCi/ML

GLYBURIDE
Tablet; Oral

DIABETA
BX	AVENTIS PHARMS	1.25MG
BX		2.5MG
BX		5MG

GLYBURIDE
AB	AMIDE PHARM	1.5MG
AB		3MG
AB		6MG
AB	COREPHARMA	1.25MG
AB		2.5MG
AB		5MG
AB	TEVA	1.25MG
AB		2.5MG
AB		5MG

GLYBURIDE (MICRONIZED)
AB	AVENTIS PHARMS	1.5MG
AB		3MG
AB		6MG
AB	CLONMEL HLTHCARE	1.5MG
AB		3MG
AB		6MG
AB	GENEVA PHARMS TECH	1.5MG
AB		3MG
AB	MYLAN	1.5MG
AB		3MG
AB		6MG
AB	TEVA	1.5MG
AB		3MG

Listing of B-rated Drugs (continued)

GLYBURIDE (continued)
Tablet; Oral

	GLYBURIDE (MICRONIZED)	
AB		4.5MG
AB		6MG
	GLYNASE	
	PHARMACIA AND UPJOHN	
AB		1.5MG
AB		3MG
+		6MG
	MICRONASE	
	PHARMACIA AND UPJOHN	
AB		1.25MG
AB		2.5MG
AB	+	5MG

HYDROCORTISONE
Tablet; Oral

	CORTEF	
	PHARMACIA AND UPJOHN	
AB		5MG
AB		10MG
AB	+	20MG
	HYDROCORTISONE	
	WEST WARD	
BP		20MG
	HYDROCORTONE	
	MERCK	
BP		10MG
BP	+	20MG

HYDROCORTISONE ACETATE; PRAMOXINE HYDROCHLORIDE
Aerosol, Metered; Topical

	EPIFOAM	
BX	SCHWARZ PHARMA	1%;1%
	HYDROCORTISONE ACETATE 1% AND PRAMOXINE HCL 1%	
	COPLEY PHARM	1%;1%
BX	PROCTOFOAM HC	
BX	SCHWARZ PHARMA	1%;1%

IBUPROFEN
Suspension; Oral

	CHILDREN'S ADVIL	
	WYETH CONS	
BX		100MG/5ML
	IBUPROFEN	
	ALPHARMA	
AB		100MG/5ML
	MOTRIN	
AB	+ MCNEIL CONS SPECLT	100MG/5ML

IRON DEXTRAN
Injectable; Injection

	DEXFERRUM	
	LUITPOLD	
BP		EQ 50MG IRON/ML

IRON DEXTRAN (continued)
Injectable; Injection

	INFED	
BP	+ SCHEIN PROFERDEX	EQ 50MG IRON/ML
BP	NEW RIVER	EQ 50MG IRON/ML

ISOSORBIDE DINITRATE
Capsule, Extended Release; Oral

	DILATRATE-SR	
BC	+ SCHWARZ PHARMA	40MG

LEUCOVORIN CALCIUM
Tablet; Oral

	LEUCOVORIN CALCIUM	
	BARR	
AB		EQ 5MG BASE
AB		EQ 25MG BASE
	GENEVA PHARMS	
	TECH	
	PAR PHARM	
AB		EQ 15MG BASE
AB		EQ 5MG BASE
AB		EQ 25MG BASE
	PHARMACHEMIE	
AB		EQ 25MG BASE
AB		EQ 5MG BASE
	ROXANE	
AB		EQ 10MG BASE
AB		EQ 15MG BASE
AB		EQ 25MG BASE
	XANODYNE PHARM	
AB	+	EQ 5MG BASE
BX		EQ 10MG BASE
AB		EQ 15MG BASE

LEVONORGESTREL
Implant; Implantation

	NORPLANT II	
	POPULATION COUNCIL	
BX	+	75MG/IMPLANT

LEVOTHYROXINE SODIUM
Tablet; Oral

	LEVO-T	
	ALARA PHARM	
BX		0.1MG
BX		0.2MG
BX	+	0.3MG
BX		0.05MG
BX		0.15MG
BX		0.025MG
BX		0.075MG
BX		0.088MG
BX		0.112MG
BX		0.125MG
BX		0.175MG
	LEVOLET	
	VINTAGE PHARMS	
BX		0.1MG
BX		0.2MG
BX		0.3MG

LEVOTHYROXINE SODIUM (continued)
Tablet; Oral

	LEVOLET	
BX		0.05MG
BX		0.15MG
BX		0.025MG
BX		0.075MG
BX		0.088MG
BX		0.112MG
BX		0.125MG
BX		0.137MG
BX		0.175MG
	LEVOTHYROXINE SODIUM	
	MYLAN	
AB		0.1MG
AB		0.2MG
AB		0.3MG
AB		0.05MG
AB		0.15MG
AB		0.025MG
AB		0.075MG
AB		0.088MG
AB		0.112MG
AB		0.125MG
AB		0.175MG
	LEVOXYL	
	JONES PHARMA	
BX		0.1MG
BX		0.2MG
BX	+	0.3MG
BX		0.05MG
BX		0.15MG
BX		0.025MG
BX		0.075MG
BX		0.088MG
BX		0.112MG
BX		0.125MG
BX		0.137MG
BX		0.175MG
	NOVOTHYROX	
	GENPHARM	
BX		0.1MG
BX		0.2MG
BX	+	0.3MG
BX		0.05MG
BX		0.15MG
BX		0.025MG
BX		0.075MG
BX		0.088MG
BX		0.112MG
BX		0.125MG
BX		0.175MG
	SYNTHROID	
	ABBOTT	
BX		0.1MG
BX		0.2MG
BX	+	0.3MG
BX		0.05MG
BX		0.15MG
BX		0.025MG

Listing of B-rated Drugs (continued)

LEVOTHYROXINE SODIUM (continued)
Tablet; Oral

SYNTHROID

BX		0.075MG
BX		0.088MG
BX		0.112MG
BX		0.125MG
BX		0.137MG
BX		0.175MG

THYRO-TABS

	LLOYD	
BX		0.1MG
BX		0.2MG
BX	+	0.3MG
BX		0.05MG
BX		0.15MG
BX		0.025MG
BX		0.075MG
BX		0.088MG
BX		0.112MG
BX		0.125MG
BX		0.175MG

UNITHROID

	STEVENS J	
AB		0.1MG
AB		0.2MG
AB	+	0.3MG
AB		0.05MG
AB		0.15MG
AB		0.025MG
AB		0.075MG
AB		0.088MG
AB		0.112MG
AB		0.125MG
AB		0.175MG

MEDROXYPROGESTERONE ACETATE
Tablet; Oral

MEDROXYPROGESTERONE ACETATE

	BARR	
AB		2.5MG
AB		5MG
AB		10MG

DURAMED PHARM

	BARR	
AB		2.5MG
AB		5MG
AB		10MG

USL PHARMA

BP		10MG

PROVERA

	PHARMACIA AND UPJOHN	
AB		2.5MG
AB		5MG
AB	+	10MG

MENOTROPINS (FSH;LH)
Injectable; Injection

PERGONAL

BX	+ SERONO	75 IU/AMP;75 IU/AMP

MENOTROPINS (FSH;LH) (continued)
Injectable; Injection

REPRONEX

BX	+ FERRING	75 IU/VIAL;75 IU/VIAL

METHYLPHENIDATE HYDROCHLORIDE
Capsule, Extended Release; Oral

METADATE CD

	CELLTECH PHARMS	
BX	+	20MG
		30MG

RITALIN LA

	NOVARTIS	
BX		20MG
		30MG
	+	40MG

METHYLPREDNISOLONE ACETATE
Injectable; Injection

DEPO-MEDROL

	PHARMACIA AND UPJOHN	
BP		20MG/ML
		40MG/ML
	+	80MG/ML

METHYLTESTOSTERONE
Capsule; Oral

TESTRED

	ICN	
BP		10MG

VIRILON

	STAR PHARMS FL	
BP		10MG

Tablet; Oral

ANDROID 10

	ICN	
AB		10MG

ANDROID 25

	ICN	
AB	+	25MG

METHYLTESTOSTERONE

	IMPAX LABS	
BP		10MG
BP		25MG

MORPHINE SULFATE
Capsule, Extended Release; Oral

AVINZA

	LIGAND	
BX	+	30MG
BX	+	60MG
	+	90MG
	+	120MG

KADIAN

	FAULDING PHARMS	
BX	+	20MG
	+	30MG
	+	50MG
BX	+	60MG
	+	100MG

Tablet, Extended Release; Oral

MORPHINE SULFATE

	AB GENERICS	
AB		15MG
AB		30MG

MORPHINE SULFATE (continued)
Tablet, Extended Release; Oral

MORPHINE SULFATE

AB		60MG
AB		100MG
AB		200MG
AB	ENDO PHARMS	15MG
AB		30MG
AB		60MG
AB		100MG
AB		200MG
AB	ESI LEDERLE	15MG
AB	WATSON LABS	100MG

MS CONTIN

	PURDUE FREDERICK	
AB		15MG
AB		30MG
AB	+	60MG
AB		100MG
AB		200MG

ORAMORPH SR

	ELAN PHARMS	
BC		15MG
BC		30MG
BC		60MG
BC		100MG

MUPIROCIN
Ointment; Topical

BACTROBAN

	GLAXOSMITHKLINE	
BX	+	2%

MUPIROCIN

	JOHNSON AND JOHNSON	
BX		2%

NIFEDIPINE
Tablet, Extended Release; Oral

ADALAT CC

	BAYER PHARMS	
AB1		30MG
AB1	+	60MG
AB1	+	90MG

NIFEDIPINE

	BIOVAIL	
AB1		30MG
AB2		30MG
AB1		60MG
AB2		60MG
AB1		90MG
AB1	ELAN PHARM	30MG
AB1		60MG

PROCARDIA XL

	PFIZER	
AB2	+	30MG
AB2	+	60MG
BC	+	90MG

Listing of B-rated Drugs (continued)

NITROGLYCERIN
Film, Extended Release; Transdermal

MINITRAN — 3M

Code		Strength
AB1		0.1MG/HR
AB1		0.2MG/HR
AB1		0.4MG/HR
AB1		0.6MG/HR

NITRO-DUR — + KEY PHARMS

Code		Strength
AB1	+	0.1MG/HR
AB1	+	0.2MG/HR
	+	0.3MG/HR
AB1	+	0.4MG/HR
AB1	+	0.6MG/HR
BX	+	0.8MG/HR

NITROGLYCERIN — HERCON LABS

Code	Strength
AB2	0.2MG/HR
AB2	0.4MG/HR
AB2	0.6MG/HR

MYLAN TECHNOLOGIES

Code	Strength
AB1	0.1MG/HR
AB2	0.1MG/HR
AB2	0.2MG/HR
AB2	0.4MG/HR
AB1	0.4MG/HR
AB1	0.6MG/HR

TRANSDERM-NITRO — + NOVARTIS

Code		Strength
AB2	+	0.1MG/HR
AB2	+	0.2MG/HR
AB2	+	0.4MG/HR
AB2	+	0.6MG/HR
BX	+	0.8MG/HR

NORTRIPTYLINE HYDROCHLORIDE
Capsule; Oral

AVENTYL HCL — LILLY

Code	Strength
BD	EQ 10MG BASE
BD	EQ 25MG BASE

NORTRIPTYLINE HCL — GENEVA PHARMS

Code	Strength
AB	EQ 10MG BASE
AB	EQ 25MG BASE
AB	EQ 50MG BASE
AB	EQ 75MG BASE

GENEVA PHARMS TECH

Code	Strength
AB	EQ 10MG BASE
AB	EQ 25MG BASE
AB	EQ 50MG BASE
AB	EQ 75MG BASE

MYLAN

Code	Strength
AB	EQ 10MG BASE
AB	EQ 25MG BASE
AB	EQ 50MG BASE
AB	EQ 75MG BASE

TARO

Code	Strength
AB	EQ 10MG BASE
AB	EQ 25MG BASE
AB	EQ 50MG BASE
AB	EQ 75MG BASE

NORTRIPTYLINE HYDROCHLORIDE (continued)
Capsule; Oral

NORTRIPTYLINE HCL — TEVA

Code	Strength
AB	EQ 10MG BASE
AB	EQ 10MG BASE
AB	EQ 25MG BASE
AB	EQ 25MG BASE
AB	EQ 50MG BASE
AB	EQ 50MG BASE
AB	EQ 75MG BASE
AB	EQ 75MG BASE

WATSON LABS

Code	Strength
AB	EQ 10MG BASE
AB	EQ 25MG BASE
AB	EQ 50MG BASE
AB	EQ 75MG BASE

PAMELOR — TYCO HLTHCARE

Code	Strength
AB	EQ 10MG BASE
AB	EQ 25MG BASE
AB	EQ 50MG BASE
AB	EQ 75MG BASE

PENICILLIN G BENZATHINE
Injectable; Injection

BICILLIN L-A — + KING PHARMS

Code	Strength
	300,000 UNITS/ML
	600,000 UNITS/ML

PERMAPEN

Code			Strength
BC	PFIZER		600,000 UNITS/ML
BC	+		

PHENDIMETRAZINE TARTRATE
Capsule, Extended Release; Oral

BONTRIL

Code		Strength
BC	MALLINCKRODT	105MG

PHENDIMETRAZINE TARTRATE

Code		Strength
BC	+ EON	105MG

X-TROZINE L.A.

Code		Strength
BC	SHIRE RICHWOOD	105MG

PHYTONADIONE
Injectable; Injection

AQUAMEPHYTON

Code		Strength
BP	+ MERCK	1MG/0.5ML
BP	+	10MG/ML

PHYTONADIONE

Code		Strength
BP	INTL MEDICATION	1MG/0.5ML

VITAMIN K1 — ABBOTT

Code	Strength
BP	1MG/0.5ML
BP	10MG/ML

POTASSIUM CHLORIDE
Tablet, Extended Release; Oral

K+8 — ALRA

Code	Strength
AB	8MEQ

POTASSIUM CHLORIDE (continued)
Tablet, Extended Release; Oral

K+10

Code		Strength
BC	ALRA	10MEQ

K-DUR 10

Code		Strength
AB	KEY PHARMS	10MEQ

K-DUR 20

Code		Strength
AB	+ KEY PHARMS	20MEQ

K-TAB

Code		Strength
BC	ABBOTT	10MEQ

KLOR-CON

Code		Strength
AB	UPSHER SMITH	8MEQ
BC	UPSHER SMITH	10MEQ

KLOR-CON M10

Code		Strength
AB	UPSHER SMITH	10MEQ

KLOR-CON M15

Code		Strength
	UPSHER SMITH	15MEQ

KLOR-CON M20

Code		Strength
AB	UPSHER SMITH	20MEQ

KLOTRIX

Code		Strength
BC	APOTHECON	10MEQ

POTASSIUM CHLORIDE

Code		Strength
BC	ABBOTT	8MEQ
AB	ANDRX PHARMS	10MEQ
AB		20MEQ
AB	COPLEY PHARM	8MEQ
AB	KV PHARM	20MEQ

SLOW-K

Code		Strength
AB	+ NOVARTIS	8MEQ

PREDNISOLONE
Tablet; Oral

PREDNISOLONE

Code		Strength
BX	EVERYLIFE	2.5MG
BX	LANNETT	5MG
BX	MARSHALL PHARMA	5MG
BX	SPERTI	1MG
BX		2.5MG
BX		5MG
BX	+ WATSON LABS	5MG

PREDNISONE
Tablet; Oral

DELTASONE — + PHARMACIA AND UPJOHN

Code		Strength
AB	+	2.5MG
AB	+	5MG
AB	+	10MG
AB	+	20MG
BX	+	50MG

PREDNISONE

Code		Strength
AB	GENEVA PHARMS	10MG
AB		20MG
AB		50MG
BX	MARSHALL PHARMA	5MG

Listing of B-rated Drugs *(continued)*

PREDNISONE *(continued)*
Tablet; Oral

PREDNISONE

AB	MUTUAL PHARM	5MG
AB		10MG
AB		20MG
AB	PVT FORM	5MG
AB	ROXANE	1MG
AB		2.5MG
AB		5MG
AB		10MG
AB		20MG
AB		50MG
AB	TRIGEN	5MG
AB		10MG
AB	VINTAGE PHARMS	5MG
AB		10MG
AB		20MG
AB	WATSON LABS	5MG
AB		10MG
AB		20MG
AB		50MG
AB	WEST WARD	5MG
AB		10MG
AB		20MG
AB		50MG

PROCAINAMIDE HYDROCHLORIDE
Tablet, Extended Release; Oral

PROCAINAMIDE HCL

AB	COPLEY PHARM	1GM
AB		500MG
AB		750MG
AB	GENEVA PHARMS	250MG
AB		500MG
AB		750MG
AB	PLIVA	500MG
AB	WATSON LABS	250MG
AB		500MG
AB		750MG

PROCANBID

AB	+ KING PHARMS	1GM
AB		500MG

PRONESTYL-SR

BC	APOTHECON	500MG

PROMETHAZINE HYDROCHLORIDE
Suppository; Rectal

PHENERGAN

AB	WYETH PHARMS INC	12.5MG
AB	+	25MG
AB		50MG

PROMETHACON

BR	POLYMEDICA	25MG

PROMETHAZINE HCL

AB	ABLE	12.5MG
AB		25MG
AB		50MG
AB	CLAY PARK	12.5MG
AB		25MG
AB	G AND W LABS	12.5MG
AB		25MG
AB	PADDOCK	12.5MG
AB		25MG

PROMETHEGAN

BR	G AND W LABS	50MG

Tablet; Oral

PHENERGAN

BP	WYETH PHARMS INC	12.5MG
BP	+	25MG
		50MG

PROMETHAZINE HCL

BP	GENEVA PHARMS	25MG
BP		50MG
BP	WATSON LABS	25MG
BP		50MG

PROPANTHELINE BROMIDE
Tablet; Oral

PRO-BANTHINE

BP	+ SHIRE LABS	7.5MG
BP	+	15MG

PROPANTHELINE BROMIDE

BP	ROXANE	7.5MG
BP		15MG

PROPRANOLOL HYDROCHLORIDE
Capsule, Extended Release; Oral

INDERAL LA

BX	WYETH PHARMS INC	60MG
BX		80MG
		120MG
		160MG

INNOPRAN XL

BX	+ RELIANT PHARMS	80MG
BX		120MG

PROPYLTHIOURACIL
Tablet; Oral

PROPYLTHIOURACIL

BD	IMPAX LABS	50MG
BD	+ LEDERLE	50MG
BD	PUREPAC PHARM	50MG
BD	WEST WARD	50MG

RESERPINE
Tablet; Oral

RESERPINE

BP	EON	0.1MG
BP		0.25MG

SERPALAN

BP	+ LANNETT	0.1MG
BP		0.25MG

SILVER SULFADIAZINE
Cream; Topical

SILVADENE

AB	+ KING PHARMS	1%

SSD

AB	BASF	1%

SSD AF

BX	BASF	1%

THERMAZENE

AB	KENDALL LP	1%

SOMATROPIN RECOMBINANT
Injectable; Injection

GENOTROPIN

	+ PHARMACIA AND UPJOHN	5.8MG/VIAL
	+	13.8MG/VIAL

GENOTROPIN PRESERVATIVE FREE

	PHARMACIA AND UPJOHN	0.2MG/VIAL
		0.4MG/VIAL
		0.6MG/VIAL
		0.8MG/VIAL
		1.2MG/VIAL
		1.4MG/VIAL
		1.5MG/VIAL
		1.6MG/VIAL
		1.8MG/VIAL
		1MG/VIAL
	+	2MG/VIAL

Listing of B-rated Drugs (continued)

SOMATROPIN RECOMBINANT (continued)
Injectable; Injection

	HUMATROPE	
BX	+ LILLY	5MG/VIAL
BX	+	6MG/VIAL
	+	12MG/VIAL
	+	24MG/VIAL
	NORDITROPIN	
	+ NOVO NORDISK	5MG/1.5ML
		10MG/1.5ML
		15MG/1.5ML
	NUTROPIN	
BX	+ GENENTECH	5MG/VIAL
		10MG/VIAL
	NUTROPIN AQ	
	+ GENENTECH	5MG/ML
	NUTROPIN AQ PEN	
	+ GENENTECH	5MG/ML
	NUTROPIN DEPOT	
BX	+ GENENTECH	13.5MG/VIAL
	+	18MG/VIAL
	+	22.5MG/VIAL
	SAIZEN	
BX	+ SERONO	5MG/VIAL
BX	+	6MG/VIAL
	+	8.8MG/VIAL
	SEROSTIM	
BX	+ SERONO	4MG/VIAL
BX	+	5MG/VIAL
BX	+	6MG/VIAL
	+	8.8MG/VIAL
	TEV-TROPIN	
BX	+ BIO TECH GEN	5MG/ML

TECHNETIUM TC-99M ALBUMIN AGGREGATED KIT
Injectable; Injection

	MACROTEC	
BS	BRACCO	N/A
	PULMOLITE	
BS	CIS	N/A
	TECHNESCAN MAA	
BS	MALLINCKRODT	N/A
	TECHNETIUM TC 99M ALBUMIN AGGREGATED KIT	N/A
BS	DRAXIMAGE	N/A

TESTOSTERONE
Film, Extended Release; Transdermal

	ANDRODERM	
BX	+ WATSON LABS	2.5MG/24HR
	+	5MG/24HR
	TESTODERM	
	+ ALZA	4MG/24HR

TESTOSTERONE (continued)
Film, Extended Release; Transdermal

	TESTODERM	
	+	6MG/24HR
	TESTODERM TTS	
BX	+ ALZA	5MG/24HR
	Gel; Topical	
	ANDROGEL	
BX	+ UNIMED PHARMS	1%
	TESTIM	
BX	+ AUXILIUM A2	1%

THEOPHYLLINE
Capsule, Extended Release; Oral

	AEROLATE III	
	+ FLEMING PHARMS	65MG
	AEROLATE JR	
	+ FLEMING PHARMS	130MG
	AEROLATE SR	
BC	+ FLEMING PHARMS	260MG
	SLO-BID	
BC	+ AVENTIS	50MG
BC		75MG
AB		100MG
AB		125MG
AB		200MG
AB		300MG
	THEO-24	
BC	+ UCB	100MG
BC		200MG
BC		300MG
BC		400MG

THEOPHYLLINE
Tablet, Extended Release; Oral

	THEOPHYLLINE	
AB	+ INWOOD LABS	100MG
AB		125MG
AB		200MG
AB		300MG
	Tablet, Extended Release; Oral	
	QUIBRON-T/SR	
BC	+ MONARCH PHARMS	300MG
	T-PHYL	
BC	+ PURDUE FREDERICK	200MG
	THEO-DUR	
AB	+ SCHERING	100MG
AB		200MG
AB		300MG
AB		450MG
	THEOCHRON	
AB	+ INWOOD LABS	100MG
AB		200MG
AB		300MG
	THEOLAIR-SR	
BC	+ 3M	200MG
		250MG
		300MG
BC	+	500MG

THEOPHYLLINE (continued)
Tablet, Extended Release; Oral

	THEOPHYLLINE	
AB	+ INWOOD LABS	450MG
AB	+ PLIVA	100MG
AB	+	200MG
AB	+	300MG
AB	+	450MG
	UNI-DUR	
BC	SCHERING	400MG
BC		600MG
	UNIPHYL	
BC	+ PURDUE FREDERICK	400MG
BC	+	600MG

TRETINOIN
Gel; Topical

	AVITA	
BT	BERTEK PHARMS	0.025%
	RETIN-A	
AB	+ JOHNSON AND JOHNSON	0.01%
		0.025%
	RETIN-A MICRO	
AB	+ JOHNSON AND JOHNSON	0.1%
		0.04%
	TRETINOIN	
AB	+ SPEAR PHARMS	0.01%
AB		0.025%

TRIAMCINOLONE
Tablet; Oral

	ARISTOCORT	
BP	FUJISAWA HLTHCARE	
	KENACORT	4MG
BP	BRISTOL MYERS SQUIBB	4MG
		8MG
	TRIAMCINOLONE	
BP	+ WATSON LABS	4MG

TRICHLORMETHIAZIDE
Tablet; Oral

	NAQUA	
BP	+ SCHERING	4MG
	TRICHLORMETHIAZIDE	
BP	ABC HOLDING	4MG
BP		2MG
BP	PAR PHARM	4MG

Listing of B-rated Drugs *(continued)*

UROFOLLITROPIN

Injectable; Intramuscular, Subcutaneous
BRAVELLE
BX + FERRING   75 IU/VIAL

Injectable; Subcutaneous
FERTINEX
BX + SERONO   75 IU/AMP

VERAPAMIL HYDROCHLORIDE

Tablet, Extended Release; Oral
COVERA-HS
BC + GD SEARLE LLC   180MG
BC +   240MG

ISOPTIN SR
AB + ABBOTT   120MG
AB +   180MG
AB +   240MG

VERAPAMIL HCL
AB   IVAX PHARMS   120MG
AB   180MG
AB   240MG
AB   MYLAN   120MG
AB   180MG
AB   240MG
AB   PLIVA   240MG

Section III

LISTING OF "PRE-1938" PRODUCTS

The Federal Food, Drug, and Cosmetic Act of 1938 required that drugs be shown to meet certain safety requirements prior to their being marketed. Drugs that were already being marketed at that time were "grandfathered" and were allowed to remain on the market without further regulatory approval if they were labeled with the same conditions of use. Many of these products remain on the market today. Because these products technically have never been *approved* by FDA, they do not appear in the listing of approved drug products with therapeutic equivalence evaluations (the "Orange Book").

The following listing identifies drug products that we believe are considered "pre-1938" or "grandfathered" and are still currently available. The list was developed by comparing an earlier general listing of frequently prescribed "pre-1938" drug entities developed by the U. S. Food and Drug Administration against current dosage form listings in the "Orange Book." The listing is not necessarily complete and comments are welcomed. Additions to or deletions from this list will be shown in future issues of *Update*. The listing of these products should not be interpreted as an attestation by USP as to their actual availability or the general recognition of safety and efficacy of the articles for medical or legal purposes or that a final determination has been made by the FDA.

Acetaminophen, Aspirin, Salicylamide,
    Codeine Phosphate, and Caffeine
  Tablets
Acetaminophen, Codeine Phosphate, and
    Caffeine
  Capsules
  Tablets
Amobarbital
  Tablets
Amobarbital Sodium
  Capsules
  Sterile
Amyl Nitrate
  Inhalant
Antipyrine and Benzocaine
  Solution, Otic
Aspirin and Codeine Phosphate
  Tablets
Chloral Hydrate
  Capsules
  Syrup
  Suppositories
Codeine and Calcium Iodide
  Syrup
Codeine Phosphate
  Injection
  Solution, Oral
  Tablets
  Tablets, Soluble
Codeine Sulfate
  Tablets
  Tablets, Soluble
Colchicine
  Injection
  Tablets
Digitoxin
  Tablets
Digoxin
  Elixir
  Tablets
Ephedrine Sulfate
  Capsules
  Injection
Ergonovine Maleate
  Injection
  Tablets
Ergotamine Tartrate
  Tablets
Erythrityl Tetranitrate
  Tablets

Hydrocodone Bitartrate
  Tablets
Hydrocodone Bitartrate, Aspirin, and Caffeine
  Tablets
Hydromorphone Hydrochloride
  Suppositories
Iodinated Glycerol
  Elixir
  Solution, Oral
  Tablets
Levothyroxine Sodium
  for Injection
Mephobarbital
  Tablets
Methenamine Mandelate
  for Solution, Oral
  Suspension, Oral
  Tablets
  Tablets (Enteric-coated)
Morphine Hydrochloride
  Suppositories
Morphine Sulfate
  Solution, Oral
  Tablets
Nitroglycerin
  Tablets (Sublingual)
Opium Alkaloids Hydrochlorides
  Injection
Opium Tincture
Oxycodone
  Tablets
Oxycodone Hydrochloride
  Solution, Oral
Paregoric
Pentaerythritol Tetranitrate
  Tablets
Phenazopyridine Hydrochloride
  Tablets
Phenobarbital
  Capsules
  Elixir
  Tablets
Phenobarbital Sodium
  Injection
  Sterile
Pilocarpine Hydrochloride
  Solution, Ophthalmic
Pilocarpine Nitrate
  Solution, Ophthalmic
Potassium Bicarbonate
  Effervescent Tablets for Oral Solution

Potassium Bicarbonate and Potassium
    Chloride
  for Effervescent Oral Solution
  Effervescent Tablets for Oral Solution
Potassium Bicarbonate and Potassium Citrate
  Effervescent Tablets for Oral Solution
Potassium Chloride
  Solution, Oral
Potassium Chloride, Potassium Bicarbonate,
    and Potassium Citrate
  Effervescent Tablets for Oral Solution
Potassium Gluconate
  Elixir
  Tablets
Potassium Gluconate and Potassium Chloride
  Solution, Oral
  for Solution, Oral
Potassium Gluconate and Potassium Citrate
  Solution, Oral
Potassium Iodide
  Solution, Oral
  Syrup
  Tablets (Enteric-coated)
Monobasic Potassium Phosphate
  Tablets for Oral Solution
Potassium Phosphates
  Capsules for Oral Solution
  for Solution, Oral
Potassium and Sodium Phosphates
  Capsules for Oral Solution
  for Solution, Oral
  Tablets for Oral Solution
Monobasic Potassium and Sodium Phosphates
  Tablets for Oral Solution
Quinine
  Capsules
Quinine Sulfate
  Tablets
Salsalate
  Capsules
  Tablets
Secobarbital Sodium and Amobarbital Sodium
  Capsules
Sodium Fluoride
  Solution, Oral
  Tablets
Thyroid
  Tablets
Trikates (Potassium Acetate, Potassium
    Bicarbonate, and Potassium Citrate)
  Solution, Oral

Section IV

CHEMISTRY AND COMPENDIAL REQUIREMENTS

ABACAVIR

Chemical name: Abacavir sulfate—(1S,cis)-4-[2-amino-6-(cyclo-propylamino)-9H-purin-9-yl]-2-cyclopentene-1-methanol sulfate (salt) (2:1).

Molecular formula: Abacavir sulfate—$(C_{14}H_{18}N_6O)_2 \cdot H_2SO_4$.

Molecular weight: Abacavir sulfate—670.76.

Description: Abacavir sulfate—White to off-white powder with a melting point around 219 °C followed by decomposition.

pKa: Abacavir sulfate—pK_1: 0.4; pK_2: 5.06.

Solubility: Abacavir sulfate—Soluble at 25 °C in 77 mg per mL distilled water (pH 3.1), in 110 mg per mL 0.1 M hydrochloride (pH 1.6), and in 22 mg per mL 0.1 M sodium hydroxide (pH 12.2).

USP requirements:
Abacavir Sulfate Oral Solution—Not in *USP–NF*.
Abacavir Sulfate Tablets—Not In *USP–NF*.

ABACAVIR, LAMIVUDINE, AND ZIDOVUDINE

For *Abacavir, Lamivudine,* and *Zidovudine*—See individual listings for chemistry information.

USP requirements: Abacavir, Lamivudine, and Zidovudine Tablets—Not in *USP–NF*.

ABCIXIMAB

Source: Derived from the murine immunoglobulin G_1 monoclonal antibody, m7E3.

Chemical name: Immunoglobulin G1, (human-mouse monoclonal c7E3 clone p7E3V$_H$hC$_{gamma4}$ Fab fragment anti-human glycoprotein IIb/IIIa receptor), disulfide with human-mouse monoclonal c7E3 clone p7E3V$_H$hC$_H$light chain.

Molecular weight: Approximately 47,600 daltons.

USP requirements: Abciximab Injection—Not in *USP–NF*.

ACACIA

Description: Acacia NF—Practically odorless. Optical rotation varies depending on the source of Acacia. For example, specific rotation values, calculated on the anhydrous basis and determined on a 1.0% (w/v) solution, usually are between −25° and −35° for *Acacia senegal* and between +35° and +60° for *Acacia seyal*.

NF category: Emulsifying and/or solubilizing agent; suspending and/or viscosity-increasing agent; tablet binder.

Solubility: Acacia NF—Insoluble in alcohol.

NF requirements:
Acacia NF—Preserve in tight containers. The dried gummy exudate from the stems and branches of *Acacia senegal* (Linné) Willdenow or of other related African species of *Acacia* (Fam. Leguminosae). Meets the requirements for Solubility and reaction, Botanic characteristics, Identification, Microbial limits, Water (not more than 15.0%), Total ash (not more than 4.0%), Acid-insoluble ash (not more than 0.5%), Insoluble residue, Arsenic (not more than 3 ppm), Lead (not more than 0.001%), Heavy metals (not more than 0.004%), Starch or dextrin, Organic volatile impurities, and Tannin-bearing gums.

Acacia Syrup NF—Preserve in tight containers, and prevent exposure to excessive heat. The label states the Latin binomial name and, following the official name, the part of the plant source from which the article was derived.

Prepare Acacia Syrup as follows: 100 grams of Acacia, granular or powdered, 1 gram of Sodium Benzoate, 5 mL of Vanilla Tincture, 800 grams of Sucrose, and Purified Water, a sufficient quantity to make 1000 mL. Mix Acacia, Sodium Benzoate, and Sucrose, add 425 mL of Purified Water, and mix. Heat the mixture on a steam bath until dissolved. When cool, remove the scum, add Vanilla Tincture, and sufficient Purified Water to make the product measure 1000 mL, and strain, if necessary.

Meets the requirement for Microbial limits.

ACARBOSE

Source: Obtained from fermentation processes of a microorganism, *Actinoplanes utahensis*.

Chemical name: D-Glucose, O-4,6-dideoxy-4-[[[1 S-(1 alpha,4 alpha,5 beta,6 alpha)]-4,5,6-trihydroxy-3-(hydroxymethyl)-2-cyclohexen-1-yl]amino]-alpha-D-glucopyranosyl-(1→4)-O-alpha-D-glucopyranosyl-(1→4)-.

Molecular formula: $C_{25}H_{43}NO_{18}$.

Molecular weight: 645.60.

Description: White to off-white powder.

pKa: 5.1.

Solubility: Soluble in water.

USP requirements: Acarbose Tablets—Not in *USP–NF*.

ACEBUTOLOL

Chemical name: Acebutolol hydrochloride—Butanamide, N-[3-acetyl-4-[2-hydroxy-3-[(1-methylethyl)amino]propoxy]phenyl]-, (±)-, monohydrochloride.

Molecular formula: Acebutolol hydrochloride—$C_{18}H_{28}N_2O_4 \cdot HCl$.

Molecular weight: Acebutolol hydrochloride—372.89.

Description: Acebutolol Hydrochloride USP—White or almost-white crystalline powder. Melts at about 141 to 144 °C.

pKa: Acebutolol hydrochloride—Apparent in water: 9.4.

Solubility: Acebutolol Hydrochloride USP—Soluble in alcohol and in water; very slightly soluble in acetone and in methylene chloride; practically insoluble in ether.

Other characteristics: Lipid solubility—Low.

USP requirements:
Acebutolol Hydrochloride USP—Preserve in tight containers, and store at controlled room temperature. Contains not less than 98.0% and not more than 102.0% of acebutolol hydrochoride, calculated on the dried basis. Meets the requirements for Identification, pH (4.5–7.0, in a solution [1 in 100]), Melting range (140–144 °C), Loss on drying (not more than 1.0%), Residue on ignition (not more than 0.1%), Heavy metals (not more than 0.002%), and Chromatographic purity.
Acebutolol Hydrochloride Capsules USP—Preserve in tight containers at a temperature not exceeding 30 °C. Contain the labeled amount, within ±10%. Meet the requirements for Identification, Dissolution (80% in 30 minutes in water in Apparatus 2 at 50 rpm), Uniformity of dosage units, and Chromatographic purity.
Acebutolol Hydrochloride Tablets—Not in *USP–NF*.

ACENOCOUMAROL

Chemical name: 2*H*-1-Benzopyran-2-one, 4-hydroxy-3-[1-(4-nitrophenyl)-3-oxobutyl]-.

Molecular formula: $C_{19}H_{15}NO_6$.

Molecular weight: 353.33.

USP requirements: Acenocoumarol Tablets—Not in *USP–NF*.

ACEPROMAZINE

Chemical name: Acepromazine maleate—Ethanone, 1-[10-[3-(dimethylamino)propyl]-10*H*-phenothiazin-2-yl]-, (*Z*)-2-butenedioate (1:1).

Molecular formula: Acepromazine maleate—$C_{19}H_{22}N_2OS \cdot C_4H_4O_4$.

Molecular weight: Acepromazine maleate—442.53.

Description: Acepromazine maleate—Yellow, odorless crystalline powder.

Solubility: Acepromazine maleate—Soluble 1 in 27 of water, 1 in 13 of alcohol, and 1 in 3 of chloroform; slightly soluble in ether.

USP requirements:
Acepromazine Maleate USP—Preserve in well-closed containers, protected from light. Label it to indicate that it is for veterinary use only. Contains not less than 98.0% and not more than 101.0% of acepromazine maleate, calculated on the anhydrous basis. Meets the requirements for Identification, Melting range (136–139 °C), pH (4.0–5.5, in a solution [1 in 100]), Water (not more than 1.0%), Residue on ignition (not more than 0.2%), and Related compounds.
Acepromazine Maleate Injection USP—Preserve in single-dose or in multiple-dose containers, preferably of Type I glass, protected from light. A sterile solution of Acepromazine Maleate in Water for Injection. Label it to indicate that it is for veterinary use only. Contains the labeled amount, within ±10%. Meets the requirements for Identification, Sterility, pH (4.5–5.8), and Injections.
Acepromazine Maleate Tablets USP—Preserve in well-closed containers, protected from light. Label Tablets to indicate that they are for veterinary use only. Contain the labeled amount, within ±10%. Meet the requirement for Identification.

ACETAMINOPHEN

Chemical name: Acetamide, *N*-(4-hydroxyphenyl)-.

Molecular formula: $C_8H_9NO_2$.

Molecular weight: 151.16.

Description: Acetaminophen USP—White, odorless, crystalline powder.

Solubility: Acetaminophen USP—Soluble in boiling water and in 1 *N* sodium hydroxide; freely soluble in alcohol.

USP requirements:
Acetaminophen USP—Preserve in tight, light-resistant containers. Contains not less than 98.0% and not more than 101.0% of acetaminophen, calculated on the anhydrous basis. Meets the requirements for Identification, Melting range (168–172 °C), Water (not more than 0.5%), Residue on ignition (not more than 0.1%), Chloride (not more than 0.014%), Sulfate (not more than 0.02%), Sulfide, Heavy metals (not more than 0.001%), Free *p*-aminophenol (not more than 0.005%), Limit of *p*-Chloroacetanilide (not more than 0.001%), Readily carbonizable substances, and Organic volatile impurities.
Acetaminophen Capsules USP—Preserve in tight containers. Contain the labeled amount, within ±10%. Meet the requirements for Identification, Dissolution (75% in 45 minutes in water in Apparatus 2 at 50 rpm), and Uniformity of dosage units.
Acetaminophen Oral Granules—Not in *USP–NF*.
Acetaminophen Oral Powders—Not in *USP–NF*.
Acetaminophen Oral Solution USP—Preserve in tight containers. Contains the labeled amount, within ±10%. Meets the requirements for Identification, pH (3.8–6.1), and Alcohol content (if present, the labeled amount, within −10% to +15%).
Acetaminophen Suppositories USP—Preserve in well-closed containers, at controlled room temperature or in a cool place. Contain the labeled amount, within ±10%. Meet the requirement for Identification.
Acetaminophen Oral Suspension USP—Preserve in tight containers. A suspension of acetaminophen in a suitable aqueous vehicle. Contains the labeled amount, within ±10%. Meets the requirements for Identification and pH (4.0–6.9).
Acetaminophen Tablets USP—Preserve in tight containers. Label Tablets that must be chewed to indicate that they are to be chewed before swallowing. Contain the labeled amount, within ±10%. Meet the requirements for Identification, Dissolution (80% in 30 minutes in phosphate buffer [pH 5.8] in Apparatus 2 at 50 rpm; and for Tablets labeled as Chewable: 75% in 45 minutes in phosphate buffer [pH 5.8] in Apparatus 2 at 75 rpm), and Uniformity of dosage units.
Acetaminophen Extended-release Tablets—Not in *USP–NF*.

ACETAMINOPHEN AND ASPIRIN

For *Acetaminophen* and *Aspirin*—See individual listings for chemistry information.

USP requirements: Acetaminophen and Aspirin Tablets USP—Preserve in tight containers. Contain the labeled amounts, within ±10%. Meet the requirements for Identification, Dissolution (75% of each active ingredient in 45 minutes in water in Apparatus 2 at 50 rpm), Uniformity of dosage units, and Salicylic acid (not more than 3.0%).

ACETAMINOPHEN, ASPIRIN, AND CAFFEINE

For *Acetaminophen, Aspirin,* and *Caffeine*—See individual listings for chemistry information.

USP requirements:

Acetaminophen, Aspirin, and Caffeine Capsules USP—Preserve in tight containers. Contain the labeled amounts, within ±10%. Meet the requirements for Identification, Dissolution (75% of each active ingredient in 45 minutes in water in Apparatus 1 at 100 rpm), Uniformity of dosage units, and Salicylic acid (not more than 3.0%).

Acetaminophen, Aspirin, and Caffeine Oral Powders—Not in *USP–NF*.

Acetaminophen, Aspirin, and Caffeine Tablets USP—Preserve in well-closed containers. Contain the labeled amounts, within ±10%. Meet the requirements for Identification, Dissolution (75% of each active ingredient in 60 minutes in water in Apparatus 2 at 100 rpm), Uniformity of dosage units, and Limit of salicylic acid (not more than 3.0%).

BUFFERED ACETAMINOPHEN, ASPIRIN, AND CAFFEINE

Source: Caffeine—Coffee, tea, cola, and cocoa or chocolate. May also be synthesized from urea or dimethylurea.

Chemical group: Caffeine—Methylated xanthine.

Chemical name:
Acetaminophen—Acetamide, *N*-(4-hydroxyphenyl)-.
Aspirin—Benzoic acid, 2-(acetyloxy)-.
Caffeine—1*H*-Purine-2,6-dione, 3,7-dihydro-1,3,7-trimethyl-.
Calcium gluconate—D-Gluconic acid, calcium salt (2:1).
Aluminum hydroxide—Aluminum hydroxide.
Magnesium hydroxide—Magnesium hydroxide.

Molecular formula:
Acetaminophen—$C_8H_9NO_2$.
Aspirin—$C_9H_8O_4$.
Caffeine—$C_8H_{10}N_4O_2$ (anhydrous); $C_8H_{10}N_4O_2 \cdot H_2O$ (monohydrate).
Calcium gluconate—$C_{12}H_{22}CaO_{14}$.
Aluminum hydroxide—$Al(OH)_3$.
Magnesium hydroxide—$Mg(OH)_2$.

Molecular weight:
Acetaminophen—151.17.
Aspirin—180.16.
Caffeine—194.19 (anhydrous); 212.21 (monohydrate).
Calcium gluconate—430.38.
Aluminum hydroxide—78.00.
Magnesium hydroxide—58.32.

Description:
Acetaminophen USP—White, odorless, crystalline powder.
Aspirin USP—White crystals, commonly tabular or needle-like, or white, crystalline powder. Is odorless or has a faint odor. Is stable in dry air; in moist air it gradually hydrolyzes to salicylic and acetic acids.
Caffeine USP—White powder or white, glistening needles, usually matted together. Is odorless. Its solutions are neutral to litmus. The hydrate is efflorescent in air.
Calcium Gluconate USP—White, crystalline, odorless granules or powder. Is stable in air. Its solutions are neutral to litmus.
Aluminum Hydroxide Gel USP—White, viscous suspension, from which small amounts of clear liquid may separate on standing.
Dried Aluminum Hydroxide Gel USP—White, odorless, amorphous powder.
Magnesium Hydroxide USP—Bulky, white powder.

pKa: Aspirin—3.5.

Solubility:
Acetaminophen USP—Soluble in boiling water and in 1 *N* sodium hydroxide; freely soluble in alcohol.
Aspirin USP—Slightly soluble in water; freely soluble in alcohol; soluble in chloroform and in ether; sparingly soluble in absolute ether.
Caffeine USP—Sparingly soluble in water and in alcohol; freely soluble in chloroform; slightly soluble in ether.
The aqueous solubility of caffeine is increased by organic acids or their alkali salts, such as citrates, benzoates, salicylates, or cinnamates, which dissociate to yield caffeine when dissolved in biological fluids.
Calcium Gluconate USP—Sparingly (and slowly) soluble in water; freely soluble in boiling water; insoluble in alcohol.
Dried Aluminum Hydroxide Gel USP—Insoluble in water and in alcohol; soluble in dilute mineral acids and in solutions of fixed alkali hydroxides.
Magnesium Hydroxide USP—Practically insoluble in water and in alcohol; soluble in dilute acids.

USP requirements: Buffered Acetaminophen, Aspirin, and Caffeine Tablets—Not in *USP–NF*.

ACETAMINOPHEN, ASPIRIN, SALICYLAMIDE, AND ALUMINUM HYDROXIDE

For *Acetaminophen, Aspirin, Salicylamide,* and *Aluminum Hydroxide*—See individual listings for chemistry information.

USP requirements: Buffered Acetaminophen, Aspirin, and Salicylamide Tablets—Not in *USP–NF*.

ACETAMINOPHEN, ASPIRIN, SALICYLAMIDE, AND CAFFEINE

For *Acetaminophen, Aspirin, Salicylamide,* and *Caffeine*—See individual listings for chemistry information.

USP requirements: Acetaminophen, Aspirin, Salicylamide, and Caffeine Tablets—Not in *USP–NF*.

ACETAMINOPHEN AND CAFFEINE

For *Acetaminophen* and *Caffeine*—See individual listings for chemistry information.

USP requirements:

Acetaminophen and Caffeine Capsules USP—Preserve in tight containers. Contain the labeled amounts, within ± 10%. Meet the requirements for Identification, Dissolution (75% of each active ingredient in 45 minutes in water in Apparatus 1 at 100 rpm), and Uniformity of dosage units.

Acetaminophen and Caffeine Tablets USP—Preserve in tight containers, and store at controlled room temperature. Contain the labeled amounts, within ±10%. Meet the requirements for Identification, Dissolution (75% of each active ingredient in 60 minutes in water in Apparatus 2 at 100 rpm), and Uniformity of dosage units.

ACETAMINOPHEN AND CODEINE

For *Acetaminophen* and *Codeine*—See individual listings for chemistry information.

USP requirements:

Acetaminophen and Codeine Phosphate Capsules USP— Preserve in tight, light-resistant containers. Contain the labeled amounts, within ±10%. Meet the requirements for Identification, Dissolution (75% of each active ingredient in 30 minutes in 0.01 *N* hydrochloric acid in Apparatus 2 at 50 rpm), and Uniformity of dosage units.

Acetaminophen and Codeine Phosphate Oral Solution USP— Preserve in tight, light-resistant containers. Contains the labeled amounts, within ±10%. Meets the requirements for Identification, pH (4.0–6.1), and Alcohol content (if present, the labeled amount, within –10% to +20%).

Acetaminophen and Codeine Phosphate Oral Suspension USP—Preserve in tight, light-resistant containers. A suspension of Acetaminophen and Codeine Phosphate in a suitable aqueous vehicle. Contains the labeled amounts, within ±10%. Meets the requirements for Identification and pH (4.0–6.1).

Acetaminophen and Codeine Phosphate Tablets USP—Preserve in tight, light-resistant containers, and store at controlled room temperature. Contain the labeled amounts, within ±10%. Meet the requirements for Identification, Dissolution (75% of each active ingredient in 30 minutes in 0.01 *N* hydrochloric acid in Apparatus 2 at 50 rpm), and Uniformity of dosage units.

ACETAMINOPHEN, CODEINE, AND CAFFEINE

For *Acetaminophen, Codeine,* and *Caffeine*—See individual listings for chemistry information.

USP requirements: Acetaminophen, Codeine Phosphate, and Caffeine Tablets—Not in *USP–NF*.

ACETAMINOPHEN, DEXTROMETHORPHAN, DOXYLAMINE, AND PSEUDOEPHEDRINE

For *Acetaminophen, Dextromethorphan, Doxylamine,* and *Pseudoephedrine*—See individual listings for chemistry information.

USP requirements:

Acetaminophen, Dextromethorphan Hydrobromide, Doxylamine Succinate, and Pseudoephedrine Hydrochloride Capsules—Not in *USP–NF*.

Acetaminophen, Dextromethorphan Hydrobromide, Doxylamine Succinate, and Pseudoephedrine Hydrochloride Oral Solution USP—Preserve in tight containers. Contains the labeled amounts, within ±10%. Meets the requirements for Identification, pH (4.5–6.3), Alcohol content, if present (within ±10%), and Microbial limits.

Acetaminophen, Dextromethorphan Hydrobromide, Doxylamine Succinate, and Pseudoephedrine Hydrochloride for Oral Solution—Not in *USP–NF*.

ACETAMINOPHEN, DIPHENHYDRAMINE, AND PSEUDOEPHEDRINE

For *Acetaminophen, Diphenhydramine,* and *Pseudoephedrine*— See individual listings for chemistry information.

USP requirements:

Acetaminophen, Diphenhydramine Hydrochloride, and Pseudoephedrine Hydrochloride for Oral Solution—Not in *USP–NF*.

Acetaminophen, Diphenhydramine Hydrochloride, and Pseudoephedrine Hydrochloride Tablets USP—Preserve in tight containers. Contain labeled amounts, within ±10%. Meet the requirements for Identification, Dissolution (75% of each active ingredient in 45 minutes in phosphate buffer [pH 5.8] in Apparatus 2 at 50 rpm, and 75% of each active ingredient in 45 minutes in phosphate buffer [pH 5.8] in Apparatus 2 at 75 rpm for tablets labeled as chewable), and Uniformity of dosage units.

ACETAMINOPHEN AND DIPHENHYDRAMINE

For *Acetaminophen* and *Diphenhydramine*—See individual listings for chemistry information.

USP requirements: Acetaminophen and Diphenhydramine Citrate Tablets USP—Preserve in tight containers. Contain the labeled amounts, within ±10%. Meet the requirements for Identification, Dissolution (75% of each active ingredient in 45 minutes in water in Apparatus 2 at 50 rpm), and Uniformity of dosage units.

ACETAMINOPHEN AND PSEUDOEPHEDRINE

For *Acetaminophen* and *Pseudoephedrine*—See individual listings for chemistry information.

USP requirements:

Acetaminophen and Pseudoephedrine Hydrochloride Capsules—Not in *USP–NF*.

Acetaminophen and Pseudoephedrine Hydrochloride Tablets USP—Preserve in tight containers. Contain the labeled amounts, within ±10%. Meet the requirements for Identification, Dissolution (75% of each active ingredient in 45 minutes in phosphate buffer [pH 5.8] in Apparatus 2 at 50 rpm and 75% of each active ingredient in 45 minutes in phosphate buffer [pH 5.8] in Apparatus 2 at 75 rpm for tablets labeled as chewable), and Uniformity of dosage units.

ACETAMINOPHEN AND SALICYLAMIDE

For *Acetaminophen* and *Salicylamide*—See individual listings for chemistry information.

USP requirements: Acetaminophen and Salicylamide Capsules—Not in *USP–NF*.

ACETAMINOPHEN, SALICYLAMIDE, AND CAFFEINE

For *Acetaminophen, Salicylamide,* and *Caffeine*—See individual listings for chemistry information.

USP requirements:
Acetaminophen, Salicylamide, and Caffeine Capsules—Not in *USP–NF*.
Acetaminophen, Salicylamide, and Caffeine Tablets—Not in *USP–NF*.

ACETAMINOPHEN, SODIUM BICARBONATE, AND CITRIC ACID

For *Acetaminophen, Sodium Bicarbonate,* and *Citric Acid*—See individual listings for chemistry information.

USP requirements: Acetaminophen for Effervescent Oral Solution USP—Preserve in tight containers. Contains, in each 100 grams, not less than 5.63 grams and not more than 6.88 grams of acetaminophen. Meets the requirements for Identification and Minimum fill (when packaged in multiple-unit containers) or Uniformity of dosage units (when packaged in single-unit containers).

ACETAZOLAMIDE

Chemical name: Acetazolamide—Acetamide, *N*-[5-(aminosulfonyl)-1,3,4-thiadiazol-2-yl]-.

Molecular formula: Acetazolamide—$C_4H_6N_4O_3S_2$.

Molecular weight: Acetazolamide—222.25.

Description: Acetazolamide USP—White to faintly yellowish white, crystalline, odorless powder.

Solubility: Acetazolamide USP—Very slightly soluble in water; sparingly soluble in practically boiling water; slightly soluble in alcohol.

USP requirements:
Acetazolamide USP—Preserve in well-closed containers. Contains not less than 98.0% and not more than 102.0% of acetazolamide, calculated on the anhydrous basis. Meets the requirements for Identification, Water (not more than 0.5%), Residue on ignition (not more than 0.1%), Chloride (not more than 0.014%), Sulfate (not more than 0.04%), Selenium (not more than 0.003%, a 200-mg specimen being used), Heavy metals (not more than 0.002%), Silver-reducing substances, Ordinary impurities, and Organic volatile impurities.
Acetazolamide Extended-release Capsules—Not in *USP–NF*.
Acetazolamide for Injection USP—Preserve in Containers for Sterile Solids, preferably of Type III glass. Prepared from Acetazolamide with the aid of Sodium Hydroxide. Suitable for parenteral use. The contents of each container, when constituted as directed in the labeling, yield a solution containing the labeled amount, within −5% to +10%. Meets the requirements for Completeness of solution, Constituted solution, Identification, Bacterial endotoxins, and

pH (9.0–10.0, in a freshly prepared solution [1 in 10]), and for Sterility tests, Uniformity of dosage units, and Labeling under Injections.
Acetazolamide Tablets USP—Preserve in well-closed containers. Contain the labeled amount, within ±5%. Meet the requirements for Identification, Dissolution (75% in 60 minutes in 0.01 *N* hydrochloric acid in Apparatus 1 at 100 rpm), and Uniformity of dosage units.

ACETIC ACID

Chemical name:
Acetic acid—Acetic acid.
Acetic acid, glacial—Acetic acid.

Molecular formula: Acetic acid, glacial—$C_2H_4O_2$.

Molecular weight: Acetic acid, glacial—60.05.

Description:
Acetic Acid NF—Clear, colorless liquid, having a strong, characteristic odor. Specific gravity is about 1.045.
NF category: Acidifying agent; buffering agent.
Glacial Acetic Acid USP—Clear, colorless liquid, having a pungent, characteristic odor. Boils at about 118 °C. Specific gravity is about 1.05.
NF category: Acidifying agent.

Solubility:
Acetic Acid NF—Miscible with water, with alcohol, and with glycerin.
Glacial Acetic Acid USP—Miscible with water, with alcohol, and with glycerin.

USP requirements:
Acetic Acid Irrigation USP—Preserve in single-dose containers, preferably of Type I or Type II glass. May be packaged in suitable plastic containers. A sterile solution of Glacial Acetic Acid in Water for Injection. Contains, in each 100 mL, not less than 237.5 mg and not more than 262.5 mg of glacial acetic acid. Meets the requirements for Identification, Bacterial endotoxins, pH (2.8–3.4), and Injections (except that the container in which it is packaged may be designed to empty rapidly and may exceed 1000 mL in capacity).
Acetic Acid Otic Solution USP—Preserve in tight containers. A solution of Glacial Acetic Acid in a suitable nonaqueous solvent. Contains an amount of glacial acetic acid equivalent to the labeled amount, within −15% to +30%. Meets the requirements for Identification and pH (2.0–4.0, when diluted with an equal volume of water).
Glacial Acetic Acid USP—Preserve in tight containers. Contains not less than 99.5% and not more than 100.5%, by weight, of glacial acetic acid. Meets the requirements for Identification, Congealing temperature (not lower than 15.6 °C), Limit of nonvolatile residue, Chloride, Sulfate, Heavy metals (not more than 5 ppm), and Readily oxidizable substances.

NF requirements:
Acetic Acid NF—Preserve in tight containers. A solution. Contains not less than 36.0% and not more than 37.0%, by weight, of acetic acid. Meets the requirements for Identification, Nonvolatile residue (not more than 0.005%), Chloride, Sulfate, Heavy metals (not more than 0.001%), Readily oxidizable substances, and Organic volatile impurities.
Diluted Acitic Acid NF—Preserve in tight containers. A solution containing, in each 200 mL, not less than 5.7 grams and not more than 6.3 grams of acetic acid.
Prepare Diluted Acetic Acid as follows: 158 mL of Acitic Acid and Purified Water, a sufficient quantity to make 1000 mL. Mix the ingredients.

Meets the requirements for Identification, Heavy metals (not more than 0.001%), Readily oxidizable substances, Limit of nonvolatile residue (not more than 0.005%), Limit of chloride, and Limit of sulfate.

ACETOHEXAMIDE

Chemical group: Sulfonylurea.

Chemical name: Benzenesulfonamide, 4-acetyl-N-[[cyclohexylamino]carbonyl]-.

Molecular formula: $C_{15}H_{20}N_2O_4S$.

Molecular weight: 324.40.

Description: Acetohexamide USP—White, crystalline, practically odorless powder.

Solubility: Acetohexamide USP—Practically insoluble in water and in ether; soluble in pyridine and in dilute solutions of alkali hydroxides; slightly soluble in alcohol and in chloroform.

USP requirements:
Acetohexamide USP—Preserve in well-closed containers. Contains not less than 97.0% and not more than 101.0% of acetohexamide, calculated on the dried basis. Meets the requirements for Identification, Melting range (182.5–187 °C), Loss on drying (not more than 1.0%), Residue on ignition (not more than 0.1%), Selenium (not more than 0.003%, a 200-mg specimen mixed with 200 mg of magnesium oxide being used), Heavy metals (not more than 0.002%), and Organic volatile impurities.
Acetohexamide Tablets USP—Preserve in well-closed containers. Contain the labeled amount, within ±7%. Meet the requirements for Identification, Dissolution (75% in 60 minutes in phosphate buffer [pH 7.6] in Apparatus 1 at 100 rpm), and Uniformity of dosage units.

ACETOHYDROXAMIC ACID

Chemical name: N-Acetyl hydroxyacetamide.

Molecular formula: $C_2H_5NO_2$.

Molecular weight: 75.07.

Description: Acetohydroxamic Acid USP—White, slightly hygroscopic, crystalline powder. Melts, after drying at about 80 °C for 2 to 4 hours, at about 88 °C.

pKa: 9.32–9.4.

Solubility: Acetohydroxamic Acid USP—Freely soluble in water and in alcohol; very slightly soluble in chloroform.

Other characteristics: Chelates metals, especially iron.

USP requirements:
Acetohydroxamic Acid USP—Preserve in tight containers, and store in a cool, dry place. Dried over phosphorus pentoxide for 16 hours, contains not less than 98.0% and not more than 101.0% of acetohydroxamic acid. Meets the requirements for Completeness of solution, Color of solution, Identification, Loss on drying (not more than 1.0%), Residue on ignition (not more than 0.1%), Heavy metals (not more than 0.002%), Limit of hydroxylamine (not more than 0.5%), and Organic volatile impurities.
Acetohydroxamic Acid Tablets USP—Preserve in tight containers. Contain the labeled amount, within ±10%. Meet the requirements for Identification, Dissolution (85% in

30 minutes in 0.01 N hydrochloric acid in Apparatus 1 at 100 rpm), Uniformity of dosage units, and Limit of hydroxylamine (not more than 0.5%).

ACETONE

Chemical name: 2-Propanone.

Molecular formula: C_3H_6O.

Molecular weight: 58.08.

Description: Acetone NF—Transparent, colorless, mobile, volatile liquid, having a characteristic odor. A solution (1 in 2) is neutral to litmus.
NF category: Solvent.

Solubility: Acetone NF—Miscible with water, with alcohol, with ether, with chloroform, and with most volatile oils.

NF requirements: Acetone NF—Preserve in tight containers, remote from fire. Contains not less than 99.0% of acetone, calculated on the anhydrous basis. Meets the requirements for Identification, Specific gravity (not more than 0.789), Water (not more than 0.5%), Nonvolatile residue (not more than 0.004%), and Readily oxidizable substances.
Caution: Acetone is very flammable. Do not use where it may be ignited.

ACETOPHENAZINE

Chemical group: Piperazine phenothiazine.

Chemical name: Acetophenazine maleate—Ethanone, 1-[10-[3-[4-(2-hydroxyethyl)-1-piperazinyl]propyl]-10H-phenothiazin-2-yl]-, (Z) 2-butenedioate (1:2) (salt).

Molecular formula: Acetophenazine maleate—$C_{23}H_{29}N_3O_2S \cdot 2C_4H_4O_4$.

Molecular weight: Acetophenazine maleate—643.71.

Description: Acetophenazine maleate—Fine, yellow powder. Melts at about 165 °C, with decomposition.

Solubility: Acetophenazine maleate—Soluble in water; slightly soluble in acetone and in alcohol.

USP requirements: Acetophenazine Maleate Tablets—Not in USP–NF.

ACETYLCHOLINE

Chemical name: Acetylcholine chloride—Ethanaminium, 2-(acetyloxy)-N,N,N-trimethyl-, chloride.

Molecular formula: Acetylcholine chloride—$C_7H_{16}ClNO_2$.

Molecular weight: Acetylcholine chloride—181.66.

Description: Acetylcholine Chloride USP—White or off-white crystals or crystalline powder.

Solubility: Acetylcholine Chloride USP—Very soluble in water; freely soluble in alcohol; insoluble in ether. Is decomposed by hot water and by alkalies.

USP requirements:
Acetylcholine Chloride USP—Preserve in tight containers. Contains not less than 98.0% and not more than 102.0% of acetylcholine chloride, calculated on the dried basis. Meets the requirements for Identification, Melting range (149–152 °C), Acidity, Loss on drying (not more than

1.0%), Residue on ignition (not more than 0.2%), Organic volatile impurities, and Chloride content (19.3–19.8%, calculated on the dried basis).

Acetylcholine Chloride for Ophthalmic Solution USP—Preserve in Containers for Sterile Solids. A sterile mixture of Acetylcholine Chloride with Mannitol or other suitable diluent, prepared by freeze-drying. Contains the labeled amount, within −10% to +15%. Meets the requirements for Constituted solution, Identification, Acidity, and Water (not more than 1.0%), and for Sterility tests and Uniformity of dosage units.

ACETYLCYSTEINE

Source: The N-acetyl derivative of the naturally occurring amino acid, L-cysteine.

Chemical name: L-Cysteine, *N*-acetyl-.

Molecular formula: $C_5H_9NO_3S$.

Molecular weight: 163.20.

Description: Acetylcysteine USP—White, crystalline powder, having a slight acetic odor.

Solubility: Acetylcysteine USP—Freely soluble in water and in alcohol; practically insoluble in chloroform and in ether.

USP requirements:

Acetylcysteine USP—Preserve in tight containers. Contains not less than 98.0% and not more than 102.0% of acetylcysteine, calculated on the dried basis. Meets the requirements for Identification, Specific rotation (+21° to +27°), pH (2.0–2.8, in a solution [1 in 100]), Loss on drying (not more than 1.0%), Residue on ignition (not more than 0.5%), Heavy metals (not more than 0.001%), and Organic volatile impurities.

Acetylcysteine Injection—Not in *USP–NF*.

Acetylcysteine Solution USP—Preserve in single-unit or in multiple-unit tight containers that effectively exclude oxygen. A sterile solution of Acetylcysteine in water, prepared with the aid of Sodium Hydroxide. Contains the labeled amount, within ±10%. Meets the requirements for Identification, Sterility, and pH (6.0–7.5).

ACETYLCYSTEINE AND ISOPROTERENOL

For *Acetylcysteine* and *Isoproterenol*—See individual listings for chemistry information.

USP requirements: Acetylcysteine and Isoproterenol Hydrochloride Inhalation Solution USP—Preserve in single-dose or in multiple-dose containers, preferably of Type I glass, tightly closed with a glass or polyethylene closure. A sterile solution of Acetylcysteine and Isoproterenol Hydrochloride in water. The label indicates that the Inhalation Solution is not to be used if its color is pinkish or darker than slightly yellow or if it contains a precipitate. Contains the labeled amounts of acetylcysteine, within ±10%, and isoproterenol hydrochloride, within −10% to +15%. Meets the requirements for Color and clarity, Identification, Sterility, and pH (6.0–7.0).

ACETYLTRIBUTYL CITRATE

Chemical name: Acetyltributyl citrate.

Molecular formula: $C_{20}H_{34}O_8$.

Molecular weight: 402.48.

Description: Acetyltributyl Citrate NF—Clear, practically colorless, oily liquid.

NF category: Plasticizer.

Solubility: Acetyltributyl Citrate NF—Insoluble in water; freely soluble in alcohol, in isopropyl alcohol, in acetone, and in toluene.

NF requirements: Acetyltributyl Citrate NF—Preserve in tight containers. Contains not less than 99.0%, calculated on the anhydrous basis. Meets the requirements for Identification, Specific gravity (1.045–1.055), Refractive index (1.4410–1.4425), Acidity, Water (not more than 0.25%), and Heavy metals (0.001%).

ACETYLTRIETHYL CITRATE

Chemical name: Acetyltriethyl citrate.

Molecular formula: $Ci1_4H_{22}O_8$.

Molecular weight: 318.32.

Description: Acetyltriethyl Citrate NF—Clear, practically colorless, oily liquid.

NF category: Plasticizer.

Solubility: Acetyltriethyl Citrate NF—Insoluble in water; freely soluble in alcohol, in isopropyl alcohol, in acetone, and in toluene.

NF requirements: Acetyltriethyl Citrate NF—Preserve in tight containers. Contains not less than 99.0%, calculated on the anhydrous basis. Meets the requirements for Identification, Specific gravity (1.135–1.139), Refractive index (1.432–1.441), Acidity, Water (not more than 0.3%), and Heavy metals (0.001%).

ACITRETIN

Source: A retinoid, an aromatic analog of vitamin A.

Chemical name: 2,4,6,8-Nonatetraenoic acid, 9-(4-methoxy-2,3,6-trimethylphenyl)-3,7-dimethyl, (*all-E*)-.

Molecular formula: $C_{21}H_{26}O_3$.

Molecular weight: 326.43.

Description: Yellow to greenish-yellow crystalline powder which may have a faint odor. Melting range is 210–220 °C.

pKa: 5.

Solubility: Slightly soluble in pH 7.5 aqueous buffer and very slightly soluble in water.

USP requirements:

Acitretin Capsules—Not in *USP–NF*.

Acitretin Tablets—Not in *USP–NF*.

ACRIVASTINE AND PSEUDOEPHEDRINE

Chemical name:

Acrivastine—2-Propenoic acid, 3-[6-[1-(4-methylphenyl)-3-(1-pyrrolidinyl)-1-propenyl]-2-pyridinyl]-, (*E,E*)-.

Pseudoephedrine hydrochloride—Benzenemethanol, alpha-[1-(methylamino)ethyl]-, [*S-(R*,R*)*]-, hydrochloride.

Molecular formula:

Acrivastine—$C_{22}H_{24}N_2O_2$.

Pseudoephedrine hydrochloride—$C_{10}H_{15}NO \cdot HCl$.

Molecular weight:

Acrivastine—348.44.

Pseudoephedrine hydrochloride—201.69.

Description:

Acrivastine—Odorless, white to pale cream crystalline powder.

Pseudoephedrine Hydrochloride USP—Fine, white to off-white crystals or powder, having a faint characteristic odor.

Solubility:

Acrivastine—Soluble in chloroform and in alcohol; slightly soluble in water.

Pseudoephedrine Hydrochloride USP—Very soluble in water; freely soluble in alcohol; sparingly soluble in chloroform.

USP requirements: Acrivastine and Pseudoephedrine Hydrochloride Capsules—Not in *USP–NF*.

ACYCLOVIR

Chemical group: Synthetic purine nucleoside analog.

Chemical name:

Acyclovir—6*H*-Purin-6-one, 2-amino-1,9-dihydro-9-[(2-hydroxyethoxy)methyl]-.

Acyclovir sodium—6*H*-Purin-6-one, 2-amino-1,9-dihydro-9-[(2-hydroxyethoxy)methyl]-, monosodium salt.

Molecular formula:

Acyclovir—$C_8H_{11}N_5O_3$.

Acyclovir sodium—$C_8H_{10}N_5NaO_3$.

Molecular weight:

Acyclovir—225.20.

Acyclovir sodium—247.19.

Description: Acyclovir USP—White to off-white, crystalline powder. Melts at temperatures higher than 250 °C, with decomposition.

Solubility: Acyclovir USP—Slightly soluble in water; soluble in diluted hydrochloric acid; insoluble in alcohol.

USP requirements:

Acyclovir USP—Preserve in tight containers. Contains not less than 98.0% and not more than 101.0% of acyclovir, calculated on the anhydrous basis. Meets the requirements for Identification, Water (not more than 6.0%), Ordinary impurities, and Organic volatile impurities.

Acyclovir Capsules USP—Preserve in tight containers. Contain labeled amount, within ±7%. Meet the requirements for Identification, Uniformity of dosage units, Dissolution (75% in 45 minutes in 0.1 *N* hydrochloric acid in Apparatus 1 at 100 rpm), and Related compunds (not more than 2.0% of guanine and not more than 0.5% of any individual impurity).

Acyclovir Cream—Not in *USP–NF*.

Acyclovir for Injection USP—Preserve in tight containers. Contains the labeled amount, within ±10%. Meets the requirements for Identification, Bacterial endotoxins, pH (11.0–12.5, in a solution containing 50 mg of acyclovir per mL), Water (not more than 5.5%), Chromatographic purity (not more than 1.0% of guanine, not more than 0.15% for any peak having a relative retention time of about 2.0, not more than 0.5% of any other individual impurity, and the total of all other impurities not more than 1.0%), and for Sterility tests, Uniformity of dosage units, and Labeling under Injection.

Acyclovir Ointment USP—Preserve in tight containers. Contains the labeled amount, within ± 10%, in a suitable ointment base. Meets the requirements for Identification, Microbial limits, Minimum fill, and Limit of guanine (not more than 2.0%).

Acyclovir Oral Suspension USP—Preserve in tight containers. Contains the labeled amount, within ±10%. Meets the requirements for Identification, pH (4.5–7.0), Microbial limits, and Limit of guanine (not more than 2.0%).

Acyclovir Tablets USP—Preserve in tight containers. Contain the labeled amount, within ±10%. Meet the requirements for Identification, Uniformity of dosage units, Dissolution (80% in 45 minutes in 0.1 *N* hydrochloric acid in Apparatus 2 at 50 rpm), and Related compunds (not more than 2.0% of guanine, and not more than 0.5% of any other impurity).

Sterile Acyclovir Sodium—Not in *USP–NF*.

ADAPALENE

Chemical name: 2-Naphthalenecarboxylic acid, 6-(4-methoxy-3-tricyclo[3.3.1.1^{3,7}]dec-1-ylphenyl)-.

Molecular formula: $C_{28}H_{28}O_3$.

Molecular weight: 412.52.

Description: White to off-white powder.

Solubility: Soluble in tetrahydrofuran; sparingly soluble in ethanol; practically insoluble in water.

USP requirements: Adapalene Gel—Not in *USP–NF*.

ADEFOVIR

Chemical group: Adefovir is an acyclic nucleotide analog of adenosine monophosphate. Adefovir dipivoxil is a diester prodrug of the active moiety adefovir.

Chemical name: Adefovir dipivoxil—Propanoic acid, 2,2-dimethyl-, [[[2-(6-amino-9*H*-purin-9-yl)ethoxy]methyl]phosphinylidene]bis(oxymethylene) ester.

Molecular formula: Adefovir dipivoxil—$C_{20}H_{32}N_5O_8P$.

Molecular weight: Adefovir dipivoxil—501.47.

Description: Adefovir dipivoxil—White to off-white crystalline powder.

Solubility: Adefovir dipivoxil—Aqueous solubility of 19 milligrams per milliliter at pH 2.0 and 0.4 milligrams per milliliter at pH 7.2.

Other requirements: Adefovir dipivoxil—Partition coefficient—Octanol/aqueous phosphate buffer (log p)—1.91.

USP requirements: Adefovir Dipivoxil Tablets—Not in *USP–NF*.

ADENINE

Chemical name: 1*H*-Purin-6-amine.

Molecular formula: $C_5H_5N_5$.

Molecular weight: 135.13.

Description: Adenine USP—White crystals or crystalline powder. Is odorless.

Solubility: Adenine USP—Very slightly soluble in water; sparingly soluble in boiling water; slightly soluble in alcohol; practically insoluble in ether and in chloroform.

USP requirements: Adenine USP—Preserve in well-closed containers. Contains not less than 98.0% and not more than 102.0% of adenine, calculated on the dried basis. Meets the requirements for Identification, Loss on drying (not more than 1.0%), Residue on ignition (not more than 0.1%), Heavy metals (not more than 0.001%), Organic impurities, Nitrogen content (50.2–53.4%, calculated on the dried basis), and Organic volatile impurities.

ADENOSINE

Chemical name: Adenosine.

Molecular formula: $C_{10}H_{13}N_5O_4$.

Molecular weight: 267.24.

Description: White, odorless, crystalline powder. Melts at about 235 °C.

Solubility: Soluble in water; practically insoluble in alcohol.

USP requirements:
Adenosine USP—Preserve in tight, light-resistant containers, and store at controlled room temperature. Contains not less than 99.0% and not more than 101.0%, calculated on the dried basis. Meets the requirements for Identification, Melting range (233°–238°), Specific rotation (between −68.0° and −72.0°), Acidity and alkalinity, Loss on drying (not more than 0.5%), Heavy metals (0.001%), Limit of ammonia (not more than 0.0004%), Limit of chloride (not more than 0.007%), Limit of sulfate (not more than 0.02%), Residue on ignition (not more than 0.1%), and Chromatographic purity (not more than 0.1% each of guanosine, inosine, and uridine, not more than 0.2% of adenine, and the total of all impurities not more than 0.5%).
Adenosine Injection USP—Preserve in tight, single-dose containers, preferably of Type I glass, and store at controlled room temperature. A sterile solution of Adenosine in Water for Injection. May contain Sodium Chloride. Contains the labeled amount, within ±10%. Meets the requirements for Identification, Bacterial endotoxins (not more than 5.95 USP Endotoxin Units per mg of adenosine), pH (4.5–7.5), Particulate matter, and Chromatographic purity, and Other requirements for Injections.

AGAR

Description: Agar NF—Odorless or has a slight odor.
NF category: Suspending and/or viscosity-increasing agent.

Solubility: Agar NF—Insoluble in cold water; soluble in boiling water.

NF requirements: Agar NF—The dried, hydrophilic, colloidal substance extracted from *Gelidium cartilagineum* (Linné) Gaillon (Fam. Gelidiaceae), *Gracilaria confervoides* (Linné) Greville (Fam. Sphaerococcaceae), and related red algae (Class Rhodophyceae). Meets the requirements for Botanic characteristics, Identification, Microbial limits, Water (not more than 20.0%), Total ash (not more than 6.5%, on a dry-weight basis), Acid-insoluble ash (not more than 0.5%, on a dry-weight basis), Foreign organic matter (not more than 1.0%), Limit of foreign insoluble matter (not more than 1.0%), Arsenic (not more than 3 ppm), Lead (not more than 0.001%), Heavy metals (not more than 0.004%), Limit of foreign starch, Organic volatile impurities, Gelatin, and Water absorption.

MEDICAL AIR

USP requirements: Medical Air USP—Preserve in cylinders or in a low pressure collecting tank. Containers used for Medical Air are not to be treated with any toxic, sleep-inducing, or narcosis-producing compounds, and are not to be treated with any compound that would be irritating to the respiratory tract when the Medical Air is used. (Note: Reduce the container pressure by means of a regulator. Measure the gases with a gas volume meter downstream from the detector tube in order to minimize contamination or change of the specimens.) A natural or synthetic mixture of gases consisting largely of nitrogen and oxygen. Where it is piped directly from the collecting tank to the point of use, label each outlet "Medical Air." Contains not less than 19.5% and not more than 23.5%, by volume, of oxygen. Meets the requirements for Water and oil, Odor, Carbon dioxide (not more than 0.05%), Carbon monoxide (not more than 0.001%), Limit of nitric oxide and nitrogen dioxide (not more than 2.5 ppm), and Sulfur dioxide (not more than 5 ppm).

ALANINE

Chemical name: L-Alanine.

Molecular formula: $C_3H_7NO_2$.

Molecular weight: 89.09.

Description: Alanine USP—White, odorless crystals or crystalline powder.

Solubility: Alanine USP—Freely soluble in water; slightly soluble in 80% alcohol; insoluble in ether.

USP requirements: Alanine USP—Preserve in tight containers, and store at controlled room temperature. Contains not less than 98.5% and not more than 101.5% of alanine, as L-alanine, calculated on the dried basis. Meets the requirements for Identification, Specific rotation (+13.7° to +15.1°), pH (5.5–7.0 in a solution [1 in 20]), Loss on drying (not more than 0.2%), Residue on ignition (not more than 0.15%), Chloride (not more than 0.05%), Sulfate (not more than 0.03%), Iron (not more than 0.003%), Heavy metals (not more than 0.0015%), Chromatographic purity, and Organic volatile impurities.

ALATROFLOXACIN

Chemical name: Alatrofloxacin mesylate—L-Alaninamide, L-alanyl-*N*-[3-[6-carboxy-8-(2,4-difluorophenyl)-3-fluoro-5,8-dihydro-5-oxo-1,8-naphthyridine-2-yl]-3-azabicyclo[3.1.0]hex-6-yl]-, monomethanesulfonate, (1 alpha,5 alpha,6 alpha).

Molecular formula: Alatrofloxacin mesylate—$C_{26}H_{25}F_3N_6O_5 \cdot CH_4O_3S$.

Molecular weight: Alatrofloxacin mesylate—654.62.

Description: Alatrofloxacin mesylate—White to light yellow powder.

USP requirements: Alatrofloxacin Mesylate Injection—Not in *USP–NF*.

ALBENDAZOLE

Chemical name: Carbamic acid, [5-(propylthio)-1*H*-benzimidazol-2-yl]-, methyl ester.

Molecular formula: $C_{12}H_{15}N_3O_2S$.

Molecular weight: 265.33.

Description: Albendazole USP—White to faintly yellowish powder.

Solubility: Albendazole USP—Freely soluble in anhydrous formic acid; very slightly soluble in ether and in methylene chloride; practically insoluble in alcohol and in water.

USP requirements:
Albendazole USP—Preserve in well-closed containers. Contains not less than 98.0% and not more than 102.0% of albendazole, calculated on the dried basis. Meets the requirements for Identification, Loss on drying (not more than 0.5%), Residue on ignition (not more than 0.2%), and Chromatographic purity.
Albendazole Oral Suspension USP—Preserve in tight containers at controlled room temperature. It is Albendazole in an aqueous vehicle. Contains one or more preservatives and dispersing or suspending agents. Label it to indicate that it is for veterinary use only. Contains the labeled amount, within ±10%. Meets the requirements for Identification and pH (4.5–5.5).
Albendazole Tablets USP—Preserve in tight containers. Contain the labeled amount, within ±10%. Tablets intended for veterinary use only are so labeled. Meet the requirements for Identification, Dissolution (80% in 30 minutes in 0.1 *N* hydrochloric acid in Apparatus 2 at 50 rpm), and Uniformity of dosage units.

ALBUMIN HUMAN

Description: Albumin Human USP—Practically odorless, moderately viscous, clear, brownish fluid.

USP requirements: Albumin Human USP—Preserve in tight containers, and store at the temperature recommended by the manufacturer or indicated on the label. A sterile, non-pyrogenic preparation of serum albumin obtained by fractionating material (source blood, plasma, serum, or placentas) from healthy human donors, the source material being tested for the absence of hepatitis B surface antigen. Made by a process that yields a product that is safe for intravenous use. Label it to state that it is not to be used if it is turbid and that it is to be used within 4 hours after the container is entered. Label it also to state the osmotic equivalent in terms of plasma, the sodium content, and the type of source material (venous plasma, placental plasma, or both) from which it was prepared. Label it also to indicate that additional fluids are needed when the 20-grams-per-100-mL or 25-grams-per-100-mL product is administered to a markedly dehydrated patient. Not less than 96% of its total protein is albumin. A solution containing, in each 100 mL, either 25 grams of serum albumin osmotically equivalent to 500 mL of normal human plasma, or 20 grams equivalent to 400 mL, or 5 grams equivalent to 100 mL, or 4 grams equivalent to 80 mL thereof, and containing not less than 93.75% and not more than 106.25% of the labeled amount in the case of the solution containing 4 grams in each 100 mL, and not less than 94.0% and not more than 106.0% of the labeled amount in the other cases. Contains no added antimicrobial agent, but may contain sodium acetyltryptophanate with or without sodium caprylate as a stabilizing agent. Has a sodium content of not less than 130 mEq per liter and not more than 160 mEq per liter. Has a heme content such that the absorbance of a solution, diluted to contain 1% of protein, in a 1-cm holding cell, measured at a wavelength of 403 nanometers, is not more than 0.25. Meets the requirements of the tests for heat stability and for pH, and for Expiration date (the expiration date is not later than 5 years after issue from manufacturer's cold storage [5 °C, 3 years] if labeling recommends storage between 2 and 10 °C; not later than 3 years after issue from manufacturer's cold storage [5 °C, 3 years] if labeling recommends storage at temperatures not higher than 37 °C; and not later than 10 years after date of manufacture if in a hermetically sealed metal container and labeling recommends storage between 2 and 10 °C). Conforms to the regulations of the U.S. Food and Drug Administration concerning biologics.

ALBUMIN MICROSPHERES SONICATED

Source: Microspheres are produced by heat treatment and sonication of appropriately diluted Albumin Human USP, in the presence of octofluoropane gas.

USP requirements: Albumin Microspheres Sonicated Injectable Suspension—Not in *USP–NF*.

ALBUTEROL

Chemical name:
Albuterol—1,3-Benzenedimethanol, alpha¹-[[(1,1-dimethylethyl)amino]methyl]-4-hydroxy-.
Albuterol sulfate—1,3-Benzenedimethanol, alpha¹-[[(1,1-dimethylethyl)amino]methyl]-4-hydroxy-, sulfate (2:1) (salt).

Molecular formula:
Albuterol—$C_{13}H_{21}NO_3$.
Albuterol sulfate—$(C_{13}H_{21}NO_3)_2 \cdot H_2SO_4$.

Molecular weight:
Albuterol—239.31.
Albuterol sulfate—576.70.

Description:
Albuterol USP—White, crystalline powder. Melts at about 156 °C.
Albuterol Sulfate USP—White or practically white powder.

Solubility:
Albuterol USP—Sparingly soluble in water; soluble in alcohol.
Albuterol Sulfate USP—Freely soluble in water; slightly soluble in alcohol, in chloroform, and in ether.

USP requirements:
Albuterol USP—Preserve in well-closed, light-resistant containers. Contains not less than 98.5% and not more than 101.0% of albuterol, calculated on the anhydrous basis. Meets the requirements for Identification, Water (not more than 0.5%), Residue on ignition (not more than 0.1%), and Chromatographic purity.
Albuterol Inhalation Aerosol—Not in *USP–NF*.
Albuterol Tablets USP—Preserve in well-closed, light-resistant containers. Contain an amount of albuterol sulfate equivalent to the labeled amount of albuterol, within ± 10%. Meet the requirements for Identification, Dissolution (80% in 30 minutes in water in Apparatus 2 at 50 rpm), Uniformity of dosage units, and Related compounds.
Albuterol Sulfate USP—Preserve in well-closed, light-resistant containers. Contains not less than 98.5% and not more than 101.0% of albuterol sulfate, calculated on the anhydrous basis. Meets the requirements for Identifica-

tion, Water (not more than 0.5%), Residue on ignition (not more than 0.1%), Chromatographic purity, and Organic volatile impurities.

Albuterol Sulfate Inhalation Aerosol—Not in *USP–NF*.
Albuterol Sulfate Injection—Not in *USP–NF*.
Albuterol Sulfate Powder for Inhalation—Not in *USP–NF*.
Albuterol Sulfate Inhalation Solution—Not in *USP–NF*.
Albuterol Sulfate Oral Solution—Not in *USP–NF*.
Albuterol Sulfate Syrup—Not in *USP–NF*.
Albuterol Sulfate Tablets—Not in *USP–NF*.
Albuterol Sulfate Extended-release Tablets—Not in *USP–NF*.

ALCLOMETASONE

Chemical name: Alclometasone dipropionate—Pregna-1,4-diene-3,20-dione, 7-chloro-11-hydroxy-16-methyl-17,21-bis(1-oxopropoxy)-, (7 alpha,11 beta,16 alpha)-.

Molecular formula: Alclometasone dipropionate—$C_{28}H_{37}ClO_7$.

Molecular weight: Alclometasone dipropionate—521.04.

Description: Alclometasone dipropionate—White powder.

Solubility: Alclometasone dipropionate—Insoluble in water; slightly soluble in propylene glycol; moderately soluble in hexylene glycol.

USP requirements:
Alclometasone Dipropionate USP—Preserve in tight containers. Contains not less than 97.0% and not more than 102.0% of alclometasone dipropionate, calculated on the dried basis. Meets the requirements for Identification, Specific rotation (+21° to +25°), Loss on drying (not more than 0.5%), Residue on ignition (not more than 0.1%), Heavy metals (not more than 0.003%), and Chromatographic purity.

Alclometasone Dipropionate Cream USP—Preserve in collapsible tubes or in tight containers. Contains the labeled amount, within ±10%, in a suitable cream base. Meets the requirements for Identification, Microbial limits, and Minimum fill.

Alclometasone Dipropionate Ointment USP—Preserve in collapsible tubes or in tight containers. Contains the labeled amount, within ±10%, in a suitable ointment base. Meets the requirements for Identification, Microbial limits, and Minimum fill.

ALCOHOL

Chemical name: Ethanol.

Molecular formula: C_2H_6O.

Molecular weight: 46.07.

Description: Alcohol USP—Clear, colorless, mobile, volatile liquid. Has a characteristic odor. Is readily volatilized even at low temperatures, and boils at about 78 °C. Is flammable.
NF category: Solvent.

Solubility: Alcohol USP—Miscible with water and with practically all organic solvents.

USP requirements: Alcohol USP—Preserve in tight containers, remote from fire. Contains not less than 92.3% and not more than 93.8%, by weight, corresponding to not less than 94.9% and not more than 96.0%, by volume, at 15.56 °C, of alcohol. Meets the requirements for Identification, Specific gravity (0.812–0.816 at 15.56 °C, indicating 92.3%–93.8%, by weight, or 94.9–96.0%, by volume, of alcohol), Acidity, Limit of nonvolatile residue, Water-insoluble substances, Aldehydes and

other foreign organic substances, Amyl alcohol and nonvolatile, carbonizable substances, etc., Limit of acetone and isopropyl alcohol, and Methanol.

DEHYDRATED ALCOHOL

Chemical name: Ethanol.

Molecular formula: C_2H_6O.

Molecular weight: 46.07.

Description: Dehydrated Alcohol USP—Clear, colorless, mobile, volatile liquid. Has a characteristic odor. Is readily volatilized even at low temperatures, and boils at about 78 °C. Is flammable.

Solubility: Dehydrated Alcohol USP— Miscible with water and with practically all organic solvents.

USP requirements:
Dehydrated Alcohol USP—Preserve in tight containers, remote from fire. Contains not less than 99.2%, by weight, corresponding to not less than 99.5%, by volume, at 15.56 °C, of alcohol. Meets the requirements for Identification, Specific gravity (not more than 0.7962 at 15.56 °C, indicating not less than 99.2% of alcohol by weight), Acidity, Limit of nonvolatile residue, Water-insoluble substances, Aldehydes and other foreign organic substances, Amyl alcohol and nonvolatile, carbonizable substances, Ultraviolet absorbance, Limit of acetone and isopropyl alcohol, and Methanol.

Dehydrated Alcohol Injection USP—Preserve in single-dose containers, preferably of Type I glass. The container may contain an inert gas in the headspace. It is Dehydrated Alcohol suitable for parenteral use. Meets the requirements for Specific gravity (not more than 0.8035 at 15.56 °C, indicating not less than 96.8%, by weight, of alcohol) and Acidity, for Identification, Limit of nonvolatile residue, Water-insoluble substances, Aldehydes and other foreign organic substances, Amyl alcohol and nonvolatile, carbonizable substances, Ultraviolet absorbance, Limit of acetone and isopropyl alcohol, and Methanol under Dehydrated Alcohol, and for Injections.

DILUTED ALCOHOL

Description: Diluted Alcohol NF—Clear, colorless, mobile liquid, having a characteristic odor.
NF category: Solvent.

NF requirements: Diluted Alcohol NF—Preserve in tight containers, remote from fire. A mixture of Alcohol and water. Contains not less than 41.0% and not more than 42.0%, by weight, corresponding to not less than 48.4% and not more than 49.5%, by volume, at 15.56 °C, of alcohol.

Prepare Diluted Alcohol as follows: 500 mL of Alcohol and 500 mL of Purified Water. Measure the Alcohol and the Purified Water separately at the same temperature, and mix. If the water and the Alcohol and the resulting mixture are measured at 25 °C, the volume of the mixture will be about 970 mL.

Meets the requirements for Specific gravity (0.935–0.937 at 15.56 °C, indicating 41.0–42.0%, by weight, or 48.4–49.5%, by volume, of alcohol), and for the tests under Alcohol (allowance being made for the difference in alcohol concentration).

MYRISTYL ALCOHOL

NF requirements:Myristyl Alcohol NF—Preserve in well-closed containers. Contains not less than 90.0% of myristyl alcohol, the remainder consisting chiefly of related alcohols. Meets the requirements for Identification, Melting range (36°–42°), Acid value (not more than 2), Iodine value (not more than 1), Hydroxyl value, and Organic volatile impurities.

RUBBING ALCOHOL

Description: Rubbing Alcohol USP—Transparent, colorless, or colored as desired, mobile, volatile liquid. Has, in the absence of added odorous constituents, a characteristic odor. Is flammable.

USP requirements: Rubbing Alcohol USP—Preserve in tight containers, remote from fire. Rubbing Alcohol and all preparations under the classification of Rubbing Alcohols are manufactured in accordance with the requirements of the U.S. Treasury Department, Bureau of Alcohol, Tobacco, and Firearms, Formula 23-H (8 parts by volume of acetone, 1.5 parts by volume of methyl isobutyl ketone, and 100 parts by volume of ethyl alcohol) being used. Label it to indicate that it is flammable. Contains not less than 68.5% and not more than 71.5% by volume of dehydrated alcohol, the remainder consisting of water and the denaturants, with or without color additives, and perfume oils. Contains, in each 100 mL, not less than 355 mg of sucrose octaacetate or not less than 1.40 mg of denatonium benzoate. Meets the requirements for Specific gravity (0.8691–0.8771 at 15.56 °C), Limit of nonvolatile residue, and Methanol. Complies with the requirements of the Bureau of Alcohol, Tobacco, and Firearms of the U.S. Treasury Department.

Note: Rubbing Alcohol is packaged, labeled, and sold in accordance with the regulations issued by the U.S. Treasury Department, Bureau of Alcohol, Tobacco, and Firearms.

ALCOHOL AND ACETONE

For *Alcohol* and *Acetone*—See individual listings for chemistry information.

USP requirements:
Alcohol and Acetone Detergent Lotion—Not in *USP–NF*.
Alcohol and Acetone Pledgets—Not in *USP–NF*.

ALCOHOL AND DEXTROSE

For *Alcohol* and *Dextrose*—See individual listings for chemistry information.

USP requirements: Alcohol in Dextrose Injection USP—Preserve in single-dose containers, preferably of Type I or Type II glass. A sterile solution of Alcohol and Dextrose in Water for Injection. The label states the total osmolarity of the solution expressed in mOsmol per liter. Contains the labeled amounts of alcohol, within ±10%, and dextrose, within ±5%. Meets the requirements for Identification, Bacterial endotoxins, pH (3.5–6.5), Heavy metals (not more than 0.0005C%, in which C is the labeled amount, in grams, of Dextrose per mL of Injection), and Limit of 5-hydroxymethylfurfural and related substances, and for Injections.

ALCOHOL AND SULFUR

For *Alcohol* and *Sulfur*—See individual listings for chemistry information.

USP requirements: Alcohol and Sulfur Lotion—Not in *USP–NF*.

ALDESLEUKIN

Chemical group: Related to naturally occurring interleukins, which are lymphokines, a subgroup of the hormone-like glycoprotein growth factors also known as cytokines.

Chemical name: 2-133-Interleukin 2 (human reduced), 125-L-serine-.

Molecular formula: $C_{690}H_{1115}N_{177}O_{203}S_6$.

Molecular weight: 15,600 daltons.

USP requirements: Aldesleukin for Injection—Not in *USP–NF*.

ALEMTUZUMAB

Source: Recombinant DNA-derived humanized monoclonal antibody that is directed against the 21–28 kD cell surface glycoprotein, CD52. The antibody is an IgG1 kappa with variable human framework and constant regions, and complementarity-determining regions from a murine (rat) monoclonal antibody. It is produced in mammalian cell (Chinese hamster overy) suspension culture containing neomycin (neomycin is not detectable in the final product).

Molecular weight: 150 kilodaltons.

Other characteristics: pH: 6.8–7.4.

USP requirements:Alemtuzumab for Injection—Not in *USP–NF*.

ALENDRONATE

Chemical name: Alendronate sodium—Phosphonic acid, (4-amino-1-hydroxybutylidene)bis-, monosodium salt, trihydrate.

Molecular formula: Alendronate sodium—$C_4H_{12}NNaO_7P_2 \cdot 3H_2O$.

Molecular weight: Alendronate sodium—325.12.

Description: Alendronate sodium—White, crystalline, nonhygroscopic powder.

Solubility: Alendronate sodium—Soluble in water; very slightly soluble in alcohol; practically insoluble in chloroform.

USP requirements: Alendronate Sodium Tablets—Not in *USP–NF*.

ALFACALCIDOL

Chemical name: (5Z,7E)-9,10-Secocholesta-5,7,10(19)-triene-1 alpha,3 beta-diol.

Molecular formula: $C_{27}H_{44}O_2$.

Molecular weight: 400.64.

USP requirements:
Alfacalcidol Capsules—Not in *USP–NF*.
Alfacalcidol Oral Drops—Not in *USP–NF*.

Alfacalcidol Injection—Not in *USP–NF*.
Alfacalcidol Oral Solution—Not in *USP–NF*.

ALFENTANIL

Chemical group: Fentanyl derivative (anilinopiperidine-derivative opioid analgesics that are chemically related to anileridine and meperidine).

Chemical name: Alfentanil hydrochloride—Propanamide, *N*-[1-[2-(4-ethyl-4,5-dihydro-5-oxo-1*H*-tetrazol-1-yl)ethyl]-4-(methoxymethyl)-4-piperidinyl]-*N*-phenyl, monohydrochloride, monohydrate.

Molecular formula: Alfentanil hydrochloride—$C_{21}H_{32}N_6O_3 \cdot$ HCl $\cdot$ H_2O.

Molecular weight: Alfentanil hydrochloride—470.99.

Description:
Alfentanil Hydrochloride USP—White to almost white powder.Melting point range, crystals from acetone: 136° – 143° (anhydrous) and reported as crystals from aqueous hydrochloric acid: 116° – 126° (monohydrate).
Alfentanil Injection USP—Clear, colorless solution.

pKa: 6.5.

Solubility: Alfentanil Hydrochloride USP—Soluble in water; freely soluble in methanol, in alcohol, and in chloroform; sparingly soluble in acetone.

Other characteristics: Partition coefficient (octanol:water)—Alfentanil hydrochloride: 130 at pH 7.4.

USP requirements:
Alfentanil Hydrochloride USP—Preserve in tight containers, and store at controlled room temperature. Contains not less than 98.0% and not more than 102.0%, calculated on the anhydrous basis. Meets the requirements for Identification, Water (not more than 4.0%), Residue on ignition (not more than 0.1%), and Chromatographic purity.
Caution: Handle Alfentanil Hydrochloride with great care since it is a potent opioid analgesic. Great care should be taken to prevent inhaling particles of Alfentanil Hydrochloride and exposing the skin to it.
Alfentanil Injection USP—Preserve in tight single-dose or in multiple-dose containers, preferably of Type I glass, and store at controlled room temperature. A sterile solution of Alfentanil Hydrochloride in Water for Injection. Contains an amount of Alfentanil Hydrochloride equivalent to the labeled amount of alfentanil, within ±10%. Meets the requirements for Identification, Bacterial endotoxins, pH (4.0–6.0), Particulate matter, and Chromatographic purity, and under Injections.
Caution: Handle Alfentanil Injection with great care since it is a potent opioid analgesic.

ALGINIC ACID

Chemical name: Alginic acid.

Description: Alginic Acid NF—White to yellowish white, fibrous powder. Odorless, or practically odorless.
NF category: Suspending and/or viscosity-increasing agent; tablet binder; tablet disintegrant.

Solubility: Alginic Acid NF—Insoluble in water and in organic solvents; soluble in alkaline solutions.

NF requirements: Alginic Acid NF—Preserve in well-closed containers. A hydrophilic colloidal carbohydrate extracted with dilute alkali from various species of brown seaweeds (Phaeophyceae). Meets the requirements for Identification, Microbial limits, pH (1.5–3.5, in a 3 in 100 dispersion in water), Loss on drying (not more than 15.0%), Ash (not more than 4.0%), Arsenic (not more than 3 ppm), Lead, Heavy metals (not more than 0.004%), and Acid value (not less than 230, calculated on the dried basis).

ALGLUCERASE

Source: Purified from a large pool of human placental tissue collected from selected donors.

Chemical name: Glucosylceramidase (human placenta isoenzyme protein moiety reduced).

Molecular formula: $C_{2532}H_{3854}N_{672}O_{711}S_{16}$ (protein moiety).

Molecular weight: 59,300 (SDS – PAGE determined).

USP requirements:
Alglucerase Injection—Not in *USP–NF*.
Alglucerase for Injection Concentrate—Not in *USP–NF*.

ALITRETINOIN

Chemical name: 9-*cis*-retinoic acid.

Molecular formula: $C_{20}H_{28}O_2$.

Molecular weight: 300.44.

Description: Alitretinoin—Yellow powder.

Solubility: Alitretinoin—Slightly soluble in ethanol at 25 °C; insoluble in water.

USP requirements: Alitretinoin Topical Gel—Not in *USP–NF*.

ALKYL (C12-15) BENZOATE

Chemical name: Benzoic acid, C12-15 alkyl ester.

Molecular formula: $C_{20}H_{32}O_2$.

Molecular weight: 304 (average).

Description: Alkyl (C12-15) Benzoate NF—Clear, practically colorless, oily liquid.
NF category: Vehicle (oleaginous); emollient.

Solubility: Alkyl (C12-15) Benzoate NF—Soluble in acetone, in alcohol, in isopropyl alcohol, in ethyl acetate, in isopropyl myristate, in isopropyl palmitate, in lanolin, in mineral oil, in vegetable oils, and in volatile silicones; insoluble in water, in glycerin, and in propylene glycol.

NF requirements: Alkyl (C12-15) Benzoate NF—Preserve in tight, light-resistant containers. Consists of esters of a mixture of C12 to C15 primary and branched alcohols and benzoic acid. Meets the requirements for Identification, Specific gravity (0.915–0.935), Acid value (not more than 0.5), Saponification value (169–182), Refractive index (1.483–1.487, determined at 20 °C), Viscosity, Water (not more than 0.3%), and Residue on ignition (not more than 0.5%).

ALLANTOIN

Chemical name: Urea, (2,5-dioxo-4-imidazolidenyl)-.

Molecular formula: $C_4H_6N_4O_3$.

Molecular weight: 158.12.

Description: White crystalline powder. Melts at about 225°, with decomposition.

Solubility: Slightly soluble in water; very slightly soluble in alcohol.

USP requirements: Allantoin USP—Contains not less than 98.5% and not more than 101.0% of allantoin. Meets the requirements for Identification, Angular rotation (−0.10° to +0.10°), Acidity or alkalinity, Loss on drying (not more than 0.1%), Residue on ignition (not more than 0.1%), Reducing substance (the solution remains violet for at least 10 minutes), and Related compounds.

ALLOPURINOL

Chemical group: A structural analogue of hypoxanthine.

Chemical name: 4H-Pyrazolo[3,4-d]pyrimidin-4-one, 1,5-dihydro-.

Molecular formula: $C_5H_4N_4O$.

Molecular weight: 136.11.

Description: Allopurinol USP—Fluffy white to off-white powder, having only a slight odor.

pKa: 10.2.

Solubility: Allopurinol USP—Very slightly soluble in water and in alcohol; soluble in solutions of potassium and sodium hydroxides; practically insoluble in chloroform and in ether.

USP requirements:
Allopurinol USP—Preserve in well-closed containers. Contains not less than 98.0% and not more than 101.0% of allopurinol, calculated on the dried basis. Meets the requirements for Identification, Loss on drying (not more than 0.5%), Chromatographic purity, and Organic volatile impurities.
Allopurinol Injection—Not in *USP–NF*.
Allopurinol Tablets USP—Preserve in well-closed containers. Contain the labeled amount, within ±7%. Meet the requirements for Identification, Dissolution (75% in 45 minutes in 0.01 N hydrochloric acid in Apparatus 2 at 75 rpm), and Uniformity of dosage units.
Allopurinol Sodium for Injection—Not in *USP–NF*.

ALLYL ISOTHIOCYANATE

Chemical name: 3-Isothiocyanato-1-propene.

Molecular formula: C_4H_5NS.

Molecular weight: 99.16.

Description: Allyl Isothiocyanate USP—Colorless to pale yellow, very refractive, liquid. Pungent, irritating odor. (Caution: Lachrymator.)

Solubility: Allyl Isothiocyanate USP—Miscible with alcohol, with carbon disulfide, and with ether. Slightly soluble in water.

USP requirements: Allyl Isothiocyanate USP—Preserve in tight containers. Contains not less than 93.0% and not more than 105.0% of allyl isothiocyanate. Meets the requirements for Identification, Specific gravity (1.013–1.020), Refractive index (1.527–1.531, determined at 20 °C), Distilling range (148–154 °C), and Limit of phenols.

Caution: Allyl Isothiocyanate is a potent lachrymator, with a pungent irritating odor. Care should be taken to protect the eyes, to prevent inhalation of fumes, and to avoid tasting.

ALMOND OIL

Description: Almond Oil NF—Clear, pale straw-colored or colorless, oily liquid. Remains clear at −10 °C, and does not congeal until cooled to almost −20 °C.

NF category: Flavors and perfumes.

Solubility: Almond Oil NF—Slightly soluble in alcohol; miscible with ether, with chloroform, with benzene, and with solvent hexane.

NF requirements: Almond Oil NF—Preserve in tight containers. The fixed oil obtained by expression from the kernels of varieties of *Prunus amygdalus* Batsch (Fam. Rosaceae). Meets the requirements for Specific gravity (0.910–0.915), Foreign kernel oils, Cottonseed oil, Sesame oil, Mineral oil and foreign fatty oils, Foreign oils, Free fatty acids, Iodine value (95–105), and Saponification value (190–200).

ALMOTRIPTAN

Source: Synthetic Almotriptan is structurally related to serotonin (5-hydroxytryptamine, 5-HT).

Chemical name: Pyrolidine, 1-[[[3-[2-(dimethylamino)ethyl]-1H-indol-5-yl]methyl]sulfonyl]-.

Molecular formula: $C_{17}H_{25}N_3O_2S$.

Molecular weight: 335.47.

Description: White to slightly yellow crystalline powder.

Solubiliuty: Soluble in water.

USP requirements: Almotriptan Tablets—Not in *USP–NF*.

ALOE

Description: Aloe USP—Has a characteristic, somewhat sour and disagreeable, odor.

USP requirements: Aloe USP—The dried latex of the leaves of *Aloe barbadensis* Miller (*Aloe vera* Linné), known in commerce as Curaçao Aloe, or of *Aloe ferox* Miller and hybrids of this species with *Aloe africana* Miller and *Aloe spicata* Baker, known in commerce as Cape Aloe (Fam. Liliaceae). Yields not less than 50.0% of water-soluble extractive. Meets the requirements for Botanic characteristics, Identification, Water (not more than 12.0%), Total ash (not more than 4.0%), and Alcohol-insoluble substances (not more than 10.0%).

ALOSETRON

Chemical name: Alosetron hydrochloride—1*H*-Pyridol[4,3-*b*]indol-1-one,2,3,4,5-tetrahydro-5-methyl-2-[5-methyl-1*H*-imidazol-4-yl)methyl]-, monohydrochloride.

Molecular formula: Alosetron hydrochloride—$C_{17}H_{18}N_4O \cdot HCl$.

Molecular weight: Alosetron hydrochloride—330.81.

Description: Alosetron hydrochloride—White to beige solid.

Solubility: Alosetron hydrochloride—Has a solubility of 61 mg/mL in water, 42 mg/mL in 0.1 *M* hydrochloric acid, 0.3 mg/mL in pH 6 phosphate buffer, and less than 0.1 mg/mL in pH 8 phosphate buffer.

USP requirements: Alosetron Tablets—Not in *USP–NF*.

ALPHA₁-PROTEINASE INHIBITOR, HUMAN

Source: Prepared from pooled human plasma of normal donors by modification and refinements of the cold ethanol method of Cohn.

Other characteristics: When alpha₁-PI is reconstituted, it has a pH of 6.6–7.4.

USP requirements: Alpha₁-proteinase Inhibitor, Human, for Injection—Not in *USP–NF*.

ALPRAZOLAM

Chemical name: 4*H*-[1,2,4]Triazolo[4,3-*a*][1,4]benzodiazepine, 8-chloro-1-methyl-6-phenyl-.

Molecular formula: $C_{17}H_{13}ClN_4$.

Molecular weight: 308.76.

Description: Alprazolam USP—A white to off-white crystalline powder. Melts at about 225 °C.

Solubility: Alprazolam USP—Insoluble in water; slightly soluble in ethyl acetate; sparingly soluble in acetone; soluble in alcohol; freely soluble in chloroform.

USP requirements:
Alprazolam USP—Preserve in well-closed containers. Contains not less than 98.0% and not more than 102.0% of alprazolam. Meets the requirements for Identification, Loss on drying (not more than 0.5%), Residue on ignition (not more than 0.5%), Heavy metals (not more than 0.002%), and Chromatographic purity.

Caution: Care should be taken to prevent inhaling particles of Alprazolam and exposing the skin to it.
Alprazolam Oral Solution—Not in *USP–NF*.
Alprazolam Tablets USP—Preserve in tight, light-resistant containers, and store at controlled room temperature. Contain the labeled amount, within ±10%. Meet the requirements for Identification, Dissolution (80% in 30 minutes in Working buffer solution in Apparatus 1 at 100 rpm), and Uniformity of dosage units.

ALPROSTADIL

Chemical name: Prost-13-en-1-oic acid, 11,15-dihydroxy-9-oxo-, (11 alpha,13*E*,15*S*)-.

Molecular formula: $C_{20}H_{34}O_5$.

Molecular weight: 354.48.

Description: Alprostadil USP—A white to off-white, crystalline powder. Melts at about 110 °C.

pKa: 6.3 in 60% ethanol in water.

Solubility: Alprostadil USP—Soluble in water; freely soluble in alcohol; soluble in acetone; slightly soluble in ethyl acetate; very slightly soluble in chloroform and in ether.

USP requirements:
Alprostadil USP—Preserve in tight containers, and store in a refrigerator. Contains not less than 95.0% and not more than 105.0% of alprostadil, calculated on the anhydrous basis. Meets the requirements for Identification, Water (not more than 0.5%, using 0.5 grams), Residue on ignition (not more than 0.5%, using 0.3 grams), Limit of chromium (not more than 0.002%), Limit of rhodium (not more than 0.002%), Limit of foreign prostaglandins (not more than 3.0% total and no single foreign prostaglandin greater than 2.0%), and Organic volatile impurities.

Caution: Great care should be taken to prevent inhaling particles of Alprostadil and exposing the skin to it.
Alprostadil for Injection—Not in *USP–NF*.
Alprostadil Injection USP—Preserve in tight, single-dose containers, preferably of Type I glass. Store in a refrigerator. A sterile solution of Alprostadil in Dehydrated Alcohol. Contains the labeled amount, within −10% to +15%. Meets the requirements for Identification, Bacterial endotoxins, Sterility, Water (not more than 0.4%), and Injections.
Alprostadil Suppositories—Not in *USP–NF*.

ALTEPLASE

Source: An enzymatic glycoprotein composed of 527 amino acids. It is produced by recombinant DNA technology using the complementary DNA for natural human tissue-type plasminogen activator obtained from a human melanoma cell line.

Chemical name: Plasminogen activator (human tissue-type 2-chain form protein moiety).

Molecular formula: $C_{2569}H_{3894}N_{746}O_{781}S_{40}$.

Molecular weight: 59,007.61.

USP requirements:
Alteplase USP—Preserve in tight containers, and store in the frozen state at a temperature of −20 °C or below. A highly purified glycosylated serine protease with fibrin-binding properties and plasminogen-specific proteolytic activities. Produced by recombinant DNA synthesis in mammalian cell culture. Has a biological potency of not less than 90.0% and not more than 115.0% of the potency stated on the label, the potency being 580,000 USP Alteplase Units per mg of protein. The presence of host cell DNA and host cell protein impurities in Alteplase is process-specific; the limits of these impurities are determined by validated methods. Meets the requirements for Identification, Peptide mapping, Bacterial endotoxins, Chromatographic purity, Single-chain content, and Protein content.
Alteplase for Injection USP—Preserve in hermetic, light-resistant containers, and store in a refrigerator. A sterile lyophilized preparation of Alteplase. Its biological activity is not less tha 90% and not more than 115% of that stated on the label in USP Alteplase Units. Label it to state the biological activity in USP Alteplase Units per vial and the amount of protein per vial. Contains the total protein content stated on the label, within −5% to +11%. Meets the requirements for Constituted solution, Identification, Bacterial endotoxins, Safety, Sterility, Uniformity of dosage units, pH (7.1–

7.5, in the solution constituted as directed in the labeling), Water (not more than 4.0%), Purity, Percent monomer, and Protein content.
Alteplase, Recombinant, for Injection—Not in *USP–NF*.

ALTRETAMINE

Source: Synthetic s-triazine derivative.

Chemical name: 1,3,5-Triazine-2,4,6-triamine, *N,N,N′,N′,-N″,N″*-hexamethyl-.

Molecular formula: $C_9H_{18}N_6$.

Molecular weight: 210.28.

Description: White, crystalline powder.

Solubility: Soluble in chloroform; insoluble in water.

USP requirements:
Altretamine USP—Preserve in well-closed containers. Contains not less than 98% and not more than 102% of altretamine, calculated on the anhydrous basis. Meets the requirements for Identification, Water (not more than 1%), Residue on ignition (not more than 0.1%), and Heavy metals (40 micrograms per gram).
Altretamine Capsules USP—Preserve in tight, light-resistant containers. Contain labeled amount of altretamine, within ±10%. Meet the requirements for Identification, Dissolution (80% in 30 minutes in 0.1 N hydrochloric acid in Apparatus 1 at 100 rpm), and Uniformity of dosage units.

ALUM

Chemical name:
Ammonium alum—Sulfuric acid, aluminum ammonium salt (2:1:1), dodecahydrate.
Potassium alum—Sulfuric acid, aluminum potassium salt (2:1:1), dodecahydrate.

Molecular formula:
Ammonium alum—$AlNH_4(SO_4)_2 \cdot 12H_2O$.
Potassium alum—$AlK(SO_4)_2 \cdot 12H_2O$.

Molecular weight:
Ammonium alum—453.33.
Potassium alum—474.39.

Description:
Ammonium Alum USP—Large, colorless crystals, crystalline fragments, or white powder. Is odorless. Its solutions are acid to litmus.
Potassium Alum USP—Large, colorless crystals, crystalline fragments, or white powder. Is odorless. Its solutions are acid to litmus.

Solubility:
Ammonium Alum USP—Freely soluble in water; very soluble in boiling water; freely but slowly soluble in glycerin; insoluble in alcohol.
Potassium Alum USP—Freely soluble in water; very soluble in boiling water; freely but slowly soluble in glycerin; insoluble in alcohol.

USP requirements:
Ammonium Alum USP—Contains not less than 99.0% and not more than 100.5% of ammonium alum, calculated on the dried basis. Meets the requirements for Identification, Loss on drying (45.0–48.0%), Alkalies and alkaline earths (not more than 0.5%), Heavy metals (not more than 0.002%), and Iron.

Potassium Alum USP—Preserve in well-closed containers. Contains not less than 99.0% and not more than 100.5% of potassium alum, calculated on the dried basis. Meets the requirements for Identification, Loss on drying (43.0–46.0%), Heavy metals (not more than 0.002%), and Iron.

ALUMINA, CALCIUM CARBONATE, AND SODIUM BICARBONATE

For *Alumina* (Alluminum Hydroxide), *Calcium Carbonate,* and *Sodium Bicarbonate*—See individual listings for chemistry information.

USP requirements: Alumina, Calcium Carbonate, and Sodium Bicarbonate Oral Suspension—Not in *USP–NF*.

ALUMINA AND MAGNESIA

For *Alumina* (Aluminum Hydroxide) and *Magnesia* (Magnesium Hydroxide)—See individual listings for chemistry information.

USP requirements:
Alumina and Magnesia Oral Suspension USP—Preserve in tight containers, and avoid freezing. A mixture containing Aluminum Hydroxide and Magnesium Hydroxide. Oral Suspension may be labeled to state the aluminum hydroxide content in terms of the equivalent amount of dried aluminum hydroxide gel, on the basis that each mg of dried gel is equivalent to 0.765 mg of aluminum hydroxide. Contains the equivalent of the labeled amounts of aluminum hydroxide and magnesium hydroxide, within ±10%. Meets the requirements for Identification, Microbial limits, Acid-neutralizing capacity, pH (7.3–8.5), Chloride (not more than 0.14%), and Sulfate (not more than 0.1%), and for Arsenic and Heavy metals under Aluminum Hydroxide Gel.
Alumina and Magnesia Tablets USP—Preserve in well-closed containers. Tablets prepared with the use of Dried Aluminum Hydroxide Gel may be labeled to state the aluminum hydroxide content in terms of the equivalent amount of dried aluminum hydroxide gel, on the basis that each mg of dried gel is equivalent to 0.765 mg of aluminum hydroxide. Contain the equivalent of the labeled amounts of aluminum hydroxide and magnesium hydroxide, within ±10%. Meet the requirements for Identification, Disintegration (10 minutes, in simulated gastric fluid TS), Uniformity of dosage units, and Acid-neutralizing capacity.

ALUMINA, MAGNESIA, AND CALCIUM CARBONATE

For *Alumina* (Aluminum Hydroxide), *Magnesia* (Magnesium Hydroxide), and *Calcium Carbonate*—See individual listings for chemistry information.

USP requirements:
Alumina, Magnesia, and Calcium Carbonate Oral Suspension USP—Preserve in tight containers, and avoid freezing. Oral Suspension may be labeled to state the aluminum hydroxide content in terms of the equivalent amount of dried aluminum hydroxide gel, on the basis that each mg of dried gel is equivalent to 0.765 mg of aluminum hydroxide. Contains the labeled amounts of aluminum hydroxide, magnesium hydroxide, and calcium carbonate, within ±10%. Meets the requirements for Identification, Microbial limits, pH (7.5–8.5), Chloride (not more than 0.14%), Sul-

fate (not more than 0.1%), and Acid-neutralizing capacity, and for Arsenic and Heavy metals under Aluminum Hydroxide Gel.

Alumina, Magnesia, and Calcium Carbonate Tablets USP— Preserve in well-closed containers. Label the Tablets to indicate that they are to be chewed before being swallowed. Tablets prepared with the use of Dried Aluminum Hydroxide Gel may be labeled to state the aluminum hydroxide content in terms of the equivalent amount of dried aluminum hydroxide gel, on the basis that each mg of dried gel is equivalent to 0.765 mg of aluminum hydroxide. Contain the labeled amounts of aluminum hydroxide, magnesium hydroxide, and calcium carbonate, within ±10%. Meet the requirements for Identification, Disintegration (45 minutes), Uniformity of dosage units, and Acid-neutralizing capacity.

ALUMINA, MAGNESIA, CALCIUM CARBONATE, AND SIMETHICONE

For *Alumina* (Aluminum Hydroxide), *Magnesia* (Magnesium Hydroxide), *Calcium Carbonate,* and *Simethicone*—See individual listings for chemistry information.

USP requirements: Alumina, Magnesia, Calcium Carbonate, and Simethicone Tablets USP—Preserve in well-closed containers. The labeling indicates that Tablets are to be chewed before swallowing. Label Tablets to state the sodium content, if it is greater than 5 mg per Tablet. Contain the equivalent of the labeled amounts of aluminum hydroxide and magnesium hydroxide, within ±10%, the labeled amount of calcium carbonate, within ±10%, and an amount of polydimethylsiloxane equivalent to the labeled amount of simethicone, within ±15%. Meet the requirements for Identification, Uniformity of dosage units, Acid-neutralizing capacity, Defoaming activity (not more than 45 seconds), Microbial limits, and Sodium content (not more than 5 mg per Tablet; where labeled as containing more than 5 mg per Tablet, not more than +10% of the labeled amount).

ALUMINA, MAGNESIA, AND MAGNESIUM CARBONATE

For *Alumina* (Aluminum Hydroxide), *Magnesia* (Magnesium Hydroxide), and *Magnesium Carbonate*—See individual listings for chemistry information.

USP requirements: Alumina, Magnesia, and Magnesium Carbonate Chewable Tablets—Not in *USP–NF*.

ALUMINA, MAGNESIA, MAGNESIUM CARBONATE, AND SIMETHICONE

For *Alumina* (Aluminum Hydroxide), *Magnesia* (Magnesium Hydroxide), *Magnesium Carbonate,* and *Simethicone*—See individual listings for chemistry information.

USP requirements: Alumina, Magnesia, Magnesium Carbonate, and Simethicone Chewable Tablets—Not in *USP–NF*.

ALUMINA, MAGNESIA, AND SIMETHICONE

For *Alumina* (Aluminum Hydroxide), *Magnesia* (Magnesium Hydroxide), and *Simethicone*—See individual listings for chemistry information.

USP requirements:

Alumina, Magnesia, and Simethicone Oral Suspension USP—Preserve in tight containers, and avoid freezing. Oral Suspension may be labeled to state the aluminum hydroxide content in terms of the equivalent amount of dried aluminum hydroxide gel, on the basis that each mg of dried gel is equivalent to 0.765 mg of aluminum hydroxide. Label it to state the sodium content if it is greater than 1 mg per mL. Contains the equivalent of the labeled amounts of aluminum hydroxide and magnesium hydroxide, within −10% to +15%. Contains an amount of polydimethylsiloxane equivalent to the labeled amount of simethicone, within ±15%. Meets the requirements for Identification, Microbial limits, Acid-neutralizing capacity, pH (7.0–8.6), Defoaming activity (not more than 45 seconds), and Sodium.

Alumina, Magnesia, and Simethicone Tablets USP—Preserve in well-closed containers. Label the Tablets to indicate that they are to be chewed before being swallowed. Label the Tablets to state the sodium content if it is greater than 5 mg per Tablet. Tablets may be labeled to state the aluminum hydroxide content in terms of the equivalent amount of dried aluminum hydroxide gel, on the basis that each mg of dried gel is equivalent to 0.765 mg of aluminum hydroxide. Contain the equivalent of the labeled amounts of aluminum hydroxide and magnesium hydroxide, within −10% to +15%. Contain an amount of polydimethylsiloxane equivalent to the labeled amount of simethicone, within ±15%. Meet the requirements for Identification, Uniformity of dosage units, Acid-neutralizing capacity, Defoaming activity (not more than 45 seconds), and Sodium.

ALUMINA, MAGNESIUM ALGINATE, AND MAGNESIUM CARBONATE

Chemical name:
  Aluminum hydroxide—Aluminum hydroxide.
  Magnesium carbonate—Carbonic acid, magnesium salt, basic; or, Carbonic acid, magnesium salt (1:1), hydrate.

Molecular formula:
  Aluminum hydroxide—$Al(OH)_3$.
  Magnesium carbonate—$MgCO_3 \cdot H_2O$.
  Magnesium carbonate, basic (approx.)—$(MgCO_3)_4 \cdot Mg(OH)_2 \cdot 5H_2O$.

Molecular weight:
  Aluminum hydroxide—78.00.
  Magnesium carbonate—102.33.
  Magnesium carbonate, basic (approx.)—485.65.

Description:
  Aluminum Hydroxide Gel USP—White, viscous suspension, from which small amounts of clear liquid may separate on standing.
  Dried Aluminum Hydroxide Gel USP—White, odorless, amorphous powder.
  Magnesium Carbonate USP—Light, white, friable masses or bulky, white powder. Is odorless, and is stable in air.

Solubility:
  Dried Aluminum Hydroxide Gel USP—Insoluble in water and in alcohol; soluble in dilute mineral acids and in solutions of fixed alkali hydroxides.
  Magnesium Carbonate USP—Practically insoluble in water to which, however, it imparts a slightly alkaline reaction; insoluble in alcohol, but is dissolved by dilute acids with effervescence.

USP requirements:
Alumina, Magnesium Alginate, and Magnesium Carbonate Oral Suspension—Not in *USP–NF*.
Alumina, Magnesium Alginate, and Magnesium Carbonate Chewable Tablets—Not in *USP–NF*.

ALUMINA AND MAGNESIUM CARBONATE

For *Alumina* (Aluminum Hydroxide) and *Magnesium Carbonate*—See individual listings for chemistry information.

USP requirements:
Alumina and Magnesium Carbonate Oral Suspension USP—Preserve in tight containers, and avoid freezing. Contains the equivalent of the labeled amounts of aluminum hydroxide and magnesium carbonate, within ±10%. Meets the requirements for Identification, Microbial limits, pH (7.5–9.5), and Acid-neutralizing capacity.
Alumina and Magnesium Carbonate Tablets USP—Preserve in tight containers. Contain the equivalent of the labeled amounts of aluminum hydroxide and magnesium carbonate, within ±10%. Meet the requirements for Identification, Disintegration (10 minutes, in simulated gastric fluid TS), Uniformity of dosage units, and Acid-neutralizing capacity.

ALUMINA, MAGNESIUM CARBONATE, AND MAGNESIUM OXIDE

For *Alumina* (Aluminum Hydroxide), *Magnesium Carbonate,* and *Magnesium Oxide*—See individual listings for chemistry information.

USP requirements: Alumina, Magnesium Carbonate, and Magnesium Oxide Tablets USP—Preserve in tight containers. Contain the equivalent of the labeled amounts of aluminum hydroxide and magnesium carbonate, within ±10%. Contain the labeled amount of magnesium oxide, within ±15%. Meet the requirements for Identification, Disintegration (10 minutes, in simulated gastric fluid TS), Uniformity of dosage units, and Acid-neutralizing capacity.

ALUMINA, MAGNESIUM CARBONATE, AND SIMETHICONE

For *Alumina* (Aluminum Hydroxide), *Magnesium Carbonate,* and *Simethicone*—See individual listings for chemistry information.

USP requirements: Alumina, Magnesium Carbonate, and Simethicone Oral Suspension—Not in *USP–NF*.

ALUMINA, MAGNESIUM CARBONATE, AND SODIUM BICARBONATE

For *Alumina* (Aluminum Hydroxide), *Magnesium Carbonate,* and *Sodium Bicarbonate*—See individual listings for chemistry information.

USP requirements: Alumina, Magnesium Carbonate, and Sodium Bicarbonate Chewable Tablets—Not in *USP–NF*.

ALUMINA AND MAGNESIUM TRISILICATE

For *Alumina* (Aluminum Hydroxide) and *Magnesium Trisilicate*—See individual listings for chemistry information.

USP requirements:
Alumina and Magnesium Trisilicate Oral Suspension USP—Preserve in tight containers. Contains the equivalent of the labeled amount of aluminum hydroxide, within ± 10%, and the labeled amount of magnesium trisilicate, within ±10%. Meets the requirements for Identification, Acid-neutralizing capacity, and pH (7.5–8.5).
Alumina and Magnesium Trisilicate Tablets USP—Preserve in well-closed containers. Tablets prepared with the use of Dried Aluminum Hydroxide Gel may be labeled to state the aluminum hydroxide content in terms of the equivalent amount of dried aluminum hydroxide gel, on the basis that each mg of dried gel is equivalent to 0.765 mg of aluminum hydroxide. Tablets intended for the temporary relief of heartburn (acid indigestion) due to acid reflux are so labeled. Tablets that must be chewed before swallowing are so labeled. Contain the equivalent of the labeled amount of aluminum hydroxide, within ±10%, and the labeled amount of magnesium trisilicate, within ±10%. Meet the requirements for Identification, Disintegration (10 minutes, in simulated gastric fluid TS [Note: Tablets that must be chewed before swallowing are exempt from this requirement]), Uniformity of dosage units, Acid-neutralizing capacity (Note: Tablets labeled for the temporary relief of heartburn [acid indigestion] due to acid reflux are exempt from this requirement), Foam (where Tablets are labeled for the temporary relief of heartburn [acid indigestion] due to acid reflux, thickness of foam not less than 10 mm), and pH (where Tablets are labeled for the temporary relief of heartburn [acid indigestion] due to acid reflux, not less than 4.5).

ALUMINA, MAGNESIUM TRISILICATE, AND SODIUM BICARBONATE

For *Alumina* (Aluminum Hydroxide), *Magnesium Trisilicate,* and *Sodium Bicarbonate*—See individual listings for chemistry information.

USP requirements: Alumina, Magnesium Trisilicate, and Sodium Bicarbonate Chewable Tablets—Not in *USP–NF*.

ALUMINA AND SIMETHICONE

For *Alumina* (Aluminum Hydroxide) and *Simethicone*—See individual listings for chemistry information.

USP requirements: Alumina and Simethicone Gel—Not in *USP–NF*.

ALUMINA AND SODIUM BICARBONATE

For *Alumina* (Aluminum Hydroxide) and *Sodium Bicarbonate*—See individual listings for chemistry information.

USP requirements: Alumina and Sodium Bicarbonate Chewable Tablets—Not in *USP–NF*.

ALUMINUM ACETATE

Chemical name: Acetic acid, aluminum salt.

Molecular formula: $C_6H_9AlO_6$.

Molecular weight: 204.11.

Description: Aluminum Acetate Topical Solution USP—Clear, colorless liquid having a faint odor of acetic acid. Specific gravity is about 1.02.

USP requirements: Aluminum Acetate Topical Solution USP—Preserve in tight containers. Yields, from each 100 mL, not less than 1.20 grams and not more than 1.45 grams of aluminum oxide, and not less than 4.24 grams and not more than 5.12 grams of acetic acid, corresponding to not less than 4.8 grams and not more than 5.8 grams of aluminum acetate. May be stabilized by the addition of not more than 0.6% of Boric Acid.

Prepare Aluminum Acetate Topical Solution as follows: 545 mL of Aluminum Subacetate Topical Solution, 15 mL of Glacial Acetic Acid, and a sufficient quantity of Purified Water to make 1000 mL. Add the Glacial Acetic Acid to the Aluminum Subacetate Topical Solution and sufficient Water to make 1000 mL. Mix, and filter, if necessary.

Meets the requirements for Identification, pH (3.6–4.4), Limit of boric acid, and Heavy metals (not more than 0.001%).

Note: Dispense only clear Aluminum Acetate Topical Solution.

BASIC ALUMINUM CARBONATE

Source: Combination of aluminum hydroxide and aluminum carbonate.

Description: Dried basic aluminum carbonate gel—White powder.

Solubility: Dried basic aluminum carbonate gel—Insoluble in water and in alcohol.

USP requirements:
Basic Aluminum Carbonate Gel (Oral Suspension)—Not in *USP–NF.*
Dried Basic Aluminum Carbonate Gel Capsules—Not in *USP–NF.*
Dried Basic Aluminum Carbonate Gel Tablets—Not in *USP–NF.*

BASIC ALUMINUM CARBONATE AND SIMETHICONE

For *Basic Aluminum Carbonate* and *Simethicone*—See individual listings for chemistry information.

USP requirements: Basic Aluminum Carbonate and Simethicone Oral Suspension—Not in *USP–NF.*

ALUMINUM CHLORIDE

Chemical name: Aluminum chloride, hexahydrate.

Molecular formula: $AlCl_3 \cdot 6H_2O$.

Molecular weight: 241.43.

Description: Aluminum Chloride USP—White, or yellowish white, deliquescent, crystalline powder. Is practically odorless. Its solutions are acid to litmus.

Solubility: Aluminum Chloride USP—Very soluble in water; freely soluble in alcohol; soluble in glycerin.

USP requirements: Aluminum Chloride USP—Preserve in tight containers. Contains not less than 95.0% and not more than 102.0% of aluminum chloride, calculated on the anhydrous basis. Meets the requirements for Identification, Water (42.0–48.0%), Sulfate, Limit of alkalies and alkaline earths (not more than 0.5%), Heavy metals (not more than 0.002%), and Iron (not more than 0.001%).

ALUMINUM CHLOROHYDRATE

Chemical name:
Aluminum chlorohydrate—Aluminum chlorohydroxide.
Aluminum chlorohydrex polyethylene glycol—Aluminum chlorohydroxide polyethylene glycol complex.
Aluminum chlorohydrex propylene glycol—Aluminum chlorohydroxide, hydrate: propylene glycol complex (1:1).
Aluminum dichlorohydrate—Aluminum chlorohydroxide.
Aluminum dichlorohydrex polyethylene glycol—Aluminum chlorohydroxide polyethylene glycol complex.
Aluminum dichlorohydrex propylene glycol—Aluminum chlorohydroxide propylene glycol complex.
Aluminum sesquichlorohydrate—Aluminum chlorohydroxide.
Aluminum sesquichlorohydrex polyethylene glycol—Aluminum chlorohydroxide polyethylene glycol complex.
Aluminum sesquichlorohydrex propylene glycol—Aluminum chlorohydroxide propylene glycol complex.

Molecular formula:
Aluminum chlorohydrate—$Al_y(OH)_{3y-z}Cl_z \cdot H_2O$.
Aluminum chlorohydrex polyethylene glycol—$Al_y(OH)_{3y-z}Cl_z \cdot nH_2O \cdot mH(OCH_2CH_2)_nOH$.
Aluminum chlorohydrex propylene glycol—$Al_y(OH)_{3y-z}Cl_z \cdot nH_2O \cdot mC_3H_8O_2$.
Aluminum dichlorohydrate—$Al_y(OH)_{3y-z}Cl_z \cdot nH_2O$.
Aluminum dichlorohydrex polyethylene glycol—$Al_y(OH)_{3y-z}Cl_z \cdot nH_2O \cdot mH(OCH_2CH_2)_nOH$.
Aluminum dichlorohydrex propylene glycol—$Al_y(OH)_{3y-z}Cl_z \cdot nH_2O \cdot mC_3H_8O_2$.
Aluminum sesquichlorohydrate—$Al_y(OH)_{3y-z}Cl_z \cdot nH_2O$.
Aluminum sesquichlorohydrex polyethylene glycol—$Al_y(OH)_{3y-z}Cl_z \cdot nH_2O \cdot mH(OCH_2CH_2)_nOH$.
Aluminum sesquichlorohydrex propylene glycol—$Al_y(OH)_{3y-z}Cl_z \cdot nH_2O \cdot mC_3H_8O_2$.

USP requirements:
Aluminum Chlorohydrate USP—Preserve in well-closed containers. Consists of complex basic aluminum chloride that is polymeric and loosely hydrated and encompasses a range of aluminum-to-chloride atomic ratios between 1.91:1 and 2.10:1. The label states the content of anhydrous aluminum chlorohydrate. Contains the equivalent of the labeled amount of anhydrous aluminum chlorohydrate, within ±10%. Meets the requirements for Identification, pH (3.0–5.0, in a solution [15 in 100 (w/w)]), Arsenic (not more than 2 mcg per gram), Heavy metals (not more than 0.002%), Limit of iron (not more than 150 mcg per gram), Content of aluminum, Content of chloride, and Aluminum/chloride atomic ratio (1.91:1–2.10:1).

Aluminum Chlorohydrate Solution USP—Preserve in well-closed containers. Consists of complex basic aluminum chloride that is polymeric and encompasses a range of aluminum-to-chloride ratios between 1.91:1 and 2.10:1. The following solvents may be used: water, propylene glycol, dipropylene glycol, or alcohol. Label Solution to state the solvent used and the claimed concentration of anhydrous aluminum chlorohydrate contained therein. Contains the equivalent of the labeled concentration of anhydrous aluminum chlorohydrate, within ±10%. Meets the requirements for Identification, pH (3.0–5.0), Arsenic (not more than 2 ppm), Heavy metals (not more than

0.001%), Limit of iron (not more than 75 mcg per gram), Content of aluminum, Content of chloride, and Aluminum/chloride atomic ratio (1.91:1–2.10:1).

Aluminum Chlorohydrex Polyethylene Glycol USP—Preserve in well-closed containers. Consists of aluminum chlorohydrate in which some of the waters of hydration have been replaced by polyethylene glycol. Encompasses a range of aluminum-to-chloride atomic ratios between 1.91:1 and 2.10:1. The label states the content of anhydrous aluminum chlorohydrate. Contains the labeled amount of anhydrous aluminum chlorohydrate, within ±10%. Meets the requirements for Identification, pH (3.0–5.0, in a solution [15 in 100 (w/w)]), Arsenic (not more than 2 mcg per gram), Heavy metals (not more than 20 mcg per gram), Limit of iron (not more than 150 mcg per gram), Content of aluminum, Content of chloride, and Aluminum/chloride atomic ratio (1.91:1–2.10:1).

Aluminum Chlorohydrex Propylene Glycol USP—Preserve in well-closed containers. A complex of aluminum chlorohydrate and propylene glycol in which some of the waters of hydration of the aluminum chlorohydrate have been replaced by propylene glycol. The label states the content of anhydrous aluminum chlorohydrate. Contains the equivalent of the labeled amount of anhydrous aluminum chlorohydrate, within ±10%. Meets the requirements for Identification, pH (3.0–5.0, in a solution [15 in 100 (w/w)]), Arsenic (not more than 2 mcg per gram), Heavy metals (not more than 20 mcg per gram), Limit of iron (not more than 150 mcg per gram), Content of aluminum, Content of chloride, and Aluminum/chloride atomic ratio (1.91:1–2.1:1).

Aluminum Dichlorohydrate USP—Preserve in well-closed containers. Consists of complex basic aluminum chloride that is polymeric and loosely hydrated and encompasses a range of aluminum-to-chloride atomic ratios between 0.90:1 and 1.25:1. The label states the content of anhydrous aluminum dichlorohydrate. Contains the labeled amount of anhydrous aluminum dichlorohydrate, within ±10%. Meets the requirements for Identification, pH (3.0–5.0, in a solution [15 in 100 (w/w)]), Arsenic (not more than 2 mcg per gram), Heavy metals (not more than 20 mcg per gram), Limit of iron (not more than 150 mcg per gram), Content of aluminum, Content of chloride, and Aluminum/chloride atomic ratio (0.90:1–1.25:1).

Aluminum Dichlorohydrate Solution USP—Preserve in well-closed containers. Consists of complex basic aluminum chloride that is polymeric and encompasses a range of aluminum-to-chloride atomic ratios between 0.90:1 and 1.25:1. The following solvents may be used: water, propylene glycol, dipropylene glycol, or alcohol. Label Solution to state the solvent used and the claimed concentration of anhydrous aluminum dichlorohydrate contained therein. Contains the equivalent of the labeled concentration of anhydrous aluminum dichlorohydrate, within ±10%. Meets the requirements for Identification, pH (3.0–5.0, in a solution prepared by diluting 3 grams of the Solution with water to obtain 10 mL), Arsenic (not more than 2 mcg per gram), Heavy metals (not more than 10 mcg per gram), Limit of iron (not more than 75 mcg per gram), Content of aluminum, Content of chloride, and Aluminum/chloride atomic ratio (0.90:1–1.25:1).

Aluminum Dichlorohydrex Polyethylene Glycol USP—Preserve in well-closed containers. Consists of aluminum dichlorohydrate in which some of the waters of hydration have been replaced by polyethylene glycol. Encompasses a range of aluminum-to-chloride atomic ratios between 0.90:1 and 1.25:1. The label states the content of anhydrous aluminum dichlorohydrate. Contains the labeled amount of anhydrous aluminum dichlorohydrate, within ±10%. Meets the requirements for Identification, pH (3.0–5.0, in a solution [15 in 100 (w/w)]), Arsenic (not more than 2 mcg per gram), Heavy metals (not more than 20

mcg per gram), Limit of iron (not more than 150 mcg per gram), Content of aluminum, Content of chloride, and Aluminum/chloride atomic ratio (0.90:1–1.25:1).

Aluminum Dichlorohydrex Propylene Glycol USP—Preserve in well-closed containers. Consists of aluminum dichlorohydrate in which some of the waters of hydration have been replaced by propylene glycol. Encompasses a range of aluminum-to-chloride atomic ratios between 0.90:1 and 1.25:1. The label states the content of anhydrous aluminum dichlorohydrate. Contains the labeled amount of anhydrous aluminum dichlorohydrate, within ±10%. Meets the requirements for Identification, pH (3.0–5.0, in a solution [15 in 100 (w/w)]), Arsenic (not more than 2 mcg per gram), Heavy metals (not more than 20 mcg per gram), Limit of iron (not more than 150 mcg per gram), Content of aluminum, Content of chloride, and Aluminum/chloride atomic ratio (0.90:1–1.25:1).

Aluminum Sesquichlorohydrate USP—Preserve in well-closed containers. Consists of complex basic aluminum chloride that is polymeric and loosely hydrated and encompasses a range of aluminum-to-chloride atomic ratios between 1.26:1 and 1.90:1. The label states the content of anhydrous aluminum sesquichlorohydrate. Contains the labeled amount of anhydrous aluminum sesquichlorohydrate, within ±10%. Meets the requirements for Identification, pH (3.0–5.0, in a solution [15 in 100 (w/w)]), Arsenic (not more than 2 mcg per gram), Heavy metals (not more than 20 mcg per gram), Limit of iron (not more than 150 mcg per gram), Content of aluminum, Content of chloride, and Aluminum/chloride atomic ratio (1.26:1–1.90:1).

Aluminum Sesquichlorohydrate Solution USP—Preserve in well-closed containers. Consists of complex basic aluminum chloride that is polymeric and encompasses a range of aluminum-to-chloride atomic ratios between 1.26:1 and 1.90:1. The following solvents may be used: water, propylene glycol, dipropylene glycol, or alcohol. Label Solution to state the solvent used and the claimed concentration of anhydrous aluminum sesquichlorohydrate contained therein. Contains the equivalent of the labeled concentration of anhydrous aluminum sesquichlorohydrate, within ±10%. Meets the requirements for Identification, pH (3.0–5.0, in a solution prepared by diluting 3 grams of the Solution with water to obtain 10 mL), Arsenic (not more than 2 mcg per gram), Heavy metals (not more than 10 mcg per gram), Limit of iron (not more than 75 mcg per gram), Content of aluminum, Content of chloride, and Aluminum/chloride atomic ratio (1.26:1–1.90:1).

Aluminum Sesquichlorohydrex Polyethylene Glycol USP—Preserve in well-closed containers. Consists of aluminum sesquichlorohydrate in which some of the waters of hydration have been replaced by polyethylene glycol. Encompasses a range of aluminum-to-chloride atomic ratios between 1.26:1 and 1.90:1. The label states the content of anhydrous aluminum sesquichlorohydrate. Contains the labeled amount of anhydrous aluminum sesquichlorohydrate, within ±10%. Meets the requirements for Identification, pH (3.0–5.0, in a solution [15 in 100 (w/w)]), Arsenic (not more than 2 mcg per gram), Heavy metals (not more than 20 mcg per gram), Limit of iron (not more than 150 mcg per gram), Content of aluminum, Content of chloride, and Aluminum/chloride atomic ratio (1.26:1–1.90:1).

Aluminum Sesquichlorohydrex Propylene Glycol USP—Preserve in well-closed containers. Consists of aluminum sesquichlorohydrate in which some of the waters of hydration have been replaced by propylene glycol. Encompasses a range of aluminum-to-chloride atomic ratios between 1.26:1 and 1.90:1. The label states the content of anhydrous aluminum sesquichlorohydrate. Contains the labeled amount of anhydrous aluminum sesquichlorohydrate, within ±10%. Meets the requirements for Identification, pH (3.0–5.0, in a solution [15 in 100 (w/w)]), Arsenic (not more than 2 mcg per gram), Heavy metals (not more than 20 mcg per gram), Limit of iron (not more

than 150 mcg per gram), Content of aluminum, Content of chloride, and Aluminum/chloride atomic ratio (1.26:1–1.90:1).

ALUMINUM HYDROXIDE

Source: An amorphous form of aluminum hydroxide in which there is a partial substitution of carbonate for hydroxide.

Chemical name: Aluminum hydroxide.

Molecular formula: $Al(OH)_3$.

Molecular weight: 78.00.

Description:
Aluminum Hydroxide Gel USP—White, viscous suspension, from which small amounts of clear liquid may separate on standing.
Dried Aluminum Hydroxide Gel USP—White, odorless, amorphous powder.

Solubility: Dried Aluminum Hydroxide Gel USP—Insoluble in water and in alcohol; soluble in dilute mineral acids and in solutions of fixed alkali hydroxides.

USP requirements:
Aluminum Hydroxide Gel USP—Preserve in tight containers, and avoid freezing. A suspension of amorphous aluminum hydroxide in which there is a partial substitution of carbonate for hydroxide. Contains the equivalent of the labeled amount of aluminum hydroxide, within ±10%. Meets the requirements for Identification, Microbial limits, Acid-neutralizing capacity, pH (5.5–8.0), Chloride, Sulfate, Arsenic (not more than 0.001%, based on the aluminum hydroxide content), and Heavy metals (not more than 0.0083%, based on the aluminum hydroxide content).
Aluminum Hydroxide Oral Suspension—Not in USP–NF.
Dried Aluminum Hydroxide Gel USP—Preserve in tight containers. An amorphous form of aluminum hydroxide in which there is a partial substitution of carbonate for hydroxide. Where the quantity of dried aluminum hydroxide gel equivalent is stated in the labeling of any preparation, this shall be understood to be on the basis that each mg of dried gel is equivalent to 0.765 mg of aluminum hydroxide. Contains the equivalent of not less than 76.5% of aluminum hydroxide, and may contain varying quantities of basic aluminum carbonate and bicarbonate. Meets the requirements for Identification, Acid-neutralizing capacity, pH (not more than 10.0, in an aqueous dispersion [1 in 25]), Chloride (not more than 0.85%), Sulfate (not more than 0.6%), Arsenic (not more than 8 ppm), and Heavy metals (not more than 0.006%).
Dried Aluminum Hydroxide Gel Capsules USP—Preserve in well-closed containers. Capsules may be labeled to state the aluminum hydroxide content in terms of the equivalent amount of dried aluminum hydroxide gel, on the basis that each mg of dried gel is equivalent to 0.765 mg of aluminum hydroxide. Contain the labeled amount, within ±10%. Meet the requirements for Identification, Disintegration (10 minutes, in simulated gastric fluid TS), Uniformity of dosage units, and Acid-neutralizing capacity.
Dried Aluminum Hydroxide Gel Tablets USP—Preserve in well-closed containers. Tablets may be labeled to state the aluminum hydroxide content in terms of the equivalent amount of dried aluminum hydroxide gel, on the basis that each mg of dried gel is equivalent to 0.765 mg of aluminum hydroxide. Contain the labeled amount, within ±10%. Meet the requirements for Identification, Disintegration (10 minutes, in simulated gastric fluid TS), Uniformity of dosage units, and Acid-neutralizing capacity.

ALUMINUM MONOSTEARATE

Chemical name: Aluminum, dihydroxy(octadecanoato-O-).

Molecular formula: $C_{18}H_{37}AlO_4$.

Molecular weight: 344.47.

Description: Aluminum Monostearate NF—Fine, white to yellowish white bulky powder, having a faint, characteristic odor.
NF category: Suspending and/or viscosity-increasing agent.

Solubility: Aluminum Monostearate NF—Insoluble in water, in alcohol, and in ether.

NF requirements: Aluminum Monostearate NF—Preserve in well-closed containers. A compound of aluminum with a mixture of solid organic acids obtained from fats, consisting chiefly of variable proportions of aluminum monostearate and aluminum monopalmitate. Contains the equivalent of not less than 14.5% and not more than 16.5% of aluminum oxide. Meets the requirements for Identification, Loss on drying (not more than 2.0%), Arsenic (not more than 4 ppm), Heavy metals (not more than 50 mcg per gram), and Organic volatile impurities.

ALUMINUM PHOSPHATE

Chemical name: Phosphoric acid, aluminum salt (1:1).

Molecular formula: $AlPO_4$.

Molecular weight: 121.95.

Description: Aluminum Phosphate Gel USP—White, viscous suspension from which small amounts of water separate on standing.

USP requirements: Aluminum Phosphate Gel USP—Preserve in tight containers. A water suspension. Contains not less than 4.0% and not more than 5.0% (w/w) of aluminum phosphate. Meets the requirements for Identification, pH (6.0–7.2), Chloride (not more than 0.16%), Soluble phosphate (not more than 0.30%), Sulfate (not more than 0.05%), Arsenic (not more than 0.6 ppm), and Heavy metals (not more than 5 ppm).

ALUMINUM SUBACETATE

Chemical name: Aluminum, bis(acetato-O)hydroxy-.

Molecular formula: $C_4H_7AlO_5$.

Molecular weight: 162.08.

Description: Aluminum Subacetate Topical Solution USP—Clear, colorless or faintly yellow liquid, having an odor of acetic acid and an acid reaction to litmus. Gradually becomes turbid on standing, through separation of a more basic salt.

USP requirements: Aluminum Subacetate Topical Solution USP—Preserve in tight containers. Yields, from each 100 mL, not less than 2.30 grams and not more than 2.60 grams of aluminum oxide, and not less than 5.43 grams and not more than 6.13 grams of acetic acid. May be stabilized by the addition of not more than 0.9% of boric acid.
Aluminum Subacetate Topical Solution may be prepared as follows: 145 grams of Aluminum Sulfate, 160 mL of Acetic Acid, 70 grams of Calcium Carbonate, and a sufficient quantity of Purified Water to make 1000 mL. Dissolve the Aluminum Sulfate in 600 mL of cold water, filter the solution, and add the Calcium Carbonate gradually, in several portions, with constant stirring. Then slowly add the Acetic Acid, mix, and set the mixture aside for 24 hours. Filter the product with the aid of vacuum if necessary, returning the first portion of the filtrate to the funnel. Wash the magma on the filter with small portions of cold water, until the total filtrate measures 1000 mL.

Meets the requirements for Identification, pH (3.8–4.6), and Limit of boric acid.

ALUMINUM SULFATE

Chemical name: Sulfuric acid, aluminum salt (3:2), hydrate.

Molecular formula: $Al_2(SO_4)_3 \cdot xH_2O$.

Molecular weight: 342.15 (anhydrous).

Description: Aluminum Sulfate USP—White, crystalline powder, shining plates, or crystalline fragments. Is stable in air. Is odorless.

Solubility: Aluminum Sulfate USP—Freely soluble in water; insoluble in alcohol.

USP requirements: Aluminum Sulfate USP—Preserve in well-closed containers. Contains not less than 54.0% and not more than 59.0% of anhydrous aluminum sulfate. Contains a varying amount of water of crystallization. Meets the requirements for Identification, pH (not less than 2.9, in a solution [1 in 20]), Water (41.0–46.0%), Heavy metals (not more than 20 mcg per gram), Alkalies and alkaline earths (not more than 0.4%), Limit of ammonium salts, Iron, and Organic volatile impurities.

ALUMINUM SULFATE AND CALCIUM ACETATE

For *Aluminum Sulfate* and *Calcium Acetate*—See individual listings for chemistry information.

USP requirements: Aluminum Sulfate and Calcium Acetate Tablets for Topical Solution USP—Preserve in tight containers, and avoid excessive heat. Contain the labeled amounts of aluminum sulfate tetradecahydrate and calcium acetate monohydrate, within ±10%. Meet the requirements for Identification, Disintegration (10 minutes), pH (4.0–4.8, in a solution [2 grams of ground Tablet powder in 500 mL of water]), Loss on drying (not more than 18%), and Uniformity of dosage units.

ALUMINUM ZIRCONIUM CHLOROHYDRATE

Chemical name:
Aluminum zirconium tetrachlorohydrex gly—Glycine aluminum-zirconium complex.
Aluminum zirconium trichlorohydrex gly—Glycine aluminum-zirconium complex.

Molecular formula:
Aluminum zirconium octachlorohydrate—$Al_yZr(OH)_{3y+4-x}Cl_x \cdot nH_2O$.
Aluminum zirconium pentachlorohydrate—$Al_yZr(OH)_{3y+4-x}Cl_x \cdot nH_2O$.
Aluminum zirconium tetrachlorohydrate—$Al_yZr(OH)_{3y+4-x}Cl_x \cdot nH_2O$.
Aluminum zirconium trichlorohydrate—$Al_yZr(OH)_{3y+4-x}Cl_x \cdot nH_2O$.

USP requirements:
Aluminum Zirconium Octachlorohydrate USP—Preserve in well-closed containers. A polymeric, loosely hydrated complex of basic aluminum zirconium chloride that encompasses a range of aluminum-to-zirconium atomic ratios between 6.0:1 and 10.0:1, and a range of (aluminum plus zirconium)-to-chloride atomic ratios between 1.5:1 and 0.9:1. The label states the content of anhydrous aluminum zirconium octachlorohydrate. Contains the labeled amount of anhydrous aluminum zirconium octachlorohy-

drate, within ±10%. Meets the requirements for Identification, pH (3.0–5.0, in a solution [15 in 100 (w/w)]), Arsenic (not more than 2 mcg per gram), Heavy metals (not more than 20 mcg per gram), Limit of iron (not more than 150 mcg per gram), Content of aluminum, Content of zirconium, Aluminum/zirconium atomic ratio (6.0:1–10.0:1), Content of chloride, and (Aluminum plus zirconium)/chloride atomic ratio (1.5:1–0.9:1).

Aluminum Zirconium Octachlorohydrate Solution USP—Preserve in well-closed containers. Consists of complex basic aluminum chloride that is polymeric and encompasses a range of aluminum-to-zirconium atomic ratios between 6.0:1 and 10.0:1, and a range of (aluminum plus zirconium)-to-chloride atomic ratios between 1.5:1 and 0.9:1. The following solvents may be used: water, propylene glycol, or dipropylene glycol. Label Solution to state the solvent used and the claimed concentration of anhydrous aluminum zirconium octachlorohydrate. Contains the equivalent of the labeled concentration of anhydrous aluminum zirconium octachlorohydrate, within ±10%. Meets the requirements for Identification, pH (3.0–5.0, in a solution prepared by diluting 3 grams of the Solution with water to obtain 10 mL), Arsenic (not more than 2 mcg per gram), Heavy metals (not more than 10 mcg per gram), Limit of iron (not more than 75 mcg per gram), Content of aluminum, Content of zirconium, Aluminum/zirconium atomic ratio (6.0:1–10.0:1), Content of chloride, and (Aluminum plus zirconium)/chloride atomic ratio (1.5:1–0.9:1).

Aluminum Zirconium Octachlorohydrex Gly USP—Preserve in well-closed containers. A derivative of Aluminum Zirconium Octachlorohydrate in which some of the water molecules have been displaced by glycine, calcium glycinate, magnesium glycinate, potassium glycinate, sodium glycinate, or zinc glycinate. Encompasses a range of aluminum-to-zirconium atomic ratios between 6.0:1 and 10.0:1, and a range of (aluminum plus zirconium)-to-chloride atomic ratios between 1.5:1 and 0.9:1. The label states the form of glycine used and the claimed content of anhydrous aluminum zirconium octachlorohydrate. Contains the labeled amount of anhydrous aluminum zirconium octachlorohydrate, within ±10%. Meets the requirements for Identification, pH (3.0–5.0, in a solution [15 in 100 (w/w)]), Arsenic (not more than 2 mcg per gram), Heavy metals (not more than 20 mcg per gram), Limit of iron (not more than 150 mcg per gram), Content of aluminum, Content of zirconium, Aluminum/zirconium atomic ratio (6.0:1–10.0:1), Content of chloride, and (Aluminum plus zirconium)/chloride atomic ratio (1.5:1–0.9:1).

Aluminum Zirconium Octachlorohydrex Gly Solution USP—Preserve in well-closed containers. A solution of Aluminum Zirconium Octachlorohydrate in which some of the waters of hydration have been displaced by glycine, calcium glycinate, magnesium glycinate, potassium glycinate, sodium glycinate, or zinc glycinate. Encompasses a range of aluminum-to-zirconium ratios between 6.0:1 and 10.0:1, and a range of (aluminum plus zirconium)-to-chloride atomic ratios between 1.5:1 and 0.9:1. The following solvents may be used: water, propylene glycol, or dipropylene glycol. Label Solution to state the solvent and form of glycine used and the claimed concentration of anhydrous aluminum zirconium octachlorohydrate. Contains the equivalent of the labeled concentration of anhydrous aluminum zirconium octachlorohydrate, within ±10%. Meets the requirements for Identification, pH (3.0–5.0, in a solution prepared by diluting 3 grams of the Solution with water to obtain 10 mL), Arsenic (not more than 2 mcg per gram), Heavy metals (not more than 10 mcg per gram), Limit of iron (not more than 75 mcg per gram), Content of aluminum, Content of zirconium, Aluminum/zirconium atomic ratio (6.0:1–10.0:1), Content of chloride, and (Aluminum plus zirconium)/chloride atomic ratio (1.5:1–0.9:1).

Aluminum Zirconium Pentachlorohydrate USP—Preserve in well-closed containers. A polymeric, loosely hydrated complex of basic aluminum zirconium chloride that en-

compasses a range of aluminum-to-zirconium atomic ratios between 6.0:1 and 10.0:1, and a range of (aluminum plus zirconium)-to-chloride atomic ratios between 2.1:1 and 1.51:1. The label states the content of anhydrous aluminum zirconium pentachlorohydrate. Contains the labeled amount of anhydrous aluminum zirconium pentachlorohydrate, within ±10%. Meets the requirements for Identification, pH (3.0–5.0, in a solution [15 in 100 (w/w)]), Arsenic (not more than 2 mcg per gram), Heavy metals (not more than 20 mcg per gram), Limit of iron (not more than 150 mcg per gram), Content of aluminum, Content of zirconium, Aluminum/zirconium atomic ratio (6.0:1–10.0:1), Content of chloride, and (Aluminum plus zirconium)/chloride atomic ratio (2.1:1–1.51:1).

Aluminum Zirconium Pentachlorohydrate Solution USP—Preserve in well-closed containers. A polymeric, loosely hydrated complex of basic aluminum zirconium chloride that encompasses a range of aluminum-to-zirconium atomic ratios between 6.0:1 and 10.0:1 and a range of (aluminum plus zirconium)-to-chloride atomic ratios between 2.1:1 and 1.51:1. The following solvents may be used: water, propylene glycol, or dipropylene glycol. Label Solution to state the solvent used and the claimed concentration of anhydrous aluminum zirconium pentachlorohydrate. Contains the equivalent of the labeled concentration of anhydrous aluminum zirconium pentachlorohydrate, within ±10%. Meets the requirements for Identification, pH (3.0–5.0, in a solution prepared by diluting 3 grams of the Solution with water to obtain 10 mL), Arsenic (not more than 2 mcg per gram), Heavy metals (not more than 10 mcg per gram), Limit of iron (not more than 75 mcg per gram), Content of aluminum, Content of zirconium, Aluminum/zirconium atomic ratio (6.0:1–10.0:1), Content of chloride, and (Aluminum plus zirconium)/chloride atomic ratio (2.1:1–1.51:1).

Aluminum Zirconium Pentachlorohydrex Gly USP—Preserve in well-closed containers. A derivative of Aluminum Zirconium Pentachlorohydrate in which some of the water molecules have been displaced by glycine, calcium glycinate, magnesium glycinate, potassium glycinate, sodium glycinate, or zinc glycinate. Encompasses a range of aluminum-to-zirconium atomic ratios between 6.0:1 and 10.0:1 and a range of (aluminum plus zirconium)-to-chloride atomic ratios between 2.1:1 and 1.51:1. The label states the form of glycine used and the claimed content of anhydrous aluminum zirconium pentachlorohydrate. Contains the labeled amount of anhydrous aluminum zirconium pentachlorohydrate, within ±10%. Meets the requirements for Identification, pH (3.0–5.0, in a solution [15 in 100 (w/w)]), Arsenic (not more than 2 mcg per gram), Heavy metals (not more than 20 mcg per gram), Limit of iron (not more than 150 mcg per gram), Content of aluminum, Content of zirconium, Aluminum/zirconium atomic ratio (6.0:1–10.0:), Content of chloride, and (Aluminum plus zirconium)/chloride atomic ratio (2.1:1–1.51:1).

Aluminum Zirconium Pentachlorohydrex Gly Solution USP—Preserve in well-closed containers. A solution of Aluminum Zirconium Pentachlorohydrate in which some of the waters of hydration have been displaced by glycine, calcium glycinate, magnesium glycinate, potassium glycinate, sodium glycinate, or zinc glycinate. Encompasses a range of aluminum-to-zirconium ratios between 6.0:1 and 10.0:1, and a range of (aluminum plus zirconium)-to-chloride atomic ratios between 2.1:1 and 1.51:1. The following solvents may be used: water, propylene glycol, or dipropylene glycol. Label Solution to state the solvent and form of glycine used and the claimed concentration of anhydrous aluminum zirconium pentachlorohydrate. Contains the equivalent of the labeled concentration of anhydrous aluminum zirconium pentachlorohydrate, within ±10%. Meets the requirements for Identification, pH (3.0–5.0, in a solution prepared by diluting 3 grams of the Solution with water to obtain 10 mL), Arsenic (not more than 2 mcg per gram), Heavy metals (not more than 10

mcg per gram), Limit of iron (not more than 75 mcg per gram), Content of aluminum, Content of zirconium, Aluminum/zirconium atomic ratio (6.0:1–10.0:1), Content of chloride, and (Aluminum plus zirconium)/chloride atomic ratio (2.1:1–1.51:1).

Aluminum Zirconium Tetrachlorohydrate USP—Preserve in well-closed containers. A polymeric, loosely hydrated complex of basic aluminum zirconium chloride that encompasses a range of aluminum-to-zirconium atomic ratios between 2.0:1 and 5.99:1 and a range of (aluminum plus zirconium)-to-chloride atomic ratios between 1.5:1 and 0.9:1. The label states the content of anhydrous aluminum zirconium tetrachlorohydrate. Contains the labeled amount of anhydrous aluminum zirconium tetrachlorohydrate, within ±10%. Meets the requirements for Identification, pH (3.0–5.0, in a solution [15 in 100 (w/w)]), Arsenic (not more than 2 mcg per gram), Heavy metals (not more than 20 mcg per gram), Limit of iron (not more than 150 mcg per gram), Content of aluminum, Content of zirconium, Aluminum/zirconium atomic ratio (2.0:1–5.99:1), Content of chloride and (Aluminum plus zirconium)/chloride atomic ratio (1.5:1–0.9:1).

Aluminum Zirconium Tetrachlorohydrate Solution USP—Preserve in well-closed containers. A polymeric, loosely hydrated complex of basic aluminum zirconium chloride that encompasses a range of aluminum-to-zirconium atomic ratios between 2.0:1 and 5.99:1 and a range of (aluminum plus zirconium)-to-chloride atomic ratios between 1.5:1 and 0.9:1. The following solvents may be used: water, propylene glycol, or dipropylene glycol. Label Solution to state the solvent used and the claimed concentration of anhydrous aluminum zirconium tetrachlorohydrate. Contains the equivalent of the labeled concentration of anhydrous aluminum zirconium tetrachlorohydrate, within ±10%. Meets the requirements for Identification, pH (3.0–5.0, in a solution prepared by diluting 3 grams of the Solution with water to obtain 10 mL), Arsenic (not more than 2 mcg per gram), Heavy metals (not more than 10 mcg per gram), Limit of iron (not more than 75 mcg per gram), Content of aluminum, Content of zirconium, Aluminum/zirconium atomic ratio (2.0:1–5.99:1), Content of chloride, and (Aluminum plus zirconium)/chloride atomic ratio (1.51:1–0.9:1).

Aluminum Zirconium Tetrachlorohydrex Gly USP—Preserve in well-closed containers. A derivative of Aluminum Zirconium Tetrachlorohydrate in which some of the water molecules have been displaced by glycine, calcium glycinate, magnesium glycinate, potassium glycinate, sodium glycinate, or zinc glycinate. Encompasses a range of aluminum-to-zirconium atomic ratios between 2.0:1 and 5.99:1 and a range of (aluminum plus zirconium)-to-chloride atomic ratios between 1.5:1 and 0.9:1. The label states the form of glycine used and the claimed content of anhydrous aluminum zirconium tetrachlorohydrate. Contains the labeled amount of anhydrous aluminum zirconium tetrachlorohydrate, within ±10%. Meets the requirements for Identification, pH (3.0–5.0, in a solution [15 in 100 (w/w)]), Arsenic (not more than 2 mcg per gram), Heavy metals (not more than 20 mcg per gram), Limit of iron (not more than 150 mcg per gram), Content of aluminum, Content of zirconium, Aluminum/zirconium atomic ratio (2.0:1–5.99:1), Content of chloride, and (Aluminum plus zirconium)/chloride atomic ratio (1.5:1–0.9:1).

Aluminum Zirconium Tetrachlorohydrex Gly Solution USP—Preserve in well-closed containers. A solution of Aluminum Zirconium Tetrachlorohydrate in which some of the waters of hydration have been displaced by glycine, calcium glycinate, magnesium glycinate, potassium glycinate, sodium glycinate, or zinc glycinate. Encompasses a range of aluminum-to-zirconium ratios between 2.0:1 and 5.99:1, and a range of (aluminum plus zirconium)-to-chloride atomic ratios between 1.5:1 and 0.9:1. The following solvents may be used: water, propylene glycol, or dipropylene glycol. Label Solution to state the solvent and

form of glycine used and the claimed concentration of anhydrous aluminum zirconium tetrachlorohydrate. Contains the equivalent of the labeled concentration of anhydrous aluminum zirconium tetrachlorohydrate, within ±10%. Meets the requirements for Identification, pH (3.0–5.0, in a solution prepared by diluting 3 grams of the Solution with water to obtain 10 mL), Arsenic (not more than 2 mcg per gram), Heavy metals (not more than 10 mcg per gram), Limit of iron (not more than 75 mcg per gram), Content of aluminum, Content of zirconium, Aluminum/zirconium atomic ratio (2.0:1–5.99:1), Content of chloride, and (Aluminum plus zirconium)/chloride atomic ratio (1.5:1–0.9:1).

Aluminum Zirconium Trichlorohydrate USP—Preserve in well-closed containers. A polymeric, loosely hydrated complex of basic aluminum zirconium chloride that encompasses a range of aluminum-to-zirconium atomic ratios between 2.0:1 and 5.99:1 and a range of (aluminum plus zirconium)-to-chloride atomic ratios between 2.1:1 and 1.51:1. The label states the content of anhydrous aluminum zirconium trichlorohydrate. Contains the labeled amount of anhydrous aluminum zirconium trichlorohydrate, within ±10%. Meets the requirements for Identification, pH (3.0–5.0, in a solution [15 in 100 (w/w)]), Arsenic (not more than 2 mcg per gram), Heavy metals (not more than 20 mcg per gram), Limit of iron (not more than 150 mcg per gram), Content of aluminum, Content of zirconium, Aluminum/zirconium atomic ratio (2.0:1–5.99:1), Content of chloride, and (Aluminum plus zirconium)/chloride atomic ratio (2.1:1–1.51:1).

Aluminum Zirconium Trichlorohydrate Solution USP—Preserve in well-closed containers. A polymeric, loosely hydrated complex of basic aluminum zirconium chloride that encompasses a range of aluminum-to-zirconium atomic ratios between 2.0:1 and 5.99:1 and a range of (aluminum plus zirconium)-to-chloride atomic ratios between 2.1:1 and 1.51:1. The following solvents may be used: water, propylene glycol, or dipropylene glycol. Label Solution to state the solvent used and the claimed concentration of anhydrous aluminum zirconium trichlorohydrate. Contains the equivalent of the labeled concentration of anhydrous aluminum zirconium trichlorohydrate, within ±10%. Meets the requirements for Identification, pH (3.0–5.0, in a solution prepared by diluting 3 grams of the Solution with water to obtain 10 mL), Arsenic (not more than 2 mcg per gram), Heavy metals (not more than 10 mcg per gram), Limit of iron (not more than 75 mcg per gram), Content of aluminum, Content of zirconium, Aluminum/zirconium atomic ratio (2.0:1–5.99:1), Content of chloride, and (Aluminum plus zirconium)/chloride atomic ratio (2.1:1–1.51:1).

Aluminum Zirconium Trichlorohydrex Gly USP—Preserve in well-closed containers. A derivative of Aluminum Zirconium Trichlorohydrate in which some of the water molecules have been displaced by glycine, calcium glycinate, magnesium glycinate, potassium glycinate, sodium glycinate, or zinc glycinate. Encompasses a range of aluminum-to-zirconium atomic ratios between 2.0:1 and 5.99:1 and a range of (aluminum plus zirconium)-to-chloride atomic ratios between 2.1:1 and 1.51:1. The label states the form of glycine used and the claimed content of anhydrous aluminum zirconium trichlorohydrate. Contains the labeled amount of anhydrous aluminum zirconium trichlorohydrate, within ±10%. Meets the requirements for Identification, pH (3.0–5.0, in a solution [15 in 100 (w/w)]), Arsenic (not more than 2 mcg per gram), Heavy metals (not more than 20 mcg per gram), Limit of iron (not more than 150 mcg per gram), Content of aluminum, Content of zirconium, Aluminum/zirconium atomic ratio (2.0:1–5.99:1), Content of chloride, and (Aluminum plus zirconium)/chloride atomic ratio (2.1:1–1.51:1).

Aluminum Zirconium Trichlorohydrex Gly Solution USP—Preserve in well-closed containers. A solution of Aluminum Zirconium Trichlorohydrate in which some of the waters of hydration have been displaced by glycine, calcium gly-

cinate, magnesium glycinate, potassium glycinate, sodium glycinate, or zinc glycinate. Encompasses a range of aluminum-to-zirconium ratios between 2.0:1 and 5.99:1, and a range of (aluminum plus zirconium)-to-chloride atomic ratios between 2.1:1 and 1.51:1. The following solvents may be used: water, propylene glycol, or dipropylene glycol. Label Solution to state the solvent and form of glycine used and the claimed concentration of anhydrous aluminum zirconium trichlorohydrate. Contains the equivalent of the labeled concentration of anhydrous aluminum zirconium trichlorohydrate, within ±10%. Meets the requirements for Identification, pH (3.0–5.0, in a solution prepared by diluting 3 grams of the Solution with water to obtain 10 mL), Arsenic (not more than 2 mcg per gram), Heavy metals (not more than 10 mcg per gram), Limit of iron (not more than 75 mcg per gram), Content of aluminum, Content of zirconium, Aluminum/zirconium atomic ratio (2.0:1–5.99:1), Content of chloride, and (Aluminum plus zirconium)/chloride atomic ratio (2.1:1–1.51:1).

AMANTADINE

Chemical name: Amantadine hydrochloride—Tricyclo[3.3.1.1^{3,7}]-decan-1-amine, hydrochloride.

Molecular formula: Amantadine hydrochloride—$C_{10}H_{17}N \cdot HCl$.

Molecular weight: Amantadine hydrochloride—187.71.

Description: Amantadine Hydrochloride USP—White or practically white, crystalline powder.

Solubility: Amantadine Hydrochloride USP—Freely soluble in water; soluble in alcohol and in chloroform.

USP requirements:

Amantadine Hydrochloride USP—Preserve in well-closed containers. Contains not less than 98.5% and not more than 101.5% of amantadine hydrochloride. Meets the requirements for Clarity and color of solution, Identification, pH (3.0–5.5, in a solution [1 in 5]), Heavy metals (not more than 0.001%), Chromatographic purity, and Organic volatile impurities.

Amantadine Hydrochloride Capsules USP—Preserve in tight containers. Contain the labeled amount, within ±5%. Meet the requirements for Identification, Dissolution (75% in 45 minutes in water in Apparatus 1 at 100 rpm), and Uniformity of dosage units.

Amantadine Hydrochloride Oral Solution USP—Preserve in tight containers. Contains the labeled amount, within ±5%. Meets the requirement for Identification.

Amantadine Hydrochloride Syrup USP—Preserve in tight containers. Contains the labeled amount, within ±5%. Meets the requirement for Identification.

Amantadine Hydrochloride Tablets—Not in *USP–NF*.

AMBENONIUM

Source: Quaternary ammonium compound.

Chemical name: Ambenonium chloride—Benzenemethanaminium, N,N'-[(1,2-dioxo-1,2-ethanediyl)bis(imino-2,1-ethanediyl)]bis[2-chloro-N,N-diethyl-, dichloride.

Molecular formula: Ambenonium chloride—$C_{28}H_{42}Cl_4N_4O_2$.

Molecular weight: Ambenonium chloride—608.47.

Description: Ambenonium chloride—White, odorless powder; melting point 196–199 °C.

Solubility: Ambenonium chloride—Soluble in water and in alcohol; slightly soluble in chloroform; practically insoluble in acetone and in ether.

USP requirements: Ambenonium Chloride Tablets—Not in *USP–NF*.

AMCINONIDE

Chemical name: Pregna-1,4-diene-3,20-dione, 21-(acetyloxy)-16,17-[cyclopentylidenebis(oxy)]-9-fluoro-11-hydroxy-, (11 beta,16 alpha)-.

Molecular formula: $C_{28}H_{35}FO_7$.

Molecular weight: 502.57.

Description: White to cream colored crystalline powder, having not more than a slight odor. Its melting point range is 248–252 °C.

USP requirements:
Amcinonide USP—Preserve in well-closed containers. Contains not less than 97.0% and not more than 102.0% of amcinonide, calculated on the dried basis. Meets the requirements for Identification, Specific rotation (+89.4° to +94.0°), Loss on drying (not more than 1.0%), and Heavy metals (not more than 0.002%).
Amcinonide Cream USP—Preserve in tight containers. It is Amcinonide in a suitable cream base. Contains the labeled amount, within −10% to +15%. Meets the requirements for Identification, Microbial limits, Minimum fill, and pH (3.5–5.2).
Amcinonide Lotion—Not in *USP–NF*.
Amcinonide Ointment USP—Preserve in tight containers. It is Amcinonide in a suitable ointment base. Contains the labeled amount, within −10% to +15%. Meets the requirements for Identification, Microbial limits, and Minimum fill.

AMDINOCILLIN

Chemical name: 4-Thia-1-azabicyclo[3.2.0]heptane-2-carboxylic acid, 6-[[(hexahydro-1*H*-azepin-1-yl)methylene]amino]-3,3-dimethyl-7-oxo-, [2*S*-(2 alpha,5 alpha,6 beta)]-.

Molecular formula: $C_{15}H_{23}N_3O_3S$.

Molecular weight: 325.43.

Description: Sterile Amdinocillin USP—White to off-white crystalline powder. Melts at 141–143 °C, with decomposition.

Solubility: Sterile Amdinocillin USP—Freely soluble in water and in methanol.

USP requirements:
Amdinocillin USP—Preserve in tight containers. Where it is intended for use in preparing injectable dosage forms, the label states that it is sterile or must be subjected to further processing during the preparation of injectable dosage forms. Contains not less than 950 mcg and not more than 1050 mcg of amdinocillin per mg, calculated on the anhydrous basis. Meets the requirements for Identification, Crystallinity, pH (4.0–6.2, in a solution [1 in 10]), Water (not more than 0.5%), and Limit of hexamethyleneimine (not more than 1.0%), for Sterility and Bacterial endotoxins under Amdinocillin for Injection (where the label states that Amdinocillin is sterile), and for Bacterial endotoxins under Amdinocillin for Injection (where the label states that Amdinocillin must be subjected to further processing during the preparation of injectable dosage forms).

Amdinocillin for Injection USP—Preserve in Containers for Sterile Solids. Contains the labeled amount, within −10% to +20%. Meets the requirements for Constituted solution, Bacterial endotoxins, Sterility, Particulate matter, and Limit of hexamethyleneimine (not more than 2.0%), for Identification, Crystallinity, pH, and Water under Amdinocillin, for Uniformity of dosage units, and for Labeling under Injections.

AMIFOSTINE

Chemical name: Ethanethiol, 2-[(3-aminopropyl)amino]-, dihydrogen phosphate (ester), trihydrate.

Molecular formula: $C_5H_{15}N_2O_3PS \cdot 3H_2O$.

Molecular weight: 268.26.

Description: White crystalline powder.

Solubility: Freely soluble in water.

USP requirements:
Amifostine USP—Preserve in tight, light-resistant containers, in a refrigerator. Contains not less than 78.0% and not more than 82.0% of amifostine, calculated on the as-is basis. Meets the requirements for Identification, X-ray diffraction, pH (6.5–7.5, in a solution [5 in 100]), Water (19.2–21.2%), Heavy metals (0.002%), Related compounds (not more than 0.1% of any individual impurity, excluding amifostine thiol and not more than 0.3% of total impurities, including amifostine thiol), and Organic volatile impurities.
Amifostine for Injection USP—Preserve in tight Containers for Sterile Solids, at controlled room temperature. It is a sterile, lyophilized crystalline substance suitable for parenteral use. Contains the labeled amount, within ±10%. Meets the requirements for Constituted solution, Bacterial endotoxins, Sterility, pH (6.5–7.5), Water (18.0–22.0%), Particulate matter, and Related compounds (for test 1: not more than 0.1% of any individual impurity, excluding amifostine thiol; for test 2: not more than 1.0% of total impurities, including amifostine thiol and amifostine disulfide), and for Uniformity of dosage units, Labeling under Injections, and tests for Identification and X-ray diffraction under Amifostine.

AMIKACIN

Source: Semi-synthetic; derived from kanamycin.

Chemical group: Aminoglycoside.

Chemical name:
Amikacin—D-Streptamine, *O*-3-amino-3-deoxy-alpha-D-glucopyranosyl-(1→6)-*O*-[6-amino-6-deoxy-alpha-D-glucopyranosyl-(1→4)]-*N'*-(4-amino-2-hydroxy-1-oxobutyl)-2-deoxy-, (*S*)-.
Amikacin sulfate—D-Streptamine, *O*-3-amino-3-deoxy-alpha-D-glucopyranosyl-(1→6)-*O*-[6-amino-6-deoxy-alpha-D-glucopyranosyl-(1→4)]-*N'*-(4-amino-2-hydroxy-1-oxobutyl)-2-deoxy-, (*S*)-, sulfate (1:2 or 1:1.8) (salt).

Molecular formula:
Amikacin—$C_{22}H_{43}N_5O_{13}$.
Amikacin sulfate—$C_{22}H_{43}N_5O_{13} \cdot 2H_2SO_4$ or $C_{22}H_{43}N_5O_{13} \cdot 1.8H_2SO_4$.

Molecular weight:
Amikacin—585.60.
Amikacin sulfate 2H₂O—781.76.
Amikacin sulfate 1.8H₂O—762.15.

Description:
    Amikacin USP—White, crystalline powder.
    Amikacin Sulfate USP—White, crystalline powder.
    Amikacin sulfate injection—Sterile, colorless to light straw colored solution. It has a pH adjusted to 4.5 with sulfuric acid.

Solubility:
    Amikacin USP—Sparingly soluble in water.
    Amikacin Sulfate USP—Freely soluble in water.

USP requirements:
    Amikacin USP—Preserve in tight containers. Has a potency of not less than 900 mcg of amikacin per mg, calculated on the anhydrous basis. Meets the requirements for Identification, Specific rotation ($+97°$ to $+105°$), Crystallinity, pH (9.5–11.5, in a solution containing 10 mg per mL), Water (not more than 8.5%), and Residue on ignition (not more than 1.0%).
    Amikacin Sulfate USP—Preserve in tight containers. Label it to indicate whether its molar ratio of amikacin to hydrogen sulfate is 1:2 or 1:1.8. Amikacin Sulfate having a molar ratio of amikacin to hydrogen sulfate of 1:2 contains an amount of amikacin sulfate equivalent to not less than 674 mcg and not more than 786 mcg of amikacin per mg, calculated on the dried basis. Amikacin Sulfate having a molar ratio of amikacin to hydrogen sulfate of 1:1.8 contains an amount of amikacin sulfate equivalent to not less than 691 mcg and not more than 806 mcg of amikacin per mg, calculated on the dried basis. Meets the requirements for Identification, Specific rotation ($+76°$ to $+84°$), Crystallinity, pH (2.0–4.0 [1:2 salt], or 6.0–7.3 [1:1.8 salt], in a solution containing 10 mg per mL), Loss on drying (not more than 13.0%), and Residue on ignition (not more than 1.0%).
    Amikacin Sulfate Injection USP—Preserve in single-dose or in multiple-dose containers, preferably of Type I or Type III glass. A sterile solution of Amikacin Sulfate in Water for Injection, or of Amikacin in Water for Injection prepared with the aid of Sulfuric Acid. Contains an amount of amikacin sulfate equivalent to the labeled amount of amikacin, within −10% to +20%. Meets the requirements for Identification, Bacterial endotoxins, pH (3.5–5.5), and Particulate matter, and for Injections.

AMILORIDE

Chemical name: Amiloride hydrochloride—Pyrazinecarboxamide, 3,5-diamino-N-(aminoiminomethyl)-6-chloro-, monohydrochloride dihydrate.

Molecular formula: Amiloride hydrochloride—$C_6H_8ClN_7O \cdot HCl \cdot 2H_2O$.

Molecular weight: Amiloride hydrochloride—302.12.

Description: Amiloride Hydrochloride USP—Yellow to greenish yellow, odorless or practically odorless powder.

pKa: 8.7.

Solubility: Amiloride Hydrochloride USP—Slightly soluble in water; insoluble in ether, in ethyl acetate, in acetone, and in chloroform; freely soluble in dimethylsulfoxide; sparingly soluble in methanol.

USP requirements:
    Amiloride Hydrochloride USP—Preserve in well-closed containers. Contains not less than 98.0% and not more than 101.0% of amiloride hydrochloride, calculated on the dried basis. Meets the requirements for Identification, Acidity, Loss on drying (11.0–13.0%), Residue on ignition (not more than 0.1%), Heavy metals (not more than 0.002%), Chromatographic purity, and Organic volatile impurities.
    Amiloride Hydrochloride Solution for Inhalation—Not in USP–NF.

    Amiloride Hydrochloride Tablets USP—Preserve in well-closed containers. Contain the labeled amount, within $\pm$ 10%. Meet the requirements for Identification, Dissolution (80% in 30 minutes in 0.1 N hydrochloric acid in Apparatus 2 at 50 rpm), and Uniformity of dosage units.

AMILORIDE AND HYDROCHLOROTHIAZIDE

For Amiloride and Hydrochlorothiazide—See individual listings for chemistry information.

USP requirements: Amiloride Hydrochloride and Hydrochlorothiazide Tablets USP—Preserve in well-closed containers. Contain the labeled amounts, within $\pm$10%. Meet the requirements for Identification, Dissolution (80% of amiloride hydrochloride and 75% of hydrochlorothiazide in 30 minutes in 0.1 N hydrochloric acid in Apparatus 2 at 50 rpm), Uniformity of dosage units, and Related compounds (not more than 1.0%).

AMILOXATE

Chemical name: 4-Methoxycinnamic acid, isoamyl ester.

Molecular formula: $C_{15}H_{20}O_3$.

Molecular weight: 248.32.

USP requirements: Amiloxate USP—Preserve in tight containers. Contains the labeld amount, within $\pm$5%. Meets the requirements for Identification, Specific gravity (1.037–1.041), Refractive index (1.556–1.560 at 20°), and Acidity (not more than 0.2 mL of titrant per mL of Amiloxate).

AMINOBENZOATE POTASSIUM

Molecular formula: $C_7H_6KNO_2$.

Molecular weight: 175.23.

Description: Aminobenzoate Potassium USP—White crystalline powder. The pH of a 1 in 100 solution in water is about 7.

Solubility: Aminobenzoate Potassium USP—Very soluble in water; soluble in alcohol; practically insoluble in ether.

USP requirements:
    Aminobenzoate Potassium USP—Preserve in well-closed containers. Contains not less than 98.5% and not more than 101.0% of aminobenzoate potassium, calculated on the dried basis. Meets the requirements for Identification, pH (8.0–9.0, in a solution [1 in 20]), Loss on drying (not more than 1.0%), Chloride (not more than 0.02%), Sulfate (not more than 0.02%), Heavy metals (not more than 0.002%), and Volatile diazotizable substances (not more than 0.002%, as p-toluidine).
    Aminobenzoate Potassium Capsules USP—Preserve in well-closed containers. Contain the labeled amount, within $\pm$ 10%. Meet the requirements for Identification, Dissolution (75% in 45 minutes in water in Apparatus 1 at 100 rpm), and Uniformity of dosage units.
    Aminobenzoate Potassium for Oral Solution USP—Preserve in tight containers. Contains the labeled amount, within $\pm$10%. Meets the requirements for Identification, pH (7.0–9.0, in a solution [1 in 10]), Minimum fill (multiple-unit containers), and Uniformity of dosage units (single-unit containers).

Aminobenzoate Potassium Tablets USP—Preserve in well-closed containers. Contain the labeled amount, within ± 10%. Meet the requirements for Identification, Dissolution (75% in 45 minutes in water in Apparatus 1 at 100 rpm), and Uniformity of dosage units.

AMINOBENZOATE SODIUM

Molecular formula: $C_7H_6NNaO_2$.

Molecular weight: 159.12.

USP requirements: Aminobenzoate Sodium USP—Preserve in well-closed containers. Contains not less than 98.5% and not more than 101.0% of aminobenzoate sodium, calculated on the dried basis. Meets the requirements for Identification, pH (8.0–9.0, in a solution [1 in 20]), Loss on drying (not more than 1.0%), Volatile diazotizable substances (not more than 0.002%, as *p*-toluidine), Chloride (not more than 0.02%), Sulfate (not more than 0.02%), and Heavy metals (not more than 0.002%).

AMINOBENZOIC ACID

Chemical name: Benzoic acid, 4-amino.

Molecular formula: $C_7H_7NO_2$.

Molecular weight: 137.14.

Description:
Aminobenzoic Acid USP—White or slightly yellow, odorless crystals or crystalline powder. Discolors on exposure to air or light.
Aminobenzoic Acid Topical Solution USP—Straw-colored solution having the odor of alcohol.

Solubility: Aminobenzoic Acid USP—Slightly soluble in water and in chloroform; freely soluble in alcohol and in solutions of alkali hydroxides and carbonates; sparingly soluble in ether.

USP requirements:
Aminobenzoic Acid USP—Preserve in tight, light-resistant containers. Contains not less than 98.5% and not more than 101.5% of aminobenzoic acid, calculated on the dried basis. Meets the requirements for Identification, Melting range (186–189 °C), Loss on drying (not more than 0.2%), Residue on ignition (not more than 0.1%), Heavy metals (not more than 0.002%), Volatile diazotizable substances (not more than 0.002%, as *p*-toluidine), and Ordinary impurities.
Aminobenzoic Acid Gel USP—Preserve in tight, light-resistant containers. Contains the labeled amount, within ±10%. Meets the requirements for Identification, Minimum fill, pH (4.0–6.0), and Alcohol content (42.3–54.0% [w/w]).
Aminobenzoic Acid Topical Solution USP—Preserve in tight, light-resistant containers. Contains, in each mL, not less than 45 mg and not more than 55 mg of aminobenzoic acid. Meets the requirements for Identification, Specific gravity (0.895–0.905), and Alcohol content (65–75%).

AMINOBENZOIC ACID, PADIMATE O, AND OXYBENZONE

For *Aminobenzoic Acid, Padimate O,* and *Oxybenzone*—See individual listings for chemistry information.

USP requirements: Aminobenzoic Acid, Padimate O, and Oxybenzone Lotion—Not in *USP–NF.*

AMINOBENZOIC ACID AND TITANIUM DIOXIDE

For *Aminobenzoic Acid* and *Titanium Dioxide*—See individual listings for chemistry information.

USP requirements:
Aminobenzoic Acid and Titanium Dioxide Cream—Not in *USP–NF.*
Aminobenzoic Acid and Titanium Dioxide Lotion—Not in *USP–NF.*

AMINOCAPROIC ACID

Chemical name: Hexanoic acid, 6-amino-.

Molecular formula: $C_6H_{13}NO_2$.

Molecular weight: 131.17.

Description: Aminocaproic Acid USP—Fine, white, crystalline powder. Is odorless, or practically odorless. Its solutions are neutral to litmus. Melts at about 205 °C.

Solubility: Aminocaproic Acid USP—Freely soluble in water, in acids, and in alkalies; slightly soluble in methanol and in alcohol; practically insoluble in chloroform and in ether.

USP requirements:
Aminocaproic Acid USP—Preserve in tight containers. Contains not less than 98.5% and not more than 101.5% of aminocaproic acid, calculated on the anhydrous basis. Meets the requirements for Identification, Water (not more than 0.5%), Residue on ignition (not more than 0.1%), and Heavy metals (not more than 0.002%).
Aminocaproic Acid Injection USP—Preserve in single-dose or in multiple-dose containers, preferably of Type I glass. A sterile solution of Aminocaproic Acid in Water for Injection. Contains the labeled amount, within –5% to +7.5%. Meets the requirements for Identification, Bacterial endotoxins, and pH (6.0–7.6), and for Injections.
Aminocaproic Acid Oral Solution USP—Preserve in tight containers. Contains the labeled amount, within –5% to +15%. Meets the requirements for Identification and pH (6.0–6.5).
Aminocaproic Acid Syrup USP—Preserve in tight containers. Contains the labeled amount, within –5% to +15%. Meets the requirements for Identification and pH (6.0–6.5).
Aminocaproic Acid Tablets USP—Preserve in tight containers. Contain the labeled amount, within ±5%. Meet the requirements for Identification, Dissolution (75% in 45 minutes in water in Apparatus 1 at 100 rpm), and Uniformity of dosage units.

AMINOGLUTETHIMIDE

Chemical name: 2,6-Piperidinedione, 3-(4-aminophenyl)-3 ethyl-.

Molecular formula: $C_{13}H_{16}N_2O_2$.

Molecular weight: 232.28.

Description: Aminoglutethimide USP—Fine, white, or creamy white, crystalline powder.

Solubility: Aminoglutethimide USP—Very slightly soluble in water; readily soluble in most organic solvents. Forms water-soluble salts with strong acids.

USP requirements:

Aminoglutethimide USP—Preserve in well-closed containers. Contains not less than 98.0% and not more than 102.0% of aminoglutethimide, calculated on the dried basis. Meets the requirements for Identification, pH (6.2–7.3, in a 1 in 1000 solution in dilute methanol [1 in 20]), Loss on drying (not more than 0.5%), Residue on ignition (not more than 0.1%), Sulfate, Heavy metals (not more than 0.001%), Chromatographic purity and limit of *m*-aminoglutethimide (not more than 1.0% total impurities, other than *m*-aminoglutethimide), Limit of azo-aminoglutethimide (not more than 0.03%), and Organic volatile impurities.

Aminoglutethimide Tablets USP—Preserve in tight, light-resistant containers. Contain the labeled amount, within ± 10%. Meet the requirements for Identification, Dissolution (70% in 30 minutes in dilute hydrochloric acid [7 in 1000] in Apparatus 1 at 100 rpm), Uniformity of dosage units, and Chromatographic purity (not more than 2.0% total impurities, other than *m*-aminoglutethimide).

AMINOHIPPURATE SODIUM

Chemical name: Glycine, *N*-(4-aminobenzoyl)-, monosodium salt.

Molecular formula: $C_9H_9N_2NaO_3$.

Molecular weight: 216.17.

pKa: 3.83.

Solubility: Soluble in water.

USP requirements: Aminohippurate Sodium Injection USP—Preserve in single-dose or in multiple-dose containers, preferably of Type I glass. A sterile solution of Aminohippuric Acid in Water for Injection prepared with the aid of Sodium Hydroxide. Contains the labeled amount, within ±5%. Meets the requirements for Identification, Bacterial endotoxins, and pH (6.7–7.6), and for Injections.

AMINOHIPPURIC ACID

Chemical name: Glycine, *N*-(4-aminobenzoyl)-.

Molecular formula: $C_9H_{10}N_2O_3$.

Molecular weight: 194.19.

Description: Aminohippuric Acid USP—White, crystalline powder. Discolors on exposure to light. Melts at about 195 °C, with decomposition.

Solubility: Aminohippuric Acid USP—Sparingly soluble in water and in alcohol; freely soluble in alkaline solutions, with some decomposition, and in diluted hydrochloric acid; very slightly soluble in carbon tetrachloride, in chloroform, and in ether.

USP requirements: Aminohippuric Acid USP—Preserve in tight, light-resistant containers. Contains not less than 98.0% and not more than 100.5% of aminohippuric acid, calculated on the dried basis. Meets the requirements for Identification, Loss on drying (not more than 0.25%), Residue on ignition (not more than 0.25%), and Heavy metals (not more than 0.001%).

AMINOLEVULINIC ACID

Chemical name: Aminolevulinic acid hydrochloride—5-aminolevulinic acid hydrochloride.

Molecular formula: Aminolevulinic acid hydrochloride—$C_5H_9NO_3 \cdot HCl$.

Molecular weight: Aminolevulinic acid hydrochloride—167.59.

Description: Aminolevulinic acid hydrochloride—A white to off-white, odorless crystalline solid.

Solubility: Aminolevulinic acid hydrochloride—Very soluble in water; slightly soluble in methanol and in ethanol; practically insoluble in chloroform, in hexane, and in mineral oil.

USP requirements: Aminolevulinic Acid Hydrochloride Topical Solution—Not in *USP–NF*.

AMINOPENTAMIDE

Chemical name: Aminopentamide sulfate—Alpha-[2-(Dimethylamino)propyl]-alpha-phenylbenzeneacetamide sulfate.

Molecular formula: Aminopentamide sulfate—$C_{19}H_{24}N_2O \cdot H_2SO_4$.

Molecular weight: Aminopentamide sulfate—394.49.

Description: Aminopentamide Sulfate USP—White, crystalline powder.

Solubility: Aminopentamide Sulfate USP—Freely soluble in water and in alcohol; very slightly soluble in chloroform; practically insoluble in ether.

USP requirements:

Aminopentamide Sulfate USP—Preserve in tight containers, at controlled room temperature. Label it to indicate that it is for veterinary use only. Contains not less than 95.0% and not more than 103.0% of aminopentamide sulfate. Meets the requirements for Clarity and color of solution, Identification, Melting range (179–186 °C), pH (1.2–3.0, in a solution [2.5 in 100]), Loss on drying (not more than 4.4%), and Residue on ignition (not more than 0.5%).

Aminopentamide Sulfate Injection—Preserve in tight single-dose or multiple-dose Containers for Injection. Store at controlled room temperature. It is a sterile solution of Aminopentamide Sulfate in Water for Injection. Label Injection to indicate that it is for veterinary use only. Contains the labeled amount, within ±10%. Meets the requirements for Identification, Bacterial endotoxins, Sterility, and pH (2.5–4.5), and for Injections.

Aminopentamide Sulfate Tablets—Preserve in tight containers, at controlled room temperature. Label Tablets to indicate that they are for veterinary use only. Contain the labeled amount, within ±5%. Meet the requirements for Identification, Disintegration (not more than 10 minutes), Uniformity of dosage units, and Loss on drying (not more than 4.0%).

AMINOPHYLLINE

Source: The ethylenediamine salt of theophylline.

Chemical name: 1*H*-Purine-2,6-dione, 3,7-dihydro-1,3-dimethyl-, compd. with 1,2-ethanediamine (2:1).

Molecular formula: $C_{16}H_{24}N_{10}O_4$.

Molecular weight: 420.43 (anhydrous).

Description:

Aminophylline USP—White or slightly yellowish granules or powder, having a slight ammoniacal odor. Upon exposure to air, it gradually loses ethylenediamine and absorbs carbon dioxide with the liberation of free theophylline. Its solutions are alkaline to litmus.

Aminophylline Tablets USP—May have a faint ammoniacal odor.

Solubility: Aminophylline USP—One gram dissolves in 25 mL of water to give a clear solution; one gram dissolved in 5 mL of water crystallizes upon standing, but redissolves when a small amount of ethylenediamine is added. Insoluble in alcohol and in ether.

USP requirements:

Aminophylline USP—Preserve in tight containers. It is anhydrous or contains not more than two molecules of water of hydration. Label it to indicate whether it is anhydrous or hydrous, and also to state the content of anhydrous theophylline. Contains not less than 84.0% and not more than 87.4% of anhydrous theophylline, calculated on the anhydrous basis. Meets the requirements for Identification, Water (not more than 0.75% for the anhydrous form and not more than 7.9% for the hydrous form), Residue on ignition (not more than 0.15%), Organic volatile impurities, and Ethylenediamine content (157–175 mg per gram of theophylline).

Aminophylline Injection USP—Preserve in single-dose containers from which carbon dioxide has been excluded, preferably of Type I glass, protected from light. A sterile solution of Aminophylline in Water for Injection, or a sterile solution of Theophylline in Water for Injection prepared with the aid of Ethylenediamine. Label the Injection to state the content of anhydrous theophylline. Contains, in each mL, an amount of aminophylline equivalent to the labeled amount of anhydrous theophylline, within ±7%. Aminophylline Injection may contain an excess of Ethylenediamine, but no other substance may be added for the purpose of pH adjustment. Meets the requirements for Identification, Bacterial endotoxins, pH (8.6–9.0), Particulate matter, and Ethylenediamine content (166–192 mg per gram of anhydrous theophylline), and for Injections.

Note: Do not use the Injection if crystals have separated.

Aminophylline Oral Solution USP—Preserve in tight containers. An aqueous solution of Aminophylline, prepared with the aid of Ethylenediamine. Label the Oral Solution to state the content of anhydrous theophylline. Contains an amount of aminophylline equivalent to the labeled amount of anhydrous theophylline, within ±10%. Aminophylline Oral Solution may contain an excess of ethylenediamine, but no other substance may be added for the purpose of pH adjustment. Meets the requirements for Identification, pH (8.5–9.7), and Ethylenediamine content (176–283 mg per gram of anhydrous theophylline).

Aminophylline Rectal Solution USP—Preserve in tight single-dose or in multiple-dose containers, at controlled room temperature. An aqueous solution of Aminophylline, prepared with the aid of Ethylenediamine. Label the Rectal Solution to state the content of anhydrous theophylline. Contains an amount of aminophylline equivalent to the labeled amount of anhydrous theophylline, within ±10%. Aminophylline Rectal Solution may contain an excess of ethylenediamine, but no other substance may be added for the purpose of pH adjustment. Meets the requirements for Identification, pH (9.0–9.5), and Ethylenediamine content (218–267 mg per gram of anhydrous theophylline).

Aminophylline Suppositories USP—Preserve in well-closed containers, in a cold place. Label the Suppositories to state the content of anhydrous theophylline. Contain an amount of aminophylline equivalent to the labeled amount of anhydrous theophylline, within ±10%. Meet the requirements for Identification and Ethylenediamine content (152–190 mg per gram of anhydrous theophylline).

Aminophylline Tablets USP—Preserve in tight containers. Label the Tablets to state the content of anhydrous theophylline. Contain an amount of aminophylline equivalent to the labeled amount of anhydrous theophylline, within ±7%. Meet the requirements for Identification, Dissolution (75% in 45 minutes in water in Apparatus 2 at 50 rpm, for uncoated or plain coated tablets), Uniformity of dosage units, and Ethylenediamine content (140–190 mg per gram of anhydrous theophylline).

Note: The ammoniacal odor present in the vapor space above Aminophylline Tablets is often quite strong, especially when bottles having suitably tight closures are newly opened. This is due to ethylenediamine vapor pressure build-up, a natural condition in the case of aminophylline.

Aminophylline Delayed-release Tablets USP—Preserve in tight containers. Label the tablets to state the content of anhydrous theophylline. Contains an amount of aminophylline equivalent to the labelled amount of anhydrous theophylline, within ±7%. Meet the requirements for Disintigration and for Identification test, Uniformity of dosage units, and Ethylenediamine content.

Note: The ammoniacal odor present in the vapor space above Aminophylline Delayed-release Tablets is often quite strong, especially when bottles having suitably tight closures are newly opened. This is due to ethylenediamine vapor pressure build-up, a natural condition in the case of aminophylline.

Aminophylline Extended-release Tablets—Not in *USP–NF*.

AMINOSALICYLATE SODIUM

Chemical name: Benzoic acid, 4-amino-2-hydroxy-, monosodium salt, dihydrate.

Molecular formula: $C_7H_6NNaO_3 \cdot 2H_2O$.

Molecular weight: 211.15.

Description: Aminosalicylate Sodium USP—White to cream-colored, crystalline powder. Is practically odorless. Its solutions decompose slowly and darken in color.

Solubility: Aminosalicylate Sodium USP—Freely soluble in water; sparingly soluble in alcohol; very slightly soluble in ether and in chloroform.

USP requirements:

Aminosalicylate Sodium USP—Preserve in tight, light-resistant containers, protected from excessive heat. Contains not less than 98.0% and not more than 101.0% of aminosalicylate sodium, calculated on the anhydrous basis. Meets the requirements for Clarity and color of solution, Identification, pH (6.5–8.5, in a solution [1 in 50]), Water (16.0–18.0%), Chloride (not more than 0.042%), Heavy metals (not more than 0.003%), Limit of *m*-aminophenol (not more than 0.25%), Hydrogen sulfide, sulfur dioxide, and amyl alcohol, and Organic volatile impurities.

Caution: Prepare solutions of Aminosalicylate Sodium within 24 hours of administration. Under no circumstances use a solution if its color is darker than that of a freshly prepared solution.

Aminosalicylate Sodium Tablets USP—Preserve in tight, light-resistant containers, protected from excessive heat. Contain the labeled amount, within ±5%. Meet the require-

ments for Identification, Dissolution (75% in 45 minutes in water in Apparatus 1 at 100 rpm), Uniformity of dosage units, and Limit of *m*-aminophenol (not more than 1.0%).

AMINOSALICYLIC ACID

Chemical name: Benzoic acid, 4-amino-2-hydroxy-.

Molecular formula: $C_7H_7NO_3$.

Molecular weight: 153.14.

Description: Aminosalicylic Acid USP—White or practically white, bulky powder, that darkens on exposure to light and to air. Is odorless, or has a slight acetous odor.

Solubility: Aminosalicylic Acid USP—Slightly soluble in water and in ether; soluble in alcohol.

USP requirements:
Aminosalicylic Acid USP—Preserve in tight, light-resistant containers, at a temperature not exceeding 30 °C. Contains not less than 98.5% and not more than 100.5% of aminosalicylic acid, calculated on the anhydrous basis. Meets the requirements for Clarity and color of solution, Identification, pH (3.0–3.7, in a saturated solution), Water (not more than 0.5%), Residue on ignition (not more than 0.2%), Chloride (not more than 0.042%), Heavy metals (not more than 0.003%), Limit of *m*-aminophenol (not more than 0.25%), and Hydrogen sulfide, sulfur dioxide, and amyl alcohol.

Caution: Under no circumstances use a solution prepared from Aminosalicylic Acid if its color is darker than that of a freshly prepared solution.

Aminosalicylic Acid Granules—Not in *USP–NF*.
Aminosalicylic Acid Tablets USP—Preserve in tight, light-resistant containers, at a temperature not exceeding 30 °C. Contain the labeled amount, within ±5%. Meet the requirements for Identification, Dissolution (75% in 45 minutes in phosphate buffer [pH 7.5] in Apparatus 1 at 100 rpm), Uniformity of dosage units, and Limit of *m*-aminophenol (not more than 1.0%).

AMIODARONE

Chemical group: Benzofuran derivative.

Chemical name: Amiodarone hydrochloride—2-Butyl-3-benzofuranyl 4-[2-(diethylamino)ethoxy]-3-5-diiodophenyl ketone, hydrochloride.

Molecular formula: Amiodarone hydrochloride—$C_{25}H_{29}I_2NO_3 \cdot HCl$.

Molecular weight: Amiodarone hydrochloride—681.77.

Description: Amiodarone hydrochloride—White to cream-colored crystalline powder.

pKa: 6.6.

Solubility: Amiodarone hydrochloride—Slightly soluble in water; soluble in alcohol; freely soluble in chloroform.

Other characteristics: Amiodarone hydrochloride—Contains 37.3% iodine by weight; highly lipophilic.

USP requirements:
Amiodarone Hydrochloride Injection—Not in *USP–NF*.
Amiodarone Hydrochloride Tablets—Not in *USP–NF*.

AMITRAZ

Chemical name: Methanimidamide, *N*-(2,4-dimethylphenyl)-*N*-[[(2,4-dimethylphenyl)imino]methyl]-*N*-methyl-.

Molecular formula: $C_{19}H_{23}N_3$.

Molecular weight: 293.41.

Description: Melting point 86–87 °C and unstable to acidic pH.

Solubility: Soluble in water (1 ppm) and in most organic solvents.

USP requirements:
Amitraz USP—Preserve in well-closed containers. Label it to indicate that it is for veterinary use only. Contains not less than 95.0% and not more than 101.5% of amitraz, calculated on the anhydrous basis. Meets the requirements for Identification, Water (not more than 0.1%), Residue on ignition (not more than 0.2%), and Related compounds.
Amitraz Concentrate for Dip USP—Preserve in well-closed containers. Contains Amitraz in a suitable vehicle. Label it to indicate that it is for veterinary use only. The label states also that it is to be diluted before use and states the name and quantity of diluent to be used, the directions for dilution, and the conditions for storage of the constituted Dip. Contains the labeled amount, within −10% to +20%. Meets the requirements for Identification and Water (not more than 0.15%).

AMITRIPTYLINE

Chemical group: Dibenzocycloheptadiene derivative.

Chemical name: Amitriptyline hydrochloride—1-Propanamine, 3-(10,11-dihydro-5*H*-dibenzo[*a,d*]cyclohepten-5-ylidene)-*N,N*-dimethyl-, hydrochloride.

Molecular formula: Amitriptyline hydrochloride—$C_{20}H_{23}N \cdot HCl$.

Molecular weight: Amitriptyline hydrochloride—313.86.

Description: Amitriptyline Hydrochloride USP—White or practically white, odorless or practically odorless, crystalline powder or small crystals.

pKa: Amitriptyline hydrochloride—9.4.

Solubility:
Amitriptyline Hydrochloride USP—Freely soluble in water, in alcohol, in chloroform, and in methanol; insoluble in ether.
Amitriptyline pamoate—Almost completely insoluble in water.

Other characteristics: Tertiary amine.

USP requirements:
Amitriptyline Hydrochloride USP—Preserve in well-closed containers. Contains not less than 99.0% and not more than 100.5% of amitriptyline hydrochloride, calculated on the dried basis. Meets the requirements for Identification, Melting range (195–199 °C), pH (5.0–6.0, in a solution [1 in 100]), Loss on drying (not more than 0.5%), Residue on ignition (not more than 0.1%), Heavy metals (not more than 0.001%), Chromatographic purity, and Organic volatile impurities.
Amitriptyline Hydrochloride Injection USP—Preserve in single-dose or in multiple-dose containers, preferably of Type I glass. A sterile solution of Amitriptyline Hydrochloride in Water for Injection. Contains the labeled amount, within ± 10%. Meets the requirements for Identification, Pyrogen, and pH (4.0–6.0), and for Injections.

Amitriptyline Hydrochloride Tablets USP—Preserve in well-closed containers. Contain the labeled amount, within ± 10%. Meet the requirements for Identification, Dissolution (75% in 45 minutes in 0.1 N hydrochloric acid in Apparatus 1 at 100 rpm), and Uniformity of dosage units.
Amitriptyline Pamoate Syrup—Not in *USP–NF*.

AMLEXANOX

Chemical name: 5H-[1]Benzopyrano[2,3-b]pyridine-3-carboxylic acid, 2-amino-7-(1-methylethyl)-5-oxo-.

Molecular formula: $C_{16}H_{14}N_2O_4$.

Molecular weight: 298.29.

Description: Odorless, white to yellowish-white crystalline powder.

USP requirements: Amlexanox Oral Paste—Not in *USP–NF*.

AMLODIPINE

Chemical name: Amlodipine besylate—3,5-Pyridinedicarboxylic acid, 2-[(2-aminoethoxy)methyl]-4-(2-chlorophenyl)-1,4-dihydro-6-methyl-, 3-ethyl 5-methyl ester, (±)-, monobenzenesulfonate.

Molecular formula: Amlodipine besylate—$C_{20}H_{25}ClN_2O_5 \cdot C_6H_6O_3S$.

Molecular weight: Amlodipine besylate—567.06.

Description: Amlodipine besylate—White crystalline powder.

Solubility: Amlodipine besylate—Slightly soluble in water; sparingly soluble in ethanol.

USP requirements: Amlodipine Besylate Tablets—Not in *USP–NF*.

AMLODIPINE AND BENAZEPRIL

For *Amlodipine* and *Benazepril*—See individual listings for chemistry information.

USP requirements: Amlodipine and Benazepril Hydrochloride Capsules—Not in *USP–NF*.

STRONG AMMONIA SOLUTION

Chemical name: Ammonia.

Molecular formula: NH_3.

Molecular weight: 17.03.

Description: Strong Ammonia Solution NF—Clear, colorless liquid, having an exceedingly pungent, characteristic odor. Specific gravity is about 0.90.
NF category: Alkalizing agent.

NF requirements: Strong Ammonia Solution NF—Preserve in tight containers at a temperature not above 25 °C. A solution of ammonia containing not less than 27.0% and not more than 31.0% (w/w) of ammonia. On exposure to air it loses ammonia rapidly. Meets the requirements for Identification, Heavy metals (not more than 0.0013%), Limit of nonvolatile residue (not more than 0.05%), and Readily oxidizable substances.

Caution: Use care in handling Strong Ammonia Solution because of the caustic nature of the Solution and the irritating properties of its vapor. Cool the container well before opening, and cover the closure with a cloth or similar material while opening. Do not taste Strong Ammonia Solution, and avoid inhalation of its vapor.

AROMATIC AMMONIA SPIRIT

Description: Aromatic Ammonia Spirit USP—Practically colorless liquid when recently prepared, but gradually acquiring a yellow color on standing. Has an aromatic and pungent odor, and is affected by light. Specific gravity is about 0.90.

USP requirements:
Aromatic Ammonia Spirit USP—Preserve in tight, light-resistant containers, at a temperature not exceeding 30 °C. A hydroalcoholic solution that contains, in each 100 mL, not less than 1.7 grams and not more than 2.1 grams of total ammonia, and Ammonium Carbonate corresponding to not less than 3.5 grams and not more than 4.5 grams. Meets the requirement for Alcohol content (62.0–68.0%).
Aromatic Ammonia Spirit Inhalant—Not in *USP–NF*.

AMMONIO METHACRYLATE COPOLYMER

Description: Ammonio Methacrylate Copolymer NF—Colorless, clear to white-opaque granules or a white powder, both with a faint amine-like odor.
NF category: Coating agent.

Solubility: Ammonio Methacrylate Copolymer NF—Soluble to freely soluble in methanol, in alcohol, and in isopropyl alcohol, each of which contains small amounts of water; soluble to freely soluble in acetone, in ethyl acetate, and in methylene chloride. The solutions are clear to slightly cloudy. Insoluble in petroleum ether and in water.

NF requirements: Ammonio Methacrylate Copolymer NF—Preserve in tight containers at a temperature not exceeding 30 °C. A fully polymerized copolymer of acrylic and methacrylic acid esters with a low content of quaternary ammonium groups. It is available in two types, which differ in content of ammonio methacrylate units. Label it to state whether it is Type A or B. Meets the requirements for Identification, Viscosity (not more than 15 centipoises), Loss on drying (not more than 3.0%), Residue on ignition (not more than 0.1%), Heavy metals (not more than 0.002%), and Limit of monomers (not more than 0.005% of methyl methacrylate and not more than 0.025% of ethyl acrylate).

AMMONIUM CARBONATE

Chemical name: Carbonic acid, monoammonium salt, mixt. with ammonium carbamate.

Molecular formula: Ammonium carbonate (normal)—$(NH_4)_2CO_3$.

Molecular weight: Ammonium carbonate (normal)—96.09.

Description: Ammonium Carbonate NF—White powder, or hard, white or translucent masses, having a strong odor of ammonia without empyreuma. Its solutions are alkaline to litmus. On exposure to air, it loses ammonia and carbon dioxide, becoming opaque, and is finally converted into friable porous lumps or a white powder of ammonium bicarbonate.
NF category: Alkalizing agent; buffering agent.

Solubility: Ammonium Carbonate NF—Freely soluble in water, but decomposed by hot water.

NF requirements: Ammonium Carbonate NF—Preserve in tight, light-resistant containers, at a temperature not above 30 °C. Consists of ammonium bicarbonate and ammonium carbamate in varying proportions. Yields not less than 30.0% and not more than 34.0% of ammonia. Meets the requirements for Identification, Residue on ignition (not more than 0.1%), Chloride (not more than 0.0035%), Sulfate (not more than 0.005%), and Heavy metals (not more than 0.001%).

AMMONIUM CHLORIDE

Chemical name: Ammonium chloride.

Molecular formula: NH_4Cl.

Molecular weight: 53.49.

Description: Ammonium Chloride USP—Colorless crystals or white, fine or coarse, crystalline powder. Is somewhat hygroscopic.

Solubility: Ammonium Chloride USP—Freely soluble in water and in glycerin, and even more so in boiling water; sparingly soluble in alcohol.

USP requirements:
Ammonium Chloride USP—Preserve in tight containers. Contains not less than 99.5% and not more than 100.5% of ammonium chloride, calculated on the dried basis. Meets the requirements for Identification, pH (4.6–6.0, in a solution [1 in 20]), Loss on drying (not more than 0.5%), Residue on ignition (not more than 0.1%), Limit of thiocyanate, and Heavy metals (not more than 0.001%).
Ammonium Chloride Injection USP—Preserve in single-dose or in multiple-dose containers, preferably of Type I or Type II glass. A sterile solution of Ammonium Chloride in Water for Injection. The label states the content of ammonium chloride in terms of weight and of milliequivalents in a given volume. The label states also the total osmolar concentration in mOsmol per liter or per mL. The label states that the Injection is not for direct injection but is to be diluted with Sodium Chloride Injection to the appropriate strength before use. Contains the labeled amount, within ±5%. Hydrochloric acid may be added to adjust the pH. Meets the requirements for Identification, Bacterial endotoxins, pH (4.0–6.0, in a concentration of not more than 100 mg of ammonium chloride per mL), Particulate matter, and Chloride content (63.0–70.3% of the labeled amount of ammonium chloride), and for Injections.
Ammonium Chloride Delayed-release Tablets USP—Preserve in tight containers. Contain the labeled amount, within ±6%. Ammonium Chloride Delayed-release Tablets are enteric-coated. Meet the requirements for Identification, Disintegration (2 hours, determined as directed for Enteric-coated Tablets), and Limit of thiocyanate.

FERRIC AMMONIUM CITRATE

USP requirements:
Ferric Ammonium Citrate USP—Preserve in tight, light-resistant containers, and store in a cool place. Contains not less than 16.5% and not more than 18.5% of iron (Fe). Meets the requirements for Identification, Ferric citrate, Sulfate (not more than 0.3%), Oxalate (no turbidity is produced within 5 minutes), Mercury (not more than 10 micrograms per gram), and Limit of lead (not more than 10 micrograms per gram).

Ferric Ammonium Citrate for Oral Solution USP—Preserve in tight, light-resistant containers, and store in a cool place. Contains Ferric Ammonium Citrate and an effervescent mixture of suitable organic acid and an alkali metal bicarbonate. Contains the labeled amount, within ±10%. May contain one or more suitable flavors, colors, or stabilizing agents. Meets the requirement for Identification.

AMMONIUM MOLYBDATE

Chemical name: Molybdate ($Mo_7O_{24}^{6-}$), hexaammonium, tetrahydrate.

Molecular formula: $(NH_4)_6Mo_7O_{24} \cdot 4H_2O$.

Molecular weight: 1235.86.

Description: Ammonium Molybdate USP—Colorless or slightly greenish or yellowish crystals.

Solubility: Ammonium Molybdate USP—Soluble in water; practically insoluble in alcohol.

USP requirements:
Ammonium Molybdate USP—Preserve in tight containers. Contains not less than 99.3% and not more than 101.8% of ammonium molybdate. Meets the requirements for Identification, Insoluble substances (not more than 0.005%), Chloride (not more than 0.002%), Limit of nitrate, Sulfate (not more than 0.02%), Arsenate, phosphate, and silicate, Phosphate (not more than 5 ppm), Magnesium and alkali salts (not more than 0.02%), and Heavy metals (not more than 10 mcg per gram).
Ammonium Molybdate Injection USP—Preserve in single-dose or in multiple-dose containers, preferably of Type I or Type II glass. A sterile solution of Ammonium Molybdate in Water for Injection. Label the Injection to indicate that it is to be diluted to the appropriate strength with Sterile Water for Injection or other suitable fluid prior to administration. Contains an amount of ammonium molybdate equivalent to the labeled amount of molybdenum, within ±15%. Meets the requirements for Identification, Pyrogen, pH (3.0–6.0), and Particulate matter, and for Injections.

AMMONIUM PHOSPHATE

Chemical name: Phosphoric acid, diammonium salt.

Molecular formula: $(NH_4)_2HPO_4$.

Molecular weight: 132.06.

Description: Ammonium Phosphate NF—Colorless or white granules or powder.
NF category: Buffering agent.

Solubility: Ammonium Phosphate NF—Freely soluble in water; practically insoluble in acetone and in alcohol.

NF requirements: Ammonium Phosphate NF—Preserve in tight containers. Contains not less than 96.0% and not more than 102.0% of ammonium phosphate. Meets the requirements for Identification, pH (7.6–8.2, in a solution [1 in 100]), Chloride (not more than 0.03%), Sulfate (not more than 0.15%), Arsenic (not more than 3 ppm), and Heavy metals (not more than 0.001%).

AMOBARBITAL

Chemical name:

Amobarbital—2,4,6(1*H*,3*H*,5*H*)-Pyrimidinetrione, 5-ethyl-5-(3-methylbutyl)-.

Amobarbital sodium—2,4,6(1*H*,3*H*,5*H*)-Pyrimidinetrione, 5-ethyl-5-(3-methylbutyl)-, monosodium salt.

Molecular formula:

Amobarbital—$C_{11}H_{18}N_2O_3$.

Amobarbital sodium—$C_{11}H_{17}N_2NaO_3$.

Molecular weight:

Amobarbital—226.27.

Amobarbital sodium—248.25.

Description:

Amobarbital—White, odorless, crystalline powder. Its saturated solution has a pH of about 5.6, determined potentiometrically.

Amobarbital Sodium USP—White, friable, granular powder. Is odorless and hygroscopic. Its solutions decompose on standing, heat accelerating the decomposition.

Solubility:

Amobarbital—Very slightly soluble in water; freely soluble in alcohol and in ether; soluble in chloroform and in solutions of fixed alkali hydroxides and carbonates.

Amobarbital Sodium USP—Very soluble in water; soluble in alcohol; practically insoluble in ether and in chloroform.

USP requirements:

Amobarbital Tablets—Not in *USP–NF*.

Amobarbital Sodium USP—Preserve in tight containers. Where it is intended for use in preparing injectable dosage forms, the label states that it is sterile or must be subjected to further processing during the preparation of injectable dosage forms. Contains not less than 98.5% and not more than 100.5% of amobarbital sodium, calculated on the dried basis. Meets the requirements for Completeness of solution, Identification, pH (not more than 11.0), Loss on drying (not more than 2.0%), Heavy metals (not more than 0.003%), and Organic volatile impurities, for Sterility and Bacterial endotoxins under Amobarbital Sodium for Injection (where the label states that Amobarbital Sodium is sterile), and for Bacterial endotoxins under Amobarbital Sodium for Injection (where the label states that Amobarbital Sodium must be subjected to further processing during the preparation of injectable dosage forms).

Amobarbital Sodium Capsules—Not in *USP–NF*.

Amobarbital Sodium for Injection USP—Preserve in Containers for Sterile Solids. It is Amobarbital Sodium suitable for parenteral use. Meets the requirements for Constituted solution, Bacterial endotoxins, and Loss on drying (not more than 1.0%), for Identification, Completeness of solution, pH, and Heavy metals under Amobarbital Sodium, and for Sterility tests, Uniformity of dosage units, and Labeling under Injections.

AMODIAQUINE

Chemical name:

Amodiaquine—Phenol, 4-[(7-chloro-4-quinolinyl)amino]-2-[(diethylamino)methyl]-.

Amodiaquine hydrochloride—Phenol, 4-[(7-chloro-4-quinolinyl)amino]-2-[(diethylamino)methyl]-, dihydrochloride, dihydrate.

Molecular formula:

Amodiaquine—$C_{20}H_{22}ClN_3O$.

Amodiaquine hydrochloride—$C_{20}H_{22}ClN_3O \cdot 2HCl \cdot 2H_2O$.

Molecular weight:

Amodiaquine—355.86.

Amodiaquine hydrochloride—464.81.

Description:

Amodiaquine USP—Very pale yellow to light tan-yellow, odorless powder.

Amodiaquine Hydrochloride USP—Yellow, crystalline powder. Is odorless.

Solubility:

Amodiaquine USP—Practically insoluble in water; sparingly soluble in 1.0 *N* hydrochloric acid; slightly soluble in alcohol.

Amodiaquine Hydrochoride USP—Soluble in water; sparingly soluble in alcohol; very slightly soluble in chloroform and in ether.

USP requirements:

Amodiaquine USP—Preserve in tight containers. Contains not less than 97.0% and not more than 103.0% of amodiaquine, calculated on the anhydrous basis. Meets the requirements for Identification, Water (not more than 0.5%), Residue on ignition (not more than 0.2%), Chromatographic purity, and Organic volatile impurities.

Amodiaquine Hydrochloride USP—Preserve in tight containers. Contains not less than 97.0% and not more than 103.0% of amodiaquine hydrochloride, calculated on the anhydrous basis. Meets the requirements for Completeness of solution, Identification, Water (7.0–9.0%), Residue on ignition (not more than 0.2%), Chromatographic purity, and Organic volatile impurities.

Amodiaquine Hydrochloride Tablets USP—Preserve in tight containers. Contain an amount of amodiaquine hydrochloride equivalent to the labeled amount of amodiaquine, within ±7%. Meet the requirements for Identification, Dissolution (75% in 30 minutes in water in Apparatus 2 at 50 rpm), and Uniformity of dosage units.

AMOXAPINE

Chemical group: Dibenzoxazepine.

Chemical name: Dibenz[*b,f*][1,4]oxazepine, 2-chloro-11-(1-piperazinyl)-.

Molecular formula: $C_{17}H_{16}ClN_3O$.

Molecular weight: 313.78.

Description: Amoxapine USP—White to yellowish crystalline powder.

pKa: 7.6 (apparent).

Solubility: Amoxapine USP—Freely soluble in chloroform; soluble in tetrahydrofuran; sparingly soluble in methanol and in toluene; slightly soluble in acetone; practically insoluble in water.

Other characteristics: Secondary amine.

USP requirements:

Amoxapine USP—Preserve in tight containers. Contains not less than 98.5% and not more than 101.0% of amoxapine, calculated on the dried basis. Meets the requirements for Identification, Melting range (177–181 °C), Loss on drying (not more than 0.5%), Residue on ignition (not more than 0.1%), and Chromatographic purity.

Amoxapine Tablets USP—Preserve in well-closed containers. Contain the labeled amount, within ±10%. Meet the requirements for Identification, Dissolution (80% in 30 minutes in simulated gastric fluid [without enzyme] in Apparatus 2 at 50 rpm), and Uniformity of dosage units.

AMOXICILLIN

Source: Semisynthetic derivative of ampicillin.

Chemical group: Semisynthetic penicillin.

Chemical name: 4-Thia-1-azabicyclo[3.2.0]heptane-2-carboxylic acid, 6-[[amino(4-hydroxyphenyl)acetyl]amino]-3,3-dimethyl-7-oxo-, trihydrate[2S-[2 alpha,5 alpha,6 beta(S*)]]-.

Molecular formula: $C_{16}H_{19}N_3O_5S \cdot 3H_2O$.

Molecular weight: 419.45.

Description: Amoxicillin USP—White, practically odorless, crystalline powder.

Solubility: Amoxicillin USP—Slightly soluble in water and in methanol; insoluble in carbon tetrachloride and in chloroform.

USP requirements:

Amoxicillin USP—Preserve in tight containers, at controlled room temperature. Where it is intended for use in preparing injectable dosage forms, the label states that it is intended for veterinary use only and that it is sterile or must be subjected to further processing during the preparation of injectable dosage forms. Label all other Amoxicillin to indicate that it is to be used in the manufacture of nonparenteral drugs only. Contains not less than 900 mcg and not more than 1050 mcg of amoxicillin per mg, calculated on the anhydrous basis. Meets the requirements for Identification, Crystallinity, pH (3.5–6.0, in a solution containing 2 mg per mL), Water (11.5–14.5%), and Dimethylaniline, for Sterility and Bacterial endotoxins under Amoxicillin for Injectable Suspension (where the label states that Amoxicillin is sterile), and for Bacterial endotoxins under Amoxicillin for Injectable Suspension (where the label states that Amoxicillin must be subjected to further processing during the preparation of injectable dosage forms).

Amoxicillin Boluses USP—Preserve in tight containers, at controlled room temperature. Label Boluses to indicate that they are for veterinary use only. Contain the labeled amount, within ±10%. Meet the requirements for Identification, Disintegration (30 minutes, simulated gastric fluid being used instead of water), and Water (not more than 7.5%).

Amoxicillin Capsules USP—Preserve in tight containers, at controlled room temperature. Contain the labeled amount, within −10% to +20%. Meet the requirements for Identification, Dissolution (80% in 60 minutes in water in Apparatus 1 at 100 rpm), Uniformity of dosage units, and Water (not more than 14.5%).

Amoxicillin Intramammary Infusion USP—Preserve in well-closed disposable syringes. A suspension of Amoxicillin in a suitable vegetable oil vehicle. Label it to indicate that it is intended for veterinary use only. Contains the labeled amount, within −10% to +20%. Contains a suitable dispersing agent and preservative. Meets the requirements for Identification and Water (not more than 1.0%).

Amoxicillin for Injectable Suspension USPm—Preserve in Containers for Sterile Solids. A sterile mixture of Amoxicillin and one or more suitable buffers, preservatives, stabilizers, and suspending agents. Label it to indicate that it is for veterinary use only. Contains the labeled amount, within −10% to +20%. Meets the requirements for Identification, Bacterial endotoxins, Sterility, pH (5.0–7.0, in the suspension constituted as directed in the labeling), and Water (11.0–14.0%).

Amoxicillin Oral Suspension USP—Preserve in multiple-dose containers equipped with a suitable dosing pump. A suspension of Amoxicillin in Soybean Oil. Label it to indicate that it is for veterinary use only. Contains the labeled amount, within −10% to +20%. Meets the requirements for Identification and Water (not more than 3.0% [except where it is labeled as containing 80 mg of amoxicillin per mL after constitution, not more than 4.0%]).

Amoxicillin for Oral Suspension USP—Preserve in tight containers, at controlled room temperature. Contains the labeled amount, within −10% to +20%. Contains one or more suitable buffers, colors, flavors, preservatives, stabilizers, sweeteners, and suspending agents. Meets the requirements for Identification, Uniformity of dosage units (single-unit containers), Deliverable volume (multiple-unit containers), pH (5.0–7.5 in the suspension constituted as directed in the labeling), and Water (not more than 3.0%).

Amoxicillin Tablets USP—Preserve in tight containers, at controlled room temperature. Label chewable Tablets to indicate that they are to be chewed before swallowing. Tablets intended solely for veterinary use are so labeled. Contain the labeled amount, within −10% to +20%. Meet the requirements for Thin-layer chromatographic identification test and Dissolution (80% in 90 minutes in water in Apparatus 2 at 75 rpm; and for products labeled as Chewable Tablets: 70% in 90 minutes in water in Apparatus 2 at 75 rpm).

Amoxicillin Tablets for Oral Suspension USP—Preserve in tight containers. Contain the labeled amount, within ± 10%. Meet the requirements for Thin-layer chromatographic identification test, Dissolution (80% in 30 minutes in water in Apparatus 2 at 75 rpm), Disintigration, Dispersion fineness, and Uniformity of dosage units.

AMOXICILLIN AND CLAVULANATE

For *Amoxicillin* and *Clavulanate*—See individual listings for chemistry information.

USP requirements:

Amoxicillin and Clavulanate Oral Suspension—Not in *USP–NF*.

Amoxicillin and Clavulanate Tablets—Not in *USP–NF*.

Amoxicillin and Clavulanate Chewable Tablets—Not in *USP–NF*.

Amoxicillin and Clavulanate Potassium for Oral Suspension USP—Preserve in tight containers, at controlled room temperature. Contains the labeled amount of amoxicillin, within −10% to +20%, and an amount of clavulanate potassium equivalent to the labeled amount of clavulanic acid, within −10% to +25%. Contains one or more suitable buffers, colors, flavors, preservatives, stabilizers, sweeteners, and suspending agents. Meets the requirements for Identification, pH (3.8–6.6, in the suspension constituted as directed in the labeling, the test being performed immediately after constitution), and Water (not more than 7.5%, where the label indicates that after constitution as directed, the suspension contains an amount of amoxicillin that is less than 40 mg per mL; not more than 8.5% where the label indicates that after constitution as directed the suspension contains an amount of amoxicillin that is equal to or more than 40 mg per mL and is less than or equal to 50 mg per mL; not more than 11.0% where the label indicates that after constitution as directed the suspension contains an amount of amoxicillin that is more than 50 mg per mL and is less than or equal to 80 mg per mL; and not more than 12.0% where the label indicates that after constitution as directed the suspension contains an amount of amoxicillin that is more than 80 mg per mL).

Amoxicillin and Clavulanate Potassium Tablets USP—Preserve in tight containers. Label chewable Tablets to include the word "chewable" in juxtaposition to the official name. The labeling indicates that chewable Tablets may be chewed before being swallowed or may be swallowed whole. Tablets intended for veterinary use only are so labeled. Contain the labeled amount of amoxicillin, within −10% to +20%, and an amount of clavulanate potassium equivalent to the labeled amount of clavulanic acid, within

−10% to +20%. Meet the requirements for Identification, Disintegration (for Tablets labeled for veterinary use only, 30 minutes, in simulated gastric fluid TS), Dissolution (85% of amoxicillin and 80% of clavulanic acid in 30 minutes [or 80% of each amoxicillin and clavulanic acid in 45 minutes where the Tablets are labeled as chewable] in water in Apparatus 2 at 75 rpm [Note: Tablets labeled for veterinary use only are exempt from this requirement]), Uniformity of dosage units, and Water (not more than 7.5% where the labeled amount of amoxicillin in each Tablet is 250 mg or less; not more than 10.0% where the labeled amount of amoxicillin in each Tablet is more than 250 mg but less than or equal to 500 mg; not more than 11.0% where the labeled amount of amoxicillin in each Tablet is more than 500 mg. Where Tablets are labeled as chewable, not more than 6.0% where the labeled amount of amoxicillin in each Tablet is 125 mg or less; not more than 8.0% where the labeled amount of amoxicillin in each Tablet is more than 125 mg. Where the Tablets are labeled for veterinary use only, not more than 10.0%).
Amoxicillin and Clavulanate Potassium Extended-release Tablets—Not in *USP–NF*.

AMPHETAMINE

Chemical name: Amphetamine sulfate—Benzeneethanamine, alpha-methyl-, sulfate (2:1), (±)-.

Molecular formula: Amphetamine sulfate—$(C_9H_{13}N)_2 \cdot H_2SO_4$.

Molecular weight: Amphetamine sulfate—368.49.

Description: Amphetamine Sulfate USP—White, odorless, crystalline powder. Its solutions are acid to litmus, having a pH of 5 to 6.

Solubility: Amphetamine Sulfate USP—Freely soluble in water; slightly soluble in alcohol; practically insoluble in ether.

USP requirements:
Amphetamine Sulfate USP—Preserve in well-closed containers. Dried at 105 °C for 2 hours, contains not less than 98.0% and not more than 102.0% of amphetamine sulfate. Meets the requirements for Identification, Loss on drying (not more than 1.0%), Residue on ignition (not more than 0.2%), Dextroamphetamine, Chromatographic purity, and Organic volatile impurities.
Amphetamine Sulfate Tablets USP—Preserve in well-closed containers. Contain the labeled amount, within ±7%. Meet the requirements for Identification, Dissolution (75% in 45 minutes in water in Apparatus 1 at 100 rpm), and Uniformity of dosage units.

AMPHETAMINE AND DEXTROAMPHETAMINE

Chemical name:
Amphetamine sulfate—Benzeneethanamine, alpha-methyl-, sulfate (2:1), (±)-.
Dextroamphetamine sulfate—Benzeneethanamine, alpha-methyl-, (S)-, sulfate (2:1).

Molecular formula:
Amphetamine sulfate—$(C_9H_{13}N)_2 \cdot H_2SO_4$.
Dextroamphetamine sulfate—$(C_9H_{13}N)_2 \cdot H_2SO_4$.

Molecular weight:
Amphetamine sulfate—368.49.
Dextroamphetamine sulfate—368.49.

Description:
Amphetamine Sulfate USP—White, odorless, crystalline powder. Its solutions are acid to litmus, having a pH of 5 to 6.

Dextroamphetamine Sulfate USP—White, odorless, crystalline powder.

Solubility:
Amphetamine Sulfate USP—Freely soluble in water; slightly soluble in alcohol; practically insoluble in ether.
Dextroamphetamine Sulfate USP—Soluble in water; slightly soluble in alcohol; insoluble in ether.

USP requirements: Amphetamine Aspartate, Amphetamine Sulfate, Dextroamphetamine Saccharate, and Dextroamphetamine Sulfate Tablets—Not in *USP–NF*.

AMPHOTERICIN B

Source:
Amphotericin B—Derived from a strain of *Streptomyces nodosus*.
Amphotericin B cholesteryl complex—A 1:1 (molar ratio) complex of amphotericin B and cholesteryl sulfate.
Amphotericin B lipid complex—A suspension of amphotericin B complexed with two phospholipids, L-alpha-dimyristroyl-phosphatidylcholine (DMPC) and L-alpha-dimyristroyl-phosphatidylglycerol (DMPG), in a 1:1 drug-to-lipid molar ratio.

Chemical name: Amphotericin B.

Molecular formula: $C_{47}H_{73}NO_{17}$.

Molecular weight: 924.08.

Description: Amphotericin B USP—Yellow to orange powder; odorless or practically so.

Solubility:
Amphotericin B USP—Insoluble in water, in anhydrous alcohol, in ether, and in toluene; soluble in dimethylformamide, in dimethyl sulfoxide, and in propylene glycol; slightly soluble in methanol.
Amphotericin B for Injection USP—It yields a colloidal dispersion in water.

Other characteristics: Solubilized by the addition of sodium desoxycholate, which yields a colloidal dispersion in water after reconstitution.

USP requirements:
Amphotericin B USP—Preserve in tight, light-resistant containers, in a cold place. Label it to state whether it is intended for use in preparing dermatological and oral dosage forms or parenteral dosage forms. Has a potency of not less than 750 mcg of amphotericin B per mg, calculated on the dried basis. Meets the requirements for Identification, Loss on drying (not more than 5.0%), Residue on ignition (not more than 0.5% [Note: Amphotericin B intended for use in preparing dermatological creams, lotions, and ointments, and oral suspensions and capsules, yields not more than 3.0%]), and Limit of amphotericin A (not more than 5.0%, calculated on the dried basis [Note: Amphotericin B intended for use in preparing dermatological creams, lotions, and ointments, and oral suspensions and capsules, contains not more than 15% of amphotericin A, calculated on the dried basis]).
Amphotericin B Cream USP—Preserve in collapsible tubes, or in other well-closed containers. Contains the labeled amount, within −10% to +25%. Meets the requirement for Minimum fill.
Amphotericin B for Injection USP—Preserve in Containers for Sterile Solids, in a refrigerator and protected from light. A sterile complex of amphotericin B and deoxycholate sodium and one or more suitable buffers. Label it to indicate that it is intended for use by intravenous infusion to hospitalized patients only, and that the solution should be protected from light during administration. Contains the

labeled amount, within −10% to +20%. Meets the requirements for Bacterial endotoxins, Sterility, pH (7.2–8.0, in an aqueous solution containing 10 mg of amphotericin B per mL), and Loss on drying (not more than 8.0%), and for Uniformity of dosage units and Labeling under Injections.

Amphotericin B Lotion USP—Preserve in well-closed containers. Contains the labeled amount, within −10% to +25%. Meets the requirements for Minimum fill and pH (5.0–7.0).

Amphotericin B Ointment USP—Preserve in collapsible tubes, or in other well-closed containers. It is Amphotericin B in a suitable ointment base. Contains the labeled amount, within −10% to +25%. Meets the requirements for Minimum fill and Water (not more than 1.0%).

Amphotericin B Cholesteryl Complex for Injection—Not in *USP–NF*.

Amphotericin B Lipid Complex Injection—Not in *USP–NF*.

Amphotericin B Liposomal Complex for Injection—Not in *USP–NF*.

Amphotericin B Liposome for Injection—Not in *USP–NF*.

AMPICILLIN

Source: Semisynthetic penicillin.

Chemical name:
Ampicillin—4-Thia-1-azabicyclo[3.2.0]heptane-2-carboxylic acid, 6-[(aminophenylacetyl)amino]-3,3-dimethyl-7-oxo-, [2S-[2 alpha,5 alpha,6 beta(S*)]]-.

Ampicillin sodium—4-Thia-1-azabicyclo[3.2.0]heptane-2-carboxylic acid, 6-[(aminophenylacetyl)amino]-3,3-dimethyl-7-oxo-, monosodium salt, [2S-[2 alpha,5 alpha,6 beta(S*)]]-.

Molecular formula:
Ampicillin—$C_{16}H_{19}N_3O_4S$.
Ampicillin sodium—$C_{16}H_{18}N_3NaO_4S$.

Molecular weight:
Ampicillin—349.41.
Ampicillin sodium—371.39.

Description:
Ampicillin USP—White, practically odorless, crystalline powder.
Ampicillin Sodium USP—White to off-white, odorless or practically odorless, crystalline powder. Is hygroscopic.

Solubility:
Ampicillin USP—Slightly soluble in water and in methanol; insoluble in benzene, in carbon tetrachloride, and in chloroform.
Ampicillin Sodium USP—Very soluble in water and in isotonic sodium chloride and dextrose solutions.

USP requirements:
Ampicillin USP—Preserve in tight containers. It is anhydrous or contains three molecules of water of hydration. Label it to indicate whether it is anhydrous or is the trihydrate. Where the quantity of ampicillin is indicated in the labeling of any preparation containing Ampicillin, this shall be understood to be in terms of anhydrous ampicillin. Where it is intended for use in preparing injectable dosage forms, the label states that it is the trihydrate and that it is sterile or must be subjected to further processing during the preparation of injectable dosage forms. Contains not less than 900 mcg and not more than 1050 mcg of ampicillin per mg, calculated on the dried basis. Meets the requirements for Identification, Crystallinity, Bacterial endotoxins, Sterility, pH (3.5–6.0, in a solution containing 10 mg per mL), Loss on drying (where it is labeled as anhydrous Ampicillin, not more than 2.0%), and Dimethylaniline.

Ampicillin Boluses USP—Preserve in tight containers. Label the Boluses to indicate that they are for veterinary use only. Contain an amount of ampicillin (as the trihydrate)

equivalent to the labeled amount of ampicillin, within −10% to +20%. Meet the requirements for Identification, Uniformity of dosage units, and Loss on drying (not more than 5.0%).

Ampicillin Capsules USP—Preserve in tight containers. Label Capsules to indicate whether the ampicillin therein is in the anhydrous form or is the trihydrate. Contain an amount of ampicillin (anhydrous or as the trihydrate) equivalent to the labeled amount of ampicillin, within −10% to +20%. Meet the requirements for Identification, Dissolution (75% in 45 minutes in water in Apparatus 1 at 100 rpm), Uniformity of dosage units, and Water (not more than 4.0% for the anhydrous and 10.0–15.0% for the trihydrate).

Ampicillin for Injection USP—Preserve in Containers for Sterile Solids. Protect the constituted solution from freezing. Contains an amount of Ampicillin Sodium equivalent to the labeled amount of ampicillin, within −10% to +15%. Meets the requirements for Constituted solution, Bacterial endotoxins, Particulate matter, Uniformity of dosage units, and for Identification tests, Crystallinity, pH, and Water under Ampicillin Sodium, and for Sterility tests, and Labeling under Injections.

Ampicillin Soluble Powder USP—Preserve in tight containers. A dry mixture of ampicillin (as the trihydrate) and one or more suitable diluents and stabilizing agents. Label it to indicate that it is for veterinary use only. Contains the labeled amount, within −10% to +20%. Meets the requirements for Identification, pH (3.5–6.0, in an aqueous solution containing the equivalent of 20 mg of ampicillin per mL), and Water (not more than 5.0%).

Ampicillin Injectable Oil Suspension USP—Preserve in single-dose or in multiple-dose containers, preferably of Type I glass. A sterile suspension of Ampicillin in a suitable oil vehicle. Label it to indicate that it is for veterinary use only. Contains an amount of ampicillin (as the trihydrate) equivalent to the labeled amount of ampicillin, within −10% to +20%. Meets the requirements for Identification, Sterility, and Water (not more than 4.0%).

Ampicillin for Injectable Suspension USP—Preserve in Containers for Sterile Solids. A dry mixture of ampicillin trihydrate and one or more suitable buffers, preservatives, stabilizers, and suspending agents. Contains the equivalent of the labeled amount of ampicillin, within −10% to +20%. Meets the requirements for Identification, Bacterial endotoxins, Sterility, pH (5.0–7.0, in the suspension constituted as directed in the labeling), and Water (11.4–14.0%), and for Uniformity of dosage units, and Labeling under Injections.

Ampicillin for Oral Suspension USP—Preserve in tight containers. Label it to indicate whether the ampicillin therein is in the anhydrous form or is the trihydrate. Contains an amount of ampicillin (anhydrous or as the trihydrate) equivalent to the labeled amount of ampicillin, within −10% to +20%, when constituted as directed. Contains one or more suitable buffers, colors, flavors, preservatives, and sweetening ingredients. Meets the requirements for Identification, Uniformity of dosage units (single-unit containers), Deliverable volume (multiple-unit containers), pH (5.0–7.5, in the suspension constituted as directed in the labeling), and Water (not more than 2.5%; not more than 5.0% if it contains ampicillin trihydrate and contains the equivalent of 100 mg of ampicillin per mL when constituted as directed in the labeling).

Ampicillin Tablets USP—Preserve in tight containers, and store at controlled room temperature. Label Tablets to indicate whether the ampicillin therein is in the anhydrous form or is the trihydrate. Label chewable Tablets to indicate that they are to be chewed before swallowing. Tablets intended for veterinary use only are so labeled. Contain an amount of Ampicillin (anhydrous form or trihydrate form) equivalent to the labeled amount of ampicillin, within −10% to +20%. Meet the requirements for Identification, Dissolution (75% in 45 minutes in water in Apparatus 1 at 100 rpm), Uniformity of dosage units, Loss on drying

(where the Tablets contain anhydrous ampicillin, not more than 4.0% for powder from nonchewable Tablets and not more than 3.0% for powder from chewable Tablets; where the Tablets contain ampicillin as the trihydrate, not more than 13.0% for powder from Tablets for veterinary use), and Water (where chewable Tablets contain ampicillin trihydrate, not more than 5.0%; where nonchewable Tablets contain ampicillin trihydrate, 9.5–12.0%).

Ampicillin Sodium USP—Preserve in tight containers. Where it is intended for use in preparing injectable dosage forms, the label states that it is sterile or must be subjected to further processing during the preparation of injectable dosage forms. Has a potency equivalent to not less than 845 mcg and not more than 988 mcg of ampicillin per mg, calculated on the anhydrous basis. Meets the requirements for Identification, Crystallinity (Note: Ampicillin Sodium in the freeze-dried form is exempt from this requirement), pH (8.0–10.0, in a solution containing 10.0 mg of ampicillin per mL), Water (not more than 2.0%), Dimethylaniline, and Limit of methylene chloride (not more than 0.2%), for Sterility and Bacterial endotoxins under Ampicillin for Injection (where the label states that Ampicillin Sodium is sterile), and for Bacterial endotoxins under Ampicillin for Injection (where the label states that Ampicillin Sodium must be subjected to further processing during the processing of injectable dosage forms).

AMPICILLIN AND PROBENECID

For *Ampicillin* and *Probenecid*—See individual listings for chemistry information.

USP requirements:

Ampicillin and Probenecid Capsules USP—Preserve in tight containers. Contain an amount of ampicillin (as the trihydrate) equivalent to the labeled amount of ampicillin, within −10% to +20%, and the labeled amount of probenecid, within ±10%. Meet the requirements for Uniformity of dosage units and Loss on drying (8.5–13.0%).

Ampicillin and Probenecid for Oral Suspension USP—Preserve in tight, unit-dose containers. Contains an amount of ampicillin (as the trihydrate) equivalent to the labeled amount of ampicillin, within −10% to +20%, and the labeled amount of probenecid, within ±10%. Contains one or more suitable colors, flavors, and suspending agents. Meets the requirements for Uniformity of dosage units (for solid packaged in single-unit containers), Deliverable volume (for solid packaged in multiple-unit containers), pH (5.0–7.5, in the suspension constituted as directed in the labeling), and Water (not more than 5.0%).

AMPICILLIN AND SULBACTAM

For *Ampicillin* and *Sulbactam*—See individual listings for chemistry information.

USP requirements: Ampicillin and Sulbactam for Injection USP—Preserve in Containers for Sterile Solids. A sterile, dry mixture of Ampicillin Sodium and Sulbactam Sodium. Contains amounts of ampicillin sodium and sulbactam sodium equivalent to the labeled amounts of ampicillin and sulbactam, within −10% to +15%, the labeled amounts representing proportions of ampicillin to sulbactam of 2:1. Contains not less than 563 mcg of ampicillin and 280 mcg of sulbactam per mg, calculated on the anhydrous basis. Meets the requirements for Constituted solution, Identification, Bacterial endotoxins, Sterility, pH (8.0–10.0, in a solution containing 10 mg of ampicillin and 5 mg of sulbactam per mL), Water (not more than 2.0%), and Particulate matter, for Uniformity of dosage units and for Labeling under Injections.

AMPRENAVIR

Chemical group: Sulfonamide.

Chemical name: [3S-[3R*(1R*,2S*)]]-[3-]](4-Aminophenyl)sulfonyl](2-methylpropyl)amino]-2-hydroxy-1-(phenylmethyl)propyl] tetrahydro-3-furanyl carbamate.

Molecular formula: $C_{25}H_{35}N_3O_6S$.

Molecular weight: 505.64.

Description: Amprenavir—White to cream-colored solid.

Solubility: Amprenavir—Soluble in approximately 0.04 mg per mL water at 25 °C.

USP requirements:
Amprenavir Capsules—Not in *USP–NF*.
Amprenavir Solution—Not in *USP–NF*.

AMPROLIUM

Chemical group: Vitamin B_1 or thiamine structural analog.

Chemical name: 1-[(4-Amino-2-propyl-5-pyrimidinyl)methyl]-2-methylpyridinium chloride monohydrochloride.

Molecular formula: $C_{14}H_{19}ClN_4 \cdot HCl$.

Molecular weight: 315.24.

Description: Amprolium USP—White to light yellow powder.

Solubility: Amprolium USP—Freely soluble in water, in methanol, in alcohol, and in dimethylformamide; sparingly soluble in dehydrated alcohol; practically insoluble in isopropyl alcohol, in butyl alcohol, and in acetone.

USP requirements:

Amprolium USP—Preserve in well-closed containers. Label it to indicate that it is for veterinary use only. Contains not less than 97.0% and not more than 101.0% of amprolium, calculated on the dried basis. Meets the requirements for Identification and Loss on drying (not more than 1.0%).

Amprolium Soluble Powder USP—Preserve in tight containers. Label it to indicate that it is for veterinary use only. Contains the labeled amount, within ±5%. Meets the requirement for Identification.

Amprolium Oral Solution USP—Preserve in tight containers. Label it to indicate that it is for veterinary use only. Contains the labeled amount, within ±7%. Meets the requirements for Identification and pH (2.5–3.0).

AMSACRINE

Chemical name: Methanesulfonamide, N-[4-(9-acridinylamino)-3-methoxyphenyl]-.

Molecular formula: $C_{21}H_{19}N_3O_3S$.

Molecular weight: 393.46.

USP requirements: Amsacrine Injection—Not in *USP–NF*.

AMYLENE HYDRATE

Chemical name: 2-Butanol, 2-methyl-.

Molecular formula: $C_5H_{12}O$.

Molecular weight: 88.15.

Description: Amylene Hydrate NF—Clear, colorless liquid, having a camphoraceous odor. Its solutions are neutral to litmus. NF category: Solvent.

Solubility: Amylene Hydrate NF—Freely soluble in water; miscible with alcohol, with chloroform, with ether, and with glycerin.

NF requirements: Amylene Hydrate NF—Preserve in tight containers. Contains not less than 99.0% and not more than 100.0% of amylene hydrate. Meets the requirements for Identification, Specific gravity (0.803–0.807), Distilling range (97–103 °C), Water (not more than 0.5%), Limit of nonvolatile residue (not more than 0.02%), Heavy metals (not more than 0.0005%), Readily oxidizable substances, Aldehyde, and Organic volatile impurities.

AMYL NITRITE

Chemical group: Mixture of nitrous acid, 2-methylbutyl ester, and nitrous acid, 3-methylbutyl ester.

Molecular formula: $C_5H_{11}NO_2$.

Molecular weight: 117.15.

Description: Amyl Nitrite USP—Clear, yellowish liquid, having a peculiar, ethereal, fruity odor. Is volatile even at low temperatures, and is flammable. Boils at about 96 °C.

Solubility: Amyl Nitrite USP—Practically insoluble in water. Miscible with alcohol and with ether.

USP requirements:
Amyl Nitrite USP—Preserve in tight containers, and store in a cool place, protected from light. A mixture of the nitrite esters of 3-methyl-1-butanol and 2-methyl-1-butanol. Contains not less than 85.0% and not more than 103.0% of amyl nitrite. Meets the requirements for Identification, Specific gravity (0.870–0.876), Acidity, Limit of nonvolatile residue (not more than 0.02%), Total nitrites (not less than 97.0%), and Organic volatile impurities.
Caution: Amyl Nitrite is very flammable. Do not use where it may be ignited.
Amyl Nitrite Inhalant USP—Preserve in tight, unit-dose glass containers, wrapped loosely in gauze or other suitable material, and store in a cool place, protected from light. Contains a mixture of the nitrite esters of 3-methyl-1-butanol and 2-methyl-1-butanol. Contains the labeled amount, within −20% to +5%. Contains a suitable stabilizer. Meets the requirements for Specific gravity (0.870–0.880) and Total nitrites (not less than 95.0%), and for Identification tests and Acidity under Amyl Nitrite.
Caution: Amyl Nitrite Inhalant is very flammable. Do not use where it may be ignited.

ANAGRELIDE

Chemical name: Anagrelide hydrochloride—Imidazo[2,1-*b*]quinazolin-2(3*H*)-one, 6,7-dichloro-1,5-dihydro-, monohydrochloride.

Molecular formula: Anagrelide hydrochloride—$C_{10}H_7Cl_2N_3O \cdot HCl$.

Molecular weight: 292.55.

Description: Off-white, nonvolatile powder.

Solubility: Practically insoluble in water; very slightly soluble in dimethyl sulfoxide and in dimethylformamide.

USP requirements:
Anagrelide Capsules—Not in *USP–NF*.
Anagrelide Hydrochloride Capsules—Not in *USP–NF*.

ANAKINRA

Source: Produced by recombinant DNA technology using an *E. coli* bacterial expression system.

Chemical name: Interleukin 1 receptor antagonist (human isoform x reduced), N^2-L-methionyl-.

Molecular formula: $C_{759}H_{1186}N_{208}O_{232}S_{10}$.

Molecular weight: 17,258 daltons.

Other characteristics: pH: 6.5 (of prepared solution).

USP requirements: Anakinra Injection–Not in *USP-NF*.

ANASTROZOLE

Chemical name: 1,3-Benzenediacetonitrile, alpha,alpha,alpha′,alpha′-tetramethyl-5-(1*H*-1,2,4-triazol-1-ylmethyl)-.

Molecular formula: $C_{17}H_{19}N_5$.

Molecular weight: 293.37.

Description: Off-white powder.

Solubility: Has moderate aqueous solubility (0.5 mg/mL at 25 °C); freely soluble in methanol, acetone, ethanol, and in tetrahydrofuran; very soluble in acetonitrile.

USP requirements: Anastrozole Tablets—Not in *USP–NF*.

ANETHOLE

Chemical name: Benzene, 1-methoxy-4-(1-propenyl)-, (*E*)-.

Molecular formula: $C_{10}H_{12}O$.

Molecular weight: 148.20.

Description: Anethole NF—Colorless or faintly yellow liquid at or above 23 °C. Has the aromatic odor of anise. Affected by light. NF category: Flavors and perfumes.

Solubility: Anethole NF—Very slightly soluble in water; freely soluble in alcohol; readily miscible with ether and with chloroform.

NF requirements: Anethole NF—Preserve in tight, light-resistant containers. Obtained from Anise Oil and other sources, or is prepared synthetically. Label it to indicate whether it is obtained from natural sources or is prepared synthetically. Meets the requirements for Specific gravity (0.983–0.988), Congealing temperature (not less than 20 °C), Distilling range (231–237 °C), Angular rotation (−0.15° to +0.15°), Refractive index (1.557–1.561), Heavy metals (20 mcg per gram), Aldehydes and ketones, Limit of phenols, and Organic volatile impurities.

ANILERIDINE

Chemical name:

Anileridine—4-Piperidinecarboxylic acid, 1-[2-(4-aminophenyl)ethyl]-4-phenyl-, ethyl ester.

Anileridine hydrochloride—4-Piperidinecarboxylic acid, 1-[2-(4-aminophenyl)ethyl]-4-phenyl-, ethyl ester, dihydrochloride.

Molecular formula:

Anileridine—$C_{22}H_{28}N_2O_2$.

Anileridine hydrochloride—$C_{22}H_{28}N_2O_2 \cdot 2HCl$.

Molecular weight:

Anileridine—352.47.

Anileridine hydrochloride—425.39.

Description:

Anileridine USP—White to yellowish white, odorless to practically odorless, crystalline powder. Is oxidized on exposure to air and light, becoming darker in color. It exhibits polymorphism, and of two crystalline forms observed, one melts at about 80 °C and the other at about 89 °C.

Anileridine Hydrochloride USP—White or nearly white, odorless, crystalline powder. Is stable in air. Melts at about 270 °C, with decomposition.

Solubility:

Anileridine USP—Very slightly soluble in water; freely soluble in alcohol and in chloroform; soluble in ether although it may show turbidity.

Anileridine Hydrochloride USP—Freely soluble in water; sparingly soluble in alcohol; practically insoluble in ether and in chloroform.

USP requirements:

Anileridine USP—Preserve in tight, light-resistant containers. Contains not less than 98.5% and not more than 101.0% of anileridine, calculated on the anhydrous basis. Meets the requirements for Identification, Water (not more than 1.0%), Residue on ignition (not more than 0.1%), and Chloride (not more than 0.040%).

Anileridine Injection USP—Preserve in single-dose or in multiple-dose containers, preferably of Type I glass, protected from light. A sterile solution of Anileridine in Water for Injection, prepared with the aid of Phosphoric Acid. Contains the labeled amount, as the phosphate, within −10% to +15%. Meets the requirements for Identification, Bacterial endotoxins, and pH (4.5–5.0), and for Injections.

Anileridine Tablets—Not in *USP–NF*.

Anileridine Hydrochloride USP—Preserve in tight, light-resistant containers. Contains not less than 96.0% and not more than 102.0% of anileridine hydrochloride, calculated on the dried basis. Meets the requirements for Identification, pH (2.5–3.0, in a solution [1 in 20]), Loss on drying (not more than 1.0%), Residue on ignition (not more than 0.1%), and Chloride content (16.0–17.2%).

Anileridine Hydrochloride Tablets USP—Preserve in tight, light-resistant containers. Contain an amount of anileridine hydrochloride equivalent to the labeled amount of anileridine, within ±5%. Meet the requirements for Identification, Dissolution (65% in 45 minutes in 0.01 *N* hydrochloric acid in Apparatus 1 at 100 rpm), and Uniformity of dosage units.

ANISE OIL

NF requirements: Anise Oil NF—Preserve in well-filled, tight containers, and avoid exposure to excessive heat. Volatile oil distilled with steam from the dried, ripe fruit of *Pimpinella ansium* L. (Fam. Apiaceae) or from the dried ripe fruit of *Illicium verum* Hook. f. (Fam. Illiciaceae). The label states the Latin bionomial name and, following the official name, the part of the plant source from which the article was derived. The la-

bel also states that if solid material has separated, carefully warm oil until it is completely liquified, and mix before using. Meets the requirements for Solubility in 90% alcohol, Specific gravity (0.978–0.988), Congealing temperature (not lower than 15°), Angular rotation (−2° to +1°), Refractive index (1.553–1.560 at 20°), Heavy metals (0.004%), and Limit of phenols.

Note—If solid material has separated, carefully warm the Anise Oil until it is completely liquified, and mix before using.

ANISINDIONE

Chemical group: Indandione derivative.

Chemical name: 2-(*p*-Methoxyphenyl)indane-1,3-dione.

Molecular formula: $C_{16}H_{12}O_3$.

Molecular weight: 252.26.

Description: White or off-white, crystalline powder.

Solubility: Practically insoluble in water.

USP requirements: Anisindione Tablets—Not in *USP–NF*.

ANISOTROPINE

Chemical group: Quaternary ammonium salt.

Chemical name: Anisotropine methylbromide—8-Azoniabicyclo[3.2.1]octane, 8,8-dimethyl-3-[(1-oxo-2-propylpentyl)oxy]-, bromide, *endo*-.

Molecular formula: Anisotropine methylbromide—$C_{17}H_{32}BrNO_2$.

Molecular weight: Anisotropine methylbromide—362.35.

Description: Anisotropine methylbromide—White, glistening powder.

Solubility: Anisotropine methylbromide—Soluble in water; sparingly soluble in alcohol.

USP requirements: Anisotropine Methylbromide Tablets—Not in *USP–NF*.

ANISTREPLASE

Source: Prepared in vitro by acylating human plasma–derived, purified, heat-treated Lys-Plasminogen and purified Streptokinase from group C beta-hemolytic streptococci.

Chemical name: Anistreplase.

Molecular weight: 131,000.

USP requirements: Anistreplase for Injection—Not in *USP–NF*.

ANTAZOLINE

Chemical name: Antazoline phosphate—1*H*-Imidazole-2-methanamine, 4,5-dihydro-*N*-phenyl-*N*-(phenylmethyl)-, phosphate (1:1).

Molecular formula: Antazoline phosphate—$C_{17}H_{19}N_3 \cdot H_3PO_4$.

Molecular weight: Antazoline phosphate—363.35.

Description: Antazoline Phosphate USP—White to off-white, crystalline powder.

USP DI

Solubility: Antazoline Phosphate USP—Soluble in water; sparingly soluble in methanol; practically insoluble in benzene and in ether.

USP requirements: Antazoline Phosphate USP—Preserve in tight containers. Contains not less than 98.0% and not more than 101.0% of antazoline phosphate, calculated on the dried basis. Meets the requirements for Identification, Melting range (194–198 °C, with decomposition), pH (4.0–5.0, in a solution [1 in 50]), Loss on drying (not more than 0.5%), and Chromatographic purity.

ANTHRALIN

Chemical name: 9(10H)-Anthracenone, 1,8-dihydroxy-.

Molecular formula: $C_{14}H_{10}O_3$.

Molecular weight: 226.23.

Description: Anthralin USP—Yellowish brown, crystalline powder. Is odorless.

Solubility: Anthralin USP—Insoluble in water; soluble in chloroform, in acetone, and in solutions of alkali hydroxides; slightly soluble in alcohol, in ether, and in glacial acetic acid.

USP requirements:

Anthralin USP—Preserve in tight containers in a cool place. Protect from light. Contains not less than 97.0% and not more than 102.0% of anthralin, calculated on the dried basis. Meets the requirements for Identification, Melting range (178–181 °C), Acidity or alkalinity, Loss on drying (not more than 0.5%), Residue on ignition (not more than 0.1%), Chloride, and Sulfate.

Anthralin Cream USP—Preserve in tight containers, in a cool place. Protect from light. It is Anthralin in an aqueous (oil-in-water) or oily (water-in-oil) cream vehicle. Label it to indicate whether the cream vehicle is aqueous or oily. If labeled to contain more than 0.1% of anthralin, contains the labeled amount, within −10% to +15%; if labeled to contain 0.1% or less of anthralin, contains the labeled amount, within −10% to +30%.

Anthralin Ointment USP—Preserve in tight containers, in a cool place. Protect from light. It is Anthralin in a petrolatum or other oleaginous vehicle. If labeled to contain more than 0.1% of anthralin, contains the labeled amount, within −10% to +15%; if labeled to contain 0.1% or less of anthralin, contains the labeled amount, within −10% to +30%.

ANTICOAGULANT CITRATE DEXTROSE

Description: Anticoagulant Citrate Dextrose Solution USP—Clear, colorless, odorless liquid. Is dextrorotatory.

USP requirements: Anticoagulant Citrate Dextrose Solution USP—Preserve in single-dose containers, of colorless, transparent, Type I or Type II glass, or of a suitable plastic material. A sterile solution of Citric Acid, Sodium Citrate, and Dextrose in Water for Injection. Label it to indicate the number of mL of Solution required per 100 mL of whole blood or the number of mL of Solution required per volume of whole blood to be collected. Contains in each 1000 mL of Solution A, not less than 20.59 grams and not more than 22.75 grams of Total Citrate, expressed as citric acid, anhydrous, not less than 23.28 grams and not more than 25.73 grams of Dextrose, and not less than 4.90 grams and not more than 5.42 grams of Sodium. Contains in each 1000 mL of Solution B, not less than 12.37 grams and not more than 13.67 grams of Total Citrate, expressed as citric acid, anhydrous, not less than 13.96 grams and not more than 15.44 grams of Dextrose, and not less than 2.94 grams and not more than 3.25 grams of Sodium. Contains no antimicrobial agents.

Prepare Anticoagulant Citrate Dextrose Solution as follows: Solution A—7.3 grams of Citric Acid (anhydrous), 22.0 grams of Sodium Citrate (dihydrate), 24.5 grams of Dextrose (monohydrate), and a sufficient quantity of Water for Injection, to make 1000 mL. Solution B—4.4 grams of Citric Acid (anhydrous), 13.2 grams of Sodium Citrate (dihydrate), 14.7 grams of Dextrose (monohydrate), and a sufficient quantity of Water for Injection, to make 1000 mL. Dissolve the ingredients, and mix. Filter the solution until clear, place immediately in suitable containers, and sterilize. If desired, 8 grams and 4.8 grams of monohydrated citric acid may be used instead of the indicated, respective amounts of anhydrous citric acid; 19.3 grams and 11.6 grams of anhydrous sodium citrate may be used instead of the indicated, respective amounts of dihydrated sodium citrate; and 22.3 grams and 13.4 grams of anhydrous dextrose may be used instead of the indicated, respective amounts of monohydrated dextrose.

Meets the requirements for Identification, Bacterial endotoxins, pH (4.5–5.5), and Chloride (not more than 0.0035%), and for Injections.

ANTICOAGULANT CITRATE PHOSPHATE DEXTROSE

Description: Anticoagulant Citrate Phosphate Dextrose Solution USP—Clear, colorless to slightly yellow, odorless liquid. Is dextrorotatory.

USP requirements: Anticoagulant Citrate Phosphate Dextrose Solution USP—Preserve in single-dose containers, of colorless, transparent, Type I or Type II glass, or of a suitable plastic material. A sterile solution of Citric Acid, Sodium Citrate, Monobasic Sodium Phosphate, and Dextrose in Water for Injection. Label it to indicate the number of mL of Solution required per 100 mL of whole blood or the number of mL of Solution required per volume of whole blood to be collected. Contains, in each 1000 mL, not less than 2.11 grams and not more than 2.33 grams of monobasic sodium phosphate; not less than 24.22 grams and not more than 26.78 grams of dextrose; not less than 19.16 grams and not more than 21.18 grams of total citrate, expressed as citric acid, anhydrous; and not less than 6.21 grams and not more than 6.86 grams of Sodium. Contains no antimicrobial agents.

Prepare Anticoagulant Citrate Phosphate Dextrose Solution as follows: 2.99 grams of Citric Acid (anhydrous), 26.3 grams of Sodium Citrate (dihydrate), 2.22 grams of Monobasic Sodium Phosphate (monohydrate), 25.5 grams of Dextrose (monohydrate), and a sufficient quantity of Water for Injection, to make 1000 mL. Dissolve the ingredients, and mix. Filter the solution until clear, place immediately in suitable containers, and sterilize. If desired, 3.27 grams of monohydrated citric acid may be used instead of the indicated amount of anhydrous citric acid; 23.06 grams of anhydrous sodium citrate may be used instead of the indicated amount of dihydrated sodium citrate; 1.93 grams of anhydrous monobasic sodium phosphate may be used instead of the indicated amount of monohydrated monobasic sodium phosphate; and 23.2 grams of anhydrous dextrose may be used instead of the indicated amount of monohydrated dextrose.

Meets the requirements for Identification, Bacterial endotoxins, pH (5.0–6.0), and Chloride (not more than 0.0035%), and for Injections.

ANTICOAGULANT CITRATE PHOSPHATE DEXTROSE ADENINE

USP requirements: Anticoagulant Citrate Phosphate Dextrose Adenine Solution USP—Preserve in single-dose containers, of colorless, transparent, Type I or Type II glass, or of a suitable plastic material. A sterile solution of Citric Acid, Sodium Citrate, Monobasic Sodium Phosphate, Dextrose, and Adenine in Water for Injection. Label it to indicate the number of mL of solution required per 100 mL of whole blood or the number of mL of solution required per volume of whole blood to be collected. Contains, in each 1000 mL, not less than 2.11 grams and not more than 2.33 grams of monobasic sodium phosphate; not less than 30.30 grams and not more than 33.50 grams of dextrose; not less than 19.16 grams and not more than 21.18 grams of total citrate, expressed as citric acid, anhydrous; not less than 6.21 grams and not more than 6.86 grams of sodium; and not less than 0.247 grams and not more than 0.303 grams of adenine. Contains no antimicrobial agents.

Prepare Anticoagulant Citrate Phosphate Dextrose Adenine Solution as follows: 2.99 grams of Citric Acid (anhydrous), 26.3 grams of Sodium Citrate (dihydrate), 2.22 grams of Monobasic Sodium Phosphate (monohydrate), 31.9 grams of Dextrose (monohydrate), 0.275 grams of Adenine, and a sufficient quantity of Water for Injection, to make 1000 mL. Dissolve the ingredients, and mix. Filter the solution until clear, place immediately in suitable containers, and sterilize. If desired, 3.27 grams of monohydrated citric acid may be used instead of the indicated amount of anhydrous citric acid; 23.06 grams of anhydrous sodium citrate may be used instead of the indicated amount of dihydrated sodium citrate; 1.93 grams of anhydrous monobasic sodium phosphate may be used instead of the indicated amount of monohydrated monobasic sodium phosphate; and 29.0 grams of anhydrous dextrose may be used instead of the indicated amount of monohydrated dextrose.

Meets the requirements for Bacterial endotoxins, pH (5.0–6.0), and Chloride (not more than 0.0035%), and for Injections.

ANTICOAGULANT HEPARIN

USP requirements: Anticoagulant Heparin Solution USP—Preserve in single-dose containers, of colorless, transparent, Type I or Type II glass, or of a suitable plastic material. A sterile solution of Heparin Sodium in Sodium Chloride Injection. Its potency is within ±10% of the potency stated on the label in terms of USP Heparin Units. Label it in terms of USP Heparin Units, and to indicate the number of mL of Solution required per 100 mL of whole blood. Contains not less than 0.85% and not more than 0.95% of sodium chloride. Contains no antimicrobial agents.

Prepare Anticoagulant Heparin Solution as follows: 75,000 Units of Heparin Sodium and a sufficient quantity of Sodium Chloride Injection to make 1000 mL. Add the Heparin Sodium, in solid form or in solution, to the Sodium Chloride Injection, mix, filter if necessary, and sterilize.

Meets the requirements for Bacterial endotoxins and pH (5.0–7.5), and for Injections.

ANTICOAGULANT SODIUM CITRATE

Description: Anticoagulant Sodium Citrate Solution USP—Clear and colorless liquid.

USP requirements: Anticoagulant Sodium Citrate Solution USP—Preserve in single-dose containers, preferably of Type I or Type II glass. A sterile solution of Sodium Citrate in Water for Injection. Contains, in each 100 mL, not less than 3.80 grams and not more than 4.20 grams of sodium citrate, dihydrate. Contains no antimicrobial agents.

Prepare Anticoagulant Sodium Citrate Solution as follows: 40 grams of Sodium Citrate (dihydrate) and a sufficient quantity of Water for Injection, to make 1000 mL. Dissolve the Sodium Citrate in sufficient Water for Injection to make 1000 mL, and filter until clear. Place the solution in suitable containers, and sterilize.

Note: Anhydrous sodium citrate (35.1 grams) may be used instead of the dihydrate.

Meets the requirements for Identification, pH (6.4–7.5), and Bacterial endotoxins, and for Injections.

ANTIHEMOPHILIC FACTOR

Description: Antihemophilic Factor USP—White or yellowish powder. On constitution is opalescent with a slight blue tinge or is a yellowish liquid.

USP requirements:

Antihemophilic Factor USP—Preserve in hermetic containers, in a refrigerator, unless otherwise indicated. A sterile, freeze-dried powder containing the Factor VIII fraction prepared from units of human venous plasma that have been tested for the absence of hepatitis B surface antigen, obtained from whole-blood donors and pooled. May contain Heparin Sodium or Sodium Citrate. Label it to state that it is to be used within 4 hours after constitution, that it is for intravenous administration, and that a filter is to be used in the administration equipment. Meets the requirements of the test for potency, by comparison with the U.S. Standard Antihemophilic Factor (Factor VIII) or with a working reference that has been calibrated with it, in containing ±20% of the potency stated on the label, the stated potency being not less than 100 Antihemophilic Factor Units per gram of protein. Meets the requirements of the test for Pyrogen, the test dose being 10 Antihemophilic Factor Units per kg, and for Expiration date (not later than 2 years from date of manufacture, within which time it may be stored at room temperature and used within 6 months of the time of such storage). Conforms to the regulations of the U.S. Food and Drug Administration concerning biologics.

Antihemophilic Factor (Human)—Not in *USP–NF*.

Antihemophilic Factor (Porcine)—Not in *USP–NF*.

Antihemophilic Factor (Recombinant)—Not in *USP–NF*.

Antihemophilic Factor (Recombinant) for Injection—Not in *USP–NF*.

CRYOPRECIPITATED ANTIHEMOPHILIC FACTOR

Description: Cryoprecipitated Antihemophilic Factor USP—Yellowish frozen solid. On thawing becomes a very viscous, yellow, gummy liquid.

USP requirements: Cryoprecipitated Antihemophilic Factor USP—Preserve in hermetic containers at a temperature of −18 °C or lower. A sterile, frozen concentrate of human antihemophilic factor prepared from the Factor VIII–rich cryoprotein fraction of human venous plasma obtained from suitable whole-blood donors from a single unit of plasma derived from whole blood or by plasmapheresis, collected and processed in a closed system. Contains no preservative. Label it to indicate the ABO blood group designation and the identification num-

ber of the donor from whom the source material was obtained. Label it also with the type and result of a serologic test for syphilis, or to indicate that it was non-reactive in such test; with the type and result of a test for hepatitis B surface antigen, or to indicate that it was non-reactive in such test; with a warning not to use it if there is evidence of breakage or thawing; with instructions to thaw it before use to a temperature between 20 and 37 °C, after which it is to be stored at room temperature and used as soon as possible but within 6 hours after thawing; to state that it is to be used within 4 hours after the container is entered; and to state that it is for intravenous administration, and that a filter is to be used in the administration equipment. Meets the requirements of the test for potency by comparison with the U.S. Standard Antihemophilic Factor (Factor VIII) or with a working reference that has been calibrated with it, in having an average potency of not less than 80 Antihemophilic Factor Units per container, made at intervals of not more than 1 month during the dating period. Meets the requirement for Expiration date (not later than 1 year from the date of collection of source material). Conforms to the regulations of the U.S. Food and Drug Administration concerning biologics.

ANTI-INHIBITOR COAGULANT COMPLEX

Source: Sterile concentrate prepared from pooled human plasma.

USP requirements: Anti-inhibitor Coagulant Complex—Not in *USP–NF*.

ANTIMONY

Chemical name:
Antimony potassium tartrate—Antimonate(2-), bis[mu-[2,3-dihydroxybutanedioato(4-)-$O^1,O^2:O^3,O^4$]]-di-, dipotassium, trihydrate, stereoisomer.
Antimony sodium tartrate—Antimonate(2-), bis[mu-[2,3-dihydroxybutanedioato(4-)-$O^1,O^2:O^3,O^4$]]di-, disodium, stereoisomer.

Molecular formula:
Antimony potassium tartrate—$C_8H_4K_2O_{12}Sb_2 \cdot 3H_2O$.
Antimony sodium tartrate—$C_8H_4Na_2O_{12}Sb_2$.

Molecular weight:
Antimony potassium tartrate—667.87.
Antimony sodium tartrate—581.61.

Description:
Antimony Potassium Tartrate USP—Colorless, odorless, transparent crystals, or white powder. The crystals effloresce upon exposure to air and do not readily rehydrate even on exposure to high humidity. Its solutions are acid to litmus.
Antimony Sodium Tartrate USP—Colorless, odorless, transparent crystals, or white powder. The crystals effloresce upon exposure to air.

Solubility:
Antimony Potassium Tartrate USP—Freely soluble in boiling water; soluble in water and in glycerin; insoluble in alcohol.
Antimony Sodium Tartrate USP—Freely soluble in water; insoluble in alcohol.

USP requirements:
Antimony Potassium Tartrate USP—Preserve in well-closed containers. Contains not less than 99.0% and not more than 103.0% of antimony potassium tartrate. Meets the requirements for Completeness of solution, Identification,

Acidity or alkalinity, Loss on drying (not more than 2.7%), Arsenic (not more than 0.015%), and Lead (not more than 0.002%).
Antimony Sodium Tartrate USP—Preserve in well-closed containers. Contains not less than 98.0% and not more than 101.0% of antimony sodium tartrate, calculated on the dried basis. Meets the requirements for Identification, Acidity or alkalinity, Loss on drying (not more than 6.0%), Arsenic (not more than 8 ppm), and Lead (not more than 0.002%).

ANTIPYRINE

Chemical name: 1,2-Dihydro-1,5-dimethyl-2-phenyl-3*H*-pyrazol-3-one.

Molecular formula: $C_{11}H_{12}N_2O$.

Molecular weight: 188.23.

Description: Antipyrine USP—Colorless crystals, or white, crystalline powder. Is odorless. Its solutions are neutral to litmus.

Solubility: Antipyrine USP—Very soluble in water; freely soluble in alcohol and in chloroform; sparingly soluble in ether.

USP requirements: Antipyrine USP—Preserve in tight containers. Contains not less than 99.0% and not more than 100.5% of antipyrine, calculated on the dried basis. Meets the requirements for Completeness and color of solution, Identification, Melting range (110–112.5 °C), Loss on drying (not more than 1.0%), Residue on ignition (not more than 0.15%), Heavy metals (not more than 0.002%), and Ordinary impurities.

ANTIPYRINE AND BENZOCAINE

For *Antipyrine* and *Benzocaine*—See individual listings for chemistry information.

USP requirements: Antipyrine and Benzocaine Otic Solution USP—Preserve in tight, light-resistant containers. A solution of Antipyrine and Benzocaine in Glycerin. Contains the labeled amounts, within ±10%. Meets the requirements for Identification and Water (not more than 1.0%).

Note: In the preparation of this Otic Solution, use Glycerin that has a low water content, in order that the Otic Solution may comply with the *Water* limit. This may be ensured by using Glycerin having a specific gravity of not less than 1.2607, corresponding to a concentration of 99.5%.

ANTIPYRINE, BENZOCAINE, AND PHENYLEPHRINE

For *Antipyrine, Benzocaine,* and *Phenylephrine*—See individual listings for chemistry information.

USP requirements: Antipyrine, Benzocaine, and Phenylephrine Hydrochloride Otic Solution USP—Preserve in tight, light-resistant containers. A solution of Antipyrine, Benzocaine, and Phenylephrine Hydrochloride in a suitable nonaqueous solvent. Contains the labeled amounts, within ±10%. Meets the requirement for Identification.

ANTITHROMBIN III

Source: Obtained from human plasma.

Chemical group: A glycoprotein.

Molecular weight: 58,000.

Description: Sterile, white powder.

Other characteristics: Antithrombin III (Human) for Injection—Has a pH of 6.5–7.5 after reconstitution.

USP requirements:

Antithrombin III for Injection Concentrate—Not in *USP–NF*.
Antithrombin III (Human) for Injection—Not in *USP–NF*.

ANTI-THYMOCYTE GLOBULIN (RABBIT)

Source: Anti-thymocyte globulin (rabbit) is a purified, pasteurized, gamma immune globulin, obtained from rabbits that are immunized with human thymocytes. Its potency is determined by lymphocytotoxicity and E-rosette inhibition assays. The amount of cross-reactive antibodies are determined by hemagglutination, platelet agglutination, anti-human serum protein antibody, antiglomerular basement membrane antibody, and fibroblast toxicity assay.

USP requirements: Anti-thymocyte Globulin (Rabbit)—Not in *USP—NF*.

ANTIVENIN (CHIRONEX FLECKERI)

Source: Prepared by hyperimmunizing sheep with the venom of the box jellyfish (*Chironex fleckeri*).

USP requirements: Antivenin (Chironex fleckeri) for Injection—Not in *USP–NF*.

ANTIVENIN (CROTALIDAE) POLYVALENT

Description: Antivenin (Crotalidae) Polyvalent USP—Solid exhibiting the characteristic structure of a freeze-dried solid; light cream in color.

USP requirements: Antivenin (Crotalidae) Polyvalent USP—Preserve in single-dose containers, and avoid exposure to excessive heat. A sterile, non-pyrogenic preparation derived by drying a frozen solution of specific venom-neutralizing globulins obtained from the serum of healthy horses immunized against venoms of four species of pit vipers, *Crotalus atrox, Crotalus adamanteus, Crotalus durissus terrificus,* and *Bothrops atrox* (Fam. Crotalidae). It is standardized by biological assay on mice, in terms of one dose of antivenin neutralizing the venoms in not less than the number of mouse LD_{50} stated, of *Crotalus atrox* (Western diamondback), 180; *Crotalus durissus terrificus* (South American rattlesnake), 1320; and *Bothrops atrox* (South American fer de lance), 780. Label it to indicate the species of snakes against which the Antivenin is to be used, and to state that it was prepared from horse serum. When constituted as specified in the labeling, it is opalescent and contains not more than 20.0% of solids, determined by drying 1 mL at 105 °C to constant weight (± 1 mg). Meets the requirements for general safety and Expiration date (for Antivenin containing a 10% excess of potency, not more than

5 years after date of issue from manufacturer's cold storage [5 °C, 1 year; or 0 °C, 2 years]). Conforms to the regulations of the U.S. Food and Drug Administration concerning biologics.

ANTIVENIN (CROTALIDAE) POLYVALENT IMMUNE FAB (OVINE)

Source: Antivenin (*Crotalidae*) polyvalent immune Fab (ovine) is a sterile, nonpyrogenic, purified, lyophilized preparation of ovine Fab (monovalent) immunoglobulin fragments obtained from the blood of healthy sheep flocks immunized with the venoms of one of the following crotalid snake species: Western Diamondback rattlesnake (*Crotalus atrox*), Eastern Diamondback rattlesnake (*C. adamanteus*), Mojave rattlesnake (*C. scutulatus*), and the Cottonmouth or Water Moccasin (*Agkistrodon piscivorus*). Each monospecific antivenin is prepared by fractionating the immunoglobulin from the ovine serum, digesting it with papain, and isolating the venom-specific Fab fragments on ion exchange and affinity chromatography columns. To obtain the final product, the four different monospecific antivenins are mixed together. The antivenin is standardized by biological assay on mice, based on its ability to neutralize the lethal action of each of the four immunogens.

USP requirements: Antivenin (Crotalidae) Polyvalent Immune Fab (Ovine) for Injection—Not in *USP–NF*.

ANTIVENIN (ENHYDRINA SCHISTOSA)

Description: Antivenin (Enhydrina schistosa)—A refined preparation of plasma from appropriately immunized horses.

USP requirements:

Antivenin (Enhydrina schistosa)—Not in *USP–NF*.
Antivenin (Enhydrina schistosa) for Injection—Not in *USP–NF*.

ANTIVENIN (LATRODECTUS MACTANS)

USP requirements: Antivenin (Latrodectus mactans) USP—Preserve in single-dose containers, and avoid exposure to excessive heat. The sterile, non-pyrogenic preparation derived by drying a frozen solution of specific venom-neutralizing globulins obtained from the serum of healthy horses immunized against venom of black widow spiders (*Latrodectus mactans*). It is standardized by biological assay on mice, in terms of one dose of antivenin neutralizing the venom of *Latrodectus mactans* in not less than 6000 mouse LD_{50}. Label it to indicate the species of spider against which the Antivenin is to be used, that it is not intended to protect against bites from other spider species, and to state that it was prepared in the horse. Thimerosal 1:10,000 is added as a preservative. When constituted as specified in the labeling, it is opalescent and contains not more than 20.0% of solids. Meets the requirement for Expiration date (for Antivenin containing a 10% excess of potency, not more than 5 years after date of issue from manufacturer's cold storage [5 °C, 1 year; or 0 °C, 2 years]). Conforms to the regulations of the U.S. Food and Drug Administration concerning biologics.

ANTIVENIN (MICRURUS FULVIUS)

Description: Antivenin (Micrurus fulvius) USP—Solid exhibiting the characteristic structure of a freeze-dried solid; light cream in color.

USP requirements: Antivenin (Micrurus fulvius) USP—Preserve in single-dose containers, and avoid exposure to excessive heat. The sterile, non-pyrogenic preparation derived by drying a frozen solution of specific venom-neutralizing globulins obtained from the serum of healthy horses immunized against venom of the Eastern Coral snake (*Micrurus fulvius*). It is standardized by biological assay on mice, in terms of one dose of antivenin neutralizing the venom of *Micrurus fulvius* in not less than 250 mouse LD_{50}. Label it to indicate the species of snake against which the Antivenin is to be used, and to state that it was prepared in the horse. When constituted as specified in the labeling, it is opalescent and contains not more than 20.0% of solids, determined by drying 1 mL at 105 °C to constant weight (±1 mg). Meets the requirements for general safety and Expiration date (for Antivenin containing a 10% excess of potency, not more than 5 years after date of issue from manufacturer's cold storage [5 °C, 1 year; or 0 °C, 2 years]). Conforms to the regulations of the U.S. Food and Drug Administration concerning biologics.

ANTIVENIN (NOTECHIS SCUTATUS)

Description: Antivenin (Notechis scutatus)—A refined, sterile concentrate of antitoxic globulins prepared from the serum of immunized horses.

USP requirements:
Antivenin (Notechis scutatus)—Not in *USP–NF*.
Antivenin (Notechis scutatus) for Injection—Not in *USP–NF*.

ANTIVENIN (PSEUDONAJA TEXTILIS)

Description: Antivenin (Pseudonaja textilis)—A refined, sterile concentrate of antitoxic globulins prepared from the serum of immunized horses.

USP requirements:
Antivenin (Pseudonaja textilis)—Not in *USP–NF*.
Antivenin (Pseudonaja textilis) for Injection—Not in *USP–NF*.

APOMORPHINE

Chemical name: Apomorphine hydrochloride—4*H*-Dibenzo[*de,g*]quinoline-10,11-diol, 5,6,6a,7-tetrahydro-6-methyl-, hydrochloride, hemihydrate, (*R*)-.

Molecular formula: Apomorphine hydrochloride—$C_{17}H_{17}NO_2 \cdot$ HCl $\cdot \frac{1}{2}H_2O$.

Molecular weight: Apomorphine hydrochloride—312.79.

Description: Apomorphine Hydrochloride USP—Minute, white or grayish white, glistening crystals or white powder. Is odorless. It gradually acquires a green color on exposure to light and to air. Its solutions are neutral to litmus.

Solubility: Apomorphine Hydrochloride USP—Sparingly soluble in water and in alcohol; soluble in water at 80 °C; very slightly soluble in chloroform and in ether.

USP requirements:
Apomorphine Hydrochloride USP—Preserve in small, tight, light-resistant containers. Containers from which Apomorphine Hydrochloride is to be taken for immediate use in compounding prescriptions contain not more than 350 mg. Contains not less than 98.5% and not more than 100.5% of apomorphine hydrochloride, calculated on the dried basis. Meets the requirements for Color of solution, Identification, Specific rotation (–60.5° to –63.0°), Loss on drying (2.0–3.5%), Residue on ignition (not more than 0.1%), Decomposition products, and Ordinary impurities.
Apomorphine Hydrochloride Injection—Not in *USP–NF*.
Apomorphine Hydrochloride Tablets USP—Preserve in tight, light-resistant containers. Contain the labeled amount, within ±10%. Meet the requirements for Color of solution, Identification, Disintegration (15 minutes), and Uniformity of dosage units.

APRACLONIDINE

Chemical name: Apraclonidine hydrochloride—1,4-Benzenediamine, 2,6-dichloro-*N*¹-2-imidazolidinylidene-, monohydrochloride.

Molecular formula: Apraclonidine hydrochloride—$C_9H_{10}Cl_2N_4 \cdot$ HCl.

Molecular weight: Apraclonidine hydrochloride—281.57.

Description: Apraclonidine Hydrochloride USP—White to off-white, odorless to practically odorless powder.

pKa: Apraclonidine hydrochloride—9.22.

Solubility: Apraclonidine Hydrochloride USP—Soluble in methanol; sparingly soluble in water and in alcohol; insoluble in chloroform, in ethyl acetate, and in hexanes.

USP requirements:
Apraclonidine Ophthalmic Solution USP—Preserve in tight, light-resistant containers. A sterile, aqueous solution of Apraclonidine Hydrochloride. Contains an amount of apraclonidine hydrochloride equivalent to the labeled amount of apraclonidine, within –10% to +15%. Meets the requirements for Identification, Sterility, and pH (4.4–7.8).
Apraclonidine Hydrochloride USP—Preserve in tight, light-resistant containers. Contains not less than 98.0% and not more than 102.0% of apraclonidine hydrochloride, calculated on the dried basis. Meets the requirements for Identification, pH (5.0–6.6, in a solution [1 in 100]), Loss on drying (not more than 1.0%), Residue on ignition (not more than 0.1%), Heavy metals (not more than 0.002%), and Chromatographic purity.
Apraclonidine Hydrochloride Ophthalmic Solution—Not in *USP–NF*.

APROBARBITAL

Chemical name: 5-Allyl-5-isopropylbarbituric acid.

Molecular formula: $C_{10}H_{14}N_2O_3$.

Molecular weight: 210.23.

Description: White crystalline powder.

Solubility: Slightly soluble in water; soluble in alcohol.

USP requirements: Aprobarbital Elixir—Not in *USP–NF*.

APROTININ

Source: Single-chain polypeptide derived from bovine tissues, consisting of 58 amino-acid residues.

Chemical name: Trypsin inhibitor, pancreatic basic.

Molecular formula: $C_{284}H_{432}N_{84}O_{79}S_7$.

Molecular weight: 6511.45.

Description: A clear colorless solution or an almost white hygroscopic powder.

Solubility: The solid is soluble in water and in solutions isotonic with blood; practically insoluble in organic solvents.

USP requirements: Aprotinin Injection—Not in *USP–NF*.

ARBUTAMINE

Chemical name: Arbutamine hydrochloride—1,2-Benzenediol, 4[1-hydroxy-2-[[4-(4-hydroxyphenyl)butyl]amino]ethyl]-, (*R*)-hydrochloride.

Molecular formula: Arbutamine hydrochloride—$C_{18}H_{23}NO_4 \cdot HCl$.

Molecular weight: Arbutamine hydrochloride—353.84.

Description: Arbutamine hydrochloride—Off-white amorphous solid.

Solubility: Arbutamine hydrochloride—Freely soluble in water and in ethanol; practically insoluble in diethyl ether and in hexane.

USP requirements:
Arbutamine Hydrochloride Injection—Not in *USP–NF*.

ARDEPARIN

Molecular weight: Ardeparin sodium—6000 ± 350 daltons.

Description: Ardeparin sodium—A low molecular weight heparin obtained by peroxide fragmentation of Heparin Sodium USP.

USP requirements: Ardeparin Sodium Injection—Not in *USP–NF*.

ARGATROBAN

Source: Argatroban is a synthetic agent which is derived from L-arginine.

Chemical name: 2-Piperidinecarboxylic acid, 1-[5-[(aminoiminomethyl)amino]-1-oxo-2-[[(1,2,3,4-tetrahydro-3-methyl-8-quinolinyl)sulfonyl]amino]pentyl]-4-methyl-, monohydrate.

Molecular formula: $C_{23}H_{36}N_6O_5S \cdot H_2O$.

Molecular weight: 526.65.

Description: White, odorless crystalline powder. Melting point 188–191°.

Solubility: Freely soluble in glacial acetic acid; slightly soluble in ethanol; insoluble in acetone, in ethyl acetate, and in ether.

USP requirements: Argatroban Injection—Not in *USP–NF*.

ARGININE

Chemical name:
Arginine—L-Arginine.
Arginine hydrochloride—L-Arginine monohydrochloride.

Molecular formula:
Arginine—$C_6H_{14}N_4O_2$.
Arginine hydrochloride—$C_6H_{14}N_4O_2 \cdot HCl$.

Molecular weight:
Arginine—174.20.
Arginine hydrochloride—210.66.

Description:
Arginine USP—White, practically odorless crystals.
Arginine Hydrochloride USP—White crystals or crystalline powder, practically odorless.

Solubility:
Arginine USP—Freely soluble in water; sparingly soluble in alcohol; insoluble in ether.
Arginine Hydrochloride USP—Freely soluble in water.

USP requirements:
Arginine USP—Preserve in well-closed containers. Contains not less than 98.5% and not more than 101.5% of arginine, as L-arginine, calculated on the dried basis. Meets the requirements for Identification, Specific rotation (+26.3° to +27.7°), Loss on drying (not more than 0.5%), Residue on ignition (not more than 0.3%), Chloride (not more than 0.05%), Sulfate (not more than 0.03%), Iron (not more than 0.003%), Heavy metals (not more than 0.0015%), Chromatographic purity, and Organic volatile impurities.

Arginine Hydrochloride USP—Preserve in well-closed containers. Contains not less than 98.5% and not more than 101.5% of arginine hydrochloride, calculated on the dried basis. Meets the requirements for Identification, Specific rotation (+21.4° to +23.6°), Loss on drying (not more than 0.2%), Residue on ignition (not more than 0.1%), Sulfate (not more than 0.03%), Heavy metals (not more than 0.002%), Chromatographic purity, Organic volatile impurities, and Chloride content (16.5–17.1%).

Arginine Hydrochloride Injection USP—Preserve in single-dose containers, preferably of Type II glass. A sterile solution of Arginine Hydrochloride in Water for Injection. The label states the total osmolar concentration in mOsmol per liter. Where the contents are less than 100 mL, or where the label states that the Injection is not for direct injection but is to be diluted before use, the label alternatively may state the total osmolar concentration in mOsmol per mL. Contains not less than 9.5% and not more than 10.5% of arginine hydrochloride. Contains no antimicrobial agents. Meets the requirements for Identification, Bacterial endotoxins, and pH (5.0–6.5), and for Injections.

Note: The chloride ion content of Arginine Hydrochloride Injection is approximately 475 mEq per liter.

AROMATIC ELIXIR

Description: Aromatic Elixir NF—NF category: Flavored and/or sweetened vehicle.

NF requirements: Aromatic Elixir NF—Preserve in tight containers.

Prepare Aromatic Elixir as follows: Suitable essential oil(s), 375 mL of Syrup, 30 grams of Talc, and a sufficient quantity of Alcohol and Purified Water to make 1000 mL. Dissolve the oil(s) in Alcohol to make 250 mL. To this solution add the Syrup in several portions, agitating vigorously after each addition, and afterwards add, in the same manner, the re-

quired quantity of Purified Water. Mix the Talc with the liquid, and filter through a filter wetted with Diluted Alcohol, returning the filtrate until a clear liquid is obtained.

Meets the requirements for Alcohol content (21.0–23.0%) and Organic volatile impurities.

ARSANILIC ACID

Chemical name: *p*-Aminobenzenearsonic acid.

Molecular formula: $C_6H_8AsNO_3$.

Molecular weight: 217.05.

Description: Arsanilic Acid USP—White to off-white crystalline powder. Melts at about 232 °C.

Solubility: Arsanilic Acid USP—Soluble in hot water, in amyl alcohol, and in solutions of alkali carbonates; sparingly soluble in concentrated mineral acids; slightly soluble in cold water, in alcohol, and in acetic acid; insoluble in acetone, in chloroform, in ether, and in dilute mineral acids.

USP requirements: Arsanilic Acid USP—Preserve in well-closed containers. Label it to indicate that it is for veterinary use only. Contains not less than 98.0% and not more than 102.0% of arsanilic acid, calculated on the dried basis. Meets the requirements for Identification, Loss on drying (not more than 0.5%), Limit of *o*-arsanilic acid (not more than 0.12%), and Limit of aniline (not more than 0.045%).

ARSENIC TRIOXIDE

Molecular formula: As_2O_3.

Molecular weight: 197.8.

Description: White to transparent, glassy, amorphous lumps or crystallized powder.

Solubility: Sparingly and extremely slowly soluble in cold water; soluble in 15 parts boiling water, in diluted hydrochloride, in alkali hydroxide or carbonate solutions; practically insoluble in alcohol, in chloroform, and in ether.

Other characteristics: pH: 7.0–9.0.

USP requirements: Arsenic Trioxide Injection—Not in *USP–NF*.

ARTICAINE AND EPINEPHRINE

Chemical name:
Articaine hydrochloride—Methyl 4-methyl-3-(2-propylamino-propionamido)thiophene-2-carboxylate hydrochloride.
Epinephrine—1,2-Benzenediol, 4-[1-hydroxy-2-(methylamino)ethyl]-, (*R*)-.

Molecular formula:
Articaine hydrochloride—$C_{13}H_{20}N_2O_3S \cdot HCl$.
Epinephrine—$C_9H_{13}NO_3$.

Molecular weight:
Articaine hydrochloride—320.8.
Epinephrine—183.20.

Description: Epinephrine USP—White to practically white, odorless, microcrystalline powder or granules, gradually darkening on exposure to light and air. With acids, it forms salts that are readily soluble in water, and the base may be recovered by the addition of ammonia water or alkali carbonates. Its solutions are alkaline to litmus.

Solubility: Epinephrine USP—Very slightly soluble in water and in alcohol; insoluble in ether, in chloroform, and in fixed and volatile oils.

USP requirements: Articaine Hydrochloride and Epinephrine Injection—Not in *USP–NF*.

ASCORBIC ACID

Chemical name: L-Ascorbic acid.

Molecular formula: $C_6H_8O_6$.

Molecular weight: 176.12.

Description: Ascorbic Acid USP—White or slightly yellow crystals or powder. On exposure to light it gradually darkens. In the dry state, is reasonably stable in air, but in solution rapidly oxidizes. Melts at about 190 °C.

NF category: Antioxidant.

pKa: 4.2 and 11.6.

Solubility: Ascorbic Acid USP—Freely soluble in water; sparingly soluble in alcohol; insoluble in chloroform and in ether.

USP requirements:
Ascorbic Acid USP—Preserve in tight, light-resistant containers. Contains not less than 99.0% and not more than 100.5% of ascorbic acid. Meets the requirements for Identification, Specific rotation (+20.5° to +21.5°), Residue on ignition (not more than 0.1%), Heavy metals (not more than 0.002%), and Organic volatile impurities.

Ascorbic Acid Extended-release Capsules—Not in *USP–NF*.

Ascorbic Acid Injection USP—Preserve in light-resistant, single-dose containers, preferably of Type I or Type II glass. A sterile solution, in Water for Injection, of Ascorbic Acid prepared with the aid of Sodium Hydroxide, Sodium Carbonate, or Sodium Bicarbonate. In addition to meeting the requirements for Labeling under Injections, fused-seal containers of the Injection in concentrations of 250 mg per mL and greater are labeled to indicate that since pressure may develop on long storage, precautions should be taken to wrap the container in a protective covering while it is being opened. Contains the labeled amount, within ± 10%. Meets the requirements for Identification, Bacterial endotoxins, pH (5.5–7.0), and Limit of oxalate, and for Injections.

Ascorbic Acid Oral Solution USP—Preserve in tight, light-resistant containers. A solution of Ascorbic Acid in a hydroxylic organic solvent or an aqueous mixture thereof. Label Oral Solution that contains alcohol to state the alcohol content. Contains the labeled amount, within ±10%. Meets the requirements for Identification and Alcohol content (the labeled amount, within ±10%).

Ascorbic Acid Syrup—Not in *USP–NF*.

Ascorbic Acid Tablets USP—Preserve in tight, light-resistant containers. Contain the labeled amount, within ±10%. Meet the requirements for Identification, Dissolution (75% in 45 minutes in water in Apparatus 2 at 50 rpm), and Uniformity of dosage units.

Ascorbic Acid Effervescent Tablets—Not in *USP–NF*.

Ascorbic Acid Extended-release Tablets—Not in *USP–NF*.

ASCORBYL PALMITATE

Chemical name: L-Ascorbic acid, 6-hexadecanoate.

Molecular formula: $C_{22}H_{38}O_7$.

Molecular weight: 414.53.

Description: Ascorbyl Palmitate NF—White to yellowish white powder, having a characteristic odor.

NF category: Antioxidant.

Solubility: Ascorbyl Palmitate NF—Very slightly soluble in water and in vegetable oils; soluble in alcohol.

NF requirements: Ascorbyl Palmitate NF—Preserve in tight containers, in a cool, dry place. Contains not less than 95.0% and not more than 100.5% of ascorbyl palmitate, calculated on the dried basis. Meets the requirements for Identification, Melting range (107–117 °C), Specific rotation (+21° to +24°), Loss on drying (not more than 2.0%), Residue on ignition (not more than 0.1%), Heavy metals (not more than 0.001%), and Organic volatile impurities.

ASPARAGINASE

Source: Commercially available asparaginase is a high molecular weight enzyme derived from *Escherichia coli.*

Chemical name: Asparaginase.

Description: White, crystalline powder; slightly hygroscopic.

Solubility: Freely soluble in water; practically insoluble in methanol, in acetone, and in chloroform.

Other characteristics: Enzyme active at pH 6.5–8.0.

USP requirements: Asparaginase for Injection—Not in *USP–NF*.

ASPARTAME

Chemical Name: L-Phenylalanine, *N*-L-alpha-aspartyl-, 1-methyl ester.

Molecular formula: $C_{14}H_{18}N_2O_5$.

Molecular weight: 294.30.

Description: Aspartame NF—White, odorless, crystalline powder. Melts at about 246 °C. The pH of an 8 in 1000 solution is about 5.

NF category: Sweetening agent.

Solubility: Aspartame NF—Sparingly soluble in water; slightly soluble in alcohol.

NF requirements: Aspartame NF—Preserve in well-closed containers. Contains not less than 98.0% and not more than 102.0% of aspartame, calculated on the dried basis. Meets the requirements for Identification, Transmittance, Specific rotation (+14.5° to +16.5°), Loss on drying (not more than 4.5%), Residue on ignition (not more than 0.2%), Heavy metals (not more than 0.001%), Limit of 5-benzyl-3,6-dioxo-2-piperazineacetic acid, Chromatographic purity, and Organic volatile impurities.

ASPARTIC ACID

Chemical name:L-Aspartic acid.

Molecular formula: $C_4H_7NO_4$.

Molecular weight: 133.10.

Description: White or almost white crystalline powder, or colorless crystals.

Solubility: Soluble in dilute solutions of alkali hydroxides and in dilute mineral acids; slightly soluble in water; practically insoluble in alcohol and in ether.

USP requirements: Aspartic Acid USP—Preserve in well-closed containers, protected from light.Contains not less than 98.5% and not more than 101.5% of aspartic acid, calculated on the dried basis. Meets the requirements for Identification, Specific rotation (+24.0° to +26.0°, at 20°), Loss on drying (not more than 0.5%), Residue on ignition (not more than 0.1%), Chloride (0.02%), Sulfate (0.03%), Iron (0.001%), Heavy metals (0.001%), Chromatographic purity, and Organic volatile impurities.

ASPIRIN

Chemical name: Benzoic acid, 2-(acetyloxy)-.

Molecular formula: $C_9H_8O_4$.

Molecular weight: 180.16.

Description: Aspirin USP—White crystals, commonly tabular or needle-like, or white, crystalline powder. Is odorless or has a faint odor. Is stable in dry air; in moist air it gradually hydrolyzes to salicylic and acetic acids.

pKa: 3.5.

Solubility: Aspirin USP—Slightly soluble in water; freely soluble in alcohol; soluble in chloroform and in ether; sparingly soluble in absolute ether.

USP requirements:

Aspirin USP—Preserve in tight containers. Contains not less than 99.5% and not more than 100.5% of aspirin, calculated on the dried basis. Meets the requirements for Identification, Loss on drying (not more than 0.5%), Readily carbonizable substances, Residue on ignition (not more than 0.05%), Substances insoluble in sodium carbonate TS, Chloride (not more than 0.014%), Sulfate (not more than 0.04%), Heavy metals (not more than 10 mcg per gram), Limit of free salicylic acid (not more than 0.1%), and Organic volatile impurities.

Aspirin Boluses USP—Preserve in tight containers. Label Boluses to indicate that they are for veterinary use only. Contain the labeled amount, within ±10%. Meet the requirements for Identification, Dissolution (80% in 45 minutes in 0.05 *M* acetate buffer [pH 4.50 ±0.05] in Apparatus 1 at 100 rpm), Uniformity of dosage units, and Limit of salicylic acid (not more than 0.3%).

Aspirin Capsules USP—Preserve in tight containers. Contain the labeled amount, within ±7%. Meet the requirements for Identification, Dissolution (80% in 30 minutes in 0.05 *M* acetate buffer [pH 4.50 ±0.05] in Apparatus 1 at 100 rpm), Uniformity of dosage units, and Limit of free salicylic acid (not more than 0.75%, calculated on the labeled aspirin content).

Note: Capsules that are enteric-coated or the contents of which are enteric-coated meet the requirements for Aspirin Delayed-release Capsules.

Aspirin Delayed-release Capsules USP—Preserve in tight containers. The label indicates that Aspirin Delayed-release Capsules or the contents thereof are enteric-coated. Contain the labeled amount, within ±7%. Meet the require-

ments for Identification, Drug release, Uniformity of dosage units, and Limit of free salicylic acid (not more than 3.0%).

Aspirin Suppositories USP—Preserve in well-closed containers, in a cool place. Contain the labeled amount, within ± 10%. Meet the requirements for Identification and Limit of free salicylic acid (not more than 3.0%).

Aspirin Tablets USP—Preserve in tight containers. Preserve flavored or sweetened Tablets of 81-mg size or smaller in containers holding not more than 36 Tablets each. Contain the labeled amount, within ±10%. Tablets of larger than 81-mg size contain no sweeteners or other flavors. Meet the requirements for Identification, Dissolution (80% in 30 minutes in 0.05 *M* acetate buffer [pH 4.50 ± 0.05] in Apparatus 1 at 50 rpm), Uniformity of dosage units, and Limit of free salicylic acid (not more than 0.3% for uncoated tablets or not more than 3.0% for coated tablets).

   Note: Tablets that are enteric-coated meet the requirements for Aspirin Delayed-release Tablets.

Aspirin Chewing Gum Tablets—Not in *USP-NF.*

Aspirin Delayed-release Tablets USP—Preserve in tight containers. The label indicates that the Tablets are enteric-coated. Contain the labeled amount, within ±5%. Meet the requirements for Identification, Drug release, Uniformity of dosage units, and Limit of free salicylic acid (not more than 3.0%).

Aspirin Extended-release Tablets USP—Preserve in tight containers. The labeling indicates the Drug Release Test with which the product complies. Contain the labeled amount, within ±5%. Meet the requirements for Identification, Drug release (20–55% in 1 hour and not less than 80% in 4 hours in 0.1 *N* hydrochloric acid in Apparatus 2 at 60 rpm for Test 1 [if the product complies with this test, the labeling indicates that it meets USP Drug Release Test 1]; 15–40% in 1 hour, 25–60% in 2 hours, 35–75% in 4 hours, and not less than 70% in 8 hours in water in Apparatus 2 at 30 rpm for Test 2 [if the product complies with this test, the labeling indicates that it meets USP Drug Release Test 2]), Uniformity of dosage units, and Free salicylic acid (not more than 3.0%).

BUFFERED ASPIRIN

Chemical name: Aspirin—Benzoic acid, 2-(acetyloxy)-.

Molecular formula: Aspirin—$C_9H_8O_4$.

Molecular weight: Aspirin—180.16.

Description: Aspirin USP—White crystals, commonly tabular or needle-like, or white, crystalline powder. Is odorless or has a faint odor. Is stable in dry air; in moist air it gradually hydrolyzes to salicylic and acetic acids.

pKa: Aspirin—3.5.

Solubility: Aspirin USP—Slightly soluble in water; freely soluble in alcohol; soluble in chloroform and in ether; sparingly soluble in absolute ether.

USP requirements: Buffered Aspirin Tablets USP—Preserve in tight containers. Contain Aspirin and suitable buffering agents. Contain the labeled amount of aspirin, within ±10%. Meet the requirements for Identification, Dissolution (80% in 30 minutes in 0.05 *M* acetate buffer [pH 4.50 ±0.05] in Apparatus 2 at 75 rpm), Uniformity of dosage units, Acid-neutralizing capacity, and Limit of free salicylic acid (not more than 3.0%).

ASPIRIN, ALUMINA, AND MAGNESIA

For *Aspirin, Alumina* (Aluminum Hydroxide), and *Magnesia* (Magnesium Hydroxide)—See individual listings for chemistry information.

USP requirements: Aspirin, Alumina, and Magnesia Tablets USP—Preserve in tight containers. Contain the labeled amount of aspirin, within ±10%, and amounts of alumina and magnesia equivalent to the labeled amounts of aluminum hydroxide and magnesium hydroxide, within ±10%. Meet the requirements for Identification, Dissolution (75% of labeled amount of aspirin in 45 minutes in 0.05 *M* acetate buffer [pH 4.50 ±0.05] in Apparatus 2 at 75 rpm), Uniformity of dosage units, Acid-neutralizing capacity, and Limit of free salicylic acid (not more than 3.0%).

ASPIRIN, ALUMINA, AND MAGNESIUM OXIDE

For *Aspirin, Alumina* (Aluminum Hydroxide), and *Magnesium Oxide*—See individual listings for chemistry information.

USP requirements: Aspirin, Alumina, and Magnesium Oxide Tablets USP—Preserve in tight containers. Contain the labeled amounts of aspirin and magnesium oxide, within ±10%, and an amount of alumina equivalent to the labeled amount of aluminum hydroxide, within ±10%. Meet the requirements for Identification, Dissolution (75% of labeled amount of aspirin in 45 minutes in 0.05 *M* acetate buffer [pH 4.50 ±0.05] in Apparatus 1 [10-mesh screen] at 100 rpm), Uniformity of dosage units, Acid-neutralizing capacity, and Limit of free salicylic acid (not more than 3.0%).

ASPIRIN AND CAFFEINE

For *Aspirin* and *Caffeine*—See individual listings for chemistry information.

USP requirements:
   Aspirin and Caffeine Capsules—Not in *USP-NF.*
   Aspirin and Caffeine Tablets—Not in *USP-NF.*

BUFFERED ASPIRIN AND CAFFEINE

Source: Caffeine—Coffee, tea, cola, and cocoa or chocolate. May also be synthesized from urea or dimethylurea.

Chemical group: Caffeine—Methylated xanthine.

Chemical name:
   Aspirin—Benzoic acid, 2-(acetyloxy)-.
   Caffeine—1*H*-Purine-2,6-dione, 3,7-dihydro-1,3,7-trimethyl-.

Molecular formula:
   Aspirin—$C_9H_8O_4$.
   Caffeine—$C_8H_{10}N_4O_2$ (anhydrous); $C_8H_{10}N_4O_2 \cdot H_2O$ (monohydrate).

Molecular weight:
   Aspirin—180.16.
   Caffeine—194.19 (anhydrous); 212.21 (monohydrate).

Description:
   Aspirin USP—White crystals, commonly tabular or needle-like, or white, crystalline powder. Is odorless or has a faint odor. Is stable in dry air; in moist air it gradually hydrolyzes to salicylic and acetic acids.

Caffeine USP—White powder or white, glistening needles, usually matted together. Is odorless. Its solutions are neutral to litmus. The hydrate is efflorescent in air.

pKa: Aspirin—3.5.

Solubility:

Aspirin USP—Slightly soluble in water; freely soluble in alcohol; soluble in chloroform and in ether; sparingly soluble in absolute ether.

Caffeine USP—Sparingly soluble in water and in alcohol; freely soluble in chloroform; slightly soluble in ether.

The aqueous solubility of caffeine is increased by organic acids or their alkali salts, such as citrates, benzoates, salicylates, or cinnamates, which dissociate to yield caffeine when dissolved in biological fluids.

USP requirements: Buffered Aspirin and Caffeine Tablets—Not in *USP–NF*.

ASPIRIN, CAFFEINE, AND DIHYDROCODEINE

For *Aspirin, Caffeine,* and *Dihydrocodeine*—See individual listings for chemistry information.

USP requirements: Aspirin, Caffeine, and Dihydrocodeine Bitartrate Capsules USP—Preserve in tight containers. Contain the labeled amounts, within ±10%. Meet the requirements for Identification, Dissolution (75% of each active ingredient in 45 minutes in 0.05 *M* acetate buffer [pH 4.50 ±0.05] in Apparatus 1 at 50 rpm), Uniformity of dosage units, and Limit of salicylic acid (not more than 3.0%).

ASPIRIN AND CODEINE

For *Aspirin* and *Codeine*—See individual listings for chemistry information.

USP requirements: Aspirin and Codeine Phosphate Tablets USP—Preserve in well-closed, light-resistant containers. Contain the labeled amounts of aspirin and codeine phosphate hemihydrate, within ±10%. Meet the requirements for Identification, Dissolution (75% of each active ingredient in 30 minutes in 0.05 *M* acetate buffer [pH 4.50 ±0.05] in Apparatus 2 at 75 rpm), Uniformity of dosage units, and Limit of free salicylic acid (not more than 3.0%).

ASPIRIN, CODEINE, ALUMINA, AND MAGNESIA

For *Aspirin, Codeine, Alumina* (Aluminum Hydroxide), and *Magnesia* (Magnesium Hydroxide)—See individual listings for chemistry information.

USP requirements: Aspirin, Codeine Phosphate, Alumina, and Magnesia Tablets USP—Preserve in well-closed, light-resistant containers. Contain the labeled amounts of aspirin and codeine phosphate hemihydrate, within ±10%, and amounts of alumina and magnesia equivalent to the labeled amounts of aluminum hydroxide and magnesium hydroxide, within ±10%. Meets the requirements for Identification, Dissolution (75% of the labeled amounts of aspirin and codeine phosphate hemihydrate in 30 minutes in 0.05 *M* acetate buffer [pH 4.50 ±0.05]

in Apparatus 2 at 75 rpm), Uniformity of dosage units, Acid-neutralizing capacity, and Limit of free salicylic acid (not more than 3.0%).

ASPIRIN, CODEINE, AND CAFFEINE

For *Aspirin, Codeine,* and *Caffeine*—See individual listings for chemistry information.

USP requirements:

Aspirin, Codeine Phosphate, and Caffeine Capsules USP—Preserve in well-closed, light-resistant containers. Contain the labeled amounts of aspirin, codeine phosphate hemihydrate, and caffeine, within ±10%. Meet the requirements for Identification, Uniformity of dosage units, and Salicylic acid (not more than 3.0%).

Aspirin, Codeine Phosphate, and Caffeine Tablets USP—Preserve in well-closed, light-resistant containers. Contain the labeled amounts of aspirin, codeine phosphate hemihydrate, and caffeine, within ±10%. Meet the requirements for Identification, Uniformity of dosage units, and Salicylic acid (not more than 3.0%).

ASPIRIN, CODEINE, CAFFEINE, ALUMINA, AND MAGNESIA

For *Aspirin, Codeine, Caffeine, Alumina* (Aluminum Hydroxide), and *Magnesia* (Magnesium Hydroxide)—See individual listings for chemistry information.

USP requirements: Aspirin, Codeine Phosphate, Caffeine, Alumina, and Magnesia Tablets—Not in *USP–NF*.

ASPIRIN, SODIUM BICARBONATE, AND CITRIC ACID

For *Aspirin, Sodium Bicarbonate,* and *Citric Acid*—See individual listings for chemistry information.

USP requirements: Aspirin Effervescent Tablets for Oral Solution USP—Preserve in tight containers. Contain Aspirin and an effervescent mixture of a suitable organic acid and an alkali metal bicarbonate and/or carbonate. Contain the labeled amount of aspirin, within ±10%. Meet the requirements for Identification, Solution time (within 5 minutes in water at 17.5 ±2.5 °C), Uniformity of dosage units, Acid-neutralizing capacity, and Limit of free salicylate (not more than 8.0%).

ASTEMIZOLE

Chemical name: 1*H*-Benzimidazol-2-amine, 1-[(4-fluorophenyl)-methyl]-*N*-[1-[2-(4-methoxyphenyl)ethyl]-4-piperidinyl]-.

Molecular formula: $C_{28}H_{31}FN_4O$.

Molecular weight: 458.57.

Description: White to slightly off-white powder. It has a melting point of 149.1 °C.

Solubility: Insoluble in water; soluble in chloroform and in methanol; slightly soluble in ethanol.

USP requirements:
  Astemizole USP—Preserve in tight containers. Contains not less than 98.0% and not more than 102.0%, calculated on the dried basis. Meets the requirements for Identification, Melting range (175°–178°), Loss on drying (not more than 0.5%), Residue on ignition (not more than 0.1%), Heavy metals (0.001%), and Chromatographic purity.
  Astemizole Oral Suspension—Not in *USP–NF*.
  Astemizole Tablets USP—Preserve in tight containers. Contain the labeled amount, within ±10%. Meet the requirements for Identification, Dissolution (80% in 45 minutes in simulated gastric fluid TS [without the enzyme] in Apparatus 2 at 100 rpm), Uniformity of dosage units, and Chromatographic purity (not more than 0.1% of any individual impurity, and the sum of all impurities not more than 1.0%).

ATENOLOL

Chemical name: Benzeneacetamide, 4-[2-hydroxy-3-[(1-methylethyl)amino]propoxy]-.

Molecular formula: $C_{14}H_{22}N_2O_3$.

Molecular weight: 266.34.

Description: White or practically white, odorless powder. Melting point 146° – 148° (crystals from ethyl acetate).

Solubility: Freely soluble in methanol; sparingly soluble in alcohol; slightly soluble in water and in isopropanol.

Other characteristics: Lipid solubility—Very low (log partition coefficient for octanol/water is 0.23).

USP requirements:
  Atenolol USP—Preserve in well-closed containers. Contains not less than 98.0% and not more than 102.0% of atenolol, calculated on the dried basis. Meets the requirements for Identification, Melting range (152–156.5 °C), Loss on drying (not more than 0.5%), Residue on ignition (not more than 0.2%), Chloride (not more than 0.1%), and Chromatographic purity.
  Atenolol Injection USP—Preserve in single-dose or in multiple-dose containers, preferably of Type I glass, in a cool place or at controlled room temperature, protected from light. Avoid freezing. A sterile solution of Atenolol in Water for Injection. Contains a suitable buffering agent. Contains the labeled amount, within ±10%. Meets the requirements for Identification, Bacterial endotoxins, Sterility, pH (5.5–6.5), and Particulate matter.
  Atenolol Tablets USP—Preserve in well-closed containers. Contain the labeled amount, within ±10%. Meet the requirements for Identification, Dissolution (80% in 30 minutes in 0.1 N acetate buffer [pH 4.6], prepared by mixing 44.9 parts [v/v] of sodium acetate TS with 55.1 parts [v/v] of 0.1 N acitic acid solution) in Apparatus 2 at 50 rpm), and Uniformity of dosage units.

ATENOLOL AND CHLORTHALIDONE

For *Atenolol* and *Chlorthalidone*—See individual listings for chemistry information.

USP requirements: Atenolol and Chlorthalidone Tablets USP—Preserve in well-closed containers. Contain the labeled amounts, within ±10%. Meet the requirements for Identification, Dissolution (80% of atenolol and 70% of chlorthalidone in 45 minutes in 0.01 N hydrochloric acid in Apparatus 2 at 50 rpm), and Uniformity of dosage units.

ATORVASTATIN

Chemical name: Atorvastatin calcium—1*H*-Pyrrole-1-heptanoic acid, 2-(4-fluorophenyl)-beta,delta-dihydroxy-5-(1-methylethyl)-3-phenyl-4-[(phenylamino]carbonyl]-, calcium salt (2:1), [*R*-(*R**,*R**)]-.

Molecular formula: Atorvastatin calcium—$C_{66}H_{68}CaF_2N_4O_{10}$.

Molecular weight: Atorvastatin calcium—1155.34.

Description: Atorvastatin calcium—White to off-white crystalline powder.

Solubility: Atorvastatin calcium—Insoluble in aqueous solutions of pH 4 and below; very slightly soluble in distilled water, in pH 7.4 phosphate buffer, and in acetonitrile; slightly soluble in ethanol; freely soluble in methanol.

USP requirements:
  Atorvastatin Calcium Tablets—Not in *USP–NF*.

ATOVAQUONE

Chemical name: 1,4-Naphthalenedione, 2-[4-(4-chlorophenyl)cyclohexyl]-3-hydroxy-, *trans*-.

Molecular formula: $C_{22}H_{19}ClO_3$.

Molecular weight: 366.84.

Description: Yellow powder.

Solubility: Freely soluble in *N*-methyl-2-pyrrolidone and in tetrahydrofuran; soluble in chloroform; sparingly soluble in acetone, in di-*n*-butyl adipate, in dimethyl sulfoxide, and in polyethylene glycol 400; slightly soluble in alcohol, in 1,3-butane-diol, in ethyl acetate, in glycerin, in octanol, and in polyethyene glycol 200; very slightly soluble in 0.1 N sodium hydroxide; insoluble in water.

USP requirements:
  Atovaquone USP—Preserve in tight, light-resistant containers. Contains not less than 97.5% and not more than 101.5% of atovaquone, calculated on the anhydrous and organic solvent-free basis. Meets the requirements for Identification, Water (not more than 1.0%), Residue on ignition (not more than 0.1%), Heavy metals (10 micrograms per gram), Limit of residual organic solvents (not more than 0.2% of methanol or of acetic acid), and Related compounds.
  Atovaquone Oral Suspension USP—Preserve in tight, light-resistant containers. Contains a leveled amount of atovaquone, within ±10%. Meets the requirements for Identification, Deliverable volume, pH (3.5–7.0), Sedimentation (not more than 1 mL of clear liquid), and Related compounds.
  Atovaquone Tablets—Not in *USP–NF*.

ATOVAQUONE AND PROGUANIL

For *Atovaquone* and *Proguanil*—See individual listings for chemistry information.

USP requirements: Atovaquone and Proguanil Hydrochloride Tablets—Not in *USP–NF*.

ATRACURIUM

Chemical name: Atracurium besylate—Isoquinolinium, 2,2′-[1,5-pentanediylbis[oxy(3-oxo-3,1-propanediyl)]]bis[1-[(3,4-dimethoxyphenyl)methyl]-1,2,3,4-tetrahydro-6,7-dimethoxy-2-methyl-, dibenzenesulfonate.

Molecular formula: Atracurium besylate—$C_{65}H_{82}N_2O_{18}S_2$.

Molecular weight: Atracurium besylate—1243.48.

Description:
Atracurium Besylate USP—White to off-white solid.
Atracurium besylate injection—Sterile, non-pyrogenic aqueous solution. The pH is adjusted to 3.25–3.65 with benzenesulfonic acid.

USP requirements:
Atracurium Besylate USP—Preserve in tight, light-resistant containers in a cold place. [Note—Atracurium Besylate is unstable at room temperature.] Contains not less than 96.0% and not more than 102.0% of atracurium besylate, calculated on the anhydrous basis. Contains not less than 5.0% and not more than 6.5% of the *trans-trans* isomer, not less than 34.5% and not more than 38.5% of the *cis-trans* isomer, and not less than 55.0% and not more than 60.0% of the *cis-cis* isomer. Meets the requirements for Identification, Water (not more than 5.0%), Residue on ignition (not more than 0.2%), Heavy metals (20 micrograms per gram), Limit of methyl benzene sulfonate (not more than 0.01%), Limit of toluene (not more than 0.5%), Chromatographic purity, and Organic volatile impurities.
Atracurium Besylate Injection USP—Preserve in single-dose or multiple-dose containers, preferably of Type I glass, in a refrigerator, and protect from freezing. Protect from light. A sterile solution containing the labeled amount, within −10% to +15%. Contains a labeled amount of atracurium besylate equivalent to the amount of *trans-trans*-isomer not less than 5.0% and not more than 6.5%, *cis-trans*-isomer not less than 34.5% and not more than 38.5%, and *cis-cis*-isomer not less than 55.0% and not more than 60.0%. Meets the requirements for Identification, Bacterial endotoxins, pH (3.00–3.65), and Related compounds, and for Injections.
Note—The Injection is unstable at room temperature. Store all samples in the refrigerator. Analyze all preparations as soon as possible, or use a refrigerated injector.

ATROPINE

Source: An alkaloid that may be extracted from belladonna root and hyoscyamine or may be produced synthetically.

Chemical group: Natural tertiary amine.

Chemical name:
Atropine—Benzeneacetic acid, alpha-(hydroxymethyl)-8-methyl-8-azabicyclo[3.2.1]oct-3-yl ester, *endo*-(±)-.
Atropine sulfate—Benzeneacetic acid, alpha-(hydroxymethyl)-, 8-methyl-8-azabicyclo[3.2.1]oct-3-yl ester, *endo*(±)-, sulfate (2:1) (salt), monohydrate.

Molecular formula:
Atropine—$C_{17}H_{23}NO_3$.
Atropine sulfate—$(C_{17}H_{23}NO_3)_2 \cdot H_2SO_4 \cdot H_2O$.

Molecular weight:
Atropine—289.37.
Atropine sulfate—694.83.

Description:
Atropine USP—White crystals, usually needle-like, or white, crystalline powder. Its saturated solution is alkaline to phenolphthalein TS. Is optically inactive, but usually contains some levorotatory hyoscyamine.
Atropine Sulfate USP—Colorless crystals, or white, crystalline powder. Odorless; effloresces in dry air; is slowly affected by light.

Solubility:
Atropine USP—Slightly soluble in water, and sparingly soluble in water at 80 °C; freely soluble in alcohol and in chloroform; soluble in glycerin and in ether.
Atropine Sulfate USP—Very soluble in water; freely soluble in alcohol and even more so in boiling alcohol; freely soluble in glycerin.

USP requirements:
Atropine USP—Preserve in tight, light-resistant containers. Contains not less than 99.0% and not more than 100.5% of atropine, calculated on the anhydrous basis. Meets the requirements for Identification, Melting range (114–118 °C), Optical rotation (−0.70° to +0.05° [limit of hyoscyamine]), Water (not more than 0.2%), Residue on ignition (not more than 0.1%), Readily carbonizable substances, Limit of foreign alkaloids and other impurities, and Organic volatile impurities.
Caution: Handle Atropine with exceptional care, since it is highly potent.
Atropine Sulfate USP—Preserve in tight containers. Contains not less than 98.5% and not more than 101.0% of atropine sulfate, calculated on the anhydrous basis. Meets the requirements for Identification, Melting temperature (not lower than 187 °C, determined after drying at 120 °C for 4 hours), Optical rotation (−0.60° to +0.05° [limit of hyoscyamine]), Acidity, Water (not more than 4.0%), Residue on ignition (not more than 0.2%), Organic volatile impurities, and Other alkaloids.
Caution: Handle Atropine Sulfate with exceptional care, since it is highly potent.
Atropine Sulfate Injection USP—Preserve in single-dose or in multiple-dose containers, preferably of Type I glass. A sterile solution of Atropine Sulfate in Water for Injection. Contains the labeled amount, within ±7%. Meets the requirements for Identification, Bacterial endotoxins, and pH (3.0–6.5), and for Injections.
Atropine Sulfate Ophthalmic Ointment USP—Preserve in collapsible ophthalmic ointment tubes. It is Atropine Sulfate in a suitable ophthalmic ointment base. Contains the labeled amount, within ±10%. It is sterile. Meets the requirements for Identification, Sterility, and Metal particles.
Atropine Sulfate Ophthalmic Solution USP—Preserve in tight containers. A sterile, aqueous solution of Atropine Sulfate. Contains the labeled amount, within ±7%. Meets the requirements for Identification, Sterility, and pH (3.5–6.0).
Atropine Sulfate Tablets USP—Preserve in well-closed containers. Contain the labeled amount, within ±10%. Meet the requirements for Identification, Disintegration (15 minutes), and Uniformity of dosage units.
Atropine Sulfate Soluble Tablets—Not in *USP–NF*.

ATROPINE, HYOSCYAMINE, METHENAMINE, METHYLENE BLUE, PHENYL SALICYLATE, AND BENZOIC ACID

Chemical name:

Atropine sulfate—Benzeneacetic acid, alpha-(hydroxymethyl)-, 8-methyl-8-azabicyclo[3.2.1]oct-3-yl ester, endo-(±)-, sulfate (2:1) (salt), monohydrate.

Hyoscyamine—Benzeneacetic acid, alpha-(hydroxymethyl)-, 8-methyl-8-azabicyclo[3.2.1]oct-3-yl ester, [3(S)-endo]-.

Methenamine—1,3,5,7-Tetraazatricyclo[3.3.1.1³,⁷]decane.

Methylene blue—Phenothiazin-5-ium, 3,7-bis(dimethylamino)-, chloride, trihydrate.

Phenyl salicylate—2-Hydroxybenzoic acid phenyl ester.

Benzoic acid—Benzoic acid.

Molecular formula:

Atropine sulfate—$(C_{17}H_{23}NO_3)_2 \cdot H_2SO_4 \cdot H_2O$.

Hyoscyamine—$C_{17}H_{23}NO_3$.

Methenamine—$C_6H_{12}N_4$.

Methylene blue—$C_{16}H_{18}ClN_3S \cdot 3H_2O$.

Phenyl salicylate—$C_{13}H_{10}O_3$.

Benzoic acid—$C_7H_6O_2$.

Molecular weight:

Atropine sulfate—694.83.

Hyoscyamine—289.37.

Methenamine—140.19.

Methylene blue—373.90.

Phenyl salicylate—214.21.

Benzoic acid—122.12.

Description:

Atropine Sulfate USP—Colorless crystals, or white, crystalline powder. Odorless; effloresces in dry air; is slowly affected by light.

Hyoscyamine USP—White, crystalline powder. Is affected by light. Its solutions are alkaline to litmus.

Methenamine USP—Colorless, lustrous crystals or white, crystalline powder. Is practically odorless. When brought into contact with fire, it readily ignites, burning with a smokeless flame. It sublimes at about 260 °C, without melting. Its solutions are alkaline to litmus.

Methylene Blue USP—Dark green crystals or crystalline powder having a bronze-like luster. Is odorless or practically so, and is stable in air. Its solutions in water and in alcohol are deep blue in color.

Phenyl salicylate—White crystals with a melting point of 40–43 °C.

Benzoic Acid USP—White crystals, scales, or needles. Has a slight odor, usually suggesting benzaldehyde or benzoin. Somewhat volatile at moderately warm temperatures. Freely volatile in steam.

NF category: Antimicrobial preservative.

Solubility:

Atropine Sulfate USP—Very soluble in water; freely soluble in alcohol and even more so in boiling alcohol; freely soluble in glycerin.

Hyoscyamine USP—Slightly soluble in water; freely soluble in alcohol, in chloroform, and in dilute acids; sparingly soluble in ether.

Methenamine USP—Freely soluble in water; soluble in alcohol and in chloroform.

Methylene Blue USP—Soluble in water and in chloroform; sparingly soluble in alcohol.

Phenyl salicylate—Very slightly soluble in water; freely soluble in alcohol.

Benzoic Acid USP—Slightly soluble in water; freely soluble in alcohol, in chloroform, and in ether.

USP requirements: Atropine Sulfate, Hyoscyamine, Methenamine, Methylene Blue, Phenyl Salicylate, and Benzoic Acid Tablets—Not in USP–NF.

ATROPINE, HYOSCYAMINE, SCOPOLAMINE, AND PHENOBARBITAL

For Atropine, Hyoscyamine, Scopolamine, and Phenobarbital—See individual listings for chemistry information.

USP requirements:

Atropine Sulfate, Hyoscyamine Sulfate (or Hyoscyamine Hydrobromide), Scopolamine Hydrobromide, and Phenobarbital Capsules—Not in USP–NF.

Atropine Sulfate, Hyoscyamine Sulfate (or Hyoscyamine Hydrobromide), Scopolamine Hydrobromide, and Phenobarbital Elixir—Not in USP–NF.

Atropine Sulfate, Hyoscyamine Sulfate (or Hyoscyamine Hydrobromide), Scopolamine Hydrobromide, and Phenobarbital Tablets—Not in USP–NF.

Atropine Sulfate, Hyoscyamine Sulfate, Scopolamine Hydrobromide, and Phenobarbital Chewable Tablets—Not in USP–NF.

Atropine Sulfate, Hyoscyamine Sulfate, Scopolamine Hydrobromide, and Phenobarbital Extended-release Tablets—Not in USP–NF.

ATROPINE AND PHENOBARBITAL

For Atropine and Phenobarbital—See individual listings for chemistry information.

USP requirements:

Atropine Sulfate and Phenobarbital Capsules—Not in USP–NF.

Atropine Sulfate and Phenobarbital Elixir—Not in USP–NF.

Atropine Sulfate and Phenobarbital Tablets—Not in USP–NF.

ATTAPULGITE

Description:

Activated Attapulgite USP—Cream-colored, micronized, non-swelling powder, free from gritty particles. The high heat treatment used in its preparation causes it to yield only moderately viscous aqueous suspensions, its dispersion consisting mainly of particle groups.

NF category: Suspending and/or viscosity-increasing agent.

Colloidal Activated Attapulgite USP—Cream-colored, micronized, non-swelling powder, free from gritty particles. Yields viscous aqueous suspensions, as a result of dispersion into its constituent ultimate particles.

NF category: Suspending and/or viscosity-increasing agent.

Solubility:

Activated Attapulgite USP—Insoluble in water.

Colloidal Activated Attapulgite USP—Insoluble in water.

USP requirements:

Activated Attapulgite USP—Preserve in well-closed containers. A highly heat-treated, processed, native magnesium aluminum silicate. Meets the requirements for Identification, Loss on drying (not more than 4.0%), Loss on ignition (between 4.0–12.0%), Volatile matter (3.0–7.5%, on the dried basis), Powder fineness, Acid-soluble matter (not more than 25%), and Organic volatile impurities, and for Microbial limit, pH, Carbonate, Arsenic and Lead, and Adsorptive capacity under Colloidal Activated Attapulgite.

Colloidal Activated Attapulgite USP—Preserve in well-closed containers. A purified native magnesium aluminum silicate. Meets the requirements for Identification, Microbial limit, pH (7.0–9.5), Loss on drying (5.0–17.0%), Loss on ignition (17.0–27.0%), Volatile matter (7.5–12.5%, on the

dried basis), Powder fineness, Acid-soluble matter (not more than 15%), Carbonate, Arsenic and Lead (not more than 2 ppm for arsenic and not more than 0.001% for lead), Adsorptive capacity, and Organic volatile impurities.

Attapulgite Oral Suspension—Not in *USP–NF*.

Attapulgite Tablets—Not in *USP–NF*.

Attapulgite Chewable Tablets—Not in *USP–NF*.

AURANOFIN

Chemical name: Gold, (2,3,4,6-tetra-*O*-acetyl-1-thio-beta-D-glu-copyranosato-*S*)(triethylphosphine)-.

Molecular formula: $C_{20}H_{34}AuO_9PS$.

Molecular weight: 678.48.

Description: White, odorless, crystalline powder.

Solubility: Very slightly soluble in water; soluble in alcohol.

USP requirements: Auranofin Capsules—Not in *USP–NF*.

AUROTHIOGLUCOSE

Chemical name: Gold, (1-thio-D-glucopyranosato)-.

Molecular formula: $C_6H_{11}AuO_5S$.

Molecular weight: 392.18.

Description: Aurothioglucose USP—Yellow, odorless or practically odorless powder. Is stable in air. An aqueous solution is unstable on long standing. The pH of its 1 in 100 solution is about 6.3.

Solubility: Aurothioglucose USP—Freely soluble in water; practically insoluble in acetone, in alcohol, in chloroform, and in ether.

USP requirements:

Aurothioglucose USP—Preserve in tight, light-resistant containers. Contains not less than 95.0% and not more than 105.0% of aurothioglucose, calculated on the dried basis. It is stabilized by the addition of a small amount of Sodium Acetate. Meets the requirements for Identification, Specific rotation (+65° to +75°), and Loss on drying (not more than 1.0%).

Aurothioglucose Injectable Suspension USP—Preserve in single-dose or in multiple-dose containers, preferably of Type I glass. Protect from light. A sterile suspension of Aurothioglucose in a suitable vegetable oil. Contains the labeled amount, within ±10%. It may contain suitable thickening agents. Meets the requirements for Identification and for Injections.

AVOBENZONE

Chemical name: 1,3-Propanedione, 1-[4-(1,1-dimethylethyl)phe-nyl]-3-(4-methoxyphenyl)-.

Molecular formula: $C_{20}H_{22}O_3$.

Molecular weight: 310.40.

USP requirements: Avobenzone USP—Preserve in tight, light-resistant containers. Contains not less than 95.0% and not more than 105.0% of avobenzone, calculated on the dried basis. Meets the requirements for Identification, Melting range

(81°–86°), Loss on drying (not more than 0.5%), and Chromatographic purity (not more than 3.0% of any individual impurity, and the sum of all the impurities not more than 4.5%).

AVOBENZONE, OCTOCRYLENE, OCTYL SALICYLATE, AND OXYBENZONE

Chemical name:

Avobenzone—1,3-Propanedione, 1-[4-(1,1-dimethylethyl)-phenyl]-3-(4-methoxyphenyl)-.

Octocrylene—2-Propenoic acid, 2-cyano-3,3-diphenyl-, 2-ethylhexyl ester.

Oxybenzone—Methanone, (2-hydroxy-4-methoxyphenyl)-phenyl-.

Molecular formula:

Avobenzone—$C_{20}H_{22}O_3$.

Octocrylene—$C_{24}H_{27}NO_2$.

Oxybenzone—$C_{14}H_{12}O_3$.

Molecular weight:

Avobenzone—310.39.

Octocrylene—361.48.

Oxybenzone—228.24.

Description: Oxybenzone USP—Pale yellow powder.

Solubility: Oxybenzone USP—Practically insoluble in water; freely soluble in alcohol and in toluene.

USP requirements: Avobenzone, Octocrylene, Octyl Salicylate, and Oxybenzone Lotion—Not in *USP–NF*.

AVOBENZONE AND OCTYL METHOXYCINNAMATE

For *Avobenzone* and *Octyl Methoxycinnamate*—See individual listings for chemistry information.

USP requirements: Avobenzone and Octyl Methoxycinnamate Lotion—Not in *USP–NF*.

AVOBENZONE, OCTYL METHOXYCINNAMATE, OCTYL SALICYLATE, AND OXYBENZONE

For *Avobenzone, Octyl Methoxycinnamate, Octyl Salicylate,* and *Oxybenzone*—See individual listings for chemistry information.

USP requirements:

Avobenzone, Octyl Methoxycinnamate, Octyl Salicylate, and Oxybenzone Cream—Not in *USP–NF*.

Avobenzone, Octyl Methoxycinnamate, Octyl Salicylate, and Oxybenzone Gel—Not in *USP–NF*.

AVOBENZONE, OCTYL METHOXYCINNAMATE, AND OXYBENZONE

For *Avobenzone, Octyl Methoxycinnamate,* and *Oxybenzone*—See individual listings for chemistry information.

USP requirements:

Avobenzone, Octyl Methoxycinnamate, and Oxybenzone Lotion—Not in *USP–NF*.

Avobenzone, Octyl Methoxycinnamate, and Oxybenzone Spray—Not in *USP–NF*.

AZAPERONE

Chemical name: 1-Butanone, 1-(4-fluorophenyl)-4-[4-(2-pyridinyl)-1-piperazinyl]-.

Molecular formula: $C_{19}H_{22}FN_3O$.

Molecular weight: 327.40.

Description: White to yellowish-white microcrystalline powder. Melting point 90–95 °C.

Solubility: Practically insoluble in water; soluble 1 in 29 of alcohol, 1 in 4 of chloroform, and 1 in 31 of ether.

USP requirements:
Azaperone USP—Preserve in well-closed containers, protected from light. Label it to indicate that it is for veterinary use only. Contains not less than 98.0% and not more than 102.0% of azaperone, calculated on the dried basis. Meets the requirements for Identification, Melting range (92–95 °C), Loss on drying (not more than 0.5%), Residue on ignition (not more than 0.1%), and Chromatographic purity.
Azaperone Injection USP—Preserve in single-dose or in multiple-dose containers, preferably of Type I glass, protected from light. A sterile solution of Azaperone in Water for Injection, prepared with the aid of Tartaric Acid. Label it to indicate that it is for veterinary use only. Contains the labeled amount, within ±10%. Meets the requirements for Identification, and pH (4.0–5.6), and for Injections.

AZATADINE

Chemical group: Piperidine derivative.

Chemical name: Azatadine maleate—5H-Benzo[5,6]cyclohepta[1,2-b]pyridine, 6,11-dihydro-11-(1-methyl-4-piperidinylidene)-, (Z)-2-butenedioate (l:2).

Molecular formula: Azatadine maleate—$C_{20}H_{22}N_2 \cdot 2C_4H_4O_4$.

Molecular weight: Azatadine maleate—522.55.

Description: Azatadine Maleate USP—White to light cream-colored, odorless powder. Melts at about 153 °C.

pKa: Azatadine maleate—8.4.

Solubility: Azatadine Maleate USP—Freely soluble in water, in alcohol, in chloroform, and in methanol; practically insoluble in ether.

USP requirements:
Azatadine Maleate USP—Preserve in well-closed containers. Contains not less than 98.0% and not more than 102.0% of azatadine maleate, calculated on the dried basis. Meets the requirements for Identification, Loss on drying (not more than 1.0%), Residue on ignition (not more than 0.1%), and Chromatographic purity.
Azatadine Maleate Tablets USP—Preserve in well-closed containers. Contain the labeled amount, within ±10%. Meet the requirements for Identification, Dissolution (80% in 30 minutes in 0.01 N hydrochloric acid in Apparatus 2 at 50 rpm), and Uniformity of dosage units.

AZATADINE AND PSEUDOEPHEDRINE

For *Azatadine* and *Pseudoephedrine*—See individual listings for chemistry information.

USP requirements: Azatadine Maleate and Pseudoephedrine Sulfate Extended-release Tablets—Not in *USP–NF*.

AZATHIOPRINE

Chemical name: 1H-Purine, 6-[(1-methyl-4-nitro-1H-imidazol-5-yl)thio]-.

Molecular formula: $C_9H_7N_7O_2S$.

Molecular weight: 277.26.

Description:
Azathioprine USP—Pale yellow, odorless powder.
Azathioprine Sodium for Injection USP—Bright yellow, hygroscopic, amorphous mass or cake.

Solubility: Azathioprine USP—Insoluble in water; soluble in dilute solutions of alkali hydroxides; sparingly soluble in dilute mineral acids; very slightly soluble in alcohol and in chloroform.

USP requirements:
Azathioprine USP—Preserve in tight, light-resistant containers. Contains not less than 98.0% and not more than 101.5% of azathioprine, calculated on the dried basis. Meets the requirements for Identification, Acidity or alkalinity, Loss on drying (not more than 1.0%), Residue on ignition (not more than 0.1%), Limit of mercaptopurine, and Organic volatile impurities.
Azathioprine Tablets USP—Protect from light. Contain the labeled amount, within ±7%. Meet the requirements for Identification, Dissolution (75% in 30 minutes in water in Apparatus 2 at 50 rpm), and Uniformity of dosage units.
Azathioprine Sodium for Injection USP—Preserve in Containers for Sterile Solids, at controlled room temperature. A sterile solid prepared by the freeze-drying of an aqueous solution of Azathioprine and Sodium Hydroxide. Contains the labeled amount, within ±7%. Meets the requirements for Completeness of solution, Identification, Bacterial endotoxins, pH (9.8–11.0), Water (not more than 7.0%), and Limit of mercaptopurine, and for Injections and Uniformity of dosage units.

AZELAIC ACID

Chemical group: Naturally occurring saturated dicarboxylic acid.

Chemical name: 1,7-heptanedicarboxylic acid.

Molecular formula: $C_9H_{16}O_4$.

Molecular weight: 188.22.

Description: Melting point 106.5 °C.

pKa: 4.53 at 25 °C and 5.33.

Solubility: One liter of water dissolves 1 gram at 1 °C, 2.4 grams at 20 °C, 8.2 grams at 50 °C, and 22 grams at 65 °C; freely soluble in boiling water and in alcohol; 1000 grams of ether dissolves 18.8 grams at 11 °C and 26.8 grams at 15 °C.

USP requirements: Azelaic Acid Cream—Not in *USP–NF*.

AZELASTINE

Chemical name: Azelastine hydrochloride—1(2*H*)-Phthalazinone, 4-[(4-chlorophenyl)methyl]-2-(hexahydro-1-methyl-1*H*-azepin-4-yl)-, monohydrochloride.

Molecular formula: Azelastine hydrochloride—$C_{22}H_{24}ClN_3O \cdot$ HCl.

Molecular weight: Azelastine hydrochloride—418.36.

Description: Azelastine hydrochloride—White, crystalline powder with a bitter taste; almost odorless.

Solubility: Azelastine hydrochloride—Sparingly soluble in ethanol, in octanol, and in glycerine.

USP requirements:
Azelastine Hydrochloride Nasal Solution—Not in *USP–NF*.
Azelastine Hydrochloride Ophthalmic Solution—Not in *USP–NF*.

AZITHROMYCIN

Chemical name: 1-Oxa-6-azacyclopentadecan-15-one, 13-[(2,6-dideoxy-3-*C*-methyl-3-*O*-methyl-alpha-L-*ribo*-hexopyranosyl)oxy]-2-ethyl-3,4,10-trihydroxy-3,5,6,8,10,12,14-heptamethyl-11-[[3,4,6-trideoxy-3-(dimethylamino)-beta-D*xylo*-hexopyranosyl]oxy]-, dihydrate, [2*R*-(2*R**,3*S**,4*R**,5*R**,8*R**,-10*R**,11*R**,12*S**,13*S**,14*R**)]-.

Molecular formula: $C_{38}H_{72}N_2O_{12}$ (anhydrous); $C_{38}H_{72}N_2O_{12} \cdot 2H_2O$ (dihydrate).

Molecular weight: 748.98 (anhydrous); 785.02 (dihydrate).

Description: White crystalline powder (for the dihydrate).

USP requirements:
Azithromycin USP—Preserve in tight containers. Contains the equivalent of not less than 945 mcg and not more than 1030 mcg of azithromycin per mg, calculated on the anhydrous basis. Meets the requirements for Identification, Specific rotation (−45° to −49°), Crystallinity, pH (9.0–11.0), Water (4.0–5.0%), Residue on ignition (not more than 0.3%), and Heavy metals (not more than 0.0025%).
Azithromycin Capsules USP—Preserve in well-closed containers. Where packaged in unit-of-use containers, each container contains six 250-mg Capsules, and the label indicates the intended sequential day of use for each Capsule. Contain the equivalent of the labeled amount of azithromycin, within ±10%. Meet the requirements for Identification, Dissolution (75% in 45 minutes in sodium phosphate buffer [pH 6.0] in Apparatus 2 at 100 rpm), Uniformity of dosage units, and Water (not more than 5.0%).
Azithromycin for Injection—Not in *USP–NF*.
Azithromycin for Oral Suspension USP—Preserve in tight containers. A dry mixture of Azithromycin and one or more buffers, sweeteners, diluents, anticaking agents, and flavors. Contains the labeled amount, within ±10%. Meets the requirements for Identification, Uniformity of dosage units (for solid packaged in single-unit containers), Deliverable volume, pH (9.0–11.0 [for solid packaged in single-unit containers], 8.5–11.0 [for solid packaged in multiple-unit containers], in the suspension constituted as directed in the labeling), and Water (not more than 1.5%).
Azithromycin Tablets—Not in *USP–NF*.

AZLOCILLIN

Chemical name:
Azlocillin—4-Thia-1-azabicyclo[3.2.0]heptane-2-carboxylic acid, 3,3-dimethyl-7-oxo-6-[[[[(2-oxo-1-imidazolidinyl)carbonyl]amino]phenylacetyl]amino]-, [2*S*-[2 alpha,5 alpha,6 beta(*S**)]]-.
Azlocillin sodium—4-Thia-1-azabicyclo[3.2.0]heptane-2-carboxylic acid, 3,3-dimethyl-7-oxo-6-[[[[(2-oxo-1-imidazolidinyl)carbonyl]amino]phenylacetyl]amino]-, monosodium salt, [2*S*-[2 alpha,5 alpha,6 beta(*S**)]]-.

Molecular formula:
Azlocillin—$C_{20}H_{23}N_5O_6S$.
Azlocillin sodium—$C_{20}H_{22}N_5NaO_6S$.

Molecular weight:
Azlocillin—461.50.
Azlocillin sodium—483.48.

Description: Sterile Azlocillin Sodium USP—White to pale yellow powder.

Solubility: Sterile Azlocillin Sodium USP—Freely soluble in water; soluble in methanol and in dimethylformamide; slightly soluble in alcohol and in isopropyl alcohol.

USP requirements:
Azlocillin for Injection USP—Preserve in Containers for Sterile Solids. Contains an amount of Azlocillin Sodium equivalent to the labeled amount of azlocillin, within −10% to +15%. Meets the requirements for Constituted solution, Bacterial endotoxins, Sterility, and Particulate matter, for Identification, Specific rotation, pH, and Water under Azlocillin Sodium, for Uniformity of dosage units, and for Labeling under Injections.
Azlocillin Sodium USP—Preserve in tight containers. Where it is intended for use in preparing injectable dosage forms, the label states that it is sterile or must be subjected to further processing during the preparation of injectable dosage forms. Has a potency equivalent to not less than 859 mcg and not more than 1000 mcg of azlocillin per mg, calculated on the anhydrous basis. Meets the requirements for Identification, Specific rotation (+170° to +200°), pH (6.0–8.0, in a solution containing the equivalent of 100 mg of azlocillin per mL), and Water (not more than 2.5%), for Sterility and Bacterial endotoxins under Azlocillin for Injection (where the label states that Azlocillin Sodium is sterile), and for Bacterial endotoxins under Azlocillin for Injection (where the label states that Azlocillin Sodium must be subjected to further processing during the preparation of injectable dosage forms).

AZTREONAM

Chemical group: Monobactams (*mono*cyclic *bac*terially produced beta-lac*tams*).

Chemical name: Propanoic acid, 2-[[[1-(2-amino-4-thiazolyl)-2-[(2-methyl-4-oxo-1-sulfo-3-azetidinyl)amino]-2-oxoethylidene]amino]oxy]-2-methyl-, [2*S*-[2 alpha,3 beta(*Z*)]]-.

Molecular formula: $C_{13}H_{17}N_5O_8S_2$.

Molecular weight: 435.44.

Description: Aztreonam USP—White, odorless, crystalline powder.

Solubility: Aztreonam USP—Soluble in dimethylformamide and in dimethyl sulfoxide; slightly soluble in methanol; very slightly soluble in dehydrated alcohol; practically insoluble in ethyl acetate, in chloroform, and in toluene.

Other characteristics: pH of aqueous solutions—4.5 to 7.5.

USP requirements:

Aztreonam USP—Preserve in tight containers. Where it is intended for use in preparing injectable dosage forms, the label states that it is sterile or must be subjected to further processing during the preparation of injectable dosage forms. Contains not less than 90.0% and not more than 105.0% of aztreonam. Meets the requirements for Identification, Bacterial endotoxins, Sterility, Water (not more than 2.0%), Residue on ignition (not more than 0.1%), and Heavy metals (not more than 0.003%).

Aztreonam Injection USP—Preserve in Containers for Sterile Solids. Maintain in the frozen state. A sterile solution of Aztreonam and Arginine and a suitable osmolality adjusting substance in Water for Injection. It meets the requirements for Labeling under Injections. The label states that it is to be thawed just prior to use, describes conditions for proper storage of the resultant solution, and directs that the solution is not to be refrozen. Contains the labeled amount, within −10% to +20%. Meets the requirements for Identification, Pyrogen, Sterility, pH (4.5–7.5), and Particulate matter.

Aztreonam for Injection USP—Preserve in Containers for Sterile Solids. A dry mixture of sterile Aztreonam and Arginine. Contains not less than 90.0% and not more than 105.0% of aztreonam, calculated on the anhydrous and arginine-free basis. Each container contains the labeled amount, within −10% to +20%. Meets the requirements for Constituted solution, Identification, Bacterial endotoxins, Sterility, pH (4.5–7.5, in a solution containing 100 mg of aztreonam per mL), Water (not more than 2.0%), Particulate matter, and Content of arginine, and for Uniformity of dosage units and Labeling under Injections.

BACAMPICILLIN

Chemical group: A semi-synthetic penicillin, an analogue of ampicillin.

Chemical name: Bacampicillin hydrochloride—4-Thia-1-azabicyclo[3.2.0]heptane-2-carboxylic acid, 6-[(aminophenylacetyl)amino]-3,3-dimethyl-7-oxo-, 1-[(ethoxycarbonyl)oxy]ethyl ester, monohydrochloride, [2S-[2 alpha,5 alpha,6 beta(S^*)]]-.

Molecular formula: Bacampicillin hydrochloride—$C_{21}H_{27}N_3O_7S$ · HCl.

Molecular weight: Bacampicillin hydrochloride—501.98.

Description: Bacampicillin Hydrochloride USP—White or practically white powder. Is hygroscopic.

Solubility: Bacampicillin Hydrochloride USP—Soluble in methylene chloride and in water; freely soluble in alcohol and in chloroform; very slightly soluble in ether.

USP requirements:

Bacampicillin Hydrochloride USP—Preserve in tight containers. Has a potency of not less than 623 mcg and not more than 727 mcg of ampicillin per mg. Meets the requirements for Identification, pH (3.0–4.5, in a solution containing 20 mg per mL), Water (not more than 1.0%), and Dimethylaniline.

Bacampicillin Hydrochloride for Oral Suspension USP—Preserve in tight containers. Contains an amount of bacampicillin hydrochloride equivalent to the labeled amount of ampicillin, when constituted as directed, within −10% to +25%. Contains one or more suitable buffers, colors, flavors, suspending agents, and sweetening ingredients. Meets the requirements for Identification, Uniformity of dosage units (single-unit containers), Deliverable volume (multiple-unit containers), pH (6.5–8.0, in the suspension constituted as directed in the labeling), and Loss on drying (not more than 2.0%).

Bacampicillin Hydrochloride Tablets USP—Preserve in tight containers. Contain an amount of bacampicillin hydrochloride equivalent to the labeled amount of ampicillin, within −10% to +25%. Meet the requirements for Identification, Dissolution (85% in 30 minutes in water in Apparatus 2 at 75 rpm), Uniformity of dosage units, and Water (not more than 2.5%).

BACILLUS CALMETTE-GUERIN (BCG) LIVE

Source: Obtained from a live culture of the bacillus Calmette-Guérin strain of *Mycobacterium tuberculosis* var. *bovis*. Commercially available strains (which are substrains of the Pasteur Institute strain) include the Armand-Frappier, Connaught, Glaxo, and Tice substrains.

Description: BCG Vaccine USP—White to creamy white, dried mass, having the characteristic texture of material dried in the frozen state.

USP requirements:

BCG Live (Connaught Strain)—Not in *USP–NF*.
BCG Live (Montreal Strain)—Not in *USP–NF*.
BCG Vaccine (Connaught Strain)—Not in *USP–NF*.
BCG Vaccine (Montreal Strain)—Not in *USP–NF*.
BCG Vaccine USP (Tice Strain)—Preserve in hermetic containers, preferably of Type I glass, at a temperature between 2 and 8 °C. A dried, living culture of the bacillus Calmette-Guérin strain of *Mycobacterium tuberculosis* var. *bovis,* grown in a suitable medium from a seed strain of known history that has been maintained to preserve its capacity for conferring immunity. Contains an amount of viable bacteria such that inoculation, in the recommended dose, of tuberculin-negative persons results in an acceptable tuberculin conversion rate. It is free from other organisms, and contains a suitable stabilizer. Contains no antimicrobial agent. Meets the requirement for expiration date (not later than 6 months after date of issue, or not later than 1 year after date of issue if stored at a temperature below 5 °C). Conforms to the regulations of the U.S. Food and Drug Administration concerning biologics.

Note: Use the Vaccine immediately after its constitution, and discard any unused portion after 2 hours.

BACITRACIN

Chemical name:

Bacitracin—Bacitracin.
Bacitracin zinc—Bacitracins, zinc complex.

Description:

Bacitracin USP—White to pale buff powder, odorless or having a slight odor. Is hygroscopic. Its solutions deteriorate rapidly at room temperature. Is precipitated from its solutions and is inactivated by salts of many of the heavy metals.
Bacitracin Zinc USP—White to pale tan powder, odorless or having a slight odor. Is hygroscopic.

Solubility:

Bacitracin USP—Freely soluble in water; soluble in alcohol, in methanol, and in glacial acetic acid, the solution in the organic solvents usually showing some insoluble residue; insoluble in acetone, in chloroform, and in ether.
Bacitracin Zinc USP—Sparingly soluble in water.

USP requirements:

Bacitracin USP—Preserve in tight containers, and store in a cool place. A polypeptide produced by the growth of an organism of the *licheniformis* group of *Bacillus subtilis* (Fam. Bacillaceae). Where it is packaged for prescription compounding, label it to indicate that it is not sterile and that the potency cannot be assured for longer than 60 days after opening, and to state the number of Bacitracin Units per milligram. Where it is intended for use in preparing injectable or other sterile dosage forms, the label states that it is sterile or must be subjected to further processing during the preparation of injectable or other sterile dosage forms. Has a potency of not less than 40 Bacitracin Units per mg. Meets the requirements for Thin-layer chromatographic identification test, pH (5.5–7.5, in a solution containing 10,000 Bacitracin Units per mL), and Loss on drying (not more than 5.0%), and for Sterility tests (where the label states that Bacitracin is sterile), for Bacterial endotoxins under Bacitracin for Injection (where intended for injectable dosage forms), and for Bacterial endotoxins under Bacitracin for Injection (where the label states that Bacitracin must be subjected to further processing during the preparation of injectable dosage forms.

Bacitracin for Injection USP—Preserve in Containers for Sterile Solids, and store in a cool place. Has a potency of not less than 50 Bacitracin Units per mg. Contains the labeled amount, within –10% to +15%. Meets the requirements for Constituted solution, Bacterial endotoxins (not more than 0.01 USP Endotoxin Unit per Bacitracin Unit), Sterility, Residue on ignition (not more than 3.0%), and Heavy metals (not more than 0.003%), Thin-layer chromatographic identification test, and for pH, and Loss on drying under Bacitracin, and for Injections and Uniformity of dosage units.

Bacitracin Ointment USP—Preserve in well-closed containers containing not more than 60 grams, unless labeled solely for hospital use, preferably at controlled room temperature. It is Bacitracin in an anhydrous ointment base. Contains the labeled amount, within –10% to +40%. Meets the requirements for Thin-layer chromatographic identification test, Minimum fill, and Water (not more than 0.5%).

Bacitracin Ophthalmic Ointment USP—Preserve in collapsible ophthalmic ointment tubes. A sterile preparation of Bacitracin in an anhydrous ointment base. Contains the labeled amount, within –10% to +40%. Meets the requirements for Thin-layer chromatographic identification test, Sterility, Water (not more than 0.5%), and Metal particles.

Soluble Bacitracin Methylene Disalicylate USP—Preserve in well-closed containers. A mixture of bacitracin methylene disalicylate and Sodium Bicarbonate. Label it to indicate that it is for veterinary use only. Has a potency of not less than 8 Bacitracin Units per mg, calculated on the dried basis. Meets the requirements for pH (8.0–9.5, in a solution containing 25 mg of specimen per mL) and Loss on drying (not more than 8.5%).

Bacitracin Methylene Disalicylate Soluble Powder USP—Preserve in tight containers. Label it to indicate that it is for veterinary use only. Label it to state the content of bacitracin in terms of grams per pound, each gram of bacitracin being equivalent to 42,000 Bacitracin Units. Contains an amount of bacitracin methylene disalicylate equivalent to the labeled amount of Bacitracin, within –10% to +20%. Meets the requirements for pH (8.0–9.5, in a solution containing 50 mg of specimen per mL) and Loss on drying (not more than 8.5%).

Bacitracin Zinc USP—Preserve in tight containers, and store in a cool place. The zinc salt of a kind of bacitracin or a mixture of two or more such salts. Label it to indicate that it is to be used in the manufacture of nonparenteral drugs only. Where it is packaged for prescription compounding, label it to indicate that it is not sterile and that the potency cannot be assured for longer than 60 days after opening, and to state the number of Bacitracin Units per mg. Where it is intended for use in preparing sterile dosage forms, the label states that it is sterile or must be subjected to further processing during the preparation of sterile dosage form. Has a potency of not less than 40 Bacitracin Units per mg. Contains not less than 2.0% and not more than 10.0% of zinc, calculated on the dried basis. Meets the requirements for Thin-layer chromatographic identification test, Sterility (where the label states that it is sterile), pH (6.0–7.5, in a [saturated] solution containing approximately 100 mg per mL), Loss on drying (not more than 5.0%), and Zinc content.

Bacitracin Zinc Ointment USP—Preserve in well-closed containers containing not more than 60 grams, unless labeled solely for hospital use, preferably at controlled room temperature. It is Bacitracin Zinc in an anhydrous ointment base. Contains an amount of bacitracin zinc equivalent to the labeled amount of bacitracin, within –10% to +40%. Meets the requirements for Thin-layer chromatographic identification test, Minimum fill, and Water (not more than 0.5%).

Bacitracin Zinc Soluble Powder USP—Preserve in tight containers. A mixture of bacitracin zinc and zinc proteinates. Label it to indicate that it is for veterinary use only. Label it to state the content of bacitracin in terms of grams per pound, each gram of bacitracin being equivalent to 42,000 Bacitracin Units. Contains an amount of bacitracin zinc equivalent to the labeled amount of bacitracin, within –10% to +20%. Meets the requirements for Loss on drying (not more than 5.0%) and Zinc content (not more than 2.0 grams of Zinc for each 42,000 Bacitracin Units).

BACITRACIN AND POLYMYXIN B

For *Bacitracin* and *Polymyxin B*—See individual listings for chemistry information.

USP requirements:

Bacitracin and Polymyxin B Sulfate Topical Aerosol USP—Preserve in pressurized containers, and avoid exposure to excessive heat. A suspension of Bacitracin and Polymyxin B Sulfate in a suitable vehicle, packaged in a pressurized container with a suitable inert propellant. Contains the labeled amount of bacitracin, within –10% to +30%, and an amount of polymyxin B sulfate equivalent to the labeled amount of polymyxin B, within –10% to +30%. May contain a suitable local anesthetic. Meets the requirements for Thin-layer chromatographic identification test and Water (not more than 0.5%), and for Pressure test, Minimum fill, and Leakage test under Aerosols, Metered-dose inhalers, and Dry powder inhalers.

Bacitracin Zinc and Polymyxin B Sulfate Ointment USP—Preserve in well-closed, light-resistant containers. Contains amounts of bacitracin zinc and polymyxin B sulfate equivalent to the labeled amounts of bacitracin and polymyxin B, within –10% to +30%. May contain a suitable local anesthetic. Meets the requirements for Thin-layer chromatographic identification test, Minimum fill, and Water (not more than 0.5%).

Bacitracin Zinc and Polymyxin B Sulfate Ophthalmic Ointment USP—Preserve in collapsible ophthalmic ointment tubes. Contains amounts of bacitracin zinc and polymyxin B sulfate equivalent to the labeled amounts of bacitracin and polymyxin B, within –10% to +30%. Meets the requirements for Thin-layer chromatographic identification test, Sterility, Minimum fill, Water (not more than 0.5%), and Metal particles.

BACLOFEN

Chemical name: Butanoic acid, 4-amino-3-(4-chlorophenyl)-.

Molecular formula: $C_{10}H_{12}ClNO_2$.

Molecular weight: 213.66.

Description: Baclofen USP—White to off-white, crystalline powder. Is odorless or practically so.

Solubility: Baclofen USP—Slightly soluble in water; very slightly soluble in methanol; insoluble in chloroform.

USP requirements:
  Baclofen USP—Preserve in tight containers. Contains not less than 99.0% and not more than 101.0% of baclofen, calculated on the anhydrous basis. Meets the requirements for Identification, Water (not more than 3.0%), Residue on ignition (not more than 0.3%), Heavy metals (not more than 0.001%), Related compounds, and Organic volatile impurities.
  Baclofen Injection—Not in *USP–NF*.
  Baclofen Tablets USP—Preserve in well-closed containers. Contain the labeled amount, within ±10%. Meet the requirements for Identification, Dissolution (75% in 30 minutes in 0.01 N hydrochloric acid in Apparatus 2 at 50 rpm), Limit of 4-(4-Chlorophenyl)-2-pyrrolidinone (not more than 4.0%), and Uniformity of dosage units.

BALSALAZIDE

Chemical name: Balsalazide disodium—Benzoic acid, 5-[[4-[[C2-carboxyethyl)amino]carbonyl]phenyl]azo]-2-hydroxy, disodium salt, dihydrate.

Molecular formula: Balsalazide disodium—$C_{17}H_{13}N_3Na_2O_6\cdot H_2O$.

Molecular weight: Balsalazide disodium—437.31.

Description: Balsalazide disodium—Stable, odorless orange to yellow microcrystalline powder.

Solubiliuty: Balsalazide disodium—Freely soluble in water and in isotonic saline; sparaingly soluble in methanol and in ethanol; practically insoluble in all other organic solvents.

USP requirements: Balsalazide Disodium Capsules—Not in *USP–NF*.

ADHESIVE BANDAGE

Description: Adhesive Bandage USP—The compress of Adhesive Bandage is substantially free from loose threads or ravelings. The adhesive strip may be perforated, and the back may be coated with a water-repellent film.

USP requirements: Adhesive Bandage USP—Package Adhesive Bandage that does not exceed 15 cm (6 inches) in width individually in such manner that sterility is maintained until the individual package is opened. Package individual packages in a second protective container. Adhesive Bandage consists of a compress of four layers of Type I Absorbent Gauze, or other suitable material, affixed to a film or fabric coated with a pressure-sensitive adhesive substance. It is sterile. The adhesive surface is protected by a suitable removable covering. The label of the second protective container bears a statement that the contents may not be sterile if the individual package has been damaged or previously opened, and it bears the names of any added antimicrobial agents. Each individual package is labeled to indicate the dimensions of the compress and the name of the manufacturer, packer, or distributor, and each protective container indicates also the address of the manufacturer, packer, or distributor. Meets the requirement for Sterility.

GAUZE BANDAGE

Description: Gauze Bandage USP—One continuous piece, tightly rolled, in various widths and lengths and substantially free from loose threads and ravelings.

USP requirements: Gauze Bandage USP—Gauze Bandage that has been rendered sterile is so packaged that the sterility of the contents of the package is maintained until the package is opened for use. It is Type I Absorbent Gauze. Its length is not less than 98.0% of that declared on the label, and its average width is not more than 1.6 mm less than the declared width. Contains no dye or other additives. The width and length of the Bandage and the number of pieces contained, and the name of the manufacturer, packer, or distributor, are stated on the package. The designation "non-sterilized" or "not sterilized" appears prominently on the package unless the Gauze Bandage has been rendered sterile, in which case it may be labeled to indicate that it is sterile and that the contents may not be sterile if the package bears evidence of damage or if the package has been previously opened.
  Note: Before determining the thread count, dimensions, and weight, hold the Bandage, unrolled for not less than 4 hours in a standard atmosphere of 65 ±2% relative humidity at 21 ±1.1 °C (70 ±2 °F).

Meets the requirements for Thread count (not more than 3 threads per inch allowed in either warp or filling, provided that the combined variations do not exceed 5 threads per square inch), Width (average of 5 measurements not more than 1.6 mm [1/16 inch] less than labeled width), Length (not less than 98.0% of labeled length), Weight (calculated weight in grams per 0.894 square meter is not less than 39.2 grams), Absorbency (complete submersion of entire bandage roll takes place in not more than 30 seconds), and Sterility, and for Ignited residue, Acid or alkali, and Dextrin or starch, in water extract, Residue on ignition, Fatty matter, and Alcohol-soluble dyes under Absorbent Gauze.

BARIUM HYDROXIDE LIME

Description: Barium Hydroxide Lime USP—White or grayish white granules. May have a color if an indicator has been added.

NF category: Sorbent, carbon dioxide.

USP requirements: Barium Hydroxide Lime USP—Preserve in tight containers. A mixture of barium hydroxide octahydrate and Calcium Hydroxide. May contain also Potassium Hydroxide and may contain an indicator that is inert toward anesthetic gases such as Ether, Cyclopropane, and Nitrous Oxide, and that changes color when the Barium Hydroxide Lime no longer can absorb carbon dioxide. If an indicator has been added, the name and color change of such indicator are stated on the container label. The container label indicates also the mesh size in terms of standard mesh sieve sizes. Meets the requirements for Identification, Size of granules, Loss on drying (11.0–16.0%), Hardness, and Carbon dioxide absorbency (not less than 19.0%).

Caution: Since Barium Hydroxide Lime contains a soluble form of barium, it is toxic if swallowed.

BARIUM SULFATE

Chemical name: Sulfuric acid, barium salt (1:1).

Molecular formula: $BaSO_4$.

Molecular weight: 233.39.

Description:
Barium Sulfate USP—Fine, white, odorless, bulky powder, free from grittiness.
Barium Sulfate for Suspension USP—White or colored, bulky or granular powder.

Solubility: Barium Sulfate USP—Practically insoluble in water, in organic solvents, and in solutions of acids and of alkalies.

USP requirements:
Barium Sulfate USP—Preserve in well-closed containers. Contains not less than 97.5% and not more than 100.5% of barium sulfate. Meets the requirements for Identification, pH (3.5–10.0, in a 10% [w/w] aqueous suspension), Limit of sulfide (not more than 0.5 mcg per gram), Limit of acid-soluble substances (not more than 0.3%), Limit of soluble barium salts (not more than 0.001%), and Heavy metals (not more than 0.001%).
Barium Sulfate Paste USP—Preserve in tight containers, protected from freezing and from excessive heat. A semisolid formulation of finely divided particles of Barium Sulfate in a suitable base. Contains a labeled amount of barium sulfate, within ±10%. May contain one or more suitable colors, flavors, suspending or dispersing agents, and preservatives. Meets the requirements for Identification, Microbial limits, and pH (3.0–10.0).
Barium Sulfate Suspension USP—Preserve in tight containers, and avoid freezing. An aqueous suspension of Barium Sulfate. Contains suitable dispersing and/or suspending agents so that when mixed as directed in the labeling, it yields a uniformly dispersed suspension. Contains the labeled amount, within ±10%. May contain one or more suitable colors, flavors, fluidizing agents, and preservatives. Meets the requirements for Identification, Microbial limits, and pH (3.5–10.0).
Barium Sulfate Oral Suspension—Not in *USP–NF*.
Barium Sulfate for Suspension USP—Preserve in well-closed containers. A dry mixture of Barium Sulfate and one or more suitable dispersing and/or suspending agents. Contains the labeled amount, within ±10%. Meets the requirements for Identification, pH (3.5–10.0, in a 60% [w/w] aqueous suspension or constituted for its intended use as directed in the labeling), and Loss on drying (not more than 1.0%).
Barium Sulfate Rectal Suspension—Not in *USP–NF*.
Barium Sulfate for Rectal Suspension—Not in *USP–NF*.
Barium Sulfate Tablets USP—Preserve in well-closed containers. Tablets are flat-sided disks between 11.5 mm and 13.5 mm in diameter. Contain the labeled amount, within ±10%. Meet the requirements for Identification, Disintegration (not less than 10 minutes and not more than 30 minutes), and Uniformity of dosage units.

BASILIXIMAB

Source: A monoclonal antibody composed of human and murine antibodies, produced through recombinant DNA technology.

Molecular weight: Approximately 144,000 daltons.

Solubility: Water soluble.

USP requirements: Basiliximab for Injection—Not in *USP–NF*.

BECAPLERMIN

Source: A human platelet–derived growth factor produced through recombinant DNA technology.

Molecular weight: Approximately 30,000 daltons.

USP requirements: Becaplermin Gel—Not in *USP–NF*.

BECLOMETHASONE

Chemical name:
Beclomethasone dipropionate—Pregna-1,4-diene-3,20-dione, 9-chloro-11-hydroxy-16-methyl-17,21-bis(1-oxopropoxy)-, (11 beta,16 beta)-.
Beclomethasone dipropionate, monohydrate—9-Chloro-11 beta, 17,21-trihydroxy-16 beta-methylpregna-1,4-diene-3,20-dione 17,21-dipropionate, monohydrate.

Molecular formula:
Beclomethasone dipropionate—$C_{28}H_{37}ClO_7$.
Beclomethasone dipropionate monohydrate—$C_{28}H_{37}ClO_7 \cdot H_2O$.

Molecular weight:
Beclomethasone dipropionate—521.04.
Beclomethasone dipropionate monohydrate—539.06.

Description:
Beclomethasone Dipropionate USP—White to cream white, odorless powder.
Beclomethasone dipropionate monohydrate—White to creamy white, odorless powder.

Solubility:
Beclomethasone Dipropionate USP—Very slightly soluble in water; very soluble in chloroform; freely soluble in acetone and in alcohol.
Beclomethasone dipropionate monohydrate—Very slightly soluble in water; very soluble in chloroform; freely soluble in acetone and in alcohol.

USP requirements:
Beclomethasone Dipropionate USP—Preserve in well-closed containers. It is anhydrous or contains one molecule of water of hydration. Contains not less than 97.0% and not more than 103.0% of beclomethasone dipropionate, calculated on the dried basis. Meets the requirements for Identification, Specific rotation (+88° to +94°), Loss on drying (not more than 0.5% for the anhydrous and 2.8–3.8% for the monohydrate), and Residue on ignition (not more than 0.1%).
Beclomethasone Dipropionate Inhalation Aerosol—Not in *USP–NF*.
Beclomethasone Dipropionate HFA Inhalation Aerosol—Not in *USP–NF*.
Beclomethasone Dipropionate Nasal Aerosol—Not in *USP–NF*.
Beclomethasone Dipropionate Capsules for Inhalation—Not in *USP–NF*.
Beclomethasone Dipropionate Cream—Not in *USP–NF*.
Beclomethasone Dipropionate Lotion—Not in *USP–NF*.
Beclomethasone Dipropionate Ointment—Not in *USP–NF*.
Beclomethasone Dipropionate Powder for Inhalation—Not in *USP–NF*.
Beclomethasone Dipropionate Monohydrate Nasal Solution—Not in *USP–NF*.
Beclomethasone Dipropionate Monohydrate Nasal Suspension—Not in *USP–NF*.

BELLADONNA

Source: The naturally occurring belladonna alkaloids are found in various solanaceous plants. Belladonna leaf is derived from the dried leaf and flowering or fruiting top of *Atropa belladonna* Linné (Fam. Solanaceae). The active alkaloids of belladonna include *l*-hyoscyamine (which probably racemizes to atropine during extraction) and scopolamine.

Description: Belladonna Leaf USP—When moistened, its odor is slight, somewhat tobacco-like.

USP requirements:
  Belladonna Extract USP—Preserve in tight containers, at a temperature not exceeding 30 °C. Contains, in each 100 grams, not less than 1.15 grams and not more than 1.35 grams of the alkaloids of belladonna leaf. Meets the requirement for Organic volatile impurities.
  Belladonna Extract Tablets USP—Preserve in tight, light-resistant containers. Contain the labeled amount of the alkaloids of belladonna leaf, within ±10%. Meet the requirements for Identification, Disintegration (30 minutes), and Uniformity of dosage units.
  Belladonna Leaf USP—Preserve in well-closed containers and avoid long exposure to direct sunlight. Preserve powdered Belladonna Leaf in light-resistant containers. Consists of the dried leaf and flowering or fruiting top of *Atropa belladonna* Linné or of its variety *acuminata* Royle ex Lindley (Fam. Solanaceae). Yields not less than 0.35% of the alkaloids of belladonna leaf. Meets the requirements for Botanic characteristics, Acid-insoluble ash (not more than 3.0%), and Belladonna stems (proportion of belladonna stems over 10 mm in diameter not more than 3.0%).
  Belladonna Tincture USP—Preserve in tight, light-resistant containers, and avoid exposure to direct sunlight and to excessive heat. Yields, from each 100 mL, not less than 27 mg and not more than 33 mg of the alkaloids of the belladonna leaf. Meets the requirement for Alcohol content (65.0–70.0%).

BELLADONNA AND BUTABARBITAL

For *Belladonna* and *Butabarbital*—See individual listings for chemistry information.

USP requirements:
  Belladonna Extract and Butabarbital Sodium Elixir—Not in *USP–NF*.
  Belladonna Extract and Butabarbital Sodium Tablets—Not in *USP–NF*.

BELLADONNA AND PHENOBARBITAL

For *Belladonna* and *Phenobarbital*—See individual listings for chemistry information.

USP requirements: Belladonna Extract and Phenobarbital Tablets—Not in *USP–NF*.

BENAZEPRIL

Chemical name: Benazepril hydrochloride—1*H*-1-Benzazepine-1-acetic acid, 3-[[1-(ethoxycarbonyl)-3-phenylpropyl]amino]2,3,4,5-tetrahydro-2-oxo-, monohydrochloride, [*S*-(*R**,*R**)]-.

Molecular formula: Benazepril hydrochloride—$C_{24}H_{28}N_2O_5 \cdot HCl$.

Molecular weight: Benazepril hydrochloride—460.95.

Description: Benazepril hydrochloride—White to off-white crystalline powder.

Solubility: Benazepril hydrochloride—Soluble in water, in ethanol, and in methanol.

USP requirements: Benazepril Hydrochloride Tablets—Not in *USP–NF*.

BENAZEPRIL AND HYDROCHLOROTHIAZIDE

For *Benazepril* and *Hydrochlorothiazide*—See individual listings for chemistry information.

USP requirements: Benazepril Hydrochloride and Hydrochlorothiazide Tablets—Not in *USP–NF*.

BENDROFLUMETHIAZIDE

Chemical name: 2*H*-1,2,4-Benzothiadiazine-7-sulfonamide, 3,4-dihydro-3-(phenylmethyl)-6-(trifluoromethyl)-, 1,1-dioxide-.

Molecular formula: $C_{15}H_{14}F_3N_3O_4S_2$.

Molecular weight: 421.42.

Description: Bendroflumethiazide USP—White to cream-colored, finely divided, crystalline powder. Is odorless or has a slight odor. Melts at about 220 °C.

pKa: 8.5.

Solubility: Bendroflumethiazide USP—Practically insoluble in water; freely soluble in alcohol and in acetone.

USP requirements:
  Bendroflumethiazide USP—Preserve in tight containers. Contains not less than 98.0% and not more than 102.0% of bendroflumethiazide, calculated on the anhydrous basis. Meets the requirements for Identification, Water (not more than 0.5%), Residue on ignition (not more than 0.2%), Heavy metals (not more than 0.002%), Selenium (not more than 0.003%), Limit of 2,4-disulfamyl-5-trifluoromethylaniline (not more than 1.5%), and Organic volatile impurities.
  Bendroflumethiazide Tablets USP—Preserve in tight containers. Contain the labeled amount, within ±10%. Meet the requirements for Identification, Dissolution (75% in 45 minutes in 0.01 *N* hydrochloric acid in Apparatus 2 at 50 rpm), and Uniformity of dosage units.

BENOXINATE

Chemical name: Benoxinate hydrochloride—Benzoic acid, 4-amino-3-butoxy-, 2-(diethylamino)ethyl ester, monohydrochloride.

Molecular formula: Benoxinate hydrochloride—$C_{17}H_{28}N_2O_3 \cdot HCl$.

Molecular weight: Benoxinate hydrochloride—344.88.

Description: Benoxinate Hydrochloride USP—White, or slightly off-white, crystals or crystalline powder. Is odorless, or has a slight characteristic odor. Its solutions are neutral to litmus, and it melts at about 158 °C.

Solubility: Benoxinate Hydrochloride USP—Very soluble in water; freely soluble in chloroform and in alcohol; insoluble in ether.

USP requirements:

Benoxinate Hydrochloride USP—Preserve in well-closed containers. Contains not less than 98.5% and not more than 101.5% of benoxinate hydrochloride, calculated on the dried basis. Meets the requirements for Identification, pH (5.0–6.0, in a solution [1 in 100]), Loss on drying (not more than 1.0%), Residue on ignition (not more than 0.2%), and Ordinary impurities.

Benoxinate Hydrochloride Ophthalmic Solution USP—Preserve in tight containers. A sterile solution of Benoxinate Hydrochloride in water. Contains the labeled amount, within ±5%. Meets the requirements for Identification, Sterility, and pH (3.0–6.0).

BENTIROMIDE

Chemical group: Synthetic peptide that contains a *p*-aminobenzoic acid (PABA) moiety as a marker.

Chemical name: Benzoic acid, 4-[[2-(benzoylamino)-3-(4-hydroxyphenyl)-1-oxopropyl]amino]-, (*S*)-.

Molecular formula: $C_{23}H_{20}N_2O_5$.

Molecular weight: 404.42.

Description: White to off-white, practically odorless powder.

pKa: 5.4.

Solubility: Practically insoluble in water, in dilute acid, and in ether; sparingly soluble in ethanol; freely soluble in dilute alkali.

USP requirements: Bentiromide Oral Solution—Not in *USP–NF*.

BENTONITE

Chemical name: Bentonite.

Description:

Bentonite NF—Very fine, odorless, pale buff or cream-colored to grayish powder, free from grit. It is hygroscopic.

NF category: Suspending and/or viscosity-increasing agent.

Purified Bentonite NF—Odorless, fine (micronized) powder or small flakes that are creamy when viewed on their flat surfaces and tan to brown when viewed on their edges.

NF category: Suspending and/or viscosity-increasing agent.

Bentonite Magma NF—NF category: Suspending and/or viscosity-increasing agent.

Solubility:

Bentonite NF—Insoluble in water, but swells to approximately twelve times its volume when added to water. Insoluble in, and does not swell in, organic solvents.

Purified Bentonite NF—Insoluble in water and in alcohol. Swells when added to water or glycerin.

NF requirements:

Bentonite NF—Preserve in tight containers. A native, colloidal, hydrated aluminum silicate. Label it to indicate that absorption of atmospheric moisture should be avoided following the opening of the original package, preferably by storage of the remainder of the contents in a tight container. Meets the requirements for Identification, Microbial limits, pH (9.5–10.5), Loss on drying (5.0–8.0%), Arsenic (not

more than 5 ppm), Lead (not more than 0.004%), Gel formation, Swelling power, Fineness of powder, and Organic volatile impurities.

Purified Bentonite NF—Preserve in tight containers. A colloidal montmorillonite that has been processed to remove grit and non-swellable ore components. Meets the requirements for Identification, Viscosity (40–200 centipoises), Microbial limits, pH (9.0–10.0, in a suspension [5 in 100] in water), Acid demand (pH not more than 4.0), Loss on drying (not more than 8.0%), Arsenic (not more than 3 ppm), Lead (not more than 0.0015%), and Organic volatile impurities.

Bentonite Magma NF—Preserve in tight containers.

Prepare Bentonite Magma as follows: 50 grams of Bentonite and a sufficient quantity of Purified Water to make 1000 grams. Sprinkle the Bentonite, in portions, upon 800 grams of hot purified water, allowing each portion to become thoroughly wetted without stirring. Allow it to stand with occasional stirring for 24 hours. Stir until a uniform magma is obtained, add Purified Water to make 1000 grams, and mix. The Magma may be prepared also by mechanical means such as by use of a blender, as follows: Place about 500 grams of Purified Water in the blender, and while the machine is running, add the Bentonite. Add Purified Water to make up to about 1000 grams or up to the operating capacity of the blender. Blend the mixture for 5 to 10 minutes, add Purified Water to make 1000 grams, and mix.

Meets the requirements for Microbial limits and Organic volatile impurities.

BENTOQUATAM

Chemical name: Quaternium-18 bentonite.

USP requirements: Bentoquatam Lotion—Not in *USP–NF*.

BENZALDEHYDE

Chemical name: Benzaldehyde.

Molecular formula: C_7H_6O.

Molecular weight: 106.12.

Description:

Benzaldehyde NF—Colorless, strongly refractive liquid, having an odor resembling that of bitter almond oil. Is affected by light.

NF category: Flavors and perfumes.

Compound Benzaldehyde Elixir NF—NF category: Flavored and/or sweetened vehicle.

Solubility: Benzaldehyde NF—Slightly soluble in water; miscible with alcohol, with ether, and with fixed and volatile oils.

NF requirements:

Benzaldehyde NF—Preserve in well-filled, tight, light-resistant containers. Contains not less than 98.0% and not more than 100.5% of benzaldehyde. Meets the requirements for Specific gravity (1.041–1.046 at 25 °C), Refractive index (1.544–1.546 at 20 °C), Limit of hydrocyanic acid, Limit of nitrobenzene, Chlorinated compounds, and Organic volatile impurities.

Compound Benzaldehyde Elixir NF—Preserve in tight, light-resistant containers. Contains 0.05% Benzaldehyde in a suitably flavored and sweetened hydroalcoholic vehicle. Meets the requirements for Alcohol content (3.0–5.0%) and Organic volatile impurities.

BENZALKONIUM CHLORIDE

Chemical name: Ammonium, alkyldimethyl(phenylmethyl)-, chloride.

Description:

Benzalkonium Chloride NF—White or yellowish white, thick gel or gelatinous pieces. Usually has a mild, aromatic odor. Its aqueous solution foams strongly when shaken, and usually is slightly alkaline.

NF category: Antimicrobial preservative; wetting and/or solubilizing agent.

Benzalkonium Chloride Solution NF—Clear liquid; colorless or slightly yellow unless a color has been added. It has an aromatic odor.

NF category: Antimicrobial preservative.

Solubility: Benzalkonium Chloride NF—Very soluble in water and in alcohol. Anhydrous form slightly soluble in ether.

USP requirements: Benzalkonium Chloride Vaginal Suppositories—Not in *USP–NF*.

NF requirements:

Benzalkonium Chloride NF—Preserve in tight containers. A mixture of alkylbenzyldimethylammonium chlorides, the composition of which is restricted within certain limits. Meets the requirements for Identification, Water (not more than 15.0%), Residue on ignition (not more than 2.0%), Water-insoluble matter, Limit of foreign amines, and Ratio of alkyl components.

Benzalkonium Chloride Solution NF—Preserve in tight containers, and prevent contact with metals. Contains the labeled amount, within ±5%, in concentrations of 1.0% or more; and contains the labeled amount, within ±7%, in concentrations of less than 1.0%. May contain a suitable coloring agent and may contain not more than 10% of alcohol. Meets the requirements for Identification, Microbial limits, Alcohol (if present, the labeled amount, within ± 5%), Ratio of alkyl components, and Limit of foreign amines.

Caution: Mixing Benzalkonium Chloride Solution with ordinary soaps and with anionic detergents may decrease or destroy the bacteriostatic activity of the Solution.

BENZETHONIUM

Chemical name: Benzethonium chloride—Benzenemethanaminium, N,N-dimethyl-N-[2-[2-[4-(1,1,3,3-tetramethylbutyl)phenoxy]ethoxy]ethyl]-, chloride.

Molecular formula: Benzethonium chloride—$C_{27}H_{42}ClNO_2$.

Molecular weight: Benzethonium chloride—448.08.

Description:

Benzethonium Chloride USP—White crystals, having a mild odor. Its solution (1 in 100) is slightly alkaline to litmus.

NF category: Antimicrobial preservative; wetting and/or solubilizing agent.

Benzethonium Chloride Solution USP—Odorless, clear liquid, slightly alkaline to litmus.

Benzethonium Chloride Tincture USP—Clear liquid, having the characteristic odor of acetone and of alcohol.

Solubility: Benzethonium Chloride USP—Soluble in water, in alcohol, and in chloroform; slightly soluble in ether.

USP requirements:

Benzethonium Chloride USP—Preserve in tight, light-resistant containers. Contains not less than 97.0% and not more than 103.0% of benzethonium chloride, calculated on the dried basis. Meets the requirements for Identification, Melting range (158–163 °C), Loss on drying (not more than 5.0%), Residue on ignition (not more than 0.1%), and Limit of ammonium compounds.

Benzethonium Chloride Concentrate USP—Preserve in tight, light-resistant containers. The label states that this article is not intended for direct administration to humans or animals. Contains the labeled amount, within ±6%. Meets the requirements for Identification, Oxidizing substances, and Limit of nitrites.

Benzethonium Chloride Topical Solution USP—Preserve in tight, light-resistant containers. Contains the labeled amount, within ±5%. Meets the requirements for Identification, Oxidizing substances, and Limit of nitrites.

Benzethonium Chloride Tincture USP—Preserve in tight, light-resistant containers. Contains, in each 100 mL, not less than 190 mg and not more than 210 mg of benzethonium chloride.

Prepare Benzethonium Chloride Tincture as follows: 2 grams of Benzethonium Chloride, 685 mL of Alcohol, 100 mL of Acetone, and a sufficient quantity of Purified Water to make 1000 mL. Dissolve the Benzethonium Chloride in a mixture of the Alcohol and the Acetone. Add sufficient Purified Water to make 1000 mL.

Meets the requirements for Identification, Specific gravity (0.868–0.876), and Alcohol and acetone content (62.0–68.0% of alcohol, and 9.0–11.0% of acetone).

Note: Benzethonium Chloride Tincture may be colored by the addition of any suitable color or combination of colors certified by the FDA for use in drugs.

BENZNIDAZOLE

Chemical group: 2-Nitroimidazole derivative.

Chemical name: N-Benzyl-2-nitroimidazole-1-acetamide.

Molecular formula: $C_{12}H_{12}N_4O_3$.

Molecular weight: 260.25.

Description: Melting point 188.5–190 °C.

Solubility: 40 mg/100 mL in water at 37 °C.

USP requirements: Benznidazole Tablets—Not in *USP–NF*.

BENZOCAINE

Chemical group: Ester of para-aminobenzoic acid (PABA).

Chemical name: Benzoic acid, 4-amino-, ethyl ester.

Molecular formula: $C_9H_{11}NO_2$.

Molecular weight: 165.19.

Description: Benzocaine USP—Small, white crystals or white, crystalline powder. Is odorless and is stable in air.

Solubility: Benzocaine USP—Very slightly soluble in water; freely soluble in alcohol, in chloroform, and in ether; sparingly soluble in almond oil and in olive oil; dissolves in dilute acids.

USP requirements:

Benzocaine USP—Preserve in well-closed containers. Dried over phosphorus pentoxide for 3 hours, contains not less than 98.0% and not more than 101.0% of benzocaine. Meets the requirements for Identification, Melting range (88–92 °C, the range between beginning and end of melting not more than 2 °C), Reaction, Loss on drying (not more than 1.0%), Residue on ignition (not more than 0.1%), Chloride, Heavy metals (not more than 0.001%), Readily carbonizable substances, and Ordinary impurities (not more than 1%).

Benzocaine Topical Aerosol USP—Preserve in pressurized containers, and avoid exposure to excessive heat. A solution of Benzocaine in a pressurized container. Contains the labeled amount, within ±10%. Meets the requirements for Identification and for Pressure test, Minimum fill, and Leakage test under Aerosols, Metered-dose inhalers, and Dry powder inhalers.

Benzocaine Cream USP—Preserve in tight containers, protected from light, and avoid prolonged exposure to temperatures exceeding 30 °C. Contains the labeled amount, within ±10%, in a suitable cream base. Meets the requirements for Identification, Microbial limits, and Minimum fill.

Benzocaine Gel USP—Preserve in well-closed containers. Contains the labeled amount, within ±10%. Meets the requirements for Identification, Microbial limits, and Minimum fill.

Benzocaine Dental Gel—Not in *USP–NF*.

Benzocaine Film-forming Gel—Not in *USP–NF*.

Benzocaine Lozenges USP—Preserve in well-closed containers. Contain the labeled amount, within –15% to +20%. Meet the requirement for Identification.

Benzocaine Ointment USP—Preserve in tight containers, protected from light, and avoid prolonged exposure to temperatures exceeding 30 °C. Contains the labeled amount, within ±10%, in a suitable ointment base. Meets the requirements for Identification, Microbial limits, and Minimum fill.

Benzocaine Dental Ointment—Not in *USP–NF*.

Benzocaine Rectal Ointment—Not in *USP–NF*.

Benzocaine Dental Paste—Not in *USP–NF*.

Benzocaine Otic Solution USP—Preserve in tight, light resistant containers. Contains the labeled amount, within ± 10%. Meets the requirements for Identification and Microbial limits.

Benzocaine Topical Solution USP—Preserve in tight containers, protected from light, and avoid prolonged exposure to temperatures exceeding 30 °C. A solution of Benzocaine in a suitable solvent. Contains the labeled amount, within ±10%. Contains a suitable antimicrobial agent. Meets the requirements for Identification and Microbial limits.

Benzocaine Dental Topical Solution—Not in *USP–NF*.

Benzocaine Topical Spray Solution—Not in *USP–NF*.

BENZOCAINE, BUTAMBEN, AND TETRACAINE

For *Benzocaine, Butamben,* and *Tetracaine*—See individual listings for chemistry information.

USP requirements:

Benzocaine, Butamben, and Tetracaine Hydrochloride Topical Aerosol USP—Preserve in pressurized containers, and avoid exposure to excessive heat. It is Benzocaine, Butamben, and Tetracaine Hydrochloride Topical Solution packaged in a pressurized container with a suitable inert propellant. Contains the labeled amounts, within ±10%. Meets the requirements for Identification and for Pressure test, Minimum fill, and Leakage test under Aerosols, Metered-dose inhalers, and Dry powder inhalers.

Benzocaine, Butamben, and Tetracaine Hydrochloride Gel USP—Preserve in tight containers, and avoid freezing. It is Benzocaine, Butamben, and Tetracaine Hydrochloride in a suitable gel base. Contains the labeled amounts, within ±10%. Meets the requirements for Identification and Minimum fill.

Benzocaine, Butamben, and Tetracaine Hydrochloride Ointment USP—Preserve in tight containers, and avoid freezing. It is Benzocaine, Butamben, and Tetracaine Hydrochloride in a suitable ointment base. Contains the labeled amounts, within ±10%. Meets the requirements for Identification and Minimum fill.

Benzocaine, Butamben, and Tetracaine Hydrochloride Topical Solution USP—Preserve in tight containers, and avoid freezing. Contains the labeled amounts, within ±10%. Meets the requirements for Identification and Minimum fill.

BENZOCAINE AND MENTHOL

For *Benzocaine* and *Menthol*—See individual listings for chemistry information.

USP requirements:

Benzocaine and Menthol Topical Aerosol USP—Preserve in tight, pressurized containers, and avoid exposure to excessive heat. A solution of Benzocaine and Menthol with suitable propellants in a pressurized container. Contains the labeled amounts, within ±10%. Meets the requirements for Identification, Microbial limits, and Minimum fill, and for Leakage test and Pressure test under Aerosols, Metered-dose inhalers, and Dry powder inhalers.

Benzocaine and Menthol Lozenges—Not in *USP–NF*.

Benzocaine and Menthol Lotion—Not in *USP–NF*.

BENZOCAINE AND PHENOL

For *Benzocaine* and *Phenol*—See individual listings for chemistry information.

USP requirements:

Benzocaine and Phenol Gel—Not in *USP–NF*.

Benzocaine and Phenol Topical Solution—Not in *USP–NF*.

BENZOIC ACID

Chemical name: Benzoic acid.

Molecular formula: $C_7H_6O_2$.

Molecular weight: 122.12.

Description: Benzoic Acid USP—White crystals, scales, or needles. Has a slight odor, usually suggesting benzaldehyde or benzoin. Somewhat volatile at moderately warm temperatures. Freely volatile in steam.

NF category: Antimicrobial preservative.

Solubility: Benzoic Acid USP—Slightly soluble in water; freely soluble in alcohol, in chloroform, and in ether.

USP requirements: Benzoic Acid USP—Preserve in well-closed containers. Contains not less than 99.5% and not more than 100.5% of benzoic acid, calculated on the anhydrous basis. Meets the requirements for Identification, Congealing range (121–123 °C), Water (not more than 0.7%), Residue on igni-

tion (not more than 0.05%), Heavy metals (not more than 10 mcg per gram), Readily carbonizable substances, and Readily oxidizable substances.

BENZOIC AND SALICYLIC ACIDS

For *Benzoic Acid* and *Salicylic Acid*—See individual listings for chemistry information.

USP requirements: Benzoic and Salicylic Acids Ointment USP—Preserve in well-closed containers, and avoid exposure to temperatures exceeding 30 °C. It is Benzoic Acid and Salicylic Acid, present in a ratio of about 2 to 1, in a suitable ointment base. Label Ointment to indicate the concentrations of Benzoic Acid and Salicylic Acid and to indicate whether the ointment base is water-soluble or water-insoluble. Contains the labeled amounts, within ±10%. Meets the requirements for Identification and Minimum fill.

BENZOIN

Description: Benzoin USP—Sumatra Benzoin has an aromatic and balsamic odor. When heated it does not emit a pinaceous odor. When Sumatra Benzoin is digested with boiling water, the odor suggests cinnamates or storax. Siam Benzoin has an agreeable, balsamic, vanilla-like odor.

USP requirements:

Benzoin USP—Preserve in well-closed containers. The balsamic resin obtained from *Styrax benzoin* Dryander or *Styrax paralleloneurus* Perkins, known in commerce as Sumatra Benzoin, or from *Styrax tonkinensis* (Piérre) Craib ex Hartwich, or other species of the Section *Anthostyrax* of the genus *Styrax*, known in commerce as Siam Benzoin (Fam. Styraceae). Label it to indicate whether it is Sumatra Benzoin or Siam Benzoin. Sumatra Benzoin yields not less than 75.0% of alcohol-soluble extractive, and Siam Benzoin yields not less than 90.0% of alcohol-soluble extractive. Meets the requirements for Botanic characteristics, Identification, Acid-insoluble ash (not more than 1.0% in Sumatra Benzoin and not more than 0.5% in Siam Benzoin), Foreign organic matter (not more than 1.0% in Siam Benzoin), and Content of benzoic acid (not less than 6.0% for Sumatra Benzoin and not less than 12.0% for Siam Benzoin).

Compound Benzoin Tincture USP—Preserve in tight, light-resistant containers, and avoid exposure to direct sunlight and to excessive heat. Label it to indicate that it is flammable.

Prepare Compound Benzoin Tincture as follows: 100 grams of Benzoin, in moderately coarse powder, 20 grams of Aloe, in moderately coarse powder, 80 grams of Storax, and 40 grams of Tolu Balsam to make 1000 mL. Prepare a Tincture by Process M, using alcohol as the menstruum.

Meets the requirements for Specific gravity (0.870–0.885), Limit of nonvolatile residue, and Alcohol content (74.0–80.0%).

BENZONATATE

Chemical name: Benzoic acid, 4-(butylamino)-, 2,5,8,11,14,-17,20,23,26-nonaoxaoctacos-28-yl ester.

Molecular formula: $C_{30}H_{53}NO_{11}$ (average).

Molecular weight: 603.00 (average).

Description: Benzonatate USP—Clear, pale yellow, viscous liquid, having a faint, characteristic odor.

Solubility: Benzonatate USP—Miscible with water in all proportions. Freely soluble in chloroform and in alcohol.

USP requirements:

Benzonatate USP—Preserve in tight, light-resistant containers. Contains not less than 95.0% and not more than 105.0% of benzonatate. Meets the requirements for Identification, Refractive index (1.509–1.511 at 20 °C), Water (not more than 0.3%), Residue on ignition (not more than 0.1%), Chloride (not more than 0.0035%), Sulfate (not more than 0.04%), Heavy metals (not more than 0.001%), and Organic volatile impurities.

Benzonatate Capsules USP—Preserve in tight, light-resistant containers. Contain the labeled amount, within ±10%. Meet the requirements for Identification and Uniformity of dosage units.

BENZOYL PEROXIDE

Chemical name: Dibenzoyl peroxide.

Molecular formula: $C_{14}H_{10}O_4$ (anhydrous).

Molecular weight: 242.23 (anhydrous).

Description:

Hydrous Benzoyl Peroxide USP—White, granular powder, having a characteristic odor.

Benzoyl Peroxide Gel USP—A soft, white gel, having a characteristic odor.

Benzoyl Peroxide Lotion USP—White, viscous, creamy lotion, having a characteristic odor.

Solubility: Hydrous Benzoyl Peroxide USP—Sparingly soluble in water and in alcohol; soluble in acetone, in chloroform, and in ether.

USP requirements:

Hydrous Benzoyl Peroxide USP—Store in the original container, at room temperature. (Note: Do not transfer Hydrous Benzoyl Peroxide to metal or glass containers fitted with friction tops. Do not return unused material to its original container, but destroy it by treatment with sodium hydroxide solution [1 in 10] until addition of a crystal of potassium iodide results in no release of free iodine.) Contains not less than 65.0% and not more than 82.0% of anhydrous benzoyl peroxide. Contains about 26% of water for the purpose of reducing flammability and shock sensitivity. Meets the requirements for Identification and Chromatographic purity.

Caution: Hydrous Benzoyl Peroxide may explode at temperatures higher than 60 °C or cause fires in the presence of reducing substances. Store it in the original container, treated to reduce static charges.

Benzoyl Peroxide Cleansing Bar—Not in *USP–NF*.

Benzoyl Peroxide Cream—Not in *USP–NF*.

Benzoyl Peroxide Gel USP—Preserve in tight containers. It is benzoyl peroxide in a suitable gel base. Contains the labeled amount, within −10% to +25%. Meets the requirements for Identification, pH (2.8–6.6), and Related compounds.

Benzoyl Peroxide Lotion USP—Preserve in tight containers. It is benzoyl peroxide in a suitable lotion base. Contains the labeled amount, within ±10%. Meets the requirements for Identification, pH (2.8–6.6), and Related compounds.
Benzoyl Peroxide Cleansing Lotion—Not in *USP–NF*.
Benzoyl Peroxide Facial Mask—Not in *USP–NF*.
Benzoyl Peroxide Stick—Not in *USP–NF*.

BENZPHETAMINE

Chemical group: Phenethylamine (amphetamine-like).

Chemical name: Benzphetamine hydrochloride—(+)-*N*-Benzyl-*N*,alpha-dimethylphenethylamine hydrochloride.

Molecular formula: Benzphetamine hydrochloride—$C_{17}H_{21}N \cdot HCl$.

Molecular weight: Benzphetamine hydrochloride—275.82.

Description: Benzphetamine hydrochloride—White crystalline powder.

Solubility: Benzphetamine hydrochloride—Readily soluble in water and in 95% ethanol.

USP requirements: Benzphetamine Hydrochloride Tablets—Not in *USP–NF*.

BENZTHIAZIDE

Chemical name: 2*H*-1,2,4-Benzothiadiazine-7-sulfonamide, 6-chloro-3-[[(phenylmethyl)thio]methyl]-, 1,1-dioxide.

Molecular formula: $C_{15}H_{14}ClN_3O_4S_3$.

Molecular weight: 431.94.

Description: Benzthiazide USP—White, crystalline powder, having a characteristic odor. Melts at about 240 °C.

Solubility: Benzthiazide USP—Practically insoluble in water; freely soluble in dimethylformamide and in solutions of fixed alkali hydroxides; slightly soluble in acetone; practically insoluble in ether and in chloroform.

USP requirements:
Benzthiazide USP—Preserve in tight containers. Contains not less than 98.0% and not more than 101.5% of benzthiazide, calculated on the dried basis. Meets the requirements for Identification, Loss on drying (not more than 1.0%), Residue on ignition (not more than 0.2%), Selenium (not more than 0.003%), Heavy metals (not more than 0.0025%), Diazotizable substances (not more than 1.0%), and Organic volatile impurities.
Benzthiazide Tablets USP—Preserve in tight containers. Contain the labeled amount, within ±10%. Meet the requirements for Identification, Disintegration (15 minutes, the use of disks being omitted), and Uniformity of dosage units.

BENZTROPINE

Chemical group: Synthetic tertiary amine.

Chemical name: Benztropine mesylate—8-Azabicyclo[3.2.1]octane, 3-(diphenylmethoxy)-, *endo*, methanesulfonate.

Molecular formula: Benztropine mesylate—$C_{21}H_{25}NO \cdot CH_4O_3S$.

Molecular weight: Benztropine mesylate—403.54.

Description: Benztropine Mesylate USP—White, slightly hygroscopic, crystalline powder.

pKa: Benztropine mesylate—10.

Solubility: Benztropine Mesylate USP—Very soluble in water; freely soluble in alcohol; very slightly soluble in ether.

USP requirements:
Benztropine Mesylate USP—Preserve in tight containers. Contains not less than 98.0% and not more than 100.5% of benztropine mesylate, calculated on the dried basis. Meets the requirements for Identification, Melting range (141–148 °C), Loss on drying (not more than 5.0%), Residue on ignition (not more than 0.1%), and Organic volatile impurities.
Benztropine Mesylate Injection USP—Preserve in single-dose or in multiple-dose containers, preferably of Type I glass. A sterile solution of Benztropine Mesylate in Water for Injection. Contains the labeled amount, within ±10%. Meets the requirements for Identification, Bacterial endotoxins, and pH (5.0–8.0), and for Injections.
Benztropine Mesylate Tablets USP—Preserve in well-closed containers. Contain the labeled amount, within ±10%. Meet the requirements for Identification, Dissolution (80% in 30 minutes in 0.1 N hydrochloric acid in Apparatus 2 at 50 rpm), and Uniformity of dosage units.

BENZYDAMINE

Chemical name: Benzydamine hydrochloride—1-Propanamine, *N*,*N*-dimethyl-3-[[1-(phenylmethyl)-1*H*-indazol-3-yl]oxy]-, monohydrochloride.

Molecular formula: Benzydamine hydrochloride—$C_{19}H_{23}N_3O \cdot HCl$.

Molecular weight: Benzydamine hydrochloride—345.87.

Description: Benzydamine hydrochloride—Melting point 160 °C.

Solubility: Benzydamine hydrochloride—Very soluble in water; rather soluble in ethanol, in chloroform, and in *n*-butanol.

USP requirements: Benzydamine Hydrochloride Oral Topical Solution—Not in *USP–NF*.

BENZYL ALCOHOL

Chemical name: Benzenemethanol.

Molecular formula: C_7H_8O.

Molecular weight: 108.14.

Description: Benzyl Alcohol NF—Clear, colorless, oily liquid. Boils at about 206 °C, without decomposition. It is neutral to litmus.
NF category: Antimicrobial preservative.

Solubility: Benzyl Alcohol NF—Sparingly soluble in water; freely soluble in 50% alcohol. Miscible with alcohol, with ether, and with chloroform.

NF requirements: Benzyl Alcohol NF—Preserve in tight containers, and prevent exposure to light. Contains not less than 97.0% and not more than 100.5% of benzyl alcohol. Meets the requirements for Identification, Specific gravity (1.042–1.047), Refractive index (1.539–1.541 at 20 °C), Acidity, Resi-

due on ignition (not more than 0.005%), Nonvolatile residue, Halogenated compounds and halides, Benzaldehyde (not more than 0.20%), and Organic volatile impurities.

BENZYL BENZOATE

Chemical name: Benzoic acid, phenylmethyl ester.

Molecular formula: $C_{14}H_{12}O_2$.

Molecular weight: 212.24.

Description: Benzyl Benzoate USP—Clear, colorless, oily liquid having a slight aromatic odor.
NF category: Solvent.

Solubility: Benzyl Benzoate USP—Practically insoluble in water and in glycerin; miscible with alcohol, with ether, and with chloroform.

USP requirements:
Benzyl Benzoate USP—Preserve in tight, well-filled, light-resistant containers, and avoid exposure to excessive heat. Contains not less than 99.0% and not more than 100.5% of benzyl benzoate. Meets the requirements for Identification, Specific gravity (1.116–1.120), Congealing temperature (not lower than 18.0 °C), Refractive index (1.568–1.570 at 20 °C), Aldehyde, Acidity, and Organic volatile impurities.
Benzyl Benzoate Emulsion—Not in USP.
Benzyl Benzoate Lotion USP—Preserve in tight containers. Contains not less than 26.0% and not more than 30.0% (w/w) of benzyl benzoate.

Prepare Benzyl Benzoate Lotion as follows: 250 mL of Benzyl Benzoate, 5 grams of Triethanolamine, 20 grams of Oleic Acid, and 750 mL of Purified Water to make about 1000 mL. Mix the Triethanolamine with the Oleic Acid, add the Benzyl Benzoate, and mix. Transfer the mixture to a suitable container of about 2000-mL capacity, add 250 mL of Purified Water, and shake the mixture thoroughly. Finally add the remaining Purified Water, and again shake thoroughly.

Meets the requirement for pH (8.5–9.2).

BENZYLPENICILLOYL POLYLYSINE

USP requirements:
Benzylpenicilloyl Polylysine Concentrate USP—Preserve in tight containers. Has a molar concentration of benzylpenicilloyl moiety of not less than 0.0125 *M* and not more than 0.020 *M*. The label states that this article is not intended for direct administration to humans or animals. Contains one or more suitable buffers. Meets the requirements for pH (6.5–8.5, the undiluted Concentrate being used), Limit of penicillenate and penamaldate, and Benzylpenicilloyl substitution (50–70%).
Benzylpenicilloyl Polylysine Injection USP—Preserve in single-dose or in multiple-dose containers, preferably of Type I glass, in a refrigerator. Has a molar concentration of benzylpenicilloyl moiety of not less than $5.4 \times 10^{-5}M$ and not more than $7.0 \times 10^{-5}M$. Contains one or more suitable buffers. Meets the requirements for Bacterial endotoxins, Sterility, and pH (6.5–8.5).

BEPRIDIL

Chemical name: Bepridil hydrochloride—1-Pyrrolideneethanamine, beta-[(2-methylpropoxy)methyl]-*N*-phenyl-*N*-(phenylmethyl)-, monohydrochloride, monohydrate.

Molecular formula: Bepridil hydrochloride—$C_{24}H_{34}N_2O \cdot HCl \cdot H_2O$.

Molecular weight: Bepridil hydrochloride—421.02.

Description: Bepridil hydrochloride—White to off-white, crystalline powder.

Solubility: Bepridil hydrochloride—Slightly soluble in water; very soluble in ethanol, in methanol, and in chloroform; freely soluble in acetone.

USP requirements: Bepridil Hydrochloride Tablets—Not in *USP–NF*.

BERACTANT

Source: A natural bovine lung extract containing phospholipids, neutral lipids, fatty acids, and surfactant-associated proteins to which colfosceril palmitate (dipalmitoylphosphatidylcholine), palmitic acid, and tripalmitin are added to standardize the composition and to mimic surface-tension lowering properties of natural lung surfactant.

Chemical name: Beractant.

USP requirements: Beractant Intratracheal Suspension—Not in *USP–NF*.

BETA CAROTENE

Chemical name: Beta,beta-carotene.

Molecular formula: $C_{40}H_{56}$.

Molecular weight: 536.87.

Description: Beta Carotene USP—Red or reddish brown to violet-brown crystals or crystalline powder.

Solubility: Beta Carotene USP—Insoluble in water and in acids and in alkalies; soluble in carbon disulfide and in chloroform; sparingly soluble in ether, in solvent hexane, and in vegetable oils; practically insoluble in methanol and in alcohol.

USP requirements:
Beta Carotene USP—Preserve in tight, light-resistant containers. Contains not less than 96.0% and not more than 101.0% of beta carotene. Meets the requirements for Identification, Melting range (176–182 °C, with decomposition), Loss on drying (not more than 0.2%), Residue on ignition (not more than 0.2%, 2 grams of specimen being used), Heavy metals (not more than 0.001%), and Organic volatile impurities.
Beta Carotene Capsules USP—Preserve in tight, light-resistant containers. Contain the labeled amount, within −10% to +25%. Meet the requirements for Identification and Uniformity of dosage units.
Beta Carotene Tablets—Not in *USP–NF*.
Beta Carotene Chewable Tablets—Not in *USP–NF*.

BETADEX

Chemical name: Beta-Cyclodextrin.

Molecular formula: $C_{42}H_{70}O_{35}$.

Molecular weight: 1134.98.

Description: Betadex NF—White, practically odorless, fine crystalline powder.

NF category: Sequestering agent.

Solubility: Betadex NF—Sparingly soluble in water.

NF requirements: Betadex NF—Preserve in tight containers. A nonreducing cyclic compound composed of 7 alpha-(1-4) linked D-glucopyranosyl units. Contains not less than 98.0% and not more than 101.0% of betadex, calculated on the anhydrous basis. Meets the requirements for Color and clarity of solution, Identification, Specific rotation (+160° to +164°), Microbial limits, Water (not more than 14.0%), Residue on ignition (not more than 0.1%), Heavy metals (not more than 5 ppm), and Reducing substances (not more than 1.0%).

BETAINE

Chemical name:
Betaine—1-Carboxy-*N,N,N*-trimethylmethanaminium inner salt.
Betaine hydrochloride—Methanaminium, 1-carboxy-*N,N,N*-trimethyl-, chloride.

Molecular formula:
Betaine—$C_5H_{11}NO_2$.
Betaine hydrochloride—$C_5H_{11}NO_2 \cdot HCl$.

Molecular weight:
Betaine—117.15
Betaine hydrochloride—153.61.

Description: White, granular, hygroscopic powder.

Solubility:
Betaine—Very soluble in water; soluble in methanol and in ethanol; sparingly soluble in ether.
Betaine hydrochloride—Soluble in water (64.7 grams/100 mL) and in ethanol (5.0 grams/100 mL) at 25 °C; practically insoluble in chloroform and in ether.

USP requirements:
Betaine Powder for Oral Solution—Not in *USP–NF*.
Betaine Hydrochloride USP—Preserve in well-closed containers. Contains not less than 98.0% and not more than 100.5% of betaine hydrochloride, calculated on the anhydrous basis. Meets the requirements for Identification, pH (0.8–1.2, in a solution [1 in 4]), Water (not more than 0.5%), Residue on ignition (not more than 0.1%), and Heavy metals (not more than 0.001%).

BETAMETHASONE

Chemical name:
Betamethasone—Pregna-1,4-diene-3,20-dione, 9-fluoro-11,17,21-trihydroxy-16-methyl-, (11 beta,16 beta)-.
Betamethasone acetate—Pregna-1,4-diene-3,20-dione, 9-fluoro-11,17-dihydroxy-16-methyl-21-(acetyloxy)-, (11 beta,16 beta)-.
Betamethasone benzoate—Pregna-1,4-diene-3,20-dione, 17-(benzoyloxy)-9-fluoro-11,21-dihydroxy-16-methyl-, (11 beta,16 beta)-.
Betamethasone dipropionate—Pregna-1,4-diene-3,20-dione, 9-fluoro-11-hydroxy-16-methyl-17,21-bis(1-oxopropoxy)-, (11 beta,16 beta).

Betamethasone sodium phosphate—Pregna-1,4-diene-3,20-dione, 9-fluoro-11,17-dihydroxy-16-methyl-21-(phosphonooxy)-, disodium salt, (11 beta,16 beta)-.
Betamethasone valerate—Pregna-1,4-diene-3,20-dione, 9-fluoro-11,21-dihydroxy-16-methyl-17-[(1-oxopentyl)oxy]-, (11 beta,16 beta)-.

Molecular formula:
Betamethasone—$C_{22}H_{29}FO_5$.
Betamethasone acetate—$C_{24}H_{31}FO_6$.
Betamethasone benzoate—$C_{29}H_{33}FO_6$.
Betamethasone dipropionate—$C_{28}H_{37}FO_7$.
Betamethasone sodium phosphate—$C_{22}H_{28}FNa_2O_8P$.
Betamethasone valerate—$C_{27}H_{37}FO_6$.

Molecular weight:
Betamethasone—392.46.
Betamethasone acetate—434.50.
Betamethasone benzoate—496.57.
Betamethasone dipropionate—504.59.
Betamethasone sodium phosphate—516.40.
Betamethasone valerate—476.58.

Description:
Betamethasone USP—White to practically white, odorless, crystalline powder. Melts at about 240 °C, with some decomposition.
Betamethasone Acetate USP—White to creamy white, odorless powder. Sinters and resolidifies at about 165 °C, and remelts at about 200 or 220 °C, with decomposition.
Betamethasone Benzoate USP—White to practically white, practically odorless powder. Melts at about 220 °C, with decomposition.
Betamethasone Dipropionate USP—White to cream-white, odorless powder.
Betamethasone Sodium Phosphate USP—White to practically white, odorless powder. Is hygroscopic.
Betamethasone Valerate USP—White to practically white, odorless powder. Melts at about 190 °C, with decomposition.

Solubility:
Betamethasone USP—Insoluble in water; sparingly soluble in acetone, in alcohol, in dioxane, and in methanol; very slightly soluble in chloroform and in ether.
Betamethasone Acetate USP—Practically insoluble in water; freely soluble in acetone; soluble in alcohol and in chloroform.
Betamethasone Benzoate USP—Insoluble in water; soluble in alcohol, in methanol, and in chloroform.
Betamethasone Dipropionate USP—Insoluble in water; freely soluble in acetone and in chloroform; sparingly soluble in alcohol.
Betamethasone Sodium Phosphate USP—Freely soluble in water and in methanol; practically insoluble in acetone and in chloroform.
Betamethasone Valerate USP—Practically insoluble in water; freely soluble in acetone and in chloroform; soluble in alcohol; slightly soluble in ether.

USP requirements:
Betamethasone USP—Preserve in well-closed containers. Contains not less than 97.0% and not more than 103.0% of betamethasone, calculated on the dried basis. Meets the requirements for Identification, Specific rotation (+118° to +126°, calculated on the dried basis), Loss on drying (not more than 1.0%), Residue on ignition (not more than 0.2%), Ordinary impurities, and Organic volatile impurities, and Other impurities .
Betamethasone Cream USP—Preserve in collapsible tubes or in tight containers. Contains the labeled amount, within −10% to +15%, in a suitable cream base. Meets the requirements for Thin-layer chromatographic identification test, Microbial limits, and Minimum fill.

Betamethasone Oral Solution USP—Preserve in well-closed containers. Contains the labeled amount, within −10% to +15%. Meets the requirement for Identification.

Betamethasone Syrup USP—Preserve in well-closed containers. Contains the labeled amount, within −10% to +15%. Meets the requirement for Identification.

Betamethasone Tablets USP—Preserve in well-closed containers. Contain the labeled amount, within ±10%. Meet the requirements for Identification, Dissolution (75% in 45 minutes in water in Apparatus 2 at 50 rpm), and Uniformity of dosage units.

Betamethasone Effervescent Tablets—Not in *USP–NF*.

Betamethasone Acetate USP—Preserve in tight containers. Contains not less than 97.0% and not more than 103.0% of betamethasone acetate, calculated on the anhydrous basis. Meets the requirements for Identification, Specific rotation (+120° to +128°), Water (not more than 4.0%), Residue on ignition (not more than 0.2%), and Ordinary impurities.

Betamethasone Benzoate USP—Preserve in tight containers. Contains not less than 98.0% and not more than 102.0% of betamethasone benzoate, calculated on the dried basis. Meets the requirements for Identification, Specific rotation (+60° to +66°), Loss on drying (not more than 0.5%), and Related steroids.

Betamethasone Benzoate Cream—Not in *USP–NF*.

Betamethasone Benzoate Gel USP—Preserve in collapsible tubes or in tight containers. Contains an amount of betamethasone benzoate equivalent to the labeled amount of betamethasone, within ±10%. Meets the requirements for Identification, Microbial limits, and Minimum fill.

Betamethasone Benzoate Lotion—Not in *USP–NF*.

Betamethasone Dipropionate USP—Preserve in well-closed containers. Contains not less than 97.0% and not more than 103.0% of betamethasone dipropionate, calculated on the dried basis. Meets the requirements for Identification, Specific rotation (+63° to +70°), Loss on drying (not more than 1.0%), Residue on ignition (not more than 0.2%), and Chromatographic purity.

Betamethasone Dipropionate Topical Aerosol USP—Preserve in tight, pressurized containers, and avoid exposure to excessive heat. A solution, in suitable propellants in a pressurized container. Contains an amount of betamethasone dipropionate equivalent to the labeled amount of betamethasone, within ±10%. Meets the requirements for Identification, and for Pressure test, Minimum fill, and Leakage test under Aerosols, Metered-dose inhalers, and Dry powder inhalers.

Betamethasone Dipropionate Cream USP—Preserve in collapsible tubes or in tight containers. Contains an amount of betamethasone dipropionate equivalent to the labeled amount of betamethasone, within ±10%, in a suitable cream base. Meets the requirements for Identification and Minimum fill.

Betamethasone Dipropionate Augmented Cream—Not in *USP–NF*.

Betamethasone Dipropionate Gel—Not in *USP–NF*.

Betamethasone Dipropionate Lotion USP—Preserve in tight containers. Contains an amount of betamethasone dipropionate equivalent to the labeled amount of betamethasone, within ±10%, in a suitable lotion base. Meets the requirements for Identification and Minimum fill.

Betamethasone Dipropionate Augmented Lotion—Not in *USP–NF*.

Betamethasone Dipropionate Ointment USP—Preserve in collapsible tubes or in well-closed containers. Contains an amount of betamethasone dipropionate equivalent to the labeled amount of betamethasone, within ±10%, in a suitable ointment base. Meets the requirements for Identification and Minimum fill.

Betamethasone Dipropionate Augmented Ointment—Not in *USP–NF*.

Betamethasone Disodium Phosphate Dental Pellets—Not in *USP–NF*.

Betamethasone Sodium Phosphate USP—Preserve in tight containers. Contains not less than 97.0% and not more than 103.0% of betamethasone sodium phosphate, calculated on the anhydrous basis. Meets the requirements for Identification, Specific rotation (+99° to +105°), Water (not more than 10.0%), Phosphate ions (not more than 1.0%), and Limit of free betamethasone (not more than 1.0%).

Betamethasone Sodium Phosphate Enema—Not in *USP–NF*.

Betamethasone Sodium Phosphate Injection USP—Preserve in single-dose or in multiple-dose containers, preferably of Type I glass. A sterile solution of Betamethasone Sodium Phosphate in Water for Injection. Contains an amount of betamethasone sodium phosphate equivalent to the labeled amount of betamethasone, within ±10%. Meets the requirements for Identification, Bacterial endotoxins, pH (8.0–9.0), and Particulate matter, and for Injections.

Betamethasone Sodium Phosphate Ophthalmic/Otic Solution—Not in *USP–NF*.

Betamethasone Sodium Phosphate Effervescent Tablets—Not in *USP–NF*.

Betamethasone Sodium Phosphate Extended-release Tablets—Not in *USP–NF*.

Betamethasone Sodium Phosphate and Betamethasone Acetate Injectable Suspension USP—Preserve in multiple-dose containers, preferably of Type I glass. A sterile preparation of Betamethasone Sodium Phosphate in solution and Betamethasone Acetate in suspension in Water for Injection. Contains an amount of betamethasone sodium phosphate equivalent to the labeled amount of betamethasone, within −10% to +15%, and the labeled amount of betamethasone acetate, within −10% to +15%. Meets the requirements for Identification, Bacterial endotoxins, and pH (6.8–7.2), and for Injections.

Betamethasone Valerate USP—Preserve in tight containers. Contains not less than 97.0% and not more than 103.0% of betamethasone valerate, calculated on the dried basis. Meets the requirements for Identification, Specific rotation (+75° to +82°), Loss on drying (not more than 0.5%), and Residue on ignition (not more than 0.2%), and Chromatographic purity.

Betamethasone Valerate Cream USP—Preserve in collapsible tubes or in tight containers. Contains an amount of betamethasone valerate equivalent to the labeled amount of betamethasone, within ±10%, in a suitable cream base. Meets the requirements for Identification, Microbial limits, and Minimum fill.

Betamethasone Valerate Foam—Not in *USP–NF*.

Betamethasone Valerate Lotion USP—Preserve in tight, light-resistant containers, and store at controlled room temperature. Contains an amount of betamethasone valerate equivalent to the labeled amount of betamethasone, within −5% to +15%. Meets the requirements for Identification, Microbial limits, Minimum fill, and pH (4.0–6.0).

Betamethasone Valerate Ointment USP—Preserve in collapsible tubes or in tight containers, and avoid exposure to excessive heat. Contains an amount of betamethasone valerate equivalent to the labeled amount of betamethasone, within ±10%, in a suitable ointment base. Meets the requirements for Identification, Microbial limits, and Minimum fill.

BETAXOLOL

Chemical name: Betaxolol hydrochloride—2-Propanol, 1-[4-[2-(cyclopropylmethoxy)ethyl]phenoxy]-3-[(1-methylethyl)amino]-, hydrochloride, (±)-.

Molecular formula: Betaxolol hydrochloride—$C_{18}H_{29}NO_3 \cdot HCl$.

Molecular weight: Betaxolol hydrochloride—343.89.

Description: Betaxolol Hydrochloride USP—White, crystalline powder.

pKa: Betaxolol hydrochloride—9.4.

Solubility: Betaxolol Hydrochloride USP—Freely soluble in water, in alcohol, in chloroform, and in methanol.

USP requirements:
Betaxolol Ophthalmic Solution USP—Preserve in tight containers. A sterile, aqueous, isotonic solution of Betaxolol Hydrochloride. Contains a suitable antimicrobial preservative. Contains the equivalent of the labeled amount of betaxolol, within ±10%. Meets the requirements for Identification, Sterility, and pH (4.0–8.0).
Betaxolol Tablets USP—Preserve in tight containers. Label Tablets to state both the content of the betaxolol active moiety and the content of betaxolol hydrochloride used in formulating them. Contain an amount of Betaxolol Hydrochloride equivalent to the labeled amount of betaxolol hydrochloride, within ±10%. Meet the requirements for Identification, Dissolution (80% in 30 minutes in 0.01 N hydrochloric acid in Apparatus 2 at 50 rpm), and Uniformity of dosage units.
Betaxolol Hydrochloride USP—Preserve in tight containers. Contains not less than 98.5% and not more than 101.5% of betaxolol hydrochloride, calculated on the dried basis. Meets the requirements for Identification, Melting range (113–117 °C), pH (4.5–6.5, in a solution [1 in 50]), Loss on drying (not more than 1.0%), Residue on ignition (not more than 0.1%), Heavy metals (not more than 0.002%), and Chromatographic purity.
Betaxolol Hydrochloride Ophthalmic Suspension—Not in *USP–NF*.

BETHANECHOL

Chemical group: Synthetic ester structurally related to acetylcholine.

Chemical name: Bethanechol chloride—1-Propanaminium, 2-[(aminocarbonyl)oxy]-N,N,N-trimethyl-, chloride.

Molecular formula: Bethanechol chloride—$C_7H_{17}ClN_2O_2$.

Molecular weight: Bethanechol chloride—196.67.

Description: Bethanechol Chloride USP—Colorless or white crystals or white, crystalline powder, usually having a slight, amine-like odor. Is hygroscopic. Exhibits polymorphism, and of two crystalline forms observed, one melts at about 211 °C and the other melts at about 219 °C.

Solubility: Bethanechol Chloride USP—Freely soluble in water and in alcohol; insoluble in chloroform and in ether.

USP requirements:
Bethanechol Chloride USP—Preserve in tight containers. Contains not less than 98.0% and not more than 101.5% of bethanechol chloride, calculated on the dried basis. Meets the requirements for Identification, pH (5.5–6.5, in a solution [1 in 100]), Loss on drying (not more than 1.0%), Residue on ignition (not more than 0.1%), Heavy metals (not more than 0.003%), Organic volatile impurities, and Chloride content (17.7–18.3%).
Bethanechol Chloride Injection USP—Preserve in single-dose containers, preferably of Type I glass. A sterile solution of Bethanechol Chloride in Water for Injection. Contains the labeled amount, within ±5%. Meets the requirements for Identification, Bacterial endotoxins, Limit of 2-hydroxypropyltrimethyl ammonium chloride (not more than 4.0%), and pH (5.5–7.5), and for Injections.
Bethanechol Chloride Tablets USP—Preserve in tight containers. Contain the labeled amount, within ±10%. Meet the requirements for Identification, Dissolution (80% in 30 minutes in 0.1 N hydrochloric acid in Apparatus 2 at 50 rpm), Limit of 2-hydroxypropyltrimethyl ammonium chloride (not more than 2.0%), and Uniformity of dosage units.

BEXAROTENE

Chemical name: 4-[1-(5,6,7,8-Tetrahydro-3,5,5,8,8-pentamethyl-2-naphthalenyl)ethenyl]benzoic acid.

Molecular formula: $C_{24}H_{28}O_2$.

Molecular weight: 348.49.

Description: Off-white to white powder.

Solubility: Insoluble in water; slightly soluble in vegetable oils and in ethanol, USP.

USP requirements:
Bexarotene Capsules—Not in *USP–NF*.
Bexarotene Gel—Not in *USP–NF*.

BICALUTAMIDE

Chemical name: Propanamide, N-[4-cyano-3-(trifluoromethyl)phenyl]-3-[(4-fluorophenyl)sulfonyl]-2-hydroxy-2-methyl-, (±)-.

Molecular formula: $C_{18}H_{14}F_4N_2O_4S$.

Molecular weight: 430.37.

Description: Fine white to off-white powder.

pKa: Approximately 12.

Solubility: Practically insoluble in water at 37 °C (5 mg/1000 mL); slightly soluble in chloroform and in absolute ethanol; sparingly soluble in methanol; soluble in acetone and in tetrahydrofuran.

USP requirements: Bicalutamide Tablets—Not in *USP–NF*.

BIMATOPROST

Chmical group: Synthetic prostaglandin analog.

Chemical name: (Z)-7-[(1R,2R,3R,5S)-3,5-Dihydroxy-2-[(1E,3S)-3-hydroxy-5-phenyl-1-pentenyl]cyclopentyl]-5-N-ethylheptenamide.

Molecular formula: $C_{25}H_{37}NO_4$.

Molecular weight: 415.58.

Description: Powder.

Solubiliuty: Very soluble in ethyl alcohol and in methyl alcohol; slightly soluble in water.

Other characteristics: pH: 6.8–7.8.

USP requirements: Bimatoprost Ophthalmic Solution—Not in *USP–NF*.

BIOLOGICAL INDICATOR FOR DRY-HEAT STERILIZATION, PAPER CARRIER

USP requirements: Biological Indicator for Dry-heat Sterilization, Paper Carrier USP—Preserve in the original package under the conditions recommended on the label, and protect from light, toxic substances, excessive heat, and moisture. The packaging and container materials do not adversely affect the performance of the article used as directed in the labeling. A defined preparation of viable spores made from a culture derived from a specified strain of *Bacillus subtilis* subspecies *niger*, on a suitable grade of paper carrier, individually packaged in a container readily penetrable by dry heat, and characterized for predictable resistance to dry-heat sterilization. Label it to state that it is a Biological Indicator for Dry-heat Sterilization, Paper Carrier; to indicate its D value and the method used to determine such D value, i.e., by spore count or fraction negative procedure after graded exposures to the sterilization conditions; the survival time and kill time under the specified sterilization conditions stated on the label; its particular total viable spore count, with a statement that such count has been determined after preliminary heat treatment; and its recommended storage conditions. State in the labeling the size of the paper carrier, the strain and ATCC number from which the spores were derived, and instructions for spore recovery and for safe disposal of the indicator. Indicate in the labeling that the stated D value is reproducible only under the exact conditions under which it was determined, that the user would not necessarily obtain the same result, and that the user should determine the suitability of the biological indicator for the particular use. The packaged Biological Indicator for Dry-heat Sterilization, Paper Carrier, has a particular labeled spore count per carrier of not less than 10^4 and not more than 10^9 spores. When labeled for and subjected to dry-heat sterilization conditions at a particular temperature, it has a survival time and kill time appropriate to the labeled spore count and to the decimal reduction value (D value, in minutes) of the preparation, specified by: Survival time (in minutes) = not less than (labeled D value) × (log labeled spore count per carrier − 2); and Kill time (in minutes) = not more than (labeled D value) × (log labeled spore count per carrier + 4). Meets the requirements for Expiration date (not less than 18 months from the date of manufacture, the date of manufacture being the date on which the first determination of the total viable spore count was made), Identification, Resistance performance tests, Purity, and Disposal.

BIOLOGICAL INDICATOR FOR ETHYLENE OXIDE STERILIZATION, PAPER CARRIER

USP requirements: Biological Indicator for Ethylene Oxide Sterilization, Paper Carrier USP—Preserve in the original package under the conditions recommended on the label, and protect it from light, toxic substances, excessive heat, and moisture. The packaging and container material shall be such that it does not adversely affect the performance of the article used as directed in the labeling. A defined preparation of viable spores made from a culture derived from a specified strain of *Bacillus subtilis* subspecies *niger* on a suitable grade of paper carrier, individually packaged in a suitable container readily penetrable by ethylene oxide sterilizing gas mixture, and characterized for predictable resistance to sterilization with such gas mixture. Label it to state that it is a Biological Indica-

tor for Ethylene Oxide Sterilization, Paper Carrier; to indicate its D value, the method used to determine such D value, i.e., by spore count or fraction negative procedure after graded exposures to the sterilization conditions; the survival time and kill time under specified sterilization conditions stated on the label; its particular total viable spore count, with a statement that such count has been determined after preliminary heat treatment; and its recommended storage conditions. State in the labeling the size of the paper carrier, the strain and ATCC number from which the spores were derived, and instructions for spore recovery and for safe disposal of the indicator. Indicate in the labeling that the stated D value is reproducible only under the exact conditions under which it was determined, that the user would not necessarily obtain the same result, and that the user should determine the suitability of the biological indicator for the particular use. The packaged Biological Indicator for Ethylene Oxide Sterilization, Paper Carrier, has a particular labeled spore count per carrier of not less than 10^4 and not more than 10^9 spores. Where labeled for and subjected to particular ethylene oxide sterilization conditions of a stated gaseous mixture, temperature, and relative humidity, it has a survival time and kill time appropriate to the labeled spore count and to the decimal reduction value (D value, in minutes) of the preparation, specified by: Survival time (in minutes) = not less than (labeled D value) × (log labeled spore count per carrier − 2); and Kill time (in minutes) = not more than (labeled D value) × (log labeled spore count per carrier + 4). Meets the requirements for Expiration date (not less than 18 months from the date of manufacture, the date of manufacture being the date on which the first determination of the total viable spore count was made), Identification, Resistance performance tests, Purity, and Stability.

BIOLOGICAL INDICATOR FOR STEAM STERILIZATION, PAPER CARRIER

USP requirements: Biological Indicator for Steam Sterilization, Paper Carrier USP—Preserve in the original package under the conditions recommended on the label, and protect it from light, toxic substances, excessive heat, and moisture. The packaging and container materials do not adversely affect the performance of the article used as directed in the labeling. A defined preparation of viable spores made from a culture derived from a specified strain of *Bacillus stearothermophilus*, on a suitable grade of paper carrier, individually packaged in a suitable container readily penetrable by steam, and characterized for predictable resistance to steam sterilization. Label it to state that it is a Biological Indicator for Steam Sterilization, Paper Carrier; to indicate its D value, the method used to determine such D value, i.e., by spore count or fraction negative procedure after graded exposures to the sterilization conditions; the survival time and kill time under specified sterilization conditions stated on the label; its particular total viable spore count, with a statement that such count has been determined after preliminary heat treatment; and its recommended storage conditions. State in the labeling the size of the paper carrier, the strain and ATCC number from which the spores were derived, and instructions for spore recovery and for safe disposal of the indicator. Indicate in the labeling that the stated D value is reproducible only under the exact conditions under which it was determined, that the user would not necessarily obtain the same result and that the user should determine the suitability of the biological indicator for the particular use. The packaged Biological Indicator for Steam Sterilization, Paper Carrier, has a particular labeled spore count per carrier of not less than 10^4 and not more than 10^9 spores. When labeled for and subjected to steam sterilization conditions at a particular temperature, it has a survival time and kill time appropriate to the labeled spore count and to the decimal reduction value (D value, in minutes) of the preparation, specified by: Survival

time (in minutes) = not less than (labeled D value) × (log labeled spore count per carrier − 2); and Kill time (in minutes) = not more than (labeled D value) × (log labeled spore count per carrier + 4). Meets the requirements for Expiration date (not less than 18 months from the date of manufacture, the date of manufacture being the date on which the first determination of the total viable spore count was made), Identification, Resistance performance tests, Purity, and Disposal.

BIOLOGICAL INDICATOR FOR STEAM STERILIZATION, SELF-CONTAINED

USP requirements: Biological Indicator for Steam Sterilization, Self-contained USP—Preserve in the original package under the conditions recommended on the label, and protect from light, from substances that may adversely affect the contained microorganisms, from excessive heat, and from moisture. A Biological Indicator for Steam Sterilization, Paper Carrier individually packaged in a suitable container readily penetrable by steam and designed to hold an appropriate bacteriological culture medium, so as to enable the packaged carrier, after subjection to saturated steam sterilization conditions, to be incubated in the supplied medium in a self-contained system. The supplied medium may contain a suitable indicator as a convenience for determining by a color change whether or not spores have survived. The design of the self-contained system is such that, after exposure to the specified sterilization conditions and inoculation of the medium under closed conditions as stated in the labeling, there is no loss of medium and inoculum during subsequent transport and handling, if done according to the provided instructions. The materials of which the self-contained system are made are such that there is no retention or release of any substance that may cause inhibition of growth of surviving spores under the incubation conditions stated in the labeling. Label it to state that it is a Biological Indicator for Steam Sterilization, Self-contained; to indicate the D value of the self-contained system, the method used to determine such D value (i.e., by spore count or fraction negative procedure after graded exposures to the sterilization conditions); the survival time and kill time under the specified conditions stated on the label; its particular total viable spore count, with a statement that such count has been determined after preliminary heat treatment; and its recommended storage conditions. State on the labeling that the supplied bacteriological medium will meet requirements for growth-promoting ability, the strain and ATCC number from which the spores were derived, and the instructions for spore recovery and for safe disposal of the indicator unit. Also indicate in the labeling that the stated resistance characteristics are reproducible only under steam sterilization conditions at the stated temperature and only under the exact conditions under which it was determined, that the user would not necessarily obtain the same result, and that the user should determine the suitability of the biological indicator for the particular use. Meets the requirements for Expiration date (not less than 18 months from the date of manufacture, the date of manufacture being the date on which the first determination of the total viable spore count was made), Identification, Resistance performance tests, Medium suitability, and Disposal.

BIOTIN

Chemical name: 1*H*-Thieno[3,4-*d*]imidazole-4-pentanoic acid, hexahydro-2-oxo-, [3a*S*-(3a alpha,4 beta,6a alpha)]-.

Molecular formula: $C_{10}H_{16}N_2O_3S$.

Molecular weight: 244.31.

Description: Biotin USP—Practically white, crystalline powder.

Solubility: Biotin USP—Very slightly soluble in water and in alcohol; insoluble in other common organic solvents.

USP requirements:
Biotin USP—Store in tight containers. Contains not less than 97.5% and not more than 100.5% of biotin. Meets the requirements for Identification, Specific rotation (+89° to +93°), and Organic volatile impurities.
Biotin Capsules—Not in *USP–NF*.
Biotin Tablets—Not in *USP–NF*.

BIPERIDEN

Chemical group: Synthetic tertiary amine.

Chemical name:
Biperiden—1-Piperidinepropanol, alpha-bicyclo[2.2.1]hept-5-en-2-yl-alpha-phenyl-.
Biperiden hydrochloride—1-Piperidinepropanol, alpha-bicyclo[2.2.1]hept-5-en-2-yl-alpha-phenyl-, hydrochloride.
Biperiden lactate—1-Piperidinepropanol, alpha-bicyclo[2.2.1]hept-5-en-2-yl-alpha-phenyl-, compd. with 2-hydroxypropanoic acid (1:1).

Molecular formula:
Biperiden—$C_{21}H_{29}NO$.
Biperiden hydrochloride—$C_{21}H_{29}NO \cdot HCl$.
Biperiden lactate—$C_{21}H_{29}NO \cdot C_3H_6O_3$.

Molecular weight:
Biperiden—311.46.
Biperiden hydrochloride—347.92.
Biperiden lactate—401.54.

Description:
Biperiden USP—White, practically odorless, crystalline powder.
Biperiden Hydrochloride USP—White, practically odorless, crystalline powder. Melts at about 275 °C, with decomposition. Is optically inactive.

Solubility:
Biperiden USP—Practically insoluble in water; freely soluble in chloroform; sparingly soluble in alcohol.
Biperiden Hydrochloride USP—Slightly soluble in water, in ether, in alcohol, and in chloroform; sparingly soluble in methanol.

USP requirements:
Biperiden USP—Preserve in well-closed, light-resistant containers. Contains not less than 98.0% and not more than 101.0% of biperiden, calculated on the dried basis. Meets the requirements for Identification, Melting range (112–116 °C), Loss on drying (not more than 1.0%), Residue on ignition (not more than 0.1%), Ordinary impurities, and Organic volatile impurities.
Biperiden Hydrochloride USP—Preserve in well-closed, light-resistant containers. Contains not less than 98.0% and not more than 101.0% of biperiden hydrochloride, calculated on the dried basis. Meets the requirements for Identification, Loss on drying (not more than 0.5%), Ordinary impurities, and Organic volatile impurities.

Biperiden Hydrochloride Tablets USP—Preserve in tight containers. Contain the labeled amount, within ±7%. Meet the requirements for Identification, Dissolution (75% in 45 minutes in 0.01 N hydrochloric acid in Apparatus 2 at 50 rpm), and Uniformity of dosage units.

Biperiden Lactate Injection USP—Preserve in single-dose containers, preferably of Type I glass, protected from light. A sterile solution of biperiden lactate in Water for Injection, prepared from Biperiden with the aid of Lactic Acid. Contains the labeled amount, within ±5%. Meets the requirements for Identification, Bacterial endotoxins, and pH (4.8–5.8), and for Injections.

BISACODYL

Chemical group: Diphenylmethane derivatives.

Chemical name: Phenol, 4,4'-(2-pyridinylmethylene)bis-, diacetate (ester).

Molecular formula: $C_{22}H_{19}NO_4$.

Molecular weight: 361.39.

Description: Bisacodyl USP—White to off-white, crystalline powder, in which the number of particles having a longest diameter smaller than 50 micrometers predominate.

Solubility: Bisacodyl USP—Practically insoluble in water; soluble in chloroform; sparingly soluble in alcohol and in methanol; slightly soluble in ether.

USP requirements:
Bisacodyl USP—Preserve in well-closed containers. Contains not less than 98.0% and not more than 101.0% of bisacodyl, calculated on the dried basis. Meets the requirements for Identification, Melting range (131–135 °C), Loss on drying (not more than 0.5%), Residue on ignition (not more than 0.1%), and Heavy metals (not more than 0.001%).

Caution: Avoid inhalation and contact with the eyes, skin, and mucous membranes.

Bisacodyl Enema—Not in USP–NF.

Bisacodyl Rectal Solution—Not in USP–NF.

Bisacodyl Suppositories USP—Preserve in well-closed containers at a temperature not exceeding 30 °C. Contain the labeled amount, within ±10%. Meet the requirement for Identification.

Bisacodyl Rectal Suspension USP—Preserve in unit-dose containers at a temperature not exceeding 30 °C. A suspension of Bisacodyl in a suitable aqueous medium. Contains the labeled amount, within −10% to +15%. Meets the requirements for Identification and pH (5.0–6.8).

Bisacodyl Delayed-release Tablets USP—Preserve in well-closed containers at a temperature not exceeding 30 °C. Label Tablets to indicate that they are enteric-coated. Contain the labeled amount, within ±10%. Bisacodyl Delayed-release Tablets are enteric-coated. Meet the requirements for Identification, Disintegration (tablets do not disintegrate after 1 hour of agitation in simulated gastric fluid TS, but then disintegrate within 45 minutes in simulated intestinal fluid TS), and Uniformity of dosage units.

BISACODYL AND DOCUSATE

For *Bisacodyl* and *Docusate*—See individual listings for chemistry information.

USP requirements: Bisacodyl and Docusate Sodium Tablets—Not in USP–NF.

BISMUTH

Chemical name:
Bismuth subgallate—Gallic acid bismuth basic salt.
Bismuth subnitrate—Bismuth hydroxide nitrate oxide $[Bi_5O(OH)_9(NO_3)_4]$.
Bismuth subsalicylate—(2-Hydroxybenzoato-O^1)-oxobismuth.

Molecular formula:
Bismuth subgallate—$C_7H_5BiO_6$.
Bismuth subnitrate—$Bi_5O(OH)_9(NO_3)_4$.
Bismuth subsalicylate—$C_7H_5BiO_4$.

Molecular weight:
Bismuth subgallate—394.09.
Bismuth subnitrate—1461.99.
Bismuth subsalicylate—362.09.

Description:
Bismuth Subcarbonate USP—White or almost white powder.
Bismuth Subgallate USP—Amorphous, bright yellow powder. Odorless. Stable in air, but affected by light.
Bismuth Subnitrate USP—White, slightly hygroscopic powder.
Bismuth Subsalicylate USP—Fine to off-white, microcrystalline, odorless powder.

Solubility:
Bismuth Subcarbonate USP—Practically insoluble in water, in alcohol, and in ether. Dissolves in dilute acids with effervescence.
Bismuth Subgallate USP—Dissolves readily with decomposition in warm, moderately dilute hydrochloric, nitric, or sulfuric acid; readily dissolved by solutions of alkali hydroxides, forming a clear, yellow liquid, which rapidly assumes a deep red color. Practically insoluble in water, in alcohol, in chloroform, and in ether; insoluble in very dilute mineral acids.
Bismuth Subnitrate USP—Practically insoluble in water and in alcohol; readily dissolved by hydrochloric acid or by nitric acid.
Bismuth Subsalicylate USP—Practically insoluble in water, in alcohol, and in ether. Reacts with alkalies and mineral acids.

USP requirements:
Bismuth Subcarbonate USP—Preserve in well-closed containers, protected from light. Contains not less than 97.6% and not more than 100.7% of bismuth subcarbonate, calculated on the dried basis. Meets the requirements for Identification, Loss on drying (not more than 1.0%), Chloride (not more than 0.05%), Limit of alkalies and alkaline earths (not more than 1.0%), Limit of nitrate (not more than 0.4%), Limit of silver (not more than 0.0025%), Arsenic (not more than 5 mcg per gram), Limit of copper (not more than 0.005%), and Limit of lead (not more than 0.002%).
Bismuth Subgallate USP—Preserve in tight, light-resistant containers. A basic salt. When dried at 105 °C for 3 hours, contains the equivalent of not less than 52.0% and not more than 57.0% of bismuth trioxide. Meets the requirements for Identification, Loss on drying (not more than 7.0%), Limit of nitrate, Arsenic (not more than 7.5 ppm), Copper, Lead, and Silver, Alkalies and alkaline earths (not more than 0.5%), and Free gallic acid (not more than 0.5%).
Bismuth Subnitrate USP—Preserve in well-closed containers. A basic salt. Contains the equivalent of not less than 79.0% of bismuth trioxide, calculated on the dried basis. Meets the requirements for Identification, Loss on drying (not more than 3.0%), Carbonate, Chloride (not more than

0.035%), Sulfate, Limit of ammonium salts, Arsenic (not more than 8 ppm), Copper, Lead, Silver, and Alkalies and alkaline earths (not more than 0.5%).

Bismuth Subsalicylate USP—Preserve in tight, light-resistant containers. A basic salt that when dried at 105 °C for 3 hours contains not less than 56.0% and not more than 59.4% of bismuth and not less than 36.5% and not more than 39.3% of total salicylates. Meets the requirements for Identification, pH (2.7–5.0), Loss on drying (not more than 1.0%), Limit of nitrate (not more than 0.4%), Arsenic (not more than 10 mcg per gram), Limit of free salicylic acid (not more than 0.2%), Limit of copper, lead, and silver (not more than 10 mcg per gram per element), and for Limit of soluble bismuth (not more than 40 mcg per gram).

Bismuth Subsalicylate Magma USP—Preserve in tight containers. Bismuth Sabsalicylate is a basic salt that when dried at 105° for 3 hours contains not less than 46.0% and not more than 59.4% bismuth and not less than 36.5% and not more than 39.3% of total salicylates. The label states that this article is not intended for direct administration to humans or animals. A suspension of Bismuth Subsalicylate in water that contains a labeled amount, within ±10%. Meets the requirements for Identification and for Limit of nitrate, Limit of free salicylic acid, Limit of copper, lead, and silver, and Limit of soluble bismuth for Bismuth Subsalicylate.

Note—Dry at 105° for 3 hours to determine the solids content and, after determining the solids content, perform all tests on a portion of the dried magma.

Bismuth Subsalicylate Oral Suspension—Not in *USP–NF*.
Bismuth Subsalicylate Tablets—Not in *USP–NF*.
Bismuth Subsalicylate Chewable Tablets—Not in *USP–NF*.

BISMUTH CITRATE

Chemical name: Bismuth citrate.

Molecular formula: $BiC_6H_5O_7$.

Molecular weight: 398.08.

Description: Bismuth Citrate USP—White, amorphous or crystalline powder. Stable in air. Melts at about 300°, with decomposition.

Solubility: Bismuth Citrate USP—Soluble in ammonia TS and in solutions of alkali citrates; insoluble in water and in alcohol.

USP requirements: Bismuth Citrate USP—Preserve in tight, light-resistant containers, store at controlled room temperature, and prevent exposure to excessive heat. Contains not less than 49% and not more than 54% of bismuth (Bi). Meets the requirements for Identification, Arsenic (not more than 10 micrograms per gram), Limit of nitrate (no brown or brownish-black color appears around the crystal), Limit of copper, lead, and silver (not more than 10 mcg per gram for each element), and Limit of soluble bismuth (not more than 40 mcg per gram).

BISMUTH, METRONIDAZOLE, AND TETRACYCLINE

For *Bismuth, Metronidazole,* and *Tetracycline*—See individual listings for chemistry information.

USP requirements: Bismuth Subsalicylate, Metronidazole, and Tetracycline Blister Card Package—Not in *USP–NF*.

MILK OF BISMUTH

Description: Milk of Bismuth USP—Thick, white, opaque suspension that separates on standing. Is odorless.

Solubility: Milk of Bismuth USP—Miscible with water and with alcohol.

USP requirements: Milk of Bismuth USP—Preserve in tight containers, and protect from freezing. Contains bismuth hydroxide and bismuth subcarbonate in suspension in water, and yields not less than 5.2% and not more than 5.8% (w/w) of bismuth trioxide.

Prepare Milk of Bismuth as follows: 80 grams of Bismuth Subnitrate, 120 mL of Nitric Acid, 10 grams of Ammonium Carbonate, and a sufficient quantity of Strong Ammonia Solution and of Purified Water, to make 1000 mL. Mix the Bismuth Subnitrate with 60 mL of Purified Water and 60 mL of the Nitric Acid in a suitable container, and agitate, warming gently until solution is effected. Pour this solution, with constant stirring, into 5000 mL of Purified Water containing 60 mL of the Nitric Acid. Dilute 160 mL of Strong Ammonia Solution with 4300 mL of Purified Water in a glazed or glass vessel of at least 12,000-mL capacity. Dissolve the Ammonium Carbonate in this solution, and then pour the bismuth solution quickly into it with constant stirring. Add sufficient 6 *N* ammonium hydroxide, if necessary, to render the mixture distinctly alkaline, allow to stand until the precipitate has settled, then pour or siphon off the supernatant liquid, and wash the precipitate twice with Purified Water, by decantation. Transfer the magma to a strainer of close texture, so as to provide continuous washing with Purified Water, the outlet tube being elevated to prevent the surface of the magma from becoming dry. When the washings no longer yield a pink color with phenolphthalein TS, drain the moist preparation, transfer to a graduated vessel, add sufficient Purified Water to make 1000 mL, and mix.

Note: This method of preparation may be varied, provided the product meets the requirements.

Meets the requirements for Identification, Microbial limits, Water-soluble substances (not more than 0.1%), Alkalies and alkaline earths (not more than 0.3%), Arsenic (not more than 0.8 ppm), and Lead.

BISOPROLOL

Chemical name: Bisoprolol fumarate—2-Propanol, 1-[4-[[2-(1-methylethoxy)ethoxy]methyl]phenoxy]-3-[(1-methylethyl)amino]-, (±)-, (*E*)-2-butenedioate (2:1) (salt).

Molecular formula: Bisoprolol fumarate—$(C_{18}H_{31}NO_4)_2 \cdot C_4H_4O_4$.

Molecular weight: Bisoprolol fumarate—766.96.

Description: Bisoprolol Fumarate USP—White crystalline powder.

Solubility: Bisoprolol Fumarate USP—Very soluble in water and in methanol; freely soluble in chloroform, in glacial acetic acid, and in alcohol; slightly soluble in acetone and in ethyl acetate.

USP requirements:
Bisoprolol Fumerate USP—Preserve in tight, light-resistant containers. Contains not less than 97.5% and not more than 102.0 of bisoprolol fumerate, calculated on the anhydrous basis. Meets the requirements for Identification, Specific rotation (−0.2° to +0.2°), Water (not more than 0.5%), Residue on ignition (not more than 0.1%), Heavy metals (0.002%), Chromatographic purity, and Content of fumeric acid (not less than 14.8% and not more than 15.4%, calculated on the anhydrous basis).
Bisoprolol Fumarate Tablets—Not in *USP–NF*.

BISOPROLOL AND HYDROCHLOROTHIAZIDE

For *Bisoprolol* and *Hydrochlorothiazide*—See individual listings for chemistry information.

USP requirements: Bisoprolol Fumarate and Hydrochlorothiazide Tablets—Not in *USP–NF*.

BITOLTEROL

Chemical name: Bitolterol mesylate—Benzoic acid, 4-methyl-, 4-[2-[(1,1-dimethylethyl)amino]-1-hydroxyethyl]-1,2-phenylene ester methanesulfonate (salt).

Molecular formula: Bitolterol mesylate—$C_{28}H_{31}NO_5 \cdot CH_4O_3S$.

Molecular weight: Bitolterol mesylate—557.66.

Description: Bitolterol mesylate—White to off-white, crystalline powder.

pKa: Bitolterol mesylate—9.1.

Solubility: Bitolterol mesylate—Sparingly soluble to soluble in water; freely soluble in alcohol.

USP requirements:
Bitolterol Mesylate Inhalation Aerosol—Not in *USP–NF*.
Bitolterol Mesylate Inhalation Solution—Not in *USP–NF*.

BIVALIRUDIN

Chemical group: A synthetic analog of hirudin.

Chemical name: L-Leucine, D-phenylalanyl-L-prolyl-L-arginyl-L-prolylglycylglycylglycylglycylglycyl-L-asparaginylglycyl-L-alpha-aspartyl-L-phenylalanyl-L-alpha-glutamyl-L-alpha-glutamyl-L-isoleucyl-L-prolyl-L-alpha-glutamyl-L-alpha-glutamyl-L-tyrosyl-.

Molecular formula: $C_{98}H_{138}N_{24}O_{33}$.

Molecular weight: 2180.29.

Other characteristics: pH: 5–6 (reconstituted solution).

USP requirements: Bivalirudin for Injection—Not in *USP–NF*.

BLEOMYCIN

Chemical name: Bleomycin sulfate—Bleomycin sulfate (salt).

Description: Bleomycin Sulfate USP—Cream-colored, amorphous powder.

Solubility: Bleomycin Sulfate USP—Very soluble in water.

Other characteristics: Inactivated in vitro by agents containing sulfhydryl groups, hydrogen peroxide, and ascorbic acid.

USP requirements:
Bleomycin Sulfate USP—Preserve in tight containers. The sulfate salt of bleomycin, a mixture of basic cytotoxic glycopeptides produced by the growth of *Streptomyces verticillus*, or produced by other means. Where it is intended for use in preparing injectable dosage forms, the label states that it is sterile or must be subjected to further processing during the preparation of injectable dosage forms. Has a potency of not less than 1.5 Bleomycin Units and not more than 2.0 Bleomycin Units per mg. Meets the requirements for Identification, pH (4.5–6.0, in a solution containing 10 Bleomycin Units per mL), Loss on drying (not more than 6.0%), Copper (not more than 0.1%), and Content of bleomycins, for Sterility and Bacterial endotoxins, under Bleomycin for Injection (where the label states that Bleomycin Sulfate is sterile), and for Bacterial endotoxins under Bleomycin for Injection (where the label states that Bleomycin Sulfate must be subjected to further processing during the preparation of injectable dosage forms).

Bleomycin for Injection USP—Preserve in Containers for Sterile Solids. Contains an amount of Bleomycin Sulfate equivalent to the labeled amount of bleomycin, within − 10% to +20%. Meets the requirements for Constituted solution, Bacterial endotoxins, Sterility, and Loss on drying (not more than 6.0%), for Identification tests, pH, Copper, and Content of bleomycins under Bleomycin Sulfate, and for Uniformity of dosage units and Labeling under Injections.

ANTI-A BLOOD GROUPING SERUM

Description: Anti-A Blood Grouping Serum USP—Liquid Serum is a clear or slightly opalescent fluid unless artificially colored blue. Dried Serum is light yellow to deep cream color, unless artificially colored as indicated for liquid Serum. The liquid Serum may develop slight turbidity on storage. The dried Serum may show slight turbidity upon reconstitution for use.

USP requirements: Anti-A Blood Grouping Serum USP—Preserve at a temperature between 2 and 8 °C. A sterile, liquid or dried preparation containing the particular blood group antibodies derived from high-titered blood plasma or serum of human subjects, with or without stimulation by the injection of Blood Group Specific Substance A (or AB). Agglutinates human red cells containing A-antigens, i.e., blood groups A and AB (including subgroups A_1, A_2, A_1B, and A_2B but not necessarily weaker subgroups). Contains a suitable antimicrobial preservative. Label it to state that the source material was not reactive for hepatitis B surface antigen, but that no known test method offers assurance that products derived from human blood will not transmit hepatitis. Label it also to state that it is for in-vitro diagnostic use. (Note: The labeling is in black lettering imprinted on paper that is white or is colored completely or in part to match the specified blue color standard.) Meets the requirements of the tests for potency, specificity, and avidity. All fresh or frozen red blood cell suspensions used for these tests are prepared under specified conditions and meet specified criteria. Meets the requirement for Expiration date (for liquid Serum, not later than 1 year, and for dried Serum, not later than 5 years after date of issue from manufacturer's cold storage [5 °C, 1 year; or 0 °C, 2 years], provided that the expiration date for dried Serum is not later than 1 year after constitution). Conforms to the regulations of the U.S. Food and Drug Administration concerning biologics.

ANTI-B BLOOD GROUPING SERUM

Description: Anti-B Blood Grouping Serum USP—Liquid Serum is a clear or slightly opalescent fluid unless artificially colored yellow. Dried Serum is light yellow to deep cream color, unless artificially colored as indicated for liquid Serum. The liquid Serum may develop a slight turbidity on storage. The dried Serum may show slight turbidity upon reconstitution for use.

USP requirements: Anti-B Blood Grouping Serum USP—Preserve at a temperature between 2 and 8 °C. A sterile, liquid or dried preparation containing the particular blood group antibodies derived from high-titered blood plasma or serum of human subjects, with or without stimulation by the injection of Blood Group Specific Substance B (or AB). Agglutinates human red cells containing B-antigens, i.e., blood groups B and AB (including subgroups A_1B and A_2B). Contains a suitable

antimicrobial preservative. Label it to state that the source material was not reactive for hepatitis B surface antigen, but that no known test method offers assurance that products derived from human blood will not transmit hepatitis. Label it also to state that it is for in-vitro diagnostic use. (Note: The labeling is in black lettering imprinted on paper that is white or is colored completely or in part to match the specified yellow color standard.) Meets the requirements of the tests for potency, specificity, and avidity. All fresh or frozen red blood cell suspensions used for these tests are prepared under specified conditions and meet specified criteria. Meets the requirement for Expiration date (for liquid Serum, not later than 1 year, and for dried Serum, not later than 5 years after date of issue from manufacturer's cold storage [5 °C, 1 year; or 0 °C, 2 years], provided that the expiration date for dried Serum is not later than 1 year after constitution). Conforms to the regulations of the U.S. Food and Drug Administration concerning biologics.

BLOOD GROUPING SERUMS

USP requirements: Blood Grouping Serums USP—Preserve at a temperature between 2 and 8 °C. Each serum is a sterile, liquid or dried preparation containing one or more of the particular blood group antibodies derived from high-titered blood plasma or serum of human subjects, with or without stimulation by the injection of red cells or other substances, or of animals after stimulation by substances that cause such antibody production. Causes either directly, or indirectly by the antiglobulin test, the visible agglutination of human red cells containing the particular antigen(s) for which it is specific. Contains a suitable antimicrobial preservative. Label each to state the source of the product if other than human and, if of human origin, to state that the source material was not reactive for hepatitis B surface antigen, but that no known test method offers assurance that products derived from human blood will not transmit hepatitis. Label each also to state that it is for in-vitro diagnostic use. Meets the requirements of the tests for potency, specificity, and avidity. All fresh or frozen red blood cell suspensions used for these tests are prepared under specified conditions and meet specified criteria. Meets the requirement for Expiration date (for liquid Serum, not later than 1 year, and for dried Serum, not later than 5 years after date of issue from manufacturer's cold storage [5 °C, 1 year; or 0 °C, 2 years], provided that the expiration date for dried Serum is not later than 1 year after constitution). Blood Grouping Serums conform to the regulations of the U.S. Food and Drug Administration concerning biologics.

Note: This monograph deals with those Blood Grouping Serums for which there are no individual monographs and which are not routinely used or required for the testing of blood or blood products for transfusion.

BLOOD GROUPING SERUMS ANTI-D, ANTI-C, ANTI-E, ANTI-c, ANTI-e

Description: Blood Grouping Serums Anti-D, Anti-C, Anti-E, Anti-c, Anti-e USP—The liquid Serums are clear, slightly yellowish fluids, that may develop slight turbidity on storage. The dried Serums are light yellow to deep cream color.

USP requirements: Blood Grouping Serums Anti-D, Anti-C, Anti-E, Anti-c, Anti-e USP—Preserve at a temperature between 2 and 8 °C. They are sterile, liquid or dried preparations derived from the blood plasma or serum of human subjects who have developed specific Rh antibodies. They are free from agglutinins for the A or B antigens and from alloantibodies other than those for which claims are made in the labeling. Contain a suit-

able antimicrobial preservative. Liquid serums are not artificially colored. Label each to state that the source material was not reactive for hepatitis B surface antigen, but that no known test method offers assurance that products derived from human blood will not transmit hepatitis. Label each to state that it is for in-vitro diagnostic use. Meet the requirements of the tests for potency, avidity, and specificity. All fresh or frozen red blood cell suspensions used for these tests are prepared under specified conditions and meet specified criteria. Meet the requirement for Expiration date (for liquid Serums, not later than 1 year, and for dried Serums, not later than 5 years, after date of issue from manufacturer's cold storage [5 °C, 1 year; or 0 °C, 2 years], provided that the expiration date for dried Serums is not later than 1 year after constitution). Conform to the regulations of the U.S. Food and Drug Administration concerning biologics.

LEUKOCYTE TYPING SERUM

USP requirements: Leukocyte Typing Serum USP—Preserve at the temperature recommended by the manufacturer. A dried or liquid preparation of serum derived from plasma or blood obtained from animals or from human donors containing an antibody or antibodies for identification of leukocyte antigens. Label it to state the source of the product if other than human and, if of human origin, to state either that the source material was found reactive for hepatitis B surface antigen and that the product may transmit hepatitis, or that the source material was not reactive for hepatitis B surface antigen but that no known test method offers assurance that products derived from human blood will not transmit hepatitis. Label it also to include the name of the specific antibody or antibodies present and the requirements for potency in relation to the antigen(s) of the corresponding specificity with which it complies; the permissible limits of error for specificity reactions with which it complies; the name of the test method or methods recommended for the product; and a statement that it is for in-vitro diagnostic use. Provide with the package enclosure the following: adequate directions for performing the tests, including a description of all recommended test methods; descriptions of all supplementary reagents, including one of a suitable complement source; description of precautions in use, including a warning against exposure of the product to carbon dioxide; a caution statement to the effect that more than one antiserum is to be used for each specificity, that the antiserum is not to be diluted, and that cross-reacting antigens exist; and directions for constitution of the product, including instructions for the use, storage, and labeling of the constituted product. Meets the requirements of the test for potency and for specificity. Meets the requirement for Expiration date (for dried Serum, not later than 2 years after date of issue from manufacturer's cold storage [5 °C, 1 year; or 0 °C, 2 years] and for liquid Serum not later than 1 year after such issue [5 °C, 1 year]). Conforms to the regulations of the U.S. Food and Drug Administration concerning biologics.

BLOOD GROUP SPECIFIC SUBSTANCES A, B, AND AB

Description: Blood Group Specific Substances A, B, and AB USP—Clear solution that may have a slight odor because of the preservative.

USP requirements: Blood Group Specific Substances A, B, and AB USP—Preserve in single-dose containers, each containing a volume of not more than 1 mL consisting of a solution containing not more than 1.25 mg of Blood Group Specific Substance powder, at a temperature between 2 and 8 °C. Dispense it in the unopened container in which it was placed by

the manufacturer. A sterile, pyrogen-free, nonanaphylactic isotonic solution of the polysaccharide-amino acid complexes that are capable of neutralizing the anti-A and the anti-B iso-agglutinins of group O blood, and are used in the immunization of plasma donors for the production of in-vitro diagnostic reagents. Contains no added preservative. Blood Group Specific Substance A is prepared from hog stomach (gastric mucin), and Blood Group Specific Substances B and AB are prepared from horse stomach (gastric mucosa). Has a total nitrogen content of not more than 8%, calculated on the moisture- and ash-free basis. Label it to state that it was derived from porcine or equine stomachs, whichever is applicable, and that it contains a single dose consisting of the stated content of dry weight of powder dissolved in the stated volume of product. Label it also to state the route of administration, and to state that it is not to be administered intravenously nor to fertile women. Label Blood Group Specific Substance B with a warning that it may contain immunogenic A activity. Meets the requirements of the test for potency (including identity). Meets the requirements for Expiration date (not more than 2 years after date of issue from manufacturer's cold storage [5 °C, 1 year; or 0 °C, 2 years]), and pH (6.0–6.8), and of the tests for safety and for anaphylaxis. Conforms to the regulations of the U.S. Food and Drug Administration concerning biologics.

RED BLOOD CELLS

Description: Red Blood Cells USP—Dark red in color when packed. May show a slight creamy layer on the surface and a small supernatant layer of yellow or opalescent plasma. Also supplied in deep-frozen form with added cryophylactic substance to extend storage time.

USP requirements: Red Blood Cells USP—Preserve in a hermetic container, which is of colorless, transparent, sterile, pyrogen-free Type I or Type II glass, or of a suitable plastic material in which it was placed by the processor. Store if unfrozen at a temperature between 1 and 6 °C, held constant within a 2 °C range except during shipment when the temperature may be between 1 and 10 °C, and store if for extended manufacturers' storage in frozen form at –65 °C or colder. The container of Red Blood Cells is accompanied by a securely attached smaller container holding an original pilot sample of blood taken from the donor at the same time as the whole human blood, or a pilot sample of Red Blood Cells removed at the time of its preparation. It is the remaining red blood cells of whole human blood that have been collected from suitable whole blood donors, and from which plasma has been removed. Red Blood Cells may be prepared at any time during the dating period of the whole blood from which it is derived, by centrifuging or undisturbed sedimentation for the separation of plasma and cells, not later than 21 days after the blood has been drawn, except that when acid citrate dextrose adenine solution has been used as the anticoagulant, such preparation may be made within 35 days therefrom. Contains a portion of the plasma sufficient to ensure optimal cell preservation or contains a cryophylactic substance if it is for extended manufacturers' storage at –65 °C or colder. In addition to labeling requirements of Whole Blood applicable to this product, label it to indicate the approved variation to which it conforms, such as "Frozen," or "Deglycerolized." Label it also with the instruction to use a filter in the administration equipment. Meets the requirement for Expiration date (for unfrozen Red Blood Cells, not later than that of the whole human blood from which it is derived if plasma has not been removed, except that if the hermetic seal of the container is broken during preparation, the expiration date is not later than 24 hours after the seal is broken; for frozen Red Blood Cells, not later than 3 years after the date of collection of the source blood when stored at –65 °C or colder and not later than 24 hours after removal from –65 °C storage provided

it is then stored at the temperature for unfrozen Red Blood Cells). Conforms to the regulations of the U.S. Food and Drug Administration concerning biologics.

WHOLE BLOOD

Description: Whole Blood USP—Deep red, opaque liquid from which the corpuscles readily settle upon standing for 24 to 48 hours, leaving a clear, yellowish or pinkish supernatant layer of plasma.

USP requirements: Whole Blood USP—Preserve in the container into which it was originally drawn. Use pyrogen-free, sterile containers of colorless, transparent, Type I or Type II glass, or of a suitable plastic material. The container is provided with a hermetic contamination-proof closure. Accessory equipment supplied with the blood is sterile and pyrogen-free. Store at a temperature between 1 and 6 °C held constant within a 2 °C range, except during shipment, when the temperature may be between 1 and 10 °C. The container of Whole Blood is accompanied by at least one securely attached smaller container holding an original pilot sample of blood, for test purposes, taken at the same time from the same donor, with the same anticoagulant. Both containers bear the donor's identification symbol or number. It is blood that has been collected from suitable whole blood human donors under rigid aseptic precautions, for transfusion to human recipients. Contains citrate ion (acid citrate dextrose or citrate phosphate dextrose or citrate phosphate dextrose with adenine) or Heparin Sodium as an anticoagulant. May consist of blood from which the antihemophilic factor has been removed, in which case it is termed "Modified." Label it to indicate the donor classification, quantity and kind of anticoagulant used and the corresponding volume of blood, the designation of ABO blood group and Rh factors, and in the case of Group O blood, whether or not iso-agglutinin titers or other tests for exclusion of specified Group O bloods were performed and to indicate any group classification of the blood resulting therefrom. If an ABO blood group color scheme is used, the labeling color used shall be: Group A (yellow), Group B (pink), Group O (blue), and Group AB (white). Label it also with the type and result of a serologic test for syphilis, or to indicate that it was non-reactive in such test; and with the type and result of a test for hepatitis B surface antigen, or to indicate that it was non-reactive in such test. If it has been issued prior to determination of test results, label it also with a warning not to use it until the test results have been received and to specify that a crossmatch be performed. Where applicable, label it as "Modified," and indicate that antihemophilic factor has been removed and that it should not be used for patients requiring that factor. Meets the requirements of tests made on a pilot sample in non-reacting in a serologic test for syphilis; for ABO blood group designation; and for classification in regard to Rh type, including those tests specified for variants and other related factors. Containers of Whole Blood shall not be entered for sterility testing prior to use of the blood for transfusion. (Note: Whole Blood may be issued prior to the results of testing, under the specified provisions.) Meets the requirement for Expiration date (not later than 21 days after the date of bleeding the donor, if it contains anticoagulant citrate dextrose solution or anticoagulant citrate phosphate dextrose solution, as the anticoagulant; or not later than 35 days if it contains anticoagulant citrate phosphate dextrose adenine solution as the anticoagulant; or not later than 48 hours after date of bleeding the donor, if it contains heparin ion as the anticoagulant). Conforms to the regulations of the U.S. Food and Drug Administration concerning biologics.

BORIC ACID

Chemical name: Boric acid (H_3BO_3).

Molecular formula: H_3BO_3.

Molecular weight: 61.83.

Description: Boric Acid NF—Colorless, odorless scales of a somewhat pearly luster, or crystals, or white powder that is slightly unctuous to the touch. Stable in air.
NF category: Buffering agent.

Solubility: Boric Acid NF—Soluble in water and in alcohol; freely soluble in glycerin, in boiling water, and in boiling alcohol.

NF requirements: Boric Acid NF—Preserve in well-closed containers. Label the container with a warning that it is not for internal use. Contains not less than 99.5% and not more than 100.5% of boric acid, calculated on the dried basis. Meets the requirements for Solubility in alcohol, Completeness of solution, Identification, Loss on drying (not more than 0.5%), and Heavy metals (not more than 0.002%).

BOSENTAN

Chemical group: Pyrimidine.

Chemical name: Benzenesulfonamide, 4-(1,1-dimethylethyl)-*N*-[6-(2-hydroxyethoxy)-5-(2-methoxyphenoxy)[2,2'-bipyrimidin]-4-yl], monohydrate.

Molecular formula: $C_{27}H_{29}N_5O_6S \cdot H_2O$.

Molecular weight: 569.63.

Description: White to yellowish powder.

Solubility: Poorly soluble in water (1.0 mg per 100 mL) and in aqueous solutions at low pH (0.1 mg per 100 mL at pH 1.1 and 4.0; 0.2 mg per 100 mL at pH 5.0). Solubility increases at higher pH values (43 mg per 100 mL at pH 7.5).

Other requirements: In the solid state, bosentan is very stable, is not hygroscopic, and is not light sensitive.

USP requirements: Bosentan Tablets—Not in *USP–NF*.

BOTULINUM TOXIN TYPE A

Source: Produced from a culture of the Hall strain of *Clostridium botulinum* grown in a medium containing N-Z amine and yeast extract.

USP requirements: Botulinum Toxin Type A for Injection—Not in *USP–NF*.

BOTULINUM TOXIN TYPE B

Source: Botulinum toxin type B is a sterile liquid form of purified botulinum toxin type B that is produced by fermentation of the bacterium *Clostridium botulinum* type B (Bean strain) and exists in a noncovalent association with hemagglutinin and non-hemagglutinin proteins as a neurotoxin complex.

Other characteristics: pH: 5.6; Specific gravity: 70–130 units per nanogram.

USP requirements: Botulinum Toxin Type B Injection USP—Not in *USP–NF*.

BOTULISM ANTITOXIN

Description: Botulism Antitoxin USP—Transparent or slightly opalescent liquid, practically colorless, and practically odorless or having an odor because of the antimicrobial agent.

USP requirements: Botulism Antitoxin USP—Preserve in single-dose containers only, at a temperature between 2 and 8 °C. A sterile, non-pyrogenic solution of the refined and concentrated antitoxic antibodies, chiefly globulins, obtained from the blood of healthy horses that have been immunized against the toxins produced by the type A and type B and/or type E strains of *Clostridium botulinum*. Label it to state that it was prepared from horse blood. Its potency is determined with the U.S. Standard Botulism Antitoxin of the relevant type, tested by neutralizing activity in mice of the corresponding U.S. Control Botulism Test Toxin. Contains not more than 20.0% of solids, and contains a suitable antimicrobial agent. Meets the requirement for Expiration date (for Antitoxin containing a 20% excess of potency, not later than 5 years after date of issue from manufacturer's cold storage [5 °C, 1 year; or 0 °C, 2 years]). Conforms to the regulations of the U.S. Food and Drug Administration concerning biologics.

BRETYLIUM

Chemical group: Bromobenzyl quaternary ammonium compound.

Chemical name: Bretylium tosylate—Benzenemethanaminium, 2-bromo-*N*-ethyl-*N*,*N*-dimethyl-, salt with 4-methylbenzenesulfonic acid (1:1).

Molecular formula: Bretylium tosylate—$C_{18}H_{24}BrNO_3S$.

Molecular weight: Bretylium tosylate—414.36.

Description: Bretylium Tosylate USP—White, crystalline powder. Is hydroscopic.

Solubility: Bretylium Tosylate USP—Freely soluble in water, in methanol, and in alcohol; practically insoluble in ether, in ethyl acetate, and in hexane.

USP requirements:
Bretylium Tosylate USP—Preserve in tight containers. Contains not less than 98.0% and not more than 101.0% of bretylium tosylate, calculated on the dried basis. Meets the requirements for Identification, Loss on drying (not more than 3.0%), Residue on ignition (not more than 0.1%), Heavy metals (not more than 0.002%), and Related compounds.
Bretylium Tosylate Injection USP—Preserve in single-dose containers, preferably of Type I glass. A sterile solution of Bretylium Tosylate in Water for Injection. Contains the labeled amount, within ±10%. Meets the requirements for Identification, Bacterial endotoxins, pH (3.5–7.0), and Particulate matter, and for Injections.

BRETYLIUM AND DEXTROSE

For *Bretylium* and *Dextrose*—See individual listings for chemistry information.

USP requirements: Bretylium Tosylate in Dextrose Injection USP—Preserve in single-dose glass or plastic containers. Glass containers are preferably of Type I or Type II glass. A sterile solution of Bretylium Tosylate and Dextrose in Water for Injection. Contains no antimicrobial agents. Contains the

labeled amounts, within ±5%. Meets the requirements for Identification, Bacterial endotoxins, and pH (3.0–6.5), and for Injections.

BRIMONIDINE

Chemical name: Brimonidine tartrate—6-Quinoxalinamine, 5-bromo-N-(4,5-dihydro-1H-imidazol-2-yl)-, [S-(R^*,R^*)]-2,3-dihydroxybutanedioate (1:1).

Molecular formula: Brimonidine tartrate—$C_{11}H_{10}BrN_5 \cdot C_4H_6O_6$.

Molecular weight: Brimonidine tartrate—442.22.

Description: Brimonidine tartrate—Off-white, pale yellow to pale pink powder.

Solubility: Brimonidine tartrate—Soluble in water (34 mg/mL).

USP requirements: Brimonidine Tartrate Ophthalmic Solution—Not in *USP–NF*.

BRINZOLAMIDE

Chemical name: 2H-Thieno[3,2-e]-1,2-thiazine-6-sulfonamide, 4-(ethylamino)-3,4-dihydro-2-(3-methoxypropyl)-, 1,1-dioxide, (R)-.

Molecular formula: $C_{12}H_{21}N_3O_5S_3$.

Molecular weight: 383.52.

Description: Brinzolamide USP—White or almost white powder. Melts at about 131 °C.

Solubility: Brinzolamide USP—Insoluble in water; slightly soluble in alcohol and in methanol.

USP requirements:
Brinzolamide USP—Preserve in well-closed containers. Contains the labeled amount, within ±2%, calculated on the dried basis. Meets the requirements for Identification, Loss on drying (not more than 0.5%), Residue on ignition (not more than 0.1%), Heavy metals (0.002%), and Related compounds.
Brinzolamide Ophthalmic Suspension USP—Preserve in tight containers. Store at a temperature between 4° and 30°. A sterile, aqueous suspension of Brinzolamide containing a suitable antimicrobial preservative. Contains the labeled amount, within ±10%. Meets the requirements for Identification, Sterility, pH (6.5–8.5), and Related compounds.

BROMAZEPAM

Chemical name: 2H-1,4-Benzodiazepin-2-one, 7-bromo-1,3-dihydro-5-(2-pyridinyl)-.

Molecular formula: $C_{14}H_{10}BrN_3O$.

Molecular weight: 316.15.

USP requirements: Bromazepam Tablets—Not in *USP–NF*.

BROMOCRIPTINE

Source: An ergot derivative.

Chemical name: Bromocriptine mesylate—Ergotaman-3″,6′,18-trione, 2-bromo-12′-hydroxy-2;″-(1-methylethyl)-5′-(2-methylpropyl)-, monomethanesulfonate (salt), (5′ alpha)-.

Molecular formula: Bromocriptine mesylate—$C_{32}H_{40}BrN_5O_5 \cdot CH_4SO_3$.

Molecular weight: Bromocriptine mesylate—750.70.

Description: Bromocriptine Mesylate USP—White or slightly colored, fine crystalline powder; odorless or having a weak, characteristic odor.

Solubility: Bromocriptine mesylate—Practically insoluble in water; sparingly soluble in methylene chloride; soluble in alcohol; freely soluble in methyl alcohol.

USP requirements:
Bromocriptine Mesylate USP—Preserve in tight, light-resistant containers, in a cold place. Contains not less than 98.0% and not more than 102.0% of bromocriptine mesylate, calculated on the dried basis. Meets the requirements for Identification, Color of solution, Specific rotation (+95° to +105°), Loss on drying (not more than 4.0%), Residue on ignition (not more than 0.1%), Heavy metals (not more than 0.002%), Limit of methanesulfonic acid content (12.5–13.4%, calculated on the dried basis), Chromatographic purity, and Organic volatile impurities.
Bromocriptine Mesylate Capsules USP—Preserve in tight, light-resistant containers. Contain an amount of bromocriptine mesylate equivalent to the labeled amount of bromocriptine, within ±10%. Meet the requirements for Identification, Dissolution (75% in 60 minutes in 0.1 N hydrochloric acid in Apparatus 2 at 50 rpm), Uniformity of dosage units, and Related compounds (not more than 5.0%).
Bromocriptine Mesylate Tablets USP—Preserve in tight, light-resistant containers. Contain an amount of bromocriptine mesylate equivalent to the labeled amount of bromocriptine, within ±10%. Meet the requirements for Identification, Dissolution (80% in 60 minutes in 0.1 N hydrochloric acid in Apparatus 1 at 120 rpm), Uniformity of dosage units, and Related compounds (not more than 5.0%).

BROMODIPHENHYDRAMINE

Chemical name: Bromodiphenhydramine hydrochloride—Ethan-amine, 2-[(4-bromophenyl)phenylmethoxy]-N,N-dimethyl-, hydrochloride.

Molecular formula: Bromodiphenhydramine hydrochloride—$C_{17}H_{20}BrNO \cdot HCl$.

Molecular weight: Bromodiphenhydramine hydrochloride—370.71.

Description: Bromodiphenhydramine Hydrochloride USP—White to pale buff, crystalline powder, having no more than a faint odor.

Solubility: Bromodiphenhydramine Hydrochloride USP—Freely soluble in water and in alcohol; soluble in isopropyl alcohol; insoluble in ether and in solvent hexane.

USP requirements:
Bromodiphenhydramine Hydrochloride USP—Preserve in tight containers. Contains not less than 98.0% and not more than 101.0% of bromodiphenhydramine hydrochloride, calculated on the dried basis. Meets the requirements for Identification, Melting range (148–152 °C), Loss on drying (not more than 0.5%), and Organic volatile impurities.

Bromodiphenhydramine Hydrochloride Capsules USP—Preserve in tight containers. Contain the labeled amount, within ±7%. Meet the requirements for Identification, Dissolution (75% in 45 minutes in water in Apparatus 1 at 100 rpm), and Uniformity of dosage units.

Bromodiphenhydramine Hydrochloride Elixir USP—Preserve in tight, light-resistant containers. Contains the labeled amount, within ±7%. Meets the requirements for Identification and Alcohol content (12.0–15.0%).

Bromodiphenhydramine Hydrochloride Oral Solution USP—Preserve in tight, light-resistant containers. Contains the labeled amount, within ±7%. Meets the requirements for Identification and Alcohol content (12.0–15.0%).

BROMODIPHENHYDRAMINE AND CODEINE

For *Bromodiphenhydramine* and *Codeine*—See individual listings for chemistry information.

USP requirements:

Bromodiphenhydramine Hydrochloride and Codeine Phosphate Oral Solution USP—Preserve in tight, light-resistant containers. Label it to indicate the alcohol content. Contains the labeled amount of bromodiphenhydramine hydrochloride and codeine phosphate hemihydrate, within ±10%. Meets the requirements for Identification, Microbial limits, pH (4.5–6.5), and Alcohol content (4.0%–6.0%).

Bromodiphenhydramine Hydrochloride and Codeine Phosphate Syrup—Not in *USP–NF*.

BROMODIPHENHYDRAMINE, DIPHENHYDRAMINE, CODEINE, AMMONIUM CHLORIDE, AND POTASSIUM GUAIACOLSULFONATE

For *Bromodiphenhydramine, Diphenhydramine, Codeine, Ammonium Chloride,* and *Potassium Guaiacolsulfonate*—See individual listings for chemistry information.

USP requirements:

Bromodiphenhydramine Hydrochloride, Diphenhydramine Hydrochloride, Codeine Phosphate, Ammonium Chloride, and Potassium Guaiacolsulfonate Oral Solution—Not in *USP–NF*.

Bromodiphenhydramine Hydrochloride, Diphenhydramine Hydrochloride, Codeine Phosphate, Ammonium Chloride, and Potassium Guaiacolsulfonate Syrup—Not in *USP–NF*.

BROMPHENIRAMINE

Chemical group: Propylamine derivative (alkylamine).

Chemical name: Brompheniramine maleate—2-Pyridinepropanamine, gamma-(4-bromophenyl)-*N,N*-dimethyl-, (*Z*)-butenedioate (1:1).

Molecular formula: Brompheniramine maleate—$C_{16}H_{19}BrN_2 \cdot C_4H_4O_4$.

Molecular weight: Brompheniramine maleate—435.31.

Description: Brompheniramine Maleate USP—White, odorless, crystalline powder.

pKa: Brompheniramine maleate—3.9 and 9.1

Solubility: Brompheniramine Maleate USP—Freely soluble in water; soluble in alcohol and in chloroform; slightly soluble in ether.

USP requirements:

Brompheniramine Maleate USP—Preserve in tight, light-resistant containers. Dried at 105 °C for 3 hours, contains not less than 98.0% and not more than 100.5% of brompheniramine maleate. Meets the requirements for Identification, Melting range (130–135 °C), pH (4.0–5.0, in a solution [1 in 100]), Loss on drying (not more than 0.5%), Residue on ignition (not more than 0.2%), Related compounds, and Organic volatile impurities.

Brompheniramine Maleate Capsules—Not in *USP–NF*.

Brompheniramine Maleate Elixir USP—Preserve in well-closed, light-resistant containers. Contains the labeled amount, within ±5%. Meets the requirements for Identification, pH (2.5–3.5), and Alcohol content (2.7–3.3%).

Brompheniramine Maleate Injection USP—Preserve in single-dose or in multiple-dose containers, preferably of Type I glass, protected from light. A sterile solution of Brompheniramine Maleate in Water for Injection. Contains the labeled amount, within ±10%. Meets the requirements for Identification, Bacterial endotoxins, and pH (6.3–7.3), and for Injections.

Brompheniramine Maleate Oral Solution USP—Preserve in well-closed, light-resistant containers. Contains the labeled amount, within ±5%. Meets the requirements for Identification, pH (2.5–3.5), and Alcohol content (2.7–3.3%).

Brompheniramine Maleate Tablets USP—Preserve in tight containers. Contain the labeled amount, within ±5%. Meet the requirements for Identification, Dissolution (75% in 45 minutes in water in Apparatus 1 at 100 rpm), and Uniformity of dosage units.

Brompheniramine Maleate Extended-release Tablets—Not in *USP–NF*.

BROMPHENIRAMINE AND PHENYLEPHRINE

For *Brompheniramine* and *Phenylephrine*—See individual listings for chemistry information.

USP requirements:

Brompheniramine Maleate and Phenylephrine Hydrochloride Elixir—Not in *USP–NF*.

Brompheniramine Maleate and Phenylephrine Hydrochloride Tablets—Not in *USP–NF*.

BROMPHENIRAMINE, PHENYLEPHRINE, AND PHENYLPROPANOLAMINE

For *Brompheniramine, Phenylephrine,* and *Phenylpropanolamine*—See individual listings for chemistry information.

USP requirements:

Brompheniramine Maleate, Phenylephrine Hydrochloride, and Phenylpropanolamine Hydrochloride Elixir—Not in *USP–NF*.

Brompheniramine Maleate, Phenylephrine Hydrochloride, and Phenylpropanolamine Hydrochloride Oral Solution—Not in *USP–NF*.

Brompheniramine Maleate, Phenylephrine Hydrochloride, and Phenylpropanolamine Hydrochloride Tablets—Not in *USP–NF*.

Brompheniramine Maleate, Phenylephrine Hydrochloride, and Phenylpropanolamine Hydrochloride Extended-release Tablets—Not in *USP–NF*.

BROMPHENIRAMINE, PHENYLEPHRINE, PHENYL-PROPANOLAMINE, AND CODEINE

For *Brompheniramine, Phenylephrine, Phenylpropanolamine, and Codeine*—See individual listings for chemistry information.

USP requirements: Brompheniramine Maleate, Phenylephrine Hydrochloride, Phenylpropanolamine Hydrochloride, and Codeine Phosphate Syrup—Not in *USP–NF*.

BROMPHENIRAMINE, PHENYLEPHRINE, PHENYL-PROPANOLAMINE, CODEINE, AND GUAIFENESIN

For *Brompheniramine, Phenylephrine, Phenylpropanolamine, Codeine,* and *Guaifenesin*—See individual listings for chemistry information.

USP requirements: Brompheniramine Maleate, Phenylephrine Hydrochloride, Phenylpropanolamine Hydrochloride, Codeine Phosphate, and Guaifenesin Oral Solution—Not in *USP–NF*.

BROMPHENIRAMINE, PHENYLEPHRINE, PHENYL-PROPANOLAMINE, AND DEXTROMETHORPHAN

For *Brompheniramine, Phenylephrine, Phenylpropanolamine, and Dextromethorphan*—See individual listings for chemistry information.

USP requirements:
Brompheniramine Maleate, Phenylephrine Hydrochloride, Phenylpropanolamine Hydrochloride, and Dextromethorphan Hydrobromide Elixir—Not in *USP–NF*.
Brompheniramine Maleate, Phenylephrine Hydrochloride, Phenylpropanolamine Hydrochloride, and Dextromethorphan Hydrobromide Tablets—Not in *USP–NF*.

BROMPHENIRAMINE, PHENYLEPHRINE, PHENYL-PROPANOLAMINE, AND GUAIFENESIN

For *Brompheniramine, Phenylephrine, Phenylpropanolamine, and Guaifenesin*—See individual listings for chemistry information.

USP requirements: Brompheniramine Maleate, Phenylephrine Hydrochloride, Phenylpropanolamine Hydrochloride, and Guaifenesin Oral Solution—Not in *USP–NF*.

BROMPHENIRAMINE, PHENYLEPHRINE, PHENYL-PROPANOLAMINE, HYDROCODONE, AND GUAIFENE-SIN

For *Brompheniramine, Phenylephrine, Phenylpropanolamine, Hydrocodone,* and *Guaifenesin*—See individual listings for chemistry information.

USP requirements: Brompheniramine Maleate, Phenylephrine Hydrochloride, Phenylpropanolamine Hydrochloride, Hydrocodone Bitartrate, and Guaifenesin Oral Solution—Not in *USP–NF*.

BROMPHENIRAMINE AND PHENYLPROPANOLAMINE

For *Brompheniramine* and *Phenylpropanolamine*—See individual listings for chemistry information.

USP requirements:
Brompheniramine Maleate and Phenylpropanolamine Hydrochloride Capsules—Not in *USP–NF*.
Brompheniramine Maleate and Phenylpropanolamine Hydrochloride Elixir—Not in *USP–NF*.
Brompheniramine Maleate and Phenylpropanolamine Hydrochloride Oral Solution—Not in *USP–NF*.
Brompheniramine Maleate and Phenylpropanolamine Hydrochloride Tablets—Not in *USP–NF*.
Brompheniramine Maleate and Phenylpropanolamine Hydrochloride Chewable Tablets—Not in *USP–NF*.
Brompheniramine Maleate and Phenylpropanolamine Hydrochloride Extended-release Tablets—Not in *USP–NF*.

BROMPHENIRAMINE, PHENYLPROPANOLAMINE, AND ACETAMINOPHEN

For *Brompheniramine, Phenylpropanolamine,* and *Acetaminophen*—See individual listings for chemistry information.

USP requirements:
Brompheniramine Maleate, Phenylpropanolamine Hydrochloride, and Acetaminophen Oral Suspension—Not in *USP–NF*
Brompheniramine Maleate, Phenylpropanolamine Hydrochloride, and Acetaminophen Tablets—Not in *USP–NF*.

BROMPHENIRAMINE, PHENYLPROPANOLAMINE, AND CODEINE

For *Brompheniramine, Phenylpropanolamine,* and *Codeine*—See individual listings for chemistry information.

USP requirements:
Brompheniramine Maleate, Phenylpropanolamine Hydrochloride, and Codeine Phosphate Oral Solution—Not in *USP–NF*.
Brompheniramine Maleate, Phenylpropanolamine Hydrochloride, and Codeine Phosphate Syrup—Not in *USP–NF*.

BROMPHENIRAMINE, PHENYLPROPANOLAMINE, AND DEXTROMETHORPHAN

For *Brompheniramine, Phenylpropanolamine,* and *Dextromethorphan*—See individual listings for chemistry information.

USP requirements:
Brompheniramine Maleate, Phenylpropanolamine Hydrochloride, and Dextromethorphan Hydrobromide Capsules—Not in *USP–NF*.

Brompheniramine Maleate, Phenylpropanolamine Hydrochloride, and Dextromethorphan Hydrobromide Elixir—
Not in *USP–NF*.

Brompheniramine Maleate, Phenylpropanolamine Hydrochloride, and Dextromethorphan Hydrobromide Oral Solution—Not in *USP–NF*.

Brompheniramine Maleate, Phenylpropanolamine Hydrochloride, and Dextromethorphan Hydrobromide Syrup—
Not in *USP–NF*.

BROMPHENIRAMINE AND PSEUDOEPHEDRINE

For *Brompheniramine* and *Pseudoephedrine*—See individual listings for chemistry information.

USP Requirements:

Brompheniramine Maleate and Pseudoephedrine Hydrochloride Extended-release Capsules—Not in *USP–NF*.

Brompheniramine Maleate and Pseudoephedrine Hydrochloride Elixir—Not in *USP–NF*.

Brompheniramine Maleate and Pseudoephedrine Hydrochloride Oral Solution—Not in *USP–NF*.

Brompheniramine Maleate and Pseudoephedrine Hydrochloride Syrup—Not in *USP–NF*.

Brompheniramine Maleate and Pseudoephedrine Hydrochloride Tablets—Not in *USP–NF*.

Brompheniramine Maleate and Pseudoephedrine Hydrochloride Chewable Tablets—Not in *USP–NF*.

Brompheniramine Maleate and Pseudoephedrine Sulfate Oral
Solution USP—Contains the labeled amounts, within ±
10%. Meets the requirement for Identification.

Brompheniramine Maleate and Pseudoephedrine Sulfate Syrup USP—Contains the labeled amounts, within ±10%.
Meets the requirement for Identification.

BROMPHENIRAMINE, PSEUDOEPHEDRINE, AND ACET-
AMINOPHEN

For *Brompheniramine, Pseudoephedrine,* and *Acetaminophen*—
See individual listings for chemistry information.

USP requirements: Brompheniramine Maleate, Pseudoephedrine Hydrochloride, and Acetaminophen Tablets—Not
in *USP–NF*.

BROMPHENIRAMINE, PSEUDOEPHEDRINE, AND DEX-
TROMETHORPHAN

For *Brompheniramine, Pseudoephedrine,* and *Dextromethorphan*—See individual listings for chemistry information.

USP requirements: Brompheniramine Maleate, Pseudoephedrine Hydrochloride, and Dextromethorphan Hydrobromide Syrup—Not in *USP–NF*.

BUCLIZINE

Chemical group: Piperazine derivative.

Chemical name: Buclizine hydrochloride—Piperazine, 1-[(4-
chlorophenyl)phenylmethyl]-4-[[4-(1,1-dimethylethyl)phenyl]-
methyl]-, dihydrochloride.

Molecular formula: Buclizine hydrochloride—$C_{28}H_{33}ClN_2 \cdot 2HCl$.

Molecular weight: Buclizine hydrochloride—505.95.

Description: Buclizine hydrochloride—White, crystalline powder.

Solubility: Buclizine hydrochloride—Slightly soluble in water; insoluble in the usual organic solvents.

USP requirements: Buclizine Hydrochloride Chewable Tablets—Not in *USP–NF*.

BUDESONIDE

Chemical name: Pregna-1,4-diene-3,20-dione, 16,17-butylide-
nebis(oxy)-11,21-dihydroxy-, [11 beta,16 alpha(*R*)], and 16 alpha,17-[(*S*)-Butylidenebis(oxy)]-11 beta,21-dihydroxypregna-
1,4-diene-3,20-dione.

Molecular formula: $C_{25}H_{34}O_6$.

Molecular weight: 430.53.

Description: White to off-white crystalline powder. Melts at 224–
231.5 °C with decomposition.

Solubility: Freely soluble in chloroform; sparingly soluble in ethanol; practically insoluble in water and in heptane.

USP requirements:

Budesonide Extended-release Capsules—Not in *USP–NF*.
Budesonide for Inhalation (Powder)—Not in *USP–NF*.
Budesonide Nasal Aerosol—Not in *USP–NF*.
Budesonide Enema—Not in *USP–NF*.
Budesonide Nasal Powder—Not in *USP–NF*.
Budesonide Nasal Solution—Not in *USP–NF*.
Budesonide Nasal Suspension—Not in *USP–NF*.
Budesonide Suspension for Inhalation—Not in *USP–NF*.
Budesonide Tablets for Suspension—Not in *USP–NF*.

BUFEXAMAC

Chemical name: 2-(*p*-Butoxyphenyl)-acetohydroxamic acid.

Molecular formula: $C_{12}H_{17}NO_3$.

Molecular weight: 223.27.

Description: Melting point 153–155 °C.

Solubility: Practically insoluble in water.

USP requirements:

Bufexamac Cream—Not in *USP–NF*.
Bufexamac Ointment—Not in *USP–NF*.

BUMETANIDE

Chemical name: Benzoic acid, 3-(aminosulfonyl)-5-(butylamino)-4-phenoxy-.

Molecular formula: $C_{17}H_{20}N_2O_5S$.

Molecular weight: 364.42.

Description: Bumetanide USP—Practically white powder.

Solubility: Bumetanide USP—Slightly soluble in water; soluble in
alkaline solutions.

USP requirements:

Bumetanide USP—Preserve in tight, light-resistant containers. Contains not less than 98.0% and not more than
102.0% of bumetanide, calculated on the dried basis.
Meets the requirements for Identification, Loss on drying

(not more than 0.5%), Residue on ignition (not more than 0.1%), Heavy metals (not more than 0.002%), and Related compounds.

Bumetanide Injection USP—Preserve in single-dose or in multiple-dose containers, preferably of Type I glass, protected from light. A sterile solution of Bumetanide in Water for Injection, prepared with the aid of Sodium Hydroxide. Contains the labeled amount, within ±10%. Meets the requirements for Identification, Bacterial endotoxins, pH (6.8–7.8), and Related compunds, and for Injections.

Bumetanide Tablets USP—Preserve in tight, light-resistant containers. Contain the labeled amount, within ±10%. Meet the requirements for Identification, Dissolution (85% in 30 minutes in water in Apparatus 2 at 50 rpm), Uniformity of dosage units, and Related compound.

BUPIVACAINE

Chemical group: Amide.

Chemical name: Bupivacaine hydrochloride—2-Piperidinecarboxamide, 1-butyl-*N*-(2,6-dimethylphenyl)-, monohydrochloride, monohydrate.

Molecular formula: Bupivacaine hydrochloride—$C_{18}H_{28}N_2O$ · HCl (anhydrous); $C_{18}H_{28}N_2O$ · HCl · H_2O (monohydrate).

Molecular weight: Bupivacaine hydrochloride—324.89 (anhydrous); 342.90 (monohydrate).

Description:
Bupivacaine Hydrochloride USP—White, odorless, crystalline powder. Melts at about 248 °C, with decomposition.
Bupivacaine Hydrochloride Injection USP—Clear, colorless solution.

pKa: 8.1.

Solubility: Bupivacaine Hydrochloride USP—Freely soluble in water and in alcohol; slightly soluble in chloroform and in acetone.

USP requirements:
Bupivacaine Hydrochloride USP—Preserve in well-closed containers. Contains not less than 98.5% and not more than 101.5% of bupivacaine hydrochloride, calculated on the anhydrous basis. Meets the requirements for Identification, pH (4.5–6.0, in a solution [1 in 100]), Water (4.0–6.0%), Residue on ignition (not more than 0.1%), Heavy metals (not more than 0.001%), Residual solvents, and Chromatographic purity.
Bupivacaine Hydrochloride Injection USP—Preserve in single-dose or in multiple-dose containers, preferably of Type I glass. Injection labeled to contain 0.5% or less of bupivacaine hydrochloride may be packaged in 50-mL multiple-dose containers. A sterile solution of Bupivacaine Hydrochloride in Water for Injection. Contains the labeled amount, within ±7%. Meets the requirements for Identification, Bacterial endotoxins, and pH (4.0–6.5), and for Injections.

BUPIVACAINE AND DEXTROSE

For *Bupivacaine* and *Dextrose*—See individual listings for chemistry information.

USP requirements: Bupivacaine Hydrochloride in Dextrose Injection USP—Preserve in single-dose containers, preferably of Type I glass. A sterile solution of Bupivacaine Hydrochloride and Dextrose in Water for Injection. Contains the labeled amounts of bupivacaine hydrochloride and dextrose, within

±7%. Contains no preservative. Meets the requirements for Identification, Bacterial endotoxins, and pH (4.0–6.5), and for Injections.

BUPIVACAINE AND EPINEPHRINE

For *Bupivacaine* and *Epinephrine*—See individual listings for chemistry information.

Description: Bupivacaine Hydrochloride and Epinephrine Injection USP—Clear, colorless solution.

USP requirements: Bupivacaine Hydrochloride and Epinephrine Injection USP—Preserve in single-dose or in multiple-dose containers, preferably of Type I glass, protected from light. Injection labeled to contain 0.5% or less of bupivacaine hydrochloride may be packaged in 50-mL multiple-dose containers. A sterile solution of Bupivacaine Hydrochloride and Epinephrine or Epinephrine Bitartrate in Water for Injection. The content of epinephrine does not exceed 0.001% (1 in 100,000). The label indicates that the Injection is not to be used if its color is pinkish or darker than slightly yellow or if it contains a precipitate. Contains the labeled amount of bupivacaine hydrochloride, within ±7%, and the equivalent of the labeled amount of epinephrine, within −10% to +15%. Meets the requirements for Color and clarity, Identification, Bacterial endotoxins, and pH (3.3–5.5), and for Injections.

BUPRENORPHINE

Chemical group: Thebaine derivative.

Chemical name: Buprenorphine hydrochloride—6,14-Ethenomorphinan-7-methanol,^17-(cyclopropylmethyl)-alpha-(1,1dimethylethyl)-4,5-epoxy-18,19-dihydro-3-hydroxy-6-methoxy-alpha-methyl-, hydrochloride, [5 alpha,7 alpha (*S*)]-.

Molecular formula: Buprenorphine hydrochloride—$C_{29}H_{41}NO_4$ · HCl.

Molecular weight: Buprenorphine hydrochloride—504.10.

Description: Buprenorphine hydrochloride—White powder.

pKa: 8.42 and 9.92.

Solubility: Buprenorphine hydrochloride—Limited solubility in water.

Other characteristics: Weakly acidic; highly lipophilic.

USP requirements:
Buprenorphine Hydrochloride USP—Preserve in tight, light-resistant containers. Contains not less than 98.5% and not more than 101.0% of buprenorphine hydrochloride, calculated on the anhydrous basis. Meets the requirements for Identification, pH (4.0–6.0, in a solution containing 10 mg per mL), Specific rotation (−92° to −98°), Water (not more than 1.0%), Residue on ignition (not more than 0.1%), and Chromatographic purity.
Buprenorphine Hydrochloride Injection—Not in *USP–NF*.

BUPROPION

Chemical group: Phenylaminoketone. Chemically unrelated to tricyclic, tetracyclic, or other antidepressants; structure closely resembles diethylpropion; related to phenylethylamines.

Chemical name: Bupropion hydrochloride—1-Propanone, 1-(3-chlorophenyl)-2-[(1,1-dimethylethyl)amino]-, hydrochloride, (±)-.

Molecular formula: Bupropion hydrochloride—$C_{13}H_{18}ClNO \cdot$ HCl.

Molecular weight: Bupropion hydrochloride—276.21.

Description: Bupropion Hydrochloride USP—White powder.

Solubility: Bupropion Hydrochloride USP—Soluble in water, in 0.1 N hydrochloric acid, and in alcohol.

USP requirements:
Bupropion Hydrochloride USP—Preserve in well-closed, light-resistant containers. Contains the labeled amount, within ±2%, calculated on the anhydrous basis. Meets the requirements for Identification, Water (not more than 0.5%), Chromatographic purity, and Content of chloride (not less than 12.6% and not more than 13.1% of chloride, calculated on the anhydrous basis).
Bupropion Hydrochloride Tablets USP—Preserve in tight containers. Contain the labeled amount, within ±10%. Meet the requirements for Identification, Dissolution (80% in 45 minutes in water in Apparatus 2 at 50 rpm), and Uniformity of dosage units.
Bupropion Hydrochloride Extended-release Tablets USP—Preserve in well-closed containers. Contain the labeled amount, within ±10%. Meet the requirements for Identification, Drug release (25–45% in one hour, 60–85% in 4 hours, and not less than 80% in water in Apparatus 2 at 50 rpm), and Related compounds.

BUSERELIN

Chemical name: Buserelin acetate—Luteinizing hormone-releasing factor (pig), 6-[*O*-(1,1-dimethylethyl)-D-serine]-9-(*N*-ethyl-L-prolinamide)-10-deglycinamide-, monoacetate (salt).

Molecular formula: Buserelin acetate—$C_{60}H_{86}N_{16}O_{13} \cdot C_2H_4O_2$.

Molecular weight: Buserelin acetate—1299.48.

Description: Buserelin acetate—Amorphous, white substance.

Solubility: Buserelin acetate—Freely soluble in water and in dilute acids.

Other characteristics: Buserelin acetate—Weak base.

USP requirements:
Buserelin Acetate Injection—Not in *USP–NF*.
Buserelin Acetate Nasal Solution—Not in *USP–NF*.

BUSPIRONE

Chemical group: Azaspirodecanedione. Not chemically related to benzodiazepines or barbiturates.

Chemical name: Buspirone hydrochloride—8-Azaspiro[4,5]decane-7,9-dione, 8-[4-[4-(2-pyrimidinyl)-1-piperazinyl]butyl]-, monohydrochloride.

Molecular formula: Buspirone hydrochloride—$C_{21}H_{31}N_5O_2 \cdot$ HCl.

Molecular weight: Buspirone hydrochloride—421.96.

Description: Buspirone Hydrochloride USP—White crystalline powder.

pKa: Buspirone hydrochloride—1.22 and 7.32.

Solubility: Buspirone Hydrochloride USP—Very soluble in water; freely soluble in methanol and in methylene chloride; sparingly soluble in ethanol and in acetonitrile; very slightly soluble in ethyl acetate; practically insoluble in hexanes.

Other characteristics: A fat-soluble, dibasic heterocyclic compound.

USP requirements:
Buspirone Hydrochloride USP—Preserve in tight, light-resistant containers, at controlled room temperature. Contains not less than 97.5% and not more than 102.5% of buspirone hydrochloride, calculated on the dried basis. Meets the requirements for Identification, Water (not more than 0.5%), Residue on ignition (not more than 0.5%), Heavy metals (not more than 0.002%), and Chloride content (8.0–8.8%).
Buspirone Hydrochloride Tablets USP—Preserve in tight, light-resistant containers, at controlled room temperature. Contain the labeled amount, within ±10%. Meet the requirements for Identification, Dissolution (80% in 30 minutes in 0.01 *N* hydrochloric acid in Apparatus 2 at 50 rpm), and Uniformity of dosage units.

BUSULFAN

Chemical name: 1,4-Butanediol, dimethanesulfonate.

Molecular formula: $C_6H_{14}O_6S_2$.

Molecular weight: 246.30.

Description: Busulfan USP—White, crystalline powder.

Solubility: Busulfan USP—Very slightly soluble in water; sparingly soluble in acetone; slightly soluble in alcohol.

USP requirements:
Busulfan USP—Preserve in tight containers. The label bears a warning that great care should be taken to prevent inhaling particles of Busulfan and exposing the skin to it. Contains not less than 98.0% and not more than 100.5% of busulfan, calculated on the dried basis. Meets the requirements for Identification, Melting range (115–118 °C), Loss on drying (not more than 2.0%), Residue on ignition (not more than 0.1%), and Organic volatile impurities.
Busulfan Injection—Not in *USP–NF*.
Busulfan Tablets USP—Preserve in well-closed containers. Contain the labeled amount, within ±7%. Meet the requirements for Identification, Disintegration (30 minutes, the use of disks being omitted), and Uniformity of dosage units.

BUTABARBITAL

Chemical name:
Butabarbital—2,4,6(1*H*,3*H*,5*H*)-Pyrimidinetrione, 5-ethyl-5-(1-methylpropyl)-.
Butabarbital sodium—2,4,6(1*H*,3*H*,5*H*)-Pyrimidinetrione, 5-ethyl-5-(1-methylpropyl)-, monosodium salt.

Molecular formula:
Butabarbital—$C_{10}H_{16}N_2O_3$.
Butabarbital sodium—$C_{10}H_{15}N_2NaO_3$.

Molecular weight:
Butabarbital—212.25.
Butabarbital sodium—234.23.

Description:
Butabarbital USP—White, odorless, crystalline powder.
Butabarbital Sodium USP—White powder.

Solubility:
Butabarbital USP—Very slightly soluble in water; soluble in alcohol, in chloroform, in ether, and in solutions of alkali hydroxides and carbonates.

Butabarbital Sodium USP—Freely soluble in water and in alcohol; practically insoluble in absolute ether.

USP requirements:

Butabarbital USP—Preserve in tight containers. Contains not less than 98.5% and not more than 101.0% of butabarbital, calculated on the dried basis. Meets the requirements for Identification, Melting range (164–167 °C), Loss on drying (not more than 1.0%), Residue on ignition (not more than 0.1%), Chromatographic purity, and Organic volatile impurities.

Butabarbital Sodium USP—Preserve in tight containers. Contains not less than 98.2% and not more than 100.5% of butabarbital sodium, calculated on the dried basis. Meets the requirements for Completeness of solution, Identification, pH (10.0–11.2), Loss on drying (not more than 5.0%), Heavy metals (not more than 0.003%), Chromatographic purity, and Organic volatile impurities.

Butabarbital Sodium Capsules USP—Preserve in well-closed containers. Contain the labeled amount, within ±10%. Meet the requirements for Identification, Dissolution (75% in 45 minutes in water in Apparatus 1 at 100 rpm), and Uniformity of dosage units.

Butabarbital Sodium Elixir USP—Preserve in tight containers. Contains the labeled amount, within ±10%. Meets the requirements for Identification and Alcohol content (the labeled amount, within –5% to +15%).

Butabarbital Sodium Oral Solution USP—Preserve in tight containers. Contains the labeled amount, within ±10%. Meets the requirements for Identification and Alcohol content (the labeled amount, within –5% to +15%).

Butabarbital Sodium Tablets USP—Preserve in well-closed containers. Contain the labeled amount, within ±10%. Meet the requirements for Identification, Dissolution (75% in 45 minutes in water in Apparatus 1 at 100 rpm), and Uniformity of dosage units.

BUTALBITAL

Chemical name: 2,4,6(1*H*,3*H*,5*H*)-Pyrimidinetrione, 5-(2-methylpropyl)-5-(2-propenyl)-.

Molecular formula: $C_{11}H_{16}N_2O_3$.

Molecular weight: 224.26.

Description: Butalbital USP—White, crystalline, odorless powder. Is stable in air. Its saturated solution is acid to litmus.

Solubility: Butalbital USP—Freely soluble in alcohol, in ether, and in chloroform; slightly soluble in cold water; soluble in boiling water, and in solutions of fixed alkalies and alkali carbonates.

USP requirements: Butalbital USP—Preserve in well-closed containers. Contains not less than 98.0% and not more than 102.0% of butalbital, calculated on the dried basis. Meets the requirements for Identification, Melting range (138–141 °C), Loss on drying (not more than 0.2%), Residue on ignition (not more than 0.1%), Heavy metals (not more than 0.002%), Chromatographic purity, and Organic volatile impurities.

BUTALBITAL AND ACETAMINOPHEN

For *Butalbital* and *Acetaminophen*—See individual listings for chemistry information.

USP requirements:

Butalbital and Acetaminophen Capsules—Not in *USP–NF*.
Butalbital and Acetaminophen Tablets—Not in *USP–NF*.

BUTALBITAL, ACETAMINOPHEN, AND CAFFEINE

For *Butalbital, Acetaminophen,* and *Caffeine*—See individual listings for chemistry information.

USP requirements:

Butalbital, Acetaminophen, and Caffeine Capsules USP—Preserve in tight containers. Contain the labeled amounts, within ±10%. Meet the requirements for Identification, Dissolution (80% of each active ingredient in 60 minutes in water in Apparatus 1 at 100 rpm), and Uniformity of dosage units.

Butalbital, Acetaminophen, and Caffeine Tablets USP—Preserve in tight containers. Contain the labeled amounts, within ±10%. Meet the requirements for Identification, Dissolution (80% of each active ingredient in 30 minutes in water in Apparatus 2 at 50 rpm), and Uniformity of dosage units.

BUTALBITAL, ACETAMINOPHEN, CAFFEINE, AND CODEINE

For *Butalbital, Acetaminophen, Caffeine,* and *Codeine*—See individual listings for chemistry information.

USP requirements: Butalbital, Acetaminophen, Caffeine, and Codeine Phosphate Capsules—Not in *USP–NF*.

BUTALBITAL AND ASPIRIN

For *Butalbital* and *Aspirin*—See individual listings for chemistry information.

USP requirements: Butalbital and Aspirin Tablets USP—Preserve in tight containers. Contain the labeled amounts, within ±10%. Meet the requirements for Identification, Dissolution (75% of each active ingredient in 60 minutes in water in Apparatus 1 at 100 rpm), Uniformity of dosage units, and Limit of free salicylic acid (not more than 3.0%).

BUTALBITAL, ASPIRIN, AND CAFFEINE

For *Butalbital, Aspirin,* and *Caffeine*—See individual listings for chemistry information.

USP requirements:

Butalbital, Aspirin, and Caffeine Capsules USP—Preserve in tight containers. Contain the labeled amounts, within ± 10%. Meet the requirements for Identification, Dissolution (75% of each active ingredient in 60 minutes in water in Apparatus 2 at 50 rpm), Uniformity of dosage units, and Free salicylic acid (not more than 2.5%).

Butalbital, Aspirin, and Caffeine Tablets USP—Preserve in tight containers. Contain the labeled amounts, within ± 10%. Meet the requirements for Identification, Dissolution

(80% of each active ingredient in 60 minutes in water in Apparatus 2 at 100 rpm), Uniformity of dosage units, and Free salicylic acid (not more than 3.0%).

BUTALBITAL, ASPIRIN, CAFFEINE, AND CODEINE

For *Butalbital, Aspirin, Caffeine,* and *Codeine*—See individual listings for chemistry information.

USP requirements:
Butalbital, Aspirin, Caffeine, and Codeine Phosphate Capsules USP—Preserve in tight, light-resistant containers. Contain the labeled amounts, within ±10%. Meet the requirements for Identification, Dissolution (75% of each active ingredient in 60 minutes in water in Apparatus 2 at 50 rpm), Uniformity of dosage units, and Free salicylic acid (not more than 3.0%).
Butalbital, Aspirin, Caffeine, and Codeine Phosphate Tablets—Not in *USP–NF.*

BUTAMBEN

Chemical group: Ester, aminobenzoic acid (PABA)–derivative.

Chemical name:
Butamben—Benzoic acid, 4-amino-, butyl ester.
Butamben picrate—Benzoic acid, 4-amino-, butyl ester, compound with 2,4,6-trinitrophenol (2:1).

Molecular formula:
Butamben—$C_{11}H_{15}NO_2$.
Butamben picrate—$(C_{11}H_{15}NO_2)_2 \cdot C_6H_3N_3O_7$.

Molecular weight:
Butamben—193.24.
Butamben picrate—615.59.

Description:
Butamben USP—White, crystalline powder. Is odorless.
Butamben picrate—Yellow powder; melting point 109–110 °C.

Solubility:
Butamben USP—Very slightly soluble in water; soluble in dilute acids, in alcohol, in chloroform, in ether, and in fixed oils. Is slowly hydrolyzed when boiled with water.
Butamben picrate—Soluble in alcohol, in chloroform, and in ether; soluble in water (1 gram/2000 mL).

USP requirements:
Butamben USP—Preserve in well-closed containers. Dried over phosphorus pentoxide for 3 hours, contains not less than 98.0% and not more than 101.0% of butamben. Meets the requirements for Completeness and color of solution, Identification, Melting range (57–59 °C), Reaction, Loss on drying (not more than 1.0%), Residue on ignition (not more than 0.2%), Chloride, and Heavy metals (not more than 0.001%).
Butamben Picrate Ointment—Not in *USP–NF.*

BUTANE

Chemical name: *n*-Butane.

Molecular formula: C_4H_{10}.

Molecular weight: 58.12.

Description: Butane NF—Colorless, flammable gas (boiling temperature is about –0.5 °C). Vapor pressure at 21 °C is about 1620 mm of mercury (17 psig).

NF category: Aerosol propellant.

Solubility: Butane NF—One volume of water dissolves 0.15 volume, and 1 volume of alcohol dissolves 18 volumes at 17 °C and 770 mm; 1 volume of ether or chloroform at 17 °C dissolves 25 or 30 volumes, respectively.

NF requirements: Butane NF—Preserve in tight cylinders, and prevent exposure to excessive heat. Contains not less than 97.0% of *n*-butane. Meets the requirements for Identification, Water (not more than 0.001%), High-boiling residues (not more than 5 ppm), Acidity of residue, and Limit of sulfur compounds.
Caution: Butane is highly flammable and explosive.

BUTENAFINE

Chemical group: Benzylamine derivative.

Molecular formula: Butenafine hydrochloride—$C_{23}H_{27}N \cdot HCl$.

Description: Butenafine hydrochloride—Melting point 200–202 °C.

Solubility: Butenafine hydrochloride—Easily soluble in methanol, in ethanol, in dichloromethane, and in chloroform; slightly soluble in water.

USP requirements: Butenafine Hydrochloride Cream—Not in *USP–NF.*

BUTOCONAZOLE

Chemical name: Butoconazole nitrate—1*H*-Imidazole, 1-[4-(4chlorophenyl)-2-[(2,6-dichlorophenyl)thio]butyl]-, mononitrate, (±)-.

Molecular formula: Butoconazole nitrate—$C_{19}H_{17}Cl_3N_2S \cdot HNO_3$.

Molecular weight: Butoconazole nitrate—474.79.

Description: Butoconazole Nitrate USP—White to off-white, crystalline powder. Melts at about 160 °C.

Solubility: Butoconazole Nitrate USP—Practically insoluble in water; very slightly soluble in ethyl acetate; slightly soluble in acetonitrile, in acetone, in dichloromethane, and in tetrahydrofuran; sparingly soluble in methanol.

USP requirements:
Butoconazole Nitrate USP—Preserve in well-closed, light-resistant containers. Contains not less than 98.0% and not more than 102.0% of butoconazole nitrate, calculated on the dried basis. Meets the requirements for Identification, Loss on drying (not more than 1.0%), Residue on ignition (not more than 0.1%), and Ordinary impurities.
Butoconazole Nitrate Vaginal Cream USP—Preserve in collapsible tubes or in tight containers. Avoid excessive heat and avoid freezing. It is Butoconazole Nitrate in a suitable cream base. Contains the labeled amount, within ±10%. Meets the requirements for Identification and Minimum fill.
Butoconazole Nitrate Vaginal Suppositories—Not in *USP–NF.*

BUTORPHANOL

Chemical name: Butorphanol tartrate—Morphinan-3,14-diol, 17-(cyclobutylmethyl)-, (–)-, [S-(R*,R*)]-2,3-dihydroxybutanedioate (1:1) (salt).

Molecular formula: Butorphanol tartrate—$C_{21}H_{29}NO_2 \cdot C_4H_6O_6$.

Molecular weight: Butorphanol tartrate—477.55.

Description: Butorphanol Tartrate USP—White powder. Its solutions are slightly acidic. Melts between 217 and 219 °C, with decomposition.

Solubility: Butorphanol Tartrate USP—Sparingly soluble in water; slightly soluble in methanol; insoluble in alcohol, in chloroform, in ethyl acetate, in ethyl ether, and in hexane; soluble in dilute acids.

USP requirements:

Butorphanol Tartrate USP—Preserve in tight containers. Contains not less than 98.0% and not more than 102.0% of butorphanol tartrate, calculated on the anhydrous basis. Meets the requirements for Identification, Specific rotation (−60° to −66°), Water (not more than 2.0%), Residue on ignition (not more than 0.1%), Heavy metals (not more than 0.003%), and Chromatographic purity.

Butorphanol Tartrate Injection USP—Preserve in single-dose or in multiple-dose containers, preferably of Type I glass, protected from light. A sterile solution of Butorphanol Tartrate in Water for Injection. Contains the labeled amount, within ±10%. Meets the requirements for Identification, Bacterial endotoxins, and pH (3.0–5.5), and for Injections.

Butorphanol Tartrate Nasal Solution—Not in *USP–NF*.

BUTYL ALCOHOL

Molecular formula: $C_4H_{10}O$.

Molecular weight: 74.12.

Description: Butyl Alcohol NF—Clear, colorless, mobile liquid, having a characteristic, penetrating vinous odor.
NF category: Solvent.

Solubility: Butyl Alcohol NF—Soluble in water. Miscible with alcohol, with ether, and with many other organic solvents.

NF requirements: Butyl Alcohol NF—Preserve in tight containers, and prevent exposure to excessive heat. It is *n*-butyl alcohol. Meets the requirements for Specific gravity (0.807–0.809), Distilling range (distils within a range of 1.5 °C, including 117.7 °C), Acidity, Water (not more than 0.1%), Limit of nonvolatile residue (not more than 0.004%), Aldehydes, and Butyl ether.

BUTYLATED HYDROXYANISOLE

Chemical name: Phenol, (1,1-dimethylethyl)-4-methoxy.

Molecular formula: $C_{11}H_{16}O_2$.

Molecular weight: 180.24.

Description: Butylated Hydroxyanisole NF—White or slightly yellow, waxy solid, having a faint, characteristic odor.
NF category: Antioxidant.

Solubility: Butylated Hydroxyanisole NF—Insoluble in water; freely soluble in alcohol, in propylene glycol, in chloroform, and in ether.

NF requirements: Butylated Hydroxyanisole NF—Preserve in well-closed containers. Contains not less than 98.5% of butylated hydroxyanisole. Meets the requirements for Identification, Residue on ignition (not more than 0.01%, determined on a 10-gram specimen), Heavy metals (not more than 0.001%), and Organic volatile impurities.

BUTYLATED HYDROXYTOLUENE

Chemical name: Phenol, 2,6-bis(1,1-dimethylethyl)-4-methyl-.

Molecular formula: $C_{15}H_{24}O$.

Molecular weight: 220.35.

Description: Butylated Hydroxytoluene NF—White, crystalline solid, having a faint characteristic odor.
NF category: Antioxidant.

Solubility: Butylated Hydroxytoluene NF—Insoluble in water and in propylene glycol; freely soluble in alcohol, in chloroform, and in ether.

NF requirements: Butylated Hydroxytoluene NF—Preserve in well-closed containers. Contains not less than 99.0% of butylated hydroxytoluene. Meets the requirements for Identification, Congealing temperature (not less than 69.2 °C, corresponding to not less than 99.0% of butylated hydroxytoluene), Residue on ignition (not more than 0.002%), Heavy metals (not more than 0.001%), and Organic volatile impurities.

BUTYLPARABEN

Chemical name: Benzoic acid, 4-hydroxy-, butyl ester.

Molecular formula: $C_{11}H_{14}O_3$.

Molecular weight: 194.23.

Description: Butylparaben NF—Small, colorless crystals or white powder.
NF category: Antimicrobial preservative.

Solubility: Butylparaben NF—Very slightly soluble in water and in glycerin; freely soluble in acetone, in alcohol, in ether, and in propylene glycol.

NF requirements: Butylparaben NF—Preserve in well-closed containers. Contains not less than 99.0% and not more than 100.5% of butylparaben, calculated on the dried basis. Meets the requirements for Identification, Melting range (68–72 °C), Acidity, Loss on drying (not more than 0.5%), Residue on ignition (not more than 0.05%), and Organic volatile impurities.

CABERGOLIN

Chemical group: An ergoline (ergot alkaloid derivative).

Chemical name: Ergoline-8 beta-carboxamide, *N*-[3-(dimethylamino)propyl]-*N*-[(ethylamino)carbonyl]-6-(2-propenyl)-.

Molecular formula: $C_{26}H_{37}N_5O_2$.

Molecular weight: 451.60.

Description: A white powder. Melting point 102–104°.

Solubility: Soluble in ethyl alcohol, in chloroform, and N, N-dimethylformamide (DMF); slightly soluble in 0.1 *N* hydrochloric acid; very slightly soluble in hexane; soluble in water.

USP requirements: Cabergolin Tablets—Not in *USP–NF*.

CAFFEINE

Source: Coffee, tea, cola, and cocoa or chocolate. May also be synthesized from urea or dimethylurea.

Chemical group: Methylated xanthine.

Chemical name: 1*H*-Purine-2,6-dione, 3,7-dihydro-1,3,7-trimethyl-.

Molecular formula: $C_8H_{10}N_4O_2$ (anhydrous); $C_8H_{10}N_4O_2 \cdot H_2O$ (monohydrate).

Molecular weight: 194.19 (anhydrous); 212.21 (monohydrate).

Description: Caffeine USP—White powder or white, glistening needles, usually matted together. Is odorless. Its solutions are neutral to litmus. The hydrate is efflorescent in air.

Solubility: Caffeine USP—Sparingly soluble in water and in alcohol; freely soluble in chloroform; slightly soluble in ether.
The aqueous solubility of caffeine is increased by organic acids or their alkali salts, such as citrates, benzoates, salicylates, or cinnamates, which dissociate to yield caffeine when dissolved in biological fluids.

USP requirements:
Caffeine USP—Preserve hydrous Caffeine in tight containers. Preserve anhydrous Caffeine in well-closed containers. It is anhydrous or contains one molecule of water of hydration. Label it to indicate whether it is anhydrous or hydrous. Contains not less than 98.5% and not more than 101.0% of caffeine, calculated on the anhydrous basis. Meets the requirements for Identification, Melting range (235–239 °C), Water (not more than 0.5% for anhydrous and not more than 8.5% for hydrous), Residue on ignition (not more than 0.1%), Heavy metals (not more than 0.001%), Readily carbonizable substances, Other alkaloids, and Organic volatile impurities, and Chromatographic purity.
Caffeine Extended-release Capsules—Not in *USP–NF*.
Caffeine Powder—Not in *USP–NF*.
Caffeine Tablets—Not in *USP–NF*.
Caffeine Chewable Tablets—Not in *USP–NF*.

CITRATED CAFFEINE

Source: Caffeine—Coffee, tea, cola, and cocoa or chocolate. May also be synthesized from urea or dimethylurea.

Chemical group: Caffeine—Methylated xanthine.

Chemical name:
Caffeine—1*H*-Purine-2,6-dione, 3,7-dihydro-1,3,7-trimethyl-.
Citric acid—1,2,3-Propanetricarboxylic acid, 2-hydroxy-.

Molecular formula:
Caffeine—$C_8H_{10}N_4O_2$ (anhydrous); $C_8H_{10}N_4O_2 \cdot H_2O$ (monohydrate).
Citric acid—$C_6H_8O_7$ (anhydrous); $C_6H_8O_7 \cdot H_2O$ (monohydrate).

Molecular weight:
Caffeine—194.19 (anhydrous); 212.21 (monohydrate).
Citric acid—192.12 (anhydrous); 210.14 (monohydrate).

Description:
Caffeine USP—White powder or white, glistening needles, usually matted together. Is odorless. Its solutions are neutral to litmus. The hydrate is efflorescent in air.
Citric Acid USP—Colorless, translucent crystals, or white, granular to fine crystalline powder. Odorless or practically odorless. The hydrous form is efflorescent in dry air.
NF category: Acidifying agent; buffering agent.

Solubility:
Caffeine USP—Sparingly soluble in water and in alcohol; freely soluble in chloroform; slightly soluble in ether.
The aqueous solubility of caffeine is increased by organic acids or their alkali salts, such as citrates, benzoates, salicylates, or cinnamates, which dissociate to yield caffeine when dissolved in biological fluids.
Citric Acid USP—Very soluble in water; freely soluble in alcohol; very slightly soluble in ether.

USP requirements:
Citrated Caffeine Injection—Not in *USP–NF*.
Citrated Caffeine Solution—Not in *USP–NF*.
Citrated Caffeine Tablets—Not in *USP–NF*.

CAFFEINE AND SODIUM BENZOATE

For *Caffeine* and *Sodium Benzoate*—See individual listings for chemistry information.

USP requirements: Caffeine and Sodium Benzoate Injection USP—Preserve in single-dose containers, preferably of Type I glass. A sterile solution containing equal amounts of Caffeine and Sodium Benzoate in Water for Injection. Contains the labeled amounts of anhydrous caffeine and sodium benzoate, within −10% to +20%. Meets the requirements for Identification, Bacterial endotoxins, and pH (6.5–8.5), and for Injections.

CALAMINE

Chemical name: Iron oxide (Fe_2O_3), mixture with zinc oxide.

Description: Calamine USP—Pink, odorless, fine powder.

Solubility: Calamine USP—Insoluble in water; practically completely soluble in mineral acids.

USP requirements:
Calamine USP—Preserve in well-closed containers. It is Zinc Oxide with a small proportion of ferric oxide. Contains, after ignition, not less than 98.0% and not more than 100.5% of zinc oxide. Meets the requirements for Identification, Microbial limits, Loss on ignition (not more than 2.0%), Acid-insoluble substances (not more than 2.0%), Alkaline substances, Arsenic (not more than 8 ppm), Calcium, Calcium or magnesium, and Lead.
Calamine Lotion USP—Preserve in tight containers.
Prepare Calamine Lotion as follows: 80 grams of Calamine, 80 grams of Zinc Oxide, 20 mL of Glycerin, 250 mL of Bentonite Magma, and a sufficient quantity of Calcium Hydroxide Topical Solution to make 1000 mL. Dilute the Bentonite Magma with an equal volume of Calcium Hydroxide Topical Solution. Mix the powders intimately with the Glycerin and about 100 mL of the diluted magma, triturating until a smooth, uniform paste is formed. Gradually incorporate the remainder of the diluted magma. Finally add enough Calcium Hydroxide Solution to make 1000 mL, and shake. If a more viscous consistency in the Lotion is desired, the quantity of Bentonite Magma may be increased to not more than 400 mL.
Meets the requirement for Microbial limits.
Note: Shake Calamine Lotion before dispensing.
Calamine Ointment—Not in *USP–NF*.

PHENOLATED CALAMINE

USP requirements: Phenolated Calamine Lotion USP—Preserve in tight containers.

Prepare Phenolated Calamine Lotion as follows: 10 mL of Liquefied Phenol and 990 mL of Calamine Lotion, to make 1000 mL. Mix the ingredients.

Note: Shake Phenolated Calamine Lotion before dispensing.

CALCIFEDIOL

Chemical name: 9,10-Secocholesta-5,7,10(19)-triene-3,25-diol monohydrate, (3 beta,5Z,7E)-.

Molecular formula: $C_{27}H_{44}O_2 \cdot H_2O$.

Molecular weight: 418.65.

Description: A white powder. It has a melting point of about 105 °C.

Solubility: Practically insoluble in water; soluble in organic solvents.

USP requirements:
Calcifediol USP—Preserve in tight, light-resistant containers at controlled room temperature. Contains not less than 97.0% and not more than 103.0% of calcifediol. Meets the requirements for Identification, Water (3.8–5.0%, determined on a 0.2-gram specimen), and Organic volatile impurities.
Calcifediol Capsules USP—Preserve in tight, light-resistant containers. Contain the labeled amount, within −10% to +20%. Meet the requirements for Identification, Dissolution (in 15 minutes in water in Apparatus 2 at 50 rpm), and Uniformity of dosage units.

CALCIPOTRIENE

Chemical group: Vitamin D derivative.

Chemical name: 9,10-Secochola-5,7,10(19),22-tetraene-1,3,24-triol, 24-cyclopropyl-, (1 alpha,3 beta,5Z,7E,22E,24S)-.

Molecular formula: $C_{27}H_{40}O_3$.

Molecular weight: 412.60.

Description: White or off-white crystalline substance.

USP requirements:
Calcipotriene Cream—Not in *USP–NF*.
Calcipotriene Ointment—Not in *USP–NF*.
Calcipotriene Solution—Not in *USP–NF*.

CALCITONIN

Source:
Calcitonin—A polypeptide hormone secreted by the parafollicular cells of the thyroid gland in mammals and by the ultimobranchial gland of birds and fish.
Calcitonin-human—A synthetic polypeptide hormone of 32 amino acids in the same linear sequence found in naturally occurring human calcitonin and differing from salmon calcitonin at 16 of the amino acid sites.
Calcitonin-salmon—A synthetic polypeptide hormone of 32 amino acids in the same linear sequence found in calcitonin of salmon origin.

Chemical name: Calcitonin (source).

Molecular formula:
Calcitonin-human—$C_{151}H_{226}N_{40}O_{45}S_3$.
Calcitonin-salmon—$C_{145}H_{240}N_{44}O_{48}S_2$.

Molecular weight:
Calcitonin-human—3527.20.
Calcitonin-salmon—3431.88.

Description:
Calcitonin-human—White to off-white amorphous powder.
Calcitonin-salmon—White or almost white, light powder.

Solubility:
Calcitonin-human—Soluble in water, in physiological salt solution, in dilute acid, and in dilute base; sparingly soluble in methanol; practically insoluble in chloroform.
Calcitonin-salmon—Freely soluble in water.

USP requirements:
Calcitonin-Human for Injection—Not in *USP–NF*.
Calcitonin-Salmon Injection—Not in *USP–NF*.
Calcitonin-Salmon Nasal Solution—Not in *USP–NF*.

CALCITRIOL

Chemical name: 9,10-Secocholesta-5,7,10(19)-triene-1,3,25-triol, (1 alpha,3 beta,5Z,7E)-.

Molecular formula: $C_{27}H_{44}O_3$.

Molecular weight: 416.64.

Description: A practically white crystalline compound with a melting range of 111–115 °C.

Solubility: Insoluble in water; soluble in organic solvents.

USP requirements:
Calcitriol Capsules—Not in *USP–NF*.
Calcitriol Injection—Not in *USP–NF*.
Calcitriol Oral Solution—Not in *USP–NF*.

CALCIUM ACETATE

Chemical name: Acetic acid, calcium salt.

Molecular formula: $C_4H_6CaO_4$.

Molecular weight: 158.17.

Description: Calcium Acetate USP—White, odorless or almost odorless, hygroscopic crystalline powder. When heated to above 160 °C, it decomposes to calcium carbonate and acetone.

Solubility: Calcium Acetate USP—Freely soluble in water; slightly soluble in methanol; practically insoluble in acetone and in dehydrated alcohol.

USP requirements:
Calcium Acetate USP—Preserve in tight containers. Where Calcium Acetate is intended for use in hemodialysis or peritoneal dialysis it is so labeled. Contains not less than 99.0% and not more than 100.5% of calcium acetate, calculated on the anhydrous basis. Meets the requirements for Identification, pH (6.3–9.6, in a solution [1 in 20]), Water (not more than 7.0%), Limit of fluoride (not more than 0.005%), Arsenic (not more than 3 ppm), Heavy metals (not more than 0.0025%), Lead (not more than 0.001%), Chloride (not more than 0.05%), Sulfate (not more than 0.06%), Limit of nitrate, Limit of aluminum (where it is labeled as intended for parenteral use or for use in hemodialysis or peritoneal dialysis, not more than 2 mcg per gram), Barium (where it is labeled as intended for use in hemodia-

lysis or peritoneal dialysis), Magnesium (where it is labeled as intended for use in hemodialysis or peritoneal dialysis, not more than 0.05%), Potassium (where it is labeled as intended for use in hemodialysis or peritoneal dialysis, not more than 0.05%), Sodium (where it is labeled as intended for use in hemodialysis or peritoneal dialysis, not more than 0.5%), Strontium (where it is labeled as intended for use in hemodialysis or peritoneal dialysis, not more than 0.05%), Readily oxidizable substances, and Organic volatile impurities.

Calcium Acetate Injection—Not in *USP–NF*.

Calcium Acetate Tablets USP—Preserve in well-closed containers. Contain the labeled amount, within ±10%. Meet the requirements for Identification, Dissolution (80% in 30 minutes in water in Apparatus 2 at 50 rpm), Uniformity of dosage units, and Limit of aluminum.

CALCIUM ASCORBATE

Chemical name: Ascorbic acid calcium salt.

Molecular formula: $C_{12}H_{14}CaO_{12} \cdot 2H_2O$.

Molecular weight: 426.34.

Description: Calcium Ascorbate USP—White to slightly yellow, practically odorless powder.

Solubility: Calcium Ascorbate USP—Freely soluble in water (approximately 50 grams per 100 mL); slightly soluble in alcohol; insoluble in ether.

USP requirements: Calcium Ascorbate USP—Preserve in tight, light-resistant containers. Contains not less than 98.0% and not more than 101.0% of calcium ascorbate calculated on as-is basis. Meets the requirements for Identification, Specific rotation ($+95°$ to $+97°$), pH (6.8–7.4, in a solution [1 in 10]), Loss on drying (not more than 0.1%), Arsenic (3 mcg per gram), Fluoride (not more than 10 ppm), and Heavy metals (not more than 0.001%).

CALCIUM CARBONATE

Chemical name: Carbonic acid, calcium salt (1:1).

Molecular formula: $CaCO_3$.

Molecular weight: 100.09.

Description: Calcium Carbonate USP—Fine, white, odorless, tasteless microcrystalline powder. Is stable in air.

NF category: Tablet and/or capsule diluent.

Solubility: Calcium Carbonate USP—Practically insoluble in water. Its solubility in water is increased by the presence of any ammonium salt or of carbon dioxide. The presence of any alkali hydroxide reduces its solubility. Insoluble in alcohol. Dissolves with effervescence in 1 *N* acetic acid, in 3 *N* hydrochloric acid, and 2 *N* nitric acid.

USP requirements:
Calcium Carbonate USP—Preserve in well-closed containers. When dried at 200 °C for 4 hours, contains an amount of calcium equivalent to not less than 98.0% and not more than 100.5% of calcium carbonate. Meets the requirements for Identification, Loss on drying (not more than 2.0%), Acid-insoluble substances (not more than 0.2%), Limit of fluoride (not more than 0.005%), Arsenic (not more than 3 ppm), Barium, Lead (not more than 3 ppm), Iron (not more than 0.1%), Mercury (not more than 0.5 mcg per gram), Magnesium and alkali salts (not more than 1.0%), Heavy metals (not more than 0.002%), and Organic volatile impurities.

Calcium Carbonate Capsules—Not in *USP–NF*.

Calcium Carbonate Chewing Gum—Not in *USP–NF*.

Calcium Carbonate Lozenges USP—Preserve in well-closed containers. Contain the labeled amount, within ±10%. Meet the requirements for Identification, Uniformity of dosage units, Acid-neutralizing capacity, and Sodium content (the declared amount, within +15%).

Calcium Carbonate Oral Suspension USP—Preserve in tight containers, and avoid freezing. Contains the labeled amount, within ±10%. Meets the requirements for Identification, Microbial limits, and pH (7.5–8.7), and for Fluoride, Arsenic, Lead, and Heavy metals under Calcium Carbonate.

Calcium Carbonate Tablets USP—Preserve in well-closed containers. Label it to indicate whether it is for use as an antacid or as a dietary supplement, or both. Contain the labeled amount, within ±10%. For Tablets labeled for any indication other than, or in addition to, antacid use the Tablets contain the labeled amount, within –10% to +15%. Meet the requirements for Identification, Dissolution (75% in 30 minutes in 0.1 *N* hydrochloric acid in Apparatus 2 at 75 rpm, for Tablets labeled for any indication other than, or in addition to, antacid use), Uniformity of dosage units, and Acid-neutralizing capacity.

Calcium Carbonate (Oyster-shell derived) Tablets—Not in *USP–NF*.

Calcium Carbonate (Oyster-shell derived) Chewable Tablets—Not in *USP–NF*.

CALCIUM CARBONATE AND MAGNESIA

For *Calcium Carbonate* and *Magnesia* (Magnesium Hydroxide)—See individual listings for chemistry information.

USP requirements:
Calcium Carbonate and Magnesia Oral Suspension—Not in *USP–NF*.

Calcium Carbonate and Magnesia Tablets USP—Preserve in well-closed containers. Label the Tablets to indicate that they are to be chewed before being swallowed. Contain the labeled amount of calcium carbonate, within ±10%, and the labeled amount of magnesium hydroxide, within –10% to +15%. Meet the requirements for Identification, Uniformity of dosage units, and Acid-neutralizing capacity.

CALCIUM CARBONATE, MAGNESIA, AND SIMETHICONE

For *Calcium Carbonate, Magnesia* (Magnesium Hydroxide), and *Simethicone*—See individual listings for chemistry information.

USP requirements:
Calcium Carbonate, Magnesia, and Simethicone Oral Suspension—Not in USP.

Calcium Carbonate, Magnesia, and Simethicone Tablets USP—Preserve in well-closed containers. Label it to indicate that the Tablets are to be chewed before swallowing. Label the Tablets to state the sodium content, in mg per Tablet, if it is greater than 5 mg per Tablet. Contain the labeled amount of calcium carbonate, within ±10%, an amount of magnesia equivalent to the labeled amount of magnesium hydroxide, within ±10%, and an amount of polydimethylsiloxane equivalent to the labeled amount of simethicone, within ±15%. Meet the requirements for Identification, Uniformity of dosage units, Acid-neutralizing capacity, Defoaming activity (not more than 45 seconds),

and Sodium content (if so labeled, each tablet contains not more than the number of mg of sodium stated on the label).

CALCIUM AND MAGNESIUM CARBONATES

For *Calcium Carbonate* and *Magnesium Carbonate*—See individual listings for chemistry information.

USP requirements:
Calcium and Magnesium Carbonates Oral Suspension USP—Preserve in tight containers, and avoid freezing. Contains labeled amount of calcium carbonate, within ±10%, and labeled amount of magnesium carbonate, within ±15%. Meets the requirements for Identification, Microbial limits, Deliverable volume, pH (7.0–8.6), and Acid-neutralizing capacity.
Calcium and Magnesium Carbonates Tablets USP—Preserve in well-closed containers. Tablets that are gelatin-coated are so labeled. Contain the labeled amount of calcium carbonate, within ±10%, and the labeled amount of magnesium carbonate, within ±15%. Meet the requirements for Identification, Disintegration (10 minutes, except that where Tablets are labeled as gelatin-coated the time is 30 minutes. simulated gastric fluid TS being substituted for water in the test), Uniformity of dosage units, and Acid-neutralizing capacity.

CALCIUM AND MAGNESIUM CARBONATES AND SODIUM BICARBONATE

For *Calcium Carbonate,Magnesium Carbonate,* and *Sodium Bicarbonate*—See individual listings for chemistry information.

USP requirements: Calcium and Magnesium Carbonates and Sodium Bicarbonate Oral Suspension—Not in *USP–NF*.

CALCIUM CARBONATE AND SIMETHICONE

For *Calcium Carbonate* and *Simethicone*—See individual listings for chemistry information.

USP requirements:
Calcium Carbonate and Simethicone Oral Suspension—Not in *USP–NF*.
Calcium Carbonate and Simethicone Chewable Tablets—Not in *USP–NF*.

CALCIUM CHLORIDE

Chemical name: Calcium chloride, dihydrate.

Molecular formula: $CaCl_2 \cdot 2H_2O$.

Molecular weight: 147.01.

Description: Calcium Chloride USP—White, hard, odorless fragments or granules; deliquescent.
NF category: Desiccant.

Solubility: Calcium Chloride USP—Freely soluble in water, in alcohol, and in boiling alcohol; very soluble in boiling water.

USP requirements:
Calcium Chloride USP—Preserve in tight containers. Where Calcium Chloride is intended for use in hemodialysis, it is so labeled. Contains an amount of anhydrous calcium chloride equivalent to not less than 99.0% and not more than 107.0% of calcium chloride dihydrate. Meets the requirements for Identification, pH (4.5–9.2, in a solution [1 in 20]), Aluminum (where it is labeled as intended for use in hemodialysis, not more than 1 mcg per gram), Iron, aluminum, and phosphate, Heavy metals (not more than 0.001%), Magnesium and alkali salts (not more than 1.0%), and Organic volatile impurities.
Calcium Chloride Injection USP—Preserve in single-dose containers, preferably of Type I glass. A sterile solution of Calcium Chloride in Water for Injection. The label states the total osmolar concentration in mOsmol per liter. Where the contents are less than 100 mL, or where the label states that the Injection is not for direct injection but is to be diluted before use, the label alternatively may state the total osmolar concentration in mOsmol per mL. Contains the labeled amount, within ±5%. Meets the requirements for Identification, Bacterial endotoxins, pH (5.5–7.5 in the undiluted Injection), and Particulate matter, and for Injections.

CALCIUM CITRATE

Chemical name: 1,2,3-Propanetricarboxylic acid, 2-hydroxy-, calcium salt (2:3), tetrahydrate.

Molecular formula: $C_{12}H_{10}Ca_3O_{14} \cdot 4H_2O$.

Molecular weight: 570.49.

Description: Calcium Citrate USP—White, odorless, crystalline powder.

Solubility: Calcium Citrate USP—Slightly soluble in water; freely soluble in diluted 3 *N* hydrochloric acid and in diluted 2 *N* nitric acid; insoluble in alcohol.

USP requirements:
Calcium Citrate USP—Preserve in well-closed containers. Contains four molecules of water of hydration. When dried at 150 °C to constant weight, contains not less than 97.5% and not more than 100.5% of anhydrous calcium citrate. Meets the requirements for Identification, Loss on drying (10.0–13.3%), Arsenic (not more than 3 ppm), Limit of fluoride (not more than 0.003%), Acid-insoluble substances (not more than 0.2%), Lead (not more than 0.001%), Heavy metals (not more than 0.002%), and Organic volatile impurities.
Calcium Citrate Tablets—Not in *USP–NF*.
Calcium Citrate Effervescent Tablets—Not in *USP–NF*.

CALCIUM GLUBIONATE

Chemical name: Calcium, (4-*O*-beta-D-galactopyranosyl-D-gluconato-O¹)(D-gluconato-O¹)-, monohydrate.

Molecular formula: $C_{18}H_{32}CaO_{19} \cdot H_2O$.

Molecular weight: 610.53.

USP requirements: Calcium Glubionate Syrup USP—Preserve in tight containers, at a temperature not exceeding 30 °C, and avoid freezing. A solution containing equimolar amounts of Calcium Gluconate and Calcium Lactobionate or with Calcium Lactobionate predominating. Contains an amount of calcium

glubionate equivalent to the labeled amount of calcium, within ±5%. Meets the requirements for Identification and pH (3.4–4.5).

CALCIUM GLUCEPTATE

Chemical name: Glucoheptonic acid, calcium salt (2:1).

Molecular formula: $C_{14}H_{26}CaO_{16}$.

Molecular weight: 490.42.

Description: Calcium Gluceptate USP—White to faintly yellow, amorphous powder. Is stable in air, but the hydrous forms may lose part of their water of hydration on standing.

Solubility: Calcium Gluceptate USP—Freely soluble in water; insoluble in alcohol and in many other organic solvents.

USP requirements:
  Calcium Gluceptate USP—Preserve in well-closed containers. It is anhydrous or contains varying amounts of water of hydration. Consists of the calcium salt of the alpha epimer of glucoheptonic acid or of a mixture of the alpha and beta epimers of glucoheptonic acid. Label it to indicate whether it is hydrous or anhydrous; if hydrous, label it to indicate also the degree of hydration. Contains not less than 95.0% and not more than 102.0% of calcium gluceptate, calculated on the dried basis. Meets the requirements for Identification, pH (6.0–8.0, in a solution [1 in 10]), Loss on drying (not more than 1.0% for anhydrous, not more than 6.9% for $2H_2O$, and not more than 11.4% for $3\frac{1}{2}H_2O$), Chloride (not more than 0.07%), Sulfate (not more than 0.05%), Heavy metals (not more than 0.002%), Reducing sugars, and Organic volatile impurities.
  Calcium Gluceptate Injection USP—Preserve in tight, single-dose containers, preferably of Type I or Type II glass. A sterile solution of Calcium Gluceptate in Water for Injection. The label states the total osmolar concentration in mOsmol per liter. Where the contents are less than 100 mL, or where the label states that the Injection is not for direct injection but is to be diluted before use, the label alternatively may state the total osmolar concentration in mOsm per mL. Contains an amount of calcium gluceptate equivalent to the labeled amount of calcium, within ±5%. Meets the requirements for Identification, Bacterial endotoxins, pH (5.6–7.0), and Particulate matter, and for Injections.

CALCIUM GLUCEPTATE AND CALCIUM GLUCONATE

For *Calcium Gluceptate* and *Calcium Gluconate*—See individual listings for chemistry information.

USP requirements: Calcium Gluceptate and Calcium Gluconate Oral Solution—Not in *USP–NF*.

CALCIUM GLUCONATE

Chemical name: D-Gluconic acid, calcium salt (2:1).

Molecular formula: $C_{12}H_{22}CaO_{14}$.

Molecular weight: 430.37.

Description: Calcium Gluconate USP—White, crystalline, odorless granules or powder. Is stable in air. Its solutions are neutral to litmus.

Solubility: Calcium Gluconate USP—Sparingly (and slowly) soluble in water; freely soluble in boiling water; insoluble in alcohol.

USP requirements:
  Calcium Gluconate USP—Preserve in well-closed containers. It is anhydrous or contains one molecule of water of hydration. Label it to indicate whether it is the anhydrous or the monohydrate. Where the quantity of calcium gluconate is indicated in the labeling of any preparation containing Calcium Gluconate, this shall be understood to be in terms of anhydrous calcium gluconate. Calcium Gluconate intended for use in preparing injectable dosage forms is so labeled. Calcium Gluconate not intended for use in preparing injectable dosage forms is so labeled; in addition, it may be labeled also as intended for use in preparing oral dosage forms. The anhydrous form contains not less than 98.0% and not more than 102.0% of calcium gluconate, calculated on the dried basis. The monohydrate form contains not less than 99.0% and not more than 101.0% of calcium gluconate (monohydrate) where labeled as intended for use in preparing injectable dosage forms, and not less than 98.5% and not more than 102.0% of calcium gluconate (monohydrate) where labeled as not intended for use in preparing injectable dosage forms. Meets the requirements for Identification, Loss on drying (for the anhydrous, not more than 3.0%; for the monohydrate, where labeled as intended for use in preparing injectable dosage forms, not more than 1.0% and where labeled as not intended for use in preparing injectable dosage forms, not more than 2.0%), Chloride (not more than 0.005%, and where labeled as not intended for use in preparation of injectable dosage forms, not more than 0.07%), Limit of oxalate (not more than 0.01% [Note: Calcium Gluconate labeled as not intended for use in preparation of injectable dosage forms is exempt from this requirement]), Limit of phosphate (not more than 0.01% [Note: Calcium Gluconate labeled as not intended for use in preparation of injectable dosage forms is exempt from this requirement]), Sulfate (not more than 0.005%, and where labeled as not intended for use in preparation of injectable dosage forms, not more than 0.05%), Arsenic (not more than 3 ppm), Heavy metals (not more than 0.001% [Note: Where Calcium Gluconate is labeled as not intended for use in preparation of injectable dosage forms, not more than 0.002%]), Limit of magnesium and alkali metals (not more than 0.4% [Note: Calcium Gluconate labeled as not intended for use in preparing injectable dosage forms is exempt from this requirement]), Limit of iron (not more than 5 ppm [Note: Calcium Gluconate labeled as not intended for use in preparation of injectable dosage forms is exempt from this requirement]), Reducing substances (not more than 1.0%), and Organic volatile impurities.
  Calcium Gluconate Gel—Not in *USP–NF*.
  Calcium Gluconate Injection USP—Preserve in single-dose containers, preferably of Type I glass. A sterile solution of Calcium Gluconate in Water for Injection. Label the Injection to indicate its content, if any, of added calcium salts, calculated as percentage of calcium in the Injection. The label states the total osmolar concentration in mOsmol per liter. Where the contents are less than 100 mL, or where the label states that the Injection is not for direct injection but is to be diluted before use, the label alternatively may state the total osmolar concentration in mOsmol per mL. The labeling indicates that the Injection must be clear at the time of use, and that if crystallization has occurred, warming may redissolve the precipitate. Injection intended for veterinary use only is so labeled. If Injection contains Boric Acid, it is so labeled. Contains the amount of total calcium, within ±5%. The calcium is in the form of calcium gluconate, except that a small amount may be replaced with an equal amount of calcium in the form of Calcium Saccharate, or other suitable calcium salts, for the purpose of stabilization. Injection intended for veterinary

use only may be prepared from Calcium Gluconate solubilized with Boric Acid, or from Glyconolactone, Boric Acid, and Calcium Carbonate. Meets the requirements for Identification, Bacterial endotoxins, pH (6.0–8.2, except that in the case where it is labeled as intended for veterinary use only and as containing boric acid, it is between 2.5 and 4.5), and Particulate matter, and for Injections.

Calcium Gluconate Tablets USP—Preserve in well-closed containers. Contain the labeled amount, within ±5%. Meet the requirements for Identification, Dissolution (75% in 45 minutes in water in Apparatus 2 at 50 rpm), and Uniformity of dosage units.

Calcium Gluconate Chewable Tablets–Not in *USP–NF*.

CALCIUM GLYCEROPHOSPHATE AND CALCIUM LACTATE

Chemical name:
  Calcium glycerophosphate—1,2,3-Propanetriol, mono(dihydrogen phosphate) calcium salt (1:1).
  Calcium lactate—Propanoic acid, 2-hydroxy-, calcium salt (2:1), hydrate.

Molecular formula:
  Calcium glycerophosphate—$C_3H_7CaO_6P$.
  Calcium lactate—$C_6H_{10}CaO_6 \cdot 5H_2O$ (pentahydrate); $C_6H_{10}CaO_6 \cdot {}_xH_2O$ (anhydrous).

Molecular weight:
  Calcium glycerophosphate—210.15.
  Calcium lactate—308.30 (pentahydrate); 218.22 (anhydrous).

Description:
  Calcium glycerophosphate—Fine, odorless, slightly hygroscopic powder.
  Calcium Lactate USP—White, practically odorless granules or powder. The pentahydrate is somewhat efflorescent and at 120 °C becomes anhydrous.

Solubility:
  Calcium glycerophosphate—Soluble in about 50 parts of water; almost insoluble in alcohol and in boiling water.
  Calcium Lactate USP—The pentahydrate is soluble in water; practically insoluble in alcohol.

USP requirements: Calcium Glycerophosphate and Calcium Lactate Injection—Not in *USP–NF*.

CALCIUM HYDROXIDE

Chemical name: Calcium hydroxide.

Molecular formula: $Ca(OH)_2$.

Molecular weight: 74.09.

Description:
  Calcium Hydroxide USP—White powder.
  Calcium Hydroxide Solution USP—Clear, colorless liquid. Is alkaline to litmus.

Solubility: Calcium Hydroxide USP—Slightly soluble in water; soluble in glycerin and in syrup; very slightly soluble in boiling water; insoluble in alcohol.

USP requirements:
  Calcium Hydroxide USP—Preserve in tight containers. Contains not less than 95.0% and not more than 100.5% of calcium hydroxide. Meets the requirements for Identification, Acid-insoluble substances (not more than 0.5%), Carbonate, Heavy metals (not more than 20 mcg per gram), Magnesium and alkali salts (not more than 4.8%), and Organic volatile impurities.

Calcium Hydroxide Topical Solution USP—Preserve in well-filled, tight containers, at a temperature not exceeding 25 °C. A solution containing, in each 100 mL, not less than 140 mg of Calcium Hydroxide.

Prepare Calcium Hydroxide Topical Solution as follows: 3 grams of Calcium Hydroxide and 1000 mL of Purified Water. Add the Calcium Hydroxide to 1000 mL of cool Purified Water, and agitate the mixture vigorously and repeatedly during 1 hour. Allow the excess calcium hydroxide to settle. Dispense only the clear, supernatant liquid.

Meets the requirements for Identification and Alkalies and their carbonates.

Note: The solubility of calcium hydroxide varies with the temperature at which the solution is stored, being about 170 mg per 100 mL at 15 °C, and less at a higher temperature. The official concentration is based upon a temperature of 25 °C. The undissolved portion of the mixture is not suitable for preparing additional quantities of Calcium Hydroxide Topical Solution.

CALCIUM LACTATE

Chemical name: Propanoic acid, 2-hydroxy-, calcium salt (2:1), hydrate.

Molecular formula: $C_6H_{10}CaO_6 \cdot 5H_2O$ (pentahydrate); $C_6H_{10}CaO_6 \cdot {}_xH_2O$ (anhydrous).

Molecular weight: 308.30 (pentahydrate); 218.22 (anhydrous).

Description: Calcium Lactate USP—White, practically odorless granules or powder. The pentahydrate is somewhat efflorescent and at 120 °C becomes anhydrous.

Solubility: Calcium Lactate USP—The pentahydrate is soluble in water; practically insoluble in alcohol.

USP requirements:
  Calcium Lactate USP—Preserve in tight containers. The label indicates whether it is the dried form or is hydrous; if the latter, the label indicates the degree of hydration. Where the quantity of Calcium Lactate is indicated in the labeling of any preparation containing Calcium Lactate, this shall be understood to be in terms of calcium lactate pentahydrate. Contains not less than 98.0% and not more than 101.0% of calcium lactate, calculated on the dried basis. Meets the requirements for Identification, Acidity, Loss on drying (22.0–27.0% for pentahydrate, 15.0–20.0% for trihydrate, 5.0–8.0% for monohydrate, and not more than 3.0% for dried form), Heavy metals (not more than 0.002%), Magnesium and alkali salts (not more than 1.0%), Volatile fatty acid, and Organic volatile impurities.
  Calcium Lactate Tablets USP—Preserve in tight containers. The quantity of calcium lactate stated in the labeling is in terms of calcium lactate pentahydrate. Contain the labeled amount, within ±6%. Meet the requirements for Identification, Dissolution (75% in 45 minutes in water in Apparatus 1 at 100 rpm), and Uniformity of dosage units.

Note: An equivalent amount of Calcium Lactate with less water of hydration may be used in place of calcium lactate pentahydrate in preparing Calcium Lactate Tablets.

CALCIUM LACTATE-GLUCONATE AND CALCIUM CARBONATE

Chemical name: Calcium carbonate—Carbonic acid, calcium salt (1:1).

Molecular formula: Calcium carbonate—$CaCO_3$.

Molecular weight: Calcium carbonate—100.09.

Description: Calcium Carbonate USP—Fine, white, odorless, microcrystalline powder. Is stable in air.

NF category: Tablet and/or capsule diluent.

Solubility: Calcium Carbonate USP—Practically insoluble in water. Its solubility in water is increased by the presence of any ammonium salt or of carbon dioxide. The presence of any alkali hydroxide reduces its solubility. Insoluble in alcohol. Dissolves with effervescence in 1 *N* acetic acid, in 3 *N* hydrochloric acid, and 2 *N* nitric acid.

USP requirements: Calcium Lactate-Gluconate and Calcium Carbonate Effervescent Tablets—Not in *USP–NF*.

CALCIUM LACTOBIONATE

Chemical name: D-Gluconic acid, 4-*O*-beta-D-galactopyranosyl-, calcium salt (2:1), dihydrate.

Molecular formula: $C_{24}H_{42}CaO_{24} \cdot 2H_2O$.

Molecular weight: 790.68.

USP requirements: Calcium Lactobionate USP—Preserve in well-closed containers. Contains not less than 96.0% and not more than 102.0% of calcium lactobionate. Meets the requirements for Identification, Specific rotation (+22.0° to +26.5°), pH (5.4–7.4, in a solution [1 in 20]), Halides (not more than 0.04%), Sulfate (not more than 0.05%), Heavy metals (not more than 0.002%), Reducing substances (not more than 1.0%), and Organic volatile impurities.

CALCIUM LEVULINATE

Chemical name: Pentanoic acid, 4-oxo-, calcium salt (2:1), dihydrate.

Molecular formula: $C_{10}H_{14}CaO_6 \cdot 2H_2O$.

Molecular weight: 306.32.

Description: Calcium Levulinate USP—White, crystalline or amorphous, powder, having a faint odor suggestive of burnt sugar.

Solubility: Calcium Levulinate USP—Freely soluble in water; slightly soluble in alcohol; insoluble in ether and in chloroform.

USP requirements:
Calcium Levulinate USP—Preserve in well-closed containers. Contains not less than 97.5% and not more than 100.5% of calcium levulinate, calculated on the dried basis. Meets the requirements for Identification, Melting range (119–125 °C), pH 7.0–8.5, in a solution [1 in 10]), Loss on drying (10.5–12.0%), Chloride (not more than 0.07%), Sulfate (not more than 0.05%), Heavy metals (not more than 0.002%), Reducing sugars, and Organic volatile impurities.
Calcium Levulinate Injection USP—Preserve in single-dose containers, preferably of Type I glass. A sterile solution of Calcium Levulinate in Water for Injection. The label states the total osmolar concentration in mOsmol per liter. Where the contents are less than 100 mL, or where the label states that the Injection is not for direct injection but is to be diluted before use, the label alternatively may state the total osmolar concentration in mOsmol per mL. Con-

tains the labeled amount, within ±5%. Meets the requirements for Identification, Bacterial endotoxins, pH (6.0–8.0), and Particulate matter, and for Injections.

CALCIUM PANTOTHENATE

Chemical name: Beta-alanine, *N*-(2,4-dihydroxy-3,3-dimethyl-1-oxobutyl)-, calcium salt (2:1), (*R*)-.

Molecular formula: $C_{18}H_{32}CaN_2O_{10}$.

Molecular weight: 476.53.

Description: Calcium Pantothenate USP—Slightly hygroscopic, white powder. Odorless.

Solubility: Calcium Pantothenate USP—Freely soluble in water; soluble in glycerin; practically insoluble in alcohol, in chloroform, and in ether.

USP requirements:
Calcium Pantothenate USP—Preserve in tight containers. The calcium salt of the dextrorotatory isomer of pantothenic acid. Contains not less than 5.7% and not more than 6.0% of nitrogen, and not less than 8.2% and not more than 8.6% of calcium, both calculated on the dried basis. Meets the requirements for Identification, Specific rotation (+25.0° to +27.5°), Alkalinity, Loss on drying (not more than 5.0%), Heavy metals (not more than 0.002%), Ordinary impurities (not more than 1.0%), Organic volatile impurities, Nitrogen content, and Calcium content.
Calcium Pantothenate Tablets USP—Preserve in tight containers. Label the Tablets to indicate the content of dextrorotatory calcium pantothenate. Contain the labeled amount of the dextrorotatory isomer of Calcium Pantothenate, within –5% to +15%. Meet the requirements for Identification, Dissolution (75% in 45 minutes in water in Apparatus 2 at 50 rpm), Uniformity of dosage units, and Calcium content.

RACEMIC CALCIUM PANTOTHENATE

Chemical name: Beta-alanine, *N*-(2,4-dihydroxy-3,3-dimethyl-1-oxobutyl)-, calcium salt (2:1), (±)-.

Molecular formula: $C_{18}H_{32}CaN_2O_{10}$.

Molecular weight: 476.53.

Description: Racemic Calcium Pantothenate USP—White, slightly hygroscopic powder, having a faint, characteristic odor. Is stable in air. Its solutions are neutral or alkaline to litmus. Is optically inactive.

Solubility: Racemic Calcium Pantothenate USP—Freely soluble in water; soluble in glycerin; practically insoluble in alcohol, in chloroform, and in ether.

USP requirements: Racemic Calcium Pantothenate USP—Preserve in tight containers. A mixture of the calcium salts of the dextrorotatory and levorotatory isomers of pantothenic acid. Label preparations containing it in terms of the equivalent amount of dextrorotatory calcium pantothenate. Contains not less than 5.7% and not more than 6.0% of nitrogen, and not less than 8.2% and not more than 8.6% of calcium, both calculated on the dried basis. Meets the requirements for Specific rotation (–0.05° to +0.05°), Alkalinity, and Organic volatile impurities, and for Identification tests, Loss on drying, Heavy metals, Nitrogen content, and Calcium content under Calcium Pantothenate.

Note: The physiological activity of Racemic Calcium Pantothenate is approximately one-half that of Calcium Pantothenate.

DIBASIC CALCIUM PHOSPHATE

Chemical name: Phosphoric acid, calcium salt (1:1).

Molecular formula: $CaHPO_4$ (anhydrous); $CaHPO_4 \cdot 2H_2O$ (dihydrate).

Molecular weight: 136.06 (anhydrous); 172.09 (dihydrate).

Description: Dibasic Calcium Phosphate USP—White, odorless powder; stable in air.
   NF category: Tablet and/or capsule diluent.

Solubility: Dibasic Calcium Phosphate USP—Practically insoluble in water; soluble in 3 *N* hydrochloric acid and in 2 *N* nitric acid; insoluble in alcohol.

USP requirements:
   Dibasic Calcium Phosphate USP—Preserve in well-closed containers. It is anhydrous or contains two molecules of water of hydration. Label it to indicate whether it is anhydrous or the dihydrate. Contains not less than 98.0% and not more than 105.0% of anhydrous dibasic calcium phosphate or of dibasic calcium phosphate dihydrate. Meets the requirements for Identification, Loss on ignition (6.6–8.5% for anhydrous Dibasic Calcium Phosphate and 24.5–26.5% for dihydrate form of Dibasic Calcium Phosphate), Limit of acid-insoluble substances (not more than 0.2%), Carbonate, Chloride (not more than 0.25%), Limit of fluoride (not more than 0.005%), Sulfate (not more than 0.5%), Arsenic (not more than 3 ppm), Barium, Heavy metals (not more than 0.003%), and Organic volatile impurities.
   Dibasic Calcium Phosphate Tablets USP—Preserve in well-closed containers. The quantity of dibasic calcium phosphate stated in the labeling is in terms of Dibasic Calcium Phosphate dihydrate. Contain the labeled amount, within ±7.5%. Meet the requirements for Identification, Dissolution (75% in 45 minutes in 0.1 *N* hydrochloric acid in Apparatus 2 at 75 rpm), and Uniformity of dosage units.
      Note: An equivalent amount of Dibasic Calcium Phosphate with less water of hydration may be used in place of Dibasic Calcium Phosphate dihydrate in preparing Dibasic Calcium Phosphate Tablets.

TRIBASIC CALCIUM PHOSPHATE

Chemical name: Calcium hydroxide phosphate $(Ca_5(OH)(PO_4)_3)$.

Molecular formula: $Ca_5(OH)(PO_4)_3$.

Molecular weight: 502.31.

Description: Tribasic Calcium Phosphate NF—White, odorless, powder. Is stable in air.
   NF category: Tablet and/or capsule diluent.

Solubility: Tribasic Calcium Phosphate NF—Practically insoluble in water; readily soluble in 3 *N* hydrochloric acid and in 2 *N* nitric acid; insoluble in alcohol.

USP requirements: Tribasic Calcium Phosphate Tablets—Not in *USP–NF*.

NF requirements: Tribasic Calcium Phosphate NF—Preserve in well-closed containers. Consists of a variable mixture of calcium phosphates having the approximate composition $10CaO \cdot 3P_2O_5 \cdot H_2O$. Contains an amount of tribasic calcium phosphate equivalent to not less than 34.0% and not more than 40.0% of calcium. Meets the requirements for Identification, Loss on ignition (not more than 8.0%), Water-soluble substances (not more than 0.5%), Acid-insoluble substances (not more than 0.2%), Carbonate, Chloride (not more than 0.14%), Sulfate (not more than 0.8%), Arsenic (not more than 3 ppm), Barium, Dibasic salt and calcium oxide, Limit of fluoride (not more than 0.0075%), Limit of nitrate, and Heavy metals (not more than 0.003%).

CALCIUM POLYCARBOPHIL

Chemical name: Calcium polycarbophil.

Description: Calcium Polycarbophil USP—White to creamy white powder.

Solubility: Calcium Polycarbophil USP—Insoluble in water, in dilute acids, in dilute alkalies, and in common organic solvents.

USP requirements:
   Calcium Polycarbophil USP—Preserve in tight containers. The calcium salt of polyacrylic acid cross-linked with divinyl glycol. Meets the requirements for Identification, Loss on drying (not more than 10.0%), Absorbing power, Calcium content (18.0–22.0%, calculated on the dried basis), and Organic volatile impurities.
   Calcium Polycarbophil Tablets—Not in *USP–NF*.
   Calcium Polycarbophil Chewable Tablets—Not in *USP–NF*.

CALCIUM SACCHARATE

Chemical name: D-Glucaric acid, calcium salt (1:1) tetrahydrate.

Molecular formula: $C_6H_8CaO_8 \cdot 4H_2O$.

Molecular weight: 320.26.

Description: Calcium Saccharate USP—White, odorless, crystalline powder.

Solubility: Calcium Saccharate USP—Very slightly soluble in cold water; slightly soluble in boiling water; very slightly soluble in alcohol; practically insoluble in ether and in chloroform; soluble in dilute mineral acids and in solutions of calcium gluconate.

USP requirements: Calcium Saccharate USP—Preserve in well-closed containers. The calcium salt of D-saccharic acid. Contains not less than 98.5% and not more than 102.0% of calcium saccharate. Meets the requirements for Identification, Specific rotation (+18.5° to +22.5°), Chloride (not more than 0.07%), Sulfate (not more than 0.12%), Heavy metals (not more than 0.002%), Sucrose and reducing sugars, and Organic volatile impurities.

CALCIUM SILICATE

Description: Calcium Silicate NF—White to off-white, free-flowing powder that remains so after absorbing relatively large amounts of water or other liquids.
   NF category: Glidant and/or anticaking agent.

Solubility: Calcium Silicate NF—Insoluble in water. Forms a gel with mineral acids.

NF requirements: Calcium Silicate NF—Preserve in well-closed containers. A compound of calcium oxide and silicon dioxide. The labeling states the claimed percentage or range of percentages for the content of calcium oxide and for the content of silicon dioxide. Contains not less than 4.0% of calcium oxide

and not less than 45.0% of silicon dioxide. Meets the requirements for Identification, pH (8.4–10.2, determined in a well-mixed aqueous suspension [1 in 20]), Loss on ignition (not more than 20.0%), Lead (not more than 0.001%), Heavy metals (not more than 20 mcg per gram), Limit of fluoride (not more than 10 mcg per gram), Ratio of silicon dioxide to calcium oxide (quotient 1.3–20), and Sum of calcium oxide, silicon dioxide, and Loss on ignition (sum of percentages of three tests not less than 90.0%).

CALCIUM STEARATE

Chemical name: Octadecanoic acid, calcium salt.

Molecular formula: $C_{36}H_{70}CaO_4$.

Molecular weight: 607.00.

Description: Calcium Stearate NF—Fine, white to yellowish white, bulky powder having a slight, characteristic odor. Is unctuous, and is free from grittiness.
  NF category: Tablet and/or capsule lubricant.

Solubility: Calcium Stearate NF—Insoluble in water, in alcohol, and in ether.

NF requirements: Calcium Stearate NF—Preserve in well-closed containers. A compound of calcium with a mixture of solid organic acids obtained from fats, consisting chiefly of variable proportions of calcium stearate and calcium palmitate. Contains the equivalent of not less than 9.0% and not more than 10.5% of calcium oxide. Meets the requirements for Identification, Loss on drying (not more than 4.0%), Heavy metals (not more than 10 mcg per gram), and Organic volatile impurities.

CALCIUM SULFATE

Chemical name: Sulfuric acid, calcium salt (1:1).

Molecular formula: $CaSO_4$.

Molecular weight: 136.14.

Description: Calcium Sulfate NF—Fine, white to slightly yellow-white, odorless powder.
  NF category: Desiccant; tablet and/or capsule diluent.

Solubility: Calcium Sulfate NF—Slightly soluble in water; soluble in 3 N hydrochloric acid.

NF requirements: Calcium Sulfate NF—Preserve in well-closed containers. It is anhydrous or contains two molecules of water of hydration. Label it to indicate whether it is anhydrous or the dihydrate. Contains not less than 98.0% and not more than 101.0% of calcium sulfate, calculated on the dried basis. Meets the requirements for Identification, Loss on drying (not more than 1.5% for anhydrous and 19.0–23.0% for dihydrate), Iron (not more than 0.01%), and Heavy metals (not more than 0.001%).

CALCIUM UNDECYLENATE

Chemical name: 10-Undecenoic acid, calcium(2+) salt.

Molecular formula: $C_{22}H_{38}O_4Ca$.

Molecular weight: 406.61.

Description: Calcium Undecylenate USP—Fine, white powder, having a characteristic odor and no grit.

Solubility: Calcium Undecylenate USP—Practically insoluble in water, in ether, in chloroform, in acetone, and in cold alcohol; slightly soluble in hot alcohol.

USP requirements: Calcium Undecylenate USP—Preserve in well-closed containers. Contains not less than 98.0% and not more than 102.0% of calcium undecylenate, calculated on the dried basis. Meets the requirements for Identification, Loss on drying (2.0–5.7%), Particle size (not less than 99.0% of it passes through a No. 100 sieve), and Free undecylenic acid (not more than 0.1%).

CALCIUM WITH VITAMIN D

USP requirements: Calcium with Vitamin D Tablets USP—Preserve in tight, light-resistant containers. The label states that the product is Calcium with Vitamin D Tablets. The label states also the quantities of calcium and Vitamin D in terms of metric units per Tablet, and the salt form of calcium and the chemical form of Vitamin D present in the Tablet. Contain the labeled amount of calcium, derived from substances generally recognized as safe, within −10% to +25%, and the labeled amount of Vitamin D, as cholecalciferol or ergocalciferol, within −10% to +65%. Contain no other vitamins or minerals for which nutritional value is claimed. May contain other labeled added substances or additional ingredients in amounts that are unobjectionable. Meet the requirements for Microbial limits, Disintegration and dissolution (75% of labeled amount of calcium in 30 minutes in 0.1 N hydrochloric acid in Apparatus 2 at 75 rpm), and Weight variation.

CALCIUM, VITAMIN D, AND MINERALS

USP requirements: Calcium and Vitamin D with Minerals Tablets USP—Preserve in tight, light-resistant containers. Contain Vitamin D as Ergocalciferol (Vitamin D_2) or Cholecalciferol (Vitamin D_3), Calcium, and one or more minerals derived from substances generally recognized as safe, furnishing one or more of the following elements in ionizable form: copper, magnesium, manganese, and zinc. The label states that the product is Calcium and Vitamin D with Minerals Tablets. The label also states the quantities of each mineral and vitamin D per dosage unit, the salt form of the mineral used as the source of each element present, and the chemical form of vitamin D present in the dosage unit. Contain the labeled amount of Vitamin D as cholecalciferol or ergocalciferol, within −10% to +65% and a labeled amount of calcium, copper, magnesium, manganese, and zinc, within −10% to +25%. May contain other labeled added substances that are generally recognized as safe, in amounts that are unobjectionable. Meet the requirements for Microbial limits, Disintigration and dissolution, and Weight variation.

CALFACTANT

Source: Natural. Extract of natural surfactant from calf lungs.

Chemical name: Calfactant.

Other characteristics: pH of a 0.9% aqueous sodium chloride solution is 5.0–6.0.

USP requirements: Calfactant Intratracheal Suspension—Not in *USP–NF*.

CAMPHOR

Chemical name: Bicyclo[2.2.1]heptane-2-one, 1,7,7-trimethyl-.

Molecular formula: $C_{10}H_{16}O$.

Molecular weight: 152.23.

Description: Camphor USP—Colorless or white crystals, granules, or crystalline masses; or colorless to white, translucent, tough masses. Has a penetrating, characteristic odor. Specific gravity is about 0.99. Slowly volatilizes at ordinary temperatures.

Solubility: Camphor USP—Slightly soluble in water; very soluble in alcohol, in chloroform, and in ether; freely soluble in carbon disulfide, in solvent hexane, and in fixed and volatile oils.

USP requirements:
Camphor USP—Preserve in tight containers, and avoid exposure to excessive heat. A ketone obtained from *Cinnamomum camphora* (Linné) Nees et Ebermaier (Fam. Lauraceae) (Natural Camphor) or produced synthetically (Synthetic Camphor). Label it to indicate whether it is obtained from natural sources or is prepared synthetically. Meets the requirements for Melting range (174–179 °C), Specific rotation (+41° to +43° for natural Camphor), Water, Limit of nonvolatile residue (not more than 0.05%), and Halogens (not more than 0.035%).
Camphor Spirit USP—Preserve in tight containers. An alcohol solution containing, in each 100 mL, not less than 9.0 grams and not more than 11.0 grams of camphor.
Prepare Camphor Spirit as follows: 100 grams of Camphor and a sufficient quantity of alcohol to make 1000 mL. Dissolve the camphor in about 800 mL of the alcohol, and add alcohol to make 1000 mL. Filter, if necessary.
Meets the requirement for Alcohol content (80.0–87.0%, the dilution to approximately 2% alcohol being made with methanol instead of with water).

CANDESARTAN CILEXETIL

Chemical name: 1*H*-Benzimidazole-7-carboxylic acid, 2-ethoxy-1-[[2'-(1*H*-tetrazole-5-yl)[1,1'biphenyl]-4-yl]methyl]-, 1-[[(cyclohexyloxy)carbonyl]oxy]ethyl ester, (±)-.

Molecular formula: $C_{33}H_{34}N_6O_6$.

Molecular weight: 610.66.

Description: Candesartan cilexetil—White to off-white powder.

Solubility: Candesartan cilexetil—Practically insoluble in water; sparingly soluble in methanol.

USP requirements: Candesartan Cilexetil Tablets—Not in *USP–NF*.

CANDESARTAN AND HYDROCHLOROTHIAZIDE

For *Candesartan* and *Hydrochlorothiazide*—See individual listings for chemistry information.

USP requirements: Candesartan Cilexetil and Hydrochlorothiazide Tablets—Not in *USP–NF*.

CANDICIDIN

Chemical name: Candicidin.

Description: Candicidin USP—Yellow to brown powder.

Solubility: Candicidin USP—Sparingly soluble in water; very slightly soluble in alcohol, in acetone, and in butyl alcohol.

USP requirements:
Candicidin USP—Preserve in tight containers, in a refrigerator. A substance produced by the growth of *Streptomyces griseus* Waksman et Henrici (Fam. Streptomycetaceae). Has a potency of not less than 1000 mcg per mg, calculated on the dried basis. Meets the requirements for Identification, pH (8.0–10.0, in an aqueous suspension containing 10 mg per mL), and Loss on drying (not more than 4.0%).
Candicidin Ointment USP—Preserve in well-closed containers, in a refrigerator. Contains the labeled amount, within −10% to +40%. Meets the requirements for Minimum fill and Water (not more than 0.1%).
Candicidin Vaginal Tablets USP—Preserve in tight containers, in a refrigerator. Contain the labeled amount, within −10% to +50%. Meet the requirements for Disintegration (30 minutes) and Loss on drying (not more than 1.0%).

CAPECITABINE

Chemical name: Carbonic acid, [1-(5-deoxy-beta-D-ribofuranosyl)-5-fluoro-1,2-dihydro-2-oxo-4-pyrimidinyl]-, pentyl ester.

Molecular formula: $C_{15}H_{22}FN_3O_6$.

Molecular weight: 259.35.

Description: Capecitabine—White to off-white crystalline powder.

Solubility: Capecitabine—Soluble in 26 mg per mL water at 20 °C.

USP requirements: Capecitabine Tablets—Not in *USP–NF*.

CAPREOMYCIN

Source: A complex of four microbiologically active components derived from *Streptomyces capreolus*.

Chemical name: Capreomycin sulfate.

Description: Capreomycin Sulfate USP—White to practically white, amorphous powder.

Solubility: Capreomycin Sulfate USP—Freely soluble in water; practically insoluble in most organic solvents.

USP requirements:
Capreomycin Sulfate USP—Preserve in tight containers. The disulfate salt of capreomycin, a polypeptide mixture produced by the growth of *Streptomyces capreolus*, suitable for parenteral use. Where it is intended for use in preparing injectable dosage forms, the label states that it is sterile or must be subjected to further processing during the preparation of injectable dosage forms. Has a potency equivalent to not less than 700 mcg and not more than 1050 mcg of capreomycin per mg. Meets the requirements for Identification, pH (4.5–7.5, in a solution containing 30 mg per mL), Loss on drying (not more than 10.0%), Residue on ignition (not more than 3.0%), Heavy metals (not more than 0.003%), and Capreomycin I content (not less than 90.0%), for and Bacterial endotoxins under Capreomycin for Injection (where the label states that Capreomycin Sulfate is sterile), and for Bacterial endotoxins under

Capreomycin for Injection (where the label states that Capreomycin Sulfate must be subjected to further processing during the preparation of injectable dosage forms).

Capreomycin for Injection USP—Preserve in Containers for Sterile Solids. Contains an amount of Capreomycin Sulfate equivalent to the labeled amount of capreomycin, within −10% to +15%. Meets the requirements for Constituted solution, Depressor substances, Bacterial endotoxins, and pH (4.5–7.5, in a solution containing 30 mg per mL), for Identification, Loss on drying, Residue on ignition, Heavy metals, and Capreomycin I content under Capreomycin Sulfate, and for Injections.

CAPSAICIN

Source: Naturally occurring substance derived from plants of the Solanaceae family.

Chemical name: 6-Nonenamide, (*E*)-*N*-[(4-hydroxy-3-methoxyphenyl)methyl]-8-methyl.

Molecular formula: $C_{18}H_{27}NO_3$.

Molecular weight: 305.41.

Description: Capsaicin USP—Off-white powder. Melts at about 65 °C.

Solubility: Capsaicin USP—Soluble in alcohol and in chloroform; slightly soluble in carbon disulfide; practically insoluble in cold water.

USP requirements:

Capsaicin USP—Preserve in tight containers, protected from light, and store in a cool place. Label it to state the percentage content of total capsaicinoids. Contains the labeled percentage of total capsaicinoids, within ±10%. The content of capsaicin is not less than 55%, and the sum of the contents of capsaicin and dihydrocapsaicin is not less than 75%, and the content of other capsaicinoids is not more than 15%, all calculated on the dried basis. Meets the requirements for Identification, Melting range (57–66 °C, the range between beginning and end of melting does not exceed 5 °C), Loss on drying (not more than 1.0%), Residue on ignition (not more than 1.0%), and Content of capsaicin, dihydrocapsaicin, and other capsaicinoids.

Caution: Handle Capsaicin with care. Prevent inhalation of particles of it and prevent its contact with any part of the body.

Capsaicin Cream—Not in *USP–NF*.

CAPSICUM

Description: Capsicum Oleoresin USP—Dark red, oily liquid.

Solubility: Capsicum Oleoresin USP—Soluble in alcohol, in acetone, in ether, in chloroform, and in volatile oils; soluble with opalescence in fixed oils.

USP requirements:

Capsicum USP—Preserve in well-closed containers. A few drops of chloroform may be added from time to time to prevent attack by insects. The dried ripe fruit of *Capsicum frutescens* Linné, known in commerce as African Chillies, or of *Capsicum annuum* Linné var. *connoides* Irish, known in commerce as Tabasco Pepper, or *Capsicum annuum* var. *longum* Sendt, known in commerce as Louisiana Long Pepper, or of a hybrid between the Honka variety of Japanese Capsicum and the Old Louisiana Sport Capsicum known in commerce as Louisiana Sport Pepper (Fam. Solanaceae). Label each container to indicate which variety of Capsicum is contained therein. Meets the requirements

for Botanic characteristics, Acid-insoluble ash (not more than 1.25%), Foreign organic matter (not more than 1%, other than stems and calyces, the proportion of which does not exceed 3%), and Nonvolatile ether-soluble extractive (not less than 12%).

Capsicum Oleoresin USP—Preserve in tight containers. An alcoholic extract of the dried ripe fruits of *Capsicum annum* var. *minimum* and small fruited varieties of *C. fruiscons* (Solanaceae). Label it to indicate that if separation occurs, it should be warmed and mixed before use. Contains not less than 8.0% of total capsaicins (capsaicin [$C_{18}H_{27}NO_3$], dihydrocapsaicin [$C_{18}H_{29}NO_3$], and nordihydrocapsaicin [$C_{17}H_{27}NO_3$]). Meets the requirement for Identification.

Caution: Capsicum Oleoresin is a powerful irritant, and even in minute quantities produces an intense burning sensation when it comes in contact with the eyes and tender parts of the skin. Care should be taken to protect the eyes and to prevent contact of the skin with Capsicum Oleoresin.

CAPTOPRIL

Chemical name: L-Proline, 1-[(2*S*)-3-mercapto-2-methyl-1-oxopropyl]-.

Molecular formula: $C_9H_{15}NO_3S$.

Molecular weight: 217.29.

Description: Captopril USP—White to off-white, crystalline powder, which may have a characteristic, sulfide-like odor. Melts in the range of 104–110 °C.

pKa: 3.7 and 9.8 (apparent).

Solubility: Captopril USP—Freely soluble in water, in methanol, in alcohol, and in chloroform.

USP requirements:

Captopril USP—Preserve in tight containers. Contains not less than 97.5% and not more than 102.0% of captopril, calculated on the dried basis. Meets the requirements for Identification, Specific rotation (−125° to −134°), Loss on drying (not more than 1.0%), Residue on ignition (not more than 0.2%), Heavy metals (not more than 0.003%), Related compounds (not more than 0.5%), and Organic volatile impurities.

Captopril Tablets USP—Preserve in tight containers. Contain the labeled amount, within ±10%. Meet the requirements for Thin-layer chromatographic identification test, Dissolution (80% in 20 minutes in 0.01 *N* hydrochloric acid in Apparatus 1 at 50 rpm), Limit of captopril disulfide (not more than 3.0%), and Uniformity of dosage units.

CAPTOPRIL AND HYDROCHLOROTHIAZIDE

For *Captopril* and *Hydrochlorothiazide*—See individual listings for chemistry information.

USP requirements: Captopril and Hydrochlorothiazide Tablets USP—Preserve in tight containers. Contain the labeled amounts, within ±10%. Meet the requirements for Identification, Dissolution (80% of the labeled amount of captopril in 20 minutes and 60% of the labeled amount of hydrochlorothiazide in 30 minutes in 0.1 *N* hydrochloric acid in Apparatus 1 at 50 rpm), Uniformity of dosage units, Limit of captopril disulfide (not more than 3.0%), and Limit of benzothiadiazine related compound (not more than 1.0%).

CARAMEL

Description: Caramel NF—Thick, dark brown liquid having the characteristic odor of burnt sugar. One part dissolved in 1000 parts of water yields a clear solution having a distinct yellowish orange color. The color of the solution is not changed and no precipitate is formed after exposure to sunlight for 6 hours. When spread in a thin layer on a glass plate, it appears homogeneous, reddish brown, and transparent.

NF category: Color.

Solubility: Caramel NF—Miscible with water. Soluble in dilute alcohol up to 55% (v/v). Immiscible with ether, with chloroform, with acetone, and with solvent hexane.

NF requirements: Caramel NF—Preserve in tight containers. A concentrated solution of the product obtained by heating sugar or glucose until the sweet taste is destroyed and a uniform dark brown mass results, a small amount of alkali or of alkaline carbonate or a trace of mineral acid being added while heating. Meets the requirements for Specific gravity (not less than 1.30), Purity, Microbial limits, Ash (not more than 8.0%), Arsenic (not more than 3 ppm), and Lead (not more than 10 ppm).

Note: Where included in articles for coloring purposes, Caramel complies with the regulations of the U.S. Food and Drug Administration concerning color additives.

CARAWAY

NF requirements:

Caraway NF—Preserve in well-closed containers. Preserve against attack by insects. Dried, ripe fruit of *Carum carvi* L. (Fam. Apiaceae). The label states the Latin binomial name and, following the official name, the part of the plant contained in the article. Meets the requirements for Botanic characteristics, Foreign organic matter (not more than 3.0%), and Acid-insoluble ash (not more than 1.5%).

Caraway Oil NF—Preserve in tight, light-resistant containers. Volatile oil distilled from the dried, ripe fruit of *Carum carvi* L. (Fam. Apiaceae). The label states the Latin binomial name and, following the official name, the part of the plant source from which the article was derived. Contains not more than 50.0% (v/v) of *d*-carvone. Meets the requirements for Solubility in 80% alcohol, Specific gravity (0.900–0.910), Angular rotation (+70° to +80°), Refractive index (1.484–1.488 at 20°), and Heavy metals (0.004%).

CARBACHOL

Chemical name: Ethanaminium, 2-[(aminocarbonyl)oxy]-*N,N,N*-trimethyl-, chloride.

Molecular formula: $C_6H_{15}ClN_2O_2$.

Molecular weight: 182.65.

Description: White or faintly yellow hygroscopic crystals or crystalline powder; odorless or with a faint amine-like odor. Its solutions in water are neutral to litmus.

Solubility: Soluble 1 in 1 of water and 1 in 50 of alcohol; practically insoluble in chloroform and in ether.

USP requirements:

Carbachol USP—Preserve in tight containers. Contains not less than 99.0% and not more than 101.0% of carbachol, calculated on the dried basis. Meets the requirements for Identification, Melting range (200–204 °C, with some de-

composition), Loss on drying (not more than 2.0%), Residue on ignition (not more than 0.1%), and Ordinary impurities.

Carbachol Intraocular Solution USP—Preserve in tight containers, at controlled room temperature, and protect from freezing. A sterile solution of Carbachol in an aqueous medium. Label it to indicate that it is for single-dose intraocular use only, and that the unused portion is to be discarded. Contains the labeled amount, within −10% to +15%. Contains no preservatives or antimicrobial agents. Meets the requirements for Identification, Sterility, and pH (5.0–7.5).

Carbachol Ophthalmic Solution USP—Preserve in tight containers. A sterile solution of Carbachol in an isotonic, aqueous medium. Contains the labeled amount, within ± 5%. Meets the requirements for Identification, Sterility, and pH (5.0–7.0).

CARBAMAZEPINE

Chemical group: Tricyclic iminostilbene derivative. Structurally resembles the psychoactive agents imipramine, chlorpromazine, and maprotiline; shares some structural features with the anticonvulsant agents phenytoin, clonazepam, and phenobarbital.

Chemical name: 5*H*-Dibenz[*b,f*]azepine-5-carboxamide.

Molecular formula: $C_{15}H_{12}N_2O$.

Molecular weight: 236.27.

Description: Carbamazepine USP—White to off-white powder.

pKa: 7.

Solubility: Carbamazepine USP—Practically insoluble in water; soluble in alcohol and in acetone.

USP requirements:

Carbamazepine USP—Preserve in tight containers. Contains not less than 98.0% and not more than 102.0% of carbamazepine, calculated on the dried basis. Meets the requirements for Identification, X-ray diffraction, Acidity, Alkalinity, Loss on drying (not more than 0.5%), Residue on ignition (not more than 0.1%), Chloride (not more than 0.014%), Heavy metals (not more than 0.001%), Chromatographic purity, and Organic volatile impurities.

Carbamazepine Extended-release Capsules—Not in *USP–NF*.

Carbamazepine Oral Suspension USP—Preserve in tight, light-resistant containers, protected from freezing and from excessive heat. Contains the labeled amount, within ±10%. Meets the requirements for Identification and Microbial limits.

Carbamazepine Tablets USP—Preserve in tight containers, preferably of glass. Dispense Carbamazepine Tablets in a container labeled "Store in a dry place. Protect from moisture." Contain the labeled amount, within ±8%. Meet the requirements for Identification, Dissolution (for product labeled as 100-mg chewable tablets: 75% in 60 minutes in water containing 1% sodium lauryl sulfate in Apparatus 2 at 75 rpm for Test 1; 75% in 0.1 *N* hydrochloric acid containing 1% sodium lauryl sulfate in Apparatus 3 at 35 dips per minutes for Test 4; and for products labeled as 200-mg tablets: 45–75% in 15 minutes and 75% in 60 minutes for Test 2; and 60–85% in 15 minutes and 75% in 60 minutes for Test 3), Water (not more than 5.0%), and Uniformity of dosage units.

Carbamazepine Extended-release Tablets USP—Preserve in tight containers at controlled room temperature. Contain the labeled amount, within ±10%. Meet the requirements for Identification, Drug release (10–35% in 3 hours, 35–65% in 6 hours, 65–90% in 12 hours, and not less than

75% in 24 hours in water in Apparatus 1 at 100 rpm), Uniformity of dosage units, Water (not more than 5.0%), Limit of residual solvents, and Chromatographic purity..

CARBAMIDE PEROXIDE

Chemical name: Urea, compd. with hydrogen peroxide (1:1).

Molecular formula: $CH_6N_2O_3$.

Molecular weight: 94.07.

Description: Carbamide Peroxide Topical Solution USP—Clear, colorless, viscous liquid, having a characteristic odor.

USP requirements:

Carbamide Peroxide USP—Preserve in tight, light-resistant containers, and avoid exposure to excessive heat. Contains not less than 96.0% and not more than 102.0% of carbamide peroxide. Meets the requirements for Identification and Organic volatile impurities.

Carbamide Peroxide Topical Solution USP—Preserve in tight, light-resistant containers, and avoid exposure to excessive heat. A solution in anhydrous glycerin of Carbamide Peroxide or of carbamide peroxide prepared from hydrogen peroxide and Urea. Contains the labeled amount, by weight, within −22% to +10%. Meets the requirements for Identification, Specific gravity (1.245–1.272), and pH (4.0–7.5).

CARBENICILLIN

Chemical name:

Carbenicillin disodium—4-Thia-1-azabicyclo[3.2.0]heptane-2-carboxylic acid, 6-[(carboxyphenylacetyl)amino]-3,3-dimethyl-7-oxo, disodium salt, [6 S-(2 alpha,5 alpha,6 beta)]-.

Carbenicillin indanyl sodium—4-Thia-1-azabicyclo[3.2.0]heptane-2-carboxylic acid, 6-[[3-[(2,3-dihydro-1 H-inden5-yl)oxy]-1,3-dioxo-2-phenylpropyl]amino]-3,3-dimethyl7-oxo-, monosodium salt, [2 S-(2 alpha,5 alpha,6 beta)]-.

Molecular formula:

Carbenicillin disodium—$C_{17}H_{16}N_2Na_2O_6S$.
Carbenicillin indanyl sodium—$C_{26}H_{25}N_2NaO_6S$.

Molecular weight:

Carbenicillin disodium—422.36.
Carbenicillin indanyl sodium—516.54.

Description:

Carbenicillin Disodium USP—White to off-white, crystalline powder.

Carbenicillin Indanyl Sodium USP—White to off-white powder.

Solubility:

Carbenicillin Disodium USP—Freely soluble in water; soluble in alcohol; practically insoluble in chloroform and in ether.

Carbenicillin Indanyl Sodium USP—Soluble in water and in alcohol.

USP requirements:

Carbenicillin Disodium USP—Preserve in tight containers. Where it is intended for use in preparing injectable dosage forms, the label states that it is sterile or must be subjected to further processing during the preparation of injectable dosage forms. Has a potency equivalent to not less than 770 mcg of carbenicillin per mg, calculated on the anhydrous basis. Meets the requirements for Identification, pH (6.5–8.0, in a solution containing 10 mg of carbenicillin per mL), and Water (not more than 6.0%), for Sterility and Bacterial endotoxins under Carbenicillin for Injection

(where the label states that Carbenicillin Disodium is sterile), and for Bacterial endotoxins under Carbenicillin for Injection (where the label states that Carbenicillin Disodium must be subjected to further processing during the preparation of injectable dosage forms).

Carbenicillin for Injection USP—Preserve in Containers for Sterile Solids. Contains an amount of Carbenicillin Disodium equivalent to the labeled amount of carbenicillin, within −10% to +20%. Meets the requirements for Identification, Bacterial endotoxins, Sterility, pH (6.5–8.0, in the solution constituted as directed in the labeling), Water (not more than 6.0%), and Particulate matter, for Uniformity of dosage units, and for Constituted solutions and Labeling under Injections.

Carbenicillin Indanyl Sodium USP—Preserve in tight containers. For periods up to 18 months, store at controlled room temperature. Has a potency equivalent to not less than 630 mcg and not more then 769 mcg of carbenicillin per mg, calculated on the anhydrous basis. Meets the requirements for Identification, pH (5.0–8.0, in a solution containing 100 mg per mL), and Water (not more than 2.0%).

Carbenicillin Indanyl Sodium Tablets USP—Preserve in tight containers. Contain the equivalent of the labeled amount of carbenicillin, within −10% to +20%. Meet the requirements for Identification, Dissolution (75% in 45 minutes in water in Apparatus 1 at 100 rpm), Uniformity of dosage units, and Water (not more than 2.0%).

CARBETAPENTANE, CHLORPHENIRAMINE, AND PHENYLEPHRINE

Description: Chlorpheniramine tannate—Light tan to buff or yellowish-tan, amorphous, fine powder having not more than a slight characteristic odor.

Solubility: Chlorpheniramine tannate—Slightly soluble in water at 25 °C.

USP requirements: Carbetapentane Tannate, Chlorpheniramine Tannate, and Phenylephrine Tennate Oral Suspension—Not in *USP–NF*.

CARBETOCIN

Source: Synthetic analog of oxytocin, a posterior pituitary hormone.

Chemical name: 1-Butyric acid-2-[3-(p-methoxyphenyl)-L-alanine]oxytocin.

Molecular formula: $C_{45}H_{69}N_{11}O_{12}S$.

Molecular weight: 988.16.

USP requirements: Carbetocin Injection—Not in *USP–NF*.

CARBIDOPA

Chemical group: Hydrazine analog of levodopa; inhibitor of aromatic amino acid decarboxylation.

Chemical name: Benzenepropanoic acid, alpha-hydrazino-3,4-dihydroxy-alpha-methyl-, monohydrate, (S).

Molecular formula: $C_{10}H_{14}N_2O_4 \cdot H_2O$.

Molecular weight: 244.24.

Description: Carbidopa USP—White to creamy white, odorless or practically odorless, powder.

Solubility: Carbidopa USP—Slightly soluble in water; freely soluble in 3 *N* hydrochloric acid; slightly soluble in methanol; practically insoluble in alcohol, in acetone, in chloroform, and in ether.

USP requirements: Carbidopa USP—Preserve in well-closed, light-resistant containers. Contains not less than 98.0% and not more than 102.0% of carbidopa. Meets the requirements for Identification, Specific rotation (–21.0° to –23.5°, calculated as the monohydrate), Loss on drying (6.9–7.9%), Residue on ignition (not more than 0.1%), Heavy metals (not more than 0.001%), Limit of methyldopa and carbidopa related compound A (not more than 0.5%), and Organic volatile impurities.

CARBIDOPA AND LEVODOPA

For *Carbidopa* and *Levodopa*—See individual listings for chemistry information.

USP requirements:
Carbidopa and Levodopa Tablets USP—Preserve in well-closed, light-resistant containers. Contain the labeled amounts, within ±10%. Meet the requirements for Identification, Dissolution (80% of each active ingredient in 30 minutes in 0.1 *N* hydrochloric acid in Apparatus 1 at 50 rpm), and Uniformity of dosage units.
Carbidopa and Levodopa Extended-release Tablets—Not in *USP–NF*.

CARBINOXAMINE

Chemical group: Ethanolamine derivative.

Chemical name: Carbinoxamine maleate—Ethanamine, 2-[(4-chlorophenyl)-2-pyridinylmethoxy]-*N,N*-dimethyl-, (*Z*)-2-butenedioate (1:1).

Molecular formula: Carbinoxamine maleate—$C_{16}H_{19}ClN_2O \cdot C_4H_4O_4$.

Molecular weight: Carbinoxamine maleate—406.86.

Description: Carbinoxamine Maleate USP—White, odorless, crystalline powder.

pKa: Carbinoxamine maleate—8.7.

Solubility: Carbinoxamine Maleate USP—Very soluble in water; freely soluble in alcohol and in chloroform; very slightly soluble in ether.

USP requirements:
Carbinoxamine Maleate USP—Preserve in tight, light-resistant containers. Dried at 105 °C for 2 hours, contains not less than 98.0% and not more than 102.0% of carbinoxamine maleate. Meets the requirements for Identification, Melting range (116–121 °C, determined after drying), pH (4.6–5.1, in a solution [1 in 100]), Loss on drying (not more than 0.5%), Residue on ignition (not more than 0.1%), Ordinary impurities, and Organic volatile impurities.
Carbinoxamine Maleate Tablets USP—Preserve in tight, light-resistant containers. Contain the labeled amount, within ± 7%. Meet the requirements for Identification, Dissolution (75% in 45 minutes in water in Apparatus 2 at 50 rpm), and Uniformity of dosage units.

CARBINOXAMINE AND PSEUDOEPHEDRINE

For *Carbinoxamine* and *Pseudoephedrine*—See individual listings for chemistry information.

USP requirements:
Carbinoxamine Maleate and Pseudoephedrine Hydrochloride Oral Solution—Not in *USP–NF*.
Carbinoxamine Maleate and Pseudoephedrine Hydrochloride Syrup—Not in *USP–NF*.
Carbinoxamine Maleate and Pseudoephedrine Hydrochloride Tablets—Not in *USP–NF*.
Carbinoxamine Maleate and Pseudoephedrine Hydrochloride Extended-release Tablets—Not in *USP–NF*.

CARBINOXAMINE, PSEUDOEPHEDRINE, AND DEXTRO-METHORPHAN

For *Carbinoxamine, Pseudoephedrine,* and *Dextromethorphan*—See individual listings for chemistry information.

USP requirements:
Carbinoxamine Maleate, Pseudoephedrine Hydrochloride, and Dextromethorphan Hydrobromide Oral Solution—Not in *USP–NF*.
Carbinoxamine Maleate, Pseudoephedrine Hydrochloride, and Dextromethorphan Hydrobromide Syrup—Not in *USP–NF*.

CARBOL-FUCHSIN

Description: Carbol-Fuchsin Topical Solution USP—Dark purple liquid, which appears purplish red when spread in a thin film.

USP requirements: Carbol-Fuchsin Topical Solution USP—Preserve in tight, light-resistant containers.

Prepare Carbol-Fuchsin Topical Solution as follows: 3 grams of Basic Fuchsin, 45 grams of Phenol, 100 grams of Resorcinol, 50 mL of Acetone, 100 mL of Alcohol, and a sufficient quantity of Purified Water, to make 1000 mL. Dissolve the Basic Fuchsin in a mixture of the Acetone and Alcohol, and add to this solution the Phenol and Resorcinol previously dissolved in 725 mL of Purified Water. Then add sufficient Purified Water to make the product measure 1000 mL, and mix.

Meets the requirements for Specific gravity (0.990–1.050) and Alcohol content (7.0–10.0%).

CARBOMER

Chemical name:
Carbomer 910—Polymer of 2-propenoic acid, cross-linked with allyl ethers of pentaerythritol.
Carbomer 934—Polymer of 2-propenoic acid, cross-linked with allyl ethers of sucrose.
Carbomer 934P—Polymer of 2-propenoic acid, cross-linked with allyl ethers of sucrose or pentaerythritol.
Carbomer 940—Polymer of 2-propenoic acid, cross-linked with allyl ethers of pentaerythritol.
Carbomer 941—Polymer of 2-propenoic acid, cross-linked with allyl ethers of pentaerythritol.

Molecular weight:
Carbomer 910—Approximately 750,000.
Carbomer 934—Approximately 3,000,000.
Carbomer 934P—Approximately 3,000,000.
Carbomer 941—Approximately 1,250,000.

Description: Carbomer 910 NF; Carbomer 934 NF; Carbomer 934P NF; Carbomer 940 NF; Carbomer 941 NF; Carbomer 1342 NF—White, fluffy powder, having a slight, characteristic odor. Hygroscopic. The pH of a 1 in 100 dispersion is about 3.

NF category: Suspending and/or viscosity-increasing agent.

Solubility: Carbomer 910 NF; Carbomer 934 NF; Carbomer 934P NF; Carbomer 940 NF; Carbomer 941 NF; Carbomer 1342 NF—When neutralized with alkali hydroxides or with amines, it dissolves in water, in alcohol, and in glycerin.

NF requirements:

Carbomer 910 NF—Preserve in tight containers. A high molecular weight polymer of acrylic acid cross-linked with allyl ethers of pentaerythritol. Label it to indicate that it is not intended for internal use. Previously dried in vacuum at 80 °C for 1 hour, contains not less than 56.0% and not more than 68.0% of carboxylic acid groups. Meets the requirements for Viscosity (3000–7000 centipoises for neutralized 1.0% aqueous dispersion) and Limit of benzene (not more than 0.5%), and for Identification, Loss on drying, and Heavy metals under Carbomer 934P.

Carbomer 934 NF—Preserve in tight containers. A high molecular weight polymer of acrylic acid cross-linked with allyl ethers of sucrose. Label it to indicate that it is not intended for internal use. Previously dried in vacuum at 80 °C for 1 hour, contains not less than 56.0% and not more than 68.0% of carboxylic acid groups. Meets the requirements for Viscosity (30,500–39,400 centipoises for neutralized 0.5% aqueous dispersion) and Limit of benzene (not more than 0.5%), and for Identification, Loss on drying, and Heavy metals under Carbomer 934P.

Carbomer 934P NF—Preserve in tight containers. A high molecular weight polymer of acrylic acid cross-linked with allyl ethers of sucrose or pentaerythritol. Previously dried in vacuum at 80 °C for 1 hour, contains not less than 56.0% and not more than 68.0% of carboxylic acid groups. Meets the requirements for Identification, Viscosity (29,400–39,400 centipoises for neutralized 0.5% aqueous dispersion), Loss on drying (not more than 2.0%), Heavy metals (not more than 0.002%), Limit of benzene (not more than 0.01%), and Organic volatile impurities.

Carbomer 940 NF—Preserve in tight containers. A high molecular weight polymer of acrylic acid cross-linked with allyl ethers of pentaerythritol. Label it to indicate that it is not intended for internal use. Previously dried in vacuum at 80 °C for 1 hour, contains not less than 56.0% and not more than 68.0% of carboxylic acid groups. Meets the requirements for Viscosity (40,000–60,000 centipoises for neutralized 0.5% aqueous dispersion) and Limit of benzene (not more than 0.5%), and for Identification, Loss on drying, and Heavy metals under Carbomer 934P.

Carbomer 941 NF—Preserve in tight containers. A high molecular weight polymer of acrylic acid cross-linked with allyl ethers of pentaerythritol. Label it to indicate that it is not intended for internal use. Previously dried in vacuum at 80 °C for 1 hour, contains not less than 56.0% and not more than 68.0% of carboxylic acid groups. Meets the requirements for Viscosity (4,000–11,000 centipoises for neutralized 0.5% aqueous dispersion) and Limit of benzene (not more than 0.5%), and for Identification, Loss on drying, and Heavy metals under Carbomer 934P.

Carbomer 1342 NF—Preserve in tight containers. A high molecular weight copolymer of acrylic acid and a long chain alkyl methacrylate cross-linked with allyl ethers of pentaerythritol. Label it to indicate that it is not intended for internal use. Previously dried in vacuum at 80 °C for 1 hour, contains not less than 52.0% and not more than 62.0% of carboxylic acid groups. Meets the requirements for Viscosity (9,500–26,500 centipoises for neutralized 1.0% aqueous dispersion) and Limit of benzene (not more than 0.2%), and for Identification, Loss on drying, and Heavy metals under Carbomer 934P.

CARBOMER COPOLYMER

NF requirements: Carbomer Copolymer NF—Preserve in tight containers, at a temperature not exceeding 45°. A high molecular weight copolymer of acrylic acid and a long chain alkyl methacrylate cross-linked with polyalkenyl ethers of polyalcohols. Label it to indicate the nominal viscosity range and the measured viscosity, the solvent or solvents used in the polymerization process, and the nominal and residual solvent levels for each solvent. Meets the requirements for Identification, Viscosity, Loss on drying (not more than 2.0%), Heavy metals (0.002%), Limit of ethyl acetate and cyclohexane (not more than 0.5% of ethyl acetate and not more than 0.3% of cyclohexane), Limit of acrylic acid (not more than 0.25%), and Content of carboxylic acid (not less than 52% and not more than 62%).

Note—Different types of Carbomer Copolymers may not have identical properties with respect to their use for specific pharmaceutical purposes, e.g. as controlled-release agents, bioadhesives, topical gels, thickening agents, and emulsifying agents. Therefore, different types of Carbomer Copolymers should not be interchanged unless performance equivalency has been ascertained.

CARBOMER INTERPOLYMER

NF requirements: Carbomer Interpolymer NF—Preserve in tight containers, at a temperature not exceeding 45°. A carbomer homopolymer or copolymer that contains a block copolymer of polyethylene glycol and a long chain alkyl acid ester. Label it to indicate the nominal viscosity range and the measured viscosity, the solvent or solvents used in the polymerization process, and the nominal and measured residual solvent levels for each solvent. Meets the requirements for Identification, Viscosity, Loss on drying (not more than 2.0%), Heavy metals (0.002%), Limit of ethyl acetate and cyclohexane (not more than 0.35% of ethyl acetate and not more than 0.15% of cyclohexane), Limit of acrylic acid (not more than 0.25%), and Content of carboxylic acid (not less than 52% and not more than 62%).

Note—Different types of Carbomer Interpolymers may not have identical properties with respect to their use for specific pharmaceutical purposes, e.g. as tablet controlled-release agents, bioadhesives, topical gels, thickening agents, and emulsifying agents. Therefore, different types of Carbomer Interpolymers should not be interchanged unless performance equivalency has been ascertained.

CARBON DIOXIDE

Chemical name: Carbon dioxide.

Molecular formula: CO_2.

Molecular weight: 44.01.

Description: Carbon Dioxide USP—Odorless, colorless gas. Its solutions are acid to litmus. One liter at 0 °C and at a pressure of 760 mm of mercury weighs 1.977 grams.

NF category: Air displacement.

Solubility: Carbon Dioxide USP—One volume dissolves in about 1 volume of water.

USP requirements: Carbon Dioxide USP—Preserve in cylinders. Contains not less than 99.0%, by volume, of carbon dioxide. Meets the requirements for Identification, Water (not more than 150 mg per cubic meter), Limit of ammonia (not more than 0.0025%), Limit of hydrogen sulfide (not more than 1 ppm), Limit of nitric oxide (not more than 2.5 ppm), Carbon monoxide (not more than 0.001%), Nitrogen dioxide (not more than 2.5 ppm), and Sulfur dioxide (not more than 5 ppm).

CARBON MONOXIDE C 11

Chemical name: Carbon-^{11}C monoxide.

Molecular formula: ^{11}CO.

USP requirements: Carbon Monoxide C 11 USP—Dispense the gas either continuously or batchwise, and preserve in a single-dose container that is adequately shielded. May also be trapped either on activated charcoal at −196 °C or on a molecular sieve at −72 °C. A colorless, odorless, nonirritating gas, suitable for administration by inhalation, in which a portion of the molecules are labeled with radioactive ^{11}C. The label must include the following: the time and date of calibration; the amount of ^{11}C as carbon monoxide expressed as total megabecquerels (or millicuries) at time of calibration; the expiration time and date; and the statement "Caution—Radioactive Material." The labeling indicates that in making dosage calculations correction is to be made for radioactive decay, and states that the radioactive half-life of ^{11}C is 20.39 minutes. Each container to hold ^{11}CO shall be independently labeled to indicate lot number and/or batch number. The labeling states that a microbiological filter (0.22 micrometer) is to be in place to remove any possible particulate matter that could be carried through to the final product. Contains the labeled amount of ^{11}C expressed in megabecquerels (or in millicuries) at the time indicated in the labeling, within ±10%. Meets the requirements for Specific activity, Radionuclide identification, Radionuclidic purity, and Radiochemical purity and mass determination.

FLUMAZENIL C 11

USP requirements: Flumazenil C 11 Injection USP—Preserve in single-dose or multiple-dose containers that are adequately shielded. A sterile solution, suitable for intravenous administration, of Flumazenil in which a portion of the molecules are labeled at the N-position with radioactive ^{11}C. Label it to include the following, in addition to the information specified for Labeling under Injections: the time and date of calibration; the amount of ^{11}C as [N-methyl-^{11}C]Flumazenil, expressed as megabecquerel (or millicurie) per micromole; the specific activity, expressed as megabecquerel (or millicurie); the concentration, expressed as megabecquerel (or millicurie) per mL, at the data and time of calibration; the expiration date and time; the lot or batch number; the name and quantity of any added preservative or stabilizer; and the statements, "Caution—Radioactive Material" and "Do not use if cloudy or if it contains particulate matter." The labeling indicates that in making dosage calculations, correction is to be made for radioactive decay, and states that the radioactive half-life of ^{11}C is 20 minutes. Contains the labeled amount of ^{11}C, within ±10%, expressed in megabecquerel (or millicurie) at the time indicated in the labeling. Specific gravity is not less than 14.8 gigabecquerel (400 millicurie) per micromol. May contain suitable buffers. Meets the requirements for Radionuclide identification, Bacterial endotoxins, pH (4.5–8.5), Radionuclidic purity, Chemical purity (not more than 0.2% of any individual impurity, and

not more than 0.9% of total impurities), Radiochemical purity, Specific activity, and for Injections (except that the Injection may be distributed or dispensed prior to completion of the test for Sterility, the latter test being started on the day following final manufacture, and except that it is not subject to the recommendation of Volume in Container).

MESPIPERONE C 11

Chemical name: $C_{23}$$^{11}CH_{28}FN_3O_2$.

Molecular formula: 8-[3-(p-Fluorobenzoyl)propyl]-3-[^{11}C]methyl-1-phenyl-1,3,8-triazaspiro[4.5]decan-4-one.

USP requirements: Mespiperone C 11 Injection USP—Preserve in single-dose or in multiple-dose containers that are adequately shielded. A sterile, isotonic solution, suitable for intravenous administration, of 3-N-[^{11}C] methylspiperone in which a portion of the molecules are labeled with radioactive ^{11}C. Its specific activity is not less that 18.5 gigabecquerels (500 millicuries) per micromole. Label it to include the following: the time and date of calibration; the amount of ^{11}C as methylspiperone expressed as total GBq (or mCi) at time of calibration; the expiration time and date; the lot or batch number; and the statements, "Caution—Radioactive Material;" and "Do not use if cloudy or if it contains particulate matter." The labeling indicates that in making dosage calculations correction is to be made for radioactive decay, and states that the radioactive half-life of ^{11}C is 20 minutes. Contains the labeled amount of ^{11}C expressed in gigabecquerels (or millicuries) at the time indicated in the labeling, within ± 10%. Meets the requirements for Specific activity, Radionuclide identification, Bacterial endotoxins, pH (4.5–7), Radionuclidic purity, Chemical purity, and Radiochemical purity, and for Injections (except that the Injection may be distributed or dispensed prior to completion of the test for Sterility, the latter test being started on the day following final manufacture, and except that it is not subject to the recommendation on Volume in Container).

METHIONINE C 11

USP requirements: Methionine C 11 Injection USP—Preserve in single-dose or in multiple-dose containers that are adequately shielded. A sterile isotonic solution, suitable for intravenous administration of L[1-^{11}C] methionine, in which a portion of the molecules are labeled with radioactive ^{11}C. Label it to include the following: the time and date of calibration; the amount of ^{11}C as methionine expressed as total megabecquerels (or millicuries) per mL at time of calibration; the expiration time and date; the name and quantity of any added preservative or stabilizer; and the statement "Caution—Radioactive Material." The labeling indicates that in making dosage calculations, correction is to be made for radioactive decay, and states that the radioactive half-life of ^{11}C is 20.4 minutes. Each container to hold ^{11}C methionine shall be independently labeled to indicate lot number and batch number. The labeling states that a microbiological filter (0.22 micrometers) is to be in place to remove any possible particulate matter that could be carried through to the final product. Contains the labeled amount of ^{11}C expressed in megabecquerels (or in millicuries), within ±10%, at the time indicated in the labeling. Meets the requirements for Specific activity (not less than 37.0 gigabecquerels [1.0 curie] per mmol), Radionuclide identification, Bacterial endotoxins, pH (6.0–8.0), Radionuclidic purity, Chemical purity, and Radiochemical purity, and for Injections (except that the Injection may be distributed or dispensed prior to completion of the tests for Sterility and Bacterial endotoxins, these

tests being started on the day of final manufacture, and except that it is not subject to the recommendation of Volume in Container).

RACLOPRIDE C 11

Chemical name: Benzamide, 3,5-dichloro-*N*-[(1-ethyl-2-pyrrolidinyl)methyl]-2-hydroxy-6-(methoxy-^{11}C)-(*S*)-.

Molecular formula: $C_{14}{}^{11}CH_{20}Cl_2N_2O_3$.

USP requirements: Raclopride C 11 Injection USP—Preserve in single-dose or in multiple-dose containers that are adequately shielded. A sterile solution, suitable for intravenous administration, of raclopride, in which a portion of the molecules are labeled at the *O*-methyl position with radioactive ^{11}C. Its specific activity is not less than 18.5 gigabecquerels (500 millicuries) per micromole. Label it to include the following, in addition to the information specified for Labeling under Injections: the time and date of calibration; the amount of ^{11}C as [*O*-methyl-^{11}C]-raclopride, expressed as total megabecquerels (or millicuries); the specific activity, expressed as megabecquerels (or millicuries) per micromole; and the concentration, expressed as megabecquerels (or millicuries) per mL, at the date and time of calibration; the expiration date and time; the lot or batch number; the name and quantity of any added preservative or stabilizer; and the statements "Caution—Radioactive Material" and "Do not use if cloudy or if it contains particulate matter." The labeling indicates that in making dosage calculations correction is to be made for radioactive decay, and states that the radioactive half-life of ^{11}C is 20 minutes. Contains the labeled amount of ^{11}C expressed in megabecquerels (or millicuries) at the time indicated in the labeling, within ±10%. Meets the requirements for Specific activity, Radionuclide identification, Bacterial endotoxins, pH (4.5–7), Radionuclidic purity, Chemical purity, and Radiochemical purity, and for Injections (except that the Injection may be distributed or dispensed prior to completion of the test for Sterility, the latter test being started on the day following final manufacture, and except that it is not subject to the recommendation on Volume in Container).

SODIUM ACETATE C 11

USP requirements: Sodium Acetate C 11 Injection USP—Preserve in single-dose or in multiple-dose containers that are adequately shielded. A sterile solution, suitable for intravenous administration, of Sodium Acetate in which a portion of the carboxyl molecules are labeled with radioactive ^{11}C. Label it to include the following, in addition to the information specified for Labeling under Injections: the time and date of calibration; the amount of ^{11}C as labeled sodium acetate expressed as total megabecquerels (or millicuries) and the concentration as megabecquerels per mL (or as millicuries per mL), on the date and time of calibration; the expiration date and time; the lot or batch number; the name and quantity of any added preservative or stabilizer; an indication on the labeling that states, "Do no use if cloudy or if it contains particulate matter;" and the statement "Caution—Radioactive Material." The labeling indicates that in making dosage calculations, correction is to be made for radioactive decay, and also indicates that the radioactive half-life of ^{11}C is 20 minutes. Contains the labeled amount of ^{11}C expressed in megabecquerels (or in microcuries or millicuries), within ±10%, at the time indicated in the labeling. Meets the requirements for Specific activity (not less than 3.7 gigabecquerels [100 millicuries] per micromol), Radionuclide identification, Bacterial endotoxins, pH (4.5–8.5), Radionuclidic purity, Chemical purity, and Radiochemical purity, and

for Injections (except that the Injection may be distributed or dispensed prior to completion of the test for Sterility, the latter test being started on the day following final manufacture, and except that it is not subject to the recommendation of Volume in Container).

UREA C 13

Chemical name: Urea.

Molecular formula: CH_4N_2O.

Molecular weight: 60.06.

Description: Urea USP—Colorless to white, prismatic crystals, or white, crystalline powder, or small white pellets. Is practically odorless, but may gradually develop a slight odor of ammonia upon long standing. Its solutions are neutral to litmus.

Solubility: Urea USP—Freely soluble in water and in boiling alcohol; practically insoluble in chloroform and in ether.

USP requirements:
Urea C 13 USP—Preserve in well-closed containers at room temperature. Contains not less than 99.0% and not more than 100.5% of urea. Meets the requirements for Limit of biuret (not more than 0.1%) and Isotopic purity (not more than 15%), and for Identification tests A and B, Melting range, Residue on ignition, Alcohol insoluble matter, Chloride, Sulfate, and Heavy metals for Urea.
Urea C 13 Oral Solution USP—Preserve in sterile, well-closed containers. A dry sterile powder prepared from Urea C 13. Label it to indicate that the solution is to be discarded if particulate matter is visible after reconstituion. [Note—It is to be reconstituted with Sterile Purified Water.] Meets the requirements for Completeness of solution, and for Identification.

UREA C 14

USP requirements: Urea C 14 Capsules USP—Preserve in tight containers, and store at controlled room temperature. Contain Urea C 14 in which a portion of the molecules are labeled with radioactive ^{14}C to provide 0.04 megabequerel (or 1 microcurie) of radioactivity per capsule. Contain the labeled amount, within ±10%. Meet the requiremetns for Expiration date, Labeling, Radionuclide identification, Dissolution (80% in 10 minutes in simulated gastric fluid TS in Apparatus 1 at 50 rpm), Uniformity of dosage units, Radionuclidic purity (not less than 99.9%), and Radiochemical purity (not less than 90%).

CARBOPLATIN

Chemical group: A platinum coordination compound.

Chemical name: Platinum, diammine[1,1-cyclobutanedicarboxylato(2-)*O,O'*]-, (*SP*-4-2).

Molecular formula: $C_6H_{12}N_2O_4Pt$.

Molecular weight: 371.25.

Description: Crystalline powder.

Solubility: Soluble in water at a rate of approximately 14 mg per mL; virtually insoluble in ethanol, in acetone, and in dimethylacetamide.

Other characteristics: pH of a 1% solution is 5–7.

USP requirements:

Carboplatin USP—Preserve in tight containers, protected from light. Contains not less than 98.0% and not more than 102.0% of carboplatin, calculated on the anhydrous basis. Meets the requirements for Identification, Crystallinity, pH (5.0–7.0, in a solution in water containing 10 mg per mL), Water (not more than 0.5%), Transmittance (not less than 97%), Water-insoluble matter (not more than 0.5%), Limit of 1,1-cyclobutanedicarboxylic acid (not more than 0.5%), Chromatographic purity, and Platinum content (52.0–53.0%, calculated on the anhydrous basis).

Caution: Great care should be taken in handling Carboplatin since it is a suspected carcinogen.

Carboplatin Injection—Not in *USP–NF*.

Carboplatin for Injection USP—Preserve in Containers for Sterile Solids, protected from light. A sterile, lyophilized mixture of Carboplatin and Mannitol. Contains the labeled amount, within ±10%. Meets the requirements for Constituted solution, Identification, Sterility, Bacterial endotoxins, pH (5.0–7.0, in a solution constituted as directed in the labeling, Sterile Water for Injection being used), Water (not more than 3.0%), Uniformity of dosage units, and Limit of 1,1-cyclobutanedicarboxylic acid (not more than 1.0%).

Caution: Great care should be taken in handling Carboplatin since it is a suspected carcinogen.

CARBOPROST

Source: Carboprost tromethamine—The tromethamine salt of the (15S)-15 methyl analogue of naturally occurring prostaglandin F$_{2\text{-alpha}}$.

Chemical name: Carboprost tromethamine—Prosta-5,13-dien-1-oic acid, 9,11,15-trihydroxy-15-methyl-, (5Z,9 alpha,11 alpha,13E,15S)-, compound with 2-amino-2-(hydroxymethyl)-1,3-propanediol (1:1).

Molecular formula: Carboprost tromethamine—C$_{21}$H$_{36}$O$_5$ · C$_4$H$_{11}$NO$_3$.

Molecular weight: Carboprost tromethamine—489.64.

Description: Carboprost Tromethamine USP—White to off-white powder. It has a melting point between 95 and 105 °C, depending on the rate of heating.

Solubility: Carboprost Tromethamine USP—Soluble in water.

USP requirements:

Carboprost Tromethamine USP—Preserve in well-closed containers, and store in a freezer. Contains not less than 95.0% and not more than 105.0% of carboprost tromethamine, calculated on the dried basis. Meets the requirements for Identification, Specific rotation (+18° to +24°), Loss on drying (not more than 1.0%), Residue on ignition (not more than 0.5%), and Limit of 15R-epimer and 5-*trans* isomer (not more than 3.0%).

Caution: Great care should be taken to prevent inhaling particles of Carboprost Tromethamine and exposing the skin to it.

Carboprost Tromethamine Injection USP—Preserve in single-dose or in multiple-dose containers, preferably of Type I glass, and store in a refrigerator. A sterile solution of Carboprost Tromethamine in aqueous solution, which may contain also benzyl alcohol, sodium chloride, and tromethamine. Contains an amount of carboprost trometha-

mine equivalent to the labeled amount of carboprost, within ±10%. Meets the requirements for Identification, Bacterial endotoxins, and pH (7.0–8.0), and for Injections.

CARBOXYMETHYLCELLULOSE

Chemical group: Semisynthetic hydrophilic derivative of cellulose.

Chemical name:

Carboxymethylcellulose calcium—Cellulose, carboxymethyl ether, calcium salt.

Carboxymethylcellulose sodium—Cellulose, carboxymethyl ether, sodium salt.

Description:

Carboxymethylcellulose Calcium NF—White to yellowish white powder. Is hygroscopic. The pH of the suspension, obtained by shaking 1 gram with 100 mL of water, is between 4.5 and 6.0.

NF category: Suspending and/or viscosity-increasing agent.

Carboxymethylcellulose Sodium USP—White to cream-colored powder or granules. The powder is hygroscopic.

NF category: Coating agent; suspending and/or viscosity-increasing agent; tablet binder.

Carboxymethylcellulose Sodium 12 NF—White to cream-colored powder or granules. The powder is hygroscopic.

NF category: Suspending and/or viscosity-increasing agent.

Solubility:

Carboxymethylcellulose Calcium NF—Practically insoluble in alcohol, in acetone, in ether, and in chloroform. It swells with water to form a suspension.

Carboxymethylcellulose Sodium USP—Is easily dispersed in water to form colloidal solutions. Insoluble in alcohol, in ether, and in most other organic solvents.

Carboxymethylcellulose Sodium 12 NF—Is easily dispersed in water to form colloidal solutions. Insoluble in alcohol, in ether, and in most other organic solvents.

USP requirements:

Carboxymethylcellulose Ophthalmic Solution—Not in *USP–NF*.

Carboxymethylcellulose Sodium USP—Preserve in tight containers. The sodium salt of a polycarboxymethyl ether of cellulose. Label it to indicate the viscosity in solutions of stated concentrations. Contains not less than 6.5% and not more than 9.5% of sodium, calculated on the dried basis. Meets the requirements for Identification, pH (6.5–8.5 in a solution [1 in 100]), Viscosity, Loss on drying (not more than 10.0%), Heavy metals (not more than 20 mcg per gram), and Organic volatile impurities.

Carboxymethylcellulose Sodium Paste USP—Preserve in well-closed containers, and avoid prolonged exposure to temperatures exceeding 30 °C. Contains not less than 16.0% and not more than 17.0% of carboxymethylcellulose sodium. Meets the requirements for Identification, Microbial limits, Loss on drying (not more than 2.0%), Heavy metals (not more than 0.005%), and Consistency.

Carboxymethylcellulose Sodium Tablets USP—Preserve in tight containers. Contain an amount of sodium equivalent to not less than 6.5% and not more than 9.5% of the labeled amount of carboxymethylcellulose sodium. Meet the requirements for Identification, Disintegration (2 hours), and Uniformity of dosage units.

NF requirements:

Carboxymethylcellulose Calcium NF—Preserve in tight containers. The calcium salt of a polycarboxymethyl ether of cellulose. Meets the requirements for Identification, Alkalinity, Loss on drying (not more than 10.0%), Residue on

ignition (10.0–20.0%), Chloride (not more than 0.36%), Silicate (not more than 1.5%), Sulfate (not more than 0.96%), Heavy metals (not more than 0.002%), Starch, and Organic volatile impurities.

Carboxymethylcellulose Sodium 12 NF—Preserve in tight containers. The sodium salt of a polycarboxymethyl ether of cellulose. Label it to indicate the viscosity in solutions of stated concentrations of either 1% (w/w) or 2% (w/w). Its degree of substitution is not less than 1.15 and not more than 1.45, corresponding to a sodium content of not less than 10.4% and not more than 12.0%, calculated on the dried basis. Meets the requirements for Identification, Viscosity, pH (6.5–8.5, in a solution [1 in 100]), Loss on drying (not more than 10.0%), Heavy metals (not more than 20 mcg per gram), Organic volatile impurities, Sodium chloride and Sodium glycolate (not more than 0.5%), and Degree of substitution.

CARDAMOM OIL

NF requirements: Cardamom Oil NF—Preserve in tight, light-resistant containers. Volatile oil distilled from the seed of *Elettaria cardamomum* (L.) Maton (Fam. Zingiberaceae). The label states the Latin binomial name and, following the official name, the part of the plant source from which the article was derived. Meets the requirements for Solubility in 7% alcohol, Specific gravity (0.917–0.947), Angular rotation (+22° to +44°), Refractive index (1.463–1.466 at 20°), Arsenic (3 mcg per gram), Lead (not more than 0.001%), and Heavy metals (0.004%).

CARDAMOM SEED

NF requirements: Cardamom Seed NF—Preserve against attack by insects. Dried ripe seed of *Elettaria cardamomum* (L.) Maton (Fam. Zingiberaceae). The label states the Latin binomial name and the official name. Meets the requirements for Botanic characteristics and Acid-insoluble ash (not more than 4.0%).

Note—Cardamom Seed should be recently removed from the capsule.

COMPOUND CARDAMOM TINCTURE

NF requirements: Compound Cardamom Tincture NF—Preserve in tight, light-resistant containers, and avoid exposer to sunlight and excessive heat.

Prepare Compound Cardamom Tincture as follows: 20 grams of Cardamom Seed, in moderately coarse powder, 25 grams of Cinnamon, in fine powder, and 12 grams of Caraway, in moderately coarse powder to make 1000 mL. Macerate the mixed powders in 750 mL of a mixture of 50 mL of Glycerin and 950 mL of Diluted Alcohol, and complete the preparation by using first the remainder of the mixture of Diluted Alcohol and Glycerin prepared as directed above, followed by Diluted Alcohol.

Meets the requirement for Alcohol content (43.0%–47.0%).

Note—Compound Cardamom Tincture may be colored with one or more colors.

CARISOPRODOL

Chemical name: 2-Methyl-2-propyl-1,3-propanediol carbamate isopropylcarbamate.

Molecular formula: $C_{12}H_{24}N_2O_4$.

Molecular weight: 260.33.

Description: Carisoprodol USP—White, crystalline powder, having a mild, characteristic odor.

Solubility: Carisoprodol USP—Very slightly soluble in water; freely soluble in alcohol, in chloroform, and in acetone.

USP requirements:
Carisoprodol USP—Preserve in tight containers. Contains not less than 98.0% and not more than 102.0% of carisoprodol, calculated on the dried basis. Meets the requirements for Identification, Melting range (91–94 °C), Loss on drying (not more than 0.5%), Heavy metals (not more than 0.001%), Limit of meprobamate (not more than 0.5%), and Organic volatile impurities.

Carisoprodol Tablets USP—Preserve in well-closed containers. Contain the labeled amount, within ±10%. Meet the requirements for Identification, Dissolution (80% in 60 minutes in 0.05 M phosphate buffer [pH 6.9] containing 5 units of alpha-amylase per mL in Apparatus 2 at 75 rpm), and Uniformity of dosage units.

CARISOPRODOL AND ASPIRIN

For *Carisoprodol* and *Aspirin*—See individual listings for chemistry information.

USP requirements: Carisoprodol and Aspirin Tablets USP—Preserve in well-closed containers. Contain the labeled amounts, within ±10%. Meet the requirements for Identification, Dissolution (75% of each active ingredient in 45 minutes in water in Apparatus 2 at 75 rpm), Uniformity of dosage units, and Limit of free salicylic acid (not more than 3.0%).

CARISOPRODOL, ASPIRIN, AND CODEINE

For *Carisoprodol, Aspirin,* and *Codeine*—See individual listings for chemistry information.

USP requirements: Carisoprodol, Aspirin, and Codeine Phosphate Tablets USP—Preserve in well-closed containers. Contain the labeled amounts, within ±10%. Meet the requirements for Identification, Dissolution (75% of each active ingredient in 45 minutes in water in Apparatus 2 at 75 rpm), Uniformity of dosage units, and Limit of free salicylic acid (not more than 3.0%).

CARMUSTINE

Chemical name: Urea, *N,N*-bis(2-chloroethyl)-*N*-nitroso-.

Molecular formula: $C_5H_9Cl_2N_3O_2$.

Molecular weight: 214.05.

Description: Lyophilized pale yellow flakes or congealed mass.

Solubility: Highly soluble in alcohol and lipids; poorly soluble in water.

USP requirements:
Carmustine Implants—Not in *USP–NF*.
Carmustine for Injection—Not in *USP–NF*.

CARRAGEENAN

Chemical name: Carrageenan.

Description: Carrageenan NF—Yellowish or tan to white, coarse to fine powder. Practically odorless.
NF category: Suspending and/or viscosity-increasing agent.

Solubility: Carrageenan NF—Soluble in water at a temperature of about 80 °C, forming a viscous, clear or slightly opalescent solution that flows readily. Disperses in water more readily if first moistened with alcohol, with glycerin, or with a saturated solution of sucrose in water.

NF requirements: Carrageenan NF—Preserve in tight containers, preferably in a cool place. The hydrocolloid obtained by extraction with water or aqueous alkali from some members of the class *Rhodophyceae* (red seaweeds). Consists chiefly of potassium, sodium, calcium, magnesium, and ammonium sulfate esters of galactose and 3,6-anhydrogalactose copolymers, which are subclassified by slight structural differences. The ester sulfate content for Carrageenan is 18 to 40%. In addition, contains inorganic salts that originate from the seaweed and from the process of recovery from the extract. Meets the requirements for Identification, Solubility in water (not more than 30 mL of water required to dissolve 1 gram at 80 °C), Viscosity (not less than 5 centipoises at 75 °C), Microbial limits, Loss on drying (not more than 12.5%), Acid-insoluble matter (not more than 2.0% of Carrageenan taken), Total ash (not more than 35.0%), Arsenic (not more than 3 ppm), Lead (not more than 0.001%), and Heavy metals (not more than 0.004%).

CARTEOLOL

Chemical name: Carteolol hydrochloride—2(1*H*)-Quinolinone, 5-[3-[(1,1-dimethylethyl)amino]-2-hydroxypropoxy]-3,4-dihydro-, monohydrochloride.

Molecular formula: Carteolol hydrochloride—$C_{16}H_{24}N_2O_3 \cdot HCl$.

Molecular weight: Carteolol hydrochloride—328.83.

Description: Carteolol hydrochloride—White crystalline powder.

pKa: 9.74.

Solubility: Carteolol hydrochloride—Soluble in water; slightly soluble in ethanol.

Other characteristics: Lipid solubility—Low.

USP requirements:
Carteolol Hydrochloride USP—Preserve in well-closed containers. Contains not less than 98.0% and not more than 101.5% of carteolol hydrochloride, calculated on the dried basis. Meets the requirements for Identification, pH (5.0–6.0, in a solution [1 in 100]), Loss on drying (not more than 0.5%), Residue on ignition (not more than 0.1%), Heavy metals (not more than 0.002%), Arsenic (not more than 3 ppm), and Chromatographic purity.
Carteolol Hydrochloride Ophthalmic Solution USP—Preserve in tight containers. A sterile, aqueous, isotonic solution of Carteolol Hydrochloride. Contains a suitable antimicrobial preservative. Contains the labeled amount, within ±10%. Meets the requirements for Identification, Sterility, and pH (6.0–8.0).

Carteolol Hydrochloride Tablets USP—Preserve in tight containers. Contain the labeled amount, within ±10%. Meet the requirements for Identification, Dissolution (80% in 30 minutes in water in Apparatus 2 at 50 rpm), Uniformity of dosage units, and Limit of dehydrocarteolol hydrochloride (not more than 1.0%).

CARVEDILOL

Chemical name: 2-Propanol, 1-(9*H*-carbazol-4-yloxy)-3-[[2-(2-methoxyphenoxy)ethyl]amino]-, (±)-.

Molecular formula: $C_{24}H_{26}N_2O_4$.

Molecular weight: 406.47.

Description: White to off-white powder.

Solubility: Freely soluble in dimethylsulfoxide; soluble in methylene chloride and in methanol; sparingly soluble in 95% ethanol and isopropanol; slightly soluble in ethyl ether; practically insoluble in water.

USP requirements: Carvedilol Tablets—Not in *USP–NF*.

CASANTHRANOL

Source: A purified mixture of the anthranol glycosides derived from *Cascara sagrada*.

Chemical group: Anthraquinones.

Chemical name: Casanthranol.

Description: Casanthranol USP—Light tan to brown, amorphous, hygroscopic powder.

Solubility: Casanthranol USP—Freely soluble in water, with some residue; partially soluble in methanol and in hot isopropyl alcohol; practically insoluble in acetone.

USP requirements:
Casanthranol USP—Preserve in tight, light-resistant containers, at a temperature not exceeding 30 °C. Obtained from Cascara Sagrada. Contains in each 100 grams not less than 20.0 grams of total hydroxyanthracene derivatives, calculated on the dried basis, calculated as cascaroside A. Not less than 80.0% of the total hydroxyanthracene derivatives consists of cascarosides, calculated as cascaroside A. Meets the requirements for Loss on drying (not more than 10.0%), Residue on ignition (not more than 4.0%), and Heavy metals (not more than 0.0025%).
Casanthranol Syrup—Not in *USP–NF*.

CASANTHRANOL AND DOCUSATE

For *Casanthranol* and *Docusate*—See individual listings for chemistry information.

USP requirements:
Casanthranol and Docusate Potassium Capsules—Not in *USP–NF*.
Casanthranol and Docusate Sodium Capsules—Not in *USP–NF*.
Casanthranol and Docusate Sodium Syrup—Not in *USP–NF*.
Casanthranol and Docusate Sodium Tablets—Not in *USP–NF*.

CASCARA SAGRADA

Source: Dried bark of *Rhamnus purshiana* (buckthorn tree); main active principles are cascarosides A and B (glycosides of barbaloin) and cascarosides C and D (glycosides of chrysaloin).

Chemical group: Anthraquinones.

Description: Cascara Sagrada USP—Has a distinct odor.

USP requirements:
Cascara Sagrada USP—The dried bark of *Rhamnus purshiana* De Candolle (Fam. Rhamnaceae). Yields not less than 7.0% of total hydroxyanthracene derivatives, calculated as cascaroside A, and calculated on the dried basis. Not less than 60% of the total hydroxyanthracene derivatives consists of cascarosides, calculated as cascaroside A. Meets the requirements for Botanic characteristics, Identification, Water (not more than 12.0%), and Foreign organic matter (not more than 4.0%).

Note: Collect Cascara Sagrada not less than one year prior to use.
Cascara Sagrada Extract USP—Preserve in tight, light-resistant containers, at a temperature not exceeding 30 °C. Contains, in each 100 grams, not less than 10.0 grams and not more than 12.0 grams of hydroxyanthracene derivatives, of which not less than 50.0% consists of cascarosides, both calculated as cascaroside A.

Prepare Cascara Sagrada Extract as follows: Mix 900 grams of Cascara Sagrada, in coarse powder, with 4000 mL of boiling water, and macerate the mixture for 3 hours. Then transfer it to a percolator, allow it to drain, exhaust it by percolation, using boiling water as the menstruum, and collect about 5000 mL of percolate. Evaporate the percolate to dryness, reduce the extract to a fine powder, and, after assaying, add sufficient starch, dried at 100 °C, or other inert, non-toxic diluents to make the product contain, in each 100 grams, 11 grams of hydroxyanthracene derivatives. Mix the powders, and pass the Extract through a number 60 sieve.
Cascara Tablets USP—Preserve in tight containers; if the Tablets are coated, well-closed containers may be used. They are prepared from Cascara Sagrada Extract. Contain an amount of hydroxyanthracene derivatives, calculated as cascaroside A, not less than 9.35% and not more than 12.65% of the labeled amount of Cascara Sagrada Extract. Not less than 50% of the hydroxyanthracene derivatives are cascarosides, calculated as cascaroside A. Meet the requirements for Disintegration (60 minutes) and Uniformity of dosage units.
Cascara Sagrada Fluidextract USP—Preserve in tight, light-resistant containers, and avoid exposure to direct sunlight and to excessive heat.

Prepare Cascara Sagrada Fluidextract as follows: To 1000 grams of coarsely ground Cascara Sagrada add 3000 mL of boiling water, mix, and allow to macerate in a suitable percolator for 2 hours. Allow the percolation to proceed at a moderate rate, gradually adding boiling water until the drug is practically exhausted of its active principles. Evaporate the percolate on a water bath or in a vacuum still to not more than 800 mL, cool, add 200 mL of alcohol and, if necessary, add sufficient water to make the product measure 1000 mL. Mix.

Meets the requirement for Alcohol content (18.0–20.0%).
Aromatic Cascara Fluidextract USP—Preserve in tight, light-resistant containers and avoid exposure to direct sunlight and to excessive heat.

Prepare Aromatic Cascara Fluidextract as follows: 1000 grams of Cascara Sagrada, in very coarse powder, 120 grams of Magnesium Oxide, Suitable sweetening agent(s), Suitable essential oils(s), Suitable flavoring agent(s), 200 mL of Alcohol, and a sufficient quantity of Purified Water, to make 1000 mL. Mix the Cascara Sagrada with the Magnesium Oxide, moisten it uniformly with 2000 mL of boiling water, and set it aside in a shallow container for 48 hours, stirring it occasionally. Pack it in a percolator, and percolate with boiling water until the drug is exhausted. Evaporate the percolate, at a temperature not exceeding 100 °C, to 750 mL, and at once dissolve in it the flavoring agent(s). When the liquid has cooled, add the Alcohol, in which the sweetening agent(s) and oils have been dissolved, add sufficient water to make the Aromatic Fluidextract measure 1000 mL, and mix.

Meets the requirement for Alcohol content (18.0–20.0%).

CASCARA SAGRADA AND ALOE

For *Cascara Sagrada* and *Aloe*—See individual listings for chemistry information.

USP requirements: Cascara Sagrada and Aloe Tablets—Not in *USP–NF*.

CASCARA SAGRADA AND PHENOLPHTHALEIN

For *Cascara Sagrada* and *Phenolphthalein*—See individual listings for chemistry information.

USP requirements: Cascara Sagrada Extract and Phenolphthalein Tablets—Not in *USP–NF*.

CASPOFUNGIN

Chemical name: Caspofungin acetate—1-[(4R,5S)-5-[2-Aminoethyl)amino-N^2-(10,12-dimethyl-1-oxotetradecyl)-4-hydroxy-L-ornithine]-5-[(3R)-3-hydroxy-L-ornithine]pneumocandin B_0, diacetate (salt).

Molecular formula: Caspofungin acetate—$C_{52}H_{88}N_{10}O_{15} \cdot 2C_2H_4O_2$.

Molecular weight: Caspofungin acetate—1213.43.

Description: Caspofungin acetate—Hygroscopic, white to off-white powder.

Solubiliuty: Caspofungin acetate—Freely soluble in water and in methanol; slightly soluble in ethanol.

Other characteristics: Caspofungin acetate—pH: Approximately 6.6.

USP requirements: Caspofungin Acetate for Injection–Not in *USP–NF*.

CASTOR OIL

Chemical group: Glycerides.

Description:
Castor Oil USP—Pale yellowish or almost colorless, transparent, viscid liquid. Has a faint, mild odor; is free from foreign and rancid odor.
NF category: Plasticizer.
Hydrogenated Castor Oil NF—White, crystalline wax.
NF category: Stiffening agent.

Solubility:
Castor Oil USP—Soluble in alcohol; miscible with dehydrated alcohol, with glacial acetic acid, with chloroform, and with ether.

Hydrogenated Castor Oil NF—Insoluble in water and in most common organic solvents.

USP requirements:

Castor Oil USP—Preserve in tight containers, and avoid exposure to excessive heat. The fixed oil obtained from the seed of *Ricinus communis* Linné (Fam. Euphorbiaceae). Contains no added substances. Meets the requirements for Specific gravity (0.957–0.961), Distinction from most other fixed oils, Heavy metals (not more than 0.001%), Free fatty acids, Hydroxyl value (160–168), Iodine value (83–88), and Saponification value (176–182).

Aromatic Castor Oil USP—Preserve in tight containers. It is Castor Oil containing suitable flavoring agents. Contains the labeled amount, within −5%. Meets the requirement for Alcohol content (not more than 4.0%).

Castor Oil Capsules USP—Preserve in tight containers, preferably at controlled room temperature. Contain the labeled amount, within ±10%, calculated from the tests for Weight variation and Specific gravity. Meet the requirements for Identification and Uniformity of dosage units, and for Specific gravity, Hydroxyl value, Iodine value, and Saponification value under Castor Oil.

Castor Oil Emulsion USP—Preserve in tight containers. Contains the labeled amount, within −10% to +20%. Meets the requirement for Identification.

NF requirements: Hydrogenated Castor Oil NF—Preserve in tight containers, and avoid exposure to excessive heat. It is refined, bleached, hydrogenated, and deodorized Castor Oil, consisting mainly of the triglyceride of hydroxystearic acid. Meets the requirements for Melting range (85–88 °C), Heavy metals (not more than 0.001%), Free fatty acids, Hydroxyl value (154–162), Iodine value (not more than 5), and Saponification value (176–182).

CEFACLOR

Chemical name: 5-Thia-1-azabicyclo[4.2.0]oct-2-ene-2-carboxylic acid, 7-[(aminophenylacetyl)amino]-3-chloro-8-oxo-, monohydrate, [6R-[6 alpha,7 beta(R*)]]-.

Molecular formula: $C_{15}H_{14}ClN_3O_4S \cdot H_2O$.

Molecular weight: 385.82.

Description: Cefaclor USP—White to off-white, crystalline powder.

Solubility: Cefaclor USP—Soluble in water; practically insoluble in methanol and in chloroform.

Other characteristics: A 2.5% aqueous suspension has a pH of 3.0–4.5.

USP requirements:

Cefaclor USP—Preserve in tight containers. Has a potency of not less than 950 mcg and not more than 1020 mcg of cefaclor, calculated on the anhydrous basis. Meets the requirements for Identification, Crystallinity, pH (3.0–4.5, in an aqueous suspension containing 25 mg per mL), Water (3.0–6.5%), and Related compounds.

Cefaclor Capsules USP—Preserve in tight containers. Contain the equivalent of the labeled amount of anhydrous cefaclor, within −10% to +20%. Meet the requirements for Identification, Dissolution (80% in 30 minutes in water in Apparatus 2 at 50 rpm), Related compounds, Uniformity of dosage units, and Water (not more than 8.0%).

Cefaclor for Oral Suspension USP—Preserve in tight containers. A dry mixture of Cefaclor and one or more suitable buffers, colors, diluents, and flavors. Contains the equivalent of the labeled amount of anhydrous cefaclor, within −10% to +20%. Meets the requirements for Identification, Uniformity of dosage units (solid packaged in single-unit containers), Deliverable volume (solid packaged in multi-ple-unit containers), pH (2.5–5.0, in the suspension constituted as directed in the labeling), Related compounds, and Water (not more than 2.0%).

Cefaclor Extended-release Tablets USP—Preserve in tight, light-resistant containers. The labeling indicates the Drug Release Test with which the product complies. Contain the labeled amount, within ±10%, Meet the requirements for Identification, Drug release (5–30% in 30 minutes, 20–50% in 60 minutes, and not less than 80% in 240 minutes in 0.1 N hydrochloric acid in Apparatus 1 [10-mesh basket] at 100 rpm), Related compounds, Uniformity of dosage units, and Water (not more than 7.0%).

CEFADROXIL

Chemical name: 5-Thia-1-azabicyclo[4.2.0]oct-2-ene-2-carboxylic acid, 7-[[amino(4-hydroxyphenyl)acetyl]amino]-3-methyl-8-oxo-, monohydrate, [6R-[6 alpha,7 beta(R*)]]-.

Molecular formula: $C_{16}H_{17}N_3O_5S \cdot H_2O$.

Molecular weight: 381.40; 372.39 (hemihydrate); 363.40 (anhydrous).

Description: Cefadroxil USP—White to off-white, crystalline powder.

Solubility: Cefadroxil USP—Slightly soluble in water; practically insoluble in alcohol, in chloroform, and in ether.

Other characteristics: Acid-stable.

USP requirements:

Cefadroxil USP—Preserve in tight containers. The hemihydrate form is so labeled. Has a potency equivalent to not less than 950 mcg and not more than 1050 mcg of cefadroxil per mg, calculated on the anhydrous basis. Meets the requirements for Identification, Specific rotation (+165.0° to +178.0°), Crystallinity, pH (4.0–6.0, in a suspension containing 50 mg per mL), Water (4.2–6.0%, except that where it is labeled as being in the hemihydrate form it is 2.4–4.5%), Chromatographic purity, and Dimethylaniline.

Cefadroxil Capsules USP—Preserve in tight containers. Capsules prepared using the hemihydrate form of Cefadroxil are so labeled. Contain the equivalent of the labeled amount of anhydrous cefadroxil, within −10% to +20%. Meet the requirements for Identification, Dissolution (80% in 30 minutes in water in Apparatus 1 at 100 rpm), Uniformity of dosage units, and Water (not more than 7.0%).

Cefadroxil for Oral Suspension USP—Preserve in tight containers. A dry mixture of Cefadroxil and one or more suitable buffers, colors, diluents, and flavors. Contains the equivalent of the labeled amount of anhydrous cefadroxil, within −10% to +20%. Meets the requirements for Identification, Uniformity of dosage units (solid packaged in single-unit containers), Deliverable volume (solid packaged in multiple-unit containers), pH (4.5–6.0, in the suspension constituted as directed in the labeling), and Water (not more than 2.0%).

Cefadroxil Tablets USP—Preserve in tight containers. The Tablets prepared using the hemihydrate form of Cefadroxil are so labeled. Contain the labeled amount of anhydrous cefadroxil, within −10% to +20%. Meet the requirements for Identification, Dissolution (75% in 30 minutes in water in Apparatus 2 at 50 rpm), Uniformity of dosage units, and Water (not more than 8.0%).

CEFAMANDOLE

Chemical name:

Cefamandole nafate—5-Thia-1-azabicyclo[4.2.0]oct-2-ene-2-carboxylic acid, 7-[[(formyloxy)phenylacetyl]amino]-3-[[(1-methyl-1*H*-tetrazol-5-yl)thio]methyl]-8-oxo-, monosodium salt, [6*R*-[6 alpha,7 beta(*R**)]]-.

Cefamandole sodium—5-Thia-1-azabicyclo[4.2.0]oct-2-ene-2-carboxylic acid, 7-[(hydroxyphenylacetyl)amino]-3-[[(1-methyl-1*H*-tetrazol-5-yl)thio]methyl]-8-oxo-, [6*R*-[6 alpha,7 beta(*R**)]]-, monosodium salt.

Molecular formula:

Cefamandole nafate—$C_{19}H_{17}N_6NaO_6S_2$.

Cefamandole sodium—$C_{18}H_{17}N_6NaO_5S_2$.

Molecular weight:

Cefamandole nafate—512.50.

Cefamandole sodium—484.49.

Description:

Cefamandole Nafate USP—White, odorless, crystalline solid.

Cefamandole nafate for injection—After addition of diluent, cefamandole nafate rapidly hydrolyzes to cefamandole. Solutions of cefamandole nafate range from light yellow to amber, depending on concentration and diluent used.

Cefamandole Sodium USP—White to light yellowish-white, odorless crystalline powder.

Solubility:

Cefamandole Nafate USP—Soluble in water and in methanol; practically insoluble in ether, in chloroform, and in cyclohexane.

Cefamandole Sodium USP—Freely soluble in water and in dimethylformamide; soluble in methanol; slightly soluble in dehydrated alcohol; very slightly soluble in acetone.

Other characteristics: Cefamandole nafate—The pH of freshly reconstituted solutions usually ranges from 6.0 to 8.5.

USP requirements:

Cefamandole Nafate USP—Preserve in tight Containers. Where it is intended for use in preparing injectable dosage forms, the label states that it is sterile or must be subjected to further processing during the preparation of injectable dosage forms. Has a potency equivalent to not less than 810 mcg and not more than 1000 mcg of cefamandole per mg, calculated on the anhydrous basis. Meets the requirements for Identification, pH (3.5–7.0, in a solution containing 100 mg per mL), and Water (not more than 2.0%), and for Sterility tests and for Bacterial endotoxins under Cefamandole Nafate for Injection (where the label states that Cefamandole Nafate is sterile), and for Bacterial endotoxins under Cefamandole Nafate for Injection (where the label states that Cefamandole Nafate must be subjected to further processing during the preparation of injectable dosage forms).

Cefamandole Nafate for Injection USP—Preserve in Containers for Sterile Solids. A sterile mixture of Sterile Cefamandole Nafate and one or more suitable buffers. Has a potency equivalent to not less than 810 mcg and not more than 1000 mcg of cefamandole per mg, calculated on the anhydrous and sodium carbonate-free basis. Contains an amount of cefamandole nafate equivalent to the labeled amount of cefamandole, within −10% to +15%. Meets the requirements for Constituted solution, Identification, Bacterial endotoxins, Sterility, pH (6.0–8.0, determined after 30 minutes in a solution containing 100 mg per mL), Uniformity of dosage units, Water (not more than 3.0%), and Particulate matter, and for Injections.

Cefamandole Sodium for Injection USP—Preserve in Containers for Sterile Solids. A sterile mixture of Sterile Cefamandole Sodium and one or more suitable buffers. Contains an amount of cefamandole sodium equivalent to the labeled amount of cefamandole, within −10% to +15%. Meets the requirements for Constituted solution, Identification, Bacterial endotoxins, Sterility, pH (6.0–8.5, in a solution containing 100 mg of cefamandole per mL), Water (not more than 3.0%), and Particulate matter, and for Uniformity of dosage units and Labeling under Injections.

Sterile Cefamandole Sodium USP—Preserve in Containers for Sterile Solids. Has a potency equivalent to not less than 860 mcg and not more than 1000 mcg of cefamandole per mg, calculated on the anhydrous basis. Meets the requirements for Identification, Bacterial endotoxins, Sterility, pH (3.5–7.0, in a solution [1 in 10]), Water (not more than 3.0%), and Particulate matter.

CEFAZOLIN

Chemical name:

Cefazolin—5-Thia-1-azabicyclo[4.2.0]oct-2-ene-2-carboxylic acid, 3-[[(5-methyl-1,3,4-thiadiazol-2-yl)thio]methyl]-8-oxo-7-[[1*H*-tetrazol-1-yl)acetyl]amino]-(6*R-trans*).

Cefazolin sodium—5-Thia-1-azabicyclo[4.2.0]oct-2-ene-2-carboxylic acid, 3-[[(5-methyl-1,3,4-thiadiazol-2-yl)thio]methyl]-8-oxo-7-[[(1*H*-tetrazol-1-yl)acetyl]amino]-, monosodium salt (6*R-trans*)-.

Molecular formula:

Cefazolin—$C_{14}H_{14}N_8O_4S_3$.

Cefazolin sodium—$C_{14}H_{13}N_8NaO_4S_3$.

Molecular weight:

Cefazolin—454.51.

Cefazolin sodium—476.49.

Description:

Cefazolin USP—White to slightly off-white, odorless, crystalline powder. Melts at about 198 to 200 °C, with decomposition.

Cefazolin Sodium USP—White to off-white, practically odorless, crystalline powder, or white to off-white solid having the characteristic appearance of products prepared by freeze-drying.

Solubility:

Cefazolin USP—Soluble in dimethylformamide and in pyridine; sparingly soluble in acetone; slightly soluble in alcohol, in methanol, and in water; very slightly soluble in ethyl acetate, in isopropyl alcohol, and in methyl isobutyl ketone; practically insoluble in chloroform, in ether, and in methylene chloride.

Cefazolin Sodium USP—Freely soluble in water, in saline TS, and in dextrose solutions; very slightly soluble in alcohol; practically insoluble in chloroform and in ether.

USP requirements:

Cefazolin USP—Preserve in tight containers. Contains not less than 95.0% and not more than 103.0% of cefazolin, calculated on the anhydrous basis. Meets the requirements for Identification, Water (not more than 2.0%), and Heavy metals (not more than 0.002%).

Cefazolin Injection USP—Preserve in Containers for Injections. Maintain in the frozen state. A sterile solution of Cefazolin and Sodium Bicarbonate in a diluent containing one or more suitable tonicity-adjusting agents. It meets the requirements for Labeling under Injections. The label states that it is to be thawed just prior to use, describes conditions for proper storage of the resultant solution, and directs that the solution is not to be refrozen. Contains the labeled amount, within −10% to +15%. Meets the requirements for Identification, Bacterial endotoxins, Sterility, pH (4.5–7.0), and Particulate matter.

Cefazolin for Injection USP—Preserve in Containers for Sterile Solids. Contains an amount of Cefazolin Sodium equivalent to the labeled amount of cefazolin, within −10% to +15%. Meets the requirements for Constituted solution, Identification, Specific rotation (−10° to −24°),

Bacterial endotoxins, Sterility, pH (4.0–6.0, in a solution containing 100 mg of cefazolin per mL), Uniformity of dosage units, Water (not more than 6.0%), and Particulate matter, and for Labeling under Injections.

Cefazolin Ophthalmic Solution USP—Preserve in tight, sterile ophthalmic containers. Store in a refrigerator. Label it to state that it is intended for use in the eye and is not to be used if a precipitate is present. Contains an amount of Cefazolin Sodium equivalent to not less than 29.7 mg and not more than 36.3 mg of cefazolin in 10.0 mL of Ophthalmic Solution. Use Cefazolin Sodium or Cefazolin for Injection that contains the designated amount of cefazolin.

Prepare Cefazolin Ophthalmic Solution as follows: 35 mg of Cefazolin Sodium, 0.2 mg Thimerosal, and Sodium Chloride Injection (0.9%), a sufficient quantity to make 10.0 mL. Dissolve accurately weighed quantities of Cefazolin Sodium and Thimerosal in Sodium Chloride Injection (0.9%), and dilute quantitatively, and stepwise if necessary, with Sodium Chloride Injection (0.9%) to obtain a solution containing, in each mL, 3.5 mg of Cefazolin Sodium and 0.02 mg of Thimerosal. Filter a 10.0-mL portion of the resulting solution to produce a clear and sterile Ophthalmic Solution. If Cefazolin for Injection is used, prepare the Ophthalmic Solution as follows. Dissolve an accurately weighed quantity of Thimerosal in Sodium Chloride Injection (0.9%), and dilute quantitatively, and stepwise if necessary, with Sodium Chloride Injection (0.9%) to obtain a solution containing 0.3 mg of Thimerosal per mL. Add 9.8 mL of the resulting solution to a vial of Cefazolin for Injection, containing 500 mg of cefazolin, and mix to obtain a stock solution. Transfer 3.3 mL of the stock solution to a 50-mL volumetric flask, dilute with Sodium Chloride Injection (0.9%) to volume, and mix. Filter a 10.0-mL portion of the resulting solution to produce a clear and sterile Ophthalmic Solution.

Meets the requirements for Sterility, pH (4.5–6.0), and Beyond use date.

Cefazolin Sodium USP—Preserve in tight containers. Where it is intended for use in preparing injectable dosage forms, the label states that it is sterile or must be subjected to further processing during the preparation of injectable dosage forms. Has a potency equivalent to not less than 89.1% and not more than 110.1% of cefazolin sodium, calculated on the anhydrous basis. Meets the requirements for Identification, Specific rotation (–10° to –24°), pH (4.0–6.0, in a solution containing 100 mg of cefazolin per mL), and Water (not more than 6.0%), for Sterility and Bacterial endotoxins under Cefazolin for Injection (where the label states that Cefazolin Sodium is sterile), and for Bacterial endotoxins under Cefazolin for Injection (where the label states that Cefazolin Sodium must be subjected to further processing during the preparation of injectable dosage forms).

CEFDINIR

Chemical name: 5-Thia-1-azabicyclo[4.2.0]oct-2-ene-2-carboxylic acid, 7-[[[(2-amino-4-thiazolyl)(hydroxyimino)acetyl]amino]3-ethenyl-8-oxo, [6R-[6 alpha,7 beta(Z)]]-.

Molecular formula: $C_{14}H_{13}N_5O_5S_2$.

Molecular weight: 395.42.

Description: White to slightly brownish-yellow solid.

Solubility: Slightly soluble in dilute hydrochloric acid; sparingly soluble in 0.1 M pH 7.0 phosphate buffer.

USP requirements:
Cefdinir Capsules—Not in *USP–NF*.
Cefdinir for Oral Suspension—Not in *USP–NF*.

CEFDITOREN

Chemical name: Cefditoren pivoxil—(-)-(6R,7R)-2,2-dimethyl-propionyloxymethyl 7-[(Z)-2-(2-aminothiazol-4-yl)-2-methoxyi-minoacitamido]-3-[(Z)-2-(4-methylthiazol-5-yl)ethenyl]-8-oxo-5-thia-1-azabicyclo[4.2.0]oct-2-ene-2-carboxylate.

Molecular formula: Cefditoren pivoxil—$C_{25}H_{28}N_6O_7S_3$.

Molecular weight: Cefditoren pivoxil—620.73.

Description: Cefditoren pivoxil—Light yellow powder. Melting point 127–129°.

Solubility: Cefditoren pivoxil—Freely soluble in dilute hydrochloric acid; soluble in ethanol at a level of 6.06 mg per mL and in water at a label less than 0.1 mg per mL.

USP requirements: Cefditoren Pivoxil Tablets—Not in *USP–NF*.

CEFEPIME

Chemical name: Cefepime hydrochloride—Pyrrolidinium, 1-[[7-[[[(2-amino-4-thiazolyl)methoxyimino)acetyl]amino]-2-carboxy-8-oxo-5-thia-1-azabicyclo[4.2.0]oct-2-en-3-yl]methyl]-1-methyl-, chloride, monohydrochloride, monohydrate, [6R-[6 alpha,7 beta(Z)]]-.

Molecular formula: Cefepime hydrochloride—$C_{19}H_{25}ClN_6O_5S_2 \cdot HCl \cdot H_2O$.

Molecular weight: Cefepime hydrochloride—571.50.

Description:
Cefepime for Injection USP—White to pale yellow powder.
Cefepime Hydrochloride USP—White to off-white crystalline, nonhygroscopic solid.

Solubility:
Cefepime for Injection USP—Freely soluble in water.
Cefepime Hydrochloride USP—Freely soluble in water.

USP requirements:
Cefepime for Injection USP—Preserve in tight, light-resistant containers for Sterile Solids as described under Injections, and store in a refrigerator or at controlled room temperature. Store reconstituted powder in a refrigerator for no more than 7 days. A sterile mixture of Cefepime Hydrochloride and Arginine. Label it to indicate that it is to be diluted with a suitable parenteral vehicle prior to intravenous infusion. Contains the equivalent of the labled amount of cefepime, within -10% to +15%. Meets the requirements for Constituted solution, Identification, Bacterial endotoxins, Sterility, Uniformity of dosage units, pH (4.0–6.0, in a solution containing about 100 mg of cefepime per mL), Water (not more than 4.0%), Limit of *N*-methylpyrrolidine, and Related compounds, and for Labeling under Injection.

Cefepime Hydrochloride USP—Preserve in tight, light-resistant containers, and store at controlled room temperature. Where it is intended for use in preparing injectable dosage forms, the label states that it is sterile or must be subjected to further processing during the preparation of injectable dosage forms. Contains the equivalent of not less than 825 micrograms and not more than 911 micrograms of cefepime per gram, calculated on the anhydrous basis. Meets the requirements for Identification, Crystallinity, Bacterial endotoxins, Water (3.0%–4.5%), Residue on ignition (not more than 0.1%), Heavy metals (0.002%),

Limit of *N*-methylpyrrolidine, and Related compounds and for Sterility under Cefepime for Injection (where the label states that Cefepime Hydrochloride is sterile). Cefepime Hydrochloride for Injection—Not in *USP–NF*.

CEFIXIME

Chemical name: 5-Thia-1-azabicyclo[4.2.0]oct-2-ene-2-carboxylic acid, 7-[[(2-amino-4-thiazolyl)[(carboxymethoxy)imino]acetyl]amino]-3-ethenyl-8-oxo-, trihydrate, [6*R*-[6 alpha,7 beta(*Z*)]]-.

Molecular formula: $C_{16}H_{15}N_5O_7S_2 \cdot 3H_2O$.

Molecular weight: 507.50.

Description: Cefixime USP—White to light yellow, crystalline powder.

Solubility: Cefixime USP—Freely soluble in methanol; soluble in propylene glycol; slightly soluble in alcohol, in acetone, and in glycerin; very slightly soluble in 70% sorbitol and in octanol; practically insoluble in ether, in ethyl acetate, in hexane, and in water.

USP requirements:
Cefixime USP—Preserve in tight containers. Label to indicate that it is the trihydrate form. Where the quantity of cefixime is indicated in the labeling of any preparation containing Cefixime, this shall be understood to be in terms of anhydrous cefixime. Contains the equivalent of not less than 950 mcg and not more than 1030 mcg of cefixime per mg, calculated on the anhydrous basis. Meets the requirements for Identification, Specific rotation (−75° to −88°), Crystallinity, pH (2.6–4.1, in a solution containing the equivalent of 0.7 mg of cefixime per mL), Chromatographic purity, and Water (9.0–12.0%).
Cefixime for Oral Suspension USP—Preserve in tight containers. A dry mixture of Cefixime and one or more suitable diluents, flavors, preservatives, and suspending agents. Label it to indicate that the cefixime contained therein is in the trihydrate form. Contains the labeled amount of anhydrous cefixime, within −10% to +20%, per mL when constituted as directed in the labeling. Meets the requirements for Identification, Uniformity of dosage units (solid packaged in single-unit containers), Deliverable volume (solid packaged in multiple-unit containers), pH (2.5–4.5, in the suspension constituted as directed in the labeling), and Water (not more than 2.0%).
Cefixime Tablets USP—Preserve in tight containers. Label Tablets to indicate that the cefixime contained therein is in the trihydrate form. Contain the labeled amount of anhydrous cefixime, within ±10%. Meet the requirements for Identification, Dissolution (75% in 45 minutes in 0.05 *M* potassium phosphate buffer [pH 7.2] in Apparatus 1 at 100 rpm), Uniformity of dosage units, and Water (not more than 10.0%).

CEFMENOXIME

Chemical name: Cefmenoxime hydrochloride—5-Thia-1-azabicyclo[4.2.0]oct-2-ene-2-carboxylic acid, 7-[[(2-amino-4-thiazolyl)(methoxyimino)acetyl]amino]-3-[[(1-methyl-1*H*-tetrazol-5-yl)thio]methyl]-8-oxo-, hydrochloride (2:1), [6*R*-[6 alpha,7 beta(*Z*)]]-.

Molecular formula: Cefmenoxime hydrochloride—$(C_{16}H_{17}N_9O_5S_3)_2 \cdot HCl$.

Molecular weight: Cefmenoxime hydrochloride—1059.58.

Description: Cefmenoxime Hydrochloride USP—White to light orange-yellow crystals or crystalline powder.

Solubility: Cefmenoxime Hydrochloride USP—Very slightly soluble in water; freely soluble in formamide; slightly soluble in methanol; practically insoluble in dehydrated alcohol and in ether.

USP requirements:
Cefmenoxime Hydrochloride USP—Preserve in tight containers. Where it is intended for use in preparing injectable dosage forms, the label states that it is sterile or must be subjected to further processing during the preparation of injectable dosage forms. Contains the equivalent of not less than 869 mcg and not more than 1015 mcg of cefmenoxime per mg, calculated on the anhydrous basis. Meets the requirements for Identification, Crystallinity, Pyrogen, Sterility, and Water (not more than 1.5%).
Cefmenoxime for Injection USP—Preserve in Containers for Sterile Solids. Contains the labeled amount, within −10% to +15%. It may contain Sodium Carbonate. Meets the requirements for Identification, Pyrogen, Sterility, pH (6.4–7.9, in a solution containing the equivalent of 100 mg of cefmenoxime per mL), Loss on drying (not more than 1.5%), and Particulate matter.

CEFMETAZOLE

Chemical name:
Cefmetazole—5-Thia-1-azabicyclo[4.2.0]oct-2-ene-2-carboxylic acid, 7-[[[(cyanomethyl)thio]acetyl]amino]-7-methoxy-3-[[(1-methyl-1*H*-tetrazol-5-yl)thio]methyl]-8-oxo-, (6*R-cis*)-.
Cefmetazole sodium—5-Thia-1-azabicyclo[4.2.0]oct-2-ene-2-carboxylic acid, 7-[[[(cyanomethyl)thio]acetyl]amino]-7-methoxy-3-[[(1-methyl-1*H*-tetrazol-5-yl)thio]methyl]-8-oxo-, monosodium salt, (6*R-cis*)-.

Molecular formula:
Cefmetazole—$C_{15}H_{17}N_7O_5S_3$.
Cefmetazole sodium—$C_{15}H_{16}N_7NaO_5S_3$.

Molecular weight:
Cefmetazole—471.54.
Cefmetazole sodium—493.52.

Description:
Cefmetazole—White solid.
Cefmetazole Sodium USP—White solid having the characteristic appearance of products prepared by freeze-drying.

Solubility:
Cefmetazole—Very soluble in water and in methanol; soluble in acetone; practically insoluble in chloroform.
Cefmetazole Sodium USP—Very soluble in water and in methanol; soluble in acetone; practically insoluble in chloroform.

USP requirements:
Cefmetazole USP—Preserve in tight containers. Contains not less than 970 mcg and not more than 1030 mcg of cefmetazole per mg, calculated on the anhydrous basis. Meets the requirements for Identification and Water (not more than 0.5%).
Cefmetazole Injection USP—Preserve in Containers for Injections. Maintain in the frozen state. A sterile isoosmotic solution of Cefmetazole and Sodium Citrate in Water for Injection. Contains one or more buffer substances and a tonicity-adjusting agent. It meets the requirements for Labeling under Injections. The label states that it is to be thawed just prior to use, describes the conditions for proper storage of the resultant solution, and directs that the solution is not to be refrozen. Contains the labeled amount,

within −10% to +20%. Meets the requirements for Identification, Bacterial endotoxins, Sterility, pH (4.2–6.2), and Particulate matter.

Cefmetazole Sodium USP—Preserve in tight containers. Where it is intended for use in preparing injectable dosage forms, the label states that it is sterile or must be subjected to further processing during the preparation of injectable dosage forms. Contains the equivalent of not less than 860 mcg and not more than 1003 mcg of cefmetazole per mg, calculated on the anhydrous basis. Meets the requirements for Identification, pH (4.2–6.2, in a solution [1 in 10]), and Water (not more than 0.5%), for Sterility tests and for Bacterial endotoxins under Cefmetazole for Injection (where the label states that Cefmetazole Sodium is sterile), and for Bacterial endotoxins under Cefmetazole for Injection (where the label states that Cefmetazole Sodium must be subjected to further processing during the preparation of injectable dosage forms).

CEFONICID

Chemical name: Cefonicid sodium—5-Thia-1-azabicyclo[4.2.0]oct-2-ene-2-carboxylic acid, 7-[(hydroxyphenylacetyl)amino]8-oxo-3-[[[1-(sulfomethyl)-1H-tetrazol-5-yl]thio]methyl]disodium salt, [6R-[6 alpha,7 beta(R^*)]].

Molecular formula: Cefonicid sodium—$C_{18}H_{16}N_6Na_2O_8S_3$.

Molecular weight: Cefonicid sodium—586.53.

Description: Cefonicid Sodium USP—White to off-white solid having the characteristic appearance of products prepared by freeze-drying.

Solubility: Cefonicid Sodium USP—Freely soluble in water, in 0.9% sodium chloride solution, and in 5% dextrose solution; soluble in methanol; very slightly soluble in dehydrated alcohol.

USP requirements:
Cefonicid Injection—Not in USP–NF.
Cefonicid for Injection USP—Preserve in Containers for Sterile Solids. Contains an amount of Cefonicid Sodium equivalent to the labeled amount of cefonicid, within −10% to +20%. Meets the requirements for Constituted solution, Bacterial endotoxins, Sterility, and Particulate matter, for Identification, Specific rotation, pH, and Water under Cefonicid Sodium, and for Uniformity of dosage units and Labeling under Injections.
Cefonicid Sodium USP—Preserve in tight containers. Where it is intended for use in preparing injectable dosage forms, the label states that it is sterile or must be subjected to further processing during the preparation of injectable dosage forms. Contains the equivalent of not less than 832 mcg and not more than 970 mcg of cefonicid per mg, calculated on the anhydrous basis. Meets the requirements for Identification, Specific rotation (−37° to −47°), pH (3.5–6.5, in a solution [1 in 20]), and Water (not more than 5.0%), for Sterility and Bacterial endotoxins under Cefonicid for Injection (where the label states that Cefonicid Sodium is sterile), and for Bacterial endotoxins under Cefonicid for Injection (where the label states that Cefonicid Sodium must be subjected to further processing during the preparation of injectable dosage forms).

CEFOPERAZONE

Chemical name: Cefoperazone sodium—5-Thia-1-azabicyclo[4.2.0]oct-2-ene-2-carboxylic acid, 7-[[[[(4-ethyl-2,3-dioxo-1piperazinyl)carbonyl]amino](4-hydroxyphenyl)acetyl]amino]3-[[(1-methyl-1H-tetrazol-5-yl)thio]methyl]-8-oxo, monosodium salt, [6R-[6 alpha,7 beta(R^*)]]-.

Molecular formula: Cefoperazone sodium—$C_{25}H_{26}N_9NaO_8S_2$.

Molecular weight: Cefoperazone sodium—667.65.

Description:
Cefoperazone Sodium USP—White to pale buff crystalline powder.

Solubility:
Cefoperazone Sodium USP—Freely soluble in water and in methanol; slightly soluble in dehydrated alcohol; insoluble in acetone, in ethyl acetate, and in ether.

USP requirements:
Cefoperazone Sodium USP—Preserve in tight containers. Where it is intended for use in preparing injectable dosage forms, the label states that it is sterile or must be subjected to further processing during the preparation of injectable dosage forms. Contains the equivalent of not less than 870 mcg and not more than 1015 mcg of cefoperazone per mg, calculated on the anhydrous basis. Meets the requirements for Identification, Crystallinity, pH (4.5–6.5, in a solution [1 in 4]), and Water (not more than 5.0%), for Sterility and Bacterial endotoxins under Cefoperazone for Injection (where the label states that Cefoperazone Sodium is sterile), and for Bacterial endotoxins under Cefoperazone for Injection (where the label states that Cefoperazone Sodium must be subjected to further processing during the preparation of injectable dosage forms.
Cefoperazone Injection USP—Preserve in Containers for Injections. Maintain in the frozen state. A sterile solution of Cefoperazone Sodium and a suitable osmolality-adjusting substance in Water for Injection. It may contain a suitable buffer. It meets the requirements for Labeling under Injections. The label states that it is to be thawed just prior to use, describes conditions for proper storage of the resultant solution, and directs that the solution is not to be refrozen. Contains the equivalent of the labeled amount, within −10% to +20%. Meets the requirements for Identification, Bacterial endotoxins, Sterility, pH (4.5–6.5), and Particulate matter.
Cefoperazone for Injection USP—Preserve in Containers for Sterile Solids. Contains an amount of Cefoperazone Sodium equivalent to the labeled amount of cefoperazone, within −10% to +20%. Meets the requirements for Constituted solution, Bacterial endotoxins, Sterility, pH (4.5–6.5, in a solution [1 in 4]), Water (not more than 5.0%, except that where it is in the freeze-dried form, not more than 2.0%), and Particulate matter, for Identification under Cefoperazone Sodium, and for Uniformity of dosage units and Labeling under Injections.

CEFORANIDE

Chemical name: 5-Thia-1-azabicyclo[4.2.0]oct-2-ene-2-carboxylic acid, 7-[[[2-(aminomethyl)phenyl]acetyl]amino]-3-[[[1-(carboxymethyl)-1H-tetrazol-5-yl]thio]methyl]-8-oxo-, (6R-trans)-.

Molecular formula: $C_{20}H_{21}N_7O_6S_2$.

Molecular weight: 519.56.

Description:
Ceforanide USP—White to off-white powder.

Ceforanide for injection—Solutions of ceforanide range in color or from light yellow to amber depending on the concentration and diluent used.

Solubility: Ceforanide USP—Practically insoluble in water, in methanol, in chloroform, and in ether; very soluble in 1 N sodium hydroxide.

Other characteristics: Ceforanide for injection—The pH of the solution ranges from 5.5 to 8.5.

USP requirements:

Ceforanide USP—Preserve in tight containers. Where it is intended for use in preparing injectable dosage forms, the label states that it is sterile or must be subjected to further processing during the preparation of injectable dosage forms. Contains not less than 900 mcg and not more than 1050 mcg of ceforanide per mg. Meets the requirements for Identification, Bacterial endotoxins, Sterility, pH (2.5–4.5, in a suspension containing 50 mg per mL), and Water (not more than 5.0%).

Ceforanide for Injection USP—Preserve in Containers for Sterile Solids. A sterile mixture of sterile Ceforanide and L-Lysine. Contains not less than 900 mcg and not more than 1050 mcg of ceforanide per mg on the L-Lysine-free basis, and the labeled amount, within −10% to +15%. Meets the requirements for Identification, Bacterial endotoxins, Sterility, pH (5.5–8.5, constituted as directed in the labeling), Water (not more than 3.0%), Particulate matter, and Content of L-lysine, for Uniformity of dosage units, and for Labeling under Injections.

CEFOTAXIME

Chemical name: Cefotaxime sodium—5-Thia-1-azabicyclo[4.2.0]oct-2-ene-2-carboxylic acid, 3-[(acetyloxy)methyl]-7-[[(2-amino-4-thiazolyl)(methoxyimino)acetyl]amino]-8-oxo-, monosodium salt, [6R-[6 alpha,7 beta(Z)]]-.

Molecular formula: Cefotaxime sodium—$C_{16}H_{16}N_5NaO_7S_2$.

Molecular weight: Cefotaxime sodium—477.45.

Description:

Cefotaxime Sodium USP—Off-white to pale yellow crystalline powder.

Solubility: Cefotaxime Sodium USP—Freely soluble in water; practically insoluble in organic solvents.

USP requirements:

Cefotaxime Sodium USP—Preserve in tight containers. Where it is intended for use in preparing injectable dosage forms, the label states that it is sterile or must be subjected to further processing during the preparation of injectable dosage forms. Contains the equivalent of not less than 916 mcg and not more than 964 mcg of cefotaxime per mg, calculated on the dried basis. Meets the requirements for Clarity and color of solution, Identification, Specific rotation (+58° to +64°), pH (4.5–6.5, in a solution [1 in 10]), Loss on drying (not more than 3.0%), and Chromatographic purity, for Sterility and Bacterial endotoxins under Cefotaxime for Injection (where the label states that Cefotaxime Sodium is sterile), and for Bacterial endotoxins under Cefotaxime for Injection (where the label states that Cefotaxime Sodium must be subjected to further processing during the preparation of injectable dosage forms).

Cefotaxime Injection USP—Preserve in single-dose containers. Maintain in the frozen state. A sterile solution of Cefotaxime Sodium in Water for Injection. Contains one or more suitable buffers. It meets the requirements for Labeling under Injections. The label states that it is to be thawed just prior to use, describes conditions for proper storage of the resultant solution, and directs that the solution is not to be refrozen. Contains an amount of cefotaxime sodium

equivalent to the labeled amount of cefotaxime, within ± 10%. Meets the requirements for Identification, Bacterial endotoxins, Sterility, pH (5.0–7.5), Particulate matter, and Chromatographic purity.

Cefotaxime for Injection USP—Preserve in Containers for Sterile Solids. Contains an amount of Cefotaxime Sodium equivalent to the labeled amount of cefotaxime, within −10% to +15%. Meets the requirements for Constituted solution, Identification, Bacterial endotoxins, Sterility, Uniformity of dosage units, Particulate matter, and Chromatographic purity, for Identification, pH, and Loss on drying under Cefotaxime Sodium, and for Labeling under Injections.

CEFOTETAN

Chemical name:

Cefotetan—5-Thia-1-azabicyclo[4.2.0]oct-2-ene-2-carboxylic acid, 7-[[[4-(2-amino-1-carboxy-2-oxoethylidene)-1,3-dithietan-2-yl]carbonyl]amino]-7-methoxy-3-[[(1-methyl-1H-tetrazol-5-yl)-thio]methyl]-8-oxo-, [6R-(6 alpha,7 alpha)]-.

Cefotetan disodium—5-Thia-1-azabicyclo[4.2.0]oct-2-ene-2-carboxylic acid, 7-[[[4-(2-amino-1-carboxy-2-oxoethylidene)-1,3-dithietan-2-yl]carbonyl]amino]-7-methoxy-3-[[(1-methyl-1H-tetrazol-5-yl)thio]methyl]-8-oxo-, disodium salt, [6R-(6 alpha,7 alpha)]-.

Molecular formula:

Cefotetan—$C_{17}H_{17}N_7O_8S_4$.

Cefotetan disodium—$C_{17}H_{15}N_7Na_2O_8S_4$.

Molecular weight:

Cefotetan—575.62.

Cefotetan disodium—619.59.

Description:

Cefotetan disodium—White to pale yellow powder.

Solubility: Cefotetan disodium—Very soluble in water.

Other characteristics: Cefotetan disodium—The pH of freshly reconstituted solutions is usually between 4.5 and 6.5.

USP requirements:

Cefotetan USP—Preserve in tight containers. Where it is intended for use in preparing injectable dosage forms, the label states that it is sterile or must be subjected to further processing during the preparation of injectable dosage forms. Contains not less than 950 mcg and not more than 1030 mcg of cefotetan per mg, calculated on the anhydrous basis. Meets the requirements for Identification, Water (not more than 2.5%), and Sterility (where it is labeled as sterile), and for Bacterial endotoxins under Cefotetan for Injection (where the label states that Cefotetan is sterile or must be subjected to further processing during the preparation of injectable dosage forms).

Cefotetan Injection USP—Preserve in Containers for Injections. Maintain in the frozen state. A sterile isoosmotic solution of Cefotetan and Sodium Bicarbonate in Water for Injection. Contains one or more buffer substances and a tonicity-adjusting agent. It meets the requirements for Labeling under Injections. The label states that it is to be thawed just prior to use, describes the conditions for proper storage of the resultant solution, and directs that the solution is not to be refrozen. Contains the labeled amount, within −10% to +20%. Meets the requirements for Identification, Bacterial endotoxins, Sterility, pH (4.0–6.5), and Particulate matter.

Cefotetan for Injection USP—Preserve in Containers for Sterile Solids. Contains an amount of Cefotetan Disodium equivalent to the labeled amount of cefotetan, within −10% to +20%. Meets the requirements for Constituted solution, Bacterial endotoxins, Sterility, and Particulate

matter, for Identification, pH, and Water under Cefotetan Disodium, for Uniformity of dosage units, and for Labeling under Injections.

Cefotetan Disodium USP—Preserve in tight containers. Where it is intended for use in preparing injectable dosage forms, the label states that it is sterile or must be subjected to further processing during the preparation of injectable dosage forms. Contains the equivalent of not less than 830 mcg and not more than 970 mcg of cefotetan per mg, calculated on the anhydrous basis. Meets the requirements for Identification, pH (4.0–6.5, in a solution [1 in 10]), and Water (not more than 1.5%), for Sterility and Bacterial endotoxins under Cefotetan for Injection (where the label states that Cefotetan Disodium is sterile), and for Bacterial endotoxins under Cefotetan for Injection (where the label states that Cefotetan Disodium must be subjected to further processing during the preparation of injectable dosage forms).

CEFOTIAM

Chemical name: Cefotiam hydrochloride—5-Thia-1-azabicyclo[4.2.0]oct-2-ene-2-carboxylic acid, 7-[[(2-amino-4-thiazolyl)acetyl]amino]-3-[[[1-[2-(dimethylamino)ethyl]-1*H*-tetrazol-5-yl]thio]methyl]-8-oxo, hydrochloride, (6*R-trans*)-.

Molecular formula: Cefotiam hydrochloride—$C_{18}H_{23}N_9O_4S_3 \cdot 2HCl$.

Molecular weight: Cefotiam hydrochloride—598.55.

Description: Cefotiam hydrochloride—White to light yellow crystals.

Solubility: Cefotiam hydrochloride—Soluble in methanol; slightly soluble in ethanol.

USP requirements:

Cefotiam Hydrochloride USP—Preserve in tight containers. Where it is intended for use in preparing injectable dosage forms, the label states that it is sterile or must be subjected to further processing during the preparation of injectable dosage forms. Contains an amount of Cefotiam Hydrochloride equivalent to not less than 790 mcg and not more than 925 mcg of cefotiam per mg, calculated on the anhydrous basis. Meets the requirements for Identification, Crystallinity, Pyrogen, Sterility, and Water (not more than 7.0%).

Cefotiam for Injection USP—Preserve in Containers for Sterile Solids. Contains an amount of Cefotiam Hydrochloride equivalent to the labeled amount of cefotiam, within −10% to +20%. It may contain Sodium Carbonate. Meets the requirements for Identification, Pyrogen, Sterility, pH (5.7–7.2, in a solution containing the equivalent of 100 mg of cefotiam per mL), Loss on drying (not more than 6.0%), and Particulate matter.

CEFOXITIN

Source: Cefoxitin sodium—Semisynthetic cephamycin derived from cephamycin C, produced by *Streptomyces lactamdurans*.

Chemical name: Cefoxitin sodium—5-Thia-1-azabicyclo[4.2.0]oct-2-ene-2-carboxylic acid, 3-[[(aminocarbonyl)oxy]methyl]-7-methoxy-8-oxo-7-[(2-thienylacetyl)amino]-, sodium salt, (6*R-cis*)-.

Molecular formula: Cefoxitin sodium—$C_{16}H_{16}N_3NaO_7S_2$.

Molecular weight: Cefoxitin sodium—449.44.

Description: Cefoxitin Sodium USP—White to off-white, granules or powder, having a slight characteristic odor. Is somewhat hygroscopic.

Solubility: Cefoxitin Sodium USP—Very soluble in water; soluble in methanol; sparingly soluble in dimethylformamide; slightly soluble in acetone; insoluble in ether and in chloroform.

USP requirements:

Cefoxitin Injection USP—Preserve in Containers for Injections. Maintain in the frozen state. A sterile solution of Cefoxitin Sodium and one or more suitable buffer substances in Water for Injection. Contains Dextrose or Sodium Chloride as a tonicity-adjusting agent. It meets the requirements for Labeling under Injections. The label states that it is to be thawed just prior to use, describes conditions for proper storage of the resultant solution, and directs that the solution is not to be refrozen. Contains an amount of cefoxitin sodium equivalent to the labeled amount of cefoxitin, within −10% to +20%. Meets the requirements for Identification, Bacterial endotoxins, Sterility, pH (4.5–8.0), and Particulate matter.

Cefoxitin for Injection USP—Preserve in Containers for Sterile Solids. Contains Cefoxitin Sodium equivalent to the labeled amount of cefoxitin, within −10% to +20%. Meets the requirements for Constituted solution, Bacterial endotoxins, Sterility, and Particulate matter, for Identification tests, pH, and Water under Cefoxitin Sodium, for Uniformity of dosage units, and for Labeling under Injections.

Cefoxitin Sodium USP—Preserve in tight containers, and store in a cold place. Where it is intended for use in preparing injectable dosage forms, the label states that it is sterile or must be subjected to further processing during the preparation of injectable dosage forms. Contains the equivalent of not less than 927 mcg and not more than 970 mcg of cefoxitin per mg, corresponding to not less than 97.5% and not more than 102.0% of cefoxitin sodium, calculated on the anhydrous and acetone- and methanol-free basis. Meets the requirements for Identification, Specific rotation (+206° to +214°, calculated on the anhydrous and acetone- and methanol-free basis), Crystallinity, pH (4.2–7.0, in a solution containing 100 mg per mL), Water (not more than 1.0%), Heavy metals (not more than 0.002%), and Limit of acetone and methanol (not more than 0.7% of acetone and 0.1% of methanol), for Sterility and Bacterial endotoxins under Cefoxitin for Injection (where the label states that Cefoxitin Sodium is sterile), and for Bacterial endotoxins under Cefoxitin for Injection (where the label states that Cefoxitin Sodium must be subjected to further processing during the preparation of injectable dosage forms).

CEFPIRAMIDE

Chemical name: 5-Thia-1-azabicyclo[4.2.0]oct-2-ene-2-carboxylic acid, 7-[[[[(4-hydroxy-6-methyl-3-pyridinyl)carbonyl]amino]-(4-hydroxyphenyl)acetyl]amino]-3-[[(1-methyl-1*H*-tetrazol-5-yl)thio]methyl]-8-oxo-, [6*R*-[6 alpha,7 beta(*R**)]]-.

Molecular formula: $C_{25}H_{24}N_8O_7S_2$.

Molecular weight: 612.64.

Description: Yellow crystals. Melting point is 213–215 °C.

USP requirements:

Cefpiramide USP—Preserve in tight containers. Where it is intended for use in preparing injectable dosage forms, the label states that it is sterile or must be subjected for further processing during the preparation of injectable dosage forms. Contains not less than 974 mcg and not more than

1026 mcg of cefpiramide per mg, calculated on the anhydrous basis. Meets the requirements for Identification, Specific rotation (−100° to −112°), Crystallinity, pH (3.0–5.0, in a suspension [1 in 200]), Water (not more than 9.0%), and Related compounds (not more than 2.0%), for Sterility and Pyrogen under Cefpiramide for Injection (where the label states that Cefpiramide is sterile) and for Pyrogen under Cefpiramide for Injection (where the label states that Cefpiramide must be subjected to further processing during the preparation of injectable dosage forms).

Cefpiramide for Injection USP—Preserve in Containers for Sterile Solids. Contains the labeled amount, within −10% to +20%. Meets the requirements for Identification, Pyrogen, Sterility, pH (6.0–8.0, in a solution containing the equivalent of 100 mg of cefpiramide per mL), Water (not more than 3.0%), and Particulate matter.

CEFPODOXIME

Chemical name: Cefpodoxime proxetil—5-Thia-1-azabicyclo[4.2.0]oct-2-ene-2-carboxylic acid, 7-[[(2-amino-4-thiazolyl)(methoxyimino)acetyl]amino]-3-(methoxymethyl)-8-oxo-, 1-[[(1-methylethoxy)carbonyl]oxy]ethyl ester, [6R-[6 alpha,7 beta(Z)]]-.

Molecular formula: Cefpodoxime proxetil—$C_{21}H_{27}N_5O_9S_2$.

Molecular weight: Cefpodoxime proxetil—557.60.

Description: Cefpodoxime Proxetil USP—White to light brownish white powder. Odorless or having a faint ordor.

Solubility: Cefpodoxime Proxetil USP—Very slightly soluble in water; soluble in acetonitrile and in methanol; freely soluble in dehydrated alcohol; slightly soluble in either.

USP requirements:
Cefpodoxime Proxetil USP—Preserve in tight containers at a temperature not exceeding 25°. Contains the equivalent of not less than 690 micrograms and not more than 805 micrograms of cefpodoxime, calculated on the anhydrous basis. Meets the requirements for Identification, Specific rotation (+35.0° to +48.0°), Water (not more than 3.0%), Residue on ignition (not more than 0.2%), Heavy metals (0.002%), Isomer ratio (0.5–0.6), and Chromatographic purity.

Cefpodoxime Proxetil for Oral Suspension USP—Preserve in tight containers, at a temperature not exceeding 30°. Store the constituted Oral Suspension in a refrigerator. Contains Cefpodoxime Proxetil and one or more buffers, suspending agents, sweetners, flavorings, and preservatives. Contains the equivalent amount of the labeled amount of cefpodoxime, within ±10%, when constituted as directed in the labeling. Meets the requirements for Identification, Uniformity of dosage units, Deliverable volume, pH (4.0–5.5, in the suspension constituted as directed in the labeling), and Water (not more than 1.5%).

Cefpodoxime Proxetil Tablets USP—Preserve in tight containers, at room temperature. Contains an equivalent amount of the labeled amount of cefpodoxime, within ±10%. Meets the requirements for Identification, Dissolution (70% in 30 minutes in a solution [pH 3.0±0.1] in Apparatus 2 at 75 rpm), Uniformity of dosage units, and Water (not more than 5.0%).

CEFPROZIL

Chemical name: 5-Thia-1-azabicyclo[4.2.0]oct-2-ene-2-carboxylic acid, 7-[[amino(4-hydroxyphenyl)acetyl]amino]-8-oxo-3-(1-propenyl)-, monohydrate, [6R-[6 alpha,7 beta(R*)]]-.

Molecular formula: $C_{18}H_{19}N_3O_5S \cdot H_2O$.

Molecular weight: 407.44.

Description: White to yellowish powder.

USP requirements:
Cefprozil USP—Preserve in tight containers. Contains not less than 900 mcg and not more than 1050 mcg of cefprozil per mg, calculated on the anhydrous basis. Meets the requirements for Identification, Crystallinity, pH (3.5–6.5, in a solution containing 5 mg per mL), Water (3.5–6.5%), and Cefprozil (E)-isomer ratio (0.06–0.11).

Cefprozil for Oral Suspension USP—Preserve in tight containers. A dry mixture of Cefprozil and one or more suitable buffers, flavors, preservatives, suspending agents, and sweeteners. Contains the labeled amount, within −10% to +20%. Meets the requirements for Identification, Uniformity of dosage units (for solids packaged in single-unit containers), pH (4.0–6.0, in the Oral Suspension constituted as directed in the labeling), and Water (not more than 3.0%).

Cefprozil Tablets USP—Preserve in tight containers. Contain the labeled amount, within −10% to +20%. Meet the requirements for Identification, Dissolution (75% in 45 minutes in water in Apparatus 1 at 100 rpm), Uniformity of dosage units, and Water (not more than 7.0%).

CEFTAZIDIME

Chemical name: Pyridinium, 1-[[7-[[(2-amino-4-thiazolyl)[(1-carboxy-1-methylethoxy)imino]acetyl]amino]-2-carboxy-8-oxo-5-thia-1-azabicyclo[4.2.0]oct-2-en-3-yl]methyl]-, hydroxide, inner salt, pentahydrate, [6R-[6 alpha,7 beta(Z)]]-.

Molecular formula: $C_{22}H_{22}N_6O_7S_2 \cdot 5H_2O$.

Molecular weight: 636.65.

Description:
Ceftazidime USP—White to cream-colored, crystalline powder.
Ceftazidime for injection—Solutions of ceftazidime range in color from light yellow to amber, depending upon the diluent and volume used.

Solubility: Ceftazidime USP—Soluble in alkali and in dimethyl sulfoxide; slightly soluble in dimethylformamide, in methanol, and in water; insoluble in acetone, in alcohol, in chloroform, in dioxane, in ether, in ethyl acetate, and in toluene.

Other characteristics: Ceftazidime for injection—The pH of freshly constituted solutions usually ranges from 5 to 8.

USP requirements:
Ceftazidime USP—Preserve in tight containers. Where it is intended for use in preparing injectable dosage forms, the label states that it is sterile or must be subjected to further processing during the preparation of injectable or other sterile dosage forms. Contains not less than 95.0% and not more than 102.0% of ceftazidime, calculated on the dried basis. Meets the requirements for Identification, Crystallinity, Steility, pH (3.0–4.0, in a solution containing 5 mg per mL), and Loss on drying (13.0–15.0%), and for Bacterial endotoxins under Ceftazidine for Injection (where the label states that Ceftazidine is sterile or that it must be subjected to further processing during the preparation of injectable or other sterile dosage forms).

Ceftazidime Injection USP—Preserve in Containers for Injections. Maintain in the frozen state. A sterile isoosmotic solution of Ceftazidime in Water for Injection. It meets the

requirements for Labeling under Injections. The label states that it is to be thawed just prior to use, describes conditions for proper storage of the resultant solution, and directs that the solution is not to be refrozen. Contains one or more suitable buffers and a tonicity-adjusting agent. Contains the labeled amount, within −10% to +20%. Meets the requirements for Identification, Pyrogen, Sterility, pH (5.0–7.5), and Particulate matter.

Ceftazidime for Injection USP—Preserve in Containers for Sterile Solids, protected from light. A sterile mixture of Sterile Ceftazidime and Sodium Carbonate or Arginine. Contains not less than 90.0% and not more than 105.0% of ceftazidime, on the dried and sodium carbonate– or arginine–free basis, and contains the labeled amount, within −10% to +20%. Meets the requirements for Identification, Bacterial endotoxins, Sterility, pH (5.0–7.5, in a solution constituted in the sealed container, taking care to relieve the pressure inside the container during constitution, containing 100 mg of ceftazidime per mL), Loss on drying (not more than 13.5%), Particulate matter, Sodium carbonate (where present), Limit of pyridine, and Content of arginine (where present), for Uniformity of dosage units, and for Labeling under Injections.

CEFTIBUTEN

Chemical name: 5-Thia-1-azabicyclo[4.2.0]oct-2-ene-2-carboxylic acid, 7-[[2-(2-amino-4-thiazolyl)-4-carboxy-1-oxo-2butenyl]amino]-8-oxo, [6R-[6 alpha,7 beta(Z)]]-.

Molecular formula: $C_{15}H_{14}N_4O_6S_2$.

Molecular weight: 410.43.

USP requirements:
Ceftibuten Capsules—Not in *USP–NF*.
Ceftibuten for Oral Suspension—Not in *USP–NF*.

CEFTIOFUR

Chemical name:
Ceftiofur hydrochloride—5-Thia-1-azabicyclo[4.2.0]oct-2-ene-2-carboxylic acid, 7-[[(2-amino-4-thiazolyl)(methoxyimino)acetyl]amino]-3-[[(2-furanylcarbonyl)thio]methyl]8-oxo-, monohydrochloride, [6R-[6 alpha,7 beta(Z)]]-.
Ceftiofur sodium—5-Thia-1-azabicyclo[4.2.0]oct-2-ene-2-carboxylic acid, 7-[[(2-amino-4-thiazolyl)(methoxyimino)acetyl]amino]-3-[[(2-furanylcarbonyl)thio]methyl]8-oxo-, monosodium salt, [6R-[6 alpha,7 beta(Z)]]-.

Molecular formula:
Ceftiofur hydrochloride—$C_{19}H_{17}N_5O_7S_3 \cdot$ HCl.
Ceftiofur sodium—$C_{19}H_{16}N_5NaO_7S_3$.

Molecular weight:
Ceftiofur hydrochloride—560.03.
Ceftiofur sodium—545.55.

USP requirements:
Sterile Ceftiofur Hydrochloride Suspension—Not in *USP–NF*.
Sterile Ceftiofur Sodium—Not in *USP–NF*.

CEFTIZOXIME

Chemical name: Ceftizoxime sodium—5-Thia-1-azabicyclo[4.2.0]oct-2-ene-2-carboxylic acid, 7-[[(2,3-dihydro-2-imino-4-thiazolyl)(methoxyimino)acetyl]amino]-8-oxomonosodium salt, [6R-[6 alpha,7 beta(Z)]]-.

Molecular formula: Ceftizoxime sodium—$C_{13}H_{12}N_5NaO_5S_2$.

Molecular weight: Ceftizoxime sodium—405.39.

Description: Ceftizoxime Sodium USP—White to pale yellow crystalline powder.

Solubility: Ceftizoxime Sodium USP—Freely soluble in water.

Other characteristics: Ceftizoxime sodium—A 10% solution in water has a pH of 6 to 8.

USP requirements:
Ceftizoxime Sodium USP—Preserve in tight containers. Where it is intended for use in preparing injectable dosage forms, the label states that it is sterile or must be subjected to further processing during the preparation of injectable dosage forms. Contains the equivalent of not less than 850 mcg and not more than 995 mcg of ceftizoxime per mg, calculated on the anhydrous basis. Meets the requirements for Identification, Crystallinity, pH (6.0–8.0, in a solution [1 in 10]), and Water (not more than 8.5%), for Sterility and Bacterial endotoxins under Ceftizoxime for Injection (where the label states that Ceftizoxime Sodium is sterile), and for Bacterial endotoxins under Ceftizoxime for Injection (where the label states that Ceftizoxime Sodium must be subjected to further processing during the preparation of injectable dosage forms).

Ceftizoxime Injection USP—Preserve in Containers for Injections. Maintain in the frozen state. A sterile solution of Ceftizoxime Sodium in a diluent containing one or more tonicity-adjusting agents in Water for Injection. It meets the requirements for Labeling under Injections. The label states that it is to be thawed just prior to use, describes conditions for proper storage of the resultant solution, and directs that the solution is not to be refrozen. Contains the equivalent of the labeled amount of ceftizoxime, within −10% to +15%. Meets the requirements for Identification, Bacterial endotoxins, Sterility, pH (5.5–8.0), and Particulate matter.

Ceftizoxime for Injection USP—Preserve in Containers for Sterile Solids. Contains an amount of Ceftizoxime Sodium equivalent to the labeled amount of ceftizoxime, within −10% to +15%. Meets the requirements for Constituted solution, Bacterial endotoxins, Sterility, and Particulate matter, for Identification, Crystallinity, pH, and Water under Ceftizoxime Sodium, and for Uniformity of Dosage Units and Labeling under Injections.

CEFTRIAXONE

Chemical name: Ceftriaxone sodium—5-Thia-1-azabicyclo[4.2.0]oct-2-ene-2-carboxylic acid, 7-[[(2-amino-4-thiazolyl)(methoxyimino)acetyl]amino]-8-oxo-3-[[(1,2,5,6-tetrahydro2-methyl-5,6-dioxo-1,2,4-triazin-3-yl)thio]methyl]-, disodium salt, [6R-[6 alpha,7 beta(Z)]]-, hydrate (2:7).

Molecular formula: Ceftriaxone sodium—$C_{18}H_{16}N_8Na_2O_7S_3 \cdot 3\frac{1}{2}H_2O$.

Molecular weight: Ceftriaxone sodium—661.60.

Description:
Ceftriaxone Sodium USP—White to yellowish-orange crystalline powder.

Solubility:
Ceftriaxone Sodium USP—Freely soluble in water; sparingly soluble in methanol; very slightly soluble in alcohol.

USP requirements:
Ceftriaxone Sodium USP—Preserve in tight containers. Where it is intended for use in preparing injectable dosage forms, the label states that it is sterile or must be subjected to further processing during the preparation of injectable dosage forms. Contains the equivalent of not less than

795 mcg of ceftriaxone per mg, calculated on the anhydrous basis. Meets the requirements for Identification, Crystallinity, pH (6.0–8.0 in a solution [1 in 10]), and Water (8.0–11.0%), for Sterility and Bacterial endotoxins under Ceftriaxone for Injection (where the label states that Ceftriaxone Sodium is sterile), and for Bacterial endotoxins under Ceftriaxone for Injection (where the label states that Ceftriaxone Sodium must be subjected to further processing during the preparation of injectable dosage forms).

Ceftriaxone Injection USP—Preserve in Containers for Injections. Maintain in the frozen state. A sterile solution of Ceftriaxone Sodium in a diluent containing one or more tonicity-adjusting agents in Water for Injection. It meets the requirements for Labeling under Injections. The label states that it is to be thawed just prior to use, describes conditions for proper storage of the resultant solution, and directs that the solution is not to be refrozen. Contains the equivalent of the labeled amount, within −10% to +15%. Meets the requirements for Identification, Bacterial endotoxins, Sterility, pH (6.0–8.0), and Particulate matter.

Ceftriaxone for Injection USP—Preserve in Containers for Sterile Solids. Contains an amount of Ceftriaxone Sodium equivalent to not less than 776 mcg of ceftriaxone per mg, calculated on the anhydrous basis, and the equivalent of the labeled amount of ceftriaxone, within −10% to +15%. Meets the requirements for Constituted solution, Bacterial endotoxins, Sterility, and Particulate matter, for Identification, Crystallinity, pH, and Water under Ceftriaxone Sodium, and for Uniformity of dosage units and Labeling under Injections.

CEFUROXIME

Chemical name:
Cefuroxime—5-Thia-1-azabicyclo[4.2.0]oct-2-ene-2-carboxylic acid, 3-[[(aminocarbonyl)oxy]methyl]-7-[[2-furanyl(methoxyimino)acetyl]amino]-8-oxo-, [6*R*-[6 alpha,7 beta(*Z*)]]-.

Cefuroxime axetil—5-Thia-1-azabicyclo[4.2.0]oct-2-ene-2-carboxylic acid, 3-[[(aminocarbonyl)oxy]methyl]-7-[[2-furanyl(methoxyimino)acetyl]amino]-8-oxo-, 1-(acetyloxy)ethyl ester, [6*R*-[6 alpha,7 beta(*Z*)]]-.

Cefuroxime sodium—5-Thia-1-azabicyclo[4.2.0]oct-2-ene-2-carboxylic acid, 3-[[(aminocarbonyl)oxy]methyl]-7-[[2-furanyl(methoxyimino)acetyl]amino]-8-oxo-, monosodium salt [6*R*-[6 alpha,7 beta(*Z*)]]-.

Molecular formula:
Cefuroxime —$C_{16}H_{16}N_4O_8S$.
Cefuroxime axetil—$C_{20}H_{22}N_4O_{10}S$.
Cefuroxime sodium—$C_{16}H_{15}N_4NaO_8S$.

Molecular weight:
Cefuroxime—424.39.
Cefuroxime axetil—510.48.
Cefuroxime sodium—446.37.

Description:
Cefuroxime Axetil USP—White to almost white powder.
Cefuroxime Sodium USP—White or faintly yellow powder.

Solubility:
Cefuroxime Axetil USP—The amorphous form is freely soluble in acetone; soluble in chloroform, in ethyl acetate, and in methanol; slightly soluble in dehydrated alcohol; insoluble in ether and in water. The crystalline form is freely soluble in acetone; sparingly soluble in chloroform, in ethyl acetate, and in methanol; slightly soluble in dehydrated alcohol; insoluble in ether and in water.
Cefuroxime Sodium USP—Freely soluble in water; soluble in methanol; very slightly soluble in alcohol, in ether, in ethyl acetate, and in chloroform.

Other characteristics: Cefuroxime—pH: 6–8.5 (freshly reconstituted solution) and 5–7.5 (thawed solutions); Osmolality: 300 mOsmol/kg.

USP requirements:
Cefuroxime Injection USP—Preserve in Containers for Injections. Maintain in the frozen state. A sterile isoosmotic solution of Cefuroxime Sodium in Water for Injection. Contains one or more suitable buffers and a tonicity-adjusting agent. It meets the requirements for Labeling under Injections. The label states that it is to be thawed just prior to use, describes conditions for proper storage of the resultant solution, and directs that the solution is not to be refrozen. Contains the labeled amount, within −10% to +20%. Meets the requirements for Identification, Bacterial endotoxins, Sterility, pH (5.0–7.5), and Particulate matter, and for Uniformity of dosage units.

Cefuroxime for Injection USP—Preserve in Containers for Sterile Solids. Contains an amount of Cefuroxime Sodium equivalent to the labeled amount of cefuroxime, within −10% to +20%. Meets the requirements for Constituted solution, Bacterial endotoxins, Sterility, Uniformity of dosage units, and Particulate matter, for Identification, pH, and Water under Cefuroxime Sodium, and for Labeling under Injections.

Cefuroxime Axetil USP—Preserve in tight containers. A mixture of the diastereoisomers of cefuroxime axetil. Label it to indicate whether it is amorphous or crystalline. Contains the equivalent of not less than 745 mcg and not more than 875 mcg of cefuroxime per mg, calculated on the anhydrous basis. Meets the requirements for Identification, Crystallinity, Water (not more than 1.5%), and Diastereoisomer ratio (0.48–0.55).

Cefuroxime Axetil for Oral Suspension USP—Preserve in well-closed containers at controlled room temperature. Contains the labeled amount, within ±10%. Meets the requirements for Identification, Dissolution (60% in 30 minutes in 0.07 M phosphate buffer [pH 7.0], prepared by dissolving 3.7 grams of monobasic sodium phosphate and 5.7 grams of dibasic sodium phosphate in 1000 mL of water, in Apparatus 2 at 50 rpm), Uniformity of dosage units, Deliverable volume, pH (3.5–7.0), and Water (not more than 6.0).

Cefuroxime Axetil Tablets USP—Preserve in well-closed containers. The labeling indicates whether the Tablets contain amorphous or crystalline Cefuroxime Axetil. If Tablets contain a mixture of amorphous and crystalline Cefuroxime Axetil, label to indicate the percentage of each contained therein. Contain an amount of cefuroxime axetil equivalent to the labeled amount of cefuroxime, within ±10%. Meet the requirements for Identification, Dissolution (60% in 15 minutes, 75% in 45 minutes; except that where Tablets are labeled to contain the equivalent of 500 mg of cefuroxime, not less than 50% in 15 minutes, and not less than 70% in 45 minutes in 0.07 *N* hydrochloric acid in Apparatus 2 at 55 rpm), Uniformity of dosage units, and Water (not more than 6.0%).

Cefuroxime Sodium USP—Preserve in tight containers. Where it is intended for use in preparing injectable dosage forms, the label states that it is sterile or must be subjected to further processing during the preparation of injectable dosage forms. Contains the equivalent of not less than 855 mcg and not more than 1000 mcg of cefuroxime, calculated on the anhydrous basis. Meets the requirements for Identification, pH (6.0–8.5, in a solution [1 in 10]), and Water (not more than 3.5%), for Sterility and Bacterial endotoxins under Cefuroxime for Injection (where the label states that Cefuroxime Sodium is sterile), and for Bacterial endotoxins under Cefuroxime for Injection (where the label

states that Cefuroxime Sodium must be subjected to further processing during the preparation of injectable dosage forms).

CELECOXIB

Chemical name: 4-[5-(4-methylphenyl)-3-(trifluoromethyl)-1H-pyrazol-1-yl]benzenesulfonamide.

Molecular formula: $C_{17}H_{14}F_3N_3O_2S$.

Molecular weight: 381.38.

Description: White powder. Melts at 160–164 °C.

pKa: 11.1.

Solubility: Practically insoluble in water.

USP requirements: Celecoxib Capsules—Not in *USP–NF*.

CELLACEFATE

Chemical name: Cellulose, acetate, 1,2-benzenedicarboxylate.

Description: Cellacefate NF—Free-flowing, white powder. May have a slight odor of acetic acid.
   NF category: Coating agent.

Solubility: Cellacefate NF—Insoluble in water and in alcohol; soluble in acetone and in dioxane.

NF requirements: Cellacefate NF—Preserve in tight containers. A reaction product of phthalic anhydride and a partial acetate ester of cellulose. Contains not less than 21.5% and not more than 26.0% of acetyl groups and not less than 30.0% and not more than 36.0% of phthalyl groups, calculated on the anhydrous, acid-free basis. Meets the requirements for Identification, Viscosity (45–90 centipoises, determined at 25 ±0.2 °C), Water (not more than 5.0%), Residue on ignition (not more than 0.1%), Heavy metals (not more than 0.001%), Limit of free acid (not more than 3.0%, calculated as phthalic acid), Organic volatile impurities, Phthalyl content, and Content of acetyl.

CELLULOSE ACETATE

Chemical name: Cellulose acetate.

Description: Cellulose Acetate NF—Fine, white powder or free-flowing pellets. Available in a range of viscosities and acetyl contents.
   NF category: Coating agent; polymer membrane, insoluble.

Solubility: Cellulose Acetate NF—High viscosity, which reflects high molecular weight, decreases solubility slightly. High acetyl content cellulose acetates generally have more limited solubility in commonly used organic solvents than low acetyl content cellulose acetates, but are more soluble in methylene chloride. All acetyl content cellulose acetates are insoluble in alcohol and in water; soluble in dioxane and in dimethylformamide.

NF requirements: Cellulose Acetate NF—Preserve in tight containers. It is partially or completely acetylated cellulose. Label it to indicate the percentage content of acetyl. Contains not less than 29.0% and not more than 44.8%, by weight, of acetyl groups. Its acetyl content is not less than 90.0% and not more than 110.0% of that indicated on the label. Meets the requirements for Identification, Loss on drying (not more than 5.0%),

Residue on ignition (not more than 0.1%), Heavy metals (not more than 0.001%), Free acid (not more than 0.1%, on the dried basis), Organic volatile impurities, and Content of acetyl.

MICROCRYSTALLINE CELLULOSE

Chemical name: Cellulose.

Description: Microcrystalline Cellulose NF—Fine, white, odorless, crystalline powder. It consists of free-flowing, nonfibrous particles that may be compressed into self-binding tablets which disintegrate rapidly in water.
   NF category: Tablet binder; tablet disintegrant; tablet and/or capsule diluent.

Solubility: Microcrystalline Cellulose NF—Insoluble in water, in dilute acids, and in most organic solvents; practically insoluble in sodium hydroxide solution (1 in 20).

NF requirements:
   Microcrystalline Cellulose NF—Preserve in tight containers. A purified, partially depolymerized cellulose prepared by treating alpha cellulose, obtained as a pulp from fibrous plant material, with mineral acids. The labeling indicates the nominal loss on drying, bulk density, and degree of polymerization values. Degree of polymerization compliance is determined using Identification test B. Where the particle size distribution is stated in the labeling, the labeling indicates the d_{10}, d_{50}, and d_{90} values and the range for each. Meets the requirements for Identification, Microbial limits, Conductivity, pH (5.0–7.0 in the supernatant solution obtained in the Conductivity test), Loss on drying (not more than 7.0%, or some other lower percentage, or is within a percentage range, as specified in the labeling), Residue on ignition (not more than 0.05%), Bulk density, Water-soluble substances (not more than 0.24%), Heavy metals (not more than 0.001%), Ether-soluble substances (not more than 0.05%), and Organic volatile impurities.

MICROCRYSTALLINE CELLULOSE AND CARBOXYMETHYLCELLULOSE SODIUM

Chemical name:
   Microcrystalline cellulose—Cellulose.
   Carboxymethylcellulose sodium—Cellulose, carboxymethyl ether, sodium salt.

Description: Microcrystalline Cellulose and Carboxymethylcellulose Sodium NF—Odorless, white to off-white, coarse to fine powder.
   NF category: Suspending and/or viscosity-increasing agent.

Solubility: Microcrystalline Cellulose and Carboxymethylcellulose Sodium NF—Swells in water, producing, when dispersed, a white, opaque dispersion or gel. Insoluble in organic solvents and in dilute acids.

NF requirements: Microcrystalline Cellulose and Carboxymethylcellulose Sodium NF—Preserve in tight containers, store in a dry place, and avoid exposure to excessive heat. A colloid-forming, attrited mixture of Microcrystalline Cellulose and Carboxymethylcellulose Sodium. Label it to indicate the percentage content of carboxymethylcellulose sodium and the viscosity of the dispersion in water of the designated weight percentage composition. Contains not less than 75.0% and not more than 125.0% of the labeled amount of carboxymethylcellulose sodium, calculated on the dried basis. The viscosity of its aqueous dispersion of percent by weight stated on the label is 60.0 to 140.0% of that stated on the label in centipoises. Meets the requirements for Identification, Visc-

osity, pH (6.0–8.0), Loss on drying (not more than 8.0%), Residue on ignition (not more than 5.0%), Heavy metals (not more than 0.001%), and Organic volatile impurities.

OXIDIZED CELLULOSE

Description: Oxidized Cellulose USP—In the form of gauze or lint. Is slightly off-white in color and has a slight, charred odor.

Solubility: Oxidized Cellulose USP—Insoluble in water and in acids; soluble in dilute alkalies.

USP requirements: Oxidized Cellulose USP—Preserve in Containers for Sterile Solids, protected from direct sunlight. Store in a cold place. The package bears a statement to the effect that the sterility of Oxidized Cellulose cannot be guaranteed if the package bears evidence of damage, or if the package has been previously opened. Oxidized Cellulose meets the requirements for Labeling under Injections. Contains not less than 16.0% and not more than 24.0% of carboxyl groups, calculated on the dried basis. It is sterile. Meets the requirements for Identification, Sterility, Loss on drying (not more than 15.0%), Residue on ignition (not more than 0.15%), Nitrogen as nitrate or nitrite (not more than 0.5%), and Formaldehyde (not more than 0.5%).

OXIDIZED REGENERATED CELLULOSE

Description: Oxidized Regenerated Cellulose USP—A knit fabric, usually in the form of sterile strips. Slightly off-white, having a slight odor.

Solubility: Oxidized Regenerated Cellulose USP—Insoluble in water and in dilute acids; soluble in dilute alkalies.

USP requirements: Oxidized Regenerated Cellulose USP—Preserve in Containers for Sterile Solids, protected from direct sunlight. Store at controlled room temperature. The package bears a statement to the effect that the sterility of Oxidized Regenerated Cellulose cannot be guaranteed if the package bears evidence of damage, or if the package has been previously opened. Oxidized Regenerated Cellulose meets the requirements for Labeling under Injections. Contains not less than 18.0% and not more than 24.0% of carboxyl groups, calculated on the dried basis. It is sterile. Meets the requirements for Identification, Sterility, Loss on drying (not more than 15%), Residue on ignition (not more than 0.15%), Nitrogen content (not more than 0.5%), and Formaldehyde (not more than 0.5%).

POWDERED CELLULOSE

Description: Powdered Cellulose NF—White, odorless substance, consisting of fibrous particles. Exhibits degrees of fineness ranging from a free-flowing dense powder to a coarse, fluffy, non-flowing material.
     NF category: Filtering aid; sorbent; tablet and/or capsule diluent.

Solubility: Powdered Cellulose NF—Insoluble in water, in dilute acids, and in nearly all organic solvents; slightly soluble in sodium hydroxide solution (1 in 20).

NF requirements: Powdered Cellulose NF—Preserve in tight containers. A purified, mechanically disintegrated cellulose prepared by processing alpha cellulose obtained as a pulp from fibrous plant materials. The labeling indicates the nom-

inal degree of polymerization value. Degree of polymerization compliance is determined using Identification test C. Meets the requirements for Identification, Microbial limits, pH (5.0–7.5), Loss on drying (not more than 6.0%), Residue on ignition (not more than 0.3%, calculated on the dried basis), Water-soluble substances (not more than 1.5%), Heavy metals (not more than 0.001%), Ether-soluble substances (not more than 0.15%), and Organic volatile impurities.

CELLULOSE SODIUM PHOSPHATE

Source: An insoluble, nonabsorbable ion-exchange resin made by phosphorylation of cellulose.

Chemical name: Cellulose, dihydrogen phosphate, disodium salt.

Description: Cellulose Sodium Phosphate USP—Free-flowing cream-colored, odorless powder.

Solubility: Cellulose Sodium Phosphate USP—Insoluble in water, in dilute acids, and in most organic solvents.

Other characteristics: Exchanges sodium for calcium and other polyvalent cations. Inorganic phosphate content is approximately 34%; sodium content is approximately 11%.

USP requirements:
     Cellulose Sodium Phosphate USP—Preserve in well-closed containers. It is prepared by phosphorylation of alpha cellulose. Has an inorganic bound phosphate content of not less than 31.0% and not more than 36.0%, calculated on the dried basis. Meets the requirements for pH (6.0–9.0, for the filtrate), Loss on drying (not more than 10.0%), Nitrogen (not more than 1.0%), Calcium binding capacity (not less than 1.8 mmol per gram, calculated on the dried basis), Heavy metals (not more than 0.004%), Free phosphate (not more than 3.5%, calculated on the dried basis), Sodium content (9.5–13.0%), and Inorganic bound phosphate.
     Cellulose Sodium Phosphate for Oral Suspension USP—Preserve in tight containers. Store in a refrigerator. Contains Cellulose Sodium Phosphate. Has an inorganic bound phosphate content not less than 28.0% and not more than 36.0% calculated on the dried basis. Meets the requirements for Loss on drying (not more than 10%), Calcium binding capacity, Free phosphate (not more than 6.0%, calculated on the dried basis), and Inorganic bound phosphate.

CEPHALEXIN

Chemical name:
     Cephalexin—5-Thia-1-azabicyclo[4.2.0]oct-2-ene-2-carboxylic acid, 7-[(aminophenylacetyl)amino]-3-methyl-8-oxo-, monohydrate [6*R*-[6 alpha,7 beta(*R**)]]-.
     Cephalexin hydrochloride—5-Thia-1-azabicyclo[4.2.0]oct-2-ene-2-carboxylic acid, 7-[(aminophenylacetyl)amino]-3-methyl-8-oxo-, monohydrochloride, monohydrate, [6*R*-[6 alpha,7 beta(*R**)]]-.

Molecular formula:
     Cephalexin—$C_{16}H_{17}N_3O_4S \cdot H_2O$.
     Cephalexin hydrochloride—$C_{16}H_{17}N_3O_4S \cdot HCl \cdot H_2O$.

Molecular weight:
     Cephalexin—365.41.
     Cephalexin hydrochloride—401.87.

Description:
     Cephalexin USP—White to off-white, crystalline powder.

Cephalexin Hydrochloride USP—White to off-white crystalline powder.

Solubility:

Cephalexin USP—Slightly soluble in water; practically insoluble in alcohol, in chloroform, and in ether.

Cephalexin Hydrochloride USP—Soluble to the extent of 10 mg per mL in water, in acetone, in acetonitrile, in alcohol, in dimethylformamide, and in methanol; practically insoluble in chloroform, in ether, in ethyl acetate, and in isopropyl alcohol.

Other characteristics: A zwitterion (contains both a basic and an acidic group); isoelectric point of cephalexin in water is approximately 4.5 to 5.

USP requirements:

Cephalexin USP—Preserve in tight containers. Has a potency of not less than 950 mcg and not more than 1030 mcg of cephalexin per mg, calculated on the anhydrous basis. Meets the requirements for Identification, Specific rotation ($+149°$ to $+158°$), Crystallinity, pH (3.0–5.5, in an aqueous suspension containing 50 mg per mL), Water (4.0–8.0%), Related compounds (not more than 5.0%), and Dimethylaniline.

Cephalexin Capsules USP—Preserve in tight containers. Contain the equivalent of the labeled amount of anhydrous cephalexin, within −10% to +20%. Meet the requirements for Identification, Dissolution (80% in 30 minutes in water in Apparatus 1 at 100 rpm), Uniformity of dosage units, and Water (not more than 10.0%).

Cephalexin for Oral Suspension USP—Preserve in tight containers. A dry mixture of Cephalexin and one or more suitable buffers, colors, diluents, and flavors. Contains the equivalent of the labeled amount of anhydrous cephalexin per mL when constituted as directed in the labeling, within −10% to +20%. Meets the requirements for Identification, Uniformity of dosage units (solid packaged in single-unit containers), Deliverable volume (solid packaged in multiple-unit containers), pH (3.0–6.0, in the suspension constituted as directed in the labeling), and Water (not more than 2.0%).

Cephalexin Tablets USP—Preserve in tight containers. They are prepared from Cephalexin or Cephalexin Hydrochloride. The label states whether the Tablets contain Cephalexin or Cephalexin Hydrochloride. Contain the equivalent of the labeled amount of anhydrous cephalexin, within −10% to +20%. Meet the requirements for Identification, Dissolution (80% in 30 minutes in water in Apparatus 1 [use 40-mesh cloth] at 100 rpm for cephalexin and 75% in 45 minutes in water in Apparatus 1 [use 10-mesh cloth] at 150 rpm for cephalexin hydrochloride), Uniformity of dosage units, and Water (not more than 9.0% where Tablets contain cephalexin; not more than 8.0% where Tablets contain cephalexin hydrochloride).

Cephalexin Tablets for Oral Suspension USP—Preserve in tight containers at controlled room temperature. Contain the labeled amount, within ±10%. Meet the requirements for Identificaton, Disintegration, Dissolution (80% in 30 minutes in water in Apparatus1 [use 40-mesh cloth] at 100 rpm), Dispersion fineness, Uniformity of dosage units, and Water (not more than 9.0%).

Cephalexin Hydrochloride USP—Preserve in tight containers. Contains the equivalent of not less than 800 mcg and not more than 880 mcg of anhydrous cephalexin per mg. Meets the requirements for Identification, Crystallinity, pH (1.5–3.0, in a solution containing 10 mg per mL), Water (3.0–6.5%), Related compounds (not more than 5.0%), and Dimethylaniline.

Cephalexin Hydrochloride Tablets—Not in *USP–NF*.

CEPHALOTHIN

Source: Cephalosporanic acid nucleus derived from cephalosporin C, produced by the fungus *Cephalosporium*.

Chemical name: Cephalothin sodium—5-Thia-1-azabicyclo[4.2.0]oct-2-ene-2-carboxylic acid, 3-[(acetyloxy)methyl]-8-oxo-7-[(2-thienylacetyl)amino]-, monosodium salt, (6R-trans)-.

Molecular formula: Cephalothin sodium—$C_{16}H_{15}N_2NaO_6S_2$.

Molecular weight: Cephalothin sodium—418.42.

Description: Cephalothin Sodium USP—White to off-white, practically odorless, crystalline powder.

Solubility: Cephalothin Sodium USP—Freely soluble in water, in saline TS, and in dextrose solutions; insoluble in most organic solvents.

USP requirements:

Cephalothin Sodium USP—Preserve in tight containers. Where it is intended for use in preparing injectable dosage forms, the label states that it is sterile or must be subjected to further processing during the preparation of injectable dosage forms. Contains the equivalent of not less than 850 mcg of cephalothin per mg, calculated on the dried basis. Meets the requirements for Identification, Specific rotation ($+124°$ to $+134°$), Crystallinity, pH (4.5–7.0, containing 250 mg per mL), Loss on drying (not more than 1.5%), and Chromatographic purity, for Sterility and Bacterial endotoxins under Cephalothin for Injection (where the label states that Cephalothin Sodium is sterile), and for Bacterial endotoxins under Cephalothin for Injection (where the label states that Cephalothin Sodium must be subjected to further processing during the preparation of injectable dosage forms).

Cephalothin Injection USP—Preserve in Containers for Injections. Maintain in the frozen state. It meets the requirements for Labeling under Injections. The label states that it is to be thawed just prior to use, describes conditions for proper storage of the resultant solution, and directs that the solution is not to be refrozen. Contains an amount of Cephalothin Sodium equivalent to the labeled amount of cephalothin, within −10% to +15%. Meets the requirements for Bacterial endotoxins, pH (6.0–8.5), and Particulate matter, for Identification test A under Cephalothin Sodium, and for Sterility under Cephalothin for Injection.

Cephalothin for Injection USP—Preserve in Containers for Sterile Solids. Contains an amount of Cephalothin Sodium equivalent to the labeled amount of cephalothin, within −10% to +15%. May contain Sodium Bicarbonate. Meets the requirements for Constituted solution, Specific rotation ($+124°$ to $+134°$, calculated on the dried and sodium bicarbonate–free basis), Content of sodium bicarbonate (if present), Bacterial endotoxins, Sterility, pH (6.0–8.5, in the solution constituted as directed in the labeling), Uniformity of dosage units, and Particulate matter, for Identification test A and Loss on drying under Cephalothin Sodium, and for Labeling under Injections.

CEPHAPIRIN

Chemical name:

Cephapirin benzathine—5-Thia-1-azabicyclo[4.2.0]oct-2-ene-2-carboxylic acid, 3-[(acetyloxy)methyl]-8-oxo-7-[[(4-pyridinylthio)acetyl]amino]-, (6R-trans)-, compd. with N,N-bis(phenylmethyl)-1,2-ethanediamine (2:1).

Cephapirin sodium—5-Thia-1-azabicyclo[4.2.0]oct-2-ene-2-carboxylic acid, 3-[(acetyloxy)methyl]-8-oxo-7-[[(4-pyridinylthio)acetyl]amino]-, monosodium salt, [6R-trans]-.

Molecular formula:

Cephapirin benzathine—$(C_{17}H_{17}N_3O_6S_2)_2 \cdot C_{16}H_{20}N_2$.

Cephapirin sodium—$C_{17}H_{16}N_3NaO_6S_2$.

Molecular weight:
Cephapirin benzathine—1087.30.
Cephapirin sodium—445.45.

Description:
Cephapirin Benzathine USP—White, crystalline powder.
Cephapirin Sodium USP—White to off-white crystalline powder, odorless or having a slight odor.

Solubility:
Cephapirin Benzathine USP—Practically insoluble in water, in ether, and in toluene; freely soluble in alcohol; soluble in 0.1 N hydrochloric acid.
Cephapirin Sodium USP—Very soluble in water; insoluble in most organic solvents.

USP requirements:
Cephapirin Benzathine USP—Preserve in well-closed containers. Label it to indicate that it is for veterinary use only. Contains the equivalent of not less than 715 mcg and not more than 820 mcg of cephapirin per mg. Meets the requirements for Identification, Crystallinity, pH (4.0–7.0, in a suspension [1 in 10]), Water (not more than 5.0%), and Benzathine content (20.0–24.0%, calculated on the anhydrous basis).
Cephapirin Benzathine Intramammary Infusion USP—Preserve in well-closed unit-dose disposable syringes at controlled room temperature. A suspension of Cephapirin Benzathine in a suitable vegetable oil vehicle. Contains a suitable dispersing agent. Label Intramammary Infusion to indicate that it is for veterinary use only. Contains an amount of cephapirin benzathine equivalent to the labeled amount of cephapirin, within −10% to +20%. Meets the requirements for Identification and Water (not more than 1.0%).
Cephapirin Sodium USP—Preserve in tight containers. Where it is intended for use in preparing injectable dosage forms, the label states that it is sterile or must be subjected to further processing during the preparation of injectable dosage forms. Has a potency equivalent to not less than 855 mcg and not more than 1000 mcg of cephapirin per mg. Meets the requirements for Identification, Crystallinity, pH (6.5–8.5, in a solution containing 10 mg of cephapirin per mL), and Water (not more than 2.0%), for Sterility and Bacterial endotoxins under Cephapirin for Injection (where the label states that Cephapirin Sodium is sterile), and for Bacterial endotoxins under Cephapirin for Injection (where the label states that Cephapirin Sodium must be subjected to further processing during the preparation of injectable dosage forms).
Cephapirin Sodium Intramammary Infusion USP—Preserve in well-closed unit-dose disposable syringes at controlled room temperature. A suspension of Cephapirin Sodium in a suitable vegetable oil vehicle. Contains a suitable dispersing agent. Label Intramammary Infusion to indicate that it is for veterinary use only. Contains an amount of cephapirin sodium equivalent to the labeled amount of cephapirin, within −10% to +20%. Meets the requirements for Identification and Water (not more than 1.0%).
Cephapirin for Injection USP—Preserve in Containers for Sterile Solids. Contains an amount of Cephapirin Sodium equivalent to the labeled amount of cephapirin, within −10% to +15%. Meets the requirements for Constituted solution, Bacterial endotoxins, Sterility, and Particulate matter, for Identification, Crystallinity, pH, and Water under Cephapirin Sodium, and for Uniformity of dosage units and Labeling under Injections.

CEPHRADINE

Chemical name: 5-Thia-1-azabicyclo[4.2.0]oct-2-ene-2-carboxylic acid, 7-[(amino-1,4-cyclohexadien-1-ylacetyl)amino]-3-methyl-8-oxo-, [6R-[6 alpha,7 beta(R*)]]-.

Molecular formula: $C_{16}H_{19}N_3O_4S$.

Molecular weight: 349.41.

Description: Cephradine USP—White to off-white, crystalline powder.

Solubility: Cephradine USP—Sparingly soluble in water; very slightly soluble in alcohol and in chloroform; practically insoluble in ether.

USP requirements:
Cephradine USP—Preserve in tight containers. Where it is the dihydrate form, the label so indicates. Where the quantity of cephradine is indicated in the labeling of any preparation containing Cephradine, this shall be understood to be in terms of anhydrous cephradine. Where it is intended for use in preparing injectable dosage forms, the label states that it is sterile or must be subjected to further processing during the preparation of injectable dosage forms. Has a potency of not less than 900 mcg and not more than 1050 mcg of total cephalosporins per mg, calculated as the sum of cephradine and cephalexin, calculated on the anhydrous basis. Meets the requirements for Identification, Crystallinity, pH (3.5–6.0, in a solution containing 10 mg per mL), Water (not more than 6.0%, except that if it is the dihydrate form, the limit is 8.5–10.5%), and Limit of cephalexin (not more than 5.0%, calculated on the anhydrous basis), for Sterility and Bacterial endotoxins under Cephradine for Injection (where the label states that Cephradine is sterile) and for Bacterial endotoxins under Cephradine for Injection (where the label states that Cephradine must be subjected to further processing during the preparation of injectable dosage forms.
Cephradine Capsules USP—Preserve in tight containers. The quantity of cephradine stated in the labeling is in terms of anhydrous cephradine. Contain the labeled amount of cephradine, within −10% to +20%, calculated as the sum of cephradine and cephalexin. Meet the requirements for Identification, Dissolution (75% in 45 minutes in 0.12 N hydrochloric acid in Apparatus 1 at 100 rpm), Uniformity of dosage units, and Loss on drying (not more than 7.0%).
Cephradine for Injection USP—Preserve in Containers for Sterile Solids. Contains the labeled amount of cephradine, within −10% to +15%, calculated as the sum of cephradine and cephalexin. Meets the requirements for Constituted solution, Identification, Bacterial endotoxins, Sterility, pH (8.0–9.6, in a solution containing 10 mg per mL), Loss on drying (not more than 5.0%), and Particulate matter, and for Uniformity of dosage units, and Labeling under Injections.
Cephradine for Oral Suspension USP—Preserve in tight containers. A dry mixture of Cephradine and one or more suitable buffers, colors, diluents, and flavors. Contains the labeled amount of cephradin, within −10% to +25%, calculated as the sum of cephradine and cephalexin. Meets the requirements for Identification, Uniformity of dosage units (solid packaged in single-unit containers), Deliverable volume (solid packaged in multiple-unit containers), pH (3.5–6.0, in the suspension constituted as directed in the labeling), and Water (not more than 1.5%).
Cephradine Tablets USP—Preserve in tight containers. Contain the labeled amount of cephradine, within −10% to +20%, calculated as the sum of cephradine and cephalexin. Meet the requirements for Identification, Dissolution (85% in 60 minutes in 0.12 N hydrochloric acid in Apparatus 2 at 75 rpm), Uniformity of dosage units, and Water (not more than 6.0%).

CERIVASTATIN

Chemical name: Cerivastatin sodium—6-Heptanoic acid, 7-[4-(4-fluorophenyl)-5-(methoxymethyl)-2,6-bis(1-methylethyl)-3-pyridinyl]-3,5-dihydroxy-[S-[R*,S*-(E)]]-, sodium salt.

Molecular formula: Cerivastatin sodium—$C_{26}H_{33}FNNaO_5$.

Molecular weight: Cerivastatin sodium—481.53.

Description: White to off-white hygroscopic amorphous powder.

Solubility: Soluble in water, in methanol, and in ethanol; very slightly soluble in acetone.

USP requirements: Cerivastatin Sodium Tablets—Not in *USP–NF*.

CETIRIZINE

Chemical name: Cetirizine hydrochloride—Acetic acid, [2-[4-[(4-chlorophenyl)phenylmethyl]-1-piperazinyl]ethoxy]-, dihydrochloride, (±)-.

Molecular formula: Cetirizine hydrochloride—$C_{21}H_{25}ClN_2O_3 \cdot 2HCl$.

Molecular weight: Cetirizine hydrochloride—461.81.

Description: Cetirizine hydrochloride—Melting point 225 °C.

USP requirements:
Cetirizine Hydrochloride Syrup—Not in *USP–NF*.
Cetirizine Hydrochloride Tablets—Not in *USP–NF*.

CETIRIZINE AND PSEUDOEPHEDRINE

For *Cetirizine* and *Pseudoephedrine*—See individual listings for chemistry information.

USP requirements: Cetirizine Hydrochloride and Pseudoephedrine Hydrochloride Extended-release Tablets—Not in *USP–NF*.

CETOSTEARYL ALCOHOL

Description: Cetostearyl Alcohol NF—Unctuous, white flakes or granules having a faint, characteristic odor.
NF category: Stiffening agent.

Solubility: Cetostearyl Alcohol NF—Insoluble in water; soluble in alcohol and in ether.

NF requirements: Cetostearyl Alcohol NF—Preserve in well-closed containers. Contains not less than 40.0% of stearyl alcohol, and the sum of the stearyl alcohol content and the cetyl alcohol content is not less than 90.0%. Meets the requirements for Identification, Melting range (48–55 °C), Acid value (not more than 2), Iodine value (not more than 4), and Hydroxyl value (208–228).

CETRORELIX

Chemical group: Cetrorelix acetate for injection—A synthetic decapeptide with gonadotropin-releasing hormone (GnRH) antagonistic activity.

Chemical name:
Cetrorelix—N-Acetyl-3-(2-naphthyl)-D-alanyl-p-chloro-D-phenylalanyl-3-(3-pyridyl)-D-alanyl-L-tyrosyl-N^5-carbamoyl-D-ornithyl-L-lencyl-L-arginyl-L-propyl-D-alaninamide.
Cetrotelix acetate for injection—Acetyl-D-3-(2'-naphtyl)-alamine-D-4-chlorophenylalamine-D-3-(3'-pyridyl)-alanine-L-serine-L-tyrosyl-D-citruline-L-leucine-L-arginine-L-proline-D-alanine-amide.

Molecular formula: Cetrorelix—$C_{70}H_{92}ClN_{17}O_{14}$.

Molecular weight:
Cetrorelix—1431.04.
Cetrorelix acetate for injection—1431.06.

Description: Cetrorelix acetate for injection—Sterile lyophilized powder.

USP requirements: Cetrorelix Acetate for Injection—Not in *USP–NF*.

CETYL ALCOHOL

Chemical name: 1-Hexadecanol.

Molecular formula: $C_{16}H_{34}O$.

Molecular weight: 242.44.

Description: Cetyl Alcohol NF—Unctuous, white flakes, granules, cubes, or castings. Has a faint characteristic odor. Usually melts in the range between 45–50 °C.
NF category: Stiffening agent.

Solubility: Cetyl Alcohol NF—Insoluble in water; soluble in alcohol and in ether, the solubility increasing with an increase in temperature.

NF requirements: Cetyl Alcohol NF—Preserve in well-closed containers. Contains not less than 90.0% of cetyl alcohol, the remainder consisting chiefly of related alcohols. Meets the requirements for Identification, Acid value (not more than 2), Iodine value (not more than 5), and Hydroxyl value (218–238).

CETYL ESTERS WAX

Description: Cetyl Esters Wax NF—White to off-white, somewhat translucent flakes, having a crystalline structure and a pearly luster when caked. Has a faint odor and a specific gravity of about 0.83 at 50 °C.
NF category: Stiffening agent.

Solubility: Cetyl Esters Wax NF—Insoluble in water; soluble in boiling alcohol, in ether, in chloroform, and in fixed and volatile oils; slightly soluble in cold solvent hexane; practically insoluble in cold alcohol.

NF requirements: Cetyl Esters Wax NF—Preserve in well-closed containers, in a dry place, and prevent exposure to excessive heat. A mixture consisting primarily of esters of saturated fatty alcohols and saturated fatty acids. Meets the requirements for Melting range (43–47 °C), Acid value (not more than 5), Iodine value (not more than 1), Saponification value (109–120), and Paraffin and free acids.

CETYL PALMITATE

Chemical name: Hexadecanoic acid hexadecyl ester.

Molecular formula: $C_{32}H_{64}O_2$.

Molecular weight: 480.87.

Description: White crystals or flakes.

NF category: Stiffening agent.

Solubility: Freely soluble in alcohol and in ether; practically insoluble in water.

NF requirements: Cetyl Palmitate NF—Preserve in tight containers at controlled room temperture, and avoid exposure to excessive heat. Consists of esters of cetyl alcohol and saturated high molecular weight fatty acids, principally palmitic acid. Meets the requirements for Identification, Melting range (46–53 °C), Acid value (not more than 1), Hydroxyl value (not more than 6), Iodine value (not more than 1), Saponification value (110–130), Loss on drying (not more than 3.0%), Residue on ignition (not more than 0.05%), Heavy metals (not more than 0.002%), and Content of palmitic acid.

CETYLPYRIDINIUM

Chemical name: Cetylpyridinium chloride—Pyridinium, 1-hexadecyl-, chloride, monohydrate.

Molecular formula: Cetylpyridinium chloride—$C_{21}H_{38}ClN \cdot H_2O$.

Molecular weight: Cetylpyridinium chloride—358.00.

Description:

Cetylpyridinium Chloride USP—White powder, having a slight, characteristic odor.

NF category: Antimicrobial preservative; wetting and/or solubilizing agent.

Cetylpyridinium Chloride Topical Solution USP—Clear liquid. Is colorless unless a color has been added; has an aromatic odor.

Solubility: Cetylpyridinium Chloride USP—Very soluble in water, in alcohol, and in chloroform; slightly soluble in ether.

USP requirements:

Cetylpyridinium Chloride USP—Preserve in well-closed containers. Contains not less than 99.0% and not more than 102.0% of cetylpyridinium chloride, calculated on the anhydrous basis. Meets the requirements for Identification, Melting range (80–84 °C), Acidity, Water (4.5–5.5%), Residue on ignition (not more than 0.2%, calculated on the anhydrous basis), Heavy metals (not more than 0.002%), Pyridine, and Organic volatile impurities.

Cetylpyridinium Chloride Lozenges USP—Preserve in well-closed containers. Contain the labeled amount, within −10% to +25%, in a suitable molded base. Meet the requirement for Identification.

Cetylpyridinium Chloride Topical Solution USP—Preserve in tight containers. Contains the labeled amount, within ± 5%. Meets the requirement for Identification.

CEVIMELINE

Source: Cevimeline hydrochloride—A quinuclidine derivative of acetylcholine.

Chemical name: Cevimeline hydrochloride—Spiro[1-azabicyclo[2.2.2]octane-3,5'-[1,3]oxathiolane], 2'-methyl-, hydrochloride, hydrate.

Molecular formula: Cevimeline hydrochloride—$C_{10}H_{17}NOS \cdot HCl \cdot 1/2H_2O$.

Molecular weight: Cevimeline hydrochloride—244.78.

Description: Cevimeline hydrochloride—A white to off-white crystalline powder. Melting point 201–203 °C.

Solubility: Cevimeline hydrochloride—Freely soluble in alcohol and in chloroform; very soluble in water; virtually insoluble in ether.

Other characteristics: Cevimeline hydrochloride—pH of a 1% solution 4.6–5.6.

USP requirements: Cevimeline Hydrochloride Capsules—Not in *USP–NF*.

CHAMOMILE

NF requirements:

Chamomile NF—Preserve in well closed containers, protected from light. Consists of the dried flower heads of *Matricaria recutita* Linné, (*Matricaria chamomilla* Linné *Matricaria chamomilla* Linné var. *courrantiana, Chamomilla recutita* Linné) Rauschert (Fam. Asteraceae alt. Compositae). The label states the Latin binomial name and, following the official name, the part of the plant contained in the article. Contains not less than 0.4% of blue volatile oil, not less than 0.3% of apigenin-7-glucoside, and not less than 0.15% of bisabolan derivatives, calculated as levomenol. Meets the requirements for Botanic characteristics, Identification, Broken flowers, Foreign organic matter (not more than 2.0%), Total ash (not more than 13.0%, determined on 1.0 gram of powdered Chamomile), Microbial limits, Pesticide residues, Volatile oil content (not less than 0.4% of blue volatile oil [Note—Retain the volatile oils for use in the test for Content of bisabolan derivatives.]), Content of apigenin-7-glucoside (not less than 0.3%), and Content of bisabolan derivatives (not less than 0.15%).

ACTIVATED CHARCOAL

Description: Activated Charcoal USP—Fine, black, odorless powder, free from gritty matter.

NF category: Sorbent.

Solubility: Practically insoluble in all usual solvents.

USP requirements:

Activated Charcoal USP—Preserve in well-closed containers. The residue from the destructive distillation of various organic materials, treated to increase its adsorptive power. Meets the requirements for Microbial limits, Reaction (neutral to litmus), Loss on drying (not more than 15.0%), Residue on ignition (not more than 4.0%), Acid-soluble substances (not more than 3.5%), Chloride (not more than 0.2%), Sulfate (not more than 0.2%), Sulfide, Cyanogen compounds, Heavy metals (not more than 0.005%), Uncarbonized constituents, and Adsorptive power.

Activated Charcoal Capsules—Not in *USP–NF*.

Activated Charcoal Oral Suspension—Not in *USP–NF*.

Activated Charcoal Tablets—Not in *USP–NF*.

ACTIVATED CHARCOAL AND SORBITOL

For *Activated Charcoal* and *Sorbitol*—See individual listings for chemistry information.

USP requirements: Activated Charcoal and Sorbitol Oral Suspension—Not in *USP–NF*.

CHENODIOL

Source: Chenodeoxycholic acid, a naturally occurring human bile acid.

Chemical name: Cholan-24-oic acid, 3,7-dihydroxy-, (3 alpha,5 beta,7 alpha)-.

Molecular formula: $C_{24}H_{40}O_4$.

Molecular weight: 392.57.

Description: White powder consisting of crystalline and amorphous particles.

Solubility: Practically insoluble in water; freely soluble in methanol, in acetone, and in acetic acid.

USP requirements: Chenodiol Tablets—Not in *USP–NF*.

CHERRY JUICE

NF requirements: Cherry Juice NF—Preserve in tight, light-resistant containers, and prevent exposure to excessive heat. Liquid expressed from the fresh ripe fruit of *Prunus cerasus* L. (Fam. Rosaceae). The label states the Latin binomial name and, following the official name, the part of the plant source from which the article was derived. Contains not less than 1.0% of malic acid. Coarsely crush washed, stemmed, un-pitted, sour cherries in a grinder so as to break the pits but not mash the kernels. Dissolve 0.1% of Benzoic Acid in the mixture, and allow to stand at room temperature until a small portion of the filtered Juice, when mixed with one-half of its volume of alcohol, does not become cloudy within 30 minutes. Press the Juice from the mixture, and filter it. Meets the requirements for Identification, Specific gravity (1.045–1.075), Refractive index (not less than 1.350), pH (3.0–4.0), Residue on ignition (0.35%–0.55%), Arsenic (0.3 mcg per gram), Lead (not more than 5 mcg per mL), Limit of nonvolatile residue (not more than 9.5%), and Limit of volatile acids (not more than 1.5 mL).

CHERRY SYRUP

NF requirements: Cherry Syrup NF—Preserve in tight, light-resistant containers, and prevent exposure to excessive heat. The label states the Latin binomial name and, following the official name, the part of the plant source from which the article was derived.

Prepare Cherry Syrup as follows: 475 mL of Cherry Juice, 800 grams of Sucrose, 20 mL of Alcohol, and Purified Water, a sufficient quantity to make 1000 mL. Dissolve Sucrose in Cherry Juice by gently heating on a steam bath, cool, and remove the foam and floating solids. Add Alcohol and sufficient Purified Water to make 1000 mL, and mix.

Meets the requirement for Alcohol content.

HORSE CHESTNUT

NF requirements:

Horse Chestnut NF—Store in a well-closed, light-resistant container, protected from moisture. Consists of the dried seeds of *Aesculus hipocastanum* L. (Fam. Hippocastanaceae). Is harvested in the fall. The label states the Latin binomial and, following the official name, the part of the plant contained in the article. Contains not less than 3.0% of triterpene glycosides, calculated on the dried basis as escin. Meets the requirements for Botanic characteristics, Thin-layer chromatographic identification test, Microbial limits, Loss on drying (not more than 10.0%), Extractable matter (not less than 18.0%), Foreign organic matter (not more than 2.0%), Total ash (not more than 4.0%), Pesticide residues, Heavy metals (not more than 20 micrograms per gram), and Content of triterpene glycosides.

Powdered Horse Chestnut NF—Preserve in well-closed, light-resistant containers, protected from moisture. It is Horse Chestnut reduced to a powder or very fine powder. The label states the Latin binomial and, following the official name, the part of the plant from which the article was derived. Contains not less than 3.0% of triterpene glycosides, calculated on the dried basis as escin. Meets the requirements for Botanic characteristics, and for Identification, Microbial limits, Loss on drying, Extractable matter, Total ash, Pesticide residues, Heavy metals, and Content of triterpene glycosides under Horse Chestnut.

Powdered Horse Chestnut Extract NF—Preserve in tight, light-resistant containers, in a cool place. Prepared from Horse Chestnut by extraction with alcohol-water mixtures or methanol-water mixtures. The ratio of starting plant material to extract is between 5:1 and 8:1. The label states the Latin binomial and, following the official name, the part of the plant from which the article was prepared. The label also indicates the content of triterpene glycosides, the extracting solvent or solvent mixture used for preparation, the ratio of the starting crude plant material to Powdered Extract, and the name and content of any added substance. It meets the requirements for labeling under *Botanical Extracts*. Contains the labeled amount of triterpene glycosides, within ±10%, calculated on the dried basis as escin. May contain suitable added substances. Meets the requirements for Thin-layer chromatographic identification test, Microbial limits, Loss on drying (not more than 5.0%), Heavy metals (not more than 20 micrograms per gram), Organic volatile impurities, and Content of triterpene glycosides, and rquirements for *Packaging and Storage*, *Residual Solvents*, and *Pesticide Residues* in *General Pharmacopeial Requirements* for powdered extracts under *Botanical Extracts*.

CHLOPHEDIANOL

Chemical name: Chlophedianol hydrochloride—Benzenemethanol, 2-chloro-alpha-[2-(dimethylamino)ethyl]-alpha-phenyl-, hydrochloride.

Molecular formula: Chlophedianol hydrochloride—$C_{17}H_{20}CINO \cdot HCl$.

Molecular weight: Chlophedianol hydrochloride—326.26.

Description: Chlophedianol hydrochloride—White, crystalline powder. Melting point 190–191 °C.

Solubility: Chlophedianol hydrochloride—Freely soluble in water, in methanol, and in ethanol. Sparingly soluble in ether and in ethyl acetate.

CHLORAL HYDRATE

Chemical name: 1,1-Ethanediol, 2,2,2-trichloro-.

Molecular formula: $C_2H_3Cl_3O_2$.

Molecular weight: 165.40.

Description: Chloral Hydrate USP—Colorless, transparent, or white crystals having an aromatic, penetrating, and slightly acrid odor. Melts at about 55 °C, and slowly volatilizes when exposed to air.

Solubility: Chloral Hydrate USP—Very soluble in water and in olive oil; freely soluble in alcohol, in chloroform, and in ether.

USP requirements:
Chloral Hydrate USP—Preserve in tight containers. Contains not less than 99.5% and not more than 102.5% of chloral hydrate. Meets the requirements for Identification, Acidity, Residue on ignition (not more than 0.1%), Chloride (not more than 0.007%), Readily carbonizable substances, and Organic volatile impurities.
Chloral Hydrate Capsules USP—Preserve in tight containers, preferably at controlled room temperature. Contain the labeled amount, within −5% to +10%. Meet the requirements for Identification and Uniformity of dosage units, and Dissolution (in 15 minutes in water in Apparatus 2 at 50 rpm).
Chloral Hydrate Oral Solution USP—Preserve in tight, light-resistant containers. Contains the labeled amount, within −5% to +10%. Meets the requirement for Identification.
Chloral Hydrate Suppositories—Not in *USP–NF*.
Chloral Hydrate Syrup USP—Preserve in tight, light-resistant containers. Contains the labeled amount, within −5% to +10%. Meets the requirement for Identification.

CHLORAMBUCIL

Chemical name: Benzenebutanoic acid, 4-[bis(2-chloroethyl)-amino]-.

Molecular formula: $C_{14}H_{19}Cl_2NO_2$.

Molecular weight: 304.21.

Description: Chlorambucil USP—Off-white, slightly granular powder.

pKa: 5.8.

Solubility: Chlorambucil USP—Very slightly soluble in water; freely soluble in acetone; soluble in dilute alkali.

USP requirements:
Chlorambucil USP—Preserve in tight, light-resistant containers. Contains not less than 98.0% and not more than 101.0% of chlorambucil, calculated on the anhydrous basis. Meets the requirements for Identification, Melting range (65–69 °C), Water (not more than 0.5%), and Organic volatile impurities.
    Caution: Great care should be taken to prevent inhaling particles of Chlorambucil and exposing the skin to it.
Chlorambucil Tablets USP—Preserve coated Tablets in well-closed containers; preserve uncoated Tablets in well-closed, light-resistant containers. Contain the labeled

amount, within −15% to +10%. Meet the requirements for Identification, Disintegration, and Uniformity of dosage units.

CHLORAMPHENICOL

Source: Originally derived from *Streptomyces venezuelae*.

Chemical name:
Chloramphenicol—Acetamide, 2,2-dichloro-N-[2-hydroxy-1-(hydroxymethyl)-2-(4-nitrophenyl)ethyl]-, [R-(R*,R*)]-.
Chloramphenicol palmitate—Hexadecanoic acid, 2-[(2,2-dichloroacetyl)amino]-3-hydroxy-3-(4-nitrophenyl) propyl ester, [R-(R*,R*)]-.
Chloramphenicol sodium succinate—Butanedioic acid, mono[2-[(2,2-dichloroacetyl)amino]-3-hydroxy-3-(4-nitrophenyl)propyl] ester, monosodium salt, [R-(R*,R*)]-.

Molecular formula:
Chloramphenicol—$C_{11}H_{12}Cl_2N_2O_5$.
Chloramphenicol palmitate—$C_{27}H_{42}Cl_2N_2O_6$.
Chloramphenicol sodium succinate—$C_{15}H_{15}Cl_2N_2NaO_8$.

Molecular weight:
Chloramphenicol—323.13.
Chloramphenicol palmitate—561.54.
Chloramphenicol sodium succinate—445.18.

Description:
Chloramphenicol USP—Fine, white to grayish white or yellowish white, needle-like crystals or elongated plates. Its solutions are practically neutral to litmus. Is reasonably stable in neutral or moderately acid solutions. Its alcohol solution is dextrorotatory and its ethyl acetate solution is levorotatory.
Chloramphenicol Palmitate USP—Fine, white, unctuous, crystalline powder, having a faint odor.
Chloramphenicol Sodium Succinate USP—Light yellow powder.

Solubility:
Chloramphenicol USP—Slightly soluble in water; freely soluble in alcohol, in propylene glycol, in acetone, and in ethyl acetate.
Chloramphenicol Palmitate USP—Insoluble in water; freely soluble in acetone and in chloroform; soluble in ether; sparingly soluble in alcohol; very slightly soluble in solvent hexane.
Chloramphenicol Sodium Succinate USP—Freely soluble in water and in alcohol.

USP requirements:
Chloramphenicol USP—Preserve in tight containers. Where it is intended for use in preparing injectable or other sterile dosage forms, the label states that it is sterile or must be subjected to further processing during the preparation of injectable or other sterile dosage forms. Contains not less than 97.0% and not more than 103.0% of chloramphenicol. Meets the requirements for Identification, Melting range (149–153 °C), Specific rotation (+17.0° to +20.0°), Crystallinity, pH (4.5–7.5, in an aqueous suspension containing 25 mg per mL), and Chromatographic purity, and for Bacterial endotoxins and Sterility.
Chloramphenicol Capsules USP—Preserve in tight containers. Contain the labeled amount, within −10% to +20%. Meet the requirements for Identification, Dissolution (85% in 30 minutes in 0.01 N hydrochloric acid in Apparatus 1 at 100 rpm), and Uniformity of dosage units.
Chloramphenicol Cream USP—Preserve in collapsible tubes or in tight containers. Contains the labeled amount, within 10% to +30%. Meets the requirements for Identification and Minimum fill.

Chloramphenicol Injection USP—Preserve in single-dose or in multiple-dose containers. A sterile solution of Chloramphenicol in one or more suitable solvents. Label it to indicate that it is for veterinary use only. Contains the labeled amount, within −10% to +15%. Meets the requirements for Identification, Bacterial endotoxins, Sterility, pH (5.0–8.0, in a solution diluted with water [1:1]), and Injections.

Chloramphenicol Ophthalmic Ointment USP—Preserve in collapsible ophthalmic ointment tubes. Contains the labeled amount, within −10% to +30%. Meets the requirements for Identification, Sterility, Minimum fill, and Metal particles.

Chloramphenicol Ophthalmic Solution USP—Preserve in tight containers, and store in a refrigerator until dispensed. The containers or individual cartons are sealed and tamperproof so that sterility is assured at time of first use. A sterile solution of Chloramphenicol. The labeling states that there is a 21-day beyond-use period after dispensing. Contains the labeled amount, within −10% to +30%. Meets the requirements for Identification, Sterility, and pH (7.0–7.5, except that in the case of Ophthalmic Solution that is unbuffered or is labeled for veterinary use it is 3.0–6.0).

Chloramphenicol for Ophthalmic Solution USP—Preserve in tight containers. A sterile, dry mixture of Chloramphenicol with or without one or more suitable buffers, diluents, and preservatives. If packaged in combination with a container of solvent, label it with a warning that it is not for injection. Contains the labeled amount, within −10% to +30%, when constituted as directed. Meets the requirements for Identification, Sterility, and pH (7.1–7.5, in an aqueous solution containing 5 mg of chloramphenicol per mL).

Chloramphenicol Oral Solution USP—Preserve in tight containers. A solution of Chloramphenicol in a suitable solvent. Label it to indicate that it is for veterinary use only and that it is not to be used in animals raised for food production. Contains the labeled amount, within −10% to +20%. Contains one or more suitable buffers and preservatives. Meets the requirements for Identification and pH (5.0–8.5, when diluted with an equal volume of water).

Chloramphenicol Otic Solution USP—Preserve in tight containers. A sterile solution of Chloramphenicol in a suitable solvent. Contains the labeled amount, within −10% to +30%. Meets the requirements for Identification, Sterility, pH (4.0–8.0, when diluted with an equal volume of water), and Water (not more than 2.0%).

Chloramphenicol Tablets USP—Preserve in tight containers. Label Tablets to indicate that they are for veterinary use only and are not to be used in animals raised for food production. Contain the labeled amount, within −10% to +20%. Meet the requirements for Identification, Disintegration (60 minutes), and Uniformity of dosage units.

Chloramphenicol Palmitate USP—Preserve in tight containers. Has a potency equivalent to not less than 555 mcg and not more than 595 mcg of chloramphenicol per mg. Meets the requirements for Identification, Melting range (87–95 °C), Specific rotation (+21° to+25°), Crystallinity, Loss on drying (not more than 0.5%), Acidity, and Free chloramphenicol.

Chloramphenicol Palmitate Oral Suspension USP—Preserve in tight, light-resistant containers. Contains an amount of chloramphenicol palmitate equivalent to the labeled amount of chloramphenicol, within −10% to +20%. Contains one or more suitable buffers, colors, flavors, preservatives, and suspending agents. Meets the requirements for Identification, Uniformity of dosage units (suspension packaged in single-unit containers), Deliverable volume (suspension packaged in multiple-unit containers), pH (4.5–7.0), and Limit of polymorph A.

Chloramphenicol Sodium Succinate USP—Preserve in tight containers. Where it is intended for use in preparing sterile dosage forms, the label states that it is sterile or must be subjected to further processing during the preparation of sterile dosage forms. Has a potency equivalent to not less than 650 mcg and not more than 765 mcg of chloramphe-

nicol per mg. Meets the requirements for Identification, Specific rotation (+5.0° to +8.0°), pH (6.4–7.0, in a solution containing the equivalent of 250 mg of chloramphenicol per mL), Water (not more than 5.0%), and Limit of free chloramphenicol (not more than 2.0%), and for Sterility and Bacterial endotoxins under Chloramphenicol Sodium Succinate for Injection (where the label states that Chloramphenicol Sodium Succinate is sterile), and for Bacterial endotoxins under Chloramphenicol Sodium Succinate for Injection (where the label states that Chloramphenicol Sodium Succinate must be subjected to further processing during the preparation of injectable dosage forms).

Chloramphenicol Sodium Succinate for Injection USP—Preserve in Containers for Sterile Solids. Contains an amount of chloramphenicol sodium succinate equivalent to the labeled amount of chloramphenicol, within −10% to +15%. Meets the requirements for Bacterial endotoxins, Sterility, Particulate matter, and Limit of free chloramphenicol (not more than 2.0%) and for Identification, Specific rotation, pH, and Water under Chloramphenicol Sodium Succinate.

CHLORAMPHENICOL AND HYDROCORTISONE

For *Chloramphenicol* and *Hydrocortisone*—See individual listings for chemistry information.

USP requirements: Chloramphenicol and Hydrocortisone Acetate for Ophthalmic Suspension USP—A sterile, dry mixture of Chloramphenicol and Hydrocortisone Acetate with or without one or more suitable buffers, diluents, and preservatives. If packaged in combination with a container of solvent, label it with a warning that it is not for injection. Contains the labeled amounts of chloramphenicol, within −10% to +30%, and hydrocortisone acetate, within −10% to +15%, when constituted as directed. Meets the requirements for Identification, Sterility, and pH (7.1–7.5, in an aqueous suspension containing 5 mg of chloramphenicol per mL).

CHLORAMPHENICOL AND POLYMYXIN B

For *Chloramphenicol* and *Polymyxin B*—See individual listings for chemistry information.

USP requirements: Chloramphenicol and Polymyxin B Sulfate Ophthalmic Ointment USP—Preserve in collapsible ophthalmic ointment tubes. Contains the labeled amount of chloramphenicol, within −10% to +20%, and an amount of polymyxin B sulfate equivalent to the labeled amount of polymyxin B, within −10% to +25%. Meets the requirements for Identification, Sterility, and Metal particles.

CHLORAMPHENICOL, POLYMYXIN B, AND HYDROCORTISONE

For *Chloramphenicol, Polymyxin B,* and *Hydrocortisone*—See individual listings for chemistry information.

USP requirements: Chloramphenicol, Polymyxin B Sulfate, and Hydrocortisone Acetate Ophthalmic Ointment USP—Preserve in collapsible ophthalmic ointment tubes. Contains the labeled amount of chloramphenicol, within −10% to +20%, an amount of polymyxin B sulfate equivalent to the labeled amount of polymyxin B, within −10% to +25%, and the labeled

amount of hydrocortisone acetate, within −10% to +15%. Meets the requirements for Identification, Sterility, Minimum fill, and Metal particles.

CHLORAMPHENICOL AND PREDNISOLONE

For *Chloramphenicol* and *Prednisolone*—See individual listings for chemistry information.

USP requirements: Chloramphenicol and Prednisolone Ophthalmic Ointment USP—Preserve in collapsible ophthalmic ointment tubes. Contains the labeled amounts of chloramphenicol, within −10% to +30%, and prednisolone, within −10% to +15%. Meets the requirements for Identification, Sterility, Minimum fill, and Metal particles.

CHLORDIAZEPOXIDE

Chemical name:
Chlordiazepoxide—3*H*-1,4-Benzodiazepin-2-amine, 7-chloro-*N*-methyl-5-phenyl, 4-oxide.
Chlordiazepoxide hydrochloride—3*H*-1,4-Benzodiazepin-2-amine, 7-chloro-*N*-methyl-5-phenyl-, 4-oxide, monohydrochloride.

Molecular formula:
Chlordiazepoxide—$C_{16}H_{14}ClN_3O$.
Chlordiazepoxide hydrochloride—$C_{16}H_{14}ClN_3O \cdot HCl$.

Molecular weight:
Chlordiazepoxide—299.75.
Chlordiazepoxide hydrochloride—336.22.

Description:
Chlordiazepoxide USP—Yellow, practically odorless, crystalline powder. Is sensitive to sunlight. Melts at about 240 °C.
Chlordiazepoxide Hydrochloride USP—White or practically white, odorless, crystalline powder. Is affected by sunlight.

Solubility:
Chlordiazepoxide USP—Insoluble in water; sparingly soluble in chloroform and in alcohol.
Chlordiazepoxide Hydrochloride USP—Soluble in water; sparingly soluble in alcohol; insoluble in solvent hexane.

USP requirements:
Chlordiazepoxide USP—Preserve in tight, light-resistant containers. Contains not less than 98.0% and not more than 102.0% of chlordiazepoxide, calculated on the dried basis. Meets the requirements for Identification, Loss on drying (not more than 0.3%), Residue on ignition (not more than 0.1%), Heavy metals (not more than 0.002%), Related compounds, and Organic volatile impurities.
Chlordiazepoxide Tablets USP—Preserve in tight, lightresistant containers. Contain the labeled amount, within ± 10%. Meet the requirements for Identification, Dissolution (85% in 30 minutes in simulated gastric fluid TS, prepared without pepsin, in Apparatus 1 at 100 rpm), Uniformity of dosage units, and Related compounds.
Chlordiazepoxide Hydrochloride USP—Preserve in tight, light-resistant containers. Where it is intended for use in preparing injectable dosage forms, the label states that it is sterile or must be subjected to further processing during the preparation of injectable dosage forms. Contains not less than 98.0% and not more than 102.0% of chlordiazepoxide hydrochloride, calculated on the dried basis. Meets the requirements for Identification, Melting range (212–218 °C, with decomposition), Loss on drying (not more than 0.5%), Residue on ignition (not more than 0.1%), Heavy metals (not more than 0.002%), Related compounds, and Organic volatile impurities, for Sterility, Label-

ing under Injections, and Bacterial endotoxins under Chlordiazepoxide Hydrochloride for Injection (where the label states that Chlordiazepoxide Hydrochloride is sterile), and for Bacterial endotoxins under Chlordiazepoxide Hydrochloride for Injection (where the label states that Chlordiazepoxide Hydrochloride must be subjected to further processing during the preparation of injectable dosage forms).
Chlordiazepoxide Hydrochloride Capsules USP—Preserve in tight, light-resistant containers. Contain the labeled amount, within ±10%. Meet the requirements for Identification, Dissolution (85% in 30 minutes in water in Apparatus 1 at 100 rpm), Uniformity of dosage units, and Related compounds.
Chlordiazepoxide Hydrochloride for Injection USP—Preserve in Containers for Sterile Solids, protected from light. It is Chlordiazepoxide Hydrochloride suitable for parenteral use. Meets the requirements for Completeness of solution, Constituted solution, Bacterial endotoxins, and pH (2.5–3.5, in a solution [1 in 100]), for Identification tests, Loss on drying and Heavy metals under Chlordiazepoxide Hydrochloride, for Related compounds under Chlordiazepoxide, and for Sterility tests, Uniformity of dosage units, and Labeling under Injections.

CHLORDIAZEPOXIDE AND AMITRIPTYLINE

For *Chlordiazepoxide* and *Amitriptyline*—See individual listings for chemistry information.

USP requirements: Chlordiazepoxide and Amitriptyline Hydrochloride Tablets USP—Preserve in tight, light-resistant containers. Contain the labeled amount of chlordiazepoxide, within ±10%, and an amount of amitriptyline hydrochloride equivalent to the labeled amount of amitriptyline, within ± 10%. Meet the requirements for Identification, Dissolution (85% of each active ingredient in 30 minutes in simulated gastric fluid TS, prepared without pepsin, in Apparatus 1 at 100 rpm), Uniformity of dosage units, and Related compounds.

CHLORDIAZEPOXIDE AND CLIDINIUM

For *Chlordiazepoxide* and *Clidinium*—See individual listings for chemistry information.

USP requirements: Chlordiazepoxide Hydrochloride and Clidinium Bromide Capsules USP—Preserve in tight, light-resistant containers. Contain the labeled amounts, within ±10%. Meet the requirements for Identification, Dissolution (75% of each active ingredient in 30 minutes in water in Apparatus 1 at 100 rpm), Uniformity of dosage units, and Related compounds.

CHLORHEXIDINE

Chemical group: Chlorhexidine gluconate—Bis-biguanide.

Chemical name:
Chlorhexidine gluconate—2,4,11,13-Tetraazatetradecanediimidamide, *N,N'*-bis(4-chlorophenyl)-3,12-diimino-, di-D-gluconate.
Chlorhexidine hydrochloride—2,4,11,13-Tetrazatetradecanediimidamide, *N,N'*-bis(4-chlorophenyl)-3,12-diimino-, dihydrochloride.

Molecular formula:
Chlorhexidine gluconate—$C_{22}H_{30}Cl_2N_{10} \cdot 2C_6H_{12}O_7$.
Chlorhexidine hydrochloride—$C_{22}H_{30}Cl_2N_{10} \cdot 2HCl$.

Molecular weight:
Chlorhexidine gluconate—897.76.
Chlorhexidine hydrochloride—578.37.

Description:
Chlorhexidine Gluconate Solution USP—Amost colorless or pale yellow, clear liquid.
Chlorhexidine Hydrochloride USP—White or almost white crystalline powder.

Solubility:
Chlorhexidine Gluconate Solution USP—Miscible with glacial acetic acid and with water; miscible with three times its volume of acetone and with five times its volume of dehydrated alcohol; further addition of acetone or dehydrated alcohol yields a white turbidity.
Chlorhexidine Hydrochloride USP—Sparingly soluble in propylene glycol and in water; very slightly soluble in alcohol.

Other characteristics: Chlorhexidine gluconate—A 5% v/v dilution in water has a pH of 5.5 to 7.0.

USP requirements:
Chlorhexidine Gluconate Periodontal Implants—Not in *USP–NF*.
Chlorhexidine Gluconate Oral Rinse USP—Preserve in tight containers, protected from light, at controlled room temperature. Prepared from Chlorhexidine Gluconate Solution. The labeling indicates that the Oral Rinse is to be expectorated and not swallowed after rinsing. Contains the labeled amount, within ±10%. Meets the requirements for Identification, pH (5.0–7.0), Limit of *p*-chloroaniline (not more than 3.0 micrograms), and Content of alcohol (within −10% to +15%).
Chlorhexidine Gluconate Solution USP—Preserve in tight containers, protected from light, at controlled room temperature. An aqueous solution of chlorhexidine gluconate. Contains not less than 19.0% and not more than 21.0% of chlorhexidine gluconate (w/v). Meets the requirements for Identification, Specific gravity (1.06–1.07), pH (5.5–7.0, when diluted 1 in 20 with water), Related compounds (not more than 3.0%), and Limit of *p*-chloroaniline.

CHLORMEZANONE

Chemical group: A substituted metathiazanone compound.

Chemical name: 2-(*p*-Chlorophenyl)tetrahydro-3-methyl-4*H*-1,3-thiazin-4-one 1,1-dioxide.

Molecular formula: $C_{11}H_{12}ClNO_3S$.

Molecular weight: 273.74.

Description: A white, crystalline powder with a faint characteristic odor.

Solubility: Soluble in water (less than 0.25% w/v); slightly soluble in alcohol.

USP requirements: Chlormezanone Tablets—Not in *USP–NF*.

CHLOROBUTANOL

Chemical name: 2-Propanol, 1,1,1-trichloro-2-methyl-.

Molecular formula: $C_4H_7Cl_3O$.

Molecular weight: 177.46.

Description: Chlorobutanol NF—Colorless to white crystals, having a characteristic, somewhat camphoraceous, odor. The anhydrous form melts at about 95 °C, and the hydrous form melts at about 76 °C.
NF category: Antimicrobial preservative.

Solubility: Chlorobutanol NF—Slightly soluble in water; freely soluble in alcohol, in ether, in chloroform, and in volatile oils; soluble in glycerin.

NF requirements: Chlorobutanol NF—Preserve in tight containers. It is anhydrous or contains not more than one-half molecule of water of hydration. Label it to indicate whether it is anhydrous or hydrous. Contains not less than 98.0% and not more than 100.5% of chlorobutanol, calculated on the anhydrous basis. Meets the requirements for Identification, Reaction, Water (for anhydrous, not more than 1.0%; for hydrous, not more than 6.0%), Chloride (not more than 0.07%), and Organic volatile impurities.

CHLOROCRESOL

Chemical name: Phenol, 4-chloro-3-methyl-.

Molecular formula: C_7H_7ClO.

Molecular weight: 142.58.

Description: Chlorocresol NF—Colorless or practically colorless crystals or crystalline powder, having a characteristic, non-tarry odor. Volatile in steam.
NF category: Antimicrobial preservative.

Solubility: Chlorocresol NF—Slightly soluble in water and more soluble in hot water; very soluble in alcohol; soluble in ether, in terpenes, in fixed oils, and in solutions of alkali hydroxides.

NF requirements: Chlorocresol NF—Preserve in tight, light-resistant containers. Contains not less than 99.0% and not more than 101.0% of chlorocresol. Meets the requirements for Completeness of solution, Identification, Melting range (63–66 °C), and Limit of nonvolatile residue (not more than 0.1%).

CHLOROPHYLLIN COPPER COMPLEX

Source: Obtained from chlorophyll by replacing the methyl and phytyl ester groups with alkali (usually sodium but sometimes sodium and potassium) and replacing the magnesium with copper.

USP requirements: Chlorophyllin Copper Complex Sodium USP—Preserve in tight, light-resistant containers. Contains no artificial coloring. Contains sodium salts of copper-chelated chlorophyll derivatives. Meets the requirements for Identification, pH (9.5–10.7, in a solution [1 in 100]), Iron (not more than 0.50%), Lead (not more than 0.001%), Arsenic (not more than 3 mcg per gram), Residue on ignition (not more than 30%, calculated on the dried basis), Loss on drying (not more than 5%), Test for fluorescence, Microbial limits, Total copper content (not less than 4.25%), Limit of ionic copper (not more than 0.25%, calculated on the dried basis), Content of chelated

copper (not less than 4.0%), Nitrogen content (not less than 4.0%), and Sodium content (5–7%, calculated on the dried basis).

CHLOROPROCAINE

Chemical group: Ester, aminobenzoic acid (PABA)-derivative.

Chemical name: Chloroprocaine hydrochloride—Benzoic acid, 4-amino-2-chloro-, 2-(diethylamino)ethyl ester, monohydrochloride.

Molecular formula: Chloroprocaine hydrochloride— $C_{13}H_{19}ClN_2O_2 \cdot HCl$.

Molecular weight: Chloroprocaine hydrochloride—307.22.

Description: Chloroprocaine Hydrochloride USP—White, crystalline powder. Is odorless, and is stable in air. Its solutions are acid to litmus.

pKa: 9.0.

Solubility: Chloroprocaine Hydrochloride USP—Soluble in water; slightly soluble in alcohol; very slightly soluble in chloroform; practically insoluble in ether.

USP requirements:
Chloroprocaine Hydrochloride USP—Preserve in well-closed containers. Contains not less than 98.0% and not more than 102.0% of chloroprocaine hydrochloride, calculated on the dried basis. Meets the requirements for Identification, Melting range (173–176 °C), Acidity, Loss on drying (not more than 1.0%), Residue on ignition (not more than 0.2%), and Related compounds (not more than 0.625%).
Chloroprocaine Hydrochloride Injection USP—Preserve in single-dose or in multiple-dose containers, preferably of Type I glass. A sterile solution of Chloroprocaine Hydrochloride in Water for Injection. Contains the labeled amount, within ±5%. Meets the requirements for Identification, pH (2.7–4.0), and Related compounds (not more than 3.0%), and for Injections.

CHLOROQUINE

Chemical name:
Chloroquine—1,4-Pentanediamine, N^4-(7-chloro-4-quinolinyl)-N^1,N^1-diethyl.
Chloroquine hydrochloride—1,4-Pentanediamine, N^4-(7-chloro-4-quinolinyl)-N^1,N^1-diethyl-, dihydrochloride.
Chloroquine phosphate—1,4-Pentanediamine, N^4-(7-chloro-4-quinolinyl)-N^1,N^1-diethyl-, phosphate (1:2).

Molecular formula:
Chloroquine—$C_{18}H_{26}ClN_3$.
Chloroquine hydrochloride—$C_{18}H_{26}ClN_3 \cdot 2HCl$.
Chloroquine phosphate—$C_{18}H_{26}ClN_3 \cdot 2H_3PO_4$.

Molecular weight:
Chloroquine—319.87.
Chloroquine hydrochloride—392.79.
Chloroquine phosphate—515.86.

Description:
Chloroquine USP—White or slightly yellow, crystalline powder. Is odorless.
Chloroquine Hydrochloride Injection USP—Colorless liquid.
Chloroquine Phosphate USP—White, crystalline powder. Is odorless and is discolored slowly on exposure to light. Its solutions have a pH of about 4.5. Exists in two polymorphic forms, one melting between 193 °C and 195 °C and the other between 210 °C and 215 °C; mixture of the forms melts between 193 °C and 215 °C.

Solubility:
Chloroquine USP—Very slightly soluble in water; soluble in dilute acids, in chloroform, and in ether.
Chloroquine Phosphate USP—Freely soluble in water; practically insoluble in alcohol, in chloroform, and in ether.

USP requirements:
Chloroquine USP—Preserve in well-closed containers. Contains not less than 98.0% and not more than 102.0% of chloroquine, calculated on the dried basis. Meets the requirements for Identification, Melting range (87–92 °C), Loss on drying (not more than 2.0%), Residue on ignition (not more than 0.2%), and Organic volatile impurities.
Chloroquine Hydrochloride Injection USP—Preserve in single-dose containers, preferably of Type I glass. A sterile solution of Chloroquine in Water for Injection prepared with the aid of Hydrochloric Acid. Contains, in each mL, not less than 47.5 mg and not more than 52.5 mg of chloroquine hydrochloride. Meets the requirements for Identification, Bacterial endotoxins, and pH (5.5–6.5), and for Injections.
Chloroquine Phosphate USP—Preserve in well-closed containers. Contains not less than 98.0% and not more than 102.0% of chloroquine phosphate, calculated on the dried basis. Meets the requirements for Identification, Loss on drying (not more than 2.0%), and Organic volatile impurities.
Chloroquine Phosphate Tablets USP—Preserve in well-closed containers. Contain the labeled amount, within ± 7%. Meet the requirements for Identification, Dissolution (75% in 45 minutes in water in Apparatus 2 at 100 rpm), and Uniformity of dosage units.

CHLOROTHIAZIDE

Chemical name:
Chlorothiazide—2H-1,2,4-Benzothiadiazine-7-sulfonamide, 6-chloro-, 1,1-dioxide.
Chlorothiazide sodium—2H-1,2,4-Benzothiadiazine-7-sulfonamide, 6-chloro-, 1,1-dioxide, monosodium salt.

Molecular formula:
Chlorothiazide—$C_7H_6ClN_3O_4S_2$.
Chlorothiazide sodium—$C_7H_5ClN_3NaO_4S_2$.

Molecular weight:
Chlorothiazide—295.73.
Chlorothiazide sodium—317.71.

Description:
Chlorothiazide USP—White or practically white, crystalline, odorless powder. Melts at about 340 °C, with decomposition.
Chlorothiazide sodium—White powder.

pKa: 6.7 and 9.5.

Solubility:
Chlorothiazide USP—Very slightly soluble in water; freely soluble in dimethylformamide and in dimethyl sulfoxide; slightly soluble in methanol and in pyridine; practically insoluble in ether and in chloroform.
Chlorothiazide sodium—Very soluble in water and in alcohol.

USP requirements:
Chlorothiazide USP—Preserve in well-closed containers. Contains not less than 98.0% and not more than 102.0% of chlorothiazide, calculated on the dried basis. Meets the requirements for Identification, Loss on drying (not more than 1.0%), Residue on ignition (not more than 0.1%), Chloride (not more than 0.05%), Selenium (not more than 0.003%), Heavy metals (not more than 0.001%), Related compounds (not more than 1.0%), and Organic volatile impurities.

Chlorothiazide Oral Suspension USP—Preserve in tight containers. Contains the labeled amount, within ±10%. Meets the requirements for Identification and pH (3.2–4.0).

Chlorothiazide Tablets USP—Preserve in well-closed containers. Contain the labeled amount, within ±10%. Meet the requirements for Identification, Dissolution (75% in 60 minutes in 0.05 *M* phosphate buffer [pH 8.0] in Apparatus 2 at 75 rpm), and Uniformity of dosage units.

Chlorothiazide Sodium for Injection USP—Preserve in Containers for Sterile Solids. A sterile, freeze-dried mixture of Chlorothiazide Sodium (prepared by the neutralization of Chlorothiazide with the aid of Sodium Hydroxide) and Mannitol. Contains an amount of chlorothiazide sodium equivalent to the labeled amount of chlorothiazide, within ±7%. Meets the requirements for Constituted solution, Identification, Bacterial endotoxins, Uniformity of dosage units, and pH (9.2–10.0, in a solution prepared as directed in the labeling), and for Injections.

CHLOROTRIANISENE

Chemical name: Benzene, 1,1′,1″-(1-chloro-1-ethenyl-2-ylidene)tris[4-methoxy]-.

Molecular formula: $C_{23}H_{21}ClO_3$.

Molecular weight: 380.86.

Description: Small, white crystals or crystalline powder. It is odorless.

Solubility: Very slightly soluble in water; slightly soluble in alcohol.

USP requirements:
Chlorotrianisene USP—Preserve in tight containers. Dried in vacuum at 60 °C for 6 hours, contains not less than 97.0% and not more than 103.0% of chlorotrianisene. Meets the requirements for Identification, Loss on drying (not more than 1.0%), Residue on ignition (not more than 1.0%), Heavy metals (not more than 0.002%), Volatile related compounds (not more than 1.0%), and Organic volatile impurities.

Chlorotrianisene Capsules USP—Preserve in well-closed containers, protected from excessive heat, cold, and moisture. Label the Capsules to indicate the vehicle used in the Capsules. Contain the labeled amount, within ±7%. Meet the requirements for Identification, Dissolution (in 15 minutes in water in Apparatus 2 at 50 rpm), and Uniformity of dosage units.

CHLOROXINE

Chemical name: 8-Quinolinol, 5,7-dichloro-.

Molecular formula: $C_9H_5Cl_2NO$.

Molecular weight: 214.05.

Description: Melting point 179–180 °C.

Solubility: Soluble in acetone; slightly soluble in cold alcohol and in acetic acid; readily soluble in sodium and potassium hydroxides and in acids, forming yellow solutions.

USP requirements: Chloroxine Lotion Shampoo—Not in *USP–NF*.

CHLOROXYLENOL

Chemical name: Phenol, 4-chloro-3,5-dimethyl-.

Molecular formula: C_8H_9ClO.

Molecular weight: 156.61.

Description: Chloroxylenol USP—White crystals or crystalline powder, having a characteristic odor. Volatile in steam.

Solubility: Chloroxylenol USP—Very slightly soluble in water; freely soluble in alcohol, in ether, in terpenes, in fixed oils, and in solutions of alkali hydroxides.

USP requirements: Chloroxylenol USP—Preserve in well-closed containers. Contains not less than 98.5% of chloroxylenol. Meets the requirements for Identification, Melting range (114–116 °C), Residue on ignition (not more than 0.1%), Iron (not more than 0.01%), Water (not more than 0.5%), and Related compounds (not more than 1.5%).

CHLORPHENESIN

Chemical name: Chlorphenesin carbamate—1,2-Propanediol, 3-(4-chlorophenoxy)-, 1-carbamate.

Molecular formula: Chlorphenesin carbamate—$C_{10}H_{12}ClNO_4$.

Molecular weight: Chlorphenesin carbamate—245.66.

Description: Chlorphenesin carbamate—White to off-white crystalline solid.

Solubility: Chlorphenesin carbamate—Almost insoluble in cold water or in cyclohexane; fairly readily soluble in dioxane; readily soluble in ethyl acetate, in 95.0% ethanol, and in acetone.

USP requirements: Chlorphenesin Carbamate Tablets—Not in *USP–NF*.

CHLORPHENIRAMINE

Chemical group: Chlorpheniramine maleate—Alkylamine derivative.

Chemical name: Chlorpheniramine maleate—2-Pyridinepropanamine, gamma-(4-chlorophenyl)-*N,N*-dimethyl-, (*Z*)-2-butenedioate (1:1).

Molecular formula: Chlorpheniramine maleate—$C_{16}H_{19}ClN_2 \cdot C_4H_4O_4$.

Molecular weight: Chlorpheniramine maleate—390.86.

Description: Chlorpheniramine Maleate USP—White, odorless, crystalline powder. Its solutions have a pH between 4 and 5.

pKa: Chlorpheniramine maleate—9.2.

Solubility: Chlorpheniramine Maleate USP—Freely soluble in water; soluble in alcohol and in chloroform; slightly soluble in ether.

USP requirements:
Chlorpheniramine Maleate USP—Preserve in tight, light-resistant containers. Contains not less than 98.0% and not more than 100.5% of chlorpheniramine maleate, calculated on the dried basis. Meets the requirements for Identification, Melting range (130–135 °C), Loss on drying (not more than 0.5%), Residue on ignition (not more than 0.2%), Related compounds, and Organic volatile impurities.

Chlorpheniramine Maleate Extended-release Capsules USP—Preserve in tight containers. Label the Capsules to indicate the Drug Release Test with which the product

complies. Contain the labeled amount, within ±10%. Meet the requirements for Identification, Drug release, and Uniformity of dosage units.

Chlorpheniramine Maleate Injection USP—Preserve in single-dose or in multiple-dose containers, preferably of Type I glass, protected from light. A sterile solution of Chlorpheniramine Maleate in Water for Injection. Contains the labeled amount, within ±10%. Meets the requirements for Identification, Bacterial endotoxins, and pH (4.0–5.2), and for Injections.

Chlorpheniramine Maleate Oral Solution USP—Preserve in tight, light-resistant containers. Contains the labeled amount, within ±10%. Meets the requirements for Identification and Alcohol content (if present, 6.0–8.0%).

Chlorpheniramine Maleate Syrup USP—Preserve in tight, light-resistant containers. Contains the labeled amount, within ±10%. Meets the requirements for Identification and Alcohol content (if present, 6.0–8.0%).

Chlorpheniramine Maleate Tablets USP—Preserve in tight containers. Contain the labeled amount, within ±10%. Meet the requirements for Identification, Dissolution (80% in 30 minutes in 0.01 N hydrochloric acid in Apparatus 2 at 50 rpm), and Uniformity of dosage units.

Chlorpheniramine Maleate Extended-release Tablets—Not in USP–NF.

CHLORPHENIRAMINE AND CODEINE

Chemical name:
Chlorpheniramine polistirex—Benzene, diethenyl-, polymer with ethenylbenzene, sulfonated, complex with gamma-(4-chlorophenyl)-N,N-dimethyl-2-pyridinepropanamine.
Codeine polistirex—Benzene, diethenyl-, polymer with ethenylbenzene, sulfonated, complex with (5 alpha,6 alpha)-7,8-didehydro-4,5-epoxy-3-methoxy-17-methylmorphinian-6-ol.

USP requirements: Chlorpheniramine and Codeine Polistirexes Oral Suspension—Not in USP–NF

CHLORPHENIRAMINE AND DEXTROMETHORPHAN

For Chlorpheniramine and Dextromethorphan—See individual listings for chemistry information.

USP requirements: Chlorpheniramine Maleate and Dextromethorphan Hydrobromide Oral Solution—Not in USP–NF.

CHLORPHENIRAMINE, DEXTROMETHORPHAN, AND ACETAMINOPHEN

For Chlorpheniramine, Dextromethorphan, and Acetaminophen—See individual listings for chemistry information.

USP requirements:
Chlorpheniramine Maleate, Dextromethorphan Hydrobromide, and Acetaminophen Capsules USP—Preserve in tight containers. The label for each article encompassed by this monograph bears a name composed of the active ingredients. The label states the name and quantity of each active ingredient and indicates its function (or purpose) in the article. Contain the labeled amounts, within ±10%. Meet the requirements for Identification, Dissolution (75% in 45 minutes in water in Apparatus 1 at 50 rpm), and Uniformity of dosage units.

Chlorpheniramine Maleate, Dextromethorphan Hydrobromide, and Acetaminophen Oral Powder USP—Preserve in tight containers. The label for each article encompassed by this monograph bears a name composed of the active ingredients contained in the article. The label states the name and quantity of each active ingredient and indicates its function (or purpose) in the article. Contains the labeled amounts, within ±10%. Meets the requirements for Identification, Minimum fill, and Uniformity of dosage units.

Chlorpheniramine Maleate, Dextromethorphan Hydrobromide, and Acetaminophen Oral Solution USP—Preserve in tight containers. The label for each article encompassed by this monograph bears a name composed of the active ingredients. The label states the name and quantity of each active ingredient and indicates its function (or purpose) in the article. Contains the labeled amounts, within ±10%. Meets the requirements for Identification, Microbial limits, pH (3.7–7.5), and Alcohol content, (if present, within ±10%).

Chlorpheniramine Maleate, Dextromethorphan Hydrobromide, and Acetaminophen Tablets USP—Preserve in tight containers, and store at controlled room temperature. The label for each article encompassed by this monograph bears a name composed of the active ingredients. The label states the name and quantity of each active ingredient and indicates its function (or purpose) in the article. Contain the labeled amounts, within ±10%. Meet the requirements for Identification, Dissolution (75% in 45 minutes in 0.1 M hydrochloric acid in Apparatus 2 at 50 rpm), and Uniformity of dosage units.

CHLORPHENIRAMINE, EPHEDRINE, AND GUAIFENESIN

For Chlorpheniramine, Ephedrine, and Guaifenesin—See individual listings for chemistry information.

USP requirements: Chlorpheniramine Maleate, Ephedrine Sulfate, and Guaifenesin Oral Solution—Not in USP–NF.

CHLORPHENIRAMINE, EPHEDRINE, PHENYLEPHRINE, AND CARBETAPENTANE

Description: Chlorpheniramine tannate—Light tan to buff or yellowish-tan, amorphous, fine powder having not more than a slight characteristic odor.

Solubility: Chlorpheniramine tannate—Slightly soluble in water at 25 °C.

USP requirements:
Chlorpheniramine Tannate, Ephedrine Tannate, Phenylephrine Tannate, and Carbetapentane Tannate Oral Suspension—Not in USP–NF.
Chlorpheniramine Tannate, Ephedrine Tannate, Phenylephrine Tannate, and Carbetapentane Tannate Tablets—Not in USP–NF.

CHLORPHENIRAMINE, EPHEDRINE, PHENYLEPHRINE, DEXTROMETHORPHAN, AMMONIUM CHLORIDE, AND IPECAC

For Chlorpheniramine, Ephedrine, Phenylephrine, Dextromethorphan, Ammonium Chloride, and Ipecac—See individual listings for chemistry information.

USP requirements: Chlorpheniramine Maleate, Ephedrine Hydrochloride, Phenylephrine Hydrochloride, Dextromethorphan Hydrobromide, Ammonium Chloride, and Ipecac Fluidextract Syrup—Not in *USP–NF*.

CHLORPHENIRAMINE AND HYDROCODONE

Chemical group: Chlorpheniramine maleate—Alkylamine derivative.

Chemical name:

Chlorpheniramine maleate—2-Pyridinepropanamine, gamma(4-chlorophenyl)-*N,N*-dimethyl-, (*Z*)-2-butenedioate (1:1).

Chlorpheniramine polistirex—Benzene, diethenyl-, polymer with ethenylbenzene, sulfonated, complex with gamma-(4-chlorophenyl)-*N,N*-dimethyl-2-pyridinepropanamine.

Hydrocodone bitartrate—Morphinan-6-one, 4,5-epoxy-3-methoxy-17-methyl-, (5 alpha)-, [*R*-(*R**,*R**)]-2,3-dihydroxybutanedioate (1:1), hydrate (2:5).

Hydrocodone polistirex—Benzene, diethenyl-, polymer with ethenylbenzene, sulfonated, complex with (5 alpha)-4,5-epoxy-3-methoxy-17-methylmorphinan-6-one.

Molecular formula:

Chlorpheniramine maleate—$C_{16}H_{19}ClN_2 \cdot C_4H_4O_4$.
Hydrocodone bitartrate—$C_{18}H_{21}NO_3 \cdot C_4H_6O_6 \cdot 2\frac{1}{2}H_2O$.

Molecular weight:

Chlorpheniramine maleate—390.86.
Hydrocodone bitartrate—494.49.

Description:

Chlorpheniramine Maleate USP—White, odorless, crystalline powder. Its solutions have a pH between 4 and 5.

Hydrocodone Bitartrate USP—Fine, white crystals or a crystalline powder. Is affected by light.

pKa: Chlorpheniramine maleate—9.2.

Solubility:

Chlorpheniramine Maleate USP—Freely soluble in water; soluble in alcohol and in chloroform; slightly soluble in ether.

Hydrocodone Bitartrate USP—Soluble in water; slightly soluble in alcohol; insoluble in ether and in chloroform.

USP requirements:

Chlorpheniramine Maleate and Hydrocodone Bitartrate Oral Solution—Not in *USP–NF*.

Chlorphenirmaine and Hydrocodone Polistirexes Oral Suspension—Not in *USP–NF*.

CHLORPHENIRAMINE, PHENINDAMINE, PHENYLEPHRINE, DEXTROMETHORPHAN, ACETAMINOPHEN, SALICYLAMIDE, CAFFEINE, AND ASCORBIC ACID

For *Chlorpheniramine, Phenindamine, Phenylephrine, Dextromethorphan, Acetaminophen, Salicylamide, Caffeine,* and *Ascorbic Acid*—See individual listings for chemistry information.

USP requirements: Chlorpheniramine Maleate, Phenindamine Tartrate, Phenylephrine Hydrochloride, Dextromethorphan Hydrobromide, Acetaminophen, Salicylamide, Caffeine, and Ascorbic Acid Tablets USP—Preserve in tight containers. The label for each article encompassed by this monograph bears a name composed of the active ingredients. The label states the name and quantity of each active ingredient and indicates its function (or purpose) in the article. Contain the labeled amounts, within ±10%. Meet the requirements for

Identification, Dissolution (75% in 45 minutes in 0.1 *M* hydrochloric acid in Apparatus 2 at 50 rpm), and Uniformity of dosage units.

CHLORPHENIRAMINE, PHENINDAMINE, AND PHENYLPROPANOLAMINE

For *Chlorpheniramine, Phenindamine,* and *Phenylpropanolamine*—See individual listings for chemistry information.

USP requirements: Chlorpheniramine Maleate, Phenindamine Tartrate, and Phenylpropanolamine Hydrochloride Extended-release Tablets—Not in *USP–NF*.

CHLORPHENIRAMINE, PHENIRAMINE, PYRILAMINE, PHENYLEPHRINE, HYDROCODONE, SALICYLAMIDE, CAFFEINE, AND ASCORBIC ACID

Source: Caffeine—Coffee, tea, cola, and cocoa or chocolate. May also be synthesized from urea or dimethylurea.

Chemical group:

Chlorpheniramine maleate—Alkylamine derivative.
Pheniramine—Alkylamine.
Pyrilamine—Ethylenediamine derivative.
Caffeine—Methylated xanthine.

Chemical name:

Chlorpheniramine maleate—2-Pyridinepropanamine, gamma-(4-chlorophenyl)-*N,N*-dimethyl-, (*Z*)-2-butenedioate (1:1).

Pheniramine maleate—2-[alpha-[2-Dimethylaminoethyl]benzyl]pyridine bimaleate.

Pyrilamine maleate—1,2-Ethanediamine, *N*-[(4-methoxyphenyl)methyl]-*N,N*-dimethyl-*N*-2-pyridinyl-, (*Z*)-2-butenedioate (1:1).

Phenylephrine hydrochloride—Benzenemethanol, 3-hydroxy-alpha-[(methylamino)methyl]-, hydrochloride.

Hydrocodone bitartrate—Morphinan-6-one, 4,5-epoxy-3-methoxy-17-methyl-, (5 alpha)-, [*R*-(*R**,*R**)]-2,3-dihydroxybutanedioate (1:1), hydrate (2:5).

Salicylamide—Benzamide, 2-hydroxy-.

Caffeine—1*H*-Purine-2,6-dione, 3,7-dihydro-1,3,7-trimethyl-.

Ascorbic acid—L-Ascorbic acid.

Molecular formula:

Chlorpheniramine maleate—$C_{16}H_{19}ClN_2 \cdot C_4H_4O_4$.
Pheniramine maleate—$C_{16}H_{20}N_2 \cdot C_4H_4O_4$.
Pyrilamine maleate—$C_{17}H_{23}N_3O \cdot C_4H_4O_4$.
Phenylephrine hydrochloride—$C_9H_{13}NO_2 \cdot HCl$.
Hydrocodone bitartrate—$C_{18}H_{21}NO_3 \cdot C_4H_6O_6 \cdot 2\frac{1}{2}H_2O$ (hydrate); $C_{18}H_{21}NO_3 \cdot C_4H_6O_6$ (anhydrous).
Salicylamide—$C_7H_7NO_2$.
Caffeine (anhydrous)—$C_8H_{10}N_4O_2$.
Ascorbic acid—$C_6H_8O_6$.

Molecular weight:

Chlorpheniramine maleate—390.86.
Pheniramine maleate—356.42.
Pyrilamine maleate—401.46.
Phenylephrine hydrochloride—203.67.
Hydrocodone bitartrate—494.49 (hydrate); 449.46 (anhydrous).
Salicylamide—137.14.
Caffeine (anhydrous)—194.19.
Ascorbic acid—176.12.

Description:

Chlorpheniramine Maleate USP—White, odorless, crystalline powder. Its solutions have a pH between 4 and 5.

Pheniramine maleate—White or almost white crystalline powder, odorless or with a slight odor.

Pyrilamine Maleate USP—White, crystalline powder, usually having a faint odor. Its solutions are acid to litmus.

Phenylephrine Hydrochloride USP—White or practically white, odorless crystals.

Hydrocodone Bitartrate USP—Fine, white crystals or a crystalline powder. Is affected by light.

Salicylamide USP—White, practically odorless, crystalline powder.

Caffeine USP—White powder, or white, glistening needles, usually matted together. Is odorless. Its solutions are neutral to litmus. The hydrate is efflorescent in air.

Ascorbic Acid USP—White or slightly yellow crystals or powder. On exposure to light it gradually darkens. In the dry state, is reasonably stable in air, but in solution rapidly oxidizes. Melts at about 190 °C.

NF category: Antioxidant.

pKa:

Chlorpheniramine maleate—9.2.

Ascorbic acid—4.2 and 11.6.

Solubility:

Chlorpheniramine Maleate USP—Freely soluble in water; soluble in alcohol and in chloroform; slightly soluble in ether.

Pheniramine maleate—Soluble 1 in 0.3 of water, 1 in 2.5 of alcohol, and 1 in 1.5 of chloroform; very slightly soluble in ether.

Pyrilamine Maleate USP—Very soluble in water; freely soluble in alcohol and in chloroform; slightly soluble in ether.

Phenylephrine Hydrochloride USP—Freely soluble in water and in alcohol.

Hydrocodone Bitartrate USP—Soluble in water; slightly soluble in alcohol; insoluble in ether and in chloroform.

Salicylamide USP—Slightly soluble in water and in chloroform; soluble in alcohol and in propylene glycol; freely soluble in ether and in solutions of alkalies.

Caffeine USP—Sparingly soluble in water and in alcohol; freely soluble in chloroform; slightly soluble in ether.

The aqueous solubility of caffeine is increased by organic acids or their alkali salts, such as citrates, benzoates, salicylates, or cinnamates, which dissociate to yield caffeine when dissolved in biological fluids.

Ascorbic Acid USP—Freely soluble in water; sparingly soluble in alcohol; insoluble in chloroform and in ether.

USP requirements: Chlorpheniramine Maleate, Pheniramine Maleate, Pyrilamine Maleate, Phenylephrine Hydrochloride, Hydrocodone Bitartrate, Salicylamide, Caffeine, and Ascorbic Acid Capsules—Not in *USP–NF*.

CHLORPHENIRAMINE AND PHENYLEPHRINE

Description: Chlorpheniramine tannate—Light tan to buff or yellowish-tan, amorphous, fine powder having not more than a slight characteristic odor.

Solubility: Chlorpheniramine tannate—Slightly soluble in water at 25 °C.

USP requirements:

Chlorpheniramine Maleate and Phenylephrine Hydrochloride Extended-release Capsules—Not in *USP–NF*.

Chlorpheniramine Maleate and Phenylephrine Hydrochloride Elixir—Not in *USP–NF*.

Chlorpheniramine Maleate and Phenylephrine Hydrochloride Oral Solution—Not in *USP–NF*.

Chlorpheniramine Maleate and Phenylephrine Hydrochloride Oral Suspension—Not in *USP–NF*.

Chlorpheniramine Maleate and Phenylephrine Hydrochloride Syrup—Not in *USP–NF*.

Chlorpheniramine Maleate and Phenylephrine Hydrochloride Tablets—Not in *USP–NF*.

Chlorpheniramine Maleate and Phenylephrine Hydrochloride Chewable Tablets—Not in *USP–NF*.

Chlorpheniramine Maleate and Phenylephrine Hydrochloride Extended-release Tablets—Not in *USP–NF*.

Chlorpheniramine Tannate and Phenylephrine Tannate Oral Suspension—Not in *USP–NF*.

Chlorpheniramine Tannate and Phenylephrine Tannate Tablets—Not in *USP–NF*.

CHLORPHENIRAMINE, PHENYLEPHRINE, AND ACETAMINOPHEN

For *Chlorpheniramine, Phenylephrine,* and *Acetaminophen*— See individual listings for chemistry information.

USP requirements:

Chlorpheniramine Maleate, Phenylephrine Hydrochloride, and Acetaminophen Capsules—Not in *USP–NF*.

Chlorpheniramine Maleate, Phenylephrine Hydrochloride, and Acetaminophen Tablets—Not in *USP–NF*.

Chlorpheniramine Maleate, Phenylephrine Hydrochloride, and Acetaminophen Extended-release Tablets—Not in *USP–NF*.

CHLORPHENIRAMINE, PHENYLEPHRINE, ACETAMINOPHEN, AND SALICYLAMIDE

For *Chlorpheniramine, Phenylephrine, Acetaminophen,* and *Salicylamide*—See individual listings for chemistry information.

USP requirements:

Chlorpheniramine Maleate, Phenylephrine Hydrochloride, Acetaminophen, and Salicylamide Capsules—Not in *USP–NF*.

Chlorpheniramine Maleate, Phenylephrine Hydrochloride, Acetaminophen, and Salicylamide Tablets—Not in *USP–NF*.

CHLORPHENIRAMINE, PHENYLEPHRINE, ACETAMINOPHEN, SALICYLAMIDE, AND CAFFEINE

For *Chlorpheniramine, Phenylephrine, Acetaminophen, Salicylamide,* and *Caffeine*—See individual listings for chemistry information.

USP requirements: Chlorpheniramine Maleate, Phenylephrine Hydrochloride, Acetaminophen, Salicylamide, and Caffeine Capsules—Not in *USP–NF*.

CHLORPHENIRAMINE, PHENYLEPHRINE, CODEINE, AND AMMONIUM CHLORIDE

For *Chlorpheniramine, Phenylephrine, Codeine,* and *Ammonium Chloride*—See individual listings for chemistry information.

USP requirements: Chlorpheniramine Maleate, Phenylephrine Hydrochloride, Codeine Phosphate, and Ammonium Chloride Oral Solution—Not in *USP–NF*.

CHLORPHENIRAMINE, PHENYLEPHRINE, CODEINE, AND POTASSIUM IODIDE

For *Chlorpheniramine, Phenylephrine, Codeine,* and *Potassium Iodide*—See individual listings for chemistry information.

USP requirements: Chlorpheniramine Maleate, Phenylephrine Hydrochloride, Codeine Phosphate, and Potassium Iodide Syrup—Not in *USP–NF*.

CHLORPHENIRAMINE, PHENYLEPHRINE, AND DEXTROMETHORPHAN

For *Chlorpheniramine, Phenylephrine,* and *Dextromethorphan*—See individual listings for chemistry information.

USP requirements:
    Chlorpheniramine Maleate, Phenylephrine Hydrochloride, and Dextromethorphan Hydrobromide Oral Solution—Not in *USP–NF*.
    Chlorpheniramine Maleate, Phenylephrine Hydrochloride, and Dextromethorphan Hydrobromide Syrup—Not in *USP–NF*.
    Chlorpheniramine Maleate, Phenylephrine Hydrochloride, and Dextromethorphan Hydrobromide Tablets—Not in *USP–NF*.

CHLORPHENIRAMINE, PHENYLEPHRINE, DEXTRO METHORPHAN, ACETAMINOPHEN, AND SALICYLAMIDE

For *Chlorpheniramine, Phenylephrine, Dextromethorphan, Acetaminophen,* and *Salicylamide*—See individual listings for chemistry information.

USP requirements: Chlorpheniramine Maleate, Phenylephrine Hydrochloride, Dextromethorphan Hydrobromide, Acetaminophen, and Salicylamide Tablets USP—Preserve in tight containers, and store at controlled room temperature. The label for each article encompassed by this monograph bears a name composed of the active ingredients. The label states the name and quantity of each active ingredient and indicates its function (or purpose) in the article. Contain the labeled amounts, within ±10%. Meet the requirements for Identification, Dissolution (75% in 45 minutes in 0.1 *M* hydrochloric acid in Apparatus 2 at 50 rpm), and Uniformity of dosage units.

CHLORPHENIRAMINE, PHENYLEPHRINE, DEXTRO METHORPHAN, AND GUAIFENESIN

For *Chlorpheniramine, Phenylephrine, Dextromethorphan,* and *Guaifenesin*—See individual listings for chemistry information.

USP requirements: Chlorpheniramine Maleate, Phenylephrine Hydrochloride, Dextromethorphan Hydrobromide, and Guaifenesin Syrup—Not in *USP–NF*.

CHLORPHENIRAMINE, PHENYLEPHRINE, DEXTRO METHORPHAN, GUAIFENESIN, AND AMMONIUM CHLORIDE

For *Chlorpheniramine, Phenylephrine, Dextromethorphan, Guaifenesin,* and *Ammonium Chloride*—See individual listings for chemistry information.

USP requirements: Chlorpheniramine Maleate, Phenylephrine Hydrochloride, Dextromethorphan Hydrobromide, Guaifenesin, and Ammonium Chloride Oral Solution—Not in *USP–NF*.

CHLORPHENIRAMINE, PHENYLEPHRINE, AND GUAIFENESIN

For *Chlorpheniramine, Phenylephrine,* and *Guaifenesin*—See individual listings for chemistry information.

USP requirements: Chlorpheniramine Maleate, Phenylephrine Hydrochloride, and Guaifenesin Oral Solution—Not in *USP–NF*.

CHLORPHENIRAMINE, PHENYLEPHRINE, AND HYDROCODONE

For *Chlorpheniramine, Phenylephrine,* and *Hydrocodone*—See individual listings for chemistry information.

USP requirements:
    Chlorpheniramine Maleate, Phenylephrine Hydrochloride, and Hydrocodone Bitartrate Oral Solution—Not in *USP–NF*.
    Chlorpheniramine Maleate, Phenylephrine Hydrochloride, and Hydrocodone Bitartrate Syrup—Not in *USP–NF*.

CHLORPHENIRAMINE, PHENYLEPHRINE, HYDRO CODONE, ACETAMINOPHEN, AND CAFFEINE

For *Chlorpheniramine, Phenylephrine, Hydrocodone, Acetaminophen,* and *Caffeine*—See individual listings for chemistry information.

USP requirements: Chlorpheniramine Maleate, Phenylephrine Hydrochloride, Hydrocodone Bitartrate, Acetaminophen, and Caffeine Tablets—Not in *USP–NF*.

CHLORPHENIRAMINE, PHENYLEPHRINE, AND METHSCOPOLAMINE

Chemical group: Chlorpheniramine maleate—Alkylamine derivative.

Chemical name:
    Chlorpheniramine maleate—2-Pyridinepropanamine, gamma-(4-chlorophenyl)-*N,N*-dimethyl-, (*Z*)-2-butenedioate (1:1).
    Phenylephrine hydrochloride—Benzenemethanol, 3-hydroxy-alpha-[(methylamino)methyl]-, hydrochloride.
    Methscopolamine nitrate—(−)-(1*S*,3*s*,5*R*,6*R*,7*S*)-6,7-Epoxy-8-methyl-3-[(*S*)-tropoyloxy]tropanium nitrate.

Molecular formula:
    Chlorpheniramine maleate—$C_{16}H_{19}ClN_2 \cdot C_4H_4O_4$.
    Phenylephrine hydrochloride—$C_9H_{13}NO_2 \cdot HCl$.
    Methscopolamine nitrate—$C_{18}H_{24}N_2O_7$.

Molecular weight:
Chlorpheniramine maleate—390.86.
Phenylephrine hydrochloride—203.67.
Methscopolamine nitrate—380.4.

Description:
Chlorpheniramine Maleate USP—White, odorless, crystalline powder. Its solutions have a pH between 4 and 5.
Phenylephrine Hydrochloride USP—White or practically white, odorless crystals.

pKa: Chlorpheniramine maleate—9.2.

Solubility:
Chlorpheniramine Maleate USP—Freely soluble in water; soluble in alcohol and in chloroform; slightly soluble in ether.
Phenylephrine Hydrochloride USP—Freely soluble in water and in alcohol.

USP requirements:
Chlorpheniramine Maleate, Phenylephrine Hydrochoride, and Methscopolamine Nitrate Extended-release Capsules—Not in *USP–NF*.
Chlorpheniramine Maleate, Phenylephrine Hydrochoride, and Methscopolamine Nitrate Syrup—Not in *USP–NF*.
Chlorpheniramine Maleate, Phenylephrine Hydrochoride, and Methscopolamine Nitrate Tablets—Not in *USP–NF*.
Chlorpheniramine Maleate, Phenylephrine Hydrochoride, and Methscopolamine Nitrate Chewable Tablets—Not in *USP–NF*.
Chlorpheniramine Maleate, Phenylephrine Hydrochoride, and Methscopolamine Nitrate Extended-release Tablets—Not in *USP–NF*.

CHLORPHENIRAMINE, PHENYLEPHRINE, AND PHE-NYLPROPANOLAMINE

For *Chlorpheniramine, Phenylephrine,* and *Phenylpropanolamine*—See individual listings for chemistry information.

USP requirements: Chlorpheniramine Maleate, Phenylephrine Hydrochloride, and Phenylpropanolamine Hydrochloride Tablets—Not in *USP–NF*.

CHLORPHENIRAMINE, PHENYLEPHRINE, PHENYLPROPANOLAMINE, ATROPINE, HYOSCYAMINE, AND SCOPOLAMINE

For *Chlorpheniramine, Phenylephrine, Phenylpropanolamine, Atropine, Hyoscyamine,* and *Scopolamine*—See individual listings for chemistry information.

USP requirements: Chlorpheniramine Maleate, Phenylephrine Hydrochloride, Phenylpropanolamine Hydrochloride, Atropine Sulfate, Hyoscyamine Sulfate, and Scopolamine Hydrobromide Extended-release Tablets—Not in *USP–NF*.

CHLORPHENIRAMINE, PHENYLEPHRINE, PHENYLPROPANOLAMINE, CARBETAPENTANE, AND POTASSIUM GUAIACOLSULFONATE

Chemical group:
Chlorpheniramine maleate—Alkylamine derivative.
Phenylpropanolamine hydrochloride—Synthetic phenylisopropanolamine.

Chemical name:
Chlorpheniramine maleate—2-Pyridinepropanamine, gamma-(4-chlorophenyl)-*N,N*-dimethyl-, (*Z*)-2-butenedioate (1:1).
Phenylephrine hydrochloride—Benzenemethanol, 3-hydroxy-alpha-[(methylamino)methyl]-, hydrochloride.
Phenylpropanolamine hydrochloride—Benzenemethanol, alpha-(1-aminoethyl)-, hydrochloride, (*R**,*S**)-, (±).
Carbetapentane citrate—2-[2-(Diethylamino)ethoxy]ethyl1-phenylcyclopentanecarboxylate citrate (1:1).
Potassium guaiacolsulfonate—Benzenesulfonic acid, hydroxymethoxy-, monopotassium salt, hemihydrate.

Molecular formula:
Chlorpheniramine maleate—$C_{16}H_{19}ClN_2 \cdot C_4H_4O_4$.
Phenylephrine hydrochloride—$C_9H_{13}NO_2 \cdot HCl$.
Phenylpropanolamine hydrochloride—$C_9H_{13}NO \cdot HCl$.
Carbetapentane citrate—$C_{20}H_{31}NO_3 \cdot C_6H_8O_7$.
Potassium guaiacolsulfonate—$C_7H_7KO_5S \cdot \frac{1}{2}H_2O$.

Molecular weight:
Chlorpheniramine maleate—390.86.
Phenylephrine hydrochloride—203.67.
Phenylpropanolamine hydrochloride—187.67.
Carbetapentane citrate—525.59.
Potassium guaiacolsulfonate—251.30.

Description:
Chlorpheniramine Maleate USP—White, odorless, crystalline powder. Its solutions have a pH between 4 and 5.
Phenylephrine Hydrochloride USP—White or practically white, odorless crystals.
Phenylpropanolamine Hydrochloride USP—White, crystalline powder, having a slight aromatic odor. Is affected by light.
Potassium guaiacolsulfonate—White, odorless crystals or crystalline powder. Gradually turns pink on exposure to air and light.

pKa:
Chlorpheniramine maleate—9.2.
Phenylpropanolamine hydrochloride—9.

Solubility:
Chlorpheniramine Maleate USP—Freely soluble in water; soluble in alcohol and in chloroform; slightly soluble in ether.
Phenylephrine Hydrochloride USP—Freely soluble in water and in alcohol.
Phenylpropanolamine Hydrochloride USP—Freely soluble in water and in alcohol; insoluble in ether.
Potassium guaiacolsulfonate—Soluble in 7.5 parts water; almost insoluble in alcohol; insoluble in ether.

USP requirements: Chlorpheniramine Maleate, Phenylephrine Hydrochloride, Phenylpropanolamine Hydrochloride, Carbetapentane Citrate, and Potassium Guaiacolsulfonate Syrup—Not in *USP–NF*.

CHLORPHENIRAMINE, PHENYLEPHRINE, PHENYLPROPANOLAMINE, AND CODEINE

For *Chlorpheniramine, Phenylephrine, Phenylpropanolamine,* and *Codeine*—See individual listings for chemistry information.

USP requirements: Chlorpheniramine Maleate, Phenylephrine Hydrochloride, Phenylpropanolamine Hydrochloride, and Codeine Phosphate Oral Solution—Not in *USP–NF*.

CHLORPHENIRAMINE, PHENYLEPHRINE, PHENYL-PROPANOLAMINE, AND DEXTROMETHORPHAN

For *Chlorpheniramine, Phenylephrine, Phenylpropanolamine, and Dextromethorphan*—See individual listings for chemistry information.

USP requirements: Chlorpheniramine Maleate, Phenylephrine Hydrochloride, Phenylpropanolamine Hydrochloride, and Dextromethorphan Hydrobromide Syrup—Not in *USP–NF*.

CHLORPHENIRAMINE, PHENYLEPHRINE, PHENYLPRO-PANOLAMINE, DEXTROMETHORPHAN, GUAIFENESIN, AND ACETAMINOPHEN

For *Chlorpheniramine, Phenylephrine, Phenylpropanolamine, Dextromethorphan, Guaifenesin,* and *Acetaminophen*—See individual listings for chemistry information.

USP requirements:
Chlorpheniramine Maleate, Phenylephrine Hydrochloride, Phenylpropanolamine Hydrochloride, Dextromethorphan Hydrobromide, Guaifenesin, and Acetaminophen Syrup—Not in *USP–NF*.
Chlorpheniramine Maleate, Phenylephrine Hydrochloride, Phenylpropanolamine Hydrochloride, Dextromethorphan Hydrobromide, Guaifenesin, and Acetaminophen Tablets USP—Preserve in tight containers, and store at controlled room temperature. The label for each article encompassed by this monograph bears a name composed of the active ingredients. The label states the name and quantity of each active ingredient and indicates its function (or purpose) in the article. Contain the labeled amounts, within ±10%. Meet the requirements for Identification, Dissolution (75% in 45 minutes in 0.1 *M* hydrochloric acid in Apparatus 2 at 50 rpm), and Uniformity of dosage units.

CHLORPHENIRAMINE, PHENYLPHRINE, PHENYLPRO-PANOLAMINE, DEXTROMETHORPHAN, POTASSIUM GUAIACOLSULFONATE, AND IPECAC

For *Chlorpheniramine, Phenylephrine, Phenylpropanolamine, Dextromethorphan, Potassium Guaiacolsulfonate* and *Ipecac*—See individual listings for chemistry information.

USP requirements: Chlorpheniramine Maleate, Phenylephrine Hydrochloride, Phenylpropanolamine Hydrochloride, Dextromethorphan Hydrobromide, Potassium Guaiacolsulfonate, and Ipecac Fluidextract Syrup—Not in *USP–NF*.

CHLORPHENIRAMINE, PHENYLEPHRINE, PHENYLPRO-PANOLAMINE, AND DIHYDROCODEINE

For *Chlorpheniramine, Phenylephrine, Phenylpropanolamine,* and *Dihydrocodeine*—See individual listings for chemistry information.

USP requirements:
Chlorpheniramine Maleate, Phenylephrine Hydrochloride, Phenylpropanolamine Hydrochloride, and Dihydrocodeine Bitartrate Oral Solution—Not in *USP–NF*.

Chlorpheniramine Maleate, Phenylephrine Hydrochloride, Phenylpropanolamine Hydrochloride, and Dihydrocodeine Bitartrate Syrup—Not in *USP–NF*.

CHLORPHENIRAMINE AND PHENYLPROPANOLAMINE

Chemical group:
Chlorpheniramine maleate—Alkylamine derivative.
Phenylpropanolamine hydrochloride—Synthetic phenyliso-propanolamine.

Chemical name:
Chlorpheniramine maleate—2-Pyridinepropanamine, gamma(4-chlorophenyl)-*N,N*-dimethyl-, (*Z*)-2-butenedioate (1:1).
Chlorpheniramine polistirex—Benzene, diethenyl-, polymer with ethenylbenzene, sulfonated, complex with gamma-(4-chlorophenyl)-*N,N*-dimethyl-2-pyridinepropanamine.
Phenylpropanolamine hydrochloride—Benzenemethanol, alpha-(1-aminoethyl)-, hydrochloride, (*R*,S**)-, (±).
Phenylpropanolamine polistirex—Benzene, diethenyl-, polymer with ethenylbenzene, sulfonated, complex with (±)-(*R*,S**)-alpha-(1-aminoethyl)benzenemethanol.

Molecular formula:
Chlorpheniramine maleate—$C_{16}H_{19}ClN_2 \cdot C_4H_4O_4$.
Phenylpropanolamine hydrochloride—$C_9H_{13}NO \cdot HCl$.

Molecular weight:
Chlorpheniramine maleate—390.86.
Phenylpropanolamine hydrochloride—187.67.

Description:
Chlorpheniramine Maleate USP—White, odorless, crystalline powder. Its solutions have a pH between 4 and 5.
Phenylpropanolamine Hydrochloride USP—White, crystalline powder, having a slight aromatic odor. Is affected by light.

pKa:
Chlorpheniramine maleate—9.2.
Phenylpropanolamine hydrochloride—9.

Solubility:
Chlorpheniramine Maleate USP—Freely soluble in water; soluble in alcohol and in chloroform; slightly soluble in ether.
Phenylpropanolamine Hydrochloride USP—Freely soluble in water and in alcohol; insoluble in ether.

USP requirements:
Chlorpheniramine Maleate and Phenylpropanolamine Hydrochloride Extended-release Capsules USP—Preserve in tight, light-resistant containers. Contain the labeled amounts, within ±10%. Meet the requirements for Identification, Drug release (20–50% in 3 hours, 45–75% in 6 hours, and not less than 75% in 12 hours in water in Apparatus 2 at 50 rpm), and Uniformity of dosage units..
Chlorpheniramine Maleate and Phenylpropanolamine Hydrochloride Granules—Not in *USP–NF*.
Chlorpheniramine Maleate and Phenylpropanolamine Hydrochloride Oral Solution—Not in *USP–NF*.
Chlorpheniramine Maleate and Phenylpropanolamine Hydrochloride Syrup—Not in *USP–NF*.
Chlorpheniramine Maleate and Phenylpropanolamine Hydrochloride Tablets—Not in *USP–NF*.
Chlorpheniramine Maleate and Phenylpropanolamine Hydrochloride Chewable Tablets—Not in *USP–NF*.
Chlorpheniramine Maleate and Phenylpropanolamine Hydrochloride Extended-release Tablets USP—Preserve in tight, light-resistant containers. Contain the labeled amounts, within ±10%. Meet the requirements for Identification, Drug release (20–50% in 3 hours, 45–75% in 6 hours, and not less than 75% in 12 hours in water in Apparatus 2 at 50 rpm), and Uniformity of dosage units..

Chlorpheniramine and Phenylpropanolamine Polistirexes Extended-release Oral Suspension—Not in *USP–NF*.

CHLORPHENIRAMINE, PHENYLPROPANOLAMINE, AND ACETAMINOPHEN

For *Chlorpheniramine, Phenylpropanolamine,* and *Acetaminophen*—See individual listings for chemistry information.

USP requirements:

Chlorpheniramine Maleate, Phenylpropanolamine Hydrochloride, and Acetaminophen Capsules USP—Preserve in tight containers. The label for each article encompassed by this monograph bears a name composed of the active ingredients. The label states the name and quantity of each active ingredient and indicates its function (or purpose) in the article. Contain the labeled amounts, within ±10%. Meet the requirements for Identification, Dissolution (75% of each active ingredient in 45 minutes in water in Apparatus 1 at 50 rpm), and Uniformity of dosage units.

Chlorpheniramine Maleate, Phenylpropanolamine Hydrochloride, and Acetaminophen Tablets USP—Preserve in tight containers. The label for each article encompassed by this monograph bears a name composed of the active ingredients. The label states the name and quantity of each active ingredient and indicates its function (or purpose) in the article. Contain the labeled amounts, within ±10%. Meet the requirements for Identification, Dissolution (75% of each active ingredient in 45 minutes in 0.1 *M* hydrochloric acid in Apparatus 2 at 50 rpm), and Uniformity of dosage units..

Chlorpheniramine Maleate, Phenylpropanolamine Hydrochloride, and Acetaminophen Effervescent Tablets—Not in *USP–NF*.

Chlorpheniramine Maleate, Phenylpropanolamine Hydrochloride, and Acetaminophen Extended-release Tablets—Not in *USP–NF*.

CHLORPHENIRAMINE, PHENYLPROPANOLAMINE, ACETAMINOPHEN, AND CAFFEINE

For *Chlorpheniramine, Phenylpropanolamine, Acetaminophen,* and *Caffeine*—See individual listings for chemistry information.

USP requirements: Chlorpheniramine Maleate, Phenylpropanolamine Hydrochloride, Acetaminophen, and Caffeine Tablets USP—Preserve in tight containers. The label for each article encompassed by this monograph bears a name composed of the active ingredients. The label states the name and quantity of each active ingredient and indicates its function (or purpose) in the article. Contain the labeled amounts, within ± 10%. Meet the requirements for Identification, Dissolution (75% in 45 minutes in 0.1 *M* hydrochloric acid in Apparatus 2 at 50 rpm), and Uniformity of dosage units.

CHLORPHENIRAMINE, PHENYLPROPANOLAMINE, AND ASPIRIN

For *Chlorpheniramine, Phenylpropanolamine,* and *Aspirin*—See individual listings for chemistry information.

USP requirements:

Chlorpheniramine Maleate, Phenylpropanolamine Bitartrate, and Aspirin Effervescent Tablets—Not in *USP–NF*.

Chlorpheniramine Maleate, Phenylpropanolamine Hydrochloride, and Aspirin for Oral Solution—Not in *USP–NF*.

Chlorpheniramine Maleate, Phenylpropanolamine Hydrochloride, and Aspirin Tablets—Not in *USP–NF*.

CHLORPHENIRAMINE, PHENYLPROPANOLAMINE, ASPIRIN, AND CAFFEINE

For *Chlorpheniramine, Phenylpropanolamine, Aspirin,* and *Caffeine*—See individual listings for chemistry information.

USP requirements:

Chlorpheniramine Maleate, Phenylpropanolamine Hydrochloride, Aspirin, and Caffeine Capsules—Not in *USP–NF*.

Chlorpheniramine Maleate, Phenylpropanolamine Hydrochloride, Aspirin, and Caffeine Tablets—Not in *USP–NF*.

CHLORPHENIRAMINE, PHENYLPROPANOLAMINE, AND CARAMIPHEN

Chemical group:

Chlorpheniramine maleate—Alkylamine derivative.

Phenylpropanolamine hydrochloride—Synthetic phenylisopropanolamine.

Chemical name:

Chlorpheniramine maleate—2-Pyridinepropanamine, gamma(4-chlorophenyl)-*N,N*-dimethyl-, (*Z*)-2-butenedioate (1:1).

Phenylpropanolamine hydrochloride—Benzenemethanol, alpha-(1-aminoethyl)-, hydrochloride, (*R**,*S**)-, (±).

Caramiphen edisylate—1-Phenylcyclopentane-1-carboxylic acid, 2-diethylaminoethyl ester, 1,2-ethanedisulfonate (2:1).

Molecular formula:

Chlorpheniramine maleate—$C_{16}H_{19}ClN_2 \cdot C_4H_4O_4$.

Phenylpropanolamine hydrochloride—$C_9H_{13}NO \cdot HCl$.

Caramiphen edisylate—$(C_{18}H_{27}NO_2)_2 \cdot C_2H_6O_6S_2$.

Molecular weight:

Chlorpheniramine maleate—390.86.

Phenylpropanolamine hydrochloride—187.67.

Caramiphen edisylate—769.03.

Description:

Chlorpheniramine Maleate USP—White, odorless, crystalline powder. Its solutions have a pH between 4 and 5.

Phenylpropanolamine Hydrochloride USP—White, crystalline powder, having a slight aromatic odor. Is affected by light.

Caramiphen edisylate—Off-white crystals. Melting point 115–116 °C.

pKa:

Chlorpheniramine maleate—9.2.

Phenylpropanolamine hydrochloride—9.

Solubility:

Chlorpheniramine Maleate USP—Freely soluble in water; soluble in alcohol and in chloroform; slightly soluble in ether.

Phenylpropanolamine Hydrochloride USP—Freely soluble in water and in alcohol; insoluble in ether.

Caramiphen edisylate—One gram dissolves in about 2 mL of water; soluble in alcohol.

USP requirements: Chlorpheniramine Maleate, Phenylpropanolamine Hydrochloride, and Caramiphen Edisylate Extended-release Capsules—Not in *USP–NF*.

CHLORPHENIRAMINE, PHENYLPROPANOLAMINE, CODEINE, GUAIFENESIN, AND ACETAMINOPHEN

For *Chlorpheniramine, Phenylpropanolamine, Codeine, Guaifenesin,* and *Acetaminophen*—See individual listings for chemistry information.

USP requirements:
Chlorpheniramine Maleate, Phenylpropanolamine Hydrochloride, Codeine Phosphate, Guaifenesin, and Acetaminophen Syrup—Not in *USP–NF.*

Chlorpheniramine Maleate, Phenylpropanolamine Hydrochloride, Codeine Phosphate, Guaifenesin, and Acetaminophen Tablets USP—Preserve in tight containers. The label for each article encompassed by this monograph bears a name composed of the active ingredients. The label states the name and quantity of each active ingredient and indicates its function (or purpose) in the article. Contain the labeled amounts, within ±10%. Meet the requirements for Identification, Dissolution (75% in 45 minutes in 0.1 *M* hydrochloric acid in Apparatus 2 at 50 rpm), and Uniformity of dosage units.

CHLORPHENIRAMINE, PHENYLPROPANOLAMINE, AND DEXTROMETHORPHAN

For *Chlorpheniramine, Phenylpropanolamine,* and *Dextromethorphan*—See individual listings for chemistry information.

USP requirements:
Chlorpheniramine Maleate, Phenylpropanolamine Hydrochloride, and Dextromethorphan Hydrobromide Capsules USP—Preserve in tight containers. The label for each article encompassed by this monograph bears a name composed of the active ingredients. The label states the name and quantity of each active ingredient and indicates its function (or purpose) in the article. Contain the labeled amounts, within ±10%. Meet the requirements for Identification, Dissolution (75% of each active ingredient in 45 minutes in water in Apparatus 1 at 50 rpm), and Uniformity of dosage units.

Chlorpheniramine Maleate, Phenylpropanolamine Hydrochloride, and Dextromethorphan Hydrobromide Oral Gel—Not in *USP–NF.*

Chlorpheniramine Maleate, Phenylpropanolamine Hydrochloride, and Dextromethorphan Hydrobromide Granules—Not in *USP–NF.*

Chlorpheniramine Maleate, Phenylpropanolamine Hydrochloride, and Dextromethorphan Hydrobromide Oral Solution USP—Preserve in tight containers. The label for each article encompassed by this monograph bears a name composed of the active ingredients. The label states the name and quantity of each active ingredient and indicates its function (or purpose) in the article. Contains the labeled amounts, within ±10%. Meets the requirements for Identification, pH (2.6–7.5), and Alcohol content, if present (within ±10%).

Chlorpheniramine Maleate, Phenylpropanolamine Hydrochloride, and Dextromethorphan Hydrobromide Syrup—Not in *USP–NF.*

Chlorpheniramine Maleate, Phenylpropanolamine Hydrochloride, and Dextromethorphan Hydrobromide Tablets USP—Preserve in tight containers. The label for each article encompassed by this monograph bears a name composed of the active ingredients. The label states the name and quantity of each active ingredient and indicates its function (or purpose) in the article. Contain the labeled amounts, within ±10%. Meet the requirements for Identifi-

cation, Dissolution (75% in 45 minutes in 0.1 *M* hydrochloric acid in Apparatus 2 at 50 rpm), and Uniformity of dosage units.

CHLORPHENIRAMINE, PHENYLPROPANOLAMINE, DEXTROMETHORPHAN, AND ACETAMINOPHEN

For *Chlorpheniramine, Phenylpropanolamine, Dextromethorphan,* and *Acetaminophen*—See individual listings for chemistry information.

USP requirements:
Chlorpheniramine Maleate, Phenylpropanolamine Hydrochloride, Dextromethorphan Hydrobromide, and Acetaminophen Capsules USP—Preserve in tight containers. The label for each article encompassed by this monograph bears a name composed of the active ingredients. The label states the name and quantity of each active ingredient and indicates its function (or purpose) in the article. Contain the labeled amounts, within ±10%. Meet the requirements for Identification, Dissolution (75% of each active ingredient in 45 minutes in water in Apparatus 1 at 50 rpm), and Uniformity of dosage units.

Chlorpheniramine Maleate, Phenylpropanolamine Hydrochloride, Dextromethorphan Hydrobromide, and Acetaminophen Oral Solution USP—Preserve in tight containers. The label for each article encompassed by this monograph bears a name composed of the active ingredients. The label states the name and quantity of each active ingredient and indicates its function (or purpose) in the article. Contains the labeled amounts, within ±10%. Meets the requirements for Identification, Microbial limits, pH (2.6–7.5), and Alcohol content, if present (within ±10%).

Chlorpheniramine Maleate, Phenylpropanolamine Hydrochloride, Dextromethorphan Hydrobromide, and Acetaminophen Tablets USP—Preserve in tight containers, and store at controlled room temperature. The label for each article encompassed by this monograph bears a name composed of the active ingredients. The label states the name and quantity of each active ingredient and indicates its function (or purpose) in the article. Contain the labeled amounts, within ±10%. Meet the requirements for Identification, Dissolution (75% of each active ingredient in 45 minutes in 0.1 *M* hydrochloric acid in Apparatus 2 at 50 rpm), and Uniformity of dosage units.

Chlorpheniramine Maleate, Phenylpropanolamine Bitartrate, Dextromethorphan Hydrobromide, and Acetaminophen Effervescent Tablets—Not in *USP–NF.*

CHLORPHENIRAMINE, PHENYLPROPANOLAMINE, DEXTROMETHORPHAN, AND AMMONIUM CHLORIDE

For *Chlorpheniramine, Phenylpropanolamine, Dextromethorphan,* and *Ammonium Chloride*—See individual listings for chemistry information.

USP requirements: Chlorpheniramine Maleate, Phenylpropanolamine Hydrochloride, Dextromethorphan Hydrobromide, and Ammonium Chloride Syrup—Not in *USP–NF.*

CHLORPHENIRAMINE, PHENYLPROPANOLAMINE, DEXTROMETHORPHAN, AND ASPIRIN

For *Chlorpheniramine, Phenylpropanolamine, Dextromethorphan,* and *Aspirin*—See individual listings for chemistry information.

USP requirements: Chlorpheniramine Maleate, Phenylpropanolamine Bitartrate, Dextromethorphan Hydrobromide, and Aspirin Effervescent Tablets—Not in *USP–NF*.

CHLORPHENIRAMINE, PHENYLPROPANOLAMINE, AND GUAIFENESIN

For *Chlorpheniramine, Phenylpropanolamine,* and *Guaifenesin*—See individual listings for chemistry information.

USP requirements: Chlorpheniramine Maleate, Phenylpropanolamine Hydrochloride, and Guaifenesin Oral Solution—Not in *USP–NF*.

CHLORPHENIRAMINE, PHENYLPROPANOLAMINE, GUAIFENESIN, AND ACETAMINOPHEN

For *Chlorpheniramine, Phenylpropanolamine, Guaifenesin,* and *Acetaminophen*—See individual listings for chemistry information.

USP requirements: Chlorpheniramine Maleate, Phenylpropanolamine Hydrochloride, Guaifenesin, and Acetaminophen Tablets USP—Preserve in tight containers. The label for each article encompassed by this monograph bears a name composed of the active ingredients. The label states the name and quantity of each active ingredient and indicates its function (or purpose) in the article. Contain the labeled amounts, within ±10%. Meet the requirements for Identification, Dissolution (75% in 45 minutes in 0.1 *M* hydrochloric acid in Apparatus 2 at 50 rpm), and Uniformity of dosage units.

CHLORPHENIRAMINE, PHENYLPROPANOLAMINE, GUAIFENESIN, SODIUM CITRATE, AND CITRIC ACID

For *Chlorpheniramine, Phenylpropanolamine, Guaifenesin, Sodium Citrate* and *Citric Acid*—See individual listings for chemistry information.

USP requirements: Chlorpheniramine Maleate, Phenylpropanolamine Hydrochloride, Guaifenesin, Sodium Citrate, and Citric Acid Oral Solution—Not in *USP–NF*.

CHLORPHENIRAMINE, PHENYLPROPANOLAMINE, AND METHSCOPOLAMINE

Chemical group:
    Chlorpheniramine maleate—Alkylamine derivative.
    Phenylpropanolamine hydrochloride—Synthetic phenylisopropanolamine.

Chemical name:
    Chlorpheniramine maleate—2-Pyridinepropanamine, gamma(4-chlorophenyl)-*N,N*-dimethyl-, (*Z*)-2-butenedioate (1:1).
    Phenylpropanolamine hydrochloride—Benzenemethanol, alpha-(1-aminoethyl)-, hydrochloride, (*R**,*S**)-, (±).

Methscopolamine nitrate—(–)-(1*S*,3*s*,5*R*,6*R*,7*S*)-6,7-Epoxy-8-methyl-3-[(*S*)-tropoyloxy]tropanium nitrate.

Molecular formula:
    Chlorpheniramine maleate—$C_{16}H_{19}ClN_2 \cdot C_4H_4O_4$.
    Phenylpropanolamine hydrochloride—$C_9H_{13}NO \cdot HCl$.
    Methscopolamine nitrate—$C_{18}H_{24}N_2O_7$.

Molecular weight:
    Chlorpheniramine maleate—390.86.
    Phenylpropanolamine hydrochloride—187.67.
    Methscopolamine nitrate—380.39.

Description:
    Chlorpheniramine Maleate USP—White, odorless, crystalline powder. Its solutions have a pH between 4 and 5.
    Phenylpropanolamine Hydrochloride USP—White, crystalline powder, having a slight aromatic odor. Is affected by light.

pKa:
    Chlorpheniramine maleate—9.2.
    Phenylpropanolamine hydrochloride—9.

Solubility:
    Chlorpheniramine Maleate USP—Freely soluble in water; soluble in alcohol and in chloroform; slightly soluble in ether.
    Phenylpropanolamine Hydrochloride USP—Freely soluble in water and in alcohol; insoluble in ether.

USP requirements: Chlorpheniramine Maleate, Phenylpropanolamine Hydrochoride, and Methscopolamine Nitrate Extended-release Tablets—Not in *USP–NF*.

CHLORPHENIRAMINE, PHENYLTOLOXAMINE, EPHEDRINE, CODEINE, AND GUAIACOL

Chemical name:
    Ephedrine—Benzenemethanol, alpha-[1-(methylamino)ethyl]-, [*R*-(*R**,*S**)]-.
    Codeine—Morphinan-6-ol, 7,8-didehydro-4,5-epoxy-3-methoxy-17-methyl-, monohydrate, (5 alpha,6 alpha)-.
    Guaiacol carbonate—Carbonic acid bis(2-methoxyphenyl) ester; guaiacol carbonic acid neutral ester; carbonic acid guaiacol ether.

Molecular formula:
    Ephedrine—$C_{10}H_{15}NO$ (anhydrous); $C_{10}H_{15}NO \cdot \frac{1}{2}H_2O$ (hemihydrate).
    Codeine—$C_{18}H_{21}NO_3 \cdot H_2O$ (monohydrate); $C_{18}H_{21}NO_3$ (anhydrous).
    Guaiacol carbonate—$C_{15}H_{14}O_5$.

Molecular weight:
    Ephedrine—165.23 (anhydrous); 174.24 (hemihydrate).
    Codeine—317.38 (monohydrate); 299.37 (anhydrous).
    Guaiacol carbonate—274.26.

Description:
    Ephedrine USP—Unctuous, practically colorless solid or white crystals or granules. Gradually decomposes on exposure to light. Melts between 33 and 40 °C, the variability of the melting point being the result of differences in the moisture content, anhydrous Ephedrine having a lower melting point than the hemihydrate of Ephedrine. Its solutions are alkaline to litmus.
    Codeine USP—Colorless or white crystals or white, crystalline powder. Effloresces slowly in dry air, and is affected by light. In acid or alcohol solutions it is levorotatory. Its saturated solution is alkaline to litmus.
    Guaiacol carbonate—Odorless needles from ethanol. It has a melting point of 88.1 °C.

Solubility:

Ephedrine USP—Soluble in water, in alcohol, in chloroform, and in ether; moderately and slowly soluble in mineral oil, the solution becoming turbid if the Ephedrine contains more than about 1% of water.

Codeine USP—Slightly soluble in water; very soluble in chloroform; freely soluble in alcohol; sparingly soluble in ether. When heated in an amount of water insufficient for complete solution, it melts to oily drops which crystallize on cooling.

Guaiacol carbonate—Practically insoluble in water; soluble in ethanol, in chloroform, and in ether; slightly soluble in liquid fatty acids.

USP requirements: Chlorpheniramine, Phenyltoloxamine, Ephedrine, Codeine, and Guaiacol Carbonate Oral Suspension—Not in *USP–NF*.

CHLORPHENIRAMINE, PHENYLTOLOXAMINE, AND PHENYLEPHRINE

Chemical group:

Chlorpheniramine maleate—Alkylamine derivative.
Phenyltoloxamine citrate—Ethanolamine derivative.

Chemical name:

Chlorpheniramine maleate—2-Pyridinepropanamine, gamma(4-chlorophenyl)-*N,N*-dimethyl-, (*Z*)-2-butenedioate (1:1).

Phenyltoloxamine citrate—2-(2-Benzylphenoxy)-*NN*-dimethylethylamine dihydrogen citrate.

Phenylephrine hydrochloride—Benzenemethanol, 3-hydroxyalpha-[(methylamino)methyl]-, hydrochloride.

Molecular formula:

Chlorpheniramine maleate—$C_{16}H_{19}ClN_2 \cdot C_4H_4O_4$.
Phenyltoloxamine citrate—$C_{17}H_{21}NO \cdot C_6H_8O_7$.
Phenylephrine hydrochloride—$C_9H_{13}NO_2 \cdot HCl$.

Molecular weight:

Chlorpheniramine maleate—390.86.
Phenyltoloxamine citrate—447.48.
Phenylephrine hydrochloride—203.67.

Description:

Chlorpheniramine Maleate USP—White, odorless, crystalline powder. Its solutions have a pH between 4 and 5.

Phenyltoloxamine citrate—It has a melting point of 138–140 °C.

Phenylephrine Hydrochloride USP—White or practically white, odorless crystals.

pKa: Chlorpheniramine maleate—9.2.

Solubility:

Chlorpheniramine Maleate USP—Freely soluble in water; soluble in alcohol and in chloroform; slightly soluble in ether.
Phenyltoloxamine citrate—Soluble in water.
Phenylephrine Hydrochloride USP—Freely soluble in water and in alcohol.

USP requirements:

Chlorpheniramine Maleate, Phenyltoloxamine Citrate, and Phenylephrine Hydrochloride Extended-release Capsules—Not in *USP–NF*.

Chlorpheniramine Maleate, Phenyltoloxamine Citrate, and Phenylephrine Hydrochloride Tablets—Not in *USP–NF*.

Chlorpheniramine Maleate, Phenyltoloxamine Citrate, and Phenylephrine Hydrochloride Extended-release Tablets—Nor in *USP–NF*.

CHLORPHENIRAMINE, PHENYLTOLOXAMINE, PHENYLEPHRINE, AND PHENYLPROPANOLAMINE

Chemical group:

Chlorpheniramine maleate—Alkylamine derivative.
Phenyltoloxamine citrate—Ethanolamine derivative.
Phenylpropanolamine hydrochloride—Synthetic phenylisopropanolamine.

Chemical name:

Chlorpheniramine maleate—2-Pyridinepropanamine, gamma(4-chlorophenyl)-*N,N*-dimethyl-, (*Z*)-2-butenedioate (1:1).

Phenyltoloxamine citrate—2-(2-Benzylphenoxy)-*NN*-dimethylethylamine dihydrogen citrate.

Phenylephrine hydrochloride—Benzenemethanol, 3-hydroxyalpha-[(methylamino)methyl]-, hydrochloride.

Phenylpropanolamine hydrochloride—Benzenemethanol, alpha-(1-aminoethyl)-, hydrochloride, (R^*,S^*)-, (±).

Molecular formula:

Chlorpheniramine maleate—$C_{16}H_{19}ClN_2 \cdot C_4H_4O_4$.
Phenyltoloxamine citrate—$C_{17}H_{21}NO \cdot C_6H_8O_7$.
Phenylephrine hydrochloride—$C_9H_{13}NO_2 \cdot HCl$.
Phenylpropanolamine hydrochloride—$C_9H_{13}NO \cdot HCl$.

Molecular weight:

Chlorpheniramine maleate—390.86.
Phenyltoloxamine citrate—447.5.
Phenylephrine hydrochloride—203.67.
Phenylpropanolamine hydrochloride—187.67.

Description:

Chlorpheniramine Maleate USP—White, odorless, crystalline powder. Its solutions have a pH between 4 and 5.

Phenyltoloxamine citrate—It has a melting point of 138–140 °C.

Phenylephrine Hydrochloride USP—White or practically white, odorless crystals.

Phenylpropanolamine Hydrochloride USP—White, crystalline powder, having a slight aromatic odor. Is affected by light.

pKa:

Chlorpheniramine maleate—9.2.
Phenylpropanolamine hydrochloride—9.

Solubility:

Chlorpheniramine Maleate USP—Freely soluble in water; soluble in alcohol and in chloroform; slightly soluble in ether.
Phenyltoloxamine citrate—Soluble in water.
Phenylephrine Hydrochloride USP—Freely soluble in water and in alcohol.
Phenylpropanolamine Hydrochloride USP—Freely soluble in water and in alcohol; insoluble in ether.

USP requirements:

Chlorpheniramine Maleate, Phenyltoloxamine Citrate, Phenylephrine Hydrochloride, and Phenylpropanolamine Hydrochloride Extended-release Capsules—Not in *USP–NF*.

Chlorpheniramine Maleate, Phenyltoloxamine Citrate, Phenylephrine Hydrochloride, and Phenylpropanolamine Hydrochloride Oral Solution—Not in *USP–NF*.

Chlorpheniramine Maleate, Phenyltoloxamine Citrate, Phenylephrine Hydrochloride, and Phenylpropanolamine Hydrochloride Syrup—Not in *USP–NF*.

Chlorpheniramine Maleate, Phenyltoloxamine Citrate, Phenylephrine Hydrochloride, and Phenylpropanolamine Hydrochloride Extended-release Tablets—Not in *USP–NF*.

CHLORPHENIRAMINE, PHENYLTOLOXAMINE, PHENYL-PROPANOLAMINE, AND ACETAMINOPHEN

Chemical group:
Chlorpheniramine maleate—Alkylamine derivative.
Phenylpropanolamine hydrochloride—Synthetic phenylisopropanolamine.

Chemical name:
Chlorpheniramine maleate—2-Pyridinepropanamine, gamma(4-chlorophenyl)-*N,N*-dimethyl-, (*Z*)-2-butenedioate (1:1).
Phenyltoloxamine dihydrogen citrate—2-(2-Benzylphenoxy)*NN*-dimethylethylamine dihydrogen citrate.
Phenylpropanolamine hydrochloride—Benzenemethanol, alpha-(1-aminoethyl)-, hydrochloride, (*R**,*S**)-, (±).
Acetaminophen—Acetamide, *N*-(4-hydroxyphenyl)-.

Molecular formula:
Chlorpheniramine maleate—$C_{16}H_{19}ClN_2 \cdot C_4H_4O_4$.
Phenyltoloxamine dihydrogen citrate—$C_{17}H_{21}NO \cdot C_6H_8O_7$.
Phenylpropanolamine hydrochloride—$C_9H_{13}NO \cdot HCl$.
Acetaminophen—$C_8H_9NO_2$.

Molecular weight:
Chlorpheniramine maleate—390.86.
Phenyltoloxamine dihydrogen citrate—447.5.
Phenylpropanolamine hydrochloride—187.67.
Acetaminophen—151.16.

Description:
Chlorpheniramine Maleate USP—White, odorless, crystalline powder. Its solutions have a pH between 4 and 5.
Phenyltoloxamine dihydrogen citrate—It has a melting point of 138–140 °C.
Phenylpropanolamine Hydrochloride USP—White, crystalline powder, having a slight aromatic odor. Is affected by light.
Acetaminophen USP—White, odorless, crystalline powder.

pKa:
Chlorpheniramine maleate—9.2.
Phenylpropanolamine hydrochloride—9.

Solubility:
Chlorpheniramine Maleate USP—Freely soluble in water; soluble in alcohol and in chloroform; slightly soluble in ether.
Phenyltoloxamine dihydrogen citrate—Soluble in water.
Phenylpropanolamine Hydrochloride USP—Freely soluble in water and in alcohol; insoluble in ether.
Acetaminophen USP—Soluble in boiling water and in 1 *N* sodium hydroxide; freely soluble in alcohol.

USP requirements: Chlorpheniramine Maleate, Phenyltoloxamine Dihydrogen Citrate, Phenylpropanolamine Hydrochloride, and Acetaminophen Capsules—Not in *USP–NF*.

CHLORPHENIRAMINE AND PSEUDOEPHEDRINE

Description: Chlorpheniramine tannate—Light tan to buff or yellowish-tan, amorphous, fine powder having not more than a slight characteristic odor.

Solubility: Chlorpheniramine tannate—Slightly soluble in water at 25 °C.

USP requirements:
Chlorpheniramine Maleate and Pseudoephedrine Hydrochloride Capsules—Not in *USP–NF*.
Chlorpheniramine Maleate and Pseudoephedrine Hydrochloride Extended-release Capsules USP—Preserve in tight, light-resistant containers, and store at controlled room temperature. The labeling indicates the Drug Release Test with which the product complies. Contain the labeled amounts, within ±10%. Meet the requirements for Identification, Drug release (for Test 1: 20–50% in 3 hours, 45–75% in 6 hours, and 75% in 12 hours in water in Apparatus

2 at 50 rpm, and for Test 2: 15–40% in 1.5 hours in simulated gastric fluid TS prepared without pepsin, and 35–75% in 3 hours and not less than 50% in 6 hours in simulated gastric fluid TS, prepared without pancreatin in Apparatus 2 at 50 rpm), and Uniformity of dosage units.
Chlorpheniramine Maleate and Pseudoephedrine Hydrochloride Oral Solution USP—Preserve in tight, light-resistant containers. Contains labeled amounts, within ±10%. Meets the requirement for Identification.
Chlorpheniramine Maleate and Pseudoephedrine Hydrochloride Oral Suspension—Not in *USP–NF*.
Chlorpheniramine Maleate and Pseudoephedrine Hydrochloride Syrup—Not in *USP–NF*.
Chlorpheniramine Maleate and Pseudoephedrine Hydrochloride Tablets—Not in *USP–NF*.
Chlorpheniramine Maleate and Pseudoephedrine Hydrochloride Chewable Tablets—Not in *USP–NF*.
Chlorpheniramine Maleate and Pseudoephedrine Sulfate Tablets—Not in *USP–NF*.
Chlorpheniramine Maleate and Pseudoephedrine Sulfate Extended-release Tablets—Not in *USP–NF*.
Chlorpheniramine Tannate and Pseudoephedrine Tannate Oral Suspension—Not in *USP–NF*.

CHLORPHENIRAMINE, PSEUDOEPHEDRINE, AND ACETAMINOPHEN

For *Chlorpheniramine, Pseudoephedrine,* and *Acetaminophen*—See individual listings for chemistry information.

USP requirements:
Chlorpheniramine Maleate, Pseudoephedrine Hydrochloride, and Acetaminophen Capsules USP—Preserve in tight containers. The label for each article encompassed by this monograph bears a name composed of the active ingredients contained in the article. The label states the name and quantity of each active ingredient and indicates its function (or purpose) in the article. Contain the labeled amounts, within ±10%. Meet the requirements for Identification, Dissolution (75% in 45 minutes in water in Apparatus 1 at 100 rpm), and Uniformity of dosage units.
Chlorpheniramine Maleate, Pseudoephedrine Hydrochloride, and Acetaminophen Oral Powder USP—Preserve in tight containers. The label for each article encompassed by this monograph bears a name composed of the active ingredients contained in the article. The label states the name and quantity of each active ingredient and indicates its function (or purpose) in the article. Contains the labeled amounts, within ±10%. Meets the requirements for Identification, Minimum fill, and Uniformity of dosage units.
Chlorpheniramine Maleate, Pseudoephedrine Hydrochloride, and Acetaminophen Oral Solution USP—Preserve in tight containers. The label for each article encompassed by this monograph bears a name composed of the active ingredients contained in the article. The label states the name and quantity of each active ingredient and indicates its function (or purpose) in the article. Contains the labeled amounts, within ±10%. Meets the requirements for Identification, pH (3.7–7.5), Alcohol content, if present (within ± 10%), and Microbial limits.
Chlorpheniramine Maleate, Pseudoephedrine Hydrochloride, and Acetaminophen for Oral Solution—Not in *USP–NF*.
Chlorpheniramine Maleate, Pseudoephedrine Hydrochloride, and Acetaminophen Tablets USP—Preserve in tight containers, and store at controlled room temperature. The label for each article encompassed by this monograph bears a name composed of the active ingredients contained in the article. The label states the name and quantity of each active ingredient and indicates its function (or purpose) in the article. Contain the labeled amounts, within ±10%.

Meet the requirements for Identification, Dissolution (75% in 45 minutes in water in Apparatus 2 at 50 rpm), and Uniformity of dosage units.
Chlorpheniramine Maleate, Pseudoephedrine Hydrochloride, and Acetaminophen Chewable Tablets—Not in *USP–NF*.

CHLORPHENIRAMINE, PSEUDOEPHEDRINE, AND CODEINE

For *Chlorpheniramine, Pseudoephedrine,* and *Codeine*—See individual listings for chemistry information.

USP requirements:
Chlorpheniramine Maleate, Pseudoephedrine Hydrochloride, and Codeine Phosphate Elixir—Not in *USP–NF*.
Chlorpheniramine Maleate, Pseudoephedrine Hydrochloride, and Codeine Phosphate Oral Solution—Not in *USP–NF*.

CHLORPHENIRAMINE, PSEUDOEPHEDRINE, CODEINE, AND ACETAMINOPHEN

For *Chlorpheniramine, Pseudoephedrine, Codeine,* and *Acetaminophen*—See individual listings for chemistry information.

USP requirements: Chlorpheniramine Maleate, Pseudoephedrine Hydrochloride, Codeine, and Acetaminophen Tablets—Not in *USP–NF*.

CHLORPHENIRAMINE, PSEUDOEPHEDRINE, AND DEXTROMETHORPHAN

For *Chlorpheniramine, Pseudoephedrine,* and *Dextromethorphan*—See individual listings for chemistry information.

USP requirements:
Chlorpheniramine Maleate, Pseudoephedrine Hydrochloride, and Dextromethorphan Hydrobromide Oral Powder USP—Preserve in tight containers. The label for each article encompassed by this monograph bears a name composed of the active ingredients contained in the article. The label states the name and quantity of each active ingredient and indicates its function (or purpose) in the article. Contains the labeled amounts, within ±10%. Meets the requirements for Identification, Minimum fill, and Uniformity of dosage units.
Chlorpheniramine Maleate, Pseudoephedrine Hydrochloride, and Dextromethorphan Hydrobromide Oral Solution USP—Preserve in tight containers. The label for each article encompassed by this monograph bears a name composed of the active ingredients. The label states the name and quantity of each active ingredient and indicates its function (or purpose) in the article. Contains the labeled amounts, within ±10%. Meets the requirements for Identification, pH (4.0–7.5), Alcohol content, if present (within ±10%), and Microbial limits.
Chlorpheniramine Maleate, Pseudoephedrine Hydrochloride, and Dextromethorphan Hydrobromide Syrup—Not in *USP–NF*.
Chlorpheniramine Maleate, Pseudoephedrine Hydrochloride, and Dextromethorphan Hydrobromide Chewable Tablets—Not in *USP–NF*.

CHLORPHENIRAMINE, PSEUDOEPHEDRINE, DEXTROMETHORPHAN, AND ACETAMINOPHEN

For *Chlorpheniramine, Pseudoephedrine, Dextromethorphan,* and *Acetaminophen*—See individual listings for chemistry information.

USP requirements:
Chlorpheniramine Maleate, Pseudoephedrine Hydrochloride, Dextromethorphan Hydrobromide, and Acetaminophen Capsules USP—Preserve in tight containers. The label for each article encompassed by this monograph bears a name composed of the active ingredients contained in the article. The label states the name and quantity of each active ingredient and indicates its function (or purpose) in the article. Contain the labeled amounts, within ±10%. Meet the requirements for Identification, Dissolution (75% of each active ingredient in 45 minutes in water in Apparatus 1 at 100 rpm), and Uniformity of dosage units.
Chlorpheniramine Maleate, Pseudoephedrine Hydrochloride, Dextromethorphan Hydrobromide, and Acetaminophen Oral Powder USP—Preserve in tight containers. The label for each article encompassed by this monograph bears a name composed of the active ingredients contained in the article. The label states the name and quantity of each active ingredient and indicates its function (or purpose) in the article. Contains the labeled amounts, within ±10%. Meets the requirements for Identification, Minimum fill, and Uniformity of dosage units.
Chlorpheniramine Maleate, Pseudoephedrine Hydrochloride, Dextromethorphan Hydrobromide, and Acetaminophen Oral Solution USP—Preserve in tight containers. The label for each article encompassed by this monograph bears a name composed of the active ingredients contained in the article. The label states the name and quantity of each active ingredient and indicates its function (or purpose) in the article. Contains the labeled amounts, within ±10%. Meets the requirements for Identification, pH (3.7–7.5), Alcohol content, if present (within ±10%), and Microbial limits.
Chlorpheniramine Maleate, Pseudoephedrine Hydrochloride, Dextromethorphan Hydrobromide, and Acetaminophen for Oral Solution—Not in *USP–NF*.
Chlorpheniramine Maleate, Pseudoephedrine Hydrochloride, Dextromethorphan Hydrobromide, and Acetaminophen Syrup—Not in *USP–NF*.
Chlorpheniramine Maleate, Pseudoephedrine Hydrochloride, Dextromethorphan Hydrobromide, and Acetaminophen Tablets USP—Preserve in tight containers, and store at controlled room temperature. The label for each article encompassed by this monograph bears a name composed of the active ingredients contained in the article. The label states the name and quantity of each active ingredient and indicates its function (or purpose) in the article. Contain the labeled amounts, within ±10%. Meet the requirements for Identification, Dissolution (75% of each active ingredient in 45 minutes in 0.1 *M* hydrochloric acid in Apparatus 2 at 50 rpm), and Uniformity of dosage units.
Chlorpheniramine Maleate, Pseudoephedrine Hydrochloride, Dextromethorphan Hydrobromide, and Acetaminophen Chewable Tablets—Not in *USP–NF*.

CHLORPHENIRAMINE, PSEUDOEPHEDRINE, DEXTROLMETHORPHAN, ACETAMINOPHEN, AND CAFFEINE

For *Chlorpheniramine, Pseudoephedrine, Dextromethorphan, Acetaminophen,* and *Caffeine*—See individual listings for chemistry information.

USP requirements: Chlorpheniramine Maleate, Pseudoephedrine Hydrochloride, Dextromethorphan Hydrobromide, Acetaminophen, and Caffeine Tablets USP—Preserve in tight containers, and store at controlled room temperature. The label for each article encompassed by this monograph bears a name composed of the active ingredients. The label states the name and quantity of each active ingredient and indicates its function (or purpose) in the article. Contain the labeled amounts, within ±10%. Meet the requirements for Identification, Dissolution (75% in 45 minutes in 0.1 *M* hydrochloric acid in Apparatus 2 at 50 rpm), and Uniformity of dosage units.

CHLORPHENIRAMINE, PSEUDOEPHEDRINE, DEXTROMETHORPHAN, AND GUAIFENESIN

For *Chlorpheniramine, Pseudoephedrine, Dextromethorphan and Guaifenesin*—See individual listings for chemistry information.

USP requirements: Chlorpheniramine Maleate, Pseudoephedrine Hydrochloride, Dextromethorphan Hydrobromide, and Guaifenesin Oral Solution—Not in *USP–NF*.

CHLORPHENIRAMINE, PSEUDOEPHEDRINE, AND GUAIFENESIN

For *Chlorpheniramine, Pseudoephedrine,* and *Guaifenesin*—See individual listings for chemistry information.

USP requirements:
Chlorpheniramine Maleate, Pseudoephedrine Hydrochloride, and Guaifenesin Extended-release Tablets—Not in *USP–NF*.
Chlorpheniramine Maleate, Pseudoephedrine Hydrochloride, and Guaifenesin Oral Solution—Not in *USP–NF*.

CHLORPHENIRAMINE, PSEUDOEPHEDRINE, AND HYDROCODONE

For *Chlorpheniramine, Pseudoephedrine,* and *Hydrocodone*—See individual listings for chemistry information.

USP requirements:
Chlorpheniramine Maleate, Pseudoephedrine Hydrochloride, and Hydrocodone Bitartrate Oral Solution—Not in *USP–NF*.
Chlorpheniramine Maleate, Pseudoephedrine Hydrochloride, and Hydrocodone Bitartrate Syrup—Not in *USP–NF*.

CHLORPHENIRAMINE, PSEUDOEPHEDRINE, AND METHSCOPOLAMINE

Chemical name:
Chlorpheniramine maleate—2-Pyridinepropanamine, gamma-(4-chlorophenyl)-*N,N*-dimethyl-, (*Z*)-2-butenedioate (1:1).
Pseudoephedrine hydrochloride—Benzenemethanol, alpha-[1-(methylamino)ethyl]-, [*S*-(*R**,*R**)]-, hydrochloride.
Methscopolamine nitrate—3-Oxa-9-azonlatricyclo [3.3.1.0²⁴] noane,7-(3-hydroxy-1-oxo-2-phenylpropoxy)-9,9-dimethyl-,nitrate,[7(*S*)-(1 alpha,2 beta,4 beta,5 alpha,7 beta)]-.

Molecular formula:
Chlorpheniramine maleate—$C_{16}H_{19}ClN_2 \cdot C_4H_4O_4$.
Pseudoephedrine hydrochloride—$C_{10}H_{15}NO \cdot HCl$.
Methscopolamine nitrate—$C_{18}H_{24}N_2O_7$.

Molecular weight:
Chlorpheniramine maleate—390.86.
Pseudoephedrine hydrochloride—201.69.
Methscopolamine nitrate—380.39.

Description:
Chlorpheniramine Maleate USP—White, odorless, crystalline powder. Its solutions have a pH between 4 and 5.
Pseudoephedrine Hydrochloride USP—Fine, white to off-white crystals or powder, having a faint characteristic odor.

pKa: Chlorpheniramine maleate—9.2.

Solubility:
Chlorpheniramine Maleate USP—Freely soluble in water; soluble in alcohol and in chloroform; slightly soluble in ether.
Pseudoephedrine Hydrochloride USP—Very soluble in water; freely soluble in alcohol; sparingly soluble in chloroform.

USP requirements: Chlorpheniramine Maleate, Pseudoephedrine Hydrochloride, and Methscopolamine Nitrate Extended-release Tablets—Not in *USP–NF*.

CHLORPHENIRAMINE, PYRILAMINE, AND PHENYLEPHRINE

Description: Chlorpheniramine tannate—Light tan to buff or yellowish-tan, amorphous, fine powder having not more than a slight characteristic odor.

Solubility: Chlorpheniramine tannate—Slightly soluble in water at 25 °C.

USP requirements:
Chlorpheniramine Tannate, Pyrilamine Tannate, and Phenylephrine Tannate Oral Suspension—Not in *USP–NF*.
Chlorpheniramine Tannate, Pyrilamine Tannate, and Phenylephrine Tannate Tablets—Not in *USP–NF*.
Chlorpheniramine Tannate, Pyrilamine Tannate, and Phenylephrine Tannate Extended-release Tablets—Not in *USP–NF*.

CHLORPHENIRAMINE, PYRILAMINE, PHENYLEPHRINE, AND ACETAMINOPHEN

For *Chlorpheniramine, Pyrilamine, Phenylephrine,* and *Acetaminophen*—See individual listings for chemistry information.

USP requirements: Chlorpheniramine Maleate, Pyrilamine Maleate, Phenylephrine Hydrochloride, and Acetaminophen Tablets—Not in *USP–NF*.

CHLORPHENIRAMINE, PYRILAMINE, PHENYLEPHRINE, AND PHENYLPROPANOLAMINE

For *Chlorpheniramine, Pyrilamine, Phenylephrine,* and *Phenylpropanolamine*—See individual listings for chemistry information.

USP requirements:
Chlorpheniramine Maleate, Pyrilamine Maleate, Phenylephrine Hydrochloride, and Phenylpropanolamine Hydrochloride Tablets—Not in *USP–NF*.

Chlorpheniramine Maleate, Pyrilamine Maleate, Phenylephrine Hydrochloride, and Phenylpropanolamine Hydrochloride Extended-release Tablets—Not in *USP–NF*.

CHLORPHENIRAMINE, PYRILAMINE, PHENYLEPHRINE, PHENYLPROPANOLAMINE, AND ACETAMINOPHEN

For *Chlorpheniramine, Pyrilamine, Phenylephrine, Phenylpropanolamine,* and *Acetaminophen*—See individual listings for chemistry information.

USP requirements: Chlorpheniramine Maleate, Pyrilamine Maleate, Phenylephrine Hydrochloride, Phenylpropanolamine Hydrochloride, and Acetaminophen Tablets USP—Preserve in tight containers. The label for each article encompassed by this monograph bears a name composed of the active ingredients. The label states the name and quantity of each active ingredient and indicates its function (or purpose) in the article. Contain the labeled amounts, within ±10%. Meet the requirements for Identification, Dissolution (75% in 45 minutes in 0.1 *M* hydrochloric acid in Apparatus 2 at 50 rpm), and Uniformity of dosage units.

CHLORPROMAZINE

Chemical group: Aliphatic phenothiazine.

Chemical name:
Chlorpromazine—10*H*-Phenothiazine-10-propanamine, 2-chloro-*N,N*-dimethyl-.
Chlorpromazine hydrochloride—10*H*-Phenothiazine-10-propanamine, 2-chloro-*N,N*-dimethyl-, monohydrochloride.

Molecular formula:
Chlorpromazine—$C_{17}H_{19}ClN_2S$.
Chlorpromazine hydrochloride—$C_{17}H_{19}ClN_2S \cdot HCl$.

Molecular weight:
Chlorpromazine—318.86.
Chlorpromazine hydrochloride—355.33.

Description:
Chlorpromazine USP—White, crystalline solid, having an amine-like odor. Darkens on prolonged exposure to light. Melts at about 60 °C.
Chlorpromazine Hydrochloride USP—White or slightly creamy white, odorless, crystalline powder. Darkens on prolonged exposure to light.

Solubility:
Chlorpromazine USP—Practically insoluble in water and in dilute alkali hydroxides; freely soluble in alcohol, in chloroform, in ether, and in dilute mineral acids.
Chlorpromazine Hydrochloride USP—Very soluble in water; freely soluble in alcohol and in chloroform; insoluble in ether.

USP requirements:
Chlorpromazine USP—Preserve in tight, light-resistant containers. Contains not less than 98.0% and not more than 101.0% of chlorpromazine, calculated on the dried basis. Meets the requirements for Identification, Loss on drying (not more than 1.0%), Other alkylated phenothiazines, and Organic volatile impurities.
Chlorpromazine Suppositories USP—Preserve in well-closed, light-resistant containers, at controlled room temperature. Contain the labeled amount, within ±10%. Meet the requirements for Identification and Other alkylated phenothiazines.

Chlorpromazine Hydrochloride USP—Preserve in tight, light-resistant containers. Contains not less than 98.0% and not more than 101.5% of chlorpromazine hydrochloride, calculated on the dried basis. Meets the requirements for Identification, Melting range (195–198 °C), Loss on drying (not more than 0.5%), Residue on ignition (not more than 0.1%), Other alkylated phenothiazines, and Organic volatile impurities.
Chlorpromazine Hydrochloride Extended-release Capsules—Not in *USP–NF*.
Chlorpromazine Hydrochloride Oral Concentrate USP—Preserve in tight, light-resistant containers. Label it to indicate that it must be diluted prior to administration. Contains the labeled amount, within ±10%. Meets the requirements for Identification, Microbial limits, pH (2.3–4.1), and Limit of chlorpromazine sulfoxide.
Chlorpromazine Hydrochloride Injection USP—Preserve in single-dose or in multiple-dose containers, preferably of Type I glass, protected from light. A sterile solution of Chlorpromazine Hydrochloride in Water for Injection. Contains, in each mL, not less than 23.75 mg and not more than 26.25 mg of chlorpromazine hydrochloride. Meets the requirements for Identification, Bacterial endotoxins, pH (3.4–5.4), and Limit of chlorpromazine sulfoxide, and for Injections.
Chlorpromazine Hydrochloride Syrup USP—Preserve in tight, light-resistant containers. Contains, in each 100 mL, not less than 190 mg and not more than 210 mg of chlorpromazine hydrochloride. Meets the requirements for Identification and Limit of chlorpromazine sulfoxide.
Chlorpromazine Hydrochloride Tablets USP—Preserve in well-closed, light-resistant containers. Contain the labeled amount, within ±5%. Meet the requirements for Identification, Dissolution (80% in 30 minutes in 0.1 *N* hydrochloric acid in Apparatus 1 at 50 rpm), Uniformity of dosage units, and Other alkylated phenothiazines.

CHLORPROPAMIDE

Chemical group: Sulfonylurea.

Chemical name: Benzenesulfonamide, 4-chloro-*N*-[(propylamino)carbonyl]-.

Molecular formula: $C_{10}H_{13}ClN_2O_3S$.

Molecular weight: 276.74.

Description: Chlorpropamide USP—White, crystalline powder, having a slight odor.

pKa: 4.8.

Solubility: Chlorpropamide USP—Practically insoluble in water; soluble in alcohol; sparingly soluble in chloroform.

USP requirements:
Chlorpropamide USP—Preserve in well-closed containers. Contains not less than 97.0% and not more than 103.0% of chlorpropamide, calculated on the dried basis. Meets the requirements for Identification, Melting range (126–129 °C), Loss on drying (not more than 1.0%), Residue on ignition (not more than 0.4%), Selenium (not more than 0.003%), Heavy metals (not more than 0.003%), and Organic volatile impurities.
Chlorpropamide Tablets USP—Preserve in well-closed containers. Contain the labeled amount, within ±10%. Meet the requirements for Identification, Dissolution (75% in 60 minutes in water in Apparatus 2 at 50 rpm), and Uniformity of dosage units.

CHLORPROTHIXENE

Chemical group: Thioxanthene derivative with general properties similar to those of the phenothiazine.

Chemical name: 1-Propanamine, 3-(2-chloro-9*H*-thioxanthen-9-ylidene)-*N,N*-dimethyl-, (*Z*)-.

Molecular formula: $C_{18}H_{18}ClNS$.

Molecular weight: 315.86.

Description: Chlorprothixene USP—Yellow, crystalline powder, having a slight amine-like odor.

Solubility: Chlorprothixene USP—Practically insoluble in water; soluble in alcohol and in ether; freely soluble in chloroform.

USP requirements:
Chlorprothixene USP—Preserve in tight, light-resistant containers. Contains not less than 99.0% and not more than 101.0% of chlorprothixene, calculated on the dried basis. Meets the requirements for Identification, Melting range (96.5–101.5 °C), Loss on drying (not more than 0.1%), Residue on ignition (not more than 0.1%), Heavy metals (not more than 0.002%), Limit of (*E*)-chlorprothixene [(*E*)-2-chloro-*N,N*-dimethylthioxanthene-Delta$^{9, \text{gamma}}$-propylamine (not more than 3.0%), and Organic volatile impurities.

Chlorprothixene Injection USP—Preserve in single-dose, low-actinic containers, protected from light. A sterile solution of Chlorprothixene in Water for Injection, prepared with the aid of Hydrochloric Acid. Contains the labeled amount, within ±5%. Meets the requirements for Identification, Bacterial endotoxins, and pH (3.0–4.0), and for Injections.

Chlorprothixene Oral Suspension USP—Preserve in tight, light-resistant containers. Contains the labeled amount, within ±10%. Meets the requirements for Identification and pH (3.5–4.5).

Chlorprothixene Tablets USP—Preserve in well-closed, light-resistant containers. Contain the labeled amount, within ± 7%. Meet the requirements for Identification, Dissolution (75% in 30 minutes in 0.1 *N* hydrochloric acid in Apparatus 1 at 100 rpm), and Uniformity of dosage units.

CHLORTETRACYCLINE

Chemical name: Chlortetracycline hydrochloride—2-Naphthacenecarboxamide, 7-chloro-4-(dimethylamino)-1,4,4a,5,5a,6,11,12a-octahydro-3,6,10,12,12a-pentahydroxy-6-methyl-1,11-dioxo-, monohydrochloride [4*S*-(4 alpha,4a alpha,5a alpha,6 beta,12a alpha)]-.

Molecular formula: Chlortetracycline hydrochloride—$C_{22}H_{23}ClN_2O_8 \cdot HCl$.

Molecular weight: Chlortetracycline hydrochloride—515.34.

Description: Chlortetracycline Hydrochloride USP—Yellow, crystalline powder. Is odorless. Is stable in air, but is slowly affected by light.

Solubility: Chlortetracycline Hydrochloride USP—Sparingly soluble in water; soluble in solutions of alkali hydroxides and carbonates; slightly soluble in alcohol; practically insoluble in acetone, in chloroform, in dioxane, and in ether.

USP requirements:
Chlortetracycline Bisulfate USP—Preserve in tight, light-resistant containers. Label it to indicate that it is intended for veterinary use only. Has a potency equivalent to not less than 760 mcg of chlortetracycline hydrochloride per mg, calculated on the dried and butyl alcohol-free basis. Meets the requirements for Identification, Crystallinity, Loss on drying (not more than 2.0%), Sulfate content (not less than 15.0%, calculated on the dried and butyl alcohol-free basis), and Butyl alcohol (not more than 15.0%).

Chlortetracycline Hydrochloride USP—Preserve in tight, light-resistant containers. Where it is intended for use in preparing sterile dosage forms, the label states that it is sterile or must be subjected to further processing during the preparation of sterile dosage forms. Has a potency of not less than 900 mcg of chlortetracycline hydrochloride per mg. Meets the requirements for Identification, Specific rotation (−235° to −250°), Crystallinity, Sterility, pH (2.3–3.3, in a solution containing 10 mg per mL), and Loss on drying (not more than 2.0%).

Note: Chlortetracycline Hydrochloride labeled solely for use in preparing oral veterinary dosage forms has a potency of not less than 820 mcg of chlortetracycline hydrochloride per mg.

Chlortetracycline Hydrochloride Capsules USP—Preserve in tight, light-resistant containers. Contain the labeled amount, within −10% to +20%. Meet the requirements for Identification, Dissolution (75% in 45 minutes in water in Apparatus 2 at 75 rpm), Uniformity of dosage units, and Loss on drying (not more than 1.0%).

Chlortetracycline Hydrochloride Ointment USP—Preserve in collapsible tubes or in well-closed, light-resistant containers. Contains the labeled amount, within −10% to +25%, in a suitable ointment base. Meets the requirements for Water (not more than 0.5%) and Minimum fill.

Chlortetracycline Hydrochloride Ophthalmic Ointment USP—Preserve in collapsible ophthalmic ointment tubes. Contains the labeled amount, within −10% to +25%. Meets the requirements for Sterility, Minimum fill, Water (not more than 0.5%), and Metal particles.

Chlortetracycline Hydrochloride Soluble Powder USP—Preserve in tight containers, protected from light. Label it to indicate that it is intended for oral veterinary use only. Contains the labeled amount, within −10% to +25%. Meets the requirement for Loss on drying (not more than 2.0%).

Chlortetracycline Hydrochloride Tablets USP—Preserve in tight containers, protected from light. Label Tablets to indicate that they are intended for veterinary use only. Contain the labeled amount, within −10% to +20%. Meet the requirements for Identification, Disintegration (1 hour, simulated gastric fluid TS being used as the test medium in place of water), Uniformity of dosage units, and Water (not more than 3.0%, or where the Tablets have a diameter of greater than 15 mm, not more than 6.0%).

CHLORTETRACYCLINE AND SULFAMETHAZINE

USP requirements: Chlortetracycline and Sulfamethazine Bisulfates Soluble Powder USP—Preserve in tight, light-resistant containers. A dry mixture of Chlortetracycline Bisulfate and Sulfamethazine Bisulfate and one or more suitable buffers and diluents. Label it to indicate that it is intended for veterinary use only. Contains amounts of chlortetracycline and sulfamethazine bisulfates equivalent to the labeled amounts of chlortetracycline hydrochloride and sulfamethazine, within −15% to +25%. Meets the requirement for Loss on drying (not more than 2.0%).

CHLORTHALIDONE

Chemical name: Benzenesulfonamide, 2-chloro-5-(2,3-dihydro-1-hydroxy-3-oxo-1H-isoindol-1-yl)-.

Molecular formula: $C_{14}H_{11}ClN_2O_4S$.

Molecular weight: 338.77.

Description: Chlorthalidone USP—White to yellowish white, crystalline powder. Melts at a temperature above 215 °C, with decomposition.

pKa: 9.4.

Solubility: Chlorthalidone USP—Practically insoluble in water, in ether, and in chloroform; soluble in methanol; slightly soluble in alcohol.

USP requirements:
Chlorthalidone USP—Preserve in well-closed containers. Contains not less than 98.0% and not more than 102.0% of chlorthalidone, calculated on the dried basis. Meets the requirements for Identification, Loss on drying (not more than 0.4%), Residue on ignition (not more than 0.1%), Chloride (not more than 0.035%), Heavy metals (not more than 0.001%), and Limit of 4'-chloro-3'-sulfamoyl-2-benzophenone carboxylic acid (CCA) (not more than 1.0%).
Chlorthalidone Tablets USP—Preserve in well-closed containers. Contain the labeled amount, within ±8%. Meet the requirements for Identification, Dissolution (70% in 60 minutes in water in Apparatus 2 at 75 rpm), and Uniformity of dosage units.

CHLORZOXAZONE

Chemical name: 2(3H)-Benzoxazolone, 5-chloro-.

Molecular formula: $C_7H_4ClNO_2$.

Molecular weight: 169.56.

Description: Chlorzoxazone USP—White or practically white, practically odorless, crystalline powder.

Solubility: Chlorzoxazone USP—Slightly soluble in water; sparingly soluble in alcohol, in isopropyl alcohol, and in methanol; soluble in solutions of alkali hydroxides and ammonia.

USP requirements:
Chlorzoxazone USP—Preserve in tight containers. Contains not less than 98.0% and not more than 102.0% of chlorzoxazone, calculated on the dried basis. Meets the requirements for Identification, Melting range (189–194 °C), Loss on drying (not more than 0.5%), Heavy metals (not more than 0.002%), Residue on ignition (not more than 0.15%), Chromatographic purity, Organic volatile impurities, and Chlorine content (20.6–21.2%, calculated on the dried basis).
Chlorzoxazone Tablets USP—Preserve in tight containers. Contain the labeled amount, within ±10%. Meet the requirements for Identification, Dissolution (75% in 60 minutes in phosphate buffer [pH 6.8] in Apparatus 2 at 75 rpm), and Uniformity of dosage units.

CHLORZOXAZONE AND ACETAMINOPHEN

For *Chlorzoxazone* and *Acetaminophen*—See individual listings for chemistry information.

USP requirements: Chlorzoxazone and Acetaminophen Tablets—Not in *USP–NF*.

CHOCOLATE

NF requirements:
Chocolate NF—Preserve in well-closed containers. A powder prepared from the roasted, cured kernels of the ripe seed of *Theobroma cacao* L. (Fam. Sterculiaceae). Yields not less than 10.0% and not more than 22.0% of nonvolatile, ether-soluble extractive. Meets the requirements for Botanic characteristics, Microbial limits, and Limit of ether-insoluble residue.
Chocolate Syrup NF—Preserve in tight containers, and avoid exposure to excessive heat. Prepare Chocolate Syrup as follows: 180 grams of Chocolate, 600 grams of Sucrose, 180 grams of Liquid Glucose, 50 mL of Glycerin, 2 grams of Sodium Chloride, 0.2 gram of Vanillin, 1 gram of Sodium Benzoate, and Purified Water, a sufficient quantity to make 1000 mL. Mix Chocolate and Sucrose, and to this mixture gradually add a solution of Liquid Glucose, Glycerin, Sodium Chloride, Vanillin, and Sodium Benzoate in 325 mL of hot Purified Water. Bring the entire mixture to a boil, and maintain at boiling temperature for 3 minutes. Allow to cool to room temperature, and add sufficient Purified Water to make the product measure 1000 mL.

Note—Chocolate containing not more than 12% of nonvolatile, ether-soluble extractive ("fat") yields a Syrup having a minimum tendency to separate. "Breakfast Chocolate" contains over 22% of "fat".

CHOLECALCIFEROL

Chemical name: 9,10-Secocholesta-5,7,10(19)-trien-3-ol, (3 beta,5Z,7E)-.

Molecular formula: $C_{27}H_{44}O$.

Molecular weight: 384.64.

Description: Cholecalciferol USP—White, odorless crystals. Is affected by air and by light. Melts at about 85 °C.

Solubility: Cholecalciferol USP—Insoluble in water; soluble in alcohol, in chloroform, and in fatty oils.

USP requirements:
Cholecalciferol USP—Preserve in hermetically sealed containers under nitrogen, in a cool place and protected from light. Contains not less than 97.0% and not more than 103.0% of cholecalciferol. Meets the requirements for Identification, Specific rotation (+105° to +112°), and Organic volatile impurities.
Cholecalciferol Solution USP—Preserve in tight, light-resistant containers. A solution of Cholecalciferol in an edible vegetable oil, in Polysorbate 80, or in Propylene Glycol. Label it to indicate the concentration, in mg per mL, of cholecalciferol. Label it also to state that it is to be used for manufacturing only. Contains the labeled amount, within −10% to +20%.

CHOLECYSTOKININ

Source: A polypeptide which occurs in two forms, one with 33 and one with 39 amino acids.

USP requirements: Cholecystokinin for Injection—Not in *USP–NF*.

CHOLESTEROL

Chemical name: Cholest-5-en-3-ol, (3 beta)-.

Molecular formula: $C_{27}H_{46}O$.

Molecular weight: 386.65.

Description: Cholesterol NF—White or faintly yellow, practically odorless, pearly leaflets, needles, powder, or granules. Acquires a yellow to pale tan color on prolonged exposure to light.
NF category: Emulsifying and/or solubilizing agent.

Solubility: Cholesterol NF—Insoluble in water; soluble in acetone, in chloroform, in dioxane, in ether, in ethyl acetate, in solvent hexane, and in vegetable oils; sparingly soluble in dehydrated alcohol; slightly (and slowly) soluble in alcohol.

NF requirements: Cholesterol NF—Preserve in well-closed, light-resistant containers. A steroid alcohol used as an emulsifying agent. Meets the requirements for Solubility in alcohol, Identification, Melting range (147–150 °C), Specific rotation (−34° to −38°), Acidity, Loss on drying (not more than 0.3%), Residue on ignition (not more than 0.1%), and Organic volatile impurities.

CHOLESTYRAMINE

Chemical name: Cholestyramine resin—Cholestyramine.

Description: Cholestyramine Resin USP—White to buff-colored, hygroscopic, fine powder. Is odorless or has not more than a slight amine-like odor.

Solubility: Cholestyramine Resin USP—Insoluble in water, in alcohol, in chloroform, and in ether.

USP requirements:
Cholestyramine Resin USP—Preserve in tight containers. A strongly basic anion-exchange resin in the chloride form, consisting of styrene-divinylbenzene copolymer with quaternary ammonium functional groups. Each gram exchanges not less than 1.8 grams and not more than 2.2 grams of sodium glycocholate, calculated on the dried basis. Meets the requirements for Identification, pH (4.0–6.0, in a slurry [1 in 100]), Loss on drying (not more than 12.0%), Residue on ignition (not more than 0.1%), Heavy metals (not more than 0.002%), Dialyzable quaternary amines, Organic volatile impurities, Chloride content (13.0–17.0%, calculated on the dried basis), and Exchange capacity.
Cholestyramine for Oral Suspension USP—Preserve in tight containers. A mixture of Cholestyramine Resin with suitable excipients and coloring and flavoring agents. Contains the labeled amount of dried cholestyramine resin, within ±15%. Meets the requirements for Identification, Uniformity of dosage units, and Exchange capacity.

CHOLINE BITARTRATE

Chemical name: 2-Hydroxyethanaminium,-*N,N,N*-trimethyl-, [*R*-(*R*,R**)]-2,3-dihydroxybutanedioate (1:1).

Molecular formula: $C_9H_{19}NO_7$.

Molecular weight: 253.25.

Description: White, hygroscopic, crystalline powder. Clear, colorless liquid in solution. Melts between 148° and 153°. Is odorless, or may have a faint trimethylamine odor.

Solubiliuty: Freely soluble in water; slightly soluble in alcohol; insoluble in ether and in chloroform.

USP requirements: Choline Bitartrate USP—Preserve in well-closed containers. Contains not less than 99.0% and not more than 100.5% of choline bitartrate, calculated on the anhydrous basis. Meets the reequirements for Identification, Specific rotation (+17.5° to +18.5°), pH (3.0–4.0, in a soulution [1 in 10]), Water (not more than 0.5%), Residue on ignition (not more than 0.1%), Arsenic (2 mcg per gram), Lead (not more than 0.3 mcg per gram), Heavy metals (10 mcg per gram), Limit of total amines (not more than 10 mcg per gram), Chromatographic purity, and Organic volatile impurities (except that the limit for 1,4-dioxane is 10 mcg per gram).

CHOLINE CHLORIDE

Chemical name: (2-Hydroxyethyl)trimethylammonium chloride.

Molecular formula: $C_5H_{14}ClNO$.

Molecular weight: 139.62.

Description: Colorless or white crystals or crystalline powder, usually having a slight odor of trimethylamine. Clear and colorless in solution. Hygroscopic.

Solubiliuty: Soluble in alcohol and in water.

USP requirements: Choline Chloride USP—Preserve in well-closed containers. Contains not less than 99.0% and not more than 100.5% of choline chloride, calculated on the anhydrous basis. Meets the requirements for Identification, pH (4.0–7.0, in a solution [1 in 10]), Water (not more than 0.5%), Residue on ignition (not more than 0.05%), Arsenic (2 mcg per gram), Lead (not more than 0.3 mcg per gram), Heavy metals (0.001%), Limit of total amines (not more than 0.001%), Chromatographic purity, and Organic volatile impurities (except that the limit for 1,4-dioxane is 10 mcg per gram).

CHOLINE SALICYLATE

Chemical name: (2-Hydroxyethyl)trimethylammonium salicylate.

Molecular formula: $C_{12}H_{19}NO_4$.

Molecular weight: 241.28.

Description: White, hygroscopic solid with a melting point of about 50 °C.

Solubility: Freely soluble in water; soluble in most hydrophilic solvents; insoluble in organic solvents.

USP requirements: Choline Salicylate Oral Solution—Not in *USP–NF*.

CHOLINE SALICYLATE AND CETYL-DIMETHYL-BENZYL-AMMONIUM CHLORIDE

Chemical name: Choline salicylate—(2-Hydroxyethyl)trimethylammonium salicylate.

Molecular formula: Choline salicylate—$C_{12}H_{19}NO_4$.

Molecular weight: Choline salicylate—241.28.

Description: Choline salicylate—White, hygroscopic solid with a melting point of about 50 °C.

Solubility: Choline salicylate—Freely soluble in water; soluble in most hydrophilic solvents; insoluble in organic solvents.

USP requirements: Choline Salicylate and Cetyl-dimethyl-ben-zyl-ammonium Chloride Gel—Not in *USP–NF*.

CHOLINE AND MAGNESIUM SALICYLATES

For *Choline Salicylate* and *Magnesium Salicylate*—See individual listings for chemistry information.

USP requirements:
Choline and Magnesium Salicylates Oral Solution—Not in *USP–NF*.
Choline and Magnesium Salicylates Tablets—Not in *USP–NF*.

CHONDROCYTE-ALGINATE

USP requirements:
Chondrocyte-Alginate Suspension—Not in *USP–NF*.
Chondrocyte-Alginate Gel—Not in *USP–NF*.

CHONDROCYTES, AUTOLOGUS CULTURED

Source: Harvested from the patient's normal, femoral cartilage and expanded via cell culture techniques.

USP requirements: Autologous Cultured Chondrocytes for Implantation—Not in *USP–NF*.

CHONDROITIN

Chemical name: Sodium chondroitin sulfate.

Molecular formula:$(C_{14}H_{19}NO_{14}SNa_2)_n$.

NF requirements:
Chondroitin Sulfate Sodium NF—Preserve in tight containers. It is the sodium salt of the sulfated linear glycosaminoglycan obtained from bovine, porcine, or avian cartilages of healthy and domestic animals used for food by humans. Consists mostly of the sodium salt of the sulfate ester of *N*-acetylchondrosamine (2-acetamido-2-deoxy-alpha-D-galactopyranose) and D-glucuronic acid copolymer. These hexoses are alternately linked beta-1,4 and beta-1,3 in the polymer. The prevalent glycosaminoglycans are designated chondroitin sulfate sodium A, containing *N*-acetyl-chondrosamine-4-*O*-sulfate, and chondroitin sulfate sodium C, containing *N*-acetylchondrosamine-6-*O*-sulfate. Label it to indicate the species of the source from which the article was derived. Contains a labeled amount of glycosaminoglycans as chondroitin sulfate sodium, within -10% and +5%, calculated on the dried basis. Meets the requirements for Clarity and color of solution (not greater than 0.35), Identification, Specific rotation (between -20.0° and -30.0°), pH (5.5–7.5, in a solution [1 in 100]), Loss on drying (not more than 10.0%), Residue on ignition (20.0–30.0°), on the dried basis, omitting the addition of sulfuric acid), Chloride (not more than 0.50%), Sulfate (not more than 0.24%), Heavy metals (0.002%), Organic volatile impurities, Microbial limits, Test for absence of *clostridium* species, Electrophoretic purity (not more than 1%), Limit of protein (not more than 60%, calculated on the dried basis), and Content of total glycosaminoglycans.

Note—Chondroitin sulfate sodium is extremely hygroscopic once dried. Avoid exposer to the atmosphere and weigh promptly.
Chondroitin Sulfate Tablets NF—Preserve in tight, light resistant containers, and store at room temperature. Prepared from Chondroitin Sulfate Sodium. Label it to indicate the species of the source from which the condroitin used to prepare the Tablets was derived. Contains the labeled amount of chondroitin sulfate sodium, within -10% to +20%. Meet the requirements for Identification, Disintigration and dissolution (75% in 60 minutes in water in Apparatus 2 at 75 rpm), Weight variation, and Content of chondroitin sulfate sodium.
Note—Chondroitin sulfate sodium is extremely hygroscopic once dried. Avoid exposer to the atmosphere and weigh promptly.

CHORIOGONADOTROPIN ALFA

Source: Produced by recombinant DNA technology using modified Chinese Hamster Ovary (CHO) cells.

Chemical name: Gonadotropin, chorionic (human alpha-subunit protein moiety reduced), complex with chorionic gonadotropin (human beta-subunit protein moiety reduced).

Molecular formula: $C_{437}H_{682}N_{122}O_{134}S_{13}$(alpha-subunit)$C_{668}H_{1090}N_{196}O_{203}S_{13}$(beta-subunit).

Molecular weight: 38,000 daltons.

Description: Sterile lyophilized powder.

Solubility: Soluble in water.

Other characteristics:pH—Reconstituted solution: 6.5 to 7.5.

USP requirements: Choriogonadotropin Alfa for Injection—Not in *USP–NF*.

SODIUM CHROMATE CR 51

Chemical name: Chromic acid ($H_2{}^{51}CrO_4$), disodium salt.

Molecular formula: $Na_2{}^{51}CrO_4$.

Description: Sodium Chromate Cr 51 Injection USP—Clear, slightly yellow solution.

USP requirements: Sodium Chromate Cr 51 Injection USP—Preserve in single-dose or in multiple-dose containers. A sterile solution of radioactive chromium (^{51}Cr) processed in the form of sodium chromate in Water for Injection. For those uses where an isotonic solution is required, Sodium Chloride may be added in appropriate amounts. Chromium 51 is produced by the neutron bombardment of enriched chromium 50. Label it to include the following, in addition to the information specified for Labeling under Injections: the time and date of calibration; the amount of sodium chromate expressed in mcg per mL; the amount of ^{51}Cr as sodium chromate expressed as total megabecquerels (or millicuries) and as megabecquerels (or millicuries) per mL at the time of calibration; a statement to indicate whether the contents are intended for diagnostic or therapeutic use; the expiration date; and the statement, "Caution—Radioactive Material." The labeling indicates that in making dosage calculations, correction is to be made for radioactive decay and the quantity of chromium, and also indicates that the radioactive half-life of ^{51}Cr is 27.8 days. Contains the labeled amount of ^{51}Cr, within ±10%, as sodium chromate expressed in megabecquerels (or millicuries) per mL at the time indicated in the labeling. The sodium chromate content is not less than 90.0% and not more than 110.0% of the labeled amount. The specific activity is not less than 370 mega-

becquerels (10 millicuries) per mg of sodium chromate at the end of the expiry period. Other chemical forms of radioactivity do not exceed 10.0% of the total radioactivity. Meets the requirements for Radionuclide identification, Bacterial endotoxins, pH (7.5–8.5), and Radiochemical purity, and for Injections (except that it is not subject to the recommendation on Volume in Container).

CHROMIC CHLORIDE

Chemical name: Chromium chloride (CrCl₃) hexahydrate.

Molecular formula: $CrCl_3 \cdot 6H_2O$.

Molecular weight: 266.45.

Description: Chromic Chloride USP—Dark green, odorless, slightly deliquescent crystals.

Solubility: Chromic Chloride USP—Soluble in water and in alcohol; slightly soluble in acetone; practically insoluble in ether.

USP requirements:
Chromic Chloride USP—Preserve in tight containers. Contains not less than 98.0% and not more than 101.0% of chromic chloride. Meets the requirements for Identification, Insoluble matter (not more than 0.01%), Substances not precipitated by ammonium hydroxide (not more than 0.20% as sulfate), Sulfate (not more than 0.01%), and Iron (not more than 0.01%).
Chromic Chloride Injection USP—Preserve in single-dose or in multiple-dose containers, preferably of Type I or Type II glass. A sterile solution of Chromic Chloride in Water for Injection. Label the Injection to indicate that it is to be diluted to the appropriate strength with Sterile Water for Injection or other suitable fluid prior to administration. Contains an amount of chromic chloride equivalent to the labeled amount of chromium, within ±10%. Meets the requirements for Identification, Bacterial endotoxins, and pH (1.5–2.5), and for Injections.

CHROMIUM

Molecular formula: Cr.

Molecular weight: 52 (elemental).

Description: Steel-gray, lustrous metal. Melting point 1900 °C.

USP requirements:
Chromium Capsules—Not in *USP–NF*.
Chromium Tablets—Not in *USP–NF*.

CHROMIUM CR 51 EDETATE

Chemical name: Glycine, *N,N*-1,2-ethanediylbis[*N*-(carboxymethyl)]-, chromium-51 complex.

USP requirements: Chromate Cr 51 Edetate Injection USP—Preserve in single-dose or multiple-dose containers, at a temperature between 2° and 8°. A sterile solution containing radioactive chromium (⁵¹Cr) in the form of a complex of chromium (III) with edetic acid, present in access. It is made isotonic by the addition of Sodium Chloride. Label it to include the following, in addition to the information specified for Labeling under Injections: the time and date of calibration; the amount of ⁵¹Cr as edetate complex expressed as total megabecquerels (or millicuries) and as megabecquerels (or millicuries) per mL at the time of calibration; the expiration date; and the statement,

"Caution—Radioactive Material." The labeling indicates that in making dosage calculations, correction is to be made for radioactive decay and the quantity of chromium, and also indicates that the radioactive half-life of ⁵¹Cr is 27.8 days. Contains the labeled amount of ⁵¹Cr, within ±10%, as edetate complex expressed in megabecquerels (or microcuries or millicuries) per mL at the time indicated in the labeling. Other chemical forms of radioactivity do not exceed 5.0% of the total radioactivity. It may contain a suitable preservative. It contains not more than 1 mg of chromium (Cr) per mL. Meets the requirements for Radionuclide identification, Bacterial endotoxins, pH (3.5–6.5), Radiochemical purity, Radionuclidic purity, Chemical purity, and Limit of free chromium, and for Injections (except that it is not subject to the recommendation on Volume in Container).

CHROMIUM PICOLINATE

Chemical name: Chromium tripicolinate.

Molecular formula: $C_{18}H_{12}N_3O_6Cr$.

Molecular weight: 418.31.

NF requirements: Chromium Picolinate NF—Preserve in tight containers. Contains not less than 98.0% and not more than 102.0%, calculated on the dried basis. Meets the requirements for Identification, Loss on drying (not more than 4.0%), Chloride (0.06%), and Sulfate (not more than 0.2%).

CHYMOPAPAIN

Source: A proteolytic enzyme isolated from the crude latex of *Carica papaya*, differing from papain in electrophoretic mobility, solubility, and substrate specificity.

Chemical name: Chymopapain.

Molecular weight: Approximately 27,000.

USP requirements: Chymopapain for Injection—Not in *USP–NF*.

CHYMOTRYPSIN

Chemical name: Chymotrypsin.

Description: Chymotrypsin USP—White to yellowish white, crystalline or amorphous, odorless, powder.

Solubility: Chymotrypsin USP—An amount equivalent to 100,000 USP Units is soluble in 10 mL of water and in 10 mL of saline TS.

USP requirements:
Chymotrypsin USP—Preserve in tight containers, and avoid exposure to excessive heat. A proteolytic enzyme crystallized from an extract of the pancreas gland of the ox, *Bos taurus* Linné (Fam. Bovidae). Contains not less than 1000 USP Chymotrypsin Units in each mg, calculated on the dried basis, and not less than 90.0% and not more than 110.0% of the labeled potency, as determined by the *Assay*. Meets the requirements for Microbial limits, Loss on drying (not more than 5.0%), Residue on ignition (not more than 2.5%), and Limit of trypsin (not more than 1%).

Chymotrypsin for Ophthalmic Solution USP—Preserve in single-dose containers, preferably of Type I glass, and avoid exposure to excessive heat. It is sterile Chymotrypsin. When constituted as directed in the labeling, yields a solution containing the labeled potency, within ±20%. Meets the requirements for Completeness of solution, Identification, pH (4.3–8.7, in the solution constituted as directed in the labeling), and Uniformity of dosage units, for the test for Trypsin under Chymotrypsin, and for Sterility tests.

CICLOPIROX

Chemical group: Synthetic pyridinone derivative; chemically unrelated to the imidazole.

Chemical name:
Ciclopirox—2(1*H*)-Pyridinone, 6-cyclohexyl-1-4-methyl.
Ciclopirox olamine—2(1*H*)-Pyridinone, 6-cyclohexyl-1-hydroxy-4-methyl-, compd. with 2-aminoethanol (1:1).

Molecular formula:
Ciclopirox—$C_{12}H_{17}NO_2$.
Ciclopirox olamine—$C_{12}H_{17}NO_2 \cdot C_2H_7NO$.

Molecular weight:
Ciclopirox—207.27.
Ciclopirox olamine—268.35.

Description: Ciclopirox olamine—White to pale yellow crystalline powder.

Solubility: Ciclopirox olamine—Soluble in methanol.

Other characteristics: Ciclopirox olamine—1% cream has a pH of 7.

USP requirements:
Ciclopirox Topical Cream—Not in *USP–NF*.
Ciclopirox Topical Lotion—Not in *USP–NF*.
Ciclopirox Olamine USP—Preserve in well-closed containers. Contains not less than 98.0% and not more than 102.0% of ciclopirox olamine, calculated on the dried basis. Meets the requirements for Identification, pH (8.0–9.0, in a solution [1 in 100]), Loss on drying (not more than 1.5%), Residue on ignition (not more than 0.1%), Heavy metals (not more than 0.002%), and Monoethanolamine content (223–230 mg per gram of ciclopirox olamine, calculated on the anhydrous basis).
Ciclopirox Olamine Cream USP—Preserve in collapsible tubes, at controlled room temperature. Contains the labeled amount, within ±10%. Meets the requirements for Identification, Minimum fill, pH (5.0–8.0), and Content of benzyl alcohol (if present, within ±10% of claimed amount).
Ciclopirox Olamine Lotion—Not in *USP–NF*.
Ciclopirox Olamine Topical Suspension USP—Preserve in tight containers. Contains the labeled amount, within ±10%. Meets the requirements for Identification, Minimum fill, pH (5.0–8.0), and Benzyl alcohol content (if present, within ±10% of claimed amount).

CIDOFOVIR

Chemical name: Phosphonic acid, [[2-(4-amino-2-oxo-1(2*H*)-pyrimidinyl)-1-(hydroxymethyl)ethoxy]methyl]-, dihydrate, (*S*)-.

Molecular formula: $C_8H_{14}N_3O_6P \cdot 2H_2O$.

Molecular weight: 315.22.

Description: White crystalline powder.

Solubility: Aqueous solubility of =170 mg/mL at pH 6–8.

Other characteristics: Log P (octanol/aqueous buffer, pH 7.1) value is –3.3.

USP requirements: Cidofovir Injection—Not in *USP–NF*.

CILASTATIN

Chemical name: Cilastatin sodium—2-Heptenoic acid, 7-[(2-amino-2-carboxyethyl)thio]-2-[[(2,2-dimethylcyclopropyl)carbonyl]amino]-, monosodium salt, [R-[R*,S*-(Z)]]-.

Molecular formula: Cilastatin sodium—$C_{16}H_{25}N_2NaO_5S$.

Molecular weight: Cilastatin sodium—380.44.

Description: Cilastatin Sodium USP—White to tan-colored powder.

Solubility: Cilastatin Sodium USP—Soluble in water and in methanol.

USP requirements: Cilastatin Sodium USP—Preserve in Containers for Sterile Solids, and store in a cold place. Where it is intended for use in preparing injectable dosage forms, the label states that it is sterile. Contains not less than 98.0% and not more than 101.5% of cilastatin sodium, calculated on the anhydrous and solvent-free basis. Meets the requirements for Identification, Specific rotation (+41.5° to +44.5°, on the anhydrous and solvent-free basis), Bacterial endotoxins (where the label states that Cilastatin Sodium is sterile, it contains not more than 0.17 USP Endotoxin Unit per mg of cilastin), Sterility (where the label states that Cilastatin Sodium is sterile), pH (6.5–7.5, in a solution [1 in 100]), Water (not more than 2.0%), Heavy metals (0.002%, Limit of solvents (not more than 1.0% of acetone, 0.5% of methanol, and 0.4% of mesityl oxide), and Chromatographic purity.

CILAZAPRIL

Chemical name: 6*H*-Pyridazino[1,2-alpha][1,2]diazepine-1-carboxylic acid, 9-[[1-(ethoxycarbonyl)-3-phenylpropyl]amino]octahydro-10-oxo-, monohydrate, [1*S*-[1 alpha,9 alpha(*R**)]]-.

Molecular formula: $C_{22}H_{31}N_3O_5 \cdot H_2O$.

Molecular weight: 435.51.

Description: White to off-white crystalline powder. Melting point 98 °C with decomposition.

pKa: pKa_1—3.3; pKa_2—6.4.

Solubility: Soluble in 0.5 gram per 100 mL water at 25 °C.

Other characteristics: Partition coefficient (Octanol)—0.8 at pH 7.4 buffer at 22 °C. The pH of 1% suspension is 4.9.

USP requirements: Cilazapril Tablets—Not in *USP–NF*.

CILOSTAZOL

Chemical name: 2(1*H*)Quinolinone, 6-[4-(1-cyclohexyl-1*H*-tetrazol-5-yl)butoxyl]-3,4-dihydro-.

Molecular formula: $C_{20}H_{27}N_5O_2$.

Molecular weight: 369.46.

Description: Colorless needle-like crystals from methanol. Melting point 159.4–160.3°.

Solubility: Freely soluble in acetic acid, in chloroform, in *n*-methyl-2-pyrrolidone, and in DMSO; practically insoluble in ether, in water, in 0.1 *N* HCl, and in 0.1 *N* NaOH.

USP requirements: Cilostazol Tablets—Not in *USP–NF*.

CIMETIDINE

Chemical group: Imidazole derivative of histamine.

Chemical name:

Cimetidine—Guanidine, *N*′-cyano-*N*-methyl-*N*-[2-[[(5-methyl-1*H*-imidazol-4-yl)methyl]thio]ethyl]-.

Cimetidine hydrochloride—Guanidine, *N*′-cyano-*N*-methyl-*N*-[2-[[(5-methyl-1*H*-imidazol-4-yl)methyl]thio]ethyl]-, monohydrochloride.

Molecular formula:

Cimetidine—$C_{10}H_{16}N_6S$.
Cimetidine hydrochloride—$C_{10}H_{16}N_6S \cdot HCl$.

Molecular weight:

Cimetidine—252.34.
Cimetidine hydrochloride—288.80.

Description:

Cimetidine USP—White to off-white, crystalline powder; odorless, or having a slight mercaptan odor.
Cimetidine hydrochloride—White crystalline powder.

pKa:

Cimetidine—6.8.
Cimetidine hydrochloride—7.11.

Solubility:

Cimetidine USP—Soluble in alcohol and in polyethylene glycol 400; freely soluble in methanol; sparingly soluble in isopropyl alcohol; slightly soluble in water and in chloroform; practically insoluble in ether.
Cimetidine hydrochloride—Freely soluble in water; soluble in alcohol; very slightly soluble in chloroform; and practically insoluble in ether.

USP requirements:

Cimetidine USP—Preserve in tight, light-resistant containers. Contains not less than 98.0% and not more than 102.0% of cimetidine, calculated on the dried basis. Meets the requirements for Identification, Melting range (139–144 °C), Loss on drying (not more than 1.0%), Residue on ignition (not more than 0.2%), Heavy metals (not more than 0.002%), Chromatographic purity, and Organic volatile impurities.

Cimetidine Injection USP—Preserve in single-dose or multiple-dose glass or plastic containers. Glass containers are preferably of Type I or Type II glass. Sterile solution of Cimetidine Hydrochloride in Water for Injection. Contains the labeled amount, within ±10%. Meets the requirements for Identification, Bacterial endotoxins, pH (3.8–6.0), and for Injections.

Cimetidine Tablets USP—Preserve in tight, light-resistant containers, at controlled room temperature. Contain the labeled amount, within ±10%. Meet the requirements for Identification, Dissolution (80% in 15 minutes in 0.01 N hydrochloric acid in Apparatus 1 at 100 rpm), and Uniformity of dosage units.

Cimetidine Hydrochloride USP—Preserve in tight, light-resistant containers. Contains not less than 98.0% and not more than 102.0% of cimetidine hydrochloride, calculated on the dried basis. Meets the requirements for Identification, Loss on drying (not more than 0.5%), Residue on igni-tion (not more than 0.2%), Heavy metals (0.002%), and Chromatographic purity (no single impurity greater than 0.2%, and the sum of all impurities not more than 1.0%).

Cimetidine Hydrochloride Injection—Not in *USP–NF*.

Cimetidine Hydrochloride Oral Solution—Not in *USP–NF*.

Cimetidine in Sodium Chloride Injection USP—Preserve in single-dose glass or plastic containers. Glass containers are preferably of Type I or Type II glass. A sterile solution of Cimetidine Hydrochloride and Sodium Chloride in Water for Injection. Contains labeled amount of cimetidine, within ±10%, and labeled amount of sodium chloride, within −5% and +10%. Meets the requirements for Identification, Bacterial endotoxins, pH (5.0–7.0), and for Injections.

CINOXACIN

Chemical group: Similar in chemical structure to nalidixic acid and oxolinic acid.

Chemical name: [1,3]Dioxolo[4,5-*g*]cinnoline-3-carboxylic acid, l-ethyl-1,4-dihydro-4-oxo-.

Molecular formula: $C_{12}H_{10}N_2O_5$.

Molecular weight: 262.22.

Description: Cinoxacin USP—White to yellowish white, crystalline solid. Is odorless.

Solubility: Cinoxacin USP—Insoluble in water and in most common organic solvents; soluble in alkaline solution.

USP requirements:

Cinoxacin USP—Preserve in tight containers. Contains not less than 97.0% and not more than 102.0% of cinoxacin, calculated on the dried basis. Meets the requirements for Identification, Loss on drying (not more than 1.0%), Related compounds (not more than 1.0%), and Organic volatile impurities.

Cinoxacin Capsules USP—Preserve in well-closed containers. Contain the labeled amount, within ±10%. Meet the requirements for Identification, Dissolution (60% in 30 minutes in phosphate buffer [pH 6.5] in Apparatus 1 at 100 rpm), and Uniformity of dosage units.

CINOXATE

Chemical name: Propenoic acid, 3-(4-methoxyphenyl)-, 2-ethoxyethyl ester.

Molecular formula: $C_{14}H_{18}O_4$.

Molecular weight: 250.29.

Description: Cinoxate USP—Slightly yellow, practically odorless, viscous liquid.

Solubility: Cinoxate USP—Very slightly soluble in water; slightly soluble in glycerin; soluble in propylene glycol. Miscible with alcohol and with vegetable oils.

USP requirements:

Cinoxate USP—Preserve in tight, light-resistant containers. Contains not less than 98.0% and not more than 101.0% of cinoxate. Meets the requirements for Identification, Specific gravity (1.100–1.105), Refractive index (1.564–1.569), and Acidity.

Cinoxate Lotion USP—Preserve in tight, light-resistant containers. It is Cinoxate in a suitable hydroalcoholic vehicle. Contains the labeled amount, within ±10%. Meets the requirements for Identification, pH (5.4–6.4), and Alcohol content (47–57%).

CIPROFLOXACIN

Chemical group: Fluoroquinolone derivative; structurally related to cinoxacin, nalidixic acid, norfloxacin, and other quinolones.

Chemical name:

Ciprofloxacin—3-Quinolinecarboxylic acid, 1-cyclopropyl-6-fluoro-1,4-dihydro-4-oxo-7-(1-piperazinyl)-.

Ciprofloxacin hydrochloride—3-Quinolinecarboxylic acid, 1-cyclopropyl-6-fluoro-1,4-dihydro-4-oxo-7-(1-piperazinyl)-, monohydrochloride, monohydrate.

Molecular formula:

Ciprofloxacin—$C_{17}H_{18}FN_3O_3$.

Ciprofloxacin hydrochloride—$C_{17}H_{18}FN_3O_3 \cdot HCl \cdot H_2O$.

Molecular weight:

Ciprofloxacin—331.34.

Ciprofloxacin hydrochloride—385.82.

Description: Ciprofloxacin Hydrochloride USP—Faintly yellowish to light yellow crystals.

Solubility: Ciprofloxacin Hydrochloride USP—Sparingly soluble in water; slightly soluble in acetic acid and in methanol; very slightly soluble in dehydrated alcohol; practically insoluble in acetone, in acetonitrile, in ethyl acetate, in hexane, and in methylene chloride.

USP requirements:

Ciprofloxacin USP—Preserve in tight, light-resistant containers. Contains not less than 98.0% and not more than 102.0% of ciprofloxacin, calculated on the dried basis. Meets the requirements for Clarity of solution, Identification, Loss on drying (not more than 1.0%), Residue on ignition (not more than 0.1%), Chloride (not more than 0.02%), Sulfate (not more than 0.04%), Heavy metals (not more than 0.002%), Limit of fluoroquinolonic acid, and Chromatographic purity.

Ciprofloxacin Injection USP—Preserve in single-dose containers, preferably of Type I glass, in a cool place or at controlled room temperature. Avoid freezing and exposure to light. A sterile solution of Ciprofloxacin in Sterile Water for Injection, in 5% Dextrose Injection, or in 0.9% Sodium Chloride Injection prepared with the aid of Lactic Acid. The label indicates whether the vehicle is Sterile Water for Injection, 5% Dextrose Injection, or 0.9% Sodium Chloride Injection. Label the Injection that has Sterile Water for Injection as the vehicle to indicate that it is a concentrated form that must be diluted to appropriate strength (1 to 2 mg per mL) with 5% Dextrose Injection or 0.9% Sodium Chloride Injection before administration, and that the resulting solution is stable for up to 14 days when stored in a cool place or at controlled room temperature. Contains the labeled amount, within ±10%. Meets the requirements for Color (where it is labeled as being in a concentrated form), Identification, Pyrogen, Sterility, pH (3.5–4.6, except that where the Injection is labeled as being a concentrated form, its pH is between 3.3 and 3.9), Particulate matter, Limit of ciprofloxacin ethylenediamine analog (not more than 0.5%), Lactic acid content (0.288–0.352 mg per mg of ciprofloxacin claimed on label, except that where the Injection is labeled as being a concentrated form, it contains between 0.335 and 0.409 mg per mg of ciprofloxacin claimed on the label), Dextrose content (if present), and Sodium chloride content (if present), and for Volume in Container under Injections.

Ciprofloxacin for Injection—Not in *USP–NF*.

Ciprofloxacin Ophthalmic Solution USP—Preserve in tight containers protected from light, at room temperature. A sterile, aqueous solution of Ciprofloxacin Hydrochloride. Contains the labeled amount, within ±10%. Meets the requirements for Identification, Sterility, and pH (3.5–5.5).

Ciprofloxacin for Oral Suspension—Not in *USP–NF*.

Ciprofloxacin Tablets USP—Preserve in well-closed containers. Contain an amount of ciprofloxacin hydrochloride equivalent to the labeled amount of ciprofloxacin, within ±10%. Meet the requirements for Identification, Dissolution (80% in 30 minutes in 0.01 N hydrochloric acid in Apparatus 2 at 50 rpm), and Uniformity of dosage units.

Ciprofloxacin Hydrochloride USP—Preserve in tight, light-resistant containers. Contains not less than 98.0% and not more than 102.0% of ciprofloxacin hydrochloride, calculated on the anhydrous basis. Meets the requirements for Identification, pH (3.0–4.5, in a solution [1 in 40]), Water (4.7–6.7%), Residue on ignition (not more than 0.1%), Sulfate (not more than 0.04%), Heavy metals (not more than 0.002%), Limit of fluoroquinolonic acid (not more than 0.2%), and Chromatographic purity.

Ciprofloxacin Hydrochloride Ophthalmic Ointment USP—Preserve in collapsible ophthalmic ointment tubes. Store at a temperature between 2° and 25°. Contains an equivalent amount of labeled amount of ciprofloxacin, within ±10%. Meets the requirements for Identification, Sterility, Minimum fill, and Metal particles.

Ciprofloxacin Hydrochloride Ophthalmic Solution—Not in *USP–NF*.

CIPROFLOXACIN AND DEXTROSE

For *Ciprofloxacin* and *Dextrose*—See individual listings for chemistry information.

USP requirements: Ciprofloxacin in Dextrose Injection—Not in *USP–NF*.

CISAPRIDE

Chemical name: Benzamide, 4-amino-5-chloro-*N*-[1-[3-(4-fluorophenoxy)propyl]-3-methoxy-4-piperidinyl]-2-methoxy-, *cis*-.

Molecular formula: $C_{23}H_{29}ClFN_3O_4$.

Molecular weight: 465.95.

Description: White to slightly beige odorless powder.

Solubility: Practically insoluble in water; sparingly soluble in methanol; soluble in acetone.

USP requirements:

Cisapride Oral Suspension—Not in *USP–NF*.

Cisapride Tablets—Not in *USP–NF*.

CISATRACURIUM

Chemical name: Cisatracurium besylate—Isoquinolinium, 2,2'-[1,5-pentanediylbis[oxy(3-oxo-3,1-propanediyl)]]bis[1-[(3,4-dimethoxyphenyl)methyl]-1,2,3,4-tetrahydro-6,7-dimethoxy-2-methyl-, dibenzenesulfonate, [1*R*-[1 alpha,2 alpha (1'*R**,2'*R**)]]-.

Molecular formula: Cisatracurium besylate—$C_{65}H_{82}N_2O_{18}S_2$.

Molecular weight: Cisatracurium besylate—1243.48.

USP requirements: Cisatracurium Besylate Injection—Not in *USP–NF*.

CISPLATIN

Chemical group: A heavy metal complex.

Chemical name: Platinum, diamminedichloro-, (*SP*-4-2)-.

Molecular formula: $Cl_2H_6N_2Pt$.

Molecular weight: 300.04.

Description: White lyophilized powder. It has a melting point of 207 °C.

Solubility: Soluble in water or saline at 1 mg per mL and in dimethylformamide at 24 mg per mL.

USP requirements:
Cisplatin USP—Preserve in tight containers. Protect from light. Contains not less than 98.0% and not more than 102.0% of cisplatin, calculated on the anhydrous basis. Meets the requirements for Identification, Crystallinity, Water (not more than 1.0%), UV purity ratio, Limit of trichloroammineplatinate (not more than 1.0%), Limit of transplatin (not more than 2.0%), and Platinum content (64.42–65.22%, on the anhydrous basis).

Caution: Cisplatin is potentially cytotoxic. Great care should be taken to prevent inhaling particles and exposing the skin to it.

Cisplatin Injection—Not in *USP–NF*.

Cisplatin for Injection USP—Preserve in Containers for Sterile Solids. Protect from light. A sterile, lyophilized mixture of Cisplatin, Mannitol, and Sodium Chloride. Contains the labeled amount, within ±10%. Meets the requirements for Constituted solution, Identification, Bacterial endotoxins, Sterility, Uniformity of dosage units, pH (3.5–6.2, in the solution constituted as directed in the labeling, using Sterile Water for Injection), Water (not more than 2.0%), Limit of trichloroammineplatinate (not more than 1.0%), and Limit of transplatin (not more than 2.0%), and for Labeling under Injections.

Caution: Cisplatin is potentially cytotoxic. Great care should be taken in handling the powder and preparing solutions.

CITALOPRAM HYDROBROMIDE

Chemical group: A racemic, bicyclic phthalane derivative, chemically unrelated to other selective serotonin reuptake inhibitors (SSRI's).

Chemical name: Citalopram hydrobromide—5-Isobenzofuran-carbonitrile, 1-[3-(dimethylamino)propyl]-1-(4-fluorophenyl)-1,3-dihydro-, monohydrobromide.

Molecular formula: Citalopram hydrobromide—$C_{20}H_{21}FN_2O \cdot HBr$.

Molecular weight: Citalopram hydrobromide—405.30.

Description: Citalopram hydrobromide—Fine white to off-white powder. Melting point 182–183 °C.

Solubility: Citalopram hydrobromide—Sparingly soluble in water; soluble in ethanol.

USP requirements: Citalopram Hydrobromide Tablets—Not in *USP–NF*.

CITRIC ACID

Chemical name: 1,2,3-Propanetricarboxylic acid, 2-hydroxy-.

Molecular formula: $C_6H_8O_7$ (anhydrous); $C_6H_8O_7 \cdot H_2O$ (monohydrate).

Molecular weight: 192.12 (anhydrous); 210.14 (monohydrate).

Description: Citric Acid USP—Colorless, translucent crystals, or white, granular to fine crystalline powder. The hydrous form is efflorescent in dry air. The anhydrous form melts at about 153°, with decomposition.
NF category: Acidifying agent; buffering agent.

Solubility: Citric Acid USP—Very soluble in water; freely soluble in alcohol; very slightly soluble in ether.

USP requirements: Citric Acid USP—Preserve in tight containers. It is anhydrous or contains one molecule of water of hydration. Label it to indicate whether it is anhydrous or hydrous. Contains not less than 99.5% and not more than 100.5% of citric acid, calculated on the anhydrous basis. Meets the requirements for Identification, Water (not more than 0.5% for anhydrous form and not more than 8.8% for hydrous form), Readily carbonizable substances, Residue on ignition (not more than 0.05%), Sulfate, Arsenic (not more than 3 ppm), Heavy metals (not more than 0.001%), Limit of oxalate, and Organic volatile impurities.

CITRIC ACID AND D-GLUCONIC ACID

Chemical name: Citric acid—1,2,3-Propanetricarboxylic acid, 2-hydroxy-.

Molecular formula:
Citric acid—$C_6H_8O_7$ (anhydrous); $C_6H_8O_7 \cdot H_2O$ (monohydrate).
D-Gluconic acid—$C_6H_{12}O_7$.

Molecular weight:
Citric acid—192.12 (anhydrous); 210.14 (monohydrate).
D-Gluconic acid—196.16.

Description:
Citric Acid USP—Colorless, translucent crystals, or white, granular to fine crystalline powder. Odorless or practically odorless. The hydrous form is efflorescent in dry air.
NF category: Acidifying agent; buffering agent.
D-Gluconic acid—Melting point 131 °C.

Solubility:
Citric Acid USP—Very soluble in water; freely soluble in alcohol; very slightly soluble in ether.
D-Gluconic acid—Freely soluble in water; slightly soluble in alcohol; insoluble in ether and most other organic solvents.

USP requirements: Citric Acid and D-Gluconic Acid for Topical Solution—Not in *USP–NF*.

CITRIC ACID, GLUCONO-DELTA-LACTONE, AND MAGNESIUM CARBONATE

Chemical name:
Citric acid—1,2,3-Propanetricarboxylic acid, 2-hydroxy-.
Magnesium carbonate—Carbonic acid, magnesium salt, basic; or, Carbonic acid, magnesium salt (1:1), hydrate.

Molecular formula:
Citric acid—$C_6H_8O_7$ (anhydrous); $C_6H_8O_7 \cdot H_2O$ (monohydrate).
Glucono-delta-lactone—$C_6H_{10}O_6$.
Magnesium carbonate—$MgCO_3 \cdot H_2O$.
Magnesium carbonate, basic (approx.)—$(MgCO_3)_4 \cdot Mg(OH)_2 \cdot 5H_2O$.

Molecular weight:
Citric acid—192.12 (anhydrous); 210.14 (monohydrate).
Glucono-delta-lactone—178.14.
Magnesium carbonate—102.33.
Magnesium carbonate, basic (approx.)—485.65.

Description:
Citric Acid USP—Colorless, translucent crystals, or white, granular to fine crystalline powder. Odorless or practically odorless. The hydrous form is efflorescent in dry air.
NF category: Acidifying agent; buffering agent.
Magnesium Carbonate USP—Light, white, friable masses or bulky, white powder. Is odorless, and is stable in air.

Solubility:
Citric Acid USP—Very soluble in water; freely soluble in alcohol; very slightly soluble in ether.
Glucono-delta-lactone—Soluble in water (59 grams/100 mL); insoluble in ether.
Magnesium Carbonate USP—Practically insoluble in water to which, however, it imparts a slightly alkaline reaction; insoluble in alcohol, but is dissolved by dilute acids with effervescence.

USP requirements: Citric Acid, Glucono-delta-lactone, and Magnesium Carbonate Solution—Not in *USP–NF*.

CITRIC ACID, MAGNESIUM OXIDE, AND SODIUM CARBONATE

For *Citric Acid, Magnesium Oxide,* and *Sodium Carbonate*—See individual listings for chemistry information.

USP requirements: Citric Acid, Magnesium Oxide, and Sodium Carbonate Irrigation USP—Preserve in single-dose containers, preferably of Type I or Type II glass. A sterile solution of Citric Acid, Magnesium Oxide, and Sodium Carbonate in Water for Injection. Contains the labeled amounts, within ± 5%. Meets the requirements for Identification, Bacterial endotoxins, and pH (3.8–4.2), and for Injections (except that the container may be designed to empty rapidly, and may exceed 1000 mL in capacity).

CLADRIBINE

Chemical name: Adenosine, 2-chloro-2'-deoxy-.

Molecular formula: $C_{10}H_{12}ClN_5O_3$.

Molecular weight: 285.69.

Description: Cladribine injection—Clear, colorless solution.

USP requirements: Cladribine Injection—Not in *USP–NF*.

CLARITHROMYCIN

Chemical name: Erythromycin, 6-*O*-methyl-.

Molecular formula: $C_{38}H_{69}NO_{13}$.

Molecular weight: 747.95.

Description: White to off-white crystalline powder.

Solubility: Soluble in acetone; slightly soluble in dehydrated alcohol, in methanol, and in acetonitrile; practically insoluble in water. Slightly soluble in phosphate buffer at pH values of 2 to 5.

USP requirements:
Clarithromycin USP—Preserve in tight containers. Contains not less than 960 mcg and not more than 1040 mcg of clarithromycin, calculated on the anhydrous basis. Meets the requirements for Identification, Specific rotation (–89° to –95°), Crystallinity, pH (7.5–10.0, determined in a 1 in 500 suspension of it in a mixture of water and methanol [19:1]), Water (not more than 2.0%), Residue on ignition (not more than 0.3%), and Heavy metals (not more than 0.002%).
Clarithromycin Oral Suspension—Not in *USP–NF*.
Clarithromycin for Oral Suspension USP—Preserve in tight containers. A dry mixture of Clarithromycin, dispersing agents, diluents, preservatives, and flavorings. Contains the labeled amount, within –10% to +15%, labeled amount being 25 mg or 50 mg per mL when constituted as directed in the labeling. Meets the requirements for Identification, pH (4.0–5.4, in the suspension constituted as directed in the labeling), Loss on drying (not more than 2.0%), and Deliverable volume.
Clarithromycin Tablets USP—Preserve in tight containers. Contain the labeled amount, within ±10%. Meet the requirements for Identification, Dissolution (80% in 30 minutes in 0.1 *M* Sodium acetate buffer in Apparatus 2 at 50 rpm), Uniformity of dosage units, and Loss on drying (not more than 6.0%).

CLAVULANATE

Chemical name:
Clavulanate potassium—4-Oxa-1-azabicyclo[3.2.0]heptane-2-carboxylic acid, 3-(2-hydroxyethylidene)-7-oxo-, monopotassium salt, [2*R*-(2 alpha,3*Z*,5 alpha)]-.
Clavulanic acid—(*Z*)-(2*R*,5*R*)-3-(2-Hydroxyethylidene)-7-oxo-4-oxa-1-azabicyclo[3.2.0]heptane-2-carboxylic acid.

Molecular formula:
Clavulanate potassium—$C_8H_8KNO_5$.
Clavulanic acid—$C_8H_9NO_5$.

Molecular weight:
Clavulanate potassium—237.25.
Clavulanic acid—199.16.

Description: Clavulanate Potassium USP—White to off-white powder. Is moisture-sensitive.

Solubility: Clavulanate Potassium USP—Freely soluble in water, but stability in aqueous solution is not good, optimum stability at a pH of 6.0 to 6.3; soluble in methanol, with decomposition.

USP requirements:
Clavulanate Potassium USP—Preserve in tight containers. Where it is intended for use in preparing injectable dosage forms, the label states that it is sterile or must be subjected to further processing during the preparation of injectable dosage forms. Contains an amount of clavulanate potassium equivalent to not less than 75.5% and not more than 92.0% of clavulanic acid, calculated on the anhydrous basis. Meets the requirements for Identification, Bacterial endotoxins (where the label states that Clavulanate

Potassium is sterile or must be subjected to further processing during the preparation of injectable dosage forms, it contains not more than 0.03 USP Endotoxin Unit per mg), Sterility (where the label states that Clavulanate Potassium is sterile), pH (5.5–8.0, in a solution [1 in 100]), Water (not more than 1.5%), Limit of clavam-2-carboxylate potassium (not more than 0.01%), Limit of methanol and *tert*-butylamine (not more than 0.1% of methanol or 0.2% of *tert*-butylamine), and Chromatographic purity.

CLEMASTINE

Chemical group: Ethanolamine derivative.

Chemical name: Clemastine fumarate—Pyrrolidine, 2-[2-[1-(4-chlorophenyl)-1-phenylethoxy]ethyl]-1-methyl-, [R-(R*,R*)]-, (E)-2-butenedioate (1:1).

Molecular formula: Clemastine fumarate—$C_{21}H_{26}ClNO \cdot C_4H_4O_4$.

Molecular weight: Clemastine fumarate—459.96.

Description: Clemastine Fumarate USP—Colorless to faintly yellow, odorless, crystalline powder. Its solutions are acid to litmus.

Solubility: Clemastine Fumarate USP—Very slightly soluble in water; slightly soluble in methanol; very slightly soluble in chloroform.

USP requirements:
Clemastine Fumarate USP—Preserve in tight, light-resistant containers, at a temperature not exceeding 25 °C. Contains not less than 98.0% and not more than 102.0% of clemastine fumarate, calculated on the dried basis. Meets the requirements for Clarity and color of solution, Identification, Specific rotation (+15.0° to 18.0°), pH (3.2–4.2, in a suspension [1 in 10]), Loss on drying (not more than 0.5%), Heavy metals (not more than 0.002%), and Chromatographic purity.
Clemastine Fumarate Syrup—Not in *USP–NF*.
Clemastine Fumarate Tablets USP—Preserve in well-closed containers. Contain the labeled amount, within ±10%. Meet the requirements for Identification, Dissolution (75% in 30 minutes in citrate buffer [pH 4.0] in Apparatus 2 at 50 rpm), and Uniformity of dosage units.

CLEMASTINE AND PHENYLPROPANOLAMINE

For *Clemastine* and *Phenylpropanolamine*—See individual listings for chemistry information.

USP requirements: Clemastine Fumarate and Phenylpropanolamine Hydrochloride Extended-release Tablets—Not in *USP–NF*.

CLIDINIUM

Chemical group: Clidinium bromide—Quaternary ammonium compound.

Chemical name: Clidinium bromide—1-Azoniabicyclo[2.2.2]octane, 3-[(hydroxydiphenylacetyl)oxy]-1-methyl-, bromide.

Molecular formula: Clidinium bromide—$C_{22}H_{26}BrNO_3$.

Molecular weight: Clidinium bromide—432.35.

Description: Clidinium Bromide USP—White to nearly white, practically odorless, crystalline powder. Is optically inactive. Melts at about 242 °C.

Solubility: Clidinium Bromide USP—Soluble in water and in alcohol; slightly soluble in ether.

USP requirements:
Clidinium Bromide USP—Preserve in tight, light-resistant containers. Contains not less than 99.0% and not more than 100.5% of clidinium bromide, calculated on the dried basis. Meets the requirements for Identification, Loss on drying (not more than 0.5%), Residue on ignition (not more than 0.1%), Heavy metals (not more than 0.002%), Related compounds, and Organic volatile impurities.
Clidinium Bromide Capsules USP—Preserve in tight, light-resistant containers. Contain the labeled amount, within ± 10%. Meet the requirements for Identification, Dissolution (80% in 15 minutes in 0.1 N hydrochloric acid in Apparatus 1 at 100 rpm), Uniformity of dosage units, and Related compounds.

CLINDAMYCIN

Source: 7(S)-Chloro derivative of lincomycin.

Chemical name:
Clindamycin hydrochloride—L-*threo*-alpha-D-*galacto*-Octopyranoside, methyl 7-chloro-6,7,8-trideoxy-6-[[(1-methyl4-propyl-2-pyrrolidinyl)carbonyl]amino]-1-thio-,(2S-trans)-, monohydrochloride.
Clindamycin palmitate hydrochloride—L-*threo*-alpha-D-*galacto*-Octopyranoside, methyl 7-chloro-6,7,8-trideoxy-6-[[(1-methyl-4-propyl-2-pyrrolidinyl)carbonyl]amino]-1-thio-2-hexadecanoate, monohydrochloride, (2S-trans)-.
Clindamycin phosphate—L-*threo*-alpha-D-*galacto*-Octopyranoside, methyl 7-chloro-6,7,8-trideoxy-6-[[(1-methyl-4-propyl-2-pyrrolidinyl)carbonyl]amino]-1-thio-, 2-(dihydrogen phosphate), (2S-trans)-.

Molecular formula:
Clindamycin hydrochloride—$C_{18}H_{33}ClN_2O_5S \cdot HCl$.
Clindamycin palmitate hydrochloride—$C_{34}H_{63}ClN_2O_6S \cdot HCl$.
Clindamycin phosphate—$C_{18}H_{34}ClN_2O_8PS$.

Molecular weight:
Clindamycin hydrochloride—461.44.
Clindamycin palmitate hydrochloride—699.85.
Clindamycin phosphate—504.96.

Description:
Clindamycin Hydrochloride USP—White or practically white, crystalline powder. Is odorless or has a faint mercaptan-like odor. Is stable in the presence of air and light. Its solutions are acidic and are dextrorotatory.
Clindamycin Palmitate Hydrochloride USP—White to off-white amorphous powder, having a characteristic odor.
Clindamycin Phosphate USP—White to off-white, hygroscopic, crystalline powder. Is odorless or practically odorless.

Solubility:
Clindamycin Hydrochloride USP—Freely soluble in water, in dimethylformamide, and in methanol; soluble in alcohol; practically insoluble in acetone.
Clindamycin Palmitate Hydrochloride USP—Very soluble in ethyl acetate and in dimethylformamide; freely soluble in water, in ether, in chloroform, and in alcohol.
Clindamycin Phosphate USP—Freely soluble in water; slightly soluble in dehydrated alcohol; very slightly soluble in acetone; practically insoluble in chloroform and in ether.

USP requirements:

Clindamycin Injection USP—Preserve in single-dose or in multiple-dose containers, preferably of Type I glass, or in suitable plastic containers. It meets the requirement for Labeling under Injections. Where it is maintained in the frozen state, the label states that it is to be thawed just prior to use, describes the conditions for proper storage of the resultant solution, and directs that the solution is not to be refrozen. Contains an amount of Clindamycin Phosphate in Water for Injection equivalent to the labeled amount of clindamycin, within –10% to +20%. It may be frozen. Meets the requirements for Identification, Bacterial endotoxins, pH (5.5–7.0), and Particulate matter, and for Injections.

Clindamycin for Injection USP—Preserve in Containers for Sterile Solids. Contains an amount of Clindamycin Phosphate having a potency equivalent to not less than 758 mcg of clindamycin per mg, calculated on the anhydrous basis. Meets the requirements for Depressor substances, Bacterial endotoxins, and Sterility, and Definition, and for Identification test, pH, Water, and Crystallinity under Clindamycin Phosphate.

Clindamycin Hydrochloride USP—Preserve in tight containers. The hydrated hydrochloride salt of clindamycin, a substance produced by the chlorination of lincomycin. Has a potency equivalent to not less than 800 mcg of clindamycin per mg. Meets the requirements for Identification, Crystallinity, pH (3.0–5.5, in a solution containing 100 mg per mL), Related compunds, and Water (3.0–6.0%).

Clindamycin Hydrochloride Capsules USP—Preserve in tight containers. Contain an amount of clindamycin hydrochloride equivalent to the labeled amount of clindamycin, within –10% to +20%. Meet the requirements for Identification, Dissolution (80% in 30 minutes in phosphate buffer [pH 6.8] in Apparatus 1 at 100 rpm), Uniformity of dosage units, and Water (not more than 7.0%).

Clindamycin Hydrochloride Oral Solution USP—Preserve in tight containers. Label oral solution to indicate that it is intended for veterinary use only. Contains the equivalent of the labeled amounts, within ±10%. Meets the requirements for Identification, Uniformity of dosage units, deliverable volume, and pH (3.0–5.5).

Clindamycin Palmitate Hydrochloride USP—Preserve in tight containers. Has a potency equivalent to not less than 540 mcg of clindamycin per mg. Meets the requirements for Identification, pH (2.8–3.8, in a solution containing 10 mg per mL), Water (not more than 3.0%), and Residue on ignition (not more than 0.5%).

Clindamycin Palmitate Hydrochloride for Oral Solution USP—Preserve in tight containers. A dry mixture of Clindamycin Palmitate Hydrochloride and one or more suitable buffers, colors, diluents, flavors, and preservatives. Contains an amount of clindamycin palmitate hydrochloride equivalent to the labeled amount of clindamycin (15 mg per mL when constituted as directed in the labeling), within –10% to +20%. Meets the requirements for Uniformity of dosage units (solid packaged in single-unit containers), Deliverable volume (solid packaged in multiple-unit containers), pH (2.5–5.0, in the solution constituted as directed in the labeling), and Water (not more than 3.0%).

Clindamycin Phosphate USP—Preserve in tight containers. Where it is intended for use in preparing injectable dosage forms, the label states that it is sterile or must be subjected to further processing during the preparation of injectable dosage forms. Has a potency equivalent to not less than 758 mcg of clindamycin per mg, calculated on the anhydrous basis. Meets the requirements for Identification, Crystallinity, pH (3.5–4.5, in a solution containing 10 mg per mL), and Water (not more than 6.0%), and for Sterility and Bacterial endotoxins under Clindamycin for Injection (where the label states that Clindamycin Phosphate is sterile), and for Bacterial endotoxins under Clindamycin for Injection (where the label states that Clindamycin Phosphate must be subjected to further processing during the preparation of injectable dosage forms.

Clindamycin Phosphate Vaginal Cream USP—Preserve in well-closed containers. Contains an amount of Clindamycin Phosphate equivalent to the labeled amount of clindamycin, within ±10%. Meets the requirements for Identification and pH (3.0–6.0, determined on the undiluted Cream).

Clindamycin Phosphate Gel USP—Preserve in tight containers. Contains an amount of clindamycin phosphate equivalent to the labeled amount of clindamycin, within ±10%. Meets the requirements for Identification, Minimum fill, and pH (4.5–6.5).

Clindamycin Phosphate Injection—Not in *USP–NF*.

Clindamycin Phosphate Topical Solution USP—Preserve in tight containers. Contains an amount of clindamycin phosphate equivalent to the labeled amount of clindamycin, within ±10%. Meets the requirements for Identification and pH (4.0–7.0).

Clindamycin Phosphate Topical Suspension USP—Preserve in tight containers. Contains an amount of clindamycin phosphate equivalent to the labeled amount of clindamycin, within ±10%. Meets the requirements for Identification, Minimum fill, and pH (4.5–6.5).

CLIOQUINOL

Chemical name: 8-Quinolinol, 5-chloro-7-iodo-.

Molecular formula: C_9H_5ClINO.

Molecular weight: 305.50.

Description: Clioquinol USP—Voluminous, spongy, yellowish white to brownish yellow powder, having a slight, characteristic odor. Darkens on exposure to light. Melts at about 180 °C, with decomposition.

Solubility: Clioquinol USP—Practically insoluble in water and in alcohol; soluble in hot ethyl acetate and in hot glacial acetic acid.

USP requirements:

Clioquinol USP—Preserve in tight, light-resistant containers. Dried over phosphorus pentoxide for 5 hours, contains not less than 93.0% and not more than 100.5% of clioquinol (the 5-chloro-7-iodo-8-quinolinol isomer). Meets the requirements for Identification, Loss on drying (not more than 0.5%), Residue on ignition (not more than 0.5%), and Free iodine and iodide.

Clioquinol Cream USP—Preserve in collapsible tubes or tight, light-resistant containers. Contains the labeled amount, within ±10%, in a suitable cream base. Meets the requirement for Identification.

Clioquinol Ointment USP—Preserve in collapsible tubes or tight, light-resistant containers. Contains the labeled amount, within ±10%, in a suitable ointment base. Meets the requirement for Identification.

Compound Clioquinol Topical Powder USP—Preserve in well-closed, light-resistant containers. Contains not less than 22.5% and not more than 27.5% of clioquinol.

Prepare Compound Clioquinol Topical Powder as follows: 250 grams of Clioquinol, 25 grams of Lactic Acid, 200 grams of Zinc Stearate, and 525 grams of Lactose to make 1000 grams. Mix the Lactic Acid with the Lactose, then add the Clioquinol and the Zinc Stearate, and mix.

Meets the requirement for Identification.

CLIOQUINOL AND FLUMETHASONE

For *Clioquinol* and *Flumethasone*—See individual listings for chemistry information.

USP requirements:
Clioquinol and Flumethasone Pivalate Cream—Not in *USP–NF*.
Clioquinol and Flumethasone Pivalate Ointment—Not in *USP–NF*.
Clioquinol and Flumethasone Pivalate Otic Solution—Not in *USP–NF*.

CLIOQUINOL AND HYDROCORTISONE

For *Clioquinol* and *Hydrocortisone*—See individual listings for chemistry information.

USP requirements:
Clioquinol and Hydrocortisone Cream USP—Preserve in collapsible tubes or in tight, light-resistant containers. Contains the labeled amounts, within ±10%, in a suitable cream base. Meets the requirements for Identification and Minimum fill.
Clioquinol and Hydrocortisone Lotion—Not in *USP–NF*.
Clioquinol and Hydrocortisone Ointment USP—Preserve in collapsible tubes or in tight, light-resistant containers. Contains the labeled amounts, within ±10%, in a suitable ointment base. Meets the requirements for Identification and Minimum fill.

CLOBAZAM

Chemical name: 1*H*-1,5-Benzodiazepine-2,4(3*H*,5*H*)-dione, 7-chloro-1-methyl-5-phenyl-.

Molecular formula: $C_{16}H_{13}ClN_2O_2$.

Molecular weight: 300.74.

Description: White, odorless, crystalline powder. Melting range of 182 ±3 °C.

Solubility: Soluble in chloroform and in methanol; very slightly soluble in water.

USP requirements: Clobazam Tablets—Not in *USP–NF*.

CLOBETASOL

Chemical name: Clobetasol propionate—Pregna-1,4-diene-3,20-dione, 21-chloro-9-fluoro-11-hydroxy-16-methyl-17-(1-oxopropoxy)-, (11 beta,16 beta)-.

Molecular formula: Clobetasol propionate—$C_{25}H_{32}ClFO_5$.

Molecular weight: Clobetasol propionate—466.97.

Description: Clobetasol propionate—White to cream-colored crystalline powder.

Solubility: Clobetasol propionate—Practically insoluble in water; slightly soluble in benzene and in diethyl ether; sparingly soluble in ethanol; soluble in acetone, in dimethyl sulfoxide, in chloroform, in methanol, and in dioxane.

USP requirements:
Clobetasol Propionate USP—Preserve in tight, light-resistant containers. Contains not less than 97.0% and not more than 102.0% of clobetasol propionate, calculated on the dried basis. Meets the requirements for Identification, Melting range (approximately 196 °C), Specific rotation (+98° to +104°), Loss on drying (not more than 2.0%), Residue on ignition (not more than 0.1%), Heavy metals (20 mcg per gram), Chromatographic purity, and Organic volatile impurities.
Clobetasol Propionate Cream USP—Preserve in collapsible tubes or in tight containers. Store at controlled room temperature. Do not refrigerate. It is Clobetasol Propionate in a suitable cream base. Contains the labeled amount, within −10% to +15%. Meets the requirements for Identification, Microbial limits, Minimum fill, and pH (4.5–7.0).
Clobetasol Propionate Ointment USP—Preserve in collapsible tubes or in tight containers. Store at controlled room temperature (15–30 °C). Do not refrigerate. It is Clobetasol Propionate in a suitable ointment base. Contains the labeled amount, within −10% to +15%. Meets the requirements for Identification, Microbial limits, and Minimum fill.
Clobetasol Propionate Topical Solution USP—Preserve in tight containers. Store at controlled room temperature. Do not refrigerate. Contains the labeled amount, within ±10%. Meets the requirements for Identification, Microbial limits, Minimum fill, and pH (4.5–6.0).

CLOBETASONE

Chemical name: Clobetasone butyrate—Pregna-1,4-diene-3,11,20-trione, 21-chloro-9-fluoro-16-methyl-17-(1-oxobutoxy)-, (16 beta)-.

Molecular formula: Clobetasone butyrate—$C_{26}H_{32}ClFO_5$.

Molecular weight: Clobetasone butyrate—478.98.

Description: Clobetasone butyrate—White to cream-colored crystalline powder.

USP requirements:
Clobetasone Butyrate Cream—Not in *USP–NF*.
Clobetasone Butyrate Ointment—Not in *USP–NF*.

CLOCORTOLONE

Chemical name: Clocortolone pivalate—Pregna-1,4-diene-3,20-dione, 9-chloro-21-(2,2-dimethyl-1-oxopropoxy)-6-fluoro-11-hydroxy-16-methyl-, (6 alpha,11 beta,16 alpha)-.

Molecular formula: Clocortolone pivalate—$C_{27}H_{36}ClFO_5$.

Molecular weight: Clocortolone pivalate—495.02.

Description: Clocortolone Pivalate USP—White to yellowish white, odorless powder. Melts at about 230 °C, with decomposition.

Solubility: Clocortolone Pivalate USP—Freely soluble in chloroform and in dioxane; soluble in acetone; sparingly soluble in alcohol; slightly soluble in ether.

USP requirements:
Clocortolone Pivalate USP—Preserve in tight, light-resistant containers. Contains not less than 97.0% and not more than 103.0% of clocortolone pivalate, calculated on the dried basis. Meets the requirements for Color and clarity of solution, Identification, Specific rotation (+125° to +135°), Loss on drying (not more than 1.0%), Residue on ignition (not more than 0.2%), and Chromatographic purity.
Clocortolone Pivalate Cream USP—Preserve in collapsible tubes or in tight, light-resistant containers. Contains the labeled amount, within ±10%, in a suitable cream base. Meets the requirements for Identification, Minimum fill,

pH (5.0–7.0, in a 1 in 10 aqueous dispersion), and Particle size determination (no particle more than 50 microns when measured in the longitudinal axis).

CLOFAZIMINE

Chemical group: Substituted iminophenazine dye.

Chemical name: 2-Phenazinamine, N,5-bis(4-chlorophenyl)-3,5-dihydro-3-[(1-methylethyl)imino]-.

Molecular formula: $C_{27}H_{22}Cl_2N_4$.

Molecular weight: 473.40.

Description: Clofazimine USP—Dark red crystals. Melts at about 217 °C, with decomposition.

Solubility: Clofazimine USP—Practically insoluble in water; soluble in chloroform; sparingly soluble in alcohol, in acetone, and in ethyl acetate.

Other characteristics: Highly lipophilic.

USP requirements:
Clofazimine USP—Preserve in tight, light-resistant containers, at room temperature. Contains not less than 98.5% and not more than 101.5% of clofazimine, calculated on the dried basis. Meets the requirements for Identification, Loss on drying (not more than 0.5%), Residue on ignition (not more than 0.1%), and Chromatographic purity.
Clofazimine Capsules USP—Preserve in well-closed containers. Contain the labeled amount, within ±10%. Meet the requirements for Identification, Dissolution (in 15 minutes in Water in Apparatus 2 at 50 rpm), Uniformity of dosage units, and Chromatographic purity.

CLOFIBRATE

Chemical name: Propanoic acid, 2-(4-chlorophenoxy)-2-methyl-,ethyl ester.

Molecular formula: $C_{12}H_{15}ClO_3$.

Molecular weight: 242.70.

Description: Clofibrate USP—Colorless to pale yellow liquid having a characteristic odor.

Solubility: Clofibrate USP—Insoluble in water; soluble in acetone, in alcohol, and in chloroform.

USP requirements:
Clofibrate USP—Preserve in tight, light-resistant containers. Contains not less than 97.0% and not more than 103.0% of clofibrate, calculated on the anhydrous basis. Meets the requirements for Identification, Refractive index (1.500–1.505, at 20 °C), Acidity, Water (not more than 0.2%), Chromatographic purity, Limit of p-chlorophenol (not more than 0.003%), and Organic volatile impurities.
Clofibrate Capsules USP—Preserve in well-closed, light-resistant containers. Contain the labeled amount, within ± 10%. Meet the requirements for Identification, Dissolution (80% in 180 minutes in sodium lauryl sulfate solution [5 in 100] in Apparatus 2 at 100 rpm), and Uniformity of dosage units.

CLOMIPHENE

Chemical name: Clomiphene citrate—Ethanamine, 2-[4-(2-chloro-1,2-diphenylethenyl)phenoxy]-N,N-diethyl-, 2-hydroxy-1,2,3-propanetricarboxylate (1:1).

Molecular formula: Clomiphene citrate—$C_{26}H_{28}ClNO \cdot C_6H_8O_7$.

Molecular weight: Clomiphene citrate—598.08.

Description: Clomiphene Citrate USP—White to pale yellow, essentially odorless powder.

Solubility: Clomiphene Citrate USP—Slightly soluble in water and in chloroform; freely soluble in methanol; sparingly soluble in alcohol; insoluble in ether.

USP requirements:
Clomiphene Citrate USP—Preserve in well-closed containers. Contains not less than 98.0% and not more than 102.0% of a mixture of the (E)- and (Z)- geometric isomers of clomiphene citrate, calculated on the anhydrous basis. Contains not less than 30.0% and not more than 50.0% of the Z-isomer, [(Z)-2-[4-(2-chloro-1,2-diphenylethenyl)phenoxy]-N,N-diethylethanamine 2-hydroxy-1,2,3-propanetricarboxylate (1:1). Meets the requirements for Identification, Water (not more than 1.0%), Heavy metals (not more than 0.002%), Content of (Z) isomer, Related compounds, and Organic volatile impurities.
Clomiphene Citrate Tablets USP—Preserve in well-closed containers, protected from light. Contain the labeled amount, within ±7%. Meet the requirements for Identification, Dissolution (75% in 30 minutes in water in Apparatus 1 at 100 rpm), and Uniformity of dosage units.

CLOMIPRAMINE

Chemical group: Dibenzazepine.

Chemical name: Clomipramine hydrochloride—5H-Dibenz[b,f]azepine-5-propanamine, 3-chloro-10,11-dihydro-N,N-dimethyl-, monohydrochloride.

Molecular formula: Clomipramine hydrochloride—$C_{19}H_{23}ClN_2 \cdot$ HCl.

Molecular weight: Clomipramine hydrochloride—351.31.

Description: Clomipramine Hydrochloride USP—White to faintly yellow, crystalline powder.

Solubility: Clomipramine Hydrochloride USP—Very soluble in water.

Other characteristics: Clomipramine hydrochloride—A 10% solution in water has a pH of 3.5–5.0.

USP requirements:
Chlomipramine Hydrochloride USP—Preserve in well-closed containers. Contains not less than 98.0% and not more than 102.0% of chlomipramine hydrochloride, calculated on the dried basis. Meets the requirements for Identification, pH (3.5–5.0, in a solution having a concentration of about 100 mg per mL), Loss on drying (not more than 1.0%), Residue on ignition (not more than 0.1%), Heavy metals (0.01%), and Chromatographic purity.
Clomipramine Hydrochloride Capsules USP—Preserve in well-closed containers. Contains the labeled amount, within ±10%. Meet the requirements for Identification, Dissolution (80% in 30 minutes in 0.1 N hydrochloric acid in Apparatus 2 at 50 rpm), and Uniformity of dosage units.
Clomipramine Hydrochloride Tablets—Not in *USP–NF*.

CLONAZEPAM

Chemical name: 2*H*-1,4-Benzodiazepin-2-one, 5-(2-chlorophenyl)-1,3-dihydro-7-nitro-.

Molecular formula: $C_{15}H_{10}ClN_3O_3$.

Molecular weight: 315.71.

Description: Clonazepam USP—Light yellow powder, having a faint odor.

Solubility: Clonazepam USP—Insoluble in water; sparingly soluble in acetone and in chloroform; slightly soluble in alcohol and in ether.

USP requirements:
Clonazepam USP—Preserve in tight, light-resistant containers, at room temperature. Contains not less than 98.0% and not more than 102.0% of clonazepam, calculated on the dried basis. Meets the requirements for Identification, Loss on drying (not more than 0.5%), Residue on ignition (not more than 0.1%), Heavy metals (not more than 0.002%), Melting range (237° to 240°), Limit of clonazepam related compound C (0.2%), Related compounds, and Organic volatile impurities.
Clonazepam Tablets USP—Preserve in tight, light-resistant containers, at room temperature. Contain the labeled amount, within ±10%. Meet the requirements for Identification, Dissolution (80% in 60 minutes in degassed water in Apparatus 2 at 100 rpm), Uniformity of dosage units, and Related compounds.

CLONIDINE

Chemical name:
Clonidine—Benzenamine, 2,6-dichloro-*N*-2-imidazolidinylidene-.
Clonidine hydrochloride—Benzenamine, 2,6-dichloro-*N*-2-imidazolidinylidene-, monohydrochloride.

Molecular formula:
Clonidine—$C_9H_9Cl_2N_3$.
Clonidine hydrochloride—$C_9H_9Cl_2N_3 \cdot HCl$.

Molecular weight:
Clonidine—230.09.
Clonidine hydrochloride—266.55.

Description: Clonidine hydrochloride—Odorless, white, crystalline substance.

Solubility: Clonidine hydrochloride—Soluble in water and in alcohol; practically insoluble in chloroform and in ether.

Other characteristics: Clonidine hydrochloride—The pH of a 10% aqueous solution is between 3 and 5.

USP requirements:
Clonidine Transdermal System—Not in *USP–NF*.
Clonidine Hydrochloride USP—Preserve in tight containers. Contains not less than 98.5% and not more than 101.0% of clonidine hydrochloride, calculated on the dried basis. Meets the requirements for Identification, pH (3.5–5.5, in a solution [1 in 20]), Loss on drying (not more than 0.5%), Residue on ignition (not more than 0.1%), and Chromatographic purity.
Clonidine Hydrochloride Injection—Not in *USP–NF*.
Clonidine Hydrochloride Tablets USP—Preserve in well-closed containers. Contain the labeled amount, within ± 10%. Meet the requirements for Identification, Dissolution (75% in 30 minutes in 0.01 *N* hydrochloric acid in Apparatus 2 at 50 rpm), and Uniformity of dosage units.

CLONIDINE AND CHLORTHALIDONE

For *Clonidine* and *Chlorthalidone*—See individual listings for chemistry information.

USP requirements: Clonidine Hydrochloride and Chlorthalidone Tablets USP—Preserve in well-closed containers. Contain the labeled amounts, within ±10%. Meet the requirements for Identification, Dissolution (80% of clonidine hydrochloride and 50% of chlorthalidone in 60 minutes in water in Apparatus 2 at 100 rpm), and Uniformity of dosage units.

CLOPIDOGREL

Chemical name: Clopidogrel bisulfate—Thieno[3,2-*c*]pyridine-5(4*H*)-acetic acid, alpha-(2-chlorophenyl)-6,7-dihydro-, methylester, (*S*)-, sulfate (1:1).

Molecular formula: Clopidogrel bisulfate—$C_{16}H_{16}ClNO_2S \cdot H_2SO_4$.

Molecular weight: Clopidogrel bisulfate—419.90.

Description: Clopidogrel bisulfate—White to off-white powder.

Solubility: Clopidogrel bisulfate—Practically insoluble in water at neutral pH; freely soluble in water at pH 1; dissolves freely in methanol; dissolves sparingly in methylene chloride; practically insoluble in ethyl ether.

USP requirements: Clopidogrel Bisulfate Tablets—Not in *USP–NF*.

CLORAZEPATE

Chemical name: Clorazepate dipotassium—1*H*-1,4-Benzodiazepine-3-carboxylic acid, 7-chloro-2,3-dihydro-2-oxo-5-phenyl-, potassium salt compd. with potassium hydroxide (1:1).

Molecular formula: Clorazepate dipotassium—$C_{16}H_{11}ClK_2N_2O_4$.

Molecular weight: Clorazepate dipotassium—408.92.

Description: Clorazepate Dipotassium USP—Light yellow, crystalline powder. Darkens on exposure to light.

Solubility: Clorazepate Dipotassium USP—Soluble in water but, upon standing, may precipitate from the solution; slightly soluble in alcohol and in isopropyl alcohol; practically insoluble in acetone, in chloroform, in ether, and in methylene chloride.

USP requirements:
Clorazepate Dipotassium USP—Preserve under nitrogen in tight, light-resistant containers. Contains not less than 98.5% and not more than 101.5% of clorazepate dipotassium, calculated on the dried basis. Meets the requirements for Identification, Loss on drying (not more than 0.5%), Heavy metals (not more than 0.002%), Related compounds, and Organic volatile impurities.
Clorazepate Dipotassium Capsules—Not in *USP–NF*.
Clorazepate Dipotassium Tablets USP—Preserve in tight, light-resistant containers. Contain the labeled amount, within ±10%. Meet the requirements for Identification, Dissolution (80% in 30 minutes in 0.01 N hydrochloric acid in Apparatus 2 at 50 rpm), Uniformity of dosage units, and Related compounds.
Clorazepate Dipotassium Extended-release Tablets—Not in *USP–NF*.

CLORSULON

Chemical name: 1,3-Benzenedisulfonamide, 4-amino-6-(tri-chloroethenyl)-.

Molecular formula: $C_6H_8Cl_3N_3O_4S_2$.

Molecular weight: 380.66.

Description: Clorsulon USP—White to off-white powder.

Solubility: Clorsulon USP—Slightly soluble in water; freely soluble in acetonitrile and in methanol; very slightly soluble in methylene chloride.

USP requirements: Clorsulon USP—Preserve in well-closed containers. Label it to indicate that it is for veterinary use only. Contains not less than 98.0% and not more than 101.0% of clorsulon, calculated on the dried basis. Meets the requirements for Identification, Melting range (197–203 °C), Loss on drying (not more than 0.5%), Residue on ignition (not more than 0.1%), Heavy metals (not more than 0.003%), and Chromatographic purity.

CLOTRIMAZOLE

Chemical name: 1H-Imidazole, 1-[(2-chlorophenyl)diphenyl-[lbmethyl]-.

Molecular formula: $C_{22}H_{17}ClN_2$.

Molecular weight: 344.84.

Description: Clotrimazole USP—White to pale yellow, crystalline powder. Melts at about 142 °C, with decomposition.

Solubility: Clotrimazole USP—Practically insoluble in water; freely soluble in methanol, in acetone, in chloroform, and in alcohol.

USP requirements:

Clotrimazole USP—Preserve in tight containers. Contains not less than 98.0% and not more than 102.0% of clotrimazole, calculated on the dried basis. Meets the requirements for Identification, Loss on drying (not more than 0.5%), Residue on ignition (not more than 0.1%), Heavy metals (not more than 0.001%), Limit of imidazole (not more than 0.5%), and Limit of clotrimazole related compound A (not more than 0.5%).

Clotrimazole Cream USP—Preserve in collapsible tubes or in tight containers, at a temperature between 2 and 30 °C. Cream that is packaged and labeled for use as a vaginal preparation shall be labeled Clotrimazole Vaginal Cream. Contains the labeled amount, within ±10%. Meets the requirement for Identification.

Clotrimazole Lotion USP—Preserve in tight containers, at a temperature between 2 and 30 °C. Contains the labeled amount, within ±10%. Meets the requirements for Identification, pH (5.0–7.0), Microbial limits, and Limit of clotrimazole related compound A (not more than 5%).

Clotrimazole Lozenges USP—Preserve in well-closed containers. Contain the labeled amount in a suitable molded base, within ±10%. Meet the requirements for Identification, Disintegration (30 minutes, but complete disintegration does not occur before 5 minutes), and Uniformity of dosage units.

Clotrimazole Topical Solution USP—Preserve in tight containers, at a temperature between 2 and 30 °C. A solution of Clotrimazole in a suitable nonaqueous, hydrophilic solvent. Contains the labeled amount, within −10% to +15%. Meets the requirement for Identification.

Clotrimazole Vaginal Tablets USP—Preserve in well-closed containers. Contain the labeled amount, within ±10%. Meet the requirements for Identification, Disintegration (20 minutes), and Uniformity of dosage units.

CLOTRIMAZOLE AND BETAMETHASONE

For *Clotrimazole* and *Betamethasone*—See individual listings for chemistry information.

USP requirements: Clotrimazole and Betamethasone Dipropionate Cream USP—Preserve in collapsible tubes or in tight containers. Contains the labeled amount of clotrimazole, within ±10%, and an amount of betamethasone dipropionate equivalent to the labeled amount of betamethasone, within ±10%, in a suitable cream base. Meets the requirements for Identification, Microbial limits, Minimum fill, and Limit of (o-chlorophenyl)diphenylmethanol (not more than 5.0% of labeled amount of clotrimazole in the Cream).

CLOVE OIL

NF requirements: Clove Oil NF—Preserve in well-filled, tight containers, and avoid exposure to excessive heat. Volatile oil distilled with steam from the dried flower buds of *Syzygium aromaticum* (L.) Merr. and L. M. Perry (Fam. Myrtaceae). The label states the Latin binomial name and, following the official name, the part of the plant source from which the article was derived. Contains not less than 85.0% (v/v) of total phenolic substances, chiefly eugenol. Meets the requirements for Solubility in 70% alcohol, Specific gravity (1.038–1.060), Angular rotation (not greater than −1.5°), Refractive index (1.527–1.535 at 20°), Heavy metals (0.004%), and Limit of phenol.

RED CLOVER

NF requirements:

Red Clover NF—Store in a well-closed, light-resistant container, protected from moisture. Consists of the dried inflorescence of *Trifolium pratense* L. (Fam. Fabaceae). The label states the Latin binomial and, following the official name, the parts of the plant contained in the article. Contains not less than 0.5% of isoflavones, calculated on the dried basis as the sum of daidzein, genistein, formononetin, and biochanin A. Meets the requirements for Botanic characteristics, Identification, Microbial limits, Loss on drying (not more than 12.0%), Foreign organic matter (no more than 2.0%), Total ash (not more than 10.0%), Acid-insoluble ash (not more than 2.0%), Water-soluble extractives (not less than 15.0%), Pesticide residues, Heavy metals (not more than 10 micrograms per gram), and Content of isoflavones.

Red Clover Tablets NF—Preserve in tight, light-resistant containers. Contain Powdered Red Clover Extract. The label states the Latin binomial and, following the official name, the article from which Tablets were prepared. The label also indicates the quantity, in mg, of Powdered Extract per Tablet. Label Tablets to indicate the content, in mg, of isoflavones per 100 mg of Powdered Extract. Contain the labeled amount of Powdered Extract, within ±10%, calculated as isoflavones. Meet the requirements for Identification, Microbial limits, Disintegration, Weight variaton, and Content of isoflavones.

Powdered Red Clover NF—Preserve in well-closed, light-resistant containers, protected from moisture. It is Red Clover reduced to powder or very fine powder. The label states the Latin binomial and, following the official name, the part of the plant from which the article was derived. Contains not less than 0.5% of isoflavones, calculated on the dried basis as the sum of daidzein, genistein, formononetin, and biochanin A. Meets the requirements for Botanic characteristics, and for Identifidation, Microbial limits, Loss on drying, Total ash, Acid-insoluble ash, Water-soluble extractives, Pesticide residues, Heavy metals, and Content of isoflavone for Red Clover.

Powdered Red Clover Extract NF—Preserve in tight, light-resistant containers, in a cool place. Prepared from Red Clover by extraction with hydroalcoholic mixtures or other suitable solvents. The ratio of plant material to extract is between 3:1 and 25:1. The label states the Latin binomial and, following the official name, the part of the plant from which the article was prepared. The label also indicates the content of isoflavones, the extracting solvent or solvent mixture used for preparation, and the ratio of the starting crude plant material to Powdered Extract. It meets the requirements for labeling under *Botanical Extracts*. Contain the labeled amount of isoflavones, within ±10%, calculated on the dried basis as the sum of daidzein, genistein, formononetin, and biochanin A. May contain suitable added substances. Meets the requirements for Identification, Microbial limits, Loss on drying (not more than 5.0%), Heavy metals (not more than 10 micrograms per gram), Organic volatile impurities, and Content of isoflavones, and for *Packaging and Storage*, *Residual Solvents*, and *Pesticide Residues* under *Botanical Extracts*.

CLOXACILLIN

Chemical name:

Cloxacillin benzathine—4-Thia-1-azabicyclo[3.2.0]heptane-2-carboxylic acid, 6-[[[3-(2-chlorophenyl)-5-methyl-4-isoxazolyl]carbonyl]amino]-3,3-dimethyl-7-oxo-, [2*S*-(2 alpha,5 alpha,6 beta)]-, compd. with *N*,*N*′-bis(phenylmethyl)-1,2-ethanediamine (2:1).

Cloxacillin sodium—4-Thia-1-azabicyclo[3.2.0]heptane-2-carboxylic acid, 6-[[[3-(2-chlorophenyl)-5-methyl-4-isoxazolyl]carbonyl]amino]-3,3-dimethyl-7-oxo-, monosodium salt, monohydrate, [2*S*-(2 alpha,5 alpha,6 beta)]-.

Molecular formula:

Cloxacillin benzathine—$(C_{19}H_{18}ClN_3O_5S)_2 \cdot C_{16}H_{20}N_2$.

Cloxacillin sodium—$C_{19}H_{17}ClN_3NaO_5S \cdot H_2O$.

Molecular weight:

Cloxacillin benzathine—1112.11.

Cloxacillin sodium—475.88.

Description:

Cloxacillin Benzathine USP—White or almost white, almost odorless, crystals or crystalline powder.

Cloxacillin Sodium USP—White, odorless, crystalline powder.

Solubility:

Cloxacillin Benzathine USP—Slightly soluble in water, in alcohol, and in isopropyl alcohol; soluble in chloroform and in methanol; sparingly soluble in acetone.

Cloxacillin Sodium USP—Freely soluble in water; soluble in alcohol; slightly soluble in chloroform.

USP requirements:

Cloxacillin Benzathine USP—Preserve in tight containers. Label it to indicate that it is for veterinary use only. Where it is intended for use in preparing sterile dosage forms, the label states that it is sterile or must be subjected to further processing during the preparation of sterile dosage forms. Has a potency equivalent to not less than 704 mcg and not more than 821 mcg of cloxacillin per mg, calculated on the anhydrous basis. Meets the requirements for Identification, Crystallinity, pH (3.0–6.5, in a suspension containing 10 mg per mL), Sterility, and Water (not more than 5.0%).

Cloxacillin Benzathine Intramammary Infusion USP—Preserve in disposable syringes that are well-closed containers, except that where the Intramammary Infusion is labeled as sterile, the individual syringes or cartons are sealed and tamperproof so that sterility is assured at time of use. A suspension of Cloxacillin Benzathine in a suitable oil vehicle. Label it to indicate that it is for veterinary use only. Intramammary Infusion that is sterile may be so labeled. Has a potency equivalent to the labeled amount of cloxacillin, within −10% to +20%. Meets the requirements for Identification, Sterility (where labeled as being sterile), and Water (not more than 1.0%).

Cloxacillin Sodium USP—Preserve in tight containers, at a temperature not exceeding 25 °C. Where it is intended for use in preparing sterile dosage forms, the label states that it is sterile or must be subjected to further processing during the preparation of sterile dosage forms. Contains the equivalent of not less than 825 mcg of cloxacillin per mg. Meets the requirements for Identification, Crystallinity, Sterility, pH (4.5–7.5, in a solution containing 10 mg per mL), Water (3.0–5.0%), and Dimethylaniline.

Cloxacillin Sodium Capsules USP—Preserve in tight containers. Contain an amount of cloxacillin sodium equivalent to the labeled amount of cloxacillin, within −10% to +20%. Meet the requirements for Dissolution (80% in 30 minutes in 0.05 M potassium phosphate buffer [pH 6.8] in Apparatus 1 at 100 rpm), Uniformity of dosage units, and Water (not more than 5.0%).

Cloxacillin Sodium Intramammary Infusion USP—Preserve in disposable syringes that are well-closed containers, except that where the Intramammary Infusion is labeled as sterile, the individual syringes or cartons are sealed and tamperproof so that sterility is assured at time of use. A suspension of Cloxacillin Sodium in a suitable natural or chemically modified vegetable oil vehicle with a suitable dispersing agent. Label it to indicate that it is for veterinary use only. Intramammary Infusion that is sterile may be so labeled. Has a potency equivalent to the labeled amount of cloxacillin, within −10% to +20%. Meets the requirements for Identification, Sterility, and Water (not more than 1.0%).

Cloxacillin Sodium Injection—Not in *USP–NF*.

Cloxacillin Sodium for Oral Solution USP—Preserve in tight containers. A dry mixture of Cloxacillin Sodium and one or more suitable buffers, colors, flavors, and preservatives. Contains an amount of cloxacillin sodium equivalent to the labeled amount of cloxacillin, within −10% to +20%. Meets the requirements for Uniformity of dosage units (solid packaged in single-unit containers), Deliverable volume (multiple-unit containers), pH (5.0–7.5, in the solution constituted as directed in the labeling), and Water (not more than 1.0%).

CLOZAPINE

Chemical name: 5*H*-Dibenzo[*b*,*e*][1,4]diazepine, 8-chloro-11-(4-methyl-1-piperazinyl)-.

Molecular formula: $C_{18}H_{19}ClN_4$.

Molecular weight: 326.82.

Description: Clozapine USP—Yellow, crystalline powder.

Solubility: Clozapine USP—Soluble in chlorform, in acetone, and in alcohol; sparingly soluble in acetonitrile; insoluble in water.

USP requirements:

Clozapine USP—Preserve in well-closed containers. Contains not less than 98.0% and not more than 102.0% of clozapine, calculated on the dried basis. Meets the requirements for Identification, Melting range (182—186°), Loss on drying (not more than 0.5%), Residue on ignition (not more than 0.1%), Heavy metals (0.002%), Chromatographic purity, and Organic volatile impurities.

Clozapine Tablets USP—Preserve in well-closed containers. Contain the labeled amount, within ±10%. Meet the requirements for Identification, Dissolution (85% in 45 minutes in pH 4.0 acetate buffer in Apparatus 2 at 100 rpm), and Chromatographic purity.

COAL TAR

Description: Coal Tar USP—Nearly black, viscous liquid, heavier than water, having a characteristic, naphthalene-like odor.

Solubility: Coal Tar USP—Slightly soluble in water, to which it imparts its characteristic odor and a faintly alkaline reaction. Partially soluble in acetone, in alcohol, in carbon disulfide, in chloroform, in ether, in methanol, and in solvent hexane.

USP requirements:

Coal Tar USP—Preserve in tight containers. The tar obtained as a by-product during the destructive distillation of bituminous coal at temperatures in the range of 900 to 1100 °C. May be processed further either by extraction with alcohol and suitable dispersing agents and maceration times or by fractional distillation with or without the use of suitable organic solvents. Meets the requirement for Residue on ignition (not more than 2.0%, from 100 mg).

Coal Tar Cleansing Bar—Not in *USP–NF*.

Coal Tar Cream—Not in *USP–NF*.

Coal Tar Gel—Not in *USP–NF*.

Coal Tar Lotion—Not in *USP–NF*.

Coal Tar Ointment USP—Preserve in tight containers.

Prepare Coal Tar Ointment as follows: 10 grams of Coal Tar, 5 grams of Polysorbate 80, and 985 grams of Zinc Oxide Paste to make 1000 grams. Blend the Coal Tar with the Polysorbate 80, and incorporate the mixture with the Zinc Oxide Paste.

Coal Tar Shampoo—Not in *USP–NF*.

Coal Tar Topical Solution USP—Preserve in tight containers.

Prepare Coal Tar Topical Solution as follows: 200 grams of Coal Tar, 50 grams of Polysorbate 80, and a sufficient quantity of Alcohol, to make 1000 mL. Mix the Coal Tar with 500 grams of washed sand, and add the Polysorbate 80 and 700 mL of Alcohol. Macerate the mixture for 7 days in a closed vessel with frequent agitation. Filter, and rinse the vessel and the filter with sufficient Alcohol to make the product measure 1000 mL.

Meets the requirement for Alcohol content (81.0–86.0%).

Coal Tar Topical Suspension—Not in *USP–NF*.

CYANOCOBALAMIN CO 57

Chemical name: Vitamin B_{12}-^{57}Co.

Molecular formula: $C_{63}H_{88}^{57}CoN_{14}O_{14}P$.

Description:

Cyanocobalamin Co 57 Capsules USP—May contain a small amount of solid or solids, or may appear empty.

Cyanocobalamin Co 57 Oral Solution USP—Clear, colorless to pink solution.

USP requirements:

Cyanocobalamin Co 57 Capsules USP—Preserve in well-closed, light-resistant containers. Contain Cyanocobalamin in which a portion of the molecules contain radioactive cobalt (^{57}Co) in the molecular structure. Label Capsules to include the following: the date of calibration; the amount of cyanocobalamin expressed in mcg per Capsule; the amount of ^{57}Co as cyanocobalamin expressed in megabecquerels (or microcuries) per Capsule at the time of calibration; the expiration date; and the statement, "Caution—Radioactive Material." The labeling indicates that in making dosage calculations, correction is to be made for radioactive decay, and also indicates that the radioactive half-life of ^{57}Co is 270.9 days. Contain the labeled amount of ^{57}Co, within ±10%, as cyanocobalamin expressed in megabecquerels (or microcuries) at the time indicated in the labeling. Contain the labeled amount of cyanocobalamin, within ±10%. The specific activity is not less than 0.02 megabecquerel (0.5 microcurie) per mcg of cyanocobalamin. Meet the requirements for Radionuclide identification, Uniformity of dosage units, Radiochemical purity, and Content of cyanocobalamin.

Cyanocobalamin Co 57 Oral Solution USP—Preserve in tight containers, and protect from light. A solution suitable for oral administration, containing Cyanocobalamin in which a portion of the molecules contain radioactive cobalt (^{57}Co) in the molecular structure. Label it to include the following: the date of calibration; the amount of ^{57}Co as cyanocobalamin expressed as total megabecquerels (or microcuries) and as megabecquerels (or microcuries) per mL at the time of calibration; the amount of cyanocobalamin expressed in mcg per mL; the name and quantity of the added preservative; the expiration date; and the statement, "Caution—Radioactive Material." The labeling indicates that in making dosage calculations, correction is to be made for radioactive decay, and also indicates that the radioactive half-life of ^{57}Co is 270.9 days, and directs that the Oral Solution be protected from light. Contains the labeled amount of ^{57}Co, within ±10%, as cyanocobalamin expressed in megabecquerels (or microcuries) per mL at the time indicated in the labeling. Contains the labeled amount of cyanocobalamin, within ±10%. The specific activity is not less than 0.02 megabecquerel (0.5 microcurie) per mcg of cyanocobalamin. Contains a suitable antimicrobial agent. Meets the requirements for Radionuclide identification, pH (4.0–5.5), Radiochemical purity (not less than 95.0%), and Content of cyanocobalamin.

CYANOCOBALAMIN CO 58

Chemical name: Vitamin B_{12}-^{58}Co.

USP requirements: Cyanocobalamin Co 58 Capsules USP—Preserve in well-closed, light-resistant containers, and store in a cold place. Capsule contains Cyanocobalamin in which a portion of the molecules contain radioactive cobalt (^{58}Co) in the molecular structure. Label it to include the following: the date of calibration; the amount of cyanocobalamin expressed in microgram per Capsule; the amount of ^{58}Co as cyanocobalamin expressed in megabecquerel (or microcurie) per Capsule at the time of calibration; the expiration date; and the statement "Caution—Radioactive Material." The labeling indicates that in making dosage calculations, correction is to be made for radioactive decay, and also indicates that the radioactive half-life of ^{58}Co is 70.9 days. Each Capsule contains a labeled amount of ^{58}Co as cyanocobalamin, within ±10%, expressed in megabecquerels (or microcuries) at the time indicated in the labeling. Contain a labeled amount of cyanocobalamin, within ±10%. Meet the requirements for Specific gravity (not less than 0.02 megabecquerel [or 0.5 microcurie] per microgram of cyanocobalamin), Disintegration,

Radionuclide identification, Uniformity of dosage units, Radiochemical purity, Radionuclidic purity, and Content of cyanocobalamin.

COCAINE

Source: An alkaloid obtained from the leaves of *Erythroxylon coca* and other species of *Erythroxylon.*

Chemical name:
Cocaine—8-Azabicyclo[3.2.1]octane-2-carboxylic acid, 3-(benzoyloxy)-8-methyl-, methyl ester, [1*R*-(*exo,exo*)]-.
Cocaine hydrochloride—8-Azabicyclo[3.2.1]octane-2-carboxylic acid, 3-(benzoyloxy)-8-methyl-, methyl ester, hydrochloride, [1*R*-(*exo,exo*)]-.

Molecular formula:
Cocaine—$C_{17}H_{21}NO_4$.
Cocaine hydrochloride—$C_{17}H_{21}NO_4 \cdot HCl$.

Molecular weight:
Cocaine—303.35.
Cocaine hydrochloride—339.81.

Description:
Cocaine USP—Colorless to white crystals or white, crystalline powder. Is levorotatory in 3 *N* hydrochloric acid solution. Its saturated solution is alkaline to litmus.
Cocaine Hydrochloride USP—Colorless crystals or white, crystalline powder.

Solubility:
Cocaine USP—Slightly soluble in water; very soluble in warm alcohol; freely soluble in alcohol, in chloroform, and in ether; soluble in olive oil; sparingly soluble in mineral oil.
Cocaine Hydrochloride USP—Very soluble in water; freely soluble in alcohol; soluble in chloroform and in glycerin; insoluble in ether.

USP requirements:
Cocaine USP—Preserve in well-closed, light-resistant containers. Dried over phosphorus pentoxide for 3 hours, contains not less than 99.0% and not more than 101.0% of cocaine. Meets the requirements for Identification, Melting range (96–98 °C), Loss on drying (not more than 1.0%), Residue on ignition (not more than 0.1%), Readily carbonizable substances, Limit of cinnamyl-cocaine and other reducing substances, and Limit of isoatropyl-cocaine.
Cocaine Hydrochloride USP—Preserve in well-closed, light-resistant containers. Contains not less than 99.0% and not more than 101.0% of cocaine hydrochloride, calculated on the dried basis. Meets the requirements for Identification, Specific rotation (−71° to −73°), Acidity, Loss on drying (not more than 1.0%), Residue on ignition (not more than 0.1%), Readily carbonizable substances, Limit of cinnamyl-cocaine and other reducing substances, and Limit of isoatropyl-cocaine.
Cocaine Hydrochloride Topical Solution—Not in *USP–NF.*
Cocaine Hydrochloride Viscous Topical Solution—Not in *USP–NF.*
Cocaine Hydrochloride Tablets for Topical Solution USP—Preserve in well-closed, light-resistant containers. Contain the labeled amount, within ±9%. Meet the requirements for Identification, Disintegration (15 minutes), and Uniformity of dosage units.

COCAINE, TETRACAINE, AND EPINEPHRINE

For *Cocaine, Tetracaine,* and *Epinephrine*—See individual listings for chemistry information.

USP requirements: Cocaine, Tetracine Hydrochloride, and Epinephrine Topical Solution USP—Preserve in sterile, tight, light-resistant containers. Store in a refrigerator. Label it to state that it is intended for external use only and that it is not to be used if a precipitate is present. The label states that it is to be protected from light. Contains not less than 3.6 grams and not more than 4.4 grams of Cocaine Hydrochloride, not less than 0.90 gram and not more than 1.10 grams of Tetracaine Hydrochloride, and not less than 20 mg and not more than 30 mg of Epinephrine in 100 mL of Topical Solution.[ql]Prepare Cocaine, Tetracaine Hydrochloride, and Epinephrine Topical Solution as follows: 4.0 grams Cocaine Hydrochloride, 1.0 gram Tetracaine Hydrochloride, 25.0 mL Epinephrine Injection (1:1000), 10 mg Benzalkonium Chloride, 6.4 mg Edetate Disodium, 35 mL Sodium Chloride Injection (0.9%), and Purified Water, a sufficient quantity to make 100 mL. Dissolve the Cocaine and Tetracaine Hydrochlorides in about 25 mL of Purified Water, and add the Epinephrine Injection (1:1000). Separately dissolve an accurately weighed quantity of Edetate Disodium in Sodium Chloride Injection (0.9%) and dilute quantitatively, and stepwise if necessary, with Sodium Chloride Injection (0.9%) to obtain 35 mL of a solution containing 6.4 mg of Edetate Disodium. Similarly, and separately, dissolve an accurately weighed quantity of Benzalkonium Chloride in Purified Water (or use an accurately measured volume of Benzolkonium Chloride Solution), and dilute quantitatively, and stepwise if necessary, with Purified Water to obtain 10 mL of a solution containing 10 mg of Benzalkonium Chloride. Combine the three solutions, add sufficient Purified Water to make the product measure 100 mL, and mix to produce the Topical Solution.[ql]Meets the requirements for pH (4.0–6.0) and Beyond-use date.

COCCIDIOIDIN

Description: Coccidioidin USP—Clear, practically colorless or amber-colored liquid.

USP requirements: Coccidioidin USP—Preserve at a temperature between 2 and 8 °C. A sterile solution containing the antigens obtained from the by-products of mycelial growth or from the spherules of the fungus *Coccidioides immitis.* Contains a suitable antimicrobial agent. Label it to state that any dilutions made of the product should be stored in a refrigerator and used within 24 hours. Label it also to state that a separate syringe and needle shall be used for each individual injection. Has a potency such that the 1:100 dilution is bioequivalent to the U.S. Reference Coccidioidin 1:100. Meets the requirement for Expiration date (not later than 3 years after date of issue from manufacturer's cold storage [5 °C, 1 year] for the mycelial product and not later than 18 months after date of issue from manufacturer's cold storage [5 °C, 18 months] for the spherule-derived product). Conforms to the regulations of the U.S. Food and Drug Administration concerning biologics.

COCOA BUTTER

Description: Cocoa Butter NF—Yellowish white solid, having a faint, agreeable odor. Usually brittle at temperatures below 25 °C.
NF category: Suppository base.

Solubility: Cocoa Butter NF—Freely soluble in ether and in chloroform; soluble in boiling dehydrated alcohol; slightly soluble in alcohol.

NF requirements: Cocoa Butter NF—Preserve in well-closed containers. The fat obtained from the seed of *Theobroma cacao* Linné (Fam. Sterculiaceae). Meets the requirements for

Melting range (clear melting point 31–35 °C), Free fatty acids, Refractive index (1.454–1.459 at 40 °C), Fatty acid composition, Iodine value (33–42), Saponification value (188–198), and Organic volatile impurities.

CODEINE

Chemical name:

Codeine—Morphinan-6-ol, 7,8-didehydro-4,5-epoxy-3-methoxy-17-methyl-, monohydrate, (5 alpha,6 alpha)-.

Codeine phosphate—Morphinan-6-ol, 7,8-didehydro-4,5-epoxy-3-methoxy-17-methyl-, (5 alpha,6 alpha)-, phosphate (1:1) (salt), hemihydrate.

Codeine sulfate—Morphinan-6-ol, 7,8-didehydro-4,5-epoxy-3-methoxy-17-methyl-, (5 alpha,6 alpha)-, sulfate (2:1) (salt), trihydrate.

Molecular formula:

Codeine—$C_{18}H_{21}NO_3 \cdot H_2O$ (monohydrate); $C_{18}H_{21}NO_3$ (anhydrous).

Codeine phosphate—$C_{18}H_{21}NO_3 \cdot H_3PO_4 \cdot \frac{1}{2}H_2O$ (hemihydrate); $C_{18}H_{21}NO_3 \cdot H_3PO_4$ (anhydrous).

Codeine sulfate—$(C_{18}H_{21}NO_3)_2 \cdot H_2SO_4 \cdot 3H_2O$ (trihydrate); $(C_{18}H_{21}NO_3)_2 \cdot H_2SO_4$ (anhydrous).

Molecular weight:

Codeine—317.38 (monohydrate); 299.37 (anhydrous).

Codeine phosphate—406.37 (hemihydrate); 397.36 (anhydrous).

Codeine sulfate—750.85 (trihydrate); 696.81 (anhydrous).

Description:

Codeine USP—Colorless or white crystals or white, crystalline powder. Effloresces slowly in dry air, and is affected by light. In acid or alcohol solutions it is levorotatory. Its saturated solution is alkaline to litmus.

Codeine Phosphate USP—Fine, white, needle-shaped crystals, or white, crystalline powder. Odorless. Is affected by light. Its solutions are acid to litmus.

Codeine Sulfate USP—White crystals, usually needle-like, or white, crystalline powder. Is affected by light.

Solubility:

Codeine USP—Slightly soluble in water; very soluble in chloroform; freely soluble in alcohol; sparingly soluble in ether. When heated in an amount of water insufficient for complete solution, it melts to oily drops which crystallize on cooling.

Codeine Phosphate USP—Freely soluble in water; very soluble in hot water; slightly soluble in alcohol but more so in boiling alcohol.

Codeine Sulfate USP—Soluble in water; freely soluble in water at 80 °C; very slightly soluble in alcohol; insoluble in chloroform and in ether.

USP requirements:

Codeine USP—Preserve in tight, light-resistant containers. Dried at 80 °C for 4 hours, contains not less than 98.5% and not more than 100.5% of anhydrous codeine. Meets the requirements for Identification, Melting range (154–158 °C, the range between beginning and end of melting not more than 2 °C), Loss on drying (not more than 6.0%), Residue on ignition (not more than 0.1%), Readily carbonizable substances, Chromatographic purity, and Limit of morphine.

Codeine Phosphate USP—Preserve in tight, light-resistant containers. Contains not less than 99.0% and not more than 101.5% of codeine phosphate, calculated on the anhydrous basis. Meets the requirements for Identification, Acidity, Water (not more than 3.0%), Chloride, Sulfate, Limit of morphine, and Chromatographic purity.

Codeine Phosphate Injection USP—Preserve in single-dose or in multiple-dose containers, preferably of Type I glass, protected from light. A sterile solution of Codeine Phosphate in Water for Injection. Contains the labeled amount of codeine phosphate (as the hemihydrate), within ±7%. Meets the requirements for Identification, Bacterial endotoxins, pH (3.0–6.0), and Limit of morphine, and for Injections.

Note: Do not use the Injection if it is more than slightly discolored or contains a precipitate.

Codeine Phosphate Oral Solution—Not in *USP–NF*.

Codeine Phosphate Tablets USP—Preserve in well-closed, light-resistant containers. Contain the labeled amount of codeine phosphate (as the hemihydrate), within ±7%. Meet the requirements for Identification, Dissolution (75% in 45 minutes in water in Apparatus 2 at 50 rpm), Uniformity of dosage units, and Limit of morphine.

Codeine Phosphate Soluble Tablets—Not in *USP–NF*.

Codeine Sulfate USP—Preserve in tight, light-resistant containers. Dried at 105 °C for 3 hours, contains not less than 98.5% and not more than 100.5% of anhydrous codeine sulfate. Meets the requirements for Identification, Specific rotation (−112.5° to −115.0°), Acidity, Water (6.0–7.5%), Readily carbonizable substances, Residue on ignition (not more than 0.1%), Limit of morphine, and Chromatographic purity.

Codeine Sulfate Tablets USP—Preserve in well-closed containers. Contain the labeled amount of codeine sulfate (as the trihydrate), within ±7%. Meet the requirements for Identification, Dissolution (75% in 45 minutes in water in Apparatus 1 at 100 rpm), and Uniformity of dosage units.

Codeine Sulfate Soluble Tablets—Not in *USP–NF*.

CODEINE, AMMONIUM CHLORIDE, AND GUAIFENESIN

For *Codeine, Ammonium Chloride,* and *Guaifenesin*—See individual listings for chemistry information.

USP requirements: Codeine Phosphate, Ammonium Chloride, and Guaifenesin Syrup—Not in *USP–NF*.

CODEINE AND CALCIUM IODIDE

Chemical name: Codeine—Morphinan-6-ol, 7,8-didehydro-4,5-epoxy-3-methoxy-17-methyl-, monohydrate, (5 alpha,6 alpha)-.

Molecular formula:

Codeine—$C_{18}H_{21}NO_3 \cdot H_2O$.

Calcium iodide—CaI_2.

Molecular weight:

Codeine—317.38.

Calcium iodide—293.9.

Description:

Codeine USP—Colorless or white crystals or white, crystalline powder. It effloresces slowly in dry air, and is affected by light. In acid or alcohol solutions it is levorotatory. Its saturated solution is alkaline to litmus.

Calcium iodide—Very hygroscopic. Aqueous solution is neutral or slightly alkaline.

Solubility:

Codeine USP—Slightly soluble in water; very soluble in chloroform; freely soluble in alcohol; sparingly soluble in ether. When heated in an amount of water insufficient for complete solution, it melts to oily drops which crystallize on cooling.

Calcium iodide—Very soluble in water, in methanol, in ethanol, and in acetone; practically insoluble in ether and in dioxane.

USP requirements: Codeine and Calcium Iodide Syrup—Not in *USP–NF*.

CODEINE AND IODINATED GLYCEROL

For *Codeine* and *Iodinated Glycerol*—See individual listings for chemistry information.

USP requirements: Codeine Phosphate and Iodinated Glycerol Oral Solution—Not in *USP–NF*.

CODEINE AND GUAIFENESIN

For *Codeine* and *Guaifenesin*—See individual listings for chemistry information.

USP requirements:
Codeine Phosphate and Guaifenesin Oral Solution—Not in *USP–NF*.
Codeine Phosphate and Guaifenesin Syrup—Not in *USP–NF*.
Codeine Phosphate and Guaifenesin Tablets—Not in *USP–NF*.

COD LIVER OIL

Description: Cod Liver Oil USP—Thin, oily liquid, having a characteristic, slightly fishy but not rancid odor.

Solubility: Cod Liver Oil USP—Slightly soluble in alcohol; freely soluble in ether, in chloroform, in carbon disulfide, and in ethyl acetate.

USP requirements: Cod Liver Oil USP—Preserve in tight containers. It may be bottled or otherwise packaged in containers from which air has been expelled by the production of a vacuum or by an inert gas. The partially destearinated fixed oil obtained from fresh livers of *Gadus morrhua* Linné and other species of Fam. Gadidae. The vitamin A potency and vitamin D potency, when designated on the label, are expressed in USP Units per gram of oil. The potencies may be expressed also in metric units, on the basis that 1 USP Vitamin A Unit = 0.3 mcg and 40 USP Vitamin D Units = 1 mcg. Contains, in each gram, not less than 255 mcg (850 USP Units) of vitamin A and not less than 2.125 mcg (85 USP Units) of vitamin D. Meets the requirements for Identification for vitamin A, Specific gravity (0.918–0.927), Color, Nondestearinated cod liver oil, Unsaponifiable matter (not more than 1.30%), Acid value, Iodine value (145–180), and Saponification value (180–192).

COLCHICINE

Chemical name: Acetamide, *N*-(5,6,7,9-tetrahydro-1,2,3,10-tetramethoxy-9-oxobenzo[*a*]heptalen-7-yl)-, (*S*)-.

Molecular formula: $C_{22}H_{25}NO_6$.

Molecular weight: 399.44.

Description: Colchicine USP—Pale yellow to pale greenish yellow, amorphous scales, or powder or crystalline powder. Is odorless or nearly so, and darkens on exposure to light.

pKa: 12.35.

Solubility: Colchicine USP—Soluble in water; freely soluble in alcohol and in chloroform; slightly soluble in ether.

USP requirements:
Colchicine USP—Preserve in tight, light-resistant containers. An alkaloid contained in various species of *Colchicum*. Contains not less than 94.0% and not more than 101.0% of colchicine, calculated on the anhydrous, solvent-free basis. Meets the requirements for Identification, Specific rotation (–240° to –250°, calculated on the anhydrous and solvent-free basis), Water (not more than 2.0%, Colchiceine, Limit of ethyl acetate (not more than 8.0%), Chromatographic purity, and Organic volatile impurities (except that the limit of chloroform is 100 ppm).

Caution: Colchicine is extremely poisonous.

Colchicine Injection USP—Preserve in single-dose containers, preferably of Type I glass, protected from light. A sterile solution of Colchicine in Water for Injection, prepared from Colchicine with the aid of Sodium Hydroxide. Contains the labeled amount, within ±10%. Meets the requirements for Identification, Bacterial endotoxins, and pH (6.0–7.2, in a solution of Injection containing 1.0 mg of potassium chloride in each mL), and for Injections.

Caution: Colchicine is extremely poisonous.

Colchicine Tablets USP—Preserve in well-closed, light-resistant containers. Contain the labeled amount, within ±10%. Meet the requirements for Identification, Dissolution (75% in 30 minutes in water in Apparatus 1 at 100 rpm), and Uniformity of dosage units.

COLESEVELAM

Chemical name: Colesevelam hydrochloride—2-propen-1-amine polymer with (chloromethyl)oxirane, *N*,*N*,*N*-trimethyl-6-(2-propenylamino)-1-hexanaminium chloride, and *N*-2-propenyl-1-decanamine, hydrochloride.

Molecular formula: Colesevelam hydrochloride—$(C_3H_7N)_m$-$(C_3H_5ClO)_n C_{12}H_{27}ClN_2)_o (C_{13}H_{27}N)_p \cdot x$HCl.

Description: Colesevelam hydrochloride—Hydrophilic.

Solubility: Colesevelam hydrochloride—Insoluble in water.

USP requirements: Colesevelam Hydrochloride Tablets—Not in *USP–NF*.

COLESTIPOL

Chemical group: An anion-exchange resin.

Chemical name: Colestipol hydrochloride—Colestipol hydrochloride. Copolymer of diethylenetriamine and 1-chloro-2,3-epoxypropane, hydrochloride (with approximately 1 out of 5 amine nitrogens protonated).

Description: Colestipol Hydrochloride USP—Yellow to orange beads.

Solubility: Colestipol Hydrochloride USP—Swells but does not dissolve in water or dilute aqueous solutions of acid or alkali. Insoluble in the common organic solvents.

USP requirements:
Colestipol Hydrochloride USP—Preserve in tight containers. An insoluble, high molecular weight basic anion-exchange copolymer of diethylenetriamine and 1-chloro-2,3-epoxypropane with approximately one out of five amino nitrogens protonated. Each gram binds not less than 1.1 mEq and not more than 1.6 mEq of sodium cholate, calcu-

lated as cholate binding capacity. Meets the requirements for Identification, pH (6.0–7.5), Loss on drying (not more than 1.0%), Residue on ignition (not more than 0.3%), Heavy metals (not more than 0.002%), Chloride content (6.5–9.0%, calculated on the dried basis), Water absorption (3.3–5.3 grams of water per gram), Cholate binding capacity (1.1–1.6 mEq per gram), Water-soluble substances (not more than 0.5%), Colestipol exchange capacity (9.0–11.0 mEq of sodium hydroxide per gram), and Organic volatile impurities.

Colestipol Hydrochloride for Oral Suspension USP—Preserve in tight, single-dose or multiple-dose containers. A mixture of Colestipol Hydrochloride with a suitable flow-promoting agent. Each gram binds not less than 1.1 mEq and not more than 1.6 mEq of sodium cholate, calculated as the cholate binding capacity. Meets the requirements for Minimum fill and Water-soluble substances (not more than 0.5%), and for Cholate binding capacity, Identification, and pH under Colestipol Hydrochloride.

COLFOSCERIL, CETYL ALCOHOL, AND TYLOXAPOL

Chemical name:
Colfosceril palmitate—3,5,9-Trioxa-4-phosphapentacosan-1-aminium, 4-hydroxy-*N,N,N*-trimethyl-10-oxo-7-[(1-oxo-hexadecyl)oxy]-, hydroxide, inner salt, 4-oxide, (*R*)-.
Cetyl alcohol—1-Hexadecanol.
Tyloxapol—Phenol, 4-(1,1,3,3-tetramethylbutyl)-, polymer with formaldehyde and oxirane.

Molecular formula:
Colfosceril palmitate—$C_{40}H_{80}NO_8P$.
Cetyl alcohol—$C_{16}H_{34}O$.

Molecular weight:
Colfosceril palmitate—734.04.
Cetyl alcohol—242.44.

Description:
Cetyl Alcohol NF—Unctuous, white flakes, granules, cubes, or castings. Has a faint characteristic odor. Usually melts in the range between 45–50 °C.
   NF category: Stiffening agent.
Tyloxapol USP—Viscous, amber liquid, having a slight, aromatic odor. May exhibit a slight turbidity.
   NF category: Wetting and/or solubilizing agent.

Solubility:
Cetyl Alcohol NF—Insoluble in water; soluble in alcohol and in ether, the solubility increasing with an increase in temperature.
Tyloxapol USP—Slowly but freely miscible with water. Soluble in glacial acetic acid, in toluene, in carbon tetrachloride, in chloroform, and in carbon disulfide.

USP requirements: Colfosceril Palmitate, Cetyl Alcohol, and Tyloxapol for Intratracheal Suspension—Not in *USP–NF*.

COLISTIMETHATE

Chemical name: Colistimethate sodium—Colistimethate sodium.

Molecular formula: Colistimethate sodium—$C_{58}H_{105}N_{16}Na_5O_{28}S_5$ (colistin A component); $C_{57}H_{103}N_{16}Na_5O_{28}S_5$ (colistin B component).

Molecular weight: Colistimethate sodium—1749.82 (colistin A component); 1735.80 (colistin B component).

Description: Colistimethate Sodium USP—White to slightly yellow, odorless, fine powder.

Solubility: Colistimethate Sodium USP—Freely soluble in water; soluble in methanol; insoluble in acetone and in ether.

USP requirements:
Colistimethate for Injection USP—Preserve in Containers for Sterile Solids. Contains an amount of Colistimethate Sodium equivalent to the labeled amount of colistin, within −10% to +20%. Meets the requirements for Constituted solution, Bacterial endotoxins, and Sterility, and for Identification, pH, Loss on drying, Heavy metals, and Free colistin under Colistimethate Sodium, for Uniformity of dosage units, and for Constituted solutions and Labeling under Injections.
Colistimethate Sodium USP—Preserve in Containers for Sterile Solids. Has a potency equivalent to not less than 390 micrograms of colistin per mg. Where it is intended for use in preparing injectable dosage forms, the label states that it is sterile or must be subjected to further processing during the preparation of injectable dosage forms. Meets the requirements for Constituted solution, Identification, pH (6.5–8.5, in a solution containing 10 mg per mL), Loss on drying (not more than 7.0%), Heavy metals (not more than 0.003%), and Free colistin, and for Sterility and Bacterial endotoxins under Colistimethate for Injection (where the label states that Colistimethate Sodium is sterile), and for Bacterial endotoxins under Colistimethate for Injection (where the label states that Colistimethate Sodium must be subjected to further processing during the preparation of injectable dosage forms).

COLISTIN

Chemical name: Colistin sulfate—Colistin, sulfate.

Molecular formula:
Sulfate, Colistin A component—$C_{53}H_{100}N_{16}O_{13} \cdot 2\frac{1}{2}H_2SO_4$.
Sulfate, Colistin B component—$C_{52}H_{98}N_{16}O_{13} \cdot 2\frac{1}{2}H_2SO_4$.

Molecular weight:
Sulfate, Colistin A component—1414.65.
Sulfate, Colistin B component—1400.63.

Description: Colistin Sulfate USP—White to slightly yellow, odorless, fine powder.

Solubility: Colistin Sulfate USP—Freely soluble in water; slightly soluble in methanol; insoluble in acetone and in ether.

USP requirements:
Colistin Sulfate USP—Preserve in tight containers. The sulfate salt of an antibacterial substance produced by the growth of *Bacillus polymyxa* var. *colistinus*. Has a potency equivalent to not less than 500 mcg of colistin per mg. Meets the requirements for Identification, pH (4.0–7.0, in a solution containing 10 mg per mL), and Loss on drying (not more than 7.0%).
Colistin Sulfate for Oral Suspension USP—Preserve in tight containers, protected from light. A dry mixture of Colistin Sulfate with or without one or more suitable buffers, colors, diluents, dispersants, and flavors. Contains an amount of colistin sulfate equivalent to the labeled amount of colistin, within −10% to +20%. Meets the requirements for Uniformity of dosage units (solid packaged in single-unit containers), Deliverable volume (solid packaged in multiple-unit containers), pH (5.0–6.0, in the suspension constituted as directed in the labeling), and Loss on drying (not more than 3.0%).

COLISTIN, NEOMYCIN, AND HYDROCORTISONE

For *Colistin, Neomycin,* and *Hydrocortisone*—See individual listings for chemistry information.

USP requirements: Colistin and Neomycin Sulfates and Hydrocortisone Acetate Otic Suspension USP—Preserve in tight containers. A sterile suspension. Contains an amount of colistin sulfate equivalent to the labeled amount of colistin, within −10% to +35%, an amount of neomycin sulfate equivalent to the labeled amount of neomycin, within −10% to +25%, and the labeled amount of hydrocortisone acetate, within ±10%. Contains one or more suitable buffers, detergents, dispersants, and preservatives. Meets the requirements for Sterility and pH (4.8–5.2).

Note: Where Colistin and Neomycin Sulfates and Hydrocortisone Acetate Otic Suspension is prescribed, without reference to the quantity of colistin, neomycin, or hydrocortisone acetate contained therein, a product containing 3.0 mg of colistin, 3.3 mg of neomycin, and 10 mg of hydrocortisone acetate per mL shall be dispensed.

COLLAGENASE (LYOPHILIZED)

Source: An enzyme derived from the fermentation of *Clostridium histolyticum.*

USP requirements: Lyophilized Collagenase—Not in *USP–NF.*

COLLODION

Description: Collodion USP—Clear, or slightly opalescent, viscous liquid. Is colorless, or slightly yellowish, and has the odor of ether.

USP requirements: Collodion USP—Preserve in tight containers, at a temperature not exceeding 30 °C, remote from fire. The label bears a caution statement to the effect that Collodion is highly flammable. Contains not less than 5.0%, by weight, of pyroxylin.

Prepare Collodion as follows: 40 grams of Pyroxylin, 750 mL of Ether, and 250 mL of Alcohol to make about 1000 mL. Add the Alcohol and Ether to the Pyroxylin contained in a suitable container, and insert the stopper into the container well. Shake the mixture occasionally until the Pyroxylin is dissolved.

Meets the requirements for Identification, Specific gravity (0.765–0.775), Acidity, and Alcohol content (22.0–26.0%).

Caution: Collodion is highly flammable.

FLEXIBLE COLLODION

Description: Flexible Collodion USP—Clear, or slightly opalescent, viscous liquid. Is colorless or slightly yellow, and has the odor of ether. The strong odor of camphor becomes noticeable as the ether evaporates.

USP requirements: Flexible Collodion USP—Preserve in tight containers, at a temperature not exceeding 30 °C, remote from fire. The label bears a caution statement to the effect that Flexible Collodion is highly flammable.

Prepare Flexible Collodion as follows: 20 grams of Camphor, 30 grams of Castor Oil, and a sufficient quantity of Collodion, to make 1000 grams. Weigh the ingredients, successively, into a dry, tared bottle, insert the stopper in the bottle, and shake the mixture until the camphor is dissolved.

Meets the requirements for Identification, Specific gravity (0.770–0.790), and Alcohol content (21.0–25.0%).

COLLOIDAL OATMEAL

USP requirements: Colloidal Oatmeal USP—Preserve in well-closed containers. The powder resulting from the grinding and further processing of whole oat grain meeting U.S. Standards for Number 1 or Number 2 oats. Meets the requirements for Identification, Viscosity (the average of three viscosities is greater than 1 and less than 100 centipoise), Microbial limits, Loss on drying (not more than 10%), Particle size, Total ash (not more than 2.5% on the dried basis), Fat content (not less than 0.2%), and Nitrogen content (not less than 2.0%).

COPPER

Chemical name: Copper gluconate—Copper, bis (D-gluconato-O^1,O^2)-.

Molecular formula: Copper gluconate—$C_{12}H_{22}CuO_{14}$.

Molecular weight: Copper gluconate—453.84.

USP requirements:

Copper Gluconate USP—Preserve in well-closed containers. Contains not less than 98.0% and not more than 102.0% of copper gluconate. Meets the requirements for Identification, Chloride (not more than 0.07%), Sulfate (not more than 0.05%), Arsenic (not more than 3 ppm), Lead (not more than 0.0025%), and Reducing substances (not more than 1.0%).

Copper Gluconate Tablets—Not in *USP–NF.*

CORN OIL

Description: Corn Oil NF—Clear, light yellow, oily liquid, having a faint, characteristic odor.

NF category: Solvent; vehicle (oleaginous).

Solubility: Corn Oil NF—Slightly soluble in alcohol; miscible with ether, with chloroform, and with solvent hexane.

NF requirements: Corn Oil NF—Preserve in tight, light-resistant containers, and avoid exposure to excessive heat. The refined fixed oil obtained from the embryo of *Zea mays* Linn;aae (Fam. Gramineae). Meets the requirements for Specific gravity (0.914–0.921), Heavy metals (not more than 0.001%), Cottonseed oil, Fatty acid composition, Free fatty acids, Iodine value (102–130), Saponification value (187–193), Unsaponifiable matter (not more than 1.5%), and Organic volatile impurities.

CORTICORELIN OVINE

Chemical name: Corticorelin ovine triflutate—Corticotropin-releasing factor (sheep), trifluoroacetate (salt).

Molecular formula: Corticorelin ovine triflutate—$C_{205}H_{339}N_{59}O_{63}S \cdot xC_2HF_3O_2$.

Molecular weight: Corticorelin ovine—4670.35 daltons.

USP requirements: Corticorelin Ovine Triflutate for Injection—Not in *USP–NF*.

CORTICOTROPIN

Chemical name:
  Corticotropin—Corticotropin.
  Corticotropin, repository—Corticotropin.
  Corticotropin zinc hydroxide—Corticotropin zinc hydroxide.

Description:
  Corticotropin Injection USP—Colorless or light straw-colored liquid.
  Corticotropin for Injection USP—White or practically white, soluble, amorphous solid having the characteristic appearance of substances prepared by freeze-drying.
  Repository Corticotropin Injection USP—Colorless or light straw-colored liquid, which may be quite viscid at room temperature. Is odorless or has an odor of an antimicrobial agent.
  Sterile Corticotropin Zinc Hydroxide Suspension USP—Flocculent, white, aqueous suspension, free from large particles following moderate shaking.

USP requirements:
  Corticotropin Injection USP—Preserve in single-dose or in multiple-dose containers, preferably of Type I glass. Store in a cold place. A sterile solution, in a suitable diluent, of the material containing the polypeptide hormone having the property of increasing the rate of secretion of adrenal corticosteroids, which is obtained from the anterior lobe of the pituitary of mammals used for food by man. If the labeling of Injection recommends intravenous administration, include specific information on dosage. Its potency is within –20% to +25% of the potency stated on the label in USP Corticotropin Units. Meets the requirements for Bacterial endotoxins, Vasopressin activity, pH (3.0–7.0), and Particulate matter, and for Injections.
  Corticotropin for Injection USP—Preserve in Containers for Sterile Solids. A sterile, dry material containing the polypeptide hormone having the property of increasing the rate of secretion of adrenal corticosteroids, which is obtained from the anterior lobe of the pituitary of mammals used for food by man. If the labeling of Corticotropin for Injection recommends intravenous administration, include specific information on dosage. Its potency is within –20% to +25% of the potency stated on the label in USP Corticotropin Units. Meets the requirements for Bacterial endotoxins, Vasopressin activity, pH (2.5–6.0, in a solution constituted as directed in the labeling supplied by the manufacturer), and Particulate matter, and for Sterility tests, Uniformity of dosage units, Constituted solutions and Labeling under Injections.
  Repository Corticotropin Injection USP—Preserve in single-dose or in multiple-dose containers, preferably of Type I glass. It is corticotropin in a solution of partially hydrolyzed gelatin. Its potency is within –20% to +25% of the potency stated on the label in USP Corticotropin Units. Meets the requirements for Bacterial endotoxins, for Vasopressin activity and pH under Corticotropin Injection, and for Injections.
  Corticotropin Zinc Hydroxide Injectable Suspension USP—Preserve in single-dose or in multiple-dose containers, preferably of Type I glass. Store at controlled room temperature. A sterile suspension of corticotropin adsorbed on zinc hydroxide. Label it to indicate that it is not recommended for intravenous use and that the suspension is to be well shaken before use. The container label and the package label state the potency in USP Corticotropin Units in each mL. Its potency is within –20% to +25% of the po-

tency stated on the label in USP Corticotropin Units. Contains not less than 1800 mcg and not more than 2200 mcg of zinc, and not less than 604 mcg and not more than 776 mcg of anhydrous dibasic sodium phosphate, for each 40 USP Corticotropin Units. Meets the requirements for Bacterial endotoxins, pH (7.5–8.5, determined potentiometrically), Zinc, and Anhydrous dibasic sodium phosphate, and for Injections.

CORTISONE

Chemical name: Cortisone acetate—Pregn-4-ene-3,11,20-trione, 21-(acetyloxy)-17-hydroxy-.

Molecular formula: Cortisone acetate—$C_{23}H_{30}O_6$.

Molecular weight: Cortisone acetate—402.48.

Description: Cortisone Acetate USP—White or practically white, odorless, crystalline powder. Is stable in air. Melts at about 240 °C, with some decomposition.

Solubility: Cortisone Acetate USP—Insoluble in water; freely soluble in chloroform; soluble in dioxane; sparingly soluble in acetone; slightly soluble in alcohol.

USP requirements:
  Cortisone Acetate USP—Preserve in well-closed containers. Contains not less than 97.0% and not more than 102.0% of cortisone acetate, calculated on the dried basis. Meets the requirements for Identification, Specific rotation (+208° to +217°), Loss on drying (not more than 1.0%), Residue on ignition (negligible, from 100 mg), Chromatographic purity, Other impurities, and Organic volatile impurities.
  Cortisone Acetate Injectable Suspension USP—Preserve in single-dose or in multiple-dose containers, preferably of Type I glass. A sterile suspension of Cortisone Acetate in a suitable aqueous medium. Contains the labeled amount, within ±10%. Meets the requirements for Identification and pH (5.0–7.0), and for Injections.
  Cortisone Acetate Tablets USP—Preserve in well-closed containers. Contain the labeled amount, within ±10%. Meet the requirements for Identification, Dissolution (75% in 45 minutes in 0.5% of sodium lauryl sulfate solution in Apparatus 2 at 50 rpm), and Uniformity of dosage units.

COSYNTROPIN

Source: Synthetic polypeptide identical to the first 24 of the 39 amino acids of corticotropin.

Chemical name: Alpha[1-24]-Corticotropin.

Molecular formula: $C_{136}H_{210}N_{40}O_{31}S$.

Molecular weight: 2933.44.

Description: White to off-white lyophilized mixture.

Solubility: Soluble in water.

USP requirements: Cosyntropin for Injection—Not in *USP–NF*.

PURIFIED COTTON

Description: Purified Cotton USP—White, soft, fine filament-like hairs appearing under the microscope as hollow, flattened and twisted bands, striate and slightly thickened at the edges. Is practically odorless.

Solubility: Purified Cotton USP—Insoluble in ordinary solvents; soluble in ammoniated cupric oxide TS.

USP requirements: Purified Cotton USP—Package it in rolls of not more than 500 grams of a continuous lap, with a lightweight paper running under the entire lap, the paper being of such width that it may be folded over the edges of the lap to a distance of at least 25 millimeters, the two together being tightly and evenly rolled, and enclosed and sealed in a well-closed container. It may be packaged also in other types of containers if these are so constructed that the sterility of the product is maintained. The hair of the seed of cultivated varieties of *Gossypium hirsutum* Linné, or of other species of *Gossypium* (Fam. Malvaceae), freed from adhering impurities, deprived of fatty matter, bleached, and sterilized in its final container. Its label bears a statement to the effect that the sterility cannot be guaranteed if the package bears evidence of damage or if the package has been opened previously. Meets the requirements for Sterility, Alkalinity or acidity, Residue on ignition (not more than 0.20%), Water-soluble substances (not more than 0.35%), Fatty matter (not more than 0.7%), Dyes, Other foreign matter, and Fiber length and Absorbency (not less than 60% of fibers, by weight, are 12.5 millimeters or greater in length and not more than 10% of fibers, by weight, are 6.25 millimeters or less in length; retains not less than 24 times its weight of water).

COTTONSEED OIL

Description: Cottonseed Oil NF—Pale yellow, oily liquid. It is odorless or nearly so. At temperatures below 10 °C particles of solid fat may separate from the Oil, and at about 0 to –5 °C, the oil becomes a solid or nearly so.

NF category: Solvent; vehicle (oleaginous).

Solubility: Cottonseed Oil NF—Slightly soluble in alcohol. Miscible with ether, with chloroform, with solvent hexane, and with carbon disulfide.

NF requirements: Cottonseed Oil NF—Preserve in tight, light-resistant containers, and avoid exposure to excessive heat. The refined fixed oil obtained from the seed of cultivated plants of various varieties of *Gossypium hirsutum* Linné or of other species of *Gossypium* (Fam. Malvaceae). Meets the requirements for Identification, Specific gravity (0.915–0.921), Free fatty acids, Iodine value (109–120), Heavy metals (not more than 0.001%), and Organic volatile impurities.

CRANBERRY LIQUID PREPARATION

NF requirements: Cranberry Liquid Preparation NF—Preserve in well-closed containers, in a refrigerator. A bright red juice derived from the fruits of *Vaccinium macrocarpon* Ait. or *Vaccinium oxycocco* Linné (Fam. Ericaceae). The label states the Latin binomial name and, following the official name, the parts of the plant source from which the article was derived. The label also states that it is for manufacturing purposes only. Contains no added substances. Meets the requirements for Identification, Refractive index (1.3435–1.3445), pH (2.5± 0.1), Limit of sorbitol and sucrose (not more than 0.05% each of sorbitol and sucrose), Content of dextrose and fructose (not less than 2.4% dextrose and not less than 0.7% of fructose), and Content of organic acids (not less than 0.9% each of quinic acid and citric acid and not less than 0.7% of malic acid, and the ratio of quinic acid to malic acid not less than 1.0).

CREATININE

Molecular formula: $C_4H_7N_3O$.

Molecular weight: 113.12.

Description: Creatinine NF—White crystals or crystalline powder. Is odorless.

NF category: Bulking agent for freeze-drying.

Solubility: Creatinine NF—Soluble in water; slightly soluble in alcohol; practically insoluble in acetone, in ether, and in chloroform.

NF requirements: Creatinine NF—Preserve in well-closed containers. Contains not less than 98.5% and not more than 102.0% of creatinine, as Creatinine, calculated on the dried basis. Meets the requirements for Identification, Loss on drying (not more than 3.0%), Residue on ignition (not more than 0.2%), and Heavy metals (not more than 0.001%).

CRESOL

Chemical name: Phenol, methyl-.

Molecular formula: C_7H_8O.

Molecular weight: 108.14.

Description: Cresol NF—Colorless, or yellowish to brownish yellow, or pinkish, highly refractive liquid, becoming darker with age and on exposure to light. It has a phenol-like, sometimes empyreumatic odor. A saturated solution of it is neutral or only slightly acid to litmus.

NF category: Antimicrobial preservative.

Solubility: Cresol NF—Sparingly soluble in water, usually forming a cloudy solution; dissolves in solutions of fixed alkali hydroxides. Miscible with alcohol, with ether, and with glycerin.

NF requirements: Cresol NF—Preserve in tight, light-resistant containers. A mixture of isomeric cresols obtained from coal tar or from petroleum. Meets the requirements for Identification, Specific gravity (1.030–1.038), Distilling range (not less than 90.0% distils between 195 and 205 °C), Hydrocarbons, and Limit of phenol (not more than 5.0%).

CORIANDER

NF requirements: Coriander Oil NF—Preserve in tight, light-resistant containers, protected from light, and store at controlled room temperature. Avoid exposure to excessive heat. The label states the Latin binomial name and, following the official name, the part of the plant source from which the article was derived. Volatile oil obtained by steam distillation from the dried ripe fruit of *Coriandrum sativum* L. (Fam. Apiaceae). Meets the requirements for Solubility in 70% alcohol, Specific gravity (0.863–0.875), Angular rotation (+8° to +15°), Refractive index (1.462–1.472 at 20°), and Heavy metals (0.004%).

CROMOLYN

Chemical name: Cromolyn sodium—4*H*-1-Benzopyran-2-carboxylic acid, 5,5'-[(2-hydroxy-1,3-propanediyl)bis(oxy)]bis[4-oxo-, disodium salt].

Molecular formula: Cromolyn sodium—$C_{23}H_{14}Na_2O_{11}$.

Molecular weight: Cromolyn sodium—512.33.

Description:
  Cromolyn Sodium USP—White, odorless, crystalline powder. Is hygroscopic.
  Cromolyn Sodium for Inhalation USP—White to creamy white, odorless, hygroscopic, and very finely divided powder.

Solubility: Cromolyn Sodium USP—Soluble in water; insoluble in alcohol and in chloroform.

USP requirements:
  Cromolyn Sodium USP—Preserve in tight containers. Contains not less than 98.0% and not more than 101.0% of cromolyn sodium, calculated on the anhydrous basis. Meets the requirements for Identification, Acidity or alkalinity, Water (not more than 10.0%), Limit of oxalate, Related compounds, Heavy metals (0.002%), and Organic volatile impurities.
  Cromolyn Sodium Inhalation Aerosol—Not in *USP–NF*.
  Cromolyn Sodium Capsules—Not in *USP–NF*.
  Cromolyn Sodium Oral Concentrate—Not in *USP–NF*.
  Cromolyn Sodium Inhalation Solution USP—Preserve in single-unit, double-ended glass ampuls or in low-density polyethylene ampuls. A sterile, aqueous solution of Cromolyn Sodium. The label indicates that the Inhalation Solution is not to be used if it contains a precipitate. Contains the labeled amount, within ±10%. Meets the requirements for Identification, Sterility, Uniformity of dosage units, pH (4.0–7.0), and Related compounds.
  Cromolyn Sodium Inhalation Powder USP (Capsules)—Preserve in tight, light-resistant containers at controlled room temperature. Avoid excessive heat. A mixture of equal parts of Lactose and Cromolyn Sodium contained in a hard gelatin capsule. Contains the labeled amount, within −5% to +25%. Meets the requirements for Identification and Uniformity of dosage units.
  Cromolyn Sodium for Nasal Insufflation—Not in *USP–NF*.
  Cromolyn Sodium Nasal Solution USP—Preserve in tight, light-resistant containers. An aqueous solution of Cromolyn Sodium. Contains the labeled amount, within ±10%. Meets the requirements for Identification, pH (4.0–7.0), and Related compounds.
  Cromolyn Sodium Ophthalmic Solution USP—Preserve in tight, light-resistant, single-dose or multiple-dose containers. Ophthalmic Solution that is packaged in multiple-dose containers contains a suitable antimicrobial agent. A sterile, aqueous solution of Cromolyn Sodium. Contains the labeled amount, within ±10%. Meets the requirements for Identification, Sterility, pH (4.0–7.0), and Related compounds.

CROSCARMELLOSE SODIUM

Description: Croscarmellose Sodium NF—White, free-flowing powder.
  NF category: Tablet disintegrant.

Solubility: Croscarmellose Sodium NF—Partially soluble in water; insoluble in alcohol, in ether, and in other organic solvents.

NF requirements: Croscarmellose Sodium NF—Preserve in tight containers. A cross-linked polymer of carboxymethylcellulose sodium. Meets the requirements for Identification, pH (5.0–7.0), Loss on drying (not more than 10.0%), Heavy metals (not more than 0.001%), Sodium chloride and sodium glycolate (not more than 0.5%), Degree of substitution (0.60–

0.85, calculated on the dried basis), Content of water-soluble material (1.0–10.0%), Settling volume, and Organic volatile impurities.

CROSPOVIDONE

Chemical name: 2-Pyrrolidinone, 1-ethenyl-, homopolymer.

Molecular formula: $(C_6H_9NO)_n$.

Description: Crospovidone NF—White to creamy-white, hygroscopic powder, having a faint odor.
  NF category: Tablet disintegrant.

Solubility: Crospovidone NF—Insoluble in water and in ordinary organic solvents.

NF requirements: Crospovidone NF—Preserve in tight containers. A water-insoluble synthetic, cross-linked homopolymer of N-vinyl-2-pyrrolidinone. Contains not less than 11.0% and not more than 12.8% of nitrogen, calculated on the anhydrous basis. Meets the requirements for Identification, pH (5.0–8.0, in an aqueous suspension [1 in 100]), Water (not more than 5.0%), Residue on ignition (not more than 0.4%), Water-soluble substances (not more than 1.50%), Heavy metals (not more than 0.001%), Vinylpyrrolidinone (not more than 0.1%), and Nitrogen content.

CROTAMITON

Chemical name: 2-Butenamide, N-ethyl-N-(2-methylphenyl)-.

Molecular formula: $C_{13}H_{17}NO$.

Molecular weight: 203.28.

Description: Crotamiton USP—Colorless to slightly yellowish oil, having a faint amine-like odor.

Solubility: Crotamiton USP—Soluble in alcohol and in methanol.

USP requirements:
  Crotamiton USP—Preserve in tight, light-resistant containers. A mixture of *cis* and *trans* isomers containing not less than 97.0% and not more than 103.0% of crotamiton. Meets the requirements for Identification, Specific gravity (1.008–1.011 at 20 °C), Refractive index (1.540–1.543 at 20 °C), Residue on ignition (not more than 0.1%), and Bound halogen.
  Crotamiton Cream USP—Preserve in collapsible tubes or in tight, light-resistant containers. Contains the labeled amount, within ±7%. Meets the requirements for Identification and Minimum fill.
  Crotamiton Lotion—Not in *USP–NF*.

CUPRIC CHLORIDE

Chemical name: Copper chloride ($CuCl_2$) dihydrate.

Molecular formula: $CuCl_2 \cdot 2H_2O$.

Molecular weight: 170.48.

Description: Cupric Chloride USP—Bluish green, deliquescent crystals.

Solubility: Cupric Chloride USP—Freely soluble in water; soluble in alcohol; slightly soluble in ether.

USP requirements:
Cupric Chloride USP—Preserve in tight containers. Contains not less than 99.0% and not more than 100.5% of cupric chloride, calculated on the dried basis. Meets the requirements for Identification, Loss on drying (20.9–21.4%), Insoluble matter (not more than 0.01%), Sulfate (not more than 0.005%), Limit of sodium (not more than 0.02%), Limit of potassium (not more than 0.01%), Limit of calcium (not more than 0.005%), Limit of iron (not more than 0.005%), Limit of nickel (not more than 0.01%), and Organic volatile impurities.
Cupric Chloride Injection USP—Preserve in single-dose or in multiple-dose containers, preferably of Type I or Type II glass. A sterile solution of Cupric Chloride in Water for Injection. Label the Injection to indicate that it is to be diluted to the appropriate strength with Sterile Water for Injection or other suitable fluid prior to administration. Contains an amount of cupric chloride equivalent to the labeled amount of copper, within ±10%. Meets the requirements for Identification, Bacterial endotoxins, pH (1.5–2.5), and Particulate matter, and for Injections.

CUPRIC SULFATE

Chemical name: Sulfuric acid, copper(2+) salt (1:1), pentahydrate.

Molecular formula: $CuSO_4 \cdot 5H_2O$.

Molecular weight: 249.69.

Description: Cupric Sulfate USP—Deep blue, triclinic crystals or blue, crystalline granules or powder. It effloresces slowly in dry air. Its solutions are acid to litmus.

Solubility: Cupric Sulfate USP—Freely soluble in water and in glycerin; very soluble in boiling water; slightly soluble in alcohol.

USP requirements:
Cupric Sulfate USP—Preserve in tight containers. Dried at 250 °C to constant weight, contains not less than 98.5% and not more than 100.5% of cupric sulfate. Meets the requirements for Identification, Loss on drying (33.0–36.5%), Limit of sodium (not more than 0.01%), Limit of potassium (not more than 0.01%), Limit of calcium (not more than 0.005%), Limit of iron (not more than 0.005%), Limit of nickel (not more than 0.01%), and Organic volatile impurities.
Cupric Sulfate Injection USP—Preserve in single-dose or in multiple-dose containers, preferably of Type I or Type II glass. A sterile solution of Cupric Sulfate in Water for Injection. Label the Injection to indicate that it is to be diluted to the appropriate strength with Sterile Water for Injection or other suitable fluid prior to administration. Contains an amount of cupric sulfate equivalent to the labeled amount of copper, within ±10%. Meets the requirements for Identification, Bacterial endotoxins, pH (2.0–3.5), and Particulate matter, and for Injections.

CYANOCOBALAMIN

Chemical name: Vitamin B_{12}.

Molecular formula: $C_{63}H_{88}CoN_{14}O_{14}P$.

Molecular weight: 1355.37.

Description: Cyanocobalamin USP—Dark red crystals or amorphous or crystalline red powder. In the anhydrous form, it is very hygroscopic and when exposed to air it may absorb about 12% of water.

Solubility: Cyanocobalamin USP—Sparingly soluble in water; soluble in alcohol; insoluble in acetone, in chloroform, and in ether.

USP requirements:
Cyanocobalamin USP—Preserve in tight, light-resistant containers. Contains not less than 96.0% and not more than 100.5% of cyanocobalamin, calculated on the dried basis. Meets the requirements for Identification, Loss on drying (not more than 12.0%), and Pseudo cyanocobalamin.
Cyanocobalamin Intranasal Gel—Not in *USP–NF*.
Cyanocobalamin Injection USP—Preserve in light-resistant, single-dose or multiple-dose containers, preferably of Type I glass. A sterile solution of Cyanocobalamin in Water for Injection, or in Water for Injection rendered isotonic by the addition of Sodium Chloride. Contains the labeled amount of anhydrous cyanocobalamin, within –5% to +15%. Meets the requirements for Identification, Bacterial endotoxins, and pH (4.5–7.0), and for Injections.
Cyanocobalamin Tablets—Not in *USP–NF*.
Cyanocobalamin Extended-release Tablets—Not in *USP–NF*.

CYCLACILLIN

Chemical name: 4-Thia-1-azabicyclo[3.2.0]heptane-2-carboxylic acid, 6-[[(1-aminocyclohexyl)carbonyl]amino]-3,3-dimethyl-7-oxo-, [2*S*-(2 alpha,5 alpha,6 beta)]-.

Molecular formula: $C_{15}H_{23}N_3O_4S$.

Molecular weight: 341.43.

Description: White, crystalline, anhydrous powder.

Solubility: Sparingly soluble in water.

USP requirements:
Cyclacillin USP—Preserve in tight containers. Contains not less than 90.0% of cyclacillin, calculated on the anhydrous basis. Has a potency of not less than 900 mcg and not more than 1050 mcg of cyclacillin per mg. Meets the requirements for Identification, Crystallinity, pH (4.0–6.5, in a solution containing 10 mg per mL), Water (not more than 1.0%), Concordance (not more than 6.0%), and Content of cyclacillin.
Cyclacillin for Oral Suspension USP—Preserve in tight containers. A dry mixture of Cyclacillin with one or more suitable buffers, colors, flavors, preservatives, sweeteners, and suspending agents. Contains the labeled amount, within –10% to +20%. Meets the requirements for Identification, Uniformity of dosage units (solid packaged in single-unit containers), Deliverable volume (multiple-unit containers), pH (4.5–6.5, in the suspension constituted as directed in the labeling), and Water (not more than 1.5%).
Cyclacillin Tablets USP—Preserve in tight containers. Contain the labeled amount, within –10% to +20%. Meet the requirements for Identification, Dissolution (75% in 45 minutes in water in Apparatus 2 at 50 rpm), and Water (not more than 5.0%).

CYCLANDELATE

Chemical name: 3,3,5-Trimethylcyclohexanol alpha-phenyl-alpha-hydroxyacetate.

Molecular formula: $C_{17}H_{24}O_3$.

Molecular weight: 276.37.

Description: White, amorphous powder having a faint menthol-like odor.

Solubility: Slightly soluble in water; highly soluble in ethyl alcohol and in organic solvents.

USP requirements:
Cyclandelate Capsules—Not in *USP–NF*.
Cyclandelate Tablets—Not in *USP–NF*.

CYCLIZINE

Chemical group: Piperazine derivative.

Chemical name:
Cyclizine—Piperazine, 1-(diphenylmethyl)-4-methyl-.
Cyclizine hydrochloride—Piperazine, 1-(diphenylmethyl)-4-methyl-, monohydrochloride.
Cyclizine lactate—Piperazine, 1-(diphenylmethyl)-4-methyl-, mono(2-hydroxypropanoate).

Molecular formula:
Cyclizine—$C_{18}H_{22}N_2$.
Cyclizine hydrochloride—$C_{18}H_{22}N_2 \cdot HCl$.
Cyclizine lactate—$C_{18}H_{22}N_2 \cdot C_3H_6O_3$.

Molecular weight:
Cyclizine—266.38.
Cyclizine hydrochloride—302.84.
Cyclizine lactate—356.46.

Description:
Cyclizine USP—White, or creamy white, crystalline, practically odorless powder.
Cyclizine Hydrochloride USP—White, crystalline powder or small, colorless crystals. Is odorless or nearly so. Melts indistinctly at about 285 °C, with decomposition.

pKa: 7.7.

Solubility:
Cyclizine USP—Slightly soluble in water; soluble in alcohol and in chloroform.
Cyclizine Hydrochloride USP—Slightly soluble in water and in alcohol; sparingly soluble in chloroform; insoluble in ether.

USP requirements:
Cyclizine USP—Preserve in tight, light-resistant containers. Contains not less than 98.0% and not more than 100.5% of cyclizine, calculated on the anhydrous basis. Meets the requirements for Clarity and color of solution, Identification, Melting range (106–109 °C), pH (7.6–8.6, in a saturated solution), Water (not more than 1.0%), Residue on ignition (not more than 0.1%), Chloride (not more than 0.014%), Ordinary impurities, and Organic volatile impurities.
Cyclizine Hydrochloride USP—Preserve in tight, light-resistant containers. Contains not less than 98.0% and not more than 100.5% of cyclizine hydrochloride, calculated on the dried basis. Meets the requirements for Identification, pH (4.5–5.5, determined potentiometrically in a 1 in 50 solution), Loss on drying (not more than 1.0%), Residue on ignition (not more than 0.2%), Ordinary impurities, and Organic volatile impurities.
Cyclizine Hydrochloride Tablets USP—Preserve in tight, light-resistant containers. Contain the labeled amount, within ± 7%. Meet the requirements for Identification, Dissolution (75% in 45 minutes in water in Apparatus 2 at 50 rpm), and Uniformity of dosage units.
Cyclizine Lactate Injection USP—Preserve in single-dose containers, preferably of Type I glass, protected from light. A sterile solution of cyclizine lactate in Water for Injection, prepared from Cyclizine with the aid of Lactic Acid. Con-

tains the labeled amount, within ±5%. Meets the requirements for Identification and pH (3.2–4.7), and for Injections.

CYCLOBENZAPRINE

Chemical name: Cyclobenzaprine hydrochloride—1-Propanamine, 3-(5H-dibenzo[a,d]cyclohepten-5-ylidene)-N,N-dimethyl-, hydrochloride.

Molecular formula: Cyclobenzaprine hydrochloride—$C_{20}H_{21}N \cdot HCl$.

Molecular weight: Cyclobenzaprine hydrochloride—311.85.

Description: Cyclobenzaprine Hydrochloride USP—White to off-white, odorless, crystalline powder.

pKa: Cyclobenzaprine hydrochloride—8.47 at 25 °C.

Solubility: Cyclobenzaprine Hydrochloride USP—Freely soluble in water, in alcohol, and in methanol; sparingly soluble in isopropanol; slightly soluble in chloroform and in methylene chloride; insoluble in hydrocarbons.

USP requirements:
Cyclobenzaprine Hydrochloride USP—Preserve in well-closed containers. Contains not less than 99.0% and not more than 101.0% of cyclobenzaprine hydrochloride, calculated on the dried basis. Meets the requirements for Identification, Melting range (215–219 °C, not more than 2 °C range between beginning and end of melting), Loss on drying (not more than 1.0%), Residue on ignition (not more than 0.1%), Heavy metals (not more than 0.001%), Chromatographic purity, and Organic volatile impurities.
Cyclobenzaprine Hydrochloride Tablets USP—Preserve in well-closed containers. Contain the labeled amount, within ±10%. Meet the requirements for Identification, Dissolution (75% in 30 minutes in 0.01 N hydrochloric acid in Apparatus 1 at 50 rpm), and Uniformity of dosage units.

CYCLOMETHICONE

Chemical name: Cyclopolydimethylsiloxane.

Molecular formula: $(C_2H_6OSi)_n$.

Description: Cyclomethicone NF—NF category: Water repelling agent.

NF requirements: Cyclomethicone NF—Preserve in tight containers. A fully methylated cyclic siloxane containing repeating units of the formula $[-(CH_3)_2SiO-]_n$, in which n is 4, 5, or 6, or a mixture of them. Label it to state, as part of the official title, the n-value of the Cyclomethicone. Where it is a mixture of 2 or 3 such cyclic siloxanes, the label states the n-value and percentage of each in the mixture. Contains not less than 98.0% of cyclomethicone, calculated as the sum of cyclomethicone 4, cyclomethicone 5, and cyclomethicone 6, and not less than 95.0% and not more than 105.0% of the labeled amount of any one or more of the individual cyclomethicone components. Meets the requirements for Identification and Limit of nonvolatile residue (not more than 0.15% [w/w]).

CYCLOPENTOLATE

Chemical name: Cyclopentolate hydrochloride—Benzeneacetic acid, alpha-(1-hydroxycyclopentyl)-, 2-(dimethylamino)ethyl ester, hydrochloride.

Molecular formula: Cyclopentolate hydrochloride—$C_{17}H_{25}NO_3 \cdot$ HCl.

Molecular weight: Cyclopentolate hydrochloride—327.85.

Description: Cyclopentolate Hydrochloride USP—White, crystalline powder, which upon standing develops a characteristic odor. Its solutions are acid to litmus. Melts at about 138 °C, the melt appearing opaque.

Solubility: Cyclopentolate Hydrochloride USP—Very soluble in water; freely soluble in alcohol; insoluble in ether.

USP requirements:
Cyclopentolate Hydrochloride USP—Preserve in tight containers, and store in a cold place. Contains not less than 98.0% and not more than 102.0% of cyclopentolate hydrochloride, calculated on the dried basis. Meets the requirements for Identification, pH (4.5–5.5, in a solution [1 in 100]), Loss on drying (not more than 0.5%), Residue on ignition (not more than 0.05%), and Chromatographic purity.

Cyclopentolate Hydrochloride Ophthalmic Solution USP—Preserve in tight containers, and store at controlled room temperature. A sterile, aqueous solution of Cyclopentolate Hydrochloride. Contains the labeled amount, within ± 10%. Meets the requirements for Identification, Sterility, and pH (3.0–5.5).

CYCLOPHOSPHAMIDE

Chemical name: 2H-1,3,2-Oxazaphosphorin-2-amine, N,N-bis(2-chloroethyl)tetrahydro-, 2-oxide, monohydrate.

Molecular formula: $C_7H_{15}Cl_2N_2O_2P \cdot H_2O$.

Molecular weight: 279.10.

Description: Cyclophosphamide USP—White, crystalline powder. Liquefies upon loss of its water of crystallization.

Solubility: Cyclophosphamide USP—Soluble in water and in alcohol.

USP requirements:
Cyclophosphamide USP—Preserve in tight containers, at a temperature between 2 and 30 °C. Contains not less than 97.0% and not more than 103.0% of cyclophosphamide, calculated on the anhydrous basis. Meets the requirements for Identification, pH (3.9–7.1, in a solution [1 in 100]), Water (5.7–6.8%), and Heavy metals (not more than 0.002%).

Caution: Great care should be taken in handling Cyclophosphamide, as it is a potent cytotoxic agent.

Cyclophosphamide for Injection USP—Preserve in Containers for Sterile Solids. Storage at a temperature not exceeding 25 °C is recommended. It will withstand brief exposure to temperatures up to 30 °C, but is to be protected from temperatures above 30 °C. A sterile mixture of Cyclophosphamide with or without a suitable diluent. Contains the labeled amount of anhydrous cyclophosphamide, within ±10%. Meets the requirements for Constituted solution, Identification, Bacterial endotoxins, and pH (3.0–9.0, the range not exceeding 3 pH units, in a solution containing the equivalent of 20 mg of anhydrous cyclophosphamide per mL), and for Sterility tests, Uniformity of dosage units, and Labeling under Injections.

Cyclophosphamide Oral Solution—Not in *USP–NF*.

Cyclophosphamide Tablets USP—Preserve in tight containers. Storage at a temperature not exceeding 25 °C is recommended. Tablets will withstand brief exposure to temperatures up to 30 °C, but are to be protected from temperatures above 30 °C. Contain the labeled amount of anhydrous cyclophosphamide, within ±10%. Meet the requirements for Identification, Disintegration (30 minutes, determined as directed under Uncoated Tablets), and Uniformity of dosage units.

CYCLOPROPANE

Chemical name: Cyclopropane.

Molecular formula: C_3H_6.

Molecular weight: 42.08.

Description: Cyclopropane USP—Colorless gas having a characteristic odor. One liter at a pressure of 760 millimeters and a temperature of 0 °C weighs about 1.88 grams.

Solubility: Cyclopropane USP—One volume dissolves in about 2.7 volumes of water at 15 °C. Freely soluble in alcohol; soluble in fixed oils.

USP requirements: Cyclopropane USP—Preserve in cylinders. The label bears a warning that cyclopropane is highly flammable and is not to be used where it may be ignited. Contains not less than 99.0%, by volume, of cyclopropane. Meets the requirements for Acidity or alkalinity, Carbon dioxide (not more than 0.03%), Halogens (not more than 0.02% as chloride), and Propylene, allene, and other unsaturated hydrocarbons.

Caution: Cyclopropane is highly flammable. Do not use where it may be ignited.

CYCLOSERINE

Source: Produced by a strain of *Streptomyces orchidaceus*; has also been synthesized.

Chemical name: 3-Isoxazolidinone, 4-amino-, (R)-.

Molecular formula: $C_3H_6N_2O_2$.

Molecular weight: 102.09.

Description: Cycloserine USP—White to pale yellow, crystalline powder. Is odorless or has a faint odor. Is hygroscopic and deteriorates upon absorbing water. Its solutions are dextrorotatory.

Solubility: Cycloserine USP—Freely soluble in water.

Other characteristics: Stable in alkaline solution, but rapidly destroyed at neutral or acid pH.

USP requirements:
Cycloserine USP—Preserve in tight containers. Has a potency of not less than 900 mcg of cycloserine per mg. Meets the requirements for Identification, Specific rotation (108° to 114°), Crystallinity, pH (5.5–6.5, in a solution [1 in 10]), Loss on drying (not more than 1.0%), Residue on ignition (not more than 0.5%), and Condensation products.

Cycloserine Capsules USP—Preserve in tight containers. Contain the labeled amount, within −10% to +20%. Meet the requirements for Identification, Dissolution (80% in 30 minutes in phosphate buffer [pH 6.8], in Apparatus 1 at 100 rpm), Uniformity of dosage units, and Loss on drying (not more than 1.0%).

CYCLOSPORINE

Chemical name: Cyclosporin A.

Molecular formula: $C_{62}H_{111}N_{11}O_{12}$.

Molecular weight: 1202.61.

Description: Cyclosporine USP—White to almost-white powder.

Solubility: Cyclosporine USP—Soluble in acetone, in alcohol, in methanol, in ether, in chloroform, and in methylene chloride; slightly soluble in saturated hydrocarbons; practically insoluble in water.

Other characteristics: Lipophilic; hydrophobic.

USP requirements:
> Cyclosporine USP—Preserve in tight, light-resistant containers. Contains not less than 98.5% and not more than 101.5% of cyclosporine A, calculated on the dried basis. Meets the requirements for Identification, Loss on drying (not more than 2.0%), Heavy metals (not more than 0.002%), and Related compounds.
> Cyclosporine Capsules USP—Preserve in tight containers, and store at controlled room temperture. Contain the labeled amount, within ±10%. Meet the requirements for Identification, Dissolution (in 15 minutes in Water in Apparatus 2 at 50 rpm, where capsules contain liquid, and 80% in 90 minutes in 0.1 N hydrochloric acid containing 0.5% of sodium lauryl sulfate in Apparatus 1 at 150 rpm, where capsules contain powder), Uniformity of dosage units, and Water (for Capsules that contain powder, not more than 3.5%).
> Cyclosporine Modified Capsules—Not in *USP–NF*.
> Cyclosporine Injection USP—Preserve in single-dose or in multiple-dose containers. A sterile solution of Cyclosporine in a suitable vehicle. Label it to indicate that it is to be diluted with a suitable parenteral vehicle prior to intravenous infusion. Contains the labeled amount, within ±10%. Meets the requirements for Identification, Bacterial endotoxins (not more than 0.84 USP Endotoxin Unit per mg of cyclosporine), Sterility, and Alcohol content (where present, the labeled amount, within ±20%).
> Cyclosporine Ophthalmic Ointment—Not in *USP–NF*.
> Cyclosporine Oral Solution USP—Preserve in tight containers. A solution of Cyclosporine in a suitable vehicle. Contains the labeled amount, within ±10%. Meets the requirements for Identification and Alcohol content (where present, the labeled amount, within ±20%).
> Cyclosporine Modified Oral Solution—Not in *USP–NF*.

CYCLOTHIAZIDE

Chemical name: 2*H*-1,2,4-Benzothiadiazine-7-sulfonamide, 3-bicyclo[2.2.1]hept-5-en-2-yl-6-chloro-3,4-dihydro-, 1,1-dioxide.

Molecular formula: $C_{14}H_{16}ClN_3O_4S_2$.

Molecular weight: 389.88.

Description: White, crystalline solid. It has a melting point of approximately 220 °C.

pKa: 10.7 in water.

Solubility: Moderately soluble in hot ethyl alcohol and in hot dilute alcohol; very soluble in cold ethyl acetate (an ethyl acetate solvate is formed); relatively insoluble in ether and in chloroform.

USP requirements: Cyclothiazide Tablets—Not in *USP–NF*.

CYPROHEPTADINE

Chemical group: Piperidine derivative.

Chemical name: Cyproheptadine hydrochloride—Piperidine, 4-(5*H*-dibenzo[*a,d*]-cyclohepten-5-ylidene)-1-methyl-, hydrochloride, sesquihydrate.

Molecular formula: Cyproheptadine hydrochloride—$C_{21}H_{21}N \cdot HCl \cdot 1\frac{1}{2}H_2O$.

Molecular weight: Cyproheptadine hydrochloride—350.88.

Description: Cyproheptadine Hydrochloride USP—White to slightly yellow, odorless or practically odorless, crystalline powder.

pKa: 9.3.

Solubility: Cyproheptadine Hydrochloride USP—Slightly soluble in water; freely soluble in methanol; soluble in chloroform; sparingly soluble in alcohol; practically insoluble in ether.

USP requirements:
> Cyproheptadine Hydrochloride USP—Preserve in well-closed containers. Contains not less than 98.5% and not more than 100.5% of cyproheptadine hydrochloride, calculated on the anhydrous basis. Meets the requirements for Identification, Acidity, Water (7.0–9.0%), Residue on ignition (not more than 0.1%), Heavy metals (not more than 0.003%), and Organic volatile impurities.
> Cyproheptadine Hydrochloride Oral Solution USP—Preserve in tight containers. Contains the labeled amount, within ±10%. Meets the requirements for Identification and pH (3.5–4.5).
> Cyproheptadine Hydrochloride Syrup USP—Preserve in tight containers. Contains the labeled amount, within ±10%. Meets the requirements for Identification and pH (3.5–4.5).
> Cyproheptadine Hydrochloride Tablets USP—Preserve in well-closed containers. Contain the labeled amount, within ±10%. Meet the requirements for Identification, Dissolution (80% in 30 minutes in 0.01 N hydrochloric acid in Apparatus 2 at 50 rpm), and Uniformity of dosage units.

CYPROTERONE

Chemical name: Cyproterone acetate—3′*H*-Cyclopropa[1,2]-pregna-1,4,6-triene-3,20-dione, 17-(acetyloxy)-6-chloro-1,2-dihydro-, (1 beta,2 beta)-.

Molecular formula: Cyproterone acetate—$C_{24}H_{29}ClO_4$.

Molecular weight: Cyproterone acetate—416.94.

Description: Cyproterone acetate—White crystals melting at about 200 °C.

USP requirements:
> Cyproterone Acetate Injection—Not in *USP–NF*.
> Cyproterone Acetate Tablets—Not in *USP–NF*.

CYSTEAMINE

Molecular formula: Cysteamine bitartrate—$C_2H_7NS \cdot C_4H_6O_6$.

Molecular weight: Cysteamine bitartrate—227.

Description: Cysteamine bitartrate—White powder.

Solubility: Cysteamine bitartrate—Highly soluble in water.

USP requirements: Cysteamine Bitartrate Capsules—Not in *USP–NF*.

CYSTEINE

Chemical name: Cysteine hydrochloride—L-Cysteine hydrochloride monohydrate.

Molecular formula: Cysteine hydrochloride—$C_3H_7NO_2S \cdot HCl \cdot H_2O$.

Molecular weight: Cysteine hydrochloride—175.64.

Description: Cysteine Hydrochloride USP—White crystals or crystalline powder.

Solubility: Cysteine Hydrochloride USP—Soluble in water, in alcohol, and in acetone.

USP requirements:
Cysteine Hydrochloride USP—Preserve in well-closed containers. Contains not less than 98.5% and not more than 101.5% of cysteine hydrochloride, as L-cysteine hydrochloride, calculated on the dried basis. Meets the requirements for Identification, Specific rotation ($+5.7°$ to $+6.8°$), Loss on drying (8.0–12.0%), Residue on ignition (not more than 0.4%), Sulfate (not more than 0.03%), Iron (not more than 0.003%), Heavy metals (not more than 0.0015%), Chromatographic purity, and Organic volatile impurities.
Cysteine Hydrochloride Injection USP—Preserve in single-dose or in multiple-dose containers, preferably of Type I glass. A sterile solution of Cysteine Hydrochloride in Water for Injection. Contains the labeled amount, within ±15%. Meets the requirements for Identification, Bacterial endotoxins, pH (1.0–2.5), and Heavy metals (not more than 2 ppm), and for Injections.

CYTARABINE

Chemical name: 2(1*H*)-Pyrimidinone, 4-amino-1-beta-D-arabinofuranosyl-.

Molecular formula: $C_9H_{13}N_3O_5$.

Molecular weight: 243.22.

Description: Cytarabine USP—Odorless, white to off-white, crystalline powder.

pKa: 4.35.

Solubility: Cytarabine USP—Freely soluble in water; slightly soluble in alcohol and in chloroform.

USP requirements:
Cytarabine USP—Preserve in well-closed, light-resistant containers. Where it is intended for use in preparing injectable dosage forms, the label states that it is sterile or must be subjected to further processing during the preparation of injectable dosage forms. Contains not less than 98.0% and not more than 102.0% of cytarabine, calculated on the dried basis. Meets the requirements for Identification, Specific rotation ($+154°$ to $+160°$), Loss on drying (not more than 1.0%), Residue on ignition (not more than 0.5%), Heavy metals (not more than 0.001%), and Chromatographic purity, for Sterility and Bacterial endotoxins under Cytarabine for Injection (where the label states that Cytarabine is sterile), and for Bacterial endotoxins under Cytarabine for Injection (where the label states that Cytarabine must be subjected to further processing during the preparation of injectable dosage forms).
Liposomal Cytarabine Injection—Not in *USP–NF*.
Cytarabine for Injection USP—Preserve in Containers for Sterile Solids. Contains the labeled amount, within ± 10%. Meets the requirements for Constituted solution, Identification, Bacterial endotoxins, pH (4.0–6.0, in a solution containing the equivalent of 10 mg of cytarabine per mL), and Water (not more than 3.0%), and for Sterility

tests, Uniformity of dosage units, and Labeling under Injections. The drug substance in the vial meets the requirements for Cytarabine.

DACARBAZINE

Chemical name: 1*H*-Imidazole-4-carboxamide, 5-(3,3-dimethyl-1-triazenyl)-.

Molecular formula: $C_6H_{10}N_6O$.

Molecular weight: 182.18.

Description: Colorless to ivory colored solid which is light sensitive.

pKa: 4.42.

Solubility: Slightly soluble in water and in alcohol.

USP requirements:
Dacarbazine USP—Preserve in tight, light-resistant containers, in a refrigerator. Contains not less than 97.0% and not more than 102.0% of dacarbazine. Meets the requirements for Identification, Residue on ignition (not more than 0.1%), and Related compounds.
Caution: Great care should be taken in handling Dacarbazine, as it is a potent cytotoxic agent.
Dacarbazine for Injection USP—Preserve in single-dose or in multiple-dose Containers for Sterile Solids, preferably of Type I glass, protected from light. A sterile, freeze-dried mixture of Dacarbazine and suitable buffers or diluents. Contains the labeled amount, within ±10%. Meets the requirements for Completeness of solution, Constituted solution, Identification, Bacterial endotoxins, pH (3.0–4.0), Water (not more than 1.5%), and Limit of 2-azahypoxanthine (not more than 1.0%), and for Sterility tests, Uniformity of dosage units, and Labeling under Injections.
Caution: Great care should be taken to prevent inhaling particles of Dacarbazine for Injection and exposing the skin to it.

DACLIZUMAB

Chemical name: Immunoglobulin G 1 (human-mouse monoclonal clone 1H4 gamma-chain anti-human interleukin 2 receptor), disulfide with human-mouse monoclonal clone 1H4 light chain, dimer.

Molecular formula: $C_{6394}H_{9888}N_{1696}O_{2012}S_{44}$(protein moiety).

Molecular weight: Approximately 150,000 daltons.

USP requirements: Daclizumab Concentrate for Injection—Not in *USP–NF*.

DACTINOMYCIN

Source: An actinomycin derived from a mixture of actinomycins produced by *Streptomyces parvullus*.

Chemical name: Actinomycin D. Specific stereoisomer of *N,N'*-[(2-amino-4,6-dimethyl-3-oxo-3*H*-phenoxazine-1,9-diyl)bis[carbonylimino(2-hydroxypropylidene)carbonyliminoisobutylidenecarbonyl-1,2-pyrrolidinediylcarbonyl(methylimino)methylenecarbonyl]]bis[*N*-methyl-L-valine] dilactone.

Molecular formula: $C_{62}H_{86}N_{12}O_{16}$.

Molecular weight: 1255.42.

Description: Dactinomycin USP—Bright red, crystalline powder. Is somewhat hygroscopic and is affected by light and heat.

Solubility: Dactinomycin USP—Soluble in water at 10 °C and slightly soluble in water at 37 °C; freely soluble in alcohol; very slightly soluble in ether.

USP requirements:
Dactinomycin USP—Preserve in tight containers, protected from light and excessive heat. Contains not less than 950 mcg and not more than 1030 mcg of dactinomycin per mg, calculated on the dried basis. Meets the requirements for Identification, Specific rotation (−292° to −317°), Crystallinity, Bacterial endotoxins, and Loss on drying (not more than 5.0%).

    Caution: Great care should be taken to prevent inhaling particles of Dactinomycin and exposing the skin to it.
Dactinomycin for Injection USP—Preserve in light-resistant Containers for Sterile Solids. A sterile mixture of Dactinomycin and Mannitol. Label it to include the statement, "Protect from light." Contains the labeled amount, within −10% to +20%, the labeled amount being 0.5 mg in each container. Meets the requirements for Constituted solution, Identification, Bacterial endotoxins, Sterility, pH (5.5–7.5, in the solution constituted as directed in the labeling), and Loss on drying (not more than 4.0%), and for Injections.

    Caution: Great care should be taken to prevent inhaling particles of Dactinomycin and exposing the skin to it.

DALTEPARIN

Source: Dalteparin sodium—Sodium salt of depolymerized heparin obtained by nitrous acid degradation of heparin from pork intestinal mucosa.

Molecular weight: 5,000 (average).

USP requirements: Dalteparin Sodium Injection—Not in *USP–NF*.

DANAPAROID

Source: Danaparoid sodium—Mixture of the sodium salts of heparin sulfate, dermatan sulfate, and chondroitin sulfate. Isolated from porcine intestinal mucosa.

Molecular weight: Danaparoid sodium—Approximately 5500 daltons.

USP requirements: Danaparoid Sodium Injection—Not in *USP–NF*.

DANAZOL

Chemical name: Pregna-2,4-dien-20-yno[2,3-*d*]isoxazol-17-ol, (17 alpha)-.

Molecular formula: $C_{22}H_{27}NO_2$.

Molecular weight: 337.46.

Description: Danazol USP—White to pale yellow, crystalline powder. Melts at about 225 °C, with some decomposition.

Solubility: Danazol USP—Practically insoluble or insoluble in water and in hexane; freely soluble in chloroform; soluble in acetone; sparingly soluble in alcohol; slightly soluble in ether.

USP requirements:
Danazol USP—Preserve in tight, light-resistant containers. Contains not less than 97.0% and not more than 102.0% of danazol, calculated on the dried basis. Meets the requirements for Identification, Specific rotation (+21° to +27°), Loss on drying (not more than 2.0%), Chromatographic purity, and Organic volatile impurities.
Danazol Capsules USP—Preserve in well-closed containers. Contain the labeled amount, within ±10%. Meet the requirements for Identification, Dissolution (75% in 30 minutes in 0.75% sodium lauryl sulfate solution in Apparatus 2 at 75 rpm), and Uniformity of dosage units.

DANTHRON AND DOCUSATE

Chemical group:
Danthron—Anthraquinones.
Docusate—Surfactants, anionic.

Chemical name:
Danthron—9,10-Anthracenedione, 1,8-dihydroxy-.
Docusate sodium—Butanedioic acid, sulfo-, 1,4-bis(2-ethylhexyl) ester, sodium salt.

Molecular formula:
Danthron—$C_{14}H_8O_4$.
Docusate sodium—$C_{20}H_{37}NaO_7S$.

Molecular weight:
Danthron—240.21.
Docusate sodium—444.56.

Description:
Danthron—Orange, odorless or almost odorless, crystalline powder.
Docusate Sodium USP—White, wax-like, plastic solid, having a characteristic odor suggestive of octyl alcohol, but no odor of other solvents.
    NF category: Wetting and/or solubilizing agent.

Solubility:
Danthron—Practically insoluble in water; very slightly soluble in alcohol; soluble in chloroform; slightly soluble in ether; dissolves in solutions of alkali hydroxides.
Docusate Sodium USP—Sparingly soluble in water; very soluble in solvent hexane; freely soluble in alcohol and in glycerin.

USP requirements:
Danthron and Docusate Sodium Capsules—Not in *USP–NF*.
Danthron and Docusate Sodium Tablets—Not in *USP–NF*.

DANTROLENE

Chemical name: Dantrolene sodium—2,4-Imidazolidinedione, 1-[[[5-(4-nitrophenyl)-2-furanyl]methylene]amino]-, sodium salt, hydrate (2:7).

Molecular formula: Dantrolene sodium—$C_{14}H_9N_4NaO_5 \cdot 3\frac{1}{2}H_2O$.

Molecular weight: Dantrolene sodium—399.29.

Description: Dantrolene sodium—Orange powder.

Solubility: Dantrolene sodium—Slightly soluble in water, but due to its slightly acidic nature the solubility increases somewhat in alkaline solution.

USP requirements:
   Dantrolene Sodium Capsules—Not in *USP–NF*.
   Dantrolene Sodium for Injection—Not in *USP–NF*.

DAPIPRAZOLE

Chemical name: Dapiprazole hydrochloride—1,2,4-Triazolo[4,3-*a*]pyridine, 5,6,7,8-tetrahydro-3-[2-[4-(2-methylphenyl)1-piperazinyl]ethyl]-, monohydrochloride.

Molecular formula: Dapiprazole hydrochloride—$C_{19}H_{27}N_5 \cdot HCl$.

Molecular weight: Dapiprazole hydrochloride—361.91.

Description: Dapiprazole hydrochloride—Sterile, white, lyophilized powder.

Solubility: Dapiprazole hydrochloride—Soluble in water.

USP requirements: Dapiprazole Hydrochloride for Ophthalmic Solution—Not in *USP–NF*.

DAPSONE

Chemical group: Sulfone.

Chemical name: Benzenamine, 4,4'-sulfonylbis-.

Molecular formula: $C_{12}H_{12}N_2O_2S$.

Molecular weight: 248.30.

Description: Dapsone USP—White or creamy white, crystalline powder. Is odorless.

Solubility: Dapsone USP—Very slightly soluble in water; freely soluble in alcohol; soluble in acetone and in dilute mineral acids.

USP requirements:
   Dapsone USP—Preserve in well-closed, light-resistant containers. Contains not less than 98.0% and not more than 102.0% of dapsone, calculated on the dried basis. Meets the requirements for Identification, Melting range (175–181 °C), Loss on drying (not more than 1.5%), Residue on ignition (not more than 0.1%), Selenium (not more than 0.003%), Chromatographic purity, and Organic volatile impurities.
   Dapsone Tablets USP—Preserve in well-closed, light-resistant containers. Contain the labeled amount, within ± 7.5%. Meet the requirements for Identification, Dissolution (75% in 60 minutes in dilute hydrochloric acid [2 in 100] in Apparatus 1 at 100 rpm), and Uniformity of dosage units.

DARBEPOETIN ALFA

Chemical name: Erythropoietin [30-asparagine, 32-threonine, 87-valine, 88-asparagine, 90-threonine] (haman).

Molecular formula: $C_{800}H_{1300}N_{228}O_{224}S_5$.

Molecular weight: 18,174 daltons.

Other characteristics: pH: Albumin solution—6±0.3; Polysorbate solution—6.2±0.2.

USP requirements: Darbepoetin Alfa Injection—Not in *USP–NF*.

DAUNORUBICIN

Source: Daunorubicin hydrochloride—An anthracycline produced by *Streptomyces coeruleorubidus or S. peucetius*.

Chemical name: Daunorubicin hydrochloride—5,12-Naphthacenedione, 8-acetyl-10-[(3-amino-2,3,6-trideoxy-alpha-L-*lyxo*-hexopyranosyl)]oxy]-7,8,9,10-tetrahydro-6,8,11-trihydroxy-1-methoxy-, (8*S-cis*)-, hydrochloride.

Molecular formula: Daunorubicin hydrochloride—$C_{27}H_{29}NO_{10} \cdot HCl$.

Molecular weight: Daunorubicin hydrochloride—563.98.

Description: Daunorubicin Hydrochloride USP—Orange-red, crystalline, hygroscopic powder.

pKa: Daunorubicin hydrochloride—10.3.

Solubility: Daunorubicin Hydrochloride USP—Freely soluble in water and in methanol; slightly soluble in alcohol; very slightly soluble in chloroform; practically insoluble in acetone.

USP requirements:
   Daunorubicin Citrate, Liposomal, Injection—Not in *USP–NF*.
   Daunorubicin Hydrochloride USP—Preserve in tight containers, protected from light and excessive heat. Has a potency equivalent to not less than 842 mcg and not more than 1030 mcg of daunorubicin per mg. Meets the requirements for Identification, Crystallinity, pH (4.5–6.5, in a solution containing 5 mg per mL), and Water (not more than 3.0%).
      Caution: Great care should be taken to prevent inhaling particles of daunorubicin hydrochloride and exposing the skin to it.
   Daunorubicin Hydrochloride for Injection USP—Preserve in light-resistant Containers for Sterile Solids. A sterile mixture of Daunorubicin Hydrochloride and Mannitol. Contains an amount of daunorubicin hydrochloride equivalent to the labeled amount of daunorubicin, within –10% to +15%. Meets the requirements for Constituted solution, Identification, Bacterial endotoxins, pH (4.5–6.5, in the solution constituted as directed in the labeling), and Water (not more than 3.0%), and for Injections.

DEBRISOQUIN

Chemical name: Debrisoquin sulfate—2(1*H*)-Isoquinolinecarboximidamide, 3,4-dihydro-, sulfate (2:1).

Molecular formula: Debrisoquin sulfate—$(C_{10}H_{13}N_3)_2 \cdot H_2SO_4$.

Molecular weight: Debrisoquin sulfate—448.54.

Description: Debrisoquin sulfate—White odorless or almost odorless crystalline powder.

Solubility: Debrisoquin sulfate—Soluble 1 in 40 of water; very slightly soluble in alcohol; almost insoluble in chloroform and in ether.

USP requirements: Debrisoquin Sulfate Tablets—Not in *USP–NF*.

DECOQUINATE

Chemical name: 3-Quinolinecarboxylic acid, 6-(decyloxy)-7-ethoxy-4-hydroxy-, ethyl ester.

Molecular formula: $C_{24}H_{35}NO_5$.

Molecular weight: 417.54.

Description: Cream to buff-colored, odorless or almost odorless, microcrystalline powder.

Solubility: Insoluble in water; practically insoluble in alcohol; very slightly soluble in chloroform and in ether.

USP requirements:

Decoquinate USP—Preserve in tight containers. Label it to indicate that it is for veterinary use only. Contains not less than 99.0% and not more than 101.0% of decoquinate, calculated on the dried basis. Meets the requirements for Identification, Loss on drying (not more than 0.5%), Residue on ignition (not more than 0.1%), and Ordinary impurities.

Decoquinate Premix USP—Preserve in well-closed containers. Label it to indicate that it is for veterinary use only. Contains the labeled amount, within ±10%, the labeled amount being between 1 gram and 10 grams per 100 grams of Premix. Meets the requirement for Identification.

DEFEROXAMINE

Source: Isolated as the iron chelate from *Streptomyces pilosus* and treated chemically to obtain the metal-free ligand.

Chemical name: Deferoxamine mesylate—Butanediamide, *N*-[5-[[4-[[5-(acetylhydroxyamino)pentyl]amino]-1,4-dioxobutyl]-hydroxyamino]pentyl]-*N*-(5-aminopentyl)-*N*-hydroxy-, monomethanesulfonate.

Molecular formula: Deferoxamine mesylate—$C_{25}H_{48}N_6O_8 \cdot CH_4O_3S$.

Molecular weight: Deferoxamine mesylate—656.79.

Description: Deferoxamine Mesylate USP—White to off-white powder.

Solubility: Deferoxamine Mesylate USP—Freely soluble in water; slightly soluble in methanol.

USP requirements:

Deferoxamine Mesylate USP—Preserve in tight containers. Where it is intended for use in preparing injectable dosage forms, the label states that it is sterile or must be subjected to further processing during the preparation of injectable dosage forms. Contains not less than 98.0% and not more than 102.0% of deferoxamine mesylate, calculated on the anhydrous basis. Meets the requirements for Identification, pH (4.0–6.0, in a solution [1 in 100]), Water (not more than 2.0%), Residue on ignition (not more than 0.1%, 2.0 grams being used for the test), Chloride (not more than 0.012%), Sulfate (not more than 0.04%), and Heavy metals (not more than 0.001%), for Sterility and Labeling under Injections, and Bacterial endotoxins under Deferoxamine Mesylate for Injection (where the label states that Deferoxamine Mesylate is sterile), and for Bacterial endotoxins under Deferoxamine Mesylate for Injection (where the label states that Deferoxamine Mesylate must be subjected to further processing during the preparation of injectable dosage forms).

Deferoxamine Mesylate for Injection USP—Preserve in single-dose or in multiple-dose containers, preferably of Type I glass. It is Deferoxamine Mesylate suitable for parenteral use. Contains the labeled amount, within ±10%. Meets the requirements for Constituted solution, Identification, pH (4.0–6.0, in a solution [1 in 100]), Bacterial endotoxins, and Water (not more than 1.5%), and for Injections and Uniformity of dosage units.

DEHYDROCHOLIC ACID

Source: Oxidized bile acid produced from the main constituent of ox bile, cholic acid.

Chemical name: Cholan-24-oic acid, 3,7,12-trioxo-, (5 beta)-.

Molecular formula: $C_{24}H_{34}O_5$.

Molecular weight: 402.52.

Description: Dehydrocholic Acid USP—White, fluffy, odorless powder.

Solubility: Dehydrocholic Acid USP—Practically insoluble in water; soluble in glacial acetic acid and in solutions of alkali hydroxides and carbonates; slightly soluble in alcohol and in ether; sparingly soluble in chloroform (the solutions in alcohol and in chloroform usually are slightly turbid).

USP requirements:

Dehydrocholic Acid USP—Preserve in well-closed containers. Contains not less than 98.5% and not more than 101.0% of dehydrocholic acid, calculated on the dried basis. Dehydrocholic Acid for parenteral use melts between 237 and 242 °C. Meets the requirements for Identification, Melting range (231–242 °C, not more than 3 °C between beginning and end of melting), Specific rotation (+29.0° to +32.5°), Loss on drying (not more than 1.0%), Residue on ignition (not more than 0.3%), Odor on boiling, Barium, Heavy metals (not more than 0.002%), and Organic volatile impurities.

Dehydrocholic Acid Tablets USP—Preserve in well-closed containers. Contain the labeled amount, within ±6%. Meet the requirements for Identification, Microbial limits, Disintegration (30 minutes), and Uniformity of dosage units.

DEHYDROCHOLIC ACID AND DOCUSATE

For *Dehydrocholic Acid* and *Docusate*—See individual listings for chemistry information.

USP requirements:

Dehydrocholic Acid and Docusate Sodium Capsules—Not in *USP–NF*.

Dehydrocholic Acid and Docusate Sodium Tablets—Not in *USP–NF*.

DEHYDROCHOLIC ACID, DOCUSATE, AND PHENOLPHTHALEIN

For *Dehydrocholic Acid, Docusate,* and *Phenolphthalein*—See individual listings for chemistry information.

USP requirements: Dehydrocholic Acid, Docusate Sodium, and Phenolphthalein Capsules—Not in *USP–NF*.

DELAVIRDINE

Chemical name: Delavirdine mesylate—Piperazine, 1-[3-[(1-methylethyl)amino]-2-pyridinyl]-4-[[5-[(methylsulfonyl)amino]-1*H*-indol-2-yl]carbonyl], monomethanesulfonate.

Molecular formula: Delavirdine mesylate—$C_{22}H_{28}N_6O_3S \cdot CH_4O_3S$.

Molecular weight: Delavirdine mesylate—552.67.

Description: Delavirdine mesylate—Odorless, white to tan crystalline powder.

DEMECARIUM

Chemical name: Demecarium bromide—Benzenaminium, 3,3′-[1,10-decanediylbis [(methylimino)carbonyloxy]]bis[*N,N,N*trimethyl-, dibromide.

Molecular formula: Demecarium bromide—$C_{32}H_{52}Br_2N_4O_4$.

Molecular weight: Demecarium bromide—716.59.

Description: Demecarium Bromide USP—White or slightly yellow, slightly hygroscopic, crystalline powder.

Solubility: Demecarium Bromide USP—Freely soluble in water and in alcohol; soluble in ether; sparingly soluble in acetone.

USP requirements:
Demecarium Bromide USP—Preserve in tight, light-resistant containers. Contains not less than 95.0% and not more than 100.5% of demecarium bromide, calculated on the anhydrous basis. Meets the requirements for Identification, pH (5.0–7.0, in a solution [1 in 100]), Water (not more than 2.0%), Residue on ignition (not more than 0.1%), Heavy metals (not more than 0.002%), and Limit of *m*-trimethylammoniophenol bromide.
Demecarium Bromide Ophthalmic Solution USP—Preserve in tight, light-resistant containers. A sterile, aqueous solution of Demecarium Bromide. Contains the labeled amount, within ±8%. Contains a suitable antimicrobial agent. Meets the requirements for Identification and Sterility.

DEMECLOCYCLINE

Chemical name:
Demeclocycline—2-Naphthacenecarboxamide, 7-chloro-4-(dimethylamino)-1,4,4a,5,5a,6,11,12a-octahydro-3,6,10,12,12a-pentahydroxy-1,11-dioxo-, [4*S*-(4 alpha,4a alpha,5a alpha,6 beta,12a alpha)]-.
Demeclocycline hydrochloride—2-Naphthacenecarboxamide, 7-chloro-4-(dimethylamino)-1,4,4a,5,5a,6,11,12a-octahydro-3,6,10,12,12a-pentahydroxy-1,11-dioxo-, monohydrochloride, [4*S*-(4 alpha,4a alpha,5a alpha,6 beta,12a alpha)]-.

Molecular formula:
Demeclocycline—$C_{21}H_{21}ClN_2O_8$.
Demeclocycline hydrochloride—$C_{21}H_{21}ClN_2O_8 \cdot HCl$.

Molecular weight:
Demeclocycline—464.85.
Demeclocycline hydrochloride—501.31.

Description:
Demeclocycline USP—Yellow, crystalline odorless powder.
Demeclocycline Hydrochloride USP—Yellow, crystalline, odorless powder.

Solubility:
Demeclocycline USP—Sparingly soluble in water; soluble in alcohol. Dissolves readily in 3 *N* hydrochloric acid and in alkaline solutions.
Demeclocycline Hydrochloride USP—Sparingly soluble in water and in solutions of alkali hydroxides and carbonates; slightly soluble in alcohol; practically insoluble in acetone and in chloroform.

USP requirements:
Demeclocycline USP—Preserve in tight, light-resistant containers. Has a potency equivalent to not less than 970 mcg of demeclocycline hydrochloride per mg, calculated on the anhydrous basis. Meets the requirements for Identification, Crystallinity, pH (4.0–5.5, in a solution containing 10 mg per mL), and Water (4.3–6.7%).
Demeclocycline Oral Suspension USP—Preserve in tight containers, protected from light. Contains the equivalent of the labeled amount of demeclocycline hydrochloride, within −10% to +25%. Meets the requirements for Identification and pH (4.0–5.8).
Demeclocycline Hydrochloride USP—Preserve in tight, light-resistant containers. Has a potency of not less than 900 mcg of demeclocycline hydrochloride per mg, calculated on the dried basis. Meets the requirements for Identification, Crystallinity, pH (2.0–3.0, in a solution containing 10 mg per mL), and Loss on drying (not more than 2.0%).
Demeclocycline Hydrochloride Capsules USP—Preserve in tight, light-resistant containers. Contain the labeled amount, within −10% to +25%. Meet the requirements for Identification, Dissolution (75% in 45 minutes in water in Apparatus 2 at 75 rpm), Uniformity of dosage units, and Loss on drying (not more than 2.0%; not more than 8.0% if the Capsules contain starch).
Demeclocycline Hydrochloride Tablets USP—Preserve in tight, light-resistant containers. Contain the labeled amount, within −10% to +25%. Meet the requirements for Identification, Dissolution (75% in 45 minutes in water in Apparatus 2 at 75 rpm), Uniformity of dosage units, and Loss on drying (not more than 2.0%).

DEMECLOCYCLINE AND NYSTATIN

For *Demeclocycline* and *Nystatin*—See individual listings for chemistry information.

USP requirements:
Demeclocycline Hydrochloride and Nystatin Capsules USP—Preserve in tight, light-resistant containers. Contain the labeled amounts of demeclocycline hydrochloride, within −10% to +25%, and USP Nystatin Units, within −10% to +35%. Meet the requirements for Identification, Dissolution (75% of the labeled amount of demeclocycline hydrochloride in 45 minutes in water in Apparatus 2 at 75 rpm), and Loss on drying (not more than 5.0%).
Demeclocycline Hydrochloride and Nystatin Tablets USP—Preserve in tight, light-resistant containers. Contain the labeled amounts of demeclocycline hydrochloride, within −10% to +25%, and USP Nystatin Units, within −10% to +35%. Meet the requirements for Identification, Dissolution (75% of the labeled amount of demeclocycline hydrochloride in 45 minutes in water in Apparatus 2 at 75 rpm), and Loss on drying (not more than 4.0%).

DENATONIUM BENZOATE

Chemical name: Benzenemethanaminium, *N*-[2-[(2,6-dimethylphenyl)amino]-2-oxoethyl]-*N,N*-diethyl-, benzoate, monohydrate.

Molecular formula: $C_{28}H_{34}N_2O_3 \cdot H_2O$ (hydrous).

Molecular weight: 464.60 (hydrous); 446.59 (anhydrous).

Description: Denatonium Benzoate NF—NF category: Alcohol denaturant.

Solubility: Denatonium Benzoate NF—Freely soluble in water and in alcohol; very soluble in chloroform and in methanol; very slightly soluble in ether.

NF requirements: Denatonium Benzoate NF—Preserve in tight containers. Dried at 105 °C for 2 hours, contains one molecule of water of hydration, or is anhydrous. Label it to indicate

whether it is hydrous or anhydrous. When dried at 105 °C for 2 hours, contains not less than 99.5% and not more than 101.0% of denatonium benzoate. Meets the requirements for Identification, Melting range (163–170 °C, on a dried specimen), pH (6.5–7.5, in a solution [3 in 100]), Loss on drying (not more than 1.0%), Residue on ignition (not more than 0.1%), and Chloride (not more than 0.2%).

DENILEUKIN DIFTITOX

Source: Produced in an *E. coli* expression system.

Chemical name: *N*-L-Methionyl-387-L-histidine-388-L-alanine-1-388-toxin (*Corynebacterium diphtheriae* strain C7) (388→2′) protein with 2-133-interleukin 2 (human clone pTIL2-21a).

Molecular formula: $C_{2560}H_{4038}N_{678}O_{799}S_{17}$.

Molecular weight: 57642.67.

USP requirements: Denileukin Diftitox Injection—Not in *USP–NF*.

DESERPIDINE

Source: Alkaloid from *Rauwolfia canescens*.

Chemical name: Methyl 17 alpha-methoxy-18 beta-[(3,4,5-trimethoxybenzoyl)oxy]-3 beta,20 alpha-yohimban-16 beta-carboxylate.

Molecular formula: $C_{32}H_{38}N_2O_8$.

Molecular weight: 578.65.

Description: White to light yellow, crystalline powder.

pKa: 5.67.

Solubility: Insoluble in water; slightly soluble in alcohol.

USP requirements: Deserpidine Tablets—Not in *USP–NF*.

DESERPIDINE AND HYDROCHLOROTHIAZIDE

For *Deserpidine* and *Hydrochlorothiazide*—See individual listings for chemistry information.

USP requirements: Deserpidine and Hydrochlorothiazide Tablets—Not in *USP–NF*.

DESERPIDINE AND METHYCLOTHIAZIDE

For *Deserpidine* and *Methyclothiazide*—See individual listings for chemistry information.

USP requirements: Deserpidine and Methyclothiazide Tablets—Not in *USP–NF*.

DESFLURANE

Chemical name: Ethane, 2-(difluoromethoxy)-1,1,1,2-tetrafluoro-, (±)-.

Molecular formula: $C_3H_2F_6O$.

Molecular weight: 168.04.

USP requirements: Desflurane USP—Preserve in tight, light-resistant containers. Contains not less than 98.0% and not more than 102.0% of desflurane. Meets the requirements for Identification, Limit of nonvolatile residue (not more than 0.075%), Limit of antimony (not more than 3 mcg per gram), Limit of fluoride (not more than 0.001%), and Related compounds.

DESIPRAMINE

Chemical group: Dibenzazepine; secondary amine.

Chemical name: Desipramine hydrochloride—5*H*-Dibenz[*b,f*]azepine-5-propanamine, 10,11-dihydro-*N*-methyl-, monohydrochloride.

Molecular formula: Desipramine hydrochloride—$C_{18}H_{22}N_2 \cdot HCl$.

Molecular weight: Desipramine hydrochloride—302.84.

Description: Desipramine Hydrochloride USP—White to off-white, crystalline powder. Melts at about 213 °C.

pKa: 1.5 and 10.2.

Solubility: Desipramine Hydrochloride USP—Soluble in water and in alcohol; freely soluble in methanol and in chloroform; insoluble in ether.

USP requirements:
Desipramine Hydrochloride USP—Preserve in tight containers. Dried in vacuum at 105 °C for 2 hours, contains not less than 98.0% and not more than 100.5% of desipramine hydrochloride. Meets the requirements for Identification, Loss on drying (not more than 0.5%), Residue on ignition (not more than 0.1%), Heavy metals (not more than 0.001%), Limit of iminodibenzyl, and Organic volatile impurities.
Desipramine Hydrochloride Capsules USP—Preserve in tight containers. Contain the labeled amount, within ±8%. Meet the requirements for Identification, Dissolution (75% in 45 minutes in water in Apparatus 1 at 100 rpm), and Uniformity of dosage units.
Desipramine Hydrochloride Tablets USP—Preserve in tight containers. Contain the labeled amount, within ±5%. Meet the requirements for Identification, Dissolution (75% in 60 minutes in 0.01 *N* hydrochloric acid in Apparatus 2 at 50 rpm), and Uniformity of dosage units.

DESLANOSIDE

Source: Obtained naturally from *Digitalis lanata* or may be produced synthetically.

Chemical name: Card-20(22)-enolide, 3-[(*O*-beta-D-glucopyranosyl-(1→4)-*O*-2,6-dideoxy-beta-D-*ribo*-hexopyranosyl-(1→4)-*O*-2,6-dideoxy-beta-D-*ribo*-hexopyranosyl-(1→4)-2,6-dideoxy-beta-D-*ribo*-hexopyranosyl)oxy]-12,14-dihydroxy-, (3 beta,5 beta,12 beta)-.

Molecular formula: $C_{47}H_{74}O_{19}$.

Molecular weight: 943.08.

Description: Hygroscopic white crystals or crystalline powder.

Solubility: Practically insoluble in water, in chloroform, and in ether; very slightly soluble in alcohol.

USP requirements:
Deslanoside USP—Preserve in tight, light-resistant containers. Contains not less than 95.0% and not more than 103.0% of deslanoside, calculated on the dried basis.

Meets the requirements for Identification, Specific rotation (+7.0° to +8.5°), Loss on drying (not more than 5.0%), and Residue on ignition (not more than 0.2%).

Caution: Handle Deslanoside with exceptional care, since it is highly potent.

Deslanoside Injection USP—Preserve in single-dose containers, preferably of Type I glass. A sterile solution of Deslanoside in a suitable solvent. Contains the labeled amount, within ±10%. Meets the requirements for Identification and pH (5.5–7.0), and for Injections.

DESLORATADINE

Chemical group: Tricyclic histamine antagonist, long-acting.

Chemical name: 8-chloro-6,11-dihydro-11-(4-piperdinylidene)-5*H*-benzo[5,6]cyclohepta[1,2-*b*]pyridine.

Molecular formula: $C_{19}H_{19}ClN_2$.

Molecular weight: 310.8.

Description: White to off-white powder.

Solubility: Slightly soluble in water; very soluble in ethanol and in propylene glycol.

USP requirements: Desloratadine Tablets—Not in *USP–NF*.

DESMOPRESSIN

Chemical group: Synthetic polypeptide structurally related to the posterior pituitary hormone arginine vasopressin (antidiuretic hormone).

Chemical name: Desmopressin acetate—Vasopressin, 1-(3-mercaptopropanoic acid)-8-D-arginine-, monoacetate (salt), trihydrate.

Molecular formula: Desmopressin acetate—$C_{48}H_{68}N_{14}O_{14}S_2 \cdot 3H_2O$.

Molecular weight: Desmopressin acetate—1183.32.

USP requirements:
Desmopressin Acetate Injection—Not in *USP–NF*.
Desmopressin Acetate Nasal Solution—Not in *USP–NF*.
Desmopressin Acetate Tablets—Not in *USP–NF*.

DESOGESTREL AND ETHINYL ESTRADIOL

Chemical name:
Desogestrel—18,19-Dinorpregn-4-en-20-yn-17-ol, 13-ethyl-11-methylene-, (17 alpha)-.
Ethinyl estradiol—19-Norpregna-1,3,5(10)-trien-20-yne-3,17-diol, (17 alpha)-.

Molecular formula:
Desogestrel—$C_{22}H_{30}O$.
Ethinyl estradiol—$C_{20}H_{24}O_2$.

Molecular weight:
Desogestrel—310.47.
Ethinyl estradiol—296.40.

Description:
Desogestrel—Melting point 109–110 °C.
Ethinyl Estradiol USP—White to creamy white, odorless, crystalline powder.

Solubility: Ethinyl Estradiol USP—Insoluble in water; soluble in alcohol, in chloroform, in ether, in vegetable oils, and in solutions of fixed alkali hydroxides.

USP requirements: Desogestrel and Ethinyl Estradiol Tablets—Not in *USP–NF*.

DESONIDE

Chemical name: Pregna-1,4-diene-3,20-dione, 11,21-dihydroxy-16,17-[(1-methylethylidene)bis(oxy)]-, (11 beta,16 alpha)-.

Molecular formula: $C_{24}H_{32}O_6$.

Molecular weight: 416.51.

Description: White to practically white, odorless powder. Melting point approximately 270 °C with decomposition.

Solubility: Practically insoluble in water; slightly soluble in methanol, in chloroform, in ether, and in dioxane.

USP requirements:
Desonide Cream—Not in *USP–NF*.
Desonide Lotion—Not in *USP–NF*.
Desonide Ointment—Not in *USP–NF*.

DESONIDE AND ACETIC ACID

For *Desonide* and *Acetic Acid*—See individual listings for chemistry information.

USP requirements: Desonide and Acetic Acid Otic Solution—Not in *USP–NF*.

DESOXIMETASONE

Chemical name: Pregna-1,4-diene-3,20-dione, 9-fluoro-11,21-dihydroxy-16-methyl-, (11 beta,16 alpha)-.

Molecular formula: $C_{22}H_{29}FO_4$.

Molecular weight: 376.46.

Description: Desoximetasone USP—White to practically white, odorless, crystalline powder.

Solubility: Desoximetasone USP—Insoluble in water; freely soluble in alcohol, in acetone, and in chloroform.

USP requirements:
Desoximetasone USP—Preserve in well-closed containers. Contains not less than 97.0% and not more than 103.0% of desoximetasone, calculated on the dried basis. Meets the requirements for Identification, Melting range (206–218 °C, not more than 4 °C between beginning and end of melting), Specific rotation (+107° to +112°), Loss on drying (not more than 1.0%), Residue on ignition (not more than 0.2%), and Heavy metals (not more than 0.002%).
Desoximetasone Cream USP—Preserve in collapsible tubes, at controlled room temperature. It is Desoximetasone in an emollient cream base. Contains the labeled amount, within ±10%. Meets the requirements for Identification, Minimum fill, and pH (4.0–8.0).
Desoximetasone Gel USP—Preserve in collapsible tubes, at controlled room temperature. Contains the labeled amount, within ±10%. Meets the requirements for Identification, Minimum fill, and Alcohol content (18.0–24.0% [w/w]).

Desoximetasone Ointment USP—Preserve in collapsible tubes, at controlled room temperature. Contains the labeled amount, within ±10%. Meets the requirements for Identification and Minimum fill.

DESOXYCORTICOSTERONE

Chemical name:

Desoxycorticosterone acetate—Pregn-4-ene-3,20-dione, 21-(acetyloxy)-.

Desoxycorticosterone pivalate—Pregn-4-ene-3,20-dione, 21-(2,2-dimethyl-1-oxopropoxy)-.

Molecular formula:

Desoxycorticosterone acetate—$C_{23}H_{32}O_4$.

Desoxycorticosterone pivalate—$C_{26}H_{38}O_4$.

Molecular weight:

Desoxycorticosterone acetate—372.50.

Desoxycorticosterone pivalate—414.58.

Description:

Desoxycorticosterone Acetate USP—White or creamy white, crystalline powder. Is odorless, and is stable in air.

Desoxycorticosterone pivalate—White or creamy white, crystalline powder. Is odorless, and is stable in air.

Solubility:

Desoxycorticosterone Acetate USP—Practically insoluble in water; sparingly soluble in alcohol, in acetone, and in dioxane; slightly soluble in vegetable oils.

Desoxycorticosterone pivalate—Practically insoluble in water; soluble in dioxane; sparingly soluble in acetone; slightly soluble in alcohol, in methanol, in ether, and in vegetable oils.

USP requirements:

Desoxycorticosterone Acetate USP—Preserve in well-closed, light-resistant containers. Contains not less than 97.0% and not more than 103.0% of desoxycorticosterone acetate, calculated on the dried basis. Meets the requirements for Identification, Melting range (155–161 °C), Specific rotation (+171° to +179°), and Loss on drying (not more than 0.5%).

Desoxycorticosterone Acetate Injection USP—Preserve in single-dose or in multiple-dose containers, preferably of Type I or Type III glass, protected from light. A sterile solution of Desoxycorticosterone Acetate in vegetable oil. Contains the labeled amount, within −10% to +15%. Meets the requirements for Identification and Bacterial endotoxins, and for Injections.

Desoxycorticosterone Acetate Pellets USP—Preserve in tight containers suitable for maintaining sterile contents, holding one pellet each. Sterile pellets composed of Desoxycorticosterone Acetate in compressed form, without the presence of any binder, diluent, or excipient. Contain the labeled amount, within ±3%. Meet the requirements for Solubility in alcohol, Identification, Melting range (155–161 °C), Specific rotation (+171° to +179°), Sterility, and Weight variation (average weight of 5 Pellets within ±5% of labeled weight; each Pellet within ±10% of labeled weight).

Desoxycorticosterone Pivalate USP—Preserve in well-closed, light-resistant containers. Label it to indicate that it is for veterinary use only. Contains not less than 97.0% and not more than 103.0% of desoxycorticosterone pivalate, calculated on the dried basis. Meets the requirements for Identification, Melting range (200–206 °C), Specific rotation (+155° to +163°), and Loss on drying (not more than 0.5%).

Desoxycorticosterone Pivalate Injectable Suspension USP—Preserve in single-dose or in multiple-dose containers, preferably of Type I glass, protected from light. A sterile suspension of Desoxycorticosterone Pivalate in an aqueous medium. Label Suspension to indicate that it is for veterinary use only. Contains the labeled amount, within ± 10%. Meets the requirements for Identification, Bacterial endotoxins, and pH (5.0–7.0), and for Injections.

DEXAMETHASONE

Chemical name:

Dexamethasone—Pregna-1,4-diene-3,20-dione, 9-fluoro-11,17,21-trihydroxy-16-methyl-, (11 beta,16 alpha)-.

Dexamethasone acetate—Pregna-1,4-diene-3,20-dione, 21-(acetyloxy)-9-fluoro-11,17-dihydroxy-16-methyl, monohydrate, (11 beta,16 alpha)-.

Dexamethasone sodium phosphate—Pregna-1,4-diene-3,20-dione, 9-fluoro-11,17-dihydroxy-16-methyl-21-(phosphonooxy)-, disodium salt, (11 beta,16 alpha)-.

Molecular formula:

Dexamethasone—$C_{22}H_{29}FO_5$.

Dexamethasone acetate—$C_{24}H_{31}FO_6 \cdot H_2O$.

Dexamethasone sodium phosphate—$C_{22}H_{28}FNa_2O_8P$.

Molecular weight:

Dexamethasone—392.46.

Dexamethasone acetate—434.51 (anhydrous); 452.51 (monohydrate).

Dexamethasone sodium phosphate—516.40.

Description:

Dexamethasone USP—White to practically white, odorless, crystalline powder. Is stable in air. Melts at about 250 °C, with some decomposition.

Dexamethasone Acetate USP—Clear, white to off-white, odorless powder.

Dexamethasone Sodium Phosphate USP—White or slightly yellow, crystalline powder. Is odorless or has a slight odor of alcohol, and is exceedingly hygroscopic.

Solubility:

Dexamethasone USP—Practically insoluble in water; sparingly soluble in acetone, in alcohol, in dioxane, and in methanol; slightly soluble in chloroform; very slightly soluble in ether.

Dexamethasone Acetate USP—Practically insoluble in water; freely soluble in methanol, in acetone, and in dioxane.

Dexamethasone Sodium Phosphate USP—Freely soluble in water; slightly soluble in alcohol; very slightly soluble in dioxane; insoluble in chloroform and in ether.

USP requirements:

Dexamethasone USP—Preserve in well-closed containers. Contains not less than 97.0% and not more than 102.0% of dexamethasone, calculated on the dried basis. Meets the requirements for Identification, Specific rotation (+72° to +80°), Loss on drying (not more than 0.5%), Residue on ignition (not more than 0.2% from 250 mg), Chromatographic purity, and Organic volatile impurities.

Dexamethasone Topical Aerosol USP—Preserve in pressurized containers, and avoid exposure to excessive heat. It is Dexamethasone in a suitable lotion base mixed with suitable propellants in a pressurized container. Delivers the labeled amount, within −10% to +20%. Meets the requirements for Identification and Microbial limits, and for Pressure test, Minimum fill, and Leakage test under Aerosols, Metered dose inhalers, and Dry powder inhalers.

Dexamethasone Elixir USP—Preserve in tight containers. Contains the labeled amount, within ±10%. Meets the requirements for Identification and Alcohol content (3.8–5.7%, *n*-propyl alcohol being used as the internal standard).

Dexamethasone Gel USP—Preserve in collapsible tubes. Keep tightly closed. Avoid exposure to temperatures exceeding 30 °C. Contains the labeled amount, within ± 10%. Meets the requirements for Identification and Minimum fill.

Dexamethasone Injection USP—Preserve in light-resistant single-dose or multiple-dose containers, preferably of Type I glass. A sterile solution of Dexamethasone in Water for Injection. Label it to indicate that it is for veterinary use only. Contains the labeled amount, within ±10%. Meets the requirements for Identification, Bacterial endotoxins, Sterility, pH (4.0–5.5), and Particulate matter, and for Injections.

Dexamethasone Ophthalmic Ointment—Not in *USP–NF*.

Dexamethasone Oral Solution USP—Preserve in tight containers. Label it concentrated Oral Solution to state that the term **Concentrate** is to appear apart from and immediately after the official title in prominent bold-face type. Label concentrated Oral Solution also to indicate that it is to be diluted to appropriate strength with a suitable diluent prior to administration unless produced for dispensing with instructions for administration by a calibrated dropper or syringe. Contains the labeled amount, within ±10%. Meets the requirements for Identification, pH (2.7–4.0), and Alcohol content (27.0–33.0%).

Dexamethasone Ophthalmic Suspension USP—Preserve in tight containers. A sterile, aqueous suspension of dexamethasone containing a suitable antimicrobial preservative. Contains the labeled amount, within ±10%. Meets the requirements for Identification, Sterility, and pH (5.0–6.0).

Dexamethasone Tablets USP—Preserve in well-closed containers. Contain the labeled amount, within ±10%. Meet the requirements for Identification, Dissolution (70% in 45 minutes in dilute hydrochloric acid [1 in 100] in Apparatus 1 at 100 rpm), and Uniformity of dosage units.

Dexamethasone Acetate USP—Preserve in well-closed containers. Contains one molecule of water of hydration or is anhydrous. Label it to indicate whether it is hydrous or anhydrous. Contains not less than 97.0% and not more than 102.0% of dexamethasone acetate, calculated on the dried basis. Meets the requirements for Identification, Chromatographic purity (not more than 1.0% of any individual impurity, and not more than 2.0% of total impurities), Specific rotation (+82° to +88°), Loss on drying (3.5–4.5% for the hydrous; not more than 0.4% for the anhydrous), Residue on ignition (not more than 0.1%), Heavy metals (not more than 0.002%), Organic volatile impurities, and Other impurities.

Dexamethasone Acetate Injectable Suspension USP—Preserve in single-dose or in multiple-dose containers, preferably of Type I glass. A sterile suspension of Dexamethasone Acetate in Water for Injection. Contains an amount of dexamethasone acetate monohydrate equivalent to the labeled amount of dexamethasone, within ±10%. Meets the requirements for Identification, Bacterial endotoxins, and pH (5.0–7.5), and for Injections.

Dexamethasone Sodium Phosphate USP—Preserve in tight containers. Contains not less than 97.0% and not more than 102.0% of dexamethasone sodium phosphate, calculated on the water-free and alcohol-free basis. Meets the requirements for Identification, Chromatographic purity (not more than 1.0% of any individual impurity, and not more than 2.0% of total impurities), Specific rotation (+74° to +82°, calculated on the water-free and alcohol-free basis), pH (7.5–10.5, in a solution [1 in 100]), Water (sum of percentages of water content and of alcohol content not more than 16.0%), Alcohol (not more than 8.0%), Phosphate ions (not more than 1.0%), Limit of free dexamethasone (not more than 1.0%), Organic volatile impurities, and Other impurities.

Dexamethasone Sodium Phosphate Inhalation Aerosol USP—Preserve in tight, pressurized containers, and avoid exposure to excessive heat. A suspension, in suitable pro-

pellants and alcohol, in a pressurized container, of dexamethasone sodium phosphate. Contains an amount of dexamethasone sodium phosphate equivalent to the labeled amount of dexamethasone phosphate, within ± 10%. Meets the requirements for Identification, Alcohol content (1.7–2.3%), and Dosage uniformity over the entire contents.

Dexamethasone Sodium Phosphate Nasal Aerosol—Not in *USP–NF*.

Dexamethasone Sodium Phosphate Cream USP—Preserve in collapsible tubes or in tight containers. Contains an amount of dexamethasone sodium phosphate equivalent to the labeled amount of dexamethasone phosphate, within −10% to +15%. Meets the requirements for Identification, Microbial limits, and Minimum fill.

Dexamethasone Sodium Phosphate Injection USP—Preserve in single-dose or in multiple-dose containers, preferably of Type I glass, protected from light. A sterile solution of Dexamethasone Sodium Phosphate in Water for Injection. Contains an amount of dexamethasone sodium phosphate equivalent to the labeled amount of dexamethasone phosphate, within −10% to +15%, present as the disodium salt. Meets the requirements for Identification, Bacterial endotoxins, and pH (7.0–8.5), and for Injections.

Dexamethasone Sodium Phosphate Ophthalmic Ointment USP—Preserve in collapsible ophthalmic ointment tubes. A sterile ointment. Contains an amount of dexamethasone sodium phosphate equivalent to the labeled amount of dexamethasone phosphate, within −10% to +15%. Meets the requirements for Identification, Minimum fill, Sterility, and Metal particles.

Dexamethasone Sodium Phosphate Ophthalmic Solution USP—Preserve in tight, light-resistant containers. A sterile, aqueous solution of Dexamethasone Sodium Phosphate. Contains an amount of dexamethasone sodium phosphate equivalent to the labeled amount of dexamethasone phosphate, within −10% to +15%. Meets the requirements for Identification, pH (6.6–7.8), and Sterility.

Dexamethasone Sodium Phosphate Otic Ophthalmic Solution—Not in *USP–NF*.

DEXBROMPHENIRAMINE

Chemical group: Propylamine derivative.

Chemical name: Dexbrompheniramine maleate—2-Pyridinepropanamine, gamma-(4-bromophenyl)-*N,N*-dimethyl-, (*S*)-, (*Z*)-2-butenedioate (1:1).

Molecular formula: Dexbrompheniramine maleate—$C_{16}H_{19}BrN_2 \cdot C_4H_4O_4$.

Molecular weight: Dexbrompheniramine maleate—435.31.

Description: Dexbrompheniramine Maleate USP—White, odorless, crystalline powder. Exists in two polymorphic forms, one melting between 106 and 107 °C and the other between 112 and 113 °C. Mixtures of the forms may melt between 105 and 113 °C. The pH of a solution (1 in 100) is about 5.

Solubility: Dexbrompheniramine Maleate USP—Freely soluble in water; soluble in alcohol and in chloroform.

USP requirements: Dexbrompheniramine Maleate USP—Preserve in tight, light-resistant containers. Contains not less than 98.0% and not more than 100.5% of dexbrompheniramine maleate, calculated on the dried basis. Meets the requirements for Identification, Specific rotation (+35.0° to +38.5°), Loss

on drying (not more than 0.5%), Residue on ignition (not more than 0.2%), Related compounds (not more than 2.0%), and Organic volatile impurities.

DEXBROMPHENIRAMINE AND PSEUDOEPHEDRINE

For *Dexbrompheniramine* and *Pseudoephedrine*—See individual listings for chemistry information.

USP requirements:
Dexbrompheniramine Maleate and Pseudoephedrine Hydrochloride Tablets—Not in *USP–NF*.
Dexbrompheniramine Maleate and Pseudoephedrine Sulfate Extended-release Capsules—Not in *USP–NF*.
Dexbrompheniramine Maleate and Pseudoephedrine Sulfate Tablets—Not in *USP–NF*.
Dexbrompheniramine Maleate and Pseudoephedrine Sulfate Extended-release Tablets—Not in *USP–NF*.
Dexbrompheniramine Maleate and Pseudoephedrine Sulfate Oral Solution USP—Contains labeled amounts, within ± 10%. Meets the requirement for Identification.

DEXBROMPHENIRAMINE, PSEUDOEPHEDRINE, AND ACETAMINOPHEN

For *Dexbrompheniramine, Pseudoephedrine,* and *Acetaminophen*—See individual listings for chemistry information.

USP requirements: Dexbrompheniramine Maleate, Pseudoephedrine Sulfate, and Acetaminophen Extended-release Tablets—Not in *USP–NF*.

DEXCHLORPHENIRAMINE

Chemical group: Propylamine derivative (alkylamine).

Chemical name: Dexchlorpheniramine maleate—2-Pyridinepropanamine, gamma-(4-chlorophenyl)-*N,N*-dimethyl-, (*S*)-, (*Z*)-2-butenedioate (1:1).

Molecular formula: Dexchlorpheniramine maleate—$C_{16}H_{19}ClN_2$ · $C_4H_4O_4$.

Molecular weight: Dexchlorpheniramine maleate—390.86.

Description: Dexchlorpheniramine Maleate USP—White, odorless, crystalline powder.

Solubility: Dexchlorpheniramine Maleate USP—Freely soluble in water; soluble in alcohol and in chloroform; slightly soluble in ether.

USP requirements:
Dexchlorpheniramine Maleate USP—Preserve in tight, light-resistant containers. Dried at 65 °C for 4 hours, contains not less than 98.0% and not more than 100.5% of dexchlorpheniramine maleate. Meets the requirements for Identification, Melting range (110–115 °C), Specific rotation (+39.5° to +43.0°), pH (4.0–5.0, in a solution [1 in 100]), Loss on drying (not more than 0.5%), Residue on ignition (not more than 0.2%), Related compounds (not more than 2.0%), and Organic volatile impurities.
Dexchlorpheniramine Maleate Oral Solution USP—Preserve in tight, light-resistant containers. Contains the labeled amount, within ±10%. Meets the requirements for Identification and Alcohol content (5.0–7.0%).

Dexchlorpheniramine Maleate Syrup USP—Preserve in tight, light-resistant containers. Contains the labeled amount, within ±10%. Meets the requirements for Identification and Alcohol content (5.0–7.0%).
Dexchlorpheniramine Maleate Tablets USP—Preserve in tight containers. Contain the labeled amount, within ±10%. Meet the requirements for Identification, Dissolution (75% in 45 minutes in water in Apparatus 2 at 50 rpm), and Uniformity of dosage units.
Dexchlorpheniramine Maleate Extended-release Tablets—Not in *USP–NF*.

DEXCHLORPHENIRAMINE, PSEUDOEPHEDRINE, AND GUAIFENESIN

For *Dexchlorpheniramine, Pseudoephedrine,* and *Guaifenesin*—See individual listings for chemistry information.

USP requirements: Dexchlorpheniramine Maleate, Pseudoephedrine Sulfate, and Guaifenesin Oral Solution—Not in *USP–NF*.

DEXFENFLURAMINE

Chemical name: Dexfenfluramine hydrochloride—Benzeneethanamine, *N*-ethyl-alpha-methyl-3-(trifluoromethyl)-, hydrochloride, (*S*)-.

Molecular formula: Dexfenfluramine hydrochloride—$C_{12}H_{16}F_3N$ · HCl.

Molecular weight: Dexfenfluramine hydrochloride—267.72.

Description: Dexfenfluramine hydrochloride—White to off-white crystalline powder.

pKa: Dexfenfluramine hydrochloride—10.

Solubility: Dexfenfluramine hydrochloride—Freely soluble in water, in alcohol, in chloroform, and in methanol.

USP requirements: Dexfenfluramine Hydrochloride Capsules—Not in *USP–NF*.

DEXMEDETOMIDINE

Chemical group: Dexmedetomidine is the S-enantiomer of medetomidine.

Chemical name: Dexmedetomidine hydrochloride—1*H*-imidazole, 4-[1-(2,3-dimethylphenyl)ethyl]-, monohydrochloride, (*S*)-.

Molecular formula: Dexmedetomidine hydrochloride—$C_{13}H_{16}N_2$ · HCl.

Molecular weight: Dexmedetomidine hydrochloride—236.70.

Description: Dexmedetomidine hydrochloride—White or almost white powder.

pKa: Dexmedetomidine hydrochloride—7.1.

Solubility: Dexmedetomidine hydrochloride—Freely soluble in water.

Other characteristics: Dexmedetomidine hydrochloride—pH of 4.5 to 7.0. Partition coefficient: 2.89 in octanol:water at pH 7.5.

USP requirements: Dexmedetomidine Hydrochloride Injection—Not in *USP–NF*.

DEXMETHYLPHENIDATE

Chemical name: Dexmethylphenidate hydrochloride—2-Piperidineacetic acid, alpha-phenyl-, methyl ester, hydrochloride, (alpha R,2R)-.

Molecular formula: Dexmethylphenidate hydrochloride—$C_{14}H_{19}NO_2 \cdot HCl$.

Molecular weight: Dexmethylphenidate hydrochloride—269.77.

Description: Dexmethylphenidate hydrochloride—White to off-white powder.

Solubility: Dexmethylphenidate hydrochloride—Freely soluble in water and in methanol; soluble in alcohol; slightly soluble in chloroform and in acetone. Its solution is acid to litmus.

USP requirements: Dexmethylphenidate Hydrochloride Tablets—Not in *USP–NF*.

DEXPANTHENOL

Chemical name: Butanamide, 2,4-dihydroxy-N-(3-hydroxypropyl)-3,3-dimethyl-, (R)-.

Molecular formula: $C_9H_{19}NO_4$.

Molecular weight: 205.25.

Description: Dexpanthenol USP—Clear, viscous, somewhat hygroscopic liquid, having a slight, characteristic odor. Some crystallization may occur on standing.

Solubility: Dexpanthenol USP—Freely soluble in water, in alcohol, in methanol, and in propylene glycol; soluble in chloroform and in ether; slightly soluble in glycerin.

USP requirements:
Dexpanthenol USP—Preserve in tight containers. Contains not less than 98.0% and not more than 102.0% of dexpanthenol, calculated on the anhydrous basis. Meets the requirements for Identification, Specific rotation (+29.0° to +31.5°), Refractive index (1.495–1.502 at 20 °C), Water (not more than 1.0%), Residue on ignition (not more than 0.1%), Limit of aminopropanol (not more than 1.0%), and Organic volatile impurities.
Dexpanthenol Preparation USP—Preserve in tight containers. Contains not less than 94.5% and not more than 98.5% of dexpanthenol, and not less than 2.7% and not more than 4.2% of pantolactone, both calculated on the anhydrous basis. Meets the requirements for Identification, Specific rotation (+27.5° to +30.0°), and Content of pantolactone, and for Refractive index, Water, Residue on ignition, and Aminopropanol under Dexpanthenol.

DEXRAZOXANE

Chemical group: Derivative of EDTA.

Chemical name: 2,6-Piperazinedione, 4,4'-(1-methyl-1,2-ethanediyl)bis-, (S)-.

Molecular formula: $C_{11}H_{16}N_4O_4$.

Molecular weight: 268.27.

Description: Whitish crystalline powder, melting at 191 to 197 °C.

pKa: 2.1.

Solubility: Sparingly soluble in water and in 0.1 N hydrochloric acid; slightly soluble in ethanol and in methanol; practically insoluble in nonpolar organic solvents.

Other characteristics: Octanol/water partition coefficient—0.025.

USP requirements: Dexrazoxane for Injection—Not in *USP–NF*.

DEXTRAN

Source:
Dextran—Polysaccharides produced by bacteria growing on a sucrose substance, containing a backbone of D-glucose units linked predominantly alpha-D(1→6).
Dextran sulfate—A prototype polyanionic compound.

USP requirements: Dextran Sulfate Aerosol Inhalation—Not in *USP–NF*.

DEXTRAN 1

Description: A white to off-white powder. Is hygroscopic.

Solubility: Very soluble in water; sparingly soluble in alcohol.

USP requirements: Dextran 1 USP—Store in well-closed containers at a temperature between 4° and 30°. A low molecular weight fraction of dextran, consisting of a mixture of isomaltooligosaccharides. Obtained by controlled hydrolysis and fractionation of dextrans produced by fermentation of *Leuconostoc mesenteroides* (strain NRRL B-512; CIP 78.59, or its substrains, for example *L. mesenteroides* B-512F; NCTC 10817), in the presence of sucrose. It is a glucose polymer in which the linkages between glucose units are almost exclusively alpha-1,6. Its weight-average molecular weight is about 1000. Where it is intended for use in preparing injectable dosage forms, the label states that it is sterile or must be subjected to further processing during the preparation of injectable dosage forms. Meets the reqirements for Identification, Absorbance, Specific rotation (+148° to +164° at 20°), Microbial limits, Bacterial endotoxins, pH (4.5–7.0, in a 15% solution in water), Loss on drying (not more than 5.0%), Heavy metals (not more than 5 mcg per gram), Limit of alcohol and related impurities, Limit of sodium chloride (not more than 1.5%), Limit of nitrogenous impurities (110 rpm, where it is labeled as intended for use in the preparation of injectables), and Molecular weight distribution and average molecular weight.

DEXTRAN 40

Source: Derived by controlled hydrolysis and fractionation of polysaccharides elaborated by the fermentative action of certain strains of *Leuconostoc mesenteroides* (NRRL, B.512 F; NCTC, 10817) on a sucrose substrate.

Chemical name: Dextrans.

Molecular weight: 35,000–45,000.

USP requirements:
Dextrans 40 USP—Preserve in well-closed containers. Where it is intended for use in preparing injectable dosage forms, the label states that it is sterile or must be subjected to further processing during the preparation of injectable dosage forms. A glucose polymer in which the linkages between glucose units are almost entirely of the alpha-1:6 type. Meets the requirements for Color of solution, Identification, Specific rotation (between +195° and +203°, [at 105° for 5 hours], determined in a solution in water), Bacterial endotoxins, Safety, pH (4.5–7.0, in a solution [1 in

10]), Loss on drying (not more than 7.0%), Sulfate (0.03%), Heavy metals (5 micrograms per gram), Limit of nitrogenous impurities (where it is labeled as intended for use in the preparation of injectables, 0.01%, as N), Limit of alcohol and related impurities, Antigenic impurities (where it is labeled as intended for use in the preparation of injectables), and Molecular weight distribution and weight and number average molecular weights.

DEXTRAN 40 AND DEXTROSE

For *Dextran 40* and *Dextrose*—See individual listings for chemistry information.

USP requirements: Dextran 40 in Dextrose Injection USP—Preserve in single-dose glass or plastic containers. A sterile solution of Dextran 40 and Dextrose in Water for Injection. The label states the total osmolar concentration in mOsmol per liter. Where the contents are less than 100 mL, the label alternatively may state the total osmolar concentration in mOsmol per mL. Contains in each 100 mL not less than 9.0 grams and not more than 11.0 grams of dextran 40 and not less than 4.1 grams and not more than 5.0 grams of dextrose. Contains no bacteriostatic agents. Meets the requirements for Color of solution, Identification (the intrinsic viscosity 18–23 mL per gram), Bacterial endotoxins, Sterility, pH (3.0–7.0), Heavy metals (5 micrograms per mL), Limit of 5-hydroxymethylfurfural and related substances (absorbance not more than 0.25), and for Injections and for Particulate matter in Injections.

DEXTRAN 40 AND SODIUM CHLORIDE

For *Dextran 40* and *Sodium Chloride*—See individual listings for chemistry information.

USP requirements: Dextran 40 in Sodium Chloride Injection USP—Preserve in single-dose glass or plastic containers. A sterile solution of Dextran 40 and Sodium Chloride in Water for Injection. The label states the total osmolar concentration in mOsmol per liter. Where the contents are less than 100 mL, the label alternatively may state the total osmolar concentration in mOsmol per mL. Contains in each 100 mL not less than 9.0 grams and not more than 11.0 grams of dextran 40; and not less than 0.81 gram and not more than 0.99 gram of sodium chloride. Contains no bacteriostatic agents. Meets the requiremetns for Color of solution, Identification (the intrinsic viscosity 18–23 mL per gram), Bacterial endotoxins, Sterility, pH (3.5–7.0), Heavy metals (5 micrograms per mL), and for Injections and for Particulate matter in Injections.

DEXTRAN 70

Source: Derived by controlled hydrolysis and fractionation of polysaccharides elaborated by the fermentative action of certain appropriate strains of *Leuconostoc mesenteroides* (NRRL, B.512 F; NCTC, 10817) on a sucrose substrate.

Chemical name: Dextrans.

Molecular weight: 63,000–77,000.

USP requirements:
Dextrans 70 USP—Preserve in well-closed containers. Where it is intended for use in preparing injectable dosage forms, the label states that it is sterile or must be subjected to further processing during the preparation of injectable dosage forms. A glucose polymer in which the linkages between glucose units are almost entirely of the alpha-1:6 type. Meets the requirements for Color of solution, Identification, Specific rotation (between +195° and +203°, calculated on the dried basis [at 105° constant weight], determined in a solution in water), Bacterial endotoxins, Safety, pH (4.5–7.0, in a solution [1 in 10]), Loss on drying (not more than 7.0%), Sulfate (0.03%), Heavy metals (5 micrograms per gram), Limit of nitrogenous impurities (where it is labeled as intended for use in the preparation of injectables), Limit of alcohol and related impurities, Antigenic impurities (where it is labeled as intended for use in the preparation of injectables), and Molecular weight distribution and weight and number average molecular weights.

DEXTRAN 70 AND DEXTROSE

For *Dextran 70* and *Dextrose*—See individual listings for chemistry information.

USP requirements: Dextran 70 in Dextrose Injection USP—Preserve in single-dose glass or plastic containers. A sterile solution of Dextran 70 and Dextrose in Water for Injection. The label states the total osmolar concentration in mOsmol per liter. Where the contents are less than 100 mL, the label alternatively may state the total osmolar concentration in mOsmol per mL. Contains in each 100 mL not less than 5.4 grams and not more than 6.6 grams of dextran 70 and not less than 4.1 grams and not more than 5.0 grams of dextrose. Contains no bacteriostatic agents. Meets the requirements for Color of solution, Identification (the intrinsic viscosity 24–29 mL per gram), Bacterial endotoxins, Sterility, pH (3.5–7.0), Heavy metals (5 micrograms per mL), Limit of 5-hydroxymethylfurfural and related substances, and for Injections and for Particulate matter in Injections.

DEXTRAN 70 AND SODIUM CHLORIDE

For *Dextran 70* and *Sodium Chloride*—See individual listings for chemistry information.

USP requirements: Dextran 70 in Sodium Chloride Injection USP—Preserve in single-dose glass or plastic containers. A sterile solution of Dextran 70 and Sodium Chloride in Water for Injection. The label states the total osmolar concentration in mOsmol per liter. Where the contents are less than 100 mL, the label alternatively may state the total osmolar concentration in mOsmol per mL. Contains in each 100 mL not less than 5.4 grams and not more than 6.6 grams of dextran 70 and not less than 0.81 gram and not more than 0.99 gram of sodium chloride. Contains no bacteriostatic agents. Meets the requiremetns for Color of solution, Identification (the intrinsic viscosity 24–29 mL per gram), Bacterial endotoxins, Sterility, pH (4.0–7.0), Heavy metals (5 micrograms per mL), and for Injections and for Particulate matter in Injections.

DEXTRATES

Description: Dextrates NF—Free-flowing, porous, white, odorless, spherical granules consisting of aggregates of microcrystals. May be compressed directly into self-binding tablets.

NF category: Sweetening agent; tablet and/or capsule diluent.

Solubility: Dextrates NF—Freely soluble in water (heating increases its solubility in water); soluble in dilute acids and alkalies and in basic organic solvents such as pyridine; insoluble in the common organic solvents.

NF requirements: Dextrates NF—Preserve in well-closed containers, in a cool, dry place. A purified mixture of saccharides resulting from the controlled enzymatic hydrolysis of starch. It is either anhydrous or hydrated. Label it to state whether it is anhydrous or hydrated. Contains dextrose equivalent to not less than 93.0% and not more than 99.0%, calculated on the dried basis. Meets the requirements for pH (3.8–5.8, determined in a 1 in 5 solution in carbon dioxide-free water), Loss on drying (not more than 2.0% for the anhydrous; 7.8–9.2% for the hydrated form), Residue on ignition (not more than 0.1%), Heavy metals (not more than 5 ppm), Organic volatile impurities, and Dextrose equivalent.

DEXTRIN

Description: Dextrin NF—Free-flowing, white, yellow, or brown powder.

NF category: Suspending and/or viscosity-increasing agent; tablet binder; tablet and/or capsule diluent.

Solubility: Dextrin NF—Its solubility in water varies; it is usually very soluble, but often contains an insoluble portion.

NF requirements: Dextrin NF—Preserve in well-closed containers. Starch, or partially hydrolyzed starch, modified by heating in a dry state, with or without acids, alkalies, or pH control agents. Meets the requirements for Botanic characteristics, Identification, Loss on drying (not more than 13.0%), Acidity, Residue on ignition (not more than 0.5%), Chloride (not more than 0.2%), Heavy metals (not more than 20 mcg per gram), Protein, Reducing sugars, and Organic volatile impurities.

DEXTROAMPHETAMINE

Chemical name: Dextroamphetamine sulfate—Benzeneethanamine, alpha-methyl-, (*S*)-, sulfate (2:1).

Molecular formula: Dextroamphetamine sulfate—$(C_9H_{13}N)_2 \cdot H_2SO_4$.

Molecular weight: Dextroamphetamine sulfate—368.49.

Description: Dextroamphetamine Sulfate USP—White, odorless, crystalline powder.

Solubility: Dextroamphetamine Sulfate USP—Soluble in water; slightly soluble in alcohol; insoluble in ether.

USP requirements:

Dextroamphetamine Sulfate USP—Preserve in well-closed containers. The dextrorotatory isomer of amphetamine sulfate. Contains not less than 98.0% and not more than 101.0% of amphetamine sulfate, calculated on the dried basis. Meets the requirements for Identification, Specific rotation (+20° to +23.5°), pH (5.0–6.0, in a solution [1 in 20]), Loss on drying (not more than 1.0%), Residue on ignition (not more than 0.1%), Chromatographic purity, and Organic volatile impurities.

Dextroamphetamine Sulfate Capsules USP—Preserve in tight containers. Contain the labeled amount, within ±10%. Meet the requirements for Identification, Dissolution (75% in 45 minutes in water in Apparatus 1 at 100 rpm), and Uniformity of dosage units.

Dextroamphetamine Sulfate Extended-release Capsules—Not in *USP–NF*.

Dextroamphetamine Sulfate Elixir USP—Preserve in tight, light-resistant containers. Contains, in each 100 mL, not less than 90.0 mg and not more than 110.0 mg of dextroamphetamine sulfate. Meets the requirements for Identification, Alcohol content (9.0–11.0%), and Isomeric purity.

Dextroamphetamine Sulfate Oral Solution USP—Preserve in tight, light-resistant containers. Contains, in each 100 mL, not less than 90.0 mg and not more than 110.0 mg of dextroamphetamine sulfate. Meets the requirements for Identification, Alcohol content (9.0–11.0%), and Isomeric purity.

Dextroamphetamine Sulfate Tablets USP—Preserve in well-closed containers. Contain the labeled amount, within ± 7%. Meet the requirements for Identification, Dissolution (75% in 45 minutes in water in Apparatus 1 at 100 rpm), Uniformity of dosage units, and Isomeric purity.

DEXTROMETHORPHAN

Source: Methylated dextroisomer of levorphanol.

Chemical group: Synthetic derivative of morphine.

Chemical name:
Dextromethorphan—Morphinan, 3-methoxy-17-methyl-, (9 alpha,13 alpha,14 alpha)-.
Dextromethorphan hydrobromide—Morphinan, 3-methoxy-17-methyl-, (9 alpha,13 alpha,14 alpha)-, hydrobromide, monohydrate.
Dextromethorphan polistirex—Benzene, diethenyl-, polymer with ethenylbenzene, sulfonated, complex with (9 alpha,13 alpha,14 alpha)-3-methoxy-17-methylmorphinan.

Molecular formula:
Dextromethorphan—$C_{18}H_{25}NO$.
Dextromethorphan hydrobromide—$C_{18}H_{25}NO \cdot HBr \cdot H_2O$.

Molecular weight:
Dextromethorphan—271.40.
Dextromethorphan hydrobromide—370.32.

Description:
Dextromethorphan USP—Practically white to slightly yellow, odorless, crystalline powder. Eleven mg of Dextromethorphan is equivalent to 15 mg of dextromethorphan hydrobromide monohydrate.
Dextromethorphan Hydrobromide USP—Practically white crystals or crystalline powder, having a faint odor. Melts at about 126 °C, with decomposition.

Solubility:
Dextromethorphan USP—Practically insoluble in water; freely soluble in chloroform.
Dextromethorphan Hydrobromide USP—Sparingly soluble in water; freely soluble in alcohol and in chloroform; insoluble in ether.

USP requirements:
Dextromethorphan USP—Preserve in tight containers. Contains not less than 98.0% and not more than 101.0% of dextromethorphan, calculated on the anhydrous basis. Meets the requirements for Identification, Melting range (109.5–112.5 °C), Specific rotation, Water (not more than 0.5%), Residue on ignition (not more than 0.1%), Heavy metals (not more than 0.002%), Limit of *N,N*-dimethylaniline (not more than 0.001%), and Limit of phenolic compounds.
Dextromethorphan Hydrobromide USP—Preserve in tight containers. Contains not less than 98.0% and not more than 102.0% of dextromethorphan hydrobromide, calculated on the anhydrous basis. Meets the requirements for Identification, Specific rotation, pH (5.2–6.5, in a solu-

tion [1 in 100]), Water (3.5–5.5%), Residue on ignition (not more than 0.1%), Limit of *N,N*-dimethylaniline, and Limit of phenolic compounds.

Dextromethorphan Hydrobromide Capsules—Not in *USP–NF*.

Dextromethorphan Hydrobromide Lozenges—Not in *USP–NF*.

Dextromethorphan Hydrobromide Oral Solution USP—Preserve in tight, light-resistant containers. Contains the labeled amount, within ±10%. Meets the requirement for Identification.

Dextromethorphan Hydrobromide Syrup USP—Preserve in tight, light-resistant containers. Contains the labeled amount, within ±10%. Meets the requirement for Identification.

Dextromethorphan Hydrobromide Chewable Tablets—Not in *USP–NF*.

Dextromethorphan Polistirex Extended-release Oral Suspension—Not in *USP–NF*.

DEXTROMETHORPHAN AND ACETAMINOPHEN

For *Dextromethorphan* and *Acetaminophen*—See individual listings for chemistry information.

USP requirements:

Dextromethorphan Hydrobromide and Acetaminiphen Capsules—Not in *USP–NF*.

Dextromethorphan Hydrobromide and Acetaminophen Oral Solution—Not in *USP–NF*.

Dextromethorphan Hydrobromide and Acetaminophen Oral Suspension—Not in *USP–NF*.

Dextromethorphan Hydrobromide and Acetaminophen Tablets—Not in *USP–NF*.

DEXTROMETHORPHAN AND GUAIFENESIN

For *Dextromethorphan* and *Guaifenesin*—See individual listings for chemistry information.

USP requirements:

Dextromethorphan Hydrobromide and Guaifenesin Capsules—Not in *USP–NF*.

Dextromethorphan Hydrobromide and Guaifenesin Extended-release Capsules—Not in *USP–NF*.

Dextromethorphan Hydrobromide and Guaifenesin Oral Gel—Not in *USP–NF*.

Dextromethorphan Hydrobromide and Guaifenesin Oral Solution—Not in *USP–NF*.

Dextromethorphan Hydrobromide and Guaifenesin Syrup—Not in *USP–NF*.

Dextromethorphan Hydrobromide and Guaifenesin Tablets—Not in *USP–NF*.

Dextromethorphan Hydrobromide and Guaifenesin Extended-release Tablets—Not in *USP–NF*.

DEXTROMETHORPHAN AND IODINATED GLYCEROL

For *Dextromethorphan* and *Iodinated Glycerol*—See individual listings for chemistry information.

USP requirements: Dextromethorphan Hydrobromide and Iodinated Glycerol Oral Solution—Not in *USP–NF*.

DEXTROSE

Chemical name: D-Glucose, monohydrate.

Molecular formula: $C_6H_{12}O_6 \cdot H_2O$ (monohydrate); $C_6H_{12}O_6$ (anhydrous).

Molecular weight: 198.17 (monohydrate); 180.16 (anhydrous).

Description: Dextrose USP—Colorless crystals or white, crystalline or granular powder. Is odorless.

NF category: Sweetening agent; tonicity agent.

Solubility: Dextrose USP—Freely soluble in water; very soluble in boiling water; soluble in boiling alcohol; slightly soluble in alcohol.

USP requirements:

Dextrose USP—Preserve in well-closed containers. A sugar usually obtained by the hydrolysis of Starch. Contains one molecule of water of hydration or is anhydrous. Label it to indicate whether it is hydrous or anhydrous. Meets the requirements for Identification, Color of solution, Specific rotation (+52.6° to +53.2°), Acidity, Water (7.5–9.5% for the hydrous form; not more than 0.5% for the anhydrous form), Residue on ignition (not more than 0.1%), Chloride (not more than 0.018%), Sulfate (not more than 0.025%), Arsenic (not more than 1 ppm), Heavy metals (not more than 5 ppm), Dextrin, and Soluble starch, sulfites.

Dextrose Injection USP—Preserve in single-dose glass or plastic containers. Glass containers are preferably of Type I or Type II glass. A sterile solution of Dextrose in Water for Injection. The label states the total osmolar concentration in mOsmol per liter. Where the contents are less than 100 mL, or where the label states that the Injection is not for direct injection but is to be diluted before use, the label alternatively may state the total osmolar concentration in mOsmol per mL. Contains the labeled amount of dextrose monohydrate, within ±5%. Contains no antimicrobial agents. Meets the requirements for Identification, Bacterial endotoxins, pH (3.2–6.5), Particulate matter, Heavy metals (not more than 0.0005*C*%), and Limit of 5-hydroxymethylfurfural and related substances, and for Injections.

DEXTROSE AND ELECTROLYTES

For *Calcium Chloride, Citric Acid, Dextrose, Dibasic Sodium Phosphate, Magnesium Chloride, Potassium Chloride, Potassium Citrate, Sodium Chloride,* and *Sodium Citrate*—See individual listings for chemistry information.

USP requirements: Dextrose and Electrolytes Solution—Not in *USP–NF*.

DEXTROSE EXCIPIENT

Description: Dextrose Excipient NF—Colorless crystals or white, crystalline or granular powder. Is odorless.

NF category: Sweetening agent; tablet and/or capsule diluent.

Solubility: Dextrose Excipient NF—Freely soluble in water; very soluble in boiling water; sparingly soluble in boiling alcohol; slightly soluble in alcohol.

NF requirements: Dextrose Excipient NF—Preserve in well-closed containers. A sugar usually obtained by hydrolysis of starch. Contains one molecule of water of hydration. Label it to indicate that it is not intended for parenteral use. Meets the requirements for Specific rotation (+52.5° to +53.5°), Water (7.5–9.5%), and Organic volatile impurities, and for Identifica-

tion test, Color of solution, Acidity, Residue on ignition, Chloride, Sulfate, Arsenic, Heavy metals, Dextrin, and Soluble starch, sulfites under Dextrose.

DEXTROSE AND SODIUM CHLORIDE

For *Dextrose* and *Sodium Chloride*—See individual listings for chemistry information.

USP requirements: Dextrose and Sodium Chloride Injection USP—Preserve in single-dose glass or plastic containers. Glass containers are preferably of Type I or Type II glass. A sterile solution of Dextrose and Sodium Chloride in Water for Injection. The label states the total osmolar concentration in mOsmol per liter. Where the contents are less than 100 mL, or where the label states that the Injection is not for direct injection but is to be diluted before use, the label alternatively may state the total osmolar concentration in mOsmol per mL. Contains the labeled amounts, within ±5%. Contains no antimicrobial agents. Meets the requirements for Identification, Bacterial endotoxins, pH (3.2–6.5), and Limit of 5-hydroxymethylfurfural and related substances, and for Injections.

DEXTROTHYROXINE

Chemical name: Dextrothyroxine sodium—D-Tyrosine, *O*-(4-hydroxy-3,5-diiodophenyl)-3,5-diiodo-, monosodium salt hydrate.

Molecular formula: Dextrothyroxine sodium—$C_{15}H_{10}I_4NNaO_4 \cdot xH_2O$.

Molecular weight: Dextrothyroxine sodium—798.85 (anhydrous).

Description: Dextrothyroxine sodium—Light yellow to buff-colored, odorless powder which may assume a slight pink color on exposure to light.

Solubility: Dextrothyroxine sodium—Soluble 1 in 700 of water and 1 in 300 of alcohol; soluble in solutions of alkali hydroxides and in hot solutions of alkali carbonates; practically insoluble in acetone, in chloroform, and in ether.

USP requirements: Dextrothyroxine Sodium Tablets—Not in *USP–NF*.

DEZOCINE

Chemical group: An opioid agonist/antagonist analgesic of the aminotetralin series.1,

Chemical name: 5,11-Methanobenzocyclodecen-3-ol, 13-amino-5,6,7,8,9,10,11,12-octahydro-5-methyl-, (5 alpha,11 alpha,13*S**)-, (–)-.

Molecular formula: $C_{16}H_{23}NO$.

Molecular weight: 245.36.

Other characteristics:*n*-Octanol:Water partition coefficient—1.7.

USP requirements: Dezocine Injection—Not in *USP–NF*.

DIACETYLATED MONOGLYCERIDES

Description: Diacetylated Monoglycerides NF—Clear liquid.
NF category: Plasticizer.

Solubility: Diacetylated Monoglycerides NF—Very soluble in 80% (w/w) aqueous alcohol, in vegetable oils, and in mineral oils; sparingly soluble in 70% alcohol.

NF requirements: Diacetylated Monoglycerides NF—Preserve in tight, light-resistant containers. Glycerin esterified with edible fat-forming fatty acids and acetic acid. May be prepared by the interesterification of edible oils with triacetin in the presence of catalytic agents, followed by molecular distillation, or by the direct acetylation of edible monoglycerides with acetic anhydride without the use of catalyst or molecular distillation. Meets the requirements for Identification, Residue on ignition (not more than 0.1%), Heavy metals (not more than 0.001%), Acid value (not more than 3), Hydroxyl value (not more than 15), and Saponification value (365–395).

DIATRIZOATE AND IODIPAMIDE

For *Diatrizoates* and *Iodipamide*—See individual listings for chemistry information.

USP requirements: Diatrizoate Meglumine and Iodipamide Meglumine Injection—Not in *USP–NF*.

DIATRIZOATES

Chemical group: Ionic, monomeric, triiodinated benzoic acid derivative.

Chemical name:
Diatrizoate meglumine—Benzoic acid, 3,5-bis(acetylamino)-2,4,6-triiodo-, compd. with 1-deoxy-1-(methylamino)-D-glucitol (1:1).
Diatrizoate sodium—Benzoic acid, 3,5-bis(acetylamino)-2,4,6-triiodo-, monosodium salt.

Molecular formula:
Diatrizoate meglumine—$C_{11}H_9I_3N_2O_4 \cdot C_7H_{17}NO_5$.
Diatrizoate sodium—$C_{11}H_8I_3N_2NaO_4$.

Molecular weight:
Diatrizoate meglumine—809.13.
Diatrizoate sodium—635.90.

Description:
Diatrizoate Meglumine USP—White, odorless powder.
Diatrizoate Meglumine Injection USP—Clear, colorless to pale yellow, slightly viscous liquid.
Diatrizoate Meglumine and Diatrizoate Sodium Injection USP—Clear, colorless to pale yellow, slightly viscous liquid. May crystallize at room temperature or below.
Diatrizoate Sodium USP—White, odorless powder.
Diatrizoate Sodium Injection USP—Clear, colorless to pale yellow, slightly viscous liquid.
Diatrizoate Sodium Solution USP—Clear, pale yellow to light brown liquid.

Solubility:
Diatrizoate Meglumine USP—Freely soluble in water.
Diatrizoate Sodium USP—Soluble in water; slightly soluble in alcohol; practically insoluble in acetone and in ether.

Other characteristics: High osmolality.

USP requirements:
Diatrizoate Meglumine USP—Preserve in well-closed containers. Contains not less than 98.0% and not more than 102.0% of diatrizoate meglumine, calculated on the dried

basis. Meets the requirements for Identification, Specific rotation (–5.65° to –6.37°), Loss on drying (not more than 1.0%), Residue on ignition (not more than 0.1%), Iodine and iodide (0.02% iodide), Heavy metals (not more than 0.002%), and Free aromatic amine.

Diatrizoate Meglumine Injection USP—Preserve Injection intended for intravascular injection either in single-dose containers, preferably of Type I or Type III glass, protected from light or, where intended for administration with a pressure injector through a suitable transfer connection, in similar glass 500-mL or 1000-mL bottles, protected from light. Injection packaged for other than intravascular use may be packaged in 100-mL multiple-dose containers, preferably of Type I or Type III glass, protected from light. A sterile solution of Diatrizoate Meglumine in Water for Injection, or a sterile solution of Diatrizoic Acid in Water for Injection prepared with the aid of Meglumine. Label containers of Injection intended for intravascular injection, where packaged in single-dose containers, to direct the user to discard any unused portion remaining in the container or, where packaged in bulk bottles to state, "Bulk Container—only for sterile filling of pressure injectors," to state that it contains no antimicrobial preservatives, and to direct the user to discard any unused portion remaining in the container after 6 hours. Indicate also in the labeling of bulk bottles that a pressure injector is to be charged with a dose just prior to administration of the Injection. Label containers of Injection intended for other than intravascular injection to show that the contents are not intended for intravascular injection. Contains the labeled amount, within ±5%. Diatrizoate Meglumine Injection intended for intravascular use contains no antimicrobial agents. Meets the requirements for Identification, Bacterial endotoxins, pH (6.0–7.7), Iodine and iodide (0.02% iodide), Heavy metals (not more than 0.002%), Free aromatic amine, and Meglumine content (22.9–25.3% of the labeled amount of diatrizoate meglumine), and for Injections.

Diatrizoate Meglumine and Diatrizoate Sodium Injection USP—Preserve either in single-dose containers, preferably of Type I or Type III glass, protected from light or, where intended for administration with a pressure injector through a suitable transfer connection, in similar glass 500-mL or 1000-mL bottles, protected from light. A sterile solution of Diatrizoate Meglumine and Diatrizoate Sodium in Water for Injection, or a sterile solution of Diatrizoic Acid in Water for Injection prepared with the aid of Sodium Hydroxide and Meglumine. Label containers of Injection intended for intravascular injection, where packaged in single-dose containers, to direct the user to discard any unused portion remaining in the container or, where packaged in bulk bottles to state, "Bulk Container—only for sterile filling of pressure injectors," to state that it contains no antimicrobial preservatives, and to direct the user to discard any unused portion remaining in the container after 6 hours. Indicate also in the labeling of bulk bottles that a pressure injector is to be charged with a dose just prior to administration of the Injection. Label containers of Injection intended for other than intravascular injection to show that the contents are not intended for intravascular injection. Contains the labeled amounts of diatrizoate meglumine and iodine, within ±5%. Diatrizoate Meglumine and Diatrizoate Sodium Injection intended for intravascular use contains no antimicrobial agents. Meets the requirements for Identification, Bacterial endotoxins, pH (6.0–7.7), Free aromatic amine, Iodine and iodide (0.02% iodide), and Heavy metals (not more than 0.002%), and for Injections.

Diatrizoate Meglumine and Diatrizoate Sodium Solution USP—Preserve in tight, light-resistant containers. A solution of Diatrizoic Acid in Purified Water prepared with the aid of Meglumine and Sodium Hydroxide. Label the con-

tainer to indicate that the contents are not intended for parenteral use. Contains the labeled amounts of diatrizoate meglumine and iodine, within ±5%. Meets the requirements for Identification, pH (6.0–7.6), and Iodine and iodide (0.02% iodide).

Diatrizoate Sodium USP—Preserve in well-closed containers. Contains not less than 98.0% and not more than 102.0% of diatrizoate sodium, calculated on the anhydrous basis. Meets the requirements for Identification, Water (not more than 10.0%), Free aromatic amine, Iodine and iodide (0.02% iodide), and Heavy metals (not more than 0.002%).

Diatrizoate Sodium Injection USP—Preserve Injection intended for intravascular injection in single-dose containers, preferably of Type I or Type III glass, protected from light. Injection intended for other than intravascular use may be packaged in 100-mL multiple-dose containers, preferably of Type I or Type III glass, protected from light. A sterile solution of Diatrizoate Sodium in Water for Injection, or a sterile solution of Diatrizoic Acid in Water for Injection prepared with the aid of Sodium Hydroxide. Label containers of Injection intended for intravascular injection to direct the user to discard any unused portion remaining in the container. Label containers of Injection intended for other than intravascular injection to show that the contents are not intended for intravascular injection. Contains the labeled amount, within ±5%. Diatrizoate Sodium Injection intended for intravascular use contains no antimicrobial agents. Meets the requirements for Identification, Bacterial endotoxins, pH (6.0–7.7), Iodine and iodide (0.02% iodide), Heavy metals (not more than 0.002%), and Free aromatic amine, and for Injections.

Diatrizoate Sodium Solution USP—Preserve in tight, light-resistant containers. A solution of Diatrizoate Sodium in Purified Water, or a solution of Diatrizoic Acid in Purified Water prepared with the aid of Sodium Hydroxide. Label the container to indicate that the contents are not intended for parenteral use. Contains the labeled amount, within ± 5%. Meets the requirements for Identification, pH (4.5–7.5), and Iodine and iodide (0.02% iodide).

DIATRIZOIC ACID

Chemical name: Benzoic acid, 3,5-bis(acetylamino)-2,4,6-triiodo-.

Molecular formula: $C_{11}H_9I_3N_2O_4$.

Molecular weight: 613.91 (anhydrous); 649.95 (dihydrate).

Description: Diatrizoic Acid USP—White, odorless powder.

Solubility: Diatrizoic Acid USP—Very slightly soluble in water and in alcohol; soluble in dimethylformamide and in alkali hydroxide solutions.

USP requirements: Diatrizoic Acid USP—Preserve in well-closed containers. It is anhydrous or contains two molecules of water of hydration. Label it to indicate whether it is anhydrous or hydrous. Contains not less than 98.0% and not more than 102.0% of diatrizoic acid, calculated on the anhydrous basis. Meets the requirements for Identification, Water (not more than 1.0% for the anhydrous form; 4.5–7.0% for the hydrous form), Residue on ignition (not more than 0.1%), Free aromatic amine, Iodine and iodide (0.02% iodide), and Heavy metals (not more than 0.002%).

DIAZEPAM

Chemical name: 2*H*-1,4-Benzodiazepin-2-one, 7-chloro-1,3dihydro-1-methyl-5-phenyl-.

Molecular formula: $C_{16}H_{13}ClN_2O$.

Molecular weight: 284.74.

Description: Diazepam USP—Off-white to yellow, practically odorless, crystalline powder.

Solubility: Diazepam USP—Practically insoluble in water; freely soluble in chloroform; soluble in alcohol.

USP requirements:
Diazepam USP—Preserve in tight, light-resistant containers. Contains not less than 95.0% and not more than 105.0% of diazepam, calculated on the dried basis. Meets the requirements for Identification, Melting range (131–135 °C), Loss on drying (not more than 0.5%), Residue on ignition (not more than 0.1%), Heavy metals (not more than 0.002%), Related compounds, and Organic volatile impurities.

Diazepam Capsules USP—Preserve in tight, light-resistant containers. Contain the labeled amount, within ±10%. Meet the requirements for Identification, Dissolution (85% in 45 minutes in 0.01 *N* hydrochloric acid in Apparatus 1 at 100 rpm), and Uniformity of dosage units.

Diazepam Extended-release Capsules USP—Preserve in tight, light-resistant containers. Contain the labeled amount, within ±10%. Meet the requirements for Identification, Drug release (15–27% in 1 hour, 49–66% in 4 hours, 76–96% in 8 hours, and 85–115% in 12 hours in simulated gastric fluid TS, prepared without enzymes, in Apparatus 1 at 100 rpm), and Uniformity of dosage units.

Sterile Diazepam Emulsion—Not in *USP–NF*.

Diazepam Rectal Gel—Not in *USP–NF*.

Diazepam Rectal Viscous Solution—Not in *USP–NF*.

Diazepam Injection USP—Preserve in single-dose or in multiple-dose containers, preferably of Type I glass, protected from light. A sterile solution of Diazepam in a suitable medium. Contains the labeled amount, within ±10%. Meets the requirements for Identification, Bacterial endotoxins and pH (6.2–6.9), and for Injections.

Diazepam Oral Solution—Not in *USP–NF*.

Diazepam for Rectal Solution—Not in *USP–NF*.

Diazepam Tablets USP—Preserve in tight, light-resistant containers. Contain the labeled amount, within ±10%. Meet the requirements for Identification, Dissolution (85% in 30 minutes in 0.1 *N* hydrochloric acid in Apparatus 1 at 100 rpm), and Uniformity of dosage units.

DIAZOXIDE

Chemical group: A nondiuretic benzothiadiazine derivative.

Chemical name: 2*H*-1,2,4-Benzothiadiazine, 7-chloro-3-methyl-, 1,1-dioxide.

Molecular formula: $C_8H_7ClN_2O_2S$.

Molecular weight: 230.67.

Description: Diazoxide USP—White or cream-white crystals or crystalline powder.

pKa: 8.5.

Solubility: Diazoxide USP—Practically insoluble to sparingly soluble in water and in most organic solvents; very soluble in strong alkaline solutions; freely soluble in dimethylformamide.

USP requirements:
Diazoxide USP—Preserve in well-closed containers. Contains not less than 97.0% and not more than 102.0% of diazoxide, calculated on the dried basis. Meets the requirements for Identification, Loss on drying (not more than 0.5%), and Residue on ignition (not more than 0.1%).

Diazoxide Capsules USP—Preserve in well-closed containers. Contain the labeled amount, within ±10%. Meet the requirements for Identification, Dissolution (75% in 45 minutes in phosphate buffer [pH 6.8] in Apparatus 1 at 100 rpm), and Uniformity of dosage units.

Diazoxide Injection USP—Preserve in single-dose containers, preferably of Type I glass, protected from light. A sterile solution of Diazoxide in Water for Injection, prepared with the aid of Sodium Hydroxide. Contains the labeled amount, within ±10%. Meets the requirements for Identification, Bacterial endotoxins, and pH (11.2–11.9), and for Injections.

Diazoxide Oral Suspension USP—Preserve in tight, light-resistant containers. Contains the labeled amount, within ±10%. Meets the requirement for Identification.

DIBUCAINE

Chemical group: Amide.

Chemical name:
Dibucaine—4-Quinolinecarboxamide, 2-butoxy-*N*-[2-(diethylamino)ethyl]-.
Dibucaine hydrochloride—4-Quinolinecarboxamide, 2-butoxy-*N*-[2-(diethylamino)ethyl]-, monohydrochloride.

Molecular formula:
Dibucaine—$C_{20}H_{29}N_3O_2$.
Dibucaine hydrochloride—$C_{20}H_{29}N_3O_2 \cdot HCl$.

Molecular weight:
Dibucaine—343.46.
Dibucaine hydrochloride—379.92.

Description:
Dibucaine USP—White to off-white powder, having a slight, characteristic odor. Darkens on exposure to light.
Dibucaine Hydrochloride USP—Colorless or white to off-white crystals or white to off-white, crystalline powder. Is odorless, is somewhat hygroscopic, and darkens on exposure to light. Its solutions have a pH of about 5.5.

pKa: 8.8.

Solubility:
Dibucaine USP—Slightly soluble in water; soluble in 1 *N* hydrochloric acid and in ether.
Dibucaine Hydrochloride USP—Freely soluble in water, in alcohol, in acetone, and in chloroform.

USP requirements:
Dibucaine USP—Preserve in tight, light-resistant containers. Contains not less than 97.0% and not more than 102.5% of dibucaine, calculated on the dried basis. Meets the requirements for Identification, Melting range (62.5–66.0 °C, determined after drying), Loss on drying (not more than 1.0%), Residue on ignition (not more than 0.2%), and Chromatographic purity.

Dibucaine Cream USP—Preserve in collapsible tubes or in tight, light-resistant containers. Contains the labeled amount, within ±10%, in a suitable cream base. Meets the requirements for Identification, Microbial limits, and Minimum fill.

Dibucaine Ointment USP—Preserve in collapsible tubes or in tight, light-resistant containers. Contains the labeled amount, within ±10%, in a suitable ointment base. Meets the requirements for Identification, Microbial limits, and Minimum fill.

Dibucaine Hydrochloride USP—Preserve in tight, light-resistant containers. Contains not less than 97.0% and not more than 100.5% of dibucaine hydrochloride, calculated on the dried basis. Meets the requirements for Identification, Loss on drying (not more than 2.0%), Residue on ignition (not more than 0.1%), and Chromatographic purity.

Dibucaine Hydrochloride Injection USP—Preserve in single-dose or in multiple-dose containers, preferably of Type I glass, and protect from light. A sterile solution of Dibucaine Hydrochloride in Water for Injection. Contains the labeled amount, within ±5%. Meets the requirements for Identification, Bacterial endotoxins, pH (4.5–7.0), and Particulate matter, and for Injections.

DIBUTYL SEBACATE

Description: Dibutyl Sebacate NF—Colorless, oily liquid of very mild odor.

NF category: Plasticizer.

Solubility: Dibutyl Sebacate NF—Soluble in alcohol, in isopropyl alcohol, and in mineral oil; very slightly soluble in propylene glycol; practically insoluble in water and in glycerin.

NF requirements: Dibutyl Sebacate NF—Preserve in tight containers. Consists of esters of *n*-butyl alcohol and saturated dibasic acids, principally sebacic acid. Contains not less than 92.0% of dibutyl sebacate. Meets the requirements for Specific gravity (0.935–0.939 at 20 °C), Refractive index (1.429–1.441), Acid value (not more than 0.1), and Saponification value (352–357).

DICHLORALPHENAZONE

Chemical name: 1,2-Dihydro-1,5-dimethyl-2-phenyl-3*H*-pyrazol-3-one, compd. with 2,2,2-trichloro-1,1-ethanediol (1:2).

Molecular formula: $C_{15}H_{18}Cl_6N_2O_5$.

Molecular weight: 519.03.

Description: Dichloralphenazone USP—White, microcrystalline powder. Has a slight odor characteristic of chloral hydrate. Decomposed by dilute alkali, liberating chloroform.

Solubility: Dichloralphenazone USP—Freely soluble in water, in alcohol, and in chloroform; soluble in dilute acids.

USP requirements: Dichloralphenazone USP—Preserve in well-closed containers. Contains not less than 97.0% and not more than 100.5% of dichloralphenazone, determined by both *Assay* procedures. Meets the requirements for Identification, Residue on ignition (not more than 0.1%), and Heavy metals (not more than 0.001%).

DICHLORODIFLUOROMETHANE

Chemical name: Methane, dichlorodifluoro-.

Molecular formula: CCl_2F_2.

Molecular weight: 120.91.

Description: Dichlorodifluoromethane NF—Clear, colorless gas having a faint ethereal odor. Its vapor pressure at 25 °C is about 4880 mm of mercury (80 psig).

NF category: Aerosol propellant.

NF requirements: Dichlorodifluoromethane NF—Preserve in tight cylinders, and avoid exposure to excessive heat. Contains not less than 99.6% and not more than 100.0% of dichlorodifluoromethane, calculated on the anhydrous basis. Meets the requirements for Identification, Boiling temperature (approximately –30 °C), Water (not more than 0.001%), High-boiling residues (not more than 0.01%), Chromatographic purity, and Inorganic chlorides.

DICHLOROTETRAFLUOROETHANE

Chemical name: Ethane, 1,2-dichloro-1,1,2,2-tetrafluoro-.

Molecular formula: $C_2Cl_2F_4$.

Molecular weight: 170.92.

Description: Dichlorotetrafluoroethane NF—Clear, colorless gas having a faint ethereal odor. Its vapor pressure at 25 °C is about 1620 mm of mercury (17 psig). Usually contains between 6% and 10% of its isomer, 1,1-dichloro-1,2,2,2-tetrafluoro ethane.

NF category: Aerosol propellant.

NF requirements: Dichlorotetrafluoroethane NF—Preserve in tight cylinders and avoid exposure to excessive heat. Contains not less than 99.6% and not more than 100.0% of dichlorotetrafluoroethane, calculated on the anhydrous basis. Meets the requirements for Identification, Boiling temperature (approximately 4 °C), Water (not more than 0.001%), High-boiling residues (not more than 0.01%), Chromatographic purity, and Inorganic chlorides.

DICHLORPHENAMIDE

Chemical name: 1,3-Benzenedisulfonamide, 4,5-dichloro-.

Molecular formula: $C_6H_6Cl_2N_2O_4S_2$.

Molecular weight: 305.16.

Description: White or practically white, crystalline compound.

Solubility: Very slightly soluble in water; soluble in dilute solutions of sodium carbonate and sodium hydroxide.

USP requirements:

Dichlorphenamide USP—Preserve in well-closed containers. Contains not less than 98.0% and not more than 101.0% of dichlorphenamide, calculated on the dried basis. Meets the requirements for Identification, Melting range (236.5–240 °C), Loss on drying (not more than 1.0%), Residue on ignition (not more than 0.2%), Chloride (not more than 0.20%), Selenium (not more than 0.003%), Heavy metals (not more than 0.001%), and Organic volatile impurities.

Dichlorphenamide Tablets USP—Preserve in well-closed containers. Contain the labeled amount, within ±8%. Meet the requirements for Identification, Dissolution (80% in 60 minutes in 0.1 *M* phosphate buffer [pH 8.0] in Apparatus 2 at 75 rpm), and Uniformity of dosage units.

DICLOFENAC

Chemical group: Phenylacetic acid derivative.

Chemical name:

Diclofenac potassium—Benzeneacetic acid, 2-[(2,6-dichlorophenyl)amino]-, monopotassium salt.
Diclofenac sodium—Benzeneacetic acid, 2-[(2,6-dichlorophenyl)amino]-, monosodium salt.

Molecular formula:
Diclofenac potassium—$C_{14}H_{10}Cl_2KNO_2$.
Diclofenac sodium—$C_{14}H_{10}Cl_2NNaO_2$.

Molecular weight:
Diclofenac potassium—334.24.
Diclofenac sodium—318.13.

Description: Diclofenac Sodium USP—White to off-white, hygroscopic, crystalline powder. Melts at about 284°.

Solubility: Diclofenac Sodium USP—Freely soluble in methanol; sparingly soluble in water; soluble in ethanol; practically insoluble in chloroform and in ether.

USP requirements:
Diclofenac Potassium Tablets—Not in *USP–NF*.
Diclofenac Sodium USP—Preserve in tight, light-resistant containers. Contains not less than 99.0% and not more than 101.0% of diclofenac sodium, calculated on the dried basis. Meets the requirements for Identification, Color of solution, Clarity of solution, pH (7.0–8.5, in a solution [1 in 100]), Loss on drying (not more than 0.5%), Heavy metals (not more than 0.001%), and Chromatographic purity.
Diclofenac Sodium Ophthalmic Solution—Not in *USP–NF*.
Diclofenac Sodium Suppositories—Not in *USP–NF*.
Diclofenac Sodium Delayed-release Tablets USP—Preserve in tight, light-resistant containers. Contain the labeled amount, within ±10%. Meet the requirements for Identification, Drug release, Uniformity of dosage units, and Chromatographic purity (not more than 1.0% of any individual Impurity and the sum of all of the impurities not more than 1.5%).
Diclofenac Sodium Extended-release Tablets—Not in *USP–NF*.

DICLOFENAC AND MISOPROSTOL

For *Diclofenac* and *Misoprostol*—See individual listings for chemistry information.

USP requirements: Diclofenac Sodium and Misoprostol Tablets—Not in *USP–NF*.

DICLOXACILLIN

Chemical name: Dicloxacillin sodium—4-Thia-1-azabicyclo[3.2.0]heptane-2-carboxylic acid, 6-[[[3-(2,6-dichlorophenyl)-5-methyl-4-isoxazolyl]carbonyl]amino]-3,3-dimethyl-7oxo-, monosodium salt, monohydrate, [2S-(2 alpha,5 alpha,6 beta)]-.

Molecular formula: Dicloxacillin sodium—$C_{19}H_{16}Cl_2N_3NaO_5S \cdot H_2O$.

Molecular weight: Dicloxacillin sodium—510.31.

Description: Dicloxacillin Sodium USP—White to off-white, crystalline powder.

Solubility: Dicloxacillin Sodium USP—Freely soluble in water.

USP requirements:
Dicloxacillin Sodium USP—Preserve in tight containers. Contains the equivalent of not less than 850 mcg of dicloxacillin per mg. Meets the requirements for Identification, Crystallinity, pH (4.5–7.5, in a solution containing 10 mg per mL), Water (3.0–5.0%), and Dimethylaniline.
Dicloxacillin Sodium Capsules USP—Preserve in tight containers. Contain an amount of dicloxacillin sodium equivalent to the labeled amount of dicloxacillin, within −10% to +20%. Meet the requirements for Identification,

Dissolution (75% in 30 minutes in water in Apparatus 1 at 100 rpm), Uniformity of dosage units, and Water (not more than 5.0%).
Dicloxacillin Sodium for Oral Suspension USP—Preserve in tight containers. A dry mixture of Dicloxacillin Sodium and one or more suitable buffers, colors, flavors, and preservatives. Contains an amount of dicloxacillin sodium equivalent to the labeled amount of dicloxacillin, within −10% to +20%. Meets the requirements for Identification, Uniformity of dosage units (solid packaged in single-unit containers), Deliverable volume (solid packaged in multiple-unit containers), pH (4.5–7.5, in the suspension constituted as directed in the labeling), and Water (not more than 2.0%).

DICUMAROL

Chemical group: Coumarin derivative.

Chemical name: 2H-1-Benzopyran-2-one], 3,3'-Methylenebis[4-hydroxy-.

Molecular formula: $C_{19}H_{12}O_6$.

Molecular weight: 336.29.

Description: White or creamy white, crystalline powder, having a faint, pleasant odor. Melts at about 290 °C.

Solubility: Practically insoluble in water, in alcohol, and in ether; readily soluble in solutions of fixed alkali hydroxides; slightly soluble in chloroform.

USP requirements: Dicumarol Tablets—Not in *USP–NF*.

DICYCLOMINE

Chemical group: Synthetic tertiary amine.

Chemical name: Dicyclomine hydrochloride—[Bicyclohexyl]-1-carboxylic acid, 2-(diethylamino)ethyl ester, hydrochloride.

Molecular formula: Dicyclomine hydrochloride—$C_{19}H_{35}NO_2 \cdot HCl$.

Molecular weight: Dicyclomine hydrochloride—345.95.

Description:
Dicyclomine Hydrochloride USP—Fine, white, crystalline powder. Is practically odorless.
Dicyclomine Hydrochloride Injection USP—Colorless solution, which may have the odor of a preservative.

pKa: Dicyclomine hydrochloride—9.0.

Solubility: Dicyclomine Hydrochloride USP—Soluble in water; freely soluble in alcohol and in chloroform; very slightly soluble in ether.

USP requirements:
Dicyclomine Hydrochloride USP—Preserve in well-closed containers. Contains not less than 99.0% and not more than 102.0% of dicyclomine hydrochloride, calculated on the dried basis. Meets the requirements for Identification, Melting range (169–174 °C), pH (5.0–5.5, in a solution [1 in 100]), Readily carbonizable substances, and Organic volatile impurities.
Dicyclomine Hydrochloride Capsules USP—Preserve in well-closed containers. Contain the labeled amount, within ± 7%. Meet the requirements for Identification, Dissolution (75% in 45 minutes in 0.01 N hydrochloric acid in Apparatus 2 at 50 rpm), and Uniformity of dosage units.
Dicyclomine Hydrochloride Injection USP—Preserve in single-dose or in multiple-dose containers, preferably of Type I glass. A sterile, isotonic solution of Dicyclomine Hydro-

chloride in Water for Injection. Contains the labeled amount, within ±7%. Meets the requirements for Identification and Bacterial endotoxins, and for Injections.

Dicyclomine Hydrochloride Syrup USP—Preserve in tight containers. Contains the labeled amount, within ±5%. Meets the requirement for Identification.

Dicyclomine Hydrochloride Tablets USP—Preserve in well-closed containers. Contain the labeled amount, within ±7%. Meet the requirements for Identification, Dissolution (75% in 45 minutes in 0.01 N hydrochloric acid in Apparatus 2 at 50 rpm), and Uniformity of dosage units.

Dicyclomine Hydrochloride Extended-release Tablets—Not in *USP–NF*.

DIDANOSINE

Chemical name: Inosine, 2',3'-dideoxy-.

Molecular formula: $C_{10}H_{12}N_4O_3$.

Molecular weight: 236.23.

Description: White, crystalline powder. Unstable in acidic solutions.

Solubility: Aqueous solubility at 25 °C and pH of approximately 6 is 27.3 mg per mL.

USP requirements:
Buffered Didanosine for Oral Solution—Not in *USP–NF*.
Didanosine for Buffered Oral Suspension—Not in *USP–NF*.
Didanosine Tablets—Not in *USP–NF*.

DIENESTROL

Chemical name: Phenol, 4,4'-(1,2-diethylidene-1,2-ethanediyl)-bis-, (*E,E*)-.

Molecular formula: $C_{18}H_{18}O_2$.

Molecular weight: 266.33.

Description: Dienestrol USP—Colorless, white or practically white, needle-like crystals, or white or practically white, crystalline powder. Is odorless.

Solubility: Dienestrol USP—Practically insoluble in water; soluble in alcohol, in acetone, in ether, in methanol, in propylene glycol, and in solutions of alkali hydroxides; slightly soluble in chloroform and in fatty oils.

USP requirements:
Dienestrol USP—Preserve in well-closed containers. Contains not less than 98.0% and not more than 100.5% of dienestrol, calculated on the dried basis. Meets the requirements for Identification, Melting range (227–234 °C, not more than 3 °C between beginning and end of melting), Loss on drying (not more than 0.5%), and Residue on ignition (not more than 0.2%).

Dienestrol Cream USP—Preserve in collapsible tubes or in tight containers. It is Dienestrol in a suitable water-miscible base. Contains the labeled amount, within ±10%. Meets the requirements for Identification and Minimum fill.

DIETHANOLAMINE

Chemical name: Ethanol, 2,2'-iminobis-.

Molecular formula: $C_4H_{11}NO_2$.

Molecular weight: 105.14.

Description: Diethanolamine NF—White or clear, colorless crystals, deliquescing in moist air; or colorless liquid.
NF category: Alkalizing agent; emulsifying and/or solubilizing agent.

Solubility: Diethanolamine NF—Miscible with water, with alcohol, with acetone, with chloroform, and with glycerin. Slightly soluble to insoluble in ether and in petroleum ether.

NF requirements: Diethanolamine NF—Preserve in tight, light-resistant containers. A mixture of ethanolamines, consisting largely of diethanolamine. Contains not less than 98.5% and not more than 101.0% of ethanolamines, calculated on the anhydrous basis as diethanolamine. Meets the requirements for Identification, Refractive index (1.473–1.476, at 30 °C), Water (not more than 0.15%), Limit of triethanolamine (not more than 1.0%), and Organic volatile impurities.

DIETHYLAMINE SALICYLATE

Molecular formula: $C_{11}H_{17}NO_3$.

Molecular weight: 211.3.

Description: White or almost white, odorless or almost odorless crystals.

Solubility: Soluble 1 in less than 1 of water, 1 in 2 of alcohol, and 1 in 1.5 of chloroform.

USP requirements: Diethylamine Salicylate Cream—Not in *USP–NF*.

DIETHYLCARBAMAZINE

Chemical group: Piperazine derivative.

Chemical name: Diethylcarbamazine citrate—1-Piperazinecarboxamide, *N,N*-diethyl-4-methyl-, 2-hydroxy-1,2,3-propanetricarboxylate.

Molecular formula: Diethylcarbamazine citrate—$C_{10}H_{21}N_3O \cdot C_6H_8O_7$.

Molecular weight: Diethylcarbamazine citrate—391.42.

Description: Diethylcarbamazine Citrate USP—White, crystalline powder. Melts at about 136 °C, with decomposition. Is odorless or has a slight odor; is slightly hygroscopic.

Solubility: Diethylcarbamazine Citrate USP—Very soluble in water; sparingly soluble in alcohol; practically insoluble in acetone, in chloroform, and in ether.

USP requirements:
Diethylcarbamazine Citrate USP—Preserve in tight containers. Contains not less than 98.0% and not more than 102.0% of diethylcarbamazine citrate, calculated on the anhydrous basis. Meets the requirements for Identification, Water (not more than 0.5%), Residue on ignition (not more than 0.1%), Heavy metals (not more than 0.002%), Ordinary impurities, and Chromatographic impurity.

Diethylcarbamazine Citrate Tablets USP—Preserve in tight containers. Contain the labeled amount, within ±5%. Meet the requirements for Identification, Disintegration (for Tablets labeled solely for veterinary use: 30 minutes), Disso-

lution (75% in 45 minutes in water in Apparatus 2 at 50 rpm), Uniformity of dosage units, and Chromatographic purity.

Note: Diethylcarbamazine Citrate Tablets labeled solely for veterinary use are exempt from the requirements of the test for *Dissolution*.

DIETHYL PHTHALATE

Chemical name: 1,2-Benzenedicarboxylic acid, diethyl ester.

Molecular formula: $C_{12}H_{14}O_4$.

Molecular weight: 222.24.

Description: Diethyl Phthalate NF—Colorless, practically odorless, oily liquid.

NF category: Plasticizer.

Solubility: Diethyl Phthalate NF—Insoluble in water. Miscible with alcohol, with ether, and with other usual organic solvents.

NF requirements: Diethyl Phthalate NF—Preserve in tight containers. Contains not less than 98.0% and not more than 102.0% of diethyl phthalate, calculated on the anhydrous basis. Meets the requirements for Identification, Specific gravity (1.118–1.122, at 20 °C), Refractive index (1.500–1.505, at 20 °C), Acidity, Water (not more than 0.2%), and Residue on ignition (not more than 0.02%).

Caution: Avoid contact.

DIETHYLENE GLYCOL MONOETHYL ETHER

Molecular formula: $C_6H_{14}O_3$.

Molecular weight: 134.18.

Description: Diethylene Glycol Monoethyl Ether NF—Clear, colorless liquid. Is hygroscopic. Specific gravity about 0.991.

Solubility: Diethylene Glycol Monoethyl Ether NF—Miscible with water, with acetone, and with alcohol; partially miscible with vegetable oils; immiscible with mineral oils.

NF requirements: Diethylene Glycol Monoethyl Ether NF—Preserve in tight containers under an atmosphere of an inert gas, at a temperature not exceeding 35°. Produced by condensation of ethylene oxide and alcohol, followed by distillation. The label indicates that it is stored under an atmosphere of an inert gas. Contains not less than 99.0% and not more than 101.0% of diethylene glycol monoethyl ether. Meets the requirements for Identification, Refractive index (1.426–1.428 at 20°), Water (not more than 0.1%, determined on a 10-gram specimen), Acid value (not more than 0.1), Peroxide value (not more than 8.0), Limit of free ethylene oxide (not more than 1 microgram per gram), and Limit of 2-methoxyethanol, 2-ethoxyethanol, ether, ethylene glycol, and diethylene glycol (not more than 500 micrograms per gram of diethylene glycol).

DIETHYLPROPION

Chemical group: Phenethylamine.

Chemical name: Diethylpropion hydrochloride—1-Propanone, 2-(diethylamino)-1-phenyl-, hydrochloride.

Molecular formula: Diethylpropion hydrochloride—$C_{13}H_{19}NO \cdot HCl$.

Molecular weight: Diethylpropion hydrochloride—241.76.

Description: Diethylpropion Hydrochloride USP—White to off-white, fine crystalline powder. Is odorless, or has a slight characteristic odor. It melts at about 175 °C, with decomposition.

Solubility: Diethylpropion Hydrochloride USP—Freely soluble in water, in chloroform, and in alcohol; practically insoluble in ether.

USP requirements:
Diethylpropion Hydrochloride USP—Preserve in well-closed, light-resistant containers. The label indicates whether it contains tartaric acid as a stabilizer. Contains not less than 97.0% and not more than 103.0% of diethylpropion hydrochloride, calculated on the anhydrous basis. Meets the requirements for Identification, Water (not more than 0.5%), Secondary amines (not more than 0.5%), Free bromine, Limit of hydrobromic acid and bromide, Chromatographic purity, and Organic volatile impurities.
Diethylpropion Hydrochloride Tablets USP—Preserve in well-closed containers. Contain the labeled amount, within ± 10%. Meet the requirements for Identification, Dissolution (75% in 45 minutes in water in Apparatus 2 at 50 rpm), and Uniformity of dosage units.
Diethylpropion Hydrochloride Extended-release Tablets—Not in *USP–NF*.

DIETHYLSTILBESTROL

Chemical name:
Diethylstilbestrol—Phenol 4,4'-(1,2-diethyl-1,2-ethenediyl) bis-,(*E*)-.
Diethylstilbestrol diphosphate—Phenol, 4,4'-(1,2-diethyl-1,2-ethenediyl)bis-, bis(dihydrogen phosphate), (*E*)-.

Molecular formula:
Diethylstilbestrol—$C_{18}H_{20}O_2$.
Diethylstilbestrol diphosphate—$C_{18}H_{22}O_8P_2$.

Molecular weight:
Diethylstilbestrol—268.35.
Diethylstilbestrol diphosphate—428.31.

Description:
Diethylstilbestrol USP—White, odorless, crystalline powder.
Diethylstilbestrol Diphosphate USP—Off-white, odorless, crystalline powder.
Diethylstilbestrol Diphosphate Injection USP—Colorless to light, straw-colored liquid.

Solubility:
Diethylstilbestrol USP—Practically insoluble in water; soluble in alcohol, in chloroform, in ether, in fatty oils, and in dilute alkali hydroxides.
Diethylstilbestrol Diphosphate USP—Sparingly soluble in water; soluble in alcohol and in dilute alkali.

USP requirements:
Diethylstilbestrol USP—Preserve in tight, light-resistant containers. Contains not less than 97.0% and not more than 100.5% of diethylstilbestrol, calculated on the dried basis. Meets the requirements for Identification, Melting range (169–175 °C, not more than 4 °C between beginning and end of melting), Acidity or alkalinity, Loss on drying (not more than 0.5%), Residue on ignition (not more than 0.05%), and Organic volatile impurities.
Diethylstilbestrol Injection USP—Preserve in light-resistant, single-dose or multiple-dose containers, preferably of Type I glass. A sterile solution of Diethylstilbestrol in a suitable vegetable oil. Contains the labeled amount, within ± 10%. Meets the requirements for Identification and Bacterial endotoxins, and for Injections.

Diethylstilbestrol Tablets USP—Preserve in well-closed containers. Contain the labeled amount, within ±10%. Meet the requirements for Identification, Disintegration (30 minutes), and Uniformity of dosage units.

Diethylstilbestrol Diphosphate USP—Preserve in tight containers, at a temperature not exceeding 21 °C. Contains not less than 95.0% and not more than 101.0% of diethylstilbestrol diphosphate, calculated on the dried basis. Meets the requirements for Identification, Loss on drying (not more than 1.0%), Chloride (not more than 1.5%), Free diethylstilbestrol (not more than 0.15%), Diethylstilbestrol monophosphate (not more than 1.5%), Pyridine, and Organic volatile impurities.

Diethylstilbestrol Diphosphate Injection USP—Preserve in single-dose or in multiple-dose containers. A sterile, buffered solution of Diethylstilbestrol Diphosphate. Contains not less than 45.0 mg and not more than 55.0 mg of diethylstilbestrol diphosphate in each mL. Meets the requirements for Identification, Bacterial endotoxins, pH (9.0–10.5), Free diethylstilbestrol (not more than 0.2 mg per mL of Injection), and Diethylstilbestrol monophosphate (not more than 2.0 mg per mL of Injection), and for Injections.

Diethylstilbestrol Diphosphate Tablets—Not in *USP–NF.*

DIETHYLSTILBESTROL AND METHYLTESTOSTERONE

For *Diethylstilbestrol* and *Methyltestosterone*—See individual listings for chemistry information.

USP requirements: Diethylstilbestrol and Methyltestosterone Tablets—Not in *USP–NF.*

DIETHYLTOLUAMIDE

Chemical name: Benzamide, *N,N*-diethyl-3-methyl-.

Molecular formula: $C_{12}H_{17}NO$.

Molecular weight: 191.27.

Description: Diethyltoluamide USP—Colorless liquid, having a faint, pleasant odor. Boils at about 111 °C under a pressure of 1 mm of mercury.

Solubility: Diethyltoluamide USP—Practically insoluble in water and in glycerin. Miscible with alcohol, with isopropyl alcohol, with ether, with chloroform, and with carbon disulfide.

USP requirements:
Diethyltoluamide USP—Preserve in tight containers. Contains not less than 95.0% and not more than 103.0% of the *meta*-isomer of diethyltoluamide, calculated on the anhydrous basis. Meets the requirements for Identification, Specific gravity (0.996–1.002), Refractive index (1.520–1.524), Acidity, and Water (not more than 0.5%).

Diethyltoluamide Topical Aerosol—Not in *USP–NF.*
Diethyltoluamide Liquid—Not in *USP–NF.*
Diethyltoluamide Lotion—Not in *USP–NF.*
Diethyltoluamide Topical Solution USP—Preserve in tight containers. A solution of Diethyltoluamide in Alcohol or Isopropyl Alcohol. Contains the labeled amount of the meta isomer of diethyltoluamide, within ±8%. If it contains Alcohol, contains the labeled amount of alcohol, within ±5%. Meets the requirements for Identification and Alcohol content (if present, 29.0–89.0%).

Diethyltoluamide Topical Spray Solution—Not in *USP–NF.*
Diethyltoluamide Towelettes—Not in *USP–NF.*

DIFENOXIN AND ATROPINE

Source: Atropine—An alkaloid that may be extracted from belladonna root and hyoscyamine or may be produced synthetically.

Chemical group:
Atropine—Natural tertiary amine.
Difenoxin—Diphenoxylic acid, principal active metabolite of diphenoxylate.

Chemical name:
Atropine sulfate—Benzeneacetic acid, alpha-(hydroxymethyl)-, 8-methyl-8-azabicyclo[3.2.1]oct-3-yl ester, *endo*-(±)-, sulfate (2:1) (salt), monohydrate.
Difenoxin hydrochloride—1-(3-Cyano-3,3-diphenylpropyl)-4-phenyl-4-piperidinecarboxylic acid monohydrochloride.

Molecular formula:
Atropine sulfate—$(C_{17}H_{23}NO_3)_2 \cdot H_2SO_4 \cdot H_2O$.
Difenoxin hydrochloride—$C_{28}H_{28}N_2O_2 \cdot HCl$.

Molecular weight:
Atropine sulfate—694.83.
Difenoxin hydrochloride—461.0.

Description:
Atropine Sulfate USP—Colorless crystals, or white, crystalline powder. Odorless; effloresces in dry air; is slowly affected by light.
Difenoxin hydrochloride—White amorphous powder. It has a melting point of 290 °C.

Solubility:
Atropine Sulfate USP—Very soluble in water; freely soluble in alcohol and even more so in boiling alcohol; freely soluble in glycerin.
Difenoxin hydrochloride—Very slightly soluble in water; sparingly soluble in chloroform, in tetrahydrofuran, in dimethylacetamide, and in dimethyl sulfoxide.

USP requirements: Difenoxin Hydrochloride and Atropine Sulfate Tablets—Not in *USP–NF.*

DIFLORASONE

Chemical name: Diflorasone diacetate—Pregna-1,4-diene-3,20-dione, 17,21-bis(acetyloxy)-6,9-difluoro-11-hydroxy-16-methyl-, (6 alpha,11 beta,16 beta)-.

Molecular formula: Diflorasone diacetate—$C_{26}H_{32}F_2O_7$.

Molecular weight: Diflorasone diacetate—494.52.

Description: Diflorasone Diacetate USP—White to pale yellow, crystalline powder.

Solubility: Diflorasone Diacetate USP—Insoluble in water; soluble in methanol and in acetone; sparingly soluble in ethyl acetate; slightly soluble in toluene; very slightly soluble in ether.

USP requirements:
Diflorasone Diacetate USP—Preserve in tight containers. Contains not less than 97.0% and not more than 103.0% of diflorasone diacetate, calculated on the dried basis. Meets the requirements for Identification, Specific rotation (+58° to +68°), Loss on drying (not more than 0.5%), and Residue on ignition (not more than 0.5%), Chromatographic purity, and Other impurities.

Diflorasone Diacetate Cream USP—Preserve in collapsible tubes, preferably at controlled room temperature. Contains the labeled amount, within ±10%. Meets the requirements for Identification, Microbial limits, and Minimum fill.

Diflorasone Diacetate Ointment USP—Preserve in collapsible tubes, preferably at controlled room temperature. Contains the labeled amount, within ±10%. Meets the requirements for Identification, Microbial limits, and Minimum fill.

DIFLUCORTOLONE

Chemical name: Diflucortolone valerate—6 alpha,9 alpha-Difluoro-11 beta,21-dihydroxy-16 alpha-methylpregna-1,4-diene-3,20-dione 21-valerate.

Molecular formula: Diflucortolone valerate—$C_{27}H_{36}F_2O_5$.

Molecular weight: Diflucortolone valerate—478.6.

Description: Diflucortolone valerate—Melting point 200–205 °C.

Solubility: Diflucortolone valerate—Soluble in chloroform; slightly soluble in methyl alcohol; practically insoluble in ether.

USP requirements:
Diflucortolone Valerate Cream—Not in *USP–NF*.
Diflucortolone Valerate Ointment—Not in *USP–NF*.

DIFLUNISAL

Chemical group: Salicylic acid derivative. However, diflunisal is not metabolized to salicylic acid in vivo.

Chemical name: [1,1'-Biphenyl]-3-carboxylic acid, 2',4'-difluoro-4-hydroxy-.

Molecular formula: $C_{13}H_8F_2O_3$.

Molecular weight: 250.20.

Description: Diflunisal USP—White to off-white, practically odorless powder.

pKa: 3.3.

Solubility: Diflunisal USP—Freely soluble in alcohol and in methanol; soluble in acetone and in ethyl acetate; slightly soluble in chloroform, in carbon tetrachloride, and in methylene chloride; insoluble in hexane and in water.

USP requirements:
Diflunisal USP—Preserve in well-closed containers. Contains not less than 98.0% and not more than 101.5% of diflunisal, calculated on the dried basis. Meets the requirements for Identification, Loss on drying (not more than 0.3%), Residue on ignition (not more than 0.1%), Heavy metals (not more than 0.001%), Chromatographic purity, and Organic volatile impurities.
Diflunisal Tablets USP—Preserve in well-closed containers. Contain the labeled amount, within ±10%. Meet the requirements for Identification, Dissolution (80% in 30 minutes in 0.1 *M* Tris buffer [pH 7.20] in Apparatus 2 at 50 rpm), and Uniformity of dosage units.

DIGITALIS

USP requirements:
Digitalis USP—Preserve in containers that protect it from absorbing moisture. Digitalis labeled to indicate that it is to be used only in the manufacture of glycosides is exempt from the moisture and storage requirements. The dried leaf of *Digitalis purpurea* Linné (Fam Scrophulariaceae). The potency of Digitalis is such that, when assayed as directed, 100 mg is equivalent to not less than 1 USP Digitalis Unit. (One USP Digitalis Unit represents the potency of 100 mg of USP Digitalis RS.) Meets the requirements for Botanic characteristics, Acid-insoluble ash (not more than 5.0%), Foreign organic matter (not more than 2.0%), Water (not more than 6.0%), and Organic volatile impurities.
Note: When Digitalis is prescribed, Powdered Digitalis is to be dispensed.
Powdered Digitalis USP—Preserve in tight, light-resistant containers. A package of suitable desiccant may be enclosed in the container. It is Digitalis dried at a temperature not exceeding 60 °C, reduced to a fine or a very fine powder, and adjusted, if necessary to conform to the official potency by admixture with sufficient Lactose, Starch or exhausted marc of digitalis, or with Powdered Digitalis having either a lower or a higher potency. The potency of Powdered Digitalis is such that, when assayed as directed, 100 mg is equivalent to 1 USP Digitalis Unit. (One USP Digitalis Unit represents the potency of 100 mg of USP Digitalis RS.) Meets the requirements for Identification, Microbial limits, Water (not more than 5.0%), Acid-insoluble ash (not more than 5.0%), and Organic volatile impurities.
Note: When Digitalis is prescribed, Powdered Digitalis is to be dispensed.
Digitalis Capsules USP—Preserve in tight containers. Contain an amount of Powdered Digitalis equivalent to the labeled potency, within −15% to +20%. Meet the requirements for Microbial limits and Uniformity of dosage units.
Digitalis Tablets USP—Preserve in tight containers. Contain an amount of Powdered Digitalis equivalent to the labeled potency, within −15% to +20%. Meet the requirements for Microbial limits, Disintegration (30 minutes), and Uniformity of dosage units.

DIGITOXIN

Chemical name: Card-20(22)-enolide, 3-[(O-2,6-dideoxy-beta-D-ribo-hexopyranosyl-(1→4)-O-2,6-dideoxy-beta-D-ribohexo-pyranosyl-(1→4)-2,6-dideoxy-beta-D-ribo-hexopyranosyl)-oxy]-14-hydroxy, (3 beta,5 beta)-.

Molecular formula: $C_{41}H_{64}O_{13}$.

Molecular weight: 764.94.

Description: Digitoxin USP—White or pale buff, odorless, microcrystalline powder.

Solubility: Digitoxin USP—Practically insoluble in water; sparingly soluble in chloroform; slightly soluble in alcohol; very slightly soluble in ether.

USP requirements:
Digitoxin USP—Preserve in tight containers. A cardiotonic glycoside obtained from *Digitalis purpurea* Linné, *Digitalis lanata* Ehrhart (Fam. Scrophulariaceae), and other suitable species of *Digitalis*. Contains not less than 92.0% and not more than 103.0% of digitoxin, calculated on the dried basis. Meets the requirements for Identification, Loss on drying (not more than 1.5%), and Residue on ignition.
Caution: Handle Digitoxin with exceptional care since it is highly potent.
Digitoxin Injection USP—Preserve in single-dose or in multiple-dose containers, preferably of Type I glass, protected from light. A sterile solution of Digitoxin in 5 to 50% (v/v) of alcohol, and may contain Glycerin or other suitable solubilizing agents. Contains the labeled amount, within ±10%. Meets the requirements for Identification, Bacterial endotoxins, and Alcohol content (the labeled percentage of alcohol, within ±10%), and for Injections.
Digitoxin Tablets USP—Preserve in well-closed containers. Contain the labeled amount, within ±10%. Meet the requirements for Identification, Dissolution (60% dissolved

in 30 minutes and 85% dissolved in 60 minutes in dilute hydrochloric acid [3 in 500] in Apparatus 1 at 120 ±5 rpm), and Uniformity of dosage units.

Note: Avoid the use of strongly adsorbing substances, such as bentonite, in the manufacture of Digitoxin Tablets.

DIGOXIN

Source: Obtained naturally from *Digitalis lanata* or may be produced synthetically.

Chemical name: Card-20(22)-enolide, 3-[(*O*-2,6-dideoxy-beta-D-*ribo*-hexopyranosyl-(1→4)-*O*-2,6-dideoxy-beta-D-*ribo*-hexopyranosyl-(1→4)-2,6-dideoxy-beta-D-*ribo*-hexopyranosyl)oxy]-12,14-dihydroxy-, (3 beta,5 beta,12 beta)-.

Molecular formula: $C_{41}H_{64}O_{14}$.

Molecular weight: 780.94.

Description: Digoxin USP—Clear to white, odorless crystals or white, odorless crystalline powder.

Solubility: Digoxin USP—Practically insoluble in water and in ether; freely soluble in pyridine; slightly soluble in diluted alcohol and in chloroform.

USP requirements:
Digoxin USP—Preserve in tight containers. A cardiotonic glycoside obtained from the leaves of *Digitalis lanata* Ehrhart (Fam. Scrophulariaceae). Contains not less than 95.0% and not more than 101.0% of digoxin, calculated on the dried basis. Meets the requirements for Identification, Loss on drying (not more than 1.0%), Residue on ignition (not more than 0.5%, a 100-mg specimen being used), Organic volatile impurities, and Related glycosides (not more than 3.0%).

Caution: Handle Digoxin with exceptional care, since it is extremely poisonous.
Digoxin Capsules—Not in *USP–NF*.
Digoxin Elixir USP—Preserve in tight containers, and avoid exposure to excessive heat. Contains, in each 100 mL, not less than 4.50 mg and not more than 5.25 mg of digoxin. Meets the requirements for Identification and Alcohol content (the labeled amount, within −10% to +15%).
Digoxin Injection USP—Preserve in single-dose containers, preferably of Type I glass. Avoid exposure to excessive heat. A sterile solution of Digoxin in Water for Injection and Alcohol or other suitable solvents. Contains the labeled amount, within −10% to +5%. Meets the requirements for Identification, Bacterial endotoxins, and Alcohol content (9.0–11.0%), and for Injections.
Digoxin Oral Suspension USP—Preserve in tight containers, and avoid exposure to excessive heat. Contains, in each 100 mL, not less than 4.50 mg and not more than 5.25 mg of digoxin. Meets the requirements for Identification and Alcohol content (the labeled amount, within −10% to +15%).
Digoxin Tablets USP—Preserve in tight containers. Contain the labeled amount, within −10% to +5%. Meet the requirements for Identification, Dissolution (80% in 60 minutes in 0.1 N hydrochloric acid in Apparatus 1 at 120 rpm), and Uniformity of dosage units.

DIGOXIN IMMUNE FAB (OVINE)

Source: Produced by a process involving immunization of sheep with digoxin that has been coupled as a hapten to human serum albumin, to stimulate production of digoxin-specific antibo-

dies. After papain digestion of the antibody, digoxin-specific antigen binding (Fab) fragments (molecular weight 50,000 daltons) are isolated and purified by affinity chromatography.

Molecular weight: 50,000.

Description: Sterile, lyophilized powder.

USP requirements: Digoxin Immune Fab (Ovine) for Injection—Not in *USP–NF*.

DIHYDROCODEINE

Chemical name: Dihydrocodeine bitartrate—Morphinan-6-ol, 4,5-epoxy-3-methoxy-17-methyl-, (5 alpha,6 alpha)-2,3-dihydroxybutanedioate (1:1) (salt).

Molecular formula: Dihydrocodeine bitartrate—$C_{18}H_{23}NO_3 \cdot C_4H_6O_6$.

Molecular weight: Dihydrocodeine bitartrate—451.47.

Description: Dihydrocodeine bitartrate—Odorless, or almost odorless, colorless crystals or white crystalline powder.

Solubility: Dihydrocodeine bitartrate—Soluble 1 in 4.5 of water; sparingly soluble in alcohol; practically insoluble in ether.

USP requirements: Dihydrocodeine Bitartrate USP—Preserve in tight containers. Contains not less than 98.5% and not more than 100.5% of dihydrocodeine bitartrate, calculated on the dried basis. Meets the requirements for Identification, Melting range (186–190 °C, not more than 2.5 °C between beginning and end of melting), Specific rotation (−72° to −75°), pH (3.2–4.2, in a solution [1 in 10]), Loss on drying (not more than 0.5%), Residue on ignition (not more than 0.1%), Ammonium salts, and Ordinary impurities.

DIHYDROCODEINE, ACETAMINOPHEN, AND CAFFEINE

For *Dihydrocodeine, Acetaminophen,* and *Caffeine*—See individual listings for chemistry information.

USP requirements: Dihydrocodeine Bitartrate, Acetaminophen, and Caffeine Capsules—Not in *USP–NF*.

DIHYDROERGOTAMINE

Chemical name: Dihydroergotamine mesylate—Ergotoman-3′,6′,18-trione,9,10-dihydro-12′-hydroxy-2′-methyl-5′-(phenylmethyl)-, (5′ alpha)-, monomethanesulfonate (salt).

Molecular formula: Dihydroergotamine mesylate—$C_{33}H_{37}N_5O_5 \cdot CH_4O_3S$.

Molecular weight: Dihydroergotamine mesylate—679.78.

Description: Dihydroergotamine Mesylate USP—White to slightly yellowish powder, or off-white to faintly red powder, having a faint odor.

pKa: 6.75.

Solubility: Dihydroergotamine Mesylate USP—Slightly soluble in water and in chloroform; soluble in alcohol.

USP requirements:
Dihydroergotamine Mesylate USP—Preserve in well-closed, light-resistant containers. Contains not less than 97.0% and not more than 103.0% of dihydroergotamine mesylate, calculated on the dried basis. Meets the requirements for Identification, Specific rotation (−16.7° to −22.7°), pH

(4.4–5.4, in a solution [1 in 1000]), Loss on drying (not more than 4.0%), and Related alkaloids (not more than 2.0%).

Dihydroergotamine Mesylate Injection USP—Preserve in single-dose containers, preferably of Type I glass, protected from light. A sterile solution of Dihydroergotamine Mesylate in Water for Injection. Contains the labeled amount, within ±10%. Meets the requirements for Identification, Bacterial endotoxins, and pH (3.4–4.9), and for Injections.

Dihydroergotamine Mesylate Nasal Solution—Not in *USP–NF*.

DIHYDROSTREPTOMYCIN

Chemical name: Dihydrostreptomycin sulfate—Dihydrostreptomycin sulfate (2:3) (salt).

Molecular formula: Dihydrostreptomycin sulfate—$(C_{21}H_{41}N_7O_{12})_2 \cdot 3H_2SO_4$.

Molecular weight: Dihydrostreptomycin sulfate—1461.42.

Description: Dihydrostreptomycin Sulfate USP—White or almost white, amorphous or crystalline powder. Amorphous form is hygroscopic.

Solubility: Dihydrostreptomycin Sulfate USP—Freely soluble in water; practically insoluble in acetone, in chloroform, and in methanol.

USP requirements:

Dihydrostreptomycin Injection USP—Preserve in single-dose or in multiple-dose containers. Label it to indicate that it is intended for veterinary use only. Contains an amount of Dihydrostreptomycin Sulfate equivalent to the labeled amount of dihydrostreptomycin, within −10% to +20%. Contains one or more suitable preservatives. Meets the requirements for Identification, Bacterial endotoxins, Sterility, and pH (5.0–8.0).

Dihydrostreptomycin Sulfate USP—Preserve in tight containers. Label it to indicate that it is intended for veterinary use only. If it is crystalline, it may be so labeled. If it is intended solely for oral use, it is so labeled. Where it is intended for use in preparing injectable dosage forms, the label states that it is sterile or must be subjected to further processing during the preparation of injectable dosage forms. Has a potency equivalent to not less than 650 mcg of dihydrostreptomycin per mg, except that if it is labeled as being crystalline, has a potency equivalent to not less than 725 mcg of dihydrostreptomycin per mg, or if it is labeled as being solely for oral use, has a potency equivalent to not less than 450 mcg of dihydrostreptomyin per mg. Meets the requirements for Identification, pH (4.5–7.0, in a solution containing 200 mg of dihydrostreptomycin per mL; 3.0–7.0, if it is labeled as being solely for oral use), Loss on drying (not more than 5.0%; not more than 14.0% if it is labeled as being solely for oral use), and Streptomycin (not more than 3.0%; not more than 1.0% if it is labeled as being crystalline; not more than 5.0% if it is labeled as being solely for oral use), and for Sterility and Bacterial endotoxins under Dihydrostreptomycin Injection (where the label states that Dihydrostreptomycin Sulfate is sterile), and for Bacterial endotoxins under Dihydrostreptomycin Injection (where the label states that Dihydrostreptomycin Sulfate must be subjected to further processing during the preparation of injectable dosage forms).

Dihydrostreptomycin Sulfate Boluses USP—Preserve in tight containers. Label Boluses to indicate that they are intended for veterinary use only. Contain an amount of Dihydrostreptomycin Sulfate equivalent to the labeled amount of dihydrostreptomycin, within −15% to +20%. Meet the requirement for Loss on drying (not more than 10.0%).

DIHYDROTACHYSTEROL

Chemical name: 9,10-Secoergosta-5,7,22-trien-3-ol, (3 beta,5*E*,7*E*,10 alpha,22*E*)-.

Molecular formula: $C_{28}H_{46}O$.

Molecular weight: 398.66.

Description: Dihydrotachysterol USP—Colorless or white, odorless crystals, or white, odorless, crystalline powder.

Solubility: Dihydrotachysterol USP—Practically insoluble in water; soluble in alcohol; freely soluble in ether and in chloroform; sparingly soluble in vegetable oils.

USP requirements:

Dihydrotachysterol USP—Preserve in light-resistant, hermetic glass containers from which air has been displaced by an inert gas. Contains not less than 97.0% and not more than 103.0% of dihydrotachysterol. Meets the requirements for Identification, Specific rotation (+100° to +103°), Residue on ignition (not more than 0.1%), and Organic volatile impurities.

Dihydrotachysterol Capsules USP—Preserve in well-closed, light-resistant containers. Contain a solution of Dihydrotachysterol in a suitable vegetable oil. Contain the labeled amount, within ±10%. Meet the requirements for Identification and Uniformity of dosage units.

Dihydrotachysterol Oral Solution USP—Preserve in tight, light-resistant glass containers. Contains the labeled amount, within ±10%. Meets the requirement for Identification.

Dihydrotachysterol Tablets USP—Preserve in well-closed, light-resistant containers. Contain the labeled amount, within ±10%. Meet the requirements for Identification, Disintegration (10 minutes), and Uniformity of dosage units.

DIHYDROXYACETONE

Source: Produced from glycerol by *Acetobacter* sp. under aerobic conditions.

Chemical name: 1,3-dihydroxy-2-propanone.

Molecular formula: $C_3H_6O_3$.

Molecular weight: 90.08.

Description: White to off-white crystalline powder. Fairly hygroscopic. Characteristic odor. Melting point about 75–80 °C.

Solubility: Monomeric form freely soluble in water, in alcohol, and in ether. Dimeric form freely soluble in water; soluble in alcohol; and sparingly soluble in ether.

USP requirements:

Dihydroxyacetone USP—Preserve in tight containers in a cool place. Contains not less than 98.0% and not more than 102.0% of dihydroxyacetone, calculated on an anhydrous basis. Meets the requirements for Identification, pH (4.0–6.0, in a solution [1 in 20]), Water (not more than 0.2%), Residue on ignition (not more than 0.1%), Heavy metals (0.001%), Limit of iron (not more than 0.002%), Chromatographic purity, and Limit of protein (the absorbance of the test solution is not more than 0.400).

DIHYDROXYALUMINUM AMINOACETATE

Source: A basic salt of aluminum and glycine.

Chemical name: Aluminum, (glycinato-*N,O*)dihydroxy-, hydrate.

Molecular formula: $C_2H_6AlNO_4 \cdot xH_2O$.

Molecular weight: 135.06 (anhydrous).

Description:
Dihydroxyaluminum Aminoacetate USP—White, odorless powder.
Dihydroxyaluminum Aminoacetate Magma USP—White, viscous suspension, from which small amounts of water may separate on standing.

Solubility: Dihydroxyaluminum Aminoacetate USP—Insoluble in water and in organic solvents; soluble in dilute mineral acids and in solutions of fixed alkalies.

USP requirements:
Dihydroxyaluminum Aminoacetate USP—Preserve in well-closed containers. Yields not less than 94.0% and not more than 102.0% of dihydroxyaluminum aminoacetate, calculated on the dried basis. Meets the requirements for Identification, pH (6.5–7.5, in a suspension of 1 gram of it, finely powdered, in 25 mL of water), Loss on drying (not more than 14.5%), Mercury (not more than 1 ppm), Isopropyl alcohol, Nitrogen (9.90–10.60%), and Organic volatile impurities.
Dihydroxyaluminum Aminoacetate Capsules USP—Preserve in well-closed containers. Contain the labeled amount, within ±10%. Meet the requirements for Identification, Disintegration (10 minutes, simulated gastric fluid TS being substituted for water in the test), Uniformity of dosage units, Acid-neutralizing capacity, and pH (6.5–7.5, in a suspension of Capsule powder equivalent to about 1 gram of dihydroxyaluminum aminoacetate in 25 mL of water).
Dihydroxyaluminum Aminoacetate Magma USP—Preserve in tight containers, and protect from freezing. A suspension that contains the labeled amount, within ±10%. Meets the requirements for Identification, Microbial limits, Acid-neutralizing capacity, and pH (6.5–7.5, in a dilution in water, equivalent to about 1 gram of dihydroxyaluminum aminoacetate in 25 mL).
Dihydroxyaluminum Aminoacetate Tablets USP—Preserve in well-closed containers. Contain the labeled amount, within ±10%. Meet the requirements for Identification, Disintegration (10 minutes, simulated gastric fluid TS being substituted for water in the test), Uniformity of dosage units, Acid-neutralizing capacity, and pH (6.5–7.5, in a suspension of ground Tablet powder in water, equivalent to about 1 gram of dihydroxyaluminum aminoacetate in 25 mL of water).

DIHYDROXYALUMINUM SODIUM CARBONATE

Chemical name: Aluminum, [carbonato(1-)-*O*]dihydroxy-, monosodium salt.

Molecular formula: $NaAl(OH)_2CO_3$.

Molecular weight: 143.99.

Description: Dihydroxyaluminum Sodium Carbonate USP—Fine, white, odorless powder.

Solubility: Dihydroxyaluminum Sodium Carbonate USP—Practically insoluble in water and in organic solvents; soluble in dilute mineral acids with the evolution of carbon dioxide.

USP requirements:
Dihydroxyaluminum Sodium Carbonate USP—Preserve in tight containers. Contains not less than 98.3% and not more than 107.9% of dihydroxyaluminum sodium carbonate, calculated on the dried basis. Meets the requirements

for Identification, pH (9.9–10.2 in a suspension [1 in 25]), Acid-neutralizing capacity, Loss on drying (not more than 14.5%), Isopropyl alcohol (not more than 1.0%), Sodium content (15.2–16.8%), Mercury (not more than 1 ppm), and Organic volatile impurities.
Dihydroxyaluminum Sodium Carbonate Tablets USP—Preserve in well-closed containers. Label the Tablets to indicate that they are to be chewed before swallowing. Contain the labeled amount, within ±10%. Meet the requirements for Identification, Uniformity of dosage units, and Acid-neutralizing capacity.

DILOXANIDE

Chemical group: Diloxanide furoate—Dichloroacetamide derivative.

Chemical name: Diloxanide furoate—4-(*N*-Methyl-2,2-dichloroacetamido)phenyl 2-furoate.

Molecular formula: Diloxanide furoate—$C_{14}H_{11}Cl_2NO_4$.

Molecular weight: Diloxanide furoate—328.20.

Description: Diloxanide Furoate USP—White or almost white, crystalline powder.

Solubility: Diloxanide Furoate USP—Freely soluble in chloroform; slightly soluble in alcohol and in ether; very slightly soluble in water.

USP requirements: Diloxanide Furoate Tablets USP—Preserve in tight, light-resistant containers. Contain not less than 98.0% and not more than 102.0% of diloxanide furoate, calculated on the dried basis. Meet the requirements for Identification, Melting range (114–116 °C), Acidity (not more than 1.3 mL of 0.1 *N* sodium hydroxide is required for neutralization), Loss on drying (not more than 0.5%), Residue on ignition (not more than 0.1%), and Related compounds.

DILTIAZEM

Chemical name: Diltiazem hydrochloride—1,5-Benzothiazepin-4(5*H*)one, 3-(acetyloxy)-5-[2-(dimethylamino)ethyl]-2,3-dihydro-2-(4-methoxyphenyl)-, monohydrochloride, (+)-*cis*-.

Molecular formula: Diltiazem hydrochloride—$C_{22}H_{26}N_2O_4S \cdot HCl$.

Molecular weight: Diltiazem hydrochloride—450.98.

Description: Diltiazem Hydrochloride USP—White, odorless, crystalline powder or small crystals. Melts at about 210 °C, with decomposition.

Solubility: Diltiazem Hydrochloride USP—Freely soluble in chloroform, in formic acid, in methanol, and in water; sparingly soluble in dehydrated alcohol; insoluble in ether.

USP requirements:
Diltiazem Hydrochloride USP—Preserve in tight, light-resistant containers. Contains not less than 98.5% and not more than 101.5% of diltiazem hydrochloride, calculated on the dried basis. Meets the requirements for Identification, Specific rotation (+110° to +116°), Loss on drying (not more than 0.5%), Residue on ignition (not more than 0.1%), Heavy metals (not more than 20 ppm), Related compounds, and Organic volatile impurities.
Diltiazem Hydrochloride Extended-release Capsules USP—Preserve in tight containers. The labeling indicates the Drug Release Test with which the product complies. Contain the labeled amount, within ±10%. Meet the requirements for Identification, Drug release (For products labeled for dosing every 12 hours: 10–25% in 3 hours,

45–85% in 9 hours, and not less than 70% in 12 hours in water in Apparatus 2 at 100 rpm for Test 1; 10–25% in 4 hours, 35–60% in 8 hours, 55–80% in 12 hours, and not less than 80% in 24 hours in water in Apparatus 2 at 100 rpm for Test 4; not more than 15% in 1 hour, 45–70% in 3 hours, and not less than 80% in 8 hours in 0.05 M phosphate buffer [pH 7.2] in Apparatus 2 at 50 rpm for Test 5; not more than 10% in 1 hour, 10–30% in 6 hours, 34–60% in 9 hours and not less than 80% in 24 hours in 0.05 M phosphate buffer [pH 6.5] in Apparatus 1 at 100 rpm for Test 10. For products labeled for dosing every 24 hours: 5–20% in 1 hour, 30–50% in 4 hours, 70–90% in 10 hours, and not less than 80% in 15 hours in water in Apparatus 2 at 100 rpm for Test 2; 20–45% in 6 hours, 25–50% in 12 hours, 35–70% in 18 hours, not less than 70% in 24 hours, and not less than 85% in 30 hours in 0.1 N hydrochloric acid in Apparatus 2 at 100 rpm for Test 3; not more than 25% in 2 hours, 25–50% in 4 hours, 60–85% in 8 hours, not less than 70% in 12 hours, and not less than 80% in 16 hours in water in Apparatus 1 at 100 rpm for Test 6; not more than 10% in 1 hour, 15–35% in 4 hours, 65–85% in 10 hours, and not less than 80% in 15 hours in acetate buffer [pH 4.2] in Apparatus 2 at 100 rpm for Test 7; and 5–20% in 1 hour, 30–50% in 4 hours, 60–90% in 10 hours, and not less than 80% in 15 hours for Test 8; 0–5% in 2 hours in 0.1 N hydrochloric acid and, 20–45% in 2 hours, 35–55% in 12 hours, not less than 60% in 18 hours, and not less than 80% in 24 hours in simulated intestinal fluid TS, prepared without enzyme and adjusted to pH of 7.5±0.1 in Apparatus 2 at 75 rpm for Test 9; not more than 10% in 1 hour, 30–40% in 6 hours, 36–58% in 12 hours, and not less than 85% in 18 hours for Test 11; not more than 20% in 2 hours, 30–55% in 8 hours, not less than 65% in 14 hours, and not less than 80% in 24 hours in water in Apparatus 1 at 100 rpm for Test 12; not more 20% in 2 hours, 30–55% in 8 hours, 60–80% in 14 hours, and not less than 80% in 24 hours in water in Apparatus 1 at 100 rpm for Test 13), and Uniformity of dosage units.

Diltiazem Hydrochloride Injection—Not in *USP–NF*.

Diltiazem Hydrochloride Tablets USP—Preserve in tight, light-resistant containers. Contain the labeled amount, within ± 10%. Meet the requirements for Identification, Dissolution (not more than 60% in 30 minutes and not less than 75% in 3 hours in water in Apparatus 2 at 75 rpm), and Uniformity of dosage units.

DIMENHYDRINATE

Chemical group: Ethanolamine derivative.

Chemical name: 1*H*-Purine-2,6-dione, 8-chloro-3,7-dihydro-1,3-dimethyl-, compd. with 2-(diphenylmethoxy)-*N,N*-dimethylethanamine (1:1).

Molecular formula: $C_{17}H_{21}NO \cdot C_7H_7ClN_4O_2$.

Molecular weight: 469.96.

Description: Dimenhydrinate USP—White, crystalline, odorless powder.

Solubility: Dimenhydrinate USP—Slightly soluble in water; freely soluble in alcohol and in chloroform; sparingly soluble in ether.

USP requirements:
Dimenhydrinate USP—Preserve in well-closed containers. Contains not less than 53.0% and not more than 55.5% of diphenhydramine, and not less than 44.0% and not more than 47.0% of 8-chlorotheophylline, calculated on the dried basis. Meets the requirements for Identification, Melting range (102–107 °C), Loss on drying (not more than 0.5%), Residue on ignition (not more than 0.3%), Bromide and iodide, Chloride, and Organic volatile impurities.

Dimenhydrinate Capsules—Not in *USP–NF*.

Dimenhydrinate Extended-release Capsules—Not in *USP–NF*.

Dimenhydrinate Elixir—Not in *USP–NF*.

Dimenhydrinate Injection USP—Preserve in single-dose or in multiple-dose containers, preferably of Type I or Type III glass. A solution of Dimenhydrinate in a mixture of Propylene Glycol and water. Contains the labeled amount, within ±5%. Meets the requirements for Identification, pH (6.4–7.2), and Content of 8-chlorotheophylline, and for Injections.

Dimenhydrinate Oral Solution USP—Preserve in tight containers. Contains the labeled amount, within ±10%. Meets the requirements for Identification, Content of 8-chlorotheophylline, and Alcohol content (4.0–6.0%)..

Dimenhydrinate Suppositories—Not in *USP–NF*.

Dimenhydrinate Syrup USP—Preserve in tight containers. Contains the labeled amount, within ±10%. Meets the requirements for Identification, Content of 8-chlorotheophylline, and Alcohol content (4.0–6.0%).

Dimenhydrinate Tablets USP—Preserve in well-closed containers. Contain the labeled amount, within ±10%. Meet the requirements for Identification, Dissolution (75% in 45 minutes in water in Apparatus 2 at 50 rpm), Uniformity of dosage units, and Content of 8-chlorotheophylline.

Dimenhydrinate Chewable Tablets—Not in *USP–NF*.

DIMERCAPROL

Chemical group: Dithiol.

Chemical name: 1-Propanol, 2,3-dimercapto.

Molecular formula: $C_3H_8OS_2$.

Molecular weight: 124.23.

Description:
Dimercaprol USP—Colorless or practically colorless liquid, having a disagreeable, mercaptan-like odor.
Dimercaprol Injection USP—Yellow, viscous solution having a pungent, disagreeable odor. Specific gravity is about 0.978.

Solubility: Dimercaprol USP—Soluble in water, in alcohol, in benzyl benzoate, and in methanol.

USP requirements:
Dimercaprol USP—Preserve in tight containers, in a cold place. Contains not less than 97.0% and not more than 100.5% of dimercaprol, and not more than 1.5% of 1,2,3-trimercaptopropane. Meets the requirements for Specific gravity (1.242–1.244), Distilling range (66–68 °C, under a pressure of 0.2 mm of mercury), Refractive index (1.567–1.573), and Limit of 1,2,3-trimercaptopropane and related impurities (not more than 1.5% of 1,2,3-trimercaptopropane).

Dimercaprol Injection USP—Preserve in single-dose or in multiple-dose containers, preferably of Type I or Type III glass. A sterile solution of Dimercaprol in a mixture of Benzyl Benzoate and vegetable oil. Contains, in each 100 grams, not less than 9.0 grams and not more than 11.0 grams of dimercaprol. Meets the requirements for Limit of 1,2,3-trimercaptopropane and related impurities, and for Injections (except that at times it may be turbid or contain small amounts of flocculent material).

DIMETHICONE

Chemical name: Dimethicone.

Description: Dimethicone NF—Clear, colorless, odorless liquid. NF category: Antifoaming agent; water repelling agent.

Solubility: Dimethicone NF—Insoluble in water, in methanol, in alcohol, and in acetone; very slightly soluble in isopropyl alcohol; soluble in chlorinated hydrocarbons, in toluene, in xylene, in n-hexane, in petroleum spirits, in ether, and in amyl acetate.

NF requirements: Dimethicone NF—Preserve in tight containers. A mixture of fully methylated linear siloxane polymers containing repeating units of the formula $[-(CH_3)_2SiO-]_n$, stabilized with trimethylsiloxy end-blocking units of the formula $[(CH_3)_3SiO-]$, wherein n has an average value such that the corresponding nominal viscosity is in a discrete range between 20 and 30,000 centistokes. Label it to indicate its nominal viscosity value. Dimethicone intended for use in coating containers that come in contact with articles for parenteral use is so labeled. Contains not less than 97.0% and not more than 103.0% of polydimethylsiloxane. The requirements for viscosity, specific gravity, refractive index, and loss on heating differ for the several types of Dimethicone. Meets the requirements for Identification, Specific gravity, Viscosity, Refractive index, Acidity, Loss on heating, Heavy metals (not more than 5 mcg per gram), and Bacterial endotoxins (where it is intended for use in coating containers that come in contact with articles for parenteral use).

DIMETHYL SULFOXIDE

Chemical name: Methane, sulfinylbis-.

Molecular formula: C_2H_6OS.

Molecular weight: 78.13.

Description: Dimethyl Sulfoxide USP—Clear, colorless, odorless, hygroscopic liquid. Melts at about 18.4 °C. Boils at about 189 °C.

Solubility: Dimethyl Sulfoxide USP—Soluble in water; practically insoluble in acetone, in alcohol, in chloroform, and in ether.

USP requirements:
Dimethyl Sulfoxide USP—Preserve in tight, light-resistant containers. Contains not less than 99.9% of dimethyl sulfoxide. Meets the requirements for Identification, Specific gravity (1.095–1.101), Congealing temperature (not less than 18.3 °C), Refractive index (1.4755–1.4775), Acidity, Water (not more than 0.1%), Ultraviolet absorbance, Substances darkened by potassium hydroxide, Limit of dimethyl sulfone, and Limit of nonvolatile residue.

Dimethyl Sulfoxide Gel USP—Preserve in tight, light-resistant containers. Label it to indicate that it is for veterinary use only. Contains the labeled concentration, within ±10%. Meets the requirements for Identification, Deliverable Volume, and pH (4.7–6.7 [determined on a mixture of 5 grams of Gel and 5 mL of water]).

Dimethyl Sulfoxide Irrigation USP—Preserve in single-dose containers, and store at controlled room temperature, protected from strong light. A sterile solution of Dimethyl Sulfoxide in Water for Injection. Label it to indicate prominently that it is not intended for injection. Contains the labeled amount, within ±5%. Meets the requirements for Identification, Bacterial endotoxins, Sterility, and pH (5.0–7.0, when diluted with water to obtain a solution containing 50 mg of dimethyl sulfoxide per mL).

Dimethyl Sulfoxide Solution—Not in *USP–NF*.

Dimethyl Sulfoxide Topical Solution USP—Preserve in tight, light-resistant containers. Label it to indicate that it is for veterinary use only. Contains the labeled concentration, within ±10%. Meets the requirement for Identification.

DINOPROST

Source: Dinoprost tromethamine—The tromethamine salt of naturally occurring prostaglandin $F_{2\text{-alpha}}$.

Chemical name: Dinoprost tromethamine—Prosta-5,13-dien-1-oic acid, 9,11,15-trihydroxy-, (5Z,9 alpha,11 alpha,13E,15S)-, compd. with 2-amino-2-(hydroxymethyl)-1,3-propanediol (1:1).

Molecular formula: Dinoprost tromethamine—$C_{20}H_{34}O_5 \cdot C_4H_{11}NO_3$.

Molecular weight: Dinoprost tromethamine—475.62.

Description: Dinoprost Tromethamine USP—White to off-white, crystalline powder.

Solubility: Dinoprost Tromethamine USP—Very soluble in water; freely soluble in dimethylformamide; soluble in methanol; slightly soluble in chloroform.

USP requirements:
Dinoprost Tromethamine USP—Preserve in tight containers. Contains not less than 95.0% and not more than 105.0% of dinoprost tromethamine, calculated on the dried basis. Meets the requirements for Identification, Specific rotation (+19° to +26°), Loss on drying (not more than 1.0%), Residue on ignition (not more than 0.5%), and Chromatographic purity.

Caution: Great care should be taken to prevent inhaling particles of Dinoprost Tromethamine and exposing the skin to it.

Dinoprost Tromethamine Injection USP—Preserve in single-dose or in multiple-dose containers, preferably of Type I glass. A sterile solution of Dinoprost Tromethamine in Water for Injection. May contain a suitable preservative, such as benzyl alcohol. Contains an amount of dinoprost tromethamine equivalent to the labeled amount of dinoprost, within ±10%. Meets the requirements for Identification, Bacterial endotoxins, and pH (7.0–9.0), for Injections, and for Sterility tests.

DINOPROSTONE

Source: The naturally occurring prostaglandin E_2.

Chemical name: Prosta-5,13-dien-1-oic acid, 11,15-dihydroxy-9-oxo-, (5Z,11 alpha,13E,15S)-.

Molecular formula: $C_{20}H_{32}O_5$.

Molecular weight: 352.47.

Description: Dinoprostone USP—White to off-white, crystalline powder. Melting point 64–71 °C.

Solubility: Dinoprostone USP—Freely soluble in acetone, in alcohol, in ether, in ethyl acetate, in isopropyl alcohol, in methanol, and in methylene chloride; soluble in toluene and in diisopropyl ether; practically insoluble in hexanes.

USP requirements:
Dinoprostone USP—Preserve in well-closed, light-resistant containers. Contains not less than 97.0% and not more than 103.0% of dinoprostone. Meets the requirements for Identification, Specific rotation (−82.0° to −90.0°, at 20°), Water (not more than 0.5%), Residue on ignition (not more than 0.5%), and Chromatographic purity.

Dinoprostone Cervical Gel—Not in *USP–NF*.
Dinoprostone Vaginal Gel—Not in *USP–NF*.
Dinoprostone Vaginal Insert—Not in *USP–NF*.
Dinoprostone Vaginal Suppositories—Not in *USP–NF*.
Dinoprostone Vaginal System—Not in *USP–NF*.

DIOXYBENZONE

Chemical name: Methanone, (2-hydroxy-4-methoxyphenyl)(2-hydroxyphenyl)-.

Molecular formula: $C_{14}H_{12}O_4$.

Molecular weight: 244.24.

Description: Dioxybenzone USP—Yellow powder.

Solubility: Dioxybenzone USP—Practically insoluble in water; freely soluble in alcohol and in toluene.

USP requirements: Dioxybenzone USP—Preserve in tight, light-resistant containers. Contains not less than 97.0% and not more than 103.0% of dioxybenzone, calculated on the dried basis. Meets the requirements for Identification, Congealing temperature (not lower than 68.0 °C), and Loss on drying (not more than 2.0%).

DIOXYBENZONE AND OXYBENZONE

For *Dioxybenzone* and *Oxybenzone*—See individual listings for chemistry information.

USP requirements: Dioxybenzone and Oxybenzone Cream USP—Preserve in tight containers. A mixture of approximately equal parts of Dioxybenzone and Oxybenzone in a suitable cream base. Contains, in each 100 grams, not less than 2.7 grams and not more than 3.3 grams each of dioxybenzone and oxybenzone. Meets the requirements for Identification and Minimum fill.

DIOXYBENZONE, OXYBENZONE, AND PADIMATE O

For *Dioxybenzone, Oxybenzone,* and *Padimate O*—See individual listings for chemistry information.

USP requirements: Dioxybenzone, Oxybenzone, and Padimate O Cream—Not in *USP–NF*.

DIPHENHYDRAMINE

Chemical group: Ethanolamine derivative.

Chemical name:
Diphenhydramine citrate—Ethanamine, 2-(diphenylmethoxy)-N,N-dimethyl-, 2-hydroxy-1,2,3-propanetricarboxylate (1:1).
Diphenhydramine hydrochloride—Ethanamine, 2-(diphenylmethoxy)-N,N-dimethyl-, hydrochloride.

Molecular formula:
Diphenhydramine citrate—$C_{17}H_{21}NO \cdot C_6H_8O_7$.

Diphenhydramine hydrochloride—$C_{17}H_{21}NO \cdot HCl$.

Molecular weight:
Diphenhydramine citrate—447.48.
Diphenhydramine hydrochloride—291.82.

Description: Diphenhydramine Hydrochloride USP—White, odorless, crystalline powder. Slowly darkens on exposure to light. Its solutions are practically neutral to litmus.

pKa: 9.

Solubility: Diphenhydramine Hydrochloride USP—Freely soluble in water, in alcohol, and in chloroform; sparingly soluble in acetone; very slightly soluble in ether.

USP requirements:
Diphenhydramine Citrate USP—Preserve in tight, light-resistant containers. Contains not less than 98.0% and not more than 100.5% of diphenhydramine citrate, calculated on the dried basis. Meets the requirements for Identification, Melting range (146–150 °C, range between beginning and end of melting not more than 2 °C), Loss on drying (not more than 0.5%), Residue on ignition (not more than 0.1%), and Organic volatile impurities.
Diphenhydramine Hydrochloride USP—Preserve in tight, light-resistant containers. Contains not less than 98.0% and not more than 102.0% of diphenhydramine hydrochloride, calculated on the dried basis. Meets the requirements for Identification, Melting range (167–172 °C), Loss on drying (not more than 0.5%), Residue on ignition (not more than 0.1%), and Organic volatile impurities.
Diphenhydramine Hydrochloride Capsules USP—Preserve in tight containers. Contain the labeled amount, within ± 10%. Meet the requirements for Identification, Dissolution (80% in 30 minutes in water in Apparatus 1 at 100 rpm), and Uniformity of dosage units.
Diphenhydramine Hydrochloride Elixir USP—Preserve in tight, light-resistant containers. Contains the labeled amount, within ±10%. Meets the requirements for Identification and Alcohol content (the labeled amount, within ± 10%).
Diphenhydramine Hydrochloride Injection USP—Preserve in single-dose or in multiple-dose containers, preferably of Type I glass, protected from light. A sterile solution of Diphenhydramine Hydrochloride in Water for Injection. Contains the labeled amount, within ±10%. Meets the requirements for Identification, Bacterial endotoxins, and pH (4.0–6.5), and for Injections.
Diphenhydramine Hydrochloride Oral Solution USP—Preserve in tight, light-resistant containers. Contains the labeled amount, within ±10%. Meets the requirements for Identification and Alcohol content (the labeled amount, within ±10%).
Diphenhydramine Hydrochloride Syrup—Not in *USP–NF*.
Diphenyhydramine Hydrochloride Tablets—Not in *USP–NF*.

DIPHENHYDRAMINE, CODEINE, AND AMMONIUM CHLORIDE

For *Diphenhydramine, Codeine,* and *Ammonium Chloride*—See individual listings for chemistry information.

USP requirements: Diphenhydramine Hydrochloride, Codeine Phosphate, and Ammonium Chloride Syrup—Not in *USP–NF*.

DIPHENHYDRAMINE, DEXTROMETHORPHAN, AND AMMONIUM CHLORIDE

For *Diphenhydramine, Dextromethorphan,* and *Ammonium Chloride*—See individual listings for chemistry information.

USP requirements: Diphenhydramine Hydrochloride, Dextromethorphan Hydrobromide, and Ammonium Chloride Syrup—Not in *USP–NF*.

DIPHENHYDRAMINE, PHENYLPROPANOLAMINE, AND ASPIRIN

For *Diphenhydramine, Phenylpropanolamine,* and *Aspirin*—See individual listings for chemistry information.

USP requirements: Diphenhydramine Citrate, Phenylpropanolamine Hydrochloride, and Aspirin Effervescent Tablets—Not in *USP–NF*.

DIPHENHYDRAMINE AND PSEUDOEPHEDRINE

For *Diphenhydramine* and *Pseudoephedrine*—See individual listings for chemistry information.

USP requirements:

Diphenhydramine and Pseudoephedrine Capsules USP— Preserve in tight containers. Label Capsules to state both the contents of the active moieties and the contents of the salts used in formulating the article. Contain the labeled amounts of diphenhydramine hydrochloride and pseudoephedrine hydrochloride, within ±10%. Meet the requirements for Identification, Dissolution (75% of each active ingredient in 30 minutes in water in Apparatus 1 at 100 rpm), Uniformity of dosage units, and Related compounds (sum of amounts of benzhydrol and benzophenone not more than 2% [w/w] of diphenhydramine hydrochloride).

Diphenhydramine and Pseudoephedrine Hydrochlorides Oral Solution—Not in *USP–NF*.

Diphenhydramine and Pseudoephedrine Hydrochlorides Tablets—Not in *USP–NF*.

DIPHENHYDRAMINE, PSEUDOEPHEDRINE, AND ACETAMINOPHEN

For *Diphenhydramine, Pseudoephedrine,* and *Acetaminophen*— See individual listings for chemistry information.

USP requirements:

Diphenhydramine Hydrochloride, Pseudoephedrine Hydrochloride, and Acetaminophen Oral Solution—Not in *USP–NF*.

Diphenhydramine Hydrochloride, Pseudoephedrine Hydrochloride, and Acetaminophen Tablets—Not in *USP–NF*.

DIPHENHYDRAMINE, PSEUDOEPHEDRINE, DEXTROMETHORPHAN, AND ACETAMINOPHEN

For *Diphenhydramine, Pseudoephedrine, Dextromethorphan,* and *Acetaminophen*—See individual listings for chemistry information.

USP requirements: Diphenhydramine Hydrochloride, Pseudoephedrine Hydrochloride, Dextromethorphan Hydrobromide, and Acetaminophen Tablets—Not in *USP–NF*.

DIPHENIDOL

Chemical name: Diphenidol hydrochloride—1-Piperidinebutanol, alpha,alpha-diphenyl, hydrochloride.

Molecular formula: Diphenidol hydrochloride—$C_{21}H_{27}NO \cdot HCl$.

Molecular weight: Diphenidol hydrochloride—345.91.

Description: Diphenidol hydrochloride—Melting point 212–214 °C.

Solubility: Diphenidol hydrochloride—Freely soluble in methanol; soluble in water and in chloroform; practically insoluble in ether.

USP requirements: Diphenidol Hydrochloride Tablets—Not in *USP–NF*.

DIPHENOXYLATE

Chemical group: Diphenoxylate hydrochloride—Similar in structure to meperidine.

Chemical name: Diphenoxylate hydrochloride—4-Piperidinecarboxylic acid, 1-(3-cyano-3,3-diphenylpropyl)-4-phenyl-, ethyl ester, monohydrochloride.

Molecular formula: Diphenoxylate hydrochloride—$C_{30}H_{32}N_2O_2 \cdot HCl$.

Molecular weight: Diphenoxylate hydrochloride—489.05.

Description: Diphenoxylate Hydrochloride USP—White, odorless, crystalline powder. Its saturated solution has a pH of about 3.3.

Solubility: Diphenoxylate Hydrochloride USP—Slightly soluble in water and in isopropanol; freely soluble in chloroform; soluble in methanol; sparingly soluble in alcohol and in acetone; practically insoluble in ether and in solvent hexane.

USP requirements: Diphenoxylate Hydrochloride USP—Preserve in well-closed containers. Contains not less than 98.0% and not more than 102.0% of diphenoxylate hydrochloride, calculated on the dried basis. Meets the requirements for Identification, Melting range (220–226 °C), Loss on drying (not more than 0.5%), and Ordinary impurities.

DIPHENOXYLATE AND ATROPINE

For *Diphenoxylate* and *Atropine*—See individual listings for chemistry information.

USP requirements:

Diphenoxylate Hydrochloride and Atropine Sulfate Oral Solution USP—Preserve in tight, light-resistant containers. Contains the labeled amount of diphenoxylate hydrochloride, within ±7%, and the labeled amount of atropine sulfate, within ±20%. Meets the requirements for Identification, pH (3.0–4.3, determined in a dilution of the Oral Solution with an equal volume of water), and Alcohol content (13.5–16.5%).

Diphenoxylate Hydrochloride and Atropine Sulfate Tablets USP—Preserve in well-closed, light-resistant containers. Contain the labeled amount of diphenoxylate hydrochloride, within ±10%, and the labeled amount of atropine sul-

fate, within ±20%. Meet the requirements for Identification, Dissolution (75% of the labeled amount of diphenoxylate hydrochloride in 45 minutes in 0.2 *M* acetic acid in Apparatus 1 at 150 rpm), and Uniformity of dosage units.

DIPHENYLPYRALINE, PHENYLEPHRINE, AND DEXTROMETHORPHAN

Chemical name:
Diphenylpyraline hydrochloride—Piperidine, 4-(diphenylmethoxy)-1-methyl-, hydrochloride.
Phenylephrine hydrochloride—Benzenemethanol, 3-hydroxy-alpha-[(methylamino)methyl]-, hydrochloride.
Dextromethorphan hydrobromide—Morphinan, 3-methoxy-17-methyl-, (9 alpha,13 alpha,14 alpha)-, hydrobromide,-monohydrate.

Molecular formula:
Diphenylpyraline hydrochloride—$C_{19}H_{23}NO \cdot HCl$.
Phenylephrine hydrochloride—$C_9H_{13}NO_2 \cdot HCl$.
Dextromethorphan hydrobromide—$C_{18}H_{25}NO \cdot HBr \cdot H_2O$.

Molecular weight:
Diphenylpyraline hydrochloride—317.85.
Phenylephrine hydrochloride—203.67.
Dextromethorphan hydrobromide—370.32.

Description:
Diphenylpyraline hydrochloride—White or almost white, odorless or almost odorless powder.
Phenylephrine Hydrochloride USP—White or practically white, odorless crystals.
Dextromethorphan Hydrobromide USP—Practically white crystals or crystalline powder, having a faint odor. Melts at about 126 °C, with decomposition.

Solubility:
Diphenylpyraline hydrochloride—Freely soluble in water, in alcohol, and in chloroform; practically insoluble in ether.
Phenylephrine Hydrochloride USP—Freely soluble in water and in alcohol.
Dextromethorphan Hydrobromide USP—Sparingly soluble in water; freely soluble in alcohol and in chloroform; insoluble in ether.

USP requirements: Diphenylpyraline Hydrochloride, Phenylephrine Hydrochloride, and Dextromethorphan Hydrobromide Oral Solution—Not in *USP–NF*.

DIPHENYLPYRALINE, PHENYLPROPANOLAMINE, ACETAMINOPHEN, AND CAFFEINE

Source: Caffeine—Coffee, tea, cola, and cocoa or chocolate. May also be synthesized from urea or dimethylurea.

Chemical group:
Phenylpropanolamine hydrochloride—Synthetic phenylisopropanolamine.
Caffeine—Methylated xanthine.

Chemical name:
Diphenylpyraline hydrochloride—Piperidine, 4-(diphenylmethoxy)-1-methyl-, hydrochloride.
Phenylpropanolamine hydrochloride—Benzenemethanol, alpha-(1-aminoethyl)-, hydrochloride, (*R**,*S**)-, (±).
Acetaminophen—Acetamide, *N*-(4-hydroxyphenyl)-.
Caffeine—1*H*-Purine-2,6-dione, 3,7-dihydro-1,3,7-trimethyl-.

Molecular formula:
Diphenylpyraline hydrochloride—$C_{19}H_{23}NO \cdot HCl$.
Phenylpropanolamine hydrochloride—$C_9H_{13}NO \cdot HCl$.
Acetaminophen—$C_8H_9NO_2$.
Caffeine—$C_8H_{10}N_4O_2$ (anhydrous); $C_8H_{10}N_4O_2 \cdot H_2O$ (monohydrate).

Molecular weight:
Diphenylpyraline hydrochloride—317.85.
Phenylpropanolamine hydrochloride—187.67.
Acetaminophen—151.16.
Caffeine—194.19 (anhydrous); 212.21 (monohydrate).

Description:
Diphenylpyraline hydrochloride—White or almost white, odorless or almost odorless powder.
Phenylpropanolamine Hydrochloride USP—White, crystalline powder, having a slight aromatic odor. Is affected by light.
Acetaminophen USP—White, odorless, crystalline powder.
Caffeine USP—White powder or white, glistening needles, usually matted together. Is odorless. Its solutions are neutral to litmus. The hydrate is efflorescent in air.

pKa: Phenylpropanolamine hydrochloride—9.

Solubility:
Diphenylpyraline hydrochloride—Freely soluble in water, in alcohol, and in chloroform; practically insoluble in ether.
Phenylpropanolamine Hydrochloride USP—Freely soluble in water and in alcohol; insoluble in ether.
Acetaminophen USP—Soluble in boiling water and in 1 *N* sodium hydroxide; freely soluble in alcohol.
Caffeine USP—Sparingly soluble in water and in alcohol; freely soluble in chloroform; slightly soluble in ether.

The aqueous solubility of caffeine is increased by organic acids or their alkali salts, such as citrates, benzoates, salicylates, or cinnamates, which dissociate to yield caffeine when dissolved in biological fluids.

USP requirements: Diphenylpyraline Hydrochloride, Phenylpropanolamine Hydrochloride, Acetaminophen, and Caffeine Tablets—Not in *USP–NF*.

DIPHTHERIA AND TETANUS TOXOIDS AND ACELLULAR PERTUSSIS VACCINE ADSORBED

Source: Acellular pertussis vaccine components are isolated from culture fluids of Phase 1 *Bordetella pertussis* grown in a modified Stainer-Scholte medium. After purification by salt precipitation, ultracentrifugation, and ultrafiltration, pertussis toxin (PT) and filamentous hemagglutinin (FHA) are combined to obtain a 1:1 ratio and treated with formaldehyde to inactivate PT.
Corynebacterium diphtheriae cultures are grown in a modified Mueller and Miller medium. *Clostridium tetani* cultures are grown in a peptone-based medium. Both toxins are detoxified with formaldehyde. The detoxified materials are then separately purified by serial ammonium sulfate fractionation and diafiltration.
The toxoids are adsorbed using aluminum potassium sulfate (alum). The adsorbed diphtheria and tetanus toxoids are combined with acellular pertussis concentrate, and diluted to a final volume using sterile phosphate-buffered physiological saline.

USP requirements: Diphtheria and Tetanus Toxoids and Acellular Pertussis Vaccine Adsorbed—Not in *USP–NF*.

DIPHTHERIA TOXIN FOR SCHICK TEST

Description: Diphtheria Toxin for Schick Test USP—Transparent liquid.

USP requirements: Diphtheria Toxin for Schick Test USP—Preserve at a temperature between 2 and 8 °C. A sterile solution of the diluted, standardized toxic products of growth of the diphtheria bacillus (*Corynebacterium diphtheriae*) of which the parent toxin contains not less than 400 MLD (minimum lethal doses) per mL or 400,000 MRD (minimum skin reaction doses) per mL in guinea pigs. Potency is determined in terms of the U.S. Standard Diphtheria Toxin for Schick Test, tested in guinea pigs. Meets the requirement for Expiration date (not later than 1 year after date of issue from manufacturer's cold storage [5 °C, 1 year]). Conforms to the regulations of the U.S. Food and Drug Administration concerning biologics.

DIPHTHERIA AND TETANUS TOXOIDS ADSORBED

Description: Diphtheria and Tetanus Toxoids Adsorbed USP—Turbid, and white, slightly gray, or slightly pink suspension, free from evident clumps after shaking.

USP requirements: Diphtheria and Tetanus Toxoids Adsorbed USP—Preserve at a temperature between 2 and 8 °C. A sterile suspension prepared by mixing suitable quantities of plain or adsorbed diphtheria toxoid and plain or adsorbed tetanus toxoid, and an aluminum adsorbing agent if plain toxoids are used. Label it to state that it is to be well shaken before use and that it is not to be frozen. The antigenicity or potency and the proportions of the toxoids are such as to provide an immunizing dose of each toxoid in the total dosage prescribed in the labeling, and each component meets the requirements for those products. Contains not more than 0.02% of residual free formaldehyde. Meets the requirement for Expiration date (not later than 2 years after date of issue from manufacturer's cold storage [5 °C, 1 year]). Conforms to the regulations of the U.S. Food and Drug Administration concerning biologics.

DIPHTHERIA AND TETANUS TOXOIDS AND PERTUSSIS VAC-
CINE ADSORBED AND HAEMOPHILUS B CONJUGATE VACCINE

Source: Diphtheria and tetanus toxoids are derived from *Corynebacterium diphtheriae* and *Clostridium tetani*, respectively.

Pertussis Vaccine is prepared by growing Phase I *Bordetella pertussis* in a modified Cohen-Wheeler broth containing acid hydrolysate of casein.

The oligosaccharides for the Haemophilus b conjugate component are derived from highly purified capsular polysaccharide, polyribosylribitol phosphate, isolated from *Haemophilus influenzae* type b grown in a chemically defined medium.

USP requirements:

Diphtheria and Tetanus Toxoids and Pertussis Vaccine Adsorbed and Haemophilus b Conjugate Vaccine (HbOC—diphtheria CRM197 protein conjugate) Injection—Not in *USP–NF*.

Diphtheria and Tetanus Toxoids and Pertussis Vaccine Adsorbed and Haemophilus b Conjugate Vaccine (PRP-D—diphtheria toxoid conjugate) Injection—Not in *USP–NF*.

DIPIVEFRIN

Source: Formed by the diesterification of epinephrine and pivalic acid.

Chemical name: Dipivefrin hydrochloride—Propanoic acid, 2,2-dimethyl-, 4-[1-hydroxy-2-(methylamino)ethyl]-1,2-phenylene ester, hydrochloride, (±)-.

Molecular formula: Dipivefrin hydrochloride—$C_{19}H_{29}NO_5 \cdot HCl$.

Molecular weight: Dipivefrin hydrochloride—387.90.

Description: Dipivefrin Hydrochloride USP—White, crystalline powder or small crystals, having a faint odor.

Solubility: Dipivefrin Hydrochloride USP—Very soluble in water.

USP requirements:

Dipivefrin Hydrochloride USP—Preserve in tight containers. Contains not less than 98.5% and not more than 101.5% of dipivefrin hydrochloride, calculated on the dried basis. Meets the requirements for Identification, Melting range (155–165 °C, range between beginning and end of melting not more than 2 °C), Loss on drying (not more than 1.0%), Residue on ignition (not more than 0.3%), Heavy metals (not more than 0.0015%), and Iron (not more than 5 ppm).

Dipivefrin Hydrochloride Ophthalmic Solution USP—Preserve in tight, light-resistant containers. A sterile, aqueous solution of Dipivefrin Hydrochloride. Contains the labeled amount, within –10% to +15%. Contains a suitable antimicrobial agent. Meets the requirements for Identification, Sterility, and pH (2.5–3.5).

DIPYRIDAMOLE

Chemical name: Ethanol, 2,2′,2″,2‴-[(4,8-di-1-piperidinylpyrimido[5,4-*d*]pyrimidine-2,6-diyl)dinitrilo]tetrakis-.

Molecular formula: $C_{24}H_{40}N_8O_4$.

Molecular weight: 504.63.

Description: Dipyridamole USP—Intensely yellow, crystalline powder or needles.

Solubility: Dipyridamole USP—Very soluble in methanol, in alcohol, and in chloroform; slightly soluble in water; very slightly soluble in acetone and in ethyl acetate.

USP requirements:

Dipyridamole USP—Preserve in tight, light-resistant containers. Contains not less than 98.0% and not more than 102.0% of dipyridamole, calculated on the dried basis. Meets the requirements for Identification, Melting range (162–168 °C, range between beginning and end of melting not more than 2 °C), Loss on drying (not more than 0.2%), Chloride, Residue on ignition (not more than 0.1%), Heavy metals (not more than 0.001%), Chromatographic purity, and Organic volatile impurities.

Dipyridamole Injection USP—Preserve in Containers for Injections as described under Injections. Protect from light, and avoid freezing. A sterile solution of Dipyridamole in Water for Injection. Contains the labeled amount of dipyridamole, within ±10%. Meets the requirements for Identification, Bacterial endotoxins, pH (2.2–3.2), and Chromatographic purity, and for Injections.

Dipyridamole Tablets USP—Preserve in tight, light-resistant containers. Contain the labeled amount, within ±10%. Meet the requirements for Identification, Dissolution (70% in 30 minutes in 0.1 N hydrochloric acid in Apparatus 2 at 50 rpm), and Uniformity of dosage units.

DIPYRIDAMOLE AND ASPIRIN

For *Dipyridamole* and *Aspirin*—See individual listings for chemistry information.

USP requirements: Dipyridamole and Aspirin Capsules—Not in *USP–NF*.

DIRITHROMYCIN

Chemical name: Erythromycin, 9-deoxo-11-deoxy-9,11-[imino[2-(2-methoxyethoxy)ethylidene]oxy]-, [9*S*(*R*)]-.

Molecular formula: $C_{42}H_{78}N_2O_{14}$.

Molecular weight: 835.07.

Description: White or practically white powder.

Solubility: Very slightly soluble in water; very soluble in methanol and in methylene chloride.

USP requirements:
Dirithromycin USP—Preserve in well-closed containers. Contains not less than 96.0% and not more than 102.0% of dirithromycin, consisting of the 16*R*- and 16*S*-epimers, calculated on the anhydrous basis. Meets the requirements for Identification, Water (not more than 1.0%), Heavy metals (0.002%), Limit of dirithromycin 16*S*-epimer (not more than 1.5%), and Chromatographic purity (not more than 1.5% of 9-(*S*)-erythromycylamine; not more than 1.0% of any other individual impurity; and not more than 4.0% of total impurities. [Note—Do not regard dirithromycin 16*S*-epimer as an impurity.]).
Dirithromycin Tablets—Not in *USP–NF*.
Dirithromycin Delayed-release Tablets USP—Preserve in tight containers. Contain the labeled amount, within ± 10%, consisting of the 16*R*- and 16*S*-epimers. Meet the requirements for Identification, Drug release (not less than 80% in 45 minutes in 0.1 *N* hydrochloride acid in Apparatus 1 10-mesh basket at 100 rpm for Acid stage, and in phosphate buffer [pH 6.8] for Buffer stage), Uniformity of dosage units, Water (not more than 5.0%), and Chromatographic purity (not more than 1.5% of 9-(*S*)-erythromycylamine; and not more than 5.0% of total impurities. [Note—Do not regard dirithromycin 16*S*-epimer as an impurity.]).

DISOPYRAMIDE

Chemical name:
Disopyramide—2-Pyridineacetamide, alpha-[2-[bis(1-methylethyl)amino]ethyl]-alpha-phenyl-.
Disopyramide phosphate—2-Pyridineacetamide, alpha-[2-[bis(1-methylethyl)amino]ethyl]-alpha-phenyl-, phosphate (1:1).

Molecular formula:
Disopyramide—$C_{21}H_{29}N_3O$.
Disopyramide phosphate—$C_{21}H_{29}N_3O \cdot H_3PO_4$.

Molecular weight:
Disopyramide—339.47.
Disopyramide phosphate—437.47.

Description:
Disopyramide—White, odorless or almost odorless powder.
Disopyramide Phosphate USP—White or practically white, odorless powder. Melts at about 205 °C, with decomposition.

pKa: 10.4.

Solubility:
Disopyramide—Slightly soluble in water; soluble 1 in 10 of alcohol, 1 in 5 of chloroform, and 1 in 5 of ether.
Disopyramide Phosphate USP—Freely soluble in water; slightly soluble in alcohol; practically insoluble in chloroform and in ether.

Other characteristics: Chloroform[hm.1]:[hm.1]water partition coefficient—3.1 at pH 7.2.

USP requirements:
Disopyramide Capsules—Not in *USP–NF*.
Disopyramide Injection—Not in *USP–NF*.
Disopyramide Phosphate USP—Preserve in tight, light-resistant containers. Contains not less than 98.0% and not more than 102.0% of disopyramide phosphate, calculated on the dried basis. Meets the requirements for Identification, pH (4.0–5.0 in a solution [1 in 20]), Loss on drying (not more than 0.5%), Heavy metals (not more than 0.002%), Chromatographic purity, and Organic volatile impurities.
Disopyramide Phosphate Capsules USP—Preserve in well-closed containers. Contain an amount of Disopyramide Phosphate equivalent to the labeled amount of disopyramide, within ±10%. Meet the requirements for Identification, Dissolution (80% in 20 minutes in water in Apparatus 2 at 50 rpm), and Uniformity of dosage units.
Disopyramide Phosphate Extended-release Capsules USP—Preserve in well-closed containers. The labeling indicates the Drug Release Test with which the product complies. Contain an amount of Disopyramide Phosphate equivalent to the labeled amount of disopyramide, within ± 10%. Meet the requirements for Identification, Drug release (5–25% in 1 hour, 17–43% in 2 hours, 50–80% in 5 hours, and not less than 85% in 12 hours in 0.1 *M* phosphate buffer [pH 2.5] in Apparatus 1 at 100 rpm for Test 1 and 5–30% in 1 hour, 40–65% in 4 hours, 60–90% in 8 hours, and not less than 75% in 12 hours in 0.1 *M* phosphate buffer [pH 2.5] in Apparatus 2 at 100 rpm for Test 2), and Uniformity of dosage units.
Disopyramide Phosphate Extended-release Tablets—Not in *USP–NF*.

DISULFIRAM

Chemical name: Thioperoxydicarbonic diamide [$(H_2N)C(S)]_2S_2$, tetraethyl-.

Molecular formula: $C_{10}H_{20}N_2S_4$.

Molecular weight: 296.54.

Description: Disulfiram USP—White to off-white, odorless, crystalline powder.

Solubility: Disulfiram USP—Very slightly soluble in water; soluble in acetone, in alcohol, in carbon disulfide, and in chloroform.

USP requirements:
Disulfiram USP—Preserve in tight, light-resistant containers. Contains not less than 98.0% and not more than 102.0% of disulfiram. Meets the requirements for Identification, Melting range (69–72 °C), Residue on ignition (not more than 0.1%), Selenium (not more than 0.003%), and Organic volatile impurities.
Disulfiram Tablets USP—Preserve in tight, light-resistant containers. Contain the labeled amount, within ±10%. Meet the requirements for Identification, Disintegration (15 minutes, the use of disks being omitted), and Uniformity of dosage units.

DIVALPROEX SODIUM

Chemical name: Pentanoic acid, 2-propyl-, sodium salt (2:1).

Molecular formula: $(C_{16}H_{31}NaO_4)_n$.

Molecular weight: 310.41.

Description: White powder, having a characteristic odor.

Solubility: Insoluble in water; very soluble in alcohol.

USP requirements:

Divalproex Sodium Delayed-release Capsules—Not in *USP–NF*.

Divalproex Sodium Delayed-release Tablets USP—Preserve in tight, light-resistant containers. Contain an equivalent amount of divalproex sodium, within −10%, and the labeled amount of valproic acid, within +10%. Meet the requirements for Identification, Drug release (80% in 1 hour and 2 hours in Apparatus 2 at 50 rpm), and Uniformity of dosage units.

DOBUTAMINE

Chemical group: A synthetic catecholamine.

Chemical name:

Dobutamine—1,2-Benzenediol, 4-[2-[[3-(4-hydroxyphenyl)-1-methylpropyl]amino]ethyl]-, (±)-.

Dobutamine hydrochloride—1,2-Benzenediol, 4-[2-[[3-(4-hydroxyphenyl)-1-methylpropyl]amino]ethyl]-, hydrochloride, (±)-.

Molecular formula:

Dobutamine—$C_{18}H_{23}NO_3$.

Dobutamine hydrochloride—$C_{18}H_{23}NO_3 \cdot HCl$.

Molecular weight:

Dobutamine—301.38.

Dobutamine hydrochloride—337.85.

Description: Dobutamine Hydrochloride USP—White to practically white, crystalline powder.

pKa: 9.4.

Solubility: Dobutamine Hydrochloride USP—Sparingly soluble in water and in methanol; soluble in alcohol and in pyridine.

USP requirements:

Dobutamine Injection USP—Preserve in single-dose or in multiple-dose containers, preferably of Type I glass. A sterile solution of Dobutamine Hydrochloride in Water for Injection. Label it to indicate that it is to be diluted to appropriate strength with a suitable parenteral vehicle prior to administration. Contains an amount of Dobutamine Hydrochloride equivalent to the labeled amount of Dobutamine, within ±10%. Meets the requirements for Identification, Bacterial endotoxins, pH (2.5–5.5), and Particulate matter, and for Injections.

Dobutamine for Injection USP—Preserve in Containers for Sterile Solids, at controlled room temperature. A sterile mixture of Dobutamine Hydrochloride with suitable diluents. Contains an amount of dobutamine hydrochloride equivalent to the labeled amount of dobutamine, within ±10%. Meets the requirements for Constituted solution (Do not use the constituted solution if it is brown or contains a precipitate.), Identification, Bacterial endotoxins (not more than 5.56), Uniformity of dosage units, pH (2.5–5.5), and Particulate matter, and for Injections.

Caution: Great care should be taken to prevent inhaling particles of Dobutamine Hydrochloride for Injection and exposing the skin to it. Protect the eyes.

Dobutamine Hydrochloride USP—Preserve in tight containers, and store at controlled room temperature. Contains not less than 98.0% and not more than 102.0% of dobutamine hydrochloride, calculated on the anhydrous basis. Meets the requirements for Color of solution, Identification, Water (not more than 1.0%), Residue on ignition (not more than 0.2%), Chromatographic purity, and Heavy metals (not more than 0.003%).

Caution: Great care should be taken to prevent inhaling particles of Dobutamine Hydrochloride and exposing the skin to it. Protect the eyes.

DOBUTAMINE AND DEXTROSE

For *Dobutamine* and *Dextrose*—See individual listings for chemistry information.

USP requirements: Dobutamine in Dextrose Injection USP—Preserve in single-dose containers, preferably of Type II glass, or a suitable plastic material, and store at room temperature, avoid excessive heat, and protect from freezing. It is a sterile solution of Dobutamine Hydrochloride and Dextrose in Water for Injection. The label states the total osmolar concentration in mOsmol per liter. Contains an amount of Dobutamine Hydrochloride equivalent to the labeled amount of dobutamine, within ±10% and the labeled amount of dextrose, within ±10%. May contain one or more suitable antioxidants or chelating agents. Meets the requirements for Identification, Bacterial endotoxins, pH (2.5–5.5), Particulate matter, Chromatographic purity, and Limit of 5-hydroxymethylfurfural, and for Injections.

DOCETAXEL

Source: Prepared by semisynthesis beginning with a precursor extracted from the renewable needle biomass of yew plants.

Chemical name: Benzenepropanoic acid, beta-[[(1,1-dimethylethoxy)carbonyl]amino]-alpha-hydroxy-, 12b-(acetyloxy)-12(benzoyloxy)-2a,3,4,4a,5,6,9,10,11,12,12a,12b-dodecahydro-4,6,11-trihydroxy-4a,8,13,13-tetramethyl-5-oxo-7,11-methano1*H*-cyclodeca[3,4]benz[1,2-*b*]oxet-9-yl ester trihydrate, [2a*R*[2a alpha,4 beta,4a beta,6 beta,9 alpha(alpha*R**, beta*S**),11 alpha,12 alpha,12a alpha,12b alpha]]-.

Molecular formula: $C_{43}H_{53}NO_{14} \cdot 3H_2O$.

Molecular weight: 861.93.

Description:

Docetaxel—White to almost-white powder.

Docetaxel for injection concentrate—Clear yellow to brownish-yellow viscous solution.

Solubility: Practically insoluble in water.

Other characteristics: Highly lipophilic.

USP requirements: Docetaxel for Injection Concentrate—Not in *USP–NF*.

DOCOSANOL

Chemical name: 1-Docosanol.

Molecular formula: $C_{22}H_{46}O$.

Molecular weight: 326.61.

USP requirements: Docosanol Topical Cream—Not in *USP–NF*.

DOCUSATE

Chemical group: Anionic surfactants.

Chemical name:
Docusate calcium—Butanedioic acid, sulfo-, 1,4-bis(2-ethylhexyl) ester, calcium salt.
Docusate potassium—Butanedioic acid, sulfo-, 1,4-bis(2-ethylhexyl) ester, potassium salt.
Docusate sodium—Butanedioic acid, sulfo-, 1,4-bis(2-ethylhexyl) ester, sodium salt.

Molecular formula:
Docusate calcium—$C_{40}H_{74}CaO_{14}S_2$.
Docusate potassium—$C_{20}H_{37}KO_7S$.
Docusate sodium—$C_{20}H_{37}NaO_7S$.

Molecular weight:
Docusate calcium—883.22.
Docusate potassium—460.67.
Docusate sodium—444.56.

Description:
Docusate Calcium USP—White, amorphous solid, having the characteristic odor of octyl alcohol. It is free of the odor of other solvents.
Docusate Potassium USP—White, amorphous solid, having a characteristic odor suggestive of octyl alcohol.
Docusate Sodium USP—White, wax-like, plastic solid, having a characteristic odor suggestive of octyl alcohol, but no odor of other solvents.
NF category: Wetting and/or solubilizing agent.

Solubility:
Docusate Calcium USP—Very slightly soluble in water; very soluble in alcohol, in polyethylene glycol 400, and in corn oil.
Docusate Potassium USP—Sparingly soluble in water; very soluble in solvent hexane; soluble in alcohol and in glycerin.
Docusate Sodium USP—Sparingly soluble in water; very soluble in solvent hexane; freely soluble in alcohol and in glycerin.

USP requirements:
Docusate Calcium USP—Preserve in well-closed containers. Contains not less than 91.0% and not more than 100.5% of docusate calcium, calculated on the anhydrous basis. Meets the requirements for Clarity of solution, Identification, Water (not more than 2.0%), Residue on ignition (14.5–16.5%, calculated on the anhydrous basis), Heavy metals (not more than 0.001%), and Limit of bis(2-ethylhexyl) maleate (not more than 0.4%).
Docusate Calcium Capsules USP—Preserve in tight containers, and store at controlled room temperature in a dry place. Contain the labeled amount, within ±15%. Meet the requirements for Identification, Dissolution (in 15 minutes in water in Apparatus 2 at 50 rpm), and Uniformity of dosage units.
Docusate Potassium USP—Preserve in well-closed containers. Contains not less than 95.0% and not more than 100.5% of docusate potassium, calculated on the dried basis. Meets the requirements for Identification, Loss on drying (not more than 3.0%), Residue on ignition (18.0–20.0%, calculated on the dried basis), Heavy metals (not more than 0.001%), and Limit of bis(2-ethylhexyl) maleate (not more than 0.4%).
Docusate Potassium Capsules USP—Preserve in tight containers, and store at controlled room temperature. Contain the labeled amount, within ±10%. Meet the requirements for Identification, Dissolution (in 15 minutes in water in Apparatus 2 at 50 rpm), and Uniformity of dosage units.
Docusate Sodium USP—Preserve in well-closed containers. Contains not less than 99.0% and not more than 100.5% of docusate sodium, calculated on the anhydrous basis. Meets the requirements for Clarity of solution, Identification, Water (not more than 2.0%), Residue on ignition

(15.5–16.5%, calculated on the anhydrous basis), Heavy metals (not more than 0.001%), and Limit of bis(2-ethylhexyl) maleate (not more than 0.4%).
Docusate Sodium Capsules USP—Preserve in tight containers, and store at controlled room temperature. Contain the labeled amount, within ±10%. Meet the requirements for Identification, Dissolution (in 15 minutes in water in Apparatus 2 at 50 rpm), and Uniformity of dosage units.
Docusate Sodium Enema—Not in *USP–NF*.
Docusate Sodium Solution USP (Oral)—Preserve in tight containers. Contains the labeled amount, within ±10%. Meets the requirements for Identification and pH (4.5–6.9).
Docusate Sodium Rectal Solution—Not in *USP–NF*.
Docusate Sodium Syrup USP—Preserve in tight, light-resistant containers. Contains the labeled amount, within ±10%. Meets the requirements for Identification and pH (5.5–6.5).
Docusate Sodium Tablets USP—Preserve in well-closed containers. Contain the labeled amount, within ±10%. Meet the requirements for Identification, Disintegration (1 hour, simulated gastric fluid TS being substituted for water in the test for Uncoated Tablets), and Uniformity of dosage units.

DOFETILIDE

Source: A methanesulfonamide derivative.

Chemical name: Methanesulfonamide, *N*-[4-[2-[methyl[2-[4-[(methylsulfonyl)amino]phenoxy]ethyl]amino]ethyl]phenyl]-.

Molecular formula: $C_{19}H_{27}N_3O_5S_2$.

Molecular weight: 441.57.

Description: White to off-white powder.

Solubility: Very slightly soluble in water and in propan-2-ol; soluble in 0.1 *M* aqueous sodium hydroxide, in acetone, and in aqueous 0.1 *M* hydrochloric acid.

USP requirements: Dofetilide Hydrochloride Injection—Not in *USP–NF*.

DOLASETRON

Chemical name: Dolasetron mesylate—1*H*-Indole-3-carboxylic acid, octahydro-3-oxo-2,6-methano-2*H*-quinolizin-8-yl ester, (2 alpha,6 alpha,8 alpha,9a beta)-, monomethanesulfonate.

Molecular formula: Dolasetron mesylate—$C_{19}H_{20}N_2O_3 \cdot CH_4O_3S \cdot H_2O$.

Molecular weight: Dolasetron mesylate—438.50.

Description: Dolasetron Mesylate USP—White to off-white powder.

Solubility: Dolasetron Mesylate USP—Freely soluble in water and in propylene glycol; slightly soluble in alcohol and in saline TS.

USP requirements:
Dolasetron Mesylate USP—Preserve in well-closed containers, protected from light. Contains not less than 98.0% and not more than 102.0% of dolasetron mesylate. Meets the requirements for Identification, Water (3.5%–4.7%), Related compounds, and Organic volatile impurities.
Dolasetron Mesylate Injection—Not in *USP–NF*.
Dolasetron Mesylate Tablets USP—Preserve in well-closed containers, protected from light. Contain the labeled amount, within ±10%. Meet the requirements for Identifi-

cation, Dissolution (80% in 30 minutes in 0.1 N hydrochloric acid in Apparatus 2 at 50 rpm), and Uniformity of dosage units.

DOMPERIDONE

Chemical name: 2*H*-Benzimidazol-2-one, 5-chloro-1-[1-[3-(2,3-dihydro-2-oxo-1*H*-benzimidazol-1-yl)propyl]-4-piperidinyl]-1,3-dihydro-.

Molecular formula: $C_{22}H_{24}ClN_5O_2$.

Molecular weight: 425.91.

USP requirements:
  Domperidone Tablets—Not in *USP–NF*
  Domperidone Maleate Tablets—Not in *USP–NF*

DONEPEZIL

Chemical name: Donepezil hydrochloride—(±)-2-[(1-Benzyl-4-piperidyl)methyl]-5,6-dimethoxy-1-indanone hydrochloride.

Molecular formula: Donepezil hydrochloride—$C_{24}H_{29}NO_3 \cdot HCl$.

Molecular weight: Donepezil hydrochloride—415.95.

Description: Donepezil hydrochloride—White crystalline powder.

Solubility: Donepezil hydrochloride—Freely soluble in chloroform; soluble in water and in glacial acetic acid; slightly soluble in ethanol and in acetonitrile; practically insoluble in ethyl acetate and in *n*-hexane.

USP requirements: Donepezil Hydrochloride Tablets—Not in *USP–NF*.

DOPAMINE

Chemical group: A naturally occurring biochemical catecholamine precursor of norepinephrine.

Chemical name: Dopamine hydrochloride—1,2-Benzenediol, 4-(2-aminoethyl)-, hydrochloride.

Molecular formula: Dopamine hydrochloride—$C_8H_{11}NO_2 \cdot HCl$.

Molecular weight: Dopamine hydrochloride—189.64.

Description: Dopamine Hydrochloride USP—White to off-white, crystalline powder. May have a slight odor of hydrochloric acid. Melts at about 240 °C, with decomposition.

Solubility: Dopamine Hydrochloride USP—Freely soluble in water and in aqueous solutions of alkali hydroxides; soluble in methanol; insoluble in ether and in chloroform.

USP requirements:
  Dopamine Hydrochloride USP—Preserve in tight containers. Contains not less than 98.0% and not more than 102.0% of dopamine hydrochloride, calculated on the dried basis. Meets the requirements for Clarity and color of solution, Identification, pH (3.0–5.5, in a solution [1 in 25]), Loss on drying (not more than 0.5%), Residue on ignition (not more than 0.1%), Heavy metals (not more than 0.002%), Sulfate, Readily carbonizable substances, and Chromatographic purity.
  Dopamine Hydrochloride Injection USP—Preserve in single-dose containers of Type I glass. A sterile solution of Dopamine Hydrochloride in Water for Injection. May contain a suitable antioxidant. Label it to indicate that the Injection

is to be diluted with a suitable parenteral vehicle prior to intravenous infusion. Contains the labeled amount, within ±5%. Meets the requirements for Identification, Bacterial endotoxins, pH (2.5–5.0), and Particulate matter, and for Injections.

Note: Do not use the Injection if it is darker than slightly yellow or discolored in any other way.

DOPAMINE AND DEXTROSE

For *Dopamine* and *Dextrose*—See individual listings for chemistry information.

USP requirements: Dopamine Hydrochloride and Dextrose Injection USP—Preserve in single-dose glass or plastic containers. Glass containers are preferably of Type I or Type II glass. A sterile solution of Dopamine Hydrochloride and Dextrose in Water for Injection. The label states the total osmolar concentration in mOsmol per liter. Where the contents are less than 100 mL, or where the label states that the Injection is not for direct injection but is to be diluted before use, the label alternatively may state the total osmolar concentration in mOsm per mL. Contains the labeled amounts, within ±5%. Meets the requirements for Identification, Bacterial endotoxins, pH (2.5–4.5), Particulate matter, and Limit of 5-hydroxymethylfurfural and related substances, and for Injections.

Note: Do not use the Injection if it is darker than slightly yellow or discolored in any other way.

DORNASE ALFA

Source: Produced by genetically engineered Chinese Hamster Ovary (CHO) cells containing DNA encoding for the native human protein, deoxyribonuclease I (DNase). The product is purified by tangential flow filtration and column chromatography. The purified glycoprotein contains 260 amino acids with an approximate molecular weight of 37,000 daltons. The primary amino acid sequence is identical to that of the native human enzyme.

Chemical name: Deoxyribonuclease (human clone 18-1 protein moiety).

Molecular formula: $C_{1321}H_{1995}N_{339}O_{396}S_9$.

Molecular weight: 29,249.62.

USP requirements: Dornase Alfa Solution for Inhalation—Not in *USP–NF*.

DORZOLAMIDE

Chemical name: Dorzolamide hydrochloride—4*H*-Thieno[2,3-*b*]thiopyran-2-sulfonamide, 4-(ethylamino)-5,6-dihydro-6-methyl-, 7,7-dioxide, monohydrochloride, (4*S-trans*)-.

Molecular formula: Dorzolamide hydrochloride—$C_{10}H_{16}N_2O_4S_3 \cdot HCl$.

Molecular weight: Dorzolamide hydrochloride—360.91.

Description: Dorzolamide Hydrochloride USP—White to off-white, crystalline powder. Melting point of about 275 °C.

Solubility: Dorzolamide Hydrochloride USP—Soluble in water.

USP requirements:

Dorzolamide Hydrochloride USP—Preserve in well-closed containers, protected from light, and store at 15° to 30°. Contains not less than 99.0% and not more than 101.0% of dorzolamide hydrochloride. Meets the requirements for Identification, Water (not more than 0.5%), Residue on ignition (not more than 0.1%, an ignition temperature of 600°), Heavy metals (0.001%), Limit of dorzolamide hydrochloride related compound A (not more than 0.5), Chromatographic purity, and Organic volatile impurities.

Dorzolamide Hydrochloride Ophthalmic Solution—Not in *USP–NF*.

DORZOLAMIDE AND TIMOLOL

For *Dorzolamide* and *Timolol*—See individual listings for chemistry information.

USP requirements: Dorzolamide Hydrochloride and Timolol Maleate Ophthalmic Solution—Not in *USP–NF*.

DOXACURIUM

Chemical name: Doxacurium chloride—Isoquinolinium, 2,2'-[(1,4-dioxo-1,4-butanediyl)bis(oxy-3,1-propanediyl)]-bis[1,2,3,4-tetrahydro-6,7,8-trimethoxy-2-methyl-1-[(3,4,5-trimethoxyphenyl)methyl]-, dichloride, [1 alpha,2 beta-(1′S*,2′R*)]-, mixture with (±)-[1 alpha,2 beta(1′R*,2′S*)]2,2'-[(1,4-dioxo-1,4-butanediyl)bis(oxy-3,1-propanediyl)]-bis[1,2,3,4-tetrahydro-6,7,8-trimethoxy-2-methyl-1-[(3,4,5-trimethoxyphenyl)methyl]isoquinolinium] dichloride.

Molecular formula: Doxacurium chloride—$C_{56}H_{78}Cl_2N_2O_{16}$.

Molecular weight: Doxacurium chloride—1106.13.

Description: Doxacurium chloride injection—Sterile, nonpyrogenic aqueous solution.

Other characteristics:

Doxacurium chloride—N-octanol:water partition coefficient: 0.

Doxacurium chloride injection—pH 3.9–5.0.

USP requirements: Doxacurium Chloride Injection—Not in *USP–NF*.

DOXAPRAM

Chemical name: Doxapram hydrochloride—2-Pyrrolidinone, 1-ethyl-4-[2-(4-morpholinyl)ethyl]-3,3-diphenyl-, monohydrochloride, monohydrate.

Molecular formula: Doxapram hydrochloride—$C_{24}H_{30}N_2O_2 \cdot HCl \cdot H_2O$.

Molecular weight: Doxapram hydrochloride—432.98.

Description: Doxapram Hydrochloride USP—White to off-white, odorless, crystalline powder. Melts at about 220 °C.

Solubility: Doxapram Hydrochloride USP—Soluble in water and in chloroform; sparingly soluble in alcohol; practically insoluble in ether.

USP requirements:

Doxapram Hydrochloride USP—Preserve in tight containers. Dried at 105 °C for 2 hours, contains not less than 98.0% and not more than 100.5% of doxapram hydrochloride. Meets the requirements for Identification, pH (3.5–5.0, in

a solution [1 in 100]), Loss on drying (3.0–4.5%), Residue on ignition (not more than 0.3%), Heavy metals (not more than 0.002%), and Chromatographic purity.

Doxapram Hydrochloride Injection USP—Preserve in single-dose or in multiple-dose containers, preferably of Type I glass. A sterile solution of Doxapram Hydrochloride in Water for Injection. Contains the labeled amount, within ±10%. Meets the requirements for Identification, Bacterial endotoxins, and pH (3.5–5.0), and for Injections.

DOXAZOSIN

Chemical name: Doxazosin mesylate—Piperazine, 1-(4-amino-6,7-dimethoxy-2-quinazolinyl)-4-[(2,3-dihydro-1,4-benzodioxin-2-yl)carbonyl]-, monomethanesulfonate.

Molecular formula: Doxazosin mesylate—$C_{23}H_{25}N_5O_5 \cdot CH_4O_3S$.

Molecular weight: Doxazosin mesylate—547.58.

Description: Doxazosin mesylate—White to off-white crystalline solid of uniform appearance. Melting point 273.7 °C.

Solubility: Doxazosin mesylate—Freely soluble in dimethylsulfoxide; soluble in dimethylformamide; slightly soluble in methanol, in ethanol, and in water (0.8% w/v at 25 °C); very slightly soluble in acetone and in methylene chloride.

USP requirements: Doxazosin Mesylate Tablets—Not in *USP–NF*.

DOXEPIN

Chemical group: Doxepin hydrochloride—Dibenzoxepin derivative.

Chemical name: Doxepin hydrochloride—1-Propanamine, 3-dibenz[b,e]oxepin-11(6H)ylidene-N,N-dimethyl-, hydrochloride.

Molecular formula: Doxepin hydrochloride—$C_{19}H_{21}NO \cdot HCl$.

Molecular weight: Doxepin hydrochloride—315.84.

Description: Doxepin hydrochloride—White, crystalline solid.

pKa: Doxepin hydrochloride—8.0.

Solubility: Doxepin hydrochloride—Readily soluble in water, in lower alcohols, and in chloroform.

Other characteristics: Tertiary amine.

USP requirements:

Doxepin Hydrochloride USP—Preserve in well-closed containers. An (E) and (Z) geometric isomer mixture. Contains the equivalent of not less than 98.0% and not more than 102.0% of doxepin hydrochloride, calculated on the dried basis. Contains not less than 13.6% and not more than 18.1% of the (Z)-isomer, and not less than 81.4% and not more than 88.2% of the (E)-isomer. Meets the requirements for Identification, Melting range (185–191 °C), Loss on drying (not more than 0.5%), Residue on ignition (not more than 0.2%), Heavy metals (not more than 0.002%), Organic volatile impurities, and Chloride content (10.9–11.6%).

Doxepin Hydrochloride Capsules USP—Preserve in well-closed containers. Contain an amount of doxepin hydrochloride equivalent to the labeled amount of doxepin, within ±10%. Meet the requirements for Identification, Dissolution (80% in 30 minutes in water in Apparatus 1 at 50 rpm), Uniformity of dosage units, and Water (not more than 9.0%).

Doxepin Hydrochloride Cream—Not in *USP–NF*.

Doxepin Hydrochloride Oral Solution USP—Preserve in tight, light-resistant containers. Label it to indicate that each dose is to be diluted with water or other suitable fluid to approximately 120 mL, just prior to administration. Contains an amount of doxepin hydrochloride equivalent to the labeled amount of doxepin, within ±10%. Meets the requirements for Identification and pH (4.0–7.0).

DOXERCALCIFEROL

Chemical group: A synthetic vitamin D analog.

Chemical name: (1 alpha,3 beta,5Z,7E,22E)-9,10 secoergosta-5,7, 10(19)22-tetraene-1,3-diol.

Molecular formula: $C_{28}H_{44}O_2$.

Molecular weight: 412.66.

Description: A colorless crystalline compound.

Solubility: Soluble in oils and in organic solvents; relatively insoluble in water.

USP requirements: Doxercalciferol Capsules—Not in *USP–NF*.

DOXORUBICIN

Source: An anthracycline glycoside obtained from *Streptomyces peucetius* var. *caesius*.

Chemical name: Doxorubicin hydrochloride—5,12-Naphthacenedione, 10-[(3-amino-2,3,6-trideoxy-alpha-L-*lyxo*-hexopyranosyl)oxy]-7,8,9,10-tetrahydro-6,8,11-trihydroxy-8-(hydroxyacetyl)-1-methoxy-, hydrochloride (8*S-cis*)-.

Molecular formula: Doxorubicin hydrochloride—$C_{27}H_{29}NO_{11}$ · HCl.

Molecular weight: Doxorubicin hydrochloride—579.98.

Description: Doxorubicin Hydrochloride USP—Red-orange, hygroscopic, crystalline powder.

Solubility: Doxorubicin Hydrochloride USP—Soluble in water, in isotonic sodium chloride solution, and in methanol; practically insoluble in chloroform, in ether, and in other organic solvents.

Other characteristics: Doxorubicin hydrochloride—Unstable in solutions with a pH less than 3 or greater than 7.

USP requirements:

Doxorubicin Hydrochloride USP—Preserve in tight containers. Contains not less than 98.0% and not more than 102.0% of doxorubicin hydrochloride, calculated on the anhydrous, solvent-free basis. Meets the requirements for Identification, Crystallinity, pH (4.0–5.5, in a solution containing 5 mg per mL), Water (not more than 4.0%), Chromatographic purity, and Limit of solvent residues (as acetone and alcohol, not more than 0.5% of acetone and total of acetone and alcohol not more than 2.5%).

Caution: Great care should be taken to prevent inhaling particles of doxorubicin hydrochloride and exposing the skin to it.

Doxorubicin Hydrochloride Injection USP—Preserve in single-dose or in multiple-dose containers, preferably of Type I glass, protected from light. Store in a refrigerator. Injection may be packaged in multiple-dose containers not exceeding 100 mL in volume. A sterile solution of Doxorubicin Hydrochloride in Sterile Water for Injection made isoosmotic with Sodium Chloride, Dextrose, or other suitable added substances. Contains the labeled amount, within −10%

to +15%. Meets the requirements for Identification, Bacterial endotoxins, Sterility, and pH (2.5–4.5), and for Injections.

Doxorubicin Hydrochloride for Injection USP—Preserve in Containers for Sterile Solids, except that multiple-dose containers may provide for the withdrawal of not more than 100 mL when constituted as directed in the labeling. A sterile mixture of Doxorubicin Hydrochloride and Lactose. Contains the labeled amount, within −10% to +15%. Meets the requirements for Constituted solution, Bacterial endotoxins, Sterility, pH (4.5–6.5, in the solution constituted as directed in the labeling, except that water is used as the diluent), and Water (not more than 4.0%), for Identification under Doxorubicin Hydrochloride, and for Uniformity of dosage units and Labeling under Injections.

Caution: Great care should be taken to prevent inhaling particles of Doxorubicin Hydrochloride and exposing the skin to it.

Doxorubicin Hydrochloride, Liposomal, Injection—Not in *USP–NF*.

DOXYCYCLINE

Chemical name:

Doxycycline—2-Naphthacenecarboxamide, 4-(dimethylamino)1,4,4a,5,5a,6,11,12a-octahydro-3,5,10,12,12a-pentahydroxy-6-methyl-1,11-dioxo-, [4*S*-(4 alpha,4a alpha,5 alpha,5a alpha,6 alpha,12a alpha)]-, monohydrate.

Doxycycline hyclate—2-Naphthacenecarboxamide, 4-(dimethyl-amino)-1,4,4a,5,5a,6,11,12a-octahydro-3,5,10,12,12a-pentahydroxy-6-methyl-1,11-dioxo-, monohydrochloride, compd. with ethanol (2:1), monohydrate, [4*S*-(4 alpha,4a alpha,5 alpha,5a alpha,6 alpha,12a alpha)]-.

Molecular formula:

Doxycycline—$C_{22}H_{24}N_2O_8 \cdot H_2O$.

Doxycycline hyclate—$(C_{22}H_{24}N_2O_8 \cdot HCl)_2 \cdot C_2H_6O \cdot H_2O$.

Molecular weight:

Doxycycline—462.45.

Doxycycline hyclate—1025.87.

Description:

Doxycycline USP—Yellow, crystalline powder.

Doxycycline Hyclate USP—Yellow, crystalline powder.

Solubility:

Doxycycline USP—Very slightly soluble in water; freely soluble in dilute acid and in alkali hydroxide solutions; sparingly soluble in alcohol; practically insoluble in chloroform and in ether.

Doxycycline Hyclate USP—Soluble in water and in solutions of alkali hydroxides and carbonates; slightly soluble in alcohol; practically insoluble in chloroform and in ether.

USP requirements:

Doxycycline USP—Preserve in tight, light-resistant containers. Has a potency equivalent to not less than 880 mcg and not more than 980 mcg of doxycycline per mg. Meets the requirements for Identification, Crystallinity, pH (5.0–6.5, in an aqueous suspension containing 10 mg per mL), Related compunds, and Water (3.6–4.6%).

Doxycycline Capsules USP—Preserve in tight, light-resistant containers. Contain the labeled amount, within −10% to +20%. Meet the requirements for Identification, Dissolution (85% in 60 minutes in 0.01 *N* hydrochloric acid in Apparatus 2 at 75 rpm), Uniformity of dosage units, and Water (not more than 5.5%, except that it is not more than 8.5% for Capsules labeled to contain the equivalent of 20 mg of doxycycline).

Doxycycline for Injection USP—Preserve in Containers for Sterile Solids, protected from light. Contains an amount of Doxycycline Hyclate equivalent to the labeled amount of doxycycline, within −10% to +20%. Meets the requirements for Constituted solution, Identification, Bacterial endotoxins, Sterility, pH (1.8–3.3, in the solution constituted as directed in the labeling), Loss on drying (not more than 4.0%), and Particulate matter.

Doxycycline for Oral Suspension USP—Preserve in tight, light-resistant containers. Contains one or more suitable buffers, colors, diluents, flavors, and preservatives. Contains the labeled amount, within −10% to +25% when constituted as directed. Meets the requirements for Identification, Uniformity of dosage units (single-unit containers), Deliverable volume, pH (5.0–6.5, in the suspension constituted as directed in the labeling), and Water (not more than 3.0%).

Doxycycline Calcium Oral Suspension USP—Preserve in tight, light-resistant containers. Prepared from Doxycycline Hyclate, and contains one or more suitable buffers, colors, diluents, flavors, and preservatives. Contains an amount of doxycycline calcium equivalent to the labeled amount of doxycycline, within −10% to +25%. Meets the requirements for Identification, Uniformity of dosage units (single-unit containers), Deliverable volume, and pH (6.5–8.0).

Doxycycline Hyclate USP—Preserve in tight containers, protected from light. Where it is intended for use in preparing injectable dosage forms, the label states that it is sterile or must be subjected to further processing during the preparation of injectable dosage forms. Has a potency equivalent to not less than 800 mcg and not more than 920 mcg of doxycycline per mg. Meets the requirements for Identification, Crystallinity, pH (2.0–3.0, in a solution containing 10 mg of doxycycline per mL), and Water (1.4–2.8%), and for Sterility and Bacterial endotoxins under Doxycycline for Injection (where the label states that Doxycycline Hyclate is sterile), and for Bacterial endotoxins for Doxycycline for Injection (where the label states that Doxycycline Hyclate must be subjected to further processing during the preparation of injectable dosage forms).

Doxycycline Hyclate Capsules USP—Preserve in tight, light-resistant containers. Contain an amount of doxycycline hyclate equivalent to the labeled amount of doxycycline, within −10% to +20%. Meet the requirements for Identification, Dissolution (80% in 30 minutes in water in Apparatus 2 at 75 rpm), Uniformity of dosage units, and Water (not more than 8.5%).

Doxycycline Hyclate Delayed-release Capsules USP—Preserve in tight, light-resistant containers. The label indicates that the contents of the Capsules are enteric-coated. Contain an amount of doxycycline hyclate equivalent to the labeled amount of doxycycline, within −10% to +20%. Meet the requirements for Identification, Drug release (Acid stage: 50% [Level 1 and Level 2] in 20 minutes in 0.06 N hydrochloric acid in Apparatus 1 at 50 rpm; Buffer stage: 85% in 30 minutes in neutralized phthalate buffer [pH 5.5] in Apparatus 1 at 50 rpm), Uniformity of dosage units, and Water (not more than 5.0%).

Doxycycline Hyclate Extended-release Periodontal Liquid—Not in *USP–NF*.

Doxycycline Hyclate Tablets USP—Preserve in tight, light-resistant containers. Contain an amount of doxycycline hyclate equivalent to the labeled amount of doxycycline, within −10% to +20%. Meet the requirements for Identification, Dissolution (85% in 90 minutes in water in Apparatus 2 at 75 rpm), Uniformity of dosage units, and Water (not more than 5.0%).

DOXYLAMINE

Chemical group: Doxylamine succinate—Ethanolamine derivative.

Chemical name: Doxylamine succinate—Ethanamine, *N,N*-dimethyl-2-[1-phenyl-1-(2-pyridinyl)ethoxy]-, butanedioate (1:1).

Molecular formula: Doxylamine succinate—$C_{17}H_{22}N_2O \cdot C_4H_6O_4$.

Molecular weight: Doxylamine succinate—388.46.

Description: Doxylamine Succinate USP—White or creamy white powder, having a characteristic odor.

pKa: Doxylamine succinate—5.8 and 9.3.

Solubility: Doxylamine Succinate USP—Very soluble in water and in alcohol; freely soluble in chloroform; very slightly soluble in ether.

USP requirements:
Doxylamine Succinate USP—Preserve in well-closed, light-resistant containers. Contains not less than 98.0% and not more than 101.0% of doxylamine succinate, calculated on the dried basis. Meets the requirements for Identification, Melting range (103–108 °C, the range between beginning and end of melting not more than 3 °C), Loss on drying (not more than 0.5%), Residue on ignition (not more than 0.1%), Volatile related compounds, and Organic volatile impurities.

Doxylamine Succinate Oral Solution USP—Preserve in tight, light-resistant containers. Contains the labeled amount, within ±8%. Meets the requirement for Identification.

Doxylamine Succinate Syrup USP—Preserve in tight, light-resistant containers. Contains the labeled amount, within ± 8%. Meets the requirement for Identification.

Doxylamine Succinate Tablets USP—Preserve in well-closed, light-resistant containers. Contain the labeled amount, within ±8%. Meet the requirements for Identification, Dissolution (80% in 30 minutes in 0.01 N hydrochloric acid in Apparatus 2 at 50 rpm), and Uniformity of dosage units.

DOXYLAMINE, CODEINE, AND ACETAMINOPHEN

For *Doxylamine, Codeine,* and *Acetaminophen*—See individual listings for chemistry information.

USP requirements: Doxylamine Succinate, Codeine Phosphate, and Acetaminophen Tablets—Not in *USP–NF*.

DOXYLAMINE, ETAFEDRINE, AND HYDROCODONE

Chemical name:
Doxylamine succinate—Ethanamine, *N,N*-dimethyl-2-[1-phenyl-1-(2-pyridinyl)ethoxy]-, butanedioate (1:1).
Etafedrine hydrochloride—Benzenemethanol, alpha-[1-(ethylmethylamino)ethyl]-, hydrochloride.
Hydrocodone bitartrate—Morphinan-6-one, 4,5-epoxy-3-methoxy-17-methyl-, (5 alpha)-, [*R*-(*R**,*R**)]-2,3-dihydroxybutanedioate (1:1), hydrate (2:5).

Molecular formula:
Doxylamine succinate—$C_{17}H_{22}N_2O \cdot C_4H_6O_4$.
Etafedrine hydrochloride—$C_{12}H_{19}NO \cdot HCL$.
Hydrocodone bitartrate—$C_{18}H_{21}NO_3 \cdot C_4H_6O_6 \cdot 2\frac{1}{2}H_2O$ (hydrate); $C_{18}H_{21}NO_3 \cdot C_4H_6O_6$ (anhydrous).

Molecular weight:
Doxylamine succinate—388.46.
Etafedrine hydrochloride—229.75.
Hydrocodone bitartrate—494.49 (hydrate); 449.46 (anhydrous).

Description:
Doxylamine Succinate USP—White or creamy white powder, having a characteristic odor.
Hydrocodone Bitartrate USP—Fine, white crystals or a crystalline powder. Is affected by light.

Solubility:
Doxylamine Succinate USP—Very soluble in water and in alcohol; freely soluble in chloroform; very slightly soluble in ether and in benzene.
Hydrocodone Bitartrate USP—Soluble in water; slightly soluble in alcohol; insoluble in ether and in chloroform.

USP requirements:
Doxylamine Succinate, Etafedrine Hydrochloride, and Hydrocodone Bitartrate Syrup—Not in *USP–NF*.
Doxylamine Succinate, Etafedrine Hydrochloride, and Hydrocodone Bitartrate Tablets—Not in *USP–NF*.

DOXYLAMINE, PHENYLPROPANOLAMINE, DEXTROMETHORPHAN, AND ASPIRIN

For *Doxylamine, Phenylpropanolamine, Dextromethorphan,* and *Aspirin*—See individual listings for chemistry information.

USP requirements: Doxylamine Succinate, Phenylpropanolamine Bitartrate, Dextromethorphan Hydrobromide, and Aspirin Effervescent Tablets—Not in *USP–NF*.

DOXYLAMINE, PSEUDOEPHEDRINE, DEXTROMETHORPHAN, AND ACETAMINOPHEN

For *Doxylamine, Pseudoephedrine, Dextromethorphan,* and *Acetaminophen*—See individual listings for chemistry information.

USP requirements:
Doxylamine Succinate, Pseudoephedrine Hydrochloride, Dextromethorphan Hydrobromide, and Acetaminophen Capsules—Not in *USP–NF*.
Doxylamine Succinate, Pseudoephedrine Hydrochloride, Dextromethorphan Hydrobromide, and Acetaminophen Oral Solution USP—Preserve in tight containers. Contains the labeled amounts, within ±10%. Meets the requirements for Identification, pH (4.5–6.3), Alcohol content, if present (within ±10%), and Microbial limits.
Doxylamine Succinate, Pseudoephedrine Hydrochloride, Dextromethorphan Hydrobromide, and Acetaminophen for Oral Solution—Not in *USP–NF*.

DRONABINOL

Chemical group: A cannabinoid; naturally-occurring and has been extracted from *Cannabis sativa* L. (marijuana).

Chemical name: 6*H*-Dibenzo[*b,d*]pyran-1-ol, 6a,7,8,10a-tetrahydro-6,6,9-trimethyl-3-pentyl-, (6a*R-trans*)-.

Molecular formula: $C_{21}H_{30}O_2$.

Molecular weight: 314.46.

Description: Viscous, oily liquid.

Solubility: Insoluble in water; soluble in 1 part of alcohol or acetone, 3 parts of glycerol; soluble in fixed oils.

USP requirements:
Dronabinol USP—Preserve in tight, light-resistant glass containers in inert atmosphere. Store in a cool place. It is Delta⁹-tetrahydrocannabinol. Contains not less than 95.0% of dronabinol. Meets the requirements for Identification and Limit of Delta⁸-tetrahydrocannabinol (not more than 2.0%).
Dronabinol Capsules USP—Preserve in well-closed, light-resistant containers, in a cool place. Contain dronabinol in sesame oil. Contain the labeled amount, within ±10%. Meet the requirements for Identification, Dissolution (in 15 minutes in water in Apparatus 2 at 50 rpm), and Uniformity of dosage units.

DROPERIDOL

Chemical name: 2*H*-Benzimidazol-2-one, 1-[1-[4-(4-fluorophenyl)-4-oxobutyl]-1,2,3,6-tetrahydro-4-pyridinyl]-1,3-dihydro-.

Molecular formula: $C_{22}H_{22}FN_3O_2$.

Molecular weight: 379.43.

Description: Droperidol USP—White to light tan, amorphous or microcrystalline powder. Melts at about 145 °C.

Solubility: Droperidol USP—Practically insoluble in water; freely soluble in chloroform; slightly soluble in alcohol and in ether.

USP requirements:
Droperidol USP—Preserve in tight, light-resistant containers, under nitrogen, in a cool place. Dried in vacuum at 70 °C for 4 hours, contains not less than 98.0% and not more than 102.0% of droperidol. Meets the requirements for Identification, Loss on drying (not more than 5.0%), Residue on ignition (not more than 0.2%), Heavy metals (not more than 0.002%), and Limit of 4,4'-bis[1,2,3,6-tetrahydro-4-(2-oxo-1-benzimidazolinyl)-1-pyridyl]butyrophenone.
Droperidol Injection USP—Preserve in single-dose or in multiple-dose containers, preferably of Type I glass, protected from light. A sterile solution of Droperidol in Water for Injection, prepared with the aid of Lactic Acid. Contains the labeled amount of droperidol, as the lactate, within ±10%. Meets the requirements for Identification, Bacterial endotoxins, pH (3.0–3.8), and Chromatographic purity, and for Injections.

DROSPIRENONE AND ETHINYL ESTRADIOL

Chemical name:
Drospirenone—(6*R*,7*R*,8*R*,9*S*,10*R*,13*S*,14*S*,15*S*,16*S*,17*S*)-1,3',4',6,6a,7,8,9,10,11,12,13,14,15,15a,16-hexadecahydro-10,13-dimethylspiro-[17*H*-dicyclopropa-6,7:15,16]cyclopenta[a]phenanthrene-17,2'(5*H*)-furan]-3,5'(2*H*)-dione).
Ethinyl estradiol—19-Norpregna-1,3,5(10)-trien-20-yne-3,17-diol, (17 alpha)-.

Molecular formula:
Drospirenone—$C_{24}H_{30}O_3$.
Ethinyl estradiol—$C_{20}H_{24}O_2$.

Molecular weight:
Drospirenone—366.49.
Ethinyl estradiol—296.40.

Description: Ethinyl Estradiol USP—White to creamy white, odorless, crystalline powder.

Solubiliuty: Ethinyl Estradiol USP—Insoluble in water; soluble in alcohol, in chloroform, in ether, in vegetable oils, and in solutions of fixed alkali hydroxides.

USP requirements: Drospirenone and Ethinyl Estradiol Tablets—Not in *USP–NF*.

DROTRECOGIN ALFA (ACTIVATED)

Source: Drotecogin alfa is a recombinant form of human Activated Protein C.

Chemical name: $C_{2071}H_{3165}N_{581}O_{640}S_{31}$.

Molecular weight: Approximately 55 kilodalton.

Description: Sterile, lyophilized, white to off-white powder.

USP requirements: Drotecogin Alfa for Injection (Activated)—Not in *USP–NF*.

ABSORBABLE DUSTING POWDER

Description: Absorbable Dusting Powder USP—White, odorless powder.

USP requirements: Absorbable Dusting Powder USP—Preserve in well-closed containers. It may be preserved in sealed paper packets. An absorbable powder prepared by processing cornstarch and intended for use as a lubricant for surgical gloves. Contains not more than 2.0% of magnesium oxide. Meets the requirements for Identification, Stability to autoclaving, Sedimentation, pH (10.0–10.8, in a 1 in 10 suspension), Loss on drying (not more than 12%), Residue on ignition (not more than 3.0%), and Heavy metals (not more than 0.001%).

DYCLONINE

Chemical name: Dyclonine hydrochloride—1-Propanone, 1-(4-butoxyphenyl)-3-(1-piperidinyl)-, hydrochloride.

Molecular formula: Dyclonine hydrochloride—$C_{18}H_{27}NO_2 \cdot HCl$.

Molecular weight: Dyclonine hydrochloride—325.87.

Description: Dyclonine Hydrochloride USP—White crystals or white crystalline powder, which may have a slight odor.

Solubility: Dyclonine Hydrochloride USP—Soluble in water, in acetone, in alcohol, and in chloroform.

USP requirements:
Dyclonine Hydrochloride USP—Preserve in tight, light-resistant containers. Contains not less than 98.0% and not more than 102.0% of dyclonine hydrochloride, calculated on the dried basis. Meets the requirements for Identification, Melting range (173–178 °C), pH (4.0–7.0, in a solution [1 in 100]), Loss on drying (not more than 1.0%), and Residue on ignition (not more than 0.2%).
Dyclonine Hydrochloride Gel USP—Preserve in collapsible, opaque plastic tubes or in tight, light-resistant glass containers. (Note: Do not use aluminum or tin tubes.) Contains the labeled amount, within ±10%. Meets the requirements for Identification and pH (2.0–4.0).
Dyclonine Hydrochloride Lozenges—Not in *USP–NF*.
Dyclonine Hydrochloride Topical Solution USP—Preserve in tight, light-resistant containers. A sterile, aqueous solution of Dyclonine Hydrochloride. Contains the labeled amount, within ±8%. Meets the requirements for Identification, Sterility, and pH (3.0–5.0).

DYDROGESTERONE

Chemical name: Pregna-4,6-diene-3,20-dione, (9 beta,10 alpha)-.

Molecular formula: $C_{21}H_{28}O_2$.

Molecular weight: 312.45.

Description: Dydrogesterone USP—White to pale yellow, crystalline powder.

Solubility: Dydrogesterone USP—Practically insoluble in water; sparingly soluble in alcohol.

USP requirements:
Dydrogesterone USP—Preserve in well-closed containers. Contains not less than 98.0% and not more than 102.0% of dydrogesterone, calculated on the dried basis. Meets the requirements for Identification, Melting range (167–171 °C), Specific rotation (−442° to −462°), Loss on drying (not more than 0.5%), Residue on ignition (not more than 0.1%), Heavy metals (not more than 0.002%), and Chromatographic purity.
Dydrogesterone Tablets USP—Preserve in well-closed containers. Contain the labeled amount, within ±10%. Meet the requirements for Identification, Dissolution (75% in 60 minutes in 0.3% sodium lauryl sulfate in Apparatus 2 at 100 rpm), and Uniformity of dosage units.

DYPHYLLINE

Source: A chemical derivative of theophylline, but not a theophylline salt as are the other agents.

Chemical name: 1*H*-Purine-2,6-dione, 7-(2,3-dihydroxypropyl)-3,7-dihydro-1,3-dimethyl-.

Molecular formula: $C_{10}H_{14}N_4O_4$.

Molecular weight: 254.24.

Description: Dyphylline USP—White, odorless, amorphous or crystalline solid.

Solubility: Dyphylline USP—Freely soluble in water; sparingly soluble in alcohol and in chloroform; practically insoluble in ether.

USP requirements:
Dyphylline USP—Preserve in tight containers. Contains not less than 98.0% and not more than 102.0% of dyphylline, calculated on the dried basis. Meets the requirements for Identification, Melting range (160–164 °C), pH (5.0–7.5, in a solution [1 in 100]), Loss on drying (not more than 0.5%), Residue on ignition (not more than 0.15%), Chloride (not more than 0.035%), Sulfate (not more than 0.010%), Heavy metals (not more than 0.002%), Limit of theophylline, Related compounds, and Organic volatile impurities.
Dyphylline Elixir USP—Preserve in tight containers. Contains the labeled amount, within ±10%. Meets the requirements for Identification and Alcohol content (within ±10% of labeled amount).
Dyphylline Injection USP—Preserve in single-dose or in multiple-dose containers, preferably of Type I glass, protected from light. To avoid precipitation, store at a temperature of not below 15 °C, but avoid excessive heat. Label it to indicate that the Injection is not to be used if crystals have separated. Contains the labeled amount, within ±10%. Meets the requirements for Identification, Bacterial endotoxins, and pH (5.0–8.0), and for Injections.
Dyphylline Oral Solution USP—Preserve in tight containers. Contains the labeled amount, within ±10%. Meets the requirements for Identification and Alcohol content (within ±10% of labeled amount).

Dyphylline Tablets USP—Preserve in tight containers. Contain the labeled amount, within ±10%. Meet the requirements for Identification, Dissolution (75% in 45 minutes in water in Apparatus 1 at 100 rpm), and Uniformity of dosage units.

DYPHYLLINE AND GUAIFENESIN

For *Dyphylline* and *Guaifenesin*—See individual listings for chemistry information.

USP requirements:
Dyphylline and Guaifenesin Capsules—Not in *USP–NF*.
Dyphylline and Guaifenesin Elixir USP—Preserve in tight containers. Contains the labeled amounts, within ±10%. Meets the requirements for Identification, pH (5.0–7.0), and Alcohol content (within ±10% of labeled amount).
Dyphylline and Guaifenesin Oral Solution USP—Preserve in tight containers. Contains the labeled amounts, within ±10%. Meets the requirements for Identification, pH (5.0–7.0), and Alcohol content (within ±10% of labeled amount).
Dyphylline and Guaifenesin Tablets USP—Preserve in tight containers. Contain the labeled amounts, within ±10%. Meet the requirements for Identification, Dissolution (75% of each active ingredient in 45 minutes in water in Apparatus 1 at 100 rpm), and Uniformity of dosage units.

ECHINACEA AUNGUSTIFOLIA

NF requirements:
Echinacea Angustifolia NF—Store in well-closed light-resistant containers. Consists of the dried rhizone and roots of *Echinacea angustifolia* DC (Fam. Asteraceae). It is harvested in the fall after 3 or more years of growth. The label states the Latin binomial and, following the official name, the parts of the plant contained in the article. Contains not less than 0.5% of total phenols, calculated on the dried basis as the sum of cafteric acid, chicoric acid, chlorogenic acid, dicaffeoylquinic acids, and echinacoside. Contains not less than 0.075% of dodecatetraenoic acid isobutylamides. Meets the requirements for Botanic characteristics, Identification, Loss on drying (not more than 10.0%), Foreign organic matter (no more than 3.0%), Total ash (not more than 7.0%), Acid-insoluble ash (not more than 4.0%), Pesticide residues, Heavy metals (0.001%), Content of total phenols, and Content of dodecatetraenoic acid isobutylamides.
Powdered Echinacea Angustifolia NF—Preserve in well-closed, light-resistant containers. It is *Echinacea angustifolia* reduced to a powder or very fine powder. The label states the Latin binomial and, following the official name, the part of the plant from which the article was derived. Meets the requirements for Botanic characteristics, and for Identification, Loss on drying, Total ash, Acid-insoluble ash, Pesticide residues, Heavy metals, Content of total phenols, and Content of dodecatetraenoic acid isobutylamides for *Ethinacea angustifolia*.
Powdered Echinacea Angustifolia Extract NF—Preserve in tight, light-resistant containers, in a cool place. Prepared from *Echinacea angustifolia* roots by extraction with hydroalcoholic mixtures or other suitable solvents. The ratio of the starting crude plant material to Powdered Extract is between 2:1 and 8:1. The label states the Latin binomial and, following the official name, the part of the plant from which the article was prepared. It meets the requirements for *Labeling for Botanical Extracts*. Contains not less than 4.0% and not more than 5.0% of total phenols, calculated

on the dried basis as the sum of caftaric acid, chicoric acid, chlorogenic acid, dicaffeoylquinic acids, and echinacoside. Contains not less than 0.6% of dodecatetraenoic acid isobutylamides. Meets the requirements for Identification, Microbial limits, Loss on drying (not more than 5.0%), Heavy metals (0.002%), Organic volatile impurities, Content of total phenols, and Content of dodecatetraenoic acid isobutylamides, and for Residual solvents and Pestiside residues under *Botanical Extracts*.

ECHINACEA PALLIDA

NF requirements:
Echinacea Pallida NF—Preserve in well-closed, light-resistant containers. Consists of the dried rhizone and roots of *Echinacea pallida* Nuttall (Fam. Asteraceae). It is harvested in the fall after 3 or more years of growth. The label states the Latin binomial and, following the official name, the parts of the plant contained in the article. Contains not less than 0.5% of total phenols, calculated on the dried basis as the sum of caftaric acid, chicoric acid, chlorogenic acid, and achinocoside. Meets the requirements for Botanic characteristics, Identification, Volatile oil of content (1.0–2.0 mL per 100 grams), and Content of total phenols, and for Loss on drying, Foreign organic matter, Total ash, Acid-insoluble ash, Pesticide residues, and Heavy metals for *Echinacea angustifolia*.
Powdered Echinacea Pallida NF—Reserve in tight, light-resistant containers. It is *Echinacea pallida* reduced to a powder or very fine powder. The label states the Latin binomial, and following the official name, the part of the plant from which the article was derived. Meets the requirements for Botanic characteristics, and for Identification, Loss on drying, Total ash, Acid-insoluble ash, Volatile oil content, Pesticide residues, Heavy metals, and Content of total phenols for *Echinacea pallida*.
Powdered Echinacea Pallida Extract NF—Preserve in tight, light-resistant containers, in a cool place. Prepared from *Echinacea pallida* roots by extraction with hydroalcoholic mixtures or other suitable solvents. The ratio of the starting crude plant material to Powdered Extract is between 2:1 and 8:1. The label states the Latin binomial and, following the official name, the parts of the plant fron which the article was prepared. It meets the requirements for Labeling under *Botanical Extracts*. Contains not less than 4.0% and not more than 5.0% of total phenols, calculated on the dried basis as the sum of caftaric acid, chicoric acid, chlorogenic acid, dicaffeoylquinic acids, and echinacoside. Meets the requirements for Identification and Content of total phenols, and for Microbial limits, Loss on drying, Heavy metals, and Organic volatile impurities for Powdered Echinacea Extract, and for residual solvents and Pesticide residues under *Botanical Extracts*.

ECHINACEA PURPUREA

NF requirements:
Echinacea Purpurea Root NF—Store in well-closed, light-resistant containers. Consists of the dried rhizone and roots of *Echinacea purpurea* (L.) Moench (Fam. Asteraceae). It is harvested in the fall after 3 or more years of growth. The label states the Latin binomial and, following the official name, the parts of the plant contained in the article. Contains not less than 0.5% of total phenols, calculated on the dried basis as the sum of caftaric acid, chicoric acid, chlorogenic acid, and echinacoside. Contains not less than 0.025% of alkamides calculated as dodecatetraenoic

acid isobutylamides. Meets the requirements for Botanic characteristics, Identification, Content of total phenols, and Content of alkamides, and for Loss on dyring, Foreign organic matter, Total ash, Acid-insoluble ash, Pesticide residues, and Heavy metals for *Echinacea angustifolia*.

Powdered Echinecea Purpurea NF—Preserve in well-closed, light-resistant containers. It is *Echinacea purpurea* Root reduced to powder or very fine powder. The label states the Latin binomial and, following the official name, the part of the plant from which the article was derived. Meets the requirements for Botanic characteristics, and for Identification, Loss on drying, Total ash, Acid-insoluble ash, Pesticide residues, Heavy metals, Content of total phenols, and Content of alkamides for *Ethinacea purpurea* Root.

Powdered Echinecea Purpurea Extract NF—Preserve in tight, light resistant containers, in a cool place. It is prepared from dried *Echinacea purpurea* Root by extraction with hydroalcoholic mixtures or other suitable solvents. The ratio of the starting crude plant material to Powdered Extract is between 2:1 and 8:1. The label states the Latin binomial and, following the official name, the parts of the plant from which the article was derived. It meets the requirements for Labeling under *Botanical Extracts*. Contains not less than 4.0% of total phenols, calculated on the dried basis as the sum of caftaric acid, chicoric acid, chlorogenic acid, and echinacoside. Contains not less than 0.025% of alkamides, calculated on the dried basis as dodecatetraenoic acid isobutylmides. Meets the requirements for Identification, Content of total phenols, and Content of alkamides, and for Microbial limits, Loss on drying, Heavy matals, and Organic volatile impurities for Powdered Echinacea Angustifolia Extract, and for Residual solvents and Pesticide residues under *Botanical Extracts*.

ECHOTHIOPHATE

Chemical name: Echothiophate iodide—Ethanaminium, 2-[(diethoxyphosphinyl)thio]-*N,N,N*-trimethyl-, iodide.

Molecular formula: Echothiophate iodide—$C_9H_{23}INO_3PS$.

Molecular weight: Echothiophate iodide—383.23.

Description:
Echothiophate Iodide USP—White, crystalline, hygroscopic solid having a slight mercaptan-like odor. Its solutions have a pH of about 4.
Echothiophate Iodide for Ophthalmic Solution USP—White, amorphous powder.

Solubility: Echothiophate Iodide USP—Freely soluble in water and in methanol; soluble in dehydrated alcohol; practically insoluble in other organic solvents.

USP requirements:
Echothiophate Iodide USP—Preserve in tight, light-resistant containers, preferably at a temperature below 0 °C. Contains not less than 95.0% and not more than 100.5% of echothiophate iodide, calculated on the dried basis. Meets the requirements for Identification and Loss on drying (not more than 1.0%).
Echothiophate Iodide for Ophthalmic Solution USP—Preserve in tight containers, preferably of Type I glass, at controlled room temperature. It is sterile Echothiophate Iodide. Contains the labeled amount, within −5% to +15%. Meets the requirements for Completeness of solution, Identification, Sterility, and Water (not more than 2.0%).

ECONAZOLE

Chemical group: Synthetic imidazole derivative, differing structurally from miconazole.

Chemical name: Econazole nitrate—1*H*-Imidazole, 1-[2-[(4-chlorophenyl)methoxy]-2-(2,4-dichlorophenyl)ethyl]-, mononitrate, (±)-.

Molecular formula: Econazole nitrate—$C_{18}H_{15}Cl_3N_2O \cdot HNO_3$.

Molecular weight: Econazole nitrate—444.70.

Description: Econazole Nitrate USP—White or practically white, crystalline powder, having not more than a slight odor.

Solubility: Econazole Nitrate USP—Very slightly soluble in water and in ether; slightly soluble in alcohol; sparingly soluble in chloroform; soluble in methanol.

USP requirements:
Econazole Nitrate USP—Preserve in well-closed containers, protected from light. Contains not less than 98.5% and not more than 101.0% of econazole nitrate, calculated on the dried basis. Meets the requirements for Identification, Melting range (162–166 °C, with decomposition), Loss on drying (not more than 0.5%), Residue on ignition (not more than 0.1%), and Chromatographic purity.
Econazole Nitrate Cream—Not in *USP–NF*.
Econazole Nitrate Vaginal Suppositories—Not in *USP–NF*.

EDETATE CALCIUM DISODIUM

Chemical name: Calciate(2-), [[*N,N*-1,2-ethanediylbis[*N*-(carboxymethyl)glycinato]](4-)-*N,N′,O,O′,O^N,O^N*], disodium, hydrate, (*OC*-6-21)-.

Molecular formula: $C_{10}H_{12}CaN_2Na_2O_8 \cdot xH_2O$.

Molecular weight: 374.27 (anhydrous).

Description: Edetate Calcium Disodium USP—White, crystalline granules or white, crystalline powder; odorless; slightly hygroscopic; stable in air.

Solubility: Edetate Calcium Disodium USP—Freely soluble in water.

USP requirements:
Edetate Calcium Disodium USP—Preserve in tight containers. A mixture of the dihydrate and trihydrate of calcium disodium ethylenediaminetetraacetate (predominantly the dihydrate). Contains not less than 97.0% and not more than 102.0% of edetate calcium disodium, calculated on the anhydrous basis. Meets the requirements for Identification, pH (6.5–8.0, in a solution [1 in 5]), Water (not more than 13.0%), Heavy metals (not more than 0.002%), Limit of nitrilotriacetic acid, and Magnesium-chelating substances.
Edetate Calcium Disodium Injection USP—Preserve in single-dose containers, preferably of Type I glass. A sterile solution of Edetate Calcium Disodium in Water for Injection. Contains, in each mL, not less than 180 mg and not more than 220 mg of edetate calcium disodium. Meets the requirements for Identification, Bacterial endotoxins, pH (6.5–8.0), and Particulate matter, and for Injections.

EDETATE DISODIUM

Chemical group: The disodium salt of ethylenediamine tetraacetic acid (EDTA).

Chemical name: Glycine, *N,N*-1,2-ethanediylbis[*N*-(carboxymethyl)-, disodium salt, dihydrate.

Molecular formula: $C_{10}H_{14}N_2Na_2O_8 \cdot 2H_2O$.

Molecular weight: 372.24.

Description: Edetate Disodium USP—White, crystalline powder.
NF category: Chelating agent; complexing agent.

Solubility: Edetate Disodium USP—Soluble in water.

USP requirements:
Edetate Disodium USP—Preserve in well-closed containers.
Contains not less than 99.0% and not more than 101.0%
of edetate disodium, calculated on the dried basis. Meets
the requirements for Identification, pH (4.0–6.0, in a solution [1 in 20]), Loss on drying (8.7–11.4%), Calcium, Heavy metals (not more than 0.005%), and Limit of
nitrilotriacetic acid.
Edetate Disodium Injection USP—Preserve in single-dose
containers, preferably of Type I glass. A sterile solution
of Edetate Disodium in Water for Injection, which as a result of pH adjustment, contains varying amounts of the disodium and trisodium salts. Contains the labeled amount,
within ±10%. Meets requirements for Identification, Bacterial endotoxins, and pH (6.5–7.5), and for Injections.
Edetate Disodium Ophthalmic Solution—Not in *USP–NF*.

EDETIC ACID

Chemical name: Glycine, *N,N'*-1,2-ethanediylbis[*N*-(carboxymethyl)-.

Molecular formula: $C_{10}H_{16}N_2O_8$.

Molecular weight: 292.24.

Description: Edetic Acid NF—White, crystalline powder. Melts
above 220 °C, with decomposition.
NF category: Chelating agent; complexing agent.

Solubility: Edetic Acid NF—Very slightly soluble in water; soluble
in solutions of alkali hydroxides.

NF requirements: Edetic Acid NF—Preserve in well-closed containers. Contains not less than 98.0% and not more than
100.5% of edetic acid. Meets the requirements for Identification, Residue on ignition (not more than 0.2%), Heavy metals
(not more than 0.003%), Iron (not more than 0.005%), and
Limit of nitrilotriacetic acid.

EDROPHONIUM

Chemical group: Synthetic quaternary ammonium compound.

Chemical name: Edrophonium chloride—Benzenaminium, *N*-
ethyl-3-hydroxy-*N,N*-dimethyl-, chloride.

Molecular formula: Edrophonium chloride—$C_{10}H_{16}ClNO$.

Molecular weight: Edrophonium chloride—201.69.

Description: Edrophonium Chloride USP—White, odorless,
crystalline powder. Its solution (1 in 10) is practically colorless.

Solubility: Edrophonium Chloride USP—Very soluble in water;
freely soluble in alcohol; insoluble in chloroform and in ether.

USP requirements:
Edrophonium Chloride USP—Preserve in well-closed containers. Contains not less than 98.0% and not more than
100.5% of edrophonium chloride, calculated on the dried
basis. Meets the requirements for Identification, Melting
range (165–170 °C, with decomposition), pH (4.0–5.0, in
a solution [1 in 10]), Loss on drying (not more than

0.5%), Residue on ignition (not more than 0.1%), Heavy
metals (not more than 0.002%), and Limit of dimethylami-
nophenol.
Edrophonium Chloride Injection USP—Preserve in single-
dose or in multiple-dose containers, preferably of Type I
glass. A sterile solution of Edrophonium Chloride in Water
for Injection. Label the Injection in multiple-dose containers to indicate an expiration date of not later than 3 years
after date of manufacture, and label the Injection in single-
dose containers to indicate an expiration date of not later
than 4 years after the date of manufacture. Contains the
labeled amount, within ±5%. Meets the requirements for
Identification, Bacterial endotoxins, and pH (5.0–5.8),
and for Injections.

EDROPHONIUM AND ATROPINE

For *Edrophonium* and *Atropine*—See individual listings for chemistry information.

USP requirements: Edrophonium Chloride and Atropine Sulfate
Injection—Not in *USP–NF*.

EFAVIRENZ

Chemical group: Benzoxazinone derivative.

Chemical name: (*S*)-6-chloro-4-(cyclopropylethynyl)-1,4-dihy-
dro-4-(trifluoromethyl)-2*H*-3,1-benzoxacin-2-one.

Molecular formula: $C_{14}H_9ClF_3NO_2$.

Molecular weight: 315.67.

Description: White to slightly pink crystalline powder.

pKa: 10.2.

Solubility: Practically insoluble in water (less than 10 micrograms per mL) at pH 1–8.

USP requirements: Efavirenz Capsules—Not in *USP–NF*.

EFLORNITHINE

Chemical name: Eflornithine hydrochloride—DL-Ornithine, 2-(di-
fluoromethyl)-, monohydrochloride, monohydrate.

Molecular formula: Eflornithine hydrochloride—$C_6H_{12}F_2N_2O_2 \cdot$
HCl $\cdot$ H_2O.

Molecular weight: Eflornithine hydrochloride—236.64.

Description: Eflornithine hydrochloride—White to off-white,
odorless, crystalline powder.

Solubility: Eflornithine hydrochloride—Freely soluble in water
and sparingly soluble in ethanol.

USP requirements:
Eflornithine Hydrochloride Cream—Not in *USP–NF*.
Eflornithine Hydrochloride Concentrate for Injection—Not in
USP–NF.

BUFFERED ELECTROLYTE AND DEXTROSE

USP requirements: Buffered Electrolyte and Dextrose Injection—Not in *USP–NF*.

MULTIPLE ELECTROLYTES

USP requirements:

Multiple Electrolytes Injection Type 1 USP—Preserve in single-dose glass or plastic containers. Glass containers are preferably of Type I or Type II glass. A sterile solution of suitable salts in Water for Injection to provide sodium, potassium, magnesium, and chloride ions. In addition, the salts may provide ions of acetate, or acetate and gluconate, or acetate, gluconate, and phosphate. The label states the content of each electrolyte in terms of milliequivalents in a given volume. The label states the total osmolar concentration in mOsmol per liter. When the contents are less than 100 mL, the label alternatively may state the total osmolar concentration in mOsmol per mL. Contains the labeled amounts of sodium, potassium, magnesium, chloride, acetate, gluconate, and phosphate, within ± 10%. Contains no antimicrobial agents. Meets the requirements for Identification, Bacterial endotoxins, and pH (4.0–8.0), and for Injections.

Multiple Electrolytes Injection Type 2 USP—Preserve in single dose glass or plastic containers. Glass containers are preferably of Type I or Type II glass. A sterile solution of suitable salts in Water for Injection to provide sodium, potassium, calcium, magnesium, and chloride ions. In addition, the salts may provide ions of either acetate and citrate, or acetate and lactate. The label states the content of each electrolyte in terms of milliequivalents in a given volume. The label states the total osmolar concentration in mOsmol per liter. When the contents are less than 100 mL, the label alternatively may state the total osmolar concentration in mOsmol per mL. Contains the labeled amounts of sodium, potassium, magnesium, calcium, chloride, acetate, citrate, and lactate, within ±10%. Contains no antimicrobial agents. Meets the requirements for Identification, Bacterial endotoxins, and pH (4.0–8.0), and for Injections.

MULTIPLE ELECTROLYTES AND DEXTROSE

USP requirements:

Multiple Electrolytes and Dextrose Injection Type 1 USP—Preserve in single-dose glass or plastic containers. Glass containers are preferably of Type I or Type II glass. A sterile solution of Dextrose and suitable salts in Water for Injection to provide sodium, potassium, magnesium, and chloride ions. In addition, the salts may provide ions of acetate, or acetate and gluconate, or acetate and phosphate, or phosphate and lactate, or phosphate and sulfate. The label states the content of each electrolyte in terms of milliequivalents in a given volume. The label states the total osmolar concentration in mOsmol per liter. When the contents are less than 100 mL, the label alternatively may state the total osmolar concentration in mOsmol per mL. Contains the labeled amounts of sodium, potassium, magnesium, acetate, gluconate, phosphate, lactate, and sulfate, within ±10%, the labeled amount of chloride, within −10% to +20%, and the labeled amount of dextrose, within −10% to +5%. Contains no antimicrobial agents. Meets the requirements for Identification, Bacterial endotoxins, and pH (4.0–6.5), and for Injections.

Multiple Electrolytes and Dextrose Injection Type 2 USP—Preserve in single-dose glass or plastic containers. Glass containers are preferably of Type I or Type II glass. A sterile solution of Dextrose and suitable salts in Water for Injection to provide sodium, potassium, magnesium, calcium, and chloride ions. In addition, the salts may provide ions of acetate, or acetate and citrate, or acetate and lactate, or gluconate and sulfate. The label states the content of each electrolyte in terms of milliequivalents in a given volume. The label states the total osmolar concentration in mOsmol per liter. When the contents are less than 100 mL, the label alternatively may state the total osmolar concentration in mOsmol per mL. Contains the labeled amounts of sodium, potassium, magnesium, calcium, acetate, citrate, lactate, gluconate, and sulfate, within ±10%, the labeled amount of chloride, within −10% to +20%, and the labeled amount of dextrose, within −10% to +5%. Contains no antimicrobial agents. Meets the requirements for Identification, Bacterial endotoxins, and pH (4.0–6.5), and for Injections.

Multiple Electrolytes and Dextrose Injection Type 3 USP—Preserve in single-dose glass or plastic containers. Glass containers are preferably of Type I or Type II glass. A sterile solution of Dextrose and suitable salts in Water for Injection to provide sodium, potassium, and chloride ions. In addition, the salts may provide ions of ammonium, or acetate and phosphate, or phosphate and lactate. The label states the content of each electrolyte in terms of milliequivalents in a given volume. The label states the total osmolar concentration in mOsmol per liter. When the contents are less than 100 mL, the label alternatively may state the total osmolar concentration in mOsmol per mL. Contains the labeled amounts of sodium, potassium, ammonium, acetate, phosphate, and lactate, within ±10%, the labeled amount of chloride, within −10% to +20%, and the labeled amount of dextrose, within −10% to +5%. Contains no antimicrobial agents. Meets the requirements for Identification, Bacterial endotoxins, and pH (4.0–6.5), and for Injections.

Multiple Electrolytes and Dextrose Injection Type 4 USP—Preserve in single-dose glass or plastic containers. Glass containers are preferably of Type I or Type II glass. A sterile solution of Dextrose and suitable salts in Water for Injection to provide sodium, magnesium, calcium, chloride, gluconate, and sulfate ions. The label states the content of each electrolyte in terms of milliequivalents in a given volume. The label states the total osmolar concentration in mOsmol per liter. When the contents are less than 100 mL, the label alternatively may state the total osmolar concentration in mOsmol per mL. Contains the labeled amounts of sodium, magnesium, calcium, gluconate, and sulfate, within ±10%, the labeled amount of chloride, within −10% to +20%, and the labeled amount of dextrose, within −10% to +5%. Contains no antimicrobial agents. Meets the requirements for Identification, Bacterial endotoxins, and pH (4.2–5.2), and for Injections.

MULTIPLE ELECTROLYTES AND INVERT SUGAR

USP requirements:

Multiple Electrolytes and Invert Sugar Injection Type 1 USP—Preserve in single-dose glass or plastic containers. Glass containers are preferably of Type I or Type II glass. A sterile solution of a mixture of equal amounts of Dextrose and Fructose, or an equivalent solution produced by the hydrolysis of Sucrose, and suitable salts in Water for Injection to provide sodium, potassium, magnesium, chloride, phosphate, and lactate ions. The label states the content of each electrolyte in terms of milliequivalents in a given volume. The label states the total osmolar concentration in

mOsmol per liter. When the contents are less than 100 mL, the label alternatively may state the total osmolar concentration in mOsmol per mL. Contains the labeled amounts of sodium, potassium, magnesium, phosphate, lactate, and invert sugar, within ±10%, and the labeled amount of chloride, within −10% to +20%. Contains no antimicrobial agents. Meets the requirements for Identification, Pyrogen, pH (3.0–6.0), and Completeness of inversion, and for Injections.

Multiple Electrolytes and Invert Sugar Injection Type 2 USP—Preserve in single-dose glass or plastic containers. Glass containers are preferably of Type I or Type II glass. A sterile solution of a mixture of equal amounts of Dextrose and Fructose, or an equivalent solution produced by the hydrolysis of Sucrose, and suitable salts in Water for Injection to provide sodium, potassium, magnesium, calcium, chloride, and lactate ions. The label states the content of each electrolyte in terms of milliequivalents in a given volume. The label states the total osmolar concentration in mOsmol per liter. When the contents are less than 100 mL, the label alternatively may state the total osmolar concentration in mOsmol per mL. Contains the labeled amounts of sodium, potassium, magnesium, calcium, lactate, and invert sugar, within ±10%, and the labeled amount of chloride, within −10% to +20%. Contains no antimicrobial agents. Meets the requirements for Identification, Pyrogen, pH (4.5–6.0), and Completeness of inversion, and for Injections.

Multiple Electrolytes and Invert Sugar Injection Type 3 USP—Preserve in single-dose glass or plastic containers. Glass containers are preferably of Type I or Type II glass. A sterile solution of a mixture of equal amounts of Dextrose and Fructose, or an equivalent solution produced by the hydrolysis of Sucrose, and suitable salts in Water for Injection to provide sodium, potassium, chloride, and ammonium ions. The label states the content of each electrolyte in terms of milliequivalents in a given volume. The label states the total osmolar concentration in mOsmol per liter. When the contents are less than 100 mL, the label alternatively may state the total osmolar concentration in mOsmol per mL. Contains the labeled amounts of sodium, potassium, ammonium, and invert sugar, within ±10%, and the labeled amount of chloride, within −10% to +20%. Contains no antimicrobial agents. Meets the requirements for Identification, Pyrogen, pH (3.0–5.5), and Completeness of inversion, and for Injections.

TRACE ELEMENTS

For *Zinc Chloride, Zinc Sulfate, Cupric Chloride, Cupric Sulfate, Chromic Chloride, Manganese Chloride, Magnesium Sulfate, Selenious Acid, Sodium Iodide,* and *Ammonium Molybdate*—See individual listings for chemistry information.

USP requirements: Trace Elements Injection USP—Preserve in single-dose or in multiple-dose containers, preferably of Type I or Type II glass. A sterile solution in Water for Injection of two or more of the following: Zinc Chloride or Zinc Sulfate, Cupric Chloride or Cupric Sulfate, Chromic Chloride, Manganese Chloride or Manganese Sulfate, Selenious Acid, Sodium Iodide, and Ammonium Molybdate. Label the Injection to specify that it is to be diluted to the appropriate strength with Sterile Water for Injection or other suitable fluid prior to administration. The label shows by an appropriate number juxtaposed to the official name, the number of trace elements contained in the Injection according to the following: zinc and copper (2), and then cumulatively, chromium (3), manganese (4), selenium (5), iodine (6), and molybdenum (7). Other combinations are indicated separately by citing the number of trace elements contained in each followed by an asterisk that is repeated with the list of labeled ingredients. Label the Injection

for its contents of zinc chloride ($ZnCl_2$), zinc sulfate ($ZnSO_4 \cdot 7H_2O$), cupric chloride ($CuCl_2$), cupric sulfate ($CuSO_4$), chromic chloride ($CrCl_2$), manganese chloride ($MnCl_2$), manganese sulfate ($MnSO_4$), selenious acid (H_2SeO_3), sodium iodide (NaI), and ammonium molybdate [$(NH_4)Mo_7 \cdot 4H_2O$], and for elemental zinc (Zn), copper (Cu), chromium (Cr), manganese (Mn), selenium (Se), iodine (I), and molybdenum (Mo), as appropriate in relation to the ingredients claimed to be present. Contains the labeled amounts of zinc (Zn), copper (Cu), chromium (Cr), manganese (Mn), selenium (Se), iodine (I), and molybdenum (Mo), within ±10%. Meets the requirements for Identification, Pyrogen, pH (1.5–3.5), and Particulate matter, and for Injections.

ELEUTHERO

NF requirements:

Eleuthero NF—Preserve in well-closed, light-resistant containers. It is the dried rhizome with roots of *Eleutherococus senticosus* (Rupr. et Maxim.) (Fam. Araliaceae) [*Acanthopanax senticosus* Harms]. The label states the Latin binomial and, following the official name, the parts of the plant contained in the article. Contains not less than 0.08% of the sum of eleutheroside B and eleutheroside E, calculated on the dried basis. Meets the requirements for Botanic characteristics, Identification, Microbial limits, Loss on drying (not more than 14.0%), Foreign organic matter (not more than 3.0%), Total ash (not more than 8.0%), Water-soluble extractives (not more than 4.0%), Pesticide residues, Heavy metals (not more than 0.002%), and Content of eleutherosides B and F.

Powdered Eleuthero NF—Preserve in well-closed, light-resistant containers. It is Eleuthero reduced to a powder or very fine powder. The label states the Latin binomial and, following the official name, the part of the plant from which the article was derived. Contains not less than 0.08% of the sum of eleutheroside B and eleutheroside E, calculated on the dried basis. Meets the requirements for botanic characteristics, and for Identification, Loss on drying, Total ash, Pesticide residues, and Content of eleutherosides B and E under Eleuthero.

Powdered Eleuthero Extract NF—Preserve in tight, light-resistant containers. It is prepared from whole or comminuted dried underground parts of *Eleutherococcus senticosus* (Rupr. et Maxim.) (Fam. Araliaceae) [Syn: *Acanthopanax senticosus* Harms] extracted with hydroalcoholic mixtures. The ratio of the starting crude plant material to Powdered Extract is between 13:1 and 25:1. The label states the Latin binomial and, following the official name, the part of the plant from which the article was prepared. The label also indicates the content of eleutherosides, the extracting solvent used for preparation, and the ratio of the starting crude plant material to Powdered Extract. It meets the requirements for *Labeling for Botanical Extracts*. Contains not less than 0.8% of eleutherosides B and E, calculated on the anhydrous basis. May contain added substances. Meets the requirements for Identification, Water (not more than 5.0%), Total ash (not more than 10.0%), Heavy metals (not more than 0.002%), Organic volatile impurities, Alcohol content (not more than 0.5%), and Content of eleutherosides B and E, and for Residual solvents and pesticide residues under *Botanical Extracts*.

ELM

USP requirements: Elm USP—Preserve in well-closed containers, and store in a cool, dry place. The dried inner bark of *Ulmus rubra* Muhlenberg (*Ulmus fulva* Michaux) (Fam. Ulmaceae). Meets the requirements for Botanic characteristics, Identification, Outer bark, Foreign organic matter (not more than 2%), Loss on drying (not more than 12%), Total ash (not more than 10%, calculated on the dried basis), and Acid-insoluble ash (not more than 0.65%, calculated on the dried basis).

EMEDASTINE

Chemical name: Emedastine difumarate—1*H*-Benzimidazole, 1-(2-ethoxyethyl)-2-(hexahydro-4-methyl-1*H*-1,4-diazepin-1-yl)-, (*E*)-2-butenedioate (1:2).

Molecular formula: Emedastine difumarate—$C_{17}H_{26}N_4O \cdot 2C_4H_4O_4$.

Molecular weight: Emedastine difumarate—534.56.

Description: Emedastine Difumarate USP—White to faintly yellow, crystalline powder. Melts at approximately 150 °C.

pKa: Emedastine difumarate—4.51 and 8.48.

Solubility: Emedastine Difumarate USP—Soluble in water.

USP requirements:
Emedastine Ophthalmic Solution USP—Preserve in tight, light-resistant containers, in a refrigerator or at controlled room temperature. Store at a temperature between 4° and 30°. A sterile, aqueous solution. Contains an equivalent amount of emedastine difumarate, within −10%, and labeled amount of emedastine, within +10%. Meets the requirements for Identification, Sterility, and pH (5.0–8.0).
Emedastine Difumarate USP—Preserve in tight, light-resistant containers, at controlled room temperature. Contains not less than 98.5% and not more than 101.0% of emedastine difumarate, calculated on the dried basis. Meets the requirements for Identification, pH (3.0–4.5, in a solution [2 in 1000]), Loss on drying (not more than 0.5%), Residue on ignition (not more than 0.1%), Heavy metals (not more than 0.002%), and Chromatographic purity.
Emedastine Difumarate Ophthalmic Solution—Not in *USP–NF*.

EMETINE

Chemical name: Emetine hydrochloride—Emetan, 6′,7′,10,11-tetramethoxy-, dihydrochloride.

Molecular formula: Emetine hydrochloride—$C_{29}H_{40}N_2O_4 \cdot 2HCl$.

Molecular weight: Emetine hydrochloride—553.56.

Description: Emetine Hydrochloride USP—White or very slightly yellowish, odorless, crystalline powder. Affected by light.

Solubility: Emetine Hydrochloride USP—Freely soluble in water and in alcohol.

USP requirements:
Emetine Hydrochloride USP—Preserve in tight, light-resistant containers. The hydrochloride of an alkaloid obtained from Ipecac, or prepared by methylation of cephaeline, or prepared synthetically. Contains not less than 98.0% and not more than 101.5% of emetine hydrochloride, calculated on the anhydrous basis. Meets the requirements for Identification, Water (15.0–19.0%), Residue on ignition (not more than 0.2%), Acidity, and Limit of cephaeline.

Emetine Hydrochloride Injection USP—Preserve in single-dose, light-resistant containers, preferably of Type I glass. A sterile solution of Emetine Hydrochloride in Water for Injection. Contains an amount of anhydrous emetine hydrochloride equivalent to the labeled amount of emetine hydrochloride, within −16% to −6%. Meets the requirements for Identification, Bacterial endotoxins, pH (3.0–5.0), and Limit of cephaeline, and for Injections.

ENALAPRIL

Chemical name: Enalapril maleate—L-Proline, 1-[*N*-[1-(ethoxycarbonyl)-3-phenylpropyl]-L-alanyl]-, (*S*)-, (*Z*)-2-butenedioate (1:1).

Molecular formula: Enalapril maleate—$C_{20}H_{28}N_2O_5 \cdot C_4H_4O_4$.

Molecular weight: Enalapril maleate—492.52.

Description: Enalapril Maleate USP—Off-white, crystalline powder. Melts at about 144 °C.

Solubility: Enalapril Maleate USP—Practically insoluble in nonpolar organic solvents; slightly soluble in semipolar organic solvents; sparingly soluble in water; soluble in alcohol; freely soluble in methanol and in dimethylformamide.

USP requirements:
Enalapril Maleate USP—Preserve in well-closed containers. Contains not less than 98.0% and not more than 102.0% of enalapril maleate, calculated on the dried basis. Meets the requirements for Identification, Specific rotation (−41.0° to −43.5°), Loss on drying (not more than 1.0%), Residue on ignition (not more than 0.2%), Heavy metals (not more than 0.001%), Related compounds, and Organic volatile impurities.
Enalapril Maleate Tablets USP—Preserve in well-closed containers. Contain the labeled amount, within ±10%. Meet the requirements for Identification, Dissolution (80% in 30 minutes in phosphate buffer [pH 6.8] in Apparatus 2 at 50 rpm), Uniformity of dosage units, and Related compounds (the sum of all related compounds including those from enalaprilat and enalapril diketopiperazine not more than 5.0%).

ENALAPRIL AND DILTIAZEM

Chemical name:
Enalapril maleate—L-Proline, 1-[*N*-[1-(ethoxycarbonyl)-3-phenylpropyl]-L-alanyl]-, (*S*)-, (*Z*)-2-butenedioate (1:1).
Diltiazem malate—1,5-Benzothiazepin-4(5*H*)-one, 3-(acetyloxy)-5-[2-(dimethylamino)ethyl]-2,3-dihydro-2-(4-methoxyphenyl)-, (2*S-cis*)-, (*S*)-hydroxybutanedioate (1:1).

Molecular formula:
Enalapril maleate—$C_{20}H_{28}N_2O_5 \cdot C_4H_4O_4$.
Diltiazem malate—$C_{22}H_{26}N_2O_4S \cdot C_4H_6O_5$.

Molecular weight:
Enalapril maleate—492.52.
Diltiazem malate—548.61.

Description: Enalapril Maleate USP—Off-white, crystalline powder. Melts at about 144 °C.

Solubility: Enalapril Maleate USP—Practically insoluble in nonpolar organic solvents; slightly soluble in semipolar organic solvents; sparingly soluble in water; soluble in alcohol; freely soluble in methanol and in dimethylformamide.

USP requirements: Enalapril Maleate and Diltiazem Malate Extended-release Tablets—Not in *USP–NF*.

ENALAPRIL AND FELODIPINE

For *Enalapril* and *Felodipine*—See individual listings for chemistry information.

USP requirements:
Enalapril Maleate and Felodipine Tablets—Not in *USP–NF*.
Enalapril Maleate and Felodipine Extended-release Tablets—Not in *USP–NF*.

ENALAPRIL AND HYDROCHLOROTHIAZIDE

For *Enalapril* and *Hydrochlorothiazide*—See individual listings for chemistry information.

USP requirements: Enalapril Maleate and Hydrochlorothiazide Tablets USP—Preserve in well-closed containers. Contain the labeled amounts, within ±10%. Meet the requirements for Identification, Dissolution (80% of enalapril maleate and 60% of hydrochlorothiazide in 30 minutes in water in Apparatus 2 at 50 rpm), Uniformity of dosage units, and Related compounds.

ENALAPRILAT

Chemical name: L-Proline, 1-[N-(1-carboxy-3-phenylpropyl)-L-alanyl]-, dihydrate, (S)-.

Molecular formula: $C_{18}H_{24}N_2O_5 \cdot 2H_2O$.

Molecular weight: 384.42.

Description: Enalaprilat USP—White to nearly white, hygroscopic, crystalline powder.

Solubility: Enalaprilat USP—Sparingly soluble in methanol and in dimethylformamide; slightly soluble in water and in isopropyl alcohol; very slightly soluble in acetone, in alcohol, and in hexane; practically insoluble in acetonitrile and in chloroform.

USP requirements:
Enalaprilat USP—Preserve in well-closed containers. Contains not less than 98.0% and not more than 101.0% of enalaprilat, calculated on the anhydrous basis. Meets the requirements for Identification, Specific rotation (−53.0° to −56.0°), Water (7.0–11.0%), Residue on ignition (not more than 0.2%), and Heavy metals (not more than 0.002%).
Enalaprilat Injection—Not in *USP–NF*.

ENCAINIDE

Chemical name: Encainide hydrochloride—Benzamide, 4-methoxy-N-[2-[2-(1-methyl-2-piperidinyl)ethyl]phenyl]-, monohydrochloride, (±)-.

Molecular formula: Encainide hydrochloride—$C_{22}H_{28}N_2O_2 \cdot HCl$.

Molecular weight: Encainide hydrochloride—388.93.

Description: White solid.

Solubility: Freely soluble in water; slightly soluble in ethanol; insoluble in heptane.

USP requirements: Encainide Hydrochloride Capsules—Not in *USP–NF*.

ENFLURANE

Chemical name: Ethane, 2-chloro-1-(difluoromethoxy)-1,1,2-trifluoro-.

Molecular formula: $C_3H_2ClF_5O$.

Molecular weight: 184.49.

Description: Enflurane USP—Clear, colorless, stable, volatile liquid, having a mild, sweet odor. Is non-flammable.

Solubility: Enflurane USP—Slightly soluble in water; miscible with organic solvents, fats, and oils.

Other characteristics:
Blood-to-Gas partition coefficient—1.91 at 37 °C.
Oil-to-Gas partition coefficient—98.5 at 37 °C.

USP requirements: Enflurane USP—Preserve in tight, light-resistant containers, and avoid exposure to excessive heat. Contains not less than 99.9% and not more than 100.0% of enflurane. Meets the requirements for Identification, Specific gravity (1.516–1.519), Refractive index (1.3020–1.3038 at 20 °C), Acidity or alkalinity, Water (not more than 0.14%), Limit of nonvolatile residue, Chloride, and Limit of fluoride ions (not more than 10 mcg per mL).

ENOXACIN

Chemical name: 1,8-Naphthyridine-3-carboxylic acid, 1-ethyl-6-fluoro-1,4-dihydro-4-oxo-7-(1-piperazinyl)-.

Molecular formula: $C_{15}H_{17}FN_4O_3$.

Molecular weight: 320.32.

Description: Ivory to slightly yellow powder. In dilute aqueous solution, unstable in strong sunlight.

USP requirements: Enoxacin Tablets—Not in *USP–NF*.

ENOXAPARIN

Source: Obtained by alkaline degradation of heparin benzyl ester derived from porcine intestinal mucosa.

Molecular weight: 4500 (average).

USP requirements: Enoxaparin Injection—Not in *USP–NF*.

ENROFLOXACIN

Chemical group: Quinolone carboxylic acid derivative.

Chemical name: 3-Quinolinecarboxylic acid, 1-cyclopropyl-7-(4-ethyl-1-piperazinyl)-6-fluoro-1,4-dihydro-4-oxo-.

Molecular formula: $C_{19}H_{22}FN_3O_3$.

Molecular weight: 359.39.

Description: Pale yellow crystals with a melting point of 219–221 °C.

Solubility: Slightly soluble in water at pH 7.

USP requirements:
Enrofloxacin Tablets—Not in *USP–NF*.
Enrofloxacin Injectable Solution—Not in *USP–NF*.

ENSULIZOLE

Chemical name: 1-*H*-Benzimidazole-5-sulfonic acid-2-phenyl-.

Molecular formula: $C_{13}H_{10}N_2O_3S$.

Molecular weight: 274.30.

USP requirements: Ensulizole USP—Preserve in tight containers in a cool place. Contains not less than 98.0% and not more than 102.0% of ensulizole, calculated on the dried basis. Meets the requirements for Identification and Loss on drying (not more than 2.0%).

ENTACAPONE

Source: Catechol-*O*-methyltransferase (COMT) inhibitor.

Chemical name: (*E*)-alpha-Cyano-*N,N*-diethyl-3,4-dihydroxy-5-nitrocinnamamide.

Molecular formula: $C_{14}H_{15}N_3O_5$.

Molecular weight: 305.29.

USP requirements: Entacapone Tablets—Not in *USP–NF*.

ENTERAL NUTRITION FORMULA

USP requirements:
Blenderized Enteral Nutrition Formula Oral Solution—Not in *USP–NF*.
Disease-specific Enteral Nutrition Formula Oral Solution—Not in *USP–NF*.
Disease-specific Enteral Nutrition Formula for Oral Solution—Not in *USP–NF*.
Fiber-containing Enteral Nutrition Formula Oral Solution—Not in *USP–NF*.
Milk-based Enteral Nutrition Formula Oral Solution—Not in *USP–NF*.
Milk-based Enteral Nutrition Formula for Oral Solution—Not in *USP–NF*.
Modular Enteral Nutrition Formula Oral Powder—Not in *USP–NF*.
Modular Enteral Nutrition Formula Oral Solution—Not in *USP–NF*.
Monomeric Enteral Nutrition Formula Oral Solution—Not in *USP–NF*.
Monomeric Enteral Nutrition Formula for Oral Solution—Not in *USP–NF*.
Polymeric Enteral Nutrition Formula Oral Solution—Not in *USP–NF*.
Polymeric Enteral Nutrition Formula for Oral Solution—Not in *USP–NF*.

ENZACAMENE

Chemical name: 3-(4-Methylbenzylidene)-camphor.

Molecular formula: $C_{18}H_{22}O$.

Molecular weight: 254.37.

USP requirements: Enzacamene USP—Preserve in tight containers. Contains not less than 98.0% and not more than 102.0% of enzacamene, calculated on the dried basis. Meets the requirements for Identification, Melting range (66–68 °C), and Loss on drying (not more than 0.2%).

EPHEDRINE

Chemical name:
Ephedrine—Benzenemethanol, alpha-[1-(methylamino)ethyl]-, [*R*-(*R*,S**)]-.
Ephedrine hydrochloride—Benzenemethanol, alpha-[1-(methylamino)ethyl]-, hydrochloride, [*R*-(*R*,S**)]-.
Ephedrine sulfate—Benzenemethanol, alpha-[1-(methylamino)ethyl]-, [*R*-(*R*,S**)]-, sulfate (2:1) (salt).

Molecular formula:
Ephedrine—$C_{10}H_{15}NO$ (anhydrous); $C_{10}H_{15}NO \cdot \frac{1}{2}H_2O$ (hemihydrate).
Ephedrine hydrochloride—$C_{10}H_{15}NO \cdot HCl$.
Ephedrine sulfate—$(C_{10}H_{15}NO)_2 \cdot H_2SO_4$.

Molecular weight:
Ephedrine—165.23 (anhydrous); 174.24 (hemihydrate).
Ephedrine hydrochloride—201.69.
Ephedrine sulfate—428.54.

Description:
Ephedrine USP—Unctuous, practically colorless solid or white crystals or granules. Gradually decomposes on exposure to light. Melts between 33 and 40 °C, the variability of the melting point being the result of differences in the moisture content, anhydrous Ephedrine having a lower melting point than the hemihydrate of Ephedrine. Its solutions are alkaline to litmus.
Ephedrine Hydrochloride USP—Fine, white, odorless crystals or powder. Is affected by light.
Ephedrine Sulfate USP—Fine, white, odorless crystals or powder. Darkens on exposure to light.
Ephedrine Sulfate Nasal Solution USP—Clear, colorless solution. Is neutral or slightly acid to litmus.

Solubility:
Ephedrine USP—Soluble in water, in alcohol, in chloroform, and in ether; moderately and slowly soluble in mineral oil, the solution becoming turbid if the Ephedrine contains more than about 1% of water.
Ephedrine Hydrochloride USP—Freely soluble in water; soluble in alcohol; insoluble in ether.
Ephedrine Sulfate USP—Freely soluble in water; sparingly soluble in alcohol.

USP requirements:
Ephedrine USP—Preserve in tight, light-resistant containers, in a cold place. It is anhydrous or contains not more than one-half molecule of water of hydration. Label it to indicate whether it is hydrous or anhydrous. Where the quantity of Ephedrine is indicated in the labeling of any preparation containing Ephedrine, this shall be understood to be in terms of anhydrous Ephedrine. Contains not less than 98.5% and not more than 100.5% of ephedrine, calculated on the anhydrous basis. Meets the requirements for Identification, Specific rotation (−40.3° to −43.3°), Water (4.5–5.5% for hydrated Ephedrine; not more than 0.5% for anhydrous Ephedrine), Residue on ignition (not more than 0.1%), Chloride (not more than 0.030%), Sulfate, Ordinary impurities, and Organic volatile impurities.

Ephedrine Hydrochloride USP—Preserve in well-closed, light-resistant containers. Contains not less than 98.0% and not more than 100.5% of ephedrine hydrochloride, calculated on the dried basis. Meets the requirements for Identification, Melting range (217–220 °C), Specific rotation (−33.0° to −35.5°), Acidity or alkalinity, Loss on drying (not more than 0.5%), Residue on ignition (not more than 0.1%), Sulfate, Ordinary impurities, and Organic volatile impurities.

Ephedrine Sulfate USP—Preserve in well-closed, light-resistant containers. Contains not less than 98.0% and not more than 101.0% of ephedrine sulfate, calculated on the dried basis. Meets the requirements for Identification, Specific rotation (−30.5° to −32.5°), Acidity or alkalinity, Loss on drying (not more than 0.5%), Residue on ignition (not more than 0.1%), Chloride (not more than 0.14%), Ordinary impurities, and Organic volatile impurities.

Ephedrine Sulfate Capsules USP—Preserve in tight, light-resistant containers. Contain the labeled amount, within ± 8%. Meet the requirements for Identification, Dissolution (80% in 30 minutes in water in Apparatus 1 at 100 rpm), and Uniformity of dosage units.

Ephedrine Sulfate Injection USP—Preserve in single-dose or in multiple-dose, light-resistant containers, preferably of Type I glass. A sterile solution of Ephedrine Sulfate in Water for Injection. Contains the labeled amount, within ±5%. Meets the requirements for Identification, Bacterial endotoxins, and pH (4.5–7.0), and for Injections.

Ephedrine Sulfate Nasal Solution USP—Preserve in tight, light-resistant containers. Contains the labeled amount, within ±7%. Meets the requirements for Identification and Microbial limits.

Ephedrine Sulfate Oral Solution USP—Preserve in tight, light-resistant containers, and avoid exposure to excessive heat. Contains, in each 100 mL, not less than 360 mg and not more than 440 mg of ephedrine sulfate. Meets the requirements for Identification and Alcohol content (2.0–4.0%).

Ephedrine Sulfate Syrup USP—Preserve in tight, light-resistant containers, and avoid exposure to excessive heat. Contains, in each 100 mL, not less than 360 mg and not more than 440 mg of ephedrine sulfate. Meets the requirements for Identification and Alcohol content (2.0–4.0%).

Ephedrine Sulfate Tablets USP—Preserve in well-closed containers. Contain the labeled amount, within ±7%. Meet the requirements for Identification, Dissolution (75% in 45 minutes in water in Apparatus 2 at 50 rpm), and Uniformity of dosage units.

EPHEDRINE, CARBETAPENTANE, AND GUAIFENESIN

Chemical name:
Ephedrine hydrochloride—Benzenemethanol, alpha-[1-(methylamino)ethyl]-, hydrochloride, [R-(R*,[hm.1]S*)]-.
Carbetapentane citrate—2-[2-(Diethylamino)ethoxy]ethyl 1-phenylcyclopentanecarboxylate citrate (1:).
Guaifenesin—1,2-Propanediol, 3-(2-methoxyphenoxy)-.

Molecular formula:
Ephedrine hydrochloride—$C_{10}H_{15}NO \cdot HCl$.
Carbetapentane citrate—$C_{20}H_{31}NO_3 \cdot C_6H_8O_7$.
Guaifenesin—$C_{10}H_{14}O_4$.

Molecular weight:
Ephedrine hydrochloride—201.69.
Carbetapentane citrate—525.59.
Guaifenesin—198.22.

Description:
Ephedrine Hydrochloride USP—Fine, white, odorless crystals or powder. Is affected by light.
Carbetapentane citrate—Crystals with a melting point of 93 °C.

Guaifenesin USP—White to slightly gray, crystalline powder. May have a slight characteristic odor.

Solubility:
Ephedrine Hydrochloride USP—Freely soluble in water; soluble in alcohol; insoluble in ether.
Carbetapentane citrate—Freely soluble in water and in chloroform; soluble in alcohol, in acetone, and in ethyl acetate; practically insoluble in ether, in petroleum ether, and in benzene.
Guaifenesin USP—Soluble in water, in alcohol, in chloroform, and in propylene glycol; sparingly soluble in glycerin.

USP requirements: Ephedrine Hydrochloride, Carbetapentane Citrate, and Guaifenesin Syrup—Not in *USP–NF*.

EPHEDRINE AND GUAIFENESIN

For *Ephedrine* and *Guaifenesin*—See individual listings for chemistry information.

USP requirements: Ephedrine Hydrochloride and Guaifenesin Syrup—Not in *USP–NF*.

EPHEDRINE AND PHENOBARBITAL

For *Ephedrine* and *Phenobarbital*—See individual listings for chemistry information.

USP requirements: Ephedrine Sulfate and Phenobarbital Capsules USP—Preserve in well-closed containers. Contain the labeled amounts, within ±9%. Meet the requirements for Identification, Dissolution (75% of each active ingredient in 45 minutes in water in Apparatus 1 at 100 rpm), and Uniformity of dosage units.

EPHEDRINE AND POTASSIUM IODIDE

For *Ephedrine* and *Potassium Iodide*—See individual listings for chemistry information.

USP requirements: Ephedrine Hydrochloride and Potassium Iodide Syrup—Not in *USP–NF*.

EPINEPHRINE

Chemical name:
Epinephrine—1,2-Benzenediol, 4-[1-hydroxy-2-(methylamino)ethyl]-, (R)-.
Epinephrine bitartrate—1,2-Benzenediol, 4-[1-hydroxy-2-(methylamino)ethyl]-, (R)-, [R-(R*,R*)]-2,3-dihydroxybutanedioate (1:1) (salt).

Molecular formula:
Epinephrine—$C_9H_{13}NO_3$.
Epinephrine bitartrate—$C_9H_{13}NO_3 \cdot C_4H_6O_6$.

Molecular weight:
Epinephrine—183.20.
Epinephrine bitartrate—333.29.

Description:
Epinephrine USP—White to practically white, odorless, microcrystalline powder or granules, gradually darkening on exposure to light and air. With acids, it forms salts that are

readily soluble in water, and the base may be recovered by the addition of ammonia water or alkali carbonates. Its solutions are alkaline to litmus.

Epinephrine Injection USP—Practically colorless, slightly acid liquid. Gradually turns dark on exposure to light and to air.

Epinephrine Inhalation Solution USP—Practically colorless, slightly acid liquid. Gradually turns dark on exposure to light and air.

Epinephrine Nasal Solution USP—Nearly colorless, slightly acid liquid. Gradually turns dark on exposure to light and air.

Epinephrine Ophthalmic Solution USP—Colorless to faint yellow solution. Gradually turns dark on exposure to light and air.

Epinephrine Bitartrate USP—White, or grayish white or light brownish gray, odorless, crystalline powder. Slowly darkens on exposure to air and light. Its solutions are acid to litmus, having a pH of about 3.5.

Epinephrine Bitartrate for Ophthalmic Solution USP—White to off-white solid.

Solubility:

Epinephrine USP—Very slightly soluble in water and in alcohol; insoluble in ether, in chloroform, and in fixed and volatile oils.

Epinephrine Bitartrate USP—Freely soluble in water; slightly soluble in alcohol; practically insoluble in chloroform and in ether.

USP requirements:

Epinephrine USP—Preserve in tight, light-resistant containers. Contains not less than 97.0% and not more than 100.5% of epinephrine, calculated on the dried basis. Meets the requirements for Identification, Specific rotation (−50.0° to −53.5°), Loss on drying (not more than 2.0%), Residue on ignition (negligible, from 100 mg), Limit of adrenalone, and Limit of norepinephrine (not more than 4.0%).

Epinephrine Inhalation Aerosol USP—Preserve in small, nonreactive, light-resistant aerosol containers equipped with metered-dose valves and provided with oral inhalation actuators. A solution of Epinephrine in propellants and Alcohol prepared with the aid of mineral acid in a pressurized container. Contains the labeled amount, within −10% to +15%. Meets the requirements for Identification and Dose uniformity over the entire contents.

Epinephrine Injection USP—Preserve in single-dose or in multiple-dose, light-resistant containers, preferably of Type I glass. A sterile solution of Epinephrine in Water for Injection prepared with the aid of Hydrochloric acid or other suitable buffers. The label indicates that the Injection is not to be used if its color is pinkish or darker than slightly yellow or if it contains a precipitate. Contains the labeled amount, within −10% to +15%. Meets the requirements for Color and clarity, Identification, Bacterial endotoxins, pH (2.2–5.0), and Total acidity, and for Injections.

Epinephrine Inhalation Solution USP—Preserve in small, well-filled, tight, light-resistant containers. A sterile solution of Epinephrine in Purified Water prepared with the aid of Hydrochloric Acid. The label indicates that the Inhalation Solution is not to be used if its color is pinkish or darker than slightly yellow or if it contains a precipitate. Contains, in each 100 mL, not less than 0.9 gram and not more than 1.15 grams of epinephrine. Meets the requirements for Sterility, Color and clarity, and Identification.

Epinephrine Nasal Solution USP—Preserve in small, well-filled, tight, light-resistant containers. A solution of Epinephrine in Purified Water prepared with the aid of Hydrochloric Acid. The label indicates that the Nasal Solution is not to be used if its color is pinkish or darker than slightly yellow or if it contains a precipitate. Contains, in each 100 mL, not less than 90 mg and not more than 115 mg of epinephrine. Meets the requirements for Color and clarity and Identification.

Epinephrine Ophthalmic Solution USP—Preserve in tight, light-resistant containers. A sterile, aqueous solution of Epinephrine prepared with the aid of Hydrochloric Acid. The label indicates that the Ophthalmic Solution is not to be used if its color is pinkish or darker than slightly yellow or if it contains a precipitate. Contains the labeled amount, within −10% to +15%. Contains a suitable antibacterial agent. Meets the requirements for Color and clarity, Identification, Sterility, and pH (2.2–4.5).

Sterile Epinephrine Suspension—Not in *USP–NF*.

Epinephrine Injectable Oil Suspension USP—Preserve in single-dose, light-resistant containers, preferably of Type I or Type III glass. A sterile suspension of Epinephrine in a suitable vegetable oil. Contains, in each mL, not less than 1.8 mg and not more than 2.4 mg of epinephrine. Meets the requirement for Injections.

Epinephrine Bitartrate USP—Preserve in tight, light-resistant containers. Contains not less than 97.0% and not more than 102.0% of epinephrine bitartrate, calculated on the dried basis. Meets the requirements for Identification, Melting range (147–152 °C, with decomposition), Loss on drying (not more than 0.5%), Residue on ignition (negligible, from 100 mg), Limit of adrenalone, and Limit of norepinephrine bitartrate (not more than 4.0%).

Epinephrine Bitartrate Inhalation Aerosol USP—Preserve in small, nonreactive, light-resistant aerosol containers equipped with metered-dose valves and provided with oral inhalation actuators. A suspension of microfine Epinephrine Bitartrate in propellants in a pressurized container. Contains the labeled amount, within ±10%. Meets the requirements for Identification, Dose uniformity over the entire contents, and Particle size.

Epinephrine Bitartrate Ophthalmic Solution USP—Preserve in small, well-filled, tight, light-resistant containers. A sterile, buffered, aqueous solution of Epinephrine Bitartrate. The label indicates that the Ophthalmic Solution is not to be used if its color is pinkish or darker than slightly yellow or if it contains a precipitate. Contains an amount of epinephrine bitartrate equivalent to the labeled amount of epinephrine, within −10% to +15%. Contains a suitable antibacterial agent. Meets the requirements for Color and clarity and pH (3.0–3.8), for Identification test for Epinephrine Nasal Solution, and for Sterility tests.

Epinephrine Bitartrate for Ophthalmic Solution USP—Preserve in Containers for Sterile Solids. A sterile, dry mixture of Epinephrine Bitartrate and suitable antioxidants, prepared by freeze-drying. Contains an amount of epinephrine bitartrate equivalent to the labeled amount of epinephrine, within ±10%. Meets the requirements for Completeness of solution and Constituted solution, for Identification test under Epinephrine Nasal Solution, and for Sterility tests and Uniformity of dosage units.

Epinephrine Hydrochloride Injection—Not in *USP–NF*.

EPINEPHRYL BORATE

Chemical name: 1,3,2-Benzodioxaborole-5-methanol, 2-hydroxy-alpha-[(methylamino)methyl]-, (*R*)-.

Molecular formula: $C_9H_{12}BNO_4$.

Molecular weight: 209.01.

Description: Epinephryl Borate Ophthalmic Solution USP—Clear, pale yellow liquid, gradually darkening on exposure to light and to air.

USP requirements: Epinephryl Borate Ophthalmic Solution USP—Preserve in small, well-filled, tight, light-resistant containers. A sterile solution in water of Epinephrine as a borate complex. The label indicates that the Ophthalmic Solution is not to be used if its color is pinkish or darker than slightly yellow or if it contains a precipitate. Contains an amount of epine-

phryl borate equivalent to the labeled amount of epinephrine, within −10% to +15%. Contains a suitable antibacterial agent and one or more suitable preservatives and buffering agents. Meets the requirements for Color and clarity, Identification, Sterility, and pH (5.5–7.6).

EPIRUBICIN

Chemical name: Epirubicin hydrochloride—5,12-Naphthacene-dione, 10-[(3-amino-2,3,6-trideoxy-alpha-L-*arabino*-hexopyranosyl)oxy]-7,8,9,10-tetrahydro-6,8,11-trihydroxy-8-(hydroxyacetyl)-1-methoxy-, hydrochloride, (8S-*cis*)-.

Molecular formula: Epirubicin hydrochloride—$C_{27}H_{29}NO_{11} \cdot HCl$.

Molecular weight: Epirubicin hydrochloride—579.98.

Description: Epirubicin hydrochloride—Red-orange crystals with a melting point of 185 °C.

USP requirements:
Epirubicin Hydrochloride Injection—Not in *USP–NF*.
Epirubicin Hydrochloride for Injection—Not in *USP–NF*.

EPITETRACYCLINE

Chemical name: Epitetracycline hydrochloride—2-Naphthacene-carboxamide, 4-(dimethylamino)-1,4,4a,5,5a,6,11,12a-octahydro-3,6,10,12,12a-pentahydroxy-6-methyl-1,11-dioxo-, monohydrochloride, [4R-(4 alpha,4a beta,5a beta,6 alpha,12a beta)]-.

Molecular formula: Epitetracycline hydrochloride—$C_{22}H_{24}N_2O_8 \cdot HCl$.

Molecular weight: Epitetracycline hydrochloride—480.90.

USP requirements: Epitetracycline Hydrochloride USP—Preserve in tight, light-resistant containers. Contains not less than 70.0% of epitetracycline hydrochloride. Meets the requirements for pH (2.3–4.0, in a solution containing 10 mg per mL), Loss on drying (not more than 6.0%), and 4-Epianhydrotetracycline (not more than 2.0%).

EPLERENONE

Chemical name: Pregn-4-ene-7,21-dicarboxylic acid, 9,11-epoxy-17-hydroxy-3-oxo-, lambda-lactone, methyl ester, (7 alpha, 11 alpha, 17 alpha)-.

Molecular formula: $C_{24}C_{30}D_6$.

Molecular weight: 414.49.

Description: Odorless, white to off-white crystalline powder.

Solubility: Very slightly soluble in water, with its solubility essentially pH independent.

Other requirements: The Octanol/water partition coefficient of eplerenone is approximately 7.1 at pH 7.0.

USP requirements: Eplerenone Tablets—Not in *USP–NF*.

EPOETIN ALFA

Chemical name: 1-165-Erythropoietin (human clone lambdaHEPOFL13 protein moiety), glycoform alpha.

Molecular formula: $C_{809}H_{1301}N_{229}O_{240}S_5$ (amino acid sequence).

Molecular weight: 18,235.72.

USP requirements: Epoetin Alfa, Recombinant, Injection—Not in *USP–NF*.

EPOPROSTENOL

Chemical group: Prostaglandin.

Chemical name: Epoprostenol sodium—Prosta-5,13-dien-1-oic acid, 6,9-epoxy-11,15-dihydroxy-, sodium salt, (5Z,9 alpha,11 alpha,13E,15S)-.

Molecular formula: Epoprostenol sodium—$C_{20}H_{31}NaO_5$.

Molecular weight: Epoprostenol sodium—374.47.

Description: Epoprostenol sodium—White to off-white powder. Has a pH of 10.2–10.8.

USP requirements: Epoprostenol Sodium for Injection—Not in *USP–NF*.

EPROSARTAN

Chemical name:
Eprosartan—2-Thiophenepropanoic acid, alpha-[[2-butyl-1-[(4-carboxyphenyl)-1H-imidazol-5-yl]methylene]-, (E)-.
Eprosartan mesylate—2-Thiophenepropanoic acid, alpha-[[2-butyl-1-[(4-carboxyphenyl)methyl]-1H-imidazol-5-yl]methylene]-, (E)-, monomethanesulfonate..

Molecular formula:
Eprosartan—$C_{23}H_{24}N_2O_4S$.
Eprosartan mesylate—$C_{23}H_{24}N_2O_4S \cdot CH_4O_3S$.

Molecular weight:
Eprosartan—424.51.
Eprosartan mesylate—520.62.

Description:
Eprosartan—Crystals. Melting point 260–261°.
Eprosartan mesylate—White to off-white free-flowing crystalline powder. Melts between 248–250 °C.

Solubility: Eprosartan mesylate—Insoluble in water; freely soluble in ethanol.

USP requirements: Eprosartan Tablets—Not in *USP–NF*.

EPTIFIBATIDE

Chemical name: N^6-(aminoiminomethyl)-N^2-(3-mercapto-1-oxopropyl-L-lysylglycyl-L-alpha-aspartyl-L-tryptophyl-L-prolyl-L-cysteinamide, cyclic (1→6)-disulfide.

Molecular formula: $C_{35}H_{49}N_{11}O_9S_2$.

Molecular weight: 831.96.

Description: A clear, colorless, sterile, nonpyrogenic solution.

USP requirements: Eptifibatide Injection—Not in *USP–NF*.

EQUILIN

Chemical name: Estra-1,3,5(10),7-tetraen-17-one, 3-hydroxy-.

Molecular formula: $C_{18}H_{20}O_2$.

Molecular weight: 268.35.

Description: Melting point 238–240 °C.

Solubility: Soluble in alcohol, in dioxane, in acetone, in ethyl acetate, and in other organic solvents; sparingly soluble in water.

USP requirements: Equilin USP—Preserve in tight, light-resistant containers. Contains not less than 97.0% and not more than 103.0% of equilin, calculated on the dried basis. Meets the requirements for Identification, Specific rotation (+300° to +316°), Loss on drying (not more than 0.5%), and Residue on ignition (not more than 0.5%).

ERGOCALCIFEROL

Chemical name: 9,10-Secoergosta-5,7,10(19),22-tetraen-3-ol, (3 beta,5*Z*,7*E*,22*E*)-.

Molecular formula: $C_{28}H_{44}O$.

Molecular weight: 396.65.

Description:
Ergocalciferol USP—White, odorless crystals. Is affected by air and light.
Ergocalciferol Oral Solution USP—Clear liquid having the characteristics of the solvent used in preparing the Solution.

Solubility: Ergocalciferol USP—Insoluble in water; soluble in alcohol, in chloroform, in ether, and in fatty oils.

USP requirements:
Ergocalciferol USP—Preserve in hermetically sealed containers under nitrogen, in a cool place and protected from light. Contains not less than 97.0% and not more than 103.0% of ergocalciferol. Meets the requirements for Identification, Melting range (115–119 °C), Specific rotation (+103° to +106°), Reducing substances, and Organic volatile impurities.
Ergocalciferol Capsules USP—Preserve in tight, light-resistant containers. Usually consist of an edible vegetable oil solution of Ergocalciferol, encapsulated with Gelatin. Label the Capsules to indicate the content of ergocalciferol in mg. The activity may be expressed also in terms of USP Units, on the basis that 40 USP Vitamin D Units = 1 mcg. Contain the labeled amount, within +20%. Meet the requirements for Disintegration (45 minutes) and Uniformity of dosage units.
Ergocalciferol Injection—Not in *USP–NF*.
Ergocalciferol Oral Solution USP—Preserve in tight, light-resistant containers. A solution of Ergocalciferol in an edible vegetable oil, in Polysorbate 80, or in Propylene Glycol. Label the Oral Solution to indicate the concentration of ergocalciferol in mg. The activity may be expressed also in terms of USP Units, on the basis that 40 USP Vitamin D Units = 1 mcg. Contains the labeled amount, within +20%.
Ergocalciferol Tablets USP—Preserve in tight, light-resistant containers. Label the Tablets to indicate the content of ergocalciferol in mg. The activity may be expressed also in terms of USP Units, on the basis that 40 USP Vitamin D Units = 1 mcg. Contain the labeled amount, within +20%. Meet the requirements for Identification, Disintegration (30 minutes), and Uniformity of dosage units.

ERGOLOID MESYLATES

Chemical name: Ergotaman-3',6',18-trione, 9,10-dihydro-12'-hydroxy-2',5'-bis(1-methylethyl)-, (5' alpha,10 alpha)-, monomethanesulfonate (salt) mixture with 9,10 alpha-dihydro-12'-hydroxy-2'-(1-methylethyl)-5'alpha-(phenylmethyl)ergotaman-3',6',18-trione monomethanesulfonate (salt), 9,10 alpha-dihydro-12'-hydroxy-2'-(1-methylethyl)-5'alpha-(2methylpropyl)ergotaman-3',6;'',18-trione monomethanesulfonate (salt), and 9,10 alpha-dihydro-12'-hydroxy-2'(1-methylethyl)-5'alpha-(1-methylpropyl)ergotaman-3',6',18-trione monomethanesulfonate (salt).

Molecular formula:
Dihydroergocornine mesylate—$C_{31}H_{41}N_5O_5 \cdot CH_4O_3S$.
Dihydroergocristine mesylate—$C_{35}H_{41}N_5O_5 \cdot CH_4O_3S$.
Dihydro-alpha-ergocryptine mesylate—$C_{32}H_{43}N_5O_5 \cdot CH_4O_3S$.
Dihydro-beta-ergocryptine mesylate—$C_{32}H_{43}N_5O_5 \cdot CH_4O_3S$.

Molecular weight:
Dihydroergocornine mesylate—659.79.
Dihydroergocristine mesylate—707.84.
Dihydro-alpha-ergocryptine mesylate—673.82.
Dihydro-beta-ergocryptine mesylate—673.82.

Description: Ergoloid Mesylates USP—White to off-white, microcrystalline or amorphous, practically odorless powder.

Solubility: Ergoloid Mesylates USP—Slightly soluble in water; soluble in methanol and in alcohol; sparingly soluble in acetone.

USP requirements:
Ergoloid Mesylates USP—Preserve in tight, light-resistant containers. A mixture of the methanesulfonate salts of the three hydrogenated alkaloids, dihydroergocristine, dihydroergocornine, and dihydroergocryptine, in an approximate weight ratio of 1:1:1. Contains not less than 97.0% and not more than 103.0% of the alkaloid methanesulfonate mixture, calculated on the anhydrous basis, and not less than 30.3% and not more than 36.3% of the methanesulfonate salt of each of the individual alkaloids. Dihydroergocryptine mesylate exists as a mixture of *alpha*- and *beta*- isomers. The ratio of *alpha*- to *beta*-isomers is not less than 1.5:1.0 and not more than 2.5:1.0. Meets the requirements for Identification, Specific rotation (+11.0° to +15.0°), pH (4.2–5.2, in a solution [1 in 200]), Water (not more than 5.0%), Limit of ergotamine, and Limit of non-hydrogenated alkaloids.
Ergoloid Mesylates Capsules USP—Preserve in tight, light-resistant containers between 15 and 25 °C. Do not freeze. Contain the labeled amount, within ±10%, consisting of not less than 30.3% and not more than 36.3% of the methane-sulfonate salt of each of the individual alkaloids (dihydroergocristine, dihydroergocornine, and dihydroergocryptine). The ratio of *alpha*- to *beta*-dihydroergocryptine mesylate is not less than 1.5:1.0 and not more than 2.5:1.0. Meet the requirements for Identification, Microbial limits, Dissolution (15 minutes in water in Apparatus 2 at 50 rpm), and Uniformity of dosage units.
Ergoloid Mesylates Oral Solution USP—Preserve in tight, light-resistant containers at a temperature not exceeding 30 °C. Contains the labeled amount, within ±10%, consisting of not less than 30.3% and not more than 36.3% of the methanesulfonate salt of each of the individual alkaloids (dihydroergocristine, dihydroergocornine, and dihydroergocryptine); the ratio of *alpha*- to *beta*-dihydroergocryptine mesylate is not less than 1.5:1.0 and not more than 2.5:1.0. Meets the requirements for Identification and Alcohol content (within ±10% of the labeled amount).
Ergoloid Mesylates Tablets USP—Preserve in tight, light-resistant containers. Label Tablets to indicate whether they are intended for sublingual administration or for swallowing. Contain the labeled amount, within ±10%, consisting of not less than 30.3% and not more than 36.3% of the methanesulfonate salt of each of the individual alkaloids (dihydroergocristine, dihydroergocornine, and dihydroer-

gocryptine); the ratio of *alpha-* to *beta*-dihydroergocryptine mesylate is not less than 1.5:1.0 and not more than 2.5:1.0. Meet the requirements for Identification, Disintegration (15 minutes, for Tablets intended for sublingual use), Dissolution (75% in 30 minutes in water in Apparatus 2 at 50 rpm, for Tablets intended to be swallowed), and Uniformity of dosage units.

ERGONOVINE

Chemical group: Ergot alkaloid.

Chemical name: Ergonovine maleate—Ergoline-8-carboxamide, 9,10-didehydro-*N*-(2-hydroxy-1-methylethyl)-6-methyl-, [8 beta(*S*)]-, (*Z*)-2-butenedioate (1:1) (salt).

Molecular formula: Ergonovine maleate—$C_{19}H_{23}N_3O_2 \cdot C_4H_4O_4$.

Molecular weight: Ergonovine maleate—441.48.

Description: Ergonovine Maleate USP—White to grayish white or faintly yellow, odorless, microcrystalline powder. Darkens with age and on exposure to light.

Solubility: Ergonovine Maleate USP—Sparingly soluble in water; slightly soluble in alcohol; insoluble in ether and in chloroform.

USP requirements:
Ergonovine Maleate USP—Preserve in tight, light-resistant containers, in a cold place. Contains not less than 97.0% and not more than 103.0% of ergonovine maleate, calculated on the dried basis. Meets the requirements for Identification, Specific rotation (+51° to +56°), Loss on drying (not more than 2.0%), and Related alkaloids.
Ergonovine Maleate Injection USP—Preserve in single-dose, light-resistant containers, preferably of Type I glass, and store in a cold place. A sterile solution of Ergonovine Maleate in Water for Injection. Contains the labeled amount, within ±10%. Meets the requirements for Identification, Bacterial endotoxins, pH (2.7–3.5), and Related alkaloids, and for Injections.
Ergonovine Maleate Tablets USP—Preserve in well-closed containers. Contain the labeled amount, within ±10%. Meet the requirements for Identification, Dissolution (75% in 45 minutes in water in Apparatus 1 at 100 rpm), Uniformity of dosage units, and Related alkaloids.

ERGOTAMINE

Chemical name: Ergotamine tartrate—Ergotaman-3',6',18-trione, 12'-hydroxy-2'-methyl-5'-(phenylmethyl)-, (5' alpha)-, [*R*-(*R**,*R**)]-2,3-dihydroxybutanedioate (2:1) (salt).

Molecular formula: Ergotamine tartrate—$(C_{33}H_{35}N_5O_5)_2 \cdot C_4H_6O_6$.

Molecular weight: Ergotamine tartrate—1313.41.

Description: Ergotamine Tartrate USP—Colorless crystals or white to yellowish white, crystalline powder. Is odorless. Melts at about 180 °C, with decomposition.

Solubility: Ergotamine Tartrate USP—One gram dissolves in about 3200 mL of water; in the presence of a slight excess of tartaric acid, 1 gram dissolves in about 500 mL of water. Slightly soluble in alcohol.

USP requirements:
Ergotamine Tartrate USP—Preserve in well-closed, light-resistant containers in a cold place. Contains not less than 97.0% and not more than 100.5% of ergotamine tartrate, calculated on the dried basis. Meets the requirements for

Identification, Specific rotation of ergotamine base (−155° to −165°), Loss on drying (not more than 5.0%), and Related alkaloids.
Ergotamine Tartrate Inhalation Aerosol USP—Preserve in small, non-reactive, light-resistant aerosol containers equipped with metered-dose valves and provided with oral inhalation actuators. A suspension of microfine Ergotamine Tartrate in propellants in a pressurized container. Contains the labeled amount, within ±10%. Meets the requirements for Identification, Dose uniformity over the entire contents, and Particle size.
Ergotamine Tartrate Injection USP—Preserve in single-dose, light-resistant containers, preferably of Type I glass. A sterile solution of Ergotamine Tartrate and the tartrates of its epimer, ergotaminine, and of other related alkaloids, in Water for Injection to which Tartaric Acid or suitable stabilizers have been added. The total alkaloid content, in each mL, is not less than 450 mcg and not more than 550 mcg. The content of ergotamine tartrate is not less than 52.0% and not more than 74.0% of the content of total alkaloid; the content of ergotaminine tartrate is not more than 45.0% of the content of total alkaloid. Meets the requirements for Bacterial endotoxins and pH (3.5–4.0) and for Injections.
Ergotamine Tartrate Tablets USP—Preserve in well-closed, light-resistant containers. Label Tablets to indicate whether they are intended for sublingual administration or for swallowing. Contain the labeled amount, within ±10%. Meet the requirements for Identification, Disintegration (5 minutes, for Tablets intended for sublingual use), Dissolution (75% in 30 minutes in tartaric acid solution [1 in 100] in Apparatus 2 at 75 rpm, for Tablets intended to be swallowed), and Uniformity of dosage units.

ERGOTAMINE, BELLADONNA ALKALOIDS, AND PHENOBARBITAL

For *Ergotamine, Belladonna Alkaloids* (Atropine, Belladonna, Hyoscyamine, and Scopolamine), and *Phenobarbital*—See individual listings for chemistry information.

USP requirements:
Ergotamine Tartrate, Belladonna Alkaloids, and Phenobarbital Sodium Tablets—Not in *USP–NF*.
Ergotamine Tartrate, Belladonna Alkaloids, and Phenobarbital Sodium Extended-release Tablets—Not in *USP–NF*.

ERGOTAMINE AND CAFFEINE

For *Ergotamine* and *Caffeine*—See individual listings for chemistry information.

USP requirements:
Ergotamine Tartrate and Caffeine Suppositories USP—Preserve in tight containers, at a temperature not above 25 °C. Do not expose unwrapped Suppositories to sunlight. Contain the labeled amounts, within ±10%. Meet the requirement for Identification.
Ergotamine Tartrate and Caffeine Tablets USP—Preserve in well-closed, light-resistant containers. Contain the labeled amounts, within ±10%. Meet the requirements for Identification, Dissolution (70% of ergotamine tartrate and 75% of caffeine in 30 minutes in tartaric acid solution [1 in 100] in Apparatus 2 at 75 rpm), and Uniformity of dosage units.

ERGOTAMINE, CAFFEINE, AND BELLADONNA ALKALOIDS

For *Ergotamine, Caffeine,* and *Belladonna Alkaloids* (Atropine, Belladonna, Hyoscyamine, and Scopolamine)—See individual listings for chemistry information.

USP requirements:
Ergotamine Tartrate, Caffeine, and Belladonna Alkaloids Suppositories—Not in *USP–NF.*
Ergotamine Tartrate, Caffeine, and Belladonna Alkaloids Tablets—Not in *USP–NF.*

ERGOTAMINE, CAFFEINE, BELLADONNA ALKALOIDS, AND PENTOBARBITAL

For *Ergotamine, Caffeine, Belladonna Alkaloids* (Anisotropine, Atropine, Belladonna, Hyoscyamine, Methscopolamine, and Scopolamine), and *Pentobarbital*—See individual listings for chemistry information.

USP requirements:
Ergotamine Tartrate, Caffeine, Belladonna Alkaloids, and Pentobarbital Suppositories—Not in *USP–NF.*
Ergotamine Tartrate, Caffeine, Belladonna Alkaloids, and Pentobarbital Sodium Tablets—Not in *USP–NF.*

ERGOTAMINE, CAFFEINE, AND CYCLIZINE

For *Ergotamine, Caffeine,* and *Cyclizine*—See individual listings for chemistry information.

USP requirements: Ergotamine Tartrate, Caffeine, and Cyclizine Hydrochloride Tablets—Not in *USP–NF.*

ERGOTAMINE, CAFFEINE, AND DIMENHYDRINATE

For *Ergotamine, Caffeine,* and *Dimenhydrinate*—See individual listings for chemistry information.

USP requirements: Ergotamine Tartrate, Caffeine, and Dimenhydrinate Capsules—Not in *USP–NF.*

ERGOTAMINE, CAFFEINE, AND DIPHENHYDRAMINE

For *Ergotamine, Caffeine,* and *Diphenhydramine*—See individual listings for chemistry information.

USP requirements: Ergotamine Tartrate, Caffeine, and Diphenhydramine Hydrochloride Capsules—Not in *USP–NF.*

ERTAPENEM

Chemical group: Ertapenem sodium—Carbapenem antibiotics; chemically similar to beta-lactam antibiotics.

Chemical name: Ertapenem sodium—1-Azabicyclo[3.2.0]hept-2-ene-2-carboxylic acd, 3-[[5-[[(3-carboxyphenyl)amino]carbonyl]-3-pyrrolidinyl]thio]-6-(1-hydroxyethyl)-4-methyl-7-oxo-, monosodium salt, [4R-[3(3S,5S), 4 alpha,5 beta,6 beta(R)]]-.

Molecular formula: Ertapenem sodium—$C_{22}N_{24}N_3NaO_7S$.

Molecular weight: Ertapenem sodium—497.50.

Description: Ertapenem sodium—White to off-white hygroscopic, weakly crystalline powder.

Solubility: Ertapenem sodium—Soluble in water and in 0.9% sodium chloride solution; practically insoluble in ethanol; insoluble in isopropyl acetate and in tetrahydrofuran.

Other requirements: Ertapenem sodium—pH: 7.5.

USP requirements: Ertapenem Sodium for Injection—Not in *USP–NF.*

ERYTHRITYL TETRANITRATE

Chemical name: 1,2,3,4-Butanetetrol, tetranitrate, (R^*, S^*)-.

Molecular formula: $C_4H_6N_4O_{12}$.

Molecular weight: 302.11.

Description: Diluted Erythrityl Tetranitrate USP—White powder, having a slight odor of nitric oxides.

Solubility: Undiluted erythrityl tetranitrate—Practically insoluble in water; soluble in acetone, in acetonitrile, and in alcohol.

USP requirements:
Diluted Erythrityl Tetranitrate USP—Preserve in tight containers, and avoid exposure to excessive heat. A dry mixture of erythrityl tetranitrate with lactose or other suitable inert excipients to permit safe handling and compliance with U.S. Interstate Commerce Commission regulations pertaining to interstate shipment. Contains not less than 90.0% and not more than 110.0% of labeled amount of erythrityl tetranitrate. Meets the requirements for Identification and Organic volatile impurities.

Caution: Undiluted erythrityl tetranitrate is a powerful explosive, and proper precautions must be taken in handling. It can be exploded by percussion or by excessive heat. Only extremely small amounts should be isolated.

Erythrityl Tetranitrate Tablets USP—Preserve in tight containers, and avoid exposure to excessive heat. Erythrityl Tetranitrate Tablets are prepared from Diluted Erythrityl Tetranitrate. Contain the labeled amount of erythrityl tetranitrate, within ±10%. Meet the requirements for Identification, Disintegration (10 minutes, determined without the use of disks), and Uniformity of dosage units.

Caution: Undiluted erythrityl tetranitrate is a powerful explosive, and proper precautions must be taken in handling. It can be exploded by percussion or by excessive heat. Only extremely small amounts should be isolated.

ERYTHROMYCIN

Source: Produced by a strain of *Streptomyces erythraeus.*

Chemical group: Macrolide group of antibiotics.

Chemical name:
Erythromycin—Erythromycin.
Erythromycin estolate—Erythromycin, 2′-propanoate, dodecyl sulfate (salt).
Erythromycin ethylsuccinate—Erythromycin 2′-(ethyl butanedioate).
Erythromycin gluceptate—Erythromycin monoglucoheptonate (salt).

Erythromycin lactobionate—Erythromycin mono(4-*O*-beta-D-galactopyranosyl-D-gluconate) (salt).

Erythromycin stearate—Erythromycin octadecanoate (salt).

Molecular formula:

Erythromycin—$C_{37}H_{67}NO_{13}$.

Erythromycin estolate—$C_{40}H_{71}NO_{14} \cdot C_{12}H_{26}O_4S$.

Erythromycin ethylsuccinate—$C_{43}H_{75}NO_{16}$.

Erythromycin gluceptate—$C_{37}H_{67}NO_{13} \cdot C_7H_{14}O_8$.

Erythromycin lactobionate—$C_{37}H_{67}NO_{13} \cdot C_{12}H_{22}O_{12}$.

Erythromycin stearate—$C_{37}H_{67}NO_{13} \cdot C_{18}H_{36}O_2$.

Molecular weight:

Erythromycin—733.94.

Erythromycin estolate—1056.39.

Erythromycin ethylsuccinate—862.05.

Erythromycin gluceptate—960.11.

Erythromycin lactobionate—1092.22.

Erythromycin stearate—1018.40.

Description:

Erythromycin USP—White or slightly yellow, crystalline powder. Is odorless or practically odorless.

Erythromycin Estolate USP—White, crystalline powder. Is odorless or practically odorless.

Erythromycin Ethylsuccinate USP—White or slightly yellow crystalline powder. Is odorless or practically odorless.

Sterile Erythromycin Gluceptate USP—White powder. Is odorless or practically odorless, and is slightly hygroscopic. Its solution (1 in 20) is neutral or slightly acid.

Erythromycin Lactobionate for Injection USP—White or slightly yellow crystals or powder, having a faint odor. Its solution (1 in 20) is neutral or slightly alkaline.

Erythromycin Stearate USP—White or slightly yellow crystals or powder. Is odorless or may have a slight, earthy odor.

Solubility:

Erythromycin USP—Slightly soluble in water; soluble in alcohol, in chloroform, and in ether.

Erythromycin Estolate USP—Soluble in alcohol, in acetone, and in chloroform; practically insoluble in water.

Erythromycin Ethylsuccinate USP—Very slightly soluble in water; freely soluble in alcohol, in chloroform, and in polyethylene glycol 400.

Sterile Erythromycin Gluceptate USP—Freely soluble in water, in alcohol, and in methanol; slightly soluble in acetone and in chloroform; practically insoluble in ether.

Erythromycin Lactobionate for Injection USP—Freely soluble in water, in alcohol, and in methanol; slightly soluble in acetone and in chloroform; practically insoluble in ether.

Erythromycin Stearate USP—Practically insoluble in water; soluble in alcohol, in chloroform, in methanol, and in ether.

USP requirements:

Erythromycin USP—Preserve in tight containers. Consists primarily of erythromycin A. The sum of the percentages of erythromycin A, erythromycin B, and erythromycin C is not less than 85.0% and not more than 100.5%, calculated on the anhydrous basis. Meets the requirements for Identification, Specific rotation (−71° to −78°), Crystallinity, Water (not more than 10.0%), Residue on ignition (not more than 0.2%), Limit of thiocyanate (not more than 0.3%), and Limit of related substances.

Erythromycin Delayed-release Capsules USP—Preserve in tight containers. Contain the labeled amount, within −10% to +15%. Meet the requirements for Identification, Drug release (Method B: 80% in 60 minutes for Acid stage and 60 minutes for Buffer stage in Apparatus 1 at 50 rpm), and Water (not more than 7.5%).

Erythromycin Topical Gel USP—Preserve in tight containers. It is Erythromycin in a suitable gel vehicle. Contains the labeled amount, within −10% to +25%. Meets the requirements for Identification and Minimum fill.

Erythromycin Intramammary Infusion USP—Preserve in single-dose disposable syringes that are well-closed containers. A solution of Erythromycin in a suitable vegetable oil vehicle. Contains one or more suitable preservatives. Label it to state that it is for veterinary use only. Contains the labeled amount, within −10% to +20%. Meets the requirements for Identification, Minimum fill, and Water (not more than 1.0%).

Erythromycin Injection USP—Preserve in multiple-dose containers. A sterile solution of Erythromycin in a polyethylene glycol vehicle. Label it to indicate that it is for veterinary use only. Label it to state that it is for intramuscular administration only. Contains the labeled amount, within −10% to +20%. Meets the requirements for Identification, Water (not more than 1.0%), and Sterility, and for Injections.

Erythromycin Ointment USP—Preserve in collapsible tubes or in other tight containers, preferably at controlled room temperature. It is Erythromycin in a suitable ointment base. Contains the labeled amount, within −10% to +25%. Meets the requirements for Identification, Minimum fill, and Water (not more than 1.0%).

Erythromycin Ophthalmic Ointment USP—Preserve in collapsible ophthalmic ointment tubes. A sterile preparation of Erythromycin in a suitable ointment base. Contains the labeled amount, within −10% to +20%. Meets the requirements for Identification, Sterility, Minimum fill, and Metal particles, and for Water under Erythromycin Ointment.

Erythromycin Pledgets USP—Preserve in tight containers. Suitable absorbent pads impregnated with Erythromycin Topical Solution. Label Pledgets to indicate that each Pledget is to be used once and then discarded. Label Pledgets also to indicate the volume, in mL, of Erythromycin Topical Solution contained in each Pledget, and the concentration, in mg of erythromycin per mL, of the Erythromycin Topical Solution. Contain the labeled volume of Erythromycin Topical Solution, within −10%. The Erythromycin Topical Solution expressed from Erythromycin Pledgets meets the requirements for Identification, Water, and Alcohol content under Erythromycin Topical Solution.

Erythromycin Topical Solution USP—Preserve in tight containers. A solution of Erythromycin in a suitable vehicle. Contains the labeled amount, within −10% to +25%. Meets the requirements for Identification, Water (not more than 8.0% [20 mg per mL]; not more than 5.0% [15 mg per mL]; or not more than 2.0% [acetone-containing solutions]), and Alcohol content (the labeled amount, within ±7.5%).

Erythromycin Tablets USP—Preserve in tight containers. Contain the labeled amount, within −10% to +20%. Meet the requirements for Identification, Dissolution (70% in 60 minutes in 0.05 *M* phosphate buffer [pH 6.8] in Apparatus 2 at 50 rpm), Uniformity of dosage units, and Loss on drying (not more than 5.0%).

Note: Tablets that are enteric-coated meet the requirements for Erythromycin Delayed-release Tablets.

Erythromycin Delayed-release Tablets USP—Preserve in tight containers. The label indicates that Erythromycin Delayed-release Tablets are enteric-coated. The labeling indicates the Drug Release Test with which the product complies. Contain the labeled amount, within −10% to +20%. Meet the requirements for Identification, Drug Release (Method B: 75% in 60 minutes for Acid stage and 60 minutes for Buffer stage in Apparatus 1 at 100 rpm for Test 1 and in Apparatus 2 at 75 rpm for Test 2), Uniformity of dosage units, and Water (not more than 6.0%).

Erythromycin Estolate USP—Preserve in tight containers. Has a potency equivalent to not less than 600 mcg of erythromycin per mg, calculated on the anhydrous basis. Meets the requirements for Identification, Crystallinity, Water (not more than 4.0%), and Free erythromycin.

Erythromycin Estolate Capsules USP—Preserve in tight containers. Contain an amount of erythromycin estolate equivalent to the labeled amount of erythromycin, within

−10% to +15%. Meet the requirements for Identification, Disintegration (30 minutes), Uniformity of dosage units, and Water (not more than 5.0%).

Erythromycin Estolate Oral Suspension USP—Preserve in tight containers, in a cool place. Contains one or more suitable buffers, colors, diluents, dispersants, and flavors. Contains an amount of erythromycin estolate equivalent to the labeled amount of erythromycin, within −10% to +15%. Meets the requirements for Identification, Uniformity of dosage units (single-unit containers), Deliverable volume, and pH (3.5–6.5).

Erythromycin Estolate for Oral Suspension USP—Preserve in tight containers. A dry mixture of Erythromycin Estolate with one or more suitable buffers, colors, diluents, dispersants, and flavors. Contains an amount of erythromycin estolate equivalent to the labeled amount of erythromycin, within −10% to +15%. Meets the requirements for Identification, Uniformity of dosage units (single-unit containers), Deliverable volume, pH (5.0–7.0 [if pediatric drops, between 5.0 and 5.5], in the suspension constituted as directed in the labeling), and Water (not more than 2.0%).

Erythromycin Estolate Tablets USP—Preserve in tight containers. Label Tablets to indicate whether they are to be chewed before swallowing. Contain an amount of erythromycin estolate equivalent to the labeled amount of erythromycin, within −10% to +20% (+15%, if chewable). Meet the requirements for Identification, Disintegration (30 minutes [Note: Chewable tablets are exempt from this requirement]), Uniformity of dosage units, and Water (not more than 5.0%; if chewable, not more than 4.0%).

Erythromycin Ethylsuccinate USP—Preserve in tight containers. Erythromycin Ethylsuccinate that is noncrystalline is labeled to indicate that it is amorphous. Any preparation containing the amorphous form of Erythromycin Ethylsuccinate is so labeled. Consists primarily of the 2′-ethylsuccinate ester of erythromycin A. Sum of erythromycin A, erythromycin B, and erythromycin C not less than 76.5%, calculated on the anhydrous basis. Meets the requirements for Identification, Crystallinity (except that when it is labeled as being in the amorphous state it does not meet the requirements), X-ray diffraction, Related compounds (not more than 3.0% of erythromycin *N*-ethylsuccinate), Water (not more than 3.0%), and Residue on ignition (not more than 1.0%).

Erythromycin Ethylsuccinate Injection USP—Preserve in single-dose or in multiple-dose containers, preferably of Type I glass. A sterile solution of Erythromycin Ethylsuccinate in Polyethylene Glycol 400, containing 2% of butyl aminobenzoate and a suitable preservative. Contains an amount of erythromycin ethylsuccinate equivalent to the labeled amount of erythromycin, within −10% to +15%. Meets the requirements for Sterility and Water (not more than 1.5%), and for Injections.

Erythromycin Ethylsuccinate Oral Suspension USP—Preserve in tight containers, and store in a cold place. A suspension of Erythromycin Ethylsuccinate containing one or more suitable buffers, colors, dispersants, flavors, and preservatives. Contains an amount of erythromycin ethylsuccinate equivalent to the labeled amount of erythromycin, within −10% to +20%. Meets the requirements for Identification, Uniformity of dosage units (single-unit containers), Deliverable volume, and pH (6.5–8.5).

Erythromycin Ethylsuccinate for Oral Suspension USP—Preserve in tight containers. A dry mixture of Erythromycin Ethylsuccinate with one or more suitable buffers, colors, diluents, dispersants, and flavors. Contains an amount of erythromycin ethylsuccinate equivalent to the labeled amount of erythromycin, within −10% to +20%. Meets the requirements for Identification, Uniformity of dosage units (single-unit containers), Deliverable volume, pH (7.0–9.0, in the suspension constituted as directed in the labeling), and Loss on drying (not more than 1.0%).

Erythromycin Ethylsuccinate Tablets USP—Preserve in tight containers. Label the chewable Tablets to indicate that they are to be chewed before swallowing. Contain an amount of erythromycin ethylsuccinate equivalent to the labeled amount of erythromycin, within −10% to +20%. Meet the requirements for Identification, Dissolution (75% in 45 minutes in 0.01 *N* hydrochloric acid in Apparatus 2 at 50 rpm for nonchewable tablets and 75% in 60 minutes in 0.1 *M* acetate buffer [pH 5.0] in Apparatus 2 at 75 rpm for Tablets labeled as chewable), Uniformity of dosage units, Loss on drying (not more than 4.0% [Note: Chewable Tablets are exempt from this requirement]), and Water (Chewable Tablets only, not more than 5.0%).

Sterile Erythromycin Ethylsuccinate USP—Preserve in Containers for Sterile Solids. It is Erythromycin Ethylsuccinate suitable for parenteral use. Has a potency equivalent to not less than 765 mcg of erythromycin per mg, calculated on the anhydrous basis. Meets the requirements for Sterility and Heavy metals (not more than 0.002%), and for Identification test, pH, Water, Residue on ignition, and Crystallinity under Erythromycin Ethylsuccinate.

Sterile Erythromycin Glucceptate USP—Preserve in Containers for Sterile Solids. It is Erythromycin Glucceptate suitable for parenteral use. Has a potency equivalent to not less than 600 mcg of erythromycin per mg, calculated on the anhydrous basis. In addition, where packaged for dispensing, contains an amount of erythromycin glucceptate equivalent to the labeled amount of erythromycin, within −10% to +15%. Meets the requirements for Identification, Bacterial endotoxins, Sterility, pH (6.0–8.0, in a solution containing 25 mg per mL), Water (not more than 5.0%), and Particulate matter, and, where packaged for dispensing, Uniformity of dosage units, Constituted solutions, and Labeling under Injections.

Erythromycin Lactobionate for Injection USP—Preserve in Containers for Sterile Solids. A sterile, dry mixture of erythromycin lactobionate and a suitable preservative. Contains an amount of erythromycin lactobionate equivalent to the labeled amount of erythromycin, within −10% to +20%. Meets the requirements for Constituted solution, Identification, Bacterial endotoxins, pH (6.5–7.5, in a solution containing the equivalent of 50 mg of erythromycin per mL), Water (not more than 5.0%), Particulate matter, and Heavy metals (not more than 0.005%), and for Injections.

Sterile Erythromycin Lactobionate USP—Preserve in Containers for Sterile Solids. Has a potency equivalent to not less than 525 mcg of erythromycin per mg, calculated on the anhydrous basis, and where packaged for dispensing, contains an amount of erythromycin lactobionate equivalent to the labeled amount of erythromycin, within −10% to +20%. Meets the requirements for Identification, Bacterial endotoxins, Sterility, pH (6.5–7.5, in a solution containing the equivalent of 50 mg of erythromycin per mL), Water (not more than 5.0%), Particulate matter, Residue on ignition (not more than 2.0%), and Heavy metals (not more than 0.005%), and where packaged for dispensing, for Uniformity of dosage units and for Constituted solutions and Labeling under Injections.

Erythromycin Stearate USP—Preserve in tight containers. The stearic acid salt of Erythromycin, with an excess of Stearic Acid. Sum of erythromycin A, erythromycin B, and erythromycin C is not less than 55.0%, calculated on the anhydrous basis. Meets the requirements for Identification, Crystallinity, Related compounds (not more than 3.0% of pseudoerythromycin A enol ether), Water (not more than 4.0%), and Residue on ignition (not more than 1.0%).

Erythromycin Stearate Oral Suspension—Not in *USP–NF*.

Erythromycin Stearate Tablets USP—Preserve in tight containers. Contain an amount of erythromycin stearate equivalent to the labeled amount of erythromycin, within −10% to +20%. Meet the requirements for Identification,

Dissolution (75% in 120 minutes in 0.05 *M* phosphate buffer [pH 6.8] in Apparatus 2 at 100 rpm), Uniformity of dosage units, and Loss on drying (not more than 5.0%).

ERYTHROMYCIN AND BENZOYL PEROXIDE

For *Erythromycin* and *Benzoyl Peroxide*—See individual listings for chemistry information.

USP requirements: Erythromycin and Benzoyl Peroxide Topical Gel USP—Before mixing, preserve the Erythromycin and the vehicle containing benzoyl peroxide in separate, tight containers. After mixing, preserve the mixture in tight containers. A mixture of Erythromycin in a suitable gel vehicle containing benzoyl peroxide and one or more suitable dispersants, stabilizers, and wetting agents. Contains the labeled amounts, within −10% to +25%. Meets the requirements for Identification, Minimum fill, and Limit of benzoyl peroxide related substances.

ERYTHROMYCIN AND SULFISOXAZOLE

For *Erythromycin* and *Sulfisoxazole*—See individual listings for chemistry information.

USP requirements:

Erythromycin Estolate and Sulfisoxazole Acetyl Oral Suspension USP—Preserve in tight containers. Contains an amount of erythromycin estolate equivalent to the labeled amount of erythromycin, within −10% to +20%, and an amount of sulfisoxazole acetyl equivalent to the labeled amount of sulfisoxazole, within −10% to +15%. Contains one or more suitable buffers, colors, diluents, emulsifiers, flavors, preservatives, and suspending agents. Meets the requirements for Identification, Uniformity of dosage units (single-unit containers), Deliverable volume, and pH (3.5–6.5).

Erythromycin Ethylsuccinate and Sulfisoxazole Acetyl for Oral Suspension USP—Preserve in tight containers. A dry mixture of Erythromycin Ethylsuccinate and Sulfisoxazole Acetyl with one or more suitable buffers, colors, flavors, surfactants, and suspending agents. Contains an amount of erythromycin ethylsuccinate equivalent to the labeled amount of erythromycin, within −10% to +20%, and an amount of sulfisoxazole acetyl equivalent to the labeled amount of sulfisoxazole, within −10% to +15%. Meets the requirements for Identification, Uniformity of dosage units (single-unit containers), Deliverable volume, pH (5.0–7.2, in the suspension constituted as directed in the labeling), and Loss on drying (not more than 1.0%).

Note: Where Erythromycin Ethylsuccinate and Sulfisoxazole Acetyl for Oral Suspension is prescribed, without reference to the quantity of erythromycin or sulfisoxazole contained therein, a product containing 40 mg of erythromycin and 120 mg of sulfisoxazole per mL when constituted as directed in the labeling shall be dispensed.

ESCITALOPRAM

Source: Escitalopram oxalate—Escitalopram is a pure S-enantiomer of the racemic, bicyclic phthalane derivative citalopram.

Chemical name: Escitalopram oxalate—*S*-(+)-5-Isobenzofurancarbonitrile, 1-[3-(dimethylamino)propyl]-1-(4-fluorophenyl)-1,3-dihydro-, oxalate.

Molecular formula: Escitalopram oxalate—$C_{20}H_{21}FN_2O \cdot C_2H_2O_4$.

Molecular weight: Escitalopram oxalate—414.40.

Description: Escitalopram oxalate—Fine white to slightly yellow powder.

Solubility: Escitalopram oxalate—Freely soluble in methanol and in dimethyl sulfoxide (DMSO); soluble in isotonic saline solution; sparingly soluble in water and ethanol; slightly soluble in ethyl acetate; insoluble in heptane.

USP requirements:
Escitalopram Tablets—Not in *USP–NF*.
Escitalopram Oxalate Tablets—Not in *USP–NF*.

ESMOLOL

Chemical name: Esmolol hydrochloride—Benzenepropanoic acid, 4-[2-hydroxy-3-[(1-methylethyl)amino]propoxy]-, methyl ester, hydrochloride, (±)-.

Molecular formula: Esmolol hydrochloride—$C_{16}H_{25}NO_4 \cdot HCl$.

Molecular weight: Esmolol hydrochloride—331.83.

Description:
Esmolol hydrochloride—White to off-white crystalline powder.
Esmolol hydrochloride injection—Clear, colorless to light yellow.

Solubility: Esmolol hydrochloride—Very soluble in water; freely soluble in alcohol.

Other characteristics: Esmolol hydrochloride—Partition coefficient: Octanol/water at pH 7.0 is 0.42.

USP requirements: Esmolol Hydrochloride Injection—Not in *USP–NF*.

ESOMEPRAZOLE

Chemical group: Esomeprazole magnesium—Substituted Benjimidazole. Esomeprazole is an enantiomer of omeprazole, especially the S-isomer.

Chemical name: Esomeprazole magnesium—1*H*-Benzimidazole, 5-methoxy-2-[(*S*)-[(4-methoxy-3,5-dimethyl-2-pyridinyl)-methyl]sulfinyl]-, magnesium salt, trihydrate.

Molecular formula: Esomeprazole magnesium—$C_{34}H_{36}$-$MgN_6O_6S_2 \cdot 3H_2O$.

Molecular weight: Esomeprazole magnesium—767.2 (hydrate); 767.2 (anhydrous).

Description: Esomeprazole magnesium—White to slightly colored crystalline powder.

Solubility: Esomeprazole magnesium—Slightly soluble in water.

Other characteristics: Esomeprazole magnesium—pH: 6.8 (buffer).

USP requirements: Esomeprazole Magnesium Delayed-release Capsules—Not in *USP–NF*.

ESTAZOLAM

Chemical group: A triazolobenzodiazepine derivative.

Chemical name: 4*H*-[1,2,4]Triazolo[4,3-*a*][1,4]benzodiazepine, 8-chloro-6-phenyl-.

Molecular formula: $C_{16}H_{11}ClN_4$.

Molecular weight: 294.74.

Description: Fine, white, odorless powder.

Solubility: Soluble in alcohol; practically insoluble in water.

USP requirements: Estazolam Tablets—Not in *USP–NF*.

ESTRADIOL

Chemical name:
Estradiol—Estra-1,3,5(10)-triene-3,17-diol, (17 beta)-.
Estradiol cypionate—Estra-1,3,5(10)-triene-3,17-diol, (17 beta)-, 17-cyclopentanepropanoate.
Estradiol valerate—Estra-1,3,5(10)-triene-3,17-diol(17 beta)-, 17-pentanoate.

Molecular formula:
Estradiol—$C_{18}H_{24}O_2$.
Estradiol cypionate—$C_{26}H_{36}O_3$.
Estradiol valerate—$C_{23}H_{32}O_3$.

Molecular weight:
Estradiol—272.38.
Estradiol cypionate—396.56.
Estradiol valerate—356.55.

Description:
Estradiol USP—White or creamy white, small crystals or crystalline powder. Is odorless, and is stable in air. Is hygroscopic.
Estradiol Cypionate USP—White to practically white, crystalline powder. Is odorless or has a slight odor.
Estradiol Valerate USP—White, crystalline powder. Is usually odorless but may have a faint, fatty odor.

Solubility:
Estradiol USP—Practically insoluble in water; soluble in alcohol, in acetone, in dioxane, in chloroform, and in solutions of fixed alkali hydroxides; sparingly soluble in vegetable oils.
Estradiol Cypionate USP—Insoluble in water; soluble in alcohol, in acetone, in chloroform, and in dioxane; sparingly soluble in vegetable oils.
Estradiol Valerate USP—Practically insoluble in water; soluble in castor oil, in methanol, in benzyl benzoate, and in dioxane; sparingly soluble in sesame oil and in peanut oil.

USP requirements: Estradiol USP—Preserve in tight, light-resistant containers. Contains not less than 97.0% and not more than 103.0% of estradiol, calculated on the anhydrous basis. Meets the requirements for Identification, Melting range (173–179 °C), Specific rotation (+76° to +83°), Chromatographic purity (not more than 0.2% of any individual impurity, and not more than 0.5% of total impurities), Water (not more than 1.0%), and Other impurities.
Estradiol Vaginal Cream USP—Preserve in collapsible tubes or in tight containers. Contains the labeled amount, within ±10%, in a suitable cream base. Meets the requirements for Identification, Microbial limits, Minimum fill, and pH (3.5–6.5).
Estradiol Vaginal Inserts—Not in *USP–NF*.
Estradiol Pellets USP—Preserve in tight containers, suitable for maintaining sterile contents, that hold 1 Pellet each. Sterile pellets composed of Estradiol in compressed form, without the presence of any binder, diluent, or excipient. Contain the labeled amount, within ±3%. Meet the requirements for Solubility in chloroform and Weight variation (for 5 pellets, average weight within ±5% of labeled weight; for each pellet, within ±10% of labeled weight), and for the requirements under Estradiol and under Sterility tests.

Estradiol Injectable Suspension USP—Preserve in single-dose or in multiple-dose containers, preferably of Type I glass. A sterile suspension of Estradiol in Water for Injection. Contains the labeled amount, within ±10%. Meets the requirements for Identification, Bacterial endotoxins, and Uniformity of dosage units, and for Injections.
Estradiol Tablets USP—Preserve in tight, light-resistant containers. Contain the labeled amount, within −10% to +15%. Meet the requirements for Identification, Dissolution (75% in 60 minutes in 0.3% sodium lauryl sulfate in water in Apparatus 2 at 100 rpm), and Uniformity of dosage units.
Estradiol Transdermal System—Not in *USP–NF*.
Estradiol Cypionate USP—Preserve in tight, light-resistant containers. Contains not less than 97.0% and not more than 103.0% of estradiol cypionate, calculated on the dried basis. Meets the requirements for Identification, Melting range (149–153 °C), Specific rotation (+39° to +44°), Loss on drying (not more than 1.0%), Other impurities, and Residue on ignition (not more than 0.2%).
Estradiol Cypionate Injection USP—Preserve in single-dose or in multiple-dose, light-resistant containers, preferably of Type I glass. A sterile solution of Estradiol Cypionate in a suitable oil. Contains the labeled amount, within ±10%. Meets the requirements for Identification and for Injections.
Estradiol Valerate USP—Preserve in tight, light-resistant containers. Contains not less than 98.0% and not more than 102.0% of estradiol valerate. Meets the requirements for Identification, Melting range (143–150 °C), Specific rotation (+41° to +47°), Water (not more than 0.1%), Limit of estradiol (not more than 1.0%), Free acid (not more than 0.5%), and Ordinary impurities.
Estradiol Valerate Injection USP—Preserve in single-dose or in multiple-dose, light-resistant containers, preferably of Type I or Type III glass. A sterile solution of Estradiol Valerate in a suitable vegetable oil. Contains the labeled amount, within −10% to +15%. Meets the requirements for Identification and Limit of estradiol (not more than 3.0%), and for Injections.

ESTRAMUSTINE

Chemical name: Estramustine phosphate sodium—Estra-1,3,5(10)-triene-3,17-diol (17 beta)-, 3-[bis(2-chloroethyl)carbamate]17-(dihydrogen phosphate), disodium salt.

Molecular formula: Estramustine phosphate sodium—$C_{23}H_{30}Cl_2NNa_2O_6P$.

Molecular weight: Estramustine phosphate sodium—564.40.

Description: Estramustine phosphate sodium—Off-white powder.

Solubility: Estramustine phosphate sodium—Readily soluble in water.

USP requirements: Estramustine Phosphate Sodium Capsules—Not in *USP–NF*.

ESTRIOL

Chemical name: Estra-1,3,5(10)-triene-3,16,17-triol, (16 alpha,17 beta)-.

Molecular formula: $C_{18}H_{24}O_3$.

Molecular weight: 288.38.

Description: Estriol USP—White to practically white, odorless, crystalline powder. Melts at about 280 °C.

Solubility: Estriol USP—Insoluble in water; sparingly soluble in alcohol; soluble in acetone, in chloroform, in dioxane, in ether, and in vegetable oils.

USP requirements: Estriol USP—Preserve in tight containers. Contains not less than 97.0% and not more than 102.0% of estriol, calculated on the dried basis. Meets the requirements for Identification, Specific rotation (+54° to +62°), Loss on drying (not more than 0.5%), Residue on ignition (not more than 0.1%), and Chromatographic purity.

CONJUGATED ESTROGENS

Description: Conjugated Estrogens USP—Conjugated estrogens obtained from natural sources is a buff-colored, amorphous powder, odorless or having a slight, characteristic odor. The synthetic form is a white to light buff, crystalline or amorphous powder, odorless or having a slight odor.

USP requirements:
Conjugated Estrogens USP—Preserve in well-closed containers. A mixture of sodium estrone sulfate and sodium equilin sulfate, derived wholly or in part from equine urine or synthetically from Estrone and Equilin. Contains other conjugated estrogenic substances of the type excreted by pregnant mares. A dispersion of the estrogenic substances on a suitable powdered diluent. Label it to state the content of Conjugated Estrogens on a weight-to-weight basis. Contains not less than 52.5% and not more than 61.5% of sodium estrone sulfate and not less than 22.5% and not more than 30.5% of sodium equilin sulfate, and the total of sodium estrone sulfate and sodium equilin sulfate is not less than 79.5% and not more than 88.0% of the labeled content of Conjugated Estrogens. Contains as concomitant components as sodium sulfate conjugates not less than 13.5% and not more than 19.5% of 17 alpha-dihydroequilin, not less than 2.5% and not more than 9.5% of 17 alpha-estradiol, and not less than 0.5% and not more than 4.0% of 17 beta-dihydroequilin, of the labeled content of Conjugated Estrogens. Meets the requirements for Identification, Content of 17 alpha-dihydroequilin, 17 beta-dihydroequilin, and 17 alpha-estradiol (concomitant components), Limits of 17 alpha-dihydroequilenin, 17 beta-dihydroequilenin, and equilenin (signal impurities), Limits of 17 beta-estradiol and Delta^{8,9}-dehydroestrone, Limit of estrone, equilin, and 17 alpha-dihydroequilin (free steroids), and Organic volatile impurities.
Conjugated Estrogens Vaginal Cream—Not in *USP–NF*.
Conjugated Estrogens for Injection—Not in *USP–NF*.
Conjugated Estrogens Tablets USP—Preserve in well-closed containers. The labeling indicates the Tablet strength and states with which in vitro Drug Release Test the product complies. Contain the labeled amount of conjugated estrogens as the total of sodium estrone sulfate and sodium equilin sulfate, within –27% to –5%. The ratio of sodium equilin sulfate to sodium estrone sulfate in the Tablets is not less than 0.35 and not more than 0.65. Meet the requirements for Identification, Drug release (for products labeled as 0.3- and 0.625-mg tablets: 19–49% in 2 hours, 66–96% in 5 hours, and not less than 80% in 8 hours in water in Apparatus 2 at 50 rpm for Test 1; for products labeled as 0.9-mg tablets: 12–37% in 2 hours, 57–85% in 5 hours, and not less than 80% in 8 hours in water in Apparatus 2 at 50 rpm for Test 2; and for products labeled as 1.25- and 2.50-mg tablets: 3–22% in 2 hours, 37–67% in 5 hours, 66–96% in 8 hours, and not less than 80% in 12 hours in water in Apparatus 2 at 50 rpm for Test 3), and Uniformity of dosage units.

CONJUGATED ESTROGENS AND MEDTROXYPROGES-TERONE

For *Conjugated Estrogens* and *Medroxyprogesterone*—See individual listings for chemistry information.

USP requirements:
Conjugated Estrogens and Medroxyprogesterone Acetate Tablets—Not in *USP–NF*.
Conjugated Estrogen, and Conjugated Estrogen and Medroxyprogesterone Tablets—Not in *USP–NF*.

CONJUGATED ESTROGENS AND METHYLTESTOSTER-ONE

For *Conjugated Estrogens* and *Methyltestosterone*—See individual listings for chemistry information.

USP requirements: Conjugated Estrogens and Methyltestosterone Tablets—Not in *USP–NF*.

ESTERIFIED ESTROGENS

Description: Esterified Estrogens USP—White or buff-colored, amorphous powder, odorless or having a slight, characteristic odor.

USP requirements:
Esterified Estrogens USP—Preserve in tight containers. A mixture of the sodium salts of the sulfate esters of the estrogenic substances, principally estrone. A dispersion of the estrogenic substances on a suitable powdered diluent. Label it to state the content of Esterified Estrogens on a weight-to-weight basis. The content of total esterified estrogens is not less than 90.0% and not more than 110.0% of the labeled amount. Contains not less than 75.0% and not more than 85.0% of sodium estrone sulfate, and not less than 6.0% and not more than 15.0% of sodium equilin sulfate, in such proportion that the total of these two components is not less than 90.0% of the labeled amount of esterified estrogens. Meets the requirements for Identification, Free steroids (not more than 3.0%), and Organic volatile impurities.
Esterified Estrogens Tablets USP—Preserve in well-closed containers. Contain the labeled amount of esterified estrogens as the total of sodium estrone sulfate and sodium equilin sulfate, within –10% to +15%. The ratio of sodium equilin sulfate to sodium estrone sulfate is not less than 0.071 and not more than 0.20. Meet the requirements for Identification, Disintegration, and Uniformity of dosage units.

ESTERIFIED ESTROGENS AND METHYLTESTOSTER-ONE

For *Esterified Estrogens* and *Methyltestosterone*—See individual listings for chemistry information.

USP requirements: Esterified Estrogens and Methyltestosterone Tablets—Not in *USP–NF*.

ESTRONE

Chemical name: Estra-1,3,5(10)-trien-17-one, 3-hydroxy-.

Molecular formula: $C_{18}H_{22}O_2$.

Molecular weight: 270.37.

Description: Estrone USP—Small, white crystals or white to creamy white, crystalline powder. Is odorless, and is stable in air. Melts at about 260 °C.

Solubility: Estrone USP—Practically insoluble in water; soluble in alcohol, in acetone, in dioxane, and in vegetable oils; slightly soluble in solutions of fixed alkali hydroxides.

USP requirements:
Estrone USP—Preserve in tight, light-resistant containers. Contains not less than 97.0% and not more than 103.0% of estrone, calculated on the dried basis. Meets the requirements for Clarity of solution, Identification, Specific rotation (+158° to +165°), Loss on drying (not more than 0.5%), Residue on ignition (not more than 0.5%), Limit of equilenin and equilin, and Ordinary impurities.
Estrone Vaginal Cream—Not in *USP–NF*.
Estrone Injection USP—Preserve in single-dose or in multiple-dose containers, preferably of Type I glass. A sterile solution of Estrone in a suitable oil. Contains the labeled amount, within −10% to +15%. Meets the requirements for Identification and for Injections.
Estrone Vaginal Suppositories—Not in *USP–NF*.
Estrone Injectable Suspension USP—Preserve in single-dose or in multiple-dose containers, preferably of Type I glass. A sterile suspension of Estrone in Water for Injection. Contains the labeled amount, within −10% to +15%. Meets the requirements for Identification, Bacterial endotoxins, and Uniformity of dosage units, and for Injections.

ESTROPIPATE

Chemical name: Estra-1,3,5(10)-trien-17-one, 3-(sulfooxy)-, compd. with piperazine (1:1).

Molecular formula: $C_{18}H_{22}O_5S \cdot C_4H_{10}N_2$.

Molecular weight: 436.57.

Description: Estropipate USP—White to yellowish white, fine crystalline powder. Is odorless, or may have a slight odor. Melts at about 190 °C to a light brown, viscous liquid which solidifies, on further heating, and finally melts at about 245 °C, with decomposition.

Solubility: Estropipate USP—Very slightly soluble in water, in alcohol, in chloroform, and in ether; soluble in warm water.

USP requirements:
Estropipate USP—Preserve in tight containers. Contains not less than 97.0% and not more than 103.0% of estropipate, calculated on the dried basis. Meets the requirements for Identification, Loss on drying (not more than 1.0%), Residue on ignition (not more than 0.5%), Free estrone (not more than 2.0%), and Organic volatile impurities.
Estropipate Vaginal Cream USP—Preserve in collapsible tubes. Contains the labeled amount, within −10% to +20%, in a suitable cream base. Meets the requirements for Identification and Minimum fill.
Estropipate Tablets USP—Preserve in well-closed containers. Contain the labeled amount, within ±10%. Meet the requirements for Identification, Dissolution (80% in 30 minutes in 0.05 M phosphate buffer [pH 6.8] in Apparatus 2 at 75 rpm), and Uniformity of dosage units.

ETANERCEPT

Source: Obtained from a Chinese hamster ovary (CHO) mammalian cell expression system via recombinant DNA technology.

Molecular formula: $C_{2224}H_{3472}N_{618}O_{701}S_{36}$ (monomer).

Molecular weight: 51,238 daltons (non-glycosylated protein, monomer).

Description: Sterile, white, preservative-free, lyophilized powder. Has a pH of 7.4 ± 0.3.

USP requirements: Etanercept Injection—Not in *USP–NF*.

ETHACRYNATE SODIUM

Chemical name: Acetic acid, [2,3-dichloro-4-(2-methylene-1-oxobutyl)phenoxy]-, sodium salt.

Molecular formula: $C_{13}H_{11}Cl_2NaO_4$.

Molecular weight: 325.12.

Description: Ethacrynate sodium for injection—White, crystalline powder or plug.

Solubility: Soluble in water at 25 °C to the extent of about 7%.

USP requirements: Ethacrynate Sodium for Injection USP—Preserve in Containers for Sterile Solids. A sterile, freeze-dried powder prepared by the neutralization of Ethacrynic Acid with the aid of Sodium Hydroxide. Label it to indicate that it was prepared by freeze-drying, having been filled into its container in the form of a true solution. Contains an amount of ethacrynate sodium equivalent to the labeled amount of ethacrynic acid, within ±10%. Meets the requirements for Constituted solution, Identification, Bacterial endotoxins, and pH (5.0–7.0), and for Sterility tests, Uniformity of dosage units, and Labeling under Injections.

ETHACRYNIC ACID

Chemical name: Acetic acid, [2,3-dichloro-4-(2-methylene-1-oxobutyl)phenoxy]-.

Molecular formula: $C_{13}H_{12}Cl_2O_4$.

Molecular weight: 303.14.

Description: Ethacrynic Acid USP—White or practically white, odorless or practically odorless, crystalline powder.

pKa: 3.5.

Solubility: Ethacrynic Acid USP—Very slightly soluble in water; freely soluble in alcohol, in chloroform, and in ether.

USP requirements:
Ethacrynic Acid USP—Preserve in well-closed containers. Contains not less than 97.0% and not more than 102.0% of ethacrynic acid, calculated on the dried basis. Meets the requirements for Identification, Loss on drying (not more than 0.25%), Residue on ignition (not more than 0.1%), Toluene extractives (not more than 2.0%), Equivalent weight (294–309, on the dried basis), Heavy metals (not more than 0.001%), and Organic volatile impurities.
Caution: Use care in handling Ethacrynic Acid, since it irritates the skin, eyes, and mucous membranes.
Ethacrynic Acid Oral Solution—Not in *USP–NF*.

Ethacrynic Acid Tablets USP—Preserve in well-closed containers. Contain the labeled amount, within ±10%. Meet the requirements for Identification, Dissolution (75% in 45 minutes in 0.1 *M* phosphate buffer [pH 8.0 ±0.05] in Apparatus 2 at 50 rpm), and Uniformity of dosage units.

ETHAMBUTOL

Chemical name: Ethambutol hydrochloride—1-Butanol, 2,2′-(1,2-ethanediyldiimino)bis-, dihydrochloride, [S-(R*,R*)]-.

Molecular formula: Ethambutol hydrochloride—$C_{10}H_{24}N_2O_2 \cdot$ 2HCl.

Molecular weight: Ethambutol hydrochloride—277.23.

Description: Ethambutol Hydrochloride USP—White, crystalline powder.

Solubility: Ethambutol Hydrochloride USP—Freely soluble in water; soluble in alcohol and in methanol; slightly soluble in ether and in chloroform.

USP requirements:
Ethambutol Hydrochloride USP—Preserve in well-closed containers. Contains not less than 98.0% and not more than 100.5% of ethambutol hydrochloride, calculated on the dried basis. Meets the requirements for Identification, Specific rotation (+6.0° to +6.7°), Loss on drying (not more than 0.5%), Heavy metals (not more than 0.002%), Limit of aminobutanol (not more than 1.0%), Ordinary impurities, and Organic volatile impurities.
Ethambutol Hydrochloride Tablets USP—Preserve in well-closed containers. Contain the labeled amount, within ± 5%. Meet the requirements for Identification, Dissolution (75% in 45 minutes in water in Apparatus 1 at 100 rpm), Uniformity of dosage units, and Limit of aminobutanol (not more than 1.0%).

ETHAMBUTOL AND ISONIAZID

For *Ethambutol* and *Isoniazid*—See individual listings for chemistry information.

USP requirements: Ethambutol and Isoniazid Tablets—Not in *USP–NF.*

ETHANOLAMINE

Chemical name: Ethanolamine oleate—9-Octadecenoic acid (Z)-, compound with 2-aminoethanol (1:1).

Molecular formula: Ethanolamine oleate—$C_{18}H_{34}O_2 \cdot C_2H_7NO$.

Molecular weight: Ethanolamine oleate—343.54.

USP requirements: Ethanolamine Oleate Injection—Not in *USP–NF.*

ETHCHLORVYNOL

Chemical name: 1-Penten-4-yn-3-ol, 1-chloro-3-ethyl-.

Molecular formula: C_7H_9ClO.

Molecular weight: 144.60.

Description: Ethchlorvynol USP—Colorless to yellow, slightly viscous liquid, having a characteristic pungent odor. Darkens on exposure to light and to air.

Solubility: Ethchlorvynol USP—Immiscible with water; miscible with most organic solvents.

USP requirements:
Ethchlorvynol USP—Preserve in tight, light-resistant glass or polyethylene containers, using polyethylene-lined closures. Contains not less than 98.0% and not more than 100.0% of *E*-ethchlorvynol, calculated on the anhydrous basis. Meets the requirements for Identification, Refractive index (1.476–1.480), Acidity, Water (not more than 0.2%), and Chromatographic purity.
Ethchlorvynol Capsules USP—Preserve in tight, light-resistant containers. Contain the labeled amount of *E*-ethchlorvynol, within ±10%. Meet the requirements for Identification, Dissolution (in 15 minutes in water in Apparatus 2 at 50 rpm), and Uniformity of dosage units.

ETHER

Chemical name: Ethane, 1,1′-oxybis-.

Molecular formula: $C_4H_{10}O$.

Molecular weight: 74.12.

Description: Ether USP—Colorless, mobile, volatile liquid, having a characteristic sweet, pungent odor. Is slowly oxidized by the action of air and light, with the formation of peroxides. Boils at about 35 °C.

Solubility: Ether USP—Soluble in water and in hydrochloric acid. Miscible with alcohol, with chloroform, with solvent hexane, and with fixed and volatile oils.

USP requirements: Ether USP—Preserve in partly filled, tight, light-resistant containers, at a temperature not exceeding 30 °C, remote from fire. Where Ether is intended for anesthetic use, the label so states. Contains not less than 96.0% and not more than 98.0% of ether, the remainder consisting of alcohol and water. Meets the requirements for Specific gravity (0.713–0.716 [indicating 96.0–98.0% of ether]), Acidity, Water (not more than 0.5%, except where labeled as intended for anesthetic use, contains not more than 0.2%), Limit of nonvolatile residue (not more than 0.003%), Aldehyde, Limit of peroxide (not more than 0.3 ppm), and Low-boiling hydrocarbons.

Caution: Ether is highly volatile and flammable. Its vapor, when mixed with air and ignited, may explode.

Note: Ether to be used for anesthesia must be preserved in tight containers of not more than 3-kg capacity, and is not to be used for anesthesia if it has been removed from the original container longer than 24 hours. Ether to be used for anesthesia may, however, be shipped in larger containers for repackaging in containers as directed above, provided the ether at the time of repackaging meets the requirements of the tests in *USP/NF.*

ETHINAMATE

Chemical name: Cyclohexanol, 1-ethynyl-, carbamate.

Molecular formula: $C_9H_{13}NO_2$.

Molecular weight: 167.21.

Description: White, essentially odorless powder. Its saturated aqueous solution has a pH of about 6.5.

Solubility: Slightly soluble in water; freely soluble in alcohol, in chloroform, and in ether.

USP requirements: Ethinamate Capsules—Not in *USP–NF*.

ETHINYL ESTRADIOL

Chemical name: 19-Norpregna-1,3,5(10)-trien-20-yne-3,17-diol, (17 alpha)-.

Molecular formula: $C_{20}H_{24}O_2$.

Molecular weight: 296.40.

Description: Ethinyl Estradiol USP—White to creamy white, odorless, crystalline powder.

Solubility: Ethinyl Estradiol USP—Insoluble in water; soluble in alcohol, in chloroform, in ether, in vegetable oils, and in solutions of fixed alkali hydroxides.

USP requirements:
Ethinyl Estradiol USP—Preserve in tight, non-metallic, light-resistant containers. Contains not less than 97.0% and not more than 102.0% of ethinyl estradiol, calculated on the dried basis. Meets the requirements for Completeness of solution, Identification, Melting range (180–186 °C; in a polymorphic modification, 142–146 °C), Specific rotation (−28.0° to −29.5°), and Loss on drying (not more than 1.0%).
Ethinyl Estradiol Tablets USP—Preserve in well-closed containers. Contain the labeled amount, within −10% to +15%. Meet the requirements for Thin-layer chromatographic identification test, Disintegration (30 minutes), Related compounds, and Uniformity of dosage units.

ETHIODIZED OIL

Description: Ethiodized Oil Injection USP—Straw-colored to amber-colored, oily liquid. May possess an alliaceous odor.

Solubility: Ethiodized Oil Injection USP—Insoluble in water; soluble in acetone, in chloroform, in ether, and in solvent hexane.

USP requirements: Ethiodized Oil Injection USP—Preserve in well-filled, light-resistant, single-dose or multiple-dose containers. An iodine addition product of the ethyl ester of the fatty acids of poppyseed oil, containing not less than 35.2% and not more than 38.9% of organically combined iodine. It is sterile. Meets the requirements for Identification, Specific gravity (1.280–1.293, at 15 °C), Viscosity (50–100 centipoises, at 15 °C), Sterility, Acidity, and Free iodine.

ETHIONAMIDE

Chemical group: Synthetic derivative of isonicotinic acid.

Chemical name: 4-Pyridinecarbothioamide, 2-ethyl-.

Molecular formula: $C_8H_{10}N_2S$.

Molecular weight: 166.24.

Description: Ethionamide USP—Bright yellow powder, having a faint to moderate sulfide-like odor.

Solubility: Ethionamide USP—Slightly soluble in water, in chloroform, and in ether; soluble in methanol; sparingly soluble in alcohol and in propylene glycol.

USP requirements:
Ethionamide USP—Preserve in tight containers. Contains not less than 98.0% and not more than 102.0% of ethionamide, calculated on the anhydrous basis. Meets the requirements for Identification, Melting range (158–164 °C), pH (6.0–7.0, in a 1 in 100 slurry in water), Water (not more than 2.0%), Residue on ignition (not more than 0.2%), Selenium (not more than 0.003%, a 200-mg test specimen being used), and Organic volatile impurities.
Ethionamide Tablets USP—Preserve in tight containers. Contain the labeled amount, within −5% to +10%. Meet the requirements for Identification, Dissolution (75% in 45 minutes in 0.1 N hydrochloric acid in Apparatus 1 at 100 rpm), and Uniformity of dosage units.

ETHOPABATE

Chemical name: Benzoic acid, 4-(acetylamino)-2-ethoxy-, methyl ester.

Molecular formula: $C_{12}H_{15}NO_4$.

Molecular weight: 237.25.

Description: Ethopabate USP—White to pinkish-white, odorless or practically odorless powder.

Solubility: Ethopabate USP—Very slightly soluble in water; soluble in acetonitrile, in acetone, in dehydrated alcohol, and in methanol; sparingly soluble in isopropyl alcohol, in dioxane, in ethyl acetate, and in methylene chloride; slightly soluble in ether.

USP requirements: Ethopabate USP—Preserve in well-closed containers, protected from light. Label it to indicate that it is for veterinary use only. Contains not less than 96.0% and not more than 101.0% of ethopabate, calculated on the dried basis. Meets the requirements for Identification, Loss on drying (not more than 1.0%), Melting range (146–151 °C), Residue on ignition (not more than 0.5%), and Chromatographic purity.

ETHOPROPAZINE

Chemical group: Phenothiazine derivative.

Chemical name: Ethopropazine hydrochloride—10*H*-Phenothiazine-10-ethanamine, *N,N*-diethyl-alpha-methyl-, monohydrochloride.

Molecular formula: Ethopropazine hydrochloride—$C_{19}H_{24}N_2S \cdot$ HCl.

Molecular weight: Ethopropazine hydrochloride—348.93.

Description: Ethopropazine Hydrochloride USP—White or slightly off-white, odorless, crystalline powder. Melts at about 210 °C, with decomposition.

Solubility: Ethopropazine Hydrochloride USP—Soluble in water at 40 °C; slightly soluble in water at 20 °C; soluble in alcohol and in chloroform; sparingly soluble in acetone; insoluble in ether.

USP requirements:

Ethopropazine Hydrochloride USP—Preserve in tight, light-resistant containers. Contains not less than 98.0% and not more than 101.5% of ethopropazine hydrochloride, calculated on the dried basis. Meets the requirements for Identification, Loss on drying (not more than 0.5%), Heavy metals (not more than 0.002%), Ordinary impurities, and Organic volatile impurities.

Ethopropazine Hydrochloride Tablets USP—Preserve in well-closed containers, protected from light. Contain the labeled amount, within ±10%. Meet the requirements for Identification, Dissolution (75% in 45 minutes in 0.1 N hydrochloric acid in Apparatus 1 at 100 rpm), Uniformity of dosage units, and Other alkylated phenothiazines.

ETHOSUXIMIDE

Chemical name: 2,5-Pyrrolidinedione, 3-ethyl-3-methyl-.

Molecular formula: $C_7H_{11}NO_2$.

Molecular weight: 141.17.

Description: Ethosuximide USP—White to off-white, crystalline powder or waxy solid, having a characteristic odor.

Solubility: Ethosuximide USP—Freely soluble in water and in chloroform; very soluble in alcohol and in ether; very slightly soluble in solvent hexane.

USP requirements:

Ethosuximide USP—Preserve in tight containers. Contains not less than 98.0% and not more than 101.0% of ethosuximide, calculated on the anhydrous basis. Meets the requirements for Identification, Melting range (47–52 °C), Water (not more than 0.5%), Residue on ignition (not more than 0.5%), Limit of cyanide, Limit of 2-ethyl-2-methylsuccinic acid and other impurities (not more than 0.5%), and Organic volatile impurities.

Ethosuximide Capsules USP—Preserve in tight containers. Contain the labeled amount, within ±7%, present in the form of a solution of Ethosuximide in Polyethylene Glycol 400 or other suitable solvent. Meet the requirements for Identification, Dissolution (80% in 30 minutes in phosphate buffer [pH 6.8] in Apparatus 1 at 50 rpm), Limit of 2-ethyl-2-methylsuccinic acid (not more than 0.5%), and Uniformity of dosage units.

Ethosuximide Oral Solution USP—Preserve in tight containers. Contains the labeled amount, within −10% to +5%. Meets the requirements for Identification, pH (4.5–5.8), and Limit of 2-ethyl-2-methylsuccinic acid (not more than 2.0%)

Ethosuximide Syrup—Not in *USP–NF*.

ETHOTOIN

Chemical group: Related to the barbiturates in chemical structure, but having a five-membered ring.

Chemical name: 3-Ethyl-5-phenylimidazolidin-2,4-dione.

Molecular formula: $C_{11}H_{12}N_2O_2$.

Molecular weight: 204.23.

Description: Ethotoin USP—White, crystalline powder.

Solubility: Ethotoin USP—Insoluble in water; freely soluble in dehydrated alcohol and in chloroform; soluble in ether.

USP requirements:

Ethotoin USP—Preserve in tight containers. Contains not less than 97.5% and not more than 102.0% of ethotoin, calculated on the dried basis. Meets the requirements for Identification, Loss on drying (not more than 1.0%), Residue on ignition (not more than 0.1%), Chloride (not more than 0.014%), Heavy metals (not more than 0.002%), Limit of 5-phenylhydantoin and related compounds (not more than 1.0%), and Organic volatile impurities.

Ethotoin Tablets USP—Preserve in tight containers. Contain the labeled amount, within ±10%. Meet the requirements for Identification, Dissolution (80% in 60 minutes in 0.1 N hydrochloric acid in Apparatus 2 at 100 rpm), and Uniformity of dosage units.

ETHYL ACETATE

Chemical name: Acetic acid, ethyl ester.

Molecular formula: $C_4H_8O_2$.

Molecular weight: 88.11.

Description: Ethyl Acetate NF—Transparent, colorless liquid, having a fragrant, refreshing, slightly acetous odor.

NF category: Flavors and perfumes; solvent.

Solubility: Ethyl Acetate NF—Soluble in water; miscible with alcohol, with ether, with fixed oils, and with volatile oils.

NF requirements: Ethyl Acetate NF—Preserve in tight containers, and avoid exposure to excessive heat. Contains not less than 99.0% and not more than 100.5% of ethyl acetate. Meets the requirements for Identification, Specific gravity (0.894–0.898), Acidity, Readily carbonizable substances, Limit of nonvolatile residue (not more than 0.02%), Limit of methyl compounds, Chromatographic purity, and Organic volatile impurities.

ETHYLCELLULOSE

Chemical name: Cellulose, ethyl ester.

Description: Ethylcellulose NF—Free-flowing, white to light tan powder. It forms films that have a refractive index of about 1.47. Its aqueous suspensions are neutral to litmus.

NF category: Coating agent; tablet binder.

Solubility: Ethylcellulose NF—Insoluble in water, in glycerin, and in propylene glycol. Ethylcellulose containing less than 46.5% of ethoxy groups is freely soluble in tetrahydrofuran, in methyl acetate, in chloroform, and in mixtures of aromatic hydrocarbons with alcohol. Ethylcellulose containing not less than 46.5% of ethoxy groups is freely soluble in alcohol, in methanol, in toluene, in chloroform, and in ethyl acetate.

NF requirements:

Ethylcellulose NF—Preserve in well-closed containers. An ethyl ether of cellulose. Label it to indicate its viscosity (under the conditions specified herein), and its ethoxy content. When dried at 105 °C for 2 hours, contains not less than 44.0% and not more than 51.0% of ethoxy ($-OC_2H_5$) groups. Meets the requirements for Identification, Viscos-

ity, Loss on drying (not more than 3.0%), Residue on ignition (not more than 0.4%), Lead (not more than 10 ppm), Heavy metals (not more than 20 mcg per gram), and Organic volatile impurities.

Ethylcellulose Aqueous Dispersion NF—Preserve in tight containers, and protect from freezing. A colloidal dispersion of Ethylcellulose in water. The labeling states the ethoxy content of the Ethylcellulose and the percentage of Ethylcellulose. Contains the labeled amount of Ethylcellulose, within ±10%. Contains suitable amounts of Cetyl Alcohol and Sodium Lauryl Sulfate, which assist in the formation and stabilization of the dispersion. Meets the requirements for Identification, Viscosity (not more than 150 centipoises), pH (4.0–7.0), Loss on drying (not more than 71.0%), Heavy metals (not more than 0.001%), and Organic volatile impurities.

ETHYL CHLORIDE

Chemical name: Ethane, chloro-.

Molecular formula: C_2H_5Cl.

Molecular weight: 64.51.

Description: Ethyl Chloride USP—Colorless, mobile, very volatile liquid at low temperatures or under pressure, having a characteristic, ethereal odor. Boils between 12–13 °C, and its specific gravity at 0 °C is about 0.921. When liberated at room temperature from its sealed container, it vaporizes immediately. Burns with a smoky, greenish flame, producing hydrogen chloride.

Solubility: Ethyl Chloride USP—Slightly soluble in water; freely soluble in alcohol and in ether.

USP requirements: Ethyl Chloride USP—Preserve in tight containers, preferably hermetically sealed, and remote from fire. Contains not less than 99.5% and not more than 100.5% of ethyl chloride. Meets the requirements for Reaction, Alcohol, Limit of nonvolatile residue and odor, and Chloride.

Caution: Ethyl Chloride is highly flammable. Do not use where it may be ignited.

ETHYLENEDIAMINE

Chemical name: 1,2-Ethanediamine.

Molecular formula: $C_2H_8N_2$.

Molecular weight: 60.10.

Description: Ethylenediamine USP—Clear, colorless or only slightly yellow liquid, having an ammonia-like odor and a strong alkaline reaction.

Solubility: Ethylenediamine USP—Miscible with water and with alcohol.

USP requirements: Ethylenediamine USP—Preserve in well-filled, tight, glass containers. Contains not less than 98.0% and not more than 100.5%, by weight, of ethylenediamine. Meets the requirements for Identification, Heavy metals (not more than 0.002%), and Organic volatile impurities.

Caution: Use care in handling Ethylenediamine because of its caustic nature and the irritating properties of its vapor.

Note: Ethylenediamine is strongly alkaline and may readily absorb carbon dioxide from the air to form a nonvolatile carbonate. Protect Ethylenediamine against undue exposure to the atmosphere.

ETHYLNOREPINEPHRINE

Chemical name: Ethylnorepinephrine hydrochloride—1,2-Benzenediol, 4-(2-amino-1-hydroxybutyl)-, hydrochloride.

Molecular formula: Ethylnorepinephrine hydrochloride—$C_{10}H_{15}NO_3 \cdot HCl$.

Molecular weight: Ethylnorepinephrine hydrochloride—233.69.

Description: Ethylnorepinephrine hydrochloride—White to practically white, crystalline powder, which gradually darkens on exposure to light. Melts at about 190 °C, with decomposition.

Solubility: Ethylnorepinephrine hydrochloride—Soluble in water and in alcohol; practically insoluble in ether.

USP requirements: Ethylnorepinephrine Hydrochloride Injection—Not in *USP–NF*.

ETHYL OLEATE

Chemical name: 9-Octadecenoic acid, (*Z*)-, ethyl ester.

Molecular formula: $C_{20}H_{38}O_2$.

Molecular weight: 310.51.

Description: Ethyl Oleate NF—Mobile, practically colorless liquid.
NF category: Vehicle (oleaginous).

Solubility: Ethyl Oleate NF—Insoluble in water; miscible with vegetable oils, with mineral oil, with alcohol, and with most organic solvents.

NF requirements: Ethyl Oleate NF—Preserve in tight, light-resistant containers. Consists of esters of ethyl alcohol and high molecular weight fatty acids, principally oleic acid. Meets the requirements for Specific gravity (0.866–0.874 at 20 °C), Viscosity (not less than 5.15 centipoises), Refractive index (1.443–1.450), Acid value (not more than 0.5), Iodine value (75–85), and Saponification value (177–188).

ETHYLPARABEN

Chemical name: Benzoic acid, 4-hydroxy-, ethyl ester.

Molecular formula: $C_9H_{10}O_3$.

Molecular weight: 166.17.

Description: Ethylparaben NF—Small, colorless crystals or white powder.
NF category: Antimicrobial preservative.

Solubility: Ethylparaben NF—Slightly soluble in water and in glycerin; freely soluble in acetone, in alcohol, in ether, and in propylene glycol.

NF requirements: Ethylparaben NF—Preserve in well-closed containers. Contains not less than 99.0% and not more than 100.5% of ethylparaben, calculated on the dried basis. Meets

the requirements for Identification, Melting range (115–118 °C), and Organic volatile impurities, and for Acidity, Loss on drying, and Residue on ignition under Butylparaben.

ETHYL VANILLIN

Chemical name: Benzaldehyde, 3-ethoxy-4-hydroxy-.

Molecular formula: $C_9H_{10}O_3$.

Molecular weight: 166.17.

Description: Ethyl Vanillin NF—Fine, white or slightly yellowish crystals. Its odor is similar to the odor of vanillin. It is affected by light. Its solutions are acid to litmus.
   NF category: Flavors and perfumes.

Solubility: Ethyl Vanillin NF—Sparingly soluble in water at 50 °C; freely soluble in alcohol, in chloroform, in ether, and in solutions of alkali hydroxides.

NF requirements: Ethyl Vanillin NF—Preserve in tight, light-resistant containers. Dried over phosphorus pentoxide for 4 hours, contains not less than 98.0% and not more than 101.0% of ethyl vanillin. Meets the requirements for Identification, Melting range (76–78 °C), Loss on drying (not more than 1.0%), Residue on ignition (not more than 0.1%), and Organic volatile impurities.

ETHYNODIOL DIACETATE

Chemical name: 19-Norpregn-4-en-20-yne-3,17-diol, diacetate, (3 beta,17 alpha)-.

Molecular formula: $C_{24}H_{32}O_4$.

Molecular weight: 384.51.

Description: Ethynodiol Diacetate USP—White, odorless, crystalline powder. Is stable in air.

Solubility: Ethynodiol Diacetate USP—Insoluble in water; very soluble in chloroform; freely soluble in ether; soluble in alcohol; sparingly soluble in fixed oils.

USP requirements: Ethynodiol Diacetate USP—Preserve in well-closed, light-resistant containers. Contains not less than 97.0% and not more than 102.0% of ethynodiol diacetate. Meets the requirements for Identification, Specific rotation (−70° to −76°), Limit of conjugated diene, Chromatographic purity, and Organic volatile impurities.

ETHYNODIOL DIACETATE AND ETHINYL ESTRADIOL

For *Ethynodiol Diacetate* and *Ethinyl Estradiol*—See individual listings for chemistry information.

USP requirements: Ethynodiol Diacetate and Ethinyl Estradiol Tablets USP—Preserve in well-closed containers. Contain the labeled amount of ethynodiol diacetate, within ±7%, and the labeled amount of ethinyl estradiol, within ±10%. Meet the requirements for Identification, Disintegration (15 minutes, the use of disks being omitted), and Uniformity of dosage units.

ETHYNODIOL DIACETATE AND MESTRANOL

For *Ethynodiol Diacetate* and *Mestranol*—See individual listings for chemistry information.

USP requirements: Ethynodiol Diacetate and Mestranol Tablets USP—Preserve in well-closed containers. Contain the labeled amounts, within ±10%. Meet the requirements for Identification, Disintegration (15 minutes, the use of disks being omitted), and Uniformity of dosage units.

ETIDOCAINE

Chemical group: Amide.

Chemical name: Etidocaine hydrochloride—Butanamide, N-(2,6-dimethylphenyl)-2-(ethylpropylamine)-, monohydrochloride.

Molecular formula: Etidocaine hydrochloride—$C_{17}H_{28}N_2O \cdot HCl$.

Molecular weight: Etidocaine hydrochloride—312.88.

Description: Etidocaine hydrochloride—White, crystalline powder.

pKa: 7.74.

Solubility: Etidocaine hydrochloride—Soluble in water; freely soluble in alcohol.

USP requirements: Etidocaine Hydrochloride Injection—Not in *USP–NF*.

ETIDOCAINE AND EPINEPHRINE

For *Etidocaine* and *Epinephrine*—See individual listings for chemistry information.

USP requirements: Etidocaine Hydrochloride and Epinephrine Injection—Not in *USP–NF*.

ETIDRONATE

Source: Synthetic analogue of inorganic pyrophosphate.

Chemical group: Diphosphonate.

Chemical name: Etidronate disodium—Phosphonic acid, (1-hydroxyethylidene)bis-, disodium salt.

Molecular formula: Etidronate disodium—$C_2H_6Na_2O_7P_2$.

Molecular weight: Etidronate disodium—249.99.

Description: Etidronate disodium—White powder.

Solubility: Etidronate disodium—Highly soluble in water.

USP requirements:
   Etidronate Disodium USP—Preserve in tight containers. Contains not less than 97.0% and not more than 101.0% of etidronate disodium, calculated on the anhydrous basis. Meets the requirements for Identification, pH (4.2–5.2, in a solution [1 in 100]), Water (not more than 5.0%), Phosphite (not more than 1.0%), Heavy metals (not more than 0.005%), and Organic volatile impurities.
   Etidronate Disodium Injection—Not in *USP–NF*.

Etidronate Disodium Tablets USP—Preserve in tight containers. Contain the labeled amount, within ±10%. Meet the requirements for Identification, Dissolution (70% in 30 minutes in water in Apparatus 1 at 100 rpm), and Uniformity of dosage units.

ETODOLAC

Chemical name: Pyrano[3,4-*b*]indole-1-acetic acid, 1,8-diethyl-1,3,4,9-tetrahydro-(±)-.

Molecular formula: $C_{17}H_{21}NO_3$.

Molecular weight: 287.36.

Description: White, crystalline compound.

pKa: 4.65.

Solubility: Insoluble in water; soluble in alcohols, in chloroform, in dimethyl sulfoxide, and in aqueous polyethylene glycol.

Other characteristics: *N*-octanol:water partition coefficient 11.4 at pH 7.4.

USP requirements:
Etodolac USP—Preserve in tight containers. Contains not less than 98.0% and not more than 102.0% of etodolac, calculated on the anhydrous basis. Meets the requirements for Identification, Water (not more than 0.5%), Residue on ignition (not more than 0.1%), Limit of chloride (not more than 0.3 mg per gram), Heavy metals (0.001%), Limit of alcohol and methanol (not more than 0.1% of each), and Chromatographic purity.
Etodolac Capsules USP—Preserve in tight containers, and store at controlled room temperature. Contain the labeled amount, within ±10%. Meet the requirements for Identification, Dissolution (75% in 30 minutes in phosphate buffer [pH 6.8] in Apparatus 1 at 100 rpm), and Uniformity of dosage units.
Etodolac Tablets USP—Preserve in tight containers. Contain the labeled amount, within ±10%. Meet the requirements for Identification, Uniformity of dosage units, and Dissolution (80% in 30 minutes in phosphate buffer [pH 6.8] in Apparatus 1 at 100 rpm).
Etodolac Extended-release Tablets—Not in *USP–NF*.

ETOMIDATE

Chemical name: 1*H*-Imidazole-5-carboxylic acid, 1-(1-phenylethyl)-, ethyl ester, (+)-.

Molecular formula: $C_{14}H_{16}N_2O_2$.

Molecular weight: 244.29.

Description: A white or yellowish crystalline or amorphous powder. Melting point about 67 °C.

Solubility: Soluble in water at 25 °C (0.0045 mg/100 mL), in chloroform, in methanol, in ethanol, in propylene glycol, and in acetone.

USP requirements: Etomidate Injection—Not in *USP–NF*.

ETOPOSIDE

Source: A semisynthetic podophyllotoxin of the mandrake plant. Also known as VP-16 or VP-16-213.

Chemical name:
Etoposide—Furo[3′,4′:6,7]naphtho[2,3-*d*]-1,3-dioxol-6(5a*H*)-one-, 9-[(4,6-*O*-ethylidene-beta-D-glucopyranosyl)oxy]5,8,8a,9-tetrahydro-5-(4-hydroxy-3,5-dimethoxyphenyl), [5*R*-[5 alpha,5a beta,8a alpha,9 beta(*R**)]]-.
Etoposide phosphate—Furo[3′,4′:6,7]naphtho[2,3-*d*]-1,3-dioxol-6(5a*H*)-one, 5-[3,5-dimethoxy-4-(phosphonooxy)phenyl]-9-[(4,6-*O*-ethylidene-beta-D-glucopyranosyl)oxy]5,8,8a,9-tetrahydro-, [5*R*-[5 alpha,5a beta,8a alpha,9 beta(*R**)]]-.

Molecular formula:
Etoposide—$C_{29}H_{32}O_{13}$.
Etoposide phosphate—$C_{29}H_{33}O_{16}P$.

Molecular weight:
Etoposide—588.56.
Etoposide phosphate—668.54.

Description: Etoposide USP—Fine, white to off-white, crystalline powder.

Solubility: Etoposide USP—Very slightly soluble in water; slightly soluble in alcohol, in chloroform, in ethyl acetate, and in methylene chloride; sparingly soluble in methanol.

Other characteristics: Lipophilic.

USP requirements:
Etoposide USP—Preserve in tight, light-resistant containers. Contains not less than 95.0% and not more than 105.0% of etoposide, calculated on the anhydrous basis. Meets the requirements for Identification, Specific rotation (−110° to −118°), Water (not more than 6.0%), Residue on ignition (not more than 0.1%), Heavy metals (not more than 0.002%), and Related compounds.
  Caution: Etoposide is potentially cytotoxic. Great care should be taken to prevent inhaling particles and exposing the skin to it.
Etoposide Capsules USP—Preserve in tight containers in a cold place. Do not freeze. Contain the labeled amount, within ±10%. Meet the requirements for Identification, Dissolution (80% in 30 minutes in acetate buffer [pH 4.5] in Apparatus 2 at 50 rpm), Uniformity of dosage units, and Related compounds.
  Caution: Etoposide is potentially cytotoxic. Great care should be taken to prevent inhaling particles of Etoposide and exposing the skin to it.
Etoposide Injection USP—Preserve in single-dose or in multiple-dose containers of Type I glass. Label it to indicate that it must be diluted with suitable parenteral vehicle prior to intravenous infusion. Contains the labeled amount, within ± 10%, in a sterile solution in a nonaqueous medium intended for dilution with a suitable parenteral vehicle prior to intravenous infusion. Meets the requirements for Identification, pH (3.0–4.0, in a solution prepared by diluting 5.0 mL with 45 mL of water), Bacterial endotoxins, Alcohol content (if present, the labeled amount, within ± 10%), Benzyl alcohol content (if present, the labeled amount, within ± 10%), and Related compounds, and for Injections.
Etoposide Phosphate for Injection—Not in *USP–NF*.

ETRETINATE

Source: Ethyl ester of an aromatic analog of retinoic acid.

Chemical group: Related to both retinoic acid and retinol (vitamin A).

Chemical name: 2,4,6,8-Nonatetraenoic acid, 9-(4-methoxy-2,3,6-trimethylphenyl)-, ethyl ester, (*all-E*-).

Molecular formula: $C_{23}H_{30}O_3$.

Molecular weight: 354.48.

Description: Greenish-yellow to yellow powder.

Solubility: Insoluble in water.

Other characteristics: Both etretinate and its pharmacologically active metabolite, acetretin (etretin), have an all-*trans* structure.

USP requirements: Etretinate Capsules—Not in *USP–NF*.

EUCALYPTOL

Chemical name: 1,3,3,-Trimethyl-2-oxabicyclo[2.2.2]octane.

Molecular formula: $C_{10}H_{18}O$.

Molecular weight: 154.25.

USP requirements: Eucalyptol USP—Preserve in tight containers. Obtained from oil of eucalyptus and from other sources. Contains not less than 98.0% and not more than 100% of eucalyptol. Meets the requirements for Identification, Specific gravity (0.921–0.924), Congealing temperature (not lower than 0 °C), Distilling range (174–177 °C), Angular rotation (−0.5° to +0.5°), Refractive index (1.455–1.460 at 20°), and Limit of phenols.

EUCATROPINE

Chemical name: Eucatropine hydrochloride—Benzeneacetic acid, alpha-hydroxy-, 1,2,2,6-tetramethyl-4-piperidinyl ester hydrochloride.

Molecular formula: Eucatropine hydrochloride—$C_{17}H_{25}NO_3 \cdot$ HCl.

Molecular weight: Eucatropine hydrochloride—327.85.

Description: Eucatropine Hydrochloride USP—White, granular, odorless powder. Its solutions are neutral to litmus.

Solubility: Eucatropine Hydrochloride USP—Very soluble in water; freely soluble in alcohol and in chloroform; insoluble in ether.

USP requirements:

Eucatropine Hydrochloride USP—Preserve in tight, light-resistant containers. Contains not less than 99.0% and not more than 100.5% of eucatropine hydrochloride, calculated on the dried basis. Meets the requirements for Identification, Melting range (183–186 °C), Loss on drying (not more than 0.5%), Residue on ignition (not more than 0.1%), and Organic volatile impurities.

Eucatropine Hydrochloride Ophthalmic Solution USP—Preserve in tight containers. A sterile, isotonic, aqueous solution of Eucatropine Hydrochloride. Contains the labeled amount, within ±5%. Meets the requirements for Identification, Sterility, and pH (4.0–5.0).

EUGENOL

Chemical name: Phenol, 2-methoxy-4-(2-propenyl)-.

Molecular formula: $C_{10}H_{12}O_2$.

Molecular weight: 164.20.

Description: Eugenol USP—Colorless or pale yellow liquid, having a strongly aromatic odor of clove. Upon exposure to air, it darkens and thickens. Is optically inactive.

Solubility: Eugenol USP—Slightly soluble in water. Miscible with alcohol, with chloroform, with ether, and with fixed oils.

USP requirements: Eugenol USP—Preserve in tight, light-resistant containers. Obtained from Clove Oil and from other sources. Meets the requirements for Solubility in 70% alcohol (1 volume dissolves in 2 volumes of 70% alcohol), Specific gravity (1.064–1.070), Distilling range (not less than 95% at 250–255 °C), Refractive index (1.540–1.542 at 20 °C), Heavy metals (not more than 0.004%), Hydrocarbons, and Limit of phenol.

EXEMESTANE

Chemical group: Steroidal aromatase inactivator.

Chemical name: 6-Methyleneandrosta-1,4-diene-3,17-dione.

Molecular formula: $C_{20}H_{24}O_2$.

Molecular weight: 296.40.

Description: White to slightly yellow crystalline powder.

Solubility: Freely soluble in N,N-dimethylformamide; soluble in methanol; practically insoluble in water.

USP requirements: Exemestane Tablets—Not in *USP–NF*.

EZETIMIBE

Chemical name: 2-Azetidinone, 1-(4-fluorophenyl)-3-[3-(4-fluorophenyl)-3-hydroxypropyl]-4-(4-hydroxyphenyl)-, [3R-[3 alpha 4(S^*), beta]]-.

Molecular formula: $C_{24}H_{21}F_2NO_3$.

Molecular weight: 409.40.

Description: White, crystalline powder. Melting point of about 163 °C. Stable at ambient temperature.

Solubility: Freely to very soluble in ethanol, methanol, and acetone; practically insoluble in water.

USP requirements: Ezetimibe Tablets—Not in *USP–NF*.

FACTOR VIIA

Source: Factor VIIa (rFVIIa) is cloned in baby hamster kidney cells (BHK cells) and secreted in its single-chain form into the culture medium (containing newborn calf serum). It is then proteolitically converted by autocatalysis to the active two-chain form (rFVIIa) in a chromatographic purification process. The purification process removes exogenous viruses, such as MuLV, SV40, Pox Virus, Reovirus, BEV, IBR virus. The production and formulation of factor VIIa does not use any human serum or proteins.

Molecular weight: 50K Dalton.

USP requirements: Factor VIIa (Recombinant)—Not in *USP–NF*.

FACTOR IX

USP requirements:

Factor IX Complex USP—Preserve in hermetic containers in a refrigerator. A sterile, freeze-dried powder consisting of partially purified Factor IX fraction, as well as concentrated Factors II, VII, and X fractions, of venous plasma obtained from healthy human donors. Contains no preservative. Label it with a warning that it is to be used within 4 hours after constitution, and to state that it is for intravenous administration and that a filter is to be used in the administration equipment. Meets the requirements of the test for potency in having within ±20% of the potency stated on the label in Factor IX Units by comparison with the U.S. Factor IX Standard or with a working reference that has been calibrated with it. Meets the requirement for Expiration date (not later than 2 years from the date of manufacture). Conforms to the regulations of the U.S. Food and Drug Administration concerning biologics.
Coagulation Factor IX (Human)—Not in *USP–NF*.
Coagulation Factor IX (Recombinant)—Not in *USP–NF*.

FAMCICLOVIR

Chemical name: 1,3-Propanediol, 2-[2-(2-amino-9*H*-purin-9-yl)ethyl]-, diacetate (ester).

Molecular formula: $C_{14}H_{19}N_5O_4$.

Molecular weight: 321.33.

Description: White to pale yellow solid.

Solubility: Freely soluble in acetone and in methanol; sparingly soluble in ethanol and in isopropanol.

USP requirements: Famciclovir Tablets—Not in *USP–NF*.

FAMOTIDINE

Chemical group: Thiazole derivative of histamine.

Chemical name: Propanimidamide, *N'*-(aminosulfonyl)-3-[[[2-[(diaminomethylene)amino]-4-thiazolyl]methyl]thio]-.

Molecular formula: $C_8H_{15}N_7O_2S_3$.

Molecular weight: 337.45.

Description: Famotidine USP—White to pale yellowish-white crystalline powder. Sensitive to light.

pKa: 7.1 in water at 25 °C.

Solubility: Famotidine USP—Freely soluble in dimethylformamide and in glacial acetic acid; slightly soluble in methanol; very slightly soluble in water; practically insoluble in acetone, in alcohol, in chloroform, in ether, and in ethyl acetate.

USP requirements:

Famotidine USP—Preserve in well-closed containers, protected from light. Contains not less than 98.5% and not more than 101.0% of famotidine, calculated on the dried basis. Meets the requirements for Identification, Loss on drying (not more than 0.5%), Residue on ignition (not more than 0.1%), Heavy metals (not more than 0.001%), Chromatographic purity, and Organic volatile impurities.
Famotidine Injection—Not in *USP–NF*.
Famotidine for Oral Suspension—Not in *USP–NF*.
Famotidine Tablets USP—Preserve in well-closed, light-resistant containers. Contain the labeled amount, within ±10%. Meet the requirements for Identification, Dissolution (75% in 30 minutes in 0.1 *M* phosphate buffer [pH 4.5] in Apparatus 2 at 50 rpm), and Uniformity of dosage units.
Famotidine Chewable Tablets—Not in *USP–NF*.
Famotidine Disintigrating Oral Tablets—Not in *USP–NF*.

HARD FAT

Description: Hard Fat NF—White mass; almost odorless and free from rancid odor; greasy to the touch. On warming, melts to give a colorless or slightly yellowish liquid. When the molten material is shaken with an equal quantity of hot water, a white emulsion is formed.

NF category: Stiffening agent; suppository base.

Solubility: Hard Fat NF—Practically insoluble in water; freely soluble in ether; slightly soluble in alcohol.

NF requirements: Hard Fat NF—Preserve in tight containers at a temperature that is 5 °C or more below the melting range stated in the labeling. A mixture of glycerides of saturated fatty acids. The labeling includes the nominal melting temperature, which is between 27 and 44 °C. Meets the requirements for Melting range (the melting temperature does not differ by more than 2° from the nominal value), Residue on ignition (not more than 0.05%), Acid value (not more than 1.0), Iodine value (not more than 7.0), Saponification value (215–255), Hydroxyl value (not more than 70), Unsaponifiable matter (not more than 3.0%), and Alkaline impurities.

FAT EMULSIONS

Source:

Egg phosphatides—A mixture of naturally occurring phospholipids which are isolated from the egg yolk.
Safflower oil—Refined fixed oil obtained from seeds of the safflower, or false (bastard) saffron, *Carthamus tinctorius* (Compositae).
Soybean oil—Obtained from soybeans by solvent extraction using petroleum hydrocarbons or, to a lesser extent, by expression using continuous screw press operations.

Chemical name:

Glycerin—1,2,3-Propanetriol.
Linoleic acid—(*Z,Z*)-9,12-Octadecadienoic acid.
Linolenic acid—(*Z,Z,Z*)-9,12,15-Octadecatrienoic acid.
Oleic acid—9-Octadecenoic acid, (*Z*)-.
Palmitic acid—Hexadecanoic acid.
Stearic acid—Octadecanoic acid.

Molecular formula:

Glycerin—$C_3H_8O_3$.
Linoleic acid—$C_{18}H_{32}O_2$.
Linolenic acid—$C_{18}H_{30}O_2$.
Oleic acid—$C_{18}H_{34}O_2$.
Palmitic acid—$C_{16}H_{32}O_2$.
Stearic acid—$C_{18}H_{36}O_2$.

Molecular weight:

Glycerin—92.09.
Linoleic acid—280.44.
Linolenic acid—278.42.
Oleic acid—282.46.

Palmitic acid—256.42.
Stearic acid—284.47.

Description:
Glycerin USP—Clear, colorless, syrupy liquid. Has not more than a slight characteristic odor, which is neither harsh nor disagreeable. Is hygroscopic. Its solutions are neutral to litmus.

NF category: Humectant; plasticizer; solvent; tonicity agent.

Linoleic acid—Colorless oil; easily oxidized by air; cannot be distilled without decomposition.

Linolenic acid—Colorless liquid.

Oleic Acid NF—Colorless to pale yellow, oily liquid when freshly prepared, but on exposure to air it gradually absorbs oxygen and darkens. It has a characteristic, lard-like odor. When strongly heated in air, it is decomposed with the production of acrid vapors.

NF category: Emulsifying and/or solubilizing agent.

Palmitic acid—White crystalline scales. Melting point 63–64 °C.

Safflower oil—Thickens and becomes rancid on prolonged exposure to air.

Soybean Oil USP—Clear, pale yellow, oily liquid having a characteristic odor.

NF category: Oleaginous vehicle.

Stearic Acid NF—Hard, white or faintly yellowish, somewhat glossy and crystalline solid, or white or yellowish white powder. Slight odor, suggesting tallow.

NF category: Emulsifying and/or solubilizing agent; tablet and/or capsule lubricant.

Solubility:
Glycerin USP—Miscible with water and with alcohol. Insoluble in chloroform, in ether, and in fixed and volatile oils.

Linoleic acid—Freely soluble in ether; soluble in absolute alcohol. One mL dissolves in 10 mL petroleum ether. Miscible with dimethylformamide, with fat solvents, and with oils.

Linolenic acid—Insoluble in water; soluble in organic solvents.

Oleic Acid NF—Practically insoluble in water. Miscible with alcohol, with chloroform, with ether, and with fixed and volatile oils.

Palmitic acid—Insoluble in water; sparingly soluble in cold alcohol or in petroleum ether; freely soluble in hot alcohol, in ether, in propyl alcohol, and in chloroform.

Safflower oil—Soluble in the usual oil and fat solvents.

Soybean Oil USP—Insoluble in water; miscible with ether and with chloroform.

Stearic Acid NF—Practically insoluble in water; freely soluble in chloroform and in ether; soluble in alcohol.

USP requirements: Fat Emulsions Injection—Not in *USP–NF*.

SHORT CHAIN FATTY ACID

Source: Produced by bacterial fermentation of dietary fiber.

USP requirements:
Short Chain Fatty Acid Enema—Not in *USP–NF*.
Short Chain Fatty Acid Solution—Not in *USP–NF*.

FELBAMATE

Chemical name: 1,3-Propanediol, 2-phenyl-, dicarbamate.

Molecular formula: $C_{11}H_{14}N_2O_4$.

Molecular weight: 238.24.

Description: White to off-white crystalline powder with a characteristic odor.

Solubility: Very slightly soluble in water; slightly soluble in ethanol; sparingly soluble in methanol; freely soluble in dimethyl sulfoxide.

USP requirements:
Felbamate Oral Suspension—Not in *USP–NF*.
Felbamate Tablets—Not in *USP–NF*.

FELODIPINE

Chemical group: Dihydropyridine derivative.

Chemical name: 3,5-Pyridinedicarboxylic acid, 4-(2,3-dichlorophenyl)-1,4-dihydro-2,6-dimethyl-, ethyl methyl ester, (±)-.

Molecular formula: $C_{18}H_{19}Cl_2NO_4$.

Molecular weight: 384.25.

Description: Light yellow to yellow, crystalline powder.

Solubility: Freely soluble in acetone and in methanol; very slightly soluble in heptane; insoluble in water.

USP requirements:
Felodipine USP—Preserve in tight, light-resistant containers, and store at controlled room temperature. Contains not less than 98.0% and not more than 101.0% of felodipine, calculated on the dried basis. Meets the requirements for Color of solution, Identification, Loss on drying (not more than 0.5%), Residue on ignition (not more than 0.1%), Heavy metals (0.002%), and Chromatographic purity.

Felodipine Extended-release Tablets USP—Preserve in tight containers. Contain the labeled amount of felodipine, within ±10%. Meet the requirements for Identification, Drug release (10–30% in 2 hours, 42–68% in 6 hours, and not less than 75% in 10 hours in 0.1 M phosphate buffer with 1% of sodium lauryl sulfate [pH 6.5]), Uniformity of dosage units, and Related compounds (not more than 2.0%).

FENBENDAZOLE

Chemical group: A benzimidazole structurally related to mebendazole.

Chemical name: Carbamic acid, [5-(phenylthio)-1*H*-benzimidazol-2-yl]-, methyl ester.

Molecular formula: $C_{15}H_{13}N_3O_2S$.

Molecular weight: 299.35.

Description: Light, brownish-gray, odorless crystalline powder with a melting point of 233 °C.

Solubility: Insoluble in water; insoluble or only very slightly soluble in the usual solvents; freely soluble in dimethylsulfoxide.

USP requirements:
Fenbendazole Granules—Not in *USP–NF*.
Fenbendazole Paste—Not in *USP–NF*.

FENFLURAMINE

Chemical group: Phenethylamine.

Chemical name: Fenfluramine hydrochloride—Benzeneethanamine, N-ethyl-alpha-methyl-3-(trifluoromethyl)-, hydrochloride.

Molecular formula: Fenfluramine hydrochloride—$C_{12}H_{16}F_3N \cdot$ HCl.

Molecular weight: Fenfluramine hydrochloride—267.72.

Description: Fenfluramine hydrochloride—White, odorless, or almost odorless, crystalline powder.

Solubility: Fenfluramine hydrochloride—Soluble 1 in 20 of water, 1 in 10 of alcohol, and 1 in 10 of chloroform; practically insoluble in ether.

USP requirements:
Fenfluramine Hydrochloride Extended-release Capsules—Not in *USP–NF*.
Fenfluramine Hydrochloride Tablets—Not in *USP–NF*.

FENNEL OIL

NF requirements: Fennel Oil NF—Preserve in tight containers. Volatile oil distilled with steam from the dried, ripe fruit of *Foeniculum vulgare* Mill. (Fam. Apiaceae). The label states the Latin binomial name and, following the official name, the part of the plant source from which the article was derived. The label also states that if solid material has separated, carefully warm Oil until it is completely liquefied, and mix before using. Meets the requirements for Solubility in 90% alcohol, Specific gravity (0.953–0.973), Congealing temperature (not lower than 3°), Angular rotation (+12° to +24°), Refractive index (1.528–1.538 at 20°), and Heavy metals (0.004%).

Note—If solid material has separated, carefully warm the Fennel Oil until it is completely liquefied, and mix before using.

FENOFIBRATE

Chemical name: Isopropyl 2-[p-(p-chlorobenzoyl)phenoxy]-2-methylpropionate.

Molecular formula: $C_{20}H_{21}ClO_4$.

Molecular weight: 360.83.

Description: A white solid with a melting point of 79 to 82 °C.

Solubility: Practically insoluble in water; slightly soluble in methanol and in ethanol; soluble in acetone, in ether, in benzene, and in chloroform.

USP requirements: Fenofibrate Micronized Capsules—Not in *USP–NF*.

FENOLDOPAM

Chemical name: Fenoldopam mesylate—1H-3-Benzazepine-7,8-diol, 6-chloro-2,3,4,5-tetrahydro-1-(4-hydroxyphenyl)-, methanesulfonate (salt).

Molecular formula: Fenoldopam mesylate—$C_{16}H_{16}ClNO_3 \cdot CH_4SO_3$.

Molecular weight: Fenoldopam mesylate—401.86.

Description: Fenoldopam Mesylate USP—White to off-white powder.

Solubility: Fenoldopam Mesylate USP—Soluble in water.

USP requirements:
Fenoldopam Mesylate USP—Preserve in tight containers, protected from moisture. Contains not less than 98.0% and not more than 102.0% of fenoldopam mesylate, calculated on the anhydrous basis. Meets the requirements for Identification, Water (not more than 1.0%), Residue on ignition (not more than 0.1%), Heavy metals (0.002%), Limit of iodide (not more than 0.2%), Related compounds, and Organic volatile impurities (not more than 0.2%).
Fenoldopam Mesylate Injection USP—Preserve in tight, single-dose Containers for Injection, preferably of Type I glass. Store in a refrigerator or at controlled room temperature. A sterile solution of Fenoldopam Mesylate. Contains the labeled amount, within ±10%. Meets the requirements for Identification, Bacterial endotoxins, Sterility, pH (2.8–3.8), Particulate matter, Related compunds (not more than 0.6%), and Content of sodium metabisulfite, and for Injections.

FENOPROFEN

Chemical group: Fenoprofen calcium—Arylacetic acid derivative.

Chemical name: Fenoprofen calcium—Benzeneacetic acid, alpha-methyl-3-phenoxy-, calcium salt dihydrate, (±)-.

Molecular formula: Fenoprofen calcium—$C_{30}H_{26}CaO_6 \cdot 2H_2O$.

Molecular weight: Fenoprofen calcium—558.63.

Description: Fenoprofen Calcium USP—White, crystalline powder.

pKa: Fenoprofen calcium—4.5 at 25 °C.

Solubility: Fenoprofen Calcium USP—Slightly soluble in n-hexanol, in methanol, and in water; practically insoluble in chloroform.

USP requirements:
Fenoprofen Calcium USP—Preserve in tight containers. Contains not less than 97.0% and not more than 103.0% of fenoprofen calcium, calculated on the anhydrous basis. Meets the requirements for Identification, Water (5.0–8.0%), Heavy metals (not more than 0.001%), Chromatographic purity, Organic volatile impurities, and Calcium content (7.3–8.0%, calculated on the anhydrous basis).
Fenoprofen Calcium Capsules USP—Preserve in well-closed containers. Contain an amount of fenoprofen calcium equivalent to the labeled amount of fenoprofen, within ± 10%. Meet the requirements for Identification, Dissolution (75% in 60 minutes in phosphate buffer [pH 7.0] in Apparatus 1 [10-mesh basket] at 100 rpm), and Uniformity of dosage units.
Fenoprofen Calcium Tablets USP—Preserve in well-closed containers. Contain an amount of fenoprofen calcium equivalent to the labeled amount of fenoprofen, within ± 10%. Meet the requirements for Identification, Dissolution (75% in 60 minutes in phosphate buffer [pH 7.0] in Apparatus 1 [10-mesh basket] at 100 rpm), and Uniformity of dosage units.

FENOTEROL

Chemical name: Fenoterol hydrobromide—1,3-Benzenediol, 5-[1-hydroxy-2-[[2-(4-hydroxyphenyl)-1-methylethyl]amino]ethyl]-, hydrobromide.

Molecular formula: Fenoterol hydrobromide—$C_{17}H_{21}NO_4 \cdot HBr$.

Molecular weight: Fenoterol hydrobromide—384.28.

Description: Fenoterol hydrobromide—White, odorless, crystalline powder. Melting point approximately 230 °C.

Solubility: Fenoterol hydrobromide—Soluble in water and in alcohol; practically insoluble in chloroform.

USP requirements:
Fenoterol Hydrobromide Inhalation Aerosol—Not in *USP–NF*.
Fenoterol Hydrobromide Inhalation Solution—Not in *USP–NF*.
Fenoterol Hydrobromide Tablets—Not in *USP–NF*.

FENTANYL

Chemical group: Fentanyl derivatives are anilinopiperidine-derivative opioid analgesics and are chemically related to anileridine and meperidine.

Chemical name:
Fentanyl—*N*-Phenyl-*N*-(1-2-phenylethyl-4-piperidyl) propanamide.
Fentanyl citrate—Propanamide, *N*-phenyl-*N*-[1-(2-phenylethyl)-4-piperidinyl]-, 2-hydroxy-1,2,3-propanetricarboxylate (1:1).

Molecular formula:
Fentanyl—$C_{22}H_{28}N_2O$.
Fentanyl citrate—$C_{22}H_{28}N_2O \cdot C_6H_8O_7$.

Molecular weight:
Fentanyl—336.5.
Fentanyl citrate—528.59.

Description: Fentanyl Citrate USP—White, crystalline powder or white, glistening crystals. Melts at about 150 °C, with decomposition.

pKa: 8.4.

Solubility: Fentanyl Citrate USP—Sparingly soluble in water; soluble in methanol; slightly soluble in chloroform.

Other characteristics: Fentanyl citrate—Partition coefficient (octanol:water): 816 at pH 7.4.

USP requirements:
Fentanyl Transmucosal Lozenges—Not in *USP–NF*.
Fentanyl Transdermal System—Not in *USP–NF*.
Fentanyl Citrate USP—Preserve in well-closed, light-resistant containers. Contains not less than 98.0% and not more than 102.0% of fentanyl citrate, calculated on the dried basis. Meets the requirements for Identification, Loss on drying (not more than 0.5%), Residue on ignition (not more than 0.5%), Heavy metals (not more than 0.002%), and Ordinary impurities.

Caution: Great care should be taken to prevent inhaling particles of Fentanyl Citrate and exposing the skin to it.
Fentanyl Citrate Injection USP—Preserve in single-dose containers, preferably of Type I glass, protected from light. A sterile solution of Fentanyl Citrate in Water for Injection. Contains the equivalent of the labeled amount of fentanyl, present as the citrate, within ±10%. Meets the requirements for Identification, Bacterial endotoxins, and pH (4.0–7.5), and for Injections.
Fentanyl Citrate Lozenges—Not in *USP–NF*.

FERRIC OXIDE

Molecular formula: Fe_2O_3.

Molecular weight: 159.69.

Description: Ferric Oxide NF—Powder exhibiting two basic colors (red and yellow) or other shades produced on blending the basic colors.
NF category: Color.

Solubility: Ferric Oxide NF—Insoluble in water and in organic solvents; dissolves in hydrochloric acid upon warming, a small amount of insoluble residue usually remaining.

NF requirements: Ferric Oxide NF—Preserve in well-closed containers. Contains not less than 97.0% and not more than 100.5% of ferric oxide, calculated on the ignited basis. Meets the requirements for Identification, Water-soluble substances (not more than 1.0%), Acid-insoluble substances (not more than 0.1%), Mercury (not more than 3 mcg per gram) Limit of arsenic (not more than 3 mcg per gram), Limit of lead (not more than 0.001%), and Organic colors and lakes.

FERRIC SUBSULFATE

Chemical name: Basic ferric sulfate solution.

Molecular formula: $Fe_4(OH)_2(SO_4)_5$.

Molecular weight: 737.71.

Description: Ferric Subsulfate Solution USP—Reddish brown liquid, odorless or nearly so. Acid to litmus, and is affected by light. Specific gravity is about 1.548.

USP requirements: Ferric Subsulfate Solution USP—Preserve Solution in tight, light-resistant containers, and store at temperatures above 22°. The label indicates that crystallization may occur if the Solution is exposed to temperatures below 22°, and that warming will redissolve the crystals. Label it to indicate that it is intended for topical and vaginal use only. Contains, in each 100 mL, basic ferric sulfate equivalent to not less than 20 grams and not more than 22 grams of iron (Fe). Ferric Subsulfate Solution may be prepared as follows. Add 55 mL of Sulfuric Acid to 800 mL of water in a porcelain dish, and heat to nearly 100°; then add 75 mL of nitric acid, and mix. Divide 1045 grams of Ferrous Sulfate, coarsely powdered, into 4 portions, and add these portions one at a time to the hot liquid, stirring after each addition until effervescence ceases. If, after the Ferrous Sulfate has dissolved, the solution has a black color, add nitric acid, a few drops at a time, with heating and stirring, until red fumes cease to be evolved. Boil the solution until it assumes a red color and is free from nitrate, as indicated by the test for *Limit of nitrate* below, maintaining the volume at about 1000 mL by the addition of water as needed. Cool, and add enough water to make the solution measure 1000 mL. Filter, if necessary, until the Solution is clear. Meets the requirements for Identification, Limit of nitrate, and Limit of ferrous salts.

FERRIC SULFATE

Chemical name: Ferric persulfate.

Molecular formula: $Fe_2(SO_4)_3 \cdot xH_2O$.

Molecular weight: 399.88 (anhydrous).

Description: Ferric Sulfate USP—Grayish white or yellowish powder or a fawn-colored pearls. Hygroscopic.

Solubility: Ferric Sulfate USP—Rapidly soluble in the presence of a trace of ferrous sulfate; slowly soluble in water; sparingly soluble in alcohol; practically insoluble in acetone and in ethyl acetate. Hydrolyzes slowly in aqueous solution.

USP requirements: Ferric Sulfate USP—Preserve in tight, light-resistant containers, and store at controlled room temperature. It is hydrated. Label it to indicate that it is intended for use in compounding topical and periodontal dosage forms only. Contains not less than 73.0% and not more than 80.0% of ferric sulfate. Meets the requirements for Identification, Limit of insoluble matter (not more than 0.02%), Limit of chloride (not more than 0.002%), Limit of ferrous iron (not more than 0.02% as Fe^{++}), Limit of copper and zinc (not more than 0.005%), Limit of nitrate (not more than 0.01%), and Substances not precipitated by ammonia (not more than 0.1%).

FERROUS CITRATE FE 59

Chemical name: 1,2,3-Propanetricarboxylic acid, 2-hydroxy-, iron(2+)-^{59}Fe salt.

Molecular formula: $C_{12}H_{10}{}^{59}Fe_3O_{14}$.

Description: Clear, slightly yellow solution.

USP requirements: Ferrous Citrate Fe 59 Injection—Not in *USP–NF*.

FERROUS FUMARATE

Chemical name: 2-Butenedioic acid, (*E*)-, iron(2+) salt.

Molecular formula: $C_4H_2FeO_4$.

Molecular weight: 169.90.

Description: Ferrous Fumarate USP—Reddish orange to red-brown, odorless powder. May contain soft lumps that produce a yellow streak when crushed.

Solubility: Ferrous Fumarate USP—Slightly soluble in water; very slightly soluble in alcohol. Its solubility in dilute hydrochloric acid is limited by the separation of fumaric acid.

USP requirements:
Ferrous Fumarate USP—Preserve in well-closed containers. Contains not less than 97.0% and not more than 101.0% of ferrous fumarate, calculated on the dried basis. Meets the requirements for Identification, Loss on drying (not more than 1.5%), Sulfate (not more than 0.2%), Arsenic (not more than 3 ppm), Limit of ferric iron (not more than 2.0%), Lead (not more than 0.001%), Mercury (not more than 3 mcg per gram), and Organic volatile impurities).
Ferrous Fumarate Capsules—Not in *USP–NF*.
Ferrous Fumarate Extended-release Capsules—Not in *USP–NF*.
Ferrous Fumarate Oral Solution—Not in *USP–NF*.
Ferrous Fumarate Oral Suspension—Not in *USP–NF*.
Ferrous Fumarate Tablets USP—Preserve in tight containers. Label the Tablets in terms of ferrous fumarate and in terms of elemental iron. Contain the labeled amount, within –5% to +10%. Meet the requirements for Identification, Dissolution (75% in 45 minutes in 0.1 *N* hydrochloric acid in 0.5% sodium lauryl sulfate in Apparatus 2 at 75 rpm), and Uniformity of dosage units.
Ferrous Fumarate Chewable Tablets—Not in *USP–NF*.

FERROUS FUMARATE AND DOCUSATE

For *Ferrous Fumarate* and *Docusate*—See individual listings for chemistry information.

USP requirements: Ferrous Fumarate and Docusate Sodium Extended-release Tablets USP—Preserve in well-closed containers. Label the Tablets in terms of the content of ferrous fumarate and in terms of the content of elemental iron. Contain the labeled amount of ferrous fumarate, within ±10%, and the labeled amount of docusate sodium, within –10% to +15%. Meet the requirement for Uniformity of dosage units.

FERROUS GLUCONATE

Chemical name: D-Gluconic acid, iron(2+) salt (2:1), dihydrate.

Molecular formula: $C_{12}H_{22}FeO_{14} \cdot 2H_2O$.

Molecular weight: 482.17.

Description: Ferrous Gluconate USP—Yellowish gray or pale greenish yellow, fine powder or granules, having a slight odor resembling that of burned sugar. Its solution (1 in 20) is acid to litmus.

Solubility: Ferrous Gluconate USP—Soluble in water, with slight heating; practically insoluble in alcohol.

USP requirements:
Ferrous Gluconate USP—Preserve in tight containers. Contains not less than 97.0% and not more than 102.0% of ferrous gluconate, calculated on the dried basis. Meets the requirements for Identification, Loss on drying (6.5–10.0%), Chloride (not more than 0.07%), Oxalic acid, Sulfate (not more than 0.1%), Arsenic (not more than 3 ppm), Limit of ferric iron (not more than 2.0%), Lead (not more than 0.001%), Mercury (not more than 3 ppm), Reducing sugars, and Organic volatile impurities.
Ferrous Gluconate Capsules USP—Preserve in tight containers. Label the Capsules in terms of the content of ferrous gluconate and in terms of the content of elemental iron. Contain the labeled amount, within ±7%. Meet the requirements for Identification, Dissolution (75% in 45 minutes in 0.1 *N* hydrochloric acid in Apparatus 1 at 100 rpm), and Uniformity of dosage units.
Ferrous Gluconate Elixir USP—Preserve in tight, light-resistant containers. Label the Elixir in terms of the content of ferrous gluconate and in terms of the content of elemental iron. Contains the labeled amount, within ±6%. Meets the requirements for Identification, pH (3.4–3.8), and Alcohol content (6.3–7.7%).
Ferrous Gluconate Oral Solution USP—Preserve in tight, light-resistant containers. Label the Elixir in terms of the content of ferrous gluconate and in terms of the content of elemental iron. Contains the labeled amount, within ± 6%. Meets the requirements for Identification, pH (3.4–3.8), and Alcohol content (6.3–7.7%).
Ferrous Gluconate Syrup—Not in *USP–NF*.
Ferrous Gluconate Tablets USP—Preserve in tight containers. Label the Tablets in terms of the content of ferrous gluconate and in terms of the content of elemental iron. Contain the labeled amount, within ±7%. Meet the requirements for Identification, Dissolution (80% in 80 minutes in simulated gastric fluid TS in Apparatus 2 at 150 rpm), and Uniformity of dosage units.
Ferrous Gluconate Extended-release Tablets—Not in *USP–NF*.

FERROUS SULFATE

Chemical name:
Ferrous sulfate—Sulfuric acid, iron(2+) salt (1:1), heptahydrate.
Ferrous sulfate, dried—Sulfuric acid, iron(2+) salt (1:1), hydrate.

Molecular formula:
Ferrous sulfate—$FeSO_4 \cdot 7H_2O$.
Ferrous sulfate, dried—$FeSO_4 \cdot xH_2O$.

Molecular weight:
Ferrous sulfate—278.02.
Ferrous sulfate, dried—151.91 (anhydrous).

Description:
Ferrous Sulfate USP—Pale, bluish green crystals or granules. Is odorless and efflorescent in dry air. Oxidizes readily in moist air to form brownish yellow basic ferric sulfate. Its solution (1 in 10) is acid to litmus, having a pH of about 3.7.
Dried Ferrous Sulfate USP—Grayish white to buff-colored powder, consisting primarily of $FeSO_4 \cdot H_2O$ with varying amounts of $FeSO_4 \cdot 4H_2O$.

Solubility:
Ferrous Sulfate USP—Freely soluble in water; very soluble in boiling water; insoluble in alcohol.
Dried Ferrous Sulfate USP—Slowly soluble in water; insoluble in alcohol.

USP requirements:
Ferrous Sulfate USP—Preserve in tight containers. Label it to indicate that it is not to be used if it is coated with brownish-yellow basic ferric sulfate. Contains an amount of anhydrous ferrous sulfate equivalent to not less than 99.5% and not more than 104.5% of ferrous sulfate heptahydrate. Meets the requirements for Identification, Arsenic (not more than 3 ppm), Lead (not more than 0.001%), Mercury (not more than 3 ppm), and Organic volatile impurities.
Ferrous Sulfate Capsules—Not in *USP–NF*.
Ferrous Sulfate (Dried) Capsules—Not in *USP–NF*.
Ferrous Sulfate (Dried) Extended-release Capsules—Not in *USP–NF*.
Ferrous Sulfate Elixir—Not in *USP–NF*.
Ferrous Sulfate Oral Solution USP—Preserve in tight, light-resistant containers. Label the Oral Solution in terms of the content of ferrous sulfate and in terms of the content of elemental iron. Contains the labeled amount, within ±6%. Meets the requirements for Identification and pH (1.4–5.3).
Ferrous Sulfate Syrup USP—Preserve in tight containers. Label Syrup in terms of the content of ferrous sulfate and in terms of the content of elemental iron. Contains, in each 100 mL, not less than 3.75 grams and not more than 4.25 grams of Ferrous Sulfate, equivalent to not less than 0.75 gram and not more than 0.85 gram of elemental iron.
Prepare Ferrous Sulfate Syrup as follows: 40 grams of Ferrous Sulfate, 2.1 grams of Citric Acid, hydrous, 2 mL of Peppermint Spirit, 825 grams of Sucrose, and a sufficient quantity of Purified Water, to make 1000 mL. Dissolve the Ferrous Sulfate, the Citric Acid, the Peppermint Spirit, and 200 grams of the Sucrose in 450 mL of Purified Water, and filter the solution until clear. Dissolve the remainder of the Sucrose in the clear filtrate, and add Purified Water to make 1000 mL. Mix, and filter, if necessary, through a pledget of cotton.
Meets the requirement for Identification.
Ferrous Sulfate Tablets USP—Preserve in tight containers. Label the Tablets in terms of ferrous sulfate and in terms of elemental iron. Contain the labeled amount, within −5% to +10%. Meet the requirements for Identification, Dissolution (75% in 45 minutes in 0.1 N hydrochloric acid in Apparatus 2 at 50 rpm), and Uniformity of dosage units.
Note: An equivalent amount of Dried Ferrous Sulfate may be used in place of ferrous sulfate heptahydrate in preparing Ferrous Sulfate Tablets.

Ferrous Sulfate (Dried) Tablets—Not in *USP–NF*.
Ferrous Sulfate Enteric-coated Tablets—Not in *USP–NF*.
Ferrous Sulfate Extended-release Tablets—Not in *USP–NF*.
Ferrous Sulfate (Dried) Extended-release Tablets—Not in *USP–NF*.
Dried Ferrous Sulfate USP—Preserve in well-closed containers. Contains not less than 86.0% and not more than 89.0% of anhydrous ferrous sulfate. Meets the requirements for Identification, Insoluble substances (not more than 0.05%), Arsenic (not more than 3 ppm), Lead (not more than 0.001%), Mercury (not more than 3 ppm), and Organic volatile impurities.

FERUMOXIDES

Source: Obtained from a reaction of ferric chloride and ferrous chloride in the presence of ammonia and dextran T-10.

Chemical group: A nonstoichiometric magnetite.

Chemical name: Iron oxide crystal is inverse spinel (X-ray data).

Molecular formula: $(Fe_2O_3)_m(FeO)_n$.

Description: Ferumoxides Injection USP—Black to reddish brown, aqueous colloid. Stable for 24 hours after dilution.

USP requirements: Ferumoxides Injection USP—Preserve in single-dose containers of Type I glass, at controlled room temperature. Avoid freezing. A sterile colloidal suspension of superparamagnetic iron oxide associated with dextran in Water for Injection. Label it to indicate that it is to be administered through a 5-micrometer filter and that it is not to be used if there are indications that the package has been exposed to freezing temperatures. Contains the labeled amount, within ± 5%. Contains, in each milliliter, not than 5.6 mg and not more than 9.1 mg of dextran and not less than 0.25 mg and not more than 0.53 mg of citrate. Also contains mannitol. Contains no antimicrobial agents. Ferumoxides is a nonstoichiometric iron oxide magnet of average formula $FeO_{1.44}$, with particles having a diameter between 100 and 250 nanometer. Meets the requirements for Identification, Specific gravity (1.031–1.041), Bacterial endotoxins, pH (5.0–9.0), Colloidal particle size, Magnetic susceptibility (not less than $17{,}100 \times 10^{-6}$ in cgs units per gram of iron), and Osmolality (325–365 mOsmol per kg), and for Injections (with the exception of Foreign matter and Particulate matter).

FERUMOXSIL

Source: Silicone polymer bonded to colloidal particles of superparamagnetic, nonstoichiometric magnetite.

Chemical name: Iron oxide crystal is inverse spinel (X-ray data).

USP requirements:
Ferumoxsil Injection—Not in *USP–NF*.
Ferumoxsil Oral Suspension USP—Preserve in tight containers, and store at controlled room temperature. An aqueous suspension of silicone-coated superparamagnetic iron oxide. Label it to indicate that it is to be well-shaken for one minute before use, and that it is not to be used if there are indications that the package has been exposed to freezing temperatures. Contains a labeled amount of iron, within ±10%. Contains a preservative and a thickening agent. May contain suitable colors, and sweetening agents. Ferumoxil is poly[N-(2-aminoethyl)-3-aminopropyl] siloxane-coated nonstichiometric magnetite [$FeO_x(C_5H_{13}N_2SiO_2)$]. Meets the requirements for Viscosity (11–60 centiposes), Osmolarity (230–270 mOsmol per kg), Microbial limits (not more than 100 per mL), pH

(5.5–9.0), Magnetic susceptibility (not less than 22,500 x 10^{-6} in cgs units per gram of iron), and Settling (not less than 80%).

FEVERFEW

NF requirements:

Feverfew NF—Preserve in well-closed containers, and store in a dry place, protected from light. The label states the Latin binomial name and, following the official name, the part of the plant contained in the article. Consists of the dried leaves of *Tanacetum parthenium* (Linné) Schultz-Bip. (Fam. Asteraceae), collected when the plant is in flower. Meets the requirements for Botanic characteristics, Identification, Total ash (not more than 12.0%), Acid-insoluble ash (not more than 3.0%), Water-soluble extractives (not less than 15.0%), Foreign organic matter (not more than 10.0%, including stalk), Pesticide residues, Heavy metals (not more than 0.002%), Loss on drying (not more than 10.0%), Microbial limits, and Content of parthenolide (not less than 0.2%).

Powdered Feverfew NF—Preserve in well-closed containers, protected from light and moisture. The label states the Latin binomial name and, following the official name, the part of the plant source from which the article was derived. Feverfew pulverized to a fine or very fine powder. Meets the requirements for Identification and for Total ash, Acid-insoluble ash, Water-soluble extractives, Pesticide residues, Heavy metals, Loss on drying, Microbial limits, and Content of parthenolide under Feverfew.

FEXOFENADINE

Chemical name: Fexofenadine hydrochloride—Benzeneacetic acid, 4-[1-hydroxy-4-[4-(hydroxydiphenylmethyl)-1-piperidinyl]butyl]-alpha,alpha-dimethyl-, hydrochloride, (±)-.

Molecular formula: Fexofenadine hydrochloride—$C_{32}H_{39}NO_4 \cdot$ HCl.

Molecular weight: Fexofenadine hydrochloride—538.12.

Description: Fexofenadine hydrochloride—White to off-white crystalline powder with a melting point of 142–143 °C.

Solubility: Fexofenadine hydrochloride—Freely soluble in methanol and in ethanol; slightly soluble in chloroform and in water; insoluble in hexane.

USP requirements:

Fexofenadine Tablets—Not in *USP–NF*.
Fexofenadine Hydrochloride Capsules—Not in *USP–NF*.

FEXOFENADINE AND PSEUDOEPHEDRINE

For *Fexofenadine* and *Pseudoephedrine*—See individual listings for chemistry information.

USP requirements: Fexofenadine Hydrochloride and Pseudoephedrine Hydrochloride Extended-release Tablets—Not in *USP–NF*.

FIBRIN SEALANT

Source: Insoluble plasma protein obtained by the action of thrombin on fibrinogen.

USP requirements: Fibrin Sealant for Solution—Not in *USP–NF*.

FILGRASTIM

Chemical name: Colony-stimulating factor (human clone 1034), *N*-L-methionyl-.

Molecular formula: $C_{845}H_{1339}N_{223}O_{243}S_9$.

Molecular weight: 18,800 daltons.

USP requirements: Filgrastim Injection—Not in *USP–NF*.

FINASTERIDE

Chemical name: 4-Azaandrost-1-ene-17-carboxamide, *N*-(1,1-dimethylethyl)-3-oxo, (5 alpha,17 beta)-.

Molecular formula: $C_{23}H_{36}N_2O_2$.

Molecular weight: 372.54.

Description: White to off-white crystalline solid. Melts at 257°.

Solubility: Freely soluble in chloroform and in alcohol; very slightly soluble in water.

USP requirements:

Finasteride USP—Preserve in tight containers, and store at controlled room temperature. Contains not less than 98.5% and not more than 101.0% of finasteride, calculated on the anhydrous basis. Meets the requirements for Identification, Specific rotation (−56.0° to −60.0°, determined at 405 nm), Water (not more than 0.3%), Residue on ignition (not more than 0.1%), Heavy metals (0.001%), and Chromatographic purity.

Finasteride Tablets USP—Preserve in tight, light-resistant containers, and store at controlled room temperature. Contain the labeled amount, within ±5%. Meet the requirements for Identification and Dissolution (75% in 45 minutes in water in Apparatus 2 at 50 rpm).

FLAVOXATE

Chemical name: Flavoxate hydrochloride—4*H*-1-Benzopyran-8-carboxylic acid, 3-methyl-4-oxo-2-phenyl-, 2-(1-piperidinyl)ethyl ester, hydrochloride.

Molecular formula: Flavoxate hydrochloride—$C_{24}H_{25}NO_4 \cdot$ HCl.

Molecular weight: Flavoxate hydrochloride—427.92.

Description: Flavoxate hydrochloride—Off-white, crystalline powder. Melts at about 230 °C, with decomposition.

Solubility: Flavoxate hydrochloride—One gram dissolves in 6 mL water or in 500 mL alcohol.

USP requirements: Flavoxate Hydrochloride Tablets—Not in *USP–NF*.

FLECAINIDE

Chemical name: Flecainide acetate—Benzamide, *N*-(2-piperidinylmethyl)-2,5-bis(2,2,2-trifluoroethoxy)-, monoacetate.

Molecular formula: Flecainide acetate—$C_{17}H_{20}F_6N_2O_3 \cdot C_2H_4O_2$.

Molecular weight: Flecainide acetate—474.39.

Description: Flecainide Acetate USP—White to slightly off-white crystalline powder.

pKa: Flecainide acetate—9.3.

Solubility: Flecainide Acetate USP—Freely soluble in alcohol; soluble in water.

USP requirements:
Flecainide Acetate USP—Preserve in well-closed containers. Contains not less than 98.0% and not more than 101.0% of flecainide acetate, calculated on the dried basis. Meets the requirements for Identification, Clarity of solution, Melting range (146–152 °C, the range between beginning and end of melting not more than 3 °C), Loss on drying (not more than 0.5%), Residue on ignition (not more than 0.2%), Heavy metals (not more than 0.002%), Chromatographic purity, and Content of acetate (12.4–12.8%, calculated on the dried basis).

Flecainide Acetate Tablets USP—Preserve in well-closed containers, protected from light. Contain the labeled amount, within ±10%. Meet the requirements for Identification, Dissolution (70% from 50-mg Tablets in 30 minutes or from 100-, 150-, or 200-mg Tablets in 60 minutes in 0.075 *N* hydrochloric acid in Apparatus 2 at 50 rpm), and Uniformity of dosage units.

FLOCTAFENINE

Chemical name: Benzoic acid, 2-[[8-(trifluoromethyl)-4-quinolinyl]amino]-, 2,3-dihydroxypropyl ester.

Molecular formula: $C_{20}H_{17}F_3N_2O_4$.

Molecular weight: 406.36.

Description: Melting point 179–180 °C.

Solubility: Soluble in alcohol and in acetone; very slightly soluble in ether, in chloroform, and in methylene chloride; insoluble in water.

USP requirements: Floctafenine Tablets—Not in *USP–NF*.

FLORFENICOL

Source: Fluorinated derivative of thiamphenicol.

Chemical name: Acetamide, 2,2-dichloro-*N*-[1-(fluoromethyl)-2-hydroxy-2-[4-(methylsulfonyl)phenyl]ethyl]-, [*R*-(*R**,*S**)]-.

Molecular formula: $C_{12}H_{14}Cl_2FNO_4S$.

Molecular weight: 358.21.

Description: Melting point 153–154 °C.

Solubility: Soluble in water.

USP requirements: Florfenicol Injection—Not in *USP–NF*.

FLOXURIDINE

Chemical group: A fluorinated pyrimidine derivative.

Chemical name: Uridine, 2'-deoxy-5-fluoro-.

Molecular formula: $C_9H_{11}FN_2O_5$.

Molecular weight: 246.19.

Description: White to off-white odorless solid.

Solubility: Freely soluble in water; soluble in alcohol.

Other characteristics: Hydrophilic.

USP requirements:
Floxuridine USP—Preserve in tight, light-resistant containers. Where it is intended for use in preparing injectable dosage forms, the label states that it is sterile or must be subjected for further processing during the preparation of injectable dosage forms. Contains not less than 98.5% and not more than 101.0% of floxuridine, calculated on the dried basis. Meets the requirements for Identification, Melting range (145–153 °C), Specific rotation (+36° to +39°), Loss on drying (not more than 0.2%), Residue on ignition (not more than 0.1%), Limit of fluoride ions (not more than 0.05%), and Heavy metals (not more than 0.002%), and for Sterile Solids under Injections and for Pyrogen under Floxuridine for Injection (where the label states that Floxuridine is sterile) and for Pyrogen under Floxuridine for Injection (where the label states that Floxuridine must be subjected to further processing during the preparation of injectable dosage forms).

Floxuridine for Injection USP—Preserve in Containers for Sterile Solids, protected from light. Store containers of constituted Floxuridine for Injection under refrigeration for not more than 2 weeks. It is lyophilized Floxuridine suitable for intraarterial infusion. Contains the labeled amount, within ±10%. Meets the requirements for Constituted solution, Identification, Pyrogen, Uniformity of dosage units, and pH (4.0–5.5 in a solution [1 in 50]), and Other requirements.

FLUCLOXACILLIN

Chemical name: (6*R*)-6-[3-(2-Chloro-6-fluorophenyl)-5-methylisoxazole-4-carboxamido]penicillanic acid.

Molecular formula:
Flucloxacillin—$C_{19}H_{17}ClFN_3O_5S$.
Flucloxacillin sodium—$C_{19}H_{16}ClFN_3NaO_5S \cdot H_2O$.

Molecular weight:
Flucloxacillin—453.9.
Flucloxacillin sodium—493.9.

Description: Flucloxacillin sodium—White or almost white crystalline hygroscopic powder.

Solubility: Flucloxacillin sodium—Soluble 1 in 1 of water and 1 in 2 of methyl alcohol; soluble in alcohol.

USP requirements:
Flucloxacillin for Oral Suspension—Not in *USP–NF*.
Flucloxacillin Sodium Capsules—Not in *USP–NF*.

FLUCONAZOLE

Chemical name: 1*H*-1,2,4-Triazole-1-ethanol, alpha-(2,4-difluorophenyl)-alpha-(1*H*-1,2,4-triazol-1-ylmethyl)-.

Molecular formula: $C_{13}H_{12}F_2N_6O$.

Molecular weight: 306.27.

Description: White crystalline solid.

Solubility: Slightly soluble in water and in saline.

USP requirements:
Fluconazole Capsules—Not in *USP–NF*.
Fluconazole Injection—Not in *USP–NF*.
Fluconazole for Oral Suspension—Not in *USP–NF*.
Fluconazole Tablets—Not in *USP–NF*.

FLUCYTOSINE

Chemical group: Fluorinated pyrimidine derivative; chemically related to fluorouracil and floxuridine.

Chemical name: Cytosine, 5-fluoro-.

Molecular formula: $C_4H_4FN_3O$.

Molecular weight: 129.09.

Description: Flucytosine USP—White to off-white, crystalline powder. Is odorless or has a slight odor.

Solubility: Flucytosine USP—Sparingly soluble in water; slightly soluble in alcohol; practically insoluble in chloroform and in ether.

USP requirements:
Flucytosine USP—Preserve in tight, light-resistant containers. Contains not less than 98.5% and not more than 101.0% of flucytosine, calculated on the dried basis. Meets the requirements for Identification, Loss on drying (not more than 1.5%), Residue on ignition (not more than 0.1%), Heavy metals (not more than 0.002%), Fluoride ions (not more than 0.05%), Fluorouracil (not more than 0.1%), and Organic volatile impurities.
Flucytosine Capsules USP—Preserve in tight, light-resistant containers. Contain the labeled amount, within ±10%. Meet the requirements for Identification, Dissolution (80% in 60 minutes in water in Apparatus 2 at 75 rpm), and Uniformity of dosage units.

FLUDARABINE

Chemical name: Fludarabine phosphate—9*H*-Purin-6-amine, 2-fluoro-9-(5-*O*-phosphono-beta-D-arabinofuranosyl)-.

Molecular formula: Fludarabine phosphate—$C_{10}H_{13}FN_5O_7P$.

Molecular weight: Fludarabine phosphate—365.21.

Description: Fludarabine Phosphate USP—White to off-white, crystalline, hygroscopic powder.

Solubility: Fludarabine Phosphate USP—Freely soluble in dimethylformamide; slightly soluble in water and in 0.1 M hydrochloric acid; practically insoluble in ethanol.

USP requirements:
Fludarabine Phosphate USP—Preserve in well-closed, light-resistant containers, and store in a refrigerator. Contains not less than 98.0% and not more than 102.0% of fludarabine phosphate, calculated on the anhydrous, solvent-free basis. Meets the requirements for Identification, Specific rotation (+10° to +14°), Microbial limits, Water (not more than 3.0%), Chloride (not more than 0.2%), Limit of ethanol (not more than 1.0%), Limit of free phosphate (0.1%), Limit of sodium (0.2%), Heavy metals (not more than 0.002%), and Chromatographic purity.

Caution—Fludarabine Phosphate is potentially cytotoxic. Great care should be taken to prevent inhaling particles and exposing the skin to it.
Fludarabine Phosphate for Injection USP—Preserve in containers for Sterile solids, as described under Injection, at 2° to 30°, or at controlled room temperature. Contains the labeled amount, within ±5%. Meets the requirements for Constituted solution, Identification, Water (not more than 5.0%), pH (7.2–8.2), Bacterial endotoxins, Sterility, Related compounds, and Uniformity of dosage units.
Caution—Fludarabine Phosphate is potentially cytotoxic. Great care should be taken to prevent inhaling particles and exposing the skin to it.

FLUDROCORTISONE

Chemical name: Fludrocortisone acetate—Pregn-4-ene-3,20-dione, 21-(acetyloxy)-9-fluoro-11,17-dihydroxy-, (11 beta)-.

Molecular formula: Fludrocortisone acetate—$C_{23}H_{31}FO_6$.

Molecular weight: Fludrocortisone acetate—422.49.

Description: Fludrocortisone Acetate USP—White to pale yellow crystals or crystalline powder. Is odorless or practically odorless. Is hygroscopic.

Solubility: Fludrocortisone Acetate USP—Insoluble in water; slightly soluble in ether; sparingly soluble in alcohol and in chloroform.

USP requirements:
Fludrocortisone Acetate USP—Preserve in well-closed containers, protected from light. Contains not less than 97.0% and not more than 103.0% of fludrocortisone acetate, calculated on the dried basis. Meets the requirements for Identification, Specific rotation (+126° to +138°), Loss on drying (not more than 3.0%), Residue on ignition (not more than 0.1%), Chromatographic purity, and Other impurities.
Fludrocortisone Acetate Tablets USP—Preserve in well-closed containers. Contain the labeled amount, within ± 10%. Meet the requirements for Identification, Dissolution (80% in 30 minutes in 0.01 N hydrochloric acid in Apparatus 2 at 75 rpm) and Uniformity of dosage units.

FLUMAZENIL

Chemical name: 4*H*-Imidazo[1,5-alpha][1,4]benzodiazepine-3-carboxylic acid, 8-fluoro-5,6-dihydro-5-methyl-6-oxo-, ethyl ester.

Molecular formula: $C_{15}H_{14}FN_3O_3$.

Molecular weight: 303.29.

Description: White to off-white crystalline compound.

Solubility: Insoluble in water; slightly soluble in acidic aqueous solutions.

Other characteristics: Octanol:buffer partition coefficient—14 to 1 at pH 7.4.

USP requirements: Flumazenil Injection—Not in *USP–NF*.

FLUMETHASONE

Chemical name: Flumethasone pivalate—Pregna-1,4-diene-3,20-dione, 21-(2,2-dimethyl-1-oxopropoxy)-6,9-difluoro-11,17-dihydroxy-16-methyl-, (6 alpha,11 beta,16 alpha)-.

Molecular formula: Flumethasone pivalate—$C_{27}H_{36}F_2O_6$.

Molecular weight: Flumethasone pivalate—494.57.

Description: Flumethasone Pivalate USP—White to off-white, crystalline powder.

Solubility: Flumethasone Pivalate USP—Insoluble in water; slightly soluble in methanol; very slightly soluble in chloroform and in methylene chloride.

USP requirements:
Flumethasone Pivalate USP—Preserve in tight, light-resistant containers. Contains not less than 97.0% and not more than 103.0% of flumethasone pivalate, calculated on the dried basis. Meets the requirements for Identification, Specific rotation (+71° to +82°), Loss on drying (not more than 1.0%), and Chromatographic purity.

Flumethasone Pivalate Cream USP—Preserve in collapsible tubes. Contains the labeled amount, within ±10%, in a suitable cream base. Meets the requirements for Identification, Microbial limits, and Minimum fill.

Flumethasone Pivalate Ointment—Not in *USP–NF*.

FLUNARIZINE

Chemical name: Flunarizine hydrochloride—Piperazine, 1-[bis(4-fluorophenyl)methyl]-4-(3-phenyl-2-propenyl)-, dihydrochloride, (*E*)-.

Molecular formula: Flunarizine hydrochloride—$C_{26}H_{26}F_2N_2 \cdot$ 2HCl.

Molecular weight: Flunarizine hydrochloride—477.42.

Description: White to pale cream colored powder.

Solubility: Soluble in dimethylsulfoxide, in polyethylene glycol (PEG) 400, in propylene glycol, in *N,N*-dimethylformamide, and in methanol; poorly soluble in water and in ethanol (0.1–1.0%).

USP requirements: Flunarizine Hydrochloride Capsules—Not in *USP–NF*.

FLUNISOLIDE

Chemical name: Pregna-1,4-diene-3,20-dione, 6-fluoro-11,21-dihydroxy-16,17-[(1-methylethylidene)bis(oxy)]-, hemihydrate, (6 alpha,11 beta,16 alpha)-.

Molecular formula: $C_{24}H_{31}FO_6 \cdot \frac{1}{2}H_2O$.

Molecular weight: 443.51; 434.51 (anhydrous).

Description: Flunisolide USP—White to creamy-white, crystalline powder. Melts at about 245 °C, with decomposition.

Solubility: Flunisolide USP—Practically insoluble in water; soluble in acetone; sparingly soluble in chloroform; slightly soluble in methanol.

USP requirements:
Flunisolide USP—Preserve in well-closed containers. Contains not less than 97.0% and not more than 102.0% of flunisolide, calculated on the anhydrous basis. Meets the requirements for Identification, Specific rotation (+103° to +111°), Loss on drying (not more than 1.0%), Water (not more than 1.0% for the anhydrous form and 1.8–2.5% for

the hemihydrate form [determined on a dried specimen]), Residue on ignition (not more than 0.1% from 250 mg), Chromatographic purity, and Organic volatile impurities.

Flunisolide Inhalation Aerosol—Not in *USP–NF*.

Flunisolide Nasal Solution USP—Preserve in tight containers, protected from light, at controlled room temperature. An aqueous, buffered solution of Flunisolide. It is supplied in a form suitable for nasal administration. Contains the labeled amount, within ±10%. Meets the requirements for Identification, pH (4.5–6.0), and Quantity delivered per spray (17–33 mcg).

FLUNIXIN

Chemical name: Flunixin meglumine—3-Pyridinecarboxylic acid, 2-[[2-methyl-3-(trifluoromethyl)phenyl]amino]-, compd. with 1-deoxy-1-(methylamino)-D-glucitol (1:1).

Molecular formula: Flunixin meglumine—$C_{14}H_{11}F_3N_2O_2 \cdot C_7H_{17}NO_5$.

Molecular weight: Flunixin meglumine—491.46.

Description: Flunixin Meglumine USP—White to off-white crystalline powder.

Solubility: Flunixin Meglumine USP—Soluble in water, in alcohol, and in methanol; practically insoluble in ethyl acetate.

USP requirements:
Flunixin Meglumine USP—Preserve in well-closed containers. Label it to indicate that it is for veterinary use only. Contains not less than 99.0% and not more than 101.0% of flunixin meglumine. Meets the requirements for Identification, Melting range (137–140 °C), pH (7.0–9.0, in a solution [1 in 20]), Loss on drying (not more than 0.5%), Specific rotation (−9° to −12°, calculated on the dried basis), Residue on ignition (not more than 0.2%), and Chromatographic purity.

Flunixin Meglumine Granules USP—Preserve in well-closed containers. Label Granules to indicate that they are for veterinary use only. Contain an amount of flunixin meglumine equivalent to the labeled amount of flunixin, within ±10%. Meet the requirements for Identification, Dissolution (75% in 30 minutes in 0.1 N hydrochloric acid in Apparatus 2 at 50 rpm), and Uniformity of dosage units.

Flunixin Meglumine Injection USP—Preserve in multiple-dose containers at controlled room temperature. A sterile solution of Flunixin Meglumine in Water for Injection. Label Injection to indicate that it is for veterinary use only. Contains an amount of flunixin meglumine equivalent to the labeled amount of flunixin, within ±10%. Meets the requirements for Identification, Bacterial endotoxins, Sterility, and pH (7.8–9.0).

Flunixin Meglumine Paste USP—Preserve in a well-closed container. Label the Paste to indicate that it is for veterinary use only. Contains an amount of flunixin meglumine equivalent to the labeled amount of flunixin, within ±10%. Meets the requirements for Identification and Microbial limits.

FLUOCINOLONE

Chemical name: Fluocinolone acetonide—Pregna-1,4-diene-3,20-dione, 6,9-difluoro-11,21-dihydroxy-16,17-[(1-methylethylidene)bis(oxy)]-, (6 alpha,11 beta,16 alpha)-.

Molecular formula: Fluocinolone acetonide—$C_{24}H_{30}F_2O_6$ (anhydrous); $C_{24}H_{30}F_2O_6 \cdot 2H_2O$ (dihydrate).

Molecular weight: Fluocinolone acetonide—452.49 (anhydrous); 488.53 (dihydrate).

Description: Fluocinolone Acetonide USP—White or practically white, odorless, crystalline powder. Is stable in air. Melts at about 270 °C, with decomposition.

Solubility: Fluocinolone Acetonide USP—Insoluble in water; soluble in methanol; slightly soluble in ether and in chloroform.

USP requirements:

Fluocinolone Acetonide USP—Preserve in well-closed containers. It is anhydrous or contains two molecules of water of hydration. Label it to indicate whether it is anhydrous or hydrous. Contains not less than 97.0% and not more than 102.0% of fluocinolone acetonide, calculated on the dried basis. Meets the requirements for Identification, Specific rotation (+98° to +108°), and Loss on drying (not more than 8.5%).

Fluocinolone Acetonide Cream USP—Preserve in collapsible tubes or in tight containers. Contains the labeled amount, within ±10%. Meets the requirements for Identification, Microbial limits, and Minimum fill.

Fluocinolone Acetonide Ointment USP—Preserve in collapsible tubes or in tight containers. Contains the labeled amount, within ±10%. Meets the requirements for Identification, Microbial limits, and Minimum fill.

Fluocinolone Acetonide Topical Solution USP—Preserve in tight containers. Contains the labeled amount, within ±10%. Meets the requirements for Identification and Microbial limits.

FLUOCINONIDE

Chemical name: Pregna-1,4-diene-3,20-dione, 21-(acetyloxy)-6,9-difluoro-11-hydroxy-16,17-[(1-methylethylidene)bis-(oxy)]-,(6 alpha,11 beta,16 alpha)-.

Molecular formula: $C_{26}H_{32}F_2O_7$.

Molecular weight: 494.52.

Description: Fluocinonide USP—White to cream-colored, crystalline powder, having not more than a slight odor.

Solubility: Fluocinonide USP—Practically insoluble in water; sparingly soluble in acetone and in chloroform; slightly soluble in alcohol, in methanol, and in dioxane; very slightly soluble in ether.

USP requirements:

Fluocinonide USP—Preserve in well-closed containers. Contains not less than 97.0% and not more than 103.0% of fluocinonide, calculated on the dried basis. Meets the requirements for Identification, Specific rotation (+81° to +89°), Loss on drying (not more than 1.0%), Residue on ignition (negligible, from 100 mg), and Chromatographic purity.

Fluocinonide Cream USP—Preserve in collapsible tubes or in tight containers. Contains the labeled amount, within ±10%. Meets the requirements for Identification, Microbial limits, and Minimum fill.

Fluocinonide Gel USP—Preserve in collapsible tubes or in tight containers. Contains the labeled amount, within ±10%. Meets the requirements for Identification and Minimum fill.

Fluocinonide Ointment USP—Preserve in collapsible tubes or in tight containers. Contains the labeled amount, within ±10%. Meets the requirements for Identification and Minimum fill.

Fluocinonide Topical Solution USP—Preserve in tight containers. Contains the labeled amount, within ±10%. Meets the requirements for Identification, Minimum fill, and Alcohol content (28.4–39.0%).

FLUOCINONIDE, PROCINONIDE, AND CIPROCINONIDE

Chemical name:

Fluocinonide—Pregna-1,4-diene-3,20-dione, 21-(acetyloxy)-6,9-difluoro-11-hydroxy-16,17-[(1-methylethylidene)bis(oxy)]-, (6 alpha,11 beta,16 alpha)-.

Procinonide—Pregna-1,4-diene-3,20-dione, 6,9-difluoro-11-hydroxy-16,17-[(1-methylethylidene)bis(oxy)]-21-(1-oxo-propoxy)-, (6 alpha,11 beta,16 alpha)-.

Ciprocinonide—Pregna-1,4-diene-3,20-dione, 21-[(cyclopropylcarbonyl)oxy]-6,9-difluoro-11-hydroxy-16,17-[(1-methylethylidene)bis(oxy)]-, (6 alpha,11 beta,16 alpha)-.

Molecular formula:

Fluocinonide—$C_{26}H_{32}F_2O_7$.

Procinonide—$C_{27}H_{34}F_2O_7$.

Ciprocinonide—$C_{28}H_{34}F_2O_7$.

Molecular weight:

Fluocinonide—494.52.

Procinonide—508.55.

Ciprocinonide—520.56.

Description: Fluocinonide USP—White to cream-colored, crystalline powder, having not more than a slight odor.

Solubility: Fluocinonide USP—Practically insoluble in water; sparingly soluble in acetone and in chloroform; slightly soluble in alcohol, in methanol, and in dioxane; very slightly soluble in ether.

USP requirements: Fluocinonide, Procinonide, and Ciprocinonide Cream—Not in *USP–NF*.

FLUORESCEIN

Chemical name:

Fluorescein—Spiro[isobenzofuran-1(3*H*),9'-[9*H*]xanthen]-3-one,3'6'-dihydroxy-.

Fluorescein sodium—Spiro[isobenzofuran-1(3*H*),9'-[9*H*]xanthene]-3-one, 3'6'-dihydroxy, disodium salt.

Molecular formula:

Fluorescein—$C_{20}H_{12}O_5$.

Fluorescein sodium—$C_{20}H_{10}Na_2O_5$.

Molecular weight:

Fluorescein—332.31.

Fluorescein sodium—376.27.

Description:

Fluorescein USP—Yellowish red to red, odorless powder.

Fluorescein Sodium USP—Orange-red, hygroscopic, odorless powder.

Fluorescein Sodium Ophthalmic Strip USP—Each Strip is a dry, white piece of paper, one end of which is rounded and is uniformly orange-red in color because of the fluorescein sodium impregnated in the paper.

Solubility:

Fluorescein USP—Insoluble in water; soluble in dilute alkali hydroxides.

Fluorescein Sodium USP—Freely soluble in water; sparingly soluble in alcohol.

USP requirements:

Fluorescein USP—Preserve in tight containers. Contains not less than 97.0% and not more than 102.0% of fluorescein, calculated on the anhydrous basis. Meets the requirements for Identification, Water (not more than 1.0%), Zinc, and Acriflavine.

Fluorescein Injection USP—Preserve in single-dose containers, preferably of Type I glass. A sterile solution, in Water for Injection, of Fluorescein prepared with the aid of Sodium Hydroxide. Contains the equivalent of the labeled amount of fluorescein sodium, within ±10%. Meets the requirements for Identification, Pyrogen, and pH (8.0–9.8), and for Injections.

Fluorescein Sodium USP—Preserve in tight containers. Contains not less than 90.0% and not more than 102.0% of fluorescein sodium, calculated on the anhydrous basis. Meets the requirements for Identification, Water (not more than 17.0%), Zinc, and Acriflavine.

Fluorescein Sodium Ophthalmic Strips USP—Package not more than 2 Strips in a single-unit container in such manner as to maintain sterility until the package is opened. Package individual packages in a second protective container. The label of the second protective container bears a statement that the contents may not be sterile if the individual package has been damaged or previously opened. The label states the amount of fluorescein sodium in each Strip. Contain the labeled amount, within +60%. Meet the requirements for Identification, Sterility, and Content uniformity (the labeled amount, within −15% to +75%).

FLUORESCEIN AND BENOXINATE

For *Fluorescein* and *Benoxinate*—See individual listings for chemistry information.

USP requirements: Fluorescein Sodium and Benoxinate Hydrochloride Ophthalmic Solution USP—Preserve in tight, light-resistant containers. A sterile aqueous solution of Fluorescein Sodium and Benoxinate Hydrochloride. Contains the labeled amounts, within −10% to +20%. Contains a suitable preservative. Meets the requirements for Identification, Sterility, and pH (4.3–5.3).

FLUORESCEIN AND PROPARACAINE

For *Fluorescein* and *Proparacaine*—See individual listings for chemistry information.

USP requirements: Fluorescein Sodium and Proparacaine Hydrochloride Ophthalmic Solution USP—Preserve in tight, light-resistant containers, preferably of Type I amber glass, and store in a refrigerator. A sterile aqueous solution of Fluorescein Sodium and Proparacaine Hydrochloride. Label it to state that it is to be stored in a refrigerator before and after the container is opened. Contains the labeled amounts, within ±10%. Contains a suitable preservative. Meets the requirements for Identification, Sterility, and pH (4.0–5.2).

FLUDEOXYGLUCOSE F 18

Source: Different methods are being used in the various clinical facilities for the on-site production of FDG injection. It can be prepared either by the electrophilic reaction of ^{18}F-enriched fluorine gas with 3,4,6-tri-O-acetyl-D-glucal or by the nucleophilic reaction of ^{18}F-labeled acetylhypofluorite with suitably protected D-mannopyranose. The fluorinated product is hydrolyzed with acid to give a mixture of 2-fluoro-2-deoxy-D-glucose and 2-fluoro-2-deoxy-D-mannose. Subsequently, it is purified by column chromatography and dissolved in an appropriate solvent, most commonly 0.9% saline. panel

Chemical group: D-glucose analog.

Chemical name: Alpha-D-glucopyranose, 2-deoxy-2-(fluoro-^{18}F)-.

Molecular formula: $C_6H_{11}{}^{18}FO_5$.

Molecular weight: 182. panelist

pKa: None between pH 1–13. panelist

Solubility: Very soluble in water. panelist

Other characteristics: Partition coefficient—Hydrocarbon:water (<0.001). panelist

USP requirements: Fludeoxyglucose F 18 Injection USP—Preserve in single-dose or in multiple-dose containers that are adequately shielded. A sterile, isotonic aqueous solution, suitable for intravenous administration, of 2-deoxy-2-[^{18}F]fluoro-D-glucose in which a portion of the molecules are labeled with radioactive ^{18}F. Label it to include the following, in addition to the information specified for Labeling under Injection: the time and date of calibration; the amount of ^{18}F as fludeoxyglucose expressed as total megabecquerels (or millicuries) per mL, at the time of calibration; the expiration date; the name and quantity of any added preservative or stabilizer; and the statement, "Caution, Radioactive Material." The labeling indicates that in making dosage calculations, correction is to be made for radioactive decay. The radioactive half-life of ^{18}F is 110 minutes. The label indicates "Do not use if cloudy or if it contains particulate matter." Contains the labeled amount of ^{18}F, within ± 10%, expressed in megabecquerels (or millicuries) per mL at the time indicated in the labeling. Meets the requirements for Specific activity (not less than 55 megabecquerels (1.5 mL per mg), 270 mCi per mmol), Radionuclide identification, Bacterial endotoxins, pH (4.5–8.5), Radiochemical purity, Isomeric purity, Radionuclidic purity, and Chemical purity, and for Injections (except that the Injection may be distributed or dispensed prior to completion of the test for Sterility, the latter test being started on the day following final manufacture).

SODIUM FLUORIDE F 18

USP requirements: Sodium Fluoride F 18 Injection USP—Preserve in single-dose or in multiple-dose containers that are adequately shielded. A sterile solution, suitable for intravenous administration, of sodium fluoride in isotonic Sodium Chloride Injection in which a portion of the molecules are labeled with radioactive ^{18}F. Label container to include the following, in addition to the information specified for Labeling under Injections: the time and date of calibration; the amount of ^{18}F as fluoride anion expressed as megabecquerels (or millicuries) per mL, at time of calibration; total activity at time of calibration; the expiration time and date; the name and quantity of any added preservative or stabilizer; and the statement "Caution—Radioactive Material." The labeling indicates that in making dosage calculations correction is to be made for radioactive decay and also indicates that the radioactive half-life of ^{18}F is 109.7 minutes. The label indicates "Do not use if cloudy or if it contains particulate matter." Contains the labeled amount of ^{18}F expressed in megabecquerels (or in millicuries) per mL at the time indicated in the labeling, within ±10%. Meets the requirements for Specific activity (not less than 37 megabecquerels [1 millicurie] per micromole at calibration time), Identification, Radionuclide identification, Bacterial endotoxins, Sterility, pH (4.5–8.0), Particulate matter, Heavy metals (not more than 5 ppm), Chemical purity, Radiochemical purity, and Radionuclide purity, and for Injections (except that

the Injection may be distributed or dispensed prior to completion of the test for Sterility, the latter test being started on the day of final manufacture, and except that it is not subject to the recommendation in Volume in Container under Injections).

FLUORODOPA F 18

Chemical name: L-Tyrosine, 2-(fluoro-^{18}F)-5-hydroxy-.

Molecular formula: $C_9H_{10}{}^{18}FNO_4$.

USP requirements: Fluorodopa F 18 Injection USP—Preserve in single-dose or in multiple-dose containers that are adequately shielded. A sterile, isotonic aqueous solution, suitable for intravenous administration of 6-[^{18}F]fluorolevodopa in which a portion of the molecules are labeled with radioactive ^{18}F. Label it to include the following, in addition to the information specified for Labeling under Injections: the time and date of calibration; the amount of ^{18}F as fluorodopa expressed as total megabecquerels (or millicuries) per mL, at time of calibration; the expiration time and date; the name and quantity of any added preservative or stabilizer; and the statement "Caution—Radioactive Material." The labeling indicates that in making dosage calculations correction is to be made for radioactive decay. The radioactive half-life of ^{18}F is 109.7 minutes. The label indicates "Do not use if cloudy or if it contains particulate matter." Contains the labeled amount of ^{18}F expressed in megabecquerels (or millicuries) per mL at the time indicated in the labeling, within ±10%. Meets the requirements for Specific activity (not less than 3.7×10^3 megabecquerels [100 millicuries] per mmol), Radionuclide identification, Bacterial endotoxins, pH (4.0–5.0), Radiochemical purity, Radionuclidic purity, Chemical purity, and Enantiomeric purity, and for Injections (except that the Injection may be distributed or dispensed prior to completion of the test for Sterility, the latter test being started within 24 hours of final manufacture, and except that it is not subject to the recommendation of Volume in Container).

FLUOROMETHOLONE

Chemical name:
   Fluorometholone—Pregna-1,4-diene-3,20-dione, 9-fluoro-11,17-dihydroxy-6-methyl-, (6 alpha,11 beta)-.
   Fluorometholone acetate—Pregna-1,4-diene-3,20-dione, 17-(acetyloxy)-9-fluoro-11-hydroxy-6-methyl-, (6 alpha,11 beta)-.

Molecular formula:
   Fluorometholone—$C_{22}H_{29}FO_4$.
   Fluorometholone acetate—$C_{24}H_{31}FO_5$.

Molecular weight:
   Fluorometholone—376.46.
   Fluorometholone acetate—418.50.

Description: Fluorometholone USP—White to yellowish white, odorless, crystalline powder. Melts at about 280 °C, with some decomposition.

Solubility: Fluorometholone USP—Practically insoluble in water; slightly soluble in alcohol; very slightly soluble in chloroform and in ether.

USP requirements:
   Fluorometholone USP—Preserve in tight, light-resistant containers. Contains not less than 97.0% and not more than 103.0% of fluorometholone, calculated on the dried basis. Meets the requirements for Identification, Specific rotation (+52° to +60°), Loss on drying (not more than 1.0%), and Residue on ignition (not more than 0.2%).

Fluorometholone Cream USP—Preserve in collapsible tubes. Contains the labeled amount, within ±10%. Meets the requirements for Identification, Microbial limits, and Minimum fill.
Fluorometholone Ophthalmic Ointment—Not in *USP–NF*.
Fluorometholone Ophthalmic Suspension USP—Preserve in tight containers. A sterile suspension of Fluorometholone in a suitable aqueous medium. Contains the labeled amount, within ±10%. Meets the requirements for Identification, Sterility, and pH (6.0–7.5).
Fluorometholone Acetate Ophthalmic Suspension—Not in *USP–NF*.

FLUOROURACIL

Chemical name: 2,4(1*H*,3*H*)-Pyrimidinedione, 5-fluoro-.

Molecular formula: $C_4H_3FN_2O_2$.

Molecular weight: 130.08.

Description: Fluorouracil USP—White to practically white, practically odorless, crystalline powder. Decomposes at about 282 °C.

pKa: 8.0 and 13.0.

Solubility: Fluorouracil USP—Sparingly soluble in water; slightly soluble in alcohol; practically insoluble in chloroform and in ether.

USP requirements:
   Fluorouracil USP—Preserve in tight, light-resistant containers. Contains not less than 98.0% and not more than 102.0% of fluorouracil, calculated on the dried basis. Meets the requirements for Identification, Loss on drying (not more than 0.5%), Residue on ignition (not more than 0.1%), Heavy metals (not more than 0.002%), and Content of fluorine (13.9–15.0%, calculated on the dried basis).
      Caution: Great care should be taken to prevent inhaling particles of Fluorouracil and exposing the skin to it.
   Fluorouracil Cream USP—Preserve in tight containers, at controlled room temperature. Contains the labeled amount, within ±10%. Meets the requirements for Identification, Microbial limits, and Minimum fill.
   Fluorouracil Injection USP—Preserve in single-dose containers, preferably of Type I glass, at controlled room temperature. Avoid freezing and exposure to light. A sterile solution of Fluorouracil in Water for Injection, prepared with the aid of Sodium Hydroxide. Label it to indicate the expiration date, which is not more than 24 months after date of manufacture. Contains, in each mL, not less than 45 mg and not more than 55 mg of fluorouracil. Meets the requirements for Identification, Bacterial endotoxins, and pH (8.6–9.4), and for Injections.
      Note: If a precipitate is formed as a result of exposure to low temperatures, redissolve it by heating to 60 °C with vigorous shaking, and allow to cool to body temperature prior to use.
   Fluorouracil Topical Solution USP—Preserve in tight containers, at controlled room temperature. Contains the labeled amount, within ±10%. Meets the requirements for Identification and Microbial limits.

FLUOXETINE

Chemical group: Cyclic, propylamine derivative. Chemically unrelated to tricyclic, tetracyclic, or other available antidepressants.

Chemical name:
Fluoxetine—Benzenepropanamine, *N*-methyl- gamma-[4-(tri-fluoromethyl)phenoxy]-, (±)-.
Fluoxetine hydrochloride—Benzenepropanamine, *N*-methyl-gamma-[4-(trifluoromethyl)phenoxy]-, hydrochloride, (±)-.

Molecular formula:
Fluoxetine—$C_{17}H_{18}F_3NO$.
Fluoxetine hydrochloride—$C_{17}H_{18}F_3NO \cdot HCl$.

Molecular weight:
Fluoxetine—309.33.
Fluoxetine hydrochloride—345.79.

Description: Fluoxetine Hydrochloride USP—White to off-white crystalline powder.

Solubility: Fluoxetine Hydrochloride USP—Sparingly soluble in water and in dichloromethane; freely soluble in alcohol and in methanol; practically insoluble in ether.

USP requirements:
Fluoxetine Capsules USP—Preserve in tight, light-resistant containers. Contain an amount of Fluoxetine Hydrochloride equivalent to the labeled amount of fluoxetine, within ± 10%. Meet the requirements for Identification, Uniform-ity of dosage units, Dissolution (80% in 30 minutes in water in Apparatus 2 at 50 rpm), and Chromatographic purity.
Fluoxetine Tablets USP—Preserve in tight containers, and store at controlled room temperature. Contain an amount of Fluoxetine Hydrochloride equivalent to the labeled amount of fluoxetine, within ±10%. Meet the requirements for Identification, Dissolution (80% in 15 minutes in 0.1 N hydrochloric acid in Apparatus 1 at 100 rpm), Uniformity of dosage units, and Chromatographic purity.
Fluoxetine Pulvules—Not in *USP–NF*.
Fluoxetine Hydrochloride USP—Preserve in tight containers. Contains not less than 98.0% and not more than 102.0% of fluoxetine hydrochloride, calculated on the anhydrous basis. Meets the requirements for Identification, Water (not more than 0.5%), Heavy metals (not more than 0.003%), Related compounds, and Organic volatile impurities.
Fluoxetine Hydrochloride Capsules—Not in *USP–NF*.
Fluoxetine Hydrochloride Oral Solution—Not in *USP–NF*.
Fluoxetine Hydrochloride Tablets—Not in *USP–NF*.

FLUOXYMESTERONE

Chemical group: Synthetic androgen; halogenated derivative of 17-alpha-methyltestosterone.

Chemical name: Androst-4-en-3-one, 9-fluoro-11,17-dihydroxy-17-methyl-, (11 beta,17 beta)-.

Molecular formula: $C_{20}H_{29}FO_3$.

Molecular weight: 336.44.

Description: Fluoxymesterone USP—White or practically white, odorless, crystalline powder. Melts at about 240 °C, with some decomposition.

Solubility: Fluoxymesterone USP—Practically insoluble in water; sparingly soluble in alcohol; slightly soluble in chloroform.

USP requirements:
Fluoxymesterone USP—Preserve in well-closed containers, protected from light. Contains not less than 97.0% and not more than 102.0% of fluoxymesterone, calculated on the dried basis. Meets the requirements for Identification, Specific rotation (+104° to +112°), Loss on drying (not more than 1.0%), Chromatographic purity, Organic volatile impurities, and Other impurities.

Fluoxymesterone Tablets USP—Preserve in well-closed containers, protected from light. Contain the labeled amount, within ±10%. Meet the requirements for Identification, Dissolution (70% in 60 minutes in 0.01 N hydrochloric acid in Apparatus 2 at 75 rpm), and Uniformity of dosage units.

FLUOXYMESTERONE AND ETHINYL ESTRADIOL

For *Fluoxymesterone* and *Ethinyl Estradiol*—See individual listings for chemistry information.

USP requirements: Fluoxymesterone and Ethinyl Estradiol Tablets—Not in *USP–NF*.

FLUPENTHIXOL

Chemical group: Thioxanthene.

Chemical name:
Flupenthixol decanoate—Cis-2-trifluoromethyl-9-(3-(4-(2-hydroxyethyl)-1-piperazinyl)-propylidene)-thioxanthene decanoate acid ester.
Flupenthixol dihydrochloride—2-Trifluoromethyl-9-(3-(4-(2-hydroxyethyl)-1-piperazinyl)-propylidene)-thioxanthene dihydrochloride.

Molecular formula:
Flupenthixol decanoate—$C_{33}H_{43}F_3N_2O_2S$.
Flupenthixol dihydrochloride—$C_{23}H_{25}F_3N_2OS \cdot lu$

Molecular weight:
Flupenthixol decanoate—588.8.
Flupenthixol dihydrochloride—507.4.

Description:
Flupenthixol decanoate—Yellow oil with a slight odor.
Flupenthixol dihydrochloride—White or yellowish white powder.

Solubility:
Flupenthixol decanoate—Very slightly soluble in water; soluble in alcohol; freely soluble in chloroform and in ether.
Flupenthixol dihydrochloride—Soluble in water and in alcohol.

Other characteristics: Structurally and pharmacologically similar to the piperazine phenothiazines, which are acetophenazine, fluphenazine, perphenazine, prochlorperazine, and trifluoperazine.

USP requirements:
Flupenthixol Decanoate Injection—Not in *USP–NF*.
Flupenthixol Dihydrochloride Tablets—Not in *USP–NF*.

FLUPHENAZINE

Chemical group: Trifluoromethyl phenothiazine derivative.

Chemical name:
Fluphenazine decanoate—2-{4-[3-(2-Trifluoromethylphe-nothiazin-10-yl)propyl]-piperazin-1-yl}ethyl decanoate.
Fluphenazine enanthate—Heptanoic acid, 2-[4-[3-[2-(trifluoro-methyl)-10*H*-phenothiazin-10-yl]propyl]-1-piperaziny-l]ethyl ester.
Fluphenazine hydrochloride—1-Piperazineethanol, 4-[3-[2-(trifluoromethyl)-10*H*-phenothiazin-10-yl]propyl]-, dihy-drochloride.

Molecular formula:
Fluphenazine decanoate—$C_{32}H_{44}F_3N_3O_2S$.
Fluphenazine enanthate—$C_{29}H_{38}F_3N_3O_2S$.
Fluphenazine hydrochloride—$C_{22}H_{26}F_3N_3OS \cdot 2HCl$.

Molecular weight:
Fluphenazine decanoate—591.8.
Fluphenazine enanthate—549.69.
Fluphenazine hydrochloride—510.44.

Description:
Fluphenazine decanoate—Pale yellow viscous liquid or a yellow crystalline oily solid with a faint ester-like odor.
Fluphenazine Enanthate USP—Pale yellow to yellow-orange, clear to slightly turbid, viscous liquid, having a characteristic odor; unstable in strong light, but stable to air at room temperature.
Fluphenazine Hydrochloride USP—White or nearly white, odorless, crystalline powder; melts, within a range of 5°, at a temperature above 225 °C.

Solubility:
Fluphenazine decanoate—Practically insoluble in water; miscible with dehydrated alcohol, with chloroform, and with ether; soluble in fixed oils.
Fluphenazine Enanthate USP—Insoluble in water; freely soluble in alcohol, in chloroform, and in ether.
Fluphenazine Hydrochloride USP—Freely soluble in water; slightly soluble in acetone, in alcohol, and in chloroform; practically insoluble in ether.

USP requirements:
Fluphenazine Decanoate USP—Preserve in tight, light-resistant containers. Contains not less than 98.0% and not more than 102.0% of fluphenazine decanoate, calculated on the dried basis. Meets the requirements for Identification, Loss on drying (not more than 1.0%), Residue on ignition (not more than 0.2%), and Ordinary impurities.
Fluphenazine Decanoate Injection USP—Preserve in single-dose or in multiple-dose containers, of Type I glass, protected from light. A sterile solution of Fluphenazine Decanoate in a suitable vegetable oil. Contains the labeled amount, within −10% to +15%. Meets the requirements for Identification and Chromatographic purity, and for Injections.
Fluphenazine Enanthate USP—Preserve in tight, light-resistant containers. Contains not less than 97.0% and not more than 103.0% of fluphenazine enanthate, calculated on the dried basis. Meets the requirements for Identification, Loss on drying (not more than 1.0%), Residue on ignition (not more than 0.2%), Heavy metals (not more than 0.003%), and Ordinary impurities.
Fluphenazine Enanthate Injection USP—Preserve in single-dose or in multiple-dose containers, preferably of Type I or Type III glass, protected from light. A sterile solution of Fluphenazine Enanthate in a suitable vegetable oil. Contains the labeled amount, within ±10%. Meets the requirements for Identification and for Injections.
Fluphenazine Hydrochloride USP—Preserve in tight, light-resistant containers. Contains not less than 97.0% and not more than 103.0% of fluphenazine hydrochloride, calculated on the dried basis. Meets the requirements for Identification, Loss on drying (not more than 1%), Residue on ignition (not more than 0.5%), Heavy metals (not more than 0.003%), Ordinary impurities, and Organic volatile impurities.
Fluphenazine Hydrochloride Elixir USP—Preserve in tight containers, protected from light. Contains the labeled amount, within ±10%. Meets the requirements for Identification, pH (5.3–5.8), and Alcohol content (within ±10% of the labeled amount, the labeled amount being not more than 15.0%).
Fluphenazine Hydrochloride Injection USP—Preserve in single-dose or in multiple-dose containers, preferably of Type I glass, protected from light. A sterile solution of Fluphenazine Hydrochloride in Water for Injection. Contains the labeled amount, within −5% to +10%. Meets the requirements for Identification, Bacterial endotoxins, and pH (4.8–5.2), and for Injections.
Fluphenazine Hydrochloride Oral Solution USP—Preserve in tight containers, protected from light. An aqueous solution of Fluphenazine Hydrochloride. Contains the labeled amount, within ±10%. Label it to indicate that it is to be diluted to appropriate strength with water or other suitable fluid prior to administration. Meets the requirements for Identification, pH (4.0–5.0), and Alcohol content (within ±10% of the labeled amount, the labeled amount being not more than 15.0%).
Fluphenazine Hydrochloride Tablets USP—Preserve in tight, light-resistant containers. Contain the labeled amount, within ±10%. Meet the requirements for Identification, Dissolution (75% in 45 minutes in 0.01 N hydrochloric acid in Apparatus 1 at 100 rpm), and Uniformity of dosage units.

FLURANDRENOLIDE

Chemical name: Pregn-4-ene-3,20-dione, 6-fluoro-11,21-dihydroxy-16,17-[(1-methylethylidene)bis(oxy)]-, (6 alpha,11 beta,16 alpha)-.

Molecular formula: $C_{24}H_{33}FO_6$.

Molecular weight: 436.51.

Description: Flurandrenolide USP—White to off-white, fluffy, crystalline powder. Is odorless.

Solubility: Flurandrenolide USP—Practically insoluble in water and in ether; freely soluble in chloroform; soluble in methanol; sparingly soluble in alcohol.

USP requirements:
Flurandrenolide USP—Preserve in tight containers in a cold place, protected from light. Contains not less than 97.0% and not more than 102.0% of flurandrenolide, calculated on the dried basis. Meets the requirements for Identification, Specific rotation (+145° to +153°), Loss on drying (not more than 1.0%), and Ordinary impurities.
Flurandrenolide Cream USP—Contains the labeled amount, within ±10%. Meets the requirements for Thin-layer chromatographic identification test, Microbial limits, and Minimum fill.
Flurandrenolide Lotion USP—Preserve in tight containers, protected from heat, light, and freezing. Contains the labeled amount, within ±10%. Meets the requirements for Identification, Microbial limits, Minimum fill, and pH (3.5–6.0).
Flurandrenolide Ointment USP—Contains the labeled amount, within ±10%. Meets the requirements for Identification, Microbial limits, and Minimum fill.
Flurandrenolide Tape USP—Preserve at controlled room temperature. A nonporous, pliable, adhesive-type tape having Flurandrenolide impregnated in the adhesive material, the adhesive material on one side being transported on a removable, protective slit-paper liner. Contains the labeled amount, within −20% to +25%. Meets the requirements for Identification and Microbial limits.

FLURAZEPAM

Chemical name:
Flurazepam hydrochloride—2H-1,4-Benzodiazepin-2-one, 7-chloro-1-[2-(diethylamino)ethyl]-5-(2-fluorophenyl)-1,3-dihydro-, dihydrochloride.

Flurazepam monohydrochloride—7-Chloro-1-(2-diethylami-
noethyl)-5-(2-fluorophenyl)-1,3-dihydro-1,4-benzodiaze-
pin-2-one hydrochloride.

Molecular formula:
Flurazepam hydrochloride—$C_{21}H_{23}ClFN_3O \cdot 2HCl$.
Flurazepam monohydrochloride—$C_{21}H_{23}ClFN_3O \cdot HCl$.

Molecular weight:
Flurazepam hydrochloride—460.80.
Flurazepam monohydrochloride—424.4.

Description:
Flurazepam Hydrochloride USP—Off-white to yellow, crystalline powder. Is odorless, or has a slight odor, and its solutions are acid to litmus. Melts at about 212 °C, with
decomposition.
Flurazepam monohydrochloride—White or almost white,
odorless or almost odorless crystalline powder.

Solubility:
Flurazepam Hydrochloride USP—Freely soluble in water and
in alcohol; slightly soluble in isopropyl alcohol and in
chloroform.
Flurazepam monohydrochloride—Very soluble in water; freely
soluble in alcohol; practically insoluble in ether.

USP requirements:
Flurazepam Hydrochloride USP—Preserve in tight, light-resistant containers. Contains not less than 99.0% and not
more than 101.0% of flurazepam hydrochloride, calculated on the dried basis. Meets the requirements for Identification, Water (not more than 0.5%), Residue on ignition
(not more than 0.1%), Heavy metals (not more than
0.002%), Limit of fluoride ion (not more than 0.05%), Related compounds, and Organic volatile impurities.
Flurazepam Hydrochloride Capsules USP—Preserve in tight,
light-resistant containers. Contain the labeled amount,
within ±10%. Meet the requirements for Identification, Dissolution (75% in 20 minutes in 0.01 N hydrochloric acid in
Apparatus 1 at 100 rpm), and Uniformity of dosage units.
Flurazepam Monohydrochloride Tablets—Not in *USP–NF*.

FLURBIPROFEN

Chemical group: A phenylalkanoic acid derivative chemically related to fenoprofen, ibuprofen, ketoprofen, naproxen, and tiaprofenic acid.

Chemical name:
Flurbiprofen—[1,1′-Biphenyl]-4-acetic acid, 2-fluoro-alpha-
methyl-, (±)-.
Flurbiprofen sodium—[1,1′-Biphenyl]-4-acetic acid, 2-fluoro-
alpha-methyl, sodium salt dihydrate, (±)-.

Molecular formula:
Flurbiprofen—$C_{15}H_{13}FO_2$.
Flurbiprofen sodium—$C_{15}H_{12}FNaO_2 \cdot 2H_2O$.

Molecular weight:
Flurbiprofen—244.26.
Flurbiprofen sodium—302.27.

Description: Flurbiprofen USP—White crystalline powder.

pKa: 4.22.

Solubility: Flurbiprofen USP—Freely soluble in acetone, in dehydrated alcohol, in ether, and in methanol; soluble in acetonitrile; practically insoluble in water. Optically inactive (1 in 50
solution in dehydrated alcohol).

Other characteristics: Acidic.

USP requirements:
Flurbiprofen USP—Preserve in tight containers. Contains not
less than 99.0% and not more than 100.5% of flurbiprofen,
calculated on the dried basis. Meets the requirements for

Identification, Melting range (114–117 °C), Loss on drying
(not more than 0.5%), Residue on ignition (not more than
0.1%), Heavy metals (not more than 0.001%), and Related
compounds.
Flurbiprofen Extended-release Capsules—Not in *USP–NF*.
Flurbiprofen Tablets USP—Preserve in well-closed containers. Contain the labeled amount, within ±10%. Meet the
requirements for Identification, Dissolution (75% in 45 minutes in phosphate buffer [pH 7.2] in Apparatus 2 at 50
rpm), and Uniformity of dosage units.
Flurbiprofen Sodium USP—Preserve in well-closed containers. Contains not less than 97.0% and not more than
103.0% of flurbiprofen sodium. Meets the requirements
for Identification, Specific rotation (−0.45° to +0.45°), Loss
on drying (11.3–12.5%), Heavy metals (not more than
0.001%), Limit of flurbiprofen related compound A (not
more than 1.5%), and Organic volatile impurities.
Flurbiprofen Sodium Ophthalmic Solution USP—Preserve in
tight containers. Contains the labeled amount of flurbiprofen sodium, within ±10%. Meets the requirements for
Identification, pH (6.0–7.0), Antimicrobial preservatives—
Effectiveness, and Sterility.

FLUSPIRILENE

Chemical name: 1,3,8-Triazaspiro[4.5]decan-4-one, 8-[4,4-
bis(4-fluorophenyl)butyl]-1-phenyl-.

Molecular formula: $C_{29}H_{31}F_2N_3O$.

Molecular weight: 475.57.

Description: White to yellowish amorphous or crystalline solid
with a melting point of 187.5–190 °C.

Solubility: Soluble in water (0.015–0.020 mg/mL).

USP requirements: Fluspirilene Injection—Not in *USP–NF*.

FLUTAMIDE

Chemical name: Propanamide, 2-methyl-N-[4-nitro-3-(trifluoromethyl)phenyl]-.

Molecular formula: $C_{11}H_{11}F_3N_2O_3$.

Molecular weight: 276.21.

Description: Flutamide USP—Pale yellow, crystalline powder.

Solubility: Flutamide USP—Freely soluble in acetone, in ethyl
acetate, and in methanol; soluble in chloroform and in ether;
practically insoluble in mineral oil, in petroleum ether, and in
water.

USP requirements:
Flutamide USP—Preserve in tight, light-resistant containers.
Contains not less than 98.0% and not more than 101.0%
of flutamide, calculated on the dried basis. Meets the requirements for Identification, Melting range (110–114 °C,
range between beginning and end of melting not more
than 2 °C), Loss on drying (not more than 1.0%), Residue
on ignition (not more than 0.1%), Heavy metals (not more
than 10 ppm), and Chromatographic purity.
Flutamide Capsules USP—Preserve in well-closed, light-resistant containers. Contain the labeled amount, within ±
7%. Meet the requirements for Identification, Dissolution
(75% in 60 minutes in 2% sodium lauryl sulfate solution
in Apparatus 2 at 75 rpm), and Uniformity of dosage units.
Flutamide Tablets—Not in *USP–NF*.

FLUTICASONE

Chemical name: Fluticasone propionate—Androsta-1,4-diene-17-carbothioic acid, 6,9-difluoro-11-hydroxy-16-methyl-3-oxo-17-(1-oxopropoxy)-, (6 alpha,11 beta,16 alpha,17 alpha)-*S*-(fluoromethyl) ester.

Molecular formula: Fluticasone propionate—$C_{25}H_{31}F_3O_5S$.

Molecular weight: Fluticasone propionate—500.57.

Description: Fluticasone propionate—White to off-white powder.

Solubility: Fluticasone propionate—Insoluble in water; freely soluble in dimethyl sulfoxide and in dimethylformamide; slightly soluble in methanol and in 95% ethanol.

USP requirements:
Fluticasone Propionate Inhalation Aerosol—Not in *USP–NF*.
Fluticasone Propionate Cream—Not in *USP–NF*.
Fluticasone Propionate Ointment—Not in *USP–NF*.
Fluticasone Propionate Powder for Inhalation—Not in *USP–NF*.
Fluticasone Propionate Nasal Suspension—Not in *USP–NF*.

FLUVASTATIN

Chemical name: Fluvastatin sodium—6-Heptenoic acid, 7-[3-(4-fluorophenyl)-1-(1-methylethyl)-1*H*-indol-2-yl]-3,5-dihydroxy-, monosodium salt, [*R**, *S**-(*E*)]-(±)-.

Molecular formula: Fluvastatin sodium—$C_{24}H_{25}FNNaO_4$.

Molecular weight: Fluvastatin sodium—433.45.

Description: Fluvastatin sodium—White to pale yellow, hygroscopic powder.

Solubility: Fluvastatin sodium—Soluble in water, in ethanol, and in methanol.

USP requirements: Fluvastatin Sodium Capsules—Not in *USP–NF*.

FLUVOXAMINE

Chemical name: Fluvoxamine maleate—1-Pentanone, 5-methoxy-1-[4-(trifluoromethyl)phenyl]-, *O*-(2-aminoethyl)oxime, (*E*)-, (*Z*)-2-butenedioate (1:1).

Molecular formula: Fluvoxamine maleate—$C_{15}H_{21}F_3N_2O_2 \cdot C_4H_4O_4$.

Molecular weight: Fluvoxamine maleate—434.41

Description: Fluvoxamine maleate—White or off-white, odorless, crystalline powder.

Solubility: Fluvoxamine maleate—Sparingly soluble in water; freely soluble in ethanol and in chloroform; practically insoluble in diethyl ether.

USP requirements: Fluvoxamine Maleate Tablets—Not in *USP–NF*.

FOLIC ACID

Chemical name: L-Glutamic acid, *N*-[4-[[(2-amino-1,4-dihydro-4-oxo-6-pteridinyl)methyl]amino]benzoyl]-.

Molecular formula: $C_{19}H_{19}N_7O_6$.

Molecular weight: 441.40.

Description:
Folic Acid USP—Yellow, yellow-brownish, or yellowish orange, odorless, crystalline powder.
Folic Acid Injection USP—Clear, yellow to orange-yellow, alkaline liquid.

Solubility:
Folic Acid USP—Very slightly soluble in water; insoluble in alcohol, in acetone, in chloroform, and in ether; readily dissolves in dilute solutions of alkali hydroxides and carbonates, and is soluble in hot, 3 *N* hydrochloric acid and in hot, 2 *N* sulfuric acid. Soluble in hydrochloric acid and in sulfuric acid, yielding very pale yellow solutions.

USP requirements:
Folic Acid USP—Preserve in well-closed, light-resistant containers. Contains not less than 97.0% and not more than 102.0% of folic acid, calculated on the anhydrous basis. Meets the requirements for Identification, Water (not more than 8.5%), Residue on ignition (not more than 0.3%), Chromatographic purity, and Organic volatile impurities.
Folic Acid Injection USP—Preserve in single-dose or in multiple-dose containers, preferably of Type I glass, protected from light. A sterile solution of Folic Acid in Water for Injection prepared with the aid of Sodium Hydroxide or Sodium Carbonate. Contains the labeled amount of folic acid, within −5% to +10%. Meets the requirements for Identification, Bacterial endotoxins, and pH (8.0–11.0), and for Injections.
Folic Acid Tablets USP—Preserve in well-closed containers. Contain the labeled amount of folic acid, within −10% to +15%. Meet the requirements for Identification, Dissolution (75% in 45 minutes in water in Apparatus 2 at 50 rpm), and Uniformity of dosage units.

FOLLITROPIN ALFA

Chemical name: Follicle-stimulating hormone, glycoform alpha.

Molecular formula: $C_{437}H_{682}N_{122}O_{134}S_{13}$ (alpha-subunit); $C_{538}H_{833}N_{145}O_{171}S_{13}$ (beta-subunit).

Molecular weight: 10,205.69 (alpha-subunit); 12,485.10 (beta-subunit).

USP requirements: Follitropin Alfa for Injection—Not in *USP–NF*.

FOLLITROPIN BETA

Chemical name: Follicle-stimulating hormone, glycoform beta.

Molecular formula: $C_{437}H_{682}N_{122}O_{134}S_{13}$ (alpha-subunit); $C_{538}H_{833}N_{145}O_{171}S_{13}$ (beta-subunit).

Molecular weight: 10,205.69 (alpha-subunit); 12,485.10 (beta-subunit).

USP requirements: Follitropin Beta for Injection—Not in *USP–NF*.

FOMEPIZOLE

Chemical name: 1*H*-Pyrazole, 4-methyl-.

Molecular formula: $C_4H_6N_2$.

Molecular weight: 82.10.

Description: Melts at 15.5 to 18.5 °C.

Solubility: Soluble in water and in alcohol.

USP requirements: Fomepizole Injection—Not in *USP–NF*.

FOMIVIRSEN

Chemical group: Phosphorothioate oligonucleotide.

Chemical name: Fomivirsen sodium—Deoxyribonucleic acid d(*P*-thio)(G-C-G-T-T-T-G-C-T-C-T-T-C-T-T-C-T-T-G-C-G), eicosasodium salt.

Molecular formula: Fomivirsen sodium—$C_{204}H_{243}N_{63}Na_{20}$-$O_{114}P_{20}S_{20}$.

Molecular weight: Fomivirsen sodium—7122.16.

Description: Fomivirsen sodium—White to off-white, hygroscopic, amorphous powder.

USP requirements: Fomivirsen Sodium Intravitreal Injection—Not in *USP–NF*.

FONDAPARINUX SODIUM

Chemical name: Methyl O-2-deoxy-6-O-sulfo-2-(sulfoamino)-alpha-D-glucopyranosyl-(1→4)-O-beta-D-glucopyranuronosyl-(1→4)-O-2-deoxy-3,6-di-O-sulfo-2-(sulfoamino)-alpha-D-glucopyranosyl-(1→4)-O-2-O-sulfo-alpha-L-idopyranuronosyl-(1→4)-2-deoxy-6-O-sulfo-2-(sulfoamino)-alpha-D-glucopyranoside, decasodium salt.

Molecular formula: $C_{31}H_{43}N_3Na_{10}O_{49}S_8$.

Molecular weight: 1728.

Other characteristics: pH: 5.0–8.0.

USP requirements: Fondaparinux Sodium Injection—Not in *USP–NF*.

FORMALDEHYDE

Chemical name: Formaldehyde.

Molecular formula: CH_2O.

Molecular weight: 30.03.

Description: Formaldehyde Solution USP—Clear, colorless or practically colorless liquid, having a pungent odor. The vapor from it irritates the mucous membrane of the throat and nose. On long standing, especially in the cold, it may become cloudy because of the separation of paraformaldehyde. This cloudiness disappears when the solution is warmed.

Solubility: Formaldehyde Solution USP—Miscible with water and with alcohol.

USP requirements: Formaldehyde Solution USP—Preserve in tight containers, preferably at a temperature not below 15 °C. The label of bulk containers of the Solution directs the drug repackager to demonstrate compliance with the USP *Assay* limit for formaldehyde of not less than 37.0%, by weight, immediately prior to repackaging. In bulk containers, contains not less than 37.0%, by weight, of formaldehyde, with methanol added to prevent polymerization. In small containers (4 liters or less), contains not less than 36.5%, by weight, of formaldehyde, with methanol present to prevent polymerization. Meets the requirements for Identification and Acidity.

FORMOTEROL

Chemical name:

Formoterol fumarate—(±)-(*R*,R**)-*N*-[2-Hydroxy-5-[1-hydroxy-2-[[2-(4-methoxyphenyl)-1-methylethyl]amino]ethyl]phenyl]formamide (*E*)-2-butenedioate (2:1) (salt).

Formoterol fumarate dihydrate—(*R*,R**)-(±)-*N*-[2-Hydroxy-5-[1-hydroxy-2-[[2-(4-methoxyphenyl)-1-methylethyl]amino]ethyl]phenyl]formamide (*E*)-2-butenedioate (2:1) dihydrate.

Molecular formula:

Formoterol fumarate—$(C_{19}H_{24}N_2O_4)_2 \cdot C_4H_4O_4$.

Formoterol fumarate dihydrate—$C_{42}H_{56}N_4O_{14}$.

Molecular weight:

Formoterol fumarate—804.88.

Formoterol fumarate dihydrate—840.9.

Description:

Formoterol fumarate—Odorless, white to yellowish crystalline powder. Melts at approximately 138 °C with decomposition.

Formoterol fumarate dihydrate—White to off-white or slightly yellow non-hygroscopic crystalline powder.

pKa:

Formoterol fumarate—7.82, 8.54.

Formoterol fumarate dihydrate—7.9 (phenolic group), 9.2 (amino group), at 25 °C.

Solubility: Formoterol fumarate—Soluble in 149 mg per mL glacial acetic acid, in 73.5 mg per mL methanol, in 4.88 mg per mL absolute ethanol, and in 0.980 mg per mL water.

Other characteristics: Formoterol fumarate dihydrate—Partition coefficient: The octanol-water partition coefficient at 25 °C is 2–6.

USP requirements:

Formoterol Fumarate Capsules for Inhalation—Not in *USP–NF*.

Formoterol Fumarate Dihydrate Powder for Inhalation—Not in *USP–NF*.

FOSCARNET

Chemical group: Pyrophosphate analog.

Chemical name: Foscarnet sodium—Phosphinecarboxylic acid, dihydroxy-, oxide, trisodium salt.

Molecular formula:

Foscarnet sodium—CNa_3O_5P.

Foscarnet sodium hexahydrate—$Na_3CO_5P \cdot 6H_2O$.

Molecular weight:

Foscarnet sodium—191.95.

Foscarnet sodium hexahydrate—300.1.

Description:

Foscarnet sodium—White, crystalline powder.

Foscarnet sodium injection—Clear and colorless solution.

Solubility: Foscarnet sodium—Soluble in water at pH 7 and 25 °C (about 5% w/w).

Other characteristics: Foscarnet sodium injection—pH is 7.4.

USP requirements: Foscarnet Sodium Injection—Not in *USP–NF*.

FOSFOMYCIN

Chemical name: Fosfomycin tromethamine—Phosphonic acid, (3-methyloxiranyl)-, (*2R-cis*)-, compd. with 2-amino-2-(hydroxymethyl-1,3-propanediol (1:1).

Molecular formula: Fosfomycin tromethamine—$C_3H_7O_4P \cdot C_4H_{11}NO_3$.

Molecular weight: Fosfomycin tromethamine—259.19.

Description: Fosfomycin tromethamine—White granular compound.

USP requirements: Fosfomycin Tromethamine for Oral Solution—Not in *USP–NF*.

FOSINOPRIL

Chemical name: Fosinopril sodium—L-Proline, 4-cyclohexyl-1-[[[2-methyl-1-(1-oxopropoxy)propoxy](4-phenylbutyl)phosphinyl]acetyl]-, sodium salt, [1[*S**(*R**)*],2 alpha,4 beta]-.

Molecular formula: Fosinopril sodium—$C_{30}H_{45}NNaO_7P$.

Molecular weight: Fosinopril sodium—585.64.

Description: Fosinopril sodium—White to off-white crystalline powder.

Solubility: Fosinopril sodium—Soluble in water (100 mg/mL), in methanol, and in ethanol; slightly soluble in hexane.

USP requirements: Fosinopril Sodium Tablets—Not in *USP–NF*.

FOSPHENYTOIN

Chemical name: Fosphenytoin sodium—2,4-Imidazolidinedione, 5,5-diphenyl-3-[(phosphonooxy)methyl]-, disodium salt.

Molecular formula: Fosphenytoin sodium—$C_{16}H_{13}N_2Na_2O_6P$.

Molecular weight: Fosphenytoin sodium—406.24.

Description: Fosphenytoin Sodium USP—White to pale yellow solid.

Solubility: Fosphenytoin Sodium USP—Freely soluble in water.

USP requirements:
Fosphenytoin Sodium USP—Preserve in tight containers. Contains not less than 98% and not more than 102.0% of fosphenytoin sodium, calculated on the anhydrous basis. Meets the requirements for Identification, pH (8.5–9.5, in a solution containing 75 mg per mL), Water (21.7% to 25.7%), Heavy metals (0.002), Chromatographic purity, and Organic volatile impurities.
Fosphenytoin Sodium Injection—Not in *USP–NF*.

FRAMYCETIN

Source: Produced by certain strains of *Streptomyces fradiae* or *Streptomyces decaris*.

Chemical name: Framycetin sulfate—2-Deoxy-4-*O*-(2,6-diamino-2,6-dideoxy-alpha-D-glucopyranosyl)-5-*O*-[3-*O*-(2,6-diamino-2,6-dideoxy-beta-L-idopyranosyl)-beta-D-ribofuranosyl]-streptamine sulfate.

Molecular formula: Framycetin sulfate—$C_{23}H_{46}N_6O_{13} \cdot 3H_2SO_4$.

Molecular weight: Framycetin sulfate—908.9.

Description: Framycetin sulfate—White or yellowish-white, odorless or almost odorless, hygroscopic powder.

Solubility: Framycetin sulfate—Soluble 1 in 1 of water; very slightly soluble in alcohol; practically insoluble in acetone, in chloroform, and in ether.

USP requirements:
Framycetin Sulfate Impregnated Gauze—Not in *USP–NF*.
Framycetin Sulfate Ophthalmic Ointment—Not in *USP–NF*.
Framycetin Sulfate Ophthalmic Solution—Not in *USP–NF*.

FRAMYCETIN AND GRAMICIDIN

For *Framycetin* and *Gramicidin*—See individual listings for chemistry information.

USP requirements: Framycetin Sulfate and Gramicidin Ointment—Not in *USP–NF*.

FRAMYCETIN, GRAMICIDIN, AND DEXAMETHASONE

For *Framycetin, Gramicidin,* and *Dexamethasone*—See individual listings for chemistry information.

USP requirements:
Framycetin Sulfate, Gramicidin, and Dexamethasone Ophthalmic Ointment—Not in *USP–NF*.
Framycetin Sulfate, Gramicidin, and Dexamethasone Otic Ointment—Not in *USP–NF*.
Framycetin Sulfate, Gramicidin, and Dexamethasone Ophthalmic Solution—Not in *USP–NF*.
Framycetin Sulfate, Gramicidin, and Dexamethasone Otic Solution—Not in *USP–NF*.

FRUCTOSE

Chemical name: D-Fructose.

Molecular formula: $C_6H_{12}O_6$.

Molecular weight: 180.16.

Description: Fructose USP—Colorless crystals or white crystalline powder. Odorless.
NF category: Sweetening agent; tablet and/or capsule diluent.

Solubility: Fructose USP—Freely soluble in water; soluble in alcohol and in methanol.

USP requirements:
Fructose USP—Preserve in well-closed containers. Dried in vacuum at 70 °C for 4 hours, contains not less than 98.0% and not more than 102.0% of fructose. Meets the requirements for Identification, Color of solution, Acidity, Loss on drying (not more than 0.5%), Residue on ignition (not more than 0.5%), Chloride (not more than 0.018%), Sulfate (not more than 0.025%), Arsenic (not more than 1 ppm), Calcium and magnesium (as calcium) (not more than 0.005% calcium), Heavy metals (not more than 5 ppm), and Limit of hydroxymethylfurfural.

Fructose Injection USP—Preserve in single-dose containers, preferably of Type I or Type II glass. A sterile solution of Fructose in Water for Injection. The label states the total osmolar concentration in mOsmol per liter. Where the contents are less than 100 mL, or where the label states that the Injection is not for direct injection but is to be diluted before use, the label alternatively may state the total osmolar concentration in mOsmol per mL. Contains the labeled amount, within ±5%. Contains no antimicrobial agents. Meets the requirements for Identification, Bacterial endotoxins, pH (3.0–6.0), Heavy metals (not more than 5 ppm), and Limit of hydroxymethylfurfural, and for Injections.

FRUCTOSE, DEXTROSE, AND PHOSPHORIC ACID

For *Fructose, Dextrose,* and *Phosphoric Acid*—See individual listings for chemistry information.

USP requirements: Fructose, Dextrose, and Phosphoric Acid Oral Solution—Not in *USP–NF*.

FRUCTOSE AND SODIUM CHLORIDE

For *Fructose* and *Sodium Chloride*—See individual listings for chemistry information.

USP requirements: Fructose and Sodium Chloride Injection USP—Preserve in single-dose containers, preferably of Type I or Type II glass. A sterile solution of Fructose and Sodium Chloride in Water for Injection. The label states the total osmolar concentration in mOsmol per liter. Where the contents are less than 100 mL, or where the label states that the Injection is not for direct injection but is to be diluted before use, the label alternatively may state the total osmolar concentration in mOsmol per mL. Contains the labeled amounts of fructose and sodium chloride, within ±5%. Contains no antimicrobial agents. Meets the requirements for Identification, Bacterial endotoxins, pH (3.0–6.0), Heavy metals (not more than 5 ppm), and Limit of hydroxymethylfurfural, and for Injections.

BASIC FUCHSIN

Chemical name: Benzenamine, 4-[(4-aminophenyl)(4-imino-2,5-cyclohexadien-1-ylidene)methyl]-2-methyl-, monohydrochloride.

Description: Basic Fuchsin USP—Dark green powder or greenish glistening crystalline fragments, having a bronze-like luster and not more than a faint odor.

Solubility: Basic Fuchsin USP—Soluble in water, in alcohol, and in amyl alcohol; insoluble in ether.

USP requirements: Basic Fuchsin USP—Preserve in well-closed containers. A mixture of rosaniline and pararosaniline hydrochlorides. Contains the equivalent of not less than 88.0% of rosaniline hydrochloride, calculated on the dried basis. Meets the requirements for Identification, Loss on drying (not more than 5.0%), Residue on ignition (not more than 0.3%), Alcohol-insoluble substances (not more than 1.0%), Arsenic (not more than 8 ppm), and Lead (not more than 30 ppm).

FULVESTRANT

Chemical group: Estrogen receptor antagonist.

Chemical name: Estra-1,3,5(10-triene-3,17-diol, 7-[9-[(4,4,5,5,5-pentafluoropentyl)sulfinyl]nonyl]-, (7 alpha, 17 beta)-.

Molecular formula: $C_{32}H_{47}F_5O_3S$.

Molecular weight: 606.77.

Description: White powder.

USP requirements: Fulvestrant Injection—Not in *USP–NF*.

FUMARIC ACID

Chemical name: 2-Butenedioic acid, [*E*]-.

Molecular formula: $C_4H_4O_4$.

Molecular weight: 116.07.

Description: Fumaric Acid NF—White, odorless granules or crystalline powder.
  NF category: Acidifying agent.

Solubility: Fumaric Acid NF—Soluble in alcohol; slightly soluble in water and in ether; very slightly soluble in chloroform.

NF requirements: Fumaric Acid NF—Preserve in well-closed containers. Contains not less than 99.5% and not more than 100.5% of fumaric acid, calculated on the anhydrous basis. Meets the requirements for Identification, Water (0.5%), Residue on ignition (not more than 0.1%), Heavy metals (not more than 0.001%), Limit of maleic acid (not more than 0.1%), and Organic volatile impurities.

FURAZOLIDONE

Chemical group: Nitrofuran.

Chemical name: 2-Oxazolidinone, 3-[[(5-nitro-2-furanyl)methylene]amino]-.

Molecular formula: $C_8H_7N_3O_5$.

Molecular weight: 225.16.

Description: Furazolidone USP—Yellow, odorless, crystalline powder.

Solubility: Furazolidone USP—Practically insoluble in water, in alcohol, and in carbon tetrachloride.

USP requirements:
  Furazolidone USP—Preserve in tight, light-resistant containers, and avoid exposure to direct sunlight. Contains not less than 97.0% and not more than 103.0% of furazolidone, calculated on the dried basis. Meets the requirements for Identification, Loss on drying (not more than 1.0%), and Residue on ignition (not more than 0.25%).
  Furazolidone Oral Suspension USP—Preserve in tight, light-resistant containers, and avoid exposure to excessive heat. A suspension of Furazolidone in a suitable aqueous vehicle. Contains the labeled amount, within ±10%. Meets the requirements for Identification and pH (6.0–8.5).
  Furazolidone Tablets USP—Preserve in tight, light-resistant containers, and avoid exposure to excessive heat. Contain the labeled amount, within ±10%. Meet the requirements for Identification and Uniformity of dosage units.

FUROSEMIDE

Chemical name: Benzoic acid, 5-(aminosulfonyl)-4-chloro-2-[(2-furanylmethyl)amino]-.

Molecular formula: $C_{12}H_{11}ClN_2O_5S$.

Molecular weight: 330.74.

Description:
Furosemide USP—White to slightly yellow, odorless, crystalline powder.
Furosemide Injection USP—Clear, colorless solution.
pKa: 3.9.

Solubility: Furosemide USP—Practically insoluble in water; freely soluble in acetone, in dimethylformamide, and in solutions of alkali hydroxides; soluble in methanol; sparingly soluble in alcohol; slightly soluble in ether; very slightly soluble in chloroform.

USP requirements:
Furosemide USP—Preserve in well-closed, light-resistant containers. Contains not less than 98.0% and not more than 101.0% of furosemide, calculated on the dried basis. Meets the requirements for Identification, Loss on drying (not more than 1.0%), Residue on ignition (not more than 0.1%), Heavy metals (not more than 0.002%), Related compounds, and Organic volatile impurities.
Furosemide Injection USP—Store in single-dose or in multiple-dose, light-resistant containers, of Type I glass. A sterile solution of Furosemide in Water for Injection prepared with the aid of Sodium Hydroxide or, where intended solely for veterinary use, Diethanolamine or Monoethanolamine Injection intended solely for veterinary use is so labeled. Contains the labeled amount, within ±10%. Meets the requirements for Identification, Bacterial endotoxins, pH (8.0–9.3 or, where labeled as intended solely for veterinary use, 7.0–7.8 if it contains diethanolamine, or 8.0–9.3 if it contains monoethanolamine), Particulate matter, and Limit of furosemide related compound B (not more than 2.5%), and for Injections.
Furosemide Oral Solution USP—Preserve in tight, light-resistant containers. Contains the labeled amount, within ±10%. Meets the requirements for Identification, Minimum fill, pH (7.0–10.0), and Limit of furosemide related compound B.
Furosemide Tablets USP—Preserve in well-closed, light-resist-ant containers. The labeling indicates with which Dissolution test the product complies. Tablets intended solely for veterinary use are so labeled. Contain the labeled amount, within ±10%. Meet the requirements for Identification, Dissolution (80% in 60 minutes in phosphate buffer [pH 5.8] in Apparatus 2 at 50 rpm for Test 1 and at 65 rpm for Test 2 [Tablets labeled as intended for veterinary use comply with Test 2]), Uniformity of dosage units, and Limit of furosemide related compound B (not more than 0.8%).

FUSIDIC ACID

Chemical name: 29-Nordammara-17(20),24-dien-21-oic acid, 16-(acetyloxy)-3,11-dihydroxy-, (3 alpha,4 alpha,8 alpha,9 beta,11 alpha,13 alpha,14 beta,16 beta,17Z)-.

Molecular formula: $C_{31}H_{48}O_6$.

Molecular weight: 516.71.

Description: White crystalline powder.

Solubility: Practically insoluble in water; soluble 1 in 5 of alcohol, 1 in 4 of chloroform, and 1 in 60 of ether.

USP requirements:
Fusidic Acid Cream—Not in *USP–NF*.
Fusidic Acid Impregnated Gauze—Not in *USP–NF*.
Fusidic Acid for Injection—Not in *USP–NF*.

Fusidic Acid Ointment—Not in *USP–NF*.
Fusidic Acid Hemihydrate Suspension—Not in *USP–NF*.
Fusidic Acid Oral Suspension—Not in *USP–NF*.
Fusidic Acid Tablets—Not in *USP–NF*.

GABAPENTIN

Chemical name: Cyclohexaneacetic acid, 1-(aminomethyl)-.

Molecular formula: $C_9H_{17}NO_2$.

Molecular weight: 171.24.

Description: White to off-white crystalline solid.

Solubility: Freely soluble in water and in both basic and acidic aqueous solutions.

USP requirements: Gabapentin Capsules—Not in *USP–NF*.

GADODIAMIDE

Chemical name: [5,8-Bis(carboxymethyl)-11-[2-(methylamino)-2-oxoethyl]-3-oxo-2,5,8,11-tetraazatridecan-13-oato(3–)]gadolinium.

Molecular formula: $C_{16}H_{28}GdN_5O_8$.

Molecular weight: 573.66 (anhydrous).

Description:
Gadodiamide USP—White, odorless powder.
Gadodiamide injection—Sterile, clear, colorless to slightly yellow, aqueous solution.

Solubility: Gadodiamide USP—Freely soluble in water and in methanol; soluble in ethyl alcohol; slightly soluble in acetone and in chloroform.

USP requirements:
Gadodiamide USP—Preserve in tight containers, and store at controlled room temperature. Contains not less than 97.0% and not more than 103.0% of gadodiamide, calculated on the anhydrous basis. Meets the requirements for Clarity of solution, Identification, Microbial limits, Bacterial endotoxins, Water (3.0–14.0%), Limit of free gadolinium (III) (not more than 0.3%, calculated on the anhydrous basis), Limit of free diethylenetriamine pentaacetic acid bis-methylamide (not more than 0.7%, calculated on the anhydrous basis), Limit of methylamine (not more than 0.05%), Limit of acetone, Ethyl alcohol, and Isopropyl alcohol, Related compounds, and Content of gadolinium (26.6–29.0%, calculated on the anhydrous basis).
Gadodiamide Injection USP—Preserve in single-dose Containers for Injections of Type I glass, protected from light. Store at controlled room temperature. It is a sterile solution of Gadodiamide in Water for Injection. Label containers of Injection to direct the user to discard any unused portion. Contains the labeled amount, within ±10%. May contain stabilizers and buffers. Gadodiamide Injection intended for intravascular use contains no antimicrobial agents. Meets the requirements for Identification, Bacterial endotoxins, pH (5.5–7.0), Osmolarity (650–1000 mOsmol per kg), and Related compounds, and for Injections..

GADOPENTETATE

Chemical name: Gadopentetate dimeglumine—Gadolinate(2–), [*N,N*-bis[2-[bis(carboxymethyl)amino]ethyl]glycinato(5–)]-, dihydrogen, compd. with 1-deoxy-1-(methylamino)-D-glucitol (1:2).

Molecular formula: Gadopentetate dimeglumine—$C_{14}H_{20}$-$GdN_3O_{10} \cdot 2C_7H_{17}NO_5$.

Molecular weight: Gadopentetate dimeglumine—1058.15.

Description: Gadopentetate dimeglumine injection—Clear, colorless to slightly yellow aqueous solution, with a pH of 6.5–8.0.

Solubility: Gadopentetate dimeglumine—Freely soluble in water.

USP requirements: Gadopentetate Dimeglumine Injection USP—Preserve in single-dose containers, preferably of Type I glass, protected from light. Store at controlled room temperature. A sterile solution of gadopentetate dimeglumine in Water for Injection. May contain small amounts of Meglumine and Pentetic Acid as stabilizers. Gadopentetate Dimeglumine Injection intended for intravascular use contains no antimicrobial agents. Label containers of Injection intended for intravascular injection to direct the user to discard any unused portion remaining in the container. Contains the labeled amount, within ±10%. Meets the requirements for Identification, Bacterial endotoxins, pH (6.5–8.0), Heavy metals (not more than 0.002%), Meglumine content (37.4–45.8%), Content of gadolinium (15.1–18.4%), and Content of pentetic acid (0.027–0.04%), and for Injections.

GADOTERIDOL

Chemical name: Gadolinium, [10-(2-hydroxypropyl)-1,4,7,10-tetraazacyclododecane-1,4,7-triacetato(3–)-$N^1,N^4,N^7,N^{10},O^1,O^4,O^7,O^{10}$]-.

Molecular formula: $C_{17}H_{29}GdN_4O_7$.

Molecular weight: 558.68.

Description: Gadoteridol USP—White to off-white, crystalline, odorless powder. Melts at about 300°.

Solubility: Gadoteridol USP—Freely soluble in water and in methyl alcohol; soluble in isopropyl alcohol.

USP requirements:
Gadoteridol USP—Preserve in tight, light-resistant containers, and store at controlled room temperature. Contains not less than 97.0% and not more than 101.0% of gadoteridol, calculated on the anhydrous basis. Meets the requirements for Identification, Water (not more than 15%), Heavy metals (not more than 0.001%), Limit of gadoteridol related compound A (not more than 0.01%, calculated on the anhydrous basis), Limit of free gadolinium (III) (not more than 0.01%), Limit of regioisomer (not more than 2.5%), and Chromatographic purity, and for Sterility tests and Bacterial endotoxins under Gadoteridol Injection (where the label states that Gadoteridol is sterile) and for Bacterial endotoxins under Gadoteridol Injection (where the label states that Gadoteridol must be subjected to further processing during the preparation of injectagle dosage form).
Gadoteridol Injection USP—Preserve in single-dose Containers for Injections, preferably of Type I glass. Store at controlled room temperature protected from light. It is a sterile solution of Gadoteridol in Water for Injection. Label containers of Injection intended for intravenous injection to direct the user to examine the product to ensure that all solids are dissolved, to discard the product if solids persist, and to discard any unused portion remaining in the container. Contains the labeled amount, within ±10%. May contain buffers and stabilizers. Gadoteridol Injection in-

tended for intravenous use contains no antimicrobial agents. Meets the requirements for Identification, Bacterial endotoxins, pH (6.5–8.0), Particulate matter, Limit of free gadolinium (III) (not more than 0.02%), and Limit of gadoteridol related compound A (not more than 0.02%), and under Injections.

GADOVERSETAMIDE

Chemical name: Gadolinium, [8,11-bis(carboxylmethyl)-14-[2-[(2-methoxyethyl)amino]-2-oxoethyl]-6-oxo-2-oxa-5,8,11,14-tetraazahexadecan-16-oato(3-)]-.

Molecular formula: $C_2H_{34}GdN_5O_{10}$.

Molecular weight: 661.76.

Other characteristics: pH: 5.5 to 7.5. Osmolality: 1110 mOsmol per kg of water at 37 °C (approximately 4 times of osmolality of plasma). Density: 1.160 grams per mL at 25 °C. Viscosity: 3.1 cP at 20 °C and 2.0 cP at 37 °C. Hypertonic under conditions of use.

USP requirements: Gadoversetamide Injection—Not in *USP–NF*.

GALAGEENAN

NF requirements: Galageenan NF—Preserve in tight containers, preferably in a cool place. It is the hydrocolloid obtained by extraction with water or aqueous alkali from the red seaweed class *Rhodophyceae* species *Eucheuma gelatinae*. Consists chiefly of potassium, sodium, calcium, magnesium, and ammonium sulfate esters of galactose and 3,6-anhydrogalactose copolymers. These hexoses are alternately linked in alpha-1,3 and beta-1,4 in the polymer. Recovered by alcohol precipitation or by freezing and pressing. The ester sulfate content ranges from 8 to 18%. In addition, contains inorganic salts that originate from the seaweed and from the process of recovery from the extract. Meets the requirements for Identification, Viscosity (at 75° not less than 15 centipoises), Microbial limits, Loss on drying (not more than 12.5%), Acidinsoluble matter (not more than 2.0%), Total ash (not more than 35.0%), Lead (not more than 0.0005%), Heavy metals (not more than 0.002%), Organic volatile impurities, and Content of sulfate (not less than 8% and not more than 18%).

GALANTAMINE

Chemical name: 6*H*-Benjofuro[3a,3,2-*ef*][2]benzazepin-6-ol,4a,5,9,10,11,12-hexahydro-3-methoxy-11-methyl-, (4a*S*,6-*R*,8a*S*)-.

Molecular formula: $C_{17}H_{21}NO_3$.

Molecular weight: 287.36.

USP requirements: Galantamine Tablets—Not in *USP–NF*.

GALLAMINE

Chemical name: Gallamine triethiodide—Ethanaminium, 2,2',2''-[1,2,3-benzenetriyltris(oxy)]tris[*N,N,N*-triethyl]-, triiodide.

Molecular formula: Gallamine triethiodide—$C_{30}H_{60}I_3N_3O_3$.

Molecular weight: Gallamine triethiodide—891.53.

Description: Gallamine Triethiodide USP—White, odorless, amorphous powder. Is hygroscopic.

Solubility: Gallamine Triethiodide USP—Very soluble in water; sparingly soluble in alcohol; very slightly soluble in chloroform.

USP requirements:
Gallamine Triethiodide USP—Preserve in tight containers, protected from light. Contains not less than 98.0% and not more than 101.0% of gallamine triethiodide, calculated on the dried basis. Meets the requirements for Clarity and color of solution, Identification, pH (5.3–7.0, in a solution [1 in 50]), Loss on drying (not more than 1.5%), Residue on ignition (not more than 0.1%), and Heavy metals (not more than 0.002%).

Gallamine Triethiodide Injection USP—Preserve in single-dose or in multiple-dose containers, preferably of Type I glass, protected from light. A sterile solution of Gallamine Triethiodide in Water for Injection. Contains the labeled amount, within ±5%. Meets the requirements for Identification, Bacterial endotoxins, and pH (6.5–7.5), and for Injections.

GALLIUM CITRATE GA 67

Chemical name: 1,2,3-Propanetricarboxylic acid, 2-hydroxy-, gallium-^{67}Ga (1:1) salt.

Molecular formula: $C_6H_5{}^{67}GaO_7$.

USP requirements: Gallium Citrate Ga 67 Injection USP—Preserve in single-dose or in multiple-dose containers. A sterile aqueous solution of radioactive, essentially carrier-free, gallium citrate Ga 67 suitable for intravenous administration. Label it to include the following, in addition to the information specified for Labeling under Injections: the time and date of calibration; the amount of ^{67}Ga as labeled gallium citrate expressed as total megabecquerels (or microcuries or millicuries) and concentration as megabecquerels (or microcuries or millicuries) per mL at the time of calibration; the expiration date and time; and the statement, "Caution—Radioactive Material." The labeling indicates that in making dosage calculations, correction is to be made for radioactive decay, and also indicates that the radioactive half-life of ^{67}Ga is 78.26 hours. Contains the labeled amount of ^{67}Ga as citrate, within ±10%, expressed in megabecquerels (or microcuries or millicuries) per mL at the time indicated in the labeling. Other chemical forms of radioactivity do not exceed 3.0% of the total radioactivity. It may contain a preservative or stabilizer. Meets the requirements for Bacterial endotoxins, pH (4.5–8.0), Radiochemical purity, Radionuclide identification, and Radionuclidic purity, and for Injections (except that the Injection may be distributed or dispensed prior to completion of the test for Sterility, the latter test being started on the day of manufacture, and except that it is not subject to the recommendation on Volume in Container).

GALLIUM NITRATE

Chemical name: Nitric acid, gallium salt, nonahydrate.

Molecular formula: $GaN_3O_9 \cdot 9H_2O$.

Molecular weight: 417.88.

Description:
Gallium nitrate—White, slightly hygroscopic, crystalline powder (nonahydrate).

Gallium nitrate injection—Clear, colorless, odorless, sterile solution.

USP requirements: Gallium Nitrate Injection—Not in *USP–NF*.

GANCICLOVIR

Source: Synthetic guanine derivative.

Chemical name:
Ganciclovir—6*H*-Purin-6-one, 2-amino-1,9-dihydro-9-[[2-hydroxy-1-(hydroxymethyl)ethoxy]methyl]-.
Ganciclovir sodium—6*H*-Purin-6-one, 2-amino-1,9-dihydro-9-[[2-hydroxy-1-(hydroxymethyl)ethoxy]methyl]-, monosodium salt.

Molecular formula:
Ganciclovir—$C_9H_{13}N_5O_4$.
Ganciclovir sodium—$C_9H_{12}N_5NaO_4$.

Molecular weight:
Ganciclovir—255.23.
Ganciclovir sodium—277.21.

Description:
Ganciclovir USP—White to off-white crystalline powder.
Ganciclovir for Injection USP—White to off-white powder.
Ganciclovir sodium—White to off-white lyophilized powder.

pKa: 2.2 and 9.4.

Solubility:
Ganciclovir—Solubility of 2.6 mg/mL in water at 25 °C.
Ganciclovir for Injection USP—Soluble in water.
Ganciclovir sodium—Aqueous solubility greater than 50 mg/mL at 25 °C.

USP requirements:
Ganciclovir USP—Preserve in well-closed containers. Contains not less than 98% and not more than 102% of ganciclovir, calculated on the previously dried basis. Meets the requirements for Identification, Water (not more than 6.0% [Note—Ganciclovir is extremely hygroscopic.]), Residue on ignition (not more than 0.1%), Heavy metals (0.002%), and Related compounds.

Ganciclovir for Injection USP—Preserve in Containers for Sterile Solids, as described under *Injections*. A freez-dried powder prepared by the neutralization of Ganciclovir with the aid of Sodium Hydroxide. Label it to state that it is to be handled with great care because it is a potent cytotoxic agent and suspected carcinogen. Contains the labeled amount, within ±10%, calculated on the anhydrous basis. Meets the requirements for Constituted solution, Identification, Bacterial endotoxins, Sterility, pH (10.8–11.4, in the solution constituted as directed in the labeling), Water (not more than 3.0%), and Particulate matter.

Ganciclovir Capsules—Not in *USP–NF*.
Ganciclovir Intravitreal Implant—Not in *USP–NF*.
Sterile Ganciclovir Sodium—Not in *USP–NF*.

GANIRELIX

Source: Ganirelix is a synthetic decapeptide, derived from native gonadatropin-releasing hormone with substitutions of amino acids in several positions.

Chemical name: Ganirelix acetate—D-Alaninamide, *N*-acetyl-3-(2-naphthalenyl)-D-alanyl-4-chloro-D-phenylalanyl-3-(3-pyridinyl)-D-alanyl-L-seryl-L-tyrosyl-*N*⁶-[(ethylamino)(ethylimino)methyl]-D-lysyl-L-leucyl*N*⁶-[(ethylamino)(ethylimino)methyl]-L-lysyl-L-prolyl-, diacetate (salt):.

Molecular formula: Ganirelix acetate—$C_{80}H_{113}CIN_{18}O_{13} \cdot 2C_2H_4O_2$.

Molecular weight: Ganirelix acetate—1690.42 and 1570.4 (anhydrous free base).

Other characteristics: Ganirelix acetate—The pH is adjusted to 5.0 with acitic acid, NF and/or sodium hydroxide, NF.

USP requirements: Ganirelix Acetate Injection—Not in *USP–NF*.

GARLIC

NF requirements:

Garlic NF—Store in well-closed containers in a cool, dry place, protected from light. Consists of the fresh or dried compound bulbs of *Allium sativum* Linné (Fam. Liliaceae). The label states the Latin binomial name and, following the official name, the part of the plant contained in the article. Contains not less than 0.5% of alliin and not less than 0.2% of gamma-glutamyl-(*S*)-allyl-L-cysteine, calculated on the dried basis. Meets the requirements for Botanic characteristics, Identification, Total ash (not more than 5.0%), Acid-insoluble ash (not more than 1.0%), Water content (not more than 65.0% for fresh bulbs, and not more than 7.0% for dried bulbs), Pesticide residues, Content of gamma-glutamyl-(*S*)-allyl-L-cysteine, and Content of alliin (not less than 0.5%, calculated on the dried basis).

Garlic Delayed-release Tablets NF—Preserve in tight containers. Prepared from Powdered Garlic or Powdered Garlic Extract. The label states the Latin binomial and, following the official name, the article from which the Tablets were prepared. Label it to indicate the amount of total alliin, in microgram per Tablet, and the amount of potential allicin, in microgram per Tablet. Contain the labeled amount of each of alliin and potential allicin, within −10% and +40%. Meet the requirements for identification, Allicin release (in buffer state in 60 minutes in Apparatus 2 at 100 rpm), Weight variation, Content of alliin, Content of potential allicin, and Alliinase activity.

Garlic Fluidextract NF—Prepared as follows: Soak 1000 grams of Garlic, whole or sliced, in a volume of a mixture of water and alcohol (between 80:20 and 50:50) sufficient to cover the cloves. Store in a suitable container for a length of time sufficient to extract the constituents, avoiding any contamination, and then filter. Concentrate the filtrate, if necessary, at the lowest possible temperature, add sufficient water or alcohol to make the product measure 1000 mL, and mix. [Note—Complete extraction may require about 30 days.] Meets the requirements for Thin-layer chromatographic identification test, Microbial limits, pH (4.5–6.5), Residue on evaporation (not less than 20%), Total ash (not more than 3.0%), Acid-insoluble ash (not more than 0.2%), Heavy metals (0.001%), and Content of *S*-allyl-L-cysteine (not less than 0.05%, calculated on the dried basis), and for Packaging and Storage, Labeling, Pesticide residues, and Alcohol content for Fluidextracts under Botanical extracts.

Powdered Garlic NF—Store in well-closed containers in a cool, dry place, protected from light. Produced from Garlic that has been cut, freeze-dried or dried at a temperature not exceeding 65 °C, and powdered. The label states the Latin binomial name and, following the official name, the part of the plant source from which the article was derived. Contains not less than 0.3% of alliin and not less than 0.1% of gamma-glutamyl-(*S*)-allyl-L-cysteine, calculated on the dried basis. Meets the requirements for Botanic characteristics, Starch, Loss on drying (not more than 7.0%), and Heavy metals (not more than 0.001%), Content of gamma-glutamyl-(*S*)-allyl-L-cysteine, for Identifica-

tion, Total ash, Acid-insoluble ash, and Pesticide residues under Garlic, and for Content of alliin (not less than 0.3%, calculated on the dried basis).

Powdered Garlic Extract NF—Preserve in tight containers, in a cool place, protected from light. Prepared from fresh Garlic bulbs by extraction with alcohol. The ratio of the starting crude plant material to Powdered Extract is between 9.5:1 and 13.5:1. The label states the Latin binomial and, following the official name, the part of the plant from which the article was prepared. The label also indicates the content of alliin, the extracting solvent or solvent mixture used for preparation, and the ratio of the starting crude plant material to Powdered Extract. Meets the requirements for *Labeling for Botanical Extracts*. Contains not less than 4.0% of alliin. May contain added Powdered Garlic or other suitable substances. Meets the rquirements for Identification, Microbial limits, Water content (not more than 5.0%), Heavy metals (0.001%), Organic volatile impurities, Content of alliin, and Alcohol content (not more than 0.5%), and for Packaging and storage and Pesticide residues under *Botanical Extracts*, and for Alliinase activity.

GATIFLOXACIN

Chemical name: (±)-1-Cyclopropyl-6-fluoro-1,4-dihydro-8-methoxy-7-(3-methyl-1-piperazinyl)-4-oxo-3-quinolinecarboxylic acid, sesquihydrate.

Molecular formula: $C_{19}H_{22}FN_3O_4 \cdot 1\,1/2H_2O$.

Molecular weight: 402.42.

Description: Sesquihydrate crystalline powder and is white to pale yellow in color.

Solubility: pH dependant. Maximum aqueous solubility (40–60 mg/mL) at pH 2–5.

USP requirements:

Gatifloxacin Intravenous Solution—Not in *USP–NF*.
Gatifloxacin Tablets—Not in *USP–NF*.

ABSORBENT GAUZE

USP requirements: Absorbent Gauze USP—Preserve in well-closed containers. Absorbent Gauze that has been rendered sterile is so packaged that the sterility of the contents of the package is maintained until the package is opened for use. It is cotton, or a mixture of cotton and not more than 53.0%, by weight, of rayon, and is in the form of a plain woven cloth conforming to the standards set forth in *USP/NF*. Absorbent Gauze that has been rendered sterile is packaged to protect it from contamination. Its type or thread count, length, and width, and the number of pieces contained, are stated on the container, and the designation "non-sterilized" or "not sterilized" appears prominently thereon unless the Gauze has been rendered sterile, in which case it may be labeled to indicate that it is sterile. The package label of sterile Gauze indicates that the contents may not be sterile if the package bears evidence of damage or has been previously opened. The name of the manufacturer, packer, or distributor is stated on the package. Meets the requirements for General characteristics, Thread count, Length (not less than 98.0% of that stated on label), Width (average of three measurements is within 1.6 mm of width stated on label), Weight, Absorbency (complete submersion takes place in not more than 30 seconds), Sterility, Dried and ignited residue, Acid or alkali, and Dextrin or starch, in water extract, Residue on ignition, Fatty matter, Alcohol-soluble dyes, and Cotton and rayon content.

Note: Condition all Absorbent Gauze for not less than 4 hours in a standard atmosphere of 65 ±2% relative humidity at 21 ±1.1 °C (70 ±2 °F), before determining the weight, thread count, and absorbency. Remove the Absorbent Gauze from its wrappings before placing it in the conditioning atmosphere, and if it is in the form of bolts or rolls, cut the quantity necessary for the various tests from the piece, excluding the first two and the last two meters when the total quantity of Gauze available so permits.

PETROLATUM GAUZE

Description: Petrolatum Gauze USP—The petrolatum recovered by draining in the *Assay* is a white or faintly yellowish, unctuous mass, transparent in thin layers even after cooling to 0 °C.

USP requirements: Petrolatum Gauze USP—Each Petrolatum Gauze unit is so packaged individually that the sterility of the unit is maintained until the package is opened for use. It is Absorbent Gauze saturated with White Petrolatum. The package label bears a statement to the effect that the sterility of the Petrolatum Gauze cannot be guaranteed if the package bears evidence of damage or has been opened previously. The package label states the width, length, and type or thread count of the Gauze. The weight of the petrolatum in the gauze is not less than 70.0% and not more than 80.0% of the weight of petrolatum gauze. Petrolatum Gauze is sterile. May be prepared by adding, under aseptic conditions, molten, sterile, White Petrolatum to dry, sterile, Absorbent Gauze, previously cut to size, in the ratio of 60 grams of petrolatum to each 20 grams of gauze. Meets the requirements for Sterility, of tests under White Petrolatum, and of tests for Thread count, Length, Width, and Weight under Absorbent Gauze.

GELATIN

Description: Gelatin NF—Sheets, flakes, or shreds, or coarse to fine powder. Faintly yellow or amber in color, the color varying in depth according to the particle size. It has a slight, characteristic, bouillon-like odor in solution. Stable in air when dry, but subject to microbic decomposition when moist or in solution. Gelatin has any suitable strength that is designated by Bloom Gelometer number. Type A Gelatin exhibits an isoelectric point between pH 7 and pH 9, and Type B Gelatin exhibits an isoelectric point between pH 4.7 and pH 5.2.

NF category: Coating agent; suspending and/or viscosity-increasing agent; tablet binder.

Solubility: Gelatin NF—Insoluble in cold water, but swells and softens when immersed in it, gradually absorbing from 5 to 10 times its own weight of water. Soluble in hot water, in 6 *N* acetic acid, and in a hot mixture of glycerin and water. Insoluble in alcohol, in chloroform, in ether, and in fixed and volatile oils.

NF requirements: Gelatin NF—Preserve in well-closed containers in a dry place. A product obtained by the partial hydrolysis of collagen derived from the skin, white connective tissue, and bones of animals. Gelatin derived from an acid-treated precursor is known as Type A, and Gelatin derived from an alkali-treated precursor is known as Type B. Gelatin, where being used in the manufacture of capsules, or for the coating of tablets, may be colored with a certified color, may contain not more than 0.15% of sulfur dioxide, and may contain a suitable concentration of sodium lauryl sulfate and suitable antimicrobial agents. Meets the requirements for Identification, Microbial limits, Residue on ignition (not more than 2.0%), Odor and

water-insoluble substances, Sulfur dioxide (not more than 0.15%), Arsenic (not more than 0.8 ppm), and Heavy metals (not more than 0.005%).

ABSORBABLE GELATIN

Description:
Absorbable Gelatin Film USP—Light amber, transparent, pliable film which becomes rubbery when moistened.
Absorbable Gelatin Sponge USP—Light, nearly white, nonelastic, tough, porous, hydrophilic solid.

Solubility:
Absorbable Gelatin Film USP—Insoluble in water.
Absorbable Gelatin Sponge USP—Insoluble in water.

USP requirements:
Absorbable Gelatin Film USP—Preserve in a hermetically sealed or other suitable container in such manner that the sterility of the product is maintained until the container is opened for use. It is Gelatin in the form of a sterile, absorbable, water-insoluble film. The package bears a statement to the effect that the sterility of Absorbable Gelatin Film cannot be guaranteed if the package bears evidence of damage, or if the package has been previously opened. Meets the requirements for Sterility, Residue on ignition (not more than 2.0%), and Proteolytic digest (average time of 3 proteolytic digest determinations, 4–8 hours).
Absorbable Gelatin Sponge USP—Preserve in a hermetically sealed or other suitable container in such manner that the sterility of the product is maintained until the container is opened for use. It is Gelatin in the form of a sterile, absorbable, water-insoluble sponge. The package bears a statement to the effect that the sterility of Absorbable Gelatin Sponge cannot be guaranteed if the package bears evidence of damage, or if the package has been previously opened. Meets the requirements for Sterility, Residue on ignition (not more than 2.0%), Digestibility (average digestion time of 3 determinations not more than 75 minutes), and Water absorption (not less than 35 times its weight of water).

GEMCITABINE

Chemical name:
Gemcitabine—Cytidine, 2′-deoxy-2′,2′-difluoro-.
Gemcitabine hydrochloride—Cytidine, 2′-deoxy-2′,2′-difluoro-, monohydrochloride.

Molecular formula:
Gemcitabine—$C_9H_{11}F_2N_3O_4$.
Gemcitabine hydrochloride—$C_9H_{11}F_2N_3O_4 \cdot HCl$.

Molecular weight:
Gemcitabine—263.20.
Gemcitabine hydrochloride—299.66.

Description: Gemcitabine hydrochloride—White to off-white solid.

Solubility: Gemcitabine hydrochloride—Soluble in water; slightly soluble in methanol; practically insoluble in ethanol and in polar organic solvents.

USP requirements:
Gemcitabine for Injection—Not in *USP–NF*.
Gemcitabine Hydrochloride for Injection—Not in *USP–NF*.

GEMFIBROZIL

Chemical name: Pentanoic acid, 5-(2,5-dimethylphenoxy)-2,2-dimethyl-.

Molecular formula: $C_{15}H_{22}O_3$.

Molecular weight: 250.33.

Description: Gemfibrozil USP—White, waxy, crystalline solid.

Solubility: Gemfibrozil USP—Practically insoluble in water; soluble in alcohol, in methanol, and in chloroform.

USP requirements:

Gemfibrozil USP—Preserve in tight containers. Contains not less than 98.0% and not more than 102.0% of gemfibrozil, calculated on the anhydrous basis. Meets the requirements for Identification, Melting range (58–61 °C), Water (not more than 0.25%), Heavy metals (not more than 0.002%), Related compounds, and Organic volatile impurities.

Gemfibrozil Capsules USP—Preserve in tight containers. Contain the labeled amount, within ±10%. Meet the requirements for Identification, Dissolution (80% in 45 minutes in 0.2 *M* phosphate buffer [pH 7.5] in Apparatus 2 at 50 rpm), and Uniformity of dosage units.

Gemfibrozil Tablets USP—Preserve in tight containers. Contain the labeled amount, within ±10%. Meet the requirements for Identification, Dissolution (80% in 30 minutes in 0.2 *M* phosphate buffer [pH 7.5] in Apparatus 2 at 50 rpm), and Uniformity of dosage units.

GEMTUZUMAB OZOGAMICIN

Source: Recombinant DNA-derived humanized monoclonal antibody conjugated with a cytotoxic antitumor antibiotic, calicheamicin, isolated from fermentation of a bacterium, *Micromonospora echinospora* sp. *calichensis*.

Molecular weight: 151–153 kilodaltons.

Description: A sterile, white, preservative-free lyophilized powder.

USP requirements: Gemtuzumab Ozogamicin for Injection—Not in *USP–NF*.

GENTAMICIN

Chemical group: Aminoglycosides.

Chemical name: Gentamicin sulfate—Gentamicin sulfate (salt).

Description:

Gentamicin Sulfate USP—White to buff powder.

Gentamicin Sulfate Injection USP—Clear, slightly yellow solution, having a faint odor.

Solubility: Gentamicin Sulfate USP—Freely soluble in water; insoluble in alcohol, in acetone, in chloroform, and in ether.

USP requirements:

Gentamicin Uterine Infusion USP—Preserve in single-dose or in multiple-dose containers, preferably of Type I glass. A sterile solution of Gentamicin Sulfate in Water for Injection. Label Uterine Infusion to indicate that it is for veterinary use only. The label states that it must be diluted with 0.9% Sodium Chloride Irrigation before aseptic uterine infusion. May contain suitable buffers, preservatives, and sequestering agents. Contains the labeled amount, within −10.0% to +25.0%. Meets the requirements for Identification, Sterility, and pH (3.0–5.5).

Gentamicin Injection USP—Preserve in single-dose or in multiple-dose containers, preferably of Type I glass. May contain suitable buffers, preservatives, and sequestering agents, unless it is intended for intrathecal use, in which case it contains only suitable tonicity agents. Contains an amount of gentamicin sulfate equivalent to the labeled amount of gentamicin, within −10% to +25%. Meets the requirements for Identification, Bacterial endotoxins, pH (3.0–5.5), and Particulate matter, and for Injections.

Gentamicin Liposome Injection—Not in *USP–NF*.

Gentamicin Sulfate USP—Preserve in tight containers. The sulfate salt, or a mixture of such salts, of the antibiotic substances produced by the growth of *Micromonospora purpurea*. Where it is intended for use in preparing injectable dosage forms, the label states that it is sterile or must be subjected to further processing during the preparation of injectable dosage forms. Has a potency equivalent to not less than 590 mcg of gentamicin per mg, calculated on the dried basis. Meets the requirements for Identification, Specific rotation (+107° to +121°), pH (3.5–5.5, in a solution [1 in 25]), Loss on drying (not more than 18.0%), Residue on ignition (not more than 1.0%), Limit of methanol (not more than 1.0%), and Content of gentamicins, and for Sterility tests and Bacterial endotoxins under Gentamicin Injection (where the label states that Gentamicin Sulfate is sterile), and for Bacterial endotoxins under Gentamicin Injection (where the label states that Gentamicin Sulfate must be subjected to further processing during the preparation of injectable dosage forms).

Gentamicin Sulfate Cream USP—Preserve in collapsible tubes or in other tight containers, and avoid exposure to excessive heat. Contains an amount of gentamicin sulfate equivalent to the labeled amount of gentamicin, within −10% to +35%. Meets the requirements for Identification and Minimum fill.

Gentamicin Sulfate Ointment USP—Preserve in collapsible tubes or in other tight containers, and avoid exposure to excessive heat. Contains an amount of gentamicin sulfate equivalent to the labeled amount of gentamicin, within −10% to +35%. Meets the requirements for Identification, Minimum fill, and Water (not more than 1.0%).

Gentamicin Sulfate Ophthalmic Ointment USP—Preserve in collapsible ophthalmic ointment tubes, and avoid exposure to excessive heat. Contains an amount of gentamicin sulfate equivalent to the labeled amount of gentamicin, within −10% to +35%. Meets the requirements for Identification, Sterility, Minimum fill, and Metal particles, and for Water under Gentamicin Sulfate Ointment.

Gentamicin Sulfate Ophthalmic Solution USP—Preserve in tight containers, and avoid exposure to excessive heat. A sterile, buffered solution of Gentamicin Sulfate with preservatives. Contains an amount of gentamicin sulfate equivalent to the labeled amount of gentamicin, within −10% to +35%. Meets the requirements for pH (6.5–7.5), for Identification test under Gentamicin Injection, and for Sterility tests.

Gentamicin Sulfate Otic Solution—Not in *USP–NF*.

GENTAMICIN AND BETAMETHASONE

For *Gentamicin* and *Betamethasone*—See individual listings for chemistry information.

USP requirements:

Gentamicin Sulfate and Betamethasone Acetate Ophthalmic Solution USP—Preserve in tight containers. Label it to indicate that it is for veterinary use only. Contains an amount of gentamicin sulfate equivalent to the labeled amount of gentamicin, within −10% to +25%, and the labeled amount

of betamethasone acetate, within ±10%. Meets the requirements for Identification, pH (5.5–7.0), and Sterility, and for Antimicrobial preservatives—Effectiveness.

Gentamicin Sulfate and Betamethasone Valerate Ointment USP—Preserve in collapsible tubes or in other tight containers. Label it to indicate that it is for veterinary use only. Contains an amount of gentamicin sulfate equivalent to the labeled amount of gentamicin, within –10% to +25%, and an amount of betamethasone valerate equivalent to the labeled amount of betamethasone, within ±10%. Meets the requirements for Identification, Microbial limits, and Minimum fill.

Gentamicin Sulfate and Betamethasone Valerate Otic Solution USP—Preserve in tight containers. Label it to indicate that it is for veterinary use only. Contains an amount of gentamicin sulfate equivalent to the labeled amount of gentamicin, within –10% to +25%, and an amount of betamethasone valerate equivalent to the labeled amount of betamethasone, within ±10%. Meets the requirements for Identification, pH (3.0–5.0), and Microbial limits.

Gentamicin Sulfate and Betamethasone Valerate Topical Solution USP—Preserve in tight containers. Label it to indicate that it is for veterinary use only. Contains an amount of gentamicin sulfate equivalent to the labeled amount of gentamicin, within –10% to +25%, and an amount of betamethasone valerate equivalent to the labeled amount of betamethasone, within ±10%. Meets the requirements for Identification, pH (3.0–4.5), and Microbial limits.

GENTAMICIN AND PREDNISOLONE

For *Gentamicin* and *Prednisolone*—See individual listings for chemistry information.

USP requirements:

Gentamicin and Prednisolone Acetate Ophthalmic Ointment USP—Preserve in collapsible ophthalmic ointment tubes, and avoid exposure to excessive heat. Contains the equivalent of the labeled amount of gentamicin, within –10% to +20%, and the labeled amount of prednisolone acetate, within ±10%. Meets the requirements for Identification, Sterility, Minimum fill, Water (not more than 2.0%), and Metal particles.

Gentamicin and Prednisolone Acetate Ophthalmic Suspension USP—Preserve in tight containers. A sterile aqueous suspension containing Gentamicin Sulfate and Prednisolone Acetate. Contains the equivalent of the labeled amount of gentamicin, within –10% to +30%, and the labeled amount of prednisolone acetate, within ±10%. Meets the requirements for Identification, Sterility, and pH (5.4–6.6).

GENTAMICIN AND SODIUM CHLORIDE

For *Gentamicin* and *Sodium Chloride*—See individual listings for chemistry information.

USP requirements: Gentamicin Sulfate in Sodium Chloride Injection—Not in *USP–NF*.

GENTIAN VIOLET

Chemical name: Methanaminium, *N*-[4-[bis[4-(dimethylamino)-phenyl]methylene]-2,5-cyclohexadien-1-ylidene]-*N*-methyl-, chloride.

Molecular formula: $C_{25}H_{30}ClN_3$.

Molecular weight: 407.98.

Description:

Gentian Violet USP—Dark green powder or greenish, glistening pieces having a metallic luster, and having not more than a faint odor.

Gentian Violet Cream USP—Dark purple, water-washable cream.

Gentian Violet Topical Solution USP—Purple liquid, having a slight odor of alcohol. A dilution (1 in 100), viewed downward through 1 cm of depth, is deep purple in color.

Solubility: Gentian Violet USP—Sparingly soluble in water; soluble in alcohol, in glycerin, and in chloroform; insoluble in ether.

USP requirements:

Gentian Violet USP—Preserve in well-closed containers. Contains not less than 96.0% and not more than 100.5% of gentian violet, calculated on the anhydrous basis. Meets the requirements for Identification, Water (not more than 7.5%), Residue on ignition (not more than 1.5%), Alcohol-insoluble substances (not more than 1.0%), Arsenic (not more than 0.001%), Lead (not more than 0.003%), Zinc, and Chromatographic purity.

Gentian Violet Cream USP—Preserve in collapsible tubes, or in other tight containers, and avoid exposure to excessive heat. It is Gentian Violet in a suitable cream base. Contains, in each 100 grams, not less than 1.20 grams and not more than 1.60 grams of gentian violet, calculated as hexamethylpararosaniline chloride. Meets the requirements for Identification and Minimum fill.

Gentian Violet Topical Solution USP—Preserve in tight containers. Contains, in each 100 mL, not less than 0.95 gram and not more than 1.05 grams of gentian violet, calculated as hexamethylpararosaniline chloride. Meets the requirements for Identification, Solution of residue in alcohol, and Alcohol content (8.0–10.0%).

Gentian Violet Vaginal Tampons—Not in *USP–NF*.

GENTISIC ACID ETHANOLAMIDE

Molecular formula: $C_9H_{11}NO_4$.

Molecular weight: 197.19.

Description: Gentisic Acid Ethanolamide NF—White to tan powder. Melts at about 149 °C.

NF category: Complexing agent.

Solubility: Gentisic Acid Ethanolamide NF—Sparingly soluble in water; freely soluble in acetone, in methanol, and in alcohol; very slightly soluble in ether; practically insoluble in chloroform.

NF requirements: Gentisic Acid Ethanolamide NF—Preserve in well-closed containers. Contains not less than 99.0% and not more than 100.5% of gentisic acid ethanolamide, calculated on the dried basis. Meets the requirements for Identification, Loss on drying (not more than 0.5%), Residue on ignition (not more than 0.1%, a 5-gram test specimen being used), Chloride (not more than 0.01%), Sulfate (not more than 0.02%), Heavy metals (not more than 0.001%), Chromatographic purity, and Organic volatile impurities.

GINGER

NF requirements:

Ginger NF—Preserve in well-closed containers, protected from light and moisture. The rhizome of *Zingiber officinale* Roscoe (Fam. Zingiberaceae), scraped or unscraped. Known in commerce as unbleached ginger. The label states the Latin binominal name and, following the official name, the part of the plant contained in the article. Meets the requirements for Botanic characteristics, Identification, Total ash (not more than 8.0%), Acid insoluble ash (not more than 2.0%), Water-soluble ash (not less than 1.9%), Water (not more than 10%), Alcohol-soluble extractives (not less than 4.5%), Water-soluble extractives (not less than 10.0%), Foreign organic matter (not more than 1.0%), Volatile oil content (not less than 1.8 mL per 100 grams), Pesticide residues, Microbial limits, Content of starch (not less than 42%), Limit of shogaols (not more than 0.18%), and Content of gingerols and gingerdiones (not less than 0.8%).

Ginger Tincture NF—Label it to indicate that it is for manufacturing purposes only, in addition to the information specified for Labeling for Tinctures under Botanical extracts. Contains not less than 0.10% of gingerols.

Prepare Ginger Tincture as follows: 200 grams Ginger and a mixture of Alcohol and Water (7:3), a sufficient quantity to make 1000 mL. Prepare a Tincture by the Maceration process as directed for Tinctures under Botanical Extracts.

Meets the requirements for Thin-layer chromatographic identification test, Specific gravity (0.90–0.95), Microbial limits, Total ash (not more than 0.5%), Pesticide residues, Arsenic (not more than 1 mcg per gram), Heavy metals (0.001%), Limit of nonvolatile residue (80–120 mg), Limit of 6-shogaol (not more than 0.034%), Content of gingerols, and Alcohol content (within ±10%), and for Packaging and Storage under Botanical Extracts.

Powdered Ginger NF—Preserve in well-closed containers, protected from light and moisture. It is Ginger reduced to a fine or a very fine powder. The label states the Latin binomial name and, following the official name, the part of the plant source from which the article was derived. Meets the requirements for Botanic characteristics and Heavy metals (not more than 0.002%), and for Identification, Total ash, Acid-insoluble ash, Water-soluble ash, Water, Alcohol-soluble extractives, Water-soluble extractives, Volatile oil content, Pesticide residues, Microbial limits, Starch content, Limit of shogaols, and Content of gingerols and gingerdiones under Ginger.

GINKGO

NF requirements: Ginkgo NF—Preserve in well-closed containers, protected from light and moisture. The label states the Latin binomial name and, following the official name, the part of the plant contained in the article. Consists of the dried leaf of *Ginkgo biloba* Linné (Fam. Ginkgoaceae). Contains not less than 0.5% of flavonoids, calculated as flavonol glycosides, with a mean molecular mass of 756.7, and not less than 0.1% of terpene lactones, calculated as the sum of bilobalide, ginkolide A, ginkolide B, ginkolide C, and ginkolide J, both on the dried basis. Meets the requirements for Botanic characteristics, Identification, Stems and other foreign organic matter (not more than 3.0% of stems and not more than 2.0% of other foreign organic matter), Pesticide residues, Loss on drying (not more than 11.0%), Total ash (not more than 11.0%, determined on 1.0 gram of finely powdered Ginkgo), Microbial limits, Content of flavonol glycosides, and Content of terpene lactones.

AMERICAN GINSENG

NF requirements:

American Ginseng NF–Store in tight, light-resistant containers, protected from heat. Consists of the dried roots of *Panax quinquefolius* Linné (Fam. Araliaceae). The label states the Latin binomial and, following the official name, the parts of the plant contained in the article. Contains not less than 4.0% of total ginsenosides, calculated on the dried basis. Meets the requirements for Botanic characteristics, Identification, Loss on drying (not more than 10.0%), Foreign organic matter (not more than 2.0%), Total ash (not more than 8%), Pesticide residues, Heavy metals (20 milligrams per gram), and Content of ginsenosides.

Powdered American Ginseng NF—Store in tight containers, protected from light, moisture, and heat. It is American Ginseng reduced to fine or a very fine powder. The label states the Latin binomial, and following the official name, the part of the plant contained in the article. Meets the requirements for Botanical characteristics and Water (not more than 7.0%), and for Identification, Loss on drying, Foreign organic matter, Total ash, Pesticide residues, Heavy metals, and Content of ginsenosides for American Ginseng.

Powdered American Ginseng Extract NF—Preserve in tight, light-resistant containers. Prepared from the pulverized dried roots of *Panax quinquefolius* Linné (Fam. Araliaceae), using suitable solvents, and dried to a powder. The label states the Latin binomial, following the official name, the part of the plant from which the article was derived. Label it to indicate the content of total ginsenosides, the extracting solvent used for preparation, and the ratio of the starting crude plant material to the Powdered Extract. It meets the labeling requirements for Botanical Extracts. Contains not less than 10.0% of total ginsenosides, calculated on the anhydrous basis. The ratio of starting crude plant material to Powdered Extract is between 3:1 and 7:1. Meets the requirements for Identification, Microbial limits, Residue in evaporation, Pesticide residues, Heavy metals (20 micrograms per gram), Content of ginsenosides, and Alcohol content (not more than 0.25%).

ASIAN GINSENG

Description:

Powdered Asian Ginseng NF—Pale yellow-brown, hygroscopic, powdery or easily pulverizable mass.

Powdered Asian Ginseng Extract NF—Pale yellow-brown, hygrospic, powdery or easily pulverizable mass.

Solubility:

Powdered Asian Ginseng NF—Soluble in water, forming a slightly cloudy solution.

Powdered Asian Ginseng Extract NF—Soluble in water, forming a slightly cloudy solution.

NF requirements:

Asian Ginseng NF—Store in cool, dry place, in well-closed containers. Consists of the dried roots of *Panax ginseng* C. A. Meyer (Fam. Araliaceae). The label states the Latin binomial name and, following the official name, the part of the plant contained in the article. Contains not less than 0.2% of ginsenoside Rg_1 and not less than 0.1% of ginsenoside Rb_1, both calculated on the dried basis. Meets the requirements for Botanic characteristics, Identification, Heavy metals (20 mcg per gram), Total ash (not more than 8.0%, determined on 1.0 gram of finely powdered Asian Ginseng), Acid-insoluble ash (not more than 1.0%), Foreign organic matter (not more than 2.0%), Pesticide residues, Loss on drying (not more than 12.0%), Alcohol-soluble extractives (not less than 14.0%), Microbial limits,

and Content of ginsenosides Rb₁ and Rg₁ (not less than 0.2% of ginsenoside Rg₁ and not less than 0.1% of ginsenoside Rb₁).

Asian ginseng Tablets NF—Preserve in tight containers, protected from light. Prepared from Powdered Asian Ginseng Extract. The label states the Latin binomial and, following the official name, the article from which the Tablets were prepared. The label also indicates the amount of Powdered Extract, in milligram per Tablet, and the content, in milligram, of ginsenosides per 100 milligrams of Powdered Extract. Contain the labeled amount of Powdered Extract, within ±10%, calculated as the sum of ginsenosides Rg₁, Re, Rb₁, Rc, Rb₂, and Rd. Meet the requirements for Identification, Microbial limits,, Disintigration and dissolution, Weight variation, and Content of ginsenosides.

Powdered Asian Ginseng NF—Preserve in well-closed containers, and store in cool, dry place. The label states the Latin binomial name and, following the official name, the part of the plant source from which the article was derived. Asian Ginseng reduced to a fine or very fine powder. Meets the requirements for Botanic characteristics and for Identification, Microbial limits, Loss on drying, Foreign organic matter, Total ash, Acid-insoluble ash, Alcohol-soluble extractives, Pesticide residues, Heavy metals, and Content of ginsenosides Rb₁ and Rg₁ for Asian Ginseng.

Powdered Asian Ginseng Extract NF—Prepared from Asian Ginseng by maceration, percolation, or both processes performed at room temperature with suitable solvents such as alcohol, methanol, water, or mixtures of these solvents, and by concentrating the fluidextract at temperatures below 50°. The ratio of the starting crude plant material to Powdered Extract is between 3:1 and 7:1. Contains not less than 3.0% of ginsenosides Rg₁, Re, Rb₁, Rb₂, and Rd combined, calculated on the anhydrous basis. May contain other added substances. Meets the requirements for Identification, Microbial limits,, Water (not more than 7.0%, determined on a 0.15 gram specimen), Pesticide residues, Heavy metals (30 micrograms per gram), Organic volatile impurities, Content of ginsenosides, and Alcohol content (not more than 0.25%), and for Packaging and storage and for Labeling under *Botanical Extracts*.

GLATIRAMER

Chemical name: Glatiramer acetate—L-Glutamic acid polymer with L-alanine, L-lysine and L-tyrosine, acetate (salt).

Molecular formula: Glatiramer acetate—(C₅H₉NO₄ · C₃H₇NO₂ · C₆H₁₄N₂O₂ · C₉H₁₁NO₃)ₓ · xC₂H₄O₂.

Molecular weight: Glatiramer acetate—4,700 to 11,000 daltons, average.

USP requirements: Glatiramer Acetate for Injection—Not in *USP–NF*.

PHARMACEUTICAL GLAZE

Description: Pharmaceutical Glaze NF—NF category: Coating agent.

NF requirements: Pharmaceutical Glaze NF—Preserve in tight, lined metal or plastic containers, protected from excessive heat, preferably at a temperature below 25 °C. A specially denatured alcoholic solution of Shellac containing between 20.0 and 57.0% of anhydrous shellac, and made with either anhydrous alcohol or alcohol containing 5% of water by volume. The solvent is a specially denatured alcohol approved for glaze manufacturing by the Internal Revenue Service. Label it to indicate the shellac type and concentration, the composi-

tion of the solvent, and the quantity of titanium dioxide, if present. Where titanium dioxide or waxes are present, the label states that the Glaze requires mixing before use. Meets the requirements for Acid value under Shellac, Wax under Shellac, and Identification, Heavy metals, and Rosin under Shellac.

GLICLAZIDE

Chemical group: Sulfonylurea.

Chemical name: 1-(3-Azabicyclo[3.3.0]oct-3-yl)-3-(*p*-tolylsulfonyl)urea.

Molecular formula: C₁₅H₂₁N₃O₃S.

Molecular weight: 323.41.

Description: White, crystalline, virtually odorless powder. Melting point approximately 168 °C.

pKa: 5.98.

Solubility: Practically insoluble in water; freely soluble in chloroform; sparingly soluble in acetone.

USP requirements: Gliclazide Tablets—Not in *USP–NF*.

GLIMEPIRIDE

Chemical group: Sulfonylurea.

Chemical name: 1*H*-Pyrrole-1-carboxamide, 3-ethyl-2,5-dihydro-4-methyl-*N*-[2-[4-[[[[(4-methylcyclohexyl)amino]carbonyl]amino]sulfonyl]phenyl]ethyl]-2-oxo-, *trans*-.

Molecular formula: C₂₄H₃₄N₄O₅S.

Molecular weight: 490.62.

Description: White to yellowish-white, crystalline, odorless to practically odorless powder.

Solubility: Practically insoluble in water.

USP requirements: Glimepiride Tablets—Not in *USP–NF*.

GLIPIZIDE

Chemical group: Sulfonylurea.

Chemical name: Pyrazinecarboxamide, *N*-[2-[4-[[[(cyclohexylamino)carbonyl]amino]sulfonyl]phenyl]ethyl]-5-methyl-.

Molecular formula: C₂₁H₂₇N₅O₄S.

Molecular weight: 445.54.

Description: Whitish, odorless powder.

pKa: 5.9.

Solubility: Insoluble in water and in alcohols; soluble in 0.1 N sodium hydroxide; freely soluble in dimethylformamide.

USP requirements:
Glipizide USP—Preserve in tight containers, and protect from light. Contains not less than 98.0% and not more than 102.0% of glipizide, calculated on the dried basis. Meets the requirements for Identification, Loss on drying (not more than 1.0%), Residue on ignition (not more than 0.4%), Heavy metals (not more than 0.005%), and Ordinary impurities.

Glipizide Tablets USP—Preserve in tight containers. Contain the labeled amount, within ±10%. Meet the requirements for Identification, Dissolution (80% in 45 minutes in simulated intestinal fluid TS [without pancreatin] in Apparatus 2 at 50 rpm), and Uniformity of dosage units.

Glipizide Extended-release Tablets—Not in *USP–NF*.

ANTI-HUMAN GLOBULIN SERUM

USP requirements: Anti-Human Globulin Serum USP—Preserve at a temperature between 2 and 8 °C. A sterile, liquid preparation of serum produced by immunizing lower animals such as rabbits or goats with human serum or plasma, or with selected human plasma proteins. It is free from agglutinins and from hemolysins to non-sensitized human red cells of all blood groups. Contains a suitable antimicrobial preservative. Label it to state the animal source of the product. Label it also to state the specific antibody activities present; to state the application for which the reagent is intended; to include a cautionary statement that it does not contain antibodies to immunoglobulins or that it does not contain antibodies to complement components, wherever and whichever is applicable; and to state that it is for in-vitro diagnostic use. (Note: The lettering on the label of the general-purpose polyspecific reagent is black on a white background. The label of all other Anti-Human Globulin Serum containers is in white lettering on a black background.) Anti-Human Globulin Serums containing Anti-IgG meet the requirements of the test for potency, in parallel with the U.S. Reference Anti-Human Globulin (Anti-IgG) Serum (at a 1:4 dilution) when tested with red cells suspended in isotonic saline sensitized with decreasing amounts of non-agglutinating Anti-D (Anti-Rh₀) serum, and with cells sensitized in the same manner with an immunoglobulin IgG Anti-Fyᵃ serum of similar potency. Anti-Human Globulin Serum containing one or more Anti-complement components meets the requirements of the tests for potency in giving a 2+ agglutination reaction (i.e., agglutinated cells dislodged into many small clumps of equal size) by the low-ionic sucrose or sucrose-trypsin procedures when tested as recommended in the labeling. Anti-Human Globulin Serum containing Anti-3Cd activity meets the requirements for stability, by potency testing of representative lots every 3 months during the dating period. Meets the requirement for Expiration date (not later than 1 year after the date of issue from manufacturer's cold storage [5 °C, 1 year; or 0 °C, 2 years]). Conforms to the regulations of the U.S. Food and Drug Administration concerning biologics.

IMMUNE GLOBULIN

Description: Immune Globulin USP—Transparent or slightly opalescent liquid, either colorless or of a brownish color due to denatured hemoglobin. Practically odorless. May develop a slight, granular deposit during storage.

USP requirements:

Immune Globulin USP—Preserve at a temperature between 2 and 8 °C. A sterile, non-pyrogenic solution of globulins that contains many antibodies normally present in adult human blood, prepared by pooling approximately equal amounts of material (source blood, plasma, serum, or placentas) from not less than 1000 donors. Label it to state that passive immunization with Immune Globulin modifies hepatitis A, prevents or modifies measles, and provides replacement therapy in persons having hypo- or agammaglobulinemia, that it is not standardized with respect to antibody titers against hepatitis B surface antigen and that it should be used for prophylaxis of viral hepatitis type B only when the specific Immune Globulin is not available,

that it may be of benefit in women who have been exposed to rubella in the first trimester of pregnancy but who would not consider a therapeutic abortion, and that it may be used in immunosuppressed patients for passive immunization against varicella if the specific Immune Globulin is not available. Label it also to state that it is not indicated for routine prophylaxis or treatment of rubella, poliomyelitis or mumps, or for allergy or asthma in patients who have normal levels of immunoglobulin, that the plasma units from which it has been derived have been tested and found non-reactive for hepatitis B surface antigen, and that it should not be administered intravenously but be given intramuscularly, preferably in the gluteal region. Contains not less than 15 grams and not more than 18 grams of protein per 100 mL, not less than 90.0% of which is gamma globulin. Contains 0.3 M glycine as a stabilizing agent and contains a suitable preservative. Has a potency of component antibodies of diphtheria antitoxin based on the U.S. Standard Diphtheria Antitoxin and a diphtheria test toxin, tested in guinea pigs (not less than 2 antitoxin units per mL), and antibodies for measles and poliovirus. Meets the requirements of the tests for heat stability in absence of gelation on heating, and for pH. Meets the requirement for Expiration date (not later than 3 years after date of issue from manufacturer's cold storage [5 °C, 3 years]). Conforms to the regulations of the U.S. Food and Drug Administration concerning biologics.

Immune Globulin Intravenous (Human) Injection—Not in *USP–NF*.

Immune Globulin Intravenous (Human) for Injection—Not in *USP–NF*.

RHO (D) IMMUNE GLOBULIN

Description: RH₀ (D) Immune Globulin USP—Transparent or slightly opalescent liquid. Practically colorless and practically odorless. May develop a slight, granular deposit during storage.

USP requirements:

RH₀ (D) Immune Globulin USP—Preserve at a temperature between 2 and 8 °C. A sterile, non-pyrogenic solution of globulins derived from human blood plasma containing antibody to the erythrocyte factor Rh₀ (D). Contains not less than 10 grams and not more than 18 grams of protein per 100 mL, not less than 90.0% of which is gamma globulin. Has a potency, determined by a suitable method, not less than that of the U.S. Reference Rh₀ (D) Immune Globulin. Contains 0.3 M glycine as a stabilizing agent and contains a suitable preservative. Meets the requirement for Expiration date (not later than 6 months from the date of issue from manufacturer's cold storage, or not later than 1 year from the date of manufacture, as indicated on the label). Conforms to the regulations of the U.S. Food and Drug Administration concerning biologics.

RH₀ (D) Immune Globulin (Human) for Injection—Not in *USP–NF*.

GLUCAGON

Chemical name: Glucagon (pig).

Molecular formula: $C_{153}H_{225}N_{43}O_{49}S$.

Molecular weight: 3482.75.

Description:

Glucagon USP—Fine, white or faintly colored, crystalline powder. Is practically odorless.

Glucagon for Injection USP—White, odorless powder.

Solubility: Glucagon USP—Soluble in dilute alkali and acid solutions; insoluble in most organic solvents.

Other characteristics: A single-chain polypeptide containing 29 amino acid residues. Chemically unrelated to insulin. One USP Unit of glucagon is equivalent to 1 International Unit of glucagon and also to about 1 mg of glucagon.

USP requirements:
Glucagon USP—Preserve in tight, glass containers, under nitrogen, in a refrigerator. A polypeptide hormone that has the property of increasing the concentration of glucose in the blood. Obtained from porcine and bovine pancreas glands. Meets the requirements for Identification, Chromatographic purity (not more than 2.5% of any individual impurity, and not more than 10.0% of total impurities), Water (not more than 10.0%), Residue on ignition (not more than 2.5%), Nitrogen content (16.0–18.5%, calculated on the anhydrous basis), and Zinc content (not more than 0.05%).
Glucagon for Injection USP—Preserve in Containers for Sterile Solids. A mixture of the hydrochloride of Glucagon with one or more suitable, dry diluents. Contains the labeled amount, within −20% to +25%. Meets the requirements for Bacterial endotoxins, Constituted solution and pH (1.7–3.0) and Clarity of solution, for Sterility tests and Labeling under Injections, and for Uniformity of dosage units.
Glucagon Recombinant for Injection—Not in *USP–NF*.

GLUCONOLACTONE

Chemical name: D-Gluconic acid delta-lactone.

Molecular formula: $C_6H_{10}O_6$.

Molecular weight: 178.14.

Description: Gluconolactone USP—Fine, white, practically odorless, crystalline powder. Melts at about 153 °C, with decomposition.

Solubility: Gluconolactone USP—Freely soluble in water; sparingly soluble in alcohol; insoluble in ether.

USP requirements: Gluconolactone USP—Preserve in wellclosed containers. Contains not less than 99.0% and not more than 101.0% of gluconolactone. Meets the requirements for Identification, Lead (not more than 0.001%), Heavy metals (not more than 0.002%), and Reducing substances.

GLUCOSAMINE

Chemical name:
Glucosamine—D-glucose, 2 amino-2-deoxy-.
Glucosamine hydrochloride—D-glucose, 2 amino-2-deoxy-, hydrochloride.
Glucosamine sulfate potassium chloride—Bis(D-glucose, 2 amino-2-deoxy-), sulfate potassium chloride complex.
Glucosamine sulfate sodium chloride—Bis(D-glucose, 2 amino-2-deoxy-), sulfate sodium chloride complex.

Molecular formula:
Glucosamine—$C_6H_{13}NO_5$.
Glucosamine hydrochloride—$C_6H_{13}NO_5 \cdot HCl$.
Glucosamine sulfate potassium chloride—$(C_6H_{14}NO_5)_2SO_4 \cdot 2KCl$.
Glucosamine sulfate sodium chloride—$(C_6H_{14}NO_5)_2SO_4 \cdot 2NaCl$.

Molecular weight:
Glucosamine—179.17.
Glucosamine hydrochloride—215.63.
Glucosamine sulfate potassium chloride—605.52.
Glucosamine sulfate sodium chloride—573.31.

NF requirements:
Glucosamine Tablets NF—Preserve in tight, light-resistant containers. Prepared from Glucosamine Hydrochloride, Glucosamine Sulfate Sodium Chloride, Glucosamine Sulfate Potassium Chloride, or a mixture of any of them. The label indicates the type of glucosamine salt contained in the article. Tablets contain the labeled amount of glucosamine, within ±10%. Meet the requirements for Identification, Disintigration and dissolution (75% in water in 45 minutes in Apparatus 2 at 50 rpm), and Weight variation.
Glucosamine Hydrochloride NF—Preserve in tight, light-resistant containers. Contains not less than 98.0% and not more than 102.0% of glucosamine hydrochloride, calculated on the dried basis. Meets the requirements for Identification, Specific rotation (+70.0° to +73.0°), pH (3.0–5.0, in a solution containing 20 milligrams per mL), Loss on drying (not more than 1.0%), Residue on ignition (not more than 0.1%), Sulfate (not more than 0.24%), Arsenic (3 milligrams per gram), Heavy metals (0.001%), and Organic volatile impurities.
Glucosamine Sulfate Potassium Chloride NF—Preserve in tight, light-resistant containers. Contains not less than 98.0% and not more than 102.0% of glucosamine sulfate potassium cholride. Meets the requirements for Identification, Specific rotation (+50.0° to +52.0°), pH (3.0–5.0, in a solution containing 20 milligrams per mL), Loss on drying (not more than 1.0%), Residue on ignition (27.0%–29.0%), Sodium, Arsenic (3 milligrams per gram), Heavy metals (0.001%), Organic volatile impurities, and Content of sulfate (15.5%–16.5%).
Glucosamine Sulfate Sodium Chloride NF—Preserve in tight, light-resistant containers. Contains not less than 98.0% and not more than 102.0% of glucosamine sulfate sodium cholride, calculated on the dried basis. Meets the requirements for Identification, Specific rotation (+52.0° to +54.0°), pH (3.0–5.0, in a solution containing 20 milligrams per mL), Loss on drying (not more than 1.0%), Residue on ignition (23.5%–25.0%), Potassium, Arsenic (3 milligrams per gram), Heavy metals (0.001%), Organic volatile impurities, and Content of sulfate (16.3%–17.3%).

GLUCOSAMINE AND CHONDROITIN

For *Glucosamine* and *Chondroitin*—See individual listings for chemistry information.

NF requirements: Glucosamine and Chondroitin Sulfate Tabalets NF—Preserve in tight, light-resistant containers. Prepared from Chondroitin Sulfate Sodium, Glucosamine Hydrochloride, Glucosamine Sulfate Sodium Chloride, Glucosamine Sulfate Potassium Chloride, or a mixture of any of them. The label indicates the types of glucosamine salts contained in the article, and the species source from which chondroitin was derived. Tablets contain a labeled amount of chondroitin sulfate sodium and glucosamine, within −10% to +20%. Meets the requirements for Identification, Disintigration and dissolution (75% in water in 60 minutes in Apparatus 2 at 75 rpm), Weight variation, Content of glucosamine, and Content of chondroitin sulfate sodium.

GLUCOSE ENZYMATIC TEST STRIP

USP requirements: Glucose Enzymatic Test Strip USP—Preserve in the original container, in a dry place, at controlled room temperature. Consists of the enzymes glucose oxidase

and horseradish peroxidase, a suitable substrate for the reaction of hydrogen peroxide catalyzed by peroxidase, and other inactive ingredients impregnated and dried on filter paper. When tested in human urine containing known glucose concentrations, it reacts in the specified times to produce colors corresponding to the color chart provided. Meets the requirements for Identification and Calibration.

LIQUID GLUCOSE

Description: Liquid Glucose NF—Colorless or yellowish, thick, syrupy liquid. Odorless or nearly odorless.
NF category: Tablet binder.

Solubility: Liquid Glucose NF—Miscible with water; sparingly soluble in alcohol.

NF requirements: Liquid Glucose NF—Preserve in tight containers. A product obtained by the incomplete hydrolysis of starch. Consists chiefly of dextrose, dextrins, maltose, and water. Meets the requirements for Identification, Acidity, Water (not more than 21.0%), Residue on ignition (not more than 0.5%), Sulfite, Heavy metals (not more than 0.001%), Starch, and Organic volatile impurities.

GLUTAMINE

Chemical name: L-Glutamine.

Molecular formula: $C_5H_{10}N_2O_3$.

Molecular weight: 146.14.

Description: Glutamine USP—White crystals or crystalline powder.

Solubility: Glutamine USP—Soluble in water; practically insoluble in alcohol and in ether.

USP requirements: Glutamine USP—Preserve in well-closed containers, and store at controlled temperature. Contains not less than 98.5% and not more than 101.5% of glutamine, calculated on the dried basis. Meets the requirements for Identification, Specific rotation (+6.3° to +7.3°, determined at 20°), Loss on drying (not more than 0.3%), Residue on ignition (not more than 0.3%), Chloride (not more than 0.05%), Sulfate (not more than 0.03%), Iron (not more than 0.003%), Heavy metals (0.0015%), Chromatogtraphic purity, and Organic volatile impurities.

GLUTARAL

Chemical name: Pentanedial.

Molecular formula: $C_5H_8O_2$.

Molecular weight: 100.12.

Description: Glutaral Concentrate USP—Clear, colorless or faintly yellow liquid, having a characteristic, irritating odor.

USP requirements: Glutaral Concentrate USP—Preserve in tight containers, protected from light, and avoid exposure to excessive heat. A solution of glutaraldehyde in Purified Water. The label states that this article is not intended for direct administration to humans or animals. Contains the labeled amount, within +4%, the labeled amount being 50.0 grams of glutaral per 100.0 grams of Concentrate. Meets the requirements for Clarity of solution, Identification, Specific gravity (1.128 to 1.135 at 20 °C/20 °C), Acidity (not more than 0.4% of acid (w/w), calculated as acetic acid), pH (3.7–4.5), and Heavy metals (not more than 0.001%).

NF requirements: Glutaral Disinfectant Solution NF—Preserve in tight, light-resistant containers, and avoid exposure to excessive heat. Contains, by weight, the labeled amount of glutaral, within +10%. Meets the requirements for Identification and pH (2.7–3.7).

GLUTETHIMIDE

Chemical name: 2,6-Piperidinedione, 3-ethyl-3-phenyl-.

Molecular formula: $C_{13}H_{15}NO_2$.

Molecular weight: 217.26.

Description: Glutethimide USP—White, crystalline powder. Its saturated solution is acid to litmus.

Solubility: Glutethimide USP—Practically insoluble in water; freely soluble in ethyl acetate, in acetone, in ether, and in chloroform; soluble in alcohol and in methanol.

USP requirements:
Glutethimide USP—Preserve in well-closed containers. Dried over phosphorus pentoxide at 45 °C to constant weight, contains not less than 98.0% and not more than 102.0% of glutethimide. Meets the requirements for Identification, Melting range (86–89 °C), Loss on drying (not more than 1.0%), Residue on ignition (not more than 0.1%), and Chromatographic purity.
Glutethimide Capsules USP—Preserve in well-closed containers. Contain the labeled amount, within ±5%. Meet the requirements for Identification, Dissolution (75% in 45 minutes in water in Apparatus 1 at 100 rpm), and Uniformity of dosage units.
Glutethimide Tablets USP—Preserve in well-closed containers. Contain the labeled amount, within ±10%. Meet the requirements for Identification, Dissolution (70% in 60 minutes in water in Apparatus 2 at 50 rpm), and Uniformity of dosage units.

GLYBURIDE

Chemical group: Sulfonylurea.

Chemical name: Benzamide, 5-chloro-N-[2-[4-[[[(cyclohexylamino)carbonyl]amino]sulfonyl]phenyl]ethyl]-2-methoxy-.

Molecular formula: $C_{23}H_{28}ClN_3O_5S$.

Molecular weight: 494.00.

Description: White, crystalline compound.

pKa: 5.3.

Solubility: Practically insoluble in water and in ether; slightly soluble in alcohol and in methyl alcohol.

USP requirements:
Glyburide USP—Preserve in tight containers. Contains not less than 98.0% and not more than 102.0% of glyburide, calculated on the dried basis. Meets the requirements for Identification, Loss on drying (not more than 1.0%), Residue on ignition (not more than 0.5%), Heavy metals (not more than 0.002%), and Chromatographic purity.

Glyburide Tablets USP—Preserve in well-closed containers. Contain the labeled amount, within ±10%. Meet the requirement for Identification.

Glyburide Tablets (Micronized)—Not in *USP–NF*.

GLYBURIDE AND METFORMIN

For *Glyburide* and *Metformin*—See individual listings for chemistry information.

USP requirements: Glyburide and Metformin Hydrochloride Tablets—Not in *USP–NF*.

GLYCERIN

Chemical name: 1,2,3-Propanetriol.

Molecular formula: $C_3H_8O_3$.

Molecular weight: 92.09.

Description: Glycerin USP—Clear, colorless, syrupy liquid. Has not more than a slight characteristic odor, which is neither harsh nor disagreeable. Is hygroscopic. Its solutions are neutral to litmus.

NF category: Humectant; plasticizer; solvent; tonicity agent.

Solubility: Glycerin USP—Miscible with water and with alcohol. Insoluble in chloroform, in ether, and in fixed and volatile oils.

USP requirements:

Glycerin USP—Preserve in tight containers. Contains not less than 99.0% and not more than 101.0% of glycerin, calculated on the anhydrous basis. Meets the requirements for Identification, Specific gravity (not less than 1.249), Color, Water (not more than 5.0%), Residue on ignition (not more than 0.01%), Chloride (not more than 0.001%), Sulfate (not more than 0.002%), Heavy metals (not more than 5 ppm), Chlorinated compounds (not more than 0.003% of chlorine), Organic volatile impurities, Fatty acids and esters, and Limit of diethylene glycol and related compounds.

Glycerin Ophthalmic Solution USP—Preserve in tight containers of glass or plastic, containing not more than 15 mL, protected from light. The container or individual carton is sealed and tamper-proof so that sterility is assured at time of first use. A sterile, anhydrous solution of Glycerin, containing not less than 98.5% of glycerin. (Note: In the preparation of this Ophthalmic Solution, use Glycerin that has a low water content, in order that the Ophthalmic Solution may comply with the Water limit. This may be ensured by using Glycerin having a specific gravity of not less than 1.2607, corresponding to a concentration of 99.5%.) Meets the requirements for Identification, Sterility, pH (4.5–7.5), and Water (not more than 1.0%).

Note: Do not use the Ophthalmic Solution if it contains crystals, or if it is cloudy, discolored, or contains a precipitate.

Glycerin Oral Solution USP—Preserve in tight containers. Contains the labeled amount, within ±5%. Meets the requirements for Identification and pH (5.5–7.5).

Glycerin Rectal Solution—Not in *USP–NF*.

Glycerin Suppositories USP—Preserve in well-closed containers. Contain Glycerin solidified with Sodium Stearate. Contain not less than 75.0% and not more than 90.0%, by weight, of glycerin. Meet the requirements for Identification and Water (not more than 15.0%).

GLYCERYL BEHENATE

Description: Glyceryl Behenate NF—Fine powder, having a faint odor. Melts at about 70 °C.

NF category: Tablet and/or capsule lubricant.

Solubility: Glyceryl Behenate NF—Practically insoluble in water and in alcohol; soluble in chloroform.

NF requirements: Glyceryl Behenate NF—Preserve in tight containers, at a temperature not higher than 35 °C. A mixture of glycerides of fatty acids, mainly behenic acid. Meets the requirements for Identification, Acid value (not more than 4), Iodine value (not more than 3), Saponification value (145–165), Residue on ignition (not more than 0.1%), Heavy metals (not more than 0.001%), Organic volatile impurities, Content of 1-monoglycerides (12.0–18.0%), and Limit of free glycerin (not more than 1.0%).

GLYCERYL MONOSTEARATE

Chemical name: Octadecanoic acid, monoester with 1,2,3-propanetriol.

Molecular formula: $C_{21}H_{42}O_4$.

Molecular weight: 358.56.

Description: Glyceryl Monostearate NF—White, wax-like solid, or white, wax-like beads or flakes. Slight agreeable fatty odor. Affected by light.

NF category: Emulsifying and/or solubilizing agent.

Solubility: Glyceryl Monostearate NF—Dissolves in hot organic solvents such as alcohol, mineral or fixed oils, ether, and acetone. Insoluble in water, but it may be dispersed in hot water with the aid of a small amount of soap or other suitable surface-active agent.

NF requirements: Glyceryl Monostearate NF—Preserve in tight, light-resistant containers. Contains not less than 90.0% of monoglycerides of saturated fatty acids, chiefly glyceryl monostearate and glyceryl monopalmitate. Meets the requirements for Melting range (not less than 55 °C), Residue on ignition (not more than 0.5%), Heavy metals (not more than 0.001%), Organic volatile impurities, Acid value (not more than 6), Iodine value (not more than 3), Saponification value (155–165), Hydroxyl value (300–330), and Free glycerin (not more than 1.2%).

GLYCINE

Chemical name: Glycine.

Molecular formula: $C_2H_5NO_2$.

Molecular weight: 75.07.

Description: Glycine USP—White, odorless, crystalline powder. Its solutions are acid to litmus.

Solubility: Glycine USP—Freely soluble in water; very slightly soluble in alcohol and in ether.

USP requirements:

Glycine USP—Preserve in well-closed containers. Contains not less than 98.5% and not more than 101.5% of glycine, calculated on the dried basis. Meets the requirements for Identification, Loss on drying (not more than 0.2%), Residue on ignition (not more than 0.1%), Chloride (not more than 0.007%), Sulfate (not more than 0.0065%), Heavy metals (not more than 0.002%), Hydrolyzable substances, and Organic volatile impurities.

Glycine Irrigation USP—Preserve in single-dose containers, preferably of Type I or Type II glass. A sterile solution of Glycine in Water for Injection. Contains the labeled amount, within ±5%. Meets the requirements for Identification, Bacterial endotoxins, and pH (4.5–6.5), and for Injections (except the container in which the solution is packaged may be designed to empty rapidly and may exceed 1000 mL in capacity).

GLYCOPYRROLATE

Chemical group: Quaternary ammonium compound.

Chemical name: Pyrrolidinium, 3-[(cyclopentylhydroxyphenylacetyl)oxy]-1,1-dimethyl-, bromide.

Molecular formula: $C_{19}H_{28}BrNO_3$.

Molecular weight: 398.33.

Description: Glycopyrrolate USP—White, odorless, crystalline powder.

Solubility: Glycopyrrolate USP—Soluble in water and in alcohol; practically insoluble in chloroform and in ether.

USP requirements:
Glycopyrrolate USP—Preserve in tight containers. Dried at 105 °C for 3 hours, contains not less than 98.0% and not more than 100.5% of glycopyrrolate. Meets the requirements for Identification, Melting range (193–198 °C, the range between beginning and end of melting not more than 2 °C), Loss on drying (not more than 0.5%), Residue on ignition (not more than 0.3%), and Ordinary impurities.
Glycopyrrolate Injection USP—Preserve in single-dose or in multiple-dose containers, preferably of Type I glass. A sterile solution of Glycopyrrolate in Water for Injection. Contains the labeled amount, within ±7%. Meets the requirements for Identification, Bacterial endotoxins, and pH (2.0–3.0), and for Injections.
Glycopyrrolate Tablets USP—Preserve in tight containers. Contain the labeled amount, within ±7%. Meet the requirements for Identification, Dissolution (75% in 45 minutes in water in Apparatus 1 at 100 rpm), and Uniformity of dosage units.

GOLDENSEAL

NF requirements:
Goldenseal NF—Store in tight containers, protected from light, moisture, and heat. Consists of the dried roots and rhizomes of *Hydrastis canadensis* (Linné) (Fam. Ranunculaceae). The label states the Latin binomial and, following the official name, the parts of the plant contained in the article. Contains not less than 2.0% of hydrastine and not less than 2.5% of berberine, calculated on the dried basis. Meets the requirements for Botanic characteristics, Thin-layer chromatographic identification test, Loss on drying (not more than 12.0%), Foreign organic matter (not more than 2.0%), Total ash (not more than 9%), Acid-insoluble ash (not more than 5%), Pesticide residues, Heavy metals (20 milligrams per gram), and Content of berberine and hydrastine.
Powdered Goldenseal NF—Store in tight containers, protected from light and moisture. It is Goldenseal reduced to a fine or very fine powder. The label states the Latin binomial, and following the official name, the parts of the plant contained in the article. Meets the requirements for Botanic characteristics, and for Thin-layer chromatographic identification test, Loss on drying, Foreign organic

matter, Total ash, Acid-insoluble ash, Pesticide residues, Heavy metals, and Content of berberine and hydrastine for Goldenseal.
Powdered Goldenseal Extract NF—Store in tight containers, protected from light and moisture. Prepared from the pulverized dried roots and rhizomes of *Hydrastis canadensis* (L.) (Fam. Ranunculaceae) using suitable solvents. The label states the Latin binomial and, following the official name, the part of the plant from which the particle was prepared. Label it to indicate the content of hydrastine and berberine, the extracting solvent used for preparation, and the ratio of the starting crude plant material to Powdered Extract. Contains not less than 5% of hydrastine and not less than 10% of total alkaloids. The ratio of starting crude plant material to Powdered Extract is 2:1. Meets the requirements for Thin-layer chromatographic identification test, Microbial limits, Loss on drying (not more than 5.0%), Pestiside residues, Heavy metals (not more than 20 milligrams per gram), and Content of total alkaloids.

GOLD SODIUM THIOMALATE

Chemical name: Butanedioic acid, mercapto-, monogold(1+) sodium salt.

Molecular formula: $C_4H_3AuNa_2O_4S + C_4H_4AuNaO_4S$.

Molecular weight: 758.17.

Description: Gold sodium thiomalate—White to yellowish white, odorless or practically odorless, lumpy solid.

Solubility: Gold sodium thiomalate—Very soluble in water; insoluble in alcohol, in ether, and in most organic solvents.

USP requirements:
Gold Sodium Thiomalate USP—Preserve in tight, light-resistant containers. A mixture of the mono- and di-sodium salts of gold thiomalic acid. Contains not less than 44.8% and not more than 49.6% of gold. Contains not less than 49.0% and not more than 52.5% of gold, on a dry, alcohol- and glycerin-free basis. Meets the requirements for Identification, pH (5.8–6.5, in a solution [1 in 10]), Loss on drying (not more than 8.0%), Limit of alcohol (not more than 4.0%), and Glycerin (not more than 5.5%).
Gold Sodium Thiomalate Injection USP—Preserve in single-dose or in multiple-dose containers, preferably of Type I glass, protected from light. A sterile solution of Gold Sodium Thiomalate in Water for Injection. Contains the labeled amount, within ±5%. Meets the requirements for Identification and pH (5.8–6.5), and for Injections.

GONADORELIN

Source: A gonad stimulating principle (luteinizing hormone-releasing factor). Source of this compound may be sheep, pig, or other species, or it could be synthetic.

Chemical name:
Gonadorelin acetate—5-Oxo-L-prolyl-L-histidyl-L-tryptophyl-L-seryl-L-tyrosylglycyl-L-leucyl-L-arginyl-L-prolylglycinamide acetate (salt) hydrate.
Gonadorelin hydrochloride—5-Oxo-L-prolyl-L-histidyl-L-tryptophyl-L-seryl-L-tyrosylglycyl-L-leucyl-L-arginyl-L-prolylglycinamide hydrochloride.

Molecular formula:
Gonadorelin acetate—$C_{55}H_{75}N_{17}O_{13} \cdot xC_2H_4O_2 \cdot yH_2O$.
Gonadorelin dihydrochloride—$C_{55}H_{75}N_{17}O_{13} \cdot 2HCl$.

Note: Gonadorelin acetate is $C_{55}H_{75}N_{17}O_{13}$ as the diacetate (as the tetrahydrate) or a mixture of monoacetate and diacetate hydrates. Gonadorelin hydrochloride is $C_{55}H_{75}N_{17}O_{13}$ as the monohydrochloride or the dihydrochloride or as a mixture of these.

Molecular weight: Gonadorelin dihydrochloride—1255.44.

Description: White powder. Hygroscopic and moisture-sensitive.

Solubility: Soluble in alcohol and in water.

USP requirements:
Gonadorelin for Injection USP—Preserve in tight, well-sealed containers. Sterile mixture of Gonadorelin Hydrochloride with suitable diluents. Contains the equivalent amount of the labeled amount of gonadorelin, within −10% to +15%. Meets the requirements for Identification, Constituted solution, Bacterial endotoxins, and pH (4.0–8.0, in a solution constituted as directed in the labeling), for Sterility tests and for Labeling under Injections.
Gonadorelin Acetate for Injection—Not in *USP–NF*.
Gonadorelin Hydrochloride USP—Preserve in tight, well-sealed containers. It is a synthetic polypeptide hormone having the property of stimulating the release of luteinizing hormone from the hypothalamus. Contains not less than 94.0% and not more than 104.0% of gonadorelin hydrochloride, calculated on the anhydrous basis. Meets the requirements for Identification, Specific rotation (−57° to −63°, calculated on the anhydrous and chloride-free basis), Water (not more than 3.0%), Limit of acetate (not more than 1.0%), Chromatographic purity (not more than 3.0% of any individual impurity, and not more than 5.0% of total impurities), and Content of chloride (4.0–6.0%).
Note: Gonadorelin Hydrochloride is extremely hygroscopic. Protect from exposure to moisture, and store in a desiccator.
Gonadorelin Hydrochloride for Injection—Not in *USP–NF*.

CHORIONIC GONADOTROPIN

Description:
Chorionic Gonadotropin USP—White or practically white, amorphous powder.
Chorionic Gonadotropin for Injection USP—White or practically white, amorphous solid having the characteristic appearance of substances prepared by freeze-drying.

Solubility: Chorionic Gonadotropin USP—Freely soluble in water.

USP requirements:
Chorionic Gonadotropin USP—Preserve in tight containers, preferably of Type I glass, in a refrigerator. A gonad-stimulating polypeptide hormone obtained from the urine of pregnant women. Its potency is not less than 1500 USP Chorionic Gonadotropin Units in each mg, and not less than 80.0% and not more than 125.0% of the potency stated on the label. Meets the requirements for Bacterial endotoxins, Acute toxicity, Water (not more than 5.0%), and Estrogenic activity.
Chorionic Gonadotropin for Injection USP—Preserve in Containers for Sterile Solids. A sterile, dry mixture of Chorionic Gonadotropin with suitable diluents and buffers. Label it to indicate the expiration date. Contains the labeled amount in USP Chorionic Gonadotropin Units, within −20% to +25%. Meets the requirements for Constituted solution, Bacterial endotoxins, pH (6.0–8.0), Estrogenic activity, and Uniformity of dosage units, and for Sterility tests and Labeling under Injections.

GOSERELIN

Source: Goserelin acetate—Synthetic decapeptide analog of luteinizing hormone-releasing hormone (LHRH).

Chemical name: Goserelin acetate—L-pyroglutamyl-L-histidyl-L-tryptophyl-L-seryl-L-tyrosyl-D-(0-tert-butyl)seryl-L-leucyl-L-arginyl-L-prolyl-azaglycine amide acetate.

Molecular formula: Goserelin acetate—$C_{61}H_{87}N_{18}O_{16}$.

Molecular weight: Goserelin acetate—1328.

Description: Goserelin acetate—Off-white powder.

Solubility: Goserelin acetate—Freely soluble in glacial acetic acid; soluble in water, in 0.1 M hydrochloric acid, in 0.1 M sodium hydroxide, in dimethylformamide, and in dimethyl sulfoxide; practically insoluble in acetone, in chloroform, and in ether.

USP requirements: Goserelin Acetate Implants—Not in *USP–NF*.

GRAMICIDIN

Chemical name: Gramicidin.

Description: Gramicidin USP—White or practically white, odorless, crystalline powder.

Solubility: Gramicidin USP—Insoluble in water; soluble in alcohol.

USP requirements: Gramicidin USP—Preserve in tight containers. An antibacterial substance produced by the growth of *Bacillus brevis* Dubos (Fam. Bacillaceae). May be obtained from tyrothricin. Has a potency of not less than 900 mcg of gramicidin per mg, calculated on the dried basis. Meets the requirements for Identification, Melting temperature (not less than 229 °C, determined after drying), Crystallinity, Loss on drying (not more than 3.0%), and Residue on ignition (not more than 1.0%).

GRANISETRON

Chemical name: 1*H*-Indazole-3-carboxamide, 1-methyl-*N*-(9-methyl-9-azabicyclo[3.3.1]non-3-yl)-, monohydrochloride, *endo*-.

Molecular formula: $C_{18}H_{24}N_4O \cdot HCl$.

Molecular weight: 348.87.

Description: Granisetron hydrochloride—White to off-white solid.

Solubility: Granisetron hydrochloride—Readily soluble in water and in normal saline at 20 °C.

USP requirements:
Granisetron Hydrochoride Injection—Not in *USP–NF*.
Granisetron Hydrochoride Tablets—Not in *USP–NF*.

GREEN SOAP

Description: Green Soap USP—Soft, unctuous, yellowish white to brownish or greenish yellow, transparent to translucent mass. Has a slight, characteristic odor, often suggesting the oil from which it was prepared. Its solution (1 in 20) is alkaline to bromothymol blue TS.

USP requirements:

Green Soap USP—Preserve in well-closed containers. A potassium soap made by the saponification of suitable vegetable oils, excluding coconut oil and palm kernel oil, without the removal of glycerin.

Green Soap may be prepared as follows: 380 grams of the Vegetable Oil, 20 grams of Oleic Acid, 91.7 grams of Potassium Hydroxide (total alkali 85%), 50 mL of Glycerin, and a sufficient quantity of Purified Water to make about 1000 grams. Mix the oil and the Oleic Acid, and heat the mixture to about 80 °C. Dissolve the Potassium Hydroxide in a mixture of the Glycerin and 100 mL of Purified Water, and add the solution, while it is still hot, to the hot oil. Stir the mixture vigorously until emulsified, then heat while continuing the stirring, until the mixture is homogeneous and a test portion will dissolve to give a clear solution in hot water. Add hot purified water to make the product weigh 1000 grams, continuing the stirring until the Soap is homogeneous.

Meets the requirements for Water (not more than 52.0%), Alcohol-insoluble substances (not more than 3.0%), Free alkali hydroxides (not more than 0.25% of potassium hydroxide), Alkali carbonates (0.35%, as potassium carbonate), Unsaponified matter, and Characteristics of the liberated fatty acids.

Green Soap Tincture USP—Preserve in tight containers.

Prepare Green Soap Tincture as follows: 650 grams of Green Soap, Suitable essential oil(s), 316 mL of Alcohol, and a sufficient quantity of Purified Water to make 1000 mL. Mix the oil(s) and Alcohol, dissolve in this the Green Soap by stirring or by agitation, set the solution aside for 24 hours, filter through paper, and add water to make 1000 mL.

Meets the requirements for Identification and Alcohol content (28.0–32.0%).

GREPAFLOXACIN

Chemical name: Grepafloxacin hydrochloride—3-Quinolinecarboxylic acid, 1-cyclopropyl-6-fluoro-1,4-dihydro-5-methyl-7-(3-methyl-1-piperazinyl)-4-oxo-, monohydrochloride, (±)-.

Molecular formula: Grepafloxacin hydrochloride—$C_{19}H_{22}FN_3O_3$ · HCl.

Molecular weight: Grepafloxacin hydrochloride—395.86.

Solubility: Grepafloxacin hydrochloride—Soluble in water; very slightly soluble in ethanol.

USP requirements: Grepafloxacin Hydrochloride Tablets—Not in *USP–NF*.

GRISEOFULVIN

Source: Derived from a species of *Penicillium*.

Chemical name: Spiro[benzofuran-2(3*H*),1'-[2]cyclohexene]-3,4'-dione, 7-chloro-2',4,6-trimethoxy-6'-methyl-, (1'*S-trans*)-.

Molecular formula: $C_{17}H_{17}ClO_6$.

Molecular weight: 352.77.

Description: Griseofulvin USP—White to creamy white, odorless powder, in which particles of the order of 4 micrometers in diameter predominate.

Solubility: Griseofulvin USP—Very slightly soluble in water; soluble in acetone, in dimethylformamide, and in chloroform; sparingly soluble in alcohol.

USP requirements:

Griseofulvin USP—Preserve in tight containers. Has a potency of not less than 900 mcg of griseofulvin per mg. Meets the requirements for Identification, Melting range (217–224 °C), Specific rotation (+348° to +364°), Crystallinity, Loss on drying (not more than 1.0%), Residue on ignition (not more than 0.2%), Permeability diameter (1.3–1.7 square meters per gram), Heavy metals (not more than 0.0025%), and Organic volatile impurities.

Griseofulvin Capsules USP (Microsize)—Preserve in tight containers. The label indicates that the griseofulvin contained is known as griseofulvin (microsize). Contain the labeled amount, within −10% to +15%. Meet the requirements for Identification, Dissolution (80% in 30 minutes in water containing 5.4 mg of sodium lauryl sulfate per mL in Apparatus 2 at 50 rpm), Uniformity of dosage units, and Loss on drying (not more than 1.0%).

Griseofulvin Oral Suspension USP (Microsize)—Preserve in tight containers. Contains one or more suitable colors, diluents, flavors, preservatives, and wetting agents. The label indicates that the griseofulvin contained is known as griseofulvin (microsize). Contains the labeled amount, within −10% to +15%. Meets the requirements for Identification, Uniformity of dosage units (single-unit containers), Deliverable volume (multiple-unit containers), and pH (5.5–7.5).

Griseofulvin Tablets USP (Microsize)—Preserve in tight containers. The label indicates that the griseofulvin contained is known as griseofulvin (microsize). Contain the labeled amount, within −10% to +15%. Meet the requirements for Identification, Dissolution (75% in 90 minutes in water containing 40.0 mg of sodium lauryl sulfate per mL in Apparatus 2 at 75 rpm), Uniformity of dosage units, and Loss on drying (not more than 5.0%).

Ultramicrosize Griseofulvin Tablets USP—Preserve in well-closed containers. Composed of ultramicrosize crystals of Griseofulvin dispersed in Polyethylene Glycol 6000 or dispersed by other suitable means. Contain the labeled amount, within −10% to +15%. Meet the requirements for Identification, Dissolution (80% in 45 minutes in water containing 5.4 mg of sodium lauryl sulfate per mL in Apparatus 2 at 75 rpm), Uniformity of dosage units, and Loss on drying (not more than 5.0%).

GUAIFENESIN

Chemical name: 1,2-Propanediol, 3-(2-methoxyphenoxy)-.

Molecular formula: $C_{10}H_{14}O_4$.

Molecular weight: 198.22.

Description: Guaifenesin USP—White to slightly gray, crystalline powder. May have a slight characteristic odor.

Solubility: Guaifenesin USP—Soluble in water, in alcohol, in chloroform, and in propylene glycol; sparingly soluble in glycerin.

USP requirements:

Guaifenesin USP—Preserve in tight containers. Contains not less than 98.0% and not more than 102.0% of guaifenesin, calculated on the dried basis. Meets the requirements for Identification, Melting range (78–82 °C, the range between beginning and end of melting not more than 3 °C), Loss on drying (not more than 0.5%), Heavy metals (not more than 0.0025%), Chromatographic purity, and Organic volatile impurities.

Guaifenesin Capsules USP—Preserve in tight containers. Contain the labeled amount, within ±10%. Meet the requirements for Identification, Dissolution (75% in 45 minutes in water in Apparatus 1 at 100 rpm), and Uniformity of dosage units.

Guaifenesin Extended-release Capsules—Not in *USP–NF*.
Guaifenesin for Injection USP—Preserve in single-dose or in multiple-dose containers, and store at controlled room temperature. It meets the requirements for Labeling under Injections. Label it to indicate that it is for veterinary use only. The label states that it is intended for injection only by the intravenous route in horses. Contains the labeled amount, within ±10%. Meets the requirements for Identification, Constituted solution, Sterility, and Bacterial endotoxins.
Guaifenesin Oral Solution USP—Preserve in tight containers. Contains the labeled amount, within ±10%. Meets the requirements for Identification, pH (2.3–3.0), and Alcohol content (if present, within −10% to +15% of labeled amount).
Guaifenesin Syrup USP—Preserve in tight containers. Contains the labeled amount, within ±10%. Meets the requirements for Identification, pH (2.3–3.0), and Alcohol content (if present, within −10% to +15% of labeled amount).
Guaifenesin Tablets USP—Preserve in tight containers. Contain the labeled amount, within ±10%. Meet the requirements for Identification, Dissolution (75% in 45 minutes in water in Apparatus 2 at 50 rpm), and Uniformity of dosage units.
Guaifenesin Extended-release Tablets—Not in *USP–NF*.

GUAIFENESIN AND CODEINE

For *Guaifenesin* and *Codeine*—See individual listings for chemistry information.

USP requirements:
Guaifenesin and Codeine Phosphate Oral Solution USP—Preserve in tight, light-resistant containers, at controlled room temperature. Contains the labeled amounts, within ±10%. Meets the requirements for Identification, pH (2.3–3.0 if it contains alcohol; 5.0–5.5 if it does not contain alcohol), and Alcohol content (if present, within −10% to +15% of labeled amount).
Guaifenesin and Codeine Phosphate Syrup USP—Preserve in tight, light-resistant containers, at controlled room temperature. Contains the labeled amounts, within ±10%. Meets the requirements for Identification, pH (2.3–3.0 if it contains alcohol; 5.0–5.5 if it does not contain alcohol), and Alcohol content (if present, within −10% to +15% of labeled amount).
Guaifenesin and Codeine Phosphate Tablets—Not in *USP–NF*.

GUAIFENESIN, PSEUDOEPHEDRINE, AND DEXTRO-METHORPHAN

For *Guaifenesin, Pseudoephedrine,* and *Dextromethorphan*— See individual listings for chemistry information.

USP requirements:
Guaifenesin, Pseudoephedrine Hydrochloride, and Dextromethorphan Hydrobromide Capsules USP—Preserve in tight, light-resistant containers. Contain the labeled amounts, within ±10%. Meet the requirements for Identification and Uniformity of dosage units.
Guaifenesin, Pseudoephedrine Hydrochloride, and Dextromethorphan Hydrobromide Oral Solution—Not in *USP–NF*.

Guaifenesin, Pseudoephedrine Hydrochloride, and Dextromethorphan Hydrobromide Syrup—Not in *USP–NF*.
Guaifenesin, Pseudoephedrine Hydrochloride, and Dextromethorphan Hydrobromide Tablets—Not in *USP–NF*.

GUANABENZ

Chemical name: Guanabenz acetate—Hydrazinecarboximidamide, 2-[(2,6-dichlorophenyl)methylene]-, monoacetate.

Molecular formula: Guanabenz acetate—$C_8H_8Cl_2N_4 \cdot C_2H_4O_2$.

Molecular weight: Guanabenz acetate—291.13.

Description: Guanabenz Acetate USP—White or almost white powder having not more than a slight odor.

Solubility: Guanabenz Acetate USP—Sparingly soluble in water and in 0.1 *N* hydrochloric acid; soluble in alcohol and in propylene glycol.

USP requirements:
Guanabenz Acetate USP—Preserve in tight, light-resistant containers. Contains not less than 98.0% and not more than 101.5% of guanabenz acetate. Meets the requirements for Identification, pH (5.5–7.0, in a solution [7 in 1000]), Loss on drying (not more than 1.0%), Residue on ignition (not more than 0.2%), Limit of 2,6-dichlorobenzaldehyde, Chromatographic purity, and Organic volatile impurities.
Guanabenz Acetate Tablets USP—Preserve in tight, light-resistant containers. Contain an amount of guanabenz acetate equivalent to the labeled amount of guanabenz, within ±10%. Meet the requirements for Identification, Dissolution (75% in 60 minutes in water in Apparatus 2 at 50 rpm), Uniformity of dosage units, and Chromatographic purity.

GUANADREL

Chemical name: Guanadrel sulfate—Guanidine (1,4-dioxaspiro[4.5]dec-2-ylmethyl)-, sulfate (2:1).

Molecular formula: Guanadrel sulfate—$(C_{10}H_{19}N_3O_2)_2 \cdot H_2SO_4$.

Molecular weight: Guanadrel sulfate—524.63.

Description: Guanadrel Sulfate USP—White to off-white, crystalline powder. Melts at about 235 °C, with decomposition.

Solubility: Guanadrel Sulfate USP—Soluble in water; sparingly soluble in methanol; slightly soluble in alcohol and in acetone.

USP requirements:
Guanadrel Sulfate USP—Preserve in well-closed containers. Contains not less than 97.0% and not more than 103.0% of guanadrel sulfate, calculated on the dried basis. Meets the requirements for Identification, Loss on drying (not more than 0.5%), Residue on ignition (not more than 0.5%), Heavy metals (not more than 0.002%), and Organic volatile impurities.
Guanadrel Sulfate Tablets USP—Preserve in tight, light-resistant containers. Contain the labeled amount, within ±10%. Meet the requirements for Identification, Dissolution (70% in 20 minutes in phosphate buffer (pH 6.8) in Apparatus 2 at 50 rpm), and Uniformity of dosage units.

GUANETHIDINE

Chemical name:
Guanethidine monosulfate—Guanidine, [2-(hexahydro-1(2H)-azocinyl)ethyl]-, sulfate (1:1).
Guanethidine sulfate—Guanidine, [2-(hexahydro-1(2H)-azocinyl)ethyl]-, sulfate (2:1).

Molecular formula:
Guanethidine monosulfate—$C_{10}H_{22}N_4 \cdot H_2SO_4$.
Guanethidine sulfate—$(C_{10}H_{22}N_4)_2 \cdot H_2SO_4$.

Molecular weight:
Guanethidine monosulfate—296.39.
Guanethidine sulfate—494.70.

Description: Guanethidine Monosulfate USP—White to off-white, crystalline powder.

pKa: 9.0 and 12.0.

Solubility: Guanethidine Monosulfate USP—Very soluble in water; sparingly soluble in alcohol; practically insoluble in chloroform.

USP requirements:
Guanethidine Monosulfate USP—Preserve in well-closed containers. Contains not less than 97.0% and not more than 103.0% of guanethidine monosulfate, calculated on the dried basis. Meets the requirements for Identification, pH (4.7–5.7, in a solution containing 20 mg per mL), Loss on drying (not more than 0.5%), Residue on ignition (not more than 0.2%), Heavy metals (not more than 0.001%), and Organic volatile impurities.
Guanethidine Monosulfate Tablets USP—Preserve in well-closed containers. Contain an amount of guanethidine monosulfate equivalent to the labeled amount of guanethidine sulfate, within ±10%. Meet the requirements for Identification, Dissolution (75% in 45 minutes in water in Apparatus 1 at 100 rpm), and Uniformity of dosage units.

GUANETHIDINE AND HYDROCHLOROTHIAZIDE

For Guanethidine and Hydrochlorothiazide—See individual listings for chemistry information.

USP requirements: Guanethidine Monosulfate and Hydrochlorothiazide Tablets—Not in USP–NF.

GUANFACINE

Chemical name: Guanfacine hydrochloride—Benzeneacetamide, N-(aminoiminomethyl)-2,6-dichloro-, monohydrochloride.

Molecular formula: Guanfacine hydrochloride—$C_9H_9Cl_2N_3O \cdot HCl$.

Molecular weight: Guanfacine hydrochloride—282.55.

Description: Guanfacine hydrochloride—White to off-white powder.

Solubility: Guanfacine hydrochloride—Sparingly soluble in water and in alcohol; slightly soluble in acetone.

USP requirements:
Guanfacine Tablets USP—Preserve in tight, light-resistant containers. Contain an amount of Guanfacine Hydrochloride equivalent to the labeled amount of guanfacine, within ±10%. Meet the requirements for Identification, Dissolution (75% in 45 minutes in water in Apparatus 2 at 50 rpm), and Uniformity of dosage units.

Guanfacine Hydrochloride USP—Preserve in tight, light-resistant containers. Contains not less than 98.0% and not more than 102.0% of guanfacine hydrochloride, calculated on the dried basis. Meets the requirements for Identification, Loss on drying (not more than 0.5%), Residue on ignition (not more than 0.1%), Heavy metals (not more than 0.002%), Related compounds, and Chromatographic purity.

Caution: Guanfacine Hydrochloride is a potent antihypertensive drug. Minimize flying dust, and avoid all bodily and respiratory contact with this substance.

GUAR GUM

Description: Guar Gum NF—White to yellowish white, practically odorless powder.
NF category: Suspending and/or viscosity-increasing agent; tablet binder.

Solubility: Guar Gum NF—Dispersible in hot or cold water, forming a colloidal solution.

NF requirements: Guar Gum NF—Preserve in well-closed containers. A gum obtained from the ground endosperms of Cyamopsis tetragonolobus (Linné) Taub. (Fam. Leguminosae). Consists chiefly of a high molecular weight hydrocolloidal polysaccharide composed of galactan and mannan units combined through glycosidic linkages, which may be described chemically as a galactomannan. Meets the requirements for Identification, Loss on drying (not more than 15.0%), Ash (not more than 1.5%), Acid-insoluble matter (not more than 7.0%), Arsenic (not more than 3 ppm), Lead (not more than 0.001%), Heavy metals (not more than 0.002%), Protein (not more than 10.0%), Starch, Content of galactomannans (not less than 66.0%), and Organic volatile impurities.

GUTTA PERCHA

Source: Trans isomer of rubber prepared from the exudate of various trees of the genus Palaquium, Fam. Sapotaceae.

Description: Gutta Percha USP—Lumps or blocks of variable size; externally brown or grayish brown to grayish white in color; internally reddish yellow or reddish gray and having a laminated or fibrous appearance. Is flexible but only slightly elastic. Has a slight, characteristic odor.

Solubility: Gutta Percha USP—Insoluble in water; about 90% soluble in chloroform; partly soluble in carbon disulfide and in turpentine oil.

USP requirements: Gutta Percha USP—Preserve under water in well-closed containers, protected from light. The coagulated, dried, purified latex of the trees of the genera Palaquium and Payena and most commonly Palaquium gutta (Hooker) Baillon (Fam. Sapotaceae). Meets the requirement for Residue on ignition (not more than 1.7%).

HAEMOPHILUS B CONJUGATE VACCINE

Source: Purified capsular polysaccharide, a polymer of ribose, ribitol, and phosphate (PRP), from the bacterium Haemophilus influenzae type b (Hib). It has been conjugated in one of the following ways—For the diphtheria toxoid conjugate, the polysaccharide has been conjugated to the diphtheria toxoid via a 6-carbon linker molecule; for the diphtheria CRM$_{197}$ protein conjugate, the oligosaccharide has been derived from the

polysaccharide and has been bound directly to CRM$_{197}$ (a nontoxic variant of diphtheria toxin) by reductive amination; for the meningococcal protein conjugate, the polysaccharide has been covalently bound to an outer membrane protein complex (OMPC) of the B11 strain of *Neisseria meningitidis* serogroup B; and for the tetanus protein conjugate, the polysaccharide has been covalently bound to tetanus toxoid protein.

USP requirements:
Haemophilus b Conjugate Vaccine Injection—Not in *USP–NF*
Haemophilus b Conjugate Vaccine (HbOC—Diphtheria CRM$_{197}$ Protein Conjugate) Injection—Not in *USP–NF*.
Haemophilus b Conjugate Vaccine (PRP-D—Diphtheria Toxoid Conjugate) Injection—Not in *USP–NF*.
Haemophilus b Conjugate Vaccine (PRP-OMP—Meningococcal Protein Conjugate) Injection—Not in *USP–NF*.
Haemophilus b Conjugate Vaccine (PRP-T—Tetanus Protein Conjugate) Injection—Not in *USP–NF*.

HAEMOPHILUS B POLYSACCHARIDE VACCINE

Source: Purified capsular polysaccharide, a polymer of ribose, ribitol, and phosphate (PRP), from the bacterium *Haemophilus influenzae* type b (Hib).

USP requirements: Haemophilus b Polysaccharide Vaccine for Injection—Not in *USP–NF*.

HALAZEPAM

Chemical name: 2*H*-1,4-Benzodiazepin-2-one, 7-chloro-1,3-dihydro-5-phenyl-1-(2,2,2-trifluoroethyl)-.

Molecular formula: C$_{17}$H$_{12}$ClF$_3$N$_2$O.

Molecular weight: 352.74.

Description: Fine, white to light cream-colored powder. Melts at about 165 °C.

Solubility: Freely soluble in chloroform; soluble in methanol; very slightly soluble in water.

USP requirements: Halazepam Tablets—Not in *USP–NF*.

HALAZONE

Chemical name: Benzoic acid, 4-[(dichloroamino)sulfonyl]-.

Molecular formula: C$_7$H$_5$Cl$_2$NO$_4$S.

Molecular weight: 270.09.

Description: Halazone USP—White, crystalline powder, having a characteristic chlorine-like odor. Affected by light. Melts at about 194 °C, with decomposition.

Solubility:
Halazone USP—Very slightly soluble in water and in chloroform; soluble in glacial acetic acid. Dissolves in solutions of alkali hydroxides and carbonates with the formation of a salt.
Halazone Tablets for Solution USP—Soluble in water.

USP requirements:
Halazone USP—Preserve in tight, light-resistant containers. Contains not less than 91.5% and not more than 100.5% of halazone, calculated on the dried basis. Meets the requirements for Identification, Loss on drying (not more than 0.5%), and Readily carbonizable substances.

Halazone Tablets for Solution USP—Preserve in tight, light-resistant containers. Label the Halazone Tablets for Solution to indicate that they are not intended to be swallowed. Contain the labeled amount, within −10% to +35%. Meet the requirements for Identification, Disintegration (10 minutes), Uniformity of dosage units, and pH (not less than 7.0, in a solution of 1 Halazone Tablet, containing 4 mg of halazone, in 200 mL of water).

HALCINONIDE

Chemical name: Pregn-4-ene-3,20-dione, 21-chloro-9-fluoro-11-hydroxy-16,17-[(1-methylethylidene)bis(oxy)]-, (11 beta,16 alpha)-.

Molecular formula: C$_{24}$H$_{32}$ClFO$_5$.

Molecular weight: 454.96.

Description: Halcinonide USP—White to off-white, odorless, crystalline powder.

Solubility: Halcinonide USP—Soluble in acetone and in chloroform; slightly soluble in alcohol and in ethyl ether; insoluble in water and in hexanes.

USP requirements:
Halcinonide USP—Preserve in well-closed containers. Contains not less than 97.0% and not more than 102.0% of halcinonide. Meets the requirements for Identification, Specific rotation (+150° to +160°), Loss on drying (not more than 1.0%), Residue on ignition (not more than 0.2%), and Chromatographic purity.
Halcinonide Cream USP—Preserve in well-closed containers. It is Halcinonide in a suitable cream base. Contains the labeled amount, within ±10%. Meets the requirements for Identification, Microbial limits, and Minimum fill.
Halcinonide Ointment USP—Preserve in well-closed containers. It is Halcinonide in a suitable ointment base. Contains the labeled amount, within ±10%. Meets the requirements for Identification, Microbial limits, and Minimum fill.
Halcinonide Topical Solution USP—Preserve in well-closed containers. It is Halcinonide in a suitable aqueous vehicle. Contains the labeled amount, within ±10%. Meets the requirements for Identification and Microbial limits.

HALOBETASOL

Chemical name: Halobetasol propionate—Pregna-1,4-diene-3,20-dione, 21-chloro-6,9-difluoro-11-hydroxy-16-methyl-17-(1-oxopropoxy)-, (6 alpha,11 beta,16 beta)-.

Molecular formula: Halobetasol propionate—C$_{25}$H$_{31}$ClF$_2$O$_5$.

Molecular weight: Halobetasol propionate—484.96.

Description: Halobetasol propionate—White crystalline powder.

Solubility: Halobetasol propionate—Insoluble in water.

USP requirements:
Halobetasol Propionate Cream—Not in *USP–NF*.
Halobetasol Propionate Ointment—Not in *USP–NF*.

HALOFANTRINE

Chemical name: Halofantrine hydrochloride—9-Phenanthrenementhanol, 1,3-dichloro-alpha-[2-(dibutylamino)ethyl]-6-(trifluoromethyl)-, hydrochloride.

Molecular formula: Halofantrine hydrochloride—$C_{26}H_{30}Cl_2F_3NO \cdot$ HCl.

Molecular weight: Halofantrine hydrochloride—536.88.

USP requirements:

Halofantrine Hydrochloride Oral Suspension—Not in *USP–NF*.

Halofantrine Hydrochloride Tablets—Not in *USP–NF*.

HALOPERIDOL

Chemical group: A butyrophenone derivative.

Chemical name:

Haloperidol—1-Butanone, 4-[4-(4-chlorophenyl)-4-hydroxy-1-piperidinyl]-1-(4-fluorophenyl)-.

Haloperidol decanoate—Decanoic acid, 4-(4-chlorophenyl)-1-[4-(4-fluorophenyl)-4-oxobutyl]-4-piperidinyl ester.

Molecular formula:

Haloperidol—$C_{21}H_{23}ClFNO_2$.

Haloperidol decanoate—$C_{31}H_{41}ClFNO_3$.

Molecular weight:

Haloperidol—375.86.

Haloperidol decanoate—530.11.

Description: Haloperidol USP—White to faintly yellowish, amorphous or microcrystalline powder. Its saturated solution is neutral to litmus.

Solubility:

Haloperidol USP—Practically insoluble in water; soluble in chloroform; sparingly soluble in alcohol; slightly soluble in ether.

Haloperidol decanoate—Practically insoluble in water; soluble in most organic solvents.

USP requirements:

Haloperidol USP—Preserve in tight, light-resistant containers. Contains not less than 98.0% and not more than 102.0% of haloperidol, calculated on the dried basis. Meets the requirements for Identification, Melting range (147–152 °C), Loss on drying (not more than 0.5%), Residue on ignition (not more than 0.1%), Limit of haloperidol related compound A, and Organic volatile impurities.

Haloperidol Injection USP—Preserve in single-dose or in multiple-dose containers, preferably of Type I glass, protected from light. A sterile solution of Haloperidol in Water for Injection, prepared with the aid of Lactic Acid. Contains the labeled amount, within ±10%. Meets the requirements for Identification, Bacterial endotoxins, and pH (3.0–3.8), and for Injections.

Haloperidol Oral Solution USP—Preserve in tight, light-resistant containers. A solution of Haloperidol in Water, prepared with the aid of Lactic Acid. Contains the labeled amount, within ±10%. Meets the requirements for Identification and pH (2.75–3.75).

Haloperidol Tablets USP—Preserve in tight, light-resistant containers. Contain the labeled amount, within ±10%. Meet the requirements for Identification, Dissolution (80% in 60 minutes in simulated gastric fluid TS, without the enzyme, in Apparatus 1 at 100 rpm), and Uniformity of dosage units.

Haloperidol Decanoate Injection—Not in *USP–NF*.

HALOPROGIN

Chemical name: Benzene, 1,2,4-trichloro-5-[(3-iodo-2-propynyl) oxy]-.

Molecular formula: $C_9H_4Cl_3IO$.

Molecular weight: 361.39.

Description: White or pale yellow crystals. Melting point is about 113–114 °C.

Solubility: Very slightly soluble in water; easily soluble in methanol and in ethanol.

USP requirements:

Haloprogin USP—Preserve in tight, light-resistant containers. Contains not less than 95.0% and not more than 102.0% of haloprogin, calculated on the dried basis. Meets the requirements for Identification, Melting range (110–114 °C), Acidity, Loss on drying (not more than 0.5%), Residue on ignition (not more than 0.1%), and Heavy metals (not more than 0.005%).

Haloprogin Cream USP—Preserve in tight, light-resistant containers, at controlled room temperature. Contains the labeled amount, within ±10%. Meets the requirements for Identification, Microbial limits, Minimum fill, and Water (not more than 3.0%).

Haloprogin Topical Solution USP—Preserve in tight, light-resistant containers, at controlled room temperature. Contains the labeled amount, within ±10%. Meets the requirements for Identification, Specific gravity (0.838–0.852), and Alcohol (within ±5% of the labeled amount).

HALOTHANE

Chemical name: Ethane, 2-bromo-2-chloro-1,1,1-trifluoro-.

Molecular formula: $C_2HBrClF_3$.

Molecular weight: 197.38.

Description: Halothane USP—Colorless, mobile, nonflammable, heavy liquid, having a characteristic odor resembling that of chloroform.

Solubility: Halothane USP—Slightly soluble in water; miscible with alcohol, with chloroform, with ether, and with fixed oils.

Other characteristics:

Blood/gas coefficient—2.5 at 37 °C.

Olive oil/water coefficient—220 at 37 °C.

USP requirements: Halothane USP—Preserve in tight, light-resistant containers, preferably of Type NP glass, and avoid exposure to excessive heat. Dispense it only in the original container. Contains 0.008% to 0.012% of thymol, by weight, as a stabilizer. Meets the requirements for Identification, Specific gravity (1.872–1.877 at 20 °C), Distilling range (not less than 95% within a 1° range between 49 and 51 °C; not less than 100% between 49 and 51 °C, a correction factor of 0.040 °C per mm being applied as necessary), Refractive index (1.369–1.371 at 20 °C), Acidity or alkalinity, Water (not more than 0.03%), Limit of nonvolatile residue, Chloride and bromide, Thymol content, and Chromatographic purity.

HAWTHORN LEAF WITH FLOWER

NF requirements:

Hawthorn Leaf with Flower NF—Store in a well-closed container, protected from light. Consists of the dried tips of the flower-bearing branches up to 7 cm in length of *Crataegus monogyna* Jacq. emend Lindman. or *Crataegus laevigata* (Poir.) DC., also known as *Crataegus oxycantha* Linné (Fam. Rosaceae). The label states the Latin binomial and, following the official name, the parts of the plant contained in the article. The label also states the following cautionary statement: "Cardiotonic Herb. Not recom-

mended for use without the advise of a health care practitioner." Contains not less than 0.6% of *C*-glycosylated flavones, expressed as vitexin, and not less than 0.45% of *O*-glycosylated flavones, expressed as hyperoside, calculated on the dried basis. Meets the requirements for Botanic characteristics, Identification, Microbial limits, Loss on drying (not more than 8.0%), Total ash (not more than 9.0%), Pesticide residues, Heavy metals (0.002%), Content of *C*-glycosylated flavones, and Content of *O*-glycosylated flavones.

Powdered Hawthorn Leaf with Flower NF—It is Hawthorn Leaf with Flower reduced to a fine or very fine powder. The Label states the latin binomial and, following the official name, the parts of the plant source from which the article was derived. The label also states the following cautionary statement: "Cardiotonic Herb. Not recommended for use without the advise of a healthcare practitioner." Meets the requirements for Botanic characteristics, Identification, Microbial limits, Loss on drying, Foreign organic matter, Total ash, Pesticide residues, Content of *C*-glycosylated flavones, and Content of *O*-glycosylated flavones for Hawthorn Leaf with Flower.

HELIUM

Chemical name: Helium.

Molecular formula: He.

Molecular weight: 4.00.

Description: Helium USP—Colorless, odorless gas, which is not combustible and does not support combustion. At 0 °C and at a pressure of 760 mm of mercury, 1000 mL of the gas weighs about 180 mg.

Solubility: Helium USP—Very slightly soluble in water.

USP requirements: Helium USP—Preserve in cylinders. Contains not less than 99.0%, by volume, of helium. Meets the requirements for Identification, Odor, Carbon monoxide (not more than 0.001%), and Air (not more than 1.0%).

HEMIN

Chemical name: Chloro[7,12-diethenyl-3,8,13,17-tetramethyl-21*H*,23*H*-porphine-2,18-dipropanoato(2-)-$N^{21},N^{22},N^{23},N^{24}$]iron.

Molecular formula: $C_{34}H_{32}ClFeN_4O_4$.

Molecular weight: 651.96.

Description: Polychromatic crystals (usually brownish to blue) which do not melt under 300 °C.

Solubility: Freely soluble in dilute base through conversion to hematin by replacement of the chlorine atom by hydroxyl; sparingly soluble in alcohol; insoluble in water.

USP requirements: Hemin for Injection—Not in *USP–NF*.

HEPARIN

Description:
Heparin calcium—White or almost white, moderately hygroscopic powder.
Heparin Sodium USP—White or pale-colored, amorphous powder. Is odorless or practically so, and is hygroscopic.

Solubility:
Heparin calcium—Soluble 1 in less than 5 of water.
Heparin Sodium USP—Soluble in water.

Other characteristics: Highly acidic.

USP requirements:
Heparin Lock Flush Solution USP—Preserve in single-dose pre-filled syringes or containers, or in multiple-dose containers, preferably of Type I glass. A sterile preparation of Heparin Sodium Injection with sufficient Sodium Chloride to make it isotonic with blood. Label it to indicate the volume of the total contents, and to indicate the potency in terms of USP Heparin Units only per mL, except that single unit-dose containers may be labeled additionally to indicate the single unit-dose volume and the total number of USP Heparin Units in the contents. Where it is labeled with total content, the label states clearly that the entire contents are to be used or, if not, any remaining portion is to be discarded. Label it to indicate the organ and species from which the heparin sodium is derived. The label states also that the Solution is intended for maintenance of patency of intravenous injection devices only, and that it is not to be used for anticoagulant therapy. The label states also that in the case of Solution having a concentration of 10 USP Heparin Units per mL, it may alter, and that in the case of higher concentrations it will alter, the results of blood coagulation tests. Exhibits the labeled potency, within −10% to +20%, stated in terms of USP Heparin Units. Contains not more than 1.00% of sodium chloride. Meets the requirements for Bacterial endotoxins, pH (5.0–7.5), and Particulate matter, and for Injections.

Heparin Calcium USP—Preserve in tight containers and store at a temperature below 40 °C, preferably at a room temperature. The calcium salt of sulfated glycosaminoglycans present as a mixture of heterogenous molecules of mixed mucopolysaccharide nature varying in molecular weights. Present in mammalian tissues and usually obtained from the intestinal mucosa or other suitable tissues of domestic mammals used for food by man. Purified to retain a combination of activities against different fractions of the blood clotting sequence. Composed of polymers of alternating derivatives of D-glycosamine (N-sulfated, O-sulfated, or N-acetylated) and uronic acid (L-iduronic acid or D-glucuronic acid) joined by glycosidic linkages. The component activities of the mixture are in ratios corresponding to those shown by the USP Heparin Sodium Reference Standard. Some of these components have the property of prolonging the clotting time of blood. This occurs through the formation of a complex of each component with the plasma proteins anti-thrombin III and heparin cofactor II to potentiate the inactivation of thrombin. Other coagulation proteases in the clotting sequence, such as activated factor X (factor X_a), are also inhibited. Label it to indicate the tissue and the animal species from which it is derived. The potency of heparin calcium, calculated on the dried basis, is not less than 140 USP Heparin Units in each mg, and not less than 90.0% and not more than 110.0% of the potency stated on the label. Heparin Calcium is essentially free from sodium. Meets the requirements for Identification, Bacterial endotoxins, pH (5.0–7.5, in a solution [1 in 100]), Loss on drying (not more than 5.0%), Residue on ignition (28.0–41.0%), Nitrogen content (1.3–2.5%, calculated on the dried basis), Protein, Heavy metals (not more than 0.003%), and Anti-factor X_a activity.

Note: The USP Heparin Unit is defined by the USP Heparin Sodium Reference Standard independent of International Units. The respective units are not equivalent. Unit for Anti-factor X_a activity is defined by the USP Heparin Sodium Reference Standard.

Heparin Calcium Injection USP—Preserve in single-dose or in multiple-dose containers, preferably of Type I glass, and store at a temperature below 40 °C, preferably at room temperature. A sterile solution of Heparin Calcium in

Water for Injection. Label it to indicate the volume of the total contents and the potency in terms of USP Heparin Units per mL, except that single-dose containers may be labeled additionally to indicate the single unit-dose volume and the total number of USP Heparin Units in the contents. Where it is labeled with total content, the label states also that the entire contents are to be used or, if not, any remaining portion is to be discarded. Label it to indicate also the tissue and the animal species from which it is derived. Exhibits the labeled potency, within ±10%, stated in terms of USP Heparin Units per mL. Meets the requirements for Bacterial endotoxins, pH (5.0–7.5), and Particulate matter, and for Injections.

Note: The USP Heparin Units defined by the USP Heparin Sodium Reference Standard independent of International Units. The respective units are not equivalent.

Heparin Sodium USP—Preserve in tight containers, and store below 40 °C, preferably at room temperature. The sodium salt of sulfated glycosaminoglycans present as a mixture of heterogeneous molecules varying in molecular weights. Present in mammalian tissues and usually obtained from the intestinal mucosa or other suitable tissues of domestic mammals used for food by man. Purified to retain a combination of activities against different fractions of the blood clotting sequence. Composed of polymers of alternating derivatives of D-glycosamine (N-sulfated, O-sulfated, or N-acetylated) and uronic acid (L-iduronic acid or D-glucuronic acid) joined by glycosidic linkages. The component activities of the mixture are in ratios corresponding to those shown by the USP Heparin Sodium Reference Standard. Some of these components have the property of prolonging the clotting time of blood. This occurs mainly through the formation of a complex of each component with the plasma proteins anti-thrombin III and heparin cofactor II to potentiate the inactivation of thrombin. Other coagulation proteases in the clotting sequence, such as activated factor X, are also inhibited. Label it to indicate the tissue and the animal species from which it is derived. The potency of heparin sodium, calculated on the dried basis, is not less than 140 USP Heparin Units in each mg, and not less than 90.0% and not more than 110.0% of the potency stated on the label. Meets the requirements for Identification, Bacterial endotoxins, pH (5.0–7.5, in a solution [1 in 100]), Loss on drying (not more than 5.0%), Residue on ignition (28.0–41.0%), Protein, Heavy metals (not more than 0.003%), Anti-factor X_a activity (within ±20%), and Nitrogen content (1.3–2.5%, calculated on the dried basis).

Note: The USP Heparin Unit is defined by the USP Heparin Sodium Reference Standard, independent of International Units. The respective units are not equivalent. The Unit for Anti-factor X_a activity is defined by the USP Heparin Sodium Reference Standard and is equivalent in potency to that Standard.

Heparin Sodium Injection USP—Preserve in single-dose or in multiple-dose containers, preferably of Type I glass, and store at a temperature below 40 °C, preferably at room temperature. A sterile solution of Heparin Sodium in Water for Injection. Label it to indicate the volume of the total contents and the potency in terms of USP Heparin Units only per mL, except that single-dose containers may be labeled additionally to indicate the single unit-dose volume and the total number of USP Heparin Units. Where it is labeled with total content, the label states also that the entire contents are to be used or, if not, any remaining portion is to be discarded. Label it to indicate also the tissue and the animal species from which it is derived. Exhibits the labeled potency, within ±10%, stated in terms of USP Heparin Units per mL. Meets the requirements for Bacterial endotoxins, pH (5.0–7.5), and Particulate matter, and for Injections.

Note: The USP Heparin Unit is defined by the USP Heparin Sodium Reference Standard, independent of International Units. The respective units are not equivalent.

HEPARIN AND DEXTROSE

For *Heparin* and *Dextrose*—See individual listings for chemistry information.

USP requirements: Heparin Sodium in Dextrose Injection—Not in *USP–NF*.

HEPARIN AND SODIUM CHLORIDE

For *Heparin* and *Sodium Chloride*—See individual listings for chemistry information.

USP requirements: Heparin Sodium in Sodium Chloride Injection—Not in *USP–NF*.

HEPATITIS A VACCINE, INACTIVATED

Source: The virus (strain HM175) is propagated in MRC_5, human diploid cells. After removal of the cell culture medium, the cells are lysed to form a suspension, then purified and concentrated by ultrafiltration and gel chromatography.

USP requirements: Hepatitis A Vaccine, Inactivated, Injection—Not in *USP–NF*.

HEPATITIS A VACCINE INACTIVATED AND HEPATITIS B VACCINE RECOMBINANT

For *Hepatitis A Vaccine Inactivated* and *Hepatitis B Vaccine Recombinant*—See indivudual listings for chemistry information.

USP requirements:Hepatitis A Vaccine Inactivated and Hepatitis B Vaccine Recombinant Injection—Not in *USP–NF*.

HEPATITIS B IMMUNE GLOBULIN

USP requirements: Hepatitis B Immune Globulin USP—Preserve at a temperature between 2 and 8 °C. A sterile, nonpyrogenic solution free from turbidity, consisting of globulins derived from the blood plasma of human donors who have high titers of antibodies against hepatitis B surface antigen. Label it to state that it is not for intravenous injection. Contains not less than 10.0 grams and not more than 18.0 grams of protein per 100 mL, of which not less than 80% is monomeric immunoglobulin G, having no ultracentrifugally detectable fragments, nor aggregates having a sedimentation coefficient greater than 12S. Contains 0.3 *M* glycine as a stabilizing agent, and contains a suitable preservative. Has a potency per mL not less than that of the U.S. Reference Hepatitis B Immune Globulin tested by an approved radioimmunoassay for the detection and measurement of antibody to hepatitis B surface antigen. Has a pH between 6.4 and 7.2, measured in a solution diluted to contain 1% of protein with 0.15 *M* sodium chloride. Meets the requirements of the test for heat stability and for Expiration date (not later than 1 year after the date

of manufacture, such date being that of the first valid potency test of the product). Conforms to the regulations of the U.S. Food and Drug Administration concerning biologics.

HEPATITIS B VACCINE RECOMBINANT

Source:

A non-infectious subunit viral vaccine derived from Hepatitis B surface antigen (HBsAg) produced in yeast cells. A portion of the hepatitis B virus gene, coding for HBsAg, is cloned into yeast, and the vaccine for hepatitis B is produced from cultures of this recombinant yeast strain according to methods developed in the Merck Research Laboratories. The antigen is harvested and purified from fermentation cultures of a recombinant strain of the yeast *Saccharomyces cerevisiae* containing the gene for the *adw* subtype of HBsAg. The HBsAg protein is released from the yeast cells by cell disruption and purified by a series of physical and chemical methods.

USP requirements: Hepatitis B Vaccine Recombinant Sterile Suspension—Not in *USP–NF.*

HEPATITIS B VIRUS VACCINE INACTIVATED

USP requirements: Hepatitis B Virus Vaccine Inactivated USP— Preserve at a temperature between 2 and 8 °C. A sterile preparation consisting of a suspension of particles of Hepatitis B surface antigen (HBsAg) isolated from the plasma of HBsAg carriers; treated with pepsin at pH 2, 8 *M* urea, and 1:4000 formalin so as to inactivate any hepatitis B virus and any representative viruses from all known virus groups that may be present; purified by ultracentrifugation and biochemical procedures and standardized to a concentration of 35 mcg to 55 mcg of Lowry (HBsAg) protein per mL. The preparation is adsorbed on aluminum hydroxide and diluted to a concentration of 20 mcg Lowry protein per mL or other appropriate concentration, depending on the intended use. Label it to state the content of HBsAg protein per recommended dose. Label it also to state that it is to be shaken before use and that it is not to be frozen. Contains not more than 0.62 mg of aluminum per mL and not more than 0.02% of residual free formaldehyde. Contains thimerosal as a preservative. Meets the requirements for potency in animal tests using mice and by a quantitative parallel line radioimmunoassay, of tests for pyrogen, for general safety, and for Expiration date (not later than 3 years from the date of manufacture, the date of manufacture being the date on which the last valid potency test was initiated).

HETACILLIN

Chemical name: Hetacillin potassium—4-Thia-1-azabicyclo[3.2.0]heptane-2-carboxylic acid, 6-(2,2-dimethyl-5-oxo-4-phen-yl-1-imidazolidinyl)-3,3-dimethyl-7-oxo-, monopotassium salt, [2*S*-[2 alpha,5 alpha,6 beta(*S**)]]-.

Molecular formula: Hetacillin potassium—$C_{19}H_{22}KN_3O_4S$.

Molecular weight: Hetacillin potassium—427.56.

Description: Hetacillin Potassium USP—White to light buff, crystalline powder.

Solubility: Hetacillin Potassium USP—Freely soluble in water; soluble in alcohol.

USP requirements:
Hetacillin Potassium USP—Preserve in tight containers. Has a potency equivalent to not less than 735 mcg of ampicillin per mg. Meets the requirements for Identification, Crystallinity, pH (7.0–9.0, in a solution containing 10 mg per mL), Water (not more than 1.0%), and Hetacillin content (82.0–95.5%).

Hetacillin Potassium Intramammary Infusion USP—Preserve in suitable, well-closed, disposable syringes. A suspension of Hetacillin Potassium in a Peanut Oil vehicle with a suitable dispersing agent. Label it to indicate that it is for veterinary use only. Contains an amount of hetacillin potassium equivalent to the labeled amount of ampicillin, within −10% to +20%. Meets the requirements for Identification and Water (not more than 1.0%).

Hetacillin Potassium Oral Suspension USP—Preserve in tight containers. It is Hetacillin Potassium suspended in a suitable nonaqueous vehicle. Label it to indicate that it is for veterinary use only. Contains an amount of hetacillin potassium equivalent to the labeled amount of ampicillin, within −10% to +20%. Contains one or more suitable colors, flavors, and gelling agents. Meets the requirements for Identification, Uniformity of dosage units (for suspension packaged in single-unit containers), Deliverable volume, pH (7.0–9.0), and Water (not more than 1.0%).

Hetacillin Potassium Tablets USP—Preserve in tight containers. Label the Tablets to indicate that they are for veterinary use only. Contain an amount of hetacillin potassium equivalent to the labeled amount of ampicillin, within −10% to ⏐20%. Meet the requirements for Identification, Disintegration (30 minutes), and Water (not more than 5.0%).

HEXACHLOROPHENE

Chemical name: Phenol, 2,2′-methylenebis[3,4,6-trichloro-.

Molecular formula: $C_{13}H_6Cl_6O_2$.

Molecular weight: 406.90.

Description:
Hexachlorophene USP—White to light tan, crystalline powder. Odorless, or has only a slight, phenolic odor.

Hexachlorophene Liquid Soap USP—Clear, amber-colored liquid, having a slight, characteristic odor. Its solution (1 in 20) is clear and has an alkaline reaction.

Solubility: Hexachlorophene USP—Insoluble in water; freely soluble in acetone, in alcohol, and in ether; soluble in chloroform and in dilute solutions of fixed alkali hydroxides.

USP requirements:
Hexachlorophene USP—Preserve in tight, light-resistant containers. Contains not less than 98.0% and not more than 100.5% of hexachlorophene, calculated on the dried basis. Meets the requirements for Identification, Melting range (161–167 °C), Loss on drying (not more than 1.0%), Residue on ignition (not more than 0.1%), and Limit of 2,3,7,8-tetrachlorodibenzo-*p*-dioxin (not more than 1 ppb).

Hexachlorophene Cleansing Emulsion USP—Preserve in tight, light-resistant, non-metallic containers. It is Hexachlorophene in a suitable aqueous vehicle. Contains the labeled amount, within ±10%. Contains no coloring agents. Meets the requirements for Identification, Microbial limits, and pH (5.0–6.0).

Hexachlorophene Liquid Soap USP—Preserve in tight, light-resistant containers. A solution of Hexachlorophene in a 10.0 to 13.0% solution of a potassium soap. Solutions of higher concentrations of hexachlorophene and potassium soap, in which the ratios of these components are consistent with the official limits, may be labeled "For the preparation of Hexachlorophene Liquid Soap, USP,"

provided that the label indicates also that the soap is a concentrate, and provided that directions are given for dilution to the official strength. Contains, in each 100 grams, not less than 225 mg and not more than 260 mg of hexachlorophene. Meets the requirements for Identification, Microbial limits, Water (86.5–90.0% by weight of the portion of Soap taken), Alcohol-insoluble substances (not more than 3.0%), Free alkali hydroxides (not more than 0.05% of potassium hydroxide), and Alkali carbonates (not more than 0.35% of potassium carbonate).

Note: The inclusion of non-ionic detergents in Hexachlorophene Liquid Soap in amounts greater than 8% on a total weight basis may decrease the bacteriostatic activity of the Soap.

HEXYLENE GLYCOL

Chemical name: 2,4-Pentanediol, 2-methyl-.

Molecular formula: $C_6H_{14}O_2$.

Molecular weight: 118.17.

Description: Hexylene Glycol NF—Clear, colorless, viscous liquid. Absorbs moisture when exposed to moist air.

NF category: Humectant; solvent.

Solubility: Hexylene Glycol NF—Miscible with water and with many organic solvents, including alcohol, ether, chloroform, acetone, and hexanes.

NF requirements: Hexylene Glycol NF—Preserve in tight containers. Hexylene Glycol is 2-methyl-2,4-pentanediol. Meets the requirements for Identification, Specific gravity (0.917–0.923), Refractive index (1.424–1.430), Acidity, and Water (not more than 0.5%).

HEXYLRESORCINOL

Chemical name: 1,3-Benzenediol, 4-hexyl-.

Molecular formula: $C_{12}H_{18}O_2$.

Molecular weight: 194.27.

Description: White or almost white needles, crystalline powder, plates, or plate aggregates composed of needle masses with a pungent odor. Acquires a brownish-pink tint on exposure to light and air. Melting point 66–68 °C.

Solubility: Very slightly soluble in water; freely soluble in alcohol, in chloroform, in ether, in glycerol, and in fixed oils; practically insoluble in petroleum spirit.

USP requirements:
Hexylresorcinol USP—Preserve in tight, light-resistant containers. Dried over silica gel for 4 hours, contains not less than 98.0% and not more than 100.5% of hexylresorcinol. Meets the requirements for Identification, Melting range (62–67 °C), Acidity, Residue on ignition (not more than 0.1%), Mercury (not more than 3 ppm), and Resorcinol and other phenols.

Caution: Hexylresorcinol is irritating to the oral mucosa and respiratory tract and to the skin, and its solution in alcohol has vesicant properties.

Hexylresorcinol Lozenges USP—Preserve in well-closed containers. Contain the labeled amount, within ±10%. Meet the requirements for Identification and Uniformity of dosage units.

HISTAMINE

Chemical name: Histamine phosphate—1*H*-Imidazole-4-ethanamine, phosphate (1:2).

Molecular formula: Histamine phosphate—$C_5H_9N_3 \cdot 2H_3PO_4$.

Molecular weight: Histamine phosphate—307.14.

Description: Histamine Phosphate USP—Colorless, odorless, long prismatic crystals. Is stable in air but is affected by light. Its solutions are acid to litmus.

Solubility: Histamine Phosphate USP—Freely soluble in water.

USP requirements:
Histamine Phosphate USP—Preserve in tight, light-resistant containers. Contains not less than 98.0% and not more than 101.0% of histamine phosphate, calculated on the dried basis. Meets the requirements for Identification and Loss on drying (not more than 3.0%).

Histamine Phosphate Injection USP—Preserve in single-dose or in multiple-dose containers, preferably of Type I glass, protected from light. A sterile solution of Histamine Phosphate in Water for Injection. Contains the labeled amount, within ±10%. Meets the requirements for Identification, Bacterial endotoxins, and pH (3.0–6.0), and for Injections.

HISTIDINE

Chemical name: L-Histidine.

Molecular formula: $C_6H_9N_3O_2$.

Molecular weight: 155.15.

Description: Histidine USP—White, odorless crystals.

Solubility: Histidine USP—Soluble in water; very slightly soluble in alcohol; insoluble in ether.

USP requirements: Histidine USP—Preserve in well-closed containers. Contains not less than 98.5% and not more than 101.5% of histidine, as L-histidine, calculated on the dried basis. Meets the requirements for Identification, Specific rotation (+12.6° to +14.0°), pH (7.0–8.5, in a solution [1 in 50]), Loss on drying (not more than 0.2%), Residue on ignition (not more than 0.4%), Chloride (not more than 0.05%), Sulfate (not more than 0.03%), Iron (not more than 0.003%), Chromatographic purity, and Heavy metals (not more than 0.0015%).

HISTOPLASMIN

Description: Histoplasmin USP—Clear, red liquid.

Solubility: Histoplasmin USP—Miscible with water.

USP requirements: Histoplasmin USP—Preserve at a temperature between 2 and 8 °C. A clear, colorless, sterile solution containing standardized culture filtrates of *Histoplasma capsulatum* grown on liquid synthetic medium. Label it to state that only the diluent supplied is to be used for making dilutions, and that it is not to be injected other than intradermally. Label it also to state that a separate syringe and needle shall be used for each individual injection. Has a potency of the 1:100 dilution equivalent to and determined in terms of the Histoplasmin Reference diluted 1:100 tested in guinea pigs. Meets the requirement for Expiration date (not later than 2 years after date of issue from manufacturer's cold storage [5 °C, 1 year]). Conforms to the regulations of the U.S. Food and Drug Administration concerning biologics.

HISTRELIN

Chemical group: Histrelin acetate—A synthetic nonapeptide gonadotropin-releasing hormone analog (GnRHa) and is of greater potency than the endogenous gonadotropin-releasing hormone (GnRh).

Chemical name:
Histrelin—Luteinizing hormone-releasing factor (pig), 6-[1-(phenylmethyl)-D-histidine]-9-(*N*-ethyl-L-prolinamide)-10-deglycinamide-.
Histrelin acetate—5-Oxo-L-prolyl-L-tryptophyl-L-seryl-L-tyrosyl-*N*-benzyl-D-histidyl-L-leucyl-L-arginyl-*N*-ethyl-L-prolinamide acetate (salt).

Molecular formula:
Histrelin—$C_{66}H_{86}N_{18}O_{12}$.
Histrelin acetate—$C_{66}H_{86}N_{18}O_{12}$ · (1.7–2.8 moles)CH_3COOH · (0.6–7.0 moles)H_2O.

Molecular weight:
Histrelin—1323.50.
Histrelin acetate—1323.52 (peptide base).

Other characteristics: Histrelin acetate—pH of 200 mcg per mL of histrelin injection: 4.5–6 (unbuffered); 500 mcg per mL and 1000 mcg per mL of histrelin injection: 4.5–6 (unbuffered).

USP requirements:
Histrelin Injection—Not in *USP–NF*.
Histrelin Acetate Injection—Not in *USP–NF*.

HOMATROPINE

Source: Semisynthetic tertiary amine derivative of mandelic acid and tropine.

Chemical group: Homatropine methylbromide—Semisynthetic quaternary ammonium compound.

Chemical name:
Homatropine hydrobromide—Benzeneacetic acid, alpha-hydroxy-, 8-methyl-8-azabicyclo[3.2.1]oct-3-yl ester, hydrobromide, *endo*-(±)-.
Homatropine methylbromide—8-Azoniabicyclo[3.2.1]octane, 3-[(hydroxyphenylacetyl)oxy]-8,8-dimethyl-, bromide, *endo*-.

Molecular formula:
Homatropine hydrobromide—$C_{16}H_{21}NO_3$ · HBr.
Homatropine methylbromide—$C_{17}H_{24}BrNO_3$.

Molecular weight:
Homatropine hydrobromide—356.25.
Homatropine methylbromide—370.28.

Description:
Homatropine Hydrobromide USP—White crystals, or white, crystalline powder. Is affected by light.
Homatropine Methylbromide USP—White, odorless powder. Slowly darkens on exposure to light. Melts at about 190 °C.

Solubility:
Homatropine Hydrobromide USP—Freely soluble in water; sparingly soluble in alcohol; slightly soluble in chloroform; insoluble in ether.
Homatropine Methylbromide USP—Very soluble in water; freely soluble in alcohol and in acetone containing about 20% of water; practically insoluble in ether and in acetone.

USP requirements:
Homatropine Hydrobromide USP—Preserve in tight, light-resistant containers. Contains not less than 98.5% and not more than 100.5% of homatropine hydrobromide, calculated on the dried basis. Meets the requirements for Identification, Melting range (214–217 °C, with slight

decomposition), pH (5.7–7.0, in a solution [1 in 50]), Loss on drying (not more than 1.5%), and Residue on ignition (not more than 0.25%).
Homatropine Hydrobromide Ophthalmic Solution USP—Preserve in tight containers. A sterile, buffered, aqueous solution of Homatropine Hydrobromide. Contains the labeled amount, within ±5%. Meets the requirements for Identification, Sterility, and pH (2.5–5.0).
Homatropine Methylbromide USP—Preserve in tight, light-resistant containers. Contains not less than 98.5% and not more than 100.5% of homatropine methylbromide, calculated on the dried basis. Meets the requirements for Identification, pH (4.5–6.5, in a solution [1 in 100]), Loss on drying (not more than 0.5%), Residue on ignition (not more than 0.2%), Homatropine, atropine, and other solanaceous alkaloids, and Organic volatile impurities.
Homatropine Methylbromide Tablets USP—Preserve in tight, light-resistant containers. Contain the labeled amount, within ±10%. Meet the requirements for Identification, Dissolution (75% in 45 minutes in water in Apparatus 2 at 50 rpm), and Uniformity of dosage units.

HOMOSALATE

Chemical name: Benzoic acid, 2-hydroxy-, 3,3,5-trimethylcyclohexyl ester.

Molecular formula: $C_{16}H_{22}O_3$.

Molecular weight: 262.34.

Description: Colorless liquid.

USP requirements:
Homosalate USP—Preserve in tight containers. Contains the labeled amount, within ±10%. Meets the requirements for Identification, Refractive index (1.516–1.519), and Specific gravity (1.049–1.053).
Homosalate Lotion—Not in *USP–NF*.
Homosalate Oil—Not in *USP–NF*.
Homosalate Spray—Not in *USP–NF*.

HOMOSALATE, MENTHYL ANTHRANILATE, AND OCTYL METHOXYCINNAMATE

Chemical name:
Homosalate—Benzoic acid, 2-hydroxy-, 3,3,5-trimethylcyclohexyl ester.
Menthyl anthranilate—Cyclohexanol, 5-Methyl-2-(1-Methylethyl)-, 2-Aminobenzoate.
Octyl methoxycinnamate—3-(4-Methoxyphenyl)-2-propenoic acid 2-ethylhexyl ester.

Molecular formula:
Homosalate—$C_{16}H_{22}O_3$.
Menthyl anthranilate—$C_{17}H_{25}NO_2$.
Octyl methoxycinnamate—$C_{18}H_{26}O_3$.

Molecular weight:
Homosalate—262.34.
Octyl methoxycinnamate—290.40.

Description: Homosalate—Colorless liquid.

USP requirements: Homosalate, Menthyl Anthranilate, and Octyl Methoxycinnamate Oil—Not in *USP–NF*.

HOMOSALATE, MENTHYL ANTHRANILATE, OCTYL METHOXYCINNAMATE, OCTYL SALICYLATE, AND OXYBENZONE

Chemical name:

Homosalate—Benzoic acid, 2-hydroxy-, 3,3,5-trimethylcyclohexyl ester.

Menthyl anthranilate—Cyclohexanol, 5-Methyl-2-(1-Methylethyl)-, 2-Aminobenzoate.

Octyl methoxycinnamate—3-(4-Methoxyphenyl)-2-propenoic acid 2-ethylhexyl ester.

Oxybenzone—Methanone, (2-hydroxy-4-methoxyphenyl)-phenyl-.

Molecular formula:

Homosalate—$C_{16}H_{22}O_3$.

Menthyl anthranilate—$C_{17}H_{25}NO_2$.

Octyl methoxycinnamate—$C_{18}H_{26}O_3$.

Oxybenzone—$C_{14}H_{12}O_3$.

Molecular weight:

Homosalate—262.34.

Octyl methoxycinnamate—290.40.

Oxybenzone—228.24.

Description:

Homosalate—Colorless liquid.

Oxybenzone USP—Pale yellow powder.

Solubility: Oxybenzone USP—Practically insoluble in water; freely soluble in alcohol and in toluene.

USP requirements:

Homosalate, Menthyl Anthranilate, Octyl Methoxycinnamate, Octyl Salicylate, and Oxybenzone Lip Balm—Not in *USP–NF*.

Homosalate, Menthyl Anthranilate, Octyl Methoxycinnamate, Octyl Salicylate, and Oxybenzone Lotion—Not in *USP–NF*.

HOMOSALATE, OCTOCRYLENE, OCTYL METHOXYCINNAMATE, AND OXYBENZONE

Chemical name:

Homosalate—Benzoic acid, 2-hydroxy-, 3,3,5-trimethylcyclohexyl ester.

Octocrylene—2-Propenoic acid, 2-cyano-3,3-diphenyl-, 2-ethylhexyl ester.

Octyl methoxycinnamate—3-(4-Methoxyphenyl)-2-propenoic acid 2-ethylhexyl ester.

Oxybenzone—Methanone, (2-hydroxy-4-methoxyphenyl)-phenyl-.

Molecular formula:

Homosalate—$C_{16}H_{22}O_3$.

Octocrylene—$C_{24}H_{27}NO_2$.

Octyl methoxycinnamate—$C_{18}H_{26}O_3$.

Oxybenzone—$C_{14}H_{12}O_3$.

Molecular weight:

Homosalate—262.34.

Octocrylene—361.48.

Octyl methoxycinnamate—290.40.

Oxybenzone—228.24.

Description:

Homosalate—Colorless liquid.

Oxybenzone USP—Pale yellow powder.

Solubility: Oxybenzone USP—Practically insoluble in water; freely soluble in alcohol and in toluene.

USP requirements: Homosalate, Octocrylene, Octyl Methoxycinnamate, and Oxybenzone Lotion—Not in *USP–NF*.

HOMOSALATE, OCTYL METHOXYCINNAMATE, OCTYL SALICYLATE, AND OXYBENZONE

Chemical name:

Homosalate—Benzoic acid, 2-hydroxy-, 3,3,5-trimethylcyclohexyl ester.

Octyl methoxycinnamate—3-(4-Methoxyphenyl)-2-propenoic acid 2-ethylhexyl ester.

Oxybenzone—Methanone, (2-hydroxy-4-methoxyphenyl)-phenyl-.

Molecular formula:

Homosalate—$C_{16}H_{22}O_3$.

Octyl methoxycinnamate—$C_{18}H_{26}O_3$.

Oxybenzone—$C_{14}H_{12}O_3$.

Molecular weight:

Homosalate—262.34.

Octyl methoxycinnamate—290.40.

Oxybenzone—228.24.

Description:

Homosalate—Colorless liquid.

Oxybenzone USP—Pale yellow powder.

Solubility: Oxybenzone USP—Practically insoluble in water; freely soluble in alcohol and in toluene.

USP requirements:

Homosalate, Octyl Methoxycinnamate, Octyl Salicylate, and Oxybenzone Lotion—Not in *USP–NF*.

Homosalate, Octyl Methoxycinnamate, Octyl Salicylate, and Oxybenzone Stick—Not in *USP–NF*.

HOMOSALATE, OCTYL METHOXYCINNAMATE, AND OXYBENZONE

Chemical name:

Homosalate—Benzoic acid, 2-hydroxy-, 3,3,5-trimethylcyclohexyl ester.

Octyl methoxycinnamate—3-(4-Methoxyphenyl)-2-propenoic acid 2-ethylhexyl ester.

Oxybenzone—Methanone, (2-hydroxy-4-methoxyphenyl)-phenyl-.

Molecular formula:

Homosalate—$C_{16}H_{22}O_3$.

Octyl methoxycinnamate—$C_{18}H_{26}O_3$.

Oxybenzone—$C_{14}H_{12}O_3$.

Molecular weight:

Homosalate—262.34.

Octyl methoxycinnamate—290.40.

Oxybenzone—228.24.

Description:

Homosalate—Colorless liquid.

Oxybenzone USP—Pale yellow powder.

Solubility: Oxybenzone USP—Practically insoluble in water; freely soluble in alcohol and in toluene.

USP requirements: Homosalate, Octyl Methoxycinnamate, and Oxybenzone Gel—Not in *USP–NF*.

HOMOSALATE AND OXYBENZONE

For *Homosalate* and *Oxybenzone*—See individual listings for chemistry information.

USP requirements: Homosalate and Oxybenzone Spray—Not in *USP–NF*.

HYALURONATE SODIUM

Chemical name: Hyaluronic acid, sodium salt.

Molecular formula: $(C_{14}H_{20}NNaO_{11})n$.

USP requirements:
Hyaluronate Sodium Injection—Not in *USP–NF*.
Hyaluronate Sodium Derivative Injection—Not in *USP–NF*.

HYALURONIDASE

Description: White or yellowish-white powder.

Solubility: Very soluble in water; practically insoluble in alcohol, in acetone, and in ether.

USP requirements:
Hyaluronidase Injection USP—Preserve in single-dose or in multiple-dose containers, preferably of Type I glass, in a refrigerator. A sterile solution of dry, soluble enzyme product, prepared from mammalian testes and capable of hydrolyzing mucopolysaccharides of the type of hyaluronic acid, in Water for Injection. Contains the labeled amount of USP Hyaluronidase Units, within –10%. Contains not more than 0.25 mcg of tyrosine for each USP Hyaluronidase Unit. Meets the requirements for Bacterial endotoxins, pH (6.4–7.4), and Limit of tyrosine (not more than 0.25 mcg for each USP Hyaluronidase Unit), and for Injections.
Hyaluronidase for Injection USP—Preserve in Containers for Sterile Solids, preferably of Type I or Type III glass, at controlled room temperature. A sterile, dry, soluble, enzyme product prepared from mammalian testes and capable of hydrolyzing mucopolysaccharides of the type of hyaluronic acid. Its potency, in USP Hyaluronidase Units, is not less than the labeled potency. Contains not more than 0.25 mcg of tyrosine for each USP Hyaluronidase Unit. Meets the requirements for Sterility, Bacterial endotoxins, and Limit of tyrosine (not more than 0.25 mcg for each USP Hyaluronidase Unit).

HYDRALAZINE

Chemical name: Hydralazine hydrochloride—Phthalazine, 1-hydrazino-, monohydrochloride.

Molecular formula: Hydralazine hydrochloride—$C_8H_8N_4 \cdot HCl$.

Molecular weight: Hydralazine hydrochloride—196.64.

Description: Hydralazine Hydrochloride USP—White to off-white, odorless, crystalline powder. Melts at about 275 °C, with decomposition.

pKa: Hydralazine hydrochloride—0.5, 7.3.

Solubility: Hydralazine Hydrochloride USP—Soluble in water; slightly soluble in alcohol; very slightly soluble in ether.

USP requirements:
Hydralazine Hydrochloride USP—Preserve in tight containers. Contains not less than 98.0% and not more than 102.0% of hydralazine hydrochloride, calculated on the dried basis. Meets the requirements for Identification, pH (3.5–4.2, in a solution [1 in 50]), Loss on drying (not more than 0.5%), Residue on ignition (not more than 0.1%), Water-insoluble substances (not more than 0.5%), Heavy metals (not more than 0.002%), Limit of hydrazine (not more than 0.001%), Chromatographic purity, and Organic volatile impurities.
Hydralazine Hydrochloride Injection USP—Preserve in single-dose or in multiple-dose containers, preferably of Type I glass. A sterile solution of Hydralazine Hydrochloride in Water for Injection. Contains the labeled amount, within ±5%. Meets the requirements for Identification, Bacterial endotoxins, pH (3.4–4.4), and Particulate matter, and for Injections.
Hydralazine Hydrochloride Oral Solution USP—Preserve in a suitable light-resistant glass or plastic bottle, with a child-resistant closure. Store in a refrigerator. Label it to state, as part of the official title, the content of Hydralazine Hydrochloride expressed as a percentage and parenthetically (mg per 5 mL). Label it to state that it is to be stored in a refrigerator. The label indicates that patients may mix the appropriate dose with fruit juice or apple sauce just prior to administration. Contains the labeled content, within ±10%.
Prepare Hydralazine Hydrochloride Oral Solution of the designated percentage strength as follows: 100 mg of Hydralazine Hydrochloride for 0.1% Oral Solution or 1.0 gram of Hydralazine Hydrochloride for 1.0% Oral Solution, 40 grams of Sorbitol Solution (70%), 65 mg of Methylparaben, 35 mg of Propylparaben, 10 grams of Propylene Glycol, 50 mg of Aspartame, and Purified Water, a sufficient quantity to make 100 mL. Dissolve the Hydralazine Hydrochloride in 30 mL of Purified Water, add the Aspartame, and shake or stir until the solids have dissolved. Add the Sorbitol Solution. In a separate container, dissolve an aliquot portion of an intimate homogeneous mixture of accurately weighed quantities of Methylparaben and Propylparaben in the Propylene Glycol and, with stirring, add this mixture to the solution containing the Hydralazine Hydrochloride. Add sufficient Purified Water to make the product measure 100 mL, and mix to produce the Oral solution.
Meets the requirements for pH (3.0–5.0) and Beyond-use date.
[Note—Hydralazine reacts with many flavors; do not add flavors when compounding.]
Hydralazine Hydrochloride Tablets USP—Preserve in tight, light-resistant containers. Contain the labeled amount, within ±10%. Meet the requirements for Identification, Dissolution (75% in 45 minutes in 0.01 N hydrochloric acid in Apparatus 1 at 100 rpm), and Uniformity of dosage units.

HYDRALAZINE AND HYDROCHLOROTHIAZIDE

For *Hydralazine* and *Hydrochlorothiazide*—See individual listings for chemistry information.

USP requirements:
Hydralazine Hydrochloride and Hydrochlorothiazide Capsules—Not in *USP–NF*.
Hydralazine Hydrochloride and Hydrochlorothiazide Tablets—Not in *USP–NF*.

HYDROCHLORIC ACID

Chemical name: Hydrochloric acid.

Molecular formula: HCl.

Molecular weight: 36.46.

Description: Hydrochloric Acid NF—Colorless, fuming liquid, having a pungent odor. It ceases to fume when it is diluted with 2 volumes of water. Specific gravity is about 1.18.
  NF category: Acidifying agent.

NF requirements: Hydrochloric Acid NF—Preserve in tight containers. Contains not less than 36.5% and not more than 38.0%, by weight, of hydrochloric acid. Meets the requirements for Identification, Residue on ignition (not more than 0.008%), Bromide or iodide, Free bromine or chlorine, Sulfate, and Sulfite, and Heavy metals (not more than 5 ppm).

DILUTED HYDROCHLORIC ACID

Description: Diluted Hydrochloric Acid NF—Colorless, odorless liquid. Specific gravity is about 1.05.
  NF category: Acidifying agent.

NF requirements: Diluted Hydrochloric Acid NF—Preserve in tight containers. Contains, in each 100 mL, not less than 9.5 grams and not more than 10.5 grams of hydrochloric acid.
  Diluted Hydrochloric Acid may be prepared as follows: 226 mL of Hydrochloric Acid and a sufficient quantity of Purified Water to make 1000 mL. Mix the ingredients.
  Meets the requirements for Identification, Residue on ignition, Sulfate, Sulfite, Heavy metals (not more than 5 ppm), and Free bromine or chlorine.

HYDROCHLOROTHIAZIDE

Chemical name: 2H-1,2,4-Benzothiadiazine-7-sulfonamide, 6-chloro-3,4-dihydro-, 1,1-dioxide.

Molecular formula: $C_7H_8ClN_3O_4S_2$.

Molecular weight: 297.74.

Description: Hydrochlorothiazide USP—White or practically white, practically odorless, crystalline powder.

pKa: 7.9 and 9.2.

Solubility: Hydrochlorothiazide USP—Slightly soluble in water; freely soluble in sodium hydroxide solution, in n-butylamine, and in dimethylformamide; sparingly soluble in methanol; insoluble in ether, in chloroform, and in dilute mineral acids.

USP requirements:
  Hydrochlorothiazide USP—Preserve in well-closed containers. Contains not less than 98.0% and not more than 102.0% of hydrochlorothiazide, calculated on the dried basis. Meets the requirements for Identification, Loss on drying (not more than 0.5%), Residue on ignition (not more than 0.1%), Chloride (not more than 0.035%), Selenium (not more than 0.003%, a 200-mg test specimen being used), Heavy metals (not more than 0.001%), Related compounds, and Organic volatile impurities.
  Hydrochlorothiazide Capsules—Not in *USP–NF*.
  Hydrochlorothiazide Oral Solution—Not in *USP–NF*.
  Hydrochlorothiazide Tablets USP—Preserve in well-closed containers. Contain the labeled amount, within ±10%. Meet the requirements for Identification, Dissolution

(60% in 60 minutes in 0.1 N hydrochloric acid in Apparatus 1 at 100 rpm), Uniformity of dosage units, and Related compounds (not more than 1.0%).

HYDROCODONE

Chemical name: Hydrocodone bitartrate—Morphinan-6-one, 4,5-epoxy-3-methoxy-17-methyl-, (5 alpha)-, [R-(R*,R*)]-2,3-dihydroxybutanedioate (1:1), hydrate (2:5).

Molecular formula: Hydrocodone bitartrate—$C_{18}H_{21}NO_3 \cdot C_4H_6O_6 \cdot 2\frac{1}{2}H_2O$ (hydrate); $C_{18}H_{21}NO_3 \cdot C_4H_6O_6$ (anhydrous).

Molecular weight: Hydrocodone bitartrate—494.49 (hydrate); 449.46 (anhydrous).

Description: Hydrocodone Bitartrate USP—Fine, white crystals or a crystalline powder. Is affected by light.

Solubility: Hydrocodone Bitartrate USP—Soluble in water; slightly soluble in alcohol; insoluble in ether and in chloroform.

USP requirements:
  Hydrocodone Bitartrate USP—Preserve in tight, light-resistant containers. Dried in vacuum at 105 °C for 2 hours, contains not less than 98.0% and not more than 102.0% of hydrocodone bitartrate. Meets the requirements for Identification, Specific rotation (−79° to −84°), pH (3.2–3.8, in a solution [1 in 50]), Loss on drying (7.5–12.0%), Residue on ignition (not more than 0.1%), Chloride, Ordinary impurities, and Organic volatile impurities.
  Hydrocodone Bitartrate Syrup—Not in *USP–NF*.
  Hydrocodone Bitartrate Tablets USP—Preserve in tight, light-resistant containers. Contain the labeled amount, within ± 10%. Meet the requirements for Identification, Dissolution (75% in 45 minutes in water in Apparatus 2 at 50 rpm), and Uniformity of dosage units.

HYDROCODONE AND ACETAMINOPHEN

For *Hydrocodone* and *Acetaminophen*—See individual listings for chemistry information.

USP requirements:
  Hydrocodone Bitartrate and Acetaminophen Capsules—Not in *USP–NF*.
  Hydrocodone Bitartrate and Acetaminophen Oral Solution—Not in *USP–NF*.
  Hydrocodone Bitartrate and Acetaminophen Tablets USP—Preserve in tight, light-resistant containers. Contain the labeled amounts, within ±10%. Meet the requirements for Identification, Dissolution (80% of each active ingredient in 30 minutes in phosphate buffer [pH 5.8 ±0.05] in Apparatus 2 at 50 rpm for Test 1 and in 0.1 N hydrochloric acid in Apparatus 1 for Test 2), and Uniformity of dosage units.

HYDROCODONE AND ASPIRIN

For *Hydrocodone* and *Aspirin*—See individual listings for chemistry information.

USP requirements: Hydrocodone Bitartrate and Aspirin Tablets—Not in *USP–NF*.

HYDROCODONE AND GUAIFENESIN

For *Hydrocodone* and *Guaifenesin*—See individual listings for chemistry information.

USP requirements:
Hydrocodone Bitartrate and Guaifenesin Oral Solution—Not in *USP–NF*.
Hydrocodone Bitartrate and Guaifenesin Syrup—Not in *USP–NF*.
Hydrocodone Bitartrate and Guaifenesin Tablets—Not in *USP–NF*.

HYDROCODONE AND HOMATROPINE

For *Hydrocodone* and *Homatropine*—See individual listings for chemistry information.

USP requirements:
Hydrocodone Bitartrate and Homatropine Methylbromide Syrup—Not in *USP–NF*.
Hydrocodone Bitartrate and Homatropine Methylbromide Tablets—Not in *USP–NF*.

HYDROCODONE AND IBUPROFEN

For *Hydrocodone* and *Ibuprofen*—See individual listings for chemistry information.

USP requirements: Hydrocodone and Ibuprofen Tablets—Not in *USP–NF*.

HYDROCODONE AND POTASSIUM GUAIACOLSULFONATE

For *Hydrocodone* and *Potassium Guaiacolsulfonate*—See individual listings for chemistry information.

USP requirements:
Hydrocodone Bitartrate and Potassium Guaiacolsulfonate Oral Solution—Not in *USP–NF*.
Hydrocodone Bitartrate and Potassium Guaiacolsulfonate Syrup—Not in *USP–NF*.

HYDROCORTISONE

Chemical name:
Hydrocortisone—Pregn-4-ene-3,20-dione, 11,17,21-trihydroxy-, (11 beta)-.
Hydrocortisone acetate—Pregn-4-ene-3,20-dione, 21-(acetyloxy)-11,17-dihydroxy-, (11 beta)-.
Hydrocortisone butyrate—Pregn-4-ene-3,20-dione, 11,21-dihydroxy-17-(1-oxobutoxy)-, (11 beta)-.
Hydrocortisone cypionate—Pregn-4-ene-3,20-dione, 21-(3-cyclopentyl-1-oxopropoxy)-11,17-dihydroxy-, (11 beta)-.
Hydrocortisone hemisuccinate—Pregn-4-ene-3,20-dione, 21-(3-carboxy-1-oxopropoxy)-11,17-dihydroxy-, (11 beta)-, monohydrate.
Hydrocortisone probutate—11 beta-Hydroxy-17-(1-oxobutoxy)-21-(1-oxopropoxy)pregan-4-ene-3,20-dione.
Hydrocortisone sodium phosphate—Pregn-4-ene-3,20-dione, 11,17-dihydroxy-21-(phosphonooxy)-, disodium salt, (11 beta)-.

Hydrocortisone sodium succinate—Pregn-4-ene-3,20-dione, 21-(3-carboxy-1-oxopropoxy)-11,17-dihydroxy-, monosodium salt, (11 beta)-.
Hydrocortisone valerate—Pregn-4-ene-3,20-dione, 11,21-dihydroxy-17-[(1-oxopentyl)oxy]-, (11 beta)-.

Molecular formula:
Hydrocortisone—$C_{21}H_{30}O_5$.
Hydrocortisone acetate—$C_{23}H_{32}O_6$.
Hydrocortisone butyrate—$C_{25}H_{36}O_6$.
Hydrocortisone cypionate—$C_{29}H_{42}O_6$.
Hydrocortisone hemisuccinate—$C_{25}H_{34}O_8 \cdot H_2O$.
Hydrocortisone probutate—$C_{28}H_{40}O_7$.
Hydrocortisone sodium phosphate—$C_{21}H_{29}Na_2O_8P$.
Hydrocortisone sodium succinate—$C_{25}H_{33}NaO_8$.
Hydrocortisone valerate—$C_{26}H_{38}O_6$.

Molecular weight:
Hydrocortisone—362.46.
Hydrocortisone acetate—404.50.
Hydrocortisone butyrate—432.55.
Hydrocortisone cypionate—486.64.
Hydrocortisone hemisuccinate—480.55.
Hydrocortisone probutate—488.61.
Hydrocortisone sodium phosphate—486.40.
Hydrocortisone sodium succinate—484.51.
Hydrocortisone valerate—446.58.

Description:
Hydrocortisone USP—White to practically white, odorless, crystalline powder. Melts at about 215 °C, with decomposition.
Hydrocortisone Acetate USP—White to practically white, odorless, crystalline powder. Melts at about 200 °C, with decomposition.
Hydrocortisone Butyrate USP—White to practically white, practically odorless, crystalline powder.
Hydrocortisone cypionate—White to practically white crystalline powder. Is odorless, or has a slight odor.
Hydrocortisone probutate—Odorless white crystalline powder.
Hydrocortisone Sodium Phosphate USP—White to light yellow, odorless or practically odorless, powder. Is exceedingly hygroscopic.
Hydrocortisone Sodium Succinate USP—White or nearly white, odorless, hygroscopic, amorphous solid.

Solubility:
Hydrocortisone USP—Very slightly soluble in water and in ether; sparingly soluble in acetone and in alcohol; slightly soluble in chloroform.
Hydrocortisone Acetate USP—Insoluble in water; slightly soluble in alcohol and in chloroform.
Hydrocortisone Butyrate USP—Practically insoluble in water; slightly soluble in ether; soluble in methanol, in alcohol, and in acetone; freely soluble in chloroform.
Hydrocortisone cypionate—Insoluble in water; very soluble in chloroform; soluble in alcohol; slightly soluble in ether.
Hydrocortisone probutate—Practically insoluble in hexane or water; slightly soluble in ether; very soluble in dichloromethienane, in methanol, and in acetone.
Hydrocortisone Sodium Phosphate USP—Freely soluble in water; slightly soluble in alcohol; practically insoluble in chloroform, in dioxane, and in ether.
Hydrocortisone Sodium Succinate USP—Very soluble in water and in alcohol; very slightly soluble in acetone; insoluble in chloroform.

USP requirements:
Hydrocortisone USP—Preserve in well-closed containers. Contains not less than 97.0% and not more than 102.0% of hydrocortisone, calculated on the dried basis. Meets the requirements for Identification, Specific rotation (+150° to +156°), Loss on drying (not more than 1.0%), Residue on ignition (negligible, from 100 mg), Chromatographic purity, and Organic volatile impurities.

Hydrocortisone Cream USP—Preserve in tight containers. It is Hydrocortisone in a suitable cream base. Contains the labeled amount, within ±10%. Meets the requirements for Identification, Microbial limits, and Minimum fill.

Hydrocortisone Gel USP—Preserve in tight containers. It is Hydrocortisone in a suitable hydroalcoholic gel base. Contains the labeled amount, within ±10%. Meets the requirements for Identification and Minimum fill.

Hydrocortisone Lotion USP—Preserve in tight containers. It is Hydrocortisone in a suitable aqueous vehicle. Contains the labeled amount, within ±10%. Meets the requirements for Identification, Microbial limits, and Minimum fill.

Hydrocortisone Ointment USP—Preserve in well-closed containers. It is Hydrocortisone in a suitable ointment base. Contains the labeled amount, within ±10%. Meets the requirements for Identification, Microbial limits, and Minimum fill.

Hydrocortisone Rectal Ointment—Not in *USP–NF*.

Hydrocortisone Topical Solution—Not in *USP–NF*.

Hydrocortisone Suppositories—Not in *USP–NF*.

Hydrocortisone Injectable Suspension USP—Preserve in single-dose or in multiple-dose containers, preferably of Type I glass. A sterile suspension of Hydrocortisone in Water for Injection. Contains the labeled amount, within ±10%. Meets the requirements for Identification, Bacterial endotoxins, and pH (5.0–7.0), and for Injections.

Hydrocortisone Rectal Suspension USP—Preserve in tight containers. Contains the labeled amount, within ±10%. Meets the requirements for Identification and pH (5.5–7.0).

Hydrocortisone Tablets USP—Preserve in well-closed containers. Contain the labeled amount, within ±10%. Meet the requirements for Identification, Dissolution (70% in 30 minutes in water in Apparatus 2 at 50 rpm), and Uniformity of dosage units.

Hydrocortisone Acetate USP—Preserve in well-closed containers. Contains not less than 97.0% and not more than 102.0% of hydrocortisone acetate, calculated on the dried basis. Meets the requirements for Identification, Specific rotation (+158° to +165°), Loss on drying (not more than 1.0%), Residue on ignition (negligible, from 100 mg), Chromatographic purity, and Other impurities.

Hydrocortisone Acetate Cream USP—Preserve in well-closed containers. It is Hydrocortisone Acetate in a suitable cream base. Contains the labeled amount, within ±10%. Meets the requirements for Identification, Microbial limits, and Minimum fill.

Hydrocortisone Acetate Foam—Not in *USP–NF*.

Hydrocortisone Acetate Rectal Aerosol Foam—Not in *USP–NF*.

Hydrocortisone Acetate Topical Aerosol Foam—Not in *USP–NF*.

Hydrocortisone Acetate Lotion USP—Preserve in tight containers. It is Hydrocortisone Acetate in a suitable aqueous vehicle. Contains the labeled amount, within ±10%. Meets the requirements for Identification and Minimum fill.

Hydrocortisone Acetate Ointment USP—Preserve in well-closed containers. It is Hydrocortisone Acetate in a suitable ointment base. Contains the labeled amount, within ±10%. Meets the requirements for Identification, Microbial limits, and Minimum fill.

Hydrocortisone Acetate Ophthalmic Ointment USP—Preserve in collapsible ophthalmic ointment tubes. It is Hydrocortisone Acetate in a suitable ophthalmic ointment base. It is sterile. Contains the labeled amount of total steroids, calculated as hydrocortisone acetate, within ±10%. Meets the requirements for Identification, Sterility, Minimum fill, and Particulate matter.

Hydrocortisone Acetate Dental Paste—Not in *USP–NF*.

Hydrocortisone Acetate Suppositories—Not in *USP–NF*.

Hydrocortisone Acetate Injectable Suspension USP—Preserve in single-dose or in multiple-dose containers, preferably of Type I glass. A sterile suspension of Hydrocortisone Acetate in a suitable aqueous medium. Contains the labeled amount of total steroids, calculated as hydrocortisone acetate, within ±10%. Meets the requirements for Identification and pH (5.0–7.0), and for Injections.

Hydrocortisone Acetate Ophthalmic Suspension USP—Preserve in tight containers. A sterile suspension of Hydrocortisone Acetate in an aqueous medium containing a suitable antimicrobial agent. Contains the labeled amount of total steroids, calculated as Hydrocortisone Acetate, within ±10%. Meets the requirements for Identification, Sterility, and pH (6.0–8.0).

Hydrocortisone Butyrate USP—Preserve in well-closed containers. Contains not less than 97.0% and not more than 102.0% of hydrocortisone butyrate, calculated on the dried basis. Meets the requirements for Clarity of solution, Identification, Specific rotation (+47° to +54°), Loss on drying (not more than 1.0%), and Chromatographic purity, and Other impurities.

Hydrocortisone Butyrate Cream USP—Preserve in well-closed containers. It is Hydrocortisone Butyrate in a suitable cream base. Contains the labeled amount, within ±10%. Meets the requirements for Identification, Microbial limits, Minimum fill, and pH (3.5–4.5).

Hydrocortisone Butyrate Ointment—Not in *USP–NF*.

Hydrocortisone Butyrate Topical Solution—Not in *USP–NF*.

Hydrocortisone Cypionate Oral Suspension—Not in *USP–NF*.

Hydrocortisone Hemisuccinate USP—Preserve in tight containers. Contains one molecule of water of hydration or is anhydrous. Label it to indicate whether it is hydrous or anhydrous. Contains not less than 97.0% and not more than 103.0% of hydrocortisone hemisuccinate, calculated on the dried basis. Meets the requirements for Identification, Specific rotation (+124° to +134°), Loss on drying (not more than 1.0% for the anhydrous form and not more than 4.0% for the hydrous form), Chromatographic purity (not more than 1.0% of any individual impurity, and not more than 2.0% of total impurities. Disregard any peak representing less than 0.05%), Residue on ignition (not more than 0.1%), and Other impurities.

Hydrocortisone Probutate Cream—Not in *USP–NF*.

Hydrocortisone Sodium Phosphate USP—Preserve in tight containers. Contains not less than 96.0% and not more than 102.0% of hydrocortisone sodium phosphate, calculated on the dried basis. Meets the requirements for Identification, Phosphate ions (not more than 1.0%), Chloride (not more than 1.00% as sodium chloride), Specific rotation, pH, and Free hydrocortisone (+121° to +129°, calculated on the dried basis, for specific rotation, and 7.5–10.5 for pH), Loss on drying (not more than 5.0%), Heavy metals (not more than 0.004%), and Organic volatile impurities.

Hydrocortisone Sodium Phosphate Injection USP—Preserve in single-dose or in multiple-dose containers, preferably of Type I glass. A sterile, buffered solution of Hydrocortisone Sodium Phosphate in Water for Injection. Contains an amount of hydrocortisone sodium phosphate equivalent to the labeled amount of hydrocortisone, within −10% to +15%. Meets the requirements for Identification, Bacterial endotoxins, pH (7.5–8.5), and Particulate matter, and for Injections.

Hydrocortisone Sodium Succinate USP—Preserve in tight, light-resistant containers. Contains not less than 97.0% and not more than 102.0% of total steroids, calculated as hydrocortisone sodium succinate, on the dried basis. Meets the requirements for Identification, Specific rotation (+140° to +150°), Loss on drying (not more than 2.0%), and Sodium content (4.60–4.84%, calculated on the dried basis).

Hydrocortisone Sodium Succinate for Injection USP—Preserve in Containers for Sterile Solids. A sterile mixture of Hydrocortisone Sodium Succinate and suitable buffers. It may be prepared from Hydrocortisone Sodium Succinate, or from Hydrocortisone Hemisuccinate with the aid of Sodium Hydroxide or Sodium Carbonate. Label it to indicate that the constituted solution prepared from Hydrocortisone

Sodium Succinate for Injection is suitable for use only if it is clear, and that the solution is to be discarded after 3 days. Label it to indicate that it was prepared by freeze-drying, having been filled into its container in the form of a true solution. Contains an amount of hydrocortisone sodium succinate equivalent to the labeled amount of hydrocortisone, within ±10%, in single-compartment containers, or in the volume of solution designated on the label of containers that are constructed to hold in separate compartments the Hydrocortisone Sodium Succinate for Injection and a solvent. Meets the requirements for Constituted solution, Identification, Bacterial endotoxins, pH (7.0–8.0 in a solution containing the equivalent of 50 mg of hydrocortisone per mL), Loss on drying (not more than 2.0%), Particulate matter, and Free hydrocortisone (not more than 6.7%), and for Sterility tests, Uniformity of dosage units, and Labeling under Injections.

Hydrocortisone Valerate USP—Preserve in well-closed containers. Contains not less than 97.0% and not more than 102.0% of hydrocortisone valerate, calculated on the dried basis. Meets the requirements for Identification, Specific rotation (37° to 43°), and Loss on drying (not more than 1.0%).

Hydrocortisone Valerate Cream USP—Preserve in well-closed containers. It is Hydrocortisone Valerate in a suitable cream base. Contains the labeled amount, within ± 10%. Meets the requirements for Identification and Minimum fill.

Hydrocortisone Valerate Ointment USP—Preserve in tight containers, and store at controlled room temperature. Contains the labeled amount, within ±10%, in a suitable ointment base. Meets the requirements for Identification, Microbial limits (not more than 100 per gram), and Minimum fill.

HYDROCORTISONE AND ACETIC ACID

For *Hydrocortisone* and *Acetic Acid*—See individual listings for chemistry information.

USP requirements: Hydrocortisone and Acetic Acid Otic Solution USP—Preserve in tight, light-resistant containers. A solution of Hydrocortisone and Glacial Acetic Acid in a suitable nonaqueous solvent. Contains the labeled amount of hydrocortisone, within –10% to +20%, and the labeled amount of acetic acid, within –15% to +30%. Meets the requirements for Identification and pH (2.0–4.0, when diluted with an equal volume of water).

HYDROCORTISONE AND UREA

For *Hydrocortisone* and *Urea*—See individual listings for chemistry information.

USP requirements: Hydrocortisone and Urea Cream—Not in *USP–NF*.

HYDROFLUMETHIAZIDE

Chemical name: 2*H*-1,2,4-Benzothiadiazine-7-sulfonamide, 3,4-dihydro-6-(trifluoromethyl)-, 1,1-dioxide.

Molecular formula: $C_8H_8F_3N_3O_4S_2$.

Molecular weight: 331.29.

Description: Hydroflumethiazide USP—White to cream-colored, finely divided, odorless, crystalline powder.

pKa: 8.9 and 10.7.

Solubility: Hydroflumethiazide USP—Very slightly soluble in water; freely soluble in acetone; soluble in alcohol.

USP requirements:

Hydroflumethiazide USP—Preserve in tight containers. Contains not less than 98.0% and not more than 102.0% of hydroflumethiazide, calculated on the anhydrous basis. Meets the requirements for Identification, Melting range (270–275 °C), pH (4.5–7.5, in a 1 in 100 dispersion in water), Water (not more than 1.0%), Residue on ignition (not more than 1.0%), Heavy metals (not more than 0.002%), Selenium (not more than 0.003%), Diazotizable substances (not more than 1.0%), and Organic volatile impurities.

Hydroflumethiazide Tablets USP—Preserve in tight containers. Contain the labeled amount, within ±5%. Meet the requirements for Identification, Dissolution (80% in 60 minutes in dilute hydrochloric acid [1 in 100] in Apparatus 2 at 50 rpm), and Uniformity of dosage units.

HYDROGEN PEROXIDE

Chemical name: Hydrogen peroxide.

Molecular formula: H_2O_2.

Molecular weight: 34.01.

Description:

Hydrogen Peroxide Concentrate USP—Clear, colorless liquid. Acid to litmus. Slowly decomposes, and is affected by light.

Hydrogen Peroxide Solution USP—Clear, colorless liquid, odorless or having an odor resembling that of ozone. Acid to litmus. Rapidly decomposes when in contact with many oxidizing as well as reducing substances. When rapidly heated, it may decompose suddenly. Affected by light. Specific gravity is about 1.01.

USP requirements:

Hydrogen Peroxide Concentrate USP—Preserve in partially-filled containers having a small vent in the closure, and store in a cool place. Label it to indicate the name and amount of any added preservative. The label states that this article is not intended for direct administration to humans or animals. Contains not less than 29.0% and not more than 32.0%, by weight, of hydrogen peroxide. Contains not more than 0.05% of a suitable preservative or preservatives. Meets the requirements for Acidity and Chloride (not more than 0.005%), and for Identification test, Nonvolatile residue, Heavy metals, and Limit of preservative under Hydrogen Peroxide Topical Solution.

Caution: Hydrogen Peroxide Concentrate is a strong oxidant.

Hydrogen Peroxide Topical Solution USP—Preserve in tight, light-resistant containers, at controlled room temperature. Contains, in each 100 mL, not less than 2.5 grams and not more than 3.5 grams of Hydrogen Peroxide. Contains not more than 0.05% of a suitable preservative or preservatives. Meets the requirements for Identification, Acidity, Barium, Heavy metals (not more than 5 ppm), Limit of nonvolatile residue, and Limit of preservative (not more than 0.05%).

HYDROMORPHONE

Chemical name: Hydromorphone hydrochloride—Morphinan-6-one, 4,5-epoxy-3-hydroxy-17-methyl-, hydrochloride, (5 alpha)-.

Molecular formula: Hydromorphone hydrochloride—$C_{17}H_{19}NO_3 \cdot$ HCl.

Molecular weight: Hydromorphone hydrochloride—321.80.

Description: Hydromorphone Hydrochloride USP—Fine, white or practically white, odorless, crystalline powder. Is affected by light.

Solubility: Hydromorphone Hydrochloride USP—Freely soluble in water; sparingly soluble in alcohol; practically insoluble in ether.

USP requirements:

Hydromorphone Hydrochloride USP—Preserve in tight, light-resistant containers. Dried at 105 °C for 2 hours, contains not less than 98.0% and not more than 101.0% of hydromorphone hydrochloride. Meets the requirements for Identification, Specific rotation (–136° to –139°), Acidity, Loss on drying (not more than 1.5%), Residue on ignition (not more than 0.3%), Sulfate, Ordinary impurities, and Organic volatile impurities.

Hydromorphone Hydrochloride Injection USP—Preserve in single-dose or in multiple-dose containers, preferably of Type I glass, protected from light. A sterile solution of Hydromorphone Hydrochloride in Water for Injection. Contains the labeled amount, within ±5%. Meets the requirements for Identification, Bacterial endotoxins, and pH (3.5–5.5), and for Injections.

Hydromorphone Hydrochloride Oral Solution—Not in *USP–NF*.

Hydromorphone Hydrochloride Suppositories—Not in *USP–NF*.

Hydromorphone Hydrochloride Tablets USP—Preserve in tight, light-resistant containers. Contain the labeled amount, within ±10%. Meet the requirements for Identification, Dissolution (75% in 45 minutes in water in Apparatus 2 at 50 rpm), and Uniformity of dosage units.

HYDROMORPHONE AND GUAIFENESIN

For *Hydromorphone* and *Guaifenesin*—See individual listings for chemistry information.

USP requirements: Hydromorphone Hydrochloride and Guaifenesin Syrup—Not in *USP–NF*.

HYDROQUINONE

Chemical name: 1,4-Benzenediol.

Molecular formula: $C_6H_6O_2$.

Molecular weight: 110.11.

Description: Hydroquinone USP—Fine white needles. Darkens upon exposure to light and to air.

Solubility: Hydroquinone USP—Freely soluble in water, in alcohol, and in ether.

USP requirements:

Hydroquinone USP—Preserve in tight, light-resistant containers. Contains not less than 99.0% and not more than 100.5% of hydroquinone, calculated on the anhydrous basis. Meets the requirements for Identification, Melting range (172–174 °C), Water (not more than 0.5%), Residue on ignition (not more than 0.5%), and Organic volatile impurities.

Hydroquinone Cream USP—Preserve in well-closed, light-resistant containers. Contains the labeled amount, within ± 6%. Meets the requirements for Identification and Minimum fill.

Hydroquinone Topical Solution USP—Preserve in tight, light-resistant containers. Contains the labeled amount, within –5% to +10%. Meets the requirements for Identification and pH (3.0–4.2).

HYDROXOCOBALAMIN

Chemical name: Cobinamide, dihydroxide, dihydrogen phosphate (ester), mono(inner salt), 3′-ester with 5,6-dimethyl-1-alpha-D-ribofuranosyl-1*H*-benzimidazole.

Molecular formula: $C_{62}H_{89}CoN_{13}O_{15}P$.

Molecular weight: 1346.36.

Description: Hydroxocobalamin USP—Dark red crystals or red crystalline powder. Is odorless, or has not more than a slight acetone odor. The anhydrous form is very hygroscopic.

Solubility: Hydroxocobalamin USP—Sparingly soluble in water, in alcohol, and in methanol; practically insoluble in acetone, in ether, and in chloroform.

USP requirements:

Hydroxocobalamin USP—Preserve in tight, light-resistant containers, and store in a cool place. Contains not less than 95.0% and not more than 102.0% of hydroxocobalamin, calculated on the dried basis. Meets the requirements for Identification, pH (8.0–10.0, in a solution [2 in 100]), Loss on drying (14.0–18.0%), pH-dependent cobalamins (within –5% to +2%, calculated on the dried basis), and Limit of cyanocobalamin (not more than 5.0%, calculated on the dried basis).

Hydroxocobalamin Injection USP—Preserve in single-dose or in multiple-dose containers, preferably of Type I glass, protected from light. A sterile solution of Hydroxocobalamin in Water for Injection. Contains the labeled amount, within –5% to +15%. Meets the requirements for Identification, Bacterial endotoxins, and pH (3.5–5.0), and for Injections.

HYDROXYAMPHETAMINE

Chemical name: Hydroxyamphetamine hydrobromide—Phenol, 4-(2-aminopropyl)-, hydrobromide.

Molecular formula: Hydroxyamphetamine hydrobromide—$C_9H_{13}NO \cdot$ HBr.

Molecular weight: Hydroxyamphetamine hydrobromide—232.12.

Description: Hydroxyamphetamine Hydrobromide USP—White, crystalline powder. Its solutions are slightly acid to litmus, having a pH of about 5.

Solubility: Hydroxyamphetamine Hydrobromide USP—Freely soluble in water and in alcohol; slightly soluble in chloroform; practically insoluble in ether.

USP requirements:

Hydroxyamphetamine Hydrobromide USP—Preserve in well-closed, light-resistant containers. Contains not less than 98.0% and not more than 101.5% of hydroxyamphetamine hydrobromide, calculated on the dried basis. Meets the requirements for Identification, Melting range (189–192 °C),

Loss on drying (not more than 0.5%), Residue on ignition (not more than 0.1%), Bromide content (33.6–35.2%, calculated on the dried basis), and Ordinary impurities.

Hydroxyamphetamine Hydrobromide Ophthalmic Solution USP—Preserve in tight, light-resistant containers. A sterile, buffered, aqueous solution of Hydroxyamphetamine Hydrobromide. Contains the labeled amount, within ± 5%. Contains a suitable antimicrobial agent. Meets the requirements for Identification, Sterility, and pH (4.2–6.0).

HYDROXYAMPHETAMINE AND TROPICAMIDE

For *Hydroxyamphetamine* and *Tropicamide*—See individual listings for chemistry information.

USP requirements: Hydroxyamphetamine Hydrobromide and Tropicamide Ophthalmic Solution—Not in *USP–NF*.

HYDROXYCHLOROQUINE

Chemical name: Hydroxychloroquine sulfate—Ethanol, 2-[[4-[(7-chloro-4-quinolinyl)amino]pentyl]ethylamino]-, sulfate (1:1) salt.

Molecular formula: Hydroxychloroquine sulfate—$C_{18}H_{26}ClN_3O \cdot H_2SO_4$.

Molecular weight: Hydroxychloroquine sulfate—433.95.

Description: Hydroxychloroquine Sulfate USP—White or practically white, crystalline powder. Is odorless. Its solutions have a pH of about 4.5. Exists in two forms, the usual form melting at about 240 °C and the other form melting at about 198 °C.

Solubility: Hydroxychloroquine Sulfate USP—Freely soluble in water; practically insoluble in alcohol, in chloroform, and in ether.

USP requirements:
  Hydroxychloroquine Sulfate USP—Preserve in well-closed, light-resistant containers. Contains not less than 98.0% and not more than 102.0% of hydroxychloroquine sulfate, calculated on the dried basis. Meets the requirements for Identification, Loss on drying (not more than 2.0%), Ordinary impurities, and Organic volatile impurities.
  Hydroxychloroquine Sulfate Tablets USP—Preserve in tight, light-resistant containers. Contain the labeled amount, within ±7%. Meet the requirements for Identification, Dissolution (70% in 60 minutes in water in Apparatus 2 at 50 rpm), and Uniformity of dosage units.

HYDROXYETHYL CELLULOSE

Chemical name: Cellulose, 2-hydroxyethyl ether.

Description: Hydroxyethyl Cellulose NF—White to light tan, practically odorless, hygroscopic powder.
  NF category: Suspending and/or viscosity-increasing agent.

Solubility: Hydroxyethyl Cellulose NF—Soluble in hot water and in cold water, giving a colloidal solution; practically insoluble in alcohol and in most organic solvents.

NF requirements: Hydroxyethyl Cellulose NF—Preserve in well-closed containers. A partially substituted poly(hydroxyethyl) ether of cellulose. It is available in several grades, varying in viscosity and degree of substitution, and some grades are modified to improve their dispersion in water. The labeling indicates its viscosity, under specified conditions, in aqueous

solution. The indicated viscosity may be in the form of a range encompassing 50% to 150% of the average value. Meets the requirements for Identification, Viscosity (not less than 50% and not more than 150% of the labeled viscosity, where stated as a single value, or it is between the maximum and minimum values, where stated as a range of viscosities), pH (6.0–8.5, in a solution [1 in 100]), Loss on drying (not more than 10.0%), Residue on ignition (not more than 5.0%), Lead (not more than 0.001%), Heavy metals (not more than 20 mcg per gram, and Organic volatile impurities.

HYDROXYPROGESTERONE

Chemical name: Hydroxyprogesterone caproate—Pregn-4-ene-3,20-dione, 17-[(1-oxohexyl)oxy]-.

Molecular formula: Hydroxyprogesterone caproate—$C_{27}H_{40}O_4$.

Molecular weight: Hydroxyprogesterone caproate—428.60.

Description: Hydroxyprogesterone Caproate USP—White or creamy white, crystalline powder. Is odorless or has a slight odor.

Solubility: Hydroxyprogesterone Caproate USP—Insoluble in water; soluble in ether.

USP requirements:
  Hydroxyprogesterone Caproate USP—Preserve in well-closed, light-resistant containers. Contains not less than 97.0% and not more than 103.0% of hydroxyprogesterone caproate, calculated on the anhydrous basis. Meets the requirements for Identification, Melting range (120–124 °C), Specific rotation (+58° to +64°), Water (not more than 0.1%), Free *n*-caproic acid, and Ordinary impurities.
  Hydroxyprogesterone Caproate Injection USP—Preserve in single-dose or in multiple-dose containers, preferably of Type I or Type III glass. A sterile solution of Hydroxyprogesterone Caproate in a suitable vegetable oil. Contains the labeled amount, within ±10%. Meets the requirements for Identification and Water (not more than 0.2%), and for Injections.

HYDROXYPROPYL CELLULOSE

Chemical name: Cellulose, 2-hydroxypropyl ether.

Description: Hydroxypropyl Cellulose NF—White to cream-colored, practically odorless, granular solid or powder. Is hygroscopic after drying.
  NF category: Coating agent; suspending and/or viscosity-increasing agent.

Solubility: Hydroxypropyl Cellulose NF—Soluble in cold water, in alcohol, in chloroform, and in propylene glycol, giving a colloidal solution; insoluble in hot water.

USP requirements: Hydroxypropyl Cellulose Ocular System USP—Preserve in single-dose containers, at a temperature not exceeding 30 °C. Contains no other substance. It is sterile. Contains the labeled amount, within ±15%. Meets the requirements for Identification, Sterility, and Weight variation.

NF requirements:Hydroxypropyl Cellulose NF—Store in well-closed containers. A partially substituted poly(hydroxypropyl) ether of cellulose. Label it to indicate the viscosity in an aqueous solution of stated concentration and temperature. The indicated viscosity may be in the form of a range encompassing 50% to 150% of the average value. May contain not more than 0.60% of silica or other suitable anticaking agents. When dried at 105 °C for 1 hour, contains not more than 80.5% of hydroxypropoxy groups. Meets the requirements for Identification,

Apparent viscosity, pH (5.0–8.0, in a solution [1 in 100]), Loss on drying (not more than 5.0%), Residue on ignition (except for silica, not more than 0.2%), Lead (not more than 0.001%), Heavy metals (not more than 20 mcg per gram), and Organic volatile impurities.

LOW-SUBSTITUTED HYDROXYPROPYL CELLULOSE

Description: Low-Substituted Hydroxypropyl Cellulose NF— White to yellowish white, practically odorless, fibrous or granular powder. Is hygroscopic. The pH of the suspension, obtained by shaking 1.0 gram with 100 mL of water, is between 5.0 and 7.5.

    NF category: Tablet disintegrant and/or tablet binder.

Solubility: Low-Substituted Hydroxypropyl Cellulose NF—Practically insoluble in ethanol and in ether. Dissolves in a solution of sodium hydroxide (1 in 10), and produces a viscous solution. Swells in water, in sodium carbonate TS, and in 2 *N* hydrochloric acid.

NF requirements: Low-Substituted Hydroxypropyl Cellulose NF—Preserve in tight containers. A low-substituted hydroxypropyl ether of cellulose. When dried at 105 °C for 1 hour, contains not less than 5.0% and not more than 16.0% of hydroxypropoxy groups (–OCH$_2$CHOHCH$_3$). Meets the requirements for Identification, Loss on drying (not more than 5.0%), Residue on ignition (not more than 0.5%), Chloride (not more than 0.36%), and Heavy metals (not more than 0.001%).

HYDROXYPROPYL METHYLCELLULOSE

Chemical name: Cellulose, 2-hydroxypropyl methyl ether.

Description:

    Hydroxypropyl Methylcellulose USP—White to slightly off-white, fibrous or granular powder. Swells in water and produces a clear to opalescent, viscous, colloidal mixture.

        NF category: Coating agent; suspending and/or viscosity-increasing agent; tablet binder.

    Hydroxypropyl Methylcellulose 2208 USP—White to slightly off-white, fibrous or granular powder. Swells in water and produces a clear to opalescent, viscous, colloidal mixture.

        NF category: Coating agent; suspending and/or viscosity-increasing agent; tablet binder.

    Hydroxypropyl Methylcellulose 2906 USP—White to slightly off-white, fibrous or granular powder. Swells in water and produces a clear to opalescent, viscous, colloidal mixture.

        NF category: Coating agent; suspending and/or viscosity-increasing agent; tablet binder.

    Hydroxypropyl Methylcellulose 2910 USP—White to slightly off-white, fibrous or granular powder. Swells in water and produces a clear to opalescent, viscous, colloidal mixture.

        NF category: Coating agent; suspending and/or viscosity-increasing agent; tablet binder.

Solubility:

    Hydroxypropyl Methylcellulose USP—Insoluble in dehydrated alcohol, in ether, and in chloroform.

    Hydroxypropyl Methylcellulose 2208 USP—Insoluble in dehydrated alcohol, in ether, and in chloroform.

    Hydroxypropyl Methylcellulose 2906 USP—Insoluble in dehydrated alcohol, in ether, and in chloroform.

    Hydroxypropyl Methylcellulose 2910 USP—Insoluble in dehydrated alcohol, in ether, and in chloroform.

USP requirements:

    Hydroxypropyl Methylcellulose USP—Preserve in well-closed containers. A propylene glycol ether of methylcellulose. Label it to indicate its substitution type and its viscosity type (viscosity of a solution [1 in 50]). When dried at 105 °C for 2 hours, contains methoxy and hydroxypropoxy groups conforming to the limits for the 4 substitution types for methoxy and hydroxypropoxy contents. Meets the requirements for Identification, Apparent viscosity, Loss on drying (not more than 5.0%), Residue on ignition (not more than 1.5% for labeled viscosity of greater than 50 centipoises, not more than 3% for labeled viscosity of 50 centipoises or less, or not more than 5% of all labeled viscosities), Heavy metals (not more than 0.001%), and Organic volatile impurities.

    Hydroxypropyl Methylcellulose Injection—Not in *USP–NF*.

    Hydroxypropyl Methylcellulose Ophthalmic Solution USP— Preserve in tight containers. A sterile solution of Hydroxypropyl Methylcellulose. Contains the labeled amount, within ±15%. Meets the requirements for Identification, Sterility, and pH (6.0–7.8).

HYDROXYUREA

Chemical name: Urea, hydroxy-.

Molecular formula: CH$_4$N$_2$O$_2$.

Molecular weight: 76.05.

Description: Hydroxyurea USP—White to off-white powder. Is somewhat hygroscopic, decomposing in the presence of moisture. Melts at a temperature exceeding 133 °C, with decomposition.

Solubility: Hydroxyurea USP—Freely soluble in water and in hot alcohol.

USP requirements:

    Hydroxyurea USP—Preserve in tight containers, in a dry atmosphere. Contains not less than 97.0% and not more than 103.0% of hydroxyurea, calculated on the dried basis. Meets the requirements for Identification, Loss on drying (not more than 1.0%), Residue on ignition (not more than 0.50%), Heavy metals (not more than 0.003%), Urea and related compounds, and Organic volatile impurities.

    Hydroxyurea Capsules USP—Preserve in tight containers, in a dry atmosphere. Contain the labeled amount, within ± 10%. Meet the requirements for Identification, Dissolution (80% in 30 minutes in water in Apparatus 2 at 50 rpm), and Uniformity of dosage units.

HYDROXYZINE

Chemical group: Piperazine derivative.

Chemical name:

    Hydroxyzine hydrochloride—Ethanol, 2-[2-[4-[(4-chlorophenyl)phenylmethyl]-1-piperazinyl]ethoxy]-, dihydrochloride.

    Hydroxyzine pamoate—Ethanol, 2-[2-[4-[(4-chlorophenyl)-phenylmethyl]-1-piperazinyl]ethoxy]-, compd. with 4,4′-methylenebis[3-hydroxy-2-naphthalenecarboxylic acid](1:1).

Molecular formula:

    Hydroxyzine hydrochloride—C$_{21}$H$_{27}$ClN$_2$O$_2$ · 2HCl.

    Hydroxyzine pamoate—C$_{21}$H$_{27}$ClN$_2$O$_2$ · C$_{23}$H$_{16}$O$_6$.

Molecular weight:

    Hydroxyzine hydrochloride—447.83.

    Hydroxyzine pamoate—763.27.

Description:
Hydroxyzine Hydrochloride USP—White, odorless powder. Melts at about 200 °C, with decomposition.
Hydroxyzine Pamoate USP—Light yellow, practically odorless powder.

pKa: Hydroxyzine hydrochloride—2.6 and 7.

Solubility:
Hydroxyzine Hydrochloride USP—Very soluble in water; soluble in chloroform; slightly soluble in acetone; practically insoluble in ether.
Hydroxyzine Pamoate USP—Practically insoluble in water and in methanol; freely soluble in dimethylformamide.

USP requirements:
Hydroxyzine Hydrochloride USP—Preserve in tight containers. Contains not less than 98.0% and not more than 100.5% of hydroxyzine hydrochloride, calculated on the dried basis. Meets the requirements for Identification, Loss on drying (not more than 5.0%), Residue on ignition (not more than 0.5%), Heavy metals (not more than 0.002%), Chromatographic purity, and Organic volatile impurities.
Hydroxyzine Hydrochloride Capsules—Not in *USP–NF.*
Hydroxyzine Hydrochloride Injection USP—Preserve in single-dose or in multiple-dose containers, protected from light. A sterile solution of Hydroxyzine Hydrochloride in Water for Injection. Contains the labeled amount, within ±10%. Meets the requirements for Identification, Bacterial endotoxins, pH (3.5–6.0), and Limit of 4-chlorobenzophenone (not more than 0.2%), and for Injections.
Hydroxyzine Hydrochloride Oral Suspension USP—Preserve in tight, light-resistant containers. Contains the labeled amount, within ±10%. Meets the requirement for Identification.
Hydroxyzine Hydrochloride Syrup USP—Preserve in tight, light-resistant containers. Contains the labeled amount, within ±10%. Meets the requirement for Identification.
Hydroxyzine Hydrochloride Tablets USP—Preserve in tight containers. Contain the labeled amount, within ±10%. Meet the requirements for Identification, Dissolution (75% in 45 minutes in water in Apparatus 3 [Drug release: 30 dips per minute]), and Uniformity of dosage units.
Hydroxyzine Pamoate USP—Preserve in tight containers. Contains not less than 97.0% and not more than 102.0% of hydroxyzine pamoate, calculated on the anhydrous basis. Meets the requirements for Identification, Water (not more than 5.0%), Residue on ignition (not more than 0.5%), Heavy metals (not more than 0.005%), Organic volatile impurities, and Pamoic acid content (49.4–51.9%, calculated on the anhydrous basis).
Hydroxyzine Pamoate Capsules USP—Preserve in well-closed containers. Contain an amount of hydroxyzine pamoate equivalent to the labeled amount of hydroxyzine hydrochloride, within ±10%. Meet the requirements for Identification, Dissolution (75% in 60 minutes in 0.1 *N* hydrochloric acid in Apparatus 2 at 50 rpm), and Uniformity of dosage units.
Hydroxyzine Pamoate Oral Suspension USP—Preserve in tight, light-resistant containers. Contains an amount of hydroxyzine pamoate equivalent to the labeled amount of hydroxyzine hydrochloride, within ±10%. Meets the requirements for Identification and pH (4.5–7.0).

HYOSCYAMINE

Source: The levo-isomer of atropine; the major active alkaloid of belladonna.

Chemical group: Natural tertiary amine.

Chemical name:
Hyoscyamine—Benzeneacetic acid, alpha-(hydroxymethyl)-, 8-methyl-8-azabicyclo[3.2.1]oct-3-yl ester, [3(*S*)-*endo*]-.
Hyoscyamine hydrobromide—Benzeneacetic acid, alpha-(hydroxymethyl)-, 8-methyl-8-azabicyclo[3.2.1]oct-3-yl ester, hydrobromide [3(*S*)-*endo*]-.
Hyoscyamine sulfate—Benzeneacetic acid, alpha-(hydroxymethyl)-, 8-methyl-8-azabicyclo[3.2.1]oct-3-yl ester, [3(*S*)-*endo*]-, sulfate (2:1), dihydrate.

Molecular formula:
Hyoscyamine—$C_{17}H_{23}NO_3$.
Hyoscyamine hydrobromide—$C_{17}H_{23}NO_3 \cdot HBr$.
Hyoscyamine sulfate—$(C_{17}H_{23}NO_3)_2 \cdot H_2SO_4 \cdot 2H_2O$.

Molecular weight:
Hyoscyamine—289.37.
Hyoscyamine hydrobromide—370.28.
Hyoscyamine sulfate—712.85.

Description:
Hyoscyamine USP—White, crystalline powder. Is affected by light. Its solutions are alkaline to litmus.
Hyoscyamine Hydrobromide USP—White, odorless crystals or crystalline powder. The pH of a solution (1 in 20) is about 5.4. Is affected by light.
Hyoscyamine Sulfate USP—White, odorless crystals or crystalline powder. Is deliquescent and is affected by light. The pH of a solution (1 in 100) is about 5.3.

Solubility:
Hyoscyamine USP—Slightly soluble in water; freely soluble in alcohol, in chloroform, and in dilute acids; sparingly soluble in ether.
Hyoscyamine Hydrobromide USP—Freely soluble in water, in alcohol, and in chloroform; very slightly soluble in ether.
Hyoscyamine Sulfate USP—Very soluble in water; freely soluble in alcohol; practically insoluble in ether.

USP requirements:
Hyoscyamine USP—Preserve in tight, light-resistant containers. Contains not less than 98.0% and not more than 101.0% of hyoscyamine, calculated on the dried basis. Meets the requirements for Identification, Melting range (106–109 °C), Specific rotation (–20° to –23°, calculated on the dried basis), Loss on drying (not more than 0.2%), Residue on ignition (not more than 0.1%), and Limit of foreign alkaloids and other impurities.
Caution: Handle Hyoscyamine with exceptional care, since it is highly potent.
Hyoscyamine Tablets USP—Preserve in well-closed, light-resistant containers. Contain the labeled amount, within ±10%. Meet the requirements for Identification, Disintegration (30 minutes, the use of disks being omitted), and Uniformity of dosage units.
Hyoscyamine Hydrobromide USP—Preserve in tight, light-resistant containers. Contains not less than 98.5% and not more than 100.5% of hyoscyamine hydrobromide, calculated on the dried basis. Meets the requirements for Identification, Melting range (not less than 149 °C), Specific rotation (not less than –24°), Loss on drying (not more than 1.0%), Residue on ignition (not more than 0.2%), and Other alkaloids.
Caution: Handle Hyoscyamine Hydrobromide with exceptional care, since it is highly potent.
Hyoscyamine Sulfate USP—Preserve in tight, light-resistant containers. Contains not less than 98.5% and not more than 100.5% of hyoscyamine sulfate, calculated on the dried basis. Meets the requirements for Identification, Melting range (not less than 200 °C), Specific rotation (not less than –24°), Loss on drying (2.0–5.5%), Residue on ignition (not more than 0.2%), Other alkaloids, Readily carbonizable substances, and Organic volatile impurities.

Caution: Handle Hyoscyamine Sulfate with exceptional care, since it is highly potent.

Hyoscyamine Sulfate Extended-release Capsules—Not in *USP–NF*.

Hyoscyamine Sulfate Elixir USP—Preserve in tight, light-resistant containers, at controlled room temperature. Contains the labeled amount, within ±10%. Meets the requirements for Identification, pH (3.0–6.5), and Alcohol content (within ±10% of labeled amount).

Hyoscyamine Sulfate Injection USP—Preserve in single-dose or in multiple-dose containers, preferably of Type I glass, at controlled room temperature. A sterile solution of Hyoscyamine Sulfate in Water for Injection. Contains the labeled amount, within ±7%. Meets the requirements for Identification, Bacterial endotoxins, and pH (3.0–6.5), and for Injections.

Hyoscyamine Sulfate Oral Solution USP—Preserve in tight, light-resistant containers, at controlled room temperature. Contains the labeled amount, within ±10%. Meets the requirements for Identification and pH (3.0–6.5).

Hyoscyamine Sulfate Tablets USP—Preserve in tight, light-resistant containers. Contain the labeled amount, within ± 10%. Meet the requirements for Identification, Disintegration (15 minutes), and Uniformity of dosage units.

Hyoscyamine Sulfate Extended-release Tablets—Not in *USP–NF*.

HYOSCYAMINE AND PHENOBARBITAL

For *Hyoscyamine* and *Phenobarbital*—See individual listings for chemistry information.

USP requirements:

Hyoscyamine Sulfate and Phenobarbital Elixir—Not in *USP–NF*.

Hyoscyamine Sulfate and Phenobarbital Oral Solution—Not in *USP–NF*.

Hyoscyamine Sulfate and Phenobarbital Tablets—Not in *USP–NF*.

HYPOPHOSPHOROUS ACID

Chemical name: Phosphinic acid.

Molecular formula: H_3PO_2.

Molecular weight: 66.00.

Description: Hypophosphorous Acid NF—Colorless or slightly yellow, odorless liquid. Specific gravity is about 1.13.

NF category: Antioxidant.

NF requirements: Hypophosphorous Acid NF—Preserve in tight containers. Contains not less than 30.0% and not more than 32.0% of hypophosphorous acid. Meets the requirements for Identification, Limit of barium and oxalate, and Heavy metals (not more than 0.002%).

HYPROMELLOSE

Chemical name: Cellulose, 2-hydroxypropyl methyl ether.

USP requirements:

Hypromellose USP—Preserve in well-closed containers. A propylene glycol ether of methylcellulose. Label it to indicate its substitution type and its viscosity type (viscosity of a solution [1 in 50]). When dried at 105 °C for 2 hours, con-

tains methoxy and hydroxypropoxy groups conforming to the limits for the 4 substitution types for hypromellose (hydroxypropyl methylcellulose) contents. Meets the requirements for Identification, Viscosity, Loss on drying (not more than 5.0%), Residue on ignition (not more than 1.5% for labeled viscosity of greater than 50 centipoises, not more than 3% for labeled viscosity of 50 centipoises or less, or not more than 5% of all labeled viscosities), Heavy metals (not more than 0.001%), and Organic volatile impurities.

Hypromellose Ophthalmic Solution USP—Preserve in tight containers. A sterile solution of Hypromellose. Contains the labeled amount, within ±15%. Meets the requirements for Identification, Sterility, and pH (6.0–7.8).

HYPROMELLOSE PHTHALATE

Description: Hypromellose Phthalate NF—White powder or granules. Is odorless.

NF category: Coating agent.

Solubility: Hypromellose Phthalate NF—Practically insoluble in water, in dehydrated alcohol, and in hexane. Produces a viscous solution in a mixture of methanol and dichloromethane (1:1), or in a mixture of dehydrated alcohol and acetone (1:1). Dissolves in 1 *N* sodium hydroxide.

NF requirements: Hypromellose Phthalate NF—Preserve in tight containers. A monophthalic acid ester of hydroxypropyl methylcellulose. Label it to indicate its viscosity and its nominal phthalyl content. Contains methoxy, hydroxypropoxy, and phthalyl groups. Contains not less than 21.0% and not more than 35.0% of phthalyl groups, calculated on the anhydrous basis. Meets the requirements for Identification, Viscosity (within ±20% of that indicated by the label), Water (not more than 5.0%), Residue on ignition (not more than 0.20%), Chloride (not more than 0.07%), Heavy metals (not more than 0.001%), Limit of free phthalic acid (not more than 1.0%), Organic volatile impurities, and Phthalyl content.

IBRITUMOMAB

Source: Ibritumomab tiuxetan—Ibritumomab tiuxetan therapeutic regimen kit for the preparation of Indium-111 (In-111) ibritumomab tiuxetan and Yttrium-90 (Y-90) ibritumomab tiuxetan. Ibritumomab tiuxetan is an immunoconjugate resulting from a stable thiourea covalent bond between the monoclonal antibody ibritumomab and the linker-chelator tiuxetan. The antibody moiety of ibritumomab, a murine IgG_1 kappa monoclonal antibody directed against the CD20 antigen, which is found on the surface of normal and malignant B lymphocytes. Ibritumomab is produced in Chinese hamster ovary cells and is composed of two kappa light chains of 213 amino acids each and two murine gamma 1 heavy chains of 445 amino acids each. Ibritumomab has an approximate apparent affinity K_D for the CD20 antigen between 14 to 18 nM. More than 90% of B-cell non-Hdgkin's lymphomas (NHL) have CD20 antigen expressed on pre-B and mature B lymphocytes. The CD20 antigen is not internalized upon antibody biding and is not shed from the cell surface. The linker-chelator, tiuxetan, provides a high affinity, conformationally restricted chelation site for Indium-111 or Yttrium-90.

Chemical name: Ibritumomab tiuxetan—Immunoglobulin G1, anti-(human DC20 (anti-gen)) (mouse monoclonal IDEC-Y2B8 gamma 1-chain), disulfide with mouse monoclonal IDEC-Y2B8 K-chain, dimer, *N*-[2-[bis(carboxymethyl)amino]-3-(4-isothiocyanatophenyl)propyl]-*N*-2-[bis(carboxymethyl)amino]propyl]glycine conjugate.

Molecular weight: Ibritumomab tiuxetan—1500 daltons.

Other characteristcs: Ibritumomab tiuxetan—Binding affinity: Ibritumomab has an approximate apparent affinity K_D for the CD20 antigen between 14 to 18 nM.

USP requirements: Ibritumomab Tiuxetan Injection—Not in *USP–NF.*

IBUPROFEN

Chemical group: Propionic acid derivative.

Chemical name: Benzeneacetic acid, alpha-methyl-4-(2-methyl-propyl), (±)-.

Molecular formula: $C_{13}H_{18}O_2$.

Molecular weight: 206.28.

Description: Ibuprofen USP—White to off-white, crystalline powder, having a slight, characteristic odor.

pKa: 5.2 (apparent).

Solubility: Ibuprofen USP—Practically insoluble in water; very soluble in alcohol, in methanol, in acetone, and in chloroform; slightly soluble in ethyl acetate.

USP requirements:
Ibuprofen USP—Preserve in tight containers. Contains not less than 97.0% and not more than 103.0% of ibuprofen, calculated on the anhydrous basis. Meets the requirements for Identification, Water (not more than 1.0%), Residue on ignition (not more than 0.5%), Heavy metals (not more than 0.002%), Chromatographic purity, Limit of 4-isobutylacetophenone (not more than 0.1%), and Organic volatile impurities.
Ibuprofen Solution for Injection—Not in *USP–NF.*
Ibuprofen Oral Suspension USP—Preserve in well-closed containers at controlled room temperature. Contains the labeled amount, within ±10%. Meets the requirements for Identification, Dissolution (80% in 60 minutes in phosphate buffer [pH 7.2] in Apparatus 2 at 50 rpm), pH (3.6–4.6), Deliverable volume, and Limit of 4-isobutylacetophenone (not more than 0.25%).
Ibuprofen Tablets USP—Preserve in well-closed containers. Where the Tablets are gelatin-coated, the label so states. Contain the labeled amount, within ±10%. Meet the requirements for Identification, Dissolution (80% in 60 minutes in phosphate buffer [pH 7.2] in Apparatus 2 at 50 rpm), Uniformity of dosage units, Water (not more than 5.0%, except that Tablets labeled as gelatin-coated are exempt from this requirement), and Limit of 4-isobutylacetophenone (not more than 0.1% per Tablet).
Ibuprofen Chewable Tablets—Not in *USP–NF.*

IBUPROFEN AND PSEUDOEPHEDRINE

For *Ibuprofen* and *Pseudoephedrine*—See individual listings for chemistry information.

USP requirements: Ibuprofen and Pseudoephedrine Hydrochloride Tablets USP—Preserve in tight containers. Contain the labeled amounts, within ±10%. Meet the requirements for Identification, Dissolution (75% of ibuprofen in 30 minutes and pseudoephedrine hydrochloride in 45 minutes in phosphate buffer [pH 7.2] in Apparatus 2 at 50 rpm), and Uniformity of dosage units.

IBUTILIDE

Chemical name: Ibutilide fumarate—Methanesulfonamide, *N*-[4-[4-(ethylheptylamino)-1-hydroxybutyl]phenyl]-, (±)-, (*E*)-2-butenedioate (2:1) (salt).

Molecular formula: Ibutilide fumarate—$(C_{20}H_{36}N_2O_3S)_2 \cdot C_4H_4O_4$.

Molecular weight: Ibutilide fumarate—885.23.

Description: Ibutilide fumarate—White to off-white powder.

Solubility: Ibutilide fumarate—Aqueous solubility of over 100 mg/mL at pH 7 or lower.

USP requirements: Ibutilide Fumarate Injection—Not in *USP–NF.*

ICHTHAMMOL

Chemical name: Ichthammol.

Description: Ichthammol USP—Reddish brown to brownish black, viscous fluid, having a strong, characteristic, empyreumatic odor.

Solubility: Ichthammol USP—Miscible with water, with glycerin, and with fixed oils and fats. Partially soluble in alcohol and in ether.

USP requirements:
Ichthammol USP—Preserve in well-closed containers. Obtained by the destructive distillation of certain bituminous schists, sulfonation of the distillate, and neutralization of the product with ammonia. Yields not less than 2.5% of ammonia and not less than 10.0% of total sulfur. Meets the requirements for Identification, Loss on drying (not more than 50.0%), Residue on ignition (not more than 0.5%), and Limit for ammonium sulfate (not more than 8.0%).
Ichthammol Ointment USP—Preserve in collapsible tubes or in tight containers, and avoid prolonged exposure to temperatures exceeding 30 °C. Contains an amount of Ichthammol equivalent to not less than 0.25% of ammonia.
    Prepare Ichthammol Ointment as follows: 100 grams of Ichthammol, 100 grams of Lanolin, 800 grams of Petrolatum, to make 1000 grams. Thoroughly incorporate the Ichthammol with the Lanolin, and combine this mixture with the Petrolatum.

IDARUBICIN

Chemical name: Idarubicin hydrochloride—5,12-Naphthacenedione, 9-acetyl-7-[(3-amino-2,3,6-trideoxy-alpha-L-*lyxo*-hexopyranosyl)oxy]-7,8,9,10-tetrahydro-6,9,11-trihydroxyhydrochloride, (7*S-cis*)-.

Molecular formula: Idarubicin hydrochloride—$C_{26}H_{27}NO_9 \cdot HCl$.

Molecular weight: Idarubicin hydrochloride—533.95.

Description: Idarubicin Hydrochloride USP—Red-orange to red-brown powder.

Solubility: Idarubicin Hydrochloride USP—Soluble in methanol; slightly soluble in water; insoluble in acetone and in ethyl ether.

USP requirements:
Idarubicin Hydrochloride USP—Preserve in tight containers. The amorphous form is so labeled. Contains not less than 960 mcg and not more than 1030 mcg of idarubicin hydrochloride per mg, calculated on the anhydrous basis. Meets the requirements for Identification, Crystallinity (except where it is labeled as amorphous, most of the particles

do not exhibit birefringence and extinction positions), pH (5.0–6.5, in a solution containing 5 mg per mL), Water (not more than 5.0%), and Chromatographic purity.

Caution: Great care should be taken to prevent inhaling particles of Idarubicin Hydrochloride and exposing the skin to it.

Idarubicin Hydrochloride for Injection USP—Preserve in Containers for Sterile Solids. A sterile mixture of Idarubicin Hydrochloride and Lactose. Contains the labeled amount, within ±10%. Meets the requirements for Constituted solution, Identification, Bacterial endotoxins, Sterility, pH (5.0–7.0, in a solution constituted as directed in the labeling, water being used as the diluent), and Water (not more than 4.0%), and for Uniformity of dosage units and Labeling under Injections.

Caution: Great care should be taken to prevent inhaling particles of Idarubicin Hydrochloride and exposing the skin to it.

IDOXURIDINE

Chemical group: An antimetabolite of thymidine.

Chemical name: Uridine, 2′-deoxy-5-iodo-.

Molecular formula: $C_9H_{11}IN_2O_5$.

Molecular weight: 354.10.

Description: Idoxuridine USP—White, crystalline, practically odorless powder.

Solubility: Idoxuridine USP—Slightly soluble in water and in alcohol; practically insoluble in chloroform and in ether.

USP requirements:
Idoxuridine USP—Preserve in tight, light-resistant containers. Contains not less than 98.0% and not more than 101.0% of idoxuridine, calculated on the dried basis. Meets the requirements for Identification and Loss on drying (not more than 1.0%).

Idoxuridine Ophthalmic Ointment USP—Preserve in collapsible ophthalmic ointment tubes in a cool place. It is Idoxuridine in a Petrolatum base. It is sterile. Contains 0.45% to 0.55% of idoxuridine. Meets the requirements for Identification, Sterility, and Metal particles.

Idoxuridine Ophthalmic Solution USP—Preserve in tight, light-resistant containers in a cold place. A sterile, aqueous solution of Idoxuridine. Contains 0.09% to 0.11% of idoxuridine. Meets the requirements for Identification, Sterility, and pH (4.5–7.0).

IFOSFAMIDE

Chemical name: 2H-1,3,2-Oxazaphosphorin-2-amine, N,3-bis(2-chloroethyl)tetrahydro-, 2-oxide.

Molecular formula: $C_7H_{15}Cl_2N_2O_2P$.

Molecular weight: 261.09.

Description: Ifosfamide USP—White, crystalline powder. Melts at about 40 °C.

Solubility: Ifosfamide USP—Freely soluble in water; very soluble in alcohol, in ethyl acetate, in isopropyl alcohol, in methanol, and in methylene chloride; very slightly soluble in hexanes.

USP requirements:
Ifosfamide USP—Preserve in tight containers at a temperature not exceeding 25 °C. Where it is intended for use in preparing injectable dosage forms, the label states that it is sterile or must be subjected to further processing during

the preparation of injectable dosage forms. Contains not less than 98.0% and not more than 102.0% of ifosfamide. Meets the requirements for Identification, pH (4.0–7.0 in a solution [1 in 10]), Water (not more than 0.3%), Heavy metals (not more than 0.002%), Ionic chloride (not more than 0.018%), Chloroform-insoluble phosphorus (not more than 0.0415%), and Limit of 2-chloroethylamine hydrochloride (not more than 0.25%), and for Sterility tests and for Bacterial endotoxins under Ifosfamide for Injection (where the label states that Ifosfamide is sterile), and for Bacterial endotoxins under Ifosfamide for Injection (where the label states that Ifosfamide must be subjected to further processing during the preparation of injectable dosage forms).

Caution: Great care should be taken in handling Ifosfamide, as it is a potent cytotoxic agent and suspected carcinogen.

Ifosfamide for Injection USP—Preserve in Containers for Sterile Solids, at controlled room temperature. Contains the labeled amount, within ±10%. Meets the requirements for Constituted solution, Identification, Bacterial endotoxins, pH (4.0–7.0, in a solution prepared as directed for Constituted Solutions under Injections, determined 30 minutes after its preparation), and Water (not more than 0.3%), and for Sterility tests, Uniformity of dosage units, and Labeling under Injections.

Caution: Great care should be taken in handling Ifosfamide, as it is a potent cytotoxic agent and suspected carcinogen.

IMATIBIN

Chemical name: Imatibin mesylate—4-[(4-Methyl-1-piperazinyl)-methyl-3-[[4-(3-pyridinyl)-2-pyrimidinyl]amino]-phenyl]benzamide methanesulfonate.

Molecular formula: Imatibin mesylate—$C_{29}H_{31}N_7O \cdot CH_4SO_3$.

Molecular weight: Imatibin mesylate—589.7.

Description: Imatibin mesylate—White to off-white to brownish or yellowish tinged crystalline powder.

Solubility: Imatibin mesylate—Very soluble in water; soluble in aqueous buffer (pH ≤ 5.5), but is very slightly soluble to insoluble in neutral/alkaline aqueous buffers. In non-aqueous solvents, freely soluble to very slightly soluble in dimethyl sulfoxide, in methol, and in ethanol, but is insoluble in n-octanol, in acetone, and in acetonitrile.

USP requirements: Imatibin Mesylate Capsules—Not in *USP-NF*.

IMIDUREA

Chemical name: N,N-Methylenebis[N-[3-(hydroxymethyl)-2,5-dioxo-4-imidazolidinyl]urea].

Molecular formula: $C_{11}H_{16}N_8O_8$.

Molecular weight: 388.29.

Description: Imidurea NF—White, odorless powder.

Solubility: Imidurea NF—Soluble in water and in glycerin; sparingly soluble in propylene glycol; insoluble in most organic solvents.

NF requirements: Imidurea NF—Preserve in tight containers. Contains not less than 26.0% and not more than 28.0% of nitrogen, calculated on the dried basis. Meets the requirements for Color and clarity of solution, Identification, pH (6.0–7.5, in a

solution [1 in 100]), Loss on drying (not more than 3.0%), Residue on ignition (not more than 3.0%), Heavy metals (not more than 0.001%), Nitrogen content, and Organic volatile impurities.

IMIGLUCERASE

Chemical name: 495-L-Histidineglucosylceramidase (human placenta isoenzyme protein moiety).

Molecular formula: $C_{2532}H_{3843}N_{671}O_{711}S_{16}$.

Molecular weight: 60,430 (determined by mass spectroscopy).

USP requirements: Imiglucerase for Injection—Not in *USP–NF*.

IMIPENEM

Source: Derivative of thienamycin, produced by the soil organism *Streptomyces cattleya*.

Chemical group: A carbapenem, which is a subclass of the beta-lactams.

Chemical name: 1-Azabicyclo[3.2.0]hept-2-ene-2-carboxylic acid, 6-(1-hydroxyethyl)-3-[[2-[(iminomethyl)amino]ethyl]thio]-7-oxo-, monohydrate, [5R-[5 alpha,6 alpha(R^*)]]-.

Molecular formula: $C_{12}H_{17}N_3O_4S \cdot H_2O$.

Molecular weight: 317.36.

Description: Imipenem USP—White to tan-colored crystalline powder.

Solubility: Imipenem USP—Sparingly soluble in water; slightly soluble in methanol.

USP requirements: Imipenem USP—Preserve in Containers for Sterile Solids, and store in a cold place. Where it is intended for use in preparing injectable dosage forms, the label states that it is sterile. Contains the equivalent of not less than 98.0% and not more than 101.0% of imipenem monohydrate. Meets the requirements for Identification, Specific rotation (+84° to +89°), Crystallinity, Bacterial endotoxins (where the label states that Imipenem is sterile), Sterility (where the label states that Imipenem is sterile), Loss on drying (5.0–8.0%), Residue on ignition (not more than 0.2%), Heavy metals (not more than 0.002%), and Solvents (not more than 0.25%).

IMIPENEM AND CILASTATIN

For *Imipenem* and *Cilastatin*—See individual listings for chemistry information.

USP requirements:

Imipenem and Cilastatin for Injection USP—Preserve in Containers for Sterile Solids and store at controlled room temperature. A sterile mixture of Imipenem, Cilastatin Sodium, and Sodium Bicarbonate. Label it to indicate that after constitution it is to be solubilized in a suitable parenteral fluid prior to intravenous infusion. Contains the labeled amounts of imipenem and cilastatin, within −10% to + 15%. Meets the requirements for Constituted solution, Identification, Bacterial endotoxins, Sterility, pH (6.5–8.5, when constituted as directed in the labeling), Loss on drying (not more than 3.5%), and Particulate matter.

Imipenem and Cilastatin for Injectable Suspension USP—Preserve in Containers for Sterile Solids and store at controlled room temperature. A sterile mixture of Imipenem and Cilastatin Sodium. Label it to indicate that the suspension obtained when constituted as directed in the labeling is for intramuscular injection only. Contains the labeled amounts of imipenem and cilastatin, within −10% to +15%. Meets the requirements for Identification, Bacterial endotoxins, Sterility, pH (6.0–7.5, when constituted as directed in the labeling), and Loss on drying (not more than 3.5%).

IMIPRAMINE

Chemical group: Dibenzazepine.

Chemical name:

Imipramine hydrochloride—5H-Dibenz[b,f]azepine-5-propanamine, 10,11-dihydro-N,N-dimethyl-, monohydrochloride.

Imipramine pamoate—5-(3-[Dimethylamino)propyl]-10,11-dihydro-5H-dibenz[b,f]azepine 4,4′-methylenebis-(3-hydroxy-2-naphthoate) (2:1).

Molecular formula:

Imipramine hydrochloride—$C_{19}H_{24}N_2 \cdot HCl$.

Imipramine pamoate—$(C_{19}H_{24}N_2)_2 \cdot C_{23}H_{16}O_6$.

Molecular weight:

Imipramine hydrochloride—316.87.

Imipramine pamoate—949.21.

Description:

Imipramine Hydrochloride USP—White to off-white, odorless or practically odorless, crystalline powder.

Imipramine pamoate—Fine, yellow, odorless powder.

pKa: Imipramine hydrochloride—9.4.

Solubility:

Imipramine Hydrochloride USP—Freely soluble in water and in alcohol; soluble in acetone; insoluble in ether.

Imipramine pamoate—Soluble in ethanol, in acetone, in ether, in chloroform, and in carbon tetrachloride. Insoluble in water.

USP requirements:

Imipramine Hydrochloride USP—Preserve in tight containers. Contains not less than 98.0% and not more than 102.0% of imipramine hydrochloride, calculated on the dried basis. Meets the requirements for Identification, Melting range (170–174 °C), Loss on drying (not more than 0.5%), Residue on ignition (not more than 0.1%), Heavy metals (not more than 0.001%), Related compounds, and Organic volatile impurities.

Imipramine Hydrochloride Injection USP—Preserve in single-dose containers, preferably of Type I glass. A sterile solution of Imipramine Hydrochloride in Water for Injection. Contains, in each mL, not less than 11.5 mg and not more than 13.5 mg of imipramine hydrochloride. Meets the requirements for Identification, Bacterial endotoxins, and pH (4.0–5.0), and for Injections.

Imipramine Hydrochloride Tablets USP—Preserve in tight containers. Contain the labeled amount, within ±7%. Meet the requirements for Identification, Dissolution (75% in 45 minutes in 0.01 N hydrochloric acid in Apparatus 1 at 100 rpm), and Uniformity of dosage units.

Imipramine Pamoate Capsules—Not in *USP–NF*.

IMIQUIMOD

Chemical name: 1*H*-Imidazo[4,5-*c*]quinolin-4-amine, 1-(2-methylpropyl).

Molecular formula: $C_{14}H_{16}N_4$.

Molecular weight: 240.30.

USP requirements: Imiquimod Cream—Not in *USP–NF*.

INAMRINONE

Chemical name: [3,4'-Bipyridin]-6(1*H*)-one, 5-amino-.

Molecular formula: $C_{10}H_9N_3O$.

Molecular weight: 187.20.

Description: Pale yellow to tan powder. It is odorless or has a faint odor.

Solubility: Slightly soluble in methanol; practically insoluble or insoluble in chloroform and in water.

USP requirements:

Inamrinone USP—Preserve in well-closed containers, protected from light. Contains not less than 98.0% and not more than 102.0% of inamrinone, calculated on the anhydrous basis. Meets the requirements for Identification, Water (not more than 1.0%), Residue on ignition (not more than 0.2%), Heavy metals (not more than 0.002%), and Chromatographic purity.

Caution: Inamrinone is a cardiotonic agent.

Inamrinone Injection USP—Preserve in single-dose containers, preferably of Type I glass, protected from light. Store at room temperature. A sterile solution of Inamrinone in Water for Injection, prepared with the aid of Lactic Acid. Contains the labeled amount, within ±10%. Meets the requirements for Identification, Bacterial endotoxins, pH (3.2–4.0), Lactic acid content (5.0–7.5 mg per mL of Injection), and Chromatographic purity, and for Injections.

Caution: Inamrinone is a cardiotonic agent.

INDAPAMIDE

Chemical name: Benzamide, 3-(aminosulfonyl)-4-chloro-*N*-(2,3-dihydro-2-methyl-1*H*-indol-1-yl)-.

Molecular formula: $C_{16}H_{16}ClN_3O_3S$.

Molecular weight: 365.84.

Description: Indapamide USP—White to off-white crystalline powder. Melts between 167 and 170 °C.

Solubility: Indapamide USP—Soluble in methanol, in alcohol, in acetonitrile, in glacial acetic acid, and in ethyl acetate; very slightly soluble in ether and in chloroform; practically insoluble in water.

USP requirements:

Indapamide USP—Preserve in well-closed containers. Contains not less than 98.0% and not more than 101.0% of indapamide, calculated on the dried basis. Meets the requirements for Identification, Loss on drying (not more than 3.0%), Residue on ignition (not more than 0.1%), Chromatographic purity, and Organic volatile impurities.

Indapamide Tablets USP—Preserve in well-closed containers. Contain the labeled amount, within ±10%. Meet the requirements for Identification, Dissolution (75% in 45 minutes in 0.05 *M* phosphate buffer (pH 6.8) in Apparatus 1 at 100 rpm), and Uniformity of dosage units.

INDIGOTINDISULFONATE

Chemical name: Indigotindisulfonate sodium—1*H*-Indole-5-sulfonic acid, 2-(1,3-dihydro-3-oxo-5-sulfo-2*H*-indol-2-ylidene)-2,3-dihydro-3-oxo-, disodium salt.

Molecular formula: Indigotindisulfonate sodium—$C_{16}H_8N_2Na_2O_8S_2$.

Molecular weight: Indigotindisulfonate sodium—466.35.

Description: Indigotindisulfonate Sodium USP—Dusky, purplish blue powder, or blue granules having a coppery luster. Affected by light. Its solutions have a blue or bluish purple color.

Solubility: Indigotindisulfonate Sodium USP—Slightly soluble in water and in alcohol; practically insoluble in most other organic solvents.

USP requirements:

Indigotindisulfonate Sodium USP—Preserve in tight, light-resistant containers. Contains not less than 96.0% and not more than 102.0% of sodium indigotinsulfonates, calculated on the dried basis as indigotindisulfonate sodium. Meets the requirements for Identification, Loss on drying (not more than 5.0%), Water-insoluble substances, Arsenic (not more than 8 ppm), Lead (not more than 0.001%), and Sulfur content (13.0–14.0%, calculated on the dried basis).

Indigotindisulfonate Sodium Injection USP—Preserve in single-dose, light-resistant containers, preferably of Type I glass. A sterile solution of Indigotindisulfonate Sodium in Water for Injection. Contains the labeled amount, within −10% to +5%. Meets the requirements for Identification, Bacterial endotoxins, and pH (3.0–6.5), and for Injections.

INDINAVIR

Chemical name: Indinavir sulfate—D-*erythro*-Pentonamide, 2,3,5-trideoxy-*N*-(2,3-dihydro-2-hydroxy-1*H*-inden-1-yl)-5-[2-[[(1,1-dimethylethyl)amino]carbonyl]-4-(3-pyridinylmethyl)-1-piperazinyl]-2-(phenylmethyl)-, [1(1*S*,2*R*,5(*S*))]-, sulfate (1:1) (salt).

Molecular formula: Indinavir sulfate—$C_{36}H_{47}N_5O_4 \cdot H_2SO_4$.

Molecular weight: Indinavir sulfate—711.87.

Description: Indinavir sulfate—White to off-white, hygroscopic, crystalline powder.

Solubility: Indinavir sulfate—Very soluble in water and in methanol.

USP requirements: Indinavir Sulfate Capsules—Not in *USP–NF*.

INDIUM IN 111 CAPROMAB PENDETIDE

USP requirements:

Indium In 111 Capromab Pendetide Injection USP—Preserve in adequately shielded single-dose containers at controlled room temperature for not more than 8 hours. A sterile, nonpyrogenic, murine monoclonal antibody, 7E11-C

5.3, (CYT-351), an immunoconjugate prepared by specific modification of the carbohydrate groups and covalent binding to the tripeptide linker chelator, glycyltyrosyl-(*N*, *E*-diethylenetriaminepentaacetic acid)-lysine hydrochloride that is complexed with ¹¹¹In. Label it to include the following in addition to the information specified for Labeling under Injections: the time and date of calibration; the amount of ¹¹¹In capromab pendetide as total megabecquerel (or millicurie) and concentration of megabecquerel (or millicurie) per mL, at the time of calibration; the expiration date and time; and the storage temperature and the statement, "Caution—Radioactive Material" The labeling indicates that, in making dosage calculations, correction is to be made for radioactive decay, and also indicates that the radioactive half-life of ¹¹¹In is 67.2 hours. Contains the specified amount of ¹¹¹In capromab pendetide, expressed in megabecquerels (or millicuries) per mL, within ±10%, at the time indicated in the labeling. Other chemical forms of radioactivity do not exceed 10.0% of the total radioactivity. Immediately prior to use, the radiolabeling is performed with Indium In 111 Chloride Solution in the presence of a sodium acetate buffer. Contains sodium chloride and buffering agents as stabilizers. The immunoreactive fraction, determined by a validated method, is not less than 70%. The monomer content is not less than 95% determined by a validated electrophoretic mobility method. Meets the requirements for Bacterial endotoxins, pH (5.0–7.0), and Radiochemical purity, and for Radionuclide identification and Radionuclidic purity under Indium In 111 Chloride Solution, and for Injections (except that the radioactive component may be distributed or dispensed prior to completion of the test for Sterility, the latter test being started on the date of manufacture).

Indium In 111 Capromab Pendetide Solution—Not in *USP–NF*.

INDIUM IN 111 CHLORIDE

Chemical name: Indium Chloride (¹¹¹InCl₃).

USP requirements: Indium In 111 Chloride Solution USP—Preserve in single-unit containers at controlled room temperature. A sterile, nonpyrogenic solution of radioactive indium (¹¹¹In) in dilute hydrochloric acid suitable for the radiolabeling of proteins such as monoclonal antibodies, peptides, or small biologically active organic molecules. The concentration of acid and ¹¹¹In per mL of Indium In 111 Chloride Solution may require adjustment for the specific antibody or peptide being labeled. Label it to include the following, in addition to the information specified for Labeling under Injections: the time and date of calibration; the amount of ¹¹¹In as labeled chloride expressed as total megabecquerels (or millicuries) and the concentration as megabecquerels per mL (or as millicuries per mL) on the date and time of calibration; the expiration date; the statement "Not for direct administration. Use only as an ingredient for radiolabeling;" and the statement "Caution—Radioactive Material." The labeling indicates that in making dosage calculations, correction is to be made for radioactive decay, and also indicates that the radioactive half-life of ¹¹¹In is 67.3 hours. Other chemical forms of radioactivity do not exceed 10.0% of the total radioactivity. (Note: Indium In 111 Chloride Solution is generally recommended for use with specific antibodies or peptides. Consult the product labeling for recommendations and applications for radiolabeling.) Contains the labeled amount of ¹¹¹In expressed as megabecquerels (or millicuries) per mL, within ±10%, at the time indicated in the labeling. Meets the requirements for Specific activity (not less than 1.85 gigabecquerels [50 millicuries] per microgram of indium at the date and time of calibration), Identification, Bacterial endotoxins, Acidity, Radionuclide identification, Radionuclidic purity, Radiochemical purity, and Chemical pur-

ity, and for Injections (except that the Solution may be distributed or dispensed prior to completion of the test for Sterility, the latter test being started on the day of final manufacture, and except that it is not subject to the recommendation of Volume in Container).

INDIUM IN 111 OXYQUINOLINE

Source: Saturated (1:3) complex of indium and oxyquinoline (oxine), a chelating agent.

Chemical name: Indium-¹¹¹*In*, tris(8-quinolinolato-*N'*,*O*⁸)-.

Molecular formula: C₂₇H₁₈¹¹¹InN₃O₃.

Molecular weight: 543.45.

USP requirements: Indium In 111 Oxyquinoline Solution USP—Preserve in single-unit containers at a temperature between 15 and 25 °C. A sterile, nonpyrogenic, isotonic aqueous solution suitable for the radiolabeling of blood cells, especially leukocytes and platelets, containing radioactive indium (¹¹¹In) in the form of a complex with 8-hydroxyquinoline, the latter being present in excess. Label it to contain the following, in addition to the information specified for Labeling under Injections: the time and date of calibration; the amount of ¹¹¹In as the 8-hydroxyquinoline complex expressed as total megabecquerels (or millicuries) and concentration as megabecquerels (or millicuries) per mL on the date and time of calibration; the expiration date; the statement, "Not for direct administration. Use only for radiolabeling of leukocytes in vitro. Administer radiolabeled cells subsequently by intravenous injection;" and the statement, "Caution—Radioactive Material." The labeling indicates that in making dosage calculations, correction is to be made for radioactive decay, and also indicates that the radioactive half-life of ¹¹¹In is 67.9 hours. Contains the labeled amount of ¹¹¹In, within ±10%, as the 8-hydroxyquinoline complex expressed as megabecquerels (or millicuries) per mL at the time indicated in the labeling. Other chemical forms of radioactivity do not exceed 10.0% of the total radioactivity. Meets the requirements for Specific activity (not less than 1.85 gigabecquerels [50 millicuries] per mcg of indium), Pyrogen, pH (6.5–7.5), Radionuclide identification, Radiochemical purity, and Radionuclidic purity.

INDIUM IN 111 PENTETATE

USP requirements: Indium In 111 Pentetate Injection USP—Preserve in single-dose containers. A sterile, isotonic solution suitable for intrathecal administration, containing radioactive indium (¹¹¹In) in the form of a chelate of pentetic acid. Label it to include the following, in addition to the information specified for Labeling under Injections: the time and date of calibration; the amount of ¹¹¹In as labeled pentetic acid complex expressed as total megabecquerels (or millicuries or microcuries) and concentration as megabecquerels (or microcuries or millicuries) per mL on the date and time of calibration; the expiration date; and the statement, "Caution—Radioactive Material." The labeling indicates that in making dosage calculations, correction is to be made for radioactive decay, and also indicates that the radioactive half-life of ¹¹¹In is 2.83 days. Contains the labeled amount of ¹¹¹In, within ±10%, as pentetic acid complex expressed in megabecquerels (or microcuries or millicuries) per mL at the time indicated in the labeling. Other chemical forms of radioactivity do not exceed 10.0% of the total radioactivity. Meets the requirements for Bacterial endotoxins, pH (7.0–8.0), Radionuclide identification, Radiochemical purity (not less than 90.0%), and Radionuclidic purity, and for Injections (except that the Injection may be distributed or dispensed prior to completion of the test for

Sterility, the latter test being started on the day of final manufacture, and except that it is not subject to the recommendation on Volume in Container).

INDIUM IN 111 PENTETREOTIDE

Chemical name: Indate (1−)-^{111}In, [N-[2-[[2-[bis(carboxymethyl)amino]ethyl](carboxymethyl)amino]ethyl]-N-(carboxymethyl)glycyl-D-phenylalanyl-L-cysteinyl-L-phenylalanyl-Dtryptophyl-L-lysyl-L-threonyl-N-[2-hydroxy-1-(hydroxymethyl)propyl]-L-cysteinamide cyclic (3→8)-disulfidato(4−)], hydrogen, stereoisomer.

Molecular formula: $C_{63}H_{84}{}^{111}InN_{13}O_{19}S_2$.

USP requirements: Indium In 111 Pentetreotide Injection USP—Preserve in single-dose containers. A sterile solution, suitable for intravenous administration, containing radioactive indium (^{111}In) in the form of a chelate of pentetreotide. Label it to include the following, in addition to the information specified for Labeling under Injections: the time and date of calibration; the amount of ^{111}In as labeled pentetreotide complex expressed as total megabecquerels (or millicuries) and the concentration as megabecquerels (or millicuries) per mL on the date and time of calibration; the expiration date; and the statement, "Caution—Radioactive Material." The labeling indicates that in making dosage calculations, correction is to be made for radioactive decay, and states that the radioactive half-life of ^{111}In is 67.3 hours. Contains the labeled amount of ^{111}In, within ±10%, as the pentetreotide complex expressed in megabecquerels (or in millicuries) per mL at the time indicated in the labeling. Other forms of radioactivity do not exceed 10.0% of the total radioactivity. Meets the requirements for Radionuclide identification, Bacterial endotoxins, pH (3.8–4.3), Radiochemical purity, and Radionuclidic purity, and for Injections (except that the Injection may be distributed or dispensed prior to the completion of the test for Sterility, the latter test being started on the day of final manufacture, and except that it is not subject to the recommendation on Volume in Container).

INDIUM IN 111 SATUMOMAB PENDETIDE

Source: The monoclonal antibody B72.3 is site-specifically labeled with ^{111}In using the linker-chelator glycyl-tyrosyl-(N,epsilon-diethylenetriaminepentaacetic acid)-lysine (GYK-DTPA). This involves conjugating B72.3 with a linker-chelator complex at oxidized carbohydrate sites on the constant region of the antibody.

Chemical name: Immunoglobulin G 1 (mouse monoclonal B72.3 anti-human glycoprotein TAG-72), disulfide with mouse monoclonal B72.3 light chain, dimer, N^6-[N-[2-[[2-[bis(carboxymethyl)amino]ethyl](carboxymethyl)amino]ethyl]-N-(carboxymethyl)glycyl]-N^2-(N-glycyl-L-tyrosyl)-L-lysine conjugate, indium-^{111}In chelate.

USP requirements: Indium In 111 Satumomab Pendetide Injection USP—Preserve in adequately shielded single-dose containers, at controlled room temperature. A sterile, nonpyrogenic, virus-free preparation of monoclonal antibody B72.3 that is labeled with ^{111}In. Satumomab pendetide is prepared by site-specific conjugation of the linker-chelator, glycyl-tyrosyl-(N,E-diethylene triamine pentaacetic acid)-lysine hydrochloride to the oxidized oligosaccharide component of the monoclonal antibody B72.3. Satumomab pendetide is radiolabeled by the addition of a sterile, nonpyrogenic solution of a buffered Indium In 111 Chloride solution. [Note: Other chemical forms of indium are not to be used in the radiolabeling.] May contain buffers and stabilizers. Label it to include the following, in addition to the information specified for Labeling under Injections: the time and date of calibration; the amount of ^{111}In as labeled satumomab pendetide expressed as total megabecquerels (or millicuries) and concentration as megabecquerels (or millicuries) per mL at the time of calibration; the expiration date; and the statement, "Caution—Radioactive Material." The labeling indicates that, in making dosage calculations, correction is to be made for radioactive decay and also indicates that the radioactive half-life of ^{111}In is 67.3 hours. Contains the labeled amount of ^{111}In as labeled satumomab pendetide expressed in megabecquerels (or in millicuries) per mL, within ± 10%, at the time indicated in the labeling. Other chemical forms of radioactivity do not exceed 10.0% of the total radioactivity. The immunoreactive fraction, as determined by a validated method, is not less than 60%. Meets the requirements for Bacterial endotoxins, pH (5.5–6.5), and Radiochemical purity, for Radionuclide identification and Radionuclidic purity under Indium In 111 Chloride Solution, and for Injections (except that it may be distributed or dispensed prior to completion of the test for Sterility, the latter test being started on the day of final manufacture, and except that it is not subject to the recommendation on Volume in Container).

INDOCYANINE GREEN

Chemical name: 1H-Benz[e]indolium, 2-[7-[1,3-dihydro-1,1-dimethyl-3-(4-sulfobutyl)-2H-benz[e]indol-2-ylidene]-1,3,5-heptatrienyl]-1,1-dimethyl-3-(4-sulfobutyl)-, hydroxide, inner salt, sodium salt.

Molecular formula: $C_{43}H_{47}N_2NaO_6S_2$.

Molecular weight: 774.96.

Description:
Indocyanine Green USP—Olive-brown, dark green, blue-green, dark blue, or black powder. Odorless, or has a slight odor. Its solutions are deep emerald-green in color. The pH of a solution (1 in 200) is about 6. Its aqueous solutions are stable for about 8 hours.

Solubility: Indocyanine Green USP—Soluble in water and in methanol; practically insoluble in most other organic solvents.

USP requirements:
Indocyanine Green USP—Preserve in well-closed containers. Where it is intended for use in preparing injectable dosage forms, the label states that it is sterile or must be subjected to further processing during the preparation of injectable dosage forms. Contains not less than 94.0% and not more than 105.0% of indocyanine green, calculated on the dried basis. Contains not more than 5.0% of sodium iodide, calculated on the dried basis. Meets the requirements for Identification, Loss on drying (not more than 6.0%), Arsenic (not more than 8 ppm), Lead (not more than 0.001%), and Sodium iodide (not more than 5.0%, calculated on the dried basis), and for Sterility tests and for Bacterial endotoxins under Indocyanine Green for Injection (where the label states that Indocyanine Green is sterile), and for Bacterial endotoxins under Indocyanine Green for Injection (where the label states that Indocyanine Green must be subjected to further processing during the preparation of injectable dosage forms).
Indocyanine Green for Injection USP—Preserve in Containers for Sterile Solids. Contains the labeled amount, within ± 10%. Meets the requirements for Constituted solutions, Bacterial endotoxins, pH (5.5–7.5, in a solution [1 in

200]), and Content variation, for Identification tests, Arsenic, Lead, and Sodium iodide under Indocyanine Green, for Sterility tests, and for Labeling under Injections.

INDOMETHACIN

Chemical group: An indoleacetic acid derivative structurally related to the pyrroleacetic acid derivative sulindac.

Chemical name:
Indomethacin—1*H*-Indole-3-acetic acid, 1-(4-chlorobenzoyl)-5-methoxy-2-methyl-.
Indomethacin sodium—1*H*-Indole-3-acetic acid, 1-(4-chlorobenzoyl)-5-methoxy-2-methyl-, sodium salt, trihydrate.

Molecular formula:
Indomethacin—$C_{19}H_{16}ClNO_4$.
Indomethacin sodium (trihydrate)—$C_{19}H_{15}ClNNaO_4 \cdot 3H_2O$.

Molecular weight:
Indomethacin—357.79.
Indomethacin sodium (trihydrate)—433.82.

Description: Indomethacin USP—Pale yellow to yellow-tan, crystalline powder, having not more than a slight odor. Is sensitive to light. Melts at about 162 °C. Exhibits polymorphism.

pKa: 4.5.

Solubility: Indomethacin USP—Practically insoluble in water; sparingly soluble in alcohol, in chloroform, and in ether.

USP requirements:
Indomethacin USP—Preserve in well-closed, light-resistant containers. Contains not less than 98.0% and not more than 101.0% of indomethacin, calculated on the dried basis. Meets the requirements for Identification, Loss on drying (not more than 0.5%), Residue on ignition (not more than 0.2%), Heavy metals (not more than 0.002%), and Organic volatile impurities.
Indomethacin Capsules USP—Preserve in well-closed containers. Contain the labeled amount, within ±10%. Meet the requirements for Identification, Dissolution (80% in 20 minutes in 1 volume of phosphate buffer [pH 7.2] mixed with 4 volumes of water in Apparatus 1 at 100 rpm), and Uniformity of dosage units.
Indomethacin Extended-release Capsules USP—Preserve in well-closed containers. The labeling indicates the Drug Release test with which the product complies. Contain the labeled amount, within ±10%. Meet the requirements for Identification, Drug release (10–25% in 1 hour, 20–40% in 2 hours, 35–55% in 4 hours, 45–65% in 6 hours, 60–80% in 12 hours, and not less than 80% in 24 hours in phosphate buffer [pH 6.2] in Apparatus 1 at 75 rpm for Test 1; 12–32% in 1 hour, 27–52% in 2 hours, 50–80% in 4 hours, and not less than 80% in 12 hours in phosphate buffer [pH 6.2] in Apparatus 1 at 75 rpm for Test 2; and 15–40% in 1 hour, 35–55% in 2 hours, 55–75% in 4 hours, 65–85% in 6 hours, not less than 75% in 12 hours, and not less than 85% in 24 hours in phosphate buffer [pH 6.8] in Apparatus 1 at 75 rpm for Test 3), Uniformity of dosage units, and Limit of 4-chlorobenzoic acid (not more than 0.44%).
Indomethacin for Injection USP—Preserve in Containers for Sterile Solids. Contains the equivalent of the labeled amount of indomethacin, within ±10%. Meets the requirements for Constituted solution, Identification, Bacterial endotoxins, pH (6.0–7.5, in a 1 in 2000 solution), Particulate matter, and Limit of 4-chlorobenzoic acid, and for Sterility tests, Uniformity of dosage units, and Labeling under Injections.
Indomethacin Suppositories USP—Preserve in well-closed containers, at controlled room temperature. Contain the labeled amount, within ±10%. Meet the requirements for

Identification, Dissolution (75% in 60 minutes in 0.1 *M* phosphate buffer [pH 7.2] in Apparatus 2 at 50 rpm), and Uniformity of dosage units.
Indomethacin Ophthalmic Suspension—Not in *USP–NF*.
Indomethacin Oral Suspension USP—Preserve in tight, light-resistant containers. Contains the labeled amount, within ±10%. Meets the requirements for Identification, Dissolution (80% in 20 minutes in 0.01 *M* phosphate buffer [pH 7.2] in Apparatus 2 at 50 rpm), pH (2.5–5.0), Limit of 4-chlorobenzoic acid (not more than 0.44%), and Sorbic acid content (where present, within ±20% of labeled amount).
Indomethacin Sodium USP—Preserve in well-closed, light-resistant containers. Where it is intended for use in preparing injectable dosage forms, the label states that it is sterile or must be subjected to further processing during the preparation of injectable dosage forms. Contains not less than 98.0% and not more than 101.0% of indomethacin sodium, calculated on the dried basis. Meets the requirements for Identification, Loss on drying (11.5–13.5%), Heavy metals (0.002%), Limit of acetone (not more than 0.1%), and Chromatographic purity, and for Sterility tests and for Pyrogen under Indomethacin for Injection (where the label states that Indomethacin Sodium is sterile), and for Pyrogen under Indomethacin for Injection (where the label states that Indomethacin Sodium must be subjected to further processing during the preparation of injectable dosage forms).

INFANT FORMULAS

USP requirements:
Hypoallergenic Infant Formula Oral Concentrate—Not in *USP–NF*.
Hypoallergenic Infant Formula Oral Solution—Not in *USP–NF*.
Hypoallergenic Infant Formula for Oral Solution—Not in *USP–NF*.
Milk-based Infant Formula Oral Concentrate—Not in *USP–NF*.
Milk-based Infant Formula Oral Powder—Not in *USP–NF*.
Milk-based Infant Formula Oral Solution—Not in *USP–NF*.
Milk-based Infant Formula for Oral Solution—Not in *USP–NF*.
Soy-based Infant Formula Oral Concentrate—Not in *USP–NF*.
Soy-based Infant Formula Oral Solution—Not in *USP–NF*.
Soy-based Infant Formula for Oral Solution—Not in *USP–NF*.

INFLIXIMAB

Source: A chimeric human-murine immunoglobulin (IgG1—$_{kappa}$) monoclonal antibody composed of human constant and murine variable regions.

Molecular weight: Approximately 149,100 daltons.

Description: A sterile, white, lyophilized powder.

USP requirements: Infliximab for Injection—Not in *USP–NF*.

INFLUENZA VIRUS VACCINE

Source: Influenza vaccine is available as either a whole-virus or split-virus preparation. The vaccine is prepared from highly purified, egg-grown influenza viruses that have been inactivated to yield a whole-virus preparation. The split-virus vaccine is produced by chemically treating a whole-virus

preparation to cause inactivation and disruption of a significant proportion of the virus into smaller subunit particles called subvirions. The preparation is then refined to remove the unwanted substances.

Description: Influenza Virus Vaccine USP—Slightly turbid liquid or suspension, which may have a slight yellow or reddish tinge and may have an odor because of the preservative.
Note: The Canadian product is more likely to be bluish.

Other characteristics: The viral antigen content of both the whole-virus vaccine and the split-virus vaccine has been standardized by immunodiffusion tests, according to current U.S. Public Health Service requirements. Each 0.5 mL dose contains the proportions and not less than the microgram amounts of hemagglutinin antigens (mcg HA) representative of the specific components recommended for the present year?s vaccine.

USP requirements: Influenza Virus Vaccine USP—Preserve at a temperature between 2 and 8 °C. A sterile, aqueous suspension of suitably inactivated influenza virus types A and B, either individually or combined, or virus sub-units prepared from the extra-embryonic fluid of influenza virus–infected chicken embryo. Label it to state that it is to be shaken before use and that it is not to be frozen. Label it also to state that it was prepared in embryonated chicken eggs. The strains of influenza virus used in the preparation of this Vaccine are those designated by the U.S. Government?s Expert Committee on Influenza and recommended by the Surgeon General of the U.S. Public Health Service. Influenza Virus Vaccine has a composition of such strains and a content of virus antigen of each, designated for the particular season, of not less than the specified weight (in micrograms) of influenza virus hemagglutinin determined in specific radial-immunodiffusion tests relative to the U.S. Reference Influenza Virus Vaccine. If formalin is used for inactivation, contains not more than 0.02% of residual free formaldehyde. Meets the requirements for Expiration date (not later than 18 months after date of issue from manufacturer's cold storage [5 °C, 1 year]). Conforms to the regulations of the U.S. Food and Drug Administration concerning biologics.

INSULIN

Source: Insuline glargine—Analog of human insulin created by replacing the amino acid at position 21 of the A-chain (asparagine) with glycine and by adding two arginines to the C-terminus of the B-chain. Synthesized by recombinant DNA process involving a genetically engineered *Escherichia coli*.

Chemical name:
Insulin—Insulin (ox), 8^A-L-threonine-10^A-L-isoleucine-.
Insulin aspart—28^B-L-Aspartic acid-insulin (human).
Insulin glargine—21^A-Glycine-30^Ba-L-arginine-30^Bb-L-arginine insulin (human).
Insulin lispro—Insulin (human), 28^B-L-lysine-29^B-L-proline-.
Insulin zinc—Insulin zinc.

Molecular formula:
Insulin—$C_{256}H_{381}N_{65}O_{76}S_6$ (pork); $C_{254}H_{377}N_{65}O_{75}S_6$ (beef).
Insulin aspart—$C_{256}H_{381}N_{65}O_{79}S_6$.
Insulin glargine—$C_{267}H_{404}N_{72}O_{78}S_6$.
Insulin human—$C_{257}H_{383}N_{65}O_{77}S_6$.
Insulin lispro—$C_{257}H_{383}N_{65}O_{77}S_6$.

Molecular weight:
Insulin—5777.55 (pork); 5733.50 (beef).
Insulin aspart—5825.55.
Insulin glargine—6062.90.
Insulin human—5807.58.
Insulin lispro—5807.58.

Description:
Insulin USP—White or practically white crystals.
Insulin Injection USP—The Injection containing, in each mL, not more than 100 USP Units is a clear, colorless or almost colorless liquid; the Injection containing, in each mL, 500 Units may be straw-colored. Contains between 0.1% and 0.25% (w/v) of either phenol or cresol. Contains between 1.4% and 1.8% (w/v) of glycerin.
Insulin Lispro USP—White or practically white crystal.
Insulin Zinc Suspension USP—Practically colorless suspension of a mixture of characteristic crystals predominantly between 10 micrometers and 40 micrometers in maximum dimension and many particles that have no uniform shape and do not exceed 2 micrometers in maximum dimension. Contains between 0.15% and 0.17% (w/v) of sodium acetate, between 0.65% and 0.75% (w/v) of sodium chloride, and between 0.09% and 0.11% (w/v) of methylparaben.
Extended Insulin Zinc Suspension USP—Practically colorless suspension of a mixture of characteristic crystals the maximum dimension of which is predominantly between 10 micrometers and 40 micrometers. Contains between 0.15% and 0.17% (w/v) of sodium acetate, between 0.65% and 0.75% (w/v) of sodium chloride, and between 0.09% and 0.11% (w/v) of methylparaben.
Isophane Insulin Suspension USP—White suspension of rod-shaped crystals, free from large aggregates of crystals following moderate agitation. Contains either (1) between 1.4% and 1.8% (w/v) of glycerin, between 0.15% and 0.17% (w/v) of metacresol, and between 0.06% and 0.07% (w/v) of phenol, or (2) between 1.4% and 1.8% (w/v) of glycerin and between 0.20% and 0.25% (w/v) of phenol. Contains between 0.15% and 0.25% (w/v) of dibasic sodium phosphate. When examined microscopically, the insoluble matter in the Suspension is crystalline, and contains not more than traces of amorphous material.
Prompt Insulin Zinc Suspension USP—Practically colorless suspension of particles that have no uniform shape and the maximum dimension of which does not exceed 2 micrometers. Contains between 0.15% and 0.17% (w/v) of sodium acetate, between 0.65% and 0.75% (w/v) of sodium chloride, and between 0.09% and 0.11% (w/v) of methylparaben.

Solubility:
Insulin USP—Soluble in solutions of dilute acids and alkalies.
Insulin Lispro USP—Soluble in solutions of dilute acids and alkalies.

Other characteristics: Insuline glargine—pH: 4.

USP requirements:
Insulin USP—Preserve in tight containers. Store, protected from light, in a freezer. A protein that affects the metabolism of glucose. It is obtained from the pancreas of healthy bovines or porcine animals, or both, used for food by humans. Label it to indicate the one or more animal species to which it is related, as pork, as beef, or as a mixture of pork and beef. If the Insulin is purified, label it as such. Its potency, calculated on the dried basis, is not less than 26.5 USP Insulin Units in each mg; Insulin labeled as purified contains not less than 27.0 USP Insulin Units in each mg, calculated on the dried basis. The proinsulin content, determined by a validated method, is not more than 10 ppm. Meets the requirements for Identification, Bioidentity, Microbial limits, Bacterial endotoxins, Loss on drying (not more than 10.0%), Zinc content (not more than 1.0%, calculated on the dried basis), Related compounds, and Limit of high molecular weight proteins (not more than 1.0%).

Note—One USP Insulin Unit is equivalent to 0.0342 mg of pure Insulin derived from beef or 0.0345 mg of pure Insulin derived from pork.

Insulin Injection USP—Preserve in the unopened multiple-dose container provided by the manufacturer. Do not repackage. Store in a refrigerator, protect from sunlight, and avoid freezing.An isotonic, sterile solution of Insulin.

Label it to indicate the one or more animal species to which it is related, as pork, as beef, or as a mixture of pork and beef. If the Insulin Injection is made from Insulin that is purified, label it as such. Label it to state that it is to be stored in a refrigerator and that freezing is to be avoided. The label states the potency in USP Insulin Units per mL. Has a potency of ±5% of the potency stated on the label, expressed in USP Insulin Units. Meets the requirements for Identification, Bacterial endotoxins, Sterility, pH (7.0–7.8, determined potentiometrically), Particulate matter, Zinc content (10–40 mcg for each 100 USP Insulin Units of appropriate species), and Limit of high molecular weight proteins (not more than 2.0%), and for Injections.

Insulin Aspart Injection—Not in *USP–NF*.

Insulin Glargine Injection—Not in *USP–NF*.

Insulin Human USP—Preserve in tight containers. Store in a freezer, and protect from light. A protein corresponding to the active principle elaborated in the human pancreas that affects the metabolism of carbohydrate (particularly glucose), fat, and protein. Derived by enzymatic modification of insulin from pork pancreas in order to change its amino acid sequence appropriately, or produced by microbial synthesis via a recombinant DNA process. Label it to indicate that it has been prepared by microbial synthesis or that it is derived by enzymatic modification of insulin from pork pancreas. Its potency, calculated on the dried basis, is not less than 27.5 USP Insulin Human Units in each mg. The proinsulin content of Insulin Human derived from pork, determined by a validated method, is not more than 10 ppm. The host cell derived proteins content of Insulin Human derived from a recombinant DNA process, determined by an appropriate and validated method, is not more than 10 ppm. The host cell or vector derived DNA content and limit of Insulin Human derived from a recombinant DNA process that utilizes eukaryotic host cells are determined by a validated method. Meets the requirements for Identification, Bioidentity, Microbial limits, Bacterial endotoxins, Loss on drying (not more than 10.0%), Related compounds, and Limit of high molecular weight proteins (not more than 1.0%), and for Zinc content under Insulin.

Note—One USP Insulin Human Unit is equivalent to 0.0347 mg of pure Insulin Human.

Insulin Human Injection USP—Preserve in a refrigerator. Protect from sunlight. Avoid freezing. Dispense it in the unopened, multiple-dose container in which it was placed by the manufacturer. An isotonic sterile solution of Insulin Human in Water for Injection. The labeling states that it has been prepared either with Insulin Human derived by enzyme modification of pork pancreas Insulin or with Insulin Human obtained from microbial synthesis, whichever is applicable. Label it to state that it is to be stored in a refrigerator and that freezing is to be avoided. The label states the potency in USP Insulin Human Units per mL. Has a potency of ±5% of the potency stated on the label, expressed in USP Insulin Human Units in each mL. Meets the requirements for Identification, Bacterial endotoxins, Sterility, and Particulate matter, and for Injections, and for pH, Zinc content, and Limit of high molecular weight proteins under Insulin Injection.

Buffered Insulin Human Injection—Not in *USP–NF*.

Isophane Insulin Suspension USP—Preserve in the unopened multiple-dose container provided by the manufacturer. Do not repackage. Store in a refrigerator, protect from sunlight, and avoid freezing. A sterile suspension of zinc-insulin crystals and Protamine Sulfate in buffered Water for Injection, combined in a manner such that the solid phase of the suspension consists of crystals composed of insulin, protamine, and zinc. The Protamine Sulfate is prepared from the sperm or from the mature testes of fish belonging to the genus *Oncorhynchus* Suckley, or *Salmo* Linn;aae (Fam. Salmonidae). Label it to indicate the one or more animal species to which it is related, as

porcine, as bovine, or as a mixture of porcine and bovine. Where it is purified, label it as such. The Suspension container label states that the Suspension is to be shaken carefully before use. The label states the potency in USP Insulin Units per mL. Label it to state that it is to be stored in a refrigerator and that freezing is to be avoided. Its potency, based on the sum of its insulin and desamido insulin components, is within ±5% of the potency stated on the label, expressed in USP Insulin Units per mL. Meets the requirements for Identification, Bacterial endotoxins, Sterility, pH (7.0–7.8, determined potentiometrically), Zinc content (0.01–0.04 mg for each 100 USP Insulin Units), Insulin in the supernatant (not more than 1.0 USP Insulin Unit per mL), and Limit of high molecular weight proteins (not more than 3.%).

Isophane Insulin Human Suspension USP—Preserve in the unopened multiple-dose container provided by the manufacturer. Do not repackage. Store in a refrigerator, protect from sunlight, and avoid freezing. A sterile suspension of zinc-insulin human crystals and Protamine Sulfate in buffered Water for Injection, combined in a manner such that the solid phase of the suspension consists of crystals composed of insulin human, protamine, and zinc. The Protamine Sulfate is prepared from the sperm or from the mature testes of fish belonging to the genus *Oncorhynchus* Suckley, or *Salmo* Linn;aae (Fam. Salmonidae). The Suspension container label states that the Suspension is to be shaken carefully before use. The labeling states also that it has been prepared with Insulin Human of semisynthetic origin (i.e., derived by enzyme modification of pork pancreas insulin) or with Insulin Human of recombinant DNA origin (i.e., obtained from microbial synthesis), whichever is applicable. Label it to state that it is to be stored in a refrigerator and that freezing is to be avoided. The label states the potency in USP Insulin Units per mL. Its potency, based on the sum of its insulin and desamido insulin components, as calculated in the *Assay*, is within ±5% of the potency stated on the label, expressed in USP Insulin Human Units in each mL. Meets the requirements for Identification, Bacterial endotoxins, Sterility, pH (7.0–7.5, determined potentiometrically), Zinc content (0.021–0.04 mg for each 100 USP Insulin Human Units), Insulin in the supernatant, and Limit of high molecular weight proteins (not more than 3.0%).

Isophane Insulin, Human, Suspension and Insulin Human Injection—Not in *USP–NF*.

Insulin Lispro USP—Preserve in tight containers, protected from light, and store in a freezer. It is identical in structure to Insulin Human, except that it has lysine and proline at positions 28 and 29, respectively, of chain B, whereas this sequence is reversed in Insulin Human. Produced by microbial synthesis via a recombinant DNA process. Label it to indicate that it has been prepared by microbial synthesis. Its potency is not less than 27.0 USP Insulin Lispro Units per mg, calculated on the dried basis. The proinsulin content of Insulin Lispro, determined by an appropriate and validated method, is not more than 10 ppm. The host cell-derived protein content, determined by an appropriate and validated method, is not more than 10 ppm. Meets the requirements for Identification, Bioidentity, Microbial limits, Bacterial endotoxins, Loss on drying (not more than 10.0%), Limit of high molecular weight proteins (not more than 0.25%), Related compounds, and Zinc content (0.30–0.60%, calculated on the dried basis).

Note—One USP Insulin Lispro Unit is equivalent to 0.0347 mg of pure Insulin Lispro.

Insulin Lispro Injection USP—Preserve in tight, multiple-dose containers, and store in a refrigerator. Avoid freezing. Protect from sunlight. Dispense it in the unopened, multiple-dose container provided by the manufacturer. It is an isotonic, sterile solution of Insulin Lispro in Water for Injection. The labeling states that it has been prepared with Insulin Lispro obtained from microbial synthesis. Label it to state

that it is to be stored in a refrigerator and that freezing is to be avoided. The label states the potency in USP Insulin Lispro Units per mL. Has a potency of not less than 95.0% and not more than 105.0% of the potency stated on the label, expressed as USP Insulin Lispro Units in each mL. Meets the requirements for Identification, Bacterial endotoxins, Sterility, pH (7.0–7.8), Particulate matter, Limit of high molecular weight proteins (not more than 1.50%), Related compounds, and Zinc content (14–35 mcg for each 100 USP Insulin Lispro Units), and the requirements under *Injections.*

Insulin Zinc Suspension USP—Preserve in the unopened multiple-dose container provided by the manufacturer. Do not repackage. Store in a refrigerator, protect from sunlight, and avoid freezing. A sterile suspension of Insulin in buffered Water for Injection, modified by the addition of a suitable zinc salt in a manner such that the solid phase of the suspension consists of a mixture of crystalline and amorphous insulin in a ratio of approximately 7 parts of crystals to 3 parts of amorphous material. Label it to indicate the one or more animal species to which it is related, as porcine, as bovine, or as a mixture of porcine and bovine. Where it is purified, label it as such. The Suspension container label states that the Suspension is to be shaken carefully before use. The label states the potency in USP Insulin Units per mL. Label it to state that it is to be stored in a refrigerator and that freezing is to be avoided. Its potency, based on the sum of its insulin and desamido insulin components, is within ±5% of the potency stated on the label, expressed in USP Insulin Units per mL. Meets the requirements for Identification, Bacterial endotoxins, pH (7.0–7.8, determined potentiometrically), Zinc content (0.12–0.25 mg for each 100 USP Insulin Units), Zinc in the supernatant (20–65%), Insulin not extracted by buffered acetone solution, and Limit of high molecular weight proteins (not more than 1.5%), and for Sterility and Insulin in the supernatant under Isophane Insulin Suspension.

Insulin Human Zinc Suspension USP—Preserve in the unopened multiple-dose container provided by the manufacturer. Do not repackage. Store in a refrigerator, protect from sunlight, and avoid freezing. A sterile suspension of Insulin Human in buffered Water for Injection, modified by the addition of a suitable zinc salt in a manner such that the solid phase of the Suspension consists of a mixture of crystalline and amorphous insulin in a ratio of approximately 7 parts of crystals to 3 parts of amorphous material. Label it to indicate that it has been prepared with Insulin Human of semisynthetic origin (i.e., derived by enzyme modification of pork pancreas insulin) or with Insulin Human of recombinant DNA origin (i.e., obtained from microbial synthesis), whichever is applicable. The Suspension container label states that the Suspension is to be shaken carefully before use. Label it to state that it is to be stored in a refrigerator and that freezing is to be avoided. The label states the potency in USP Insulin Human Units per mL. Its potency, based on the sum of its insulin and desamido insulin components as calculated in the *Assay* is within ± 5% of the potency stated on the label, expressed in USP Insulin Human Units in each mL. Meets the requirements for Bacterial endotoxins, pH (7.0–7.8, determined potentiometrically), Insulin activity in supernatant liquid, and Limit of high molecular weight proteins (not more than 1.5%), and for Identification, Sterility, and Insulin in the supernatant under Isophane Insulin Human Suspension and for Zinc content, Zinc in the supernatant, and Insulin not extracted by buffered acetone solution under Insulin Zinc Suspension.

Extended Insulin Zinc Suspension USP—Preserve in the unopened multiple-dose container provided by the manufacturer. Do not repackage. Store in a refrigerator, protect from sunlight, and avoid freezing. A sterile suspension of Insulin in buffered Water for Injection, modified by the addition of a suitable zinc salt in a manner such that the solid phase of the suspension is predominantly crystalline. La-

bel it to indicate the one or more animal species to which it is related, as porcine, as bovine, or as a mixture of porcine and bovine. When it is purified, label it as such. Its container label states that the Suspension is to be shaken carefully before use. The container label states the potency in USP Insulin Units per mL. Label it to state that it is to be stored in a refrigerator and that freezing is to be avoided. Its potency, based on the sum of its insulin and desamido insulin components, is within ±5% of the potency stated on the label, expressed in USP Insulin Units per mL. Meets the requirements for Identification, Bacterial endotoxins, pH (7.0–7.8, determined potentiometrically), Insulin not extracted by buffered acetone solution, and Limit of high molecular weight proteins (not more than 1.5%), and Sterility, Insulin in the supernatant under Isophane Insulin Suspension, and for Zinc content and Zinc in the supernatant under Insulin Zinc Suspension.

Extended Insulin Human Zinc Suspension USP—Preserve in the unopened multiple-dose container provided by the manufacturer. Do not repackage. Store in a refrigerator, protect from sunlight, and avoid freezing. A sterile suspension of Insulin Human in buffered Water for Injection, modified by the addition of a suitable zinc salt in a manner such that the solid phase of the Suspension is predominantly crystalline. Label it to indicate that it has been prepared with Insulin Human of semisynthetic origin (i.e., derived by enzyme modification of pork pancreas insulin) or with Insulin Human of recombinant DNA origin (i.e., obtained from microbial synthesis), whichever is applicable. The Suspension container label states that the Suspension is to be shaken carefully before use. Label it to state that it is to be stored in a refrigerator and that freezing is to be avoided. The label states the potency in USP Insulin Human Units per mL. Its potency, based on the sum of its insulin and desamido insulin components, is within ±5% of the potency stated on the label, expressed in USP Insulin Human Units per mL. Meets the requirements for Bacterial endotoxins, pH (7.0–7.8, determined potentiometrically), Limit of high molecular weight proteins (not more than 1.5%), and for Identification, Sterility, and Insulin in supernatant under Isophane Insulin Human Suspension and for Zinc content, Zinc in the supernatant, and Insulin not extracted by buffered acetone solution under Insulin Zinc Suspension.

Prompt Insulin Zinc Suspension USP—Preserve in the unopened multiple-dose container provided by the manufacturer. Do not repackage. Store in a refrigerator, protect from sunlight, and avoid freezing. A sterile suspension of Insulin in buffered Water for Injection, modified by the addition of a suitable zinc salt in a manner such that the solid phase of the suspension is amorphous. Label it to indicate the one or more animal species to which it is related, as porcine, as bovine, or as a mixture of porcine and bovine. Where it is purified, label it as such. Its container label states that the Suspension is to be shaken carefully before use. The label states the potency in USP Insulin Units per mL. Label it to state that it is to be stored in a refrigerator and that freezing is to be avoided. Its potency, based on the sum of its insulin and desamido insulin components, is within ±5% of the potency stated on the label, expressed in USP Insulin Units per mL. Meets the requirements for Identification, Bacterial endotoxins, pH (7.0–7.8, determined potentiometrically), Insulin not extracted by buffered acetone solution (no crystalline residue remains), and Limit of high molecular weight proteins (not more than 1.5%), and Sterility, Insulin in the supernatant under Isophane Insulin Suspension, for Zinc content, and Zinc in the supernatant under Insulin Zinc Suspension.

INTERFERON ALFA

Source:

    Interferon Alfa-2a, recombinant—Synthetic. A protein chain of 165 amino acids produced by a recombinant DNA process involving genetically engineered *Escherichia coli*. Recombinant interferon alfa-2a has a lysine group at position 23. Purification procedure for recombinant interferon alfa-2a includes affinity chromatography using a murine monoclonal antibody.

    Interferon Alfa-2b, recombinant—Synthetic. A protein chain of 165 amino acids produced by a recombinant DNA process involving genetically engineered *Escherichia coli*. Recombinant interferon alfa-2b has an arginine group at position 23. Purification of recombinant interferon alfa-2b is done by proprietary methods.

    Interferon Alfa-n1 (lns)—A highly purified blend of natural human alpha interferons, obtained from human lymphoblastoid cells following induction with Sendai virus.

    Interferon Alfa-n3—A protein chain of approximately 166 amino acids. Manufactured from pooled units of human leukocytes that have been induced by incomplete infection with an avian virus (Sendai virus) to produce interferon alfa-n3. The manufacturing process includes immunoaffinity chromatography with a murine monoclonal antibody, acidification (pH 2) for 5 days at 4 °C, and gel filtration chromatography.

    Interferon alfacon-1—Synthetic. A protein chain of 166 amino acids produced by a recombinant DNA process involving genetically engineered *Escherichia coli*. The amino acid sequence was derived by comparison of the sequences of several natural interferon alpha subtypes and assigning the most frequently observed amino acid in each corresponding position. Four additional amino acid changes were made to facilitate molecular construction. Interferon alfacon-1 differs from interferon alfa-2 at 20/166 amino acids (88% homology), and is 30% identical to interferon beta, which is closer than any natural alpha interferon subtype.

    Following oxidation of recombinatant interferon alfacon-1 to its native state, the purification procedure includes sequential passage over a series of chromatograph columns.

Chemical group:

    Interferon alfa—Related to naturally occurring alfa interferons. Interferons are produced and secreted by cells in response to viral infections or various synthetic and biologic inducers; alfa interferons are produced mainly by leukocytes.

    Interferon alfacon-1—Type-I interferon, related to naturally occuring alpha and beta interferons.

Chemical name:

    Interferon Alfa-2a—Interferon alphaA (human leukocyte protein moiety reduced).

    Interferon Alfa-2b—Interferon alpha2b (human leukocyte clone Hif-SN206 protein moiety reduced).

    Interferon Alfa-n1—alpha-Interferons.

    Interferon Alfa-n3—Interferons, alpha-.

Molecular formula:

    Interferon Alfa-2a—$C_{860}H_{1353}N_{227}O_{255}S_9$.

    Interferon Alfa-2b—$C_{860}H_{1353}N_{229}O_{255}S_9$.

    Interferon Alfacon-1—$C_{870}H_{1366}N_{236}O_{259}S_9$.

Molecular weight:

    Interferon Alfa-2a—19,240.92.

    Interferon Alfa-2b—19,268.93.

    Interferon alfacon-1—19,564.18.

Solubility: Water-soluble.

Other characteristics: Interferon alfacon-1—pH: 7±0.2.

USP requirements:

    Interferon Alfa-2a, Recombinant, Injection—Not in *USP–NF*.

    Interferon Alfa-2a, Recombinant, for Injection—Not in *USP–NF*.

    Interferon Alfa-2b, Recombinant, for Injection—Not in *USP–NF*.

    Interferon Alfa-n1 (lns) Injection—Not in *USP–NF*.

    Interferon Alfa-n3 Injection—Not in *USP–NF*.

    Interferon Alfacon-1, Recombinant, Injection—Not in *USP–NF*.

INTERFERON BETA

Source:

    Interferon beta-1a—Produced from cultured Chinese Hamster ovary cells containing the engineered gene for human interferon beta.

    Interferon beta-1b—Manufactured by bacterial fermentation of a strain of *Escherichia coli* that bears a genetically engineered plasmid containing the gene for human interferon beta$_{ser17}$.

Chemical name:

    Interferon beta-1a—Interferon beta1 (human fibroblast protein moiety).

    Interferon beta-1b—2-166-Interferon beta1 (human fibroblast reduced), 17-L-serine-.

Molecular formula:

    Interferon beta-1a—$C_{908}H_{1406}N_{246}O_{252}S_7$.

    Interferon beta-1b—$C_{903}H_{1399}N_{245}O_{252}S_5$.

Molecular weight:

    Interferon beta-1a—20,024.85.

    Interferon beta-1b—19,879.60.

USP requirements:

    Interferon Beta-1a Injection—Not in *USP–NF*.

    Interferon Beta-1a for Injection—Not in *USP–NF*.

    Interferon Beta-1b for Injection—Not in *USP–NF*.

INTERFERON GAMMA

Chemical name: Interferon gamma-1b—1-139-Interferon gamma (human lymphocyte protein moiety reduced), N^2-L-methionyl-.

Molecular formula: Interferon gamma-1b—$C_{734}H_{1166}N_{204}O_{216}S_5$.

Molecular weight: Interferon gamma-1b—16,464.69.

Description: Interferon gamma-1b injection—Sterile, clear, colorless solution.

USP requirements: Interferon Gamma-1b, Recombinant, Injection—Not in *USP–NF*.

INULIN

Source: A polysaccharide obtained from the tubers of *Dahlia variabilis, Helianthus tuberosus,* and other genera of the family Compositae.

Chemical name: Inulin.

Molecular formula: $C_6H_{11}O_5(C_6H_{10}O_5)_nOH$.

Description: Inulin USP—White, friable, chalk-like, amorphous, odorless powder.

Solubility: Inulin USP—Soluble in hot water; slightly soluble in cold water and in organic solvents.

Other characteristics: Hygroscopic.

USP requirements:

Inulin USP—Preserve in well-closed containers. A polysaccharide which, on hydrolysis, yields mainly fructose. Contains not less than 94.0% and not more than 102.0% of inulin, calculated on the dried basis. Meets the requirements for Completeness of solution, Specific rotation (−32° to −40°), Microbial limits, Loss on drying (not more than 10.0%), Residue on ignition (not more than 0.05%), pH, Chloride, Sulfate, Iron, and Reducing sugars (4.5–7.0 for pH and not more than 0.014% for chloride), Calcium (not more than 0.10%), Heavy metals (not more than 5 ppm), Free fructose (not more than 2.0%, calculated on the dried basis), and Content of combined glucose (2.0–5.0%, calculated on the dried basis).

Inulin Injection—Not in *USP–NF*.

INULIN AND SODIUM CHLORIDE

For *Inulin* and *Sodium Chloride*—See individual listings for chemistry information.

USP requirements: Inulin in Sodium Chloride Injection USP—Preserve in single-dose containers, preferably of Type I or Type II glass. A sterile solution, which may be supersaturated, of Inulin and Sodium Chloride in Water for Injection. May require heating before use if crystallization has occurred. Contains the labeled amounts of inulin, within ±10%, and sodium chloride, within ±5%. Contains no antimicrobial agents. Meets the requirements for Clarity, Bacterial endotoxins, pH (4.0–7.0), and Free fructose (2.2 mg per mL), and for Injections.

IOBENGUANE I 123

Chemical name: [[3-(Iodo-^{123}I)-phenyl]methyl]guanidine sulfate (2:1).

Molecular formula: $(C_8H_{10}^{123}IN_3)_2 \cdot H_2SO_4$.

USP requirements: Iobenguane I 123 Injection USP—Preserve in single-dose or in multiple-dose containers that are adequately shielded. Store in a freezer. A sterile solution containing iobenguane sulfate in which a portion of the molecules contain radioactive iodine (^{123}I) in the molecular structure. Label it to include the following: the time and date of calibration; the amount of ^{123}I as iobenguane expressed as total megabecquerels (or millicuries) per mL at the time of calibration; the name and quantity of any added preservative or stabilizer; the expiration time; and the statement "Caution—Radioactive Material." The labeling indicates that in making dosage calculations, correction is to be made for radioactive decay, and also indicates that the radioactive half-life of ^{123}I is 13.2 hours. Contains the labeled amount of I 123 as iobenguane, within ±10%, expressed in megabecquerels (or in millicuries) per mL at the time indicated in the labeling. Contains the labeled amount of iobenguane, within ±10%. Meets the requirements for Radionuclidic identification, Bacterial endotoxins, pH (6.0–7.5), Radionuclidic purity, and Radiochemical purity, and for Injections (except that the Injection may be distributed or dispensed prior to the completion of the test for Sterility, the latter test being started on the day of final manufacture, and except that it is not subject to the recommendation on Volume in Container).

IOBENGUANE I 131

Chemical name: Iobenguane sulfate I 131—[[3-(Iodo-^{131}I)-phenyl]methyl]guanidine sulfate (2:1).

Molecular formula: Iobenguane sulfate I 131—$(C_8H_{10}^{131}IN_3)_2 \cdot H_2SO_4$.

USP requirements: Iobenguane I 131 Injection USP—Preserve in single-dose or in multiple-dose containers that are adequately shielded. Store in a freezer. A sterile solution containing iobenguane sulfate in which a portion of the molecules contain radioactive iodine (^{131}I) in the molecular structure. May contain preservatives or stabilizers. Label it to include the following: the date of calibration; the amount of ^{131}I as iobenguane sulfate expressed as total megabecquerels (or millicuries) per mL at the time of calibration; the name and quantity of any added preservative or stabilizer; the expiration date; and the statement, "Caution—Radioactive Material" The labeling indicates that, in making dosage calculations, correction is to be made for radioactive decay, and also indicates that the radioactive half-life of ^{131}I is 8.04 days. Contains the labeled amount of ^{131}I, within ± 10%, as iobenguane sulfate expressed in megabecquerels (or in millicuries) per mL at the time indicated in the labeling. Meets the requirements for Radionuclidic identification, Bacterial endotoxins, pH (4.5–7.5), Radionuclidic purity, and Radiochemical purity, and for Injections (except that the Injection may be distributed or dispensed prior to the completion of the test for Sterility, the latter test being started on the day of final manufacture, and except that it is not subject to the recommendation for Volume in Container).

IOCETAMIC ACID

Chemical group: Ionic, triiodinated benzoic acid derivative.

Chemical name: Propanoic acid, 3-[acetyl(3-amino-2,4,6-triiodophenyl)amino]-2-methyl-.

Molecular formula: $C_{12}H_{13}I_3N_2O_3$.

Molecular weight: 613.96.

Description: White to light cream-colored powder. Melting point 224–225 °C.

pKa: 4.10 and 4.25.

Solubility: Practically insoluble in water; very slightly soluble in ether and in ethanol; slightly soluble in acetone and in chloroform.

USP requirements:

Iocetamic Acid USP—Preserve in well-closed containers. Contains not less than 98.0% and not more than 102.0% of iocetamic acid, calculated on the dried basis. Meets the requirements for Identification, Loss on drying (not more than 1.0%), Residue on ignition (not more than 0.1%), Iodide (not more than 0.005%), and Heavy metals (not more than 0.002%).

Iocetamic Acid Tablets USP—Preserve in tight containers. Contain the labeled amount, within ±10%. Meet the requirements for Identification, Dissolution (35% in 30 minutes and 50% in 60 minutes in simulated intestinal fluid TS, prepared without pancreatin, in Apparatus 1 at 150 rpm), and Uniformity of dosage units.

IODINATED GLYCEROL

Chemical group: An isomeric mixture formed by the interaction of iodine and glycerol, the active ingredient thought to be iodopropylidene glycerol; contains about 50% of organically bound iodine.

Chemical name: 1,3-Dioxolane-4-methanol, 2-(1-iodoethyl)-.

Molecular formula: $C_6H_{11}IO_3$.

Molecular weight: 258.05.

Description: Viscous, amber liquid stable in acid media, including gastric juice, which contains virtually no inorganic iodide and no free iodine.

Solubility: Miscible with water, with alcohol, and with glycerin; soluble in ether, in chloroform, in isobutyl alcohol, in methyl acetate, in ethyl acetate, in methyl formate, and in tetrahydrofuran.

USP requirements:
Iodinated Glycerol Elixir—Not in *USP–NF.*
Iodinated Glycerol Oral Solution—Not in *USP–NF.*
Iodinated Glycerol Tablets—Not in *USP–NF.*

IODINATED I 125 ALBUMIN

Description: Iodinated I 125 Albumin Injection USP—Clear, colorless to slightly yellow solution. Upon standing, both the Albumin and the glass container may darken as a result of the effects of the radiation.

USP requirements: Iodinated I 125 Albumin Injection USP—Preserve in single-dose or in multiple-dose containers, at a temperature between 2 and 8 °C. A sterile, buffered, isotonic solution containing normal human albumin adjusted to provide not more than 37 megabecquerels (or 1 millicurie) of radioactivity per mL. Derived by mild iodination of normal human albumin with the use of radioactive iodine (^{125}I) to introduce not more than one gram-atom of iodine for each gram-molecule (60,000 grams) of albumin. Label it to include the following, in addition to the information specified for Labeling under Injections: the date of calibration; the amount of ^{125}I as iodinated albumin, expressed as total megabecquerels (or microcuries or millicuries), and concentration as megabecquerels (or microcuries or millicuries) per mL on the date of calibration; the expiration date; and the statement, "Caution—Radioactive Material" The labeling indicates that in making dosage calculations, correction is to be made for radioactive decay, and also indicates that the radioactive half-life of ^{125}I is 60 days. Contains the labeled amount of ^{125}I, within ±5%, as iodinated albumin, expressed in megabecquerels (or microcuries or millicuries) per mL at the time indicated in the labeling. Other forms of radioactivity do not exceed 3% of the total radioactivity. Its production and distribution are subject to federal regulations. Meets the requirements for Radionuclide identification, Bacterial endotoxins, pH (7.0–8.5), and Radiochemical purity, and for Biologics and Injections (except that it is not subject to the recommendation on Volume in Container and meets all other applicable requirements of the U.S. Food and Drug Administration).

IODIXANOL

Chemical name: 1,3-Benzenedicarboxamide, 5,5'-[(2-hydroxy-1,3-propanediyl)bis(acetylimino)]bis[*N,N*-bis(2,3-dihydroxypropyl)-2,4,6-triiodo-.

Molecular formula: $C_{35}H_{44}I_6N_6O_{15}$.

Molecular weight: 1550.18.

Description: Iodixanol USP—White to off-white amorphous, ordorless, hygroscopic powder.

Solubility: Iodixanol USP—Freely soluble in water.

USP requirements:
Iodixanol USP—Preserve in well-closed, light-resistant containers. Contains not less than 98.6% and not more than 101.0% of iodixanol, calculated on the anhydrous basis. Meets the requirements for Identificatioin, Specific rotation (−0.5° to +0.5°), Microbial limits (not more than 100 cfu per gram), Water (not more than 4.0%), Heavy metals (0.001%), Free iodine (the toluene layer shows no red or pink color), Limit of free iodine (not more than 10 milligrams of iodine per gram), Limit of free aromatic amine (not more than 0.05%), Limit of calcium (not more than 5 milligrams per gram), Limit of ionic compounds (not more than 0.02%), Limit of methanol, isopropyl alcohol, and methoxyethanol (not more than 50 milligrams per gram of each of methanol, isopropyl alcohol, and methoxyethanol), and Related compounds.
Iodixanol Injection USP—Preserve in single-dose containers of Type I glass, protected from light, or in plastic containers. A sterile solution of iodixanol in Water for Injection. Contains the labeled amount, within ±5%, as organically bound iodine. May contain stabilizers and buffers. Contains no antimicrobial agents. Meets the reequirements for Identification, Bacterial endotoxins, pH (6.8–7.7), Osmolarity (270–310 mOsmol per kg), Heavy metals (0.002%), Limit of free iodide (not more than 20 mg of iodide per gram), and Chromatographic purity, and the requirements under *Injections*.

IODOFORM

Chemical name: Triiodomethane.

Molecular formula: CHI_3.

Molecular weight: 393.85.

Description: Iodoform USP—Lustroush greenish yellow powder, or lustrous crystals. It is slightly volatile even at ordinary temperatures, and distills slowly with steam. Melts to a brown liquid at about 115 °C, and decomposes at a higher temperature, emitting vapors of iodine.

Solubility: Iodoform USP—Freely soluble in ether and in chloroform; soluble in boiling alcohol; sparingly soluble in alcohol, in glycerin, and in olive oil; practically insoluble in water.

USP requirements: Iodoform USP—Preserve in tight, light-resistant containers, store at controlled room temperature, and prevent exposure to excessive heat. Label it to indicate that it is intended for use in compounding dosage forms for topical, periodontal, nasal, and intracavitary use only. Iodoform, previously dried over silica gel for 24 hours, contains not more than 99.0% and not less than 100.5% of iodoform. Meets the requirements for Identification, Loss on drying (not more than 0.5%), Residue on ignition (not more than 0.1%), Coloring matter, acids, and alkalies, Chloride (not more than 0.011%), and Sulfate (not more than 0.017%).

IOTHALAMATE SODIUM I 125

Chemical name: Benzoic acid, 3-(acetylamino)diiodoiodo-^{125}I-5-[(methylamino)carbonyl]-, monosodium salt.

Molecular formula: $C_{11}H_8{}^{125}I_3N_2NaO_4$.

USP requirements: Iothalamate Sodium I 125 Injection USP—Preserve in single-dose or in multiple-dose containers that are adequately shielded. A sterile solution of Iothalamic Acid in Water for Injection prepared with the aid of Sodium Bicarbonate. A portion of the molecules contain radioactive iodine (^{125}I) in the molecular structure. Label it to include the following, in addition to the information specified for Labeling under Injections: the time and date of calibration; the amount of ^{125}I as iothalamate sodium expressed as total megabecquerels (or microcuries or millicuries equivalent) per mL at the time of calibration; the expiration date; and the statement "Caution—Radioactive Material." The labeling indicates that in making dosage calculations, correction is to be made for radioactive decay, and also indicates that the radioactive half-life of ^{125}I is 60 days. Contains the concentration of Iothalamate Sodium and the labeled amount of ^{125}I as Iothalamate Sodium, within ± 10%, expressed in kilobecquerels (or in microcuries) per mL at the time indicated in the labeling. Other chemical forms of radioactivity do not exceed 2.0% of the total radioactivity. Meets the requirements for Bacterial endotoxins, pH (7.0–8.5), Radionuclide identification, and Radiochemical purity, and for Injections (except that it is not subject to the recommendation in Volume in Container).

IODINATED I 131 ALBUMIN

Description:

Iodinated I 131 Albumin Injection USP—Clear, colorless to slightly yellow solution. Upon standing, both the albumin and the glass container may darken as a result of the effects of the radiation.

Iodinated I 131 Albumin Aggregated Injection USP—Dilute suspension of white to faintly yellow particles, which may settle on standing. The glass container may darken on standing, as a result of the effects of the radiation.

USP requirements:

Iodinated I 131 Albumin Injection USP—A sterile, buffered, isotonic solution containing normal human albumin adjusted to provide not more than 37 megabecquerels (1 millicurie) of radioactivity per mL. Derived by mild iodination of normal human albumin with the use of radioactive iodine (^{131}I) to introduce not more than one gram-atom of iodine for each gram-molecule (60,000 grams) of albumin. Label it to include the following, in addition to the information specified for Labeling under Injections: the date of calibration; the amount of ^{131}I as iodinated albumin expressed as total megabecquerels (or millicuries or microcuries), and concentration as megabecquerels (or millicuries or microcuries) per mL on the date of calibration; the expiration date; and the statement, "Caution—Radioactive Material." The labeling indicates that in making dosage calculations, correction is to be made for radioactive decay, and also indicates that the radioactive half-life of ^{131}I is 8.08 days. Contains the labeled amount of ^{131}I, within ±5%, as iodinated albumin, expressed in megabecquerels (or millicuries or microcuries) per mL at the time indicated in the labeling. Other forms of radioactivity do not exceed 3% of the total radioactivity. Its production and distribution are subject to federal regulations. Meets the requirements for Radionuclide identification, for Packaging and storage, Bacterial endotoxins, pH (7.0–8.5), and Radiochemical purity under Iodinated I 125 Albumin Injection USP, and for Biologics and Injections (except that it is not subject to the recommendation on Volume in Container and meets all other applicable requirements of the U.S. Food and Drug Administration).

Iodinated I 131 Albumin Aggregated Injection USP—Preserve in single-dose or in multiple-dose containers, at a temperature between 2 and 8 °C. A sterile aqueous suspension of Albumin Human that has been iodinated with ^{131}I and denatured to produce aggregates of controlled particle size. Label it to include the following, in addition to the information specified for Labeling under Injections: the time and date of calibration; the amount of ^{131}I as aggregated albumin expressed as total megabecquerels (or microcuries or millicuries) and as aggregated albumin in mg per mL on the date of calibration; the expiration date; and the statement, "Caution—Radioactive Material." The labeling indicates that in making dosage calculations, correction is to be made for radioactive decay, and also indicates that the radioactive half-life of ^{131}I is 8.08 days; in addition, the labeling states that it is not to be used if clumping of the albumin is observed and directs that the container be agitated before the contents are withdrawn into a syringe. Each mL of the suspension contains not less than 300 mcg and not more than 3.0 mg of aggregated albumin with a specific activity of not less than 7.4 megabecquerels (200 microcuries) per mg and not more than 44.4 megabecquerels (1.2 millicuries) per mg of aggregated albumin. Contains the labeled amount of ^{131}I, within ±5%, as aggregated albumin, expressed in megabecquerels (or microcuries) per mL or megabecquerels (or millicuries) per mL at the time indicated in the labeling. Other chemical forms of radioactivity do not exceed 6% of the total radioactivity. Its production and distribution are subject to federal regulations. Meets the requirements for Radionuclide identification and pH (5.0–6.0), for Biologics and Injections (except that it is not subject to the recommendation on Volume in Container), and for Particle size, Bacterial endotoxins, and Radiochemical purity under Technetium Tc 99m Albumin Aggregated Injection (except that in the test for Radiochemical purity, not more than 6% of the radioactivity is found in the supernaturant liquid following centrifugation).

IODINE

Chemical name: Iodine.

Molecular formula: I_2.

Molecular weight: 253.81.

Description:

Iodine USP—Heavy, grayish black plates or granules, having a metallic luster and a characteristic odor.

Iodine Topical Solution USP—Transparent, reddish brown liquid, having the odor of iodine.

Iodine Tincture USP—Transparent liquid having a reddish brown color and the odor of iodine and of alcohol.

Solubility: Iodine USP—Very slightly soluble in water; freely soluble in carbon disulfide, in chloroform, in carbon tetrachloride, and in ether; soluble in alcohol and in solutions of iodides; sparingly soluble in glycerin.

USP requirements:

Iodine USP—Preserve in tight containers. Contains not less than 99.8% and not more than 100.5% of iodine. Meets the requirements for Identification, Limit of nonvolatile residue (not more than 0.05%), and Chloride or bromide (not more than 0.028% as chloride).

Iodine Topical Solution USP—Preserve in tight, light-resistant containers, at a temperature not exceeding 35 °C. Contains, in each 100 mL, not less than 1.8 grams and not more than 2.2 grams of iodine, and not less than 2.1 grams and not more than 2.6 grams of sodium iodide.

Prepare Iodine Topical Solution as follows: 20 grams of Iodine, 24 grams of Sodium Iodide, and a sufficient quantity of Purified Water to make 1000 mL. Dissolve the Iodine and the Sodium Iodide in 50 mL of Purified Water, then add Purified Water to make 1000 mL.

Meets the requirement for Identification.

Iodine Tincture USP—Preserve in tight containers. Contains, in each 100 mL, not less than 1.8 grams and not more than 2.2 grams of iodine, and not less than 2.1 grams and not more than 2.6 grams of sodium iodide.

Iodine Tincture may be prepared by dissolving 20 grams of iodine and 24 grams of Sodium Iodide in 500 mL of Alcohol and then adding Purified Water to make the product measure 1000 mL.

Meets the requirements for Identification and Alcohol content (44.0–50.0%).

STRONG IODINE

Description: Strong Iodine Solution USP—Transparent liquid having a deep brown color and having the odor of iodine.

USP requirements:
Strong Iodine Solution USP—Preserve in tight containers, preferably at a temperature not exceeding 35 °C. Contains, in each 100 mL, not less than 4.5 grams and not more than 5.5 grams of iodine, and not less than 9.5 grams and not more than 10.5 grams of potassium iodide.

Strong Iodine Solution may be prepared by dissolving 50 grams of Iodine and 100 grams of Potassium Iodide in 100 mL of Purified Water, then adding Purified Water to make the product measure 1000 mL.

Strong Iodine Tincture may be prepared by dissolving 50 grams of Potassium Iodide in 50 mL of Purified Water, adding 70 grams of Iodine, and agitating until solution is effected, and then adding Alcohol to make the product measure 1000 mL.

Meets the requirements for Identification and Alcohol content (82.5–88.5%).

IODOHIPPURATE SODIUM I 123

Chemical name: Glycine, *N*-[2-(iodo-^{123}*I*)benzoyl]-, monosodium salt.

Molecular formula: $C_9H_7{}^{123}INNaO_3$.

USP requirements: Iodohippurate Sodium I 123 Injection USP—Preserve in single-dose or in multiple-dose containers that are adequately shielded. A sterile, aqueous solution containing *o*-iodohippurate sodium in which a portion of the molecules contain radioactive iodine (^{123}I) in the molecular structure. Label it to include the following, in addition to the information specified for Labeling under Injections: the time and date of calibration; the amount of I^123 as iodohippurate sodium expressed as total megabecquerels (or microcuries or millicuries) per mL at the time of calibration; the name and quantity of any added preservative or stabilizer; the expiration time; and the statement, "Caution—Radioactive Material." The labeling indicates that in making dosage calculations, correction is to be made for radioactive decay, and also indicates that the radioactive half-life of I 123 is 13.2 hours. Contains the labeled amount of I 123, within ±10%, as iodohippurate sodium expressed in megabecquerels (or microcuries or millicuries) per mL at the time indicated in the labeling. Contains the labeled amount of *o*-iodohippuric acid, within ±10%. Other chemical forms of radioactivity do not exceed 3.0% of total radioactivity. Meets the requirements for Radionuclidic identification, Bacterial endotoxins, pH (7.0–8.5), Radionuclidic purity, Radiochemical purity, and Biological distribution, and for Injections (except that the Injection may be distributed or dispensed prior to completion of the test for Sterility, the latter test being started on the day of final manufacture, and except that it is not subject to the recommendation on Volume in Container).

IODOHIPPURATE SODIUM I 131

Chemical name: Glycine, *N*-[2-(iodo-^{131}*I*)benzoyl]-, monosodium salt.

Molecular formula: $C_9H_7{}^{131}INNaO_3$.

Description: Iodohippurate Sodium I 131 Injection USP—Clear, colorless solution. Upon standing, both the Injection and the glass container may darken as a result of the effects of the radiation.

USP requirements: Iodohippurate Sodium I 131 Injection USP—Preserve in single-dose or in multiple-dose containers. A sterile solution containing *o*-iodohippurate sodium in which a portion of the molecules contain radioactive iodine (^{131}I) in the molecular structure. Label it to include the following, in addition to the information specified for Labeling under Injections: the time and date of calibration; the amount of ^{131}I as iodohippurate sodium expressed as total megabecquerels (or microcuries or millicuries) and as megabecquerels (or microcuries or millicuries) per mL at the time of calibration; the expiration date; and the statement, "Caution—Radioactive Material." The labeling indicates that in making dosage calculations, correction is to be made for radioactive decay, and also indicates that the radioactive half-life of ^{131}I is 8.08 days. Contains the labeled amount of ^{131}I, within ±10%, as iodohippurate sodium expressed in megabecquerels (or microcuries or millicuries) per mL at the time indicated in the labeling. Other chemical forms of radioactivity do not exceed 3.0% of the total radioactivity. Meets the requirements for Radionuclide identification, Bacterial endotoxins, pH (7.0–8.5), and Radiochemical purity, and for Injections (except that the Injection may be distributed or dispensed prior to the completion of the test for Sterility, the latter test being started on the day of final manufacture and except that it is not subject to the recommendation on Volume in Container).

SODIUM IODIDE I 123

Chemical name: Sodium iodide (Na^{123}I).

Description:
Sodium Iodide I 123 Capsules USP—Capsules may contain a small amount of solid or solids, or may appear empty.
Sodium Iodide I 123 Solution USP—Clear, colorless solution. Upon standing, both the Solution and the glass container may darken as a result of the effects of the radiation.

USP requirements:
Sodium Iodide I 123 Capsules USP—Preserve in well-closed containers that are adequately shielded. Contain radioactive iodine (^{123}I) processed in the form of Sodium Iodide obtained from the bombardment of enriched tellurium 124 with protons or of enriched tellurium 122 with deuterons or by the decay of xenon 123 in such manner that it is carrier-free. Label Capsules to include the following: the name of the Capsules; the name, address, and batch or lot number of the manufacturer; the time and date of calibration; the amount of ^{123}I as iodide expressed in megabecquerels (or microcuries or millicuries) per Capsule at the time of calibration; the name and quantity of any added preservative or stabilizer; a statement indicating that the Capsules are for oral use only; the expiration date and time; and the statement, "Caution—Radioactive Material." The labeling indicates that in making dosage calculations,

correction is to be made for radioactive decay, and also indicates that the radioactive half-life of ¹²³I is 13.2 hours. Contain the labeled amount of ¹²³I, within ±10%, as iodide expressed in megabecquerels (or microcuries or millicuries) at the time indicated in the labeling. Other chemical forms of radioactivity do not exceed 5% of the total radioactivity. Meet the requirements for Radionuclide identification, Uniformity of dosage units, Radionuclidic purity, and Radiochemical purity.

Sodium Iodide I 123 Solution USP—Preserve in single-dose or in multiple-dose containers that previously have been treated to prevent adsorption, if necessary. A solution, suitable for oral or for intravenous administration, containing radioactive iodine (¹²³I) processed in the form of Sodium Iodide, obtained from the bombardment of enriched tellurium 124 with protons or of enriched tellurium 122 with deuterons, or by the decay of xenon 123 in such manner that it is carrier-free. Label it to include the following: the time and date of calibration; the amount of ¹²³I as iodide expressed as total megabecquerels (or microcuries or millicuries) per mL at the time of calibration; the name and quantity of any added preservative or stabilizer; a statement indicating whether the contents are intended for oral or for intravenous use; the expiration date and time; and the statement, "Caution—Radioactive Material." The labeling indicates that in making dosage calculations, correction is to be made for radioactive decay, and also indicates that the radioactive half-life of ¹²³I is 13.2 hours. Contains the labeled amount of ¹²³I, within ±10%, as iodide expressed in megabecquerels (or microcuries or in millicuries) per mL at the time indicated in the labeling. Other chemical forms of radioactivity do not exceed 5% of the total radioactivity. Meets the requirements for Radionuclide identification, Radionuclidic purity, Bacterial endotoxins, pH (7.5–9.0), and Radiochemical purity, and for Injections (if for intravenous use, except that it may be distributed or dispensed prior to completion of the test for Sterility, the latter test being started on the day of final manufacture, and except that it is not subject to the recommendation on Volume in Container).

SODIUM IODIDE I 131

Chemical name: Sodium iodide (Na¹³¹I).

Molecular formula: Na¹³¹I.

Description:

Sodium Iodide I 131 Capsules USP—May contain a small amount of solid or solids, or may appear empty.

Sodium Iodide I 131 Solution USP—Clear, colorless solution. Upon standing, both the Solution and the glass container may darken as a result of the effects of the radiation.

USP requirements:

Sodium Iodide I 131 Capsules USP—Preserve in well-closed containers. Contain radioactive iodine (¹³¹I) processed in the form of Sodium Iodide from products of uranium fission or the neutron bombardment of tellurium in such a manner that it is essentially carrier-free and contains only minute amounts of naturally occurring iodine 127. Label Capsules to include the following: the date of calibration; the amount of ¹³¹I as iodide expressed in megabecquerels (or microcuries or in millicuries) per Capsule at the time of calibration; a statement of whether the contents are intended for diagnostic or therapeutic use; the expiration date; and the statement, "Caution—Radioactive Material." The labeling indicates that in making dosage calculations, correction is to be made for radioactive decay, and also indicates that the radioactive half-life of ¹³¹I is 8.08 days. Contain the labeled amount of ¹³¹I, within ±10%, as iodide expressed in megabecquerels (or microcuries or in millicuries) at the

time indicated in the labeling. Other chemical forms of radioactivity do not exceed 5% of the total radioactivity. Meet the requirements for Radionuclide identification, Uniformity of dosage units, and Radiochemical purity.

Sodium Iodide I 131 Solution USP—Preserve in single-dose or in multiple-dose containers that previously have been treated to prevent adsorption. A solution suitable for either oral or intravenous administration, containing radioactive iodine (¹³¹I) processed in the form of Sodium Iodide from the products of uranium fission or the neutron bombardment of tellurium in such a manner that it is essentially carrier-free and contains only minute amounts of naturally occurring iodine 127. Label it to include the following: the time and date of calibration; the amount of ¹³¹I as iodide expressed as total megabecquerels (or microcuries or millicuries) and as megabecquerels (or microcuries or millicuries) per mL at the time of calibration; the name and quantity of any added preservative or stabilizer; a statement of the intended use, whether oral or intravenous; a statement of whether the contents are intended for diagnostic or therapeutic use; the expiration date; and the statement, "Caution—Radioactive Material." The labeling indicates that in making dosage calculations, correction is to be made for radioactive decay, and also indicates that the radioactive half-life of ¹³¹I is 8.08 days. Contains the labeled amount of ¹³¹I, within ±10%, as iodide expressed in megabecquerels (or microcuries or in millicuries) per mL at the time indicated in the labeling. Other chemical forms of radioactivity do not exceed 5% of the total radioactivity. Meets the requirements for Radionuclide identification, Bacterial endotoxins (if intended for intravenous use), pH (7.5–9.0), and Radiochemical purity, and for Injections (if for intravenous use, except that the Solution may be distributed or dispensed prior to completion of the test for Sterility, the latter test being started on the day of final manufacture, and except that it is not subject to the recommendation on Volume in Container).

ROSE BENGAL SODIUM I 131

Chemical name: Spiro[isobenzofuran-1(3H),9'-[9H]-xanthene]-3-one, 4,5,6,7-tetrachloro-3',6'-dihydroxy-2',4',5',7'-tetraiodo-, disodium salt, labeled with iodine-131.

Molecular formula: $C_{20}H_2Cl_4{}^{131}I_4Na_2O_5$.

Description: Sodium Rose Bengal I 131 Injection USP—Clear, deep-red solution.

USP requirements: Rose Bengal Sodium I 131 Injection USP—Preserve in single-dose or in multiple-dose containers. A sterile solution containing rose bengal sodium in which a portion of the molecules contain radioactive iodine (¹³¹I) in the molecular structure. Label it to include the following, in addition to the information specified for Labeling under Injections: the time and date of calibration; the amount of ¹³¹I as rose bengal sodium expressed as total megabecquerels (or microcuries or millicuries) and as megabecquerels (or microcuries or millicuries) per mL on the date of calibration; the expiration date; and the statement, "Caution—Radioactive Material." The labeling indicates that in making dosage calculations, correction is to be made for radioactive decay, and also indicates that the radioactive half-life of ¹³¹I is 8.08 days. Contains the labeled amount of ¹³¹I, within ±10%, as rose bengal sodium expressed in megabecquerels (or microcuries or millicuries) per mL at the time indicated in the labeling. Contains the labeled amount of rose bengal sodium, within ±10%. Other chemical forms of radioactivity do not exceed 10.0% of the total radioactivity. Meets the requirements for Radionuclide identification, Bacterial endotoxins, pH (7.0–8.5), and Radiochemical purity, and for Injections (except that the Injection may be distributed or dispensed prior to the completion of the test for Sterility, the

latter test being started on the day of final manufacture, and except that it is not subject to the recommendation on Volume in Container).

IODIPAMIDE

Chemical group: Ionic, dimeric, triiodinated benzoic acid derivative.

Chemical name:
Iodipamide—Benzoic acid, 3,3'-[(1,6-dioxo-1,6-hexanediyl)-diimino]bis[2,4,6-triiodo-.
Iodipamide meglumine—Benzoic acid, 3,3'-[(1,6-dioxo-1,6-hexanediyl)diimino]bis[2,4,6-triiodo-, compd. with 1-deoxy-1-(methylamino)-D-glucitol (1:2).

Molecular formula:
Iodipamide—$C_{20}H_{14}I_6N_2O_6$.
Iodipamide meglumine—$C_{20}H_{14}I_6N_2O_6 \cdot 2C_7H_{17}NO_5$.

Molecular weight:
Iodipamide—1139.76.
Iodipamide meglumine—1530.19.

Description:
Iodipamide USP—White, practically odorless, crystalline powder.
Iodipamide Meglumine Injection USP—Clear, colorless to pale yellow, slightly viscous liquid.

Solubility: Iodipamide USP—Very slightly soluble in water, in chloroform, and in ether; slightly soluble in alcohol.

USP requirements:
Iodipamide USP—Preserve in well-closed containers. Contains not less than 98.0% and not more than 102.0% of iodipamide, calculated on the anhydrous basis. Meets the requirements for Identification, Water (not more than 1.0%), Residue on ignition (not more than 0.1%), and Free aromatic amine, and for Iodine and iodide and Heavy metals under Diatrizoic Acid.
Iodipamide Meglumine Injection USP—Preserve in single-dose containers, preferably of Type I or Type III glass, protected from light. A sterile solution of Iodipamide in Water for Injection, prepared with the aid of Meglumine. Label containers of Injection intended for intravascular injection to direct the user to discard any unused portion remaining in the container. Label containers of Injection intended for other than intravascular injection to show that the contents are not intended for intravascular injection. Contains the labeled amount, within ±5%. Iodipamide Meglumine Injection intended for intravascular use contains no antimicrobial agents. Meets the requirements for Identification, Bacterial endotoxins, pH (6.5–7.7), Free aromatic amine, and Meglumine content (23.5–26.8% of the labeled amount of iodipamide meglumine), for the tests for Iodine and iodide and Heavy metals under Diatrizoate Meglumine Injection, and for Injections.

IODIXANOL

Chemical name: 1,3-Benzenedicarboxamide, 5,5'-[(2-hydroxy-1,3-propanediyl)bis(acetylimino)]bis[*N,N*-bis(2,3-dihydroxypropyl)-2,4,6-triiodo-.

Molecular formula: $C_{35}H_{44}I_6N_6O_{15}$.

Molecular weight: 1550.18.

USP requirements: Iodixanol Injection—Not in *USP–NF*.

IODOQUINOL

Chemical group: Halogenated 8-hydroxyquinoline.

Chemical name: 8-Quinolinol, 5,7-diiodo-.

Molecular formula: $C_9H_5I_2NO$.

Molecular weight: 396.95.

Description: Iodoquinol USP—Light yellowish to tan, microcrystalline powder not readily wetted by water. Is odorless or has a faint odor; is stable in air. Melts with decomposition.

Solubility: Iodoquinol USP—Practically insoluble in water; sparingly soluble in alcohol and in ether.

USP requirements:
Iodoquinol USP—Preserve in well-closed containers. Contains not less than 96.0% and not more than 100.5% of iodoquinol, calculated on the dried basis. Meets the requirements for Identification, Loss on drying (not more than 0.5%), Residue on ignition (not more than 0.5%), and Free iodine and iodide.
Iodoquinol Tablets USP—Preserve in well-closed containers. Contain the labeled amount, within ±5%. Meet the requirements for Identification, Disintegration (1 hour), Uniformity of dosage units, and Soluble iodides.

IOFETAMINE I 123

Chemical name: Iofetamine hydrochloride I 123—Benzeneethanamine, 4-(iodo-^{123}I)-alpha-methyl-*N*-(1-methylethyl)-, hydrochloride, (±)-.

Molecular formula: Iofetamine hydrochloride I 123—$C_{12}H_{18}{}^{123}IN \cdot HCl$.

Molecular weight: Iofetamine hydrochloride I 123—335.74.

Description: Iofetamine hydrochloride I 123—Melting point 156–158 °C.

USP requirements: Iofetamine Hydrochloride I 123 Injection—Not in *USP–NF*.

IOHEXOL

Chemical group: Non-ionic, monomeric, triiodinated benzoic acid derivative.

Chemical name: 1,3-Benzenedicarboxamide, 5-[acetyl(2,3-dihydroxypropyl)amino]-*N,N*-bis(2,3-dihydroxypropyl)-2,4,6-triiodo-.

Molecular formula: $C_{19}H_{26}I_3N_3O_9$.

Molecular weight: 821.14.

Description:
Iohexol USP—White to off-white, hygroscopic, odorless powder.
Iohexol Injection USP—Clear, colorless to pale yellow liquid.

Solubility: Iohexol USP—Very soluble in water and in methanol; practically insoluble or insoluble in ether and in chloroform.

Other characteristics: Low osmolality. The osmolality of iohexol injection with iodine concentrations of 180, 240, 300, and 350 mg per mL is 408, 520, 672, and 844 mOsmol per kg of water, respectively.

USP requirements:

Iohexol USP—Preserve in well-closed, light-resistant containers. Contains not less than 98.0% and not more than 102.0% of iohexol, calculated on the anhydrous basis. Meets the requirements for Identification, Color of solution, Specific rotation (−0.5° to +0.5°), Water (not more than 4.0%), Heavy metals (not more than 0.002%), Free aromatic amine, Free iodine, Free iodide (not more than 0.001%), Ionic compounds (not more than 0.0002% solution of sodium chloride [equivalent to 0.01% ionic compounds]), Limit of methanol, isopropyl alcohol, and methoxyethanol (not more than 0.005% each of methanol and isopropyl alcohol, and not more than 0.002% of methoxyethanol), Limit of 3-chloro-1,2-propanediol (not more than 0.0025%), Limit of O-alkylated compounds (not more than 0.6%), and Related compounds.

Iohexol Injection USP—Preserve Injection intended for intravascular or intrathecal use in single-dose containers of Type I glass, protected from light. A sterile solution of Iohexol in Water for Injection. Label containers of Injection to direct the user to discard any unused portion. The labeling states also that it is not to be used if it is discolored or contains a precipitate. Label it also to state its routes of administration. Contains the labeled amount of Iohexol as organically bound iodine, within ±5%. Iohexol Injection intended for intravascular or intrathecal use contains no antimicrobial agents. Meets the requirements for Identification, Bacterial endotoxins, pH (6.8–7.7), Particulate matter, and Free iodide (not more than 0.02%, based on the content of iohexol), and the requirements under Injections, and for Heavy metals and Related compounds for Iohexol.

IOPAMIDOL

Chemical group: A nonionic contrast medium.

Chemical name: 1,3-Benzenedicarboxamide, *N,N*-bis[2-hydroxy1-(hydroxymethyl)ethyl]-5-[(2-hydroxy-1-oxopropyl)amino]2,4,6-triiodo-, (*S*)-.

Molecular formula: $C_{17}H_{22}I_3N_3O_8$.

Molecular weight: 777.09.

Description: Iopamidol USP—Practically odorless, white to off-white powder.

Solubility: Iopamidol USP—Very soluble in water; sparingly soluble in methanol; practically insoluble in alcohol and in chloroform.

Other characteristics: Low osmolality. The osmolality of iopamidol injection with iodine concentrations of 200, 300, and 370 mg per mL is 413, 616, and 796 mOsmol per kg of water, respectively.

USP requirements:

Iopamidol USP—Preserve in well-closed, light-resistant containers. Contains not less than 98.0% and not more than 101.0% of iopamidol, calculated on the dried basis. Meets the requirements for Identification, Specific rotation (−4.6° to −5.2°), Loss on drying (not more than 0.5%), Residue on ignition (not more than 0.1%), Free aromatic amine (not more than 0.02%), Free iodine, Limit of free iodide (not more than 0.001%), Free acid or alkali, Heavy metals (not more than 0.001%), and Related compounds (not more than 0.25%).

Iopamidol Injection USP—Preserve Injection intended for intravascular or intrathecal use in single-dose containers, preferably of Type I glass, and protected from light. A sterile solution of Iopamidol in Water for Injection. Label containers of Injection to direct the user to discard any unused portion remaining in the container and to check for the presence of particulate matter before using. Label it also to state its routes of administration. Contains the labeled amount, within ±5%. Iopamidol Injection intended for intravascular or intrathecal use contains no antimicrobial agents. Meets the requirements for Identification, Bacterial endotoxins, pH (6.5–7.5), Particulate matter, Free aromatic amine (not more than 0.05%), Free iodine, and Limit of free iodide (not more than 0.04 mg of iodide per mL), and for Injections.

IOPANOIC ACID

Chemical group: Ionic, triiodinated benzoic acid derivative.

Chemical name: Benzenepropanoic acid, 3-amino-alpha-ethyl-2,4,6-triiodo-.

Molecular formula: $C_{11}H_{12}I_3NO_2$.

Molecular weight: 570.93.

Description: Iopanoic Acid USP—Cream-colored powder. Has a faint, characteristic odor. Affected by light.

pKa: 4.8.

Solubility: Iopanoic Acid USP—Insoluble in water; soluble in alcohol, in chloroform, and in ether; soluble in solutions of alkali hydroxides and carbonates.

USP requirements:

Iopanoic Acid USP—Preserve in tight, light-resistant containers. Contains an amount of iodine equivalent to not less than 97.0% and not more than 101.0% of iopanoic acid, calculated on the dried basis. Meets the requirements for Identification, Melting range (152–158 °C, with decomposition), Loss on drying (not more than 1.0%), Residue on ignition (not more than 0.1%), Free iodine, Halide ions, and Heavy metals (not more than 0.002%).

Iopanoic Acid Tablets USP—Preserve in tight, light-resistant containers. Contain the labeled amount, within ±5%. Meet the requirements for Identification, Disintegration (30 minutes), Uniformity of dosage units, and Halide ions.

IOPHENDYLATE

Chemical group: Ionic organic iodine compound.

Chemical name: Benzenedecanoic acid, iodo-iota-methyl-, ethyl ester.

Molecular formula: $C_{19}H_{29}IO_2$.

Molecular weight: 416.34.

Description:

Iophendylate USP—Colorless to pale yellow, viscous liquid, the color darkening on long exposure to air. Is odorless or has a faintly ethereal odor.

Iophendylate Injection USP—Colorless to pale yellow, viscous liquid, the color darkening on long exposure to air. Is odorless or has a faintly ethereal odor.

Solubility:

Iophendylate USP—Very slightly soluble in water; freely soluble in alcohol, in chloroform, and in ether.

Iophendylate Injection USP—Very slightly soluble in water; freely soluble in alcohol, in chloroform, and in ether.

Other characteristics: Iophendylate injection—Immiscible with CSF; high specific gravity in relation to that of CSF.

USP requirements:

Iophendylate USP—Preserve in tight, light-resistant containers. A mixture of isomers of ethyl iodophenylundecanoate, consisting chiefly of ethyl 10-(iodophenyl)undecanoate. Contains not less than 98.0% and not more than 102.0% of iophendylate. Meets the requirements for Identification, Specific gravity (1.248–1.257), Refractive index (1.524–1.526), Residue on ignition (not more than 0.1%), Free acids, Free iodine, and Saponification value (132–142).

Iophendylate Injection USP—Preserve in single-dose containers, preferably of Type I glass, protected from light. It is sterile Iophendylate. Meets the requirements for Bacterial endotoxins, for Identification, Specific gravity, Refractive index, Residue on ignition, Free acids, Free iodine, and Saponification value under Iophendylate, and for Injections.

IOPROMIDE

Chemical name: 1,3-Benzenedicarboxamide, *N,N'*-bis(2,3-dihydroxypropyl)-2,4,6-triiodo-5-[(methoxyacetyl)amino]-*N*-methy-.

Molecular formula: $C_{18}H_{24}I_3N_3O_8$.

Molecular weight: 791.11.

Description: White to slightly yellow powder.

Solubility: Freely soluble in water and in dimethyl sulfoxide; practically insoluble in alcohol, in acetone, and in ether.

USP requirements:

Iopromide USP—Preserve in well closed, light-resistant containers. Contains not less than 97.0% and not more than 102.5% of iopromide, calculated on the anhydrous and solvent-free basis. Meets the requirements for Identification, Water (not more than 1.5%), Residue on ignition (not more than 0.1%), Heavy metals (not more than 0.002%), Free iodine (the toluene layer shows no red color), Limit of free iodide (not more than 0.002%), Limit of free aromatic amine (not more than 0.1%), Limit of alcohol (not more than 0.4%), Limit of *N*-acetyl compound, iopromide related compound B (not more than 1.5%), Oridinary impurities (not more than 3.0%), Organic volatile impurities, and Isomer distribution (49.0% to 60.0% *E*2- and *Z*2-isomers).

Iopromide Injection USP—Preserve in single-dose glass containers, and protect from light. A sterile solution of iopromide in Water for Injection. Contains no antimicrobial agents. Label Injection to state that it is not to be used if it contains particulate matter and that after use any unused portion remaining in the container is to be discarded. It is labeled also to state that it is not for intrathecal use. Contains not less than 94.0% and not more 105.0% of the labeled amount of iopromide. May contain small amounts of suitable buffers and of Edetate Calcium Disodium as a stabilizer. Meets the requirements for Identification, Bacterial endotoxins, pH (6.5–8.0), Free iodine, Limit of free iodide (not more than 80 mcg per gram), Limit of free aromatic amine (not more than 0.2%), Limit of *N*-acetyl compound (not more than 1.5%), and Isomer distribution, and for Injection, and for Ordinary impurities and Heavy metals under Iopromide..

IOTHALAMATE

Chemical group: Ionic, monomeric, triiodinated benzoic acid derivative.

Chemical name:

Iothalamate meglumine—Benzoic acid, 3-(acetylamino)-2,4,6-triiodo-5-[(methylamino)carbonyl]-, compd. with 1-deoxy-1-(methylamino)-D-glucitol (1:1).

Iothalamate sodium—Benzoic acid, 3-(acetylamino)-2,4,6-triiodo-5-[(methylamino)carbonyl]-, monosodium salt.

Molecular formula:

Iothalamate meglumine—$C_{11}H_9I_3N_2O_4 \cdot C_7H_{17}NO_5$.

Iothalamate sodium—$C_{11}H_8I_3N_2NaO_4$.

Molecular weight:

Iothalamate meglumine—809.13.

Iothalamate sodium—635.90.

Description:

Iothalamate Meglumine Injection USP—Clear, colorless to pale yellow, slightly viscous liquid.

Iothalamate Meglumine and Iothalamate Sodium Injection USP—Clear, colorless to pale yellow, slightly viscous liquid.

Iothalamate Sodium Injection USP—Clear, colorless to pale yellow, slightly viscous liquid.

USP requirements:

Iothalamate Meglumine Injection USP—Preserve in single-dose containers, preferably of Type I glass, protected from light. A sterile solution of Iothalamic Acid in Water for Injection, prepared with the aid of Meglumine. Label containers of Injection intended for intravascular injection to direct the user to discard any unused portion remaining in the container. Label containers of Injection intended for other than intravascular injection to show that the contents are not intended for intravascular injection. Contains the labeled amount, within ±5%. Iothalamate Meglumine Injection intended for intravascular use contains no antimicrobial agents. Meets the requirements for Identification, Bacterial endotoxins, pH (6.5–7.7), Free aromatic amine, Iodine and iodide, Heavy metals (not more than 0.002%), and Meglumine content (22.9% to 25.3% of the labeled amount of iothalamate meglumine), and for Injections.

Iothalamate Meglumine and Iothalamate Sodium Injection USP—Preserve in single-dose containers, preferably of Type I glass, protected from light. A sterile solution of Iothalamic Acid in Water for Injection, prepared with the aid of Meglumine and Sodium Hydroxide. Label containers of Injection intended for intravascular injection to direct the user to discard any unused portion remaining in the container. Label containers of Injection intended for other than intravascular injection to show that the contents are not intended for intravascular injection. Contains the labeled amounts of iothalamate meglumine and iothalamate sodium, within ±5%. Iothalamate Meglumine and Iothalamate Sodium Injection intended for intravascular use contains no antimicrobial agents. Meets the requirements for Identification, Bacterial endotoxins, pH (6.5–7.7), Free aromatic amine, Iodine and iodide (not more than 0.02% iodide), and Heavy metals (not more than 0.002%), and for Injections.

Iothalamate Sodium Injection USP—Preserve in single-dose containers, preferably of Type I glass, protected from light. A sterile solution of Iothalamic Acid in Water for Injection prepared with the aid of Sodium Hydroxide. Label containers of the Injection intended for intravascular injection to direct the user to discard any unused portion remaining in the container. Label containers of the Injection intended for other than intravascular injection to show that the contents are not intended for intravascular injection. Contains the labeled amount, within ±5%. Iothalamate Sodium Injection intended for intravascular use contains no antimicrobial agents. Meets the requirements for Identification,

Bacterial endotoxins, pH (6.5–7.7), Free aromatic amine, Iodine and iodide (not more than 0.02% of iodide), and Heavy metals (not more than 0.002%), and for Injections.

IOTHALAMIC ACID

Chemical name: Benzoic acid, 3-(acetylamino)-2,4,6-triiodo-5-[(methylamino)carbonyl]-.

Molecular formula: $C_{11}H_9I_3N_2O_4$.

Molecular weight: 613.91.

Description: Iothalamic Acid USP—White, odorless powder.

Solubility: Iothalamic Acid USP—Slightly soluble in water and in alcohol; soluble in solutions of alkali hydroxides.

USP requirements: Iothalamic Acid USP—Preserve in well-closed containers. Contains not less than 98.0% and not more than 102.0% of iothalamic acid, calculated on the anhydrous basis. Meets the requirements for Identification, Water (not more than 1.0%), Residue on ignition (not more than 0.1%), Free aromatic amine, Iodine and iodide, and Heavy metals (not more than 0.002%).

IOVERSOL

Chemical name: 1,3-Benzenedicarboxamide, *N,N*-bis(2,3-dihydroxypropyl)-5-[(hydroxyacetyl)(2-hydroxyethyl)amino]-2,4,6-triiodo-.

Molecular formula: $C_{18}H_{24}I_3N_3O_9$.

Molecular weight: 807.11.

USP requirements:
  Ioversol USP—Preserve in well-closed containers. Contains not less than 97.0% and not more than 101.0% of ioversol, calculated on the anhydrous basis. Meets the requirements for Identification, Water (not more than 5%), Residue on ignition (not more than 0.1%), Related compounds, Iodine and iodide (not more than 0.02% of iodide), and Heavy metals (not more than 20 mcg per gram).
  Ioversol Injection USP—Preserve in single-dose containers, preferably of Type I glass, protected from light. A sterile solution of ioversol in Water for Injection. Ioversol Injection intended for intravascular use contains no antimicrobial agents. Label containers of Injection intended for intravascular injection to direct the user to discard any unused portion remaining in the container. Contains the labeled amounts of ioversol and iodine, within ±5%. Meets the requirements for Identification, Bacterial endotoxins, pH (6.0–7.4), Heavy metals (not more than 20 mcg per gram), and Related compounds, and for Injections.

IOXAGLATE

Chemical group: Ionic, dimeric, contrast agent; benzoic acid salt.

Chemical name:
  Ioxaglate meglumine—Benzoic acid, 3-[[[[3-(acetylmethylamino)-2,4,6-triiodo-5-[(methylamino)carbonyl]benzoyl]amino]acetyl]amino]-5-[[(2-hydroxyethyl)amino]carbonyl]-2,4,6-triiodo-, compound with 1-deoxy-1-(methylamino)-D-glucitol (1:1).

  Ioxaglate sodium—Benzoic acid, 3-[[[[3-(acetylmethylamino)-2,4,6-triiodo-5-[(methylamino)carbonyl]benzoyl]amino]acetyl]amino]-5-[[(2-hydroxyethyl)amino]carbonyl]-2,4,6-triiodo-, sodium salt.

Molecular formula:
  Ioxaglate meglumine—$C_{24}H_{21}I_6N_5O_8 \cdot C_7H_{17}NO_5$.
  Ioxaglate sodium—$C_{24}H_{20}I_6N_5NaO_8$.

Molecular weight:
  Ioxaglate meglumine—1464.09.
  Ioxaglate sodium—1290.86.

Other characteristics:
  Ioxaglate meglumine—Contains approximately 52% of iodine.
  Ioxaglate sodium—Contains approximately 59% of iodine.

USP requirements: Ioxaglate Meglumine and Ioxaglate Sodium Injection USP—Preserve in single-dose containers, preferably of Type I glass, protected from light. A sterile solution of Ioxaglic Acid in Water for Injection, prepared with the aid of Meglumine and Sodium Hydroxide. May contain small amounts of Edetate Calcium Disodium as a stabilizer. Ioxaglate Meglumine and Ioxaglate Sodium Injection intended for intravascular use contains no antimicrobial agents. Label containers of Injection intended for intravascular injection to direct the user to discard any unused portion remaining in the container. Label containers of Injection intended for other than intravascular injection to indicate that the contents are not intended for intravascular injection. Contains the labeled amounts of ioxaglate meglumine and iodine, within ±5%. Meets the requirements for Identification, pH (6.0–7.6), Heavy metals (not more than 0.002%), and Free iodine and iodide (not more than 0.02% of iodide), and for Injections.

IOXAGLIC ACID

Chemical name: Benzoic acid, 3-[[[[3-(acetylmethylamino)-2,4,6-triiodo-5-[(methylamino)carbonyl]benzoyl]amino]acetyl]amino]-5-[[(2-hydroxyethyl)amino]carbonyl]-2,4,6-triiodo-.

Molecular formula: $C_{24}H_{21}I_6N_5O_8$.

Molecular weight: 1268.88.

Other characteristics: Contains approximately 60% of iodine.

USP requirements: Ioxaglic Acid USP—Preserve in well-closed containers. Contains not less than 98.5% and not more than 101.5% of ioxaglic acid, calculated on the anhydrous basis. Meets the requirements for Identification, Water (not more than 5%), Residue on ignition (not more than 0.1%), Heavy metals (not more than 0.002%), and Free iodine and iodide (not more than 0.02% of iodide).

IOXILAN

Chemical name: 1,3-Benzenedicarboxamide, 5-[acetyl(2,3-dihydroxypropyl)amino]-*N*-(2,3-dihydroxypropyl)-*N'*-(2-hydroxyethyl)-2,4,6-triiodo-.

Molecular formula: $C_{18}H_{24}I_3N_3O_8$.

Molecular weight: 791.11.

Description:
  Ioxilan USP—White to off-white, practically odorless powder.
  Ioxilan Injection USP—Clear, colorless to pale yellow liquid.

Solubility: Ioxilan USP—Soluble in water and in methanol.

USP requirements:
  Ioxilan USP—Preserve in well-closed, light-resistant containers. Contains not less than 98.0% and not more than 102.0% of ioxilan, calculated on the anhydrous and

methanol-free basis. Meets the requirements for Identification, Bacterial endotoxins, Heavy metals (0.002%), pH (5.0–7.5, in a solution [1 in 10]), Water (not more than 4.0%), Free iodine, Free iodide (not more than 30 microgram), Free aromatic amine (not more than 0.05%), Residual method (not more than 2.0%), Limit of serinol impurity (not more than 0.5%), and Chromatographic purity (not more than 0.5% of any individual impurity is found, and the total of all impurities not more than 1.5%).

Ioxilan Injection USP—Preserve injection in single-dose containers of Type I glass, protected from light. A sterile solution of Ioxilan in Water for Injection. Label containers of the Injection to direct the user to discard any unused portion. The label states that it is not to be used if it is discolored or contains a precipitate and states also that it is not for intrathecal use. Contains the labeled amount, within ±5% as organically bound iodide. May contain small amounts of suitable buffers and of Edetate Calcium Disodium as a stabilizer. Contains no antimicrobial agents. Meets the requirements for Identification, Bacterial endotoxins, Heavy metals (not more than 0.002%), pH (6.0–7.5), Free iodine, Free iodide (not more than 200 microgram), Residual methanol (not more than 0.005%), and for Injections.

IPECAC

Description: Powdered Ipecac USP—Pale brown, weak yellow, or light olive-gray powder.

USP requirements:

Ipecac USP—Consists of the dried rhizome and roots of *Cephaëlis acuminata* Karsten, or of *Cephaëlis ipecacuanha* (Brotero) A. Richard (Fam. Rubiaceae). Yields not less than 2.0% of the total ether-soluble alkaloids of ipecac. Its content of emetine and cephaeline together is not less than 90.0% of the amount of the total ether-soluble alkaloids. The content of cephaeline varies from an amount equal to, to an amount not more than 2.5 times, the content of emetine. Meets the requirements for Botanic characteristics, Overground stems (not more than 5%), and Foreign organic matter (not more than 2.0%).

Powdered Ipecac USP—Preserve in tight containers. It is Ipecac reduced to a fine or a very fine powder and adjusted to a potency of not less than 1.9% and not more than 2.1% of the total ether-soluble alkaloids of ipecac, by the addition of exhausted marc of ipecac or of other suitable inert diluent or by the addition of powdered ipecac of either a lower or a higher potency. The content of emetine and cephaeline together is not less than 90.0% of the total amount of the ether-soluble alkaloids. The content of cephaeline varies from an amount equal to, to an amount not more than 2.5 times, the content of emetine. Meets the requirement for Botanic characteristics.

Ipecac Oral Solution USP—Preserve in tight containers, preferably at a temperature not exceeding 25 °C. Containers intended for sale to the public without prescription contain not more than 30 mL of Oral Solution. Yields, from each 100 mL, not less than 123 mg and not more than 157 mg of the total ether-soluble alkaloids of ipecac. The content of emetine and cephaeline together is not less than 90.0% of the amount of the total ether-soluble alkaloids. The content of cephaeline varies from an amount equal to, to an amount not more than 2.5 times, the content of emetine.

Prepare Ipecac Oral Solution as follows: 70 grams of Powdered Ipecac, 100 mL of Glycerin, and a sufficient quantity of Syrup to make 1000 mL. Exhaust the powdered Ipecac by percolation, using a mixture of 3 volumes of alcohol and 1 volume of water as the menstruum, macerating for 72 hours, and percolating slowly. Reduce the entire percolate to a volume of 70 mL by evaporation at a temperature not exceeding 60 °C and preferably in vacuum, and add 140 mL of water. Allow the mixture to stand overnight, filter, and wash the residue on the filter with water. Evaporate the filtrate and washings to 40 mL, and to this add 2.5 mL of hydrochloric acid and 20 mL of alcohol, mix, and filter. Wash the filter with a mixture of 30 volumes of alcohol, 3.5 volumes of hydrochloric acid, and 66.5 volumes of water, using a volume sufficient to produce 70 mL of the filtrate. Add 100 mL of Glycerin and enough Syrup to make the product measure 1000 mL, and mix.

Meets the requirements for Microbial limits and Alcohol content (1.0–2.5%).

Ipecac Syrup USP—Preserve in tight containers, preferably at a temperature not exceeding 25 °C. Containers intended for sale to the public without prescription contain not more than 30 mL of Syrup. Yields, from each 100 mL, not less than 123 mg and not more than 157 mg of the total ether-soluble alkaloids of ipecac. The content of emetine and cephaeline together is not less than 90.0% of the amount of the total ether-soluble alkaloids. The content of cephaeline varies from an amount equal to, to an amount not more than 2.5 times, the content of emetine.

Prepare Ipecac Syrup as follows: 70 grams of Powdered Ipecac, 100 mL of Glycerin, and a sufficient quantity of Syrup to make 1000 mL. Exhaust the powdered Ipecac by percolation, using a mixture of 3 volumes of alcohol and 1 volume of water as the menstruum, macerating for 72 hours, and percolating slowly. Reduce the entire percolate to a volume of 70 mL by evaporation at a temperature not exceeding 60 °C and preferably in vacuum, and add 140 mL of water. Allow the mixture to stand overnight, filter, and wash the residue on the filter with water. Evaporate the filtrate and washings to 40 mL, and to this add 2.5 mL of hydrochloric acid and 20 mL of alcohol, mix, and filter. Wash the filter with a mixture of 30 volumes of alcohol, 3.5 volumes of hydrochloric acid, and 66.5 volumes of water, using a volume sufficient to produce 70 mL of the filtrate. Add 100 mL of Glycerin and enough Syrup to make the product measure 1000 mL, and mix.

Meets the requirements for Microbial limits and Alcohol content (1.0–2.5%).

IPODATE

Chemical group: Triiodinated benzoic acid derivative.

Chemical name:

Ipodate calcium—Benzenepropanoic acid, 3-[[(dimethylamino)methylene]amino]-2,4,6-triiodo-, calcium salt.

Ipodate sodium—Benzenepropanoic acid, 3-[[(dimethylamino)methylene]amino]-2,4,6-triiodo-, sodium salt.

Molecular formula:

Ipodate calcium—$C_{24}H_{24}CaI_6N_4O_4$.

Ipodate sodium—$C_{12}H_{12}I_3N_2NaO_2$.

Molecular weight:

Ipodate calcium—1233.98.

Ipodate sodium—619.94.

Description:

Ipodate Calcium USP—White to off-white, odorless, fine, crystalline powder.

Ipodate Sodium USP—White to off-white, odorless, fine, crystalline powder.

Solubility:

Ipodate Calcium USP—Slightly soluble in water, in alcohol, in chloroform, and in methanol.

Ipodate Sodium USP—Freely soluble in water, in alcohol, and in methanol; very slightly soluble in chloroform.

USP requirements:

Ipodate Calcium USP—Preserve in tight containers. Contains not less than 97.5% and not more than 102.5% of ipodate calcium, calculated on the anhydrous basis. Meets the requirements for Identification, Water (not more than 3.5%), Iodide or iodine, and Heavy metals (not more than 0.003%).

Ipodate Calcium for Oral Suspension USP—Preserve in well-closed containers. A dry mixture of Ipodate Calcium and one or more suitable suspending, dispersing, and flavoring agents. Contains the labeled amount, within ±15%. Meets the requirements for Identification and Minimum fill.

Ipodate Sodium USP—Preserve in tight containers. Contains not less than 97.5% and not more than 102.5% of ipodate sodium, calculated on the dried basis. Meets the requirements for Identification, Loss on drying (not more than 0.5%), Iodide or iodine, and Heavy metals (not more than 0.003%).

Ipodate Sodium Capsules USP—Preserve in tight containers. Contain the labeled amount, within ±10%. Meet the requirements for Identification and Uniformity of dosage units.

IPRATROPIUM

Source: A synthetic quaternary ammonium derivative of atropine.

Chemical name: Ipratropium bromide—8-Azoniabicyclo[3.2.1]-octane, 3-(3-hydroxy-1-oxo-2-phenylpropoxy)-8-methyl-8-(1-methylethyl)-, bromide, monohydrate(*endo,syn*)-, (±)-.

Molecular formula: Ipratropium bromide—$C_{20}H_{30}BrNO_3 \cdot H_2O$.

Molecular weight: Ipratropium bromide—430.38.

Description: Ipratropium bromide—A white, crystalline substance.

Solubility: Ipratropium bromide—Freely soluble in water and in lower alcohols; insoluble in lipophilic solvents such as chloroform, ether, and fluorocarbons. Has a low lipid solubility.

Other characteristics: Ipratropium bromide—Fairly stable in neutral solutions and in acid solutions; rapidly hydrolyzed in alkaline solutions.

USP requirements:

Ipratropium Bromide Inhalation Aerosol—Not in *USP–NF*.
Ipratropium Bromide Nasal Aerosol—Not in *USP–NF*.
Ipratropium Bromide Inhalation Solution—Not in *USP–NF*.
Ipratropium Bromide Nasal Solution—Not in *USP–NF*.

IPRATROPIUM AND ALBUTEROL

For *Ipratropium* and *Albuterol*—See individual listings for chemistry information.

USP requirements:

Ipratropium Bromide and Albuterol Sulfate Inhalation Aerosol—Not in *USP–NF*.
Ipratropium Bromide and Albuterol Sulfate Solution—*USP–NF*.

IRBESARTAN

Chemical name: 1,3-Diazaspiro[4.4]non-1-en-4-one, 2-butyl-3-[[2'-(1*H*-tetrazol-5-yl)[1,1'-biphenyl]-4-yl]methyl]-.

Molecular formula: $C_{25}H_{28}N_6O$.

Molecular weight: 428.53.

Description: White to off-white crystalline powder.

Solubility: Slightly soluble in alcohol and in methylene chloride; practically insoluble in water.

USP requirements: Irbesartan Tablets—Not in *USP–NF*.

IRINOTECAN

Source: Irinotecan hydrochloride—Semisynthetic derivative of camptothecin, an alkaloid extract from plants such as *Camptotheca acuminata*.

Chemical name: Irinotecan hydrochloride—[1,4'-Bipiperidine]-1'-carboxylic acid, 4,11-diethyl-3,4,12,14-tetrahydro-4-hydroxy-3,14-dioxo-1*H*-pyrano[3',4':6,7]indolizino[1,2-*b*]quinolin-9-yl ester, monohydrochloride, trihydrate, (*S*)-.

Molecular formula: Irinotecan hydrochloride—$C_{33}H_{38}N_4O_6 \cdot$ HCl $\cdot$ $3H_2O$.

Molecular weight: Irinotecan hydrochloride—677.18.

Description: Irinotecan hydrochloride—Pale yellow to yellow crystalline powder.

Solubility: Irinotecan hydrochloride—Slightly soluble in water and in organic solvents.

USP requirements: Irinotecan Hydrochloride Injection—Not in *USP–NF*.

FERROUS CITRATE FE 59

Chemical name: 1,2,3-Propanetricarboxylic acid, 2-hydroxy-, iron(2+)-^{59}Fe salt.

Molecular formula: $C_{12}H_{10}{}^{59}Fe_3O_{14}$.

USP requirements: Ferrous Citrate Fe 59 Injection—Not in USP.

IRON DEXTRAN

Source: A complex of ferric oxyhydroxide and a low-molecular weight dextran derivative.

Description: Iron Dextran Injection USP—Dark brown, slightly viscous liquid.

USP requirements: Iron Dextran Injection USP—Preserve in single-dose or in multiple-dose containers, preferably of Type I or Type II glass. A sterile, colloidal solution of ferric hydroxide in complex with partially hydrolyzed Dextran of low molecular weight, in Water for Injection. Contains the labeled amount of iron, within ±5%. Meets the requirements for Identification, Bacterial endotoxins, Acute toxicity, Absorption from injection site, pH (4.5–7.0), Nonvolatile residue, Chloride content, and Limit of phenol (not more than 0.5%), and for Injections.

IRON-POLYSACCHARIDE

Source: A complex of ferric iron and a low-molecular weight polysaccharide.

Description: Polysaccharide-iron complex—An amorphous brown powder.

Solubility: Polysaccharide-iron complex—Very soluble in water; insoluble in alcohol.

USP requirements:
Iron-Polysaccharide Capsules—Not in *USP–NF*.
Iron-Polysaccharide Elixir—Not in *USP–NF*.
Iron-Polysaccharide Tablets—Not in *USP–NF*.

IRON SORBITEX

Source: A sterile, colloidal solution of a complex of trivalent iron, sorbitol, and citric acid, stabilized with dextrin and sorbitol.

Chemical name: Iron sorbitex.

Molecular weight: Average of complex less than 5000.

Description: Iron Sorbitex Injection USP—Clear liquid, having a dark brown color.

USP requirements:
Iron Sorbitex Injection USP—Preserve in single-dose containers, preferably of Type I glass. A sterile solution of a complex of iron, Sorbitol, and Citric Acid that is stabilized with the aid of Dextrin and an excess of Sorbitol. Label it to indicate its expiration date, which is not more than 24 months after date of manufacture. Contains an amount of iron sorbitex equivalent to the labeled amount of iron, within −6% to +4%. Meets the requirements for Identification, Specific gravity (1.17–1.19 at 20 °C), Viscosity (8–13 centipoises, determined at 20 °C with a capillary tube viscosimeter), Bacterial endotoxins, pH (7.2–7.9), and Limit of ferrous iron (not more than 8.5 mg per mL), and for Injections.
Iron Sorbitol Injection—Not in *USP–NF*.

IRON SUCROSE

Chemical name: Iron saccharate.

Molecular formula: $[Na_2Fe_5O_8(OH)\cdot3(H_2O)]_n\cdot m(C_{12}H_{22}O_{11})$.

Molecular weight: 34,000–60,000 daltons.

Other characteristics: pH:10.5–11.1.

USP requirements:
Iron Sucrose Injection USP—Preserve in single-dose containers of Type I glass. Store at controlled room temperature. Do not freeze. A sterile, colloidal solution of ferric hydroxide in complex with Sucrose in Water for Injection. Label it to state that it is for intravenous use only. Label it to indicate that when administered by intravenous infusion, the Injection must be diluted with 0.9% Sodium Chloride Injection to a concentration of 0.5 to 2.0 mg of elemental iron per mL. Label it also to state the total osmolarity of the solution expressed in mOsmol per liter. Contains the labeld amount, within ±5%. Sodium Hydroxide may be added to adjust the pH. It contains no antimicrobial agent, chelating agent, dextran, gluconate, or other added substances. Meets the requirements for Identification, Specific gravity (1.135–1.165 at 20 °C, Bacterial endotoxins (not more than 3.7), Alkalinity (not less than 0.5 mL or not more than 0.8 mL of 0.1 N hydrochloric acid), pH (10.5–11.1 at 20°), Osmolarity (not less than 1150 and not more than 1350 mOsmol per liter), Absence of low-molecular weight Fe (II) and Fe (III) complexes, Turbidity (not less than 4.4 and not more than 5.3), Particulate matter, Limit of iron

(II) (not more than 0.4% [w/v]), and Content of chloride (not less than 0.012% and not more than 0.025%), and for Injection.
Iron Sucrose for Injection—Not in *USP–NF*.

ISOAMYL METHOXYCINNAMATE

Chemical name: 4-Methoxycinnamic acid, isoamyl ester.

Molecular formula: $C_{15}H_{20}O_3$.

Molecular weight: 248.32.

USP requirements: Isoamyl Methoxycinnamate USP—Preserve in tight containers. Contains not less than 95.0% and not more than 105.0% of isoamyl methoxycinnamate. Meets the requirements for Identification, Specific gravity (1.037–1.041), Refractive index (1.556–1.560 at 20°), Acidity (not more than 0.2 mL of titrant per mL of Isoamyl Methoxycinnamate), and Chromatographic purity.

ISOBUTANE

Molecular formula: C_4H_{10}.

Molecular weight: 58.12.

Description: Isobutane NF—Colorless, flammable gas (boiling temperature is about −11 °C). Vapor pressure at 21 °C is about 2950 mm of mercury (31 psig).
NF category: Aerosol propellant.

NF requirements: Isobutane NF—Preserve in tight cylinders and prevent exposure to excessive heat. Contains not less than 95.0% of isobutane. Meets the requirements for Identification, Water (not more than 0.001%), High-boiling residues (not more than 5 ppm), Acidity of residue, and Limit of sulfur compounds.
Caution: Isobutane is highly flammable and explosive.

ISOBUTYRAMIDE

USP requirements: Isobutyramide Oral Solution—Not in *USP–NF*.

ISOCARBOXAZID

Chemical group: Hydrazine derivative, structurally similar to amphetamine.

Chemical name: 3-Isoxazolecarboxylic acid, 5-methyl-, 2-(phenylmethyl)hydrazide.

Molecular formula: $C_{12}H_{13}N_3O_2$.

Molecular weight: 231.25.

Description: Isocarboxazid USP—White, or practically white, crystalline powder, having a slight characteristic odor.

Solubility: Isocarboxazid USP—Slightly soluble in water; very soluble in chloroform; soluble in alcohol.

USP requirements:
Isocarboxazid USP—Preserve in well-closed containers. Contains not less than 98.5% and not more than 100.5% of isocarboxazid, calculated on the dried basis. Meets the re-

quirements for Identification, Melting range (105–108 °C), Loss on drying (not more than 0.3%), Residue on ignition (not more than 0.1%), Chloride (not more than 0.2%), Limit of methyl 5-methyl-3-isoxazolecarboxylate and 1-benzyl-3-methyl-5-aminopyrazole, and Organic volatile impurities.

Isocarboxazid Tablets USP—Preserve in well-closed, light-resistant containers. Contain the labeled amount, within ± 5%. Meet the requirements for Identification, Dissolution (80% in 45 minutes in 0.1 N hydrochloric acid in Apparatus 2 at 50 rpm), and Uniformity of dosage units.

ISOETHARINE

Chemical name:
Isoetharine hydrochloride—1,2-Benzenediol, 4-[1-hydroxy-2-[(1-methylethyl)amino]butyl]-, hydrochloride.
Isoetharine mesylate—1,2-Benzenediol, 4-[1-hydroxy-2-[(1-methylethyl)amino]butyl]-, methanesulfonate (salt).

Molecular formula:
Isoetharine hydrochloride—$C_{13}H_{21}NO_3 \cdot HCl$.
Isoetharine mesylate—$C_{13}H_{21}NO_3 \cdot CH_4O_3S$.

Molecular weight:
Isoetharine hydrochloride—275.77.
Isoetharine mesylate—335.42.

Description:
Isoetharine Inhalation Solution USP—Colorless or slightly yellow, slightly acid liquid, gradually turning dark on exposure to air and light.
Isoetharine Hydrochloride USP—White to off-white, odorless, crystalline solid. Melts between 196 and 208 °C, with decomposition.
Isoetharine Mesylate USP—White or practically white, odorless crystals.

Solubility:
Isoetharine Hydrochloride USP—Soluble in water; sparingly soluble in alcohol; practically insoluble in ether.
Isoetharine Mesylate USP—Freely soluble in water; soluble in alcohol; practically insoluble in acetone and in ether.

USP requirements:
Isoetharine Inhalation Solution USP—Preserve in small, tight containers that are well-filled or otherwise protected from oxidation. Protect from light. A sterile solution of Isoetharine Hydrochloride in Purified Water. The label indicates that the Inhalation Solution is not to be used if its color is pinkish or darker than slightly yellow or if it contains a precipitate. Contains the labeled amount of isoetharine hydrochloride, within ±8%. Meets the requirements for Color and clarity, Identification, Sterility, and pH (2.5–5.5).
Isoetharine Hydrochloride USP—Preserve in tight containers. Contains not less than 97.0% and not more than 102.0% of isoetharine hydrochloride, calculated on the dried basis. Meets the requirements for Identification, pH (4.0–5.6, in a solution [1 in 100]), Loss on drying (not more than 1.0%), and Aromatic ketones.
Isoetharine Mesylate USP—Preserve in tight containers. Contains not less than 97.0% and not more than 102.0% of isoetharine mesylate, calculated on the dried basis. Meets the requirements for Identification, Melting range (162–168 °C), pH (4.5–5.5, in a solution [1 in 100]), Loss on drying (not more than 1.0%), and Limit of keto precursor.
Isoetharine Mesylate Inhalation Aerosol USP—Preserve in small, nonreactive, light-resistant, aerosol containers equipped with metered-dose valves and provided with oral inhalation actuators. A solution of Isoetharine Mesylate in Alcohol in an inert propellant base. Contains the labeled

amount, within ±10%. Meets the requirements for Identification, Alcohol content (25.9–35.0% [w/w]), and Dosage uniformity over the entire contents.

ISOFLUPREDONE

Chemical name: Isoflupredone acetate—Pregna-1,4-diene-3,20-dione, 21-(acetyloxy)-9-fluoro-11,17-dihydroxy-, (11 beta)-.

Molecular formula: Isoflupredone acetate—$C_{23}H_{29}FO_6$.

Molecular weight: Isoflupredone acetate—420.48.

Description: Isoflupredone acetate—Melting point 244–246 °C.

USP requirements:
Isoflupredone Acetate USP—Preserve in well-closed, light-resistant containers. Label it to indicate that it is intended for veterinary use only. Where it is intended to use in preparing injectable dosage forms, the label states that it is sterile or must be subjected to further processing during the preparation of injectable dosage forms. Contains not less than 97.0% and not more than 103.0% of isoflupredone acetate, calculated on the dried basis. Meets the requirements for Identification, Specific rotation (+110° to +120°), Bacterial endotoxins, Loss on drying (not more than 1.0%), Residue on ignition (not more than 0.5%), and Chromatographic purity, and for Sterility test (where the label states that it is sterile).
Sterile Isoflupredone Acetate Injection—Not in *USP–NF*.
Sterile Isoflupredone Acetate Aqueous Suspension—Not in *USP–NF*.
Isoflupredone Acetate Injectable Suspension USP—Preserve in single-dose or multiple-dose containers, preferably Type I glass. Label it to indicate that it is intended for veterinary use only. Contains the labeled amount, within –10% to +15%. Meets the requirements for Identification, Bacterial endotoxins, Sterility, and pH (5.0–7.5), and requirements under *Injections*.

ISOFLURANE

Chemical name: Ethane, 2-chloro-2-(difluoromethoxy)-1,1,1-trifluoro-.

Molecular formula: $C_3H_2ClF_5O$.

Molecular weight: 184.49.

Description: Isoflurane USP—Clear, colorless, volatile liquid, having a slight odor. Boils at about 49 °C.

Solubility: Isoflurane USP—Insoluble in water; miscible with common organic solvents and with fats and oils.

Other characteristics:
Blood-to-Gas partition coefficient at 37 °C—1.43.
Oil-to-Gas partition coefficient at 37 °C—90.8.

USP requirements: Isoflurane USP—Preserve in tight containers. Contains not less than 99.9% of isoflurane. Meets the requirements for Identification, Refractive index (1.2990–1.3005 at 20 °C), Water (not more than 0.10%), Chloride (not more than 0.001%), Nonvolatile residue, Limit of fluoride (not more than 0.001% [w/v]), and Related compounds.

ISOFLUROPHATE

Chemical name: Phosphorofluoridic acid, bis(1-methylethyl) ester.

Molecular formula: $C_6H_{14}FO_3P$.

Molecular weight: 184.15.

Description: Isoflurophate USP—Clear, colorless or faintly yellow, liquid. Its vapor is extremely irritating to the eye and mucous membranes. Is decomposed by moisture, with the formation of hydrogen fluoride. Specific gravity is about 1.05.

Solubility: Isoflurophate USP—Sparingly soluble in water; soluble in alcohol and in vegetable oils.

USP requirements:
Isoflurophate USP—Preserve in glass, fuse-sealed containers, or in other suitable sealed containers, in a cool place. Label it to indicate that in the handling of Isoflurophate in open containers, the eyes, nose, and mouth are to be protected with a suitable mask, and contact with the skin is to be avoided. Contains not less than 95.0% of isoflurophate. Meets the requirements for Identification, Acidity (not more than 0.01%), and Ionic fluorine (not more than 0.15%).
Caution—Handle Isoflurophate with exceptional care since it is very toxic. Wear full-face breathing apparatus and gloves. Open the container only in a hood.
Isoflurophate Ophthalmic Ointment USP—Preserve in collapsible ophthalmic ointment tubes. Label it to indicate the expiration date, which is not later than 2 years after date of manufacture. Contains not less than 0.0225% and not more than 0.0275% of isoflurophate, in a suitable anhydrous ointment base. It is sterile. Meets the requirements for Identification, Irritation, Sterility, Minimum fill, Water (not more than 0.03%), and Metal particles.

ISOLEUCINE

Chemical name: L-Isoleucine.

Molecular formula: $C_6H_{13}NO_2$.

Molecular weight: 131.17.

Description: Isoleucine USP—White, practically odorless crystals.

Solubility: Isoleucine USP—Soluble in water; slightly soluble in hot alcohol; insoluble in ether.

USP requirements: Isoleucine USP—Preserve in well-closed containers. Contains not less than 98.5% and not more than 101.5% of isoleucine, as L-isoleucine, calculated on the dried basis. Meets the requirements for Identification, Specific rotation ($+38.9°$ to $+41.8°$), pH (5.5–7.0, in a solution [1 in 100]), Loss on drying (not more than 0.3%), Residue on ignition (not more than 0.3%), Chloride (not more than 0.05%), Sulfate (not more than 0.03%), Iron (not more than 0.003%), Heavy metals (0.0015%), Chromatographic purity, and Organic volatile impurities.

ISOMETHEPTENE

Chemical name: Isometheptene mucate—Isometheptene, galactarate (2:1) (salt).

Molecular formula: Isometheptene mucate—$(C_9H_{19}N)_2 \cdot C_6H_{10}O_8$.

Molecular weight: Isometheptene mucate—492.65.

Description: Isometheptene Mucate USP—White, crystalline powder.

Solubility: Isometheptene Mucate USP—Freely soluble in water; soluble in alcohol; practically insoluble in chloroform and in ether.

USP requirements: Isometheptene Mucate USP—Preserve in well-closed containers. Contains not less than 99.0% and not more than 103.0% of isometheptene mucate, calculated on the dried basis. Meets the requirements for Identification, pH (6.0–7.5, in a solution [1 in 20]), Loss on drying (not more than 1.0%), and Residue on ignition (not more than 0.1%).

ISOMETHEPTENE, DICHLORALPHENAZONE, AND ACETAMINOPHEN

For *Isometheptene, Dichloralphenazone,* and *Acetaminophen*— See individual listings for chemistry information.

USP requirements: Isometheptene Mucate, Dichloralphenazone, and Acetaminophen Capsules USP—Preserve in well-closed containers. Contain the labeled amounts of isometheptene mucate and dichloralphenazone, within −15% to +10%, and the labeled amount of acetaminophen, within ±10%. Meet the requirements for Identification, Dissolution (65% of each active ingredient in 60 minutes in water in Apparatus 1 at 100 rpm), and Uniformity of dosage units.

ISONIAZID

Chemical group: Hydrazide derivative of isonicotinic acid.

Chemical name: 4-Pyridinecarboxylic acid, hydrazide.

Molecular formula: $C_6H_7N_3O$.

Molecular weight: 137.14.

Description:
Isoniazid USP—Colorless or white crystals or white, crystalline powder. Is odorless and is slowly affected by exposure to air and to light.
Isoniazid Injection USP—Clear, colorless to faintly greenish yellow liquid. Gradually darkens on exposure to air and to light. Tends to crystallize at low temperatures.

Solubility: Isoniazid USP—Freely soluble in water; sparingly soluble in alcohol; slightly soluble in chloroform; and very slightly soluble in ether.

USP requirements:
Isoniazid USP—Preserve in tight, light-resistant containers. Contains not less than 98.0% and not more than 102.0% of isoniazid, calculated on the dried basis. Meets the requirements for Identification, Melting range (170–173 °C), pH (6.0–7.5, in a solution [1 in 10]), Loss on drying (not more than 1.0%), Residue on ignition (not more than 0.2%), Heavy metals (not more than 0.002%), and Organic volatile impurities.
Isoniazid Injection USP—Preserve in single-dose or in multiple-dose containers, preferably of Type I glass, protected from light. A sterile solution of Isoniazid in Water for Injection. Its package label states that if crystallization has occurred, the Injection should be warmed to redissolve the crystals prior to use. Contains the labeled amount, within ±10%. Meets the requirements for Identification, Bacterial endotoxins, and pH (6.0–7.0), and for Injections.
Isoniazid Oral Solution USP—Preserve in tight, light-resistant containers. Contains, in each 100 mL, not less than 0.93 gram and not more than 1.10 grams of isoniazid. Meets the requirement for Identification.

Isoniazid Syrup USP—Preserve in tight, light-resistant containers. Contains, in each 100 mL, not less than 0.93 gram and not more than 1.10 grams of isoniazid. Meets the requirement for Identification.

Isoniazid Tablets USP—Preserve in well-closed, light-resistant containers. Contain the labeled amount, within ± 10%. Meet the requirements for Identification, Dissolution (80% in 45 minutes in 0.01 N hydrochloric acid in Apparatus 1 at 100 rpm), and Uniformity of dosage units.

ISONIAZID AND THIACETAZONE

Chemical group: Isoniazid—Hydrazide derivative of isonicotinic acid.

Chemical name:
Isoniazid—4-Pyridinecarboxylic acid, hydrazide.
Thiacetazone—4-Acetamidobenzaldehyde thiosemicarbazone.

Molecular formula:
Isoniazid—$C_6H_7N_3O$.
Thiacetazone—$C_{10}H_{12}N_4OS$.

Molecular weight:
Isoniazid—137.14.
Thiacetazone—236.3.

Description:
Isoniazid USP—Colorless or white crystals or white, crystalline powder. Is odorless and is slowly affected by exposure to air and to light.
Thiacetazone—Minute, pale yellow crystals. Darkens on exposure to light.

Solubility:
Isoniazid USP—Freely soluble in water; sparingly soluble in alcohol; slightly soluble in chloroform; and very slightly soluble in ether.
Thiacetazone—Soluble in hot alcohol; very sparingly soluble in cold alcohol; insoluble in water, in acetone, in carbon tetrachloride, in chloroform, in carbon disulfide, and in petroleum ether; practically insoluble in other common organic solvents except glycols; solubility in propylene glycol about 1%.

USP requirements: Isoniazid and Thiacetazone Tablets—Not in *USP–NF*.

ISOPROPAMIDE

Chemical group: Quaternary ammonium compound, synthetic.

Chemical name: Isopropamide iodide—Benzenepropanaminium, gamma-(aminocarbonyl)-N-methyl-N,N-bis(1-methylethyl)-gamma-phenyl-, iodide.

Molecular formula: Isopropamide iodide—$C_{23}H_{33}IN_2O$.

Molecular weight: Isopropamide iodide—480.43.

Description: Isopropamide Iodide USP—White to pale yellow, crystalline powder.

Solubility: Isopropamide Iodide USP—Sparingly soluble in water; freely soluble in chloroform and in alcohol; very slightly soluble in ether.

USP requirements:
Isopropamide Iodide USP—Preserve in well-closed, light-resistant containers. Dried in vacuum at 60 °C for 2 hours, contains not less than 98.0% and not more than 101.0% of isopropamide iodide. Meets the requirements for Identification, Loss on drying (not more than 1.0%), Residue on

ignition (not more than 0.5%), Heavy metals (not more than 0.002%), Ordinary impurities, and Organic volatile impurities.

Isopropamide Iodide Tablets USP—Preserve in well-closed containers. Contain an amount of isopropamide iodide equivalent to the labeled amount of isopropamide, within ±7%. Meet the requirements for Identification, Dissolution (70% in 60 minutes in water in Apparatus 2 at 100 rpm), and Uniformity of dosage units.

ISOPROPYL ALCOHOL

Chemical name: 2-Propanol.

Molecular formula: C_3H_8O.

Molecular weight: 60.10.

Description: Isopropyl Alcohol USP—Transparent, colorless, mobile, volatile liquid, having a characteristic odor. Is flammable.
NF category: Solvent.

Solubility: Isopropyl Alcohol USP—Miscible with water, with alcohol, with ether, and with chloroform.

USP requirements: Isopropyl Alcohol USP—Preserve in tight containers, remote from heat. Contains not less than 99.0% of isopropyl alcohol. Meets the requirements for Identification, Specific gravity (0.783–0.787), Refractive index (1.376–1.378 at 20 °C), Acidity, and Limit of nonvolatile residue (not more than 0.005%).

AZEOTROPIC ISOPROPYL ALCOHOL

Description: Azeotropic Isopropyl Alcohol USP—Transparent, colorless, mobile, volatile liquid, having a characteristic odor. Is flammable.

Solubility: Azeotropic Isopropyl Alcohol USP—Miscible with water, with alcohol, with ether, and with chloroform.

USP requirements: Azeotropic Isopropyl Alcohol USP—Preserve in tight containers, remote from heat. Contains not less than 91.0% and not more than 93.0% of isopropyl alcohol, by volume, the remainder consisting of water. Meets the requirements for Identification, Specific gravity (0.815–0.810, indicating 91.0–93.0% by volume of isopropyl alcohol), Refractive index (1.376–1.378 at 20 °C), Acidity, Limit of nonvolatile residue (not more than 0.005%), and Volatile impurities.

ISOPROPYL MYRISTATE

Chemical name: Tetradecanoic acid, 1-methylethyl ester.

Molecular formula: $C_{17}H_{34}O_2$.

Molecular weight: 270.45.

Description: Isopropyl Myristate NF—Clear, practically colorless, oily liquid. It is practically odorless and congeals at about 5 °C.
NF category: Vehicle (oleaginous).

Solubility: Isopropyl Myristate NF—Insoluble in water, in glycerin, and in propylene glycol; freely soluble in 90% alcohol; miscible with most organic solvents and with fixed oils.

NF requirements: Isopropyl Myristate NF—Preserve in tight, light-resistant containers. Consists of esters of isopropyl alcohol and saturated high molecular weight fatty acids, principally myristic acid. Contains not less than 90.0% of isopropyl myristate. Meets the requirements for Identification, Specific gravity (0.846–0.854), Refractive index (1.432–1.436 at 20 °C), Residue on ignition (not more than 0.1%), Organic volatile impurities, Acid value (not more than 1), Saponification value (202–212), and Iodine value (not more than 1).

ISOPROPYL PALMITATE

Chemical name: Hexadecanoic acid, 1-methylethyl ester.

Molecular formula: $C_{19}H_{38}O_2$.

Molecular weight: 298.50.

Description: Isopropyl Palmitate NF—Colorless, mobile liquid having a very slight odor.
NF category: Vehicle (oleaginous).

Solubility: Isopropyl Palmitate NF—Soluble in acetone, in castor oil, in chloroform, in cottonseed oil, in ethyl acetate, in alcohol, and in mineral oil; insoluble in water, in glycerin, and in propylene glycol.

NF requirements: Isopropyl Palmitate NF—Preserve in tight, light-resistant containers. Consists of esters of isopropyl alcohol and saturated high molecular weight fatty acids. Contains not less than 90.0% of isopropyl palmitate. Meets the requirements for Identification, Specific gravity (0.850–0.855), Refractive index (1.435–1.438), Residue on ignition (not more than 0.1%), Organic volatile impurities, Acid value (not more than 1), Iodine value (not more than 1), and Saponification value (183–193).

ISOPROPYL RUBBING ALCOHOL

USP requirements: Isopropyl Rubbing Alcohol USP—Preserve in tight containers, remote from heat. Label it to indicate that it is flammable. Contains not less than 68.0% and not more than 72.0% of isopropyl alcohol, by volume, the remainder consisting of water, with or without suitable stabilizers, perfume oils, and color additives certified by the U.S. Food and Drug Administration for use in drugs. Meets the requirements for Specific gravity (0.872–0.883 at 20 °C), Acidity, and Limit of nonvolatile residue (not more than 0.01%).

ISOPROTERENOL

Chemical name:
Isoproterenol hydrochloride—1,2-Benzenediol, 4-[1-hydroxy-2-[(1-methylethyl)amino]ethyl]-, hydrochloride.
Isoproterenol sulfate—1,2-Benzenediol, 4-[1-hydroxy-2-[(methylethyl)amino]ethyl]-, sulfate (2:1) (salt), dihydrate.

Molecular formula:
Isoproterenol hydrochloride—$C_{11}H_{17}NO_3 \cdot HCl$.
Isoproterenol sulfate—$(C_{11}H_{17}NO_3)_2 \cdot H_2SO_4 \cdot 2H_2O.(C_{11}H_{17}NO_3)_2 \cdot H_2SO_4 \cdot 2H_2O$.

Molecular weight:
Isoproterenol hydrochloride—247.73.
Isoproterenol sulfate—556.64.

Description:
Isoproterenol Inhalation Solution USP—Colorless or practically colorless, slightly acid liquid, gradually turning dark on exposure to air and to light.
Isoproterenol Hydrochloride USP—White to practically white, odorless, crystalline powder. Gradually darkens on exposure to air and to light. Its solutions become pink to brownish pink on standing exposed to air, and almost immediately so when rendered alkaline. Its solution (1 in 100) has a pH of about 5.
Isoproterenol Hydrochloride Injection USP—Colorless or practically colorless liquid, gradually turning dark on exposure to air and to light.
Isoproterenol Sulfate USP—White to practically white, odorless, crystalline powder. It gradually darkens on exposure to air and to light. Its solutions become pink to brownish pink on standing exposed to air, doing so almost immediately when rendered alkaline. A solution (1 in 100) has a pH of about 5.

Solubility:
Isoproterenol Hydrochloride USP—Freely soluble in water; sparingly soluble in alcohol and less soluble in dehydrated alcohol; insoluble in chloroform and in ether.
Isoproterenol Sulfate USP—Freely soluble in water; very slightly soluble in alcohol and in ether.

USP requirements:
Isoproterenol Inhalation Solution USP—Preserve in small, tight containers that are well-filled or otherwise protected from oxidation. Protect from light. A sterile solution of Isoproterenol Hydrochloride in Purified Water. Label it to indicate that the Inhalation Solution is not to be used if its color is pinkish or darker than slightly yellow or if it contains a precipitate. Contains the labeled amount of isoproterenol hydrochloride, within −10% to +15%. It may contain Sodium Chloride. Meets the requirements for Color and clarity, Identification, Sterility, and pH (2.5–5.5).
Isoproterenol Hydrochloride USP—Preserve in tight, light-resistant containers. Contains not less than 97.0% and not more than 101.5% of isoproterenol hydrochloride, calculated on the dried basis. Meets the requirements for Identification, Melting range (165–170 °C), Loss on drying (not more than 1.0%), Residue on ignition (not more than 0.2%), Sulfate (not more than 0.2%), Limit of isoproterenone, Organic volatile impurities, and Chloride content (13.9–14.6%, calculated on the dried basis).
Isoproterenol Hydrochloride Inhalation Aerosol USP—Preserve in small, nonreactive, light-resistant aerosol containers equipped with metered-dose valves and provided with oral inhalation actuators. A solution of Isoproterenol Hydrochloride in Alcohol in an inert propellant base. Contains the labeled amount, within −10% to +15%. Meets the requirements for Identification, Alcohol content (28.5–38.5% [w/w]), and Dosage uniformity over the entire contents.
Isoproterenol Hydrochloride Injection USP—Preserve in single-dose containers, preferably of Type I glass, protected from light. Label it to indicate that the Injection is not to be used if its color is pinkish or darker than slightly yellow or if it contains a precipitate. A sterile solution of Isoproterenol Hydrochloride in Water for Injection. Contains the labeled amount, within −10% to +15%. Meets the requirements for Color and clarity, Identification, Bacterial endotoxins, pH (2.5–4.5), and Particulate matter, and for Injections.
Isoproterenol Hydrochloride Tablets USP—Preserve in well-closed, light-resistant containers. Contain the labeled amount, within ±7%. Meet the requirements for Identification, Dissolution (75% in 45 minutes in water in Apparatus 2 at 50 rpm), and Uniformity of dosage units.
Isoproterenol Sulfate USP—Preserve in tight, light-resistant containers. Contains not less than 97.0% and not more than 103.0% of isoproterenol sulfate, calculated on the anhydrous basis. Meets the requirements for Identification,

Water (not more than 7.0%), Residue on ignition (not more than 0.2%), Chloride (not more than 0.14%), Limit of isoproterenone, and Organic volatile impurities.

Isoproterenol Sulfate Inhalation Aerosol USP—Preserve in small, nonreactive, light-resistant aerosol containers equipped with metered-dose valves and provided with oral inhalation actuators. A suspension of microfine Isoproterenol Sulfate in fluorochlorohydrocarbon propellants in a pressurized container. Contains the labeled amount within ±10%, and delivers the labeled dose per inhalation, within ±25%, through an oral inhalation actuator. Meets the requirements for Identification, Microbial limits, Unit spray content, and Particle size, and for Leak testing under Aerosols.

Isoproterenol Sulfate Inhalation Solution USP—Store in small, tight containers that are well-filled or otherwise protected from oxidation. Protect from light. A sterile solution of Isoproterenol Sulfate in Purified Water. Label it to indicate that the Inhalation Solution is not to be used if its color is pinkish or darker than slightly yellow or if it contains a precipitate. Contains the labeled amount, within −10% to +15%. Meets the requirements for Color and clarity, Sterility, and Identification.

ISOPROTERENOL AND PHENYLEPHRINE

Chemical name: Isoproterenol hydrochloride—1,2-Benzenediol, 4-[1-hydroxy-2-[(1-methylethyl)amino]ethyl]-, hydrochloride.

Molecular formula:
Isoproterenol hydrochloride—$C_{11}H_{17}NO_3 \cdot HCl$.
Phenylephrine bitartrate—$C_9H_{13}NO_2 \cdot C_4H_6O_6$.

Molecular weight:
Isoproterenol hydrochloride—247.72.
Phenylephrine bitartrate—317.29.

Description:
Isoproterenol Hydrochloride USP—White to practically white, odorless, crystalline powder. Gradually darkens on exposure to air and to light. Its solutions become pink to brownish pink on standing exposed to air, and almost immediately so when rendered alkaline. Its solution (1 in 100) has a pH of about 5.
Phenylephrine bitartrate—White, crystalline powder.

Solubility:
Isoproterenol Hydrochloride USP—Freely soluble in water; sparingly soluble in alcohol and less soluble in dehydrated alcohol; insoluble in chloroform and in ether.
Phenylephrine bitartrate—Soluble in water; insoluble in alcohol.

USP requirements: Isoproterenol Hydrochloride and Phenylephrine Bitartrate Inhalation Aerosol USP—Preserve in small, non-reactive, light-resistant aerosol containers equipped with metered-dose valves and provided with oral inhalation actuators. A suspension of microfine Isoproterenol Hydrochloride and Phenylephrine Bitartrate in suitable propellants in a pressurized container. Contains the labeled amounts, within ±10%. Meets the requirements for Identification, Particle size, and Dosage uniformity over the entire contents.

ISOSORBIDE

Chemical name:
Isosorbide—D-Glucitol, 1,4:3,6-dianhydro-.
Isosorbide dinitrate—D-Glucitol, 1,4:3,6-dianhydro-, dinitrate.
Isosorbide mononitrate—D-Glucitol, 1,4:3,6-dianhydro-, 5-nitrate.

Molecular formula:
Isosorbide—$C_6H_{10}O_4$.
Isosorbide dinitrate—$C_6H_8N_2O_8$.
Isosorbide mononitrate—$C_6H_9NO_6$.

Molecular weight:
Isosorbide—146.14.
Isosorbide dinitrate—236.14.
Isosorbide mononitrate—191.14.

Description:
Isosorbide Concentrate USP—Colorless to slightly yellow liquid.
Diluted Isosorbide Dinitrate USP—Ivory-white, odorless powder. (Note: Undiluted isosorbide dinitrate occurs as white, crystalline rosettes.)

Solubility:
Isosorbide Concentrate USP—Soluble in water and in alcohol.
Undiluted isosorbide dinitrate—Very slightly soluble in water; very soluble in acetone; freely soluble in chloroform; sparingly soluble in alcohol.

USP requirements:
Isosorbide Concentrate USP—Preserve in tight, light-resistant containers. An aqueous solution. The label states that this article is not intended for direct administration to humans or animals. Contains, in each 100 grams, not less than 70.0 grams and not more than 80.0 grams of isosorbide. Meets the requirements for Identification, Specific rotation (+44.5° to +47.0°), Water (24.0–26.0%), Residue on ignition (not more than 0.01%), Heavy metals (not more than 5 ppm, calculated on the anhydrous basis), Periodate consumption, Acid value (not more than 0.5, calculated on the anhydrous basis), and Methyl ethyl ketone (not more than 0.05 mg per mL).

Isosorbide Oral Solution USP—Preserve in tight containers. Contains the labeled amount, within ±10%. Meets the requirements for Identification and pH (3.2–3.8).

Diluted Isosorbide Dinitrate USP—Preserve in tight containers. A dry mixture of isosorbide dinitrate with Lactose, Mannitol, or suitable inert excipients to permit safe handling. Contains the labeled amount of isosorbide dinitrate, within ±5%. Usually contains approximately 25% of isosorbide dinitrate. Meets the requirements for Identification, Loss on drying (not more than 1.0%), Heavy metals (not more than 0.001%), and Organic volatile impurities.

Caution: Exercise proper precautions in handling undiluted isosorbide dinitrate, which is a powerful explosive and can be exploded by percussion or excessive heat. Only exceedingly small amounts should be isolated.

Isosorbide Dinitrate Capsules—Not in *USP–NF*.

Isosorbide Dinitrate Extended-release Capsules USP—Preserve in well-closed containers. Contain the labeled amount, within ±10%. Meet the requirements for Identification, Drug release, and Uniformity of dosage units.

Isosorbide Dinitrate Tablets USP—Preserve in well-closed containers. Contain the labeled amount, within ±10%. Meet the requirements for Identification, Dissolution (70% in 45 minutes in water in Apparatus 2 at 75 rpm), and Uniformity of dosage units.

Isosorbide Dinitrate Chewable Tablets USP—Preserve in well-closed containers. Contain the labeled amount, within ±10%. Meet the requirements for Identification and Uniformity of dosage units.

Isosorbide Dinitrate Extended-release Tablets USP—Preserve in well-closed containers. Contain the labeled amount, within ±10%. Meet the requirements for Identification, Drug release (15–30% in 1 hour, 50–70% in 2 hours, 65–85% in 4 hours, and not less than 75% in 6 hours in water in Apparatus 2 at 50 rpm), and Uniformity of dosage units.

Isosorbide Dinitrate Sublingual Tablets USP—Preserve in well-closed containers. Contain the labeled amount, within ±10%. Meet the requirements for Identification, Disinte-

gration (2 minutes), Dissolution (80% in 20 minutes in water in Apparatus 2 at 50 rpm), and Uniformity of dosage units.

Isosorbide Mononitrate Tablets—Not in *USP–NF*.

Isosorbide Mononitrate Extended-release Tablets—Not in *USP–NF*.

ISOTRETINOIN

Chemical group: Vitamin A derivative (retinoid).

Chemical name: Retinoic acid, 13-*cis*-.

Molecular formula: $C_{20}H_{28}O_2$.

Molecular weight: 300.44.

Description: Isotretinoin USP—Yellow crystals.

Solubility: Isotretinoin USP—Practically insoluble in water; soluble in chloroform; sparingly soluble in alcohol, in isopropyl alcohol, and in polyethylene glycol 400.

USP requirements:

Isotretinoin USP—Preserve in tight containers, under an atmosphere of an inert gas, protected from light. Contains not less than 98.0% and not more than 102.0% of isotretinoin, calculated on the dried basis. Meets the requirements for Identification, Loss on drying (not more than 0.5%), Residue on ignition (not more than 0.1%), Heavy metals (not more than 0.002%), Limit of tretinoin (not more than 1.0%), and Organic volatile impurities.

Caution—Isotretinoin is teratogenic. Avoid inhalation and skin contact.

Isotretinoin Capsules USP—Preserve in tight containers, protected from light. Store at controlled room temperature, in a dry place. Contain the labeled amount, within ±10%. Meet the requirements for Identification, Uniformity of dosage units, and Chromatographic purity.

Caution—Isotretinoin is teratogenic. Avoid inhalation and skin contact.

Isotretinoin Gel—Not in *USP–NF*.

ISOXSUPRINE

Chemical name: Isoxsuprine hydrochloride—Benzenemethanol, 4-hydroxy-alpha-[1-[(1-methyl-2-phenoxyethyl)amino]ethyl]-, hydrochloride, stereoisomer.

Molecular formula: Isoxsuprine hydrochloride—$C_{18}H_{23}NO_3 \cdot HCl$.

Molecular weight: Isoxsuprine hydrochloride—337.84.

Description: Isoxsuprine Hydrochloride USP—White, odorless, crystalline powder. Melts, with decomposition, at about 200 °C.

Solubility: Isoxsuprine Hydrochloride USP—Slightly soluble in water; sparingly soluble in alcohol.

USP requirements:

Isoxsuprine Hydrochloride USP—Preserve in tight containers. Contains not less than 97.0% and not more than 103.0% of isoxsuprine hydrochloride, calculated on the dried basis. Meets the requirements for Identification, pH (4.5–6.0, in a solution [1 in 100]), Loss on drying (not more than 0.5%), Residue on ignition (not more than 0.2%), Heavy metals (not more than 0.002%), Related compounds (not more than 2.0%), and Organic volatile impurities.

Isoxsuprine Hydrochloride Injection USP—Preserve in single-dose or in multiple-dose containers, preferably of Type I glass. A sterile solution of Isoxsuprine Hydrochloride in Water for Injection. Contains the labeled amount, within ±5%. Meets the requirements for Identification, Bacterial endotoxins, and pH (4.9–6.0), and for Injections.

Isoxsuprine Hydrochloride Tablets USP—Preserve in tight containers. Contain the labeled amount, within ±7%. Meet the requirements for Identification, Dissolution (75% in 45 minutes in water in Apparatus 1 at 100 rpm), and Uniformity of dosage units.

ISRADIPINE

Chemical name: 3,5-Pyridinedicarboxylic acid, 4-(4-benzofuranzanyl)-1,4-dihydro-2,6-dimethyl-, methyl 1-methylethyl ester, (±)-.

Molecular formula: $C_{19}H_{21}N_3O_5$.

Molecular weight: 371.39.

Description: Isradipine USP—Yellow, fine crystalline powder.

Solubility: Practically insoluble in water; soluble in ethanol; freely soluble in acetone, in chloroform, and in methylene chloride.

USP requirements:

Isradipine USP—Preserve in well-closed, light-resistant containers. Contains not less than 98.0% and not more than 102.0%, calculated on the dried basis. Meets the requirements for Identification, Melting range (166–170 °C), Loss on drying (not more than 0.2%), Residue on ignition (not more than 0.1%), Heavy metals (not more than 0.002%), and Chromatographic purity.

Isradipine Capsules—Not in *USP–NF*.

Isradipine Extended-release Tablets—Not in *USP–NF*.

ITRACONAZOLE

Chemical name: 3*H*-1,2,4-Triazol-3-one, 4-[4-[4-[4-[[2-(2,4-dichlorophenyl)-2-(1*H*-1,2,4-triazol-1-ylmethyl)-1,3-dioxolan-4-yl]methoxy]phenyl]-1-piperazinyl]phenyl]-2,4-dihydro-2-(1-methylpropyl)-.

Molecular formula: $C_{35}H_{38}Cl_2N_8O_4$.

Molecular weight: 705.63.

Description: White to slightly yellowish powder.

pKa: 3.70.

Solubility: Insoluble in water at pH 1–12; very slightly soluble in alcohols; freely soluble in dichloromethane.

Other characteristics: Log (n-octanol/water partition coefficient)—5.66 at pH 8.1.

USP requirements:

Itraconazole Capsules—Not in *USP–NF*.

Intraconazole Injection—Not in *USP–NF*.

Itraconazole Oral Solution—Not in *USP–NF*.

IVERMECTIN

Source: Semisynthetic macrocyclic lactone produced by the actinomycete *Streptomyces avermitilis.*

Chemical group: Avermectins.

Other characteristics: A mixture of Ivermectin component B_{1a} and Ivermectin component B_{1b}.

USP requirements: Ivermectin Tablets—Not in *USP–NF.*

JAPANESE ENCEPHALITIS VIRUS VACCINE INACTIVATED

Source: Prepared by inoculating mice intracerebrally with Japanese encephalitis (JE) virus, "Nakayama-NIH" strain, manufactured by The Research Foundation for Microbial Diseases of Osaka University. Infected brains are harvested and homogenized in phosphate buffer saline, pH 8.0. The homogenate is centrifuged and the supernatant inactivated with formaldehyde, then processed to yield a partially purified, inactivated virus suspension. This is further purified by ultracentrifugation through 40 w/v% sucrose.

USP requirements: Japanese Encephalitis Virus Vaccine Inactivated for Injection—Not in *USP–NF.*

JAPANESE ENCEPHALITIS VIRUS VACCINE (LIVE, ATTENUATED)

Source: Derived from primary hamster kidney (PHK) cells and produced from the SA14-14-2 viral strain.

USP requirements: Japanese encephalitis Virus Vaccine (Live, Attenuated)—Not in *USP–NF.*

JUNIPER TAR

Description: Juniper Tar USP—Dark brown, clear, thick liquid, having a tarry odor.

Solubility: Juniper Tar USP—Very slightly soluble in water; partially soluble in solvent hexane. One volume dissolves in 9 volumes of alcohol. Dissolves in 3 volumes of ether, leaving only a slight, flocculent residue. Miscible with amyl alcohol, with chloroform, and with glacial acetic acid.

USP requirements: Juniper Tar USP—Preserve in tight, light-resistant containers, and avoid exposure to excessive heat. The empyreumatic volatile oil obtained from the woody portions of *Juniperus oxycedrus* Linné (Fam. Pinaceae). Meets the requirements for Identification, Specific gravity (0.950–1.055), Reaction, and Rosin or rosin oils.

KANAMYCIN

Source: Derived from *Streptomyces kanamyceticus.*

Chemical group: Aminoglycosides.

Chemical name: Kanamycin sulfate—D-Streptamine, *O*-3-amino-3-deoxy-alpha-D-glucopyranosyl(1→6)-*O*-[6-amino-6-deoxy-alpha-D-glucopyranosyl(1→4)]-2-deoxy-, sulfate (1:1) (salt).

Molecular formula: Kanamycin sulfate—$C_{18}H_{36}N_4O_{11} \cdot H_2SO_4$.

Molecular weight: Kanamycin sulfate—582.58.

Description: Kanamycin Sulfate USP—White, odorless, crystalline powder.

Solubility: Kanamycin Sulfate USP—Freely soluble in water; insoluble in acetone and in ethyl acetate.

USP requirements:

Kanamycin Injection USP—Preserve in single-dose or in multiple-dose containers, preferably of Type I or Type III glass. Contains suitable buffers and preservatives. Contains an amount of Kanamycin Sulfate equivalent to the labeled amount of kanamycin, within −10% to +15%. Meets the requirements for Identification, Bacterial endotoxins, Sterility, pH (3.5–5.0), and Particulate matter and for Injections.

Kanamycin Sulfate USP—Preserve in tight containers. Where it is intended for use in preparing injectable dosage forms, the label states that it is sterile or must be subjected to further processing during the preparation of injectable dosage forms. Has a potency equivalent to not less than 750 mcg of kanamycin per mg, calculated on the dried basis. Meets the requirements for Identification, Crystallinity, pH (6.5–8.5, in a solution [1 in 100]), Loss on drying (not more than 4.0%), Residue on ignition (not more than 1.0%), and Chromatographic purity, and for Sterility and Bacterial endotoxins under Kanamycin Injection (where the label states that Kanamycin Sulfate is sterile) and for Bacterial endotoxins under Kanamycin Injection (where the label states that Kanamycin Sulfate must be subjected to further processing during the preparation of injectable dosage forms).

Kanamycin Sulfate Capsules USP—Preserve in tight containers. Contain an amount of kanamycin sulfate equivalent to the labeled amount of kanamycin, within −10% to +15%. Meet the requirements for Thin-layer chromatographic identification test, Dissolution (75% in 45 minutes in 0.01 *N* hydrochloric acid in Apparatus 1 at 100 rpm), and Loss on drying (not more than 4.0%).

KAOLIN

Description: Kaolin USP—Soft, white or yellowish white powder or lumps. When moistened with water, it assumes a darker color and develops a marked clay-like odor.

NF category: Tablet and/or capsule diluent.

Solubility: Kaolin USP—Insoluble in water, in cold, dilute acids, and in solutions of alkali hydroxides.

USP requirements: Kaolin USP—Preserve in well-closed containers. A native hydrated aluminum silicate, powdered and freed from gritty particles by elutriation. Meets the requirements for Identification, Microbial limit, Loss on ignition (not more than 15.0%), Acid-soluble substances (not more than 2.0%), Carbonate, Iron, Lead (not more than 0.001%), and Organic volatile impurities.

KAOLIN AND PECTIN

For *Kaolin* and *Pectin*—See individual listings for chemistry information.

USP requirements: Kaolin and Pectin Oral Suspension—Not in *USP–NF.*

KAOLIN, PECTIN, HYOSCYAMINE, ATROPINE, AND SCOPOLAMINE

For *Kaolin, Pectin, Hyoscyamine, Atropine,* and *Scopolamine*— See individual listings for chemistry information.

USP requirements: Kaolin, Pectin, Hyoscyamine Sulfate, Atropine Sulfate, and Scopolamine Hydrobromide Oral Suspension—Not in *USP–NF*.

KAOLIN, PECTIN, AND PAREGORIC

For *Kaolin, Pectin,* and *Paregoric*—See individual listings for chemistry information.

USP requirements: Kaolin, Pectin, and Paregoric Oral Suspension—Not in *USP–NF*.

KETAMINE

Chemical name: Ketamine hydrochloride—Cyclohexanone, 2-(2-chlorophenyl)-2-(methylamino)-, hydrochloride.

Molecular formula: Ketamine hydrochloride—$C_{13}H_{16}ClNO \cdot HCl$.

Molecular weight: Ketamine hydrochloride—274.19.

Description: Ketamine Hydrochloride USP—White, crystalline powder, having a slight, characteristic odor.

Solubility: Ketamine Hydrochloride USP—Freely soluble in water and in methanol; soluble in alcohol; sparingly soluble in chloroform.

USP requirements:
Ketamine Hydrochloride USP—Preserve in well-closed containers. Contains not less than 98.0% and not more than 102.0% of ketamine hydrochloride. Meets the requirements for Clarity and color of solution, Identification, pH (3.5–4.1, in a solution [1 in 10]), Residue on ignition (not more than 0.1%), Heavy metals (not more than 0.002%), and Related compounds.
Ketamine Hydrochloride Injection USP—Preserve in single-dose or in multiple-dose containers, preferably of Type I glass, protected from light and heat. A sterile solution of Ketamine Hydrochloride in Water for Injection. Contains an amount of ketamine hydrochloride equivalent to the labeled amount of ketamine, within ±5%. Meets the requirements for Identification, Bacterial endotoxins, and pH (3.5–5.5), and for Injections.

KETAZOLAM

Chemical name: 4*H*-[1,3]-Oxazino[3,2-*d*][1,4]benzodiazepine-4,7(6*H*)-dione, 11-chloro-8,12b-dihydro-2,8-dimethyl-.

Molecular formula: $C_{20}H_{17}ClN_2O_3$.

Molecular weight: 368.81.

Description: Melting point 182–183.5 °C.

USP requirements: Ketazolam Capsules—Not in *USP–NF*.

KETOCONAZOLE

Chemical group: Imidazoles.

Chemical name: Piperazine, 1-acetyl-4-[4-[[2-(2,4-dichlorophenyl)-2-(1*H*-imidazol-1-ylmethyl)-1,3-dioxolan-4-yl]methoxy]phenyl]-, *cis*-.

Molecular formula: $C_{26}H_{28}Cl_2N_4O_4$.

Molecular weight: 531.43.

Description: Almost white to slightly beige powder.

Solubility: Freely soluble in chloroform, in methanol, and in diluted hydrochloric acid; sparingly soluble in isopropyl alcohol and in acetone; practically insoluble in water.

Other characteristics: Weakly dibasic; requires acidity for dissolution and absorption.

USP requirements:
Ketoconazole USP—Preserve in well-closed containers. Contains not less than 98.0% and not more than 102.0% of ketoconazole, calculated on the dried basis. Meets the requirements for Identification, Melting range (148–152 °C), Specific rotation (−1° to +1°, at 20 °C), Loss on drying (not more than 0.5%), Residue on ignition (not more than 0.1% from 2 grams), Heavy metals (not more than 0.002%), Chromatographic purity, and Organic volatile impurities.
Ketoconazole Cream—Not in *USP–NF*.
Ketoconazole Shampoo—Not in *USP–NF*.
Ketoconazole Oral Suspension USP—Preserve in tight, light-resistant amber containers. Store at controlled room temperature. Label it to state that it is to be well shaken before using and that it is to be protected from light. Contains not less than 1.8 grams and not more than 2.2 grams of Ketoconazole in 100 mL of Oral Suspension. Use Ketoconazole or the number of Ketoconazole Tablets that contain the designated amount of Ketoconazole, and prepare Ketoconazole Oral Suspension as follows: 2.0 grams Ketoconazole, 10 mg Cetylpyridinium Chloride, 0.15 gram Xanthan Gum, 30 mL Purified Water, and Suspension Structured Vehicle or Sugar-free Suspension Structured Vehicle, a sufficient quantity, to make 100 mL. Transfer the Ketoconazole, or Ketoconazole Tablets, to a glass mortar. If Tablets are used, finely powder the Tablets such that they pass through a 40-mesh or 45-mesh sieve, and place the sieved portion in the glass mortar. Dissolve an accurately weighed quantity of Cetylpyridinium Chloride in Purified Water and dilute quantitatively, and stepwise if necessary, with Purified Water to obtain 10 mL of a solution containing 10 mg of Cetylpyridinium Chloride. Transfer this solution, in divided portions, to the mortar containing the powder, and mix to form a smooth paste. Place 20 mL of Purified Water in a beaker. Using moderate heat, stir to form a vortex, and slowly sprinkle the Xanthan Gum into the vortex to obtain a uniform dispersion. Add the dispersion to the wetted powder paste, and mix until smooth. Add a sufficient quantity of the Suspension Structured Vehicle or Sugar-free Suspension Structured Vehicle to make a final volume of 100 mL, and mix. Meets the requirement for Beyond use date.
Ketoconazole Tablets USP—Preserve in well-closed containers. Contain the labeled amount, within ±10%. Meet the requirements for Identification, Disintegration (10 minutes), and Uniformity of dosage units.

KETOPROFEN

Chemical group: Propionic acid derivative.

Chemical name: Benzeneacetic acid, 3-benzoyl-alpha-methyl-, (±)-.

Molecular formula: $C_{16}H_{14}O_3$.

Molecular weight: 254.28.

Description: White or off-white, odorless, nonhygroscopic, fine to granular powder. Melts at about 95 °C.

Solubility: Freely soluble in ethanol, in chloroform, in acetone, and in ether; soluble in strong alkali; practically insoluble in water at 20 °C.

Other characteristics: Highly lipophilic.

USP requirements:

Ketoprofen USP—Preserve in tight containers. Contains not less than 98.5% and not more than 101.0% of ketoprofen, calculated on the dried basis. Meets the requirements for Identification, Melting range (92.0–97.0 °C), Loss on drying (not more than 0.5%), Specific rotation (+1° to –1°), Residue on ignition (not more than 0.2%), Heavy metals (not more than 0.002%), Chromatographic purity (not more than 0.2% of any individual impurity, and the sum of all impurities not more than 1.0%), and Organic volatile impurities.

Ketoprofen Capsules—Not in *USP–NF*.

Ketoprofen Extended-release Capsules—Not in *USP–NF*.

Ketoprofen Suppositories—Not in *USP–NF*.

Ketoprofen Tablets—Not in *USP–NF*.

Ketoprofen Delayed-release Tablets—Not in *USP–NF*.

Ketoprofen Extended-release Tablets—Not in *USP–NF*.

KETOROLAC

Chemical name: Ketorolac tromethamine—1*H*-Pyrrolizine-1-carboxylic acid, 5-benzoyl-2,3-dihydro, (±)-, compound with 2-amino-2-(hydroxymethyl)-1,3-propanediol (1:1).

Molecular formula: Ketorolac tromethamine—$C_{15}H_{13}NO_3 \cdot C_4H_{11}NO_3$.

Molecular weight: Ketorolac tromethamine—376.40.

Description:

Ketorolac Tromethamine USP—White to off-white, crystalline powder. Melts at 165°–170°, with decomposition.

Ketorolac tromethamine injection—Clear and slightly yellow in color.

pKa: Ketorolac tromethamine—3.54.

Solubility: Ketorolac Tromethamine USP—Freely soluble in water and in methanol; slightly soluble in alcohol, in dehydrated alcohol, and in tetrahydrofuran; practically insoluble in acetone, in dichloronmethane, in toluene, in ethyl acetate, in dioxane, in hexane, in butyl alcohol, and in acetonitrile.

Other characteristics: Ketorolac tromethamine—*n*-Octanol: water partition coefficient: 0.26.

USP requirements:

Ketorolac Tromethamine USP—Preserve in tight, light-resistant containers. Contains not less than 98.5% and not more than 101.5% of ketorolac tromethamine, calculated on the dried basis. Meets the requirements for Identification, pH (5.7–6.7, in a solution [1 in 100]), Loss on drying (not more than 0.5%), Residue on ignition (not more than 0.1%), Heavy metals (not more than 0.002%), Organic volatile impurities, and Chromatographic purity.

Ketorolac Tromethamine Injection USP—Preserve in single-dose containers, preferably of Type I glass, at controlled room temperature, protected from light. A sterile solution of Ketorolac Tromethamine. Contains the labeled amount, within ±10%. Meets the requirements for Identification, Bacterial endotoxins, Sterility, pH (6.9–7.9), and Particulate matter, and for Injections.

Ketorolac Tromethamine Ophthalmic Solution—Not in *USP–NF*.

Ketorolac Tromethamine Tablets USP—Preserve in well-closed containers at controlled room temperature, protected from light and excessive humidity. Contain the labeled amount, within ±10%. Meet the requirements for Identification, Dissolution (75% in 45 minutes in water in Apparatus 2 at 50 rpm), and Uniformity of dosage units.

KETOTIFEN

Chemical name:

Ketotifen—4,9-Dihydro-4-1-(1-methyl-4-piperidinylidene)-10*H*-benzo[4,5]cyclohepta[1,2-*b*]thiophen-10-one.

Ketotifen fumarate—10*H*-Benzo[4,5]cyclohepta[1,2-*b*]thiophen-10-one, 4,9-dihydro-4-(1-methyl-4-piperidinylidene)-, (*E*)-2-butenedioate (1:1).

Molecular formula:

Ketotifen—$C_{19}H_{19}NOS$.

Ketotifen fumarate—$C_{19}H_{19}NOS \cdot C_4H_4O_4$.

Molecular weight:

Ketotifen—309.43.

Ketotifen fumarate—425.50.

Description:

Ketotifen—Crystals from ethyl acetate. Melting point 152–153°.

Ketotifen fumarate—Fine crystalline, yellowish-gray powder. Melting point 192°.

Solubility: Ketotifen fumarate—Readily soluble in water.

USP requirements:

Ketotifen Ophthalmic Solution—Not in *USP–NF*.

Ketotifen Fumarate Syrup—Not in *USP–NF*.

Ketotifen Fumarate Tablets—Not in *USP–NF*.

KRYPTON KR 81M

Chemical name: Krypton, isotope of mass 81 (metastable).

Molecular formula: Kr 81m.

USP requirements: Krypton Kr 81m USP—The generator column is enclosed in a lead container. The unit is stored at room temperature. A gas suitable only for inhalation in diagnostic studies, obtained from a generator that contains rubidium 81 adsorbed on an immobilized suitable column support. Rubidium 81 decays with a half-life of 4.58 hours and forms its radioactive daughter $^{81}_mKr$, which is eluted from the generator by passage of humidified oxygen or air through the column. Rubidium 81 is produced in an accelerator by proton bombardment of Kr 82. Other radioisotopes of rubidium are produced and are present on the generator column. These other radioisotopes do not decay to $^{81}_mKr$. The labeling indicates the name and address of the manufacturer, the name of the generator, the quantity of ^{81}Rb at the date and time of calibration, and the statement, "Caution—Radioactive Material." The labeling indicates that in making dosage calculations, correction is to be made for radioactive decay, and also indicates that the radioactive half-life of $^{81}_mKr$ is 13.1 seconds. The column contains the labeled amount of Rb 81, within ±10%, at the date and time indicated in the labeling, and on elution yields not less than 80.0% of $^{81}_mKr$. Meets the requirements for Radionuclide identification and Radionuclidic purity.

LABETALOL

Chemical name: Labetalol hydrochloride—Benzamide, 2-hydroxy-5-[1-hydroxy-2-[(1-methyl-3-phenylpropyl)amino]ethyl]-, monohydrochloride.

Molecular formula: Labetalol hydrochloride—$C_{19}H_{24}N_2O_3 \cdot HCl$.

Molecular weight: Labetalol hydrochloride—364.87.

Description: Labetalol Hydrochloride USP—White to off-white powder. Melts at about 180 °C, with decomposition.

pKa: 9.45.

Solubility: Labetalol Hydrochloride USP—Soluble in water and in alcohol; insoluble in ether and in chloroform.

Other characteristics: Lipid solubility—Low.

USP requirements:
Labetalol Hydrochloride USP—Preserve in tight, light-resistant containers. Contains not less than 97.5% and not more than 101.0% of labetalol hydrochloride, calculated on the dried basis. Meets the requirements for Identification, pH (4.0–5.0, in a solution [1 in 100]), Loss on drying (not more than 1.0%), Residue on ignition (not more than 0.1%), Heavy metals (not more than 0.002%), Chromatographic purity, Organic volatile impurities, and Diastereoisomer ratio.
Labetalol Hydrochloride Injection USP—Preserve in single-dose containers, or in multiple-dose containers not exceeding 60 mL in volume, preferably of Type I glass, at a temperature between 2 and 30 °C. Avoid freezing and exposure to light. A sterile solution of Labetalol Hydrochloride in Water for Injection. Contains the labeled amount, within ±10%. Meets the requirements for Identification, Bacterial endotoxins, and pH (3.0–4.5), and for Injections.
Labetalol Hydrochloride Tablets USP—Preserve in tight, light-resistant containers, at a temperature between 2 and 30 °C. Contain the labeled amount, within ±10%. Meet the requirements for Identification, Dissolution (80% in 45 minutes in water in Apparatus 2 at 50 rpm), and Uniformity of dosage units.

LACTASE

USP requirements: Lactase USP—Preserve in tight containers at room temperature. A hydrolytic enzyme derived from the mold *Aspergillus oryzae*. Label it to indicate lactase activity in USP Units. Contains not less than 30,000 USP Lactase Units in each gram. Meets the requirements for Microbial limits, Loss on drying (not more than 6.0%), Arsenic (not more than 3 mcg per gram), Lead (not more than 5 mcg per gram), and Heavy metals (not more than 30 mcg per gram).
Note: One USP Lactase Unit is the lactase activity contained in the amount of enzyme that hydrolyses one microequivalent of galactosidic linkage per minute at a pH of 4.5 and at 37 °C as directed under Assay for lactase activity.

LACTIC ACID

Chemical name: Propanoic acid, 2-hydroxy-.

Molecular formula: $C_3H_6O_3$.

Molecular weight: 90.08.

Description: Lactic Acid USP—Colorless or yellowish, practically odorless, syrupy liquid. Is hygroscopic. When it is concentrated by boiling, lactic acid lactate is formed. Specific gravity is about 1.20.

NF category: Buffering agent.

Solubility: Lactic Acid USP—Miscible with water, with alcohol, and with ether. Insoluble in chloroform.

USP requirements: Lactic Acid USP—Preserve in tight containers. A mixture of lactic acid and lactic acid lactate equivalent to a total of not less than 88.0% and not more than 92.0%, by weight, of lactic acid. Obtained by the lactic fermentation of sugars or prepared synthetically. Lactic Acid obtained by fermentation of sugars is levorotatory, while that prepared synthetically is racemic. (Note: Lactic Acid prepared by fermentation becomes dextrorotatory on dilution, which hydrolyzes L(−) lactic acid lactate to L(+) lactic acid.) Label it to indicate whether it is levorotatory or racemic. Meets the requirements for Identification, Specific rotation (−0.05° to +0.05°, for racemic Lactic Acid), Readily carbonizable substances, Residue on ignition (not more than 0.05%), Sugars, Chloride, Sulfate, Heavy metals (not more than 0.001%), and Limit of citric, oxalic, phosphoric, or tartaric acid.

LACTITOL

Chemical name: 4-*O*-beta-D-Galactopyranosyl-D-glucitol.

Molecular formula: $C_{12}H_{24}O_{11}$.

Molecular weight: 344.31; 362.34 (Monohydrate); 380.35 (Dihydrate).

NF requirements: Lactitol NF—Preserve in well-closed containers. Label it to indicate whether it is the monohydrate, the dihydrate, or the anhydrous form. Contains not less than 98.0% and not more than 101.0% of lactitol, calculated on the anhydrous basis. Meets the requirements for Identification, Water (not more than 0.5% for the anhydrous form), Residue on ignition (not more than 0.5%), Heavy metals (not more than 5 micrograms per gram), Reducing sugars (not more than 0.2%, as dextrose), Organic volatile impurities, and Related compounds (not more than 1.5%).

ANHYDROUS LACTOSE

Description: Anhydrous Lactose NF—White or almost white powder.
NF category: Tablet and/or capsule diluent.

Solubility: Anhydrous Lactose NF—Freely soluble in water; practically insoluble in alcohol.

NF requirements: Anhydrous Lactose NF—It is primarily beta lactose or a mixture of alpha and beta lactose. Where the labeling indicates the relative quantities of alpha and beta lactose, determine compliance using Content of alpha and beta anomers. Meets the requirements for Identification, Loss on drying (not more than 0.5%), Water (not more than 1.0%), Heavy metals (not more than 5 mcg per gram), and Content of alpha and beta anomers, and for Packaging and storage, Labeling, Clarity and color of solution, Specific rotation, Microbial limits, Acidity or alkalinity, Residue on ignition, and Protein and light-absorbing impurities under Lactose Monohydrate.

LACTOSE MONOHYDRATE

Chemical name: D-Glucose, 4-*O*-beta-D-galactopyranosyl-, monohydrate.

Molecular formula: $C_{12}H_{22}O_{11} \cdot H_2O$.

Molecular weight: 360.31.

Description: Lactose Monohydrate NF—White, free-flowing powder.

NF category: Tablet and/or capsule diluent.

Solubility: Lactose Monohydrate NF—Freely but slowly soluble in water; practically insoluble in alcohol.

NF requirements: Lactose Monohydrate NF—Preserve in tight containers. A natural disaccharide, obtained from milk, which consists of one glucose and one galactose moiety. (Note: Lactose Monohydrate may be modified as to its physical characteristics. May contain varying proportions of amorphous lactose.) Where the labeling states the particle size distribution, it also indicates the d_{10}, d_{50}, and d_{90} values and the range for each. For modified Lactose Monohydrate, also label it to indicate the method of modification. Meets the requirements for Clarity and color of solution, Identification, Specific rotation (+54.4° to +55.9°, calculated on the anhydrous basis at 20 °C), Microbial limits, Acidity or alkalinity, Loss on drying (not more than 0.5% for the monohydrate form and not more than 1.0% for the modified monohydrate form), Water (4.5–5.5%), Residue on ignition (not more than 0.1%), Heavy metals (not more than 5 ppm), and Protein and light-absorbing impurities.

LACTULOSE

Chemical name: D-Fructose, 4-*O*-beta-D-galactopyranosyl-.

Molecular formula: $C_{12}H_{22}O_{11}$.

Molecular weight: 342.30.

Description: Lactulose Concentrate USP—Colorless to amber syrupy liquid, which may exhibit some precipitation and darkening upon standing.

Solubility: Lactulose Concentrate USP—Miscible with water.

USP requirements:
Lactulose Concentrate USP—Preserve in tight containers, preferably at a temperature between 2 and 30 °C. Avoid subfreezing temperatures. A solution of sugars prepared from Lactose. Consists principally of lactulose together with minor quantities of lactose and galactose, and traces of other related sugars and water. The label states that this article is not intended for direct administration to humans or animals. Contains the labeled amount, within ±5%. Contains no added substances. Meets the requirements for Identification, Related compounds, Refractive index (not less than 1.451, at 20 °C), and Residue on ignition (not more than 0.1%).
Lactulose Solution USP—Preserve in tight containers, preferably at a temperature between 2 and 30 °C. Avoid subfreezing temperatures. A solution in water prepared from Lactulose Concentrate. Contains the labeled amount, within ±10%. Meets the requirements for Microbial limits and pH (2.5–6.5, after 15 minutes of contact with the electrodes), and for Identification tests and Related compounds under Lactulose Concentrate.

LAMIVUDINE

Chemical name: 2(1*H*)-Pyrimidinone, 4-amino-1-[2-(hydroxymethyl)-1,3-oxathiolan-5-yl]-, (2*R-cis*)-.

Molecular formula: $C_8H_{11}N_3O_3S$.

Molecular weight: 229.26.

Description: White to off-white solid. Melts between 178° and 182°.

Solubility: Soluble in water.

USP requirements:
Lamivudine USP—Preserve in well-closed, light-resistant containers, at controlled room temperature. Contains not less than 98.0% and not more than 102.0% of lamivudine, calculated on the anhydrous and solvent-free basis. Meets the requirements for Identification, Light absorption (not more than 0.0015), Water (not more than 0.2%), Limit of lamivudine enantiomer (not more than 0.3%), Limit of residual solvents, and Chromatographic purity.
Lamivudine Oral Solution—Not in *USP–NF*.
Lamivudine Tablets—Not in *USP–NF*.

LAMIVUDINE AND ZIDOVUDINE

For *Lamivudine* and *Zidovudine*—See individual listings for chemistry information.

USP requirements: Lamivudine and Zidovudine Tablets—Not in *USP–NF*.

LAMOTRIGINE

Chemical group: Phenyltriazine.

Chemical name: 1,2,4-Triazine-3,5-diamine, 6-(2,3-dichlorophenyl)-.

Molecular formula: $C_9H_7Cl_2N_5$.

Molecular weight: 256.09.

Description: Melting point 216–218 °C.

USP requirements:
Lamotrigine Tablets—Not in *USP–NF*.
Lamotrigine Chewable/Dispersible Tablets—Not in *USP–NF*.

LANOLIN

Description: Lanolin USP—Yellow, tenacious, unctuous mass, having a slight characteristic odor.

NF category: Ointment base.

Solubility: Lanolin USP—Insoluble in water, but mixes without separation with about twice its weight of water. Sparingly soluble in cold alcohol; more soluble in hot alcohol; freely soluble in ether and in chloroform.

USP requirements: Lanolin USP—Preserve in well-closed containers, preferably at controlled room temperature. The purified, wax-like substance from the wool of sheep, *Ovis aries* Linné (Fam. Bovidae), that has been cleaned, decolorized, and deodorized. The label states that it is not to be used undiluted. Contains not more than 0.25% of water. May contain not more than 0.02% of a suitable antioxidant. Meets the requirements for Melting range (38–44 °C), Acidity, Alkalinity, Water (not more than 0.25%), Residue on ignition (not more than 0.1%), Water-soluble acids and alkalies, Water-soluble

oxidizable substances, Chloride (not more than 0.035%), Ammonia, Iodine value (18–36), Petrolatum, and Foreign substances (not more than 10 ppm of any individual specified residue and not more than 40 ppm for total of all specified residues).

LANOLIN ALCOHOLS

Description: Lanolin Alcohols NF—Hard, waxy, amber solid, having a characteristic odor.

NF category: Emulsifying and/or solubilizing agent.

Solubility: Lanolin Alcohols NF—Insoluble in water; slightly soluble in alcohol; freely soluble in chloroform, in ether, and in petroleum ether.

NF requirements: Lanolin Alcohols NF—Preserve in well-closed, light-resistant containers, preferably at controlled room temperature. A mixture of aliphatic alcohols, triterpenoid alcohols, and sterols, obtained by the hydrolysis of Lanolin. Meets the requirements for Identification, Melting range (not below 56 °C), Acidity and alkalinity, Loss on drying (not more than 0.5%), Residue on ignition (not more than 0.15%), Copper (not more than 5 ppm), Acid value (not more than 2), Saponification value (not more than 12), and Content of sterols (as cholesterol, not less than 30% of sterol).

MODIFIED LANOLIN

USP requirements: Modified Lanolin USP—Preserve in tight, preferably rust-proof containers, preferably at controlled room temperature. The purified wax-like substance from the wool of sheep, *Ovis aries* Linné (Fam. Bovidae), that has been processed to reduce the contents of free lanolin alcohols and detergent and pesticide residues. Contains not more than 0.25% of water. May contain not more than 0.02% of a suitable antioxidant. Meets the requirements for Acidity, Alkalinity, Water (not more than 0.25%), Water-soluble acids and alkalies, Ammonia, Limit of free lanolin alcohols (not more than 6%), Foreign substances (not more than 3 ppm for total specified residues and not more than 1 ppm for individual specified residue), and Petrolatum.

LANSOPRAZOLE

Chemical name: 1*H*-Benzimidazole, 2-[[[3-methyl-4-(2,2,2-trifluoroethoxy)-2-pyridinyl]methyl]sulfinyl]-.

Molecular formula: $C_{16}H_{14}F_3N_3O_2S$.

Molecular weight: 369.36.

Description: White to brownish-white odorless crystalline powder which melts with decomposition at approximately 166 °C.

Solubility: Freely soluble in dimethylformamide; soluble in methanol; sparingly soluble in ethanol; slightly soluble in ethyl acetate, in dichloromethane, and in acetonitrile; very slightly soluble in ether; practically insoluble in hexane and in water.

USP requirements:

Lansoprazole USP—Preserve in well-closed, light-resistant containers. Contains not less than 99.0% and not more than 101.0% of lansoprazole. Meets the requirements for

Identification, Water (not more than 0.10%, determined on a 1.0 gram specimen, 50 mL of a dehydrated mixture of pyridine, and ethylene glycol [9:1 to 8:2]), Residue of ignition (not more than 0.10%), and Chromatographic purity.

Lansoprazole Delayed-release Capsules USP—Store in a tight container at controlled room temperature. Contain the labeled amount of lansoprazole, within ±10%. Meet the requirements for Identification, Drug release (Acid stage: 10% in 60 minutes in 0.1 N hydrochloric acid in Apparatus 2 at 75 rpm, and Buffer stage: 80% in 60 minutes in a solution [ph 6.8] in Apparatus 2 at 75 rpm), Uniformity of dosage units, and Loss on drying (not more than 5.0%).

LATANOPROST

Source: Synthetic analogue of dinoprost (prostaglandin $F_{2\ alpha}$).

Chemical name: 5-Heptenoic acid, 7-[3,5-dihydroxy-2-(3-hydroxy-5-phenylpentyl)cyclopentyl]-1-methylethyl ester, [1*R*-[1 alpha(*Z*),2 beta(*R**),3 alpha,5 alpha]]-.

Molecular formula: $C_{26}H_{40}O_5$.

Molecular weight: 432.59.

Description: Colorless to slightly yellow oil.

Solubility: Very soluble in acetonitrile; freely soluble in acetone, in ethanol, in ethyl acetate, in ispropanol, in methanol, and in octanol; practically insoluble in water.

USP requirements: Latanoprost Ophthalmic Solution—Not in *USP–NF*.

LECITHIN

Description: Lecithin NF—The consistency of both natural grades and refined grades of lecithin may vary from plastic to fluid, depending upon free fatty acid and oil content, and upon the presence or absence of other diluents. Its color varies from light yellow to brown, depending on the source, on crop variations, and on whether it is bleached or unbleached. Odorless, or has a characteristic, slight, nutlike odor.

NF category: Emulsifying and/or solubilizing agent.

Solubility: Lecithin NF—Partially soluble in water, but it readily hydrates to form emulsions. The oil-free phosphatides are soluble in fatty acids, but are practically insoluble in fixed oils. When all phosphatide fractions are present, lecithin is partially soluble in alcohol and practically insoluble in acetone.

NF requirements: Lecithin NF—Preserve in well-closed containers. A complex mixture of acetone-insoluble phosphatides, which consist chiefly of phosphatidyl choline, phosphatidyl ethanolamine, phosphatidyl serine, and phosphatidyl inositol, combined with various amounts of other substances such as triglycerides, fatty acids, and carbohydrates, as separated from the crude vegetable oil source. Contains not less than 50.0% of acetone-insoluble matter. Meets the requirements for Acid value, Water (not more than 1.5%), Hexane-insoluble matter (not more than 0.3%), Lead (not more than 0.001%), Heavy metals (not more than 20 mcg per gram), Organic volatile impurities, and Content of acetone-insoluble matter.

LEFLUNOMIDE

Chemical name: 4-Isoxazolecarboxamide, 5-methyl-*N*-[4-(tri-fluoromethyl)phenyl]-.

Molecular formula: $C_{12}H_9F_3N_2O_2$.

Molecular weight: 270.21.

USP requirements: Leflunomide Tablets—Not in *USP–NF*.

LEMON OIL

NF requirements: Lemon Oil NF—Preserve in well-filled, tight containers, and avoid exposure to excessive heat. The volatile oil obtained by expression, without the aid of heat, from the fresh peel of the fruit of *Citrus x limon* (L.) Osbeck (Fam. Rutaceae), with or without the previous separation of the pulp and the peel. The label states the Latin binomial name and, following the official name, the part of the plant source from which the article was derived. Label it to also indicate whether it is California-type or Italian-type Lemon Oil. The label indicates that Oil is not to be used if it has a terebinthine ordor. Total aldehyde contain, calculated as citral, is not less than 2.2% and not more than 3.8% for California-type Lemon Oil, and not less than 3.0% and not more than 5.5% for Italian-type Lemon Oil. Meets the requirements for Specific gravity (0.849–0.855), Angular rotation (+57° to +65.6°), Refractive index (1.473–1.476 at 20°), Ultraviolet absorbance (not less than 0.20 for California-type Lemon Oil, or not less than 0.49 for Italian Lemon Oil), Heavy metals (0.004%), and Foreign oils.

Note—Do not use Lemon Oil that has a terebinthine odor.

LEMON TINCTURE

NF requirements:

Lemon Tinctue NF—Preserve Lemon Tincture in tight, light-resistant containers, and avoid exposure to direct sunlight and to excessive heat. Store at controlled room temperature. The label states the Latin binomial name and, following the official name, the part of the plant source from which the article was derived.

Prepared from lemon peel, which is the outer yellow rind of the fresh, ripe fruit of *Citrus x Limon* Osbeck (Fam. Rutaceae): 500 grams of Lemon peel, 900 mL of alcohol, and alcohol, sufficient quantity to make 1000 mL. Prepare peel as directed for Process M in Tinctures under Pharmaceutical Dosage Forms. Macerate 500 grams of the lemon peel in 900 mL of alcohol in a closed container, and store in a warm place. Agitate the container frequently for 3 days or until the soluble matter is dissolved. Transfer the mixture to a filter, using talc as the filtering medium, and when most of the liquid has drained away, wash the residue on the filter with a sufficient amount of alcohol, and combine the filtrates so that the preparation is brought to a final volume of 1000 mL.

Meets the rquirements for Heavy metals (not more than 0.004%) and Alcohol content (62–72%).

LEPIRUDIN

Source: Synthetic. Recombinant form of hirudin (a naturally occurring family of highly homologous isopolypeptides produced by the leech *Hirudo medicinalis*) that is produced by a recombinant DNA process involving yeast cells. A polypeptide com-posed of 65 amino acids, which differs from naturally occurring hirudin by substitution of leucine for isoleucine at the N-terminal end of the molecule and by absence of a sulfate group on the tyrosine at position 63.

Chemical name: 1-L-Leucine-2-L-threonine-63-desulfohirudin-(*Hirudo medicinalis* isoform HV1).

Molecular formula: $C_{287}H_{440}N_{80}O_{111}S_6$.

Molecular weight: 6979.43.

Other characteristics: pH: Approximately 7.

USP requirements: Lepirudin for Injection—Not in *USP–NF*.

LETROZOLE

Chemical name: Benzonitrile, 4,4′-(1*H*-1,2,4-triazole-1-ylmethy-lene)bis-.

Molecular formula: $C_{17}H_{11}N_5$.

Molecular weight: 285.31.

Description: Letrozole USP—White to yellowish crystalline powder. Practically orderless.

Solubility: Letrozole USP—Freely soluble in dichloromethane; slightly soluble in alcohol; practically insoluble in water. Melting range 184–185 °C.

pKa: 0.7±0.2 in water at 22 °C.

USP requirements:

Letrozole USP—Preserve in tight containers at controlled room temperature. Contains not less than 98.0% and not more than 102.0% of letrozole, calculated on the anhydrous basis. Meets the requirements for Identification, Water (not more than 0.3%), Residue on ignition (not more than 0.1%), Heavy metals (not more than 0.001%), Related compounds, and Organic volatile impurities.

Letrozole Tablets USP—Preserve in tight containers at controlled room temperature. Contain the labeled amount, within ±5%. Meet the requirements for Identification, Dissolution (80% in 30 minutes in 0.1 *N* hydrochloric acid in Apparatus 2 at 75 rpm), Uniformity of dosage units, and Related compounds.

LEUCINE

Chemical name: L-Leucine.

Molecular formula: $C_6H_{13}NO_2$.

Molecular weight: 131.17.

Description: Leucine USP—White, practically odorless crystals.

Solubility: Leucine USP—Sparingly soluble in water; insoluble in ether.

USP requirements: Leucine USP—Preserve in well-closed containers. Contains not less than 98.5% and not more than 101.5% of leucine, as L-leucine, calculated on the dried basis. Meets the requirements for Identification, Specific rotation (+14.9° to +17.3°), pH (5.5–7.0, in a solution [1 in 100]), Loss on drying (not more than 0.2%), Residue on ignition (not more than 0.4%), Chloride (not more than 0.05%), Sulfate (not more than 0.03%), Iron (not more than 0.003%), Heavy metals (not more than 0.0015%), Chromatographic purity, and Organic volatile impurities.

LEUCOVORIN

Chemical name: Leucovorin calcium—L-Glutamic acid, *N*-[4-[[(2-amino-5-formyl-1,4,5,6,7,8-hexahydro-4-oxo-6-pteridinyl)-methyl]amino]benzoyl]-, calcium salt (1:1).

Molecular formula: Leucovorin calcium—$C_{20}H_{21}CaN_7O_7$.

Molecular weight: Leucovorin calcium—511.50.

Description:
Leucovorin Calcium USP—Yellowish white or yellow, odorless powder.
Leucovorin Calcium Injection USP—Clear, yellowish solution.

pKa: Leucovorin calcium—3.8, 4.8, and 10.4.

Solubility: Leucovorin Calcium USP—Very soluble in water; practically insoluble in alcohol.

USP requirements:
Leucovorin Calcium USP—Preserve in well-closed, light-resistant containers. Contains not less than 95.0% and not more than 105.0% of leucovorin calcium, calculated on the anhydrous basis. Meets the requirements for Identification, Water (not more than 17.0%), and Heavy metals (not more than 0.005%).
Leucovorin Calcium Injection USP—Preserve in single-dose, light-resistant containers, preferably of Type I glass. A sterile solution of Leucovorin Calcium in Water for Injection. Contains an amount of leucovorin calcium equivalent to the labeled amount of leucovorin, within −10% to +20%. Meets the requirements for Identification, Bacterial endotoxins, and pH (6.5–8.5), and for Injections.
Leucovorin Calcium for Injection—Not in *USP–NF*.
Leucovorin Calcium Tablets USP—Preserve in well-closed containers, protected from light, at controlled room temperature. Contain an amount of leucovorin calcium equivalent to the labeled amount of leucovorin, within ±10%. Meet the requirements for Identification, Dissolution (75% in 30 minutes in water in Apparatus 2 at 50 rpm), Uniformity of dosage units, and Chromatographic purity.

LEUPROLIDE

Source: Synthetic nonapeptide analog of naturally occurring gonadotropin releasing hormone.

Chemical name: Leuprolide acetate—Luteinizing hormone–releasing factor (pig), 6-D-leucine-9-(*N*-ethyl-L-prolinamide)-10-deglycinamide-, monoacetate (salt).

Molecular formula: Leuprolide acetate—$C_{59}H_{84}N_{16}O_{12} \cdot C_2H_4O_2$.

Molecular weight: Leuprolide acetate—1269.45.

Description: Leuprolide acetate—White to off-white powder.

Solubility: Leuprolide acetate—Solubility greater than 250 mg/mL in water and greater than 1 g/mL in alcohol at 25 °C.

USP requirements:
Leuprolide Acetate Injection—Not in *USP–NF*.
Leuprolide Acetate for Injection—Not in *USP–NF*.

LEVALBUTEROL

Chemical name: Levalbuterol hydrochloride—(R)-alpha¹-[(*tert*-Butylamino)methyl]-4-hydroxy-*m*-xylene-alpha,alpha¹-diol hydrochloride.

Molecular formula: Levalbuterol hydrochloride—$C_{13}H_{21}NO_3 \cdot$ HCl.

Molecular weight: Levalbuterol hydrochloride—275.77.

Description: Levalbuterol hydrochloride—An off-white, crystalline solid and is the (R)-enantiomer of the drug substance racemic albuterol. Melting point approximately 187 °C.

Solubility: Levalbuterol hydrochloride—Soluble approximately 180 mg per mL in water.

Other characteristics: Levalbuterol hydrochloride—pH: 4 (3.3–4.5).

USP requirements: Levalbuterol Hydrochloride Inhalation Solution—Not in *USP–NF*.

LEVAMISOLE

Chemical name: Levamisole hydrochloride—Imidazo[2,1-*b*]thiazole, 2,3,5,6-tetrahydro-6-phenyl-, monohydrochloride, (*S*)-.

Molecular formula: Levamisole hydrochloride—$C_{11}H_{12}N_2S \cdot HCl$.

Molecular weight: Levamisole hydrochloride—240.75.

Description: Levamisole Hydrochloride USP—White or almost white crystalline powder.

Solubility: Levamisole Hydrochloride USP—Freely soluble in water; soluble in alcohol; slightly soluble in methylene chloride; practically insoluble in ether.

USP requirements:
Levamisole Hydrochloride USP—Preserve in well-closed containers, protected from light. Contains not less than 98.5% and not more than 101.0% of levamisole hydrochloride, calculated on the dried basis. Meets the requirements for Completeness of solution, Color of solution, Identification, Melting range (226–231 °C), Light absorption, Specific rotation (−121.5° to −128.0°), pH (3.0–4.5, in a solution [1 in 20]), Loss on drying (not more than 0.5%), Residue on ignition (not more than 0.1%), Heavy metals (not more than 0.001%), and Chromatographic purity.
Levamisole Hydrochloride Tablets USP—Preserve in well-closed containers. Label Tablets to state both the content of the active moiety and the content of the salt used in formulating the article. Contain an amount of Levamisole Hydrochloride equivalent to the labeled amount of levamisole, within ±10%. Meet the requirements for Identification, Dissolution (80% in 45 minutes in 0.01 *N* hydrochloric acid in Apparatus 2 at 50 rpm), Uniformity of dosage units, and Chromatographic purity.

LEVETIRACETAM

Source: Pyrrolidine derivative.

Chemical name: (*S*)-alpha-Ethyl-2-oxo-1-pyrrolidineacetamide.

Molecular formula: $C_{18}H_{14}N_2O_2$.

Molecular weight: 170.21.

Description: A white to off-white crystalline powder with a faint odor.

Solubility: Very soluble in water (104 grams/100 mL); freely soluble in chloroform (65.3 grams/100 mL) and in methanol (53.6 grams/100 mL); soluble in ethanol (16.5 grams/100 mL); sparingly soluble in acetonitrile (5.7 grams/100 mL); practically insoluble in n-hexane.

USP requirements: Levetiracetam Tablets—Not in *USP–NF*.

LEVMETAMFETAMINE

Chemical name: Benzeneethanamine, N, alpha-dimethyl-, (R)-.

Molecular formula: $C_{10}H_{15}N$.

Molecular weight: 149.23.

Description: Clear, practically colorless liquid.

USP requirements: Levmetamfetamine USP—Preserve in tight, light-resistant containers. Contains not less than 98.0% and not more than 100.5% of levmetamfetamine. Meets the requirements for Identification, Specific rotation (−18.5° to −21.5°), Limit of methamphetamine (not more than 0.1%), Limit of nonvolatile residue (not more than 0.5%), Ordinary impurities, and Organic volatile impurities.

LEVOBETAXOLOL

Chemical name: Levobetaxolol hydrochloride—2-Propanol, 1-[4-[2-(cyclopropylmethoxy)ethyl]phenoxy]-3-[(-methylethyl)amino]-, hydrochloride, (S)-.

Molecular formula: Levobetaxolol hydrochloride—$C_{18}H_{29}NO_3 \cdot$ HCl.

Molecular weight: Levobetaxolol hydrochloride—343.89.

Description: Levobetaxolol hydrochloride—White, crystalline powder.

Other characteristics:: Levobetaxolol hydrochloride—pH: 5.5–7.5. An osmolality of 260–340 mOsm per kg.

USP requirements:
Levobetaxolol Ophthalmic Suspension—Not in USP–NF.
Levobetaxolol Hydrochloride Ophthalmic Suspension—Not in USP–NF.

LEVOBUNOLOL

Chemical name: Levobunolol hydrochloride—1(2H)-Naphthalenone, 5-[3-[(1,1-dimethylethyl)amino]-2-hydroxypropoxy]-3,4-dihydro-, hydrochloride, (−)-.

Molecular formula: Levobunolol hydrochloride—$C_{17}H_{25}NO_3 \cdot$ HCl.

Molecular weight: Levobunolol hydrochloride—327.85.

Description: Levobunolol Hydrochloride USP—White crystalline, odorless powder.

pKa: Levobunolol hydrochloride—9.4.

Solubility: Levobunolol Hydrochloride USP—Soluble in water and in methanol; slightly soluble in alcohol and in chloroform.

USP requirements:
Levobunolol Hydrochloride USP—Preserve in well-closed containers. Contains not less than 98.5% and not more than 101.0% of levobunolol hydrochloride, calculated on the dried basis. Meets the requirements for Identification, Melting range (206–211 °C, within a range of 3 °C, determined after drying), Specific rotation (−19° to −20°), pH (4.5–6.5, in a solution [1 in 20]), Loss on drying (not more than 0.5%), and Residue on ignition (not more than 0.1%).
Levobunolol Hydrochloride Ophthalmic Solution USP—Preserve in tight containers. Contains the labeled amount, within ±10%. Meets the requirements for Identification, Antimicrobial preservatives—effectiveness, Sterility, and pH (5.5–7.5).

LEVOBUPIVACAINE

Chemical group; Amides.

Chemical name:
Levobupivacaine—(S)-1-Butyl-2′,6′-pipecoloxylidide.
Levobupivacaine hydrochloride—(S)-1-Butyl-N-(2,6-dimethylphenyl)-2-piperidinecarboxamide monohydrochloride.

Molecular formula:
Levobupivacaine—$C_{18}H_{28}N_2O$.
Levobupivacaine hydrochloride—$C_{18}H_{28}N_2O \cdot$ HCl.

Molecular weight:
Levobupivacaine—288.43.
Levobupivacaine hydrochloride—324.90.

Description: Levobupivacaine hydrochloride—White crystalline powder.

pKa: Levobupivacaine hydrochloride—8.09.

Solubility: Levobupivacaine hydrochloride—Soluble in water (10 mg/mL) at 20 °C.

Other characteristics: Levobupivacaine hydrochloride—pH: 4.0–6.5. Partition coefficient (oleyl alcohol/water) is 1624.

USP requirements: Levobupivacaine Injection—Not in USP–NF.

LEVOCABASTINE

Chemical name: Levocabastine hydrochloride—4-Piperidinecarboxylic acid, 1-[4-cyano-4-(4-fluorophenyl)cyclohexyl]-3-methyl-4-phenyl-, monohydrochloride, (−)-[1(cis),3 alpha,4 beta]-.

Molecular formula: Levocabastine hydrochloride—$C_{26}H_{29}FN_2O_2 \cdot$ HCl.

Molecular weight: Levocabastine hydrochloride—456.98.

Description: Levocabastine hydrochloride—White to almost white powder with a melting temperature of less than 300 °C.

pKa: Levocabastine hydrochloride—3.1 and 9.7.

Solubility: Levocabastine hydrochloride—Freely soluble in dimethylsulfoxide; soluble in N,N-dimethylformamide and in methanol; slightly soluble in propylene glycol, in polyethylene glycol, and in ethanol. In aqueous medium the solubility is a function of pH, with minimum solubility at pH 4.1 to 9.8.

Other characteristics: Levocabastine hydrochloride—Log-partition coefficient (n-octanol/aqueous buffer at pH 8.0): 1.82.

USP requirements:
Levocabastine Hydrochloride Nasal Suspension—Not in USP–NF.
Levocabastine Hydrochloride Ophthalmic Suspension—Not in USP–NF.

LEVOCARNITINE

Source: Naturally occurring amino acid derivative.

Chemical name: 1-Propanaminium, 3-carboxy-2-hydroxy-N,N,N-trimethyl-, hydroxide, inner salt, (R)-.

Molecular formula: $C_7H_{15}NO_3$.

Molecular weight: 161.20.

Description: Levocarnitine USP—White crystals or crystalline powder. Hygroscopic.

Solubility: Levocarnitine USP—Freely soluble in water and in hot alcohol; practically insoluble in acetone and in ether.

USP requirements:

Levocarnitine USP—Preserve in tight containers. Contains not less than 97.0% and not more than 103.0% of levocarnitine, calculated on the anhydrous basis. Meets the requirements for Identification, Specific rotation (−29° to −32°), pH (5.5–9.5, in a solution [1 in 20]), Water content (not more than 4.0%), Residue on ignition (not more than 0.5%), Chloride (not more than 0.4%), Limit of potassium (not more than 0.2%), Limit of sodium (not more than 0.1%), and Heavy metals (not more than 0.002%).

Levocarnitine Injection USP—Preserve in single-dose containers, preferably of Type I glass. Store below 25°. Do not freeze. A sterile solution of Levocarnitine in Water for Injection. Contains labeled amount, within ±10%. Meets the requirements for Identification, Bacterial endotoxins, pH (6.0–6.5), Particulate matter, and for Injections..

Levocarnitine Oral Solution USP—Preserve in tight containers. A solution of Levocarnitine in water. Contains suitable antimicrobial agents. Contains the labeled amount, within ±10%. Meets the requirements for Identification and pH (4.0–6.0).

Levocarnitine Tablets USP—Preserve in tight containers. Contain the labeled amount, within ±10%. Meet the requirements for Identification, Uniformity of dosage units, and Dissolution (75% in 30 minutes in water in Apparatus 2 at 75 rpm).

LEVODOPA

Chemical group: L-Dihydroxyphenylalanine; precursor of dopamine.

Chemical name: L-Tyrosine, 3-hydroxy-.

Molecular formula: $C_9H_{11}NO_4$.

Molecular weight: 197.19.

Description: Levodopa USP—White to off-white, odorless, crystalline powder. In the presence of moisture, is rapidly oxidized by atmospheric oxygen and darkens.

Solubility: Levodopa USP—Slightly soluble in water; freely soluble in 3 N hydrochloric acid; insoluble in alcohol.

USP requirements:

Levodopa USP—Preserve in tight, light-resistant containers, in a dry place, and prevent exposure to excessive heat. Contains not less than 98.0% and not more than 102.0% of levodopa, calculated on the dried basis. Meets the requirements for Identification, Specific rotation (−160° to −167°), Loss on drying (not more than 0.5%), Residue on ignition (not more than 0.1%), Heavy metals (not more than 0.002%), Related compounds, and Organic volatile impurities.

Levodopa Capsules USP—Preserve in tight, light-resistant containers, in a dry place, and prevent exposure to excessive heat. Contain the labeled amount, within ±10%. Meet the requirements for Identification, Dissolution (75% in 30 minutes in 0.01 N hydrochloric acid in Apparatus 1 at 100 rpm), Related compounds, and Uniformity of dosage units.

Levodopa Tablets USP—Preserve in tight, light-resistant containers, in a dry place, and prevent exposure to excessive heat. Contain the labeled amount, within ±10%. Meet the requirements for Identification, Dissolution (75% in 30 minutes in 0.01 N hydrochloric acid in Apparatus 1 at 100 rpm), Related compounds, and Uniformity of dosage units.

LEVODOPA AND BENSERAZIDE

Chemical group: Levodopa—L-Dihydroxyphenylalanine; precursor of dopamine.

Chemical name:

Levodopa—L-Tyrosine, 3-hydroxy-.

Benserazide—DL-Serine, 2-[(2,3,4-trihydroxyphenyl)methyl]-hydrazide.

Molecular formula:

Levodopa—$C_9H_{11}NO_4$.

Benserazide—$C_{10}H_{15}N_3O_5$.

Molecular weight:

Levodopa—197.19.

Benserazide—257.24.

Description:

Levodopa USP—White to off-white, odorless, crystalline powder. In the presence of moisture, is rapidly oxidized by atmospheric oxygen and darkens.

Benserazide—Unstable in a neutral, alkaline, or strongly acidic medium.

Solubility:

Levodopa USP—Slightly soluble in water; freely soluble in 3 N hydrochloric acid; insoluble in alcohol.

Benserazide—Highly soluble in water.

USP requirements: Levodopa and Benserazide Capsules—Not in *USP–NF*.

LEVOFLOXACIN

Chemical name: 7H-Pyrido[1,2,3-de]-1,4-benzoxazine-6-carboxylic acid, 9-fluoro-2,3-dihydro-3-methyl-10-(4-methyl-1-piperazinyl)-7-oxo-hydrate (2:1), (S)-.

Molecular formula: $C_{18}H_{20}FN_3O_4 \cdot \frac{1}{2}H_2O$.

Molecular weight: 370.38.

Description: Light yellowish-white to yellow-white crystal or crystalline powder.

USP requirements:

Levofloxacin Injection—Not in *USP–NF*.

Levofloxacin Concentrate for Injection—Not in *USP–NF*.

Levofloxacin Ophthalmic Solution—Not in *USP–NF*.

Levofloxacin Tablets—Not in *USP–NF*.

LEVOMETHADYL

Chemical name: Levomethadyl acetate hydrochloride—Benzeneethanol, beta-[2-(dimethylamino)propyl]-alpha-ethyl-beta-phenyl-, acetate (ester), hydrochloride, [S-(R*,R*)]-.

Molecular formula: Levomethadyl acetate hydrochloride—$C_{23}H_{31}NO_2 \cdot HCl$.

Molecular weight: Levomethadyl acetate hydrochloride—389.96.

Description: Levomethadyl acetate hydrochloride—White crystalline powder.

Solubility: Levomethadyl acetate hydrochloride—Soluble in water (>15 mg/mL), in ethanol, and in methyl ethyl ketone.

Other characteristics: Levomethadyl acetate hydrochloride—Octanol:water partition coefficient: 405:1 at physiologic pH.

USP requirements: Levomethadyl Acetate Hydrochloride Oral Solution—Not in *USP–NF*.

LEVONORDEFRIN

Chemical name: 1,2-Benzenediol, 4-(2-amino-1-hydroxypropyl)-, [R-(R*,S*)]-.

Molecular formula: $C_9H_{13}NO_3$.

Molecular weight: 183.20.

Description: Levonordefrin USP—White to buff-colored, odorless, crystalline solid. Melts at about 210 °C.

Solubility: Levonordefrin USP—Practically insoluble in water; freely soluble in aqueous solutions of mineral acids; slightly soluble in acetone, in chloroform, in alcohol, and in ether.

USP requirements: Levonordefrin USP—Preserve in well-closed containers. Dried in vacuum at 60 °C for 15 hours, contains not less than 98.0% and not more than 102.0% of levonordefrin. Meets the requirements for Identification, Specific rotation (−28° to −31°), Loss on drying (not more than 1.0%), Residue on ignition (not more than 0.2%), and Chromatographic purity.

LEVONORGESTREL

Chemical name: 18,19-Dinorpregn-4-en-20-yn-3-one, 13-ethyl-17-hydroxy-, (17 alpha)-(−)-.

Molecular formula: $C_{21}H_{28}O_2$.

Molecular weight: 312.45.

Description: Levonorgestrel USP—White or practically white, odorless powder.

Solubility: Levonorgestrel USP—Practically insoluble in water; soluble in chloroform; slightly soluble in alcohol.

USP requirements:
Levonorgestrel USP—Preserve in well-closed, light-resistant containers. Contains not less than 98.0% and not more than 102.0% of levonorgestrel, calculated on the dried basis. Meets the requirements for Identification, Melting range (232–239 °C, the range between beginning and end of melting not more than 4 °C), Specific rotation (−30° to −35°), Loss on drying (not more than 0.5%), Residue on ignition (not more than 0.3%), Limit of ethynyl group (7.81–8.18%), and Chromatographic purity.
Levonorgestrel Implant Capsules—Not in *USP–NF*.
Levonorgestrel Implants—Not in *USP–NF*.
Levonorgestrel Tablets—Not in *USP–NF*.

LEVONORGESTREL AND ETHINYL ESTRADIOL

For *Levonorgestrel* and *Ethinyl Estradiol*—See individual listings for chemistry information.

USP requirements: Levonorgestrel and Ethinyl Estradiol Tablets USP—Preserve in well-closed containers. Contain the labeled amounts, within ±10%. Meet the requirements for Identification, Dissolution (for uncoated tablets, 80% of levonorgestrel in 60 minutes and 75% of ethinyl estradiol in 60 minutes; for coated tablets, 60% of levonorgestrel in 60 minutes and 60%

of ethinyl estradiol in 60 minutes; both, in polysorbate 80 [5 mcg per gram] in water in Apparatus 2 at 75 rpm), and Uniformity of dosage units.

LEVORPHANOL

Chemical name: Levorphanol tartrate—Morphinan-3-ol, 17-methyl-, [R-(R*,R*)]-2,3-dihydroxybutanedioate (1:1) (salt), dihydrate.

Molecular formula: Levorphanol tartrate—$C_{17}H_{23}NO \cdot C_4H_6O_6 \cdot 2H_2O$ (dihydrate); $C_{17}H_{23}NO \cdot C_4H_6O_6$ (anhydrous).

Molecular weight: Levorphanol tartrate—443.49 (dihydrate); 407.46 (anhydrous).

Description: Levorphanol Tartrate USP—Practically white, odorless, crystalline powder. Melts, in a sealed tube, at about 110 °C, with decomposition.

Solubility: Levorphanol Tartrate USP—Sparingly soluble in water; slightly soluble in alcohol; insoluble in chloroform and in ether.

USP requirements:
Levorphanol Tartrate USP—Preserve in well-closed containers. Contains not less than 99.0% and not more than 101.0% of levorphanol tartrate, calculated on the anhydrous basis. Meets the requirements for Identification, Specific rotation (−14.7° to −16.3°), Water (7.0–9.0%), Residue on ignition (not more than 0.1%), and Ordinary impurities.
Levorphanol Tartrate Injection USP—Preserve in single-dose or in multiple-dose containers, preferably of Type I glass. A sterile solution of Levorphanol Tartrate in Water for Injection. Contains the labeled amount, within ±7%. Meets the requirements for Identification, Bacterial endotoxins, and pH (4.1–4.5), and for Injections.
Levorphanol Tartrate Tablets USP—Preserve in well-closed containers. Contain the labeled amount, within ±7%. Meet the requirements for Identification, Dissolution (75% in 30 minutes in water in Apparatus 2 at 50 rpm), and Uniformity of dosage units.

LEVOTHYROXINE

Chemical name: Levothyroxine sodium—L-Tyrosine, O-(4-hydroxy-3,5-diiodophenyl)-3,5-diiodo-, monosodium salt, hydrate.

Molecular formula: Levothyroxine sodium—$C_{15}H_{10}I_4NNaO_4 \cdot xH_2O$.

Molecular weight: Levothyroxine sodium—798.85 (anhydrous).

Description: Levothyroxine Sodium USP—Light yellow to buff-colored, odorless, hygroscopic powder. Is stable in dry air but may assume a slight pink color upon exposure to light. The pH of a saturated solution is about 8.9.

Solubility: Levothyroxine Sodium USP—Very slightly soluble in water; soluble in solutions of alkali hydroxides and in hot solutions of alkali carbonates; slightly soluble in alcohol; insoluble in acetone, in chloroform, and in ether.

USP requirements:
Levothyroxine Sodium USP—Preserve in tight containers, protected from light. The sodium salt of the levo isomer of thyroxine, an active physiological principle obtained from the thyroid gland of domesticated animals used for food by man or prepared synthetically. Contains not less than 97.0% and not more than 103.0% of levothyroxine sodium, calculated on the anhydrous basis. Meets the re-

quirements for Identification, Specific rotation (–5° to –6°), Water (not more than 11.0%), Limit of inorganic iodides (not more than 0.08%), and Limit of liothyronine sodium (not more than 2.0%).

Levothyroxine Sodium Injection—Not in *USP–NF*.

Levothyroxine Sodium for Injection—Not in *USP–NF*.

Levothyroxine Sodium Oral Powder USP—Preserve in tight, light-resistant containers. Label it to indicate that it is for veterinary use only. Contains the labeled amount, within ±10%. Meets the requirement for Loss on drying (not more than 2.0%).

Levothyroxine Sodium Tablets USP—Preserve in tight, light-resistant containers. When more than one Dissolution test is given, the labeling states the Dissolution test used only if Test 1 is not used. Contain the labeled amount, within ± 10%. Meet the requirements for Identification, Dissolution (70% in 45 minutes for Test 1, and 80% in 15 minutes for Test 2 in 0.01 *N* hydrochloric acid containing 0.2% sodium lauryl sulfate in Apparatus 2 at 50 rpm), Uniformity of dosage units, and Limit of liothyronine sodium (not more than 2.0%).

LICORICE

NF requirements:

Licorice NF—Preserve in well-closed containers. Store in a cool, dry place. Consists of the roots, rhizomes, and stolons of *Glycyrrhiza glabra* Linné or *Glycyrrhiza uralensis* Fisher (Fam. Leguminosae). The label states the Latin binomial name and, following the official name, the part of the plant contained in the article. Contains not less than 2.5% of glycyrrhizic acid, calculated on the dried basis. Meets the requirements for Botanic characteristics, Thin-layer chromatographic identification test, Loss on drying (not more than 12.0%), Foreign organic matter (not more than 2.0%), Total ash (not more than 7.0%), Acid-insoluble ash (not more than 2.0%), Alcohol-soluble extractives (not less than 25.0%), Pesticide residues, Heavy metals (0.003%), and Content of glycyrrhizic acid.

Licorice Fluidextract NF—Preserve in tight, light-resistant containers, and avoid exposure to direct sunlight and to excessive heat. The label states the Latin binomial name and, following the official name, the part of the plant source from which the article was derived.

Prepare Licorice Fluidextract as follows: To 1000 grams of coarsely ground Licorice add about 3000 mL of boiling Purified Water, mix, and allow to macerate in a suitable, covered percolator for 2 hours. Allow the percolation to proceed at a rate of 1 to 3 mL per minute, gradually adding boiling Purified Water until the glycyrrhiza is exhausted. Add enough diluted ammonia solution to the percolate to impart a distinctly ammoniacal odor, and boil the liquid actively under normal atmospheric pressure until it is reduced in volume to about 1500 mL. Filter the liquid, evaporate the filtrate on a steam bath until the residue measures 750 mL, cool, gradually add 250 mL of Alcohol and enough Purified Water to make the product measure 1000 mL, and mix.

Meets the requirement for Alcohol content (20.0–24.0%).

Powdered Licorice NF—Store in well-closed containers in a cool, dry place. It is Licorice reduced to a fine or very fine powder. The label states the Latin binomial name and, following the official name, the part of the plant contained in the article. Contains not less than 2.5% of glycyrrhizic acid, calculated on the dried basis. Meets the requirements for Botanic characteristics, and for Thin-layer chromatographic identification test and the tests for Loss on drying, Foreign organic matter, Total ash, Acid-insoluble ash, Alcohol-soluble extractives, Pesticide residues, Heavy metals, and Content of glycyrrhizic acid for Licorice.

Powdered Licorice Extract NF—Preserve in tight containers, protected from light. Prepared from comminuted Licorice extracted with water or suitable solvents such as alcohol, water, or mixtures of these solvents. The ratio of the crude plant material of Powdered Extract is between 5:1 and 7:1. The label states the Latin binomial name and, following the official name, the part of the plant from which the article was derived. The label also indicates the content of glycyrrhizic acid, the extracting solvent or solvent mixture used for preparation, and the ratio of the starting material to final product. It meets the requirements for Labeling under *Botanical Extracts*. Contains not less than 6.0% of glycyrrhizic acid, calculated on the dried basis. Meets the requirements for Thin-layer chromatographic identificatin test, Loss on drying (not more than 10.0%), Total ash (not more than 12.0%), Pesticide residues, Heavy metals (0.003%), Organic volatile impurities, and Content of glycyrrhizic acid.

LIDOCAINE

Chemical group: Amide.

Chemical name:

Lidocaine—Acetamide, 2-(diethylamino)-*N*-(2,6-dimethylphenyl)-.

Lidocaine hydrochloride—Acetamide, 2-(diethylamino)-*N*-(2,6-dimethylphenyl)-, monohydrochloride, monohydrate.

Molecular formula:

Lidocaine—$C_{14}H_{22}N_2O$.

Lidocaine hydrochloride—$C_{14}H_{22}N_2O \cdot HCl \cdot H_2O$.

Molecular weight:

Lidocaine—234.34.

Lidocaine hydrochloride—288.81.

Description:

Lidocaine USP—White or slightly yellow, crystalline powder. Has a characteristic odor and is stable in air.

Lidocaine Hydrochloride USP—White, odorless, crystalline powder.

pKa: Lidocaine—7.86.

Solubility:

Lidocaine USP—Practically insoluble in water; very soluble in alcohol and in chloroform; freely soluble in ether; dissolves in oils.

Lidocaine Hydrochloride USP—Very soluble in water and in alcohol; soluble in chloroform; insoluble in ether.

USP requirements:

Lidocaine USP—Preserve in well-closed containers. Contains not less than 97.5% and not more than 102.5% of lidocaine. Meets the requirements for Identification, Melting range (66–69 °C), Residue on ignition (not more than 0.1%), Chloride (not more than 0.0035%), Sulfate, and Heavy metals (not more than 0.002%).

Lidocaine Topical Aerosol USP (Solution)—Preserve in nonreactive aerosol containers equipped with metered-dose valves. A solution of Lidocaine in a suitable flavored vehicle with suitable propellants in a pressurized container equipped with a metering valve. Contains the labeled amount, within ±10%, and delivers within ±15% of the labeled amount per actuation. Meets the requirements for Identification and Microbial limits, and for Total number of Discharges per Container and Uniformity of dosage units for Topical Aerosols under Aerosols, Metered-dose inhalers, and Dry powder inhalers.

Lidocaine Ointment USP—Preserve in tight containers. It is Lidocaine in a suitable hydrophilic ointment base. Contains the labeled amount, within ±5%. Meets the requirements for Identification, Microbial limits, and Minimum fill.

Lidocaine Oral Topical Solution USP—Preserve in tight containers. Contains the labeled amount, within ±5%. Contains a suitable flavor. Meets the requirement for Identification.

Lidocaine Topical Spray Solution—Not in *USP–NF*.

Lidocaine Topical System—Not in *USP–NF*.

Lidocaine Hydrochloride USP—Preserve in well-closed containers. Where it is intended for use in preparing injectable dosage forms, the label states that it is sterile or must be subjected to further processing during the preparation of injectable dosage forms. Contains not less than 97.5% and not more than 102.5% of lidocaine hydrochloride, calculated on the anhydrous basis. Meets the requirements for Identification, Melting range (74–79 °C), Water (5.0–7.0%), Residue on ignition (not more than 0.1%), Sulfate, and Heavy metals (not more than 0.002%), and for Sterility tests and for Bacterial endotoxins under Lidocaine Hydrochloride Injection (where the label states that Lidocaine Hydrochloride is sterile) and for Bacterial endotoxins under Lidocaine Hydrochloride Injection (where the label states that Lidocaine Hydrochloride must be subjected to further processing during the preparation of injectable dosage forms).

Lidocaine Hydrochloride Topical Aerosol—Not in *USP–NF*.

Lidocaine Hydrochloride Film-forming Gel—Not in *USP–NF*.

Lidocaine Hydrochloride Injection USP—Preserve in single-dose or in multiple-dose containers, preferably of Type I glass. Injection may be packaged in 50-mL multiple-dose containers. A sterile solution of Lidocaine Hydrochloride in Water for Injection, or a sterile solution prepared from Lidocaine with the aid of Hydrochloric Acid in Water for Injection. Injections that are of such concentration that they are not intended for direct injection into tissues are labeled to indicate that they are to be diluted prior to administration. Contains the labeled amount, within ±5%. Meets the requirements for Identification, Bacterial endotoxins, pH (5.0–7.0), and Particulate matter, and for Injections.

Lidocaine Hydrochloride Injection for Continuous Intravenous Infusion—Not in *USP–NF*.

Lidocaine Hydrochloride Injection for Direct Intravenous Injection—Not in *USP–NF*.

Lidocaine Hydrochloride Jelly USP—Preserve in tight containers. It is Lidocaine Hydrochloride in a suitable, water-soluble, sterile, viscous base. Contains the labeled amount, within ±5%. Meets the requirements for Identification, Sterility, Minimum fill, and pH (6.0–7.0).

Lidocaine Hydrochloride Ointment—Not in *USP–NF*.

Lidocaine Hydrochloride Topical Solution USP—Preserve in tight containers. Contains the labeled amount, within ±5%. Meets the requirements for Identification and pH (5.0–7.0).

Lidocaine Hydrochloride Topical Spray Solution—Not in *USP–NF*.

Lidocaine Hydrochloride Oral Topical Solution USP—Preserve in tight containers. Contains the labeled amount, within ±5%. Contains a suitable flavor and/or sweetening agent. Meets the requirements for Identification and pH (5.0–7.0).

LIDOCAINE AND DEXTROSE

For *Lidocaine* and *Dextrose*—See individual listings for chemistry information.

USP requirements:

Lidocaine Hydrochloride and Dextrose Injection USP—Preserve in single-dose glass or plastic containers. Glass containers are preferably of Type I or Type II glass. A sterile solution of Lidocaine Hydrochloride and Dextrose in Water for Injection. Contains the labeled amounts, within ±5%. Meets the requirements for Identification, Bacterial endotoxins, and pH (3.0–7.0), and for Injections.

Lidocaine Hydrochloride and Dextrose Injection for Continuous Intravenous Infusion—Not in *USP–NF*.

LIDOCAINE AND EPINEPHRINE

For *Lidocaine* and *Epinephrine*—See individual listings for chemistry information.

USP requirements: Lidocaine Hydrochloride and Epinephrine Injection USP—Preserve in single-dose or in multiple-dose, light-resistant containers, preferably of Type I glass. A sterile solution prepared from Lidocaine Hydrochloride and Epinephrine with the aid of Hydrochloric Acid in Water for Injection, or a sterile solution prepared from Lidocaine and Epinephrine with the aid of Hydrochloric Acid in Water for Injection, or a sterile solution of Lidocaine Hydrochloride and Epinephrine Bitartrate in Water for Injection. The content of epinephrine does not exceed 0.002% (1 in 50,000). The label indicates that the Injection is not to be used if its color is pinkish or darker than slightly yellow or if it contains a precipitate. Contains the labeled amount of lidocaine hydrochloride, within ±5%, and the labeled amount of epinephrine, within –10% to +15%. Meets the requirements for Color and clarity, Bacterial endotoxins, and pH (3.3–5.5), for Identification test under Lidocaine Hydrochloride Injection, and for Injections.

LIDOCAINE AND PRILOCAINE

For *Lidocaine* and *Prilocaine*—See individual listings for chemistry information.

USP requirements:

Lidocaine and Prilocaine Cream—Not in *USP–NF*.

Lidocaine and Prilocaine Topical Disc—Not in *USP–NF*.

LIME

Chemical name: Calcium oxide.

Molecular formula: CaO.

Molecular weight: 56.08.

Description: Lime USP—Hard, white or grayish white masses or granules, or white or grayish white powder. Is odorless.

Solubility: Lime USP—Slightly soluble in water; very slightly soluble in boiling water.

USP requirements: Lime USP—Preserve in tight containers. When freshly ignited to constant weight, contains not less than 95.0% of lime. Meets the requirements for Identification, Loss on ignition (not more than 10.0%), Insoluble substances (not more than 1.0%), Carbonate, Magnesium and alkali salts, and Organic volatile impurities.

SULFURATED LIME

Source: Mixture of sublimed sulfur, lime, and water resulting in formation of calcium pentasulfide and calcium thiosulfate.

Description: Sulfurated lime solution—Clear orange liquid with a slight odor of hydrogen sulfide.

USP requirements:
 Sulfurated Lime Mask—Not in *USP–NF*.
 Sulfurated Lime Topical Solution—Not in *USP–NF*.

LINCOMYCIN

Source: Produced by the growth of a member of the *lincolnensis* group of *Streptomyces lincolnensis* (Fam. *Streptomycetaceae*).

Chemical name:
 Lincomycin—D-*erythro*-alpha-D-*galacto*-Octopyranoside, methyl 6,8-dideoxy-6-[[(1-methyl-4-propyl-2-pyrrolidinyl)carbonyl]amino]-1-thio-, (2S-*trans*)-.
 Lincomycin hydrochloride—D-*erythro*-alpha-D-*galacto*-Octopyranoside, methyl 6,8-dideoxy-6-[[(1-methyl-4-propyl-2-pyrrolidinyl)carbonyl]amino]-1-thio-, monohydrochloride, monohydrate, (2S-*trans*)-.

Molecular formula:
 Lincomycin—$C_{18}H_{34}N_2O_6S$.
 Lincomycin hydrochloride—$C_{18}H_{34}N_2O_6S \cdot HCl \cdot H_2O$.

Molecular weight:
 Lincomycin—406.54.
 Lincomycin hydrochloride—461.01.

Description:
 Lincomycin Hydrochloride USP—White or practically white, crystalline powder. Is odorless or has a faint odor. Is stable in the presence of air and light. Its solutions are acid and are dextrorotatory.
 Lincomycin Hydrochloride Injection USP—Clear, colorless to slightly yellow solution, having a slight odor.
 Lincomycin Hydrochloride Soluble Powder USP—White to off-white, or light tan free-flowing, fine powder.

Solubility: Lincomycin Hydrochloride USP—Freely soluble in water; soluble in dimethylformamide; very slightly soluble in acetone.

USP requirements:
 Lincomycin Injection USP—Preserve in single-dose or in multiple-dose containers, preferably of Type I glass. Contains benzyl alcohol as a preservative. Contains an amount of Lincomycin Hydrochloride in Water for Injection equivalent to the labeled amount of lincomycin, within –10% to +20%. Meets the requirements for Bacterial endotoxins, Sterility, pH (3.0–5.5), and Particulate matter, and for Injections.
 Lincomycin Oral Solution USP—Preserve in tight containers. Contains an amount of Lincomycin Hydrochloride equivalent to the labeled amount of lincomycin, within –10% to +20%, and one or more suitable colors, flavors, preservatives, and sweeteners in water. Meets the requirements for Uniformity of dosage units (for oral solution packaged in single-unit containers), Deliverable volume , and pH (3–5.5).
 Lincomycin Hydrochloride USP—Preserve in tight containers. Where it is intended for use in preparing injectable dosage forms, the label states that it is sterile or must be subjected to further processing during the preparation of injectable dosage forms. Has a potency equivalent to not less than 790 mcg of lincomycin per mg. Meets the requirements for Identification, Specific rotation (+135° to +150°), Crystallinity, pH (3.0–5.5, in a solution [1 in 10]), Water (3.0–6.0%), and Limit of lincomycin B, and for Sterility and Bacterial endotoxins under Lincomycin Injection (where the label states that Lincomycin Hydrochloride is sterile), and for Bacterial endotoxins under Lincomycin Injection (where the label states that Lincomycin Hydrochloride must be subjected to further processing during the preparation of injectable dosage forms).

 Lincomycin Hydrochloride Capsules USP—Preserve in tight containers. Contain an amount of lincomycin hydrochloride equivalent to the labeled amount of lincomycin, within –10% to +20%. Meet the requirements for Dissolution (75% in 45 minutes in water in Apparatus 1 at 100 rpm), Uniformity of dosage units, and Water (not more than 7.0%).
 Lincomycin Hydrochloride Soluble Powder USP—Preserve in tight containers. Label it to indicate that it is for veterinary use only. Contains an amount of Lincomycin Hydrochloride equivalent to the labeled amount of lincomycin, within ±10%. Meets the requirements for Identification, Water, and Minimum fill.
 Lincomycin Hydrochloride Syrup USP—Preserve in tight containers. Contains an amount of Lincomycin Hydrochloride equivalent to the labeled amount of lincomycin, within –10% to +20%, and one or more suitable colors, flavors, preservatives, and sweeteners in water. Meets the requirements for Uniformity of dosage units (for syrup packaged in single-unit containers), Deliverable volume, and pH (3–5.5).

LINDANE

Chemical name: Cyclohexane, 1,2,3,4,5,6-hexachloro-, (1 alpha,2 alpha,3 beta,4 alpha,5 alpha,6 beta)-.

Molecular formula: $C_6H_6Cl_6$.

Molecular weight: 290.83.

Description: Lindane USP—White, crystalline powder, having a slight, musty odor.

Solubility: Lindane USP—Practically insoluble in water; freely soluble in chloroform; soluble in dehydrated alcohol; sparingly soluble in ether; slightly soluble in ethylene glycol.

USP requirements:
 Lindane USP—Preserve in well-closed containers. The gamma isomer of hexachlorocyclohexane. Contains not less than 99.0% and not more than 100.5% of lindane. Meets the requirements for Identification, Congealing temperature (not less than 112 °C), Water (not more than 0.5%), and Chloride ion.
 Lindane Cream USP—Preserve in tight containers. It is Lindane in a suitable cream base. Contains the labeled amount, within ±10%. Meets the requirements for Identification and pH (8.0–9.0, in a 1 in 5 dilution).
 Lindane Lotion USP—Preserve in tight containers. It is Lindane in a suitable aqueous vehicle. Contains the labeled amount, within ±10%. Meets the requirements for Identification and pH (6.5–8.5).
 Lindane Shampoo USP—Preserve in tight containers. It is Lindane in a suitable vehicle. Contains the labeled amount, within ±10%. Meets the requirements for Identification and pH (6.2–7.0).

LINEZOLID

Source: A synthetic antibacterial agent.

Chemical group: Oxazolidinone.

Chemical name: Acetamide, *N*-[[3-[3-fluoro-4-(4-morpholinyl)phenyl]-2-oxo-5-oxazolidinyl]methyl]-, (*S*)-.

Molecular formula: $C_{16}H_{20}FN_3O_4$.

Molecular weight: 337.35.

USP requirements:
 Linezolid Injection—Not in *USP–NF*.

Linezolid for Oral Suspension—Not in *USP–NF*.
Linezolid Tablets—Not in *USP–NF*.

LIOTHYRONINE

Chemical name: Liothyronine sodium—L-Tyrosine, *O*-(4-hydroxy-3-iodophenyl)-3,5-diiodo-, monosodium salt.

Molecular formula: Liothyronine sodium—$C_{15}H_{11}I_3NNaO_4$.

Molecular weight: Liothyronine sodium—672.96.

Description: Liothyronine Sodium USP—Light tan, odorless, crystalline powder.

Solubility: Liothyronine Sodium USP—Very slightly soluble in water; slightly soluble in alcohol; practically insoluble in most other organic solvents.

USP requirements:
Liothyronine Sodium USP—Preserve in tight containers. The sodium salt of L-3,3′,5-triiodothyronine. Contains not less than 95.0% and not more than 101.0% of liothyronine sodium, calculated on the dried basis. Meets the requirements for Identification, Specific rotation (+18° to +22°), Loss on drying (not more than 4.0%), Limit of inorganic iodide (not more than 0.08%), Limit of levothyroxine sodium (not more than 5.0%), Chloride content (not more than 1.2%), and Sodium content (2.9–4.0%).
Liothyronine Sodium Injection—Not in *USP–NF*.
Liothyronine Sodium Tablets USP—Preserve in tight containers. Contain an amount of liothyronine sodium equivalent to the labeled amount of liothyronine, within ±10%. Meet the requirements for Identification, Dissolution (70% in 45 minutes in alkaline borate buffer [pH 10.0±0.05] in Apparatus 3), and Uniformity of dosage units.

LIOTRIX

Source: A mixture of liothyronine sodium and levothyroxine sodium, in a ratio of 1:1 in terms of biological activity, or in a ratio of 1:4 in terms of weight.

Chemical name: L-Tyrosine, *O*-(4-hydroxy-3,5-diiodophenyl)-3,5-diiodo-, monosodium salt, hydrate, mixt. with *O*-(4-hydroxy-3-iodophenyl)-3,5-diiodo-L-tyrosine monosodium salt.

USP requirements: Liotrix Tablets USP—Preserve in tight containers. Contain the labeled amounts of Levothyroxine Sodium and Liothyronine Sodium in a ratio by weight of 4 to 1, respectively, within ±10%. Meet the requirements for Identification, Disintegration (30 minutes), and Uniformity of dosage units.

ALPHA LIPOIC ACID

Chemical name: Thioctic Acid.

Molecular formula: $C_8H_{14}O_2S_2$.

Molecular weight: 206.33.

NF requirements:
Alpha Lipoic Acid NF—Preserve in well-closed containers. Contains not less than 99.0% and not more than 101.0% of alpha lipoic acid, calculated on the dried basis. Meets the requirements for Identification, Melting range (60.0°–62.0°), Specific rotation (−1.0° to +1.0°), Loss on drying (not more than 0.2%), Residue on ignition (less than

0.1%), Heavy metals (0.001%), Limit of 6,8-epitrithiooctanoic acid (not more than 0.1%), and Limit of polymer content (not more than 2%).
Alpha Lipoic Acid Capsules NF—Reserve in well-closed containers. Contain the labeled amount, within −10% to +15%. Meet the requirements for Identification, Disintigration and dissolution (70% in 60 minutes in water in Apparatus 1 at 100 rpm [for hard gelatin capsules] and in Apparatus 2 at 75 rpm [for soft gelatin capsules]), Weight variation, and Content of alpha lipic acid.
Alpha Lipoic Acid Tablets NF—Preserve in well-closed containers. Tablets that are coated are so labeled. Contain the labeled amount, within −10% to +15%. Meet the requirements for Identification, Disintigration and dissolution (70% in 60 minutes in water in Apparatus 2 at 75 rpm), Weight variation, and Content of alpha lipoic acid.

LISADIMATE, OXYBENZONE, AND PADIMATE O

Chemical name:
Lisadimate—1,2,3-Propanetriol, 1-(4-aminobenzoate), (±)-.
Oxybenzone—Methanone, (2-hydroxy-4-methoxyphenyl)-phenyl-.
Padimate O—Benzoic acid, 4-(dimethylamino)-, 2-ethylhexyl ester.

Molecular formula:
Lisadimate—$C_{10}H_{13}NO_4$.
Oxybenzone—$C_{14}H_{12}O_3$.
Padimate O—$C_{17}H_{27}NO_2$.

Molecular weight:
Lisadimate—211.21.
Oxybenzone—228.24.
Padimate O—277.40.

Description:
Lisadimate—Waxy semisolid or syrup.
Oxybenzone USP—Pale yellow powder.
Padimate O USP—Light yellow, mobile liquid having a faint, aromatic odor.

Solubility:
Lisadimate—Insoluble in water, in oils, or in fats; soluble in alcohol, in isopropyl alcohol, or in propylene glycol.
Oxybenzone USP—Practically insoluble in water; freely soluble in alcohol and in toluene.
Padimate O USP—Practically insoluble in water; soluble in alcohol, in isopropyl alcohol, and in mineral oil; practically insoluble in glycerin and in propylene glycol.

USP requirements: Lisadimate, Oxybenzone, and Padimate O Lotion—Not in *USP–NF*.

LISADIMATE AND PADIMATE O

Chemical name:
Lisadimate—1,2,3-Propanetriol, 1-(4-aminobenzoate), (±)-.
Padimate O—Benzoic acid, 4-(dimethylamino)-, 2-ethylhexyl ester.

Molecular formula:
Lisadimate—$C_{10}H_{13}NO_4$.
Padimate O—$C_{17}H_{27}NO_2$.

Molecular weight:
Lisadimate—211.21.
Padimate O—277.40.

Description:
Lisadimate—Waxy semisolid or syrup.

Padimate O USP—Light yellow, mobile liquid having a faint, aromatic odor.

Solubility:
Lisadimate—Insoluble in water, in oils, or in fats; soluble in alcohol, in isopropyl alcohol, or in propylene glycol.
Padimate O USP—Practically insoluble in water; soluble in alcohol, in isopropyl alcohol, and in mineral oil; practically insoluble in glycerin and in propylene glycol.

USP requirements: Lisadimate and Padimate O Lotion—Not in *USP–NF*.

LISINOPRIL

Chemical name: L-Proline, 1-[N^2-(1-carboxy-3-phenylpropyl)-L-lysyl]-, dihydrate, (*S*)-.

Molecular formula: $C_{21}H_{31}N_3O_5 \cdot 2H_2O$.

Molecular weight: 441.52.

Description: Lisinopril USP—White, crystalline powder. Melts at about 160 °C, with decomposition.

Solubility: Lisinopril USP—Soluble in water; sparingly soluble in methanol; practically insoluble in alcohol, in acetone, in acetonitrile, and in chloroform.

USP requirements:
Lisinopril USP—Preserve in well-closed containers. Contains not less than 98.0% and not more than 102.0% of lisinopril, calculated on the anhydrous basis. Meets the requirements for Identification, Specific rotation (−115.3° to −122.5°), Water (8.0–9.5%), Residue on ignition (not more than 0.1%), and Heavy metals (not more than 0.001%).
Lisinopril Tablets USP—Preserve in tight containers. Contain the labeled amount, within ±10%. Meet the requirements for Identification, Dissolution (80% in 30 minutes in 0.1 *N* hydrochloric acid in Apparatus 2 at 50 rpm), Uniformity of dosage units, and Related compounds.

LISINOPRIL AND HYDROCHLOROTHIAZIDE

For *Lisinopril* and *Hydrochlorothiazide*—See individual listings for chemistry information.

USP requirements: Lisinopril and Hydrochlorothiazide Tablets—Not in *USP–NF*.

LITHIUM

Chemical name:
Lithium carbonate—Carbonic acid, dilithium salt.
Lithium citrate—1,2,3-Propanetricarboxylic acid, 2-hydroxy-, trilithium salt tetrahydrate.
Lithium hydroxide—Lithium hydroxide monohydrate.

Molecular formula:
Lithium carbonate—Li_2CO_3.
Lithium citrate—$C_6H_5Li_3O_7 \cdot 4H_2O$.
Lithium hydroxide—$LiOH \cdot H_2O$.

Molecular weight:
Lithium carbonate—73.89.
Lithium citrate—281.98.
Lithium hydroxide—41.96.

Description:
Lithium Carbonate USP—White, granular, odorless powder.
Lithium Citrate USP—White, odorless, deliquescent powder or granules.
Lithium hydroxide—Small crystals.

Solubility:
Lithium Carbonate USP—Sparingly soluble in water; very slightly soluble in alcohol. Dissolves, with effervescence, in dilute mineral acids.
Lithium Citrate USP—Freely soluble in water; slightly soluble in alcohol.
Lithium hydroxide—Solubility in water (w/w) at 0 °C: 10.7%, at 20 °C: 10.9%, and at 100 °C: 14.8%; slightly soluble in alcohol.

Other characteristics: A monovalent cation; salts share some chemical characteristics with salts of sodium and potassium.

USP requirements:
Lithium Oral Solution USP—Preserve in tight containers. Prepared from Lithium Citrate or Lithium Hydroxide to which an excess of Citric Acid has been added. Contains an amount of lithium citrate equivalent to the labeled amount of lithium, within ±10%. Meets the requirements for Identification and pH (4.0–5.0).
Lithium Carbonate USP—Preserve in well-closed containers. Contains not less than 99.0% of lithium carbonate, calculated on the dried basis. Meets the requirements for Identification, Reaction, Loss on drying (not more than 1.0%), Insoluble substances, Chloride (not more than 0.07%), Sulfate (not more than 0.1%), Aluminum and iron, Calcium (not more than 0.15%), Sodium (not more than 0.1%), Heavy metals (not more than 0.002%), and Organic volatile impurities.
Lithium Carbonate Capsules USP—Preserve in well-closed containers. Contain the labeled amount, within ±5%. Meet the requirements for Identification, Dissolution (80% in 30 minutes in water in Apparatus 1 at 100 rpm), and Uniformity of dosage units.
Lithium Carbonate Slow-release Capsules—Not in *USP–NF*.
Lithium Carbonate Tablets USP—Preserve in well-closed containers. Contain the labeled amount, within ±5%. Meet the requirements for Identification, Dissolution (80% in 30 minutes in water in Apparatus 1 at 100 rpm), and Uniformity of dosage units.
Lithium Carbonate Extended-release Tablets USP—Preserve in well-closed containers. The labeling indicates the Drug Release Test with which the product complies. Contain the labeled amount, within ±10%. Meet the requirements for Identification, Drug release (2–16% in 15 minutes, 25–45% in 45 minutes, 60–85% in 90 minutes, and not less than 85% in 120 minutes in dilute hydrochloric acid (7:1000) in Apparatus 1 at 100 rpm for Test 1; not more than 40% in 1 hour, 45–75% in 3 hours, and not less than 70% in 7 hours in water in Apparatus 1 at 100 rpm for Test 2; and 10–45% in 1 hour, 25–75% in 2 hours, and not less than 70% in 6 hours in water in Apparatus 3, 6 dips per minute, 20–mesh top screen and 100–mesh bottom screen for Test 3), and Uniformity of dosage units.
Lithium Citrate USP—Preserve in tight containers. Contains not less than 98.0% and not more than 102.0% of lithium citrate, calculated on the anhydrous basis. Meets the requirements for Identification, pH (7.0–10.0, in a solution [1 in 20]), Water (24.0–28.0%), Carbonate, Heavy metals (not more than 0.001%), and Organic volatile impurities.
Lithium Citrate Syrup USP—Preserve in tight containers. Prepared from Lithium Citrate or Lithium Hydroxide to which an excess of Citric Acid has been added. Contains an amount of lithium citrate equivalent to the labeled amount of lithium, within ±10%. Meets the requirements for Identification and pH (4.0–5.0).
Lithium Hydroxide USP—Preserve in tight containers. Contains not less than 98.0% and not more than 102.0% of lithium hydroxide, calculated on the anhydrous basis. Meets the requirements for Identification, Water (41.0–43.5%), Carbonate (not more than 0.7%), Sulfate (not

more than 0.05%), Calcium (not more than 0.20%), Heavy metals (not more than 0.002%), Organic volatile impurities, and Lithium content (28.4–29.1%, calculated on the anhydrous basis).

Caution: Exercise great care in handling Lithium Hydroxide, as it rapidly destroys tissues.

LODOXAMIDE

Chemical name: Lodoxamide tromethamine—Acetic acid, 2,2'-[(2-chloro-5-cyano-1,3-phenylene)diimino]bis[2-oxo-, compound with 2-amino-2-(hydroxymethyl)-1,3-propanediol (1:2).

Molecular formula: Lodoxamide tromethamine—$C_{11}H_6ClN_3O_6$ · $2C_4H_{11}NO_3$.

Molecular weight: Lodoxamide tromethamine—553.90.

Description: Lodoxamide tromethamine—White, crystalline powder.

Solubility: Lodoxamide tromethamine—Soluble in water.

USP requirements: Lodoxamide Tromethamine Ophthalmic Solution—Not in *USP–NF*.

LOMEFLOXACIN

Chemical name: Lomefloxacin hydrochloride—3-Quinolinecarboxylic acid, 1-ethyl-6,8-difluoro-1,4-dihydro-7-(3-methyl-1-piperazinyl)-4-oxo, monohydrochloride, (±)-.

Molecular formula: Lomefloxacin hydrochloride—$C_{17}H_{19}F_2N_3O_3$ · HCl.

Molecular weight: Lomefloxacin hydrochloride—387.81.

Description: Lomefloxacin hydrochloride—White to pale yellow powder. Stable to heat and moisture but sensitive to light in dilute aqueous solution.

Solubility: Lomefloxacin hydrochloride—Slightly soluble in water; practically insoluble in alcohol.

USP requirements: Lomefloxacin Hydrochloride Tablets—Not in *USP–NF*.

LOMUSTINE

Chemical name: Urea, N-(2-chloroethyl)-N'-cyclohexyl-N-nitroso-.

Molecular formula: $C_9H_{16}ClN_3O_2$.

Molecular weight: 233.70.

Description: Yellow powder.

Solubility: Soluble in 10% ethanol and in absolute alcohol; relatively insoluble in water; highly soluble in lipids.

USP requirements: Lomustine Capsules—Not in *USP–NF*.

LOPERAMIDE

Source: Synthetic piperidine derivative.

Chemical group: Opiate agonist.

Chemical name: Loperamide hydrochloride—1-Piperidinebutanamide, 4-(4-chlorophenyl)-4-hydroxy-N,N-dimethyl-alpha,alpha-diphenyl-, monohydrochloride.

Molecular formula: Loperamide hydrochloride—$C_{29}H_{33}ClN_2O_2$ · HCl.

Molecular weight: Loperamide hydrochloride—513.50.

Description: Loperamide Hydrochloride USP—White to slightly yellow powder. Melts at about 225 °C, with some decomposition.

pKa: Loperamide hydrochloride—8.6.

Solubility: Loperamide Hydrochloride USP—Freely soluble in methanol, in isopropyl alcohol, and in chloroform; slightly soluble in water and in dilute acids.

USP requirements:

Loperamide Hydrochloride USP—Preserve in well-closed containers. Contains not less than 98.0% and not more than 102.0% of loperamide hydrochloride, calculated on the dried basis. Meets the requirements for Identification, Loss on drying (not more than 0.5%), Residue on ignition (not more than 0.2%), Heavy metals (not more than 0.002%), Chromatographic purity, and Chloride content (13.52–14.20%).

Loperamide Hydrochloride Capsules USP—Preserve in well-closed containers. Contain the labeled amount, within ± 10%. Meet the requirements for Identification, Dissolution (80% in 30 minutes in acetate buffer [pH 4.7] in Apparatus 1 at 100 rpm), and Uniformity of dosage units.

Loperamide Hydrochloride Oral Solution USP—Preserve in tight, light-resistant containers. Store below 40°, preferably between 15° and 30°, unless otherwise specified by the manufacturer. Contains the labeled amount, within ± 10%. Meets the requirements for Identification, pH (2.7–5.0), and Alcohol content (within ±10%).

Loperamide Hydrochloride Tablets USP—Preserve in well-closed, light-resistant containers. Contain the labeled amount, within ±10%. Meet the requirements for Identification, Dissolution (80% in 30 minutes in 0.01 N hydrochloric acid in Apparatus 2 at 50 rpm), and Uniformity of dosage units.

LOPERAMIDE AND SIMETHICONE

For *Loperamide* and *Simethicone*—See individual listings for chemistry information.

USP requirements: Loperamide and Simethicone Chewable Tablets—Not in *USP–NF*.

LOPINAVIR AND RITONAVIR

Chemical name:

Lopinavir—[1S-[1R*(R*),3R*,4R*]]-N-[4-[[(2,6-Dimethylphenoxy)acetyl]amino]-3-hydroxy-5-phenyl-1-(phenylmethyl)-pentyl]tetrahydro-alpha-(1-methylethyl)-2-oxo-1(2H)-pyrimidineacetamide.

Ritonavir—2,4,7,12-Tetraazatridecan-13-oic acid, 10-hydroxy-2-methyl-5-(1-methylethyl)-1-[2-(1-methylethyl)-4-thiazolyl]-3,6-dioxo-8,11-bis(phenylmethyl)-5-thiazolylmethyl ester [5S-(5R*,8R*,10R*,11R*)]-.

Molecular formula:
  Lopinavir—$C_{37}H_{48}N_4O_5$.
  Ritonavir—$C_{37}H_{48}N_6O_5S_2$.

Molecular weight:
  Lopinavir—628.82.
  Ritonavir—720.95.

Description:
  Lopinavir—White to light tan powder.
  Ritonavir—White-to-light-tan powder.

Solubility:
  Lopinavir—Freely soluble in methanol and in ethanol; soluble in isopropanol; practically insoluble in water.
  Ritonavir—Freely soluble in methanol and in ethanol; soluble in isopropanol; practically insoluble in water.

USP requirements:
  Lopinavir and Ritonavir Capsules—Not in *USP–NF*.
  Lopinavir and Ritonavir Oral Solution—Not in *USP–NF*.

LORACARBEF

Chemical name: 1-Azabicyclo[4.2.0]oct-2-ene-2-carboxylic acid, 7-[(aminophenylacetyl)amino]-3-chloro-8-oxo-, monohydrate, [6*R*-[6 alpha,7 beta(*R**)]]-.

Molecular formula: $C_{16}H_{16}ClN_3O_4 \cdot H_2O$.

Molecular weight: 367.78.

Description: White crystalline compound.

USP requirements:
  Loracarbef USP—Preserve in tight containers. Contains not less than 960 mcg and not more than 1020 mcg of anhydrous loracarbef per mg, calculated on the anhydrous basis. Meets the requirements for Identification, Specific rotation (+27° to +33°, calculated on the anhydrous basis), Crystallinity, pH (3.0–5.5, in a suspension [1 in 10]), Related compounds (not more than 0.15% of phenylglycine, not more than 0.5% of any other related compound, and the sum of all other related compounds not more than 2.0%), and Water (3.5–6.0%).
  Loracarbef Capsules USP—Preserve in well-closed containers. Contain the labeled amount of anhydrous loracarbef, within ±10%. Meet the requirements for Identification, Dissolution (75% in 30 minutes in water in Apparatus 2 at 50 rpm), Uniformity of dosage units, Related compounds (not more than 1.0% of any individual related compound, and the sum of all related compounds not more than 3.0%), and Water (not more than 8.5%).
  Loracarbef for Oral Suspension USP—Preserve in tight containers. A dry mixture of Loracarbef and one or more suitable suspending agents, preservatives, coloring agents, antifoaming agents, flavorings, and sweeteners. Contains the labeled amount of anhydrous loracarbef, within −10% to +15%. Meets the requirements for Identification, Uniformity of dosage units, Deliverable volume, pH (3.0–5.5, in the Loracarbef for Oral Suspension constituted as directed in the labeling), Related compounds (not more than 1.0% of any individual related compound, and the sum of all related compounds not more than 4.0%), and Water (not more than 2.0%).

LORATADINE

Chemical name: 1-Piperidinecarboxylic acid, 4-(8-chloro-5,6-dihydro-11*H*-benzo[5,6]cyclohepta[1,2-*b*]pyridin-11-ylidene)-, ethyl ester.

Molecular formula: $C_{22}H_{23}ClN_2O_2$.

Molecular weight: 382.88.

Description: White to off-white powder. Melting point 134–136 °C.

Solubility: Very soluble in acetone, in alcohol, and in chloroform; not soluble in water.

USP requirements:
  Loratadine Syrup—Not in *USP–NF*.
  Loratadine Tablets—Not in *USP–NF*.

LORATADINE AND PSEUDOEPHEDRINE

For *Loratadine* and *Pseudoephedrine*—See individual listings for chemistry information.

USP requirements:
  Loratadine and Pseudoephedrine Sulfate Tablets—Not in *USP–NF*.
  Loratadine and Pseudoephedrine Sulfate Extended-release Tablets—Not in *USP–NF*.

LORAZEPAM

Chemical name: 2*H*-1,4-Benzodiazepin-2-one, 7-chloro-5-(2-chlorophenyl)-1,3-dihydro-3-hydroxy-.

Molecular formula: $C_{15}H_{10}Cl_2N_2O_2$.

Molecular weight: 321.16.

Description: Lorazepam USP—White or practically white, practically odorless powder.

Solubility: Lorazepam USP—Insoluble in water; sparingly soluble in alcohol; slightly soluble in chloroform.

USP requirements:
  Lorazepam USP—Preserve in tight, light-resistant containers. Contains not less than 98.0% and not more than 102.0% of lorazepam, calculated on the dried basis. Meets the requirements for Identification, Loss on drying (not more than 0.5%), Residue on ignition (not more than 0.3%), Heavy metals (not more than 0.002%), and Related compounds.
  Lorazepam Injection USP—Preserve in a single-dose or in multiple-dose containers, preferably of Type I glass, protected from light. A sterile solution of Lorazepam in a suitable medium. Contains the labeled amount, within ±10%. Meets the requirements for Identification, Bacterial endotoxins, and Related compounds, and for Injections.
  Lorazepam Oral Concentrate USP—Preserve in well-closed, light-resistant containers. Contains the labeled amount, within ±10%. Meets the requirements for Identification and Related compounds.
  Lorazepam Tablets USP—Preserve in tight, light-resistant containers. Contain the labeled amount, within ±10%. Meet the requirements for Identification, Dissolution (60% in 30 minutes and 80% in 60 minutes in water in Apparatus 1 at 100 rpm), Uniformity of dosage units, and Related compounds.
  Lorazepam Sublingual Tablets—Not in *USP–NF*.

LOSARTAN

Chemical name: Losartan potassium—1*H*-Imidazole-5-methanol, 2-butyl-4-chloro-1-[[2′-(1*H*-tetrazol-5-yl)[1,1′-biphenyl]-4-yl]methyl]-, monopotassium salt.

Molecular formula: Losartan potassium—$C_{22}H_{22}ClKN_6O$.

Molecular weight: Losartan potassium—461.00.

Description: Losartan potassium—White to off-white free-flowing crystalline powder.

Solubility: Losartan potassium—Freely soluble in water; soluble in alcohols; slightly soluble in common organic solvents such as acetonitrile and methyl ethyl ketone.

USP requirements: Losartan Potassium Tablets—Not in *USP–NF*.

LOSARTAN AND HYDROCHLOROTHIAZIDE

For *Losartan* and *Hydrochlorothiazide*—See individual listings for chemistry information.

USP requirements: Losartan Potassium and Hydrochlorothiazide Tablets—Not in *USP–NF*.

LOTEPREDNOL

Chemical name: Loteprednol etabonate—Androsta-1,4-diene-17-carboxylic acid, 17-[(ethoxycarbonyl)oxy]-11-hydroxy-3-oxo-, chloromethyl ester, (11 beta,17 alpha)-.

Molecular formula: Loteprednol etabonate—$C_{24}H_{31}ClO_7$.

Molecular weight: Loteprednol etabonate—466.95.

Description: Loteprednol etabonate—White to off-white powder.

USP requirements: Loteprednol Etabonate Ophthalmic Suspension—Not in *USP–NF*.

LOVASTATIN

Source: Isolated from a strain of *Aspergillus terreus*.

Chemical name: Butanoic acid, 2-methyl-, 1,2,3,7,8,8a-hexahydro-3,7-dimethyl-8-[2-(tetrahydro-4-hydroxy-6-oxo-2*H*-pyran-2-yl)ethyl]-1-naphthalenyl ester, [1*S*-[1 alpha(*R**), 3 alpha,7 beta,8 beta(2*S**,4*S**)8a beta]]-.

Molecular formula: $C_{24}H_{36}O_5$.

Molecular weight: 404.54.

Description: Lovastatin USP—White to off-white, crystalline powder.

Solubility: Lovastatin USP—Freely soluble in choroform; soluble in acetone, in acetonitrile, and in methanol; sparingly soluble in alcohol; practically insoluble in hexane; insoluble in water.

USP requirements:
Lovastatin USP—Preserve in tight containers under nitrogen in a cold place. Contains not less than 98.5% and not more than 101.0% of lovastatin, calculated on the dried basis. Meets the requirements for Identification, Specific rotation (+324° to +338°), Loss on drying (not more than 0.3%), Residue on ignition (not more than 0.2%), Heavy metals (not more than 0.002%), Limit of lovastatin related compound A, and Chromatographic purity.

Lovastatin Tablets USP—Preserve in well-closed light-resistant containers. Protect from light and store either in a cool place or at controlled room temperature. Contain the labeled amount, within ±10%. Meet the requirements for Identification, Dissolution (80% in 30 minutes in buffer solution in Apparatus 2 at 50 rpm), and Uniformity of dosage units.

LOXAPINE

Chemical group: A tricyclic dibenzoxazepine derivative.

Chemical name:
Loxapine—Dibenz[*b,f*][1,4]oxazepine, 2-chloro-11-(4-methyl1-piperazinyl)-.
Loxapine succinate—Butanedioic acid, compd. with 2-chloro-11-(4-methyl-1-piperazinyl)dibenz[*b,f*][1,4]oxazepine (1:1).

Molecular formula:
Loxapine—$C_{18}H_{18}ClN_3O$.
Loxapine hydrochloride—$C_{18}H_{18}ClN_3O \cdot HCl$.
Loxapine succinate—$C_{18}H_{18}ClN_3O \cdot C_4H_6O_4$.

Molecular weight:
Loxapine—327.81.
Loxapine hydrochloride—364.3.
Loxapine succinate—445.90.

Description: Loxapine Succinate USP—White to yellowish, crystalline powder. Is odorless.

pKa: 6.6.

Solubility: Loxapine succinate—Slightly soluble in water and in alcohol.

USP requirements:
Loxapine Capsules USP—Preserve in tight containers. Contain an amount of loxapine succinate equivalent to the labeled amount of loxapine, within ±10%. Meet the requirements for Identification, Dissolution (75% in 45 minutes in water in Apparatus 1 at 100 rpm), and Uniformity of dosage units.
Loxapine Hydrochloride Injection—Not in *USP–NF*.
Loxapine Hydrochloride Oral Solution—Not in *USP–NF*.
Loxapine Succinate USP—Preserve in tight containers. Contains not less than 98.5% and not more than 101.0% of loxapine succinate, calculated on the dried basis. Meets the requirements for Identification, Melting range (150–153 °C), Loss on drying (not more than 0.5%), Residue on ignition (not more than 0.1%), Heavy metals (not more than 0.002%), Chromatographic purity, and Organic volatile impurities.
Loxapine Succinate Capsules—Not in *USP–NF*.
Loxapine Succinate Tablets—Not in *USP–NF*.

LYME DISEASE VACCINE

Source: Contains lipoprotein OspA, an outer surface protein of *Borrelia burgdorferi sensu stricto* ZS7, as expressed by *Escherichia coli*. Lipoprotein OspA is a single polypeptide chain of 270 amino acids with lipids covalently bonded to the N terminus. No substance of animal origin is used in the manufacturing process. The fermentation media consist primarily of inorganic salts and vitamins, with small quantities of antifoam containing silicon, kanamycin sulfate, and yeast extract. Silicon and kanamycin are removed to levels below detection. The vaccine is adsorbed onto aluminum hydroxide.

USP requirements: Lyme Disease Vaccine Injection—Not in *USP–NF*.

LYPRESSIN

Source: A synthetic vasopressin analog.

Chemical name: Vasopressin, 8-L-lysine-.

Molecular formula: $C_{46}H_{65}N_{13}O_{12}S_2$.

Molecular weight: 1056.22.

Description: Hygroscopic, crystalline powder.

Solubility: Freely soluble in water.

USP requirements: Lypressin Nasal Solution USP—Preserve in containers suitable for administering the contents by spraying into the nasal cavities in a controlled individualized dosage. A solution, in a suitable diluent, of the polypeptide hormone, prepared synthetically and free from foreign proteins, which has the properties of causing the contraction of vascular and other smooth muscle and of producing antidiuresis, and which is present in the posterior lobe of the pituitary of healthy pigs. Contains suitable preservatives, and is packaged in a form suitable for nasal administration so that the required dosage can be controlled as required. Label it to indicate that it is for intranasal administration only. Label it also to state that the package insert should be consulted for instructions to regulate the dosage according to symptoms. Each mL of Lypressin Nasal Solution possesses a pressor activity of that stated on the label in USP Posterior Pituitary Units, within −15% to +20%. Meets the requirements for pH (3.0–4.3) and Limit of oxytocic activity.

LYSINE

Chemical name:
   Lysine acetate—L-Lysine monoacetate.
   Lysine hydrochloride—L-Lysine monohydrochloride.

Molecular formula:
   Lysine acetate—$C_6H_{14}N_2O_2 \cdot C_2H_4O_2$.
   Lysine hydrochloride—$C_6H_{14}N_2O_2 \cdot HCl$.

Molecular weight:
   Lysine acetate—206.24.
   Lysine hydrochloride—182.65.

Description:
   Lysine Acetate USP—White, odorless crystals or crystalline powder.
   Lysine Hydrochloride USP—White, odorless powder.

Solubility:
   Lysine Acetate USP—Freely soluble in water.
   Lysine Hydrochloride USP—Freely soluble in water.

USP requirements:
   Lysine Acetate USP—Preserve in well-closed containers. Contains not less than 98.0% and not more than 102.0% of lysine acetate, as L-lysine acetate, calculated on the dried basis. Meets the requirements for Identification, Specific rotation (+8.4° to +9.9°), Loss on drying (not more than 0.2%), Residue on ignition (not more than 0.4%), Chloride (not more than 0.05%), Sulfate (not more than 0.03%), Iron (not more than 0.003%), Heavy metals (0.0015%), Chromatographic purity, and Organic volatile impurities.
   Lysine Hydrochloride USP—Preserve in well-closed containers. Contains not less than 98.5% and not more than 101.5% of lysine hydrochloride, as L-lysine hydrochloride,

calculated on the dried basis. Meets the requirements for Identification, Specific rotation (+20.4° to +21.4°), Loss on drying (not more than 0.4%), Residue on ignition (not more than 0.1%), Sulfate (not more than 0.03%), Iron (not more than 0.003%), Heavy metals (not more than 0.0015%), Organic volatile impurities, and Chloride content (19.0–19.6%).

MAFENIDE

Chemical group: Methylated sulfonamide.

Chemical name: Mafenide acetate—Benzenesulfonamide, 4-(aminomethyl)-, monoacetate.

Molecular formula: Mafenide acetate—$C_7H_{10}N_2O_2S \cdot C_2H_4O_2$.

Molecular weight: Mafenide acetate—246.28.

Description: Mafenide Acetate USP—White to pale yellow, crystalline powder.

Solubility: Mafenide Acetate USP—Freely soluble in water.

Other characteristics: Sulfonamides have certain chemical similarities to some goitrogens, diuretics (acetazolamide and thiazides), and oral antidiabetic agents.

USP requirements:
   Mafenide Acetate USP—Preserve in tight, light-resistant containers. Contains not less than 98.0% and not more than 102.0% of mafenide acetate, calculated on the anhydrous basis. Meets the requirements for Identification, Melting range (162–171 °C, the range between beginning and end of melting not more than 4 °C), pH (6.4–6.8, in a solution [1 in 10]), Water (not more than 1.0%), Residue on ignition (not more than 0.2%), Selenium (not more than 0.003%, a 200-mg test specimen being used), Heavy metals (not more than 0.002%), Chromatographic purity, and Organic volatile impurities.
   Mafenide Acetate Cream USP—Preserve in tight, light-resistant containers, and avoid exposure to excessive heat. It is Mafenide Acetate in a water-miscible, oil-in-water cream base, containing suitable preservatives. Contains an amount of mafenide acetate equivalent to the labeled amount of mafenide, within ±10%. Meets the requirement for Identification.
   Mafenide Acetate Solution—Not in *USP–NF*.
   Mafenide Acetate for Topical Solution USP—Preserve in tight, light-resistant containers, at controlled room temperature. For prepared solution, use within 48 hours of preparation. Contains not less than 98.0% and not more than 102.0% of mafenide acetate, calculated on the anhydrous basis. Meets the requirements for Identification, Chromatographic purity, and Content of acetic acid, and for pH and Water under Mafenide Acetate.

MAGALDRATE

Source: A combination of aluminum and magnesium hydroxides and sulfate.

Chemical name: Aluminum magnesium hydroxide sulfate.

Molecular formula: $Al_5Mg_{10}(OH)_{31}(SO_4)_2 \cdot xH_2O$.

Molecular weight: 1097.31 (anhydrous, approx.).

Description: Magaldrate USP—White, odorless, crystalline powder.

Solubility: Magaldrate USP—Insoluble in water and in alcohol; soluble in dilute solutions of mineral acids.

USP requirements:

Magaldrate USP—Preserve in well-closed containers. A chemical combination of aluminum and magnesium hydroxides and sulfate, corresponding approximately to the formula: $Al_5Mg_{10}(OH)_{31}(SO_4)_2 \cdot xH_2O$. Contains the equivalent of not less than 90.0% and not more than 105.0% of magaldrate, calculated on the dried basis. Meets the requirements for Identification, Microbial limits, Loss on drying (10.0–20.0%), Soluble chloride (not more than 3.5%), Soluble sulfate (not more than 1.9%), Sodium (not more than 0.11%), Arsenic (not more than 8 ppm), Heavy metals (not more than 0.006%), Organic volatile impurities, Magnesium hydroxide content (49.2–66.6%, calculated on the dried basis), Aluminum hydroxide content (32.1–45.9%, calculated on the dried basis), and Sulfate content (16.0–21.0%, calculated on the dried basis).

Magaldrate Oral Suspension USP—Preserve in tight containers. Contains the labeled amount, within ±10%. Meets the requirements for Identification, Microbial limits, Acid-neutralizing capacity, Magnesium hydroxide content (492–666 mg per gram of labeled amount of magaldrate), and Aluminum hydroxide content (321–459 mg per gram of labeled amount of magaldrate), and for Arsenic and Heavy metals under Magaldrate.

Magaldrate Tablets USP—Preserve in well-closed containers. Label the Tablets to indicate whether they are to be swallowed or to be chewed. Contain the labeled amount, within ±10%. Meet the requirements for Identification, Microbial limits, Disintegration (2 minutes, for Magaldrate Tablets labeled to be swallowed), Uniformity of dosage units, Acid-neutralizing capacity, Magnesium hydroxide content (492–666 mg per gram of labeled amount of magaldrate), and Aluminum hydroxide content (321–459 mg per gram of labeled amount of magaldrate).

MAGALDRATE AND SIMETHICONE

For *Magaldrate* and *Simethicone*—See individual listings for chemistry information.

USP requirements:

Magaldrate and Simethicone Oral Suspension USP—Preserve in tight containers, and keep from freezing. Contains the labeled amount of magaldrate, within ±10%. Contains an amount of polydimethylsiloxane equivalent to the labeled amount of simethicone, within ±15%. Meets the requirements for Identification, Microbial limits, Acid-neutralizing capacity, Defoaming activity, Magnesium hydroxide content (492–666 mg per gram of labeled amount of magaldrate), and Aluminum hydroxide content (321–459 mg per gram of labeled amount of magaldrate), and for Arsenic and Heavy metals under Magaldrate.

Magaldrate and Simethicone Tablets USP—Preserve in well-closed containers. Label the Tablets to indicate that they are to be chewed before being swallowed. Contain the labeled amount of magaldrate, within ±10%. Contain an amount of polydimethylsiloxane equivalent to the labeled amount of simethicone, within ±15%. Meet the requirements for Identification, Microbial limits, Uniformity of dosage units, Acid-neutralizing capacity, Defoaming activity (not more than 45 seconds), Magnesium hydroxide content (492–666 mg per gram of labeled amount of magaldrate), and Aluminum hydroxide content (321–459 mg per gram of labeled amount of magaldrate).

MAGNESIUM ALUMINOMETASILICATE

Description: Magnesium Aluminometasilicate NF—White powder or granules having an amorphous structure.

Solubility: Magnesium Aluminometasilicate NF—Practically soluble in acids and in alkalies; practically insoluble in water and in alcohol.

NF requirements: Magnesium Aluminometasilicate NF—Preserve in tight containers, and prevent exposure to excessive heat. A synthetic material that exists in two forms, Type I-A and Type I-B, having different pH requirements. Label it to indicate whether it is Type I-A or Type I-B. The required contents for both forms are the same: not less than 29.1% and not more than 35.5% of aluminum oxide, not less than 11.4% and not more than 14.0% of magnesium oxide, and not less than 29.2% and not more than 35.6% of silicon dioxide, calculated on the dried basis. Meets the requirements for Identification, Acid-consuming capacity (not less than 210 mL of 0.1 N hydrochloric acid per gram, calculated on the dried basis), Alkalinity, pH (6.5–8.5 for Type I-A, and 8.5–10.5 for Type I-B), Loss on drying (not more than 20.0%), Soluble salts (not more than 1.6%), and Chloride (not more than 0.053%), Sulfate (not more than 0.480%), Arsenic (3 mcg per gram), Iron (0.03%), and Heavy metals (30 mcg per gram).

MAGNESIUM ALUMINOSILICATE

Description: Magnesium Aluminosilicate NF—White powder or granules having an amorphous structure.

Solubility: Magnesium Aluminosilicate NF—Practically soluble in water and in alcohol.

NF requirements: Magnesium Aluminosilicate NF—Preserve in tight containers, and prevent exposer to excessive heat. A synthesized material that contains not less than 20.5% and not more than 27.7% of magnesium oxide, not less than 27.0% and not more than 34.3% of aluminum oxide, and not less than 14.4% and not more than 21.7% of silicon dioxide, calculated on the dried basis. Meets the requirements for Acid-consuming capacity (not less than 250 mL of 0.1 N hydrochloric acid per gram, calculated on the dried basis) and pH (8.5–10.5), and for Identification, Loss on drying, Soluble salts, Alkalinity, Chloride, Sulfate, Arsenic, Iron, and Heavy metals for Magnesium Aluminometasilicate.

MAGNESIUM ALUMINUM SILICATE

Description: Magnesium Aluminum Silicate NF—Odorless, fine (micronized) powder, small cream to tan granules, or small flakes that are creamy when viewed on their flat surfaces and tan to brown when viewed on their edges.

NF category: Suspending and/or viscosity-increasing agent.

Solubility: Magnesium Aluminum Silicate NF—Insoluble in water and in alcohol. Swells when added to water or glycerin.

NF requirements: Magnesium Aluminum Silicate NF—Preserve in tight containers. A blend of colloidal montmorillonite and saponite that has been processed to remove grit and non-swellable ore components. It is available in 4 types that differ in requirements for viscosity and ratio of aluminum content to magnesium content. Label it to indicate its type. Meets the requirements for Identification, Viscosity, Microbial limits, pH (9.0–10.0, in a suspension [5 in 100] in water), Loss on drying

(not more than 8.0%), Acid demand (pH not more than 4.0), Arsenic (not more than 3 ppm), and Lead (not more than 0.0015%).

MAGNESIUM CARBONATE

Chemical name: Carbonic acid, magnesium salt, basic; or, Carbonic acid, magnesium salt (1:1), hydrate.

Molecular formula:
Magnesium carbonate—$MgCO_3 \cdot H_2O$.
Magnesium carbonate, basic (approx.)—$(MgCO_3)_4 \cdot Mg(OH)_2 \cdot 5H_2O$.

Molecular weight:
Magnesium carbonate—102.33.
Magnesium carbonate, basic (approx.)—485.65.

Description: Magnesium Carbonate USP—Light, white, friable masses or bulky, white powder. Is odorless, and is stable in air.

Solubility: Magnesium Carbonate USP—Practically insoluble in water to which, however, it imparts a slightly alkaline reaction; insoluble in alcohol, but is dissolved by dilute acids with effervescence.

USP requirements: Magnesium Carbonate USP—Preserve in well-closed containers. A basic hydrated magnesium carbonate or a normal hydrated magnesium carbonate. Contains the equivalent of not less than 40.0% and not more than 43.5% of magnesium oxide. Meets the requirements for Identification, Microbial limits, Soluble salts (not more than 1.0%), Acid-insoluble substances (not more than 0.05%), Arsenic (not more than 4 ppm), Limit of calcium (not more than 0.45%), Heavy metals (not more than 0.003%), and Iron (not more than 0.02%).

MAGNESIUM CARBONATE AND CITRIC ACID

For *Magnesium Carbonate* and *Citric Acid*—See individual listings for chemistry information.

USP requirements: Magnesium Carbonate and Citric Acid for Oral Solution USP—Preserve in tight containers. The label contains directions for constitution of the powder and states the equivalent amount of magnesium citrate in a given volume of the Oral Solution obtained after constitution. Contains a dry mixture of Magnesium Carbonate and Citric Acid that when constituted as directed in the labeling yields a solution that contains labeled amount of magnesium citrate, within ±10%. Meets the requirements for Microbial limits, Uniformity of dosage units, Content of anhydrous citric acid (76.6–107.8%), and for Identification and for Chloride, Sulfate, and Tartaric acid under Magnesium Citrate Oral Solution.

MAGNESIUM CARBONATE AND SODIUM BICARBONATE

For *Magnesium Carbonate* and *Sodium Bicarbonate*—See individual listings for chemistry information.

USP requirements:
Magnesium Carbonate and Sodium Bicarbonate for Oral Suspension USP—Preserve in tight containers. Contains the labeled amounts, within ±10%. Meets the requirements for Identification, Acid-neutralizing capacity, and Minimum fill.

Magnesium Carbonate and Sodium Bicarbonate Chewable Tablets—Not in *USP–NF*.

MAGNESIUM CHLORIDE

Chemical name: Magnesium chloride, hexahydrate.

Molecular formula: $MgCl_2 \cdot 6H_2O$.

Molecular weight: 203.30.

Description: Magnesium Chloride USP—Colorless, odorless, deliquescent flakes or crystals, which lose water when heated to 100 °C and lose hydrochloric acid when heated to 110 °C.

Solubility: Magnesium Chloride USP—Very soluble in water; freely soluble in alcohol.

USP requirements:
Magnesium Chloride USP—Preserve in tight containers. Where Magnesium Chloride is intended for use in hemodialysis, it is so labeled. Contains not less than 98.0% and not more than 101.0% of magnesium chloride. Meets the requirements for Identification, pH (4.5–7.0, in a 1 in 20 solution in carbon dioxide–free water), Insoluble matter (not more than 0.005%), Sulfate (not more than 0.005%), Aluminum (where it is labeled as intended for use in hemodialysis, not more than 1 mcg per gram), Barium, Limit of calcium (not more than 0.01%), Potassium, Heavy metals (not more than 0.001%), and Organic volatile impurities.
Magnesium Chloride Injection—Not in *USP–NF*.
Magnesium Chloride Tablets—Not in *USP–NF*.
Magnesium Chloride Enteric-coated Tablets—Not in *USP–NF*.
Magnesium Chloride Extended-release Tablets—Not in *USP–NF*.

MAGNESIUM CITRATE

Chemical name: 1,2,3-Propanetricarboxylic acid, hydroxy-, magnesium salt (2:3).

Molecular formula: $C_{12}H_{10}Mg_3O_{14}$.

Molecular weight: 451.12.

Description: Magnesium Citrate Oral Solution USP—Colorless to slightly yellow, clear, effervescent liquid.

USP requirements:
Magnesium Citrate USP—Preserve in tight containers. Magnesium Citrate that loses not more than 2.0% of its weight in the test for Loss on drying may be labeled as Anhydrous Magnesium Citrate. Contains not less than 14.5% and not more than 16.4% of magnesium, calculated on the dried basis. Meets the requirements for Identification, pH (5.0–9.0, in a suspension [50 mg per mL]), Loss on drying (not more than 29%, except where it is labeled as anhydrous, not more than 2.0%), Chloride (not more than 0.05%), Sulfate (not more than 0.2%), Arsenic (not more than 3 mcg per gram), Heavy metals (not more than 50 mcg per gram), Iron (not more than 200 mcg per gram), Limit of calcium (not more than 1.0%, calculated on the dried basis), and Organic volatile impurities.
Magnesium Citrate Oral Solution USP—Preserve at controlled room temperature or in a cool place, in bottles containing not less than 200 mL. A sterilized or pasteurized solution. Contains, in each 100 mL, not less than 7.59 grams of anhydrous citric acid and an amount of magnesium citrate equivalent to not less than 1.55 grams and not more than 1.9 grams of magnesium oxide.

Prepare Magnesium Citrate Oral Solution as follows: 15 grams of Magnesium Carbonate, 27.4 grams of Anhydrous Citric Acid, 60 mL of Syrup, 5 grams of Talc, 0.1 mL of Lemon Oil, 2.5 grams of Potassium Bicarbonate, and a sufficient quantity of Purified Water to make 350 mL. Dissolve the anhydrous Citric Acid in 150 mL of hot Purified Water in a suitable dish, slowly add the Magnesium Carbonate, previously mixed with 100 mL of Purified Water, and stir until it is dissolved. Then add the Syrup, heat the mixed liquids to the boiling point, immediately add the Lemon Oil, previously triturated with the Talc, and filter the mixture, while hot, into a strong bottle (previously rinsed with boiling Purified Water) of suitable capacity. Add boiled Purified Water to make the product measure 350 mL. Use Purified Cotton as a stopper for the bottle, allow to cool, add the Potassium Bicarbonate, and immediately insert the stopper in the bottle securely. Finally, shake the solution occasionally until the Potassium Bicarbonate is dissolved, cap the bottle, and sterilize or pasteurize the solution.

Note: An amount (30 grams) of citric acid containing 1 molecule of water of hydration, equivalent to 27.4 grams of anhydrous citric acid, may be used in the foregoing formula. In this process the 2.5 grams of potassium bicarbonate may be replaced by 2.1 grams of sodium bicarbonate, preferably in tablet form. The Oral Solution may be further carbonated by the use of carbon dioxide under pressure.

Meets the requirements for Identification, Chloride (not more than 0.01%), Sulfate (not more than 0.015%), and Tartaric acid.

Magnesium Citrate for Oral Solution USP—Preserve in tight containers. The label contains directions for constitution of the powder and states the equivalent amount of magnesium citrate in a given volume of the Oral Solution obtained after constitution. When constituted as directed in the labeling, yields a solution that contains labeled amount of magnesium citrate, within ±10%. Meets the requirements for Microbial limits, Uniformity of dosage units, Content of anhydrous citric acid (76.6–93.7%), Identification tests, and for Chloride, Sulfate, and Tartaric acid under Magnesium Citrate Oral Solution.

MAGNESIUM GLUCEPTATE

Molecular formula: $C_{14}H_{26}MgO_{16}$.

Molecular weight: 474.7.

USP requirements: Magnesium Gluceptate Oral Solution—Not in *USP–NF*.

MAGNESIUM GLUCONATE

Chemical name: D-Gluconic acid, magnesium salt (2:1), hydrate.

Molecular formula: $C_{12}H_{22}MgO_{14}$ (anhydrous); $C_{12}H_{22}MgO_{14} \cdot 2H_2O$ (dihydrate).

Molecular weight: 414.60 (anhydrous); 450.63 (dihydrate).

Description: Magnesium Gluconate USP—Colorless crystals or white powder or granules. Odorless.

Solubility: Magnesium Gluconate USP—Freely soluble in water; very slightly soluble in alcohol; insoluble in ether.

USP requirements:

Magnesium Gluconate USP—Preserve in well-closed containers. Contains not less than 98.0% and not more than 102.0% of magnesium gluconate, calculated on the anhydrous basis. Meets the requirements for Identification, pH (6.0–7.8, in a solution [1 in 20]), Water (3.0–12.0%), Chloride (not more than 0.05%), Sulfate (not more than 0.05%), Heavy metals (not more than 0.002%), Reducing substances (not more than 1.0%), and Organic volatile impurities.

Magnesium Gluconate Oral Solution—Not in *USP–NF*.

Magnesium Gluconate Tablets USP—Preserve in well-closed containers. Contain the labeled amount, within ±5%. Meet the requirements for Identification, Dissolution (80% in 30 minutes in water in Apparatus 2 at 50 rpm), and Uniformity of dosage units.

MAGNESIUM HYDROXIDE

Chemical name: Magnesium hydroxide.

Molecular formula: $Mg(OH)_2$.

Molecular weight: 58.32.

Description:

Magnesium Hydroxide USP—Bulky, white powder.

Milk of Magnesia USP—White, opaque, more or less viscous suspension from which varying proportions of water usually separate on standing. pH is about 10.

Solubility: Magnesium Hydroxide USP—Practically insoluble in water and in alcohol; soluble in dilute acids.

USP requirements:

Magnesium Hydroxide USP—Preserve in tight containers. Dried at 105 °C for 2 hours, contains not less than 95.0% and not more than 100.5% of magnesium hydroxide. Meets the requirements for Identification, Microbial limits, Loss on drying (not more than 2.0%), Loss on ignition (30.0–33.0%), Soluble salts, Carbonate, Limit of calcium (not more than 1.5%), Heavy metals (not more than 20 mcg per gram), and Lead (not more than 0.001%).

Magnesium Hydroxide Paste USP—Preserve in tight containers. An aqueous paste of magnesium hydroxide, each 100 grams of which contains not less than 29.0 grams and not more than 33.0 grams of magnesium hydroxide. Meets the requirements for Identification, Microbial limits, Soluble alkalies, Soluble salts (not more than 12 mg from 1.67 grams of Paste), Carbonate and acid-insoluble matter, Limit of calcium (not more than 1.5%), and Heavy metals (not more than 5 ppm, based on amount of diluted Paste taken).

Magnesium Hydroxide Tablets—Not in *USP–NF*.

Magnesia Tablets USP—Preserve in well-closed containers. Contain an amount of magnesia equivalent to the labeled amount of magnesium hydroxide, within ±7%. Meet the requirements for Identification, Disintegration (10 minutes, simulated gastric fluid TS being substituted for water in the test), Uniformity of dosage units, and Acid-neutralizing capacity.

Milk of Magnesia USP—Preserve in tight containers, preferably at a temperature not exceeding 35 °C. Avoid freezing. A suspension of Magnesium Hydroxide. Double- or Triple-strength Milk of Magnesia is so labeled, or may be labeled as 2X or 3X Concentrated Milk of Magnesia, respectively. Milk of Magnesia, Double-strength Milk of Magnesia, and Triple-strength Milk of Magnesia contain an amount of magnesia equivalent to the labeled amount of magnesium hydroxide, within −10% to +15%, the labeled amount being 80, 160, and 240 mg of magnesium hydroxide per mL, respectively. Meets the requirements for Identification, Microbial limits, Acid-neutralizing capacity, Soluble alkalies, Carbonate and acid-insoluble matter,

Limit of calcium (not more than 0.07%), and Heavy metals (not more than 20/*W* ppm, the *W* being the weight, in grams, of specimen taken).

MAGNESIUM HYDROXIDE AND CASCARA SAGRADA

For *Magnesium Hydroxide* and *Cascara Sagrada*—See individual listings for chemistry information.

USP requirements: Magnesium Hydroxide and Cascara Sagrada Oral Suspension—Not in *USP–NF*.

MAGNESIUM HYDROXIDE AND MINERAL OIL

For *Magnesium Hydroxide* and *Mineral Oil*—See individual listings for chemistry information.

USP requirements: Milk of Magnesia and Mineral Oil Emulsion—Not in *USP–NF*.

MAGNESIUM LACTATE

Chemical name: 2-Hydroxypropanoic acid magnesium salt.

Molecular formula: $C_6H_{10}MgO_6$.

Molecular weight: 202.4.

USP requirements: Magnesium Lactate Extended-release Tablets—Not in *USP–NF*.

MAGNESIUM OXIDE

Chemical name: Magnesium oxide.

Molecular formula: MgO.

Molecular weight: 40.30.

Description: Magnesium Oxide USP—Very bulky, white powder known as Light Magnesium Oxide or relatively dense, white powder known as Heavy Magnesium Oxide. Five grams of Light Magnesium Oxide occupies a volume of approximately 40 to 50 mL, while 5 grams of Heavy Magnesium Oxide occupies a volume of approximately 10 to 20 mL.

Solubility: Magnesium Oxide USP—Practically insoluble in water; soluble in dilute acids; insoluble in alcohol.

USP requirements:
Magnesium Oxide USP—Preserve in tight containers. Label it to indicate whether it is Light Magnesium Oxide or Heavy Magnesium Oxide. After ignition, contains not less than 96.0% and not more than 100.5% of magnesium oxide. Meets the requirements for Identification, Loss on ignition (not more than 10.0%), Free alkali and soluble salts (not more than 2.0%), Acid-insoluble substances (not more than 0.1%), Limit of calcium (not more than 1.1%), Heavy metals (not more than 20 mcg per gram), and Iron (not more than 0.05%).
Magnesium Oxide Capsules USP—Preserve in well-closed containers. Contain the labeled amount, within ±10%. Meet the requirements for Identification, Dissolution (75% in 45 minutes in 0.1 *N* hydrochloric acid in Apparatus 1 at 100 rpm), Uniformity of dosage units, and Acid-neutralizing capacity.

Magnesium Oxide Tablets USP—Preserve in well-closed containers. Contain the labeled amount, within ±10%. Meet the requirements for Dissolution (75% in 45 minutes in 0.1 *N* hydrochloric acid in Apparatus 2 at 75 rpm), Uniformity of dosage units, and Acid-neutralizing capacity (where Tablets are labeled as intended for antacid use), and for Identification test under Magnesium Oxide Capsules.

MAGNESIUM PHOSPHATE

Chemical name: Phosphoric acid, magnesium salt (2:3), pentahydrate.

Molecular formula: $Mg_3(PO_4)_2 \cdot 5H_2O$.

Molecular weight: 352.93.

Description: Magnesium Phosphate USP—White, odorless powder.

Solubility: Magnesium Phosphate USP—Almost insoluble in water; readily soluble in diluted mineral acids.

USP requirements: Magnesium Phosphate USP—Preserve in well-closed containers. Ignited at 425 °C to constant weight, contains not less than 98.0% and not more than 101.5% of magnesium phosphate. Meets the requirements for Identification, Microbial limits, Loss on ignition (20.0–27.0%), Acid-insoluble substances (not more than 0.2%), Soluble substances (not more than 1.5%), Carbonate, Chloride (not more than 0.14%), Limit of nitrate, Sulfate (not more than 0.6%), Arsenic (not more than 3 ppm), Barium, Calcium, Heavy metals (not more than 0.003%), Dibasic salt and magnesium oxide, and Lead (not more than 5 ppm).

MAGNESIUM PIDOLATE

Molecular formula: $(C_5H_6NO_3)_2Mg$.

Molecular weight: 280.5.

USP requirements: Magnesium Pidolate for Oral Solution—Not in *USP–NF*.

MAGNESIUM SALICYLATE

Chemical name: Magnesium, bis(2-hydroxybenzoato-O^1,O^2)-, tetrahydrate.

Molecular formula: $C_{14}H_{10}MgO_6 \cdot 4H_2O$ (tetrahydrate); $C_{14}H_{10}MgO_6$ (anhydrous).

Molecular weight: 370.59 (tetrahydrate); 298.53 (anhydrous).

Description: Magnesium Salicylate USP—White, odorless, efflorescent, crystalline powder.

Solubility: Magnesium Salicylate USP—Freely soluble in methanol; soluble in alcohol and in water; slightly soluble in ether.

USP requirements:
Magnesium Salicylate USP—Store in tight containers. Contains not less than 98.0% and not more than 103.0% of magnesium salicylate. Meets the requirements for Identification, Water (17.5–21.0%), Heavy metals (not more than 0.004%), Magnesium content (6.3–6.7%), and Organic volatile impurities.
Magnesium Salicylate Tablets USP—Preserve in tight containers. Contain an amount of magnesium salicylate tetrahydrate equivalent to the labeled amount of anhydrous

magnesium salicylate, within ±5%. Meet the requirements for Identification, Dissolution (80% in 120 minutes in water in Apparatus 2 at 50 rpm), and Uniformity of dosage units.

MAGNESIUM SILICATE

Description: Magnesium Silicate NF—Fine, white, odorless powder, free from grittiness.
NF category: Glidant and/or anticaking agent.

Solubility: Magnesium Silicate NF—Insoluble in water and in alcohol. Readily decomposed by mineral acids.

NF requirements: Magnesium Silicate NF—Preserve in well-closed containers. A compound of magnesium oxide and silicon dioxide. Contains not less than 15.0% of magnesium oxide and not less than 67.0% of silicon dioxide, calculated on the ignited basis. Meets the requirements for Identification, pH (7.0–10.8, determined in a well-mixed aqueous suspension [1 in 10]), Loss on drying (not more than 15.0%), Loss on ignition (not more than 15%), Soluble salts (not more than 3.0%), Fluoride (not more than 10 ppm), Free alkali, Lead (not more than 0.001%), Ratio of silicon dioxide to magnesium oxide (quotient 2.50–4.50), Heavy metals (not more than 20 mcg per gram), and Organic volatile impurities.

MAGNESIUM STEARATE

Chemical name: Octadecanoic acid, magnesium salt.

Molecular formula: $C_{36}H_{70}MgO_4$.

Molecular weight: 591.24.

Description: Magnesium Stearate NF—Very fine, light, white powder, slippery to touch.
NF category: Tablet and/or capsule lubricant.

Solubility: Magnesium Stearate NF—Insoluble in water, in alcohol, and in ether.

NF requirements: Magnesium Stearate NF—Preserve in tight containers. A compound of magnesium with a mixture of solid organic acids, consisting chiefly of variable proportions of magnesium stearate and magnesium palmitate. The fatty acids are derived from edible sources. Where the labeling states the specific surface area, it also indicates which method specified under Specific Surface Area is used. Contains not less than 4.0% and not more than 5.0% of magnesium, calculated on the dried basis. Meets the requirements for Identification, Microbial limits, Acidity or alkalinity, Loss on drying (not more than 6.0%), Specific surface area, Limit of chloride (not more than 0.1%), Limit of sulfate (not more than 1.0%), Lead (not more than 0.001%), Organic volatile impurities, and Relative content of stearic acid and palmitic acid.

MAGNESIUM SULFATE

Chemical name: Sulfuric acid magnesium salt (1:1), heptahydrate.

Molecular formula: $MgSO_4 \cdot 7H_2O$.

Molecular weight: 246.48.

Description: Magnesium Sulfate USP—Small, colorless crystals, usually needle-like. It effloresces in warm, dry air.

Solubility: Magnesium Sulfate USP—Freely soluble in water; freely (and slowly) soluble in glycerin; very soluble in boiling water; sparingly soluble in alcohol.

USP requirements:
Magnesium Sulfate USP (Crystals)—Preserve in well-closed containers. The label states whether it is the monohydrate, the dried form, or the heptahydrate. Magnesium Sulfate intended for use in preparing parenteral dosage forms is so labeled. Magnesium Sulfate not intended for use in preparing parenteral dosage forms is so labeled; in addition, it may be labeled also as intended for use in preparing nonparenteral dosage forms. When rendered anhydrous by ignition, contains not less than 99.0% and not more than 100.5% of magnesium sulfate. Meets the requirements for Identification, pH (5.0–9.2, in a solution [1 in 20]), Loss on drying (the anhydrous form losses not more than 2%), Loss on ignition (monohydrate, 13.0–16.0%; dried form, 22.0–28.0%; heptahydrate, 40.0–52.0%), Chloride (not more than 0.014%), Iron (not more than 20 mcg per gram, when intended for use in preparing nonparenteral dosage forms; not more than 0.5 mcg per gram, when intended for use in preparing parenteral dosage forms), Heavy metals (not more than 0.001%), Selenium (not more than 0.003%), and Organic volatile impurities.
Magnesium Sulfate Injection USP—Preserve in single-dose or in multiple-dose containers, preferably of Type I glass. A sterile solution of Magnesium Sulfate in Water for Injection. The label states the total osmolar concentration in mOsmol per liter. Where the contents are less than 100 mL, or where the label states that the Injection is not for direct injection but is to be diluted before use, the label alternatively may state the total osmolar concentration in mOsmol per mL. Contains the labeled amount, within ± 7%. Meets the requirements for Identification, Bacterial endotoxins, pH (5.5–7.0, when diluted to a concentration of 5% [w/v]), and Particulate matter, and for Injections.
Magnesium Sulfate Tablets—Not in *USP–NF*.

MAGNESIUM SULFATE AND DEXTROSE

For *Magnesium Sulfate* and *Dextrose*—See individual listings for chemistry information.

USP requirements: Magnesium Sulfate in Dextrose Injection USP—Preserve in single-dose glass or plastic containers. Glass containers are preferably of Type I or Type II glass. A sterile solution of Magnesium Sulfate and Dextrose in Water for Injection. Contains the labeled amounts of magnesium sulfate and dextrose, within ±7% and ±10%, respectively. Meets the requirements for Identification, Bacterial endotoxins, pH (3.5–6.5), and Limit of 5-hydroxymethylfurfural and related substances, and for Injections.

MAGNESIUM TRISILICATE

Chemical name: Silicic acid ($H_4Si_3O_8$), magnesium salt (1:2), hydrate.

Molecular formula: $2MgO \cdot 3SiO_2 \cdot xH_2O$ (hydrate); $Mg_2Si_3O_8$ (anhydrous).

Molecular weight: 260.86 (anhydrous).

Description: Magnesium Trisilicate USP—Fine, white, odorless powder, free from grittiness.

Solubility: Magnesium Trisilicate USP—Insoluble in water and in alcohol. Is readily decomposed by mineral acids.

USP requirements:

Magnesium Trisilicate USP—Preserve in well-closed containers. A compound of Magnesium Oxide and silicon dioxide with varying proportions of water. Contains not less than 20.0% of magnesium oxide and not less than 45.0% of silicon dioxide. Meets the requirements for Identification, Water (17.0–34.0%), Soluble salts (not more than 1.5%), Chloride (not more than 0.055%), Sulfate (not more than 0.5%), Free alkali, Arsenic (not more than 8 ppm), Heavy metals (not more than 0.003%), Acid-consuming capacity, and Ratio of silicon dioxide to magnesium oxide (quotient 2.10–2.37).

Magnesium Trisilicate Tablets USP—Preserve in well-closed containers. Contain the labeled amount, within ±10%. Meet the requirements for Identification, Disintegration (10 minutes, simulated gastric fluid TS being substituted for water in the test), Uniformity of dosage units, and Acid-neutralizing capacity.

MALATHION

Chemical name: Butanedioic acid, [(dimethoxyphosphinothioyl)-thio]-, diethyl ester.

Molecular formula: $C_{10}H_{19}O_6PS_2$.

Molecular weight: 330.36.

Description: Malathion USP—Yellow to deep brown liquid, having a characteristic odor. Congeals at about 2.9 °C.

Solubility: Malathion USP—Slightly soluble in water. Miscible with alcohols, with esters, with ketones, with ethers, with aromatic and alkylated aromatic hydrocarbons, and with vegetable oils.

USP requirements:

Malathion USP—Preserve in tight, light-resistant containers. Contains not less than 98.0% and not more than 102.0% of malathion. Meets the requirements for Identification, Specific gravity (1.220–1.240), Water (not more than 0.1%), and Limit of isomalathion (not more than 0.3%).

Malathion Lotion USP—Preserve in tight, glass containers. It is Malathion in a suitable isopropyl alcohol vehicle. The labeling states the percentage (v/v) of isopropyl alcohol in the Lotion. Contains the labeled amount, within ±10%. Meets the requirements for Identification and Isopropyl alcohol content (within ±10% of labeled amount).

MALIC ACID

Chemical name: Hydroxybutanedioic acid.

Molecular formula: $C_4H_6O_5$.

Molecular weight: 134.09.

Description: Malic Acid NF—White, or practically white, crystalline powder or granules. Melts at about 130 °C.

NF category: Acidifying agent.

Solubility: Malic Acid NF—Very soluble in water; freely soluble in alcohol.

NF requirements: Malic Acid NF—Preserve in well-closed containers. Contains not less than 99.0% and not more than 100.5% of malic acid. Meets the requirements for Identification, Residue on ignition (not more than 0.1%), Water-insoluble substances (not more than 0.1%), Heavy metals (not more than 0.002%), Fumaric and maleic acids (not more than 1.0% of fumaric acid; not more than 0.05% of maleic acid), and Organic volatile impurities.

MALTITOL SOLUTION

NF requirements: Maltitol Solution NF—Preserve in tight containers. A water solution of a hydrogenated, partially hydrolyzed starch. Contains, on the anhydrous basis, not less than 50.0% of D-maltitol (w/w), and not more than 16.0% of D-sorbitol (w/w). Amounts of total sugars, other polyhydric alcohols, and any polyol anhydrides, if detected, are not included in the requirements nor the calculated amount under Other Impurities. Meets the requirements for Identification, Water (not more than 30.0%), Residue on ignition (not more than 0.1%), Chloride (not more than 0.005%), Sulfate (not more than 0.010%), Heavy metals (not more than 0.001%), and Reducing sugars.

MALTODEXTRIN

Description: Maltodextrin NF—White, hygroscopic powder or granules.

NF category: Tablet and/or capsule diluent; coating agent; tablet binder; viscosity-increasing agent.

Solubility: Maltodextrin NF—Freely soluble or readily dispersible in water; slightly soluble to insoluble in anhydrous alcohol.

NF requirements: Maltodextrin NF—Preserve in tight containers, or in well-closed containers at a temperature not exceeding 30 °C and a relative humidity not exceeding 50%. A nonsweet, nutritive saccharide mixture of polymers that consists of D-glucose units, with a Dextrose Equivalent less than 20. Prepared by the partial hydrolysis of a food grade starch with suitable acids and/or enzymes. May be physically modified to improve its physical and functional characteristics. Meets the requirements for Microbial limits, pH (4.0–7.0, in a 1 in 5 solution in carbon dioxide-free water), Loss on drying (not more than 6.0%), Residue on ignition (not more than 0.5%), Heavy metals (not more than 5 ppm), Protein (not more than 0.1%), Sulfur dioxide (not more than 0.004%), and Dextrose equivalent (less than 20).

MALT SOUP EXTRACT

Source: Obtained from the grain of one or more varieties of barley; contains 73% maltose, 12% other polymeric carbohydrates, 7% protein, 1.5% potassium, and small amounts of calcium, magnesium, phosphorus, and vitamins.

USP requirements:

Malt Soup Extract Powder—Not in *USP–NF*.
Malt Soup Extract Oral Solution—Not in *USP–NF*.
Malt Soup Extract Tablets—Not in *USP–NF*.

MALT SOUP EXTRACT AND PSYLLIUM

For *Malt Soup Extract* and *Psyllium*—See individual listings for chemistry information.

USP requirements: Malt Soup Extract and Psyllium Powder—Not in *USP–NF*.

MANDELIC ACID

Chemical name: Mandelic acid—Alpha-hydroxyphenylacetic acid.

Molecular formula: Mandelic acid—$C_8H_8O_3$.

Molecular weight: Mandelic acid—152.15.

Description: Mandelic Acid USP—White to yellowish-white crystals or crystalline powder. Almost odorless. Gradually turns yellow and decomposes on prolonged exposure to light.

Solubility: Mandelic Acid USP—Freely soluble in ether, in isopropyl alcohol, and in water; very soluble in alcohol; soluble in chloroform.

USP requirements: Mandelic Acid USP—Preserve in well-closed, light-resistant containers. Previously dried in vacuum at 75 °C for 4 hours, contains not less than 98.0% and not more than 102.0% of mandelic acid. Meets the requirements for Identification, Melting range (118–121 °C), Turbidity, Water (not more than 0.5%), Chloride (not more than 0.01%), Residue on ignition (not more than 0.1%), Heavy metals (not more than 20 mcg per gram), Related compounds (not more than 0.1% of benzoylformic acid, 1.0% of benzoic acid, 0.05% of benzaldehyde, and 0.01% of acetophenone), and Organic volatile impurities.

MANGAFODIPIR

Chemical group: Complex formed between a chelating agent (fodipir) and a paramagnetic metal ion (manganese [II]).

Chemical name: Mangafodipir trisodium—Trisodium trihydrogen (*OC*-6-13)-[[*N,N*-1,2-ethanediylbis[*N*-[[3-hydroxy-2-methyl-5-[phosphonooxy)methyl]-4-pyridinyl]methyl]glycinato]](8-)manganate(6-).

Molecular formula: Mangafodipir trisodium—$C_{27}H_{27}MnN_4Na_3O_{14}P_2$.

Molecular weight: Mangafodipir trisodium—757.33.

Description: Mangafodipir Trisodium USP—Pale yellow crystals or crystalline powder.

Solubility: Mangafodipir Trisodium USP—Freely soluble in water; sparingly soluble in methanol; slightly soluble in chloroform; very slightly soluble in alcohol and in acetone.

Other characteristics: Mangafodipir trisodium—Osmolality: 298 mOsmol per kg of water; pH: 8.8.

USP requirements:
Mangafodipir Trisodium USP—Preserve in well-closed containers. Contains not less than 97.0% and not more than 103.0% of mangafodipir trisodium, calculated on the anhydrous basis. Meets the requirements for Identification, Microbial limits (not more than 500 cfu per gram), Bacterial endotoxins, pH (5.5–7.0, in a solution [1 in 100]), Water (not more than 20%), Limit of residual solvents, Limit of free manganese and free fodipir, and Related compounds.
Mangafodipir Trisodium Injection—Not in *USP–NF*.

MANGANESE

Chemical name:
Manganese chloride—Manganese chloride ($MnCl_2$) tetrahydrate.
Manganese gluconate—Bis(D-gluconato-O^1,O^2)manganese.
Manganese sulfate—Sulfuric acid, manganese(2+) salt (1:1) monohydrate.

Molecular formula:
Manganese chloride—$MnCl_2 \cdot 4H_2O$.
Manganese gluconate—$C_{12}H_{22}MnO_{14}$.
Manganese sulfate—$MnSO_4 \cdot H_2O$.

Molecular weight:
Manganese chloride—197.90.
Manganese gluconate—445.23.
Manganese sulfate—169.02.

Description:
Manganese Chloride USP—Large, irregular, pink, odorless, translucent crystals.
Manganese Chloride for Oral Solution USP—Off-white to tan-colored powder with a strawberry ordor.
Manganese Sulfate USP—Pale red, slightly efflorescent crystals, or purple, odorless powder.

Solubility:
Manganese Chloride USP—Soluble in water and in alcohol; insoluble in ether.
Manganese Chloride for Oral Solution USP—Soluble in water.
Manganese Sulfate USP—Soluble in water; insoluble in alcohol.

USP requirements:
Manganese Chloride USP—Preserve in tight containers. Contains not less than 98.0% and not more than 101.0% of manganese chloride, calculated on the dried basis. Meets the requirements for Identification, pH (3.5–6.0), Loss on drying (36.0–38.5%), Insoluble matter (not more than 0.005%), Sulfate (not more than 0.005%), Substances not precipitated by ammonium sulfide (not more than 0.2% as sulfate), Iron (not more than 5 ppm), Zinc, Heavy metals (not more than 5 ppm), and Organic volatile impurities.
Manganese Chloride Injection USP—Preserve in single-dose or in multiple-dose containers, preferably of Type I or Type II glass. A sterile solution of Manganese Chloride in Water for Injection. Label the Injection to indicate that it is to be diluted to the appropriate strength with Sterile Water for Injection or other suitable fluid prior to administration. Contains an amount of manganese chloride equivalent to the labeled amount of manganese, within ±10%. Meets the requirements for Identification, Bacterial endotoxins, pH (1.5–2.5), and Particulate matter, and for Injections.
Manganese Chloride for Oral Solution USP—Preserve in tight, light-resistant, single-dose containers. The label contains directions for constitution of the powder and states the amount of manganese in a given volume of the Oral Solution obtained after constituion. Contains the labeled amount of manganese, within ±10%. May contain one or more suitable flavors, sweetening agents, thickening agents, and stabilizers. Meets the requirements for Identification, pH (6.0–8.0, when constituted to 300 mL with water), and Osmolarity (230 mOsmol at pH 6.0 to 8.0).
Manganese Gluconate USP—Preserve in well-closed containers. It is dried or contains two molecules of water of hydration. The label indicates whether it is the dried or the dihydrate form. Contains not less than 98.0% and not more than 102.0% of manganese gluconate, calculated on the anhydrous basis. Meets the requirements for Identification, Water (3.0–9.0% where labeled as the dried form and 6.0–9.0% where labeled as the dihydrate form), Chloride (not more than 0.05%), Sulfate (not more than 0.2%), Lead (not more than 0.001%), Heavy metals (not more than 20 mcg per gram), Reducing substances (not more than 1.0%), and Organic volatile impurities.

Manganese Sulfate USP—Preserve in tight containers. Contains not less than 98.0% and not more than 102.0% of manganese sulfate. Meets the requirements for Identification, Loss on ignition (10.0–13.0%), Substances not precipitated by ammonium sulfide (not more than 0.5%), and Organic volatile impurities.

Manganese Sulfate Injection USP—Preserve in single-dose or in multiple-dose containers, preferably of Type I or Type II glass. A sterile solution of Manganese Sulfate in Water for Injection. Label the Injection to indicate that it is to be diluted to the appropriate strength with Sterile Water for Injection or other suitable fluid prior to administration. Contains an amount of manganese sulfate equivalent to the labeled amount of manganese, within ±10%. Meets the requirements for Identification, Bacterial endotoxins, pH (2.0–3.5), and Particulate matter, and for Injections.

MANNITOL

Chemical name: D-Mannitol.

Molecular formula: $C_6H_{14}O_6$.

Molecular weight: 182.17.

Description: Mannitol USP—White, crystalline powder or free-flowing granules. Is odorless.

NF category: Sweetening agent; tablet and/or capsule diluent; tonicity agent; bulking agent for freeze-drying.

Solubility: Mannitol USP—Freely soluble in water; soluble in alkaline solutions; slightly soluble in pyridine; very slightly soluble in alcohol; practically insoluble in ether.

USP requirements:

Mannitol USP—Preserve in well-closed containers. Contains not less than 96.0% and not more than 101.5% of mannitol, calculated on the dried basis. The amounts of total sugars, other polyhydric alcohols, and any hexitol anhydrides, if detected, are not included in the requirements nor the calculated amount under Other impurities. Meets the requirements for Identification, Melting range (164–169 °C), Specific rotation (+137° to +145°), Acidity, Loss on drying (not more than 0.3%), Chloride (not more than 0.007%), Sulfate (not more than 0.01%), Arsenic (not more than 1 ppm), and Reducing sugars.

Mannitol Injection USP—Preserve in single-dose glass or plastic containers. Glass containers are preferably of Type I or Type II glass. A sterile solution, which may be supersaturated, of Mannitol in Water for Injection. Contains no antimicrobial agents. May require warming or autoclaving before use if crystallization has occurred. The label states the total osmolar concentration in mOsmol per liter. Where the contents are less than 100 mL, or where the label states that the Injection is not for direct injection but is to be diluted before use, the label alternatively may state the total osmolar concentration in mOsmol per mL. Contains the labeled amount, within ±5%. Meets the requirements for Identification, Specific rotation, Bacterial endotoxins, pH (4.5–7.0, determined potentiometrically), and Particulate matter, and for Injections.

MANNITOL AND SODIUM CHLORIDE

For *Mannitol* and *Sodium Chloride*—See individual listings for chemistry information.

USP requirements: Mannitol in Sodium Chloride Injection USP—A sterile solution of Mannitol and Sodium Chloride in Water for Injection. Contains no antimicrobial agents. The label states the total osmolar concentration in mOsmol per liter. Where the contents are less than 100 mL, or where the label states that the Injection is not for direct injection but is to be diluted before use, the label alternatively may state the total osmolar concentration in mOsmol per mL. Contains the labeled amounts, within ±5%. Meets the requirements for Identification, Bacterial endotoxins, and pH (4.5–7.0), for Packaging and storage under Mannitol Injection, and for Injections.

MAPROTILINE

Chemical group: Dibenzo-bicyclo-octadiene.

Chemical name: Maprotiline hydrochloride—9,10-Ethanoanthracene-9(10H)-propanamine, N-methyl-, hydrochloride.

Molecular formula: Maprotiline hydrochloride—$C_{20}H_{23}N \cdot HCl$.

Molecular weight: Maprotiline hydrochloride—313.86.

Description: Maprotiline Hydrochloride USP—Fine, white to off-white, crystalline powder. Is practically odorless.

Solubility: Maprotiline Hydrochloride USP—Freely soluble in methanol and in chloroform; slightly soluble in water; practically insoluble in isooctane.

USP requirements:

Maprotiline Hydrochloride USP—Preserve in tight containers. Contains not less than 99.0% and not more than 101.0% of maprotiline hydrochloride, calculated on the dried basis. Meets the requirements for Identification, Loss on drying (not more than 1.0%), Residue on ignition (not more than 0.1%), Heavy metals (not more than 0.001%), Chromatographic purity, and Organic volatile impurities.

Maprotiline Hydrochloride Tablets USP—Preserve in well-closed containers. Contain the labeled amount, within ± 10%. Meet the requirements for Identification, Dissolution (75% in 60 minutes in dilute hydrochloric acid [7 in 1000] in Apparatus 2 at 50 rpm), and Uniformity of dosage units.

MARITIME PINE

NF requirements:

Maritime Pine NF—Store at room temperature. Protect from moisture and excessive heat. Consists of the bark of stems of *Pinus pinaster* Aiton (*Pinus maritima* Poir.) Fam. Pinaceae. The label states the Latin binomial and, following the official name, the part of the plant contained in the article. Contains not less than 8.0% and not more than 12.0% of procyanidins, calculated on the dried basis. Meets the requirements for Botanical characteristics, Identification, Water content (not more than 35.0%), Foreign organic matter (not more than 5%), Total ash (not more than 1.5%), and Content of procyanidins.

Note—This article is intended to be used in the preparation of extracts only and is not for direct human consumption.

Maritime Pine Extract NF—Store in tight containers, protected from light. Prepared from the pulverized Martime Pine using suitable solvents. The label states the official name of the article, the Latin binomial, and the part of the plant from which the article was prepared, in addition to the information required for Labeling under Botanical extracts. Contains between 65% and 75% of procyanidins, calculated on the dried basis. Meets the requirements for Identification, Microbial limits, Loss on drying (not more than

8.0%), Total ash (not more than 0.7%), Pesticide residue, Limit of water-insoluble substances, and Content of procyanidins, and for Heavy metals under Botanical extracts.

MASOPROCOL

Source: Compound isolated from the plant *Larrea divaricata*.

Chemical name: 1,2-Benzenediol, 4,4'-(2,3-dimethyl-1,4-butanediyl)bis-, (R*,S*)-.

Molecular formula: $C_{18}H_{22}O_4$.

Molecular weight: 302.36.

Description: White to off-white crystalline powder.

USP requirements: Masoprocol Cream—Not in *USP-NF*.

MAZINDOL

Chemical group: Imidazoisoindole.

Chemical name: 3*H*-Imidazo[2,1-*a*]isoindol-5-ol, 5-(4-chlorophenyl)-2,5-dihydro-.

Molecular formula: $C_{16}H_{13}ClN_2O$.

Molecular weight: 284.74.

Description: Mazindol USP—White to off-white, crystalline powder, having not more than a faint odor.

Solubility: Mazindol USP—Insoluble in water; slightly soluble in methanol and in chloroform.

USP requirements:

Mazindol USP—Preserve in tight containers. Contains not less than 98.0% and not more than 102.0% of mazindol, calculated on the dried basis. Meets the requirements for Clarity and color of solution, Identification, Loss on drying (not more than 0.5%), Residue on ignition (not more than 0.1%), Heavy metals (not more than 0.002%), Sulfate (not more than 0.04%), and Chromatographic purity.

Mazindol Tablets USP—Preserve in tight containers, at a temperature not exceeding 25 °C. Contain the labeled amount, within ±10%. Meet the requirements for Identification, Dissolution (80% in 120 minutes in 0.01 *N* hydrochloric acid in Apparatus 2 at 50 rpm), and Uniformity of dosage units.

MEASLES, MUMPS, AND RUBELLA VIRUS VACCINE LIVE

Description: Measles, Mumps, and Rubella Virus Vaccine Live USP—Solid having the characteristic appearance of substances dried from the frozen state. The Vaccine is to be constituted with a suitable diluent just prior to use. Constituted vaccine undergoes loss of potency on exposure to sunlight.

USP requirements: Measles, Mumps, and Rubella Virus Vaccine Live USP—Preserve in single-dose containers, or in light-resistant, multiple-dose containers, at a temperature between 2 and 8 °C. Multiple-dose containers for 50 doses are adapted for use only in jet injectors, and those for 10 doses for use by jet or syringe injection. A bacterially sterile preparation of a combination of live measles virus, live mumps virus, and live rubella virus such that each component is prepared in conformity with and meets the requirements for Measles Virus Vaccine Live, for Mumps Virus Vaccine Live, and for Rubella Virus Vaccine Live, whichever is applicable. Each component

provides an immunizing dose and meets the requirements of the corresponding Virus Vaccine in the total dosage prescribed in the labeling. Label the Vaccine in multiple-dose containers to indicate that the contents are intended solely for use by jet injector or for use by either jet or syringe injection, whichever is applicable. Label the Vaccine in single-dose containers, if such containers are not light-resistant, to state that it should be protected from sunlight. Label it also to state that constituted Vaccine should be discarded if not used within 8 hours. Meets the requirement for Expiration date (1 to 2 years, depending on the manufacturerā s data, after date of issue from manufacturer's cold storage [–20 °C, 1 year]). Conforms to the regulations of the U.S. Food and Drug Administration concerning biologics.

MEASLES AND RUBELLA VIRUS VACCINE LIVE

Description: Measles and Rubella Virus Vaccine Live USP—Solid having the characteristic appearance of substances dried from the frozen state. The Vaccine is to be constituted with a suitable diluent just prior to use. Constituted vaccine undergoes loss of potency on exposure to sunlight.

USP requirements: Measles and Rubella Virus Vaccine Live USP—Preserve in single-dose containers, or in light-resistant, multiple-dose containers, at a temperature between 2 and 8 °C. Multiple-dose containers for 50 doses are adapted for use only in jet injectors, and those for 10 doses for use by jet or syringe injection. A bacterially sterile preparation of a combination of live measles virus and live rubella virus such that each component is prepared in conformity with and meets the requirements for Measles Virus Vaccine Live and for Rubella Virus Vaccine Live, whichever is applicable. Each component provides an immunizing dose and meets the requirements of the corresponding Virus Vaccine in the total dosage prescribed in the labeling. Label the Vaccine in multiple-dose containers to indicate that the contents are intended solely for use by jet injector or for use by either jet or syringe injection, whichever is applicable. Label the Vaccine in single-dose containers, if such containers are not light-resistant, to state that it should be protected from sunlight. Label it also to state that constituted Vaccine should be discarded if not used within 8 hours. Meets the requirement for Expiration date (1 to 2 years, depending on the manufacturer's data, after date of issue from manufacturerā s cold storage [–20 °C, 1 year]). Conforms to the regulations of the U.S. Food and Drug Administration concerning biologics.

MEASLES VIRUS VACCINE LIVE

Source: The currently available vaccine in the U.S. (*Attenuvax*, MSD) contains a lyophilized preparation of a more attenuated line of live measles virus derived from Endersā attenuated Edmonston strain. Further modification of the virus was achieved by multiple passage of Edmonston virus in cell cultures of chick embryo at low temperature. *Attenuvax*, Morson (UK) and Measles Virus Vaccine, Live Attenuated (Dried), Connaught (Canada) brands of live measles virus vaccine also contain the Endersā attenuated Edmonston strain.

Description: Measles Virus Vaccine Live USP—Solid having the characteristic appearance of substances dried from the frozen state. Undergoes loss of potency on exposure to sunlight. The Vaccine is to be constituted with a suitable diluent just prior to use.

Other characteristics: Slightly acidic, pH 6.2 to 6.6.

USP requirements: Measles Virus Vaccine Live USP—Preserve in single-dose containers, or in light-resistant, multiple-dose containers, at a temperature between 2 and 8 °C. Multiple-dose containers for 50 doses are adapted for use only in jet injectors, and those for 10 doses for use by jet or syringe injection. A bacterially sterile preparation of live virus derived from a strain of measles virus tested for neurovirulence in monkeys, for safety, and for immunogenicity, free from all demonstrable viable microbial agents except unavoidable bacteriophage, and found suitable for human immunization. The strain is grown for purposes of vaccine production on chicken embryo primary cell tissue cultures derived from pathogen-free flocks, meets the requirements of the specific safety tests in adult and suckling mice; the requirements of the tests in monkey kidney, chicken embryo and human tissue cell cultures and embryonated eggs; and the requirements of the tests for absence of *Mycobacterium tuberculosis* and of avian leucosis, unless the production cultures were derived from certified avian leucosis-free sources and the control fluids were tested for avian leucosis. The strain cultures are treated to remove all intact tissue cells. The Vaccine meets the requirements of the specific tissue culture test for live virus titer, in a single immunizing dose, of not less than the equivalent of 1000 TCID$_{50}$ (quantity of virus estimated to infect 50% of inoculated cultures × 1000) when tested in parallel with the U.S. Reference Measles Virus, Live Attenuated. Label the Vaccine in multiple-dose containers to indicate that the contents are intended solely for use by jet injector or for use by either jet or syringe injection, whichever is applicable. Label the Vaccine in single-dose containers, if such containers are not light-resistant, to state that it should be protected from sunlight. Label it also to state that constituted Vaccine should be discarded if not used within 8 hours. Meets the requirement for Expiration date (1 to 2 years, depending on the manufacturer's data, after date of issue from manufacturerā s cold storage [−20 °C, 1 year]). Conforms to the regulations of the U.S. Food and Drug Administration concerning biologics.

MEBENDAZOLE

Chemical group: Benzimidazole carbamate derivative.

Chemical name: Carbamic acid, (5-benzoyl-1*H*-benzimidazol-2-yl)-, methyl ester.

Molecular formula: $C_{16}H_{13}N_3O_3$.

Molecular weight: 295.29.

Description: Mebendazole USP—White to slightly yellow powder. Is almost odorless. Melts at about 290 °C.

Solubility: Mebendazole USP—Practically insoluble in water, in dilute solutions of mineral acids, in alcohol, in ether, and in chloroform; freely soluble in formic acid.

USP requirements:
Mebendazole USP—Preserve in well-closed containers. Contains not less than 98.0% and not more than 102.0% of mebendazole, calculated on the dried basis. Meets the requirements for Identification, Loss on drying (not more than 0.5%), Residue on ignition (not more than 0.1%), Heavy metals (not more than 0.002%), and Chromatographic purity.
Mebendazole Oral Suspension USP—Preserve in tight containers at controlled room temperature. It is Mebendazole in an aqueous vehicle. Label it to indicate that it is for veterinary use only. Contains the labeled amount, within ± 10%. Meets the requirements for Identification and pH (6.0–7.0).

Mebendazole Tablets USP—Preserve in well-closed containers. Contain the labeled amount, within ±10%. Meet the requirements for Identification, Dissolution (75% in 120 minutes in 0.1 N hydrochloric acid containing 1.0% sodium lauryl sulfate in Apparatus 2 at 75 rpm), and Uniformity of dosage units.

MEBROFENIN

Chemical name: Glycine, N-[2-[(3-bromo-2,4,6-trimethylphenyl)-amino]-2-oxoethyl]-N-(carboxymethyl)-.

Molecular formula: $C_{15}H_{19}BrN_2O_5$.

Molecular weight: 387.23.

USP requirements: Mebrofenin USP—Preserve in tight containers. Contains not less than 97.0% and not more than 101.0% of mebrofenin, calculated on the dried basis. Meets the requirements for Identification, Melting range (185–200 °C, the range between beginning and end of melting not more than 4 °C), Loss on drying (not more than 0.3%), Residue on ignition (not more than 0.1%), Heavy metals (not more than 0.003%), Limit of nitrilotriacetic acid (not more than 0.1%), and Chromatographic purity.

MECAMYLAMINE

Chemical name: Mecamylamine hydrochloride—Bicyclo[2.2.1]heptan-2-amine, N,2,3,3-tetramethyl-, hydrochloride.

Molecular formula: Mecamylamine hydrochloride—$C_{11}H_{21}N \cdot HCl$.

Molecular weight: Mecamylamine hydrochloride—203.75.

Description: Mecamylamine hydrochloride—White, odorless or practically odorless, crystalline powder. Melts at about 245 °C, with decomposition.

pKa: Mecamylamine hydrochloride—11.2.

Solubility: Mecamylamine hydrochloride—Freely soluble in water and in chloroform; soluble in isopropyl alcohol; practically insoluble in ether.

USP requirements:
Mecamylamine Hydrochloride USP—Preserve in tight containers. Contains not less than 95.0% and not more than 100.5% of mecamylamine hydrochloride, calculated on the dried basis. Meets the requirements for Identification, Acidity, Loss on drying (not more than 1.0%), Residue on ignition (not more than 0.5%), Heavy metals (not more than 0.005%), Organic volatile impurities, and Chloride content (17.0–17.8%).
Mecamylamine Hydrochloride Tablets USP—Preserve in well-closed containers. Contain the labeled amount, within ±10%. Meet the requirements for Identification, Dissolution (75% in 30 minutes in water in Apparatus 2 at 50 rpm), and Uniformity of dosage units.

MECHLORETHAMINE

Chemical name: Mechlorethamine hydrochloride—Ethanamine,2-chloro-N-(2-chloroethyl)-N-methyl-, hydrochloride.

Molecular formula: Mechlorethamine hydrochloride—$C_5H_{11}Cl_2N \cdot HCl$.

Molecular weight: Mechlorethamine hydrochloride—192.51.

Description: Mechlorethamine Hydrochloride USP—White, crystalline powder. Is hygroscopic.

pKa: Mechlorethamine hydrochloride—6.1.

Solubility: Mechlorethamine hydrochloride—Very soluble in water; soluble in alcohol.

USP requirements:

Mechlorethamine Hydrochloride USP—Preserve in tight, light-resistant containers. The label bears a warning that great care should be taken to prevent inhaling particles of Mechlorethamine Hydrochloride and exposing the skin to it. Contains not less than 97.5% and not more than 100.5% of mechlorethamine hydrochloride, calculated on the anhydrous basis. Meets the requirements for Identification, Melting range (108–111 °C), pH (3.0–5.0, in a solution [1 in 500]), Water (not more than 0.4%), and Ionic chloride content (18.0–19.3%).

Mechlorethamine Hydrochloride for Injection USP—Preserve in Containers for Sterile Solids. A sterile mixture of Mechlorethamine Hydrochloride with Sodium Chloride or other suitable diluent. It meets the requirements for Labeling under Injections. The label bears a warning that great care should be taken to prevent inhaling particles of Mechlorethamine Hydrochloride for Injection and exposing the skin to it. Contains the labeled amount, within ±10%. Meets the requirements for Completeness of solution, Constituted solution, Identification, Bacterial endotoxins, pH (3.0–5.0, in a solution [1 in 50]), Water (not more than 1.0%), and Particulate matter, and for Sterility tests and Uniformity of dosage units.

Mechlorethamine Hydrochloride Ointment—Not in *USP–NF*.

Mechlorethamine Hydrochloride Topical Solution—Not in *USP–NF*.

MECLIZINE

Chemical group: Piperazine derivative.

Chemical name: Meclizine hydrochloride—Piperazine, 1-[(4-chlorophenyl)phenylmethyl]-4-[(3-methylphenyl)methyl]-, dihydrochloride, monohydrate.

Molecular formula: Meclizine hydrochloride—$C_{25}H_{27}ClN_2 \cdot 2HCl \cdot H_2O$.

Molecular weight: Meclizine hydrochloride—481.88.

Description: Meclizine Hydrochloride USP—White or slightly yellowish, crystalline powder. Has a slight odor.

Solubility: Meclizine Hydrochloride USP—Practically insoluble in water and in ether; freely soluble in chloroform, in pyridine, and in acid-alcohol-water mixtures; slightly soluble in dilute acids and in alcohol.

USP requirements:

Meclizine Hydrochloride USP—Preserve in tight containers. Contains not less than 97.0% and not more than 100.5% of meclizine hydrochloride, calculated on the anhydrous basis. Meets the requirements for Identification, Water (not more than 5.0%), Residue on ignition (not more than 0.1%), Chromatographic purity, and Organic volatile impurities.

Meclizine Hydrochloride Capsules—Not in *USP–NF*.

Meclizine Hydrochloride Tablets USP—Preserve in well-closed containers. Contain the labeled amount, within –5% to +10%. Meet the requirements for Identification,

Dissolution (75% in 45 minutes in 0.01 N hydrochloric acid in Apparatus 1 at 100 rpm), and Uniformity of dosage units.

Meclizine Hydrochloride Chewable Tablets—Not in *USP–NF*.

MECLOCYCLINE

Chemical name: Meclocycline sulfosalicylate—2-Naphthacenecarboxamide, 7-chloro-4-(dimethylamino)-1,4,4a,5,5a,6,11,12a-octahydro-3,5,10,12,12a-pentahydroxy-6-methylene-1,11-dioxo-, [4S-(4 alpha,4a alpha,5 alpha,5a alpha,12a alpha)]-, mono(2-hydroxy-5-sulfobenzoate) (salt).

Molecular formula: Meclocycline sulfosalicylate—$C_{22}H_{21}ClN_2O_8 \cdot C_7H_6O_6S$.

Molecular weight: Meclocycline sulfosalicylate—695.05.

Description: Meclocycline sulfosalicylate—Yellow, crystalline powder.

USP requirements:

Meclocycline Sulfosalicylate USP—Preserve in tight containers, protected from light. Has a potency equivalent to not less than 620 mcg of meclocycline per mg. Meets the requirements for Identification, Crystallinity, pH (2.5–3.5, in a solution containing 10 mg per mL), and Water (not more than 4.0%).

Meclocycline Sulfosalicylate Cream USP—Preserve in tight containers, protected from light. Contains an amount of meclocycline sulfosalicylate equivalent to the labeled amount of meclocycline, within –10% to +25%. Meets the requirement for Minimum fill.

MECLOFENAMATE

Chemical group: Fenamate derivative.

Chemical name: Meclofenamate sodium—Benzoic acid, 2-[(2,6-dichloro-3-methylphenyl)amino]-, monosodium salt, monohydrate.

Molecular formula: Meclofenamate sodium—$C_{14}H_{10}Cl_2NNaO_2 \cdot H_2O$.

Molecular weight: Meclofenamate sodium—336.15.

Description: Meclofenamate Sodium USP—White to creamy white, odorless to almost odorless, crystalline powder.

Solubility: Meclofenamate Sodium USP—Soluble in methanol; slightly soluble in chloroform; practically insoluble in ether. Freely soluble in water, the solution sometimes being somewhat turbid due to partial hydrolysis and absorption of carbon dioxide; the solution is clear above pH 11.5.

USP requirements:

Meclofenamate Sodium USP—Preserve in tight, light-resistant containers. Contains not less than 97.0% and not more than 103.0% of meclofenamate sodium, calculated on the anhydrous basis. Meets the requirements for Identification, Water (4.8–5.8%), Copper (not more than 0.003%), Chromatographic purity, and Organic volatile impurities.

Meclofenamate Sodium Capsules USP—Preserve in tight, light-resistant containers. Contain an amount of meclofenamate sodium equivalent to the labeled amount of meclofenamic acid, within ±10%. Meet the requirements for Identification, Dissolution (75% in 45 minutes in 0.05 M phosphate buffer [pH 7.5] in Apparatus 2 at 50 rpm), and Uniformity of dosage units.

MEDROGESTONE

Chemical group: Synthetic progestogen structurally related to progesterone.

Chemical name: Pregna-4,6-diene-3,20-dione, 6,17-dimethyl-.

Molecular formula: $C_{23}H_{32}O_2$.

Molecular weight: 340.50.

Description: Melting point 144–146 °C.

USP requirements: Medrogestone Tablets—Not in *USP–NF*.

MEDROXYPROGESTERONE

Chemical name: Medroxyprogesterone acetate—Pregn-4-ene-3,20-dione, 17-(acetyloxy)-6-methyl-, (6 alpha)-.

Molecular formula: Medroxyprogesterone acetate—$C_{24}H_{34}O_4$.

Molecular weight: Medroxyprogesterone acetate—386.52.

Description: Medroxyprogesterone Acetate USP—White to off-white, odorless, crystalline powder. Melts at about 205 °C. Is stable in air.

Solubility: Medroxyprogesterone Acetate USP—Insoluble in water; freely soluble in chloroform; soluble in acetone and in dioxane; sparingly soluble in alcohol and in methanol; slightly soluble in ether.

USP requirements:

Medroxyprogesterone Acetate USP—Preserve in tight, light-resistant containers. Contains not less than 97.0% and not more than 103.0% of medroxyprogesterone acetate, calculated on the dried basis. Meets the requirements for Identification, Specific rotation (+45° to +51°), Chromatographic purity, Limit of medroxyprogesterone acetate related compound A (not more than 0.5%), Loss on drying (not more than 1.0%), and Other impurities.

Medroxyprogesterone Acetate Injectable Suspension USP—Preserve in single-dose or in multiple-dose containers, preferably of Type I glass. A sterile suspension of Medroxyprogesterone Acetate in a suitable aqueous medium. Contains the labeled amount, within ±10%. Meets the requirements for Identification and pH (3.0–7.0), and for Injections.

Medroxyprogesterone Acetate Tablets USP—Preserve in well-closed containers. Contain the labeled amount, within ±7%. Meet the requirements for Identification, Dissolution (50% in 45 minutes in 0.5% sodium lauryl sulfate in Apparatus 2 at 50 rpm), and Uniformity of dosage units.

MEDROXYPROGESTERONE AND ESTRADIOL

For *Medroxyprogesterone* and *Estradiol*—See individual listings for chemistry information.

USP requirements: Medroxyprogesterone Acetate and Estradiol Cypionate for Injection—Not in *USP–NF*.

MEDRYSONE

Chemical name: Pregn-4-ene-3,20-dione, 11-hydroxy-6-methyl-,(6 alpha,11 beta)-.

Molecular formula: $C_{22}H_{32}O_3$.

Molecular weight: 344.49.

Description: White to off-white, crystalline powder. Is odorless or may have a slight odor. Melts at about 158 °C, with decomposition.

Solubility: Sparingly soluble in water; soluble in methylene chloride and in chloroform.

USP requirements: Medrysone Ophthalmic Suspension—Not in *USP–NF*.

MEFENAMIC ACID

Chemical group: Fenamate derivative.

Chemical name: Benzoic acid, 2-[(2,3-dimethylphenyl)amino]-.

Molecular formula: $C_{15}H_{15}NO_2$.

Molecular weight: 241.29.

Description: Mefenamic Acid USP—White to off-white, crystalline powder. Melts at about 230 °C, with decomposition.

pKa: 4.2 (apparent).

Solubility: Mefenamic Acid USP—Soluble in solutions of alkali hydroxides; sparingly soluble in chloroform; slightly soluble in alcohol and in methanol; practically insoluble in water.

USP requirements:

Mefenamic Acid USP—Preserve in tight, light-resistant containers. Contains not less than 98.0% and not more than 102.0% of mefenamic acid, calculated on the dried basis. Meets the requirements for Identification, Loss on drying (not more than 1.0%), Residue on ignition (not more than 0.1%), Heavy metals (not more than 0.002%), and Chromatographic purity.

Mefenamic Acid Capsules USP—Preserve in tight containers. Contain the labeled amount, within ±10%. Meet the requirements for Identification, Dissolution (75% in 45 minutes in 0.05 *M* tris buffer in Apparatus 1 at 100 rpm), and Uniformity of dosage units.

MEFLOQUINE

Chemical name: Mefloquine hydrochloride—4-Quinolinemethanol, alpha-2-piperidinyl-2,8-bis(trifluoromethyl)-, monohydrochloride, (R^*,S^*)- (±)-.

Molecular formula: Mefloquine hydrochloride—$C_{17}H_{16}F_6N_2O \cdot$ HCl.

Molecular weight: Mefloquine hydrochloride—414.77.

Description: Mefloquine hydrochloride—White to almost white crystalline compound.

Solubility: Mefloquine hydrochloride—Slightly soluble in water.

USP requirements: Mefloquine Hydrochloride Tablets—Not in *USP–NF*.

MEGESTROL

Chemical name: Megestrol acetate—Pregna-4,6-diene-3,20-dione, 17-(acetyloxy)-6-methyl-.

Molecular formula: Megestrol acetate—$C_{24}H_{32}O_4$.

Molecular weight: Megestrol acetate—384.51.

Description: Megestrol Acetate USP—White to creamy white, essentially odorless, crystalline powder. Is unstable under aqueous conditions at pH 7 or above.

Solubility: Megestrol Acetate USP—Insoluble in water; sparingly soluble in alcohol; slightly soluble in ether and in fixed oils; soluble in acetone; very soluble in chloroform.

USP requirements:
Megestrol Acetate USP—Preserve in well-closed containers, protected from light. Contains not less than 97.0% and not more than 103.0% of megestrol acetate, calculated on the anhydrous basis. Meets the requirements for Completeness of solution, Identification, Melting range (213–220 °C, the range between beginning and end of melting not more than 3 °C), Specific rotation (+8.8° to +12.0°), Water (not more than 0.5%), Residue on ignition (not more than 0.2%), Heavy metals (not more than 0.002%), and Organic volatile impurities.
Megestrol Acetate Suspension—Not in *USP–NF*.
Megestrol Acetate Oral Suspension USP—Preserve in well-closed, light-resistant containers. Contains the labeled amount, within ±10%. Meets the requirements for Thin-layer chromatographic identification test, Deliverable volume, and pH (3.0–4.7).
Megestrol Acetate Tablets USP—Preserve in well-closed containers. Tablets intended solely for veterinary use are so labeled. Contain the labeled amount, within ±7%. Meet the requirements for Identification, Disintegration (for Tablets labeled solely for veterinary use, 30 minutes), Dissolution (75% in 60 minutes in 1% sodium lauryl sulfate in Apparatus 2 at 75 rpm), and Uniformity of dosage units.
Note: Megestrol Acetate Tablets labeled solely for veterinary use are exempt from the requirements of the test for Dissolution.

MEGLUMINE

Chemical name:
Meglumine—D-Glucitol, 1-deoxy-1-(methylamino)-.
Meglumine antimoniate—1-Deoxy-1-methylamino-D-glucitol antimonate.

Molecular formula:
Meglumine—$C_7H_{17}NO_5$.
Meglumine antimoniate—$C_7H_{18}NO_8Sb$.

Molecular weight:
Meglumine—195.21.
Meglumine antimoniate—366.0.

Description: Meglumine USP—White to faintly yellowish white, odorless crystals or powder.

Solubility: Meglumine USP—Freely soluble in water; sparingly soluble in alcohol.

USP requirements:
Meglumine USP—Preserve in well-closed containers. Contains not less than 99.0% and not more than 100.5% of meglumine, calculated on the dried basis. Meets the requirements for Identification, Melting range (128–132 °C), Specific rotation (−15.7° to −17.3°), Loss on drying (not more than 1.0%), Residue on ignition (not more than 0.1%), Absence of reducing substances, and Heavy metals (not more than 0.002%).
Meglumine Antimoniate for Injection—Not in *USP–NF*.

MELARSOMINE

Chemical name: Melarsomine dihydrochloride—4-[(4,6-diamino-1,3,5-triazon-2-yl)amino]phenyl-dithioarsenite of di(2-aminoethyl), dihydrochloride.

Molecular weight: Melarsomine dihydrochloride—501.34.

Solubility: Melarsomine dihydrochloride—Freely soluble in water.

USP requirements: Melarsomine Dihydrochloride for Injection—Not in *USP–NF*.

MELARSOPROL

Source: Trivalent arsenical derivative.

Chemical name: 2-[p-(4,6-Diamino-s-triazin-2-ylamino)phenyl]-1,3,2-dithiarsolane-4-methanol.

Molecular formula: $C_{12}H_{15}AsN_6OS_2$.

Molecular weight: 398.34.

Description: Slightly cream-colored or greyish cream-colored, odorless powder containing 18.5% of arsenic.

Solubility: Practically insoluble in water, in alcohol, and in ether; slowly soluble in propylene glycol but more readily soluble on warming.

USP requirements: Melarsoprol for Injection—Not in *USP–NF*.

MELOXICAM

Chemical group: An oxicam derivative.

Chemical name: 4-hydroxy-2-methyl-N-(5-methyl-2-thiazolyl)-2H-1,2-benzothiazine-3-carboxamide 1,1-dioxide.

Molecular formula: $C_{14}H_{13}N_3O_4S_2$.

Molecular weight: 351.40.

Description: A yellow solid.

pKa: 1.1 and 4.2.

Solubility: Practically insoluble in water, in strong acids, and in bases; slightly soluble in methanol.

Other characteristics: Partition coefficient: 0.1 in n-octanol/buffer pH 7.5.

USP requirements: Meloxicam Tablets—Not in *USP–NF*.

MELPHALAN

Chemical name: L-Phenylalanine, 4-[bis(2-chloroethyl)amino]-.

Molecular formula: $C_{13}H_{18}Cl_2N_2O_2$.

Molecular weight: 305.20.

Description: Melphalan USP—Off-white to buff powder, having a faint odor. Melts at about 180 °C, with decomposition.

Solubility: Melphalan USP—Practically insoluble in water, in chloroform, and in ether; soluble in dilute mineral acids; slightly soluble in alcohol and in methanol.

USP requirements:
Melphalan USP—Preserve in tight, light-resistant, glass containers. Contains not less than 93.0% and not more than 100.5% of melphalan, calculated on the dried and ionizable chlorine-free basis. Meets the requirements for Iden-

tification, Specific rotation (−30° to −36°), Loss on drying (not more than 7.0%), Residue on ignition (not more than 0.3%), Ionizable chlorine, Nitrogen content (8.90–9.45%), and Organic volatile impurities.

Caution: Handle Melphalan with exceptional care since it is a highly potent agent.

Melphalan for Injection—Not in *USP–NF*.

Melphalan Tablets USP—Preserve in well-closed, light-resistant, glass containers. Contain the labeled amount, within ±10%. Meet the requirements for Identification, Dissolution (80% in 45 minutes in water in Apparatus 2 at 50 rpm), and Uniformity of dosage units.

Melphalan Hydrochloride for Injection—Not in *USP–NF*.

MENADIOL

Chemical name: Menadiol sodium diphosphate—1,4-Naphthalenediol, 2-methyl-, bis(dihydrogen phosphate), tetrasodium salt, hexahydrate.

Molecular formula: Menadiol sodium diphosphate—$C_{11}H_8$-$Na_4O_8P_2 \cdot 6H_2O$.

Molecular weight: Menadiol sodium diphosphate—530.17.

Description: Menadiol Sodium Diphosphate USP—White to pink powder, having a characteristic odor. Is hygroscopic. Its solutions are neutral or slightly alkaline to litmus, having a pH of about 8.

Solubility: Menadiol Sodium Diphosphate USP—Very soluble in water; insoluble in alcohol.

USP requirements:

Menadiol Sodium Diphosphate USP—Preserve in tight, light-resistant containers, and store in a cold place. Contains not less than 97.5% and not more than 102.0% of menadiol sodium diphosphate, calculated on the anhydrous basis. Meets the requirements for Identification and Water (19.0–21.5%).

Menadiol Sodium Diphosphate Injection USP—Preserve in single-dose, light-resistant containers, preferably of Type I glass. A sterile solution of Menadiol Sodium Diphosphate in Water for Injection. Contains the labeled amount, within −5% to +10%. Meets the requirements for Identification, Bacterial endotoxins, and pH (7.5–8.5), and for Injections.

Menadiol Sodium Diphosphate Tablets USP—Preserve in well-closed, light-resistant containers. Contain the labeled amount, within −5% to +10%. Meet the requirements for Identification, Dissolution (75% in 30 minutes in 0.1 *N* hydrochloric acid in Apparatus 1 at 100 rpm), and Uniformity of dosage units.

MENADIONE

Chemical name: 1,4-Naphthalenedione, 2-methyl.

Molecular formula: $C_{11}H_8O_2$.

Molecular weight: 172.18.

Description: Menadione USP—Bright yellow, crystalline, practically odorless powder. Affected by sunlight.

Solubility: Menadione USP—Practically insoluble in water; soluble in vegetable oils; sparingly soluble in chloroform and in alcohol.

USP requirements:

Menadione USP—Preserve in well-closed, light-resistant containers. Contains not less than 98.5% and not more than 101.0% of menadione, calculated on the dried basis. Meets the requirements for Identification, Melting range

(105–107 °C), Loss on drying (not more than 0.3%), Residue on ignition (not more than 0.1%), and Ordinary impurities.

Caution: Menadione powder is irritating to the respiratory tract and to the skin, and a solution of it in alcohol is a vesicant.

Menadione Injection USP—Preserve in single-dose or in multiple-dose containers, preferably of Type I glass. A sterile solution of Menadione in oil. Contains the labeled amount, within −10% to +20%. Meets the requirements for Bacterial endotoxins and for Injections.

MENOTROPINS

Chemical name: Follicle stimulating hormone.

USP requirements:

Menotropins USP—Preserve in tight containers, preferably of Type I glass, in a refrigerator. An extract of human postmenopausal urine containing both follicle-stimulating hormone and luteinizing hormone, having the property in females of stimulating growth and maturation of ovarian follicles and the properties in males of maintaining and stimulating testicular interstitial cells (Leydig tissue) related to testosterone production and of being responsible for the full development and maturation of spermatozoa in the seminiferous tubules. Has a potency of not less than 40 USP Follicle-stimulating Hormone Units and not less than 40 USP Luteinizing Hormone Units per mg, and contains each of the hormone potencies stated on the label, within −20% to +25%. The ratio of units of Follicle-stimulating Hormone to units of Luteinizing Hormone is approximately 1. When necessary, Chorionic Gonadotropin obtained from the urine of pregnant women may be added to achieve this ratio. Not more than 30% of the luteinizing hormone activity is contributed by Chorionic Gonadotropin, as determined by a validated method. Meets the requirements for Bacterial endotoxins, Safety, and Water (not more than 5.0%).

Menotropins for Injection USP—Preserve in Containers for Sterile Solids. A sterile, freeze-dried mixture of menotropins and suitable excipients. Contains labeled potencies of Follicle-stimulating Hormone and Luteinizing Hormone, within −20% to +25%. Meets the requirements for Constituted solution, Bacterial endotoxins, pH (6.0–7.0, in the solution constituted as directed in the labeling), and Uniformity of dosage units, and for Sterility tests and Labeling under Injections.

MENTHOL

Chemical name: Cyclohexanol, 5-methyl-2-(1-methylethyl)-.

Molecular formula: $C_{10}H_{20}O$.

Molecular weight: 156.27.

Description: Menthol USP—Colorless, hexagonal crystals, usually needle-like, or in fused masses, or crystalline powder. It has a pleasant, peppermint-like odor.

NF category: Flavors and perfumes.

Solubility: Menthol USP—Slightly soluble in water; very soluble in alcohol, in chloroform, in ether, and in solvent hexane; freely soluble in glacial acetic acid, in mineral oil, and in fixed and volatile oils.

USP requirements:

Menthol USP—Preserve in tight containers, preferably at controlled room temperature. An alcohol obtained from diverse mint oils or prepared synthetically. Menthol may be levorotatory (*l*-Menthol), from natural or synthetic sources, or racemic (*dl*-Menthol). Label it to indicate whether it is levorotatory or racemic. Meets the requirements for Identification, Melting range of *l*-Menthol (41–44 °C), Congealing range of *dl*-Menthol, Specific rotation (−45° to −51° for *l*-Menthol; −2° to +2° for *dl*-Menthol), Limit of nonvolatile residue (not more than 0.05%), Chromatographic purity, Readily oxidizable substances in *dl*-Menthol, and Organic volatile impurities.

Menthol Lozenges USP—Preserve in well-closed containers. Contain the labeled amount in a suitable molded base, within -10% to +25%. Meet the requirement for Identification.

MENTHYL ANTHRANILATE

Chemical name: Menthyl-*O*-aminobenzoate.

Molecular formula: $C_{17}H_{25}NO_2$.

Molecular weight: 275.39.

USP requirements:

Menthyl Anthranilate USP—Preserve in tight containers. Contains not less than 95.0% and not more than 105.0% of menthyl anthranilate. Meets the requirements for Identification, Specific rotation (−4° to +4°), Refractive index (1.540–1.544 at 20 °C),, Acidity (not more than 0.2 mL of titrant per mL of Menthyl Anthranilate), and Chromatographic purity.

Menthyl Anthranilate Cream—Not in *USP–NF*.

MENTHYL ANTHRANILATE, OCTOCRYLENE, AND OCTYL METHOXYCINNAMATE

For *Menthyl Anthranilate, Octocrylene,* and *Octyl Methoxycinnamate*—See individual listings for chemistry information.

USP requirements: Menthyl Anthranilate, Octocrylene, and Octyl Methoxycinnamate Cream—Not in *USP–NF*.

MENTHYL ANTHRANILATE, OCTOCRYLENE, OCTYL METHOXYCINNAMATE, AND OXYBENZONE

For *Menthyl Anthranilate, Octocrylene, Octyl Methoxycinnamate,* and *Oxybenzone*—See individual listings for chemistry information.

USP requirements: Menthyl Anthranilate, Octocrylene, Octyl Methoxycinnamate, and Oxybenzone Gel—Not in *USP–NF*.

MENTHYL ANTHRANILATE AND OCTYL METHOXYCINNAMATE

For *Menthyl Anthranilate* and *Octyl Methoxycinnamate*—See individual listings for chemistry information.

USP requirements:

Menthyl Anthranilate and Octyl Methoxycinnamate Cream—Not in *USP–NF*.

Menthyl Anthranilate and Octyl Methoxycinnamate Lotion—Not in *USP–NF*.

MENTHYL ANTHRANILATE, OCTYL METHOXYCINNAMATE, AND OCTYL SALICYLATE

For *Menthyl Anthranilate, octyl Methoxycinnamate,* and *Octyl Salicylate*—See individual listings for chemistry information.

USP requirements: Menthyl Anthranilate, Octyl Methoxycinnamate, and Octyl Salicylate Cream—Not in *USP–NF*.

MENTHYL ANTHRANILATE, OCTYL METHOXYCINNAMATE, OCTYL SALICYLATE, AND OXYBENZONE

For *Menthyl Anthranilate, Octyl Methoxycinnamate, Octyl Salicylate,* and *Oxybenzone*—See individual listings for chemistry information.

USP requirements: Menthyl Anthranilate, Octyl Methoxycinnamate, Octyl Salicylate, and Oxybenzone Lotion—Not in *USP–NF*.

MENTHYL ANTHRANILATE, OCTYL METHOXYCINNAMATE, AND OXYBENZONE

For *Menthyl Anthranilate, Octyl Methoxycinnamate,* and *Oxybenzone*—See individual listings for chemistry information.

USP requirements:

Menthyl Anthranilate, Octyl Methoxycinnamate, and Oxybenzone Gel—Not in *USP–NF*.

Menthyl Anthranilate, Octyl Methoxycinnamate, and Oxybenzone Lip Balm—Not in *USP–NF*.

Menthyl Anthranilate, Octyl Methoxycinnamate, and Oxybenzone Lotion—Not in *USP–NF*.

MENTHYL ANTHRANILATE AND PADIMATE O

For *Menthyl Anthranilate* and *Padimate O*—See individual listings for chemistry information.

USP requirements: Menthyl Anthranilate and Padimate O Lip Balm—Not in *USP–NF*.

MENTHYL ANTHRANILATE AND TITANIUM DIOXIDE

For *Menthyl Anthranilate* and *Titanium Dioxide*—See individual listings for chemistry information.

USP requirements: Menthyl Anthranilate and Titanium Dioxide Cream—Not in *USP–NF*.

MEPENZOLATE

Chemical group: Quaternary ammonium compound.

Chemical name: Mepenzolate bromide—Piperidinium, 3-[(hydroxydiphenylacetyl)oxy]-1,1-dimethyl-, bromide.

Molecular formula: Mepenzolate bromide—$C_{21}H_{26}BrNO_3$.

Molecular weight: Mepenzolate bromide—420.34.

Description: Mepenzolate bromide—White or light cream-colored powder.

Solubility: Mepenzolate bromide—Slightly soluble in water and in chloroform; freely soluble in methanol; practically insoluble in ether.

USP requirements:
Mepenzolate Bromide USP—Preserve in tight containers. Contains not less than 98.0% and not more than 101.0% of mepenzolate bromide, calculated on the dried basis. Meets the requirements for Identification, Loss on drying (not more than 0.5%), Residue on ignition (not more than 0.2%), Heavy metals (not more than 0.002%), Organic volatile impurities, and Bromide content (18.60–19.40%).
Mepenzolate Bromide Tablets USP—Preserve in well-closed containers. Contain the labeled amount, within ±7%. Meet the requirements for Identification, Disintegration (30 minutes), and Uniformity of dosage units.

MEPERIDINE

Chemical name: Meperidine hydrochloride—4-Piperidinecarboxylic acid, 1-methyl-4-phenyl-, ethyl ester, hydrochloride.

Molecular formula: Meperidine hydrochloride—$C_{15}H_{21}NO_2 \cdot HCl$.

Molecular weight: Meperidine hydrochloride—283.79.

Description: Meperidine Hydrochloride USP—Fine, white, crystalline, odorless powder. The pH of a solution (1 in 20) is about 5.

Solubility: Meperidine Hydrochloride USP—Very soluble in water; soluble in alcohol; sparingly soluble in ether.

USP requirements:
Meperidine Hydrochloride USP—Preserve in well-closed, light-resistant containers. Contains not less than 98.0% and not more than 102.0% of meperidine hydrochloride, calculated on the dried basis. Meets the requirements for Identification, Melting range (186–189 °C), Loss on drying (not more than 1.0%), Residue on ignition (not more than 0.1%), Chromatographic purity, Organic volatile impurities, and Chloride content (12.2–12.7%).
Meperidine Hydrochloride Injection USP—Preserve in single-dose or in multiple-dose containers, preferably of Type I glass. A sterile solution of Meperidine Hydrochloride in Water for Injection. Contains the labeled amount, within ±5%. Meets the requirements for Identification, Bacterial endotoxins, and pH (3.5–6.0), and for Injections.
Meperidine Hydrochloride Oral Solution USP—Preserve in tight, light-resistant containers. Contains the labeled amount, within ±5%. Meets the requirements for Identification and pH (3.5–4.1).
Meperidine Hydrochloride Syrup USP—Preserve in tight, light-resistant containers. Contains the labeled amount, within ±5%. Meets the requirements for Identification and pH (3.5–4.1).

Meperidine Hydrochloride Tablets USP—Preserve in well-closed, light-resistant containers. Contain the labeled amount, within ±5%. Meet the requirements for Identification, Dissolution (75% in 45 minutes in water in Apparatus 1 at 100 rpm), and Uniformity of dosage units.

MEPHENTERMINE

Chemical group: Structurally similar to methamphetamine.

Chemical name: Mephentermine sulfate—Benzeneethanamine, N,alpha,alpha-trimethyl-, sulfate (2:1).

Molecular formula: Mephentermine sulfate—$(C_{11}H_{17}N)_2 \cdot H_2SO_4$.

Molecular weight: Mephentermine sulfate—424.60.

Description: Mephentermine Sulfate USP—White, odorless crystals or crystalline powder. Its solutions are slightly acid to litmus, having a pH of about 6.

pKa: 10.11.

Solubility: Mephentermine Sulfate USP—Soluble in water; slightly soluble in alcohol; insoluble in chloroform.

USP requirements:
Mephentermine Sulfate USP—Preserve in well-closed, light-resistant containers. It is anhydrous or contains two molecules of water of hydration. Label it to indicate whether it is anhydrous or hydrous. Contains not less than 98.0% and not more than 102.0% of mephentermine sulfate, calculated on the anhydrous basis. Meets the requirements for Identification, Water (not more than 0.2% for the anhydrous and 6.8–8.8% for the hydrated form), Residue on ignition (not more than 0.1%), and Chromatographic purity.
Mephentermine Sulfate Injection USP—Preserve in single-dose or in multiple-dose containers, preferably of Type I glass. A sterile solution of Mephentermine Sulfate in Water for Injection. Contains an amount of mephentermine sulfate equivalent to the labeled amount of mephentermine, within ±5%. Meets the requirements for Identification, Bacterial endotoxins, pH (4.0–6.5), and Particulate matter, and for Injections.

MEPHENYTOIN

Chemical group: Related to the barbiturates in chemical structure, but having a five-membered ring.

Chemical name: 2,4-Imidazolidinedione, 5-ethyl-3-methyl-5-phenyl-, (±)-.

Molecular formula: $C_{12}H_{14}N_2O_2$.

Molecular weight: 218.25.

Description: Mephenytoin USP—White, crystalline powder.

Solubility: Mephenytoin USP—Very slightly soluble in water; freely soluble in chloroform; soluble in alcohol and in aqueous solutions of alkali hydroxides; sparingly soluble in ether.

USP requirements:
Mephenytoin USP—Preserve in tight containers, and store at controlled room temperature. Contains not less than 98.0% and not more than 102.0% of mephenytoin, calculated on the dried basis. Meets the requirements for Identification, Melting range (136–140 °C), Loss on drying (not more than 1.0%), Residue on ignition (not more than 0.1%), Heavy metals (not more than 0.002%), Chromatographic purity, and Organic volatile impurities.

Mephenytoin Tablets USP—Preserve in tight containers, and store at controlled room temperature. Contain the labeled amount, within ±10%. Meet the requirements for Dissolution (70% in 60 minutes in water in Apparatus 2 at 75 rpm), Uniformity of dosage units, and Chromatographic purity.

MEPHOBARBITAL

Chemical name: 2,4,6(1*H*,3*H*,5*H*)-Pyrimidinetrione, 5-ethyl-1-methyl-5-phenyl-.

Molecular formula: $C_{13}H_{14}N_2O_3$.

Molecular weight: 246.26.

Description: Mephobarbital USP—White, odorless, crystalline powder. Its saturated solution is acid to litmus.

Solubility: Mephobarbital USP—Slightly soluble in water, in alcohol, and in ether; soluble in chloroform and in solutions of fixed alkali hydroxides and carbonates.

USP requirements:

Mephobarbital USP—Preserve in well-closed containers. Contains not less than 98.0% and not more than 100.5% of mephobarbital, calculated on the dried basis. Meets the requirements for Identification, Melting range (176–181 °C), Loss on drying (not more than 1.0%), Residue on ignition (not more than 0.1%), and Organic volatile impurities.

Mephobarbital Tablets USP—Preserve in well-closed containers. Contain the labeled amount, within −5% to +10%. Meet the requirements for Identification, Dissolution (70% in 75 minutes in phosphate buffer [pH 6.8] in Apparatus 2 at 75 rpm), and Uniformity of dosage units.

MEPIVACAINE

Chemical group: Amide.

Chemical name: Mepivacaine hydrochloride—2-Piperidinecarboxamide, *N*-(2,6-dimethylphenyl)-1-methyl-, monohydrochloride.

Molecular formula: Mepivacaine hydrochloride—$C_{15}H_{22}N_2O \cdot$ HCl.

Molecular weight: Mepivacaine hydrochloride—282.81.

Description: Mepivacaine Hydrochloride USP—White, odorless, crystalline solid. The pH of a solution (1 in 50) is about 4.5.

pKa: Mepivacaine hydrochloride—7.73 ±0.08.

Solubility: Mepivacaine Hydrochloride USP—Freely soluble in water and in methanol; very slightly soluble in chloroform; practically insoluble in ether.

USP requirements:

Mepivacaine Hydrochloride USP—Preserve in well-closed containers. Contains not less than 98.0% and not more than 102.0% of mepivacaine hydrochloride, calculated on the dried basis. Meets the requirements for Identification, Loss on drying (not more than 1.0%), Residue on ignition (not more than 0.1%), and Chromatographic purity.

Mepivacaine Hydrochloride Injection USP—Preserve in single-dose or in multiple-dose containers, preferably of Type I glass. Injection labeled to contain 2% or less of mepivacaine hydrochloride may be packaged in 50-mL multiple-dose containers. A sterile solution of Mepivacaine Hydrochloride in Water for Injection. Contains the labeled amount, within ±5%. Meets the requirements for Identification, Bacterial endotoxins, and pH (4.5–6.8), and for Injections.

MEPIVACAINE AND LEVONORDEFRIN

For *Mepivacaine* and *Levonordefrin*—See individual listings for chemistry information.

USP requirements: Mepivacaine Hydrochloride and Levonordefrin Injection USP—Preserve in single-dose or in multiple-dose containers, preferably of Type I glass. A sterile solution of Mepivacaine Hydrochloride and Levonordefrin in Water for Injection. The label indicates that the Injection is not to be used if its color is pinkish or darker than slightly yellow or if it contains a precipitate. Contains the labeled amount of mepivacaine hydrochloride, within ±5%, and the labeled amount of levonordefrin, within ±10%. Meets the requirements for Color and clarity, Identification, Bacterial endotoxins, and pH (3.3–5.5), and for Injections.

MEPREDNISONE

Chemical name: Pregna-1,4-diene-3,11,20-trione, 17,21-dihydroxy-16-methyl-, (16 beta)-.

Molecular formula: $C_{22}H_{28}O_5$.

Molecular weight: 372.45.

Description: Melting point 200–205°C.

USP requirements: Meprednisone USP—Preserve in tight, light-resistant containers, and avoid exposure to excessive heat. Contains not less than 97.5% and not more than 102.5% of meprednisone, calculated on the dried basis. Meets the requirements for Identification, Specific rotation (+180° to +188°), Loss on drying (not more than 1.0%), and Residue on ignition (not more than 0.1%).

MEPROBAMATE

Chemical group: A carbamate derivative.

Chemical name: 1,3-Propanediol, 2-methyl-2-propyl-, dicarbamate.

Molecular formula: $C_9H_{18}N_2O_4$.

Molecular weight: 218.25.

Description: Meprobamate USP—White powder, having a characteristic odor.

Solubility: Meprobamate USP—Slightly soluble in water; freely soluble in acetone and in alcohol; practically insoluble or insoluble in ether.

USP requirements:

Meprobamate USP—Preserve in tight containers. Contains not less than 97.0% and not more than 101.0% of meprobamate, calculated on the dried basis. Meets the requirements for Identification, Melting range (103–107 °C, the range between beginning and end of melting not more than 2 °C), Loss on drying (not more than 0.5%), Chromatographic purity, Limit of methyl carbamate (not more than 0.5%), and Organic volatile impurities.

Meprobamate Extended-release Capsules—Not in *USP–NF*.

Meprobamate Oral Suspension USP—Preserve in tight containers. Contains the labeled amount, within −5% to +10%. Meets the requirement for Identification.

Meprobamate Tablets USP—Preserve in well-closed containers. Contain the labeled amount, within ±10%. Meet the requirements for Identification, Dissolution (75% in 30 minutes in deaerated water in Apparatus 1 at 100 rpm), and Uniformity of dosage units.

MEPROBAMATE AND ASPIRIN

For *Meprobamate* and *Aspirin*—See individual listings for chemistry information.

USP requirements: Meprobamate and Aspirin Tablets—Not in *USP–NF*.

MEQUINOL AND TRETINOIN

Chemical name:
Mequinol—Phenol, 4 methoxy.
Tretinoin—Retinoic acid.

Molecular formula:
Mequinol—$C_7H_8O_2$.
Tretinoin—$C_{20}H_{28}O_2$.

Molecular weight:
Mequinol—124.14.
Tretinoin—300.44.

Description: Tretinoin USP—Yellow to light-orange, crystalline powder.

Solubility: Tretinoin USP—Insoluble in water; slightly soluble in alcohol and in chloroform.

USP requirements: Mequinol and Tretinoin Topical Solution—Not in *USP–NF*.

MERADIMATE

Chemical name: Menthyl-*O*-aminobenzoate.

Molecular formula: $C_{17}H_{25}NO_2$.

Molecular weight: 275.39.

USP requirements:
Meradimate USP—Preserve in tight containers. Contains the labeled amount, within ±5%. Meets the requirements for Identification, Specific rotation (−4° to +4°), Refractive index (1.540–1.544 at 20 °C), and Acidity (not more than 0.2 mL of titrant per mL of Meradimate).

MERCAPTOPURINE

Chemical name: 6*H*-Purine-6-thione, 1,7-dihydro-, monohydrate.

Molecular formula: $C_5H_4N_4S \cdot H_2O$.

Molecular weight: 170.19.

Description: Mercaptopurine USP—Yellow, odorless or practically odorless, crystalline powder. Melts at a temperature exceeding 308 °C, with decomposition.

pKa: 7.77 and 11.17.

Solubility: Mercaptopurine USP—Insoluble in water, in acetone, and in ether; soluble in hot alcohol and in dilute alkali solutions; slightly soluble in 2 *N* sulfuric acid.

USP requirements:
Mercaptopurine USP—Preserve in well-closed containers. Contains not less than 97.0% and not more than 102.0% of mercaptopurine, calculated on the anhydrous basis. Meets the requirements for Identification, Water (not more than 12.0%), Phosphorus (not more than 0.010%), and Organic volatile impurities.

Mercaptopurine Tablets USP—Preserve in well-closed containers. Contain the labeled amount, within −7% to +10%. Meet the requirements for Identification, Disintegration (30 minutes), and Uniformity of dosage units.

AMMONIATED MERCURY

Chemical name: Mercury amide chloride.

Molecular formula: $Hg(NH_2)Cl$.

Molecular weight: 252.07.

Description: Ammoniated Mercury USP—White, pulverulent pieces or white, amorphous powder. Is odorless, and is stable in air, but darkens on exposure to light.

Solubility: Ammoniated Mercury USP—Insoluble in water, and in alcohol; readily soluble in warm hydrochloric, nitric, and acetic acids.

USP requirements:
Ammoniated Mercury USP—Preserve in well-closed, light-resistant containers. Contains not less than 98.0% and not more than 100.5% of ammoniated mercury. Meets the requirements for Identification, Residue on ignition (not more than 0.2%), and Mercurous compounds (not more than 0.2%).

Ammoniated Mercury Ointment USP—Preserve in collapsible tubes or in well-closed, light-resistant containers. Contains the labeled amount, within ±10%, in a suitable oleaginous ointment base. Meets the requirements for Identification and Minimum fill.

Ammoniated Mercury Ophthalmic Ointment USP—Preserve in collapsible ophthalmic ointment tubes. A sterile ointment. Contains the labeled amount, within ±10%, in a suitable oleaginous ointment base. Meets the requirements for Sterility and Metal particles, and for Identification tests and Minimum fill under Ammoniated Mercury Ointment.

MEROPENEM

Chemical name: 1-Azabicyclo[3.2.0]hept-2-ene-2-carboxylic acid,3-[[5-[(dimethylamino)carbonyl]-3-pyrrolidinyl]thio]-6-(1-hydroxyethyl)-4-methyl-7-oxo-, trihydrate, [4*R*-[3(3*S**,5*S**),4 alpha,5 beta,6 beta(*R**)]]-.

Molecular formula: $C_{17}H_{25}N_3O_5S \cdot 3H_2O$.

Molecular weight: 437.51.

Description: Colorless to white crystals.

Solubility: Soluble in dimethylformamide and in 5% monobasic potassium phosphate solution; sparingly soluble in water; very slightly soluble in alcohol; practically insoluble in acetone and in ether.

USP requirements:

Meropenem USP—Preserve in tight containers. Store the dry powder at controlled room temperature. Where it is intended for use in preparing injectable dosage forms, the label states that it is sterile or must be subjected to further processing during the preparation of injectable dosage forms. Contains not less than 98.0% and not more than 101.0% of meropenem, calculated on the anhydrous basis. Meets the requirements for Identification, Specific rotation (between −17° to −21°, measured at 20°), pH (4.0–6.0, in a solution [1 in 100]), Water (11.4–13.4%), Residue on ignition (not more than 0.1%, igniting at 500 ±50°, instead of at 800 ±50°), Heavy metals (not more than 0.001%), and Chromatographic purity, and for Sterility and for Bacterial endotoxins under Meropenem for Injection (where the label states that Meropenem is sterile) and for Bacterial endotoxins under Meropenem for Injection (where the label states that Meropenem must be subjected to further processing during the preparation of injectable dosage forms).

Meropenem for Injection USP—Preserve in tight Containers for Sterile Solids. Store at controlled room temperature. A sterile dry mixture of Meropenem and Sodium Carbonate. Meets the requirements for Labeling under Injections. Label it to state the quantity, in mg, of sodium (Na) in a Given dosage of meropenem. Contains the labeled amount, within −10% to +20%. Meets the requirements for Constituted solution, Identification, Bacterial endotoxins, Sterility, Uniformity of dosage units, pH (7.3–8.3, in a solution [1 in 20]), Loss on drying (between 9.0–12.0%), Particulate matter, Chromatographic purity, and Content of sodium (80–120% of the labeled amount of sodium).

MESALAMINE

Chemical group: The active moiety of the prodrug sulfasalazine, which belongs to the salicylate and sulfonamide groups.

Chemical name: Benzoic acid, 5-amino-2-hydroxy-.

Molecular formula: $C_7H_7NO_3$.

Molecular weight: 153.14.

Description: Mesalamine USP—Light tan to pink colored needle-shaped crystals. Color may darken on exposure to air. Odorless or may have a slight characteristic odor.

Solubility: Mesalamine USP—Slightly soluble in water; very slightly soluble in methanol, in dehydrated alcohol, and in acetone; practically insoluble in n-butyl alcohol, in chloroform, in ether, in ethyl acetate, in n-hexane, in methylene chloride, and in n-propyl alcohol; soluble in dilute hydrochloric acid and in dilute alkali hydroxides.

USP requirements:

Mesalamine USP—Preserve in tight, light-resistant containers. Contains not less than 98.5% and not more than 101.5% of mesalamine, calculated on the dried basis. Meets the requirements for Clarity of solution, Identification, pH (3.5–4.5, in a suspension [1 in 40]), Loss on drying (not more than 0.5%), Residue on ignition (not more than 0.2%), Chloride (0.1%), Heavy metals (not more than 0.002%), Hydrogen sulfide and sulfur dioxide, Sulfate (0.2%), and Related compounds.

Mesalamine Extended-release Capsules USP—Preserve in tight, light-resistant containers. Contain the labeled amount, within ±10%. Meet the requirements for Identification, Drug release, and Uniformity of dosage units.

Mesalamine Suppositories—Not in USP–NF.

Mesalamine Rectal Suspension USP—Preserve in tight, light-resistant containers. A suspension of Mesalamine in a suitable aqueous vehicle. Contains one or more suitable preservatives. Contains the labeled amount, within ±

10%. Meets the requirements for Identification, Uniformity of dosage units, pH (3.5–5.5, when diluted 1 to 10 with water), Related compounds, and Content of sodium benzoate (0.05–0.125%).

Mesalamine Delayed-release Tablets USP—Preserve in tight containers. Contain the labeled amount, within ±10%. Meet the requirements for Identification, Drug release, Uniformity of dosage units, and Chromatographic purity..

Mesalamine Extended-release Tablets—Not in USP–NF.

MESNA

Chemical name: Ethanesulfonic acid, 2-mercapto-, monosodium salt.

Molecular formula: $C_2H_5NaO_3S_2$.

Molecular weight: 164.18.

Description: Mesna injection—Clear and colorless aqueous solution, with a pH of 6.5–8.5.

USP requirements: Mesna Injection—Not in USP–NF.

MESORIDAZINE

Chemical group: Mesoridazine besylate—Salt of a metabolite of thioridazine, a phenothiazine derivative.

Chemical name: Mesoridazine besylate—10 H-Phenothiazine, 10-[2-(1-methyl-2-piperidinyl)ethyl]-2-(methylsulfinyl)-, mono-benzenesulfonate.

Molecular formula: Mesoridazine besylate—$C_{21}H_{26}N_2OS_2 \cdot C_6H_6O_3S$.

Molecular weight: Mesoridazine besylate—544.75.

Description: Mesoridazine Besylate USP—White to pale yellowish powder, having not more than a faint odor. Melts at about 178 °C, with decomposition.

Solubility: Mesoridazine Besylate USP—Freely soluble in water, in chloroform, and in methanol.

USP requirements:

Mesoridazine Besylate USP—Preserve in tight, light-resistant containers. Contains not less than 98.0% and not more than 102.0% of mesoridazine besylate, calculated on the dried basis. Meets the requirements for Identification, pH (4.2–5.7, in a freshly prepared solution [1 in 100]), Loss on drying (not more than 0.5%), Residue on ignition (not more than 0.2%), Heavy metals (not more than 0.002%), Selenium (not more than 0.003%), Ordinary impurities, and Organic volatile impurities.

Mesoridazine Besylate Injection USP—Preserve in single-dose containers, preferably of Type I glass, protected from light. A sterile solution of Mesoridazine Besylate in Water for Injection. Contains an amount of mesoridazine besylate equivalent to the labeled amount of mesoridazine, within ±10%. Meets the requirements for Identification, Bacterial endotoxins, and pH (4.0–5.0), and for Injections.

Mesoridazine Besylate Oral Solution USP—Preserve in tight, light-resistant containers, at a temperature not exceeding 25 °C. Label it to indicate that it is to be diluted to the appropriate strength with water or other suitable fluid prior to administration. Contains an amount of mesoridazine besylate equivalent to the labeled amount of mesoridazine, within ±10%. Meets the requirements for Identification and Alcohol content (0.25–1.0%).

Mesoridazine Besylate Tablets USP—Preserve in well-closed, light-resistant containers. Preserve Tablets having an opaque coating in well-closed containers. Contain an

amount of mesoridazine besylate equivalent to the labeled amount of mesoridazine, within ±10%. Meet the requirements for Identification, Dissolution (80% in 60 minutes in 0.01 N hydrochloric acid in Apparatus 2 at 100 rpm), and Uniformity of dosage units.

MESTRANOL

Chemical name: 19-Norpregna-1,3,5(10)-trien-20-yn-17-ol, 3-methoxy-, (17 alpha)-.

Molecular formula: $C_{21}H_{26}O_2$.

Molecular weight: 310.43.

Description: Mestranol USP—White to creamy white, odorless, crystalline powder.

Solubility: Mestranol USP—Insoluble in water; freely soluble in chloroform; soluble in dioxane; sparingly soluble in dehydrated alcohol; slightly soluble in methanol.

USP requirements: Mestranol USP—Preserve in well-closed, light-resistant containers. Contains not less than 97.0% and not more than 102.0% of mestranol, calculated on the dried basis. Meets the requirements for Identification, Melting range (146–154 °C, the range between beginning and end of melting not more than 4 °C), Specific rotation (+2° to +8°), and Loss on drying (not more than 1.0%).

METACRESOL

Chemical name: 3-Methylphenol.

Molecular formula: C_7H_8O.

Molecular weight: 108.14.

USP requirements: Metacresol USP—Preserve in tight, light-resistant containers. Contains not less than 95.0% and not more than 101.0% of metacresol. Meets the requirements for Clarity of solution and Identification.

METAPROTERENOL

Chemical name: Metaproterenol sulfate—1,3-Benzenediol, 5-[1-hydroxy-2-[(1-methylethyl)amino]ethyl]-, sulfate (2:1) (salt).

Molecular formula: Metaproterenol sulfate—$(C_{11}H_{17}NO_3)_2 \cdot H_2SO_4$.

Molecular weight: Metaproterenol sulfate—520.59.

Description: Metaproterenol Sulfate USP—White to off-white, crystalline powder.

Solubility: Metaproterenol Sulfate USP—Freely soluble in water.

USP requirements:
Metaproterenol Sulfate USP—Preserve in tight, light-resistant containers. Contains not less than 98.0% and not more than 102.0% of metaproterenol sulfate, calculated on the anhydrous, isopropyl alcohol-free, and methanol-free basis. Meets the requirements for Identification, pH (4.0–5.5, in a solution containing 100 mg per mL), Water (not more than 2.0%), Residue on ignition (not more than 0.1%), Heavy metals (not more than 0.001%), Iron (not more than 5 ppm), Limit of metaproterenone sulfate (not more than 0.1%), Isopropyl alcohol and methanol (not more than 0.3% of isopropyl alcohol and not more than 0.1% of methanol), and Organic volatile impurities.

Metaproterenol Sulfate Inhalation Aerosol USP—Preserve in small, nonreactive, light-resistant aerosol containers equipped with metered-dose valves and provided with oral inhalation actuators. A suspension of microfine Metaproterenol Sulfate in fluorochlorohydrocarbon propellants in a pressurized container. Contains the labeled amount, within ±10%. Meets the requirements for Identification, Dose uniformity over the entire contents,, Particle size, and Water (not more than 0.075%).

Metaproterenol Sulfate Inhalation Solution USP—Store in small, tight containers that are well-filled or otherwise protected from oxidation. Protect from light. A sterile solution of Metaproterenol Sulfate in Purified Water. Label it to indicate that the Inhalation Solution is not to be used if its color is pinkish or darker than slightly yellow or if it contains a precipitate. Contains the labeled amount, within ±10%. Meets the requirements for Color and clarity, Identification, Sterility, and pH (2.8–4.0).

Metaproterenol Sulfate Oral Solution USP—Preserve in tight, light-resistant containers. Contains the labeled amount, within ±10%. Meets the requirements for Identification and pH (2.5–4.0, in a solution obtained by mixing 1 volume of Oral Solution and 4 volumes of water).

Metaproterenol Sulfate Syrup USP—Preserve in tight, light-resistant containers. Contains the labeled amount, within ±10%. Meets the requirements for Identification and pH (2.5–4.0, in a solution obtained by mixing 1 volume of Syrup and 4 volumes of water).

Metaproterenol Sulfate Tablets USP—Preserve in well-closed, light-resistant containers. Contain the labeled amount, within ±8%. Meet the requirements for Identification, Dissolution (70% in 30 minutes in water in Apparatus 2 at 50 rpm), and Uniformity of dosage units.

METARAMINOL

Chemical name: Metaraminol bitartrate—Benzenemethanol, alpha-(1-aminoethyl)-3-hydroxy-, [R-(R*,S*)]-, [R-(R*,R*)]-2,3-dihydroxybutanedioate (1:1) (salt).

Molecular formula: Metaraminol bitartrate—$C_9H_{13}NO_2 \cdot C_4H_6O_6$.

Molecular weight: Metaraminol bitartrate—317.29.

Description: Metaraminol bitartrate—White, practically odorless, crystalline powder.

Solubility: Metaraminol bitartrate—Freely soluble in water; slightly soluble in alcohol; practically insoluble in chloroform and in ether.

USP requirements:
Metaraminol Bitartrate USP—Preserve in well-closed containers. Contains not less than 99.0% and not more than 100.5% of metaraminol bitartrate, calculated on the dried basis. Meets the requirements for Identification, Melting range (171–175 °C), Specific rotation (−31.5° to −33.5°), pH (3.2–3.5, in a solution [1 in 20]), Loss on drying (not more than 1.0%), Residue on ignition (not more than 0.1%), and Heavy metals (not more than 0.002%).

Metaraminol Bitartrate Injection USP—Preserve in single-dose or in multiple-dose containers, preferably of Type I glass, protected from light. A sterile solution of Metaraminol Bitartrate in Water for Injection. Contains, in each mL, an amount of metaraminol bitartrate equivalent to not less than 9.0 mg and not more than 11.0 mg of metaraminol. Meets the requirements for Identification, Bacterial endotoxins, pH (3.2–4.5), and Particulate matter, and for Injections.

METAXALONE

Chemical name: 2-Oxazolidinone, 5-[(3,5-dimethylphenoxy)-methyl]-.

Molecular formula: $C_{12}H_{15}NO_3$.

Molecular weight: 221.25.

Description: White, crystalline powder. Melts at about 123 °C.

Solubility: Very slightly soluble in water; soluble in alcohol; freely soluble in chloroform.

USP requirements: Metaxalone Tablets—Not in *USP–NF*.

METFORMIN

Chemical name: Metformin hydrochloride—Imidodicarbonimidic diamide, *N,N*-dimethyl-, monohydrochloride.

Molecular formula: Metformin hydrochloride—$C_4H_{11}N_5 \cdot HCl$.

Molecular weight: Metformin hydrochloride—165.62.

Description: Metformin hydrochloride—White to off-white crystalline compound.

pKa: 12.4.

Solubility: Metformin hydrochloride—Freely soluble in water; practically insoluble in acetone, in chloroform, and in ether.

USP requirements:
Metformin Hydrochloride Tablets—Not in *USP–NF*.
Metformin Hydrochloride Extended-release Tablets—Not in *USP–NF*.

METHACHOLINE

Chemical name: Methacholine chloride—1-Propanaminium, 2-(acetyloxy)-*N,N,N*-trimethyl-, chloride.

Molecular formula: Methacholine chloride—$C_8H_{18}ClNO_2$.

Molecular weight: Methacholine chloride—195.69.

Description: Methacholine Chloride USP—Colorless or white crystals, or white, crystalline powder. Is odorless or has a slight odor, and is very hygroscopic. Its solutions are neutral to litmus.

Solubility: Methacholine Chloride USP—Very soluble in water; freely soluble in alcohol and in chloroform.

USP requirements:
Methacholine Chloride USP—Preserve in tight containers. Dried at 105 °C for 4 hours, contains not less than 98.0% and not more than 101.0% of methacholine chloride. Meets the requirements for Identification, Melting range (170–173 °C), Loss on drying (not more than 1.5%), Residue on ignition (not more than 0.1%), Acetylcholine chloride, and Heavy metals (not more than 0.002%).
Methacholine Chloride for Inhalation—Not in *USP–NF*.

METHACRYLIC ACID COPOLYMER

Description:
Methacrylic Acid Copolymer NF—White powder, having a faint characteristic odor.
NF category: Coating agent.

Methacrylic Acid Copolymer Dispersion NF—Milky-white liquid of low viscosity.

Solubility:
Methacrylic Acid Copolymer NF—The polymer is insoluble in water, in diluted acids, in simulated gastric fluid TS, and in buffer solutions of up to pH 5; soluble in diluted alkali, in simulated intestinal fluid TS, and in buffer solutions of pH 7 and above. The solubility between pH 5.5 and pH 7 depends on the content of methacrylic acid units in the copolymer. Soluble to freely soluble in methanol, in alcohol, in isopropyl alcohol, and in acetone, each of which contains not less than 3% of water.
Methacrylic Acid Copolymer Dispersion NF—It is miscible with water in any proportion; the milky-white appearance is retained. A clear or slightly opalescent, viscous solution is obtained on mixing one part with five parts of acetone, alcohol, or isopropyl alcohol; the polymer substance is first precipitated, but then dissolves in the excess organic solvent. A clear or slightly opalescent, viscous solution is obtained on mixing one part with two parts of 1 N sodium hydroxide.

NF requirements:
Methacrylic Acid Copolymer NF—Preserve in tight containers. A fully polymerized copolymer of methacrylic acid and an acrylic or methacrylic ester. It is available in 3 types, which differ in content of methacrylic acid units and viscosity. Label it to state whether it is Type A, B, or C. Meets the requirements for Identification, Viscosity, Loss on drying (not more than 5.0%), Residue on ignition (not more than 0.1% for Types A and B; not more than 0.4% for Type C), Heavy metals (not more than 0.002%), Limit of monomers (not more than 0.05%), and Organic volatile impurities.
Methacrylic Acid Copolymer Dispersion NF—Preserve in tight containers, at a temperature not exceeding 30 °C. Protect from freezing. An aqueous dispersion of Methacrylic Acid Copolymer Type C in water. The label indicates the name and amount of any substance added as a surface-active agent. Contains, on the basis of the calculated amount of dry substance in the Dispersion, not less than 46.0 percent and not more than 50.6 percent of methacrylic acid units. May contain suitable surface-active agents. Meets the requirements for Identification, Viscosity (not more than 15 centipoises), pH (2.0–3.0), Loss on drying (68.5%–71.5%), Residue on ignition (not more than 0.2%, calculated on the undried Dispersion basis), Heavy metals (not more than 0.002%), Limit of monomers (not more than 0.01%), and Coagulum content.

METHACYCLINE

Chemical name: Methacycline hydrochloride—2-Naphthacenecarboxamide, 4-(dimethylamino)-1,4,4a,5,5a,6,11,12a-octahydro-3,5,10,12,12a-pentahydroxy-6-methylene-1,11-dioxo-, monohydrochloride, [4*S*-(4 alpha,4a alpha,5 alpha,5a alpha,12a alpha)]-.

Molecular formula: Methacycline hydrochloride—$C_{22}H_{22}N_2O_8 \cdot HCl$.

Molecular weight: Methacycline hydrochloride—478.88.

Description: Methacycline Hydrochloride USP—Yellow to dark yellow, crystalline powder.

Solubility: Methacycline Hydrochloride USP—Soluble in water.

USP requirements:
Methacycline Hydrochloride USP—Preserve in tight, light-resistant containers. Has a potency equivalent to not less than 832 mcg and not more than 970 mcg of methacycline

per mg. Meets the requirements for Identification, Crystallinity, pH (2.0–3.0, in a solution containing 10 mg of methacycline per mL), and Water (not more than 2.0%).

Methacycline Hydrochloride Capsules USP—Preserve in tight, light-resistant containers. Contain an amount of methacycline hydrochloride equivalent to the labeled amount of methacycline, within −10% to +20%. Meet the requirements for Identification, Dissolution (70% in 60 minutes in water in Apparatus 1 at 100 rpm), Uniformity of dosage units, and Water (not more than 7.5%).

Methacycline Hydrochloride Oral Suspension USP—Preserve in tight, light-resistant containers. Contains an amount of methacycline hydrochloride equivalent to the labeled amount of methacycline, within −10% to +25%. Contains one or more suitable and harmless buffers, colors, diluents, dispersants, flavors, and preservatives. Meets the requirements for Identification, pH (6.5–8.0), Deliverable volume (for Suspension packaged in multiple-unit containers), and Uniformity of dosage units (for Suspension packaged in single-unit containers).

METHADONE

Chemical name: Methadone hydrochloride—3-Heptanone, 6-(dimethylamino)-4,4-diphenyl-, hydrochloride.

Molecular formula: Methadone hydrochloride—$C_{21}H_{27}NO \cdot HCl$.

Molecular weight: Methadone hydrochloride—345.91.

Description:
Methadone Hydrochloride USP—Colorless crystals or white, crystalline, odorless powder.
Methadone Hydrochloride Oral Concentrate USP—Clear to slightly hazy, syrupy liquid.

Solubility: Methadone Hydrochloride USP—Soluble in water; freely soluble in alcohol and in chloroform; practically insoluble in ether and in glycerin.

USP requirements:
Methadone Hydrochloride USP—Preserve in tight, light-resistant containers. Contains not less than 98.5% and not more than 100.5% of methadone hydrochloride, calculated on the dried basis. Meets the requirements for Identification, pH (4.5–6.5, in a solution [1 in 100]), Loss on drying (not more than 0.3%), Residue on ignition (not more than 0.1%), Ordinary impurities, and Organic volatile impurities.
Methadone Hydrochloride Oral Concentrate USP—Preserve in tight containers, protected from light, at controlled room temperature. Label it to indicate that it is to be diluted with water or other liquid to 30 mL or more prior to administration. Contains, in each mL, not less than 9.0 mg and not more than 11.0 mg of methadone hydrochloride. Contains a suitable preservative. Meets the requirements for Identification and pH (1.0–6.0).
Methadone Hydrochloride Injection USP—Preserve in single-dose or in multiple-dose, light-resistant containers, preferably of Type I glass. A sterile solution of Methadone Hydrochloride in Water for Injection. Contains, in each mL, not less than 9.5 mg and not more than 10.5 mg of methadone hydrochloride. Meets the requirements for Identification, Bacterial endotoxins, and pH (3.0–6.5), and for Injections.
Methadone Hydrochloride Oral Solution USP—Preserve in tight containers, protected from light, at controlled room temperature. Contains the labeled amount, within ±10%. Meets the requirements for Identification, pH (1.0–4.0), and Alcohol content (if present, the labeled amount, within −10% to +15%, determined by the gas-liquid chromatographic procedure, acetone being used as the internal standard).

Methadone Hydrochloride Tablets USP—Preserve in well-closed containers. Contain the labeled amount, within ± 7%. Meet the requirements for Identification, Dissolution (75% in 45 minutes in water in Apparatus 1 at 100 rpm), and Uniformity of dosage units.

Methadone Hydrochloride Tablets for Oral Suspension USP—Preserve in well-closed containers. Label the Tablets for Oral Suspension to indicate that they are intended for dispersion in a liquid prior to oral administration of the prescribed dose. Contain the labeled amount, within ±7%. Meet the requirements for Identification, Disintegration (15 minutes), and Uniformity of dosage units.

METHAMPHETAMINE

Chemical name: Methamphetamine hydrochloride—Benzeneethanamine, N, alpha-dimethyl-, hydrochloride, (S)-.

Molecular formula: Methamphetamine hydrochloride—$C_{10}H_{15}N \cdot HCl$.

Molecular weight: Methamphetamine hydrochloride—185.76.

Description: Methamphetamine Hydrochloride USP—White crystals or white, crystalline powder. Is odorless or practically so. Its solutions have a pH of about 6.

Solubility: Methamphetamine Hydrochloride USP—Freely soluble in water, in alcohol, and in chloroform; very slightly soluble in absolute ether.

USP requirements:
Methamphetamine Hydrochloride USP—Preserve in tight, light-resistant containers. Contains not less than 98.5% and not more than 100.5% of methamphetamine hydrochloride, calculated on the dried basis. Meets the requirements for Identification, Melting range (171–175 °C), Specific rotation (+16° to +19°), Loss on drying (not more than 0.5%), Residue on ignition (not more than 0.1%), Ordinary impurities, and Organic volatile impurities.
Methamphetamine Hydrochloride Tablets USP—Preserve in tight, light-resistant containers. Contain the labeled amount, within ±10%. Meet the requirements for Identification, Dissolution (75% in 45 minutes in water in Apparatus 2 at 50 rpm), and Uniformity of dosage units.
Methamphetamine Hydrochloride Extended-release Tablets—Not in *USP–NF*.

METHANTHELINE

Chemical group: Quaternary ammonium compound.

Chemical name: Methantheline bromide—Ethanaminium, N,N-diethyl-N-methyl-2-[(9H-xanthen-9-ylcarbonyl)oxy]-, bromide.

Molecular formula: Methantheline bromide—$C_{21}H_{26}BrNO_3$.

Molecular weight: Methantheline bromide—420.34.

Description: Methantheline bromide—White or nearly white, practically odorless powder. Its solutions have a pH of about 5.

Solubility: Methantheline bromide—Very soluble in water; freely soluble in alcohol and in chloroform; practically insoluble in ether. Its water solution decomposes on standing.

USP requirements: Methantheline Bromide Tablets—Not in *USP–NF*.

METHARBITAL

Chemical name: 2,4,6(1H,3H,5H)-Pyrimidinetrione, 5,5-diethyl-1-methyl-.

Molecular formula: $C_9H_{14}N_2O_3$.

Molecular weight: 198.22.

Description: White to nearly white, crystalline powder, having a faint aromatic odor. The pH of a saturated solution is about 6.

Solubility: Slightly soluble in water; soluble in alcohol; sparingly soluble in ether.

USP requirements: Metharbital Tablets—Not in USP–NF.

METHAZOLAMIDE

Chemical name: Acetamide, N-[5-(aminosulfonyl)-3-methyl-1,3,-4-thiadiazol-2(3H)-ylidene]-.

Molecular formula: $C_5H_8N_4O_3S_2$.

Molecular weight: 236.27.

Description: Methazolamide USP—White or faintly yellow, crystalline powder having a slight odor. Melts at about 213 °C.

Solubility: Methazolamide USP—Very slightly soluble in water and in alcohol; soluble in dimethylformamide; slightly soluble in acetone.

USP requirements:

Methazolamide USP—Preserve in well-closed, light-resistant containers. Contains not less than 98.0% and not more than 102.0% of methazolamide, calculated on the dried basis. Meets the requirements for Identification, Loss on drying (not more than 0.5%), Residue on ignition (not more than 0.1%), Selenium (not more than 0.003%), Heavy metals (not more than 0.002%, a 200-mg specimen being used), and Organic volatile impurities.

Methazolamide Tablets USP—Preserve in well-closed containers. Contain the labeled amount, within ±10%. Meet the requirements for Identification, Dissolution (75% in 45 minutes in acetate buffer [pH 4.5] in Apparatus 2 at 75 rpm), and Uniformity of dosage units.

METHDILAZINE

Chemical name:

Methdilazine—10H-Phenothiazine, 10-[(1-methyl-3-pyrrolidinyl)methyl]-.

Methdilazine hydrochloride—10H-Phenothiazine, 10-[(1-methyl-3-pyrrolidinyl)methyl]-, monohydrochloride.

Molecular formula:

Methdilazine—$C_{18}H_{20}N_2S$.

Methdilazine hydrochloride—$C_{18}H_{20}N_2S \cdot HCl$.

Molecular weight:

Methdilazine—296.43.

Methdilazine hydrochloride—332.89.

Description:

Methdilazine USP—Light tan, crystalline powder, having a characteristic odor.

Methdilazine Hydrochloride USP—Light tan, crystalline powder, having a slight, characteristic odor.

Solubility:

Methdilazine USP—Practically insoluble in water; freely soluble in 3 N hydrochloric acid; soluble in alcohol and in chloroform.

Methdilazine Hydrochloride USP—Freely soluble in water, in alcohol, and in chloroform.

USP requirements:

Methdilazine USP—Preserve in tight, light-resistant containers. Contains not less than 97.0% and not more than 103.0% of methdilazine, calculated on the dried basis. Meets the requirements for Identification, Melting range (83–88 °C, the range between beginning and end of melting not more than 2 °C), Loss on drying (not more than 1.0%), Residue on ignition (not more than 0.5%), Selenium (not more than 0.003%), Heavy metals (not more than 0.002%), and Organic volatile impurities.

Methdilazine Tablets USP—Preserve in tight, light-resistant containers. Contains the labeled amount, within ±7%. Meets the requirements for Identification, Disintegration (30 minutes), and Uniformity of dosage units.

Methdilazine Hydrochloride USP—Preserve in tight, light-resistant containers. Contains not less than 97.0% and not more than 103.0% of methdilazine hydrochloride, calculated on the dried basis. Meets the requirements for Identification, Melting range (184–190 °C), pH (4.8–6.0, in a solution [1 in 100]), Loss on drying (not more than 1.0%), Selenium (not more than 0.003%), Residue on ignition (not more than 0.5%), Heavy metals (not more than 0.002%), Ordinary impurities, and Organic volatile impurities.

Methdilazine Hydrochloride Oral Solution USP—Preserve in tight, light-resistant containers. Contains the labeled amount, within ±7%. Meets the requirements for Identification, pH (3.3–4.1), and Alcohol content (6.5–7.5%).

Methdilazine Hydrochloride Syrup USP—Preserve in tight, light-resistant containers. Contains the labeled amount, within ±7%. Meets the requirements for Identification, pH (3.3–4.1), and Alcohol content (6.5–7.5%).

Methdilazine Hydrochloride Tablets USP—Preserve in tight, light-resistant containers. Contain the labeled amount, within ±7%. Meet the requirements for Identification, Dissolution (75% in 45 minutes in water in Apparatus 1 at 100 rpm), and Uniformity of dosage units.

Methdilazine Hydrochloride Chewable Tablets–Not in USP–NF.

METHENAMINE

Chemical name:

Methenamine—1,3,5,7-Tetraazatricyclo[3.3.1.1³,⁷]decane.

Methenamine hippurate—Glycine, N-benzoyl, compd. with 1,3,5,7-tetraazatricyclo[3.3.1.1³,⁷]decane (1:1).

Methenamine mandelate—Benzeneacetic acid, alphahydroxy-, compd. with 1,3,5,7-tetraazatricyclo[3.3.1.1³,⁷]-decane (1:1).

Molecular formula:

Methenamine—$C_6H_{12}N_4$.

Methenamine hippurate—$C_6H_{12}N_4 \cdot C_9H_9NO_3$.

Methenamine mandelate—$C_6H_{12}N_4 \cdot C_8H_8O_3$.

Molecular weight:

Methenamine—140.19.

Methenamine hippurate—319.36.

Methenamine mandelate—292.33.

Description:

Methenamine USP—Colorless, lustrous crystals or white, crystalline powder. Is practically odorless. When brought into contact with fire, it readily ignites, burning with a smokeless flame. It sublimes at about 260 °C, without melting. Its solutions are alkaline to litmus.

Methenamine hippurate—Fine, white, crystalline powder; practically odorless. Melts at about 115 °C.

Methenamine Mandelate USP—White crystalline powder. Is practically odorless. Its solutions have a pH of about 4. Melts at about 127 °C, with decomposition.

Solubility:

Methenamine USP—Freely soluble in water; soluble in alcohol and in chloroform.

Methenamine hippurate—Freely soluble in water, in alcohol, and in chloroform.

Methenamine Mandelate USP—Very soluble in water; soluble in alcohol and in chloroform; slightly soluble in ether.

USP requirements:

Methenamine USP—Preserve in well-closed containers. Dried over phosphorus pentoxide for 4 hours, contains not less than 99.0% and not more than 100.5% of methenamine. Meets the requirements for Identification, Loss on drying (not more than 2.0%), Residue on ignition (not more than 0.1%), Chloride (not more than 0.014%), Sulfate, Ammonium salts, Heavy metals (not more than 0.001%), and Organic volatile impurities.

Methenamine Elixir USP—Preserve in tight containers. Contains the labeled amount, within ±10%. Meets the requirements for Identification and Alcohol content (the labeled amount, within ±10%).

Methenamine Oral Solution USP—Preserve in tight containers. Contains the labeled amount, within ±10%. Meets the requirements for Identification and Alcohol content (the labeled amount, within ±10%).

Methenamine Tablets USP—Preserve in well-closed containers. Contain the labeled amount, within ±5%. Meet the requirements for Identification, Dissolution (75% in 45 minutes in water in Apparatus 1 at 100 rpm), and Uniformity of dosage units.

Methenamine Hippurate USP—Preserve in well-closed containers. Dried in vacuum at 60 °C for 1 hour, contains not less than 95.5% and not more than 102.0% of methenamine hippurate, and contains not less than 54.0% and not more than 58.0% of hippuric acid. Meets the requirements for Identification, Loss on drying (not more than 1.0%), Residue on ignition (not more than 0.1%), Sulfate, Heavy metals (not more than 0.0015%), Organic volatile impurities, and Hippuric acid content.

Methenamine Hippurate Tablets USP—Preserve in well-closed containers. Contain the labeled amount, within ± 5%. Meet the requirements for Identification, Disintegration (30 minutes), and Uniformity of dosage units.

Methenamine Mandelate USP—Preserve in well-closed containers. Contains not less than 95.5% and not more than 102.0% of methenamine mandelate, and contains not less than 50.0% and and not more than 53.0% of mandelic acid, calculated on the dried basis. Meets the requirements for Identification, Loss on drying (not more than 1.5%), Residue on ignition (not more than 0.1%), Chloride (not more than 0.01%), Sulfate, Heavy metals (not more than 0.0015%), Organic volatile impurities, and Mandelic acid content.

Methenamine Mandelate for Oral Solution USP (Granules)—Preserve in well-closed containers. Label Methenamine Mandelate for Oral Solution that contains insoluble ingredients to indicate that the aqueous constituted Oral Solution contains dissolved methenamine mandelate but may remain turbid because of the presence of added substances. Contains the labeled amount, within ±10%. Meets the requirements for Identification, pH (4.0–4.5 in a mixture of 1 gram with 30 mL of water), and Water (not more than 0.5%).

Methenamine Mandelate Oral Suspension USP—Preserve in tight containers. It is Methenamine Mandelate suspended in vegetable oil. Contains the labeled amount, within ± 10%. Meets the requirements for Identification and Water (not more than 0.1%).

Methenamine Mandelate Tablets USP—Preserve in well-closed containers. Contain the labeled amount, within ± 5%. Meet the requirements for Identification, Dissolution (for uncoated or plain coated Tablets, 75% in 45 minutes in water in Apparatus 1 at 100 rpm), and Uniformity of dosage units.

Methenamine Mandelate Delayed-release Tablets USP—Preserve in well-closed containers. Contain the labeled amount, within ±5%. Meet the requirements for Disintegration (2 hours and 30 minutes, determined as directed under Delayed-release [enteric coated] Tablets) and for Identification test and Uniformity of dosage units.

METHENAMINE AND MONOBASIC SODIUM PHOSPHATE

For *Methenamine* and *Monobasic Sodium Phosphate*—See individual listings for chemistry information.

USP requirements: Methenamine and Monobasic Sodium Phosphate Tablets USP—Preserve in tight containers. Contain the labeled amounts, within ±7.5%. Meet the requirements for Identification, Dissolution (75% of labeled amount of methenamine in 45 minutes in water in Apparatus 1 at 100 rpm), Uniformity of dosage units, and Ammonium salts.

METHICILLIN

Chemical name: Methicillin sodium—4-Thia-1-azabicyclo[3.2.0]-heptane-2-carboxylic acid, 6-[(2,6-dimethoxybenzoyl)amino]3,3-dimethyl-7-oxo-, monosodium salt, monohydrate, [2*S*-(2 alpha,5 alpha,6 beta)]-.

Molecular formula: Methicillin sodium—$C_{17}H_{19}N_2NaO_6S \cdot H_2O$.

Molecular weight: Methicillin sodium—420.41.

Description: Methicillin for Injection USP—Fine, white, crystalline powder, odorless or having a slight odor.

Solubility: Methicillin for Injection USP—Freely soluble in water, in methanol, and in pyridine; slightly soluble in propyl and amyl alcohols, in chloroform, and in ethylene chloride; insoluble in acetone and in ether.

USP requirements:

Methicillin Sodium—Preserve in tight containers, at controlled room temperature. Where it is intended for use in preparing injectable dosage forms, the label states that it is sterile or must be subjected to further processing during the preparation of injectable dosage forms. Has a potency equivalent to not less than 815 mcg of methicillin per mg. Meets the requirements for Identification, Cristallinity, pH (5.0–7.5, in a solution containing 10 mg per mL, and Water (3.0%–6.0%), and for Sterility and Bacterial endotoxins under Methicillin for Injection (where the label states that Methicillin Sodium is sterile) and for Bacterial endotoxins under Methicillin for Injection (where the label states that Methicillin Sodium must be subjected to further processing during the preparation of injectable dosage forms).

Methicillin for Injection USP—Preserve in Containers for Sterile Solids, at controlled room temperature. Contains an amount of methicillin sodium equivalent to the labeled amount of methicillin, within −10% to +15%. May contain Sodium Citrate and one or more suitable preservatives. Meets the requirements for Constituted solution, Identification, Bacterial endotoxins, Sterility, pH (6.0–8.5, in a solution containing 10 mg per mL), Water (not more than 6.0%), and Particulate matter, and for Uniformity of dosage units and Labeling under Injections.

METHIMAZOLE

Chemical group: Thioimidazole derivative.

Chemical name: 2H-Imidazole-2-thione, 1,3-dihydro-1-methyl-.

Molecular formula: $C_4H_6N_2S$.

Molecular weight: 114.17.

Description: Methimazole USP—White to pale buff, crystalline powder, having a faint, characteristic odor. Its solutions are practically neutral to litmus.

Solubility: Methimazole USP—Freely soluble in water, in alcohol, and in chloroform; slightly soluble in ether.

USP requirements:
Methimazole USP—Preserve in well-closed, light-resistant containers. Contains not less than 98.0% and not more than 101.0% of methimazole, calculated on the dried basis. Meets the requirements for Identification, Melting range (143–146 °C), Loss on drying (not more than 0.5%), Residue on ignition (not more than 0.1%), Selenium (not more than 0.003%, a 200-mg specimen being used), Ordinary impurities, and Organic volatile impurities.
Methimazole Suppositories—Not in *USP–NF*.
Methimazole Tablets USP—Preserve in well-closed, light-resistant containers. Contain the labeled amount, within ± 6%. Meet the requirements for Identification, Dissolution (80% in 30 minutes in water in Apparatus 1 at 100 rpm), and Uniformity of dosage units.

METHIONINE

Chemical name: L-Methionine.

Molecular formula: $C_5H_{11}NO_2S$.

Molecular weight: 149.21.

Description: Methionine USP—White crystals, having a characteristic odor.

Solubility: Methionine USP—Soluble in water, in warm dilute alcohol, and in dilute mineral acids; insoluble in ether, in absolute alcohol, and in acetone (L-form).

USP requirements: Methionine USP—Preserve in well-closed containers. Contains not less than 98.5% and not more than 101.5% of methionine, as L-methionine, calculated on the dried basis. Meets the requirements for Identification, Specific rotation (+22.4° to +24.7°), pH (5.6–6.1 in a solution [1 in 100]), Loss on drying (not more than 0.3%), Residue on ignition (not more than 0.4%), Chloride (not more than 0.05%), Sulfate (not more than 0.03%), Iron (not more than 0.003%), Heavy metals (0.0015%), Chromatographic purity, and Organic volatile impurities.

METHOCARBAMOL

Chemical name: 1,2-Propanediol, 3-(2-methoxyphenoxy)-, 1-carbamate.

Molecular formula: $C_{11}H_{15}NO_5$.

Molecular weight: 241.24.

Description: Methocarbamol USP—White powder, odorless, or having a slight characteristic odor. Melts at about 94 °C, or, if previously ground to a fine powder, melts at about 90 °C.

Solubility: Methocarbamol USP—Sparingly soluble in water and in chloroform; soluble in alcohol only with heating; insoluble in n-hexane.

USP requirements:
Methocarbamol USP—Preserve in tight containers. Contains not less than 98.5% and not more than 101.5% of methocarbamol, calculated on the dried basis. Meets the requirements for Identification, Loss on drying (not more than 0.5%), Residue on ignition (not more than 0.1%), Heavy metals (not more than 0.002%), Organic volatile impurities, and Chromatographic purity.
Methocarbamol Injection USP—Preserve in single-dose containers, preferably of Type I glass. A sterile solution of Methocarbamol in an aqueous solution of Polyethylene Glycol 300. Contains the labeled amount, within ±5%. Meets the requirements for Identification, Bacterial endotoxins, pH (3.5–6.0), Particulate matter (under Small-volume Injections), and Aldehydes (not more than 0.01%, as formaldehyde), and for Injections.
Methocarbamol Tablets USP—Preserve in tight containers. Contain the labeled amount, within ±5%. Meet the requirements for Identification, Dissolution (75% in 45 minutes in water in Apparatus 2 at 50 rpm), and Uniformity of dosage units.

METHOHEXITAL

Chemical group: Methohexital sodium—A methylated oxybarbiturate; differs chemically from the established barbiturate anesthetics in that it contains no sulfur.

Chemical name:
Methohexital—2,4,6(1H,3H,5H)-Pyrimidinetrione, 1-methyl-5-(1-methyl-2-pentynyl)-5-(2-propenyl)-, (±)-.
Methohexital sodium—2,4,6(1H,3H,5H)-Pyrimidinetrione, 1-methyl-5-(1-methyl-2-pentynyl)-5-(2-propenyl)-, (±)-, monosodium salt.

Molecular formula:
Methohexital—$C_{14}H_{18}N_2O_3$.
Methohexital sodium—$C_{14}H_{17}N_2NaO_3$.

Molecular weight:
Methohexital—262.30.
Methohexital sodium—284.29.

Description:
Methohexital USP—White to faintly yellowish white, crystalline odorless powder.
Methohexital Sodium for Injection USP—White to off-white hygroscopic powder. Is essentially odorless.

Solubility:
Methohexital USP—Very slightly soluble in water; slightly soluble in alcohol, in chloroform, and in dilute alkalies.
Methohexital sodium—Freely soluble in water.

Other characteristics:
Methohexital sodium—75% un-ionized at pH 7.4.
Methohexital sodium for injection—A 1% solution in sterile water has a pH of 10 to 11; a 0.2% solution in 5% dextrose has a pH of 9.5 to 10.5.

USP requirements:
Methohexital USP—Preserve in well-closed containers. Contains not less than 98.0% and not more than 101.0% of methohexital, calculated on the anhydrous basis. Meets the requirements for Identification, Melting range (92–96 °C, but the range between beginning and end of melting not more than 3 °C), Water (not more than 2.0%), Chloride (not more than 0.03%), Heavy metals (not more than 0.001%), and Ordinary impurities.
Methohexital Sodium for Injection USP—Preserve in tight Containers for Sterile Solids. Store at controlled room temperature. Injection may be packaged in 50-mL multiple-dose containers. A freeze-dried, sterile mixture of methohexital sodium and anhydrous Sodium Carbonate as a

buffer, prepared from an aqueous solution of Methohexital, Sodium Hydroxide, and Sodium Carbonate. Contains the labeled amount, within ±10%. Meets the requirements for Completeness of solution, Constituted solution, Identification, Bacterial endotoxins, Uniformity of dosage units, pH (10.6–11.6), Loss on drying (not more than 2.0%), and Heavy metals (not more than 0.001%), and for Injections.
Methohexital Sodium for Rectal Solution—Not in *USP–NF*.

METHOTREXATE

Chemical name: L-Glutamic acid, *N*-[4-[[(2,4-diamino-6-pteridinyl)methyl]methylamino]benzoyl]-.

Molecular formula: $C_{20}H_{22}N_8O_5$.

Molecular weight: 454.44.

Description: Methotrexate USP—Orange-brown, or yellow, crystalline powder.

Solubility: Methotrexate USP—Practically insoluble in water, in alcohol, in chloroform, and in ether; freely soluble in dilute solutions of alkali hydroxides and carbonates; slightly soluble in 6 *N* hydrochloric acid.

USP requirements:
Methotrexate USP—Preserve in tight, light-resistant containers. A mixture of 4-amino-10-methylfolic acid and closely related compounds. Contains not less than 98.0% and not more than 102.0% of methotrexate, calculated on the anhydrous basis. Meets the requirements for Identification, Specific rotation (+19° to +24°, calculated on the anhydrous basis), Water (not more than 12.0%), Residue on ignition (not more than 0.1%), Chromatographic purity, and Organic volatile impurities.
    Caution: Great care should be taken to prevent inhaling particles of Methotrexate and exposing the skin to it.
Methotrexate Injection USP—Preserve in single-dose or in multiple-dose containers, preferably of Type I glass, protected from light. A sterile solution of Methotrexate in Water for Injection prepared with the aid of Sodium Hydroxide. Contains the labeled amount of methotrexate, within ±10%. Meets the requirements for Identification, Bacterial endotoxins, and pH (7.0–9.0), and for Injections.
Methotrexate for Injection USP—Preserve in Containers for Sterile Solids, protected from light. A sterile, freeze-dried preparation of methotrexate sodium with or without suitable added substances, buffers, and/or diluents. Contains the labeled amount of methotrexate, within −5% to +15%. Meets the requirements for Constituted solution, Identification, Bacterial endotoxins, and pH (7.0–9.0 in a solution constituted as directed in the labeling, except that water is used as the diluent), and for Labeling under Injections, Sterility tests, and Uniformity of dosage units.
    Caution: Great care should be taken to prevent inhaling particles of methotrexate sodium and exposing the skin to it.
Methotrexate Tablets USP—Preserve in well-closed containers. A unit-of-use container contains a quantity of Tablets sufficient to provide one week's therapy as indicated in the labeling. When packaged in a unit-of-use container, the label indicates the total amount of methotrexate present as one week's supply. Contain the labeled amount, within ±10%. Meet the requirements for Identification, Dissolution (75% in 45 minutes in 0.1 *N* hydrochloric acid in Apparatus 2 at 50 rpm), and Uniformity of dosage units.
Methotrexate Sodium Injection—Not in *USP–NF*.
Methotrexate Sodium for Injection—Not in *USP–NF*.

METHOTRIMEPRAZINE

Chemical group: Phenothiazine derivative.

Chemical name: 10*H*-Phenothiazine-10-propanamine, 2-methoxy-*N,N*,beta-trimethyl-, (–)-.

Molecular formula:
    Methotrimeprazine—$C_{19}H_{24}N_2OS$.
    Methotrimeprazine hydrochloride—$C_{19}H_{24}N_2OS \cdot HCl$.
    Methotrimeprazine maleate—$C_{19}H_{24}N_2OS \cdot C_4H_4O_4$.

Molecular weight:
    Methotrimeprazine—328.47.
    Methotrimeprazine hydrochloride—364.9.
    Methotrimeprazine maleate—444.5.

Description:
    Methotrimeprazine USP—Fine, white, practically odorless, crystalline powder. Melts at about 126 °C.
    Methotrimeprazine hydrochloride—White or slightly yellow, slightly hygroscopic crystalline powder. It deteriorates on exposure to air and light.

Solubility:
    Methotrimeprazine USP—Practically insoluble in water; freely soluble in chloroform and in ether; sparingly soluble in methanol; sparingly soluble in alcohol at 25 °C; freely soluble in boiling alcohol.
    Methotrimeprazine hydrochloride—Freely soluble in water, in alcohol, and in chloroform; practically insoluble in ether.
    Methotrimeprazine maleate—Sparingly soluble in water and in ethanol.

USP requirements:
Methotrimeprazine USP—Preserve in well-closed, light-resistant containers. Contains not less than 98.0% and not more than 101.0% of methotrimeprazine, calculated on the dried basis. Meets the requirements for Identification, Specific rotation (–15° to –18°), Loss on drying (not more than 0.5%), and Selenium (not more than 0.003%).
Methotrimeprazine Injection USP—Preserve in single-dose or in multiple-dose containers, preferably of Type I glass, protected from light. A sterile solution of Methotrimeprazine in Water for Injection, prepared with the aid of hydrochloric acid. Contains the labeled amount, as the hydrochloride, within ±10%. Meets the requirements for Identification, Bacterial endotoxins, and pH (3.0–5.0), and for Injections.
Methotrimeprazine Hydrochloride Oral Solution—Not in *USP–NF*.
Methotrimeprazine Hydrochloride Syrup—Not in *USP–NF*.
Methotrimeprazine Maleate Tablets—Not in *USP–NF*.

METHOXAMINE

Chemical name: Methoxamine hydrochloride—Benzenemethanol, alpha-(1-aminoethyl)-2,5-dimethoxy-, hydrochloride.

Molecular formula: Methoxamine hydrochloride—$C_{11}H_{17}NO_3 \cdot HCl$.

Molecular weight: Methoxamine hydrochloride—247.72.

Description: Methoxamine hydrochloride—Colorless or white, plate-like crystals or white, crystalline powder. Is odorless or has only a slight odor. Its solutions have a pH of about 5.

Solubility: Methoxamine hydrochloride—Freely soluble in water; soluble in alcohol; practically insoluble in chloroform and in ether.

USP requirements: Methoxamine Hydrochloride Injection—Not in *USP–NF*.

METHOXSALEN

Source: Methoxsalem (Extracorpreal)—Found in the seeds of the Ammi majus (Umbelliferae) plant.

Chemical group; Methoxsalen (Extracorpreal)—Psoralens or Furocumarins.

Chemical name: 7*H*-Furo[3,2-*g*][1]benzopyran-7-one, 9-methoxy-.

Molecular formula: $C_{12}H_8O_4$.

Molecular weight: 216.19.

Description:
Methoxsalen USP—White to cream-colored, fluffy, needle-like crystals. Is odorless.
Methoxsalen Topical Solution USP—Clear, colorless liquid.

Solubility: Methoxsalen USP—Practically insoluble in water; freely soluble in chloroform; soluble in boiling alcohol, in acetone, in acetic acid, and in propylene glycol; sparingly soluble in boiling water and in ether.

USP requirements:
Methoxsalen USP—Preserve in well-closed, light-resistant containers. Contains not less than 98.0% and not more than 102.0% of methoxsalen, calculated on the anhydrous basis. Meets the requirements for Identification, Melting range (143–148 °C), Water (not more than 0.5%), Residue on ignition (not more than 0.1%, a 1-gram specimen being used), Heavy metals (not more than 0.002%), Chromatographic impurities, and Organic volatile impurities.
Caution: Avoid contact with the skin.
Methoxsalen Capsules USP—Preserve in tight, light-resistant containers. Label the Capsules to state that Methoxsalen Hard Gelatin Capsules may not be interchangeable with Methoxsalen Soft Gelatin Capsules without retitration of the patient. Contain the labeled amount, within ±10%. Meet the requirements for Identification, Dissolution (75% in 45 minutes in water in Apparatus 2 at 50 rpm for Soft Gelatin Capsules and 75% in 90 minutes in water in Apparatus 1 at 150 rpm for Hard Gelatin Capsules), and Uniformity of dosage units.
Sterile Methoxsalen Extracorporeal Solution—Not in *USP–NF*.
Methoxsalen Topical Solution USP—Store in tight, light-resistant containers. A solution of Methoxsalen in a suitable vehicle. Contains not less than 9.2 mg and not more than 10.8 mg of methoxsalen per mL. Meets the requirements for Identification and Alcohol content, if present (66.5–77.0%).

METHOXYFLURANE

Chemical name: Ethane, 2,2-dichloro-1,1-difluoro-1-methoxy-.

Molecular formula: $C_3H_4Cl_2F_2O$.

Molecular weight: 164.97.

Description: Methoxyflurane USP—Clear, practically colorless, mobile liquid, having a characteristic odor. Boils at about 105 °C.

Solubility: Methoxyflurane USP—Miscible with alcohol, with acetone, with chloroform, with ether, and with fixed oils.

Other characteristics:
Blood-to-Gas (mean range) partition coefficient at 37 °C— 10.20 to 14.06.
Oil-to-Gas partition coefficient at 37 °C—825.

USP requirements: Methoxyflurane USP—Preserve in tight, light-resistant containers, and avoid exposure to excessive heat. Contains not less than 99.9% and not more than 100.0% of methoxyflurane. Meets the requirements for Identi-

fication, Specific gravity (1.420–1.425), Acidity, Water (not more than 0.1%), Foreign odor, and Limit of nonvolatile residue (not more than 1 mg per 50 mL).

METHSCOPOLAMINE

Source: Quaternary ammonium derivative of scopolamine.

Chemical name: Methscopolamine bromide—3-Oxa-9-azoniatricyclo[3.3.1.0²,⁴]nonane, 7-(3-hydroxy-1-oxo-2-phenylpropoxy)-9,9-dimethyl-, bromide, [7(*S*)-(1 alpha,2 beta,4 beta,5 alpha,7 beta)]-.

Molecular formula: Methscopolamine bromide—$C_{18}H_{24}BrNO_4$.

Molecular weight: Methscopolamine bromide—398.29.

Description: Methscopolamine bromide—White crystals or white, odorless, crystalline powder. Melts at about 225 °C, with decomposition.

Solubility: Methscopolamine bromide—Freely soluble in water; slightly soluble in alcohol; insoluble in acetone and in chloroform.

USP requirements: Methscopolamine Bromide Tablets—Not in *USP–NF*.

METHSUXIMIDE

Chemical name: 2,5-Pyrrolidinedione, 1,3-dimethyl-3-phenyl-.

Molecular formula: $C_{12}H_{13}NO_2$.

Molecular weight: 203.24.

Description: Methsuximide USP—White to grayish white, crystalline powder. Is odorless, or has not more than a slight odor.

USP requirements:
Methsuximide USP—Preserve in tight containers. Contains not less than 97.0% and not more than 103.0% of methsuximide, calculated on the dried basis. Meets the requirements for Identification, Melting range (50–56 °C), Loss on drying (not more than 0.5%), Residue on ignition (not more than 0.2%), Limit of cyanide, Chromatographic purity, and Organic volatile impurities.
Methsuximide Capsules USP—Preserve in tight containers, and avoid exposure to excessive heat. Contain the labeled amount, within ±8%. Meet the requirements for Identification, Dissolution (75% in 120 minutes in water in Apparatus 1 at 100 rpm), and Uniformity of dosage units.

METHYCLOTHIAZIDE

Chemical name: 2*H*-1,2,4-Benzothiadiazine-7-sulfonamide, 6-chloro-3-(chloromethyl)-3,4-dihydro-2-methyl-, 1,1-dioxide.

Molecular formula: $C_9H_{11}Cl_2N_3O_4S_2$.

Molecular weight: 360.24.

Description: Methyclothiazide USP—White or practically white, crystalline powder. Is odorless, or has a slight odor.

pKa: 9.4.

Solubility: Methyclothiazide USP—Very slightly soluble in water and in chloroform; freely soluble in acetone and in pyridine; sparingly soluble in methanol; slightly soluble in alcohol.

USP requirements:

Methyclothiazide USP—Preserve in well-closed containers. Contains not less than 97.0% and not more than 102.0% of methyclothiazide, calculated on the dried basis. Meets the requirements for Identification, Loss on drying (not more than 0.5%), Residue on ignition (not more than 0.2%), Chloride (not more than 0.02%), Selenium (not more than 0.003%), Heavy metals (not more than 0.002%), and Diazotizable substances (not more than 1.0%).

Methyclothiazide Tablets USP—Preserve in well-closed containers. Contain the labeled amount, within ±10%. Meet the requirements for Identification, Dissolution (70% in 60 minutes in 0.01 N hydrochloric acid in Apparatus 2 at 50 rpm), and Uniformity of dosage units.

METHYL ALCOHOL

Chemical name: Methanol.

Molecular formula: CH_4O.

Molecular weight: 32.04.

Description: Methyl Alcohol NF—Clear, colorless liquid, having a characteristic odor. Is flammable.

NF category: Solvent.

Solubility: Methyl Alcohol NF—Miscible with water, with alcohol, with ether, and with most other organic solvents.

NF requirements: Methyl Alcohol NF—Preserve in tight containers, remote from heat, sparks, and open flames. Contains not less than 99.5% of methyl alcohol. Meets the requirements for Identification, Acidity, Alkalinity (as ammonia, not more than 3 ppm), Water (not more than 0.1%), Nonvolatile residue (not more than 0.001% [w/w]), Readily carbonizable substances, Readily oxidizable substances, Acetone and aldehydes (as acetone, not more than 0.003%), and Organic volatile impurities.

Caution: Methyl Alcohol is poisonous.

METHYLBENZETHONIUM

Chemical name: Methylbenzethonium chloride—Benzenemethanaminium, *N,N*-dimethyl-*N*-[2-[2-[methyl-4-(1,1,3,3-tetramethylbutyl)phenoxy]ethoxy]ethyl]-, chloride, monohydrate.

Molecular formula: Methylbenzethonium chloride—$C_{28}H_{44}ClNO_2 \cdot H_2O$.

Molecular weight: Methylbenzethonium chloride—480.12.

Description: Methylbenzethonium Chloride USP—White, hygroscopic crystals, having a mild odor. Its solutions are neutral or slightly alkaline to litmus.

Solubility: Methylbenzethonium Chloride USP—Very soluble in water, in alcohol, and in ether; practically insoluble in chloroform.

USP requirements:

Methylbenzethonium Chloride USP—Preserve in tight containers. Contains not less than 97.0% and not more than 103.0% of methylbenzethonium chloride, calculated on the dried basis. Meets the requirements for Identification, Melting range (159–163 °C, the specimen having been previously dried), Loss on drying (not more than 5.0%), Residue on ignition (not more than 0.1%), and Limit of ammonium compounds.

Methylbenzethonium Chloride Lotion USP—Preserve in tight containers. An emulsion containing the labeled amount, within ±10%. Meets the requirements for Identification and pH (5.2–6.0).

Methylbenzethonium Chloride Ointment USP—Preserve in collapsible tubes or in tight containers. Contains the labeled amount, within ±10%. Meets the requirements for Identification and pH (5.0–7.0, in a dispersion of it in carbon dioxide-free water [1 in 100]).

Methylbenzethonium Chloride Topical Powder USP—Preserve in well-closed containers. Contains the labeled amount, within ±15%, in a suitable fine powder base, free from grittiness. Meets the requirements for Identification, pH (9.0–10.5, in a dispersion of it in carbon dioxide-free water [1 in 100]), and Powder fineness (not less than 99% of it passes through a No. 200 sieve).

METHYLCELLULOSE

Chemical group: Semisynthetic hydrophilic derivative of cellulose.

Chemical name: Cellulose, methyl ether.

Description: Methylcellulose USP—White, fibrous powder or granules. Its aqueous suspensions are neutral to litmus. It swells in water and produces a clear to opalescent, viscous colloidal suspension.

NF category: Coating agent; suspending and/or viscosity-increasing agent; tablet binder.

Solubility: Methylcellulose USP—Insoluble in alcohol, in ether, and in chloroform; soluble in glacial acetic acid and in a mixture of equal volumes of alcohol and chloroform.

USP requirements:

Methylcellulose Capsules—Not in *USP–NF*.

Methylcellulose USP (Granules or Powder)—Preserve in well-closed containers. A methyl ether of cellulose. When dried at 105 °C for 2 hours, contains not less than 27.5% and not more than 31.5% of methoxy (OCH_3) groups. Label it to indicate its viscosity type (viscosity of a solution [1 in 50]). Meets the requirements for Identification, Apparent viscosity (within ±20% of labeled viscosity when 100 centipoises or less, within −25% to +40% of labeled viscosity when greater than 100 centipoises), Loss on drying (not more than 5.0%), Residue on ignition (not more than 1.5%), Heavy metals (not more than 0.001%), and Organic volatile impurities.

Methylcellulose Ophthalmic Solution USP—Preserve in tight containers. A sterile solution of Methylcellulose. Contains the labeled amount, within ±15%. Meets the requirements for Identification, Sterility, and pH (6.0–7.8).

Methylcellulose Oral Solution USP—Preserve in tight, light-resistant containers, and avoid exposure to direct sunlight and to excessive heat. Avoid freezing. A flavored solution of Methylcellulose. Contains the labeled amount, within ± 15%. Meets the requirements for Identification, Microbial limits, and Alcohol content (3.5–6.5%).

Methylcellulose Tablets USP—Preserve in well-closed containers. Contain the labeled amount, within ±10%. Meet the requirements for Identification, Disintegration (30 minutes), and Uniformity of dosage units.

METHYLDOPA

Chemical name:
Methyldopa—L-Tyrosine, 3-hydroxy-alpha-methyl-, sesquihydrate.
Methyldopate hydrochloride—L-Tyrosine, 3-hydroxy-alpha-methyl-, ethyl ester, hydrochloride.

Molecular formula:
Methyldopa—$C_{10}H_{13}NO_4 \cdot 1\frac{1}{2}H_2O$.
Methyldopate hydrochloride—$C_{12}H_{17}NO_4 \cdot HCl$.

Molecular weight:
Methyldopa—238.24.
Methyldopate hydrochloride—275.73.

Description:
Methyldopa USP—White to yellowish white, odorless, fine powder, which may contain friable lumps.
Methyldopate Hydrochloride USP—White or practically white, odorless or practically odorless, crystalline powder.

Solubility:
Methyldopa USP—Sparingly soluble in water; very soluble in 3 N hydrochloric acid; slightly soluble in alcohol; practically insoluble in ether.
Methyldopate Hydrochloride USP—Freely soluble in water, in alcohol, and in methanol; slightly soluble in chloroform; practically insoluble in ether.

USP requirements:
Methyldopa USP—Preserve in well-closed, light-resistant containers. Contains not less than 98.0% and not more than 101.0% of methyldopa, calculated on the anhydrous basis. Meets the requirements for Identification, Specific rotation (−25° to −28°), Acidity, Water (10.0–13.0%), Residue on ignition (not more than 0.1%), Heavy metals (not more than 0.001%), Limit of 3-o-methylmethyldopa (not more than 0.5%), and Organic volatile impurities.
Methyldopa Oral Suspension USP—Preserve in tight, light-resistant containers, at a temperature not exceeding 26 °C. An aqueous suspension of Methyldopa. Contains one or more suitable flavors, wetting agents, and preservatives. Contains the labeled amount, within ±10%. Meets the requirements for Identification, pH (3.0–5.0; 3.2–3.8 if sucrose is present), and Limit of methyldopa-glucose reaction product (if sucrose is present).
Methyldopa Tablets USP—Preserve in well-closed containers. Contain the labeled amount, within ±10%. Meet the requirements for Identification, Dissolution (80% in 20 minutes in 0.1 N hydrochloric acid in Apparatus 2 at 50 rpm), and Uniformity of dosage units.
Methyldopate Hydrochloride USP—Preserve in well-closed containers. Contains not less than 98.0% and not more than 101.0% of methyldopate hydrochloride, calculated on the dried basis. Meets the requirements for Identification, Specific rotation (−13.5° to −14.9°), pH (3.0–5.0, in a solution [1 in 100]), Loss on drying (not more than 0.5%), Residue on ignition (not more than 0.1%), and Heavy metals (not more than 0.001%).
Methyldopate Hydrochloride Injection USP—Preserve in single-dose containers, preferably of Type I glass. A sterile solution of Methyldopate Hydrochloride in Water for Injection. Contains the labeled amount, within ±10%. Meets the requirements for Identification, Bacterial endotoxins, pH (3.0–4.2), and Particulate matter, and for Injections.

METHYLDOPA AND CHLOROTHIAZIDE

For *Methyldopa* and *Chlorothiazide*—See individual listings for chemistry information.

USP requirements: Methyldopa and Chlorothiazide Tablets USP—Preserve in well-closed containers. Contain the labeled amounts, within ±10%. Meet the requirements for Identification, Dissolution (80% of methyldopa in 30 minutes in 0.1 N hydrochloric acid in Apparatus 2 at 75 rpm; and 75% of chlorothiazide in 60 minutes in 0.05 M phosphate buffer [pH 8.0] in Apparatus 2 at 75 rpm), and Uniformity of dosage units.

METHYLDOPA AND HYDROCHLOROTHIAZIDE

For *Methyldopa* and *Hydrochlorothiazide*—See individual listings for chemistry information.

USP requirements: Methyldopa and Hydrochlorothiazide Tablets USP—Preserve in well-closed containers. Contain the labeled amounts, within ±10%. Meet the requirements for Identification, Dissolution (80% of methyldopa in 30 minutes and 80% of hydrochlorothiazide in 60 minutes in 0.1 N hydrochloric acid in Apparatus 2 at 50 rpm), and Uniformity of dosage units.

METHYLENE BLUE

Chemical name: Phenothiazin-5-ium, 3,7-bis(dimethylamino)-, chloride, trihydrate.

Molecular formula: $C_{16}H_{18}ClN_3S \cdot 3H_2O$.

Molecular weight: 373.90.

Description: Methylene Blue USP—Dark green crystals or crystalline powder having a bronze-like luster. Odorless or practically so. Stable in air. Its solutions in water and in alcohol are deep blue in color.

Solubility: Methylene Blue USP—Soluble in water and in chloroform; sparingly soluble in alcohol.

USP requirements:
Methylene Blue USP—Preserve in well-closed containers. Contains not less than 98.0% and not more than 103.0% of methylene blue, calculated on the dried basis. Meets the requirements for Identification, Loss on drying (8.0–18.0%), Residue on ignition (not more than 1.2%), Arsenic (not more than 8 ppm), Copper or zinc (not more than 0.02% of copper), Chromatographic purity, and Organic volatile impurities.
Methylene Blue Injection USP—Preserve in single-dose containers, preferably of Type I glass. A sterile solution of Methylene Blue in Water for Injection. Contains, in each mL, not less than 9.5 mg and not more than 10.5 mg of methylene blue. Meets the requirements for Identification, Bacterial endotoxins, and pH (3.0–4.5), and for Injections.
Methylene Blue Tablets—Not in *USP–NF*.

METHYLENE CHLORIDE

Chemical name: Methane, dichloro-.

Molecular formula: CH_2Cl_2.

Molecular weight: 84.93.

Description: Methylene Chloride NF—Clear, colorless, mobile liquid, having an odor resembling that of chloroform.
NF category: Solvent.

Solubility: Methylene Chloride NF—Miscible with alcohol, with ether, and with fixed and volatile oils.

NF requirements: Methylene Chloride NF—Preserve in tight containers. Contains not less than 99.0% of methylene chloride. Meets the requirements for Identification, Specific gravity (1.318–1.322), Water (not more than 0.02%), Limit of hydrogen chloride (not more than 0.001%), Limit of nonvolatile residue (not more than 0.002%), Heavy metals (not more than 1 ppm), and Free chlorine.

Caution: Perform all steps involving evaporation of methylene chloride in a well-ventilated fume hood.

METHYLERGONOVINE

Chemical group: Semi-synthetic ergot alkaloid.

Chemical name: Methylergonovine maleate—Ergoline-8-carboxamide, 9,10-didehydro-*N*-[1-(hydroxymethyl)propyl]-6-methyl-, [8 beta(*S*)]-, (*Z*)-2-butenedioate (1:1) (salt).

Molecular formula: Methylergonovine maleate—$C_{20}H_{25}N_3O_2 \cdot C_4H_4O_4$.

Molecular weight: Methylergonovine maleate—455.50.

Description: Methylergonovine Maleate USP—White to pinkish tan, microcrystalline powder. Is odorless.

Solubility: Methylergonovine Maleate USP—Slightly soluble in water and in alcohol; very slightly soluble in chloroform and in ether.

USP requirements:

Methylergonovine Maleate USP—Preserve in tight, light-resistant containers, and store in a cold place. Contains not less than 97.0% and not more than 103.0% of methylergonovine maleate, calculated on the dried basis. Meets the requirements for Identification, Specific rotation (+44° to +50°), pH (4.4–5.2, in a solution [1 in 5000]), Loss on drying (not more than 2.0%), Residue on ignition (not more than 0.1%), and Related alkaloids.

Methylergonovine Maleate Injection USP—Preserve in single-dose, light-resistant containers, preferably of Type I glass. A sterile solution of Methylergonovine Maleate in Water for Injection. Contains, in each mL, the labeled amount, within ±10%. Meets the requirements for Identification, Bacterial endotoxins, pH (2.7–3.5), and Related alkaloids, and for Injections.

Methylergonovine Maleate Tablets USP—Preserve in tight, light-resistant containers. Contain the labeled amount, within ±10%. Meet the requirements for Identification, Dissolution (70% in 30 minutes in tartaric acid solution [1 in 200] in Apparatus 2 at 75 rpm), Uniformity of dosage units, and Related alkaloids.

METHYL ISOBUTYL KETONE

Chemical name: 2-Pentanone, 4-methyl-.

Molecular formula: $C_6H_{12}O$.

Molecular weight: 100.16.

Description: Methyl Isobutyl Ketone NF—Transparent, colorless, mobile, volatile liquid, having a faint ketonic and camphoraceous odor.

NF category: Alcohol denaturant; solvent.

Solubility: Methyl Isobutyl Ketone NF—Slightly soluble in water; miscible with alcohol and with ether.

NF requirements: Methyl Isobutyl Ketone NF—Preserve in tight containers. Contains not less than 99.0% of methyl isobutyl ketone. Meets the requirements for Identification, Specific gravity (not more than 0.799), Distilling range (114–117 °C), Acidity, and Limit of nonvolatile residue (not more than 0.008%).

METHYLPARABEN

Chemical name:
Methylparaben—Benzoic acid, 4-hydroxy-, methyl ester.
Methylparaben sodium—Benzoic acid, 4-hydroxy-, methyl ester, sodium salt.

Molecular formula:
Methylparaben—$C_8H_8O_3$.
Methylparaben sodium—$C_8H_7NaO_3$.

Molecular weight:
Methylparaben—152.15.
Methylparaben sodium—174.13.

Description:
Methylparaben NF—White, crystalline powder or colorless crystals.
NF category: Antimicrobial preservative.
Methylparaben Sodium NF—White, hygroscopic powder.
NF category: Antimicrobial preservative.

Solubility:
Methylparaben NF—Slightly soluble in water; freely soluble in alcohol and in methanol.
Methylparaben Sodium NF—Freely soluble in water; sparingly soluble in alcohol; insoluble in fixed oils.

NF requirements:
Methylparaben NF—Preserve in well-closed containers. Contains not less than 99.0% and not more than 100.5% of methylparaben. Meets the requirements for Identification, Color of solution, Melting range (125–128 °C), Acidity, Residue on ignition (not more than 0.1%), Chromatographic purity, and Organic volatile impurities.
Methylparaben Sodium NF—Preserve in tight containers. Contains not less than 98.5% and not more than 101.5% of methylparaben sodium. Meets the requirements for Completeness of solution, Identification, pH (9.5–10.5, in a solution [1 in 1000]), Water (not more than 5.0%), Chloride (not more than 0.035%), Sulfate (not more than 0.12%), and Organic volatile impurities.

METHYLPHENIDATE

Chemical name: Methylphenidate hydrochloride—2-Piperidineacetic acid, alpha-phenyl-, methyl ester, hydrochloride, (*R*,R**)-(±)-.

Molecular formula: Methylphenidate hydrochloride—$C_{14}H_{19}NO_2 \cdot HCl$.

Molecular weight: Methylphenidate hydrochloride—269.77.

Description: Methylphenidate Hydrochloride USP—White, odorless, fine, crystalline powder. Its solutions are acid to litmus.

Solubility: Methylphenidate Hydrochloride USP—Freely soluble in water and in methanol; soluble in alcohol; slightly soluble in chloroform and in acetone.

USP requirements:

Methylphenidate Hydrochloride USP—Preserve in well-closed containers. Contains not less than 98.0% and not more than 100.5% of methylphenidate hydrochloride, calculated on the dried basis. Meets the requirements for Identification, Loss on drying (not more than 0.5%), Residue on ignition (not more than 0.1%), Heavy metals (not

more than 0.001%), Limit of erythro [(*R**,*S**)] isomer, Limit of alpha-phenyl-2-piperidineacetic acid hydrochloride, and Organic volatile impurities.

Methylphenidate Hydrochloride Tablets USP—Preserve in tight containers. Contain the labeled amount, within ± 7%. Meet the requirements for Identification, Dissolution (75% in 45 minutes in water in Apparatus 1 at 100 rpm), and Uniformity of dosage units.

Methylphenidate Hydrochloride Extended-release Tablets USP—Preserve in tight containers. Contain the labeled amount, within ±10%. Meet the requirements for Identification, Drug release (25 to 45% in 1 hour, 40 to 65% in 2 hours, 55 to 80% in 3.5 hours, 70 to 90% in 5 hours, not less than 80% in 7 hours, in water in Apparatus 2 at 50 rpm), and Uniformity of dosage units.

METHYLPREDNISOLONE

Chemical name:

Methylprednisolone—Pregna-1,4-diene-3,20-dione, 11,17,21-trihydroxy-6-methyl-, (6 alpha,11 beta)-.

Methylprednisolone acetate—Pregna-1,4-diene-3,20-dione, 21-(acetyloxy)-11,17-dihydroxy-6-methyl-, (6 alpha,11 beta)-.

Methylprednisolone hemisuccinate—Pregna-1,4-diene-3,20-dione, 21-(3-carboxy-1-oxopropoxy)-11,17-dihydroxy-6-methyl-, (6 alpha,11 beta)-.

Methylprednisolone sodium succinate—Pregna-1,4-diene-3,20-dione, 21-(3-carboxy-1-oxopropoxy)-11,17-dihydroxy-6-methyl-, monosodium salt, (6 alpha,11 beta)-.

Molecular formula:

Methylprednisolone—$C_{22}H_{30}O_5$.
Methylprednisolone acetate—$C_{24}H_{32}O_6$.
Methylprednisolone hemisuccinate—$C_{26}H_{34}O_8$.
Methylprednisolone sodium succinate—$C_{26}H_{33}NaO_8$.

Molecular weight:

Methylprednisolone—374.47.
Methylprednisolone acetate—416.51.
Methylprednisolone hemisuccinate—474.54.
Methylprednisolone sodium succinate—496.53.

Description:

Methylprednisolone USP—White to practically white, odorless, crystalline powder. Melts at about 240 °C, with some decomposition.

Methylprednisolone Acetate USP—White or practically white, odorless, crystalline powder. Melts at about 225 °C, with some decomposition.

Methylprednisolone Hemisuccinate USP—White or nearly white, odorless or nearly odorless, hygroscopic solid.

Methylprednisolone Sodium Succinate USP—White or nearly white, odorless, hygroscopic, amorphous solid.

Solubility:

Methylprednisolone USP—Practically insoluble in water; sparingly soluble in alcohol, in dioxane, and in methanol; slightly soluble in acetone and in chloroform; very slightly soluble in ether.

Methylprednisolone Acetate USP—Practically insoluble in water; soluble in dioxane; sparingly soluble in acetone, in alcohol, in chloroform, and in methanol; slightly soluble in ether.

Methylprednisolone Hemisuccinate USP—Very slightly soluble in water; freely soluble in alcohol; soluble in acetone.

Methylprednisolone Sodium Succinate USP—Very soluble in water and in alcohol; very slightly soluble in acetone; insoluble in chloroform.

USP requirements:

Methylprednisolone USP—Preserve in tight, light-resistant containers. Contains not less than 97.0% and not more than 103.0% of methylprednisolone, calculated on the dried basis. Meets the requirements for Identification, Specific rotation (+79° to +86°), Loss on drying (not more than 1.0%), Residue on ignition (not more than 0.2%), Chromatographic purity (not more than 1.0% of any individual impurity, and not more than 2.0% of total impurities), and Other impurities.

Methylprednisolone Tablets USP—Preserve in tight containers. Contain the labeled amount, within ±7.5%. Meet the requirements for Identification, Dissolution (70% in 30 minutes in water in Apparatus 2 at 50 rpm), and Uniformity of dosage units.

Methylprednisolone Acetate USP—Preserve in tight, light-resistant containers. Contains not less than 97.0% and not more than 103.0% of methylprednisolone acetate, calculated on the dried basis. Meets the requirements for Identification, Specific rotation (+97° to +105°), Loss on drying (not more than 1.0%), Residue on ignition (not more than 0.2%), Chromatographic purity (not more than 1.0% of any individual impurity is found, and not more than 2.0% of total impurities is found), and Other impurities.

Methylprednisolone Acetate Cream USP—Preserve in collapsible tubes or in tight containers, protected from light. Contains the labeled amount, within ±10%. Meets the requirements for Identification and Minimum fill.

Methylprednisolone Acetate Injectable Suspension USP—Preserve in single-dose or in multiple-dose containers, preferably of Type I glass. A sterile suspension of Methylprednisolone Acetate in a suitable aqueous medium. Contains the labeled amount, within ±10%. Meets the requirements for Identification, Uniformity of dosage units, pH (3.0–7.0), and Particle size (not less than 99% are less than 20 micrometers in length [measured on longest axis] and not less than 75% are less than 10 micrometers in length, using 400x magnification), and for Injections.

Methylprednisolone Hemisuccinate USP—Preserve in tight containers. Contains not less than 97.0% and not more than 103.0% of methylprednisolone hemisuccinate, calculated on the dried basis. Meets the requirements for Identification, Specific rotation (+87° to +95°), Loss on drying (not more than 1.0%), Residue on ignition (not more than 0.2%), Chromatographic purity, and Other impurities.

Methylprednisolone Sodium Succinate USP—Preserve in tight, light-resistant containers. Contains not less than 97.0% and not more than 103.0% of methylprednisolone sodium succinate, calculated on the dried basis. Meets the requirements for Identification, Specific rotation (+96° to +104°), Loss on drying (not more than 3.0%), and Sodium content (4.49–4.77%, calculated on the dried basis).

Methylprednisolone Sodium Succinate for Injection USP—Preserve in Containers for Sterile Solids. A sterile mixture of Methylprednisolone Sodium Succinate with suitable buffers. May be prepared from Methylprednisolone Sodium Succinate or from Methylprednisolone Hemisuccinate with the aid of Sodium Hydroxide or Sodium Carbonate. Contains an amount of methylprednisolone sodium succinate equivalent to the labeled amount of methylprednisolone, within ±10%, in the volume of constituted solution designated on the label. Meets the requirements for Constituted solution, Identification, Bacterial endotoxins, pH (7.0–8.0, in a solution containing about 50 mg of methylprednisolone sodium succinate per mL), Loss on drying (not more than 2.0%), Particulate matter, and Free methylprednisolone (not more than 6.6% of labeled amount of methylprednisolone), and for Sterility tests, Uniformity of dosage units, and Labeling under Injections.

METHYL SALICYLATE

Chemical name: Benzoic acid, 2-hydroxy-, methyl ester.

Molecular formula: $C_8H_8O_3$.

Molecular weight: 152.15.

Description: Methyl Salicylate NF—Colorless, yellowish, or reddish liquid, having the characteristic odor of wintergreen. It boils between 219 and 224 °C, with some decomposition. NF category: Flavors and perfumes.

Solubility: Methyl Salicylate NF—Slightly soluble in water; soluble in alcohol and in glacial acetic acid.

NF requirements: Methyl Salicylate NF—Preserve in tight containers. It is produced synthetically or is obtained by maceration and subsequent distillation with steam from the leaves of *Gaultheria procumbens* Linné (Fam. Ericaceae) or from the bark of *Betula lenta* Linné (Fam. Betulaceae). Label it to indicate whether it was made synthetically or distilled from either of the plants mentioned above. Contains not less than 98.0% and not more than 100.5% of methyl salicylate. Meets the requirements for Solubility in 70% alcohol (if it is synthetic, one volume dissolves in 7 volumes of 70% alcohol; if it is natural, one volume dissolves in 7 volumes of 70% alcohol, the solution having not more than a slight cloudiness), Identification, Specific gravity (for the synthetic, 1.180–1.185; for the natural, 1.176–1.182), Angular rotation, Refractive index (1.535–1.538 at 20 °C), Heavy metals (not more than 20 mcg per gram), and Organic volatile impurities.

METHYLTESTOSTERONE

Chemical group: Synthetic derivative of testosterone.

Chemical name: Androst-4-en-3-one, 17-hydroxy-17-methyl-, (17 beta)-.

Molecular formula: $C_{20}H_{30}O_2$.

Molecular weight: 302.45.

Description: Methyltestosterone USP—White or creamy white crystals or crystalline powder. Is odorless and is stable in air, but is slightly hygroscopic. Is affected by light.

Solubility: Methyltestosterone USP—Practically insoluble in water; soluble in alcohol, in methanol, in ether, and in other organic solvents; sparingly soluble in vegetable oils.

USP requirements:
Methyltestosterone USP—Preserve in well-closed, light-resistant containers. Contains not less than 97.0% and not more than 103.0% of methyltestosterone, calculated on the dried basis. Meets the requirements for Identification, Melting range (162–167 °C), Specific rotation (+79° to +85°), Loss on drying (not more than 2.0%), Organic volatile impurities, Chromatographic purity, and Other impurities.
Methyltestosterone Capsules USP—Preserve in well-closed containers. Contain the labeled amount, within ±10%. Meet the requirements for Identification, Dissolution (70% in 45 minutes in water in Apparatus 1 at 100 rpm), and Uniformity of dosage units.
Methyltestosterone Tablets USP—Preserve in well-closed containers. Contain the labeled amount, within ±10%. Meet the requirements for Identification, Disintegration (30 minutes. Tablets intended for buccal administration meet the requirements for Buccal Tablets), and Uniformity of dosage units.

METHYPRYLON

Chemical name: 2,4-Piperidinedione, 3,3-diethyl-5-methyl-.

Molecular formula: $C_{10}H_{17}NO_2$.

Molecular weight: 183.25.

Description: White, or practically white, crystalline powder, having a slight, characteristic odor.

Solubility: Soluble in water; freely soluble in alcohol, in chloroform, and in ether.

USP requirements:
Methyprylon Capsules—Not in *USP–NF*.
Methyprylon Tablets—Not in *USP–NF*.

METHYSERGIDE

Chemical name: Methysergide maleate—Ergoline-8-carboxamide, 9,10-didehydro-*N*-[1-(hydroxymethyl)propyl]-1,6-dimethyl-, (8 beta)-, (*Z*)-2-butenedioate (1:1) (salt).

Molecular formula: Methysergide maleate—$C_{21}H_{27}N_3O_2 \cdot C_4H_4O_4$.

Molecular weight: Methysergide maleate—469.53.

Description: Methysergide Maleate USP—White to yellowish white or reddish white, crystalline powder. Is odorless or has not more than a slight odor.

Solubility: Methysergide Maleate USP—Slightly soluble in water and in alcohol; very slightly soluble in chloroform; practically insoluble in ether.

USP requirements:
Methysergide Maleate USP—Preserve in tight, light-resistant containers, in a cold place. Contains not less than 97.0% and not more than 103.0% of methysergide maleate, calculated on the dried basis. Meets the requirements for Identification, Specific rotation (+35° to +45°), pH (3.7–4.7, in a 1 in 500 solution in carbon dioxide-free water), Loss on drying (not more than 7.0%), and Ordinary impurities.
Methysergide Maleate Tablets USP—Preserve in tight containers. Contain the labeled amount, within ±10%. Meet the requirements for Identification, Dissolution (70% in 30 minutes in tartaric acid solution [1 in 200] in Apparatus 2 at 100 rpm), and Uniformity of dosage units.

METIPRANOLOL

Chemical name: Metipranolol hydrochloride—Phenol, (±)-4-[2-hydroxy-3-[(1-methylethyl)amino]propoxy]-2,3,6-trimethyl-,1-acetate, hydrochloride.

Molecular formula: Metipranolol hydrochloride—$C_{17}H_{27}NO_4 \cdot$ HCl.

Molecular weight: Metipranolol hydrochloride—345.86.

Description: White, odorless, crystalline powder.

Solubility: Metipranolol hydrochloride—Soluble in water.

USP requirements: Metipranolol Hydrochloride Ophthalmic Solution—Not in *USP–NF*.

METOCLOPRAMIDE

Source: p-Aminobenzoic acid derivative, structurally related to procainamide.

Chemical name: Metoclopramide hydrochloride—Benzamide, 4-amino-5-chloro-N-[2-(diethylamino)ethyl]-2-methoxy-, monohydrochloride, monohydrate.

Molecular formula: Metoclopramide hydrochloride—$C_{14}H_{22}ClN_3O_2 \cdot HCl \cdot H_2O$.

Molecular weight: Metoclopramide hydrochloride—354.27.

Description: Metoclopramide Hydrochloride USP—White or practically white, crystalline, odorless or practically odorless powder.

pKa: Metoclopramide hydrochloride—0.6 and 9.3.

Solubility: Metoclopramide Hydrochloride USP—Very soluble in water; freely soluble in alcohol; sparingly soluble in chloroform; practically insoluble in ether.

USP requirements:

Metoclopramide Injection USP—Preserve in single-dose or in multiple-dose containers, preferably of Type I glass, protected from light. (Note: Injection containing an antioxidant agent does not require protection from light.) A sterile solution of Metoclopramide Hydrochloride in Water for Injection. Contains the labeled amount, within ±10%. Meets the requirements for Identification, Bacterial endotoxins, pH (2.5–6.5), and Particulate matter, and for Injections.

Metoclopramide Oral Solution USP—Store in tight, light-resistant containers at controlled room temperature. Protect from freezing. Contains an amount of Metoclopramide Hydrochloride equivalent to the labeled amount of metoclopramide, within ±10%. Meets the requirements for Identification and pH (2.0–5.5).

Metoclopramide Tablets USP—Preserve in tight, light-resistant containers. Contain an amount of metoclopramide hydrochloride equivalent to the labeled amount of metoclopramide, within ±10%. Meet the requirements for Identification, Dissolution (75% in 30 minutes in water in Apparatus 1 at 50 rpm), and Uniformity of dosage units.

Metoclopramide Hydrochloride USP—Preserve in tight, light-resistant containers. Contains not less than 98.0% and not more than 101.0% of metoclopramide hydrochloride, calculated on the anhydrous basis. Meets the requirements for Identification, Water (4.5–6.0%), Residue on ignition (not more than 0.1%), Chromatographic purity, and Organic volatile impurities.

Metoclopramide Hydrochloride Oral Solution (Concentrate)—Not in USP–NF.

Metoclopramide Hydrochloride Tablets—Not in USP–NF.

METOCURINE

Chemical name: Metocurine iodide—Tubocuraranium, 6,6',7',12'-tetramethoxy-2,2,2',2'-tetramethyl-, diiodide.

Molecular formula: Metocurine iodide—$C_{40}H_{48}I_2N_2O_6$.

Molecular weight: Metocurine iodide—906.63.

Description: Metocurine Iodide USP—White or pale yellow, crystalline powder.

Solubility: Metocurine Iodide USP—Slightly soluble in water, in 3 N hydrochloric acid, and in dilute solutions of sodium hydroxide; very slightly soluble in alcohol; practically insoluble in chloroform and in ether.

USP requirements:

Metocurine Iodide USP—Preserve in tight containers. Contains not less than 95.0% and not more than 105.0% of metocurine iodide, calculated on the anhydrous basis.

Meets the requirements for Identification, Specific rotation (+148° to +158°), Water (not more than 7.0%), and Related compounds.

Caution: Handle Metocurine Iodide with exceptional care since it is a highly potent skeletal muscle relaxant.

Metocurine Iodide Injection USP—Preserve in single-dose or in multiple-dose containers, preferably of Type I glass. Phenol, 0.5%, or some other suitable bacteriostatic substance, is added to the Injection in multiple-dose containers. A sterile solution of Metocurine Iodide in isotonic sodium chloride solution. Contains the labeled amount, within ±7%. Meets the requirements for Identification and Bacterial endotoxins, and for Injections.

METOLAZONE

Chemical name: 6-Quinazolinesulfonamide, 7-chloro-1,2,3,4-tetrahydro-2-methyl-3-(2-methylphenyl)-4-oxo.

Molecular formula: $C_{16}H_{16}ClN_3O_3S$.

Molecular weight: 365.84.

Description: Colorless, odorless crystalline powder; is light-sensitive. Melts between 253–259 °C.

pKa: 9.72.

Solubility: Sparingly soluble in water; more soluble in plasma, in blood, in alkali, and in organic solvents.

USP requirements:

Metolazone USP—Preserve in tight, light-resistant containers. Contains not less than 97.0% and not more than 102.0% of metolazone, calculated on the dried basis. Meets the requirements for Identification, Loss on drying (not more than 1.0%), Residue on ignition (not more than 0.1%), Heavy metals (not more than 0.0015%), and Chromatographic purity.

Metolazone Tablets USP—Preserve in tight, light-resistant containers. Contain the labeled amount, within ±10%. Meet the requirements for Identification and Uniformity of dosage units.

Extended Metolazone Tablets—Not in USP–NF.

Prompt Metolazone Tablets—Not in USP–NF.

METOPROLOL

Chemical name:

Metoprolol fumarate—2-Propanol, 1-[4-(2-methoxyethyl)phenoxy]-3-[(1-methylethyl)amino]-, (±)-, (E)-2-butanedioate (2:1) (salt).

Metoprolol succinate—2-Propanol, 1-[4-(2-methoxyethyl)phenoxy]-3-[(1-methylethyl)amino]-, (±)-, butanedioate (2:1) (salt).

Metoprolol tartrate—2-Propanol, 1-[4-(2-methoxyethyl)phenoxy]-3-[(1-methylethyl)amino]-, (±)-, [R-(R*,R*)]-2,3-dihydroxybutanedioate (2:1) (salt).

Molecular formula:

Metoprolol fumarate—$(C_{15}H_{25}NO_3)_2 \cdot C_4H_4O_4$.

Metoprolol succinate—$(C_{15}H_{25}NO_3)_2 \cdot C_4H_6O_4$.

Metoprolol tartrate—$(C_{15}H_{25}NO_3)_2 \cdot C_4H_6O_6$.

Molecular weight:

Metoprolol fumarate—650.80.

Metoprolol succinate—652.82.

Metoprolol tartrate—684.81.

Description:

Metoprolol Succinate USP—White to off-white powder.

Metoprolol Tartrate USP—White, crystalline powder.

pKa: Metoprolol tartrate—9.68.

Solubility:
Metoprolol Succinate USP—Freely soluble in water; soluble in methanol; sparingly soluble in alcohol; slightly soluble in isopropyl alcohol.
Metoprolol Tartrate USP—Very soluble in water; freely soluble in methylene chloride, in chloroform, and in alcohol; slightly soluble in acetone; insoluble in ether.

Other characteristics: Lipid solubility—Moderate.

USP requirements:
Metoprolol Fumarate USP—Preserve in tight, light-resistant containers. Contains not less than 99.0% and not more than 100.5% of metoprolol fumarate, calculated on the dried basis. Meets the requirements for Identification, Melting range (145–148 °C), pH (5.5–6.5, in a solution [1 in 10]), Loss on drying (not more than 0.5%), Residue on ignition (not more than 0.1%), Heavy metals (not more than 0.001%), Organic volatile impurities, and Chromatographic purity.
Metoprolol Succinate USP—Preserve in tight containers at controlled room temperature. Contains not less than 98.0% and not more than 102.0% of metoprolol succinate, calculated on the dried basis. Meets the requirements for Clarity and color of solution, Identification, pH (7.0–7.6, in a solution containing 65 mg per mL), Loss on drying (not more than 0.2%), Residue in ignition (not more than 0.1%), Heavy metals (not more than 0.001%), and Related compound.
Metoprolol Succinate Extended-release Tablets USP—Preserve in tight containers at controlled room temperature. Store at a temperature between 15–30 °C. Label it to indicate the content of metoprolol succinate and its equivalent, expressed as metoprolol tartrate. Contain the labeled amount, within ±10%. Meet the requirements for Identification, Drug release (not more than 25% in one hour, 20–40% in 4 hours, 40–60% in 8 hours, and not less than 80% in 20 hours in phosphate buffer [pH 6.8] in Apparatus 2 at 50 rpm, and Uniformity of dosage units.
Metoprolol Tartrate USP—Preserve in tight, light-resistant containers. Contains not less than 99.0% and not more than 101.0% of metoprolol tartrate, calculated on the dried basis. Meets the requirements for Identification, Specific rotation (+6.5° to +10.5°), pH (6.0–7.0, in a solution [1 in 10]), Loss on drying (not more than 0.5%), Residue on ignition (not more than 0.1%), Heavy metals (not more than 0.001%), Chromatographic purity, and Organic volatile impurities.
Metoprolol Tartrate Injection USP—Preserve in single-dose, light-resistant containers, preferably of Type I or Type II glass. A sterile solution of Metoprolol Tartrate in Water for Injection. Contains Sodium Chloride as a tonicity-adjusting agent. Contains the labeled amount, within ±10%. Meets the requirements for Identification, Bacterial endotoxins, Sterility, and pH (5.0–8.0), and for Injections.
Metoprolol Tartrate Tablets USP—Preserve in tight, light-resistant containers. Contain the labeled amount, within ±10%. Meet the requirements for Identification, Dissolution (75% in 30 minutes in simulated gastric fluid TS [without enzyme] in Apparatus 1 at 100 rpm), and Uniformity of dosage units.
Metoprolol Tartrate Extended-release Tablets—Not in *USP–NF.*

METOPROLOL AND HYDROCHLOROTHIAZIDE

For *Metoprolol* and *Hydrochlorothiazide*—See individual listings for chemistry information.

USP requirements: Metoprolol Tartrate and Hydrochlorothiazide Tablets USP—Preserve in tight, light-resistant containers. Contain the labeled amounts, within ±10%. Meet the requirements for Identification, Dissolution (80% of each active ingredient in 30 minutes in simulated gastric fluid TS [without enzyme] in Apparatus 1 at 100 rpm), Uniformity of dosage units, and Diazotizable substances (not more than 1.0%).

METRIFONATE

Chemical name: Phosphonic acid, (2,2,2-trichloro-1-hydroxyethyl)phosphonate.

Molecular formula: $C_4H_8Cl_3O_4P$.

Molecular weight: 257.44.

USP requirements: Metrifonate USP—Preserve in well-closed containers at a temperature not exceeding 25 °C. Metrifonate itended for veterinary use only is so labeled. Contains not less than 98.0% and not more than 100.5% of metrifonate, calculated on the anhydrous basis. Meets the requirements for Completeness of solution, Color of solution, Identification, Acidity, Water (not more than 0.3%), Heavy metals (not more than 0.001%), Limit of free chloride (0.05%), and Chromatographic purity.

METRIZAMIDE

Chemical group: Non-ionic, monomeric, triiodinated benzoic acid derivative.

Chemical name: D-Glucose, 2-[[3-(acetylamino)-5-(acetylmethylamino)-2,4,6-triiodobenzoyl]amino]-2-deoxy-.

Molecular formula: $C_{18}H_{22}I_3N_3O_8$.

Molecular weight: 789.10.

Description: White crystals.

Solubility: Very soluble in water (50% w/v) at room temperature.

Other characteristics: Low osmolality. The osmolality of metrizamide injection with iodine concentrations of 200 and 300 mg per mL is 340 and 484 mOsmol per kg of water, respectively.

USP requirements: Metrizamide for Injection—Not in *USP–NF.*

METRONIDAZOLE

Chemical group: Nitroimidazoles.

Chemical name:
Metronidazole—1*H*-Imidazole-1-ethanol, 2-methyl-5-nitro-.
Metronidazole hydrochloride—1*H*-Imidazole-1-ethanol, 2-methyl-5-nitro-, hydrochloride.

Molecular formula:
Metronidazole—$C_6H_9N_3O_3$.
Metronidazole hydrochloride—$C_6H_9N_3O_3 \cdot$ HCl.

Molecular weight:
Metronidazole—171.15.
Metronidazole hydrochloride—207.61.

Description: Metronidazole USP—White to pale yellow, odorless crystals or crystalline powder. Is stable in air, but darkens on exposure to light.

Solubility: Metronidazole USP—Sparingly soluble in water and in alcohol; slightly soluble in ether and in chloroform.

USP requirements:

Metronidazole USP—Preserve in well-closed, light-resistant containers. Contains not less than 99.0% and not more than 101.0% of metronidazole, calculated on the dried basis. Meets the requirements for Identification, Melting range (159–163 °C), Loss on drying (not more than 0.5%), Residue on ignition (not more than 0.1%), Heavy metals (not more than 0.005%), Non-basic substances, and Chromatographic purity.

Metronidazole Capsules—Not in *USP–NF*.

Metronidazole Cream—Not in *USP–NF*.

Metronidazole Vaginal Cream—Not in *USP–NF*.

Metronidazole Gel USP—Preserve in laminated collapsible tubes at controlled room temperature. Contains the labeled amount, within ±10%. Meets the requirements for Identification, Minimum fill, and pH (4.0–6.5, determined potentiometrically).

Metronidazole Topical Gel—Not in *USP–NF*.

Metronidazole Vaginal Gel—Not in *USP–NF*.

Metronidazole Injection USP—Preserve in single-dose containers of Type I or Type II glass, or in suitable plastic containers, protected from light. A sterile, isotonic, buffered solution of Metronidazole in Water for Injection. Contains the labeled amount, within ±10%. Meets the requirements for Identification, Bacterial endotoxins, pH (4.5–7.0), and Particulate matter, and for Injections.

Metronidazole Vaginal Inserts—Not in *USP–NF*.

Metronidazole Topical Lotion—Not in *USP–NF*.

Metronidazole Tablets USP—Preserve in well-closed, light-resistant containers. Contain the labeled amount, within ± 10%. Meet the requirements for Identification, Dissolution (85% in 60 minutes in 0.1 *N* hydrochloric acid in Apparatus 1 at 100 rpm), and Uniformity of dosage units.

Metronidazole Extended-release Tablets—Not in *USP–NF*.

Metronidazole Vaginal Tablets—Not in *USP–NF*.

Metronidazole Hydrochloride for Injection—Not in *USP–NF*.

METRONIDAZOLE AND NYSTATIN

For *Metronidazole* and *Nystatin*—See individual listings for chemistry information.

USP requirements:

Metronidazole and Nystatin Vaginal Cream—Not in *USP–NF*.

Metronidazole and Nystatin Vaginal Suppositories—Not in *USP–NF*.

Metronidazole and Nystatin Vaginal Tablets—Not in *USP–NF*.

METYRAPONE

Chemical name: 1-Propanone, 2-methyl-1,2-di-3-pyridinyl-.

Molecular formula: $C_{14}H_{14}N_2O$.

Molecular weight: 226.27.

Description: Metyrapone USP—White to light amber, fine, crystalline powder, having a characteristic odor. Darkens on exposure to light.

Solubility: Metyrapone USP—Sparingly soluble in water; soluble in methanol and in chloroform. It forms water-soluble salts with acids.

USP requirements:

Metyrapone USP—Preserve in tight containers, protected from heat and light. Contains not less than 98.0% and not more than 102.0% of metyrapone, calculated on the dried basis. Meets the requirements for Identification, Loss

on drying (not more than 0.5%), Heavy metals (not more than 0.001%), Residue on ignition (not more than 0.1%), and Chromatographic purity.

Metyrapone Tablets USP—Preserve in tight, light-resistant containers, and avoid exposure to excessive heat. Contain the labeled amount, within ±5%. Meet the requirements for Identification, Dissolution (60% in 45 minutes in 0.1 *N* hydrochloric acid in Apparatus 1 at 100 rpm), and Uniformity of dosage units.

METYROSINE

Chemical name: L-Tyrosine, alpha-methyl-, (–)-.

Molecular formula: $C_{10}H_{13}NO_3$.

Molecular weight: 195.22.

Description: White, crystalline compound.

pKa: 2.7 and 10.1.

Solubility: Very slightly soluble in water, in acetone, and in methanol; soluble in acidic aqueous solutions; soluble in alkaline aqueous solutions, but is subject to oxidative degradation in them; insoluble in chloroform.

USP requirements:

Metyrosine USP—Preserve in well-closed containers. Contains not less than 98.6% and not more than 101.0% of metyrosine, calculated on the dried basis. Meets the requirements for Identification, Specific rotation (+185° to +195°), Loss on drying (not more than 1.0%), Residue on ignition (not more than 0.1%), Heavy metals (not more than 0.003%), Chromatographic purity, and Organic volatile impurities.

Metyrosine Capsules USP—Preserve in well-closed containers. Contain the labeled amount, within ±10%. Meet the requirements for Identification, Dissolution (75% in 60 minutes in 0.1 *N* hydrochloric acid in Apparatus 1 at 100 rpm), and Uniformity of dosage units.

MEXILETINE

Chemical name: Mexiletine hydrochloride—2-Propanamine, 1-(2,6-dimethylphenoxy)-, hydrochloride.

Molecular formula: Mexiletine hydrochloride—$C_{11}H_{17}NO \cdot HCl$.

Molecular weight: Mexiletine hydrochloride—215.72.

Description: Mexiletine Hydrochloride USP—White powder.

pKa: 9.2.

Solubility: Mexiletine Hydrochloride USP—Freely soluble in dehydrated alcohol and in water; slightly soluble in acetonitrile; practically insoluble in ether. Optically inactive (1 in 20 solution in water).

USP requirements:

Mexiletine Hydrochloride USP—Preserve in tight containers. Contains not less than 98.0% and not more than 102.0% of mexiletine hydrochloride, calculated on the dried basis. Meets the requirements for Identification, pH (3.5–5.5, in a solution [1 in 10]), Loss on drying (not more than 0.5%), Residue on ignition (not more than 0.1%), Heavy metals (not more than 0.001%), Chromatographic purity, and Organic volatile impurities.

Mexiletine Hydrochloride Capsules USP—Preserve in tight
containers. Contain the labeled amount, within ±10%.
Meet the requirements for Identification, Dissolution
(80% in 30 minutes in water in Apparatus 2 at 50 rpm), Uniformity of dosage units, and Chromatographic purity.

MEZLOCILLIN

Chemical name: Mezlocillin sodium—4-Thia-1-azabicy-
clo[3.2.0]heptane-2-carboxylic acid, 3,3-dimethyl-6-[[[[[3-
(methylsulfonyl)-2-oxo-1-imidazolidinyl]carbonyl]amino]phe-
nylacetyl]amino]-7-oxo-, monosodium salt, [2S[2 alpha,5 alpha,6 beta(S*)]]-.

Molecular formula: Mezlocillin sodium—$C_{21}H_{24}NaN_5O_8S_2$.

Molecular weight: Mezlocillin sodium—561.57.

Description: Mezlocillin Sodium USP—White to pale yellow,
crystalline powder.

Solubility: Mezlocillin Sodium USP—Freely soluble in water.

USP requirements:
Mezlocillin Sodium USP—Preserve in tight containers. Where
it is intended for use in preparing injectable dosage forms,
the label states that it is sterile or must be subjected to
further processing during the preparation of injectable dosage forms. Contains the equivalent of not less than 838
micrograms and not more than 978 micrograms of mezlocillin per mg, calculated on the anhydrous basis. Meets the
requirements for Identification, Specific rotation (175°–
195°), pH (4.5–8.0, in a solution [1 in 10]), Water (not more
than 6.0%), and for Sterility and Bacterial endotoxins under Mezlocillin for Injection (where the label states that Mezlocillin Sodium is sterile), and for Bacterial endotoxins
under Mezlocillin for Injection (where the label states that
Mezlocillin Sodium must be subjected to further processing during the preparation of injectable dosage forms).
Mezlocillin Sodium for Injection USP—Preserve in Containers
for Sterile Solids. Contains an amount of mezlocillin sodium equivalent to the labeled amount of mezlocillin, within −10% to +15%. Meets the requirements for Constituted
solution, Bacterial endotoxins, Sterility, and Particulate
matter, for Identification tests, and for Specific rotation,
pH, and Water under Mezlocillin Sodium, and for Uniformity of dosage units and Labeling under Injections.

MIBEFRADIL

Chemical name: Mibefradil dihydrochloride—Acetic acid, me-
thoxy-, 2-[2-[[3-(1H-benzimidazol-2-yl)propyl]methylami-
no]ethyl]-6-fluoro-1,2,3,4-tetrahydro-1-(1-methylethyl)-2-
naphthalenyl ester, dihydrochloride, (1S-cis)-.

Molecular formula: Mibefradil dihydrochloride—$C_{29}H_{38}FN_3O_3 \cdot$
2HCl.

Molecular weight: Mibefradil dihydrochloride—568.55.

Description: Mibefradil dihydrochloride—Odorless, white to off-
white crystalline powder.

pKa: Mibefradil dihydrochloride—4.8; 5.5.

Solubility: Mibefradil dihydrochloride—Readily soluble in water.

USP requirements: Mibefradil Dihydrochloride Tablets—Not in
USP–NF.

MIBOLERONE

Chemical name: Ester-4-en-3-one, 17-hydroxy-7, 17-dimethyl-,
(7 alpha,17 beta)-.

Molecular formula: $C_{20}H_{30}O_2$.

Molecular weight: 302.45.

USP requirements:
Mibolerone USP—Preserve in well-closed containers. Label it
to indicate that it is for veterinary use only. Contains not
less than 96.0% and not more than 106.0% of mibolerone,
calculated on the dried basis. Meets the requirements for
Identification, Specific rotation (+34° to +40°), Loss on
drying (not more than 0.5%), and Residue on ignition
(not more than 0.5%).
Mibolerone Oral Solution—Preserve in tight containers, protected from light. Label it to indicate that it is for veterinary
use only. Contains the labeled amount of mibolerone,
within −10% to +15%. Meets the requirements for Identification and Specific gravity (1.030–1.045).

MICONAZOLE

Chemical group: Imidazoles.

Chemical name:
Miconazole—1H-Imidazole, 1-[2-(2,4-dichlorophenyl)-2-[(2,4-
dichlorophenyl)methoxy]ethyl]-.
Miconazole nitrate—1H-Imidazole, 1-[2-(2,4-dichlorophenyl)-
2-[(2,4-dichlorophenyl)methoxy]ethyl]-, mononitrate.

Molecular formula:
Miconazole—$C_{18}H_{14}Cl_4N_2O$.
Miconazole nitrate—$C_{18}H_{14}Cl_4N_2O \cdot HNO_3$.

Molecular weight:
Miconazole—416.13.
Miconazole nitrate—479.14.

Description:
Miconazole USP—White to pale cream powder. Melts in the
range of 78 °C to 88 °C. May exhibit polymorphism.
Miconazole Nitrate USP—White or practically white, crystalline powder, having not more than a slight odor. Melts in
the range of 178 °C to 183 °C, with decomposition.

Solubility:
Miconazole USP—Insoluble in water; soluble in ether; freely
soluble in alcohol, in methanol, in isopropyl alcohol, in
acetone, in propylene glycol, in chloroform, and in dimethylformamide.
Miconazole Nitrate USP—Insoluble in ether; very slightly soluble in water and in isopropyl alcohol; slightly soluble in
alcohol, in chloroform, and in propylene glycol; sparingly
soluble in methanol; soluble in dimethylformamide; freely
soluble in dimethyl sulfoxide.

USP requirements:
Miconazole USP—Preserve in well-closed containers, protected from light. Contains not less than 98.0% and not
more than 102.0% of miconazole, calculated on the dried
basis. Meets the requirements for Identification, Loss on
drying (not more than 0.5%), Residue on ignition (not more
than 0.2%), and Chromatographic purity.
Miconazole Injection USP—Preserve in single-dose containers, preferably of Type I glass, at controlled room temperature. A sterile solution of Miconazole in Water for Injection.
Contains the labeled amount, within ±10%. Meets the requirements for Identification, Bacterial endotoxins, pH
(3.7–5.7), and Particulate matter, and for Injections.
Miconazole Nitrate USP—Preserve in well-closed containers,
protected from light. Contains not less than 98.0% and not
more than 102.0% of miconazole nitrate, calculated on the

dried basis. Meets the requirements for Identification, Loss
on drying (not more than 0.5%), Residue on ignition (not
more than 0.2%), and Related compounds (0.5%).
Miconazole Nitrate Topical Aerosol Powder—Not in *USP–NF*.
Miconazole Nitrate Topical Aerosol Solution—Not in *USP–NF*.
Miconazole Nitrate Cream USP—Preserve in collapsible
tubes or in tight containers. Cream that is packaged and
labeled for use as a vaginal preparation shall be labeled
Miconazole Nitrate Vaginal Cream. Contains the labeled
amount, within ±10%. Meets the requirements for Identification and Minimum fill.
Miconazole Nitrate Vaginal Cream—Not in *USP–NF*.
Miconazole Nitrate Lotion—Not in *USP–NF*.
Miconazole Nitrate Topical Powder USP—Preserve in well-
closed containers. Contains the labeled amount, within
±10%. Meets the requirements for Identification, Microbial
limits, and Minimum fill.
Miconazole Nitrate Vaginal Suppositories USP—Preserve in
tight containers, at controlled room temperature. Contain
the labeled amount, within ±10%. Meet the requirement
for Identification.
Miconazole Nitrate Vaginal Tampons—Not in *USP–NF*.

MIDAZOLAM

Chemical group: Benzodiazepine.

Chemical name: Midazolam hydrochloride—4*H*-Imidazo[1,5-
a][1,4]benzodiazepine, 8-chloro-6-(2-fluorophenyl)-1-methyl-,
monohydrochloride.

Molecular formula: Midazolam hydrochloride—$C_{18}H_{13}ClFN_3$ ·
HCl.

Molecular weight: Midazolam hydrochloride—362.23.

Description: White to light yellow crystalline compound.

pKa: Midazolam hydrochloride—6.2.

Solubility: Midazolam hydrochloride—Soluble in aqueous solutions. At physiologic pH, midazolam becomes highly lipophilic,
and is one of the most lipid soluble of the benzodiazepines.

Other characteristics: Midazolam hydrochloride injection—An
aqueous solution with an acidic pH of approximately 3.

USP requirements:
Midazolam Hydrochloride Injection—Not in *USP–NF*.
Midazolam Hydrochloride Oral Solution—Not in *USP–NF*.

MIDODRINE

Chemical name: Midodrine hydrochloride—Acetamide, 2-ami-
no-*N*-[2-(2,5-dimethoxyphenyl)-2-hydroxyethyl]-, monohydrochloride, (±)-.

Molecular formula: Midodrine hydrochloride—$C_{12}H_{18}N_2O_4$ · HCl.

Molecular weight: Midodrine hydrochloride—290.74.

Description: Midodrine hydrochloride—Odorless, white, crystalline powder; melts between 200 and 203 °C.

pKa: Midodrine hydrochloride—7.8 (0.3% aqueous solution).

Solubility: Midodrine hydrochloride—Soluble in water; sparingly
soluble in methanol.

USP requirements: Midodrine Hydrochloride Tablets—Not in
USP–NF.

MIFEPRISTONE

Chemical name: (11 beta,17 beta)-11-[4-(Dimethylamino)phe-
nyl]-17-hydroxy-17-(1-propynyl)-estra-4,9-dien-3-one.

Molecular formula: $C_{29}H_{35}NO_2$.

Molecular weight: 429.59.

Description: Yellow powder. Melting point 191–196 °C.

Solubility: Very soluble in methanol, in chloroform, and in acetone; poorly soluble in water, in hexane, and in isopropyl.

USP requirements: Mifepristone Tablets—Not in *USP–NF*.

MIGLITOL

Chemical name: 3,4,5-Piperadinetriol, 1-(2-hydroxyethyl)-2-(hydroxymethyl)-, [2*R*(2 alpha,3 beta,4 alpha,5 beta)]-.

Molecular formula: $C_8H_{17}NO_5$.

Molecular weight: 207.22.

Description: White to pale-yellow powder.

pKa: 5.9.

Solubility: Soluble in water.

USP requirements: Miglitol Tablets—Not in *USP–NF*.

MILK THISTLE

NF requirements:
Milk Thistle NF—Preserve in well-closed containers, protected
from light and moisture. Consists of the dried ripe fruit of
Silybum marianum (L.) Gaertn. (Fam. Asteraceae), the
pappus having been removed. The label states the Latin
binomial and, following the official name, the part of the
plant contained in the article. Contains not less than
2.0% of silymarin, calculated as silybin, on the dried basis.
Meets the requirements for Botanic characteristics, Inden-
tification, Foreign organic matter (not more than 2.0%), Total ash (not more than 8.0%, determined on 1.0 gram of
finely powdered Milk Thistle), Pesticide residues, Loss
on drying (not more than 8.0%), Heavy metals (not more
than 0.001%), Microbial limits, and Content of silymarin.
Milk Thistle Capsules NF—Preserve in tight, light-resistant containers. Prepared from Powdered Milk Thistle Extract. The
label states the Latin binomial and, following the official
name, the article from which the Capsules were prepared.
The label also indicates the content of silymarin, in mg per
Capsule. Contains the labeled amount silymarin as silybin,
within ±10%, calculated on the sum of silydianin, silychristin, silybin A, silybin B, isosilybin A, and isosilybin B. Meet
the requirements for Identification, Microbial limits, Disintigration and dissolution (75% in 45 minutes in Phosphate
buffer [pH 7.5] containing 2% lauryl sulfate in Apparatus 2
at 100 rpm), Weight variation, and Content of silymarin.
Milk Thistle Tablets NF–Preserve in tight, light-resistant containers. Prepared from Powdered Milk Thistle Extract.
The label states the Latin binomial and, following the official name, the article from which the Tablets were prepared. The label also indicates the content of silymarin,
in mg per Tablet. Contain the label amount of silymarin
as silybin, within ±10%, calculated as the sum of silydianin, silychristin, silybin A, silybin B, isosylibin A, and isosylibin B. Meet the requirements for Identification, Microbial
limits, Disintigration and dissolution, Weight variation, and
Content of silymarin.

Powdered Milk Thistle NF—Preserve in well-closed containers, protected from light and moisture. Milk Thistle reduced to a fine or very fine powder. The label states the Latin binomial and, following the official name, the part of the plant source from which the article was derived. Contains not less than 2.0% of silymarin, calculated as silybin, on the dried basis. Meets the requirements for Botanic characteristics and Heavy metals (20 milligrams per gram), and the requirements for Identification, Foreign organic matter, Total ash, Pesticide residues, Loss on drying, Microbial limits, and Content of silymarin under Milk Thistle.

Powdered Milk Thistle Extract NF–Preserve in tight, light-resistant containers, in a cool place. Prepared from Milk Thistle fruits or seeds by fat removal and subsequent extraction with suitable solvents. The label states the Latin binomial and, following the official name, the part of the plant from which the article was prepared. It meets the requirements for *Labeling for Botanical Extracts*. Contains the labeled amount of silymarin, within ±10%, calculated as silybin, on the dried basis, consisting of not less than 20.0% and not more than 45.0% for the sum of silydianin and silychristin, not less than 40.0% and not more than 65.0% for the sum of silybin A and silybin B, and not less than 10.0% and not more than 20.0% for the sum of isosilybin A and isosilybin B. Meets the requirements for Identification, Microbial limits, Loss on drying (not nore than 5.0%), Heavy metals (20 micrograms per gram), Organic volatile impurities, and Content of silymarin, and for Residual solvents and Pesticide residues under *Botanical Extracts*.

MILRINONE

Chemical name: Milrinone lactate—1,6-Dihydro-2-methyl-6-oxo-[3,4′-bipyridine]-5-carbonitrile lactate.

Molecular formula: $C_{12}H_9N_3O$.

Molecular weight: 211.22.

Description: Off-white to tan crystalline compound.

Solubility: Slightly soluble in methanol; very slightly soluble in chloroform and in water.

USP requirements: Milrinone Lactate Injection—Not in *USP–NF*.

MINERAL OIL

Source: Complex mixture of hydrocarbons derived from crude petroleum; aromatic amines and unsaturated hydrocarbons are removed when refined for human use, leaving various saturated hydrocarbons behind.

Description: Mineral Oil USP—Colorless, transparent, oily liquid, free, or practically free from fluorescence. Is odorless when cold, and develops not more than a faint odor of petroleum when heated.

NF category: Solvent; vehicle (oleaginous).

Solubility: Mineral Oil USP—Insoluble in water and in alcohol; soluble in volatile oils. Miscible with most fixed oils, but not with castor oil.

USP requirements:

Mineral Oil USP—Preserve in tight containers. A mixture of liquid hydrocarbons obtained from petroleum. Label it to indicate the name of any substance added as a stabilizer. Meets the requirements for Specific gravity (0.845–0.905), Viscosity (not less than 34.5 centistokes at 40.0 °C), Neutrality, Readily carbonizable substances, Limit of polynuclear compounds, and Solid paraffin.

Mineral Oil Emulsion USP—Preserve in tight containers.

Prepare Mineral Oil Emulsion as follows: 500 mL of Mineral Oil, 125 grams of Acacia in very fine powder, 100 mL of Syrup, 40 mg of Vanillin, 60 mL of Alcohol, and a sufficient quantity of Purified Water to make 1000 mL. Mix the Mineral Oil with the Powdered Acacia in a dry mortar, add 250 mL of Purified Water all at once, and emulsify the mixture. Then add, in divided portions, triturating after each addition, a mixture of the Syrup, 50 mL of Purified Water, and the Vanillin dissolved in the alcohol. Finally add Purified Water to make the product measure 1000 mL, and mix. The Vanillin may be replaced by not more than 1% of any other official flavoring substance or any mixture of official flavoring substances. Sixty mL of sweet orange peel tincture or 2 grams of benzoic acid may be used as a preservative in place of the Alcohol.

Meets the requirement for Alcohol content (4.0–6.0%).

Mineral Oil, Rectal USP—Preserve in tight, single-unit containers. It is Mineral Oil that has been suitably packaged. Meets the requirements for Specific gravity (0.845–0.905), Viscosity (not less than 34.5 centistokes at 40.0 °C), and Neutrality.

Mineral Oil Gel—Not in *USP–NF*.

Mineral Oil Oral Suspension—Not in *USP–NF*.

LIGHT MINERAL OIL

Description: Light Mineral Oil NF—Colorless, transparent, oily liquid, free, or practically free, from fluorescence. Odorless when cold, and develops not more than a faint odor of petroleum when heated.

NF category: Tablet and/or capsule lubricant; vehicle (oleaginous).

Solubility: Light Mineral Oil NF—Insoluble in water and in alcohol; soluble in volatile oils. Miscible with most fixed oils, but not with castor oil.

USP requirements: Topical Light Mineral Oil USP—Preserve in tight containers. It is Light Mineral Oil that has been suitably packaged. Label it to indicate the name of any substance added as a stabilizer, and label packages intended for direct use by the public to indicate that it is not intended for internal use. Meets the requirements for Specific gravity (0.818–0.880) and Viscosity (not more than 33.5 centistokes at 40 °C), and for Neutrality and Solid paraffin under Mineral Oil.

NF requirements: Light Mineral Oil NF—Preserve in tight containers. A mixture of liquid hydrocarbons obtained from petroleum. Label it to indicate the name of any substance added as a stabilizer, and label packages intended for direct use by the public to indicate that it is not intended for internal use. Meets the requirements for Specific gravity (0.818–0.880) and Viscosity (not more than 33.5 centistokes at 40 °C), and for Neutrality, Readily carbonizable substances, Limit of polynuclear compounds, and Solid paraffin under Mineral Oil.

MINERAL OIL AND GLYCERIN

For *Mineral Oil* and *Glycerin*—See individual listings for chemistry information.

USP requirements: Mineral Oil and Glycerin Emulsion—Not in *USP–NF*.

MINERAL OIL, GLYCERIN, AND PHENOLPHTHALEIN

For *Mineral Oil, Glycerin,* and *Phenolphthalein*—See individual listings for chemistry information.

USP requirements: Mineral Oil, Glycerin, and Phenolphthalein Emulsion—Not in *USP–NF*.

MINERAL OIL AND PHENOLPHTHALEIN

For *Mineral Oil* and *Phenolphthalein*—See individual listings for chemistry information.

USP requirements:
Mineral Oil and Phenolphthalein Emulsion—Not in *USP–NF*.
Mineral Oil and Phenolphthalein Oral Suspension—Not in *USP–NF*.

MINERALS

USP requirements:
Minerals Capsules USP—Preserve in tight, light-resistant containers. Contain two or more minerals derived from substances generally recognized as safe, furnishing two or more of the following elements in ionizable form: calcium, chromium, copper, fluorine, iodine, iron, magnesium, manganese, molybdenum, phosphorus, potassium, selenium, and zinc. The label states that the product is Minerals Capsules. The label states also the salt form of the mineral used as the source of each element. Where more than one *Assay* method is given for a particular mineral, the labeling states the *Assay* method used only if *Method 1* is not used. Contain the labeled amounts of calcium, copper, iron, magnesium, manganese, phosphorus, potassium, and zinc, within −10% to +25%, and the labeled amounts of chromium, fluorine, iodine, molybdenum, and selenium, within −10% to +100%. Contain no vitamins. May contain other labeled added substances in amounts that are unobjectionable. Meet the requirements for Microbial limits, Disintegration and dissolution, and Weight variation.
Minerals Tablets USP—Preserve in tight, light-resistant containers. Contain two or more minerals derived from substances generally recognized as safe, furnishing two or more of the following elements in ionizable form: calcium, chromium, copper, fluorine, iodine, iron, magnesium, manganese, molybdenum, phosphorus, potassium, selenium, and zinc. The label states that the product is Minerals Tablets. The label states also the salt form of the mineral used as the source of each element. Where more than one *Assay* method is given for a particular mineral, the labeling states the *Assay* method used only if *Method 1* is not used. Contain the labeled amounts of calcium, copper, iron, magnesium, manganese, phosphorus, potassium, and zinc, within −10% to +25%, and the labeled amounts of chromium, fluorine, iodine, molybdenum, and selenium, within −10% to +100%. Contain no vitamins. May contain other labeled added substances in amounts that are unobjectionable. Meet the requirements for Microbial limits, Disintegration and dissolution, and Weight variation.

MINOCYCLINE

Chemical name: Minocycline hydrochloride—2-Naphthacenecarboxamide, 4,7-bis(dimethylamino)-1,4,4a,5,5a,6,11,12aoctahydro-3,10,12,12a-tetrahydroxy-1,11-dioxo-, monohydrochloride, [4S-(4 alpha,4a alpha,5a alpha,12a alpha)]-.

Molecular formula: Minocycline hydrochloride—$C_{23}H_{27}N_3O_7 \cdot$ HCl.

Molecular weight: Minocycline hydrochloride—493.94.

Description: Minocycline Hydrochloride USP—Yellow, crystalline powder.

Solubility: Minocycline Hydrochloride USP—Sparingly soluble in water; soluble in solutions of alkali hydroxides and carbonates; slightly soluble in alcohol; practically insoluble in chloroform and in ether.

USP requirements:
Minocycline for Injection USP—Preserve in Containers for Sterile Solids, protected from light. It is sterile, freeze-dried Minocycline Hydrochloride suitable for parenteral use. Contains an amount of minocycline hydrochloride equivalent to the labeled amount of minocycline, within −10% to +20%. Meets the requirements for Constituted solution, Identification, Bacterial endotoxins, pH (2.0–3.5, in a solution containing the equivalent of 10 mg of minocycline per mL), Water (not more than 3.0%), Particulate matter, and Limit of epiminocycline (not more than 6.0%), and for Sterility tests, Uniformity of dosage units, and Labeling under Injections.
Minocycline Hydrochloride USP—Preserve in tight containers, protected from light. Where it is intended for use in preparing injectable dosage forms, the label states that it is sterile or must be subjected to further processing during the preparation of injectable dosage forms. Contains the equivalent of not less than 890 mcg and not more than 950 mcg of minocycline per mg, calculated on the anhydrous basis. Meets the requirements for Identification, Crystallinity, pH (3.5–4.5, in a solution containing the equivalent of 10 mg of minocycline per mL), Water (4.3–8.0%), Residue on ignition (not more than 0.15%), Heavy metals (not more than 0.005%), and Chromatographic purity, and for Sterility tests and Bacterial endotoxins under Minocycline for Injection (where the label states that Minocycline Hydrochloride is sterile), and for Bacterial endotoxins under Minocycline for Injection (where the label states that Minocycline Hydrochloride must be subjected to further processing during the preparation of injectable dosage forms).
Minocycline Hydrochloride Capsules USP—Preserve in tight, light-resistant containers. Contain an amount of minocycline hydrochloride equivalent to the labeled amount of minocycline, within −10% to +15%. Meet the requirements for Identification, Dissolution (75% in 45 minutes in water in Apparatus 2 at 50 rpm), Uniformity of dosage units, and Water (not more than 12.0%).
Minocycline Hydrochloride Oral Suspension USP—Preserve in tight, light-resistant containers. Contains one or more suitable diluents, flavors, preservatives, and wetting agents in an aqueous vehicle. Contains an amount of minocycline hydrochloride equivalent to the labeled amount of minocycline, within −10% to +30%. Meets the requirements for Identification, Uniformity of dosage units (single-unit containers), Deliverable volume (multiple-unit containers), and pH (7.0–9.0).

Minocycline Hydrochloride Tablets USP—Preserve in tight, light-resistant containers. Contain an amount of minocycline hydrochloride equivalent to the labeled amount of minocycline, within −10% to +15%. Meet the requirements for Identification, Dissolution (75% in 45 minutes in water in Apparatus 2 at 50 rpm), Uniformity of dosage units, and Water (not more than 12.0%).

Minocycline Periodontal System—Not in *USP–NF*.

MINOXIDIL

Chemical name: 2,4-Pyrimidinediamine, 6-(1-piperidinyl)-, 3-oxide.

Molecular formula: $C_9H_{15}N_5O$.

Molecular weight: 209.25.

Description:
Minoxidil USP—White to off-white, crystalline powder. Melts in the approximate range of between 248 and 268 °C, with decomposition.
Minoxidil topical solution—Clear, colorless to slightly yellow solution.

pKa: 4.61.

Solubility: Minoxidil USP—Soluble in alcohol and in propylene glycol; sparingly soluble in methanol; slightly soluble in water; practically insoluble in chloroform, in acetone, in ethyl acetate, and in hexane.

USP requirements:
Minoxidil USP—Preserve in well-closed containers. Contains not less than 97.0% and not more than 103.0% of minoxidil, calculated on the dried basis. Meets the requirements for Identification, Loss on drying (not more than 0.5%), Residue on ignition (not more than 0.5%), Heavy metals (not more than 0.002%), Organic volatile impurities, and Chromatographic purity.
Minoxidil Topical Solution USP—Preserve in tight containers. Contains labeled amount, within ±10%. Meets the requirements for Identification.
Minoxidil Tablets USP—Preserve in tight containers. Contain the labeled amount, within ±10%. Meet the requirements for Identification, Dissolution (75% in 15 minutes in phosphate buffer [pH 7.2] in Apparatus 1 at 75 rpm), and Uniformity of dosage units.

MIRTAZAPINE

Chemical group: Piperazino-azepine.

Chemical name: Pyrazino[2,1-a]pyrido[2,3-c][2]benzazepine, 1,2,3,4,10,14b-hexahydro-2-methyl-.

Molecular formula: $C_{17}H_{19}N_3$.

Molecular weight: 265.35.

Description: White to creamy white crystalline powder.

Solubility: Slightly soluble in water.

USP requirements:
Mirtazapine Tablets—Not in *USP–NF*.
Mirtazapine Oral Disintigrating Tablets—Not in *USP–NF*.

MISOPROSTOL

Chemical group: Synthetic prostaglandin E₁ analog.

Chemical name: Prost-13-en-1-oic acid, 11,16-dihydroxy-16-methyl-9-oxo-, methyl ester, (11 alpha,13E)-(±)-.

Molecular formula: $C_{22}H_{38}O_5$.

Molecular weight: 382.53.

Description: Light yellow, viscous liquid with a musty odor.

Solubility: Soluble in water.

USP requirements: Misoprostol Tablets—Not in *USP–NF*.

MITOMYCIN

Source: Isolated from the broth of *Streptomyces caespitosus*.

Chemical name: Azirino[2′,3′:3,4]pyrrolo[1,2-a]indole-4,7-dione, 6-amino-8-[[(aminocarbonyl)oxy]methyl]-1,1a,2,8,8a,8b-hexahydro-8a-methoxy-5-methyl-, [1aR-(1a alpha,8 beta,8a alpha,8b alpha)]-.

Molecular formula: $C_{15}H_{18}N_4O_5$.

Molecular weight: 334.33.

Description: Mitomycin USP—Blue-violet, crystalline powder.

Solubility: Mitomycin USP—Slightly soluble in water; soluble in acetone, in methanol, in butyl acetate, and in cyclohexanone.

USP requirements:
Mitomycin USP—Preserve in tight, light-resistant containers. Has a potency of not less than 970 mcg of mitomycin per mg. Meets the requirements for Identification, Crystallinity, pH (6.0–7.5, in an aqueous suspension containing 5 mg per mL), and Water (not more than 2.5%).
Mitomycin for Injection USP—Preserve in Containers for Sterile Solids, protected from light. A dry mixture of Mitomycin and Mannitol. Contains the labeled amount, within −10% to +20%. Meets the requirements for Constituted solution, Identification, Bacterial endotoxins, Sterility, pH (6.0–8.0, in the solution constituted as directed in the labeling), and Water (not more than 5.0%), and for Injections and Uniformity of dosage units.

MITOTANE

Chemical name: Benzene, 1-chloro-2-[2,2-dichloro-1-(4-chlorophenyl)ethyl]-.

Molecular formula: $C_{14}H_{10}Cl_4$.

Molecular weight: 320.04.

Description: Mitotane USP—White, crystalline powder, having a slight aromatic odor.

Solubility: Mitotane USP—Practically insoluble in water; soluble in alcohol, in ether, in solvent hexane, and in fixed oils and fats.

USP requirements:
Mitotane USP—Preserve in tight, light-resistant containers. Contains not less than 97.0% and not more than 103.0% of mitotane, calculated on the dried basis. Meets the requirements for Identification, Melting range (75–81 °C), Loss on drying (not more than 0.5%), Residue on ignition (not more than 0.5%), and Organic volatile impurities.
Caution: Handle Mitotane with exceptional care, since it is a highly potent agent.

Mitotane Tablets USP—Preserve in tight, light-resistant containers. Contain the labeled amount, within ±10%. Meet the requirements for Identification, Disintegration (15 minutes, the use of disks being omitted), and Uniformity of dosage units.

MITOXANTRONE

Chemical group: Synthetic anthracenedione.

Chemical name: Mitoxantrone hydrochloride—9,10-Anthracenedione, 1,4-dihydroxy-5,8-bis-[[2-[(2-hydroxyethyl)amino]ethyl]amino]-, dihydrochloride.

Molecular formula: Mitoxantrone hydrochloride—$C_{22}H_{28}N_4O_6 \cdot 2HCl$.

Molecular weight: Mitoxantrone hydrochloride—517.40.

Description:
Mitoxantrone Hydrochloride USP—Dark blue powder.
Mitoxantrone hydrochloride concentrate for injection—Dark blue aqueous solution.

Solubility: Mitoxantrone Hydrochloride USP—Sparingly soluble in water; slightly soluble in methanol; practically insoluble in acetone, in acetonitrile, and in chloroform.

USP requirements:
Mitoxantrone Hydrochloride USP—Preserve in tight containers. Contains not less than 97.0% and not more than 102.0% of mitoxantrone hydrochloride, calculated on the anhydrous basis. Meets the requirements for Identification, Water (not more than 6.0%), Alcohol (not more than 1.5%), Heavy metals (not more than 0.002%), and Chromatographic purity.
Mitoxantrone Injection USP—Preserve in single-dose containers, preferably of Type I glass. A sterile solution of Mitoxantrone Hydrochloride in Water for Injection. Label Injection to state both the content of the active moiety and the name of the salt used in formulating the article. Label Mitoxantrone Injection to indicate that it is to be diluted to appropriate strength with water or other suitable fluid prior to administration. Contains the equivalent of the labeled amount of mitoxantrone, within −10% to +5%. Meets the requirements for Identification, Bacterial endotoxins, Sterility, pH (3.0–4.5), and Chromatographic purity, and for Injections.

MIVACURIUM

Chemical name: Mivacurium chloride—Isoquinolinium, 2,2′-[(1,8-dioxo-4-octene-1,8-diyl)bis(oxy-3,1-propanediyl)]-bis[1,2,3,4-tetrahydro-6,7-dimethoxy-2-methyl-1-[(3,4,5-trimethoxyphenyl)methyl]-, dichloride, [R-[R*,R*-(E)]]-.

Molecular formula: Mivacurium chloride—$C_{58}H_{80}Cl_2N_2O_{14}$.

Molecular weight: Mivacurium chloride—1100.17.

USP requirements: Mivacurium Chloride Injection—Not in *USP–NF*.

MIVACURIUM AND DEXTROSE

For *Mivacurium* and *Dextrose*—See individual listings for chemistry information.

USP requirements: Mivacurium Chloride in Dextrose Injection—Not in *USP–NF*.

MOCLOBEMIDE

Chemical name: Benzamide, 4-chloro-N-[2-(4-morpholinyl)ethyl]-.

Molecular formula: $C_{13}H_{17}ClN_2O_2$.

Molecular weight: 268.74.

Description: Almost white crystalline powder with a faint odor. Melting point approximately 138 °C.

pKa: 6.2 (approximate).

Solubility: Slightly soluble in water.

USP requirements: Moclobemide Tablets—Not in *USP–NF*.

MODAFINIL

Chemical name: Acetamide, 2-[(diphenylmethyl)sulfinyl]-.

Molecular formula: $C_{15}H_{15}NO_2S$.

Molecular weight: 273.35.

Description: A white to off-white, crystalline powder.

Solubility: Practically soluble in water and in cyclohexane; sparingly to slightly soluble in methanol and in acetone.

USP requirements: Modafinil Tablets—Not in *USP–NF*.

MOEXIPRIL

Chemical name: Moexipril hydrochloride—3-Isoquinolinecarboxylic acid, 2-[2-[[1-(ethoxycarbonyl)-3-phenylpropyl]amino]-1-oxopropyl]-1,2,3,4-tetrahydro-6,7-dimethoxy-, monohydrochloride, [3S-[2[R*(R*)], 3R*]]-.

Molecular formula: Moexipril hydrochloride—$C_{27}H_{34}N_2O_7 \cdot HCl$.

Molecular weight: Moexipril hydrochloride—535.03.

Description: Moexipril hydrochloride—Fine white to off-white powder.

Solubility: Moexipril hydrochloride—Soluble (about 10% weight-to-volume) in distilled water at room temperature.

USP requirements: Moexipril Hydrochloride Tablets—Not in *USP–NF*.

MOEXIPRIL AND HYDROCHLOROTHIAZIDE

For *Moexipril* and *Hydrochlorothiazide*—See individual listings for chemistry information.

USP requirements: Moexipril Hydrochloride and Hydrochlorothiazide Tablets—Not in *USP–NF*.

MOLINDONE

Chemical group: Dihydroindolone.

Chemical name: Molindone hydrochloride—4*H*-Indol-4-one, 3-ethyl-1,5,6,7-tetrahydro-2-methyl-5-(4-morpholinylmethyl)-, monohydrochloride.

Molecular formula: Molindone hydrochloride—C$_{16}$H$_{24}$N$_2$O$_2$ · HCl.

Molecular weight: Molindone hydrochloride—312.83.

Description: Molindone hydrochloride—White, crystalline powder.

pKa: 6.94.

Solubility: Molindone hydrochloride—Freely soluble in water and in alcohol.

USP requirements:
Molindone Hydrochloride USP—Preserve in tight, light-resistant containers. Contains not less than 98.0% and not more than 101.5% of molindone hydrochloride, calculated on the anhydrous basis. Meets the requirements for Identification, pH (4.0–5.0, in a solution [1 in 100]), Water (not more than 0.5%), Residue on ignition (not more than 0.25%), Heavy metals (not more than 0.003%), and Chromatographic purity.
Molindone Hydrochloride Oral Solution—Not in *USP–NF*.
Molindone Hydrochloride Tablets USP—Preserve in tight, light-resistant containers. Contain the labeled amount, within ±10%. Meet the requirements for Identification, Dissolution (80% in 30 minutes in 0.1 *N* hydrochloric acid in Apparatus 1 at 100 rpm), and Uniformity of dosage units.

MOMETASONE

Chemical name: Mometasone furoate—Pregna-1,4-diene-3,20-dione, 9,21-dichloro-17-[(2-furanylcarbonyl)oxy]-11-hydroxy-16-methyl-, (11 beta,16 alpha)-.

Molecular formula: Mometasone furoate—C$_{27}$H$_{30}$Cl$_2$O$_6$.

Molecular weight: Mometasone furoate—521.43.

Description: Mometasone Furoate USP—White to off-white powder. Melts at about 220 °C, with decomposition.

Solubility: Mometasone Furoate USP—Soluble in acetone and in methylene chloride.

USP requirements:
Mometasone Furoate USP—Preserve in well-closed containers. Contains not less than 97.0% and not more than 102.0% of mometasone furoate, calculated on the dried basis. Meets the requirements for Identification, Specific rotation (+56° to +62°), Loss on drying (not more than 0.5%), Residue on ignition (not more than 0.1%), Heavy metals (not more than 30 ppm), and Chromatographic purity.
Mometasone Furoate Cream USP—Preserve in well-closed containers. It is Mometasone Furoate in a suitable cream base. Contains the labeled amount, within ±10%. Meets the requirements for Identification, Microbial limits, and Minimum fill.
Mometasone Furoate Lotion—Not in *USP–NF*.
Mometasone Furoate Ointment USP—Preserve in well-closed containers. It is Mometasone Furoate in a suitable ointment base. Contains the labeled amount, within ± 10%. Meets the requirements for Identification, Microbial limits, and Minimum fill.

Mometasone Furoate Topical Solution USP—Preserve in well-closed containers. It is Mometasone Furoate in a suitable aqueous vehicle. Contains the labeled amount, within ±10%. Meets the requirements for Identification, Microbial limits, and pH (4.0–5.0).
Mometasone Furoate Nasal Suspension—Not in *USP–NF*.

MONENSIN

Chemical name:
Monensin—Monensin.
Monensin sodium—Monensin, sodium salt.

Molecular formula:
Monensin—C$_{36}$H$_{62}$O$_{11}$ (monensin A); C$_{35}$H$_{60}$O$_{11}$ (monensin B); C$_{37}$H$_{64}$O$_{11}$ (monensin C).
Monensin sodium—C$_{36}$H$_{61}$NaO$_{11}$ (monensin A sodium); C$_{35}$H$_{59}$NaO$_{11}$ (monensin B sodium); C$_{37}$H$_{63}$NaO$_{11}$ (monensin C sodium).

Molecular weight:
Monensin—670.87 (monensin A); 656.84 (monensin B); 684.90 (monensin C).
Monensin sodium—692.85 (monensin A sodium); 678.83 (monensin B sodium); 706.88 (monensin C sodium).

Description: Monensin Sodium USP—Off-white to tan, crystalline powder.

Solubility:
Monensin—Slightly soluble in water; more soluble in hydrocarbons; very soluble in organic solvents.
Monensin Sodium USP—Slightly soluble in water; soluble in chloroform and in methanol; practically insoluble in solvent hexane.

USP requirements:
Monensin USP—Preserve in well-closed containers. Avoid moisture and excessive heat. A mixture of antibiotic substances produced by the growth of *Streptomyces cinnamonensis*. Label it to indicate that it is for veterinary use only. Label it also to state that it is for manufacturing, processing, or repackaging. Has a potency of not less than 110 mcg of monensin per mg. Meets the requirements for Identification, Loss on drying (not more than 10%), and Content of monensin A and B activity (not less than 95%).
Monensin Granulated USP—Preserve in well-closed containers. Avoid moisture and excessive heat. May contain added Monensin Sodium. Contains Monensin mixed with suitable diluents, carriers, and inactive ingredients prepared in a granulated form that is free-flowing and free from aggregates. Label it to indicate that it is for veterinary use only. Label it also to state that it is for manufacturing, processing, or repackaging. Contains not less than 140 mg of monensin per gram. Meets the requirements for Identification, Loss on drying (not more than 10%), and Content of monensin A and B activity (not less than 95%).
Monensin Premix USP—Preserve in well-closed containers. Avoid moisture and excessive heat. Contains Monensin Granulated mixed with suitable diluents and inactive ingredients. Label it to indicate that it is for veterinary use only. The label bears the statement "Do not feed undiluted." Contains the equivalent of the labeled amount of monensin, within ±15%. Meets the requirements for Identification and Loss on drying (not more than 10%).
Monensin Sodium USP—Preserve in well-closed containers. Avoid moisture and excessive heat. Label it to indicate that it is for veterinary use only. Label it also to state that it is for manufacturing, processing, or repackaging. Has a potency of not less than 800 mcg per mg. Meets the require-

ments for Identification, Loss on drying (not more than 4%), and Content of monensin A and B activity (not less than 95%).

MONOBENZONE

Chemical name: Phenol, 4-(phenylmethoxy)-.

Molecular formula: $C_{13}H_{12}O_2$.

Molecular weight: 200.23.

Description: Monobenzone USP—White, odorless, crystalline powder.

Solubility:
Monobenzone USP—Practically insoluble in water; soluble in alcohol, in chloroform, in ether, and in acetone.
Monobenzone Ointment USP—Dispersible with, but not soluble in, water.

USP requirements:
Monobenzone USP—Preserve in tight, light-resistant containers, and avoid exposure to temperatures above 30 °C. Dried at 105° C for 3 hours, contains not less than 98.0% and not more than 102.0% of monobenzone. Meets the requirements for Identification, Melting range (117–120 °C), Loss on drying (not more than 1.0%), Residue on ignition (not more than 0.5%), and Organic volatile impurities.
Monobenzone Cream USP—Preserve in tight containers, and avoid exposure to temperatures above 30 °C. Contains the labeled amount, within ±6%. Meets the requirement for Identification.

MONOCTANOIN

Source: A semisynthetic mixture of glycerol esters, containing 80–85% of glyceryl mono-octanoate, 10–15% of glyceryl mono-decanoate and glyceryl di-octanoate, and a maximum of 2.5% of free glycerol.

Chemical group: Mono- and diglycerides of medium chain length fatty acids.

Chemical name: Octanoic acid monoester with 1,2,3-propanetriol.

USP requirements: Monoctanoin Irrigation—Not in *USP–NF*.

MONO- AND DI-ACETYLATED MONOGLYCERIDES

Description: Mono- and Di-acetylated Monoglycerides NF—White to pale yellow waxy solid, melting at about 45 °C.
NF category: Plasticizer.

Solubility: Mono- and Di-acetylated Monoglycerides NF—Soluble in ether and in chloroform; slightly soluble in carbon disulfide; insoluble in water.

NF requirements: Mono- and Di-acetylated Monoglycerides NF—Preserve in tight, light-resistant containers. It is glycerin esterified with edible fat-forming fatty acids and acetic acid. May be prepared by the inter-esterification of edible oils with triacetin or a mixture of triacetin and glycerin in the presence of catalytic agents, followed by molecular distillation, or by direct acetylation of edible monoglycerides and diglycerides with acetic anhydride with or without the use of catalysts or molecular distillation. Meets the requirements for Identification, Residue on ignition (not more than 0.5%), Heavy metals (not

more than 0.001%), Acid value (not more than 3), Hydroxyl value (133–152), Saponification value (279–292), Free glycerin (not more than 1.5%), and Organic volatile impurities.

MONO- AND DI-GLYCERIDES

Description: Mono- and Di-glycerides NF—Varies in consistency from yellow liquids through ivory-colored plastics to hard ivory-colored solids having a bland odor.
NF category: Emulsifying and/or solubilizing agent.

Solubility: Mono- and Di-glycerides NF—Insoluble in water; soluble in alcohol, in ethyl acetate, in chloroform, and in other chlorinated hydrocarbons.

NF requirements: Mono- and Di-glycerides NF—Preserve in tight, light-resistant containers. A mixture of glycerol mono- and di-esters, with minor amounts of tri-esters, of fatty acids from edible oils. Contains not less than 40.0% of monoglycerides. The labeling indicates the monoglyceride content, hydroxyl value, iodine value, saponification value, and the name and quantity of any stabilizers. The monoglyceride content is within ±10% of the value indicated in the labeling. Meets the requirements for Residue on ignition (not more than 0.1%), Arsenic (not more than 3 ppm), Heavy metals (not more than 0.001%), Acid value (not more than 4), Hydroxyl value (within ±10.0% of value indicated in labeling), Iodine value (within ± 10.0% of value indicated in labeling), Saponification value (within ±10% of value indicated in labeling), Limit of free glycerin (not more than 7.0%), and Organic volatile impurities.

MONOETHANOLAMINE

Chemical name: Ethanol, 2-amino-.

Molecular formula: C_2H_7NO.

Molecular weight: 61.08.

Description: Monoethanolamine NF—Clear, colorless, moderately viscous liquid, having a distinctly ammoniacal odor.
NF category: Emulsifying and/or solubilizing agent (adjunct).

Solubility: Monoethanolamine NF—Miscible with water, with acetone, with alcohol, with glycerin, and with chloroform. Immiscible with ether, with solvent hexane, and with fixed oils, although it dissolves in many essential oils.

NF requirements: Monoethanolamine NF—Preserve in tight, light-resistant containers. Contains not less than 98.0% and not more than 100.5%, by weight, of monoethanolamine. Meets the requirements for Specific gravity (1.013–1.016), Distilling range (not less than 95% distils at 167–173 °C), Residue on ignition (not more than 0.1%), and Organic volatile impurities.

MONOSODIUM GLUTAMATE

Molecular formula: $C_5H_8NNaO_4 \cdot H_2O$.

Molecular weight: 187.13.

Description: Monosodium Glutamate NF—White, practically odorless, free-flowing crystals or crystalline powder.
NF category: Flavors and perfumes.

Solubility: Monosodium Glutamate NF—Freely soluble in water; sparingly soluble in alcohol.

NF requirements: Monosodium Glutamate NF—Preserve in tight containers. Contains not less than 99.0% and not more than 100.5% of monosodium glutamate. Meets the requirements for Clarity and color of solution, Identification, Specific rotation (+24.8° to +25.3° at 20 °C), pH (6.7–7.2, in a solution [1 in 20]), Loss on drying (not more than 0.5%), Chloride (not more than 0.25%), Lead (not more than 10 ppm), Heavy metals (not more than 0.002%), and Organic volatile impurities.

MONOTHIOGLYCEROL

Chemical name: 1,2-Propanediol, 3-mercapto-.

Molecular formula: $C_3H_8O_2S$.

Molecular weight: 108.16.

Description: Monothioglycerol NF—Colorless or pale yellow viscous liquid, having a slight sulfidic odor. Hygroscopic.
   NF category: Antioxidant.

Solubility: Monothioglycerol NF—Miscible with alcohol. Freely soluble in water; insoluble in ether.

NF requirements: Monothioglycerol NF—Preserve in tight containers. Contains not less than 97.0% and not more than 101.0% of monothioglycerol, calculated on the anhydrous basis. Meets the requirements for Specific gravity (1.241–1.250), Refractive index (1.521–1.526), pH (3.5–7.0, in a solution [1 in 10]), Water (not more than 5.0%), Residue on ignition (not more than 0.1%), Selenium (not more than 0.003%), Heavy metals (not more than 0.002%), and Organic volatile impurities.

MONTELUKAST

Chemical name: Montelukast sodium—Cyclopropaneacetic acid, 1-[[[1-[3-[2-(7-chloro-2-quinolinyl)-ethenyl]phenyl]-3-[2-(1-hydroxy-1-methylethyl)phenyl]-propyl]thio]methyl]-, sodium salt, [R-(E)]-.

Molecular formula: Montelukast sodium—$C_{35}H_{35}ClNNaO_3S$.

Molecular weight: Montelukast sodium—608.17.

Description: Montelukast sodium—White to off-white powder.

Solubility: Montelukast sodium—Freely soluble in ethanol, in methanol, and in water; practically insoluble in acetonitrile.

USP requirements:
   Montelukast Sodium Tablets—Not in *USP–NF*.
   Montelukast Sodium Chewable Tablets—Not in *USP–NF*.

MORICIZINE

Chemical name: Moricizine hydrochloride—Carbamic acid, [10-[3-(4-morpholinyl)-1-oxopropyl]-10*H*-phenothiazin-2-yl]-, ethyl ester, hydrochloride.

Molecular formula: Moricizine hydrochloride—$C_{22}H_{25}N_3O_4S \cdot$ HCl.

Molecular weight: Moricizine hydrochloride—463.98.

Description: Moricizine Hydrochloride USP—White to off-white, crystalline powder. Melts at about 189 °C, with decomposition.

pKa: Moricizine hydrochloride—6.4 (weak base).

Solubility: Moricizine Hydrochloride USP—Soluble in water and in alcohol.

USP requirements:
   Moricizine Hydrochloride USP—Preserve in tight containers. Contains not less than 98.0% and not more than 102.0% of moricizine hydrochloride, calculated on the anhydrous and alcohol-free basis. Meets the requirements for Identification, Clarity of solution, Loss on drying (not more than 1.0%), Water (not more than 1.0%), Residue on ignition (not more than 0.1%), Heavy metals (not more than 10 mcg per gram), Organic volatile impurities, Chromatographic purity, Limit of alcohol (not more than 0.25%), and Content of chloride (7.49–7.80%, calculated on the anhydrous and alcohol-free basis).
   Moricizine Hydrochloride Tablets USP—Preserve in tight containers. Contain the labeled amount, within ±10%. Meet the requirements for Identification, Dissolution (75% in 30 minutes in 0.1 N hydrochloric acid in Apparatus 2 at 50 rpm), Uniformity of dosage units, and Limit of degradation products.

MORPHINE

Chemical name:
   Morphine hydrochloride—Morphinan-3,6-diol, 7,8-didehydro-4,5-epoxy-17-methyl, (5 alpha,6 alpha)-, hydrochloride (1:1) (salt), trihydrate.
   Morphine sulfate—Morphinan-3,6-diol, 7,8-didehydro-4,5-epoxy-17-methyl, (5 alpha,6 alpha)-, sulfate (2:1) (salt), pentahydrate.

Molecular formula:
   Morphine hydrochloride—$C_{17}H_{19}NO_3 \cdot HCl \cdot 3H_2O$.
   Morphine sulfate—$(C_{17}H_{19}NO_3)_2 \cdot H_2SO_4 \cdot 5H_2O$ (pentahydrate); $(C_{17}H_{19}NO_3)_2 \cdot H_2SO_4$ (anhydrous).

Molecular weight:
   Morphine hydrochloride—375.8.
   Morphine sulfate—758.83 (pentahydrate); 668.76 (anhydrous).

Description:
   Morphine hydrochloride—Colorless, silky crystals, cubical masses, or a white or almost white, crystalline powder.
   Morphine Sulfate USP—White, feathery, silky crystals, cubical masses of crystals, or white, crystalline powder. Is odorless, and when exposed to air it gradually loses water of hydration. Darkens on prolonged exposure to light.

Solubility:
   Morphine hydrochloride—Soluble 1 in 24 of water and 1 in 10 of boiling alcohol (90%); practically insoluble in chloroform and in ether.
   Morphine Sulfate USP—Soluble in water; freely soluble in hot water; slightly soluble in alcohol but more so in hot alcohol; insoluble in chloroform and in ether.

USP requirements:
   Morphine Hydrochloride Suppositories—Not in *USP–NF*.
   Morphine Hydrochloride Syrup—Not in *USP–NF*.
   Morphine Hydrochloride Tablets—Not in *USP–NF*.
   Morphine Hydrochloride Extended-release Tablets—Not in *USP–NF*.
   Morphine Sulfate USP—Preserve in tight, light-resistant containers. Contains not less than 98.0% and not more than 102.0% of morphine sulfate, calculated on the anhydrous basis. Meets the requirements for Identification, Specific rotation (−107° to −109.5°), Acidity, Water (10.4–13.4%), Residue on ignition (not more than 0.1%, from 500 mg), Chloride, Ammonium salts, Limit of foreign alkaloids, and Organic volatile impurities.
   Morphine Sulfate Capsules—Not in *USP–NF*.
   Morphine Sulfate Extended-release Capsules—Not in *USP–NF*.

Morphine Sulfate Concentrate (Preservative-free)—Not in *USP–NF*.

Morphine Sulfate Injection USP—Preserve in single-dose or in multiple-dose containers, preferably of Type I glass, protected from light. Preserve Injection labeled "Preservative-free" in single-dose containers. A sterile solution of Morphine Sulfate in Water for Injection. It meets the requirements for Labeling under Injections. Label it to state that the Injection is not to be used if it is darker than pale yellow, if it is discolored in any other way, or if it contains a precipitate. Injection containing no antioxidant or antimicrobial agents prominently bears on its label the words "Preservative-free" and includes, in its labeling, its routes of administration and the statement that it is not to be heat-sterilized. Injection containing antioxidant or antimicrobial agents includes in its labeling its routes of administration and the statement that it is not for intrathecal or epidural use. Contains the labeled amount, within ±10%. Injection intended for intramuscular or intravenous administration may contain sodium chloride as a tonicity-adjusting agent, and suitable antioxidants and antimicrobial agents. Injection intended for intrathecal or epidural use may contain sodium chloride as a tonicity-adjusting agent, but contains no other added substances. Meets the requirements for Identification, Bacterial endotoxins, pH (2.5–6.5), and Particulate matter, and for Injections.

Morphine Sulfate Oral Solution—Not in *USP–NF*.

Morphine Sulfate Suppositories USP—For suppositories compounded in fatty acid base: Preserve in tight containers, and store in refrigerator. Label Suppositories to state that they are Morphine Sulfate Suppositories in a Fatty Acid Base and to state that they are for rectal use only. Label Suppositories to state that they are to be stored in a refrigerator (2–8 °C). The label also bears a warning that the Suppositories are a specially formulated strength to be used only by the patient for whom they were prescribed, and that wrappers are to be removed prior to use. Contain the labeled amount, within ±10%. Prepare Morphine Sulfate Suppositories in Fatty Acid Base as follows: 50 mg Morphine Sulfate, Silica Gel, and Fatty Acid Base, a sufficient quantity to make one suppository. Calibrate the actual molds with the Fatty Acid Base that is used for preparing the Suppositories, and adjust the formula accordingly. Mix thoroughly the Morphine Sulfate and Silica Gel to obtain a uniform powder. Heat the Fatty Acid Base slowly and evenly until melted. Slowly add the powder to the melted base, with stirring. Mix thoroughly, and pour into molds. Cool, trim, and wrap. Meet the requirements for Uniformity of dosage units and Beyond-use date.

For suppositories compounded in polyethylene glycol base: Preserve in tight containers, and store in refrigerator. Do not dispense or store polyethylene glycol-base suppositories in polystyrene containers. Label Suppositories to state that they are Morphine Sulfate Suppositories in a Polyethylene Glycol Base and to state that they are for rectal use only. Label Suppositories to state that they are to be stored in a refrigerator (2–8 °C). The label also bears a warning that the Suppositories are a specially formulated strength to be used only by the patient for whom they were prescribed, and that wrappers are to be removed prior to use. Prepare Morphine Sulfate Suppositories in Polyethylene Glycol Base as follows: 50 mg of Morphine Sulfate, 25 mg of Silica Gel, and Polyethylene Glycol Gel, a sufficient quantity to make one suppository. Calibrate the actual molds with Polyethylene Glycol Base that is used for preparing the Suppositories, and adjust the formula accordingly. Mix thoroughly the Morphine Sulfate and Silica Gel to obtain a uniform powder. Heat the Polyethylene Glycol Base slowly and evenly until melted. Slowly add the powder to the melted base, with stirring. Mix thoroughly, and pour into molds. Cool, trim, and wrap. Meet the requirements for Uniformity of dosage units and Beyond-use date.

Morphine Sulfate Syrup—Not in *USP–NF*.
Morphine Sulfate Tablets—Not in *USP–NF*.
Morphine Sulfate Extended-release Tablets—Not in *USP–NF*.
Morphine Sulfate Soluble Tablets—Not in *USP–NF*.

MORRHUATE SODIUM

Description: Pale-yellowish, granular powder with a slight fishy odor.

Solubility: Soluble in water and in alcohol.

USP requirements: Morrhuate Sodium Injection USP—Preserve in single-dose or in multiple-dose containers, preferably of Type I glass. May be packaged in 50-mL multiple-dose containers. A sterile solution of the sodium salts of the fatty acids of Cod Liver Oil. Contains, in each mL, not less than 46.5 mg and not more than 53.5 mg of morrhuate sodium. A suitable antimicrobial agent, not to exceed 0.5%, and ethyl alcohol or benzyl alcohol, not to exceed 3.0%, may be added. Meets the requirements for Identification, Bacterial endotoxins, Acidity and alkalinity, and Iodine value of the fatty acids (not less than 130), and for Injections (except that at times it may show a slight turbidity or precipitate).

Note: Morrhuate Sodium Injection may show a separation of solid matter on standing. Do not use the material if such solid does not dissolve completely upon warming.

MOXALACTAM

Source: Semisynthetic 1-oxa-beta-lactam antibiotic structurally related to cephalosporins, cephamycins, and penicillins.

Chemical name: Moxalactam disodium—5-Oxa-1-azabicyclo[4.2.0]oct-2-ene-2-carboxylic acid, 7-[[carboxy(4-hydroxyphenyl)acetyl]amino]-7-methoxy-3-[[(1-methyl-1 *H*-tetrazol-5-yl)thio]methyl]-8-oxo-, disodium salt.

Molecular formula: Moxalactam disodium—$C_{20}H_{18}N_6Na_2O_9S$.

Molecular weight: Moxalactam disodium—564.44.

Description: Moxalactam disodium—White to off-white powder with a faint characteristic odor.

Solubility: Moxalactam disodium—Very soluble in water.

USP requirements: Moxalactam Disodium for Injection USP—Preserve in Containers for Sterile Solids. A sterile mixture of moxalactam disodium and Mannitol. The mixture has a potency equivalent to not less than 722 mcg of moxalactam per mg. Contains an amount of moxalactam disodium equivalent to the labeled amount of moxalactam, within −10% to +20%. Meets the requirements for Constituted solution, Identification, Bacterial endotoxins, Sterility, pH (4.5–7.0 in a solution [1 in 10]), Water (not more than 3.0%), Particulate matter, and Isomer ratio (response ratio of R-isomer to S-isomer 0.8–1.4), and for Uniformity of dosage units and Labeling under Injections.

MOXIFLOXACIN

Chemical name:
Moxifloxacin—1-Cyclopropyl-6-fluoro-1,4-dihydro-8-methoxy-7-[(4a*S*,7a*S*)-octahydro-6*H*-pyrrolo[3,4-*b*]pyridin-6-yl]-4-oxo-3-quinolinecarboxylic acid.

Moxifloxacin hydrochloride—(4a*S*-cis)-1-Cyclopropyl-6-fluoro-1,4-dihydro-8-methoxy-7-(octahydro-6*H*-pyrrolo[3,4-*b*]pyridin-6-yl)-4-oxo-3-quinolinecarboxylic acid, monohydrochloride.

Molecular formula:
Moxifloxacin—$C_{21}H_{24}FN_3O_4$.
Moxifloxacin hydrochloride—$C_{21}H_{24}FN_3O_4 \cdot HCl$.

Molecular weight:
Moxifloxacin—401.43.
Moxifloxacin hydrochloride—437.90.

Description: Moxifloxacin hydrochloride—Slightly yellow to yellow crystalline substance.

USP requirements:
Moxifloxacin Injection—Not in *USP–NF*.
Moxifloxacin Tablets—Not in *USP–NF*.

MUMPS SKIN TEST ANTIGEN

Description: Mumps Skin Test Antigen USP—Slightly turbid liquid.

USP requirements: Mumps Skin Test Antigen USP—Preserve at a temperature between 2 and 8 °C. A sterile suspension of formaldehyde-inactivated mumps virus prepared from the extra-embryonic fluids of the mumps virus–infected chicken embryo, concentrated and purified by differential centrifugation, and diluted with isotonic sodium chloride solution. Label it to state that it was prepared in embryonated chicken eggs and that a separate syringe and needle are to be used for each individual injection. Contains not less than 20 complement-fixing units in each mL. Contains approximately 0.006 *M* glycine as a stabilizing agent, and contains a preservative. Meets the requirement for Expiration date (not later than 18 months after date of manufacture or date of issue from manufacturer's cold storage [5 °C, 1 year]). Conforms to the regulations of the U.S. Food and Drug Administration concerning biologics.

MUMPS VIRUS VACCINE LIVE

Source: The vaccine currently available in the U.S. (*Mumpsvax*, MSD) contains a lyophilized preparation of the Jeryl Lynn (B level) strain of mumps virus. This virus was adapted to and propagated in cell cultures of chick embryo free of avian leukosis virus and other adventitious agents. *Mumpsvax*, MSD (Canada) and Morson (U.K.) brands of mumps virus vaccine live, also contain the Jeryl Lynn strain of mumps virus.

Description: Mumps Virus Vaccine Live USP—Solid having the characteristic appearance of substances dried from the frozen state. The vaccine is to be constituted with a suitable diluent just prior to use. Constituted vaccine undergoes loss of potency on exposure to sunlight.

USP requirements: Mumps Virus Vaccine Live USP (for Injection)—Preserve in single-dose containers, or in light-resistant, multiple-dose containers, at a temperature between 2 and 8 °C. Multiple-dose containers for 50 doses are adapted for use only in jet injectors, and those for 10 doses for use by jet or syringe injection. A bacterially sterile preparation of live virus derived from a strain of mumps virus tested for neurovirulence in monkeys, and for immunogenicity, free from all demonstrable viable microbial agents except unavoidable bacteriophage, and found suitable for human immunization. The strain is grown for the purpose of vaccine production on chicken embryo primary cell tissue cultures derived from pathogen-free flocks, meets the requirements of the specific safety tests in adult and suckling mice; the requirements of the tests in monkey kidney, chicken embryo and human tissue cell cultures and embryonated eggs; and the requirements of the tests for absence of *Mycobacterium tuberculosis* and of avian leucosis, unless the production cultures were derived from certified avian leucosis-free sources and the control fluids were tested for avian leucosis. The strain cultures are treated to remove all intact tissue cells. The Vaccine meets the requirements of the specific tissue culture test for live virus titer, in a single immunizing dose, of not less than the equivalent of 5000 $TCID_{50}$ (quantity of virus estimated to infect 50% of inoculated cultures × 5000) when tested in parallel with the U.S. Reference Mumps Virus, Live. Label the Vaccine in multiple-dose containers to indicate that the contents are intended solely for use by jet injector or for use by either jet or syringe injection, whichever is applicable. Label the Vaccine in single-dose containers, if such containers are not light-resistant, to state that it should be protected from sunlight. Label it also to state that constituted Vaccine should be discarded if not used within 8 hours. Meets the requirement for Expiration date (1 to 2 years, depending on the manufacturer's data, after date of issue from manufacturer's cold storage [–20 °C, 1 year]). Conforms to the regulations of the U.S. Food and Drug Administration concerning biologics.

MUPIROCIN

Source: Produced by fermentation of *Pseudomonas fluorescens*.

Chemical name:
Mupirocin—Nonanoic acid, 9-[[3-methyl-1-oxo-4-[tetrahydro-3,4-dihydroxy-5-[[3-(2-hydroxy-1-methylpropyl)oxiranyl]methyl]-2*H*-pyran-2-yl]-2-butenyl]oxy]-, [2*S*-[2 alpha(*E*),3 beta,4 beta,5 alpha[2*R**,3*R**(1*R**,2*R**)]]]-.
Mupirocin calcium—Nonanoic acid, 9-[[3-methyl-1-oxo-4-[tetrahydro-3,4-dihydroxy-5-[[3-(2-hydroxy-1-methylpropyl)oxiranyl]methyl]-2*H*-pyran-2-yl]-2-butenyl]oxy]-, calcium salt (2:1), dihydrate, [2*S*-[2 alpha(*E*),3 beta,4 beta,5 alpha[2*R**,3*R**(1*R**,2*R**)]]]-.

Molecular formula:
Mupirocin—$C_{26}H_{44}O_9$.
Mupirocin calcium—$C_{52}H_{86}CaO_{18} \cdot 2H_2O$.

Molecular weight:
Mupirocin—500.62.
Mupirocin calcium—1075.34.

Description: Mupirocin USP—White to off-white, crystalline solid.

Solubility: Mupirocin USP—Freely soluble in acetone, in chloroform, in dehydrated alcohol, and in methanol; slightly soluble in ether; very slightly soluble in water.

USP requirements:
Mupirocin USP—Preserve in tight containers. Contains not less than 920 mcg and not more than 1020 mcg of mupirocin per mg, calculated on the anhydrous basis. Meets the requirements for Identification, Crystallinity, pH (3.5–4.5, in a saturated aqueous solution), and Water (not more than 1.0%).
Mupirocin Ointment USP—Preserve in collapsible tubes or in well-closed containers. Contains the labeled amount, within ±10%. Meets the requirements for Identification and Minimum fill.
Mupirocin Calcium Cream—Not in *USP–NF*.
Mupirocin Calcium Nasal Ointment—Not in *USP–NF*.

MUROMONAB-CD3

Source: Produced by a process involving fusion of mouse myeloma cells to lymphocytes from immunized animals to produce a hybridoma which secretes antigen-specific antibodies (murine monoclonal antibodies). Muromonab-CD3 is a biochemically purified $IgG_{2 \; alpha}$ immunoglobulin with a heavy chain of approximately 50,000 daltons and a light chain of approximately 25,000 daltons.

USP requirements: Muromonab-CD3 Injection—Not in *USP–NF*.

MYCOPHENOLATE

Chemical name:
  Mycophenolate mofetil—4-Hexenoic acid, 6-(1,3-dihydro-4-hydroxy-6-methoxy-7-methyl-3-oxo-5-isobenzofuranyl)-4-methyl-, 2-(4-morpholinyl)ethyl ester, (*E*)-.
  Mycophenolate mofetil hydrochloride—2-(4-Morpholinyl)ethyl ester (*E*)-6-(1,3-dihydro-4-hydroxy-6-methoxy-7-methyl-3-oxo-5-isobenzofuranyl)-4-methyl-4-hexenoic acid, hydrochloride.

Molecular formula:
  Mycophenolate mofetil—$C_{23}H_{31}NO_7$.
  Mycophenolate mofetil hydrochloride—$C_{23}H_{31}NO_7 \cdot HCl$.

Molecular weight:
  Mycophenolate mofetil—433.49.
  Mycophenolate mofetil hydrochloride—469.96.

Description: Mycophenolate mofetil—White to off-white crystalline powder.

pKa: Mycophenolate mofetil—5.6 for morpholino group; 8.5 for phenolic group.

Solubility: Mycophenolate mofetil—Slightly soluble in water (43 mcg/mL at pH 7.4); solubility increases in acidic medium (4.27 mg/mL at pH 3.6); freely soluble in acetone; soluble in methanol; sparingly soluble in ethanol.

USP requirements:
  Mycophenolate Mofetil Capsules—Not in *USP–NF*.
  Mycophenolate Mofetil Tablets—Not in *USP–NF*.
  Mycophenolate Mofetil Hydrochloride for Injection—Not in *USP–NF*.

MYRISTYL ALCOHOL

Molecular formula: $C_{14}H_{30}O$.

Molecular weight: 214.39.

Description: Myristyl Alcohol NF—White wax-like mass.
  NF category: Oleaginous vehicle.

Solubility: Myristyl Alcohol NF—Soluble in ether; slightly soluble in alcohol; insoluble in water.

NF requirements: Myristyl Alcohol NF—Preserve in well-closed containers. Contains not less than 90.0% of myristyl alcohol, the remainder consisting chiefly of related alcohols. Meets the requirements for Identification, Melting range (36–42 °C), Acid value (not more than 2), Iodine value (not more than 1), Hydroxyl value (250–267), and Organic volatile impurities.

MYRRH

USP requirements:
  Myrrh USP—Preserve in tight containers and store at controlled room temperature in a dry place. It is the oleo-gum resin obtained from stems and branches of *Commiphora molmol* Engler and other related species of *Commiphora* other than *Commiphora mukul* (Fam. Burseraceae). Label it to indicate the species of *Commiphora* from which the oleo-gum resin was obtained. Label it also to indicate that it is intended for topical and oropharyngeal use only. Meets the requirements for Botanic characteristics, Identification, Loss on drying (not more than 15.0%), Foreign organic matter (not more than 2%), Total ash (not more than 10.0%), Acid insoluble ash (not more than 5.0%), Alcohol-soluble extractives (not less than 40% and not more than 70%), Water soluble extractives (not less than 50%), Heavy metals (not more than 0.002%), and Volatile oil content (not less than 6.0%).
  Myrrh Topical Solution USP—Prepare Myrrh Topical Solution as follows: 200 grams of Myrrh, 900 mL of a mixture of Alcohol and Water (85:15), and Alcohol, a sufficient quantity, to make 1000 mL. Macerate about 200 grams of coarsely ground Myrrh with an alcohol–water mixture for 48 hours at room temperature in a suitable vessel, which is fitted with a lid and a mechanical stirrer, agitating the mixture with the stirrer. Allow the resulting mixture to stand overnight. Decant the mixture, filter, dilute the filtrate with Alcohol to 1000 mL, and mix. Label it to indicate that it is intended for topical and oropharyngeal use only. Meets the requirements for Identification and Alcohol content, and for Packaging and Storage and Labeling for Tinctures under Botanical extracts.

NABILONE

Chemical group: Synthetic cannabinoid. Resembles the cannabinols but is not a tetrahydrocannabinol.

Chemical name: 9*H*-Dibenzo[*b,d*]pyran-9-one, 3-(1,1-dimethylheptyl)-6,6a,7,8,10,10a-hexahydro-1-hydroxy-6,6-dimethyl-, *trans*-, (±)-.

Molecular formula: $C_{24}H_{36}O_3$.

Molecular weight: 372.54.

Description: White, polymorphic crystalline powder.

Solubility: In aqueous media, solubility less than 0.5 mg/L.

USP requirements: Nabilone Capsules—Not in *USP–NF*.

NABUMETONE

Chemical name: 2-Butanone, 4-(6-methoxy-2-naphthalenyl)-.

Molecular formula: $C_{15}H_{16}O_2$.

Molecular weight: 228.29.

Description: Nabumetone USP—A white or almost white crystalline powder.

Solubility: Nabumetone USP—Freely soluble in acetone; sparingly soluble in alcohol and in methanol; practically insoluble in water.

Other characteristics: N-octanol:phosphate buffer partition coefficient—2400 at pH 7.4.

USP requirements:
  Nabumetone USP—Preserve in tight, light-resistant containers. Contais not less than 98.0% and not more than 101.0% of nabumetone, calculated on the anhydrous ba-

sis. Meets the requirements for Identification, Water (not more than 0.2%, determined on a 1-gram specimen), Residue on ignition (not more than 0.1%), Heavy metals (0.001%), and Related compounds.

Nabumetone Tablets USP—Preserve in tight containers. Contain the labeled amount, within ±5%. Meet the requirements for Identification, Dissolution (75% in 45 minutes in sodium lauryl sulfate solution [2 in 100] in Apparatus 2 at 50 rpm), and Uniformity of dosage units.

NADOLOL

Chemical name: 2,3-Naphthalenediol, 5-[3-[(1,1-dimethylethyl) amino]-2-hydroxypropoxy]-1,2,3,4-tetrahydro-, *cis-*.

Molecular formula: $C_{17}H_{27}NO_4$.

Molecular weight: 309.40.

Description: Nadolol USP—White to off-white, practically odorless, crystalline powder.

pKa: 9.67.

Solubility: Nadolol USP—Freely soluble in alcohol and in methanol; soluble in water at pH 2; slightly soluble in chloroform, in methylene chloride, in isopropyl alcohol, and in water (between pH 7 and pH 10); insoluble in acetone, in ether, in hexane, and in trichloroethane.

Other characteristics: Lipid solubility—Low.

USP requirements:
Nadolol USP—Preserve in well-closed containers. Contains not less than 98.0% and not more than 101.5% of nadolol, calculated on the dried basis. Meets the requirements for Identification, Loss on drying (not more than 2.0%), Residue on ignition (not more than 0.1%), Heavy metals (not more than 0.003%), Racemate composition, Chromatographic purity, and Organic volatile impurities.
Nadolol Tablets USP—Preserve in tight containers. Contain the labeled amount, within ±10%. Meet the requirements for Identification, Dissolution (80% in 50 minutes in 0.01 *N* hydrochloric acid in Apparatus 1 at 100 rpm), and Uniformity of dosage units.

NADOLOL AND BENDROFLUMETHIAZIDE

For *Nadolol* and *Bendroflumethiazide*—See individual listings for chemistry information.

USP requirements: Nadolol and Bendroflumethiazide Tablets USP—Preserve in tight containers. Contain the labeled amounts, within ±10%. Meet the requirements for Identification, Dissolution (80% of each active ingredient in 30 minutes in 0.1 *N* hydrochloric acid in Apparatus 2 at 50 rpm), and Uniformity of dosage units.

NAFARELIN

Source: Nafarelin acetate—Synthetic analog of the naturally occurring gonadotropin releasing hormone (GnRH).

Chemical name: Nafarelin acetate—Luteinizing hormone-releasing factor (pig), 6-[3-(2-naphthalenyl)-D-alanine]-, acetate (salt), hydrate.

Molecular formula: Nafarelin acetate—$C_{66}H_{83}N_{17}O_{13} \cdot xC_2H_4O_2 \cdot yH_2O$.

Description: Nafarelin acetate—Fine white to off-white amorphous powder.

Solubility: Nafarelin acetate—Slightly soluble in water; slightly soluble in 0.02 *M* phosphate buffer (pH 7.58), in methanol, and in ethanol; practically insoluble in acetonitrile and in dichloromethane.

USP requirements: Nafarelin Acetate Nasal Solution—Not in *USP–NF.*

NAFCILLIN

Chemical name: Nafcillin sodium—4-Thia-1-azabicyclo[3.2.0]-heptane-2-carboxylic acid, 6-[[(2-ethoxy-1-naphthalenyl)carbonyl]amino]-3,3-dimethyl-7-oxo-, monosodium salt, monohydrate, [2*S*-(2 alpha,5 alpha,6 beta)].

Molecular formula: Nafcillin sodium—$C_{21}H_{21}N_2NaO_5S \cdot H_2O$.

Molecular weight: Nafcillin sodium—454.47.

Description:
Nafcillin Sodium USP—White to yellowish white powder, having not more than a slight characteristic odor.

Solubility:
Nafcillin Sodium USP—Freely soluble in water and in chloroform; soluble in alcohol.

USP requirements:
Nafcillin Injection USP—Preserve in Containers for Injections. Maintain in the frozen state. A sterile isoosmotic solution of Nafcillin Sodium and one or more buffer substances in Water for Injection. Contains dextrose as a tonicity-adjusting agent. It meets the requirements for Labeling under Injections. The label states that it is to be thawed just prior to use, describes conditions for proper storage of the resultant solution, and directs that the solution is not to be refrozen. Contains an amount of nafcillin sodium equivalent to the labeled amount of nafcillin, within −10% to +20%. Contains no antimicrobial preservatives. Meets the requirements for Identification, Bacterial endotoxins, Sterility, pH (6.0–8.5), and Particulate matter.
Nafcillin for Injection USP—Preserve in Containers for Sterile Solids. Contains an amount of nafcillin sodium equivalent to the labeled amount of nafcillin, within −10% to +20%. Meets the requirements for Constituted solution, Identification, Bacterial endotoxins, Sterility, pH (6.0–8.5, in the solution constituted as directed in the labeling), Water (3.5–5.3%), and Particulate matter, and for Uniformity of dosage units and Labeling under Injections.
Nafcillin Sodium USP—Preserve in tight containers. Where it is intended for use in preparing injectable dosage forms, the label states that it is sterile or must be subjected to further processing during the preparation of injectable dosage forms. Has a potency equivalent to not less than 820 mcg of nafcillin per mg. Meets the requirements for Identification, Crystallinity, pH (5.0–7.0, in a solution containing 30 mg per mL), and Water (3.5–5.3%), and for Sterility tests and for Bacterial endotoxins under Nafcillin for Injection (where the label states that Nafcillin Sodium is sterile), and for Bacterial endotoxins under Nafcillin for Injection (where the label states that Nafcillin Sodium must be subjected to further processing during the preparation of injectable dosage forms).
Nafcillin Sodium Capsules USP—Preserve in tight containers. Contain an amount of nafcillin sodium equivalent to the labeled amount of nafcillin, within −10% to +20%. Meet the requirements for Dissolution (75% in 45 minutes in water in Apparatus 1 at 100 rpm), Uniformity of dosage units, and Water (not more than 5.0%).

Nafcillin Sodium for Oral Solution USP—Preserve in tight containers. Contains an amount of nafcillin sodium equivalent to the labeled amount of nafcillin, within −10% to +20%. Contains one or more suitable buffers, colors, diluents, dispersants, flavors, and preservatives. Meets the requirements for Uniformity of dosage units (single-unit containers), Deliverable volume (multiple-unit containers), pH (5.5–7.5, in the solution constituted as directed in the labeling), and Water (not more than 5.0%).

Nafcillin Sodium Tablets USP—Preserve in tight, light-resistant containers. Contain an amount of nafcillin sodium equivalent to the labeled amount of nafcillin, within −10% to +20%. Meet the requirements for Dissolution (75% in 45 minutes in pH 4.0 buffer in Apparatus 2 at 50 rpm), Uniformity of dosage units, and Water (not more than 5.0%).

NAFTIFINE

Chemical group: Allylamine derivative.

Chemical name: Naftifine hydrochloride—1-Naphthalenemethanamine, N-methyl-N-(3-phenyl-2-propenyl)-, hydrochloride, (E)-.

Molecular formula: Naftifine hydrochloride—$C_{21}H_{21}N \cdot HCl$.

Molecular weight: Naftifine hydrochloride—323.86.

Description: Naftifine hydrochloride—White to yellow, fine, crystalline powder.

pKa: Naftifine hydrochloride—6.82.

Solubility: Naftifine hydrochloride—0.68 mg/mL in water and 3.4 mg/mL in alcohol at 25 °C.

USP requirements:
Naftifine Hydrochloride USP—Preserve in tight containers. Contains not less than 99.0% and not more than 101.0% of naftifine hydrochloride, calculated on the dried basis. Meets the requirements for Identification, Melting range (175–179 °C), Loss on drying (not more than 0.5%), Residue on ignition (not more than 0.1%), Heavy metals (not more than 0.001%), and Chromatographic purity.
Naftifine Hydrochloride Cream USP—Preserve in tight containers. Contains the labeled amount, within ±10%, in a water-miscible base. Meets the requirements for Identification, Microbial limits, Minimum fill, and pH (4.0–6.0).
Naftifine Hydrochloride Gel USP—Preserve in tight containers. Contains the labeled amount, within ±10%, in a water-miscible base. Meets the requirements for Identification, Microbial limits, Minimum fill, pH (5.5–7.5), and Content of alcohol (40–45%).

NALBUPHINE

Chemical name: Nalbuphine hydrochloride—Morphinan-3,6,14-triol, 17-(cyclobutylmethyl)-4,5-epoxy-, hydrochloride, (5 alpha,6 alpha)-.

Molecular formula: Nalbuphine hydrochloride—$C_{21}H_{27}NO_4 \cdot HCl$.

Molecular weight: Nalbuphine hydrochloride—393.90.

Description: Nalbuphine hydrochloride—White to slightly off-white powder.

pKa: Nalbuphine hydrochloride—8.71 and 9.96.

Solubility: Nalbuphine hydrochloride—Soluble in water; slightly soluble in alcohol.

USP requirements: Nalbuphine Hydrochloride Injection—Not in *USP–NF.*

NALIDIXIC ACID

Chemical group: Closely related to cinoxacin.

Chemical name: 1,8-Naphthyridine-3-carboxylic acid, 1-ethyl-1,4-dihydro-7-methyl-4-oxo-.

Molecular formula: $C_{12}H_{12}N_2O_3$.

Molecular weight: 232.24.

Description: Nalidixic Acid USP—White to very pale yellow, odorless, crystalline powder.

Solubility: Nalidixic Acid USP—Soluble in chloroform, in methylene chloride, and in solutions of fixed alkali hydroxides and carbonates; slightly soluble in acetone, in alcohol, in methanol, and in toluene; very slightly soluble in ether and in water.

USP requirements:
Nalidixic Acid USP—Preserve in tight containers. Contains not less than 99.0% and not more than 101.0% of nalidixic acid, calculated on the dried basis. Meets the requirements for Identification, Melting range (225–231 °C), Loss on drying (not more than 0.5%), Residue on ignition (not more than 0.1%), Heavy metals (not more than 0.002%), and Chromatographic purity.
Nalidixic Acid Oral Suspension USP—Preserve in tight containers. Contains the labeled amount, within ±5%, in a suitable aqueous vehicle. Meets the requirement for Identification.
Nalidixic Acid Tablets USP—Preserve in tight containers. Contain the labeled amount, within ±7%. Meet the requirements for Identification, Dissolution (80% in 30 minutes in pH 8.60 buffer in Apparatus 2 at 60 rpm), and Uniformity of dosage units.

NALMEFENE

Chemical name: Nalmefene hydrochloride—17-(Cyclopropylmethyl)-4,5 alpha-epoxy-6-methylenemorphinan-3, 14-diol, hydrochloride salt.

Molecular formula: Nalmefene hydrochloride—$C_{21}H_{25}NO_3 \cdot HCl$.

Molecular weight: Nalmefene hydrochloride—375.9.

Description: Nalmefene hydrochloride—White to off-white crystalline powder.

pKa: Nalmefene hydrochloride—7.6.

Solubility: Nalmefene hydrochloride—Freely soluble in water up to 130 mg/mL; slightly soluble in chloroform up to 0.13 mg/mL.

USP requirements: Nalmefene Hydrochloride Injection—Not in *USP–NF.*

NALORPHINE

Chemical name: Nalorphine hydrochloride—Morphinan-3,6-diol, 7,8-didehydro-4,5-epoxy-17-(2-propenyl)-(5 alpha,6 alpha)-, hydrochloride.

Molecular formula: Nalorphine hydrochloride—$C_{19}H_{21}NO_3 \cdot HCl$.

Molecular weight: Nalorphine hydrochloride—347.84.

Description: Nalorphine hydrochloride—White or practically white, odorless, crystalline powder, slowly darkening on exposure to air and light. Melting point about 261 °C.

Solubility: Nalorphine hydrochloride—1 gram in about 8 mL of water or about 35 mL of alcohol; insoluble in chloroform or in ether; soluble in diluted alkali hydroxide solution.

USP requirements:
Nalorphine Hydrochloride USP—Preserve in tight, light-resistant containers. Contains not less than 97.0% and not more than 103.0% of nalorphine hydrochloride, calculated on the dried basis. Meets the requirements for Identification, Specific rotation (−122° to −125°), Loss on drying (not more than 0.5%), and Residue on ignition (not more than 0.1%).

Nalorphine Hydrochloride Injection USP—Preserve in single-dose or in multiple-dose containers, preferably of Type I glass. A suitably buffered, sterile solution of Nalorphine Hydrochloride in Water for Injection. Contains the labeled amount, within ±10%. Meets the requirements for Identification, Bacterial endotoxins, and pH (6.0–7.5), and for Injections.

NALOXONE

Chemical name: Naloxone hydrochloride—Morphinan-6-one, 4,5-epoxy-3,14-dihydroxy-17-(2-propenyl)-, hydrochloride, (5 alpha)-.

Molecular formula: Naloxone hydrochloride—$C_{19}H_{21}NO_4 \cdot HCl$.

Molecular weight: Naloxone hydrochloride—363.84.

Description:
Naloxone Hydrochloride USP—White to slightly off-white powder. Its aqueous solution is acidic.
Naloxone Hydrochloride Injection USP—Clear, colorless liquid.

Solubility: Naloxone Hydrochloride USP—Soluble in water, in dilute acids, and in strong alkali; slightly soluble in alcohol; practically insoluble in ether and in chloroform.

USP requirements:
Naloxone Hydrochloride USP—Preserve in tight, light-resistant containers. It is anhydrous or contains two molecules of water of hydration. Contains not less than 98.0% and not more than 100.5% of naloxone hydrochloride, calculated on the dried basis. Meets the requirements for Identification, Specific rotation (−170° to −181°), Loss on drying (not more than 0.5% for the anhydrous form and not more than 11.0% for the hydrous form), Noroxymorphone hydrochloride and other impurities, and Chloride content (9.54–9.94%, calculated on the dried basis).

Naloxone Hydrochloride Injection USP—Preserve in single-dose or in multiple-dose containers of Type I glass, protected from light. A sterile, isotonic solution of Naloxone Hydrochloride in Water for Injection. Contains the labeled amount, within ±10%. Meets the requirements for Identification, Bacterial endotoxins, pH (3.0–6.5), and Limit of 2,2′-bisnaloxone (not more than 4.0%), and for Injections.

NALTREXONE

Chemical group: A synthetic congener of oxymorphone; technically a thebaine derivative; also chemically related to the opioid antagonist naloxone.

Chemical name: Naltrexone hydrochloride—Morphinan-6-one, 17-(cyclopropylmethyl)-4,5-epoxyl-3,14-dihydroxy-, hydrochloride, (5 alpha)-.

Molecular formula: Naltrexone hydrochloride—$C_{20}H_{23}NO_4 \cdot HCl$.

Molecular weight: Naltrexone hydrochloride—377.87.

Description: Naltrexone hydrochloride—White, crystalline compound.

Solubility: Naltrexone hydrochloride—Soluble in water to the extent of about 100 mg per mL.

USP requirements:
Naltrexone Hydrochloride USP—Preserve in tight containers. Contains not less than 98.0% and not more than 102.0% of naltrexone hydrochloride, calculated on the anhydrous, solvent-free basis. Meets the requirements for Completeness of solution, Identification, Specific rotation (−187° to −197°, calculated on the anhydrous, solvent-free basis), Water, Residue on ignition (not more than 0.1%), Heavy metals (not more than 0.002%), Limit of total solvents (the sum of water and alcohol solvents is not more than 5.0% for the anhydrous form and not more than 11.0% for the dihydrate form), Related compounds (not more than 0.5% of any individual related compound, and the total of all related compounds not more than 1.5%), and Content of chloride (9.20% to 9.58%, calculated on the anhydrous, solvent-free basis).

Naltrexone Hydrochloride Tablets USP—Preserve in tight containers. Contain labeled amount, within ±10%. Meet the requirements for Identification, Dissolution (80% in 60 minutes in water in Apparatus 2 at 50 rpm), and Uniformity of dosage units.

NANDROLONE

Chemical name:
Nandrolone decanoate—Estr-4-en-3-one, 17-[(1-oxodecyl)oxy]-, (17 beta)-.
Nandrolone phenpropionate—Estr-4-en-3-one, 17-(1-oxo-3-phenylpropoxy)-, (17 beta)-.

Molecular formula:
Nandrolone decanoate—$C_{28}H_{44}O_3$.
Nandrolone phenpropionate—$C_{27}H_{34}O_3$.

Molecular weight:
Nandrolone decanoate—428.65.
Nandrolone phenpropionate—406.56.

Description:
Nandrolone Decanoate USP—Fine, white to creamy white, crystalline powder. Is odorless, or may have a slight odor.
Nandrolone phenpropionate—Fine, white to creamy white, crystalline powder, having a slight, characteristic odor.

Solubility:
Nandrolone Decanoate USP—Practically insoluble in water; soluble in chloroform, in alcohol, in acetone, and in vegetable oils.
Nandrolone phenpropionate—Practically insoluble in water; soluble in alcohol, in chloroform, in dioxane, and in vegetable oils.

USP requirements:
Nandrolone Decanoate USP—Preserve in tight, light-resistant containers, and store in a refrigerator. Contains not less than 97.0% and not more than 103.0% of nandrolone decanoate, calculated on the dried basis. Meets the requirements for Completeness and clarity of solution, Identification, Melting range (33–37 °C), Specific rotation (+32° to +36°), Loss on drying (not more than 0.5%), Chromatographic purity (the sum of all impurities not more than 3.0%), and Organic volatile impurities.

Nandrolone Decanoate Injection USP—Preserve in single-dose or in multiple-dose containers, preferably of Type I glass, protected from light. A sterile solution of Nandrolone Decanoate in Sesame Oil, with a suitable preservative. Contains the labeled amount, within ±10%. Meets the requirements for Identification and Limit of nandrolone (not more than 1.0%), and for Injections.

Nandrolone Phenpropionate USP—Preserve in tight, light-resistant containers. Contains not less than 97.0% and not more than 103.0% of nandrolone phenpropionate, calculated on the dried basis. Meets the requirements for Identification, Melting range (95–99 °C), Specific rotation (+48° to +51°), Loss on drying (not more than 0.5%), and Organic volatile impurities.

Nandrolone Phenpropionate Injection USP—Preserve in single-dose or in multiple-dose containers, preferably of Type I glass, protected from light. A sterile solution of Nandrolone Phenpropionate in a suitable oil. Contains the labeled amount, within ±10%. Meets the requirements for Identification and Limit of nandrolone, and for Injections.

NAPHAZOLINE

Chemical name: Naphazoline hydrochloride—1*H*-Imidazole, 4,5-dihydro-2-(1-naphthalenylmethyl)-, monohydrochloride.

Molecular formula: Naphazoline hydrochloride—$C_{14}H_{14}N_2 \cdot HCl$.

Molecular weight: Naphazoline hydrochloride—246.74.

Description: Naphazoline Hydrochloride USP—White, crystalline powder. Is odorless. Melts at a temperature of about 255 °C, with decomposition.

Solubility: Naphazoline Hydrochloride USP—Freely soluble in water and in alcohol; very slightly soluble in chloroform; practically insoluble in ether.

USP requirements:

Naphazoline Hydrochloride USP—Preserve in tight, light-resistant containers. Contains not less than 98.0% and not more than 100.5% of naphazoline hydrochloride, calculated on the dried basis. Meets the requirements for Identification, pH (5.0–6.6, in a 1 in 100 solution in carbon dioxide-free water), Loss on drying (not more than 0.5%), Residue on ignition (not more than 0.2%), and Ordinary impurities.

Naphazoline Hydrochloride Nasal Solution USP—Preserve in tight, light-resistant containers. A solution of Naphazoline Hydrochloride in water adjusted to a suitable pH and tonicity. Contains the labeled amount, within ±10%. Meets the requirement for Identification.

Naphazoline Hydrochloride Ophthalmic Solution USP—Preserve in tight containers. A sterile, buffered solution of Naphazoline Hydrochloride in water adjusted to a suitable tonicity. Contains the labeled amount, within −10% to +15%. Contains a suitable preservative. Meets the requirements for Identification, Sterility, and pH (5.5–7.0).

NAPHAZOLINE AND PHENIRAMINE

For *Naphazoline* and *Pheniramine*—See individual listings for chemistry information.

USP requirements: Naphazoline Hydrochloride and Pheniramine Maleate Ophthalmic Solution USP—Preserve in tight containers, and store at a temperature between 20° and 25°, protected from light. A sterile, buffered solution of Naphazoline Hydrochloride and Pheniramine Maleate in water adjusted to a suitable tonicity. Contains the labeled amount of each ingredient, within ±10%. contains a suitable preservative. Meets the requirements for Identification, Sterility, and pH (5.7–6.3).

NAPROXEN

Chemical group: Propionic acid derivative.

Chemical name:

Naproxen—2-Naphthaleneacetic acid, 6-methoxy-alpha-methyl-, (*S*)-.

Naproxen sodium—2-Naphthaleneacetic acid, 6-methoxy-alpha-methyl-, sodium salt, (*S*)-.

Molecular formula:

Naproxen—$C_{14}H_{14}O_3$.

Naproxen sodium—$C_{14}H_{13}NaO_3$.

Molecular weight:

Naproxen—230.26.

Naproxen sodium—252.24.

Description:

Naproxen USP—White to off-white, practically odorless, crystalline powder.

Naproxen Sodium USP—White to creamy crystalline powder. Melts at about 255 °C, with decomposition.

pKa: 4.15 (apparent).

Solubility:

Naproxen USP—Practically insoluble in water; freely soluble in chloroform and in dehydrated alcohol; soluble in alcohol; sparingly soluble in ether.

Naproxen Sodium USP—Soluble in water and in methanol; sparingly soluble in alcohol; very slightly soluble in acetone; practically insoluble in chloroform and in toluene.

USP requirements:

Naproxen USP—Preserve in tight containers. Contains not less than 98.5% and not more than 101.5% of naproxen, calculated on the dried basis. Meets the requirements for Identification, Specific rotation (+63.0° to +68.5°), Loss on drying (not more than 0.5%), Heavy metals (not more than 0.002%), Chromatographic purity, and Organic volatile impurities.

Naproxen Suppositories—Not in *USP–NF*.

Naproxen Oral Suspension USP—Preserve in tight, light-resistant containers. Store at room temperature. Contains the labeled amount, within ±10%. Meets the requirements for Identification and pH (2.2–3.7).

Naproxen Tablets USP—Preserve in well-closed containers. Contain the labeled amount, within ±10%. Meet the requirements for Identification, Dissolution (80% in 45 minutes in 0.1 *M* phosphate buffer [pH 7.4] in Apparatus 2 at 50 rpm), and Uniformity of dosage units.

Naproxen Delayed-release Tablets—Not in *USP–NF*.

Naproxen Extended-release Tablets—Not in *USP–NF*.

Naproxen Sodium USP—Preserve in tight containers. Contains not less than 98.0% and not more than 102.0% of naproxen sodium, calculated on the dried basis. Meets the requirements for Identification, Specific rotation (−15.3° to −17.0°), Loss on drying (not more than 1.0%), Heavy metals (not more than 0.002%), Free naproxen (not more than 1.0%), Chromatographic purity, and Organic volatile impurities.

Naproxen Sodium Tablets USP—Preserve in well-closed containers. Contain the labeled amount, within ±10%. Meet the requirements for Identification, Dissolution (80% in 45 minutes in 0.1 *M* phosphate buffer [pH 7.4] in Apparatus 2 at 50 rpm), and Uniformity of dosage units.

Naproxen Sodium Extended-release Tablets—Not in *USP–NF*.

NARASIN

Chemical name: 2*H*-Pyran-2-acetic acid, alpha-ethyl-6-[5-[2-(5-ethyltetrahydro-5-hydroxy-6-methyl-2*H*-pyran-2-yl)-15-hydroxy-2,10,12-trimethyl-1,6,8-trioxadispiro[4.1.5.3]pentadec-13-en-9-yl]-2-hydroxy-1,3-dimethyl-4-oxoheptyl]tetrahydro-3,5-dimethyl-.

Molecular formula:
Narasin A—$C_{43}H_{72}O_{11}$.
Narasin B—$C_{43}H_{71}O_{11}$.
Narasin D—$C_{44}H_{74}O_{11}$.
Narasin I—$C_{44}H_{74}O_{11}$.

Molecular weight:
Narasin A—765.03.
Narasin B—764.03.
Narasin D—779.07.
Narasin I—779.07.

Description: White to off-white, crystalline powder. Melts at about 217 °C, with decomposition.

Solubility: Soluble in methanol and in water.

USP requirements:
Narasin Granular USP—Preserve in well-closed containers. Avoid moisture and excessive heat. Contains narasin mixed with suitable carriers and inactive ingredients prepared in a granular form that is free-flowing and free of aggregates. Label it to indicate that it is for animal use only. Label it also to indicate that it is for manufacturing, processing, or repackaging. Contains not less than 100 mg and not more than 160 mg of narasin per gram. Meets the requirements for Identification, Loss on drying (not more than 10%), Powder fineness (not less than 99% passes a No. 30 sieve, and not more than 15% passes a No. 140 sieve), and Content of narasin A (not less than 85%).
Narasin Premix USP—Preserve in well-closed containers. Avoid moisture and excessive heat. Contains Narasin Granular mixed with suitable diluents and inactive ingredients. Label it to indicate that it is for animal use only. The label bears the statement, "Do not feed undiluted." Contains labeled amount of narasin, within ±10%. Meets the requirements for Identification and Loss on drying (not more than 12%).

NARATRIPTAN

Chemical name: Naratriptan hydrochloride—1*H*-Indole-5-ethanesulfonamide, *N*-methyl-3-(1-methyl-4-piperidinyl)-, monohydrochloride.

Molecular formula: Naratriptan hydrochloride—$C_{17}H_{25}N_3O_2S$ · HCl.

Molecular weight: Naratriptan hydrochloride—371.93.

Description: Naratriptan hydrochloride—White to pale yellow powder. It melts at 246 °C.

pKa: Naratriptan hydrochloride—9.7 (piperidinyl nitrogen).

Solubility: Naratriptan hydrochloride—Readily soluble in water.

USP requirements: Naratriptan Hydrochloride Tablets—Not in *USP–NF*.

NATAMYCIN

Source: Derived from *Streptomyces natalensis*.

Chemical group: Tetraene polyene antifungal.

Chemical name: Pimaricin.

Molecular formula: $C_{33}H_{47}NO_{13}$.

Molecular weight: 665.73.

Description: Natamycin USP—Off-white to cream-colored powder, which may contain up to 3 moles of water.

Solubility: Natamycin USP—Practically insoluble in water; slightly soluble in methanol; soluble in glacial acetic acid and in dimethylformamide.

USP requirements:
Natamycin USP—Preserve in tight, light-resistant containers. Contains not less than 90.0% and not more than 102.0% of natamycin, calculated on the anhydrous basis. Meets the requirements for Identification, Crystallinity, pH (5.0–7.5, in an aqueous suspension containing 10 mg per mL), and Water (6.0–9.0%).
Natamycin Ophthalmic Suspension USP—Preserve in tight, light-resistant containers. The containers or individual cartons are sealed and tamper-proof so that sterility is assured at time of first use. A sterile suspension of Natamycin in a suitable aqueous vehicle. Contains one or more suitable preservatives. Contains the labeled amount, within −10% to +25%. Meets the requirements for Identification, Sterility, and pH (5.0–7.5).

NATEGLINIDE

Chemical name: D-Phenylalamine, *N*-[[*trans*-4-(1-methylethyl)-cyclohexyl]carbonyl].

Molecular formula: $C_{19}H_{27}NO_3$.

Molecular weight: 317.43.

Description: White powder.

Solubility: Freely soluble in methanol, in ethanol, and in chloroform; soluble in ether; sparingly soluble in acetonitrile and in octanol; practically insoluble in water.

USP requirements: Nateglinide Tablets—Not in *USP–NF*.

NEDOCROMIL

Chemical group: Nedocromil sodium—Pyranoquinoline.

Chemical name:
Nedocromil—4*H*-Pyrano[3,2-*g*]quinoline-2,8-dicarboxylic acid, 9-ethyl-6,9-dihydro-4,6-dioxo-10-propyl-.
Nedocromil sodium—4*H*-Pyrano[3,2-*g*]quinoline-2,8-dicarboxylic acid, 9-ethyl-6,9-dihydro-4,6-dioxo-10-propyl, disodium salt.

Molecular formula:
Nedocromil—$C_{19}H_{17}NO_7$.
Nedocromil sodium—$C_{19}H_{15}NNa_2O_7$.

Molecular weight:
Nedocromil—371.34.
Nedocromil sodium—415.31.

Description: Nedocromil sodium—Yellow powder. Melting point over 300 °C with decomposition.

pKa: 2.

Solubility: Nedocromil sodium—Soluble in water. Greater than 26 mg/mL at 24 °C in aqueous buffer at pH 4.4–7.4.

USP requirements:
Nadocromil Inhalation Aerosol—Not in *USP–NF*.
Nedocromil Sodium Inhalation Aerosol—Not in *USP–NF*.
Nedocromil Sodium Ophthalmic Solution—Not in *USP–NF*.

NEFAZODONE

Chemical group: Nefazodone hydrochloride—Synthetic phenylpiperazine derivative.

Chemical name:
Nefazodone—2-[3-[4-(3-Chlorophenyl)-1-piperazinyl]propyl]-5-ethyl-2,4-dihydro-4-(2-phenoxyethyl)-3*H*-1,2,4-triazol-3-one.
Nefazodone hydrochloride—3*H*-1,2,4-Triazol-3-one, 2-[3-[4-(3-chlorophenyl)-1-piperazinyl)]propyl-5-ethyl-2,4-dihydro-4-(2-phenoxyethyl)-, monohydrochloride.

Molecular formula:
Nefazodone—$C_{25}H_{32}ClN_5O_2$.
Nefazodone hydrochloride—$C_{25}H_{32}ClN_5O_2 \cdot HCl$.

Molecular weight:
Nefazodone—470.01.
Nefazodone hydrochloride—506.47.

Description:
Nefazodone—Melting point 83–84 °C.
Nefazodone hydrochloride—Nonhygroscopic, white crystalline solid.

Solubility: Nefazodone hydrochloride—Freely soluble in chloroform; soluble in propylene glycol; slightly soluble in polyethylene glycol and in water.

USP requirements:
Nefazodone Tablets—Not in *USP–NF*.
Nefazodone Hydrochloride Tablets—Not in *USP–NF*.

NELFINAVIR

Chemical name: Nelfinavir mesylate—3-Isoquinolinecarboxamide, *N*-(1,1-dimethylethyl)decahydro-2-[2-hydroxy-3-[(3-hydroxy-2-methylbenzoyl)amino]-4-(phenylthio)butyl], [3*S*-[2(2*S**,3*S**),3 alpha,4a beta,8a beta]]-, monomethanesulfonate (salt).

Molecular formula: Nelfinavir mesylate—$C_{32}H_{45}N_3O_4S \cdot CH_4O_3S$.

Molecular weight: Nelfinavir mesylate—663.89.

USP requirements:
Nelfinavir Mesylate Oral Powder—Not in *USP–NF*.
Nelfinavir Mesylate Tablets—Not in *USP–NF*.

NEOMYCIN

Chemical group: Aminoglycosides.

Chemical name: Neomycin sulfate.

Description: Neomycin Sulfate USP—White to slightly yellow powder, or cryodesiccated solid. Is odorless or practically so and is hygroscopic. Its solutions are dextrorotatory.

Solubility: Neomycin Sulfate USP—Freely soluble in water; very slightly soluble in alcohol; insoluble in acetone, in chloroform, and in ether.

USP requirements:
Neomycin Boluses USP—Preserve in tight containers. Label Boluses to indicate that they are for veterinary use only. Contain an amount of Neomycin Sulfate equivalent to the labeled amount of neomycin, within −10% to +25%. Meet the requirements for Identification, Uniformity of dosage units, and Disintegration (60 minutes).
Neomycin for Injection USP—Preserve in Containers for Sterile Solids. Contains an amount of neomycin sulfate equivalent to the labeled amount of neomycin within −10% to +20%. Meets the requirements for Bacterial endotoxins, Thin-layer chromatographic identification test, and Sterility, and requirements for pH and Loss on drying under Neomycin Sulfate, and for Uniformity of dosage units and Labeling under Injections.
Neomycin Sulfate USP—Preserve in tight, light-resistant containers. The sulfate salt of a kind of neomycin, an antibacterial substance produced by the growth of *Streptomyces fradiae* Waksman (Fam. Streptomycetaceae), or a mixture of two or more such salts. Where it is intended for use in preparing injectable or other sterile dosage forms, the label states that it is sterile or must be subjected to further processing during the preparation of injectable or other sterile dosage forms. Has a potency equivalent to not less than 600 mcg of neomycin per mg, calculated on the dried basis. Meets the requirements for Identification, pH (5.0–7.5, in a solution containing 33 mg of neomycin per mL), and Loss on drying (not more than 8.0%), and for Sterility and Bacterial endotoxins under Neomycin for Injection (where the label states that Neomycin Sulfate is sterile), and for Bacterial endotoxins under Neomycin for Injection (where the label states that Neomycin Sulfate must be subjected to further processing during the preparation of injectable dosage forms. It is exempt from the requirements for Bacterial endotoxins (where it is intended for use in preparing nonparenteral sterile dosage forms).
Neomycin Sulfate Cream USP—Preserve in well-closed containers, preferably at controlled room temperature. Contains an amount of neomycin sulfate equivalent to the labeled amount of neomycin, within −10% to +35%. Meets the requirements for Thin-layer chromatographic identification test and Minimum fill.
Neomycin Sulfate Ointment USP—Preserve in well-closed containers, preferably at controlled room temperature. Contains an amount of neomycin sulfate equivalent to the labeled amount of neomycin, within −10% to +35%. Meets the requirements for Thin-layer chromatographic identification test, Minimum fill, and Water (not more than 1.0%).
Neomycin Sulfate Ophthalmic Ointment USP—Preserve in collapsible ophthalmic ointment tubes. A sterile preparation of Neomycin Sulfate in a suitable ointment base. Contains an amount of neomycin sulfate equivalent to the labeled amount of neomycin, within −10% to +35%. Meets the requirements for Thin-layer chromatographic identification test, Sterility, Minimum fill, Water (not more than 1.0%), and Metal particles.
Neomycin Sulfate Oral Solution USP—Preserve in tight, light-resistant containers, preferably at controlled room temperature. Contains an amount of neomycin sulfate equivalent to the labeled amount of neomycin, within −10% to +25%. Meets the requirements for Thin-layer chromatographic identification test and pH (5.0–7.5).
Neomycin Sulfate Tablets USP—Preserve in tight containers. Contain an amount of neomycin sulfate equivalent to the labeled amount of neomycin, within −10% to +25%. Meet the requirements for Thin-layer chromatographic identification test, Disintegration (60 minutes), Uniformity of dosage units, and Loss on drying (not more than 10.0%).

NEOMYCIN AND BACITRACIN

For *Neomycin* and *Bacitracin*—See individual listings for chemistry information.

USP requirements:
Neomycin Sulfate and Bacitracin Ointment USP—Preserve in tight, light-resistant containers, preferably at controlled room temperature. Contains amounts of neomycin sulfate and bacitracin equivalent to the labeled amounts of neomycin and bacitracin, within −10% to +30%. Meets the requirements for Thin-layer chromatographic identification test, Minimum fill, and Water (not more than 0.5%).

Neomycin Sulfate and Bacitracin Zinc Ointment USP—Preserve in collapsible tubes or in well-closed containers. Contains amounts of neomycin sulfate and bacitracin zinc equivalent to the labeled amounts of neomycin and bacitracin, within −10% to +30%. Meets the requirements for Thin-layer chromatographic identification test, Minimum fill, and Water (not more than 0.5%).

NEOMYCIN AND DEXAMETHASONE

For *Neomycin* and *Dexamethasone*—See individual listings for chemistry information.

USP requirements:
Neomycin Sulfate and Dexamethasone Sodium Phosphate Cream USP—Preserve in collapsible tubes or in tight containers. Contains an amount of neomycin sulfate equivalent to the labeled amount of neomycin, within −10% to +35%, and an amount of dexamethasone sodium phosphate equivalent to the labeled amount of dexamethasone phosphate, within ±10%. Meets the requirements for Identification and Minimum fill.

Neomycin Sulfate and Dexamethasone Sodium Phosphate Ophthalmic Ointment USP—Preserve in collapsible ophthalmic ointment tubes. A sterile ointment containing Neomycin Sulfate and Dexamethasone Sodium Phosphate. Contains an amount of neomycin sulfate equivalent to the labeled amount of neomycin, within −10% to +35%, and an amount of dexamethasone sodium phosphate equivalent to the labeled amount of dexamethasone phosphate, within ±10%. Meets the requirements for Identification, Sterility, Minimum fill, Water (not more than 1.0%), and Metal particles.

Note: Where Neomycin Sulfate and Dexamethasone Sodium Phosphate Ophthalmic Ointment is prescribed without reference to the quantity of neomycin or dexamethasone phosphate contained therein, a product containing 3.5 mg of neomycin and 0.5 mg of dexamethasone phosphate per gram shall be dispensed.

Neomycin Sulfate and Dexamethasone Sodium Phosphate Ophthalmic Solution USP—Preserve in tight, light-resistant containers, and avoid exposure to excessive heat. A sterile, aqueous solution of Neomycin Sulfate and Dexamethasone Sodium Phosphate. Contains an amount of neomycin sulfate equivalent to the labeled amount of neomycin, within −10% to +30%, and an amount of dexamethasone sodium phosphate equivalent to the labeled amount of dexamethasone phosphate, within −10% to +15%. Meets the requirements for Identification, Sterility, and pH (6.0–8.0).

Note: Where Neomycin Sulfate and Dexamethasone Sodium Phosphate Ophthalmic Solution is prescribed, without reference to the amount of neomycin or dexamethasone phosphate contained therein, a product containing 3.5 mg of neomycin and 1.0 mg of dexamethasone phosphate per mL shall be dispensed.

NEOMYCIN AND FLUOCINOLONE

For *Neomycin* and *Fluocinolone*—See individual listings for chemistry information.

USP requirements: Neomycin Sulfate and Fluocinolone Acetonide Cream USP—Preserve in collapsible tubes or in tight containers. Contains an amount of neomycin sulfate equivalent to the labeled amount of neomycin, within −10% to +35%, and the labeled amount of fluocinolone acetonide, within ±10%. Meets the requirements for Identification and Minimum fill.

NEOMYCIN AND FLUOROMETHOLONE

For *Neomycin* and *Fluorometholone*—See individual listings for chemistry information.

USP requirements: Neomycin Sulfate and Fluorometholone Ointment USP—Preserve in collapsible tubes or in well-closed containers. Contains an amount of neomycin sulfate equivalent to the labeled amount of neomycin, within −10% to: +35%, and the labeled amount of fluorometholone, within ± 10%. Meets the requirements for Identification, Minimum fill, and Water (not more than 1.0%).

NEOMYCIN AND FLURANDRENOLIDE

For *Neomycin* and *Flurandrenolide*—See individual listings for chemistry information.

USP requirements:
Neomycin Sulfate and Flurandrenolide Cream USP—Preserve in collapsible tubes or in tight containers, protected from light. Contains an amount of neomycin sulfate equivalent to the labeled amount of neomycin, within −10% to +35%, and the labeled amount of flurandrenolide, within ±10%. Meets the requirements for Identification and Minimum fill.

Neomycin Sulfate and Flurandrenolide Lotion USP—Preserve in tight containers, protected from light. Contains an amount of neomycin sulfate equivalent to the labeled amount of neomycin, within −10% to +30%, and the labeled amount of flurandrenolide, within ±10%. Meets the requirements for Identification, Microbial limits, and Minimum fill.

Neomycin Sulfate and Flurandrenolide Ointment USP—Preserve in collapsible tubes or in tight containers, protected from light. Contains an amount of neomycin sulfate equivalent to the labeled amount of neomycin, within −10% to +35%, and the labeled amount of flurandrenolide, within ±10%. Meets the requirements for Identification, Minimum fill, and Water (not more than 1.0%).

NEOMYCIN AND GRAMICIDIN

For *Neomycin* and *Gramicidin*—See individual listings for chemistry information.

USP requirements: Neomycin Sulfate and Gramicidin Ointment USP—Preserve in collapsible tubes or in well-closed containers. Contains amounts of neomycin sulfate and gramicidin

equivalent to the labeled amounts of neomycin and gramicidin, within −10% to +40%. Meets the requirements for Identification, Minimum fill, and Water (not more than 1.0%).

NEOMYCIN AND HYDROCORTISONE

For *Neomycin* and *Hydrocortisone*—See individual listings for chemistry information.

USP requirements:

Neomycin Sulfate and Hydrocortisone Cream USP—Preserve in collapsible tubes or in well-closed containers. Contains an amount of neomycin sulfate equivalent to the labeled amount of neomycin, within −10% to +35%, and the labeled amount of hydrocortisone, within ±10%. Meets the requirements for Identification and Minimum fill.

Neomycin Sulfate and Hydrocortisone Ointment USP—Preserve in collapsible tubes or in well-closed containers. Contains an amount of neomycin sulfate equivalent to the labeled amount of neomycin, within −10% to +35%, and the labeled amount of hydrocortisone, within ±10%. Meets the requirements for Identification, Minimum fill, and Water (not more than 1.0%).

Neomycin Sulfate and Hydrocortisone Otic Suspension USP—Preserve in tight, light-resistant containers. A sterile suspension. Contains an amount of neomycin sulfate equivalent to the labeled amount of neomycin, within −10% to +30%, and the labeled amount of hydrocortisone, within ±10%. Contains Acetic Acid. Meets the requirements for Sterility and pH (4.5–6.0).

Note: Where Neomycin Sulfate and Hydrocortisone Otic Suspension is prescribed, without reference to the quantity of neomycin or hydrocortisone contained therein, a product containing 3.5 mg of neomycin and 10 mg of hydrocortisone per mL shall be dispensed.

Neomycin Sulfate and Hydrocortisone Acetate Cream USP—Preserve in well-closed containers. Contains an amount of neomycin sulfate equivalent to the labeled amount of neomycin, within −10% to +35%, and the labeled amount of hydrocortisone acetate, within ±10%. Meets the requirements for Identification and Minimum fill.

Neomycin Sulfate and Hydrocortisone Acetate Lotion USP—Preserve in well-closed containers. Contains an amount of neomycin sulfate equivalent to the labeled amount of neomycin, within −10% to +30%, and the labeled amount of hydrocortisone acetate, within ±10%. Meets the requirements for Identification and Minimum fill.

Neomycin Sulfate and Hydrocortisone Acetate Ointment USP—Preserve in collapsible tubes or in well-closed containers. Contains an amount of neomycin sulfate equivalent to the labeled amount of neomycin, within −10% to +35%, and the labeled amount of hydrocortisone acetate, within ±10%. Meets the requirements for Identification, Minimum fill, and Water (not more than 1.0%).

Neomycin Sulfate and Hydrocortisone Acetate Ophthalmic Ointment USP—Preserve in collapsible ophthalmic ointment tubes. Contains an amount of neomycin sulfate equivalent to the labeled amount of neomycin, within −10% to +35%, and the labeled amount of hydrocortisone acetate, within ±10%. Meets the requirements for Identification, Sterility, Minimum fill, Water (not more than 1.0%), and Metal particles.

Neomycin Sulfate and Hydrocortisone Acetate Ophthalmic Suspension USP—Preserve in tight containers. The containers or individual cartons are sealed and tamper-proof so that sterility is assured at time of first use. A sterile, aqueous suspension. Contains an amount of neomycin sulfate equivalent to the labeled amount of neomycin,

within −10% to +30%, and the labeled amount of hydrocortisone acetate, within ±10%. Meets the requirements for Identification, Sterility, and pH (5.5–7.5).

NEOMYCIN AND METHYLPREDNISOLONE

For *Neomycin* and *Methylprednisolone*—See individual listings for chemistry information.

USP requirements: Neomycin Sulfate and Methylprednisolone Acetate Cream USP—Preserve in collapsible tubes or in tight containers, protected from light. Contains an amount of neomycin sulfate equivalent to the labeled amount of neomycin, within −10% to +35%, and the labeled amount of methylprednisolone acetate, within ±10%. Meets the requirements for Identification and Minimum fill.

NEOMYCIN AND POLYMYXIN B

For *Neomycin* and *Polymyxin B*—See individual listings for chemistry information.

USP requirements:

Neomycin and Polymyxin B Sulfates Cream USP—Preserve in well-closed containers, preferably at controlled room temperature. Contains amounts of neomycin sulfate and polymyxin B sulfate equivalent to the labeled amounts of neomycin and polymyxin B, within −10% to +30%. May contain a suitable local anesthetic. Meets the requirements for Thin-layer chromatographic identification test and Minimum fill.

Neomycin and Polymyxin B Sulfates Ophthalmic Ointment USP—Preserve in collapsible ophthalmic ointment tubes. A sterile ointment containing Neomycin Sulfate and Polymyxin B Sulfate. Contains amounts of neomycin sulfate and polymyxin B sulfate equivalent to the labeled amounts of neomycin and polymyxin B, within −10% to +30%. Meets the requirements for Thin-layer chromatographic identification test, Sterility, Minimum fill, Water (not more than 0.5%), and Metal particles.

Neomycin and Polymyxin B Sulfates Solution for Irrigation USP—Preserve in tight containers. A sterile, aqueous solution. Label it to indicate that it is to be diluted for use in a urinary bladder irrigation and is not intended for injection. Contains amounts of neomycin sulfate and polymyxin B sulfate equivalent to the labeled amounts of neomycin and polymyxin B, within −10% to +30%. Meets the requirements for Thin-layer chromatographic identification test, Sterility, and pH (4.5–6.0).

Neomycin and Polymyxin B Sulfates Ophthalmic Solution USP—Preserve in tight containers, and avoid exposure to excessive heat. Contains amounts of neomycin sulfate and polymyxin B sulfate equivalent to the labeled amounts of neomycin and polymyxin B, within −10% to +30%. Meets the requirements for Thin-layer chromatographic identification test, Sterility, and pH (5.0–7.0).

NEOMYCIN, ISOFLUPREDONE, AND TETRACAINE

For *Neomycin*, *Isoflupredone*, and *Tetracaine*—See individual listings for chemistry information.

USP requirements:

Neomycin Sulfate, Isoflupredone Acetate, and Tetracaine Hydrochloride Ointment USP—Preserve in collapsible tubes or well-closed containers. Label it to indicate that it is in-

tended for veterinary use only. Contains the equivalent of the labeled amount of neomycin, within −10% to +20%, and a labeled amount of isoflupredone acetate and tetracaine hydrochloride, within −7.5% to +17.5%, in a suitable ointment base. Meets the requirements for Identification, Minimum fill, and Water (not more than 1.0%).

Neomycin Sulfate, Isoflupredone Acetate, and Tetracaine Hydrochloride Topical Powder USP—Preserve in well-closed containers. Label it to indicate that it is intended for veterinary use only. Contains an amount equivalent to the labeled amount of neomycin, within −10% to +25%, and labeled amount of isoflupredone acetate and tetracaine hydrochloride, within −10% to +20%. Meets the requirements for Identification, Minimum fill, and Loss on drying (not more than 8.0%).

NEOMYCIN, POLYMYXIN B, AND BACITRACIN

For *Neomycin, Polymyxin B,* and *Bacitracin*—See individual listings for chemistry information.

USP requirements:

Neomycin and Polymyxin B Sulfates and Bacitracin Ointment USP—Preserve in tight, light-resistant containers, preferably at controlled room temperature. Contains amounts of neomycin sulfate, polymyxin B sulfate, and bacitracin equivalent to the labeled amounts of neomycin, polymyxin B, and bacitracin, within −10% to +30%. May contain a suitable local anesthetic. Meets the requirements for Thin-layer chromatographic identification test, Minimum fill, and Water (not more than 0.5%).

Neomycin and Polymyxin B Sulfates and Bacitracin Ophthalmic Ointment USP—Preserve in collapsible ophthalmic ointment tubes. A sterile ointment containing Neomycin Sulfate, Polymyxin B Sulfate, and Bacitracin. Contains amounts of neomycin sulfate, polymyxin B sulfate, and bacitracin equivalent to the labeled amounts of neomycin, polymyxin B, and bacitracin, within −10% to +40%. Meets the requirements for Thin-layer chromatographic identification test, Sterility, Minimum fill, Water (not more than 0.5%), and Metal particles.

Neomycin and Polymyxin B Sulfates and Bacitracin Zinc Ointment USP—Preserve in well-closed containers, preferably at controlled room temperature. Contains amounts of neomycin sulfate, polymyxin B sulfate, and bacitracin zinc equivalent to the labeled amounts of neomycin, polymyxin B, and bacitracin, within −10% to +30%. May contain a suitable local anesthetic. Meets the requirements for Thin-layer chromatographic identification test, Minimum fill, and Water (not more than 0.5%).

Neomycin and Polymyxin B Sulfates and Bacitracin Zinc Ophthalmic Ointment USP—Preserve in collapsible ophthalmic ointment tubes. Contains amounts of neomycin sulfate, polymyxin B sulfate, and bacitracin zinc equivalent to the labeled amounts of neomycin, polymyxin B, and bacitracin, within −10% to +40%. Meets the requirements for Thin-layer chromatographic identification test, Sterility, Minimum fill, Water (not more than 0.5%), and Metal particles.

NEOMYCIN, POLYMYXIN B, BACITRACIN, AND HYDROCORTISONE

For *Neomycin, Polymyxin B, Bacitracin,* and *Hydrocortisone*—See individual listings for chemistry information.

USP requirements:

Neomycin and Polymyxin B Sulfates, Bacitracin, and Hydrocortisone Acetate Ointment USP—Preserve in collapsible tubes or in well-closed containers. Contains amounts of neomycin sulfate, polymyxin B sulfate, and bacitracin equivalent to the labeled amounts of neomycin, polymyxin B, and bacitracin, within −10% to +30%, and the labeled amount of hydrocortisone acetate, within ±10%, in a suitable ointment base. Meets the requirements for Identification, Minimum fill, and Water (not more than 0.5%).

Neomycin and Polymyxin B Sulfates, Bacitracin, and Hydrocortisone Acetate Ophthalmic Ointment USP—Preserve in collapsible ophthalmic ointment tubes. Contains amounts of neomycin sulfate, polymyxin B sulfate, and bacitracin equivalent to the labeled amounts of neomycin, polymyxin B, and bacitracin, within −10% to +40%, and the labeled amount of hydrocortisone acetate, within ±10%, in a suitable ointment base. Meets the requirements for Identification, Sterility, Minimum fill, Water (not more than 0.5%), and Metal particles.

Neomycin and Polymyxin B Sulfates, Bacitracin Zinc, and Hydrocortisone Ointment USP—Preserve in well-closed containers, preferably at controlled room temperature. Contains amounts of neomycin sulfate, polymyxin B sulfate, and bacitracin zinc equivalent to the labeled amounts of neomycin, polymyxin B, and bacitracin, within −10% to +30%, and the labeled amount of hydrocortisone, within ±10%. Meets the requirements for Identification, Minimum fill, and Water (not more than 0.5%).

Neomycin and Polymyxin B Sulfates, Bacitracin Zinc, and Hydrocortisone Ophthalmic Ointment USP—Preserve in collapsible ophthalmic ointment tubes. A sterile ointment containing Neomycin Sulfate, Polymyxin B Sulfate, Bacitracin Zinc, and Hydrocortisone. Contains amounts of neomycin sulfate, polymyxin B sulfate, and bacitracin zinc equivalent to the labeled amounts of neomycin, polymyxin B, and bacitracin, within −10% to +40%, and the labeled amount of hydrocortisone, within ±10%. Meets the requirements for Identification, Sterility, Minimum fill, Water (not more than 0.5%), and Metal particles.

Neomycin and Polymyxin B Sulfates, Bacitracin Zinc, and Hydrocortisone Acetate Ophthalmic Ointment USP—Preserve in collapsible ophthalmic ointment tubes. A sterile ointment containing Neomycin Sulfate, Polymyxin B Sulfate, Bacitracin Zinc, and Hydrocortisone Acetate. Contains amounts of neomycin sulfate, polymyxin B sulfate, and bacitracin zinc equivalent to the labeled amounts of neomycin, polymyxin B, and bacitracin, within −10% to +40%, and the labeled amount of hydrocortisone acetate, within ±10%. Meets the requirements for Identification, Sterility, Minimum fill, Water (not more than 0.5%), and Metal particles.

NEOMYCIN, POLYMYXIN B, BACITRACIN, AND LIDOCAINE

For *Neomycin, Polymyxin B, Bacitracin,* and *Lidocaine*—See individual listings for chemistry information.

USP requirements:

Neomycin and Polymyxin B Sulfates, Bacitracin, and Lidocaine Ointment USP—Preserve in well-closed containers, preferably at controlled room temperature. Contains amounts of neomycin sulfate, polymyxin B sulfate, and bacitracin equivalent to the labeled amounts of neomycin, polymyxin B, and bacitracin, within −10% to +30%, and the labeled amount of lidocaine, within ±10%. Meets the requirements for Identification, Minimum fill, and Water (not more than 0.5%).

Neomycin and Polymyxin B Sulfates, Bacitracin Zinc, and Lidocaine Ointment USP—Preserve in well-closed containers, preferably at controlled room temperature. Contains amounts of neomycin sulfate, polymyxin B sulfate, and bacitracin zinc equivalent to the labeled amounts of neomycin, polymyxin B, and bacitracin, within −10% to +30%, and the labeled amount of lidocaine, within ±10%. Meets the requirements for Identification, Minimum fill, and Water (not more than 0.5%).

NEOMYCIN, POLYMYXIN B, AND DEXAMETHASONE

For *Neomycin, Polymyxin B,* and *Dexamethasone*—See individual listings for chemistry information.

USP requirements:

Neomycin and Polymyxin B Sulfates and Dexamethasone Ophthalmic Ointment USP—Preserve in collapsible ophthalmic ointment tubes. Contains amounts of neomycin sulfate and polymyxin B sulfate equivalent to the labeled amounts of neomycin and polymyxin B, within −10% to +30%, and the labeled amount of dexamethasone, within ±10%. Meets the requirements for Identification, Sterility, Minimum fill, Water (not more than 0.5%), and Metal particles.

Neomycin and Polymyxin B Sulfates and Dexamethasone Ophthalmic Suspension USP—Preserve in tight, light-resistant containers in a cool place or at controlled room temperature. The containers or individual cartons are sealed and tamper-proof so that sterility is assured at time of first use. Contains amounts of neomycin sulfate and polymyxin B sulfate equivalent to the labeled amounts of neomycin and polymyxin B, within −10% to +30%, and the labeled amount of dexamethasone, within ±10%. Meets the requirements for Identification, Sterility, and pH (3.5–6.0).

NEOMYCIN, POLYMYXIN B, AND GRAMICIDIN

For *Neomycin, Polymyxin B,* and *Gramicidin*—See individual listings for chemistry information.

USP requirements:

Neomycin and Polymyxin B Sulfates and Gramicidin Cream USP—Preserve in collapsible tubes or in well-closed containers. Contains amounts of neomycin sulfate, polymyxin B sulfate, and gramicidin equivalent to the labeled amounts of neomycin, polymyxin B, and gramicidin, within −10% to +30%. Meets the requirement for Minimum fill.

Neomycin and Polymyxin B Sulfates and Gramicidin Ophthalmic Solution USP—Preserve in tight containers. The containers or individual cartons are sealed and tamper-proof so that sterility is assured at time of first use. A sterile, isotonic aqueous solution of Neomycin Sulfate, Polymyxin B Sulfate, and Gramicidin. Contains amounts of neomycin sulfate, polymyxin B sulfate, and gramicidin equivalent to the labeled amounts of neomycin, polymyxin B, and gramicidin, within −10% to +30%. Meets the requirements for Identification, Sterility, and pH (4.7–6.0).

NEOMYCIN, POLYMYXIN B, GRAMICIDIN, AND HYDROCORTISONE

For *Neomycin, Polymyxin B, Gramicidin,* and *Hydrocortisone*—See individual listings for chemistry information.

USP requirements: Neomycin and Polymyxin B Sulfates, Gramicidin, and Hydrocortisone Acetate Cream USP—Preserve in well-closed containers. Contains amounts of neomycin sulfate, polymyxin B sulfate, and gramicidin equivalent to the labeled amounts of neomycin, polymyxin B, and gramicidin, within −10% to +30%, and the labeled amount of hydrocortisone acetate, within ±10%. Meets the requirement for Minimum fill.

NEOMYCIN, POLYMYXIN B, AND HYDROCORTISONE

For *Neomycin, Polymyxin B,* and *Hydrocortisone*—See individual listings for chemistry information.

USP requirements:

Neomycin and Polymyxin B Sulfates and Hydrocortisone Otic Solution USP—Preserve in tight, light-resistant containers. The containers or individual cartons are sealed and tamper-proof so that sterility is assured at time of first use. A sterile solution. Contains amounts of neomycin sulfate and polymyxin B sulfate equivalent to the labeled amounts of neomycin and polymyxin B, within −10% to +30%, and the labeled amount of hydrocortisone, within ±10%. Meets the requirements for Sterility and pH (2.0–4.5).

Neomycin and Polymyxin B Sulfates and Hydrocortisone Ophthalmic Suspension USP—Preserve in tight containers. The containers or individual cartons are sealed and tamper-proof so that sterility is assured at time of first use. A sterile, aqueous suspension. Contains amounts of neomycin sulfate and polymyxin B sulfate equivalent to the labeled amounts of neomycin and polymyxin B, within −10% to +30%. Meets the requirements for Identification, Sterility, and pH (4.1–7.0).

Neomycin and Polymyxin B Sulfates and Hydrocortisone Otic Suspension USP—Preserve in tight, light-resistant containers. The containers or individual cartons are sealed and tamper-proof so that sterility is assured at time of first use. A sterile suspension. Contains amounts of neomycin sulfate and polymyxin B sulfate equivalent to the labeled amounts of neomycin and polymyxin B, within −10% to +30%, and the labeled amount of hydrocortisone, within ±10%. Meets the requirements for Identification, Sterility, and pH (3.0–7.0).

Neomycin and Polymyxin B Sulfates and Hydrocortisone Acetate Cream USP—Preserve in well-closed containers. Contains amounts of neomycin sulfate and polymyxin B sulfate equivalent to the labeled amounts of neomycin and polymyxin B, within −10% to +30%, and the labeled amount of hydrocortisone acetate, within ±10%. Meets the requirements for Identification and Minimum fill.

Neomycin and Polymyxin B Sulfates and Hydrocortisone Acetate Ophthalmic Suspension USP—Preserve in tight containers. The containers or individual cartons are sealed and tamper-proof so that sterility is assured at time of first use. A sterile suspension of Hydrocortisone Acetate in an aqueous solution of Neomycin Sulfate and Polymyxin B Sulfate. Contains amounts of neomycin sulfate and polymyxin B sulfate equivalent to the labeled amounts of neomycin and polymyxin B, within −10% to +25%, and the labeled amount of hydrocortisone acetate, within ±10%. Meets the requirements for Sterility and pH (5.0–7.0).

NEOMYCIN, POLYMYXIN B, AND LIDOCAINE

For *Neomycin, Polymyxin B,* and *Lidocaine*—See individual listings for chemistry information.

USP requirements: Neomycin and Polymyxin B Sulfates and Lidocaine Cream USP—Preserve in well-closed containers, preferably at controlled room temperature. Contains amounts of neomycin sulfate and polymyxin B sulfate equivalent to the labeled amounts of neomycin and polymyxin B, within −10% to +30%, and the labeled amount of lidocaine, within ±10%. Meets the requirements for Identification and Minimum fill.

NEOMYCIN, POLYMYXIN B, AND PRAMOXINE

For *Neomycin, Polymyxin B,* and *Pramoxine*—See individual listings for chemistry information.

USP requirements:Neomycin and Polymyxin B Sulfates and Pramoxine Hydrochloride Cream USP—Preserve in well-closed containers, preferably at controlled room temperature. Contains the equivalent of the labeled amount of neomycin and polymyxin B, within -10% to +30%, and pramoxine hydrochloride, within ±10%. Meets the requirements for Identification and pH (3.3–6.0).

NEOMYCIN, POLYMYXIN B, AND PREDNISOLONE

For *Neomycin, Polymyxin B,* and *Prednisolone*—See individual listings for chemistry information.

USP requirements: Neomycin and Polymyxin B Sulfates and Prednisolone Acetate Ophthalmic Suspension USP—Preserve in tight containers. The containers or individual cartons are sealed and tamper-proof so that sterility is assured at time of first use. A sterile suspension of Prednisolone Acetate in an aqueous solution of Neomycin Sulfate and Polymyxin B Sulfate. Contains amounts of neomycin sulfate and polymyxin B sulfate equivalent to the labeled amounts of neomycin and polymyxin B, within −10% to +25%, and the labeled amount of prednisolone acetate, within ±10%. Meets the requirements for Identification, Sterility, and pH (5.0–7.0).

NEOMYCIN AND PREDNISOLONE

For *Neomycin* and *Prednisolone*—See individual listings for chemistry information.

USP requirements:
Neomycin Sulfate and Prednisolone Acetate Ointment USP—Preserve in collapsible tubes or in tight containers, protected from light. Contains an amount of neomycin sulfate equivalent to the labeled amount of neomycin, within −10% to +35%, and the labeled amount of prednisolone acetate, within ±10%. Meets the requirements for Identification, Minimum fill, and Water (not more than 1.0%).
Neomycin Sulfate and Prednisolone Acetate Ophthalmic Ointment USP—Preserve in collapsible ophthalmic ointment tubes. A sterile ointment containing Neomycin Sulfate and Prednisolone Acetate. Contains an amount of neomycin sulfate equivalent to the labeled amount of neomycin, within −10% to +35%, and the labeled amount of prednisolone acetate, within ±10%. Meets the requirements for Identification, Sterility, Minimum fill, Water (not more than 1.0%), and Metal particles.

Neomycin Sulfate and Prednisolone Acetate Ophthalmic Suspension USP—Preserve in tight containers. The containers or individual cartons are sealed and tamper-proof so that sterility is assured at time of first use. Contains an amount of neomycin sulfate equivalent to the labeled amount of neomycin, within −10% to +30%, and the labeled amount of prednisolone acetate, within ±10%. Meets the requirements for Identification, Sterility, and pH (5.5–7.5).
Neomycin Sulfate and Prednisolone Sodium Phosphate Ophthalmic Ointment USP—Preserve in collapsible ophthalmic ointment tubes. A sterile ointment containing Neomycin Sulfate and Prednisolone Sodium Phosphate. Contains amounts of neomycin sulfate and prednisolone sodium phosphate equivalent to the labeled amounts of neomycin, within −10% to +35%, and prednisolone phosphate, within −10% to +15%. Meets the requirements for Identification, Sterility, Minimum fill, Water (not more than 1.0%), and Metal particles.
Note: Where Neomycin Sulfate and Prednisolone Sodium Phosphate Ophthalmic Ointment is prescribed without reference to the quantity of neomycin or prednisolone phosphate contained therein, a product containing 3.5 mg of neomycin and 2.5 mg of prednisolone phosphate per gram shall be dispensed.

NEOMYCIN, SULFACETAMIDE, AND PREDNISOLONE

For *Neomycin, Sulfacetamide,* and *Prednisolone*—See individual listings for chemistry information.

USP requirements: Neomycin Sulfate, Sulfacetamide Sodium, and Prednisolone Acetate Ophthalmic Ointment USP—Preserve in collapsible ophthalmic ointment tubes. Contains an amount of neomycin sulfate equivalent to the labeled amount of neomycin, within −10% to +35%, and the labeled amounts of sulfacetamide sodium and prednisolone acetate, within ± 10%. Meets the requirements for Identification, Sterility, Minimum fill, and Metal particles.

NEOMYCIN AND TRIAMCINOLONE

For *Neomycin* and *Triamcinolone*—See individual listings for chemistry information.

USP requirements:
Neomycin Sulfate and Triamcinolone Acetonide Cream USP—Preserve in collapsible tubes or in tight containers. Contains an amount of neomycin sulfate equivalent to the labeled amount of neomycin, within −10% to +35%, and the labeled amount of triamcinolone acetonide, within ± 10%. Meets the requirements for Identification and Minimum fill.
Neomycin Sulfate and Triamcinolone Acetonide Ophthalmic Ointment USP—Preserve in collapsible ophthalmic ointment tubes. Contains an amount of neomycin sulfate equivalent to the labeled amount of neomycin, within −10% to +35%, and the labeled amount of triamcinolone acetonide, within ±10%. Meets the requirements for Identification, Sterility, Minimum fill, Water (not more than 1.0%), and Metal particles.

NEOSTIGMINE

Chemical name:
Neostigmine bromide—Benzenaminium, 3-[[(dimethylamino)-carbonyl]oxy]-*N,N,N*-trimethyl-, bromide.
Neostigmine methylsulfate—Benzenaminium, 3-[[(dimethyla-mino)carbonyl]oxy]-*N,N,N*-trimethyl-, methyl sulfate.

Molecular formula:
Neostigmine bromide—$C_{12}H_{19}BrN_2O_2$.
Neostigmine methylsulfate—$C_{13}H_{22}N_2O_6S$.

Molecular weight:
Neostigmine bromide—303.20.
Neostigmine methylsulfate—334.39.

Description:
Neostigmine bromide—White, crystalline powder. Odorless. Its solutions are neutral to litmus.
Neostigmine methylsulfate—White, crystalline powder. Odorless. Its solutions are neutral to litmus.

Solubility
Neostigmine bromide—Very soluble in water; soluble in alcohol; practically insoluble in ether.
Neostigmine methylsulfate—Very soluble in water; soluble in alcohol.

USP requirements:
Neostigmine Bromide USP—Preserve in tight containers. Contains not less than 98.0% and not more than 102.0% of neostigmine bromide, calculated on the dried basis. Meets the requirements for Identification, Melting range (171–176 °C, with decomposition), Loss on drying (not more than 2.0%), Residue on ignition (not more than 0.15%), and Sulfate.
Neostigmine Bromide Tablets USP—Preserve in tight containers. Contain the labeled amount, within ±7%. Meet the requirements for Identification, Dissolution (75% in 45 minutes in water in Apparatus 2 at 50 rpm), and Uniformity of dosage units.
Neostigmine Methylsulfate USP—Preserve in tight containers. Contains not less than 98.0% and not more than 102.0% of neostigmine methylsulfate, calculated on the dried basis. Meets the requirements for Identification, Melting range (144–149 °C), Loss on drying (not more than 1.0%), Residue on ignition (not more than 0.1%), Chloride, and Sulfate ion.
Neostigmine Methylsulfate Injection USP—Preserve in single-dose or in multiple-dose containers, protected from light. A sterile solution of Neostigmine Methylsulfate in Water for Injection. Contains the labeled amount, within ±10%. Meets the requirements for Identification and pH (5.0–6.5), and for Injections.

NESIRITIDE

Source: Nesiritide is a sterile, purified preparation of human B-type natriuretic peptide (hBNP) manufactured from *Escherichia coli* using recombinant DNA technology. It has the same 32-amino acid sequence as the endogenous peptide, which is produced by the ventricular myocardium.

Chemical name: Natriuretic factor-32 (human brain clone lambda hBNP57).

Molecular formula: $C_{143}H_{244}N_{50}O_{42}S_4$.

Molecular weight: 3464 grams per mol.

Description: White- to off-white lyophilized powder.

USP requirements: Nesiritide for Injection—Not in *USP–NF*.

NETILMICIN

Source: Semi-synthetic derivative of sisomicin.

Chemical name: Netilmicin sulfate—D-Streptamine, *O*-3-deoxy-4-*C*-methyl-3-(methylamino)-beta-L-arabinopyranosyl-(1→6)-*O*-[2,6-diamino-2,3,4,6-tetradeoxy-alpha-D-*glycero*-hex-4-en-opyranosyl-(1→4)]-2-deoxy-*N'*-ethyl-, sulfate (2:5) (salt).

Molecular formula: Netilmicin sulfate—$(C_{21}H_{41}N_5O_7)_2 \cdot 5H_2SO_4$.

Molecular weight: Netilmicin sulfate—1441.56.

Description: Netilmicin Sulfate USP—White- to pale yellowish-white powder.

Solubility: Netilmicin Sulfate USP—Freely soluble in water; practically insoluble in dehydrated alcohol and in ether.

USP requirements:
Netilmicin Sulfate USP—Preserve in tight containers. Has a potency equivalent to not less than 595 mcg of netilmicin per mg, calculated on the dried basis. Meets the requirements for Identification, Specific rotation (+88° to +96°), pH (3.5–5.5, in a solution containing 40 mg of netilmicin per mL), Loss on drying (not more than 15.0%), and Residue on ignition (not more than 1.0%).
Netilmicin Sulfate Injection USP—Preserve in single-dose or in multiple-dose containers, preferably of Type I glass. A sterile solution of Netilmicin Sulfate in Water for Injection. Contains an amount of netilmicin sulfate equivalent to the labeled amount of netilmicin, within −10% to +15%. Meets the requirements for Identification, Bacterial endotoxins, Sterility, pH (3.5–6.0), and Particulate matter, and for Injections.

NEVIRAPINE

Chemical name: 6*H*-Dipyrido[3,2-*b*:2',3'-*e*][1,4]diazepin-6-one, 11-cyclopropyl-5,11-dihydro-4-methyl-.

Molecular formula: $C_{15}H_{14}N_4O$.

Molecular weight: 266.30.

Description: White to off-white crystalline powder.

USP requirements:
Nevirapine Oral Suspension—Not in *USP–NF*.
Nevirapine Tablets—Not in *USP–NF*.

NIACIN

Chemical name: 3-Pyridinecarboxylic acid.

Molecular formula: $C_6H_5NO_2$.

Molecular weight: 123.11.

Description: Niacin USP—White crystals or crystalline powder. Is odorless, or has a slight odor. Melts at about 235 °C.

pKa: 4.85.

Solubility: Niacin USP—Sparingly soluble in water; freely soluble in boiling water, in boiling alcohol, and in solutions of alkali hydroxides and carbonates; practically insoluble in ether.

USP requirements:
Niacin USP—Preserve in well-closed containers. Contains not less than 99.0% and not more than 101.0% of niacin, calculated on the dried basis. Meets the requirements for Identification, Loss on drying (not more than 1.0%), Residue on ignition (not more than 0.1%), Chloride (not more than 0.02%), Sulfate (not more than 0.02%), Heavy metals (not more than 0.002%), Ordinary impurities, and Organic volatile impurities.

Niacin Extended-release Capsules—Not in *USP–NF*.

Niacin Injection USP—Preserve in single-dose or in multiple-dose containers, preferably of Type I glass. A sterile solution of Niacin and niacin sodium in Water for Injection, made with the aid of Sodium Carbonate or Sodium Hydroxide. Contains the labeled amount, within −5% to +10%. Meets the requirements for Identification, Bacterial endotoxins, and pH (4.0–6.0), and for Injections.

Niacin Oral Solution—Not in *USP–NF*.

Niacin Tablets USP—Preserve in well-closed containers. Contain the labeled amount, within ±10%. Meet the requirements for Identification, Dissolution (65% in 60 minutes in 0.1 *N* hydrochloric acid in Apparatus 1 at 100 rpm) , and Uniformity of dosage units.

Niacin Extended-release Tablets—Not in *USP–NF*.

NIACIN AND LOVASTATIN

For *Niacin* and *Lovastatin*—See individual listings for chemistry information.

USP requirements: Niacin Extended-release and Lovastatin Tablets—Not in *USP–NF*.

NIACINAMIDE

Chemical name: 3-Pyridinecarboxamide.

Molecular formula: $C_6H_6N_2O$.

Molecular weight: 122.12.

Description: Niacinamide USP—White, crystalline powder. Is odorless or practically so. Its solutions are neutral to litmus.

pKa: 0.5 and 3.35.

Solubility: Niacinamide USP—Freely soluble in water and in alcohol; soluble in glycerin.

USP requirements:

Niacinamide USP—Preserve in tight containers. Contains not less than 98.5% and not more than 101.5% of niacinamide, calculated on the dried basis. Meets the requirements for Identification, Melting range (128–131 °C), Loss on drying (not more than 0.5%), Residue on ignition (not more than 0.1%), Heavy metals (not more than 0.003%), Readily carbonizable substances, and Organic volatile impurities.

Niacinamide Gel—Not in *USP–NF*.

Niacinamide Injection USP—Preserve in single-dose or in multiple-dose containers, preferably of Type I glass. A sterile solution of Niacinamide in Water for Injection. Contains the labeled amount, within −5% to +10%. Meets the requirements for Identification, Bacterial endotoxins, and pH (5.0–7.0), and for Injections.

Niacinamide Tablets USP—Preserve in tight containers. Contain the labeled amount, within ±10%. Meet the requirements for Identification, Dissolution (75% in 45 minutes in water in Apparatus 2 at 50 rpm), and Uniformity of dosage units.

NICARDIPINE

Chemical name: Nicardipine hydrochloride—3,5-Pyridinedicarboxylic acid, 1,4-dihydro-2,6-dimethyl-4-(3-nitrophenyl)-, methyl 2-[methyl(phenylmethyl)amino]ethyl ester, monohydrochloride.

Molecular formula: Nicardipine hydrochloride—$C_{26}H_{29}N_3O_6$ · HCl.

Molecular weight: Nicardipine hydrochloride—515.99.

Description: Nicardipine hydrochloride—Greenish-yellow, odorless, crystalline powder. Melts at about 169 °C.

Solubility: Nicardipine hydrochloride—Freely soluble in chloroform, in methanol, and in glacial acetic acid; sparingly soluble in anhydrous ethanol; slightly soluble in n-butanol, in water, in 0.01 *M* potassium dihydrogen phosphate, in acetone, and in dioxane; very slightly soluble in ethyl acetate; practically insoluble in ether and in hexane.

USP requirements:

Nicardipine Hydrochloride Capsules—Not in *USP–NF*.

Nicardipine Hydrochloride Extended-release Capsules—Not in *USP–NF*.

NICLOSAMIDE

Chemical group: Derivative of salicylanilide.

Chemical name: Benzamide, 5-chloro-*N*-(2-chloro-4-nitrophenyl)-2-hydroxy-.

Molecular formula: $C_{13}H_8Cl_2N_2O_4$.

Molecular weight: 327.12.

Description: Pale yellow crystals with a melting point of 225–230 °C.

Solubility: Practically insoluble in water; sparingly soluble in ethanol, in chloroform, and in ether.

USP requirements: Niclosamide Chewable Tablets—Not in *USP–NF*.

NICOTINAMIDE

Source: Active form of niacin and chemical form of vitamin B_2.

USP requirements: Nicotinamide Topical Gel—Not in *USP–NF*.

NICOTINE

Chemical name:

Nicotine—3-(1-Methyl-2-pyrrolidinyl)pyridine.

Nicotine polacrilex—2-Propenoic acid, 2-methyl-, polymer with diethenylbenzene, complex with (*S*)-3-(1-methyl-2-pyrrolidinyl)pyridine.

Molecular formula:

Nicotine—$C_{10}H_{14}N_2$.

Nicotine polacrilex—$[(C_4H_6O_2)_x(C_{10}H_{10})_y](C_{10}H_{14}N_2)$.

Molecular weight: 162.23.

Description: Colorless to pale yellow, strongly alkaline, oily, volatile, hygroscopic liquid; has a characteristic pungent odor; turns brown on exposure to air or light.

Solubility: Freely soluble in water.

USP requirements:

Nicotine USP—Store under nitrogen in well-closed containers below 25 °C, protected from light and moisture. Contains not less than 99.0% and not more than 101.0% of nicotine, calculated on the anhydrous basis. Meets the require-

ments for Identification, Specific rotation (–130° to –143°), Water (not more than 0.5%), Heavy metals (not more than 0.002%), and Chromatographic purity.

Nicotine for Inhalation—Not in *USP–NF*.

Nicotine Nasal Solution—Not in *USP–NF*.

Nicotine Transdermal System USP—Preserve in the hermetic, light-resistant, unit-dose pouch. The labeling indicates the Drug Release Test with which the product complies. Contains the labeled amount, within ±10%. Meets the requirements for Identification, Drug release (31–87% in 2 hours, 62–191% in 12 hours, and 85–261% in 24 hours in phosphoric acid solution [1 in 1000] in Apparatus 7 for Test 1; 71–157% in 6 hours and 156–224% in 24 hours in phosphate buffer in Apparatus 6 at 50 rpm for Test 2; 35–75% in 1 hour, 55–95% in 2 hours, and not less than 73% in 4 hours in water in Apparatus 5 at 50 rpm for Test 3; 36–66% in 4 hours and 72–112% in 16 hours in 0.025 N hydrochloric acid in Apparatus 5 at 50 rpm for Test 4; and 79–112% in 3 hours, 108–141% in 6 hours, and 156–202% in 24 hours in phosphate buffer and Apparatus for Test 5), and Uniformity of dosage units.

Nicotine Polacrilex USP—Preserve in tight containers. A weak carboxylic cation-exchange resin prepared from methacrylic acid and divinylbenzene, in complex with nicotine. Contains not less than 95.0% and not more than 115.0% of the labeled amount of nicotine, calculated on the anhydrous basis. Meets the requirements for Identification, Nicotine release (not less than 70% released in 10 minutes), Water (not more than 5.0%), and Chromatographic purity.

Nicotine Polacrilex Gum USP—Contains an amount of Nicotine Polacrilex equivalent to the labeled amount of nicotine, within –10% to +20%. Meets the requirements for Identification and Uniformity of dosage units.

NICOTINYL ALCOHOL

Chemical name: 3-Pyridinemethanol.

Molecular formula: Nicotinyl alcohol tartrate—$C_6H_7NO \cdot C_4H_6O_6$.

Molecular weight: Nicotinyl alcohol tartrate—259.21.

Description: Nicotinyl alcohol tartrate—White or almost white, odorless or almost odorless, crystalline powder.

Solubility: Nicotinyl alcohol tartrate—Freely soluble in water; slightly soluble in alcohol; practically insoluble in chloroform and in ether.

USP requirements: Nicotinyl Alcohol Tartrate Extended-release Tablets—Not in *USP–NF*.

NIFEDIPINE

Chemical name: 3,5-Pyridinedicarboxylic acid, 1,4-dihydro-2,6-dimethyl-4-(2-nitrophenyl)-, dimethyl ester.

Molecular formula: $C_{17}H_{18}N_2O_6$.

Molecular weight: 346.33.

Description: Nifedipine USP—Yellow powder; affected by exposure to light.

Solubility: Nifedipine USP—Practically insoluble in water; freely soluble in acetone.

USP requirements:

Nifedipine USP—Preserve in tight, light-resistant containers. Contains not less than 98.0% and not more than 102.0% of nifedipine, calculated on the dried basis. Meets the requirements for Identification, Melting range (171–175 °C), Loss on drying (not more than 0.5%), Residue on ignition (not more than 0.1%), Heavy metals (not more than 0.001%), Perchloric acid titration, Chloride and sulfate, Related compounds, and Organic volatile impurities.

Nifedipine Capsules USP—Preserve in tight, light-resistant containers at a temperature between 15 and 25 °C. Contain the labeled amount, within ±10%. Meet the requirements for Identification, Dissolution (80% in 20 minutes in simulated gastric fluid TS [without pepsin] in Apparatus 2 at 50 rpm), Uniformity of dosage units, and Related compounds.

Nifedipine Tablets—Not in *USP–NF*.

Nifedipine Extended-release Tablets USP—Preserve in tight, light-resistant containers, and store at controlled room temperature. The labeling indicates the Drug release test with which the product complies. Contain the labeled amount, within ±10%. Meet the requirements for Identification, Drug release (for Test 1: 5–17% in 4 hours, 43–80% in 12 hours, and not less than 80% in 24 hours in water in Apparatus 7, and for Test 2: 10–30% in 3 hours, 40–65% in 6 hours, and not less than 80% in 12 hours in a mixture of 125.0 mL of Buffer concentrate and 1 liter of 10% sodium lauryl sulfate solution in Apparatus 2 at 50 rpm; for Test 3: for Tablets labeled to contain 30 mg of nifedipine: Phae 1: in one hour in 0.05 M phosphate buffer [pH 7.5] in Apparatus 2 at 100 rpm, and Phase 2: not more than 30% in one hour, 30–55% in 4 hours, not less than 60% in 8 hours, and not less than 80% in 12 hours in 0.5% sodium lauryl sulfate in simulated gastric fluid without enzyme [pH 1.2] in Apparatus 2 at 100 rpm; for Tablets labeled to contain 60 mg of nifedipine: Phase 1: in 25 minutes in 0.05 M phosphate buffer [pH 7.5] in apparatus 2 at 100 rpm, and Phase 2: not more than 30% in one hour, 40–70% in 4 hours, not less than 70% in 8 hours, and not less than 80% in 12 hours in 0.5% sodium lauryl sulfate in simulated gastric fluid without enzyme [pH 1.2] in Apparatus 2 at 100 rpm; for Test 4: for Tablets labeled to contain 30 mg of nifedipine: 12–35% in one hour, 44–67% in 4 hours, and not less than 80% in 12 hours, and for Tablets labeled to contain 60 mg of nifedipine: 10–30% in one hour, 40–63% in 4 hours, and not less than 80% in 12 hours in 0.5% sodium lauryl sulfate in simulated gastric fluid without enzyme [pH 1.2] in apparatus 2 at 100 rpm), Uniformity of dosage units, and Related compounds (not more than 2.0% of nifedipine nitrophenylpyridine analog and not more than 0.5% of nifedipine nitrosophenylpyridine analog, both relative to the nifedipine content).

NIFURTIMOX

Source: Nitrofuran derivative.

Chemical name: 4-[(5-Nitrofurfurylidene)amino]-3-methylthiomorpholine 1,1-dioxide.

Molecular formula: $C_{10}H_{13}N_3O_5S$.

Molecular weight: 287.29.

Description: Orange-red crystals melting at about 181 °C.

Solubility: Soluble in water.

USP requirements: Nifurtimox Tablets—Not in *USP–NF*.

NILUTAMIDE

Chemical name: 5,5-Dimethyl-3-(alpha,alpha,alpha-trifluoro-4-nitro-*m*-tolyl)hydantoin.

Molecular formula: $C_{12}H_{10}F_3N_3O_4$.

Molecular weight: 317.22.

Description: White to off-white powder. Melts between 153–156 °C.

Solubility: Soluble in ethyl acetate, in acetone, in chloroform, in ethyl alcohol, in dichloromethane, and in methanol; slightly soluble in water (less than 0.1% w/v) at 25 °C.

USP requirements: Nilutamide Tablets—Not in *USP–NF*.

NIMODIPINE

Chemical name: 3,5-Pyridinedicarboxylic acid, 1,4-dihydro-2,6-dimethyl-4-(3-nitrophenyl)-, 2-methoxyethyl 1-methylethyl ester.

Molecular formula: $C_{21}H_{26}N_2O_7$.

Molecular weight: 418.44.

Description: Yellow crystalline substance.

Solubility: Practically insoluble in water.

USP requirements: Nimodipine Capsules—Not in *USP–NF*.

NISOLDIPINE

Chemical name: 3,5-Pyridinedicarboxylic acid, 1,4-dihydro-2,6-dimethyl-4-(2-nitrophenyl)-, methyl 2-methylpropyl ester, (±)-.

Molecular formula: $C_{20}H_{24}N_2O_6$.

Molecular weight: 488.41.

Description: Yellow crystalline substance. Melting point 151–152 °C.

Solubility: Practically insoluble in water; soluble in ethanol.

USP requirements: Nisoldipine Extended-release Tablets—Not in *USP–NF*.

NITAZOXANIDE

Source: Synthetic antiprotozoal agent.

Chemical name: 2-acetyloxy-*N*-(5-nitro-2-thiazolyl)benzamide.

Molecular formula: $C_{12}H_9N_3O_5S$.

Molecular weight: 307.3.

Description: Light yellow crystalline powder.

Solubility: Poorly soluble in ethanol; practically insoluble in water.

USP requirements: Nitazoxanide for Oral Suspension—Not in *USP–NF*.

NITISINONE

Chemical name: 2-(alpha,alpha,alpha-Trifluoro-2-nitro-*p*-toluoyl)-1,3-cyclohexanedione.

Molecular formula: $C_{14}H_{10}F_3NO_5$.

Molecular weight: 329.23.

Description: Yellowish-white crystalline powder.

Solubility: Practically insoluble in water; soluble in 2M sodium hydroxide and in methanol; sparingly soluble in alcohol.

USP requirements: Nitisinone Capsules—Not in *USP–NF*.

NITRAZEPAM

Chemical name: 2*H*-1,4-Benzodiazepin-2-one, 1,3-dihydro-7-nitro-5-phenyl-.

Molecular formula: $C_{15}H_{11}N_3O_3$.

Molecular weight: 281.27.

Description: Yellow, crystalline powder.

Solubility: Practically insoluble in water; slightly soluble in alcohol and in ether; sparingly soluble in chloroform.

USP requirements: Nitrazepam Tablets—Not in *USP–NF*.

NITRIC ACID

Chemical name: Nitric acid.

Molecular formula: HNO_3.

Molecular weight: 63.01.

Description: Nitric Acid NF—Highly corrosive, fuming liquid, having a characteristic, highly irritating odor. Stains animal tissue yellow. Boils at about 120 °C. Specific gravity is about 1.41.
    NF category: Acidifying agent.

NF requirements: Nitric Acid NF—Preserve in tight containers. Contains not less than 69.0% and not more than 71.0%, by weight, of nitric acid. Meets the requirements for Clarity and color, Identification, Residue on ignition (not more than 5 ppm), Chloride (not more than 0.5 ppm), Sulfate (not more than 1 ppm), Iron (not more than 0.2 ppm), and Heavy metals (not more than 0.2 ppm).
    Caution: Avoid contact, since Nitric Acid rapidly destroys tissues.

NITRIC OXIDE

Chemical group: Nitric oxide is a gas with the chemical formula NO.

Chemical name: Nitrogen monoxide.

Molecular formula: NO.

Molecular weight: 30.01.

USP requirements: Nitric Oxide Gas—Not in *USP–NF*.

NITROFURANTOIN

Chemical group: Nitrofuran derivative.

Chemical name: 2,4-Imidazolidenedione, 1-[[(5-nitro-2-furanyl)methylene]amino]-.

Molecular formula: $C_8H_6N_4O_5$.

Molecular weight: 238.16.

Description: Nitrofurantoin USP—Lemon-yellow, odorless crystals or fine powder.

Solubility: Nitrofurantoin USP—Very slightly soluble in water and in alcohol; soluble in dimethylformamide.

USP requirements:

Nitrofurantoin USP—Preserve in tight, light-resistant containers. It is anhydrous or contains one molecule of water of hydration. Label it to indicate whether it is anhydrous or hydrous. Nitrofurantoin in the form of macrocrystals is so labeled. The labeling states the specific surface area and which method, specified under *Specific Surface Area*, is used. Contains not less than 98.0% and not more than 102.0% of nitrofurantoin, calculated on the anhydrous basis. Meets the requirements for Identification, Water (not more than 1.0% for the anhydrous form and 6.5–7.5% for the hydrous form), Specific surface area (0.045 m² to 0.20 m² per gram), Limit of nitrofurfural diacetate (not more than 1.0%), and Limit of nitrofurazone.

Caution: Nitrofurantoin and solutions of it are discolored by alkali and by exposure to light, and are decomposed upon contact with metals other than stainless steel and aluminum.

Nitrofurantoin Capsules USP—Preserve in tight, light-resistant containers. Capsules that contain the macrocrystalline form of Nitrofurantoin are so labeled. Contain the labeled amount, within ±10%. Meet the requirements for Identification, Dissolution (where labeled as containing Nitrofurantoin macrocrystals: 20–60% in 1 hour, not less than 45% in 3 hours, and not less than 60% in 8 hours in phosphate buffer [pH 7.2 (±0.05)] in Apparatus 1, at 100 rpm), Uniformity of dosage units, and Limit of nitrofurazone (not more than 0.01%).

Nitrofurantoin Extended-release Capsules—Not in *USP–NF*.

Nitrofurantoin Oral Suspension USP—Preserve in tight, light-resistant containers. A suspension of Nitrofurantoin in a suitable, aqueous vehicle. Contains, in each 100 mL, not less than 460 mg and not more than 540 mg of nitrofurantoin. Meets the requirements for Identification, pH (4.5–6.5), and Limit of N-(aminocarbonyl)-N-[((5-nitro-2-furanyl]methylene)amino]glycine.

Nitrofurantoin Tablets USP—Preserve in tight, light-resistant containers. Contain the labeled amount, within ±10%. Meet the requirements for Identification, Dissolution (25% in 60 minutes and 85% in 120 minutes in phosphate buffer [pH 7.2] in Apparatus 1 at 100 rpm), Uniformity of dosage units, and Nitrofurazone (not more than 0.01%).

Solubility:

Nitrofurazone USP—Very slightly soluble in alcohol and in water; soluble in dimethylformamide; slightly soluble in propylene glycol and in polyethylene glycol mixtures; practically insoluble in chloroform and in ether.

Nitrofurazone Cream USP—Miscible with water.

Nitrofurazone Ointment USP—Miscible with water.

Nitrofurazone Topical Solution USP—Miscible with water.

USP requirements:

Nitrofurazone USP—Preserve in tight, light-resistant containers, and avoid exposure to direct sunlight and to excessive heat. Dried at 105 °C for 1 hour, contains not less than 98.0% and not more than 102.0% of nitrofurazone. Meets the requirements for Identification, pH (5.0–7.5), Loss on drying (not more than 0.5%), Residue on ignition (not more than 0.1%), Ordinary impurities, and Limit of 5-nitro-2-furfuraldazine.

Note: Where Neomycin Sulfate and Prednisolone Sodium Phosphate Ophthalmic Ointment is prescribed without reference to the quantity of neomycin or prednisolone phosphate, a product containing 3.5 mg of neomycin and 2.5 mg of prednisolone phosphate per gram shall be dispensed.

Nitrofurazone Cream USP—Preserve in tight, light-resistant containers. Avoid exposure to direct sunlight, strong fluorescent lighting, and excessive heat. It is Nitrofurazone in a suitable, emulsified water-miscible base. Contains the labeled amount, within ±10%. Meets the requirements for Identification and Minimum fill.

Note: Avoid exposure at all times to direct sunlight, excessive heat, strong fluorescent lighting, and alkaline materials.

Nitrofurazone Soluble Dressing—Not in *USP–NF*.

Nitrofurazone Ointment USP—Preserve in tight, light-resistant containers. Avoid exposure to direct sunlight, strong fluorescent lighting, and excessive heat. It is Nitrofurazone in a suitable water-miscible base. Contains the labeled amount, within ±10%. Meets the requirements for Completeness of solution and Identification.

Note: Avoid exposure at all times to direct sunlight, excessive heat, strong fluorescent lighting, and alkaline materials.

Nitrofurazone Topical Solution USP—Preserve in tight, light-resistant containers. Avoid exposure to direct sunlight and excessive heat. Contains the labeled amount, within ±5% (w/w). Meets the requirement for Identification.

Note: Avoid exposure at all times to direct sunlight, excessive heat, and alkaline materials.

NITROFURAZONE

Chemical name: Hydrazinecarboxamide, 2-[(5-nitro-2-furanyl)methylene]-.

Molecular formula: $C_6H_6N_4O_4$.

Molecular weight: 198.14.

Description:

Nitrofurazone USP—Lemon yellow, odorless, crystalline powder. Darkens slowly on exposure to light. Melts at about 236 °C, with decomposition.

Nitrofurazone Cream USP—Yellow, opaque cream.

Nitrofurazone Ointment USP—Yellow, opaque, and has ointment-like consistency.

Nitrofurazone Topical Solution USP—Light yellow, clear, somewhat viscous liquid, having a faint, characteristic odor.

NITROGEN

Chemical name: Nitrogen.

Molecular formula: N_2.

Molecular weight: 28.01.

Description: Nitrogen NF—Colorless, odorless gas. It is nonflammable and does not support combustion. One liter at 0 °C and at a pressure of 760 mm of mercury weighs about 1.251 grams.

NF category: Air displacement.

Solubility: Nitrogen NF—One volume dissolves in about 65 volumes of water and in about 9 volumes of alcohol at 20 °C and at a pressure of 760 mm of mercury.

NF requirements: Nitrogen NF—Preserve in cylinders. Contains not less than 99.0%, by volume, of nitrogen. Meets the requirements for Identification, Odor, Carbon monoxide (not more than 0.001%), and Limit of oxygen (not more than 1.0%).

NITROGEN 97 PERCENT

NF requirements: Nitrogen 97 Percent NF—Preserve in cylinders or in a low-pressure collecting tank. It is Nitrogen produced from air by physical separation methods. Where it is piped directly from the collecting tank to the point of use, label each outlet "Nitrogen 97 Percent." Contains not less than 97.0%, by volume, of nitrogen. Meets the requirements for Identification, Odor, Carbon dioxide (not more than 0.03%), Carbon monoxide (not more than 0.001%), Sulfur dioxide (not more than 5 ppm), Limit of nitric oxide and nitrogen dioxide (not more than 2.5 ppm), and Limit of oxygen (not more than 3.0%).

AMMONIA N 13

Source: Different methods are being used in the various clinical facilities for the on-site production of $^{13}NH_3$. It can be produced by irradiation of ^{16}O-water with protons and subsequent reduction using De Varda's alloy or titanium (III) salts. The resultant $^{13}NH_3$ is collected as the ammonium ion in saline solution.

Chemical name: Ammonia-^{13}N.

Molecular formula: $H_3$$^{13}N$.

USP requirements: Ammonia N 13 Injection USP—Preserve in single-dose or in multiple-dose containers that are adequately shielded. A sterile, aqueous solution, suitable for intravenous administration, of $^{13}NH_3$ in which a portion of the molecules are labeled with radioactive ^{13}N. Label it to include the following, in addition to the information specified for Labeling under Injections: the time and date of calibration; the amount of ^{13}N as ammonia expressed as total megabecquerels (or millicuries) per mL, at time of calibration; the expiration time and date; the name and quantity of any added preservative or stabilizer; and the statement "Caution—Radioactive Material." The labeling indicates that in making dosage calculations correction is to be made for radioactive decay and also indicates that the radioactive half-life of ^{13}N is 9.96 minutes. The label indicates "Do not use if cloudy or if it contains particulate matter." Contains the labeled amount of ^{13}N expressed in megabecquerels (or millicuries) per mL, within ±10%, at the time indicated in the labeling. Meets the requirements for Specific activity (not less than 37×10^4 megabecquerels [10 curies] per mmol), Radionuclide identification, Bacterial endotoxins, pH (4.5–8.5), Radiochemical purity, Radionuclidic purity, and Chemical purity, and for Injections (except that the Injection may be distributed or dispensed prior to completion of the test for Sterility, the latter test being started on the day following final manufacture, and except that it is not subject to the recommendation in Volume in Container).

NITROGLYCERIN

Chemical name: 1,2,3-Propanetriol, trinitrate.

Molecular formula: $C_3H_5N_3O_9$.

Molecular weight: 227.09.

Description: Diluted Nitroglycerin USP—White, odorless powder, when diluted with lactose. When diluted with propylene glycol or alcohol, it is a clear, colorless, or pale yellow liquid. (Note: Undiluted nitroglycerin is a white to pale yellow, thick, flammable, explosive liquid.)

Solubility: Undiluted nitroglycerin—Slightly soluble in water; soluble in methanol, in alcohol, in carbon disulfide, in acetone, in ethyl ether, in ethyl acetate, in glacial acetic acid, in toluene, in phenol, in chloroform, and in methylene chloride.

USP requirements:
Diluted Nitroglycerin USP—Preserve in tight, light-resistant containers, and prevent exposure to excessive heat. A mixture of nitroglycerin with lactose, dextrose, alcohol, propylene glycol, or other suitable inert excipient to permit safe handling. Contains the labeled amount of nitroglycerin, within ±10%. Usually contains not more than 10% of nitroglycerin. Meets the requirements for Identification and Chromatographic purity.

Caution: Taking into consideration the concentration and amount of nitroglycerin in Diluted Nitroglycerin, exercise appropriate precautions when handling this material. Nitroglycerin is a powerful explosive and can be detonated by percussion or excessive heat. Do not isolate nitroglycerin.

Nitroglycerin Lingual Aerosol—Not in *USP–NF*.

Nitroglycerin Extended-release Capsules—Not in *USP–NF*.

Nitroglycerin Injection USP—Preserve in single-dose or in multiple-dose containers, preferably of Type I or Type II glass. A sterile solution prepared from Diluted Nitroglycerin; the solvent may contain Alcohol, Propylene Glycol, and Water for Injection. Where necessary, label it to indicate that it is to be diluted before use. Contains the labeled amount, within ±10%. Meets the requirements for Identification, Bacterial endotoxins, pH (3.0–6.5), Particulate matter, and Alcohol content (labeled amount, within ± 10%), and for Injections.

Nitroglycerin Ointment USP—Preserve in tight containers. It is Diluted Nitroglycerin in a suitable ointment base. Label multiple-dose containers with a direction to close tightly, immediately after each use. Contains the labeled amount, within −10% to +15%. Meets the requirements for Identification, Minimum fill, and Homogeneity (within ±10% of mean value).

Nitroglycerin Transdermal System—Not in *USP–NF*.

Nitroglycerin Tablets USP (Sublingual)—Preserve in tight containers, preferably of glass, at controlled room temperature. Each container holds not more than 100 Tablets. The labeling indicates that the Tablets are for sublingual use, and the label directs that the Tablets be dispensed in the original, unopened container, labeled with the following statement directed to the patient. "Warning: to prevent loss of potency, keep these tablets in the original container or in a supplemental Nitroglycerin container specifically labeled as being suitable for Nitroglycerin Tablets. Close tightly immediately after each use." Contain the labeled amount, within −10% to +15%. Meet the requirements for Identification, Disintegration (2 minutes), and Uniformity of dosage units.

Nitroglycerin Extended-release Tablets—Not in *USP–NF*.

Nitroglycerin Extended-release Buccal Tablets—Not in *USP–NF*.

NITROMERSOL

Chemical name: 7-Oxa-8-mercurabicyclo[4.2.0]octa-1,3,5-triene, 5-methyl-2-nitro.

Molecular formula: $C_7H_5HgNO_3$.

Molecular weight: 351.71.

Description:
Nitromersol USP—Brownish yellow to yellow granules or brownish yellow to yellow powder. Odorless. Affected by light.
Nitromersol Topical Solution USP—Clear, reddish orange solution. Affected by light.

Solubility: Nitromersol USP—Very slightly soluble in water, in alcohol, in acetone, and in ether; soluble in solutions of alkalies and of ammonia by opening of the anhydride ring and the formation of a salt.

USP requirements:
Nitromersol USP—Preserve in tight, light-resistant containers. Dried at 105 °C for 2 hours, contains not less than 98.0% and not more than 100.5% of nitromersol. Meets the requirements for Identification, Loss on drying (not more than 1.0%), Residue on ignition (not more than 0.1%), Mercury ions, Alkali-insoluble substances (not more than 0.1%), and Uncombined nitrocresol (not more than 1%).
Nitromersol Topical Solution USP—Preserve in tight, light-resistant containers. Yields, from each 100 mL, not less than 180.0 mg and not more than 220.0 mg of Nitromersol.

Prepare Nitromersol Topical Solution as follows: 2 grams of Nitromersol, 0.4 gram of Sodium Hydroxide, 4.25 grams of Sodium Carbonate, monohydrate, and a sufficient quantity of Purified Water to make 1000 mL. Dissolve the Sodium Hydroxide and the monohydrated Sodium Carbonate in 50 mL of Purified Water, add the Nitromersol, and stir until dissolved. Gradually add Purified Water to make 1000 mL.

Meets the requirements for Identification, Specific gravity (1.005–1.010), and Mercury ions.

Note: Prepare dilutions of Nitromersol Topical Solution as needed, since they tend to precipitate on standing.

NITROUS OXIDE

Chemical name: Nitrogen oxide (N_2O).

Molecular formula: N_2O.

Molecular weight: 44.01.

Description: Nitrous Oxide USP—Colorless gas, without appreciable odor. One liter at 0 °C and at a pressure of 760 mm of mercury weighs about 1.97 grams.

Solubility: Nitrous Oxide USP—One volume dissolves in about 1.4 volumes of water at 20 °C and at a pressure of 760 mm of mercury; freely soluble in alcohol; soluble in ether and in oils.

Other characteristics:
Blood-to-Gas partition coefficient at 37 °C—0.47.
Oil-to-Gas partition coefficient at 37 °C—1.4.

USP requirements: Nitrous Oxide USP—Preserve in cylinders. Contains not less than 99%, by volume, of nitrous oxide. Meets the requirements for Identification, Water (not more than 150 mg per cubic meter), Limit of ammonia (not more than 0.0025%), Limit of nitric oxide (not more than 1 ppm), Carbon monoxide (not more than 0.001%), Nitrogen dioxide (not more than 1 ppm), Halogens (not more than 1 ppm), Carbon dioxide (not more than 0.03%), and Air (not more than 1.0%).

NIZATIDINE

Chemical name: 1,1-Ethenediamine, *N*-[2-[[[2-[(dimethylamino)methyl]-4-thiazolyl]methyl]thio]ethyl]-*N*-methyl-2-nitro-.

Molecular formula: $C_{12}H_{21}N_5O_2S_2$.

Molecular weight: 331.46.

Description: Off-white to buff crystalline solid.

Solubility: Freely soluble in chloroform; soluble in methanol; sparingly soluble in water.

USP requirements:
Nizatidine USP—Preserve in tight, light-resistant containers. Contains not less than 98.0% and not more than 101.0% of nizatidine, calculated on the dried basis. Meets the requirements for Identification, Loss on drying (not more than 1.0%), Residue on ignition (not more than 0.1%), Heavy metals (not more than 0.001%), and Chromatographic purity.
Nizatidine Capsules USP—Preserve in tight, light-resistant containers. Store at controlled room temperature. Contain the labeled amount, within ±10%. Meet the requirements for Identification, Dissolution (75% in 30 minutes in water in Apparatus 2 at 50 rpm), Uniformity of dosage units, and Chromatographic purity.
Nizatidine Tablets—Not in *USP–NF*.

NONOXYNOL 9

Chemical name: Poly(oxy-1,2-ethanediyl), alpha-(4-nonylphenyl)-omega-hydroxy-.

Molecular formula: $C_{15}H_{24}O(C_2H_4O)_n$ (*n* = approximately 9).

Description: Nonoxynol 9 USP—Clear, colorless to light yellow viscous liquid.
NF category: Wetting and/or solubilizing agent.

Solubility: Nonoxynol 9 USP—Soluble in water, in alcohol, and in corn oil.

USP requirements:
Nonoxynol 9 USP—Preserve in tight containers. An anhydrous liquid mixture consisting chiefly of mononononylphenyl ethers of polyethylene glycols corresponding to the formula $C_9H_{19}C_6H_4(OCH_2CH_2)_nOH$, in which the average value of *n* is about 9. Contains not less than 90.0% and not more than 110.0% of nonoxynol 9. Meets the requirements for Identification, Acid value (not more than 0.2), Water (not more than 0.5%), Polyethylene glycol (not more than 1.0%), Cloud point (52–56 °C), Free ethylene oxide (not more than 1 ppm), and Limit of dioxane.
Nonoxynol 9 Vaginal Cream—Not in *USP–NF*.
Nonoxynol 9 Vaginal Film—Not in *USP–NF*.
Nonoxynol 9 Vaginal Foam—Not in *USP–NF*.
Nonoxynol 9 Vaginal Gel—Not in *USP–NF*.
Nonoxynol 9 Vaginal Jelly—Not in *USP–NF*.
Nonoxynol 9 Vaginal Sponge—Not in *USP–NF*.
Nonoxynol 9 Vaginal Suppositories—Not in *USP–NF*.

NONOXYNOL 10

Chemical name: Poly(oxy-1,2-ethanediyl), alpha-(4-nonylphenyl)-omega-hydroxy-.

Description: Nonoxynol 10 NF—Colorless to light amber viscous liquid, having an aromatic odor.
NF category: Wetting and/or solubilizing agent.

Solubility: Nonoxynol 10 NF—Soluble in polar organic solvents and in water.

NF requirements: Nonoxynol 10 NF—Preserve in tight containers. An anhydrous liquid mixture consisting chiefly of mononylphenyl ethers of polyethylene glycols corresponding to the formula $C_9H_{19}C_6H_4(OCH_2CH_2)_nOH$, in which the average value of *n* is about 10. The labeling includes a cloud point range that is not greater than 6 °C and that is between 52 °C and 67 °C. Meets the requirements for Identification, Cloud point, Hydroxyl value (81–97), Water (not more than 0.5%), Residue on ignition (not more than 0.4%), Heavy metals (not more than 0.002%), and Organic volatile impurities.

NORELGESTROMIN AND ETHINYL ESTRADIOL

Chemical name:
Norelgestromin—18,19-Dinopregn-4-en-20-yn-3-one, 13-ethyl-17-hydroxy-, oxiome, (17 alpha)-.
Ethinyl estradiol—19-Norpregna-1,3,5(10)-trien-20-yne-3,17-diol, (17 alpha)-.

Molecular formula:
Norelgestromin—$C_{21}H_{29}NO_2$.
Ethinyl estradiol—$C_{20}H_{20}O_2$.

Molecular weight:
Norelgestromin—327.47.
Ethinyl estradiol—296.40.

Description: Ethinyl Estradiol USP—White to creamy white, odorless, crystalline powder.

Solubility: Ethinyl Estradiol USP—Insoluble in water; soluble in alcohol, in chloroform, in ether, in vegetable oils, and in solutions of fixed alkali hydroxides.

USP requirements: Norelgestromin and Ethinyl Estradiol Transdermal System—Not in *USP–NF*.

NOREPINEPHRINE

Chemical group: A primary amine, differing from epinephrine by the absence of a methyl group on the nitrogen atom.

Chemical name: Norepinephrine bitartrate—1,2-Benzenediol, 4-(2-amino-1-hydroxyethyl)-, (*R*)-[*R*-(*R**,*R**)]-2,3-dihydroxybutanedioate (1:1) (salt), monohydrate.

Molecular formula: Norepinephrine bitartrate—$C_8H_{11}NO_3 \cdot C_4H_6O_6 \cdot H_2O$.

Molecular weight: Norepinephrine bitartrate—337.28.

Description:
Norepinephrine Bitartrate USP—White or faintly gray, odorless, crystalline powder. Slowly darkens on exposure to air and light. Its solutions are acid to litmus, having a pH of about 3.5. Melts between 98 and 104 °C, without previous drying of the specimen, the melt being turbid.
Norepinephrine Bitartrate Injection USP— Colorless or practically colorless liquid, gradually turning dark on exposure to air and light.

Solubility: Norepinephrine Bitartrate USP—Freely soluble in water; slightly soluble in alcohol; practically insoluble in chloroform and in ether.

USP requirements:
Norepinephrine Bitartrate USP—Preserve in tight, light-resistant containers. Contains not less than 97.0% and not more than 102.0% of norepinephrine bitartrate, calculated on the anhydrous basis. Meets the requirements for Identification, Specific rotation (–10° to –12°), Water (4.5–5.8%), Residue on ignition (negligible, from 200 mg), and Limit of arterenone.

Norepinephrine Bitartrate Injection USP—Preserve in single-dose, light-resistant containers, preferably of Type I glass. A sterile solution of Norepinephrine Bitartrate in Water for Injection. Label the Injection in terms of mg of norepinephrine per mL, and, where necessary, label it to indicate that it must be diluted prior to use. The label indicates that the Injection is not to be used if its color is pinkish or darker than slightly yellow or if it contains a precipitate. Contains an amount of norepinephrine bitartrate equivalent to the labeled amount of norepinephrine, within –10% to +15%. Meets the requirements for Color and clarity, Identification, Bacterial endotoxins, pH (3.0–4.5), and Particulate matter, and for Injections.

NORETHINDRONE

Chemical name:
Norethindrone—19-Norpregn-4-en-20-yn-3-one, 17-hydroxy-, (17 alpha)-.
Norethindrone acetate—19-Norpregn-4-en-20-yn-3-one, 17-(acetyloxy)-, (17 alpha).

Molecular formula:
Norethindrone—$C_{20}H_{26}O_2$.
Norethindrone acetate—$C_{22}H_{28}O_3$.

Molecular weight:
Norethindrone—298.42.
Norethindrone acetate—340.46.

Description:
Norethindrone USP—White to creamy white, odorless, crystalline powder. Is stable in air.
Norethindrone Acetate USP—White to creamy white, odorless, crystalline powder.

Solubility:
Norethindrone USP—Practically insoluble in water; soluble in chloroform and in dioxane; sparingly soluble in alcohol; slightly soluble in ether.
Norethindrone Acetate USP—Practically insoluble in water; very soluble in chloroform; freely soluble in dioxane; soluble in ether and in alcohol.

USP requirements:
Norethindrone USP—Preserve in well-closed containers. Contains not less than 97.0% and not more than 102.0% of norethindrone, calculated on the dried basis. Meets the requirements for Completeness of solution, Identification, Melting range (202–208 °C), Specific rotation (–30° to –38°), Loss on drying (not more than 0.5%), Chromatographic purity, Limit of ethynyl group (8.18–8.43%), and Organic volatile impurities.
Norethindrone Tablets USP—Preserve in well-closed containers. Contain the labeled amount, within ±10%. Meet the requirements for Identification, Disintegration (15 minutes, the use of disks being omitted), and Uniformity of dosage units.
Norethindrone Acetate USP—Preserve in well-closed containers. Contains not less than 97.0% and not more than 103.0% of norethindrone acetate, calculated on the dried basis. Meets the requirements for Completeness of solution, Identification, Specific rotation (–32° to –38°), Loss on drying (not more than 0.5%), Limit of ethynyl group (7.13–7.57%), Chromatographic purity, and Organic volatile impurities.
Norethindrone Acetate Tablets USP— Preserve in well-closed containers. Contain the labeled amount, within ±10%. Meet the requirements for Identification, Dissolution

(70% in 60 minutes in dilute hydrochloric acid [1 in 100] containing 0.02% of sodium lauryl sulfate in Apparatus 1 at 100 rpm), and Uniformity of dosage units.

NORETHINDRONE AND ESTRADIOL

For *Norethindrone* and *Estradiol*—See individual listings for chemistry information.

USP requirements: Norethindrone and Estradiol Tablets—Not in *USP–NF*.

NORETHINDRONE AND ETHINYL ESTRADIOL

For *Norethindrone* and *Ethinyl Estradiol*—See individual listings for chemistry information.

USP requirements:
Norethindrone and Ethinyl Estradiol Tablets USP—Preserve in well-closed containers. Contain the labeled amounts of norethindrone and ethinyl estradiol, within ±10%. Meet the requirements for Identification, Dissolution (75% of each active ingredient in 60 minutes in 0.09% sodium lauryl sulfate in 0.1 N hydrochloric acid in Apparatus 2 at 75 rpm), and Uniformity of dosage units.
Norethindrone Acetate and Ethinyl Estradiol Tablets USP—Preserve in well-closed containers. Contain the labeled amount of norethindrone acetate, within ±10%, and the labeled amount of ethinyl estradiol, within ±12%. Meet the requirements for Identification, Dissolution (80% of each active ingredient in 60 minutes in 0.025 M acetate buffer [pH 5.0] with 0.15% sodium lauryl sulfate in Apparatus 2 at 75 rpm), and Uniformity of dosage units.

NORETHINDRONE, ETHINYL ESTRADIOL, AND FERROUS FUMARATE

For *Norethindrone, Ethinyl Estradiol,* and *Ferrous Fumarate*—See individual listings for chemistry information.

USP requirements: Norethindrone Acetate, Ethinyl Estradiol, and Ferrous Fumarate Tablets—Not in *USP–NF*.

NORETHINDRONE AND MESTRANOL

For *Norethindrone* and *Mestranol*—See individual listings for chemistry information.

USP requirements: Norethindrone and Mestranol Tablets USP—Preserve in well-closed containers. Contain the labeled amounts, within ±10%. Meet the requirements for Identification, Dissolution (75% of each active ingredient in 60 minutes in 0.09% sodium lauryl sulfate in 0.1 N hydrochloric acid in Apparatus 2 at 75 rpm), and Uniformity of dosage units.

NORETHYNODREL

Chemical name: 19-Norpregn-5(10)-en-20-yn-3-one, 17-hydroxy-, (17 alpha)-.

Molecular formula: $C_{20}H_{26}O_2$.

Molecular weight: 298.42.

Description: Norethynodrel USP—White or practically white, odorless, crystalline powder. Melts at about 175 °C, over a range of about 3 C°. Is stable in air.

Solubility: Norethynodrel USP—Very slightly soluble in water and in solvent hexane; freely soluble in chloroform; soluble in acetone; sparingly soluble in alcohol.

USP requirements: Norethynodrel USP—Preserve in well-closed containers. Contains not less than 97.0% and not more than 101.0% of norethynodrel. Meets the requirements for Identification, Specific rotation (+119° to +125°), Limit of ethynyl group (8.18–8.43%), Limit of norethindrone, Ordinary impurities, and Organic volatile impurities.

NORFLOXACIN

Chemical group: Fluoroquinolone derivative; structurally related to nalidixic acid.

Chemical name: 3-Quinolinecarboxylic acid, 1-ethyl-6-fluoro-1,4-dihydro-4-oxo-7-(1-piperazinyl)-.

Molecular formula: $C_{16}H_{18}FN_3O_3$.

Molecular weight: 319.33.

Description: Norfloxacin USP—White to pale yellow crystalline powder. Sensitive to light and moisture.

Solubility: Norfloxacin USP—Slightly soluble in acetone, in water, and in alcohol; freely soluble in acetic acid; sparingly soluble in chloroform; very slightly soluble in methanol and in ethyl acetate; insoluble in ether.

USP requirements:
Norfloxacin USP—Preserve in tight, light-resistant containers. Contains not less than 99.0% and not more than 101.0% of norfloxacin, calculated on the dried basis. Meets the requirements for Identification, Loss on drying (not more than 1.0%), Residue on ignition (not more than 0.1%, a platinum crucible being used), Heavy metals (not more than 0.0015%), and Chromatographic purity.
Norfloxacin Ophthalmic Solution USP—Preserve in tight, light-resistant containers, stored at controlled room temperature. A sterile aqueous solution of Norfloxacin. Contains the labeled amount, within ±10%. Meets the requirements for Identification, Sterility, and pH (5.0–5.4).
Norfloxacin Tablets USP—Preserve in well-closed containers. Contain the labeled amount, within ±10%. Meet the requirements for Identification, Dissolution (80% in 30 minutes in pH 4.0 buffer in Apparatus 2 at 50 rpm), and Uniformity of dosage units.

NORGESTIMATE

Chemical name: 18,19-Dinor-17-pregan-4-2n-20-yn-3-one, 17-(acetyloxy)-13-ethyl-, oxime, (17 alpha)- (+)-.

Molecular formula: $C_{23}H_{31}NO_3$.

Molecular weight: 369.50.

Description: Norgestimate USP—White to pale yellow powder. Melting and decomposition begin at 221 °C.

Solubility: Norgestimate USP—Freely to very soluble in methylene chloride; insoluble in water; sparingly soluble in acetonitrile.

USP requirements: Norgestimate USP—Preserve in well-closed containers. A mixture of (*E*)- to (*Z*)-isomer between 1.27 and 1.78. Contains not less than 98.0% and not more than 1.2.0% of norgestimate, calculated on the dried basis. Meets the requirements for Identification, Specific rotation (between +40° to +46°), Loss on drying (not more than 0.5%), Residue on ignition (not more than 0.3%), Heavay metals (0.002%), Limit of residual solvents, Chromatographic purity, and organic volatile impurities.

NORGESTIMATE AND 17 BETA-ESTRADIOL

Chemical name:
17 beta-estradiol—estra-1,3,5(10)-triene,17 beta-diol.
Norgestimate—18,19-Dinor-17-pregn-4-en-20-yn-3-one, 17-(acetyloxy)-13-ethyl, oxime, (17 alpha)- (+)-.

Molecular formula:
17 beta-estradiol—$C_{18}H_{24}O_2$.
Norgestrimte—$C_{23}H_{31}NO_3$.

Molecular weight:
17 beta-estradiol—272.39.
Norgestimate—369.50.

Description:
17 beta-estradiol—White, crystalline solid.
Norgestimate USP—White to pale yellow powder. Melting and decomposition begin at 221 °C.

Solubility: Norgestimate USP—Freely to very soluble in methylene chloride; insoluble in water; sparingly soluble in acetonitrile.

USP requirements: Norgestimate and 17 Beta-Estradiol Tablets—Not in *USP-NF*.

NORGESTIMATE AND ETHINYL ESTRADIOL

Chemical name:
Norgestimate—18,19-Dinor-17-pregn-4-en-20-yn-3-one, 17-(acetyloxy)-13-ethyl-, oxime, (17 alpha)- (+)-.
Ethinyl estradiol—19-Norpregna-1,3,5(10)-trien-20-yne-3,17diol, (17 alpha)-.

Molecular formula:
Norgestimate—$C_{23}H_{31}NO_3$.
Ethinyl estradiol—$C_{20}H_{24}O_2$.

Molecular weight:
Norgestimate—369.50.
Ethinyl estradiol—296.40.

Description:
Norgestimate USP—White to pale yellow powder. Melting and decomposition begin at 221 °C.
Ethinyl Estradiol USP—White to creamy white, odorless, crystalline powder.

Solubility:
Norgestimate USP—Freely to very soluble in methylene chloride; insoluble in water; sparingly soluble in acetonitrile.
Ethinyl Estradiol USP—Insoluble in water; soluble in alcohol, in chloroform, in ether, in vegetable oils, and in solutions of fixed alkali hydroxides.

USP requirements: Norgestimate and Ethinyl Estradiol Tablets—Not in *USP-NF*.

NORGESTREL

Chemical name: 18,19-Dinorpregn-4-en-20-yn-3-one, 13-ethyl-17-hydroxy-, (17 alpha)-(±)-.

Molecular formula: $C_{21}H_{28}O_2$.

Molecular weight: 312.45.

Description: Norgestrel USP—White or practically white, practically odorless, crystalline powder.

Solubility: Norgestrel USP—Insoluble in water; freely soluble in chloroform; sparingly soluble in alcohol.

USP requirements:
Norgestrel USP—Preserve in well-closed containers. Contains not less than 98.0% and not more than 102.0% of norgestrel, calculated on the dried basis. Meets the requirements for Identification, Melting range (205–212 °C, the range between beginning and end of melting not more than 4 °C), Optical rotation (−0.1° to +0.1°), Loss on drying (not more than 0.5%), Residue on ignition (not more than 0.3%), Chromatographic purity, and Limit of ethynyl group (7.81–8.18%).
Norgestrel Tablets USP—Preserve in well-closed containers. Contain the labeled amount, within ±10%. Meet the requirements for Identification, Disintegration (15 minutes, the use of disks being omitted), and Uniformity of dosage units.

NORGESTREL AND ETHINYL ESTRADIOL

For *Norgestrel* and *Ethinyl Estradiol*—See individual listings for chemistry information.

USP requirements: Norgestrel and Ethinyl Estradiol Tablets USP—Preserve in well-closed containers. Contain the labeled amounts, within ±10%. Meet the requirements for Identification, Disintegration (15 minutes, the use of disks being omitted), and Uniformity of dosage units.

NORTRIPTYLINE

Chemical group: Dibenzocycloheptadiene.

Chemical name: Nortriptyline hydrochloride—1-Propanamine, 3-(10,11-dihydro-5*H*-dibenzo[*a,d*]cyclohepten-5-ylidene)-*N*-methyl-, hydrochloride.

Molecular formula: Nortriptyline hydrochloride—$C_{19}H_{21}N \cdot HCl$.

Molecular weight: Nortriptyline hydrochloride—299.84.

Description: Nortriptyline Hydrochloride USP—White to off-white powder, having a slight, characteristic odor. Its solution (1 in 100) has a pH of about 5.

pKa: Nortriptyline hydrochloride—9.73.

Solubility: Nortriptyline Hydrochloride USP—Soluble in water and in chloroform; sparingly soluble in methanol; practically insoluble in ether and in most other organic solvents.

USP requirements:
Nortriptyline Hydrochloride USP—Preserve in tight, light-resistant containers. Contains not less than 97.0% and not more than 101.5% of nortriptyline hydrochloride, calculated on the dried basis. Meets the requirements for Identification, Melting range (215–220 °C, the range between beginning and end of melting not more than 3 °C), Loss on drying (not more than 0.5%), Residue on ignition (not more than 0.1%), Heavy metals (not more than 0.001%), Chromatographic purity, and Organic volatile impurities.

Nortriptyline Hydrochloride Capsules USP—Preserve in tight containers. Contain an amount of nortriptyline hydrochloride equivalent to the labeled amount of nortriptyline, within ±10%. Meet the requirements for Identification, Dissolution (80% in 30 minutes in water in Apparatus 1 at 100 rpm), and Uniformity of dosage units.

Nortriptyline Hydrochloride Oral Solution USP—Preserve in tight, light-resistant containers. Contains an amount of nortriptyline hydrochloride equivalent to the labeled amount of nortriptyline, within ±10%. Meets the requirements for Identification, pH (2.5–4.0), and Alcohol content (3.0–5.0%).

NOSCAPINE

Chemical name: 1(3H)-Isobenzofuranone, 6,7-dimethoxy-3-(5,6,7,8-tetrahydro-4-methoxy-6-methyl-1,3-dioxolo[4,5-g]isoquinolin-5-yl), [S-(R*,S*)]-.

Molecular formula: $C_{22}H_{23}NO_7$.

Molecular weight: 413.42.

Description: Noscapine USP—Fine, white or practically white, crystalline powder.

Solubility: Noscapine USP—Freely soluble in chloroform; soluble in acetone; slightly soluble in alcohol and in ether; practically insoluble in water.

USP requirements: Noscapine USP—Preserve in well-closed containers. Contains not less than 99.0% and not more than 100.5% of noscapine, calculated on the anhydrous basis. Meets the requirements for Identification, Melting range (174–176 °C), Specific rotation (+42° to +48°), Water (not more than 1.0%), Residue on ignition (not more than 0.1%), Chloride (not more than 0.02%), Limit of morphine, and Ordinary impurities.

NOVOBIOCIN

Chemical name: Novobiocin sodium—Benzamide, N-[7-[[3-O-(aminocarbonyl)-6-deoxy-5-C-methyl-4-O-methyl-beta-L-lyxo-hexopyranosyl]oxy]-4-hydroxy-8-methyl-2-oxo-2H-1-benzo-pyran-3-yl]-4-hydroxy-3-(3-methyl-2-butenyl)-, monosodium salt.

Molecular formula: Novobiocin sodium—$C_{31}H_{35}N_2NaO_{11}$.

Molecular weight: Novobiocin sodium—634.61.

Description: Novobiocin Sodium USP—White or yellowishwhite, odorless, hygroscopic crystalline powder.

Solubility: Novobiocin Sodium USP—Freely soluble in water, in alcohol, in methanol, in glycerin, and in propylene glycol; slightly soluble in butyl acetate; practically insoluble in acetone, in chloroform, and in ether.

USP requirements:

Novobiocin Sodium USP—Preserve in tight containers. Has a potency equivalent to not less than 850 mcg of novobiocin per mg, calculated on the dried basis. Meets the requirements for Identification, Specific rotation (−50° to −58°), Crystallinity, pH (6.5–8.5, in a solution containing 25 mg per mL), Loss on drying (not more than 6.0%), and Residue on ignition (10.5–12.0%).

Novobiocin Sodium Capsules USP—Preserve in tight, light-resistant containers. Contain an amount of novobiocin sodium equivalent to the labeled amount of novobiocin, within −10% to +20%. Meet the requirements for Identification and Loss on drying (not more than 6.0%).

Novobiocin Sodium Intramammary Infusion USP—Preserve in disposable syringes that are well-closed containers. A suspension of Novobiocin Sodium in a suitable vegetable oil vehicle. Contains suitable preservative and suspending agents. Label it to indicate that it is for veterinary use only. Contains an amount of novobiocin sodium equivalent to the labeled amount of novobiocin, within −10% to +25%. Meets the requirement for Water (not more than 1.0%).

NYLIDRIN

Chemical name: Nylidrin hydrochloride—Benzenemethanol, 4-hydroxy-alpha-[1-[(1-methyl-3-phenylpropyl)amino]ethyl]-, hydrochloride.

Molecular formula: Nylidrin hydrochloride—$C_{19}H_{25}NO_2 \cdot HCl$.

Molecular weight: Nylidrin hydrochloride—335.87.

Description: Nylidrin hydrochloride—White, odorless, crystalline powder.

Solubility: Nylidrin hydrochloride—Sparingly soluble in water and in alcohol; slightly soluble in chloroform and in ether.

USP requirements: Nylidrin Hydrochloride Tablets—Not in USP.

NYSTATIN

Chemical name: Nystatin.

Description: Nystatin USP—Yellow to light tan powder, having an odor suggestive of cereals. Is hygroscopic, and is affected by long exposure to light, heat, and air.

Solubility: Nystatin USP—Freely soluble in dimethylformamide and dimethyl sulfoxide; slightly to sparingly soluble in methanol, in n-propyl alcohol, and in n-butyl alcohol; practically insoluble in water and in alcohol; insoluble in chloroform and in ether.

USP requirements:

Nystatin USP—Preserve in tight, light-resistant containers. A substance, or a mixture of two or more substances, produced by the growth of *Streptomyces noursei* Brown et al. (Fam. Streptomycetaceae). Where packaged for use in the extemporaneous preparation of oral suspensions, the label so states. Has a potency of not less than 4400 USP Nystatin Units per mg, or, where intended for use in the extemporaneous preparation of oral suspensions, not less than 5000 USP Nystatin Units per mg. Meets the requirements for Identification, Suspendibility (where packaged for use in the extemporaneous preparation of oral suspensions), Crystallinity, pH (6.0–8.0, in a 3% aqueous suspension), and Loss on drying (not more than 5.0%).

Nystatin Cream USP—Preserve in collapsible tubes, or in other tight containers, and avoid exposure to excessive heat. Contains the labeled amount of USP Nystatin Units, within −10% to +30%. Meets the requirement for Minimum fill.

Nystatin Vaginal Cream—Not in *USP–NF*.

Nystatin Lotion USP—Preserve in tight containers, at controlled room temperature. Contains the labeled amount of USP Nystatin Units, within −10% to +40%. Meets the requirement for pH (5.5–7.5).

Nystatin Lozenges USP—Preserve in tight, light-resistant containers. Contain the labeled amount of USP Nystatin Units, within −10% to +25%. Meet the requirements for Disintegration (90 minutes, determined as set forth under Uncoated Tablets) and pH (5.0–7.5).

Nystatin Ointment USP—Preserve in well-closed containers, preferably at controlled room temperature. Contains the labeled amount of USP Nystatin Units, within −10% to +30%. Meets the requirements for Minimum fill and Water (not more than 0.5%).

Nystatin Topical Powder USP—Preserve in well-closed containers. A dry powder composed of Nystatin and Talc. Contains the labeled amount of USP Nystatin Units, within −10% to +30%. Meets the requirement for Loss on drying (not more than 2.0%).

Nystatin Vaginal Suppositories USP—Preserve in tight, light-resistant containers, at controlled room temperature. Contain the labeled amount of USP Nystatin Units, within −10% to +30%. Meet the requirement for Water (not more than 1.5%).

Nystatin Oral Suspension USP—Preserve in tight, light-resistant containers. Contains suitable dispersants, flavors, preservatives, and suspending agents. Contains the labeled amount of USP Nystatin Units, within −10% to +30%. Meets the requirements for Uniformity of dosage units (single-unit containers), Deliverable volume (multiple-dose units), and pH (4.5–6.0; or 5.3–7.5 if it contains glycerin).

Nystatin for Oral Suspension USP—Preserve in tight containers. A dry mixture of Nystatin with one or more suitable colors, diluents, suspending agents, flavors, and preservatives. Contains the labeled amount of USP Nystatin Units, within −10% to +40%. Meets the requirements for pH (4.9–5.5, in the suspension constituted as directed in the labeling) and Water (not more than 7.0%).

Nystatin Tablets USP—Preserve in tight, light-resistant containers. Label the Tablets to indicate that they are intended for oral use only (as distinguished from Vaginal Tablets). Contain the labeled amount of USP Nystatin Units, within −10% to +30%. Meet the requirements for Disintegration (120 minutes for plain-coated) and Loss on drying (not more than 5.0% for plain-coated; not more than 8.0% for film-coated).

Nystatin Vaginal Tablets USP—Preserve in tight, light-resistant containers and, where so specified in the labeling, in a refrigerator. Tablets composed of Nystatin with suitable binders, diluents and lubricants. Contain the labeled amount of USP Nystatin Units, within −10% to +40%. Meet the requirements for Disintegration (60 minutes) and Loss on drying (not more than 5.0%).

NYSTATIN, NEOMYCIN, GRAMICIDIN, AND TRIAMCINOLONE

For *Nystatin, Neomycin, Gramicidin,* and *Triamcinolone*—See individual listings for chemistry information.

USP requirements:

Nystatin, Neomycin Sulfate, Gramicidin, and Triamcinolone Acetonide Cream USP—Preserve in tight containers. Contains amounts of nystatin, neomycin sulfate, and gramicidin equivalent to the labeled amounts of nystatin, neomycin, and gramicidin, within −10% to +40%, and the labeled amount of triamcinolone acetonide, within ±10%. Meets the requirements for Identification and Minimum fill.

Nystatin, Neomycin Sulfate, Gramicidin, and Triamcinolone Acetonide Ointment USP—Preserve in tight containers. Contains amounts of nystatin, neomycin sulfate, and gramicidin equivalent to the labeled amounts of nystatin, neomycin, and gramicidin, within −10% to +40%, and the labeled amount of triamcinolone acetonide, within ±10%. Meets the requirements for Identification, Water (not more than 0.5%), and Minimum fill.

NYSTATIN, NEOMYCIN, THIOSTREPTON, AND TRIAMCINOLONE

For *Nystatin, Neomycin, Thiostrepton,* and *Triamcinolone*—See individual listings for chemistry information.

USP requirements:

Nystatin, Neomycin Sulfate, Thiostrepton, and Triamcinolone Acetonide Cream USP—Preserve in tight containers. Label it to indicate that it is for veterinary use only. Contains the labeled amounts of nystatin and thiostrepton, within −10% to +30%, an amount of neomycin sulfate equivalent to the labeled amount of neomycin, within −10% to +30%, and the labeled amount of triamcinolone acetonide, within ±10%. Meets the requirements for Identification and Minimum fill.

Nystatin, Neomycin Sulfate, Thiostrepton, and Triamcinolone Acetonide Ointment USP—Preserve in tight containers. Label it to indicate that it is for veterinary use only. Contains the labeled amounts of nystatin and thiostrepton, within −10% to +30%, an amount of neomycin sulfate equivalent to the labeled amount of neomycin, within −10% to +30%, and the labeled amount of triamcinolone acetonide, within ±10%. Meets the requirements for Identification and Minimum fill.

NYSTATIN AND TRIAMCINOLONE

For *Nystatin* and *Triamcinolone*—See individual listings for chemistry information.

USP requirements:

Nystatin and Triamcinolone Acetonide Cream USP—Preserve in tight containers. Contains the labeled amount of USP Nystatin Units, within −10% to +40%, and the labeled amount of triamcinolone acetonide, within ±10%. Meets the requirements for Identification and Minimum fill.

Nystatin and Triamcinolone Acetonide Ointment USP—Preserve in tight containers. Contains the labeled amount of USP Nystatin Units, within −10% to +40%, and the labeled amount of triamcinolone acetonide, within ±10%. Meets the requirements for Identification, Minimum fill, and Water (not more than 0.5%).

OCTINOXATE

Chemical name: 2-Ethylhexyl 3-(4-methoxyphenyl)-2-propenoate.

Molecular formula: $C_{18}H_{26}O_3$.

Molecular weight: 290.40.

USP requirements: Octinoxate USP—Preserve in tight containers, in a cool place. Contains the labeled amount, within ±5%, calculated on the as-is basis. Meets the requirements for Identification, Specific gravity (1.005–1.013), Refractive index (1542–1548), Acidity (not more than 0.8 mL consumed), and Chromatographic purity .

OCTISALATE

Chemical name: 2-Ethylhexyl salicylate.

Molecular formula: $C_{15}H_{22}O_3$.

Molecular weight: 250.33.

USP requirements: Octyl Salicylate USP—Preserve in tight containers. Contains the labeled amount, within ±5.%. Meets the requirements for Identification, Specific gravity (1.011–1.016), Refractive index (1.500–1.503 at 20°), Acidity (not more than 0.2 mL of 0.1 N sodium hydroxide per mL of Octisalate for neutralization), and Chromatographic purity.

OCTOCRYLENE

Chemical name: 2-Propenoic acid, 2-cyano-3,3-diphenyl, 2-ethylhexyl ester.

Molecular formula: $C_{24}H_{27}NO_2$.

Molecular weight: 361.48.

USP requirements: Octocrylene USP—Preserve in tight containers. Contains not less than 95.0% and not more than 105.0% of octocrylene. Meets the requirements for Identification, Specific gravity (1.045–1.055), Acidity (not more than 0.18 mL of titrant per mg of Octocrylene is necessary to obtain a persistent pink endpoint), Refractive index (1.561–1.571 at 20°), and Chromatographic purity.

OCTOCRYLENE AND OCTYL METHOXYCINNAMATE

For *Octocrylene* and *Octyl Methoxycinnamate*—See individual listings for chemistry information.

USP requirements: Octocrylene and Octyl Methoxycinnamate Lotion—Not in *USP–NF*.

OCTOCRYLENE, OCTYL METHOXYCINNAMATE, OCTYL SALICYLATE, AND OXYBENZONE

For *Octocrylene, Octyl Methoxycinnamate Octyl Salicylate,* and *Oxybenzone*—See individual listings for chemistry information.

USP requirements: Octocrylene, Octyl Methoxycinnamate, Octyl Salicylate, and Oxybenzone Lotion—Not in *USP–NF*.

OCTOCRYLENE, OCTYL METHOXYCINNAMATE, OCTYL SALICYLATE, OXYBENZONE, AND TITANIUM DIOXIDE

For *Octocrylene, Octyl Methoxycinnamate, Octyl Salicylate, Oxybenzone,* and *Titanium Dioxide*—See individual listings for chemistry information.

USP requirements: Octocrylene, Octyl Methoxycinnamate, Octyl Salicylate, Oxybenzone, and Titanium Dioxide Lotion—Not in *USP–NF*.

OCTOCRYLENE, OCTYL METHOXYCINNAMATE, AND OXYBENZONE

For *Octocrylene, Octyl Methoxycinnamate,* and *Oxybenzone*—See individual listings for chemistry information.

USP requirements:
Octocrylene, Octyl Methoxycinnamate, and Oxybenzone Cream—Not in *USP–NF*.
Octocrylene, Octyl Methoxycinnamate, and Oxybenzone Gel—Not in *USP–NF*.
Octocrylene, Octyl Methoxycinnamate, and Oxybenzone Lotion—Not in *USP–NF*.

OCTOCRYLENE, OCTYL METHOXYCINNAMATE, OXYBENZONE, AND TITANIUM DIOXIDE

For *Octocrylene, Octyl Methoxycinnamate, Oxybenzone,* and *Titanium Dioxide*—See individual listings for chemistry information.

USP requirements: Octocrylene, Octyl Methoxycinnamate, Oxybenzone, and Titanium Dioxide Lotion—Not in *USP–NF*.

OCTOCRYLENE, OCTYL METHOXYCINNAMATE, AND TITANIUM DIOXIDE

For *Octocrylene, Octyl Methoxycinnamate,* and *Titaninum Dioxide*—See individual listings for chemistry information.

USP requirements: Octocrylene, Octyl Methoxycinnamate, and Titanium Dioxide Lotion—Not in *USP–NF*.

OCTOXYNOL 9

Chemical name: Poly(oxy-1,2-ethanediyl), alpha-(octylphenyl)-omega-hydroxy-.

Molecular Formula: $C_{34}H_{62}O_{11}$ (average).

Molecular Weight: 647.00 (average).

Description: Octoxynol 9 NF—Clear, pale yellow, viscous liquid, having a faint odor.
NF category: Wetting and/or solubilizing agent.

Solubility: Octoxynol 9 NF—Miscible with water, with alcohol, and with acetone; soluble in toluene; practically insoluble in solvent hexane.

USP requirements:
Octoxynol 9 Vaginal Cream—Not in *USP–NF*.
Octoxynol 9 Vaginal Jelly—Not in *USP–NF*.

NF requirements: Octoxynol 9 NF—Preserve in tight containers. An anhydrous liquid mixture consisting chiefly of monooctylphenyl ethers of polyethylene glycols, corresponding to the formula $C_8H_{17}C_6H_4(OCH_2CH_2)_nOH$, in which the average value of n is 9. Meets the requirements for Identification, Water (not more than 0.5%), Residue on ignition (not more than 0.4%), Heavy metals (not more than 0.002%), Hydroxyl value (85–101), Cloud point (63–69 °C), Organic volatile impurities, Free ethylene oxide (not more than 5 ppm), and Limit of dioxane.

OCTREOTIDE

Source: Synthetic octapeptide analog of somatostatin.

Chemical name: Octreotide acetate—L-Cysteinamide, D-phenylalanyl-L-cysteinyl-L-phenylalanyl-D-tryptophyl-L-lysyl-L-threonyl-N-[2-hydroxy-1-(hydroxymethyl)propyl]-, cyclic (2→7)disulfide, [R-(R*,R*)]-, acetate (salt).

Molecular formula: Octreotide acetate—$C_{49}H_{66}N_{10}O_{10}S_2 \cdot xC_2H_4O_2$.

Description: Octreotide acetate injection—Clear sterile solution.

USP requirements:
　　Octreotide Acetate Injection—Not in *USP–NF*.
　　Octreotide Acetate for Injectable Suspension—Not in *USP–NF*.

OCTYLDODECANOL

Molecular formula: $C_{20}H_{42}O$.

Molecular weight: 298.55.

Description: Octyldodecanol NF—Clear, water-white, free-flowing liquid.
　　NF category: Oleaginous vehicle.

Solubility: Octyldodecanol NF—Insoluble in water; soluble in alcohol and in ether.

NF requirements: Octyldodecanol NF—Preserve in tight containers. Contains not less than 90.0% of 2-octyldodecanol, the remainder consisting chiefly of related alcohols. Meets the requirements for Identification, Acid value (not more than 0.5), Iodine value (not more than 8), Hydroxyl value (175–190), Saponification value (not more than 5), and Organic volatile impurities.

OCTYL METHOXYCINNAMATE

Chemical name: 2-Ethylhexyl 3-(4-methoxyphenyl)-2-propenoate.

Molecular formula: $C_{18}H_{26}O_3$.

Molecular weight: 290.40.

Description: Octyl Methoxycinnamate USP—Pale yellow oil.

Solubility: Octyl Methoxycinnamate USP—Insoluble in water.

USP requirements:
　　Octyl Methoxycinnamate USP—Preserve in tight containers, in a cool place. Contains not less than 95.0% and not more than 105.0% of octyl methoxycinnamate, calculated on the as-is basis. Meets the requirements for Identification, Specific gravity (1.005–1.013), Acidity (not more than 0.8 mL consumed), and Chromatographic purity (not more than 0.5% of any individual impurity, and not more than 2.0% of total impurities).
　　Octyl Methoxycinnamate Gel—Not in *USP–NF*.
　　Octyl Methoxycinnamate Lotion—Not in *USP–NF*.

OCTYL METHOXYCINNAMATE AND OCTYL SALICYLATE

For *Octyl Methoxcinnamate* and *Octyl Salicylate*—See individual listings for chemistry information.

USP requirements:
　　Octyl Methoxycinnamate and Octyl Salicylate Gel—Not in *USP–NF*.
　　Octyl Methoxycinnamate and Octyl Salicylate Lotion—Not in *USP–NF*.
　　Octyl Methoxycinnamate and Octyl Salicylate Oil—Not in *USP–NF*.

OCTYL METHOXYCINNAMATE, OCTYL SALICYLATE, AND OXYBENZONE

For *Octyl Methoxycinnamate, Octyl Salicylate,* and *Oxybenzone*—See individual listings for chemistry information.

USP requirements:
　　Octyl Methoxycinnamate, Octyl Salicylate, and Oxybenzone Cream—Not in *USP–NF*.
　　Octyl Methoxycinnamate, Octyl Salicylate, and Oxybenzone Gel—Not in *USP–NF*.
　　Octyl Methoxycinnamate, Octyl Salicylate, and Oxybenzone Lip Balm—Not in *USP–NF*.
　　Octyl Methoxycinnamate, Octyl Salicylate, and Oxybenzone Lotion—Not in *USP–NF*.
　　Octyl Methoxycinnamate, Octyl Salicylate, and Oxybenzone Spray—Not in *USP–NF*.
　　Octyl Methoxycinnamate, Octyl Salicylate, and Oxybenzone Stick—Not in *USP–NF*.

OCTYL METHOXYCINNAMATE, OCTYL SALICYLATE, OXYBENZONE, AND PADIMATE O

For *Octyl Methoxycinnamate, Octyl Salicylate, Oxybenzone,* and *Padimate O*—See individual listings for chemistry information.

USP requirements:
　　Octyl Methoxycinnamate, Octyl Salicylate, Oxybenzone, and Padimate O Lotion—Not in *USP–NF*.
　　Octyl Methoxycinnamate, Octyl Salicylate, Oxybenzone, and Padimate O Spray—Not in *USP–NF*.

OCTYL METHOXYCINNAMATE, OCTYL SALICYLATE, OXYBENZONE, PADIMATE O, AND TITANIUM DIOXIDE

For *Octyl Methoxycinnamate, Octyl Salicylate, Oxybenzone, Padimate O,* and *Titanium Dioxide*—See individual listings for chemistry information.

USP requirements: Octyl Methoxycinnamate, Octyl Salicylate, Oxybenzone, Padimate O, and Titanium Dioxide Lotion—Not in *USP–NF*.

OCTYL METHOXYCINNAMATE, OCTYL SALICYLATE, OXYBENZONE, PHENYLBENZIMIDAZOLE, AND TITANIUM DIOXIDE

For *Octyl Methoxycinnamate, Octyl Salicylate, Oxybenzone, Phenylbenzimidazole,* and *Titanium Dioxide*—See individual listings for chemistry information.

USP requirements: Octyl Methoxycinnamate, Octyl Salicylate, Oxybenzone, Phenylbenzimidazole, and Titanium Dioxide Lotion—Not in *USP–NF*.

OCTYL METHOXYCINNAMATE, OCTYL SALICYLATE, OXYBENZONE, AND TITANIUM DIOXIDE

For *Octyl Methoxycinnamate, Octyl Salicylate, Oxybenzone,* and *Titanium Dioxide*—See individual listings for chemistry information.

USP requirements:
- Octyl Methoxycinnamate, Octyl Salicylate, Oxybenzone, and Titanium Dioxide Cream—Not in *USP–NF*.
- Octyl Methoxycinnamate, Octyl Salicylate, Oxybenzone, and Titanium Dioxide Lotion—Not in *USP–NF*.

OCTYL METHOXYCINNAMATE, OCTYL SALICYLATE, PHENYLBENZIMIDAZOLE, AND TITANIUM DIOXIDE

For *Octyl Methoxycinnamate, Octyl Salicylate, Phenylbenzimidazole,* and *Titanium Dioxide*—See individual listings for chemistry information.

USP requirements: Octyl Methoxycinnamate, Octyl Salicylate, Phenylbenzimidazole, and Titanium Dioxide Lotion—Not in *USP–NF*.

OCTYL METHOXYCINNAMATE, OCTYL SALICYLATE, AND TITANIUM DIOXIDE

For *Octyl Methoxycinnamate, Octyl Salicylate,* and *Titanium Dioxide*—See individual listings for chemistry information.

USP requirements: Octyl Methoxycinnamate, Octyl Salicylate, and Titanium Dioxide Lotion —Not in *USP–NF*.

OCTYL METHOXYCINNAMATE AND OXYBENZONE

For *Octyl Methoxycinnamate* and *Oxybenzone*—See individual listings for chemistry information.

USP requirements:
- Octyl Methoxycinnamate and Oxybenzone Cream—Not in *USP–NF*.
- Octyl Methoxycinnamate and Oxybenzone Gel—Not in *USP–NF*.
- Octyl Methoxycinnamate and Oxybenzone Lip Balm—Not in *USP–NF*.
- Octyl Methoxycinnamate and Oxybenzone Lotion—Not in *USP–NF*.
- Octyl Methoxycinnamate and Oxybenzone Stick—Not in *USP–NF*.

OCTYL METHOXYCINNAMATE, OXYBENZONE, AND PADIMATE O

For *Octyl Methoxycinnamate, Oxybenzone,* and *Padimate O*—See individual listings for chemistry information.

USP requirements: Octyl Methoxycinnamate, Oxybenzone, and Padimate O Lotion—Not in *USP–NF*.

OCTYL METHOXYCINNAMATE, OXYBENZONE, PADIMATE O, AND TITANIUM DIOXIDE

For *Octyl Methoxycinnamate, Oxybenzone, Padimate O,* and *Titanium Dioxide*—See individual listings for chemistry information.

USP requirements: Octyl Methoxycinnamate, Oxybenzone, Padimate O, and Titanium Dioxide Stick—Not in *USP–NF*.

OCTYL METHOXYCINNAMATE, OXYBENZONE, AND TITANIUM DIOXIDE

For *Octyl Methoxycinnamate, Oxybenzone,* and *Titanium Dioxide*—See individual listings for chemistry information.

USP requirements: Octyl Methoxycinnamate, Oxybenzone, and Titanium Dioxide Lotion—Not in *USP–NF*.

OCTYL METHOXYCINNAMATE AND PADIMATE O

For *Octyl Methoxycinnamate* and *Padimate O*—See individual listings for chemistry information.

USP requirements: Octyl Methoxycinnamate and Padimate O Oil—Not in *USP–NF*.

OCTYL METHOXYCINNAMATE AND PHENYLBENZIMIDAZOLE

For *Octyl Methoxycinnamate* and *Phenylbenzimidazole*—See individual listings for chemistry information.

USP requirements:
- Octyl Methoxycinnamate and Phenylbenzimidazole Cream—Not in *USP–NF*.
- Octyl Methoxycinnamate and Phenylbenzimidazole Lotion—Not in *USP–NF*.

OCTYL SALICYLATE

Chemical name: 2-Ethylhexyl salicylate.

Molecular formula: $C_{15}H_{22}O_3$.

Molecular weight: 250.33.

USP requirements:
- Octyl Salicylate USP—Preserve in tight containers. Contains not less than 95.0% and not more than 105.0% of octyl salicylate. Meets the requirements for Identification, Specific gravity (1.011–1.016), Refractive index (1.500–1.503 at 20°), Acidity (not more than 0.2 mL of titrant per mL of Octyl Salicylate necessary), and Chromatographic purity.
- Octyl Salicylate Spray—Not in *USP–NF*.

OCTYL SALICYLATE AND PADIMATE O

For *Octyl Salicylate* and *Padimate O*—See individual listings for chemistry information.

USP requirements: Octyl Salicylate and Padimate O Lotion—Not in *USP–NF*.

OFLOXACIN

Chemical name: 7*H*-Pyrido[1,2,3-*de*]-1,4-benzoxazine-6-carboxylic acid, 9-fluoro-2,3-dihydro-3-methyl-10-(4-methyl-1-piperazinyl)-7-oxo-, (±)-.

Molecular formula: $C_{18}H_{20}FN_3O_4$.

Molecular weight: 361.37.

Description: Pale yellowish white to light yellowish white crystals or crystalline powder.

Solubility: Slightly soluble in alcohol, in methanol, and in water; sparingly soluble in chloroform.

USP requirements:
Ofloxacin USP—Preserve in well-closed containers, protected from light. Contains not less than 98.5% and not more than 101.5% of ofloxacin, calculated on the dried basis. Meets the requirements for Identification, Specific rotation (+1° to −1°), Loss on drying (not more than 0.2%), Residue on ignition (not more than 0.1%), Arsenic (not more than 1 mcg per gram), Heavy metals (not more than 0.001%), Chromatographic purity, and Limit of methanol and ethanol (not more than 0.005% of methanol and not more than 0.05% of ethanol).
Ofloxacin Injection—Not in *USP–NF*.
Ofloxacin Ophthalmic Solution USP—Preserve in tight containers at controlled room temperature. A sterile aqueous solution of Ofloxacin. Contains the labeled amount, within ±10%. Meets the requirements for Identification, Sterility, and pH (6.0–6.8).
Ofloxacin Otic Solution—Not in *USP–NF*.
Ofloxacin Tablets—Not in *USP–NF*.

OFLOXACIN AND DEXTROSE

For *Ofloxacin* and *Dextrose*—See individual listings for chemistry information.

USP requirements: Ofloxacin in Dextrose Injection—Not in *USP–NF*.

BLAND LUBRICATING OPHTHALMIC OINTMENT

USP requirements: Bland Lubricating Ophthalmic Ointment USP—Preserve in suitable collapsible ophthalmic ointment tubes. A sterile ointment of white petrolatum and mineral oil. May contain Lanolin, Modified Lanolin, or Lanolin Alcohols. Meets the requirements for Appearance, Color, Sterility, Homogeneity, Acidity or alkalinity, and Metal particles.

HYDROPHILIC OINTMENT

Description: Hydrophilic Ointment USP—NF category: Ointment base.

USP requirements: Hydrophilic Ointment USP—Preserve in tight containers.

Prepare Hydrophilic Ointment as follows: 0.25 gram of Methylparaben, 0.15 gram of Propylparaben, 10 grams of Sodium Lauryl Sulfate, 120 grams of Propylene Glycol, 250 grams of Stearyl Alcohol, 250 grams of White Petrolatum, and 370 grams of Purified Water, to make about 1000 grams. Melt the Stearyl Alcohol and the White Petrolatum on a steam bath, and warm to about 75 °C. Add the other ingredients, previously dissolved in the water and warmed to 75 °C, and stir the mixture until it congeals.

WHITE OINTMENT

Description: White Ointment USP—NF category: Ointment base.

USP requirements: White Ointment USP—Preserve in well-closed containers.

Prepare White Ointment as follows: 50 grams of White Wax and 950 grams of White Petrolatum, to make 1000 grams. Melt the White Wax in a suitable dish on a water bath, add the White Petrolatum, warm until liquefied, then discontinue the heating, and stir the mixture until it begins to congeal.

YELLOW OINTMENT

Description: Yellow Ointment USP—NF category: Ointment base.

USP requirements: Yellow Ointment USP—Preserve in well-closed containers.

Prepare Yellow Ointment as follows: 50 grams of Yellow Wax and 950 grams of Petrolatum, to make 1000 grams. Melt the Yellow Wax in a suitable dish on a steam bath, add the Petrolatum, warm until liquefied, then discontinue the heating, and stir the mixture until it begins to congeal.

OLANZAPINE

Chemical group: Thienobenzodiazepine.

Chemical name: 10*H*-Thieno[2,3-*b*][1,5]benzodiazepine, 2-methyl-4-(4-methyl-1-piperazinyl)-.

Molecular formula: $C_{17}H_{20}N_4S$.

Molecular weight: 312.43.

Description: Yellow crystalline solid.

Solubility: Practically insoluble in water.

USP requirements: Olanzapine Tablets—Not in *USP–NF*.

OLEIC ACID

Chemical name: 9-Octadecenoic acid, (*Z*)-.

Molecular formula: $C_{18}H_{34}O_2$.

Molecular weight: 282.46.

Description: Oleic Acid NF—Colorless to pale yellow, oily liquid when freshly prepared, but on exposure to air it gradually absorbs oxygen and darkens. It has a characteristic, lard-like odor. When strongly heated in air, it is decomposed with the production of acrid vapors.

NF category: Emulsifying and/or solubilizing agent.

Solubility: Oleic Acid NF—Practically insoluble in water. Miscible with alcohol, with chloroform, with ether, and with fixed and volatile oils.

NF requirements: Oleic Acid NF—Preserve in tight containers. It is manufactured from fats and oils derived from edible sources, animal and vegetable, and consists chiefly of (*Z*)-9-octadecenoic acid [CH_3-(CH_2)$_7$CH:CH(CH_2)$_7$COOH]. If it is for external use only, the labeling so indicates. Label it to indicate whether it is derived from animal or vegetable sources. Meets the requirements for Specific gravity (0.889–0.895), Congealing temperature (between 3° and 10° for Oleic Acid derived from animal sources; between 10° and 16° for Oleic Acid derived from vegetable sources), Residue on ignition (not more than 0.01% [about]), Mineral acids, Neutral fat or mineral oil, Acid value (196–204), Iodine value (85–95), and Organic volatile impurities.

Note: Oleic Acid labeled solely for external use is exempt from the requirement that it be prepared from edible sources.

OLEOVITAMIN A AND D

Description:

Oleovitamin A and D USP—Yellow to red, oily liquid, practically odorless or having a fish-like odor, and having no rancid odor. It is a clear liquid at temperatures exceeding 65 °C, and may crystallize on cooling. Unstable in air and in light.

Oleovitamin A and D Capsules USP—The oil contained in Oleovitamin A and D Capsules is a yellow to red, oily liquid, practically odorless or having a fish-like odor, and having no rancid odor. Is a clear liquid at temperatures exceeding 65 °C, and may crystallize on cooling. Is unstable in air and in light.

Solubility: Oleovitamin A and D USP—Insoluble in water and in glycerin; very soluble in ether and in chloroform; soluble in dehydrated alcohol and in vegetable oils.

USP requirements:

Oleovitamin A and D USP—Preserve in tight containers, protected from light and air, preferably under an atmosphere of an inert gas. Store in a dry place. A solution of vitamin A and vitamin D in fish liver oil or in an edible vegetable oil. The vitamin D is present as ergocalciferol or cholecalciferol obtained by the activation of ergosterol or 7-dehydrocholesterol or from natural sources. Label it to indicate the content of vitamin A in mg per gram. The vitamin A content may also be expressed in USP Vitamin A Units per gram. Label it to show whether it contains ergocalciferol, cholecalciferol, or vitamin D from a natural source. Label it to indicate also the vitamin D content in mcg per gram. Its vitamin D content may be expressed also in USP Vitamin D Units per gram. Contains not less than 90.0% of the labeled amounts of vitamins A and D. Meets the requirement for Organic volatile impurities.

Oleovitamin A and D Capsules USP—Preserve in tight, light-resistant containers. Store in a dry place. Label the Capsules to indicate the content, in mg, of vitamin A in each capsule. The vitamin A content in each capsule may be expressed also in USP Vitamin A Units. Label the Capsules to show whether they contain ergocalciferol, cholecalciferol, or vitamin D from a natural source. Label the Capsules to indicate also the vitamin D content, in mcg, in each capsule. The vitamin D content may be expressed also in USP Vitamin D Units in each capsule. Contain the labeled amounts of vitamins A and D, within −10%. The oil in Oleovitamin A and D Capsules conforms to the definition for Oleovitamin A and D.

OLEYL ALCOHOL

Chemical name: 9-Octadecen-1-ol, (*Z*)-.

Molecular formula: $C_{18}H_{36}O$.

Molecular weight: 268.48.

Description: Oleyl Alcohol NF—Clear, colorless to light yellow, oily liquid. Has a faint characteristic odor.

NF category: Emulsifying and/or solubilizing agent.

Solubility: Oleyl Alcohol NF—Insoluble in water; soluble in alcohol, in ether, in isopropyl alcohol, and in light mineral oil.

NF requirements: Oleyl Alcohol NF—Preserve in well-filled, tight containers, and store at controlled room temperature. A mixture of unsaturated and saturated high molecular weight fatty alcohols consisting chiefly of oleyl alcohol. Meets the requirements for Cloud point (not above 10 °C), Refractive index (1.458–1.460), Acid value (not more than 1), Hydroxyl value (205–215), and Iodine value (85–95).

OLIVE OIL

Description: Olive Oil NF—Pale yellow, or light greenish yellow, oily liquid, having a slight characteristic odor.

NF category: Oleaginous vehicle.

Solubility: Olive Oil NF—Slightly soluble in alcohol. Miscible with ether, with chloroform, and with carbon disulfide.

NF requirements: Olive Oil NF—Preserve in tight containers, and prevent exposure to excessive heat. The fixed oil obtained from the ripe fruit of *Olea europaea* Linné (Fam. Oleaceae). Meets the requirements for Specific gravity (0.910–0.915), Heavy metals (not more than 0.001%), Cottonseed oil, Peanut oil, Sesame oil, Teaseed oil, Solidification range of fatty acids (17–26 °C), Free fatty acids, Iodine value (79–88), Saponification value (190–195), and Organic volatile impurities.

OLMESARTAN

Chemical name: Olmesartan medoxomil—1*H*-Imidazol-5-carboxylic acid, 4-(1-hydroxy-1-methylethyl)-2-propyl-1-[[2'-(1*H*-tetrazol-5-yl) [1,1'-biphenyl]-4-yl]methyl]-, (5-methyl-2-oxo-1,3-dioxol-4-yl) methyl ester.

Molecular formula: Olmesartan medoxomil—$C_{29}H_{30}N_6O_6$.

Molecular weight: Olmesartan medoxomil—558.59.

Description: Olmesartan medoxomil—White to light yellowish-white powder or crystalline powder.

Solubility: Olmesartan medoxomil—Practically insoluble in water; sparingly soluble in methanol.

USP requirements: Olmesartan Medoxomil Tablets—Not in *USP–NF*.

OLOPATADINE

Chemical name: Olopatadine hydrochloride—Dibenz[*b,e*]oxepin-2-acetic acid, 11-[3-(dimethylamino)-propylidene]-6,11-dihydro-, hydrochloride, (*Z*)-.

Molecular formula: Olopatadine hydrochloride—$C_{21}H_{23}NO_3 \cdot HCl$.

Molecular weight: Olopatadine hydrochloride—373.87.

Description: Olopatadine hydrochloride—White, crystalline powder.

Solubility: Olopatadine hydrochloride—Soluble in water.

USP requirements: Olopatadine Hydrochloride Ophthalmic Solution—Not in *USP–NF*.

OLSALAZINE

Chemical name: Olsalazine sodium—Benzoic acid, 3,3'-azobis[6-hydroxy-, disodium salt.

Molecular formula: Olsalazine sodium—$C_{14}H_8N_2Na_2O_6$.

Molecular weight: Olsalazine sodium—346.20.

Description: Olsalazine sodium—Yellow crystalline powder; melts with decomposition at 240 °C.

Solubility: Olsalazine sodium—Soluble in water and in dimethyl sulfoxide; practically insoluble in ethanol, in chloroform, and in ether.

USP requirements: Olsalazine Sodium Capsules—Not in *USP–NF*.

OMEPRAZOLE

Chemical group: Substituted benzimidazole.

Chemical name: 1*H*-Benzimidazole, 5-methoxy-2-[[(4-methoxy-3,5-dimethyl-2-pyridinyl)methyl]sulfinyl]-.

Molecular formula: $C_{17}H_{19}N_3O_3S$.

Molecular weight: 345.42.

Description: Omeprazole USP—White to off-white powder. Melts between 150 and 160 °C, with decomposition.

pKa: 4.0 and 8.7.

Solubility: Omeprazole USP—Soluble in dichloromethane; sparingly soluble in methanol and in alcohol; very slightly soluble in water.

Other characteristics: The stability of omeprazole is a function of pH; omeprazole is rapidly degraded in acid media, but has acceptable stability under alkaline conditions.

USP requirements:
Omeprazole USP—Preserve in tight containers and store in a cold place, protected from moisture. Contains not less than 98.0% and not more than 102.0% of omeprazole, calculated on the dried basis. Meets the requirements for Identification, Completeness of solution, Color of solution, Loss on drying (not more than 0.5%), Residue on ignition (not more than 0.1%), Heavy metals (not more than 0.002%), Organic volatile impurities, and Chromatographic purity.
Omeprazole Delayed-release Capsules—Not in *USP–NF*.
Omeprazole Tablets—Not in *USP–NF*.
Omeprazole Magnesium Delayed-release Tablets—Not in *USP–NF*.

ONDANSETRON

Chemical name: Ondansetron hydrochloride—4*H*-Carbazol-4-one, 1,2,3,9-tetrahydro-9-methyl-3-[(2-methyl-1*H*-imidazol-1-yl)methyl]-, monohydrochloride, (±)-, dihydrate.

Molecular formula: Ondansetron hydrochloride—$C_{18}H_{19}N_3O \cdot HCl \cdot 2H_2O$.

Molecular weight: Ondansetron hydrochloride—365.85.

Description: Ondansetron hydrochloride—White to off-white powder.

Solubility: Ondansetron hydrochloride—Sparingly soluble in water and in alcohol; soluble in methanol; slightly soluble in isopropyl alcohol and in dichloromethane; very slightly soluble in acetone, in chloroform, and in ethyl acetate.

USP requirements:
Ondansetron Injection USP—Preserve in single-dose or in multiple-dose containers, preferably of Type I glass, at a temperature between 2° and 30°, protected from light. A sterile solution of Ondansetron Hydrochloride in Water for Injection. Contains an amount equivalent to the labeled amount of ondansetron, within ±5%. Meets the requirements for Identification, Bacterial endotoxins, pH (3.3–4.0), Particulate matter, Limit of ondansetron related compound D (not more than 0.12%), and Chromatographic purity (not more than 0.2% of any individual impurity, and the total of all impurities not more than 0.5%), and for Injections.
Ondansetron Oral Disintegrating Tablets—Not in *USP–NF*.
Ondansetron Hydrochloride USP—Preserve in tight, lightresistant containers. Contains not less than 98.0% and not more than 102.0% of ondansetron hydrochloride, calculated on the anhydrous basis. Meets the requirements for Identification, Water (9.0–10.5%), Residue on ignition (not more than 0.1%), Limit of ondansetron related compound D (not more than 0.10%), and Chromatographic purity (not more than 0.2% of any individual impurity, and the total of all impurities not more than 0.5%).
Ondansetron Hydrochloride Injection—Not in *USP–NF*.
Ondansetron Hydrochloride Oral Solution—Not in *USP–NF*.
Ondansetron Hydrochloride Tablets—Not in *USP–NF*.

ONDANSETRON AND DEXTROSE

For *Ondansetron* and *Dextrose*—See individual listings for chemistry information.

USP requirements: Ondansetron in Dextrose Injection—Not in *USP–NF*.

OPIUM

Description:

Opium USP—Has a very characteristic odor.

Powdered Opium USP—Light brown or moderately yellowish brown powder.

USP requirements:

Opium USP—The air-dried milky exudate obtained by incising the unripe capsules of *Papaver somniferum* Linné or its variety *album* De Candolle (Fam. Papaveraceae). Yields not less than 9.5% of anhydrous morphine. Meets the requirement for Botanic characteristics.

Powdered Opium USP—Preserve in well-closed containers. It is Opium dried at a temperature not exceeding 70 °C, and reduced to a very fine powder. Yields not less than 10.0% and not more than 10.5% of anhydrous morphine. Meets the requirement for Botanic characteristics.

Opium Tincture USP (Laudanum)—Preserve in tight, light-resistant containers, and avoid exposure to direct sunlight and to excessive heat. Contains, in each 100 mL, not less than 0.90 gram and not more than 1.10 grams of anhydrous morphine.

Opium Tincture may be prepared as follows: Place 100 grams of granulated or sliced Opium in a suitable vessel. (Note: Do not use Powdered Opium.) Add 500 mL of boiling water, and allow to stand, with frequent stirring, for 24 hours. Transfer the mixture to a percolator, allow it to drain, percolate with water as the menstruum to complete extraction, and evaporate the percolate to a volume of 400 mL. Boil actively for not less than 15 minutes, and allow to stand overnight. Heat the mixture to 80 °C, add 50 grams of paraffin, and heat until the paraffin is melted. Beat the mixture thoroughly, and cool. Remove the paraffin, and filter the concentrate, washing the paraffin and the filter with sufficient water to make the filtrate measure 750 mL. Add 188 mL of alcohol to the filtrate, mix, and assay a 10-mL portion of the resulting solution as directed. Dilute the remaining solution with a mixture of 1 volume of alcohol and 4 volumes of water to obtain a Tincture containing 1 gram of anhydrous morphine in each 100 mL. Mix.

Meets the requirement for Alcohol content (17.0–21.0%).

Opium Alkaloids Hydrochlorides Injection—Not in *USP–NF*.

OPRELVEKIN

Chemical name: 2-178-Interleukin 11 (human clone pXM/IL-11).

Molecular formula: $C_{854}H_{1411}N_{253}O_{235}S_2$.

Molecular weight: 19,047.04.

Description: Sterile, white, preservative-free, lyophilized powder.

USP requirements: Oprelvekin for Injection—Not in *USP–NF*.

ORANGE OIL

NF requirements: Orange Oil NF—Preserve in well-filled, tight containers, and avoid exposure to excessive heat. The volatile oil obtained by expression from the fresh peel of the ripe fruit of *Citrus sinensis* L. Osbeck (Fam. Rutaceae). The label states the Latin binomial name and, following the official name, the part of the plant source from which the article was derived. Label it also to indicate whether it is California-type or Florida-type Orange Oil. The label indicates that Oil is not to be used if it has a terebinathine ordor. Total aldehyde content, calculated as decanal, is not less than 1.2% and not more than 2.5%. It may contain a suitable antioxidant. Meets the require-

ments for Specific gravity (0.842–0.846), Angular rotation (+94° to +99°), Refractive index (1.472–1.474 at 20°), Ultraviolet absorbance (not less than 0.130 for California-type Orange Oil, or not less than 0.240 for Florida-type Orange Oil), Heavy metals (0.004%), and Foreign oils.

Note—Do not use Orange Oil that has a terebinthine odor.

ORANGE SYRUP

NF requirements: Orange Syrup NF—Preserve in tight containers, and store in a cold place. The label states the Latin binomial name and, following the official name, the part of the plant source from which the article was derived. The label indicates that Syrup is not to be used if it has a terebinthine odor or taste or shows other indications of deterioration. Contains, in each 100 mL, not less than 450 mg and not more than 540 mg of citric acid.

Prepare Orange Syrup as follows: 50 mL of Sweet Orange Peel Tincture, 5 grams of Citric Acid (anhydrous), 15 grams of Talc, 820 grams of Sucrose, and Purified water, a sufficient quantity, to make 1000 mL. Triturate Talc with Tincture and Citric Acid, and gradually add 400 mL of Purified Water. Filter, returning the first portions of the filtrate until it becomes clear, and wash the mortar and the filter with sufficient Purified Water to make the filtrate measure 450 mL. Dissolve Sucrose in this filtrate by agitation, without heating, and add Purified Water to make the product measure 1000 mL. Mix, and strain.

Meets the requirement for Alcohol content (2.0%–5.0%).

Note—Do not use Orange Syrup that has a terebinthine odor or taste or shows other indications of deterioration.

SWEET ORANGE PEEL TINCTURE

NF requirements: Sweet Orange Peel Tincture NF—Preserve in tight, light-resistant containers. Avoid exposure to direct sunlight and excessive heat. Prepared from sweet orange peel, which is the outer rind of the non-artificially colored, fresh, ripe fruit of *Citrus sinesis* (L.) Osbeck (Fam. Rutaceae). The label states the Latin binomial name and the official name.

Prepare Sweet Orange Peel Tincture as follows: Macerate 500 grams of sweet orange peel in 900 mL of alcohol, and dilute the preparation with alcohol to make the product measure 1000 mL. [Note—Exclude the inner, white portion of the rind.] Use Talc as the filtering medium.

Meets the requirement for Alcohol content (62.0–72.0%).

ORGOTEIN

Source: Water-soluble protein congeners derived from red blood cells, liver, and other tissues. Produced from beef liver as Cu-Zn mixed chelate having superoxide dismutase activity.

Chemical name: Orgotein.

Molecular weight: 33,000 with compact conformation maintained by about 4 gram-atoms of divalent metal.

USP requirements: Orgotein for Injection—Not in *USP–NF*.

ORLISTAT

Chemical name:L-Leucine, *N*-formyl-, 1-[(3-hexyl-4-oxo-2oxeta-nyl)methyl]dodecyl ester, [2*S*-[2 alpha(*R**),3 beta]]-.

Molecular formula: $C_{29}H_{53}NO_5$.

Molecular weight: 495.73.

Description: White to off-white crystalline powder. Melting point 43 °C.

Solubility: Practically soluble in water; freely soluble in chloroform; very soluble in methanol and in ethanol.

USP requirements: Orlistat Capsules—Not in *USP–NF*.

ORPHENADRINE

Chemical name:
Orphenadrine citrate—Ethanamine, *N,N*-dimethyl-2-[(2-methylphenyl)phenylmethoxy]-, 2-hydroxy-1,2,3-propane-tricarboxylate (1:1).
Orphenadrine hydrochloride—2-Dimethylaminoethyl 2-methylbenzhydryl ether hydrochloride.

Molecular formula:
Orphenadrine citrate—$C_{18}H_{23}NO \cdot C_6H_8O_7$.
Orphenadrine hydrochloride—$C_{18}H_{23}NO \cdot HCl$.

Molecular weight:
Orphenadrine citrate—461.50.
Orphenadrine hydrochloride—305.83.

Description:
Orphenadrine Citrate USP—White, practically odorless, crystalline powder.
Orphenadrine hydrochloride—White or almost white, odorless or almost odorless, crystalline powder.

Solubility:
Orphenadrine Citrate USP—Sparingly soluble in water; slightly soluble in alcohol; insoluble in chloroform and in ether.
Orphenadrine hydrochloride—Soluble 1 in 1 of water and of alcohol and 1 in 2 of chloroform; practically insoluble in ether.

USP requirements:
Orphenadrine Citrate USP—Preserve in tight, light-resistant containers. Contains not less than 98.0% and not more than 101.5% of orphenadrine citrate, calculated on the dried basis. Meets the requirements for Clarity and color of solution, Identification, Melting range (134–138 °C), Loss on drying (not more than 0.5%), Residue on ignition (not more than 0.1%), Chromatographic purity, Organic volatile impurities, and Isomer content (not more than 3.0%).
Orphenadrine Citrate Injection USP—Preserve in single-dose or in multiple-dose containers, preferably of Type I glass, protected from light. A sterile solution of Orphenadrine Citrate in Water for Injection, prepared with the aid of Sodium Hydroxide. Contains the labeled amount, within ±7%. Meets the requirements for Identification, Bacterial endotoxins, and pH (5.0–6.0), and for Injections.
Orphenadrine Citrate Extended-release Tablets—Not in *USP–NF*.
Orphenadrine Hydrochloride Tablets—Not in *USP–NF*.

ORPHENADRINE, ASPIRIN, AND CAFFEINE

For *Orphenadrine, Aspirin,* and *Caffeine*—See individual listings for chemistry information.

USP requirements: Orphenadrine Citrate, Aspirin, and Caffeine Tablets—Not in *USP–NF*.

OSELTAMIVIR PHOSPHATE

Chemical name: [3*R*-(3 alpha,4 beta,5 alpha)]-Ethyl 4-(acetyla-mino)-5-amino-3-(1-ethylpropoxy)-1-cyclohexene-1-carboxyl-ate phosphate (1:1).

Molecular formula: $C_{16}H_{28}N_2O_4 \cdot H_3PO_4$ (Oseltamivir phosphate); $C_{16}H_{28}N_2O_4$ (Oseltamivir phosphate free base).

Molecular weight: 410.41 (Oseltamivir phosphate); 312.4 (Oseltamivir phosphate free base).

Description: White crystalline solid.

USP requirements: Oseltamivir Phosphate Capsules—Not in *USP–NF*.

OXACILLIN

Chemical name: Oxacillin sodium—4-Thia-1-azabicyclo[3.2.0]-heptane-2-carboxylic acid, 3,3-dimethyl-6-[[(5-methyl-3-phe-nyl-4-isoxazolyl)carbonyl]amino]-7-oxo-, monosodium salt, monohydrate, [2*S*-(2 alpha,5 alpha,6 beta)] .

Molecular formula: Oxacillin sodium—$C_{19}H_{18}N_3NaO_5S \cdot H_2O$.

Molecular weight: Oxacillin sodium—441.43.

Description:
Oxacillin for Injection USP—Fine, white, crystalline powder, odorless or having a slight odor.
Oxacillin Sodium USP—Fine, white, crystalline powder, odorless or having a slight odor.

Solubility:
Oxacillin for Injection USP—Freely soluble in water, in methanol, and in dimethylsulfoxide; slightly soluble in absolute alcohol, in chloroform, in pyridine, and in methyl acetate; insoluble in ethyl acetate, in ether, and in ethylene chloride.
Oxacillin Sodium USP—Freely soluble in water, in methanol, and in dimethylsulfoxide; slightly soluble in absolute alcohol, in chloroform, in pyridine, and in methyl acetate; insoluble in ethyl acetate, in ether, and in ethylene chloride.

USP requirements:
Oxacillin Injection USP—Preserve in Containers for Injections. Maintain in the frozen state. A sterile isoosmotic solution of Oxacillin Sodium in Water for Injection. Contains dextrose as a tonicity-adjusting agent and one or more suitable buffer substances. Contains no preservatives. It meets the requirements for Labeling under Injections. The label states that it is to be thawed just prior to use, describes conditions for proper storage of the resultant solution, and directs that the solution is not to be refrozen. Contains an amount of oxacillin sodium equivalent to the labeled amount of oxacillin, within −10% to +15%. Meets the requirements for Identification, Pyrogen, Sterility, pH (6.0–8.5), and Particulate matter.
Oxacillin for Injection USP—Preserve in Containers for Sterile Solids, at controlled room temperature. Contains an amount of oxacillin sodium equivalent to the labeled amount of oxacillin, within −10% to +15%. Meets the requirements for Constituted solution, Identification, Bacterial endotoxins, Sterility, Uniformity of dosage units, pH (6.0–8.5, in the solution constituted as directed in the labeling), Water (not more than 6.0%), and Particulate matter.

Oxacillin Sodium USP—Preserve in tight containers, at controlled room temperature. Where it is intended for use in preparing injectable dosage forms, the label states that it is sterile or must be subjected to further processing during the preparation of injectable dosage forms. Contains the equivalent of not less than 815 mcg and not more than 950 mcg of oxacillin per mg. Meets the requirements for Identification, Crystallinity, pH (4.5–7.5, in a solution containing 30 mg per mL), and Water (3.5–5.0%), and for Sterility and Bacterial endotoxins under Oxacillin for Injection) and for Bacterial endotoxins under Oxacillin for Injection (where the label states that Oxacillin Sodium must be subjected to further processing during the preparation of injectable dosage forms.

Oxacillin Sodium Capsules USP—Preserve in tight containers, at controlled room temperature. Contain an amount of oxacillin sodium equivalent to the labeled amount of oxacillin, within −10% to +20%. Meet the requirements for Identification, Dissolution (75% in 45 minutes in water in Apparatus 1 at 100 rpm), Uniformity of dosage units, and Water (not more than 6.0%).

Oxacillin Sodium for Oral Solution USP—Preserve in tight containers at controlled room temperature. Contains one or more suitable buffers, colors, flavors, preservatives, and stabilizers. Contains an amount of oxacillin sodium equivalent to the labeled amount of oxacillin, within −10% to +20%. Meets the requirements for Identification, Uniformity of dosage units (single-unit containers), Deliverable volume (multiple-unit containers), pH (5.0–7.5, in the solution constituted as directed in the labeling), and Water (not more than 1.0%).

OXALIPLATIN

Chemical name: [SP-4-2-(1 R-trans)]-(1,2-cyclohexanediamine-N,N)[ethanedioato(2-)-O,O']platinum.

Molecular formula: $C_8H_{14}N_2O_4Pt$.

Molecular weight: 397.29.

Description: Sterile, preservative-free lyophilized powder.

Solubility: Slightly soluble in water at 6 mg/mL; very slightly soluble in methanol; practically insoluble in ethanol and in acetone.

USP requirements: Oxaliplatin for Injection—Not in *USP–NF*.

OXAMNIQUINE

Chemical group: Tetrahydroquinoline derivative.

Chemical name: 6-Quinolinemethanol, 1,2,3,4-tetrahydro-2-[[(1-methylethyl)amino]methyl]-7-nitro-.

Molecular formula: $C_{14}H_{21}N_3O_3$.

Molecular weight: 279.33.

Description: Oxamniquine USP—Yellow-orange crystalline solid.

Solubility: Oxamniquine USP—Sparingly soluble in water; soluble in methanol, in chloroform, and in acetone.

USP requirements:

Oxamniquine USP—Preserve in well-closed containers. Contains not less than 97.0% and not more than 103.0% of oxamniquine, calculated on the anhydrous basis. Meets the requirements for Identification, Melting range (145–152 °C), Specific rotation (−4° to +4°), pH (8.0–10.0 in a suspension [1 in 100]), Water (not more than 1.0%), Residue on ignition (not more than 0.2%, determined on a 2.0-gram test specimen), Iron (not more than 0.005%), Heavy metals (not more than 0.005%), Limit of methyl isobutyl ketone (not more than 0.10%), Related compounds, and Alcohol.

Oxamniquine Capsules USP—Preserve in tight containers. Contain the labeled amount, within ±10%. Meet the requirements for Identification, Dissolution (70% in 60 minutes in 0.1 N hydrochloric acid in Apparatus 2 at 50 rpm), and Uniformity of dosage units.

OXANDROLONE

Chemical group: 17-alpha alkylated anabolic steroid.

Chemical name: 2-Oxaandrostan-3-one, 17-hydroxy-17-methyl-,(5 alpha,17 beta)-.

Molecular formula: $C_{19}H_{30}O_3$.

Molecular weight: 306.44.

Description: Oxandrolone USP—White, odorless, crystalline powder. Is stable in air, but darkens on exposure to light. Melts at about 225 °C.

Solubility: Oxandrolone USP—Practically insoluble in water; freely soluble in chloroform; sparingly soluble in alcohol and in acetone.

USP requirements:

Oxandrolone USP—Preserve in well-closed, light-resistant containers. Contains not less than 97.0% and not more than 100.5% of oxandrolone, calculated on the dried basis. Meets the requirements for Identification, Specific rotation (−18° to −24°), Loss on drying (not more than 1.0%), Residue on ignition (not more than 0.2%), Ordinary impurities, and Organic volatile impurities.

Oxandrolone Tablets USP—Preserve in tight, light-resistant containers. Contain the labeled amount, within ±8%. Meet the requirements for Identification, Disintegration (15 minutes), and Uniformity of dosage units.

OXAPROZIN

Chemical name: 2-Oxazolepropanoic acid, 4,5-diphenyl-.

Molecular formula: $C_{18}H_{15}NO_3$.

Molecular weight: 293.32.

Description: White to off-white powder with a slight odor and a melting point of 162–163 °C.

pKa: 4.3 in water.

Solubility: Slightly soluble in alcohol; insoluble in water.

Other characteristics: Octanol/water partition coefficient—4.8 at physiologic pH (7.4).

USP requirements: Oxaprozin Tablets—Not in *USP–NF*.

OXAZEPAM

Chemical name: 2*H*-1,4-Benzodiazepin-2-one, 7-chloro-1,3-dihydro-3-hydroxy-5-phenyl-.

Molecular formula: $C_{15}H_{11}ClN_2O_2$.

Molecular weight: 286.71.

Description: Oxazepam USP—Creamy white to pale yellow powder. Is practically odorless.

Solubility: Oxazepam USP—Practically insoluble in water; slightly soluble in alcohol and in chloroform; very slightly soluble in ether.

USP requirements:
Oxazepam USP—Preserve in well-closed containers. Contains not less than 98.0% and not more than 102.0% of oxazepam, calculated on the dried basis. Meets the requirements for Identification, pH (4.8–7.0, in an aqueous suspension [1 in 50]), Loss on drying (not more than 2.0%), Residue on ignition (not more than 0.3%), and Organic volatile impurities.
Oxazepam Capsules USP—Preserve in well-closed containers. Contain the labeled amount, within ±10%. Meet the requirements for Identification, Dissolution (75% in 60 minutes in 0.1 *N* hydrochloric acid in Apparatus 2 at 75 rpm), and Uniformity of dosage units.
Oxazepam Tablets USP—Preserve in well-closed containers. Contain the labeled amount, within ±10%. Meet the requirements for Identification, Dissolution (80% in 60 minutes in 0.1 *N* hydrochloric acid in Apparatus 2 at 50 rpm), and Uniformity of dosage units.

OXCARBAZEPINE

Chemical name: 10,11-Dihydro-10-oxo-5*H*-dibenz[b,f]azepine-5-carboxamide.

Molecular formula: $C_{15}H_{12}N_2O_2$.

Molecular weight: 252.27.

Description: White to faintly orange crystalline powder.

Solubility: Slightly soluble in chloroform, in dichloromethane, in acetone, and in methanol; practically insoluble in ethanol, in ether, and in water.

USP requirements: Oxcarbazepine Tablets—Not in *USP–NF*.

OXFENDAZOLE

Chemical name: Carbamic acid, [5-phenylsulfinyl)-1*H*-benzimidazol-2-yl]-, methyl ester.

Molecular formula: $C_{15}H_{13}N_3O_3S$.

Molecular weight: 315.35.

Description: Oxfendazole USP—White or almost white powder.

Solubility: Oxfendazole USP—Slightly soluble in alcohol and in methylene chloride; practically insoluble in water.

USP requirements:
Oxfendazole USP—Preserve in well-closed, light-resistant containers. Label it to indicate that it is for veterinary use only. Contains not less than 98.0% and not more than 100.5% of oxfendazole, calculated on the dried basis. Meets the requirements for Identification, Loss on drying (not more than 1.0%), Residue on ignition (not more than 0.1%), and Related compounds (not more than 2%).

Oxfendazole Oral Suspension USP—Preserve in tight containers, and protect from excessive heat. Label the Suspension to indicate that it is for veterinary use only. Contains the labeled amount, within ±10%. Meets the requirements for Identification and pH (4.3–4.9).

OXICONAZOLE

Chemical name: Oxiconazole nitrate—Ethanone, 1-(2,4-dichlorophenyl)-2-(1*H*-imidazol-1-yl)-, *O*-[(2,4-dichlorophenyl)methyl]oxime, (*Z*)-, mononitrate.

Molecular formula: Oxiconazole nitrate—$C_{18}H_{13}Cl_4N_3O \cdot HNO_3$.

Molecular weight: Oxiconazole nitrate—492.14.

Description: Oxiconazole nitrate—Nearly white crystalline powder.

Solubility: Oxiconazole nitrate—Soluble in methanol; sparingly soluble in ethanol, in chloroform, and in acetone; very slightly soluble in water.

USP requirements:
Oxiconazole Nitrate Cream—Not in *USP–NF*.
Oxiconazole Nitrate Lotion—Not in *USP–NF*.

OXPRENOLOL

Chemical name: Oxprenolol hydrochloride—2-Propanol, 1-(*o*-allyloxyphenoxy)-3-isopropylamino-, hydrochloride.

Molecular formula: Oxprenolol hydrochloride—$C_{15}H_{23}NO_3 \cdot HCl$.

Molecular weight: Oxprenolol hydrochloride—301.81.

Description: Oxprenolol Hydrochloride USP—White, crystalline powder.

Solubility: Oxprenolol Hydrochloride USP—Freely soluble in alcohol, in chloroform, and in water; sparingly soluble in acetone; practically insoluble in ether.

Other characteristics: Lipid solubility—Moderate.

USP requirements:
Oxprenolol Hydrochloride USP—Preserve in well-closed containers. Contains not less than 98.5% and not more than 101.0% of oxprenolol hydrochloride, calculated on the dried basis. Meets the requirements for Clarity of solution, Identification, pH (4.0–6.0, in a solution [1 in 10]), Loss on drying (not more than 0.5%), Residue on ignition (not more than 0.1%), Heavy metals (not more than 0.001%), Chromatographic purity, and Organic volatile impurities.
Oxprenolol Hydrochloride Tablets USP—Preserve in well-closed, light-resistant containers. Contain the labeled amount, within ±10%. Meet the requirements for Identification, Dissolution (80% in 30 minutes in 0.1 *N* hydrochloric acid in Apparatus 1 at 100 rpm), and Uniformity of dosage units.
Oxprenolol Hydrochloride Extended-release Tablets USP—Preserve in well-closed, light-resistant containers. Contain the labeled amount, within ±10%. Meet the requirements for Identification, Drug release (15–45% in 1 hour in 0.1 *N* hydrochloric acid, 30–60% in 1 hour in Dissolution medium, 50–80% in 3 hours in Dissolution medium, and not less than 75% in 7 hours in Dissolution medium, in Apparatus 1 at 100 rpm, the Dissolution medium being simulated intestinal fluid TS without enzyme), and Uniformity of dosage units.

OXTRIPHYLLINE

Source: The choline salt of theophylline.

Chemical name: Ethanaminium, 2-hydroxy-*N,N,N*-trimethyl-, salt with 3,7-dihydro-1,3-dimethyl-1*H*-purine-2,6-dione.

Molecular formula: $C_{12}H_{21}N_5O_3$.

Molecular weight: 283.33.

Description: Oxtriphylline USP—White, crystalline powder, having an amine-like odor. A solution (1 in 100) has a pH of about 10.3.

Solubility: Oxtriphylline USP—Freely soluble in water and in alcohol; very slightly soluble in chloroform.

USP requirements:
Oxtriphylline USP—Preserve in tight containers. Contains not less than 61.7% and not more than 65.5% of anhydrous theophylline, calculated on the dried basis. Meets the requirements for Identification, Melting range (185–189 °C), Loss on drying (not more than 1.0%), Residue on ignition (not more than 0.3%), Chloride (not more than 0.02%), Ordinary impurities, Organic volatile impurities, and Choline content.

Oxtriphylline Oral Solution USP—Preserve in tight containers. Label Oral Solution to state both the content of oxtriphylline and the content of anhydrous theophylline. Contains an amount of oxtriphylline equivalent to the labeled amount of anhydrous theophylline, within ±10%. Meets the requirements for Identification, pH (6.4–9.0), and Alcohol content (if present, within −10% to +15% of labeled amount, the labeled amount being not more than 20.0%).

Oxtriphylline Syrup—Not in *USP–NF*.

Oxtriphylline Tablets USP—Preserve in tight containers. Label Tablets to state both the content of oxtriphylline and the content of anhydrous theophylline. Contain an amount of Oxtriphylline equivalent to the labeled amount of anhydrous theophylline, within ±10%. Meet the requirements for Identification, Dissolution (80% in 30 minutes in water in Apparatus 2 at 50 rpm), and Uniformity of dosage units.

Oxtriphylline Delayed-release Tablets USP—Preserve in tight containers. Label the Tablets to state both the content of oxtriphylline and the content of anhydrous theophylline. The label indicates that the Tablets are enteric-coated. Contain an amount of oxtriphylline equivalent to the labeled amount of anhydrous theophylline, within ±10%. Meet the requirements for Identification, Disintegration, and Uniformity of dosage units.

Oxtriphylline Extended-release Tablets USP—Preserve in tight containers. Label the Tablets to state both the content of oxtriphylline and the content of anhydrous theophylline. Contain an amount of oxtriphylline equivalent to the labeled amount of anhydrous theophylline, within ±10%. Meet the requirements for Identification, Drug release (5–30% in 1 hour, 50–70% in 3 hours, 65–85% in 5 hours, and not less than 75% in 7 hours for Test 1 [for products labeled as 400-mg tablets] and 15–40% in 1 hour, 50–70% in 3 hours, and not less than 75% in 7 hours for Test 2 [for products labeled as 600-mg tablets] in 0.1 *N* hydrochloric acid for the first hour, then buffer [pH 7.5] in Apparatus 2 at 50 rpm), and Uniformity of dosage units.

OXTRIPHYLLINE AND GUAIFENESIN

For *Oxtriphylline* and *Guaifenesin*—See individual listings for chemistry information.

USP requirements: Oxtriphylline and Guaifenesin Elixir—Not in *USP–NF*.

OXYBENZONE

Chemical name: Methanone, (2-hydroxy-4-methoxyphenyl)phenyl-.

Molecular formula: $C_{14}H_{12}O_3$.

Molecular weight: 228.24.

Description: Oxybenzone USP—Pale yellow powder.

Solubility: Oxybenzone USP—Practically insoluble in water; freely soluble in alcohol and in toluene.

USP requirements: Oxybenzone USP—Preserve in tight, light-resistant containers. Contains not less than 97.0% and not more than 103.0% of oxybenzone, calculated on the dried basis. Meets the requirements for Identification, Congealing temperature (not lower than 62.0 °C), and Loss on drying (not more than 2.0%).

OXYBENZONE AND PADIMATE O

For *Oxybenzone* and *Padimate O*—See individual listings for chemistry information.

USP requirements:
Oxybenzone and Padimate O Cream—Not in *USP–NF*.
Oxybenzone and Padimate O Lip Balm—Not in *USP–NF*.
Oxybenzone and Padimate O Lotion—Not in *USP–NF*.
Oxybenzone and Padimate O Oil—Not in *USP–NF*.
Oxybenzone and Padimate O Stick—Not in *USP–NF*.

OXYBENZONE AND ROXADIMATE

For *Oxybenzone* and *Roxadimate*—See individual listings for chemistry information.

USP requirements:
Oxybenzone and Roxadimate Cream—Not in *USP–NF*.
Oxybenzone and Roxadimate Lotion—Not in *USP–NF*.

OXYBUTYNIN

Chemical group: Synthetic tertiary amine.

Chemical name: Oxybutynin chloride—Benzeneacetic acid, alpha-cyclohexyl-alpha-hydroxy-, 4-(diethylamino)-2-butynyl ester hydrochloride.

Molecular formula: Oxybutynin chloride—$C_{22}H_{31}NO_3 \cdot HCl$.

Molecular weight: Oxybutynin chloride—393.95.

Description: Oxybutynin Chloride USP—White, crystalline, practically odorless powder.

pKa: Oxybutynin chloride—6.96.

Solubility: Oxybutynin Chloride USP—Freely soluble in water and in alcohol; very soluble in methanol and in chloroform; soluble in acetone; slightly soluble in ether; very slightly soluble in hexane.

USP requirements:
Oxybutynin Chloride USP—Preserve in well-closed containers. Contains not less than 97.0% and not more than 101.0% of oxybutynin chloride, calculated on the dried basis. Meets the requirements for Identification, Melting range (124–129 °C), Loss on drying (not more than 3%), Residue on ignition (not more than 0.1%), Heavy metals (not more than 0.002%), Chromatographic purity, Organic volatile impurities, and Chloride content (8–10%).

Oxybutynin Chloride Oral Solution USP—Preserve in tight, light-resistant containers. Contains the labeled amount, within ±10%. Meets the requirement for Identification.

Oxybutynin Chloride Syrup USP—Preserve in tight, light-resistant containers. Contains the labeled amount, within ±10%. Meets the requirement for Identification.

Oxybutynin Chloride Tablets USP—Preserve in tight, light-resistant containers. Contain the labeled amount, within ± 10%. Meet the requirements for Identification, Dissolution (80% in 30 minutes in water in Apparatus 2 at 50 rpm), and Uniformity of dosage units.

OXYCODONE

Chemical name:

Oxycodone hydrochloride—Morphinan-6-one, 4,5-epoxy-14-hydroxy-3-methoxy-17-methyl-, hydrochloride, (5 alpha)-.

Oxycodone terephthalate—Morphinan-6-one, 4,5-epoxy-14-hydroxy-3-methoxy-17-methyl-, 1,4-benzenedicarboxylate(2:1 salt), (5 alpha).

Molecular formula:

Oxycodone hydrochloride—$C_{18}H_{21}NO_4 \cdot HCl$.

Oxycodone terephthalate—$(C_{18}H_{21}NO_4)_2 \cdot C_8H_6O_4$.

Molecular weight:

Oxycodone hydrochloride—351.82.

Oxycodone terephthalate—796.86.

Description: Oxycodone Hydrochloride USP—White to off-white, hygroscopic crystals or powder. Is odorless.

Solubility: Oxycodone Hydrochloride USP—Soluble in water; slightly soluble in alcohol.

USP requirements:

Oxycodone Hydrochloride USP—Preserve in tight containers. Contains not less than 97.0% and not more than 103.0% of oxycodone hydrochloride, calculated on the anhydrous, solvent-free basis. Meets the requirements for Identification, Specific rotation (−137° to −149°), Water (not more than 7.0%), Residue on ignition (not more than 0.05%), Limit of alcohol (not more than 1.0%), Chloride content (9.8–10.4%, calculated on the anhydrous, solvent-free basis), and Chromatographic purity.

Oxycodone Hydrochloride Oral Solution USP—Preserve in tight, light-resistant containers. Contains the labeled amount, within ±10%. Meets the requirements for Identification, pH (1.4–4.0), and Alcohol content (if present, 85.0–115.0%).

Oxycodone Hydrochloride Suppositories—Not in *USP–NF*.

Oxycodone Hydrochloride Tablets USP—Preserve in tight, light-resistant containers. Contain the labeled amount, within ±10%. Meet the requirements for Identification, Dissolution (70% in 45 minutes in water in Apparatus 2 at 50 rpm), and Uniformity of dosage units.

Oxycodone Hydrochloride Extended-release Tablets—Not in *USP–NF*.

Oxycodone Terephthalate USP—Preserve in tight containers. Contains not less than 97.0% and not more than 103.0% of oxycodone terephthalate, calculated on the dried basis. Meets the requirements for Identification, Loss on drying (not more than 1.5%), Residue on ignition (not more than 1%), Related compounds, and Terephthalic acid content (20.2–21.5%, calculated on the dried basis).

OXYCODONE AND ACETAMINOPHEN

For *Oxycodone* and *Acetaminophen*—See individual listings for chemistry information.

USP requirements:

Oxycodone and Acetaminophen Capsules USP—Preserve in tight, light-resistant containers. Contain Oxycodone Hydrochloride and Acetaminophen, or Oxycodone Hydrochloride, Oxycodone Terephthalate, and Acetaminophen. Contain the labeled amounts of oxycodone hydrochloride or oxycodone hydrochloride and oxycodone terephthalate, calculated as total oxycodone, and the labeled amount of acetaminophen, within ±10%. Meet the requirements for Identification, Dissolution (75% of each active ingredient in 45 minutes in 0.1 N hydrochloric acid in Apparatus 2 at 50 rpm), and Uniformity of dosage units.

Oxycodone and Acetaminophen Oral Solution—Not in *USP–NF*.

Oxycodone and Acetaminophen Tablets USP—Preserve in tight, light-resistant containers. Contain Oxycodone Hydrochloride and Acetaminophen. Tablets may be labeled to indicate the content of oxycodone hydrochloride equivalent. Each mg of oxycodone is equivalent to 1.116 mg of oxycodone hydrochloride. Contain the labeled amounts of oxycodone and acetaminophen, within ±10%. Meet the requirements for Identification, Dissolution (75% of each active ingredient in 45 minutes in 0.1 N hydrochloric acid in Apparatus 2 at 50 rpm), and Uniformity of dosage units.

OXYCODONE AND ASPIRIN

For *Oxycodone* and *Aspirin*—See individual listings for chemistry information.

USP requirements: Oxycodone and Aspirin Tablets USP—Preserve in tight, light-resistant containers. Contain Oxycodone Hydrochloride and Aspirin, or Oxycodone Hydrochloride, Oxycodone Terephthalate, and Aspirin. Label Tablets to state both the content of the oxycodone active moiety and the content or contents of the salt or salts of oxycodone used in formulating the article. Contain the labeled amount of oxycodone, within ±7%, and the labeled amount of aspirin, within ±10%. Meet the requirements for Identification, Dissolution (80% of oxycodone and 75% of aspirin in 30 minutes in 0.05 M acetate buffer [pH 4.50 ±0.05] in Apparatus 1 at 50 rpm), Uniformity of dosage units, and Salicylic acid (not more than 3.0%).

OXYGEN

Chemical name: Oxygen.

Molecular formula: O_2.

Molecular weight: 32.00.

Description: Oxygen USP—Colorless, odorless gas, which supports combustion more energetically than does air. One liter at 0 °C and at a pressure of 760 mm of mercury weighs about 1.429 grams.

Solubility: Oxygen USP—One volume dissolves in about 32 volumes of water and in about 7 volumes of alcohol at 20 °C and at a pressure of 760 mm of mercury.

USP requirements: Oxygen USP—Preserve in cylinders or in a pressurized storage tank. Containers used for Oxygen must not be treated with any toxic, sleep-inducing, or narcosis-producing compounds, and must not be treated with any compound that will be irritating to the respiratory tract when the Oxygen is used. Label it to indicate whether or not it has been produced by the air-liquefaction process. Where it is piped directly from the cylinder or storage tank to the point of use, label each outlet "Oxygen." Contains not less than 99.0%, by volume, of oxygen. (Note: Oxygen that is produced by the air-liquefaction process is exempt from the requirements of the

tests for Carbon dioxide and Carbon monoxide.) Meets the requirements for Identification, Odor, Carbon dioxide (not more than 0.03%), and Carbon monoxide (not more than 0.001%).

OXYGEN 93 PERCENT

USP requirements: Oxygen 93 Percent USP—Preserve in cylinders or in a low pressure collecting tank. Containers used for Oxygen 93 Percent must not be treated with any toxic, sleep-inducing, or narcosis-producing compounds, and must not be treated with any compound that will be irritating to the respiratory tract when the Oxygen 93 Percent is used. It is Oxygen produced from air by the molecular sieve process. Where it is piped directly from the collecting tank to the point of use, label each outlet "Oxygen 93 Percent." Contains not less than 90.0% and not more than 96.0%, by volume, of oxygen, the remainder consisting mostly of argon and nitrogen. Meets the requirements for Identification, Odor, Carbon dioxide (not more than 0.03%), and Carbon monoxide (not more than 0.001%).

WATER O 15

Chemical name: Water-^{15}O.

Molecular formula: H$_2$^{15}O.

USP requirements: Water O 15 Injection USP—Preserve in a single-dose container that is adequately shielded. A sterile solution of Water O 15 in isotonic Sodium Chloride Injection in which a portion of the molecules are labeled with radioactive ^{15}O. Label container to include the following, in addition to the information specified for Labeling under Injections: the time and date of calibration; the amount of ^{15}O as water expressed as megabecquerels (or millicuries) per mL, at time of calibration; total activity at time of calibration; the expiration time and date; the name and quantity of any added preservative or stabilizer; and the statement "Caution—Radioactive Material." The labeling indicates that in making dosage calculations, correction is to be made for radioactive decay and also indicates that the radioactive half-life of ^{15}O is 123 seconds. The label indicates "Do not use if cloudy or if it contains particulate matter." Contains the labeled amount of ^{15}O, within ±10%, expressed in megabecquerels (or millicuries) per mL at the time indicated in the labeling. Meets the requirements for Specific activity, Identification, Radionuclide identification, Bacterial endotoxins, Sterility, pH (4.5–8.0), Particulate matter, Radiochemical purity, Radionuclidic purity, and Heavy metals (not more than 5 ppm), and for Injections (except that the Injection may be distributed or dispensed prior to completion of the test for Sterility, the latter test being started on the day of final manufacture, and except that it is not subject to the recommendation for Volume in Container under Injections).

OXYMETAZOLINE

Source: Prepared from (4-*tert*-butyl-2,6-dimethyl-3-hydroxyphenyl)acetonitrile and ethylenediamine.

Chemical name: Oxymetazoline hydrochloride—Phenol, 3-[(4,5-dihydro-1*H*-imidazol-2-yl)methyl]-6-(1,1-dimethylethyl)-2,4-dimethyl-, monohydrochloride.

Molecular formula: Oxymetazoline hydrochloride—C$_{16}$H$_{24}$N$_2$O · HCl.

Molecular weight: Oxymetazoline hydrochloride—296.84.

Description: Oxymetazoline Hydrochloride USP—White to practically white, fine crystalline powder. Is hygroscopic. Melts at about 300 °C, with decomposition.

Solubility: Oxymetazoline Hydrochloride USP—Soluble in water and in alcohol; practically insoluble in chloroform and in ether.

USP requirements:
Oxymetazoline Hydrochloride USP—Preserve in tight containers. Contains not less than 98.5% and not more than 101.5% of oxymetazoline hydrochloride, calculated on the dried basis. Meets the requirements for Identification, pH (4.0–6.5, in a solution [1 in 20]), Loss on drying (not more than 1.0%), Residue on ignition (not more than 0.1%), and Heavy metals (not more than 0.001%).
Oxymetazoline Hydrochloride Nasal Solution USP—Preserve in tight containers. A solution of Oxymetazoline Hydrochloride in water adjusted to a suitable tonicity. Contains the labeled amount, within ±10%. Meets the requirements for Identification and pH (4.0–6.5).
Oxymetazoline Hydrochloride Ophthalmic Solution USP—Preserve in tight containers. A sterile, buffered solution of Oxymetazoline Hydrochloride in water adjusted to a suitable tonicity. Contains the labeled amount, within ± 10%. Contains a suitable preservative. Meets the requirements for Identification, Sterility, and pH (5.8–6.8).

OXYMETHOLONE

Chemical group: 17-alpha alkylated anabolic steroid.

Chemical name: Androstan-3-one, 17-hydroxy-2-(hydroxymethylene)-17-methyl-, (5 alpha,17 beta)-.

Molecular formula: C$_{21}$H$_{32}$O$_3$.

Molecular weight: 332.48.

Description: Oxymetholone USP—White to creamy white, crystalline powder. Is odorless, and is stable in air.

Solubility: Oxymetholone USP—Practically insoluble in water; freely soluble in chloroform; soluble in dioxane; sparingly soluble in alcohol; slightly soluble in ether.

USP requirements:
Oxymetholone USP—Preserve in well-closed containers. Contains not less than 97.0% and not more than 103.0% of oxymetholone, calculated on the dried basis. Meets the requirements for Completeness of solution, Identification, Melting range (172–180 °C), Specific rotation (+34° to +38°), Loss on drying (not more than 1.0%), and Organic volatile impurities.
Oxymetholone Tablets USP—Preserve in well-closed containers. Contain the labeled amount, within ±10%. Meet the requirements for Identification, Dissolution (75% in 45 minutes in 0.05 *M* alkaline borate buffer [pH 8.5] in Apparatus 1 at 100 rpm), and Uniformity of dosage units.

OXYMORPHONE

Chemical name: Oxymorphone hydrochloride—Morphinan-6-one, 4,5-epoxy-3,14-dihydroxy-17-methyl-, hydrochloride, (5 alpha)-.

Molecular formula: Oxymorphone hydrochloride—C$_{17}$H$_{19}$NO$_4$ · HCl.

Molecular weight: Oxymorphone hydrochloride—337.80.

Description: Oxymorphone Hydrochloride USP—White or slightly off-white, odorless powder. Darkens on exposure to light. Its aqueous solutions are slightly acidic.

Solubility: Oxymorphone Hydrochloride USP—Freely soluble in water; sparingly soluble in alcohol and in ether.

USP requirements:

Oxymorphone Hydrochloride USP—Preserve in tight, light-resistant containers. Contains not less than 97.0% and not more than 102.0% of oxymorphone hydrochloride, calculated on the dried basis. Meets the requirements for Identification, Specific rotation (–145° to –155°), Acidity, Loss on drying (not more than 8.0%), Residue on ignition (not more than 0.3%), Limit of nonphenolic substances, Ordinary impurities, and Chloride content (10.2–10.8%, calculated on the dried basis).

Oxymorphone Hydrochloride Injection USP—Preserve in single-dose or in multiple-dose containers of Type I glass, protected from light. A sterile solution of Oxymorphone Hydrochloride in Water for Injection. Contains the labeled amount, within ±7%. Meets the requirements for Identification, Bacterial endotoxins, and pH (2.7–4.5), and for Injections.

Oxymorphone Hydrochloride Suppositories USP—Preserve in well-closed containers, and store in a refrigerator. Contain the labeled amount, within ±7%. Meet the requirement for Identification.

OXYPHENBUTAZONE

Chemical name: 3,5-Pyrazolidinedione, 4-butyl-1-(4-hydroxyphenyl)-2-phenyl-, monohydrate.

Molecular formula: $C_{19}H_{20}N_2O_3 \cdot H_2O$.

Molecular weight: 342.39.

Description: Oxyphenbutazone USP—White to yellowish white, odorless, crystalline powder. Melts over a wide range between about 85 and 100 °C.

Solubility: Oxyphenbutazone USP—Very slightly soluble in water; soluble in alcohol; freely soluble in acetone and in ether.

USP requirements:

Oxyphenbutazone USP—Preserve in tight containers. Contains not less than 98.0% and not more than 100.5% of oxyphenbutazone, calculated on the anhydrous basis. Meets the requirements for Identification, Water (5.0–6.0%), Residue on ignition (not more than 0.1%), Chloride, and Chromatographic purity.

Oxyphenbutazone Tablets USP—Preserve in tight containers. Contain the labeled amount, within ±6%. Meet the requirements for Identification, Dissolution (60% in 30 minutes in phosphate buffer [pH 7.5] in Apparatus 1 at 100 rpm), and Uniformity of dosage units.

OXYQUINOLINE SULFATE

Chemical name: 8-Quinolinol sulfate (2:1) (salt).

Molecular formula: $(C_9H_7NO)_2 \cdot H_2SO_4$.

Molecular weight: 388.40.

Description: Oxyquinoline Sulfate NF—Yellow powder. Melts at about 185 °C.

NF category: Complexing agent.

Solubility: Oxyquinoline Sulfate NF—Very soluble in water; freely soluble in methanol; slightly soluble in alcohol; practically insoluble in acetone and in ether.

NF requirements: Oxyquinoline Sulfate NF—Preserve in well-closed containers. It is 8-hydroxyquinoline sulfate. Contains not less than 97.0% and not more than 101.0% of oxyquinoline sulfate, calculated on the anhydrous basis. Meets the requirements for Identification, Water (4.0–6.0%), Residue on ignition (not more than 0.3%), Heavy metals (not more than 20 mcg per gram), and Organic volatile impurities.

OXYTETRACYCLINE

Chemical name:

Oxytetracycline—2-Naphthacenecarboxamide, 4-(dimethylamino)-1,4,4a,5,5a,6,11,12a-octahydro-3,5,6,10,12,12-ahexahydroxy-6-methyl-1,11-dioxo-, [4S-(4 alpha,4a alpha,5 alpha,5a alpha,6 beta,12a alpha)]-, dihydrate.

Oxytetracycline calcium—2-Naphthacenecarboxamide, 4-(dimethylamino)-1,4,4a,5,5a,6,11,12a-octahydro-3,5,6,10,12,12a-hexahydroxy-6-methyl-1,11-dioxo-, calcium salt, [4S-(4 alpha,4a alpha,5 alpha,5a alpha,6 beta,12a alpha)]-.

Oxytetracycline hydrochloride—2-Naphthacenecarboxamide, 4-(dimethylamino)-1,4,4a,5,5a,6,11,12a-octahydro-3,5,6,10,12,12a-hexahydroxy-6-methyl-1,11-dioxo-, monohydrochloride, [4S-(4 alpha,4a alpha,5 alpha,5a alpha,6 beta,12a alpha)]-.

Molecular formula:

Oxytetracycline—$C_{22}H_{24}N_2O_9 \cdot 2H_2O$.

Oxytetracycline calcium—$C_{44}H_{46}CaN_4O_{18}$.

Oxytetracycline hydrochloride—$C_{22}H_{24}N_2O_9 \cdot HCl$.

Molecular weight:

Oxytetracycline—496.46.

Oxytetracycline calcium—958.93.

Oxytetracycline hydrochloride—496.89.

Description:

Oxytetracycline USP—Pale yellow to tan, odorless, crystalline powder. Is stable in air, but exposure to strong sunlight causes it to darken. It loses potency in solutions of pH below 2, and is rapidly destroyed by alkali hydroxide solutions.

Oxytetracycline Calcium USP—Yellow to light brown, crystalline powder.

Oxytetracycline Hydrochloride USP—Yellow, odorless, crystalline powder. Is hygroscopic. Decomposes at a temperature exceeding 180 °C, and exposure to strong sunlight or to temperatures exceeding 90 °C in moist air causes it to darken. Its potency is diminished in solutions having a pH below 2, and is rapidly destroyed by alkali hydroxide solutions.

Solubility:

Oxytetracycline USP—Very slightly soluble in water; freely soluble in 3 N hydrochloric acid and in alkaline solutions; sparingly soluble in alcohol.

Oxytetracycline Calcium USP—Insoluble in water.

Oxytetracycline Hydrochloride USP—Freely soluble in water, but crystals of oxytetracycline base separate as a result of partial hydrolysis of the hydrochloride. Sparingly soluble in alcohol and in methanol, and even less soluble in dehydrated alcohol; insoluble in chloroform and in ether.

USP requirements:

Oxytetracycline USP—Preserve in tight, light-resistant containers. Where it is intended for use in preparing injectable dosage forms, the label states that it is sterile or must be subjected to further processing during the preparation of injectable dosage forms. Has a potency equivalent to not less than 832 mcg of oxytetracycline per mg. Meets the

requirements for Identification, Crystallinity, pH (4.5–7.0, in an aqueous suspension containing 10 mg per mL), and Water (6.0–9.0%), and for Sterility and Bacterial endotoxins under Oxytetracycline for Injection (where the label states that Oxytetracycline is sterile), and for Bacterial endotoxins under Oxytetracycline for Injection (where the label states that Oxytetracycline must be subjected to further processing during the preparation of injectable dosage forms).

Oxytetracycline Injection USP—Preserve in single-dose or in multiple-dose containers, protected from light. A sterile solution of Oxytetracycline with or without one or more suitable anesthetics, antioxidants, buffers, complexing agents, preservatives, and solvents. Contains the labeled amount, within −10% to +20%. Meets the requirements for Identification, Bacterial endotoxins, Sterility, and pH (8.0–9.0).

Oxytetracycline for Injection USP—Preserve in Containers for Sterile Solids, protected from light. Contains an amount of oxytetracycline hydrochloride equivalent to the labeled amount of oxytetracycline, within −10% to +15%. Meets the requirements for Constituted solution, Bacterial endotoxins, Sterility, pH (1.8–2.8, in a solution containing 25 mg per mL), Loss on drying (not more than 3.0%), and Particulate matter, for Identification test B under Oxytetracycline Hydrochloride, and for Uniformity of dosage units and Labeling under Injections.

Oxytetracycline Tablets USP—Preserve in tight, light-resistant containers. Contain the labeled amount, within −10% to +20%. Meet the requirements for Identification, Dissolution (75% in 45 minutes in 0.1 N hydrochloric acid in Apparatus 1 at 100 rpm), Uniformity of dosage units, and Water (not more than 7.5%).

Oxytetracycline Calcium USP—Preserve in tight, light-resistant containers, and store in a cool place. Has a potency equivalent to not less than 865 mcg of oxytetracycline per mg, calculated on the anhydrous basis. Meets the requirements for Identification, Crystallinity, pH (6.0–8.0, in an aqueous suspension containing 25 mg per mL), Water (8.0–14.0%), and Calcium content (3.85–4.35%, calculated on the anhydrous basis).

Oxytetracycline Calcium Oral Suspension USP—Preserve in tight, light-resistant containers. Contains an amount of oxytetracycline calcium equivalent to the labeled amount of oxytetracycline, within −10% to +20%. Contains one or more suitable buffers, colors, flavors, preservatives, stabilizers, and suspending agents. Meets the requirements for Identification, pH (5.0–8.0), Deliverable volume (for Suspension packaged in multiple-unit containers), and Uniformity of dosage units (for Suspension packaged in single-unit containers).

Oxytetracycline Hydrochloride USP—Preserve in tight, light-resistant containers. Where it is intended for use in preparing injectable or ophthalmic dosage forms, the label states that it is sterile or must be subjected to further processing during the preparation of injectable or ophthalmic dosage forms. Has a potency equivalent to not less than 835 mcg of oxytetracycline per mg, calculated on the dried basis. Meets the requirements for Identification, Crystallinity, pH (2.0–3.0, in a solution containing 10 mg per mL), and Loss on drying (not more than 2.0%), and for Sterility and Bacterial endotoxins under Oxytetracycline for Injection (where the label states that Oxytetracycline Hydrochloride is sterile), and for Bacterial endotoxins under Oxytetracycline for Injection (where the label states that Oxytetracycline Hydrochloride must be subjected to further processing during the preparation of injectable dosage forms). It is exempt from the requirements for Bacterial endotoxins (where it is intended for use in preparing ophthalmic dosage forms).

Oxytetracycline Hydrochloride Capsules USP—Preserve in tight, light-resistant containers. Contain an amount of oxytetracycline hydrochloride equivalent to the labeled amount of oxytetracycline, within −10% to +20%. Meet

the requirements for Identification, Dissolution (80% in 60 minutes in water in Apparatus 2 at 75 rpm), Uniformity of dosage units, and Loss on drying (not more than 5.0%).

Oxytetracycline Hydrochloride Soluble Powder USP—Preserve in well-closed containers. A mixture of Oxytetracycline Hydrochloride and one or more suitable excipients. Label it to indicate that it is for oral veterinary use only. Contains the labeled amount, within ±10%. Meets the requirements for Identification, pH (1.5–3.0, in the solution obtained as directed in the labeling), Loss on drying (not more than 3.0%, and Minimum fill.

OXYTETRACYCLINE AND HYDROCORTISONE

For *Oxytetracycline* and *Hydrocortisone*—See individual listings for chemistry information.

USP requirements:

Oxytetracycline Hydrochloride and Hydrocortisone Ointment USP—Preserve in collapsible tubes or in well-closed, light-resistant containers. Contains an amount of oxytetracycline hydrochloride equivalent to the labeled amount of oxytetracycline, within −10% to +15%, and the labeled amount of hydrocortisone, within ±10%. Meets the requirements for Minimum fill and Water (not more than 1.0%).

Oxytetracycline Hydrochloride and Hydrocortisone Acetate Ophthalmic Suspension USP—Preserve in tight, light-resistant containers. The containers are sealed and tamper-proof so that sterility is assured at time of first use. A sterile suspension of Oxytetracycline Hydrochloride and Hydrocortisone Acetate in a suitable oil vehicle with one or more suitable suspending agents. Contains an amount of oxytetracycline hydrochloride equivalent to the labeled amount of oxytetracycline, within −10% to +15%, and the labeled amount of hydrocortisone acetate, within ±10%. Meets the requirements for Sterility and Water (not more than 1.0%).

OXYTETRACYCLINE AND NYSTATIN

For *Oxytetracycline* and *Nystatin*—See individual listings for chemistry information.

USP requirements:

Oxytetracycline and Nystatin Capsules USP—Preserve in tight, light-resistant containers. Contain the labeled amount of oxytetracycline, within −10% to +20%, and the labeled amount of USP Nystatin Units, within −10% to +35%. Meet the requirements for Identification, Dissolution (75% of oxytetracycline in 45 minutes in 0.1 N hydrochloric acid in Apparatus 1 at 100 rpm), Uniformity of dosage units, and Water (not more than 7.5%).

Oxytetracycline and Nystatin for Oral Suspension USP—Preserve in tight, light-resistant containers, at controlled room temperature. A dry mixture of Oxytetracycline and Nystatin with one or more suitable buffers, colors, diluents, flavors, suspending agents, and preservatives. When constituted as directed in the labeling, contains the labeled amount of oxytetracycline, within −10% to +20%, and the labeled amount of USP Nystatin Units, within −10% to +35%. Meets the requirements for Identification, Uniformity of dosage units (for solid packaged in single-unit containers), Deliverable volume (for solid packaged in multiple-unit

containers), pH (4.5–7.5, in the suspension constituted as directed in the labeling), and Water (not more than 2.0%).

OXYTETRACYCLINE, PHENAZOPYRIDINE, AND SULFA-METHIZOLE

For *Oxytetracycline, Phenazopyridine,* and *Sulfamethizole*—See individual listings for chemistry information.

USP requirements: Oxytetracycline and Phenazopyridine Hydrochlorides and Sulfamethizole Capsules USP—Preserve in tight, light-resistant containers. Contain an amount of oxytetracycline hydrochloride equivalent to the labeled amount of oxytetracycline, within −10% to +20%, and the labeled amounts of phenazopyridine hydrochloride, within −10% to +15%, and sulfamethizole, within ±10%. Meet the requirements for Uniformity of dosage units and Loss on drying (not more than 5.0%).

OXYTETRACYCLINE AND POLYMYXIN B

For *Oxytetracycline* and *Polymyxin B*—See individual listings for chemistry information.

USP requirements:
Oxytetracycline Hydrochloride and Polymyxin B Sulfate Ointment USP—Preserve in collapsible tubes or in well-closed, light-resistant containers. Contains amounts of oxytetracycline hydrochloride and polymyxin B sulfate equivalent to the labeled amounts of oxytetracycline, within −10% to +20%, and polymyxin B, within −10% to +25%. Meets the requirements for Minimum fill and Water (not more than 1.0%).

Oxytetracycline Hydrochloride and Polymyxin B Sulfate Ophthalmic Ointment USP—Preserve in collapsible ophthalmic ointment tubes. A sterile ointment containing Oxytetracycline Hydrochloride and Polymyxin B Sulfate. Contains amounts of oxytetracycline hydrochloride and polymyxin B sulfate equivalent to the labeled amounts of oxytetracycline, within −10% to +20%, and polymyxin B, within −10% to +25%. Meets the requirements for Sterility, Minimum fill, Water (not more than 1.0%), and Metal particles.

Oxytetracycline Hydrochloride and Polymyxin B Sulfate Topical Powder USP—Preserve in well-closed containers. Contains amounts of oxytetracycline hydrochloride and polymyxin B sulfate equivalent to the labeled amounts of oxytetracycline and polymyxin B, within −10% to +20%, in a suitable fine powder base. Meets the requirements for Minimum fill and Loss on drying (not more than 2.0%).

Oxytetracycline Hydrochloride and Polymyxin B Sulfate Vaginal Tablets USP—Preserve in well-closed containers. Contain amounts of oxytetracycline hydrochloride and polymyxin B sulfate equivalent to the labeled amounts of oxytetracycline and polymyxin B, within −10% to +20%. Meet the requirement for Loss on drying (not more than 3.0%).

OXYTOCIN

Chemical name: Oxytocin.

Molecular formula: $C_{43}H_{66}N_{12}O_{12}S_2$.

Molecular weight: 1007.19.

Description: White powder.

Solubility: Soluble in water.

USP requirements:
Oxytocin USP—Preserve in tight containers, preferably of Type I glass, in a refrigerator. A nonapeptide hormone having the property of causing the contraction of uterine smooth muscle and of the myoepithelial cells within the mammary gland. Prepared by synthesis or obtained from the posterior lobe of the pituitary of healthy domestic animals used for food by man. Its oxytocic activity is not less than 400 USP Oxytocin Units per mg. Meets the requirements for Microbial limits, Identification, Vasopressor activity, and Ordinary impurities.

Oxytocin Injection USP—Preserve in single-dose or in multiple-dose containers, preferably of Type I glass. Do not freeze. A sterile solution of Oxytocin in a suitable diluent. Label it to indicate its oxytocic activity in USP Oxytocin Units per mL. Label it also to state the animal source if naturally derived, or to state that it is synthetic. Each mL of Oxytocin Injection possesses an oxytocic activity of that stated on the label in USP Oxytocin Units, within ±10%. Meets the requirements for Bacterial endotoxins, pH (3.0–5.0), and Particulate matter, and for Injections.

Oxytocin Nasal Solution USP—Preserve in containers suitable for administering the contents by spraying into the nasal cavities with the patient in the upright position, or for instillation in drop form. A solution of Oxytocin in a suitable diluent. Contains suitable preservatives, and is packaged in a form suitable for nasal administration. Label it to indicate that it is for intranasal administration only. Label it to state the origin (animal or synthetic), and the animal source of the product if of animal origin. Each mL of Oxytocin Nasal Solution possesses an oxytocic activity of that stated on the label in USP Oxytocin Units, within −15% to +20%. Meets the requirements for pH (3.7–4.3) and Vasopressor activity.

PACLITAXEL

Chemical name: Benzenepropanoic acid, beta-(benzoylamino)-alpha-hydroxy-, 6,12b-bis(acetyloxy)-12-(benzoyloxy)-2a,3,4,4a,5,6,9,10,11,12,12a,12b-dodecahydro-4,11-dihydroxy-4a,8,13,13-tetramethyl-5-oxo-7,11-methano-1*H*-cyclodeca[3,4]benz[1,2-b]-oxet-9-yl ester, [2a*R*-[2a alpha,4 beta,4a beta,6 beta,9 alpha(alpha*R**,beta*S**),11 alpha,12 alpha, 12a alpha,12b alpha]]-.

Molecular formula: $C_{47}H_{51}NO_{14}$.

Molecular weight: 853.91.

Description: Paclitaxel USP—White to off-white powder. Melts at around 216–217 °C.

Solubility: Paclitaxel USP—Insoluble in water; soluble in alcohol.

Other characteristics: Highly lipophilic.

USP requirements:
Paclitaxel USP—Preserve in tight, light-resistant containers, and store between 20° and 25°. The labeling indicates the type of process used to produce the material and the Related compounds test with which the material complies. Contains not less than 97.0% not more than 102.0% of paclitaxel, calculated on the anhydrous, solvent-free basis. Meets the requirements for Identification, Specific rotation (−49.0° to −55.0° at 20°, calculated on the anhydrous, sol-

vent-free basis), Microbial limits (not more than 100 cfu per gram), Bacterial endotoxins, Water (not more than 4.0%), Residue on ignition (not more than 0.2%), Heavy metals (0.002%), Related compounds, and Organic volatile impurities.

Caution—Paclitaxel is cytotoxic. Great care should be taken to prevent inhaling particles of Paclitaxel and exposing the skin to it.

Paclitaxel Concentrate for Injection USP—Preserve in single-dose or multiple-dose containers, probably of Type I glass, at controlled room temperature. A sterile, stabilized solution of Paclitaxel, suitable for dilution for intravenous administration. Label to indicate that it is to be diluted with a suitable parenteral vehicle prior to intravenous infusion. Contains the labeled amount, within ±10%. Meets the requirements for Identification, Bacterial endotoxins, pH (3.0–7.0, in a solution [1 in 10]), and Limit of degradation products, and for Injections.

PADIMATE O

Chemical name: Benzoic acid, 4-(dimethylamino)-, 2-ethylhexyl ester.

Molecular formula: $C_{17}H_{27}NO_2$.

Molecular weight: 277.40.

Description: Padimate O USP—Light yellow, mobile liquid having a faint, aromatic odor.

Solubility: Padimate O USP—Practically insoluble in water; soluble in alcohol, in isopropyl alcohol, and in mineral oil; practically insoluble in glycerin and in propylene glycol.

USP requirements:
Padimate O USP—Preserve in tight, light-resistant containers. Contains not less than 97.0% and not more than 103.8% of padimate O. Meets the requirements for Identification, Specific gravity (0.990–1.000), Refractive index (1.5390–1.5430), Acid value (not more than 1.0), Saponification value (195–215), and Chromatographic purity.
Padimate O Lip Balm—Not in *USP–NF*.
Padimate O Lotion USP—Preserve in tight, light-resistant containers. Contains the labeled amount, within ±10%. Meets the requirement for Identification.
Padimate O Oil—Not in *USP–NF*.

PALIVIZUMAB

Source: A humanized monoclonal antibody (IgG1k) produced by recombinant DNA technology, directed to an epitope in the A antigenic site of the F protein of respiratory syncytial virus (RSV); a composite of 95% human and 5% murine antibody sequences.

Molecular weight: Approximately 148,000 daltons.

USP requirements: Palivizumab Injection—Not in *USP–NF*.

PAMABROM

Chemical name: 8-Bromo-3,7-dihydro-1,3-dimethyl-1-*H*-purine-2,6-dione compound with 2-amino-2-methyl-1-propanol (1:1).

Molecular formula: $C_{11}H_{18}BrN_5O_3$.

Molecular weight: 348.20.

USP requirements: Pamabrom USP—Preserve in well-closed containers. Contains not less than 72.2% and not more than 76.6% of 8-bromotheophylline, calculated on the anhydrous basis; and not less than 24.6% and not more than 26.6% of 2-amino-2-methyl-1-propanol, calculated on the anhydrous basis. Meets the requirements for Identification, Water (not more than 3%), Heavy metals (not more than 20 mcg per gram), and Limit of theophylline (not more than 0.5%).

PAMIDRONATE

Chemical name: Pamidronate disodium—Phosphonic acid, (3-amino-1-hydroxypropylidene)bis-, disodium salt, pentahydrate.

Molecular formula: Pamidronate disodium—$C_3H_9NNa_2O_7P_2 \cdot 5H_2O$.

Molecular weight: Pamidronate disodium—369.11.

Description: Pamidronate disodium—White to practically white powder.

Solubility: Pamidronate disodium—Soluble in water and in 2 *N* sodium hydroxide; sparingly soluble in 0.1 *N* hydrochloric acid and in 0.1 *N* acetic acid; practically insoluble in organic solvents.

USP requirements: Pamidronate Disodium for Injection—Not in *USP–NF*.

PANCREATIN

Chemical name: Pancreatin.

Description: Pancreatin USP—Cream-colored, amorphous powder, having a faint, characteristic, but not offensive odor. It hydrolyzes fats to glycerol and fatty acids, changes protein into proteoses and derived substances, and converts starch into dextrins and sugars. Its greatest activities are in neutral or faintly alkaline media; more than traces of mineral acids or large amounts of alkali hydroxides make it inert. An excess of alkali carbonate also inhibits its action.

USP requirements:
Pancreatin USP—Preserve in tight containers, at a temperature not exceeding 30 °C. A substance containing enzymes, principally amylase, lipase, and protease, obtained from the pancreas of the hog, *Sus scrofa* Linné var. *domesticus* Gray (Fam. Suidae) or of the ox, *Bos taurus* Linné (Fam. Bovidae). Contains, in each mg, not less than 25 USP Units of amylase activity, not less than 2.0 USP Units of lipase activity, and not less than 25 USP Units of protease activity. Pancreatin of a higher digestive power may be labeled as a whole-number multiple of the three minimum activities or may be diluted by admixture with lactose, or with sucrose containing not more than 3.25% of starch, or with pancreatin of lower digestive power. Meets the requirements for Microbial limits, Loss on drying (not more than 5.0%), and Fat.
Note: One USP Unit of amylase activity is contained in the amount of pancreatin that decomposes starch at an initial rate such that 0.16 microequivalent of glycosidic linkage is hydrolyzed per minute under the conditions of the *Assay for amylase activity*. One USP Unit of lipase activity is contained in the amount of pancreatin that liberates 1.0 microequivalent of acid per minute at a pH of 9.0 and 37 °C under the conditions of the *As-*

say for lipase activity. One USP Unit of protease activity is contained in the amount of pancreatin that under the conditions of the *Assay for protease activity* hydrolyzes casein at an initial rate such that there is liberated per minute an amount of peptides not precipitated by trichloroacetic acid that gives the same absorbance at 280 nanometers as 15 nanomoles of tyrosine.

Pancreatin Capsules USP—Preserve in tight containers, preferably at a temperature not exceeding 30 °C. Label the Capsules to indicate minimum pancreatin fat digestive power; i.e., single strength, double strength, triple strength. Contain the labeled amount, within −10%. Meet the requirement for Microbial limits.

Pancreatin Tablets USP—Preserve in tight containers, preferably at a temperature not exceeding 30 °C. Label the Tablets to indicate minimum pancreatin fat digestive power; i.e., single strength, double strength, triple strength. Contain the labeled amount, within −10%. Meet the requirements for Microbial limits and Disintegration (60 minutes).

PANCRELIPASE

Chemical name: Lipase, triacylglycerol.

Description:

Pancrelipase USP—Cream colored, amorphous powder, having a faint, characteristic, but not offensive odor. It hydrolyzes fats to glycerol and fatty acids, changes protein into proteoses and derived substances, and converts starch into dextrins and sugars. Its greatest activities are in neutral or faintly alkaline media; more than traces of mineral acids or large amounts of alkali hydroxides make it inert. An excess of alkali carbonate also inhibits its action.

Pancrelipase Capsules USP—The contents of the Capsules conform to the Description under Pancrelipase, except that the odor may vary with the flavoring agent used.

USP requirements:

Pancrelipase USP—Preserve in tight containers, preferably at a temperature not exceeding 25 °C. A substance containing enzymes, principally lipase, with amylase and protease, obtained from the pancreas of the hog, *Sus scrofa* Linné var. *domesticus* Gray (Fam. Suidae). Label it to indicate lipase activity in USP Units. Contains, in each mg, not less than 24 USP Units of lipase activity, not less than 100 USP Units of amylase activity, and not less than 100 USP Units of protease activity. Meets the requirements for Microbial limits, Loss on drying (not more than 5.0%), and Fat (not more than 5.0%).

Note: One USP Unit of amylase activity is contained in the amount of pancrelipase that decomposes starch at an initial rate such that 0.16 microequivalent of glycosidic linkage is hydrolyzed per minute under the conditions of the *Assay for amylase activity,* One USP Unit of lipase activity is contained in the amount of pancrelipase that liberates 1.0 microequivalent of acid per minute at pH 9.0 and 37 °C under the conditions of the *Assay for lipase activity.* One USP Unit of protease activity is contained in the amount of pancrelipase that under the conditions of the *Assay for protease activity* hydrolyzes casein at an initial rate such that there is liberated per minute an amount of peptides not precipitated by trichloroacetic acid that gives the same absorbance at 280 nanometers as 15 nanomoles of tyrosine.

Pancrelipase Capsules USP—Preserve in tight containers, preferably with a desiccant, at a temperature not exceeding 25 °C. Label the Capsules to indicate lipase activity in USP Units. Contain an amount of Pancrelipase equivalent to the labeled lipase activity, within −10% to +50%, ex-

pressed in USP Units, the labeled activity being not less than 8000 USP Units per Capsule. They contain, in each Capsule, the pancrelipase equivalent of not less than 30,000 USP Units of amylase activity, and not less than 30,000 USP Units of protease activity. Meet the requirements for Microbial limits and Loss on drying (not more than 5.0%).

Pancrelipase Delayed-release Capsules USP—Preserve in tight containers at controlled room temperature. Label the Capsules to indicate lipase, amylase, and protease activities in USP Units. The label also indicates that the Capsule contents are enteric-coated. Contain an amount of Pancrelipase equivalent to the labeled amount of lipase, within −10% to +65%, and the labeled activities of amylase and protease, within −10%, expressed in the respective USP Units. Meet the requirements for Microbial limits, Dissolution (75% of the labeled USP Units of lipase activity in 60 minutes in simulated gastric fluid TS, without enzyme, in Apparatus 1 at 100 rpm for Part 1 and in 30 minutes in phosphate buffer [pH 6.0] in Apparatus 2 at 100 rpm for Part 2), and Loss on drying (not more than 5.0%).

Pancrelipase Powder—Not in *USP–NF.*

Pancrelipase Tablets USP—Preserve in tight containers, preferably with a desiccant, at a temperature not exceeding 25 °C. Label the Tablets to indicate the lipase activity in USP Units. Contain an amount of Pancrelipase equivalent to the labeled lipase activity, within −10% to +50%, expressed in USP Units, the labeled activity being not less than 8000 USP Units per Tablet. They contain, in each Tablet, the pancrelipase equivalent of not less than 30,000 USP Units of amylase activity, and not less than 30,000 USP Units of protease activity. Meet the requirements for Microbial limits, Disintegration (75 minutes), and Loss on drying (not more than 5.0%).

PANCURONIUM

Chemical name: Pancuronium bromide—Piperidinium, 1,1′-[(2 beta,3 alpha,5 alpha,16 beta,17 beta)-3,17-bis(acetyloxy)androstane-2,16-diyl]bis[1-methyl]-, dibromide.

Molecular formula: Pancuronium bromide—$C_{35}H_{60}Br_2N_2O_4$.

Molecular weight: Pancuronium bromide—732.67.

Description: Pancuronium bromide—White or almost white, hygroscopic crystalline powder.

Solubility: Pancuronium bromide—Freely or very soluble in water; freely soluble in alcohol and in chloroform; practically insoluble in ether.

USP requirements: Pancuronium Bromide Injection—Not in *USP–NF.*

PANTHENOL

Chemical name: Butanamide, 2,4-dihydroxy-*N*-(3-hydroxypropyl)-3,3-dimethyl-, (±)-.

Molecular formula: $C_9H_{19}NO_4$.

Molecular weight: 205.25.

Description: Panthenol USP—White to creamy white, crystalline powder having a slight, characteristic odor.

Solubility: Panthenol USP—Freely soluble in water, in alcohol, and in propylene glycol; soluble in chloroform and in ether; slightly soluble in glycerin.

USP requirements: Panthenol USP—Preserve in tight containers. A racemic mixture of the dextrorotatory and levorotatory isomers of panthenol. Contains not less than 99.0% and not more than 102.0% of panthenol, calculated on the dried basis. Meets the requirements for Identification, Melting range (64.5–68.5 °C), Specific rotation (−0.05° to +0.05°), Loss on drying (not more than 0.5%), Residue on ignition (not more than 0.1%), Limit of aminopropanol (not more than 0.10%), and Organic volatile impurities.

PANTOPRAZOLE

Chemical name: 1*H*-Benzimidazole, 5-(difluoromethoxy)-2-[[(3,-4-dimethoxy-2-pyridinyl)methyl]sulfinyl]-.

Molecular formula: $C_{16}H_{15}F_2N_3O_4S$.

Molecular weight: 383.37.

Description: White to off-white powder.

pKa: 3.92 pyridine; 8.19 benzimidazole.

Solubility: Freely soluble in ethanol; soluble in water; slightly soluble in hexane.

USP requirements:
Pantoprazole Tablets—Not in *USP–NF*.
Pantoprazole Enteric-coated Tablets—Not in *USP–NF*.

PANTOTHENIC ACID

Chemical name: (+)-(*R*)-3-(2,4-Dihydroxy-3,3-dimethylbutyramido)propionic acid.

Molecular formula: $C_9H_{17}NO_5$.

Molecular weight: 219.24.

Description: Unstable, viscous oil. Extremely hygroscopic.

Solubility: Freely soluble in water, in ethyl acetate, in dioxane, and in glacial acetic acid; moderately soluble in ether and in amyl alcohol; practically insoluble in chloroform.

USP requirements:
Pantothenic Acid Capsules—Not in *USP–NF*.
Pantothenic Acid Oral Solution—Not in *USP–NF*.
Pantothenic Acid Tablets—Not in *USP–NF*.
Pantothenic Acid Extended-release Tablets—Not in *USP–NF*.

PAPAIN

Description: Papain USP—White to light tan, amorphous powder.

Solubility: Papain USP—Soluble in water, the solution being colorless to light yellow and more or less opalescent; practically insoluble in alcohol, in chloroform, and in ether.

USP requirements:
Papain USP—Preserve in tight, light-resistant containers, in a cool place. A purified proteolytic substance derived from *Carica papaya* Linné (Fam. Caricaceae). Papain, when assayed as directed in *USP–NF*, contains not less than 6000 Units per mg. Papain of a higher digestive power may be reduced to the official standard by admixture with papain of lower activity, lactose, or other suitable diluents. One USP Unit of Papain activity is the activity that releases the equivalent of 1 mcg of tyrosine from a specified casein substrate under the conditions of the *Assay*, using the enzyme concentration that liberates 40 mcg of tyrosine per mL of test solution. Meets the requirements for pH (4.8–6.2, in a solution [1 in 50]) and Loss on drying (not more than 7.0%).
Papain Tablets for Topical Solution USP—Preserve in tight, light-resistant containers in a cool place. Contain not less than 100.0% of the labeled potency. Meet the requirements for Completeness of solution, Microbial limits, Disintegration (not more than 15 minutes at 23 ±2 °C), and pH (6.9–8.0, determined in a solution of 1 Tablet in 10 mL).

PAPAVERINE

Chemical name: Papaverine hydrochloride—Isoquinoline, 1-[(3,-4-dimethoxyphenyl)methyl]-6,7-dimethoxy-, hydrochloride.

Molecular formula: Papaverine hydrochloride—$C_{20}H_{21}NO_4 \cdot HCl$.

Molecular weight: Papaverine hydrochloride—375.85.

Description: Papaverine Hydrochloride USP—White crystals or white, crystalline powder. Odorless. Optically inactive. Its solutions are acid to litmus. Melts at about 220 °C, with decomposition.

Solubility: Papaverine Hydrochloride USP—Soluble in water and in chloroform; slightly soluble in alcohol; practically insoluble in ether.

USP requirements:
Papaverine Hydrochloride USP—Preserve in tight, light-resistant containers. Contains not less than 98.5% and not more than 100.5% of papaverine hydrochloride, calculated on the dried basis. Meets the requirements for Completeness of solution, Identification, pH (3.0–4.5, in a solution [1 in 50]), Loss on drying (not more than 0.5%), Residue on ignition (not more than 0.1%), Limit of cryptopine, thebaine, or other organic impurities, and Organic volatile impurities .
Papaverine Hydrochloride Extended-release Capsules—Not in *USP–NF*.
Papaverine Hydrochloride Injection USP—Preserve in single-dose or in multiple-dose containers, preferably of Type I glass. A sterile solution of Papaverine Hydrochloride in Water for Injection. Contains the labeled amount, within ±5%. Meets the requirements for Identification, Bacterial endotoxins, and pH (not less than 3.0), and for Injections.
Papaverine Hydrochloride Tablets USP—Preserve in tight containers. Contain the labeled amount, within ±7%. Meet the requirements for Identification, Dissolution (80% in 30 minutes in water in Apparatus 1 at 100 rpm), and Uniformity of dosage units.

PARACHLOROPHENOL

Chemical name: Phenol, 4-chloro-.

Molecular formula: C_6H_5ClO.

Molecular weight: 128.56.

Description: Parachlorophenol USP—White or pink crystals having a characteristic phenolic odor. When undiluted, it whitens and cauterizes the skin and mucous membranes. Melts at about 42 °C.

Solubility: Parachlorophenol USP—Sparingly soluble in water and in liquid petrolatum; very soluble in alcohol, in glycerin, in chloroform, in ether, and in fixed and volatile oils; soluble in petrolatum.

USP requirements: Parachlorophenol USP—Preserve in tight, light-resistant containers. Contains not less than 99.0% and not more than 100.5% of parachlorophenol. Meets the requirements for Clarity and reaction of solution, Identification, Congealing temperature (42–44 °C), Limit of nonvolatile residue (not more than 0.1%), and Chloride.

CAMPHORATED PARACHLOROPHENOL

USP requirements: Camphorated Parachlorophenol USP—Preserve in tight, light-resistant containers. A triturated mixture. Contains not less than 33.0% and not more than 37.0% of parachlorophenol and not less than 63.0% and not more than 67.0% of camphor. The sum of the percentages of parachlorophenol and camphor is not less than 97.0% and not more than 103.0%.

PARAFFIN

Description: Paraffin NF—Colorless or white, more or less translucent mass showing a crystalline structure. Odorless. Slightly greasy to the touch.
NF category: Stiffening agent.

Solubility: Paraffin NF—Insoluble in water and in alcohol; freely soluble in chloroform, in ether, in volatile oils, and in most warm fixed oils; slightly soluble in dehydrated alcohol.

NF requirements: Paraffin NF—Preserve in well-closed containers, and avoid exposure to excessive heat. A purified mixture of solid hydrocarbons obtained from petroleum. Meets the requirements for Identification, Congealing range (47–65 °C), Reaction, and Readily carbonizable substances.

SYNTHETIC PARAFFIN

Description: Synthetic Paraffin NF—Very hard, white, practically odorless wax. Contains mostly long-chain, unbranched, saturated hydrocarbons, with a small amount of branched hydrocarbons. Is represented by the formula C_nH_{2n+2}, in which n may range from 20 to about 100. The average molecular weight may range from 400 to 1400.
NF category: Stiffening agent.

Solubility: Synthetic Paraffin NF—Insoluble in water; very slightly soluble in aliphatic, oxygenated, and halogenated hydrocarbon solvents; slightly soluble in aromatic and normal paraffinic solvents.

NF requirements: Synthetic Paraffin NF—Preserve in well-closed containers. Synthesized by the Fischer-Tropsch process from carbon monoxide and hydrogen, which are catalytically converted to a mixture of paraffin hydrocarbons; the lower molecular weight fractions are removed by distillation, and the residue is hydrogenated and further treated by percolation through activated charcoal. This mixture may be fractionated into its components by a solvent separation method, using a suitable synthetic isoparaffinic petroleum hydrocarbon solvent. The labeling indicates its congealing temperature, viscosity, and needle penetration range under specified conditions. Meets the requirements for Identification, Absorptivity (not more than 0.01), Heavy metals (not more than 0.002%), and Oil content (not more than 0.5%).

PARALDEHYDE

Chemical name: 1,3,5-Trioxane, 2,4,6-trimethyl-.

Molecular formula: $C_6H_{12}O_3$.

Molecular weight: 132.16.

Description: Paraldehyde USP—Colorless, transparent liquid. Has a strong, characteristic but not unpleasant or pungent odor. Specific gravity is about 0.99.

Solubility: Paraldehyde USP—Soluble in water, but less soluble in boiling water. Miscible with alcohol, with chloroform, with ether, and with volatile oils.

USP requirements:
Paraldehyde USP—Preserve in well-filled, tight, light-resistant containers, preferably of Type I or Type II glass, holding not more than 30 mL, at a temperature not exceeding 25 °C. Paraldehyde may be shipped in bulk containers holding a minimum of 22.5 kg (50 lb) to commercial drug repackagers only. The label of all containers of Paraldehyde, including those dispensed by the pharmacist, includes a statement directing the user to discard the unused contents of any container that has been opened for more than 24 hours. (Note: The label of bulk containers of Paraldehyde directs the commercial drug repackager to demonstrate compliance with the USP purity tests for Paraldehyde immediately prior to repackaging, and not to repackage from a container that has been opened longer than 24 hours.) Meets the requirements for Identification, Congealing temperature (not lower than 11 °C), Distilling range (120–126 °C), Acidity (not more than 0.5% as acetic acid), Chloride, Sulfate, Limit of nonvolatile residue (not more than 0.06%), and Limit of acetaldehyde (not more than 0.4%).
Note: Paraldehyde is subject to oxidation to form acetic acid. It may contain a suitable stabilizer.
Sterile Paraldehyde—Not in *USP–NF*.

PARAMETHADIONE

Chemical group: Oxazolidinedione.

Chemical name: 2,4-Oxazolidinedione, 5-ethyl-3,5-dimethyl-.

Molecular formula: $C_7H_{11}NO_3$.

Molecular weight: 157.17.

Description: Clear, colorless liquid. May have an aromatic odor. A solution (1 in 40) has a pH of about 6.

Solubility: Sparingly soluble in water; freely soluble in alcohol, in chloroform, and in ether.

USP requirements: Paramethadione Capsules—Not in *USP–NF*.

PARAMETHASONE

Chemical name: Paramethasone acetate—Pregna-1,4-diene-3,20-dione, 21-(acetyloxy)-6-fluoro-11,17-dihydroxy-16-methyl-, (6 alpha,11 beta,16 alpha)-.

Molecular formula: Paramethasone acetate—$C_{24}H_{31}FO_6$.

Molecular weight: Paramethasone acetate—434.50.

Description: Paramethasone Acetate USP—Fluffy, white to creamy white, odorless, crystalline powder. Melts at about 240 °C, with decomposition.

Solubility: Paramethasone Acetate USP—Insoluble in water; soluble in chloroform, in ether, and in methanol.

USP requirements:
  Paramethasone Acetate USP—Preserve in tight containers. Contains not less than 95.0% and not more than 101.0% of paramethasone acetate, calculated on the dried basis. Meets the requirements for Identification, Specific rotation (+67° to +77°), X-ray diffraction, and Loss on drying (not more than 1.0%).
  Paramethasone Acetate Tablets USP—Preserve in well-closed containers. Contain the labeled amount, within ± 15%. Meet the requirements for Identification, Disintegration (15 minutes, the use of disks being omitted), and Uniformity of dosage units.

PAREGORIC

USP requirements: Paregoric USP—Preserve in tight, light-resistant containers, and avoid exposure to direct sunlight and to excessive heat. Yields, from each 100 mL, not less than 35 mg and not more than 45 mg of anhydrous morphine.

Paregoric may be prepared as follows: 4.3 grams of Powdered Opium, Suitable essential oil(s), 3.8 grams of Benzoic Acid, 900 mL of Diluted Alcohol, and 38 mL of Glycerin to make about 950 mL. Macerate for 5 days the Powdered Opium, Benzoic Acid, and essential oil(s), with occasional agitation, in a mixture of 900 mL of Diluted Alcohol and 38 mL of Glycerin. Then filter, and pass enough Diluted Alcohol through the filter to obtain 950 mL of total filtrate. Assay a portion of this filtrate as directed, and dilute the remainder with a sufficient quantity of Diluted Alcohol containing, in each 100 mL, 400 mg of Benzoic Acid, 4 mL of Glycerin, and sufficient essential oil(s) to yield a solution containing, in each 100 mL, 40 mg of anhydrous morphine.

Meets the requirements for alcoholic content (43.0–47.01).

Note: Paregoric may be prepared also by using Opium or Opium Tincture instead of Powdered Opium, the anhydrous morphine content being adjusted to 40 mg in each 100 mL and the alcohol content being adjusted to 45%.

PARICALCITOL

Chemical name: 19-nor-1 alpha,3 beta,25-trihydroxy-9,10-secoergosta-5(Z),7(E),22(E)-triene.

Molecular formula: $C_{27}H_{44}O_3$.

Molecular weight: 416.65.

Description: White powder.

USP requirements: Paricalcitol Injection—Not in *USP–NF*.

PAROMOMYCIN

Chemical name: Paromomycin sulfate—D-Streptamine, *O*-2-amino-2-deoxy-alpha-D-glucopyranosyl-(1→4)-*O*-[*O*-2,6-diamino-2,6-dideoxy-beta-L-idopyranosyl-(1→3)-beta-D-ribofuranosyl-(1→5)]-2-deoxy-, sulfate (salt).

Molecular formula: Paromomycin sulfate—$C_{23}H_{45}N_5O_{14} \cdot xH_2SO_4$.

Molecular weight: 615.63 (base).

Description: Paromomycin Sulfate USP—Creamy white to light yellow powder. Odorless or practically so. Very hygroscopic.

Solubility: Paromomycin Sulfate USP—Very soluble in water; insoluble in alcohol, in chloroform, and in ether.

USP requirements:
  Paromomycin Sulfate USP—Preserve in tight containers. The sulfate salt of an antibiotic substance or substances produced by the growth of *Streptomyces rimosus* var. *paromomycinus,* or a mixture of two or more such salts. Has a potency equivalent to not less than 675 mcg of paromomycin per mg, calculated on the dried basis. Meets the requirements for Identification, Specific rotation (+50° to +55°), pH (5.0–7.5, in a solution [3 in 100]), Loss on drying (not more than 5.0%), and Residue on ignition (not more than 2.0%).
  Paromomycin Sulfate Capsules USP—Preserve in tight containers. Contain an amount of paromomycin sulfate equivalent to the labeled amount of paromomycin, within −10% to +25%. Meet the requirements for Identification, Disintegration (15 minutes, the use of disks being omitted), Uniformity of dosage units, and Loss on drying (not more than 7.0%).
  Paromomycin Sulfate Oral Solution USP—Preserve in tight containers. Contains an amount of Paromomycin Sulfate equivalent to the labeled amount of paromomycin, within −10% to +30%. Meets the requirements for Uniformity of dosage units (single-unit containers), Deliverable volume (multiple-unit containers), and pH (7.5–8.5).
  Paromomycin Sulfate Syrup USP—Preserve in tight containers. Contains an amount of Paromomycin Sulfate equivalent to the labeled amount of paromomycin, within −10% to +30%. Meets the requirements for Uniformity of dosage units (single-unit containers), Deliverable volume (multiple-unit containers), and pH (7.5–8.5).

PAROXETINE

Chemical name: Paroxetine hydrochloride—(−)-*trans*-5-(4-*p*-Fluorophenyl-3-piperidylmethoxy)-1,3-benzodioxole hydrochloride.

Molecular formula: Paroxetine hydrochloride—$C_{19}H_{20}FNO_3 \cdot$ HCl.

Molecular weight: Paroxetine hydrochloride—365.83.

Description: Paroxetine hydrochloride—Odorless, off-white powder, having a melting point range of 120–138 °C.

Solubility: Paroxetine hydrochloride—Soluble in water (5.4 mg/mL).

USP requirements:
  Paroxetine Hydrochloride Oral Suspension—Not in *USP–NF*.
  Paroxetine Hydrochloride Tablets—Not in *USP–NF*.
  Paroxetine Hydrochloride Extended-release Tablets—Not in *USP–NF*.

PEANUT OIL

Description: Peanut Oil NF—Colorless or pale yellow oily liquid. May have a characteristic, nutty odor.

  NF category: Solvent; vehicle (oleaginous).

Solubility: Peanut Oil NF—Very slightly soluble in alcohol. Miscible with ether, with chloroform, and with carbon disulfide.

NF requirements: Peanut Oil NF—Preserve in tight, light-resistant containers, and prevent exposure to excessive heat. The refined fixed oil obtained from the seed kernels of one or more of the cultivated varieties of *Arachis hypogaea* Linné (Fam. Leguminosae). Meets the requirements for Identification, Specific gravity (0.912–0.920), Refractive index (1.462–1.464 at 40 °C), Heavy metals (not more than 0.001%), Cottonseed oil, Rancidity, Solidification range of fatty acids (26–33 °C), Free

fatty acids, Iodine value (84–100), Saponification value (185–195), Unsaponifiable matter (not more than 1.5%), and Organic volatile impurities.

PECTIN

Chemical name: Pectin.

Description: Pectin USP—Coarse or fine powder, yellowish white in color, almost odorless.

NF category: Suspending and/or viscosity-increasing agent.

Solubility: Pectin USP—Almost completely soluble in 20 parts of water, forming a viscous, opalescent, colloidal solution that flows readily and is acid to litmus. Is practically insoluble in alcohol or in diluted alcohol and in other organic solvents. Pectin dissolves in water more readily if first moistened with alcohol, glycerin, or simple syrup, or if first mixed with 3 or more parts of sucrose.

USP requirements: Pectin USP—Preserve in tight containers. A purified carbohydrate product obtained from the dilute acid extract of the inner portion of the rind of citrus fruits or from apple pomace. Consists chiefly of partially methoxylated polygalacturonic acids. Label it to indicate whether it is of apple or of citrus origin. Pectin yields not less than 6.7% of methoxy groups and not less than 74.0% of galacturonic acid, calculated on the dried basis. Meets the requirements for Identification, Microbial limits, Loss on drying (not more than 10.0%), Arsenic (not more than 3 ppm), Lead, Sugars and organic acids, and Organic volatile impurities.

Note: Commercial pectin for the production of jellied food products is standardized to the convenient "150 jelly grade" by addition of dextrose or other sugars, and sometimes contains sodium citrate or other buffer salts. This monograph refers to the pure pectin to which no such additions have been made.

PEG 3350 AND ELECTROLYTES

For *Polyethylene Glycol, Sodium Bicarbonate, Sodium Chloride, Sodium Sulfate,* and *Potassium Chloride*—See individual listings for chemistry information.

USP requirements:

PEG 3350 and Electrolytes for Oral Solution USP—Preserve in tight containers. A mixture of Polyethylene Glycol 3350, Sodium Bicarbonate, Sodium Chloride, Sodium Sulfate (anhydrous), and Potassium Chloride. When constituted as directed in the labeling it contains the labeled amounts of polyethylene glycol 3350, potassium, sodium, bicarbonate, chloride, and sulfate, within ±10%, the labeled amounts per liter being 10 mmol (10 mEq) of potassium, 125 mmol (125 mEq) of sodium, 20 mmol (20 mEq) of bicarbonate, 35 mmol (35 mEq) of chloride, and 40 mmol (80 mEq) of sulfate. Meets the requirements for Completeness of solution, Identification, pH (7.5–9.5, in the solution prepared as directed in the labeling), Uniformity of dosage units, and Osmolarity (235–304 mOsmol, in the solution prepared as directed in the labeling).

Polyethylene Glycol 3350 and Electrolytes Oral Solution—Not in *USP–NF*.

PEGADEMASE

Source: Pegademase bovine—A conjugate of numerous strands of monomethoxypolyethylene glycol (PEG), covalently attached to the enzyme adenosine deaminase (ADA); ADA used in the manufacture of pegademase bovine injection is derived from bovine intestine.

Chemical name: Pegademase bovine—Deaminase, adenosine, cattle, reaction product with succinic anhydride, esters with polyethylene glycol, mono-Me ether.

Description: Pegademase bovine injection—Clear, colorless solution; pH 7.2–7.4.

USP requirements: Pegademase Bovine Injection—Not in *USP–NF*.

PEGASPARGASE

Source: Modified version of the enzyme ʟ-asparaginase.

Chemical name: Pegaspargase.

USP requirements: Pegaspargase Injection—Not in *USP–NF*.

PEGINTERFERON ALFA-2B

Source: Synthetic. Peginterferon alfa-2b is a covalent conjugate of recombinant alfa-2b interferon with monomethoxy polyethylene glycol (PEG). It is manufactured by bacterial fermentation of a strain of *Escherichia coli* that bears a genetically engineered plasmid containing the gene for human interferon. The native gene was obtained from human leukocytes.

Chemical name: Interferon Alfa-2b—Interferon alpha2b (human leukocyte clone Hif-SN206 protein moiety reduced).

Molecular formula: Interferon Alfa-2b— $C_{860}H_{1353}N_{229}O_{255}S_9$.

Molecular weight:
Interferon Alfa-2b—19,268.93 daltons.
Peginterferon alfa-2b—31,000 daltons.

Description: Peginterferon alfa-2b—White to off-white lyophilized powder.

Solubility: Interferon Alfa-2b—Soluble in water.

Other characteristics: Peginterferon alfa-2b—Specific activity: Approximately 0.7×10^8 International Units (IU) per mg of protein.

USP requirements: Peginterferon Alfa-2b for Injection—Not in *USP–NF*.

PEGFILGRASTIM

Source: A covalent conjugate of recombinant methionyl human G-CSF (Filgrastim) and monomethoxypolyethylene glycol. Filgrastin is obtained from the bacterial fermentation of a strain of *Escherichia coli.*

Molecular weight: 39 kilodaltons.

Solubility: Soluble in water.

USP requirements: Pegfilgrastim Injection—Not in *USP–NF*.

PEMIROLAST

Chemical name: Pemirolast potassium—4*H*-Pyridol[1,2-*a*]pyrimidin-4-one, 9-methyl-3-(1*H*-tetrazol-5-yl), potassium salt.

Molecular formula: Pemirlast potassium—$C_{10}H_7KN_6O$.

Molecular weight: Pemirolast potassium—266.30.

Description: Pemirolast potassium—Slightly yellow powder.

Solubility: Pemirolast potassium—Freely soluble in water.

Other characteristics: Pemirolat potassium—pH 8.0.

USP requirements: Pemirolast Potassium Ophthalmic Solution—Not in *USP–NF*.

PEMOLINE

Chemical group: Oxazolidine.

Chemical name: 4(5*H*)-Oxazolone, 2-amino-5-phenyl-.

Molecular formula: $C_9H_8N_2O_2$.

Molecular weight: 176.17.

Description: White, odorless powder.

Solubility: Relatively insoluble (less than 1 mg/mL) in water, in chloroform, in ether, and in acetone; solubility in 95% ethyl alcohol 2.2 mg/mL.

USP requirements:
Pemoline Tablets—Not in *USP–NF*.
Pemoline Chewable Tablets—Not in *USP–NF*.

PENBUTOLOL

Chemical name: Penbutolol sulfate—2-Propanol, 1-(2-cyclopentylphenoxy)-3-[(1,1-dimethylethyl)amino]-, (*S*)-, sulfate (2:1) (salt).

Molecular formula: Penbutolol sulfate—$(C_{18}H_{29}NO_2)_2 \cdot H_2SO_4$.

Molecular weight: Penbutolol sulfate—680.94.

Description: Penbutolol Sulfate USP—White to off-white, crystalline powder. Melts at about 217 °C, with decomposition.

pKa: 9.3.

Solubility: Penbutolol Sulfate USP—Soluble in water and in methanol.

Other characteristics: Lipid solubility—Moderate.

USP requirements:
Penbutolol Sulfate USP—Preserve in tight, light-resistant containers. Contains not less than 98.0% and not more than 102.0% of penbutolol sulfate, calculated on the anhydrous basis. Meets the requirements for Identification, Loss on drying (not more than 1.0%), Residue on ignition (not more than 0.2%), Specific rotation (−22° to −26°), and Chromatographic purity.
Penbutolol Sulfate Tablets USP—Preserve in well-closed, light-resistant containers. Contain the labeled amount, within ±10%. Meet the requirements for Identification, Dissolution (75% in 30 minutes in water in Apparatus 2 at 50 rpm), and Chromatographic purity.

PENCICLOVIR

Chemical group: Synthetic acyclic guanine derivative.

Chemical name: 6*H*-Purin-6-one, 2-amino-1,9-dihydro-9-[4-hydroxy-3-(hydroxymethyl)butyl]-.

Molecular formula: $C_{10}H_{15}N_5O_3$.

Molecular weight: 253.26.

Description: White to pale yellow solid.

Solubility: Solubility at 20 °C: 0.2 mg/mL in methanol, 1.3 mg/mL in propylene glycol, 1.7 mg/mL in water, and 10.0 mg/mL in aqueous buffer (pH 2).

Other characteristics: Not hygroscopic. Partition coefficient in *n*-octanol/water at pH 7.5 is 0.024.

USP requirements: Penciclovir Cream—Not in *USP–NF*.

PENICILLAMINE

Chemical name: D-Valine, 3-mercapto-.

Molecular formula: $C_5H_{11}NO_2S$.

Molecular weight: 149.21.

Description: Penicillamine USP—White or practically white, crystalline powder, having a slight, characteristic odor.

Solubility: Penicillamine USP—Freely soluble in water; slightly soluble in alcohol; insoluble in chloroform and in ether.

USP requirements:
Penicillamine USP—Preserve in tight containers. Contains not less than 97.0% and not more than 102.0% of penicillamine, calculated on the dried basis. Meets the requirements for Identification, Specific rotation (−60.5° to −64.5°), pH (4.5–5.5, in a solution [1 in 100]), Loss on drying (not more than 0.5%), Residue on ignition (not more than 0.1%), Heavy metals (not more than 0.002%), Limit of penicillin activity, Mercury (not more than 0.002%), and Limit of penicillamine disulfide (not more than 1.0%).
Penicillamine Capsules USP—Preserve in tight containers. Contain the labeled amount, within ±10%. Meet the requirements for Identification, Dissolution (80% in 30 minutes in 0.1 N hydrochloric acid in Apparatus 1 at 100 rpm), Uniformity of dosage units, Loss on drying (not more than 1.0%), and Limit of penicillamine disulfide (not more than 2.0%).
Penicillamine Tablets USP—Preserve in tight containers. Contain the labeled amount, within ±10%. Meet the requirements for Identification, Dissolution (80% in 60 minutes in 0.5% edetate disodium and 0.05% sodium lauryl sulfate in Apparatus 1 at 100 rpm), Uniformity of dosage units, Loss on drying (not more than 3.0%), and Penicillamine disulfide (not more than 3.0%).

PENICILLIN G

Chemical name:
Penicillin G benzathine—4-Thia-1-azabicyclo[3.2.0]heptane2-carboxylic acid, 3,3-dimethyl-7-oxo-6-[(phenylacetyl)amino]-, [2*S*-(2 alpha,5 alpha,6 beta)]-, compd. with *N*,*N*-bis(phenylmethyl)-1,2-ethanediamine (2:1), tetrahydrate.
Penicillin G potassium—4-Thia-1-azabicyclo[3.2.0]heptane-2-carboxylic acid, 3,3-dimethyl-7-oxo-6-[(phenylacetyl)amino]-, monopotassium salt, [2*S*-(2 alpha,5 alpha,6 beta)]-.
Penicillin G procaine—4-Thia-1-azabicyclo[3.2.0]heptane-2-carboxylic acid, 3,3-dimethyl-7-oxo-6-[(phenylacetyl)amino]-, [2*S*-(2 alpha,5 alpha,6 beta)]-, compd. with 2-(diethylamino)ethyl 4-aminobenzoate (1:1) monohydrate.

Penicillin G sodium—4-Thia-1-azabicyclo[3.2.0]-heptane-2-carboxylic acid, 3,3-dimethyl-7-oxo-6-[(phenylacetyl)amino]-, [2*S*-(2 alpha,5 alpha,6 beta)]-, monosodium salt.

Molecular formula:

Penicillin G benzathine—($C_{16}H_{18}N_2O_4S)_2 \cdot C_{16}H_{20}N_2 \cdot 4H_2O$.

Penicillin G potassium—$C_{16}H_{17}KN_2O_4S$.

Penicillin G procaine—$C_{16}H_{18}N_2O_4S \cdot C_{13}H_{20}N_2O_2 \cdot H_2O$.

Penicillin G sodium—$C_{16}H_{17}N_2NaO_4S$.

Molecular weight:

Penicillin G benzathine—981.19.

Penicillin G potassium—372.48.

Penicillin G procaine—588.72.

Penicillin G sodium—356.37.

Description:

Penicillin G Benzathine USP—White, odorless, crystalline powder.

Penicillin G Potassium USP—Colorless or white crystals, or white, crystalline powder. Is odorless or practically so, and is moderately hygroscopic. Its solutions are dextrorotatory. Its solutions retain substantially full potency for several days at temperatures below 15 °C, but are rapidly inactivated by acids, alkali hydroxides, glycerin, and oxidizing agents.

Penicillin G Procaine USP—White crystals or white, very fine, microcrystalline powder. Is odorless or practically odorless, and is relatively stable in air. Its solutions are dextrorotatory. Is rapidly inactivated by acids, by alkali hydroxides, and by oxidizing agents.

Penicillin G Sodium USP—Colorless or white crystals or white to slightly yellow, crystalline powder. Is odorless or practically odorless, and is moderately hygroscopic. Its solutions are dextrorotatory. Is relatively stable in air, but is inactivated by prolonged heating at about 100 °C, especially in the presence of moisture. Its solutions lose potency fairly rapidly at room temperature, but retain substantially full potency for several days at temperatures below 15 °C. Its solutions are rapidly inactivated by acids, alkali hydroxides, oxidizing agents, and penicillinase.

Solubility:

Penicillin G Benzathine USP—Very slightly soluble in water; sparingly soluble in alcohol.

Penicillin G Potassium USP—Very soluble in water, in saline TS, and in dextrose solutions; sparingly soluble in alcohol.

Penicillin G Procaine USP—Slightly soluble in water; soluble in alcohol and in chloroform.

USP requirements:

Penicillin G Benzathine USP—Preserve in tight containers. Where it is intended for use in preparing injectable dosage forms, the label states that it is sterile or must be subjected to further processing during the preparation of injectable dosage forms. Has a potency of not less than 1090 Penicillin G Units and not more than 1272 Penicillin G Units per mg. Meets the requirements for Identification, Crystallinity, Bacterial endotoxins, Sterility, pH (4.0–6.5), Water (5.0–8.0%), and Benzathine content (24.0–27.0%, calculated on the anhydrous basis).

Penicillin G Benzathine Injectable Suspension USP—Preserve in single-dose or in multiple-dose containers, preferably of Type I or Type II glass, in a refrigerator. A sterile suspension of Penicillin G Benzathine in Water for Injection with one or more suitable buffers, dispersants, preservatives, and suspending agents. Contains an amount of penicillin G benzathine equivalent to the labeled amount of penicillin G, within −10% to +15%. Meets the requirements for Identification, Bacterial endotoxins, Sterility, and pH (5.0–7.5), and for Injections.

Penicillin G Benzathine Oral Suspension USP—Preserve in tight containers. Contains an amount of penicillin G benzathine equivalent to the labeled amount of penicillin G, within −10% to +20%. Contains one or more suitable buffers, colors, dispersants, flavors, and preservatives. Meets the requirements for Identification, Uniformity of dosage units (single-unit containers), Deliverable volume (multiple-unit containers), and pH (6.0–7.0).

Penicillin G Benzathine Tablets USP—Preserve in tight containers. Contain an amount of penicillin G benzathine equivalent to the labeled amount of penicillin G, within −10% to +20%. Meet the requirements for Identification, Disintegration (60 minutes, simulated gastric fluid TS being used in place of water as the test medium), Uniformity of dosage units, and Water (not more than 8.0%).

Penicillin G Benzathine and Penicillin G Procaine Injectable Suspension USP—Preserve in single-dose or in multiple-dose containers, preferably of Type I or Type III glass. A sterile suspension of Penicillin G Benzathine and Penicillin G Procaine or when labeled for veterinary use only, of Penicillin G Benzathine and Penicillin G Procaine, in Water for Injection. Where it is intended for veterinary use only, it is so labeled. May contain one or more suitable buffers, preservatives, and suspending agents. Contains the labeled amounts, within −10% to +15%. Meets the requirements for Identification, Crystallinity , pH (5.0–7.5), Limit of soluble penicillin G and procaine (where it is prepared from penicillin G procaine and is labeled for veterinary use only, not more than 1%), for Bacterial endotoxins, and Sterility under Penicillin G Procaine Injectable Suspension, and for Injections.

Penicillin G Potassium USP—Preserve in tight containers. Where it is intended for use in preparing injectable dosage forms, the label states that is is sterile or must be subjected to further processing during the preparation of injectable dosage forms. Has a potency of not less than 1440 Penicillin G Units and not more than 1680 Penicillin G Units per mg. Meets the requirements for Identification, Crystallinity, pH (5.0–7.5, in a solution containing 60 mg per mL), and Loss on drying (not more than 1.5%), for Sterility and Bacterial endotoxins under Penicillin G Potassium for Injection (where the label states that Penicillin G Potassium is sterile), and for Bacterial endotoxins under Penicillin G Potassium for Injection (where the label states that Penicillin G Potassium must be subjected to further processing during the preparation of injectable dosage forms).

Penicillin G Potassium Capsules USP—Preserve in tight containers. Contain the labeled number of Penicillin G Units, within −10% to +20%. Meet the requirements for Identification, Dissolution (75% in 45 minutes in phosphate buffer [pH 6.0] in Apparatus 1 at 100 rpm), Uniformity of dosage units, and Loss on drying (not more than 1.5%).

Penicillin G Potassium Injection USP—Preserve in single-dose containers. Maintain in the frozen state. A sterile isoosmotic solution of Penicillin G Potassium in Water for Injection. Contains one or more suitable buffers and a tonicity-adjusting agent. It meets the requirements for Labeling under Injections. The label states that it is to be thawed just prior to use, describes conditions for proper storage of the resultant solution, and directs that the solution is not to be refrozen. Contains the labeled number of Penicillin G Units, within −10% to +15%. Meets the requirements for Identification, Bacterial endotoxins, Sterility, pH (5.5–8.0), and Particulate matter.

Penicillin G Potassium for Injection USP—Preserve in Containers for Sterile Solids. It is sterile Penicillin G Potassium or a sterile, dry mixture of Penicillin G Potassium with not less than 4.0% and not more than 5.0% of Sodium Citrate, of which not more than 0.15% may be replaced by Citric Acid. Has a potency of the labeled number of Penicillin G Units, within −10% to +20%. In addition, where it contains Sodium Citrate it has a potency of not less than 1335 and not more than 1595 Penicillin G Units per mg. Meets the requirements for Constituted solution, Identification, Crystallinity, Bacterial endotoxins, Sterility, pH (6.0–8.5, in a solution containing 60 mg per mL, or, where packaged for dispensing, in the solution constituted as directed in

the labeling), Loss on drying (not more than 1.5%), and Particulate matter, and for Uniformity of dosage units and Labeling under Injections.

Penicillin G Potassium for Oral Solution USP—Preserve in tight containers. A dry mixture of Penicillin G Potassium and one or more suitable buffers, colors, diluents, flavors, and preservatives. Contains the labeled number of Penicillin G Units when constituted as directed in the labeling, within −10% to +30%. Meets the requirements for Identification, Uniformity of dosage units (single-unit containers), Deliverable volume (multiple-unit containers), pH (5.5–7.5, in the solution constituted as directed in the labeling), and Water (not more than 1.0%).

Penicillin G Potassium Tablets USP—Preserve in tight containers. Contain the labeled number of Penicillin G Units, within −10% to +20%. Meet the requirements for Identification, Dissolution (70% in 60 minutes in phosphate buffer [pH 6.0] in Apparatus 2 at 75 rpm), Uniformity of dosage units, and Loss on drying (not more than 1.0%).

Penicillin G Potassium Tablets for Oral Solution USP—Preserve in tight containers. Contain the labeled number of Penicillin G Units, within −10% to +20%. Meet the requirements for Identification and Loss on drying (not more than 1.0%), and for Uniformity of dosage units under Penicillin G Potassium Tablets.

Penicillin G Procaine USP—Preserve in Containers for Sterile Solids. Where it is intended for use in preparing injectable dosage forms, the label states that it is sterile or must be subjected to further processing during the preparation of injectable dosage forms. Has a potency of not less than 900 Penicillin G Units and not more than 1050 Penicillin G Units per mg. Meets the requirements for Identification, Crystallinity, Bacterial endotoxins, Sterility, pH (5.0–7.5, in a [saturated] solution containing about 300 mg per mL), Water (2.8–4.2%), and Content of Penicillin G and procaine (37.5–43.0%).

Penicillin G Procaine Intramammary Infusion USP—Preserve in well-closed disposable syringes. A suspension of Penicillin G Procaine in a suitable vegetable oil vehicle. Label it to indicate that it is for veterinary use only. Contains an amount of penicillin G procaine equivalent to the labeled amount of penicillin G, within −10% to +15%. Meets the requirements for Identification and Water (not more than 1.4%).

Penicillin G Procaine Injectable Suspension USP—Preserve in single-dose or in multiple-dose containers, preferably of Type I or Type III glass, in a refrigerator. A sterile suspension of Penicillin G Procaine or, where labeled for veterinary use only, of sterile penicillin G procaine, in Water for Injection and contains one or more suitable buffers, dispersants, or suspending agents, and a suitable preservative. It may contain procaine hydrochloride in a concentration not exceeding 2.0%. Where it is intended for veterinary use, the label so states. Contains an amount of penicillin G procaine equivalent to the labeled amount of penicillin G, within −10% to +15%, the labeled amount being not less than 300,000 Penicillin G Units per mL or per container. Meets the requirements for Identification, Crystallinity, Bacterial endotoxins, Sterility, pH (5.0–7.5), and Penicillin G and procaine contents, and for Injections.

Penicillin G Procaine for Injectable Suspension USP—Preserve in single-dose or in multiple-dose containers, preferably of Type I or Type III glass. A sterile mixture of Penicillin G Procaine and one or more suitable buffers, dispersants, or suspending agents, and preservatives. Contains an amount of penicillin G procaine equivalent to the labeled amount of penicillin G, within −10% to +15%, the labeled amount being not less than 300,000 Penicillin G Units per container or per mL of constituted Suspension. Meets the requirements for Identification, pH (5.0–7.5, when constituted as directed in the labeling), and Water (2.8–4.2%), for Bacterial endotoxins and Sterility under Penicillin G Procaine Injectable Suspension, and for Injections and Uniformity of dosage units.

Penicillin G Sodium USP—Preserve in tight containers. Where it is intended for use in preparing injectable dosage forms, the label states that it is sterile or must be subjected to further processing during the preparation of injectable dosage forms. Has a potency of not less than 1500 Penicillin G Units and not more than 1750 Penicillin G Units per mg. Meets the requirements for Identification, Crystallinity, pH (5.0–7.5, in a solution containing 60 mg per mL), and Loss on drying (not more than 1.5%), for Sterility and Bacterial endotoxins under Penicillin G Sodium for Injection (where the label states that Penicillin G Sodium is sterile), and for Bacterial endotoxins under Penicillin G Sodium for Injection (where the label states that Penicillin G Sodium must be subjected to further processing during the preparation of injectable dosage forms).

Penicillin G Sodium for Injection USP—Preserve in Containers for Sterile Solids. It is sterile Penicillin G Sodium or a sterile mixture of penicillin G sodium and not less than 4.0% and not more than 5.0% of Sodium Citrate, of which not more than 0.15% may be replaced by Citric Acid. Contains the labeled amount of Penicillin G, within −10% to +20%, and where it contains Sodium Citrate it has a potency of not less than 1420 and not more than 1667 Penicillin G Units per mg. Meets the requirements for Constituted solution, Identification, Crystallinity, Bacterial endotoxins, Sterility, pH (6.0–7.5, in a solution containing 60 mg per mL), Loss on drying (not more than 1.5%), and Particulate matter, and for Uniformity of dosage units and Labeling under Injections.

PENICILLIN G AND ALUMINUM STEARATE

Chemical name:

Penicillin G procaine—4-Thia-1-azabicyclo[3.2.0]heptane-2-carboxylic acid, 3,3-dimethyl-7-oxo-6-[(phenylacetyl)amino]-, [2S-(2 alpha,5 alpha,6 beta)-, compd. with 2-(diethylamino)ethyl 4-aminobenzoate (1:1) monohydrate.

Aluminum stearate—Octadecanoic acid aluminum salt.

Molecular formula:

Penicillin G procaine—$C_{16}H_{18}N_2O_4S \cdot C_{13}H_{20}N_2O_2 \cdot H_2O$.

Aluminum stearate—$C_{54}H_{105}AlO_6$.

Molecular weight:

Penicillin G procaine—588.72.

Aluminum stearate—877.35.

Description:

Penicillin G Procaine USP—White crystals or white, very fine, microcrystalline powder. Is odorless or practically odorless, and is relatively stable in air. Its solutions are dextrorotatory. Is rapidly inactivated by acids, by alkali hydroxides, and by oxidizing agents.

Aluminum stearate—Melting point 117–120 °C.

Solubility:

Penicillin G Procaine USP—Slightly soluble in water; soluble in alcohol and in chloroform.

Aluminum stearate—Practically insoluble in water; when freshly made, soluble in alcohol, in oil turpentine, and in mineral oils.

USP requirements: Penicillin G Procaine with Aluminum Stearate Injectable Oil Suspension USP—Preserve in single-dose or in multiple-dose containers, preferably of Type I or Type III glass. A sterile suspension of Sterile Penicillin G Procaine in a refined vegetable oil with one or more suitable dispersants and hardening agents. Contains an amount of penicillin G procaine

equivalent to the labeled amount of penicillin G, within −10% to +15%. Meets the requirements for Bacterial endotoxins, Sterility, and Water (not more than 1.4%), and for Injections.

PENICILLIN G AND DIHYDROSTREPTOMYCIN

For *Penicillin G* and *Dihydrostreptomycin*—See individual listings for chemistry information.

USP requirements:

Penicillin G Procaine and Dihydrostreptomycin Sulfate Intramammary Infusion USP—Preserve in well-closed, disposable syringes. A suspension of Penicillin G Procaine and Dihydrostreptomycin Sulfate in a suitable vegetable oil vehicle. Label it to indicate that it is intended for veterinary use only. Contains amounts of penicillin G procaine and dihydrostreptomycin sulfate equivalent to the labeled amounts of Penicillin G Units and dihydrostreptomycin, within −10% to +20%. Meets the requirements for Identification and Water (not more than 1.4%).

Penicillin G Procaine and Dihydrostreptomycin Sulfate Injectable Suspension USP—Preserve in single-dose or in multiple-dose, tight containers. A sterile suspension of Penicillin G Procaine in a solution of Dihydrostreptomycin Sulfate in Water for Injection, and contains one or more suitable buffers, preservatives, and dispersing or suspending agents. May contain Procaine Hydrochloride in a concentration not exceeding 2.0%. Label it to indicate that it is intended for veterinary use only. Contains amounts of penicillin G procaine and dihydrostreptomycin sulfate equivalent to the labeled amounts of Penicillin G Units and dihydrostreptomycin, within −10% to +15%. Meets the requirements for Identification, Bacterial endotoxins, Sterility, and pH (5.0–8.0).

PENICILLIN G, DIHYDROSTREPTOMYCIN, CHLORPHENIRAMINE, AND DEXAMETHASONE

For *Penicillin G, Dihydrostreptomycin, Chlorpheniramine,* and *Dexamethasone*—See individual listings for chemistry information.

USP requirements: Penicillin G Procaine, Dihydrostreptomycin Sulfate, Chlorpheniramine Maleate, and Dexamethasone Injectable Suspension USP—Preserve in single-dose or in multiple-dose, tight containers, in a cool place. A sterile suspension of Penicillin G Procaine and Dexamethasone in a solution of Sterile Dihydrostreptomycin Sulfate and Chlorpheniramine Maleate in Water for Injection. Contains one or more suitable buffers, preservatives, and dispersing or suspending agents. May contain Procaine Hydrochloride in a concentration not exceeding 2.0%. Label it to indicate that it is intended for veterinary use only. Contains amounts of penicillin G procaine and dihydrostreptomycin sulfate equivalent to the labeled amounts of Penicillin G Units and dihydrostreptomycin, within −10% to +15%, and the labeled amounts of chlorpheniramine maleate and dexamethasone, within ± 10%. Meets the requirements for Identification, Bacterial endotoxins, and pH (5.0–6.0), for Sterility under Penicillin G Procaine and Dihydrostreptomycin Sulfate Injectable Suspension, and for Injections.

PENICILLIN G, DIHYDROSTREPTOMYCIN, AND PREDNISOLONE

For *Penicillin G, Dihydrostreptomycin,* and *Prednisolone*—See individual listings for chemistry information.

USP requirements: Penicillin G Procaine, Dihydrostreptomycin Sulfate, and Prednisolone Injectable Suspension USP—Preserve in single-dose or in multiple-dose, tight containers. A sterile suspension of Penicillin G Procaine and Prednisolone in a solution of Dihydrostreptomycin Sulfate in Water for Injection. Contains one or more suitable buffers, dispersants, preservatives, and suspending agents. May contain not more than 2.0% of procaine hydrochloride. Label it to indicate that it is intended for veterinary use only, and is not to be used in animals to be slaughtered for human consumption. Contains amounts of penicillin G procaine and dihydrostreptomycin sulfate equivalent to the labeled number of Penicillin G Units and the labeled amount of dihydrostreptomycin, within −10% to +15%, and the labeled amount of prednisolone, within ± 10%. Meets the requirements for Identification and Bacterial endotoxins, and for Sterility and pH under Penicillin G Procaine and Dihydrostreptomycin Sulfate Injectable Suspension.

PENICILLIN G, NEOMYCIN, POLYMYXIN B, AND HYDROCORTISONE

For *Penicillin G, Neomycin, Polymyxin B,* and *Hydrocortisone*—See individual listings for chemistry information.

USP requirements: Penicillin G Procaine, Neomycin and Polymyxin B Sulfates, and Hydrocortisone Acetate Topical Suspension USP—Preserve in well-closed containers. A suspension of Penicillin G Procaine, Neomycin Sulfate, Polymyxin B Sulfate, and Hydrocortisone Acetate in Peanut Oil or Sesame Oil. Label it to indicate that it is intended for veterinary use only. Contains amounts of penicillin G procaine, neomycin sulfate, and polymyxin B sulfate equivalent to the labeled amounts of Penicillin G Units, neomycin, and polymyxin B Units, within −10% to +40%, and the labeled amount of hydrocortisone acetate, within ±10%. Meets the requirement for Water (not more than 1.0%).

PENICILLIN G AND NOVOBIOCIN

For *Penicillin G* and *Novobiocin*—See individual listings for chemistry information.

USP requirements: Penicillin G Procaine and Novobiocin Sodium Intramammary Infusion USP—Preserve in disposable syringes that are well-closed containers. A suspension of Penicillin G Procaine and Novobiocin Sodium in a suitable vegetable oil vehicle. Contains a suitable preservative and suspending agent. Label it to indicate that it is for veterinary use only. Contains amounts of penicillin G procaine and novobiocin sodium equivalent to the labeled amounts of Penicillin G Units and novobiocin, within −10% to +25%. Meets the requirement for Water (not more than 1.0%).

PENICILLIN V

Chemical name:

Penicillin V—4-Thia-1-azabicyclo[3.2.0]heptane-2-carboxylic acid, 3,3-dimethyl-7-oxo-6-[(phenoxyacetyl)amino]-, [2S-(2 alpha,5 alpha,6 beta)]-.

Penicillin V benzathine—4-Thia-1-azabicyclo[3.2.0]heptane-2-carboxylic acid, 3,3-dimethyl-7-oxo-6-[(2-phenoxyacetyl)amino]-, [2S-(2 alpha,5 alpha,6 beta)]-, compd. with N,N-bis(phenylmethyl)-1,2-ethanediamine (2:1).

Penicillin V potassium—4-Thia-1-azabicyclo[3.2.0]heptane-2-carboxylic acid, 3,3-dimethyl-7-oxo-6-[(phenoxyacetyl)amino]-, monopotassium salt, [2S-(2 alpha,5 alpha,6 beta)]-.

Molecular formula:

Penicillin V—$C_{16}H_{18}N_2O_5S$.

Penicillin V benzathine—$(C_{16}H_{18}N_2O_5S)_2 \cdot C_{16}H_{20}N_2$.

Penicillin V potassium—$C_{16}H_{17}KN_2O_5S$.

Molecular weight:

Penicillin V—350.39.

Penicillin V benzathine—941.12.

Penicillin V potassium—388.48.

Description:

Penicillin V USP—White, odorless, crystalline powder.

Penicillin V Benzathine USP—Practically white powder, having a characteristic odor.

Penicillin V Potassium USP—White, odorless, crystalline powder.

Solubility:

Penicillin V USP—Very slightly soluble in water; freely soluble in alcohol and in acetone; insoluble in fixed oils.

Penicillin V Benzathine USP—Very slightly soluble in water; slightly soluble in alcohol and in ether; sparingly soluble in chloroform.

Penicillin V Potassium USP—Very soluble in water; slightly soluble in alcohol; insoluble in acetone.

USP requirements:

Penicillin V USP—Preserve in tight containers. Label it to indicate that it is to be used in the manufacture of nonparenteral drugs only. Has a potency of not less than 1525 and not more than 1780 Penicillin V Units per mg. Meets the requirements for Identification, Crystallinity, pH (2.5–4.0, in a suspension containing 30 mg per mL), Water (not more than 2.0%), Phenoxyacetic acid (not more than 0.5%), and Limit of p-hydroxypenicillin V (not more than 5.0%).

Penicillin V for Oral Suspension USP—Preserve in tight containers. A dry mixture of Penicillin V with or without one or more suitable buffers, colors, flavors, and suspending agents. It may be labeled in terms of the weight of penicillin V contained therein, in addition to or instead of Units, on the basis that 1600 Penicillin V Units are equivalent to 1 mg of penicillin V. Contains the labeled number of Penicillin V Units, within −10% to +20%, when constituted as directed. Meets the requirements for Identification, Uniformity of dosage units (single-unit containers), Deliverable volume (multiple-unit containers), pH (2.0–4.0, in the suspension constituted as directed in the labeling), and Water (not more than 1.0%).

Penicillin V Tablets USP—Preserve in tight containers. The Tablets may be labeled in terms of the weight of penicillin V contained therein, in addition to or instead of Units, on the basis that 1600 Penicillin V Units are equivalent to 1 mg of penicillin V. Contain the labeled number of Penicillin V Units, within −10% to +20%. Meet the requirements for Identification, Dissolution (75% in 45 minutes in water in Apparatus 2 at 50 rpm), Uniformity of dosage units, and Water (not more than 3.0%).

Penicillin V Benzathine USP—Preserve in tight containers. Has a potency of not less than 1060 and not more than 1240 Penicillin V Units per mg. Meets the requirements for Crystallinity, pH (4.0–6.5, in a suspension containing about 30 mg per mL), Water (5.0–8.0%), and Penicillin V content (62.3–72.5%).

Penicillin V Benzathine Oral Suspension USP—Preserve in tight containers, and store in a refrigerator. Contains one or more suitable buffers, colors, dispersants, flavors, and preservatives. It may be labeled in terms of the weight of penicillin V contained therein, in addition to or instead of Units, on the basis that 1600 Penicillin V Units are equivalent to 1 mg of penicillin V. Contains the labeled number of Penicillin V Units, within −10% to +20%. Meets the requirements for Uniformity of dosage units (single-unit containers), Deliverable volume (multiple-unit containers), and pH (6.0–7.0).

Penicillin V Potassium USP—Preserve in tight containers. Label it to indicate that it is to be used in the manufacture of nonparenteral drugs only. Has a potency of not less than 1380 and not more than 1610 Penicillin V Units per mg. Meets the requirements for Identification, Crystallinity, Specific rotation (+220° to +235°), pH (4.0–7.5, in a solution containing 30 mg per mL), Loss on drying (not more than 1.5%), Phenoxyacetic acid (not more than 0.5%), and Limit of p-hydroxypenicillin V (not more than 5.0%).

Penicillin V Potassium for Oral Solution USP—Preserve in tight containers. A dry mixture of Penicillin V Potassium with or without one or more suitable buffers, colors, flavors, preservatives, and suspending agents. It may be labeled in terms of the weight of penicillin V contained therein, in addition to or instead of Units, on the basis that 1600 Penicillin V Units are equivalent to 1 mg of penicillin V. Contains the labeled number of Penicillin V Units, within −10% to +35%, when constituted as directed. Meets the requirements for Identification, Uniformity of dosage units (single-unit containers), Deliverable volume (multiple-unit containers), pH (5.0–7.5, when constituted as directed in the labeling), and Water (not more than 1.0%).

Penicillin V Potassium Tablets USP—Preserve in tight containers. Label the chewable Tablets to indicate that they are to be chewed before swallowing. The Tablets may be labeled in terms of the weight of penicillin V contained therein, in addition to or instead of Units, on the basis that 1600 Penicillin V Units are equivalent to 1 mg of penicillin V. Contain the labeled number of Penicillin V Units, within −10% to +20%. Meet the requirements for Identification, Dissolution (75% in 45 minutes in phosphate buffer [pH 6.0] in Apparatus 2 at 50 rpm), Uniformity of dosage units, and Loss on drying (not more than 1.5%).

PENTAERYTHRITOL TETRANITRATE

Chemical name: 1,3-Propanediol, 2,2-bis[(nitrooxy) methyl]-, dinitrate (ester).

Molecular formula: $C_5H_8N_4O_{12}$.

Molecular weight: 316.14.

Description: Diluted Pentaerythritol Tetranitrate USP—White to ivory-colored powder, having a faint, mild odor.

Solubility: Undiluted pentaerythritol tetranitrate—Soluble in acetone; slightly soluble in alcohol and in ether; practically insoluble in water.

USP requirements:

Diluted Pentaerythritol Tetranitrate USP—Preserve in tight containers, and prevent exposure to excessive heat. A dry mixture of pentaerythritol tetranitrate with Lactose or Mannitol or other suitable inert excipients, to permit safe handling and compliance with U.S. Interstate Commerce Commission regulations pertaining to interstate shipment.

Contains the labeled amount of pentaerythritol tetranitrate, within ±5%. Meets the requirements for Identification and Organic volatile impurities.

Caution: Undiluted pentaerythritol tetranitrate is a powerful explosive; take proper precautions in handling. It can be exploded by percussion or by excessive heat. Only exceedingly small amounts should be isolated.

Pentaerythritol Tetranitrate Extended-release Capsules—Not in *USP–NF*.

Pentaerythritol Tetranitrate Tablets USP—Preserve in tight containers. Prepared from Diluted Pentaerythritol Tetranitrate. Contain the labeled amount of Diluted Pentaerythritol Tetranitrate, within ±7%. Meet the requirements for Identification, Disintegration (10 minutes), and Uniformity of dosage units.

Caution: Undiluted pentaerythritol tetranitrate is a powerful explosive; take proper precautions in handling. It can be exploded by percussion or by excessive heat. Only exceedingly small amounts should be isolated.

Pentaerythritol Tetranitrate Extended-release Tablets—Not in *USP–NF*.

PENTAGASTRIN

Chemical name: L-Phenylalaninamide, *N*-[(1,1-dimethylethoxy)-carbonyl]-beta-alanyl-L-tryptophyl-L-methionyl-L-alpha-aspartyl-.

Molecular formula: $C_{37}H_{49}N_7O_9S$.

Molecular weight: 767.89.

Description: Colorless crystalline solid.

Solubility: Soluble in dimethylformamide and in dimethylsulfoxide; almost insoluble in water, in ethanol, in ether, in chloroform, and in ethyl acetate.

USP requirements: Pentagastrin Injection—Not in *USP–NF*.

PENTAMIDINE

Chemical group: Diamidine derivative, related to hydroxystilbamidine.

Chemical name: Pentamidine isethionate—4,4'-diamidinodiphenoxypentane di-(beta-hydroxyethanesulfonate).

Molecular formula: Pentamidine isethionate—$C_{19}H_{24}N_4O_2 \cdot 2C_2H_6O_4S$.

Molecular weight: Pentamidine isethionate—592.68.

Description: Pentamidine isethionate—White crystalline powder.

Solubility: Pentamidine isethionate—Soluble in water and in glycerin; insoluble in acetone, in chloroform, and in ether.

USP requirements:
Pentamidine Isethionate for Inhalation Solution—Not in *USP–NF*.
Sterile Pentamidine Isethionate—Not in *USP–NF*.

PENTASTARCH AND SODIUM CHLORIDE

Source: Pentastarch—A starch composed of more than 90% amylopectin that has been etherified to the extent that an average of 4 to 5 of the OH groups present in every 10 D-glucopyranose units of the starch polymer have been converted to OCH_2CH_2OH groups.

Chemical name:
Pentastarch—Starch 2-hydroxyethyl ether.
Sodium chloride—Sodium chloride.

Molecular formula: Sodium chloride—NaCl.

Molecular weight:
Pentastarch—Average approximately 264,000 with a range of 150,000 to 350,000 and with 80% of the polymers falling between 10,000 and 2,000,000.
Sodium chloride—58.44.

Description:
Pentastarch in sodium chloride injection—Clear, pale yellow to amber solution.
Sodium Chloride USP—Colorless, cubic crystals or white crystalline powder.
NF category: Tonicity agent.

Solubility: Sodium Chloride USP—Freely soluble in water; and slightly more soluble in boiling water; soluble in glycerin; slightly soluble in alcohol.

USP requirements: Pentastarch in Sodium Chloride Injection—Not in *USP–NF*.

PENTAZOCINE

Chemical name:
Pentazocine—2,6-Methano-3-benzazocin-8-ol, 1,2,3,4,5,6-hexahydro-6,11-dimethyl-3-(3-methyl-2-butenyl)-, (2 alpha,6 alpha,11*R**)-.
Pentazocine hydrochloride—2,6-Methano-3-benzazocin-8-ol, 1,2,3,4,5,6-hexahydro-6,11-dimethyl-3-(3-methyl-2-butenyl)-, hydrochloride, (2 alpha,6 alpha,11*R**)-.
Pentazocine lactate—2,6-Methano-3-benzazocin-8-ol, 1,2,3,4,5,6-hexahydro-6,11-dimethyl-3-(3-methyl-2-butenyl)-, (2 alpha,6 alpha,11*R**)-, compd. with 2-hydroxypropanoic acid (1:1).

Molecular formula:
Pentazocine—$C_{19}H_{27}NO$.
Pentazocine hydrochloride—$C_{19}H_{27}NO \cdot HCl$.
Pentazocine lactate—$C_{19}H_{27}NO \cdot C_3H_6O_3$.

Molecular weight:
Pentazocine—285.42.
Pentazocine hydrochloride—321.88.
Pentazocine lactate—375.50.

Description:
Pentazocine USP—White or very pale, tan-colored powder.
Pentazocine Hydrochloride USP—White, crystalline powder. It exhibits polymorphism, one form melting at about 254 °C and the other at about 218 °C.
Pentazocine lactate—White, crystalline substance.

Solubility:
Pentazocine USP—Practically insoluble in water; freely soluble in chloroform; soluble in alcohol, in acetone, and in ether; sparingly soluble in ethyl acetate.
Pentazocine Hydrochloride USP—Freely soluble in chloroform; soluble in alcohol; sparingly soluble in water; very slightly soluble in acetone and in ether.
Pentazocine lactate—Soluble in acidic aqueous solutions.

USP requirements:

Pentazocine USP—Preserve in tight, light-resistant containers. Contains not less than 98.0% and not more than 101.5% of pentazocine, calculated on the dried basis. Meets the requirements for Identification, Melting range (147–158 °C, with slight darkening), Loss on drying (not more than 1.0%), Residue on ignition (not more than 0.2%), and Ordinary impurities.

Pentazocine Injection USP—Preserve in single-dose or in multiple-dose containers, preferably of Type I glass. A sterile solution of Pentazocine in Water for Injection, prepared with the aid of Lactic Acid. Contains the labeled amount, within ±5%. Meets the requirements for Identification, Bacterial endotoxins, and pH (4.0–5.0), and for Injections.

Pentazocine Hydrochloride USP—Preserve in tight, light-resistant containers. Contains not less than 98.0% and not more than 102.0% of pentazocine hydrochloride, calculated on the dried basis. Meets the requirements for Identification, Loss on drying (not more than 1.0%), Residue on ignition (not more than 0.2%), and Ordinary impurities.

Pentazocine Hydrochloride Tablets USP—Preserve in tight, light-resistant containers. Contain an amount of pentazocine hydrochloride equivalent to the labeled amount of pentazocine, within ±10%. Meet the requirements for Identification, Dissolution (75% in 45 minutes in water in Apparatus 2 at 50 rpm), and Uniformity of dosage units.

Pentazocine Lactate Injection USP—Preserve in single-dose or in multiple-dose containers, preferably of Type I glass. A sterile solution of pentazocine lactate in Water for Injection, prepared from Pentazocine with the aid of Lactic Acid. Contains an amount of pentazocine lactate equivalent to the labeled amount of pentazocine, within ±5%. Meets the requirements for Identification, Bacterial endotoxins, and pH (4.0–5.0), and for Injections.

PENTAZOCINE AND ACETAMINOPHEN

For *Pentazocine* and *Acetaminophen*—See individual listings for chemistry information.

USP requirements: Pentazocine Hydrochloride and Acetaminophen Tablets—Not in *USP–NF*.

PENTAZOCINE AND ASPIRIN

For *Pentazocine* and *Aspirin*—See individual listings for chemistry information.

USP requirements:

Pentazocine and Aspirin Tablets USP—Preserve in tight, light-resistant containers. Contain an amount of Pentazocine Hydrochloride equivalent to the labeled amount of pentazocine, within ±10%, and the labeled amount of aspirin, within ±10%. Meet the requirements for Thin-layer chromatographic identification test, Nonaspirin salicylates (not more than 3.0%), Dissolution (80% of pentazocine and 70% of aspirin in 30 minutes in water in Apparatus 1 at 80 rpm), and Uniformity of dosage units.

Pentazocine Hydrochloride and Aspirin Tablets USP—Preserve in tight, light-resistant containers. Contain an amount of pentazocine hydrochloride equivalent to the labeled amount of pentazocine, within ±10%, and the labeled amount of aspirin, within ±10%. Meet the requirements for Identification, Non-aspirin salicylates (not more than 3.0%), Dissolution (80% of pentazocine and 70% of aspirin in 30 minutes in water in Apparatus 1 at 80 rpm), and Uniformity of dosage units.

PENTAZOCINE AND NALOXONE

For *Pentazocine* and *Naloxone*—See individual listings for chemistry information.

USP requirements:

Pentazocine and Naloxone Tablets USP—Preserve in tight, light-resistant containers. Contain amounts of Pentazocine Hydrochloride and Naloxone Hydrochloride equivalent to the labeled amounts of pentazocine and naloxone, within ±10%. Meet the requirements for Identification, Dissolution (75% of pentazocine in 45 minutes in water in Apparatus 2 at 50 rpm), and Uniformity of dosage units.

Pentazocine and Naloxone Hydrochlorides Tablets USP—Preserve in tight, light-resistant containers. Contain amounts of pentazocine hydrochloride and naloxone hydrochloride equivalent to the labeled amounts of pentazocine and naloxone, within ±10%. Meet the requirements for Identification, Dissolution (75% of pentazocine in 45 minutes in water in Apparatus 2 at 50 rpm), and Uniformity of dosage units.

PENTETIC ACID

Chemical name: Glycine, *N,N*-bis[2-[bis(carboxymethyl)amino]ethyl]-.

Molecular formula: $C_{14}H_{23}N_3O_{10}$.

Molecular weight: 393.35.

Description: Pentetic Acid USP—White, odorless or almost odorless powder. Melts with foaming and degradation at 220 °C.

USP requirements: Pentetic Acid USP—Preserve in well-closed containers. Contains not less than 98.0% and not more than 100.5% of pentetic acid. Meets the requirements for Identification, Residue on ignition (not more than 0.2%), Heavy metals (not more than 0.005%), Limit of nitrilotriacetic acid (not more than 0.1%), and Iron (not more than 0.01%).

PENTOBARBITAL

Chemical name:

Pentobarbital—2,4,6(1*H*,3*H*,5*H*)-Pyrimidinetrione, 5-ethyl-5-(1-methylbutyl)-.

Pentobarbital sodium—2,4,6(1*H*,3*H*,5*H*)-Pyrimidinetrione, 5ethyl-5-(1-methylbutyl), monosodium salt.

Molecular formula:

Pentobarbital—$C_{11}H_{18}N_2O_3$.

Pentobarbital sodium—$C_{11}H_{17}N_2NaO_3$.

Molecular weight:

Pentobarbital—226.27.

Pentobarbital sodium—248.25.

Description:

Pentobarbital USP—White to practically white, fine, practically odorless powder. May occur in a polymorphic form that melts at about 116 °C. This form gradually reverts to the more stable higher-melting form upon being heated at about 110 °C.

Pentobarbital Sodium USP—White, crystalline granules or white powder. Is odorless or has a slight characteristic odor. Its solutions decompose on standing, heat accelerating the decomposition.

Solubility:

Pentobarbital USP—Very slightly soluble in water and in carbon tetrachloride; very soluble in alcohol, in methanol, in ether, in chloroform, and in acetone.

Pentobarbital Sodium USP—Very soluble in water; freely soluble in alcohol; practically insoluble in ether.

USP requirements:

Pentobarbital USP—Preserve in tight containers. Contains not less than 98.5% and not more than 101.0% of pentobarbital, calculated on the dried basis. Meets the requirements for Identification, Melting range (127–133 °C), Loss on drying (not more than 1.0%), Residue on ignition (not more than 0.1%), Heavy metals (not more than 0.002%), Organic volatile impurities, and Isomer content.

Pentobarbital Elixir USP—Preserve in tight containers. Contains the labeled amount, within ±7.5%. Meets the requirements for Identification and Alcohol content (16.0–20.0%).

Pentobarbital Sodium USP—Preserve in tight containers. Contains not less than 98.5% and not more than 101.0% of pentobarbital sodium, calculated on the dried basis. Meets the requirements for Completeness of solution, Identification, pH (9.8–11.0, in the solution prepared in the test for Completeness of solution), Loss on drying (not more than 3.5%), Heavy metals (not more than 0.003%), Organic volatile impurities, and Isomer content.

Pentobarbital Sodium Capsules USP—Preserve in tight containers. Contain the labeled amount, within ±7.5%. Meet the requirements for Identification, Dissolution (75% in 45 minutes in water in Apparatus 1 at 100 rpm), and Uniformity of dosage units.

Pentobarbital Sodium Injection USP—Preserve in single-dose or in multiple-dose containers, preferably of Type I glass. The Injection may be packaged in 50-mL containers. A sterile solution of Pentobarbital Sodium in a suitable solvent. Pentobarbital may be substituted for the equivalent amount of Pentobarbital Sodium, for adjustment of the pH. The label indicates that the Injection is not to be used if it contains a precipitate. Contains the equivalent of the labeled amount, within ±8%. Meets the requirements for Identification, Bacterial endotoxins, and pH (9.0–10.5), and for Injections.

Pentobarbital Oral Solution USP—Preserve in tight containers. Contains the labeled amount, within ±7.5%. Meets the requirements for Identification and Alcohol content (16.0–20.0%).

Pentobarbital Sodium Suppositories—Not in *USP–NF*.

PENTOSAN

Chemical name: Pentosan polysulfate sodium—beta-D-Xylan, (1→4), 2,3-bis(hydrogen sulfate), sodium salt.

Molecular formula: Pentosan polysulfate sodium—$[C_5H_6Na_2O_{10}S_2]_n$ (n = 6 to 12).

Molecular weight: 4000 to 6000 daltons.

Description: Pentosan polysulfate sodium—White, odorless, slightly hygroscopic powder.

Solubility: Pentosan polysulfate sodium—Soluble in water to 50% at pH 6.

USP requirements: Pentosan Polysulfate Sodium Capsules—Not in *USP–NF*.

PENTOSTATIN

Chemical name: Imidazo[4,5-*d*][1,3]diazepin-8-ol, 3-(2-deoxy-beta-D-*erythro*-pentofuranosyl)-3,6,7,8-tetrahydro-, (*R*)-.

Molecular formula: $C_{11}H_{16}N_4O_4$.

Molecular weight: 268.27.

Description: White to off-white solid.

Solubility: Freely soluble in distilled water.

USP requirements: Pentostatin for Injection—Not in *USP–NF*.

PENTOXIFYLLINE

Chemical group: A trisubstituted xanthine derivative.

Chemical name: 1*H*-purine-2,6-dione, 3,7-dihydro-3,7-dimethyl-1-(5-oxohexyl)-.

Molecular formula: $C_{13}H_{18}N_4O_3$.

Molecular weight: 278.31.

Description: Pentoxifylline USP—White to almost white crystalline powder.

Solubility: Pentoxifylline USP–Freely soluble in chloroform and in methanol; soluble in water; sparingly soluble in alcohol; slightly soluble in ether.

USP requirements:

Pentoxifylline USP—Preserve in well-closed containers. Contains not less than 98.0% and not more than 102.0% of pentoxifylline. Meets the requirements for Completeness of solution, Identification, Melting range (104°–107°), Acidity (not more than 0.2 mL of 0.01 N sodium hydroxide required), Loss on drying (not more than 0.5%), Residue on ignition (not more than 0.1%), Chloride (0.011%), Sulfate (0.02%), Heavy metals (0.001%), Chromatographic purity, and Organic volatile impurities.

Pentoxifylline Extended-release Tablets USP—Preserve in well-closed containers. Protect from light, and store between 15° and 30°. The labeling indicates the Drug Release Test with which the product complies. Contain the labeled amount, within ±5%. Meet the requirements for Identification, Drug release (for Test 1: not more than 30% in one hour, 30–55% in 4 hours, not less than 60% in 8 hours, and not less than 80% in 12 hours in water in Apparatus 2 at 100 rpm; for Test 2: 8–30% in one hour, 35–60% in 6 hours, 53–80% in 10 hours, and not less than 80% in 20 hours in water in Apparatus 2 at 75 rpm; for Test 3: 15–35% in 2 hour, 55–75% in 8 hours, 75–95% in 12 hours, and not less than 85% in 20 hours in water in Apparatus 1 at 100 rpm; for Test 4: 0–20% in one hour, 35–65% in 8 hours, and not less than 80% in 24 hours in water in Apparatus 2 at 50 rpm; for Test 5: 5–25% in one hour, 10–35% in 2 hours, 20–50% in 4 hours, 30–60% in 6 hours, and not less than 80% in 20 hours in water in Apparatus 2 at 75 rpm; for Test 6: 10–30% in 2 hours, 40–60% in 8 hours, 55–75% in 12 hours, and not less than 85% in 24 hours in simulated gastric fluid [without enzymes] in Apparatus 2 at 50 rpm; for Test 7: not more than 25% in one hour, 25–45% in 3 hours, 55–75% in 8 hours, and not less than 80% in 18 hours in water at Apparatus 2 at 50 rpm; for Test 8: 10–20% in one hour, 15–35% in 2 hours, 25–45% in 4 hours, 55–75% in 10 hours, and not less than 80% in 16 hours in water in Apparatus 2 at 75 rpm; for Test 9: 0–20% in one hour, 20–40% in 3 hours, 30–60% in 6 hours 50–80% in 12 hours, and not less than 80% in 18 hours in water in Apparatus 2 at 50 rpm; for Test 10: not more than 20% in one hour, 35–65% in 6 hours,

60–90% in 12 hours, and not less than 80% in 20 hours in water in Apparatus 2 at 75 rpm), Uniformity of dosage units, and Chromatographic purity.

PEPPERMINT

Description: Peppermint NF—Has an aromatic, characteristic odor.

NF category: Flavors and perfumes.

NF requirements: Peppermint NF—Consists of the dried leaf and flowering top of Mentha piperita Linnéae (Fam. Labiatae). Meets the requirements for Stems and other foreign organic matter, Botanic characteristics, and Organic volatile impurities.

PEPPERMINT OIL

Description: Peppermint Oil NF—Colorless or pale yellow liquid, having a strong, penetrating, characteristic odor.

NF category: Flavors and perfumes.

NF requirements: Peppermint Oil NF—Preserve in tight containers, and prevent exposure to excessive heat. The volatile oil distilled with steam from the fresh overground parts of the flowering plant of Mentha piperita Linnéae (Fam. Labiatae), rectified by distillation and neither partially nor wholly dementholized. Yields not less than 5.0% of esters, calculated as menthyl acetate, and not less than 50.0% of total menthol, free and as esters. Meets the requirements for Solubility in 70% alcohol (one volume dissolves in 3 volumes of 70% alcohol, with not more than slight opalescence), Identification, Specific gravity (0.896–0.908), Angular rotation (–18° to –32°), Refractive index (1.459–1.465 at 20 °C), Heavy metals (not more than 20 mcg per gram), and Limit of dimethyl sulfide.

PEPPERMINT SPIRIT

Description: Peppermint Spirit USP—NF category: Flavors and perfumes.

USP requirements: Peppermint Spirit USP—Preserve in tight containers, protected from light. Contains, in each 100 mL, not less than 9.0 mL and not more than 11.0 mL of peppermint oil.

Prepare Peppermint Spirit as follows: 100 mL of Peppermint Oil, 10 grams of Peppermint, in coarse powder, and a sufficient quantity of Alcohol to make 1000 mL. Macerate the peppermint leaves, freed as much as possible from stems and coarsely powdered, for 1 hour in 500 mL of purified water, and then strongly express them. Add the moist, macerated leaves to 900 mL of alcohol, and allow the mixture to stand for 6 hours with frequent agitation. Filter, and to the filtrate add the oil and add alcohol to make the product measure 1000 mL.

Meets the requirement for Alcohol content (79.0–85.0%).

PEPPERMINT WATER

Description: Peppermint Water NF—NF category: Flavored and/or sweetened vehicle.

NF requirements: Peppermint Water NF—Preserve in tight containers. A clear, saturated solution of Peppermint Oil in Purified Water, prepared by one of the processes described under Aromatic Waters. Meets the requirement for Organic volatile impurities.

PERFLUBRON

Chemical name: Octane, 1-bromo-1,1,2,2,3,3,4,4,5,5,6,6, 7,7,8,8,8-heptadecafluoro-.

Molecular formula: C_8BrF_{17}.

Molecular weight: 498.96.

Description: Perflubron USP—Clear, colorless, practically odorless liquid.

Solubility: Not miscible with water.

USP requirements:

Perflubron USP—Preserve in tight, light-resistant containers. Contains not less than 98.0% and not more than 100.0% of perflubron. Meets the requirements for Identification, Specific gravity (1.916–1.919), Chromatographic purity, and Nonvolatile residue (not more than 0.002%).

Perflubron Oral Solution—Not in USP–NF.

PERFLUOROCHEMICAL EMULSION

Molecular formula:

Perfluorodecalin—$C_{10}F_{18}$.

Perfluorotri-n-propylamine—$C_9F_{21}N$.

Description: Stable emulsion of synthetic perfluorochemicals (perfluorodecalin, perfluorotri-n-propylamine) in Water for Injection. Also contains Poloxamer 188 (a nonionic surfactant which is a polyoxyethylene [160]-polyoxypropylene [30] glycol block copolymer), glycerin, egg yolk phospholipids (a mixture of naturally occurring phospholipids isolated from egg yolk), dextrose (a naturally occurring sugar), and the potassium salt of oleic acid (a naturally occurring fatty acid), plus electrolytes in physiologic concentrations.

Other characteristics:

Osmolarity—Approximately 410 mOsmol per liter.

Mean particle diameter—Less than 270 nanometers as determined by laser light scattering spectrophotometry. The content of particles greater than 400 nanometers is less than 10%.

pH—After preparation for administration: 7.3.

Solubility of oxygen—At 37 °C and at partial pressure of oxygen (pO_2) of 760 mm Hg: 7 volume %. Increases with decreasing temperature; at 10 °C and pO_2 of 760 mm Hg, is 9 volume %.

Solubility of carbon dioxide—At 37 °C and at partial pressure of carbon dioxide (pCO_2) of 760 mm Hg: 66 volume %.

Viscosity—Less viscous than whole blood at 37 °C and at physiological shear rates.

USP requirements: Perfluorochemical Emulsion for Injection—Not in USP–NF.

PERFLUTREN PROTEIN-TYPE A MICROSPHERES

USP requirements:

Perflutren Protein-Type A Microspheres for Injection USP—Preserve in single-dose, tight containers that contain perflutren gas in the headspace, and store in a refrigerator. A

sterile, nonpyrogenic suspension of microspheres produced by dispersing perflutren (octafluoropropane) gas in an aqueous solution of diluted sterile Albumin Human. Label it to indicate that perflutren gas is contained within the microspheres. The labeling also provides the following warnings: Do not use if lower layer is cloudy or turbid, contains visible foreign matter, or if the contents do not appear as a homogeneous, opaque, milky-white suspension after mixing. Do not use if the upper white layer of product is absent. Do not inject air into the vial. Invert the vial, and gently rotate to resuspend the microspheres. Do not use if, after resuspension, the solution appears to be clear rather than opaque milky-white. Contains not less than 0.8 % and not more than 1.2% protein. May contain stabilizers, but contains no preservatives. Meets the requirements for Bacterial endotoxins, Safety, Sterility, pH (6.4–7.4), Microsphere size and concentration, Container headspace content, and Microsphere perflutren content (0.11–0.33 mg per mL), and for Injections (except that it is not subject to the requirement for Particulate matter for Constituted solutions).

Perflutren Protein-Type A Microspheres Injectable Suspension USP—Preserve in single-dose, tight containers that contain perflutren gas in the headspace, and store in a refrigerator. A sterile, nonpyrogenic suspension of microspheres produced by dispersing perflutren (octafluoropropane) gas in an aqueous solution of diluted sterile Albumin Human. Label it to indicate that perflutren gas is contained within the microspheres. The labeling also provides the following warnings: "Do not use if lower layer is cloudy or turbid, contains visible foreign matter, or if the contents do not appear as a homogeneous, opaque, milky-white suspension after mixing. Do not use if the upper white layer of product is absent. Do not inject air into the vial. Invert the vial, and gently rotate to resuspend the microspheres. Do not use if, after resuspension, the solution appears to be clear rather than opaque milky-white." Contains not less than 0.8 % and not more than 1.2% protein. May contain stabilizers, but contains no preservatives. Meets the requirements for Bacterial endotoxins, Safety, Sterility, pH (6.4–7.4), Microsphere size and concentration, Container headspace content, and Microsphere perflutren content (0.11–0.33 mg per mL), and for Injections (except that it is not subject to the requirement for Particulate matter for Constituted solutions).

PERGOLIDE

Source: Ergot derivative.

Chemical name: Pergolide mesylate—Ergoline, 8-[(methylthio)-methyl]-6-propyl-, monomethanesulfonate, (8 beta)-.

Molecular formula: Pergolide mesylate—$C_{19}H_{26}N_2S \cdot CH_4O_3S$.

Molecular weight: Pergolide mesylate—410.60.

Description: Pergolide Mesylate USP—White to off-white powder.

Solubility: Pergolide Mesylate USP—Sparingly soluble in methanol; slightly soluble in water, in dehydrated alcohol, and in chloroform; very slightly soluble in acetone; practically insoluble in ether.

USP requirements:
Pergolide Tablets USP—Preserve in tight, light-resistant containers. Contain an amount of Pergolide Mesylate equivalent to the labeled amount of pergolide, within ±10%. Meet the requirements for Thin-layer chromatographic identification test, Dissolution (75% in 30 minutes in simulated gastric fluid TS [without enzyme] containing 20 mcg of L-cyteine per mL in Apparatus 2 at 50 rpm), Uniformity of dosage units, and Chromatographic purity.

Pergolide Mesylate USP—Preserve in tight, light-resistant containers. Contains not less than 97.5% and not more than 102.0% of pergoloid mesylate, calculated on the dried basis. Meets the requirements for Identification, Specific rotation (−17° to −23° at 20°), Loss on drying (not more than 0.5%), Residue on ignition (not more than 0.1%), Heavy metals (0.001%), Chromatographic purity, and Organic volatile impurieis.

Pergolide Mesylate Tablets—Not in *USP–NF*

PERICYAZINE

Chemical group: Piperidine.

Chemical name: 10-[3-(4-Hydroxypiperidino)propyl]phenothiazine-2-carbonitrile.

Molecular formula: $C_{21}H_{23}N_3OS$.

Molecular weight: 365.49.

Description: A yellow almost odorless powder. Melts at 115 °C.

Solubility: Practically insoluble in water; soluble in alcohol and in acetone; freely soluble in chloroform; slightly soluble in ether.

USP requirements:
Pericyazine Capsules—Not in *USP–NF*.
Pericyazine Oral Solution—Not in *USP–NF*.

PERINDOPRIL

Chemical name: Perindopril erbumine—1*H*-Indole-2-carboxylic acid, 1-[2-[[1-(ethoxycarbonyl)butyl]amino]-1-oxopropyl]octahydro-, [2*S*-[1[*R**(*R**)], 2 alpha,3 alpha beta,7 alpha beta]]-, compd. with 2-methyl-2-propanamine (1:1).

Molecular formula: Perindopril erbumine—$C_{19}H_{32}N_2O_5 \cdot C_4H_{11}N_1$.

Molecular weight: Perindopril erbumine—368.47 (free acid); 441.61 (salt form).

Description: Perindopril erbumine—White crystalline powder.

Solubility: Perindopril erbumine—Freely soluble in water (60% w/w), in alcohol, and in chloroform.

USP requirements: Perindopril Erbumine Tablets—Not in *USP–NF*.

PERMETHRIN

Source: A mixture of the *cis* and *trans* isomers of a synthetic pyrethroid. Permethrin is the first pyrethroid formulated for human use.

Chemical name: Cyclopropanecarboxylic acid, 3-(2,2-dichloroethenyl)-2,2-dimethyl-, (3-phenoxyphenyl)methyl ester.

Molecular formula: $C_{21}H_{20}Cl_2O_3$.

Molecular weight: 391.29.

Description: A yellow to light orange-brown, low-melting solid or viscous liquid.

Solubility: Practically insoluble in water; soluble in nonpolar organic solvents.

USP requirements:
Permethrin Cream—Not in *USP–NF*.
Permethrin Lotion—Not in *USP–NF*.

PERPHENAZINE

Chemical group: Piperazinyl phenothiazine.

Chemical name: Piperazineethanol, 4-[3-(2-chloro-10*H*-phenothiazin-10-yl)propyl]-.

Molecular formula: $C_{21}H_{26}ClN_3OS$.

Molecular weight: 403.97.

Description: Perphenazine USP—White to creamy white, odorless powder.

Solubility: Perphenazine USP—Practically insoluble in water; freely soluble in alcohol and in chloroform; soluble in acetone.

USP requirements:
Perphenazine USP—Preserve in tight, light-resistant containers. Contains not less than 98.0% and not more than 102.0% of perphenazine, calculated on the dried basis. Meets the requirements for Clarity and color of solution, Identification, Melting range (94–100 °C), Loss on drying (not more than 0.5%), Residue on ignition (not more than 0.1%), Ordinary impurities, and Organic volatile impurities.
Perphenazine Injection USP—Preserve in single-dose or in multiple-dose containers, preferably of Type I glass, protected from light. A sterile solution of Perphenazine in Water for Injection, prepared with the aid of Citric Acid. Contains the labeled amount, as the citrate, within ± 10%. Meets the requirements for Identification, Bacterial endotoxins, and pH (4.2–5.6), and for Injections.
Perphenazine Oral Solution USP—Preserve in well-closed, light-resistant containers. Contains the labeled amount, within ±10%. Meets the requirements for Identification and Limit of perphenazine sulfoxide (not more than 5.0%).
Perphenazine Syrup USP—Preserve in well-closed, light-resistant containers. Contains the labeled amount, within ±10%. Meets the requirement for Identification.
Perphenazine Tablets USP—Preserve in tight, light-resistant containers. Contain the labeled amount, within ±10%. Meet the requirements for Identification, Dissolution (75% in 45 minutes in 0.1 *N* hydrochloric acid in Apparatus 2 at 50 rpm), and Uniformity of dosage units.

PERPHENAZINE AND AMITRIPTYLINE

For *Perphenazine* and *Amitriptyline*—See individual listings for chemistry information.

USP requirements: Perphenazine and Amitriptyline Hydrochloride Tablets USP—Preserve in well-closed containers. Contain the labeled amounts, within ±10%. Meet the requirements for Identification, Dissolution (75% of each active ingredient in 60 minutes in 0.1 *N* hydrochloric acid in Apparatus 2 at 50 rpm), and Uniformity of dosage units.

PERTUSSIS IMMUNE GLOBULIN

Description: Pertussis Immune Globulin USP—Transparent or slightly opalescent liquid, practically colorless, free from turbidity or particles, and practically odorless. May develop a slight, granular deposit during storage. Is standardized for agglutinating activity with the U.S. Standard Antipertussis Serum.

USP requirements: Pertussis Immune Globulin USP—Preserve at a temperature between 2 and 8 °C. A sterile, non-pyrogenic solution of globulins derived from the blood plasma of adult human donors who have been immunized with pertussis vaccine such that each 1.25 mL contains not less than the amount of immune globulin to be equivalent to 25 mL of human hyperimmune serum. Contains a suitable preservative. Label it to state that it is not intended for intravenous injection. Meets the requirement for Expiration date (not later than 3 years after date of issue from manufacturer's cold storage [5 °C, 3 years]). Conforms to the regulations of the U.S. Food and Drug Administration concerning biologics.

PETROLATUM

Description: Petrolatum USP—Unctuous, yellowish to light amber mass, having not more than a slight fluorescence, even after being melted. It is transparent in thin layers. Free or practically free from odor.

NF category: Ointment base.

Solubility: Petrolatum USP—Insoluble in water; freely soluble in carbon disulfide, in chloroform, and in turpentine oil; soluble in ether, in solvent hexane, and in most fixed and volatile oils; practically insoluble in cold alcohol and hot alcohol and in cold dehydrated alcohol.

USP requirements: Petrolatum USP—Preserve in well-closed containers. A purified mixture of semisolid hydrocarbons obtained from petroleum. Label it to indicate the name and proportion of any added stabilizer. Meets the requirements for Specific gravity (0.815–0.880 at 60 °C), Melting range (38–60 °C), Consistency (value of 100–300), Alkalinity, Acidity, Residue on ignition (not more than 0.1%), Organic acids, Fixed oils, fats, and rosin, and Color.

HYDROPHILIC PETROLATUM

Description: Hydrophilic Petrolatum USP—NF category: Ointment base.

USP requirements: Hydrophilic Petrolatum USP—Prepare Hydrophilic Petrolatum as follows: 30 grams of Cholesterol, 30 grams of Stearyl Alcohol, 80 grams of White Wax, and 860 grams of White Petrolatum to make 1000 grams. Melt the Stearyl Alcohol and White Wax together on a steam bath, then add the Cholesterol, and stir until completely dissolved. Add the White Petrolatum, and mix. Remove from the bath, and stir until the mixture congeals.

WHITE PETROLATUM

Description: White Petrolatum USP—White or faintly yellowish, unctuous mass, transparent in thin layers even after cooling to 0 °C.

NF category: Ointment base.

Solubility: White Petrolatum USP—Insoluble in water; slightly soluble in cold or hot alcohol, and in cold dehydrated alcohol; freely soluble in carbon disulfide and in chloroform; soluble in ether, in solvent hexane, and in most fixed and volatile oils.

USP requirements: White Petrolatum USP—Preserve in well-closed containers. A purified mixture of semisolid hydrocarbons obtained from petroleum, and wholly or nearly decolorized. Label it to indicate the name and proportion of any added stabilizer. Meets the requirements for Residue on ignition (not more than 0.05%) and Color, and for Specific gravity, Melting range, Consistency, Alkalinity, Acidity, Organic acids, and Fixed oils, fats, and rosin under Petrolatum.

PHENACEMIDE

Chemical group: Substituted acetylurea derivative.

Chemical name: Benzeneacetamide, *N*-(aminocarbonyl)-.

Molecular formula: $C_9H_{10}N_2O_2$.

Molecular weight: 178.19.

Description: Phenacemide USP—White to practically white, fine crystalline powder. Is odorless, or practically odorless, and melts at about 213 °C.

Solubility: Phenacemide USP—Very slightly soluble in water, in alcohol, in chloroform, and in ether; slightly soluble in acetone and in methanol.

USP requirements:
Phenacemide USP—Preserve in tight containers. Contains not less than 98.0% and not more than 100.5% of phenacemide, calculated on the dried basis. Meets the requirements for Identification, Loss on drying (not more than 1.0%), Residue on ignition (not more than 0.1%), Heavy metals (not more than 0.002%), Ordinary impurities, and Organic volatile impurities.
Phenacemide Tablets USP—Preserve in well-closed containers. Contain the labeled amount, within ±5%. Meet the requirements for Identification, Dissolution (35% in 60 minutes in 0.1 N hydrochloric acid in Apparatus 2 at 100 rpm), and Uniformity of dosage units.

PHENAZOPYRIDINE

Chemical name: Phenazopyridine hydrochloride—2,6-Pyridinediamine, 3-(phenylazo)-, monohydrochloride.

Molecular formula: Phenazopyridine hydrochloride—$C_{11}H_{11}N_5 \cdot$ HCl.

Molecular weight: Phenazopyridine hydrochloride—249.70.

Description: Phenazopyridine Hydrochloride USP—Light or dark red to dark violet, crystalline powder. Is odorless, or has a slight odor. Melts at about 235 °C, with decomposition.

Solubility: Phenazopyridine Hydrochloride USP—Slightly soluble in water, in alcohol, and in chloroform.

USP requirements:
Phenazopyridine Hydrochloride USP—Preserve in tight containers. Contains not less than 99.0% and not more than 101.0% of phenazopyridine hydrochloride, calculated on the dried basis. Meets the requirements for Identification, Loss on drying (not more than 1.0%), Residue on ignition (not more than 0.2%), Water-insoluble substances (not more than 0.1%), Heavy metals (not more than 0.002%), and Ordinary impurities.

Phenazopyridine Hydrochloride Tablets USP—Preserve in tight containers. Contain the labeled amount, within ± 10%. Meet the requirements for Identification, Dissolution (75% in 45 minutes in water in Apparatus 2 at 50 rpm), and Uniformity of dosage units.

PHENDIMETRAZINE

Chemical group: Morpholine.

Chemical name: Phendimetrazine tartrate—Morpholine, 3,4-dimethyl-2-phenyl-, (2S-*trans*)-, [R-(R*,R*)]-2,3-dihydroxybutanedioate (1:1).

Molecular formula: Phendimetrazine tartrate—$C_{12}H_{17}NO \cdot C_4H_6O_6$.

Molecular weight: Phendimetrazine tartrate—341.36.

Description: Phendimetrazine Tartrate USP—White, odorless, crystalline powder.

Solubility: Phendimetrazine Tartrate USP—Freely soluble in water; sparingly soluble in warm alcohol; insoluble in chloroform, in acetone, and in ether. Phendimetrazine base is extracted by organic solvents from alkaline solution.

USP requirements:
Phendimetrazine Tartrate USP—Preserve in tight containers. Contains not less than 98.0% and not more than 102.0% of phendimetrazine tartrate, calculated on the dried basis. Meets the requirements for Identification, Melting range (182–188 °C, with decomposition, the range between beginning and end of melting not more than 3 °C), Specific rotation (+32° to +36°), pH (3.0–4.0, in a solution [1 in 40]), Loss on drying (not more than 0.5%), Residue on ignition (not more than 0.1%), Chloride (not more than 0.035%), Sulfate (not more than 0.01%), Heavy metals (not more than 0.001%), Chromatographic purity, Organic volatile impurities, and L-*erythro* isomer (not more than 0.1%).
Phendimetrazine Tartrate Capsules USP—Preserve in tight containers. Contain the labeled amount, within ±5%. Meet the requirements for Identification, Dissolution (70% in 60 minutes in water in Apparatus 1 at 100 rpm), and Uniformity of dosage units.
Phendimetrazine Tartrate Extended-release Capsules—Not in *USP–NF*.
Phendimetrazine Tartrate Tablets USP—Preserve in well-closed containers. Contain the labeled amount, within ± 10%. Meet the requirements for Identification, Dissolution (70% in 60 minutes in water in Apparatus 1 at 100 rpm), and Uniformity of dosage units.
Phendimetrazine Tartrate Extended-release Tablets—Not in *USP–NF*.

PHENELZINE

Chemical group: Hydrazine derivative.

Chemical name: Phenelzine sulfate—Hydrazine, (2-phenylethyl)-, sulfate (1:1).

Molecular formula: Phenelzine sulfate—$C_8H_{12}N_2 \cdot H_2SO_4$.

Molecular weight: Phenelzine sulfate—234.27.

Description: Phenelzine Sulfate USP—White to yellowish white powder, having a characteristic odor.

Solubility: Phenelzine Sulfate USP—Freely soluble in water; practically insoluble in alcohol, in chloroform, and in ether.

USP requirements:

Phenelzine Sulfate USP—Preserve in tight containers, protected from heat and light. Contains not less than 98.0% and not more than 102.0% of phenelzine sulfate, calculated on the dried basis. Meets the requirements for Identification, Melting range (164–168 °C), pH (1.4–1.9, in a solution [1 in 100]), Loss on drying (not more than 1.0%), Heavy metals (not more than 0.002%), Limit of hydrazine (not more than 0.1%), Ordinary impurities, and Organic volatile impurities.

Phenelzine Sulfate Tablets USP—Preserve in tight containers, protected from heat and light. Contain an amount of phenelzine sulfate equivalent to the labeled amount of phenelzine, within ±10%. Meet the requirements for Identification, Disintegration, and Uniformity of dosage units.

PHENINDAMINE

Chemical group: Piperidine derivative.

Chemical name: Phenindamine tartrate—2,3,4,9-Tetrahydro-2-methyl-9-phenyl-1*H*-indeno[2,1-*c*]pyridine.

Molecular formula: Phenindamine tartrate—$C_{19}H_{19}N \cdot C_4H_6O_6$.

Molecular weight: Phenindamine tartrate—411.45.

Description: Phenindamine tartrate—White or almost white, odorless or almost odorless, voluminous powder. A 1% solution in water has a pH of 3.4 to 3.9.

Solubility: Phenindamine tartrate—Soluble 1 in 70 of water; slightly soluble in alcohol; practically insoluble in chloroform and in ether.

USP requirements: Phenindamime Tartrate Tablets—Not in *USP–NF*.

PHENIRAMINE

Chemical name: Pheniramine maleate—2-[Alpha-[2-dimethylaminoethyl]benzyl]pyridine bimaleate.

Molecular formula: Pheniramine maleate—$C_{16}N_{20}N_2 \cdot C_4H_4O_4$

Molecular weight: Pheniramine maleate—356.42

Description: Pheniramine Maleate USP—White, crystalline powder having a faint amine-like odor.

Solubility: Pheniramine Maleate USP—Soluble in water and in alcohol.

USP requirements: Pheniramine Maleate USP—Preserve in well-closed containers. Contains not less than 98.0% and not more than 102.0% of pheniramine maleate, calculated on the dried basis. Meets the requirements for Identification, Melting range (104–109 °C), pH (4.5–5.5, in a solution [10 mg per mL]), Loss on drying (not more than 0.5%), Residue on ignition (not more than 0.5%), Heavy metals (not more than 0.002%), Chromatographic purity, and Organic volatile impurities.

PHENIRAMINE, CODEINE, AND GUAIFENESIN

Chemical group: Pheniramine—Alkylamine derivative.

Chemical name:

Pheniramine maleate—2-[alpha-[2-Dimethylaminoethyl]benzyl]pyridine bimaleate.

Codeine phosphate—Morphinan-6-ol, 7,8-didehydro-4,5-epoxy-3-methoxy-17-methyl-, (5 alpha,6 alpha)-, phosphate (1:1) (salt), hemihydrate.

Guaifenesin—1,2-Propanediol, 3-(2-methoxyphenoxy)-.

Molecular formula:

Pheniramine maleate—$C_{16}H_{20}N_2 \cdot C_4H_4O_4$.

Codeine phosphate—$C_{18}H_{21}NO_3 \cdot H_3PO_4 \cdot \frac{1}{2}H_2O$ (hemihydrate); $C_{18}H_{21}NO_3 \cdot H_3PO_4$ (anhydrous).

Guaifenesin—$C_{10}H_{14}O_4$.

Molecular weight:

Pheniramine maleate—356.42.

Codeine phosphate—406.37 (hemihydrate); 397.36 (anhydrous).

Guaifenesin—198.22.

Description:

Pheniramine maleate—White crystalline powder having a faint amine-like odor.

Codeine Phosphate USP—Fine, white, needle-shaped crystals, or white, crystalline powder. Is odorless, and is affected by light. Its solutions are acid to litmus.

Guaifenesin USP—White to slightly gray, crystalline powder. May have a slight characteristic odor.

Solubility:

Pheniramine maleate—Soluble in water and in alcohol.

Codeine Phosphate USP—Freely soluble in water; very soluble in hot water; slightly soluble in alcohol but more so in boiling alcohol.

Guaifenesin USP—Soluble in water, in alcohol, in chloroform, and in propylene glycol; sparingly soluble in glycerin.

USP requirements: Pheniramine Maleate, Codeine Phosphate, and Guaifenesin Syrup—Not in *USP–NF*.

PHENIRAMINE AND PHENYLEPHRINE

Chemical group: Pheniramine—Alkylamine derivative.

Chemical name:

Pheniramine maleate—2-[alpha-[2-Dimethylaminoethyl]benzyl]pyridine bimaleate.

Phenylephrine hydrochloride—Benzenemethanol, 3-hydroxy-alpha-[(methylamino)methyl]-, hydrochloride.

Molecular formula:

Pheniramine maleate—$C_{16}H_{20}N_2 \cdot C_4H_4O_4$.

Phenylephrine hydrochloride—$C_9H_{13}NO_2 \cdot HCl$.

Molecular weight:

Pheniramine maleate—356.42.

Phenylephrine hydrochloride—203.67.

Description:

Pheniramine maleate—White crystalline powder having a faint amine-like odor.

Phenylephrine Hydrochloride USP—White or practically white, odorless crystals.

Solubility:

Pheniramine maleate—Soluble in water and in alcohol.

Phenylephrine Hydrochloride USP—Freely soluble in water and in alcohol.

USP requirements: Pheniramine Maleate and Phenylephrine Hydrochloride for Oral Solution—Not in *USP–NF*.

PHENIRAMINE, PHENYLEPHRINE, AND ACETAMINO-PHEN

Chemical group: Pheniramine—Alkylamine derivative.

Chemical name:

Pheniramine maleate—2-[alpha-[2-Dimethylaminoethyl]benzyl]pyridine bimaleate.

Phenylephrine hydrochloride—Benzenemethanol, 3-hydroxy-alpha-[(methylamino)methyl]-, hydrochloride.

Acetaminophen—Acetamide, *N*-(4-hydroxyphenyl)-.

Molecular formula:

Pheniramine maleate—$C_{16}H_{20}N_2 \cdot C_4H_4O_4$.

Phenylephrine hydrochloride—$C_9H_{13}NO_2 \cdot HCl$.

Acetaminophen—$C_8H_9NO_2$.

Molecular weight:

Pheniramine maleate—356.42.

Phenylephrine hydrochloride—203.67.

Acetaminophen—151.16.

Description:

Pheniramine maleate—White crystalline powder having a faint amine-like odor.

Phenylephrine Hydrochloride USP—White or practically white, odorless crystals.

Acetaminophen USP—White, odorless, crystalline powder.

Solubility:

Pheniramine maleate—Soluble in water and in alcohol.

Phenylephrine Hydrochloride USP—Freely soluble in water and in alcohol.

Acetaminophen USP—Soluble in boiling water and in 1 *N* sodium hydroxide; freely soluble in alcohol.

USP requirements: Pheniramine Maleate, Phenylephrine Hydrochloride, and Acetaminophen for Oral Solution—Not in *USP–NF*.

PHENIRAMINE, PHENYLEPHRINE, CODEINE, SODIUM CITRATE, SODIUM SALICYLATE, AND CAFFEINE

Source: Caffeine—Coffee, tea, cola, and cocoa or chocolate. May also be synthesized from urea or dimethylurea.

Chemical group:

Pheniramine—Alkylamine derivative.

Caffeine—Methylated xanthine.

Chemical name:

Pheniramine maleate—2-[alpha-[2-Dimethylaminoethyl]benzyl]pyridine bimaleate.

Phenylephrine hydrochloride—Benzenemethanol, 3-hydroxy-alpha-[(methylamino)methyl]-, hydrochloride.

Codeine phosphate—Morphinan-6-ol, 7,8-didehydro-4,5epoxy-3-methoxy-17-methyl-, (5 alpha,6 alpha)-, phosphate (1:1) (salt), hemihydrate.

Sodium citrate—1,2,3-Propanetricarboxylic acid, 2-hydroxy-, trisodium salt.

Sodium salicylate—Benzoic acid, 2-hydroxy-, monosodium salt.

Caffeine—1*H*-Purine-2,6-dione, 3,7-dihydro-1,3,7-trimethyl-.

Citric Acid—1,2,3-Propanetricarboxylic acid, 2-hydroxy-.

Molecular formula:

Pheniramine maleate—$C_{16}H_{20}N_2 \cdot C_4H_4O_4$.

Phenylephrine hydrochloride—$C_9H_{13}NO_2 \cdot HCl$.

Codeine phosphate—$C_{18}H_{21}NO_3 \cdot H_3PO_4 \cdot \frac{1}{2}H_2O$ (hemihydrate); $C_{18}H_{21}NO_3 \cdot H_3PO_4$ (anhydrous).

Sodium citrate—$C_6H_5Na_3O_7$.

Sodium salicylate—$C_7H_5NaO_3$.

Caffeine—$C_8H_{10}N_4O_2$ (anhydrous); $C_8H_{10}N_4O_2 \cdot H_2O$ (monohydrate).

Citric acid—$C_6H_8O_7$ (anhydrous); $C_6H_8O_7 \cdot H_2O$ (monohydrate).

Molecular weight:

Pheniramine maleate—356.42.

Phenylephrine hydrochloride—203.67.

Codeine phosphate—406.37 (hemihydrate); 397.36 (anhydrous).

Sodium citrate—258.07 (anhydrous).

Sodium salicylate—160.10.

Caffeine—194.19 (anhydrous); 212.21 (monohydrate).

Citric acid—192.12 (anhydrous); 210.14 (monohydrate).

Description:

Pheniramine maleate—White crystalline powder having a faint amine-like odor.

Phenylephrine Hydrochloride USP—White or practically white, odorless crystals.

Codeine Phosphate USP—Fine, white, needle-shaped crystals, or white, crystalline powder. Is odorless, and is affected by light. Its solutions are acid to litmus.

Sodium Citrate USP—Colorless crystals or white, crystalline powder.

NF category: Buffering agent.

Sodium Salicylate USP—Amorphous or microcrystalline powder or scales. Is colorless, or has not more than a faint, pink tinge. Is odorless, or has a faint, characteristic odor, and is affected by light. A freshly made solution (1 in 10) is neutral or acid to litmus.

Caffeine USP—White powder or white, glistening needles, usually matted together. Is odorless. Its solutions are neutral to litmus. The hydrate is efflorescent in air.

Citric Acid USP—Colorless, translucent crystals, or white, granular to fine crystalline powder. Odorless or practically odorless. The hydrous form is efflorescent in dry air.

NF category: Acidifying agent; buffering agent.

Solubility:

Pheniramine maleate—Soluble in water and in alcohol.

Phenylephrine Hydrochloride USP—Freely soluble in water and in alcohol.

Codeine Phosphate USP—Freely soluble in water; very soluble in hot water; slightly soluble in alcohol but more so in boiling alcohol.

Sodium Citrate USP—Hydrous form freely soluble in water and very soluble in boiling water; insoluble in alcohol.

Sodium Salicylate USP—Freely (and slowly) soluble in water and in glycerin; very soluble in boiling water and in boiling alcohol; slowly soluble in alcohol.

Caffeine USP—Sparingly soluble in water and in alcohol; freely soluble in chloroform; slightly soluble in ether.

The aqueous solubility of caffeine is increased by organic acids or their alkali salts, such as citrates, benzoates, salicylates, or cinnamates, which dissociate to yield caffeine when dissolved in biological fluids.

Citric Acid USP—Very soluble in water; freely soluble in alcohol; very slightly soluble in ether.

USP requirements:

Pheniramine Maleate, Phenylephrine Hydrochloride, Codeine Phosphate, Sodium Citrate, Sodium Salicylate, and Caffeine Citrate Syrup—Not in *USP–NF*.

Pheniramine Maleate, Phenylephrine Hydrochloride, Codeine Phosphate, Sodium Citrate, Sodium Salicylate, and Caffeine Citrate Oral Solution—Not in *USP–NF*.

PHENIRAMINE, PHENYLEPHRINE, AND DEXTRO-METHORPHAN

Source: Dextromethorphan—Methylated dextroisomer of levorphanol.

Chemical group:

Pheniramine—Alkylamine derivative.

Dextromethorphan—Synthetic derivative of morphine.

Chemical name:

Pheniramine maleate—2-[alpha-[2-Dimethylaminoethyl]benzyl]pyridine bimaleate.

Phenylephrine hydrochloride—Benzenemethanol, 3-hydroxy-alpha-[(methylamino)methyl]-, hydrochloride.

Dextromethorphan hydrobromide—Morphinan, 3-methoxy17-methyl-, (9 alpha,13 alpha,14 alpha)-, hydrobromide, monohydrate.

Molecular formula:

Pheniramine maleate—$C_{16}H_{20}N_2 \cdot C_4H_4O_4$.

Phenylephrine hydrochloride—$C_9H_{13}NO_2 \cdot HCl$.

Dextromethorphan hydrobromide—$C_{18}H_{25}NO \cdot HBr \cdot H_2O$.

Molecular weight:

Pheniramine maleate—356.42.

Phenylephrine hydrochloride—203.67.

Dextromethorphan hydrobromide—370.32.

Description:

Pheniramine maleate—White crystalline powder having a faint amine-like odor.

Phenylephrine Hydrochloride USP—White or practically white, odorless crystals.

Dextromethorphan Hydrobromide USP—Practically white crystals or crystalline powder, having a faint odor. Melts at about 126 °C, with decomposition.

Solubility:

Pheniramine maleate—Soluble in water and in alcohol.

Phenylephrine Hydrochloride USP—Freely soluble in water and in alcohol.

Dextromethorphan Hydrobromide USP—Sparingly soluble in water; freely soluble in alcohol and in chloroform; insoluble in ether.

USP requirements: Pheniramine Maleate, Phenylephrine Hydrochloride, and Dextromethorphan Hydrobromide for Oral Solution—Not in *USP–NF*.

PHENIRAMINE, PHENYLEPHRINE, PHENYLPROPANOLAMINE, HYDROCODONE, AND GUAIFENESIN

Chemical group:

Pheniramine—Alkylamine derivative.

Phenylpropanolamine hydrochloride—Synthetic phenylisopropanolamine.

Chemical name:

Pheniramine maleate—2-[alpha-[2-Dimethylaminoethyl]benzyl]pyridine bimaleate.

Phenylephrine hydrochloride—Benzenemethanol, 3-hydroxy-alpha-[(methylamino)methyl]-, hydrochloride.

Phenylpropanolamine hydrochloride—Benzenemethanol, alpha-(1-aminoethyl)-, hydrochloride, (R^*,S^*)-, ($\pm$).

Hydrocodone bitartrate—Morphinan-6-one, 4,5-epoxy-3-methoxy-17-methyl-, (5 alpha)-, $[R\text{-}(R^*,R^*)]$-2,3-dihydroxybutanedioate (1:1), hydrate (2:5).

Guaifenesin—1,2-Propanediol, 3-(2-methoxyphenoxy)-.

Molecular formula:

Pheniramine maleate—$C_{16}H_{20}N_2 \cdot C_4H_4O_4$.

Phenylephrine hydrochloride—$C_9H_{13}NO_2 \cdot HCl$.

Phenylpropanolamine hydrochloride—$C_9H_{13}NO \cdot HCl$.

Hydrocodone bitartrate—$C_{18}H_{21}NO_3 \cdot C_4H_6O_6 \cdot 2\frac{1}{2}H_2O$ (hydrate); $C_{18}H_{21}NO_3 \cdot C_4H_6O_6$ (anhydrous).

Guaifenesin—$C_{10}H_{14}O_4$.

Molecular weight:

Pheniramine maleate—356.42.

Phenylephrine hydrochloride—203.67.

Phenylpropanolamine hydrochloride—187.67.

Hydrocodone bitartrate—494.49 (hydrate); 449.46 (anhydrous).

Guaifenesin—198.22.

Description:

Pheniramine maleate—White crystalline powder having a faint amine-like odor.

Phenylephrine Hydrochloride USP—White or practically white, odorless crystals.

Phenylpropanolamine Hydrochloride USP—White, crystalline powder, having a slight aromatic odor. Is affected by light.

Hydrocodone Bitartrate USP—Fine, white crystals or a crystalline powder. Is affected by light.

Guaifenesin USP—White to slightly gray, crystalline powder. May have a slight characteristic odor.

pKa: Phenylpropanolamine hydrochloride—9.

Solubility:

Pheniramine maleate—Soluble in water and in alcohol.

Phenylephrine Hydrochloride USP—Freely soluble in water and in alcohol.

Phenylpropanolamine Hydrochloride USP—Freely soluble in water and in alcohol; insoluble in ether.

Hydrocodone Bitartrate USP—Soluble in water; slightly soluble in alcohol; insoluble in ether and in chloroform.

Guaifenesin USP—Soluble in water, in alcohol, in chloroform, and in propylene glycol; sparingly soluble in glycerin.

USP requirements:

Pheniramine Maleate, Phenylephrine Hydrochloride, Phenylpropanolamine Hydrochloride, Hydrocodone Bitartrate, and Guaifenesin Oral Solution—Not in *USP–NF*.

Pheniramine Maleate, Phenylephrine Hydrochloride, Phenylpropanolamine Hydrochloride, Hydrocodone Bitartrate, and Guaifenesin Syrup—Not in *USP–NF*.

PHENIRAMINE, PHENYLEPHRINE, SODIUM SALICYLATE, AND CAFFEINE

Source: Caffeine—Coffee, tea, cola, and cocoa or chocolate. May also be synthesized from urea or dimethylurea.

Chemical group:

Pheniramine—Alkylamine derivative.

Caffeine—Methylated xanthine.

Chemical name:

Pheniramine maleate—2-[alpha-[2-Dimethylaminoethyl]benzyl]pyridine bimaleate.

Phenylephrine hydrochloride—Benzenemethanol, 3-hydroxy-alpha-[(methylamino)methyl]-, hydrochloride.

Sodium salicylate—Benzoic acid, 2-hydroxy-, monosodium salt.

Caffeine—1*H*-Purine-2,6-dione, 3,7-dihydro-1,3,7-trimethyl-.

Citric Acid—1,2,3-Propanetricarboxylic acid, 2-hydroxy-.

Molecular formula:

Pheniramine maleate—$C_{16}H_{20}N_2 \cdot C_4H_4O_4$.

Phenylephrine hydrochloride—$C_9H_{13}NO_2 \cdot HCl$.

Sodium salicylate—$C_7H_5NaO_3$.

Caffeine—$C_8H_{10}N_4O_2$ (anhydrous); $C_8H_{10}N_4O_2 \cdot H_2O$ (monohydrate).

Citric acid—$C_6H_8O_7$ (anhydrous); $C_6H_8O_7 \cdot H_2O$ (monohydrate).

Molecular weight:

Pheniramine maleate—356.42.

Phenylephrine hydrochloride—203.67.

Sodium salicylate—160.10.

Caffeine—194.19 (anhydrous); 212.21 (monohydrate).

Citric acid—192.12 (anhydrous); 210.14 (monohydrate).

Description:

Pheniramine maleate—White crystalline powder having a faint amine-like odor.

Phenylephrine Hydrochloride USP—White or practically white, odorless crystals.

Sodium Salicylate USP—Amorphous or microcrystalline powder or scales. Is colorless, or has not more than a faint, pink tinge. Is odorless, or has a faint, characteristic odor, and is affected by light. A freshly made solution (1 in 10) is neutral or acid to litmus.

Caffeine USP—White powder or white, glistening needles, usually matted together. Is odorless. Its solutions are neutral to litmus. The hydrate is efflorescent in air.

Citric Acid USP—Colorless, translucent crystals, or white, granular to fine crystalline powder. Odorless or practically odorless. The hydrous form is efflorescent in dry air.

    NF category: Acidifying agent; buffering agent.

Solubility:

Pheniramine maleate—Soluble in water and in alcohol.

Phenylephrine Hydrochloride USP—Freely soluble in water and in alcohol.

Sodium Salicylate USP—Freely (and slowly) soluble in water and in glycerin; very soluble in boiling water and in boiling alcohol; slowly soluble in alcohol.

Caffeine USP—Sparingly soluble in water and in alcohol; freely soluble in chloroform; slightly soluble in ether.

    The aqueous solubility of caffeine is increased by organic acids or their alkali salts, such as citrates, benzoates, salicylates, or cinnamates, which dissociate to yield caffeine when dissolved in biological fluids.

Citric Acid USP—Very soluble in water; freely soluble in alcohol; very slightly soluble in ether.

USP requirements:

Pheniramine Maleate, Phenylephrine Hydrochloride, Sodium Salicylate, and Caffeine Citrate Oral Solution—Not in *USP–NF*.

Pheniramine Maleate, Phenylephrine Hydrochloride, Sodium Salicylate, and Caffeine Citrate Syrup—Not in *USP–NF*.

PHENIRAMINE, PHENYLTOLOXAMINE, PYRILAMINE, AND PHENYLPROPANOLAMINE

Chemical group:

Pheniramine—Alkylamine derivative.

Phenyltoloxamine citrate—Ethanolamine derivative.

Pyrilamine—Ethylenediamine derivative.

Phenylpropanolamine hydrochloride—Synthetic phenylisopropanolamine.

Chemical name:

Pheniramine maleate—2-[alpha-[2-Dimethylaminoethyl]benzyl]pyridine bimaleate.

Phenyltoloxamine citrate—2-(2-Benzylphenoxy)-*N*,*N*-dimethylethylamine dihydrogen citrate.

Pyrilamine maleate—1,2-Ethanediamine, *N*-[(4-methoxyphenyl)methyl]-*N*,*N*-dimethyl-*N*-2-pyridinyl-, (*Z*)-2-butenedioate (1:1).

Phenylpropanolamine hydrochloride—Benzenemethanol, alpha-(1-aminoethyl)-, hydrochloride, (*R**,*S**)-, ($\pm$).

Molecular formula:

Pheniramine maleate—$C_{16}H_{20}N_2 \cdot C_4H_4O_4$.

Phenyltoloxamine citrate—$C_{17}H_{21}NO \cdot C_6H_8O_7$.

Pyrilamine maleate—$C_{17}H_{23}N_3O \cdot C_4H_4O_4$.

Phenylpropanolamine hydrochloride—$C_9H_{13}NO \cdot HCl$.

Molecular weight:

Pheniramine maleate—356.42.

Phenyltoloxamine citrate—447.5.

Pyrilamine maleate—401.46.

Phenylpropanolamine hydrochloride—187.67.

Description:

Pheniramine maleate—White crystalline powder having a faint amine-like odor.

Pyrilamine Maleate USP—White, crystalline powder, usually having a faint odor. Its solutions are acid to litmus.

Phenyltoloxamine citrate—It has a melting point of 138–140 °C.

Phenylpropanolamine Hydrochloride USP—White, crystalline powder, having a slight aromatic odor. Affected by light.

pKa: Phenylpropanolamine hydrochloride—9.

Solubility:

Pheniramine maleate—Soluble in water and in alcohol.

Pyrilamine Maleate USP—Very soluble in water; freely soluble in alcohol and in chloroform; slightly soluble in ether.

Phenyltoloxamine citrate—Soluble in water.

Phenylpropanolamine Hydrochloride USP—Freely soluble in water and in alcohol; insoluble in ether.

USP requirements:

Pheniramine Maleate, Phenyltoloxamine Citrate, Pyrilamine Maleate, and Phenylpropanolamine Hydrochloride Extended-release Capsules—Not in *USP–NF*.

Pheniramine Maleate, Phenyltoloxamine Citrate, Pyrilamine Maleate, and Phenylpropanolamine Hydrochloride Elixir—Not in *USP–NF*.

PHENIRAMINE, PYRILAMINE, HYDROCODONE, POTASSIUM CITRATE, AND ASCORBIC ACID

Chemical group:

Pheniramine—Alkylamine derivative.

Pyrilamine—Ethylenediamine derivative.

Chemical name:

Pheniramine maleate—2-[alpha-[2-Dimethylaminoethyl]benzyl]pyridine bimaleate.

Pyrilamine maleate—1,2-Ethanediamine, *N*-[(4-methoxyphenyl)methyl]-*N*,*N*-dimethyl-*N*-2-pyridinyl-, (*Z*)-2-butenedioate (1:1).

Hydrocodone bitartrate—Morphinan-6-one, 4,5-epoxy-3-methoxy-17-methyl-, (5 alpha)-, [*R*-(*R**,*R**)]-2,3-dihydroxybutanedioate (1:1), hydrate (2:5).

Potassium citrate—1,2,3-Propanetricarboxylic acid, 2-hydroxy-, tripotassium salt, monohydrate.

Ascorbic acid—L-Ascorbic acid.

Molecular formula:

Pheniramine maleate—$C_{16}H_{20}N_2 \cdot C_4H_4O_4$.

Pyrilamine maleate—$C_{17}H_{23}N_3O \cdot C_4H_4O_4$.

Hydrocodone bitartrate—$C_{18}H_{21}NO_3 \cdot C_4H_6O_6 \cdot 2\frac{1}{2}H_2O$ (hydrate); $C_{18}H_{21}NO_3 \cdot C_4H_6O_6$ (anhydrous).

Potassium citrate—$C_6H_5K_3O_7 \cdot H_2O$.

Ascorbic acid—$C_6H_8O_6$.

Molecular weight:

Pheniramine maleate—356.42.

Pyrilamine maleate—401.46.

Hydrocodone bitartrate—494.49 (hydrate); 449.46 (anhydrous).

Potassium citrate—324.41.

Ascorbic acid—176.12.

Description:

Pheniramine maleate—White crystalline powder having a faint amine-like odor.

Pyrilamine Maleate USP—White, crystalline powder, usually having a faint odor. Its solutions are acid to litmus.

Hydrocodone Bitartrate USP—Fine, white crystals or a crystalline powder. Is affected by light.

Potassium Citrate USP—Transparent crystals or white, granular powder. Is odorless and is deliquescent when exposed to moist air.

Ascorbic Acid USP—White or slightly yellow crystals or powder. On exposure to light it gradually darkens. In the dry state, is reasonably stable in air, but in solution rapidly oxidizes. Melts at about 190 °C.

NF category: Antioxidant.

Solubility:
Pheniramine maleate—Soluble in water and in alcohol.
Pyrilamine Maleate USP—Very soluble in water; freely soluble in alcohol and in chloroform; slightly soluble in ether.
Hydrocodone Bitartrate USP—Soluble in water; slightly soluble in alcohol; insoluble in ether and in chloroform.
Potassium Citrate USP—Freely soluble in water; almost insoluble in alcohol.
Ascorbic Acid USP—Freely soluble in water; sparingly soluble in alcohol; insoluble in chloroform and in ether.

USP requirements: Pheniramine Maleate, Pyrilamine Maleate, Hydrocodone Bitartrate, Potassium Citrate, and Ascorbic Acid Syrup—Not in *USP–NF*.

PHENIRAMINE, PYRILAMINE, PHENYLEPHRINE, PHENYLPROPANOLAMINE, AND HYDROCODONE

Chemical group:
Pheniramine—Alkylamine derivative.
Pyrilamine—Ethylenediamine derivative.
Phenylpropanolamine hydrochloride—Synthetic phenylisopro-panolamine.

Chemical name:
Pheniramine maleate—2-[alpha-[2-Dimethylaminoethyl]benzyl]pyridine bimaleate.
Pyrilamine maleate—1,2-Ethanediamine, N-[(4-methoxyphenyl)methyl]-N,N-dimethyl-N-2-pyridinyl-, (Z)-2-butenedioate (1:1).
Phenylephrine hydrochloride—Benzenemethanol, 3-hydroxy-alpha-[(methylamino)methyl]-, hydrochloride.
Phenylpropanolamine hydrochloride—Benzenemethanol, alpha-(1-aminoethyl)-, hydrochloride, (R*,S*)-, (±).
Hydrocodone bitartrate—Morphinan-6-one, 4,5-epoxy-3-methoxy-17-methyl-, (5 alpha)-, [R-(R*,R*)]-2,3-dihydroxybutanedioate (1:1), hydrate (2:5).

Molecular formula:
Pheniramine maleate—$C_{16}H_{20}N_2 \cdot C_4H_4O_4$.
Pyrilamine maleate—$C_{17}H_{23}N_3O \cdot C_4H_4O_4$.
Phenylephrine hydrochloride—$C_9H_{13}NO_2 \cdot HCl$.
Phenylpropanolamine hydrochloride—$C_9H_{13}NO \cdot HCl$.
Hydrocodone bitartrate—$C_{18}H_{21}NO_3 \cdot C_4H_6O_6 \cdot 2\frac{1}{2}H_2O$ (hydrate); $C_{18}H_{21}NO_3 \cdot C_4H_6O_6$ (anhydrous).

Molecular weight:
Pheniramine maleate—356.42.
Pyrilamine maleate—401.46.
Phenylephrine hydrochloride—203.67.
Phenylpropanolamine hydrochloride—187.67.
Hydrocodone bitartrate—494.49 (hydrate); 449.46 (anhydrous).

Description:
Pheniramine maleate—White crystalline powder having a faint amine-like odor.
Pyrilamine Maleate USP—White, crystalline powder, usually having a faint odor. Its solutions are acid to litmus.
Phenylephrine Hydrochloride USP—White or practically white, odorless crystals.
Phenylpropanolamine Hydrochloride USP—White, crystalline powder, having a slight aromatic odor. Is affected by light.
Hydrocodone Bitartrate USP—Fine, white crystals or a crystalline powder. Is affected by light.

pKa: Phenylpropanolamine hydrochloride—9.

Solubility:
Pheniramine maleate—Soluble in water and in alcohol.
Pyrilamine Maleate USP—Very soluble in water; freely soluble in alcohol and in chloroform; slightly soluble in ether.
Phenylephrine Hydrochloride USP—Freely soluble in water and in alcohol.
Phenylpropanolamine Hydrochloride USP—Freely soluble in water and in alcohol; insoluble in ether.
Hydrocodone Bitartrate USP—Soluble in water; slightly soluble in alcohol; insoluble in ether and in chloroform.

USP requirements: Pheniramine Maleate, Pyrilamine Maleate, Phenylephrine Hydrochloride, Phenylpropanolamine Hydrochloride, and Hydrocodone Bitartrate Oral Solution—Not in *USP–NF*.

PHENIRAMINE, PYRILAMINE, AND PHENYLPROPANOLAMINE

Chemical group:
Pheniramine—Alkylamine derivative.
Pyrilamine—Ethylenediamine derivative.
Phenylpropanolamine hydrochloride—Synthetic phenyliso-pro-panolamine.

Chemical name:
Pheniramine maleate—2-[alpha-[2-Dimethylaminoethyl]benzyl]pyridine bimaleate.
Pyrilamine maleate—1,2-Ethanediamine, N-[(4-methoxyphenyl)methyl]-N,N-dimethyl-N-2-pyridinyl-, (Z)-2-butenedioate (1:1).
Phenylpropanolamine hydrochloride—Benzenemethanol, alpha-(1-aminoethyl)-, hydrochloride, (R*,S*)-, (±).

Molecular formula:
Pheniramine maleate—$C_{16}H_{20}N_2 \cdot C_4H_4O_4$.
Pyrilamine maleate—$C_{17}H_{23}N_3O \cdot C_4H_4O_4$.
Phenylpropanolamine hydrochloride—$C_9H_{13}NO \cdot HCl$.

Molecular weight:
Pheniramine maleate—356.42.
Pyrilamine maleate—401.46.
Phenylpropanolamine hydrochloride—187.67.

Description:
Pheniramine maleate—White crystalline powder having a faint amine-like odor.
Pyrilamine Maleate USP—White, crystalline powder, usually having a faint odor. Its solutions are acid to litmus.
Phenylpropanolamine Hydrochloride USP—White, crystalline powder, having a slight aromatic odor. Affected by light.

pKa: Phenylpropanolamine hydrochloride—9.

Solubility:
Pheniramine maleate—Soluble in water and in alcohol.
Pyrilamine Maleate USP—Very soluble in water; freely soluble in alcohol and in chloroform; slightly soluble in ether.
Phenylpropanolamine Hydrochloride USP—Freely soluble in water and in alcohol; insoluble in ether.

USP requirements:
Pheniramine Maleate, Pyrilamine Maleate, and Phenylpropanolamine Hydrochloride Oral Solution—Not in *USP–NF*.
Pheniramine Maleate, Pyrilamine Maleate, and Phenylpropanolamine Hydrochloride Extended-release Tablets—Not in *USP–NF*.

PHENIRAMINE, PYRILAMINE, PHENYLPROPANOLAMINE, AND CODEINE

Chemical group:
Pheniramine—Alkylamine derivative.
Pyrilamine—Ethylenediamine derivative.
Phenylpropanolamine hydrochloride—Synthetic phenyliso-
propanolamine.

Chemical name:
Pheniramine maleate—2-[alpha-[2-Dimethylaminoethyl]ben-
zyl]pyridine bimaleate.
Pyrilamine maleate—1,2-Ethanediamine, N-[(4-methoxyphe-
nyl)methyl]-N,N-dimethyl-N-2-pyridinyl-, (Z)-2-butenedio-
ate (1:1).
Phenylpropanolamine hydrochloride—Benzenemethanol, al-
pha-(1-aminoethyl)-, hydrochloride, (R^*,S^*)-, ($\pm$).
Codeine phosphate—Morphinan-6-ol, 7,8-didehydro-4,5-ep-
oxy-3-methoxy-17-methyl-, (5 alpha,6 alpha)-, phosphate
(1:1) (salt), hemihydrate.

Molecular formula:
Pheniramine maleate—$C_{16}H_{20}N_2 \cdot C_4H_4O_4$.
Pyrilamine maleate—$C_{17}H_{23}N_3O \cdot C_4H_4O_4$.
Phenylpropanolamine hydrochloride—$C_9H_{13}NO \cdot HCl$.
Codeine phosphate—$C_{18}H_{21}NO_3 \cdot H_3PO_4 \cdot \frac{1}{2}H_2O$ (hemihydrate);
$C_{18}H_{21}NO_3 \cdot H_3PO_4$ (anhydrous).

Molecular weight:
Pheniramine maleate—356.42.
Pyrilamine maleate—401.46.
Phenylpropanolamine hydrochloride—187.67.
Codeine phosphate—406.37 (hemihydrate); 397.36 (anhy-
drous).

Description:
Pheniramine maleate—White crystalline powder having a fine
amine-like odor.
Pyrilamine Maleate USP—White, crystalline powder, usually
having a faint odor. Its solutions are acid to litmus.
Phenylpropanolamine Hydrochloride USP—White, crystalline
powder, having a slight aromatic odor. Affected by light.
Codeine Phosphate USP—Fine, white, needle-shaped crystals, or white, crystalline powder. Is odorless, and is affected by light. Its solutions are acid to litmus.

pKa: Phenylpropanolamine hydrochloride—9.

Solubility:
Pheniramine maleate—Soluble in water and in alcohol.
Pyrilamine Maleate USP—Very soluble in water; freely soluble
in alcohol and in chloroform; slightly soluble in ether.
Phenylpropanolamine Hydrochloride USP—Freely soluble in
water and in alcohol; insoluble in ether.
Codeine Phosphate USP—Freely soluble in water; very soluble in hot water; slightly soluble in alcohol but more so in
boiling alcohol.

USP requirements: Pheniramine Maleate, Pyrilamine Maleate,
Phenylpropanolamine Hydrochloride and Codeine Phosphate
Syrup—Not in *USP–NF*.

PHENIRAMINE, PYRILAMINE, PHENYLPROPANOLAMINE, CODEINE, ACETAMINOPHEN, AND CAFFEINE

Source: Caffeine—Coffee, tea, cola, and cocoa or chocolate.
May also be synthesized from urea or dimethylurea.

Chemical group:
Pheniramine—Alkylamine derivative.
Pyrilamine—Ethylenediamine derivative.
Phenylpropanolamine hydrochloride—Synthetic phenyliso-
propanolamine.
Caffeine—Methylated xanthine.

Chemical name:
Pheniramine maleate—2-[alpha-[2-Dimethylaminoethyl]ben-
zyl]pyridine bimaleate.
Pyrilamine maleate—1,2-Ethanediamine, N-[(4-methoxyphe-
nyl)methyl]-N,N-dimethyl-N-2-pyridinyl-, (Z)-2-butenedio-
ate (1:1).
Phenylpropanolamine hydrochloride—Benzenemethanol, al-
pha-(1-aminoethyl)-, hydrochloride, (R^*,S^*)-, ($\pm$).
Codeine phosphate—Morphinan-6-ol, 7,8-didehydro-4,5-ep-
oxy-3-methoxy-17-methyl-, (5 alpha,6 alpha)-, phosphate
(1:1) (salt), hemihydrate.
Acetaminophen—Acetamide, N-(4-hydroxyphenyl)-.
Caffeine—1H-Purine-2,6-dione, 3,7-dihydro-1,3,7-trimethyl-.

Molecular formula:
Pheniramine maleate—$C_{16}H_{20}N_2 \cdot C_4H_4O_4$.
Pyrilamine maleate—$C_{17}H_{23}N_3O \cdot C_4H_4O_4$.
Phenylpropanolamine hydrochloride—$C_9H_{13}NO \cdot HCl$.
Codeine phosphate—$C_{18}H_{21}NO_3 \cdot H_3PO_4 \cdot \frac{1}{2}H_2O$ (hemihydrate);
$C_{18}H_{21}NO_3 \cdot H_3PO_4$ (anhydrous).
Acetaminophen—$C_8H_9NO_2$.
Caffeine—$C_8H_{10}N_4O_2$ (anhydrous); $C_8H_{10}N_4O_2 \cdot H_2O$ (monohy-
drate).

Molecular weight:
Pheniramine maleate—356.42.
Pyrilamine maleate—401.46.
Phenylpropanolamine hydrochloride—187.67.
Codeine phosphate—406.37 (hemihydrate); 397.36 (anhy-
drous).
Acetaminophen—151.16.
Caffeine—194.19 (anhydrous); 212.21 (monohydrate).

Description:
Pheniramine maleate—White crystalline powder having a faint
amine-like odor.
Pyrilamine Maleate USP—White, crystalline powder, usually
having a faint odor. Its solutions are acid to litmus.
Phenylpropanolamine Hydrochloride USP—White, crystalline
powder, having a slight aromatic odor. Is affected by light.
Codeine Phosphate USP—Fine, white, needle-shaped crystals, or white, crystalline powder. Is odorless, and is affected by light. Its solutions are acid to litmus.
Acetaminophen USP—White, odorless, crystalline powder.
Caffeine USP—White powder, or white, glistening needles,
usually matted together. Is odorless. Its solutions are neutral to litmus. The hydrate is efflorescent in air.

pKa: Phenylpropanolamine hydrochloride—9.

Solubility:
Pheniramine maleate—Soluble in water and in alcohol.
Pyrilamine Maleate USP—Very soluble in water; freely soluble
in alcohol and in chloroform; slightly soluble in ether.
Phenylpropanolamine Hydrochloride USP—Freely soluble in
water and in alcohol; insoluble in ether.
Codeine Phosphate USP—Freely soluble in water; very soluble in hot water; slightly soluble in alcohol but more so in
boiling alcohol.
Acetaminophen USP—Soluble in boiling water and in 1 N sodium hydroxide; freely soluble in alcohol.
Caffeine USP—Sparingly soluble in water and in alcohol;
freely soluble in chloroform; slightly soluble in ether.

The aqueous solubility of caffeine is increased by organic
acids or their alkali salts, such as citrates, benzoates, salicylates, or cinnamates, which dissociate to yield caffeine
when dissolved in biological fluids.

USP requirements: Pheniramine Maleate, Pyrilamine Maleate,
Phenylpropanolamine Hydrochloride, Codeine Phosphate,
Acetaminophen, and Caffeine Tablets—Not in *USP–NF*.

PHENIRAMINE, PYRILAMINE, PHENYLPROPANOLAMINE, AND DEXTROMETHORPHAN

Source: Dextromethorphan—Methylated dextroisomer of levorphanol.

Chemical group:
Pheniramine—Alkylamine derivative.
Pyrilamine—Ethylenediamine derivative.
Phenylpropanolamine hydrochloride—Synthetic phenylisopropanolamine.
Dextromethorphan—Synthetic derivative of morphine.

Chemical name:
Pheniramine maleate—2-[alpha-[2-Dimethylaminoethyl]benzyl]pyridine bimaleate.
Pyrilamine maleate—1,2-Ethanediamine, N-[(4-methoxyphenyl)methyl]-N,N-dimethyl-N-2-pyridinyl-, (Z)-2-butenedioate (1:1).
Phenylpropanolamine hydrochloride—Benzenemethanol, alpha-(1-aminoethyl)-, hydrochloride, (R*,S*)-, (±).
Dextromethorphan hydrobromide—Morphinan, 3-methoxy-17-methyl-, (9 alpha,13 alpha,14 alpha)-, hydrobromide, monohydrate.

Molecular formula:
Pheniramine maleate—$C_{16}H_{20}N_2 \cdot C_4H_4O_4$.
Pyrilamine maleate—$C_{17}H_{23}N_3O \cdot C_4H_4O_4$.
Phenylpropanolamine hydrochloride—$C_9H_{13}NO \cdot HCl$.
Dextromethorphan hydrobromide—$C_{18}H_{25}NO \cdot HBr \cdot H_2O$.

Molecular weight:
Pheniramine maleate—356.42.
Pyrilamine maleate—401.46.
Phenylpropanolamine hydrochloride—187.67.
Dextromethorphan hydrobromide—370.32.

Description:
Pheniramine maleate—White crystalline powder having a faint amine-like odor.
Pyrilamine Maleate USP—White, crystalline powder, usually having a faint odor. Its solutions are acid to litmus.
Phenylpropanolamine Hydrochloride USP—White, crystalline powder, having a slight aromatic odor. Is affected by light.
Dextromethorphan Hydrobromide USP—Practically white crystals or crystalline powder, having a faint odor. Melts at about 126 °C, with decomposition.

pKa: Phenylpropanolamine hydrochloride—9.

Solubility:
Pheniramine maleate—Soluble in water and in alcohol.
Pyrilamine Maleate USP—Very soluble in water; freely soluble in alcohol and in chloroform; slightly soluble in ether.
Phenylpropanolamine Hydrochloride USP—Freely soluble in water and in alcohol; insoluble in ether.
Dextromethorphan Hydrobromide USP—Sparingly soluble in water; freely soluble in alcohol and in chloroform; insoluble in ether.

USP requirements: Pheniramine Maleate, Pyrilamine Maleate, Phenylpropanolamine Hydrochloride, and Dextromethorphan Hydrobromide Syrup—Not in USP–NF.

PHENIRAMINE, PYRILAMINE, PHENYLPROPANOLAMINE, DEXTROMETHORPHAN, AND AMMONIUM CHLORIDE

Source: Dextromethorphan—Methylated dextroisomer of levorphanol.

Chemical group:
Pheniramine—Alkylamine derivative.
Pyrilamine—Ethylenediamine derivative.

Phenylpropanolamine hydrochloride—Synthetic phenylisopropanolamine.
Dextromethorphan—Synthetic derivative of morphine.

Chemical name:
Pheniramine maleate—2-[alpha-[2-Dimethylaminoethyl]benzyl]pyridine bimaleate.
Pyrilamine maleate—1,2-Ethanediamine, N-[(4-methoxyphenyl)methyl]-N,N-dimethyl-N-2-pyridinyl-, (Z)-2-butenedioate (1:1).
Phenylpropanolamine hydrochloride—Benzenemethanol, alpha-(1-aminoethyl)-, hydrochloride, (R*,S*)-, (±).
Dextromethorphan hydrobromide—Morphinan, 3-methoxy-17-methyl-, (9 alpha,13 alpha,14 alpha)-, hydrobromide, monohydrate.
Ammonium chloride—Ammonium chloride.

Molecular formula:
Pheniramine maleate—$C_{16}H_{20}N_2 \cdot C_4H_4O_4$.
Pyrilamine maleate—$C_{17}H_{23}N_3O \cdot C_4H_4O_4$.
Phenylpropanolamine hydrochloride—$C_9H_{13}NO \cdot HCl$.
Dextromethorphan hydrobromide—$C_{18}H_{25}NO \cdot HBr \cdot H_2O$.
Ammonium chloride—NH_4Cl.

Molecular weight:
Pheniramine maleate—356.42.
Pyrilamine maleate—401.46.
Phenylpropanolamine hydrochloride—187.67.
Dextromethorphan hydrobromide—370.32.
Ammonium chloride—53.49.

Description:
Pheniramine maleate—White crystalline powder having a faint amine-like odor.
Pyrilamine Maleate USP—White, crystalline powder, usually having a faint odor. Its solutions are acid to litmus.
Phenylpropanolamine Hydrochloride USP—White, crystalline powder, having a slight aromatic odor. Is affected by light.
Dextromethorphan Hydrobromide USP—Practically white crystals or crystalline powder, having a faint odor. Melts at about 126 °C, with decomposition.
Ammonium Chloride USP—Colorless crystals or white, fine or coarse, crystalline powder. Is somewhat hygroscopic.

pKa: Phenylpropanolamine hydrochloride—9.

Solubility:
Pheniramine maleate—Soluble in water and in alcohol.
Pyrilamine Maleate USP—Very soluble in water; freely soluble in alcohol and in chloroform; slightly soluble in ether.
Phenylpropanolamine Hydrochloride USP—Freely soluble in water and in alcohol; insoluble in ether.
Dextromethorphan Hydrobromide USP—Sparingly soluble in water; freely soluble in alcohol and in chloroform; insoluble in ether.
Ammonium Chloride USP—Freely soluble in water and in glycerin, and even more so in boiling water; sparingly soluble in alcohol.

USP requirements: Pheniramine Maleate, Pyrilamine Maleate, Phenylpropanolamine Hydrochloride, Dextromethorphan Hydrobromide, and Ammonium Chloride Syrup—Not in USP–NF.

PHENIRAMINE, PYRILAMINE, PHENYLPROPANOLAMINE, DEXTROMETHORPHAN, AND GUAIFENESIN

Source: Dextromethorphan—Methylated dextroisomer of levorphanol.

Chemical group:
Pheniramine—Alkylamine derivative.
Pyrilamine—Ethylenediamine derivative.

Phenylpropanolamine hydrochloride—Synthetic phenylisopropanolamine.
Dextromethorphan—Synthetic derivative of morphine.

Chemical name:
Pheniramine maleate—2-[alpha-[2-Dimethylaminoethyl]ben-
zyl]pyridine bimaleate.
Pyrilamine maleate—1,2-Ethanediamine, *N*-[(4-methoxyphe-
nyl)methyl]-*N*,*N*-dimethyl-*N*-2-pyridinyl-, (*Z*)-2-butenedio-
ate (1:1).
Phenylpropanolamine hydrochloride—Benzenemethanol, al-
pha-(1-aminoethyl)-, hydrochloride, (*R**,*S**)-, (±).
Dextromethorphan hydrobromide—Morphinan, 3-methoxy-
17-methyl-, (9 alpha,13 alpha,14 alpha)-, hydrobromide,-
monohydrate.
Guaifenesin—1,2-Propanediol, 3-(2-methoxyphenoxy)-.

Molecular formula:
Pheniramine maleate—$C_{16}H_{20}N_2 \cdot C_4H_4O_4$.
Pyrilamine maleate—$C_{17}H_{23}N_3O \cdot C_4H_4O_4$.
Phenylpropanolamine hydrochloride—$C_9H_{13}NO \cdot HCl$.
Dextromethorphan hydrobromide—$C_{18}H_{25}NO \cdot HBr \cdot H_2O$.
Guaifenesin—$C_{10}H_{14}O_4$.

Molecular weight:
Pheniramine maleate—356.42.
Pyrilamine maleate—401.46.
Phenylpropanolamine hydrochloride—187.67.
Dextromethorphan hydrobromide—370.32.
Guaifenesin—198.22.

Description:
Pheniramine maleate—White crystalline powder having a faint
amine-like odor.
Pyrilamine Maleate USP—White, crystalline powder, usually
having a faint odor. Its solutions are acid to litmus.
Phenylpropanolamine Hydrochloride USP—White, crystalline
powder, having a slight aromatic odor. Is affected by light.
Dextromethorphan Hydrobromide USP—Practically white
crystals or crystalline powder, having a faint odor. Melts
at about 126 °C, with decomposition.
Guaifenesin USP—White to slightly gray, crystalline powder.
May have a slight characteristic odor.

pKa: Phenylpropanolamine hydrochloride—9.

Solubility:
Pheniramine maleate—Soluble in water and in alcohol.
Pyrilamine Maleate USP—Very soluble in water; freely soluble
in alcohol and in chloroform; slightly soluble in ether.
Phenylpropanolamine Hydrochloride USP—Freely soluble in
water and in alcohol; insoluble in ether.
Dextromethorphan Hydrobromide USP—Sparingly soluble in
water; freely soluble in alcohol and in chloroform; insoluble
in ether.
Guaifenesin USP—Soluble in water, in alcohol, in chloroform,
and in propylene glycol; sparingly soluble in glycerin.

USP requirements: Pheniramine Maleate, Pyrilamine Maleate,
Phenylpropanolamine Hydrochloride, Dextromethorphan Hydrobromide, and Guaifenesin Oral Solution—Not in *USP–NF*.

PHENIRAMINE, PYRILAMINE, PHENYLPROPANOLAMINE, AND GUAIFENESIN

Chemical group:
Pheniramine—Alkylamine derivative.
Pyrilamine—Ethylenediamine derivative.
Phenylpropanolamine hydrochloride—Synthetic phenyliso-
propanolamine.

Chemical name:
Pheniramine maleate—2-[alpha-[2-Dimethylaminoethyl]ben-
zyl]pyridine bimaleate.

Pyrilamine maleate—1,2-Ethanediamine, *N*-[(4-methoxyphe-
nyl)methyl]-*N*,*N*-dimethyl-*N*-2-pyridinyl-, (*Z*)-2-butenedio-
ate (1:1).
Phenylpropanolamine hydrochloride—Benzenemethanol, al-
pha-(1-aminoethyl)-, hydrochloride, (*R**,*S**)-, (±).
Guaifenesin—1,2-Propanediol, 3-(2-methoxyphenoxy)-.

Molecular formula:
Pheniramine maleate—$C_{16}H_{20}N_2 \cdot C_4H_4O_4$.
Pyrilamine maleate—$C_{17}H_{23}N_3O \cdot C_4H_4O_4$.
Phenylpropanolamine hydrochloride—$C_9H_{13}NO \cdot HCl$.
Guaifenesin—$C_{10}H_{14}O_4$.

Molecular weight:
Pheniramine maleate—356.42.
Pyrilamine maleate—401.46.
Phenylpropanolamine hydrochloride—187.67.
Guaifenesin—198.22.

Description:
Pheniramine maleate—White crystalline powder having a faint
amine-like odor.
Pyrilamine Maleate USP—White, crystalline powder, usually
having a faint odor. Its solutions are acid to litmus.
Phenylpropanolamine Hydrochloride USP—White, crystalline
powder, having a slight aromatic odor. Is affected by light.
Guaifenesin USP—White to slightly gray, crystalline powder.
May have a slight characteristic odor.

pKa: Phenylpropanolamine hydrochloride—9.

Solubility:
Pheniramine maleate—Soluble in water and in alcohol.
Pyrilamine Maleate USP—Very soluble in water; freely soluble
in alcohol and in chloroform; slightly soluble in ether.
Phenylpropanolamine Hydrochloride USP—Freely soluble in
water and in alcohol; insoluble in ether.
Guaifenesin USP—Soluble in water, in alcohol, in chloroform,
and in propylene glycol; sparingly soluble in glycerin.

USP requirements: Pheniramine Maleate, Pyrilamine Maleate,
Phenylpropanolamine Hydrochloride, and Guaifenesin Oral
Solution—Not in *USP–NF*.

PHENIRAMINE, PYRILAMINE, PHENYLPROPANOLAMINE, AND HYDROCODONE

Chemical group:
Pheniramine—Alkylamine derivative.
Pyrilamine—Ethylenediamine derivative.
Phenylpropanolamine hydrochloride—Synthetic phenyliso-
propanolamine.

Chemical name:
Pheniramine maleate—2-[alpha-[2-Dimethylaminoethyl]ben-
zyl]pyridine bimaleate.
Pyrilamine maleate—1,2-Ethanediamine, *N*-[(4-methoxyphe-
nyl)methyl]-*N*,*N*-dimethyl-*N*-2-pyridinyl-, (*Z*)-2-butenedio-
ate (1:1).
Phenylpropanolamine hydrochloride—Benzenemethanol, al-
pha-(1-aminoethyl)-, hydrochloride, (*R**,*S**)-, (±).
Hydrocodone bitartrate—Morphinan-6-one, 4,5-epoxy-3-me-
thoxy-17-methyl-, (5 alpha)-, [*R*-(*R**,*R**)]-2,3-dihydroxybu-
tanedioate (1:1), hydrate (2:5).

Molecular formula:
Pheniramine maleate—$C_{16}H_{20}N_2 \cdot C_4H_4O_4$.
Pyrilamine maleate—$C_{17}H_{23}N_3O \cdot C_4H_4O_4$.
Phenylpropanolamine hydrochloride—$C_9H_{13}NO \cdot HCl$.
Hydrocodone bitartrate—$C_{18}H_{21}NO_3 \cdot C_4H_6O_6 \cdot 2\frac{1}{2}H_2O$ (hy-
drate); $C_{18}H_{21}NO_3 \cdot C_4H_6O_6$ (anhydrous).

Molecular weight:
Pheniramine maleate—356.42.
Pyrilamine maleate—401.46.

Phenylpropanolamine hydrochloride—187.67.
Hydrocodone bitartrate—494.49 (hydrate); 449.46 (anhydrous).

Description:
Pheniramine maleate—White crystalline powder having a faint amine-like odor.
Pyrilamine Maleate USP—White, crystalline powder, usually having a faint odor. Its solutions are acid to litmus.
Phenylpropanolamine Hydrochloride USP—White, crystalline powder, having a slight aromatic odor. Is affected by light.
Hydrocodone Bitartrate USP—Fine, white crystals or a crystalline powder. Is affected by light.

pKa: Phenylpropanolamine hydrochloride—9.

Solubility:
Pheniramine maleate—Soluble in water and in alcohol.
Pyrilamine Maleate USP—Very soluble in water; freely soluble in alcohol and in chloroform; slightly soluble in ether.
Phenylpropanolamine Hydrochloride USP—Freely soluble in water and in alcohol; insoluble in ether.
Hydrocodone Bitartrate USP—Soluble in water; slightly soluble in alcohol; insoluble in ether and in chloroform.

USP requirements:
Pheniramine Maleate, Pyrilamine Maleate, Phenylpropanolamine Hydrochloride, and Hydrocodone Bitartrate Oral Solution—Not in USP-NF.
Pheniramine Maleate, Pyrilamine Maleate, Phenylpropanolamine Hydrochloride, and Hydrocodone Bitartrate Syrup—Not in USP-NF.

PHENIRAMINE, PYRILAMINE, PHENYLPROPANOLAMINE, HYDROCODONE, AND GUAIFENESIN

Chemical group:
Pheniramine—Alkylamine derivative.
Pyrilamine—Ethylenediamine derivative.
Phenylpropanolamine hydrochloride—Synthetic phenylisopropanolamine.

Chemical name:
Pheniramine maleate—2-[alpha-[2-Dimethylaminoethyl]benzyl]pyridine bimaleate.
Pyrilamine maleate—1,2-Ethanediamine, N-[(4-methoxyphenyl)methyl]-N,N-dimethyl-N-2-pyridinyl-, (Z)-2-butenedioate (1:1).
Phenylpropanolamine hydrochloride—Benzenemethanol, alpha-(1-aminoethyl)-, hydrochloride, $(R*,S*)$-, ($\pm$).
Hydrocodone bitartrate—Morphinan-6-one, 4,5-epoxy-3-methoxy-17-methyl-, (5 alpha)-, $[R-(R*,R*)]$-2,3-dihydroxybutanedioate (1:1), hydrate (2:5).
Guaifenesin—1,2-Propanediol, 3-(2-methoxyphenoxy)-.

Molecular formula:
Pheniramine maleate—$C_{16}H_{20}N_2 \cdot C_4H_4O_4$.
Pyrilamine maleate—$C_{17}H_{23}N_3O \cdot C_4H_4O_4$.
Phenylpropanolamine hydrochloride—$C_9H_{13}NO \cdot HCl$.
Hydrocodone bitartrate—$C_{18}H_{21}NO_3 \cdot C_4H_6O_6 \cdot 2\frac{1}{2}H_2O$ (hydrate); $C_{18}H_{21}NO_3 \cdot C_4H_6O_6$ (anhydrous).
Guaifenesin—$C_{10}H_{14}O_4$.

Molecular weight:
Pheniramine maleate—356.42.
Pyrilamine maleate—401.46.
Phenylpropanolamine hydrochloride—187.67.
Hydrocodone bitartrate—494.49 (hydrate); 449.46 (anhydrous).
Guaifenesin—198.22.

Description:
Pheniramine maleate—White crystalline powder having a faint amine-like odor.
Pyrilamine Maleate USP—White, crystalline powder, usually having a faint odor. Its solutions are acid to litmus.
Phenylpropanolamine Hydrochloride USP—White, crystalline powder, having a slight aromatic odor. Is affected by light.
Hydrocodone Bitartrate USP—Fine, white crystals or a crystalline powder. Is affected by light.
Guaifenesin USP—White to slightly gray, crystalline powder. May have a slight characteristic odor.

pKa: Phenylpropanolamine hydrochloride—9.

Solubility:
Pheniramine maleate—Soluble in water and in alcohol.
Pyrilamine Maleate USP—Very soluble in water; freely soluble in alcohol and in chloroform; slightly soluble in ether.
Phenylpropanolamine Hydrochloride USP—Freely soluble in water and in alcohol; insoluble in ether.
Hydrocodone Bitartrate USP—Soluble in water; slightly soluble in alcohol; insoluble in ether and in chloroform.
Guaifenesin USP—Soluble in water, in alcohol, in chloroform, and in propylene glycol; sparingly soluble in glycerin.

USP requirements:
Pheniramine Maleate, Pyrilamine Maleate, Phenylpropanolamine Hydrochloride, Hydrocodone Bitartrate, and Guaifenesin Elixir—Not in USP-NF.
Pheniramine Maleate, Pyrilamine Maleate, Phenylpropanolamine Hydrochloride, Hydrocodone Bitartrate, and Guaifenesin Oral Solution—Not in USP-NF.

PHENMETRAZINE

Chemical group: Morpholine.

Chemical name: Phenmetrazine hydrochloride—Morpholine, 3-methyl-2-phenyl-, hydrochloride.

Molecular formula: Phenmetrazine hydrochloride—$C_{11}H_{15}NO \cdot HCl$.

Molecular weight: Phenmetrazine hydrochloride—213.70.

Description: Phenmetrazine Hydrochloride USP—White to off-white, crystalline powder.

Solubility: Phenmetrazine Hydrochloride USP—Very soluble in water; freely soluble in alcohol and in chloroform.

USP requirements:
Phenmetrazine Hydrochloride USP—Preserve in tight containers. Dried at 105 °C for 2 hours, contains not less than 98.0% and not more than 102.0% of phenmetrazine hydrochloride. Meets the requirements for Identification, Melting range (172–182 °C, the range between beginning and end of melting not more than 3 °C), pH (4.5–5.5, in a solution [1 in 40]), Loss on drying (not more than 0.5%), Residue on ignition (not more than 0.1%), Sulfate (not more than 0.01%), Chloride content (16.3–17.0%), Heavy metals (not more than 0.001%), Ordinary impurities, and Organic volatile impurities.
Phenmetrazine Hydrochloride Tablets USP—Preserve in tight containers. Contain the labeled amount, within ±7%. Meet the requirements for Identification, Dissolution (75% in 45 minutes in water in Apparatus 2 at 50 rpm), and Uniformity of dosage units.

PHENOBARBITAL

Chemical name:
Phenobarbital—2,4,6(1*H*,3*H*,5*H*)-Pyrimidinetrione, 5-ethyl-5-phenyl-.
Phenobarbital sodium—2,4,6(1*H*,3*H*,5*H*)-Pyrimidinetrione, 5ethyl-5-phenyl-, monosodium salt.

Molecular formula:
Phenobarbital—$C_{12}H_{12}N_2O_3$.
Phenobarbital sodium—$C_{12}H_{11}N_2NaO_3$.

Molecular weight:
Phenobarbital—232.24.
Phenobarbital sodium—254.22.

Description:
Phenobarbital USP—White, odorless, glistening, small crystals, or white, crystalline powder, which may exhibit polymorphism. Is stable in air. Its saturated solution has a pH of about 5.
Phenobarbital Sodium USP—Flaky crystals, or white, crystalline granules, or white powder. Is odorless and is hygroscopic. Its solutions are alkaline to phenolphthalein TS, and decompose on standing.

Solubility:
Phenobarbital USP—Very slightly soluble in water; soluble in alcohol, in ether, and in solutions of fixed alkali hydroxides and carbonates; sparingly soluble in chloroform.
Phenobarbital Sodium USP—Very soluble in water; soluble in alcohol; practically insoluble in ether and in chloroform.

USP requirements:
Phenobarbital USP—Preserve in well-closed containers. Contains not less than 98.0% and not more than 101.0% of phenobarbital, calculated on the dried basis. Meets the requirements for Identification, Melting range (174–178 °C, the range between beginning and end of melting not more than 2 °C), Loss on drying (not more than 1.0%), Residue on ignition (not more than 0.15%), and Organic volatile impurities.
Phenobarbital Capsules—Not in *USP–NF*.
Phenobarbital Elixir USP—Preserve in tight, light-resistant containers. Contains the labeled amount, within ±10%. Meets the requirements for Identification and Alcohol content (12.0–15.0%).
Phenobarbital Oral Solution USP—Preserve in tight, light-resistant containers. Contains the labeled amount, within ± 10%. Meets the requirements for Identification and Alcohol content (12.0–15.0%).
Phenobarbital Tablets USP—Preserve in well-closed containers. Contain the labeled amount, within ±10%. Meet the requirements for Identification, Dissolution (75% in 45 minutes in water in Apparatus 2 at 50 rpm), and Uniformity of dosage units.
Phenobarbital Sodium USP—Preserve in tight containers. Where it is intended for use in preparing injectable dosage forms, the label states that it is sterile or must be subjected to further processing during the preparation of injectable dosage forms. Contains not less than 98.5% and not more than 101.0% of phenobarbital sodium, calculated on the dried basis. Meets the requirements for Completeness of solution, Identification, pH (9.2–10.2, in the solution prepared in the test for Completeness of solution), Loss on drying (not more than 7.0%), Heavy metals (not more than 0.003%), and Organic volatile impurities, for Sterility tests and for Bacterial endotoxins under Phenobarbital Sodium for Injection (where the label states that Phenobarbital Sodium is sterile), and for Bacterial endotoxins under Phenobarbital Sodium for Injection (where the label states that Phenobarbital Sodium must be subjected to further processing during the preparation of injectable dosage forms).
Phenobarbital Sodium Injection USP—Preserve in single-dose or in multiple-dose containers, preferably of Type I glass. A sterile solution of Phenobarbital Sodium in a suitable solvent. Phenobarbital may be substituted for the equivalent amount of Phenobarbital Sodium, for adjustment of the pH. The label indicates that the Injection is not to be used if it contains a precipitate. Contains the labeled amount, within –10% to +5%. Meets the requirements for Identification, Bacterial endotoxins, and pH (9.2–10.2), and for Injections.
Phenobarbital Sodium for Injection USP—Preserve in Containers for Sterile Solids. It is Phenobarbital Sodium suitable for parenteral use. Meets the requirements for Constituted solution and Bacterial endotoxins, for Identification tests, Completeness of solution, pH, Loss on drying, and Heavy metals under Phenobarbital Sodium, and for Sterility tests, Uniformity of dosage units, and Labeling under Injections.

PHENOBARBITAL, ASPIRIN, AND CODEINE

For *Phenobarbital, Aspirin* (ASA), and *Codeine*—See individual listings for chemistry information.

USP requirements: Phenobarbital, ASA, and Codeine Phosphate Capsules—Not in *USP–NF*.

PHENOL

Chemical name: Phenol.

Molecular formula: C_6H_6O.

Molecular weight: 94.11.

Description: Phenol USP—Colorless to light pink, interlaced or separate, needleshaped crystals, or white to light pink, crystalline mass. It has a characteristic odor. Liquefied by warming, and by the addition of 10% of water. Boils at about 182 °C, and its vapor is flammable. Gradually darkens on exposure to light and air.

NF category: Antimicrobial preservative.

Solubility: Phenol USP—Soluble in water. Very soluble in alcohol, in glycerin, in chloroform, in ether, and in fixed and volatile oils; sparingly soluble in mineral oil.

USP requirements: Phenol USP—Preserve in tight, light-resistant containers. Label it to indicate the name and amount of any substance added as a stabilizer. Contains not less than 99.0% and not more than 100.5% of phenol, calculated on the anhydrous basis. Meets the requirements for Clarity of solution and reaction, Identification, Congealing temperature (not lower than 39 °C), Water (not more than 0.5%), Limit of nonvolatile residue (not more than 0.05%), and Organic volatile impurities.

Caution: Avoid contact with skin, since serious burns may result.

LIQUEFIED PHENOL

Description: Liquefied Phenol USP—Colorless to pink liquid, which may develop a red tint upon exposure to air or light. Has a characteristic, somewhat aromatic odor. It whitens and cauterizes the skin and mucous membranes. Specific gravity is about 1.065.

Solubility: Liquefied Phenol USP—Miscible with alcohol, with ether, and with glycerin. A mixture of equal volumes of Liquefied Phenol and glycerin is miscible with water.

USP requirements: Liquefied Phenol USP—Preserve in tight, light-resistant glass containers. It is Phenol maintained in a liquid condition by the presence of about 10% of water. Label it to indicate the name and amount of any substance added as a stabilizer. Contains not less than 89.0% by weight of phenol. Meets the requirements for Distilling range (not higher than 182.5 °C) and Organic volatile impurities, and for Identification tests, Clarity of solution and reaction, and Nonvolatile residue under Phenol.

Caution: Avoid contact with skin, since serious burns may result.

Note: When phenol is to be mixed with a fixed oil, mineral oil, or white petrolatum, use crystalline Phenol, not Liquefied Phenol.

PHENOLPHTHALEIN

Chemical group: Diphenylmethane derivative.

Chemical name: 1(3*H*)-Isobenzofuranone, 3,3-bis(4-hydroxyphenyl)-.

Molecular formula: $C_{20}H_{14}O_4$.

Molecular weight: 318.32.

Description: Phenolphthalein USP—White or faintly yellowish white, crystalline powder. Is odorless, and is stable in air.

Solubility: Phenolphthalein USP—Practically insoluble in water; soluble in alcohol; sparingly soluble in ether.

USP requirements:

Phenolphthalein USP—Preserve in well-closed containers. Contains not less than 98.0% and not more than 101.0% of phenolphthalein, calculated on the dried basis. Meets the requirements for Color of solution, Identification, Melting temperature (not lower than 258 °C), Loss on drying (not more than 1.0%), Residue on ignition (not more than 0.1%), Heavy metals (not more than 0.0015%), Limit of fluoran, Chromatographic purity, and Organic volatile impurities.

Phenolphthalein Tablets USP—Preserve in tight containers. Where Tablets contain Yellow Phenolphthalein, the labeling so indicates. Contain the labeled amount, within ± 10%. Meet the requirements for Identification, Disintegration (30 minutes), and Uniformity of dosage units.

YELLOW PHENOLPHTHALEIN

USP requirements: Yellow Phenolphthalein USP—Preserve in well-closed containers. Contains not less than 93.0% and not more than 100.0% of phenolphthalein, calculated on the dried basis. Meets the requirements for Color of solution, Melting temperature (not lower than 255 °C), and Chromatographic purity, and for Identification tests, Loss on drying, Residue on ignition, Arsenic, and Heavy metals under Phenolphthalein.

PHENOLPHTHALEIN AND DOCUSATE

For *Phenolphthalein* and *Docusate*—See individual listings for chemistry information.

USP requirements:

Phenolphthalein and Docusate Calcium Capsules—Not in *USP-NF*.

Phenolphthalein and Docusate Sodium Capsules—Not in *USP-NF*.

Phenolphthalein and Docusate Sodium Tablets—Not in *USP-NF*.

PHENOLPHTHALEIN AND SENNA

For *Phenolphthalein* and *Senna*—See individual listings for chemistry information.

USP requirements: Phenolphthalein and Senna Tablets—Not in *USP-NF*.

PHENOLSULFONPHTHALEIN

Chemical name: Phenol, 4,4′-(3*H*-2,1-benzoxathiol-3-ylidene)-bis-, (*S,S*-dioxide).

Molecular formula: $C_{19}H_{14}O_5S$.

Molecular weight: 354.38.

Description: Bright to dark red, odorless, crystalline powder.

pKa: 7.9.

Solubility: Very slightly soluble in water; slightly soluble in alcohol.

USP requirements: Phenolsulfonphthalein Injection—Not in *USP-NF*.

PHENOXYBENZAMINE

Chemical name: Phenoxybenzamine hydrochloride—Benzenemethanamine, *N*-(2-chloroethyl)-*N*-(1-methyl-2-phenoxyethyl)-, hydrochloride.

Molecular formula: Phenoxybenzamine hydrochloride—$C_{18}H_{22}ClNO \cdot HCl$.

Molecular weight: Phenoxybenzamine hydrochloride—340.29.

Description: Phenoxybenzamine hydrochloride—Colorless, crys-talline powder. Melting point is 136 to 141 °C.

pKa: Phenoxybenzamine hydrochloride—4.4.

Solubility: Phenoxybenzamine hydrochloride—Soluble in water, in alcohol, and in chloroform; insoluble in ether.

USP requirements:

Phenoxybenzamine Hydrochloride USP—Preserve in well-closed containers. Contains not less than 98.0% and not more than 101.0% of phenoxybenzamine hydrochloride, calculated on the dried basis. Meets the requirements for Identification, Melting range (136–141 °C), Loss on drying (not more than 0.5%), Ordinary impurities, and Organic volatile impurities.

Phenoxybenzamine Hydrochloride Capsules USP—Preserve in well-closed containers. Contain the labeled amount, within ±10%. Meet the requirements for Identification, Dissolution (75% in 45 minutes in 0.1 *N* hydrochloric acid in Apparatus 1 at 100 rpm), and Uniformity of dosage units.

PHENSUXIMIDE

Chemical name: 2,5-Pyrrolidinedione, 1-methyl-3-phenyl-, (±)-.

Molecular formula: $C_{11}H_{11}NO_2$.

Molecular weight: 189.21.

Description: Phensuximide USP—White to off-white crystalline powder. Is odorless, or has not more than a slight odor.

Solubility: Phensuximide USP—Slightly soluble in water; very soluble in chloroform; soluble in alcohol.

USP requirements:
Phensuximide USP—Preserve in tight containers. Contains not less than 97.0% and not more than 103.0% of phensuximide, calculated on the anhydrous basis. Meets the requirements for Identification, Melting range (68–74 °C), Water (not more than 1.0%), Residue on ignition (not more than 0.5%), Limit of cyanide, Ordinary impurities, and Organic volatile impurities.

Phensuximide Capsules USP—Preserve in tight containers. Contain the labeled amount, within ±7%. Meet the requirements for Identification, Dissolution (75% in 120 minutes in water in Apparatus 1 at 100 rpm), and Uniformity of dosage units.

PHENTERMINE

Chemical group: Phenethylamine.

Chemical name: Phentermine hydrochloride—Benzeneethanamine, alpha,alpha-dimethyl-, hydrochloride.

Molecular formula: Phentermine hydrochloride—$C_{10}H_{15}N \cdot HCl$.

Molecular weight: Phentermine hydrochloride—185.69.

Description:
Phentermine Hydrochloride USP—White, odorless, hygroscopic, crystalline powder.
Phentermine resin—Coarse granular substance.

Solubility:
Phentermine Hydrochloride USP—Soluble in water and in the lower alcohols; slightly soluble in chloroform; insoluble in ether.
Phentermine resin—Practically insoluble in water.

USP requirements:
Phentermine Hydrochloride USP—Preserve in tight containers. Contains not less than 98.0% and not more than 101.0% of phentermine hydrochloride, calculated on the dried basis. Meets the requirements for Identification, Melting range (202–205 °C), pH (5.0–6.0, in a solution [1 in 50]), Loss on drying (not more than 2.0%), Residue on ignition (not more than 0.1%), Chromatographic purity, and Organic volatile impurities.

Phentermine Hydrochloride Capsules USP—Preserve in tight containers. Contain the labeled amount, within ±10%. Meet the requirements for Identification, Dissolution (75% in 45 minutes in water in Apparatus 2 at 50 rpm), and Uniformity of dosage units.

Phentermine Hydrochloride Tablets USP—Preserve in tight containers. Contain the labeled amount, within ±10%. Meet the requirements for Identification, Dissolution (75% in 45 minutes in water in Apparatus 2 at 50 rpm), and Uniformity of dosage units.

Phentermine Resin Capsules—Not in *USP–NF*.

PHENTOLAMINE

Chemical name: Phentolamine mesylate—Phenol, 3-[[(4,5-dihydro-1*H*-imidazol-2-yl)methyl](4-methylphenyl)amino]-, monomethanesulfonate (salt).

Molecular formula: Phentolamine mesylate—$C_{17}H_{19}N_3O \cdot CH_4O_3S$.

Molecular weight: Phentolamine mesylate—377.46.

Description: Phentolamine Mesylate USP—White or off-white, odorless, crystalline powder. Its solutions are acid to litmus, having a pH of about 5, and slowly deteriorate. Melts at about 178 °C.

Solubility: Phentolamine Mesylate USP—Freely soluble in water and in alcohol; slightly soluble in chloroform.

USP requirements:
Phentolamine Mesylate USP—Preserve in tight, light-resistant containers. Contains not less than 98.0% and not more than 102.0% of phentolamine mesylate, calculated on the dried basis. Meets the requirements for Identification, Loss on drying (not more than 0.5%), Residue on ignition (not more than 0.1%), Sulfate (not more than 0.2%), and Chromatographic purity.

Phentolamine Mesylate for Injection USP—Preserve in Containers for Sterile Solids. It is sterile Phentolamine Mesylate or a sterile mixture of Phentolamine Mesylate with a suitable buffer or suitable diluents. Contains the labeled amount, within ±10%. Meets the requirements for Constituted solution, Identification, Bacterial endotoxins, Uniformity of dosage units, and pH (4.5–6.5 in a freshly prepared solution having a concentration of about 1 in 100), and for Sterility tests and Labeling under Injections.

PHENYLALANINE

Chemical name: L-Phenylalanine.

Molecular formula: $C_9H_{11}NO_2$.

Molecular weight: 165.19.

Description: Phenylalanine USP—White, odorless crystals.

Solubility: Phenylalanine USP—Sparingly soluble in water; very slightly soluble in methanol, in alcohol, and in dilute mineral acids.

USP requirements: Phenylalanine USP—Preserve in well-closed containers. Contains not less than 98.5% and not more than 101.5% of phenylalanine, calculated on the dried basis. Meets the requirements for Identification, Specific rotation (−32.7° to −34.7°), pH (5.4–6.0, in a solution [1 in 100]), Loss on drying (not more than 0.3%), Residue on ignition (not more than 0.4%), Chloride (not more than 0.05%), Sulfate (not more than 0.03%), Iron (not more than 0.003%), Heavy metals (0.0015%), Chromatographic purity, and Organic volatile impurities.

PHENYLBENZIMIDAZOLE

USP requirements:
Phenylbenzimidazole Gel—Not in *USP–NF*.
Phenylbenzimidazole Lotion—Not in *USP–NF*.

PHENYLBENZIMIDAZOLE AND SULISOBENZONE

For *Phenylbenzimidazole* and *Sulisobenzone*—See individual listings for chemistry information.

USP requirements: Phenylbenzimidazole and Sulisobenzone Gel—Not in *USP–NF*.

PHENYLBUTAZONE

Chemical group: Pyrazole derivative.

Chemical name: 3,5-Pyrazolidinedione, 4-butyl-1,2-diphenyl-.

Molecular formula: $C_{19}H_{20}N_2O_2$.

Molecular weight: 308.37.

Description: Phenylbutazone USP—White to off-white, odorless, crystalline powder.

Solubility: Phenylbutazone USP—Very slightly soluble in water; freely soluble in acetone and in ether; soluble in alcohol.

USP requirements:

Phenylbutazone USP—Preserve in tight containers. Contains not less than 98.0% and not more than 102.0% of phenylbutazone, calculated on the dried basis. Meets the requirements for Identification, Melting range (104–107 °C), Loss on drying (not more than 0.5%), Residue on ignition (not more than 0.1%), Chloride (not more than 0.007%), Sulfate (not more than 0.01%), Heavy metals (not more than 0.001%), and Organic volatile impurities.

Phenylbutazone Boluses USP—Preserve in well-closed containers. Label Boluses to indicate that they are for veterinary use only. Contain the labeled amount, within ±10%. Meet the requirements for Identification, Disintegration (45 minutes with disks), and Uniformity of dosage units.

Phenylbutazone Capsules USP—Preserve in tight containers. Contain the labeled amount, within ±10%. Meet the requirements for Identification, Dissolution (70% in 30 minutes in phosphate buffer [pH 7.5] in Apparatus 1 at 100 rpm), and Uniformity of dosage units.

Phenylbutazone Injection USP—Preserve in single-dose or in multiple-dose containers, preferably of Type I glass. Protect from light, and store in a refrigerator. A sterile solution of Phenylbutazone in Sterile Water for Injection. Label Injection to indicate that it is for veterinary use only. Contains the labeled amount, within ±10%. Meets the requirements for Clarity of solution, Identification, Sterility, Bacterial endotoxins, and pH (9.5–10.0), and for Injections.

Phenylbutazone Tablets USP—Preserve in tight containers. Contain the labeled amount, within ±7%. Meet the requirements for Identification, Dissolution (70% in 30 minutes in simulated intestinal fluid TS [without the enzyme] in Apparatus 1 at 100 rpm), and Uniformity of dosage units.

Phenylbutazone Buffered Tablets—Not in *USP–NF*.

BUFFERED PHENYLBUTAZONE

Chemical group: Phenylbutazone—Pyrazole derivative.

Chemical name:

Phenylbutazone—3,5-Pyrazolidinedione, 4-butyl-1,2-diphenyl-.

Magnesium trisilicate—Silicic acid ($H_4Si_3O_8$), magnesium salt (1:2), hydrate.

Molecular formula:

Phenylbutazone—$C_{19}H_{20}N_2O_2$.

Magnesium trisilicate—$2MgO \cdot 3SiO_2 \cdot xH_2O$ (hydrate); $Mg_2Si_3O_8$ (anhydrous).

Molecular weight:

Phenylbutazone—308.37.

Magnesium trisilicate—260.86 (anhydrous).

Description:

Phenylbutazone USP—White to off-white, odorless, crystalline powder.

Magnesium Trisilicate USP—Fine, white, odorless powder, free from grittiness.

Dried Aluminum Hydroxide Gel USP—White, odorless, amorphous powder.

Solubility:

Phenylbutazone USP—Very slightly soluble in water; freely soluble in acetone and in ether; soluble in alcohol.

Magnesium Trisilicate USP—Insoluble in water and in alcohol. Is readily decomposed by mineral acids.

Dried Aluminum Hydroxide Gel USP—Insoluble in water and in alcohol; soluble in dilute mineral acids and in solutions of fixed alkali hydroxides.

USP requirements: Buffered Phenylbutazone Tablets—Not in *USP–NF*.

PHENYLEPHRINE

Chemical name: Phenylephrine hydrochloride—Benzenemethanol, 3-hydroxy-alpha-[(methylamino)methyl]-, hydrochloride.

Molecular formula: Phenylephrine hydrochloride—$C_9H_{13}NO_2 \cdot HCl$.

Molecular weight: Phenylephrine hydrochloride—203.67.

Description:

Phenylephrine Hydrochloride USP—White or practically white, odorless crystals.

Phenylephrine Hydrochloride Nasal Solution USP—Clear, colorless or slightly yellow, odorless liquid. Is neutral or acid to litmus.

Phenylephrine Hydrochloride Ophthalmic Solution USP—Clear, colorless or slightly yellow liquid, depending on the concentration.

Solubility: Phenylephrine Hydrochloride USP—Freely soluble in water and in alcohol.

USP requirements:

Phenylephrine Hydrochloride USP—Preserve in tight, light-resistant containers. Contains not less than 97.5% and not more than 102.5% of phenylephrine hydrochloride, calculated on the dried basis. Meets the requirements for Identification, Melting range (140–145 °C), Specific rotation (−42° to −47.5°), Loss on drying (not more than 1.0%), Residue on ignition (not more than 0.2%), Sulfate (not more than 0.20%), Limit of ketones, Chromatographic purity, and Chloride content (17.0–17.7%, calculated on the dried basis).

Phenylephrine Hydrochloride Injection USP—Preserve in single-dose or in multiple-dose containers, preferably of Type I glass, protected from light. A sterile solution of Phenylephrine Hydrochloride in Water for Injection. Contains the labeled amount, within −10% to +15%. Meets the requirements for Identification, Bacterial endotoxins, and pH (3.0–6.5), and for Injections.

Phenylephrine Hydrochloride Nasal Jelly USP—Preserve in tight containers. Contains the labeled amount, within ±10%. Meets the requirements for Identification and Minimum fill.

Phenylephrine Hydrochloride Nasal Solution USP—Preserve in tight, light-resistant containers. Contains the labeled amount, within −10% to +15%. Meets the requirement for Identification.

Phenylephrine Hydrochloride Ophthalmic Solution USP—Preserve in tight, light-resistant containers of not more than 15-mL size. A sterile, aqueous solution of Phenylephrine Hydrochloride. Contains the labeled amount, within −10% to +15%. Meets the requirements for Identification, Sterility, and pH (4.0–7.5 for buffered Ophthalmic Solution; 3.0–4.5 for unbuffered Ophthalmic Solution).

PHENYLEPHRINE AND ACETAMINOPHEN

For *Phenylephrine* and *Acetaminophen*—See individual listings for chemistry information.

USP requirements:
Phenylephrine Hydrochloride and Acetaminophen for Oral Solution—Not in *USP–NF*.
Phenylephrine Hydrochloride and Acetaminophen Chewable Tablets—Not in *USP–NF*.

PHENYLEPHRINE AND CODEINE

For *Phenylephrine* and *Codeine*—See individual listings for chemistry information.

USP requirements: Phenylephrine Hydrochloride and Codeine Phosphate Oral Solution—Not in *USP–NF*.

PHENYLEPHRINE, DEXTROMETHORPHAN, AND GUAIFENESIN

For *Phenylephrine, Dextromethorphan,* and *Guaifenesin*—See individual listings for chemistry information.

USP requirements:
Phenylephrine Hydrochloride, Dextromethorphan Hydrobromide, and Guaifenesin Oral Solution—Not in *USP–NF*.
Phenylephrine Hydrochloride, Dextromethorphan Hydrobromide, and Guaifenesin Syrup—Not in *USP–NF*.

PHENYLEPHRINE AND GUAIFENESIN

For *Phenylephrine* and *Guaifenesin*—See individual listings for chemistry information.

USP requirements:
Phenylephrine Hydrochloride and Guaifenesin Extended-release Capsules—Not in *USP–NF*.
Phenylephrine Hydrochloride and Guaifenesin Oral Solution—Not in *USP–NF*.
Phenylephrine Hydrochloride and Guaifenesin Extended-release Tablets—Not in *USP–NF*.

PHENYLEPHRINE, GUAIFENESIN, ACETAMINOPHEN, SALICYLAMIDE, AND CAFFEINE

For *Phenylephrine, Guaifenesin, Acetaminophen, Salicylamide,* and *Caffeine*—See individual listings for chemistry information.

USP requirements: Phenylephrine Hydrochloride, Guaifenesin, Acetaminophen, Salicylamide, and Caffeine Tablets—Not in *USP–NF*.

PHENYLEPHRINE AND HYDROCODONE

For *Phenylephrine* and *Hydrocodone*—See individual listings for chemistry information.

USP requirements:
Phenylephrine Hydrochloride and Hydrocodone Bitartrate Elixir—Not in *USP–NF*.
Phenylephrine Hydrochloride and Hydrocodone Bitartrate Oral Solution—Not in *USP–NF*.

PHENYLEPHRINE, HYDROCODONE, AND GUAIFENESIN

For *Phenylephrine, Hydrocodone,* and *Guaifenesin*—See individual listings for chemistry information.

USP requirements:
Phenylephrine Hydrochloride, Hydrocodone Bitartrate, and Guaifenesin Oral Solution—Not in *USP–NF*.
Phenylephrine Hydrochloride, Hydrocodone Bitartrate, and Guaifenesin Syrup—Not in *USP–NF*.

PHENYLEPHRINE, PHENYLPROPANOLAMINE, AND ACETAMINOPHEN

For *Phenylephrine, Phenylpropanolamine,* and *Acetaminophen*—See individual listings for chemistry information.

USP requirements: Phenylephrine Hydrochloride, Phenylpropanolamine Hydrochloride, and Acetaminophen Tablets—Not in *USP–NF*.

PHENYLEPHRINE, PHENYLPROPANOLAMINE, CARBETAPENTANE, AND POTASSIUM GUAIACOLSULFONATE

Chemical group: Phenylpropanolamine hydrochloride—Synthetic phenylisopropanolamine.

Chemical name:
Phenylephrine hydrochloride—Benzenemethanol, 3-hydroxyalpha-[(methylamino)methyl]-, hydrochloride.
Phenylpropanolamine hydrochloride—Benzenemethanol, alpha-(1-aminoethyl)-, hydrochloride, (R^*,S^*)-, (±).
Carbetapentane citrate—2-[2-(Diethylamino)ethoxy]ethyl 1phenylcyclopentanecarboxylate citrate (1:1).
Potassium guaiacolsulfonate—Benzenesulfonic acid, hydroxymethoxy-, monopotassium salt, hemihydrate.

Molecular formula:
Phenylephrine hydrochloride—$C_9H_{13}NO_2 \cdot HCl$.
Phenylpropanolamine hydrochloride—$C_9H_{13}NO \cdot HCl$.
Carbetapentane citrate—$C_{20}H_{31}NO_3 \cdot C_6H_8O_7$.
Potassium guaiacolsulfonate—$C_7H_7KO_5S \cdot \frac{1}{2}H_2O$.

Molecular weight:
Phenylephrine hydrochloride—203.67.
Phenylpropanolamine hydrochloride—187.67.
Carbetapentane citrate—525.59.
Potassium guaiacolsulfonate—251.30.

Description:

Phenylephrine Hydrochloride USP—White or practically white, odorless crystals.

Phenylpropanolamine Hydrochloride USP—White, crystalline powder, having a slight aromatic odor. Is affected by light.

Potassium guaiacolsulfonate—White, odorless crystals or crystalline powder. Gradually turns pink on exposure to air and light.

pKa: Phenylpropanolamine hydrochloride—9.

Solubility:

Phenylephrine Hydrochloride USP—Freely soluble in water and in alcohol.

Phenylpropanolamine Hydrochloride USP—Freely soluble in water and in alcohol; insoluble in ether.

Potassium guaiacolsulfonate—Soluble in 7.5 parts water; almost insoluble in alcohol; insoluble in ether.

USP requirements: Phenylephrine Hydrochloride, Phenylpropanolamine Hydrochloride, Carbetapentane Citrate, and Potassium Guaiacolsulfonate Capsules—Not in *USP–NF*.

PHENYLEPHRINE, PHENYLPROPANOLAMINE, AND GUAIFENESIN

For *Phenylephrine, Phenylpropanolamine,* and *Guaifenesin*—See individual listings for chemistry information.

USP requirements:

Phenylephrine Hydrochloride, Phenylpropanolamine Hydrochloride, and Guaifenesin Capsules—Not in *USP–NF*.

Phenylephrine Hydrochloride, Phenylpropanolamine Hydrochloride, and Guaifenesin Oral Solution—Not in *USP–NF*.

PHENYLETHYL ALCOHOL

Chemical name: Benzeneethanol.

Molecular formula: $C_8H_{10}O$.

Molecular weight: 122.16.

Description: Phenylethyl Alcohol USP—Colorless liquid, having a rose-like odor.

NF category: Antimicrobial preservative.

Solubility: Phenylethyl Alcohol USP—Sparingly soluble in water; very soluble in alcohol, in fixed oils, in glycerin, and in propylene glycol; slightly soluble in mineral oil.

USP requirements: Phenylethyl Alcohol USP—Preserve in tight, light-resistant containers, and store in a cool, dry place. Meets the requirements for Identification, Specific gravity (1.017–1.020), Refractive index (1.531–1.534 at 20 °C), Residue on ignition (not more than 0.005%), Chlorinated compounds, Aldehyde (no yellow color appears in the organic [top] layer), and Organic volatile impurities.

PHENYLMERCURIC ACETATE

Chemical name: Mercury, (acetato-*O*)phenyl-.

Molecular formula: $C_8H_8HgO_2$.

Molecular weight: 336.74.

Description: Phenylmercuric Acetate NF—White to creamy white crystalline powder, or small, white prisms or leaflets. Odorless.

NF category: Antimicrobial preservative.

Solubility: Phenylmercuric Acetate NF—Slightly soluble in water; soluble in alcohol and in acetone.

NF requirements: Phenylmercuric Acetate NF—Preserve in tight, light-resistant containers. Contains not less than 98.0% and not more than 100.5% of phenylmercuric acetate. Meets the requirements for Identification, Melting range (149–153 °C), Residue on ignition (not more than 0.2%), Mercuric salts and Heavy metals, Polymercurated benzene compounds (not more than 1.5%), and Organic volatile impurities.

PHENYLMERCURIC NITRATE

Chemical name: Mercury, (nitrato-*O*)phenyl-.

Molecular formula: $C_6H_5HgNO_3$.

Molecular weight: 339.70.

Description: Phenylmercuric Nitrate NF—White, crystalline powder. Affected by light. Its saturated solution is acid to litmus.

NF category: Antimicrobial preservative.

Solubility: Phenylmercuric Nitrate NF—Very slightly soluble in water; slightly soluble in alcohol and in glycerin. It is more soluble in the presence of either nitric acid or alkali hydroxides.

NF requirements: Phenylmercuric Nitrate NF—Preserve in tight, light-resistant containers. A mixture of phenylmercuric nitrate and phenylmercuric hydroxide containing not less than 87.0% and not more than 87.9% of phenylmercuric ion, and not less than 62.75% and not more than 63.50% of mercury. Meets the requirements for Identification, Residue on ignition (not more than 0.1%), Mercury ions, and Organic volatile impurities.

PHENYLPROPANOLAMINE

Chemical group: Phenylpropanolamine hydrochloride—Synthetic phenylisopropanolamine.

Chemical name:

Phenylpropanolamine bitartrate—(R^*,S^*)-$(\pm)$-alpha-(1-Aminoethyl)benzenemethanol bitartrate.

Phenylpropanolamine hydrochloride—Benzenemethanol, alpha-(1-aminoethyl)-, hydrochloride, (R^*,S^*)-, $(\pm)$.

Molecular formula:

Phenylpropanolamine bitartrate—$C_9H_{13}NO \cdot C_4H_6O_6$.

Phenylpropanolamine hydrochloride—$C_9H_{13}NO \cdot HCl$.

Molecular weight:

Phenylpropanolamine bitartrate—301.29.

Phenylpropanolamine hydrochloride—187.67.

Description:

Phenylpropanolamine Bitartrate USP—White, crystalline powder.

Phenylpropanolamine Hydrochloride USP—White, crystalline powder, having a slight aromatic odor. Is affected by light.

pKa: Phenylpropanolamine hydrochloride—9.

Solubility: Phenylpropanolamine Hydrochloride USP—Freely soluble in water and in alcohol; insoluble in ether.

Other characteristics: Similar in structure and action to ephedrine but with less central nervous system (CNS) stimulation.

USP requirements:

Phenylpropanolamine Bitartrate USP—Preserve in tight, light-resistant containers. Contains not less than 98.0% and not more than 101.0% of phenylpropanolamine bitartrate, calculated on the dried basis. Meets the requirements for

Identification, Melting range (150–164 °C), pH (3.1–3.7, in a solution [3 in 100]), Loss on drying (not more than 1.0%), Residue on ignition (not more than 0.1%), Heavy metals (not more than 0.002%), Limit of cathinone hydrochloride, Limit of amphetamine hydrochloride (not more than 0.001%), and phenylpropanediol, and Organic volatile impurities.

Phenylpropanolamine Hydrochloride USP—Preserve in tight, light-resistant containers. Contains not less than 98.0% and not more than 101.0% of phenylpropanolamine hydrochloride, calculated on the dried basis. Meets the requirements for Identification, Melting range (191–196 °C), pH (4.2–5.5, in a solution [3 in 100]), Loss on drying (not more than 0.5%), Residue on ignition (not more than 0.1%), Heavy metals (not more than 0.002%), Limit of cathinone hydrochloride, Limit of amphetamine hydrochloride (not more than 0.001%), and Organic volatile impurities.

Phenylpropanolamine Hydrochloride Capsules USP—Preserve in tight, light-resistant containers. Contain the labeled amount, within ±10%. Meet the requirements for Identification, Dissolution (75% in 45 minutes in water in Apparatus 1 at 100 rpm), and Uniformity of dosage units.

Phenylpropanolamine Hydrochloride Extended-release Capsules USP—Preserve in tight, light-resistant containers. The labeling indicates the Drug Release Test with which the product complies. Contain the labeled amount, within ±10%. Meet the requirements for Identification, Drug release (15–45% in 3 hours, 40–70% in 6 hours, and not less than 70% in 12 hours in water in Apparatus 1 at 100 rpm), and Uniformity of dosage units.

Phenylpropanolamine Hydrochloride Oral Solution USP—Preserve in tight containers. Contains the labeled amount, within ±10%. Meets the requirements for Identification and Alcohol content (within ±10%).

Phenylpropanolamine Hydrochloride Tablets USP—Preserve in tight, light-resistant containers. Contain the labeled amount, within ±10%. Meet the requirements for Identification, Dissolution (75% in 45 minutes in water in Apparatus 2 at 50 rpm), and Uniformity of dosage units.

Phenylpropanolamine Hydrochloride Extended-release Tablets USP—Preserve in tight, light-resistant containers. The labeling states the in-vitro Drug release test conditions of times and tolerances, as directed under Drug release. Contain the labeled amount, within ±10%. Meet the requirements for Identification, Drug release, and Uniformity of dosage units.

PHENYLPROPANOLAMINE AND ACETAMINOPHEN

For *Phenylpropanolamine* and *Acetaminophen*—See individual listings for chemistry information.

USP requirements:
Phenylpropanolamine Hydrochloride and Acetaminophen Capsules—Not in *USP–NF*.
Phenylpropanolamine Hydrochloride and Acetaminophen Oral Solution—Not in *USP–NF*.
Phenylpropanolamine Hydrochloride and Acetaminophen Tablets—Not in *USP–NF*.

PHENYLPROPANOLAMINE, ACETAMINOPHEN, AND ASPIRIN

For *Phenylpropanolamine, Acetaminophen,* and *Aspirin*—See individual listings for chemistry information.

USP requirements: Phenylpropanolamine Hydrochloride, Acetaminophen, and Aspirin Capsules—Not in *USP–NF*.

PHENYLPROPANOLAMINE, ACETAMINOPHEN, AND CAFFEINE

For *Phenylpropanolamine, Acetaminophen,* and *Caffeine*—See individual listings for chemistry information.

USP requirements: Phenylpropanolamine Hydrochloride, Acetaminophen, and Caffeine Tablets—Not in *USP–NF*.

PHENYLPROPANOLAMINE, ACETAMINOPHEN, SALICYLAMIDE, AND CAFFEINE

For *Phenylpropanolamine, Acetaminophen, Salicylamide,* and *Caffeine*—See individual listings for chemistry information.

USP requirements: Phenylpropanolamine Hydrochloride, Acetaminophen, Salicylamide, and Caffeine Capsules—Not in *USP–NF*.

PHENYLPROPANOLAMINE AND ASPIRIN

For *Phenylpropanolamine* and *Aspirin*—See individual listings for chemistry information.

USP requirements:
Phenylpropanolamine Bitartrate and Aspirin Effervescent Tablets—Not in *USP–NF*.
Phenylpropanolamine Hydrochloride and Aspirin for Oral Solution—Not in *USP–NF*.
Phenylpropanolamine Hydrochloride and Aspirin Tablets—Not in *USP–NF*.

PHENYLPROPANOLAMINE AND CARAMIPHEN

Chemical group: Phenylpropanolamine hydrochloride—Synthetic phenylisopropanolamine.

Chemical name:
Phenylpropanolamine hydrochloride—Benzenemethanol, alpha(1-aminoethyl)-, hydrochloride, (*R*,S**)-, (±).
Caramiphen edisylate—1-Phenylcyclopentane-1-carboxylic acid, 2-diethylaminoethyl ester, 1,2-ethanedisulfonate (2:1).

Molecular formula:
Phenylpropanolamine hydrochloride—$C_9H_{13}NO \cdot HCl$.
Caramiphen edisylate—$(C_{18}H_{27}NO_2)_2 \cdot C_2H_6O_6S_2$.

Molecular weight:
Phenylpropanolamine hydrochloride—187.67.
Caramiphen edisylate—769.03.

Description:
Phenylpropanolamine Hydrochloride USP—White, crystalline powder, having a slight aromatic odor. Is affected by light.
Caramiphen edisylate—Off-white crystals with a melting point of 115–116 °C.

pKa: Phenylpropanolamine hydrochloride—9.

Solubility:
Phenylpropanolamine Hydrochloride USP—Freely soluble in water and in alcohol; insoluble in ether.

Caramiphen edisylate—1 gram dissolves in about 2 mL of water; soluble in alcohol.

USP requirements: Phenylpropanolamine Hydrochloride and Caramiphen Edisylate Extended-release Capsules—Not in *USP–NF*.

PHENYLPROPANOLAMINE, CODEINE, AND GUAIFENE-SIN

For *Phenylpropanolamine, Codeine,* and *Guaifenesin*—See individual listings for chemistry information.

USP requirements:
Phenylpropanolamine Hydrochloride, Codeine Phosphate, and Guaifenesin Oral Solution—Not in *USP–NF*.
Phenylpropanolamine Hydrochloride, Codeine Phosphate, and Guaifenesin Oral Suspension—Not in *USP–NF*.
Phenylpropanolamine Hydrochloride, Codeine Phosphate, and Guaifenesin Syrup—Not in *USP–NF*.

PHENYLPROPANOLAMINE AND DEXTROMETHOR-PHAN

For *Phenylpropanolamine* and *Dextromethorphan*—See individual listings for chemistry information.

USP requirements:
Phenylpropanolamine Hydrochloride and Dextromethorphan Hydrobromide Oral Gel—Not in *USP–NF*.
Phenylpropanolamine Hydrochloride and Dextromethorphan Hydrobromide Granules—Not in *USP–NF*.
Phenylpropanolamine Hydrochloride and Dextromethorphan Hydrobromide Oral Solution—Not in *USP–NF*.
Phenylpropanolamine Hydrochloride and Dextromethorphan Hydrobromide Syrup—Not in *USP–NF*.

PHENYLPROPANOLAMINE, DEXTROMETHORPHAN, AND ACETAMINOPHEN

For *Phenylpropanolamine, Dextromethorphan,* and *Acetaminophen*—See individual listings for chemistry information.

USP requirements:
Phenylpropanolamine Hydrochloride, Dextromethorphan Hydrobromide, and Acetaminophen Capsules USP—Preserve in tight containers. The label for each article encompassed by this monograph bears a name composed of the active ingredients. The label states the name and quantity of each active ingredient and indicates its function (or purpose) in the article. Contain the labeled amounts, within ±10%. Meet the requirements for Identification, Dissolution (75% in 45 minutes in water in Apparatus 1 at 50 rpm), and Uniformity of dosage units.
Phenylpropanolamine Hydrochloride, Dextromethorphan Hydrobromide, and Acetaminophen Oral Solution USP—Preserve in tight containers. The label for each article encompassed by this monograph bears a name composed of the active ingredients. The label states the name and quantity of each active ingredient and indicates its function (or purpose) in the article. Contains the labeled amounts, within ±10%. Meets the requirements for Identification, Microbial limits, pH (2.6–7.5), and Alcohol content, (if present, within ±10%).

Phenylpropanolamine Hydrochloride, Dextromethorphan Hydrobromide, and Acetaminophen Tablets USP—Preserve in tight containers. The label for each article encompassed by this monograph bears a name composed of the active ingredients. The label states the name and quantity of each active ingredient and indicates its function (or purpose) in the article. Contain the labeled amounts, within ±10%. Meet the requirements for Identification, Dissolution (75% in 45 minutes in 0.1 *M* hydrochloric acid in Apparatus 2 at 50 rpm), and Uniformity of dosage units.

PHENYLPROPANOLAMINE, DEXTROMETHORPHAN, AND GUAIFENESIN

For *Phenylpropanolamine, Dextromethorphan,* and *Guaifenesin*—See individual listings for chemistry information.

USP requirements:
Phenylpropanolamine Hydrochloride, Dextromethorphan Hydrobromide, and Guaifenesin Oral Solution—Not in *USP–NF*.
Phenylpropanolamine Hydrochloride, Dextromethorphan Hydrobromide, and Guaifenesin Syrup—Not in *USP–NF*.

PHENYLPROPANOLAMINE AND GUAIFENESIN

For *Phenylpropanolamine* and *Guaifenesin*—See individual listings for chemistry information.

USP requirements:
Phenylpropanolamine Hydrochloride and Guaifenesin Granules—Not in *USP–NF*.
Phenylpropanolamine Hydrochloride and Guaifenesin Oral Solution—Not in *USP–NF*.
Phenylpropanolamine Hydrochloride and Guaifenesin Syrup—Not in *USP–NF*.
Phenylpropanolamine Hydrochloride and Guaifenesin Tablets—Not in *USP–NF*.
Phenylpropanolamine Hydrochloride and Guaifenesin Extended-release Tablets—Not in *USP–NF*.

PHENYLPROPANOLAMINE, DEXTROMETHORPHAN, GUAIFENESIN, AND ACETAMINOPHEN

For *Phenylpropanolamine, Dextromethorphan, Guaifenesin,* and *Acetaminophen*—See individual listings for chemistry information.

USP requirements:
Phenylpropanolamine Hydrochloride, Dextromethorphan Hydrobromide, Guaifenesin, and Acetaminophen Syrup—Not in *USP–NF*.
Phenylpropanolamine Hydrochloride, Dextromethorphan Hydrobromide, Guaifenesin, and Acetaminophen Tablets USP—Preserve in tight containers. The label for each article encompassed by this monograph bears a name composed of the active ingredients. The label states the name and quantity of each active ingredient and indicates its function (or purpose) in the article. Contain the labeled amounts, within ±10%. Meet the requirements for Identification, Dissolution (75% in 45 minutes in 0.1 *M* hydrochloric acid in Apparatus 2 at 50 rpm), and Uniformity of dosage units.

PHENYLPROPANOLAMINE AND HYDROCODONE

For *Phenylpropanolamine* and *Hydrocodone*—See individual listings for chemistry information.

USP requirements:
   Phenylpropanolamine Hydrochloride and Hydrocodone Bitartrate Oral Solution—Not in *USP–NF*.
   Phenylpropanolamine Hydrochloride and Hydrocodone Bitartrate Syrup—Not in *USP–NF*.

PHENYLPROPANOLAMINE, HYDROCODONE, GUAIFENESIN, AND SALICYLAMIDE

For *Phenylpropanolamine, Hydrocodone, Guaifenesin,* and *Salicylamide*—See individual listings for chemistry information.

USP requirements: Phenylpropanolamine Hydrochloride, Hydrocodone Bitartrate, Guaifenesin, and Salicylamide Tablets—Not in *USP–NF*.

PHENYLTOLOXAMINE AND HYDROCODONE

USP requirements:
   Phenyltoloxamine Resin Complex and Hydrocodone Resin Complex Oral Suspension—Not in *USP–NF*.
   Phenyltoloxamine Resin Complex and Hydrocodone Resin Complex Tablets—Not in *USP–NF*.

PHENYLTOLOXAMINE, PHENYLPROPANOLAMINE, AND ACETAMINOPHEN

Chemical group: Phenylpropanolamine hydrochloride—Synthetic phenylisopropanolamine.

Chemical name:
   Phenyltoloxamine citrate—2-(2-Benzylphenoxy)-*N,N*-dimethylethylamine dihydrogen citrate.
   Phenylpropanolamine hydrochloride—Benzenemethanol, alpha-(1-aminoethyl)-, hydrochloride, (*R*,S**)-, (±).
   Acetaminophen—Acetamide, *N*-(4-hydroxyphenyl)-.

Molecular formula:
   Phenyltoloxamine citrate—$C_{17}H_{21}NO \cdot C_6H_8O_7$.
   Phenylpropanolamine hydrochloride—$C_9H_{13}NO \cdot HCl$.
   Acetaminophen—$C_8H_9NO_2$.

Molecular weight:
   Phenyltoloxamine citrate—447.5.
   Phenylpropanolamine hydrochloride—187.67.
   Acetaminophen—151.16.

Description:
   Phenyltoloxamine citrate—It has a melting point of 138–140 °C.
   Phenylpropanolamine Hydrochloride USP—White, crystalline powder, having a slight aromatic odor. Affected by light.
   Acetaminophen USP—White, odorless, crystalline powder.

pKa: Phenylpropanolamine hydrochloride—9.

Solubility:
   Phenyltoloxamine citrate—Soluble in water.
   Phenylpropanolamine Hydrochloride USP—Freely soluble in water and in alcohol; insoluble in ether.
   Acetaminophen USP—Soluble in boiling water and in 1 *N* sodium hydroxide; freely soluble in alcohol.

USP requirements: Phenyltoloxamine Citrate, Phenylpropanolamine Hydrochloride, and Acetaminophen Extended-release Tablets—Not in *USP–NF*.

PHENYTOIN

Chemical group: Related to the barbiturates in chemical structure, but has a five-membered ring.

Chemical name:
   Phenytoin—2,4-Imidazolidinedione, 5,5-diphenyl-.
   Phenytoin sodium—2,4-Imidazolidinedione, 5,5-diphenyl-, monosodium salt.

Molecular formula:
   Phenytoin—$C_{15}H_{12}N_2O_2$.
   Phenytoin sodium—$C_{15}H_{11}N_2NaO_2$.

Molecular weight:
   Phenytoin—252.27.
   Phenytoin sodium—274.25.

Description:
   Phenytoin USP—White, odorless powder. Melts at about 295 °C.
   Phenytoin Sodium USP—White, odorless powder. Is somewhat hygroscopic and on exposure to air gradually absorbs carbon dioxide.

pKa: 8.06–8.33 (apparent).

Solubility:
   Phenytoin USP—Practically insoluble in water; soluble in hot alcohol; slightly soluble in cold alcohol, in chloroform, and in ether.
   Phenytoin Sodium USP—Freely soluble in water, the solution usually being somewhat turbid due to partial hydrolysis and absorption of carbon dioxide. Soluble in alcohol; practically insoluble in ether and in chloroform.

USP requirements:
   Phenytoin USP—Preserve in tight containers. Contains not less than 98.0% and not more than 102.0% of phenytoin, calculated on the dried basis. Meets the requirements for Clarity and color of solution, Identification, Loss on drying (not more than 1.0%), Heavy metals (not more than 0.002%), Chromatographic purity, Limit of benzophenone (not more than 0.1%), and Organic volatile impurities.
   Phenytoin Oral Suspension USP—Preserve in tight containers. Avoid freezing. It is Phenytoin suspended in a suitable medium. The label bears a statement that the patient must use an accurately calibrated measuring device with multiple-dose containers. Contains the labeled amount, within ±5%. Meets the requirements for Identification and Dissolution (80% in 60 minutes in 0.05 *M* tris buffer in Apparatus 2 at 35 rpm).
   Phenytoin Tablets USP—Preserve in well-closed containers. Label the Tablets to indicate that they are to be chewed. Contain the labeled amount, within ±5%. Meet the requirements for Identification, Dissolution (70% in 120 minutes in 0.05 *M* Tris buffer in Apparatus 2 at 100 rpm), and Uniformity of dosage units.
   Phenytoin Sodium USP—Preserve in tight containers. Contains not less than 98.0% and not more than 102.0% of phenytoin sodium, calculated on the dried basis. Meets the requirements for Clarity and color of solution, Identification, Loss on drying (not more than 2.5%), Heavy metals (not more than 0.002%), Related compounds, and Organic volatile impurities.
   Extended Phenytoin Sodium Capsules USP—Preserve in tight, light-resistant containers. Protect from moisture. Store at controlled room temperature. When more than one Dissolution test is given, the labeling states the Dissolution test used only if Test 1 is not used. Contain the la-

beled amount, within ±5%. Meet the requirements for Identification, Dissolution (for Test 1: for products labeled as 30-mg capsules: not more than 40% in 30 minutes, 56% in 60 minutes, and not less than 65% in 120 minutes in water in Apparatus 1 at 50 rpm; for products labeled as 100-mg capsules: not more than 45% in 30 minutes, 60% in 60 minutes, and not less than 70% in 120 minutes in water in Apparatus 1 at 50 rpm; for Test 2: for products labeled as 100-mg capsules: not more than 45% in 30 minutes, 65% in 60 minutes, and not more than 70% in 120 minutes in water in Apparatus 2 at 75 rpm; for Test 3: for products labeled as 200-mg and 300-mg capsules: not more than 30% in 30 minutes, 50% in 60 minutes, and not less than 60% in 120 minutes in water in Apparatus 1 at 75 rpm), and Uniformity of dosage units.

Prompt Phenytoin Sodium Capsules USP—Preserve in tight containers. Label the Capsules with the statement, "Not for once-a-day dosing," printed immediately under the official name, in a bold and contrasting color and/or enclosed within a box. Contain the labeled amount, within ±5%. Meet the requirements for Identification, Dissolution (85% in 30 minutes in water in Apparatus 1 at 50 rpm), Uniformity of dosage units, and Related compounds.

Phenytoin Sodium Injection USP—Preserve in single-dose or in multiple-dose containers, preferably of Type I glass, at controlled room temperature. A sterile solution of Phenytoin Sodium with Propylene Glycol and Alcohol in Water for Injection. Contains the labeled amount, within ±5%. Meets the requirements for Identification, Bacterial endotoxins, pH (10.0–12.3), Alcohol and propylene glycol content (9–11% alcohol; 37–43% propylene glycol), and Particulate matter, and for Injections.

Note: Do not use the Injection if it is hazy or contains a precipitate.

CHROMIC PHOSPHATE P 32

Chemical name: Phosphoric-^{32}P acid, chromium(3+) salt (1:1).

Molecular formula: $Cr^{32}PO_4$.

Description: Chromic phosphate P 32 suspension—Grayish-green to brownish-green suspension.

USP requirements: Chromic Phosphate P 32 Suspension USP—Preserve in single-dose or in multiple-dose containers. A sterile, aqueous suspension of radioactive chromic phosphate P 32 in a 30% Dextrose solution suitable for intraperitoneal, intrapleural, or interstitial administration. Label it to include the following, in addition to the information specified for Labeling under Injections: the time and date of calibration; the amount of ^{32}P as labeled chromic phosphate expressed as total megabecquerels (or millicuries) and concentration as megabecquerels (or millicuries) per mL at the time of calibration; the expiration date; and the statements, "Caution—Radioactive Material," and "For intracavitary use only." The labeling indicates that in making dosage calculations, correction is to be made for radioactive decay, and also indicates that the radioactive half-life of ^{32}P is 14.3 days. Contains the labeled amount of ^{32}P as chromic phosphate expressed in megabecquerels (or millicuries) per mL at the time indicated in the labeling, within ±10%. Other chemical forms of radioactivity do not exceed 5.0% of the total radioactivity. Meets the requirements for Radionuclide identification, Bacterial endotoxins, pH (3.0–5.0), and Radiochemical purity, and for Injections (except that the Suspension may be distributed or dispensed prior to the completion of the test for Sterility, the

latter test being started on the day of final manufacture, and except that it is not subject to the recommendations on Volume in Container).

SODIUM PHOSPHATE P 32

Chemical name: Phosphoric-^{32}P acid, disodium salt.

Description: Sodium Phosphate P 32 Solution USP—Clear, colorless solution. Upon standing, both the solution and the glass container may darken as a result of the effects of the radiation.

USP requirements: Sodium Phosphate P 32 Solution USP—Preserve in single-dose or in multiple-dose containers that previously have been treated to prevent adsorption. A solution suitable for either oral or intravenous administration, containing radioactive phosphorus (^{32}P) processed in the form of Dibasic Sodium Phosphate from the neutron bombardment of elemental sulfur. Nonradioactive Dibasic Sodium Phosphate may be added during the processing. Label it to include the following: the time and date of calibration; the amount of ^{32}P as phosphate expressed in total megabecquerels (or microcuries or millicuries) and in megabecquerels (or microcuries or in millicuries) per mL at the time of calibration; the name and quantity of any added preservative or stabilizer; a statement of the intended use, whether oral or intravenous; a statement of whether the contents are intended for diagnostic or therapeutic use; the expiration date; and the statements, "Caution—Radioactive Material" and "Not for intracavitary use." The labeling indicates that in making dosage calculations, correction is to be made for radioactive decay, and also indicates that the radioactive half-life of ^{32}P is 14.3 days. Contains the labeled amount of ^{32}P as phosphate expressed in megabecquerels (or microcuries or millicuries) per mL at the time indicated in the labeling, within ±10%. Other chemical forms of radioactivity are absent. Meets the requirements for Radionuclide identification, Bacterial endotoxins, pH (5.0–6.0), and Radiochemical purity, and for Injections (if for intravenous use, except that the Solution may be distributed or dispensed prior to completion of the test for Sterility, the latter test being started on the day of final manufacture, and except that it is not subject to the recommendation on Volume in Container).

PHOSPHORIC ACID

Chemical name: Phosphoric acid.

Molecular formula: H_3PO_4.

Molecular weight: 98.00.

Description: Phosphoric Acid NF—Colorless, odorless liquid of syrupy consistency. Specific gravity is about 1.71.

NF category: Acidifying agent; buffering agent.

Solubility: Phosphoric Acid NF—Miscible with water and with alcohol.

NF requirements: Phosphoric Acid NF—Preserve in tight containers. Contains not less than 85.0% and not more than 88.0%, by weight, of phosphoric acid. Meets the requirements for Identification, Sulfate, Heavy metals (not more than 0.001%), Alkali phosphates, Limit of nitrate, and Phosphorous or hypophosphorous acid.

Caution: Avoid contact, as Phosphoric Acid rapidly destroys tissues.

DILUTED PHOSPHORIC ACID

Description: Diluted Phosphoric Acid NF—Clear, colorless, odorless liquid. Specific gravity is about 1.057.

NF category: Acidifying agent.

NF requirements: Diluted Phosphoric Acid NF—Preserve in tight containers. Contains, in each 100 mL, not less than 9.5 grams and not more than 10.5 grams of phosphoric acid.

Prepare Diluted Phosphoric Acid as follows: 69 mL of Phosphoric Acid and a sufficient quantity of Purified Water to make 1000 mL. Mix the ingredients.

Meets the requirements for Alkali phosphates and Heavy metals (not more than 5 ppm), and for Identification test, Nitrate, Phosphorous or hypophosphorous acid, and Sulfate under Phosphoric Acid.

PHYSOSTIGMINE

Source: Derivative of Calabar bean.

Chemical name:

Physostigmine—Pyrrolo[2,3-*b*]indol-5-ol, 1,2,3,3a,8,8a-hexahydro-1,3a,8-trimethyl-, methylcarbamate (ester), (3a*S-cis*).

Physostigmine salicylate—Pyrrolo[2,3-*b*]indol-5-ol, 1,2,3,3a,8,8a-hexahydro-1,3a,8-trimethyl-, methylcarbamate (ester), (3a*S-cis*)-, mono(2-hydroxybenzoate).

Physostigmine sulfate—Pyrrolo[2,3-*b*]indol-5-ol, 1,2,3,3a,8,8ahexahydro-1,3a,8-trimethyl-, methylcarbamate (ester), (3a*S-cis*)-, sulfate (2:1).

Molecular formula:

Physostigmine—$C_{15}H_{21}N_3O_2$.

Physostigmine salicylate—$C_{15}H_{21}N_3O_2 \cdot C_7H_6O_3$.

Physostigmine sulfate—$(C_{15}H_{21}N_3O_2)_2 \cdot H_2SO_4$.

Molecular weight:

Physostigmine—275.35.

Physostigmine salicylate—413.47.

Physostigmine sulfate—648.77.

Description:

Physostigmine USP—White, odorless, microcrystalline powder. Acquires a red tint when exposed to heat, light, air, or contact with traces of metals. Melts at a temperature not lower than 103 °C.

Physostigmine Salicylate USP—White, shining, odorless crystals or white powder. Acquires a red tint when exposed to heat, light, air, or contact with traces of metals for long periods. Melts at about 184 °C.

Physostigmine Sulfate USP—White, odorless, microcrystalline powder. Is deliquescent in moist air and acquires a red tint when exposed to heat, light, air, or contact with traces of metals for long periods. Melts at about 143 °C.

Solubility:

Physostigmine USP—Slightly soluble in water; very soluble in chloroform and in dichloromethane; freely soluble in alcohol; soluble in fixed oils.

Physostigmine Salicylate USP—Sparingly soluble in water; freely soluble in chloroform; soluble in alcohol; slightly soluble in ether.

Physostigmine Sulfate USP—Freely soluble in water; very soluble in alcohol; very slightly soluble in ether.

USP requirements:

Physostigmine USP—Preserve in tight, light-resistant containers. An alkaloid usually obtained from the dried ripe seed of *Physostigma venenosum* Balfour (Fam. Leguminosae). Contains not less than 97.0% and not more than 102.0% of physostigmine, calculated on the dried basis. Meets the requirements for Identification, Specific rotation (−236° to −246°), Loss on drying (not more than 1.0%), Residue on ignition (negligible, from 100 mg), and Readily carbonizable substances.

Physostigmine Salicylate USP—Preserve in tight, light-resistant containers. Contains not less than 97.0% and not more than 102.0% of physostigmine salicylate, calculated on the dried basis. Meets the requirements for Identification, Specific rotation (−91° to −94°), Loss on drying (not more than 1.0%), Residue on ignition (negligible, from 100 mg), Sulfate, and Readily carbonizable substances.

Physostigmine Salicylate Injection USP—Preserve in single-dose containers, preferably of Type I glass, protected from light. A sterile solution of Physostigmine Salicylate in Water for Injection. Contains the labeled amount, within ±10%. Meets the requirements for Identification, Bacterial endotoxins, and pH (3.5–5.0), and for Injections.

Note: Do not use the Injection if it is more than slightly discolored.

Physostigmine Salicylate Ophthalmic Solution USP—Preserve in tight, light-resistant containers. A sterile, aqueous solution of Physostigmine Salicylate. Contains the labeled amount, within ±10%. Meets the requirements for Identification, Sterility, and pH (2.0–4.0).

Physostigmine Sulfate USP—Preserve in tight, light-resistant containers. Contains not less than 97.0% and not more than 102.0% of physostigmine sulfate, calculated on the dried basis. Meets the requirements for Identification, Specific rotation (−116° to −120°), Loss on drying (not more than 1.0%), Residue on ignition (negligible, from 100 mg), and Readily carbonizable substances.

Physostigmine Sulfate Ophthalmic Ointment USP—Preserve in collapsible ophthalmic ointment tubes. It is sterile. Contains the labeled amount, within ±10%. Meets the requirements for Identification, Sterility, and Metal particles.

PHYTONADIONE

Chemical name: 1,4-Naphthalenedione, 2-methyl-3-(3,7,11,15-tetramethyl-2-hexadecenyl)-, [R-[R*,R*-(E)]]-.

Molecular formula: $C_{31}H_{46}O_2$.

Molecular weight: 450.70.

Description: Phytonadione USP—Clear, yellow to amber, very viscous, odorless or practically odorless liquid, having a specific gravity of about 0.967. Is stable in air, but decomposes on exposure to sunlight.

Solubility: Phytonadione USP—Insoluble in water; soluble in dehydrated alcohol, in chloroform, in ether, and in vegetable oils; slightly soluble in alcohol.

USP requirements:

Phytonadione USP—Preserve in tight, light-resistant containers. A mixture of *E* and *Z* isomers. Contains not less than 97.0% and not more than 103.0% of phytonadione. Contains not more than 21.0% of the *Z* isomer. Meets the requirements for Identification, Refractive index (1.523–1.526), Reaction, Limit of menadione, and *Z* isomer content.

Phytonadione Injectable Emulsion USP—Preserve in single-dose or in multiple-dose containers, preferably of Type I glass, protected from light. A sterile, aqueous dispersion of Phytonadione. Contains suitable solubilizing and/or dispersing agents. Contains the labeled amount, within ± 10%. Meets the requirements for Identification, Bacterial endotoxins, and pH (3.5–7.0), and for Injections.

Phytonadione Injection USP—Preserve in single-dose or in multiple-dose containers, preferably of Type I glass, protected from light. A sterile, aqueous dispersion of Phytonadione. Contains suitable solubilizing and/or dispersing

agents. Contains the labeled amount, within ±10%. Meets the requirements for Identification, Bacterial endotoxins, and pH (3.5–7.0), and for Injections.

Phytonadione Tablets USP—Preserve in well-closed, light-resistant containers. Contain the labeled amount, within ±10%. Meet the requirements for Identification, Disintegration (30 minutes), and Uniformity of dosage units.

PILOCARPINE

Chemical name:

Pilocarpine—2(3*H*)-Furanone, 3-ethyldihydro-4-[(1-methyl-1*H*-imidazol-5-yl)methyl]-, (3*S-cis*)-.

Pilocarpine hydrochloride—2(3*H*)-Furanone, 3-ethyldihydro-4[(1-methyl-1*H*-imidazol-5-yl)methyl]-, monohydrochloride, (3*S-cis*)-.

Pilocarpine nitrate—2(3*H*)-Furanone, 3-ethyldihydro-4-[(1-methyl-1*H*-imidazol-5-yl)methyl]-, (3*S-cis*)-, mononitrate.

Molecular formula:

Pilocarpine—$C_{11}H_{16}N_2O_2$.
Pilocarpine hydrochloride—$C_{11}H_{16}N_2O_2 \cdot HCl$.
Pilocarpine nitrate—$C_{11}H_{16}N_2O_2 \cdot HNO_3$.

Molecular weight:

Pilocarpine—208.26.
Pilocarpine hydrochloride—244.72.
Pilocarpine nitrate—271.27.

Description:

Pilocarpine USP—A viscous, oily liquid, or crystals melting at about 34 °C. Exceedingly hygroscopic.

Pilocarpine Hydrochloride USP—Colorless, translucent, odorless crystals. Is hygroscopic and is affected by light. Its solutions are acid to litmus.

Pilocarpine Nitrate USP—Shining, white crystals. Is stable in air but is affected by light. Its solutions are acid to litmus.

Solubility:

Pilocarpine USP—Soluble in water, in alcohol, and in chloroform; practically insoluble in petroleum ether; sparingly soluble in ether.

Pilocarpine Hydrochloride USP—Very soluble in water; freely soluble in alcohol; slightly soluble in chloroform; insoluble in ether.

Pilocarpine Nitrate USP—Freely soluble in water; sparingly soluble in alcohol; insoluble in chloroform and in ether.

USP requirements:

Pilocarpine USP—Preserve in tight, light-resistant containers, in a cold place. Contains not less than 95.0% and not more than 100.5% of pilocarpine, calculated on the anhydrous basis. Meets the requirements for Identification, Specific rotation (+102° to +107°), Refractive index (1.5170–1.5210 at 25 °C), Water (not more than 0.5%), Chloride (not more than 0.25%), Sulfate (not more than 0.004%), Limit of nitrate, and Related substances (not more than 5.0%).

Pilocarpine Ocular System USP—Preserve in single-dose containers, in a cold place. It is sterile. Contains the labeled amount, within ±15%. Meets the requirements for Identification, Sterility, Uniformity of dosage units (for capsules), and Drug release pattern (the labeled release pattern, within ±20%).

Pilocarpine Ophthalmic System—Not in *USP–NF*.

Pilocarpine Hydrochloride USP—Preserve in tight, light-resistant containers. Contains not less than 98.5% and not more than 101.0% of pilocarpine hydrochloride, calculated on the dried basis. Meets the requirements for Identification, Melting range (199–205 °C, the range between beginning and end of melting not more than 3 °C), Specific

rotation (+88.5° to 91.5°), Loss on drying (not more than 3.0%), Readily carbonizable substances, Ordinary impurities, and Other alkaloids.

Pilocarpine Hydrochloride Ophthalmic Gel—Not in *USP–NF*.

Pilocarpine Hydrochloride Ophthalmic Solution USP—Preserve in tight containers. A sterile, buffered, aqueous solution of Pilocarpine Hydrochloride. Contains the labeled amount, within ±10%. Meets the requirements for Identification, Sterility, and pH (3.5–5.5).

Pilocarpine Hydrochloride Tablets—Not in *USP–NF*.

Pilocarpine Nitrate USP—Preserve in tight, light-resistant containers. Contains not less than 98.5% and not more than 101.0% of pilocarpine nitrate, calculated on the dried basis. Meets the requirements for Identification, Melting range (171–176 °C, with decomposition, the range between beginning and end of melting not more than 3 °C), Specific rotation (+79.5° to +82.5°), Loss on drying (not more than 2.0%), Readily carbonizable substances, Chloride, and Other alkaloids.

Pilocarpine Nitrate Ophthalmic Solution USP—Preserve in tight, light-resistant containers. A sterile, buffered, aqueous solution of Pilocarpine Nitrate. Contains the labeled amount, within ±10%. Meets the requirements for Identification, Sterility, and pH (4.0–5.5).

PIMECROLIMUS

Chemical name:15,19-Epoxy-3*H*-pyrido[2,1-*c*][1,4]oxaazacyclotricosine-1,17,20,21(4*H*,23*H*)-tetrone, 3-[(1*E*)-2-[(1*R*,3*R*,4*S*)-4-chloro-3-methoxycyclohexyl]-1-methylethenyl]-8-ethyl-5,6,8,11,12,13,14,15,16,17,18,19,24,26,26a-hexadecahydro-5,19-dihydroxy-14,16-dimethoxy-4,10,12,18-tetramethyl-, (3*S*,4*R*,5*S*,8*R*,9*E*,12*S*,14*S*,15*R*,16*S*,18*R*,19*R*,26a*S*)-.

Molecular formula:$C_{43}H_{68}ClNO_{11}$.

Molecular weight:913.92.

Description: White to off-white fine crystalline powder.

Solubility: Soluble in methanol and in ethanol; insoluble in water.

USP requirements: Pimecrolimus Cream—Not in *USP–NF*.

PIMOZIDE

Chemical group: A diphenylbutylpiperidine derivative.

Chemical name: 2*H*-Benzimidazol-2-one, 1-[1-[4,4-bis(4-fluorophenyl)butyl]-4-piperidinyl]-1,3-dihydro-.

Molecular formula: $C_{28}H_{29}F_2N_3O$.

Molecular weight: 461.55.

Description: Pimozide USP—White, crystalline powder.

Solubility: Pimozide USP—Insoluble in water; slightly soluble in ether and in alcohol; freely soluble in chloroform.

USP requirements:

Pimozide USP—Preserve in tight, light-resistant containers. Contains not less than 98.0% and not more than 102.0% of pimozide, calculated on the dried basis. Meets the requirements for Identification, Melting range (216–220 °C), Loss on drying (not more than 0.5%), Residue on ignition (not more than 0.2%), Heavy metals (not more than 0.002%), Ordinary impurities, and Organic volatile impurities.

Pimozide Tablets USP—Preserve in tight, light-resistant containers. Contain the labeled amount, within ±10%. Meet the requirements for Identification, Dissolution (80% in 30 minutes in 0.01 N hydrochloric acid in Apparatus 2 at 50 rpm), and Uniformity of dosage units.

PINDOLOL

Chemical name: 2-Propanol, 1-(1*H*-indol-4-yloxy)-3-[(1-methylethyl)amino]-.

Molecular formula: $C_{14}H_{20}N_2O_2$.

Molecular weight: 248.32.

Description: Pindolol USP—White to off-white, crystalline powder, having a faint odor.

Solubility: Pindolol USP—Practically insoluble in water; slightly soluble in methanol; very slightly soluble in chloroform.

Other characteristics: Lipid solubility—Moderate.

USP requirements:
Pindolol USP—Preserve in well-closed containers, protected from light. Contains not less than 98.5% and not more than 101.0% of pindolol, calculated on the dried basis. Meets the requirements for Identification, Melting range (169–173 °C, the range between beginning and end of melting not more than 3 °C), Loss on drying (not more than 0.5%), Residue on ignition (not more than 0.1%), Heavy metals (not more than 0.002%), Chromatographic purity, and Organic volatile impurities.
Pindolol Tablets USP—Preserve in well-closed containers, protected from light. Contain the labeled amount, ±10%. Meet the requirements for Identification, Dissolution (80% in 15 minutes in 0.1 N hydrochloric acid in Apparatus 2 at 50 rpm), Uniformity of dosage units, and Chromatographic purity.

PINDOLOL AND HYDROCHLOROTHIAZIDE

For *Pindolol* and *Hydrochlorothiazide*—See individual listings for chemistry information.

USP requirements: Pindolol and Hydrochlorothiazide Tablets—Not in *USP–NF*.

PIOGLITAZONE

Chemical name: Pioglitazone hydrochloride—2,4-Thiazolidinedione, 5-[[4-[2-(5-ethyl-2-pyridinyl)ethoxy]phenyl]methyl]-, monohydrochloride, (±)-.

Molecular formula: Pioglitazone hydrochloride—$C_{19}H_{20}N_2O_3S \cdot$ HCl.

Molecular weight: Pioglitazone hydrochloride—392.90.

Description: Pioglitazone hydrochloride—Odorless white crystalline powder. Melting point 193–194 °C.

Solubility: Pioglitazone hydrochloride—Soluble in *N,N*-dimethylformamide; slightly soluble in anhydrous ethanol; very slightly soluble in acetone and in acetonitrile; practically insoluble in water and in ether.

USP requirements:
Pioglitazone Tablets—Not in *USP–NF*.
Pioglitazone Hydrochloride Tablets—Not in *USP–NF*.

PIPECURONIUM

Chemical name: Pipecuronium bromide—Piperazinium, 4,4′-[(2 beta,3 alpha,5 alpha,16 beta,17 beta)-3,17-bis(acetyloxy)androstane-2,16-diyl]bis[1,1-dimethyl-, dibromide.

Molecular formula: Pipecuronium bromide—$C_{35}H_{62}Br_2N_4O_4$.

Molecular weight: Pipecuronium bromide—762.70.

Description: Pipecuronium bromide—Melting point 262–264 °C.

USP requirements: Pipecuronium Bromide for Injection—Not in *USP–NF*.

PIPERACILLIN

Chemical name:
Piperacillin—4-Thia-1-azabicyclo[3.2.0]heptane-2-carboxylic acid, 6-[[[[(4-ethyl-2,3-dioxo-1-piperazinyl)carbonyl]amino]phenylacetyl]amino]-3,3-dimethyl-7-oxo-, monohydrate, [2*S*-[2 alpha,5 alpha,6 beta(*S**)]].
Piperacillin sodium—4-Thia-1-azabicyclo[3.2.0]heptane-2-carboxylic acid, 6-[[[[(4-ethyl-2,3-dioxo-1-piperazinyl)carbon-yl]amino]phenylacetyl]amino]-3,3-dimethyl-7-oxo-, monosodium salt, [2*S*-[2 alpha,5 alpha,6 beta(*S**)]].

Molecular formula:
Piperacillin—$C_{23}H_{27}N_5O_7S \cdot H_2O$.
Piperacillin sodium—$C_{23}H_{26}N_5NaO_7S$.

Molecular weight:
Piperacillin—535.57.
Piperacillin sodium—539.54.

Description:
Piperacillin USP—White to off-white crystalline powder.
Piperacillin Sodium USP—White to off-white solid having the characteristic appearance of products prepared by freeze-drying.

Solubility:
Piperacillin USP—Very slightly soluble in water; very soluble in methanol; sparingly soluble in isopropyl alcohol; slightly soluble in ethyl acetate.
Piperacillin Sodium USP—Freely soluble in water and in alcohol.

USP requirements:
Piperacillin USP—Preserve in well-closed containers. Where it is intended for use in preparing injectable dosage forms, the label states that it is sterile or must be subjected to further processing during the preparation of injectable dosage forms. Contains not less than 960 mcg and not more than 1030 mcg of piperacillin per mg, calculated on the anhydrous basis. Meets the requirements for Identification, Water (2.0–4.0%), Heavy metals (not more than 0.002%), Specific rotation (+155° to +175°), and Related compounds, for Sterility and Bacterial endotoxins under Piperacillin for Injection (where the label states that Piperacillin is sterile), and for Bacterial endotoxins under Piperacillin for Injection (where the label states that Piperacillin must be subjected to further processing during the preparation of injectable dosage forms).
Piperacillin for Injection USP—Preserve in Containers for Sterile Solids. Contains an amount of piperacillin sodium equivalent to the labeled amount of piperacillin within −10% to +20%. Meets the requirements for Constituted

solution, Bacterial endotoxins, Sterility, pH (4.8–6.8, in a solution containing 200 mg of piperacillin per mL), Water (not more than 0.9%), Particulate matter, and Related compounds, and for Identification under Piperacillin, Uniformity of dosage units, and Labeling under Injections.

Piperacillin Sodium USP—Preserve in tight containers. Where it is intended for use in preparing injectable dosage forms, the label states that it is sterile or must be subjected to further processing during the preparation of injectable dosage forms. Has a potency equivalent to not less than 863 mcg and not more than 1007 mcg of piperacillin per mg, calculated on the anhydrous basis. Meets the requirements for Identification, pH (5.5–7.5, in a solution containing 400 mg per mL), Water (not more than 1.0%), and Related compounds, for Sterility and Bacterial endotoxins under Piperacillin for Injection (where the label states that Piperacillin Sodium is sterile), and for Bacterial endotoxins under Piperacillin for Injection (where the label states that Piperacillin Sodium must be subjected to further processing during the preparation of injectable dosage forms).

PIPERACILLIN AND TAZOBACTAM

Chemical group: Tazobactam—A penicillanic acid sulphone derivative similar to sulbactam.

Chemical name:
Piperacillin sodium—4-Thia-1-azabicyclo[3.2.0]heptane-2carboxylic acid, 6-[[[[(4-ethyl-2,3-dioxo-1-piperazinyl)carbonyl]amino]phenylacetyl]amino]-3,3-dimethyl-7-oxo-,monosodium salt, [2S-[2 alpha,5 alpha,6 beta(S*)]].
Tazobactam sodium—4-Thia-1-azabicyclo[3.2.0]heptane-2-carboxylic acid, 3-methyl-7-oxo-3-(1H-1,2,3-triazol-1-ylmethyl)-, 4,4-dioxide, sodium salt, [2S-(2 alpha,3 beta,5 alpha)]-.

Molecular formula:
Piperacillin sodium—$C_{23}H_{26}N_5NaO_7S$.
Tazobactam sodium—$C_{10}H_{11}N_4NaO_5S$.

Molecular weight:
Piperacillin sodium—539.54.
Tazobactam sodium—322.27.

Description: Piperacillin Sodium USP—White to off-white solid having the characteristic appearance of products prepared by freeze-drying.

Solubility: Piperacillin Sodium USP—Freely soluble in water and in alcohol.

USP requirements:
Piperacillin Sodium and Tazobactam Sodium Injection—Not in *USP–NF*.
Sterile Piperacillin Sodium and Tazobactam Sodium—Not in *USP–NF*.

PIPERAZINE

Chemical name:
Piperazine—Piperazine.
Piperazine adipate—Hexanedioic acid compd. with piperazine (1:1).
Piperazine citrate—Piperazine, 2-hydroxy-1,2,3-propanetricarboxylate (3:2), hydrate.

Molecular formula:
Piperazine—$C_4H_{10}N_2$.
Piperazine adipate—$C_4H_{10}N_2 \cdot C_6H_{10}O_4$.
Piperazine citrate—$(C_4H_{10}H_2)_3 \cdot 2C_6H_8O_7$ (anhydrous).

Molecular weight:
Piperazine—86.14.
Piperazine adipate—232.3.
Piperazine citrate (anhydrous)—642.65.

Description:
Piperazine USP—White to slightly off-white lumps or flakes, having an ammoniacal odor.
Piperazine adipate—White, crystalline powder. Melts at about 150°, with decomposition.
Piperazine Citrate USP—White, crystalline powder, having not more than a slight odor. Its solution (1 in 10) has a pH of about 5.

Solubility:
Piperazine USP—Soluble in water and in alcohol; insoluble in ether.
Piperazine adipate—Soluble in water; sparingly soluble in methanol; practically insoluble in dehydrated alcohol, in dioxane, and in isopropyl alcohol.
Piperazine Citrate USP—Soluble in water; insoluble in alcohol and in ether.

USP requirements:
Piperazine USP—Preserve in tight containers, protected from light. Contains not less than 98.0% and not more than 101.0% of piperazine, calculated on the anhydrous basis. Meets the requirements for Color of solution, Identification, Melting range (109–113 °C), Water (not more than 2.0%), and Primary amines and ammonia (not more than 0.7%).
Piperazine Adipate Granules for Oral Solution—Not in *USP–NF*.
Piperazine Adipate Oral Suspension—Not in *USP–NF*.
Piperazine Citrate USP—Preserve in well-closed containers. Contains not less than 98.0% and not more than 100.5% of piperazine citrate, calculated on the anhydrous basis. Meets the requirements for Identification, Water (not more than 12.0%), and Primary amines and ammonia (not more than 0.7%).
Piperazine Citrate Syrup USP—Preserve in tight containers. Prepared from Piperazine Citrate or from Piperazine to which an equivalent amount of Citric Acid is added. Contains an amount of piperazine citrate equivalent to the labeled amount of piperazine hexahydrate, within ±7%. Meets the requirement for Identification.
Piperazine Citrate Tablets USP—Preserve in tight containers. Contain an amount of piperazine citrate equivalent to the labeled amount of piperazine hexahydrate, within ±7%. Meet the requirements for Identification, Dissolution (75% in 45 minutes in water in Apparatus 2 at 50 rpm), and Uniformity of dosage units.

PIPOTIAZINE

Chemical group: Piperidine phenothiazine.

Chemical name: Pipotiazine palmitate—Hexadecanoic acid, 2-[1-[3-[2-[(dimethylamino)sulfonyl]-10H-phenothiazin-10-yl]propyl]-4-piperidinyl]ethyl ester.

Molecular formula: Pipotiazine palmitate—$C_{40}H_{63}N_3O_4S_2$.

Molecular weight: Pipotiazine palmitate—714.08.

USP requirements: Pipotiazine Palmitate Injection—Not in *USP–NF*.

PIRBUTEROL

Chemical name: Pirbuterol acetate—2,6-Pyridinedimethanol, alpha^6-[[(1,1-dimethylethyl)amino]methyl]-3-hydroxy-, monoacetate (salt).

Molecular formula: Pirbuterol acetate—$C_{12}H_{20}N_2O_3 \cdot C_2H_4O_2$.

Molecular weight: Pirbuterol acetate—300.35.

Description: Pirbuterol acetate—A white, crystalline powder.

Solubility: Pirbuterol acetate—Freely soluble in water.

USP requirements: Pirbuterol Acetate Inhalation Aerosol—Not in *USP–NF*.

PIRENZEPINE

Chemical group: Synthetic tertiary amine.

Chemical name: Pirenzepine hydrochloride—6*H*-Pyrido[2,3-*b*][1,4]benzodiazepin-6-one, 5,11-dihydro-11-[(4-methyl-1-piperazinyl)acetyl]-, dihydrochloride.

Molecular formula: Pirenzepine hydrochloride—$C_{19}H_{21}N_5O_2 \cdot$ 2HCl.

Molecular weight: Pirenzepine hydrochloride—424.32.

Solubility: Pirenzepine hydrochloride—Soluble in water; slightly soluble in methanol; practically Insoluble in ether.

USP requirements: Pirenzepine Hydrochloride Tablets—Not in *USP–NF*.

PIROXICAM

Chemical group: Oxicam derivative.

Chemical name: 2*H*-1,2-Benzothiazine-3-carboxamide, 4-hydroxy-2-methyl-*N*-2-pyridinyl-, 1,1-dioxide.

Molecular formula: $C_{15}H_{13}N_3O_4S$.

Molecular weight: 331.35.

Description: Piroxicam USP—Off-white to light tan or light yellow, odorless powder. Forms a monohydrate that is yellow.

pKa: 1.8 and 5.1.

Solubility: Piroxicam USP—Very slightly soluble in water, in dilute acids, and in most organic solvents; slightly soluble in alcohol and in aqueous alkaline solutions.

USP requirements:
Piroxicam USP—Preserve in tight, light-resistant containers. Contains not less than 97.0% and not more than 103.0% of piroxicam. Meets the requirements for Identification, Water (not more than 0.5%), Residue on ignition (not more than 0.3%), Heavy metals (not more than 0.005%), and Organic volatile impurities.
Piroxicam Capsules USP—Preserve in tight, light-resistant containers. Contain the labeled amount, within ±7.5%. Meet the requirements for Identification, Dissolution (75% in 45 minutes in simulated gastric fluid TS, prepared without pepsin, in Apparatus 1 at 50 rpm), Uniformity of dosage units, and Water (not more than 8.0%).
Piroxicam Suppositories—Not in *USP–NF*.

POSTERIOR PITUITARY

USP requirements: Posterior Pituitary Injection USP—Preserve in single-dose or in multiple-dose containers, preferably of Type I glass. Do not freeze. A sterile solution, in a suitable diluent, of material containing the polypeptide hormones having the property of causing the contraction of uterine, vascular, and other smooth muscle, which is prepared from the posterior lobe of the pituitary body of healthy, domestic animals used for food by man. Each mL of Posterior Pituitary Injection possesses oxytocic and pressor activities of not less than 85.0% and not more than 120.0% of those stated on the label in USP Posterior Pituitary Units. Meets the requirements for Bacterial endotoxins and pH (2.5–4.5), and for Injections.

PIVAMPICILLIN

Chemical name: Pivaloyloxymethyl (6*R*)-6(alpha-D-phenylglycylamino)penicillanate.

Molecular formula: $C_{22}H_{29}N_3O_6S$.

Molecular weight: 463.55.

USP requirements:
Pivampicillin for Oral Suspension—Not in *USP–NF*.
Pivampicillin Tablets—Not in *USP–NF*.

PIVMECILLINAM

Chemical name: Pivmecillinam hydrochloride—[2*s*-(2 alpha,5 alpha,6 beta)]-6*E*-{[Hexahydro-1*H*-azepin-1-yl)methylene]amino}-3,3-dimethyl-7-oxo-4-thia-1-azabicyclo[3.2.0]heptane2-carboxylic acid (2,2-dimethyl-1-oxopropoxy)methyl ester monohydrochloride.

Molecular formula: Pivmecillinam hydrochloride—$C_{21}H_{33}N_3O_5S \cdot$ HCl.

Molecular weight: Pivmecillinam hydrochloride—476.04.

Description: Pivmecillinam hydrochloride—White crystalline powder.

USP requirements: Pivmecillinam Hydrochloride Tablets—Not in *USP–NF*.

PIZOTYLINE

Chemical name: Pizotyline malate—9,10-Dihydro-4-(1-methyl-4-piperidylidene)-4*H*-benzo[4,5]cycloheptal[1,2-*b*]thiophene malate.

Molecular formula: Pizotyline malate—$C_{19}H_{21}NS \cdot C_4H_6O_5$.

Molecular weight: Pizotyline malate—429.53.

Description: Pizotyline malate—White or slightly yellowishwhite, odorless or almost odorless, crystalline powder.

Solubility: Pizotyline malate—Very slightly soluble in water; slightly soluble in alcohol and in chloroform; sparingly soluble in methyl alcohol.

USP requirements: Pizotyline Malate Tablets—Not in *USP–NF*.

PLANTAGO SEED

Description: Plantago Seed USP—All varieties are practically odorless.

USP requirements: Plantago Seed USP—Preserve in well-closed containers, secure against insect attack. The cleaned, dried, ripe seed of *Plantago psyllium* Linn;aae, or of *Plantago indica* Linné (*Plantago arenaria* Waldstein et Kitaibel), known in commerce as Spanish or French Psyllium Seed; or of *Plantago ovata* Forskal, known in commerce as Blond Psyllium or Indian Plantago Seed (Fam. Plantaginaceae). Meets the requirements for Botanic characteristics, Water absorption, Total ash (not more than 4.0%), Acid-insoluble ash (not more than 1.0%), and Foreign organic matter (not more than 0.50%).

PLASMA PROTEIN FRACTION

USP requirements: Plasma Protein Fraction USP—Preserve at the temperature indicated on the label. A sterile preparation of serum albumin and globulin obtained by fractionating material (source blood, plasma, or serum) from healthy human donors, the source material being tested for the absence of hepatitis B surface antigen. Made by a process that yields a product having protein components of approved composition and sedimentation coefficient content. Label it to state that it is not to be used if it is turbid and that it is to be used within 4 hours after the container is entered. Label it also to state the osmotic equivalent in terms of plasma and the sodium content. Not less than 83% of its total protein is albumin and not more than 17% of its total protein consists of alpha and beta globulins. Not more than 1% of its total protein has the electrophoretic properties of gamma globulin. A solution containing, in each 100 mL, 5 grams of protein, and contains the labeled amount, within ±6%. Contains no added antimicrobial agent, but contains sodium acetyltryptophanate with or without sodium caprylate as a stabilizing agent. Has a sodium content of not less than 130 mEq per liter and not more than 160 mEq per liter and a potassium content of not more than 2 mEq per liter. Has a pH between 6.7 and 7.3, measured in a solution diluted to contain 1% of protein with 0.15 *M* sodium chloride. Meets the requirements of the test for heat stability and for Expiration date (minimum date not later than 5 years after issue from manufacturer's cold storage [5 °C, 1 year] if labeling recommends storage between 2 and 10 °C; not later than 3 years after issue from manufacturer's cold storage [5 °C, 1 year] if labeling recommends storage at temperatures not higher than 30 °C). Conforms to the regulations of the U.S. Food and Drug Administration concerning biologics.

PLATELET CONCENTRATE

USP requirements: Platelet Concentrate USP—Preserve in hermetic containers of colorless, transparent, sterile, pyrogen-free Type I or Type II glass, or of a suitable plastic material. Preserve at the temperature relevant to the volume of resuspension plasma, either between 20 and 24 °C or between 1 and 6 °C, the latter except during shipment, when the temperature may be between 1 and 10 °C. In addition to the labeling requirements of Whole Blood applicable to this product, label it to state the volume of original plasma present, the kind and volume of anticoagulant solution present in the original plasma, the blood group designation of the source blood, and the hour of expiration on the stated expiration date. Where labeled for storage at 20 to 24 °C, label it also to state that a continuous gentle agitation shall be maintained, or where labeled for storage at 1 to 6 °C, to state that such agitation is optional. Label it also with the type and result of a serologic test for syphilis, or to indicate that it was nonreactive in such test; with the type and result of a test for hepatitis B surface antigen, or to indicate that it was nonreactive in such test; with a warning that it is to be used as soon as possible but not more than 4 hours after entering the container; to state that a filter is to be used in the administration equipment; and to state that the instruction circular provided is to be consulted for directions for use. Contains the platelets taken from plasma obtained by whole blood collection, by plasmapheresis, or by plateletpheresis, from a single suitable human donor of whole blood; or from a plasmapheresis donor; or from a plateletpheresis donor who meets the criteria described in the product license application (in which case the collection procedure is as described therein), except where a licensed physician has determined that the recipient is to be transfused with the platelets from a specific donor (in which case the plateletpheresis procedure is performed under the supervision of a licensed physician who is aware of the health status of the donor and has certified that the donor's health permits such procedure). In all cases, the collection of source material is made by a single, uninterrupted venipuncture with minimal damage to and manipulation of the donor's tissue. Concentrate consists of such platelets suspended in a specified volume of the original plasma, the separation of plasma and resuspension of the platelets being done in a closed system, within 4 hours of collection of the whole blood or plasma. The separation of platelets is by a procedure shown to yield an unclumped product without visible hemolysis, with a content of not less than 5.5×10^{10} platelets per unit in not less than 75% of the units tested, and the volume of original plasma used for resuspension of the separated platelets is such that the product has a pH of not less than 6 during the storage period when kept at the selected storage temperature, the selected storage temperature and corresponding volume of resuspension plasma being either 30 to 50 mL of plasma for storage at 20 to 24 °C, or 20 to 30 mL of plasma for storage at 1 to 6 °C. Meets the aforementioned requirements for platelet count, pH, and actual plasma volume, when tested 72 hours after preparation, and for Expiration date (not more than 72 hours from the time of collection of the source material). Conforms to the regulations of the U.S. Food and Drug Administration concerning biologics.

PLICAMYCIN

Source: Antibiotic produced by *Streptomyces argillaceus, Streptomyces tanashiensis,* and *Streptomyces plicatus.*

Chemical name: Plicamycin.

Molecular formula: $C_{52}H_{76}O_{24}$.

Molecular weight: 1085.15.

Description: Plicamycin USP—Yellow, odorless, hygroscopic, crystalline powder.

Solubility: Plicamycin USP—Slightly soluble in water and in methanol; very slightly soluble in alcohol; freely soluble in ethyl acetate.

USP requirements:
Plicamycin USP—Preserve in tight, light-resistant containers, at a temperature between 2 and 8 °C. Has a potency of not less than 900 mcg of plicamycin per mg, calculated on the dried basis. Meets the requirements for Identification, Crystallinity, pH (4.5–5.5, in a solution containing 0.5 mg per mL), and Loss on drying (not more than 8.0%).

Plicamycin for Injection USP—Preserve in light-resistant Containers for Sterile Solids, at a temperature between 2 and 8 °C. A sterile, dry mixture of Plicamycin and Mannitol. Label it with the mandatory instruction to consult the professional information for dosage and warnings, and with the warning that it is intended for hospital use only, under the direct supervision of a physician. Contains the labeled amount, within ±10%. Meets the requirements for Constituted solution, Identification, Bacterial endotoxins, Sterility, pH (5.0–7.5, in the solution constituted as directed in the labeling), and Water (not more than 2.0%).

PNEUMOCOCCAL CONJUGATE VACCINE

Source: The 7-valent conjugate vaccine contains the saccharides of the capsular antigens of the 7 *Streptococcus pneumoniae* serotypes 4, 6B, 9V, 14, 18C, 19F, and 23F, which cause 80% of invasive pneumococcal disease in children under 6 years of age in the U.S. Polysaccharides derived from the serotypes are purified and chemically activated to make saccharides, which are then conjugated to the protein carrier CRM_{197} to form the glycoconjugate. CRM_{197} is a nontoxic variant of diphtheria toxin isolated from cultures of *Corynebacterium diphtheriae*. The individual glycoconjugates are compounded to formulate the 7-valent conjugate vaccine, which provides 2 mcg of each saccharide of serotypes 4, 9V, 14, 18C, 19F, and 23F, and 4 mcg of serotype 6B per 0.5 mL dose. Each 0.5 mL dose also contains 20 mcg of CRM_{197} and 0.125 mg of aluminum as aluminum phosphate adjuvant.

USP requirements: Pneumococcal Conjugate Vaccine Injection—Not in *USP–NF*.

PNEUMOCOCCAL VACCINE POLYVALENT

Source:

The currently available vaccines in the U.S. and Canada contain a mixture of purified capsular polysaccharides from the 23 most prevalent pneumococcal types responsible for 85 to 90% of serious pneumococcal disease. Each of the pneumococcal polysaccharide types is produced separately. The resultant 23 polysaccharides are separated from the cells, purified, and combined to give 25 mcg of each type per 0.5-mL dose of the final vaccine.

Other characteristics:

The U.S. nomenclature for these 23 types is: 1, 2, 3, 4, 5, 26, 51, 8, 9, 68, 34, 43, 12, 14, 54, 17, 56, 57, 19, 20, 22, 23, 70.

The Danish nomenclature for these 23 types is: 1, 2, 3, 4, 5, 6B, 7F, 8, 9N, 9V, 10A, 11A, 12F, 14, 15B, 17F, 18C, 19A, 19F, 20, 22F, 23F, 33F.

USP requirements: Pneumococcal Vaccine Polyvalent Injection—Not in *USP–NF*.

PODOFILOX

Source: Chemically synthesized or purified from the plant families *Coniferae* and *Berberidaceae* (e.g. species of *Juniperus* and *Podophyllum*).

Chemical name: Furo[3′,4′:6,7]naphtho[2,3-*d*]-1,3-dioxol-6(5a*H*)one, 5,8,8a,9-tetrahydro-9-hydroxy-5-(3,4,5-trimethoxyphenyl)-, [5*R*-(5 alpha,5a beta,8a alpha,9 alpha)]-.

Molecular formula: $C_{22}H_{22}O_8$.

Molecular weight: 414.41.

Solubility: Soluble in alcohol; sparingly soluble in water.

USP requirements:
Podofilox Gel—Not in *USP–NF*.
Podofilox Topical Solution—Not in *USP–NF*.

PODOPHYLLUM

Source: Podophyllum resin—Dried resin from the roots and rhizomes of *Podophyllum peltatum* (mandrake or May apple plant), the North American variety; active constituents are lignans including podophyllotoxin (20%), alpha-peltatin (10%), and beta-peltatin (5%).

Description:
Podophyllum USP—Has a slight odor.
Podophyllum Resin USP—Amorphous powder, varying in color from light brown to greenish yellow, turning darker when subjected to a temperature exceeding 25 °C or when exposed to light. Its alcohol solution is acid to moistened litmus paper.

Solubility: Podophyllum Resin USP—Soluble in alcohol with a slight opalescence; partially soluble in ether and in chloroform. The major active constituent of podophyllum, podophyllotoxin, is lipid soluble.

USP requirements:
Podophyllum USP—Consists of the dried rhizomes and roots of *Podophyllum peltatum* Linné (Fam. Berberidaceae). Yields not less than 5.0% of podophyllum resin. Meets the requirements for Botanic characteristics, Indian podophyllum, Acid-insoluble ash (not more than 2.0%), Foreign organic matter (not more than 2.0%), and Organic volatile impurities.
Podophyllum Resin USP—Preserve in tight, light-resistant containers. The powdered mixture of resins extracted from Podophyllum by percolation with Alcohol and subsequent precipitation from the concentrated percolate upon addition to acidified water. Contains not less than 40.0% and not more than 50.0% of hexane-insoluble matter. Meets the requirements for Identification, Residue on ignition (not more than 1.5%), Distinction from resin of Indian podophyllum, and Hexane-insoluble matter.
Caution: Podophyllum Resin is highly irritating to the eye and to mucous membranes in general.
Podophyllum Resin Topical Solution USP—Preserve in tight, light-resistant containers. A solution in Alcohol consisting of Podophyllum Resin and an alcoholic extract of Benzoin. Contains, in each 100 mL, not less than 10 grams and not more than 13 grams of hexane-insoluble matter. Meets the requirements for Identification, Alcohol content (69.0–72.0%), and Hexane-insoluble matter.
Caution: Podophyllum Resin Topical Solution is highly irritating to the eye and to mucous membranes in general.

POLACRILIN POTASSIUM

Chemical name: 2-Propenoic acid, 2-methyl-, polymer with divinylbenzene, potassium salt.

Description: Polacrilin Potassium NF—White to off-white, free-flowing powder. It has a faint odor or is odorless.

NF category: Tablet disintegrant.

Solubility: Polacrilin Potassium NF—Insoluble in water and in most liquids.

NF requirements: Polacrilin Potassium NF—Preserve in well-closed containers. The potassium salt of a unifunctional low-cross-linked carboxylic cation-exchange resin prepared from methacrylic acid and divinylbenzene. When previously dried at 105 °C for 6 hours, contains not less than 20.6% and not more than 25.1% of potassium. Meets the requirements for Identification, Loss on drying (not more than 10.0%), Powder fineness, Iron (not more than 0.01%), Sodium (not more than 0.20%), Heavy metals (not more than 0.002%), and Organic volatile impurities.

POLIOVIRUS VACCINE

Source: Produced from a mixture of 3 types of attenuated polioviruses that have been propagated in monkey kidney cell culture.
Poliovirus vaccine inactivated (IPV) and Poliovirus vaccine inactivated enhanced potency (enhanced-potency IPV): The polioviruses are inactivated with formaldehyde.
Poliovirus vaccine live oral (OPV): Contains the live, attenuated polioviruses.

Description:
Poliovirus Vaccine Inactivated USP—Clear, reddish-tinged or yellowish liquid, that may have a slight odor because of the preservative.

USP requirements:
Poliovirus Vaccine Inactivated USP (Injection)—Preserve at a temperature between 2 and 8 °C. A sterile aqueous suspension of inactivated poliomyelitis virus of Types 1, 2, and 3. Label it to state that it is to be well shaken before use. Label it also to state that it was prepared in monkey tissue cultures. The virus strains are grown separately in primary cell cultures of monkey kidney tissue, and from a virus suspension with a virus titer of not less than $10^{6.5}$ $TCID_{50}$ measured in comparison with the U.S. Reference Poliovirus of the corresponding type, are inactivated so as to reduce the virus titer by a factor of 10^{-8}, and after inactivation are combined in suitable proportions. No extraneous protein, capable of producing allergenic effects upon injection into human subjects, is added to the final virus production medium. If animal serum is used at any stage, its calculated concentration in the final medium does not exceed 1 part per million. Suitable antimicrobial agents may be used during the production. Meets the requirements of the specific monkey potency test by virus neutralizing antibody production, based on the U.S. Reference Poliovirus Antiserum, such that the ratio of the geometric mean titer of the group of monkey serums representing the vaccine to the mean titer value of the reference serum is not less than 1.29 for Type 1, 1.13 for Type 2, and 0.72 for Type 3. Meets the requirement for Expiration date (not later than 1 year after date of issue from manufacturerãs cold storage [5 °C, 1 year]). Conforms to the regulations of the U.S. Food and Drug Administration concerning biologics.
Poliovirus Vaccine Inactivated Enhanced Potency (Injection)—Not in *USP–NF*.

POLOXALENE

Chemical name: Oxirane, methyl-, polymer with oxirane.

Molecular weight: Approximately 3000.

Description: Poloxalene USP—Colorless or pale yellow liquid.

Solubility: Poloxalene USP—Soluble in water, in chloroform, and in ethylene dichloride.

USP requirements: Poloxalene USP—Preserve in tight containers. A synthetic block copolymer of ethylene oxide and propylene oxide. Label it to indicate that it is for veterinary use only. Contains not less than 98.0% and not more than 103.0% of poloxalene. Meets the requirements for Identification, Average molecular weight (2850–3150), pH (5.0–7.5, in a solution [1 in 40]), Water (not more than 0.4%), Hydroxyl value (36.0–40.0), and Cloud point (42.5–46.5 °C).

POLOXAMER

Chemical group: Nonionic surfactants.

Chemical name: Oxirane, methyl-, polymer with oxirane.

Molecular formula: $HO(C_2H_4O)_a(C_3H_6O)_b(C_2H_4O)_aH$.

Molecular weight: Average—
Poloxamer 124: 2090–2360.
Poloxamer 188: 7680–9510.
Poloxamer 237: 6840–8830.
Poloxamer 338: 12700–17400.
Poloxamer 407: 9840–14600.

Description: Poloxamer NF—Poloxamer 124 is a colorless liquid, having a mild odor. When solidified, it melts at about 16 °C. Poloxamer 188 (melting at about 52 °C), Poloxamer 237 (melting at about 49 °C), Poloxamer 338 (melting at about 57 °C), and Poloxamer 407 (melting at about 56 °C), are white, prilled or cast solids, odorless, or having a very mild odor.
NF category: Emulsifying and/or solubilizing agent.

Solubility: Poloxamer NF—Poloxamer 124 is freely soluble in water, in alcohol, in isopropyl alcohol, in propylene glycol, and in xylene. Poloxamer 188 is freely soluble in water and in alcohol. Poloxamer 237 is freely soluble in water and in alcohol; sparingly soluble in isopropyl alcohol and in xylene. Poloxamer 338 is freely soluble in water and in alcohol; sparingly soluble in propylene glycol. Poloxamer 407 is freely soluble in water, in alcohol, and in isopropyl alcohol.

USP requirements: Poloxamer 188 Capsules—Not in *USP–NF*.

NF requirements: Poloxamer NF—Preserve in tight containers. A synthetic block copolymer of ethylene oxide and propylene oxide. It is available in several types. May contain a suitable antioxidant. Label it to state, as part of the official title, the Poloxamer number. Label it to indicate the name and quantity of any antioxidant. Meets the requirements for Average molecular weight, Weight percent oxyethylene, pH (5.0–7.5, in a solution [1 in 40]), Unsaturation, Heavy metals (not more than 0.002%), Organic volatile impurities, and Limit of free ethylene oxide, propylene oxide, and 1,4-dioxane (not more than 1 mcg of ethylene oxide per gram, not more than 5 mcg of propylene oxide per gram, and not more than 5 mcg of 1,4-dioxane per gram).

POLYACRYLAMIDE

Source: A homopolymer of acrylamide, made of long chains of carbon atoms which are commonly found in fatty acids, carotinoids, and natural rubber.

USP requirements: Polyacrylamide Injection—Not in *USP–NF*.

POLYCARBOPHIL

Chemical name: Polycarbophil.

Description: Polycarbophil UPS—White to creamy white granules, having a characteristic, ester-like odor. Swells in water to a range of volumes, depending primarily on the pH.

Solubility: Polycarbophil USP—Insoluble in water, in dilute acids, in dilute alkalies, and in common organic solvents.

USP requirements: Polycarbophil USP—Preserve in tight containers. Polyacrylic acid cross-linked with divinyl glycol. Meets the requirements for Identification, pH (not more than 4.0), Loss on drying (not more than 1.5%), Residue on ignition (not more than 4.0%), Absorbing power, Limit of acrylic acid (not more than 0.3%), Limit of ethyl acetate (not more than 0.45%), and Organic volatile impurities.

POLYETHYLENE GLYCOL

Chemical name: Poly(oxy-1,2-ethanediyl, alpha-hydro-omega-hydroxy-.

Molecular formula: $H(OCH_2CH_2)_nOH$.

Description:

Polyethylene Glycol NF—Polyethylene Glycol is usually designated by a number that corresponds approximately to its average molecular weight. As the average molecular weight increases, the water solubility, vapor pressure, hygroscopicity, and solubility in organic solvents decrease, while congealing temperature, specific gravity, flash point, and viscosity increase. Liquid grades occur as clear to slightly hazy, colorless or practically colorless, slightly hygroscopic, viscous liquids, having a slight, characteristic odor, and a specific gravity at 25 °C of about 1.12. Solid grades occur as practically odorless white, waxy, plastic material having a consistency similar to beeswax, or as creamy white flakes, beads, or powders. The accompanying table states the approximate congealing temperatures that are characteristic of commonly available grades.

Nominal Molecular Weight Polyethylene Glycol	Approximate Congealing Temperature (°C)
300	−11
400	6
600	20
900	34
1000	38
1450	44
3350	56
4500	58
8000	60

NF category: Coating agent; plasticizer; solvent; suppository base; tablet and/or capsule lubricant.
Polyethylene Glycol Ointment NF—NF category: Ointment base.

Solubility: Polyethylene Glycol NF—Liquid grades are miscible with water; solid grades are freely soluble in water; and all are soluble in acetone, in alcohol, in chloroform, in ethylene glycol monoethyl ether, in ethyl acetate, and in toluene; all are insoluble in ether and in hexane.

NF requirements:

Polyethylene Glycol NF—Preserve in tight containers. An addition polymer of ethylene oxide and water, represented by the formula $H(OCH_2CH_2)_nOH$, in which *n* represents the average number of oxyethylene groups. The average molecular weight is not less than 95.0% and not more than 105.0% of the labeled nominal value if the labeled nominal value is below 1000; it is not less than 90.0% and not more than 110.0% of the labeled nominal value if the labeled nominal value is between 1000 and 7000; it is not less than 87.5% and not more than 112.5% of the labeled nominal value if the labeled nominal value is above 7000. May contain a suitable antioxidant. Label it to state, as part of the official title, the average nominal molecular weight of the Polyethylene Glycol. Label it to indicate the name and quantity of any added antioxidant. Meets the requirements for Completeness and color of solution, Viscosity, Average molecular weight, pH (4.5–7.5, determined potentiometrically), Residue on ignition (not more than 0.1%), Heavy metals (not more than 5 ppm), Limit of free ethylene oxide and 1,4-dioxane (not more than 10 mcg per gram of each), Limit of ethylene glycol and diethylene glycol (not more than 0.25%), and Organic volatile impurities.

Polyethylene Glycol Ointment NF—Preserve in well-closed containers.

Prepare Polyethylene Glycol Ointment as follows: 400 grams of Polyethylene Glycol 3350 and 600 grams of Polyethylene Glycol 400 to make 1000 grams. Heat the two ingredients on a water bath to 65 °C. Allow to cool, and stir until congealed. If a firmer preparation is desired, replace up to 100 grams of the polyethylene glycol 400 with an equal amount of polyethylene glycol 3350.

Note: If 6% to 25% of an aqueous solution is to be incorporated in Polyethylene Glycol Ointment, replace 50 grams of the polyethylene glycol 3350 with an equal amount of stearyl alcohol.

POLYETHYLENE GLYCOL MONOMETHYL ETHER

Chemical name: Poly(oxy-1,2-ethanediyl), alpha-methyl-omega-hydroxy-.

Description: Polyethylene Glycol Monomethyl Ether NF—Polyethylene Glycol Monomethyl Ether is usually designated by a number that corresponds approximately to its average molecular weight. As the average molecular weight increases, the water solubility, vapor pressure, hygroscopicity, and solubility in organic solvents decrease, while congealing temperature, specific gravity, flash point, and viscosity increase. Liquid grades occur as clear to slightly hazy, colorless or practically colorless, slightly hygroscopic, viscous liquids, having a slight, characteristic odor, and a specific gravity at 25 °C of about 1.09–1.10. Solid grades occur as practically odorless, white, waxy, plastic material having a consistency similar to beeswax, or as creamy white flakes, beads, or powders. The accompanying table states the approximate congealing temperatures that are characteristic of commonly available grades.

Nominal Molecular Weight Polyethylene Glycol Monomethyl Ether	Approximate Congealing Temperature (°C)
350	−7
550	17
750	28
1000	35
2000	51
5000	59
8000	60
10000	61

NF category: Ointment base; solvent; plasticizer.

Solubility: Polyethylene Glycol Monomethyl Ether NF—Liquid grades are miscible with water; solid grades are freely soluble in water; and all are soluble in acetone, in alcohol, in chloroform, in ethylene glycol monoethyl ether, in ethyl acetate, and in toluene; all are insoluble in ether and in hexane.

NF requirements: Polyethylene Glycol Monomethyl Ether NF—Preserve in tight containers. An addition polymer of ethylene oxide and methanol, represented by the formula $CH_3(OCH_2CH_2)_nOH$, in which n represents the average number of oxyethylene groups. The average molecular weight is not less than 95.0% and not more than 105.0% of the labeled nominal value if the labeled nominal value is below 1000; it is not less than 90.0% and not more than 110.0% of the labeled nominal value if the labeled nominal value is between 1000 and 4750; it is not less than 87.5% and not more than 112.5% of the labeled nominal value if the labeled nominal value is above 4750. Label it to state, as part of the official title, the average nominal molecular weight of the Polyethylene Glycol Monomethyl Ether. Meets the requirements for Completeness and color of solution, Viscosity, Average molecular weight, pH (4.5–7.5, determined potentiometrically), Residue on ignition (not more than 0.1%), Heavy metals (not more than 5 ppm), Free ethylene oxide and 1,4-dioxane (not more than 10 ppm of each), Limit of ethylene glycol and diethylene glycol (not more than 0.25%), and Limit of 2-methoxyethanol (not more than 10 ppm).

POLYETHYLENE GLYCOL 3350

Molecular formula: Polyethylene Glycol 3350 NF—HO(-C_2H_4O)$_n$H.

Molecular weight: Polyethylene Glycol 3350 NF—3350.

Description: Polyethylene Glycol 3350 NF—A free flowing white powder below 55 °C.

Solubility: Polyethylene Glycol 3350 NF—Freely soluble in water.

NF requirements: Polyethylene Glycol 3350 Powder NF—Not in *USP–NF*.

POLYETHYLENE OXIDE

Description: Polyethylene Oxide NF—Polyethylene oxide resins are high molecular weight polymers having the common structure (–O–CH_2CH_2–)$_n$, in which n, the degree of polymerization, varies from about 2000 to over 100,000. Polyethylene oxide, being a polyether, strongly hydrogen, bonds with water. It is nonionic and undergoes salting-out effects associated with neutral molecules in solutions of high dielectric media. Salting-out effects manifest themselves in depressing the upper temperature limit of solubility, and in reducing the viscosity of both dilute and concentrated solutions of the polymers. All molecular weight grades are powdered or granular solids.

NF category: Suspending and/or viscosity-increasing agent; tablet binder.

Solubility: Polyethylene Oxide NF—Soluble in water, but, because of the high solution viscosities obtained (see table), solutions over 1% in water may be difficult to prepare.

Approximate Molecular Weight	Typical Solution Viscosity (cps), 25 °C	
	5 % Solution	1% Solution
100,000	40	
200,000	100	
300,000	800	
400,000	3000	
600,000	6000	
900,000	15000	
4,000,000		3500
5,000,000		5500

The water solubility, hygroscopicity, solubility in organic solvents, and melting point do not vary in the specified molecular weight range. At room temperature polyethylene oxide is miscible with water in all proportions. At concentrations of about 20% polymer in water the solutions are nontacky, reversible, elastic gels. At higher concentrations, the solutions are tough, elastic materials with the water acting as a plasticizer. Polyethylene oxide is also freely soluble in acetonitrile, in ethylene dichloride, in trichloroethylene, and in methylene chloride. Heating may be required to obtain solutions in many other organic solvents. It is insoluble in aliphatic hydrocarbons, in ethylene glycol, in diethylene glycol, and in glycerol.

NF requirements: Polyethylene Oxide NF—Preserve in tight, light-resistant containers. A nonionic homopolymer of ethylene oxide, represented by the formula $(OCH_2CH_2)_n$, in which n represents the average number of oxyethylene groups. It is a white to off-white powder obtainable in several grades, varying in viscosity profile in an aqueous isopropyl alcohol solution. It may contain a suitable antioxidant. The labeling indicates its viscosity profile in aqueous isopropyl alcohol solution. Label it to indicate the name and quantity of any added antioxident. Meets the requirements for Identification, Loss on drying (not more than 1.0%), Silicon dioxide and nonsilicon dioxide residue on ignition, Heavy metals (not more than 0.001%), Limit of free ethylene oxide (not more than 0.001%), and Organic volatile impurities.

POLYMYXIN B

Chemical group: Polypeptide.

Chemical name: Polymyxin B sulfate—Polymyxin B, sulfate.

Description:
Polymyxin B for Injection USP—White to buff-colored powder. Odorless or has a faint odor.
Polymyxin B Sulfate USP—White to buff-colored powder. Odorless or has a faint odor.

Solubility:
Polymyxin B for Injection USP—Freely soluble in water; slightly soluble in alcohol.
Polymyxin B Sulfate USP—Freely soluble in water; slightly soluble in alcohol.

USP requirements:

Polymyxin B for Injection USP—Preserve in Containers for Sterile Solids, protected from light. Label it to indicate that where it is administered intramuscularly and/or intrathecally, it is to be given only to patients hospitalized so as to provide constant supervision by a physician. Contains an amount of Polymyxin B Sulfate equivalent to the labeled amount of polymyxin B, within −10% to +20%. Meets the requirements for Thin-layer chromatographic identification test, Constituted solution, Pyrogen, Sterility, Particulate matter, Residue on ignition (not more than 5.0%), and Heavy metals (not more than 0.01%), pH and Loss on drying under Polymyxin B Sulfate, and for Uniformity of dosage units and for Labeling under Injections.

Polymyxin B Sulfate USP—Preserve in tight, light-resistant containers. The sulfate salt of a kind of polymyxin, a substance produced by the growth of *Bacillus polymyxa* (Prazmowski) Migula (Fam. Bacillaceae), or a mixture of two or more such salts. Where packaged for prescription compounding, the label states the number of Polymyxin B Units in the container and per milligram, that it is not intended for manufacturing use, that it is not sterile, and that its potency cannot be assured for longer than 60 days after opening. Where it is intended for use in preparing injectable or other sterile dosage forms, the label states that it is sterile or must be subjected to further processing during the preparation of injectable or other sterile dosage forms. Has a potency of not less than 6000 Polymyxin B Units per mg, calculated on the dried basis. Meets the requirements for Identification, Content of phenylalamine (9–12% of phenylalamine, calculated on the dried basis), pH (5.0–7.5, in a solution containing 5 mg per mL), and Loss on drying (not more than 7.0%), and for Residue on ignition under Polymyxin B for Injection (if for prescription compounding), and for Sterility tests (where the label states that Polymyxin B Sulfate is sterile) and Pyrogen Polymyxin B for Injection (where intended for injectable dosage forms), and for Pyrogen under Polymyxin B for Injection (where the label states that Polymyxin Sulfate must be subjected to further processing during the preparation of injectable dosage forms.

Polymyxin B Sulfate for Ophthalmic Solution—Not in *USP–NF.*

POLYMYXIN B AND BACITRACIN

For *Polymyxin B* and *Bacitracin*—See individual listings for chemistry information.

USP requirements:

Polymyxin B Sulfate and Bacitracin Zinc Topical Aerosol USP—Preserve in pressurized containers, and avoid exposure to excessive heat. Contains amounts of polymyxin B sulfate and bacitracin zinc equivalent to the labeled amounts of polymyxin B and bacitracin, within −10% to +30%. Meets the requirements for Identification, Microbial limits, and Water (not more than 0.5%), and for Pressure test, Minimum fill, and Leakage test under Aerosols, Metered-dose inhalers, and Dry powder inhalers.

Polymyxin B Sulfate and Bacitracin Zinc Topical Powder USP—Preserve in well-closed containers. Contains amounts of polymyxin B sulfate and bacitracin zinc equivalent to the labeled amounts of polymyxin B and bacitracin, within −10% to +30%. Meets the requirements for Microbial limits and Water (not more than 7.0%).

POLYMYXIN B AND HYDROCORTISONE

For *Polymyxin B* and *Hydrocortisone*—See individual listings for chemistry information.

USP requirements: Polymyxin B Sulfate and Hydrocortisone Otic Solution USP—Preserve in tight, light-resistant containers. A sterile solution. Contains an amount of polymyxin B sulfate equivalent to the labeled amount of polymyxin B, within −10% to +30%, and the labeled amount of hydrocortisone, within ±10%. Meets the requirements for Sterility and pH (3.0–5.0).

Note: Where Polymyxin B Sulfate and Hydrocortisone Otic Solution is prescribed, without reference to the quantity of polymyxin B or hydrocortisone contained therein, a product containing 10,000 Polymyxin B Units and 5 mg of hydrocortisone per mL shall be dispensed.

POLYMYXIN B AND TRIMETHOPRIM

For *Polymyxin B* and *Trimethoprim*—See individual listings for chemistry information.

USP requirements: Polymyxin B Sulfate and Trimethoprim Ophthalmic Solution USP—Preserve in tight, light-resistant containers, and store at controlled room temperature. A sterile, isotonic, aqueous solution of Polymixin B Sulfate and Trimethoprim Sulfate or of Polymyxin B Sulfate and Trimethoprim that has been solubilized with sulfuric acid. Label it to indicate that it is to be stored at 15° to 25°, protected from light. Contains the labeled amount of polymyxin B, within −10% to +30% and the amount equivalent to the labeled amount of trimethoprim, within ±10%. Contains one or more preservatives. Meets the requirements for Identification, Sterility, and pH (4.0–6.2).

POLYOXYL 10 OLEYL ETHER

Chemical name: Polyoxy-1,2-ethanediyl, alpha-[(*Z*)-9-octadecenyl-omega-hydroxy-.

Description: Polyoxyl 10 Oleyl Ether NF—White, soft semisolid, or pale yellow liquid, having a bland odor.

NF category: Emulsifying and/or solubilizing agent; wetting and or solubilizing agent.

Solubility: Polyoxyl 10 Oleyl Ether NF—Soluble in water and in alcohol; dispersible in mineral oil and in propylene glycol, with possible separation on standing.

NF requirements: Polyoxyl 10 Oleyl Ether NF—Preserve in tight containers, in a cool place. A mixture of the monooleyl ethers of mixed polyoxyethylene diols, the average polymer length being equivalent to not less than 8.6 and not more than 10.4 oxyethylene units. Label it to indicate the names and proportions of any added stabilizers. Meets the requirements for Identification, Water (not more than 3.0%), Residue on ignition (not more than 0.4%), Heavy metals (not more than 0.002%), Acid value (not more than 1.0), Hydroxyl value (75–95), Iodine value (23–40), Saponification value (not more than 3), Free polyethylene glycols (not more than 7.5%), Free ethylene oxide (not more than 0.01%), Average polymer length, and Organic volatile impurities.

POLYOXYL 20 CETOSTEARYL ETHER

Description: Polyoxyl 20 Cetostearyl Ether NF—Cream-colored, waxy, unctuous mass, melting, when heated, to a clear, brownish yellow liquid.

NF category: Emulsifying and/or solubilizing agent; wetting and/or solubilizing agent.

Solubility: Polyoxyl 20 Cetostearyl Ether NF—Soluble in water, in alcohol, and in acetone; insoluble in solvent hexane.

NF requirements: Polyoxyl 20 Cetostearyl Ether NF—Preserve in tight containers, in a cool place. A mixture of monocetostearyl (mixed hexadecyl and octadecyl) ethers of mixed polyoxyethylene diols, the average polymer length being equivalent to not less than 17.2 and not more than 25.0 oxyethylene units. Meets the requirements for Identification, pH (4.5–7.5, determined in a solution [1 in 10]), Water (not more than 1.0%), Residue on ignition (not more than 0.4%), Heavy metals (not more than 0.002%), Acid value (not more than 0.5%), Hydroxyl value (42–60), Saponification value (not more than 2), Free polyethylene glycols (not more than 7.5%), Free ethylene oxide (not more than 0.01%), Average polymer length, and Organic volatile impurities.

POLYOXYL 35 CASTOR OIL

Description: Polyoxyl 35 Castor Oil NF—Yellow, oily liquid, having a faint, characteristic odor.

NF category: Emulsifying and/or solubilizing agent; wetting and/or solubilizing agent.

Solubility: Polyoxyl 35 Castor Oil NF—Very soluble in water, producing a practically odorless and colorless solution; soluble in alcohol and in ethyl acetate; insoluble in mineral oils.

NF requirements: Polyoxyl 35 Castor Oil NF—Preserve in tight containers. Contains mainly the tri-ricinoleate ester of ethoxylated glycerol, with smaller amounts of polyethylene glycol ricinoleate and the corresponding free glycols. Results from the reaction of glycerol ricinoleate with about 35 moles of ethylene oxide. Meets the requirements for Identification, Specific gravity (1.05–1.06), Viscosity (650–850 centipoises at 25 °C), Water (not more than 3.0%), Residue on ignition (not more than 0.3%), Heavy metals (not more than 0.001%), Acid value (not more than 2.0), Hydroxyl value (65–80), Iodine value (25–35), Saponification value (60–75), and Organic volatile impurities.

POLYOXYL 40 HYDROGENATED CASTOR OIL

Description: Polyoxyl 40 Hydrogenated Castor Oil NF—White to yellowish paste or pasty liquid, having a faint odor.

NF category: Emulsifying and/or solubilizing agent; wetting and/or solubilizing agent.

Solubility: Polyoxyl 40 Hydrogenated Castor Oil NF—Very soluble in water, producing a practically odorless and colorless solution; soluble in alcohol and in ethyl acetate; insoluble in mineral oils.

NF requirements: Polyoxyl 40 Hydrogenated Castor Oil NF—Preserve in tight containers. Contains mainly the tri-hydroxystearate ester of ethoxylated glycerol, with smaller amounts of polyethylene glycol tri-hydroxystearate and of the corresponding free glycols. Results from the reaction of glycerol tri-hydroxystearate with about 40 to 45 moles of ethylene oxide. Meets the requirements for Identification, Congealing temperature (16–26 °C), Water (not more than 3.0%), Residue on ignition (not more than 0.3%), Heavy metals (not more than 0.001%), Acid value (not more than 2.0), Hydroxyl value (60–80), Iodine value (not more than 2.0), Saponification value (45–69), and Organic volatile impurities.

POLYOXYL 40 STEARATE

Chemical name: Poly(oxy-1,2-ethanediyl), alpha-hydro-omega-hydroxy-, octadecanoate.

Description: Polyoxyl 40 Stearate NF—Waxy, white to light tan solid. It is odorless or has a faint fat-like odor.

NF category: Emulsifying and/or solubilizing agent; wetting and/or solubilizing agent.

Solubility: Polyoxyl 40 Stearate NF—Soluble in water, in alcohol, in ether, and in acetone; insoluble in mineral oil and in vegetable oils.

NF requirements: Polyoxyl 40 Stearate NF—Preserve in tight containers. A mixture of the monoesters and di-esters of Stearic Acid or Purified Stearic Acid with mixed polyoxyethylene diols, the average polymer length being about 40 oxyethylene units. Meets the requirements for Identification, Congealing temperature (37–47 °C), Water (not more than 3.0%), Heavy metals (not more than 0.001%), Acid value (not more than 2), Hydroxyl value (25–40), Saponification value (25–35), Free polyethylene glycols (17–27%), and Organic volatile impurities.

POLYOXYL 50 STEARATE

Chemical name: Poly(oxy-1,2-ethanediyl), alpha-(1-oxooctadecyl)-omega-hydroxy-.

Description: Polyoxyl 50 Stearate NF—Soft, cream-colored, waxy solid, having a faint, fat-like odor. Melts at about 45 °C.

NF category: Wetting and/or solubilizing agent.

Solubility: Polyoxyl 50 Stearate NF—Soluble in water and in isopropyl alcohol.

NF requirements: Polyoxyl 50 Stearate NF—Preserve in tight containers. A mixture of the monostearate and distearate esters of mixed polyoxyethylene diols and the corresponding free diols. The average polymer length is equivalent to about 50 oxyethylene units. Meets the requirements for Identification, Acid value (not more than 2), Hydroxyl value (23–35), Saponification value (20–28), Free polyethylene glycols (17–27%), and Organic volatile impurities, and for Water and Heavy metals under Polyoxyl 40 Stearate.

POLYSORBATE 20

Chemical name: Sorbitan, monododecanoate, poly(oxy-1,2-ethanediyl) derivs.

Molecular formula: $C_{58}H_{114}O_{26}$ (approximate).

Description: Polysorbate 20 NF—Lemon to amber liquid, having a faint characteristic odor.

NF category: Emulsifying and/or solubilizing agent; wetting and/or solubilizing agent.

Solubility: Polysorbate 20 NF—Soluble in water, in alcohol, in ethyl acetate, in methanol, and in dioxane; insoluble in mineral oil.

NF requirements: Polysorbate 20 NF—Preserve in tight containers. A laurate ester of sorbitol and its anhydrides copolymerized with approximately 20 moles of ethylene oxide for each mole of sorbitol and sorbitol anhydrides. Meets the requirements for Identification, Hydroxyl value (96–108), Saponification value (40–50), and Organic volatile impurities, and for Water, Residue on ignition, Heavy metals, and Acid value under Polysorbate 80.

POLYSORBATE 40

Chemical name: Sorbitan, monohexadecanoate, poly(oxy-1,2-ethanediyl) derivs.

Molecular formula: $C_{62}H_{122}O_{26}$ (approximate).

Description: Polysorbate 40 NF—Yellow liquid, having a faint, characteristic odor.

    NF category: Emulsifying and/or solubilizing agent; wetting and/or solubilizing agent.

Solubility: Polysorbate 40 NF—Soluble in water and in alcohol; insoluble in mineral oil and in vegetable oils.

NF requirements: Polysorbate 40 NF—Preserve in tight containers. A palmitate ester of sorbitol and its anhydrides copolymerized with approximately 20 moles of ethylene oxide for each mole of sorbitol and sorbitol anhydrides. Meets the requirements for Identification, Hydroxyl value (89–105), Saponification value (41–52), and Organic volatile impurities, and for Water, Residue on ignition, Heavy metals, and Acid value under Polysorbate 80.

POLYSORBATE 60

Chemical name: Sorbitan, monooctadecanoate, poly(oxy-1,2-ethanediyl) derivs.

Molecular formula: $C_{64}H_{126}O_{26}$ (approximate).

Description: Polysorbate 60 NF—Lemon- to orange-colored, oily liquid or semi-gel, having a faint, characteristic odor.

    NF category: Emulsifying and/or solubilizing agent; wetting and/or solubilizing agent.

Solubility: Polysorbate 60 NF—Soluble in water, in ethyl acetate, and in toluene; insoluble in mineral oil and in vegetable oils.

NF requirements: Polysorbate 60 NF—Preserve in tight containers. A mixture of stearate and palmitate esters of sorbitol and its anhydrides copolymerized with approximately 20 moles of ethylene oxide for each mole of sorbitol and sorbitol anhydrides. Meets the requirements for Identification, Hydroxyl value (81–96), and Saponification value (45–55), and for Water, Residue on ignition, Heavy metals, Acid value under Polysorbate 80, and Organic volatile impurities.

POLYSORBATE 80

Chemical name: Sorbitan, mono-9-octadecenoate, poly(oxy-1,2-ethanediyl) derivs., (Z)-.

Description: Polysorbate 80 NF—Lemon- to amber-colored, oily liquid, having a faint, characteristic odor.

    NF category: Emulsifying and/or solubilizing agent; wetting and/or solubilizing agent.

Solubility: Polysorbate 80 NF—Very soluble in water, producing an odorless and practically colorless solution; soluble in alcohol and in ethyl acetate; insoluble in mineral oil.

NF requirements: Polysorbate 80 NF—Preserve in tight containers. An oleate ester of sorbitol and its anhydrides copolymerized with approximately 20 moles of ethylene oxide for each mole of sorbitol and sorbitol anhydrides. Meets the requirements for Identification, Specific gravity (1.06–1.09), Viscosity (300–500 centistokes when determined at 25 °C), Water (not more than 3.0%), Residue on ignition (not more than 0.25%), Heavy metals (not more than 0.001%), Acid value (2.2), Hydroxyl value (65–80), Saponification value (45–55), and Organic volatile impurities.

POLYTHIAZIDE

Chemical name: 2H-1,2,4-Benzothiadiazine-7-sulfonamide, 6-chloro-3,4-dihydro-2-methyl-3-[[(2,2,2-trifluoroethyl)thio]-methyl]-, 1,1-dioxide.

Molecular formula: $C_{11}H_{13}ClF_3N_3O_4S_3$.

Molecular weight: 439.88.

Description: Polythiazide USP—White, crystalline powder, having a characteristic odor.

Solubility: Polythiazide USP—Practically insoluble in water and in chloroform; soluble in methanol and in acetone.

USP requirements:

    Polythiazide USP—Preserve in tight, light-resistant containers. Dried in vacuum at 60 °C for 2 hours, contains not less than 97.0% and not more than 101.0% of polythiazide. Meets the requirements for Identification, Melting range (207–217 °C, with decomposition), Loss on drying (not more than 1.0%), Residue on ignition (not more than 0.2%), Selenium (not more than 0.003%), Heavy metals (not more than 0.0025%), and Diazotizable substances (not more than 1.0%).

    Polythiazide Tablets USP—Preserve in tight, light-resistant containers. Contain the labeled amount, within ±10%. Meet the requirements for Identification, Dissolution (50% in 90 minutes in dilute hydrochloric acid [1 in 100] in Apparatus 2 at 50 rpm), and Uniformity of dosage units.

POLYVINYL ACETATE PHTHALATE

Description: Polyvinyl Acetate Phthalate NF—Free-flowing, white powder. May have a slight odor of acetic acid.

    NF category: Coating agent.

Solubility: Polyvinyl Acetate Phthalate NF—Insoluble in water, in methylene chloride, and in chloroform. Soluble in methanol and in alcohol.

NF requirements: Polyvinyl Acetate Phthalate NF—Preserve in tight containers. A reaction product of phthalic anhydride and partially hydrolyzed polyvinyl acetate. Contains not less than 55.0% and not more than 62.0% of phthalyl (o-carboxybenzoyl, $C_8H_5O_3$) groups, calculated on an anhydrous acid-free basis. Meets the requirements for Identification, Viscosity (7–11 centipoises, determined at 25 °C ±0.2 °C [apparent]), Water (not more than 5.0%), Residue on ignition (not more than 1.0%), Free phthalic acid (not more than 0.6%, on the anhydrous basis), Free acid other than phthalic (not more than 0.6%, on the anhydrous basis), Phthalyl content, and Organic volatile impurities.

POLYVINYL ALCOHOL

Chemical name: Ethenol, homopolymer.

Molecular formula: $(C_2H_4O)_n$.

Description: Polyvinyl Alcohol USP—White to cream-colored granules, or white to cream-colored powder. Is odorless.
NF category: Suspending and/or viscosity-increasing agent.

Solubility: Polyvinyl Alcohol USP—Freely soluble in water at room temperature. Solution may be effected more rapidly at somewhat higher temperatures.

USP requirements: Polyvinyl Alcohol USP—Preserve in well-closed containers. A water-soluble synthetic resin, represented by the formula: $(C_2H_4O)_n$, in which the average value of *n* lies between 500 and 5000. Prepared by 85 to 89% hydrolysis of polyvinyl acetate. The apparent viscosity, in centipoises, at 20 °C, of a solution containing 4 grams of Polyvinyl Alcohol in each 100 grams, is within ±15% of that stated on the label. Meets the requirements for Viscosity, pH (5.0–8.0, in a solution [1 in 25]), Loss on drying (not more than 5.0%), Residue on ignition (not more than 2.0%), Water-insoluble substances (not more than 0.1%), Degree of hydrolysis (85–89%), and Organic volatile impurities.

PORACTANT ALFA

Source: An extract of procine (pig) lung containing not less than 90% of phospholipids, about 1% of hydrophobic proteins (SP-B and SP-C) and about 90% of other lipids.

Other characteristics: pH of 6.2 (5.5–6.5), adjusted with salium bicarbonate.

USP requirements: Poractant Alfa Intratracheal Suspension—Not in *USP–NF*.

PORFIMER

Source: Porfimer sodium—A mixture of oligomers formed by ether and ester linkages of up to eight porphyrin units.

Chemical name: Porfimer sodium—Photofrin II.

Molecular weight: Porfimer sodium—1178–4659 depending on the number of porphyrin units.

Description: Porfimer sodium—When freeze-dried, dark red to reddish-brown cake or crystalline powder which is hygroscopic. Has no melting point and decomposes above 250 °C.

Solubility: Porfimer sodium—Aqueous solubility at least 25 mg/mL at pH 7–8; soluble in methanol; insoluble in methylene chloride.

USP requirements: Sterile Porfimer Sodium for Injection—Not in *USP–NF*.

SULFURATED POTASH

Chemical name: Thiosulfuric acid, dipotassium salt, mixt. with potassium sulfide (K_2S_x).

Description: Sulfurated Potash USP—Irregular, liver-brown pieces when freshly made, changing to a greenish-yellow. Has an odor of hydrogen sulfide and decomposes on exposure to air. A solution (1 in 10) is light brown in color and is alkaline to litmus.

Solubility: Sulfurated Potash USP—Freely soluble in water, usually leaving a slight residue. Alcohol dissolves only the sulfides.

USP requirements: Sulfurated Potash USP—Preserve in tight containers. Containers from which it is to be taken for immediate use in compounding prescriptions contain not more than 120 grams. A mixture composed chiefly of potassium polysulfides and potassium thiosulfate. Contains not less than 12.8% of sulfur in combination as sulfide. Meets the requirements for Identification and Organic volatile impurities.

POTASSIUM ACETATE

Chemical name: Acetic acid, potassium salt.

Molecular formula: $C_2H_3KO_2$.

Molecular weight: 98.14.

Description: Potassium Acetate USP—Colorless, monoclinic crystals or white, crystalline powder. Is odorless, or has a faint acetous odor. Deliquesces on exposure to moist air.

Solubility: Potassium Acetate USP—Very soluble in water; freely soluble in alcohol.

USP requirements:
Potassium Acetate USP—Preserve in tight containers. Contains not less than 99.0% and not more than 100.5% of potassium acetate, calculated on the dried basis. Meets the requirements for Identification, pH (7.5–8.5, in a solution [1 in 20]), Loss on drying (not more than 1.0%), Heavy metals (not more than 0.002%), and Sodium (not more than 0.03%).
Potassium Acetate Injection USP—Preserve in single-dose or in multiple-dose containers, preferably of Type I or Type II glass. A sterile solution of Potassium Acetate in Water for Injection. The label states the potassium acetate content in terms of weight and of milliequivalents in a given volume. Label the Injection to indicate that it is to be diluted to appropriate strength with water or other suitable fluid prior to administration. The label states also the total osmolar concentration in mOsmol per liter. Where the contents are less than 100 mL, or where the label states that the Injection is not for direct injection but is to be diluted before use, the label alternatively may state the total osmolar concentration in mOsmol per mL. Contains the labeled amount, within ±5%. Meets the requirements for Identification, Bacterial endotoxins, pH (5.5–8.0, when diluted with water to 1.0% of potassium acetate), and Particulate matter, and for Injections.

POTASSIUM BENZOATE

Chemical name: Benzoic acid, potassium salt.

Molecular formula: $C_7H_5KO_2$.

Molecular weight: 160.21.

Description: Potassium Benzoate NF—White, odorless, or practically odorless, granular or crystalline powder. Stable in air.
NF category: Antimicrobial preservative.

Solubility: Potassium Benzoate NF—Freely soluble in water; sparingly soluble in alcohol and somewhat more soluble in 90% alcohol.

NF requirements: Potassium Benzoate NF—Preserve in well-closed containers. Contains not less than 99.0% and not more than 100.5% of potassium benzoate, calculated on the anhy-

drous basis. Meets the requirements for Identification, Alkalinity, Water (not more than 1.5%), Heavy metals (not more than 0.001%), and Organic volatile impurities.

the labeled amounts of potassium and chloride, within ± 10%. Meet the requirements for Identification and Uniformity of dosage units.

POTASSIUM BICARBONATE

Chemical name: Carbonic acid, monopotassium salt.

Molecular formula: $KHCO_3$.

Molecular weight: 100.12.

Description: Potassium Bicarbonate USP—Colorless, transparent, monoclinic prisms or as a white, granular powder. Is odorless, and is stable in air. Its solutions are neutral or alkaline to phenolphthalein TS.

Solubility: Potassium Bicarbonate USP—Freely soluble in water; practically insoluble in alcohol.

USP requirements:
Potassium Bicarbonate USP—Preserve in well-closed containers. Contains not less than 99.5% and not more than 101.5% of potassium bicarbonate, calculated on the dried basis. Meets the requirements for Identification, Loss on drying (not more than 0.3%), Normal carbonate (not more than 2.5%), Heavy metals (not more than 0.001%), and Organic volatile impurities.
Potassium Bicarbonate Effervescent Tablets for Oral Solution USP—Preserve in tight containers, protected from excessive heat. The label states the potassium content in terms of weight and in terms of milliequivalents. Where the Tablets are packaged in individual pouches, the label instructs the user not to open until the time of use. Contain an amount of potassium bicarbonate equivalent to the labeled amount of potassium, within ±10%. Meet the requirements for Identification and Uniformity of dosage units.

POTASSIUM BICARBONATE AND POTASSIUM CHLORIDE

For *Potassium Bicarbonate* and *Potassium Chloride*—See individual listings for chemistry information.

USP requirements:
Potassium Bicarbonate and Potassium Chloride for Effervescent Oral Solution USP—Preserve in tight containers, protected from excessive heat. The label states the potassium and chloride contents in terms of weight and in terms of milliequivalents. Where packaged in individual pouches, the label instructs the user not to open until the time of use. Contains amounts of potassium bicarbonate and potassium chloride equivalent to the labeled amounts of potassium and chloride, within ±10%. Meets the requirements for Identification, Uniformity of dosage units (single-unit containers), and Minimum fill (multiple-unit containers).
Potassium Bicarbonate and Potassium Chloride Effervescent Tablets for Oral Solution USP—Preserve in tight containers, protected from excessive heat. The label states the potassium and chloride contents in terms of weight and in terms of milliequivalents. Where the Tablets are packaged in individual pouches, the label instructs the user not to open until the time of use. Contain amounts of potassium bicarbonate and potassium chloride equivalent to

POTASSIUM BICARBONATE AND POTASSIUM CITRATE

For *Potassium Bicarbonate* and *Potassium Citrate*—See individual listings for chemistry information.

USP requirements: Potassium Bicarbonate and Potassium Citrate Effervescent Tablets for Oral Solution—Not in *USP–NF*.

POTASSIUM AND SODIUM BICARBONATES AND CITRIC ACID

For *Potassium Bicarbonate, Sodium Bicarbonate,* and *Citric Acid*—See individual listings for chemistry information.

USP requirements: Potassium and Sodium Bicarbonates and Citric Acid Effervescent Tablets for Oral Solution USP—Preserve in tight containers. Label it to state the sodium content. The label states also that the Tablets are to be dissolved in water before being taken. Contain the labeled amounts of potassium bicarbonate, sodium bicarbonate, and anhydrous citric acid, within ±10%. Meet the requirements for Identification and Acid-neutralizing capacity.

POTASSIUM BITARTRATE

Chemical name: Butanedioic acid, 2,3-dihydroxy-, [R-(R*,R*)]-, monopotassium salt.

Molecular formula: $C_4H_5KO_6$.

Molecular weight: 188.18.

Description: Potassium Bitartrate USP—Colorless or slightly opaque crystals, or white crystalline powder. A saturated solution is acid to litmus.

Solubility: Potassium Bitartrate USP—Soluble in boiling water; slightly soluble in water; very slightly soluble in alcohol.

USP requirements: Potassium Bitartrate USP—Preserve in tight containers. Dried at 105 °C for 3 hours, contains not less than 99.0% and not more than 101.0% of potassium bitartrate. Meets the requirements for Identification, Insoluble matter, Ammonia, and Heavy metals (not more than 0.002%).

POTASSIUM BITARTRATE AND SODIUM BICARBONATE

For *Potassium Bitartrate* and *Sodium Bicarbonate*—See individual listings for chemistry information.

USP requirements: Potassium Bitartrate and Sodium Bicarbonate Suppositories—Not in *USP–NF*.

POTASSIUM CARBONATE

Chemical name: Carbonic acid, dipotassium salt.

Molecular formula: K_2CO_3.

Molecular weight: 138.21.

Description: Hygroscopic, odorless granules or granular powder.

Solubility: Soluble in 1 part cold, 0.7 part boiling water; practically insoluble in alcohol.

USP requirements: Potassium Carbonate USP—Preserve in well-closed containers. Contains not less than 99.5% and not more than 100.5% of potassium carbonate, calculated on the dried basis. Meets the requirements for Identification, Loss on drying (not more than 0.5%), Insoluble substances, Heavy metals (not more than 0.0005%), and Organic volatile impurities.

POTASSIUM CHLORIDE

Chemical name: Potassium chloride.

Molecular formula: KCl.

Molecular weight: 74.55.

Description: Potassium Chloride USP—Colorless, elongated, prismatic, or cubical crystals, or white, granular powder. Is odorless and is stable in air. Its solutions are neutral to litmus. NF category: Tonicity agent.

Solubility: Potassium Chloride USP—Freely soluble in water and even more soluble in boiling water; insoluble in alcohol.

USP requirements:

Potassium Chloride USP—Preserve in well-closed containers. Where Potassium Chloride is intended for use in hemodialysis, it is so labeled. Contains not less than 99.0% and not more than 100.5% of potassium chloride, calculated on the dried basis. Meets the requirements for Identification, Acidity or alkalinity, Loss on drying (not more than 1.0%), Iodide or bromide, Aluminum (not more than 1 mcg per gram), Calcium and magnesium, Sodium, Heavy metals (not more than 0.001%), and Organic volatile impurities.

Potassium Chloride Extended-release Capsules USP—Preserve in tight containers at a temperature not exceeding 30 °C. Contain the labeled amount, within ±10%. Meet the requirements for Identification, Dissolution (not more than 35% of labeled amount in 2 hours in water in Apparatus 1 at 100 rpm), and Uniformity of dosage units.

Potassium Chloride for Injection Concentrate USP—Preserve in single-dose or in multiple-dose containers, preferably of Type I or Type II glass. A sterile solution of Potassium Chloride in Water for Injection. The label states the potassium chloride content in terms of weight and of milliequivalents in a given volume. Label the Concentrate to indicate that it is to be diluted to appropriate strength with water or other suitable fluid prior to administration. Immediately following the name, the label bears the boxed warning: **Concentrate Must be Diluted Before Use.** This warning is not required when the liquid preparation is in a *Pharmacy bulk package* and the label thereon states prominently "Pharmacy Bulk Package—Not for direct infusion." The cap of the container and the overseal of the cap must be black and both bear the words: "Must be Diluted" in readily legible type, in a color that stands out from its background OR the overseal may be of a clear plastic material through which the black cap is visible and the printing is readily legible. When the nature of the container-closure system prevents compliance, the design shall follow the intent of this requirement as closely as possible, the black color

being used beneath the words "Must be Diluted," which are so placed that words are readily visible as the contents of the container are being removed. Ampuls shall be identified by a black band or a series of black bands above the constriction. The label states also the total osmolar concentration in mOsmol per liter. Where the contents are less than 100 mL, the label alternatively may state the total osmolar concentration in mOsmol per mL. Contains the labeled amount, within ±5%. Meets the requirements for Identification, Bacterial endotoxins, pH (4.0–8.0), and Particulate matter, and for Injections.

Potassium Chloride Oral Solution USP—Preserve in tight containers. Contains the labeled amount, within ±5%. May contain alcohol. Meets the requirements for Identification and Alcohol content (within −10% to +15% of the labeled amount which is not more than 7.5%).

Potassium Chloride for Oral Solution USP—Preserve in tight containers. A dry mixture of Potassium Chloride and one or more suitable colors, diluents, and flavors. The label states the Potassium Chloride content in terms of weight and in terms of milliequivalents. Contains the labeled amount, within ±10%. Meets the requirements for Identification, Minimum fill (multiple-unit containers), and Uniformity of dosage units (single-unit containers).

Potassium Chloride for Oral Suspension—Not in *USP–NF*.

Potassium Chloride Extended-release Tablets USP—Preserve in tight containers at a temperature not exceeding 30 °C. The labeling states with which Assay Preparation the product complies only if Assay Preparation 1 is not used. Contain the labeled amount, within ±10%. Meet the requirements for Identification, Dissolution (35% in water in 2 hours in Apparatus 2 at 50 rpm), and Uniformity of dosage units.

POTASSIUM CHLORIDE AND DEXTROSE

For *Potassium Chloride* and *Dextrose*—See individual listings for chemistry information.

USP requirements: Potassium Chloride in Dextrose Injection USP—Preserve in single-dose glass or plastic containers. Glass containers are preferably of Type I or Type II glass. A sterile solution of Potassium Chloride and Dextrose in Water for Injection. The label states the total osmolar concentration in mOsmol per liter. Where the contents are less than 100 mL, or where the label states that the Injection is not for direct injection but is to be diluted before use, the label alternatively may state the total osmolar concentration in mOsmol per mL. The content of potassium, in milliequivalents, is prominently displayed on the label. Contains the labeled amounts of potassium chloride, within −5% to +10%, and dextrose, within ±5%. Contains no antimicrobial agents. Meets the requirements for Identification, Bacterial endotoxins, pH (3.5–6.5, determined on a portion diluted with water, if necessary, to a concentration of not more than 5% of dextrose), and Limit of 5-hydroxymethylfurfural and related substances, for Heavy metals under Dextrose Injection, and for Injections.

POTASSIUM CHLORIDE, DEXTROSE, AND SODIUM CHLORIDE

For *Potassium Chloride, Dextrose,* and *Sodium Chloride*—See individual listings for chemistry information.

USP requirements: Potassium Chloride in Dextrose and Sodium Chloride Injection USP—Preserve in single-dose containers, preferably of Type I or Type II glass, or of a suitable plastic. A sterile solution of Potassuim Chloride, Dextrose, and So-

dium Chloride in Water for Injection. The label states the potassium, sodium, and chloride contents in terms of milliequivalents in a given volume. The label states also the total osmolar concentration in mOsmol per liter. Where the contents are less than 100 mL, the label alternatively may state the total osmolar concentration in mOsmol per mL. Contains the equivalent of the labeled amounts of potassium and chloride, within −5% to +10%, and the equivalent of the labeled amounts of dextrose and sodium, within ±5%. Contains no antimicrobial agents. Meets the requirements for Identification, Bacterial endotoxins, pH (3.5–6.5), Heavy metals, and 5-Hydroxymethylfurfural and related substances, and for Injections.

POTASSIUM CHLORIDE, LACTATED RINGER'S, AND DEXTROSE

For *Potassium Chloride, Calcium Chloride, Sodium Chloride, Sodium Lactate,* and *Dextrose*—See individual listings for chemistry information.

USP requirements: Potassium Chloride in Lactated Ringer's and Dextrose Injection USP—Preserve in single-dose glass or plastic containers. Glass containers are preferably of Type I or Type II glass. A sterile solution of Calcium Chloride, Potassium Chloride, Sodium Chloride, and Sodium Lactate in Water for Injection. The label states the total osmolar concentration in mOsmol per liter. Where the contents are less than 100 mL, the label alternatively may state the total osmolar concentration in mOsmol per mL. The label includes also the warning: "Not for use in the treatment of lactic acidosis." Contains, in each 100 mL, not less than 285.0 mg and not more than 315.0 mg of sodium (as sodium chloride and sodium lactate), not less than 4.90 mg and not more than 6.00 mg of calcium (calcium, equivalent to not less than 18.0 mg and not more than 22.0 mg of hydrous calcium chloride), and not less than 231.0 mg and not more than 261.0 mg of lactate (lactate, equivalent to not less than 290.0 mg and not more than 330.0 mg of sodium lactate). Contains the labeled amount of Potassium Chloride, within ±5%, the labeled amount of dextrose, within −10% to +15%, and the equivalent of the labeled amount of chloride (chloride, as sodium chloride, potassium chloride, and hydrous calcium chloride), within ±10%. Contains no antimicrobial agents. Meets the requirements for Identification, Bacterial endotoxins, pH (3.5–6.5), Heavy metals, and Limit of 5-hydroxymethylfurfural and related substances, and for Injections.

POTASSIUM CHLORIDE, POTASSIUM BICARBONATE, AND POTASSIUM CITRATE

For *Potassium Chloride, Potassium Bicarbonate,* and *Potassium Citrate*—See individual listings for chemistry information.

USP requirements: Potassium Chloride, Potassium Bicarbonate, and Potassium Citrate Effervescent Tablets for Oral Solution USP—Preserve in tight containers, protected from excessive heat. The label states the potassium and chloride contents in terms of weight and in terms of milliequivalents. Where Tablets are packaged in individual pouches, the label instructs the user not to open until the time of use. Contain the equivalent of the labeled amounts of potassium and chloride, within ±10%. Meet the requirements for Identification and Uniformity of dosage units.

POTASSIUM CHLORIDE AND SODIUM CHLORIDE

For *Potassium Chloride* and *Sodium Chloride*—See individual listings for chemistry information.

USP requirements: Potassium Chloride in Sodium Chloride Injection USP—Preserve in single-dose containers, preferably of Type I or Type II glass, or of a suitable plastic. A sterile solution of Potassium Chloride and Sodium Chloride in Water for Injection. The label states the potassium, sodium, and chloride contents in terms of milliequivalents in a given volume. The label states also the total osmolar concentration in mOsmol per liter. Where the contents are less than 100 mL, the label may alternatively state the total osmolar concentration in mOsmol per mL. Contains the equivalent of the labeled amounts of potassium and chloride, within −5% to +10%, and the equivalent of the labeled amount of sodium, within ±5%. Contains no antimicrobial agents. Meets the requirements for Identification, Bacterial endotoxins, pH (3.5–6.5), and Heavy metals, and for Injections.

POTASSIUM CITRATE

Chemical name: 1,2,3-Propanetricarboxylic acid, 2-hydroxy-, tripotassium salt, monohydrate.

Molecular formula: $C_6H_5K_3O_7 \cdot H_2O$.

Molecular weight: 324.41.

Description: Potassium Citrate USP—Transparent crystals or white, granular powder. Is odorless and is deliquescent when exposed to moist air.

NF category: Buffering agent.

Solubility: Potassium Citrate USP—Freely soluble in water; almost insoluble in alcohol.

USP requirements:

Potassium Citrate USP—Preserve in tight containers. Contains not less than 99.0% and not more than 100.5% of potassium citrate, calculated on the dried basis. Meets the requirements for Identification, Alkalinity, Loss on drying (3.0–6.0%), Tartrate, Heavy metals (not more than 0.001%), and Organic volatile impurities.

Potassium Citrate Tablets—Not in *USP–NF*.

Potassium Citrate Extended-release Tablets USP—Preserve in tight containers. Contain the labeled amount, within ± 10%. Meet the requirements for Identification, Dissolution (not more than 45% in 30 minutes, not more than 60% in 1 hour, and not less than 80% in 3 hours, in water in Apparatus 2 at 50 rpm), Uniformity of dosage units, and Potassium content (36.4–40.2%).

POTASSIUM CITRATE AND CITRIC ACID

For *Potassium Citrate* and *Citric Acid*—See individual listings for chemistry information.

USP requirements:

Potassium Citrate and Citric Acid Oral Solution USP—Preserve in tight containers. A solution of Potassium Citrate and Citric Acid in a suitable aqueous medium. Contains, in each 100 mL, not less than 7.55 grams and not more than 8.35 grams of potassium; not less than 12.18 grams and not more than 13.46 grams of citrate, equivalent to not less than 20.9 grams and not more than 23.1 grams of potassium citrate monohydrate; and not less than 6.34 grams and not more than 7.02 grams of citric acid monohydrate. Meets the requirements for Identification and pH (4.9–5.4).

Note: The potassium ion content of Potassium Citrate and Citric Acid Oral Solution is approximately 2 mEq per mL.
Potassium Citrate and Citric Acid for Oral Solution—Not in *USP–NF.*

POTASSIUM CITRATE AND SODIUM CITRATE

For *Potassium Citrate* and *Sodium Citrate*—See individual listings for chemistry information.

USP requirements: Potassium Citrate and Sodium Citrate Tablets—Not in *USP–NF.*

POTASSIUM GLUCONATE

Chemical name: D-Gluconic acid, monopotassium salt.

Molecular formula: $C_6H_{11}KO_7$.

Molecular weight: 234.25.

Description: Potassium Gluconate USP—White to yellowish white, crystalline powder or granules. Is odorless and is stable in air. Its solutions are slightly alkaline to litmus.

Solubility: Potassium Gluconate USP—Freely soluble in water; practically insoluble in dehydrated alcohol, in ether, and in chloroform.

USP requirements:
Potassium Gluconate USP—Preserve in tight containers. It is anhydrous or contains one molecule of water of hydration. Label it to indicate whether it is anhydrous or the monohydrate. Contains not less than 97.0% and not more than 103.0% of potassium gluconate, calculated on the dried basis. Meets the requirements for Identification, Loss on drying (not more than 3.0% for the anhydrous form and 6.0–7.5% for the monohydrate form), Heavy metals (not more than 0.002%), Reducing substances (not more than 1.0%), and Organic volatile impurities.
Potassium Gluconate Elixir USP—Preserve in tight, light-resistant containers. Contains the labeled amount, within ±5%. Meets the requirements for Identification and Alcohol content (4.5–5.5%).
Potassium Gluconate Oral Solution USP—Preserve in tight, light-resistant containers. Contains the labeled amount, within ±5%. Meets the requirements for Identification and Alcohol content (4.5–5.5%).
Potassium Gluconate Tablets USP—Preserve in tight containers. Contain the labeled amount, within ±5%. Meet the requirements for Identification, Dissolution (75% in 45 minutes in water in Apparatus 2 at 100 rpm), and Uniformity of dosage units.

POTASSIUM GLUCONATE AND POTASSIUM CHLORIDE

For *Potassium Gluconate* and *Potassium Chloride*—See individual listings for chemistry information.

USP requirements:
Potassium Gluconate and Potassium Chloride Oral Solution USP—Preserve in tight containers. A solution of Potassium Gluconate and Potassium Chloride in a suitable aqueous medium. Label it to state the potassium and chloride contents in terms of milliequivalents of each in a given vol-

ume of Oral Solution. Contains the equivalent of the labeled amounts of potassium and chloride, within ±10%. Meets the requirement for Identification.
Potassium Gluconate and Potassium Chloride for Oral Solution USP—Preserve in tight containers. A dry mixture of Potassium Gluconate and Potassium Chloride and one or more suitable colors, diluents, and flavors. Label it to state the potassium and chloride contents in terms of milliequivalents. Where packaged in unit-dose pouches, the label instructs the user not to open until the time of use. Contains the equivalent of the labeled amounts of potassium and chloride, within ±10%. Meets the requirements for Identification and Minimum fill.

POTASSIUM GLUCONATE AND POTASSIUM CITRATE

For *Potassium Gluconate* and *Potassium Citrate*—See individual listings for chemistry information.

USP requirements: Potassium Gluconate and Potassium Citrate Oral Solution USP—Preserve in tight containers. A solution of Potassium Gluconate and Potassium Citrate in a suitable aqueous medium. Label it to state the potassium content in terms of milliequivalents in a given volume of Oral Solution. Contains the equivalent of the labeled amount of potassium, within ±10%. Meets the requirement for Identification.

POTASSIUM GLUCONATE, POTASSIUM CITRATE, AND AMMONIUM CHLORIDE

For *Potassium Gluconate, Potassium Citrate,* and *Ammonium Chloride*—See individual listings for chemistry information.

USP requirements: Potassium Gluconate, Potassium Citrate, and Ammonium Chloride Oral Solution USP—Preserve in tight containers. A solution of Potassium Gluconate, Potassium Citrate, and Ammonium Chloride in a suitable aqueous medium. Label it to state the potassium and chloride contents in terms of milliequivalents of each in a given volume of Oral Solution. Contains the equivalent of the labeled amounts of potassium and chloride, within ±10%. Meets the requirement for Identification.

POTASSIUM GUAIACOLSULFONATE

Chemical name: Benzenesulfonic acid, hydroxymethoxy-, monopotassium salt, hemihydrate.

Molecular formula: $C_7H_7KO_5S \cdot \frac{1}{2}H_2O$.

Molecular weight: 251.30 (hemihydrate); 242.29 (anhydrous).

Description: White, odorless crystals or crystalline powder. Gradually turns pink on exposure to air and light.

Solubility: Soluble in 7.5 parts water; almost insoluble in alcohol; insoluble in ether.

USP requirements: Potassium Guaiacolsulfonate USP—Preserve in well-closed, light-resistant containers. Contains not less than 98.0% and not more than 102.0% of potassium guaiacolsulfonate, calculated on the anhydrous basis. Meets the requirements for Identification, Water (3.0–6.0%), Selenium (not more than 0.003%), Sulfate, and Heavy metals (not more than 0.002%).

POTASSIUM HYDROXIDE

Chemical name: Potassium hydroxide.

Molecular formula: KOH.

Molecular weight: 56.11.

Description: Potassium Hydroxide NF—White or practically white fused masses, or small pellets, or flakes, or sticks, or other forms. It is hard and brittle and shows a crystalline fracture. Exposed to air, it rapidly absorbs carbon dioxide and moisture, and deliquesces.
NF category: Alkalizing agent.

Solubility: Potassium Hydroxide NF—Freely soluble in water, in alcohol, and in glycerin; very soluble in boiling alcohol.

NF requirements: Potassium Hydroxide NF—Preserve in tight containers. Contains not less than 85.0% of total alkali, calculated as potassium hydroxide, including not more than 3.5% of anhydrous potassium carbonate. Meets the requirements for Identification, Insoluble substances, and Heavy metals (not more than 0.003%).
Caution: Exercise great care in handling Potassium Hydroxide, as it rapidly destroys tissues.

POTASSIUM IODIDE

Chemical group: Inorganic iodides.

Chemical name: Potassium iodide.

Molecular formula: KI.

Molecular weight: 166.00.

Description:
Potassium Iodide USP—Hexahedral crystals, either transparent and colorless or somewhat opaque and white, or a white, granular powder. Is slightly hygroscopic. Its solutions are neutral or alkaline to litmus.
Potassium Iodide Oral Solution USP—Clear, colorless, odorless liquid. Is neutral or alkaline to litmus. Specific gravity is about 1.70.

Solubility: Potassium Iodide USP—Very soluble in water and even more soluble in boiling water; freely soluble in glycerin; soluble in alcohol.

USP requirements:
Potassium Iodide USP—Preserve in well-closed containers. Contains not less than 99.0% and not more than 101.5% of potassium iodide, calculated on the dried basis. Meets the requirements for Identification, Alkalinity, Loss on drying (not more than 1.0%), Iodate (not more than 4 ppm), Limit of nitrate, nitrite, and ammonia, Thiosulfate and barium, Heavy metals (not more than 0.001%), and Organic volatile impurities.
Potassium Iodide Oral Solution USP—Preserve in tight, light-resistant containers. Contains the labeled amount, within ±6%. Meets the requirement for Identification.
Note: If Potassium Iodide Oral Solution is not to be used within a short time, add 0.5 mg of sodium thiosulfate for each gram of potassium iodide. Crystals of potassium iodide may form in Potassium Iodide Oral Solution under normal conditions of storage, especially if refrigerated.
Potassium Iodide Syrup—Not in *USP–NF*.
Potassium Iodide Tablets USP—Preserve in tight containers. Contain the labeled amount, within ±6% for Tablets of 300 mg or more; within ±7.5% for Tablets of less than 300 mg. Meet the requirements for Identification, Dissolution (for uncoated Tablets, 75% in 15 minutes in water in Apparatus 2 at 50 rpm), and Uniformity of dosage units.

Potassium Iodide Delayed-release Tablets USP—Preserve in tight containers. Contain not less than 94.0% and not more than 106.0% of labeled amount of Potassium Iodide for Tablets of 300 mg or more, and not less than 92.5% and not more than 107.5% for Tablets of less than 300 mg. Meet the requirements for Disintegration (the tablets do not disintegrate after 1 hour of agitation in simulated gastric fluid TS, but they disintegrate within 90 minutes in simulated intestinal fluid TS), Identification test, and for Uniformity of dosage units for Potassium Iodide Tablets.

POTASSIUM METABISULFITE

Chemical name: Disulfurous acid, dipotassium salt.

Molecular formula: $K_2S_2O_5$.

Molecular weight: 222.33.

Description: Potassium Metabisulfite NF—White or colorless, free-flowing crystals, crystalline powder, or granules, usually having an odor of sulfur dioxide. Gradually oxidizes in air to the sulfate. Its solutions are acid to litmus.
NF category: Antioxidant.

Solubility: Potassium Metabisulfite NF—Soluble in water; insoluble in alcohol.

NF requirements: Potassium Metabisulfite NF—Preserve in well-fitted, tight containers, and avoid exposure to excessive heat. Contains an amount of potassium metabisulfite equivalent to not less than 51.8% and not more than 57.6% of sulfur dioxide. Meets the requirements for Identification, Iron (not more than 0.001%), Heavy metals (not more than 0.001%), and Organic volatile impurities.

POTASSIUM METAPHOSPHATE

Chemical name: Metaphosphoric acid (HPO_3), potassium salt.

Molecular formula: KPO_3.

Molecular weight: 118.07.

Description: Potassium Metaphosphate NF—White, odorless powder.
NF category: Buffering agent.

Solubility: Potassium Metaphosphate NF—Insoluble in water; soluble in dilute solutions of sodium salts.

NF requirements: Potassium Metaphosphate NF—Preserve in well-closed containers. A straight-chain polyphosphate, having a high degree of polymerization. Contains the equivalent of not less than 59.0% and not more than 61.0% of phosphorus pentoxide. Meets the requirements for Identification, Viscosity (6.5–15 centipoises), Lead (not more than 5 ppm), Heavy metals (not more than 0.002%), and Limit of fluoride (not more than 0.001%).

POTASSIUM NITRATE

Chemical name: Potassium nitrate.

Molecular formula: KNO_3.

Molecular weight: 101.10.

Description: Potassium Nitrate USP—White, crystalline powder or colorless crystals.

Solubility: Potassium Nitrate USP—Freely soluble in water; very soluble in boiling water; soluble in glycerin; practically insoluble in alcohol.

USP requirements:

Potassium Nitrate USP—Preserve in tight containers. Contains not less than 99.0% and not more than 100.5% of potassium nitrate. Meets the requirements for Identification, Chloride (not more than 0.03%), Sulfate (not more than 0.1%), Arsenic (not more than 3 ppm), Lead (not more than 0.001%), Heavy metals (not more than 0.002%), Iron (not more than 0.001%), Limit of sodium (not more than 0.1%), and Limit of nitrite (not more than 5 mcg per gram).

Potassium Nitrate Solution USP—Preserve in tight containers. Contains the labeled amount, within ±2%. Meets the requirements, based on the potassium nitrate content of the Solution, for Identification, Chloride (not more than 0.03%), Sulfate (not more than 0.1%), Arsenic (not more than 3 ppm), Lead (not more than 0.001%), Heavy metals (not more than 0.002%), Iron (not more than 0.001%), Limit of sodium (not more than 0.1%), and Limit of nitrite (not more than 5 mcg per gram).

POTASSIUM PERCHLORATE

USP requirements:

Potassium Perchlorate USP—Preserve in well-closed containers. Contains not less 99.0% and not more than 100.5% of potassium perchlorate, calculated on the dried basis. Meets the requirements for Identification, pH (5.0–6.5, in a 0.1 M solution), Loss on drying (not more than 0.5%), Insoluble substances (not more than 0.005%), Chloride (not more than 0.003%), Heavy metals (not more than 0.001%), Limit of sodium (no pronounced yellow color imparted to the flame), and Organic volatile impurities.

Caution—Great care should be taken in handling Potassium Perchlorate in solution or in the dry state, as explosions may occur if it is brought into contact with organic or other readily oxidizable substances.

Potassium Perchlorate Capsules USP—Preserve in tight, light-resistant containers. Contain the labeled amount, within ±10%. Meet the requirements for Identification, Disintegration, and Uniformity of dosage units.

POTASSIUM PERMANGANATE

Chemical name: Permanganic acid ($HMnO_4$), potassium salt.

Molecular formula: $KMnO_4$.

Molecular weight: 158.03.

Description: Potassium Permanganate USP—Dark purple crystals, almost opaque by transmitted light and of a blue metallic luster by reflected light. Its color is sometimes modified by a dark bronze-like appearance. Is stable in air.

Solubility: Potassium Permanganate USP—Soluble in water; freely soluble in boiling water.

USP requirements: Potassium Permanganate USP—Preserve in well-closed containers. Contains not less than 99.0% and not more than 100.5% of potassium permanganate, calculated on the dried basis. Meets the requirements for Identification, Loss on drying (not more than 0.5%), and Insoluble substances (not more than 0.2%).

Caution: Observe great care in handling Potassium Permanganate, as dangerous explosions may occur if it is brought into contact with organic or other readily oxidizable substances, either in solution or in the dry state.

DIBASIC POTASSIUM PHOSPHATE

Chemical name: Phosphoric acid, dipotassium salt.

Molecular formula: K_2HPO_4.

Molecular weight: 174.18.

Description: Dibasic Potassium Phosphate USP—Colorless or white, somewhat hygroscopic, granular powder. The pH of a solution (1 in 20) is about 8.5 to 9.6.

NF category: Buffering agent.

Solubility: Dibasic Potassium Phosphate USP—Freely soluble in water; very slightly soluble in alcohol.

USP requirements: Dibasic Potassium Phosphate USP—Preserve in well-closed containers. Contains not less than 98.0% and not more than 100.5% of dibasic potassium phosphate, calculated on the dried basis. Meets the requirements for Identification, pH (8.5–9.6, in a solution [1 in 20]), Loss on drying (not more than 1.0%), Insoluble substances (not more than 0.2%), Carbonate, Chloride (not more than 0.03%), Sulfate (not more than 0.1%), Arsenic (not more than 3 ppm), Iron (not more than 0.003%), Sodium, Heavy metals (not more than 0.001%), Limit of fluoride (not more than 0.001%), and Limit of monobasic or tribasic salt.

MONOBASIC POTASSIUM PHOSPHATE

Chemical name: Phosphoric acid, monopotassium salt.

Molecular formula: KH_2PO_4.

Molecular weight: 136.09.

Description: Monobasic Potassium Phosphate NF—Colorless crystals or white, granular or crystalline powder. Is odorless, and is stable in air. The pH of a solution (1 in 100) is about 4.5.

NF category: Buffering agent.

Solubility: Monobasic Potassium Phosphate NF—Freely soluble in water; practically insoluble in alcohol.

USP requirements: Monobasic Potassium Phosphate Tablets for Oral Solution—Not in USP.

NF requirements: Monobasic Potassium Phosphate NF—Preserve in tight containers. Dried at 105 °C for 4 hours, contains not less than 98.0% and not more than 100.5% of monobasic potassium phosphate. Meets the requirements for Identification, Loss on drying (not more than 1.0%), Insoluble substances (not more than 0.2%), Arsenic (not more than 3 ppm), Lead (not more than 5 ppm), Heavy metals (not more than 0.002%), Limit of fluoride (not more than 0.001%), and Organic volatile impurities.

POTASSIUM PHOSPHATES

For *Monobasic Potassium Phosphate* and *Dibasic Potassium Phosphate*—See individual listings for chemistry information.

USP requirements:

Potassium Phosphates Capsules for Oral Solution—Not in *USP–NF*.

Potassium Phosphates Injection USP—Preserve in single-dose containers, preferably of Type I glass. A sterile solution of Monobasic Potassium Phosphate and Dibasic Potassium Phosphate in Water for Injection. The label states the potassium content in terms of milliequivalents in a given volume, and states also the elemental phosphorus content in terms of millimoles in a given volume. Label the Injection to indicate that it is to be diluted to appropriate strength with water or other suitable fluid prior to administration, and that once opened any unused portion is to be discarded. The label states also the total osmolar concentration in mOsmol per liter. Where the contents are less than 100 mL, or where the label states that the Injection is not for direct injection but is to be diluted before use, the label alternatively may state the total osmolar concentration in mOsmol per mL. Contains the labeled amounts of monobasic potassium phosphate and dibasic potassium phosphate, within ±5%. Contains no bacteriostat or other preservative. Meets the requirements for Identification, Bacterial endotoxins, and Particulate matter, and for Injections.

Potassium Phosphates for Oral Solution—Not in *USP–NF*.

POTASSIUM AND SODIUM PHOSPHATES

For *Dibasic Potassium Phosphate, Dibasic Sodium Phosphate, Monobasic Potassium Phosphate,* and *Monobasic Sodium Phosphate*—See individual listings for chemistry information.

USP requirements:
Potassium and Sodium Phosphates Capsules for Oral Solution—Not in *USP–NF*.
Potassium and Sodium Phosphates for Oral Solution—Not in *USP–NF*.
Potassium and Sodium Phosphates Tablets for Oral Solution—Not in *USP–NF*.

MONOBASIC POTASSIUM AND SODIUM PHOSPHATES

For *Monobasic Potassium Phosphate* and *Monobasic Sodium Phosphate*—See individual listings for chemistry information.

USP requirements: Monobasic Potassium and Sodium Phosphates Tablets for Oral Solution—Not in *USP–NF*.

POTASSIUM SODIUM TARTRATE

Chemical name: Butanedioic acid, 2,3-dihydroxy-, [R-(R*,R*)]-, monopotassium monosodium salt, tetrahydrate.

Molecular formula: $C_4H_4KNaO_6 \cdot 4H_2O$.

Molecular weight: 282.22 (tetrahydrate); 210.16 (anhydrous).

Description: Potassium Sodium Tartrate USP—Colorless crystals or white, crystalline powder. As it effloresces slightly in warm, dry air, the crystals are often coated with a white powder.

Solubility: Potassium Sodium Tartrate USP—Freely soluble in water; practically insoluble in alcohol.

USP requirements: Potassium Sodium Tartrate USP—Preserve in tight containers. Contains not less than 99.0% and not more than 102.0% of potassium sodium tartrate, calculated on the anhydrous basis. Meets the requirements for Identification, Alkalinity, Water (21.0–27.0%), Limit of ammonia, and Heavy metals (not more than 0.001%).

POTASSIUM SORBATE

Chemical name: 2,4-Hexadienoic acid, (*E,E'*)- potassium salt; 2,4-Hexadienoic acid, potassium salt.

Molecular formula: $C_6H_7KO_2$.

Molecular weight: 150.22.

Description: Potassium Sorbate NF—White crystals or powder, having a characteristic odor. Melts at about 270 °C, with decomposition.

NF category: Antimicrobial preservative.

Solubility: Potassium Sorbate NF—Freely soluble in water; soluble in alcohol.

NF requirements:Potassium Sorbate NF—Preserve in tight containers, protected from light, and avoid exposure to excessive heat. Contains not less than 98.0% and not more than 101.0% of potassium sorbate, calculated on the dried basis. Meets the requirements for Identification, Acidity or alkalinity, Loss on drying (not more than 1.0%), Heavy metals (not more than 0.001%), and Organic volatile impurities.

POVIDONE

Chemical name: 2-Pyrrolidinone, 1-ethenyl-, homopolymer.

Molecular formula: $(C_6H_9NO)_n$.

Description: Povidone USP—White to slightly creamy white powder. Is hygroscopic.

NF category: Suspending and/or viscosity-increasing agent; tablet binder.

Solubility: Povidone USP—Freely soluble in water, in methanol and in alcohol; slightly soluble in acetone; practically insoluble in ether .

USP requirements: Povidone USP—Preserve in tight containers. A synthetic polymer consisting essentially of linear 1-vinyl-2-pyrrolidinone groups, the degree of polymerization of which results in polymers of various molecular weights. Characterized by its viscosity in aqueous solution, relative to that of water, expressed as a K-value, ranging from 10 to 120. Label it to state, as part of the official title, the K-value or K-value range of the Povidone. The K-value of Povidone having a nominal K-value of 15 or less is not less than 85.0% and not more than 115.0% of the nominal K-value, and the K-value of Povidone having a nominal K-value or nominal K-value range with an average of more than 15 is not less than 90.0% and not more than 108.0% of the nominal K-value or average of the nominal K-value range. Meets the requirements for Identification, pH (3.0–7.0, in a solution [1 in 20]), Water (not more than 5.0%), Residue on ignition (not more than 0.1%), Lead (not more than 10 ppm), Limit of aldehydes, Limit of hydrazine (not more than 1 ppm), Vinylpyrrolidinone (not more than 0.2%), K-value, and Nitrogen content (11.5–12.8%, on the anhydrous basis).

POVIDONE-IODINE

Chemical name: 2-Pyrrolidinone, 1-ethenyl-, homopolymer, compd. with iodine.

Molecular formula: $(C_6H_9NO)_n \cdot xI$.

Description:
Povidone-Iodine USP—Yellowish brown to reddish-brown, amorphous powder, having a slight characteristic odor. Its solution is acid to litmus.
Povidone-Iodine Topical Aerosol Solution USP—The liquid obtained from Povidone-Iodine Topical Aerosol Solution is transparent, having a reddish-brown color.

Solubility: Povidone-Iodine USP—Soluble in water and in alcohol; practically insoluble in chloroform, in carbon tetrachloride, in ether, in solvent hexane, and in acetone.

USP requirements:
Povidone-Iodine USP—Preserve in tight containers. A complex of Iodine with Povidone. Contains not less than 9.0% and not more than 12.0% of available iodine, calculated on the dried basis. Meets the requirements for Identification, Loss on drying (not more than 8.0%), Residue on ignition (negligible, from 2 grams), Iodide ion (not more than 6.6%, calculated on the dried basis), Heavy metals (not more than 0.002%), and Nitrogen content (9.5%–11.5%, calculated on the dried basis).
Povidone-Iodine Topical Aerosol USP—Preserve in pressurized containers, and avoid exposure to excessive heat. A solution of Povidone-Iodine under nitrogen in a pressurized container. Contains an amount of povidone-iodine equivalent to the labeled amount of iodine, within –15% to +20%. Meets the requirements for Identification and pH (not more than 6.0), and for Pressure test, Minimum fill, and Leakage test under Aerosols, Metered-dose inhalers, and Dry powder inhalers.
Povidone-Iodine Ointment USP—Preserve in tight containers. An emulsion, solution, or suspension of Povidone-Iodine in a suitable water-soluble ointment base. Contains an amount of povidone-iodine equivalent to the labeled amount of iodine, within –15% to +20%. Meets the requirements for Identification, Minimum fill, and pH (1.5–6.5, determined in a solution [1 in 20]).
Povidone-Iodine Cleansing Solution USP—Preserve in tight containers. A solution of Povidone-Iodine with one or more suitable surface-active agents. May contain a small amount of alcohol. Contains an amount of povidone-iodine equivalent to the labeled amount of iodine, within –15% to +20%. Meets the requirements for Identification, pH (1.5–6.5), and Alcohol content (if present, within ±10% of labeled amount).
Povidone-Iodine Topical Solution USP—Preserve in tight containers. A solution of Povidone-Iodine. May contain a small amount of alcohol. Contains an amount of povidone-iodine equivalent to the labeled amount of iodine, within –15% to +20%. Meets the requirements for Identification, pH (1.5–6.5), and Alcohol content (if present, within ±10% of the labeled amount).

PRALIDOXIME

Chemical name: Pralidoxime chloride—Pyridinium, 2-[(hydroxyimino)methyl]-1-methyl-, chloride.

Molecular formula: Pralidoxime chloride—$C_7H_9ClN_2O$.

Molecular weight: Pralidoxime chloride—172.61.

Description:
Pralidoxime Chloride USP—White to pale-yellow, crystalline powder. Odorless and stable in air.

Solubility:
Pralidoxime Chloride USP—Freely soluble in water.

USP requirements:
Pralidoxime Chloride USP—Preserve in well-closed containers. Where it is intended for use in preparing injectable dosage forms, the label states that it is sterile or must be subjected to further processing during the preparation of injectable dosage forms. Contains not less than 97.0% and not more than 102.0% of pralidoxime chloride, calculated on the dried basis. Meets the requirements for Identification, Melting range (215–225 °C, with decomposition), Loss on drying (not more than 2.0%), Residue on ignition (not more than 0.5%), Heavy metals (not more than 0.002%), and Chloride content (20.2–20.8%, calculated on the dried basis), for Sterility tests and for Bacterial endotoxins under Pralidoxime Chloride for Injection (where the label states that Pralidoxime Chloride is sterile), and for Bacterial endotoxins under Pralidoxime Chloride for Injection (where the label states that Pralidoxime Chloride must be subjected to further processing during the preparation of injectable dosage forms).
Pralidoxime Chloride for Injection USP—Preserve in Containers for Sterile Solids. Contains the labeled amount, within ±10%. Meets the requirements for Completeness of solution, Constituted solution, Bacterial endotoxins, and pH (3.5–4.5, in a solution [1 in 20]), for Identification tests, Loss on drying, and Heavy metals under Pralidoxime Chloride, and for Sterility tests, Uniformity of dosage units, and Labeling under Injections.
Pralidoxime Chloride Tablets USP—Preserve in well-closed containers. Contain the labeled amount, within ±5%. Meet the requirements for Identification, Dissolution (55% in 60 minutes in water in Apparatus 1 at 100 rpm), and Uniformity of dosage units.

PRAMIPEXOLE

Chemical name:
Pramipexole—2,6-Benzothiazolediamine, 4,5,6,7-tetrahydro-N^6-propyl-, (S)-.
Pramipexole dihydrochloride—(S)-2-amino-4,5,6,7-tetrahydro-6-propylamino-benzothiazole dihydrochloride monohydrate.

Molecular formula:
Pramipexole—$C_{10}H_{17}N_3S$.
Pramipexole dihydrochloride—$C_{10}H_{17}N_3S \cdot 2HCl \cdot H_2O$.

Molecular weight:
Pramipexole—211.33.
Pramipexole dihydrochloride—302.76.

Description: Pramipexole dihydrochloride—White to off-white powder. Melts at 296 to 301 °C, with decomposition.

pKa: Pramipexole dihydrochloride—5.0 and 9.6.

Solubility: Pramipexole dihydrochloride—More than 20% soluble in water; about 8% soluble in methanol; about 0.5% soluble in ethanol; practically insoluble in dichloromethane.

USP requirements:
Pramipexole Tablets—Not in USP–NF.
Pramipexole Dihydrochloride Tablets—Not in USP–NF.
Pramipexole Hydrochloride Tablets—Not in USP–NF.

PRAMOXINE

Chemical name: Pramoxine hydrochloride—Morpholine, 4-[3-(4-butoxyphenoxy)propyl]-, hydrochloride.

Molecular formula: Pramoxine hydrochloride—$C_{17}H_{27}NO_3 \cdot HCl$.

Molecular weight: Pramoxine hydrochloride—329.86.

Description: Pramoxine Hydrochloride USP—White to practically white, crystalline powder. May have a slight aromatic odor. The pH of a solution (1 in 100) is about 4.5.

Solubility: Pramoxine Hydrochloride USP—Freely soluble in water and in alcohol; soluble in chloroform; very slightly soluble in ether.

USP requirements:
Pramoxine Hydrochloride USP—Preserve in tight containers. Contains not less than 98.0% and not more than 102.0% of pramoxine hydrochloride, calculated on the dried basis. Meets the requirements for Identification, Melting range (170–174 °C), Loss on drying (not more than 1.0%), and Residue on ignition (not more than 0.1%).
Pramoxine Hydrochloride Cream USP—Preserve in tight containers. Contains the labeled amount, within ±10%, in a suitable water-miscible base. Meets the requirements for Identification, Microbial limits, and Minimum fill.
Pramoxine Hydrochloride Aerosol Foam—Not in *USP–NF*.
Pramoxine Hydrochloride Jelly USP—Preserve in tight containers, preferably in collapsible tubes. Contains the labeled amount, within ±6%. Meets the requirements for Identification and Microbial limits.
Pramoxine Hydrochloride Lotion—Not in *USP–NF*.
Pramoxine Hydrochloride Ointment—Not in *USP–NF*.

PRAMOXINE AND MENTHOL

For *Pramoxine* and *Menthol*—See individual listings for chemistry information.

USP requirements:
Pramoxine Hydrochloride and Menthol Gel—Not in *USP–NF*.
Pramoxine Hydrochloride and Menthol Lotion—Not in *USP–NF*.

PRAVASTATIN

Chemical name: Pravastatin sodium—1-Naphthalene-heptanoic acid, 1,2,6,7,8,8a-hexahydro-beta,delta,6-trihydroxy-2-methyl-8-(2-methyl-1-oxobutoxy)-, monosodium salt, [1*S*-[1 alpha(beta*S**,delta*S**),2 alpha,6 alpha,8 beta(*R**),8a alpha]]-.

Molecular formula: Pravastatin sodium—$C_{23}H_{35}NaO_7$.

Molecular weight: Pravastatin sodium—446.51.

Description: Pravastatin sodium—Odorless, white to off-white, fine or crystalline powder.

Solubility: Pravastatin sodium—Soluble in methanol and in water; slightly soluble in isopropanol; practically insoluble in acetone, in acetonitrile, in chloroform, and in ether.

Other characteristics: Pravastatin sodium—Partition coefficient (octanol/water) 0.59 at pH 7.0.

USP requirements: Pravastatin Sodium Tablets—Not in *USP–NF*.

PRAZEPAM

Chemical name: 2*H*-1,4-Benzodiazepin-2-one, 7-chloro-1-(cyclopropylmethyl)-1,3-dihydro-5-phenyl-.

Molecular formula: $C_{19}H_{17}ClN_2O$.

Molecular weight: 324.80.

Description: Prazepam USP—White to off-white crystalline powder.

Solubility: Prazepam USP—Freely soluble in acetone; soluble in dilute mineral acids, in alcohol, and in chloroform.

USP requirements:
Prazepam USP—Preserve in tight, light-resistant containers. Contains not less than 98.5% and not more than 101.0% of prazepam, calculated on the dried basis. Meets the requirements for Identification, Melting range (143–148 °C, the range between beginning and end of melting not more than 3 °C), Loss on drying (not more than 0.5%), Residue on ignition (not more than 0.1%), Heavy metals (not more than 0.002%), Related compounds, and Organic volatile impurities.
Prazepam Capsules USP—Preserve in tight, light-resistant containers. Contain the labeled amount, within ±10%. Meet the requirements for Identification, Dissolution (80% in 60 minutes in 0.1 *N* hydrochloric acid in Apparatus 1 at 50 rpm), and Uniformity of dosage units.
Prazepam Tablets USP—Preserve in tight, light-resistant containers. Contain the labeled amount, within ±10%. Meet the requirements for Identification, Dissolution (80% in 60 minutes in 0.1 *N* hydrochloric acid in Apparatus 1 at 50 rpm), and Uniformity of dosage units.

PRAZIQUANTEL

Chemical group: Pyrazinoisoquinoline derivative.

Chemical name: 4*H*-Pyrazino[2,1-*a*]isoquinolin-4-one, 2-(cyclohexylcarbonyl)-1,2,3,6,7,11b-hexahydro-.

Molecular formula: $C_{19}H_{24}N_2O_2$.

Molecular weight: 312.41.

Description: Praziquantel USP—White or practically white, crystalline powder; odorless or having a faint characteristic odor.

Solubility: Praziquantel USP—Very slightly soluble in water; freely soluble in alcohol and in chloroform.

Other characteristics: Hygroscopic.

USP requirements:
Praziquantel USP—Preserve in well-closed, light-resistant containers. Contains not less than 98.5% and not more than 101.0% of praziquantel, calculated on the dried basis. Meets the requirements for Identification, Melting range (136–142 °C), Loss on drying (not more than 0.5%), Residue on ignition (not more than 0.1%), Heavy metals (not more than 0.002%), Related compounds, and Phosphate.
Praziquantel Tablets USP—Preserve in tight containers. Contain the labeled amount, within ±10%. Meet the requirements for Identification, Dissolution (75% in 60 minutes in 0.1 *N* hydrochloric acid containing 2.0 mg of sodium lauryl sulfate per mL in Apparatus 2 at 50 rpm), and Uniformity of dosage units.

PRAZOSIN

Chemical name: Prazosin hydrochloride—Piperazine, 1-(4-amino-6,7-dimethoxy-2-quinazolinyl)-4-(2-furanylcarbonyl)-, monohydrochloride.

Molecular formula: Prazosin hydrochloride—$C_{19}H_{21}N_5O_4 \cdot HCl$.

Molecular weight: Prazosin hydrochloride—419.86.

Description: Prazosin Hydrochloride USP—White to tan powder.

pKa: 6.5 in 1:1 water-ethanol solution.

Solubility: Prazosin Hydrochloride USP—Slightly soluble in water, in methanol, in dimethylformamide, and in dimethylacetamide; very slightly soluble in alcohol; practically insoluble in chloroform and in acetone.

USP requirements:
Prazosin Hydrochloride USP—Preserve in tight, light-resistant containers. Label it to indicate whether it is anhydrous or is the polyhydrate. Contains not less than 97.0% and not more than 103.0% of prazosin hydrochloride, calculated on the anhydrous basis. Meets the requirements for Identification, Water (not more than 2.0% for the anhydrous form and 8.0–15.0% for the polyhydrate form), Residue on ignition (not more than 0.4%), Heavy metals (not more than 0.005%), Iron (not more than 0.010%), Nickel (not more than 0.010%), Ordinary impurities, and Organic volatile impurities.
  Caution: Care should be taken to prevent inhaling particles of Prazosin Hydrochloride and to prevent its contacting any part of the body.
Prazosin Hydrochloride Capsules USP—Preserve in well-closed, light-resistant containers. Contain an amount of prazosin hydrochloride equivalent to the labeled amount of prazosin, within ±10%. Meet the requirements for Identification, Dissolution (75% in 60 minutes in 0.1 N hydrochloric acid containing 3% sodium lauryl sulfate in Apparatus 1 at 100 rpm), and Uniformity of dosage units.
  Caution: Care should be taken to prevent inhaling particles of Prazosin Hydrochloride and to prevent its contacting any part of the body.
Prazosin Hydrochloride Tablets—Not in *USP–NF*.

PRAZOSIN AND POLYTHIAZIDE

For *Prazosin* and *Polythiazide*—See individual listings for chemistry information.

USP requirements: Prazosin Hydrochloride and Polythiazide Capsules—Not in *USP–NF*.

PREDNICARBATE

Chemical group: Nonhalogenated prednisolone derivative.

Chemical name: Pregna-1,4-diene-3,20-dione, 17-[(ethoxycarbonyl)oxy]-11-hydroxy-21-(1-oxopropoxy)-, (11 beta)-.

Molecular formula: $C_{27}H_{36}O_8$.

Molecular weight: 488.57.

USP requirements: Prednicarbate Emollient Cream—Not in *USP–NF*.

PREDNISOLONE

Chemical name:
  Prednisolone—Pregna-1,4-diene-3,20-dione, 11,17,21-trihydroxy-, (11 beta)-.
  Prednisolone acetate—Pregna-1,4-diene-3,20-dione, 21-(acetyloxy)-11,17-dihydroxy-, (11 beta)-.
  Prednisolone hemisuccinate—Pregna-1,4-diene-3,20-dione,21(3-carboxy-1-oxopropoxy)-11,17-dihydroxy-, (11 beta)-.
  Prednisolone sodium phosphate—Pregna-1,4-diene-3,20-dione, 11,17-dihydroxy-21-(phosphonooxy)-, disodium salt, (11 beta)-.
  Prednisolone sodium succinate—Pregna-1,4-diene-3,20-dione, 21-(3-carboxyl-1-oxopropoxy)-11,17-dihydroxy-, monosodium salt, (11 beta)-.
  Prednisolone tebutate—Pregna-1,4-diene-3,20-dione, 11,17-dihydroxy-21-[(3,3-dimethyl-1-oxobutyl)oxy]-, (11 beta)-.

Molecular formula:
  Prednisolone—$C_{21}H_{28}O_5$.
  Prednisolone acetate—$C_{23}H_{30}O_6$.
  Prednisolone hemisuccinate—$C_{25}H_{32}O_8$.
  Prednisolone sodium phosphate—$C_{21}H_{27}Na_2O_8P$.
  Prednisolone sodium succinate—$C_{25}H_{31}NaO_8$.
  Prednisolone tebutate—$C_{27}H_{38}O_6$.

Molecular weight:
  Prednisolone—360.44.
  Prednisolone acetate—402.48.
  Prednisolone hemisuccinate—460.52.
  Prednisolone sodium phosphate—484.39.
  Prednisolone sodium succinate—482.50.
  Prednisolone tebutate—458.59.

Description:
  Prednisolone USP—White to practically white, odorless, crystalline powder. Melts at about 235 °C, with some decomposition.
  Prednisolone Acetate USP—White to practically white, odorless, crystalline powder. Melts at about 235 °C, with some decomposition.
  Prednisolone Hemisuccinate USP—Fine, creamy white powder with friable lumps; practically odorless. Melts at about 205 °C, with decomposition.
  Prednisolone Sodium Phosphate USP—White or slightly yellow, friable granules or powder. Is odorless or has a slight odor. Is slightly hygroscopic.
  Prednisolone Sodium Succinate for Injection USP—Creamy white powder with friable lumps, having a slight odor.
  Prednisolone Tebutate USP—White to slightly yellow, free-flowing powder, which may show some soft lumps. Is odorless or has not more than a moderate, characteristic odor. Is hygroscopic.

Solubility:
  Prednisolone USP—Very slightly soluble in water; soluble in methanol and in dioxane; sparingly soluble in acetone and in alcohol; slightly soluble in chloroform.
  Prednisolone Acetate USP—Practically insoluble in water; slightly soluble in acetone, in alcohol, and in chloroform.
  Prednisolone Hemisuccinate USP—Very slightly soluble in water; freely soluble in alcohol; soluble in acetone.
  Prednisolone Sodium Phosphate USP—Freely soluble in water; soluble in methanol; slightly soluble in alcohol and in chloroform; very slightly soluble in acetone and in dioxane.
  Prednisolone Tebutate USP—Very slightly soluble in water; freely soluble in chloroform and in dioxane; soluble in acetone; sparingly soluble in alcohol and in methanol.

USP requirements:
  Prednisolone USP—Preserve in well-closed containers. It is anhydrous or contains one and one-half molecules of water of hydration. Label it to indicate whether it is anhydrous or hydrous. Contains not less than 97.0% and not more than 102.0% of prednisolone, calculated on the dried

basis. Meets the requirements for Identification, Specific rotation (+97° to +103°), Loss on drying (not more than 1.0% for anhydrous Prednisolone and not more than 7.0% for hydrous Prednisolone), Residue on ignition (negligible, from 100 mg), and Selenium (not more than 0.003%, a 200-mg test specimen being used), and Chromatographic purity.

Prednisolone Cream USP—Preserve in collapsible tubes or in tight containers. Contains the labeled amount, within ± 10%, in a suitable cream base. Meets the requirements for Identification and Minimum fill.

Prednisolone Oral Solution USP—Preserve in tight, light-resistant containers. Contains the labeled amount, within ±10%. May contain alcohol. Meets the requirements for Identification, pH (3.0–4.5), and Alcohol content (if present, within −10% to +15%).

Prednisolone Syrup USP—Preserve in tight, light-resistant containers. Contains the labeled amount, within ±10%. Prednisolone Syrup may contain alcohol. Meets the requirements for Identification, pH (3.0–4.5), and Alcohol content (if present, within −10% to +15%).

Prednisolone Tablets USP—Preserve in well-closed containers. Contain the labeled amount, within ±10%. Meet the requirements for Identification, Dissolution (70% in 30 minutes in water in Apparatus 2 at 50 rpm), and Uniformity of dosage units.

Prednisolone Acetate USP—Preserve in well-closed containers. Contains not less than 97.0% and not more than 102.0% of prednisolone acetate, calculated on the dried basis. Meets the requirements for Identification, Specific rotation (+112° to +119°), Loss on drying (not more than 1.0%), Chromatographic purity (not more than 1.0% of any individual impurity, and not more than 2.0% of total impurities), and Other impurities.

Prednisolone Acetate Injectable Suspension USP—Preserve in single-dose or in multiple-dose containers, preferably of Type I glass. A sterile suspension of Prednisolone Acetate in a suitable aqueous medium. Contains the labeled amount, within ±10%. Meets the requirements for Identification and pH (5.0–7.5), and for Injections.

Prednisolone Acetate Ophthalmic Suspension USP—Preserve in tight containers. A sterile, aqueous suspension of prednisolone acetate containing a suitable antimicrobial preservative. Contains the labeled amount, within −10% to +15%. Meets the requirements for Identification, Sterility, and pH (5.0–6.0).

Prednisolone Acetate and Prednisolone Sodium Phosphate Injectable Suspension—Not in *USP–NF*.

Sterile Prednisolone Acetate and Prednisolone Sodium Phosphate Suspension—Not in *USP–NF*.

Prednisolone Hemisuccinate USP—Preserve in tight containers. Contains not less than 98.0% and not more than 102.0% of prednisolone hemisuccinate, calculated on the dried basis. Meets the requirements for Identification, Specific rotation (+99° to +104°), Loss on drying (not more than 0.5%), and Residue on ignition (negligible, from 100 mg).

Prednisolone Sodium Phosphate USP—Preserve in tight containers. Contains not less than 96.0% and not more than 102.0% of prednisolone sodium phosphate, calculated on the dried basis. Meets the requirements for Identification, Specific rotation (+95° to +102°), pH (7.5–10.5, in a solution [1 in 100]), Water (not more than 6.5%), Phosphate ions (not more than 1.0%), Selenium (not more than 0.003%, a 200-mg test specimen being used), and Free prednisolone (not more than 1.0%).

Prednisolone Sodium Phosphate Injection USP—Preserve in single-dose or in multiple-dose containers, preferably of Type I glass, protected from light. A sterile solution of Prednisolone Sodium Phosphate in Water for Injection. Contains an amount of prednisolone sodium phosphate equivalent to the labeled amount of prednisolone phos-

phate, present as the disodium salt, within ±10%. Meets the requirements for Identification, Bacterial endotoxins, pH (7.0–8.0), and Particulate matter, and for Injections.

Prednisolone Sodium Phosphate Ophthalmic Solution USP—Preserve in tight, light-resistant containers. A sterile solution of Prednisolone Sodium Phosphate in a buffered, aqueous medium. Contains an amount of prednisolone sodium phosphate equivalent to the labeled amount of prednisolone phosphate, present as the disodium salt, within −10% to +15%. Meets the requirements for Identification, Sterility, and pH (6.2–8.2).

Prednisolone Sodium Phosphate Oral Solution—Not in *USP–NF*.

Prednisolone Sodium Succinate for Injection USP—Preserve in Containers for Sterile Solids. It is sterile prednisolone sodium succinate prepared from Prednisolone Hemisuccinate with the aid of Sodium Hydroxide or Sodium Carbonate. Contains suitable buffers. Contains an amount of prednisolone sodium succinate equivalent to the labeled amount of prednisolone, within ±10%. Meets the requirements for Constituted solution, Identification, Bacterial endotoxins, pH (6.7–8.0, determined in the solution constituted as directed in the labeling), Loss on drying (not more than 2.0%), and Particulate matter, and for Sterility tests, Uniformity of dosage units, and Labeling under Injections.

Prednisolone Tebutate USP—Preserve in tight containers sealed under sterile nitrogen, in a cold place. Contains not less than 97.0% and not more than 103.0% of prednisolone tebutate, calculated on the dried basis. Meets the requirements for Identification, Specific rotation (+100° to +115°), Loss on drying (not more than 5.0%), Residue on ignition (not more than 0.1%), and Selenium (not more than 0.003%, a 200-mg specimen being used).

Prednisolone Tebutate Injectable Suspension USP—Preserve in single-dose or in multiple-dose containers, preferably of Type I glass. A sterile suspension of Prednisolone Tebutate in a suitable aqueous medium. Contains the labeled amount, within ±10%. Meets the requirements for Identification, Bacterial endotoxins, and pH (6.0–8.0), and for Injections.

PREDNISONE

Chemical name: Pregna-1,4-diene-3,11,20-trione monohydrate, 17,21-dihydroxy-.

Molecular formula: $C_{21}H_{26}O_5 \cdot H_2O$.

Molecular weight: 376.44.

Description: Prednisone USP—White to practically white, odorless, crystalline powder. Melts at about 230 °C, with some decomposition.

Solubility: Prednisone USP—Very slightly soluble in water; slightly soluble in alcohol, in chloroform, in dioxane, and in methanol.

USP requirements:

Prednisone USP—Preserve in well-closed containers. Label to indicate whether it is hydrous or anhydrous. Contains one molecule of water of hydration or is anhydrous. Contains not less than 97.0% and not more than 102.0% of prednisone, calculated on the anhydrous basis. Meets the requirements for Identification, Specific rotation (+167° to +175°), Water (not more than 5.0% for Prednisone monohydrate and not more than 1.0% for anhydrous Prednisone), Residue on ignition (negligible, from 100 mg), Chromatographic purity (not more than 1.5% of any individual impurity, and not more than 2.0% of total impurities), and Other impurities.

Prednisone Oral Solution USP—Preserve in tight containers. Contains the labeled amount, within ±10%. Meets the requirements for Identification, pH (2.6–4.5), and Alcohol content (2.0–6.0%).

Prednisone Injectable Suspension USP—Preserve in multiple-dose containers, preferably of Type I glass. A sterile suspension of Prednisone in a suitable aqueous medium. Label it to indicate that it is for veterinary use only. Label it to indicate that it is for intramuscular administration only. Contains the labeled amount, within ±10%. Meets the requirements for Identification, pH (3.0–7.0), Sterility, and Bacterial endotoxins, and for Injections.

Prednisone Tablets USP—Preserve in well-closed containers. Contain the labeled amount, within ±10%. Meet the requirements for Identification, Dissolution (80% in 30 minutes in water in Apparatus 2 at 50 rpm), and Uniformity of dosage units.

PRILOCAINE

Chemical group: Amide.

Chemical name: Prilocaine hydrochloride—Propanamide, N-(2-methylphenyl)-2-(propylamino)-, monohydrochloride.

Molecular formula: Prilocaine hydrochloride—$C_{13}H_{20}N_2O \cdot HCl$.

Molecular weight: Prilocaine hydrochloride—256.77.

Description: Prilocaine Hydrochloride USP—White, odorless, crystalline powder.

pKa: Prilocaine hydrochloride—7.89.

Solubility: Prilocaine Hydrochloride USP—Freely soluble in water and in alcohol; slightly soluble in chloroform; very slightly soluble in acetone; practically insoluble in ether.

USP requirements:
Prilocaine Hydrochloride USP—Preserve in well-closed containers. Contains not less than 99.0% and not more than 101.0% of prilocaine hydrochloride, calculated on the dried basis. Meets the requirements for Identification, Melting range (166–169 °C), Loss on drying (not more than 0.3%), Residue on ignition (not more than 0.1%), and Heavy metals (not more than 0.002%).

Prilocaine Hydrochloride Injection USP—Preserve in single-dose or in multiple-dose containers, preferably of Type I glass. A sterile solution of Prilocaine Hydrochloride in Water for Injection. Contains the labeled amount, ±5%. Meets the requirements for Identification, Bacterial endotoxins, and pH (6.0–7.0), and for Injections.

PRILOCAINE AND EPINEPHRINE

For *Prilocaine* and *Epinephrine*—See individual listings for chemistry information.

USP requirements: Prilocaine and Epinephrine Injection USP—Preserve in single-dose or in multiple-dose, light-resistant containers, preferably of Type I glass. A sterile solution prepared from Prilocaine Hydrochloride and Epinephrine with the aid of Hydrochloric Acid in Water for Injection, or a sterile solution of Prilocaine Hydrochloride and Epinephrine Bitartrate in Water for Injection. The content of epinephrine does not exceed 0.002% (1 in 50,000). The label indicates that the Injection is not to be used if its color is pinkish or darker than slightly yellow or if it contains a precipitate. Contains the labeled amount of prilocaine hydrochloride, within ±5%, and the labeled amount of epinephrine, within −10% to +15%. Meets the requirements for Color and clarity, Identification, Bacterial endotoxins, and pH (3.3–5.5), and for Injections.

PRIMAQUINE

Chemical group: 8-Aminoquinolines.

Chemical name: Primaquine phosphate—1,4-Pentanediamine, N⁴-(6-methoxy-8-quinolinyl)-, phosphate (1:2).

Molecular formula: Primaquine phosphate—$C_{15}H_{21}N_3O \cdot 2H_3PO_4$.

Molecular weight: Primaquine phosphate—455.34.

Description: Primaquine Phosphate USP—Orange-red, crystalline powder. Is odorless. Its solutions are acid to litmus. Melts at about 200 °C.

Solubility: Primaquine Phosphate USP—Soluble in water; insoluble in chloroform and in ether.

USP requirements:
Primaquine Phosphate USP—Preserve in well-closed, lightresistant containers. Contains not less than 98.0% and not more than 102.0% of primaquine phosphate, calculated on the dried basis. Meets the requirements for Identification, Loss on drying (not more than 1.0%), and Organic volatile impurities.

Primaquine Phosphate Tablets USP—Preserve in wellclosed, light-resistant containers. Contain the labeled amount, within ±7%. Meet the requirements for Identification, Dissolution (80% in 60 minutes in 0.01 N hydrochloric acid in Apparatus 2 at 50 rpm), and Uniformity of dosage units.

PRIMIDONE

Chemical group: A congener of phenobarbital in which the carbonyl oxygen of the urea moiety is replaced by two hydrogen atoms.

Chemical name: 4,6(1H,5H)-Pyrimidinedione, 5-ethyldihydro-5-phenyl-.

Molecular formula: $C_{12}H_{14}N_2O_2$.

Molecular weight: 218.25.

Description: Primidone USP—White, crystalline powder. Is odorless.

Solubility: Primidone USP—Very slightly soluble in water and in most organic solvents; slightly soluble in alcohol.

Other characteristics: Highly stable compound; no acidic properties, in contrast to its barbiturate analog.

USP requirements:
Primidone USP—Preserve in well-closed containers. Contains not less than 98.0% and not more than 102.0% of primidone, calculated on the dried basis. Meets the requirements for Identification, Melting range (279–284 °C), Loss on drying (not more than 0.5%), Residue on ignition (not more than 0.2%), Ordinary impurities, and Organic volatile impurities.

Primidone Oral Suspension USP—Preserve in tight, light-resistant containers. A suspension of Primidone in a suitable aqueous vehicle. Contains, in each 100 mL, not less than 4.5 grams and not more than 5.5 grams of primidone. Meets the requirements for Identification and pH (5.5–8.5).

Primidone Tablets USP—Preserve in well-closed containers. Tablets intended solely for veterinary use are so labeled. Contain the labeled amount, within ±5%. Meet the require-

ments for Identification, Dissolution (75% in 60 minutes in water in Apparatus 2 at 50 rpm), and Uniformity of dosage units.

Primidone Chewable Tablets—Not in *USP–NF*.

PROBENECID

Chemical name: Benzoic acid, 4-[(dipropylamino)sulfonyl]-.

Molecular formula: $C_{13}H_{19}NO_4S$.

Molecular weight: 285.36.

Description: Probenecid USP—White or practically white, fine, crystalline powder. Is practically odorless.

pKa: 3.4.

Solubility: Probenecid USP—Practically insoluble in water and in dilute acids; soluble in dilute alkali, in chloroform, in alcohol, and in acetone.

USP requirements:
Probenecid USP—Preserve in well-closed containers. Contains not less than 98.0% and not more than 101.0% of probenecid, calculated on the dried basis. Meets the requirements for Identification, Melting range (198–200 °C), Acidity, Loss on drying (not more than 0.5%), Residue on ignition (not more than 0.1%), Selenium (not more than 0.003%, a 100-mg test specimen, mixed with 100 mg of magnesium oxide, being used), Heavy metals (not more than 0.002%), Chromatographic purity, and Organic volatile impurities.

Probenecid Tablets USP—Preserve in well-closed containers. Contain the labeled amount, within ±7%. Meet the requirements for Identification, Dissolution (80% in 30 minutes in simulated intestinal fluid TS [pH 7.5 ±0.1], prepared without pancreatin, in Apparatus 2 at 75 rpm), and Uniformity of dosage units.

PROBENECID AND COLCHICINE

For *Probenecid* and *Colchicine*—See individual listings for chemistry information.

USP requirements: Probenecid and Colchicine Tablets USP—Preserve in well-closed, light-resistant containers. Contain the labeled amount of colchicine, within −10% to +15%, and the labeled amount of probenecid, within ±10%. Meet the requirements for Identification, Dissolution (80% of each active ingredient in 30 minutes in phosphate buffer [pH 6.8] in Apparatus 2 at 50 rpm), and Uniformity of dosage units.

PROBUCOL

Chemical name: Phenol, 4,4′-[(1-methylethylidene)bis(thio)]-bis[2,6-bis(1,1-dimethylethyl)-.

Molecular formula: $C_{31}H_{48}O_2S_2$.

Molecular weight: 516.84.

Description: Probucol USP—White to off-white, crystalline powder.

Solubility: Probucol USP—Insoluble in water; freely soluble in chloroform and in *n*-propyl alcohol; soluble in alcohol and in solvent hexane.

USP requirements:
Probucol USP—Preserve in well-closed, light-resistant containers. Contains not less than 98.0% and not more than 102.0% of probucol, calculated on the dried basis. Meets the requirements for Identification, Melting range (124–127 °C, a dried specimen being used), Loss on drying (not more than 1.0%), Residue on ignition (not more than 0.1%), Heavy metals (not more than 0.002%), Related compounds, and Organic volatile impurities.

Probucol Tablets USP—Preserve in well-closed, light-resistant containers. Contain the labeled amount, within ± 10%. Meet the requirements for Identification and Uniformity of dosage units.

PROCAINAMIDE

Chemical name: Procainamide hydrochloride—Benzamide, 4-amino-*N*-[2-(diethylamino)ethyl]-, monohydrochloride.

Molecular formula: Procainamide hydrochloride—$C_{13}H_{21}N_3O \cdot$ HCl.

Molecular weight: Procainamide hydrochloride—271.79.

Description:
Procainamide Hydrochloride USP—White to tan, crystalline powder. Is odorless. Its solution (1 in 10) has a pH of 5.0–6.5.

Procainamide Hydrochloride Injection USP—Colorless, or having not more than a slight yellow color.

pKa: 9.23.

Solubility: Procainamide Hydrochloride USP—Very soluble in water; soluble in alcohol; slightly soluble in chloroform; very slightly soluble in ether.

USP requirements:
Procainamide Hydrochloride USP—Preserve in tight containers. Contains not less than 98.0% and not more than 102.0% of procainamide hydrochloride, calculated on the dried basis. Meets the requirements for Identification, Melting range (165–169 °C), Loss on drying (not more than 0.3%), Residue on ignition (not more than 0.1%), Heavy metals (not more than 0.002%), Limit of free *p*-aminobenzoic acid (not more than 0.1%), Ordinary impurities, and Organic volatile impurities.

Procainamide Hydrochloride Capsules USP—Preserve in tight containers. Contain the labeled amount, within ± 5%. Meet the requirements for Identification, Dissolution (75% in 90 minutes in 0.01 *N* hydrochloric acid in Apparatus 2 at 50 rpm), and Uniformity of dosage units.

Procainamide Hydrochloride Injection USP—Preserve in single-dose or in multiple-dose containers, preferably of Type I glass. A sterile solution of Procainamide Hydrochloride in Water for Injection. Label it to indicate that the Injection is not to be used if it is darker than slightly yellow, or is discolored in any other way. Contains the labeled amount, within ±5%. Meets the requirements for Identification, Bacterial endotoxins, pH (4.0–6.0), and Particulate matter, and for Injections.

Procainamide Hydrochloride Tablets USP—Preserve in tight containers. Contain the labeled amount, within ±5%. Meet the requirements for Identification, Dissolution (80% in 60 minutes in 0.1 *N* hydrochloric acid in Apparatus 2 at 50 rpm), and Uniformity of dosage units.

Procainamide Hydrochloride Extended-release Tablets USP—Preserve in tight containers. The labeling indicates the Drug Release Test with which the product complies. Contain the labeled amount, within ±7%. Meet the requirements for Identification, Drug release (for Test 1: 30–60% in one hour, 60–90% in 4 hours, and not less than 75% in 6 hours in 0.1 N hydrochloric acid in Apparatus 2 at 50 rpm; for Test 2: 30–60% in one hour, 60–90% in 4 hours, and

not less than 80% in 8 hours in Apparatus 2 at 5 rpm; for Test 3: 25–50% in one hour, 40–75% in 3 hours, 65–90% in 6 hours, and not less than 80% in 8 hours in Apparatus 2 at 50 rpm; for Test 4: not more than 30% in one hour, 25–45% in 2 hours, 45–75% in 4 hours, 70–90% in 8 hours, and not less than 80% in 14 hours in 0.1 N hydrochloric acid in Apparatus 1 at 50 rpm; for Test 5: for 500 mg tablets: 30–45% in 1 hour, 55–75% in 4 hours, not less than 60% in 6 hours, and not less than 75% in 8 hours, and for 750 and 1000 mg tablets: 30–50% in one hour, 60–80% in 4 hours, 70–90% in 6 hours, and not less than 75% in 8 hours in Apparatus 2 at 50 rpm; for Test 6: for 250 mg tablets: 30–60% in one hour, 60–90% in 4 hours, and not less than 80% in 8 hours; for 500 mg tablets: 30–50% in one hour, 60–80% in 4 hours, and not less than 85% in 8 hours; for 750 mg tablets: 30–50% in one hour, 60–80% in 4 hours, and not less than 80% in 8 hours in Apparatus 2 at 50 rpm; and for Test 8: 33–50% in one hour, 70–85% in 4 hours, not less than 80% in 6 hours, and not less than 85% in 8 hours in Apparatus 2 at 50 rpm) , and Uniformity of dosage units.

PROCAINE

Chemical group: Ester.

Chemical name: Procaine hydrochloride—Benzoic acid, 4-amino-, 2-(diethylamino)ethyl ester, monohydrochloride.

Molecular formula: Procaine hydrochloride—$C_{13}H_{20}N_2O_2 \cdot HCl$.

Molecular weight: Procaine hydrochloride—272.78.

Description:
Procaine Hydrochloride USP—Small, white crystals or white, crystalline powder. Is odorless.
Procaine Hydrochloride Injection USP—Clear, colorless liquid.

pKa: 8.7.

Solubility:
Procaine Hydrochloride USP—Freely soluble in water; soluble in alcohol; slightly soluble in chloroform; practically insoluble in ether.

USP requirements:
Procaine Hydrochloride USP—Preserve in well-closed containers. Where it is intended for use in preparing injectable dosage forms, the label states that it is sterile or must be subjected to further processing during the preparation of injectable dosage forms. Contains not less than 99.0% and not more than 101.0% of procaine hydrochloride, calculated on the dried basis. Meets the requirements for Identification, Bacterial endotoxins, Melting range (153–158 °C), Acidity, Loss on drying (not more than 1.0%), Residue on ignition (not more than 0.15%), Heavy metals (not more than 0.002%), Sterility, and Chromatographic purity.
Procaine Hydrochloride Injection USP—Preserve in single-dose or in multiple-dose containers, preferably of Type I or Type II glass. The Injection may be packaged in 100-mL multiple-dose containers. A sterile solution of Procaine Hydrochloride in Water for Injection. Contains the labeled amount, within ±5%. Meets the requirements for Identification, Bacterial endotoxins, pH (3.0–5.5), and Particulate matter, and for Injections.

PROCAINE AND EPINEPHRINE

For *Procaine* and *Epinephrine*—See individual listings for chemistry information.

USP requirements: Procaine Hydrochloride and Epinephrine Injection USP—Preserve in single-dose or in multiple-dose, light-resistant containers, preferably of Type I or Type II glass. A sterile solution of Procaine Hydrochloride and epinephrine hydrochloride in Water for Injection. The content of epinephrine does not exceed 0.002% (1 in 50,000). The label indicates that the Injection is not to be used if its color is pinkish or darker than slightly yellow or if it contains a precipitate. Contains the labeled amounts of procaine hydrochloride, within ±5%, and epinephrine, within −10% to +15%. Meets the requirements for Color and clarity, Identification, Bacterial endotoxins, pH (3.0–5.5), and Content of epinephrine, and for Injections.

PROCAINE AND PHENYLEPHRINE

For *Procaine* and *Phenylephrine*—See individual listings for chemistry information.

USP requirements: Procaine and Phenylephrine Hydrochlorides Injection USP—Preserve in single-dose or in multiple-dose containers, preferably of Type I glass. A sterile solution of Procaine Hydrochloride and Phenylephrine Hydrochloride in Water for Injection. Contains the labeled amounts of procaine hydrochloride, within ±5%, and phenylephrine hydrochloride, within ±10%. Meets the requirements for Identification, Bacterial endotoxins, and pH (3.0–5.5), and for Injections.

PROCAINE, TETRACAINE, AND LEVONORDEFRIN

For *Procaine, Tetracaine,* and *Levonordefrin*—See individual listings for chemistry information.

USP requirements: Procaine and Tetracaine Hydrochlorides and Levonordefrin Injection USP—Preserve in single-dose or in multiple-dose containers, preferably of Type I glass. A sterile solution of Procaine Hydrochloride, Tetracaine Hydrochloride, and Levonordefrin in Water for Injection. The label indicates that the Injection is not to be used if its color is pinkish or darker than slightly yellow or if it contains a precipitate. Contains the labeled amounts of procaine hydrochloride and tetracaine hydrochloride, within ±5%, and levonordefrin, within ±10%. Meets the requirements for Color and clarity, Identification, Bacterial endotoxins, and pH (3.5–5.0), and for Injections.

PROCARBAZINE

Chemical name: Procarbazine hydrochloride—Benzamide, N-(1-methylethyl)-4-[(2-methylhydrazino)methyl]-, monohydrochloride.

Molecular formula: Procarbazine hydrochloride—$C_{12}H_{19}N_3O \cdot HCl$.

Molecular weight: Procarbazine hydrochloride—257.76.

Description: Procarbazine hydrochloride—White to pale yellow, crystalline powder.

Solubility: Procarbazine hydrochloride—Soluble but unstable in water or in aqueous solutions.

USP requirements:
Procarbazine Hydrochloride USP—Preserve in tight, light-resistant containers. Contains not less than 98.5% and not more than 100.5% of procarbazine hydrochloride. Meets

the requirements for Identification, Residue on ignition (not more than 0.1%), Heavy metals (not more than 0.002%), and Organic volatile impurities.

Caution: Handle Procarbazine Hydrochloride with exceptional care, since it is a highly potent agent.

Procarbazine Hydrochloride Capsules USP—Preserve in tight, light-resistant containers. Contain the labeled amount, within ±10%. Meet the requirements for Identification, Dissolution (75% in 45 minutes in water in Apparatus 2 at 50 rpm), and Uniformity of dosage units.

PROCATEROL

Chemical name: Procaterol hydrochloride hemihydrate—8-hydroxy-5-[1-hydroxy-2[(1-methylethyl)amino]butyl]-2-(1*H*)quinolone, monohydrochloride, hemihydrate, racemic mixture of (±) (*R**,*S**) isomers.

Molecular formula: Procaterol hydrochloride hemihydrate—$C_{16}H_{22}N_2O_3 \cdot HCl \cdot \frac{1}{2}H_2O$.

Molecular weight: Procaterol hydrochloride hemihydrate—335.83.

Description: Procaterol hydrochloride hemihydrate—White to off-white powder, unstable to light.

Solubility: Procaterol hydrochloride hemihydrate—Soluble in water and in methanol; slightly soluble in ethanol; practically insoluble in acetone, in ether, in ethyl acetate, and in chloroform.

USP requirements: Procaterol Hydrochloride Hemihydrate Inhalation Aerosol—Not in *USP–NF*.

PROCHLORPERAZINE

Chemical group: Phenothiazine derivative of piperazine group.

Chemical name:

Prochlorperazine—10*H*-Phenothiazine, 2-chloro-10-[3-(4methyl-1-piperazinyl)propyl]-.

Prochlorperazine edisylate—10*H*-Phenothiazine, 2-chloro-10-[3-(4-methyl-1-piperazinyl)propyl]-, 1,2-ethanedisulfonate (1:1).

Prochlorperazine maleate—10*H*-Phenothiazine, 2-chloro-10-[3-(4-methyl-1-piperazinyl)propyl]-, (*Z*)-2-butenedioate (1:2).

Prochlorperazine mesylate—10*H*-Phenothiazine, 2-chloro-10[3-(4-methyl-1-piperazinyl)propyl]-, dimethanesulphonate.

Molecular formula:

Prochlorperazine—$C_{20}H_{24}ClN_3S$.

Prochlorperazine edisylate—$C_{20}H_{24}ClN_3S \cdot C_2H_6O_6S_2$.

Prochlorperazine maleate—$C_{20}H_{24}ClN_3S \cdot 2C_4H_4O_4$.

Prochlorperazine mesylate—$C_{20}H_{24}ClN_3S \cdot 2CH_3SO_3H$.

Molecular weight:

Prochlorperazine—373.94.

Prochlorperazine edisylate—564.14.

Prochlorperazine maleate—606.09.

Prochlorperazine mesylate—566.1.

Description:

Prochlorperazine USP—Clear, pale yellow, viscous liquid. Is sensitive to light.

Prochlorperazine Edisylate USP—White to very light yellow, odorless, crystalline powder. Its solutions are acid to litmus.

Prochlorperazine Maleate USP—White or pale yellow, practically odorless, crystalline powder. Its saturated solution is acid to litmus.

Prochlorperazine mesylate—White or almost white, odorless or almost odorless, powder.

Solubility:

Prochlorperazine USP—Very slightly soluble in water; freely soluble in alcohol, in chloroform, and in ether.

Prochlorperazine Edisylate USP—Freely soluble in water; very slightly soluble in alcohol; insoluble in ether and in chloroform.

Prochlorperazine Maleate USP—Practically insoluble in water and in alcohol; slightly soluble in warm chloroform.

Prochlorperazine mesylate—Soluble 1 in less than 0.5 of water and 1 in 40 of alcohol; slightly soluble in chloroform; practically insoluble in ether.

USP requirements:

Prochlorperazine USP—Preserve in tight, light-resistant containers. Contains not less than 98.0% and not more than 101.0% of prochlorperazine. Meets the requirements for Identification, Residue on ignition (not more than 0.1%), and Ordinary impurities.

Prochlorperazine Oral Solution USP—Preserve in tight, light-resistant containers. Contains an amount of prochlorperazine edisylate equivalent to the labeled amount of prochlorperazine, within ±8%. Meets the requirement for Identification.

Prochlorperazine Suppositories USP—Preserve in tight containers at a temperature below 37 °C. Do not expose the unwrapped Suppositories to sunlight. Contain the labeled amount, within ±10%. Meet the requirement for Identification.

Prochlorperazine Edisylate USP—Preserve in tight, light-resistant containers. Contains not less than 98.0% and not more than 101.5% of prochlorperazine edisylate, calculated on the dried basis. Meets the requirements for Identification, Loss on drying (not more than 0.5%), Residue on ignition (not more than 0.1%), Selenium (not more than 0.003%, a 100-mg test specimen, mixed with 100 mg of magnesium oxide, being used), Ordinary impurities, and Organic volatile impurities.

Prochlorperazine Edisylate Injection USP—Preserve in single-dose or in multiple-dose containers, preferably of Type I glass, protected from light. A sterile solution of Prochlorperazine Edisylate in Water for Injection. Contains an amount of prochlorperazine edisylate equivalent to the labeled amount of prochlorperazine, within ±10%. Meets the requirements for Identification, Bacterial endotoxins, and pH (4.2–6.2), and for Injections.

Prochlorperazine Edisylate Syrup USP—Preserve in tight, light-resistant containers. Contains, in each 100 mL, an amount of prochlorperazine edisylate equivalent to not less than 92.0 mg and not more than 108.0 mg of prochlorperazine. Meets the requirements for Identification.

Prochlorperazine Maleate USP—Preserve in tight, light-resistant containers. Contains not less than 98.0% and not more than 101.5% of prochlorperazine maleate, calculated on the dried basis. Meets the requirements for Identification, Loss on drying (not more than 0.5%), Residue on ignition (not more than 0.1%), Ordinary impurities, and Organic volatile impurities.

Prochlorperazine Maleate Extended-release Capsules—Not in *USP–NF*.

Prochlorperazine Maleate Tablets USP—Preserve in well-closed containers, protected from light. Contain an amount of prochlorperazine maleate equivalent to the labeled amount of prochlorperazine, within ±5%. Meet the requirements for Identification, Dissolution (75% in 60 minutes in 0.1 *N* hydrochloric acid in Apparatus 2 at 75 rpm), and Uniformity of dosage units.

Prochlorperazine Mesylate Injection—Not in *USP–NF*.
Prochlorperazine Mesylate Oral Solution—Not in *USP–NF*.
Prochlorperazine Mesylate Syrup—Not in *USP–NF*.

PROCYCLIDINE

Chemical group: Synthetic tertiary amine.

Chemical name: Procyclidine hydrochloride—1-Pyrrolidinepropanol, alpha-cyclohexyl-alpha-phenyl-, hydrochloride.

Molecular formula: Procyclidine hydrochloride—$C_{19}H_{29}NO \cdot HCl$.

Molecular weight: Procyclidine hydrochloride—323.90.

Description: Procyclidine Hydrochloride USP—White, crystalline powder, having a moderate, characteristic odor. Melts at about 225 °C, with decomposition.

Solubility: Procyclidine Hydrochloride USP—Soluble in water and in alcohol; insoluble in ether and in acetone.

USP requirements:
Procyclidine Hydrochloride USP—Preserve in tight, light-resistant containers, and store in a dry place. Contains not less than 99.0% and not more than 101.0% of procyclidine hydrochloride, calculated on the dried basis. Meets the requirements for Identification, pH (5.0–6.5, in a solution [1 in 100]), Loss on drying (not more than 0.5%), Residue on ignition (not more than 0.1%), Related compounds (not more than 4.0%), and Organic volatile impurities.
Procyclidine Hydrochloride Elixir—Not in *USP–NF*.
Procyclidine Hydrochloride Tablets USP—Preserve in tight containers, and store in a dry place. Contain the labeled amount, within ±7%. Meet the requirements for Identification, Dissolution (75% in 45 minutes in water in Apparatus 2 at 50 rpm), Related compounds, and Uniformity of dosage units.

PROGESTERONE

Chemical name: Pregn-4-ene-3,20-dione.

Molecular formula: $C_{21}H_{30}O_2$.

Molecular weight: 314.46.

Description: Progesterone USP—White or creamy white, odorless, crystalline powder. Is stable in air.

Solubility: Progesterone USP—Practically insoluble in water; soluble in alcohol, in acetone, and in dioxane; sparingly soluble in vegetable oils.

USP requirements:
Progesterone USP—Preserve in tight, light-resistant containers. Contains not less than 97.0% and not more than 103.0% of progesterone, calculated on the dried basis. Meets the requirements for Identification, Melting range (126–131 °C; if existing in a polymorphic modification, melting at about 121 °C), Specific rotation (+175° to +183°), and Loss on drying (not more than 0.5%), and Other impurities.
Progesterone Capsules (Micronized)—Not in *USP–NF*.
Progesterone Gel (Micronized)—Not in *USP–NF*.
Progesterone Injection USP—Preserve in single-dose or in multiple-dose containers, preferably of Type I or Type III glass. A sterile solution of Progesterone in a suitable solvent. Contains the labeled amount, within ±10%. Meets the requirements for Identification and for Injections.
Progesterone Vaginal Suppositories USP—For Suppositories compounded in Fatty Acid Base: Preserve in well-closed, light-resistant containers. Store in a refrigerator. Label Suppositories to state that they are Progesterone Vaginal Suppositories in a Fatty Acid Base and to state the content, in mg, of progesterone per suppository. Label Suppositories to state that they are to be stored in a refrigerator (2° to 8°). Label them to state that they are to be used only as directed, and that wrappers are to be removed prior to use. Prepare Progesterone Vaginal Suppositories in Fatty Acid Base as follows: 25 mg to 600 mg of micronized Progesterone, 25 mg of Silica Gel, and Fatty Acid Base, a sufficient quantity to make one suppository. Calibrate the actual molds with the Fatty Acid Base that is used for preparing the suppositories, and adjust the formula accordingly. Mix thoroughly the Progesterone and Silica Gel to obtain a uniform powder. Heat the Fatty Acid Base slowly and evenly until melted. Slowly add the powder to the melted base, with stirring. Mix thoroughly, and pour into molds. Cool in a refrigerator until solidified, trim, and wrap. Meet the requirements for Uniformity of dosage units and Beyond-use date.
For Suppositories compounded in Polyethylene Glycol Base: Preserve in tight, light-resistant containers. Do not dispense or store polyethylene glycol-base suppositories in polystyrene containers. Store in a refrigerator. Label Suppositories to state that they are Progesterone Vaginal Suppositories in a Polyethylene Glycol Base and to state the content, in mg, of progesterone per suppository. Label Suppositories to state that they are to be stored in a refrigerator (2° to 8°). Label them to state that they are to be used only as directed, and that wrappers are to be removed prior to use, and that, if necessary, they may be moistened prior to insertion. Prepare Progesterone Vaginal Suppositories in Polyethylene Glycol Base as follows: 25 mg to 600 mg of micronized Progesterone, 25 mg of Silica Gel, and Polyethylene Glycol Base, a sufficient quantity to make one suppository. Calibrate the actual molds with the Polyethylene Glycol Base that is used for preparing the suppositories, and adjust the formula accordingly. Mix thoroughly the Progesterone and Silica Gel to obtain a uniform powder. Heat the Polyethylene Glycol Base slowly and evenly until melted. Slowly add the powder to the melted base, with stirring. Mix thoroughly, and pour into molds. Cool, trim, and wrap. Meet the requirements for Uniformity of dosage units and Beyond-use date.
Progesterone Injectable Suspension USP—Preserve in single-dose or in multiple-dose containers, preferably of Type I glass. A sterile suspension of Progesterone in Water for Injection. Contains the labeled amount, within ±7%. Meets the requirements for Identification and pH (4.0–7.5), and for Injections.
Progesterone Intrauterine Contraceptive System USP—Preserve in sealed, single-unit containers. It is sterile. Contains the labeled amount, within ±10%. Meets the requirements for Identification, Sterility, Uniformity of dosage units, Chromatographic purity, and Drug-release pattern.

PROGUANIL

Chemical name: Proguanil hydrochloride—1-(4-Chlorophenyl)-5-isopropylbiguanide hydrochloride.

Molecular formula: Proguanil hydrochloride—$C_{11}H_{16}ClN_5 \cdot HCl$.

Molecular weight: Proguanil hydrochloride—290.2.

Description: Proguanil hydrochloride—White or odorless or almost odorless crystalline powder.

Solubility: Proguanil hydrochloride—Slightly soluble in water; more soluble in hot water; soluble 1 in 40 of alcohol; practically insoluble in chloroform and in ether.

USP requirements: Proguanil Hydrochloride Tablets—Not in *USP–NF*.

PROLINE

Chemical name: L-Proline.

Molecular formula: $C_5H_9NO_2$.

Molecular weight: 115.13.

Description: Proline USP—White, odorless crystals.

Solubility: Proline USP—Freely soluble in water and in absolute alcohol; insoluble in ether, in butanol, and in isopropanol.

USP requirements: Proline USP—Preserve in well-closed containers. Contains not less than 98.5% and not more than 101.5% of proline, as L-proline, calculated on the dried basis. Meets the requirements for Identification, Specific rotation (–84.3° to –86.3°), Loss on drying (not more than 0.4%), Residue on ignition (not more than 0.4%), Chloride (not more than 0.05%), Sulfate (not more than 0.03%), Iron (not more than 0.003%), Heavy metals (not more than 0.0015%), Chromatographic purity, and Organic volatile impurities.

PROMAZINE

Chemical group: Phenothiazine.

Chemical name: Promazine hydrochloride—10*H*-Phenothiazine-10-propanamine, *N,N*-dimethyl-, monohydrochloride.

Molecular formula: Promazine hydrochloride—$C_{17}H_{20}N_2S \cdot HCl$.

Molecular weight: Promazine hydrochloride—320.88.

Description: Promazine Hydrochloride USP—White to slightly yellow, practically odorless, crystalline powder. It oxidizes upon prolonged exposure to air and acquires a blue or pink color.

Solubility: Promazine Hydrochloride USP—Freely soluble in water and in chloroform.

USP requirements:
Promazine Hydrochloride USP—Preserve in tight, light-resistant containers. Dried at 105 °C for 2 hours, contains not less than 98.0% and not more than 102.0% of promazine hydrochloride. Meets the requirements for Completeness and clarity of solution, Identification, Melting range (172–182 °C, the range between beginning and end of melting not more than 3 °C), pH (4.2–5.2, in a solution [1 in 20]), Loss on drying (not more than 0.5%), Residue on ignition (not more than 0.1%), Selenium (not more than 0.003%), Heavy metals (not more than 0.005%), Chromatographic purity, and Organic volatile impurities.
Promazine Hydrochloride Injection USP—Preserve in single-dose or in multiple-dose containers, preferably of Type I glass, protected from light. A sterile solution of Promazine Hydrochloride in Water for Injection. Contains the labeled amount, within –5% to +10%. Meets the requirements for Identification, Bacterial endotoxins, and pH (4.0–5.5), and for Injections.
Promazine Hydrochloride Oral Solution USP—Preserve in tight, light-resistant containers. Contains the labeled amount, within –5% to +10%. Meets the requirements for Identification and pH (5.0–5.5).
Promazine Hydrochloride Syrup USP—Preserve in tight, light-resistant containers. Contains the labeled amount, within –5% to +10%. Meets the requirement for Identification.

Promazine Hydrochloride Tablets USP—Preserve in tight, light-resistant containers. Contain the labeled amount, within –5% to +10%. Meet the requirements for Identification, Disintegration (30 minutes, with disks), and Uniformity of dosage units.

PROMETHAZINE

Chemical group: Phenothiazine derivative.

Chemical name: Promethazine hydrochloride—10*H*-Phenothiazine-10-ethanamine, *N,N*,alpha-trimethyl-, monohydrochloride.

Molecular formula: Promethazine hydrochloride—$C_{17}H_{20}N_2S \cdot HCl$.

Molecular weight: Promethazine hydrochloride—320.88.

Description: Promethazine Hydrochloride USP—White to faint yellow, practically odorless, crystalline powder. Slowly oxidizes, and acquires a blue color, on prolonged exposure to air.

pKa: Promethazine hydrochloride—9.1.

Solubility: Promethazine Hydrochloride USP—Freely soluble in water, in hot dehydrated alcohol, and in chloroform; practically insoluble in ether, in acetone, and in ethyl acetate.

USP requirements:
Promethazine Hydrochloride USP—Preserve in tight, light-resistant containers. Contains not less than 97.0% and not more than 101.5% of promethazine hydrochloride, calculated on the dried basis. Meets the requirements for Completeness and clarity of solution, Identification, pH (4.0–5.0, in a solution [1 in 20]), Loss on drying (not more than 0.5%), Residue on ignition (not more than 0.1%), and Related substances.
Promethazine Hydrochloride Injection USP—Preserve in single-dose or in multiple-dose containers, preferably of Type I glass, protected from light. A sterile solution of Promethazine Hydrochloride in Water for Injection. Contains the labeled amount, within –5% to +10%. Meets the requirements for Identification, Bacterial endotoxins, and pH (4.0–5.5), and for Injections.
Promethazine Hydrochloride Suppositories USP—Preserve in tight, light-resistant containers, and store in a cold place. Contain the labeled amount, within –5% to +10%. Meet the requirement for Identification.
Promethazine Hydrochloride Oral Solution USP—Preserve in tight, light-resistant containers. Contains the labeled amount, within ±10%. Meets the requirement for Identification.
Promethazine Hydrochloride Syrup USP—Preserve in tight, light-resistant containers. Contains the labeled amount, within ±10%. Meets the requirement for Identification.
Promethazine Hydrochloride Tablets USP—Preserve in tight, light-resistant containers. Contain the labeled amount, within –5% to +10%. Meet the requirements for Identification, Dissolution (75% in 45 minutes in 0.01 *N* hydrochloric acid in Apparatus 1 at 100 rpm), and Uniformity of dosage units.

PROMETHAZINE AND CODEINE

For *Promethazine* and *Codeine*—See individual listings for chemistry information.

USP requirements:
Promethazine Hydrochloride and Codeine Phosphate Oral Solution—Not in *USP–NF*.

Promethazine Hydrochloride and Codeine Phosphate Syrup—Not in *USP–NF*.

PROMETHAZINE, CODEINE, AND POTASSIUM GUAIACOLSULFONATE

For *Promethazine, Codeine,* and *Potassium Guaiacolsulfonate*—See individual listings for chemistry information.

USP requirements: Promethazine Hydrochloride, Codeine Phosphate, and Potassium Guaiacolsulfonate Syrup—Not in *USP–NF*.

PROMETHAZINE AND DEXTROMETHORPHAN

For *Promethazine* and *Dextromethorphan*—See individual listings for chemistry information.

USP requirements:
Promethazine Hydrochloride and Dextromethorphan Hydrobromide Oral Solution—Not in *USP–NF*.
Promethazine Hydrochloride and Dextromethorphan Hydrobromide Syrup—Not in *USP–NF*.

PROMETHAZINE AND PHENYLEPHRINE

For *Promethazine* and *Phenylephrine*—See individual listings for chemistry information.

USP requirements: Promethazine Hydrochloride and Phenylephrine Hydrochloride Syrup—Not in *USP–NF*.

PROMETHAZINE, PHENYLEPHRINE, AND CODEINE

For *Promethazine, Phenylephrine,* and *Codeine*—See individual listings for chemistry information.

USP requirements:
Promethazine Hydrochloride, Phenylephrine Hydrochloride, and Codeine Phosphate Oral Solution—Not in *USP–NF*.
Promethazine Hydrochloride, Phenylephrine Hydrochloride, and Codeine Phosphate Syrup—Not in *USP–NF*.

PROMETHAZINE, PHENYLEPHRINE, CODEINE, AND POTASSIUM GUAIACOLSULFONATE

For *Promethazine, Phenylephrine, Codeine,* and *Potassium Guaiacolsulfonate*—See individual listings for chemistry information.

USP requirements: Promethazine Hydrochloride, Phenylephrine Hydrochloride, Codeine Phosphate, and Potassium Guaiacolsulfonate Syrup—Not in *USP–NF*.

PROMETHAZINE, PHENYLEPHRINE, AND POTASSIUM GUAIACOLSULFONATE

For *Promethazine, Phenylephrine,* and *Potassium Guaiacolsulfonate*—See individual listings for chemistry information.

USP requirements: Promethazine Hydrochloride, Phenylephrine Hydrochloride, and Potassium Guaiacolsulfonate Syrup—Not in *USP–NF*.

PROMETHAZINE AND POTASSIUM GUAIACOLSULFONATE

For *Promethazine* and *Potassium Guaiacolsulfonate*—See individual listings for chemistry information.

USP requirements: Promethazine Hydrochloride and Potassium Guaiacolsulfonate Syrup—Not in *USP–NF*.

PROMETHAZINE, PSEUDOEPHEDRINE, AND DEXTROMETHORPHAN

For *Promethazine, Pseudoephedrine,* and *Dextromethorphan*—See individual listings for chemistry information.

USP requirements: Promethazine Hydrochloride, Pseudoephedrine Hydrochloride, and Dextromethorphan Hydrobromide Syrup—Not in *USP–NF*.

PROPAFENONE

Chemical name: Propafenone hydrochloride—1-Propanone, 1-[2-[2-hydroxy-3-(propylamino)propoxy]phenyl]-3-phenyl-, hydrochloride.

Molecular formula: Propafenone hydrochloride—$C_{21}H_{27}NO_3 \cdot HCl$.

Molecular weight: Propafenone hydrochloride—377.90.

Description: Propafenone Hydrochloride USP—White powder.

Solubility: Propafenone Hydrochloride USP—Soluble in methanol and in hot water; slightly soluble in alcohol and in chloroform; very slightly soluble in acetone; insoluble in diethyl ether and in toluene.

USP requirements:
Propafenone Hydrochloride USP—Preserve in tight, light-resistant containers. Contains not less than 98.0% and not more than 102.0% of propafenone hydrochloride, calculated on the dried basis. Meets the requirements for Clarity of solution, Identification, Melting range (171–175 °C), pH (5.0–6.2, in a solution [1 in 200]), Loss on drying (not more than 0.5%), Residue on ignition (not more than 0.1%), Heavy metals (not more than 20 ppm), Limit of methanol and acetone (not more than 100 ppm of methanol and not more than 1000 ppm of acetone), and Chromatographic purity.
Propafenone Hydrochloride Tablets—Not in *USP–NF*.

PROPAMIDINE

Chemical name: Propamidine isotheonate—4,4'-Trimethylene-dioxydibenzamidine bis(2-hydroxyethanesulphonate).

Molecular formula: Propamidine isotheonate—$C_{17}H_{20}N_4O_2 \cdot 2C_2H_6O_4S$.

Molecular weight: Propamidine isotheonate—564.6.

Description: Propamidine isotheonate—Hygroscopic, very bitter crystals or granular powder. Melting point ~ 235 °C.

Solubility: Propamidine isotheonate—Soluble in water (~ 1 in 5), in glycerol, and in 95% alcohol (~ 1 in 33); practically insoluble in ether, in chloroform, in fixed oils, and in liquid petrolatum.

Other characteristics: Propamidine isotheonate— pH of a 5% w/v solution in water 4.5–6.5.

USP requirements: Propamidine Isotheonate 1% Ophthalmic Solution—Not in *USP–NF*.

PROPANE

Molecular formula: C_3H_8.

Molecular weight: 44.10.

Description: Propane NF—Colorless, flammable gas (boiling temperature is about –42 °C). Vapor pressure at 21 °C is about 10290 mm of mercury (108 psig).

NF category: Aerosol propellant.

Solubility: Propane NF—One hundred volumes of water dissolves 6.5 volumes at 17.8 °C and 753 mm pressure; 100 volumes of anhydrous alcohol dissolves 790 volumes at 16.6 °C and 754 mm pressure; 100 volumes of ether dissolves 926 volumes at 16.6 °C and 757 mm pressure; 100 volumes of chloroform dissolves 1299 volumes at 21.6 °C and 757 mm pressure.

NF requirements: Propane NF—Preserve in tight cylinders, and prevent exposure to excessive heat. Contains not less than 98.0% of propane. Meets the requirements for Identification, Water (not more than 0.001%), High-boiling residues (not more than 5 ppm), Acidity of residue, and Limit of sulfur compounds.

Caution: Propane is highly flammable and explosive.

PROPANTHELINE

Chemical group: Synthetic quaternary ammonium compound.

Chemical name: Propantheline bromide—2-Propanaminium, *N*-methyl-*N*-(1-methylethyl)-*N*-[2-[(9*H*-xanthen-9-ylcarbonyl)oxy]ethyl]-, bromide.

Molecular formula: Propantheline bromide—$C_{23}H_{30}BrNO_3$.

Molecular weight: Propantheline bromide—448.39.

Description:
Propantheline Bromide USP—White or practically white crystals. Is odorless. Melts at about 160 °C, with decomposition.
Sterile Propantheline Bromide USP—White or practically white crystals. Is odorless.

Solubility:
Propantheline Bromide USP—Very soluble in water, in alcohol, and in chloroform; practically insoluble in ether.
Sterile Propantheline Bromide USP—Very soluble in water, in alcohol, and in chloroform; practically insoluble in ether.

USP requirements:
Propantheline Bromide USP—Preserve in well-closed containers. Contains not less than 98.0% and not more than 102.0% of propantheline bromide, calculated on the dried basis. Meets the requirements for Identification, Loss on drying (not more than 0.5%), Residue on ignition (not more than 0.1%), Related compounds (not more than 3.0%), Organic volatile impurities, and Bromide content (17.5–18.2%, calculated on the dried basis).
Sterile Propantheline Bromide USP—Preserve in Containers for Sterile Solids. It is Propantheline Bromide suitable for parenteral use. Meets the requirements for Completeness of solution, Constituted solution, and Bacterial endotoxins, for Identification tests, Loss on drying, Residue on ignition, Related compounds, and Bromide content under Propantheline Bromide, and for Sterility tests, Uniformity of dosage units, and Labeling under Injections.
Propantheline Bromide Tablets USP—Preserve in well-closed containers. Contain the labeled amount, within ±10%. Meet the requirements for Identification, Dissolution (75% in 45 minutes in Acetate buffer [pH 4.5 ±0.05] in Apparatus 2 at 50 rpm), Uniformity of dosage units, and Related compounds.

PROPARACAINE

Chemical name: Proparacaine hydrochloride—Benzoic acid, 3-amino-4-propoxy-, 2-(diethylamino)ethyl ester, monohydrochloride.

Molecular formula: Proparacaine hydrochloride—$C_{16}H_{26}N_2O_3 \cdot$ HCl.

Molecular weight: Proparacaine hydrochloride—330.85.

Description:
Proparacaine Hydrochloride USP—White to off-white, or faintly buff-colored, odorless, crystalline powder. Its solutions are neutral to litmus.
Proparacaine Hydrochloride Ophthalmic Solution USP—Colorless or faint yellow solution.

Solubility: Proparacaine Hydrochloride USP—Soluble in water, in warm alcohol, and in methanol; insoluble in ether.

USP requirements:
Proparacaine Hydrochloride USP—Preserve in well-closed containers. Contains not less than 97.0% and not more than 103.0% of proparacaine hydrochloride, calculated on the dried basis. Meets the requirements for Identification, Melting range (178–185 °C, the range between beginning and end of melting not more than 2 °C), Loss on drying (not more than 0.5%), Residue on ignition (not more than 0.15%), and Ordinary impurities.
Proparacaine Hydrochloride Ophthalmic Solution USP—Preserve in tight, light-resistant containers. A sterile, aqueous solution of Proparacaine Hydrochloride. Label it to indicate that it is to be stored in a refrigerator after the container is opened. Contains the labeled amount, within –5% to +10%. Meets the requirements for Identification, Sterility, and pH (3.5–6.0).

PROPIOMAZINE

Chemical name: Propiomazine hydrochloride—1-Propanone, 1-[10-[2-(dimethylamino)propyl]-10*H*-phenothiazin-2-yl]-, monohydrochloride.

Molecular formula: Propiomazine hydrochloride—$C_{20}H_{24}N_2OS \cdot$ HCl.

Molecular weight: Propiomazine hydrochloride—376.94.

Description: Propiomazine hydrochloride—Yellow, practically odorless powder.

Solubility: Propiomazine hydrochloride—Very soluble in water; freely soluble in alcohol.

USP requirements: Propiomazine Hydrochloride Injection—Not in *USP–NF*.

PROPIONIC ACID

Molecular formula: $C_3H_6O_2$.

Molecular weight: 74.08.

Description: Propionic Acid NF—Oily liquid, having a slight, pungent, rancid odor.
NF category: Acidifying agent.

Solubility: Propionic Acid NF—Miscible with water and with alcohol and with various other organic solvents.

NF requirements: Propionic Acid NF—Preserve in tight containers. Contains not less than 99.5% and not more than 100.5%, by weight, of propionic acid. Meets the requirements for Specific gravity (0.988–0.993), Distilling range (138.5–142.5 °C), Heavy metals (not more than 0.001%), Limit of nonvolatile residue, Readily oxidizable substances, Limit of aldehydes, and Organic volatile impurities.

PROPOFOL

Chemical group: Alkyl phenol.

Chemical name: Phenol, 2,6-bis(1-methylethyl).

Molecular formula: $C_{12}H_{18}O$.

Molecular weight: 178.27.

Description:
Propofol—Exists as an oil at room temperature.
Propofol injection—Formulated as a white, oil-in-water emulsion with a pH of 7–8.5.

pKa: 11.

Solubility: Very slightly soluble in water.

USP requirements: Propofol Injection—Not in *USP–NF*.

PROPOXYCAINE

Chemical name: Propoxycaine hydrochloride—Benzoic acid, 4-amino-2-propoxy-, 2-(diethylamino)ethyl ester, monohydrochloride.

Molecular formula: Propoxycaine hydrochloride—$C_{16}H_{26}N_2O_3 \cdot$ HCl.

Molecular weight: Propoxycaine hydrochloride—330.85.

Description: Propoxycaine Hydrochloride USP—White, odorless, crystalline solid which discolors on prolonged exposure to light and to air. The pH of a solution (1 in 50) is about 5.4.

Solubility: Propoxycaine Hydrochloride USP—Freely soluble in water; soluble in alcohol; sparingly soluble in ether; practically insoluble in acetone and in chloroform.

USP requirements: Propoxycaine Hydrochloride USP—Preserve in well-closed, light-resistant containers. Dried at 105 °C for 3 hours, contains not less than 98.0% and not more than

102.0% of propoxycaine hydrochloride. Meets the requirements for Identification, Melting range (146–151 °C), Loss on drying (not more than 0.5%), Residue on ignition (not more than 0.2%), and Chromatographic purity.

PROPOXYCAINE, PROCAINE, AND LEVONORDEFRIN

For *Propoxycaine, Procaine,* and *Levonordefrin*—See individual listings for chemistry information.

USP requirements: Propoxycaine and Procaine Hydrochlorides and Levonordefrin Injection USP—Preserve in single-dose containers, preferably of Type I glass. A sterile solution of Propoxycaine Hydrochloride, Procaine Hydrochloride, and Levonordefrin in Water for Injection. The label indicates that the Injection is not to be used if its color is pinkish or darker than slightly yellow or if it contains a precipitate. Contains the labeled amounts of propoxycaine hydrochloride and procaine hydrochloride, within ±5%, and the labeled amount of levonordefrin, within ±10%. Meets the requirements for Color and clarity, Identification, Bacterial endotoxins, and pH (3.5–5.0), and for Injections.

PROPOXYCAINE, PROCAINE, AND NOREPINEPHRINE

For *Propoxycaine, Procaine,* and *Norepinephrine*—See individual listings for chemistry information.

USP requirements: Propoxycaine and Procaine Hydrochlorides and Norepinephrine Bitartrate Injection USP—Preserve in single-dose or in multiple-dose containers, preferably of Type I glass. A sterile solution of Propoxycaine Hydrochloride, Procaine Hydrochloride, and Norepinephrine Bitartrate in Water for Injection. The label indicates that the Injection is not to be used if its color is pinkish or darker than slightly yellow or if it contains a precipitate. Contains the labeled amounts of propoxycaine hydrochloride and procaine hydrochloride, within ±5%, and an amount of norepinephrine bitartrate equivalent to the labeled amount of norepinephrine, within ±10%. Meets the requirements for Color and clarity, Identification, Bacterial endotoxins, and pH (3.5–5.0), and for Injections.

PROPOXYPHENE

Chemical name:
Propoxyphene hydrochloride—Benzeneethanol, alpha-[2-(dimethylamino)-1-methylethyl]-alpha-phenyl-, propanoate (ester), hydrochloride, [S-(R*,S*)]-.
Propoxyphene napsylate—Benzeneethanol, alpha-[2-(dimethylamino)-1-methylethyl]-alpha-phenyl-, propanoate (ester), [S-(R*,S*)]-, compd. with 2-naphthalenesulfonic acid (1:1), monohydrate.

Molecular formula:
Propoxyphene hydrochloride—$C_{22}H_{29}NO_2 \cdot$ HCl.
Propoxyphene napsylate—$C_{22}H_{29}NO_2 \cdot C_{10}H_8O_3S \cdot H_2O$ (monohydrate); $C_{22}H_{29}NO_2 \cdot C_{10}H_8O_3S$ (anhydrous).

Molecular weight:
Propoxyphene hydrochloride—375.93.
Propoxyphene napsylate—565.72 (monohydrate); 547.71 (anhydrous).

Description:
Propoxyphene Hydrochloride USP—White, crystalline powder. Is odorless.

Propoxyphene Napsylate USP—White powder, having essentially no odor.

Solubility:

Propoxyphene Hydrochloride USP—Freely soluble in water; soluble in alcohol, in chloroform, and in acetone; practically insoluble in ether.

Propoxyphene Napsylate USP—Very slightly soluble in water; soluble in methanol, in alcohol, in chloroform, and in acetone.

USP requirements:

Propoxyphene Hydrochloride USP—Preserve in tight containers. Contains not less than 98.0% and not more than 101.0% of propoxyphene hydrochloride, calculated on the dried basis. Meets the requirements for Identification, Melting range (163.5–168.5 °C, the range between beginning and end of melting not more than 3 °C), Specific rotation (+52° to +57°), Loss on drying (not more than 1.0%), Related compounds (not more than 0.6%), and Organic volatile impurities.

Propoxyphene Hydrochloride Capsules USP—Preserve in tight containers. Contain the labeled amount, within ± 7.5%. Meet the requirements for Identification, Dissolution (85% in 60 minutes in acetate buffer [pH 4.5] in Apparatus 1 at 100 rpm), and Uniformity of dosage units.

Propoxyphene Hydrochloride Tablets—Not in *USP–NF*.

Propoxyphene Napsylate USP—Preserve in tight containers. Contains not less than 97.0% and not more than 103.0% of propoxyphene napsylate, calculated on the anhydrous basis. Meets the requirements for Identification, Melting range (158–165 °C, the range between beginning and end of melting not more than 4 °C, determined after drying at 105 °C for 3 hours), Specific rotation (+35° to +43°), Water (2.5–5.0%), Residue on ignition (not more than 0.5%), Heavy metals (not more than 0.003%), Related compounds (not more than 0.6%), and Organic volatile impurities.

Propoxyphene Napsylate Capsules—Not in *USP–NF*.

Propoxyphene Napsylate Oral Suspension USP—Preserve in tight containers, protected from light. Avoid freezing. Contains the labeled amount, within ±10%. Meets the requirements for Identification and Alcohol content (0.5–1.5%).

Propoxyphene Napsylate Tablets USP—Preserve in tight containers. Contain the labeled amount, within ±10%. Meet the requirements for Identification, Dissolution (75% in 60 minutes in acetate buffer [pH 4.5] in Apparatus 1 at 100 rpm), and Uniformity of dosage units.

PROPOXYPHENE AND ACETAMINOPHEN

For *Propoxyphene* and *Acetaminophen*—See individual listings for chemistry information.

USP requirements:

Propoxyphene Hydrochloride and Acetaminophen Tablets USP—Preserve in tight containers. Contain the labeled amounts, within ±10%. Meet the requirements for Identification, Dissolution (80% of each active ingredient in 30 minutes in acetate buffer [pH 4.5] in Apparatus 2 at 50 rpm), and Uniformity of dosage units (with respect to propoxyphene hydrochloride).

Propoxyphene Napsylate and Acetaminophen Tablets USP—Preserve in tight containers, at controlled room temperature. Contain the labeled amounts, within ±10%. Meet the requirements for Identification, Dissolution (75% of each active ingredient in 60 minutes in acetate buffer

[pH 4.5] in Apparatus 1 at 100 rpm), and Uniformity of dosage units (with respect to propoxyphene napsylate and acetaminophen).

PROPOXYPHENE AND ASPIRIN

For *Propoxyphene* and *Aspirin*—See individual listings for chemistry information.

USP requirements:

Propoxyphene Napsylate and Aspirin Capsules—Not in *USP–NF*.

Propoxyphene Napsylate and Aspirin Tablets USP—Preserve in tight containers, at controlled room temperature. Contain the labeled amounts, within ±10%. Meet the requirements for Identification, Dissolution (75% of each active ingredient in 60 minutes in acetate buffer [pH 4.5] in Apparatus 1 at 100 rpm), Uniformity of dosage units (with respect to propoxyphene napsylate), and Free salicylic acid (not more than 3.0%, calculated on the basis of labeled amount of aspirin).

PROPOXYPHENE, ASPIRIN, AND CAFFEINE

For *Propoxyphene, Aspirin,* and *Caffeine*—See individual listings for chemistry information.

USP requirements:

Propoxyphene Hydrochloride, Aspirin, and Caffeine Capsules USP—Preserve in tight containers at controlled room temperature. Contain the labeled amounts, within ±10%. Meet the requirements for Identification, Dissolution (75% of the aspirin and 85% of the propoxyphene hydrochloride in 60 minutes in acetate buffer [pH 4.5] in Apparatus 1 at 100 rpm), Free salicylic acid (not more than 3.0%, calculated on the basis of labeled amount of aspirin), and Uniformity of dosage units (with respect to propoxyphene hydrochloride and caffeine).

Note: Where Propoxyphene Hydrochloride, Aspirin, and Caffeine Capsules are prescribed, the quantity of propoxyphene hydrochloride is to be specified. Where the Capsules are prescribed without reference to the quantity of aspirin or caffeine contained therein, a product containing 389 mg of aspirin and 32.4 mg of caffeine shall be dispensed.

Propoxyphene Hydrochloride, Aspirin, and Caffeine Tablets—Not in *USP–NF*.

Propoxyphene Napsylate, Aspirin, and Caffeine Capsules—Not in *USP–NF*.

PROPRANOLOL

Chemical name: Propranolol hydrochloride—2-Propanol, 1-[(1-methylethyl)amino]-3-(1-naphthalenyloxy)-, hydrochloride.

Molecular formula: Propranolol hydrochloride—$C_{16}H_{21}NO_2 \cdot HCl$.

Molecular weight: Propranolol hydrochloride—295.80.

Description: Propranolol Hydrochloride USP—White to off-white, crystalline powder. Is odorless. Melts at about 164 °C.

Solubility: Propranolol Hydrochloride USP—Soluble in water and in alcohol; slightly soluble in chloroform; practically insoluble in ether.

Other characteristics: Lipid solubility—High.

USP requirements:

Propranolol Hydrochloride USP—Preserve in well-closed containers. Contains not less than 98.0% and not more than 101.5% of propranolol hydrochloride, calculated on the dried basis. Meets the requirements for Identification, Melting range (162–165 °C), Specific rotation (–1.0° to +1.0°), Loss on drying (not more than 0.5%), Residue on ignition (not more than 0.1%), and Organic volatile impurities.

Propranolol Hydrochloride Extended-release Capsules USP—Preserve in well-closed containers. The labeling states the Drug Release Test with which the product complies. Contain the labeled amount, within ±10%. Meet the requirements for Identification, Drug release (for Test 1: not more than 30% in 1.5 hours in buffer solution [pH 1.2 for the Acid stage], and 35–60% in 4 hours, 55–80% in 8 hours, 70–95% in 14 hours, and 81–110% in 24 hours in buffer solution [pH 6.8 for the Buffer stage] in Apparatus 1 at 100 rpm; for Test 2: not more than 20% in 1 hour in buffer solution [pH 1.2 for the Acid stage], and 20–45% in 3 hours, 45–80% in 6 hours, and not less than 80% in 12 hours in buffer solution [pH 7.5 for the Buffer stage] in Apparatus 1 at 50 rpm), and Uniformity of dosage units.

Propranolol Hydrochloride Injection USP—Preserve in single-dose, light-resistant containers, preferably of Type I glass. A sterile solution of Propranolol Hydrochloride in Water for Injection. Contains the labeled amount, within ±10%. Meets the requirements for Identification, Bacterial endotoxins, and pH (2.8–4.0), and for Injections.

Propranolol Hydrochloride Oral Solution—Not in USP–NF.

Propranolol Hydrochloride Tablets USP—Preserve in well-closed, light-resistant containers. Contain the labeled amount, within ±10%. Meet the requirements for Identification, Dissolution (75% in 30 minutes in dilute hydrochloric acid [1 in 100] in Apparatus 1 at 100 rpm), and Uniformity of dosage units.

PROPRANOLOL AND HYDROCHLOROTHIAZIDE

For Propranolol and Hydrochlorothiazide—See individual listings for chemistry information.

USP requirements:

Propranolol Hydrochloride and Hydrochlorothiazide Extended-release Capsules USP—Preserve in well-closed containers. Contain the labeled amounts, within ±10%. Meet the requirements for Identification, Drug release (propranolol hydrochloride: not more than 30% in 1.5 hours in buffer solution [pH 1.5 for the Acid stage], 35–60% in 4 hours, 55–80% in 8 hours, 70–95% in 14 hours, and 83–108% in 24 hours in buffer solution [pH 6.8 for the Buffer stage]; hydrochlorothiazide: not less than 80% in 30 minutes in buffer solution [pH 1.5], in Apparatus 1 at 100 rpm), Uniformity of dosage units, and Related compounds (not more than 1.0%).

Propranolol Hydrochloride and Hydrochlorothiazide Tablets USP—Preserve in well-closed containers. Contain the labeled amounts, within ±10%. Meet the requirements for Identification, Dissolution (80% of each active ingredient in 30 minutes in 0.01 N hydrochloric acid in Apparatus 1 at 100 rpm), Related compounds (not more than 1.0%), Uniformity of dosage units, and Limit of 4-amino-6-chloro-1,3-benzenesulfonamide.

PROPYLENE CARBONATE

Chemical name: 4-Methyl-1,3-dioxolan-2-one.

Molecular formula: $C_4H_6O_3$.

Molecular weight: 102.09.

Description: Propylene Carbonate NF—Clear, colorless, mobile liquid.

NF category: Solvent.

Solubility: Propylene Carbonate NF—Freely soluble in water; insoluble in hexane; miscible with alcohol and with chloroform.

NF requirements: Propylene Carbonate NF—Preserve in tight containers. Contains not less than 99.0% and not more than 100.5% of propylene carbonate. Meets the requirements for Identification, Specific gravity (1.203–1.210 at 20 °C), pH (6.0–7.5), Residue on ignition (not more than 0.01%), and Organic volatile impurities.

PROPYLENE GLYCOL

Chemical name: 1,2-Propanediol.

Molecular formula: $C_3H_8O_2$.

Molecular weight: 76.09.

Description: Propylene Glycol USP—Clear, colorless, viscous liquid. It is practically odorless. It absorbs moisture when exposed to moist air.

NF category: Humectant; plasticizer; solvent.

Solubility: Propylene Glycol USP—Miscible with water, with acetone, and with chloroform. Soluble in ether and will dissolve many essential oils, but is immiscible with fixed oils.

USP requirements: Propylene Glycol USP—Preserve in tight containers. Contains not less than 99.5% of propylene glycol. Meets the requirements for Identification, Specific gravity (1.035–1.037), Acidity, Water (not more than 0.2%), Residue on ignition, Chloride (not more than 0.007%), Sulfate (not more than 0.006%), Heavy metals (not more than 5 ppm), and Organic volatile impurities.

PROPYLENE GLYCOL ALGINATE

Description: Propylene Glycol Alginate NF—White to yellowish fibrous or granular powder. Practically odorless.

NF category: Suspending and/or viscosity-increasing agent.

Solubility: Propylene Glycol Alginate NF—Soluble in water, in solutions of dilute organic acids, and, depending on the degree of esterification, in hydroalcoholic mixtures containing up to 60% by weight of alcohol to form stable, viscous colloidal solutions at a pH of 3.

NF requirements: Propylene Glycol Alginate NF—Preserve in well-closed containers. A propylene glycol ester of alginic acid. Each gram yields not less than 0.16 and not more than 0.20 gram of carbon dioxide, calculated on the dried basis. Meets the requirements for Identification, Microbial limits, Loss on drying (not more than 20.0%), Ash (not more than 10.0%, calculated on the dried basis), Arsenic (not more than 3 ppm), Lead (not more than 0.001%), Heavy metals (not more than 0.004%), Free carboxyl groups, and Esterified carboxyl groups.

PROPYLENE GLYCOL DIACETATE

Molecular formula: $C_7H_{12}O_4$.

Molecular weight: 160.17.

Description: Propylene Glycol Diacetate NF—Clear, colorless liquid, having a mild, fruity odor.
NF category: Emulsifying and/or solubilizing agent.

Solubility: Propylene Glycol Diacetate NF—Soluble in water.

NF requirements: Propylene Glycol Diacetate NF—Preserve in tight containers, and avoid contact with metal. Contains not less than 98.0% and not more than 102.0% of propylene glycol diacetate. Meets the requirements for Identification, Specific gravity (1.040–1.060), Refractive index (1.4130–1.4150 at 20 °C), pH (4.0–6.0, in a solution [1 in 20]), Limit acetic acid (not more than 0.2%), Chromatographic purity, and Organic volatile impurities.

PROPYLENE GLYCOL MONOSTEARATE

Chemical name: Octadecanoic acid, monoester with 1,2-propanediol.

Molecular formula: $C_{21}H_{42}O_3$.

Molecular weight: 342.56.

Description: Propylene Glycol Monostearate NF—White, wax-like solid, or white, wax-like beads or flakes. It has a slight, agreeable, fatty odor.
NF category: Emulsifying and/or solubilizing agent.

Solubility: Propylene Glycol Monostearate NF—Insoluble in water, but may be dispersed in hot water with the aid of a small amount of soap or other suitable surface-active agent; soluble in organic solvents, such as alcohol, mineral or fixed oils, ether, and acetone.

NF requirements: Propylene Glycol Monostearate NF—Preserve in well-closed containers. A mixture of the propylene glycol mono- and di-esters of stearic and palmitic acids. Contains not less than 90.0% of monoesters of saturated fatty acids, chiefly propylene glycol monostearate and propylene glycol monopalmitate. Meets the requirements for Congealing temperature (not lower than 45 °C), Residue on ignition (not more than 0.5%), Acid value (not more than 4), Saponification value (155–165), Hydroxyl value (160–175), Iodine value (not more than 3), Free glycerin and propylene glycol, Propylene glycol monoesters, and Organic volatile impurities.

PROPYL GALLATE

Chemical name: Benzoic acid, 3,4,5-trihydroxy-, propyl ester.

Molecular formula: $C_{10}H_{12}O_5$.

Molecular weight: 212.20.

Description: Propyl Gallate NF—White, crystalline powder, having a very slight, characteristic odor.
NF category: Antioxidant.

Solubility: Propyl Gallate NF—Slightly soluble in water; freely soluble in alcohol.

NF requirements: Propyl Gallate NF—Preserve in tight containers, protected from light, and avoid contact with metals. Contains not less than 98.0% and not more than 102.0% of propyl gallate, calculated on the dried basis. Meets the requirements for Identification, Melting range (146–150 °C), Loss on drying (not more than 0.5%), Residue on ignition (not more than 0.1%), Heavy metals (not more than 0.001%), and Organic volatile impurities.

PROPYLHEXEDRINE

Chemical name: Cyclohexaneethanamine, *N*,alpha-dimethyl-, (±).

Molecular formula: $C_{10}H_{21}N$.

Molecular weight: 155.28.

Description: Propylhexedrine USP—Clear, colorless liquid, having a characteristic, amine-like odor. Volatilizes slowly at room temperature. Absorbs carbon dioxide from the air, and its solutions are alkaline to litmus. Boils at about 205 °C.

Solubility: Propylhexedrine USP—Very slightly soluble in water. Miscible with alcohol, with chloroform, and with ether.

USP requirements:
Propylhexedrine USP—Preserve in tight containers. Contains not less than 98.0% and not more than 101.0% of propylhexedrine. Meets the requirements for Identification and Specific gravity (0.848–0.852).
Propylhexedrine Inhalant USP—Preserve in tight containers (inhalers), and avoid exposure to excessive heat. Consists of cylindrical rolls of suitable fibrous material impregnated with Propylhexedrine, usually aromatized, and contained in a suitable inhaler. Inhaler contains the labeled amount, within −10% to +25%. Meets the requirement for Identification.

PROPYLIODONE

Chemical name: 1(4*H*)-Pyridineacetic acid, 3,5-diiodo-4-oxo-, propyl ester.

Molecular formula: $C_{10}H_{11}I_2NO_3$.

Molecular weight: 447.01.

Description: Propyliodone USP—White or almost white, crystalline powder. Odorless or has a faint odor.

Solubility: Propyliodone USP—Practically insoluble in water; soluble in acetone, in alcohol, and in ether.

USP requirements:
Propyliodone USP—Preserve in tight, light-resistant containers. Contains not less than 99.0% and not more than 101.0% of propyliodone, calculated on the dried basis. Meets the requirements for Identification, Melting range (187–190 °C), Acidity, Loss on drying (not more than 0.5%), Residue on ignition (not more than 0.1%), Iodine and iodide, and Heavy metals (not more than 0.002%).
Propyliodone Injectable Oil Suspension USP—Preserve in single-dose, light-resistant containers. A sterile suspension of Propyliodone in Peanut Oil. Contains not less than 57.0% and not more than 63.0% of propyliodone. Meets the requirements for Identification, Weight per mL (1.236–1.276 grams), and Iodine and iodide, and for Injections.

PROPYLPARABEN

Chemical name: Benzoic acid, 4-hydroxy-, propyl ester.

Molecular formula: $C_{10}H_{12}O_3$.

Molecular weight: 180.20.

Description: Propylparaben NF—Small, colorless crystals or white powder.
NF category: Antimicrobial preservative.

Solubility: Propylparaben NF—Very slightly soluble in water; freely soluble in alcohol and in ether; slightly soluble in boiling water.

NF requirements: Propylparaben NF—Preserve in well-closed containers. Contains not less than 99.0% and not more than 100.5% of propylparaben, calculated on the dried basis. Meets the requirements for Identification, Melting range (95–98 °C), and Organic volatile impurities, and for Acidity, Loss on drying, and Residue on ignition under Butylparaben.

PROPYLPARABEN SODIUM

Chemical name: Benzoic acid, 4-hydroxy-, propyl ester, sodium salt.

Molecular formula: $C_{10}H_{11}NaO_3$.

Molecular weight: 202.18.

Description: Propylparaben Sodium NF—White powder. It is odorless and hygroscopic.
NF category: Antimicrobial preservative.

Solubility: Propylparaben Sodium NF—Freely soluble in water; sparingly soluble in alcohol; insoluble in fixed oils.

NF requirements: Propylparaben Sodium NF—Preserve in tight containers. Contains not less than 98.5% and not more than 101.5% of propylparaben sodium, calculated on the anhydrous basis. Meets the requirements for Completeness of solution, Identification, pH (9.5–10.5, in a solution [1 in 1000]), Water (not more than 5.0%), Chloride (not more than 0.035%), Sulfate (not more than 0.12%), and Organic volatile impurities.

PROPYLTHIOURACIL

Chemical group: Thiourea derivative.

Chemical name: 4(1*H*)-Pyrimidinone, 2,3-dihydro-6-propyl-2thioxo-.

Molecular formula: $C_7H_{10}N_2OS$.

Molecular weight: 170.23.

Description: Propylthiouracil USP—White, powdery, crystalline substance; starch-like in appearance and to the touch.

Solubility: Propylthiouracil USP—Slightly soluble in water; sparingly soluble in alcohol; slightly soluble in chloroform and in ether; soluble in ammonium hydroxide and in alkali hydroxides.

USP requirements:
Propylthiouracil USP—Preserve in well-closed, light-resistant containers. Contains not less than 98.0% and not more than 100.5% of propylthiouracil, calculated on the dried basis. Meets the requirements for Identification, Melting range (218–221 °C), Loss on drying (not more than 0.5%), Residue on ignition (not more than 0.1%), Sele-

nium (not more than 0.003%, a 200-mg specimen being used), Heavy metals (not more than 0.002%), Ordinary impurities, and Organic volatile impurities.
Propylthiouracil Enema—Not in *USP–NF*.
Propylthiouracil Suppositories—Not in *USP–NF*.
Propylthiouracil Tablets USP—Preserve in well-closed containers. Contain the labeled amount, within ±7%. Meet the requirements for Identification, Dissolution (85% in 30 minutes in water in Apparatus 1 at 100 rpm), and Uniformity of dosage units.

PROSTAGLANDIN E₁, LIPOSOMAL

Chemical name: Prostaglandin E₁—(11 alpha,13*E*,15*S*)-11,15-Dihydroxy-9-oxoprost-13-en-1-oic acid.

Molecular formula: Prostaglandin E₁—$C_{20}H_{34}O_5$.

Molecular weight: Prostaglandin E₁—354.49.

Description: Prostaglandin E₁—Crystals from ethyl acetate and heptane. Melting point 115–116 °C.

Other characteristics: Prostaglandin E₁—Easily dehydrated in solution at pHs less than 4 and greater than 8.

USP requirements: Liposomal Prostaglandin E₁ Injection—Not in *USP–NF*.

PROTAMINE

Description:
Protamine Sulfate Injection USP—Colorless solution, which may have the odor of a preservative.
Protamine Sulfate for Injection USP—White, odorless powder, having the characteristic appearance of solids dried from the frozen state.

USP requirements:
Protamine Sulfate USP—Preserve in tight containers, in a refrigerator. A purified mixture of simple protein principles obtained from the sperm or testes of suitable species of fish, which has the property of neutralizing heparin. Each mg of Protamine Sulfate, calculated on the dried basis, neutralizes not less than 100 USP Heparin Units. Meets the requirements for Loss on drying (not more than 5%), Sulfate (16–22%, calculated on the dried basis), Ultraviolet absorbance (not more than 0.1), and Nitrogen content (22.5–25.5%, calculated on the dried basis).
Protamine Sulfate Injection USP—Preserve in single-dose containers, preferably of Type I glass. Store in a refrigerator. A sterile, isotonic solution of Protamine Sulfate. Label it to indicate the approximate neutralization capacity in USP Heparin Units. Contains the labeled amount, within −10% to +20%. Meets the requirements for Identification (tests for Sulfate) and Bacterial endotoxins, and for Injections.
Protamine Sulfate for Injection USP—Preserve in Containers for Sterile Solids. Preserve the accompanying solvent in single-dose or in multiple-dose containers, preferably of Type I glass. A sterile mixture of Protamine Sulfate with one or more suitable, dry diluents. Label it to indicate the approximate neutralization capacity in USP Heparin Units. Contains the labeled amount, within −10% to +20%. Meets the requirements for Constituted solution (under Injections at time of use), Bacterial endotoxins, and pH and clarity of solution (6.5–7.5, and the solution is clear), for

Uniformity of dosage units, and both the medication and the accompanying solvent meet the requirements for Sterility tests and Labeling under Injections.

PROTEIN HYDROLYSATE

Description: Protein Hydrolysate Injection USP—Yellowish to reddish amber, transparent liquid.

USP requirements: Protein Hydrolysate Injection USP—Preserve in single-dose containers, preferably of Type I or Type II glass, and avoid excessive heat. A sterile solution of amino acids and short-chain peptides which represent the approximate nutritive equivalent of the casein, lactalbumin, plasma, fibrin, or other suitable protein from which it is derived by acid, enzymatic, or other method of hydrolysis. May be modified by partial removal and restoration or addition of one or more amino acids. May contain alcohol, dextrose, or other carbohydrate suitable for intravenous infusion. Not less than 50.0% of the total nitrogen present is in the form of alpha-amino nitrogen. The label of the immediate container bears in a subtitle the name of the protein from which the hydrolysate has been derived and the word "modified" if one or more of the "essential" amino acids has been partially removed, restored, or added. The label bears a statement of the pH range; the name and percentage of any added other nutritive ingredient; the method of hydrolysis; the nature of the modification, if any, in amino acid content after hydrolysis; the percentage of each essential amino acid or its equivalent; the approximate protein equivalent, in grams per liter; the approximate number of calories per liter; the percentage of the total nitrogen in the form of alpha-amino nitrogen; and the quantity of the sodium and of the potassium ions present in each 100 mL of the Injection. Injection that contains not more than 30 mg of sodium per 100 mL may be labeled "Protein Hydrolysate Injection, Low Sodium," or by a similar title the approximate equivalent thereof. The label states the total osmolar concentration in mOsmol per liter. Where the contents are less than 100 mL, or where the label states that the Injection is not for direct injection but is to be diluted before use, the label alternatively may state the total osmolar concentration in mOsmol per mL. Meets the requirements for Non-antigenicity, Bacterial endotoxins, Biological adequacy (for Protein), pH (4.0–7.0, determined potentiometrically, but the variation from the pH range stated on the label is not greater than ±0.5 pH unit), Content of alpha-amino nitrogen, Nitrogen content, Potassium content, and Sodium content, and for Injections.

PROTIRELIN

Source: A synthetic tripeptide thought to be structurally identical to the naturally occurring thyrotropin-releasing hormone produced by the hypothalamus.

Chemical name: L-Prolinamide, 5-oxo-L-prolyl-L-histidyl-.

Molecular formula: $C_{16}H_{22}N_6O_4$.

Molecular weight: 362.38.

Description: Slightly yellowish hygroscopic powder.

Solubility: Very soluble in water and in methanol; soluble in isopropanol.

USP requirements: Protirelin Injection—Not in *USP–NF*.

PROTRIPTYLINE

Chemical group: Protriptyline hydrochloride—Dibenzocycloheptene derivative.

Chemical name: Protriptyline hydrochloride—5H-Dibenzo[a,d]-cycloheptene-5-propanamine, N-methyl-, hydrochloride.

Molecular formula: Protriptyline hydrochloride—$C_{19}H_{21}N \cdot HCl$.

Molecular weight: Protriptyline hydrochloride—299.85.

Description: Protriptyline Hydrochloride USP—White to yellowish powder. Is odorless, or has not more than a slight odor. Melts at about 168 °C.

Solubility: Protriptyline Hydrochloride USP—Freely soluble in water, in alcohol, and in chloroform; practically insoluble in ether.

Other characteristics: Secondary amine.

USP requirements:
Protriptyline Hydrochloride USP—Preserve in well-closed containers. Contains not less than 99.0% and not more than 101.0% of protriptyline hydrochloride, calculated on the dried basis. Meets the requirements for Identification, pH (5.0–6.5, in a solution [1 in 100]), Loss on drying (not more than 0.3%), Residue on ignition (not more than 0.1%), Heavy metals (not more than 0.001%), and Organic volatile impurities.
Protriptyline Hydrochloride Tablets USP—Preserve in tight containers. Contain the labeled amount, within ±10%. Meet the requirements for Identification, Dissolution (75% in 45 minutes in water in Apparatus 1 at 100 rpm), and Uniformity of dosage units.

PRUSSIAN BLUE

Chemical name: Ferric (III) hexacyanoferrate (II).

Molecular formula: $Fe_4[Fe(CN)_6]_3$.

Molecular weight: 859.2

Solubility: Insoluble in water and in diluted acids.

USP requirements: Prussian Blue Capsules—Not in *USP–NF*.

PSEUDOEPHEDRINE

Chemical name:
Pseudoephedrine hydrochloride—Benzenemethanol, alpha-[1-(methylamino)ethyl]-, [S-(R*,R*)]-, hydrochloride.
Pseudoephedrine sulfate—Benzenemethanol, alpha-[1(methylamino)ethyl]-, [S-(R*,R*)]-, sulfate (2:1) (salt).

Molecular formula:
Pseudoephedrine hydrochloride—$C_{10}H_{15}NO \cdot HCl$.
Pseudoephedrine sulfate—$(C_{10}H_{15}NO)_2 \cdot H_2SO_4$.

Molecular weight:
Pseudoephedrine hydrochloride—201.69.
Pseudoephedrine sulfate—428.54.

Description:
Pseudoephedrine Hydrochloride USP—Fine, white to offwhite crystals or powder, having a faint characteristic odor.
Pseudoephedrine Sulfate USP—White crystals or crystalline powder. Is odorless.

Solubility:
Pseudoephedrine Hydrochloride USP—Very soluble in water; freely soluble in alcohol; slightly soluble in chloroform.
Pseudoephedrine Sulfate USP—Freely soluble in alcohol.

USP requirements:

Pseudoephedrine Hydrochloride USP—Preserve in tight, light-resistant containers. Contains not less than 98.0% and not more than 100.5% of pseudoephedrine hydrochloride, calculated on the dried basis. Meets the requirements for Identification, Melting range (182–186 °C, the range between beginning and end of melting not more than 2 °C), Specific rotation (+61.0° to +62.5°), pH (4.6–6.0, in a solution [1 in 20]), Loss on drying (not more than 0.5%), Residue on ignition (not more than 0.1%), Ordinary impurities, and Organic volatile impurities.

Pseudoephedrine Hydrochloride Capsules—Not in *USP–NF*.

Pseudoephedrine Hydrochloride Extended-release Capsules USP—Preserve in tight containers. Contain a labeled amount, within ±10%. Meet the requirements for Identification, Drug release (20–50% in 3 hours, 45–75% in 6 hours, and not less than 75% in 12 hours in water in Apparatus 2 at 50 rpm), and Uniformity of dosage units.

Pseudoephedrine Hydrochloride Oral Solution USP—Preserve in tight, light-resistant containers. Contains the labeled amount, within ±10%. Meets the requirements for Identification and Reaction (acid to litmus).

Pseudoephedrine Hydrochloride Syrup USP—Preserve in tight, light-resistant containers. Contains the labeled amount, within ±10%. Meets the requirements for Identification and Reaction (acid to litmus).

Pseudoephedrine Hydrochloride Tablets USP—Preserve in tight containers. Contain the labeled amount, within ±10%. Meet the requirements for Identification, Dissolution (75% in 45 minutes in water in Apparatus 2 at 50 rpm), and Uniformity of dosage units.

Pseudoephedrine Hydrochloride Extended-release Tablets USP—Preserve in tight containers. Contain the labeled amount, within ±10%. Meet the requirements for Identification and Uniformity of dosage units.

Pseudoephedrine Sulfate USP—Preserve in tight, light-resistant containers. Contains not less than 98.0% and not more than 100.5% of pseudoephedrine sulfate, calculated on the dried basis. Meets the requirements for Identification, Melting range (174–179 °C, the range between beginning and end of melting not more than 2 °C), Specific rotation (+56.0° to +59.0°), pH (5.0–6.5, in a solution [1 in 20]), Loss on drying (not more than 2.0%), Residue on ignition (not more than 0.1%), Chloride (not more than 0.14%), Heavy metals, and Ordinary impurities.

Pseudoephedrine Sulfate Tablets—Not in *USP–NF*.

Pseudoephedrine Sulfate Extended-release Tablets—Not in *USP–NF*.

PSEUDOEPHEDRINE AND ASPIRIN

For *Pseudoephedrine* and *Aspirin*—See individual listings for chemistry information.

USP requirements: Pseudoephedrine Hydrochloride and Aspirin Tablets—Not in *USP–NF*.

PSEUDOEPHEDRINE AND CODEINE

For *Pseudoephedrine* and *Codeine*—See individual listings for chemistry information.

USP requirements:

Pseudoephedrine Hydrochloride and Codeine Phosphate Capsules—Not in *USP–NF*.

Pseudoephedrine Hydrochloride and Codeine Phosphate Syrup—Not in *USP–NF*.

Pseudoephedrine Hydrochloride and Codeine Phosphate Tablets—Not in *USP–NF*.

PSEUDOEPHEDRINE, CARBINOXAMINE, AND DEXTRO-METHORPHAN

For *Pseudoephedrine*, *Carbinoxamine*, and *Dextromethorphan*—See individual listings for chemistry information.

USP requirements: Pseudoephedrine Hydrochloride, Carbinoxamine Maleate, and Dextromethorphan Hydrobromide Oral Solution USP—Preserve in tight light-resistant containers, and store at controlled room temperature. Contains the labeled amounts, within ±10%. Meets the requirements for Identification, Microbial limits, pH (3.0–5.0), and Alcohol content (within ±10%).

PSEUDOEPHEDRINE, CODEINE, AND GUAIFENESIN

For *Pseudoephedrine*, *Codeine*, and *Guaifenesin*—See individual listings for chemistry information.

USP requirements:

Pseudoephedrine Hydrochloride, Codeine Phosphate, and Guaifenesin Oral Solution—Not in *USP–NF*.

Pseudoephedrine Hydrochloride, Codeine Phosphate, and Guaifenesin Syrup—Not in *USP–NF*.

PSEUDOEPHEDRINE AND DEXTROMETHORPHAN

For *Pseudoephedrine* and *Dextromethorphan*—See individual listings for chemistry information.

USP requirements:

Pseudoephedrine Hydrochloride and Dextromethorphan Hydrobromide Capsules—Not in *USP–NF*.

Pseudoephedrine Hydrochloride and Dextromethorphan Hydrobromide Oral Solution—Not in *USP–NF*.

Pseudoephedrine Hydrochloride and Dextromethorphan Hydrobromide Syrup—Not in *USP–NF*.

Pseudoephedrine Hydrochloride and Dextromethorphan Hydrobromide Chewable Tablets—Not in *USP–NF*.

PSEUDOEPHEDRINE, DEXTROMETHORPHAN, AND ACETAMINOPHEN

For *Pseudoephedrine*, *Dextromethorphan*, and *Acetaminophen*—See individual listings for chemistry information.

USP requirements:

Pseudoephedrine Hydrochloride, Dextromethorphan Hydrobromide, and Acetaminophen Capsules USP—Preserve in tight containers. The label for each article encompassed by this monograph bears a name composed of the active ingredients contained in the article. The label states the name and quantity of each active ingredient and indicates its function (or purpose) in the article. Contain the labeled amounts, within ±10%. Meet the requirements for Identification, Dissolution (75% in 45 minutes in water in Apparatus 1 at 100 rpm), and Uniformity of dosage units.

Pseudoephedrine Hydrochloride, Dextromethorphan Hydrobromide, and Acetaminophen Oral Powder USP—Preserve in tight containers. The label for each article

encompassed by this monograph bears a name composed of the active ingredients. The label states the name and quantity of each active ingredient and indicates its function (or purpose) in the article. Contains the labeled amounts, within ±10%. Meets the requirements for Identification, Minimum fill, and Uniformity of dosage units.

Pseudoephedrine Hydrochloride, Dextromethorphan Hydrobromide, and Acetaminophen Oral Solution USP—Preserve in tight containers. The label for each article encompassed by this monograph bears a name composed of the active ingredients. The label states the name and quantity of each active ingredient and indicates its function (or purpose) in the article. Contains the labeled amounts, within ±10%. Meets the requirements for Identification, pH (3.7–7.5), Alcohol content, if present (within ± 10%), and Microbial limits.

Pseudoephedrine Hydrochloride, Dextromethorphan Hydrobromide, and Acetaminophen for Oral Solution—Not in *USP–NF*.

Pseudoephedrine Hydrochloride, Dextromethorphan Hydrobromide, and Acetaminophen Oral Suspension—Not in *USP–NF*.

Pseudoephedrine Hydrochloride, Dextromethorphan Hydrobromide, and Acetaminophen Tablets USP—Preserve in tight containers, and store at controlled room temperature. The label for each article encompassed by this monograph bears a name composed of the active ingredients. The label states the name and quantity of each active ingredient and indicates its function (or purpose) in the article. Contain the labeled amounts, within ±10%. Meet the requirements for Identification, Dissolution (75% in 45 minutes in water in Apparatus 2 at 50 rpm), and Uniformity of dosage units.

PSEUDOEPHEDRINE, DEXTROMETHORPHAN, GUAIFENESIN, AND ACETAMINOPHEN

For *Pseudoephedrine, Dextromethorphan, Guaifenesin,* and *Acetaminophen*—See individual listings for chemistry information.

USP requirements:
Pseudoephedrine Hydrochloride, Dextromethorphan Hydrobromide, Guaifenesin, and Acetaminophen Capsules—Not in *USP–NF*.

Pseudoephedrine Hydrochloride, Dextromethorphan Hydrobromide, Guaifenesin, and Acetaminophen Oral Solution—Not in *USP–NF*.

Pseudoephedrine Hydrochloride, Dextromethorphan Hydrobromide, Guaifenesin, and Acetaminophen Syrup—Not in *USP–NF*.

PSEUDOEPHEDRINE AND GUAIFENESIN

For *Pseudoephedrine* and *Guaifenesin*—See individual listings for chemistry information.

USP requirements:
Pseudoephedrine Hydrochloride and Guaifenesin Capsules USP—Preserve in tight, light-resistant containers. Contain the labeled amounts, within ±10%. Meet the requirements for Identification and Uniformity of dosage units.

Pseudoephedrine Hydrochloride and Guaifenesin Extended-release Capsules—Not in *USP–NF*.

Pseudoephedrine Hydrochloride and Guaifenesin Oral Solution—Not in *USP–NF*.

Pseudoephedrine Hydrochloride and Guaifenesin Syrup—Not in *USP–NF*.

Pseudoephedrine Hydrochloride and Guaifenesin Tablets—Not in *USP–NF*.

Pseudoephedrine Hydrochloride and Guaifenesin Extended-release Tablets—Not in *USP–NF*.

PSEUDOEPHEDRINE AND HYDROCODONE

For *Pseudoephedrine* and *Hydrocodone*—See individual listings for chemistry information.

USP requirements:
Pseudoephedrine Hydrochloride and Hydrocodone Bitartrate Oral Solution—Not in *USP–NF*.

Pseudoephedrine Hydrochloride and Hydrocodone Bitartrate Syrup—Not in *USP–NF*.

Pseudoephedrine Hydrochloride and Hydrocodone Bitartrate Tablets—Not in *USP–NF*.

PSEUDOEPHEDRINE, HYDROCODONE, AND GUAIFENESIN

For *Pseudoephedrine, Hydrocodone,* and *Guaifenesin*—See individual listings for chemistry information.

USP requirements:
Pseudoephedrine Hydrochloride, Hydrocodone Bitartrate, and Guaifenesin Elixir—Not in *USP–NF*.

Pseudoephedrine Hydrochloride, Hydrocodone Bitartrate, and Guaifenesin Oral Solution—Not in *USP–NF*.

Pseudoephedrine Hydrochloride, Hydrocodone Bitartrate, and Guaifenesin Syrup—Not in *USP–NF*.

Pseudoephedrine Hydrochloride, Hydrocodone Bitartrate, and Guaifenesin Tablets—Not in *USP–NF*.

PSEUDOEPHEDRINE, HYDROCODONE, AND POTASSIUM GUAIACOLSULFONATE

For *Pseudoephedrine, Hydrocodone,* and *Potassium Guaiacolsulfonate*—See individual listings for chemistry information.

USP requirements: Pseudoephedrine Hydrochloride, Hydrocodone Bitartrate, and Potassium Guaiacolsulfonate Oral Solution—Not in *USP–NF*.

PSYLLIUM

Source: Psyllium seed—Cleaned, dried, ripe seed of *Plantago psyllium* and related species having a high content of hemicellulose mucilages.

USP requirements:
Psyllium Caramels—Not in *USP–NF*.
Psyllium Granules—Not in *USP–NF*.
Psyllium Powder—Not in *USP–NF*.

PSYLLIUM HUSK

USP requirements: Psyllium Husk USP—Preserve in well-closed containers, secured against insect attack. The cleaned, dried seed coat (epidermis) separated by winnowing and thrashing from the seeds of *Plantago ovata* Forskal, known in commerce as Blond Psyllium or Indian Psyllium or Ispaghula, or from *Plantago psyllium* Linné or from *Plantago indica* Linné (*Plantago arenaria* Waldstein et Kitaibel) known in commerce as Spanish or French Psyllium (Fam. Plantaginaceae), in whole or in powdered form. Meets the requirements for Botanic characteristics, Identification, Microbial limits, Total ash (not more than 4.0%), Acid-insoluble ash (not more than 1.0%), Water (not more than 12.0%), Light extraneous matter (not more than 15%), Heavy extraneous matter (not more than 1.1%), Insect infestation, and Swell volume.

PSYLLIUM HYDROPHILIC MUCILLOID

Source: Obtained from the coating of *Plantago ovata*; contains about 50% hemicellulose.

Description: White to cream-colored, slightly granular powder with little or no odor.

USP requirements:
Psyllium Hydrophilic Mucilloid Granules—Not in *USP–NF*.
Psyllium Hydrophilic Mucilloid Powder—Not in *USP–NF*.
Psyllium Hydrophilic Mucilloid Effervescent Powder—Not in *USP–NF*.
Psyllium Hydrophilic Mucilloid Oral Powder—Not in *USP–NF*.
Psyllium Hydrophilic Mucilloid for Oral Suspension USP—Preserve in tight containers. A dry mixture of Psyllium Husk with suitable additives. Meets the requirements for Identification, Microbial limits, and Swell volume.
Psyllium Hydrophilic Mucilloid Wafers—Not in *USP–NF*.

PSYLLIUM HYDROPHILIC MUCILLOID AND CARBOXY-METHYLCELLULOSE

For *Psyllium Hydrophilic Mucilloid* and *Carboxymethylcellulose*—See individual listings for chemistry information.

USP requirements: Psyllium Hydrophilic Mucilloid and Carboxymethylcellulose Sodium Granules—Not in *USP–NF*.

PSYLLIUM HYDROPHILIC MUCILLOID AND SENNA

For *Psyllium Hydrophilic Mucilloid* and *Senna*—See individual listings for chemistry information.

USP requirements: Psyllium Hydrophilic Mucilloid and Senna Granules—Not in *USP–NF*.

PSYLLIUM HYDROPHILIC MUCILLOID AND SENNOSIDES

For *Psyllium Hydrophilic Mucilloid* and *Sennosides*—See individual listings for chemistry information.

USP requirements: Psyllium Hydrophilic Mucilloid and Sennosides Powder—Not in *USP–NF*.

PSYLLIUM AND SENNA

For *Psyllium* and *Senna*—See individual listings for chemistry information.

USP requirements: Psyllium and Senna Granules—Not in *USP–NF*.

PUMICE

Description: Pumice USP—Very light, hard, rough, porous, grayish masses or gritty, grayish powder. Is odorless and stable in air.

Solubility: Pumice USP—Practically insoluble in water; is not attacked by acids.

USP requirements: Pumice USP—Preserve in well-closed containers. A substance of volcanic origin, consisting chiefly of complex silicates of aluminum, potassium, and sodium. Label powdered Pumice to indicate, in descriptive terms, the fineness of the powder. Powdered Pumice meets requirements for several sizes (Pumice Flour or Superfine Pumice, Fine Pumice, and Coarse Pumice). Meets the requirements for Water-soluble substances (not more than 0.20%), Acid-soluble substances (not more than 6.0%), and Iron.

PYRANTEL

Chemical name: Pyrantel pamoate—Pyrimidine, 1,4,5,6-tetrahydro-1-methyl-2-[2-(2-thienyl)ethenyl]-, (*E*)-, compd. with 4,4′methylenebis[3-hydroxy-2-naphthalenecarboxylic acid] (1:1).

Molecular formula: Pyrantel pamoate—$C_{11}H_{14}N_2S \cdot C_{23}H_{16}O_6$.

Molecular weight: Pyrantel pamoate—594.68.

Description: Pyrantel Pamoate USP—Yellow to tan solid.

Solubility: Pyrantel Pamoate USP—Practically insoluble in water and in methanol; soluble in dimethylsulfoxide; slightly soluble in dimethylformamide.

USP requirements:
Pyrantel Pamoate USP—Preserve in well-closed, light-resistant containers. Contains not less than 97.0% and not more than 103.0% of pyrantel pamoate, calculated on the dried basis. Meets the requirements for Identification, Loss on drying (not more than 2.0%), Residue on ignition (not more than 0.5%, from 1.33 grams), Heavy metals (not more than 0.005%), Iron (not more than 0.0075%), Related compounds, and Content of pamoic acid (63.4–67.3%, calculated on the dried basis).
Pyrantel Pamoate Oral Suspension USP—Preserve in tight, light-resistant containers. A suspension of Pyrantel Pamoate in a suitable aqueous vehicle. Contains an amount of pyrantel pamoate equivalent to the labeled amount of pyrantel, within ±10%. Meets the requirements for Identification and pH (4.5–6.0).
Pyrantel Pamoate Tablets—Not in *USP–NF*.

PYRAZINAMIDE

Source: Pyrazine analogue of nicotinamide.

Chemical name: Pyrazinecarboxamide.

Molecular formula: $C_5H_5N_3O$.

Molecular weight: 123.11.

Description: Pyrazinamide USP—White to practically white, odorless or practically odorless, crystalline powder.

Solubility: Pyrazinamide USP—Sparingly soluble in water; slightly soluble in alcohol, in ether, and in chloroform.

USP requirements:

Pyrazinamide USP—Preserve in well-closed containers. Contains not less than 99.0% and not more than 101.0% of pyrazinamide, calculated on the anhydrous basis. Meets the requirements for Identification, Melting range (188–191 °C), Water (not more than 0.5%), Residue on ignition (not more than 0.1%), Heavy metals (not more than 0.001%), and Organic volatile impurities.

Pyrazinamide Tablets USP—Preserve in well-closed containers. Contain the labeled amount, within ±7%. Meet the requirements for Identification, Dissolution (75% in 45 minutes in water in Apparatus 2 at 50 rpm), and Uniformity of dosage units.

PYRETHRINS AND PIPERONYL BUTOXIDE

Source:

Pyrethrins—Obtained from flowers of the pyrethrum plant, *Chrysanthemum cincerariaefolium,* which is related to the ragweed plant; esters formed by the combination of chrysanthenic and pyrethric acids and pyrethrolone, cinerolone, and jasmolone alcohols.

Piperonyl butoxide—Synthetic piperic acid derivative.

Chemical name: Piperonyl butoxide—5-[2-(2-Butoxyethoxy)ethoxymethyl]-6-propyl-1,3-benzodioxole.

Molecular formula: Piperonyl butoxide—$C_{19}H_{30}O_5$.

Molecular weight: Piperonyl butoxide—338.44.

Description:

Pyrethrins—Viscous liquid.

Piperonyl butoxide—Yellow or pale brown oily liquid with a faint characteristic odor.

Solubility:

Pyrethrins—Practically insoluble in water; soluble in alcohol, in petroleum ether, in kerosene, in carbon tetrachloride, in ethylene dichloride, and in nitromethane.

Piperonyl butoxide—Very slightly soluble in water; miscible with alcohol, with chloroform, with ether, with petroleum oils, and with liquefied aerosol propellants.

USP requirements:

Pyrethrins and Piperonyl Butoxide Gel—Not in *USP–NF*.

Pyrethrins and Piperonyl Butoxide Solution Shampoo—Not in *USP–NF*.

Pyrethrins and Piperonyl Butoxide Topical Solution—Not in *USP–NF*.

PYRETHRUM EXTRACT

Description: Pyrethrum Extract USP—Pale yellow liquid having a bland, flowery odor. *Pyrethrins I* denotes the group containing pyrethrin 1, cinerin 1, and jasmolin 1; *Pyrethrins II* denotes the group containing pyrethrin 2, cinerin 2, and jasmolin 2.

Solubility: Pyrethrum Extract USP—Insoluble in water; soluble in mineral oil and in most organic solvents.

USP requirements: Pyrethrum Extract USP—Preserve in tight, light-resistant containers. A mixture of three naturally occurring, closely related insecticidal esters of chrysanthemic acid (Pyrethrins I: jasmolin I, cinerin I, and pyrethrin I) and three closely related esters of pyrethric acid (Pyrethrins II: jasmolin II, cinerin II, and pyrethrin II). Contains the labeled amount of pyrethrins (sum of Pyrethrins I and Pyrethrins II), within ±10%. The ratio of Pyrethrins I to Pyrethrins II in the Extract is not less than 0.8 and not more than 2.8. May contain pigments characteristic of chrysanthemum species, triglyceride oils, terpenoids, and carotenoid. May also contain suitable solvents and antioxidants. Contains no other added substances. Meets the requirement for Identification.

PYRIDOSTIGMINE

Source: Synthetic quaternary ammonium compound.

Chemical name: Pyridostigmine bromide—Pyridinium, 3-[[(dimethylamino)carbonyl]oxy]-1-methyl-, bromide.

Molecular formula: Pyridostigmine bromide—$C_9H_{13}BrN_2O_2$.

Molecular weight: Pyridostigmine bromide—261.12.

Description: Pyridostigmine Bromide USP—White or practically white, crystalline powder, having an agreeable, characteristic odor. Hygroscopic.

Solubility: Pyridostigmine Bromide USP—Freely soluble in water, in alcohol, and in chloroform; slightly soluble in solvent hexane; practically insoluble in ether.

USP requirements:

Pyridostigmine Bromide USP—Preserve in tight containers. Contains not less than 98.5% and not more than 100.5% of pyridostigmine bromide, calculated on the dried basis. Meets the requirements for Identification, Melting range (154–157 °C, the test specimen having been previously dried), Loss on drying (not more than 2.0%), Residue on ignition (not more than 0.1%), Ordinary impurities, and Organic volatile impurities.

Pyridostigmine Bromide Injection USP—Preserve in single-dose containers, preferably of Type I glass, protected from light. A sterile solution of Pyridostigmine Bromide in a suitable medium. Contains the labeled amount, within ±10%. Meets the requirements for Identification, Bacterial endotoxins, and pH (4.5–5.5), and for Injections.

Pyridostigmine Bromide Oral Solution USP—Preserve in tight, light-resistant containers. Contains, in each 100 mL, not less than 1.08 grams and not more than 1.32 grams of pyridostigmine bromide. Meets the requirement for Identification.

Pyridostigmine Bromide Syrup USP—Preserve in tight, light-resistant containers. Contains, in each 100 mL, not less than 1.08 grams and not more than 1.32 grams of pyridostigmine bromide. Meets the requirement for Identification.

Pyridostigmine Bromide Tablets USP—Preserve in tight containers. Contain the labeled amount, within ±5%. Meet the requirements for Identification, Dissolution (80% in 60 minutes in water in Apparatus 2 at 50 rpm), and Uniformity of dosage units.

Pyridostigmine Bromide Extended-release Tablets—Not in *USP–NF*.

PYRIDOXINE

Chemical name: Pyridoxine hydrochloride—3,4-Pyridinedimethanol, 5-hydroxy-6-methyl-, hydrochloride.

Molecular formula: Pyridoxine hydrochloride—$C_8H_{11}NO_3 \cdot HCl$.

Molecular weight: Pyridoxine hydrochloride—205.64.

Description: Pyridoxine Hydrochloride USP—White to practically white crystals or crystalline powder. Is stable in air, and is slowly affected by sunlight. Its solutions have a pH of about 3.

Solubility: Pyridoxine Hydrochloride USP—Freely soluble in water; slightly soluble in alcohol; insoluble in ether.

USP requirements:
Pyridoxine Hydrochloride USP—Preserve in tight, light-resistant containers. Contains not less than 98.0% and not more than 102.0% of pyridoxine hydrochloride, calculated on the dried basis. Meets the requirements for Identification, Loss on drying (not more than 0.5%), Residue on ignition (not more than 0.1%), Heavy metals (not more than 0.003%), Organic volatile impurities, and Chloride content (16.9–17.6%, calculated on the dried basis).
Pyridoxine Hydrochloride Extended-release Capsules—Not in *USP–NF*.
Pyridoxine Hydrochloride Injection USP—Preserve in single-dose or in multiple-dose containers, preferably of Type I glass, protected from light. A sterile solution of Pyridoxine Hydrochloride in Water for Injection. Contains the labeled amount, within −5% to +15%. Meets the requirements for Identification, Bacterial endotoxins, and pH (2.0–3.8), and for Injections.
Pyridoxine Hydrochloride Tablets USP—Preserve in well-closed containers, protected from light. Contain the labeled amount, within −5% to +15%. Meet the requirements for Identification, Dissolution (75% in 45 minutes in water in Apparatus 2 at 50 rpm), and Uniformity of dosage units.
Pyridoxine Hydrochloride Extended-release Tablets—Not in *USP–NF*.

PYRILAMINE

Chemical group: Ethylenediamine derivative.

Chemical name: Pyrilamine maleate—1,2-Ethanediamine, *N*-[(4-methoxyphenyl)methyl]-*N′*,*N*-dimethyl-*N*-2-pyridinyl-, (*Z*)-2-butenedioate (1:1).

Molecular formula: Pyrilamine maleate—$C_{17}H_{23}N_3O \cdot C_4H_4O_4$.

Molecular weight: Pyrilamine maleate—401.46.

Description: Pyrilamine Maleate USP—White, crystalline powder, usually having a faint odor. Its solutions are acid to litmus.

Solubility: Pyrilamine Maleate USP—Very soluble in water; freely soluble in alcohol and in chloroform; slightly soluble in ether.

USP requirements:
Pyrilamine Maleate USP—Preserve in tight, light-resistant containers. Dried in vacuum over phosphorus pentoxide for 5 hours, contains not less than 98.0% and not more than 100.5% of pyrilamine maleate. Meets the requirements for Identification, Melting range (99–103 °C), Loss on drying (not more than 0.5%), Residue on ignition (not more than 0.1%), Related compounds, and Organic volatile impurities.

Pyrilamine Maleate Tablets USP—Preserve in well-closed containers. Contain the labeled amount, within ±7%. Meet the requirements for Identification, Dissolution (75% in 45 minutes in water in Apparatus 2 at 50 rpm), and Uniformity of dosage units.

PYRILAMINE AND CODEINE

For *Pyrilamine* and *Codeine*—See individual listings for chemistry information.

USP requirements: Pyrilamine Maleate and Codeine Phosphate Oral Solution—Not in *USP–NF*.

PYRILAMINE, PHENYLEPHRINE, ASPIRIN, AND CAFFEINE

For *Pyrilamine, Phenylephrine, Aspirin,* and *Caffeine*—See individual listings for chemistry information.

USP requirements: Pyrilamine Maleate, Phenylephrine Hydrochloride, Aspirin, and Caffeine Tablets—Not in *USP–NF*.

PYRILAMINE, PHENYLEPHRINE, AND CODEINE

For *Pyrilamine, Phenylephrine,* and *Codeine*—See individual listings for chemistry information.

USP requirements: Pyrilamine Maleate, Phenylephrine Hydrochloride, and Codeine Phosphate Syrup—Not in *USP–NF*.

PYRILAMINE, PHENYLEPHRINE, AND DEXTROMETHORPHAN

For *Pyrilamine, Phenylephrine,* and *Dextromethorphan*—See individual listings for chemistry information.

USP requirements: Pyrilamine Maleate, Phenylephrine Hydrochloride, and Dextromethorphan Hydrobromide Syrup—Not in *USP–NF*.

PYRILAMINE, PHENYLEPHRINE, AND HYDROCODONE

For *Pyrilamine, Phenylephrine,* and *Hydrocodone*—See individual listings for chemistry information.

USP requirements: Pyrilamine Maleate, Phenylephrine Hydrochloride, and Hydrocodone Bitartrate Syrup—Not in *USP–NF*.

PYRILAMINE, PHENYLEPHRINE, HYDROCODONE, AND AMMONIUM CHLORIDE

For *Pyrilamine, Phenylephrine, Hydrocodone,* and *Ammonium Chloride*—See individual listings for chemistry information.

USP requirements: Pyrilamine Maleate, Phenylephrine Hydrochloride, Hydrocodone Bitartrate, and Ammonium Chloride Syrup—Not in *USP–NF*.

PYRILAMINE, PHENYLPROPANOLAMINE, ACETAMINOPHEN, AND CAFFEINE

For *Pyrilamine, Phenylpropanolamine, Acetaminophen,* and *Caffeine*—See individual listings for chemistry information.

USP requirements: Pyrilamine Maleate, Phenylpropanolamine Hydrochloride, Acetaminophen, and Caffeine Tablets—Not in *USP–NF*.

PYRILAMINE, PHENYLPROPANOLAMINE, DEXTROMETHORPHAN, GUAIFENESIN, POTASSIUM CITRATE, AND CITRIC ACID

For *Pyrilamine, Phenylpropanolamine, Dextromethorphan, Guaifenesin, Potassium Citrate,* and *Citric Acid*—See individual listings for chemistry information.

USP requirements: Pyrilamine Maleate, Phenylpropanolamine Hydrochloride, Dextromethorphan Hydrobromide, Guaifenesin, Potassium Citrate, and Citric Acid Syrup—Not in *USP–NF*.

PYRILAMINE, PHENYLPROPANOLAMINE, DEXTROMETHORPHAN, AND SODIUM SALICYLATE

For *Pyrilamine, Phenylpropanolamine, Dextromethorphan,* and *Sodium Salicylate*—See individual listings for chemistry information.

USP requirements: Pyrilamine Maleate, Phenylpropanolamine Hydrochloride, Dextromethorphan Hydrobromide, and Sodium Salicylate Oral Solution—Not in *USP–NF*.

PYRILAMINE, PSEUDOEPHEDRINE, DEXTROMETHORPHAN, AND ACETAMINOPHEN

For *Pyrilamine, Pseudoephedrine, Dextromethorphan,* and *Acetaminophen*—See individual listings for chemistry information.

USP requirements: Pyrilamine Maleate, Pseudoephedrine Hydrochloride, Dextromethorphan Hydrobromide, and Acetaminophen Oral Solution—Not in *USP–NF*.

PYRIMETHAMINE

Chemical group: Structurally related to trimethoprim.

Chemical name: 2,4-Pyrimidinediamine, 5-(4-chlorophenyl)-6-ethyl-.

Molecular formula: $C_{12}H_{13}ClN_4$.

Molecular weight: 248.71.

Description: Pyrimethamine USP—White, odorless, crystalline powder.

Solubility: Pyrimethamine USP—Practically insoluble in water; slightly soluble in acetone, in alcohol, and in chloroform.

USP requirements:
Pyrimethamine USP—Preserve in tight, light-resistant containers. Contains not less than 99.0% and not more than 101.0% of pyrimethamine, calculated on the dried basis. Meets the requirements for Identification, Melting range (238–242 °C), Loss on drying (not more than 0.5%), Residue on ignition (not more than 0.1%), Ordinary impurities, and Organic volatile impurities.
Pyrimethamine Tablets USP—Preserve in tight, light-resistant containers. Contain the labeled amount, within ±7%. Meet the requirements for Identification, Dissolution (75% in 45 minutes in 0.01 *N* hydrochloric acid in Apparatus 2 at 50 rpm), and Uniformity of dosage units.

PYRITHIONE

Chemical name: Pyrithione zinc—Zinc, bis(1-hydroxy-2(1*H*)-pyridinethionato-*O,S*)-(T-4)-.

Molecular formula: Pyrithione zinc—$C_{10}H_8N_2O_2S_2Zn$.

Molecular weight: Pyrithione zinc—317.70.

Description: Pyrithione zinc—Off-white to gray colored powder with not more than a mild characteristic odor.

Solubility: Pyrithione zinc—Soluble in dimethylsulfoxide; practically insoluble in acetone, in alcohol, and in water.

USP requirements:
Pyrithione Zinc Bar Shampoo—Not in *USP–NF*.
Pyrithione Zinc Cream Shampoo—Not in *USP–NF*.
Pyrithione Zinc Lotion Shampoo—Not in *USP–NF*.

PYROXYLIN

Chemical name: Cellulose, nitrate.

Description: White to light yellow cuboid granules or fibrous material resembling cotton wool but harsher to the touch and more powdery.

Solubility: Soluble in acetone and in glacial acetic acid.

USP requirements: Pyroxylin USP—Preserve loosely packed in cartons, protected from light. A product obtained by the action of a mixture of nitric and sulfuric acids on cotton and consists chiefly of cellulose tetranitrate. The label bears a caution statement to the effect that Pyroxylin is highly flammable. Meets the requirements for Viscosity (110–147 poises), Residue on ignition (not more than 0.3%), Acidity and water-soluble substances, and Organic volatile impurities.

Note: Dry Pyroxylin is a light yellow, matted mass of filaments, resembling raw cotton in appearance, but harsh to the touch. *It is exceedingly flammable,* burning, when unconfined, very rapidly and with a luminous flame. When kept in well-closed bottles and exposed to light, it is decomposed with the evolution of nitrous vapors, leaving a carbonaceous residue. Pyroxylin available commercially is moistened with about 30% of alcohol or other suitable solvent. The alcohol or other solvent must be allowed to evaporate from the Pyroxylin to yield the dried substance described in *USP–NF*. Pyroxylin moistened with alcohol or other solvent may be used in these tests, provided the weight of test specimen taken corresponds to the specified amount of dry Pyroxylin.

PYRVINIUM

Chemical name: Pyrvinium pamoate—Quinolinium, 6-(dimethy-lamino)-2-[2-(2,5-dimethyl-1-phenyl-1H-pyrrol-3-yl)ethenyl]-1-methyl-, salt with 4,4'-methylenebis[3-hydroxy-2-naphthalene-carboxylic acid] (2:1).

Molecular formula: Pyrvinium pamoate—$C_{75}H_{70}N_6O_6$.

Molecular weight: Pyrvinium pamoate—1151.40.

Description:
  Pyrvinium Pamoate USP—Bright orange or orange-red to practically black, crystalline powder.
  Pyrvinium Pamoate Oral Suspension USP—Dark red, opaque suspension of essentially very fine, amorphous particles or aggregates, usually less than 10 micrometers in size. Larger particles, some of which may be crystals, up to 100 micrometers in size also may be present.

Solubility: Pyrvinium Pamoate USP—Practically insoluble in water and in ether; freely soluble in glacial acetic acid; slightly soluble in chloroform and in methoxyethanol; very slightly soluble in methanol.

USP requirements:
  Pyrvinium Pamoate USP—Preserve in tight, light-resistant containers. Contains not less than 96.0% and not more than 104.0% of pyrvinium pamoate, calculated on the anhydrous basis. Meets the requirements for Identification, Water (not more than 6.0%), and Residue on ignition (not more than 0.5%).
  Pyrvinium Pamoate Oral Suspension USP—Preserve in tight, light-resistant containers. Contains, in each 100 mL, an amount of pyrvinium pamoate equivalent to not less than 0.90 gram and not more than 1.10 grams of pyrvinium. Meets the requirements for Identification and pH (6.0–8.0, determined potentiometrically).
  Pyrvinium Pamoate Tablets USP—Preserve in tight, light-resistant containers. Contain an amount of pyrvinium pamoate equivalent to the labeled amount of pyrvinium, within ± 8%. Meet the requirements for Identification, Disintegration (30 minutes), and Uniformity of dosage units.

QUAZEPAM

Chemical name: 2H-1,4-Benzodiazepine-2-thione, 7-chloro-5-(2-fluorophenyl)-1,3-dihydro-1-(2,2,2-trifluoroethyl)-.

Molecular formula: $C_{17}H_{11}ClF_4N_2S$.

Molecular weight: 386.80.

Description: Quazepam USP—Off-white to yellowish powder.

Solubility: Soluble in ethanol; insoluble in water.

USP requirements:
  Quazepam USP—Preserve in well-closed containers. Contains not less than 98.5% and not more than 101.5% of quazepam, calculated on the dried basis. Meets the requirements for Identification, Melting range (146–151 °C, the range between beginning and end of melting does not exceed 2 °C), Loss on drying (not more than 0.5%), Residue onignition (not more than 0.2%), Heavy metals (not more than 20 mcg per gram), and Related compounds.
  Quazepam Tablets USP—Preserve in a well-closed container. Contain the labeled amount, within ±10%. Meets the requirements for Identification, Dissolution (80% in 30 minutes in 1% sodium lauryl sulfate in Apparatus 2 at 50 rpm), Uniformity of dosage units, and Related compounds.

QUETIAPINE

Chemical name: Quetiapine fumarate—Ethanol, 2-[2-(4-dibenzo[b,f][1,4]thiazepin-11-yl-1-piperazinyl)ethoxy]-, (E)-2-butenedioate (2:1) (salt).

Molecular formula: Quetiapine fumarate—$(C_{21}H_{25}N_3O_2S)_2 \cdot C_4H_4O_4$.

Molecular weight: Quetiapine fumarate—883.09.

Description: Quetiapine fumarate—White to off-white crystalline powder. Melting point 172.0–174 °C.

pKa: Quetiapine fumarate—6.83 in phosphate buffer at 22 °C; 3.32 in formic buffer at 22 °C.

Solubility: Quetiapine fumarate—Very slightly soluble in ether; slightly soluble in water; soluble in 0.1 NHCl.

USP requirements: Quetiapine Fumarate Tablets—Not in *USP–NF*.

QUINACRINE

Chemical group: Acridine derivative.

Chemical name: Quinacrine hydrochloride—1,4-Pentanediamine, N⁴-(6-chloro-2-methoxy-9-acridinyl)-N',N'-diethyl-, dihydrochloride, dihydrate.

Molecular formula: Quinacrine hydrochloride—$C_{23}H_{30}ClN_3O \cdot 2HCl \cdot 2H_2O$.

Molecular weight: Quinacrine hydrochloride—508.91.

Description: Quinacrine hydrochloride—Bright yellow, crystalline powder. Is odorless. Its solution (1 in 100) has a pH of about 4.5. Melts at about 250 °C, with decomposition.

Solubility: Quinacrine hydrochloride—Sparingly soluble in water; soluble in alcohol.

USP requirements: Quinacrine Hydrochloride Tablets—Not in USP.

QUINAPRIL

Chemical name: Quinapril hydrochloride—3-Isoquinolinecarboxylic acid, 2-[2-[[1-(ethoxycarbonyl)-3-phenylpropyl]amino]-1-oxopropyl]-1,2,3,4-tetrahydro-, monohydrochloride, [3S-[2[R*(R*)],3R*]].

Molecular formula: Quinapril hydrochloride—$C_{25}H_{30}N_2O_5 \cdot HCl$.

Molecular weight: Quinapril hydrochloride—474.98.

Description: Quinapril hydrochloride—White to off-white amorphous powder.

Solubility: Quinapril hydrochloride—Freely soluble in aqueous solvents.

USP requirements: Quinapril Hydrochloride Tablets—Not in USP.

QUINAPRIL AND HYDROCHLOROTHIAZIDE

For *Quinapril* and *Hydrochlorothiazide*—See individual listings for chemistry information.

USP requirements: Quinapril Hydrochloride and Hydrochlorothiazide Tablets—Not in *USP–NF*.

QUINESTROL

Chemical name: 19-Norpregna-1,3,5(10)-trien-20-yn-17-ol, 3-(cyclopentyloxy)-, (17 alpha)-.

Molecular formula: $C_{25}H_{32}O_2$.

Molecular weight: 364.52.

Description: White, practically odorless powder.

Solubility: Insoluble in water; soluble in alcohol, in chloroform, and in ether.

USP requirements: Quinestrol Tablets—Not in USP.

QUINETHAZONE

Chemical name: 6-Quinazolinesulfonamide, 7-chloro-2-ethyl-1,2,3,4-tetrahydro-4-oxo-.

Molecular formula: $C_{10}H_{12}ClN_3O_3S$.

Molecular weight: 289.74.

Description: White to yellowish white, crystalline powder.

pKa: 9.3 and 10.7.

Solubility: Very slightly soluble in water; freely soluble in solutions of alkali hydroxides and carbonates; sparingly soluble in pyridine; slightly soluble in alcohol.

USP requirements: Quinethazone Tablets—Not in USP.

QUINIDINE

Source: Quinidine polygalacturonate—A polymer of quinidine and polygalacturonic acid.

Chemical name:
Quinidine gluconate—Cinchonan-9-ol, 6′-methoxy-, (9S)-, mono-D-gluconate (salt).
Quinidine sulfate—Cinchonan-9-ol, 6′-methoxy-, (9S)-, sulfate (2:1) (salt), dihydrate.

Molecular formula:
Quinidine gluconate—$C_{20}H_{24}N_2O_2 \cdot C_6H_{12}O_7$.
Quinidine polygalacturonate—$(C_{20}H_{24}N_2O_2 \cdot C_6H_{10}O_7 \cdot H_2O)_x$.
Quinidine sulfate—$(C_{20}H_{24}N_2O_2)_2 \cdot H_2SO_4 \cdot 2H_2O$.

Molecular weight:
Quinidine gluconate—520.57.
Quinidine sulfate—782.94.

Description:
Quinidine Gluconate USP—White powder. Odorless.
Quinidine polygalacturonate—Creamy white, amorphous powder.
Quinidine Sulfate USP—Fine, needle-like, white crystals, frequently cohering in masses, or fine, white powder. Is odorless, and darkens on exposure to light. Its solutions are neutral or alkaline to litmus.

Solubility:
Quinidine Gluconate USP—Freely soluble in water; slightly soluble in alcohol.
Quinidine polygalacturonate—Sparingly soluble in water; freely soluble in hot 40% alcohol.
Quinidine Sulfate USP—Slightly soluble in water; soluble in alcohol; sparingly soluble in chloroform; insoluble in ether.

USP requirements:
Quinidine Bisulfate Extended-release Tablets—Not in *USP–NF*.
Quinidine Gluconate USP—Preserve in well-closed, light-resistant containers. The gluconate of an alkaloid that may be obtained from various species of *Cinchona* and their hybrids, or from *Remijia pedunculata* Fl;auuckiger (Fam. Rubiaceae), or prepared from quinine. Contains not less than 99.0% and not more than 100.5% of total alkaloid salt, calculated as quinidine gluconate, on the dried basis. Meets the requirements for Identification, Loss on drying (not more than 0.5%), Residue on ignition (not more than 0.15%), Heavy metals (not more than 0.001%), Limit of dihydroquinidine gluconate, Chromatographic purity, and Organic volatile impurities.
Quinidine Gluconate Injection USP—Preserve in single-dose or in multiple-dose containers, preferably of Type I glass. A sterile solution of Quinidine Gluconate in Water for Injection. Contains, in each mL, amounts of quinidine gluconate and dihydroquinidine gluconate totaling not less than 76 mg and not more than 84 mg of quinidine gluconate, calculated as quinidine gluconate. Meets the requirements for Identification, Bacterial endotoxins, and Chromatographic purity, and for Injections.
Quinidine Gluconate Tablets—Not in *USP–NF*.
Quinidine Gluconate Extended-release Tablets USP—Preserve in well-closed, light-resistant containers. The labeling indicates the Drug Release test with which the product complies. Contain amounts of quinidine gluconate and dihydroquinidine gluconate totaling the labeled amount of quinidine gluconate, calculated as quinidine gluconate, within ±10%. Meet the requirements for Identification, Drug release (30–50% in 1 hour, 45–65% in 2 hours, 60–85% in 4 hours, and not less than 85% in 8 hours in 0.1 *M* acetate buffer [pH 5.4] in Apparatus 2 at 75 rpm for Test 1; and 30–45% in 1 hour, 45–60% in 2 hours, 60–80% in 4 hours, and not less than 85% in 8 hours in 0.1 *N* hydrochloric acid in Apparatus 2 at 75 rpm for Test 4), Uniformity of dosage units, and Chromatographic purity.
Quinidine Polygalacturonate Tablets—Not in *USP–NF*.
Quinidine Sulfate USP—Preserve in well-closed, light-resistant containers. The sulfate of an alkaloid obtained from various species of *Cinchona* and their hybrids and from *Remijia pedunculata* Fl;auuckiger (Fam. Rubiaceae), or prepared from quinine. Contains not less than 99.0% and not more than 101.0% of total alkaloid salt, calculated as quinidine sulfate, on the anhydrous basis. Meets the requirements for Identification, Specific rotation (+275° to +288°, calculated on the anhydrous basis), Water (4.0–5.5%), Residue on ignition (not more than 0.1%), Chloroform-alcohol-insoluble substances (not more than 0.1%), Heavy metals (not more than 0.001%), Limit of dihydroquinidine sulfate, Chromatographic purity, and Organic volatile impurities.
Quinidine Sulfate Capsules USP—Preserve in tight, light-resistant containers. Contain amounts of quinidine sulfate and dihydroquinidine sulfate totaling the labeled amount of quinidine sulfate, calculated as quinidine sulfate, within ±10%. Meet the requirements for Identification, Dissolution (85% in 30 minutes in 0.01 *N* hydrochloric acid in Apparatus 1 at 100 rpm), Uniformity of dosage units, and Chromatographic purity.
Quinidine Sulfate Injection—Not in *USP–NF*.
Quinidine Sulfate Tablets USP—Preserve in well-closed, light-resistant containers. Contain amounts of quinidine sulfate and dihydroquinidine sulfate totaling the labeled amount of quinidine sulfate, within ±10%. Meet the requirements for Identifica-

tion, Dissolution (85% in 30 minutes in 0.01 N hydrochloric acid in Apparatus 1 at 100 rpm), Uniformity of dosage units, and Chromatographic purity.

Quinidine Sulfate Extended-release Tablets USP—Preserve in well-closed, light-resistant containers. The labeling indicates the Drug Release test with which the product complies. Contain amounts of quinidine sulfate and dihydroquinidine sulfate totaling the labeled amount of quinidine sulfate, calculated as quinidine sulfate, within ± 10%. Meet the requirements for Identification, Drug release (20–50% in 1 hour, 43–73% in 4 hours, and not less than 70% in 12 hours for Test 1 and 10–35% in 1 hour, 30–55% in 4 hours, and not less than 75% in 12 hours for Test 2 in 0.1 N hydrochloric acid in Apparatus 1 at 100 rpm), Uniformity of dosage units, and Chromatographic purity.

QUININE

Chemical name: Quinine sulfate—Cinchonan-9-ol, 6′-methoxy-, (8 alpha,9R)-, sulfate (2:1) (salt), dihydrate.

Molecular formula: Quinine sulfate—$(C_{20}H_{24}N_2O_2)_2 \cdot H_2SO_4 \cdot 2H_2O$.

Molecular weight: Quinine sulfate—782.94.

Description: Quinine Sulfate USP—White, fine, needle-like crystals, usually lusterless, making a light and readily compressible mass. Is odorless. It darkens on exposure to light. Its saturated solution is neutral or alkaline to litmus.

Solubility: Quinine Sulfate USP—Slightly soluble in water, in alcohol, and in chloroform; very slightly soluble in ether; freely soluble in alcohol at 80 °C, and in a mixture of 2 volumes of chloroform and 1 volume of dehydrated alcohol; sparingly soluble in water at 100 °C.

USP requirements:

Quinine Dihydrochloride Injection—Not in *USP–NF*.

Quinine Sulfate USP—Preserve in well-closed, light-resistant containers. The sulfate of an alkaloid obtained from the bark of species of *Cinchona*. Contains not less than 99.0% and not more than 101.0% of total alkaloid salt, calculated as quinine sulfate, on the anhydrous basis. Meets the requirements for Identification, Specific rotation (−235° to −245°), Water (4.0–5.5%), Residue on ignition (not more than 0.1%), Heavy metals (not more than 0.001%), Chloroform-alcohol-insoluble substances (not more than 0.1%), Chromatographic purity, Limit of dihydroquinine sulfate, and Organic volatile impurities.

Quinine Sulfate Capsules USP—Preserve in tight containers. Contain amounts of quinine sulfate and dihydroquinine sulfate totaling the labeled amount of quinine sulfate, calculated as quinine sulfate dihydrate, within ±10%. Meet the requirements for Identification, Dissolution (75% in 45 minutes in 0.1 N hydrochloric acid in Apparatus 1 at 100 rpm), Uniformity of dosage units, and Chromatographic purity.

Quinine Sulfate Tablets USP—Preserve in well-closed containers. Contain amounts of quinine sulfate and dihydroquinine sulfate totaling the labeled amount of quinine sulfate, calculated as quinine sulfate dihydrate, within ± 10%. Meet the requirements for Identification, Dissolution (75% in 45 minutes in 0.01 N hydrochloric acid in Apparatus 1 at 100 rpm), Uniformity of dosage units, and Chromatographic purity.

QUINUPRISTIN AND DALFOPRISTIN

Source: Quinupristin and dalfopristin combination, a streptogamin antibacterial agent for intravenous administration, is a sterile lyophilized formulation of two semisynthetic pristinamycin derivatives. Quinupristin is derived from pristinamycin I, while dalfopristin is derived from pristinamycin IIA. Quinupristin and dalfopristin are present in a ratio of 30 parts quinupristin to 70 parts of dalfopristin.

Chemical group: Pristinamycin.

Chemical name:

Quinupristin—N-[(6R,9S,10R,13S,15aS,18R,22S,24aS)-22-[p(Dimethylamino)benzyl]-6-ethyldocosahydro-10,23-dimethyl-5,8,12,15,17,21,24-heptaoxo-13-phenyl-18-[[(3S)3-quinuclidinylthio]-12H-pyrido[2,1-f]pyrrolo[2,1-f][1,4,7,10,13,16]oxapentaazacyclononadecin-9-yl]3-hydroxypicolinamide.

Dalfopristin—(3R,4R,5E,10E,12E,14S,26R,26aS)-26-[[2-Diethylamino)ethyl]sulfonyl]-8,9,14,15,24,25,26,26a-octahydro-14-hydroxy-3-isopropyl-4,12-dimethyl-3H-21,18nitrilo-1H,22H-pyrrolo[2,1-c][1,8,4,19]dioxadiazacyclotetracosine-1,7,16,22-(4H,17H)-tetrone.

Molecular formula:

Quinupristin—$C_{53}H_{67}N_9O_{10}S$.

Dalfopristin—$C_{34}H_{50}N_4O_9S$.

Molecular weight:

Quinupristin—1022.22.

Dalfopristin—690.85.

Description:

Quinupristin—A white to very slightly yellow, hygroscopic powder.

Dalfopristin—A slightly yellow to yellow, hygroscopic powder.

USP requirements: Quinupristin and Dalfopristin for Injection—Not in *USP–NF*.

RABEPRAZOLE

Chemical group: Substituted benzimidazole.

Chemical name:

Rabeprazole—2-[[[4-(3-Methoxypropoxy)-3-methyl-2-pyridinyl]methyl]sulfinyl]-1H-benzimidazole.

Rabeprazole sodium—1H-Benzimidazole, 2-[[[4-(3-methoxypropoxy)-3-methyl-2-pyridinyl]methyl]sulfinyl]-, sodium salt.

Molecular formula:

Rabeprazole—$C_{18}H_{21}N_3O_3S$.

Rabeprazole Sodium—$C_{18}H_{20}N_3NaO_3S$.

Molecular weight:

Rabeprazole—359.45.

Rabeprazole sodium—381.43.

Description:

Rabeprazole—White crystals. Melting point 99–100°.

Rabeprazole sodium—White to slightly yellowish-white solid. Melting point 140–141°.

Solubility: Rabeprazole sodium—Very soluble in water and in methanol; freely soluble in ethanol and in n-hexane.

USP requirements: Rabeprazole Delayed-release Tablets—Not in *USP–NF*.

RABIES IMMUNE GLOBULIN

Description: Rabies Immune Globulin USP—Transparent or slightly opalescent liquid, practically colorless and practically odorless. May develop a slight, granular deposit during storage.

USP requirements: Rabies Immune Globulin USP—Preserve at a temperature between 2 and 8 °C. A sterile, non-pyrogenic, slightly opalescent solution consisting of globulins derived from blood plasma or serum that has been tested for the absence of hepatitis B surface antigen, derived from selected adult human donors who have been immunized with rabies vaccine and have developed high titers of rabies antibody. Label it to state that it is not for intravenous injection. Has a potency such that when labeled as 150 International Units (IU) per mL, it has a geometric mean lower limit (95% confidence) potency value of not less than 110 IU per mL, and proportionate lower limit potency values for other labeled potencies, based on the U.S. Standard Rabies Immune Globulin and using the CVS Virus challenge, by neutralization test in mice or tissue culture. Contains not less than 10 grams and not more than 18 grams of protein per 100 mL, of which not less than 80% is monomeric immunoglobilin G, having a sedimentation coefficient in the range of 6.0 to 7.5S, with no fragments having a sedimentation coefficient less than 6S and no aggregates having a sedimentation coefficient greater than 12S. Contains 0.3 *M* glycine as a stabilizing agent, and contains a suitable preservative. Has a pH of 6.4–7.2, measured in a solution diluted to contain 1% of protein with 0.15 *M* sodium chloride. Meets the requirements of the test for heat stability and for Expiration date (not later than 1 year after date of issue from manufacturer's cold storage [5 °C, 1 year]). Conforms to the regulations of the U.S. Food and Drug Administration concerning biologics.

RABIES VACCINE

Description: Rabies Vaccine USP—White to straw-colored, amorphous pellet, which may or may not become fragmented when shaken.

USP requirements:

Rabies Vaccine USP—Preserve at a temperature between 2 and 8 °C. A sterile preparation, in dried or liquid form, of inactivated rabies virus harvested from inoculated diploid cell cultures. Label it to state that it contains rabies antigen equivalent to not less than 2.5 IU per dose and that it is intended for intramuscular injection only. The cell cultures are shown to consist of diploid cells by tests of karyology, to be non-tumorigenic by tests in hamsters treated with anti-lymphocytic serum (ALS), and to be free from extraneous agents by tests in animals or cell-culture systems. The harvested virus meets the requirements for identity by serological tests, for absence of infectivity by tests in mice or cell-culture systems, and for absence of extraneous agents by tests in animals or cell-culture systems. The Vaccine meets the requirements for absence of live virus by tests using a suitable virus amplification system involving inoculation and incubation of sensitive cell cultures for not less than 14 days followed by inoculation of the cell-culture fluid thereafter into not less than 20 adult mice. Has a potency of rabies antigen equivalent to not less than 2.5 International Units for Rabies Vaccine, per dose, determined with the specific mouse protection test using the U.S. Standard Rabies Vaccine. Meets the requirements for general safety and for Expiration date (not later than 2 years after date of issue from manufacturer's cold storage [5 °C, 1 year]). Conforms to the regulations of the U.S. Food and Drug Administration concerning biologics.

Rabies Vaccine, Human Diploid Cell (For Intradermal Injection) (HDCV)—Not in USP.

Rabies Vaccine, Human Diploid Cell (For Intramascular Injection) (HDCV)—Not in USP.

RABIES VACCINE ADSORBED

Source: RVA is prepared from the CVS Kissling/MDPH strain of rabies virus grown in a diploid cell line derived from fetal rhesus monkey lung cells. The vaccine virus is inactivated by betapropiolactone and concentrated by adsorption to aluminum phosphate.

USP requirements: Rabies Vaccine Adsorbed Suspension (RVA)—Not in *USP–NF*.

RACEMETHIONINE

Chemical name: Methionine, DL-.

Molecular formula: $C_5H_{11}NO_2S$.

Molecular weight: 149.21.

Description: White, crystalline powder or platelets.

Solubility: Soluble in water; very slightly soluble in alcohol.

USP requirements:

Racemethionine Capsules—Not in *USP–NF*.
Racemethionine Oral Solution—Not in *USP–NF*.
Racemethionine Tablets—Not in *USP–NF*.

RACEPINEPHRINE

Chemical name: 1,2-Benzenediol, 4-[1-hydroxy-2-(methylamino)ethyl]-, (±)-.

Molecular formula:

Racepinephrine—$C_9H_{13}NO_3$.
Racepinephrine hydrochloride—$C_9H_{13}NO_3 \cdot HCl$.

Molecular weight:

Racepinephrine—183.20.
Racepinephrine hydrochloride—219.67.

Description:

Racepinephrine USP—White to nearly white, crystalline, odorless powder, gradually darkening on exposure to light and air. With acids, it forms salts that are readily soluble in water, and the base may be recovered by the addition of ammonium hydroxide.

Racepinephrine Hydrochloride USP—Fine, white, odorless powder. Darkens on exposure to light and air. Its solutions are acid to litmus. Melts at about 157 °C.

Solubility:

Racepinephrine USP—Very slightly soluble in water and in alcohol; insoluble in ether, in chloroform, and in fixed and volatile oils.

Racepinephrine Hydrochloride USP—Freely soluble in water; sparingly soluble in alcohol.

USP requirements:

Racepinephrine USP—Preserve in tight, light-resistant containers. A racemic mixture of the enantiomorphs of epinephrine. Contains not less than 97.0% and not more than 102.0% of racepinephrine, calculated on the dried basis. Meets the requirements for Identification, Specific rotation (−1° to +1°), Loss on drying (not more than 2.0%),

Residue on ignition (not more than 0.5%), Limit of adrenalone, Limit of norepinephrine (not more than 4.0%), and Organic volatile impurities.

Racepinephrine Inhalation Solution USP—Preserve in tight, light-resistant containers. Do not freeze. A sterile solution of Racepinephrine in Purified Water prepared with the aid of Hydrochloric Acid or of Racepinephrine Hydrochloride in Purified Water. The label indicates that the Inhalation Solution is not to be used if its color is pinkish or darker than slightly yellow or if it contains a precipitate. Contains the labeled amount, within ±10%. Meets the requirements for Color and clarity, Identification, Sterility, and pH (2.0–3.5).

Racepinephrine Hydrochloride USP—Preserve in tight, light-resistant containers. A racemic mixture of the hydrochlorides of the enantiomorphs of epinephrine. Contains not less than 97.0% and not more than 102.0% of racepinephrine hydrochloride, calculated on the anhydrous basis. Meets the requirements for Identification, Specific rotation (−1° to +1°), Water (not more than 0.5%), Residue on ignition (not more than 0.5%), and Organic volatile impurities, and for Adrenalone and Limit of norepinephrine under Racepinephrine.

RALOXIFENE

Chemical name: Raloxifene hydrochloride—Methanone, [6-hydroxy-2-(4-hydroxyphenyl)benzo[*b*]thien-3-yl]-[4-[2-(1-piperidinyl)ethoxy]phenyl]-, hydrochloride.

Molecular formula: Raloxifene hydrochloride—$C_{28}H_{27}NO_4S \cdot HCl$.

Molecular weight: Raloxifene hydrochloride—510.04.

Description: Raloxifene hydrochloride—Off-white to pale yellow solid.

Solubility: Raloxifene hydrochloride—Very slightly soluble in water.

USP requirements: Raloxifene Hydrochloride Tablets—Not in *USP–NF*.

RALTITREXED

Chemical name: L-Glutamic acid, *N*-[[5-[[1,4-dihydro-2-methyl-4-oxo-6-quinazolinyl)methyl]methylamino]-2-thienyl]carbonyl].

Molecular formula: $C_{21}H_{22}N_4O_6S$.

Molecular weight: 458.49.

Description: Raltitrexed disodium—Pale yello-brown to brown powder. Melting point 179–181 °C.

pKa: Raltitrexed disodium—The estimated pKa values of the two carboxylic acid groups are 4.5 and 5.7 at 25 °C.

Solubility: Raltitrexed disodium—Solubility is susceptible to pH.

USP requirements: Raltitrexed Disodium Injection—Not in *USP–NF*.

RAMIPRIL

Chemical name: Cyclopenta[*b*]pyrrole-2-carboxylic acid, 1-[2-[[1-(ethoxycarbonyl)-3-phenylpropyl]amino]-1-oxopropyl]octahydro-, [2*S*-[1[*R**(*R**)]],2 alpha,3a beta,6a beta]]-.

Molecular formula: $C_{23}H_{32}N_2O_5$.

Molecular weight: 416.51.

Description: Ramipril USP—White to almost white crystalline powder. Melts between 105–112 °C.

Solubility: Ramipril USP—Freely soluble in methanol; sparingly soluble in water.

USP requirements:

Ramipril USP—Preserve in tight containers. contains not less than 98.0% and not more than 101.0% of ramipril, calculated on the dried basis. Meets the requirements for Identification, Melting range (105°–112°), Specific rotation (between +32.0° to +38.0, determined at 20°), Loss on drying (not more than 0.2%), Residue on ignition (not more than 0.1%), Limit of palladium (0.002%), and Related compounds.

Ramipril Capsules—Not in *USP–NF*.

RANITIDINE

Chemical group: Amino-alkyl furan derivative of histamine.

Chemical name:

Ranitidine—1,1-Ethenediamine, *N*-[2-[[[5-[(dimethylamino)methyl]-2-furanyl]methyl]thio]ethyl]-*N*-methyl-2-nitro-.

Ranitidine bismuth citrate—1,2,3-Propanetricarboxylic acid, 2-hydroxy-, bismuth(3+) salt (1:1), compd. with *N*-[2-[[[5-[(dimethylamino)methyl]-2-furanyl]methyl]thio]ethyl]-*N*-methyl-2-nitro-1,1-ethenediamine (1:1).

Ranitidine hydrochloride—1,1-Ethenediamine, *N*-[2-[[[5-[(dimethylamino)methyl]-2-furanyl]methyl]thio]ethyl]-*N*-methyl-2-nitro-, monohydrochloride.

Molecular formula:

Ranitidine—$C_{13}H_{22}N_4O_3S$.

Ranitidine bismuth citrate—$C_{13}H_{22}N_4O_3S \cdot C_6H_5BiO_7$.

Ranitidine hydrochloride—$C_{13}H_{22}N_4O_3S \cdot HCl$.

Molecular weight:

Ranitidine—314.41.

Ranitidine bismuth citrate—712.49.

Ranitidine hydrochloride—350.87.

Description:

Ranitidine bismuth citrate—White to off-white amorphous powder.

Ranitidine Hydrochloride USP—White to pale yellow, crystalline, practically odorless powder. Is sensitive to light and moisture. Melts at about 140 °C, with decomposition.

pKa: Ranitidine hydrochloride—8.2 and 2.7.

Solubility:

Ranitidine bismuth citrate—Readily soluble in water.

Ranitidine Hydrochloride USP—Very soluble in water; sparingly soluble in chloroform.

USP requirements:

Ranitidine Bismuth Citrate Tablets—Not in *USP–NF*.

Ranitidine Hydrochloride USP—Preserve in tight, light-resistant containers. Contains not less than 97.5% and not more than 102.0% of ranitidine hydrochloride, calculated on the dried basis. Meets the requirements for Identification, pH (4.5–6.0, in a solution [1 in 100]), Loss on drying (not more than 0.75%), Residue on ignition (not more than 0.1%), Chromatographic purity, and Organic volatile impurities.

Ranitidine Hydrochloride Capsules—Not in *USP–NF*.

Ranitidine Hydrochloride Effervescent Granules—Not in *USP–NF*.

Ranitidine Hydrochloride Injection USP—Preserve in single-dose or in multiple-dose containers of Type I glass, protected from light. Store below 30 °C. Do not freeze. A sterile solution of Ranitidine Hydrochloride in Water for

Injection. Label Injection to state both the content of the active moiety and the content of the salt used in formulating the article. Contains the equivalent of the labeled amount of ranitidine, within ±10%. Meets the requirements for Identification, Bacterial endotoxins, pH (6.7–7.3), Particulate matter, and Chromatographic purity, and for Injections.

Ranitidine Oral Solution USP—Preserve in tight, light-resistant containers. Store below 25 °C. Do not freeze. A solution of Ranitidine Hydrochloride in water. Contains the equivalent of the labeled amount of ranitidine, within ± 10%. Meets the requirements for Identification, Antimicrobial effectiveness testing, Microbial limits, pH (6.7–7.5), and Chromatographic purity.

Ranitidine Hydrochloride Syrup—Not in *USP–NF.*

Ranitidine Hydrochloride Tablets USP—Preserve in tight, light-resistant containers. Contain an amount of ranitidine hydrochloride equivalent to the labeled amount of ranitidine, within ±10%. Meet the requirements for Identification, Dissolution (80% in 45 minutes in water in Apparatus 2 at 50 rpm), Uniformity of dosage units, and Chromatographic purity.

Ranitidine Hydrochloride Effervescent Tablets—Not in *USP–NF.*

RANITIDINE AND SODIUM CHLORIDE

For *Ranitidine* and *Sodium Chloride*—See individual listings for chemistry information.

USP requirements: Ranitidine in Sodium Chloride Injection USP—Preserve in glass containers, preferably of Type I or Type II glass, or in containers of suitable plastic, protected from light. Store at a temperature between 2 and 25 °C. Do not freeze. A sterile solution of Ranitidine Hydrochloride and Sodium Chloride in Water for Injection. Contains the labeled amounts of both ranitidine and sodium chloride, within ± 10%. Meets the requirements for Identification, Bacterial endotoxins, pH (6.7–7.3), and Chromatographic purity, and for Injections.

RAPACURONIUM

Chemical group: Propenyl bromide ammonium salt with a basic steroid backbone.

Chemical name: Rapacuronium bromide—1-Allyl-1-(3 alpha,17 beta-dihydroxy-2 beta-piperidino-5 alpha-androstan-16 beta-yl)piperidinium bromide, 3-acetate 17-propionate.

Molecular formula: Rapacuronium bromide—$C_{37}H_{61}BrN_2O_4$.

Molecular weight: Rapacuronium bromide—677.80.

USP requirements: Rapacuronium Bromide for Injection—Not in *USP–NF.*

RAUWOLFIA SERPENTINA

Description: Powdered rauwolfia serpentina—Light tan to light brown powder.

Solubility: Powdered rauwolfia serpentina—Slightly soluble in water; sparingly soluble in alcohol.

USP requirements:
Rauwolfia Serpentina USP—Preserve in well-closed containers, and store at controlled room temperature, in a dry place, secure against insect attack. The dried root of *Rauwolfia serpentina* (Linné) Bentham ex Kurz (Fam. Apocynaceae), sometimes having fragments of rhizome and aerial stem bases attached. Contains not less than 0.15% of reserpine-rescinnamine group alkaloids, calculated as reserpine. Meets the requirements for Botanic characteristics, Microbial limits, Loss on drying (not more than 12.0%), Acid-insoluble ash (not more than 2.0%), Stems and other foreign organic matter (not more than 2.0% of stems and not more than 3.0% of other foreign organic matter), Chemical identification, and Organic volatile impurities.

Powdered Rauwolfia Serpentina USP—Preserve in well-closed containers, and store at controlled room temperature, in a dry place, secure against insect attack. It is Rauwolfia Serpentina reduced to a fine or a very fine powder, and adjusted, if necessary, to conform to the requirements for reserpine-rescinnamine group alkaloids by admixture with lactose or starch or with a powdered rauwolfia serpentina containing a higher or lower content of these alkaloids. Contains not less than 0.15% and not more than 0.20% of reserpine-rescinnamine group alkaloids, calculated as reserpine. Meets the requirements for Identification, Microbial limit, and Acid-insoluble ash (not more than 2.0%).

Rauwolfia Serpentina Tablets USP—Preserve in tight, light-resistant containers. Contain an amount of reserpine-rescinnamine group alkaloids, calculated as reserpine, equivalent to not less than 0.15% and not more than 0.20% of the labeled amount of powdered rauwolfia serpentina. Meet the requirements for Identification, Microbial limits, Disintegration (1 hour, with disks using simulated gastric fluid TS, without enzyme), and Uniformity of dosage units.

RAUWOLFIA SERPENTINA AND BENDROFLUMETHIAZIDE

For *Rauwolfia Serpentina* and *Bendroflumethiazide*—See individual listings for chemistry information.

USP requirements: Rauwolfia Serpentina and Bendroflumethiazide Tablets—Not in *USP–NF.*

PURIFIED RAYON

Description: Purified Rayon USP—White, lustrous or dull, fine, soft, filamentous fibers, appearing under the microscope as round, oval, or slightly flattened translucent rods, straight or crimped, striate and with serrate cross-sectional edges. Is practically odorless.

Solubility: Purified Rayon USP—Very soluble in ammoniated cupric oxide TS and in dilute sulfuric acid (3 in 5); insoluble in ordinary solvents.

USP requirements: Purified Rayon USP—A fibrous form of bleached, regenerated cellulose. Meets the requirements for Alkalinity or acidity, Residue on ignition (not more than 1.50%, determined on a 5.0-gram test specimen), Acid-insoluble ash (not more than 1.25%), Water-soluble substances (not more than 1.0%), and Fiber length and absorbency, and for Dyes and Other foreign matter under Purified Cotton.

ORAL REHYDRATION SALTS

For *Dextrose, Potassium Chloride, Sodium Bicarbonate, Sodium Chloride,* and *Sodium Citrate*—See individual listings for chemistry information.

USP requirements: Oral Rehydration Salts USP (For Oral Solution)—Preserve in tight containers, and avoid exposure to temperatures in excess of 30 °C. The Sodium Bicarbonate or Sodium Citrate component may be omitted from the mixture and packaged in a separate, accompanying container. A dry mixture of Sodium Chloride, Potassium Chloride, Sodium Bicarbonate, and Dextrose (anhydrous). Alternatively, may contain Sodium Citrate (anhydrous or dihydrate) instead of Sodium Bicarbonate. May contain Dextrose (monohydrate) instead of Dextrose (anhydrous), provided that the Sodium Bicarbonate or Sodium Citrate is packaged in a separate, accompanying container. Contains the equivalent of the amounts of sodium, potassium, chloride, and bicarbonate or citrate, calculated from the labeled amounts of Sodium Chloride, Potassium Chloride, and Sodium Bicarbonate (or Sodium Citrate [anhydrous or dihydrate]), within ±10%. Contains the labeled amounts of anhydrous dextrose or dextrose monohydrate, within ±10%. The label indicates prominently whether Sodium Bicarbonate or Sodium Citrate is a component by the placement of the word "'Bicarbonate" or "Citrate," as appropriate, in juxtaposition to the official title. The label states the name and quantity, in grams, of each component in each unit-dose container, or in a stated quantity, in grams, of Salts in a multiple-unit container. The label states the net weight in each container, and provides directions for constitution. Where packaged in individual unit-dose pouches, the label instructs the user not to open until the time of use. The label states also that any solution that remains unused 24 hours after constitution is to be discarded. Meets the requirements for Identification, Loss on drying (not more than 1.0%), Minimum fill, and pH (7.0–8.8, in the solution constituted as directed in labeling).

REMIFENTANIL

Chemical name: Remifentanil hydrochloride—1-Piperidinepropanoic acid, 4-(methoxycarbonyl)-4-[(1-oxopropyl)phenylamino]-, methyl ester, monohydrochloride.

Molecular formula: Remifentanil hydrochloride—$C_{20}H_{28}N_2O_5 \cdot$ HCl.

Molecular weight: Remifentanil hydrochloride—412.92.

Description: Remifentanil hydrochloride—White to off-white solid. Melting point approximately 205 °C.

pKa: 7.07.

USP requirements: Remifentanil Hydrochloride for Injection—Not in *USP–NF*.

REPAGLINIDE

Chemical name: (*S*)-2-Ethyoxy-4-[2-[[methyl-1-[2-[(1-piperidinyl)phenyl]butyl]amino]-2-oxoethyl]-benzoic acid.

Molecular formula: $C_{27}H_{36}N_2O_4$.

Molecular weight: 452.59.

Description: Repaglinide USP—White to off-white solid. Melts at about 132° to 136°.

Solubility: Repaglinide USP—Soluble in methanol.

USP requirements:
Repaglinide USP—Preserve in tight containers. Contains not less than 98.0% and not more than 101.0% of repaglinide, calculated on the dried basis. Meets the requirements for Identification, Specific rotation (between +6.3° to +7.3°, at 20°), Loss on drying (not more than 0.7%), Residue on ignition (not more than 0.1%, an ignition temperature of 600 ± 25°), Heavy metals (0.001%), and Chromatographic purity.
Repaglinide Tablets USP—Preserve in tight containers. Contain the labeled amount, within ±5%. Meet the requirements for Identification, Dissolution (70% in 30 minutes in pH 5.0 buffer in Apparatus 2 at 75 rpm), Uniformity of dosage units, Loss on drying (not more than 6.0%), and Chromatographic purity.

RESERPINE

Chemical source: A crystalline alkaloid derived from *Rauwolfia serpentina.*

Chemical name: Yohimban-16-carboxylic acid, 11,17-dimethoxy18-[(3,4,5-trimethoxybenzoyl)oxy]-, methyl ester, (3 beta,16 beta,17 alpha,18 beta,20 alpha)-.

Molecular formula: $C_{33}H_{40}N_2O_9$.

Molecular weight: 608.69.

Description: Reserpine USP—White or pale buff to slightly yellowish, odorless, crystalline powder. Darkens slowly on exposure to light, but more rapidly when in solution.

pKa: 6.6.

Solubility: Reserpine USP—Insoluble in water; freely soluble in acetic acid and in chloroform; very slightly soluble in alcohol and in ether.

USP requirements:
Reserpine USP—Preserve in tight, light-resistant containers. Contains not less than 97.0% and not more than 101.0% of reserpine, calculated on the dried basis. Meets the requirements for Identification, Loss on drying (not more than 0.5%), and Residue on ignition (not more than 0.1%).
Reserpine Elixir USP—Preserve in tight, light-resistant containers. Contains the labeled amount, within ±10%. Meets the requirements for Identification and Alcohol content (11.0–13.0%).
Reserpine Injection USP—Preserve in single-dose (or, if stabilizers are present, in multiple-dose), light-resistant containers, preferably of Type I glass. A sterile solution of Reserpine in Water for Injection, prepared with the aid of a suitable acid. Contains the labeled amount, within ± 10%. Contains suitable antioxidants. Meets the requirements for Identification, Bacterial endotoxins, pH (3.0–4.0), and Other alkaloids, and for Injections.
Reserpine Oral Solution USP—Preserve in tight, light-resistant containers. Contains the labeled amount, within ± 10%. Meets the requirements for Identification and Alcohol content (11.0–13.0%).
Reserpine Tablets USP—Preserve in tight, light-resistant containers. Contain the labeled amount, within ±10%. Meet the requirements for Identification, Dissolution (75% in 45 minutes in 0.1 *N* acetic acid in Apparatus 1 at 100 rpm), Uniformity of dosage units, and Other alkaloids.

RESERPINE AND CHLOROTHIAZIDE

For *Reserpine* and *Chlorothiazide*—See individual listings for chemistry information.

USP requirements: Reserpine and Chlorothiazide Tablets USP—Preserve in tight, light-resistant containers. Contain the labeled amount of reserpine, within ±10%, and the labeled amount of chlorothiazide, within ±7%. Meet the requirements for Identification, Dissolution (75% of each active ingredient in 60 minutes in mixture of phosphate buffer [pH 8.0] and *n*-propyl alcohol [3:2] in Apparatus 2 at 75 rpm), and Uniformity of dosage units.

RESERPINE AND CHLORTHALIDONE

For *Reserpine* and *Chlorthalidone*—See individual listings for chemistry information.

USP requirements: Reserpine and Chlorthalidone Tablets—Not in *USP–NF*.

RESERPINE, HYDRALAZINE, AND HYDROCHLOROTHIAZIDE

For *Reserpine, Hydralazine*, and *Hydrochlorothiazide*—See individual listings for chemistry information.

USP requirements: Reserpine, Hydralazine Hydrochloride, and Hydrochlorothiazide Tablets USP—Preserve in tight, light-resistant containers. Contain the labeled amount of reserpine, within ±10%, and the labeled amounts of hydralazine hydrochloride and hydrochlorothiazide, within ±7%. Meet the requirements for Identification, Disintegration (30 minutes), Uniformity of dosage units, and Diazotizable substances.

Note: Where Reserpine, Hydralazine Hydrochloride, and Hydrochlorothiazide Tablets are prescribed, without reference to the quantity of reserpine, hydralazine hydrochloride, or hydrochlorothiazide contained therein, a product containing 0.1 mg of reserpine, 25 mg of hydralazine hydrochloride, and 15 mg of hydrochlorothiazide shall be dispensed.

RESERPINE AND HYDROCHLOROTHIAZIDE

For *Reserpine* and *Hydrochlorothiazide*—See individual listings for chemistry information.

USP requirements: Reserpine and Hydrochlorothiazide Tablets USP—Preserve in tight, light-resistant containers. Contain the labeled amount of reserpine, within ±10%, and the labeled amount of hydrochlorothiazide, within ±7%. Meet the requirements for Identification, Dissolution (80% of reserpine in 45 minutes and 80% of hydrochlorothiazide in 60 minutes in mixture of 0.1 N hydrochloric acid and *n*-propyl alcohol [3:2] in Apparatus 2 at 50 rpm), Diazotizable substances, and Uniformity of dosage units.

RESERPINE AND HYDROFLUMETHIAZIDE

For *Reserpine* and *Hydroflumethiazide*—See individual listings for chemistry information.

USP requirements: Reserpine and Hydroflumethiazide Tablets—Not in *USP–NF*.

RESERPINE AND METHYCLOTHIAZIDE

For *Reserpine* and *Methyclothiazide*—See individual listings for chemistry information.

USP requirements: Reserpine and Methyclothiazide Tablets—Not in *USP–NF*.

RESERPINE AND POLYTHIAZIDE

For *Reserpine* and *Polythiazide*—See individual listings for chemistry information.

USP requirements: Reserpine and Polythiazide Tablets—Not in *USP–NF*.

RESERPINE AND TRICHLORMETHIAZIDE

For *Reserpine* and *Trichlormethiazide*—See individual listings for chemistry information.

USP requirements: Reserpine and Trichlormethiazide Tablets—Not in *USP–NF*.

RESORCINOL

Chemical name:
Resorcinol—1,3-Benzenediol.
Resorcinol monoacetate—1,3-Benzenediol, monoacetate.

Molecular formula:
Resorcinol—$C_6H_6O_2$.
Resorcinol monoacetate—$C_8H_8O_3$.

Molecular weight:
Resorcinol—110.11.
Resorcinol monoacetate—152.15.

Description:
Resorcinol USP—White, or practically white, needle-shaped crystals or powder. Has a faint, characteristic odor. Acquires a pink tint on exposure to light and air. Its solution (1 in 20) is neutral or acid to litmus.

Solubility:
Resorcinol USP—Freely soluble in water, in alcohol, in glycerin, and in ether; slightly soluble in chloroform.

USP requirements:
Resorcinol USP—Preserve in well-closed, light-resistant containers. Contains not less than 99.0% and not more than 100.5% of resorcinol, calculated on the dried basis. Meets the requirements for Identification, Melting range (109–111 °C), Loss on drying (not more than 1.0%), Residue on ignition (not more than 0.05%), Phenol, Catechol, Ordinary impurities, and Organic volatile impurities.
Resorcinol Lotion—Not in USP.
Resorcinol Ointment—Not in USP.
Compound Resorcinol Ointment USP—Preserve in tight containers and avoid prolonged exposure to temperatures exceeding 30 °C.

Prepare Compound Resorcinol Ointment as follows: 60 grams of Resorcinol, 60 grams of Zinc Oxide, 60 grams of Bismuth Subnitrate, 20 grams of Juniper Tar, 100 grams of Yellow Wax, 290 grams of Petrolatum, 280 grams of Lanolin, and 130 grams of Glycerin, to make 1000 grams of Compound Resorcinol Ointment. Melt the Yellow Wax and the Lanolin in a dish on a steam bath. Triturate the Zinc Oxide and the Bismuth Subnitrate with the Petrolatum until smooth, and add it to the melted mixture. Dissolve the Resorcinol in the Glycerin, incorporate the solution with the warm mixture just prepared, then add the Juniper Tar, and stir the Ointment until it congeals.

Resorcinol Monoacetate USP—Preserve in tight, light-resistant containers. Meets the requirements for Identification, Specific gravity (1.203–1.207), Acidity, Loss on drying (not more than 2.5%), Residue on ignition (not more than 0.1%), and Organic volatile impurities.

RESORCINOL AND SULFUR

For *Resorcinol* and *Sulfur*—See individual listings for chemistry information.

USP requirements:

Resorcinol and Sulfur Cake—Not in *USP–NF*.
Resorcinol and Sulfur Cream—Not in *USP–NF*.
Resorcinol and Sulfur Gel—Not in *USP–NF*.
Resorcinol and Sulfur Lotion USP—Preserve in tight containers. It is Resorcinol and Sulfur in a suitable hydroalcoholic vehicle. Contains the labeled amount of resorcinol, within ±10%, and the labeled amount of sulfur, within −5% to +10%. Meets the requirements for Identification and Alcohol content (within ±10% of labeled amount).
Resorcinol and Sulfur Stick—Not in *USP–NF*.

RESPIRATORY SYNCYTIAL VIRUS IMMUNE GLOBULIN INTRAVENOUS (HUMAN)

Source: A sterile solution of immune globulin G (IgG) purified from pooled adult human plasma selected for high titers of neutralizing antibody against respiratory syncytial virus (RSV). The product is purified using Cohn-Oncley cold ethanol fractionation and a solvent detergent partitioning method to inactivate blood-borne pathogens.

USP requirements: Respiratory Syncytial Virus Immune Globulin Intravenous (Human) Injection—Not in *USP–NF*.

RETEPLASE

Source: Reteplase is a nonglycosylated deletion mutein of tissue plasminogen activator produced by recombinant DNA technology in *Escherichia coli*, and purified by chromatographic separation.

Chemical name: 173-L-Serine-174-L-tyrosine-175-L-glutamine-173-527-plasminogen activator (human tissue-type).

Molecular formula: $C_{1736}H_{2653}N_{499}O_{522}S_{22}$.

Molecular weight: 39,571.14.

USP requirements:
Reteplase for Injection—Not in *USP–NF*
Reteplase Recombinant for Injection—Not in *USP–NF*.

RIBAVIRIN

Chemical group: A synthetic nucleoside; structurally related to inosine, guanosine, and xanthosine.

Chemical name: 1*H*-1,2,4-Triazole-3-carboxamide, 1-beta-D-ribofuranosyl-.

Molecular formula: $C_8H_{12}N_4O_5$.

Molecular weight: 244.21.

Description: Ribavirin USP—White, crystalline powder.

Solubility: Ribavirin USP—Freely soluble in water; slightly soluble in dehydrated alcohol.

USP requirements:
Ribavirin USP—Preserve in tight containers. Contains not less than 98.9% and not more than 101.5% of ribavirin, calculated on the dried basis. Meets the requirements for Identification, Specific rotation (−33.5° to −37.0°), pH (4.0–6.5, in a solution [1 in 50]), Loss on drying (not more than 0.5%), Residue on ignition (not more than 0.25%), Heavy metals (not more than 0.001%), and Chromatographic purity.
Ribavirin for Injection—Not in *USP–NF*.
Ribavirin for Inhalation Solution USP—Preserve in tight containers, in a dry place at controlled room temperature. A sterile, freeze-dried form of ribavirin. The labeling indicates that Ribavirin for Inhalation Solution must be constituted with a measured volume of Sterile Water for Injection or with Sterile Water for Inhalation containing no preservatives, and that the constituted solution is to be administered only by a small-particle aerosol generator. When constituted as directed in the labeling, the inhalation solution so obtained contains the labeled amount, within ±5%. Meets the requirements for Identification, Sterility, pH (4.0–6.5, in the solution constituted as directed in the labeling), and Chromatographic purity, and for Specific rotation, Loss on drying, Residue on ignition, and Heavy metals under Ribavirin.
Ribavirin for Oral Solution—Not in *USP–NF*.

RIBAVIRIN AND INTERFERON ALFA

For *Ribavirin* and *Interferon alfa*—See individual listings for chemistry information.

USP requirements:
Ribavirin and Interferon Alfa-2b Capsules—Not in *USP–NF*.
Ribavirin and Interferon Alfa-2b Injection—Not in *USP–NF*.

RIBAVIRIN AND PEGINTERFERON ALFA-2B

For *Ribavirin* and *Peginterferon alfa-2b*—See individual listings for chemistry information.

USP requirements: Ribavirin Capsules and Peginterferon alfa-2b Powder for Solution—Not in *USP–NF*.

RIBOFLAVIN

Chemical name:
Riboflavin—Riboflavine.
Riboflavin 5′-phosphate sodium—Riboflavin 5′-(dihydrogen phosphate), monosodium salt, dihydrate.

Molecular formula:
Riboflavin—$C_{17}H_{20}N_4O_6$.
Riboflavin 5′-phosphate sodium—$C_{17}H_{20}N_4NaO_9P \cdot 2H_2O$.

Molecular weight:
Riboflavin—376.37.
Riboflavin 5′-phosphate sodium—514.36.

Description:
Riboflavin USP—Yellow to orange-yellow, crystalline powder having a slight odor. Melts at about 280 °C. Its saturated solution is neutral to litmus. When dry, it is not appreciably affected by diffused light, but when in solution, light induces quite rapid deterioration, especially in the presence of alkalies.
Riboflavin 5′-Phosphate Sodium USP—Fine, orange-yellow, crystalline powder, having a slight odor. When dry, it is not affected by diffused light, but when in solution, light induces deterioration rapidly. Is hygroscopic.

pKa: 10.2.

Solubility:
Riboflavin USP—Very slightly soluble in water, in alcohol, and in isotonic sodium chloride solution; soluble in dilute solutions of alkalies; insoluble in ether and in chloroform.
Riboflavin 5′-Phosphate Sodium USP—Sparingly soluble in water.

USP requirements:
Riboflavin USP—Preserve in tight, light-resistant containers. Contains not less than 98.0% and not more than 102.0% of riboflavin, calculated on the dried basis. Meets the requirements for Identification, Specific rotation (+56.5° to +59.5°), Loss on drying (not more than 1.5%), Residue on ignition (not more than 0.3%), Limit of lumiflavin, and Organic volatile impurities.
Riboflavin Injection USP—Preserve in light-resistant, in single-dose or in multiple-dose containers, preferably of Type I glass. A sterile solution of Riboflavin in Water for Injection. Contains the labeled amount, within −5% to +20%. Meets the requirements for Identification, Bacterial endotoxins, and pH (4.5–7.0), and for Injections.
Riboflavin Tablets USP—Preserve in tight, light-resistant containers. Contain the labeled amount, within −5% to +15%. Meet the requirements for Dissolution (75% in 45 minutes in water in Apparatus 2 at 50 rpm) and Uniformity of dosage units.
Riboflavin 5′-Phosphate Sodium USP—Preserve in tight, light-resistant containers. Contains not less than the equivalent of 73.0% and not more than the equivalent of 79.0% of riboflavin, calculated on the dried basis. Meets the requirements for Identification, Specific rotation (+37.0° to +42.0°), pH (5.0–6.5, in a solution [1 in 100]), Loss on drying (not more than 7.5%), Residue on ignition (not more than 25.0%), Free phosphate, Free riboflavin and riboflavin diphosphates (not more than 6.0% of free riboflavin and not more than 6.0% of riboflavin diphosphates, as riboflavin, calculated on the dried basis), Limit of lumiflavin, and Organic volatile impurities.

RICE SYRUP SOLIDS AND ELECTROLYTES

Chemical name:
Sodium chloride—Sodium chloride.
Potassium citrate—1,2,3-Propanetricarboxylic acid, 2-hydroxy-, tripotassium salt, monohydrate.
Sodium citrate—1,2,3-Propanetricarboxylic acid, 2-hydroxy-, trisodium salt.
Citric acid—1,2,3-Propanetricarboxylic acid, 2-hydroxy-.

Molecular formula:
Sodium chloride—NaCl.
Potassium citrate—$C_6H_5K_3O_7 \cdot H_2O$.

Sodium citrate—$C_6H_5Na_3O_7$.
Citric acid—$C_6H_8O_7$ (anhydrous); $C_6H_8O_7 \cdot H_2O$ (monohydrate).

Molecular weight:
Sodium chloride—58.44.
Potassium citrate—324.41.
Sodium citrate—258.07 (anhydrous).
Citric acid—192.13 (anhydrous); 210.14 (monohydrate).

Description:
Sodium Chloride USP—Colorless, cubic crystals or white crystalline powder.
NF category: Tonicity agent.
Potassium Citrate USP—Transparent crystals or white, granular powder. Is odorless and is deliquescent when exposed to moist air.
NF category: Buffering agent.
Sodium Citrate USP—Colorless crystals or white, crystalline powder.
NF category: Buffering agent.
Citric Acid USP—Colorless, translucent crystals, or white, granular to fine crystalline powder. Odorless or practically odorless. The hydrous form is efflorescent in dry air.
NF category: Acidifying agent; buffering agent.

Solubility:
Sodium Chloride USP—Freely soluble in water; and slightly more soluble in boiling water; soluble in glycerin; slightly soluble in alcohol.
Potassium Citrate USP—Freely soluble in water; almost insoluble in alcohol.
Sodium Citrate USP—Hydrous form freely soluble in water and very soluble in boiling water. Insoluble in alcohol.
Citric Acid USP—Very soluble in water; freely soluble in alcohol; very slightly soluble in ether.

USP requirements: Rice Syrup Solids and Electrolytes Solution—Not in *USP–NF*.

RIFABUTIN

Chemical name: (9*S*,12*E*,14*S*,15*R*,16*S*,17*R*,18*R*,19*R*,20*S*,-21*S*,2*E*,24*Z*)-6,16,18,20-tetrahydroxy-1′-isobutyl-14-methoxy-7,9,15,17,19,21,25-heptamethylspiro[9,4-(epoxypentadeca[1,11,13]trienimino)-2*H*-furo[2′,3′:7,8]naphth[1,2-*d*]imidazole-2,4′-piperidine]-5,10,26-(3*H*,9*H*)-trione-16-acetate.

Molecular formula: $C_{46}H_{62}N_4O_{11}$.

Molecular weight: 847.00.

Description: Rifabutin USP—Amorphous red-violet powder.

Solubility: Rifabutin USP—Soluble in chloroform and in methanol; sparingly soluble in alcohol; very slightly soluble in water.

USP requirements:
Rifabutin USP—Preserve in well-closed containers, protected from light and from excessive heat. Contains not less than 950 mcg and not more than 1020 mcg of rifabutin per mg, calculated on the anhydrous basis. Meets the requirements for Identification, Water (not more than 2.5%), Limit of *N*-isobutylpiperidone (not more than 0.5%), and Chromatographic purity.
Rifabutin Capsules USP—Preserve in well-closed containers, protected from light and from excessive heat. Contain the labeled amount, within ±10%. Meet the requirements for Identification, Dissolution (75% in 45 minutes in 0.01 *N* hydrochloric acid in Apparatus 1 at 100 rpm), and Chromatographic purity.

RIFAMPIN

Source: Semisynthetic derivative of rifamycin B.

Chemical name: Rifamycin, 3-[[(4-methyl-1-piperazinyl)imino]-methyl]-.

Molecular formula: $C_{43}H_{58}N_4O_{12}$.

Molecular weight: 822.94.

Description: Rifampin USP—Red-brown, crystalline powder.

Solubility: Rifampin USP—Very slightly soluble in water; freely soluble in chloroform; soluble in ethyl acetate and in methanol.

USP requirements:
Rifampin USP—Preserve in tight, light-resistant containers, protected from excessive heat. Contains not less than 95.0% and not more than 103.0% of rifampin, calculated on the dried basis. Meets the requirements for Identification, Crystallinity, pH (4.5–6.5, in a suspension [1 in 100]), Loss on drying (not more than 2.0%), and Related substances.
Rifampin Capsules USP—Preserve in tight, light-resistant containers, protected from excessive heat. Contain the labeled amount, within ±10%. Meet the requirements for Identification, Dissolution (75% in 45 minutes in 0.1 N hydrochloric acid in Apparatus 1 at 100 rpm), Uniformity of dosage units, and Loss on drying (not more than 3.0%).
Rifampin for Injection USP—Preserve in Containers for Sterile Solids. Contains the labeled amount, within −10% to +15%. Meets the requirements for Identification, Bacterial endotoxins, Sterility, pH (7.8–8.8, in a solution containing 60 mg of rifampin per mL), Water (not more than 1.0%), and Particulate matter.
Rifampin Oral Suspension USP—Preserve in a tight, light-resistant glass or plastic prescription bottle, with a child-resistant closure. Store at controlled room temperature. Label it to state that the Suspension is to be well shaken. Label it to state that it contains 50 mg of rifampin in 5 mL of Oral Suspension. Contains the labeled amount, within ± 10%. Use Rifampin or the number of Rifampin Capsules that contain the designated amount of Rifampin, and prepare Rifampin Oral Suspension as follows: 1.20 gram of Rifampin Syrup, a sufficient quantity to make 120 mL. Transfer 1.20 gram of Rifampin, or the contents of Rifampin Capsules, into a mortar. [Note—If necessary, gently crush the Capsule contents with a pestle to produce a fine powder.] Add about 2 mL of Syrup to the mortar, and triturate until a smooth paste is formed. Add about 10 mL of Syrup, and triturate to form a suspension. Continue to add Syrup, until about 80 mL has been added. Transfer this suspension to a 120-mL precalibrated light-resistant glass or plastic prescription bottle. Rinse the mortar and pestle with successive small portions of Syrup, and add the rinses to the bottle. Shake vigorously. If necessary, add Citric Acid or Sodium Citrate to adjust to a pH of 5.0. Add a suitable flavor if desired. Add sufficient Syrup to make the product measure 120 mL, and shake vigorously to produce the Oral Suspension. Meets the requirements for pH (4.5–5.5) and Beyond-use date.

RIFAMPIN AND ISONIAZID

For *Rifampin* and *Isoniazid*—See individual listings for chemistry information.

USP requirements: Rifampin and Isoniazid Capsules USP—Preserve in tight, light-resistant containers, and avoid exposure to excessive heat. Contain the labeled amount of rifampin, within −10% to +30%, and the labeled amount of isoniazid, within ±10%. Meet the requirements for Identification, Loss on drying (not more than 3.0%) and Dissolution (75% of rifampin and 80% of isoniazid in 45 minutes in 0.1 N hydrochloric acid in Apparatus 1 at 100 rpm).

Note: Where Rifampin and Isoniazid Capsules are prescribed without reference to the quantity of rifampin or isoniazid contained therein, a product containing 300 mg of rifampin and 150 mg of isoniazid shall be dispensed.

RIFAMPIN, ISONIAZID, AND PYRAZINAMIDE

For *Rifampin, Isoniazid,* and *Pyrazinamide*—See individual listings for chemistry information.

USP requirements: Rifampin, Isoniazid, and Pyrazinamide Tablets USP—Preserve in tight, light-resistant containers at controlled room temperature. Contain the labeled amount of each ingrediant, within ±10%. Meet the requirements for Identification, Dissolution (80% of the labeled amount of isoniazid and 75% of the labeled amount of pyrazinamide in 30 minutes in simulated gastric fluid TS, without pepsin, in Apparatus 1 at 100 rpm), Uniformity of dosage units, and Loss on drying (not more than 3.0%).

RIFAMPIN, ISONIAZID, PYRAZINAMIDE, AND ETHAMBUTOL

For *Rifampin, Isoniazid, Pyrazinamide,* and *Ethambutol*—See individual listings for chemistry information.

USP requirements: Rifampin, Isoniazid, Pyrazinamide, and Ethambutal Hydrochloride Tablets USP—Preserve in tight, light-resistant containers, and store at controlled room temperature. Contain the labeled amount of each active ingredient, within ±10%. Meet the requirements for Identification, Dissolution (75% of each active ingredient in 10 mM sodium phosphate buffer [pH 6.8] in 45 minutes in Apparatus 2 at 100 rpm), and Loss on drying (not more 3.0%).

RIFAPENTINE

Chemical name: Rifamycin, 3-[[(4-cyclopentyl-1-piperazinyl)imino]methyl]-.

Molecular formula: $C_{47}H_{64}N_4O_{12}$.

Molecular weight: 877.03.

USP requirements: Rifapentine Tablets—Not in *USP–NF*.

RILUZOLE

Chemical group: Benzothiazole.

Chemical name: 2-Benzothiazolamine, 6-(trifluoromethoxy)-.

Molecular formula: $C_8H_5F_3N_2OS$.

Molecular weight: 234.20.

Description: White to slightly yellow powder.

Solubility: Very soluble in dimethylformamide, in dimethylsulfoxide, and in methanol; freely soluble in dichloromethane; sparingly soluble in 0.1 *N* hydrochloric acid; very slightly soluble in water and in 0.1 *N* sodium hydroxide.

USP requirements: Riluzole Tablets—Not in *USP–NF*.

RIMANTADINE

Chemical name: Rimantadine hydrochloride—Tricyclo[3.3.1.1^{3,7}]-decane-1-methanamine, alpha-methyl-, hydrochloride.

Molecular formula: Rimantadine hydrochloride—$C_{12}H_{21}N \cdot HCl$.

Molecular weight: Rimantadine hydrochloride—215.76.

Description: Rimantadine hydrochloride—White to off-white crystalline powder.

Solubility: Rimantadine hydrochloride—Freely soluble in water (50 mg/mL at 20 °C).

USP requirements:
Rimantadine Hydrochloride Syrup—Not in *USP–NF*.
Rimantadine Hydrochloride Tablets—Not in *USP–NF*.

RIMEXOLONE

Chemical name: Androsta-1,4-dien-3-one, 11-hydroxy-16,17-dimethyl-17-(1-oxopropyl)-, (11 beta,16 alpha,17 beta)-.

Molecular formula: $C_{24}H_{34}O_3$.

Molecular weight: 370.52.

USP requirements:
Rimexolone USP—Preserve in well-closed containers. Contains not less than 97.0% and not more than 102.0% of rimexolone, calculated on the dried basis. Meets the requirements for Identification, Specific rotation (+47° to +54°), Loss on drying (not more than 1.0%), Residue in ignition (not more than 0.1%), Heavy metals (0.002%), Chromatographic purity (not more than 1.0% of any individual impurity and the sum of all impurities not more than 2.0%), and Organic volatile impurities.
Rimexolone Ophthalmic Suspension USP—Preserve in well-closed containers. A sterile suspension of Rimexolone in a suitable aqueous medium. Contains labeled amount, within ±10%. May contain suitable stabilizers, buffers, and antimicrobial agents. Meets the requirements for Identification, Viscosity (50–350 centipoises), Sterility, and pH (6.0–8.0).

RINGER'S

For *Sodium Chloride, Potassium Chloride,* and *Calcium Chloride*—See individual listings for chemistry information.

USP requirements:
Ringer's Injection USP—Preserve in single-dose glass or plastic containers. Glass containers are preferably of Type I or Type II glass. A sterile solution of Sodium Chloride, Potassium Chloride, and Calcium Chloride in Water for Injection. Contains no antimicrobial agents. The label states the total osmolar concentration in mOsmol per liter. Where the contents are less than 100 mL, the label alternatively may state the total osmolar concentration in mOsmol per mL. Contains, in each 100 mL, not less than 323.0 mg and not more than 354.0 mg of sodium (equivalent to not less

than 820.0 mg and not more than 900.0 mg of sodium chloride); not less than 14.9 mg and not more than 16.5 mg of potassium (equivalent to not less than 28.5 mg and not more than 31.5 mg of potassium chloride); not less than 8.20 mg and not more than 9.80 mg of calcium (equivalent to not less than 30.0 mg and not more than 36.0 mg of calcium chloride dihydrate); and not less than 523.0 mg and not more than 580.0 mg of chloride (as sodium chloride, potassium chloride, and calcium chloride dihydrate).
Prepare Ringer's Injection as follows: Combine 8.6 grams of Sodium Chloride, 0.3 grams of Potassium Chloride, 0.33 grams of Calcium Chloride, and a sufficient quantity of Water for Injection, to make 1000 mL. Dissolve the three salts in the Water for Injection, filter until clear, place in suitable containers, and sterilize.
Meets the requirements for Identification, Bacterial endotoxins, pH (5.0–7.5), and Heavy metals (not more than 0.3 ppm), and for Injections.
Note: The calcium, chloride, potassium, and sodium ion contents of Ringer's Injection are approximately 4.5, 156, 4, and 147.5 milliequivalents per liter, respectively.
Ringer's Irrigation USP—Preserve in single-dose glass or plastic containers. Glass containers are preferably of Type I or Type II glass. The container may be designed to empty rapidly and may contain a volume of more than 1 liter. It is Ringer's Injection that has been suitably packaged, and contains no antimicrobial agents. The designation "not for injection" appears prominently on the label. Meets the requirements for Bacterial endotoxins and Sterility, and for Identification tests, pH, and Heavy metals under Ringer's Injection.

RINGER'S AND DEXTROSE

For *Sodium Chloride, Potassium Chloride, Calcium Chloride,* and *Dextrose*—See individual listings for chemistry information.

USP requirements: Ringer's and Dextrose Injection USP—Preserve in single-dose glass or plastic containers. Glass containers are preferably of Type I or Type II glass. A sterile solution of Sodium Chloride, Potassium Chloride, Calcium Chloride, and Dextrose in Water for Injection. Contains no antimicrobial agents. The label states the total osmolar concentration in mOsmol per liter. Where the contents are less than 100 mL, the label alternatively may state the total osmolar concentration in mOsmol per mL. The label includes also the warning: "Not for use in the treatment of lactic acidosis." Contains, in each 100 mL, not less than 323.0 mg and not more than 354.0 mg of sodium (equivalent to not less than 820.0 mg and not more than 900.0 mg of sodium chloride), not less than 14.9 mg and not more than 16.5 mg of potassium (equivalent to not less than 28.5 mg and not more than 31.5 mg of potassium chloride), not less than 8.20 mg and not more than 9.80 mg of calcium (equivalent to not less than 30.0 mg and not more than 36.0 mg of calcium chloride dihydrate), and not less than 523.0 mg and not more than 608.5 mg of chloride (as sodium choride, potassium chloride, and calcium chloride dihydrate). Contains the labeled amount of dextrose, within ±5%. Meets the requirements for Identification, Bacterial endotoxins, pH (3.5–6.5), Heavy metals, and Limit of 5-hydroxymethylfurfural and related substances, and for Injections.
Note: The calcium, chloride, potassium, and sodium ion contents of Ringer's and Dextrose Injection are approximately 4.5, 156, 4, and 147.5 milliequivalents per liter, respectively.

LACTATED RINGER'S

For *Calcium Chloride, Potassium Chloride, Sodium Chloride,* and *Sodium Lactate*—See individual listings for chemistry information.

USP requirements: Lactated Ringer's Injection USP—Preserve in single-dose glass or plastic containers. Glass containers are preferably of Type I or Type II glass. A sterile solution of Calcium Chloride, Potassium Chloride, Sodium Chloride, and Sodium Lactate in Water for Injection. Contains no antimicrobial agents. The label states the total osmolar concentration in mOsmol per liter. Where the contents are less than 100 mL, the label alternatively may state the total osmolar concentration in mOsmol per mL. The label includes also the warning: "Not for use in the treatment of lactic acidosis." Contains, in each 100 mL, not less than 285.0 mg and not more than 315.0 mg of sodium (as sodium chloride and sodium lactate), not less than 14.2 mg and not more than 17.3 mg of potassium (equivalent to not less than 27.0 mg and not more than 33.0 mg of potassium chloride), not less than 4.90 mg and not more than 6.00 mg of calcium (equivalent to not less than 18.0 mg and not more than 22.0 mg of calcium chloride dihydrate), not less than 368.0 mg and not more than 408.0 mg of chloride (as sodium chloride, potassium chloride, and calcium chloride dihydrate), and not less than 231.0 mg and not more than 261.0 mg of lactate (equivalent to not less than 290.0 mg and not more than 330.0 mg of sodium lactate). Meets the requirements for Identification, Bacterial endotoxins, pH (6.0–7.5), and Heavy metals (not more than 0.3 ppm), and for Injections.

Note: The calcium, potassium, and sodium contents of Lactated Ringerās Injection are approximately 2.7, 4, and 130 milliequivalents per liter, respectively.

LACTATED RINGER'S AND DEXTROSE

For *Calcium Chloride, Potassium Chloride, Sodium Chloride, Sodium Lactate,* and *Dextrose*—See individual listings for chemistry information.

USP requirements:

Lactated Ringer's and Dextrose Injection USP—Preserve in single-dose glass or plastic containers. Glass containers are preferably of Type I or Type II glass. A sterile solution of Calcium Chloride, Potassium Chloride, Sodium Chloride, Sodium Lactate, and Dextrose in Water for Injection. Contains no antimicrobial agents. The label states the total osmolar concentration in mOsmol per liter. Where the contents are less than 100 mL, the label alternatively may state the total osmolar concentration in mOsmol per mL. The label includes also the warning: "Not for use in the treatment of lactic acidosis." Contains, in each 100 mL, not less than 285.0 mg and not more than 315.0 mg of sodium (as sodium chloride and sodium lactate), not less than 14.2 mg and not more than 17.3 mg of potassium (equivalent to not less than 27.0 mg and not more than 33.0 mg of potassium chloride), not less than 4.90 mg and not more than 6.00 mg of calcium (equivalent to not less than 18.0 mg and not more than 22.0 mg of calcium chloride dihydrate), not less than 368.0 mg and not more than 428.0 mg of chloride (as sodium chloride, potassium chloride, and calcium chloride dihydrate), and not less than 231.0 mg and not more than 261.0 mg of lactate (equivalent to not less than 290.0 mg and not more than 330.0 mg of sodium lactate). Contains the labeled amount of dextrose, within −10% to +5%. Meets the requirements for Identification, Bacterial endotoxins, pH (4.0–6.5), 5-Hydroxymethylfurfural and related substances, and Heavy metals, and for Injections.

Note: The calcium, potassium, and sodium contents of Lactated Ringer's and Dextrose Injection are approximately 2.7, 4, and 130 milliequivalents per liter, respectively.

Half-strength Lactated Ringer's and Dextrose Injection USP—Preserve in single-dose glass or plastic containers. Glass containers are preferably of Type I or Type II glass. A sterile solution of Calcium Chloride, Potassium Chloride, Sodium Chloride, Sodium Lactate, and Dextrose in Water for Injection. Contains no antimicrobial agents. The label states the total osmolar concentration in mOsmol per liter. Where the contents are less than 100 mL, the label alternatively may state the total osmolar concentration in mOsmol per mL. The label includes also the warning: "Not for use in the treatment of lactic acidosis." Contains, in each 100 mL, not less than 142.5 mg and not more than 157.5 mg of sodium (as sodium chloride and sodium lactate), not less than 7.08 mg and not more than 8.65 mg of potassium (equivalent to not less than 13.5 mg and not more than 16.5 mg of potassium chloride), not less than 2.45 mg and not more than 3.00 mg of calcium (equivalent to not less than 9.0 mg and not more than 11.0 mg of calcium chloride dihydrate), not less than 184.0 mg and not more than 214.0 mg of chloride (as sodium chloride, potassium chloride, and calcium chloride dihydrate), and not less than 115.5 mg and not more than 130.5 mg of lactate (equivalent to not less than 145.0 mg and not more than 165.0 mg of sodium lactate). Contains the labeled amount of dextrose, within −10% to +5%. Meets the requirements for Identification, Bacterial endotoxins, pH (4.0–6.5), Heavy metals, and 5-Hydroxymethylfurfural and related substances, and for Injections.

Note: The calcium, potassium, and sodium contents of Half-strength Lactated Ringer's and Dextrose Injection are approximately 1.4, 2, and 65 milliequivalents per liter, respectively.

Modified Lactated Ringer's and Dextrose Injection USP—Preserve in single-dose glass or plastic containers. Glass containers are preferably of Type I or Type II glass. A sterile solution of Calcium Chloride, Potassium Chloride, Sodium Chloride, Sodium Lactate, and Dextrose in Water for Injection. Contains no antimicrobial agents. The label states the total osmolar concentration in mOsmol per liter. Where the contents are less than 100 mL, the label alternatively may state the total osmolar concentration in mOsmol per mL. The label includes also the warning: "Not for use in the treatment of lactic acidosis." Contains, in each 100 mL, not less than 57.0 mg and not more than 63.0 mg of sodium (as sodium chloride and sodium lactate), not less than 2.82 mg and not more than 3.46 mg of potassium (equivalent to not less than 5.4 mg and not more than 6.6 mg of potassium chloride), not less than 0.98 mg and not more than 1.20 mg of calcium (equivalent to not less than 3.6 mg and not more than 4.4 mg of calcium chloride dihydrate), not less than 73.6 mg and not more than 85.6 mg of chloride (as sodium chloride, potassium chloride, and calcium chloride dihydrate), and not less than 46.2 mg and not more than 52.20 mg of lactate (equivalent to not less than 58.0 mg and not more than 66.0 mg of sodium lactate). Contains the labeled amount of dextrose, within −10% to +5%. Meets the requirements for Identification, Bacterial endotoxins, pH (4.0–6.5), Heavy metals, and Limit of 5-hydroxymethylfurfural and related substances, and for Injections.

Note: The calcium, potassium, and sodium contents of Modified Lactated Ringer's and Dextrose Injection are approximately 0.5, 0.8, and 26 milliequivalents per liter, respectively.

RISEDRONATE

Chemical name: Risedronate sodium—Phosphonic acid, [1-hydroxy-2-(3-pyridinyl)ethylidene]bis-, monosodium salt.

Molecular formula: Risedronate sodium—$C_7H_{10}NNaO_7P_2$.

Molecular weight: Risedronate sodium—305.09 (Anhydrous); 350.13 (Hemi-pentahydrate).

Description: Fine, white to off-white, orderless, crystalline powder.

Solubility: Risedronate sodium—Soluble in water; soluble in aqueous solutions; essentially insoluble in common organic solvents.

USP requirements: Risedronate Sodium Tablets—Not in *USP–NF*.

RISPERIDONE

Chemical group: Benzisoxazole derivative.

Chemical name: 4*H*-Pyrido[1,2-*a*]pyrimidin-4-one, 3-[2-[4-(6-fluoro-1,2-benzisoxazol-3-yl)-1-piperidinyl]ethyl]-6,7,8,9-tetrahydro-2-methyl-.

Molecular formula: $C_{23}H_{27}FN_4O_2$.

Molecular weight: 410.48.

Description: Slightly beige to almost white powder. Melting point 169–173 °C.

Solubility: Practically insoluble in water (pH 8.7); freely soluble in dichloromethane; soluble in methanol and in 0.1 N hydrochloric acid.

USP requirements:
  Risperidone Oral Solution—Not in *USP–NF*.
  Risperidone Tablets—Not in *USP–NF*.

RITODRINE

Chemical name: Ritodrine hydrochloride—Benzenemethanol, 4-hydroxy-alpha-[1-[[2-(4-hydroxyphenyl)ethyl]amino]ethyl]-,hydrochloride, (*R**, *S**)-.

Molecular formula: Ritodrine hydrochloride—$C_{17}H_{21}NO_3 \cdot HCl$.

Molecular weight: Ritodrine hydrochloride—323.82.

Description: Ritodrine Hydrochloride USP—White to nearly white, odorless or practically odorless, crystalline powder. Melts at about 200 °C.

Solubility: Ritodrine Hydrochloride USP—Freely soluble in water and in alcohol; soluble in *n*-propyl alcohol; practically insoluble in ether.

USP requirements:
  Ritodrine Hydrochloride USP—Preserve in tight containers. Contains not less than 97.0% and not more than 103.0% of ritodrine hydrochloride, calculated on the dried basis. Meets the requirements for Identification, pH (4.5–6.0, in a solution [1 in 50]), Loss on drying (not more than 1.0%), Residue on ignition (not more than 0.2%), Heavy metals (not more than 0.002%), Related compounds, and Organic volatile impurities.
  Ritodrine Hydrochloride Extended-release Capsules—Not in USP.
  Ritodrine Hydrochloride Injection USP—Preserve in single-dose containers, preferably of Type I glass. Store at room temperature, preferably below 30 °C. A sterile solution of Ritodrine Hydrochloride in Water for Injection. Contains

the labeled amount, within ±10%. Meets the requirements for Identification, Bacterial endotoxins, and pH (4.8–5.5), and for Injections.
  Ritodrine Hydrochloride Tablets USP—Preserve in tight containers. Store at room temperature, preferably below 30 °C. Contain the labeled amount, within ±10%. Meet the requirements for Identification, Dissolution (80% in 30 minutes in 0.01 N hydrochloric acid in Apparatus 2 at 50 rpm), and Uniformity of dosage units.

RITODRINE AND DEXTROSE

For *Ritodrine* and *Dextrose*—See individual listings for chemistry information.

USP requirements: Ritodrine Hydrochloride in 5% Dextrose Injection—Not in *USP–NF*.

RITONAVIR

Chemical name: 10-Hydroxy-2-methyl-5-(1-methylethyl)-1-[2-(1-methylethyl)-4-thiazolyl]-3,6-dioxo-8,11-bis(phenylmethyl)-2,4,7,12-tetraazatridecan-13-oic acid, 5-thiazolylmethyl ester, [5*S*-(5*R**,8*R**,10*R**,11*R**)].

Molecular formula: $C_{37}H_{48}N_6O_5S_2$.

Molecular weight: 720.95.

Description: White-to-light-tan powder.

Solubility: Freely soluble in methanol and in ethanol; soluble in isopropanol; practically insoluble in water.

USP requirements:
  Ritonavir Capsules—Not in *USP–NF*.
  Ritonavir Oral Solution—Not in *USP–NF*.

RITUXIMAB

Source: Synthetic (genetically engineered) chimeric murine/human monoclonal antibody, an IgG1-kappa immunoglobulin containing murine light- and heavy-chain variable region sequences and human constant region sequences. It is composed of two heavy chains of 451 amino acids and two light chains of 213 amino acids (based on cDNA analysis). The chimeric anti-CD20 antibody is produced by mammalian cell (Chinese hamster ovary) suspension culture in a nutrient medium containing gentamicin (although gentamicin does not appear in the final product). Purification procedure includes affinity and ion exchange chromatography, as well as specific viral inactivation and removal procedures.

Chemical name: Immunoglobulin G 1 (human-mouse monoclonal IDEC-C2B8 gamma 1-chain anti-human antigen CD 20), disulfide with human-mouse monoclonal IDEC-C2B8 kappa-chain, dimer.

Molecular weight: 144,187 daltons.

USP requirements: Rituximab Concentrate for Injection—Not in *USP–NF*.

RIVASTIGMINE

Chemical name:
Rivastigmine—(S)-3-[1-(Dymethylamino)ethyl]phenyl ethyl-methylcarbamate.
Rivastigmine tartrate—(S)-N-Ethyl-N-methyl-3-[1-(dimethyla-mino)ethyl]phenyl.

Molecular formula:
Rivastigmine—$C_{14}H_{22}N_2O_2$.
Rivastigmine tartrate—$C_{14}H_{22}N_2O_2 \cdot C_4H_6O_6$.

Molecular weight:
Rivastigmine—250.34.
Rivastigmine tartrate—400.43.

Description: Rivastigmine tartrate—White to off-white, fine crystalline powder.

Solubility: Rivastigmine tartrate—Very soluble in water; soluble in ethanol and in acetonitrile; slightly soluble in n-octanol; very slightly soluble in ethyl acetate.

Other characteristics: Rivastigmine tartrate—The distribution coefficient at 37 °C in *n*-octanol/phosphate buffer solution pH 7 is 3.0.

USP requirements: Rivastigmine Capsules—Not in *USP–NF*.

RIZATRIPTAN

Chemical name: Rizatriptan benzoate—1*H*-Indole-3-ethanamine, *N,N*-dimethyl-5-(1*H*-1,2,4-triazole-1-ylmethyl)-, mono-benzoate.

Molecular formula: Rizatriptan benzoate—$C_{15}H_{19}N_5 \cdot C_7H_6O_2$.

Molecular weight: Rizatriptan benzoate—391.47.

Description: Rizatriptan benzoate—White to off-white crystalline solid.

Solubility: Rizatriptan benzoate—Soluble in water at about 42 mg per mL (expressed as free base) at 25 °C.

USP requirements:
Rizatriptan Benzoate Tablets—Not in *USP–NF*.
Rizatriptan Benzoate Orally Disintegrating Tablets—Not in *USP–NF*.

ROCURONIUM

Chemical name: Rocuronium bromide—Pyrrolidinium, 1-[(2 beta,3 alpha,5 alpha,16 beta,17 beta)-17-(acetyloxy)-3-hydroxy-2-(4-morpholinyl)androstan-16-yl]-1-(2-propenyl)-, bromide.

Molecular formula: Rocuronium bromide—$C_{32}H_{53}BrN_2O_4$.

Molecular weight: Rocuronium bromide—609.68.

Other characteristics: Rocuronium bromide—Partition coefficient in n-octanol/water at 20 °C: 0.5.

USP requirements: Rocuronium Bromide Injection—Not in *USP–NF*.

ROFECOXIB

Chemical name: 4-[4-(methylsulfonyl)phenyl]-3-phenyl-2(5*H*)-furanone.

Molecular formula: $C_{17}H_{14}O_4S$.

Molecular weight: 314.36.

Description: White to off-white to light yellow powder.

Solubility: Soluble in acetone; slightly soluble in methanol and in isopropyl acetate; very slightly soluble in ethanol; practically insoluble in octanol; insoluble in water.

USP requirements:
Rofecoxib Oral Suspension—Not in *USP–NF*.
Rofecoxib Tablets—Not in *USP–NF*.

ROPINIROLE

Chemical name: Ropinirole hydrochloride—2(*H*)-Indol-2-one, 4-[2-(dipropylamino)ethyl]-1,3-dihydro-, monohydrochloride.

Molecular formula: Ropinirole hydrochloride—$C_{16}H_{24}N_2O \cdot HCl$.

Molecular weight: Ropinirole hydrochloride—296.84.

Description: Ropinirole hydrochloride—White to pale greenish-yellow powder.

Solubility: Ropinirole hydrochloride—133 mg/mL in water.

USP requirements: Ropinirole Hydrochloride Tablets—Not in *USP–NF*.

ROPIVACAINE

Chemical group: Ropivacaine hydrochloride—Amino amide.

Chemical name: Ropivacaine hydrochloride—*S*-(–)-1-propyl-2′,6′-pipecoloxylidide hydrochloride monohydrate.

Molecular formula: Ropivacaine hydrochloride—$C_{17}H_{26}N_2O \cdot HCl \cdot H_2O$.

Molecular weight: Ropivacaine hydrochloride—328.89.

Description: Ropivacaine hydrochloride—White crystalline powder.

pKa: 8.07 in 0.1 *M* potassium chloride solution.

Solubility: Ropivacaine hydrochloride—Soluble in water 53.8 mg/mL at 25 °C.

USP requirements: Ropivacaine Hydrochloride Injection—Not in *USP–NF*.

ROSE OIL

Description: Rose Oil NF—Colorless or yellow liquid, having the characteristic odor of rose. At 25 °C it is a viscous liquid. Upon gradual cooling, it changes to a translucent, crystalline mass, easily liquefied by warming.
NF category: Flavors and perfumes.

NF requirements: Rose Oil NF—Preserve in well-filled, tight containers. A volatile oil distilled with steam from the fresh flowers of *Rosa gallica* Linné, *Rosa damascena* Miller, *Rosa alba* Linné, *Rosa centifolia* Linné, and varieties of these species (Fam. Rosaceae). Meets the requirements for Solubility test (1 mL is miscible with 1 mL of chloroform without turbidity. Add 20 mL of 90% alcohol to this mixture: the resulting liquid is neutral or acid to moistened litmus paper and, upon standing at 20 °C, deposits crystals within 5 minutes), Specific grav-

ity (0.848–0.863 at 30 °C compared with water at 15 °C), Angular rotation (–1° to –4°), and Refractive index (1.457–1.463 at 30 °C).

ROSE WATER OINTMENT

Description: Rose Water Ointment USP—NF category: Ointment base.

USP requirements: Rose Water Ointment USP—Preserve in tight, light-resistant containers.

Prepare Rose Water Ointment as follows: 125 grams of Cetyl Esters Wax, 120 grams of White Wax, 560 grams of Almond Oil, 5 grams of Sodium Borate, 25 mL of Stronger Rose Water, 165 mL of Purified Water, and 200 microliters of Rose Oil, to make about 1000 grams of Rose Water Ointment. Reduce the cetyl esters wax and the white wax to small pieces, melt them on a steam bath, add the almond oil, and continue heating until the temperature of the mixture reaches 70 °C. Dissolve the sodium borate in the purified water and the stronger rose water, warmed to 70 °C, and gradually add the warm aqueous phase to the melted oil phase, stirring rapidly and continuously until it has cooled to about 45 °C. Then incorporate the rose oil.

Note: Rose Water Ointment is free from rancidity. If the Ointment has been chilled, warm it slightly before attempting to incorporate other ingredients.

ROSIGLITAZONE

Chemical name: Rosiglitazone maleate—(±)-5-[[4-[2-(methyl-2-pyridinylamino)ethoxy]phenyl]methyl]-2,4-thiazolidinedione, (Z)-2-butenedioate (1:1).

Molecular formula: Rosiglitazone maleate—$C_{18}H_{19}N_3O_3S \cdot C_4H_4O_4$.

Molecular weight: Rosiglitazone maleate—473.52 (357.44 free base).

Description: Rosiglitazone maleate—White to off-white solid. Melting point 122–123 °C.

pKa: Rosiglitazone maleate—6.8; 6.1.

Solubility: Rosiglitazone maleate—Readily soluble in ethanol and in a buffered aqueous solution with pH 2.3. Solubility decreases with increasing pH in the physiological range.

USP requirements: Rosiglitazone Maleate Tablets—Not in *USP–NF*.

ROTAVIRUS VACCINE LIVE ORAL

Source: Rotavirus vaccine live oral is a rhesus-based tetravalent rotavirus vaccine. The vaccine virus strains are grown in FRhL-2 cells.

USP requirements: Rotavirus Vaccine Live Oral (Oral Solution)—Not in *USP–NF*.

ROXADIMATE

Chemical name: Benzoic acid, 4-[bis(2-hydroxypropyl)amino]-, ethyl ester.

Molecular formula: $C_{15}H_{23}NO_4$.

Molecular weight: 281.35.

ROXARSONE

Chemical name: Arsonic acid, (4-hydroxy-3-nitrophenyl)-.

Molecular formula: $C_6H_6AsNO_6$.

Molecular weight: 263.04.

Description: Roxarsone USP—Pale yellow crystalline powder.

Solubility: Roxarsone USP—Slightly soluble in cold water; soluble in boiling water; freely soluble in acetic acid, in acetone, in alkalies, in methanol, and in dehydrated alcohol; sparingly soluble in dilute mineral acids; insoluble in ether and in ethyl acetate. Puffs up and deflagrates on heating.

USP requirements: Roxarsone USP—Preserve in well-closed containers. Label it to indicate that it is for veterinary use only. Contains not less than 98.0% and not more than 101.0% of roxarsone, calculated on the dried basis. Meets the requirements for Identification, Loss on drying (not more than 1.0%), Residue on ignition (not more than 0.5%), Limit of trivalent arsenic (not more than 0.05%), and Content of total arsenic (28.0–28.8%, calculated on the dried basis).

STRONGER ROSE WATER

Description: Stronger Rose Water NF—Practically colorless and clear, having the pleasant odor of fresh rose blossoms. It is free from empyreuma, mustiness, and fungal growths.

NF category: Flavors and perfumes.

NF requirements: Stronger Rose Water NF—The odor of Stronger Rose Water is best preserved by allowing a limited access of fresh air to the container. A saturated solution of the odoriferous principles of the flowers of *Rosa centifolia* Linné (Fam. Rosaceae) prepared by distilling the fresh flowers with water and separating the excess volatile oil from the clear, water portion of the distillate. Meets the requirements for Reaction (neutral or acid to litmus), Residue on evaporation (not more than 0.015%), Heavy metals (not more than 2 ppm), and Organic volatile impurities.

Note: Stronger Rose Water, diluted with an equal volume of purified water, may be supplied when "Rose Water" is required.

RUBELLA AND MUMPS VIRUS VACCINE LIVE

Description: Rubella and Mumps Virus Vaccine Live USP—Solid having the characteristic appearance of substances dried from the frozen state. The Vaccine is to be constituted with a suitable diluent just prior to use. Constituted vaccine undergoes loss of potency on exposure to sunlight.

USP requirements: Rubella and Mumps Virus Vaccine Live USP—Preserve in single-dose containers, or in light-resistant, multiple-dose containers, at a temperature between 2 and 8 °C. Multiple-dose containers for 50 doses are adapted for use only in jet injectors, and those for 10 doses for use by jet or syringe injection. A bacterially sterile preparation of a combination of live rubella virus and live mumps virus such that each component is prepared in conformity with and meets the requirements for Rubella Virus Vaccine Live, and for Mumps Virus Vaccine Live, whichever is applicable. Label

the Vaccine in multiple-dose containers to indicate that the contents are intended solely for use by jet injector or for use by either jet or syringe injection, whichever is applicable. Label the Vaccine in single-dose containers, if such containers are not light-resistant, to state that it should be protected from sunlight. Label it also to state that constituted Vaccine should be discarded if not used within 8 hours. Meets the requirement for Expiration date (1 to 2 years, depending on the manufacturera's data, after date of issue from manufacturer's cold storage [−20 °C, 1 year]). Conforms to the regulations of the U.S. Food and Drug Administration concerning biologics.

RUBELLA VIRUS VACCINE LIVE

Source:
The vaccine currently available in the U.S. contains a sterile, lyophilized preparation of live, attenuated Wistar Institute RA 27/3 strain of rubella virus. The virus is propagated in human diploid (WI-38) cell culture.

The vaccines currently available in Canada also contain the RA 27/3 strain of rubella virus.

Description: Rubella Virus Vaccine Live USP—Solid having the characteristic appearance of substances dried from the frozen state. Undergoes loss of potency on exposure to sunlight. The vaccine is to be constituted with a suitable diluent just prior to use.

Other characteristics: Slightly acidic, pH 6.2 to 6.6.

USP requirements: Rubella Virus Vaccine Live USP (for Injection)—Preserve in single-dose containers, or in light-resistant, multiple-dose containers, at a temperature between 2 and 8 °C. Multiple-dose containers for 50 doses are adapted for use only in jet injectors, and those for 10 doses for use by jet or syringe injection. A bacterially sterile preparation of live virus derived from a strain of rubella virus that has been tested for neurovirulence in monkeys, and for immunogenicity, that is free from all demonstrable viable microbial agents except unavoidable bacteriophage, and that has been found suitable for human immunization. The strain is grown, for purposes of vaccine production, on primary cell cultures of duck embryo tissue, derived from pathogen-free flocks, or on primary cell cultures of a designated strain of human tissue, provided that the same cell culture system is used as that in which the strain was tested. The strain meets the requirements of the specific safety tests in adult and suckling mice; and the requirements of the tests in monkey kidney, chicken embryo, and human tissue cell cultures and embryonated eggs. In the case of virus grown in duck embryo cell cultures, the strain meets the requirements of the test by inoculation of embryonated duck eggs, and of the tests for absence of *Mycobacterium tuberculosis* and of avian leucosis. In the case of virus grown in rabbit kidney cell cultures, the strain meets the requirements of the tests by inoculation of rabbits and guinea pigs, and of the tests for absence of *Mycobacterium tuberculosis* and of known adventitious agents of rabbits. In the case of virus grown in human tissue cell cultures, the strain meets the requirements of the specific safety tests and tests for absence of *Mycobacterium tuberculosis* or other adventitious agents tests by inoculation of rabbits and guinea pigs and the requirements for karyology and of the tests for absence of adventitious and other infective agents, including hemadsorption viruses and *Mycoplasma,* in human diploid cell cultures. The strain cultures are treated to remove all intact tissue cells. The Vaccine meets the requirements of the specific tissue culture test for live virus titer, in a single immunizing dose, of not less than the equivalent of 1000 TCID$_{50}$ (quantity of virus estimated to infect 50% of inoculated cultures × 1000) when tested in parallel with the U.S. Reference Rubella Virus, Live. Label the Vaccine in multiple-dose containers to indicate that the contents are intended solely for use by jet injector or for use by

either jet or syringe injection, whichever is applicable. Label the Vaccine in single-dose containers, if such containers are not light-resistant, to state that it should be protected from sunlight. Label it also to state that constituted Vaccine should be discarded if not used within 8 hours. Meets the requirement for Expiration date (1 to 2 years, depending on the manufacturer's data, after date of issue from manufacturer's cold storage [−20 °C, 1 year]). Conforms to the regulations of the U.S. Food and Drug Administration concerning biologics.

RUBIDIUM RB 82

Chemical name: Rubidium chloride Rb 82—Rubidium chloride (^{82}RbCl).

Molecular formula: Rubidium chloride Rb 82—Cl^{82}Rb.

USP requirements: Rubidium Chloride Rb 82 Injection USP—Requirements for packaging, storage, and labeling do not apply; Rubidium Chloride Rb 82 Injection is obtained by elution from the generator and is administered by direct infusion. A sterile solution, suitable for intravenous administration. Contains the labeled amount of ^{82}Rb, within ±10%, expressed in megabecquerels (or in millicuries) per mL at the time indicated in the labeling. Obtained by elution from a strontium 82-rubidium 82 generator system. ^{82}Rb, with a half-life of 76 seconds, is a short-lived positron-emitting radionuclide formed by the radioactive decay of the parent nuclide ^{82}Sr. Strontium Sr 82 with a half-life of 25.5 days is produced by the proton irradiation of rubidium or spallation of molybdenum. The chemical form of the Injection is ^{82}RbCl. (Note: Elute with additive-free Sodium Chloride Injection only. Discard the first 50 mL of the eluate each day the generator is eluted.) Meets the requirements for Bacterial endotoxins, Radionuclide identification, pH (4.0–8.0), Radionuclidic purity, and Chemical purity, and for Injections (except that the Injection may be distributed or dispensed prior to completion of the test for Sterility, the latter test being started on the day of final manufacture, and except that it is not subject to the recommendation for Volume in Container under Injections).

SACCHARIN

Chemical name:
Saccharin—1,2-Benzisothiazol-3(2*H*)-one, 1,1-dioxide.
Saccharin calcium—1,2-Benzisothiazol-3(2*H*)-one, 1,1-dioxide, calcium salt, hydrate (2:7).
Saccharin sodium—1,2-Benzisothiazol-3(2*H*)-one, 1,1-dioxide, sodium salt, dihydrate.

Molecular formula:
Saccharin—$C_7H_5NO_3S$.
Saccharin calcium—$C_{14}H_8CaN_2O_6S_2 \cdot 3\frac{1}{2}H_2O$.
Saccharin sodium—$C_7H_4NNaO_3S \cdot 2H_2O$.

Molecular weight:
Saccharin—183.19.
Saccharin calcium—467.49.
Saccharin sodium—241.20.

Description:
Saccharin NF—White crystals or white crystalline powder. Odorless or has a faint, aromatic odor. Its solutions are acid to litmus.

NF category: Sweetening agent.
Saccharin Calcium USP—White crystals or white, crystalline powder. Odorless or has a faint aromatic odor.

NF category: Sweetening agent.

Saccharin Sodium USP—White crystals or white crystalline powder. Odorless or has a faint aromatic odor. When in powdered form it usually contains about the theoretical amount of water of hydration as a result of efflorescence.

NF category: Sweetening agent.

Saccharin Sodium Oral Solution USP—Clear, colorless, odorless liquid.

Solubility:

Saccharin NF—Slightly soluble in water, in chloroform, and in ether; soluble in boiling water; sparingly soluble in alcohol. Readily dissolved by dilute solutions of ammonia, by solutions of alkali hydroxides, and by solutions of alkali carbonates with the evolution of carbon dioxide.

Saccharin Calcium USP—Freely soluble in water.

Saccharin Sodium USP—Freely soluble in water; sparingly soluble in alcohol.

USP requirements:

Saccharin Calcium USP—Preserve in well-closed containers. Where the quantity of saccharin calcium is indicated in the labeling of any preparation containing Saccharin Calcium, this shall be expressed in terms of saccharin. Contains not less than 98.0% and not more than 101.0% of saccharin calcium, calculated on the anhydrous basis. Meets the requirements for Identification, Water (not more than 15.0%), Readily carbonizable substances, Selenium (not more than 0.003%), Toluenesulfonamides, Heavy metals (not more than 0.001%), Limit of benzoate and salicylate, and Organic volatile impurities.

Saccharin Sodium USP—Preserve in well-closed containers. Where the quantity of saccharin sodium is indicated in the labeling of any preparation containing Saccharin Sodium, this shall be expressed in terms of saccharin. Contains not less than 98.0% and not more than 101.0% of saccharin sodium, calculated on the anhydrous basis. Meets the requirements for Identification, Alkalinity, Toluenesulfonamides, Heavy metals (not more than 0.001%), and Organic volatile impurities, and for Identification tests, Water, Benzoate and salicylate, Selenium, and Readily carbonizable substances under Saccharin Calcium.

Saccharin Sodium Oral Solution USP—Preserve in tight containers. Contains an amount of saccharin sodium equivalent to the labeled amount of saccharin, within ±5%. Meets the requirements for Identification and pH (3.0–5.0).

Saccharin Sodium Tablets USP—Preserve in well-closed containers. Contain an amount of saccharin sodium equivalent to the labeled amount of saccharin, within −5% to +10%. Meet the requirements for Completeness of solution, Identification, and Limit of ammonium salts.

NF requirements: Saccharin NF—Preserve in well-closed containers. Contains not less than 98.0% and not more than 101.0% of saccharin, calculated on the dried basis. Meets the requirements for Identification, Melting range (226–230°C), Loss on drying (not more than 1.0%), Readily carbonizable substances, Residue on ignition (not more than 0.2%), Toluenesulfonamides, Selenium (not more than 0.003%, a 100-mg specimen, mixed with 100 mg of magnesium oxide, being used), Heavy metals (not more than 0.001%), Benzoic and salicylic acids, and Organic volatile impurities.

SACROSIDASE

Source: Enzyme derived from bakera's yeast (*Saccharomyces cerevisiae*).

Chemical name: Beta-Fructofuranoside (*Saccharomyces cerevisiae* clone F14 protein moiety reduced).

Molecular weight: Approximately 140,000 daltons.

USP requirements: Sacroside Oral solution—Not in *USP–NF*.

SAFFLOWER OIL

Description: Safflower Oil USP—Light yellow oil. Thickens and becomes rancid on prolonged exposure to air.

NF category: Vehicle (oleaginous).

Solubility: Safflower Oil USP—Insoluble in water. Miscible with ether and with chloroform.

USP requirements: Safflower Oil USP—Preserve in tight, light-resistant containers. The refined fixed oil yielded by the seed of *Carthamus tinctorius* Linné (Fam. Compositae). Meets the requirements for Fatty acid composition, Free fatty acids, Iodine value (135–150), Heavy metals (not more than 0.001%), Unsaponifiable matter (not more than 1.5%), and Peroxide (not more than 10.0).

SALICYLAMIDE

Chemical name: Benzamide, 2-hydroxy-.

Molecular formula: $C_7H_7NO_2$.

Molecular weight: 137.14.

Description: Salicylamide USP—White, practically odorless, crystalline powder.

Solubility: Salicylamide USP—Slightly soluble in water and in chloroform; soluble in alcohol and in propylene glycol; freely soluble in ether and in solutions of alkalies.

USP requirements: Salicylamide USP—Preserve in well-closed containers. Contains not less than 98.0% and not more than 102.0% of salicylamide, calculated on the anhydrous basis. Meets the requirements for Identification, Melting range (139–142 °C), Water (not more than 0.5%), Residue on ignition (not more than 0.1%), Heavy metals (not more than 0.001%), Chromatographic purity, and Organic volatile impurities.

SALICYLIC ACID

Chemical name: Benzoic acid, 2-hydroxy-.

Molecular formula: $C_7H_6O_3$.

Molecular weight: 138.12.

Description: Salicylic Acid USP—White crystals, usually in fine needles, or fluffy, white, crystalline powder. Is stable in air. The synthetic form is white and odorless. When prepared from natural methyl salicylate, it may have a slightly yellow or pink tint, and a faint, mint-like odor.

Solubility: Salicylic Acid USP—Slightly soluble in water; freely soluble in alcohol and in ether; soluble in boiling water; sparingly soluble in chloroform.

USP requirements:

Salicylic Acid USP—Preserve in well-closed containers. Contains not less than 99.5% and not more than 101.0% of salicylic acid, calculated on the dried basis. Meets the requirements for Identification, Melting range (158–161 °C), Loss on drying (not more than 0.5%), Residue on ignition

(not more than 0.05%), Chloride (not more than 0.014%), Sulfate (not more than 0.02%), Heavy metals (not more than 20 mcg per gram), and Related compounds.

Salicylic Acid Collodion USP—Preserve in tight containers, at controlled room temperature, remote from fire. Contains not less than 9.5% and not more than 11.5% of salicylic acid.

Prepare Salicylic Acid Collodion as follows: 100 grams of Salicylic Acid and a sufficient quantity of Flexible Collodion to make 1000 mL. Dissolve the Salicylic Acid in about 750 mL of Flexible Collodion, add sufficient of the latter to make the product measure 1000 mL, and mix.

Salicylic Acid Cream—Not in *USP–NF*.

Salicylic Acid Topical Foam USP—Preserve in tight containers. Contains the labeled amount, within ±10%. Meets the requirements for Identification and pH (5.0–6.0).

Salicylic Acid Gel USP—Preserve in collapsible tubes or in tight containers, preferably at controlled room temperature. It is Salicylic Acid in a suitable viscous hydrophilic vehicle. Contains the labeled amount, within ±10%. Meets the requirements for Identification and Alcohol content (if present, within ±10% of labeled amount).

Salicylic Acid Lotion—Not in *USP–NF*.

Salicylic Acid Ointment—Not in *USP–NF*.

Salicylic Acid Pads—Not in *USP–NF*.

Salicylic Acid Plaster USP—Preserve in well-closed containers, preferably at controlled room temperature. A uniform mixture of Salicylic Acid in a suitable base, spread on paper, cotton cloth, or other suitable backing material. The plaster mass contains the labeled amount, within ±10%.

Salicylic Acid Shampoo—Not in *USP–NF*.

Salicylic Acid Soap—Not in *USP–NF*.

Salicylic Acid Topical Solution—Not in *USP–NF*.

SALICYLIC ACID AND SULFUR

For *Salicylic Acid* and *Sulfur*—See individual listings for chemistry information.

USP requirements:

Salicylic Acid and Sulfur Cream—Not in *USP–NF*.

Salicylic Acid and Sulfur Cleansing Cream—Not in *USP–NF*.

Salicylic Acid and Sulfur Lotion—Not in *USP–NF*.

Salicylic Acid and Sulfur Cleansing Lotion—Not in *USP–NF*.

Salicylic Acid and Sulfur Cream Shampoo—Not in *USP–NF*.

Salicylic Acid and Sulfur Lotion Shampoo—Not in *USP–NF*.

Salicylic Acid and Sulfur Suspension Shampoo—Not in *USP–NF*.

Salicylic Acid and Sulfur Bar Soap—Not in *USP–NF*.

Salicylic Acid and Sulfur Cleansing Suspension—Not in *USP–NF*.

Salicylic Acid and Sulfur Topical Suspension—Not in *USP–NF*.

SALICYLIC ACID, SULFUR, AND COAL TAR

For *Salicylic Acid, Sulfur,* and *Coal Tar*—See individual listings for chemistry information.

USP requirements:

Salicylic Acid, Sulfur, and Coal Tar Cream Shampoo—Not in *USP–NF*.

Salicylic Acid, Sulfur, and Coal Tar Lotion Shampoo—Not in *USP–NF*.

SALMETEROL

Chemical name: Salmeterol xinafoate—1,3-Benzenedimethanol, 4-hydroxy-alpha¹-[[[6-(4-phenylbutoxy)hexyl]amino]-methyl]-, (±)-, 1-hydroxy-2-naphthalenecarboxylate (salt).

Molecular formula: Salmeterol xinafoate—$C_{25}H_{37}NO_4 \cdot C_{11}H_8O_3$.

Molecular weight: Salmeterol xinafoate—603.75.

Description: Salmeterol xinafoate—White to off-white powder.

Solubility: Salmeterol xinafoate—Freely soluble in methanol; slightly soluble in ethanol, in chloroform, and in isopropanol; sparingly soluble in water.

USP requirements:

Salmeterol Xinafoate Inhalation Aerosol—Not in *USP–NF*.

Salmeterol Xinafoate Powder for Inhalation—Not in *USP–NF*.

SALSALATE

Chemical name: Benzoic acid, 2-hydroxy-, 2-carboxyphenyl ester.

Molecular formula: $C_{14}H_{10}O_5$.

Molecular weight: 258.23.

Description: Odorless or almost odorless, white or almost white powder.

Solubility: Very slightly soluble in water; soluble 1 in 6 of alcohol, 1 in 8 of chloroform, and 1 in 12 of ether.

USP requirements:

Salsalate USP—Preserve in tight containers. Contains not less than 98.0% and not more than 102.0% of total salicylates, expressed as the sum of the percentages of salsalate, salicylic acid, and trisalicylic acid, calculated on the dried basis. Meets the requirements for Identification, Loss on drying (not more than 0.5%), Residue on ignition (not more than 0.10%), Chloride (not more than 0.01%), Sulfate (not more than 0.05%), Heavy metals (not more than 10 mcg per gram), Limit of dimethylaniline (not more than 0.05%), Isopropyl, ethyl, and methyl salicylates, Chromatographic purity, Related compounds (not more than 0.5% of salicylic acid and not more than 2.5% of trisalicylic acid), and Organic volatile impurities.

Salsalate Capsules USP—Preserve in tight containers. Contain the labeled amount, within ±10%. Meet the requirements for Identification, Disintegration (30 minutes, simulated gastric fluid TS [without pepsin] being used), Uniformity of dosage units, and Limit of salicylic acid (not more than 1.5%).

Salsalate Tablets USP—Preserve in tight containers. Contain the labeled amount, within ±10%. Meet the requirements for Identification, Dissolution (70% in 60 minutes in 0.25 *M* phosphate buffer [pH 7.4] in Apparatus 2 at 50 rpm for Test 1; 70% in 60 minutes in 0.05 *M* phosphate buffer [pH 7.5] in Apparatus 2 at 100 rpm for Test 2), Uniformity of dosage units, and Limit of salicylic acid (not more than 3.0%).

SAMARIUM SM 153 LEXIDRONAM

Source: Sm 153: Neutron irradiation of isotopically enriched Sm 152 oxide.

Chemical name: Samarium Sm 153 Lexidronam Pentasodium—Samarate-(5-)-¹⁵³*Sm*, [[[1,2-ethanediylbis[nitrilobis(methylene)]]tetrakis[phosphonato]](8-)-[sp*N,N′,O*ᵖ,*O*ᵖ′,*O*ᵖ″,*O*ᵖ‴]-, pentasodium, (*OC*-6-21)-.

Molecular formula: $C_6H_{12}N_2Na_5O_{12}P_4{}^{153}Sm$ (pentasodium form); $^{153}Sm^{+3}[CH_2N(CH_2PO_3^{-2})2]2$ (ionic formula).

Molecular weight: 696.01 (pentasodium form); 581.1 (ionic formula).

Other characteristics: pH of the solution (7.0–8.5).

USP requirements: Samarium Sm 153 Lexidronam Injection USP—Preserve in adequately shielded single-dose containers in a freezer. A sterile aqueous solution suitable for intravenous injection that contains ^{153}Sm in the form of a complex with ethylenediaminetetramethylenephosphonic acid (EDTMP). Not less than 99% of the Sm-153 is complexed by EDTMP. Contains no antimicrobial agents. Label it to include the following, in addition to the information specified for Labeling under Injections: the time and date of calibration; the amount of ^{153}Sm complexed with EDTMP expressed as total megabecquerels (or millicuries) and the concentration as megabecquerels per mL (or millicuries per mL) at the time of calibration; the expiration date and time; and the statement, "Caution—Radioactive Material." The labeling indicates that in making dosage calculations, correction is to be made for radioactive decay, and also indicates that the radioactive half-life of ^{153}Sm is 46.3 hours. The labeling indicates that it should not be diluted or mixed with other solutions, that it is to be thawed at room temperature before administration, and that it is to be used within 8 hours of thawing. Contains the labeled amount of ^{153}Sm, within ±10%, expressed in megabecquerels per mL (or millicuries per mL) at the date and time indicated in the labeling. Meets the requirements for Radionuclide identification, Bacterial endotoxins, pH (7.0–8.5), Radionuclidic purity, and Radiochemical purity (not less than 99% of the Sm-153 is complexed by EDTMP), and for Injections (except that it is not subject to the recommendation on Volume in Container).

SAQUINAVIR

Chemical name:
Saquinavir—[3*S*-[2[1*R**(*R**)],2*S**],3l,4a theta,8a theta]]-*N*'-[3-[3-[[(1,1-Dimethylethyl)amino]carbonyl]octahydro-2(1*H*)-isoquinolinyl]-2-hydroxy-1-(phenylmethyl)propyl]2-[(2-quinolinylcarbonyl)amino]butanediamide.
Saquinavir mesylate—Butanediamide, *N*'-[3-[3-[[(1,1-dimethylethyl)amino]carbonyl]octahydro-2(1*H*)-isoquinolinyl]-2-hydroxy-1-(phenylmethyl)propyl]-2-[(2-quinolinylcarbonyl)amino]-, [3*S*-[2[1*R**(*R**),2*S**],3 alpha,4a beta,8a beta]]-, monomethanesulfonate (salt).

Molecular formula:
Saquinavir—$C_{38}H_{50}N_6O_5$.
Saquinavir mesylate—$C_{38}H_{50}N_6O_5 \cdot CH_4O_3S$.

Molecular weight:
Saquinavir—670.86.
Saquinavir mesylate—766.95.

Description: Saquinavir mesylate—White to off-white, very fine powder.

Solubility: Saquinavir mesylate—Aqueous solubility of 2.22 mg per mL at 25 °C.

USP requirements:
Saquinavir Soft Gelatin Capsules—Not in *USP–NF*.
Saquinavir Shampoo—Not in *USP–NF*.
Saquinavir Capsules USP—Preserve in tight containers, and store at controlled room temperature. Contain not less than 95.0% and not more than 105.0% of saquinavir. Meet the requirements for Identification, Dissolution (75% in 45 minutes in Citrate buffer in Apparatus 2 at 50 rpm), Uniformity of dosage units, Water (not more than 3.0%), and Chromatographic purity.

Saquinavir Mesylate USP—Preserve in tight containers, and store at controlled room temperature. Contains not less than 98.5% and not more than 101.0% of saquinavir mesylate, calculated on the anhydrous basis. Meets the requirements for Identification, Specific rotation (−66.8° to −69.6° [lambda = 436 nanometer at 20°]), Water (not more than 1.0%), Residue on ignition (not more than 0.1%), Heavy metals (not more than 0.002%), and Chromatographic purity.
Saquinavir Mesylate Shampoo—Not in *USP–NF*.

SARAFLOXACIN

Chemical name: Sarafloxacin hydrochloride—3-Quinolinecarboxylic acid, 6-fluoro-1-(4-fluorophenyl)-1,4-dihydro-4-oxo-7-(1-piperazinyl)-, monohydrochloride.

Molecular formula: Sarafoxacin hydrochloride—$C_{20}H_{17}F_2N_3O_3 \cdot HCl$.

Molecular weight: Sarafloxacin hydrochloride—421.82.

USP requirements: Sarafloxacin Hydrochloride Soluble Powder—Not in *USP–NF*.

SARGRAMOSTIM

Source: A single chain, glycosylated polypeptide of 127 amino acid residues expressed from *Saccharomyces cerevisiae*.

Chemical name: Colony-stimulating factor 2 (human clone pHG$_{25}$ protein moiety), 23-L-leucine-.

Molecular formula: $C_{639}H_{1002}N_{168}O_{196}S_8$.

Molecular weight: 15,500–19,500 daltons.

Description: White, crystalline powder.

Solubility: In water, 500 mcg per mL.

USP requirements:
Sargramostim USP—Preserve in sealed containers, at a temperature of -20 °C or below. A highly purified glycosylated protein consisting of 127 amino acids. Has the property to generate granulocyte, macrophage, and mixed granulocyte-macrophage colonies from hematopoietic progenitor cells found in bone marrow. Produced by recombinant DNA synthesis in yeast culture, and possesses the primary sequence of the natural form of granulocyte-macrophage colony-stimulating factor with a substitution in the amino acid residue at position 23 (Leu$_{23}$ in place of Arg$_{23}$). Has a biological potency of not less than 73.0 percent and not more than 146.0 percent of the potency stated on the label, the potency being 5.6 million USP Sargramostim Units per mg of protein. The presence of host cell DNA and host cell protein impurities in Sargramostim is process-specific; the limits of these impurities are determined by validated methods. Meets the requirements for Identification, Peptide mapping, Bacterial endotoxins, Microbial limits, Chromatographic purity, and Protein content.
Sargramostim Injection—Not in *USP–NF*.
Sargramostim for Injection USP—Preserve in hermetic containers at a temperature between 2–8 °C. A sterile, lyophilized preparation of Sargramostim. Label it to state the biological activity in USP Sargramostim Units per vial and the amount of protein per vial. Contains the labeled total protein content, within ±10%. Biological activity is not less than 73.0% and not more than 146.0% of that stated on the label in USP Sargramostim Units. Meets the requirements for Constituted solution, Identification,

Bacterial endotoxins, Safety, Sterility, Uniformity of dosage units, pH (7.1–7.7, in the solution constituted as directed in the labeling), Water (not more than 2.0%), and Chromatographic purity.

SAW PALMETTO

NF requirements:

Saw Palmetto NF—Preserve in tight containers, protected from light. The label states the Latin binomial name and, following the official name, the part of the plant contained in the article. Consists of partially dried, ripe fruit of *Serenoa repens* (Bartram) Small (Fam. Arecaceae) [*Serenoa serrulatum* Schultes; *Sabal serrulata* (Michaux) Nichols]. Meets the requirements for Botanic characteristics, Identification, Foreign organic matter (not more than 2.0%), Loss on drying (not more than 12.0%), Total ash (not more than 5.0%), Acid-insoluble ash (not more than 1.0%), Heavy metals (not more than 0.001%), Volatile oil content, Pesticide residues, Microbial limits, Content of lipophilic extract (not less than 7%), and Content of fatty acids.

Saw Palmetto Extract NF—Obtained from comminuted Saw Palmetto by extraction with hydroalcoholic mixtures or solvent hexane, or by supercritical extraction with carbon dioxide. The ratio of starting crude plant material to Extract is between 8.0:1 and 14:3:1. The label states the Latin binomial and, following the official name, the part of the plant from which the article was prepared. The label also indicates the content of fatty acids and sterols and the ratio of the starting crude plant material to Extract. It meets the requirements for *Labeling* under *Botanical Extracts*. Contains not less than 70.0% and not more than 95.0% of fatty acids and not less than 0.2% and not more than 0.5% of sterols, calculated on the anhydrous basis. The lipophilic Extract contains not less than 0.15% and not more than 0.35% of long-chain alcohols. The hydroalcoholic Extract contains not less than 0.01% and not more than 0.15% of long-chain alcohols. Contains no added substances. Meets the requirements for Identification, Iodine value (40–50), Saponification value (210–250), Unsaponifiable matter (1.8%–3.5%), Water (not more than 3%, in the hydroalcoholic Extract), Heavy metals (40 micrograms per gram), Organic volatile impurities, Content of fatty acids, Content of long chain alcohols and sterols, and Alcohol content (not more than 1%), and for the tests for Packaging and Storage and Pesticide residues under Botanical extracts.

Saw Palmetto Capsules NF—Preserve in tight, light-resistant containers. The label states the Latin binomial and, following the official name, the name of article from which the Capsules were prepared. Label it to indicate the amount of Extract in milligram per Capsule. Contain not less than 22.0% of lauric acid and not more than 34.0% of the labeled amount of Saw Palmetto Extract. The ratio of the concentrations of lauric acid to caprylic acid is not less than 10 and not more than 17.5. The ratio of the concentrations of lauric acid to myristic acid is not less than 2.2 and not more than 2.8. Meet the requirements for Identification, Microbial Limits, Rupture (in 15 minutes in simulated gastric fluid TS in Apparatus 2 at 50 rpm), Weight variation, and Content of lauric acid and the ratios of the concentrations of lauric acid to caprylic acid and lauric acid to myristic acid.

Powdered Saw Palmetto NF—Preserve in tight containers, protected from light. The label states the Latin binomial name and, following the official name, the part of the plant source from which the article was derived. It is Saw Palmetto reduced to a fine or very fine powder. Meets the requirements for Identification test and for Foreign organic matter, Loss on drying, Total ash, Acid-insoluble ash, Pes-

ticide residues, Heavy metals, Volatile oil content, Microbial limits, Content of lipophilic extract, and Content of fatty acids under Saw Palmetto.

SCHICK TEST CONTROL

Description: Schick Test Control USP—Transparent liquid.

USP requirements: Schick Test Control USP—Preserve at a temperature between 2 and 8 °C. It is Diphtheria Toxin for Schick Test that has been inactivated by heat for use as control for the Schick Test. Meets the requirements of the specific guinea pig test for detoxification by injection of not less than 2.0 mL into each of at least four guinea pigs. The animals are observed daily for 30 days and during this period show no evidence of diphtheria toxin poisoning (extensive necrosis, paralysis, or specific lethality). Meets the requirement for Expiration date (not later than 1 year after date of issue from manufacturer's cold storage [5 °C, 1 year]). Conforms to the regulations of the U.S. Food and Drug Administration concerning biologics.

SCOPOLAMINE

Chemical group: Natural tertiary amine.

Chemical name:

Scopolamine butylbromide—(–)-(1S,3s,5R,6R,7S,8r)-6,7-Epoxy-8-butyl-3-[(S)-tropoyloxy]tropanium bromide.

Scopolamine hydrobromide—Benzeneacetic acid, alpha-(hydroxymethyl)-, 9-methyl-3-oxa-9-azatricyclo[3.3.1.0^{2,4}]-non7-yl ester, hydrobromide, trihydrate, [7(S)-(1 alpha,2 beta,4 beta,5 alpha,7 beta)]-.

Molecular formula:

Scopolamine butylbromide—$C_{21}H_{30}BrNO_4$.

Scopolamine hydrobromide—$C_{17}H_{21}NO_4 \cdot HBr \cdot 3H_2O$.

Molecular weight:

Scopolamine butylbromide—440.4.

Scopolamine hydrobromide—438.31.

Description:

Scopolamine butylbromide—White or almost white, odorless or almost odorless, crystalline powder.

Scopolamine Hydrobromide USP—Colorless or white crystals or white, granular powder. Melts at about 197 °C, with decomposition. Is odorless, and slightly efflorescent in dry air.

pKa: 7.55 (23 °C)–7.81 (25 °C).

Solubility:

Scopolamine butylbromide—Soluble 1 in 1 of water, 1 in 50 of alcohol, and 1 in 5 of chloroform.

Scopolamine Hydrobromide USP—Freely soluble in water; soluble in alcohol; slightly soluble in chloroform; insoluble in ether.

USP requirements:

Scopolamine Transdermal System—Not in *USP–NF*.

Scopolamine Butylbromide Injection—Not in *USP–NF*.

Scopolamine Butylbromide Suppositories—Not in *USP–NF*.

Scopolamine Butylbromide Tablets—Not in *USP–NF*.

Scopolamine Hydrobromide USP—Preserve in tight, light-resistant containers. Contains not less than 98.5% and not more than 102.0% of scopolamine hydrobromide, calculated on the anhydrous basis. Meets the requirements for Identification, Specific rotation (–24° to –26°), pH (4.0–5.5, in a solution [1 in 20]), Water (not more than

13.0%), Residue on ignition (negligible, from 100 mg), Limit of apoatropine, Other foreign alkaloids, and Organic volatile impurities.

Caution: Handle Scopolamine Hydrobromide with exceptional care, since it is highly potent.

Scopolamine Hydrobromide Injection USP—Preserve in light-resistant, single-dose or multiple-dose containers, preferably of Type I glass. A sterile solution of Scopolamine Hydrobromide in Water for Injection. Contains the labeled amount, within ±10%. Meets the requirements for Identification, Bacterial endotoxins, and pH (3.5–6.5), and for Injections.

Scopolamine Hydrobromide Ophthalmic Ointment USP—Preserve in collapsible ophthalmic ointment tubes. It is Scopolamine Hydrobromide in a suitable ophthalmic ointment base. It is sterile. Contains the labeled amount, within ±10%. Meets the requirements for Identification, Sterility, and Metal particles.

Scopolamine Hydrobromide Ophthalmic Solution USP—Preserve in tight containers. A sterile, buffered, aqueous solution of Scopolamine Hydrobromide. Contains the labeled amount, within ±10%. Meets the requirements for Identification, Sterility, and pH (4.0–6.0).

Scopolamine Hydrobromide Tablets USP—Preserve in tight, light-resistant containers. Contain the labeled amount, within ±10%. Meet the requirements for Identification, Disintegration (15 minutes, the use of disks being omitted), and Uniformity of dosage units.

SECOBARBITAL

Chemical name:

Secobarbital—2,4,6(1*H*,3*H*,5*H*)-Pyrimidinetrione, 5-(1-methylbutyl)-5-(2-propenyl)-.

Secobarbital sodium—2,4,6(1*H*,3*H*,5*H*)-Pyrimidinetrione, 5(1-methylbutyl)-5-(2-propenyl)-, monosodium salt.

Molecular formula:

Secobarbital—$C_{12}H_{18}N_2O_3$.

Secobarbital sodium—$C_{12}H_{17}N_2NaO_3$.

Molecular weight:

Secobarbital—238.28.

Secobarbital sodium—260.26.

Description:

Secobarbital USP—White, amorphous or crystalline, odorless powder. Its saturated solution has a pH of about 5.6.

Secobarbital Sodium USP—White powder. Is odorless and is hygroscopic. Its solutions decompose on standing, heat accelerating the decomposition.

Solubility:

Secobarbital USP—Very slightly soluble in water; freely soluble in alcohol, in ether, and in solutions of fixed alkali hydroxides and carbonates; soluble in chloroform.

Secobarbital Sodium USP—Very soluble in water; soluble in alcohol; practically insoluble in ether.

USP requirements:

Secobarbital USP—Preserve in tight containers. Contains not less than 97.5% and not more than 100.5% of secobarbital, calculated on the dried basis. Meets the requirements for Identification, Loss on drying (not more than 1.0%), Residue on ignition (not more than 0.1%), Organic volatile impurities, and Isomer content.

Secobarbital Elixir USP—Preserve in tight containers. Contains, in each 100 mL, not less than 417 mg and not more than 461 mg of secobarbital, in a suitable, flavored vehicle. Meets the requirements for Identification and Alcohol content (10.0–14.0%).

Secobarbital Oral Solution USP—Preserve in tight containers. Contains, in each 100 mL, not less than 417 mg and not more than 461 mg of secobarbital, in a suitable, flavored vehicle. Meets the requirements for Identification and Alcohol content (10.0–14.0%).

Secobarbital Sodium USP—Preserve in tight containers. Where it is intended for use in preparing injectable dosage forms, the label states that it is sterile or must be subjected to further processing during the preparation of injectable dosage forms. Contains not less than 98.5% and not more than 100.5% of secobarbital sodium, calculated on the dried basis. Meets the requirements for Completeness of solution, Identification, pH (9.7–10.5, in the solution prepared in the test for Completeness of solution), Loss on drying (not more than 3.0%), Heavy metals (not more than 0.003%), Organic volatile impurities, and Isomer content, for Sterility tests and for Bacterial endotoxins under Secobarbital Sodium for Injection (where the label states that Secobarbital Sodium is sterile), and for Bacterial endotoxins under Secobarbital Sodium for Injection (where the label states that Secobarbital Sodium must be subjected to further processing during the preparation of injectable dosage forms).

Secobarbital Sodium Capsules USP—Preserve in tight containers. Contain the labeled amount, within ±7.5%. Meet the requirements for Identification, Dissolution (75% in 60 minutes in water in Apparatus 1 at 100 rpm), and Uniformity of dosage units.

Secobarbital Sodium Injection USP—Preserve in single-dose or in multiple-dose containers, preferably of Type I glass, protected from light, in a refrigerator. A sterile solution of Secobarbital Sodium in a suitable solvent. The label indicates that the Injection is not to be used if it contains a precipitate. Contains the labeled amount, within ±10%. Meets the requirements for Identification, Bacterial endotoxins, and pH (9.0–10.5), and for Injections.

Secobarbital Sodium for Injection USP—Preserve in Containers for Sterile Solids. It is Secobarbital Sodium suitable for parenteral use. Contains the labeled amount, within ±10%. Meets the requirements for Constituted solution and Bacterial endotoxins, for Identification tests, pH, Completeness of solution, Loss on drying, and Heavy metals under Secobarbital Sodium, and for Sterility tests, Uniformity of dosage units, and Labeling under Injections.

SECOBARBITAL AND AMOBARBITAL

For *Secobarbital* and *Amobarbital*—See individual listings for chemistry information.

USP requirements: Secobarbital Sodium and Amobarbital Sodium Capsules USP—Preserve in well-closed containers. Contain the labeled amounts, within ±10%. Meet the requirements for Identification, Dissolution (60% of each active ingredient in 60 minutes in water in Apparatus 1 at 100 rpm), and Uniformity of dosage units.

SELEGILINE

Chemical name: Selegiline hydrochloride—Benzeneethanamine,*N*,alpha-dimethyl-*N*-2-propynyl-, hydrochloride, (*R*)-.

Molecular formula: Selegiline hydrochloride—$C_{13}H_{17}N \cdot HCl$.

Molecular weight: Selegiline hydrochloride—223.74.

Description: Selegiline Hydrochloride USP—White, odorless, crystalline powder.

Solubility: Selegiline Hydrochloride USP—Freely soluble in water, in chloroform, and in methanol.

USP requirements:

Selegiline Hydrochloride USP—Preserve in tight, light-resistant containers. Contains not less than 98.0% and not more than 101.0% of selegiline hydrochloride, calculated on the dried basis. Meets the requirements for Identification, Melting range (not greater than 2 °C, within the limits of 141–145 °C), Specific rotation (−10.0° to −12.0°), Loss on drying (not more than 1.0%), Residue on ignition (not more than 0.2%), Heavy metals (not more than 0.002%), and Chromatographic purity.

Selegiline Hydrochloride Capsules—Not in *USP–NF*.

Selegiline Hydrochloride Tablets USP—Preserve in tight, light-resistant containers. Contain the labeled amount, within ±10%. Meet the requirements for Identification, Dissolution (80% in 20 minutes in water in Apparatus 1 at 50 rpm), Chromatographic purity, Uniformity of dosage units, and Limit of methamphetamine hydrochloride (not more than 2.0%).

SELENIOUS ACID

Chemical name: Selenium dioxide, monohydrated.

Molecular formula: H_2SeO_3.

Molecular weight: 128.97.

USP requirements:

Selenious Acid USP—Preserve in tight containers. Contains not less than 93.0% and not more than 101.0% of selenious acid. Meets the requirements for Identification, Residue on ignition (not more than 0.01%), Insoluble matter, Selenate and sulfate, and Organic volatile impurities.

Selenious Acid Injection USP—Preserve in single-dose or in multiple-dose containers, preferably of Type I or Type II glass. A sterile solution in Water for Injection of Selenious Acid or of selenium dissolved in nitric acid. Label the Injection to indicate that it is to be diluted to the appropriate strength with Sterile Water for Injection or other suitable fluid prior to administration. Contains an amount of selenious acid equivalent to the labeled amount of selenium, within ±5%. Meets the requirements for Identification, Bacterial endotoxins, pH (1.8–2.4), and Particulate matter, and for Injections.

SELENIUM

Molecular formula: Se.

Molecular weight: 78.96.

Description: Dark-red amorphous, or bluish black crystalline, powder.

Solubility: Insoluble in water; soluble in solutions of sodium and potassium hydroxides or sulfides.

USP requirements: Selenium Tablets—Not in *USP–NF*.

SELENIUM SULFIDE

Chemical name: Selenium sulfide (SeS_2).

Molecular formula: SeS;l2.

Molecular weight: 143.09.

Description: Selenium Sulfide USP—Reddish brown to bright orange powder, having not more than a faint odor.

Solubility: Selenium Sulfide USP—Practically insoluble in water and in organic solvents.

USP requirements:

Selenium Sulfide USP—Preserve in well-closed containers. Contains not less than 52.0% and not more than 55.5% of selenium. Meets the requirements for Identification, Residue on ignition (not more than 0.2%), and Soluble selenium compounds (not more than 5 ppm).

Selenium Sulfide Lotion USP—Preserve in tight containers. An aqueous, stabilized suspension of Selenium Sulfide. Contains suitable buffering and dispersing agents. Contains the labeled amount, within ±10%. Meets the requirements for Identification and pH (2.0–6.0).

Note: Where labeled for use as a shampoo, contains a detergent. Where labeled for other uses, may contain a detergent.

SELENOMETHIONINE

Chemical name: Butanoic acid, 2-amino-4-(methylseleno)-, (*S*)-.

Molecular formula: $C_5H_{11}NO_2Se$.

Molecular weight: 196.11.

USP requirements: Selenomethionine USP—Preserve in well-closed containers. Contains not less than 97.0% and not more than 103.0% of selenomethionine and contains not less than 39.0% and not more than 41.0% of selenium, calculated on the as-is basis. Meets the requirements for Identification, Specific rotation (+17.0 to +19.5 °C), Heavy metals (not more than 0.002%), Limit of sodium (not more than 0.1%), Chromatographic purity (not more than 1.0%), and Content of selenium.

SENNA

Chemical group: Anthraquinones.

USP requirements:

Senna USP—Preserve against attack by insects and rodents. Consists of the dried leaflet of *Cassia acutifolia* Delile, known in commerce as Alexandria Senna, or of *Cassia angustifolia* Vahl, known in commerce as Tinnevelly Senna (Fam. Leguminosae). Meets the requirements for Botanic characteristics, Identification, Senna stems, pods, or other foreign organic matter (not more than 2.0%), and Acid-insoluble ash (not more than 3.0%).

Senna Fluidextract USP—Preserve in tight, light-resistant containers, and avoid exposure to direct sunlight and to excessive heat.

Prepare Senna Fluidextract as follows: Mix 1000 grams of Senna, in coarse powder, with a sufficient quantity (600 mL to 800 mL) of menstruum consisting of a mixture of 1 volume of alcohol and 2 volumes of water to make it evenly and distinctly damp. After 15 minutes, pack the mixture firmly into a suitable percolator, and cover the drug with additional menstruum. Macerate for 24 hours, then percolate at a moderate rate, adding fresh menstruum, until the drug is practically exhausted of its active principles. Re-

serve the first 800 mL of percolate, and use it to dissolve the residue from the additional percolate that has been concentrated to a soft extract at a temperature not to exceed 60 °C. Add water and alcohol to make the product measure 1000 mL, and mix.

Meets the requirement for Alcohol content (23.0–27.0%).

Senna Granules—Not in *USP–NF*.

Senna Oral Solution USP—Preserve in tight containers, at a temperature not exceeding 25 °C.

Prepare Senna Syrup as follows: 250 mL of Senna Fluidextract, Suitable essential oil(s), 635 grams of Sucrose, and a sufficient quantity of Purified Water to make 1000 mL. Mix the oil(s) with the Senna Fluidextract, and gradually add 330 mL of Purified Water. Allow the mixture to stand for 24 hours in a cool place, with occasional agitation, then filter, and pass enough Purified Water through the filter to obtain 580 mL of filtrate. Dissolve the Sucrose in this liquid, and add sufficient Purified Water to make the product measure 1000 mL. Mix, and strain.

Meets the requirement for Alcohol content (within ±10% of labeled amount).

Senna for Oral Solution—Not in *USP–NF*.

Senna Suppositories—Not in *USP–NF*.

Senna Syrup USP—Preserve in tight containers, at a temperature not exceeding 25 °C.

Prepare Senna Syrup as follows: 250 mL of Senna Fluidextract, Suitable essential oil(s), 635 grams of Sucrose, and a sufficient quantity of Purified Water to make 1000 mL. Mix the oil(s) with the Senna Fluidextract, and gradually add 330 mL of Purified Water. Allow the mixture to stand for 24 hours in a cool place, with occasional agitation, then filter, and pass enough Purified Water through the filter to obtain 580 mL of filtrate. Dissolve the Sucrose in this liquid, and add sufficient Purified Water to make the product measure 1000 mL. Mix, and strain.

Meets the requirement for Alcohol content (within ±10% of labeled amount).

Senna Tablets—Not in *USP–NF*.

SENNOSIDES

Chemical group: Anthraquinones.

Description: Sennosides USP—Brownish powder.

Solubility: Soluble 1 in 35 of water, 1 in 2100 of alcohol, 1 in 3700 of chloroform, and 1 in 6100 of ether.

USP requirements:

Sennosides USP—Preserve in well-closed containers. A partially purified natural complex of anthraquinone glucosides found in senna, isolated from *Cassia angustifolia* or *C. acutifolia* as calcium salts. Contains not less than 90.0% and not more than 110.0% of sennosides, calculated on the dried basis, or, if the sennosides is in higher concentration, not less than 90.0% and not more than 110.0% of the concentration indicated on the label. Meets the requirements for Identification, pH (6.3–7.3, in a solution [1 in 10]), Loss on drying (not more than 5.0%), Residue on ignition (5.0–8.0%), and Heavy metals (not more than 0.006%).

Sennosides Granules—Not in *USP–NF*.

Sennosides Oral Solution—Not in *USP–NF*.

Sennosides Syrup—Not in *USP–NF*.

Sennosides Tablets USP—Preserve in well-closed containers. Contain the labeled amount, within ±10%. Meet the requirements for Identification, Dissolution (75% in 120 minutes in water in Apparatus 1 at 100 rpm), and Uniformity of dosage units.

SENNOSIDES AND DOCUSATE

For *Sennosides* and *Docusate*—See individual listings for chemistry information.

USP requirements: Sennosides and Docusate Sodium Tablets—Not in *USP–NF*.

SERINE

Chemical name: $C_3H_7NO_3$.

Molecular formula: L-Serine.

Molecular weight: 105.09.

Description: Serine USP—White, odorless crystals.

Solubility: Serine USP—Soluble in water; practically insoluble in absolute alcohol and in ether.

USP requirements: Serine USP—Preserve in well-closed containers. Contains not less than 98.5% and not more than 101.5% of serine, as L-serine, calculated on the dried basis. Meets the requirements for Identification, Specific rotation (+14.0° to +15.6°), Loss on drying (not more than 0.2%), Residue on ignition (not more than 0.1%), Chloride (not more than 0.05%), Sulfate (not more than 0.03%), Iron (not more than 0.003%), Heavy metals (not more than 0.0015%), Chromatographic purity, and Organic volatile impurities.

SERMORELIN

Chemical name: Sermorelin acetate—Somatoliberin (human pancreatic islet), 29-L-argininamide-30-de-L-glutamine-31-de-L-glutamine-32-deglycine-33-de-L-glutamic acid-34-de-L-serine-35-de-L-asparagine-36-de-L-glutamine-37-de-L-glutamic acid-38-de-L-arginine-39-deglycine-40-de-L-alanine-41-de-L-arginine-42-de-L-alanine-43-de-L-arginine-44-de-L-leucinamide-, acetate (salt), hydrate.

Molecular formula: Sermorelin acetate—$C_{149}H_{246}N_{44}O_{42}S \cdot xC_2H_4O_2 \cdot yH_2O$.

USP requirements: Sermorelin Acetate Injection—Not in *USP–NF*.

SERTRALINE

Chemical name: Sertraline hydrochloride—1-Naphthalenamine, 4-(3,4-dichlorophenyl)-1,2,3,4-tetrahydro-*N*-methyl-, hydrochloride, (1*S-cis*)-.

Molecular formula: Sertraline hydrochloride—$C_{17}H_{17}Cl_2N \cdot HCl$.

Molecular weight: Sertraline hydrochloride—342.69.

Description: Sertraline hydrochloride—White, crystalline powder.

Solubility: Sertraline hydrochloride—Slightly soluble in water and in isopropyl alcohol; sparingly soluble in ethanol.

USP requirements:

Sertraline Hydrochloride Capsules—Not in *USP–NF*.

Sertraline Hydrochloride Tablets—Not in *USP–NF*.

SESAME OIL

Description: Sesame Oil NF—Pale yellow, oily liquid. Practically odorless.

NF category: Solvent; vehicle (oleaginous).

Solubility: Sesame Oil NF—Slightly soluble in alcohol. Miscible with ether, with chloroform, with solvent hexane, and with carbon disulfide.

NF requirements: Sesame Oil NF—Preserve in tight, light-resistant containers, and prevent exposure to excessive heat. The refined fixed oil obtained from the seed of one or more cultivated varieties of *Sesamum indicum* Linnée (Fam. Pedaliaceae). Meets the requirements for Identification, Triglyceride composition, Specific gravity (0.916–0.921), Heavy metals (not more than 0.001%), Cottonseed oil, Solidification range of fatty acids (20–25 °C), Free fatty acids, Iodine value (103–116), Saponification value (188–195), Unsaponifiable matter (not more than 1.5%), and Organic volatile impurities.

SEVELAMER

Chemical name: Sevelamer hydrochloride—2-Propen-1-amine polymer with (chloromethyl)oxirane, hydrochloride.

Molecular formula: Sevelamer hydrochloride—$(C_3H_7N)_m$ $(C_3H_5ClO)_n \cdot {}_xHCl$.

Description: Sevelamer hydrochloride—White to off-white powder.

Solubility: Sevelamer hydrochloride—Hydrophilic, but insoluble in water.

USP requirements: Sevelamer Hydrochloride Capsules—Not in *USP–NF*.

SEVOFLURANE

Chemical name: Propane, 1,1,1,3,3,3-hexafluoro-2-(fluoromethoxy)-.

Molecular formula: $C_4H_3F_7O$.

Molecular weight: 200.05.

Description: Clear, colorless, stable liquid.

Solubility: Miscible with ethanol, with ether, and with chloroform; slightly soluble in water.

Other characteristics:
Blood/gas partition coefficient at 37 °C—0.63–0.69.
Water/gas partition coefficient at 37 °C—0.36.
Olive oil/gas partition coefficient at 37 °C—47–54.
Brain/gas partition coefficient at 37 °C—1.15.

USP requirements: Sevoflurane Inhalation—Not in *USP–NF*.

SHELLAC

Description: Shellac NF—
Orange Shellac: Thin, hard, brittle, transparent, pale lemon-yellow to brownish orange flakes, having little or no odor.
Bleached Shellac: Opaque, amorphous cream to yellow granules or coarse powder, having little or no odor.
NF category: Coating agent.

Solubility: Shellac NF—Insoluble in water; very slowly soluble in alcohol, 85 to 95% (w/w); in ether, 13 to 15%; in petroleum ether, 2 to 6%; soluble in aqueous solutions of ethanolamines, alkalies, and borax; sparingly soluble in oil of turpentine.

NF requirements: Shellac NF—Preserve in well-closed containers, preferably in a cold place. Obtained by the purification of Lac, the resinous secretion of the insect *Laccifer Lacca Kerr* (Fam. Coccidae). Orange Shellac is produced either by a process of filtration in the molten state, or by hot solvent process, or both. Orange Shellac may retain most of its wax or be dewaxed, and may contain lesser amounts of the natural color than originally present. Bleached (White) Shellac is prepared by dissolving the Lac in aqueous sodium carbonate, bleaching the solution with sodium hypochlorite and precipitating the Bleached Shellac with 2 *N* sulfuric acid. Removal of the wax, by filtration, during the process results in Refined Bleached Shellac. Label it to indicate whether it is bleached or is orange, and whether it is dewaxed or wax-containing. Meets the requirements for Identification, Loss on drying, Heavy metals (not more than 0.001%), Acid value, Wax, and Rosin. Shellac conforms to the specifications in the accompanying table.

	Acid value (on dried basis)	Loss on drying	Wax
Orange Shellac	between 68 and 76	not more than 2.0%	not more than 5.5%
Dewaxed Orange Shellac	between 71 and 79	not more than 2.0%	not more than 0.2%
Regular Bleached Shellac	between 73 and 89	not more than 6%	not more than 5.5%
Refined Bleached Shellac	between 75 and 91	not more than 6.0%	not more than 0.2%

SIBUTRAMINE

Chemical name: Sibutramine hydrochloride monohydrate—Cyclobutanemethanamine, 1-(4-chlorophenyl)-*N,N*-dimethyl-alpha-(2-methylpropyl)-, hydrochloride, monohydrate, (±)-.

Molecular formula: Sibutramine hydrochloride monohydrate—$C_{17}H_{26}ClN \cdot HCl \cdot H_2O$.

Molecular weight: Sibutramine hydrochloride monohydrate—334.32.

Description: Sibutramine hydrochloride monohydrate—White to cream crystalline powder.

Solubility: Sibutramine hydrochloride monohydrate—2.9 mg/mL in pH 5.2 water.

USP requirements: Sibutramine Hydrochloride Monohydrate Capsules—Not in *USP–NF*.

SILDENAFIL

Chemical name: Sildenafil citrate—Piperazine, 1-[[3-(6,7-dihydro-1-methyl-7-oxo-3-propyl-1*H*-pyrazolo[4,3-*d*]pyrimidin-5-yl)-4-ethoxyphenyl]sulfonyl]-4-methyl-,2-hydroxy-1,2,3-propanetricarboxylate (1:1).

Molecular formula: Sildenafil citrate—$C_{22}H_{30}N_6O_4S \cdot C_6H_8O_7$.

Molecular weight: Sildenafil citrate—666.70.

Description: Sildenafil citrate—White to off-white crystalline powder.

Solubility: Sildenafil citrate—3.5 mg/mL in water.

USP requirements: Sildenafil Citrate Tablets—Not in *USP–NF*.

DENTAL-TYPE SILICA

Description: Dental-Type Silica NF—Fine, white, hygroscopic, odorless, amorphous powder, in which the diameter of the average particle ranges between 0.5 micrometer and 40 micrometers.

  NF category: Glidant and/or anticaking agent; suspending and/or viscosity-increasing agent.

Solubility: Dental-Type Silica NF—Insoluble in water, in alcohol, and in acid (except hydrofluoric acid); soluble in hot solutions of alkali hydroxides.

NF requirements: Dental-Type Silica NF—Preserve in tight containers. Obtained from sodium silicate solution by destabilizing with acid in such a way as to yield very fine particles. The sum of the Assay value and the Sodium Sulfate content is not less than 98.0%. Label it to indicate the maximum percentage of Loss on drying. Meets the requirements for pH (4.0–8.5 in a slurry [1 in 20]), Loss on drying, and Sodium sulfate (not more than 4.0%), and for Loss on ignition, Chloride, Arsenic, and Heavy metals under Silicon Dioxide.

PURIFIED SILICEOUS EARTH

Description: Purified Siliceous Earth NF—Very fine, white, light gray, or pale buff mixture of amorphous powder and lesser amounts of crystalline polymorphs, including quartz and cristobalite. It is gritty, readily absorbs moisture, and retains about 4 times its weight of water without becoming fluid.

  NF category: Filtering aid; sorbent.

Solubility: Purified Siliceous Earth NF—Insoluble in water, in acids, and in dilute solutions of alkali hydroxides.

NF requirements: Purified Siliceous Earth NF—Preserve in well-closed containers. A form of silica (SiO_2) consisting of the frustules and fragments of diatoms, purified by calcining. Meets the requirements for Loss on drying (not more than 0.5%), Loss on ignition (not more than 2.0%), Acid-soluble substances (not more than 2.0%), Water-soluble substances (not more than 0.2%), Leachable arsenic (not more than 0.001%), Leachable lead (not more than 0.001%), and Limit of nonsiliceous substances.

SILICON DIOXIDE

Molecular formula: $SiO_2 \cdot xH_2O$.

Molecular weight: 60.08 (anhydrous).

Description: Silicon Dioxide NF—Fine, white, hygroscopic, odorless, amorphous powder, in which the diameter of the average particles ranges between 2 and 10 micrometers.

  NF category: Desiccant; suspending and/or viscosity-increasing agent.

Solubility: Silicon Dioxide NF—Insoluble in water, in alcohol, and in other organic solvents; soluble in hot solutions of alkali hydroxides.

NF requirements: Silicon Dioxide NF—Preserve in tight containers, protected from moisture. Obtained by insolubilizing the dissolved silica in sodium silicate solution. Where obtained by addition of sodium silicate to a mineral acid, the product is termed silica gel; where obtained by the destabilization of a solution of sodium silicate in such manner as to yield very fine particles, the product is termed precipitated silica. Label it to state whether it is silica gel or precipitated silica. After ignition at 1000 °C for not less than 1 hour, contains not less than 99.0% of anhydrous silicon dioxide. Meets the requirements for Identification, pH (4–8, in a slurry [1 in 20]), Loss on drying (not more than 5.0%), Loss on ignition (not more than 8.5%), Chloride (not more than 0.1%), Sulfate (not more than 0.5%), Arsenic (not more than 3 ppm), Heavy metals (not more than 0.003%), and Organic volatile impurities.

COLLOIDAL SILICON DIOXIDE

Chemical name: Silica.

Molecular formula: SiO_2.

Molecular weight: 60.08.

Description: Colloidal Silicon Dioxide NF—Light, white, nongritty powder of extremely fine particle size (about 15 nm).

  NF category: Glidant and/or anticaking agent; suspending and/or viscosity-increasing agent.

Solubility: Colloidal Silicon Dioxide NF—Insoluble in water and in acid (except hydrofluoric); soluble in hot solutions of alkali hydroxides.

NF requirements: Colloidal Silicon Dioxide NF—Preserve in well-closed containers. A submicroscopic fumed silica prepared by the vapor-phase hydrolysis of a silicon compound. When ignited at 1000 °C for 2 hours, contains not less than 99.0% and not more than 100.5% of silicon dioxide. Meets the requirements for Identification, pH (3.5–5.5, in a 1 in 25 dispersion), Loss on drying (not more than 2.5%), Loss on ignition (not more than 2.0%), Arsenic (not more than 8 mcg per gram), and Organic volatile impurities.

SILICONE OIL

Source: Silicones are polymers with a structure consisting of alternate atoms of silicon and oxygen, with organic groups attached to the silicon atoms. As the degree of polymerization increases, the products become more viscous and the various grades are distinguished by a number, approximately corresponding to the viscosity of the particular grade. Silicones may be fluids (or oils), greases, waxes, resins, or rubbers depending on the degree of polymerization.

USP requirements: Silicone Oil 5000 Centistokes for Injection—Not in *USP–NF*.

SILVER NITRATE

Chemical name: Nitric acid silver(1+) salt.

Molecular formula: AgNO₃.

Molecular weight: 169.87.

Description:

Silver Nitrate USP—Colorless or white crystals. The pH of its solutions is about 5.5. On exposure to light in the presence of organic matter, it becomes gray or grayish black.

Toughened Silver Nitrate USP—White, crystalline masses generally molded as pencils or cones. It breaks with a fibrous fracture. Its solutions are neutral to litmus. It becomes gray or grayish black upon exposure to light.

Solubility:

Silver Nitrate USP—Very soluble in water and even more so in boiling water; sparingly soluble in alcohol; freely soluble in boiling alcohol; slightly soluble in ether.

Toughened Silver Nitrate USP—Soluble in water to the extent of its nitrate content (there is always a residue of silver chloride). Partially soluble in alcohol; slightly soluble in ether.

USP requirements:

Silver Nitrate USP—Preserve in tight, light-resistant containers. Powdered and then dried in the dark over silica gel for 4 hours, contains not less than 99.8% and not more than 100.5% of silver nitrate. Meets the requirements for Clarity and color of solution, Identification, and Copper.

Silver Nitrate Ophthalmic Solution USP—Preserve it protected from light, in inert, collapsible capsules or in other suitable single-dose containers. A solution of Silver Nitrate in a water medium. The solution may be buffered by the addition of Sodium Acetate. Contains the labeled amount, within ±5%. Meets the requirements for Clarity and color of solution, Identification, Sterility, and pH (4.5–6.0).

Toughened Silver Nitrate USP—Preserve in tight, light-resistant containers. Contains not less than 94.5% of silver nitrate, the remainder consisting of silver chloride. Meets the requirements for Identification and Copper.

SIMETHICONE

Chemical name: Simethicone.

Description: Simethicone USP—Translucent, gray, viscous fluid.

NF category: Antifoaming agent; water-repelling agent.

Solubility: Simethicone USP—Insoluble in water and in alcohol. The liquid phase is soluble in chloroform and in ether, but silicon dioxide remains as a residue in these solvents.

USP requirements:

Simethicone USP—Preserve in tight containers. A mixture of fully methylated linear siloxane polymers containing repeating units of the formula [–(CH₃)₂SiO–]ₘ stabilized with trimethylsiloxy end-blocking units of the formula [(CH₃)₃SiO–], and silicon dioxide. Contains not less than 90.5% and not more than 99.0% of polydimethylsiloxane, and not less than 4.0% and not more than 7.0% of silicon dioxide. Meets the requirements for Identification, Loss on heating (not more than 18.0%), Heavy metals (not more than 5 mcg per gram), Defoaming activity (not more than 15 seconds), Organic volatile impurities, and Content of silicon dioxide.

Simethicone Capsules USP—Preserve in well-closed containers. Contain an amount of polydimethylsiloxane equivalent to the labeled amount of simethicone, within ±15%. Meet the requirements for Identification, Disintegration (30 minutes), Uniformity of dosage units, and Defoaming activity.

Simethicone Emulsion USP—Preserve in tight containers. A water-dispersible form of Simethicone composed of Simethicone, suitable emulsifiers, preservatives, and water. Contains an amount of polydimethylsiloxane equivalent to the labeled amount of simethicone, within –15% to +10%. Meets the requirements for Identification, Microbial limits, Heavy metals (not more than 5 mcg per gram), and Defoaming activity (not more than 15 seconds).

Simethicone Oral Suspension USP—Preserve in tight, light-resistant containers. A suspension of Simethicone in Water. Contains an amount of polydimethylsiloxane equivalent to the labeled amount of simethicone, within ±15%. Meets the requirements for Identification, pH (3.5–4.6), and Defoaming activity (not more than 45 seconds).

Simethicone Tablets USP—Preserve in well-closed containers. Tablets that are gelatin-coated are so labeled. Contain an amount of polydimethylsiloxane equivalent to the labeled amount of simethicone, within ±15%. Meet the requirements for Identification, Disintegration (30 minutes; 60 minutes for plain-coated Tablets; and 45 minutes for Tablets labeled as gelatin-coated, simulated gastric fluid being used as the medium), Uniformity of dosage units, and Defoaming activity (not more than 45 seconds).

SIMVASTATIN

Source: Derived synthetically from a fermentation product of *Aspergillus terreus*.

Chemical name: Butanoic acid, 2,2-dimethyl-, 1,2,3,7,8,8a-hexahydro-3,7-dimethyl-8-[2-(tetrahydro-4-hydroxy-6-oxo-2*H*pyran-2-yl)ethyl]-1-naphthalenyl ester, [1 *S*-[1 alpha,3 alpha,7 beta,8 beta(2*S**,4*S**),8a beta]]-.

Molecular formula: C₂₅H₃₈O₅.

Molecular weight: 418.57.

Description: Simvastatin USP—White to off-white powder.

Solubility: Simvastatin USP—Practically insoluble in water; freely soluble in chloroform, in methanol, and in alcohol; sparingly soluble in propylene glycol; very slightly soluble in hexane.

USP requirements:

Simvastatin USP—Preserve in well-closed containers, under nitrogen. Contains not less than 98.0% and not more than 101.0% of simvastatin, calculated on the dried basis. May contain a suitable antioxidant. Meets the requirements for Identification, Specific rotation (+285° to +298°), Loss on drying (not more than 0.5%), Residue on ignition (not more than 0.1%), Heavy metals (not more than 0.002%), Chromatographic purity, and Limit of lovastatin (not more than 1%).

Simvastatin Tablets USP—Preserve in tight containers. Contain the labeled amount, within ±10%. Meet the requirements for Identification, Dissolution (75% in 30 minutes in buffer solution containing 0.5% sodium dodecyl sulfate in 0.01 *M* sodium phosphate [pH 7.0] in Apparatus 2 at 50 rpm), and Uniformity of dosage units.

SINCALIDE

Chemical name: Caerulein, 1-de(5-oxo-L-proline)-2-de-L-gluta-mine-5-L-methionine-.

Molecular formula: $C_{49}H_{62}N_{10}O_{16}S_3$.

Molecular weight: 1143.27.

Description: White to off-white, fluffy powder.

Solubility: Very slightly soluble in water; practically insoluble in alcohol.

USP requirements: Sincalide for Injection USP—Preserve in single-dose containers, preferably of Type I glass. It is a sterile, synthetically prepared C-terminal octapeptide of cholecystokinin and sodium chloride. Label it to state that it is to be used within 24 hours after constitution. Contains the labeled amount, within −15.0% to +25.0%. Meets the requirements for Constituted solution, Bacterial endotoxins, pH (5.0–7.5, the contents of 1 vial being dissolved in 5 mL of water), and Particulate matter, and for Injections.

SIROLIMUS

Source: *Streptomyces hygroscopicus.*

Chemical group: Macrocyclic lactone.

Chemical name: (3S,6R,7E,9R,10R,12R,14S,15E,17E, 19E,21S,23S,26R,27R,34aS)-9,10,12,13,14,21,22,23,24,25, 26,27,31,33,34,34a-Hexadecahydro-9,27-dihydroxy-3-[(1R)-2[(1S,3R,4R)-4-hydroxy-3-methoxycyclohexyl]-1methylethyl]-10,21-dimethoxy-6,8,12,14,20,26-hexamethyl-23,27-epoxy-3H-pyridol[2,1-c][1,4]oxaazacyclohentriacontine-1,5,11,28,29 (4H,6H,31H)-pentone.

Molecular formula: $C_{51}H_{79}NO_{13}$.

Molecular weight: 914.17.

Description: White to off-white powder.

Solubility: Insoluble in water; freely soluble in benzyl alcohol, in chloroform, in acetone, and in acetonitrile.

USP requirements: Sirolimus Oral Solution—Not in *USP–NF*.

SISOMICIN

Chemical name: Sisomicin sulfate—D-Streptamine, (2S-cis)-4-O-[3-amino-6-(aminomethyl)-3,4-dihydro-2H-pyran-2-yl]-2-deoxy-6-O-[3-deoxy-4-C-methyl-3-(methylamino)-beta-L-ara-binopyranosyl]-, sulfate (2:5) (salt).

Molecular formula: Sisomicin sulfate—$(C_{19}H_{37}N_5O_7)_2 \cdot 5H_2SO_4$.

Molecular weight: Sisomicin sulfate—1385.45.

USP requirements:

Sisomicin Sulfate USP—Preserve in tight containers. Has a potency equivalent to not less than 580 mcg of sisomicin per mg, calculated on the dried basis. Meets the requirements for Identification, Specific rotation (+100° to +110°), pH (3.5–5.5, in a solution containing 40 mg of sisomicin per mL), Loss on drying (not more than 15.0%), and Residue on ignition (not more than 1.0%).

Sisomicin Sulfate Injection USP—Preserve in single-dose or in multiple-dose containers, preferably of Type I glass. A sterile solution of Sisomicin Sulfate in Water for Injection. Contains an amount of sisomicin sulfate equivalent to the labeled amount of sisomicin, within −10% to +20%. Meets the requirements for Identification, Bacterial endotoxins, and pH (2.5–5.5), and for Injections.

SMALLPOX VACCINE

Description: Smallpox Vaccine USP—Liquid vaccine is a turbid, whitish to greenish suspension, which may have a slight odor due to the antimicrobial agent. Dried vaccine is a yellow to grayish pellet, which may or may not become fragmented when shaken.

USP requirements: Smallpox Vaccine USP—Preserve and dispense in the containers in which it was placed by the manufacturer. Keep liquid Vaccine during storage and in shipment at a temperature below 0 °C. Keep dried Vaccine at a temperature between 2 and 8 °C. A suspension or solid containing the living virus of vaccinia of a strain of approved origin and manipulation, that has been grown in the skin of a vaccinated bovine calf. Label it to state that it contains not more than 200 microorganisms per mL in the case of Vaccine intended for multiple-puncture administration, or that it contains not more than 1 microganism per 100 doses in the case of Vaccine intended for jet injection, unless it meets the requirements for sterility. In the case of Vaccine intended for jet injection, so state on the label. In the case of dried Vaccine, label it to state that after constitution it is to be well shaken before use. Label it also to state that it was prepared in the bovine calf. Meets the requirements of the specific potency test using embryonated chicken eggs in comparison with the U.S. Reference Smallpox Vaccine in the case of Vaccine intended for multiple-puncture administration or with such Reference Vaccine diluted (1:30) in the case of Vaccine intended for jet injection, and the requirements for the tests for absence of specific microorganisms. Meets the requirement for Expiration date (for liquid Vaccine, not later than 3 months after date of issue from manufacturer's cold storage [−10° C, 9 months as glycerinated or equivalent preparation]; for dried Vaccine, not later than 18 months after date of issue from manufacturerã s cold storage [5 °C, 6 months]). Conforms to the regulations of the U.S. Food and Drug Administration concerning biologics.

SODA LIME

Description: Soda Lime NF—White or grayish white granules. It may have a color if an indicator has been added.

NF category: Sorbent, carbon dioxide.

NF requirements: Soda Lime NF—A mixture of Calcium Hydroxide and Sodium or Potassium Hydroxide or both. May contain an indicator that is inert toward anesthetic gases such as Ether, Cyclopropane, and Nitrous Oxide, and that changes color when the Soda Lime no longer can absorb Carbon Dioxide. Meets the requirements for Identification, Loss on drying (12.0–19.0%), Moisture absorption (increase in weight not more than 7.5%), Hardness, and Carbon dioxide absorbency (not less than 19.0%), and for Packaging and storage, Labeling, and Size of granules under Barium Hydroxide Lime.

SODIUM ACETATE

Chemical name: Acetic acid, sodium salt, trihydrate.

Molecular formula: $C_2H_3NaO_2 \cdot 3H_2O$ (trihydrate); $C_2H_3NaO_2$ (anhydrous).

Molecular weight: 136.08 (trihydrate); 82.03 (anhydrous).

Description: Sodium Acetate USP—Colorless, transparent crystals, or white, granular crystalline powder, or white flakes. It is odorless, or has a faint, acetous odor. Efflorescent in warm, dry air.

NF category: Buffering agent.

Solubility: Sodium Acetate USP—Very soluble in water; soluble in alcohol.

USP requirements:

Sodium Acetate USP—Preserve in tight containers. Contains three molecules of water of hydration, or is anhydrous. Contains not less than 99.0% and not more than 101.0% of sodium acetate, calculated on the dried basis. Label it to indicate whether it is the trihydrate or is anhydrous. Where Sodium Acetate is intended for use in hemodialysis, it is so labeled. Meets the requirements for Identification, pH (7.5–9.2, in a solution in carbon dioxide–free water containing the equivalent of 30 mg of anhydrous sodium acetate per mL), Loss on drying (38.0–41.0% for the hydrous, not more than 1.0% for the anhydrous), Insoluble matter (not more than 0.05%), Chloride (not more than 0.035%), Sulfate (not more than 0.005%), Calcium and magnesium, Potassium, Aluminum (where it is labeled as intended for use in hemodialysis, not more than 0.2 mcg per gram), Heavy metals (not more than 0.001%), and Organic volatile impurities.

Sodium Acetate Injection USP—Preserve in single-dose containers, preferably of Type I glass. A sterile solution of Sodium Acetate in Water for Injection. The label states the sodium acetate content in terms of weight and of milliequivalents in a given volume. Label the Injection to indicate that it is to be diluted to appropriate strength with water or other suitable fluid prior to administration. The label states also the total osmolar concentration in mOsmol per liter. Where the contents are less than 100 mL, or where the label states that the Injection is not for direct injection but is to be diluted before use, the label alternatively may state the total osmolar concentration in mOsmol per mL. Contains the labeled amount, within ± 5%. Meets the requirements for Identification, Bacterial endotoxins, pH (6.0–7.0), and Particulate matter, and for Injections.

Sodium Acetate Solution USP—Preserve in tight containers. An aqueous solution of Sodium Acetate. Contains the labeled amount, within ±3% (w/w). Meets the requirements for Identification, pH (7.5–9.2, when diluted with carbon dioxide–free water to contain 5% of solids), Insoluble matter (not more than 0.005%), Chloride (not more than 0.035%), Sulfate (not more than 0.005%), Calcium and magnesium, Potassium, and Heavy metals (not more than 0.001%).

SODIUM ALGINATE

Chemical name: Alginic acid, sodium salt.

Description: Sodium Alginate NF—Practically odorless, coarse or fine powder, yellowish white in color.

NF category: Suspending and/or viscosity-increasing agent.

Solubility: Sodium Alginate NF—Soluble in water, forming a viscous, colloidal solution; insoluble in alcohol and in hydroalcoholic solutions in which the alcohol content is greater than about 30% by weight; insoluble in chloroform, in ether, and in acids when the pH of the resulting solution becomes lower than about 3.

NF requirements: Sodium Alginate NF—Preserve in tight containers. The purified carbohydrate product extracted from brown seaweeds by the use of dilute alkali. Consists chiefly of the sodium salt of Alginic Acid, a polyuronic acid composed of beta-D-mannuronic acid residues linked so that the carboxyl group of each unit is free while the aldehyde group is shielded by a glycosidic linkage. Contains not less than 90.8% and not more than 106.0% of sodium alginate of average equivalent weight 222.00, calculated on the dried basis. Meets the requirements for Identification, Microbial limits, Loss on drying (not more than 15.0%), Total ash (18.0–27.0%, calculated on the dried basis), Arsenic (not more than 1.5 ppm), Lead (not more than 0.001%), and Heavy metals (not more than 0.004%).

SODIUM ASCORBATE

Chemical name: L-Ascorbic acid, monosodium salt.

Molecular formula: $C_6H_7NaO_6$.

Molecular weight: 198.11.

Description: Sodium Ascorbate USP—White or very faintly yellow crystals or crystalline powder. Is odorless or practically odorless. Is relatively stable in air. On exposure to light it gradually darkens.

Solubility: Sodium Ascorbate USP—Freely soluble in water; very slightly soluble in alcohol; insoluble in chloroform and in ether.

USP requirements:

Sodium Ascorbate USP—Preserve in tight, light-resistant containers. Contains not less than 99.0% and not more than 101.0% of sodium ascorbate, calculated on the dried basis. Meets the requirements for Identification, Specific rotation (+103° to +108°), pH (7.0–8.0, in a solution [1 in 10]), Loss on drying (not more than 0.25%), Heavy metals (not more than 0.002%), and Organic volatile impurities.

Sodium Ascorbate Injection—Not in USP–NF.

SODIUM BENZOATE

Chemical name: Benzoic acid, sodium salt.

Molecular formula: $C_7H_5NaO_2$.

Molecular weight: 144.10.

Description: Sodium Benzoate NF—White, odorless or practically odorless, granular or crystalline powder. It is stable in air.

NF category: Antimicrobial preservative.

Solubility: Sodium Benzoate NF—Freely soluble in water; sparingly soluble in alcohol, and somewhat more soluble in 90% alcohol.

NF requirements: Sodium Benzoate NF—Preserve in well-closed containers. Contains not less than 99.0% and not more than 100.5% of sodium benzoate. Meets the requirements for Identification, Alkalinity, Water (not more than 1.5%), Heavy metals (not more than 0.001%), and Organic volatile impurities.

SODIUM BENZOATE AND SODIUM PHENYLACETATE

Chemical name:

Sodium benzoate—Benzoic acid, sodium salt.
Sodium phenylacetate—Benzeneacetic acid, sodium salt.

Molecular formula:

Sodium benzoate—$C_7H_5NaO_2$.
Sodium phenylacetate—$C_8H_7NaO_2$.

Molecular weight:
 Sodium benzoate—144.10.
 Sodium phenylacetate—158.13.

Description: Sodium Benzoate NF—White, odorless or practically odorless, granular or crystalline powder. It is stable in air.
 NF category: Antimicrobial preservative.

Solubility: Sodium Benzoate NF—Freely soluble in water; sparingly soluble in alcohol, and somewhat more soluble in 90% alcohol.

Other characteristics: The pH of the undiluted sodium benzoate and sodium phenylacetate combination solution is approximately 6.0.

USP requirements: Sodium Benzoate and Sodium Phenylacetate Oral Solution—Not in *USP–NF*.

SODIUM BICARBONATE

Chemical name: Carbonic acid monosodium salt.

Molecular formula: $NaHCO_3$.

Molecular weight: 84.01.

Description: Sodium Bicarbonate USP—White, crystalline powder. Is stable in dry air, but slowly decomposes in moist air. Its solutions, when freshly prepared with cold water, without shaking, are alkaline to litmus. The alkalinity increases as the solutions stand, as they are agitated, or as they are heated.
 NF category: Alkalizing agent.

Solubility: Sodium Bicarbonate USP—Soluble in water; insoluble in alcohol.

USP requirements:
 Sodium Bicarbonate USP—Preserve in well-closed containers. Where Sodium Bicarbonate is intended for use in hemodialysis, it is so labeled. Contains not less than 99.0% and not more than 100.5% of sodium bicarbonate, calculated on the dried basis. Meets the requirements for Identification, Loss on drying (not more than 0.25%), Insoluble substances, Carbonate (where it is labeled as intended for use in hemodialysis, not more than 0.23%), Normal carbonate, Chloride (not more than 0.015%), Limit of sulfur compunds (not more than 0.015%), Aluminum (where it is labeled as intended for use in hemodialysis, not more than 2 mcg per gram), Arsenic (not more than 2 ppm), Calcium and magnesium (where it is labeled as intended for use in hemodialysis, not more than 0.01% for calcium, and not more than 0.004% for magnesium), Copper (where it is labeled as intended for use in hemodialysis, not more than 1 ppm), Iron (where it is labeled as intended for use in hemodialysis, not more than 5 ppm), Heavy metals (not more than 5 ppm), Limit of organics (where it is labeled as intended for use in hemodialysis, not more than 0.01%), and Organic volatile impurities.
 Effervescent Sodium Bicarbonate—Not in *USP–NF*.
 Sodium Bicarbonate Injection USP—Preserve in single-dose containers, of Type I glass. A sterile solution of Sodium Bicarbonate in Water for Injection, the pH of which may be adjusted by means of Carbon Dioxide. The label states the total osmolar concentration in mOsmol per liter. Where the contents are less than 100 mL, or where the label states that the Injection is not for direct injection but is to be diluted before use, the label alternatively may state the total osmolar concentration in mOsmol per mL. Contains the labeled amount, within ±5%. Meets the requirements for Identification, Bacterial endotoxins, pH (7.0–8.5), and Particulate matter, and for Injections.
 Note: Do not use the Injection if it contains a precipitate.

Sodium Bicarbonate Oral Powder USP—Preserve in well-closed containers. Contains Sodium Bicarbonate and suitable added substances. Label Oral Powder to indicate that it is for oral use only. Contains not less than 98.5% and not more than 100.5% of sodium bicarbonate, calculated on the dried basis. Meets the requirements for Identification and Loss on drying under Sodium Bicarbonate.
Sodium Bicarbonate Tablets USP—Preserve in well-closed containers. Contain the labeled amount, within ±5%. Meet the requirements for Identification, Disintegration (30 minutes, simulated gastric fluid TS being substituted for water in the test), and Uniformity of dosage units.

SODIUM BORATE

Chemical name: Borax.

Molecular formula: $Na_2B_4O_7 \cdot 10H_2O$.

Molecular weight: 381.37.

Description: Sodium Borate NF—Colorless, transparent crystals or white, crystalline powder. It is odorless. Its solutions are alkaline to phenolphthalein TS. As it effloresces in warm, dry air, the crystals are often coated with white powder.
 NF category: Alkalizing agent.

Solubility: Sodium Borate NF—Soluble in water; freely soluble in boiling water and in glycerin; insoluble in alcohol.

NF requirements: Sodium Borate NF—Preserve in tight containers. Contains an amount of anhydrous sodium borate equivalent to not less than 99.0% and not more than 105.0% of hydrous sodium borate. Meets the requirements for Identification, Carbonate and bicarbonate, Heavy metals (not more than 0.002%), and Organic volatile impurities.

SODIUM BUTYRATE

Chemical name: Butyric acid, sodium salt.

Molecular formula: $C_4H_7NaO_2$.

Molecular weight: 110.10.

Description: Sodium Butyrate USP—Clear, colorless, hygroscopic powder. Melting range is about 250° to 253°.

Solubility: Sodium Butyrate USP—Soluble in water and in methanol.

USP requirements: Sodium Butyrate USP—Preserve in tight containers, and store at controlled room temperature. Label it to indicate that it is intended for use in compounding dosage forms for rectal use only. Contains not less than 98.0% and not more than 101.0% of sodium butyrate, calculated on the anhydrous basis. Meets the requirements for Identification, Alkalinity, Water (not more than 1.0%), Heavy metals (not more than 0.001%), and Organic volatile impurities.

SODIUM CARBONATE

Chemical name: Carbonic acid, disodium salt.

Molecular formula: Na_2CO_3 (anhydrous); $Na_2CO_3 \cdot H_2O$ (monohydrate).

Molecular weight: 105.99 (anhydrous); 124.00 (monohydrate).

Description: Sodium Carbonate NF—Colorless crystals, or white crystalline powder or granules. Stable in air under ordinary conditions. When exposed to air above 50 °C, the hydrous salt effloresces and, at 100 °C, becomes anhydrous.

NF category: Alkalizing agent.

Solubility: Sodium Carbonate NF—Freely soluble in water, but still more soluble in boiling water.

NF requirements: Sodium Carbonate NF—Preserve in well-closed containers. It is anhydrous or contains one molecule of water of hydration. Label it to indicate whether it is anhydrous or hydrous. Contains not less than 99.5% and not more than 100.5% of sodium carbonate, calculated on the anhydrous basis. Meets the requirements for Identification, Water (for the anhydrous form, not more than 0.5%; for the hydrous form, 12.0–15.0%), Heavy metals (not more than 0.001%), and Organic volatile impurities.

SODIUM CHLORIDE

Chemical name: Sodium chloride.

Molecular formula: NaCl.

Molecular weight: 58.44.

Description:

Sodium Chloride USP—Colorless, cubic crystals or white crystalline powder.

NF category: Tonicity agent.

Sodium Chloride Inhalation Solution USP—Clear, colorless solution.

Bacteriostatic Sodium Chloride Injection USP—Clear, colorless solution, odorless or having the odor of the bacteriostatic substance.

NF category: Vehicle (sterile).

Sodium Chloride Irrigation USP—Clear, colorless solution.

Solubility: Sodium Chloride USP—Freely soluble in water; and slightly more soluble in boiling water; soluble in glycerin; slightly soluble in alcohol.

USP requirements:

Sodium Chloride USP—Preserve in well-closed containers. Contains no added substance. Where Sodium Chloride is intended for use in the manufacture of injectable dosage forms, peritoneal dialysis solutions, hemodialysis solutions, or hemofiltration solutions, it is so labeled. Contains not less than 99.0% and not more than 100.5% of sodium chloride, calculated on the dried basis. Meets the requirements for Appearance of solution, Identification, Acidity or alkalinity, Loss on drying (not more than 0.5%), Aluminum (where it is labeled as intended for use in the manufacture of peritoneal dialysis solutions, hemodialysis solutions, or hemofiltration solutions, not more than 0.2 mcg per gram), Arsenic (1 mcg per gram), Iron (not more than 2 ppm), Barium, Sulfate (not more than 0.020%), Heavy metals (not more than 5 ppm), Limit of bromides (not more than 0.010%), Iodides, Magnesium and alkaline-earth metals, Ferrocyanides, Nitrates, Limit of phosphates (not more than 0.0025%), and Limit of potassium (not more than 0.05%).

Sodium Chloride Injection USP—Preserve in single-dose glass or plastic containers. Glass containers are preferably of Type I or Type II glass. A sterile solution of Sodium Chloride in Water for Injection. Contains no antimicrobial agents. The label states the total osmolar concentration in mOsmol per liter. Where the contents are less than 100 mL, or where the label states that the Injection is not for direct injection but is to be diluted before use, the label alternatively may state the total osmolar con-

centration in mOsmol per mL. Contains the labeled amount, within ±5%. Meets the requirements for Identification, Bacterial endotoxins, pH (4.5–7.0), Particulate matter, Iron (not more than 2 ppm), and Heavy metals (not more than 0.001%, based on amount of sodium chloride), and for Injections.

Bacteriostatic Sodium Chloride Injection USP—Preserve in single-dose or in multiple-dose containers, of not larger than 30-mL size, preferably of Type I or Type II glass. A sterile, isotonic solution of Sodium Chloride in Water for Injection, containing one or more suitable antimicrobial agents. Label it to indicate the name(s) and proportion(s) of the added antimicrobial agent(s). Label it also to include the statement, "NOT FOR USE IN NEWBORNS," in boldface capital letters, on the label immediately under the official name, printed in a contrasting color, preferably red. Alternatively, the statement may be placed prominently elsewhere on the label if the statement is enclosed within a box. Label it also to include the statement "NOT FOR INHALATION." Contains not less than 0.85% and not more than 0.95% of sodium chloride. Meets the requirements for Antimicrobial agent(s), Bacterial endotoxins, and Particulate matter, for Identification test, pH, Iron, and Heavy metals under Sodium Chloride Injection, and for Injections.

Note: Use Bacteriostatic Sodium Chloride Injection with due regard for the compatibility of the antimicrobial agent or agents it contains with the particular medicinal substance that is to be dissolved or diluted.

Sodium Chloride Irrigation USP—Preserve in single-dose glass or plastic containers. Glass containers are preferably of Type I or Type II glass. The container may be designed to empty rapidly and may contain a volume of more than 1 liter. It is Sodium Chloride Injection that has been suitably packaged, and contains no antimicrobial agents. The designation "not for injection" appears prominently on the label. Contains the labeled amount, within ±5%. Meets the requirements for Identification, Bacterial endotoxins, and Sterility, and for pH, Iron, and Heavy metals under Sodium Chloride Injection.

Sodium Chloride Ophthalmic Ointment USP—Preserve in collapsible ophthalmic ointment tubes. It is Sodium Chloride in a suitable ophthalmic ointment base. It is sterile. Contains the labeled amount, within ±10%. Meets the requirements for Identification, Sterility, Minimum fill, and Metal particles.

Sodium Chloride Inhalation Solution USP—Preserve in single-dose containers. A sterile solution of Sodium Chloride in water purified by distillation or by reverse osmosis and rendered sterile. Contains the labeled amount, within ± 10%. Contains no antimicrobial agents or other added substances. Meets the requirements for Identification, Sterility, and pH (4.5–7.0).

Sodium Chloride Ophthalmic Solution USP—Preserve in tight containers. A sterile solution of Sodium Chloride. Contains a buffer. Contains the labeled amount, within ±10%. Meets the requirements for Identification, Sterility, and pH (6.0–8.0).

Sodium Chloride Tablets USP—Preserve in well-closed containers. Contain the labeled amount, within ±5%. Meet the requirements for Identification, Disintegration (30 minutes), Uniformity of dosage units, Iodide or bromide, Barium, and Calcium and magnesium.

Sodium Chloride Tablets for Solution USP—Composed of Sodium Chloride in compressed form, containing no added substance. Contain the labeled amount, within ±5%. Meet the requirements for Identification test, Packaging and storage, Iodide or bromide, Barium, Calcium and magnesium, Disintegration, and Uniformity of dosage units under Sodium Chloride Tablets.

SODIUM CHLORIDE AND DEXTROSE

For *Sodium Chloride* and *Dextrose*—See individual listings for chemistry information.

USP requirements: Sodium Chloride and Dextrose Tablets USP—Preserve in well-closed containers. Contain the labeled amounts, within ±7.5%. Meet the requirements for Identification, Disintegration (30 minutes), and Uniformity of dosage units.

SODIUM CITRATE

Chemical name: 1,2,3-Propanetricarboxylic acid, 2-hydroxy-, trisodium salt.

Molecular formula: $C_6H_5Na_3O_7$ (anhydrous); $C_6H_5Na_3O_7 \cdot 2H_2O$ (hydrous).

Molecular weight: 258.07 (anhydrous); 294.10 (hydrous).

Description: Sodium Citrate USP—Colorless crystals or white, crystalline powder.
  NF category: Buffering agent.

Solubility: Sodium Citrate USP—Hydrous form freely soluble in water and very soluble in boiling water. Insoluble in alcohol.

USP requirements: Sodium Citrate USP—Preserve in tight containers. It is anhydrous or contains two molecules of water of hydration. Label it to indicate whether it is anhydrous or hydrous. Contains not less than 99.0% and not more than 100.5% of sodium citrate, calculated on the anhydrous basis. Meets the requirements for Identification, Alkalinity, Water (10.0–13.0% for the hydrous form, not more than 1.0% for the anhydrous form), Tartrate, and Heavy metals (not more than 0.001%).

SODIUM CITRATE AND CITRIC ACID

For *Sodium Citrate* and *Citric Acid*—See individual listings for chemistry information.

Description: Sodium Citrate and Citric Acid Oral Solution USP—Clear solution having the color of any added preservative or flavoring agents.

USP requirements: Sodium Citrate and Citric Acid Oral Solution USP—Preserve in tight containers. A solution of Sodium Citrate and Citric Acid in a suitable aqueous medium. Contains, in each 100 mL, not less than 2.23 grams and not more than 2.46 grams of sodium, and not less than 6.11 grams and not more than 6.75 grams of citrate, equivalent to not less than 9.5 grams and not more than 10.5 grams of sodium citrate dihydrate; and not less than 6.34 grams and not more than 7.02 grams of citric acid monohydrate. Meets the requirements for Identification and pH (4.0–4.4).

SODIUM DEHYDROACETATE

Chemical name: 2*H*-Pyran-2,4(3*H*)-dione, 3-acetyl-6-methyl-, monosodium salt.

Molecular formula: $C_8H_7NaO_4$.

Molecular weight: 190.13.

Description: Sodium Dehydroacetate NF—White or practically white odorless powder.
  NF category: Antimicrobial preservative.

Solubility: Sodium Dehydroacetate NF—Freely soluble in water, in propylene glycol, and in glycerin.

NF requirements: Sodium Dehydroacetate NF—Preserve in well-closed containers. Contains not less than 98.0% and not more than 100.5% of sodium dehydroacetate, calculated on the anhydrous basis. Meets the requirements for Identification, Water (8.5–10.0%), Heavy metals (not more than 0.001%), and Organic volatile impurities.

SODIUM FERRIC GLUCONATE AND SUCROSE

Chemical name: Sucrose–Alpha-D-glucopyranoside, beta-D-fructofuranosyl-.

Molecular formula: Sucrose—$C_{12}H_{22}O_{11}$.

Molecular weight:
  Sodium ferric gluconate—350,000 daltons.
  Sucrose—342.30.

Description: Sucrose NF—White, crystalline powder or lustrous, dry, colorless or white crystals.

Solubility: Sucrose NF—Very soluble in water; slightly soluble in alcohol; practically insoluble in dehydrated alcohol.

Other charcteristics: Sodium ferric gluconate—pH 7.7–9.7.

USP requirements: Sodium Ferric Gluconate Complex in Sucrose Injection—Not in *USP–NF*.

SODIUM FLUORIDE

Chemical name: Sodium fluoride.

Molecular formula: NaF.

Molecular weight: 41.99.

Description: Sodium Fluoride USP—White, odorless powder.

Solubility: Sodium Fluoride USP—Soluble in water; insoluble in alcohol.

USP requirements:
  Sodium Fluoride USP—Preserve in well-closed containers. Contains not less than 98.0% and not more than 102.0% of sodium fluoride, calculated on the dried basis. Meets the requirements for Identification, Acidity or alkalinity, Loss on drying (not more than 1.0%), Fluosilicate, Chloride (not more than 0.012%), Heavy metals (not more than 0.003%), and Organic volatile impurities.
  Sodium Fluoride Lozenges—Not in *USP–NF*.
  Sodium Fluoride Oral Solution USP—Preserve in tight containers, plastic containers being used for Oral Solution having a pH below 7.5. Label Oral Solution in terms of the content of sodium fluoride (NaF) and in terms of the content of fluoride ion. Contains the labeled amount, within ±10%. Meets the requirement for Identification.
  Sodium Fluoride Tablets USP—Preserve in tight containers. Label the Tablets in terms of the content of sodium fluoride (NaF) and in terms of the content of fluoride ion. The Tablets that are to be chewed may be labeled as Sodium Fluoride Chewable Tablets. Contain the labeled amount, within ±10%. Meet the requirements for Identification, Disintegration (15 minutes), and Uniformity of dosage units.

SODIUM FLUORIDE AND PHOSPHORIC ACID

For *Sodium Fluoride* and *Phosphoric Acid*—See individual listings for chemistry information.

USP requirements:

Sodium Fluoride and Phosphoric Acid Gel USP—Preserve in tight, plastic containers. Label Gel in terms of the content of sodium fluoride (NaF) and in terms of the content of fluoride ion. Contains the labeled amount of fluoride ion, within ±10%, in an aqueous medium containing a suitable viscosity-inducing agent. Meets the requirements for Identification, Viscosity (7,000–20,000 centipoises), and pH (3.0–4.0).

Sodium Fluoride and Phosphoric Acid Topical Solution USP—Preserve in tight, plastic containers. Label Topical Solution in terms of the content of sodium fluoride (NaF) and in terms of the content of fluoride ion. Contains the labeled amount of fluoride ion, within ±10%. Meets the requirements for pH (3.0–4.5), and for Identification tests under Sodium Fluoride and Phosphoric Acid Gel.

Sodium Fluoride and Acidulated Phosphate Topical Solution USP—Preserve in tight plastic containers. Label Topical Solution in terms of the content of sodium fluoride (NaF) and in terms of the content of fluoride ion. Contains the labeled amount of fluoride ion, within ±10%. Meets the requirements for pH (3.0–4.5), and for Identification tests under Sodium Fluoride and Phosphoric Acid Gel.

SODIUM FLUORIDE AND TRICLOSAN

Chemical name:

Sodium fluoride—Sodium fluoride.
Triclosan—Phenol, 5-chloro-2-(2,4-dichlorophenoxy)-.

Molecular formula:

Sodium fluoride—NaF.
Triclosan—$C_{12}H_7Cl_3O_2$.

Molecular weight:

Sodium fluoride—41.99.
Triclosan—289.54.

Description: Sodium Fluoride USP—White, odorless powder.

Solubility: Sodium Fluoride USP—Soluble in water; insoluble in alcohol.

USP requirements: Sodium Fluoride and Triclosan Dental Paste—Not in *USP–NF*.

SODIUM FORMALDEHYDE SULFOXYLATE

Chemical name: Methanesulfinic acid, hydroxy-, monosodium salt.

Molecular formula: CH_3NaO_3S.

Molecular weight: 118.09.

Description: Sodium Formaldehyde Sulfoxylate NF—White crystals or hard white masses, having the characteristic odor of garlic.

NF category: Antioxidant.

Solubility: Sodium Formaldehyde Sulfoxylate NF—Freely soluble in water; slightly soluble in alcohol, in ether, and in chloroform.

NF requirements: Sodium Formaldehyde Sulfoxylate NF—Preserve in well-closed, light-resistant containers, and store at controlled room temperature. Contains an amount of sodium formaldehyde sulfoxylate equivalent to not less than 45.5% and not more than 54.5% of sulfur dioxide, calculated on the dried basis. Meets the requirements for Clarity and color of solution, Identification, Alkalinity, pH (9.5–10.5, in a solution [1 in 50]), Loss on drying (not more than 27.0%), Sulfide, Iron (not more than 0.0025%), Sodium sulfite (not more than 5.0%, calculated on the dried basis), and Organic volatile impurities.

SODIUM FUSIDATE

Chemical name: 29-Nordammara-17(20),24-dien-21-oic acid, 16-(acetyloxy)-3,11-dihydroxy-, monosodium salt.

Molecular formula: $C_{31}H_{47}NaO_4$.

Molecular weight: 506.69.

Description: A white or almost white, slightly hydroscoic, crystalline powder.

Solubility: Freely soluble in water and in alcohol.

Other charecteristics: pH 7.5–9.0 of 1.25% solution in water.

USP requirements: Sodium Fusidate Injection—Not in *USP–NF*. Sodium Fusidate Tablet—Not in *USP–NF*.

SODIUM GLUCONATE

Chemical name: D-Gluconic acid, monosodium salt.

Molecular formula: $C_6H_{11}NaO_7$.

Molecular weight: 218.14.

Description: Crystals. Technical grade may have a pleasant odor.

Solubility: Soluble in water at 25 °C: 59 grams/100 mL; sparingly soluble in alcohol; insoluble in ether.

USP requirements: Sodium Gluconate USP—Preserve in well-closed containers. Contains not less than 98.0% and not more than 102.0% of sodium gluconate. Meets the requirements for Identification, Chloride (not more than 0.07%), Sulfate (not more than 0.05%), Lead (not more than 0.001%), Heavy metals (not more than 0.002%), and Reducing substances (not more than 0.5%).

SODIUM HYDROXIDE

Chemical name: Sodium hydroxide.

Molecular formula: NaOH.

Molecular weight: 40.00.

Description: Sodium Hydroxide NF—White or practically white, fused masses, in small pellets, in flakes, or sticks, and in other forms. It is hard and brittle and shows a crystalline fracture. Exposed to the air, it rapidly absorbs carbon dioxide and moisture.

NF category: Alkalizing agent.

Solubility: Sodium Hydroxide NF—Freely soluble in water and in alcohol.

NF requirements: Sodium Hydroxide NF—Preserve in tight containers. Contains not less than 95.0% and not more than 100.5% of total alkali, calculated as sodium hydroxide, including not more than 3.0% of anhydrous sodium carbonate. Meets the requirements for Identification, Insoluble substances and organic matter, Potassium, and Heavy metals (not more than 0.003%).

Caution: Exercise great care in handling Sodium Hydroxide, as it rapidly destroys tissues.

SODIUM HYPOCHLORITE

Chemical name: Hypochlorous acid, sodium salt.

Molecular formula: NaClO.

Molecular weight: 74.44.

Description: Sodium Hypochlorite Solution USP—Clear, pale greenish yellow liquid, having the odor of chlorine. Affected by light.

USP requirements:

Sodium Hypochlorite Solution USP—Preserve in tight, light-resistant containers, at a temperature not exceeding 25 °C. Contains not less than 4.0% and not more than 6.0%, by weight, of sodium hypochlorite. Meets the requirement for Identification.

Caution: This Solution is not suitable for application to wounds.

Sodium Hypochlorite Topical Solution USP—Preserve in tight, light-resistant 1-liter plastic containers, and store at controlled room temperature. Label it to indicate that its strength is 0.025%, and to state the correct beyond-use date. (Note: For external use only; it may be applied to wounds and burns.) Contains not less than 0.20 gram and not more than 0.32 gram of Sodium Hypochlorite in 1000 mL of Topical Solution. Prepare Sodium Hypochlorite Topical Solution as follows: 5.0 mL Sodium Hypochlorite Solution, 1.02 gram Monobasic Sodium Phosphate monohydrate, 17.61 gram Dibasic Sodium Phosphate anhydrous, and Purified Water, a sufficient quantity to make 1000 mL. Dissolve the Dibasic Sodium Phosphate anhydrous and the Monobasic Sodium Phosphate monohydrate in about 500 mL of Purified Water. Add the Sodium Hypochlorite Solution and sufficient Purified Water to make the product measure 1000 mL, and mix to produce the Topical Solution.

Note—The source of the Sodium Hypochlorite Solution may be commercial unscented laundry bleach (nominally 5.25% w/v) provided that the commercial laundry bleach was recently acquired.

Meets the requirements for pH (7.8–8.2) and Beyond-use date.

SODIUM IODIDE

Chemical name: Sodium iodide.

Molecular formula: NaI.

Molecular weight: 149.89.

Description: Sodium Iodide USP—Colorless, odorless crystals, or white, crystalline powder. Is deliquescent in moist air, and develops a brown tint upon decomposition.

Solubility: Sodium Iodide USP—Very soluble in water; freely soluble in alcohol and in glycerin.

USP requirements:

Sodium Iodide USP—Preserve in tight containers. Contains not less than 99.0% and not more than 101.5% of sodium iodide, calculated on the anhydrous basis. Meets the requirements for Identification, Alkalinity, Water (not more

than 2.0%), Iodate, Thiosulfate and barium, Potassium, Heavy metals (not more than 0.001%), Limit of nitrate, nitrite, and ammonia, and Organic volatile impurities.
Sodium Iodide Injection—Not in *USP–NF*.

SODIUM LACTATE

Chemical name: Sodium lactate—Propanoic acid, 2-hydroxy-, monosodium salt.

Molecular formula: Sodium lactate—$C_3H_5NaO_3$.

Molecular weight: Sodium lactate—112.06.

Description: Sodium Lactate Solution USP—Clear, colorless or practically colorless, slightly viscous liquid, odorless, or having a slight, not unpleasant odor.

NF category: Buffering agent.

Solubility: Sodium Lactate Solution USP—Miscible with water.

USP requirements:

Sodium Lactate Injection USP—Preserve in single-dose glass or plastic containers. Glass containers are preferably of Type I or Type II glass. It is sterile Sodium Lactate Solution in Water for Injection, or a sterile solution of Lactic Acid in Water for Injection prepared with the aid of Sodium Hydroxide. The label states the total osmolar concentration in mOsmol per liter. Where the contents are less than 100 mL, or where the label states that the Injection is not for direct injection but is to be diluted before use, the label alternatively may state the total osmolar concentration in mOsmol per mL. The label includes also the warning: "Not for use in the treatment of lactic acidosis." Contains the labeled amount, within −5% to +10%. Meets the requirements for Identification, Bacterial endotoxins, pH (6.0–7.3, the Injection being diluted with water, if necessary, to approximately 0.16 *M* [20 mg per mL]), Particulate matter, and Heavy metals (not more than 0.001%), and for Injections.

Sodium Lactate Solution USP—Preserve in tight containers. An aqueous solution containing not less than 50.0%, by weight, of monosodium lactate. Label it to indicate its content of sodium lactate. Contains the labeled amount, within ±2%. Meets the requirements for Identification, pH (5.0–9.0), Chloride (not more than 0.05%), Sulfate, Heavy metals (not more than 0.001%), Sugars, Limit of citrate, oxalate, phosphate, or tartrate, and Limit of methanol and methyl esters.

SODIUM LAURYL SULFATE

Chemical name: Sulfuric acid monododecyl ester sodium salt.

Molecular formula: $C_{12}H_{25}NaO_4S$.

Molecular weight: 288.38.

Description: Sodium Lauryl Sulfate NF—Small, white or light yellow crystals having a slight characteristic odor.

NF category: Emulsifying and/or solubilizing agent; wetting and/or solubilizing agent.

Solubility: Sodium Lauryl Sulfate NF—Freely soluble in water, forming an opalescent solution.

NF requirements: Sodium Lauryl Sulfate NF—Preserve in well-closed containers. A mixture of sodium alkyl sulfates consisting chiefly of sodium lauryl sulfate [$CH_3(CH_2)_{10}CH_2OSO_3Na$]. The combined content of sodium chloride and sodium sulfate is not more than 8.0%. Meets the requirements for Identifica-

tion, Alkalinity, Heavy metals (not more than 0.002%), Organic volatile impurities, Sodium chloride, Sodium sulfate, Unsulfated alcohols, and Total alcohols.

SODIUM METABISULFITE

Chemical name: Disulfurous acid, disodium salt.

Molecular formula: $Na_2S_2O_5$.

Molecular weight: 190.11.

Description: Sodium Metabisulfite NF—White crystals or white to yellowish crystalline powder, having the odor of sulfur dioxide.

NF category: Antioxidant.

Solubility: Sodium Metabisulfite NF—Freely soluble in water and in glycerin; slightly soluble in alcohol.

NF requirements: Sodium Metabisulfite NF—Preserve in well-filled, tight containers, and avoid exposure to excessive heat. Contains an amount of sodium metabisulfite equivalent to not less than 65.0% and not more than 67.4% of sulfur dioxide. Meets the requirements for Identification, Limit of chloride (not more than 0.05%), Iron (not more than 0.002%), Limit of thiosulfate (not more than 0.05%), and Heavy metals (not more than 0.002%).

SODIUM MONOFLUOROPHOSPHATE

Chemical name: Phosphorofluoridic acid, disodium salt.

Molecular formula: Na_2PFO_3.

Molecular weight: 143.95.

Description: Sodium Monofluorophosphate USP—White to slightly gray, odorless powder.

Solubility: Sodium Monofluorophosphate USP—Freely soluble in water.

USP requirements: Sodium Monofluorophosphate USP—Preserve in well-closed containers. Contains not less than 91.7% and not more than 100.5% of sodium monofluorophosphate, calculated on the dried basis. Meets the requirements for Identification, pH (6.5–8.0, in a solution [1 in 50]), Loss on drying (not more than 0.2%), Arsenic (not more than 3 ppm), Limit of fluoride ion (not more than 1.2%), Heavy metals (not more than 0.005%), and Organic volatile impurities.

SODIUM NITRITE

Chemical name: Nitrous acid, sodium salt.

Molecular formula: $NaNO_2$.

Molecular weight: 69.00.

Description:
Sodium Nitrite USP—White to slightly yellow, granular powder, or white or practically white, opaque, fused masses or sticks. Deliquescent in air. Its solutions are alkaline to litmus.
Sodium Nitrite Injection USP—Clear, colorless liquid.

Solubility: Sodium Nitrite USP—Freely soluble in water; sparingly soluble in alcohol.

USP requirements:
Sodium Nitrite USP—Preserve in tight containers. Contains not less than 97.0% and not more than 101.0% of sodium nitrite, calculated on the dried basis. Meets the requirements for Identification, Loss on drying (not more than 0.25%), and Heavy metals (not more than 0.002%).
Sodium Nitrite Injection USP—Preserve in single-dose containers, of Type I glass. A sterile solution of Sodium Nitrite in Water for Injection. Contains the labeled amount, within ±5%. Meets the requirements for Identification, Bacterial endotoxins, and pH (7.0–9.0), and for Injections.

SODIUM NITROPRUSSIDE

Chemical name: Ferrate(2-), pentakis(cyano-*C*)nitrosyl-, disodium, dihydrate, (*OC*-6-22)-.

Molecular formula: $Na_2[Fe(CN)_5NO] \cdot 2H_2O$.

Molecular weight: 297.95.

Description:
Sodium Nitroprusside USP—Reddish brown, practically odorless, crystals or powder.
Sodium Nitroprusside for Injection USP—Reddish brown, practically odorless, crystals or powder.

Solubility:
Sodium Nitroprusside USP—Freely soluble in water; slightly soluble in alcohol; very slightly soluble in chloroform.
Sodium Nitroprusside for Injection USP—Freely soluble in water; slightly soluble in alcohol; very slightly soluble in chloroform.

USP requirements:
Sodium Nitroprusside USP—Preserve in tight, light-resistant containers. Where it is intended for use in preparing injectable dosage forms, the label states that it is sterile or must be subjected to further processing during the preparation of injectable dosage forms. Contains not less than 99.0% of sodium nitroprusside. Meets the requirements for Identification, Water (9.0–15.0%), Insoluble substances (not more than 0.01%), Chloride (not more than 0.02%), Limit of ferricyanide (not more than 0.02%), Limit of ferrocyanide (not more than 0.02%), and Sulfate (not more than 0.01%), and for Sterility tests and for Bacterial endotoxins under Sodium Nitroprusside for Injection (where the label states that Sodium Nitroprusside is sterile), and for Bacterial endotoxins under Sodium Nitroprusside for Injection (where the label states that Sodium Nitroprusside must be subjected to further processing during the preparation of injectable dosage forms).
Sodium Nitroprusside for Injection USP—Preserve protected from light in Containers for Sterile Solids. It is Sodium Nitroprusside suitable for parenteral use. Contains the labeled amount, within ±10%. Meets the requirements for Constituted solution, Identification, Bacterial endotoxins, and Water (not more than 15.0%), for Identification test under Sodium Nitroprusside, and for Sterility tests, Uniformity of dosage units, and Labeling under Injections.

SODIUM PHENYLBUTYRATE

Chemical name: Benzenebutanoic acid, sodium salt.

Molecular formula: $C_{10}H_{11}NaO_2$.

Molecular weight: 186.18.

Description: Off-white crystalline substance.

Solubility: Soluble in water; freely soluble in methanol; practically insoluble in acetone and in diethyl ester.

USP requirements:
Sodium Phenylbutyrate for Oral Solution—Not in *USP–NF*.
Sodium Phenylbutyrate Tablets—Not in *USP–NF*.

DIBASIC SODIUM PHOSPHATE

Chemical name: Phosphoric acid, disodium salt, heptahydrate.

Molecular formula: $Na_2HPO_4 \cdot 7H_2O$.

Molecular weight: 268.07.

Description:
Dibasic Sodium Phosphate USP (dried)—White powder that readily absorbs moisture.
  NF category: Buffering agent.
Dibasic Sodium Phosphate USP (heptahydrate)—Colorless or white, granular or caked salt. Effloresces in warm, dry air. Its solutions are alkaline to phenolphthalein TS, a 0.1 *M* solution having a pH of about 9.
  NF category: Buffering agent.

Solubility:
Dibasic Sodium Phosphate USP (dried)—Freely soluble in water; insoluble in alcohol.
Dibasic Sodium Phosphate USP (heptahydrate)—Freely soluble in water; very slightly soluble in alcohol.

USP requirements:
Dibasic Sodium Phosphate USP—Preserve in tight containers. It is dried or contains one, two, seven, or twelve molecules of water of hydration. Label it to indicate whether it is dried or is the monohydrate, the dihydrate, the heptahydrate, or the dodecahydrate. Contains not less than 98.0% and not more than 100.5% of dibasic sodium phosphate, calculated on the dried basis. Meets the requirements for Identification, Loss on drying (not more than 5.0% for the dried form, 10.3–12.0% for the monohydrate, 18.5–21.5% for the dihydrate, 43.0–50.0% for the heptahydrate, and 55.0–64.0% for the dodecahydrate), Insoluble substances (not more than 0.4%), Chloride (not more than 0.06%), Sulfate (not more than 0.2%), Arsenic (not more than 16 ppm), and Heavy metals (not more than 0.002%).
Sodium Phosphate Effervescent Powder—Not in *USP–NF*.

MONOBASIC SODIUM PHOSPHATE

Chemical name: Phosphoric acid, monosodium salt, monohydrate; phosphoric acid, monosodium salt, dihydrate.

Molecular formula: $NaH_2PO_4 \cdot xH_2O$.

Molecular weight: 137.99 (monohydrate); 119.98 (anhydrous); 156.01 (dihydrate).

Description: Monobasic Sodium Phosphate USP—Colorless crystals or white, crystalline powder. Odorless and slightly deliquescent. Its solutions are acid to litmus and effervesce with sodium carbonate.
  NF category: Buffering agent.

Solubility: Monobasic Sodium Phosphate USP—Freely soluble in water; practically insoluble in alcohol.

USP requirements: Monobasic Sodium Phosphate USP—Preserve in well-closed containers. Contains one or two molecules of water of hydration, or is anhydrous. Label it to indicate whether it is anhydrous or is the monohydrate or the dihydrate. Contains not less than 98.0% and not more than 103.0% of monobasic sodium phosphate, calculated on the anhydrous basis. Meets the requirements for Identification, pH (4.1–4.5, in a solution containing the equivalent of 1.0 gram of monobasic sodium phosphate [monohydrate] in 20 mL of water), Water (less than 2.0% for the anhydrous form, 10.0–15.0% for the monohydrate, 18.0–26.5% for the dihydrate), Insoluble substances (not more than 0.2%), Chloride (not more than 0.014%), Sulfate (not more than 0.15%), Aluminum, calcium, and related elements, Arsenic (not more than 8 ppm), Heavy metals (not more than 0.002%), and Organic volatile impurities.

SODIUM PHOSPHATES

For *Dibasic Sodium Phosphate* and *Monobasic Sodium Phosphate*—See individual listings for chemistry information.

USP requirements:
Sodium Phosphates Injection USP—Preserve in single-dose containers, preferably of Type I glass. A sterile solution of Monobasic Sodium Phosphate and Dibasic Sodium Phosphate in Water for Injection. Contains no bacteriostat or other preservative. The label states the sodium content in terms of milliequivalents in a given volume, and states also the phosphorus content in terms of millimoles in a given volume. Label the Injection to indicate that it is to be diluted to appropriate strength with water or other suitable fluid prior to administration, and that once opened any unused portion is to be discarded. The label states also the total osmolar concentration in mOsmol per liter. Where the contents are less than 100 mL, or where the label states that the Injection is not for direct injection but is to be diluted before use, the label alternatively may state the total osmolar concentration in mOsmol per mL. Contains the labeled amounts of monobasic sodium phosphate and dibasic sodium phosphate, within ±5%. Meets the requirements for Identification, Bacterial endotoxins, and Particulate matter, and for Injections.
Sodium Phosphates Oral Solution USP—Preserve in tight containers. A solution of Dibasic Sodium Phosphate and Monobasic Sodium Phosphate, or Dibasic Sodium Phosphate and Phosphoric Acid, in Purified Water. Contains, in each 100 mL, not less than 16.2 grams and not more than 19.8 grams of dibasic sodium phosphate (heptahydrate), and not less than 43.2 grams and not more than 52.8 grams of monobasic sodium phosphate (monohydrate). Meets the requirements for Identification, Specific gravity (1.333–1.366), and pH (4.4–5.2).
Sodium Phosphates Rectal Solution USP—Preserve in tight, single-unit containers, at controlled room temperature. A solution of Dibasic Sodium Phosphate and Monobasic Sodium Phosphate, or Dibasic Sodium Phosphate and Phosphoric Acid, in Purified Water. Contains, in each 100 mL, not less than 5.4 grams and not more than 6.6 grams of dibasic sodium phosphate (heptahydrate), and not less than 14.4 grams and not more than 17.6 grams of monobasic sodium phosphate (monohydrate). Meets the requirements for Identification, Specific gravity (1.112–1.136), and pH (5.0–5.8).

SODIUM POLYSTYRENE SULFONATE

Chemical name: Benzene, diethenyl-, polymer with ethenylbenzene, sulfonated, sodium salt.

Description: Sodium Polystyrene Sulfonate USP—Golden brown, fine powder. Is odorless.

Solubility: Sodium Polystyrene Sulfonate USP—Insoluble in water.

USP requirements:

Sodium Polystyrene Sulfonate USP (for Suspension)—Preserve in well-closed containers. A cation-exchange resin prepared in the sodium form. Sodium Polystyrene Sulfonate that is intended for preparing suspensions for oral or rectal administration may be labeled Sodium Polystyrene Sulfonate for Suspension. Each gram exchanges not less than 110 mg and not more than 135 mg of potassium, calculated on the anhydrous basis. Meets the requirements for Water (not more than 10.0%), Limit of ammonium salts, Sodium content (9.4–11.5%, calculated on the anhydrous basis), and Potassium exchange capacity.

Sodium Polystyrene Sulfonate Suspension USP—Preserve in well-closed containers, protected from freezing and from excessive heat. A suspension of Sodium Polystyrene Sulfonate in an aqueous vehicle containing a suitable quantity of sorbitol. Label it to state the quantity of sorbitol in a given volume of Suspension. Contains the labeled amount of sorbitol, within ±10%. Each gram of the labeled amount of sodium polystyrene sulfonate exchanges not less than 110 mg and not more than 135 mg of potassium. Meets the requirements for Microbial limits, Sodium content (9.4–11.5%, based on the labeled amount) and Potassium exchange capacity.

SODIUM PROPIONATE

Chemical name: Propanoic acid, sodium salt, hydrate.

Molecular formula: $C_3H_5NaO_2 \cdot xH_2O$.

Molecular weight: 96.06 (anhydrous).

Description: Sodium Propionate NF—Colorless, transparent crystals or granular, crystalline powder. Odorless, or has a faint acetic-butyric odor. Deliquescent in moist air.

NF category: Antimicrobial preservative.

Solubility: Sodium Propionate NF—Very soluble in water; soluble in alcohol.

NF requirements: Sodium Propionate NF—Preserve in tight containers. Dried at 105 °C for 2 hours, contains not less than 99.0% and not more than 100.5% of anhydrous sodium propionate. Meets the requirements for Identification, Alkalinity, Water (not more than 1.0%), Heavy metals (not more than 0.001%), and Organic volatile impurities.

SODIUM SALICYLATE

Chemical name: Benzoic acid, 2-hydroxy-, monosodium salt.

Molecular formula: $C_7H_5NaO_3$.

Molecular weight: 160.10.

Description: Sodium Salicylate USP—Amorphous or microcrystalline powder or scales. Is colorless, or has not more than a faint, pink tinge. Is odorless, or has a faint, characteristic odor, and is affected by light. A freshly made solution (1 in 10) is neutral or acid to litmus.

Solubility: Sodium Salicylate USP—Freely (and slowly) soluble in water and in glycerin; very soluble in boiling water and in boiling alcohol; slowly soluble in alcohol.

USP requirements:

Sodium Salicylate USP—Preserve in well-closed, light-resistant containers. Contains not less than 99.5% and not more than 100.5% of sodium salicylate, calculated on the anhydrous basis. Meets the requirements for Identification, Water (not more than 0.5%), Sulfite or thiosulfate, Heavy metals (not more than 0.002%), and Organic volatile impurities.

Sodium Salicylate Tablets USP—Preserve in well-closed containers. Contain the labeled amount, within ±5%. Meet the requirements for Identification, Dissolution (75% in 45 minutes in water in Apparatus 1 at 100 rpm), and Uniformity of dosage units.

Sodium Salicylate Delayed-release Tablets—Not in *USP–NF*.

SODIUM STARCH GLYCOLATE

Chemical name: Starch carboxymethyl ether, sodium salt.

Description: Sodium Starch Glycolate NF—White, odorless, relatively free-flowing powder; available in several different viscosity grades. A 2% (w/v) dispersion in cold water settles, on standing, in the form of a highly hydrated layer.

NF category: Tablet disintegrant.

NF requirements: Sodium Starch Glycolate NF—Preserve in well-closed containers, preferably protected from wide variations in temperature and humidity, which may cause caking. The sodium salt of a carboxymethyl ether of starch. The labeling indicates the pH range. Contains not less than 2.8% and not more than 4.2% of sodium on the dried, alcohol-washed basis. May contain not more than 7.0% of Sodium Chloride. Meets the requirements for Identification, Microbial limits, pH (3.0–5.0 or 5.5–7.5), Loss on drying (not more than 10.0%), Iron (not more than 0.002%), Heavy metals (not more than 0.002%), and Sodium chloride.

SODIUM STEARATE

Chemical name: Octadecanoic acid, sodium salt.

Molecular formula: $C_{18}H_{35}NaO_2$.

Molecular weight: 306.46.

Description: Sodium Stearate NF—Fine, white powder, soapy to the touch, usually having a slight tallow-like odor. It is affected by light. Its solutions are alkaline to phenolphthalein TS.

NF category: Emulsifying and/or solubilizing agent.

Solubility: Sodium Stearate NF—Slowly soluble in cold water and in cold alcohol; readily soluble in hot water and in hot alcohol.

NF requirements: Sodium Stearate NF—Preserve in well-closed, light-resistant containers. A mixture of sodium stearate and sodium palmitate, which together constitute not less than 90.0% of the total content. The content of sodium stearate is not less than 40.0% of the total. Contains small amounts of the sodium salts of other fatty acids. Meets the requirements for Identification, Acidity, Loss on drying (not more than 5.0%), Alcohol-insoluble substances, Iodine value of fatty acids (not more than 4.0), Acid value of fatty acids (196–211), and Organic volatile impurities.

SODIUM STEARYL FUMARATE

Description: Sodium Stearyl Fumarate NF—Fine, white powder. NF category: Tablet and/or capsule lubricant.

Solubility: Sodium Stearyl Fumarate NF—Slightly soluble in methanol; practically insoluble in water.

NF requirements: Sodium Stearyl Fumarate NF—Preserve in well-closed containers. Contains not less than 99.0% and not more than 101.5% of sodium stearyl fumarate, calculated on the anhydrous basis. Meets the requirements for Identification, Water (not more than 5.0%), Lead (not more than 0.001%), Heavy metals (not more than 0.002%), Saponification value (142.2–146.0, calculated on the anhydrous basis), Limit of sodium stearyl maleate and stearyl alcohol (not more than 0.25% of sodium stearyl maleate and not more than 0.5% of stearyl alcohol), and Organic volatile impurities.

SODIUM SULFATE

Chemical name: Sulfuric acid disodium salt, decahydrate.

Molecular formula: $Na_2SO_4 \cdot 10H_2O$.

Molecular weight: 322.20.

Description: Sodium Sulfate USP—Large, colorless, odorless, transparent crystals, or granular powder. Effloresces rapidly in air, liquifies in its water of hydration at about 33 °C, and loses all of its water of hydration at about 100 °C.

Solubility: Sodium Sulfate USP—Freely soluble in water; soluble in glycerin; insoluble in alcohol.

USP requirements:
Sodium Sulfate USP—Preserve in tight containers, preferably at a temperature not exceeding 30 °C. Contains ten molecules of water of hydration, or is anhydrous. Label it to indicate whether it is the decahydrate or is anhydrous. Contains not less than 99.0% of sodium sulfate, calculated on the dried basis. Meets the requirements for Identification, Acidity or alkalinity, Loss on drying (51.0–57.0% for the decahydrate and not more than 0.5% for the anhydrous form), Chloride (not more than 0.02%), and Heavy metals (not more than 0.001%).
Sodium Sulfate Injection USP—Preserve in single-dose containers, preferably of Type I glass. A sterile, concentrated solution of Sodium Sulfate in Water for Injection, which upon dilution is suitable for parenteral use. Label it to indicate that it is to be diluted before injection to render it isotonic (3.89% of sodium sulfate decahydrate). Contains the labeled amount, within ±5%. Meets the requirements for Identification, Pyrogen, and pH (5.0–6.5), and for Injections.

SODIUM SULFIDE

Chemical name: Sodium sulfide nonhydrate.

Molecular formula: $Na_2S \cdot 9H_2O$.

Molecular weight: 240.18.

USP requirements:
Sodium Sulfide USP—Preserve in tight containers, and store in a cool place. Contains not less than 98.0% and not more than 103.0% of sodium sulfide. Meets the requirements for Identification, Limit of iron (the solution is clear and colorless), and Limit of sulfite and thiosulfate (not more than 3.0 mL).

Sodium Sulfide Topical Gel USP—Preserve in tight containers at controlled room temperature or in a cool place. Contains the labeled amount, within −10% to +20%. Meets the requirements for Identification and pH (11.5–13.5).

SODIUM THIOSULFATE

Chemical name: Thiosulfuric acid, disodium salt, pentahydrate.

Molecular formula: $Na_2S_2O_3 \cdot 5H_2O$.

Molecular weight: 248.19.

Description: Sodium Thiosulfate USP—Large, colorless crystals or coarse, crystalline powder. Is deliquescent in moist air and effloresces in dry air at temperatures exceeding 33 °C. Its solutions are neutral or faintly alkaline to litmus.
NF category: Antioxidant.

Solubility: Sodium Thiosulfate USP—Very soluble in water; insoluble in alcohol.

USP requirements:
Sodium Thiosulfate USP—Preserve in tight containers. Contains not less than 99.0% and not more than 100.5% of sodium thiosulfate, calculated on the anhydrous basis. Meets the requirements for Identification, Water (32.0–37.0%), Calcium, and Heavy metals (not more than 0.002%).
Sodium Thiosulfate Injection USP—Preserve in single-dose containers, of Type I glass. A sterile solution of Sodium Thiosulfate in freshly boiled Water for Injection. Contains the labeled amount, within ±5%. Meets the requirements for Identification, Bacterial endotoxins, and pH (6.0–9.5), and for Injections.

SODIUM OXYBATE

Chemical name: Butanoic acid, 4-hydroxy-, sodium salt.

Molecular formula: $C_4H_7NaO_3$.

Molecular weight: 126.09 grams/mole.

Description: White to off-white crystalline powder.

Solubility: Very soluble in aqueous solutions.

USP requirements: Sodium Oxybate Oral Solution—Not in *USP–NF*.

SOMATREM

Source: Biosynthetic. A single polypeptide chain of 192 amino acids, one more (methionine) than naturally occurring human growth hormone, produced by a recombinant DNA process in *Escherichia coli*.

Chemical name: Somatotropin (human), *N*-L-methionyl-.

Molecular formula: $C_{995}H_{1537}N_{263}O_{301}S_8$.

Molecular weight: 22,255.97.

USP requirements: Somatrem for Injection—Not in *USP–NF*.

SOMATROPIN

Source: Somatropin, recombinant—Biosynthetic, produced by a recombinant DNA process in *Escherichia coli*; same amino acid sequence as pituitary-derived somatropin. A single polypeptide chain of 191 amino acids.

Chemical name: Growth hormone (human).

Molecular formula: $C_{990}H_{1528}N_{262}O_{300}S_7$.

Molecular weight: 22,124.77.

USP requirements:
Somatropin Injection—Not in *USP–NF*.
Somatropin for Injection—Not in *USP–NF*.
Somatropin, Recombinant, Injection—Not in *USP–NF*.
Somatropin, Recombinant, for Injection—Not in *USP–NF*.

SORBIC ACID

Chemical name: 2,4-Hexadienoic acid, (*E,E*)-; 2,4-Hexadienoic acid.

Molecular formula: $C_6H_8O_2$.

Molecular weight: 112.13.

Description: Sorbic Acid NF—Free-flowing, white, crystalline powder, having a characteristic odor.
NF category: Antimicrobial preservative.

Solubility: Sorbic Acid NF—Slightly soluble in water; soluble in alcohol and in ether.

NF requirements: Sorbic Acid NF—Preserve in tight containers, protected from light, and avoid exposure to excessive heat. Contains not less than 99.0% and not more than 101.0% of sorbic acid, calculated on the anhydrous basis. Meets the requirements for Identification, Melting range (132–135 °C), Water (not more than 0.5%), Residue on ignition (not more than 0.2%), Heavy metals (not more than 0.001%), and Organic volatile impurities.

SORBITAN MONOLAURATE

Chemical name: Sorbitan, esters, monododecanoate.

Description: Sorbitan Monolaurate NF—Yellow to amber oily liquid, having a bland, characteristic odor.
NF category: Emulsifying and/or solubilizing agent; wetting and/or solubilizing agent.

Solubility: Sorbitan Monolaurate NF—Insoluble in water; soluble in mineral oil; slightly soluble in cottonseed oil and in ethyl acetate.

NF requirements: Sorbitan Monolaurate NF—Preserve in tight containers. A partial ester of lauric acid with Sorbitol and its mono- and dianhydrides. Yields, upon saponification, not less than 55.0% and not more than 63.0% of fatty acids, and not less than 39.0% and not more than 45.0% of polyols (w/w). Meets the requirements for Identification, Water (not more than 1.5%), Residue on ignition (not more than 0.5%), Heavy metals (not more than 0.001%), Acid value (not more than 8), Hydroxyl value (330–358), Saponification value (158–170), and Organic volatile impurities.

SORBITAN MONOOLEATE

Chemical name: Sorbitan esters, mono(*Z*)-9-octadecenoate.

Molecular formula: $C_{24}H_{44}O_6$ (approximate).

Description: Sorbitan Monooleate NF—Viscous, yellow to amber-colored, oily liquid, having a bland, characteristic odor.
NF category: Emulsifying and/or solubilizing agent; wetting and/or solubilizing agent.

Solubility: Sorbitan Monooleate NF—Insoluble in water and in propylene glycol. Miscible with mineral and vegetable oils.

NF requirements: Sorbitan Monooleate NF—Preserve in tight containers. A partial oleate ester of Sorbitol and its mono- and dianhydrides. Yields, upon saponification, not less than 72.0% and not more than 78.0% of fatty acids, and not less than 25.0% and not more than 31.0% of polyols (w/w). Meets the requirements for Identification, Water (not more than 1.0%), Residue on ignition (not more than 0.5%), Heavy metals (not more than 0.001%), Acid value (not more than 8), Hydroxyl value (190–215), Iodine value (62–76), Saponification value (145–160), and Organic volatile impurities.

SORBITAN MONOPALMITATE

Chemical name: Sorbitan, esters, monohexadecanoate.

Molecular formula: $C_{22}H_{42}O_6$ (approximate).

Description: Sorbitan Monopalmitate NF—Cream-colored, waxy solid, having a faint fatty odor.
NF category: Emulsifying and/or solubilizing agent; wetting and/or solubilizing agent.

Solubility: Sorbitan Monopalmitate NF—Insoluble in water; soluble in warm absolute alcohol; soluble, with haze, in warm peanut oil and in warm mineral oil.

NF requirements: Sorbitan Monopalmitate NF—Preserve in well-closed containers. A partial ester of palmitic acid with Sorbitol and its mono- and dianhydrides. Yields, upon saponification, not less than 63.0% and not more than 71.0% of fatty acids, and not less than 32.0% and not more than 38.0% of polyols (w/w). Meets the requirements for Identification, Water (not more than 1.5%), Residue on ignition (not more than 0.5%), Heavy metals (not more than 0.001%), Acid value (not more than 8), Hydroxyl value (275–305), Saponification value (140–150), and Organic volatile impurities.

SORBITAN MONOSTEARATE

Chemical name: Sorbitan, esters, monooctadecanoate.

Molecular formula: $C_{24}H_{46}O_6$ (approximate).

Description: Sorbitan Monostearate NF—Cream-colored to tan, hard, waxy solid, having a bland odor.
NF category: Emulsifying and/or solubilizing agent; wetting and/or solubilizing agent.

Solubility: Sorbitan Monostearate NF—Insoluble in cold water and in acetone; dispersible in warm water; soluble, with haze, above 50 °C in mineral oil and in ethyl acetate.

NF requirements: Sorbitan Monostearate NF—Preserve in well-closed containers. A partial ester of Stearic Acid with Sorbitol and its mono- and dianhydrides. Yields, upon saponification, not less than 68.0% and not more than 76.0% of fatty acids, and not less than 27.0% and not more than 34.0% of polyols (w/w). Meets the requirements for Identification, Water (not more than 1.5%), Residue on ignition (not more than 0.5%),

Heavy metals (not more than 0.001%), Acid value (not more than 10), Hydroxyl value (235–260), Saponification value (147–157), and Organic volatile impurities.

SORBITAN SESQUIOLEATE

Chemical name: Sorbitan, esters, sesqui-9-octadecenoate, (*Z*)-.

Molecular formula: $C_{33}H_{60}O_{6.5}$ (approximate).

Description: Sorbitan Sesquioleate NF—Viscous, yellow to amber-colored, oily liquid.
  NF category: Emulsifying and/or solubilizing agent; wetting and/or solubilizing agent.

Solubility: Sorbitan Sesquioleate NF—Insoluble in water and in propylene glycol; soluble in alcohol, in isopropyl alcohol, in cottonseed oil, and in mineral oil.

NF requirements: Sorbitan Sesquioleate NF—Preserve in tight containers. A partial oleate ester of Sorbitol and its mono- and dianhydrides. Yields, upon saponification, not less than 74.0% and not more than 80.0% of fatty acids, and not less than 22.0% and not more than 28.0% of polyols (w/w). Meets the requirements for Identification, Water (not more than 1.0%), Residue on ignition (not more than 1.4%), Heavy metals (not more than 0.001%), Acid value (not more than 14), Hydroxyl value (182–220), Iodine value (65–75), and Saponification value (143–165).

SORBITAN TRIOLEATE

Chemical name: Sorbitan, esters, tri-9-octadecenoate, (*Z,Z,Z*)-.

Molecular formula: $C_{60}H_{108}O_8$ (approximate).

Description: Sorbitan Trioleate NF—Yellow to amber-colored, oily liquid.
  NF category: Emulsifying and/or solubilizing agent; wetting and/or solubilizing agent.

Solubility: Sorbitan Trioleate NF—Insoluble in water, in ethylene glycol, and in propylene glycol; soluble in methyl alcohol, in alcohol, in isopropyl alcohol, in corn oil, in cottonseed oil, and in mineral oil.

NF requirements: Sorbitan Trioleate NF—Preserve in tight containers. The triester of Oleic Acid and Sorbitol and its mono- and dianhydrides. Yields, upon saponification, not less than 85.5% and not more than 90.0% of fatty acids, and not less than 13.0% and not more than 19.0% of polyols (w/w). Meets the requirements for Identification, Water (not more than 0.7%), Residue on ignition (not more than 0.25%), Heavy metals (not more than 0.001%), Acid value (not more than 17), Hydroxyl value (50–75), Iodine value (77–85), and Saponification value (169–183).

SORBITOL

Chemical name: D-Glucitol.

Molecular formula: $C_6H_{14}O_6$.

Molecular weight: 182.17.

Description:
  Sorbitol NF—White, hygroscopic powder, granules, or flakes.
    NF category: Humectant; sweetening agent; tablet and/or capsule diluent.

Sorbitol Solution USP—Clear, colorless, syrupy liquid. Neutral to litmus.
  NF category: Sweetening agent; vehicle (flavored and/or sweetened).

Solubility: Sorbitol NF—Very soluble in water; slightly soluble in alcohol, in methanol, and in acetic acid.

USP requirements: Sorbitol Solution USP—Preserve in tight containers. A water solution containing, in each 100.0 grams, not less than 64.0 grams of D–1.465 at 20 °C), Water (28.5–31.5%), Residue on ignition (not more than 0.1%), Chloride (not more than 0.0035%), Sulfate (not more than 0.008%), Arsenic (not more than 2.5 ppm), Heavy metals (not more than 0.001%), and Reducing sugars.

NF requirements:
  Sorbitol NF—Preserve in tight containers. Contains not less than 91.0% and not more than 100.5% of sorbitol, calculated on the anhydrous basis. The amounts of other polyhydric alcohols, and any hexitol anhydrides, if detected, are not included in the requirements, nor the calculated amount under Other impurities. Meets the requirements for Identification, Water (not more than 1.0%), Residue on ignition (not more than 0.1%), Chloride (not more than 0.0050%), Sulfate (not more than 0.010%), Arsenic (not more than 3 ppm), Heavy metals (not more than 0.001%), Reducing sugars, Total sugars, and Organic volatile impurities.
  Noncrystallizing Sorbitol Solution NF—Preserve in tight containers. An aqueous solution of hydrogenated, fully and partially hydrolyzed starches. Contains not less than 45.0% of D-sorbitol (w/w). The amounts of total sugars, other polyhydric alcohols, and any hexitol anhydrides, if detected, are not included in the requirements nor the calculated amount under Other impurities. Meets the requirements for Identification, Specific gravity (not less than 1.290), Refractive index (1.457–1.467), Heavy metals (not more than 0.001%), and Reducing sugars, and for Water, Residue on ignition, Chloride, Sulfate, and Arsenic under Sorbitol Solution.

SOTALOL

Chemical name: Sotalol hydrochloride—Methanesulfonamide, *N*-[4-[1-hydroxy-2-[(1-methylethyl)amino]ethyl]phenyl]-, monohydrochloride.

Molecular formula: Sotalol hydrochloride—$C_{12}H_{20}N_2O_3S \cdot HCl$.

Molecular weight: Sotalol hydrochloride—308.83.

Description: Sotalol Hydrochloride USP—White to off-white powder.

Solubility: Sotalol Hydrochloride USP—Freely soluble in water; soluble in alcohol; very slightly soluble in chloroform.

Other characteristics: Lipid solubility—Low.

USP requirements:
  Sotalol Hydrochloride USP—Preserve in well-closed containers. Contains not less than 98.5% and not more than 101.5% of sotalol hydrochloride. Meets the requirements for Identification, Specific rotation (−0.7° to +0.7°), Water (not more than 0.5%), Residue on ignition (not more than 0.5%), Heavy metals (0.002%), Limit of methanol, isopropyl alcohol, and acetone, Related compounds, Organic volatile impurities, and Content of chloride (11.1–11.9%).

Sotalol Hydrochloride Tablets USP—Preserve in well-closed, light-resistant containers. Contain the labeled amount, within ±5%. Meet the requirements for Identification, Dissolution (80% in 30 minutes in water in Apparatus 2 at 50 rpm), and Uniformity of dosage units.

SOYBEAN OIL

Description: Soybean Oil USP—Clear, pale yellow, oily liquid having a characteristic odor.

NF category: Vehicle (oleaginous).

Solubility: Soybean Oil USP—Insoluble in water. Miscible with ether and with chloroform.

USP requirements: Soybean Oil USP—Preserve in tight, light-resistant containers, and avoid exposure to excessive heat. The refined fixed oil obtained from the seeds of the soya plant *Glycine soja* (Fam. Leguminosae). Meets the requirements for Specific gravity (0.916–0.922), Refractive index (1.465–1.475), Heavy metals (not more than 0.001%), Free fatty acids, Fatty acid composition, Iodine value (120–141), Saponification value (180–200), Unsaponifiable matter (not more than 1.0%), Cottonseed oil, and Peroxide.

SPARFLOXACIN

Chemical name: 3-Quinolinecarboxylic acid, 5-amino-1-cyclopropyl-7-(3,5-dimethyl-1-piperazinyl)-6,8-difluoro-1,4-dihydro-4-oxo-, *cis*-.

Molecular formula: $C_{19}H_{22}F_2N_4O_3$.

Molecular weight: 392.40.

Description: Yellow crystalline powder.

Solubility: Sparingly soluble in glacial acetic acid and in chloroform; very slightly soluble in ethanol; practically insoluble in water and in ether.

USP requirements: Sparfloxacin Tablets—Not in *USP–NF*.

SPECTINOMYCIN

Source: Produced by a species of the soil microorganism *Streptomyces spectabilis*.

Chemical name: Spectinomycin hydrochloride—4*H*-Pyrano[2,3*b*][1,4]benzodioxin-4-one, decahydro-4a,7,9-trihydroxy-2-methyl-6,8-bis(methylamino)-, dihydrochloride, pentahydrate.

Molecular formula: Spectinomycin hydrochloride—$C_{14}H_{24}N_2O_7 \cdot$ 2HCl · 5H₂O.

Molecular weight: Spectinomycin hydrochloride—495.35.

Description: Spectinomycin Hydrochloride USP—White to pale-buff crystalline powder.

Solubility: Spectinomycin Hydrochloride USP—Freely soluble in water; practically insoluble in alcohol, in chloroform, and in ether.

USP requirements:
Spectinomycin Hydrochloride USP—Preserve in tight containers. Where it is intended for use in preparing injectable dosage forms, the label states that it is sterile or must be subjected to further processing during the preparation of injectable dosage forms. Has a potency equivalent to not

less than 603 mcg of spectinomycin per mg. Meets the requirements for Identification, Crystallinity, Bacterial endotoxins (where the label states that Spectinomycin Hydrochloride is sterile or that it must be subjected to further processing during the preparation of injectable dosage forms), Sterility (where the label states that Spectinomycin Hydrochloride is sterile), pH (3.8–5.6, in a solution containing 10 mg per mL), Water (16.0–20.0%), and Residue on ignition (not more than 1.0%).

Spectinomycin for Injectable Suspension USP—Preserve in Containers for Sterile Solids. Contains an amount of Spectinomycin Hydrochloride equivalent to the labeled amount of spectinomycin, within −10% to +20%. Meets the requirement for pH (4.0–7.0), in the suspension constituted as directed in the labeling. Conforms to the definition and meets the requirements for Identification test, Crystallinity, Bacterial endotoxins, Sterility, Water, and Residue on ignition under Spectinomycin Hydrochloride, and for Uniformity of dosage units and Labeling under Injections.

SPIRAMYCIN

Source: Produced by *Streptomyces ambofaciens*.

Chemical name: Leucomycin.

Molecular formula: $C_{43}H_{74}N_2O_{14}$.

Molecular weight: 843.1.

Description: White or slightly yellowish, slightly hygroscopic powder.

Solubility: Slightly soluble in water; freely soluble in alcohol, in acetone, and in methyl alcohol; sparingly soluble in ether.

USP requirements:
Spiramycin Capsules—Not in *USP–NF*.
Spiramycin Tablets—Not in *USP–NF*.
Spiramycin Adipate Injection—Not in *USP–NF*.
Spiramycin Adipate Suppositories—Not in *USP–NF*.

SPIRONOLACTONE

Chemical name: Pregn-4-ene-21-carboxylic acid, 7-(acetylthio)-17-hydroxy-3-oxo-, gamma-lactone, (7 alpha,17 alpha)-.

Molecular formula: $C_{24}H_{32}O_4S$.

Molecular weight: 416.57.

Description: Spironolactone USP—Light cream-colored to light tan, crystalline powder. Has a faint to mild mercaptan-like odor; is stable in air.

Solubility: Spironolactone USP—Practically insoluble in water; freely soluble in chloroform; soluble in ethyl acetate and in alcohol; slightly soluble in methanol and in fixed oils.

USP requirements:
Spironolactone USP—Preserve in well-closed containers. Contains not less than 97.0% and not more than 103.0% of spironolactone, calculated on the dried basis. Meets the requirements for Identification, Melting range (198–209 °C, with decomposition), Specific rotation (−33° to −37°), Loss on drying (not more than 0.5%), Limit of mercapto compounds, Ordinary impurities, and Organic volatile impurities.

Spironolactone Tablets USP—Preserve in tight, light-resistant containers. Contain the labeled amount, within ±5%. Meet the requirements for Identification, Dissolution (75% in 60

minutes in 0.1 *N* hydrochloric acid containing 0.1% of sodium lauryl sulfate in Apparatus 2 at 75 rpm), and Uniformity of dosage units.

SPIRONOLACTONE AND HYDROCHLOROTHIAZIDE

For *Spironolactone* and *Hydrochlorothiazide*—See individual listings for chemistry information.

USP requirements: Spironolactone and Hydrochlorothiazide Tablets USP—Preserve in tight, light-resistant containers. Contain the labeled amounts, within ±10%. Meet the requirements for Identification, Dissolution (75% of each active ingredient in 60 minutes in 0.1 *N* hydrochloric acid containing 0.1% sodium lauryl sulfate in Apparatus 2 at 75 rpm), and Uniformity of dosage units.

SQUALANE

Chemical name: Tetracosane, 2,6,10,15,19,23-hexamethyl-.

Molecular formula: $C_{30}H_{62}$.

Molecular weight: 422.81.

Description: Squalane NF—Colorless, practically odorless transparent oil.
NF category: Ointment base; vehicle (oleaginous).

Solubility: Squalane NF—Insoluble in water; very slightly soluble in absolute alcohol; slightly soluble in acetone. Miscible with ether and with chloroform.

NF requirements: Squalane NF—Preserve in tight containers. A saturated hydrocarbon obtained by hydrogenation of squalene, an aliphatic triterpene occurring in some fish oils. Meets the requirements for Identification, Specific gravity (0.807–0.810 at 20 °C), Refractive index (1.4510–1.4525 at 20 °C), Residue on ignition (not more than 0.5%), Acid value (not more than 0.2), Iodine value (not more than 4), Saponification value (not more than 2), and Chromatographic purity.

STANNOUS FLUORIDE

Chemical name: Tin fluoride (SnF_2).

Molecular formula: SnF_2.

Molecular weight: 156.71.

Description: Stannous Fluoride USP—White, crystalline powder. Melts at about 213 °C.

Solubility: Stannous Fluoride USP—Freely soluble in water; practically insoluble in alcohol, in ether, and in chloroform.

USP requirements:
Stannous Fluoride USP—Preserve in well-closed containers. Contains not less than 71.2% of stannous tin, and not less than 22.3% and not more than 25.5% of fluoride, calculated on the dried basis. Meets the requirements for Identification, pH (2.8–3.5, in a freshly prepared 0.4% solution), Loss on drying (not more than 0.5%), Water-insoluble substances (not more than 0.2%), and Antimony (not more than 0.005%).
Stannous Fluoride Gel USP—Preserve in well-closed containers. Contains the labeled amount, within −5% to +15%, in a suitable medium containing a suitable viscosity-inducing agent. Meets the requirements for Identification, Viscosity

(600–170,000 centipoises), pH (2.8–4.0, in a freshly prepared mixture with water [1:1]), Total tin content, and Stannous ion content.
Note: If Glycerin is used as the medium in the preparation of this Gel, use Glycerin that has a low water content, that is, Glycerin having a specific gravity of not less than 1.2607, corresponding to a concentration of 99.5%.

STANOZOLOL

Chemical group: 17-alpha alkylated anabolic steroid.

Chemical name: 2'*H*-Androst-2-eno[3,2-*c*]pyrazol-17-ol, 17-methyl-, (5 alpha,17 beta)-.

Molecular formula: $C_{21}H_{32}N_2O$.

Molecular weight: 328.49.

Description: Stanozolol USP—Odorless, crystalline powder, occurring in two forms: as needles, melting at about 155 °C, and as prisms, melting at about 235 °C.

Solubility: Stanozolol USP—Insoluble in water; soluble in dimethylformamide; sparingly soluble in alcohol and in chloroform; slightly soluble in ethyl acetate and in acetone.

USP requirements:
Stanozolol USP—Preserve in tight, light-resistant containers. Contains not less than 98.0% and not more than 100.5% of stanozolol, calculated on the dried basis. Meets the requirements for Identification, Specific rotation (+34° to +40°), Loss on drying (not more than 1.0%), Chromatographic purity, and Organic volatile impurities.
Stanozolol Tablets USP—Preserve in tight, light-resistant containers. Contain the labeled amount, within ±10%. Meet the requirements for Identification, Dissolution (75% in 45 minutes in 0.1 *N* hydrochloric acid in Apparatus 2 at 50 rpm), and Uniformity of dosage units.

STARCH

Chemical name: Starch.

Description: Starch NF—Irregular, angular, white masses or fine powder. Odorless.
NF category: Tablet and/or capsule diluent; tablet disintegrant.

Solubility: Starch NF—Insoluble in cold water and in alcohol.

NF requirements: Starch NF—Preserve in well-closed containers. Consists of the granules separated from the mature grain of corn (*Zea mays* Linné [Fam. Gramineae]) or of wheat (*Triticum aestivum* Linné [Fam. Gramineae]), or from tubers of the potato (*Solanum tuberosum* Linné [Fam. Solanaceae]) or of tapioca (*Manihot utilissima* Pehl [Fam. Euphorbi Aceae]). Label it to indicate the botanical source from which it was derived. Meets the requirements for Botanic characteristics, Identification, Microbial limits, pH (4.5–7.0 for Corn starch, Tapioca starch, and Wheat starch, and 5.0–8.0 for Potato starch), Loss on drying (not more than 14.0%), Residue on ignition (not more than 0.5%), Iron (not more than 0.002%), Oxidizing substances (not more than 0.002%), Sulfur dioxide (not more than 0.008%), and Organic volatile impurities.

Note: Starches obtained from different botanical sources may not have identical properties with respect to their use for specific pharmaceutical purposes, e.g., as a tablet-disinte-

grating agent. Therefore, types of starch should not be interchanged unless performance equivalency has been ascertained.

PREGELATINIZED STARCH

Description: Pregelatinized Starch NF—Moderately coarse to fine, white to off-white powder. Odorless.
  NF category: Tablet binder; tablet and/or capsule diluent; tablet disintegrant.

Solubility: Pregelatinized Starch NF—Slightly soluble to soluble in cold water; insoluble in alcohol.

NF requirements: Pregelatinized Starch NF—Starch that has been chemically and/or mechanically processed to rupture all or part of the granules in the presence of water and subsequently dried. Some types of Pregelatinized Starch may be modified to render them compressible and flowable in character. Meets the requirements for pH (4.5–7.0, determined potentiometrically), Iron (not more than 0.002%), Oxidizing substances, Sulfur dioxide (not more than 0.008%), and Organic volatile impurities, and for Identification test B, Packaging and storage, Labeling, Microbial limits, Loss on drying, and Residue on ignition under Starch.

TOPICAL STARCH

USP requirements: Topical Starch USP—Preserve in well-closed containers. Consists of the granules separated from the mature grain of corn (*Zea mays* Linné [Fam. Gramineae]). Meets the requirements for Botanic characteristics, Identification, Microbial limits, pH (4.5–7.0, determined potentiometrically), Loss on drying (not more than 14.0%), Residue on ignition (not more than 0.5%), Iron (not more than 0.001%), Oxidizing substances (not more than 0.018%), and Sulfur dioxide (not more than 0.008%).

STAVUDINE

Chemical name: Thymidine, 2′,3′-didehydro-3′-deoxy-.

Molecular formula: $C_{10}H_{12}N_2O_4$.

Molecular weight: 224.21.

Description: White to off-white crystalline solid.

Solubility: At 23 °C, approximately 83 mg/mL in water and 30 mg/mL in propylene glycol.

Other characteristics: *N*-octanol/water partition coefficient at 23 °C—0.144.

USP requirements:
  Stavudine Capsules—Not in *USP–NF*.
  Stavudine for Oral Solution—Not in *USP–NF*.

STEARIC ACID

Chemical name: Octadecanoic acid.

Molecular formula: $C_{18}H_{36}O_2$.

Molecular weight: 284.48.

Description: Stearic Acid NF—Hard, white or faintly yellowish, somewhat glossy and crystalline solid, or white or yellowish-white powder. Slight odor, suggesting tallow.
  NF category: Emulsifying and/or solubilizing agent; tablet and/or capsule lubricant.

Solubility: Stearic Acid NF—Practically insoluble in water; freely soluble in chloroform and in ether; soluble in alcohol.

NF requirements: Stearic Acid NF—Preserve in well-closed containers. Manufactured from fats and oils derived from edible sources and is a mixture of Stearic Acid and palmitic acid. The content of Stearic Acid is not less than 40.0%, and the sum of the two is not less than 90.0%. If it is for external use only, the labeling so indicates. Meets the requirements for Congealing temperature (not lower than 54 °C), Residue on ignition (not more than 0.1%), Heavy metals (not more than 0.001%), Mineral acid, Neutral fat or paraffin, Iodine value (not more than 4), and Organic volatile impurities.
  Note: Stearic Acid labeled solely for external use is exempt from the requirement that it be prepared from edible sources.

PURIFIED STEARIC ACID

Description: Purified Stearic Acid NF—Hard, white or faintly yellowish, somewhat glossy and crystalline solid, or white or yellowish-white powder. Its odor is slight, suggesting tallow.
  NF category: Tablet and/or capsule lubricant.

Solubility: Purified Stearic Acid NF—Practically insoluble in water; freely soluble in chloroform and in ether; soluble in alcohol.

NF requirements: Purified Stearic Acid NF—Preserve in well-closed containers. Manufactured from fats and oils derived from edible sources and is a mixture of Stearic Acid and palmitic acid, which together constitute not less than 96.0% of the total content. The content of Stearic Acid is not less than 90.0% of the total. If it is for external use only, the labeling so indicates. Meets the requirements for Congealing temperature (66–69 °C), Acid value (195–200), Iodine value (not more than 1.5), and Organic volatile impurities, and for Residue on ignition, Heavy metals, Mineral acid, and Neutral fat or paraffin under Stearic Acid.
  Note: Purified Stearic Acid labeled solely for external use is exempt from the requirement that it be prepared from edible sources.

STEARYL ALCOHOL

Chemical name: 1-Octadecanol.

Molecular formula: $C_{18}H_{38}O$.

Molecular weight: 270.49.

Description: Stearyl Alcohol NF—Unctuous, white flakes or granules. Has a faint, characteristic odor.
  NF category: Stiffening agent.

Solubility: Stearyl Alcohol NF—Insoluble in water; soluble in alcohol and in ether.

NF requirements: Stearyl Alcohol NF—Preserve in well-closed containers. Contains not less than 90.0% of stearyl alcohol, the remainder consisting chiefly of related alcohols. Meets the requirements for Identification, Melting range (55–60 °C), Acid value (not more than 2), Iodine value (not more than 2), and Hydroxyl value (195–220).

ST. JOHN'S WORT

NF requirements:

St. John's Wort NF—Store in tight containers, protected from light and moisture. The label states the Latin binomial name and, following the official name, the parts of the plant contained in the article. Consists of the dried flowering tops or aerial parts of *Hypericum perforatum* Linné (Fam. Hypericaceae), gathered shortly before or during flowering. Contains not less than 0.04% of the combined total of hypericin and pseudohypericin and not less than 0.6% of hyperforin. Meets the requirements for Botanical characteristics, Identificaton, Total ash (not more than 5.0%), Water content (not more than 10.0%), Foreign organic matter (not more than 2.0%), Pesticide residues, Microbial limits, and Content of hypericin and pseudohypericin, and Content of hyperforin.

Powdered St. John's Wort NF—Store in tight containers, protected from light and moisture. It is St. John's Wort reduced to a fine or a very fine powder. The label states the Latin binomial name and, following the official name, the parts of the plant source from which the article was derived. Contains not less than 0.6% of hyperforin and not less than 0.04% of hypericin and pseudohypericin combined. Meets the requirements for Botanic characteristics and Heavy metals (not more than 0.002%), and for Identification, Total ash, Water content, Foreign organic matter, Pestiside residues, Microbial limits, Content of hypericin and pseudohypericin, and Content of hyperforin under St. John's Wort.

Powdered St. John's Wort Extract NF—Preserve in tight containers, protected from moisture and light. Prepared from comminuted St. John's Wort extracted with 80% methanol or other suitable solvents. The ratio of the starting crude plant material to Powdered Extract is between 3:1 and 7:1. The label states the Latin binomial and, following the official name, the part of the plant from which the article was prepared. The label also indicates the content of hypericin, pseudohypericin, and hyperforin; the extracting solvent or solvent mixture used for preparation; and the ratio of the starting crude plant material to Powdered Extract. Contains not less than 0.2% of the combined total of hypericin and pseudohypericin and not less than 3.0% of hyperforin. Meets the requirements for Identification, Water (not more than 5.0%), Total ash (not more than 7.0%), Pesticide residues, Heavy metals (0.005%), Organic volatile impurities, Content of hypericin and pseudohypericin, and Content of hyperforin, and for Residue on evaporation, Residual solvents, and Heavy metals for Botanical Extracts.

STORAX

Description: Storax USP—Semiliquid, grayish to grayish-brown, sticky, opaque mass depositing on standing a heavy dark brown layer (Levant Storax); or semisolid, sometimes a solid mass, softened by gently warming (American Storax). Is transparent in thin layers, has a characteristic odor, and is more dense than water.

Solubility: Storax USP—Insoluble in water; soluble, usually incompletely, in an equal weight of warm alcohol; soluble in acetone, in carbon disulfide, and in ether, some insoluble residue usually remaining.

USP requirements: Storax USP—Preserve in well-closed containers. A balsam obtained from the trunk of *Liquidambar orientalis* Miller, known in commerce as Levant Storax, or of *Liquidambar styraciflua* Linné, known in commerce as American Storax (Fam. Hamamelidaceae). Meets the requirements for Loss on drying (not more than 20.0%), Alcohol-insoluble substances (not more than 5.0%), Alcohol-soluble substances, Acid value, Saponification value, Cinnamic acid (acid value 50–85 for Levant Storax and 36–85 for American Storax and saponification value 160–200), and Organic volatile impurities.

STREPTOKINASE

Source: A protein obtained from culture filtrates of certain strains of *Streptococcus haemolyticus* group C.

Molecular weight: About 46,000 daltons.

Description: Hygroscopic white powder or friable solid.

Solubility: Freely soluble in water.

USP requirements: Streptokinase for Injection—Not in *USP–NF*.

STREPTOMYCIN

Source: Derived from *Streptomyces griseus.*

Chemical name: Streptomycin sulfate—D-Streptamine, *O*-2-deoxy-2-(methylamino)-alpha-L-glucopyranosyl-(1→2)-*O*-5-deoxy-3-*C*-formyl-alpha-L-lyxofuranosyl-(1→4)-*N*,*N*′bis(aminoiminomethyl)-, sulfate (2:3) (salt).

Molecular formula: Streptomycin sulfate—$(C_{21}H_{39}N_7O_{12})_2 \cdot 3H_2SO_4$.

Molecular weight: Streptomycin sulfate—1457.39.

Description:

Streptomycin Injection USP—Clear, colorless to yellow, viscous liquid. Is odorless or has a slight odor.

Streptomycin Sulfate USP—White or practically white powder. Is odorless or has not more than a faint odor. Is hygroscopic, but is stable in air and on exposure to light. Its solutions are acid to practically neutral to litmus.

Solubility: Streptomycin Sulfate USP—Freely soluble in water; very slightly soluble in alcohol; practically insoluble in chloroform.

USP requirements:

Streptomycin Injection USP—Preserve in single-dose or in multiple-dose containers, preferably of Type I glass. Contains an amount of streptomycin sulfate equivalent to the labeled amount of streptomycin, within −10% to +15%. Meets the requirements for Bacterial endotoxins and pH (5.0–8.0), for Identification test A, and Sterility under Streptomycin for Injection, and for Injections.

Streptomycin for Injection USP—Preserve in Containers for Sterile Solids. Contains an amount of streptomycin sulfate equivalent to the labeled amount of streptomycin, within −10% to +15%. Meets the requirements for Constituted solution, Identification, Bacterial endotoxins, Sterility, pH (4.5–7.0, in a solution containing 200 mg of streptomycin per mL), and Loss on drying (not more than 5.0%), and for Uniformity of dosage units and Labeling under Injections.

Streptomycin Sulfate USP—Preserve in tight containers. Where it is intended for use in preparing injectable dosage forms, the label states that it is sterile or must be subjected to further processing during the preparation of injectable dosage forms. Has a potency equivalent to not less than 650 mcg and not more than 850 mcg of streptomycin per mg. Meets the requirements for Identification, pH (4.5–7.0, in a solution containing 200 mg of streptomycin per mL), and Loss on drying (not more than 5.0%), and for Sterility tests and Bacterial endotoxins under Streptomycin for Injection (where the label states that Streptomycin Sulfate is sterile) and for Bacterial endotoxins under Streptomycin for Injection (where the label states that Streptomycin Sulfate must be subjected to further processing during the preparation of injectable dosage forms), and for Uniformity of dosage units and Labeling under Injections.

STREPTOZOCIN

Chemical name: D-Glucopyranose, 2-deoxy-2-[[(methylnitrosoamino)carbonyl]amino]-.

Molecular formula: $C_8H_{15}N_3O_7$.

Molecular weight: 265.22.

Description: Ivory-colored crystalline powder.

Solubility: Very soluble in water or in physiological saline; soluble in alcohol.

USP requirements: Streptozocin for Injection—Not in *USP–NF*.

STRONTIUM CHLORIDE SR 89

Chemical name: Strontium chloride ($^{89}SrCl_2$).

Molecular formula: $^{89}SrCl_2$.

Molecular weight: 159.9.

USP requirements: Strontium Chloride Sr 89 Injection USP—Preserve in single-dose containers that are adequately shielded. A sterile solution of radioactive strontium (^{89}Sr) processed in the form of strontium chloride in Water for Injection. Label it to include the following, in addition to the information specified for Labeling under Injections: the time and date of calibration; the amount of strontium chloride expressed as mg of strontium per mL; the amount of ^{89}Sr as labeled strontium chloride expressed as total megabecquerels (or millicuries) and concentration as megabecquerels per mL (or as millicuries per mL) on the date and time of calibration; the expiration date; and the statement "Caution—Radioactive Material." The labeling indicates that in making dosage calculations, correction is to be made for radioactive decay, and also indicates that the radioactive half-life of ^{89}Sr is 50.5 days. Contains the labeled amount of ^{89}Sr as strontium chloride, within ±10%, expressed in megabecquerels (or in millicuries) per mL at the time indicated in the labeling. Meets the requirements for Specific activity, Radionuclide identification, Bacterial endotoxins, pH (4.0–7.5), Radionuclidic purity, and Chemical purity (limit of aluminum, not more than 2 micrograms per gram), and for Injections (except that it is not subject to the recommendation on Volume in Container).

SUCCIMER

Chemical name: Butanedioic acid, 2,3-dimercapto-, (R*,S*)-.

Molecular formula: $C_4H_6O_4S_2$.

Molecular weight: 182.22.

Description: White, crystalline powder with an unpleasant, characteristic mercaptan odor.

USP requirements: Succimer Capsules—Not in *USP–NF*.

SUCCINYLCHOLINE

Chemical name: Succinylcholine chloride—Ethanaminium, 2,2′-[(1,4-dioxo-1,4-butanediyl)bis(oxy)]bis[N,N,N-trimethyl-], dichloride.

Molecular formula: Succinylcholine chloride—$C_{14}H_{30}Cl_2N_2O_4$.

Molecular weight: Succinylcholine chloride—361.30.

Description:
Succinylcholine Chloride USP—White, odorless, crystalline powder. Its solutions have a pH of about 4. The dihydrate form melts at about 160 °C; the anhydrous form melts at about 190 °C, and is hygroscopic.
Succinylcholine Chloride for Injection USP—White, odorless, crystalline powder. Its solutions have a pH of about 4. The dihydrate form melts at about 160 °C; the anhydrous form melts at about 190 °C, and is hygroscopic.

Solubility:
Succinylcholine Chloride USP—Freely soluble in water; slightly soluble in alcohol and in chloroform; practically insoluble in ether.
Succinylcholine Chloride for Injection USP—Freely soluble in water; slightly soluble in alcohol and in chloroform; practically insoluble in ether.

USP requirements:
Succinylcholine Chloride USP—Preserve in tight containers. Usually contains approximately two molecules of water of hydration. Label it in terms of its anhydrous equivalent. Where it is intended for use in preparing injectable or other sterile dosage forms, the label states that it is sterile or must be subjected to further processing during the preparation of injectable dosage forms. Contains not less than 96.0% and not more than 102.0% of succinylcholine chloride, calculated on the anhydrous basis. Meets the requirements for Identification, Water (not more than 10.0%), Residue on ignition (not more than 0.2%), Limit of ammonium salts, Chromatographic purity, and Chloride content (19.3–19.8%), and for Sterility tests and for Bacterial endotoxins under Succinylcholine Chloride for Injection (where the label states that Succinylcholine Chloride is sterile), and for Bacterial endotoxins under Succinylcholine Chloride for Injection (where the label states that Succinylcholine Chloride must be subjected to further processing during the preparation of injectable dosage forms).
Succinylcholine Chloride Injection USP—Preserve in single-dose or in multiple-dose containers, preferably of Type I or Type II glass, in a refrigerator. A sterile solution of Succinylcholine Chloride in a suitable aqueous vehicle. Label it to indicate, as its expiration date, the month and year not more than 2 years from the month during which the Injection was last assayed and released by the manufacturer. Contains an amount of succinylcholine chloride equivalent to the labeled amount of anhydrous succinylcholine chloride, within ±10%. Meets the requirements for Identification, Bacterial endotoxins, and pH (3.0–4.5), and for Injections.

Succinylcholine Chloride for Injection USP—Preserve in Containers for Sterile Solids. It is Succinylcholine Chloride suitable for parenteral use. Meets the requirements for Completeness of solution, Constituted solution, Bacterial endotoxins, and Chromatographic purity (not more than 2.0%), for Identification, Water, Residue on ignition, Limit of ammonium salts, and Chloride content under Succinylcholine Chloride, and for Sterility tests, Uniformity of dosage units, and Labeling under Injections.

SUCRALFATE

Chemical name: Alpha-D-glucopyranoside, beta-D-fructofuranosyl-, octakis(hydrogen sulfate), aluminum complex.

Molecular formula: $C_{12}H_mAl_{16}O_nS_8$.

Description: Whitish or white, odorless, amorphous powder.

Solubility: Soluble in dilute hydrochloric acid and in sodium hydroxide; practically insoluble in water, in boiling water, in ethanol, and in chloroform.

Other characteristics: Metal salt of a sulfated disaccharide.

USP requirements:
Sucralfate USP—Preserve in tight containers. The hydrous basic aluminum salt of sucrose octasulfate. Contains the equivalent of not less than 30.0% and not more than 38.0% of sucrose octasulfate. Meets the requirements for Clarity and color of solution, Identification, Acid neutralizing capacity (not less than 12 milliequivalent), Chloride (not more than 0.50%), Arsenic (not more than 4 ppm), Heavy metals (not more than 0.002%), Limit of pyridine and 2-methylpyridine (not more than 0.05% of each), Limit of sucrose heptasulfate (not more than 0.1), Aluminum content (15.5–18.5%, calculated on an "as is" basis), and Organic volatile impurities.
Sucralfate Suspension—Not in *USP–NF*.
Sucralfate Oral Suspension–Not in *USP–NF*.
Sucralfate Tablets USP—Preserve in tight containers. Contain the labeled amount, within ±10%, corresponding to not less than 30.6% and not more than 37.4% of sucrose octasulfate. Meet the requirements for Identification, Disintegration (15 minutes), Uniformity of dosage units, and Acid neutralizing capacity (not less than 12 milliequivalent).

SUCRALOSE

Chemical name: 1,6-Dichloro-1,6-dideoxy-beta-D-fructofuranosyl-4-chloro-4-deoxy-alpha-D-galactopyranoside.

Molecular formula: $C_{12}H_{19}Cl_3O_8$.

Molecular weight: 397.64.

Description: Sucralose NF—White to off-white crystalline powder.
NF category: Sweetening agent.

Solubility: Sucralose NF—Freely soluble in water, in methanol, and in alcohol; slightly soluble in ethyl acetate.

NF requirements: Preserve in well-closed containers, in a cool, dry place, at a temperature not exceeding 21 °C. Contains not less than 98.0% and not more than 102.0% of sucralose, calculated on an anhydrous basis. Meets the requirements for Identification, Specific rotation (+84.0° to +87.5°, determined at 20°), Water (not more than 2.0%), Residue on ignition (not more than 0.7%), Heavy metals (not more than 0.001%), Limit of hydrolysis products (not more than 0.1%), Limit of methanol (not more than 0.1%), and Related compounds (not more than 0.5%).

SUCROSE

Chemical name: Alpha-D-glucopyranoside, beta-D-fructofuranosyl-.

Molecular formula: $C_{12}H_{22}O_{11}$.

Molecular weight: 342.30.

Description: Sucrose NF—White, crystalline powder or lustrous, dry, colorless or white crystals.

Solubility: Sucrose NF—Very soluble in water; slightly soluble in alcohol; practically insoluble in dehydrated alcohol.

NF requirements: Sucrose NF—Preserve in well-closed containers. A sugar obtained from *Saccharum officinarum* Linné (Fam. Gramineae), *Beta vulgaris* Linné (Fam. Chenopodiaceae), and other sources. Contains no added substances. Meets the requirements for Specific rotation (not less than +65.9°), Residue on ignition (not more than 0.05%, a 5-gram specimen being used), Chloride (not more than 0.0035%), Sulfate (not more than 0.006%), Calcium, Heavy metals (not more than 5 ppm), Invert sugar, and Organic volatile impurities.

SUCROSE OCTAACETATE

Chemical name: Alpha-D-glucopyranoside, 1,3,4,6-tetra-*O*-acetyl-beta-D-fructofuranosyl, tetraacetate.

Molecular formula: $C_{28}H_{38}O_{19}$.

Molecular weight: 678.59.

Description: Sucrose Octaacetate NF—White, practically odorless powder. Hygroscopic.
NF category: Alcohol denaturant.

Solubility: Sucrose Octaacetate NF—Very slightly soluble in water; very soluble in methanol and in chloroform; soluble in alcohol and in ether.

NF requirements: Sucrose Octaacetate NF—Preserve in tight containers. Contains not less than 98.0% and not more than 100.5% of sucrose octaacetate, calculated on the anhydrous basis. Meets the requirements for Melting temperature (not lower than 78 °C), Acidity, Water (not more than 1.0%), and Residue on ignition (not more than 0.1%).

SUFENTANIL

Chemical group: Fentanyl derivatives are anilinopiperidine-derivative opioid analgesics and are chemically related to anileridine and meperidine.

Chemical name: Sufentanil citrate—Propanamide, *N*-[4-(methoxymethyl)-1-[2-(thienyl)ethyl]-4-piperidinyl]-*N*-phenyl-, 2-hydroxy-1,2,3-propanetricarboxylate (1:1).

Molecular formula: Sufentanil citrate—$C_{22}H_{30}N_2O_2S \cdot C_6H_8O_7$.

Molecular weight: Sufentanil citrate—578.68.

Description: Sufentanil Citrate USP—White powder. Melts between 133 and 140 °C.

pKa: Sufentanil citrate—8.01.

Solubility: Sufentanil Citrate USP—Soluble in water; freely soluble in methanol; sparingly soluble in acetone, in alcohol, and in chloroform.

Other characteristics: Log partition coefficient (*n*-octanol/aqueous buffer solution at pH 10.8)—3.95.

USP requirements:
Sufentanil Citrate USP—Preserve in well-closed containers. Contains not less than 98.0% and not more than 101.0% of sufentanil citrate, calculated on the dried basis. Meets the requirements for Identification, Loss on drying (not more than 0.5%), Heavy metals (not more than 0.002%), Limit of acetone (not more than 0.5%), and Chromatographic purity.

Caution: Handle Sufentanil Citrate with great care since it is a potent opioid analgesic. Great care should be taken to prevent inhaling particles of Sufentanil Citrate and exposing the skin to it.

Sufentanil Citrate Injection USP—Preserve in single-dose or in multiple-dose containers, preferably of Type I glass. A sterile solution of Sufentanil Citrate in Water for Injection. Contains an amount of sufentanil citrate equivalent to the labeled amount of sufentanil, within ±10%, as the citrate. Meets the requirements for Identification, Bacterial endotoxins, pH (3.5–6.0), and Particulate matter, and for Injections.

Caution: Handle Sufentanil Citrate Injection with great care since it is a potent opioid analgesic.

COMPRESSIBLE SUGAR

Description: Compressible Sugar NF—Practically white, crystalline, odorless powder. Stable in air.

NF category: Sweetening agent; tablet and/or capsule diluent.

Solubility: Compressible Sugar NF—The sucrose portion of Compressible Sugar is very soluble in water.

NF requirements: Compressible Sugar NF—Preserve in well-closed containers. Previously dried at 105 °C for 4 hours, contains not less than 95.0% and not more than 98.0% of sucrose. Meets the requirements for Identification, Microbial limits, Loss on drying (0.25–1.0%), Residue on ignition (not more than 0.1%), Chloride, Sulfate, Calcium, Heavy metals (not more than 0.014% for chloride, not more than 0.010% for sulfate, and not more than 5 ppm for heavy metals), and Organic volatile impurities.

CONFECTIONER'S SUGAR

Description: Confectioner≈s Sugar NF—Fine, white, odorless powder. Stable in air.

NF category: Sweetening agent; tablet and/or capsule diluent.

Solubility: Confectioner's Sugar NF—The sucrose portion of Confectioner's Sugar is soluble in cold water. Freely soluble in boiling water.

NF requirements: Confectioner's Sugar NF—Preserve in well-closed containers. It is Sucrose ground together with corn starch to a fine powder. Contains not less than 95.0% of sucrose, calculated on the dried basis. Meets the requirements for Identification, Specific rotation, Chloride, Calcium, Sulfate, and Heavy metals (not less than +62.6°, calculated on the dried basis, for specific rotation, not more than 0.014% for chloride, not more than 0.006% for sulfate, and not more than

5 ppm for heavy metals), Microbial limits, Loss on drying (not more than 1.0%), Residue on ignition (not more than 0.08%), and Organic volatile impurities.

INVERT SUGAR

USP requirements: Invert Sugar Injection USP—Preserve in single-dose containers, preferably of Type I or Type II glass, or of a suitable plastic material. A sterile solution of a mixture of equal amounts of Dextrose and Fructose in Water for Injection, or an equivalent sterile solution produced by the hydrolysis of Sucrose, in Water for Injection. Contains no antimicrobial agents. The label states the total osmolar concentration in mOsmol per liter. Contains the labeled amount of fructose, within ±5%. Meets the requirements for Identification, Bacterial endotoxins, pH (3.0–6.5), Chloride (not more than 0.012%), Heavy metals, Limit of 5-hydroxymethylfurfural and related substances, and Completeness of inversion, and for Injections.

Note: Invert Sugar Injection that is produced by mixing Dextrose and Fructose is exempt from the requirement of the test for Completeness of inversion.

SUGAR SPHERES

Description: Sugar Spheres NF—Hard, brittle, free-flowing, spherical masses ranging generally in size from 10- to 60-mesh. Usually white, but may be colored.

NF category: Vehicle (solid carrier).

Solubility: Sugar Spheres NF—Solubility in water varies according to the sugar-to-starch ratio.

NF requirements: Sugar Spheres NF—Preserve in well-closed containers. The label states the nominal particle size range. Contain not less than 62.5% and not more than 91.5% of sucrose, calculated on the dried basis, the remainder consisting chiefly of starch. Consist of approximately spherical particles of a labeled nominal size range. Meet the requirements for Identification and Specific rotation (+41° to +61°, calculated on the dried basis, for specific rotation), Microbial limits, Loss on drying (not more than 4.0%), Residue on ignition (not more than 0.25%), Particle size, Heavy metals (not more than 5 ppm), and Organic volatile impurities.

SULBACTAM

Chemical name: Sulbactam sodium—4-Thia-1-azabicyclo[3.2.0]-heptane-2-carboxylic acid, 3,3-dimethyl-7-oxo-, 4,4-dioxide, sodium salt, (2*S-cis*)-.

Molecular formula: Sulbactam sodium—$C_8H_{10}NNaO_5S$.

Molecular weight: Sulbactam sodium—255.22.

Description: Sterile Sulbactam Sodium USP—White to off-white crystalline powder.

Solubility: Sterile Sulbactam Sodium USP—Freely soluble in water and in dilute acid; sparingly soluble in acetone, in ethyl acetate, and in chloroform.

USP requirements: Sulbactam Sodium USP—Preserve in tight containers. Where it is intended for use in preparing injectable dosage forms, the label states that it is sterile or must be subjected to further processing during the preparation of injectable dosage forms. Contains not less than 886 mcg and not more than 941 mcg of sulbactam, calculated on the anhydrous

basis. Meets the requirements for Identification, Crystallinity, Bacterial endotoxins, Sterility, and Water (not more than 1.0%).

SULCONAZOLE

Chemical name: Sulconazole nitrate—1*H*-Imidazole, 1-[2-[[(4-chlorophenyl)methyl]thio]-2-(2,4-dichlorophenyl)ethyl]-, mononitrate, (±)-.

Molecular formula: Sulconazole nitrate—$C_{18}H_{15}Cl_3N_2S \cdot HNO_3$.

Molecular weight: Sulconazole nitrate—460.76.

Description: Sulconazole Nitrate USP—White to off-white, crystalline powder. Melts at about 130 °C, with decomposition.

Solubility: Sulconazole Nitrate USP—Very slightly soluble in water, in toluene, and in dioxane; slightly soluble in alcohol, in chloroform, in acetone, and in methylene chloride; sparingly soluble in methanol; freely soluble in pyridine.

USP requirements:
Sulconazole Nitrate USP—Preserve in well-closed containers, protected from light. Contains not less than 98.0% and not more than 102.0% of sulconazole nitrate, calculated on the dried basis. Meets the requirements for Identification, Loss on drying (not more than 1.0%), Residue on ignition (not more than 0.1%), and Ordinary impurities.
Sulconazole Nitrate Topical Cream—Not in *USP–NF*.
Sulconazole Nitrate Topical Solution—Not in *USP–NF*.

TRIPLE SULFA

For *Sulfathiazole, Sulfacetamide,* and *Sulfabenzamide*—See individual listings for chemistry information.

USP requirements:
Triple Sulfa Vaginal Cream USP—Preserve in well-closed, light-resistant containers, or in collapsible tubes. Contains the labeled amounts of sulfathiazole, sulfacetamide, and sulfabenzamide, within ±10%. Meets the requirements for Identification, Minimum fill, and pH (3.0–4.0).
Triple Sulfa Vaginal Tablets USP—Preserve in well-closed, light-resistant containers. Contain the labeled amounts of sulfathiazole, sulfacetamide, and sulfabenzamide, within ±10%. Meet the requirements for Identification, Disintegration (30 minutes), and Uniformity of dosage units.

SULFABENZAMIDE

Chemical name: Benzamide, *N*-[(4-aminophenyl)sulfonyl]-.

Molecular formula: $C_{13}H_{12}N_2O_3S$.

Molecular weight: 276.31.

Description: Sulfabenzamide USP—Fine, white, practically odorless powder.

Solubility: Sulfabenzamide USP—Insoluble in water and in ether; soluble in alcohol, in acetone, and in sodium hydroxide TS.

USP requirements: Sulfabenzamide USP—Preserve in well-closed, light-resistant containers. Contains not less than 99.0% and not more than 100.5% of sulfabenzamide, calculated on the dried basis. Meets the requirements for Color and clarity of solution, Identification, Melting range (180–184 °C), Loss on drying (not more than 0.5%), Selenium (not more

than 0.001%, a 300-mg test specimen and 3 mL of Stock Solution being used), Heavy metals (not more than 0.002%), and Ordinary impurities.

SULFACETAMIDE

Chemical name:
Sulfacetamide—Acetamide, *N*-[(4-aminophenyl)sulfonyl]-.
Sulfacetamide sodium—Acetamide, *N*-[(4-aminophenyl)sulfonyl]-, monosodium salt, monohydrate.

Molecular formula:
Sulfacetamide—$C_8H_{10}N_2O_3S$.
Sulfacetamide sodium—$C_8H_9N_2NaO_3S \cdot H_2O$.

Molecular weight:
Sulfacetamide—214.24.
Sulfacetamide sodium—254.24.

Description:
Sulfacetamide USP—White, crystalline, odorless powder. Its aqueous solutions are sensitive to light, and are unstable when acidic or strongly alkaline.
Sulfacetamide Sodium USP—White, crystalline powder. Is odorless.

Solubility:
Sulfacetamide USP—Slightly soluble in water and in ether; freely soluble in dilute mineral acids and in solutions of potassium and sodium hydroxides; soluble in alcohol; very slightly soluble in chloroform.
Sulfacetamide Sodium USP—Freely soluble in water; sparingly soluble in alcohol; practically insoluble in chloroform and in ether.

USP requirements:
Sulfacetamide USP—Preserve in well-closed, light-resistant containers. Contains not less than 99.0% and not more than 100.5% of sulfacetamide, calculated on the dried basis. Meets the requirements for Clarity and color of solution, Identification, Melting range (181–184 °C), Reaction (a solution [1 in 150] is acid to litmus), Loss on drying (not more than 0.5%), Residue on ignition (not more than 0.1%), Sulfate (not more than 0.04%), Selenium (not more than 0.003%, a 200-mg test specimen being used), and Heavy metals (not more than 0.002%).
Sulfacetamide Sodium USP—Preserve in tight, light-resistant containers. Contains not less than 99.0% and not more than 100.5% of sulfacetamide sodium, calculated on the anhydrous basis. Meets the requirements for Identification, pH (8.0–9.5, in a solution [1 in 20]), Water (not more than 8.1%), Selenium (not more than 0.003%, a 200-mg test specimen being used), Heavy metals (not more than 0.002%), and Ordinary impurities.
Sulfacetamide Sodium Ophthalmic Ointment USP— Preserve in collapsible ophthalmic ointment tubes. It is sterile. Contains the labeled amount, within ±10%. Meets the requirements for Identification, Sterility, and Metal particles.
Sulfacetamide Sodium Ophthalmic Solution USP—Preserve in tight, light-resistant containers, in a cool place. A sterile solution. Contains the labeled amount, within ±10%. Meets the requirements for Identification and Sterility.
Sulfacitamide Sodium Topical Suspension USP—Preserve in well-closed containers, at controlled room temperature. Contains the labeled amount, within ±10%. Meets the requirements for Identification, Microbial limits, Minimum fill, and pH (6.5–7.5).

SULFACETAMIDE AND PREDNISOLONE

For *Sulfacetamide* and *Prednisolone*—See individual listings for chemistry information.

USP requirements:

Sulfacetamide Sodium and Prednisolone Acetate Ophthalmic Ointment USP—Preserve in collapsible ophthalmic ointment tubes that are tamper-proof so that sterility is assured at time of first use. A sterile ointment. Contains the labeled amounts, within ±10%. Meets the requirements for Identification, Minimum fill, Sterility, and Metal particles.

Sulfacetamide Sodium and Prednisolone Acetate Ophthalmic Suspension USP—Preserve in tight containers. The containers or individual cartons are sealed and tamper-proof so that sterility is assured at time of first use. A sterile, aqueous suspension. Contains the labeled amounts, within ±10%. Meets the requirements for Identification, Sterility, and pH (6.0–7.4).

SULFACHLORPYRIDAZINE

Chemical name: N^1-(6-Chloro-3-pyridazinyl)sulfanilamide.

Molecular formula: $C_{10}H_9ClN_4O_2S$.

Molecular weight: 284.72.

USP requirements: Sulfachlorpyridazine USP—Preserve in well-closed, light-resistant containers. Label it to indicate that it is for veterinary use only. Contains not less than 97.0% and not more than 103.0% of sulfachlorpyridazine, calculated on the dried basis. Meets the requirements for Identification, Clarity and color of solution, Acidity, Loss on drying (not more than 0.5%), Residue on ignition (not more than 0.1%), and Heavy metals (not more than 0.002%).

SULFADIAZINE

Chemical name:

Sulfadiazine—Benzenesulfonamide, 4-amino-*N*-2-pyrimidinyl-.

Sulfadiazine sodium—Benzenesulfonamide, 4-amino-*N*-2-pyrimidinyl-, monosodium salt.

Molecular formula:

Sulfadiazine—$C_{10}H_{10}N_4O_2S$.

Sulfadiazine sodium—$C_{10}H_9N_4NaO_2S$.

Molecular weight:

Sulfadiazine—250.28.

Sulfadiazine sodium—272.26.

Description:

Sulfadiazine USP—White or slightly yellow powder. Odorless or nearly odorless and stable in air, but slowly darkens on exposure to light.

Sulfadiazine Sodium USP—White powder. On prolonged exposure to humid air it absorbs carbon dioxide with liberation of sulfadiazine and becomes incompletely soluble in water. Its solutions are alkaline to phenolphthalein. Affected by light.

Solubility:

Sulfadiazine USP—Practically insoluble in water; freely soluble in dilute mineral acids, in solutions of potassium and sodium hydroxides, and in ammonia TS; sparingly soluble in alcohol and in acetone; slightly soluble in human serum at 37 °C.

Sulfadiazine Sodium USP—Freely soluble in water; slightly soluble in alcohol.

USP requirements:

Sulfadiazine USP—Preserve in well-closed, light-resistant containers. Contains not less than 98.0% and not more than 102.0% of sulfadiazine, calculated on the dried basis. Meets the requirements for Clarity and color of solution, Identification, Acidity, Loss on drying (not more than 0.5%), Residue on ignition (not more than 0.1%), Selenium (not more than 0.003%, a 200-mg test specimen being used), Heavy metals (not more than 0.002%), and Ordinary impurities.

Sulfadiazine Tablets USP—Preserve in well-closed, light-resistant containers. Contain the labeled amount, within ± 5%. Meet the requirements for Identification, Dissolution (70% in 90 minutes in 0.1 *N* hydrochloric acid in Apparatus 2 at 75 rpm), and Uniformity of dosage units.

Sulfadiazine Sodium USP—Preserve in tight, light-resistant containers. Contains not less than 99.0% and not more than 100.5% of sulfadiazine sodium, calculated on the dried basis. Meets the requirements for Identification, Loss on drying (not more than 0.5%), Selenium (not more than 0.003%, a 200-mg test specimen being used), and Heavy metals (not more than 0.002%).

Sulfadiazine Sodium Injection USP—Preserve in single-dose, light-resistant containers, of Type I glass. A sterile solution of Sulfadiazine Sodium in Water for Injection. Contains, in each mL, not less than 237.5 mg and not more than 262.5 mg of sulfadiazine sodium. Meets the requirements for Identification, Bacterial endotoxins, pH (8.5–10.5), and Particulate matter, and for Injections.

SILVER SULFADIAZINE

Chemical group: Metal sulfanilamide derivative.

Chemical name: Benzenesulfonamide, 4-amino-*N*-2-pyrimidinyl-, monosilver(1+) salt.

Molecular formula: $C_{10}H_9AgN_4O_2S$.

Molecular weight: 357.14.

Description: Silver Sulfadiazine USP—White to creamy-white, crystalline powder, odorless to having a slight odor. Is stable in air, but turns yellow on exposure to light.

Solubility: Silver Sulfadiazine USP—Slightly soluble in acetone; practically insoluble in alcohol, in chloroform, and in ether; freely soluble in 30% ammonium solution; decomposes in moderately strong mineral acids.

Other characteristics: Sulfonamides have certain chemical similarities to some goitrogens, diuretics (acetazolamide and thiazides), and oral antidiabetic agents.

USP requirements:

Silver Sulfadiazine USP—Preserve in well-closed, light-resistant containers. Contains not less than 98.0% and not more than 102.0% of silver sulfadiazine, calculated on the dried basis. Meets the requirements for Identification, Particle size, Loss on drying (not more than 0.5%), Limit of nitrate (not more than 0.1%), Chromatographic purity, and Silver content (29.3–30.5%).

Silver Sulfadiazine Cream USP—Preserve in collapsible tubes or in tight, light-resistant containers. Contains the labeled amount, within ±10%. Meets the requirements for Identification, Microbial limits, Minimum fill, and pH (4.0–7.0).

SULFADIAZINE AND TRIMETHOPRIM

For *Sulfadiazine* and *Trimethoprim*—See individual listings for chemistry information.

USP requirements:
Sulfadiazine and Trimethoprim Oral Suspension—Not in *USP–NF*.
Sulfadiazine and Trimethoprim Tablets—Not in *USP–NF*.

SULFADIMETHOXINE

Chemical name:
Sulfadimethoxine—Benzenesulfonamide, 4-amino-*N*-(2,6-dimethoxy-4-pyrimidinyl)-.
Sulfadimethoxine sodium—Benzenesulfonamide, 4-amino-*N*-(2,6-dimethoxy-4-pyrimidinyl)-, monosodium salt.

Molecular formula:
Sulfadimethoxine—$C_{12}H_{14}N_4O_4S$.
Sulfadimethoxine sodium—$C_{12}H_{13}N_4NaO_4S$.

Molecular weight:
Sulfadimethoxine—310.34.
Sulfadimethoxine sodium—332.31.

Description: Sulfadimethoxine USP—Practically white, crystalline powder.

Solubility: Sulfadimethoxine USP—Soluble in 2 *N* sodium hydroxide; sparingly soluble in 2 *N* hydrochloric acid; slightly soluble in alcohol, in ether, in chloroform, and in hexane; practically insoluble in water.

USP requirements:
Sulfadimethoxine USP—Preserve in tight, light-resistant containers, and store at controlled room temperature. Label it to indicate that it is for veterinary use only. Contains not less than 98.0% and not more than 102.0% of sulfadimethoxine, calculated on the dried basis. Meets the requirements for Identification, Melting range (197–202 °C), Loss on drying (not more than 0.5%), Residue on ignition (not more than 0.1%), and Heavy metals (not more than 0.002%).
Sulfadimethoxine Soluble Powder USP—Preserve in tight, light-resistant containers, and store at controlled room temperature. Label it to indicate that it is for veterinary use only. Contains the labeled amount, within ±10%. Meets the requirements for Identification, Minimum fill, and pH (7.0–8.0, in a solution [1 in 20]).
Sulfadimethoxine Oral Suspension USP—Preserve in tight, light-resistant containers, and store at controlled room temperature. Label it to indicate that it is for veterinary use only. Contains the labeled amount, within ±10%. Meets the requirements for Identification and pH (5.0–7.0).
Sulfadimethoxine Tablets USP—Preserve in tight, light-resistant containers, and store at controlled room temperature. Label the Tablets to indicate that they are for veterinary use only. Contain the labeled amount, within ±10%. Meet the requirements for Identification, Disintegration (30 minutes), and Uniformity of dosage units.
Sulfadimethoxine Sodium USP—Preserve in tight, light-resistant containers, and store at controlled room temperature. Label it to indicate that it is for veterinary use only. Contains not less than 98.0% and not more than 102.0% of sulfadimethoxine sodium, calculated on the dried basis. Meets the requirements for Identification, pH (8.0–9.5, in a solution [1 in 20]), Loss on drying (not more than 5.0%), and Heavy metals (not more than 0.002%).

SULFADOXINE

Chemical name: Benzenesulfonamide, 4-amino-*N*-(5,6-dimethoxy-4-pyrimidinyl)-.

Molecular formula: $C_{12}H_{14}N_4O_4S$.

Molecular weight: 310.33.

Description: White or yellowish-white crystalline powder, melting at 197–200 °C.

Solubility: Very slightly soluble in water; slightly soluble in alcohol and in methyl alcohol; practically insoluble in ether. Dissolves in solutions of alkali hydroxides and in dilute mineral acids.

USP requirements: Sulfadoxine USP—Preserve in well-closed, light-resistant containers. Contains not less than 99.0% and not more than 101.0% of sulfadoxine, calculated on the dried basis. Meets the requirements for Identification, Melting range (197–200 °C), Loss on drying (not more than 0.5%), Residue on ignition (not more than 0.1%), Heavy metals (not more than 0.002%), and Chromatographic purity.

SULFADOXINE AND PYRIMETHAMINE

For *Sulfadoxine* and *Pyrimethamine*—See individual listings for chemistry information.

USP requirements: Sulfadoxine and Pyrimethamine Tablets USP—Preserve in well-closed, light-resistant containers. Contain the labeled amounts, within ±10%. Meet the requirements for Identification, Dissolution (60% of each active ingredient in 30 minutes in phosphate buffer [pH 6.8] in Apparatus 2 at 75 rpm), and Uniformity of dosage units.

SULFAMERAZINE

Chemical name: Benzenesulfonamide, 4-amino-*N*-(4-methyl-2-pyrimidinyl)-.

Molecular formula: $C_{11}H_{12}N_4O_2S$.

Molecular weight: 264.30.

Description: Sulfamerazine USP—White or faintly yellowish white crystals or powder. Odorless or practically odorless. Stable in air, but slowly darkens on exposure to light.

Solubility: Sulfamerazine USP—Very slightly soluble in water; sparingly soluble in acetone; slightly soluble in alcohol; very slightly soluble in ether and in chloroform.

USP requirements:
Sulfamerazine USP—Preserve in well-closed, light-resistant containers. Contains not less than 99.0% and not more than 100.5% of sulfamerazine, calculated on the dried basis. Meets the requirements for Clarity and color of solution, Identification, Melting range (234–239 °C), Acidity, Loss on drying (not more than 0.5%), Residue on ignition (not more than 0.1%), Selenium (not more than 0.003%, a 200-mg test specimen being used), Heavy metals (not more than 0.002%), and Ordinary impurities.
Sulfamerazine Tablets USP—Preserve in well-closed containers. Contain the labeled amount, within ±5%. Meet the requirements for Identification, Dissolution (75% in 45 minutes in water in Apparatus 1 at 100 rpm), and Uniformity of dosage units.

SULFAMETHAZINE

Chemical name: Benzenesulfonamide, 4-amino-*N*-(4,6-dimethyl-2-pyrimidinyl)-.

Molecular formula: $C_{12}H_{14}N_4O_2S$.

Molecular weight: 278.33.

Description: Sulfamethazine USP—White to yellowish white powder, which may darken on exposure to light. Practically odorless.

Solubility: Sulfamethazine USP—Very slightly soluble in water and in ether; soluble in acetone; slightly soluble in alcohol.

USP requirements:
Sulfamethazine USP—Preserve in well-closed, light-resistant containers. Avoid moisture and excessive heat. Contains not less than 99.0% and not more than 100.5% of sulfamethazine, calculated on the dried basis. Meets the requirements for Clarity and color of solution, Identification, Melting range (197–200 °C), Acidity, Loss on drying (not more than 0.5%), Residue on ignition (not more than 0.1%), Selenium (not more than 0.003%, a 200-mg test specimen being used), Heavy metals (not more than 0.002%), and Ordinary impurities.

Sulfamethazine Granulated USP—Preserve in well-closed containers. Contains Sulfamethazine mixed with suitable diluents, carriers, and inactive ingredients. Label it to indicate that it is for veterinary use only. Label it also to indicate that it is for manufacturing, processing, or repackaging. Contains the labeled amount, within ±10%. Meets the requirements for Identification, Loss on drying (not more than 10%), and Powder fineness.

SULFAMETHIZOLE

Chemical name: Benzenesulfonamide, 4-amino-*N*-(5-methyl-1,3,4-thiadiazol-2-yl)-.

Molecular formula: $C_9H_{10}N_4O_2S_2$.

Molecular weight: 270.33.

Description: Sulfamethizole USP—White crystals or powder. Practically odorless, and has no odor of hydrogen sulfide.

Solubility: Sulfamethizole USP—Very slightly soluble in water, in chloroform, and in ether; freely soluble in solutions of ammonium, potassium, and sodium hydroxides; soluble in dilute mineral acids and in acetone; sparingly soluble in alcohol.

USP requirements:
Sulfamethizole USP—Preserve in well-closed, light-resistant containers. Contains not less than 98.0% and not more than 101.0% of sulfamethizole, calculated on the dried basis. Meets the requirements for Clarity and color of solution, Identification, Melting range (208–212 °C), Acidity, Loss on drying (not more than 0.5%), Residue on ignition (not more than 0.1%), Chloride (not more than 0.014%), Sulfate (not more than 0.04%), Selenium (not more than 0.003%), Heavy metals (not more than 0.002%), and Ordinary impurities.

Sulfamethizole Oral Suspension USP—Preserve in tight, light-resistant containers. Contains the labeled amount, within ±10%, in a buffered aqueous suspension. Meets the requirement for Identification.

Sulfamethizole Tablets USP—Preserve in well-closed containers. Contain the labeled amount, within ±5%. Meet the requirements for Identification, Dissolution (75% in 30 minutes in 0.01 *N* hydrochloric acid in Apparatus 2 at 50 rpm), and Uniformity of dosage units.

SULFAMETHOXAZOLE

Chemical name: Benzenesulfonamide, 4-amino-*N*-(5-methyl-3-isoxazolyl)-.

Molecular formula: $C_{10}H_{11}N_3O_3S$.

Molecular weight: 253.28.

Description: Sulfamethoxazole USP—White to off-white, practically odorless, crystalline powder.

Solubility: Sulfamethoxazole USP—Practically insoluble in water, in ether, and in chloroform; freely soluble in acetone and in dilute solutions of sodium hydroxide; sparingly soluble in alcohol.

Other characteristics: Sulfonamides have certain chemical similarities to some goitrogens, diuretics (acetazolamide and thiazides), and oral antidiabetic agents.

USP requirements:
Sulfamethoxazole USP—Preserve in well-closed, light-resistant containers. Contains not less than 99.0% and not more than 101.0% of sulfamethoxazole, calculated on the dried basis. Meets the requirements for Identification, Melting range (168–172 °C), Loss on drying (not more than 0.5%), Residue on ignition (not more than 0.1%), Selenium (not more than 0.003%, a 200-mg test specimen being used), Sulfanilamide and sulfanilic acid (not more than 0.2%), and Organic volatile impurities.

Sulfamethoxazole Oral Suspension USP—Preserve in tight, light-resistant containers. Contains the labeled amount, within −5% to + 10%. Meets the requirement for Identification.

Sulfamethoxazole Tablets USP—Preserve in well-closed, light-resistant containers. Contain the labeled amount, within ±5%. Meet the requirements for Identification, Dissolution (80% in 30 minutes in dilute hydrochloric acid [7 in 100] in Apparatus 1 at 100 rpm), and Uniformity of dosage units.

SULFAMETHOXAZOLE AND PHENAZOPYRIDINE

For *Sulfamethoxazole* and *Phenazopyridine*—See individual listings for chemistry information.

USP requirements: Sulfamethoxazole and Phenazopyridine Hydrochloride Tablets—Not in *USP–NF*.

SULFAMETHOXAZOLE AND TRIMETHOPRIM

For *Sulfamethoxazole* and *Trimethoprim*—See individual listings for chemistry information.

USP requirements:
Sulfamethoxazole and Trimethoprim Injection USP—Preserve in single-dose, light-resistant containers, preferably of Type I glass. May be packaged in 50-mL multiple-dose containers. A sterile solution of Sulfamethoxazole and Trimethoprim in Water for Injection which, when diluted with Dextrose Injection, is suitable for intravenous infusion. Label it to indicate that it is to be diluted with 5% Dextrose Injection prior to administration. Contains the labeled amounts, within ±10%. Meets the requirements for Identification, Pyrogen, pH (9.5–10.5), Particulate matter, and Related compounds, and for Injections.

Sulfamethoxazole and Trimethoprim Oral Suspension USP—Preserve in tight, light-resistant containers. Contains the labeled amounts, within ±10%. Meets the requirements for Identification, pH (5.0–6.5), Chromatographic purity, and Alcohol content (not more than 0.5%).

Sulfamethoxazole and Trimethoprim Tablets USP—Preserve in well-closed, light-resistant containers. Contain the labeled amounts, within ±7%. Meet the requirements for Identification, Dissolution (70% of each active ingredient in 60 minutes in 0.1 *N* hydrochloric acid in Apparatus 2 at 75 rpm), and Uniformity of dosage units.

SULFANILAMIDE

Chemical name: *p*-Aminobenzenesulfonamide.

Molecular formula: $C_6H_8N_2O_2S$.

Molecular weight: 172.21.

Description: White, odorless, crystalline powder.

Solubility: Slightly soluble in water, in alcohol, in acetone, in glycerin, in propylene glycol, in hydrochloric acid, and in solutions of potassium and sodium hydroxide; practically insoluble in chloroform, in ether, and in petroleum ether.

USP requirements:
Sulfanilamide Vaginal Cream—Not in *USP–NF*.
Sulfanilamide Vaginal Suppositories—Not in *USP–NF*.

SULFANILAMIDE, AMINACRINE, AND ALLANTOIN

Chemical name:
Sulfanilamide—*p*-Aminobenzenesulfonamide.
Aminacrine hydrochloride—9-Acridinamine monohydrochloride.
Allantoin—Urea, (2,5-dioxo-4-imidazolidinyl)-.

Molecular formula:
Sulfanilamide—$C_6H_8N_2O_2S$.
Aminacrine hydrochloride—$C_{13}H_{10}N_2 \cdot HCl$.
Allantoin—$C_4H_6N_4O_3$.

Molecular weight:
Sulfanilamide—172.21.
Aminacrine hydrochloride—230.69.
Allantoin—158.12.

Description:
Sulfanilamide—White, odorless crystalline powder.
Aminacrine hydrochloride—Pale yellow, crystalline powder; highly fluorescent.
Allantoin—Colorless crystals, melting at 238 °C.

Solubility:
Sulfanilamide—Slightly soluble in water, in alcohol, in acetone, in glycerin, in propylene glycol, in hydrochloric acid, and in solutions of potassium and sodium hydroxide; practically insoluble in chloroform, in ether, and in petroleum ether.
Aminacrine hydrochloride—1 gram soluble in 300 mL of water and in 150 mL of alcohol; soluble in glycerin.
Allantoin—1 gram dissolves in 190 mL of water or in 500 mL of alcohol; nearly insoluble in ether.

USP requirements:
Sulfanilamide, Aminacrine Hydrochloride, and Allantoin Vaginal Cream—Not in *USP–NF*.
Sulfanilamide, Aminacrine Hydrochloride, and Allantoin Vaginal Suppositories—Not in *USP–NF*.

SULFAPYRIDINE

Chemical group: Sulfonamide.

Chemical name: Benzenesulfonamide, 4-amino-*N*-2-pyridinyl-.

Molecular formula: $C_{11}H_{11}N_3O_2S$.

Molecular weight: 249.29.

Description: Sulfapyridine USP—White or faintly yellowish white crystals, granules, or powder. Is odorless or practically odorless, and is stable in air, but slowly darkens on exposure to light.

Solubility: Sulfapyridine USP—Very slightly soluble in water; freely soluble in dilute mineral acids and in solutions of potassium and sodium hydroxides; sparingly soluble in acetone; slightly soluble in alcohol.

Other characteristics: Sulfonamides have certain chemical similarities to some goitrogens, diuretics (acetazolamide and thiazides), and oral hypoglycemic agents.

USP requirements:
Sulfapyridine USP—Preserve in well-closed, light-resistant containers. Contains not less than 99.0% and not more than 100.5% of sulfapyridine, calculated on the dried basis. Meets the requirements for Clarity and color of solution, Identification, Melting range (190–193 °C), Acidity, Loss on drying (not more than 0.5%), Residue on ignition (not more than 0.1%), Selenium (not more than 0.003%, a 200-mg test specimen being used), Heavy metals (not more than 0.002%), and Organic volatile impurities.
Sulfapyridine Tablets USP—Preserve in well-closed, light-resistant containers. Contain the labeled amount, within ± 5%. Meet the requirements for Identification, Dissolution (70% in 60 minutes in 0.01 *N* hydrochloric acid in Apparatus 2 at 50 rpm), and Uniformity of dosage units.

SULFAQUINOXALINE

Chemical name: *N*'-2-Quinoxalinylsulfanilamide.

Molecular formula: $C_{14}H_{12}N_4O_2S$.

Molecular weight: 300.34.

Description: Yellow, odorless powder.

Solubility: Practically insoluble in water; very slightly soluble in alcohol; practically insoluble in ether; freely soluble in aqueous solutions of alkalis.

USP requirements:
Sulfaquinoxaline USP—Preserve in well-closed containers, protected from light. Contains not less than 98.0% and not more than 101.0% of sulfaquinoxaline, calculated on the dried basis. Meets the requirements for Identification, Acidity, Loss on drying (not more than 1.0%), Residue on ignition (not more than 0.1%), Heavy metals (not more than 0.002%), and Related compounds.
Sulfaquinoxaline Oral Solution USP—Preserve in tight, light-resistant containers. Label it to indicate that it is for veterinary use only. Contains the equivalent of the labeled concentration of sulfaquinoxaline, within ±10%. Meets the requirements for Identification, Deliverable volume, and pH (not less than 12).

SULFASALAZINE

Source: Synthesized by the diazotization of sulfapyridine and the coupling of the diazonium salt with salicylic acid.

Chemical name: Benzoic acid, 2-hydroxy-5-[[4-[(2-pyridinylamino)sulfonyl]phenyl]azo]-.

Molecular formula: $C_{18}H_{14}N_4O_5S$.

Molecular weight: 398.39.

Description: Sulfasalazine USP—Bright yellow or brownish yellow, odorless, fine powder. Melts at about 255 °C, with decomposition.

Solubility: Sulfasalazine USP—Very slightly soluble in alcohol; practically insoluble in water, in ether, and in chloroform; soluble in aqueous solutions of alkali hydroxides.

USP requirements:
Sulfasalazine USP—Preserve in tight, light-resistant containers. Contains not less than 97.0% and not more than 101.5% of sulfasalazine, calculated on the dried basis. Meets the requirements for Identification, Loss on drying (not more than 1.0%), Residue on ignition (not more than 0.5%), Chloride (not more than 0.014%), Sulfate (not more than 0.04%), Heavy metals (not more than 0.002%), Chromatographic purity, and Organic volatile impurities.
Sulfasalazine Capsules—Not in *USP–NF*.
Sulfasalazine Oral Suspension—Not in *USP–NF*.
Sulfasalazine Rectal Suspension—Not in *USP–NF*.
Sulfasalazine Tablets USP—Preserve in well-closed containers. Contain the labeled amount, within ±5%. Meet the requirements for Identification, Dissolution (85% in 60 minutes in phosphate buffer [pH 7.5] in Apparatus 1 at 100 rpm), and Uniformity of dosage units.
Sulfasalazine Delayed-release Tablets USP—Preserve in well-closed containers. Contain the labeled amount, within ±5%. Meet the requirements for Disintegration (15 minutes [enteric coated]), for Identification test, and for Uniformity of dosage units under Sulfasalazine Tablets.

SULFATHIAZOLE

Chemical name: Benzenesulfonamide, 4-amino-N-2-thiazolyl-.

Molecular formula: $C_9H_9N_3O_2S_2$.

Molecular weight: 255.32.

Description: Sulfathiazole USP—Fine, white or faintly yellowish white, practically odorless powder.

Solubility: Sulfathiazole USP—Very slightly soluble in water; soluble in acetone, in dilute mineral acids, in solutions of alkali hydroxides, and in 6 N ammonium hydroxide; slightly soluble in alcohol.

USP requirements: Sulfathiazole USP—Preserve in well-closed, light-resistant containers. Contains not less than 99.0% and not more than 100.5% of sulfathiazole, calculated on the dried basis. Meets the requirements for Identification, Melting range (200–204 °C), Acidity, Loss on drying (not more than 0.5%), Residue on ignition (not more than 0.1%), Chloride (not more than 0.014%), Sulfate (not more than 0.04%), Heavy metals (not more than 0.002%), and Ordinary impurities.

SULFINPYRAZONE

Chemical group: A pyrazole compound chemically related to phenylbutazone.

Chemical name: 3,5-Pyrazolidinedione, 1,2-diphenyl-4-[2-(phenylsulfinyl)ethyl]-.

Molecular formula: $C_{23}H_{20}N_2O_3S$.

Molecular weight: 404.48.

Description: Sulfinpyrazone USP—White to off-white powder.

pKa: 2.8.

Solubility: Sulfinpyrazone USP—Practically insoluble in water and in solvent hexane; soluble in alcohol and in acetone; sparingly soluble in dilute alkali.

USP requirements:
Sulfinpyrazone USP—Preserve in well-closed containers. Contains not less than 98.5% and not more than 101.5% of sulfinpyrazone, calculated on the dried basis. Meets the requirements for Solubility in acetone, Solubility in 0.50 N sodium hydroxide, Identification, Melting range (130.5–134.5 °C), Loss on drying (not more than 0.5%), Residue on ignition (not more than 0.1%), Heavy metals (not more than 0.001%), Chromatographic purity, and Organic volatile impurities.
Sulfinpyrazone Capsules USP—Preserve in well-closed containers. Contain the labeled amount, within ±7%. Meet the requirements for Identification, Dissolution (75% in 45 minutes in phosphate buffer [pH 6.8] in Apparatus 1 at 100 rpm), and Uniformity of dosage units.
Sulfinpyrazone Tablets USP—Preserve in well-closed containers. Contain the labeled amount, within ±7%. Meet the requirements for Identification, Dissolution (75% in 45 minutes in phosphate buffer [pH 6.8] in Apparatus 1 at 100 rpm), and Uniformity of dosage units.

SULFISOXAZOLE

Chemical name:
Sulfisoxazole—Benzenesulfonamide, 4-amino-N-(3,4-dimethyl5-isoxazolyl)-.
Sulfisoxazole acetyl—Acetamide, N-[(4-aminophenyl)sulfonyl]N-(3,4-dimethyl-5-isoxazolyl)-.
Sulfisoxazole diolamine—Benzenesulfonamide, 4-amino-N-(3,4-dimethyl-5-isoxazolyl)-, compd. with 2,2'-iminobis[ethanol] (1:1).

Molecular formula:
Sulfisoxazole—$C_{11}H_{13}N_3O_3S$.
Sulfisoxazole acetyl—$C_{13}H_{15}N_3O_4S$.
Sulfisoxazole diolamine—$C_{11}H_{13}N_3O_3S \cdot C_4H_{11}NO_2$.

Molecular weight:
Sulfisoxazole—267.31.
Sulfisoxazole acetyl—309.34.
Sulfisoxazole diolamine—372.44.

Description:
Sulfisoxazole USP—White to slightly yellowish, odorless, crystalline powder.
Sulfisoxazole Acetyl USP—White or slightly yellow, crystalline powder.
Sulfisoxazole Diolamine USP—White to off-white, fine crystalline, odorless powder.

Solubility:
Sulfisoxazole USP—Very slightly soluble in water; soluble in boiling alcohol and in 3 N hydrochloric acid.
Sulfisoxazole Acetyl USP—Practically insoluble in water; sparingly soluble in chloroform; slightly soluble in alcohol.
Sulfisoxazole Diolamine USP—Freely soluble in water; soluble in alcohol.

Other characteristics: Sulfonamides have certain chemical similarities to some goitrogens, diuretics (acetazolamide and thiazides), and oral antidiabetic agents.

USP requirements:

Sulfisoxazole USP—Preserve in tight, light-resistant containers. Contains not less than 99.0% and not more than 101.0% of sulfisoxazole, calculated on the dried basis. Meets the requirements for Identification, Melting range (194–199 °C), Loss on drying (not more than 0.5%), Residue on ignition (not more than 0.1%), Selenium (not more than 0.003%, a 200-mg test specimen being used), Heavy metals (not more than 0.002%), and Ordinary impurities.

Sulfisoxazole Tablets USP—Preserve in well-closed, light-resistant containers. Contain the labeled amount, within ± 5%. Meet the requirements for Identification, Dissolution (70% in 30 minutes in dilute hydrochloric acid [1 in 12.5] in Apparatus 1 at 100 rpm), and Uniformity of dosage units.

Sulfisoxazole Acetyl USP—Preserve in tight, light-resistant containers. Contains not less than 98.0% and not more than 100.5% of sulfisoxazole acetyl, calculated on the dried basis. Meets the requirements for Identification, Melting range (192–195 °C), Loss on drying (not more than 0.5%), Ordinary impurities, and Organic volatile impurities, and for Residue on ignition, Selenium, and Heavy metals under Sulfisoxazole.

Sulfisoxazole Acetyl Oral Suspension USP—Preserve in tight, light-resistant containers. Contains an amount of sulfisoxazole acetyl equivalent to the labeled amount of sulfisoxazole, within ±7%. Meets the requirements for Identification and pH (5.0–5.5).

Sulfisoxazole Acetyl Oral Syrup—Not in *USP–NF*.

Sulfisoxazole Diolamine USP—Preserve in tight, light-resistant containers. Contains not less than 99.0% and not more than 101.0% of sulfisoxazole diolamine, calculated on the dried basis. Meets the requirements for Identification, Melting range (119–124 °C), Loss on drying (not more than 0.2%), Residue on ignition (not more than 0.1%), and Heavy metals (not more than 0.002%).

Sulfisoxazole Diolamine Injection USP—Preserve in single-dose or in multiple-dose containers, preferably of Type I glass, protected from light. A sterile solution of Sulfisoxazole Diolamine in Water for Injection. Contains an amount of sulfisoxazole diolamine equivalent to the labeled amount of sulfisoxazole, within ±10%. Meets the requirements for Identification, Pyrogen, pH (7.0–8.5), and Particulate matter, and for Injections.

Sulfisoxazole Diolamine Ophthalmic Ointment USP—Preserve in collapsible ophthalmic ointment tubes. A sterile ointment. Contains an amount of sulfisoxazole diolamine equivalent to the labeled amount of sulfisoxazole, within ± 10%. Meets the requirements for Identification, Sterility, Minimum fill, Leakage, and Metal particles.

Sulfisoxazole Diolamine Ophthalmic Solution USP—Preserve in tight, light-resistant containers. A sterile solution. Contains an amount of sulfisoxazole diolamine equivalent to the labeled amount of sulfisoxazole, within −10% to + 15%. Meets the requirements for Identification, Sterility, and pH (7.2–8.2).

SULFISOXAZOLE AND PHENAZOPYRIDINE

For *Sulfisoxazole* and *Phenazopyridine*—See individual listings for chemistry information.

USP requirements: Sulfisoxazole and Phenazopyridine Hydrochloride Tablets—Not in *USP–NF*.

SULFUR

Chemical name: Precipitated sulfur—Sulfur.

Molecular formula: Precipitated sulfur—S.

Molecular weight: Precipitated sulfur—32.07.

Description: Precipitated Sulfur USP—Very fine, pale yellow, amorphous or microcrystalline powder. Is odorless.

Solubility: Precipitated Sulfur USP—Practically insoluble in water; very soluble in carbon disulfide; slightly soluble in olive oil; very slightly soluble in alcohol.

USP requirements:

Precipitated Sulfur USP—Preserve in well-closed containers. Contains not less than 99.5% and not more than 100.5% of sulfur, calculated on the anhydrous basis. Meets the requirements for Identification, Reaction, Water (not more than 0.5%), Residue on ignition (not more than 0.3%), and Other forms of sulfur.

Sulfur Cream—Not in *USP–NF*.

Sulfur Lotion—Not in *USP–NF*.

Sulfur Ointment USP—Preserve in well-closed containers, and avoid prolonged exposure to excessive heat. Contains not less than 9.5% and not more than 10.5% of Sulfur.

Prepare Sulfur Ointment as follows: 100 grams of Precipitated Sulfur, 100 grams of Mineral Oil, and 800 grams of White Ointment, to make 1000 grams. Levigate the sulfur with the Mineral Oil to a smooth paste, and then incorporate with the White Ointment.

Sulfur Bar Soap—Not in *USP–NF*.

SUBLIMED SULFUR

Chemical name: Sulfur.

Molecular formula: S.

Molecular weight: 32.07.

Description: Sublimed Sulfur USP—Fine, yellow, crystalline powder, having a faint odor.

Solubility: Sublimed Sulfur USP—Practically insoluble in water and in alcohol; sparingly soluble in olive oil.

USP requirements: Sublimed Sulfur USP—Preserve in well-closed containers. Dried over phosphorus pentoxide for 4 hours, contains not less than 99.5% and not more than 100.5% of sulfur. Meets the requirements for Solubility in carbon disulfide, Identification, Residue on ignition (not more than 0.5%), and Arsenic (not more than 4 ppm).

SULFUR DIOXIDE

Chemical name: Sulfur dioxide.

Molecular formula: SO_2.

Molecular weight: 64.06.

Description: Sulfur Dioxide NF—Colorless, non-flammable gas, possessing a strong suffocating odor characteristic of burning sulfur. Under pressure, it condenses readily to a colorless liquid that boils at −10 °C and has a density of approximately 1.5.

NF category: Antioxidant.

Solubility: Sulfur Dioxide NF—At 20 °C and at standard pressure, approximately 36 volumes dissolve in 1 volume of water, and approximately 114 volumes dissolve in 1 volume of alcohol. Soluble also in ether and in chloroform.

NF requirements: Sulfur Dioxide NF—Preserve in cylinders. Note: Sulfur Dioxide is used most in the form of a gas in pharmaceutical applications, and the monograph deals with it for such purposes. However, it is usually packaged under pressure; hence, the NF specifications are designed for testing it in liquid form. Contains not less than 97.0%, by volume, of sulfur dioxide. Meets the requirements for Water (not more than 2.0%), Limit of nonvolatile residue (not more than 0.0025%), and Sulfuric acid (about 0.002%).

Caution: Sulfur Dioxide is poisonous.

SULFURIC ACID

Chemical name: Sulfuric acid.

Molecular formula: H_2SO_4.

Molecular weight: 98.08.

Description: Sulfuric Acid NF—Clear, colorless, oily liquid. Very caustic and corrosive. Specific gravity is about 1.84.
NF category: Acidifying agent.

Solubility: Sulfuric Acid NF—Miscible with water and with alcohol with the generation of much heat.

NF requirements: Sulfuric Acid NF—Preserve in tight containers. Contains not less than 95.0% and not more than 98.0%, by weight, of sulfuric acid. Meets the requirements for Identification, Residue on ignition (not more than 0.005%), Chloride (not more than 0.005%), Arsenic (not more than 1 ppm), Heavy metals (not more than 5 ppm), and Reducing substances.

Caution: When Sulfuric Acid is to be mixed with other liquids, always add it to the diluent, and exercise great caution.

SULINDAC

Chemical group: Indeneacetic acid derivative.

Chemical name: 1H-Indene-3-acetic acid, 5-fluoro-2-methyl-1-[[4-(methylsulfinyl)phenyl]methylene]-, (Z)-.

Molecular formula: $C_{20}H_{17}FO_3S$.

Molecular weight: 356.41.

Description: Sulindac USP—Yellow, crystalline powder, which is odorless or practically so.

Solubility: Sulindac USP—Slightly soluble in methanol, in alcohol, in acetone, and in chloroform; very slightly soluble in isopropanol and in ethyl acetate; practically insoluble in hexane and in water.

USP requirements:
Sulindac USP—Preserve in well-closed containers. Contains not less than 99.0% and not more than 101.0% of sulindac, calculated on the dried basis. Meets the requirements for Identification, Loss on drying (not more than 0.5%), Residue on ignition (not more than 0.1%), Heavy metals (not more than 0.001%), Chromatographic purity, and Organic volatile impurities.
Sulindac Tablets USP—Preserve in well-closed containers. Contain the labeled amount, within ±10%. Meet the requirements for Identification, Dissolution (80% in 45 minutes in 0.1 M phosphate buffer [pH 7.2] in Apparatus 2 at 50 rpm), Uniformity of dosage units, and Related compounds.

SULISOBENZONE

Chemical name: Benzenesulfonic acid, 5-benzoyl-4-hydroxy-2-methoxy-.

Molecular formula: $C_{14}H_{12}O_6S$.

Molecular weight: 308.31.

Description: Sulisobenzone USP—Light tan powder, with a melting point of about 145°.

Solubility: Sulisobenzone USP—Freely soluble in methanol, in alcohol, and in water; sparingly soluble in ethyl acetate.

USP requirements: Sulisobenzone USP—Preserve in tight, light-resistant containers. Contains the labeled amount, within ±5%, calculated on the as-is basis. Meets the requirements for Identification.

SUMATRIPTAN

Chemical name: Sumatriptan succinate—1H-Indole-5-methanesulfonamide, 3-[2-(dimethylamino)ethyl]-N-methyl-, butanedioate (1:1).

Molecular formula: Sumatriptan succinate—$C_{14}H_{21}N_3O_2S \cdot C_4H_6O_4$.

Molecular weight: Sumatriptan succinate—413.49.

Description: Sumatriptan succinate—White to off-white powder.

Solubility: Sumatriptan succinate—Readily soluble in water and in saline.

USP requirements:
Sumatriptan Succinate Injection—Not in *USP–NF*.
Sumatriptan Succinate Nasal Spray—Not in *USP–NF*.
Sumatriptan Succinate Tablets—Not in *USP–NF*.

SUPROFEN

Chemical name: Benzeneacetic acid, alpha-methyl-4-(2-thienyl-carbonyl)-.

Molecular formula: $C_{14}H_{12}O_3S$.

Molecular weight: 260.31.

Description: Suprofen USP—White to off-white powder, odorless to having a slight odor.

Solubility: Suprofen USP—Sparingly soluble in water.

USP requirements:
Suprofen USP—Preserve in well-closed containers. Contains not less than 98.0% and not more than 102.0% of suprofen, calculated on the dried basis. Meets the requirements for Clarity of solution, Identification, Melting range (118–125 °C, within a range of less than 4 °C), Loss on drying (not more than 0.5%), Residue on ignition (not more than 0.2%), Heavy metals (not more than 0.002%), and Ordinary impurities.
Suprofen Ophthalmic Solution USP—Preserve in tight containers. A sterile, buffered, aqueous solution of Suprofen adjusted to a suitable tonicity. Contains a suitable antimicrobial preservative. Contains the labeled amount, within −10% to +15%. Meets the requirements for Identification, Sterility, and pH (6.5–8.0).

SURAMIN

Molecular formula: Suramin sodium—$C_{51}H_{34}N_6Na_6O_{23}S_6$.

Molecular weight: Suramin sodium—1429.20.

Description: Suramin sodium—White, pinkish-white, or slightly cream-colored, odorless or almost odorless, hygroscopic powder.

Solubility: Suramin sodium—Soluble 1 in less than 1 of water; very slightly soluble in alcohol; practically insoluble in chloroform and in ether.

USP requirements: Suramin Sodium for Injection—Not in *USP–NF*.

SUSPENSION STRUCTURED VEHICLE

NF requirements: Suspension Structured Vehicle NF—Preserve in tight, light-resistant containers. Store at room temperature, and avoid freezing. Label it to state that it must be well shaken before using.

Prepare Suspension Structured Vehicle as follows: 0.15 gram of Potassium Sorbate, 0.15 gram of Xanthan Gum, 0.15 gram of Citric Acid, Anhydrous, 20 grams of Sucrose, and Purified Water, a sufficient quantity to make 100 mL. Transfer the Potassium Sorbate to a suitable beaker, and dissolve in 50 mL of Purified Water. Place the beaker on an electric hot plate and stirrer, and add into the vortex, slowly stirring, the Xanthan Gum. Apply minimal heat, and incorporate the Citric Acid and the Sucrose. Add a sufficient quantity of Purified Water to obtain a final volume of 100 mL, and mix.

Meets the requirement for Beyond-use date.

SUGAR-FREE SUSPENSION STRUCTURED VEHICLE

NF requirements: Sugar-free Suspension Structured Vehicle NF—Preserve in tight, light-resistant containers. Store at room temperature and avoid freezing. Label it to state that it must be well shaken before using.

Prepare Sugar-free Suspension Structured Vehicle as follows: 0.20 gram of Xanthan Gum, 0.20 gram of Saccharin Sodium, 0.15 gram of Potassium Sorbate, 0.10 gram of Citric Acid, 2.0 grams of Sorbitol, 2.0 grams of Mannitol, 2.0 mL of Glycerin, and Purified Water, a sufficient quantity to make 100 mL. Transfer 30 mL of Purified Water to a beaker, placing it on an electric hot plate and stirrer. Using moderate heat, stir to form a vortex, and slowly sprinkle the Xanthan Gum into the vortex. In a separate beaker, dissolve the Saccharin Sodium, Potassium Sorbate, and Citric Acid in 50 mL of Purified Water. Using moderate heat, incorporate the Sorbitol, Mannitol, and Glycerin into this mixture. Add to this mixture the previously prepared Xanthan Gum dispersion. Add a sufficient quantity of Purified Water to obtain a final volume of 100 mL, and mix. Meets the requirement for Beyond-use date.

SUTILAINS

Chemical name: Sutilains.

Description: Sutilains USP—Cream-colored powder.

USP requirements:

Sutilains USP—Preserve in tight containers, and store in a refrigerator. Allow to reach room temperature before opening container. A substance, containing proteolytic enzymes, derived from the bacterium *Bacillus subtilis*. When assayed as in *USP/NF*, contains not less than 2,500,000 USP Casein Units of proteolytic activity per gram, calculated on the dried basis. Meets the requirements for Solubility test, pH (6.1–7.1, in a solution [1 in 100]), Loss on drying (not more than 5.0%), Nitrogen (11.0–13.5%), and Organic volatile impurities.

Note: One USP Casein Unit of proteolytic activity is contained in the amount of sutilains which, when incubated with 35 mg of denatured casein at 37 °C, produces in 1 minute a hydrolysate whose absorbance at 275 nanometers is equal to that of a tyrosine solution containing 1.5 mcg of USP Tyrosine Reference Standard per mL.

Sutilains Ointment USP—Preserve in collapsible tubes or in tight containers, and store in a refrigerator. Contains the labeled potency of sutilains, within −15% to +25%, in a suitable ointment base. Meets the requirement for Sterility.

Note: One USP Casein Unit of proteolytic activity is contained in the amount of sutilains which, when incubated with 35 mg of denatured casein at 37 °C, produces in 1 minute a hydrolysate whose absorbance at 275 nanometers is equal to that of a tyrosine solution containing 1.5 mcg of USP Tyrosine Reference Standard per mL.

ABSORBABLE SURGICAL SUTURE

USP requirements: Absorbable Surgical Suture USP—Preserve dry or in fluid, in containers (packets) so designed that sterility is maintained until the container is opened. A number of such containers may be placed in a box. A sterile, flexible strand prepared from collagen derived from healthy mammals, or from a synthetic polymer. Suture prepared from synthetic polymer may be in either monofilament or multifilament form. It is capable of being absorbed by living mammalian tissue, but may be treated to modify its resistance to absorption. Its diameter and tensile strength correspond to the size designation indicated on the label, within the limits prescribed in *USP-NF*. May be modified with respect to body or texture. May be impregnated or treated with a suitable coating, softening, or antimicrobial agent. May be colored by a color additive approved by the U.S. Food and Drug Administration. The collagen suture is designated as either *Plain Suture* or *Chromic Suture*. Both types consist of processed strands of collagen, but *Chromic Suture* is processed by physical or chemical means so as to provide greater resistance to absorption in living mammalian tissue. The label of each individual container (packet) of Suture indicates the size, length, type of Suture, kind of needle (if a needle is included), number of sutures (if multiple), lot number, and name of the manufacturer or distributor. If removable needles are used, the labeling so indicates. Suture size is designated by the metric size (gauge number) and the corresponding USP size. The label of the box indicates also the address of the manufacturer, packer, or distributor, and the composition of any packaging fluids used. Note: If the Suture is packaged with a fluid, make the required measurements for the following tests within 2 minutes after removing it from the fluid—Length, Diameter, Tensile strength, and Needle attachment. Meets the requirements for Length (not less than 95.0% of length stated on label), Diameter, Tensile strength, Needle attachment, Sterility, Extractable color (if Suture is dyed), and Soluble chromium compounds.

NONABSORBABLE SURGICAL SUTURE

USP requirements: Nonabsorbable Surgical Suture USP—Preserve nonsterilized Suture in well-closed containers. Preserve sterile Suture dry or in fluid, in containers (packets) so designed that sterility is maintained until the container is opened. A number of such containers may be placed in a box. A flexible strand of material that is suitably resistant to the action of living mammalian tissue. It may be in either monofilament or multifilament form. If it is a multifilament strand, the individual filaments may be combined by spinning, twisting, braiding, or any combination thereof. May be either sterile or nonsterile. Its diameter and tensile strength correspond to the size designation indicated on the label, within the limits prescribed in *USP-NF*. May be modified with respect to body or texture, or to reduce capillarity, and may be suitably bleached. May be impregnated or treated with a suitable coating, softening, or antimicrobial agent. May be colored by a color additive approved by the U.S. Food and Drug Administration. Nonabsorbable Surgical Suture is classed and typed as follows: *Class I* Suture is composed of silk or synthetic fibers of monofilament, twisted or braided construction where the coating, if any, does not significantly affect thickness (e.g., braided silk, polyester, or nylon; microfilament nylon, or polypropylene). *Class II* Suture is composed of cotton or linen fibers or coated natural or synthetic fibers where the coating significantly affects thickness but does not contribute significantly to strength (e.g., virgin silk sutures). *Class III* Suture is composed of monofilament or multifilament metal wire. The label of each individual container (packet) of Suture indicates the material from which the Suture is made, the size, construction, and length of the Suture, whether it is sterile or non-sterile, kind of needle (if a needle is included), number of sutures (if multiple), lot number, and name of the manufacturer or distributor. If removable needles are used, the labeling so indicates. Suture size is designated by the metric size (gauge number) and the corresponding USP size. The label of the box indicates also the address of the manufacturer, packer, or distributor, and the composition of any packaging fluids used. Note: If the Suture is packaged with a fluid, make the required measurements for the following tests within 2 minutes after removing it from the fluid—Length, Diameter, Tensile strength, and Needle attachment. Meets the requirements for Length (not less than 95.0% of length stated on label), Diameter, Tensile strength, Needle attachment, Sterility, and Extractable color (if Suture is dyed).

SYRUP

Description: Syrup NF—NF category: Sweetening agent; tablet binder; flavored and/or sweetened vehicle.

NF requirements: Syrup NF—Preserve in tight containers, preferably in a cool place. A solution of Sucrose in Purified Water. Contains a preservative unless it is used when freshly prepared.

Prepare Syrup as follows: 850 grams of Sucrose and a sufficient quantity of Purified Water to make 1000 mL. May be prepared by the use of boiling water or, preferably, without heat, by the following process. Place the Sucrose in a suitable percolator, the neck of which is nearly filled with loosely packed cotton, moistened after packing with a few drops of water. Pour carefully about 450 mL of Purified Water upon the Sucrose, and regulate the outflow to a steady drip of percolate. Return the percolate, if necessary, until all of the Sucrose has been dissolved. Then wash the inside of the percolator and the cotton with sufficient Purified Water to bring the volume of the percolate to 1000 mL, and mix.

Meets the requirements for Specific gravity (not less than 1.30) and Organic volatile impurities.

TACRINE

Chemical name: Tacrine hydrochloride—9-Acridinamine, 1,2,3,4-tetrahydro-, monohydrochloride.

Molecular formula: Tacrine hydrochloride—$C_{13}H_{14}N_2 \cdot HCl$.

Molecular weight: Tacrine hydrochloride—234.72.

Description: Tacrine Hydrochloride USP—White powder.

Solubility: Tacrine Hydrochloride USP—Freely soluble in water, in 0.1 N hydrochloric acid, in acetate buffer (pH 4.0), in phosphate buffer (pH 7.0–7.4), in methanol, in dimethylsulfoxide, in alcohol, and in propylene glycol; sparingly soluble in linoleic acid and in polyethylene glycol 400.

USP requirements:
Tacrine Capsules USP—Preserve in well-closed containers. Contain Tacrine Hydrochloride equivalent to the labeled amount of tacrine, within ±10%. Meet the requirements for Identification, Dissolution (85% in 30 minutes in 0.1 N hydrochloric acid in Apparatus 2 at 50 rpm), and Uniformity of dosage units.
Tacrine Hydrochloride USP—Preserve in well-closed containers. Contains not less than 98.5% and not more than 101.5% of tacrine hydrochloride. Meets the requirements for Identification, Water (6.0–8.0%), Residue on ignition (not more than 0.1%), Heavy metals (not more than 0.001%), Chromatographic purity, and Content of chloride (13.6–14.4%).
Tacrine Hydrochloride Capsules—Not in *USP–NF*.

TACROLIMUS

Chemical name: 15,19-Epoxy-3H-pyrido[2,1-c][1,4]oxaazacyclo-tricosine-1,7,20,21(4H,23H)-tetrone, 5,6,8,11,12,13,14,15,16,17,18,19,24,25,26,26a-hexadecahydro-5,19-dihydroxy-3-[2-(4-hydroxy-3-methoxycyclohexyl)-1-methylethenyl]-14,16-dimethoxy-4,10,12,18-tetramethyl-8-(2-propenyl)-, monohydrate, [3S-[3R*,[E(1S*,3S*,4S*)],4S*,5R*,8-S*,9E,12R*,14R*,15S*,16R*,18S*,19S*,26aR*]]-.

Molecular formula: $C_{44}H_{69}NO_{12} \cdot H_2O$.

Molecular weight: 822.03.

Description: White crystals or crystalline powder.

Solubility: Practically insoluble in water; freely soluble in ethanol; very soluble in methanol and in chloroform.

USP requirements:
Tacrolimus Capsules—Not in *USP–NF*.
Tacrolimus Injection—Not in *USP–NF*.
Tacrolimus for Injection—Not in *USP–NF*.
Tacrolimus Ointment—Not in *USP–NF*.

TALC

Molecular formula: Talc intrapleural aerosol—$Mg_3Si_4O_{10}(OH)_2$.

Molecular weight: Talc intrapleural aerosol—379.3.

Description:
Talc USP—Very fine, white or grayish-white, crystalline powder. It is unctuous, adheres readily to the skin, and is free from grittiness.

NF category: Glidant and/or anticaking agent; tablet and/or capsule lubricant.

Talc intrapleural aersol—White or off-white to light grey, as-bestos-free, and brucite-free grade of talc of controlled granulometry.

Solubility: Talc intrapleural aerosol—Practically insoluble in water, and in dilute solutions of acids and alkali hydroxide.

USP requirements:

Talc USP—Preserve in well-closed containers. A native, hy-drous magnesium silicate, sometimes containing a small proportion of aluminum silicate. Meets the requirements for Identification, Microbial limits, Loss on ignition (not more than 6.5%), Acid-soluble substances (not more than 2.0%), Reaction and soluble substances (not more than 0.1%), Water-soluble iron, Arsenic, Heavy metals, and Lead (not more than 3 ppm for arsenic, not more than 0.004% for heavy metals, and not more than 0.001% for lead).

Talc Intrapleural Aerosol Powder—Not in *USP–NF*.

TAMOXIFEN

Chemical name: Tamoxifen citrate—Ethanamine, 2-[4-(1,2-di-phenyl-1-butenyl)phenoxy]-*N,N*-dimethyl, (*Z*)-, 2-hydroxy-1,2,3-propanetricarboxylate (1:1).

Molecular formula: Tamoxifen citrate—$C_{26}H_{29}NO \cdot C_6H_8O_7$.

Molecular weight: Tamoxifen citrate—563.64.

Description: Tamoxifen Citrate USP—White, fine, crystalline powder. Melts at about 142 °C, with decomposition.

pKa: Tamoxifen citrate—8.85.

Solubility: Tamoxifen Citrate USP—Very slightly soluble in water, in acetone, in chloroform, and in alcohol; soluble in methanol.

USP requirements:

Tamoxifen Citrate USP—Preserve in well-closed, light-resis-tant containers. Contains not less than 99.0% and not more than 101.0% of tamoxifen citrate, calculated on the dried basis. Meets the requirements for Identification, Loss on drying (not more than 0.5%), Residue on ignition (not more than 0.2%), Limit of *E-isomer* (not more than 0.3% of tamoxifen citrate), Iron (not more than 0.005%), Heavy metals (not more than 0.001%), Related impurities, and Organic volatile impurities.

Tamoxifen Citrate Tablets USP—Preserve in well-closed, light-resistant containers. Contain an amount of tamoxifen citrate equivalent to the labeled amount of tamoxifen, with-in ±10%. Meet the requirements for Identification, Disso-lution (75% in 30 minutes in 0.02 *N* hydrochloric acid in Apparatus 1 at 100 rpm), and Uniformity of dosage units.

Tamoxifen Citrate Enteric-coated Tablets—Not in *USP–NF*.

TAMSULOSIN

Chemical name: Tamsulosin hydrochloride—Benzenesulfona-mide, 5-[2-[[2-(2-ethoxyphenoxy)ethyl]amino]-propyl]-2-me-thoxy-, monohydrochloride, (*R*)-.

Molecular formula: Tamsulosin hydrochloride—$C_{20}H_{28}N_2O_5S \cdot$ HCl.

Molecular weight: Tamsulosin hydrochloride—444.97.

Description: Tamsulosin hydrochloride—White crystals. Melt with decomposition at approximately 230 °C.

Solubility: Tamsulosin hydrochloride—Sparingly soluble in water and in methanol; slightly soluble in glacial acetic acid and in ethanol; practically insoluble in ether.

USP requirements: Tamsulosin Hydrochloride Capsules—Not in *USP–NF*.

TANNIC ACID

Chemical name: Tannin.

Description: Tannic Acid USP—Amorphous powder, glistening scales, or spongy masses, varying in color from yellowish white to light brown. Is odorless or has a faint, characteristic odor.

Solubility: Tannic Acid USP—Very soluble in water, in acetone, and in alcohol; freely soluble in diluted alcohol, and only slightly soluble in dehydrated alcohol; practically insoluble in chloroform, in ether, and in solvent hexane; 1 gram dissolves in about 1 mL of warm glycerin.

USP requirements: Tannic Acid USP—Preserve in tight, light-re-sistant containers. A tannin usually obtained from nutgalls, the excrescences produced on the young twigs of *Quercus infec-toria* Oliver, and allied species of *Quercus* Linné (Fam. Faga-ceae), from the seed pods of Tara (*Caesalpinia spinosa*), or from the nutgalls or leaves of sumac (any of a genus *Rhus*). Meets the requirements for Identification, Loss on drying (not more than 12.0%), Residue on ignition (not more than 1.0%), Arsenic (not more than 3 ppm), Heavy metals (not more than 0.004%), Gum or dextrin, Resinous substances, and Organic volatile impurities.

ADHESIVE TAPE

USP requirements: Adhesive Tape USP—Preserve in well-closed containers, and prevent exposure to excessive heat and to sunlight. Tape that has been rendered sterile is so packaged that the sterility of the contents of the package is maintained until the package is opened for use. Consists of fabric and/or film evenly coated on one side with a pressure-sensitive, adhesive mixture. Its length is not less than 98.0% of that declared on the label, and its average width is not less than 95.0% of the declared width. If Adhesive Tape has been rendered sterile, it is protected from contamination by appro-priate packaging. The package label of Tape that has been rendered sterile indicates that the contents may not be sterile if the package bears evidence of damage or previously has been opened. The package label indicates the length and width of the Tape, and the name of the manufacturer, packer, or distributor. Meets the requirements for Dimensions (length, not less than 98.0% of labeled length; width, average of 5 measurements not less than 95% of the labeled width of Tape), Tensile strength, Adhesive strength, and Sterility.

TARTARIC ACID

Chemical name: Butanedioic acid, 2,3-dihydroxy-; Butanedioic acid, 2,3-dihydroxy-, [*R*-(*R*,R**)]-.

Molecular formula: $C_4H_6O_6$.

Molecular weight: 150.09.

Description: Tartaric Acid NF—Colorless or translucent crystals, or white, fine to granular, crystalline powder. Odorless. Stable in air.

NF category: Acidifying agent.

Solubility: Tartaric Acid NF—Very soluble in water; freely soluble in alcohol.

NF requirements: Tartaric Acid NF—Preserve in well-closed containers. Dried over phosphorus pentoxide for 3 hours, contains not less than 99.7% and not more than 100.5% of tartaric acid. Meets the requirements for Identification, Specific rotation ($+12.0°$ to $+13.0°$), Loss on drying (not more than 0.5%), Residue on ignition (not more than 0.1%), Limit of oxalate, Sulfate, Heavy metals (not more than 0.001%), and Organic volatile impurities.

TAURINE

Chemical name: Taurine.

Molecular formula: $C_2H_7NO_3S$.

Molecular weight: 125.15.

Description: Taurine USP—White crystals or crystalline powder.

Solubility: Taurine USP—Soluble in water.

USP requirements: Taurine USP—Preserve in well-closed containers. Contains not less than 98.5% and not more than 101.5% of taurine, calculated on the dried basis. Meets the requirements for Identification, Loss on drying (not more than 0.3%), Residue on ignition (not more than 0.3%), Chloride (not more than 0.05%), Sulfate (not more than 0.03%), Iron (0.003%), Heavy metals (0.0015%), Chromatographic purity, and Organic volatile impurities.

TAZAROTENE

Chemical name: 3-Pyridinecarboxylic acid, 6-[(3,4-dihydro-4,4-dimethyl-2H-1-benzothiopyran-6-yl)ethnyl]-, ethyl ester.

Molecular formula: $C_{21}H_{21}NO_2S$.

Molecular weight: 351.46.

USP requirements: Tazarotene Gel—Not in *USP–NF*.

TECHNETIUM TC 99M ALBUMIN

USP requirements: Technetium Tc 99m Albumin Injection USP—Preserve in single-dose or in multiple-dose containers, at a temperature between 2 and 8 °C. A sterile, aqueous solution, suitable for intravenous administration, of Albumin Human that is labeled with ^{99m}Tc. Label it to include the following in addition to the information specified for Labeling under Injections: the time and date of calibration; the amount of ^{99m}Tc as albumin expressed as total megabecquerels (or microcuries or millicuries) and concentration as megabecquerels (or microcuries or millicuries) per mL at the time of calibration; the expiration date; and the statement, "Caution—Radioactive Material." The labeling indicates that in making dosage calculations, correction is to be made for radioactive decay, and also indicates that the radioactive half-life of ^{99m}Tc is 6.0 hours. Its production and distribution are subject to U.S. regulations. Contains the labeled amount of ^{99m}Tc, within ±10%, as albumin expressed in megabecquerels (or microcuries or millicuries) per mL at the time indicated in the labeling. Other chemical forms of radioactivity do not exceed 10.0% of the total radioactivity. Meets the requirements for Bacterial endotoxins, pH (2.5–5.0), Radiochemical purity, and Biological distribution, for Radionuclide identification and Radionuclidic purity under Sodium Pertechnetate Tc 99m Injection, and for Injections (except that it may be distributed or dispensed prior to completion of the test for Sterility, the latter test being started on the day of final manufacture, and except that it is not subject to the recommendation on Volume in Container).

TECHNETIUM TC 99M ALBUMIN AGGREGATED

Description: Technetium Tc 99m Albumin Aggregated Injection USP—Milky suspension, from which particles settle upon standing.

USP requirements: Technetium Tc 99m Albumin Aggregated Injection USP—Preserve in single-dose or in multiple-dose containers, at a temperature between 2 and 8 °C. A sterile, aqueous suspension of Albumin Human that has been denatured to produce aggregates of controlled particle size that are labeled with ^{99m}Tc. Suitable for intravenous administration. Label it to include the following, in addition to the information specified for Labeling under Injections: the time and date of calibration; the amount of ^{99m}Tc as aggregated albumin expressed as total megabecquerels (or millicuries or microcuries) and concentration as megabecquerels (or microcuries or millicuries) per mL at the time of calibration; the expiration date; and the statement, "Caution—Radioactive Material." The labeling indicates that in making dosage calculations, correction is to be made for radioactive decay, and also indicates that the radioactive half-life of ^{99m}Tc is 6.0 hours. In addition, the labeling states that it is not to be used if clumping of the albumin is observed and directs that the container be agitated before the contents are withdrawn into a syringe. Its production and distribution are subject to U.S. regulations. Contains the labeled amount of ^{99m}Tc, within ±10%, as aggregated albumin expressed in megabecquerels (or microcuries or millicuries) per mL at the time indicated in the labeling. Other chemical forms of radioactivity do not exceed 10.0% of the total radioactivity. Meets the requirements for Particle size, Bacterial endotoxins, pH (3.8–8.0), Radiochemical purity, Protein concentration, and Biological distribution, for Radionuclide identification and Radionuclidic purity under Sodium Pertechnetate Tc 99m Injection, and for Injections (except that it may be distributed or dispensed prior to completion of the test for Sterility, the latter test being started on the day of final manufacture, and except that it is not subject to the recommendation on Volume in Container).

TECHNETIUM TC 99M ALBUMIN COLLOID

USP requirements: Technetium Tc 99m Albumin Colloid Injection USP—Preserve in single-dose or in multiple-dose containers, at a temperature between 2 and 8 °C. A sterile, pyrogen-free, aqueous suspension of Albumin Human that has been denatured to produce colloids of controlled particle size and that are labeled with $^{99}{}_mTc$. Label it to include the following, in addition to the information specified for Labeling under Injections: the time and date of calibration; the amount of ^{99m}Tc expressed as total megabecquerels (or millicuries) and concentration as megabecquerels (or millicuries) per mL at the time of calibration; the expiration date and time and a statement, "Caution—Radioactive Material." The labeling indicates that in making dosage calculations, correction is to be made for radioactive decay, and also indicates that the radioactive half-life of ^{99m}Tc is 6.0 hours. In addition, the labeling states that it is not to be used if clumping of the albumin is observed, and directs that the container be agitated before the contents are withdrawn into a syringe. The vials are sealed under a suitable inert atmosphere. Its production and distribution are subject to U.S. regulations. Contains the labeled amount

of ^{99m}Tc, within ±10%, as albumin colloid complex, expressed in megabecquerels (or millicuries) per mL at the time indicated on the labeling. Other chemical forms of radioactivity do not exceed 10.0% of the total radioactivity. Meets the requirements for Bacterial endotoxins, pH (7.5–8.5), Radiochemical purity, Particle size distribution, Biological distribution, and Albumin content, for Radionuclide identification and Radionuclidic purity under Sodium Pertechnetate Tc 99m Injection, and for Injections (except that it may be distributed or dispensed prior to completion of the test for Sterility, the latter test being started on the date of manufacture, and except that it is not subject to the recommendation on Volume in Container).

TECHNETIUM TC 99M APCITIDE

Chemical name: 13, 13′-[Oxybis[methylene(2,5-dioxo-1,3-pyrro-lidinediyl)]]bis[N-(mercaptoacetyl)-D-tyrosyl-S-(3-aminopropyl)-L-cysteinylglycyl-L-alpha-aspartyl-L-cysteinylglycylglycyl-S-[(acetylamino)methyl]-L-cysteinylglycyl-S-[(acetylamino)-methyl]-L-cysteinylglycylglycyl-L-cysteinamide], cyclic (1→5), (1′→5′)-bis(sulfide).

Molecular formula: $C_{112}H_{162}N_{36}O_{43}S_{10}$.

Molecular weight: 3021.4.

Description: Lyophilized powder.

USP requirements: Technetium Tc 99m Apcitide Injection USP—Preserve in single-dose containers at controlled room temperature. A sterile aqueous solution for intavenous injection that contains ^{99m}Tc in the form of an apcitide complex. May contain reducing agents, stabilizing agents, and buffers. Contains no antimicrobial agents. Label it to include the following, in addition to the information specified for Labeling under Injections: the time and date of calibration; the amount of ^{99m}Tc as labeled apcitide complex expressed as total megabecquerels per mL (or millicuries per mL) at the time of calibration; the expiration date and time; the storage temperature; and the statement, "Caution—Radioactive Material." The labeling indicates that in making dosage calculations, correction is to be made for radioactive decay, and also indicates that the radioactive half-life of ^{99m}Tc is 6.0 hours. Contains the labeled amount of ^{99m}Tc, within ±10%, as the apcitide complex expressed in megabecquerels per mL (or millicuries per mL) at the time indicated in the labeling. Other chemical forms of radioactivity do not exceed 10.0% of the total radioactivity. Meets the requirements for Bacterial endotoxins, pH (6.0–8.0), and Radiochemical purity (the sum of hydrophilic and immobile impurities not more than 10%), and for Radionuclide identification and Radionuclidic purity under Sodium Pertechnetate Tc 99m Injection, and for Injections (except that it is not subject to the recommendation on Volume in Container and that it may be distributed or dispensed prior to completion of the test for Sterility, the latter test being started on the date of manufacture).

TECHNETIUM TC 99M ARCITUMOMAB

USP requirements: Technetium Tc 99m Arcitumomab Injection USP—Preserve in single-dose Containers for Injections that are adequately shielded as described for Injections, and store at controlled room temperature. It is a sterile, nonpyrogenic preparation of the 50,000-dalton Fab′ fragment generated from the murine IgG monoclonal antibody Immu-4, suitable for intravenous administration that is labeled with ^{99m}Tc. Label it to include the following, in addition to the information specified for Labeling under Injections: the time and date of calibration; the amount of ^{99m}Tc as labeled arcitumomab expressed as total megabequerel (or millicurie) per mL, at the time of ca-

libration; the expiration date and time; the storage temperature; and the statement "Caution—Radioactive Material." The labeling indicates that, in making dosage calculations, correction is to be made for radioactive decay, and also indicates that the radioactive half-life of ^{99m}Tc is 6.0 hours. The labeling also states that it should be used within 4 hours following constitution. Contains the labeled amount of ^{99m}Tc, within ±10%, as an arcitumomab complex, expressed in megabecquerels (or millicuries) per mL at the time indicated in the labeling. Other chemical forms of radioactivity do not exceed 10.0% of the total radioactivity. The immunoreactive fraction determined by a validated method is not less than 75%. The Fab′ fragment content is not less than 90% as determined by size-exclusion HPLC. Meets the requirements for Bacterial endotoxins, pH (5.0–7.0), and Radiochemical purity (not more than 5.0% of the total radioactivity at the solvent front as unbound pertechnetate), and for Radionuclide identification and Radionuclidic purity under Sodium Pertechnetate Tc 99m Injection, and for Injections (except that it may be distributed or dispensed prior to completion of the test for Sterility, the latter test being started on the date of manufacture).

TECHNETIUM TC 99M BICISATE

Chemical name: Technetium-^{99m}TC, [[diethyl N,N-1,2-ethane-diylbis[L-cysteinato]](3–)-N,N,S,S′]oxo-, (SP-5-35)-.

Molecular formula: $C_{12}H_{21}N_2O_5S_2{}^{99m}Tc$.

USP requirements: Technetium Tc 99m Bicisate Injection USP—Preserve in single-dose or multiple-dose containers, at controlled room temperature. A sterile, clear, colorless solution, suitable for intravenous administration, of bicisate dihydrochloride complexed to radioactive technetium (^{99m}Tc). Label it to include the following, in addition to the information specified for Labeling under Injections: the time and date of calibration; the amount of ^{99m}Tc as labeled bicisate expressed as total megabecquerels (or millicuries) per mL at the time of calibration; the expiration date and time; the lot number; and the statement "Caution—Radioactive Material." The labeling indicates that in making dosage calculations, correction is to be made for radioactive decay, and also indicates that the radioactive half-life of ^{99m}Tc is 6.0 hours. Contains the labeled amount of ^{99m}Tc, within ±10%, as a complex with bicisate, expressed in megabecquerels (or in millicuries) per mL at the time indicated in the labeling. Other chemical forms of radioactivity do not exceed 10% of the total radioactivity. Meets the requirements for Bacterial endotoxins, Radiochemical purity, and Related radiochemical compounds, for Radionuclide identification and Radionuclidic purity under Sodium Pertechnetate Tc 99m Injection, and for Injections, (except that the Injection may be distributed or dispensed prior to the completion of the test for Sterility, the latter test being started on the day of manufacture).

TECHNETIUM TC 99M DEPREOTIDE

USP requirements:Technetium Tc 99m Depreotide Injection USP—Preserve in single-dose containers, at controlled room temperature. A sterile, aqueous solution suitable for intravenous injection that contains ^{99m}Tc in the form of a depreotide complex. Label it to include the following, in addition to the information specified for Labeling under Injections: the time and date of calibration; the amount of ^{99m}Tc as labeled depreotide complex expressed as total megabecquerels (or millicuries) per mL at the time of calibration; the expiration date and time; the storage temperature; and the statement 'Caution—Radioactive Material'. The labeling indicates that, in making dosage

calculations, correction is to be made for radioactive decay, and also indicates that the radioactive half-life of ^{99m}Tc is 6.0 hours. Contains the labeld amount of ^{99m}Tc, within ±10%, as the depreotide complex expressed in megabecquerels (or in millicuries) per mL at the time indicated in the labeling. May contain reducing agents, stabilizing agents, and buffers. Contains no antimicrobial agents. Other chemical forms of radioactivity do not exceed 10.0% of the total radioactivity. Meets the requirements for Bacterial endotoxines, pH (6.0–8.0), and Radiochemical purity (not more than 10%), and for Radionuclide identification and Radionuclidic purity for Sodium Pertechnetate Tc 99m Injection (except that the Injection is not subject to the recommendation on Volume in Container, and except that it may be distributed or dispensed prior to completion of the test for Sterility, the latter test being started on the date of manufacture).

TECHNETIUM TC 99M DISOFENIN

Chemical group: Disofenin—derivative of iminodiacetic acid (IDA).

Chemical name: Disofenin—Glycine, *N*-[2-[[2,6-bis(1-methylethyl)phenyl]amino]-2-oxoethyl]-*N*-(carboxymethyl)-.

Molecular formula: Disofenin—$C_{18}H_{26}N_2O_5$.

Molecular weight: Disofenin—350.42.

USP requirements: Technetium Tc 99m Disofenin Injection USP—Preserve in single-dose or in multiple-dose containers sealed under a suitable inert atmosphere. A sterile, aqueous solution, suitable for intravenous administration, of disofenin that is labeled with ^{99m}Tc. Contains a suitable reducing agent. Label it to include the following, in addition to the information specified for Labeling under Injections: the time and date of preparation; the amount of ^{99m}Tc expressed as total megabecquerels (or microcuries or millicuries) and concentration as megabecquerels (or microcuries or millicuries) per mL at the time of preparation; the expiration date and time; and a statement, "Caution—Radioactive Material." The labeling indicates that in making dosage calculations, correction is to be made for radioactive decay, and also indicates that the radioactive half-life of ^{99m}Tc is 6.0 hours. Contains the labeled amount of ^{99m}Tc, within ±10%, as a disofenin complex, expressed in megabecquerels (or microcuries or millicuries) per mL at the time indicated on the labeling. Meets the requirements for pH (4.0–5.0), Radiochemical purity, and Biological distribution, for Radionuclide identification, Radionuclidic purity, and Bacterial endotoxins under Sodium Pertechnetate Tc 99m Injection, and for Injections (except that it may be distributed or dispensed prior to completion of the test for Sterility, the latter test being started on the date of preparation, and except that it is not subject to the recommendation on Volume in Container).

TECHNETIUM TC 99M ETIDRONATE

USP requirements: Technetium Tc 99m Etidronate Injection USP—Preserve in single-dose or in multiple-dose containers. A sterile, clear, colorless solution, suitable for intravenous administration, of radioactive technetium (^{99m}Tc) in the form of a chelate of etidronate sodium. Label it to include the following, in addition to the information specified for Labeling under Injections: the time and date of calibration; the amount of ^{99m}Tc as labeled etidronate expressed as total megabecquerels (or microcuries or millicuries) and concentration as megabecquerels (or microcuries or millicuries) per mL at the time of calibration; the expiration date and time; and the statement, "Caution—Radioactive Material." The labeling indicates that in making dosage calculations, correction is to be made for ra-

dioactive decay, and also indicates that the radioactive half-life of ^{99m}Tc is 6.0 hours. Contains the labeled amount of ^{99m}Tc, within ±10%, as chelate expressed in megabecquerels (or microcuries or millicuries) per mL at the time indicated in the labeling. Other chemical forms of radioactivity do not exceed 10.0% of the total radioactivity. Meets the requirements for pH (2.5–7.0), and for Bacterial endotoxins, Radiochemical purity, Biological distribution, and Other requirements under Technetium Tc 99m Pyrophosphate Injection.

TECHNETIUM TC 99M EXAMETAZIME

Chemical name: 2-Butanone, 3,3′-[(2,2-dimethyl-1,3-propanediyl)diimino]bis-dioxime-^{99m}Tc.

USP requirements: Technetium Tc 99m Exametazime Injection USP—Preserve in single-dose or in multiple-dose containers, at controlled room temperature. A sterile, aqueous solution, suitable for intravenous administration, composed of the primary lipophilic complex of exametazime that is labeled with radioactive ^{99m}Tc. Label it to include the following, in addition to the information specified for Labeling under Injections: the time and date of calibration; the amount of ^{99m}Tc as labeled exametazime expressed as total megabecquerels (or as total microcuries or millicuries) and concentration as megabecquerels (or as microcuries or millicuries) per mL at the time of calibration; the expiration date and time; and the statement, "Caution—Radioactive Material." The labeling indicates that in making dosage calculations, correction is to be made for radioactive decay, and also indicates that the radioactive half-life of ^{99m}Tc is 6.0 hours. (Note: The label states that upon constitution with Sodium Pertechnetate Tc 99m Injection, the beyond-use time is 30 minutes for the unstabilized Injection and between 4 hours and 6 hours for the stabilized Injection.) Contains the labeled amount of ^{99m}Tc, within ±10%, as primary lipophilic exametazime complex expressed in megabecquerels (or in microcuries or millicuries) per mL at the date and time indicated in the labeling. Other chemical forms of radioactivity (^{99m}Tc pertechnetate, ^{99m}Tc hydrolyzed reduced species, and ^{99m}Tc secondary exametazime complex) do not exceed 20.0% of the total radioactivity. Meets the requirements for pH (9.0–9.8 for unstabilized Injection, and 6.5–7.5 for stabilized Injection), Radiochemical purity, and Biological distribution, for Radionuclidic identification, Radionuclide purity, and Bacterial endotoxins under Sodium Pertechnetate Tc 99m Injection, and for Injections (except that it may be distributed or dispensed prior to completion of the test for Sterility, the latter test being started on the day of manufacture, and except that it is not subject to the recommendation on Volume in Container).

TECHNETIUM TC 99M GLUCEPTATE

Chemical name: D-*glycero[sp*-[rpD-*gulo*-Heptonic acid, technetium-^{99m}*Tc* complex.

USP requirements: Technetium Tc 99m Gluceptate Injection USP—Preserve in single-dose or in multiple-dose containers, at a temperature between 2 and 8 °C. A sterile, aqueous solution, suitable for intravenous administration, of sodium gluceptate and stannous chloride that is labeled with ^{99m}Tc. Label it to include the following, in addition to the information specified for Labeling under Injections: the time and date of calibration; the amount of ^{99m}Tc as labeled stannous gluceptate expressed as total megabecquerels (or microcuries or millicuries) and concentration as megabecquerels (or microcuries or millicuries) per mL at the time of calibration; the expiration date and time; and the statement, "Caution—Radioactive Material." The labeling indicates that in making dosage calculations,

correction is to be made for radioactive decay, and also indicates that the radioactive half-life of ^{99m}Tc is 6.0 hours. Contains the labeled amount of ^{99m}Tc, within ±10%, as stannous gluceptate complex expressed in megabecquerels (or microcuries or millicuries) per mL at the time indicated in the labeling. Other chemical forms of radioactivity do not exceed 10.0% of the total radioactivity. Meets the requirements for Bacterial endotoxins, pH (4.0–8.0), Radiochemical purity, and Biological distribution, for Radionuclide identification and Radionuclidic purity under Sodium Pertechnetate Tc 99m Injection, and for Injections (except that it may be distributed or dispensed prior to completion of the test for Sterility, the latter test being started on the date of manufacture, and except that it is not subject to the recommendation on Volume in Container).

TECHNETIUM TC 99M LIDOFENIN

Chemical group: Lidofenin—Derivative of iminodiacetic acid (IDA).

Chemical name: Lidofenin—Glycine, *N*-(carboxymethyl)-*N*-[2-[(2,6-dimethylphenyl)amino]-2-oxoethyl]-.

Molecular formula: Lidofenin—$C_{14}H_{18}N_2O_5$.

Molecular weight: Lidofenin—294.31.

Description: Lidofenin—Possesses both a lipophilic component and a hydrophilic group; forms an anionic bis-complex with Tc 99m.

USP requirements: Technetium Tc 99m Lidofenin Injection USP—Preserve in single-dose or in multiple-dose containers at a temperature between 2 and 8 °C. A sterile, clear, colorless solution of lidofenin complexed to radioactive technetium (^{99m}Tc) in the form of a chelate. Suitable for intravenous injection. Label it to include the following, in addition to the information specified for Labeling under Injections: the time and date of calibration; the amount of ^{99m}Tc as labeled lidofenin expressed as total megabecquerels (or millicuries) per mL at the time of calibration; the expiration date and time; the storage temperature and the statement, "Caution—Radioactive Material." The labeling indicates that, in making dosage calculations, correction is to be made for radioactive decay, and also indicates that the radioactive half-life of ^{99m}Tc is 6.0 hours. Contains the labeled amount of ^{99m}Tc, within ±10%, as the lidofenin chelate, expressed in megabecquerels (or millicuries) per mL at the time indicated in the labeling. Other chemical forms of radioactivity do not exceed 10.0% of the total radioactivity. Meets the requirements for Bacterial endotoxins, pH (3.5–5.0), Radiochemical purity, and Biological distribution, for Radionuclide identification and Radionuclidic purity under Sodium Pertechnetate Tc 99m Injection, and for Injections (except that it may be distributed or dispensed prior to completion of the test for Sterility, the latter test being started on the day of manufacture, and except that it is not subject to the recommendation on Volume in Container).

TECHNETIUM TC 99M MEBROFENIN

Chemical group: Mebrofenin—Derivative of iminodiacetic acid (IDA).

Chemical name: Mebrofenin—Glycine, *N*-[2-[(3-bromo-2,4,6-trimethylphenyl)amino]-2-oxoethyl]-*N*-(carboxymethyl)-.

Molecular formula: Mebrofenin—$C_{15}H_{19}BrN_2O_5$.

Molecular weight: Mebrofenin—387.23.

Description: Mebrofenin—Possesses both a lipophilic component and a hydrophilic group; forms an anionic bis-complex with Tc 99m.

USP requirements: Technetium Tc 99m Mebrofenin Injection USP—Preserve in single-dose or in multiple-dose containers, at controlled room temperature. A sterile aqueous solution of Stannous Fluoride and Mebrofenin labeled with radioactive technetium Tc 99m suitable for intravenous administration. Label it to include the following, in addition to the information specified for Labeling under Injections: the time and date of calibration; the amount of ^{99m}Tc as labeled mebrofenin expressed as total megabecquerels (or millicuries) and the concentration as megabecquerels per mL (or as millicuries per mL) on the date and time of calibration; the expiration date and time; and the statement, "Caution—Radioactive Material." The labeling indicates that in making dosage calculations, correction is to be made for radioactive decay, and also indicates that the radioactive half-life of ^{99m}Tc is 6.0 hours. Contains the labeled amount of ^{99m}Tc, within ±10%, as the complex with mebrofenin, expressed in megabecquerels (or in millicuries) per mL at the time indicated in the labeling. Other chemical forms of radioactivity do not exceed 10.0% of the total radioactivity. Meets the requirements for pH (4.2–5.7), Radiochemical purity, and Biological distribution, for Radionuclide identification, Radionuclidic purity, and Bacterial endotoxins under Sodium Pertechnetate Tc 99m Injection, and for Injections (except that it may be distributed and dispensed prior to the completion of the test for Sterility, the latter test being started on the day of manufacture, and except that it is not subject to the recommendation on Volume in Container).

TECHNETIUM TC 99M MEDRONATE

Chemical group: Sodium medronate—A biphosphonate compound.

USP requirements: Technetium Tc 99m Medronate Injection USP—Preserve in single-dose or in multiple-dose containers at a temperature specified in the labeling. A sterile, aqueous solution, suitable for intravenous administration, of sodium medronate and stannous chloride or stannous fluoride that is labeled with radioactive Tc 99m. Contains the labeled amount of Tc 99m, within ±10%, as stannous medronate complex expressed in megabecquerels (or microcuries or millicuries) per mL at the date and time indicated in the labeling. Other chemical forms of radioactivity do not exceed 10.0% of the total radioactivity. Meets the requirements for Bacterial endotoxins, pH (4.0–7.8), and Radiochemical purity, for Radionuclide identification and Radionuclidic purity under Sodium Pertechnetate Tc 99m Injection, for Labeling and Biological distribution under Technetium Tc 99m Pyrophosphate Injection, and for Injections (except that it may be distributed or dispensed prior to completion of the test for Sterility, the latter test being started on the day of manufacture, and except that it is not subject to the recommendation on Volume in Container).

TECHNETIUM TC 99M MERTIATIDE

Chemical name: Technetate(2–)-^{99m}*Tc*, [*N*-[*N*-[*N*-(mercaptoacetyl)glycyl]glycyl]glycinato(5–)-*N*,*N'*, *N''*,*S*]-oxo-, disodium, (*SP*-5-25)-.

Molecular formula: $C_8H_8N_3Na_2O_6S^{99m}Tc$.

USP requirements: Technetium Tc 99m Mertiatide Injection USP—Preserve in single-dose or in multiple-dose containers. A sterile aqueous solution, suitable for intravenous injection, that contains ^{99m}Tc in the form of a chelate of mertiatide. Label it to include the following, in addition to the information specified for Labeling under Injections: the time and date of calibration; the amount of ^{99m}Tc as labeled mertiatide expressed as total megabecquerels (or millicuries) and the concentration as megabecquerels per mL (or as millicuries per mL) on the date and time of calibration; the expiration date and time; and the statement, "Caution—Radioactive Material." The labeling indicates that in making dosage calculations, correction is to be made for radioactive decay, and also indicates that the radioactive half-life of ^{99m}Tc is 6.0 hours. Contains uncomplexed betiatide, a suitable ^{99m}Tc reducing agent, a transfer ligand, and stabilizers. Contains the labeled amount of ^{99m}Tc, within ±10%, as mertiatide complex expressed in megabecquerels (or in microcuries or millicuries) per mL at the date and time indicated in the labeling. Meets the requirements for Bacterial endotoxins, pH (5.0–6.0), and Radiochemical purity, for Radionuclide identification and Radionuclidic purity under Sodium Pertechnetate Tc 99m Injection, and for Injections (except that it may be distributed or dispensed prior to completion of the test for Sterility, the latter test being started on the day of final manufacture, and except that it is not subject to the recommendation on Volume in Container).

TECHNETIUM TC 99M NOFETUMOMAB MERPENTAN

USP requirements: Technetium Tc 99m Nofetumomab Merpentan Injection USP—Preserve in single-dose containers. A sterile, nonpyrogenic preparation of the Fab fragment of IgG2b murine monoclonal antibody NRLU-10 that is labeled with ^{99m}Tc and is suitable for intravenous administration. Label it to include the following, in addition to the information specified for Labeling under Injections: the time and date of calibration; the amount of ^{99m}Tc as labeled nofetumomab merpentan expressed in megabecquerels (or millicuries) per mL at the time of calibration; the expiration date and time; the storage temperature; and the statement, "Caution—Radioactive Material." The labeling indicates that the radioactive half-life of ^{99m}Tc is 6.0 hours and that, in making dosage calculations, correction is to be made for radioactive decay. The labeling also states that the Injection is to be used within 6 hours following constitution. Contains the labeled amount of ^{99m}Tc, within ±10%, as nofetumomab complex, expressed in megabecquerels (or millicuries) per mL at the time indicated in the labeling. It may contain reducing agents, buffers, and stabilizers. It contains no antimicrobial agents. Other chemical forms of radioactivity do not exceed 10.0% of the total radioactivity. The immunoreactive fraction, as determined by a validated method, is not less than 85%. Meets the requirements for Bacterial endotoxins, pH (7.0–8.0), and Radiochemical purity, and for Radionuclide identification and Radionuclidic purity under Sodium Pertechnetate Tc 99m Injection, and for Injections (except that it may be distributed or dispensed prior to completion of the test for Sterility, the latter test being started on the date of manufacture.

Caution: Components of the commercial kit that are used to prepare the Injection are not to be administered directly to the patient.

TECHNETIUM TC 99M OXIDRONATE

Chemical group: Oxidronate sodium—A biphosphonate compound.

USP requirements: Technetium Tc 99m Oxidronate Injection USP—Preserve in single-dose or in multiple-dose containers. A sterile, clear, colorless solution, suitable for intravenous administration, of radioactive technetium (^{99m}Tc) in the form of a chelate of oxidronate sodium. Label it to include the following, in addition to the information specified for Labeling under Injections: the time and date of calibration; the amount of ^{99m}Tc as labeled oxidronate expressed as total megabecquerels (or microcuries or millicuries) and concentration as megabecquerels (or microcuries or millicuries) per mL at the time of calibration; the expiration date and time; and the statement, "Caution—Radioactive Material." The labeling indicates that in making dosage calculations, correction is to be made for radioactive decay, and also indicates that the radioactive half-life of ^{99m}Tc is 6.0 hours. Contains the labeled amount of ^{99m}Tc, within ±10%, as chelate expressed in megabecquerels (or microcuries or millicuries) per mL at the date and time indicated in the labeling. Other chemical forms of radioactivity do not exceed 10.0% of the total radioactivity. Meets the requirements for pH (2.5–7.0), and for Bacterial endotoxins, Radiochemical purity, Biological distribution, and Other requirements under Technetium Tc 99m Pyrophosphate Injection.

TECHNETIUM TC 99M PENTETATE

Chemical name: Technetate(1-)^{99m}Tc, [N,N-bis[2-bis(carboxymethyl)amino]ethyl]glycinato(5-)]-, sodium.

Molecular formula: $C_{14}H_{18}N_3NaO_{10}^{99m}Tc$.

Description: Technetium Tc 99m Pentetate Injection USP—Clear, colorless solution.

USP requirements: Technetium Tc 99m Pentetate Injection USP—Preserve in single-dose or in multiple-dose containers, at a temperature between 2 and 8 °C. A sterile solution of pentetic acid that is complexed with ^{99m}Tc in Sodium Chloride Injection. Suitable for intravenous administration. Label it to include the following, in addition to the information specified for Labeling under Injections: the time and date of calibration; the amount of ^{99m}Tc as labeled pentetic acid complex expressed as total megabecquerels (or millicuries or microcuries) and concentration as megabecquerels (or microcuries or millicuries) per mL at the time of calibration; the expiration date; and the statement, "Caution—Radioactive Material." The labeling indicates that in making dosage calculations, correction is to be made for radioactive decay, and also indicates that the radioactive half-life of ^{99m}Tc is 6.0 hours. Contains the labeled amount of ^{99m}Tc, within ±10%, as the pentetic acid complex, expressed in megabecquerels (or microcuries or millicuries) per mL at the time indicated on the labeling. Other chemical forms of radioactivity do not exceed 10.0% of the total radioactivity. Meets the requirements for Bacterial endotoxins, pH (3.8–7.5), Biological distribution, and Radiochemical purity, for Radionuclide identification and Radionuclidic purity under Sodium Pertechnetate Tc 99m Injection, and for Injections (except that it may be distributed or dispensed prior to completion of the test for Sterility, the latter test being started on the day of manufacture, and except that it is not subject to the recommendation on Volume in Container).

SODIUM PERTECHNETATE TC 99M

Chemical name: Pertechnetic acid ($H^{99m}TcO_4$), sodium salt.

Molecular formula: $Na^{99m}TcO_4$.

Description: Sodium Pertechnetate Tc 99m Injection USP—Clear, colorless solution.

USP requirements: Sodium Pertechnetate Tc 99m Injection USP—Preserve in single-dose or in multiple-dose containers. A sterile solution, suitable for intravenous or oral administration, containing radioactive technetium (^{99m}Tc) in the form of sodium pertechnetate and sufficient Sodium Chloride to make the solution isotonic. Technetium 99m is a radioactive nuclide formed by the radioactive decay of molybdenum 99. Molybdenum 99 is a radioactive isotope of molybdenum and may be formed by the neutron bombardment of molybdenum 98 or as a product of uranium fission. If intended for intravenous use, label it with the information specified for Labeling under Injections. Label it also to include the following: the time and date of calibration; the amount of ^{99m}Tc as sodium pertechnetate expressed as total megabecquerels (or millicuries) and as megabecquerels (or millicuries) per mL on the date and at the time of calibration; a statement of the intended use, whether oral or intravenous; the expiration date; and the statement, "Caution—Radioactive Material." If the Injection has been prepared from molybdenum 99 produced from uranium fission, the label so states. The labeling indicates that in making dosage calculations, correction is to be made for radioactive decay, and also indicates that the radioactive half-life of ^{99m}Tc is 6.0 hours. Contains the labeled amount of ^{99m}Tc, within ±10%, at the date and hour stated on the label. Other chemical forms of ^{99m}Tc do not exceed 5% of the total radioactivity. Meets the requirements for Radionuclide identification, Bacterial endotoxins, pH (4.5–7.5), Radiochemical purity, Radionuclidic purity, and Chemical purity, and for Injections (except that the Injection may be distributed or dispensed prior to the completion of the test for Sterility, the latter test being started on the day of manufacture, and except that it is not subject to the recommendation on Volume in Container).

TECHNETIUM TC 99M PYROPHOSPHATE

USP requirements: Technetium Tc 99m Pyrophosphate Injection USP—Preserve in single-dose or in multiple-dose containers, at a temperature between 2 and 8 °C. A sterile aqueous solution, suitable for intravenous administration, of pyrophosphate that is labeled with ^{99m}Tc. Label it to include the following, in addition to the information specified for Labeling under Injections: the time and date of calibration; the amount of ^{99m}Tc as labeled tetrasodium pyrophosphate expressed as total megabecquerels (or microcuries or millicuries) and concentration as megabecquerels (or microcuries or millicuries) per mL at the time of calibration; the expiration date and time; and the statement, "Caution—Radioactive Material." The labeling indicates that in making dosage calculations, correction is to be made for radioactive decay, and also indicates that the radioactive half-life of ^{99m}Tc is 6.0 hours. Contains the labeled amount of ^{99m}Tc, within ±10%, as pyrophosphate expressed in megabecquerels (or microcuries or millicuries) per mL at the time indicated in the labeling. Other chemical forms of radioactivity do not exceed 10.0% of the total radioactivity. Meets the requirements for Bacterial endotoxins, pH (4.0–7.5), Radiochemical purity, and Biological distribution, for Radionuclide identification and Radionuclidic purity under Sodium Pertechnetate Tc 99m Injection, and for Injections (except that it may be distributed or dispensed prior to completion of the test for Sterility, the latter test being started on the day of final manufacture, and except that it is not subject to the recommendation on Volume in Container).

TECHNETIUM TC 99M (PYRO- AND TRIMETA-) PHOSPHATES

Chemical name:
Sodium pyrophosphate—Diphosphoric acid, tetrasodium salt.
Sodium trimetaphosphate—Metaphosphoric acid ($H_3P_3O_9$), trisodium salt.
Stannous chloride—Tin chloride ($SnCl_2$) dihydrate.

Molecular formula:
Sodium pyrophosphate—$Na_4P_2O_7$.
Sodium trimetaphosphate—$Na_3P_3O_9$.
Stannous chloride—$SnCl_2 \cdot 2H_2O$.

Molecular weight:
Sodium pyrophosphate—265.90.
Sodium trimetaphosphate—305.89.
Stannous chloride—225.65.

Description: Technetium Tc 99m (Pyro- and Trimeta-) Phosphates Injection USP—Clear solution.

USP requirements: Technetium Tc 99m (Pyro- and trimeta-) Phosphates Injection USP—A sterile, aqueous solution, suitable for intravenous administration, composed of sodium pyrophosphate, sodium trimetaphosphate, and stannous chloride labeled with radioactive Tc 99m. Contains the labeled amount of ^{99m}Tc, within ±10%, as phosphate expressed in megabecquerels (or microcuries or millicuries) per mL at the time indicated in the labeling. Other chemical forms of radioactivity do not exceed 10.0% of the total radioactivity. Meets the requirements for pH (4.0–7.0) and Radiochemical purity, for Radionuclide identification and Radionuclidic purity under Sodium Pertechnetate Tc 99m Injection, for Packaging and storage, Labeling, Bacterial endotoxins, and Biological distribution under Technetium Tc 99m Pyrophosphate Injection, and for Injections (except that it may be distributed or dispensed prior to completion of the test for Sterility, the latter test being started on the day of final manufacture, and except that it is not subject to the recommendation on Volume in Container).

TECHNETIUM TC 99M RED BLOOD CELLS

USP requirements: Technetium Tc 99m Red Blood Cells Injection USP—Preserve in adequately shielded single-dose or multiple-dose containers, at controlled room temperature. A preparation of anticoagulated whole blood that is labeled with ^{99m}Tc. The cells are prepared for labeling by collection of an autologous sample of whole blood, which is anticoagulated with Heparin Sodium or anticoagulant dextrose solution. Label it to include the following, in addition to the information specified for Labeling under Injections: the patient's name and identification number; the type of anticoagulant used; the time and date of calibration; the amount expressed as total megabecquerels (or microcuries or millicuries) and concentration as megabecquerels (or microcuries or millicuries) per mL at the time of calibration; the expiration date; and the statement "Caution—Radioactive Material." The labeling indicates that in making dosage calculations, correction is to be made for radioactive decay, and also indicates that the radioactive half-life of ^{99m}Tc is 6.0 hours. May contain anticoagulants, such as heparin or anticoagulant citrate solution, chelating agents, stannous chloride, and sodium hypochlorite. Other chemical forms of radioactivity do not exceed 10.0% of the total radioactivity. When derived from donor blood, its production and distribution derived from donor blood are subject to federal regulations. Contains the labeled concentration of ^{99m}Tc, within ±10%, as labeled blood cells expressed in megabecquerels (or in microcuries or millicuries) per mL at the time indicated in the labeling. Meets the requirements for Bacterial endotoxins, pH (5.5–8.0), Radiochemical purity, and Clarity and color of solution, for Radionuclide identification and Radionuclidic purity under Sodium Pertechnetate Tc 99m Injection, and for

Injections (except that it may be distributed or dispensed prior to completion of the test for Sterility, the latter test being started on the day of final manufacture, and except that it is not subject to the recommendation on Volume in Container).

Caution: A strict aseptic technique must be followed for collection of the blood sample, along with the processing steps required to label it with Technetium Tc 99m. The blood samples must be labeled with the name of the patient and patient's identification code to prevent administration of the sample to other than the intended patient. In the event that donor blood is used, it must first be tested for viral contaminants and carefully typed and cross-matched to ensure compatibility with that of the recipient.

TECHNETIUM TC 99M SESTAMIBI

Chemical name: Technetium(1+)-^{99m}*Tc*, hexakis(1-isocyano-2-methoxy-2-methylpropane)-, (*OC*-6-11)-.

Molecular formula: $C_{36}H_{66}N_6O_6{}^{99m}Tc$.

USP requirements: Technetium Tc 99m Sestamibi Injection USP—Preserve in single-dose or in multiple-dose containers. A sterile, aqueous solution of tetrakis(2-methoxy-isobutyl isonitrile) copper(I) tetrafluoroborate that is labeled with ^{99m}Tc suitable for intravenous administration. Contains reducing agents, a buffer, and an inert filler. Label it to include the following, in addition to the information specified for Labeling under Injections: the time and date of constitution; the volume of constitution; the amount of ^{99m}Tc as labeled sestamibi expressed as total megabecquerels (or millicuries) per mL at the time of constitution; the expiration date and time; the lot number; and the statement, "Caution—Radioactive Material." The labeling indicates that in making dosage calculations, correction is to be made for radioactive decay, and also indicates that the radioactive half-life of ^{99m}Tc is 6.0 hours. Contains the labeled amount of ^{99m}Tc, within ±10%, as a complex with sestamibi, expressed in megabecquerels (or in millicuries) per mL at the time indicated in the labeling. Other chemical forms of radioactivity do not exceed 10.0% of the total radioactivity. Meets the requirements for Bacterial endotoxins, pH (5–6), and Radiochemical purity, for Radionuclide identification and Radionuclidic purity under Sodium Pertechnetate Tc 99m Injection, and for Injections (except that it may be distributed and dispensed prior to the completion of the test for Sterility, the latter being started on the day of manufacture, and except that it is not subject to the recommendation on Volume in Container).

TECHNETIUM TC 99M SUCCIMER

Chemical name: meso-2,3-Dimercaptosuccinic acid, ^{99m}*Tc* complex.

USP requirements: Technetium Tc 99m Succimer Injection USP—Preserve in single-dose containers, at a temperature between 15 and 30 °C. Do not freeze or store above 30 °C. Protect from light. A sterile, clear, colorless, aqueous solution of succimer complexed with ^{99m}Tc. Suitable for intravenous administration. Label it to include the following, in addition to the information specified for Labeling under Injections: the time and date of calibration; the amount of ^{99m}Tc as labeled succimer expressed as total megabecquerels (or microcuries or millicuries) and concentration as megabecquerels (or microcuries or millicuries) per mL at the time of calibration; the expiration date and time; and the statement, "Caution—Radioactive Material." The labeling indicates that in making dosage calculations, correction is to be made for radioactive decay, and also indicates that the radioactive half-life of

^{99m}Tc is 6.0 hours. In addition, the labeling states that it is not to be used if discoloration or particulate matter is observed. (Note: A beyond-use time of 30 minutes shall be stated on the label upon constitution with Sodium Pertechnetate Tc 99m Injection.) Contains the labeled amount of ^{99m}Tc, within −15%, as the succimer complex expressed in megabecquerels (or microcuries or millicuries) per mL at the time indicated in the labeling. Other chemical forms of radioactivity do not exceed 15.0% of the total radioactivity. Meets the requirements for Bacterial endotoxins, pH (2.0–3.0), Radiochemical purity, and Biological distribution, for Radionuclide identification and Radionuclidic purity under Sodium Pertechnetate Tc 99m Injection, and for Injections (except that it may be distributed or dispensed prior to completion of the test for Sterility, the latter test being started on the day of final manufacture, and except that it is not subject to the recommendation on Volume in Container).

TECHNETIUM TC 99M SULFUR COLLOID

Description: Technetium Tc 99m Sulfur Colloid Injection USP—Colloidal dispersion. Slightly opalescent, colorless to light tan liquid.

USP requirements: Technetium Tc 99m Sulfur Colloid Injection USP—Store in single-dose or in multiple-dose containers. A sterile, colloidal dispersion of sulfur labeled with radioactive ^{99m}Tc, suitable for intravenous administration. Label it to include the following, in addition to the information specified for Labeling under Injections: the time and date of calibration; the amount of ^{99m}Tc as sulfur colloid expressed as total megabecquerels (or microcuries or millicuries) and concentration as megabecquerels (or microcuries or millicuries) per mL at the time of calibration; the expiration date; and the statement, "Caution—Radioactive Material." The labeling indicates that in making dosage calculations, correction is to be made for radioactive decay, and also indicates that the radioactive half-life of ^{99m}Tc is 6.0 hours; in addition, the labeling states that it is not to be used if flocculent material is visible and directs that the container be agitated before the Injection is withdrawn into a syringe. Contains the labeled concentration of ^{99m}Tc, within ±10%, as sulfur colloid expressed in megabecquerels (or microcuries or millicuries) per mL at the time indicated in the labeling. Other chemical forms of radioactivity do not exceed 8% of the total radioactivity. Meets the requirements for Radionuclide identification, Bacterial endotoxins, pH (4.5–7.5), Radionuclidic purity under Sodium Pertechnetate Tc 99m Injection, Radiochemical purity, and Biological distribution, and for Injections (except that the Injection may be distributed or dispensed prior to completion of the test for Sterility, the latter test being started on the day of final manufacture, and except that it is not subject to the recommendation on Volume in Container).

Note: Agitate the container before withdrawing the Injection into a syringe.

TECHNETIUM TC 99M TEBOROXIME

Chemical name: Technetium-^{99m}*Tc*, [bis[(1,2-cyclohexanedione dioximato)(1-)-*O*][(1,2-cyclohexanedione dioximato)(2-)-*O*]methylborato(2-)-*N,N′,N″,N‴,N‴,N‴*]-chloro-, (*TPS*-7-1-232′4′54)-.

Molecular formula: $C_{19}H_{29}BClN_6O_6{}^{99m}Tc$.

USP requirements: Technetium Tc 99m Teboroxime Injection—Not in *USP–NF*.

TECHNETIUM TC 99M TETROFOSMIN

USP requirements: Technetium Tc 99m Tetrofosmin Injection USP—Preserve in adequately shielded single-dose or in multiple-dose containers. Protect from light. Store at a temperature not exceeding 25 °C. A sterile aqueous solution, suitable for intravenous injection, that contains ^{99m}Tc in the form of a complex of tetrofosmin. May contain reducing agents, stabilizers, and buffers. Contains no antimicrobial agents. Label it to include the following, in addition to the information specified for Labeling under Injections: the time and date of calibration; the amount of ^{99m}Tc as labeled tetrofosmin expressed as total megabecquerels (or millicuries) and concentration as megabecquerels per mL (or as millicuries per mL) on the date and time of calibration; the expiration date and time; and a statement, "Caution—Radioactive Material." The labeling indicates that in making dosage calculations, correction is to be made for radioactive decay, and also indicates that the radioactive half-life of ^{99m}Tc is 6.0 hours. Contains the labeled amount of ^{99m}Tc, within ±10%, as the tetrofosmin complex expressed in megabecquerels (or millicuries) per mL at the date and time indicated in the labeling. Other chemical forms of radioactivity do not exceed 10.0% of the total. Meets the requirements for Bacterial endotoxins, pH (8.3–9.1), and Radiochemical purity (the sum of radioactivity at the solvent front [unbound pertechnetate] and the origin [reduced hydrolyzed technetium and hydrophilic impurities] not more than 10%), for Radionuclide identification and Radionuclidic purity under Sodium Pertechnetate Tc 99m Injection, and for Injections (except that it may be distributed or dispensed prior to completion of the test for Sterility, the latter test being started on the date of manufacture).

TELMISARTAN

Chemical name: [1,1'-Biphenyl]-2-carboxylic acid, 4'-[(1,4'-dimethyl-2'-propyl[2,6'-bi-1*H*-benzimidazol]-1'-yl)methyl]-.

Molecular formula: $C_{33}H_{30}N_4O_2$.

Molecular weight: 514.62.

Description: White to off-white, odorless crystalline powder.

Solubility: Practically insoluble in water and in the pH range of 3–9; sparingly soluble in strong acid (except insoluble in hydrochloric acid); soluble in strong base.

USP requirements: Telmisartan Tablets—Not in *USP–NF*.

TELMISARTAN AND HYDROCHLOROTHIAZIDE

For *Telmisartan* and *Hydrochlorothiazide*—See individual listings for chemistry information.

USP requirements: Telmisartan and Hydrochlorothiazide Tablets—Not in *USP–NF*.

TEMAZEPAM

Chemical name: 2*H*-1,4-Benzodiazepin-2-one, 7-chloro-1,3-dihydro-3-hydroxy-1-methyl-5-phenyl-.

Molecular formula: $C_{16}H_{13}ClN_2O_2$.

Molecular weight: 300.75.

Description: Temazepam USP—White or nearly white crystalline powder. Melts between 157 and 163 °C, within a 3 °C range.

Solubility: Temazepam USP—Very slightly soluble in water; sparingly soluble in alcohol.

USP requirements:
Temazepam USP—Preserve in well-closed, light-resistant containers. Contains not less than 98.0% and not more than 102.0% of temazepam, calculated on the dried basis. Meets the requirements for Identification, Loss on drying (not more than 0.5%), Residue on ignition (not more than 0.1%), Heavy metals (not more than 20 ppm), and Chromatographic purity.
  Caution: Temazepam is a potent sedative—its powder should not be inhaled.
Temazepam Capsules USP—Preserve in well-closed, light-resistant containers. Contain the labeled amount, within ±10%. Meet the requirements for Identification, Dissolution (80% in 30 minutes in sodium acetate buffer with 0.05% polysorbate 80 in Apparatus 2 at 75 rpm), and Uniformity of dosage units.
  Caution: Temazepam is a potent sedative—its powder should not be inhaled.
Temazepam Tablets—Not in *USP–NF*.

TEMOZOLOMIDE

Chemical group: Imidazotetrazine derivative.

Chemical name: Imidazo[5,1-*d*]-1,2,3,5-tetrazine-8-carboxamide, 3,4-dihydro-3-methyl-4-oxo-.

Molecular formula: $C_6H_6N_6O_2$.

Molecular weight: 194.15.

Description: White to light tan/light pink powder. Melting point 212°.

Other characteristics: Temozolomide is a prodrug, which hydrolyzes to 5-(3-methyltriazen-1-yl)imidazole-4-carboxamide (MTIC) at neutral and alkaline pH values. MTIC is the active form of the drug.

USP requirements: Temozolomide Capsules—Not in *USP–NF*.

TENECTEPLASE

Source: Tenecteplase is a tissue plasminogen activator (tPA) produced by recombinant DNA technology using an established mammalian cell line (Chinese Hamster Ovary cells).

Chemical name: 103-L-Asperagine-117-L-glutamine-296-L-alanine-297-L-alanine-298-L-alanine-299-L-alanineplasminogen activator (human tissue type).

Molecular formula: $C_{2558}H_{3872}N_{738}O_{781}S_{40}$.

Molecular weight: 58,742 daltons (polypeptide portion only).

USP requirements: Tenecteplase for Injection—Not in *USP–NF*.

TENIPOSIDE

Source: Semisynthetic derivative of podophyllotoxin.

Chemical name: Furo[3',4':6,7]naphtho[2,3-*d*]-1,3-dioxol-6(5a*H*)-one, 5,8,8a,9-tetrahydro-5-(4-hydroxy-3,5-dimethoxyphenyl)-9-[[4,6-*O*-(2-thienylmethylene)-beta-D-glucopyranosyl]-oxy]-, [5*R*-[5 alpha,5a beta,8a alpha,9 beta(*R**)]]-.

Molecular formula: $C_{32}H_{32}O_{13}S$.

Molecular weight: 656.65.

Description: White to off-white crystalline powder.

Solubility: Insoluble in water and in ether; slightly soluble in methanol; very soluble in acetone and in dimethylformamide.

USP requirements: Teniposide Injection—Not in *USP–NF*.

TENOFOVIR

Chemical name: Tenofovir disoproxil fumarate—(*R*)-5-[[2-(6-Amino-9*H*-purin-9-yl)-1-methylethoxy]methyl]-2,4,6,8-tetra-oxa-5-phosphanonanedioic acid, bis(1-methylethyl) ester, 5-oxide, (*E*)-2-butenedioate (1:1).

Molecular formula: Tenofovir disoproxil fumarate—$C_{19}H_{30}N_5O_{10}P \cdot C_4H_4O_4$.

Molecular weight: Tenofovir disoproxil fumarate—635.52.

Description: Tenofovir disoproxil fumarate—White to off-white powder.

Solubility: Tenofovir disoproxil fumarate—Soluble 13.4 mg per mL in distilled water at 25 °C.

Other characteristics: Tenofovir disoproxil fumarate—pH: 6.5; Partition coefficient: 1.25 at 25 °C.

USP requirements: Tenofovir Disoproxil Fumarate Tablets—Not in *USP–NF*.

TENOXICAM

Chemical name: 2*H*-Thieno[2,3-*e*]-1,2-thiazine-3-carboxamide, 4-hydroxy-2-methyl-*N*-2-pyridinyl-, 1,1-dioxide.

Molecular formula: $C_{13}H_{11}N_3O_4S_2$.

Molecular weight: 337.38.

Description: Yellow, practically odorless, crystalline powder which melts with decomposition at approximately 205 °C.

pKa: Approximately 1.1 and 5.3.

Solubility: Quite insoluble in water and in common organic solvents.

USP requirements: Tenoxicam Tablets—Not in *USP–NF*.

TERAZOSIN

Chemical group: Quinazoline derivative.

Chemical name: Terazosin hydrochloride—Piperazine, 1-(4-amino-6,7-dimethoxy-2-quinazolinyl)-4-[(tetrahydro-2-fura-nyl)carbonyl]-, monohydrochloride, dihydrate. Is a racemic mixture, both components of which are active.

Molecular formula: Terazosin hydrochloride—$C_{19}H_{25}N_5O_4 \cdot 2H_2O$.

Molecular weight: Terazosin hydrochloride—459.92.

Description: Terazosin hydrochloride—White, crystalline substance.

pKa: 7.04.

Solubility: Terazosin hydrochloride—Freely soluble in water and in isotonic saline.

USP requirements: Terazosin Hydrochloride Capsules—Not in *USP–NF*.

TERBINAFINE

Chemical name: Terbinafine hydrochloride—(E)-*N*-(6,6-di-methyl-2-hepten-4-ynyl)-*N*-methyl-1-naphthalenemethana-mine hydrochloride.

Molecular formula: Terbinafine hydrochloride—$C_{21}H_{26}ClN$.

Molecular weight: Terbinafine hydrochloride—327.90.

Description: Terbinafine hydrochloride—White to off-white fine crystalline powder.

Solubility: Terbinafine hydrochloride—Freely soluble in metha-nol and in methylene chloride; soluble in ethanol; slightly solu-ble in water.

USP requirements:
Terbinafine Hydrochloride Cream—Not in *USP–NF*.
Terbinafine Hydrochloride Solution—Not in *USP–NF*.
Terbinafine Hydrochloride Tablets—Not in *USP–NF*.

TERBUTALINE

Chemical name: Terbutaline sulfate—1,3-Benzenediol, 5-[2-[(1,1-dimethylethyl)amino]-1-hydroxyethyl]-, sulfate (2:1) (salt).

Molecular formula: Terbutaline sulfate—$(C_{12}H_{19}NO_3)_2 \cdot H_2SO_4$.

Molecular weight: Terbutaline sulfate—548.65.

Description: Terbutaline Sulfate USP—White to gray-white, crystalline powder. Is odorless or has a faint odor of acetic acid.

Solubility: Terbutaline Sulfate USP—Soluble in water and in 0.1 *N* hydrochloric acid; slightly soluble in methanol; insoluble in chloroform.

USP requirements:
Terbutaline Sulfate USP—Preserve in well-closed, light-resis-tant containers, at controlled room temperature. Contains not less than 98.0% and not more than 101.0% of terbuta-line sulfate, calculated on the dried basis. Meets the re-quirements for Identification, Acidity, Loss on drying (not more than 0.5%), Residue on ignition (not more than 0.2%), Heavy metals (not more than 0.0025%), Chromato-graphic purity, and Organic volatile impurities.
Terbutaline Sulfate Inhalation Aerosol USP—Preserve in small, nonreactive, light-resistant aerosol containers equipped with metered-dose valves and provided with oral inhalation actuators. Store at controlled room temperature. A suspension of microfine Terbutaline Sulfate in suitable propellants in a pressurized container. Contains the la-beled amount, within ±10%. Meets the requirements for Identification, Water (not more than 0.02%), Dosage uni-formity over the entire contents, and Particle size.
Terbutaline Sulfate Injection USP—Preserve in single-dose containers, preferably of Type I glass, protected from light, at controlled room temperature. A sterile solution of Terbu-taline Sulfate in Water for Injection. Contains the labeled amount, within ±10%. Meets the requirements for Identifi-cation, Bacterial endotoxins, and pH (3.0–5.0), and for In-jections.
Note: Do not use the Injection if it is discolored.

Terbutaline Sulfate Tablets USP—Preserve in tight containers, at controlled room temperature. Contain the labeled amount, within ±10%. Meet the requirements for Identification, Dissolution (75% in 45 minutes in water in Apparatus 1 at 100 rpm), and Uniformity of dosage units.

TERCONAZOLE

Chemical name: Piperazine, 1-[4-[[2-(2,4-dichlorophenyl)-2-(1*H*-1,2,4-triazol-1-ylmethyl)-1,3-dioxolan-4-yl]methoxy]phenyl]-4-(1-methylethyl)-, *cis*-.

Molecular formula: $C_{26}H_{31}Cl_2N_5O_3$.

Molecular weight: 532.46.

Description: White to almost white powder.

Solubility: Soluble in butanol; sparingly soluble in ethanol; insoluble in water.

USP requirements:
Terconazole Vaginal Cream—Not in *USP–NF*.
Terconazole Vaginal Suppositories—Not in *USP–NF*.

TERFENADINE

Chemical group: Butyrophenone derivative.

Chemical name: 1-Piperidinebutanol, alpha-[4-(1,1-dimethylethyl)phenyl]-4-(hydroxydiphenylmethyl)-.

Molecular formula: $C_{32}H_{41}NO_2$.

Molecular weight: 471.67.

Description: Terfenadine USP—White to off-white, crystalline powder.

Solubility: Terfenadine USP—Slightly soluble in water, in hexane, and in 0.1 *N* hydrochloric acid; freely soluble in chloroform; soluble in alcohol, in methanol, in octanol, and in toluene.

USP requirements:
Terfenadine USP—Preserve in tight, light-resistant containers. Contains not less than 98.0% and not more than 101.5% of terfenadine, calculated on the dried basis. Meets the requirements for Identification, Melting range (145–151 °C), Loss on drying (not more than 0.5%), Residue on ignition (not more than 0.1%), and Chromatographic purity.
Terfenadine Oral Suspension—Not in USP.
Terfenadine Tablets USP—Preserve in tight, light-resistant containers. Contain the labeled amount, within ±10%. Meet the requirements for Identification, Dissolution (75% in 45 minutes in 0.1 *N* hydrochloric acid in Apparatus 2 at 50 rpm), Uniformity of dosage units, and Related compounds.

TERFENADINE AND PSEUDOEPHEDRINE

For *Terfenadine* and *Pseudoephedrine*—See individual listings for chemistry information.

USP requirements: Terfenadine and Pseudoephedrine Hydrochloride Extended-release Tablets—Not in *USP–NF*.

TERIPARATIDE

Source: Teriparatide acetate—A synthetic polypeptide hormone consisting of the 1–34 fragment of human parathyroid hormone, the biologically active N-terminal region of the 84-amino-acid native hormone.

Chemical name: Teriparatide acetate—L-Phenylalanine, L-seryl-L-valyl-L-seryl-L-alpha-glutamyl-L-isoleucyl-L-glutaminyl-L-leucyl-L-methionyl-L-histidyl-L-asparaginyl-L-leucylglycyl-L-lysyl-L-histidyl-L-leucyl-L-asparaginyl-L-seryl-L-methionyl-L-alpha-glutamyl-L-arginyl-L-valyl-L-alpha-glutamyl-L-tryptophyl-L-leucyl-L-arginyl-L-lysyl-L-lysyl-L-leucyl-L-glutaminyl-L-alpha-aspartyl-L-valyl-L-histidyl-L-asparaginyl-, acetate (salt) hydrate.

Molecular formula: Teriparatide acetate—$C_{181}H_{291}N_{55}O_{51}S_2 \cdot xH_2O \cdot yC_2H_4O_2$.

USP requirements: Teriparatide Acetate for Injection—Not in *USP–NF*.

TERPIN HYDRATE

Chemical name: Cyclohexanemethanol, 4-hydroxy-alpha,alpha,4-trimethyl-, monohydrate.

Molecular formula: $C_{10}H_{20}O_2 \cdot H_2O$.

Molecular weight: 190.28.

Description: Terpin Hydrate USP—Colorless, lustrous crystals or white powder. Has a slight odor, and effloresces in dry air. A hot solution (1 in 100) is neutral to litmus. When dried in vacuum at 60 °C for 2 hours, it melts at about 103 °C.

Solubility: Terpin Hydrate USP—Slightly soluble in water, in chloroform, and in ether; very soluble in boiling alcohol; soluble in alcohol; sparingly soluble in boiling water.

USP requirements:
Terpin Hydrate USP—Preserve in tight containers. Contains not less than 98.0% and not more than 100.5% of terpin hydrate, calculated on the anhydrous basis. Meets the requirements for Identification, Water (9.0–10.0%), Residue on ignition (not more than 0.1%), and Residual turpentine.
Terpin Hydrate Elixir USP—Preserve in tight containers. Contains, in each 100 mL, not less than 1.53 grams and not more than 1.87 grams of terpin hydrate. Meets the requirement for Alcohol content (within ±10% of labeled amount).
Terpin Hydrate Oral Solution USP—Preserve in tight containers. Contains, in each 100 mL, not less than 1.53 grams and not more than 1.87 grams of terpin hydrate. Meets the requirement for Alcohol content (within ±10% of labeled amount).

TERPIN HYDRATE AND CODEINE

For *Terpin Hydrate* and *Codeine*—See individual listings for chemistry information.

USP requirements:
Terpin Hydrate and Codeine Elixir USP—Preserve in tight containers. Contains, in each 100 mL, not less than 1.53 grams and not more than 1.87 grams of terpin hydrate, and not less than 180 mg and not more than 220 mg of codeine. Meets the requirements for Identification and Alcohol content (within ±10% of labeled amount).
Terpin Hydrate and Codeine Oral Solution USP—Preserve in tight containers. Contains, in each 100 mL, not less than 1.53 grams and not more than 1.87 grams of terpin hy-

drate, and not less than 180 mg and not more than 220 mg of codeine. Meets the requirements for Identification and Alcohol content (within ±10% of labeled amount).

TERPIN HYDRATE AND DEXTROMETHORPHAN

For *Terpin Hydrate* and *Dextromethorphan*—See individual listings for chemistry information.

USP requirements: Terpin Hydrate and Dextromethorphan Hydrobromide Elixir USP—Preserve in tight containers. Contains, in each 100 mL, not less than 1.53 grams and not more than 1.87 grams of terpin hydrate, and not less than 180 mg and not more than 220 mg of dextromethorphan hydrobromide. Meets the requirements for Identification and Alcohol content (within ±10% of labeled amount).

TESTOLACTONE

Chemical name: D-Homo-17a-oxaandrosta-1,4-diene-3,17-dione.

Molecular formula: $C_{19}H_{24}O_3$.

Molecular weight: 300.39.

Description: Testolactone USP—White to off-white, practically odorless, crystalline powder. Melts at about 218 °C.

Solubility: Testolactone USP—Slightly soluble in water and in benzyl alcohol; soluble in alcohol and in chloroform; insoluble in ether and in solvent hexane.

USP requirements:
Testolactone USP—Preserve in tight containers. Contains not less than 95.0% and not more than 105.0% of testolactone, calculated on the dried basis. Meets the requirements for Identification, Specific rotation (−44° to −52°), Loss on drying (not more than 1.0%), Residue on ignition (not more than 0.1%), Heavy metals (not more than 0.003%), Chromatographic purity, Ordinary impurities, and Organic volatile impurities, and Other impurities.
Testolactone Tablets USP—Preserve in tight containers. Contain the labeled amount, within ±10%. Meet the requirements for Identification, Dissolution (80% in 120 minutes in 0.01 N hydrochloric acid in Apparatus 2 at 75 rpm), and Uniformity of dosage units.

TESTOSTERONE

Chemical group: Naturally occurring androgen.

Chemical name:
Testosterone—Androst-4-en-3-one, 17-hydroxy-, (17 beta)-.
Testosterone cypionate—Androst-4-en-3-one, 17-(3-cyclopentyl-1-oxopropoxy)-, (17 beta)-.
Testosterone enanthate—Androst-4-en-3-one, 17-[(1-oxoheptyl)oxy]-, (17 beta)-.
Testosterone propionate—Androst-4-en-3-one, 17-(1-oxopropoxy)-, (17 beta)-.
Testosterone undecanoate—17 beta-undecanoyloxy-androst-4-en-3-one.

Molecular formula:
Testosterone—$C_{19}H_{28}O_2$.
Testosterone cypionate—$C_{27}H_{40}O_3$.
Testosterone enanthate—$C_{26}H_{40}O_3$.
Testosterone propionate—$C_{22}H_{32}O_3$.
Testosterone undecanoate—$C_{30}H_{48}O_3$.

Molecular weight:
Testosterone—288.42.
Testosterone cypionate—412.60.
Testosterone enanthate—400.59.
Testosterone propionate—344.49.
Testosterone undecanoate—456.7.

Description:
Testosterone USP—White or slightly creamy white crystals or crystalline powder. Is odorless, and is stable in air.
Testosterone Cypionate USP—White or creamy white, crystalline powder. Is odorless or has a slight odor, and is stable in air.
Testosterone Enanthate USP—White or creamy white, crystalline powder. Is odorless or has a faint odor characteristic of heptanoic acid.
Testosterone Propionate USP—White or creamy white crystals or crystalline powder. Is odorless and is stable in air.
Testosterone undecanoate—Creamy-white crystalline powder.

Solubility:
Testosterone USP—Practically insoluble in water; freely soluble in dehydrated alcohol and in chloroform; soluble in dioxane and in vegetable oils; slightly soluble in ether.
Testosterone Cypionate USP—Insoluble in water; freely soluble in alcohol, in chloroform, in dioxane, and in ether; soluble in vegetable oils.
Testosterone Enanthate USP—Insoluble in water; very soluble in ether; soluble in vegetable oils.
Testosterone Propionate USP—Insoluble in water; freely soluble in alcohol, in dioxane, in ether, and in other organic solvents; soluble in vegetable oils.
Testosterone undecanoate—Insoluble in water; soluble in oleic acid = 160 mg/mL.

USP requirements:
Testosterone USP—Preserve in well-closed containers. Contains not less than 97.0% and not more than 103.0% of testosterone, calculated on the dried basis. Meets the requirements for Identification, Melting range (153–157 °C), Specific rotation (+101° to +105°), Loss on drying (not more than 1.0%), and Organic volatile impurities.
Testosterone Implants—Not in *USP–NF*.
Testosterone Pellets—Not in *USP–NF*.
Testastone Sublingual—Not in *USP–NF*.
Testosterone Injectable Suspension USP—Preserve in single-dose or in multiple-dose containers, preferably of Type I glass. A sterile suspension of Testosterone in an aqueous medium. Contains the labeled amount, within ±10%. Meets the requirements for Identification, Bacterial endotoxins, Uniformity of dosage units, and pH (4.0–7.5), and for Injections.
Testosterone Transdermal System—Not in *USP–NF*.
Testosterone Cypionate USP—Preserve in well-closed, light-resistant containers. Contains not less than 97.0% and not more than 103.0% of testosterone cypionate, calculated on the dried basis. Meets the requirements for Identification, Melting range (98–104 °C), Specific rotation (+85° to +92°), Loss on drying (not more than 0.5%), Residue on ignition (not more than 0.2%), Free cyclopentanepropionic acid (not more than 0.20%), and Organic volatile impurities, and Other impurities.
Testosterone Cypionate Injection USP—Preserve in single-dose or in multiple-dose containers, preferably of Type I glass, protected from light. A sterile solution of Testosterone Cypionate in a suitable vegetable oil. Contains the labeled amount, within ±10%. Meets the requirements for Identification and for Injections.
Testosterone Enanthate USP—Preserve in well-closed containers, in a cool place. Contains not less than 97.0% and not more than 103.0% of testosterone enanthate. Meets the requirements for Identification, Melting range (34–39 °C), Specific rotation (+77° to +82°), Water (not

more than 0.05%), Free heptanoic acid (not more than 0.16%), Ordinary impurities, and Organic volatile impurities.

Testosterone Enanthate Injection USP—Preserve in single-dose or in multiple-dose containers, preferably of Type I glass. A sterile solution of Testosterone Enanthate in a suitable vegetable oil. Contains the labeled amount, within ±10%. Meets the requirements for Identification and for Injections.

Testosterone Propionate USP—Preserve in well-closed, light-resistant containers. Contains not less than 97.0% and not more than 103.0% of testosterone propionate, calculated on the dried basis. Meets the requirements for Identification, Melting range (118–123 °C), Specific rotation (+83° to +90°), Loss on drying (not more than 0.5%), and Organic volatile impurities.

Testosterone Propionate Injection USP—Preserve in single-dose or in multiple-dose containers, preferably of Type I glass. A sterile solution of Testosterone Propionate in a suitable vegetable oil. Contains the labeled amount, within ±12%. Meets the requirements for Identification and for Injections.

Testosterone Propionate Ointment—Not in *USP–NF*.
Testosterone Undecanoate Capsules—Not in *USP–NF*.

TESTOSTERONE AND ESTRADIOL

Chemical name:
Testosterone cypionate—Androst-4-en-3-one, 17-(3-cyclopentyl-1-oxopropoxy)-, (17 beta)-.
Testosterone enanthate—Androst-4-en-3-one, 17-[(1-oxoheptyl)oxy]-, (17 beta)-.
Estradiol cypionate—Estra-1,3,5(10)-triene-3,17-diol, (17 beta)-, 17-cyclopentanepropanoate.
Estradiol valerate—Estra-1,3,5(10)-triene-3,17-diol(17 beta)-, 17-pentanoate.
Estradiol benzoate—Estra-1,3,5(10)-triene-3,17-diol, (17 beta)-, 3-benzoate.

Molecular formula:
Testosterone cypionate—$C_{27}H_{40}O_3$.
Testosterone enanthate—$C_{26}H_{40}O_3$.
Estradiol cypionate—$C_{26}H_{36}O_3$.
Estradiol valerate—$C_{23}H_{32}O_3$.
Estradiol benzoate—$C_{25}H_{28}O_3$.

Molecular weight:
Testosterone cypionate—412.60.
Testosterone enanthate—400.59.
Estradiol cypionate—396.56.
Estradiol valerate—356.50.
Estradiol benzoate—376.49.

Description:
Testosterone Cypionate USP—White or creamy white, crystalline powder. Is odorless or has a slight odor, and is stable in air.
Testosterone Enanthate USP—White or creamy white, crystalline powder. Is odorless or has a faint odor characteristic of heptanoic acid.
Estradiol Cypionate USP—White to practically white, crystalline powder. Is odorless or has a slight odor.
Estradiol Valerate USP—White, crystalline powder. Is usually odorless but may have a faint, fatty odor.
Estradiol benzoate—Colorless crystals or a white or almost white crystalline powder.

Solubility:
Testosterone Cypionate USP—Insoluble in water; freely soluble in alcohol, in chloroform, in dioxane, and in ether; soluble in vegetable oils.
Testosterone Enanthate USP—Insoluble in water; very soluble in ether; soluble in vegetable oils.

Estradiol Cypionate USP—Insoluble in water; soluble in alcohol, in acetone, in chloroform, and in dioxane; sparingly soluble in vegetable oils.
Estradiol Valerate USP—Practically insoluble in water; soluble in castor oil, in methanol, in benzyl benzoate, and in dioxane; sparingly soluble in sesame oil and in peanut oil.
Estradiol benzoate—Practically insoluble in water; slightly soluble in alcohol and in fixed oils; soluble 1 in 50 of acetone.

USP requirements:
Testosterone Cypionate and Estradiol Cypionate Injection—Not in *USP–NF*.
Testosterone Enanthate and Estradiol Valerate Injection—Not in *USP–NF*.
Testosterone Enanthate Benzilic Acid Hydrazone, Estradiol Dienanthate, and Estradiol Benzoate Injection—Not in *USP–NF*.

TETANUS IMMUNE GLOBULIN

Description: Tetanus Immune Globulin USP—Transparent or slightly opalescent liquid, practically colorless and practically odorless. May develop a slight granular deposit during storage.

USP requirements: Tetanus Immune Globulin Injection USP—Preserve at a temperature between 2 and 8 °C. A sterile, non-pyrogenic solution of globulins derived from the blood plasma of adult human donors who have been immunized with tetanus toxoid. Label it to state that it is not for intravenous injection. Has a potency of not less than 50 antitoxin units per mL based on the U.S. Standard Tetanus Antitoxin and the U.S. Control Tetanus Test Toxin, tested in guinea pigs. Contains not less than 10 grams and not more than 18 grams of protein per 100 mL, of which not less than 90% is gamma globulin. Contains 0.3 M glycine as a stabilizing agent, and contains a suitable preservative. Meets the requirement for Expiration date (for Tetanus Immune Globulin containing a 10% excess of potency, not later than 3 years after date of issue from manufacturer's cold storage [5 °C, 1 year]). Conforms to the regulations of the U.S. Food and Drug Administration concerning biologics.

TETANUS TOXOID

Source: Tetanus toxoid adsorbed and fluid are prepared by growing the tetanus bacilli *Clostridium tetani* on a protein-free, semi-synthetic medium. The tetanus toxin produced by these bacilli is detoxified using formaldehyde and forms the tetanus toxoid. Thimerosal is added as a preservative. In addition, for tetanus toxoid adsorbed, aluminum phosphate or aluminum potassium sulfate is used as a mineral adjuvant to adsorb the tetanus antigens. This prolongs and enhances the antigenic properties by retarding the rate of absorption of the injected toxoid into the body.

Description:
Tetanus Toxoid USP—Clear, colorless to brownish yellow, or slightly turbid liquid, free from evident clumps or particles, having a characteristic odor or an odor of formaldehyde.
Tetanus Toxoid Adsorbed USP—Turbid, white, slightly gray, or slightly pink suspension, free from evident clumps after shaking.

USP requirements:
Tetanus Toxoid USP (Fluid)—Preserve at a temperature between 2 and 8 °C. A sterile solution of the formaldehyde-treated products of growth of the tetanus bacillus (*Clostridium tetani*). Label it to state that it is not to be frozen. Meets the requirements of the specific guinea pig potency

test of antitoxin production based on the U.S. Standard Tetanus Antitoxin and the U.S. Control Tetanus Test Toxin. Meets the requirements of the specific guinea pig detoxification test. Contains not more than 0.02% of residual free formaldehyde. Contains a preservative other than a phenoloid compound. Meets the requirement for Expiration date (not later than 2 years after date of issue from manufacturer's cold storage [5 °C, 1 year]). Conforms to the regulations of the U.S. Food and Drug Administration concerning biologics.

Tetanus Toxoid Adsorbed USP (Injection)—Preserve at a temperature between 2 and 8 °C. A sterile preparation of plain tetanus toxoid that meets all of the requirements for that product with the exception of those for potency, and that has been precipitated or adsorbed by alum, aluminum hydroxide, or aluminum phosphate adjuvants. Label it to state that it is to be well shaken before use and that it is not to be frozen. Meets the requirements of the specific mouse or guinea pig potency test of antitoxin production based on the U.S. Standard Tetanus Antitoxin and the U.S. Control Test Tetanus Toxin. Meets the requirements of the specific guinea pig detoxification test. Meets the requirements for Expiration date (not later than 2 years after date of issue from manufacturerãs cold storage [5 °C, 1 year]) and Aluminum content. Conforms to the regulations of the U.S. Food and Drug Administration concerning biologics.

TETANUS AND DIPHTHERIA TOXOIDS ADSORBED FOR ADULT USE

Description: Tetanus and Diphtheria Toxoids Adsorbed for Adult Use USP—Turbid, white, slightly gray, or cream-colored suspension, free from evident clumps after shaking.

USP requirements: Tetanus and Diphtheria Toxoids Adsorbed for Adult Use USP—Preserve at a temperature between 2 and 8 °C. A sterile suspension prepared by mixing suitable quantities of adsorbed diphtheria toxoid and adsorbed tetanus toxoid using the same precipitating or adsorbing agent for both toxoids. The antigenicity or potency and the proportions of the toxoids are such as to provide, in each dose prescribed in the labeling, an immunizing dose of Tetanus Toxoid Adsorbed as defined for that product, and one-tenth of the immunizing dose of Diphtheria Toxoid Adsorbed as defined for that product for children, such that in the specific guinea pig antigenicity test it meets the requirement of production of not less than 0.5 unit of diphtheria antitoxin per mL and each immunizing dose has an antigen content of not more than 2 Lf (flocculating units) value as measured with the U.S. Reference Diphtheria Antitoxin for Flocculation Test. Each component meets the other requirements for those products. Contains not more than 0.02% of residual free formaldehyde. Label it to state that it is to be well-shaken before use and that it is not to be frozen. Meets the requirement for Expiration date (not later than 2 years after date of issue from manufacturer's cold storage [5 °C, 1 year]). Conforms to the regulations of the U.S. Food and Drug Administration concerning biologics.

TETRACAINE

Chemical group: Ester, aminobenzoic acid (PABA)–derivative.

Chemical name:

Tetracaine—Benzoic acid, 4-(butylamino)-, 2-(dimethylamino)ethyl ester.
Tetracaine hydrochloride—Benzoic acid, 4-(butylamino)-, 2-(dimethylamino)ethyl ester, monohydrochloride.

Molecular formula:

Tetracaine—$C_{15}H_{24}N_2O_2$.
Tetracaine hydrochloride—$C_{15}H_{24}N_2O_2 \cdot HCl$.

Molecular weight:

Tetracaine—264.36.
Tetracaine hydrochloride—300.82.

Description:

Tetracaine USP—White or light yellow, waxy solid.
Tetracaine Hydrochloride USP—Fine, white, crystalline, odorless powder. Its solutions are neutral to litmus. Melts at about 148 °C, or may occur in either of two other polymorphic modifications that melt at about 134 °C and 139 °C, respectively. Mixtures of the forms may melt within the range of 134 to 147 °C. Is hygroscopic.
Tetracaine Hydrochloride for Injection USP—Fine, white, crystalline, odorless powder. Its solutions are neutral to litmus. Melts at about 148 °C, or may occur in either of two other polymorphic modifications that melt at about 134 °C and 139 °C, respectively. Mixtures of the forms may melt within the range of 134 to 147 °C. Is hygroscopic.

pKa: Tetracaine hydrochloride—8.39.

Solubility:

Tetracaine USP—Very slightly soluble in water; soluble in alcohol, in ether, and in chloroform.
Tetracaine Hydrochloride USP—Very soluble in water; soluble in alcohol; insoluble in ether.
Sterile Tetracaine Hydrochloride USP—Very soluble in water; soluble in alcohol; insoluble in ether.

USP requirements:

Tetracaine USP—Preserve in tight, light-resistant containers. Contains not less than 98.0% and not more than 101.0% of tetracaine, calculated on the dried basis. Meets the requirements for Identification, Melting range (41–46 °C), Loss on drying (not more than 0.5%), Residue on ignition (not more than 0.1%), and Chromatographic purity.
Tetracaine Topical Aerosol—Not in *USP–NF*.
Tetracaine Ointment USP—Preserve in collapsible ointment tubes. Contains the labeled amount, within ± 10%, in a suitable ointment base. Meets the requirements for Identification, Microbial limits, and Minimum fill.
Tetracaine Ophthalmic Ointment USP—Preserve in collapsible ophthalmic ointment tubes. A sterile ointment. Contains not less than 0.45% and not more than 0.55% of Tetracaine in White Petrolatum. Meets the requirements for Identification, Sterility, Minimum fill, and Metal particles.
Tetracaine Hydrochloride USP—Preserve in tight, light-resistant containers. Where it is intended for use in preparing injectable dosage forms, the label states that it is sterile or must be subjected to further processing during the preparation of injectable or other sterile dosage forms. Contains not less than 98.5% and not more than 101.0% of tetracaine hydrochloride, calculated on the anhydrous basis. Meets the requirements for Identification, Water (not more than 2.0%), Residue on ignition (not more than 0.1%), and Chromatographic purity, and for Sterility tests and Bacterial endotoxins under Tetracaine Hydrochloride for Injection is sterile), and for Bacterial endotoxins under Tetracaine Hydrochloride for Injection (where the label states that Tetracaine Hydrochloride must be subjected to further processing during the preparation of injectable or other sterile dosage forms).
Tetracaine Hydrochloride Cream USP—Preserve in collapsible, lined metal tubes. Contains an amount of tetracaine hydrochloride equivalent to the labeled amount of tetracaine, within ±10%, in a suitable water-miscible base. Meets the requirements for Identification, Microbial limits, Minimum fill, and pH (3.2–3.8).
Tetracaine Hydrochloride Injection USP—Preserve in single-dose or in multiple-dose containers, preferably of Type I glass, under refrigeration and protected from light. It may be packaged in 100-mL multiple-dose containers. Injec-

tion supplied as a component of spinal anesthesia trays may be stored at room temperature for 12 months. A sterile solution of Tetracaine Hydrochloride in Water for Injection. Label it to indicate that the Injection is not to be used if it contains crystals, or if it is cloudy or discolored. Contains the labeled amount, within ±5%. Meets the requirements for Identification, Bacterial endotoxins, pH (3.2–6.0), and Particulate matter, and for Injections.

Tetracaine Hydrochloride for Injection USP—Preserve in Containers for Sterile Solids, preferably of Type I glass. Contains the labeled amount, within ±10 Meets the requirements for Completeness of solution, Constituted solution, Identification, Bacterial endotoxins, Uniformity of dosage units, pH (5.0–6.0, in a solution [1 in 100]), Water (not more than 2.0%), Residue on ignition (not more than 0.1%), and Chromatographic purity, and for Sterility tests and Labeling under Injections.

Tetracaine Hydrochloride Ophthalmic Solution USP—Preserve in tight, light-resistant containers. A sterile, aqueous solution of Tetracaine Hydrochloride. Label it to indicate that the Ophthalmic Solution is not to be used if it contains crystals, or if it is cloudy or discolored. Contains the labeled amount, within ±10%. Meets the requirements for Identification, Sterility, and pH (3.7–6.0).

Tetracaine Hydrochloride Topical Solution USP—Preserve in tight, light-resistant containers. An aqueous solution of Tetracaine Hydrochloride. Contains a suitable antimicrobial agent. Label it to indicate that the Topical Solution is not to be used if it contains crystals, or if it is cloudy or discolored. Contains the labeled amount, within ±5%. Meets the requirements for Identification and pH (4.5–6.0).

TETRACAINE AND DEXTROSE

For *Tetracaine* and *Dextrose*—See individual listings for chemistry information.

USP requirements: Tetracaine Hydrochloride in Dextrose Injection USP—Preserve in single-dose or in multiple-dose containers, preferably of Type I glass, under refrigeration and protected from light. It may be packaged in 100-mL multiple-dose containers. Injection supplied as a component of spinal anesthesia trays may be stored at room temperature for 12 months. A sterile solution of Tetracaine Hydrochloride and Dextrose in Water for Injection. Label it to indicate that the Injection is not to be used if it contains crystals, or if it is cloudy or discolored. Contains the labeled amounts, within ±5%. Meets the requirements for Identification, Bacterial endotoxins, pH (3.5–6.0), and Particulate matter under Small-volume injections, and for Injections.

TETRACAINE AND MENTHOL

For *Tetracaine* and *Menthol*—See individual listings for chemistry information.

USP requirements: Tetracaine and Menthol Ointment USP—Preserve in collapsible ointment tubes. Contains the labeled amounts, within ±10%, in a suitable ointment base. Meets the requirements for Identification and Minimum fill.

TETRACYCLINE

Chemical name:
Tetracycline—2-Naphthacenecarboxamide, 4-(dimethylamino)1,4,4a,5,5a,6,11,12a-octahydro-3,6,10,12,12a-pentahydroxy-6-methyl-1,11-dioxo-, [4*S*-(4 alpha,4a alpha,5a alpha,6 beta,12a alpha)]-.

Tetracycline hydrochloride—2-Naphthacenecarboxamide, 4-(dimethylamino)-1,4,4a,5,5a,6,11,12a-octahydro-3,6,10,12,12a-pentahydroxy-6-methyl-1,11-dioxo-, monohydrochloride, [4*S*-(4 alpha,4a alpha,5a alpha,6 beta,12a alpha)]-.

Tetracycline phosphate complex—2-Naphthacenecarboxamide, 4-(dimethylamino)-1,4,4a,5,5a,6,11,12a-octahydro-3,6,10,12,12a-pentahydroxy-6-methyl-1,11-dioxo, [4*S*-(4 alpha,4a alpha,5a alpha,6 beta,12a alpha)]-, phosphate complex.

Molecular formula:
Tetracycline—$C_{22}H_{24}N_2O_8$.
Tetracycline hydrochloride—$C_{22}H_{24}N_2O_8 \cdot HCl$.

Molecular weight:
Tetracycline—444.43.
Tetracycline hydrochloride—480.90.

Description:
Tetracycline USP—Yellow, odorless, crystalline powder. Is stable in air, but exposure to strong sunlight causes it to darken. It loses potency in solutions of pH below 2, and is rapidly destroyed by alkali hydroxide solutions.

Tetracycline Hydrochloride USP—Yellow, odorless, crystalline powder. Is moderately hygroscopic. Is stable in air, but exposure to strong sunlight in moist air causes it to darken. It loses potency in solution at a pH below 2, and is rapidly destroyed by alkali hydroxide solutions.

Tetracycline Phosphate Complex USP—Yellow, crystalline powder, having a faint, characteristic odor.

Solubility:
Tetracycline USP—Very slightly soluble in water; freely soluble in dilute acid and in alkali hydroxide solutions; sparingly soluble in alcohol; practically insoluble in chloroform and in ether.

Tetracycline Hydrochloride USP—Soluble in water and in solutions of alkali hydroxides and carbonates; slightly soluble in alcohol; practically insoluble in chloroform and in ether.

Tetracycline Phosphate Complex USP—Sparingly soluble in water; slightly soluble in methanol; very slightly soluble in acetone.

USP requirements:
Tetracycline USP—Preserve in tight, light-resistant containers. Label it to indicate that it is to be used in the manufacture of nonparenteral drugs only. Has a potency equivalent to not less than 975 mcg of tetracycline hydrochloride per mg, calculated on the anhydrous basis. Meets the requirements for Identification, Specific rotation (–260° to –280°, calculated on the anhydrous basis), Crystallinity, pH (3.0–7.0, in an aqueous suspension containing 10 mg per mL), Water (not more than 13.0%), Heavy metals (not more than 0.005%), and Limit of 4-epianhydrotetracycline (not more than 2.0%).

Tetracycline Boluses USP—Preserve in tight containers. Label Boluses to indicate that they are intended for veterinary use only. Contain the equivalent of the labeled amount of tetracycline hydrochloride, within –10% to +20%. Meet the requirements for Identification, Uniformity of dosage units, and Loss on drying (not more than 3.0%; or for Boluses greater than 15 mm in diameter, not more than 6.0%).

Tetracycline Periodontal Fibers—Not in *USP–NF*.

Tetracycline Oral Suspension USP—Preserve in tight, light-resistant containers. It is Tetracycline with or without one or more suitable buffers, preservatives, stabilizers, and suspending agents. Contains the equivalent of the labeled

amount of tetracycline hydrochloride, within −10% to +25%. Meets the requirements for Identification, Uniformity of dosage units (single-unit containers), Deliverable volume, pH (3.5–6.0), and Limit of 4-epianhydrotetracycline (not more than 5.0%).

Tetracycline Hydrochloride USP—Preserve in tight, light-resistant containers. Where it is intended for use in preparing injectable or other sterile dosage forms, the label states that it is sterile or must be subjected to further processing during the preparation of injectable or other sterile dosage forms. Has a potency of not less than 900 mcg of tetracycline hydrochloride per mg. Meets the requirements for Identification, Specific rotation (−240° to −255°, calculated on the dried basis), Crystallinity, pH (1.8–2.8, in a solution containing 10 mg per mL), Loss on drying (not more than 2.0%), Heavy metals (not more than 0.005%), and Limit of 4-epianhydrotetracycline (not more than 2.0%), and for Sterility and Bacterial endotoxins under Tetracycline Hydrochloride for Injection (where the label states that Tetracycline Hydrochloride is sterile), and for Bacterial endotoxins under tetracycline Hydrochloride for Injection (where the label states that Tetracycline Hydrochloride must be subjected to further processing during the preparation of injectable dosage forms). It is exempt from requirements for Bacterial endotoxins (where it is intended for use in preparing nonparenteral sterile dosage forms).

Tetracycline Hydrochloride Capsules USP—Preserve in tight, light-resistant containers. Contain the labeled amount, within −10% to +25%. Meet the requirements for Identification, Dissolution (80% in 60 minutes, 90 minutes for 500-mg capsules, in water in Apparatus 2 at 75 rpm), Uniformity of dosage units, Loss on drying (not more than 4.0%), and Limit of 4-epianhydrotetracycline (not more than 3.0%).

Tetracycline Hydrochloride for Injection USP—Preserve in Containers for Sterile Solids, protected from light. It is sterile Tetracycline Hydrochloride or a sterile, dry mixture of Sterile Tetracycline Hydrochloride, one form of which contains Magnesium Chloride or magnesium ascorbate and one or more suitable buffers, and may contain one or more suitable preservatives, solubilizers, stabilizers, and anesthetic agents, and the other form of which contains one or more suitable stabilizing agents. Label Tetracycline Hydrochloride for Injection that contains an anesthetic agent to indicate that it is intended for intramuscular administration only. Contains the labeled amount, within −10% to +15%. Meets the requirements for Constituted solution, Identification, Bacterial endotoxins, Sterility, pH (2.0–3.0, in a solution containing 10 mg per mL), Loss on drying (not more than 5.0%), Particulate matter, and Limit of 4-epianhydrotetracycline (not more than 3.0%), and for Uniformity of dosage units and for Labeling under Injections.

Tetracycline Hydrochloride Ointment USP—Preserve in well-closed containers, preferably at controlled room temperature. Contains the labeled amount, within −10% to +25%. Meets the requirements for Identification, Minimum fill, and Water (not more than 1.0%).

Tetracycline Hydrochloride Ophthalmic Ointment USP—Preserve in collapsible ophthalmic ointment tubes. Contains the labeled amount, within −10% to +25%. Meets the requirements for Sterility, Minimum fill, Water (not more than 0.5%), and Metal particles.

Tetracycline Hydrochloride Soluble Powder USP—Preserve in tight containers. Label it to indicate that it is intended for veterinary use only. Contains the labeled amount, within −10% to +25%. Meets the requirements for Identification and Loss on drying (not more than 2.0%).

Tetracycline Hydrochloride for Topical Solution USP—Preserve in tight, light-resistant containers. A dry mixture of Tetracycline Hydrochloride and Epitetracycline Hydrochloride with Sodium Metabisulfite packaged in conjunction with a suitable aqueous vehicle. Contains the labeled amount of tetracycline hydrochloride, within −10% to +30%, when constituted as directed. Meets the requirements for Identification, pH (1.9–3.5, in the solution constituted as directed in the labeling), Loss on drying (not more than 5.0%), and Content of epitetracycline hydrochloride.

Tetracycline Hydrochloride Ophthalmic Suspension USP—Preserve in tight, light-resistant containers of glass or plastic, containing not more than 15 mL. The containers or individual cartons are sealed and tamper-proof so that sterility is assured at time of first use. A sterile suspension of sterile Tetracycline Hydrochloride in a suitable oil. Contains the labeled amount, within −10% to +25%. Meets the requirements for Identification, Sterility, and Water (not more than 0.5%).

Tetracycline Hydrochloride Oral Suspension USP—Preserve in tight, light-resistant containers. Store at controlled room temperature, and protect from freezing. Label it to state that it should not be frozen and that it is to be well shaken before using. Contains not less than 2.25 grams and not more than 2.75 grams of tetracycline hydrochloride in 100 mL of Oral Suspension.

Prepare Tetracycline Hydrochloride Oral Suspension as follows: 2.50 grams of Tetracycline Hydrochloride, 10 mg of Cetylpyridinium Chloride, 0.15 gram of Xanthan Gum, 60 mg of Dibasic Sodium Phosphate, 0.65 gram of Monobasic Sodium Phosphate, 0.30 gram of Sodium Hydroxide, 35 mL of Purified Water, and Suspension Structured Vehicle or Sugar-free Suspension Structured Vehicle, a sufficient quantity, to make 100 mL. Dissolve the Dibasic Sodium Phosphate and the Monobasic Sodium Phosphate in 25 mL of Purified Water. Separately dissolve an accurately weighed quantity of Cetylpyridinium Chloride in Purified Water and dilute quantitatively, and stepwise if necessary, with Purified Water to obtain 5 mL of a solution containing 10 mg of Cetylpyridinium Chloride. Mix this solution with 5 mL of the aqueous phosphate solution and add the resulting solution, in divided portions, with mixing, to the Tetracycline Hydrochloride in a glass mortar to completely wet the powder, and make a smooth paste. Transfer the remaining 20 mL of the aqueous phosphate solution to a beaker. Using moderate heat, stir to form a vortex, and slowly sprinkle the Xanthan Gum into the vortex to produce a uniform dispersion. Add this dispersion to the paste in the glass mortar, and mix until smooth; then add 20 mL of the Suspension Structured Vehicle or Sugar-free Suspension Vehicle to the mixture. Dissolve the Sodium Hydroxide in 5 mL of Purified Water, and while mixing, slowly add this solution to the prepared mixture. Complete the suspension by adding a sufficient quantity of the Suspension Structured Vehicle or Sugar-free Suspension Vehicle to make a final volume of 100 mL, and pass this final dispersion through a hand homogenizer prior to transferring it to the dispensing container.

Meets the requirements for pH (3.5–6.0) and Beyond-use date.

Tetracycline Hydrochloride Tablets USP—Preserve in tight, light-resistant containers. Contain the labeled amount, within −10% to +25%. Meet the requirements for Identification, Dissolution (80% in 60 minutes in water in Apparatus 2 at 75 rpm), Uniformity of dosage units, Loss on drying (not more than 3.0%), and Limit of 4-epianhydrotetracycline (not more than 3.0%).

Tetracycline Phosphate Complex USP—Preserve in tight, light-resistant containers. Label it to indicate that it is to be used in the manufacture of nonparenteral drugs only. Has a potency equivalent to not less than 750 mcg of tetracycline hydrochloride per mg, calculated on the anhydrous basis. Meets the requirements for Identification, Crystallinity, pH (2.0–4.0, in an aqueous suspension containing 10 mg per mL), Water (not more than 9.0%), Chloride (not more than 0.2%), Limit of tetracycline (not more than 1.0%), and Limit of 4-epianhydrotetracycline (not more than 2.0%).

Tetracycline Phosphate Complex Capsules USP—Preserve in tight, light-resistant containers. Contain an amount of tetracycline phosphate complex equivalent to the labeled amount of tetracycline hydrochloride, within −10% to +25%. Meet the requirements for Identification, Dissolution (75% in 30 minutes in 0.1 N hydrochloric acid in Apparatus 1 at 100 rpm), Uniformity of dosage units, Loss on drying (not more than 9.0%), and Limit of 4-epianhydrotetracycline (not more than 3.0%).

Tetracycline Phosphate Complex for Injection USP—Preserve in Containers for Sterile Solids, protected from light. A sterile, dry mixture of Sterile Tetracycline Phosphate Complex and Magnesium Chloride or magnesium ascorbate, and one or more suitable buffers. Contains an amount of tetracycline phosphate complex equivalent to the labeled amount of tetracycline hydrochloride, within −10% to +15%. Meets the requirements for Constituted solution, Identification, Bacterial endotoxins, Sterility, pH (2.0–3.0, in a solution containing 10 mg per mL), Loss on drying (not more than 5.0%), Particulate matter, and Limit of 4-epianhydrotetracycline (not more than 3.0%), and for Uniformity of dosage units and Labeling under Injections.

Sterile Tetracycline Phosphate Complex USP—Preserve in Containers for Sterile Solids, protected from light. It is Tetracycline Phosphate Complex suitable for parenteral use. Has a potency equivalent to not less than 750 mcg of tetracycline hydrochloride per mg, calculated on the anhydrous basis. Meets the requirements for Sterility, and for Identification tests, pH, Water, Chloride, Crystallinity, Tetracycline, and 4-Epianhydrotetracycline under Tetracycline Phosphate Complex.

TETRACYCLINE AND NOVOBIOCIN

For *Tetracycline* and *Novobiocin*—See individual listings for chemistry information.

USP requirements:

Tetracycline Hydrochloride and Novobiocin Sodium Tablets USP—Preserve in tight containers. Label the Tablets to indicate that they are intended for veterinary use only. Contain amounts of tetracycline hydrochloride and novobiocin sodium equivalent to the labeled amounts of tetracycline hydrochloride and novobiocin, within −10% to +25%. Meet the requirements for Identification, Disintegration (60 minutes, simulated gastric fluid TS being substituted for water in the test), Uniformity of dosage units, Loss on drying (not more than 6.0%), and Limit of 4-epianhydrotetracycline (not more than 2.0%).

Tetracycline Phosphate Complex and Novobiocin Sodium Capsules USP—Preserve in tight containers. Label the Capsules to indicate that they are intended for veterinary use only. Contain amounts of tetracycline phosphate complex and novobiocin sodium equivalent to the labeled amounts of tetracycline hydrochloride and novobiocin, within −10% to +20%. Meet the requirements for Identification, Uniformity of dosage units, Loss on drying (not more than 9.0%), and Limit of 4-epianhydrotetracycline (not more than 3.0%).

TETRACYCLINE, NOVOBIOCIN, AND PREDNISOLONE

For *Tetracycline, Novobiocin,* and *Prednisolone*—See individual listings for chemistry information.

USP requirements: Tetracycline Hydrochloride, Novobiocin Sodium, and Prednisolone Tablets USP—Preserve in tight containers. Label the Tablets to indicate that they are intended for veterinary use only. Contain amounts of tetracycline hydrochloride and novobiocin sodium equivalent to the labeled amounts of tetracycline hydrochloride and novobiocin, within −10% to +25%, and the labeled amount of prednisolone, within ±10%. Meet the requirements for Disintegration (60 minutes, simulated gastric fluid TS being substituted for water in the test), Uniformity of dosage units, and Limit of 4-epianhydrotetracycline (not more than 2.0%), and for Identification test and Loss on drying under Tetracycline Hydrochloride and Novobiocin Sodium Tablets.

TETRACYCLINE AND NYSTATIN

For *Tetracycline* and *Nystatin*—See individual listings for chemistry information.

USP requirements: Tetracycline Hydrochloride and Nystatin Capsules USP—Preserve in tight, light-resistant containers. Contain the labeled amount of tetracycline hydrochloride, within −10% to +25%, and the labeled amount of USP Nystatin Units, within −10% to +35%. Meet the requirements for Identification, Dissolution (70% in 60 minutes in water in Apparatus 2 at 75 rpm), Loss on drying (not more than 4.0%), and Limit of 4-epianhydrotetracycline (not more than 3.0%).

TETRAHYDROZOLINE

Chemical name: Tetrahydrozoline hydrochloride—1H-Imidazole, 4,5-dihydro-2-(1,2,3,4-tetrahydro-1-naphthalenyl)-, monohydrochloride.

Molecular formula: Tetrahydrozoline hydrochloride—$C_{13}H_{16}N_2 \cdot HCl$.

Molecular weight: Tetrahydrozoline hydrochloride—236.74.

Description: Tetrahydrozoline Hydrochloride USP—White, odorless solid. Melts at about 256 °C, with decomposition.

Solubility: Tetrahydrozoline Hydrochloride USP—Freely soluble in water and in alcohol; very slightly soluble in chloroform; practically insoluble in ether.

USP requirements:

Tetrahydrozoline Hydrochloride USP—Preserve in tight containers. Contains not less than 98.0% and not more than 100.5% of tetrahydrozoline hydrochloride, calculated on the dried basis. Meets the requirements for Identification, Loss on drying (not more than 1.0%), Residue on ignition (not more than 0.1%), Heavy metals (not more than 0.005%), and Ordinary impurities.

Tetrahydrozoline Hydrochloride Nasal Solution USP—Preserve in tight containers. A solution of Tetrahydrozoline Hydrochloride in water adjusted to a suitable tonicity. Contains the labeled amount, within ±10%. Meets the requirements for Identification, Microbial limits, and pH (5.3–6.5).

Tetrahydrozoline Hydrochloride Ophthalmic Solution USP—Preserve in tight containers. A sterile, isotonic solution of Tetrahydrozoline Hydrochloride in water. Contains the labeled amount, within ±10%. Meets the requirements for Identification, Sterility, and pH (5.8–6.5).

THALIDOMIDE

Chemical name: 1*H*-Isoindole-1,3(2*H*)-dione, 2-(2,6-dioxo-3-piperidinyl)-, (±)-.

Molecular formula: $C_{13}H_{10}N_2O_4$.

Molecular weight: 258.23.

Description: Thalidomide USP—White to off-white powder. Melting point 269–271 °C.

Solubility: Thalidomide USP—Very soluble in dimethylformamide, in dioxane, and in pyridine; sparingly soluble in acetone, in butyl acetate, in ethanol, in ethyl acetate, in glacial acetic acid, in methanol, and in water; practically insoluble in benzene, in chloroform, and in ether.

USP requirements:

Thalidomide USP—Preserve in tight containers, protected from light, at controlled room temperature. Contains not less than 98.0% and not more than 101.5% of thalidomide, calculated on the anhydrous basis. Meets the requirements for Identification, Microbial limits, Water (not more than 0.5%), Heavy metals (not more than 0.002%), Chromatographic purity, Ordinary impurities, and Organic volatile impurities.

Thalidomide Capsules USP—Preserve in tight containers, protected from light, at controlled room temperature. Do not repackage. Contain the labeled amount, within ± 10%. Meet the requirements for Identification, Dissolution (70% in 60 minutes in 1.0 mL of polyoxyethylene (23) lauryl ether solution, prepared by dissolving 50 grams in 100 mL of water, to 0.225 *M* hydrochloric acid in Apparatus 2 at 75 rpm), and Uniformity of dosage units.

THALLOUS CHLORIDE TL 201

Chemical name: Thallium chloride (^{201}TlCl).

Molecular formula: ^{201}TlCl.

USP requirements: Thallous Chloride Tl 201 Injection USP—Preserve in single-dose or in multiple-dose containers. A sterile, isotonic, aqueous solution of radioactive thallium (^{201}Tl) in the form of thallous chloride suitable for intravenous administration. Label it to include the following, in addition to the information specified for Labeling under Injections: the time and date of calibration; the amount of ^{201}Tl as labeled thallous chloride expressed as total megabecquerels (or microcuries or millicuries) and concentration as megabecquerels (or microcuries or millicuries) per mL at the time of calibration; the expiration date and time; and the statement, "Caution—Radioactive Material." The labeling indicates that in making dosage calculations, correction is to be made for radioactive decay, and also indicates that the radioactive half-life of ^{201}Tl is 73.1 hours. Contains the labeled amount of ^{201}Tl, within ± 10%, as chloride, expressed in megabecquerels (or microcuries or millicuries) per mL, at the time indicated in the labeling. Other chemical forms of radioactivity do not exceed 5.0% of the total radioactivity. Meets the requirements for Radionuclide identification, Bacterial endotoxins, pH (4.5–7.5), Radiochemical purity, Radionuclidic purity, Content of thallium, Iron, and Copper, and for Injections (except that the Injection may be distributed or dispensed prior to completion of the test for Sterility, the latter test being started on the day of final manufacture, and except that it is not subject to the recommendation on Volume in Container).

THEOPHYLLINE

Source: Theophylline sodium glycinate—An equimolar mixture of theophylline sodium and glycine buffered by an additional mole of the essential amino acid, glycine.

Chemical name:

Theophylline—1*H*-Purine-2,6-dione, 3,7-dihydro-1,3-dimethyl-, monohydrate.

Theophylline sodium glycinate—Glycine, mixt. with 3,7-dihydro-1,3-dimethyl-1*H*-purine-2,6-dione, monosodium salt.

Molecular formula: $C_7H_8N_4O_2 \cdot H_2O$ (hydrous); $C_7H_8N_4O_2$ (anhydrous).

Molecular weight: 198.18 (hydrous); 180.17 (anhydrous).

Description:

Theophylline USP—White, odorless, crystalline powder. Is stable in air.

Theophylline Sodium Glycinate USP—White, crystalline powder having a slight ammoniacal odor.

Solubility:

Theophylline USP—Slightly soluble in water, but more soluble in hot water; freely soluble in solutions of alkali hydroxides and in ammonia; sparingly soluble in alcohol, in chloroform, and in ether.

Theophylline Sodium Glycinate USP—Freely soluble in water; very slightly soluble in alcohol; practically insoluble in chloroform.

USP requirements:

Theophylline USP—Preserve in well-closed containers. Contains one molecule of water of hydration or is anhydrous. Label it to indicate whether it is hydrous or anhydrous. Contains not less than 97.0% and not more than 102.0% of theophylline, calculated on the dried basis. Meets the requirements for Identification, Melting range (270–274 °C, the range between beginning and end of melting not more than 3 °C), Acidity, Loss on drying (7.5–9.5% for the hydrous form and not more than 0.5% for the anhydrous form), Residue on ignition (not more than 0.15%), and Organic volatile impurities.

Theophylline Capsules USP—Preserve in well-closed containers. Contain the labeled amount of anhydrous theophylline, within ±10%. Meet the requirements for Identification, Dissolution (80% in 60 minutes in water in Apparatus 2 at 50 rpm), and Uniformity of dosage units.

Theophylline Extended-release Capsules USP—Preserve in well-closed containers. The labeling indicates whether the product is intended for dosing every 12 or 24 hours, and states with which in-vitro *Drug Release Test* the product complies. Contain the labeled amount of anhydrous theophylline, within ±10%. Meet the requirements for Identification, Drug release, and Uniformity of dosage units.

Theophylline Elixir—Not in *USP–NF*.

Theophylline Oral Solution USP—Preserve in tight, light-resistant containers, and avoid exposer to excessive heat. Label it to indicate the alcohol content (if present). Contains the labeled amount, within ±5%. Meets the requirements for Identification, Microbial limits, pH (4.3–4.7), and Alcohol content (90.0%–115.0%).

Theophylline Syrup—Not in *USP–NF*.

Theophylline Tablets USP—Preserve in well-closed containers. Contain the labeled amount of anhydrous theophylline, within ±6%. Meet the requirements for Identification, Dissolution (80% in 45 minutes in water in Apparatus 2 at 50 rpm), and Uniformity of dosage units.

Theophylline Extended-release Tablets—Not in *USP–NF*.

Theophylline Sodium Glycinate USP—Preserve in tight containers. An equilibrium mixture containing Theophylline Sodium and Glycine in approximately equimolecular proportions buffered with an additional mole of Glycine. Dried at 105 °C for 4 hours, contains theophylline sodium glycinate equivalent to not less than 44.5% and not more than

47.3% of anhydrous theophylline. Meets the requirements for Identification, pH (8.5–9.5, in a saturated solution), Loss on drying (not more than 2.0%), Glycine content (42.0–48.0%, on the dried basis), and Organic volatile impurities.

Theophylline Sodium Glycinate Elixir USP—Preserve in tight containers. Label Elixir to state both the content of theophylline sodium glycinate and the content of anhydrous theophylline. Contains an amount of theophylline sodium glycinate equivalent to the labeled amount of anhydrous theophylline, within ±7%. Meets the requirements for Identification, pH (8.3–9.1), and Alcohol content (17.0–23.0%).

Theophylline Sodium Glycinate Oral Solution USP—Preserve in tight containers. Label Elixir to state both the content of theophylline sodium glycinate and the content of anhydrous theophylline. Contains an amount of theophylline sodium glycinate equivalent to the labeled amount of anhydrous theophylline, within ±7%. Meets the requirements for Identification, pH (8.3–9.1), and Alcohol content (17.0–23.0%).

Theophylline Sodium Glycinate Tablets USP—Preserve in well-closed containers. Label Tablets to state both the content of theophylline sodium glycinate and the content of anhydrous theophylline. Contain an amount of theophylline sodium glycinate equivalent to the labeled amount of anhydrous theophylline, within ±7%. Meet the requirements for Identification, Dissolution (75% in 45 minutes in water in Apparatus 1 at 100 rpm), and Uniformity of dosage units.

THEOPHYLLINE AND DEXTROSE

For *Theophylline* and *Dextrose*—See individual listings for chemistry information.

USP requirements: Theophylline in Dextrose Injection USP—Preserve in single-dose containers, preferably of Type I or Type II glass, or of a suitable plastic material. A sterile solution of Theophylline and Dextrose in Water for Injection. Contains the labeled amount of anhydrous theophylline, within ±7%, and the labeled amount of dextrose, within ±5%. Meets the requirements for Identification, Bacterial endotoxins, pH (3.5–6.5), and Limit of 5-hydroxymethylfurfural and related substances, and for Injections.

THEOPHYLLINE, EPHEDRINE, GUAIFENESIN, AND PHENOBARBITAL

For *Theophylline, Ephedrine, Guaifenesin,* and *Phenobarbital*—See individual listings for chemistry information.

USP requirements:
Theophylline, Ephedrine Hydrochloride, Guaifenesin, and Phenobarbital Elixir—Not in *USP–NF*.
Theophylline, Ephedrine Hydrochloride, Guaifenesin, and Phenobarbital Tablets—Not in *USP–NF*.
Theophylline, Ephedrine Sulfate, Guaifenesin, and Phenobarbital Elixir—Not in *USP–NF*.
Theophylline, Ephedrine Sulfate, Guaifenesin, and Phenobarbital Tablets—Not in *USP–NF*.

THEOPHYLLINE, EPHEDRINE, AND HYDROXYZINE

For *Theophylline, Ephedrine,* and *Hydroxyzine*—See individual listings for chemistry information.

USP requirements:
Theophylline, Ephedrine Sulfate, and Hydroxyzine Hydrochloride Syrup—Not in *USP–NF*.
Theophylline, Ephedrine Sulfate, and Hydroxyzine Hydrochloride Tablets—Not in *USP–NF*.

THEOPHYLLINE, EPHEDRINE, AND PHENOBARBITAL

For *Theophylline, Ephedrine,* and *Phenobarbital*—See individual listings for chemistry information.

USP requirements: Theophylline, Ephedrine Hydrochloride, and Phenobarbital Tablets USP—Preserve in tight containers. Contain the labeled amounts of anhydrous theophylline, ephedrine hydrochloride, and phenobarbital, within ±10%. Meet the requirements for Identification, Dissolution (75% of each active ingredient in 30 minutes in water in Apparatus 1 at 100 rpm), and Uniformity of dosage units.

THEOPHYLLINE AND GUAIFENESIN

For *Theophylline* and *Guaifenesin*—See individual listings for chemistry information.

USP requirements:
Theophylline and Guaifenesin Capsules USP—Preserve in tight containers. Contain the labeled amounts of anhydrous theophylline and guaifenesin, within ±10%. Meet the requirements for Identification, Dissolution (75% of each active ingredient in 45 minutes in simulated gastric fluid in Apparatus 1 at 100 rpm), and Uniformity of dosage units.
Theophylline and Guaifenesin Elixir—Not in *USP–NF*.
Theophylline and Guaifenesin Oral Solution USP—Preserve in tight containers. Contains the labeled amount of anhydrous theophylline, within ±10%, and the labeled amount of guaifenesin, within ±13.3%. Meets the requirements for Identification and Alcohol content (if present, within ±10% of labeled amount).
Theophylline and Guaifenesin Syrup—Not in *USP–NF*.
Theophylline and Guaifenesin Tablets—Not in *USP–NF*.
Theophylline Sodium Glycinate and Guaifenesin Elixir—Not in *USP–NF*.
Theophylline Sodium Glycinate and Guaifenesin Syrup—Not in *USP–NF*.
Theophylline Sodium Glycinate and Guaifenesin Tablets—Not in *USP–NF*.

THIABENDAZOLE

Chemical group: Benzimidazole derivative; structurally related to mebendazole.

Chemical name: 1*H*-Benzimidazole, 2-(4-thiazolyl)-.

Molecular formula: $C_{10}H_7N_3S$.

Molecular weight: 201.25.

Description: Thiabendazole USP—White to practically white, odorless or practically odorless powder.

Solubility: Thiabendazole USP—Practically insoluble in water; slightly soluble in acetone and in alcohol; very slightly soluble in chloroform and in ether.

USP requirements:

Thiabendazole USP—Preserve in well-closed containers. Contains not less than 98.0% and not more than 101.0% of thiabendazole, calculated on the dried basis. Meets the requirements for Identification, Melting range (296–303 °C), Loss on drying (not more than 0.5%), Residue on ignition (not more than 0.1%), Selenium (not more than 0.003%, a 200-mg test specimen being used), Heavy metals (not more than 0.001%), and Chromatographic purity.

Note: Thiabendazole labeled solely for veterinary use is exempt from the requirements of the tests for Residue on igniton, Selenium, Heavy metals, and Chromatographic purity.

Thiabendazole Oral Suspension USP—Preserve in tight containers. Contains the labeled amount, within ±10%. Meets the requirements for Identification and pH (3.4–4.2).

Thiabendazole Topical Suspension—Not in *USP–NF*.

Thiabendazole Tablets USP—Preserve in tight containers. Label the Tablets to indicate that they are to be chewed before swallowing. Contain the labeled amount, within ±10%. Meet the requirements for Identification and Uniformity of dosage units.

THIACETARSAMIDE

Chemical name: Benzamide, *p*-[bis(carboxymethylmercapto)arsino]-.

Molecular formula: $C_{11}H_{12}AsNO_5S_2$.

Molecular weight: 377.27.

Description: Thiacetarsamide USP—White to yellowish crystalline powder.

Solubility: Thiacetarsamide USP—Sparingly soluble in cold dehydrated alcohol, in cold methanol, and in cold water; more soluble in water above 90 °C; soluble in warm dehydrated alcohol and in warm methanol; insoluble in warm isopropyl alcohol.

pKa: 4.

USP requirements:

Thiacetarsamide USP—Preserve in well-closed containers. Label it to indicate that it is for veterinary use only. Contains not less than 95.0% and not more than 102.0% of thiacetarsamide, calculated on the dried basis. Meets the requirements for Identification, Melting range (160–168 °C), Loss on drying (not more than 2.0%), and Limit of ammonium salts (not more than 1.0%).

Thiacetarsamide Sodium Injection USP—Preserve in Containers for Injections. A sterile solution of Thiacetarsamide in Water for Injection and solubilized with the aid of Sodium Hydroxide. Label it to indicate that it is for veterinary use only. Contains the equivalent of the labeled amount of sodium thiacetarsamide, within ±10%. Meets the requirements for Identification, Pyrogen, Sterility, pH (6.8–7.2), and Particulate matter and for Injections.

THIAMINE

Chemical name:

Thiamine hydrochloride—Thiazolium, 3-[(4-amino-2-methyl-5-pyrimidinyl)methyl]-5-(2-hydroxyethyl)-4-methyl-, chloride, monohydrochloride.

Thiamine mononitrate—Thiazolium, 3-[(4-amino-2-methyl-5-pyrimidinyl)methyl]-5-(2-hydroxyethyl)-4-methyl-, nitrate (salt).

Molecular formula:

Thiamine hydrochloride—$C_{12}H_{17}ClN_4OS \cdot HCl$.

Thiamine mononitrate—$C_{12}H_{17}N_5O_4S$.

Molecular weight:

Thiamine hydrochloride—337.27.

Thiamine mononitrate—327.36.

Description:

Thiamine Hydrochloride USP—White crystals or crystalline powder, usually having a slight, characteristic odor. When exposed to air, the anhydrous product rapidly absorbs about 4% of water. Melts at about 248 °C, with some decomposition.

Thiamine Mononitrate USP—White crystals or crystalline powder, usually having a slight, characteristic odor.

pKa: 4.8 and 9.0.

Solubility:

Thiamine Hydrochloride USP—Freely soluble in water; soluble in glycerin; slightly soluble in alcohol; insoluble in ether.

Thiamine Mononitrate USP—Sparingly soluble in water; slightly soluble in alcohol; very slightly soluble in chloroform.

USP requirements:

Thiamine Hydrochloride USP—Preserve in tight, light-resistant containers. Contains not less than 98.0% and not more than 102.0% of thiamine hydrochloride, calculated on the anhydrous basis. Meets the requirements for Identification, pH (2.7–3.4, in a solution [1 in 100]), Water (not more than 5.0%), Residue on ignition (not more than 0.2%), Absorbance of solution (not more than 0.025), Limit of nitrate, Chromatographic purity, and Organic volatile impurities.

Thiamine Hydrochloride Elixir USP—Preserve in tight, light-resistant containers. Contains the labeled amount, within –5% to +35%. Meets the requirements for Identification and Alcohol content (within ±10% of labeled amount).

Thiamine Hydrochloride Injection USP—Preserve in single-dose or in multiple-dose containers, preferably of Type I glass, protected from light. A sterile solution of Thiamine Hydrochloride in Water for Injection. Contains the labeled amount, within ±10%. Meets the requirements for Identification, Bacterial endotoxins, and pH (2.5–4.5), and for Injections.

Thiamine Hydrochloride Oral Solution USP—Preserve in tight, light-resistant containers. Contains the labeled amount, within –5% to +35%. Meets the requirements for Identification and Alcohol content (within ±10% of labeled amount).

Thiamine Hydrochloride Tablets USP—Preserve in tight, light-resistant containers. Contain the labeled amount, within ±10%. Meet the requirements for Identification, Dissolution (75% in 45 minutes in water in Apparatus 2 at 50 rpm), and Uniformity of dosage units.

Thiamine Mononitrate USP—Preserve in tight, light-resistant containers. Contains not less than 98.0% and not more than 102.0% of thiamine mononitrate, calculated on the dried basis. Meets the requirements for Identification, pH (6.0–7.5, in a solution [1 in 50]), Loss on drying (not more than 1.0%), Residue on ignition (not more than 0.2%), Chloride (not more than 0.06%), Chromatographic purity, and Organic volatile impurities.

Thiamine Mononitrate Elixir USP—Preserve in tight, light-resistant containers. Contains the labeled amount, within –5% to +15%. Meets the requirements for Identification and Alcohol content (within ±10% of labeled amount).

Thiamine Mononitrate Oral Solution USP—Preserve in tight, light-resistant containers. Contains the labeled amount, within −5% to +15%. Meets the requirements for Identification and Alcohol content (within ±10% of labeled amount).

THIAMYLAL

Chemical group: Thiamylal sodium—A thiobarbiturate.

Chemical name:
Thiamylal—Dihydro-5-(1-methylbutyl)-5-(2-propenyl)-2-thioxo-4,6-(1*H*,5*H*)-pyrimidinedione.
Thiamylal sodium—4,6-(1*H*,5*H*)-Pyrimidinedione, dihydro-5-(1-methylbutyl)-5-(2-propenyl)-2-thioxo-, monosodium salt.

Molecular formula:
Thiamylal—$C_{12}H_{18}N_2O_2S$.
Thiamylal sodium—$C_{12}H_{17}N_2NaO_2S$.

Molecular weight:
Thiamylal—254.35.
Thiamylal sodium—276.33.

Description: Thiamylal Sodium for Injection USP—Pale yellow, hygroscopic powder, having a disagreeable odor.

USP requirements:
Thiamylal USP—Preserve in well-closed containers. Contains not less than 98.0% and not more than 102.0% of thiamylal, calculated on the dried basis. Meets the requirements for Identification, Melting range (135–139 °C), Loss on drying (not more than 1.0%), and Ordinary impurities.
Thiamylal Sodium for Injection USP—Preserve in Containers for Sterile Solids. A sterile mixture of thiamylal with anhydrous Sodium Carbonate as a buffer. Contains the labeled amount, within ±7%. It meets the requirements for Labeling under Injections. Meets the requirements for Completeness of solution, Constituted solution, Identification, Bacterial endotoxins, Sterility, Uniformity of dosage units, pH (10.7–11.5, in the solution prepared as directed in the test for Completeness of solution), Loss on drying (not more than 2.0%), and Heavy metals (not more than 0.003%).

THIETHYLPERAZINE

Chemical name:
Thiethylperazine malate—10*H*-Phenothiazine, 2-(ethylthio)-10-[3-(4-methyl-1-piperazinyl)propyl]-, 2-hydroxy-1,4-butanedioate (1:2).
Thiethylperazine maleate—10*H*-Phenothiazine, 2-(ethylthio)-10-[3-(4-methyl-1-piperazinyl)propyl]-, (*Z*)-2-butenedioate (1:2).

Molecular formula:
Thiethylperazine malate—$C_{22}H_{29}N_3S_2 \cdot 2C_4H_6O_5$.
Thiethylperazine maleate—$C_{22}H_{29}N_3S_2 \cdot 2C_4H_4O_4$.

Molecular weight:
Thiethylperazine malate—667.79.
Thiethylperazine maleate—631.76.

Description:
Thiethylperazine malate—White to faintly yellow crystalline powder with not more than a slight odor.
Thiethylperazine Maleate USP—Yellowish, granular powder. Odorless or has not more than a slight odor. Melts at about 183 °C, with decomposition.

Solubility:
Thiethylperazine malate—Soluble 1 in 40 of water, 1 in 90 of alcohol, 1 in 525 of chloroform, and 1 in 3400 of ether.
Thiethylperazine Maleate USP—Practically insoluble in water; slightly soluble in methanol; practically insoluble in chloroform.

USP requirements:
Thiethylperazine Malate USP—Preserve in tight, light-resistant containers. Contains not less than 98.0% and not more than 101.5% of thiethylperazine malate, calculated on the dried basis. Meets the requirements for Identification, pH (2.8–3.8, in a freshly prepared solution [1 in 100]), Loss on drying (not more than 0.5%), Residue on ignition (not more than 0.1%), Selenium (not more than 0.003%), and Organic volatile impurities.
Thiethylperazine Malate Injection USP—Preserve in single-dose containers, preferably of Type I glass, protected from light. A sterile solution of Thiethylperazine Malate in Water for Injection. Contains the labeled amount, within ±10%. Meets the requirements for Identification, Bacterial endotoxins, and pH (3.0–4.0), and for Injections.
Thiethylperazine Maleate USP—Preserve in tight, light-resistant containers. Contains not less than 98.0% and not more than 101.5% of thiethylperazine maleate, calculated on the dried basis. Meets the requirements for Identification, pH (2.8–3.8), Loss on drying (not more than 0.5%), Residue on ignition (not more than 0.1%), Selenium (not more than 0.003%), Chromatographic purity, and Organic volatile impurities.
Thiethylperazine Maleate Suppositories USP—Preserve in tight containers at temperatures below 25 °C. Do not expose unwrapped Suppositories to sunlight. Contain the labeled amount, within ±10%. Meet the requirements for Identification, Uniformity of dosage units, and Chromatographic purity.
Thiethylperazine Maleate Tablets USP—Preserve in tight, light-resistant containers. Contain the labeled amount, within ±10%. Meet the requirements for Identification, Dissolution (75% in 30 minutes in 0.01 *N* hydrochloric acid in Apparatus 1 at 120 rpm), and Uniformity of dosage units.

THIMEROSAL

Chemical name: Mercury, ethyl (2-mercaptobenzoato-*S*)-, sodium salt.

Molecular formula: $C_9H_9HgNaO_2S$.

Molecular weight: 404.81.

Description:
Thimerosal USP—Light cream-colored, crystalline powder, having a slight characteristic odor. Affected by light. The pH of a solution (1 in 100) is about 6.7.
NF category: Antimicrobial preservative.
Thimerosal Topical Solution USP—Clear liquid, having a slight characteristic odor. Affected by light.
Thimerosal Tincture USP—Transparent, mobile liquid, having the characteristic odor of alcohol and acetone. Affected by light.

Solubility: Thimerosal USP—Freely soluble in water; soluble in alcohol; practically insoluble in ether.

USP requirements:
Thimerosal USP—Preserve in tight, light-resistant containers. Contains not less than 97.0% and not more than 101.0% of thimerosal, calculated on the dried basis. Meets the requirements for Identification, Loss on drying (not more than 0.5%), Ether-soluble substances (not more than 0.8%), Mercury ions (not more than 0.70%), and Readily carbonizable substances.

Thimerosal Topical Aerosol USP—Preserve in tight, light-resistant, pressurized containers, and avoid exposure to excessive heat. An alcoholic solution of Thimerosal mixed with suitable propellants in a pressurized container. Contains the labeled amount, within ±15%. Meets the requirements for Identification and Alcohol content (18.7–25.3% [w/w]), and for Pressure test, Minimum fill, and Leakage test under Aerosols, Metered-dose inhalers, and Dry powder inhalers.

Note: Thimerosal Topical Aerosol is sensitive to some metals.

Thimerosal Topical Solution USP—Preserve in tight, light-resistant containers, and avoid exposure to excessive heat. Contains, in each 100 mL, not less than 95 mg and not more than 105 mg of thimerosal. Meets the requirements for Identification and pH (9.6–10.2).

Note: Thimerosal Topical Solution is sensitive to some metals.

Thimerosal Tincture USP—Preserve in tight, light-resistant containers, and avoid exposure to excessive heat. Contains, in each 100 mL, not less than 90 mg and not more than 110 mg of thimerosal. Meets the requirements for Identification and Alcohol content (45.0–55.0%).

Note: Thimerosal Tincture is sensitive to some metals.

THIOGUANINE

Chemical name: 6*H*-Purine-6-thione, 2-amino-1,7-dihydro-.

Molecular formula: $C_5H_5N_5S \cdot xH_2O$.

Molecular weight: 167.19 (anhydrous).

Description: Thioguanine USP—Pale yellow, odorless or practically odorless, crystalline powder.

pKa: 8.1.

Solubility: Thioguanine USP—Insoluble in water, in alcohol, and in chloroform; freely soluble in dilute solutions of alkali hydroxides.

USP requirements:
Thioguanine USP—Preserve in tight containers. It is anhydrous or contains one-half molecule of water of hydration. Label it to indicate its state of hydration. Contains not less than 97.0% and not more than 100.5% of thioguanine, calculated on the dried basis. Meets the requirements for Identification, Loss on drying (not more than 6.0%), Selenium (not more than 0.003%, 200 mg being used for the test), Phosphorus-containing substances, Free sulfur, Organic volatile impurities, and Nitrogen content (40.6–43.1%, calculated on the dried basis).
Thioguanine Tablets USP—Preserve in tight containers. Contain the labeled amount, within ±7%. Meet the requirements for Identification, Dissolution (75% in 45 minutes in water in Apparatus 2 at 50 rpm), and Uniformity of dosage units.

THIOPENTAL

Chemical group: A thiobarbiturate, the sulfur analog of pentobarbital sodium.

Chemical name: Thiopental sodium—4,6(1*H*,5*H*)-Pyrimidinedione, 5-ethyldihydro-5-(1-methylbutyl)-2-thioxo-, monosodium salt.

Molecular formula: Thiopental sodium—$C_{11}H_{17}N_2NaO_2S$.

Molecular weight: Thiopental sodium—264.32.

Description:
Thiopental Sodium USP—White to off-white, crystalline powder, or yellowish-white to pale greenish-yellow, hygroscopic powder. May have a disagreeable odor. Its solutions are alkaline to litmus. Its solutions decompose on standing, and on boiling precipitation occurs.
Thiopental Sodium for Injection USP—White to off-white, crystalline powder, or yellowish-white to pale greenish-yellow, hygroscopic powder. May have a disagreeable odor. Its solutions are alkaline to litmus. Its solutions decompose on standing, and on boiling precipitation occurs.

pKa: Thiopental sodium—7.4.

Solubility: Thiopental Sodium USP—Soluble in water and in alcohol; insoluble in absolute ether and in solvent hexane.

USP requirements:
Thiopental Sodium USP—Preserve in tight containers. Contains not less than 97.0% and not more than 102.0% of thiopental sodium, calculated on the dried basis. Meets the requirements for Identification, Loss on drying (not more than 2.0%), Heavy metals (not more than 0.002%), and Ordinary impurities.
Thiopental Sodium for Injection USP—Preserve in Containers for Sterile Solids, preferably of Type III glass. A sterile mixture of Thiopental Sodium and anhydrous Sodium Carbonate as a buffer. Contains the labeled amount, within ±7%. Meets the requirements for Completeness of solution, Constituted solution, Bacterial endotoxins, and pH (10.2–11.2), for Identification tests and Heavy metals under Thiopental Sodium, and for Sterility tests, Uniformity of dosage units, and Labeling under Injections.
Thiopental Sodium for Rectal Solution—Not in *USP–NF*.
Thiopental Sodium Rectal Suspension—Not in *USP–NF*.

THIOPROPAZATE

Chemical group: Piperazine phenothiazine derivative.

Chemical name: Thiopropazate hydrochloride—4-[3-(2-Chlorophenothiazin-10-yl)propyl]-1-piperazineethanol acetate dihydrochloride.

Molecular formula: Thiopropazate hydrochloride—$C_{23}H_{28}ClN_3O_2S \cdot 2HCl$.

Molecular weight: Thiopropazate hydrochloride—518.93.

Description: Thiopropazate hydrochloride—White or pale yellow crystalline powder with a faint odor.

Solubility: Thiopropazate hydrochloride—Soluble 1 in 4 of water, 1 in 130 of alcohol, and 1 in 65 of chloroform; practically insoluble in ether.

USP requirements: Thiopropazate Hydrochloride Tablets—Not in *USP–NF*.

THIOPROPERAZINE

Chemical group: Phenothiazine.

Chemical name: Thioproperazine mesylate—*NN*-Dimethyl-10-[3-(4-methylpiperazin-1-yl)propyl]phenothiazine-2-sulphonamide dimethanesulphonate.

Molecular formula: Thioproperazine mesylate—$C_{22}H_{30}N_4O_2S_2 \cdot 2CH_4O_3S$.

Molecular weight: Thioproperazine mesylate—638.8.

Description: Thioproperazine mesylate—Slightly hygroscopic white powder with a yellowish tint.

Solubility: Thioproperazine mesylate—Readily soluble in water; slightly soluble in ethanol; practically insoluble in methanol and in dimethylformamide.

USP requirements: Thioproperazine Mesylate Tablets—Not in *USP–NF*.

THIORIDAZINE

Chemical group: Phenothiazine.

Chemical name:
Thioridazine—10*H*-Phenothiazine, 10-[2-(1-methyl-2-piperidinyl)ethyl]-2-(methylthio)-.
Thioridazine hydrochloride—10*H*-Phenothiazine, 10-[2-(1-methyl-2-piperidinyl)ethyl]-2-(methylthio)-, monohydrochloride.

Molecular formula:
Thioridazine—$C_{21}H_{26}N_2S_2$.
Thioridazine hydrochloride—$C_{21}H_{26}N_2S_2 \cdot HCl$.

Molecular weight:
Thioridazine—370.58.
Thioridazine hydrochloride—407.04.

Description:
Thioridazine USP—White to slightly yellow, crystalline or micronized powder, odorless or having a faint odor.
Thioridazine Hydrochloride USP—White to slightly yellow, granular powder, having a faint odor.

Solubility:
Thioridazine USP—Practically insoluble in water; freely soluble in dehydrated alcohol and in ether; very soluble in chloroform.
Thioridazine Hydrochloride USP—Freely soluble in water, in methanol, and in chloroform; insoluble in ether.

USP requirements:
Thioridazine USP—Preserve in well-closed, light-resistant containers. Contains not less than 99.0% and not more than 101.0% of thioridazine, calculated on the dried basis. Meets the requirements for Identification, Loss on drying (not more than 0.5%), Residue on ignition (not more than 0.1%), Chromatographic purity, and Organic volatile impurities.
Thioridazine Oral Suspension USP—Preserve in tight, light-resistant containers, at a temperature not exceeding 30 °C. Contains the labeled amount, within ±10%. Meets the requirements for Identification, Specific gravity (1.180–1.310), and pH (8.0–10.0).
Thioridazine Hydrochloride USP—Preserve in tight, light-resistant containers. Contains not less than 99.0% and not more than 101.0% of thioridazine hydrochloride, calculated on the dried basis. Meets the requirements for Identification, Melting range (159–165 °C, the range between beginning and end of melting not more than 3 °C), pH (4.2–5.2, in a solution [1 in 100]), Loss on drying (not more than 0.4%), Residue on ignition (not more than 0.1%), Selenium (not more than 0.003%, a 100-mg specimen being used, 100 mg of magnesium oxide being added to the *Test Solution*), Chromatographic purity, and Organic volatile impurities.
Thioridazine Hydrochloride Oral Solution USP—Preserve in tight, light-resistant containers, at controlled room temperature. Label it to indicate that it is to be diluted to appropriate strength with water or other suitable fluid prior to administration. Contains the labeled amount, within ± 10%. Meets the requirements for Identification and Alcohol content (not more than 4.75%).
Thioridazine Hydrochloride Tablets USP—Preserve in tight, light-resistant containers. Contain the labeled amount, within ±10%. Meet the requirements for Identification, Dissolution (75% in 60 minutes in 0.01 *N* hydrochloric acid in Apparatus 2 at 75 rpm), and Uniformity of dosage units.

THIOSTREPTON

Molecular formula: $C_{72}H_{85}N_{19}O_{18}S_5$.

Molecular weight: 1664.89.

Description: Thiostrepton USP—White to off-white, crystalline solid.

Solubility: Thiostrepton USP—Practically insoluble in water, in the lower alcohols, in nonpolar organic solvents, and in dilute aqueous acids or alkali; soluble in glacial acetic acid, in chloroform, in dimethylformamide, in dimethyl sulfoxide, in dioxane, and in pyridine.

USP requirements: Thiostrepton USP—Preserve in tight containers. An antibacterial substance produced by the growth of strains of *Streptomyces azureus* (Fam. Streptomycetaceae). Has a potency of not less than 900 USP Thiostrepton Units per mg, calculated on the dried basis. Meets the requirements for Identification, Loss on drying (not more than 5.0%), and Residue on ignition (not more than 1.0%).

THIOTEPA

Chemical name: Aziridine,1,1′,1″-phosphinothioylidynetris-.

Molecular formula: $C_6H_{12}N_3PS$.

Molecular weight: 189.22.

Description:
Thiotepa USP—Fine, white, crystalline flakes, having a faint odor.
Thiotepa for Injection USP—White powder.

Solubility: Thiotepa USP—Freely soluble in water, in alcohol, in chloroform, and in ether.

USP requirements:
Thiotepa USP—Preserve in tight, light-resistant containers, and store in a refrigerator. Contains not less than 97.0% and not more than 102.0% of thiotepa, calculated on the anhydrous basis. Meets the requirements for Identification, Melting range (52–57 °C), and Water (not more than 2.0%).
   Caution: Great care should be taken to prevent inhaling particles of Thiotepa or exposing the skin to it.
Thiotepa for Injection USP—Preserve in Containers for Sterile Solids, and store in a refrigerator, protected from light. It is Thiotepa, with or without added substances, that is suitable for parenteral use. Contains the labeled amount, within −5% to +10%. Meets the requirements for Completeness of solution, Identification, pH (5.5–7.5, in a solution, constituted as directed in the labeling, containing 10 mg of thiotepa per mL), Water (not more than 0.5%), and Bacterial endotoxins, and for Sterility tests, Uniformity of dosage units, and Labeling under Injections.

THIOTHIXENE

Chemical group: Thioxanthene derivative.

Chemical name:

Thiothixene—9*H*-Thioxanthene-2-sulfonamide, *N,N*-dimethyl-9-[3-(4-methyl-1-piperazinyl)propylidene]-, (*Z*)-.

Thiothixene hydrochloride—9*H*-Thioxanthene-2-sulfonamide, *N,N*-dimethyl-9-[3-(4-methyl-1-piperazinyl)propylidene]-, dihydrochloride, dihydrate (*Z*)-.

Molecular formula:

Thiothixene—$C_{23}H_{29}N_3O_2S_2$.

Thiothixene hydrochloride—$C_{23}H_{29}N_3O_2S_2 \cdot 2HCl \cdot 2H_2O$.

Molecular weight:

Thiothixene—443.63.

Thiothixene hydrochloride—552.58.

Description:

Thiothixene USP—White to tan, practically odorless crystals. Is affected by light.

Thiothixene Hydrochloride USP—White, or practically white, crystalline powder, having a slight odor. Is affected by light.

Solubility:

Thiothixene USP—Practically insoluble in water; very soluble in chloroform; slightly soluble in methanol and in acetone.

Thiothixene Hydrochloride USP—Soluble in water; slightly soluble in chloroform; practically insoluble in acetone and in ether.

Other characteristics: Structurally and pharmacologically similar to the piperazine phenothiazines.

USP requirements:

Thiothixene USP—Preserve in tight, light-resistant containers. Contains not less than 96.0% and not more than 101.5% of thiothixene, calculated on the dried basis. Meets the requirements for Identification, Melting range (147–153.5 °C), Loss on drying (not more than 2.0%), Residue on ignition (not more than 0.2%), Selenium (not more than 0.003%), Heavy metals (not more than 0.0025%), Limit of (*E*)-thiothixene (not more than 1.0%), and Organic volatile impurities.

Thiothixene Capsules USP—Preserve in well-closed, light-resistant containers. Contain the labeled amount, within ± 10%. Meet the requirements for Identification, Dissolution (80% in 20 minutes in solution of 2.0 grams of sodium chloride and 7 mL of hydrochloric acid in water to make 1000 mL in Apparatus 1 at 100 rpm), and Uniformity of dosage units.

Thiothixene Hydrochloride USP—Preserve in tight, light-resistant containers. Contains two molecules of water of hydration or is anhydrous. Contains not less than 97.0% and not more than 102.5% of thiothixene hydrochloride, calculated on the anhydrous basis. Meets the requirements for Identification, Water (6.2–7.5% for the dihydrate and not more than 1.0% for the anhydrous form), Residue on ignition (not more than 0.2%), Heavy metals (not more than 0.0025%), Selenium (not more than 0.003%), Limit of (*E*)-thiothixene (not more than 1.0%), and Organic volatile impurities.

Thiothixene Hydrochloride Injection USP—Preserve in single-dose containers, preferably of Type I glass, protected from light. A sterile solution of Thiothixene Hydrochloride in Water for Injection. Contains an amount of thiothixene hydrochloride equivalent to the labeled amount of thiothixene, within ±10%. Meets the requirements for Identification, Bacterial endotoxins, and pH (2.5–3.5), and for Injections.

Thiothixene Hydrochloride for Injection USP—Preserve in light-resistant Containers for Sterile Solids. A sterile, dry mixture of Thiothixene Hydrochloride and Mannitol. Contains an amount of thiothixene hydrochloride equivalent to the labeled amount of thiothixene, within ±10%. Meets the requirements for Identification, Bacterial endotoxins,

pH (2.3–3.7, in the solution constituted as directed in the labeling), and Water (not more than 4.0%), and for Injections.

Thiothixene Hydrochloride Oral Solution USP—Preserve in tight, light-resistant containers. Contains an amount of thiothixene hydrochloride equivalent to the labeled amount of thiothixene, within ±10%. Meets the requirements for Identification, pH (2.0–3.0), and Alcohol content (if present, within ±10% of the labeled amount, the labeled amount being not more than 7.0%).

THREONINE

Chemical name: L-Threonine.

Molecular formula: $C_4H_9NO_3$.

Molecular weight: 119.12.

Description: Threonine USP—White, odorless crystals.

Solubility: Threonine USP—Freely soluble in water; insoluble in absolute alcohol, in ether, and in chloroform.

USP requirements: Threonine USP—Preserve in well-closed containers. Contains not less than 98.5% and not more than 101.5% of threonine, as L-threonine, calculated on the dried basis. Meets the requirements for Identification, Specific rotation (−26.7° to −29.1°), pH (5.0–6.5, in a solution [1 in 20]), Loss on drying (not more than 0.2%), Residue on ignition (not more than 0.4%), Chloride (not more than 0.05%), Sulfate (not more than 0.03%), Iron (not more than 0.003%), Heavy metals (not more than 0.0015%), Chromatographic purity, and Organic volatile impurities.

THROMBIN

Description: Thrombin USP—White to grayish, amorphous substance dried from the frozen state.

USP requirements: Thrombin USP—Preserve at a temperature between 2 and 8 °C. Dispense it in the unopened container in which it was placed by the manufacturer. A sterile, freeze-dried powder derived from bovine plasma containing the protein substance prepared from prothrombin through interaction with added thromboplastin in the presence of calcium. It is capable, without the addition of other substances, of causing the clotting of whole blood, plasma, or a solution of fibrinogen. Its potency is determined in U.S. Units in terms of the U.S. Standard Thrombin in a test comparing clotting times of fibrinogen solution. Label it to indicate that solutions of Thrombin are to be used within a few hours after preparation, and are not to be injected into or otherwise allowed to enter large blood vessels. Meets the requirement for Expiration date (not more than 3 years after date of manufacture). Conforms to the regulations of the U.S. Food and Drug Administration concerning biologics.

THYMOL

Chemical name: Phenol, 5-methyl-2-(1-methylethyl)-.

Molecular formula: $C_{10}H_{14}O$.

Molecular weight: 150.22.

Description: Thymol NF—Colorless, often large, crystals, or white, crystalline powder, having an aromatic, thyme-like odor. Affected by light. Its alcohol solution is neutral to litmus.

NF category: Antimicrobial preservative; flavors and perfumes.

Solubility: Thymol NF—Very slightly soluble in water; freely soluble in alcohol, in chloroform, in ether, and in olive oil; soluble in glacial acetic acid and in fixed and volatile oils.

NF requirements: Thymol NF—Preserve in tight, light-resistant containers. Contains not less than 99.0% and not more than 101.0% of thymol. Meets the requirements for Identification, Melting range (48–51 °C, but when melted, Thymol remains liquid at a considerably lower temperature), Limit of nonvolatile residue (not more than 0.05%), and Organic volatile impurities.

THYROGLOBULIN

Chemical name: Thyroglobulin.

Description: Cream to tan-colored, free-flowing powder, having a slight, characteristic odor.

Solubility: Insoluble in water, in dimethylformamide, in alcohol, in hydrochloric acid, in chloroform, and in carbon tetrachloride.

USP requirements: Thyroglobulin Tablets—Not in *USP–NF*.

THYROID

Description: Thyroid USP—Yellowish to buff-colored, amorphous powder, having a slight, characteristic, meat-like odor.

USP requirements:
Thyroid USP—Preserve in tight containers. The cleaned, dried, and powdered thyroid gland previously deprived of connective tissue and fat. Obtained from domesticated animals that are used for food by humans. On hydrolysis, yields the labeled amounts of levothyroxine and liothyronine, within ±10%, calculated on the dried basis. It is free from iodine in inorganic or any form of combination other than that peculiar to the thyroid gland. Meets the requirements for Identification, Microbial limits, Loss on drying (not more than 6.0%), and Limit of inorganic iodides (not more than 0.01%).
Thyroid Tablets USP—Preserve in tight containers. Contain the labeled amounts of levothyroxine and liothyronine, within ±10%, the labeled amounts being 38 mcg of levothyroxine and 9 mcg of liothyronine for each 65 mg of the labeled content of thyroid. Meet the requirements for Microbial limits, Disintegration (15 minutes with disks), and Uniformity of dosage units.

THYROTROPIN

Source:
Thyrotropin—Thyroid stimulating hormone (TSH) isolated from bovine anterior pituitary.
Thyrotropin alpha—Recombinant thyroid stimulating hormone (TSH), a heterodimeric glycoprotein, synthesized in a genitically modified Chinese hamster ovary cell line.

Molecular weight: Thyrotropin—Range of 28,000–30,000.

Description: Thyrotropin alpha—A sterile, non-pyrogenic, white to off-white lyophilized product.

Solubility: Thyrotropin—Dissolves readily in physiologic saline.

Other characteristics: Thyrotropin alpha—The pH of reconstituted solution is approximately 7.0.

USP requirements:
Thyrotropin for Injection—Not in *USP–NF*.
Thyrotropin Alfa for Injection—Not in *USP–NF*.

TIAGABINE

Chemical name: Tiagabine hydrochloride—3-Piperidinecarboxylic acid, 1-[4,4-bis(3-methyl-2-thienyl)-3-butenyl]-, hydrochloride, (*R*)-.

Molecular formula: Tiagabine hydrochloride—$C_{20}H_{25}NO_2S_2 \cdot$ HCl.

Molecular weight: Tiagabine hydrochloride—412.01.

Description: Tiagabine Hydrochloride USP—White to off-white powder.

Solubility: Tiagabine Hydrochloride USP—Very slightly soluble in chloroform; practically insoluble in *n*-heptane.

USP requirements:
Tiagabine Hydrochloride USP—Preserve in tight, light-resistant containers at a temperature not higher than 30°. Contains not less than 97.5% and not more than 102.5% of tiagabine hydrochloride, calculated on the anhydrous basis. Meets the requirements for Identification, Water (not more than 6.0%), Residue on ignition (not more than 0.2%), Heavy metals (0.002%), Limit of (*S*)-(+) isomer (not more than 0.5%), and Chromatographic purity.
Tiagabine Hydrochloride Tablets—Not in *USP–NF*.

TIAMULIN

Chemical name: Tiamulin fumarate—Acetic acid, [[2-(diethylaminoethyl]thio]-, 6- ethenyl-decahydro-5-hydroxy-4,6,9,10-tetramethyl-1-oxo-3a,9-propano-3a*H*-cyclopentacycloocten-8-yl ester [3a*S*-(3a alpha,4 beta,5 alpha,6 alpha,8 beta,9 alpha,9a beta,10*S**)]-, (*E*-2-butenedioate (1:1) (salt).

Molecular formula: Tiamulin fumarate—$C_{28}H_{47}NO_4S \cdot C_4H_4O_4$.

Molecular weight: Tiamulin fumarate—609.82.

USP requirements: Tiamulin Fumarate USP—Preserve in tight, light-resistant containers, and store at room temperature. Label to indicate that is for veterinary use only. Contains not less than 98% and not more than 102.0% of tiamulin fumarate, calculated on the dried basis. Meets the requirements for Color and clarity of solution, Identification, Melting temperature (143°–149°), Specific rotation (+24° to +28°, on the dried basis, measured at 20°), pH (3.1–4.1), Loss on drying (not more than 0.5%), Residue on ignition (not more than 0.1%), Heavy metals (not more than 0.001%), Limit of residual solvents, Chromatographic purity, and Content of fumarate (83.7–87.3 mg).

TIAPROFENIC ACID

Chemical group: Propionic acid derivative.

Chemical name: 5-Benzoyl-alpha-methyl-2-thiopheneacetic acid.

Molecular formula: $C_{14}H_{12}O_3S$.

Molecular weight: 260.31.

Description: White, microcrystalline powder. Melts at about 95 °C.

pKa: 3.0.

Solubility: Readily soluble in alcohol, in chloroform, and in acetone; sparingly soluble in water.

USP requirements:
Tiaprofenic Acid Extended-release Capsules—Not in *USP–NF*.

Tiaprofenic Acid Tablets—Not in *USP–NF*.

TICARCILLIN

Chemical name:
Ticarcillin disodium—4-Thia-1-azabicyclo[3.2.0]heptane-2-carboxylic acid, 6-[(carboxy-3-thienylacetyl)amino]-3,3-dimethyl-7-oxo-, disodium salt, [2S-[2 alpha,5 alpha,6 beta(S*)]]-.

Ticarcillin monosodium—4-Thia-1-azabicyclo[3.2.0]heptane-2-carboxylic acid, 6-[(carboxy-3-thienylacetyl)amino]-3,3-dimethyl-7-oxo, monosodium salt, [2S-[2 alpha,5 alpha,6 beta(S*)]]-, monohydrate.

Molecular formula:
Ticarcillin disodium—$C_{15}H_{14}N_2Na_2O_6S_2$.
Ticarcillin monosodium—$C_{15}H_{15}N_2NaO_6S_2 \cdot H_2O$.

Molecular weight:
Ticarcillin disodium—428.39.
Ticarcillin monosodium—424.43.

Description: Ticarcillin Disodium USP—White to pale yellow powder, or white to pale yellow solid having the characteristic appearance of products prepared by freeze-drying.

Solubility: Ticarcillin Disodium USP—Freely soluble in water.

USP requirements:
Ticarcillin Disodium USP—Preserve in tight containers. Where it is intended for use in preparing injectable dosage forms, the label states that it is sterile or must be subjected to further processing during the preparation of injectable dosage forms. Has a potency equivalent to not less than 800 mcg of ticarcillin per mg, calculated on the anhydrous basis. Meets the requirements for Identification, Specific rotation (+172° to +187°), pH (6.0–8.0, in a solution containing 10 mg of ticarcillin per mL, Water (not more than 6.0%), Dimethylaniline, and Ticarcillin content (80.0–94.0%, calculated on the anhydrous basis), for Sterility tests and for Bacterial endotoxins under Ticarcillin for Injection (where the label states that Ticarcillin Disodium is sterile), and for Bacterial endotoxins under Ticarcillin for Injection (where the label states that Ticarcillin Disodium must be subjected to further processing during the preparation of injectable dosage forms).

Ticarcillin for Injection USP—Preserve in Containers for Sterile Solids. Contains an amount of ticarcillin disodium equivalent to the labeled amount of ticarcillin, within –10% to +15%. Meets the requirements for Constituted solution, Bacterial endotoxins, Sterility, pH (6.0–8.0, in the solution constituted as directed in the labeling), Water (not more than 6.0%), and Particulate matter, for Identification tests and for Water and Dimethylaniline under Ticarcillin Disodium, and for Uniformity of dosage units and Labeling under Injections. Ticarcillin for Injection that contains no added substances meets the requirements for Specific rotation and Ticarcillin content under Ticarcillin Disodium.

Ticarcillin Monosodium USP—Preserve in tight containers. Where it is intended for use in preparing injectable dosage forms, the label states that it is sterile or must be subjected to further processing during the preparation of injectable dosage forms. Contains the equivalent of not less than 890 mcg of ticarcillin per mg, calculated on the anhydrous basis. Meets the requirements for Identification, Specific

rotation (+181° to +197°, calculated on the anhydrous basis), Crystallinity, pH (2.5–4.0, in a solution containing the equivalent of 10 mg of ticarcillin per mL), Water (4.0–6.0%), and Dimethylaniline, for Sterility and for Bacterial endotoxins under Ticarcillin for Injection (where the label states that Ticarcillin Monosodium is sterile), and for Bacterial endotoxins under Ticarcillin for Injection (where the label states that Ticarcillin Monosodium must be subjected to further processing during the preparation of injectable dosage forms).

TICARCILLIN AND CLAVULANATE

For *Ticarcillin* and *Clavulanate*—See individual listings for chemistry information.

USP requirements:
Ticarcillin and Clavulanate Acid Injection USP—Preserve in Containers for Injections. Maintain in the frozen state. A sterile isoosmotic solution of Ticarcillin Monosodium and Clavulanate Potassium in Water for Injection. Contains one or more suitable buffering agents and a tonicity-adjusting agent. It meets the requirements for Labeling under Injections. The label states that it is to be thawed just prior to use, describes conditions for proper storage of the resultant solution, and directs that the solution is not to be refrozen. Contains an amount of ticarcillin disodium equivalent to the labeled amount of ticarcillin, within –10 to +15%, and an amount of clavulanate potassium equivalent to the labeled amount of clavulanic acid, within –15% to +20%. Meets the requirements for Identification, Bacterial endotoxins, Sterility, pH (5.5–7.5), and Particulate matter, for Uniformity of dosage units, and for Labeling under Injections.

Ticarcillin and Clavulanate Acid for Injection USP—Preserve in Containers for Sterile Solids. A sterile, dry mixture of Sterile Ticarcillin Disodium and Sterile Clavulanate Potassium. Contains amounts of ticarcillin disodium and clavulanate potassium equivalent to the labeled amount of ticarcillin, within –10% to +15%, and clavulanic acid, within –15% to +20%, the labeled amounts representing proportions of ticarcillin to clavulanic acid of 15:1 or 30:l. Meets the requirements for Constituted solution, Identification, Bacterial endotoxins, Sterility, pH (5.5–7.5, in a solution [1 in 10]), Water (not more than 4.2%), and Particulate matter, for Uniformity of dosage units, and for Labeling under Injections.

TICLOPIDINE

Chemical name: Ticlopidine hydrochloride—Thieno[3,2-c]pyridine, 5-[(2-chlorophenyl)methyl]-4,5,6,7-tetrahydro-, hydrochloride.

Molecular formula: Ticlopidine hydrochloride—$C_{14}H_{14}ClNS \cdot HCl$.

Molecular weight: Ticlopidine hydrochloride—300.25.

Description: Ticlopidine hydrochloride—White crystalline solid.

Solubility: Ticlopidine hydrochloride—Freely soluble in water and in self buffers to a pH of 3.6, and in methanol; sparingly soluble in methylene chloride and in ethanol; slightly soluble in acetone; insoluble in a buffer solution of pH 6.3.

USP requirements: Ticlopidine Hydrochloride Tablets—Not in *USP–NF*.

TILETAMINE

Chemical name: Tiletamine hydrochloride—Cyclohexanone, 2-(ethylamino)-2-(2-thienyl)-.

Molecular formula: Tiletamine hydrochloride—$C_{12}H_{17}NOS \cdot HCl$.

Molecular weight: Tiletamine hydrochloride—259.80.

Description: Tiletamine Hydrochloride USP—White to off-white crystalline powder.

Solubility: Tiletamine Hydrochloride USP—Freely soluble in water and in 0.1 N hydrochloric acid; soluble in methanol; slightly soluble in chloroform; practically insoluble in ether.

USP requirements: Tiletamine Hydrochloride USP—Preserve in tight containers. Label it to indicate that it is for veterinary use only. Where it is intended for use in preparing injectable dosage forms, the label states that it is sterile or must be subjected to further processing during the preparation of injectable dosage forms. Contains not less than 97.0% and not more than 103.0% of tiletamine hydrochloride. Meets the requirements for Identification, Melting range (190–195 °C, within 2° range), pH (3.0–5.0, in a solution [1 in 10]), Water (not more than 1.0%), Residue on ignition (not more than 0.5%), Heavy metals (not more than 0.002%), Chromatographic purity, and Chloride content (13.24–14.06%), for Bacterial endotoxins (where the label states that Tiletamine Hydrochloride is sterile or must be subjected to further processing during the preparation of injectable dosage forms), and for Sterility (where the label states that Tiletamine Hydrochloride is sterile).

TILETAMINE AND ZOLAZEPAM

For *Tiletamine* and *Zolazepam*—See individual listings for chemistry information.

USP requirements: Tiletamine and Zolazepam for Injection USP—Preserve in Containers for Sterile Solids. A sterile dry mixture of Tiletamine Hydrochloride and Zolazepam Hydrochloride. Contains the equivalent amount of the labeled amount of tiletamine and zolazepam, within ±10%. Meets the requirements for Identification, Bacterial endotoxins, Sterility, pH (2.0–3.5, when constituted as directed in the labeling), and Water (not more than 20 mg in a container containing the equivalent of 250 mg of tiletamine and 250 mg of zolazepam), for Injections, and for Uniformity of dosage units.

TILMICOSIN

Chemical name: Tylosin, 4^A^-O-de(2,6-dideoxy-3-C-methyl-alpha-L-*ribo*-hexopyranosyl)-20-deoxo-20-(3,5-dimethyl-1-piperidinyl)-, 20(*cis*)-.

Molecular formula: $C_{46}H_{80}N_2O_{13}$.

Molecular weight: 869.13.

Description: Tilmicosin USP—White to off-white amorphous solid.

Solubility: Tilmicosin USP—Slightly soluble in water and in *n*-hexane.

USP requirements:

Tilmicosin USP—Preserve in well-closed, light-resistant containers. Avoid excessive heat. Label it to indicate that it is for veterinary use only. Contains not less than 85.0% of tilmicosin, calculated on the anhydrous basis. The content of tilmicosin *cis*-isomers is between 82.0% and 88.0%, and the content of tilmicosin *trans*-isomers is between 12.0% and 18.0%. Meets the requirements for Identification, Water (not more than 5.0%), and Related compounds.

Caution: Tilmicosin is irritating to the eyes and may cause allergic reaction. Avoid contact.

Tilmicosin Injection USP—Preserve in light-resistant Containers for Injections. Store at or below 30°. A sterile solution of Tilmicosin in a mixture of Propylene Glycol and Water for Injection, solubilized with the aid of Phosphoric Acid. Label the Injection to indicate that it is for veterinary use only. Contains the labeled amount, within ±10%. Meets the requirements for Identification, Bacterial endotoxins, Sterility, pH (5.5–6.5), Particulate matter, and Content of propylene glycol (within ±20% of labeled amount).

TILUDRONATE

Chemical name: Tiludronate disodium—Phosphonic acid, [[(4-chlorophenyl)thio]methylene]bis-, disodium salt.

Molecular formula: Tiludronate disodium—$C_7H_7ClNa_2O_6P_2S$.

Molecular weight: Tiludronate disodium—362.57.

USP requirements: Tiludronate Disodium Tablets—Not in *USP–NF*.

TIMOLOL

Chemical name: Timolol maleate—2-Propanol, 1-[(1,1-dimethylethyl)amino]-3-[[4-(4-morpholinyl)-1,2,5-thiadiazol-3-yl]oxy]-, (*S*)-, (*Z*)-2-butenedioate (1:1) (salt).

Molecular formula: Timolol maleate—$C_{13}H_{24}N_4O_3S \cdot C_4H_4O_4$.

Molecular weight: Timolol maleate—432.49.

Description:
Timolol hemihydrate—White, odorless, crystalline powder.
Timolol Maleate USP—White to practically white, odorless or practically odorless, powder.

pKa: Timolol maleate—Approximately 9 in water at 25 °C.

Solubility:
Timolol hemihydrate—Slightly soluble in water; freely soluble in ethanol.
Timolol Maleate USP—Soluble in water, in alcohol, and in methanol; sparingly soluble in chloroform and in propylene glycol; insoluble in ether and in cyclohexane.

Other characteristics: Lipid solubility—Moderate.

USP requirements:
Timolol Hemihydrate Ophthalmic Solution—Not in *USP–NF*.
Timolol Maleate USP—Preserve in well-closed containers. Contains not less than 98.0% and not more than 101.0% of timolol maleate, calculated on the dried basis. Meets the requirements for Identification, Specific rotation (–11.7° to –12.5°), pH (3.8–4.3, in a solution containing 20 mg per mL), Loss on drying (not more than 0.5%), Residue on ignition (not more than 0.1%), Heavy metals (not more than 0.002%), Chromatographic purity, and Organic volatile impurities.
Timolol Maleate Ophthalmic Solution USP—Preserve in tight, light-resistant containers. A sterile, aqueous solution of Timolol Maleate. Contains an amount of timolol maleate equivalent to the labeled amount of timolol, within ±10%. Meets the requirements for Identification, Sterility, and pH (6.5–7.5).
Timolol Maleate Ophthalmic Gel-forming Solution—Not in *USP–NF*.

Timolol Maleate Tablets USP—Preserve in well-closed containers. Contain the labeled amount, within ±10%. Meet the requirements for Identification, Dissolution (80% in 20 minutes in 0.1 N hydrochloric acid in Apparatus 1 at 100 rpm), and Uniformity of dosage units.

TIMOLOL AND HYDROCHLOROTHIAZIDE

For *Timolol* and *Hydrochlorothiazide*—See individual listings for chemistry information.

USP requirements: Timolol Maleate and Hydrochlorothiazide Tablets USP—Preserve in well-closed, light-resistant containers. Contain the labeled amounts, within ±10%. Meet the requirements for Identification, Dissolution (80% of each active ingredient in 20 minutes in 0.1 N hydrochloric acid in Apparatus 2 at 50 rpm), Limit of 4-amino-6-chloro-1,3-benzenedisulfonamide (not more than 1.0%), Related compounds (not more than 1.0%), and Uniformity of dosage units.

TINIDAZOLE

Chemical name: 1H-Imidazole, 1-[2-(ethylsulfonyl)ethyl]-2-methyl-5-nitro-.

Molecular formula: $C_{18}H_{13}N_3O_4S$.

Molecular weight: 247.28.

Description: Tinidazole USP—Almost white or pale yellow, crystalline powder.

Solubility: Tinidazole USP—Soluble in acetone and in methylene chloride; sparingly soluble in methanol; practically insoluble in water.

USP requirements: Tinidazole USP—Preserve in tight containers, protected from light, at controlled room temperature. Contains not less than 98.0% and not more than 101.0% of tinidazole, calculated on the dried basis. Meets the requirements for Identification, Melting range (125–128 °C), Loss on drying (not more than 0.5%), Residue on ignition (not more than 0.1%), Heavy metals (not more than 0.002%), and Related compounds.

TINZAPARIN

Source: Tinzaparin sodium—Tinzaparin is obtained by enzymatic depolymerization of unfractionated heparin from porcine intestinal mucosa using heparinase from *Flavobacterium heparinum*.

Molecular weight: Tinzaparin sodium—Average between 5500 and 7500 daltons.

USP requirements: Tinzaparin Sodium Injection—Not in *USP–NF*.

TIOCONAZOLE

Chemical name: 1H-Imidazole, 1-[2-[(2-chloro-3-thienyl)-methoxy]-2-(2,4-dichlorophenyl)ethyl]-.

Molecular formula: $C_{16}H_{13}Cl_3N_2OS$.

Molecular weight: 387.71.

Description: White to off-white crystalline solid.

Solubility: Moderately soluble in chloroform, in methanol, in ethanol, and in ethyl acetate; virtually insoluble in water.

USP requirements:
Tioconazole USP—Preserve in tight containers. Contains not less than 97.0% and not more than 103.0% of tioconazole. Meets the requirements for Identification, Water (not more than 0.5%), Residue on ignition (not more than 0.2%), Chloride (not more than 0.05%), Heavy metals (not more than 0.005%), and Related compounds (not more than 1.0% for each related compound).
Tioconazole Cream USP—Preserve in tight containers. Contains the labeled amount, within ±10%, in a suitable cream base. Meets the requirements for Identification, Microbial limits, Minimum fill, and pH (3.0–6.0, in a 1:1 aqueous suspension of the Cream).
Tioconazole Vaginal Ointment—Not in *USP–NF*.
Tioconazole Vaginal Suppositories—Not in *USP–NF*.

TIOPRONIN

Chemical name: N-(2-Mercaptopropionyl)glycine.

Molecular formula: $C_5H_9NO_3S$.

Molecular weight: 163.20.

Description: A white, crystalline powder with a characteristic sulphurous odor.

Solubility: Soluble in water.

Other characteristics: Chemically similar to penicillamine.

USP requirements: Tiopronin Tablets—Not in *USP–NF*.

TIROFIBAN

Chemical name: Tirofiban hydrochloride—L-Tyrosine, N-(butylsulfonyl)-O-[4-(4-piperidinyl)butyl]-, monohydrochloride, monohydrate.

Molecular formula: Tirofiban hydrochloride—$C_{22}H_{36}N_2O_5S \cdot HCl \cdot H_2O$.

Molecular weight: Tirofiban hydrochloride—495.07.

Description: Tirofiban hydrochloride—White to off-white, non-hygroscopic, free-flowing powder.

Solubility: Tirofiban hydrochloride—Very slightly soluble in water.

USP requirements: Tirofiban Hydrochloride Injection—Not in *USP–NF*.

TITANIUM DIOXIDE

Chemical name: Titanium oxide (TiO_2).

Molecular formula: TiO_2.

Molecular weight: 79.87.

Description: Titanium Dioxide USP—White, odorless powder. Its 1 in 10 suspension in water is neutral to litmus.
NF category: Coating agent.

Solubility: Titanium Dioxide USP—Insoluble in water, in hydrochloric acid, in nitric acid, and in 2 *N* sulfuric acid. Dissolves in hydrofluoric acid and in hot sulfuric acid. It is rendered soluble by fusion with potassium bisulfate or with alkali carbonates or hydroxides.

USP requirements:

Titanium Dioxide USP—Preserve in well-closed containers. If intended for UV-attenuation, the material must be labeled as attenuation grade. If intended for UV-attenuation, and any added coatings, stabilizers, or treatments are used, the labeling shall include the name and amount of the additives. If labeled as attenuation grade, then Titanium Dioxide contains not less than 99.0% and not more than 100.5% of titanium dioxide, calculated on the ignited basis. Attenuation grade material may contain suitable coatings, stabilizers, and treatments to assist formulation. Contains not less than 99.0% and not more than 100.5% of titanium dioxide, calculated on the dried basis. Meets the requirements for Identification, Loss on drying (not more than 0.5%), Loss on ignition (not more than 0.5%; if labeled as attenuation grade, not more than 13%), Water-soluble substances (not more than 0.25%), Acid-soluble substances (not more than 0.5%), Arsenic (not more than 1 ppm), and Organic volatile impurities.

Note: If labeled as attenuation grade, then all tests and assays are conducted on uncoated, untreated material. For UV attenuation grade, the test for Loss on drying does not apply. The U.S. Food and Drug Administration requires the content of lead to be not more than 10 ppm, that of antimony to be not more than 2 ppm, and that of mercury to be not more than 1 ppm.

Titanium Dioxide Lotion—Not in *USP–NF*.

TITANIUM DIOXIDE AND ZINC OXIDE

For *Titanium Dioxide* and *Zinc Oxide*—See individual listings for chemistry information.

USP requirements: Titanium Dioxide and Zinc Oxide Lotion—Not in *USP–NF*.

TIXOCORTOL

Chemical name: Pregn-4-ene-3,20-dione,21-[(2,2-dimethyl-1-oxopropyl)thio]-11,17-dihydroxy-, (11 beta)-.

Molecular formula: $C_{26}H_{38}O_5S$.

Molecular weight: 462.64.

Description: Crystals from ethanol. Melting point 195–200 °C.

USP requirements: Tixocortol Pivalate Enema—Not in *USP–NF*.

TIZANIDINE

Chemical name: Tizanidine hydrochloride—2,1,3-Benzothiadiazol-4-amine, 5-chloro-*N*-(4,5-dihydro-1*H*-imidazol-2-yl)-, monohydrochloride.

Molecular formula: Tizanidine hydrochloride—$C_9H_8ClN_5S \cdot HCl$.

Molecular weight: Tizanidine hydrochloride—290.17.

USP requirements: Tizanidine Hydrochloride Tablets—Not in *USP–NF*.

TOBRAMYCIN

Source: Derived from *Streptomyces tenebrarius*.

Chemical group: Aminoglycoside.

Chemical name:

Tobramycin—D-Streptamine, *O*-3-amino-3-deoxy-alpha-Dglucopyranosyl-(1→6)-*O*-[2,6-diamino-2,3,6-trideoxy-alpha-D-*ribo*-hexopyranosyl-(1→4)]-2-deoxy-.

Tobramycin sulfate—D-Streptamine, *O*-3-amino-3-deoxy-alpha-D-glucopyranosyl-(1→6)-*O*-[2,6-diamino-2,3,6-trideoxy-alpha-D-*ribo*-hexopyranosyl-(1→4)]-2-deoxy-, sulfate (2:5) (salt).

Molecular formula:

Tobramycin—$C_{18}H_{37}N_5O_9$.

Tobramycin sulfate—$(C_{18}H_{37}N_5O_9)_2 \cdot 5H_2SO_4$.

Molecular weight:

Tobramycin—467.51.

Tobramycin sulfate—1425.43.

Description:

Tobramycin USP—White to off-white, hygroscopic powder.

Tobramycin Sulfate Injection USP—Clear, colorless solution.

Solubility: Tobramycin USP—Freely soluble in water; very slightly soluble in alcohol; practically insoluble in chloroform and in ether.

USP requirements:

Tobramycin USP—Preserve in tight containers. Where it is intended for use in preparing injectable or ophthalmic dosage forms, the label states that it is sterile or must be subjected to further processing during the preparation of injectable or ophthalmic dosage forms. Has a potency of not less than 900 mcg of tobramycin per mg, calculated on the anhydrous basis. Meets the requirements for Identification, pH (9–11, in a solution [1 in 10]), Water (not more than 8.0%), Residue on ignition (not more than 1.0%), Heavy metals (not more than 0.003%), and Chromatographic purity (not more than 1.0%), for Sterility and Bacterial endotoxins under Tobramycin for Injection (where the label states that Tobramycin is sterile), and for Bacterial endotoxins under Tobramycin for Injection (where the label states that Tobramycin must be subjected to further processing during the preparation of injectable dosage forms). Where it is intended for use in preparing ophthalmic dosage forms, it is exempt from the requirements for Bacterial endotoxins.

Tobramycin for Inhalation—Not in *USP–NF*.

Tobramycin Injection USP—Preserve in single-dose or in multiple-dose glass or plastic containers. Glass containers are preferably of Type I glass. A sterile solution of Tobramycin Sulfate or of Tobramycin in Water for Injection prepared with the aid of Sulfuric Acid. Contains an amount of tobramycin sulfate equivalent to the labeled amount of tobramycin, within −10% to +20%. Meets the requirements for Identification, Bacterial endotoxins, Sterility, pH (3.0–6.5), and Particulate matter, and for Injections.

Tobramycin for Injection USP—Preserve in Containers for Sterile Solids. Contains an amount of tobramycin sulfate equivalent to the labeled amount of tobramycin within −10% to +15%. Meets the requirements for Constituted solution, Identification, Bacterial endotoxins, Sterility, pH (6.0–8.0, in a solution containing 40 mg per mL [or, where packaged for dispensing, in the solution constituted as di-

rected in the labeling]), Water (not more than 2.0%), and Particulate matter, for Residue on ignition and Heavy metals under Tobramycin, and for Uniformity of dosage units (where packaged for dispensing) and Labeling under Injections.

Tobramycin Ophthalmic Ointment USP—Preserve in collapsible ophthalmic ointment tubes. Contains the labeled amount, within −10% to +20%. Meets the requirements for Identification, Sterility, Minimum fill, Water (not more than 1.0%), and Metal particles.

Tobramycin Ophthalmic Solution USP—Preserve in tight containers, and avoid exposure to excessive heat. Contains the labeled amount, within −10% to +20%. Meets the requirements for Identification, Sterility, and pH (7.0–8.0).

Tobramycin Sulfate USP—Preserve in tight containers. Where it is intended for use in preparing injectable dosage forms, the label states that it is sterile or must be subjected to further processing during the preparation of injectable dosage forms. Has a potency of not less than 634 mcg and not more than 739 mcg of tobramycin per mg. Meets the requirements for Identification, pH (6.0–8.0, in a solution containing 40 mg per mL), and Water (not more than 2.0%), and for Residue on ignition, Heavy metals, and Chromatographic purity under Tobramycin, for Sterility tests and for Bacterial endotoxins under Tobramycin for Injection (where the label states that Tobramycin Sulfate is sterile), and for Bacterial endotoxins under Tobramycin for Injection (where the label states that Tobramycin Sulfate must be subjected to further processing during the preparation of injectable dosage forms).

TOBRAMYCIN AND DEXAMETHASONE

For *Tobramycin* and *Dexamethasone*—See individual listings for chemistry information.

USP requirements:

Tobramycin and Dexamethasone Ophthalmic Ointment USP—Preserve in collapsible ophthalmic ointment tubes. Contains the labeled amount of tobramycin, within −10% to +20%, and the labeled amount of dexamethasone, within ±10%. Meets the requirements for Identification, Sterility, Minimum fill, Water (not more than 1.0%), and Metal particles.

Tobramycin and Dexamethasone Ophthalmic Suspension USP—Preserve in tight containers. A sterile aqueous suspension containing Tobramycin and Dexamethasone. Contains the labeled amount of tobramycin, within −10% to +20%, and the labeled amount of dexamethasone, within ±10%. Meets the requirements for Identification, Sterility, and pH (5.0–6.0).

TOBRAMYCIN AND FLUOROMETHOLONE

For *Tobramycin* and *Fluorometholone*—See individual listings for chemistry information.

USP requirements: Tobramycin and Fluorometholone Acetate Ophthalmic Suspension USP—Preserve in tight containers. A sterile aqueous suspension of Tobramycin and Fluorometholone Acetate. Contains the labeled amount of tobramycin, within −10% to +20%, and the labeled amount of fluorometholone acetate, within −10% to +15%. Meets the requirements for Identification, Sterility, and pH (6.0–7.0).

TOBRAMYCIN AND SODIUM CHLORIDE

For *Tobramycin* and *Sodium Chloride*—See individual listings for chemistry information.

USP requirements: Tobramycin Sulfate in Sodium Chloride Injection—Not in *USP–NF*.

TOCAINIDE

Chemical name: Tocainide hydrochloride—Propanamide, 2-amino-*N*-(2,6-dimethylphenyl)-, hydrochloride.

Molecular formula: Tocainide hydrochloride—$C_{11}H_{16}N_2O \cdot HCl$.

Molecular weight: Tocainide hydrochloride—228.72.

Description: Tocainide Hydrochloride USP—Fine, white, odorless powder.

pKa: Tocainide hydrochloride—7.7.

Solubility: Tocainide Hydrochloride USP—Freely soluble in water and in alcohol; practically insoluble in chloroform and in ether.

USP requirements:

Tocainide Hydrochloride USP—Preserve in well-closed containers. Contains not less than 98.0% and not more than 101.0% of tocainide hydrochloride, calculated on the dried basis. Meets the requirements for Identification, Loss on drying (not more than 0.5%), Residue on ignition (not more than 0.1%), Heavy metals (not more than 0.002%), Chromatographic purity, and Organic volatile impurities.

Tocainide Hydrochloride Tablets USP—Preserve in well-closed containers. Contain the labeled amount, within ± 5%. Meet the requirements for Identification, Dissolution (80% in 30 minutes in water in Apparatus 2 at 50 rpm), and Uniformity of dosage units.

TOCOPHEROLS EXCIPIENT

Description: Tocopherols Excipient NF—Brownish red to red, clear, viscous oil, having a mild, characteristic odor. May show a slight separation of waxlike constituents in microcrystalline form. Oxidizes and darkens slowly in air and on exposure to light, particularly in alkaline media.

NF category: Antioxidant.

Solubility: Tocopherols Excipient NF—Insoluble in water; soluble in alcohol; miscible with acetone, with chloroform, with ether, and with vegetable oils.

NF requirements: Tocopherols Excipient NF—Preserve in tight containers, protected from light. Protect with a blanket of an inert gas. A vegetable oil solution. Label it to indicate the content, in mg per gram, of total tocopherols and of the sum of beta, gamma, and delta tocopherols. Contains not less than 50.0% of total tocopherols, of which not less than 80.0% consists of varying amounts of beta, gamma, and delta tocopherols. Meets the requirements for Identification, Acidity, and Organic volatile impurities.

TOLAZAMIDE

Chemical group: Sulfonylurea.

Chemical name: Benzenesulfonamide, *N*-[[(hexahydro-1*H*-azepin-1-yl)amino]carbonyl]-4-methyl-.

Molecular formula: $C_{14}H_{21}N_3O_3S$.

Molecular weight: 311.40.

Description: Tolazamide USP—White to off-white, crystalline powder, odorless or having a slight odor. Melts with decomposition in the approximate range of 161 to 173 °C.

pKa: 3.6 at 25 °C and 5.68 at 37.5 °C.

Solubility: Tolazamide USP—Very slightly soluble in water; freely soluble in chloroform; soluble in acetone; slightly soluble in alcohol.

USP requirements:
Tolazamide USP—Preserve in well-closed containers. Contains not less than 97.5% and not more than 102.5% of tolazamide, calculated on the dried basis. Meets the requirements for Identification, Loss on drying (not more than 0.5%), Residue on ignition (not more than 0.2%), Selenium (not more than 0.003%, a 200-mg specimen being used), Heavy metals (not more than 0.002%), Limit of *N*-aminohexamethyleneimine (not more than 0.005%), Chromatographic purity, and Organic volatile impurities, and Other impurities.
Tolazamide Tablets USP—Preserve in tight containers. Contain the labeled amount, within ±5%. Meet the requirements for Identification, Dissolution (70% in 30 minutes in 0.05 *M* Tris(hydroxymethyl)aminomethane, adjusted, if necessary, with hydrochloric acid to a pH of 7.6, in Apparatus 2 at 75 rpm), and Uniformity of dosage units.

TOLAZOLINE

Chemical group: Imidazoline derivative, structurally related to phentolamine.

Chemical name: Tolazoline hydrochloride—1*H*-Imidazole, 4,5-dihydro-2-(phenylmethyl)-, monohydrochloride.

Molecular formula: Tolazoline hydrochloride—$C_{10}H_{12}N_2 \cdot HCl$.

Molecular weight: Tolazoline hydrochloride—196.68.

Description: Tolazoline Hydrochloride USP—White to off-white, crystalline powder. Its solutions are slightly acid to litmus.

pKa: 10.5.

Solubility: Tolazoline Hydrochloride USP—Freely soluble in water and in alcohol.

USP requirements:
Tolazoline Hydrochloride USP—Preserve in well-closed containers. Contains not less than 98.0% and not more than 101.0% of tolazoline hydrochloride, calculated on the dried basis. Meets the requirements for Identification, Melting range (172.0–176.0 °C), Loss on drying (not more than 0.2%), Residue on ignition (not more than 0.1%), Heavy metals (not more than 0.001%), and Chromatographic purity.
Tolazoline Hydrochloride Injection USP—Preserve in single-dose or in multiple-dose containers, preferably of Type^I glass. A sterile solution of Tolazoline Hydrochloride in Water for Injection. Contains the labeled amount, within ±5%. Meets the requirements for Identification, Bacterial endotoxins, and pH (3.0–4.0), and for Injections.

TOLBUTAMIDE

Chemical group: Sulfonylurea.

Chemical name:
Tolbutamide—Benzenesulfonamide, *N*-[(butylamino)carbonyl]4-methyl-.

Tolbutamide sodium—Benzenesulfonamide, *N*-[(butylamino)carbonyl]-4-methyl-, monosodium salt.

Molecular formula:
Tolbutamide—$C_{12}H_{18}N_2O_3S$.
Tolbutamide sodium—$C_{12}H_{17}N_2NaO_3S$.

Molecular weight:
Tolbutamide—270.35.
Tolbutamide sodium—292.33.

Description:
Tolbutamide USP—White, or practically white, crystalline powder. Is practically odorless.
Tolbutamide for Injection USP—White to off-white, practically odorless, crystalline powder.

pKa: 5.3.

Solubility:
Tolbutamide USP—Practically insoluble in water; soluble in alcohol and in chloroform.
Tolbutamide for Injection USP—Freely soluble in water; soluble in alcohol and in chloroform; very slightly soluble in ether.

USP requirements:
Tolbutamide USP—Preserve in well-closed containers. Where it is intended for use in preparing injectable dosage forms, the label states that it is sterile or must be subjected to further processing during the preparation of injectable dosage forms. Contains not less than 97.0% and not more than 103.0% of tolbutamide, calculated on the dried basis. Meets the requirements for Identification, Melting range (126–130 °C), Loss on drying (not more than 0.5%), Selenium (not more than 0.003%, a 100-mg specimen, mixed with 100 mg of magnesium oxide, being used), Heavy metals (not more than 0.002%), Organic volatile impurities, and Limit of non-sulfonyl urea, and for Sterility tests and for Bacterial endotoxins under Tolbutamide for Injection (where the label states that Tolbutamide is sterile), and for Bacterial endotoxins under Tolbutamide for Injection (where the label states that Tolbutamide must be subjected for further processing during the preparation of injectable dosage forms).
Tolbutamide for Injection USP—Preserve in Containers for Sterile Solids. Prepared from Tolbutamide with the aid of Sodium Hydroxide. Contains an amount of tolbutamide sodium equivalent to the labeled amount of tolbutamide, within ±5%. Meets the requirements for Constituted solution, Identification, Bacterial endotoxins, pH (8.0–9.8, in a solution containing 50 mg per mL), and Loss on drying (not more than 1.0%), and for Sterility, Uniformity of dosage units, and Labeling under Injections.
Tolbutamide Tablets USP—Preserve in well-closed containers. Contain the labeled amount, within ±10%. Meet the requirements for Identification, Dissolution (70% in 30 minutes in phosphate buffer [pH 7.4] in Apparatus 2 at 75 rpm), and Uniformity of dosage units.

TOLCAPONE

Chemical name: Methanone, (3,4-dihydroxy-5-nitrophenyl)(4-methylphenyl)-.

Molecular formula: $C_{14}H_{11}NO_5$.

Molecular weight: 273.24.

Description: Yellow, odorless, nonhygroscopic, crystalline powder.

pKa: 4.3.

Solubility: Practically insoluble in water and in acidic aqueous medium; easily soluble in most organic solvents.

USP requirements: Tolcapone Tablets—Not in *USP–NF*.

TOLMETIN

Chemical group: Pyrroleacetic acid derivative.

Chemical name: Tolmetin sodium—1*H*-Pyrrole-2-acetic acid, 1-methyl-5-(4-methylbenzoyl)-, sodium salt, dihydrate.

Molecular formula: Tolmetin sodium—$C_{15}H_{14}NNaO_3 \cdot 2H_2O$.

Molecular weight: Tolmetin sodium—315.30.

Description: Tolmetin Sodium USP—Light yellow to light orange, crystalline powder.

pKa: 3.5.

Solubility: Tolmetin Sodium USP—Freely soluble in water and in methanol; slightly soluble in alcohol; very slightly soluble in chloroform.

USP requirements:

Tolmetin Sodium USP—Preserve in well-closed containers. Contains not less than 98.0% and not more than 102.0% of tolmetin sodium, calculated on the dried basis. Meets the requirements for Identification, Loss on drying (10.4–12.4%), Heavy metals (not more than 0.002%), Chromatographic purity, and Organic volatile impurities.

Tolmetin Sodium Capsules USP—Preserve in tight containers. Contain an amount of tolmetin sodium equivalent to the labeled amount of tolmetin, within ±7%. Meet the requirements for Identification, Dissolution (85% in 30 minutes in phosphate buffer [pH 4.5] in Apparatus 2 at 50 rpm), and Uniformity of dosage units.

Tolmetin Sodium Tablets USP—Preserve in well-closed containers. Contain an amount of tolmetin sodium equivalent to the labeled amount of tolmetin, within ±10%. Meet the requirements for Identification, Dissolution (75% in 30 minutes in phosphate buffer [pH 4.5] in Apparatus 2 at 50 rpm), and Uniformity of dosage units.

TOLNAFTATE

Chemical name: Carbamothioic acid, methyl(3-methylphenyl)-, *O*-2-naphthalenyl ester.

Molecular formula: $C_{19}H_{17}NOS$.

Molecular weight: 307.41.

Description: Tolnaftate USP—White to creamy white, fine powder, having a slight odor.

Solubility: Tolnaftate USP—Practically insoluble in water; freely soluble in acetone and in chloroform; sparingly soluble in ether; slightly soluble in alcohol.

USP requirements:

Tolnaftate USP—Preserve in tight containers. Contains not less than 98.0% and not more than 102.0% of tolnaftate, calculated on the dried basis. Meets the requirements for Identification, Melting range (110–113 °C), Loss on drying (not more than 0.5%), Residue on ignition (not more than 0.1%), and Heavy metals (not more than 0.002%).

Tolnaftate Topical Aerosol USP—Preserve in tight, pressurized containers. Store at controlled room temperature, and avoid exposure to excessive heat. A suspension of

powder in suitable propellants in a pressurized container. Contains the labeled amount, within ±10%. Meets the requirements for Identification and for Pressure test, Minimum fill, and Leakage test under Aerosols, Metered-dose inhalers, and Dry powder inhalers.

Tolnaftate Cream USP—Preserve in tight containers. Contains the labeled amount, within ±10%. Meets the requirements for Identification and Minimum fill.

Tolnaftate Gel USP—Preserve in tight containers. Contains the labeled amount, within ±10%. Meets the requirements for Identification and Minimum fill.

Tolnaftate Topical Powder USP—Preserve in tight containers. Contains the labeled amount, within ±10%. Meets the requirements for Identification and Minimum fill.

Tolnaftate Topical Solution USP—Preserve in tight containers. Contains the labeled amount, within −10% to +15%. Meets the requirement for Identification.

Tolnaftate Topical Aerosol Solution—Not in *USP–NF*.

TOLTERODINE

Chemical name: Tolterodine tartrate—(*R*)-N,N-diisopropyl-3-(2-hydroxy-5-methylphenyl)-3-phenylpropanamine L-hydrogen tartrate.

Molecular formula: Tolterodine tartrate—$C_{26}H_{37}NO_7$.

Molecular weight: Tolterodine tartrate—475.6.

Description: Tolterodine tartrate—White crystalline powder.

Solubility: Tolterodine tartrate—Soluble at 12 mg/mL in water at room temperature and in methanol; slightly soluble in ethanol; practically insoluble in toluene.

USP requirements: Tolterodine Tartrate Tablets—Not in *USP–NF*.

TOLU BALSAM

Description: Tolu Balsam USP—Brown or yellowish-brown, plastic solid, transparent in thin layers and brittle when old, dried, or exposed to cold temperatures. Has a pleasant, aromatic odor resembling that of vanilla.

NF category: Flavors and perfumes.

Solubility: Tolu Balsam USP—Practically insoluble in water and in solvent hexane; soluble in alcohol, in chloroform, and in ether, sometimes with a slight residue or turbidity.

USP requirements: Tolu Balsam USP—Preserve in tight containers, and avoid exposure to excessive heat. A balsam obtained from *Myroxylon balsamum* (Linné) Harms (Fam. Leguminosae). Meets the requirements for Rosin, rosin oil, and copaiba, Acid value (112–168), and Saponification value (154–220).

TOPIRAMATE

Chemical name: Beta-D-Fructopyranose, 2,3:4,5-bis-*O*-(1-methylethylidene)-, sulfamate.

Molecular formula: $C_{12}H_{21}NO_8S$.

Molecular weight: 339.36.

Description: White crystalline powder with a bitter taste.

Solubility: Soluble in alkaline solutions containing sodium hydroxide or sodium phosphate and having a pH of 9 to 10; freely soluble in acetone, in chloroform, in dimethylsulfoxide, and in ethanol; soluble in water 9.8 mg/mL.

USP requirements: Topiramate Tablets—Not in *USP–NF*.

TOPOTECAN

Source: Topotecan hydrochloride—Semisynthetic derivative of camptothecin.

Chemical name: Topotecan hydrochloride—1*H*-Pyrano[3′,4′:6,7]indolizino[1,2-*b*]quinoline-3,14(4*H*,12*H*)-dione, 10-[(dimethylamino)methyl]-4-ethyl-4,9-dihydroxy-, monohydrochloride, (*S*)-.

Molecular formula: Topotecan hydrochloride—$C_{23}H_{23}N_3O_5 \cdot HCl$.

Molecular weight: Topotecan hydrochloride—457.91.

Description: Topotecan hydrochloride—Melts with decomposition at 213–218 °C.

Solubility: Topotecan hydrochloride—Soluble in water.

USP requirements: Topotecan Hydrochloride for Injection—Not in *USP–NF*.

TOREMIFENE

Chemical name: Toremifene citrate—Ethanamine, 2-[4-(4-chloro-1,2-diphenyl-1-butenyl)phenoxy]-*N*,*N*-dimethyl-, (*Z*)-, 2-hydroxy-1,2,3-propanetricarboxylate (1:1).

Molecular formula: Toremifene citrate—$C_{26}H_{28}ClNO \cdot C_6H_8O_7$.

Molecular weight: Toremifene citrate—598.08.

pKa: Toremifene citrate—8.0.

Solubility: Toremifene citrate—Soluble in water 0.63 mg/mL at 0.37 °C and in 0.02N HCl 0.38 mg/mL at 37 °C.

USP requirements: Toremifene Citrate Tablets—Not in *USP–NF*.

TORSEMIDE

Chemical name: 3-Pyridinesulfonamide, *N*-[[(1-methylethyl)amino]carbonyl]-4-[(3-methylphenyl)amino]-.

Molecular formula: $C_{16}H_{20}N_4O_3S$.

Molecular weight: 348.42.

Description: Torsemide USP—White to off-white crystalline powder.

Solubility: Torsemide USP—Slightly soluble in 0.1 N sodium hydroxide, in 0.1 N hydrochloric acid, in alcohol, and in methanol; very slightly soluble in acetone and in chloroform; practically insoluble in water and in ethel.

pKa: 7.1.

USP requirements:
Torsemide USP—Preserve in well-closed containers. Contains not less than 98.0% and not more than 102.0% of torsemide, calculated on the anhydrous basis. Meets the requirements for Identification, Water (not more than 0.8%), Residue on ignition (not more than 0.1%), Heavy metals (0.001%), and Related compounds.

Torsemide Injection—Not in *USP–NF*.
Torsemide Tablets—Not in *USP–NF*.

TRAGACANTH

Description: Tragacanth NF—Odorless.
NF category: Suspending and/or viscosity-increasing agent.

NF requirements: Tragacanth NF—Preserve in well-closed containers. The dried gummy exudation from *Astragalus gummifer* Labillardiére, or other Asiatic species of *Astragalus* (Fam. Leguminosae). Meets the requirements for Botanic characteristics, Identification, Microbial limits, Lead (not more than 0.001%), Heavy metals (not more than 20 mcg per gram), Karaya gum, and Organic volatile impurities.

TRAMADOL

Chemical name: Tramadol hydrochloride—($\pm$)-*cis*-2-[(Dimethylamino)methyl]-1-(3-methoxyphenyl)cyclohexanol hydrochloride.

Molecular formula: Tramadol hydrochloride—$C_{16}H_{25}NO_2 \cdot HCl$.

Molecular weight: Tramadol hydrochloride—299.84.

Description: Tramadol hydrochloride—White, crystalline, odorless powder. Has a melting point of 180–181 °C.

pKa: Tramadol hydrochloride—9.41.

Solubility: Tramadol hydrochloride—Readily soluble in water and in ethanol.

USP requirements: Tramadol Hydrochloride Tablets—Not in *USP–NF*.

TRAMADOL AND ACETAMINOPHEN

For *Tramadol* and *Acetaminophen*—See individual listings for chemistry information.

USP requirements: Tramadol Hydrochloride and Acetaminophen Tablets—Not in *USP–NF*.

TRANDOLAPRIL

Chemical name: (2*S*,3a*R*,7a*S*)-1-[(*S*)-*N*-[(*S*)-1-Carboxy-3-phenylpropyl]alanyl]hexahydro-2-indolinecarboxylic acid, 1-ethyl ester.

Molecular formula: $C_{24}H_{34}N_2O_5$.

Molecular weight: 430.54.

Description: Colorless, crystalline substance with a melting point of 125 °C.

Solubility: Soluble (>100 mg/mL) in chloroform, in dichloromethane, and in methanol.

USP requirements: Trandolapril Tablets—Not in *USP–NF*.

TRANDOLAPRIL AND VERAPAMIL

For *Trandolapril* and *Verapamil*—See individual listings for chemistry information.

USP requirements: Trandolapril and Verapamil Hydrochloride Extended-release Tablets—Not in *USP–NF.*

TRANEXAMIC ACID

Chemical name: Cyclohexanecarboxylic acid, 4-(aminomethyl)-, *trans-*.

Molecular formula: $C_8H_{15}NO_2$.

Molecular weight: 157.21.

Description: White, odorless or almost odorless, crystalline powder.

Solubility: Freely soluble in water and in glacial acetic acid; practically insoluble in alcohol and in ether.

USP requirements:
Tranexamic Acid Injection—Not in *USP–NF.*
Tranexamic Acid Oral Solution—Not in *USP–NF.*
Tranexamic Acid Tablets—Not in *USP–NF.*

TRANYLCYPROMINE

Chemical group: Nonhydrazine derivative structurally similar to amphetamine, with the exception of a cyclopropyl rather than an isopropyl side chain.

Chemical name: Tranylcypromine sulfate—Cyclopropanamine, 2-phenyl-, *trans-*(±)-, sulfate (2:1).

Molecular formula: Tranylcypromine sulfate—$(C_9H_{11}N)_2 \cdot H_2SO_4$.

Molecular weight: Tranylcypromine sulfate—364.46.

Description: Tranylcypromine sulfate—White or almost white crystalline powder, odorless or having a faint odor of cinnamaldehyde.

Solubility: Tranylcypromine sulfate—Soluble 1 in 20 of water; very slightly soluble in alcohol and in ether; practically insoluble in chloroform.

USP requirements: Tranylcypromine Sulfate Tablets—Not in *USP–NF.*

TRASTUZUMAB

Chemical name: Recombinant DNA-derived humanized monoclonal antibody derived from a mammalian cell (Chinese Hamster Ovary) suspension culture in a nutrient medium containing gentamicin (although gentamicin does not appear in the final product).

Description: Sterile, white to pale yellow, preservative-free lyophilized powder.

Other characteristics: pH—Approximately 6 (after reconstitution). Binding affinity—High for the extracellular domain of the human epidermal growth factor receptor 2 [HER2] protein.

USP requirements: Trastuzumab for Injection—Not in *USP–NF.*

TRAVOPROST

Source: Synthetic prostaglandin $F_{2\ alpha}$ analog.

Chemical name: [1*R*-[1 alpha(*Z*),2 beta(1*E*,3*R**),3 alpha,5 alpha]]-7-[3,5-Dihydroxy-2-[3-hydroxy-4-[3-(trifluoromethyl)phenoxy]-1-butenyl]cyclopentyl]-5-heptenoic acid, 1-methylethyl ester.

Molecular formula: $C_{26}H_{35}F_3O_6$.

Molecular weight: 500.56.

Description: Clear, colorless to slightly yellow oil.

Solubility: Very soluble in acetonitrile, in methanol, in octanol, and in chloroform; practically insoluble in water.

Other characteristics: pH—6.0; Osmolality approximately 290 mOsmol per kilogram.

USP requirements:
Travoprost Ophthalmic Solution—Not in *USP-NF.*
Travoprost Ophthalmic Suspension—Not in *USP-NF.*

TRAZODONE

Chemical group: Triazolopyridine derivative.

Chemical name: Trazodone hydrochloride—1,2,4-Triazolo[4,3-*a*]pyridin-3(2*H*)-one, 2-[3-[4-(3-chlorophenyl)-1-piperazinyl]-propyl]-, monohydrochloride.

Molecular formula: Trazodone hydrochloride—$C_{19}H_{22}ClN_5O \cdot HCl$.

Molecular weight: Trazodone hydrochloride—408.32.

Description: Trazodone Hydrochloride USP—White to off-white crystalline powder. Melts between 231 and 234 °C when the melting point determination is carried out in an evacuated capillary tube; otherwise melts with decomposition over a broad range below 230 °C.

Solubility: Trazodone Hydrochloride USP—Sparingly soluble in chloroform and in water.

Other characteristics: Not chemically related to tricyclic, tetracyclic, or other known antidepressants.

USP requirements:
Trazodone Hydrochloride USP—Preserve in tight, light-resistant containers. Contains not less than 97.0% and not more than 102.0% of trazodone hydrochloride, calculated on the dried basis. Meets the requirements for Identification, Loss on drying (not more than 0.5%), Residue on ignition (not more than 0.2%), Chromatographic purity, and Ordinary impurities.
Trazodone Hydrochloride Tablets USP—Preserve in tight, light-resistant containers. Contain the labeled amount, within ±10%. Meet the requirements for Identification, Dissolution (80% in 60 minutes in 0.01 *N* hydrochloric acid in Apparatus 2 at 50 rpm), and Uniformity of dosage units.

TRENBOLONE ACETATE

Chemical name: Estra-4,9,11-trien-3-one, 17-(acetyloxy)-, (17 beta)-.

Molecular formula: $C_{20}H_{24}O_3$.

Molecular weight: 312.40.

USP requirements:
Trenbolone Acetate USP—Preserve in tight containers, and store in a refrigerator. Label it to indicate that it is for veterinary use only. Contains not less than 97.0% and not

more than 101.0% of trenbolone acetate. Meets the requirements for Identification, Absorbance, Specific rotation (+39° to +43°), Loss on drying (not more than 0.5%), Residue on ignition (not more than 0.1%), Limit of trenbolone acetate 17alpha-isomer, Chromatographic purity, and Organic volatile impurities.

TREPROSTINIL

Chemical name: Acitic acid, [[(1*R*,2*R*,3a*S*,9a*S*)-2,3,3a,4.9,9a-hexahydro-2-hydroxy-1-[(3*S*)-3-hydroxyoctyl]-1*H*-benz[*f*]inden-5-yl]oxyl]-.

Molecular formula: $C_{23}H_{34}O_5$.

Molecular weight: 390.62.

Other characteristics: pH: 6.0–7.2.

USP requirements: Treprostinil Sodium Injection—Not in *USP–NF*.

TRETINOIN

Chemical name: Retinoic acid.

Molecular formula: $C_{20}H_{28}O_2$.

Molecular weight: 300.44.

Description: Tretinoin USP—Yellow to light-orange, crystalline powder.

Solubility: Tretinoin USP—Insoluble in water; slightly soluble in alcohol and in chloroform.

USP requirements:
Tretinoin USP—Preserve in tight containers, preferably under an atmosphere of an inert gas, protected from light. Contains not less than 97.0% and not more than 103.0% of tretinoin, calculated on the dried basis. Meets the requirements for Identification, Loss on drying (not more than 0.5%), Residue on ignition (not more than 0.1%), Heavy metals (not more than 0.002%), and Limit of isotretinoin (not more than 5.0%).
Tretinoin Capsules—Not in *USP–NF*.
Tretinoin Cream USP—Preserve in collapsible tubes or in tight, light-resistant containers. Contains the labeled amount, within −10% to +20%. Meets the requirements for Identification and Minimum fill.
Tretinoin Emollient Cream—Not in *USP–NF*.
Tretinoin Gel USP—Preserve in tight containers, protected from light. Contains the labeled amount, within −10% to +30%. Meets the requirements for Identification and Minimum fill.
Tretinoin Gel (Aqueous)—Not in *USP–NF*.
Tretinoin Topical Solution USP—Preserve in tight, light-resistant containers. A solution of Tretinoin in a suitable nonaqueous, hydrophilic solvent. Contains the labeled amount (w/w), within −10% to +35%. Meets the requirements for Identification and Alcohol content (within ±10% of labeled amount).

TRIACETIN

Chemical name: 1,2,3-Propanetriol triacetate.

Molecular formula: $C_9H_{14}O_6$.

Molecular weight: 218.20.

Description: Triacetin USP—Colorless, somewhat oily liquid having a slight fatty odor.
NF category: Plasticizer.

Solubility: Triacetin USP—Soluble in water; slightly soluble in carbon disulfide. Miscible with alcohol, with ether, and with chloroform.

USP requirements: Triacetin USP—Preserve in tight containers. Contains not less than 97.0% and not more than 100.5% of triacetin, calculated on the anhydrous basis. Meets the requirements for Identification, Specific gravity (1.152–1.158), Refractive index (1.429–1.430), Acidity, and Water (not more than 0.2%).

TRIAMCINOLONE

Chemical name:
Triamcinolone—Pregna-1,4-diene-3,20-dione, 9-fluoro-11,16,17,21-tetrahydroxy-, (11 beta,16 alpha).
Triamcinolone acetonide—Pregna-1,4-diene-3,20-dione, 9-fluoro-11,21-dihydroxy-16,17-[(1-methylethylidene)bis(oxy)]-, (11 beta,16 alpha)-.
Triamcinolone diacetate—Pregna-1,4-diene-3,20-dione, 16,21-bis(acetyloxy)-9-fluoro-11,17-dihydroxy-, (11 beta,16 alpha)-.
Triamcinolone hexacetonide—Pregna-1,4-diene-3,20-dione, 21-(3,3-dimethyl-1-oxobutoxy)-9-fluoro-11-hydroxy-16,17[(1-methylethylidene)bis(oxy)]-, (11 beta,16 alpha)-.

Molecular formula:
Triamcinolone—$C_{21}H_{27}FO_6$.
Triamcinolone acetonide—$C_{24}H_{31}FO_6$.
Triamcinolone diacetate—$C_{25}H_{31}FO_8$.
Triamcinolone hexacetonide—$C_{30}H_{41}FO_7$.

Molecular weight:
Triamcinolone—394.43.
Triamcinolone acetonide—434.50.
Triamcinolone diacetate—478.51.
Triamcinolone hexacetonide—532.64.

Description:
Triamcinolone USP—White or practically white, odorless, crystalline powder.
Triamcinolone Acetonide USP—White to cream-colored, crystalline powder, having not more than a slight odor.
Triamcinolone Diacetate USP—Fine, white to off-white, crystalline powder, having not more than a slight odor.
Triamcinolone Hexacetonide USP—White to cream-colored powder.

Solubility:
Triamcinolone USP—Very slightly soluble in water, in chloroform, and in ether; slightly soluble in alcohol and in methanol.
Triamcinolone Acetonide USP—Practically insoluble in water; sparingly soluble in dehydrated alcohol, in chloroform, and in methanol.
Triamcinolone Diacetate USP—Practically insoluble in water; soluble in chloroform; sparingly soluble in alcohol and in methanol; slightly soluble in ether.
Triamcinolone Hexacetonide USP—Practically insoluble in water; soluble in chloroform; slightly soluble in methanol.

USP requirements:

Triamcinolone USP—Preserve in well-closed containers. Contains not less than 97.0% and not more than 102.0% of triamcinolone, calculated on the dried basis. Meets the requirements for Identification, Specific rotation (+65° to +72°), Loss on drying (not more than 2.0%), Residue on ignition (not more than 0.5%), Heavy metals (not more than 0.0025%), and Other impurities.

Triamcinolone Tablets USP—Preserve in well-closed containers. Contain the labeled amount, within ±10%. Meet the requirements for Identification, Dissolution (75% in 45 minutes in 0.01 *N* hydrochloric acid in Apparatus 1 at 100 rpm), and Uniformity of dosage units.

Triamcinolone Acetonide USP—Preserve in well-closed containers. Contains not less than 97.0% and not more than 102.0% of triamcinolone acetonide, calculated on the dried basis. Meets the requirements for Identification, Specific rotation (+118° to +130°), Loss on drying (not more than 1.5%), Heavy metals (not more than 0.0025%), Chromatographic purity, and Other impurities.

Triamcinolone Acetonide Inhalation Aerosol—Not in *USP–NF*.

Triamcinolone Acetonide Nasal Aerosol—Not in *USP–NF*.

Triamcinolone Acetonide Topical Aerosol USP—Preserve in pressurized containers, and avoid exposure to excessive heat. A solution of Triamcinolone Acetonide in a suitable propellant in a pressurized container. Contains the labeled amount, within –10% to +15%. Meets the requirements for Identification and Microbial limits, and for Pressure test, Minimum fill, and Leakage test under Aerosols, Metered-dose inhalers, and Dry powder inhalers.

Triamcinolone Acetonide Cream USP—Preserve in tight containers. It is Triamcinolone Acetonide in a suitable cream base. Contains the labeled amount, within –10% to +15%. Meets the requirements for Identification, Microbial limits, and Minimum fill.

Triamcinolone Acetonide Lotion USP—Preserve in tight containers. It is Triamcinolone Acetonide in a suitable lotion base. Contains the labeled amount, within ±10%. Meets the requirements for Identification, Microbial limits, and Minimum fill.

Triamcinolone Acetonide Ointment USP—Preserve in well-closed containers. It is Triamcinolone Acetonide in a suitable ointment base. Contains the labeled amount, within –10% to +15%. Meets the requirements for Identification, Microbial limits, and Minimum fill.

Triamcinolone Acetonide Dental Paste USP—Preserve in tight containers. It is Triamcinolone Acetonide in a suitable emollient paste. Contains the labeled amount, within –10% to +15%. Meets the requirements for Identification, Microbial limits, and Minimum fill.

Triamcinolone Acetonide Nasal Solution—Not in *USP–NF*.

Triamcinolone Acetonide Injectable Suspension USP—Preserve in single-dose or in multiple-dose containers, preferably of Type I glass, protected from light. A sterile suspension of Triamcinolone Acetonide in a suitable aqueous medium. Contains the labeled amount, within –10% to +15%. Meets the requirements for Identification, Bacterial endotoxins, and pH (5.0–7.5), and for Injections.

Triamcinolone Acetonide Nasal Suspension—Not in *USP–NF*.

Triamcinolone Diacetate USP—Preserve in well-closed containers. Contains not less than 97.0% and not more than 103.0% of triamcinolone diacetate, calculated on the dried basis. Meets the requirements for Identification, Specific rotation (+39° to +45°), Loss on drying (not more than 6.0%), Residue on ignition (not more than 0.5%), Water (not more than 6.0%), Heavy metals (not more than 0.0025%), and Other impurities.

Triamcinolone Diacetate Injectable Suspension USP—Preserve in single-dose or in multiple-dose containers, preferably of Type I glass. A sterile suspension of

Triamcinolone Diacetate in a suitable aqueous medium. Contains the labeled amount, within –10% to +15%. Meets the requirements for Identification, Bacterial endotoxins, Uniformity of dosage units, and pH (4.5–7.5), and for Injections.

Triamcinolone Diacetate Oral Solution USP—Preserve in tight, light-resistant containers. Contains a suitable preservative. Contains the labeled amount, within ±10%. Meets the requirement for Identification.

Triamcinolone Diacetate Syrup USP—Preserve in tight, light-resistant containers. Contains a suitable preservative. Contains the labeled amount, within ±10%. Meets the requirement for Identification.

Triamcinolone Hexacetonide USP—Preserve in well-closed containers. Contains not less than 97.0% and not more than 102.0% of triamcinolone hexacetonide, calculated on the dried basis. Meets the requirements for Identification, Specific rotation (+85° to +95°), Loss on drying (not more than 2.0%), Heavy metals (not more than 0.002%), and Limit of triamcinolone acetonide (not more than 1.0%).

Triamcinolone Hexacetonide Injectable Suspension USP—Preserve in single-dose or in multiple-dose containers, preferably of Type I glass. A sterile suspension of Triamcinolone Hexacetonide in a suitable aqueous medium. Contains the labeled amount, within –10% to +15%. Meets the requirements for Identification, Bacterial endotoxins, pH (4.0–8.0), and Limit of triamcinolone acetonide (not more than 1.0%), and for Injections.

TRIAMTERENE

Chemical name: 2,4,7-Pteridinetriamine, 6-phenyl-.

Molecular formula: $C_{12}H_{11}N_7$.

Molecular weight: 253.26.

Description: Triamterene USP—Yellow, odorless, crystalline powder.

pKa: 6.2.

Solubility: Triamterene USP—Practically insoluble in water, in chloroform, in ether, and in dilute alkali hydroxides; soluble in formic acid; sparingly soluble in methoxyethanol; very slightly soluble in acetic acid, in alcohol, and in dilute mineral acids.

USP requirements:

Triamterene USP—Preserve in tight, light-resistant containers. Contains not less than 98.0% and not more than 102.0% of triamterene, calculated on the dried basis. Meets the requirements for Identification, Loss on drying (not more than 1.0%), Ordinary impurities, Limit of 2,4,6-triamino-5-nitrosopyrimidine (not more than 0.1%), and Organic volatile impurities.

Triamterene Capsules USP—Preserve in tight, light-resistant containers. When more than one Dissolution test is given, the labeling states the Dissolution test used only if Test 1 is not used. Contain the labeled amount, within ±7%. Meet the requirements for Identification, Dissolution (for Test 1: 75% in 45 minutes in 0.1 *N* hydrochloric acid in Apparatus 1 at 100 rpm; for Test 2: 80% in 120 minutets in 1% w/v of polysorbate 20 in 0.1 N acetic acid in Apparatus 2 at 100 rpm), and Uniformity of dosage units.

Triamterene Tablets—Not in *USP–NF*.

TRIAMTERENE AND HYDROCHLOROTHIAZIDE

For *Triamterene* and *Hydrochlorothiazide*—See individual listings for chemistry information.

USP requirements:

Triamterene and Hydrochlorothiazide Capsules USP—Preserve in tight, light-resistant containers. Label the Capsules to indicate the Dissolution test with which the product complies. Contain the labeled amounts, within ± 10%. Meet the requirements for Identification, Dissolution (80% of each active ingredient in 120 minutes in 0.1 *M* acetic acid containing 1% polysorbate 20 in Apparatus 2 at 100 rpm for Test 1; 70% of triamterene and 80% of hydrochlorothiazide in 8 hours in 4.0% tetrasodium ethylenediaminetetraacetate, 2.0% polysorbate 40, 0.05% pancreatin in Apparatus 1 [use 10-mesh baskets] at 100 rpm for Test 2; and 75% of each active ingredient in 45 minutes in 0.1 *N* hydrochloric acid in Apparatus 1 at 100 rpm for Test 3), Uniformity of dosage units, and Related compounds (not more than 1.0%).

Note: The Capsules and Tablets dosage forms should not be considered bioequivalent. If patients are to be transferred from one dosage form to the other, retitration and appropriate changes in dosage may be necessary.

Triamterene and Hydrochlorothiazide Tablets USP—Preserve in tight, light-resistant containers. Contain the labeled amounts, within ±10%. Meet the requirements for Identification, Dissolution (80% of each active ingredient in 30 minutes in 0.1 *N* hydrochloric acid in Apparatus 2 at 75 rpm), Uniformity of dosage units, and Related compounds (not more than 1.0%).

Note: The Capsules and Tablets dosage forms should not be considered bioequivalent. If patients are to be transferred from one dosage form to the other, retitration and appropriate changes in dosage may be necessary.

TRIAZOLAM

Chemical name: 4*H*-[1,2,4]Triazolo[4,3-*a*][1,4]benzodiazepine, 8-chloro-6-(2-chlorophenyl)-1-methyl-.

Molecular formula: $C_{17}H_{12}Cl_2N_4$.

Molecular weight: 343.21.

Description: Triazolam USP—White to off-white, practically odorless, crystalline powder.

Solubility: Triazolam USP—Soluble in chloroform; slightly soluble in alcohol; practically insoluble in ether and in water.

USP requirements:

Triazolam USP—Preserve in well-closed containers. Contains not less than 97.0% and not more than 103.0% of triazolam, calculated on the dried basis. Meets the requirements for Identification, Loss on drying (not more than 0.5%), Residue on ignition (not more than 0.5%), Heavy metals (not more than 0.002%), Chromatographic purity, and Other impurities.

Caution: Exercise care to prevent inhaling particles of triazolam and to prevent its contacting any part of the body.

Triazolam Tablets USP—Preserve in tight, light-resistant containers. Contain the labeled amount, within ±10%. Meet the requirements for Identification, Dissolution (70% in 30 minutes in water in Apparatus 2 at 50 rpm), and Uniformity of dosage units.

TRIBUTYL CITRATE

Molecular formula: $C_{18}H_{32}O_7$.

Molecular weight: 360.45.

Description: Tributyl Citrate NF—Clear, practically colorless, oily liquid.

NF category: Plasticizer.

Solubility: Tributyl Citrate NF—Insoluble in water; freely soluble in alcohol, in isopropyl alcohol, in acetone, and in toluene.

NF requirements: Tributyl Citrate NF—Preserve in tight containers. Contains not less than 99.0% of tributyl citrate, calculated on the anhydrous basis. Meets the requirements for Identification, Specific gravity (1.037–1.045), Refractive index (1.443—1.445), Acidity, Water (not more than 0.2%), and Heavy metals (not more than 0.001%).

TRICHLORFON

Chemical name: Dimethyl(2,2,2-trichloro-1-hydroxyethyl)phosphonate.

Molecular formula: $C_4H_8Cl_3O_4P$.

Molecular weight: 257.44.

Description: Trichlorfon USP—White crystalline powder. Decomposed by alkali. Melts at about 78 °C with decomposition.

Solubility: Trichlorfon USP—Freely soluble in acetone, in alcohol, in chloroform, in ether, and in water; very soluble in methylene chloride; very slightly soluble in hexane and in pentane.

USP requirements: Trichlorfon USP—Preserve in well-closed containers at a temperature not exceeding 25 °C. Label it to indicate that it is for veterinary use only. Contains not less than 98.0% and not more than 100.5% of trichlorfon, calculated on the anhydrous basis. Meets the requirements for Completeness of solution, Color of solution, Identification, Acidity, Limit of free chloride, Water (not more than 0.3%), Heavy metals (not more than 0.001%), and Chromatographic purity.

TRICHLORMETHIAZIDE

Chemical name: 2*H*-1,2,4-Benzothiadiazine-7-sulfonamide, 6-chloro-3-(dichloromethyl)-3,4-dihydro-, 1,1-dioxide.

Molecular formula: $C_8H_8Cl_3N_3O_4S_2$.

Molecular weight: 380.66.

Description: Trichlormethiazide USP—White or practically white, crystalline powder. Is odorless, or has a slight characteristic odor. Melts at about 274 °C, with decomposition.

pKa: 8.6.

Solubility: Trichlormethiazide USP—Very slightly soluble in water, in ether, and in chloroform; freely soluble in acetone; soluble in methanol; sparingly soluble in alcohol.

USP requirements:

Trichlormethiazide USP—Preserve in well-closed containers. Dried at 105 °C for 3 hours, contains not less than 98.0% and not more than 102.0% of trichlormethiazide. Meets the requirements for Identification, Loss on drying (not more than 0.5%), Residue on ignition (not more than 0.1%), Selenium (not more than 0.003%), Heavy metals (not more than 0.002%), and Diazotizable substances (not more than 2.5%).

Trichlormethiazide Tablets USP—Preserve in tight containers. Contain the labeled amount, within ±10%. Meet the requirements for Identification, Dissolution (65% in 60 minutes in water in Apparatus 2 at 50 rpm), and Uniformity of dosage units.

TRICHLOROMONOFLUOROMETHANE

Chemical name: Methane, trichlorofluoro-.

Molecular formula: CCl_3F.

Molecular weight: 137.37.

Description: Trichloromonofluoromethane NF—Clear, colorless gas, having a faint, ethereal odor. Its vapor pressure at 25 °C is about 796 mm of mercury (1 psig).
NF category: Aerosol propellant.

NF requirements: Trichloromonofluoromethane NF—Preserve in tight cylinders, and avoid exposure to excessive heat. Meets the requirements for Identification, Boiling temperature (approximately 24 °C), Water (not more than 0.001%), High-boiling residues (not more than 0.01%), Chromatographic purity, and Inorganic chlorides.

TRICITRATES

For *Sodium Citrate, Potassium Citrate,* and *Citric Acid*—See individual listings for chemistry information.

USP requirements: Tricitrates Oral Solution USP—Preserve in tight containers. A solution of Sodium Citrate, Potassium Citrate, and Citric Acid in a suitable aqueous medium. Contains, in each 100 mL, not less than 2.23 grams and not more than 2.46 grams of sodium, equivalent to not less than 9.5 grams and not more than 10.5 grams of sodium citrate dihydrate; not less than 3.78 grams and not more than 4.18 grams of potassium, equivalent to not less than 10.45 grams and not more than 11.55 grams of potassium citrate monohydrate; not less than 12.20 grams and not more than 13.48 grams of citrate as sodium citrate and potassium citrate; and not less than 6.34 grams and not more than 7.02 grams of citric acid monohydrate. Meets the requirements for Identification and pH (4.9–5.4).
Note: The sodium and potassium ion contents of Tricitrates Oral Solution are each approximately 1 mEq per mL.

TRICLABENDAZOLE

Source: Related to the benzimidazole-2-carbamate anthelmintics.

Chemical name: 5-Chloro-6-(2,3-dichlorophenoxy)-2-(methylthio)benzimidazole.

Molecular formula: $C_{14}H_9Cl_3N_2OS$.

Molecular weight: 359.66.

Description: Crystal. Melting point 175–176 °C.

USP requirements: Triclabendazole Tablets—Not in *USP–NF*.

TRICLOSAN

Chemical name: Penol, 5-chloro-2-(2,4-dichlorophenoxy)-.

Molecular formula: $C_{12}H_7Cl_3O_2$.

Molecular weight: 289.55.

Description: Triclosan USP—Fine, whitish crystalline powder. Melts at about 57 °C.

Solubility: Triclosan USP—Practically insoluble in water; soluble in methanol, in alcohol, and in acetone; slightly soluble in hexane.

USP requirements: Triclosan USP—Preserve in tight, light-resistant containers. Contains not less than 97.0% and not more than 103.0% of triclosan, calculated on the anhydrous basis. Meets the requirements for Identification, Water (not more than 0.1%), Residue on ignition (not more than 0.1%), Heavy metals (not more than 0.002%), Related compounds (not more than 0.1% of any individual impurity, and not more than 0.5% of total impurities), Limit of monochlorophenols and 2,4-dichlorophenol, Limit of 1,3,7-trichlorodibenzo-*p*-dioxin, 2,8-dichlorodibenzo-*p*-dioxin, 2,8-dichlorodibenzofuran, and 2,4,8-trichlorodibenzofuran, and Limit of 2,3,7,8-tetrachlorodibenzo-*p*-dioxin and 2,3,7,8-tetrachlorodibenzofuran.

TRIENTINE

Chemical name: Trientine hydrochloride—1,2-Ethanediamine, *N,N*-bis(2-aminoethyl)-, dihydrochloride.

Molecular formula: Trientine hydrochloride—$C_6H_{18}N_4 \cdot 2HCl$.

Molecular weight: Trientine hydrochloride—219.16.

Description: Trientine Hydrochloride USP—White to pale yellow, crystalline powder. Melts at about 117 °C.

Solubility: Trientine Hydrochloride USP—Insoluble in chloroform and in ether; slightly soluble in alcohol; soluble in methanol; freely soluble in water.

USP requirements:
Trientine Hydrochloride USP—Preserve under an inert gas in tight, light-resistant containers, and store in a refrigerator. Contains not less than 97.0% and not more than 103.0% of trientine hydrochloride, calculated on the dried basis. Meets the requirements for Identification, pH (7.0–8.5, in a solution [1 in 100]), Loss on drying (not more than 2.0%), Residue on ignition (not more than 0.15%), Heavy metals (not more than 0.001%), Chromatographic purity, and Organic volatile impurities.
Trientine Hydrochloride Capsules USP—Preserve in tight containers, and store in a refrigerator. Contain the labeled amount, within ±10%. Meet the requirements for Identification, Dissolution (80% in 30 minutes in water in Apparatus 2 at 50 rpm), and Uniformity of dosage units.

TRIETHANOLAMINE

Chemical name: 2,2′,2″-Nitrilotrisethanol.

Molecular formula: $C_6H_{15}NO_3$.

Molecular weight: 149.19.

Description: Very hygroscopic, viscous liquid. Slight ammoniacal odor. Turns brown on exposure to air and light. Melting point 21.57 °C.

Solubility: Miscible with water, with methanol, and with acetone. Soluble at 25 °C in ether 1.6%, in carbon tetrachloride 0.4%, and in *n*-heptane <0.1%.

USP requirements: Triethanolamine Salicylate Cream—Not in *USP–NF*.

TRIETHYL CITRATE

Molecular formula: $C_{12}H_{20}O_7$.

Molecular weight: 276.28.

Description: Triethyl Citrate NF—Practically colorless, oily liquid. NF category: Plasticizer.

Solubility: Triethyl Citrate NF—Soluble in water; miscible with alcohol and with ether.

NF requirements: Triethyl Citrate NF—Preserve in tight containers. Contains not less than 99.0% and not more than 100.5% of triethyl citrate, calculated on the anhydrous basis. Meets the requirements for Specific gravity (1.135–1.139), Refractive index (1.439–1.441), Acidity, Heavy metals (not more than 0.001%), and Water (not more than 0.25%).

TRIFLUOPERAZINE

Chemical group: Phenothiazine derivative of piperazine.

Chemical name: Trifluoperazine hydrochloride—10*H*-Phenothiazine, 10-[3-(4-methyl-1-piperazinyl)propyl]-2-(trifluoromethyl)-, dihydrochloride.

Molecular formula: Trifluoperazine hydrochloride—$C_{21}H_{24}F_3N_3S \cdot 2HCl$.

Molecular weight: Trifluoperazine hydrochloride—480.42.

Description: Trifluoperazine Hydrochloride USP—White to pale yellow, crystalline powder. Is practically odorless. Melts at about 242 °C, with decomposition.

Solubility: Trifluoperazine Hydrochloride USP—Freely soluble in water; soluble in alcohol; sparingly soluble in chloroform; insoluble in ether.

USP requirements:
Trifluoperazine Oral Solution USP—Preserve in tight, light-resistant containers. Contains an amount of trifluoperazine hydrochloride equivalent to the labeled amount of trifluoperazine, within ±7%. Meets the requirements for Identification and pH (2.0–3.2).
Trifluoperazine Hydrochloride USP—Preserve in tight, light-resistant containers. Dried in vacuum at 60 °C for 4 hours, contains not less than 98.0% and not more than 101.0% of trifluoperazine hydrochloride. Meets the requirements for Identification, pH (1.7–2.6, in a solution [1 in 20]), Loss on drying (not more than 1.5%), Residue on ignition (not more than 0.1%), and Organic volatile impurities.
Trifluoperazine Hydrochloride Injection USP—Preserve in multiple-dose containers, preferably of Type I glass, protected from light. A sterile solution of Trifluoperazine Hydrochloride in Water for Injection. Contains an amount of trifluoperazine hydrochloride equivalent to the labeled amount of trifluoperazine, within ±10%. Meets the requirements for Identification, Bacterial endotoxins, and pH (4.0–5.0), and for Injections.
Trifluoperazine Hydrochloride Oral Solution—Not in *USP–NF*.
Trifluoperazine Hydrochloride Syrup USP—Preserve in tight, light-resistant containers. Contains an amount of trifluoperazine hydrochloride equivalent to the labeled amount of trifluoperazine, within ±7%. Meets the requirements for Identification and pH (2.0–3.2).
Trifluoperazine Hydrochloride Tablets USP—Preserve in well-closed, light-resistant containers. Contain an amount of trifluoperazine hydrochloride equivalent to the labeled

amount of trifluoperazine, within ±7%. Meet the requirements for Identification, Dissolution (75% in 30 minutes in 0.1 *N* hydrochloric acid in Apparatus 1 at 50 rpm), and Uniformity of dosage units.

TRIFLUPROMAZINE

Chemical group: Phenothiazine.

Chemical name:
Triflupromazine—10*H*-Phenothiazine-10-propanamine, *N,N*-dimethyl-2-(trifluoromethyl)-.
Triflupromazine hydrochloride—10*H*-Phenothiazine-10-propanamine, *N,N*-dimethyl-2-(trifluoromethyl)-, monohydrochloride.

Molecular formula:
Triflupromazine—$C_{18}H_{19}F_3N_2S$.
Triflupromazine hydrochloride—$C_{18}H_{19}F_3N_2S \cdot HCl$.

Molecular weight:
Triflupromazine—352.42.
Triflupromazine hydrochloride—388.89.

Description:
Triflupromazine USP—Viscous, light amber-colored, oily liquid, which crystallizes on prolonged standing into large, irregular crystals.
Triflupromazine Hydrochloride USP—White to pale tan, crystalline powder, having a slight characteristic odor. Melts between 170 and 178 °C.

Solubility:
Triflupromazine USP—Practically insoluble in water.
Triflupromazine Hydrochloride USP—Soluble in water, in alcohol, and in acetone; insoluble in ether.

USP requirements:
Triflupromazine USP—Preserve in tight, light-resistant containers. Contains not less than 97.0% and not more than 103.0% of triflupromazine. Meets the requirements for Identification, Residue on ignition (not more than 0.2%), Ordinary impurities, and Organic volatile impurities.
Triflupromazine Oral Suspension USP—Preserve in tight, light-resistant, glass containers. Contains an amount of triflupromazine equivalent to the labeled amount of triflupromazine hydrochloride, within ±10%. Meets the requirement for Identification.
Triflupromazine Hydrochloride USP—Preserve in well-closed, light-resistant glass containers. Contains not less than 97.0% and not more than 103.0% of triflupromazine hydrochloride, calculated on the dried basis. Meets the requirements for Identification, Loss on drying (not more than 0.5%), Residue on ignition (not more than 0.1%), Ordinary impurities, and Organic volatile impurities.
Triflupromazine Hydrochloride Injection USP—Preserve in single-dose or in multiple-dose containers, preferably of Type I glass, protected from light. A sterile solution of Triflupromazine Hydrochloride in Water for Injection. Contains the labeled amount, within −10% to +12%. Meets the requirements for Identification, Bacterial endotoxins, and pH (3.5–5.2), and for Injections.
Triflupromazine Hydrochloride Tablets USP—Preserve in well-closed, light-resistant containers. Contain the labeled amount, within ±10%. Meet the requirements for Identification, Dissolution (75% in 45 minutes in 0.01 *N* hydrochloric acid in Apparatus 1 at 100 rpm), and Uniformity of dosage units.

TRIFLURIDINE

Chemical group: Fluorinated pyrimidine nucleoside.

Chemical name: Thymidine, alpha,alpha,alpha-trifluoro-.

Molecular formula: $C_{10}H_{11}F_3N_2O_5$.

Molecular weight: 296.20.

Description: Trifluridine USP—Odorless, white powder appearing under the microscope as rodlike crystals; melts at 175 °C, with sublimation.

Solubility: Soluble in water and in alcohol.

USP requirements:
Trifluridine USP—Preserve in tight, light-resistant containers. Contains not less than 98.0% and not more than 102.0% of trifluridine, calculated on the dried basis. Meets the requirements for Identification, Loss on drying (not more than 1.0%), Specific rotation (+47° to +51°), and Related compounds.
Trifluridine Ophthalmic Solution—Not in *USP–NF*.

TRIHEXYPHENIDYL

Chemical group: Tertiary amine.

Chemical name: Trihexyphenidyl hydrochloride—1-Piperidinepropanol, alpha-cyclohexyl-alpha-phenyl-, hydrochloride.

Molecular formula: Trihexyphenidyl hydrochloride—$C_{20}H_{31}NO \cdot HCl$.

Molecular weight: Trihexyphenidyl hydrochloride—337.93.

Description: Trihexyphenidyl Hydrochloride USP—White or slightly off-white, crystalline powder, having not more than a very faint odor. Melts at about 250 °C.

Solubility: Trihexyphenidyl Hydrochloride USP—Slightly soluble in water; soluble in alcohol and in chloroform.

USP requirements:
Trihexyphenidyl Hydrochloride USP—Preserve in tight containers. Contains not less than 98.0% and not more than 102.0% of trihexyphenidyl hydrochloride, calculated on the dried basis. Meets the requirements for Identification, Loss on drying (not more than 0.5%), Residue on ignition (not more than 0.1%), Heavy metals (not more than 0.002%), Chloride content (10.3–10.7%, calculated on the dried basis), Chromatographic purity, and Organic volatile impurities.
Trihexyphenidyl Hydrochloride Extended-release Capsules USP—Preserve in tight containers. Contain the labeled amount, within ±10%. Meet the requirements for Identification, Drug release (20–50% in 3 hours, 40–70% in 6 hours, and not less than 70% in 12 hours in water in Apparatus 1 at 100 rpm), and Uniformity of dosage units.
Trihexyphenidyl Hydrochloride Elixir USP—Preserve in tight containers. Contains the labeled amount, within ±10%. Meets the requirements for Identification, pH (2.0–3.0), and Alcohol content (within ±10% of labeled amount).
Trihexyphenidyl Hydrochloride Oral Solution USP—Preserve in tight containers. Contains the labeled amount, within ± 10%. Meets the requirements for Identification, pH (2.0–3.0), and Alcohol content (within ±10% of labeled amount).
Trihexyphenidyl Hydrochloride Tablets USP—Preserve in tight containers. Contain the labeled amount, within ± 10%. Meet the requirements for Identification, Dissolution (75% in 45 minutes in acetate buffer [pH 4.5] in Apparatus 1 at 100 rpm), and Uniformity of dosage units.

TRIKATES

For *Potassium Acetate, Potassium Bicarbonate,* and *Potassium Citrate*—See individual listings for chemistry information.

USP requirements: Trikates Oral Solution USP—Preserve in tight, light-resistant containers. A solution of Potassium Acetate, Potassium Bicarbonate, and Potassium Citrate in Purified Water. Contains the labeled amount of potassium, within ±10%. Meets the requirement for Identification.

TRILOSTANE

Chemical name: Androst-2-ene-2-carbonitrile, 4,5-epoxy-3,17-dihydroxy-, (4 alpha,5 alpha,17 beta)-.

Molecular formula: $C_{20}H_{27}NO_3$.

Molecular weight: 329.43.

Description: White to nearly white crystalline powder.

Solubility: Practically insoluble in water.

USP requirements: Trilostane Capsules—Not in *USP–NF*.

TRIMEPRAZINE

Chemical group: Phenothiazine derivative.

Chemical name: Trimeprazine tartrate—10H-Phenothiazine-10-propanamine N,N,beta-trimethyl-, [R-(R*,R*)]-2,3-dihydroxy-butanedioate (2:1).

Molecular formula: Trimeprazine tartrate—$(C_{18}H_{22}N_2S)_2 \cdot C_4H_6O_6$.

Molecular weight: Trimeprazine tartrate—747.98.

Description: Trimeprazine Tartrate USP—White to off-white, odorless, crystalline powder.

Solubility: Trimeprazine Tartrate USP—Freely soluble in water and in chloroform; soluble in alcohol; very slightly soluble in ether.

USP requirements:
Trimeprazine Oral Solution USP—Preserve in tight, light-resistant containers. Contains an amount of trimeprazine tartrate equivalent to the labeled amount of trimeprazine, within ±10%. Meets the requirements for Identification, Alcohol content (4.5–6.5%), and Limit of trimeprazine sulfoxide (not more than 0.036 mg per mL).
Trimeprazine Tartrate USP—Preserve in tight, light-resistant containers. Contains not less than 98.0% and not more than 101.0% of trimeprazine tartrate, calculated on the dried basis. Meets the requirements for Identification, Loss on drying (not more than 0.5%), Residue on ignition (not more than 0.1%), Heavy metals (not more than 0.002%), and Ordinary impurities.
Trimeprazine Tartrate Extended-release Capsules—Not in *USP–NF*.
Trimeprazine Tartrate Syrup USP—Preserve in tight, light-resistant containers. Contains an amount of trimeprazine tartrate equivalent to the labeled amount of trimeprazine, within ±10%. Meets the requirements for Identification, Alcohol content (4.5–6.5%), and Limit of trimeprazine sulfoxide (not more than 0.036 mg per mL).
Trimeprazine Tartrate Tablets USP—Preserve in well-closed, light-resistant containers. Contain an amount of trimeprazine tartrate equivalent to the labeled amount of trimeprazine, within ±7%. Meet the requirements for Identification,

Dissolution (75% in 45 minutes in 0.01 *N* hydrochloric acid in Apparatus 1 at 100 rpm), and Uniformity of dosage units.

TRIMETHADIONE

Chemical group: Oxazolidinedione.

Chemical name: 2,4-Oxazolidinedione, 3,5,5-trimethyl-.

Molecular formula: $C_6H_9NO_3$.

Molecular weight: 143.14.

Description: Trimethadione USP—White, crystalline granules. Has a slight camphor-like odor.

Solubility: Trimethadione USP—Soluble in water; freely soluble in alcohol, in ether, and in chloroform.

USP requirements:
Trimethadione USP—Preserve in tight containers, preferably at controlled room temperature. Contains not less than 98.0% and not more than 102.0% of trimethadione, calculated on the dried basis. Meets the requirements for Identification, Melting range (45–47 °C), Loss on drying (not more than 0.5%), Residue on ignition (not more than 0.1%), Urethane (not more than 1 ppm), and Organic volatile impurities.
Trimethadione Capsules USP—Preserve in tight containers, preferably at controlled room temperature. Contain the labeled amount, within ±6%. Meet the requirements for Identification, Dissolution (80% in 30 minutes in water in Apparatus 1 at 100 rpm), and Uniformity of dosage units.
Trimethadione Oral Solution USP—Preserve in tight containers, preferably at controlled room temperature. An aqueous solution of trimethadione. Contains the labeled amount, within ±6%. Meets the requirements for Identification and pH (3.0–5.0).
Trimethadione Tablets USP—Preserve in tight containers, preferably at a temperature not exceeding 25 °C. Contain the labeled amount, within ±6%. Meet the requirements for Identification, Disintegration (30 minutes), and Uniformity of dosage units.

TRIMETHAPHAN

Chemical name: Trimethaphan camsylate—Thieno[1′,2′:1,2]thieno[3,4-*d*]imidazol-5-ium, decahydro-2-oxo-1,3-bis(phenylmethyl)-, salt with (+)-7,7-dimethyl-2-oxobicyclo[2.2.1]heptane-1-methanesulfonic acid (1:1).

Molecular formula: Trimethaphan camsylate—$C_{32}H_{40}N_2O_5S_2$.

Molecular weight: Trimethaphan camsylate—596.80.

Description: Trimethaphan Camsylate USP—White crystals or white, crystalline powder. Is odorless or has a slight odor. Its solution (1 in 10) is clear and practically colorless. Melts at about 232 °C, with decomposition.

Solubility: Trimethaphan Camsylate USP—Freely soluble in water, in alcohol, and in chloroform; insoluble in ether.

USP requirements:
Trimethaphan Camsylate USP—Preserve in tight containers, in a cold place. Contains not less than 99.0% and not more than 101.5% of trimethaphan camsylate, calculated on the dried basis. Meets the requirements for Identification, Specific rotation (+20° to +23°), Loss on drying (not more than 0.1%), Residue on ignition (not more than 0.1%), and Selenium (not more than 0.003%, a 100-mg specimen, mixed with 100 mg of magnesium oxide, being used).

Trimethaphan Camsylate Injection USP—Preserve in single-dose or in multiple-dose containers, preferably of Type I glass. Store in a refrigerator, but avoid freezing. A sterile solution of Trimethaphan Camsylate in Water for Injection. Label it to indicate that it is to be appropriately diluted prior to administration. Contains the labeled amount, within ± 7%. Meets the requirements for Identification, Bacterial endotoxins, pH (4.9–5.6), and Particulate matter, and for Injections.

TRIMETHOBENZAMIDE

Chemical group: Trimethobenzamide hydrochloride—Ethanolamine derivative.

Chemical name: Trimethobenzamide hydrochloride—Benzamide, *N*-[[4-[2-(dimethylamino)ethoxy]phenyl]methyl]-3,4,5trimethoxy-, monohydrochloride.

Molecular formula: Trimethobenzamide hydrochloride—$C_{21}H_{28}N_2O_5 \cdot HCl$.

Molecular weight: Trimethobenzamide hydrochloride—424.92.

Description: Trimethobenzamide Hydrochloride USP—White, crystalline powder having a slight phenolic odor.

Solubility: Trimethobenzamide Hydrochloride USP—Soluble in water and in warm alcohol; insoluble in ether.

USP requirements:
Trimethobenzamide Hydrochloride USP—Preserve in well-closed containers. Dried at 105 °C for 4 hours, contains not less than 98.5% and not more than 100.5% of trimethobenzamide hydrochloride. Meets the requirements for Identification, Melting range (186–190 °C), Loss on drying (not more than 0.5%), Residue on ignition (not more than 0.1%), and Heavy metals (not more than 0.002%).
Trimethobenzamide Hydrochloride Capsules USP—Preserve in well-closed containers. Contain the labeled amount, within ±10%. Meet the requirements for Identification, Dissolution (75% in 45 minutes in water in Apparatus 1 at 100 rpm), and Uniformity of dosage units.
Trimethobenzamide Hydrochloride Injection USP—Preserve in single-dose or in multiple-dose containers, preferably of Type I glass. A sterile solution of Trimethobenzamide Hydrochloride in Water for Injection. Contains the labeled amount, within ±5%. Meets the requirements for Identification, Bacterial endotoxins, and pH (4.5–5.5), and for Injections.
Trimethobenzamide Hydrochloride Suppositories—Not in *USP–NF*.

TRIMETHOPRIM

Chemical name:
Trimethoprim—2,4-Pyrimidinediamine, 5-[(3,4,5-trimethoxyphenyl)methyl]-.
Trimethoprim sulfate—2,4-Pyrimidinediamine, 5-[(3,4,5-trimethoxyphenyl)methyl]-, sulfate (2:1) (salt).

Molecular formula:
Trimethoprim—$C_{14}H_{18}N_4O_3$.
Trimethoprim sulfate—$(C_{14}H_{18}N_4O_3)_2 \cdot H_2SO_4$.

Molecular weight:
Trimethoprim—290.32.
Trimethoprim sulfate—678.72.

Description:
Trimethoprim USP—White to cream-colored, odorless crystals, or crystalline powder.

Trimethoprim Sulfate USP—White to off-white crystalline powder.

Solubility:

Trimethoprim USP—Very slightly soluble in water; soluble in benzyl alcohol; sparingly soluble in chloroform and in methanol; slightly soluble in alcohol and in acetone; practically insoluble in ether and in carbon tetrachloride.

Trimethoprim Sulfate USP—Soluble in water, in alcohol, in dilute mineral acids, and in fixed alkalies.

USP requirements:

Trimethoprim USP—Preserve in tight, light-resistant containers. Contains not less than 98.5% and not more than 101.0% of trimethoprim, calculated on the dried basis. Meets the requirements for Identification, Melting range (199–203 °C), Loss on drying (not more than 0.5%), Residue on ignition (not more than 0.1%), and Chromatographic purity.

Trimethoprim Tablets USP—Preserve in tight, light-resistant containers. Contain the labeled amount, within ±10%. Meet the requirements for Identification, Dissolution (75% in 45 minutes in 0.01 N hydrochloric acid in Apparatus 2 at 50 rpm), and Uniformity of dosage units.

Trimethoprim Sulfate USP—Preserve in well-closed containers. Contains not less than 98.5% and not more than 101.0% of trimethoprim sulfate, calculated on the anhydrous basis. Meets the requirements for Identification, Melting range (210–215 °C), pH (7.5–8.5, in a solution [0.5 mg per mL]), Water (not more than 3.0%), and Chromatographic purity.

TRIMETREXATE

Chemical group: A dihydrofolate reductase inhibitor with general properties similar to those of methotrexate.

Chemical name: Trimetrexate glucuronate—2,4-Quinazolinediamine, 5-methyl-6-[[(3,4,5-trimethoxyphenyl)amino]methyl]-, mono-D-glucuronate.

Molecular formula: Trimetrexate glucuronate—$C_{19}H_{23}N_5O_3 \cdot C_6H_{10}O_7$.

Molecular weight: Trimetrexate glucuronate—563.56.

Description:

Trimetrexate glucuronate—Tan-colored solid.

Trimetrexate glucuronate for injection—Pale greenish-yellow powder or cake.

pKa: 8.0 in 50% methanol/water.

Solubility: Trimetrexate glucuronate—Soluble in water.

USP requirements: Trimetrexate Glucuronate for Injection—Not in *USP–NF*.

TRIMIPRAMINE

Chemical group: Dibenzazepine.

Chemical name: Trimipramine maleate—5H-Dibenz[b,f]azepine5-propanamine, 10,11-dihydro-N,N,beta-trimethyl-, (Z)-2-butenedioate (1:1).

Molecular formula: Trimipramine maleate—$C_{20}H_{26}N_2 \cdot C_4H_4O_4$.

Molecular weight: Trimipramine maleate—410.51.

Description: Trimipramine maleate—Almost odorless, white or slightly cream-colored, crystalline substance, melting at 140–144 °C.

pka: Trimipramine maleate—7.72.

Solubility: Trimipramine maleate—Very slightly soluble in ether and in water; slightly soluble in ethyl alcohol and in acetone; freely soluble in chloroform and in methanol at 20 °C.

Other characteristics: Tertiary amine.

USP requirements:

Trimipramine Maleate Capsules—Not in *USP–NF*.

Trimipramine Maleate Tablets—Not in *USP–NF*.

TRIOXSALEN

Chemical name: 7H-Furo[3,2-g][1]benzopyran-7-one, 2,5,9-trimethyl-.

Molecular formula: $C_{14}H_{12}O_3$.

Molecular weight: 228.24.

Description: Trioxsalen USP—White to off-white or grayish, odorless, crystalline solid. Melts at about 230 °C.

Solubility: Trioxsalen USP—Practically insoluble in water; sparingly soluble in chloroform; slightly soluble in alcohol.

USP requirements:

Trioxsalen USP—Preserve in well-closed, light-resistant containers. Contains not less than 97.0% and not more than 103.0% of trioxsalen, calculated on the dried basis. Meets the requirements for Identification, Loss on drying (not more than 0.5%), Residue on ignition (not more than 0.5%), Related compounds, and Organic volatile impurities.

Caution: Avoid exposing the skin to Trioxsalen.

Trioxsalen Tablets USP—Preserve in well-closed, light-resistant containers. Contain the labeled amount, within ±7%. Meet the requirements for Identification, Dissolution (75% in 60 minutes in dilute simulated intestinal fluid [1 in 12 solution of simulated intestinal fluid TS and water] in Apparatus 2 at 100 rpm), and Uniformity of dosage units.

TRIPELENNAMINE

Chemical group: Ethylenediamine derivative.

Chemical name:

Tripelennamine citrate—1,2-Ethanediamine, N,N-dimethyl-N'-(phenylmethyl)-N'-2-pyridinyl-, 2-hydroxy-1,2,3-propanetricarboxylate (1:1).

Tripelennamine hydrochloride—1,2-Ethanediamine, N,N-dimethyl-N'-(phenylmethyl)-N'-2-pyridinyl-, monohydrochloride.

Molecular formula:

Tripelennamine citrate—$C_{16}H_{21}N_3 \cdot C_6H_8O_7$.

Tripelennamine hydrochloride—$C_{16}H_{21}N_3 \cdot HCl$.

Molecular weight:

Tripelennamine citrate—447.48.

Tripelennamine hydrochloride—291.82.

Description:

Tripelennamine Citrate USP—White, crystalline powder. Its solutions are acid to litmus. Melts at about 107 °C.

Tripelennamine Hydrochloride USP—White, crystalline powder. Slowly darkens on exposure to light. Its solutions are practically neutral to litmus.

pKa: 3.9 and 9.0.

Solubility:

Tripelennamine Citrate USP—Freely soluble in water and in alcohol; very slightly soluble in ether; practically insoluble in chloroform.

Tripelennamine Hydrochloride USP—Freely soluble in water, in alcohol, and in chloroform; slightly soluble in acetone; insoluble in ether and in ethyl acetate.

USP requirements:

Tripelennamine Citrate USP—Preserve in well-closed, light-resistant containers. Contains not less than 98.0% and not more than 100.5% of tripelennamine citrate, calculated on the dried basis. Meets the requirements for Identification, Loss on drying (not more than 0.5%), Residue on ignition (not more than 0.1%), Ordinary impurities, and Organic volatile impurities.

Tripelennamine Citrate Elixir USP—Preserve in tight, light-resistant containers. Contains, in each 100 mL, not less than 705 mg and not more than 795 mg of tripelennamine citrate. Meets the requirements for Identification and Alcohol content (11.0–13.0%).

Tripelennamine Hydrochloride USP—Preserve in well-closed, light-resistant containers. Contains not less than 98.0% and not more than 100.5% of tripelennamine hydrochloride, calculated on the dried basis. Meets the requirements for Identification, Melting range (188–192 °C), Loss on drying (not more than 1.0%), Residue on ignition (not more than 0.1%), Chromatographic purity, and Organic volatile impurities.

Tripelennamine Hydrochloride Injection USP—Preserve in tight, single-dose or multiple-dose Containers for Injections, as described for Injections. Store at a controlled room temperature, and protect from light. A sterile solution of Tripelennamine Hydrochloride in Water for Injection. Label it to indicate that it is for veterinary use only. Contains the labeled amount, within ±10%. Meets the requirements for Identification, Bacterial endotoxins, Sterility, pH (6.0–7.0), and Particulate matter, and for Injections.

Tripelennamine Hydrochloride Tablets USP—Preserve in well-closed containers. Contain the labeled amount, within ±5%. Meet the requirements for Identification, Dissolution (75% in 45 minutes in water in Apparatus 1 at 100 rpm), and Uniformity of dosage units.

Tripelennamine Hydrochloride Extended-release Tablets—Not in *USP–NF*.

TRIPROLIDINE

Chemical group: Propylamine derivative (alkylamine).

Chemical name: Triprolidine hydrochloride—Pyridine, 2-[1-(4-methylphenyl)-3-(1-pyrrolidinyl)-1-propenyl]-, monohydrochloride, monohydrate, (*E*)-.

Molecular formula: Triprolidine hydrochloride—$C_{19}H_{22}N_2 \cdot HCl \cdot H_2O$.

Molecular weight: Triprolidine hydrochloride—332.87.

Description: Triprolidine Hydrochloride USP—White, crystalline powder, having no more than a slight, unpleasant odor. Its solutions are alkaline to litmus, and it melts at about 115 °C.

pKa: Triprolidine hydrochloride—3.6 and 9.3.

Solubility: Triprolidine Hydrochloride USP—Soluble in water, in alcohol, and in chloroform; insoluble in ether.

USP requirements:

Triprolidine Hydrochloride USP—Preserve in tight, light-resistant containers. Contains not less than 98.0% and not more than 101.0% of triprolidine hydrochloride, calculated on the anhydrous basis. Meets the requirements for Iden-

tification, Water (4.0–6.0%), Residue on ignition (not more than 0.1%), Heavy metals (not more than 0.002%), Chromatographic purity, and Organic volatile impurities.

Triprolidine Hydrochloride Oral Solution USP—Preserve in tight, light-resistant containers. Contains the labeled amount, within ±10%. Meets the requirements for Identificatio8, pH (5.6–6.6), and Alcohol content (3.0–5.0%).

Triprolidine Hydrochloride Syrup USP—Preserve in tight, light-resistant containers. Contains the labeled amount, within ±10%. Meets the requirements for Identification, pH (5.6–6.6), and Alcohol content (3.0–5.0%).

Triprolidine Hydrochloride Tablets USP—Preserve in tight, light-resistant containers. Contain the labeled amount, within ±10%. Meet the requirements for Identification, Dissolution (80% in 30 minutes in acetate buffer [pH 4.0 ± 0.05] in Apparatus 1 at 50 rpm), and Uniformity of dosage units.

TRIPROLIDINE AND PSEUDOEPHEDRINE

For *Triprolidine* and *Pseudoephedrine*—See individual listings for chemistry information.

USP requirements:

Triprolidine Hydrochloride and Pseudoephedrine Hydrochloride Capsules—Not in *USP–NF*.

Triprolidine and Pseudoephedrine Hydrochlorides Oral Solution USP—Preserve in tight, light-resistant containers. Contains the labeled amounts, within ±10%. Meets the requirement for Identification.

Triprolidine and Pseudoephedrine Hydrochlorides Syrup USP—Preserve in tight, light-resistant containers. Contains the labeled amounts, within ±10%. Meets the requirement for Identification.

Triprolidine and Pseudoephedrine Hydrochlorides Tablets USP—Preserve in tight, light-resistant containers. Contain the labeled amounts, within ±10%. Meet the requirements for Identification, Dissolution (75% of each active ingredient in 45 minutes in water in Apparatus 2 at 50 rpm), and Uniformity of dosage units.

TRIPROLIDINE, PSEUDOEPHEDRINE, AND ACETAMINOPHEN

For *Triprolidine, Pseudoephedrine,* and *Acetaminophen*—See individual listings for chemistry information.

USP requirements: Triprolidine Hydrochloride, Pseudoephedrine Hydrochloride, and Acetaminophen Tablets—Not in *USP–NF*.

TRIPROLIDINE, PSEUDOEPHEDRINE, AND CODEINE

For *Triprolidine, Pseudoephedrine,* and *Codeine*—See individual listings for chemistry information.

USP requirements:

Triprolidine Hydrochloride, Pseudoephedrine Hydrochloride, and Codeine Phosphate Oral Solution—Not in *USP–NF*.

Triprolidine Hydrochloride, Pseudoephedrine Hydrochloride, and Codeine Phosphate Syrup—Not in *USP–NF*.

Triprolidine Hydrochloride, Pseudoephedrine Hydrochloride, and Codeine Phosphate Tablets—Not in *USP–NF*.

TRIPROLIDINE, PSEUDOEPHEDRINE, CODEINE, AND GUAIFENESIN

For *Triprolidine, Pseudoephedrine, Codeine,* and *Guaifenesin*—
See individual listings for chemistry information.

USP requirements: Triprolidine Hydrochloride, Pseudoephedrine Hydrochloride, Codeine Phosphate, and Guaifenesin Oral Solution—Not in *USP–NF.*

TRIPROLIDINE, PSEUDOEPHEDRINE, AND DEXTRO-METHORPHAN

For *Triprolidine, Pseudoephedrine,* and *Dextromethorphan*—See
individual listings for chemistry information.

USP requirements:

Triprolidine Hydrochloride, Pseudoephedrine Hydrochloride,
and Dextromethorphan Hydrobromide Oral Solution—
Not in *USP–NF.*

Triprolidine Hydrochloride, Pseudoephedrine Hydrochloride,
and Dextromethorphan Hydrobromide Tablets—Not in
USP–NF.

TRIPTORELIN

Chemical name:

Triptorelin—Luteinizing hormone-releasing factor (pig), 6-D-
tryptophan.

Triptorelin pamoate—Luteinizing hormone-releasing factor
(swine), 6-D-tryptophan-, 4,4'-methylenebis[3-hydroxy-2-
naphthalenecarboxylate] (salt).

Molecular formula:

Triptorelin—$C_{64}H_{82}N_{18}O_{13}$.

Triptorelin pamoate—$C_{64}H_{82}N_{18}O_{13} \cdot C_{23}H_{16}O_6$.

Molecular weight:

Triptorelin—1311.45.

Triptorelin pamoate—1699.90.

USP requirements:

Triptorelin for Injection—Not in *USP–NF*

Triptorelin Pamoate for Injectable Suspension—Not in *USP–
NF.*

TRISODIUM CITRATE

Source: Trisodium citrate dihydrate—A tribasic salt of citric acid.

Molecular formula: Trisodium citrate dihydrate—$C_6H_5Na_3O_7 \cdot 2H_2O$.

Description: Trisodium citrate dihydrate—White, granular crystals or white, crystalline powder. An odorless substance with
a pleasant, salty taste.

Solubility: Trisodium citrate dihydrate—Slightly deliquescent in
moist air; freely soluble in water; partially insoluble in ethanol
(96%).

USP requirements: Trisodium Citrate Concentrate—Not in
USP–NF.

TRISULFAPYRIMIDINES

For *Sulfadiazine, Sulfamerazine,* and *Sulfamethazine*—See individual listings for chemistry information.

USP requirements:

Trisulfapyrimidines Oral Suspension USP—Preserve in tight
containers, at a temperature above freezing. Its label indicates the presence and proportion of any sodium citrate or
sodium lactate and any antimicrobial agent. Contains, in
each 100 mL, not less than 3.0 grams and not more than
3.7 grams of sulfadiazine, of sulfamerazine, and of sulfamethazine. May contain either Sodium Citrate or Sodium
Lactate, and may contain a suitable antimicrobial agent.
Meets the requirement for Identification.

Trisulfapyrimidines Tablets USP—Preserve in well-closed
containers. Contain the labeled amount of each of the sulfapyrimidines, consisting of equal amounts of sulfadiazine,
sulfamerazine, and sulfamethazine, within ±5%. Meet the
requirements for Identification, Dissolution (70% of labeled
amount of total sulfapyrimidines in 60 minutes in 0.01 *N*
hydrochloric acid in Apparatus 2 at 50 rpm), and Uniformity
of dosage units.

TROGLITAZONE

Chemical name: 2,4-Thiazolidinedione, 5-[[4-[(3,4-dihydro-6-hy-
droxy-2,5,7,8-tetramethyl-2*H*-1-benzopyran-2-yl)methoxy]-
phenyl]methyl]-.

Molecular formula: $C_{24}H_{27}NO_5S$.

Molecular weight: 441.54.

Description: White to yellowish crystalline compound; it may
have a faint, characteristic odor.

Solubility: Soluble in *N,N*-dimethylformamide or in acetone;
sparingly soluble in ethyl acetate; slightly soluble in acetonitrile, in anhydrous ethanol, or in ether; practically insoluble in
water.

USP requirements: Troglitazone Tablets—Not in *USP–NF.*

TROLAMINE

Chemical name: Ethanol, 2,2',2''-nitrilotris-.

Molecular formula: $C_6H_{15}NO_3$.

Molecular weight: 149.19.

Description: Trolamine NF—Colorless to pale yellow, viscous,
hygroscopic liquid, having a slight ammoniacal odor.

NF category: Alkalizing agent; emulsifying and/or solubilizing
agent.

Solubility: Trolamine NF—Miscible with water and with alcohol.
Soluble in chloroform.

NF requirements: Trolamine NF—Preserve in tight, light-resistant containers. A mixture of alkanolamines consisting largely
of triethanolamine containing some diethanolamine and
monoethanolamine. Contains not less than 99.0% and not
more than 107.4% of alkanolamines, calculated on the anhydrous basis as triethanolamine. Meets the requirements for
Identification, Specific gravity (1.120–1.128), Refractive index
(1.481–1.486 at 20 °C), Water (not more than 0.5%), Residue
on ignition (not more than 0.05%), and Organic volatile impurities.

TROLAMINE SALICYLATE

Chemical name: Triethanolamine salicylate.

Molecular formula: $C_{13}H_{21}NO_6$.

Molecular weight: 287.32.

USP requirements: Trolamine Salicylate USP—Preserve in tight containers in a cool place. A compounded mixture of Trolamine and Salicylic Acid in propylene glycol. Contains the labeled amount, within ±5%. Meets the requirements for Identification, Specific gravity (1.190–1.220), Refractive index (1.505–1.535 at 20 °C), pH (6.5–7.5, in a 50 mg per mL solution in water), Limit of free salicylic acid (not more than 0.02%), and Chromatographic purity (not more than 1.0% of any individual impurity, and not more than 2.0% of total impurities). Trolamine Salicylate Oil—Not in *USP–NF*.

TROLEANDOMYCIN

Chemical name: Oleandomycin, triacetate (ester).

Molecular formula: $C_{41}H_{67}NO_{15}$.

Molecular weight: 813.97.

Description: Troleandomycin USP—White, odorless, crystalline powder.

Solubility: Troleandomycin USP—Freely soluble in alcohol; soluble in chloroform; slightly soluble in ether and in water.

USP requirements:
Troleandomycin USP—Preserve in tight containers. Contains the equivalent of not less than 750 mcg of oleandomycin per mg. Meets the requirements for Identification, Crystallinity, pH (7.0–8.5, in a solution of alcohol and water [1:1] containing 100 mg per mL), Loss on drying (not more than 1.0%), Residue on ignition (not more than 0.1%), and Content of acetyl (15.3–16.0%).
Troleandomycin Capsules USP—Preserve in tight containers. Contain an amount of troleandomycin equivalent to the labeled amount of oleandomycin, within −10% to +20%. Meet the requirements for Identification and Loss on drying (not more than 5.0%).

TROMETHAMINE

Chemical name: 1,3-Propanediol, 2-amino-2-(hydroxymethyl)-.

Molecular formula: $C_4H_{11}NO_3$.

Molecular weight: 121.14.

Description: Tromethamine USP—White, crystalline powder, having a slight characteristic odor.

Solubility: Tromethamine USP—Freely soluble in water and in low molecular weight aliphatic alcohols; practically insoluble in chloroform and in carbon tetrachloride.

USP requirements:
Tromethamine USP—Preserve in tight containers. Contains not less than 99.0% and not more than 101.0% of tromethamine, calculated on the dried basis. Meets the requirements for Identification, Melting range (168–172 °C), pH (10.0–11.5, in a solution [1 in 20]), Loss on drying (not more than 1.0%), Residue on ignition (not more than 0.1%), Heavy metals (0.001%), and Organic volatile impurities.
Tromethamine for Injection USP—Preserve in Containers for Sterile Solids. A sterile, lyophilized mixture of tromethamine with Potassium Chloride and Sodium Chloride. Contains the labeled amount of tromethamine, within ±7%,

and the labeled amounts of potassium chloride and sodium chloride, within ±10%. Meets the requirements for Constituted solution, Identification, Bacterial endotoxins, pH (10.0–11.5, in a solution constituted as directed in the labeling), Water (not more than 1.0%), Particulate matter, Potassium chloride content, and Sodium chloride content, and for Sterility tests, Uniformity of dosage units, and Labeling under Injections.

TROPICAMIDE

Chemical name: Benzeneacetamide, *N*-ethyl-alpha-(hydroxymethyl)-*N*-(4-pyridinylmethyl)-.

Molecular formula: $C_{17}H_{20}N_2O_2$.

Molecular weight: 284.35.

Description: Tropicamide USP—White or practically white, crystalline powder, odorless or having not more than a slight odor.

Solubility: Tropicamide USP—Slightly soluble in water; freely soluble in chloroform and in solutions of strong acids.

USP requirements:
Tropicamide USP—Preserve in tight, light-resistant containers. Contains not less than 99.0% and not more than 101.0% of tropicamide, calculated on the dried basis. Meets the requirements for Identification, Melting range (96–100 °C), Loss on drying (not more than 0.5%), and Heavy metals (not more than 0.002%).
Tropicamide Ophthalmic Solution USP—Preserve in tight containers, and avoid freezing. A sterile, aqueous solution of Tropicamide. Contains a suitable antimicrobial agent, and may contain suitable substances to increase its viscosity. Contains the labeled amount, within ±5%. Meets the requirements for Identification, Sterility, and pH (4.0–5.8).

TROVAFLOXACIN

Chemical name: Trovafloxacin mesylate—1,8-Naphthyridine-3-carboxylic acid, 7-(6-amino-3-azabicyclo[3.1.0]hex-3-yl)-1-(2,4-difluorophenyl)-6-fluoro-1,4-dihydro-4-oxo-(1 alpha,5 alpha,6 alpha)-, monomethanesulfonate.

Molecular formula: Trovafloxacin mesylate—$C_{20}H_{15}F_3N_4O_3 \cdot CH_4O_3S$.

Molecular weight: Trovafloxacin mesylate—512.46.

Description: Trovafloxacin mesylate—White to off-white powder.

USP requirements: Trovafloxacin Mesylate Tablets—Not in *USP–NF*.

CRYSTALLIZED TRYPSIN

Description:
Crystallized Trypsin USP—White to yellowish white, odorless, crystalline or amorphous powder.
Crystallized Trypsin for Inhalation Aerosol—White to yellowish white, crystalline or amorphous powder.

USP requirements:
Crystallized Trypsin USP—Preserve in tight containers, and avoid exposure to excessive heat. A proteolytic enzyme crystallized from an extract of the pancreas gland of the ox, *Bos taurus* Linné (Fam. Bovidae). When assayed as directed in *USP-NF*, contains not less than 2500 USP

Trypsin Units in each mg, calculated on the dried basis, and not less than 90.0% and not more than 110.0% of the labeled potency. Meets the requirements for Solubility test, Microbial limits, Loss on drying (not more than 5.0%), Residue on ignition (not more than 2.5%), and Limit of chymotrypsin (not more than approximately 5%).

Note: Determine the suitability of the substrates and check the adjustment of the spectrophotometer by performing the Assay using USP Crystallized Trypsin Reference Standard.

TRYPTOPHAN

Chemical name: L-Tryptophan.

Molecular formula: $C_{11}H_{12}N_2O_2$.

Molecular weight: 204.23.

Description: Tryptophan USP—White to slightly yellowish white crystals or crystalline powder.

Solubility: Tryptophan USP—Soluble in hot alcohol and in dilute hydrochloric acid.

USP requirements:
Tryptophan USP—Preserve in well-closed containers. Contains not less than 98.5% and not more than 101.5% of tryptophan, as L-tryptophan, calculated on the dried basis. Meets the requirements for Identification, Specific rotation (−29.4° to −32.8°), pH (5.5–7.0, in a solution [1 in 100]), Loss on drying (not more than 0.3%), Residue on ignition (not more than 0.1%), Chloride (not more than 0.05%), Sulfate (not more than 0.03%), Iron (not more than 0.003%), Heavy metals (not more than 0.0015%), and Organic volatile impurities.
L-Tryptophan Capsules—Not in *USP–NF.*
L-Tryptophan Tablets–Not in *USP–NF.*

TUBERCULIN

Description: Tuberculin USP—Old Tuberculin is a clear, brownish liquid and has a characteristic odor. Purified Protein Derivative (PPD) of Tuberculin is a very slightly opalescent, colorless solution. Old Tuberculin and PPD concentrates contain 50% of glycerin for use with various application devices. Old Tuberculin and PPD are also dried on the tines of multiple-puncture devices.

Solubility: Tuberculin USP—Old Tuberculin is readily miscible with water.

USP requirements: Tuberculin USP—Preserve at a temperature between 2 and 8 °C. Multiple-puncture devices may be stored at a temperature not exceeding 30 °C. A sterile solution derived from the concentrated, soluble products of growth of the tubercle bacillus (*Mycobacterium tuberculosis* or *Mycobacterium bovis*) prepared in a special medium. Provided either as Old Tuberculin, a culture filtrate adjusted to the standard potency based on the U.S. Standard Tuberculin, Old, by addition of glycerin and isotonic sodium chloride solution, or as Purified Protein Derivative (PPD), a further purified protein fraction standardized with the U.S. Standard Tuberculin, Purified Protein Derivative. Has a potency, tested by comparison with the corresponding U.S. Standard Tuberculin, on intradermal injection of sensitized guinea pigs, of between 80–120% of that stated on the label. Free from viable *Mycobacteria* as shown by injection into guinea pigs. Meets the requirement for Expiration date (for concentrated Old Tuberculin containing 50% of glycerin, not later than 5 years after date of issue from manufacturerã s cold storage [5 °C, 1 year; or 0 °C, 2 years];

for diluted Old Tuberculin, not later than 1 year after date of issue from manufacturer's cold storage [5 °C, 1 year; or 0 °C, 2 years]; for concentrated PPD containing 50% of glycerin, not later than 2 years after date of issue from manufacturer's cold storage [5 °C, 1 year]; for diluted PPD, not later than 1 year after date of issue by the manufacturer; for Old Tuberculin and PPD dried on multiple-puncture devices, not later than 2 years after date of issue from manufacturer's cold storage [30 °C, 1 year], provided the recommended storage is at a temperature not exceeding 30 °C). Conforms to the regulations of the U.S. Food and Drug Administration concerning biologics.

TUBOCURARINE

Chemical name: Tubocurarine chloride—Tubocuraranium, 7′,12′-dihydroxy-6,6′-dimethoxy-2,2′,2′-trimethyl-, chloride, hydrochloride, pentahydrate.

Molecular formula: Tubocurarine chloride—$C_{37}H_{41}ClN_2O_6 \cdot HCl \cdot 5H_2O$ (pentahydrate); $C_{37}H_{41}ClN_2O_6 \cdot HCl$ (anhydrous).

Molecular weight: Tubocurarine chloride—771.72 (pentahydrate); 681.65 (anhydrous).

Description: Tubocurarine Chloride USP—White or yellowish white to grayish white, crystalline powder. Melts at about 270 °C, with decomposition.

Solubility: Tubocurarine Chloride USP—Soluble in water; sparingly soluble in alcohol.

USP requirements:
Tubocurarine Chloride USP—Preserve in tight containers. Contains not less than 95.0% and not more than 105.0% of tubocurarine chloride, calculated on the anhydrous basis. Meets the requirements for Identification, Specific rotation (+210° to +224°), Water (not more than 12.0%), Residue on ignition (not more than 0.25%), Related compounds, and Chloride content (9.9–10.7%, calculated on the anhydrous basis).
Tubocurarine Chloride Injection USP—Preserve in single-dose or in multiple-dose containers. A sterile solution of Tubocurarine Chloride in Water for Injection. Contains the labeled amount, within ±7%. Meets the requirements for Identification, Angular rotation (+0.32° to +0.48° for each mg of tubocurarine chloride per mL claimed on the label), Bacterial endotoxins, and pH (2.5–5.0), and for Injections.

TYLOSIN

Chemical name: (10*E*,12*E*)-(3*R*,4*S*,5*S*,6*R*,8*R*,14*S*,15*R*)-14-[(6-deoxy-2,3-di-*O*-methyl-beta-D-allopyranosyl)oxymethyl]-5-[[3,6-dideoxy-4-*O*-(2,6-dideoxy-3-*C*-methyl-alpha-L-ribo-hexopyranosyl)-3-dimethylamino-beta-D-glucopyranosyl]- oxy]-6-formylmethyl-3-hydroxy-4,8,12-trimethyl-9-oxoheptadeca-10,12-dien-15-olide.

Molecular formula: $C_{46}H_{77}NO_{17}$.

Molecular weight: 916.1.

Description: Tylosin USP—White to buff-colored powder.

Solubility: Tylosin USP—Freely soluble in methanol; soluble in alcohol, in amyl acetate, in chloroform, and in dilute mineral acids; slightly soluble in water.

USP requirements:
Tylosin USP—Preserve in well-closed containers, protected from light, moisture, and excessive heat. The macrolide antibiotic substance, or the mixture of such substances,

produced by the growth of *Streptomyces fradiae*, or by any other means. Label it to indicate that it is for use in animals only. Potency is not less than 900 mcg of tylosin per mg, calculated on the dried basis. Meets the requirements for Identification, Loss on drying (not more than 5%), Residue on ignition (not more than 3.0%), Heavy metals (not more than 0.003%), Limit of tyramine, and Content of tylosins.

Tylosin Granulated USP—Preserve in well-closed, polyethylene-lined or polypropylene-lined containers, protected from moisture and excessive heat. Contains tylosin phosphate mixed with suitable carriers and inactive ingredients. Label it to indicate that it is for animal use only. Label it also to indicate that it is for manufacturing, processing, or repackaging. Contains the labeled amount, within ±20%. Meets the requirements for Identification, Loss on drying (not more than 12.0%), Powder fineness, and Content of tylosins.

TYLOXAPOL

Chemical name: Phenol, 4-(1,1,3,3-tetramethylbutyl)-, polymer with formaldehyde and oxirane.

Description: Tyloxapol USP—Viscous, amber liquid, having a slight, aromatic odor. May exhibit a slight turbidity.

NF category: Wetting and/or solubilizing agent.

Solubility: Tyloxapol USP—Slowly but freely miscible with water. Soluble in glacial acetic acid, in toluene, in carbon tetrachloride, in chloroform, and in carbon disulfide.

USP requirements: Tyloxapol USP—Preserve in tight containers. A nonionic liquid polymer of the alkyl aryl polyether alcohol type. Meets the requirements for Identification, Cloud point (92–97 °C), pH (4.0–7.0, in a solution [1 in 20]), Residue on ignition (not more than 1.0%), Free phenol, Limit of anionic detergents (not more than 0.075%), Absence of cationic detergents, Limit of formaldehyde (not more than 0.0075%), Limit of ethylene oxide (not more than 10 ppm), and Organic volatile impurities.

Note: Precautions should be exercised to prevent contact of Tyloxapol with metals.

TYPHOID VACCINE LIVE ORAL

Source: Typhoid vaccine Ty21a is a live attenuated vaccine for oral administration. The vaccine contains the attenuated strain *Salmonella typhi* Ty21a. The vaccine strain is grown under controlled conditions in a medium containing dextrose, galactose, a digest of bovine tissues, and an acid digest of casein. The bacteria are collected by centrifugation, mixed with a stabilizer containing lactose and amino acids, and then lyophilized. The lyophilized bacteria mixture is placed in gelatin capsules, which are coated with an organic solution to render them resistant to dissolution by stomach acids.

USP requirements: Typhoid Vaccine Live Oral Enteric-coated Capsules—Not in *USP–NF*.

TYPHOID VI POLYSACCHARIDE VACCINE

Source: Typhoid Vi polysaccharide vaccine is a sterile solution for intramuscular administration. The vaccine contains the cell surface Vi polysaccharide extracted from *Salmonella typhi* Ty2 strain. The vaccine strain is grown in a semisynthetic medium without animal proteins. The capsular polysaccharide

is precipitated from the concentrated culture supernatant by the addition of hexadecyltrimethylammonium bromide and purified by differential centrifugation and precipitation. The potency of the purified polysaccharide is assessed by molecular size and O-acetyl content.

USP requirements: Typhoid Vi Polysaccharide Vaccine—Not in *USP–NF*.

TYROPANOATE

Chemical group: Triiodinated benzoic acid derivative.

Chemical name: Tyropanoate sodium—Benzenepropanoic acid, alpha-ethyl-2,4,6-triiodo-3-[(1-oxobutyl)amino]-, monosodium salt.

Molecular formula: Tyropanoate sodium—$C_{15}H_{17}I_3NNaO_3$.

Molecular weight: Tyropanoate sodium—663.01.

Description: Tyropanoate Sodium USP—White, hygroscopic, odorless powder.

Solubility: Tyropanoate Sodium USP—Soluble in water, in alcohol, and in dimethylformamide; very slightly soluble in acetone and in ether.

USP requirements:

Tyropanoate Sodium USP—Preserve in tight, light-resistant containers. Contains not less than 98.0% and not more than 102.0% of tyropanoate sodium, calculated on the anhydrous basis. Meets the requirements for Identification, Water (not more than 3.0%), Iodine and iodide, and Heavy metals (not more than 0.003%).

Tyropanoate Sodium Capsules USP—Preserve in tight, light-resistant containers. Contain the labeled amount, within ± 6%. Meet the requirements for Identification, Iodine and iodide, and Uniformity of dosage units.

TYROSINE

Chemical name: L-Tyrosine.

Molecular formula: $C_9H_{11}NO_3$.

Molecular weight: 181.19.

Description: Tyrosine USP—White, odorless crystals or crystalline powder.

Solubility: Tyrosine USP—Very slightly soluble in water; insoluble in alcohol and in ether.

USP requirements: Tyrosine USP—Preserve in well-closed containers. Contains not less than 98.5% and not more than 101.5% of tyrosine, as L-tyrosine, calculated on the dried basis. Meets the requirements for Identification, Specific rotation (−9.8° to −11.2°), Loss on drying (not more than 0.3%), Residue on ignition (not more than 0.4%), Chloride (not more than 0.04%), Sulfate (not more than 0.04%), Iron (not more than 0.003%), Heavy metals (not more than 0.0015%), Chromatographic purity, and Organic volatile impurities.

TYROTHRICIN

USP requirements: Tyrothricin USP—Preserve in tight containers. An antibacterial substance produced by the growth of *Bacillus brevis* Dubos (Fam. *Bacteriaceae*). Consists principally of gramicidin and tyrocidine, the tyrocidine usually being present as the hydrochloride. Contains not less than 900 mcg and

not more than 1400 mcg of tyrothricin per mg. Meets the requirements for Identification and Loss on drying (not more than 5.0%).

UBIDECARENONE

Chemical name: 2,5-Cyclohexadiene-1,4-dione, 2-[(2*E*,6*E*,10*E*,-14*E*,18*E*,22*E*,26*E*,30*E*,34*E*)-3,7,11,15,19,23,27,31,35,39-decamethyl-2,6,10,14,18,22,26,30,34,38-tetracontadecaenyl]-5,6-dimethoxy-3-methyl.

Molecular formula: $C_{59}H_{90}O_4$.

Molecular weight: 863.37.

Description: Yellow to orange crystalline powder. Melts at about 48°.

Solubility: Soluble in ether; very slightly soluble in dehydrated alcohol; practically insoluble in water.

USP requirements:
Ubidecarenone NF—Preserve in well-closed, light-resistant containers. Contains not less than 98.0% and not more than 101.0% of ubidecarenone, calculated on the anhydrous basis. Meets the requirements for Identification, Water (not more than 0.2%), Residue on ignition (not more than 0.1%), Heavy metals (0.002%), and Chromatographic purity.
Ubidecarenone Capsules NF—Preserve in tight, light-resistant containers. Contain a labeled amount, within -10% to +15%. Meet the requirements for Identification, Disintigration and dissolution, and Weight variation.
Ubidecarenone Tablets NF—Preserve in tight, light-resistant containers. Contain the labeled amount, within -10% to +15%. Meet the requirements for Identification, Disintigration and dissolution, and Weight variation.

UNDECYLENIC ACID

Chemical name: 10-Undecenoic acid.

Molecular formula: $C_{11}H_{20}O_2$.

Molecular weight: 184.28.

Description: Undecylenic Acid USP—Clear, colorless to pale yellow liquid having a characteristic odor.

Solubility: Undecylenic Acid USP—Practically insoluble in water; miscible with alcohol, with chloroform, with ether, and with fixed and volatile oils.

USP requirements: Undecylenic Acid USP—Preserve in tight, light-resistant containers. Contains not less than 97.0% and not more than 100.5% of undecylenic acid. Meets the requirements for Identification, Specific gravity (0.910–0.913), Congealing range (not lower than 21 °C), Refractive index (1.447–1.448), Residue on ignition (not more than 0.15%), Water-soluble acids, Heavy metals (not more than 0.001%), and Iodine value (131–138).

COMPOUND UNDECYLENIC ACID

USP requirements:
Compound Undecylenic Acid Cream—Not in *USP–NF*.
Compound Undecylenic Acid Topical Aerosol Foam—Not in *USP–NF*.

Compound Undecylenic Acid Ointment USP—Preserve in tight containers, and avoid prolonged exposure to temperatures exceeding 30 °C. Contains undecylenic acid, calcium undecylenate, copper undecylenate, or zinc undecylenate, individually or in combination, in a suitable ointment base. Contains the labeled amount of total undecylenic acid, within ±10%.
Compound Undecylenic Acid Topical Powder—Not in *USP–NF*.
Compound Undecylenic Acid Topical Aerosol Powder—Not in *USP–NF*.
Compound Undecylenic Acid Topical Solution—Not in *USP–NF*.

UNOPROSTONE

Chemical name:
Unoprostone—(+)-(*Z*)-7-[1*R*,2*R*,3*R*,5*S*]-3,5-Dihydroxy-2-(3-oxodecyl)cyclopentyl]-5-heptenoic acid.
Unoprostone isopropyl—(+)-(*Z*)-7-[1*R*,2*R*,3*R*,5*S*]-3,5-Dihydroxy-2-(3-oxodecyl)cyclopentyl]-5-heptenoate.

Molecular formula:
Unoprostone—$C_{22}H_{38}O_5$.
Unoprostone isopropyl—$C_{22}H_{44}O_5$.

Molecular weight:
Unoprostone—382.53.
Unoprostone isopropyl—424.62.

Description: Unoprostone isopropyl—Clear, colorless viscous liquid.

Solubility: Unoprostone isopropyl—Very soluble in acetonitrile, in ethanol, in ethyl acetate, in isopropanol, in dioxane, in ether, and in hexane; practically insoluble in water.

Other characteristcs: Unoprostone isopropyl—pH 5.0–6.5. Osmolality 235–300 mOsmo/kg.

USP requirements: Unoprostone Isopropyl Ophthalmic Solution—Not in *USP–NF*.

URACIL MUSTARD

Chemical name: 2,4(1*H*,3*H*)-Pyrimidinedione, 5-[bis(2-chloroethyl)amino]-.

Molecular formula: $C_8H_{11}Cl_2N_3O_2$.

Molecular weight: 252.10.

Description: Off-white, odorless, crystalline powder. Melts at about 200 °C, with decomposition.

Solubility: Very slightly soluble in water; slightly soluble in acetone and in alcohol; practically insoluble in chloroform.

USP requirements: Uracil Mustard Capsules—Not in *USP–NF*.

UREA

Chemical name: Urea.

Molecular formula: CH_4N_2O.

Molecular weight: 60.06.

Description:
Urea USP—Colorless to white, prismatic crystals, or white, crystalline powder, or small white pellets. Is practically odorless, but may gradually develop a slight odor of ammonia upon long standing. Its solutions are neutral to litmus.

Solubility: Urea USP—Freely soluble in water and in boiling alcohol; practically insoluble in chloroform and in ether.

USP requirements:
Urea USP—Preserve in well-closed containers. Where it is intended for use in preparing injectable dosage forms, the label states that it is sterile or must be subjected to further processing during the preparation of injectable dosage forms. Contains not less than 99.0% and not more than 100.5% of urea. Meets the requirements for Identification, Melting range (132–135 °C), Residue on ignition (not more than 0.1%), Alcohol-insoluble matter (not more than 0.04%), Chloride (not more than 0.007%), Sulfate (not more than 0.010%), and Heavy metals (not more than 0.002%), and for Sterility tests and for Bacterial endotoxins under Urea for Injection (where the label states that Urea is sterile), and for Bacterial endotoxins under Urea for Injection (where the label states that Urea must be subjected for further processing during the preparation of injectable dosage forms).
Urea for Injection USP—Preserve in Containers for Sterile Solids. It is Urea suitable for parenteral use. Meets the requirements for Completeness of solution, Constituted solution, and Bacterial endotoxins, and for Identification tests, Melting range, Residue on ignition, Alcohol-insoluble matter, Chloride, Sulfate, Heavy metals, and for Sterility tests, Uniformity of dosage units, and Labeling under Injections.

UROFOLLITROPIN

Source: A preparation of purified extract of human postmenopausal urine containing follicle-stimulating hormone (FSH).

Chemical name: Urofollitropin.

Description: Urofollitropin for injection—White to off-white powder or pellets.

USP requirements: Urofollitropin for Injection—Not in *USP–NF*.

UROKINASE

Source: An enzyme obtained from human kidney cells by tissue culture techniques.

Chemical name: Kinase (enzyme-activating), uro-.

Molecular weight: 34,000 daltons.

Solubility: Soluble in water.

USP requirements: Urokinase for Injection—Not in *USP–NF*.

URSODIOL

Source: Ursodeoxycholic acid, a naturally occurring human bile acid found in small quantities in normal human bile and in larger quantities in the biles of certain species of bears.

Chemical name: Cholan-24-oic acid, 3,7-dihydroxy-, (3 alpha,5 beta,7 beta)-.

Molecular formula: $C_{24}H_{40}O_4$.

Molecular weight: 392.57.

Description: Ursodiol USP—White or almost white, crystalline powder.

Solubility: Ursodiol USP—Practically insoluble in water; freely soluble in alcohol and in glacial acetic acid; sparingly soluble in chloroform; slightly soluble in ether.

USP requirements:
Ursodiol USP—Preserve in tight containers. Contains not less than 98.5% and not more than 101.5% of ursodiol, calculated on the dried basis. Meets the requirements for Identification, Melting range (200–205 °C), Specific rotation (57° to 62°), Loss on drying (not more than 0.5%), Residue on ignition (not more than 0.1%), Heavy metals (not more than 0.001%), and Related compounds.
Ursodiol Capsules USP—Preserve in well-closed containers. Contain the labeled amount, within ±10%. Meet the requirements for Identification, Dissolution (80% in 30 minutes in 0.2 M phosphate buffer [pH 8.4] in Apparatus 2 at 75 rpm), and Uniformity of dosage units.
Ursodiol Tablets USP—Preserve in well-closed containers, and store at temperature between 20° and 25°. Contain the labeled amount, within ±10%. Meet the requirements for Identification, Dissolution (80% in 45 minutes in simulated intenstinal fluid TS, prepared without pancreatin and adjusted with 0.1 N sodium hydroxide or 0.1 N hydrochloric acid to a pH of 8.0 in Apparatus 2 at 75 rpm), Uniformity of dosage units, and Related compounds.

VACCINIA IMMUNE GLOBULIN

Description: Vaccinia Immune Globulin USP—Transparent or slightly opalescent liquid. Practically colorless and practically odorless. May develop a slight granular deposit during storage.

USP requirements: Vaccinia Immune Globulin USP—Preserve at a temperature between 2 and 8 °C. A sterile, non-pyrogenic solution of globulins derived from the blood plasma of adult human donors who have been immunized with vaccinia virus (Smallpox Vaccine). It is standardized for viral neutralizing activity in eggs or tissue culture with the U.S. Reference Vaccinia Immune Globulin and a specified vaccinia virus. Label it to state that it is not intended for intravenous injection. Contains not less than 15 grams and not more than 18 grams of protein per 100 mL, not less than 90.0% of which is gamma globulin. Contains 0.3 M glycine as a stabilizing agent, and contains a suitable antimicrobial agent. Meets the requirement for Expiration date (not later than 3 years after date of issue). Conforms to the regulations of the U.S. Food and Drug Administration concerning biologics.

VALACYCLOVIR

Chemical name: Valacyclovir hydrochloride—L-Valine, 2-[(2-amino-1,6-dihydro-6-oxo-9H-purin-9-yl)methoxy]ethyl ester, monohydrochloride.

Molecular formula: Valacyclovir hydrochloride—$C_{13}H_{20}N_6O_4 \cdot$ HCl.

Molecular weight: Valacyclovir hydrochloride—360.80.

Description: Valacyclovir hydrochloride—White to off-white powder.

pKa: Valacyclovir hydrochloride—1.90, 7.47, 9.43.

Solubility: Valacyclovir hydrochloride—Maximum solubility in water at 25 °C is 174 mg/mL.

USP requirements: Valacyclovir Hydrochloride Tablets—Not in *USP–NF*.

VALDECOXIB

Chemical name: 4-(5-Methyl-3-phenyl-4-isoxazolyl)benzenesulfonamide.

Molecular formula: $C_{16}H_{14}N_2O_3S$.

Molecular weight: 314.36.

Description: White crystalline powder.

Solubility: Relatively insoluble in water at 25 °C and pH 7.0; soluble in methanol and in ethanol; freely soluble in organic solvents and in alkaline (pH = 12) aqueous solutions.

USP requirements: Valdecoxib Tablets—Not in *USP–NF*.

VALERIAN

Description: Powdered Valerian Extract NF—Brown, hygroscopic, powdery or easily pulverizable mass.

Solubility: Powdered Valerian Extract NF—Soluble in water to form a slightly cloudy solution; sparingly soluble in 70% alcohol; practically insoluble in alcohol.

NF requirements:

Valerian NF—Store in tight containers, protected from light and moisture. Consists of the subterranean parts of *Valeriana officinalis* Linné (Fam. Valerianaceae) including the rhizome, roots, and stolons. The label states the Latin binomial name and, following the official name, the parts of the plant contained in the article. Contains not less than 0.5% of volatile oil and not less than 0.05% of valerenic acid, calculated on the dried basis. Meets the requirements for Botanic characteristics, Identification, Total ash (not more than 12.0%), Acid-insoluble ash (not more than 5.0%), Water content (not more than 12.0%), Extractable matter (not less than 20%), Volatile oil (not less than 0.5%), Pesticide residues, Foreign organic matter (not more than 2.0%), Microbial limits, and Content of valerenic acid (not less than 0.05%).

Valerian Tablets NF—Preserve in tight, light-resistant containers. Contain Powdered Valerian Extract. The label states the Latin binomial and, following the official name, the article from which the Tablets were prepared. The label also indicates the quantity, in mg, of Powdered Valerian Extract per Tablet and the content, in mg, of valerenic acid per 100 mg of Powdered Valerian Extract. Contain the labeled amount, within −10% to +20%, calculated as valerenic acid. Meet the requirements for Identification, Microbial limits, Disintigration andn dissolution, Weight variation, and Content of valerenic acid.

Powdered Valerian NF—Preserve in well-closed containers, protected from light and moisture. It is Valerian reduced to a fine or a very fine powder. The label states that the Latin binomial name and, following the official name, the parts of the plant source from which the article was de-

rived. Contains no calcium oxalate crystals and no foreign starch granules. Contains not less than 0.3% of volatile oil and not less than 0.04% of valerenic acid. Meets the requirements for Botanic characteristics, Water content (not more than 5.0%), and Heavy metals (not more than 0.005%), for Identification, Total ash, Acid-insoluble ash, Extractable matter, Pesticide residues, and Microbial limits under Valerian, and for Volatile oil (not less than 0.3%) and Content of valerenic acid (not less than 0.04%). Powdered Valerian Extract NF—Preserve in tight containers, store at controlled temperature, and protected from moisture and light. It is prepared from comminuted Valerian and with 70% alcohol or other suitable solvents. The ratio of the starting crude plant material to the Extract is between 4:1 and 7:1. The label states the official name of the article and states also the Latin binomial name and the part of the plant from which the article was prepared. Label it to indicate the content of valerenic acid, the extracting solvent used for preparation, and the ratio of the starting crude plant material to the Extract. Contains not less than 0.3% of valerenic acid. Meets the requirements for Identification, Microbial limits, Loss on drying (not more than 9.0%), Total ash (not more than 7.0%), Pesticide residues, Organic volatile impurities, Alcohol content (not more than 2.0%), and Content of valerenic acid (not more than 0.3%).

POWDERED VALERIAN EXTRACT

Description: Powdered Valerian Extract NF—Brown, hygroscopic, powdery or easily pulverizable mass.

Solubility: Powdered Valerian Extract NF—Soluble in water to form a slightly cloudy solution; sparingly soluble in 70% alcohol; practically insoluble in alcohol.

NF requirements: Powdered Valerian Extract NF—Preserve in tight containers, protected from moisture and light. It is prepared from comminuted Valerian and with 70% alcohol or other suitable solvents. The ratio of the starting crude plant material to the Extract is between 4:1 and 7:1. The label states the official name of the article and states also the Latin binomial name and the part of the plant from which the article was prepared. Label it to indicate the content of valerenic acid, the extracting solvent used for preparation, and the ratio of the starting crude plant material to the Extract. Contains not less than 0.3% of valerenic acid. Meets the requirements for Identification, Microbial limits, Loss on drying (not more than 9.0%), Total ash (not more than 7.0%), Pesticide residues, Organic volatile impurities, Alcohol content (not more than 2.0%), and Content of valerenic acid (not more than 0.3%).

VALGANCICLOVIR

Chemical name: Valganciclovir hydrochloride—L-Valine, easter with 9-[[2-hydroxy-1-(hydroxymethyl)ethoxy]methyl]guanine, monohydrochloride.

Molecular formula: Valganciclovir hydrochloride—$C_{14}H_{22}N_6O_5 \cdot$ HCL.

Molecular weight: Valganciclovir hydrochloride—390.82.

Description: Valganciclovir hydrochloride—White to off-white crystalline powder.

pKa: Valganciclovir hydrochloride—7.6.

Solubility: Valganciclovir hydrochloride—Soluble in 70 mg per mL water at 20 °C at an n-octano/water partition coefficient of 0.0095.

USP requirements: Valganciclovir Hydrochloride Tablets—Not in *USP–NF*.

VALINE

Chemical name:L-Valine.

Molecular formula: $C_5H_{11}NO_2$.

Molecular weight: 117.15.

Description: Valine USP—White, odorless crystals.

Solubility: Valine USP—Soluble in water; practically insoluble in ether, in alcohol, and in acetone.

USP requirements: Valine USP—Preserve in well-closed containers. Contains not less than 98.5% and not more than 101.5% of valine, as L-valine, calculated on the dried basis. Meets the requirements for Identification, Specific rotation (+26.6° to +28.8°), pH (5.5–7.0, in a solution [1 in 20]), Loss on drying (not more than 0.3%), Residue on ignition (not more than 0.1%), Chloride (not more than 0.05%), Sulfate (not more than 0.03%), Iron (not more than 0.003%), Heavy metals (not more than 0.0015%), Chromatographic purity, and Organic volatile impurities.

VALPROIC ACID

Chemical name:
Valproate sodium—Pentanoic acid, 2-propyl-, sodium salt.
Valproic acid—Pentanoic acid, 2-propyl-.

Molecular formula:
Valproate sodium—$C_8H_{15}NaO_2$.
Valproic acid—$C_8H_{16}O_2$.

Molecular weight:
Valproate sodium—166.20.
Valproic acid—144.21.

Description:
Valproate sodium—Essentially white and odorless, crystalline, deliquescent powder.
Valproic Acid USP—Colorless to pale yellow, slightly viscous, clear liquid, having a characteristic odor. Refractive index: about 1.423 at 20 °C.

pKa:
Valproate sodium—4.95.
Valproic acid—4.8.

Solubility:
Valproate sodium—Very soluble in water and in alcohol; practically insoluble in ether.
Valproic Acid USP—Slightly soluble in water; freely soluble in 1 *N* sodium hydroxide, in methanol, in alcohol, in acetone, in chloroform, in ether, and in *n*-heptane; slightly soluble in 0.1 *N* hydrochloric acid.

Other characteristics: Valproate sodium—pH adjusted to 7.6 with sodium hydroxide and/or hydrochloric acid.

USP requirements:
Valproate Sodium Injection—Not in *USP–NF*.
Valproic Acid USP—Preserve in tight, glass, stainless steel or polyethylene (HDPE) containers. Contains not less than 98.0% and not more than 102.0% of valproic acid, calculated on the anhydrous basis. Meets the requirements for Identification, Water (not more than 1.0%), Residue on ignition (not more than 0.1%), Heavy metals (not more than 0.002%), Chromatographic purity, and Organic volatile impurities.

Valproic Acid Capsules USP—Preserve in tight containers, at controlled room temperature. Contain the labeled amount, within ±10%. Meet the requirements for Identification, Disintegration (15 minutes, determined as directed for Soft Gelatin Capsules), Dissolution (85% in 60 minutes in a solution containing 5 mg per mL of sodium lauryl sulfate in simulated intestinal fluid TS [prepared without the enzyme and with monobasic sodium phosphate instead of monobasic potassium phosphate], adjusted with 5 *M* sodium hydroxide [pH 7.5] in Apparatus 2 at 50 rpm), and Uniformity of dosage units.

Valproic Acid Oral Solution USP—Preserve in tight containers. Contains the labeled amount, within ±10%. It is prepared with the aid of Sodium Hydroxide. Meets the requirements for Identification and pH (7.0–8.0).

Valproic Acid Syrup USP—Preserve in tight containers. Contains the labeled amount, within ±10%. It is prepared with the aid of Sodium Hydroxide. Meets the requirements for Identification and pH (7.0–8.0).

VALRUBICIN

Chemical name: (2*S-cis*)-2-[1,2,3,4,6,11-hexahydro-2,5,12-trihydroxy-7-methoxy-6,11-dioxo-4-[[2,3,6,-trideoxy-3-[(trifluoroacetyl)amino]-alpha-L-*lyxo*-hexopyranosyl]oxyl]-2-naphthacenyl]-2-oxoethyl pentanoate.

Molecular formula: $C_{34}H_{36}F_3NO_{13}$.

Molecular weight: 723.65.

Description: Valrubicin USP—Orange or orange-red, crystallined powder.

Solubility: Valrubicin USP—Soluble in methylene chloride in dehydrated alcohol, in methanol, and in acetone; very slightly soluble in water, in hexane, and in patroleum ether.

USP requirements:
Valrubicin USP—Preserve in tight, light-resistant containers at controlled room temperature. Contains not less than 95.0% and not more 103.0% of valrubicin, calculated on the dried basis. Meets the requirements for Identification, Loss on drying (not more than 3.0%), Residue on ignition (not more than 0.2%), Limit of residual solvents, and Related compounds.

Caution—Great care should be taken to prevent inhaling particles of Valrubicin and exposing the skin to it.

Valrubicin Intravesical Solution USP—Preserve in single-dose or multiple-dose containers, preferably of Type I glass. Store in a refrigerator. A sterile solution of Valrubicin in a suitable vehicle. Label it to indicate that it is not intended for intravenous or intramascular injection, but is to be used for intravesical instillation. Contains the labeled amount, within ±5%. Meets the requirements for Identification, Bacterial endotoxins, pH (4.0–7.0, in a solution of 0.9% sodium chloride [1 in 15], and Related compounds, and for Injection. Sterile Valrubicin Solution—Not in *USP–NF*.

VALSARTAN

Chemical name:L-Valine, *N*-(1-oxopentyl)-*N*-[[2′-(1*H*-tetrazol-5-yl)[1,1′-biphenyl]-4-yl]methyl]-.

Molecular formula: $C_{24}H_{29}N_5O_3$.

Molecular weight: 435.52.

Description: White to practically white fine powder. Practically odorless.

pKa: 4.73; 3.90.

Solubility: Soluble in ethanol and in methanol; slightly soluble in water.

USP requirements: Valsartan Capsules—Not in *USP–NF*.

VALSARTAN AND HYDROCHLOROTHIAZIDE

For *Valsartan* and *Hydrochlorothiazide*—See individual listings for chemistry information.

USP requirements: Valsartan and Hydrochlorothiazide Tablets—Not in *USP–NF*.

VANCOMYCIN

Source: Derived from *Amycolatopsis orientalis* (formerly *Nocardia orientalis*).

Chemical group: High-molecular-weight tricyclic glycopeptide.

Chemical name:
Vancomycin—Vancomycin.
Vancomycin hydrochoride—Vancomycin, monohydrochloride.

Molecular formula:
Vancomycin—$C_{66}H_{75}Cl_2N_9O_{24}$.
Vancomycin hydrochloride—$C_{66}H_{75}Cl_2N_9O_{24} \cdot HCl$.

Molecular weight:
Vancomycin—1449.25.
Vancomycin hydrochloride—1485.71.

Description:
Vancomycin Hydrochloride USP—Tan to brown, free-flowing powder, odorless.
Sterile Vancomycin Hydrochloride USP—Tan to brown, free-flowing powder, odorless.

Solubility:
Vancomycin Hydrochloride USP—Freely soluble in water; insoluble in ether and in chloroform.
Sterile Vancomycin Hydrochloride USP—Freely soluble in water; insoluble in ether and in chloroform.

USP requirements:
Vancomycin USP—Preserve in tight containers. Has a potency equivalent to not less than 950 mcg of vancomycin per mg, calculated on the anhydrous basis. Meets the requirements for Identification, Water (not more than 20%), Heavy metals (not more than 0.003%), and Chromatographic purity.
Vancomycin Injection USP—Preserve in Containers for Injections. Maintain in the frozen state. A sterile isoosmotic solution of Vancomycin Hydrochloride in Water for Injection. Contains a suitable tonicity-adjusting agent. It meets the requirements for Labeling under Injections. The label states that it is to be thawed just prior to use, describes conditions for proper storage of the resultant solution, and directs that the solution is not to be refrozen. Contains the labeled amount, within −10% to +15%. Meets the requirements for Identification, Bacterial endotoxins, Sterility, pH (3.0–5.0), Particulate matter, and Chromatographic purity, and for Injections.
Vancomycin Hydrochloride USP—Preserve in tight containers. The hydrochloride salt of a kind of vancomycin, a substance produced by the growth of *Streptomyces orientalis* (Fam. Streptomycetaceae), or a mixture of two or more such salts. Has a potency equivalent to not less than 900 mcg of vancomycin per mg, calculated on the anhy-

drous basis. Meets the requirements for Identification, pH (2.5–4.5, in a solution containing 50 mg per mL), Water (not more than 5.0%), and Chromatographic purity.
Vancomycin Hydrochloride Capsules USP—Preserve in tight containers. Contain an amount of vancomycin hydrochloride equivalent to the labeled amount of vancomycin, within −10% to +15%. Meet the requirements for Identification, Dissolution (85% in 45 minutes in water in Apparatus 1 at 100 rpm), Uniformity of dosage units, and Water (not more than 8.0%).
Vancomycin Hydrochloride for Injection USP—Preserve in Containers for Sterile Solids. A sterile dry mixture of Vancomycin Hydrochloride and a suitable stabilizing agent. Has a potency equivalent to not less than 925 mcg of vancomycin per mg, calculated on the anhydrous basis. In addition, contains an amount of vancomycin hydrochloride equivalent to the labeled amount of vancomycin, within −10% to +15%. Meets the requirements for Constituted solution, Bacterial endotoxins, Sterility, Particulate matter, Heavy metals (not more than 0.003%), and Chromatographic purity, for Identification test, pH, and Water under Vancomycin Hydrochloride, and for Uniformity of dosage units and Labeling under Injections.
Vancomycin Hydrochloride for Oral Solution USP—Preserve in tight containers. Contains an amount of vancomycin hydrochloride equivalent to the labeled amount of vancomycin, within −10% to +15%. Meets the requirements for pH (2.5–4.5, for the solution constituted as directed in the labeling) and Water (not more than 5.0%).
Sterile Vancomycin Hydrochloride USP—Preserve in Containers for Sterile Solids. Has a potency equivalent to not less than 900 mcg per mg, calculated on the anhydrous basis and, where packaged for dispensing, contains an amount of vancomycin hydrochloride equivalent to the labeled amount of vancomycin, within −10% to +15%. Meets the requirements for Constituted solution, Bacterial endotoxins, Sterility, Particulate matter, and Heavy metals (not more than 0.003%), for Identification test, pH, Water, and Chromatographic purity under Vancomycin Hydrochloride, and for Uniformity of dosage units and Labeling under Injections.

VANILLA

NF requirements: Vanilla USP—Preserve in tight containers, and store in a cold place. Cured, full-grown, unripe fruit of *Vanilla planifolia* Jacks., often known in commerce as Mexican, Bourbon, or Madagascar vanilla, or of *Vanilla tahitensis* J.W. Moore, known in commerce as Tahitian vanilla (Fam. Orchidaceae). The label states the Latin binomial name and, following the official name, the part of the plant contained in the article. The commercial variety of Vanilla, whether Mexican, Bourbon, Madagascar, or Tahitian, is also stated on the label. The label states that Vanilla that has become brittle is not to be used. Yields not less than 12.0% of anhydrous, diluted, alcohol-soluble extractive. Meets the requirements for Botanic characteristics and Test for vanillin.

VANILLA TINCTURE

NF requirements: Vanilla Tincture NF—Preserve in tight, light-resistant containers, and avoid exposure to direct sunlight and excessive heat. The label states the Latin binomial name and, following the official name, the part of the plant source from which the article was derived.

Prepare Vanilla Tincture as follows: 100 grams of Vanilla, cut into small pieces, 200 mL of Purified Water, 207 mL of Alcohol, 200 grams of Sucrose, in coarse granules, and Diluted Alcohol, a sufficient quantity to make 1000 mL. Add Purified Water to the comminuted Vanilla in a suitable covered container, and macerate for 12 hours, preferably in a warm place. Add Alcohol to the mixture, mix, and macerate for about 3 days. Transfer the mixture to a percolator containing Sucrose, and drain. Pack the drug firmly, and percolate slowly, using diluted Alcohol as the menstruum.

Meets the requirement for Alcohol content (38.0–42.0%).

VANILLIN

Chemical name: Benzaldehyde, 4-hydroxy-3-methoxy-.

Molecular formula: $C_8H_8O_3$.

Molecular weight: 152.15.

Description: Vanillin NF—Fine, white to slightly yellow crystals, usually needle-like, having an odor suggestive of vanilla. It is affected by light. Its solutions are acid to litmus.

NF category: Flavors and perfumes.

Solubility: Vanillin NF—Slightly soluble in water; freely soluble in alcohol, in chloroform, in ether, and in solutions of the fixed alkali hydroxides; soluble in glycerin and in hot water.

NF requirements: Vanillin NF—Preserve in tight, light-resistant containers. Contains not less than 97.0% and not more than 103.0% of vanillin, calculated on the dried basis. Meets the requirements for Identification, Melting range (81–83 °C), Loss on drying (not more than 1.0%), Residue on ignition (not more than 0.05%), and Organic volatile impurities.

VARICELLA VIRUS VACCINE LIVE

Source: Preparation of the Oka/Merck strain of live, attenuated varicella virus. The virus was initially obtained from a child with natural varicella, then introduced into human embryonic lung cell cultures, adapted to and propagated in embryonic guinea pig cell cultures and finally propagated in human diploid cell cultures.

USP requirements: Varicella Virus Vaccine Live Injection—Not in *USP–NF*.

VARICELLA-ZOSTER IMMUNE GLOBULIN

USP requirements: Varicella-Zoster Immune Globulin USP—Preserve at a temperature between 2 and 8 °C. A sterile 15 to 18% solution of pH 7.0 containing the globulin fraction of human plasma consisting of not less than 99% of immunoglobulin G with traces of immunoglobulin A and immunoglobulin M, in 0.3 *M* glycine as a stabilizer and 1:10,000 thimerosal as a preservative. Derived from adult human plasma selected for high titers of varicella-zoster antibodies. Each unit of blood or plasma has been found non-reactive for hepatitis B surface antigen by a suitable method. The proteins of the plasma pools are fractionated by the cold ethanol precipitation method. The content of specific antibody is not less than 125 units, deliverable from a vial containing not more than 2.5 mL solution. The unit is defined as equivalent to 0.01 mL of a Varicella-Zoster Immune Globulin lot found effective in clinical trials and used as a reference for potency determinations, based on a fluorescent-antibody membrane antigen (FAMA) method for antibody titration. Label it to state that it is to be administered by intramuscular injection, in the recommended dose based on body weight. Meets the requirement for Expiration date (not later than 2 years after date of issue from manufacturer's cold storage). Conforms to the regulations of the U.S. Food and Drug Administration concerning biologics.

VASOPRESSIN

Chemical name: Vasopressin, 8-L-arginine- (arginine form); Vasopressin, 8-L-lysine- (lysine form).

Molecular formula: $C_{46}H_{65}N_{15}O_{12}S_2$ (arginine form); $C_{46}H_{65}N_{13}O_{12}S_2$ (lysine form).

Molecular weight: 1084.23 (arginine form); 1056.22 (lysine form).

Description: Vasopressin Injection USP—Clear, colorless or practically colorless liquid, having a faint, characteristic odor.

USP requirements:
Vasopressin USP—Preserve in tight containers, preferably of Type I glass, in a refrigerator. A polypeptide hormone having the properties of causing the contraction of vascular and other smooth muscles, and of antidiuresis. Prepared by synthesis or obtained from the posterior lobe of the pituitary of healthy, domestic animals used for food by humans. Its vasopressor activity is not less than 300 USP Vasopressin Units per mg. Meets the requirements for Microbial limits, Identification, Oxytocic activity, and Ordinary impurities.

Vasopressin Injection USP—Preserve in single-dose or in multiple-dose containers, preferably of Type I glass. Do not freeze. A sterile solution of Vasopressin in a suitable diluent. Label it to indicate its origin (animal or synthetic). Label it also to state the potency in USP Vasopressin Units per mL. Each mL of Vasopressin Injection possesses an activity of that stated on the label in USP Vasopressin Units, within ±10%. Meets the requirements for Bacterial endotoxins, pH (2.5–4.5), and Particulate matter, and for Injections.

VECURONIUM

Chemical name: Vecuronium bromide—Piperidinium, 1-[(2 beta,3 alpha,5 alpha,16 beta,17 beta)-3,17-bis(acetyloxy)-2-(1-piperidinyl)androstan-16-yl]-1-methyl-, bromide.

Molecular formula: Vecuronium bromide—$C_{34}H_{57}BrN_2O_4$.

Molecular weight: Vecuronium bromide—637.73.

Description: Vecuronium bromide—White crystals melting at about 230 °C.

pKa: Vecuronium bromide—8.97 in distilled water at 25 °C.

Solubility: Vecuronium bromide—Solubilities of 9 and 23 mg/mL in water and in alcohol, respectively.

USP requirements: Vecuronium Bromide for Injection—Not in *USP–NF*.

HYDROGENATED VEGETABLE OIL

Description: Hydrogenated Vegetable Oil NF—Type I Hydrogenated Vegetable Oil—Fine, white powder, beads, or small flakes. Type II Hydrogenated Vegetable Oil—Plastic (semi-solid) or flakes having a softer consistency than Type I.

NF category:
Type I Hydrogenated Vegetable Oil—Tablet and/or capsule lubricant.
Type II Hydrogenated Vegetable Oil—Ointment base.

Solubility: Hydrogenated Vegetable Oil NF—Insoluble in water; soluble in hot isopropyl alcohol, in hexane, and in chloroform.

NF requirements: Hydrogenated Vegetable Oil NF—Preserve in tight containers, in a cool place. A mixture of triglycerides of fatty acids. The melting range, heavy metals limit, iodine value, and saponification value differ, depending on Type, as set forth in the accompanying table.

	Type I	Type II
Melting range	57–85	20–50°C
Heavy metals	0.001%	0.001%
Iodine value	0–5	55–80
Saponification value	175–200	175–200

Label it to state whether it is Type I or Type II. Meets the requirements for Loss on drying (not more than 0.1%), Acid value (not more than 4.0), Unsaponifiable matter (not more than 0.8%), and Organic volatile impurities.

VENLAFAXINE

Chemical group: Phenethylamine.

Chemical name: Venlafaxine hydrochloride—Cyclohexanol, 1-[2-(dimethylamino)-1-(4-methoxyphenyl)ethyl]-, hydrochloride.

Molecular formula: Venlafaxine hydrochloride—$C_{17}H_{27}NO_2 \cdot$ HCl.

Molecular weight: Venlafaxine hydrochloride—313.86.

Description: Venlafaxine hydrochloride—White to off-white crystalline solid.

pKa: Venlafaxine hydrochloride—9.4.

Solubility: Venlafaxine hydrochloride—Solubility of 572 mg/mL in water (adjusted to ionic strength of 0.2 *M* with sodium chloride).

Other characteristics: Venlafaxine hydrochloride—Octanol: water (0.2 *M* sodium chloride) partition coefficient: 0.43.

USP requirements:
Venlafaxine Hydrochloride Extended-release Capsules—Not in USP.
Venlafaxine Hydrochloride Tablets—Not in *USP–NF*.

VERAPAMIL

Chemical name: Verapamil hydrochloride—Benzeneacetonitrile, alpha-[3-[[2-(3,4-dimethoxyphenyl)ethyl]methylamino]propyl]-3,4-dimethoxy-alpha-(1-methylethyl)-, monohydrochloride.

Molecular formula: Verapamil hydrochloride—$C_{27}H_{38}N_2O_4 \cdot$ HCl.

Molecular weight: Verapamil hydrochloride—491.06.

Description: Verapamil Hydrochloride USP—White or practically white, crystalline powder. It is practically odorless.

Solubility: Verapamil Hydrochloride USP—Soluble in water; freely soluble in chloroform; sparingly soluble in alcohol; practically insoluble in ether.

USP requirements:
Verapamil Hydrochloride USP—Preserve in tight, light-resistant containers. Contains not less than 99.0% and not more than 100.5% of verapamil hydrochloride, calculated on the dried basis. Meets the requirements for Identification, Melting range (140–144 °C), pH (4.5–6.5, in a solution, prepared with gentle heating, containing 50 mg per mL), Loss on drying (not more than 0.5%), Residue on ignition (not more than 0.1%), Chromatographic purity, and Organic volatile impurities.
Verapamil Hydrochloride Extended-release Capsules—Not in *USP–NF*.
Verapamil Hydrochloride Injection USP—Preserve in single-dose containers, preferably of Type I glass, protected from light. A sterile solution of Verapamil Hydrochloride in Water for Injection. Contains the labeled amount, within ±10%. Meets the requirements for Identification, Bacterial endotoxins, pH (4.0–6.5), Particulate matter, and Related compounds, and for Injections.
Verapamil Hydrochloride Tablets USP—Preserve in tight, light-resistant containers. Contain the labeled amount, within ±10%. Meet the requirements for Identification, Dissolution (75% in 30 minutes in 0.01 *N* hydrochloric acid in Apparatus 2 at 50 rpm), Uniformity of dosage units, and Related compounds.
Verapamil Hydrochloride Extended-release Tablets USP—Preserve in tight, light-resistant containers. The labeling indicates the Drug Release Test with which the product complies. Contain the labeled amount, within ±10%. Meet the requirements for Identification, Drug release (Test 1: for products labeled to contain 180 mg or 240 mg, 7–15% in 1 hour, 16–30% in 2 hours, 31–50% in 3.5 hours, 51–75% in 5 hours, and not less than 85% in 8 hours; for products labeled to contain 120 mg, 10–21% in 1 hour, 18–33% in 2 hours, 35–60% in 3.5 hours, 50–82% in 5 hours, and not less than 85% in 8 hours in simulated gastric fluid TS [without enzyme] for Acid stage and simulated intestinal fluid TS [without enzyme] for Buffer stage in Apparatus 2 at 50 rpm. Test 2: for products labeled to contain 240 mg, 8–20% in 1 hour, 15–35% in 2 hours, 35–65% in 3.5 hours, 55–85% in 5 hours, and not less than 80% in 8 hours; for products labeled to contain 180 mg, 10–25% in 1 hour, 20–40% in 2 hours, 40–75% in 3.5 hours, and not less than 80% in 8 hours in simulated gastric fluid TS [without enzyme] for Acid stage and simulated intestinal fluid TS [without enzyme] for Buffer stage in Apparatus 2 at 50 rpm. Test 3: 8–20% in 1 hour, 15–35% in 2 hours, 27–57% in 3.5 hours, 45–75% in 5 hours, and not less than 80% in 8 hours in simulated gastric fluid TS [without enzyme] for Acid stage and simulated intestinal fluid TS [without enzyme] for Buffer stage in Apparatus 2 at 50 rpm. Test 4: not more than 10% in 3 hours, 20–50% in 6 hours, 52.5–82.5% in 9 hours, and not less than 85% in 14 hours in phosphate buffer solution in Apparatus 7 at 20 cycles per minute. Test 5: 2–12% in 1 hour, 10–25% in 2 hours, 25–50% in 4 hours, and not less than 80% in 8 hours in phosphate buffer solution in Apparatus 2 at 50 rpm), Uniformity of dosage units, and Chromatographic purity.

VERTEPORFIN

Source: Benzoprophyrin derivative.

Chemical name: 23*H*,25*H*-Benzo[*b*]porphine-9,13-dipropanoic acid, 18-ethenyl-4,4a-dihydro-3,4-bis(methoxycarbonyl)-4a,8,14,19-tetramethyl, monomethyl ester, *trans*-.

Molecular formula: $C_{41}H_{42}N_4O_8$.

Molecular weight: 718.79.

USP requirements: Verteporfin for Injection—Not in *USP–NF*.

VIDARABINE

Source: Obtained from fermentation cultures of *Streptomyces antibioticus*.

Chemical group: Purine nucleoside.

Chemical name: 9*H*-Purin-6-amine, 9-beta-D-arabinofuranosyl-, monohydrate.

Molecular formula: $C_{10}H_{13}N_5O_4 \cdot H_2O$.

Molecular weight: 285.26.

Description: Sterile Vidarabine USP—White to off-white powder.

Solubility: Sterile Vidarabine USP—Very slightly soluble in water; slightly soluble in dimethylformamide.

USP requirements:
Vidarabine USP—Preserve in tight containers. Where it is intended for use in preparing injectable or other sterile dosage forms, the label states that it is sterile or must be subjected to further processing during the preparation of injectable or other sterile forms. Has a potency equivalent to not less than 845 mcg and not more than 985 mcg of vidarabine per mg. Meets the requirements for Identification, Specific rotation (−56.0° to −65.0°), Bacterial endotoxins, Sterility, and Loss on drying (5.0–7.0%).

Vidarabine Concentrate for Injection USP—Preserve in single-dose or in multiple-dose containers, preferably of Type I glass. Contains suitable buffers and preservatives. Label it to indicate that it is to be solubilized in a suitable parenteral vehicle prior to intravenous infusion. Contains an amount of vidarabine equivalent to the labeled amount of anhydrous vidarabine, within −10% to +20%, in a sterile, aqueous suspension intended for solubilization with a suitable parenteral vehicle prior to intravenous infusion. Meets the requirements for Bacterial endotoxins, Sterility, and pH (5.0–6.2, in the undiluted suspension).

Vidarabine Ophthalmic Ointment USP—Preserve in collapsible ophthalmic ointment tubes. Contains an amount of vidarabine equivalent to the labeled amount of anhydrous vidarabine, within −10% to +20%. Meets the requirements for Sterility, Minimum fill, and Metal particles.

VINBLASTINE

Source: Salt of an alkaloid extracted from *Vinca rosea* Linn, a common flowering herb known as the periwinkle.

Chemical name: Vinblastine sulfate—Vincaleukoblastine, sulfate (1:1) (salt).

Molecular formula: Vinblastine sulfate—$C_{46}H_{58}N_4O_9 \cdot H_2SO_4$.

Molecular weight: Vinblastine sulfate—909.05.

Description: Vinblastine Sulfate USP—White or slightly yellow, odorless, amorphous or crystalline powder. Is hygroscopic.

pKa: 5.4 and 7.4 in water.

Solubility: Vinblastine Sulfate USP—Freely soluble in water.

USP requirements:
Vinblastine Sulfate USP—Preserve in tight, light-resistant containers, in a freezer. Where it is intended for use in preparing injectable dosage forms, the label states that it is sterile or must be subjected to further processing during the preparation of injectable dosage forms. Contains not less than 96.0% and not more than 102.0% of vinblastine sulfate, corrections being applied for loss in weight. Meets the requirements for Identification, pH (3.5–5.0, in a solution prepared by dissolving 3 mg in 2 mL of water), Loss on drying (not more than 15.0%), and Related compounds, for Sterility and Bacterial endotoxins under Vinblastine Sulfate for Injection (where the label states that Vinblastine Sulfate is sterile), and for Bacterial endotoxins under Vinblastine Sulfate for Injection (where the label states that Vinblastine Sulfate must be subjected to further processing during the preparation of injectable dosage forms).

Caution: Handle Vinblastine Sulfate with great care since it is a potent cytotoxic agent.

Vinblastine Sulfate Injection—Not in *USP–NF*.

Vinblastine Sulfate for Injection USP—Preserve in Containers for Sterile Solids, in a refrigerator. It is Vinblastine Sulfate suitable for parenteral use. The label states: "FATAL IF GIVEN INTRATHECALLY. FOR INTRAVENOUS USE ONLY." When dispensed, the container or syringe (holding the individual dose prepared for administration to the patient) must be enclosed in an overwrap bearing the statement "DO NOT REMOVE COVERING UNTIL MOMENT OF INJECTION. FATAL IF GIVEN INTRATHECALLY. FOR INTRAVENOUS USE ONLY." Contains the labeled amount, within ±10%. Meets the requirements for Completeness of solution, Constituted solution, Bacterial endotoxins, Sterility, Uniformity of dosage units, and Related compounds, for Identification test under Vinblastine Sulfate, and for Labeling under Injections.

Caution: Handle Vinblastine Sulfate for Injection with great care since it is a potent cytotoxic agent.

VINCRISTINE

Source: Salt of an alkaloid extracted from *Vinca rosea* Linn, a common flowering herb known as the periwinkle.

Chemical name: Vincristine sulfate—Vincaleukoblastine, 22 oxo-,sulfate (1:1) (salt).

Molecular formula: Vincristine sulfate—$C_{46}H_{56}N_4O_{10} \cdot H_2SO_4$.

Molecular weight: Vincristine sulfate—923.04.

Description:
Vincristine Sulfate USP—White to slightly yellow, odorless, amorphous or crystalline powder. Is hygroscopic.
Vincristine Sulfate for Injection USP—Yellowish white solid, having the characteristic appearance of products prepared by freeze-drying.

pKa: 5.1 and 7.5 in water.

Solubility: Vincristine Sulfate USP—Freely soluble in water; soluble in methanol; slightly soluble in alcohol.

USP requirements:
Vincristine Sulfate USP—Preserve in tight, light-resistant containers, in a freezer. Contains not less than 95.0% and not more than 105.0% of vincristine sulfate, corrections being applied for loss in weight. Meets the requirements for Identification, pH (3.5–4.5, in a solution [1 in 1000]), Loss on drying (not more than 12.0%), and Related compounds.

Caution: Handle Vincristine Sulfate with great care since it is a potent cytotoxic agent.

Vincristine Sulfate Injection USP—Preserve in light-resistant, glass containers, in a refrigerator. A sterile solution of Vincristine Sulfate in Water for Injection. The label states: "FATAL IF GIVEN INTRATHECALLY. FOR INTRAVENOUS USE ONLY." Where labeled as containing more than 2 mg, it must also be labeled as a Pharmacy bulk package. The labeling directs that the drug be dispensed only in containers enclosed in an overwrap labeled as directed below. When

packaged in a Pharmacy bulk package, it is exempt from the requirement under Injections, that the closure be penetrated only one time after constitution with a suitable sterile transfer device or dispensing set, when it contains a suitable substance or mixture of substances to prevent the growth of microorganisms. When dispensed, the container or syringe (holding the individual dose prepared for administration to the patient) must be enclosed in an overwrap bearing the statement "DO NOT REMOVE COVERING UNTIL MOMENT OF INJECTION. FATAL IF GIVEN INTRATHECALLY. FOR INTRAVENOUS USE ONLY." Contains the labeled amount, within ± 10%. Meets the requirements for Identification, Bacterial endotoxins, pH (3.5–5.5), and Related compounds, for Sterility tests, and for Labeling under Injections.

Caution: Handle Vincristine Sulfate Injection with great care since it is a potent cytotoxic agent.

Vincristine Sulfate for Injection USP—Preserve in Containers for Sterile Solids, in a refrigerator. A sterile mixture of Vincristine Sulfate with suitable diluents. The label states: "FATAL IF GIVEN INTRATHECALLY. FOR INTRAVENOUS USE ONLY." Where labeled as containing more than 2 mg, it must also be labeled as a Pharmacy bulk package. The labeling directs that the drug be dispensed only in containers enclosed in an overwrap labeled as directed below. When packaged in a Pharmacy bulk package, it is exempt from the requirement under Injections, that the closure be penetrated only one time after constitution with a suitable sterile transfer device or dispensing set, when it contains a suitable substance or mixture of substances to prevent the growth of microorganisms. When dispensed, the container or syringe (holding the individual dose prepared for administration to the patient) must be enclosed in an overwrap bearing the statement "DO NOT REMOVE COVERING UNTIL MOMENT OF INJECTION. FATAL IF GIVEN INTRATHECALLY. FOR INTRAVENOUS USE ONLY." Contains the labeled amount, within ± 10%. Meets the requirements for Constituted solution, Identification, Bacterial endotoxins, Uniformity of dosage units, and Related compounds, for Sterility tests, and for Labeling under Injections.

Caution: Handle Vincristine Sulfate for Injection with great care since it is a potent cytotoxic agent.

VINDESINE

Chemical name:
Vindesine—Vincaleukoblastine, 23-amino-O^4-deacetyl-23-demethoxy-.
Vindesine sulfate—Vincaleukoblastine, 3-(aminocarbonyl)-O^4-deacetyl-3-de(methoxycarbonyl)sulfate (1:1) (salt).

Molecular formula:
Vindesine—$C_{43}H_{55}N_5O_7$.
Vindesine sulfate—$C_{43}H_{55}N_5O_7 \cdot H_2SO_4$.

Molecular weight:
Vindesine—753.93.
Vindesine sulfate—852.01.

Description: Vindesine sulfate—Amorphous solid melting at less than 250 °C.

USP requirements:
Vindesine Injection—Not in *USP–NF*.
Vindesine Sulfate for Injection—Not in *USP–NF*.

VINORELBINE

Chemical group: Semisynthetic derivative of vinblastine.

Chemical name: Vinorelbine tartrate—C'-Norvincaleukoblastine, 3′,4′-didehydro-4′-deoxy-, [R-(R^*,R^*)]-2,3-dihydroxybutanedioate (1:2) (salt).

Molecular formula: Vinorelbine tartrate—$C_{45}H_{54}N_4O_8 \cdot 2C_4H_6O_6$.

Molecular weight: Vinorelbine tartrate—1079.11.

Description: Vinorelbine Tartrate USP—White to yellow or light brown, amorphous powder.

Solubility: Vinorelbine Tartrate USP—Freely soluble in water.

USP requirements:
Vinorelbine Tartrate USP—Preserve in tight, light-resistant containers. Store in a freezer. Contains not less than 98.0% and not more than 102.0% of vinorelbine tartrate, calculated on the anhydrous basis. Meets the requirements for Clarity of solution, Color of solution, Identification, pH (3.3–3.8, in a solution [10 mg per mL]), Water (not more than 4.0%), Residue on ignition (not more than 0.1%), and Related compounds.

Caution—Vinorelbine Tartrate is cytotoxic. Great care should be taken to prevent inhaling particles and exposing the skin to it.

Vinorelbine Tartrate Injection—Not in *USP–NF*.

VITAMIN A

Chemical name: Retinol—3,7-Dimethyl-9-(2,6,6-trimethyl-1cyclohexen-1-yl)-2,4,6,8-nonate-traen-1-ol.

Molecular formula: Retinol—$C_{20}H_{30}O$.

Molecular weight: Retinol—286.46.

Description: Vitamin A USP—In liquid form, a light-yellow to red oil that may solidify upon refrigeration. In solid form, has the appearance of any diluent that has been added. May be practically odorless or may have a mild fishy odor, but has no rancid odor. Is unstable to air and light.

Solubility: Vitamin A USP—In liquid form, insoluble in water and in glycerin; very soluble in chloroform and in ether; soluble in absolute alcohol and in vegetable oils. In solid form, may be dispersible in water.

USP requirements:
Vitamin A USP—Preserve in tight containers, preferably under an atmosphere of an inert gas, protected from light. Label it to indicate the form in which the vitamin is present, and to indicate the presence of any antimicrobial agent, dispersant, antioxidant, or other added substance, and to indicate the vitamin A activity in terms of the equivalent amount of retinol, in mg per gram. The vitamin A activity may be stated also in USP Units, on the basis that 1 USP Vitamin A Unit equals the biological activity of 0.3 mcg of the all-*trans* isomer of retinol. Contains a suitable form of retinol (vitamin A alcohol) and possesses vitamin A activity equivalent to not less than 95.0% of that declared on the label. May consist of retinol or esters of retinol formed from edible fatty acids, principally acetic and palmitic acids. May be diluted with edible oils, or it may be incorporated in solid, edible carriers or excipients. Meets the requirements for Identification for vitamin A and Absorbance ratio.

Vitamin A Capsules USP—Preserve in tight, light-resistant containers. Label the Capsules to indicate the form in which the vitamin is present, and to indicate the vitamin A activity in terms of the equivalent amount of retinol in mg. The vitamin A activity may be stated also in USP Units per Capsule, on the basis that 1 USP Vitamin A Unit equals the biological activity of 0.3 mcg of the all-*trans* iso-

mer of retinol. Contain the labeled amount, within –5% to +20%. Meet the requirements for Disintegration (45 minutes) and Uniformity of dosage units, for Identification tests for vitamin A, and for the Absorbance ratio test under Vitamin A.

Vitamin A Injection—Not in *USP–NF*.

Vitamin A Oral Solution—Not in *USP–NF*.

Vitamin A Tablets—Not in *USP–NF*.

VITAMIN E

Molecular formula:

d- or *dl-*Alpha tocopherol—$C_{29}H_{50}O_2$.

d- or *dl-*Alpha tocopheryl acetate—$C_{31}H_{52}O_3$.

d- or *dl-*Alpha tocopheryl acid succinate—$C_{33}H_{54}O_5$.

Description:

Vitamin E USP—Practically odorless. The alpha tocopherols and alpha tocopheryl acetates occur as clear, yellow, or greenish-yellow, viscous oils. *d-*Alpha tocopheryl acetate may solidify in the cold. Alpha tocopheryl acid succinate occurs as a white powder; the *d-*isomer melts at about 75 °C, and the *dl-*form melts at about 70 °C. The alpha tocopherols are unstable to air and to light, particularly when in alkaline media. The esters are stable to air and to light, but are unstable to alkali; the acid succinate is also unstable when held molten.

Vitamin E Preparation USP—The liquid forms are clear, yellow to brownish-red, viscous oils. The solid forms are white to tan-white granular powders.

Solubility:

Vitamin E USP—Alpha tocopheryl acid succinate is insoluble in water; slightly soluble in alkaline solutions; soluble in alcohol, in ether, in acetone, and in vegetable oils; very soluble in chloroform. The other forms of Vitamin E are insoluble in water; soluble in alcohol; miscible with ether, with acetone, with vegetable oils, and with chloroform.

Vitamin E Preparation USP—The liquid forms are insoluble in water; soluble in alcohol; and miscible with ether, with acetone, with vegetable oils, and with chloroform. The solid forms disperse in water to give cloudy suspensions.

USP requirements:

Vitamin E USP—Preserve in tight containers, protected from light. Protect *d-* or *dl-*alpha tocopherol with a blanket of an inert gas. A form of alpha tocopherol. Includes the following: *d-* or *dl-*alpha tocopherol; *d-* or *dl-*alpha tocopheryl acetate; *d-* or *dl-*alpha tocopheryl acid succinate. Label Vitamin E to indicate the chemical form and to indicate whether it is the *d-* or the *dl-* form. The Vitamin E activity may be expressed in terms of the equivalent amount of *d-*alpha tocopherol, in mg per gram, based on the relationship between the former USP Units (equal to the former International Units) and mass. Contains not less than 96.0% and not more than 102.0% of *d-* or *dl-*alpha tocopherol, *d-* or *dl-*alpha tocopheryl acetate, or *d-* or *dl-*alpha tocopheryl acid succinate, respectively. Meets the requirements for Identification, Acidity, and Organic volatile impurities.

Vitamin E Preparation USP—Preserve in tight containers, protected from light. Protect Preparation containing *d-* or *dl-*alpha tocopherol with a blanket of an inert gas. A combination of a single form of Vitamin E with one or more inert substances. May be in a liquid or solid form. Label it to indicate the chemical form of Vitamin E present, and to indicate whether the *d-* or the *dl-*form is present, excluding any different forms that may be introduced as a minor constituent of the vehicle. Designate the quantity of Vitamin E present. Contains the labeled amount of Vitamin E, within –5% to +20%. Vitamin E Preparation labeled to contain a *dl-*form of Vitamin E may contain also a small amount of a *d-*form occurring as a minor constituent of an added substance. Meets the requirements for Identification and Acidity.

Vitamin E Capsules USP—Preserve in tight containers, and store at room temperature. Protect Capsules containing *d-* or *dl-*alpha tocopherol from light. Contain Vitamin E or Vitamin E Preparation. The Capsules meet the requirements for Labeling under Vitamin E Preparation. Contain the labeled amount, within –5% to +20%. Meet the requirements for Identification, Disintegration (45 minutes), and Uniformity of dosage units.

Vitamin E Oral Solution—Not in *USP–NF*.

Vitamin E Tablets—Not in *USP–NF*.

Vitamin E Chewable Tablets—Not in *USP–NF*.

VITAMIN E POLYETHYLENE GLYCOL SUCCINATE

NF requirements: Vitamin E Polyethylene Glycol Succinate NF—Preserve in tight containers, protected from light. It is a mixture formed by the esterification of *d-*alpha tocopheryl acid succinate and polyethylene glycol. The ester mixture consists primarily of the mono-esterified polyethylene glycol and a small amount of di-esterified polyethylene glycol. The labeling indicates the *d-*alpha tocopherol content, expressed in mg per gram. Contains not less than 25.0% of *d-*alpha tocopherol. Meets the requirements for Identification, Solubility in water, Acid value, Organic volatile impurities, Specific rotation (not less than +24.0°), and Content of alpha tocopherol.

VITAMINS A, D, AND C AND FLUORIDE

Chemical name:

Retinol—3,7-Dimethyl-9-(2,6,6-trimethyl-1-cyclohexen-1-yl)-2,4,6,8-nonate-traen-1-ol.

Calcifediol—9,10-Secocholesta-5,7,10(19)-triene-3,25-diol monohydrate, (3 beta,5*Z*,7*E*)-.

Calcitriol—9,10-Secocholesta-5,7,10(19)-triene-1,3,25-triol, (1 alpha,3 beta,5*Z*,7*E*)-.

Ergocalciferol—9,10-Secoergosta-5,7,10(19),22-tetraen-3-ol, (3 beta,5*Z*,7*E*,22*E*)-.

Ascorbic acid—L-Ascorbic acid.

Sodium fluoride—Sodium fluoride.

Pyridoxine hydrochloride—3,4-Pyridinedimethanol, 5-hydroxy-6-methyl-, hydrochloride.

Molecular formula:

Retinol—$C_{20}H_{30}O$.

Calcifediol—$C_{27}H_{44}O_2 \cdot H_2O$.

Calcitriol—$C_{27}H_{44}O_3$.

Ergocalciferol—$C_{28}H_{44}O$.

Ascorbic acid—$C_6H_8O_6$.

Sodium fluoride—NaF.

Potassium fluoride—FK.

Pyridoxine hydrochloride—$C_8H_{11}NO_3 \cdot HCl$.

d- or *dl-*Alpha tocopherol—$C_{29}H_{50}O_2$.

d- or *dl-*Alpha tocopheryl acetate—$C_{31}H_{52}O_3$.

d- or *dl-*Alpha tocopheryl acid succinate—$C_{33}H_{54}O_5$.

Molecular weight:

Retinol—286.45.

Calcifediol—418.65.

Calcitriol—416.64.

Ergocalciferol—396.65.

Ascorbic acid—176.12.

Sodium fluoride—41.99.

Potassium fluoride—58.10.

Pyridoxine hydrochloride—205.64.

Description:

Vitamin A USP—In liquid form, a light-yellow to red oil that may solidify upon refrigeration. In solid form, has the appearance of any diluent that has been added. May be practically odorless or may have a mild fishy odor, but has no rancid odor. Is unstable to air and light.

Calcifediol—A white powder. It has a melting point of about 105 °C.

Calcitriol—A practically white crystalline compound with a melting range of 111–115 °C.

Ergocalciferol USP—White, odorless crystals. Is affected by air and by light.

Ascorbic Acid USP—White or slightly yellow crystals or powder. On exposure to light it gradually darkens. In the dry state, is reasonably stable in air, but in solution rapidly oxidizes. Melts at about 190 °C.

NF category: Antioxidant.

Sodium Fluoride USP—White, odorless powder.

Potassium fluoride—White, deliquescent powder or solid. Melting point 859.9 °C.

Pyridoxine Hydrochloride USP—White to practically white crystals or crystalline powder. Is stable in air, and is slowly affected by sunlight. Its solutions have a pH of about 3.

Vitamin E USP—Practically odorless. The alpha tocopherols and alpha tocopheryl acetates occur as clear, yellow, or greenish-yellow, viscous oils. *d*-Alpha tocopheryl acetate may solidify in the cold. Alpha tocopheryl acid succinate occurs as a white powder; the *d*-isomer melts at about 75 °C, and the *dl*-form melts at about 70 °C. The alpha tocopherols are unstable to air and to light, particularly when in alkaline media. The esters are stable to air and to light, but are unstable to alkali; the acid succinate is also unstable when held molten.

Solubility:

Vitamin A USP—In liquid form, insoluble in water and in glycerin; very soluble in chloroform and in ether; soluble in absolute alcohol and in vegetable oils. In solid form, may be dispersible in water.

Calcifediol—Practically insoluble in water; soluble in organic solvents.

Calcitriol—Insoluble in water; soluble in organic solvents.

Ergocalciferol USP—Insoluble in water; soluble in alcohol, in chloroform, in ether, and in fatty oils.

Ascorbic Acid USP—Freely soluble in water; sparingly soluble in alcohol; insoluble in chloroform and in ether.

Sodium Fluoride USP—Soluble in water; insoluble in alcohol.

Potassium fluoride—Soluble in water (92.3 grams per 100 mL at 18 °C and 96.4 grams per 100 mL at 21 °C); very freely soluble in boiling water; insoluble in alcohol unless water is present.

Pyridoxine Hydrochloride USP—Freely soluble in water; slightly soluble in alcohol; insoluble in ether.

Vitamin E USP—Alpha tocopheryl acid succinate is insoluble in water; slightly soluble in alkaline solutions; soluble in alcohol, in ether, in acetone, and in vegetable oils; very soluble in chloroform. The other forms of Vitamin E are insoluble in water; soluble in alcohol; miscible with ether, with acetone, with vegetable oils, and with chloroform.

USP requirements:

Vitamins A, D, and C and Sodium or Potassium Fluoride Oral Solution—Not in *USP–NF*.

Vitamins A, D, and C and Sodium or Potassium Fluoride Chewable Tablets—Not in *USP–NF*.

MULTIPLE VITAMINS AND FLUORIDE

Chemical name:

Ascorbic acid—L-Ascorbic acid.
Cyanocobalamin—Vitamin B$_{12}$.

Folic acid—L-Glutamic acid, *N*-[4-[[(2-amino-1,4-dihydro-4oxo-6-pteridinyl)methyl]amino]benzoyl]-.

Niacin—3-Pyridinecarboxylic acid.

Pyridoxine hydrochloride—3,4-Pyridinedimethanol, 5-hydroxy-6-methyl-, hydrochloride.

Riboflavin—Riboflavine.

Thiamine hydrochloride—Thiazolium, 3-[(4-amino-2-methyl-5-pyrimidinyl)methyl]-5-(2-hydroxyethyl)-4-methyl-, chloride, monohydrochloride.

Retinol—3,7-Dimethyl-9-(2,6,6-trimethyl-1-cyclohexen-1-yl)-2,4,6,8-nonate-traen-1-ol.

Calcifediol—9,10-Secocholesta-5,7,10(19)-triene-3,25-diol monohydrate, (3 beta,5*Z*,7*E*)-.

Calcitriol—9,10-Secocholesta-5,7,10(19)-triene-1,3,25-triol, (1 alpha,3 beta,5*Z*,7*E*)-.

Ergocalciferol—9,10-Secoergosta-5,7,10(19),22-tetraen-3-ol, (3 beta,5*Z*,7*E*,22*E*)-.

Sodium fluoride—Sodium fluoride.

Molecular formula:

Ascorbic acid—C$_6$H$_8$O$_6$.
Cyanocobalamin—C$_{63}$H$_{88}$CoN$_{14}$O$_{14}$P.
Folic acid—C$_{19}$H$_{19}$N$_7$O$_6$.
Niacin—C$_6$H$_5$NO$_2$.
Pyridoxine hydrochloride—C$_8$H$_{11}$NO$_3$ · HCl.
Riboflavin—C$_{17}$H$_{20}$N$_4$O$_6$.
Thiamine hydrochloride—C$_{12}$H$_{17}$ClN$_4$OS · HCl.
Retinol—C$_{20}$H$_{30}$O.
Calcifediol—C$_{27}$H$_{44}$O$_2$ · H$_2$O.
Calcitriol—C$_{27}$H$_{44}$O$_3$.
Ergocalciferol—C$_{28}$H$_{44}$O.
d- or *dl*-Alpha tocopherol—C$_{29}$H$_{50}$O$_2$.
d- or *dl*-Alpha tocopheryl acetate—C$_{31}$H$_{52}$O$_3$.
d- or *dl*-Alpha tocopheryl acid succinate—C$_{33}$H$_{54}$O$_5$.
Sodium fluoride—NaF.
Potassium fluoride—FK.

Molecular weight:

Ascorbic acid—176.12.
Cyanocobalamin—1355.37.
Folic acid—441.40.
Niacin—123.11.
Pyridoxine hydrochloride—205.64.
Riboflavin—376.36.
Thiamine hydrochloride—337.27.
Retinol—286.45.
Calcifediol—418.65.
Calcitriol—416.64.
Ergocalciferol—396.65.
Sodium fluoride—41.99.
Potassium fluoride—58.10.

Description:

Ascorbic Acid USP—White or slightly yellow crystals or powder. On exposure to light it gradually darkens. In the dry state, is reasonably stable in air, but in solution rapidly oxidizes. Melts at about 190 °C.

NF category: Antioxidant.

Cyanocobalamin USP—Dark red crystals or amorphous or crystalline red powder. In the anhydrous form, it is very hygroscopic and when exposed to air it may absorb about 12% of water.

Folic Acid USP—Yellow, yellow-brownish, or yellowish orange, odorless, crystalline powder.

Niacin USP—White crystals or crystalline powder. Is odorless, or has a slight odor. Melts at about 235 °C.

Pyridoxine Hydrochloride USP—White to practically white crystals or crystalline powder. Is stable in air, and is slowly affected by sunlight. Its solutions have a pH of about 3.

Riboflavin USP—Yellow to orange-yellow, crystalline powder having a slight odor. Melts at about 280 °C. Its saturated solution is neutral to litmus. When dry, it is not appreciably affected by diffused light, but when in solution, light induces quite rapid deterioration, especially in the presence of alkalies.

Thiamine Hydrochloride USP—White crystals or crystalline powder, usually having a slight, characteristic odor. When exposed to air, the anhydrous product rapidly absorbs about 4% of water. Melts at about 248 °C, with some decomposition.

Vitamin A USP—In liquid form, a light-yellow to red oil that may solidify upon refrigeration. In solid form, has the appearance of any diluent that has been added. May be practically odorless or may have a mild fishy odor, but has no rancid odor. Is unstable to air and light.

Calcifediol—A white powder. It has a melting point of about 105 °C.

Calcitriol—A practically white crystalline compound with a melting range of 111–115 °C.

Ergocalciferol USP—White, odorless crystals. Is affected by air and by light.

Vitamin E USP—Practically odorless. The alpha tocopherols and alpha tocopheryl acetates occur as clear, yellow, or greenish-yellow, viscous oils. d-Alpha tocopheryl acetate may solidify in the cold. Alpha tocopheryl acid succinate occurs as a white powder; the d-isomer melts at about 75 °C, and the dl-form melts at about 70 °C. The alpha tocopherols are unstable to air and to light, particularly when in alkaline media. The esters are stable to air and to light, but are unstable to alkali; the acid succinate is also unstable when held molten.

Sodium Fluoride USP—White, odorless powder.

Potassium fluoride—White, deliquescent powder or solid. Melting point 859.9 °C.

Solubility:

Ascorbic Acid USP—Freely soluble in water; sparingly soluble in alcohol; insoluble in chloroform and in ether.

Cyanocobalamin USP—Sparingly soluble in water; soluble in alcohol; insoluble in acetone, in chloroform, and in ether.

Folic Acid USP—Very slightly soluble in water; insoluble in alcohol, in acetone, in chloroform, and in ether; readily dissolves in dilute solutions of alkali hydroxides and carbonates, and is soluble in hot, 3 N hydrochloric acid and in hot, 2 N sulfuric acid. Soluble in hydrochloric acid and in sulfuric acid, yielding very pale yellow solutions.

Niacin USP—Sparingly soluble in water; freely soluble in boiling water, in boiling alcohol, and in solutions of alkali hydroxides and carbonates; practically insoluble in ether.

Pyridoxine Hydrochloride USP—Freely soluble in water; slightly soluble in alcohol; insoluble in ether.

Riboflavin USP—Very slightly soluble in water, in alcohol, and in isotonic sodium chloride solution; very soluble in dilute solutions of alkalies; insoluble in ether and in chloroform.

Thiamine Hydrochloride USP—Freely soluble in water; soluble in glycerin; slightly soluble in alcohol; insoluble in ether.

Vitamin A USP—In liquid form, insoluble in water and in glycerin; very soluble in chloroform and in ether; soluble in absolute alcohol and in vegetable oils. In solid form, may be dispersible in water.

Calcifediol—Practically insoluble in water; soluble in organic solvents.

Calcitriol—Insoluble in water; soluble in organic solvents.

Ergocalciferol USP—Insoluble in water; soluble in alcohol, in chloroform, in ether, and in fatty oils.

Vitamin E USP—Alpha tocopheryl acid succinate is insoluble in water; slightly soluble in alkaline solutions; soluble in alcohol, in ether, in acetone, and in vegetable oils; very soluble in chloroform. The other forms of Vitamin E are insoluble in water; soluble in alcohol; miscible with ether, with acetone, with vegetable oils, and with chloroform.

Sodium Fluoride USP—Soluble in water; insoluble in alcohol.

Potassium fluoride—Soluble in water (92.3 grams per 100 mL at 18 °C and 96.4 grams per 100 mL at 21 °C); very freely soluble in boiling water; insoluble in alcohol unless water is present.

USP requirements:

Multiple Vitamins and Sodium or Potassium Fluoride Oral Solution—Not in USP–NF.

Multiple Vitamins and Sodium or Potassium Fluoride Chewable Tablets—Not in USP–NF.

OIL-SOLUBLE VITAMINS

For Vitamin A, Vitamin D (Cholecalciferol or Ergocalciferol), Vitamin E, Phytonadione, and Beta Carotene—See individual listings for chemistry information.

USP requirements:

Oil-soluble Vitamins Capsules USP—Preserve in tight, light-resistant containers. Contain two or more of the following oil-soluble vitamins: Vitamin A, Vitamin D as Ergocalciferol (Vitamin D2) or Cholecalciferol (Vitamin D3), Vitamin E, Phytonadione (Vitamin K1), and Beta Carotene. Oil-soluble Vitamins Capsules contain no other vitamins, or any minerals. May contain other labeled added substances that are generally recognized as safe, in amounts that are unobjectionable. Label the Capsules to state that the product is Oil-soluble Vitamins Capsules. The label states also the quantity of each vitamin per dosage unit and, where necessary, the chemical form in which it is present. Where the product contains vitamin E, the label indicates also whether it is the d- or dl- form. Where more than one Assay method is given for a particular vitamin, the labeling states the Assay method used only if Method 1 is not used. Capsules contain the labeled amounts of Vitamin A, as retinol or esters of retinol in the form of retinyl acetate or retinyl palmitate; Vitamin D, as ergocalciferol or cholecalciferol; Vitamin E as alpha tocopherol, alpha tocopheryl acetate, or alpha tocopheryl acid succinate; phytonadione; and beta carotene, within −10% to +65%. Meet the requirements for Microbial limits, Disintegration and dissolution, and Weight variation.

Oil-soluble Vitamins Tablets USP—Preserve in tight, light-resistant containers. Contain two or more of the following oil-soluble vitamins: Vitamin A, Vitamin D as Ergocalciferol (Vitamin D2) or Cholecalciferol (Vitamin D3), Vitamin E, Phytonadione (Vitamin K1), and Beta Carotene. Oil-soluble Vitamins Tablets contain no other vitamins or any minerals. May contain other labeled added substances that are generally recognized as safe, in amounts that are unobjectionable. Label the Tablets to state that the product is Oil-soluble Vitamins Tablets. The label states also the quantity of each vitamin per dosage unit and where necessary the chemical form in which it is present. Where the product contains Vitamin E, the label indicates whether it is the d- or dl- form. Where more than one Assay method is given for a particular vitamin, the labeling states the Assay method used only if Method 1 is not used. Tablets contain the labeled amounts of Vitamin A, as retinol or esters of retinol in the form of retinyl acetate or retinyl palmitate; Vitamin D, as ergocalciferol or cholecalciferol; Vitamin E as alpha tocopherol, alpha tocopheryl acetate, or alpha tocopheryl acid succinate; phytonadione; and beta carotene, within − 10% to +65%. Meet the requirements for Microbial limits, Disintegration and dissolution, and Weight variation.

OIL- AND WATER-SOLUBLE VITAMINS

For Vitamin A, Vitamin D (Cholecalciferol or Ergocalciferol), Vitamin E, Phytonadione, Beta Carotene, Ascorbic Acid or Calcium Ascorbate or Sodium Ascorbate, Biotin, Cyanocobalamin, Folic Acid, Niacin or Niacinamide, Dex-

panthenol or *Panthenol, Pantothenic Acid* (Calcium Pantothenate or Racemic Calcium Pantothenate), *Pyridoxine, Riboflavin,* and *Thiamine*—See individual listings for chemistry information.

USP requirements:

Oil- and Water-soluble Vitamins Capsules USP—Preserve in tight, light-resistant containers. Contain one or more of the following oil-soluble vitamins: Vitamin A, Vitamin D as Ergocalciferol (Vitamin D_2) or Cholecalciferol (Vitamin D_3), Vitamin E, Phytonadione (Vitamin K_1), and Beta Carotene, and one or more of the following water-soluble vitamins: Ascorbic Acid or its equivalent as Calcium Ascorbate or Sodium Ascorbate, Biotin, Cyanocobalamin, Folic Acid, Niacin or Niacinamide, Dexpanthenol or Panthenol, Pantothenic Acid (as Calcium Pantothenate or Racemic Calcium Pantothenate), Pyridoxine Hydrochloride, Riboflavin, and Thiamine Hydrochloride or Thiamine Mononitrate. Do not contain any minerals. May contain other labeled added substances that are generally recognized as safe, in amounts that are unobjectionable. The label states that the product is Oil- and Water-soluble Vitamins Capsules. The label states also the quantity of each vitamin per dosage unit and where necessary the chemical form in which it is present. Where the product contains vitamin E, the label indicates whether it is the *d-* or *dl-* form. Where more than one *Assay* method is given for a particular vitamin, the labeling states with which *Assay* method the product complies only if *Method 1* is not used. Contain the labeled amounts of vitamin A as retinol or esters of retinol in the form of retinyl acetate or retinyl palmitate; Vitamin D as ergocalciferol or cholecalciferol; Vitamin E as alpha tocopherol, alpha tocopheryl acetate, or alpha tocopheryl acid succinate; phytonadione; and beta carotene, within −10% to +65%. Contain the labeled amounts of ascorbic acid or its salts as calcium ascorbate or sodium ascorbate, biotin, cyanocobalamin, folic acid, niacin or niacinamide, dexpanthenol or panthenol, calcium pantothenate, pyridoxine hydrochloride, riboflavin, and thiamine as thiamine hydrochoride or thiamine mononitrate, within −10% to +50%. Meet the requirements for Microbial limits, Disintegration and dissolution, and Weight variation.

Oil- and Water-soluble Vitamins Oral Solution USP—Preserve in tight, light-resistant containers, under an inert gas or with a minimum of headspace. Contains one or more of the following oil-soluble vitamins: Vitamin A, Vitamin D as Ergocalciferol (Vitamin D_2) or Cholecalciferol (Vitamin D_3), and Vitamin E; and one or more of the following water-soluble vitamins: Ascorbic Acid or its equivalent as Calcium Ascorbate or Sodium Ascorbate, Cyanocobalamin, Niacin or Niacinamide, Dexpanthenol or Panthenol, Pantothenic Acid (as Calcium Pantothenate or Racemic Calcium Pantothenate), Pyridoxine Hydrochloride, Riboflavin or Riboflavin-5'-Phosphate Sodium, and Thiamine Hydrochloride or Thiamine Mononitrate. The label states that the product is Oil- and Water-soluble Vitamins Oral Solution. The label states the quantity of each vitamin present in a given volume of Oral Solution and, where necessary, the chemical form in which a vitamin is present. Where the product contains vitamin E, the label indicates whether it is the *d-* or *dl-* form. Where the product is labeled to contain panthenol, the label states the equivalent content of dexpanthenol. Where more than one *Assay* method is given for a particular vitamin, the labeling states with which *Assay* method the product complies only if *Method 1* is not used. Contains the labeled amounts of vitamin A as retinol or esters of retinol in the form of retinyl acetate or retinyl palmitate, Vitamin D as ergocalciferol or cholecalciferol, Vitamin E as alpha tocopherol or alpha tocopheryl acetate or alpha tocopheryl acid succinate, ascorbic acid or its salts as calcium ascorbate or sodium ascorbate, and thiamine as thiamine hydrochoride or thiamine mononitrate, within −10% to +150%; the labeled amounts of niacin or niacinamide, dexpanthenol or panthenol, calcium

pantothenate, pyridoxine hydrochloride, and riboflavin or riboflavin-5'-phosphate sodium, within −10% to +50%; and the labeled amount of cyanocobalamin, within −10% to +350%. Meets the requirements for Alcohol content (if present, within −10% to +20% of labeled amount) and Microbial limits.

Oil- and Water-soluble Vitamins Tablets USP—Preserve in tight, light-resistant containers. Contain one or more of the following oil-soluble vitamins: Vitamin A, Vitamin D as Ergocalciferol (Vitamin D_2) or Cholecalciferol (Vitamin D_3), Vitamin E, Phytonadione (Vitamin K_1), and Beta Carotene, and one or more of the following water-soluble vitamins: Ascorbic Acid or its equivalent as Calcium Ascorbate or Sodium Ascorbate, Biotin, Cyanocobalamin, Folic Acid, Niacin or Niacinamide, Pantothenic Acid (as Calcium Pantothenate or Racemic Calcium Pantothenate), Pyridoxine Hydrochloride, Riboflavin, and Thiamine Hydrochloride or Thiamine Mononitrate. Do not contain any minerals. May contain other labeled added substances that are generally recognized as safe, in amounts that are unobjectionable. The label states that the product is Oil- and Water-soluble Vitamins Tablets. The label states also the quantity of each vitamin per dosage unit and where necessary the chemical form in which it is present. Where the product contains vitamin E, the label indicates whether it is the *d-* or *dl-* form. Where more than one *Assay* method is given for a particular vitamin, the labeling states with which *Assay* method the product complies only if *Method 1* is not used. Contain the labeled amounts of vitamin A as retinol or esters of retinol in the form of retinyl acetate or retinyl palmitate; Vitamin D as ergocalciferol or cholecalciferol; Vitamin E as alpha tocopherol, alpha tocopheryl acetate, or alpha tocopheryl acid succinate; phytonadione; and beta carotene, within −10% to +65%. Contain the labeled amounts of ascorbic acid or its salts, as calcium ascorbate or sodium ascorbate, biotin, cyanocobalamin, folic acid, niacin or niacinamide, calcium pantothenate, pyridoxine hydrochloride, riboflavin, and thiamine as thiamine hydrochoride or thiamine mononitrate, within −10% to +50%. Meet the requirements for Microbial limits, Disintegration and dissolution, and Weight variation.

OIL- AND WATER-SOLUBLE VITAMINS WITH MINERALS

USP requirements:

Oil- and Water-soluble Vitamins with Minerals Capsules USP—Preserve in tight, light-resistant containers. Contain one or more of the following oil-soluble vitamins: Vitamin A, Vitamin D as Ergocalciferol (Vitamin D_2) or Cholecalciferol (Vitamin D_3), Vitamin E, Phytonadione (Vitamin K_1), and Beta Carotene; one or more of the following water-soluble vitamins: Ascorbic Acid or its equivalent as Calcium Ascorbate or Sodium Ascorbate, Biotin, Cyanocobalamin, Folic Acid, Niacin or Niacinamide, Dexpanthenol or Panthenol, Pantothenic Acid (as Calcium Pantothenate or Racemic Calcium Pantothenate), Pyridoxine Hydrochloride, Riboflavin, and Thiamine Hydrochloride or Thiamine Mononitrate; and one mineral or more, furnishing one or more of the following elements in ionizable form: calcium, chromium, copper, fluorine, iodine, iron, magnesium, manganese, molybdenum, phosphorus, potassium, selenium, and zinc, derived from substances generally recognized as safe. May contain other labeled added substances that are generally recognized as safe, in amounts that are unobjectionable. The label states that the product is Oil- and Water-soluble Vitamins with Minerals Capsules. The label states also the quantity of each vitamin and mineral per dosage unit and where necessary the chemical form in which a vitamin is present and states

also the salt form of the mineral used as the source of each element. Where the product contains vitamin E, the label indicates whether it is the *d*- or *dl*- form. Where more than one *Assay* method is given for a particular vitamin or mineral, the labeling states with which *Assay* method the product complies only if *Method 1* is not used. Contain the labeled amounts of vitamin A as retinol or esters of retinol in the form of retinyl acetate or retinyl palmitate, vitamin D as ergocalciferol or cholecalciferol, vitamin E as alpha tocopherol or alpha tocopheryl acetate or alpha tocopheryl acid succinate, phytonadione, and beta carotene, within −10% to +65%; the labeled amounts of ascorbic acid or its salts as calcium ascorbate or sodium ascorbate, biotin, cyanocobalamin, folic acid, niacin or niacinamide, dexpanthenol or panthenol, calcium pantothenate, pyridoxine hydrochloride, riboflavin, and thiamine as thiamine hydrochloride or thiamine mononitrate, within −10% to +50%; the labeled amounts of calcium, copper, iron, magnesium, manganese, phosphorus, potassium, and zinc, within −10% to +25%; and the labeled amounts of chromium, fluorine, iodine, molybdenum, and selenium, within −10% to +100%. Meet the requirements for Microbial limits, Disintegration and dissolution, and Weight variation.

Oil- and Water-soluble Vitamins with Minerals Oral Solution USP—Preserve in tight, light-resistant containers, under an inert gas or with a minimum of headspace. Contains one or more of the following oil-soluble vitamins: Vitamin A, Vitamin D as Ergocalciferol (Vitamin D$_2$) or Cholecalciferol (Vitamin D$_3$), and Vitamin E; one or more of the following water-soluble vitamins: Ascorbic Acid or its equivalent as Calcium Ascorbate or Sodium Ascorbate, Biotin, Cyanocobalamin, Niacin or Niacinamide, Dexpanthenol or Panthenol, Pantothenic Acid (as Calcium Pantothenate or Racemic Calcium Pantothenate), Pyridoxine Hydrochloride, Riboflavin or Riboflavin-5′-Phosphate Sodium, and Thiamine Hydrochloride or Thiamine Mononitrate; and one or more minerals, derived from substances generally recognized as safe, furnishing one or more of the following elements in ionizable form: chromium, fluorine, iodine, iron, magnesium, manganese, molybdenum, and zinc. The label states that the product is Oil- and Water-soluble Vitamins with Minerals Oral Solution. The label states the quantity of each vitamin and mineral in a given volume of the Oral Solution and, where necessary, the chemical form in which a vitamin is present, and states also the salt form of the mineral used as the source of each element. Where the product contains vitamin E, the label indicates whether it is the *d*- or *dl*- form. Where the product is labeled to contain panthenol, the label states the equivalent content of dexpanthenol. Where more than one *Assay* method is given for a particular vitamin or mineral the labeling states with which *Assay* method the product complies only if *Method 1* is not used. Contains the labeled amounts of vitamin A as retinol or esters of retinol in the form of retinyl acetate or retinyl palmitate, vitamin D as ergocalciferol or cholecalciferol, vitamin E as alpha tocopherol or alpha tocopheryl acetate or alpha tocopheryl acid succinate, ascorbic acid or its salts as calcium ascorbate or sodium ascorbate, and thiamine as thiamine hydrochloride or thiamine mononitrate, within −10% to +100%; the labeled amounts of biotin, niacin or niacinamide, dexpanthnol or panthenol, calcium pantothenate, pyridoxine hydrochloride, and riboflavin or riboflavin-5′-phosphate sodium, within −10% to +50%; the labeled amount of cyanocobalamin, within −10% to +350%; and the labeled amounts of chromium, fluorine, iodine, iron, magnesium, manganese, molybdenum, and zinc, within −10% to +25%. Meets the requirements for Microbial limits and Alcohol content (if present, within −10% to +20% of labeled amount).

Oil- and Water-soluble Vitamins with Minerals Tablets USP—Preserve in tight, light-resistant containers. Contain one or more of the following oil-soluble vitamins: Vitamin A, Vita-

min D as Ergocalciferol (Vitamin D$_2$) or Cholecalciferol (Vitamin D$_3$), Vitamin E, Phytonadione (Vitamin K$_1$), and Beta Carotene; one or more of the following water-soluble vitamins: Ascorbic Acid or its equivalent as Calcium Ascorbate or Sodium Ascorbate, Biotin, Cyanocobalamin, Folic Acid, Niacin or Niacinamide, Pantothenic Acid (as Calcium Pantothenate or Racemic Calcium Pantothenate), Pyridoxine Hydrochloride, Riboflavin, and Thiamine Hydrochloride or Thiamine Mononitrate; and one or more minerals derived from substances generally recognized as safe, furnishing one or more of the following elements in ionizable form: calcium, chromium, copper, fluorine, iodine, iron, magnesium, manganese, molybdenum, phosphorus, potassium, selenium, and zinc. May contain other labeled added substances that are generally recognized as safe, in amounts that are unobjectionable. The label states that the product is Oil- and Water-soluble Vitamins with Minerals Tablets. The label states also the quantity of each vitamin and mineral per dosage unit and where necessary the chemical form in which a vitamin is present and states also the salt form of the mineral used as the source of each element. Where the product contains vitamin E, the label indicates whether it is the *d*- or *dl*- form. Where more than one *Assay* method is given for a particular vitamin, the labeling states with which *Assay* method the product complies only if *Method 1* is not used. Contain the labeled amounts of Vitamin A as retinol or esters of retinol in the form of retinyl acetate or retinyl palmitate, vitamin D as ergocalciferol or cholecalciferol, Vitamin E as alpha tocopherol or alpha tocopheryl acetate or alpha tocopheryl acid succinate, phytonadione, and beta carotene, within −10% to +65%; the labeled amounts of ascorbic acid or its salts as calcium ascorbate or sodium ascorbate, biotin, cyanocobalamin, folic acid, niacin or niacinamide, calcium pantothenate, pyridoxine hydrochloride, riboflavin, and thiamine as thiamine hydrochloride or thiamine mononitrate, within −10% to +50%; the labeled amounts of calcium, copper, iron, manganese, magnesium, phosphorus, potassium, and zinc, within −10% to +25%; and the labeled amounts of chromium, fluorine, iodine, molybdenum, and selenium, within −10% to +100%. Meet the requirements for Microbial limits, Disintegration and dissolution, and Weight variation.

WATER-SOLUBLE VITAMINS

For *Ascorbic Acid* or *Sodium Ascorbate* or *Calcium Ascorbate, Biotin, Cyanocobalamin, Folic Acid, Niacin* or *Niacinamide, Dexpanthenol* or *Panthenol, Pantothenic Acid* (Calcium Pantothenate or Racemic Calcium Pantothenate), *Pyridoxine, Riboflavin,* and *Thiamine*—See individual listings for chemistry information.

USP requirements:

Water-soluble Vitamins Capsules USP—Preserve in tight, light-resistant containers. Contain two or more of the following water-soluble vitamins: Ascorbic Acid or its equivalent as Sodium Ascorbate or Calcium Ascorbate, Biotin, Cyanocobalamin, Folic Acid, Niacin or Niacinamide, Dexpanthenol or Panthenol, Pantothenic Acid (as Calcium Pantothenate or Racemic Calcium Pantothenate), Pyridoxine Hydrochloride, Riboflavin, and Thiamine Hydrochloride or Thiamine Mononitrate. Do not contain any form of Vitamins A, D, E, K, or Beta Carotene. Do not contain any minerals for which nutritional value is claimed. May contain other labeled added substances in amounts that are unobjectionable. The label states that the product is Water-soluble Vitamins Capsules. The label states also the quantity of each vitamin in terms of metric units per dosage unit and where necessary the salt form in which it is

present. Where more than one *Assay* method is given for a particular vitamin, the labeling states which *Assay* method is used only if *Method I* is not used. Where products are labeled to contain panthenol, the label states the equivalent content of dexpanthenol. Contain the labeled amounts of ascorbic acid, biotin, cyanocobalamin, folic acid, niacin or niacinamide, dexpanthenol or panthenol, calcium pantothenate, pyridoxine hydrochloride, riboflavin, and thiamine as the hydrochloride or mononitrate, within −10% to +50%. Meet the requirements for Microbial limits, Disintegration and dissolution, and Weight variation.

Water-soluble Vitamins Tablets USP—Preserve in tight, light-resistant containers. Contain two or more of the following water-soluble vitamins: Ascorbic Acid or its equivalent as Sodium Ascorbate or Calcium Ascorbate, Biotin, Cyanocobalamin, Folic Acid, Niacin or Niacinamide, Pantothenic Acid (as Calcium Pantothenate or Racemic Calcium Pantothenate), Pyridoxine Hydrochloride, Riboflavin, and Thiamine Hydrochloride or Thiamine Mononitrate. Do not contain any form of Vitamins A, D, E, K, or Beta Carotene. Do not contain any minerals for which nutritional value is claimed. May contain other labeled added substances in amounts that are unobjectionable. The label states that the product is Water-soluble Vitamins Tablets. The label states also the quantity of each vitamin in terms of metric units per dosage unit and where necessary the salt form in which it is present. Where more than one *Assay* method is given for a particular vitamin, the labeling states which *Assay* method is used only if *Method I* is not used. Contain the labeled amounts of ascorbic acid or its equivalent as sodium ascorbate or calcium ascorbate, biotin, thiamine as the hydrochloride or mononitrate, cyanocobalamin, folic acid, niacin or niacinamide, calcium pantothenate, pyridoxine hydrochloride, and riboflavin, within −10% to +50%. Meet the requirements for Microbial limits, Disintegration and dissolution, and Weight variation.

WATER-SOLUBLE VITAMINS WITH MINERALS

USP requirements:

Water-soluble Vitamins with Minerals Capsules USP—Preserve in tight, light-resistant containers. Contain one or more of the following water-soluble vitamins: Ascorbic Acid or its equivalent as Calcium Ascorbate or Sodium Ascorbate, Biotin, Cyanocobalamin, Folic Acid, Niacin or Niacinamide, Dexpanthenol or Panthenol, Pantothenic Acid (as Calcium Pantothenate or Racemic Calcium Pantothenate), Pyridoxine Hydrochloride, Riboflavin, and Thiamine Hydrochloride or Thiamine Mononitrate; and one mineral or more, furnishing one or more of the following elements in ionizable form: calcium, chromium, copper, fluorine, iodine, iron, magnesium, manganese, molybdenum, phosphorus, potassium, selenium, and zinc, derived from substances generally recognized as safe. Do not contain any form of Vitamins A, D, E, or K, or Beta Carotene. May contain other labeled added substances that are generally recognized as safe, in amounts that are unobjectionable. The label states that the product is Water-soluble Vitamins with Minerals Capsules. The label states also the quantity of each vitamin and mineral in terms of metric units per dosage unit and where necessary the chemical form in which a vitamin is present and states also the salt form of the mineral used as the source of each element. Where more than one *Assay* method is given for a particular vitamin or mineral, the labeling states with which *Assay* method the product complies only if *Method 1* is not used. Contain the labeled amounts of ascorbic acid or its salts as calcium ascorbate or sodium ascorbate, biotin, cyanocobalamin, folic acid, niacin or niacinamide, dexpanthenol or panthenol, calcium pantothenate,

pyridoxine hydrochloride, riboflavin, and thiamine as thiamine hydrochoride or thiamine mononitrate, within −10% to +50%; the labeled amounts of calcium, copper, iron, magnesium, manganese, phosphorus, potassium, and zinc, within −10% to +25%; and the labeled amounts of chromium, fluorine, iodine, molybdenum, and selenium, within −10% to +100%. Meet the requirements for Microbial limits, Disintegration and dissolution, and Weight variation.

Water-soluble Vitamins with Minerals Oral Solution USP—Preserve in tight, light-resistant containers, under an inert gas or with a minimum of headspace. Contains one or more of the following water-soluble vitamins: Cyanocobalamin, Niacin or Niacinamide, Dexpanthenol or Panthenol, Pantothenic Acid (as Calcium Pantothenate or Racemic Calcium Pantothenate), Pyridoxine Hydrochloride, Riboflavin or Riboflavin-5′-Phosphate Sodium, and Thiamine Hydrochloride or Thiamine Mononitrate; and one or more minerals derived from substances generally recognized as safe, furnishing one or more of the following elements in ionizable form: iodine, iron, magnesium, manganese, and zinc. The label states that the product is Water-soluble Vitamins with Minerals Oral Solution. The label states the quantity of each vitamin and mineral present in terms of metric units in a given volume of the Oral Solution and, where necessary, the chemical form in which a vitamin is present, and states also the salt form of the mineral used as the source of each element. Where products are labeled to contain panthenol, the label states the equivalent content of dexpanthenol. Where more than one *Assay* method is given for a particular vitamin or mineral, the labeling states with which *Assay* method the product complies only if *Method 1* is not used. Contains the labeled amount of cyanocobalamin, within −10% to +350%; the labeled amount of thiamine as thiamine hydrochoride or thiamine mononitrate, within −10% to +150%; the labeled amounts of niacin or niacinamide, dexpanthenol or panthenol, calcium pantothenate, pyridoxine hydrochloride, and riboflavin or riboflavin-5′-phosphate sodium, within −10% to +50%; and the labeled amounts of iodine, iron, magnesium, manganese, and zinc, within −10% to +25%. Meets the requirements for Microbial limits and Alcohol content (if present, within −10% to +20% of the labeled amount).

Water-soluble Vitamins with Minerals Tablets USP—Preserve in tight, light-resistant containers. Contain one or more of the following water-soluble vitamins: Ascorbic Acid or its equivalent as Calcium Ascorbate or Sodium Ascorbate, Biotin, Cyanocobalamin, Folic Acid, Niacin or Niacinamide, Pantothenic Acid (as Calcium Pantothenate or Racemic Calcium Pantothenate), Pyridoxine Hydrochloride, Riboflavin, and Thiamine Hydrochloride or Thiamine Mononitrate; and one or more minerals derived from substances generally recognized as safe, furnishing one or more of the following elements in ionizable form: calcium, chromium, copper, fluorine, iodine, iron, magnesium, manganese, molybdenum, phosphorus, potassium, selenium, and zinc. Do not contain any form of Vitamins A, D, E, K, or Beta Carotene. May contain other labeled added substances that are generally recognized as safe, in amounts that are unobjectionable. The label states that the product is Water-soluble Vitamins with Minerals Tablets. The label states also the quantity of each vitamin and mineral in terms of metric units per dosage unit and where necessary the chemical form in which a vitamin is present and states also the salt form of the mineral used as the source of each element. Where more than one *Assay* method is given for a particular vitamin, the labeling states which *Assay* method is used only if *Method 1* is not used. Contain the labeled amounts of ascorbic acid or its salts as calcium ascorbate or sodium ascorbate, biotin, cyanocobalamin, folic acid, niacin or niacinamide, calcium pantothenate, pyridoxine hydrochloride, riboflavin, and thiamine as thiamine hydrochoride or thiamine mononitrate, within −10% to +50%;

the labeled amounts of calcium, copper, iron, manganese, magnesium, phosphorus, potassium, and zinc, within −10% to +25%; and the labeled amounts of chromium, fluorine, iodine, molybdenum, and selenium, within −10% to +100%. Meet the requirements for Microbial limits, Disintegration and dissolution, and Weight variation.

WARFARIN

Chemical group: Coumarin derivative.

Chemical name: Warfarin sodium—2*H*-1-Benzopyran-2-one, 4-hydroxy-3-(3-oxo-1-phenylbutyl)-, sodium salt.

Molecular formula: Warfarin sodium—$C_{19}H_{15}NaO_4$.

Molecular weight: Warfarin sodium—330.31.

Description: Warfarin Sodium USP—White, odorless, amorphous or crystalline powder. Is discolored by light.

Solubility: Warfarin Sodium USP—Very soluble in water; freely soluble in alcohol; very slightly soluble in chloroform and in ether.

USP requirements:
Warfarin Sodium USP—Preserve in well-closed, light-resistant containers. An amorphous solid or a crystalline clathrate. Label it to indicate whether it is the amorphous or the crystalline form. The clathrate form consists principally of warfarin sodium and isopropyl alcohol, in a 2:1 molecular ratio; contains not less than 8.0% and not more than 8.5% of isopropyl alcohol. Contains not less than 97.0% and not more than 102.0% of warfarin sodium, calculated on the anhydrous basis for the amorphous form or on the anhydrous and isopropyl alcohol-free basis for the crystalline form. Meets the requirements for Identification, pH (7.2–8.3, in a solution [1 in 100]), Water (not more than 4.5% for the amorphous form and not more than 0.3% for the crystalline clathrate form), Absorbance in alkaline solution, Heavy metals (not more than 0.001%), Isopropyl alcohol content, Chromatographic purity, and Organic volatile impurities.
Warfarin Sodium for Injection USP—Preserve in light-resistant Containers for Sterile Solids. A sterile, freeze-dried mixture of Warfarin Sodium and suitable added substances. Contains the labeled amount, within ±5%. Meets the requirements for Completeness of solution, Constituted solution, Bacterial endotoxins, and Water (not more than 4.5%), for Identification tests A and B, pH, and Heavy metals under Warfarin Sodium, and for Sterility tests, Uniform-ity of dosage units, and Labeling under Injections.
Warfarin Sodium Tablets USP—Preserve in tight, light-resistant containers. Contain the labeled amount, within ±5%. Meet the requirements for Identification, Dissolution (80% in 30 minutes in water in Apparatus 2 at 50 rpm), and Uniformity of dosage units.

WATER

Chemical name: Purified water—Water.

Molecular formula: Purified water—H_2O.

Molecular weight: Purified water—18.02.

Description:
Water for Injection USP—Clear, colorless, odorless liquid.
 NF category: Solvent.
Bacteriostatic Water for Injection USP—Clear, colorless liquid, odorless, or having the odor of the antimicrobial substance.

 NF category: Vehicle (sterile).
Sterile Water for Inhalation USP—Clear, colorless solution.
Sterile Water for Injection USP—Clear, colorless, odorless liquid.
 NF category: Solvent.
Sterile Water for Irrigation USP—Clear, colorless, odorless liquid.
 NF category: Solvent.
Purified Water USP—Clear, colorless, odorless liquid.
 NF category: Solvent.

USP requirements:
Water for Injection USP—It is water purified by distillation or by other suitable process. Prepared from water complying with the U.S. Environmental Protection Agency National Primary Drinking Water Regulations or comparable regulations of the European Union or Japan. Contains no added substance. Meets the requirements for Bacterial endotoxins, Total organic carbon, and Water conductivity.
 Note: Water for Injection is intended for use in the preparation of parenteral solutions. Where used for the preparation of parenteral solutions subject to final sterilization, use suitable means to minimize microbial growth, or first render the Water for Injection sterile and thereafter protect it from microbial contamination. For parenteral solutions that are prepared under aseptic conditions and are not sterilized by appropriate filtration or in the final container, first render the Water for Injection sterile and, thereafter, protect it from microbial contamination. The tests for Total organic carbon and Conductivity apply to Water for Injection produced on site for use in manufacturing. Water for Injection packaged in bulk for commercial use elsewhere meets the requirements of the test for Bacterial endotoxin as indicated below and the requirements of all the tests under Sterile Purified Water, except Labeling.
Bacteriostatic Water for Injection USP—Preserve in single-dose or in multiple-dose glass or plastic containers. Glass containers are preferably of Type I or Type II glass, of not larger than 30-mL size. It is prepared from Water for Injection that is sterilized and suitably packaged, containing one or more suitable antimicrobial agents. Label it to indicate the name(s) and proportion(s) of the added antimicrobial agent(s). Label it also to include the statement, "**NOT FOR USE IN NEWBORNS**," in boldface capital letters on the label immediately under the official name, printed in a contrasting color, preferably red. Alternatively, the statement may be placed prominently elsewhere on the label if the statement is enclosed within a box. Meets the requirements for Antimicrobial agent(s), Bacterial endotoxins, and pH (4.5–7.0, in a solution containing 0.3 mL of saturated potassium chloride solution per 100 mL), for Particulate matter under Sterile Water for Injection, and for all of the tests under Sterile Purified Water, except pH, Ammonia, Chloride, and Oxidizable substances.
 Note: Use Bacteriostatic Water for Injection with due regard for the compatibility of the antimicrobial agent or agents it contains with the particular medicinal substance that is to be dissolved or diluted.
Sterile Water for Inhalation USP—Preserve in glass or plastic containers. Glass containers are preferably of Type I or Type II glass. It is prepared from Water for Injection that is sterilized and suitably packaged. Contains no antimicrobial agents, except where used in humidifiers or other similar devices and where liable to contamination over a period of time, or other added substances. Label it to indicate that it is for inhalation therapy only and that it is not for parenteral administration. Meets the requirements for Bacterial endotoxins and pH (4.5–7.5. in a solution containing 0.3 mL of saturated potassium chloride solution per 100 mL), and for all of the tests under Sterile Purified Water except pH.

Note: Do not use Sterile Water for Inhalation for parenteral administration or for other sterile compendial dosage forms.

Sterile Water for Injection USP—Preserve in single-dose glass or plastic containers, of not larger than 1-liter size. Glass containers are preferably of Type I or Type II glass. It is prepared from Water for Injection that is sterilized and suitably packaged. Contains no antimicrobial agent or other added substance. Label it to indicate that no antimicrobial or other substance has been added, and that it is not suitable for intravascular injection without its first having been made approximately isotonic by the addition of a suitable solute. Meets the requirements for Bacterial endotoxins and Particulate matter, and for all of the tests under Sterile Purified Water.

Sterile Water for Irrigation USP—Preserve in single-dose glass or plastic containers. Glass containers are preferably of Type I or Type II glass. The container may contain a volume of more than 1 liter, and may be designed to empty rapidly. It is prepared from Water for Injection that is sterilized and suitably packaged. Contains no antimicrobial agent or other added substance. Label it to indicate that no antimicrobial or other substance has been added. The designations "For irrigation only" and "Not for injection" appear prominently on the label. Meets the requirements of all of the tests under Sterile Purified Water and for Bacterial endotoxins under Water for Injection.

Purified Water USP—It is water obtained by a suitable process. Prepared from water complying with the U.S. Environmental Protection Agency National Primary Drinking Water Regulations or comparable regulations of the European Union or Japan. Contains no added substance. Meets the requirements for Total organic carbon and Water conductivity.

Note: Purified Water is intended for use as an ingredient of official preparations and in tests and assays unless otherwise specified (see Water in Ingredients and Processes and in Tests and Assays under General Notices and Requirements). Where used for sterile dosage forms, other than for parenteral administration, process the article to meet the requirements under Sterility tests, or first render the Purified Water sterile and thereafter protect it from microbial contamination. Do not use Purified Water in preparations intended for parenteral administration. For such purposes use Water for Injection, Bacteriostatic Water for Injection, or Sterile Water for Injection. The tests for Total organic carbon and Conductivity apply to Purified Water produced on site for use as an ingredient of official preparations and in tests and assays. Purified Water packaged in bulk for commercial use elsewhere meets the requirements of all of the tests under Sterile Purified Water, except Labeling and Sterility.

Sterile Purified Water USP—Preserve in suitable, tight containers. It is Purified Water sterilized and suitably packaged. Label it to indicate the method of preparation and that it is not for parenteral administration. Meets the requirements for Sterility, pH (5.0–7.0), Ammonia, Calcium, Carbon dioxide, Chloride, Sulfate, and Oxidizable substances.

Note: Do not use Sterile Purified Water in preparations intended for parenteral administration. For such purposes use Water for Injection, Bacteriostatic Water for Injection, or Sterile Water for Injection.

CARNAUBA WAX

Description: Carnauba Wax NF—Light brown to pale yellow, moderately coarse powder or flakes, possessing a characteristic bland odor, and free from rancidity. Specific gravity is about 0.99.

NF category: Coating agent.

Solubility: Carnauba Wax NF—Insoluble in water; soluble in warm chloroform and in warm toluene; slightly soluble in boiling alcohol.

NF requirements: Carnauba Wax NF—Preserve in well-closed containers. Obtained from the leaves of *Copernicia cerifera* Mart. (Fam. Palmae). Meets the requirements for Melting range (80–86 °C), Residue on ignition (not more than 0.25%), Heavy metals (not more than 20 mcg per gram), Acid value (2–7), Saponification value (78–95), and Organic volatile impurities.

EMULSIFYING WAX

Description: Emulsifying Wax NF—Creamy white, wax-like solid, having a mild characteristic odor.

NF category: Emulsifying and/or solubilizing agent; stiffening agent.

Solubility: Emulsifying Wax NF—Insoluble in water; freely soluble in ether, in chloroform, in most hydrocarbon solvents, and in aerosol propellants; soluble in alcohol.

NF requirements: Emulsifying Wax NF—Preserve in well-closed containers. A waxy solid prepared from Cetostearyl Alcohol containing a polyoxyethylene derivative of a fatty acid ester of sorbitan. Meets the requirements for Melting range (50–54 °C), pH (5.5–7.0), Hydroxyl value (178–192), Iodine value (not more than 3.5), and Saponification value (not more than 14).

MICROCRYSTALLINE WAX

Description: Microcrystalline Wax NF—White or cream-colored, odorless, waxy solid.

NF category: Coating agent.

Solubility: Microcrystalline Wax NF—Insoluble in water; sparingly soluble in dehydrated alcohol; soluble in chloroform, in ether, in volatile oils, and in most warm fixed oils.

NF requirements: Microcrystalline Wax NF—Preserve in tight containers. A mixture of straight-chain, branched-chain, and cyclic hydrocarbons, obtained by solvent fractionation of the still bottom fraction of petroleum by suitable dewaxing or deoiling means. Label it to indicate the name and proportion of any added stabilizer. Meets the requirements for Color, Melting range (54–102 °C), Consistency (0.3–10.0 mm), Acidity, Alkalinity, Residue on ignition (not more than 0.1%), Organic acids, Fixed oils, fats, and rosin, and Organic volatile impurities.

WHITE WAX

Description: White Wax NF—Yellowish white solid, somewhat translucent in thin layers. Has a faint, characteristic odor, and is free from rancidity. Specific gravity is about 0.95.

NF category: Stiffening agent.

Solubility: White Wax NF—Insoluble in water; sparingly soluble in cold alcohol. Boiling alcohol dissolves the cerotic acid and a portion of the myricin, which are constituents of White Wax.

Completely soluble in chloroform, in ether, and in fixed and volatile oils. Partly soluble in cold carbon disulfide, and completely soluble in this liquid at about 30 °C.

NF requirements: White Wax NF—Preserve in well-closed containers. The product of bleaching and purifying Yellow Wax that is obtained from the honeycomb of the bee (*Apis mellifera* Linné [Fam. Apidae]) and that meets the requirements for the Saponification cloud test. Meets the requirements for Melting range (62–65 °C), Saponification cloud test, Fats or fatty acids, Japan wax, rosin, and soap, Acid value (17–24), and Ester value (72–79).

YELLOW WAX

Description: Yellow Wax NF—Solid varying in color from yellow to grayish brown. Has an agreeable, honey-like odor. Somewhat brittle when cold, and presents a dull, granular, noncrystalline fracture when broken. It becomes pliable from the heat of the hand. Specific gravity is about 0.95.

NF category: Stiffening agent.

Solubility: Yellow Wax NF—Insoluble in water; sparingly soluble in cold alcohol. Boiling alcohol dissolves the cerotic acid and a portion of the myricin, which are constituents of Yellow Wax. Completely soluble in chloroform, in ether, in fixed oils, and in volatile oils. Partly soluble in cold carbon disulfide, and completely soluble in this liquid at about 30 °C.

NF requirements: Yellow Wax NF—Preserve in well-closed containers. The purified wax from the honeycomb of the bee (*Apis mellifera* Linné [Fam. Apidae]). Meets the requirements for Melting range, Saponification cloud test, Fats or fatty acids, Japan wax, rosin, and soap, Acid value, and Ester value under White Wax.

Note: To meet specifications of this monograph, the crude beeswax used to prepare Yellow Wax conforms to the Saponification cloud test.

WHEAT BRAN

Description: Light tan powder having a characteristic aroma. Available in a variety of particle sizes depending upon the degree of milling to which it is subjected. Color and flavor development variable, depending on the extent to which it is heat-stabilized.

Solubility: Practically insoluble in cold water and in alcohol.

USP requirements: Wheat Bran USP—Preserve in well-closed containers, secured against insect attack. It is the outer fraction of the cereal grain comprising the pericarp, seed coat (testa), nucellar tissue, and aleuronic layer, and is derived from *Triticum aestivum* Linné, *T. compactum* Host, *T. durum* Desf., and other common einkorn and emmer wheat cultivars. Obtained by the milling and processing of the whole wheat grain meeting U.S. Standards for Number 1 wheat (7 CFR 810.2201). Contains not less than 36.0% of dietary fiber. Meets the requirements for Identification, Microbial limits, Water (not more than 12%), Total ash (not more than 8%), Heavy metals (not more than 0.004%), Absence of peroxidase activity (no color change is observed, indicating the absence of peroxidase activity), Limit of fat (not more than 6%), Limit of insect infestation (not more than 25 insect fragments), Limit of protein (not more than 18.5%), and content of total dietary fiber (not less than 36.0%).

WHITE LOTION

USP requirements: White Lotion USP—Dispense in tight containers.

Prepare White Lotion as follows: 40 grams of Zinc Sulfate, 40 grams of Sulfurated Potash, and a sufficient quantity of Purified Water to make 1000 mL. Dissolve the Zinc Sulfate and the Sulfurated Potash separately, each in 450 mL of Purified Water, and filter each solution. Add the sulfurated potash solution slowly to the zinc sulfate solution with constant stirring. Then add the required amount of purified water, and mix.

Note: Prepare the Lotion fresh, and shake it thoroughly before dispensing.

WITCH HAZEL

USP requirements: Witch Hazel USP—Preserve in tight containers, and avoid exposure to excessive heat. A clear, colorless distillate prepared from recently cut and partially dried dormant twigs of *Hamamelis virginiana* Linné.

Prepare Witch Hazel as follows. Macerate a weighed amount of the twigs for about 24 hours in about twice their weight of water, then distil until not less than 800 mL and not more than 850 mL of clear, colorless distillate is obtained from each 1000 grams of the twigs taken. Add 150 mL of Alcohol to each 850 mL of distillate, and mix thoroughly.

Meets the requirements for Specific gravity (0.979–0.983), pH (3.0–5.0), Nonvolatile residue (not more than 0.025%), Limit of tannins, and Alcohol content (14.0–15.0%).

XANTHAN GUM

Description: Xanthan Gum NF—Cream-colored powder. Its solutions in water are neutral to litmus.

NF category: Suspending and/or viscosity-increasing agent.

Solubility: Xanthan Gum NF—Soluble in hot or cold water.

NF requirements:

Xanthan Gum NF—Preserve in well-closed containers. A high molecular weight polysaccharide gum produced by a pure-culture fermentation of a carbohydrate with *Xanthomonas campestris*, then purified by recovery with Isopropyl Alcohol, dried, and milled. Contains D-glucose and D-mannose as the dominant hexose units, along with D-glucuronic acid, and is prepared as the sodium, potassium, or calcium salt. Yields not less than 4.2% and not more than 5.0% of carbon dioxide, calculated on the dried basis, corresponding to not less than 91.0% and not more than 108.0% of Xanthan Gum. Meets the requirements for Identification, Viscosity (not less than 600 centipoises at 24 °C), Microbial limits, Loss on drying (not more than 15.0%), Ash (6.5–16.0%, calculated on the dried basis), Arsenic (not more than 3 ppm), Heavy metals (not more than 0.003%), Lead (not more than 5 ppm), Isopropyl alcohol (not more than 0.075%), Pyruvic acid (not less than 1.5%), and Organic volatile impurities.

Xanthan Gum Solution NF—Preserve in tight, light-resistant containers, and store at controlled room temperature. Label it to state, as part of the official title, the percentage content of xanthan gum.

Prepare Xanthan Gum Solution of the designated percentage strength as follows: 100 mg of Xanthan Gum for 0.1% Solution or 1.0 gram of Xanthan Gum for 1.0% Solution, 100 mg of Methylparaben, 20 mg of Propylparaben, and Purified Water, a sufficient quantity to make 100 mL. Dissolve an accurately weighed quantity of Propylparaben in Purified Water with heating to about 50° and stirring. Cool,

and dilute quantitatively, and stepwise if necessary, with Purified Water to obtain 90 mL of solution containing 20 mg of Propylparaben. Heat to about 50°, and add the Methylparaben, with stirring, to dissolve. Cool, stir with a blender, slowly sift the Xanthan Gum into the vortex, and continue to blend for 2 minutes after the Xanthan Gum has been added. Add 10 mL of Purified Water, and blend for 5 minutes. Allow to stand for 1 hour for excess foam to subside, and remove most of the remaining foam by passing the solution through a strainer. Add Purified Water, if necessary, to make the final volume 100 mL, and stir. [Note—Depending on the volume needed and the equipment available, adjust the formula proportionally.]

Meets the requirement for Beyond-use date.

XENOGENEIC HEPATOCYTES

USP requirements: Xenogeneic Hepatocytes Liver Assist System—Not in *USP–NF*.

XENON XE 127

Description: Xenon Xe 127 USP—Clear, colorless gas.

USP requirements: Xenon Xe 127 USP—Preserve in single-dose vials having leak-proof stoppers, at room temperature. The vials are enclosed in appropriate lead radiation shields. The vial content may be diluted with air and is packaged at atmospheric pressure. A gas suitable for inhalation in diagnostic studies. Xenon 127 is a radioactive nuclide that may be prepared from the bombardment of a cesium 133 target with high-energy protons. Label it to include the following: the name of the preparation; the container volume, megabecquerels (or millicuries) of ^{127}Xe per container; the amount of ^{127}Xe expressed as megabecquerels (or millicuries) per mL; the intended route of administration; recommended storage conditions; the date of calibration; the expiration date; the name, address, and batch number of the manufacturer; the statement "Caution—Radioactive Material"; and a radioactive symbol. The labeling contains a statement of radionuclide purity, identifies probable radionuclidic impurities, and indicates permissible quantities of each impurity. The labeling indicates that in making dosage calculations, correction is to be made for radioactive decay, and also indicates that the radioactive half-life of ^{127}Xe is 36.41 days. Contains the labeled amount of ^{127}Xe, within ±15%, at the calibration date indicated in the labeling. Meets the requirements for Radionuclide identification and Radionuclidic purity.

XENON XE 133

Chemical name: Xenon, isotope of mass 133.

Description: Xenon Xe 133 Injection USP—Clear, colorless solution.

USP requirements:

Xenon Xe 133 USP—Preserve in single-dose or in multiple-dose vials having leak-proof stoppers, at room temperature. A gas suitable for inhalation in diagnostic studies. Xenon 133 is a radioactive nuclide that may be prepared from the fission of uranium 235. Contains the labeled amount of ^{133}Xe, within ±15%, at the date and time indicated in the labeling. Meets the requirements for Labeling (except for the information specified for Labeling under Injections), for

Radionuclide identification, and for Radionuclidic purity under Xenon 133 Injection (except to determine the radioactivity in megabecquerels [or millicuries] per container).

Xenon Xe 133 Injection USP—Preserve in single-dose containers that are totally filled, so that any air present occupies not more than 0.5% of the total volume of the container. Store at a temperature between 2 and 8 °C. If there is free space above the solution, a significant amount of the xenon 133 is present in the gaseous phase. Glass containers may darken under the effects of radiation. A sterile, isotonic solution of Xenon 133 in Sodium Chloride Injection suitable for intravenous administration. Xenon 133 is a radioactive nuclide prepared from the fission of uranium 235. Label it to include the following, in addition to the information specified for Labeling under Injections: the time and date of calibration; the amount of xenon 133 expressed as total megabecquerels (or microcuries or millicuries), and concentration as megabecquerels (or microcuries or millicuries), per mL at the time of calibration; the expiration date; the name and amount of any added bacteriostatic agent; and the statement, "Caution—Radioactive Material." The labeling indicates that in making dosage calculations, correction is to be made for radioactive decay, and also indicates that the radioactive half-life of ^{133}Xe is 5.24 days. Contains the labeled amount of Xenon 133, within ±10%, at the date and time stated on the label. Meets the requirements for Radionuclide identification, Bacterial endotoxins, pH (4.5–8.0), and Radionuclidic purity, and for Injections (except that the Injection may be distributed or dispensed prior to the completion of the test for Sterility, the latter test being started on the day of manufacture, and except that it is not subject to the recommendation on Volume in Container).

XYLAZINE

Chemical name:
Xylazine—4*H*-1,3-Thiazin-2-amine, *N*-(2,6-dimethylphenyl)-5,6-dihydro-.
Xylazine hydrochloride—4*H*-1,3-Thiazin-2-amine, *N*-(2,6-dimethylphenyl)-5,6-dihydro-, monohydrochloride.

Molecular formula:
Xylazine—$C_{12}H_{16}N_2S$.
Xylazine hydrochloride—$C_{12}H_{16}N_2S \cdot HCl$.

Molecular weight:
Xylazine—220.34.
Xylazine hydrochloride—256.80.

Description:
Xylazine USP—Colorless to white crystals.
Xylazine Hydrochloride USP—Colorless to white crystals.

Solubility:
Xylazine USP—Sparingly soluble in dilute acid, in acetone, and in chloroform; insoluble in dilute alkali.
Xylazine Hydrochloride USP—Sparingly soluble in dilute acid, in acetone, and in methanol; insoluble in dilute alkali.

USP requirements:
Xylazine USP—Preserve in tight containers. Where it is intended for veterinary use only, the label so states. Contains not less than 98.0% and not more than 102.0% of xylazine. Meets the requirements for Identification, Melting range (136°–142°), Loss on drying (not more than 0.5%), Residue on ignition (not more than 0.1%), Heavy metals (20 micrograms per gram), Limit of 3-amino-1-propanol (not more than 0.5%), Limit of acetone and isopropyl alcohol (not more than 0.02% of acetone and not more than 0.2% of isopropyl alcohol), and chromatographic purity (not more than 0.5% of any individual impurity, and the sum of all impurities not more than 1%).

Xylazine Injection USP—Preserve in single-dose or multiple-dose containers. A sterile solution of Xylazine in Water for Injection prepared with the aid of Hydrochloric Acid or a sterile solution of Xylazine Hydrochloride in Water for Injection. Where it is intended for veterinary use only, the label so states. Contains the equivalent of the labeled amount of xylazine, within ±10%. Meets the requirements for Identification, Bacterial endotoxins, Sterility, and pH (4.5–5.5), and for Injections.

Xylazine Hydrochloride USP—Preserve in tight containers. Where it is intended for veterinary use only, the label so states. Contains not less than 98.0% and not more than 102.0% of xylazine hydrochloride. Meets the requirements for Identification, Melting range (164°–168°), pH (4.0–6.0, in a solution [1 in 100]), Loss on drying (not more than 1.0%), Residue on ignition (not more than 0.1%), Heavy metals (20 micrograms per gram), and Chromatographic purity (the sum of the impurity not greater than 2.0%).

XYLITOL

Chemical name: Xylitol.

Molecular formula: $C_5H_{12}O_5$.

Molecular weight: 152.15.

Description: Xylitol NF—White crystals or crystalline powder. Crystalline xylitol has a melting range between 92 and 96 °C.

Solubility: Xylitol NF—One gram dissolves in about 0.65 mL of water. Sparingly soluble in alcohol.

NF requirements: Xylitol NF—Preserve in well-closed containers. Contains not less than 98.5% and not more than 101.0% of xylitol, calculated on the anhydrous basis. Meets the requirements for Identification, Water (not more than 0.5%), Residue on ignition (not more than 0.5%), Heavy metals (not more than 0.001%), Reducing sugars, Organic volatile impurities, and Limit of other polyols (not more than 2.0%).

XYLOMETAZOLINE

Chemical name: Xylometazoline hydrochloride—1*H*-Imidazole, 2-[[4-(1,1-dimethylethyl)-2,6-dimethylphenyl]methyl]-4,5-dihydro-, monohydrochloride.

Molecular formula: Xylometazoline hydrochloride—$C_{16}H_{24}N_2 \cdot$ HCl.

Molecular weight: Xylometazoline hydrochloride—280.84.

Description: Xylometazoline Hydrochloride USP—White to off-white, odorless, crystalline powder. Melts above 300 °C, with decomposition.

Solubility: Xylometazoline Hydrochloride USP—Soluble in water; freely soluble in alcohol; sparingly soluble in chloroform; practically insoluble in ether.

USP requirements:
Xylometazoline Hydrochloride USP—Preserve in tight, light-resistant containers. Contains not less than 99.0% and not more than 101.0% of xylometazoline hydrochloride, calculated on the dried basis. Meets the requirements for Identification, pH (5.0–6.6, in a solution [1 in 20]), Loss on drying (not more than 0.5%), Residue on ignition (not more than 0.1%), and Chromatographic purity.

Xylometazoline Hydrochloride Nasal Solution USP—Preserve in tight, light-resistant containers. An isotonic solution of Xylometazoline Hydrochloride in Water. Contains the labeled amount, within ±10%. Meets the requirements for Identification and pH (5.0–7.5).

XYLOSE

Chemical name: D-Xylose.

Molecular formula: $C_5H_{10}O_5$.

Molecular weight: 150.13.

Description: Xylose USP—Colorless needles or white, crystalline powder. Is odorless.

Solubility: Xylose USP—Very soluble in water; slightly soluble in alcohol.

USP requirements: Xylose USP—Preserve in tight containers at controlled room temperature. Contains not less than 98.0% and not more than 102.0% of xylose, calculated on the dried basis. Meets the requirements for Color of solution, Identification, Specific rotation (+18.2° to +19.4°), Loss on drying (not more than 0.1%), Residue on ignition (not more than 0.05%), Iron (not more than 5 ppm), Heavy metals (not more than 0.001%), Chromatographic purity, and Organic volatile impurities.

YELLOW FEVER VACCINE

Description: Yellow Fever Vaccine USP—Slightly dull, light-orange colored, flaky or crustlike, desiccated mass.

USP requirements: Yellow Fever Vaccine USP (for Injection)—Preserve in nitrogen-filled, flame-sealed ampuls or suitable stoppered vials at a temperature preferably below 0 °C but never above 5 °C, throughout the dating period. Preserve it during shipment in a suitable container adequately packed in solid carbon dioxide, or provided with other means of refrigeration, so as to insure a temperature constantly below 0 °C. The attenuated strain that has been tested in monkeys for viscerotropism, immunogenicity, and neurotropism, of living yellow fever virus selected for high antigenic activity and safety. Prepared by the culturing of the virus in the living embryos of chicken eggs, from which a suspension is prepared, processed with aseptic precautions, and finally dried from the frozen state. It is sterile and contains no human serum and no antimicrobial agent. Yellow Fever Vaccine is constituted, with Sodium Chloride Injection containing no antimicrobial agent, just prior to use. Label it to state that it is to be well shaken before use and that the constituted vaccine is to be used entirely or discarded within 1 hour of opening the container. Label it also to state that it is the living yellow fever vaccine virus prepared from chicken embryos and that the dose is the same for persons of all ages, but that it is not recommended for infants under six months of age. Meets the requirements of the specific mouse potency test in titer of mouse LD_{50} (quantity of virus estimated to produce fatal specific encephalitis in 50% of the mice) or the requirements for plaque-forming units in a suitable cell-culture system, such as a Vero cell system for which the relationship between mouse LD_{50} and plaque-forming units has been established, in which cell monolayers in 35 mm petri dishes are inoculated for a specified time with dilutions of Vaccine, after which the dilutions are replaced with 0.5% agarose-containing medium. Following adsorption and incubation for five days an overlay is added of the 0.5% agarose medium containing 1:50,000 neutral red and the plaques are counted on the sixth day following inoculation. Meets the requirement for Expiration date (not later than 1 year after the

date of issue from manufacturerã s cold storage [–20 °C, 1 year]). Conforms to the regulations of the U.S. Food and Drug Administration concerning biologics.

YOHIMBINE

Source: Yohimbine hydrochloride—Obtained from the principal alkaloid of the bark of the yohimbe tree.

Chemical name: Yohimbine hydrochloride—17 alpha-Hydroxy-20-alpha-yohimban-16-beta-carboxylic acid, methyl ester, hydrochloride.

Molecular formula: Yohimbine hydrochloride—$C_{21}H_{26}N_2O_3 \cdot HCl$.

Molecular weight: Yohimbine hydrochloride—390.91.

Description: Yohimbine Hydrochloride USP—White to yellow powder. Melts at about 295 °C, with decomposition.

Solubility: Yohimbine Hydrochloride USP—Slightly soluble in water and in alcohol; soluble in boiling water.

USP requirements:
Yohimbine Hydrochloride USP—Preserve in tight containers, and store at controlled room temperature. Where it is intended for veterinary use only, it is so labeled. Contains not less than 98.0% and not more than 102.0% of yohimbine hydrochloride, calculated on the dried basis. Meets the requirements for Identification, Specific rotation (100–105 °C), Loss on drying (not more than 1.0%), and Chromatographic purity.
Yohimbine Hydrochloride Tablets—Not in *USP–NF*.
Yohimbine Injection USP—Preserve in single-dose or multi-dose Containers for Injections as described for Injections, and store at controlled room temperature. It is a sterile solution of Yohimbine Hydrochloride in Water for Injection. Where it is intended for veterinary use only, it is so labeled. Contains the labeled amount of yohimbine, within ±10%. Meets the requirements for Identification, Bacterial endotoxins, Sterility, and pH (3.7–4.3), and for Injections.

ZAFIRLUKAST

Chemical name: Carbamic acid, [3-[[2-methoxy-4-[[[2-methyl-phenyl)sulfonyl]amino]carbonyl]phenyl]methyl]-1-methyl-1H-indol-5-yl], cyclopentyl ester.

Molecular formula: $C_{31}H_{33}N_3O_6S$.

Molecular weight: 575.68.

Description: Fine white to pale yellow amorphous powder.

Solubility: Practically insoluble in water; slightly soluble in methanol; freely soluble in tetrahydrofuran, in dimethylsulfoxide, and in acetone.

USP requirements: Zafirlukast Tablets—Not in *USP–NF*.

ZALCITABINE

Chemical name: Cytidine, 2′,3′-dideoxy-.

Molecular formula: $C_9H_{13}N_3O_3$.

Molecular weight: 211.22.

Description: Zalcitabine USP—White to off-white crystalline powder.

Solubility: Zalcitabine USP—Soluble in water and in methanol; sparingly soluble in alcohol, in acetonitrile, in chloroform, and in methylene chloride; slightly soluble in cyclohexane.

USP requirements:
Zalcitabine USP—Preserve in tight, light-resistant containers. Contains not less than 98.0% and not more than 102.0%, calculated on the dried basis. Meets the requirements for Identification, Specific rotation (+73° to +77°), Water (not more than 0.3%), Residue on ignition (not more than 0.1%), Heavy metals (not more than 0.002%), Chromatographic purity, and Ordinary impurities.
Caution: Great care should be taken to prevent inhaling particles of Zalcitabine and exposing it to the skin.
Zalcitabine Tablets USP—Preserve in tight, light-resistant containers. Contain the labeled amount, within ±10%. Meet the requirements for Identification, Dissolution (80% in 20 minutes in water in Apparatus 2 at 50 rpm), and Uniformity of dosage units.
Caution: Great care should be taken to prevent inhaling particles of zalcitabine and exposing it to the skin.

ZALEPLON

Chemical group: Pyrazolopyrimidine, structurally unrelated to benzodiazepines, barbiturates, or other drugs with known hypnotic properties.

Chemical name: Acetmide, N-[3-(3-cyanopyrazolo[1,5 alpha]-pyrimidin-7-yl)phenyl-N-ethyl-.

Molecular formula: $C_{17}H_{15}N_5O$.

Molecular weight: 305.33.

Description: White to off-white powder.

Solubility: Practically insoluble in water; sparingly soluble in alcohol or in propylene glycol.

Other characteristics: Partition coefficient: Log partition coefficient is 1.23 in octanol/water over a pH range of 1 to 7.

USP requirements: Zaleplon Capsules—Not in *USP–NF*.

ZANAMIVIR

Source: A sialic acid derivative.

Chemical name: D-glycero-D-galacto-Non-2-enomic acid, 5-(acetylamino)-4-[(aminoiminomethyl)amino]-2,6-anhydro-3,4,5-trideoxy-.

Molecular formula: $C_{12}H_{20}N_4O_7$.

Molecular weight: 332.31.

Description: White to off-white powder.

Solubility: Soluble approximately 18 mg/mL in water at 20 °C.

USP requirements: Zanamivir Powder for Inhalation—Not in *USP–NF*.

ZEIN

Description: Zein NF—White to yellow powder.
NF category: Coating agent.

Solubility: Zein NF—Soluble in aqueous alcohols, in glycols, in ethylene glycol ethyl ether, in furfuryl alcohol, in tetrahydrofurfuryl alcohol, and in aqueous alkaline solutions of pH 11.5 or

greater. Insoluble in water and in acetone; readily soluble in acetone-water mixtures between the limits of 60% and 80% of acetone by volume; insoluble in all anhydrous alcohols except methanol.

NF requirements: Zein NF—Preserve in tight containers. A prolamine derived from corn (*Zea mays* Linnéae [Fam. Gramineae]). Meets the requirements for Identification, Microbial limits, Loss on drying (not more than 8.0%), Residue on ignition (not more than 2.0%), Heavy metals (not more than 0.002%), Nitrogen content (13.1–17.0%, on the dried basis), and Organic volatile impurities.

ZIDOVUDINE

Chemical group: Dideoxynucleoside analog; also a thymidine analog.

Chemical name: Thymidine, 3'-azido-3'-deoxy-.

Molecular formula: $C_{10}H_{13}N_5O_4$.

Molecular weight: 267.24.

Description: Zidovudine USP— White to yellowish powder. Melts at about 124 °C. Exhibits polymorphism.

Solubility: Zidovudine USP—Sparingly soluble in water; freely soluble in alcohol.

USP requirements:
Zidovudine USP—Preserve in tight, light-resistant containers. Contains not less than 97.0% and not more than 102.0% of zidovudine, calculated on the anhydrous basis. Meets the requirements for Identification, Specific rotation (+60.5° to +63°), Water (not more than 1.0%), Residue on ignition (not more than 0.25%), Chromatographic purity, and Organic volatile impurities.
Zidovudine Capsules USP—Preserve in tight, light-resistant containers. Contain the labeled amount, within ±10%, calculated on the anhydrous basis. Meet the requirements for Identification, Dissolution (75% in 45 minutes in water in Apparatus 2 at 50 rpm), Uniformity of dosage units, and Related compounds.
Zidovudine Injection USP—Preserve in tight, light-resistant containers. A sterile solution of Zidovudine in Water for Injection. Contains the labeled amount, within ±10%. Meets the requirements for Identification, Sterility, pH (3.5–7.0, in a mixture containing a volume of Injection equivalent to 150 mg of zidovudine and 5 mL of 0.12 *M* potassium chloride), Bacterial endotoxins, and Related compounds (not more than 1.0%) and for Injections.
Zidovudine Oral Solution USP—Preserve in tight, lightresistant containers. Contains the labeled amount, within ± 10%. Meets the requirements for Identification, Microbial limits, pH (3.0–4.0, in a mixture containing a volume of Oral Solution equivalent to 150 mg of zidovudine and 5 mL of 0.12 *M* potassium chloride [3:1]), and Related compounds.
Zidovudine Syrup—Not in *USP–NF*.
Zidovudine Tablets USP—Preserve in tight, light-resistant containers, and store at controlled room temperature. Contain the labeled amount, within ±10%. Meet the requirements for Identification, Dissolution (80% in 30 minutes in water in Apparatus 2 at 50 rpm), Uniformity of dosage units, and Related compounds.

ZILEUTON

Chemical name: Urea, *N*-(1-benzo[*b*]thien-2-ylethyl)-*N*-hydroxy-,(±)-.

Molecular formula: $C_{11}H_{12}N_2O_2S$.

Molecular weight: 236.29.

Description: Zileuton USP—White to off-white powder.

Solubility: Soluble in methanol and in ethanol; slightly soluble in acetonitrile; practically insoluble in water and in hexane.

USP requirements:
Zileuton USP—Preserve in tight, light-resistant containers. Contains not less than 98.5% and not ore than 101.5% of zileuton, calculated on the anhydrous basis. Meets the requirements for Identification, Specific rotation (– 0.5° to +0.5°), Water (not more than 1.5%), Residue on ignition (not more than 0.2%), Heavy metals (0.002%), and Chromatographic purity.
Zileuton Tablets—Not in *USP–NF*.

ZINC ACETATE

Chemical name: Acetic acid, zinc salt, dihydrate.

Molecular formula: $C_4H_6O_4Zn \cdot 2H_2O$.

Molecular weight: 219.51.

Description: Zinc Acetate USP—White crystals or granules, having a slight acetous odor. Is slightly efflorescent.

Solubility: Zinc Acetate USP—Freely soluble in water and in boiling alcohol; slightly soluble in alcohol.

USP requirements:
Zinc Acetate USP—Preserve in tight containers. Contains not less than 98.0% and not more than 102.0% of zinc acetate. Meets the requirements for Identification, pH (6.0–8.0, in a solution [1 in 20]), Insoluble matter (not more than 0.005%), Arsenic (not more than 3 ppm), Lead (not more than 0.002%), Chloride (not more than 0.005%), Sulfate (not more than 0.010%), Alkalies and alkaline earths (not more than 0.2%), and Organic volatile impurities.
Zinc Acetate Capsules—Not in *USP–NF*.

ZINC CARBONATE

Chemical name: Bis[carbonato(2–)]hexahydroxypentazinc.

Molecular formula: $3Zn(OH)_2 \cdot 2ZnCO_3$.

Molecular weight: 549.01.

USP requirements: Zinc Carbonate USP—Preserve in tight containers. Contains the equivalent of not less than 70.0% of zinc oxide. Meets the requirements for Identification, Insoluble matter (not more than 0.02%), Chloride (not more than 0.002%), Sulfate (not more than 0.01%), Iron (not more than 0.002%), Lead (not more than 5 ppm), and Substances not precipitated by ammonium sulfide (not more than 0.4%).

ZINC CHLORIDE

Chemical name: Zinc chloride.

Molecular formula: $ZnCl_2$.

Molecular weight: 136.30.

Description: Zinc Chloride USP—White or practically white, odorless, crystalline powder, or white or practically white crystalline granules. May also be in porcelain-like masses or molded into cylinders. Very deliquescent. A solution (1 in 10) is acid to litmus.

Solubility: Zinc Chloride USP—Very soluble in water; freely soluble in alcohol and in glycerin. Its solution in water or in alcohol is usually slightly turbid, but the turbidity disappears when a small quantity of hydrochloric acid is added.

USP requirements:

Zinc Chloride USP—Preserve in tight containers. Contains not less than 97.0% and not more than 100.5% of zinc chloride. Meets the requirements for Identification, Limit of oxychloride, Sulfate (not more than 0.03%), Limit of ammonium salts, Lead (not more than 0.005%), Alkalies and alkaline earths (not more than 1.0%), and Organic volatile impurities.

Zinc Chloride Injection USP—Preserve in single-dose or in multiple-dose containers, preferably of Type I or Type II glass. A sterile solution of Zinc Chloride in Water for Injection. Label the Injection to indicate that it is to be diluted with Water for Injection or other suitable fluid to appropriate strength prior to administration. Contains an amount of zinc chloride equivalent to the labeled amount of zinc, within ±10%. Meets the requirements for Identification, Bacterial endotoxins, pH (1.5–2.5), and Particulate matter, and for Injections.

ZINC GLUCONATE

Chemical name: Bis(D-gluconato-O^1,O^2) zinc.

Molecular formula: $C_{12}H_{22}O_{14}Zn$.

Molecular weight: 455.68.

Description: Zinc Gluconate USP—White or practically white powder or granules.

Solubility: Zinc Gluconate USP—Soluble in water; very slightly soluble in alcohol.

USP requirements:

Zinc Gluconate USP—Preserve in well-closed containers. Contains not less than 97.0% and not more than 102.0% of zinc gluconate, calculated on the anhydrous basis. Meets the requirements for Identification, pH (5.5–7.5, in a solution [1 in 100]), Water (not more than 11.6%), Chloride (not more than 0.05%), Sulfate (not more than 0.05%), Arsenic (not more than 3 ppm), Reducing substances (not more than 1.0%), Cadmium (not more than 5 ppm), Lead (not more than 0.001%), and Organic volatile impurities.

Zinc Gluconate Lozenges—Not in *USP–NF*.

Zinc Gluconate Tablets—Not in *USP–NF*.

ZINC OXIDE

Chemical name: Zinc oxide.

Molecular formula: ZnO.

Molecular weight: 81.39.

Description: Zinc Oxide USP—Very fine, odorless, amorphous, white or yellowish white powder, free from gritty particles. Gradually absorbs carbon dioxide from air.

Solubility: Zinc Oxide USP—Insoluble in water and in alcohol; soluble in dilute acids.

USP requirements:

Zinc Oxide USP—Preserve in well-closed containers. Freshly ignited, contains not less than 99.0% and not more than 100.5% of zinc oxide. Meets the requirements for Identification, Alkalinity, Loss on ignition (not more than 1.0%), Carbonate and color of solution, Arsenic (not more than 6 ppm), Iron and other heavy metals, and Lead.

Zinc Oxide Ointment USP—Preserve in well-closed containers, and avoid prolonged exposure to temperatures exceeding 30 °C. Contains not less than 18.5% and not more than 21.5% of zinc oxide.

Zinc Oxide Ointment may be prepared as follows: 200 grams of Zinc Oxide, 150 grams of Mineral Oil, and 650 grams of White Ointment, to make 1000 grams. Levigate the Zinc Oxide with the Mineral Oil to a smooth paste, and then incorporate the White Ointment.

Meets the requirements for Identification, Minimum fill, and Calcium, magnesium, and other foreign substances.

Zinc Oxide Paste USP—Preserve in well-closed containers, and avoid prolonged exposure to temperatures exceeding 30 °C. Contains not less than 24.0% and not more than 26.0% of zinc oxide.

Zinc Oxide Paste may be prepared as follows: 250 grams of Zinc Oxide, 250 grams of Starch, and 500 grams of White Petrolatum, to make 1000 grams. Mix the ingredients.

Meets the requirements for Identification and Minimum fill.

ZINC OXIDE AND SALICYLIC ACID

For *Zinc Oxide* and *Salicylic Acid*—See individual listings for chemistry information.

USP requirements: Zinc Oxide and Salicylic Acid Paste USP—Preserve in well-closed containers. Contains not less than 23.5% and not more than 25.5% of zinc oxide, and not less than 1.9% and not more than 2.1% of salicylic acid.

Zinc Oxide and Salicylic Acid Paste may be prepared as follows: 20 grams of Salicylic Acid, in fine powder, and a sufficient quantity of Zinc Oxide Paste to make 1000 grams. Thoroughly triturate the Salicylic Acid with a portion of the paste, then add the remaining paste, and triturate until a smooth mixture is obtained.

Meets the requirements for Identification and Minimum fill.

ZINC STEARATE

Chemical name: Octadecanoic acid, zinc salt.

Description: Zinc Stearate USP—Fine, white, bulky powder, free from grittiness. Has a faint, characteristic odor. Is neutral to moistened litmus paper.

NF category: Tablet and/or capsule lubricant.

Solubility: Zinc Stearate USP—Insoluble in water, in alcohol, and in ether.

USP requirements: Zinc Stearate USP—Preserve in well-closed containers. A compound of zinc with a mixture of solid organic acids obtained from fats, consisting chiefly of variable proportions of zinc stearate and zinc palmitate. Contains the equivalent of not less than 12.5% and not more than 14.0% of zinc oxide. Meets the requirements for Identification, Arsenic (not more than 1.5 ppm), Lead (not more than 0.001%), Alkalies and alkaline earths (not more than 1.0%), and Organic volatile impurities.

ZINC SULFATE

Chemical name: Sulfuric acid, zinc salt (1:1), hydrate.

Molecular formula: $ZnSO_4 \cdot xH_2O$.

Molecular weight: 179.46 (monohydrate); 287.56 (heptahydrate); 161.46 (anhydrous).

Description: Zinc Sulfate USP—Colorless, transparent prisms, or small needles. May occur as a white, granular, crystalline powder. Odorless; efflorescent in dry air. Its solutions are acid to litmus.

Solubility: Zinc Sulfate USP—Very soluble in water (heptahydrate); freely soluble in water (monohydrate); freely soluble in glycerin (heptahydrate); practically insoluble in alcohol (monohydrate); insoluble in alcohol (heptahydrate).

USP requirements:
Zinc Sulfate USP—Preserve in tight containers. Contains one or seven molecules of water of hydration. The label indicates whether it is the monohydrate or the heptahydrate. Label any oral or parenteral preparations containing Zinc Sulfate to state the content of elemental zinc. The monohydrate contains not less than 89.0% and not more than 90.4% of anhydrous zinc sulfate, corresponding to not less than 99.0% and not more than 100.5% of zinc sulfate (monohydrate), and the heptahydrate contains not less than 55.6% and not more than 61.0% of anhydrous zinc sulfate, corresponding to not less than 99.0% and not more than 108.7% of zinc sulfate (heptahydrate). Meets the requirements for Identification, Acidity, Arsenic (not more than 14 ppm), Lead (not more than 0.002%), and Alkalies and alkaline earths (not more than 0.9%).
Zinc Sulfate Capsules—Not in *USP–NF*.
Zinc Sulfate Injection USP—Preserve in single-dose or in multiple-dose containers. A sterile solution of Zinc Sulfate in Water for Injection. Label the Injection in terms of its content of anhydrous zinc sulfate and in terms of its content of elemental zinc. Label it to state that it is not intended for direct injection but is to be added to other intravenous solutions. Contains an amount of zinc sulfate equivalent to the labeled amount of zinc, within ±10%. Meets the requirements for Identification, Bacterial endotoxins, pH (2.0–4.0), and Particulate matter, and for Injections.
Zinc Sulfate Ophthalmic Solution USP—Preserve in tight containers. A sterile solution of Zinc Sulfate in Water rendered isotonic by the addition of suitable salts. Contains the labeled amount, within ±5%. Meets the requirements for Identification, Sterility, and pH (5.8–6.2; or, if it contains sodium citrate, 7.2–7.8).
Zinc Sulfate Tablets—Not in *USP–NF*.
Zinc Sulfate Extended-release Tablets—Not in *USP–NF*.

ZINC UNDECYLENATE

Chemical name: 10-Undecenoic acid, zinc(2+) salt.

Molecular formula: $C_{22}H_{38}O_4Zn$.

Molecular weight: 431.92.

Description: Zinc Undecylenate USP—Fine, white powder.

Solubility: Zinc Undecylenate USP—Practically insoluble in water and in alcohol.

USP requirements: Zinc Undecylenate USP—Preserve in well-closed containers. Contains not less than 98.0% and not more than 102.0% of zinc undecylenate, calculated on the dried basis. Meets the requirements for Identification, Loss on drying (not more than 1.25%), and Alkalies and alkaline earths (not more than 1.0%).

ZIPRASIDONE

Chemical name: Ziprasidone hydrochloride—2*H*-Indol-2-one, 5-[2-[4-(1,2-benzisothiazol-3-yl)-1-piperazinyl]ethyl]-6-chloro-1,3-dihydro, monohydrochloride.

Molecular formula: Ziprasidone hydrochloride—$C_{21}H_{21}ClN_4OS \cdot HCl \cdot H_2O$; $C_{21}H_{21}ClN_4OS$ (free base).

Molecular weight: Ziprasidone hydrochloride—467.41; 419.94 (free base).

Description: Ziprasidone hydrochloride—White to slightly pink powder.

USP requirements: Ziprasidone Hydrochloride Capsules—Not in *USP–NF*.

ZOLAZEPAM

Chemical name: Zolazepam hydrochloride—Pyrazolo[3,4-*e*][1,4]diazepin-7(1*H*-one, 4-(2-fluorophenyl)-6,8-dihydro-1,38-trimethyl-, monohydrochloride.

Molecular formula: Zolazepam hydrochloride—$C_{15}H_{15}FN_4O \cdot HCl$.

Molecular weight: Zolazepam hydrochloride—322.77.

Description: Zolazepam Hydrochloride USP—White to off-white crystalline powder.

Solubility: Zolazepam Hydrochloride USP—Freely soluble in water and in 0.1 N hydrochloric acid; soluble in methanol; slightly soluble in chloroform; practically insoluble in ether.

USP requirements: Zolazepam Hydrochloride USP—Preserve in tight containers. Label it to indicate that it is for veterinary use only. Where it is intended for use in preparing injectable dosage forms, the label states that it is sterile or must be subjected to further processing during the preparation of injectable dosage forms. Contains not less than 97.0% and not more than 103.0% of zolazepam hydrochloride. Meets the rquirements for Identification, pH (1.5–3.5, in a solution [1 in 10]), Loss on drying (not more than 1.0%), Residue on ignition (not more than 0.5%), Heavy metals (not more than 0.002%), Chromatographic purity, Bacterial endotoxins (where the label states that Zolazepam Hydrochloride is sterile or must be subjected to further processing during the preparation of injectable dosage forms), Sterility (where the label states that Zolazepam Hydrochloride is sterile), and Chloride content.

ZOLEDRONIC ACID

Chemical name: Phosphonic acid, [1-hydroxy-2-(1*H*-imidazol-1-yl)-ethylidene]bis-, monohydrate.

Molecular formula: $C_5H_{10}N_2O_7P_2 \cdot H_2O$.

Molecular weight: 290.10 grams per mol.

Description: White crystalline powder.

Solubility: Highly soluble in 0.1 N sodium hydroxide solution; sparingly soluble in water and in 0.1 N hydrochloric acid; practically insoluble in solvents.

Other characteristics: The pH of a 0.7% solution of zoledronic acid in water is approximately 2.0.

USP requirements: Zoledronic Acid for Injection—Not in *USP–NF*.

ZOLMITRIPTAN

Chemical name: 2-Oxazolidinone, 4-[[3-[2-(dimethylamino)ethyl]-1*H*-indol-5-yl]methyl]-, (*S*)-.

Molecular formula: $C_{16}H_{21}N_3O_2$.

Molecular weight: 287.36.

Description: White to almost white powder.

Solubility: Readily soluble in water.

USP requirements: Zolmitriptan Tablets—Not in *USP–NF*.

ZOLPIDEM

Chemical name: Zolpidem tartrate—Imidazo[1,2-*a*]pyridine-3-acetamide, *N,N,*6-trimethyl-2-(4-methylphenyl)-, [*R*-(*R*,R**)]2,3-dihydroxybutanedioate (2:1).

Molecular formula: Zolpidem tartrate—$(C_{19}H_{21}N_3O)_2 \cdot C_4H_6O_6$.

Molecular weight: Zolpidem tartrate—764.87.

Description: Zolpidem tartrate—White to off-white crystalline powder.

Solubility: Zolpidem tartrate—Sparingly soluble in water, in alcohol, and in propylene glycol.

USP requirements: Zolpidem Tartrate Tablets—Not in *USP–NF*.

ZONISAMIDE

Source: Benzisoxazole derivative.

Chemical group: Sulfonamide.

Chemical name: 1,2-Benzisoxazole-3-methanesulfonamide.

Molecular formula: $C_8H_8N_2O_3S$.

Molecular weight: 212.23.

Description: White powder. Odorless. Melting point 160–163°.

pKa: 10.2.

Solubility: Moderately soluble in water (0.80 mg/mL) and in 0.1 N HCl (0.50 mg/mL); sparingly soluble in chloroform and in n-hexane; soluble in methanol, in ethanol, in ethyl acetate, and in acetic acid.

USP requirements: Zonisamide Capsules—Not in *USP–NF*.

ZOPICLONE

Chemical name: 4-Methyl-1-piperazinecarboxylic acid ester with 6-(5-chloro-2-pyridyl)-6,7-dihydro-7-hydroxy-5*H*-pyrrolo[3,4-*b*]pyrazin-5-one.

Molecular formula: $C_{17}H_{17}ClN_6O_3$.

Molecular weight: 388.81.

Description: Fine white odorless non-hygroscopic powder with a melting point of 178 °C.

Solubility: Freely soluble in chloroform and in methylene chloride; soluble in dimethylformamide and in 0.1 *N* hydrochloric acid; slightly soluble in acetone; practically insoluble in water, in ethanol, and in ethyl ether.

USP requirements: Zopiclone Tablets—Not in *USP–NF*.

Section V: USP Reference Tables

CONTAINERS FOR DISPENSING CAPSULES AND TABLETS

The following table is provided as a reminder for the pharmacist engaged in the typical dispensing situation who already is acquainted with the *Packaging and storage* requirements set forth in the individual monographs. It lists the capsules and tablets that are official in the United States Pharmacopeia and indicates the relevant tight (T), well-closed (W), and light-resistant (LR) specifications applicable to containers in which the drug that is repackaged should be dispensed.

This table is not intended to replace, nor should it be interpreted as replacing, the definitive requirements stated in the individual monographs.

Container Specifications for Capsules and Tablets

Monograph Title	Container Specification
Acebutolol Hydrochloride Capsules	T
Acepromazine Maleate Tablets	W, LR
Acetaminophen Capsules	T
Acetaminophen Tablets	T
Acetaminophen and Aspirin Tablets	T
Acetaminophen, Aspirin, and Caffeine Tablets	W
Acetaminophen and Caffeine Tablets	T
Acetaminophen and Salts of Chlorpheniramine, Dextromethorphan, and Phenylpropanolamine, Capsules Containing at Least Three of the following—	T
Acetaminophen and Salts of Chlorpheniramine, Dextromethorphan, and Phenylpropanolamine, Tablets Containing at Least Three of the following—	T
Acetaminophen and Salts of Chlorpheniramine, Dextromethorphan, and Pseudoephedrine, Capsules Containing at Least Three of the following—	T
Acetaminophen and Salts of Chlorpheniramine, Dextromethorphan, and Pseudoephedrine, Tablets Containing at Least Three of the following—	T
Acetaminophen and Codeine Phosphate Capsules	T, LR
Acetaminophen and Codeine Phosphate Tablets	T, LR
Acetaminophen and Diphenhydramine Citrate Tablets	T
Acetaminophen, Diphenhydramine Hydrochloride, and Pseudoephedrine Hydrochloride Tablets	T
Acetaminophen and Pseudoephedrine Hydrochloride Tablets	T
Acetazolamide Tablets	W
Acetohexamide Tablets	W
Acetohydroxamic Acid Tablets	T
Acyclovir Capsules	T
Acyclovir Tablets	T
Albendazole Tablets	T

Change to read:

Monograph Title	Container Specification
Albuterol Tablets	▲T, ▲USP27 LR
Allopurinol Tablets	W
Alprazolam Tablets	T, LR
Altretamine Capsules	T, LR
Alumina and Magnesia Tablets	W
Alumina, Magnesia, and Calcium Carbonate Tablets	W

Monograph Title	Container Specification
Alumina, Magnesia, Calcium Carbonate, and Simethicone Tablets	W
Alumina, Magnesia, and Simethicone Tablets	W
Alumina and Magnesium Carbonate Tablets	T
Alumina, Magnesium Carbonate, and Magnesium Oxide Tablets	T
Alumina and Magnesium Trisilicate Tablets	W
Aluminum Carbonate Gel, Dried Basic, Capsules	W
Aluminum Carbonate Gel, Dried Basic, Tablets	W
Aluminum Hydroxide Gel, Dried, Capsules	W
Aluminum Hydroxide Gel, Dried, Tablets	W
Amantadine Hydrochloride Capsules	T
Amiloride Hydrochloride Tablets	W
Amiloride Hydrochloride and Hydrochlorothiazide Tablets	W
Aminobenzoate Potassium Capsules	W
Aminobenzoate Potassium Tablets	W
Aminocaproic Acid Tablets	T
Aminoglutethimide Tablets	T, LR
Aminopentamide Sulfate Tablets	W
Aminophylline Tablets	T
Aminophylline Tablets, Delayed-Release	T
Aminosalicylate Sodium Tablets	T, LR
Aminosalicylic Acid Tablets	T, LR
Amitriptyline Hydrochloride Tablets	W
Ammonium Chloride Tablets, Delayed-Release	T
Amoxapine Tablets	W
Amodiaquine Hydrochloride Tablets	T
Amoxicillin Capsules	T
Amoxicillin Tablets	T
Amoxicillin and Clavulanate Potassium Tablets	T
Amphetamine Sulfate Tablets	W
Ampicillin Capsules	T
Ampicillin Tablets	T
Anileridine Hydrochloride Tablets	T, LR
Apomorphine Hydrochloride Tablets	T, LR
Ascorbic Acid Tablets	T, LR
Aspirin Capsules	T
Aspirin Capsules, Delayed-Release	T
Aspirin Tablets	T
Aspirin Tablets, Buffered	T
Aspirin Tablets, Delayed-Release	T
Aspirin Tablets, Effervescent for Oral Solution	T
Aspirin Tablets, Extended-Release	T
Aspirin, Alumina, and Magnesia Tablets	T
Aspirin, Alumina, and Magnesium Oxide Tablets	T
Aspirin, Caffeine, and Dihydrocodeine Bitartrate Capsules	T

Monograph Title	Container Specification	Monograph Title	Container Specification
Aspirin and Codeine Phosphate Tablets	W, LR	Cefadroxil Tablets	T
Aspirin, Codeine Phosphate, Alumina, and Magnesia Tablets	W, LR	Cefixime Tablets	T
		Cefpodoxime Proxetil Tablets	T
Astemizole Tablets	T	Cefprozil Tablets	T
Atenolol Tablets	W	Cefuroxime Axetil Tablets	W
Atenolol and Chlorthalidone Tablets	W	Cephalexin Capsules	T
Atropine Sulfate Tablets	W	Cephalexin Tablets	T
Azatadine Maleate Tablets	W	Cephradine Capsules	T
Azathioprine Tablets	LR	Cephradine Tablets	T
Azithromycin Capsules	W	Chloral Hydrate Capsules	T
Bacampicillin Hydrochloride Tablets	T	Chlorambucil Tablets	W, LR
Baclofen Tablets	W	Chloramphenicol Capsules	T
Barium Sulfate Tablets	W	Chloramphenicol Tablets	T
Belladonna Extract Tablets	T, LR	Chlordiazepoxide Tablets	T, LR
Bendroflumethiazide Tablets	T	Chlordiazepoxide and Amitriptyline Hydrochloride Tablets	T, LR
Benzonatate Capsules	T, LR		
Benztropine Mesylate Tablets	W	Chlordiazepoxide Hydrochloride Capsules	T, LR
Beta Carotene Capsules	T, LR	Chlordiazepoxide Hydrochloride and Clidinium Bromide Capsules	T, LR
Betamethasone Tablets	W		
Betaxolol Tablets	T	Chloroquine Phosphate Tablets	W
Bethanechol Chloride Tablets	T	Chlorothiazide Tablets	W
Biperiden Hydrochloride Tablets	T	Chlorpheniramine Maleate Capsules, Extended-Release	T
Bisacodyl Tablets	T		
Bisacodyl Tablets, Delayed-Release	W	Chlorpheniramine Maleate Tablets	T
Bromocriptine Mesylate Capsules	T, LR	Chlorpheniramine Maleate and Phenylpropanolamine Hydrochloride Capsules, Extended-Release	T, LR
Bromocriptine Mesylate Tablets	T, LR		
Brompheniramine Maleate Tablets	T		
Bumetanide Tablets	T, LR	Chlorpheniramine Maleate and Phenylpropanolamine Hydrochloride Tablets, Extended-Release	T, LR
Bupropion Hydrochloride Tablets, Extended-Release	W		
Buspirone Hydrochloride Tablets	T, LR	Chlorpheniramine Maleate and Pseudoephedrine Hydrochloride Capsules, Extended-Release	T, LR
Busulfan Tablets	W		
Butabarbital Sodium Tablets	W	Chlorpromazine Hydrochloride Tablets	W, LR
Butalbital, Acetaminophen, and Caffeine Capsules	T	Chlorpropamide Tablets	W
		Chlortetracycline Hydrochloride Tablets	T, LR
Butalbital, Acetaminophen, and Caffeine Tablets	T	Chlorthalidone Tablets	W
Butalbital and Aspirin Tablets	T	Chlorzoxazone Tablets	T
Butalbital, Aspirin, and Caffeine Capsules	T	Chlorzoxazone and Acetaminophen Capsules	T
Butalbital, Aspirin, and Caffeine Tablets	T	Chondroitin Sulfate Sodium Tablets	T, LR
Butalbital, Aspirin, Caffeine, and Codeine Phosphate Capsules	T, LR	Cimetidine Tablets	T, LR
		Cinoxacin Capsules	W
Calcifediol Capsules	T, LR	Ciprofloxacin Tablets	W
Calcium with Vitamin D Tablets	T, LR	Clarithromycin Tablets	T
Calcium Acetate Tablets	W	Clemastine Fumarate Tablets	W
Calcium Carbonate Tablets	W	Clindamycin Hydrochloride Capsules	T
Calcium Carbonate and Magnesia Tablets	W	Clofazimine Capsules	W
Calcium and Magnesium Carbonates Tablets	W	Clofibrate Capsules	W, LR
Calcium Gluconate Tablets	W	Clomiphene Citrate Tablets	W
Calcium Lactate Tablets	T	Clomipramine Hydrochloride Capsules	W
Calcium Pantothenate Tablets	T	Clonazepam Tablets	T, LR
Calcium Phosphate, Dibasic, Tablets	W	Clonidine Hydrochloride Tablets	W
Captopril Tablets	T	Clonidine Hydrochloride and Chlorthalidone Tablets	W
Captopril and Hydrochlorothiazide Tablets	T		
Carbamazepine Tablets	T	Clorazepate Dipotassium Tablets	T, LR
Carbamazepine Tablets, Extended-Release	T	Clotrimazole Vaginal Tablets	W
Carbenicillin Indanyl Sodium Tablets	T	Red Clover Tablets	T, LR
Carbidopa and Levodopa Tablets	W, LR	Cloxacillin Sodium Capsules	T
Carbinoxamine Maleate Tablets	T, LR	Clozapine Tablets	W
Urea C14 Capsules	T	Cyanocobalamin Co 57 Capsules	W, LR
Carboxymethylcellulose Sodium Tablets	T	Cyanocobalamin Co 58 Capsules	W, LR
Carisoprodol Tablets	W	Cocaine Hydrochloride Tablets for Topical Solution	W, LR
Carisoprodol and Aspirin Tablets	W		
Carisoprodol, Aspirin, and Codeine Phosphate Tablets	W	Codeine Phosphate Tablets	W, LR
		Codeine Sulfate Tablets	W
Carteolol Hydrochloride Tablets	T	Cortisone Acetate Tablets	W
Cascara Tablets	T, W	Cromolyn Sodium for Inhalation (in capsules)	T, LR
Castor Oil Capsules	T	Cyclizine Hydrochloride Tablets	T, LR
Cefaclor Capsules	T	Cyclobenzaprine Hydrochloride Tablets	W
Cefaclor Tablets, Extended-Release	T, LR	Cyclophosphamide Tablets	T
Cefadroxil Capsules	T	Cycloserine Capsules	T

Monograph Title	Container Specification
Cyclosporine Capsules	T
Cyproheptadine Hydrochloride Tablets	W
Danazol Capsules	W
Dapsone Tablets	W, LR
Dehydrocholic Acid Tablets	W
Demeclocycline Hydrochloride Capsules	T, LR
Demeclocycline Hydrochloride Tablets	T, LR
Desipramine Hydrochloride Tablets	T
Dexamethasone Tablets	W
Dexchlorpheniramine Maleate Tablets	T
Dextroamphetamine Sulfate Capsules	T
Dextroamphetamine Sulfate Tablets	W
Diazepam Capsules	T, LR
Diazepam Capsules, Extended-Release	T, LR
Diazepam Tablets	T, LR
Diazoxide Capsules	W
Dichlorphenamide Tablets	W
Diclofenac Sodium Tablets, Delayed-Release	T, LR
Dicloxacillin Sodium Capsules	T
Dicyclomine Hydrochloride Capsules	W
Dicyclomine Hydrochloride Tablets	W
Diethylcarbamazine Citrate Tablets	T
Diethylpropion Hydrochloride Tablets	W
Diethylstilbestrol Tablets	W
Diflunisal Tablets	W
Digitalis Capsules	T
Digitalis Tablets	T
Digitoxin Tablets	W
Digoxin Tablets	T
Dihydrotachysterol Capsules	W, LR
Dihydrotachysterol Tablets	W, LR
Dihydroxyaluminum Sodium Carbonate Tablets	W
Diltiazem Hydrochloride Tablets	T, LR
Diltiazem Hydrochloride Capsules, Extended-Release	T
Dimenhydrinate Tablets	W
Diphenhydramine Hydrochloride Capsules	T
Diphenhydramine and Pseudoephedrine Capsules	T
Diphenoxylate Hydrochloride and Atropine Sulfate Tablets	W, LR
Dipyridamole Tablets	T, LR
Dirithromycin Tablets, Delayed-Release	T
Disopyramide Phosphate Capsules	W
Disopyramide Phosphate Capsules, Extended-Release	W
Disulfiram Tablets	T, LR
Divalproex Sodium Tablets, Delayed-Release	T, LR
Docusate Calcium Capsules	T
Docusate Potassium Capsules	T
Docusate Sodium Capsules	T
Docusate Sodium Tablets	W
Dolasetron Mesylate Tablets	W
Doxepin Hydrochloride Capsules	W
Doxycycline Capsules	T, LR
Doxycycline Hyclate Capsules	T, LR
Doxycycline Hyclate Capsules, Delayed-Release	T, LR
Doxycycline Hyclate Tablets	T, LR
Doxylamine Succinate Tablets	W, LR
Dronabinol Capsules	W, LR
Dydrogesterone Tablets	W
Dyphylline Tablets	T
Dyphylline and Guaifenesin Tablets	T
Enalapril Maleate Tablets	W
Enalapril Maleate and Hydrochlorothiazide Tablets	W
Ephedrine Sulfate Capsules	T, LR
Ergocalciferol Capsules	T, LR
Ergocalciferol Tablets	T, LR
Ergoloid Mesylates Capsules	T, LR

Monograph Title	Container Specification
Ergoloid Mesylates Tablets	T, LR
Ergonovine Maleate Tablets	W
Ergotamine Tartrate Tablets	W, LR
Ergotamine Tartrate and Caffeine Tablets	W, LR
Erythromycin Capsules, Delayed-Release	T
Erythromycin Tablets	T
Erythromycin Tablets, Delayed-Release	T
Erythromycin Estolate Capsules	T
Erythromycin Estolate Tablets	T
Erythromycin Ethylsuccinate Tablets	T
Erythromycin Stearate Tablets	T
Estradiol Tablets	T, LR
Estrogens, Conjugated, Tablets	W
Estrogens, Esterified, Tablets	W
Estropipate Tablets	W
Ethacrynic Acid Tablets	W
Ethambutol Hydrochloride Tablets	W
Ethchlorvynol Capsules	T, LR
Ethinyl Estradiol Tablets	W
Ethionamide Tablets	W
Ethosuximide Capsules	T
Ethotoin Tablets	T
Ethynodiol Diacetate and Ethinyl Estradiol Tablets	W
Ethynodiol Diacetate and Mestranol Tablets	W
Etidronate Disodium Tablets	T
Etodolac Capsules	T
Etodolac Tablets	T
Famotidine Tablets	W, LR
Felodipine Tablets, Extended-Release	T
Fenoprofen Calcium Capsules	W
Fenoprofen Calcium Tablets	W
Ferrous Fumarate Tablets	T
Ferrous Fumarate and Docusate Sodium Tablets, Extended-Release	W
Ferrous Gluconate Capsules	T
Ferrous Gluconate Tablets	T
Ferrous Sulfate Tablets	T
Finasteride Tablets	T, LR
Flecainide Acetate Tablets	W
Flucytosine Capsules	T, LR
Fludrocortisone Acetate Tablets	W
Fluoxetine Capsules	T, LR
Fluoxetine Tablets	T
Fluoxymesterone Tablets	W
Fluphenazine Hydrochloride Tablets	T, LR
Flurazepam Hydrochloride Capsules	T, LR
Flurbiprofen Tablets	W
Flutamide Capsules	W, LR
Folic Acid Tablets	W
Furazolidone Tablets	T, LR
Furosemide Tablets	W, LR
Garlic Tablets, Delayed-Release	T
Gemfibrozil Capsules	T
Gemfibrozil Tablets	T
Asian Ginseng Capsules	T, LR
Asian Ginseng Tablets	T, LR
Glipizide Tablets	T
Glucosamine Tablets	T, LR
Glucosamine and Chondroitin Sulfate Tablets	T, LR
Glyburide Tablets	W
Glycopyrrolate Tablets	T
Griseofulvin Capsules	T
Griseofulvin Tablets	T
Griseofulvin, Ultramicrosize, Tablets	W
Guaifenesin Capsules	T
Guaifenesin Tablets	T
Guaifenesin and Pseudoephedrine Hydrochloride Capsules	T, LR

Monograph Title	Container Specification
Guaifenesin, Pseudoephedrine Hydrochloride, and Dextromethorphan Hydrobromide Capsules	T, LR
Guanabenz Acetate Tablets	T, LR
Guanadrel Sulfate Tablets	T, LR
Guanethidine Monosulfate Tablets	W
Guanfacine Tablets	T, LR
Halazone Tablets for Solution	T, LR
Haloperidol Tablets	T, LR
Hexylresorcinol Lozenges	W
Homatropine Methylbromide Tablets	T, LR
Hydralazine Hydrochloride Tablets	T, LR
Hydrochlorothiazide Tablets	W
Hydrocodone Bitartrate Tablets	T, LR
Hydrocodone Bitartrate and Acetaminophen Tablets	T, LR
Hydrocortisone Tablets	W
Hydroflumethiazide Tablets	T
Hydromorphone Hydrochloride Tablets	T, LR
Hydroxychloroquine Sulfate Tablets	T, LR
Hydroxyurea Capsules	T
Hydroxyzine Hydrochloride Tablets	T
Hydroxyzine Pamoate Capsules	W
Hyoscyamine Tablets	W, LR
Hyoscyamine Sulfate Tablets	T, LR
Ibuprofen Tablets	W
Ibuprofen and Pseudoephedrine Hydrochloride Tablets	T
Imipramine Hydrochloride Tablets	T
Indapamide Tablets	W
Indomethacin Capsules	W
Indomethacin Capsules, Extended-Release	W
Sodium Iodide I 123 Capsules	W
Sodium Iodide I 131 Capsules	W
Iodoquinol Tablets	W
Iopanoic Acid Tablets	T, LR
Ipodate Sodium Capsules	T
Isoniazid Tablets	W, LR
Isopropamide Iodide Tablets	W
Isoproterenol Hydrochloride Tablets	W, LR
Isosorbide Dinitrate Capsules, Extended-Release	W
Isosorbide Dinitrate Tablets	W
Isosorbide Dinitrate Tablets, Chewable	W
Isosorbide Dinitrate Tablets, Extended-Release	W
Isosorbide Dinitrate Tablets, Sublingual	W
Isotretinoin Capsules	T
Isoxsuprine Hydrochloride Tablets	T
Kanamycin Sulfate Capsules	T
Ketoconazole Tablets	W
Ketorolac Tromethamine Tablets	W
Labetalol Hydrochloride Tablets	T, LR
Lansoprazole Capsules, Delayed-Release	T
Letrozole Tablets	W
Leucovorin Calcium Tablets	W, LR
Levamisole Hydrochloride Tablets	W
Levocarnitine Tablets	T
Levodopa Capsules	T, LR
Levodopa Tablets	T, LR
Levonorgestrel and Ethinyl Estradiol Tablets	W
Levorphanol Tartrate Tablets	W
Levothyroxine Sodium Tablets	T, LR
Lincomycin Hydrochloride Capsules	T
Alpha Lipoic Acid Capsules	W
Alpha Lipoic Acid Tablets	W
Liothyronine Sodium Tablets	T
Liotrix Tablets	T
Lithium Carbonate Capsules	W
Lithium Carbonate Tablets	W
Lithium Carbonate Tablets, Extended-Release	W
Loperamide Hydrochloride Capsules	W

Monograph Title	Container Specification
Loracarbef Capsules	W
Lorazepam Tablets	T, LR
Lovastatin Tablets	W
Loxapine Capsules	T
Magaldrate Tablets	W
Magaldrate and Simethicone Tablets	W
Magnesia Tablets	W
Magnesia and Alumina Tablets	W
Magnesium Gluconate Tablets	W
Magnesium Oxide Capsules	W
Magnesium Oxide Tablets	W
Magnesium Salicylate Tablets	T
Magnesium Trisilicate Tablets	W
Maprotiline Hydrochloride Tablets	W
Mazindol Tablets	T
Mebendazole Tablets	W
Mecamylamine Hydrochloride Tablets	W
Meclizine Hydrochloride Tablets	W
Meclofenamate Sodium Capsules	T, LR
Medroxyprogesterone Acetate Tablets	W
Mefenamic Acid Capsules	T
Megestrol Acetate Tablets	W
Melphalan Tablets	W, LR
Menadiol Sodium Diphosphate Tablets	W, LR
Meperidine Hydrochloride Tablets	W, LR
Mephenytoin Tablets	W
Mephobarbital Tablets	W
Meprobamate Tablets	W
Mercaptopurine Tablets	W
Mesalamine Capsules, Extended-Release	T, LR
Mesalamine Tablets, Delayed-Release	T
Mesoridazine Besylate Tablets	W, LR
Metaproterenol Sulfate Tablets	W, LR
Methacycline Hydrochloride Capsules	T, LR
Methadone Hydrochloride Tablets	W
Methamphetamine Hydrochloride Tablets	T, LR
Methazolamide Tablets	W
Methdilazine Hydrochloride Tablets	T, LR
Methenamine Tablets	W
Methenamine Hippurate Tablets	W
Methenamine Mandelate Tablets	W
Methenamine Mandelate Tablets, Delayed-Release	W
Methimazole Tablets	W, LR
Methocarbamol Tablets	T
Methotrexate Tablets	W
Methoxsalen Capsules	T, LR
Methsuximide Capsules	T
Methyclothiazide Tablets	W
Methylcellulose Tablets	W
Methyldopa Tablets	W
Methyldopa and Chlorothiazide Tablets	W
Methyldopa and Hydrochlorothiazide Tablets	W
Methylergonovine Maleate Tablets	T, LR
Methylphenidate Hydrochloride Tablets	T
Methylphenidate Hydrochloride Tablets, Extended-Release	T
Methylprednisolone Tablets	W
Methyltestosterone Capsules	W
Methyltestosterone Tablets	W
Methysergide Maleate Tablets	W
Metoclopramide Tablets	T, LR
Metoprolol Succinate Tablets, Extended-Release	W
Metoprolol Tartrate Tablets	T, LR
Metoprolol Tartrate and Hydrochlorothiazide Tablets	T, LR
Metronidazole Tablets	W, LR
Metyrapone Tablets	T, LR
Metyrosine Capsules	W
Mexiletine Hydrochloride Capsules	T

Monograph Title	Container Specification
Minerals Capsules	T, LR
Minerals Tablets	T, LR
Minocycline Hydrochloride Capsules	T, LR
Minocycline Hydrochloride Tablets	T, LR
Minoxidil Tablets	T
Mitotane Tablets	T, LR
Molindone Hydrochloride Tablets	T, LR
Moricizine Hydrochloride Tablets	T
Change to read:	
Nabumetone Tablets	▲W▲USP27
Nadolol Tablets	T
Nadolol and Bendroflumethiazide Tablets	T
Nafcillin Sodium Capsules	T
Nafcillin Sodium Tablets	T, LR
Nalidixic Acid Tablets	T
Naltrexone Hydrochloride Tablets	T
Naproxen Tablets	W
Naproxen Sodium Tablets	W
Neomycin Sulfate Tablets	T
Neostigmine Bromide Tablets	T
Niacin Tablets	W
Niacinamide Tablets	T
Nifedipine Capsules	T, LR
Nifedipine Tablets, Extended-Release	T, LR
Nitrofurantoin Capsules	T, LR
Nitrofurantoin Tablets	T, LR
Nitroglycerin Tablets	T
Norethindrone Tablets	W
Norethindrone and Ethinyl Estradiol Tablets	W
Norethindrone and Mestranol Tablets	W
Norethindrone Acetate Tablets	W
Norethindrone Acetate and Ethinyl Estradiol Tablets	W
Norfloxacin Tablets	W
Norgestrel Tablets	W
Norgestrel and Ethinyl Estradiol Tablets	W
Nortriptyline Hydrochloride Capsules	T
Nystatin Tablets	T, LR
Nystatin Vaginal Tablets	W, LR
Oleovitamin A and D Capsules	T, LR
Oxacillin Sodium Capsules	T
Oxandrolone Tablets	T, LR
Oxazepam Capsules	W
Oxazepam Tablets	W
Oxprenolol Hydrochloride Tablets	W, LR
Oxprenolol Hydrochloride Tablets, Extended-Release	W, LR
Oxtriphylline Tablets	T
Oxtriphylline Tablets, Delayed-Release	T
Oxtriphylline Tablets, Extended-Release	T
Oxybutynin Chloride Tablets	T, LR
Oxycodone Hydrochloride Tablets	T, LR
Oxycodone and Acetaminophen Capsules	T, LR
Oxycodone and Acetaminophen Tablets	T, LR
Oxycodone and Aspirin Tablets	T, LR
Oxymetholone Tablets	W
Oxytetracycline Tablets	T, LR
Oxytetracycline and Nystatin Capsules	T, LR
Oxytetracycline Hydrochloride Capsules	T, LR
Oxytetracycline Hydrochloride and Polymyxin B Sulfate Vaginal Tablets	W
Pancreatin Tablets	T
Pancrelipase Capsules	T
Pancrelipase Capsules, Delayed-Release	T
Pancrelipase Tablets	T
Papain Tablets for Topical Solution	T, LR
Papaverine Hydrochloride Tablets	T
Paramethasone Acetate Tablets	W
Paromomycin Sulfate Capsules	T

Monograph Title	Container Specification
Penbutolol Sulfate Tablets	W, LR
Penicillamine Capsules	T
Penicillamine Tablets	T
Penicillin G Benzathine Tablets	T
Penicillin G Potassium Tablets	T
Penicillin V Tablets	T
Penicillin V Potassium Tablets	T
Pentazocine Hydrochloride and Aspirin Tablets	T, LR
Pentazocine and Naloxone Hydrochlorides Tablets	T, LR
Pentobarbital Sodium Capsules	T
Pentoxifylline Tablets, Extended-Release	W
Perphenazine Tablets	T, LR
Perphenazine and Amitriptyline Hydrochloride Tablets	W
Phenazopyridine Hydrochloride Tablets	T
Phendimetrazine Tartrate Capsules	T
Phendimetrazine Tartrate Tablets	W
Phenelzine Sulfate Tablets	T
Phenmetrazine Hydrochloride Tablets	T
Phenobarbital Tablets	W
Phenoxybenzamine Hydrochloride Capsules	W
Phensuximide Capsules	T
Phentermine Hydrochloride Capsules	T
Phentermine Hydrochloride Tablets	T
Phenylbutazone Tablets	T
Phenylpropanolamine Hydrochloride Capsules	T, LR
Phenylpropanolamine Hydrochloride Capsules, Extended-Release	T, LR
Phenylpropanolamine Hydrochloride Tablets	T, LR
Phenylpropanolamine Hydrochloride Tablets, Extended-Release	T, LR
Phenytoin Tablets	W
Phenytoin Sodium Capsules, Extended	T
Phenytoin Sodium Capsules, Prompt	T
Phytonadione Tablets	W, LR
Pimozide Tablets	T, LR
Pindolol Tablets	W, LR
Piperazine Citrate Tablets	T
Piroxicam Capsules	T, LR
Potassium Bicarbonate Effervescent Tablets for Oral Solution	T
Potassium Bicarbonate and Potassium Chloride Effervescent Tablets for Oral Solution	T
Potassium and Sodium Bicarbonates and Citric Acid Effervescent Tablets for Oral Solution	T
Potassium Chloride Capsules, Extended-Release	T
Potassium Chloride Tablets, Extended-Release	T
Potassium Chloride, Potassium Bicarbonate, and Potassium Citrate Effervescent Tablets for Oral Solution	T
Potassium Citrate Tablets, Extended-Release	T
Potassium Gluconate Tablets	T
Potassium Iodide Tablets	T
Potassium Iodide Tablets, Delayed-Release	T
Potassium Perchlorate Capsules	T, LR
Praziquantel Tablets	T
Prazosin Hydrochloride Capsules	W, LR
Prednisolone Tablets	W
Prednisone Tablets	W
Primaquine Phosphate Tablets	W, LR
Primidone Tablets	W
Probenecid and Colchicine Tablets	W, LR
Probucol Tablets	W, LR
Procainamide Hydrochloride Capsules	T
Procainamide Hydrochloride Tablets	T
Procarbazine Hydrochloride Capsules	T, LR
Prochlorperazine Maleate Tablets	W
Procyclidine Hydrochloride Tablets	T
Promazine Hydrochloride Tablets	T, LR

Monograph Title	Container Specification
Promethazine Hydrochloride Tablets	T, LR
Propantheline Bromide Tablets	W
Propoxyphene Hydrochloride Capsules	T
Propoxyphene Hydrochloride and Acetaminophen Tablets	T
Propoxyphene Hydrochloride, Aspirin, and Caffeine Capsules	T
Propoxyphene Napsylate Tablets	T
Propoxyphene Napsylate and Acetaminophen Tablets	T
Propoxyphene Napsylate and Aspirin Tablets	T
Propranolol Hydrochloride Capsules, Extended-Release	W
Propranolol Hydrochloride Tablets	W, LR
Propranolol Hydrochloride and Hydrochlorothiazide Capsules, Extended-Release	W
Propranolol Hydrochloride and Hydrochlorothiazide Tablets	W
Propylthiouracil Tablets	W
Protriptyline Hydrochloride Tablets	T
Pseudoephedrine Hydrochloride Tablets	T
Pseudoephedrine Hydrochloride Tablets, Extended-Release	T
Pyrazinamide Tablets	W
Pyridostigmine Bromide Tablets	T
Pyridoxine Hydrochloride Tablets	W
Pyrilamine Maleate Tablets	W
Pyrimethamine Tablets	T, LR
Pyrvinium Pamoate Tablets	T, LR
Quazepam Tablets	W
Quinidine Gluconate Tablets, Extended-Release	W, LR
Quinidine Sulfate Capsules	T, LR
Quinidine Sulfate Tablets	W, LR
Quinidine Sulfate Tablets, Extended-Release	W, LR
Quinine Sulfate Capsules	T
Quinine Sulfate Tablets	W
Ranitidine Tablets	T, LR
Rauwolfia Serpentina Tablets	T, LR
Reserpine Tablets	T, LR
Reserpine and Chlorothiazide Tablets	T, LR
Reserpine, Hydralazine Hydrochloride, and Hydrochlorothiazide Tablets	T, LR
Reserpine and Hydrochlorothiazide Tablets	T, LR
Riboflavin Tablets	T, LR
Rifabutin Capsules	W
Rifampin Capsules	T, LR
Rifampin and Isoniazid Capsules	T, LR
Rifampin, Isoniazid, and Pyrazinamide Tablets	T, LR
Rifampin, Isoniazid, Pyrazinamide, and Ethambutol Hydrochloride Tablets	T, LR
Ritodrine Hydrochloride Tablets	T
Saccharin Sodium Tablets	W
Salsalate Capsules	T
Salsalate Tablets	T
Saquinavir Capsules	T
Saw Palmetto Capsules	T, LR
Scopolamine Hydrobromide Tablets	T, LR
Secobarbital Sodium Capsules	T
Secobarbital Sodium and Amobarbital Sodium Capsules	W
Selegiline Hydrochloride Tablets	T, LR
Sennosides Tablets	W
Simethicone Capsules	W
Simethicone Tablets	W
Simvastatin Tablets	T
Sodium Bicarbonate Tablets	W
Sodium Chloride Tablets	W
Sodium Chloride Tablets for Solution	W
Sodium Chloride and Dextrose Tablets	W

Monograph Title	Container Specification
Sodium Fluoride Tablets	T
Sodium Salicylate Tablets	W
Sotalol Hydrochloride Tablets	W, LR
Spironolactone Tablets	T, LR
Spironolactone and Hydrochlorothiazide Tablets	T, LR
Stanozolol Tablets	T, LR
Sulfadiazine Tablets	W, LR
Sulfadimethoxine Tablets	T, LR
Sulfadoxine and Pyrimethamine Tablets	W, LR
Sulfamethizole Tablets	W
Sulfamethoxazole Tablets	W, LR
Sulfamethoxazole and Trimethoprim Tablets	W, LR
Sulfapyridine Tablets	W, LR
Sulfasalazine Tablets	W
Sulfasalazine Tablets, Delayed-Release	W
Sulfinpyrazone Capsules	W
Sulfinpyrazone Tablets	W
Sulfisoxazole Tablets	W, LR
Sulindac Tablets	W
Tamoxifen Citrate Tablets	W, LR
Temazepam Capsules	W, LR
Terbutaline Sulfate Tablets	T
Testolactone Tablets	T
Tetracycline Hydrochloride Capsules	T, LR
Tetracycline Hydrochloride Tablets	T, LR
Tetracycline Hydrochloride and Novobiocin Sodium Tablets	T
Tetracycline Hydrochloride, Novobiocin Sodium, and Prednisolone Tablets	T
Tetracycline Hydrochloride and Nystatin Capsules	T, LR
Thalidomide Capsules	W
Theophylline Capsules	W
Theophylline Capsules, Extended-Release	W
Theophylline Tablets	W
Theophylline, Ephedrine Hydrochloride, and Phenobarbital Tablets	T
Theophylline and Guaifenisin Capsules	T
Theophylline Sodium Glycinate Tablets	W
Thiabendazole Tablets	T
Thiamine Hydrochloride Tablets	T, LR
Thiethylperazine Maleate Tablets	T, LR
Thioguanine Tablets	T
Thioridazine Hydrochloride Tablets	T, LR
Thiothixene Capsules	W, LR
Thyroid Tablets	T
Timolol Maleate Tablets	W
Timolol Maleate and Hydrochlorothiazide Tablets	W, LR
Tocainide Hydrochloride Tablets	W
Tolazamide Tablets	T
Tolazoline Hydrochloride Tablets	W
Tolbutamide Tablets	W
Tolmetin Sodium Capsules	T
Tolmetin Sodium Tablets	W
Trazodone Hydrochloride Tablets	T, LR
Triamcinolone Tablets	W
Triamterene Capsules	T, LR
Triamterene and Hydrochlorothiazide Capsules	T, LR
Triamterene and Hydrochlorothiazide Tablets	T, LR
Triazolam Tablets	T, LR
Trichlormethiazide Tablets	T
Trientine Hydrochloride Capsules	T
Trifluoperazine Hydrochloride Tablets	W, LR
Triflupromazine Hydrochloride Tablets	W, LR
Trihexyphenidyl Hydrochloride Capsules, Extended-Release	T
Trihexyphenidyl Hydrochloride Tablets	T
Trimeprazine Tartrate Tablets	W, LR
Trimethobenzamide Hydrochloride Capsules	W
Trimethoprim Tablets	T, LR

Monograph Title	Container Specification
Trioxsalen Tablets	W, LR
Tripelennamine Hydrochloride Tablets	W
Triple Sulfa Vaginal Tablets	W, LR
Triprolidine Hydrochloride Tablets	T, LR
Triprolidine and Pseudoephedrine Hydrochlorides Tablets	T, LR
Trisulfapyrimidines Tablets	W
Troleandomycin Capsules	T
Ubidecarenone Capsules	T, LR
Ubidecarenone Tablets	T, LR
Ursodiol Capsules	W
Ursodiol Tablets	W
Valerian Tablets	T, LR
Valproic Acid Capsules	T
Vancomycin Hydrochloride Capsules	T
Verapamil Hydrochloride Tablets	T, LR
Verapamil Hydrochloride Tablets, Extended-Release	T, LR

Monograph Title	Container Specification
Vitamin A Capsules	T, LR
Vitamin E Capsules	T
Oil-Soluble Vitamins Capsules	T, LR
Oil-Soluble Vitamins Tablets	T, LR
Oil- and Water-Soluble Vitamins Capsules	T, LR
Oil- and Water-Soluble Vitamins Tablets	T, LR
Oil- and Water-Soluble Vitamins with Minerals Capsules	T, LR
Oil- and Water-Soluble Vitamins with Minerals Tablets	T, LR
Water-Soluble Vitamins Capsules	T, LR
Water-Soluble Vitamins Tablets	T, LR
Water-Soluble Vitamins with Minerals Capsules	T, LR
Water-Soluble Vitamins with Minerals Tablets	T, LR
Warfarin Sodium Tablets	T, LR
Zalcitabine Tablets	T, LR
Zidovudine Capsules	T, LR
Zidovudine Tablets	T, LR

Section VI

SELECTED USP GENERAL NOTICES AND CHAPTERS

This Section is intended to provide convenient access to portions of the *USP–NF* that are most often used by Volume III subscribers. The information is arranged in the following manner:

Selected General Notices and Requirements

Selected Chapters

⟨1⟩ Injections
⟨71⟩ Sterility Tests
⟨85⟩ Bacterial Endotoxins Tests
⟨661⟩ Containers
⟨671⟩ Containers—Permeation
⟨751⟩ Metal Particles in Ophthalmic Ointments
⟨771⟩ Ophthalmic Ointments
⟨785⟩ Osmolarity
⟨795⟩ Pharmaceutical Compounding—Nonsterile Preparations
⟨797⟩ Pharmaceutical Compounding—Sterile Preparations
⟨1091⟩ Labeling of Inactive Ingredients
⟨1101⟩ Medicine Dropper
⟨1121⟩ Nomenclature
⟨1146⟩ Packaging Practice—Repackaging a Single Solid Oral Drug Product into a Unit-Dose Container
⟨1151⟩ Pharmaceutical Dosage Forms
⟨1160⟩ Pharmaceutical Calculations in Prescription Compounding
⟨1176⟩ Prescription Balances and Volumetric Apparatus
⟨1191⟩ Stablity Considerations in Dispensing Practice
⟨1211⟩ Sterilization and Sterility Assurance of Compendial Articles
⟨1221⟩ Teaspoon
⟨1231⟩ Water for Pharmaceutical Purposes

Guide to USP General Chapters

Selected General Notices and Requirements

Applying to Standards, Tests, Assays, and Other Specifications of the United States Pharmacopeia

Change to read:

"OFFICIAL" AND "OFFICIAL ARTICLES"

The word "official", as used in this Pharmacopeia or with reference hereto, is synonymous with "Pharmacopeial", with "USP", and with "compendial".

The designation "USP" in conjunction with the official title or elsewhere on the label of an article ▲indicates that a monograph is included in the *USP* and that the article▲*USP27* purports to comply with ▲all applicable▲*USP27* USP standards. ▲The▲*USP27* designation ▲"USP"▲*USP27* on the label ▲may not and▲*USP27* does not constitute a representation, endorsement, or incorporation by the manufac-

turer's labeling of the informational material contained in the USP monograph, nor does it constitute assurance by USP that the article is known to comply with USP standards. An article may only purport to comply with a USP standard ▲or other requirements▲*USP27* when the article is recognized in the *USP*. The standards apply equally to articles bearing the official titles or names derived by transposition of the definitive words of official titles or transposition in the order of the names of two or more active ingredients in official titles, whether or not the added designation "USP" is used. Names considered to be synonyms of the official titles may not be used for official titles.

Although both compendia, the *United States Pharmacopeia* and the *National Formulary*, currently are published under one cover, they remain separate compendia. The designation *USP–NF* or similar combination may be used on the label of an article, provided the label also bears a statement such as "Meets *NF* standards as published by the USP," indicating the particular compendium to which the article purports to apply.

Where an article differs from the standards of strength, quality, and purity, as determined by the application of the assays and tests set forth for it in the Pharmacopeia, its difference shall be plainly stated on its label. Where an article fails to comply in identity with the identity prescribed in the *USP*, or contains an added substance that interferes with the prescribed assays and tests, such article shall be designated by a name that is clearly distinguishing and differentiating from any name recognized in the Pharmacopeia.

Articles listed herein are official and the standards set forth in the monographs apply to them only when the articles are intended or labeled for use as drugs, as nutritional or dietary supplements, or as medical devices and when bought, sold, or dispensed for these purposes or when labeled as conforming to this Pharmacopeia.

An article is deemed to be recognized in this Pharmacopeia when a monograph for the article is published in it, including its supplements, addenda, or other interim revisions, and an official date is generally or specifically assigned to it.

The following terminology is used for distinguishing the articles for which monographs are provided: an *official substance* is an active drug entity, a recognized nutrient, a dietary supplement ingredient, or a pharmaceutic ingredient (see also *NF 22*) or a component of a finished device for which the monograph title includes no indication of the nature of the finished form; an *official preparation* is a *drug product*, a *nutritional supplement, dietary supplement*, or a *finished device*. It is the finished or partially finished (e.g., as in the case of a sterile solid to be constituted into a solution for administration) preparation or product of one or more official substances formulated for use on or for the patient or consumer; an *article* is an item for which a monograph is provided, whether an official substance or an official preparation.

▲*Designating Conformance with Official Standards*—When the letters "USP" or "NF" or "USP–NF" are utilized on the label of an article to indicate compliance with compendial standards, the letters shall appear in conjunction with the official title of the article or when appropriate, with the ingredients contained therein. The letters are not to be enclosed in any symbol such as a circle, square, etc., and must appear in block capital letters.

If a dietary supplement purports to be or is represented as an official product and such claim is determined by USP not to be made in good faith, it is the policy of the USP to seek appropriate legal redress.▲*USP27*

Products Not Marketed in the United States—Interest in the USP outside the United States has always existed. From time to time, monographs may be adopted for articles not legally marketed in the United States as a service to authorities in other countries where USP standards are recognized and applied. Appearance of any such monograph does not grant any marketing rights whatsoever, and the status of the article in the United States must be checked with the U.S. Food and Drug Administration in the event of any question.

Nutritional and Other Dietary Supplements—The designation of an official preparation containing one or more recognized nutrients or dietary supplement ingredients as "USP" or the use of the designation "USP" in conjunction with the title of such nutritional or dietary supplement preparation may be made only if the preparation meets ▲all▲*USP27* the applicable requirements contained in the individual monograph and general chapters.

▲Any language modifying or limiting this representation shall be accompanied by a statement indicating that the article is "not USP", and indicating how the article differs from the standards of strength, quality, or purity as determined by the application of the tests and assays set forth in the compendia.▲*USP27* Any additional ingredient in such article that is not recognized in the Pharmacopeia and for which nutritional value is claimed shall not be represented nor imply that such ingredient is of USP quality or recognized by USP. If a preparation does not comply with ▲all▲*USP27* applicable requirements but contains nutrients or dietary supplement ingredients that are recognized in the *USP*, the article may not designate the individual nutrients or ingredients as complying with USP standards or being of USP quality without designating on the label that the article itself does not comply with USP standards.

ATOMIC WEIGHTS AND CHEMICAL FORMULAS

The atomic weights used in computing molecular weights and the factors in the assays and elsewhere are those recommended in 1997 by the IUPAC Commission on Atomic Weights and Isotopic Abundances. Chemical formulas, other than those in the Definitions, tests, and assays, are given for purposes of information and calculation. The format within a given monograph is such that after the official title, the primarily informational portions of the text appear first, followed by the text comprising requirements, the latter section of the monograph being introduced by a boldface double-arrow symbol ». (Graphic formulas and chemical nomenclature provided as information in the individual monographs are discussed in the *Preface*.)

ABBREVIATIONS

The term RS refers to a USP Reference Standard as stated under *Reference Standards* in these *General Notices* (see also *USP Reference Standards* ⟨11⟩ for a comprehensive discussion of reference materials).

The terms CS and TS refer to Colorimetric Solution and Test Solution, respectively (see under *Reagents, Indicators, and Solutions*). The term VS refers to Volumetric Solution as stated under *Solutions* in the *General Notices*.

The term *PF* refers to *Pharmacopeial Forum*, the journal of standards development and official compendia revision (see *Pharmacopeial Forum* in these *General Notices*).

Abbreviations for the names of many institutions, organizations, and publications are used for convenience throughout *USP* and *NF*. An alphabetized tabulation follows.

Abbreviation	Institution, Organization, or Publication
AAMI	Association for the Advancement of Medical Instrumentation
ACS	American Chemical Society
ANSI	American National Standards Institute
AOAC	AOAC International (formerly Association of Official Analytical Chemists)
ASTM	American Society for Testing and Materials
ATCC	American Type Culture Collection
CAS	Chemical Abstracts Service
CFR	U.S. Code of Federal Regulations
EP	European Pharmacopoeia
EPA	U.S. Environmental Protection Agency
FCC	Food Chemicals Codex
FDA	U.S. Food and Drug Administration
HIMA	Health Industry Manufacturers Association
ISO	International Organization for Standardization
IUPAC	International Union of Pure and Applied Chemistry
JP	Japanese Pharmacopoeia
NIST	National Institute of Standards and Technology
USAN	United States Adopted Names
WHO	World Health Organization

Abbreviated Statements in Monographs—Incomplete sentences are employed in various portions of the monographs for directness and brevity. Where the limit tests are so abbreviated, it is to be understood that the chapter numbers (shown in angle brackets) designate the respective procedures to be followed, and that the values specified after the colon are the required limits.

SIGNIFICANT FIGURES AND TOLERANCES

Where limits are expressed numerically herein, the upper and lower limits of a range include the two values themselves and all intermediate values, but no values outside the limits. The limits expressed in monograph definitions and tests, regardless of whether the values are expressed as percentages or as absolute numbers, are considered significant to the last digit shown.

Equivalence Statements in Titrimetric Procedures—The directions for titrimetric procedures conclude with a statement of the weight of the analyte that is equivalent to each mL of the standardized titrant. In such an equivalence statement, it is to be understood that the number of significant figures in the concentration of the titrant corresponds to the number of significant figures in the weight of the analyte. Blank corrections are to be made for all titrimetric assays where appropriate (see *Titrimetry* ⟨541⟩).

Tolerances—The limits specified in the monographs for Pharmacopeial articles are established with a view to the use of these articles as drugs, nutritional or dietary supplements, or devices, except where it is indicated otherwise. The use of the molecular formula for the active ingredient(s) named in defining the required strength of a Pharmacopeial article is intended to designate the chemical entity or entities, as given in the complete chemical name of the article, having absolute (100 percent) purity.

A dosage form shall be formulated with the intent to provide 100 percent of the quantity of each ingredient declared on the label. The tolerances and limits stated in the definitions in the monographs for Pharmacopeial articles allow for analytical error, for unavoidable variations in manufacturing and compounding, and for deterioration to an extent considered acceptable under practical conditions. Where the minimum amount of a

substance present in a nutritional or dietary supplement is required to be higher than the lower tolerance limit allowed for in the monograph because of applicable legal requirements, then the upper tolerance limit contained in the monograph shall be increased by a corresponding amount.

The specified tolerances are based upon such attributes of quality as might be expected to characterize an article produced from suitable raw materials under recognized principles of good manufacturing practice.

The existence of compendial limits or tolerances does not constitute a basis for a claim that an official substance that more nearly approaches 100 percent purity "exceeds" the Pharmacopeial quality. Similarly, the fact that an article has been prepared to closer tolerances than those specified in the monograph does not constitute a basis for a claim that the article "exceeds" the Pharmacopeial requirements.

Interpretation of Requirements—Analytical results observed in the laboratory (or calculated from experimental measurements) are compared with stated limits to determine whether there is conformance with compendial assay or test requirements. The observed or calculated values usually will contain more significant figures than there are in the stated limit, and an observed or calculated result is to be rounded off to the number of places that is in agreement with the limit expression by the following procedure. [NOTE—Limits, which are fixed numbers, are not rounded off.]

When rounding off is required, consider only one digit in the decimal place to the right of the last place in the limit expression. If this digit is smaller than 5, it is eliminated and the preceding digit is unchanged. If this digit is greater than 5, it is eliminated and the preceding digit is increased by one. If this digit equals 5, the 5 is eliminated and the preceding digit is increased by one.

Illustration of Rounding Numerical Values for Comparison with Requirements

Compendial Requirement	Unrounded Value	Rounded Result	Conforms
Assay limit ≥98.0%	97.96%	98.0%	Yes
	97.92%	97.9%	No
	97.95%	98.0%	Yes
Assay limit ≤101.5%	101.55%	101.6%	No
	101.46%	101.5%	Yes
	101.45%	101.5%	Yes
Limit test ≤0.02%	0.025%	0.03%	No
	0.015%	0.02%	Yes
	0.027%	0.03%	No
Limit test ≤3 ppm	0.00035%	0.0004%	No
	0.00025%	0.0003%	Yes
	0.00028%	0.0003%	Yes

GENERAL CHAPTERS

Each general chapter is assigned a number that appears in brackets adjacent to the chapter name (e.g., ⟨621⟩ *Chromatography*). General chapters that include general *requirements* for tests and assays are numbered from ⟨1⟩ to ⟨999⟩, chapters that are *informational* are numbered from ⟨1000⟩ to ⟨1999⟩, and chapters pertaining to *nutritional supplements* are numbered above ⟨2000⟩.

The use of the general chapter numbers is encouraged for the identification and rapid access to general tests and information. It is especially helpful where monograph section headings and chapter names are not the same (e.g., *Ultraviolet Absorption* ⟨197U⟩ in a monograph refers to method ⟨197U⟩ under general tests chapter ⟨197⟩ *Spectrophotometric Identification Tests*; *Specific rotation* ⟨781S⟩ in a monograph refers to method ⟨781S⟩ under general tests chapter ⟨781⟩ *Optical Rotation*; and *Calcium* ⟨191⟩ in a monograph refers to the tests for *Calcium* under general tests chapter ⟨191⟩ *Identification Tests—General*).

PHARMACOPEIAL FORUM

Pharmacopeial Forum (*PF*) is the USP journal of standards development and official compendia revision. *Pharmacopeial Forum* is the working document of the USP Committee of Revision. It is intended to provide public portions of communications within the General Committee of Revision and public notice of proposed new and revised standards of the *USP* and *NF* and to afford opportunity for comment thereon. The organization of *PF* includes, but is not limited to, the following sections. Subsections occur where needed for Drugs and Pharmaceutic Ingredients (Excipients) and for Nutritional Supplements.

Pharmacopeial Previews—Possible revisions or new monographs or chapters that are considered to be in a preliminary stage of development.

In-Process Revision—New or revised monographs or chapters that are proposed for adoption as official USP or NF standards.

Stimuli to the Revision Process—Reports, statements, articles, or commentaries relating to compendial issues.

Nomenclature—Articles and announcements relevant to compendial nomenclature issues and listings of suggested and new United States Adopted Names (USAN) and International Nonproprietary Names (INN).

Interim Revision Announcement (if present)—Official revisions and their effective dates, announcement of the availability of new USP Reference Standards, and announcement of assays or tests that are held in abeyance pending availability of required USP Reference Standards.

Official Reference Standards—Catalog of current lots of USP Reference Standards with ordering information and names and addresses of worldwide suppliers.

SUPPLEMENT

Supplements to official text are published periodically and include text previously published in *PF*, which is ready to be made official.

REAGENT STANDARDS

The proper conduct of the Pharmacopeial tests and assays and the reliability of the results depend, in part, upon the quality of the reagents used in the performance of the procedures. Unless otherwise specified, reagents are to be used that conform to the specifications set forth in the current edition of *Reagent Chemicals* published by the American Chemical Society. Where such ACS reagent specifications are not available or where for various reasons the required purity differs, compendial specifications for reagents of acceptable quality are provided (see *Reagents, Indicators, and Solutions*). Listing of these reagents, including the indicators and solutions employed as reagents, in no way implies that they have therapeutic utility; furthermore, any reference to USP or NF in their labeling shall include also the term "reagent" or "reagent grade."

REFERENCE REAGENTS

Some compendial tests or assays require the use of specific reagents. These are supplied by USP when they might not be generally commercially available or because they are necessary for the testing and are available only to the originator of the tests or assay.

USP REFERENCE STANDARDS

USP Reference Standards are authentic specimens that have been approved by the USP Reference Standards Committee as suitable for use as comparison standards in USP or NF tests and

assays. (See *USP Reference Standards* ⟨11⟩.) Currently official lots of USP Reference Standards are published in *Pharmacopeial Forum*.

Where a USP Reference Standard is referred to in a monograph or chapter, the words "Reference Standard" are abbreviated to "RS" (see *USP Reference Standards* ⟨11⟩).

Where a test or an assay calls for the use of a compendial article rather than for a USP Reference Standard as a material standard of reference, a substance meeting all of the compendial monograph requirements for that article is to be used.

The requirements for any new USP or NF standards, tests, or assays for which a new USP Reference Standard is specified are not in effect until the specified USP Reference Standard is available. The availability of new USP Reference Standards and the official dates of the USP or NF standards, tests, or assays requiring their use are announced via *Supplements* or *Interim Revision Announcements*.

UNITS OF POTENCY

For substances that cannot be completely characterized by chemical and physical means, it may be necessary to express quantities of activity in biological units of potency, each defined by an authoritative, designated reference standard.

Units of biological potency defined by the World Health Organization (WHO) for International Biological Standards and International Biological Reference Preparations are termed International Units (IU). Units defined by USP Reference Standards are USP Units, and the individual monographs refer to these. Unless otherwise indicated, USP Units are equivalent to the corresponding International Units, where such exist. Such equivalence is usually established on the basis solely of the compendial assay for the substance.

For biological products, whether or not International Units or USP Units do exist (see *Biologics* ⟨1041⟩), units of potency are defined by the corresponding US Standard established by the FDA.

Change to read:

INGREDIENTS AND PROCESSES

Official drug products and finished devices are prepared from ingredients that meet the requirements of the compendial monographs for those individual ingredients for which monographs are provided (see also *NF 22*). Generally, nutritional and dietary supplements are prepared from ingredients that meet requirements of the compendial monographs for those ingredients for which monographs are provided, except that substances of acceptable food grade quality may be utilized in the event of a difference.

Official substances are prepared according to recognized principles of good manufacturing practice and from ingredients complying with specifications designed to assure that the resultant substances meet the requirements of the compendial monographs (see also *Foreign Substances and Impurities* under *Tests and Assays*).

Preparations for which a complete composition is given in this Pharmacopeia, unless specifically exempted herein or in the individual monograph, are to contain only the ingredients named in the formulas. However, there may be deviation from the specified processes or methods of compounding, though not from the ingredients or proportions thereof, provided the finished preparation conforms to the relevant standards laid down herein and to preparations produced by following the specified process.

The tolerances specified in individual monographs and in the general chapters for compounded preparations are based on those attributes of quality as might be expected to characterize an article compounded from suitable bulk drug substances and ingredients in accordance with the procedures provided or under

recognized principles of good pharmaceutical practice as described in this Pharmacopeia (see ▲*Pharmaceutical Compounding—Nonsterile Preparations*▲*USP27* ⟨795⟩) and elsewhere.

Monographs for preparations intended to be compounded pursuant to prescription may contain assay methods. Assay methods are not intended for evaluating a compounded preparation prior to dispensing. Assay methods are intended to serve as the official test methods in the event of a question or dispute as to whether or not the compounded preparation complies with official standards.

Where a monograph on a preparation calls for an ingredient in an amount expressed on the dried basis, the ingredient need not be dried prior to use if due allowance is made for the water or other volatile substances present in the quantity taken.

Unless specifically exempted elsewhere in this Pharmacopeia, the identity, strength, quality, and purity of an official article are determined by the definition, physical properties, tests, assays, and other specifications relating to the article, whether incorporated in the monograph itself, in the *General Notices*, or in the section *General Chapters*.

Water —Water used as an ingredient of official preparations meets the requirements for *Purified Water*, for *Water for Injection*, or for one of the sterile forms of water covered by a monograph in this Pharmacopeia.

Potable water meeting the requirements for drinking water as set forth in the regulations of the U.S. Environmental Protection Agency may be used in the preparation of official substances.

Alcohol —All statements of percentages of alcohol, such as under the heading *Alcohol content* refer to percentage, by volume, of C_2H_5OH at 15.56°. Where reference is made to "C_2H_5OH," the chemical entity possessing absolute (100 percent) strength is intended.

Alcohol—Where "alcohol" is called for in formulas, tests, and assays, the monograph article *Alcohol* is to be used.

Dehydrated Alcohol—Where "dehydrated alcohol" (absolute alcohol) is called for in tests and assays, the monograph article *Dehydrated Alcohol* is to be used.

Denatured Alcohol—Specially denatured alcohol formulas are available for use in accordance with federal statutes and regulations of the Internal Revenue Service. A suitable formula of specially denatured alcohol may be substituted for Alcohol in the manufacture of Pharmacopeial preparations intended for internal or topical use, provided that the denaturant is volatile and does not remain in the finished product. A finished product that is intended for topical application to the skin may contain specially denatured alcohol, provided that the denaturant is either a normal ingredient or a permissible added substance; in either case the denaturant must be identified on the label of the topical preparation. Where a process is given in the individual monograph, the preparation so made must be identical with that prepared by the given process.

Added Substances —An official substance, as distinguished from an official preparation, contains no added substances except where specifically permitted in the individual monograph. Where such addition is permitted, the label indicates the name(s) and amount(s) of any added substance(s).

Unless otherwise specified in the individual monograph, or elsewhere in the *General Notices*, suitable substances such as antimicrobial agents, bases, carriers, coatings, colors, flavors, preservatives, stabilizers, and vehicles may be added to an official preparation to enhance its stability, usefulness, or elegance or to facilitate its preparation. Such substances are regarded as unsuitable and are prohibited unless (a) they are harmless in the amounts used, (b) they do not exceed the minimum quantity required to provide their intended effect, (c) their presence does not impair the bioavailability or the therapeutic efficacy or safety of the official preparation, and (d) they do not interfere with the assays and tests prescribed for determining compliance with the Pharmacopeial standards.

Nutritional and Dietary Supplements—Unless otherwise specified in the individual monograph, or elsewhere in the *General Notices*, consistent with applicable regulatory requirements,

suitable added substances such as bases, carriers, coatings, colors, flavors, preservatives, and stabilizers may be added to a nutritional supplement preparation to enhance its stability, usefulness, or elegance, or to facilitate its preparation. Such added substances shall be regarded as suitable and shall be permitted unless they interfere with the assays and tests prescribed for determining compliance with Pharmacopeial standards.

Additional Ingredients—Additional ingredients, including excipients, may be added to nutritional supplement preparations containing recognized nutrients, consistent with applicable regulatory requirements, provided that they do not interfere with the assays and tests prescribed for determining compliance with Pharmacopeial standards.

Inert Headspace Gases—The air in a container of an article for parenteral use may be evacuated or be replaced by carbon dioxide, helium, or nitrogen, or by a mixture of these gases, which fact need not be declared in the labeling.

Colors—Added substances employed solely to impart color may be incorporated into official preparations, except those intended for parenteral or ophthalmic use, in accordance with the regulations pertaining to the use of colors issued by the FDA provided such added substances are otherwise appropriate in all respects. (See also *Added Substances* under *Injections* ⟨1⟩.)

Ointments and Suppositories—In the preparation of ointments and suppositories, the proportions of the substances constituting the base may be varied to maintain a suitable consistency under different climatic conditions, provided the concentrations of active ingredients are not varied and the bioavailability, therapeutic efficacy or safety of the preparation is not impaired.

TESTS AND ASSAYS

Apparatus—A specification for a definite size or type of container or apparatus in a test or assay is given solely as a recommendation. Where volumetric flasks or other exact measuring, weighing, or sorting devices are specified, this or other equipment of at least equivalent accuracy shall be employed. (See also *Thermometers* ⟨21⟩, *Volumetric Apparatus* ⟨31⟩, and *Weights and Balances* ⟨41⟩.) Where low-actinic or light-resistant containers are specified, clear containers that have been rendered opaque by application of a suitable coating or wrapping may be used.

Where an instrument for physical measurement, such as a spectrophotometer, is specified in a test or assay by its distinctive name, another instrument of equivalent or greater sensitivity and accuracy may be used. In order to obtain solutions having concentrations that are adaptable to the working range of the instrument being used, solutions of proportionately higher or lower concentrations may be prepared according to the solvents and proportions thereof that are specified for the procedure.

Where a particular brand or source of a material, instrument, or piece of equipment, or the name and address of a manufacturer or distributor, is mentioned (ordinarily in a footnote), this identification is furnished solely for informational purposes as a matter of convenience, without implication of approval, endorsement, or certification. Items capable of equal or better performance may be used if these characteristics have been validated.

Where the use of a centrifuge is indicated, unless otherwise specified, the directions are predicated upon the use of apparatus having an effective radius of about 20 cm (8 inches) and driven at a speed sufficient to clarify the supernatant layer within 15 minutes.

Unless otherwise specified, for chromatographic tubes and columns the diameter specified refers to internal diameter (ID); for other types of tubes and tubing the diameter specified refers to outside diameter (OD).

Steam Bath—Where the use of a steam bath is directed, exposure to actively flowing steam or to another form of regulated heat, corresponding in temperature to that of flowing steam, may be used.

Water Bath—Where the use of a water bath is directed without qualification with respect to temperature, a bath of vigorously boiling water is intended.

Foreign Substances and Impurities—Tests for the presence of foreign substances and impurities are provided to limit such substances to amounts that are unobjectionable under conditions in which the article is customarily employed (see also *Impurities in Official Articles* ⟨1086⟩).

While one of the primary objectives of the Pharmacopeia is to assure the user of official articles of their identity, strength, quality, and purity, it is manifestly impossible to include in each monograph a test for every impurity, contaminant, or adulterant that might be present, including microbial contamination. These may arise from a change in the source of material or from a change in the processing, or may be introduced from extraneous sources. Tests suitable for detecting such occurrences, the presence of which is inconsistent with applicable good manufacturing practice or good pharmaceutical practice, should be employed in addition to the tests provided in the individual monograph.

Other Impurities—Official substances may be obtained from more than one process, and thus may contain impurities not considered during preparation of monograph assays or tests. Wherever a monograph includes a chromatographic assay or purity test based on chromatography, other than a test for organic volatile impurities, and that monograph does not detect such an impurity, solvents excepted, the impurity shall have its amount and identity, where both are known, stated under the heading *Other Impurity(ies)* by the labeling (certificate of analysis) of the official substance.

The presence of any unlabeled impurity in an official substance is a variance from the standard if the content is 0.1% or greater. Tests suitable for detection and quantitating unlabeled impurities, when present as the result of process change or other identifiable, consistent occurrence, shall be submitted to the USP for inclusion in the individual monograph. Otherwise, the impurity shall be identified, preferably by name, and the amount listed under the heading *Other Impurity(ies)* in the labeling (certificate of analysis) of the official substance. The sum of all *Other Impurities* combined with the monograph-detected impurities does not exceed 2.0% (see *Ordinary Impurities* ⟨466⟩), unless otherwise stated in the monograph.

Categories of drug substances excluded from *Other Impurities* requirements are fermentation products and semi-synthetics derived therefrom, radiopharmaceuticals, biologics, biotechnology-derived products, peptides, herbals, and crude products of animal or plant origin. Any substance known to be toxic must not be listed under *Other Impurities*.

Procedures—Assay and test procedures are provided for determining compliance with the Pharmacopeial standards of identity, strength, quality, and purity.

In performing the assay or test procedures in this Pharmacopeia, it is expected that safe laboratory practices will be followed. This includes the utilization of precautionary measures, protective equipment, and work practices consistent with the chemicals and procedures utilized. Prior to undertaking any assay or procedure described in this Pharmacopeia, the individual should be aware of the hazards associated with the chemicals and the procedures and means of protecting against them. This Pharmacopeia is not designed to describe such hazards or protective measures.

Every compendial article in commerce shall be so constituted that when examined in accordance with these assay and test procedures, it meets all of the requirements in the monograph defining it. However, it is not to be inferred that application of every analytical procedure in the monograph to samples from every production batch is necessarily a prerequisite for assuring compliance with Pharmacopeial standards before the batch is released for distribution. Data derived from manufacturing *process validation* studies and from *in-process controls* may provide greater assurance that a batch meets a particular monograph requirement than analytical data derived from an examination of finished units drawn from that batch. On the basis

of such assurances, the analytical procedures in the monograph may be omitted by the manufacturer in judging compliance of the batch with the Pharmacopeial standards.

Automated procedures employing the same basic chemistry as those assay and test procedures given in the monograph are recognized as being equivalent in their suitability for determining compliance. Conversely, where an automated procedure is given in the monograph, manual procedures employing the same basic chemistry are recognized as being equivalent in their suitability for determining compliance. Compliance may be determined also by the use of alternative methods, chosen for advantages in accuracy, sensitivity, precision, selectivity, or adaptability to automation or computerized data reduction or in other special circumstances. Such alternative or automated procedures or methods shall be validated. However, Pharmacopeial standards and procedures are interrelated; therefore, where a difference appears or in the event of dispute, only the result obtained by the procedure given in this Pharmacopeia is conclusive.

In the performance of assay or test procedures, not less than the specified number of dosage units should be taken for analysis. Proportionately larger or smaller quantities than the specified weights and volumes of assay or test substances and Reference Standards may be taken, provided the measurement is made with at least equivalent accuracy and provided that any subsequent steps, such as dilutions, are adjusted accordingly to yield concentrations equivalent to those specified and are made in such manner as to provide at least equivalent accuracy. To minimize environmental impact or contact with hazardous materials, apparatus and chemicals specified in Pharmacopeial procedures also may be proportionally changed.

Where it is directed in an assay or a test that a certain quantity of substance or a counted number of dosage units is to be examined, the specified quantity or number is a minimal figure (the singlet determination) chosen only for convenience of analytical manipulation; it is not intended to restrict the total quantity of substance or number of units that may be subjected to the assay or test or that should be tested in accordance with good manufacturing practices.

Where it is directed in the assay of Tablets to "weigh and finely powder not less than" a given number, usually 20, of the Tablets, it is intended that a counted number of Tablets shall be weighed and reduced to a powder. The portion of the powdered tablets taken for assay is representative of the whole Tablets and is, in turn, weighed accurately. The result of the assay is then related to the amount of active ingredient per Tablet by multiplying this result by the average Tablet weight and dividing by the weight of the portion taken for the assay.

Similarly, where it is directed in the assay of Capsules to remove, as completely as possible, the contents of not less than a given number, usually 20, of the Capsules, it is intended that a counted number of Capsules should be carefully opened and the contents quantitatively removed, combined, mixed, and weighed accurately. The portion of mixed Capsules contents taken for the assay is representative of the contents of the Capsules and is, in turn, weighed accurately. The result of the assay is then related to the amount of active ingredient per Capsule by multiplying this result by the average weight of Capsule content and dividing by the weight of the portion taken for the assay.

Where the definition in a monograph states the tolerances as being "calculated on the dried (or anhydrous or ignited) basis," the directions for drying or igniting the sample prior to assaying are generally omitted from the *Assay* procedure. Assay and test procedures may be performed on the undried or unignited substance and the results calculated on the dried, anhydrous, or ignited basis, provided a test for *Loss on drying*, or *Water*, or *Loss on ignition*, respectively, is given in the monograph. Where the presence of moisture or other volatile material may interfere with the procedure, previous drying of the substance is specified in the individual monograph and is obligatory.

Throughout a monograph that includes a test for *Loss on drying* or *Water*, the expression "previously dried" without qualification signifies that the substance is to be dried as directed under *Loss on drying* or *Water* (gravimetric determination).

Unless otherwise directed in the test or assay in the individual monograph or in a general chapter, USP Reference Standards are to be dried before use, or used without prior drying, specifically in accordance with the instructions given in the chapter *USP Reference Standards* ⟨11⟩, and on the label of the Reference Standard. Where the label instructions differ in detail from those in the chapter, the label text is determinative.

In stating the appropriate quantities to be taken for assays and tests, the use of the word "about" indicates a quantity within 10% of the specified weight or volume. However, the weight or volume taken is accurately determined and the calculated result is based upon the exact amount taken. The same tolerance applies to specified dimensions.

Where the use of a pipet is directed for measuring a specimen or an aliquot in conducting a test or an assay, the pipet conforms to the standards set forth under *Volumetric Apparatus* ⟨31⟩, and is to be used in such manner that the error does not exceed the limit stated for a pipet of its size. Where a pipet is specified, a suitable buret, conforming to the standards set forth under *Volumetric Apparatus* ⟨31⟩, may be substituted. Where a "to contain" pipet is specified, a suitable volumetric flask may be substituted.

Expressions such as "25.0 mL" and "25.0 mg," used with respect to volumetric or gravimetric measurements, indicate that the quantity is to be "accurately measured" or "accurately weighed" within the limits stated under *Volumetric Apparatus* ⟨31⟩ or under *Weights and Balances* ⟨41⟩.

The term "transfer" is used generally to specify a quantitative manipulation.

The term "concomitantly," used in such expressions as "concomitantly determine" or "concomitantly measured," in directions for assays and tests, is intended to denote that the determinations or measurements are to be performed in immediate succession. See also *Use of Reference Standards* under *Spectrophotometry and Light-Scattering* ⟨851⟩.

Blank Determination—Where it is directed that "any necessary correction" be made by a blank determination, the determination is to be conducted using the same quantities of the same reagents treated in the same manner as the solution or mixture containing the portion of the substance under assay or test, but with the substance itself omitted.

Desiccator—The expression "in a desiccator" specifies the use of a tightly closed container of suitable size and design that maintains an atmosphere of low moisture content by means of silica gel or other suitable desiccant.

A "vacuum desiccator" is one that maintains the low-moisture atmosphere at a reduced pressure of not more than 20 mm of mercury or at the pressure designated in the individual monograph.

Dilution—Where it is directed that a solution be diluted "quantitatively and stepwise," an accurately measured portion is to be diluted by adding water or other solvent, in the proportion indicated, in one or more steps. The choice of apparatus to be used should take into account the relatively larger errors generally associated with using small-volume volumetric apparatus (see *Volumetric Apparatus* ⟨31⟩).

Drying to Constant Weight—The specification "dried to constant weight" means that the drying shall be continued until two consecutive weighings do not differ by more than 0.50 mg per g of substance taken, the second weighing following an additional hour of drying.

Filtration—Where it is directed to "filter," without further qualification, the intent is that the liquid be filtered through suitable filter paper or equivalent device until the filtrate is clear.

Identification Tests—The Pharmacopeial tests headed *Identification* are provided as an aid in verifying the identity of articles as they are purported to be, such as those taken from labeled containers. Such tests, however specific, are not necessarily sufficient to establish proof of identity; but failure of an article taken from a labeled container to meet the requirements of a prescribed identification test indicates that the article may be

mislabeled. Other tests and specifications in the monograph often contribute to establishing or confirming the identity of the article under examination.

Ignition to Constant Weight—The specification "ignite to constant weight" means that the ignition shall be continued, at $800 \pm 25°$ unless otherwise indicated, until two consecutive weighings do not differ by more than 0.50 mg per g of substance taken, the second weighing following an additional 15-minute ignition period.

Indicators—Where the use of a test solution ("TS") as an indicator is specified in a test or an assay, approximately 0.2 mL, or 3 drops, of the solution shall be added, unless otherwise directed.

Logarithms—Logarithms used in the assays are to the base 10.

Microbial Strains—Where a microbial strain is cited and identified by its ATCC catalog number, the specified strain shall be used directly or, if subcultured, shall be used not more than five passages removed from the original strain.

Negligible—This term indicates a quantity not exceeding 0.50 mg.

Odor—Terms such as "odorless," "practically odorless," "a faint characteristic odor," or variations thereof, apply to examination, after exposure to the air for 15 minutes, of either a freshly opened package of the article (for packages containing not more than 25 g) or (for larger packages) of a portion of about 25 g of the article that has been removed from its package to an open evaporating dish of about 100-mL capacity. An odor designation is descriptive only and is not to be regarded as a standard of purity for a particular lot of an article.

Pressure Measurements—The term "mm of mercury" used with respect to measurements of blood pressure, pressure within an apparatus, or atmospheric pressure refers to the use of a suitable manometer or barometer calibrated in terms of the pressure exerted by a column of mercury of the stated height.

Solutions—Unless otherwise specified in the individual monograph, all solutions called for in tests and assays are prepared with *Purified Water*.

An expression such as "(1 in 10)" means that 1 part *by volume* of a liquid is to be diluted with, or 1 part *by weight* of a solid is to be dissolved in, sufficient of the diluent or solvent to make the volume of the finished solution 10 parts *by volume*.

An expression such as "(20 : 5 : 2)" means that the respective numbers of parts, by volume, of the designated liquids are to be mixed, unless otherwise indicated.

The notation "VS" after a specified volumetric solution indicates that such solution is standardized in accordance with directions given in the individual monograph or under *Volumetric Solutions* in the section *Reagents, Indicators, and Solutions*, and is thus differentiated from solutions of approximate normality or molarity.

Where a standardized solution of a specific concentration is called for in a test or an assay, a solution of other normality or molarity may be used, provided allowance is made for the difference in concentration and provided the error of measurement is not increased thereby.

Specific Gravity—Unless otherwise stated, the specific gravity basis is $25°/25°$, i.e., the ratio of the weight of a substance in air at $25°$ to the weight of an equal volume of water at the same temperature.

Temperatures—Unless otherwise specified, all temperatures in this Pharmacopeia are expressed in centigrade (Celsius) degrees, and all measurements are made at $25°$. Where moderate heat is specified, any temperature not higher than $45°$ ($113°$ F) is indicated. See *Storage Temperature* under *Preservation, Packaging, Storage, and Labeling* for other definitions.

Time Limit—In the conduct of tests and assays, 5 minutes shall be allowed for the reaction to take place unless otherwise specified.

Vacuum—The term "in vacuum" denotes exposure to a pressure of less than 20 mm of mercury unless otherwise indicated.

Where drying in vacuum over a desiccant is directed in the individual monograph, a vacuum desiccator or a vacuum drying pistol, or other suitable vacuum drying apparatus, is to be used.

Water—Where water is called for in tests and assays, *Purified Water* is to be used unless otherwise specified. For special kinds of water such as "carbon dioxide–free water," see the introduction to the section *Reagents, Indicators, and Solutions*. For *High-purity Water* see *Containers* ⟨661⟩.

Water and Loss on Drying—Where the water of hydration or adsorbed water of a Pharmacopeial article is determined by the titrimetric method, the test is generally given under the heading *Water*. Monograph limits expressed as a percentage are figured on a weight/weight basis unless otherwise specified. Where the determination is made by drying under specified conditions, the test is generally given under the heading *Loss on drying*. However, *Loss on drying* is most often given as the heading where the loss in weight is known to represent residual volatile constituents including organic solvents as well as water.

Test Results, Statistics, and Standards—Interpretation of results from official tests and assays requires an understanding of the nature and style of compendial standards, in addition to an understanding of the scientific and mathematical aspects of laboratory analysis and quality assurance for analytical laboratories.

Confusion of compendial standards with release tests and with statistical sampling plans occasionally occurs. Compendial standards define what is an acceptable article and give test procedures that demonstrate that the article is in compliance. These standards apply at any time in the life of the article from production to consumption. The manufacturer's release specifications, and compliance with good manufacturing practices generally, are developed and followed to assure that the article will indeed comply with compendial standards until its expiration date, when stored as directed. Thus, when tested from the viewpoint of commercial or regulatory compliance, any specimen tested as directed in the monograph for that article shall comply.

Tests and assays in this Pharmacopeia prescribe operation on a single specimen, that is, the singlet determination, which is the minimum sample on which the attributes of a compendial article should be measured. Some tests, such as those for *Dissolution* and *Uniformity of dosage units*, require multiple dosage units in conjunction with a decision scheme. These tests, albeit using a number of dosage units, are in fact the singlet determinations of those particular attributes of the specimen. These procedures should not be confused with statistical sampling plans. Repeats, replicates, statistical rejection of outliers, or extrapolations of results to larger populations are neither specified nor proscribed by the compendia; such decisions are dependent on the objectives of the testing. Commercial or regulatory compliance testing, or manufacturer's release testing, may or may not require examination of additional specimens, in accordance with predetermined guidelines or sampling strategies. Treatments of data handling are available from organizations such as ISO, IUPAC, and AOAC.

Description—Information on the "description" pertaining to an article, which is relatively general in nature, is provided in the reference table *Description and Relative Solubility of USP and NF Articles* in this Pharmacopeia for those who use, prepare, and dispense drugs and/or related articles, solely to indicate properties of an article complying with monograph standards. The properties are not in themselves standards or tests for purity even though they may indirectly assist in the preliminary evaluation of an article.

Solubility—The statements concerning solubilities given in the reference table *Description and Relative Solubility of USP and NF Articles* for Pharmacopeial articles are not standards or tests for purity but are provided primarily as information for those who use, prepare, and dispense drugs and/or related articles. Only where a quantitative solubility test is given, and is designated as such, is it a test for purity.

The approximate solubilities of Pharmacopeial substances are indicated by the descriptive terms in the accompanying table. Soluble Pharmacopeial articles, when brought into solution, may show traces of physical impurities, such as minute fragments of filter paper, fibers, and other particulate matter, unless limited or excluded by definite tests or other specifications in the individual monographs.

Descriptive Term	Parts of Solvent Required for 1 Part of Solute
Very soluble	Less than 1
Freely soluble	From 1 to 10
Soluble	From 10 to 30
Sparingly soluble	From 30 to 100
Slightly soluble	From 100 to 1000
Very slightly soluble	From 1000 to 10,000
Practically insoluble, or Insoluble	Greater than or equal to 10,000

Interchangeable Methods—Certain general chapters contain a statement that the text in question is harmonized with the corresponding text of the *European Pharmacopoeia* and/or the *Japanese Pharmacopoeia* and that these texts are interchangeable. Therefore, if a substance or preparation is found to comply with a requirement using an interchangeable method from one of these pharmacopeias, it should comply with the requirements of the *United States Pharmacopeia*. However, where a difference appears, or in the event of dispute, only the result obtained by the procedure given in this Pharmacopeia is conclusive.

PRESCRIBING AND DISPENSING

Prescriptions for compendial articles shall be written to state the quantity and/or strength desired in metric units unless otherwise indicated in the individual monograph (see also *Units of Potency* in these *General Notices*). If an amount is prescribed by any other system of measurement, only an amount that is the metric equivalent of the prescribed amount shall be dispensed.

Change to read:

PRESERVATION, PACKAGING, STORAGE, AND LABELING

Containers—The *container* is that which holds the article and is or may be in direct contact with the article. The *immediate container* is that which is in direct contact with the article at all times. The *closure* is a part of the container.

Prior to its being filled, the container should be clean. Special precautions and cleaning procedures may be necessary to ensure that each container is clean and that extraneous matter is not introduced into or onto the article.

The container does not interact physically or chemically with the article placed in it so as to alter the strength, quality, or purity of the article beyond the official requirements.

The Pharmacopeial requirements for the use of specified containers apply also to articles as packaged by the pharmacist or other dispenser, unless otherwise indicated in the individual monograph.

Tamper-Evident Packaging —The container or individual carton of a sterile article intended for ophthalmic or otic use, except where extemporaneously compounded for immediate dispensing on prescription, shall be so sealed that the contents cannot be used without obvious destruction of the seal.

Articles intended for sale without prescription are also required to comply with the tamper-evident packaging and labeling requirements of the FDA where applicable.

Preferably, the immediate container and/or the outer container or protective packaging utilized by a manufacturer or distributor for all dosage forms that are not specifically exempt is designed so as to show evidence of any tampering with the contents.

Light-Resistant Container (see *Light Transmission* under *Containers* ⟨661⟩)—A light-resistant container protects the contents from the effects of light by virtue of the specific properties of the material of which it is composed, including any coating applied to it. Alternatively, a clear and colorless or a translucent container may be made light-resistant by means of an opaque covering, in which case the label of the container bears a statement that the opaque covering is needed until the contents are to be used or administered. Where it is directed to "protect from light" in an individual monograph, preservation in a light-resistant container is intended.

Where an article is required to be packaged in a light-resistant container, and if the container is made light-resistant by means of an opaque covering, a single-use, unit-dose container or mnemonic pack for dispensing may not be removed from the outer opaque covering prior to dispensing.

Well-Closed Container—A well-closed container protects the contents from extraneous solids and from loss of the article under the ordinary or customary conditions of handling, shipment, storage, and distribution.

Tight Container—A tight container protects the contents from contamination by extraneous liquids, solids, or vapors, from loss of the article, and from efflorescence, deliquescence, or evaporation under the ordinary or customary conditions of handling, shipment, storage, and distribution, and is capable of tight re-closure. Where a tight container is specified, it may be replaced by a hermetic container for a single dose of an article.

A gas cylinder is a metallic container designed to hold a gas under pressure. As a safety measure, for carbon dioxide, cyclopropane, helium, nitrous oxide, and oxygen, the Pin-index Safety System of matched fittings is recommended for cylinders of Size E or smaller.

NOTE—Where packaging and storage in a *tight container* or a *well-closed container* is specified in the individual monograph, the container utilized for an article when dispensed on prescription meets the requirements under *Containers—Permeation* ⟨671⟩.

Hermetic Container—A hermetic container is impervious to air or any other gas under the ordinary or customary conditions of handling, shipment, storage, and distribution.

Single-Unit Container—A single-unit container is one that is designed to hold a quantity of drug product intended for administration as a single dose or a single finished device intended for use promptly after the container is opened. Preferably, the immediate container and/or the outer container or protective packaging shall be so designed as to show evidence of any tampering with the contents. Each single-unit container shall be labeled to indicate the identity, quantity and/or strength, name of the manufacturer, lot number, and expiration date of the article.

Single-Dose Container (see also *Containers for Injections* under *Injections* ⟨1⟩)—A single-dose container is a single-unit container for articles intended for parenteral administration only. A single-dose container is labeled as such. Examples of single-dose containers include pre-filled syringes, cartridges, fusion-sealed containers, and closure-sealed containers when so labeled.

Unit-Dose Container—A unit-dose container is a single-unit container for articles intended for administration by other than the parenteral route as a single dose, direct from the container.

Unit-of-Use Container—A unit-of-use container is one that contains a specific quantity of a drug product and that is intended to be dispensed as such without further modification except for the addition of appropriate labeling. A unit-of-use container is labeled as such.

Multiple-Unit Container—A multiple-unit container is a container that permits withdrawal of successive portions of the contents without changing the strength, quality, or purity of the remaining portion.

Multiple-Dose Container (see also *Containers for Injections* under *Injections* ⟨1⟩)—A multiple-dose container is a multiple-unit container for articles intended for parenteral administration only.

Storage Temperature and Humidity—Specific directions are stated in some monographs with respect to the temperatures and humidity at which Pharmacopeial articles shall be stored and distributed (including the shipment of articles to the consumer) when stability data indicate that storage and distribution at a lower or a higher temperature and a higher humidity produce undesirable results. Such directions apply except where the label on an article states a different storage temperature on the basis of stability studies of that particular formulation. Where no specific storage directions or limitations are provided in the individual monograph, but the label of an article states a storage temperature that is based on stability studies of that particular formulation, such labeled storage directions apply (see also *Stability* under *Pharmaceutical Dosage Forms* ⟨1151⟩). The conditions are defined by the following terms.

Freezer—A place in which the temperature is maintained thermostatically between −25° and −10° (−13° and 14 °F).

Cold—Any temperature not exceeding 8° (46 °F). A *refrigerator* is a cold place in which the temperature is maintained thermostatically between 2° and 8° (36° and 46 °F).

Cool—Any temperature between 8° and 15° (46° and 59 °F). An article for which storage in a *cool place* is directed may, alternatively, be stored and distributed in a *refrigerator*, unless otherwise specified by the individual monograph.

Room Temperature—The temperature prevailing in a working area.

Controlled Room Temperature—A temperature maintained thermostatically that encompasses the usual and customary working environment of 20° to 25° (68° to 77 °F); that results in a mean kinetic temperature calculated to be not more than 25°; and that allows for excursions between 15° and 30° (59° and 86 °F) that are experienced in pharmacies, hospitals, and warehouses. Provided the mean kinetic temperature remains in the allowed range, transient spikes up to 40° are permitted as long as they do not exceed 24 hours. Spikes above 40° may be permitted if the manufacturer so instructs. Articles may be labeled for storage at "controlled room temperature" or at "up to 25°", or other wording based on the same mean kinetic temperature. The mean kinetic temperature is a calculated value that may be used as an isothermal storage temperature that simulates the nonisothermal effects of storage temperature variations. (See also *Stability* under *Pharmaceutical Dosage Forms* ⟨1151⟩.)

An article for which storage at *Controlled room temperature* is directed may, alternatively, be stored and distributed in a *cool place*, unless otherwise specified in the individual monograph or on the label.

Warm—Any temperature between 30° and 40° (86° and 104 °F).

Excessive Heat—Any temperature above 40° (104 °F).

Protection from Freezing—Where, in addition to the risk of breakage of the container, freezing subjects an article to loss of strength or potency, or to destructive alteration of its characteristics, the container label bears an appropriate instruction to protect the article from freezing.

Dry Place—The term "dry place" denotes a place that does not exceed 40% average relative humidity at *Controlled Room Temperature* or the equivalent water vapor pressure at other temperatures. The determination may be made by direct measurement at the place or may be based on reported climatic conditions. Determination is based on not less than 12 equally spaced measurements that encompass either a season, a year, or, where recorded data demonstrate, the storage period of the article. There may be values of up to 45% relative humidity provided that the average value is 40% relative humidity.

Storage in a container validated to protect the article from moisture vapor, including storage in bulk, is considered a dry place.

Storage under Nonspecific Conditions—▲Where no specific directions or limitations are provided in the packaging and storage section of individual monographs or in the article's labeling, the conditions of storage shall include storage at controlled room temperature, protection from moisture, and, where necessary, protection from light. Articles shall be protected from moisture, freezing, and excessive heat, and, where necessary, from light during shipping and distribution. Active pharmaceutical ingredients are exempt from this requirement.▲*USP27*

Labeling—The term "labeling" designates all labels and other written, printed, or graphic matter upon an immediate container of an article or upon, or in, any package or wrapper in which it is enclosed, except any outer shipping container. The term "label" designates that part of the labeling upon the immediate container.

A shipping container containing a single article, unless such container is also essentially the immediate container or the outside of the consumer package, is labeled with a minimum of product identification (except for controlled articles), lot number, expiration date, and conditions for storage and distribution.

Articles in this Pharmacopeia are subject to compliance with such labeling requirements as may be promulgated by governmental bodies in addition to the Pharmacopeial requirements set forth for the articles.

Amount of Ingredient per Dosage Unit—The strength of a drug product is expressed on the container label in terms of micrograms or milligrams or grams or percentage of the therapeutically active moiety or drug substance, whichever form is used in the title, unless otherwise indicated in an individual monograph. Both the active moiety and drug substance names and their equivalent amounts are then provided in the labeling.

Pharmacopeial articles in capsule, tablet, or other unit dosage form shall be labeled to express the quantity of each active ingredient or recognized nutrient contained in each such unit; except that, in the case of unit-dose oral solutions or suspensions, whether supplied as liquid preparations or as liquid preparations that are constituted from solids upon addition of a designated volume of a specific diluent, the label shall express the quantity of each active ingredient or recognized nutrient delivered under the conditions prescribed in *Deliverable Volume* ⟨698⟩. Pharmacopeial drug products not in unit dosage form shall be labeled to express the quantity of each active ingredient in each milliliter or in each gram, or to express the percentage of each such ingredient (see *Percentage Measurements*), except that oral liquids or solids intended to be constituted to yield oral liquids may, alternatively, be labeled in terms of each 5-mL portion of the liquid or resulting liquid. Unless otherwise indicated in a monograph or chapter, such declarations of strength or quantity shall be stated only in metric units (see also *Units of Potency* in these *General Notices*).

Use of Leading and Terminal Zeros—In order to help minimize the possibility of errors in the dispensing and administration of drugs, the quantity of active ingredient when expressed in whole numbers shall be shown without a decimal point that is followed by a terminal zero (e.g., express as 4 mg [not 4.0 mg]). The quantity of active ingredient when expressed as a decimal number smaller than one shall be shown with a zero preceding the decimal point (e.g., express as 0.2 mg [not .2 mg]).

Labeling of Salts of Drugs—It is an established principle that Pharmacopeial articles shall have only one official name. For purposes of saving space on labels, and because chemical symbols for the most common inorganic salts of drugs are well known to practitioners as synonymous with the written forms, the following alternatives are permitted in labeling official articles that are salts: HCl for hydrochloride; HBr for hydrobromide; Na for sodium; and K for potassium. The symbols Na and K are intended for use in abbreviating names of the salts of organic acids; but these symbols are not used where the word Sodium or Potassium appears at the beginning of an official title (e.g., Phenobarbital Na is acceptable, but Na Salicylate is not to be written).

Labeling Vitamin-Containing Products—The vitamin content of an official drug product shall be stated on the label in metric units per dosage unit. The amounts of vitamins A, D, and E may be

stated also in USP Units. Quantities of vitamin A declared in metric units refer to the equivalent amounts of retinol (vitamin A alcohol). The label of a nutritional supplement shall bear an identifying lot number, control number, or batch number.

Labeling Parenteral and Topical Preparations—The label of a preparation intended for parenteral or topical use states the names of all added substances (see *Added Substances* in these *General Notices and Requirements*, and see *Labeling* under *Injections* ⟨1⟩), and, in the case of parenteral preparations, also their amounts or proportions, except that for substances added for adjustment of pH or to achieve isotonicity, the label may indicate only their presence and the reason for their addition.

Labeling Electrolytes—The concentration and dosage of electrolytes for replacement therapy (e.g., sodium chloride or potassium chloride) shall be stated on the label in milliequivalents (mEq). The label of the product shall indicate also the quantity of ingredient(s) in terms of weight or percentage concentration.

Labeling Alcohol—The content of alcohol in a liquid preparation shall be stated on the label as a percentage (v/v) of C_2H_5OH.

Special Capsules and Tablets—The label of any form of Capsule or Tablet intended for administration other than by swallowing intact bears a prominent indication of the manner in which it is to be used.

Expiration Date and Beyond-Use Date—The label of an official drug product, nutritional or dietary supplement product shall bear an expiration date. All articles shall display the expiration date so that it can be read by an ordinary individual under customary conditions of purchase and use. The expiration date shall be prominently displayed in high contrast to the background or sharply embossed, and easily understood (e.g., "EXP 6/89," "Exp. June 89," or "Expires 6/89"). [NOTE—For additional information and guidance, refer to the Nonprescription Drug Manufacturers Association's *Voluntary Codes and Guidelines of the OTC Medicines Industry*.]

The monographs for some preparations state how the expiration date that shall appear on the label is to be determined. In the absence of a specific requirement in the individual monograph for a drug product or nutritional supplement, the label shall bear an expiration date assigned for the particular formulation and package of the article, with the following exception: the label need not show an expiration date in the case of a drug product or nutritional supplement packaged in a container that is intended for sale without prescription and the labeling of which states no dosage limitations, and which is stable for not less than 3 years when stored under the prescribed conditions.

Where an official article is required to bear an expiration date, such article shall be dispensed solely in, or from, a container labeled with an expiration date, and the date on which the article is dispensed shall be within the labeled expiry period. The expiration date identifies the time during which the article may be expected to meet the requirements of the Pharmacopeial monograph, provided it is kept under the prescribed storage conditions. The expiration date limits the time during which the article may be dispensed or used. Where an expiration date is stated only in terms of the month and the year, it is a representation that the intended expiration date is the last day of the stated month. The beyond-use date is the date after which an article must not be used. The dispenser shall place on the label of the prescription container a suitable beyond-use date to limit the patient's use of the article based on any information supplied by the manufacturer and the *General Notices and Requirements* of this Pharmacopeia. The beyond-use date placed on the label shall not be later than the expiration date on the manufacturer's container.

For articles requiring constitution prior to use, a suitable beyond-use date for the constituted product shall be identified in the labeling.

For all other dosage forms, in determining an appropriate period of time during which a prescription drug may be retained by a patient after its dispensing, the dispenser shall take into account, in addition to any other relevant factors, the nature of the drug; the container in which it was packaged by the manufacturer and the expiration date thereon; the characteristics of the patient's container, if the article is repackaged for dispensing; the expected storage conditions to which the article may be exposed; any unusual storage conditions to which the article may be exposed; and the expected length of time of the course of therapy. The dispenser shall, on taking into account the foregoing, place on the label of a multiple-unit container a suitable beyond-use date to limit the patient's use of the article. Unless otherwise specified in the individual monograph, or in the absence of stability data to the contrary, such beyond-use date shall be not later than (a) the expiration date on the manufacturer's container, or (b) one year from the date the drug is dispensed, whichever is earlier. For nonsterile solid and liquid dosage forms that are packaged in single-unit and unit-dose containers, the beyond-use date shall be one year from the date the drug is packaged into the single-unit or unit-dose container or the expiration date on the manufacturer's container, whichever is earlier, unless stability data or the manufacturer's labeling indicates otherwise.

The dispenser must maintain the facility where the dosage forms are packaged and stored, at a temperature such that the mean kinetic temperature is not greater than 25°. The plastic material used in packaging the dosage forms must afford better protection than polyvinyl chloride, which does not provide adequate protection against moisture permeation. Records must be kept of the temperature of the facility where the dosage forms are stored, and of the plastic materials used in packaging.

Pharmaceutical Compounding—The label on the container or package of an official compounded preparation shall bear a beyond-use date. The beyond-use date is the date after which a compounded preparation is not to be used. Because compounded preparations are intended for administration immediately or following short-term storage, their beyond-use dates may be assigned based on criteria different from those applied to assigning expiration dates to manufactured drug products.

The monograph for an official compounded preparation typically includes a beyond-use requirement that states the time period following the date of compounding during which the preparation, properly stored, is to be used. In the absence of stability information that is applicable to a specific drug and preparation, recommendations for maximum beyond-use dates have been devised for nonsterile compounded drug preparations that are packaged in tight, light-resistant containers and stored at controlled room temperature unless otherwise indicated (see *Stability Criteria and Beyond-Use Dating* under *Stability of Compounded Preparations* in the general tests chapter ▲*Pharmaceutical Compounding—Nonsterile Preparations*▲USP27 ⟨795⟩).

VEGETABLE AND ANIMAL SUBSTANCES

The requirements for vegetable and animal substances apply to the articles as they enter commerce; however, lots of such substances intended solely for the manufacture or isolation of volatile oils, alkaloids, glycosides, or other active principles may depart from such requirements.

Statements of the distinctive microscopic structural elements in powdered substances of animal or vegetable origin may be included in the individual monograph as a means of determining identity, quality, or purity.

Foreign Matter—Vegetable and animal substances are to be free from pathogenic organisms (see *Microbiological Attributes of Nonsterile Pharmaceutical Products* ⟨1111⟩), and are to be as free as reasonably practicable from microorganisms, insects, and other animal contamination, including animal excreta. They shall show no abnormal discoloration, abnormal odor, sliminess, or other evidence of deterioration.

The amount of foreign inorganic matter in vegetable or animal substances, estimated as *Acid-insoluble ash*, shall not exceed 2 percent of the weight of the substance, unless otherwise specified in the individual monograph.

Before vegetable substances are ground or powdered, stones, dust, lumps of soil, and other foreign inorganic matter are to be removed by mechanical or other suitable means.

In commerce it is seldom possible to obtain vegetable substances that are without some adherent or admixed, innocuous, foreign matter, which usually is not detrimental. No poisonous, dangerous, or otherwise noxious foreign matter or residues may be present. Foreign matter includes any part of the plant not specified as constituting the substance.

Preservation—Vegetable or animal substances may be protected from insect infestation or microbiological contamination by means of suitable agents or processes that leave no harmful residues.

WEIGHTS AND MEASURES

The International System of Units (SI) is used in this Pharmacopeia. The SI metric and other units, and the symbols commonly employed, are as follows.

Bq = becquerel	L = liter
kBq = kilobecquerel	mL = milliliter, ‡
MBq = megabecquerel	μL = microliter
GBq = gigabecquerel	Eq = gram-equivalent weight
Ci = curie	mEq = milliequivalent
mCi = millicurie	mol = gram-molecular weight (mole)
μCi = microcurie	Da = dalton (relative molecular mass)
nCi = nanocurie	mmol = millimole
Gy = gray	Osmol = osmole
mGy = milligray	mOsmol = milliosmole
m = meter	Hz = hertz
	kHz = kilohertz
	MHz = megahertz
	V = volts
dm = decimeter	MeV = million electron volts
cm = centimeter	keV = kilo-electron volt
mm = millimeter	mV = millivolt
μm = micrometer (0.001m)	psi = pounds per square inch
nm = nanometer *	Pa = pascal
kg = kilogram	kPa = kilopascal
g = gram **	g = gravity (in centrifugation)
mg = milligram	
μg; mcg = microgram †	
ng = nanogram	
pg = picogram	
fg = femtogram	
dL = deciliter	

* Formerly the symbol mμ (for millimicron) was used.
** The gram is the unit of mass that is used to measure quantities of materials. Weight, which is a measure of the gravitational force acting on the mass of a material, is proportional to, and may differ slightly from, its mass due to the effects of factors such as gravity, temperature, latitude, and altitude. The difference between mass and weight is considered to be insignificant for compendial assays and tests, and the term "weight" is used throughout *USP* and *NF*.
† Formerly the abbreviation mcg was used in the Pharmacopeial monographs; however, the symbol μg now is more widely accepted and thus is used in this Pharmacopeia. The term "gamma," symbolized by γ, is frequently used for microgram in biochemical literature.

NOTE—The abbreviation mcg is still commonly employed to denote microgram(s) in labeling and in prescription writing. Therefore, for purposes of labeling, "mcg" may be used to denote microgram(s).
‡ One milliliter (mL) is used herein as the equivalent of 1 cubic centimeter(cc).

CONCENTRATIONS

Molal, molar, and normal solution concentrations are indicated throughout this Pharmacopeia for most chemical assay and test procedures (see also *Volumetric Solutions* in the section, *Reagents, Indicators, and Solutions*). Molality is designated by the symbol *m* preceded by a number that is the number of moles of the designated solute contained in one kilogram of the designated solvent. Molarity is designated by the symbol M preceded by a number that is the number of moles of the designated solute contained in an amount of the designated solvent that is sufficient to prepare one liter of solution. Normality is designated by the symbol N preceded by a number that is the number of equivalents of the designated solute contained in an amount of the designated solvent that is sufficient to prepare one liter of solution.

Percentage Measurements—Percentage concentrations are expressed as follows:

Percent Weight in Weight—(w/w) expresses the number of g of a constituent in 100 g of solution or mixture.

Percent Weight in Volume—(w/v) expresses the number of g of a constituent in 100 mL of solution, and is used regardless of whether water or another liquid is the solvent.

Percent Volume in Volume—(v/v) expresses the number of mL of a constituent in 100 mL of solution.

The term *percent* used without qualification means, for mixtures of solids and semisolids, percent weight in weight; for solutions or suspensions of solids in liquids, percent weight in volume; for solutions of liquids in liquids, percent volume in volume; and for solutions of gases in liquids, percent weight in volume. For example, a 1 percent solution is prepared by dissolving 1 g of a solid or semisolid, or 1 mL of a liquid, in sufficient solvent to make 100 mL of the solution.

In the dispensing of prescription medications, slight changes in volume owing to variations in room temperatures may be disregarded.

Guide to General Chapters

General Tests and Assays

General Requirements for Tests and Assays

⟨1⟩ Injections
⟨11⟩ USP Reference Standards

Apparatus for Tests and Assays

⟨16⟩ Automated Methods of Analysis
⟨21⟩ Thermometers
⟨31⟩ Volumetric Apparatus
⟨41⟩ Weights and Balances

Microbiological Tests

⟨51⟩ Antimicrobial Effectiveness Testing
⟨55⟩ Biological Indicators—Resistance Performance Tests
⟨61⟩ Microbial Limit Tests
⟨71⟩ Sterility Tests

Biological Tests and Assays

⟨81⟩ Antibiotics—Microbial Assays
⟨85⟩ Bacterial Endotoxins Test
⟨87⟩ Biological Reactivity Tests, In Vitro

⟨88⟩ Biological Reactivity Tests, In Vivo
⟨91⟩ Calcium Pantothenate Assay
⟨111⟩ Design and Analysis of Biological Assays
⟨115⟩ Dexpanthenol Assay
⟨121⟩ Insulin Assays
⟨141⟩ Protein—Biological Adequacy Test
⟨151⟩ Pyrogen Test
⟨161⟩ Transfusion and Infusion Assemblies and Similar
Medical Devices
⟨171⟩ Vitamin B_{12} Activity Assay

Chemical Tests and Assays

IDENTIFICATION TESTS

⟨181⟩ Identification—Organic Nitrogenous Bases
⟨191⟩ Identification Tests—General
⟨193⟩ Identification—Tetracyclines
⟨197⟩ Spectrophotometric Identification Tests
⟨201⟩ Thin-Layer Chromatographic Identification Test

LIMIT TESTS

⟨206⟩ Aluminum
⟨211⟩ Arsenic
⟨221⟩ Chloride and Sulfate
⟨223⟩ Dimethylaniline
⟨226⟩ 4-Epianhydrotetracycline
⟨231⟩ Heavy Metals
⟨241⟩ Iron
⟨251⟩ Lead
⟨261⟩ Mercury
⟨271⟩ Readily Carbonizable Substances Test
⟨281⟩ Residue on Ignition
⟨291⟩ Selenium

OTHER TESTS AND ASSAYS

⟨301⟩ Acid-Neutralizing Capacity
⟨311⟩ Alginates Assay
⟨331⟩ Amphetamine Assay
⟨341⟩ Antimicrobial Agents—Content
⟨351⟩ Assay for Steroids
⟨361⟩ Barbiturate Assay
⟨371⟩ Cobalamin Radiotracer Assay
⟨381⟩ Elastomeric Closures for Injections
⟨391⟩ Epinephrine Assay
⟨401⟩ Fats and Fixed Oils
⟨411⟩ Folic Acid Assay
⟨425⟩ Iodometric Assay—Antibiotics
⟨431⟩ Methoxy Determination
⟨441⟩ Niacin or Niacinamide Assay
⟨451⟩ Nitrite Titration
⟨461⟩ Nitrogen Determination
⟨466⟩ Ordinary Impurities
⟨467⟩ Organic Volatile Impurities
⟨471⟩ Oxygen Flask Combustion
⟨481⟩ Riboflavin Assay
⟨501⟩ Salts of Organic Nitrogenous Bases
⟨511⟩ Single-Steroid Assay
⟨521⟩ Sulfonamides
⟨531⟩ Thiamine Assay
⟨541⟩ Titrimetry
⟨551⟩ Alpha Tocopherol Assay
⟨561⟩ Articles of Botanical Origin
⟨563⟩ Identification of Articles of Botanical Origin
⟨565⟩ Botanical Extracts
⟨571⟩ Vitamin A Assay
⟨581⟩ Vitamin D Assay
⟨591⟩ Zinc Determination

Physical Tests and Determinations

⟨601⟩ Aerosols, Metered-Dose Inhalers, and Dry Powder
⟨611⟩ Alcohol Determination
⟨616⟩ Bulk Density and Tapped Density
⟨621⟩ Chromatography
⟨631⟩ Color and Achromicity
⟨641⟩ Completeness of Solution
⟨643⟩ Total Organic Carbon
⟨645⟩ Water Conductivity
⟨651⟩ Congealing Temperature
⟨661⟩ Containers
⟨671⟩ Containers—Permeation
⟨691⟩ Cotton
⟨695⟩ Crystallinity
⟨696⟩ Crystallinity Determination by Solution Calorimetry
⟨698⟩ Deliverable Volume
⟨699⟩ Density of Solids
⟨701⟩ Disintegration
⟨711⟩ Dissolution
⟨721⟩ Distilling Range
⟨724⟩ Drug Release
⟨726⟩ Electrophoresis
⟨727⟩ Capillary Electrophoresis
⟨731⟩ Loss on Drying
⟨733⟩ Loss on Ignition
⟨736⟩ Mass Spectrometry
⟨741⟩ Melting Range or Temperature
⟨751⟩ Metal Particles in Ophthalmic Ointments
⟨755⟩ Minimum Fill
⟨761⟩ Nuclear Magnetic Resonance
⟨771⟩ Ophthalmic Ointments
⟨776⟩ Optical Microscopy
⟨781⟩ Optical Rotation
⟨785⟩ Osmolarity
⟨786⟩ Particle Size Distribution Estimation by Analytical
Sieving
⟨788⟩ Particulate Matter in Injections
⟨791⟩ pH
⟨795⟩ Pharmaceutical Compounding—Nonsterile
Preparations
⟨797⟩ Pharmaceutical Compounding—Sterile
Preparations
⟨801⟩ Polarography
⟨811⟩ Powder Fineness
⟨821⟩ Radioactivity
⟨823⟩ Radiopharmaceuticals for Positron Emission
Tomography—Compounding
⟨831⟩ Refractive Index
⟨841⟩ Specific Gravity
⟨846⟩ Specific Surface Area
⟨851⟩ Spectrophotometry and Light-Scattering
⟨861⟩ Sutures—Diameter
⟨871⟩ Sutures—Needle Attachment
⟨881⟩ Tensile Strength
⟨891⟩ Thermal Analysis
⟨905⟩ Uniformity of Dosage Units
⟨911⟩ Viscosity
⟨921⟩ Water Determination
⟨941⟩ X-Ray Diffraction

General Information

⟨1015⟩ Automated Radiochemical Synthesis Apparatus
⟨1031⟩ The Biocompatibility of Materials Used in Drug
Containers, Medical Devices, and Implants
⟨1035⟩ Biological Indicators for Sterilization
⟨1041⟩ Biologics

Guide to General Chapters— Dietary Supplements

⟨1⟩ INJECTIONS

INTRODUCTION

Parenteral articles are preparations intended for injection through the skin or other external boundary tissue, rather than through the alimentary canal, so that the active substances they contain are administered, using gravity or force, directly into a blood vessel, organ, tissue, or lesion. Parenteral articles are prepared scrupulously by methods designed to ensure that they meet Pharmacopeial requirements for sterility, pyrogens, particulate matter, and other contaminants, and, where appropriate, contain inhibitors of the growth of microorganisms. An Injection is a preparation intended for parenteral administration and/or for constituting or diluting a parenteral article prior to administration.

NOMENCLATURE AND DEFINITIONS

Nomenclature*

The following nomenclature pertains to five general types of preparations, all of which are suitable for, and intended for, parenteral administration. They may contain buffers, preservatives, or other added substances.

1. [DRUG] *Injection*—Liquid preparations that are drug substances or solutions thereof.
2. [DRUG] *for Injection*—Dry solids that, upon the addition of suitable vehicles, yield solutions conforming in all respects to the requirements for *Injections*.
3. [DRUG] *Injectable Emulsion*—Liquid preparations of drug substances dissolved or dispersed in a suitable emulsion medium.
4. [DRUG] *Injectable Suspension*—Liquid preparations of solids suspended in a suitable liquid medium.
5. [DRUG] *for Injectable Suspension*—Dry solids that, upon the addition of suitable vehicles, yield preparations conforming in all respects to the requirements for *Injectable Suspensions*.

Definitions

PHARMACY BULK PACKAGE

A *Pharmacy bulk package* is a container of a sterile preparation for parenteral use that contains many single doses. The contents are intended for use in a pharmacy admixture program and are restricted to the preparation of admixtures for infusion or, through a sterile transfer device, for the filling of empty sterile syringes.

---

* This nomenclature has been adopted by the USP Drug Nomenclature Committee for implementation by supplemental revisions of *USP 23-NF 18*. For currently official monograph titles in the form *Sterile [DRUG]* that have not yet been revised, the following nomenclature continues in use in this Pharmacopeia: (1) medicaments or solutions or emulsions thereof suitable for injection, bearing titles of the form [DRUG] *Injection;* (2) dry solids or liquid concentrates containing no buffers, diluents, or other added substances, and which, upon the addition of suitable solvents, yield solutions conforming in all respects to the requirements for Injections, and which are distinguished by titles of the form *Sterile [DRUG]*; (3) preparations the same as those described under (2) except that they contain one or more buffers, diluents, or other added substances, and which are distinguished by titles of the form [DRUG] *for Injection;* (4) solids which are suspended in a suitable fluid medium and which are not to be injected intravenously or into the spinal canal, distinguished by titles of the form *Sterile [DRUG] Suspension;* and (5) dry solids which, upon the addition of suitable vehicles, yield preparations conforming in all respects to the requirements for Sterile Suspensions, and which are distinguished by titles of the form *Sterile [DRUG] for Suspension.*

The closure shall be penetrated only one time after constitution with a suitable sterile transfer device or dispensing set which allows measured dispensing of the contents. The *Pharmacy bulk package* is to be used only in a suitable work area such as a laminar flow hood (or an equivalent clean air compounding area).

Designation as a *Pharmacy bulk package* is limited to preparations from *Nomenclature* categories 1, 2, or 3 as defined above. *Pharmacy bulk packages*, although containing more than one single dose, are exempt from the multiple-dose container volume limit of 30 mL and the requirement that they contain a substance or suitable mixture of substances to prevent the growth of microorganisms.

Where a container is offered as a *Pharmacy bulk package*, the label shall (a) state prominently "Pharmacy Bulk Package—Not for direct infusion," (b) contain or refer to information on proper techniques to help assure safe use of the product, and (c) bear a statement limiting the time frame in which the container may be used once it has been entered, provided it is held under the labeled storage conditions.

LARGE- AND SMALL-VOLUME INJECTIONS

Where used in this Pharmacopeia, the designation *Large-volume intravenous solution* applies to a single-dose injection that is intended for intravenous use and is packaged in containers labeled as containing more than 100 mL. The designation *Small-volume Injection* applies to an Injection that is packaged in containers labeled as containing 100 mL or less.

BIOLOGICS

The Pharmacopeial definitions for sterile preparations for parenteral use generally do not apply in the case of the biologics because of their special nature and licensing requirements (see *Biologics* ⟨1041⟩).

INGREDIENTS

Vehicles and Added Substances

Aqueous Vehicles—The vehicles for aqueous Injections meet the requirements of the *Pyrogen Test* ⟨151⟩ or the *Bacterial Endotoxins Test* ⟨85⟩, whichever is specified. *Water for Injection* generally is used as the vehicle, unless otherwise specified in the individual monograph. Sodium chloride may be added in amounts sufficient to render the resulting solution isotonic; and *Sodium Chloride Injection*, or *Ringer's Injection*, may be used in whole or in part instead of *Water for Injection*, unless otherwise specified in the individual monograph. For conditions applying to other adjuvants, see *Added Substances* in this chapter.

Other Vehicles—Fixed oils used as vehicles for nonaqueous Injections are of vegetable origin, are odorless or nearly so, and have no odor suggesting rancidity. They meet the requirements of the test for *Solid paraffin* under *Mineral Oil*, the cooling bath being maintained at 10°, have a *Saponification Value* between 185 and 200 (see *Fats and Fixed Oils* ⟨401⟩), have an *Iodine Value* between 79 and 141 (see *Fats and Fixed Oils* ⟨401⟩), and meet the requirements of the following tests.

Unsaponifiable Matter—Reflux on a steam bath 10 mL of the oil with 15 mL of sodium hydroxide solution (1 in 6) and 30 mL of alcohol, with occasional shaking until the mixture becomes clear. Transfer the solution to a shallow dish, evaporate the alcohol on a steam bath, and mix the residue with 100 mL of water: a clear solution results.

Free Fatty Acids—The free fatty acids in 10 g of oil require for neutralization not more than 2.0 mL of 0.020 N sodium hydroxide (see *Fats and Fixed Oils* ⟨401⟩).

Synthetic mono- or diglycerides of fatty acids may be used as vehicles, provided they are liquid and remain clear when cooled to 10° and have an *Iodine Value* of not more than 140 (see *Fats and Fixed Oils* ⟨401⟩).

These and other nonaqueous vehicles may be used, provided they are safe in the volume of Injection administered, and also provided they do not interfere with the therapeutic efficacy of the preparation or with its response to prescribed assays and tests.

Added Substances—Suitable substances may be added to preparations intended for injection to increase stability or usefulness, unless proscribed in the individual monograph, provided they are harmless in the amounts administered and do not interfere with the therapeutic efficacy or with the responses to the specified assays and tests. No coloring agent may be added, solely for the purpose of coloring the finished preparation, to a solution intended for parenteral administration (see also *Added Substances* under *General Notices* and *Antimicrobial Effectiveness Testing* ⟨51⟩).

Observe special care in the choice and use of added substances in preparations for injection that are administered in a volume exceeding 5 mL. The following maximum limits prevail unless otherwise directed: for agents containing mercury and the cationic, surface-active compounds, 0.01%; for chlorobutanol, cresol, phenol, and similar types of substances, 0.5%; and for sulfur dioxide, or an equivalent amount of the sulfite, bisulfite, or metabisulfite of potassium or sodium, 0.2%.

A suitable substance or mixture of substances to prevent the growth of microorganisms must be added to preparations intended for injection that are packaged in multiple-dose containers, regardless of the method of sterilization employed, unless one of the following conditions prevails: (1) there are different directions in the individual monograph; (2) the substance contains a radionuclide with a physical half-life of less than 24 hours; and (3) the active ingredients are themselves antimicrobial. Such substances are used in concentrations that will prevent the growth of or kill microorganisms in the preparations for injection. Such substances also meet the requirements of *Antimicrobial Effectiveness Testing* ⟨51⟩ and *Antimicrobial Agents—Content* ⟨341⟩. Sterilization processes are employed even though such substances are used (see also *Sterilization and Sterility Assurance of Compendial Articles* ⟨1211⟩). The air in the container may be evacuated or be displaced by a chemically inert gas. Where specified in a monograph, information regarding sensitivity of the article to oxygen is to be provided in the labeling.

LABELS AND LABELING

Labeling—[NOTE—See definitions of "label" and "labeling" under *Labeling* in the section *Preservation, Packaging, Storage, and Labeling* of the *General Notices and Requirements*.]

The label states the name of the preparation; in the case of a liquid preparation, the percentage content of drug or amount of drug in a specified volume; in the case of a dry preparation, the amount of *active* ingredient; the route of administration; a statement of storage conditions and an expiration date; the name and place of business of the manufacturer, packer, or distributor; and an identifying lot number. The lot number is capable of yielding the complete manufacturing history of the specific package, including all manufacturing, filling, sterilizing, and labeling operations.

Where the individual monograph permits varying concentrations of active ingredients in the large-volume parenteral, the concentration of each ingredient named in the official title is stated as if part of the official title, e.g., Dextrose Injection 5%, or Dextrose (5%) and Sodium Chloride (0.2%) Injection.

The labeling includes the following information if the complete formula is not specified in the individual monograph: (1) In the case of a liquid preparation, the percentage content of each ingredient or the amount of each ingredient in a specified volume, except that ingredients added to adjust to a given pH or to make the solution isotonic may be declared by name and a statement of their effect; and (2) in the case of a dry preparation or other

preparation to which a diluent is intended to be added before use, the amount of each ingredient, the composition of recommended diluent(s) [the name(s) alone, if the formula is specified in the individual monograph], the amount to be used to attain a specific concentration of active ingredient and the final volume of solution so obtained, a brief description of the physical appearance of the constituted solution, directions for proper storage of the constituted solution, and an expiration date limiting the period during which the constituted solution may be expected to have the required or labeled potency if it has been stored as directed.

Containers for Injections that are intended for use as dialysis, hemofiltration, or irrigation solutions and that contain a volume of more than 1 liter are labeled to indicate that the contents are not intended for use by intravenous infusion.

Injections intended for veterinary use are labeled to that effect.

The container is so labeled that a sufficient area of the container remains uncovered for its full length or circumference to permit inspection of the contents.

PACKAGING

Containers for Injections

Containers, including the closures, for preparations for injections do not interact physically or chemically with the preparations in any manner to alter the strength, quality, or purity beyond the official requirements under the ordinary or customary conditions of handling, shipment, storage, sale, and use. The container is made of material that permits inspection of the contents. The type of glass preferable for each parenteral preparation is usually stated in the individual monograph. Unless otherwise specified in the individual monograph, plastic containers may be used for packaging injections (see *Containers* ⟨661⟩).

For definitions of single-dose and multiple-dose containers, see *Containers* in the *General Notices and Requirements.* Containers meet the requirements under *Containers* ⟨661⟩.

Containers are closed or sealed in such a manner as to prevent contamination or loss of contents. Validation of container integrity must demonstrate no penetration of microbial contamination or chemical or physical impurities. In addition, the solutes and the vehicle must maintain their specified total and relative quantities or concentrations when exposed to anticipated extreme conditions of manufacturing and processing, and storage, shipment, and distribution. Closures for multiple-dose containers permit the withdrawal of the contents without removal or destruction of the closure. The closure permits penetration by a needle and, upon withdrawal of the needle, closes at once, protecting the container against contamination. Validation of the multiple-dose container integrity must include verification that such a package prevents microbial contamination or loss of product contents under anticipated conditions of multiple entry and use.

Piggyback containers are usually intravenous infusion containers used to administer a second infusion through a connector of some type or an injection port on the administration set of the first fluid, thereby avoiding the need for another injection site on the patient's body. Piggyback containers are also known as secondary infusion containers.

Potassium Chloride for Injection Concentrate

The use of a black closure system on a vial (e.g., a black flip-off button and a black ferrule to hold the elastomeric closure) or the use of a black band or series of bands above the constriction on an ampul is prohibited, except for *Potassium Chloride for Injection Concentrate.*

Containers for Sterile Solids

Containers, including the closures, for dry solids intended for parenteral use do not interact physically or chemically with the preparation in any manner to alter the strength, quality, or purity beyond the official requirements under the ordinary or customary conditions of handling, shipment, storage, sale, and use.

A container for a sterile solid permits the addition of a suitable solvent and withdrawal of portions of the resulting solution or suspension in such manner that the sterility of the product is maintained.

Where the *Assay* in a monograph provides a procedure for the *Assay preparation*, in which the total withdrawable contents are to be withdrawn from a single-dose container with a hypodermic needle and syringe, the contents are to be withdrawn as completely as possible into a dry hypodermic syringe of a rated capacity not exceeding three times the volume to be withdrawn and fitted with a 21-gauge needle not less than 2.5 cm (1 inch) in length, with care being taken to expel any air bubbles, and discharged into a container for dilution and assay.

Volume in Container

Each container of an Injection is filled with sufficient excess of the labeled "size" or that volume which is to be withdrawn. See *Injections* under *Pharmaceutical Dosage Forms* ⟨1151⟩.

DETERMINATION OF VOLUME OF INJECTION IN CONTAINERS

Select one or more containers if the volume of the container is 10 mL or more, three or more if the volume is more than 3 mL and less than 10 mL, or five or more if the volume is 3 mL or less. Individually take up the contents of each container selected into a dry hypodermic syringe of a rated capacity not exceeding three times the volume to be measured and fitted with a 21-gauge needle not less than 2.5 cm (1 inch) in length. Expel any air bubbles from the syringe and needle, and then discharge the contents of the syringe, without emptying the needle, into a standardized, dry cylinder (graduated to contain rather than to deliver the designated volumes) of such size that the volume to be measured occupies at least 40% of the cylinder's rated volume. Alternatively, the contents of the syringe may be discharged into a dry, tared beaker, the volume, in mL, being calculated as the weight, in g, of Injection taken divided by its density. The contents of up to five 1- or 2-mL containers may be pooled for the measurement, provided that a separate dry syringe assembly is used for each container. The content of containers holding 10 mL or more may be determined by means of opening them and emptying the contents directly into the graduated cylinder or tared beaker.

The volume is not less than the labeled volume in the case of containers examined individually or, in the case of 1- and 2-mL containers, is not less than the sum of the labeled volumes of the containers taken collectively.

For Injections in multiple-dose containers labeled to yield a specific number of doses of a stated volume, proceed as directed in the foregoing, using the same number of separate syringes as the number of doses specified. The volume is such that each syringe delivers not less than the stated dose.

For Injections containing oil, warm the containers, if necessary, and thoroughly shake them immediately before removing the contents. Cool to 25° before measuring the volume.

For Injections in cartridges or prefilled syringes, assemble the container with any required accessories such as a needle or plunger. Following the same procedure as above, and without emptying the needle, transfer the entire contents of each container to a dry, tared beaker by slowly and constantly depressing the plunger. Weigh, and calculate the volume as described above. The volume of each container is not less than the labeled volume.

For large-volume intravenous solutions, select 1 container, and transfer the contents into a dry measuring cylinder of such size that the volume to be measured occupies at least 40% of its rated volume. The volume is not less than the labeled volume.

Packaging and Storage

The volume of Injection in single-dose containers provides the amount specified for parenteral administration at one time and in no case is more than sufficient to permit the withdrawal and administration of 1 liter.

Preparations intended for intraspinal, intracisternal, or peridural administration are packaged only in single-dose containers.

Unless otherwise specified in the individual monograph, a multiple-dose container contains a volume of Injection sufficient to permit the withdrawal of not more than 30 mL.

Injections packaged for use as irrigation solutions, for hemofiltration or dialysis, or for parenteral nutrition are exempt from the 1-liter restriction of the foregoing requirements relating to packaging. Containers for Injections packaged for use as hemofiltration or irrigation solutions may be designed to empty rapidly and may contain a volume of more than 1 liter.

Injections labeled for veterinary use are exempt from packaging and storage requirements concerning the limitation to single-dose containers and the limitation on the volume of multiple-dose containers.

FOREIGN MATTER AND PARTICLES

Foreign Matter

Every care should be exercised in the preparation of all products intended for injection to prevent contamination with microorganisms and foreign material. Good pharmaceutical practice requires also that each final container of Injection be subjected individually to a physical inspection, whenever the nature of the container permits, and that every container whose contents shows evidence of contamination with visible foreign material be rejected.

Particulate Matter

All large-volume Injections for single-dose infusion, and those small-volume Injections for which the monographs specify such requirements, are subject to the particulate matter limits set forth under *Particulate Matter in Injections* ⟨788⟩. An article packaged as both a large-volume and a small-volume Injection meets the requirements set forth for small-volume Injections where the container is labeled as containing 100 mL or less if the individual monograph includes a test for *Particulate Matter;* it meets the requirements set forth for large-volume Injections for single-dose infusion where the container is labeled as containing more than 100 mL. Injections packaged and labeled for use as irrigating solutions are exempt from requirements for *Particulate Matter.*

STERILITY

Sterility Tests—Preparations for injection meet the requirements under *Sterility Tests* ⟨71⟩.

CONSTITUTED SOLUTIONS

Dry solids from which constituted solutions are prepared for injection bear titles of the form [DRUG] for Injection. Since these dosage forms are constituted at the time of use by the health care practitioner, tests and standards pertaining to the solution as constituted for administration are not included in the individual monographs on sterile dry solids or liquid concentrates. However,

in the interest of assuring the quality of injection preparations as they are actually administered, the following nondestructive tests are provided for demonstrating the suitability of constituted solutions when they are prepared just prior to use.

Completeness and Clarity of Solution—Constitute the solution as directed in the labeling supplied by the manufacturer for the sterile dry dosage form.

A: The solid dissolves completely, leaving no visible residue as undissolved matter.

B: The constituted solution is not significantly less clear than an equal volume of the diluent or of Purified Water contained in a similar vessel and examined similarly.

Particulate Matter—Constitute the solution as directed in the labeling supplied by the manufacturer for the sterile dry dosage form: the solution is essentially free from particles of foreign matter that can be observed on visual inspection.

⟨71⟩ STERILITY TESTS

▲♦Portions of this general chapter have been harmonized with the corresponding texts of the European Pharmacopeia and/or the Japanese Pharmacopeia. Those portions that are not harmonized are marked with symbols (♦♦) to specify this fact.♦

The following procedures are applicable for determining whether a Pharmacopeial article purporting to be sterile complies with the requirements set forth in the individual monograph with respect to the test for sterility. Pharmacopeial articles are to be tested by the *Membrane Filtration* method under *Test for Sterility of the Product to be Examined* where the nature of the product permits. If the membrane filtration technique is unsuitable, use the *Direct Inoculation of the Culture Medium* method under *Test for Sterility of the Product to be Examined*. All devices, with the exception of *Devices with Pathways Labeled Sterile*, are tested using the *Direct Inoculation of the Culture Medium* method. Provisions for retesting are included under *Observation and Interpretation of Results*.

Because sterility testing is a very exacting procedure, where asepsis of the procedure must be ensured for a correct interpretation of results, it is important that personnel be properly trained and qualified. The test for sterility is carried out under aseptic conditions. In order to achieve such conditions, the test environment has to be adapted to the way in which the sterility test is performed. The precautions taken to avoid contamination are such that they do not affect any microorganisms that are to be revealed in the test. The working conditions in which the tests are performed are monitored regularly by appropriate sampling of the working area and by carrying out appropriate controls.

These Pharmacopeial procedures are not by themselves designed to ensure that a batch of product is sterile or has been sterilized. This is accomplished primarily by validation of the sterilization process or of the aseptic processing procedures.

When evidence of microbial contamination in the article is obtained by the appropriate Pharmacopeial method, the result so obtained is conclusive evidence of failure of the article to meet the requirements of the test for sterility, even if a different result is obtained by an alternative procedure. For additional information on sterility testing, see *Sterilization and Sterility Assurance of Compendial Articles* ⟨1211⟩.

MEDIA

Prepare media for the tests as described below, or dehydrated formulations may be used provided that, when reconstituted as directed by the manufacturer or distributor, they meet the requirements of the *Growth Promotion Test of Aerobes, Anaerobes, and Fungi*. Media are sterilized using a validated process.

The following culture media have been found to be suitable for the test for sterility. *Fluid Thioglycollate Medium* is primarily intended for the culture of anaerobic bacteria. However, it will also detect aerobic bacteria. *Soybean–Casein Digest Medium* is suitable for the culture of both fungi and aerobic bacteria.

Fluid Thioglycollate Medium . . . .

L-Cystine	0.5 g
Sodium Chloride.	2.5 g
Dextrose ($C_6H_{12}O_6 \cdot H_2O$)	5.5/5.0 g
Agar, granulated (moisture content not exceeding 15%)	0.75 g
Yeast Extract (water-soluble)	5.0 g
Pancreatic Digest of Casein	15.0 g
Sodium Thioglycollate	0.5 g
or Thioglycolic Acid	0.3 mL
Resazurin Sodium Solution (1 in 1000), freshly prepared	1.0 mL
Purified Water	1000 mL

Mix the L-cystine, sodium chloride, dextrose, yeast extract, and pancreatic digest of casein with the purified water, and heat until solution is effected. Dissolve the sodium thioglycollate or thioglycolic acid in the solution and, if necessary, add 1 N sodium hydroxide so that, after sterilization, the solution will have a pH of 7.1 ± 0.2. If filtration is necessary, heat the solution again without boiling, and filter while hot through moistened filter paper. Add the resazurin sodium solution, mix, and place the medium in suitable vessels that provide a ratio of surface to depth of medium such that not more than the upper half of the medium has undergone a color change indicative of oxygen uptake at the end of the incubation period. Sterilize using a validated process. If the medium is stored, store at a temperature between 2° and 25° in a sterile, airtight container. If more than the upper one-third of the medium has acquired a pink color, the medium may be restored once by heating the containers in a water-bath or in free-flowing steam until the pink color disappears and by cooling quickly, taking care to prevent the introduction of nonsterile air into the container.

Fluid Thioglycollate Medium is to be incubated at 32.5 ± 2.5°.

◆Alternative Thioglycollate Medium

Prepare a mixture having the same composition as that of the *Fluid Thioglycollate Medium*, but omitting the agar and the resazurin sodium solution, sterilize as directed above, and allow to cool prior to use. The pH after sterilization is 7.1 ± 0.2. Incubate under anaerobic conditions for the duration of the incubation period.

Alternative Fluid Thioglycollate Medium is to be incubated at 32.5 ± 2.5°.◆

Soybean–Casein Digest Medium . . . .

Pancreatic Digest of Casein	17.0 g
Papaic Digest of Soybean Meal	3.0 g
Sodium Chloride.	5.0 g
Dibasic Potassium Phosphate	2.5 g
Dextrose ($C_6H_{12}O_6 \cdot H_2O$)	2.5/2.3 g
Purified Water	1000 mL

Dissolve the solids in the *Purified water*, heating slightly to effect a solution. Cool the solution to room temperature, and adjust the pH with 1 N sodium hydroxide so that, after sterilization, it will have a pH of 7.3 ± 0.2. Filter, if necessary to clarify, dispense into suitable containers, and sterilize using a validated filtration process. Store at a temperature between 2° and 25° in a sterile well-closed container, unless it is intended for immediate use.

Soybean–Casein Digest Medium is to be incubated at 22.5 ± 2.5°.◆

◆Media for Penicillins or Cephalosporins

Where sterility test media are to be used in the *Direct Inoculation of the Culture Medium* method under *Test for Sterility of the Product to be Examined*, modify the preparation of *Fluid Thioglycollate Medium* and the *Soybean–Casein Digest Medium* as follows. To the containers of each medium, transfer aseptically a quantity of β-lactamase sufficient to inactivate the amount of antibiotic in the specimen under test. Determine the quantity of β-lactamase required to inactivate the antibiotic by using a β-lactamase preparation that has been assayed previously for its penicillin- or cephalosporin-inactivating power. [NOTE—Supplemented β-lactamase media can also be used in the membrane filtration test.]

Alternatively (in an area completely separate from that used for sterility testing), confirm that an appropriate amount of β-lactamase is incorporated into the medium, following either method under *Validation Test*, using less than 100 colony-forming units (cfu) of *Staphylococcus aureus* (see *Table 1*) as the challenge. Typical microbial growth of the inoculated culture must be observed as a confirmation that the β-lactamase concentration is appropriate.◆

Suitability Tests

The media used comply with the following tests, carried out before, or in parallel, with the test on the product to be examined.

STERILITY

Confirm the sterility of each sterilized batch of medium by incubating a portion of the media at the specified incubation temperature for 14 days. No growth of microorganisms occurs.

GROWTH PROMOTION TEST OF AEROBES, ANAEROBES, AND FUNGI

Test each lot of of ready-prepared medium and each batch of medium prepared either from dehydrated medium or from ingredients ◆[1]◆. Suitable strains of microorganisms are indicated in *Table 1*.

Inoculate portions of *Fluid Thioglycollate Medium* with a small number (not more than 100 cfu) of the following microorganisms, using a separate portion of medium for each of the following species of microorganism: *Clostridium sporogenes*, *Pseudomonas aeruginosa*, and *Staphylococcus aureus*. ◆Inoculate portions of *Alternative Fluid Thioglycollate Medium* with a small number (not more than 100 cfu) of *Clostridium sporogenes*.◆ Inoculate portions of *Soybean–Casein Digest Medium* with a small number (not more than 100 cfu) of the following microorganisms, using a separate portion of medium for each of the following species of microorganism: *Aspergillus niger*, *Bacillus subtilis*, and *Candida albicans*. Incubate for not more than 3 days in the case of bacteria and not more than 5 days in the case of fungi.

The media are suitable if a clearly visible growth of the microorganisms occurs.

◆STORAGE

If prepared media are stored in unsealed containers, they can be used for 1 month, provided that they are tested for growth promotion within 2 weeks of the time of use and that color indicator requirements are met. If stored in tight containers, the

---

◆[1] In appropriate cases, periodic testing of the different batches prepared from the same lot of dehydrated medium is acceptable.◆

media can be used for 1 year, provided that they are tested for growth promotion within 3 months of the time of use and that the color indicator requirements are met.◆

Table 1. Strains of the Test Microorganisms Suitable for Use in the Growth Promotion Test and the Validation Test

Aerobic bacteria
Staphylococcus aureus◆1.   ATCC 6538, CIP 4.83, NCTC 10788, NCIMB 9518
Bacillus subtilis   ATCC 6633, CIP 52.62, NCIMB 8054
Pseudomonas aeruginosa◆2.   ATCC 9027, NCIMB 8626, CIP 82.118
Anaerobic bacterium
Clostridium sporogenes◆3.   ATCC 19404, CIP 79.3, NCTC 532 or ATCC 11437
Fungi
Candida albicans   ATCC 10231, IP 48.72, NCPF 3179
Aspergillus niger   ATCC 16404, IP 1431.83, IMI 149007

◆1 An alternative to *Staphylococcus aureus* is *Bacillus subtilis* (ATCC 6633).◆
◆2 An alternative microorganism is *Micrococcus luteus* (*Kocuria rhizophila*), ATCC 9341.◆
◆3 An alternative to *Clostridium sporogenes*, when a nonspore-forming microorganism is desired, is *Bacetroides vulgatus* (ATCC 8482).◆
[NOTE—Seed-lot culture maintenance techniques (seed-lot systems) are used so that the viable microorganisms used for inoculation are not more than five passages removed from the original master seed lot.]

◆DILUTING AND RINSING FLUIDS FOR MEMBRANE FILTRATION

Fluid A

PREPARATION

Dissolve 1 g of peptic digest of animal tissue in water to make 1 liter, filter or centrifuge to clarify, if necessary, and adjust to a pH of 7.1 ± 0.2. Dispense into containers, and sterilize using a validated process.

PREPARATION FOR PENICILLINS OR CEPHALOSPORINS

Aseptically add to the above *Preparation*, if necessary, a quantity of sterile β-lactamase sufficient to inactivate any residual antibiotic activity on the membranes after the solution of the test specimen has been filtered (see *Media for Penicillins or Cephalosporins*).

Fluid D

To each liter of *Fluid A* add 1 mL of polysorbate 80, adjust to a pH of 7.1 ± 0.2, dispense into containers, and sterilize using a validated process. Use this fluid for articles containing lecithin or oil, or for devices labeled as "sterile pathway."

Fluid K

Dissolve 5.0 g of peptic digest of animal tissue, 3.0 g of beef extract, and 10.0 g of polysorbate 80 in water to make 1 liter. Adjust the pH to obtain, after sterilization, a pH of 6.9 ± 0.2. Dispense into containers, and sterilize using a validated process.◆

VALIDATION TEST

Carry out a test as described below under *Test for Sterility of the Product to be Examined* using exactly the same methods, except for the following modifications.

Membrane Filtration

After transferring the content of the container or containers to be tested to the membrane, add an inoculum of a small number of viable microorganisms (not more than 100 cfu) to the final portion of sterile diluent used to rinse the filter.

Direct Inoculation

After transferring the contents of the container or containers to be tested (for catgut and other surgical sutures for veterinary use: strands) to the culture medium, add an inoculum of a small number of viable microorganisms (not more than 100 cfu) to the medium.

In both cases use the same microorganisms as those described above under *Growth Promotion Test of Aerobes, Anaerobes, and Fungi*. Perform a growth promotion test as a positive control. Incubate all the containers containing medium for not more than 5 days.

If clearly visible growth of microorganisms is obtained after the incubation, visually comparable to that in the control vessel without product, either the product possesses no antimicrobial activity under the conditions of the test or such activity has been satisfactorily eliminated. The test for sterility may then be carried out without further modification.

If clearly visible growth is not obtained in the presence of the product to be tested, visually comparable to that in the control vessels without product, the product possesses antimicrobial activity that has not been satisfactorily eliminated under the conditions of the test. Modify the conditions in order to eliminate the antimicrobial activity, and repeat the validation test.

This validation is performed (a) when the test for sterility has to be carried out on a new product; and (b) whenever there is a change in the experimental conditions of the test. The validation may be performed simultaneously with the *Test for Sterility of the Product to be Examined*.

TEST FOR STERILITY OF THE PRODUCT TO BE EXAMINED

◆Number of Articles to Be Tested

Unless otherwise specified elsewhere in this chapter or in the individual monograph, test the number of articles specified in *Table 3*. If the contents of each article are of sufficient quantity (see *Table 2*), they may be divided so that equal appropriate portions are added to each of the specified media. [NOTE—Perform sterility testing employing two or more of the specified media.] If each article does not contain sufficient quantities for each medium, use twice the number of articles indicated in *Table 3*.◆

The test may be carried out using the technique of *Membrane Filtration* or by *Direct Inoculation of the Culture Medium* with the product to be examined. Appropriate negative controls are included. The technique of membrane filtration is used whenever the nature of the product permits; that is, for filterable aqueous preparations, for alcoholic or oily preparations, and for preparations miscible with, or soluble in, aqueous or oily solvents, provided these solvents do not have an antimicrobial effect in the conditions of the test.

Membrane Filtration

Use membrane filters having a nominal pore size not greater than 0.45 μm whose effectiveness to retain microorganisms has been established. Cellulose nitrate filters, for example, are used for aqueous, oily, and weakly alcoholic solutions; and cellulose acetate filters, for example, are used for strongly alcoholic solutions. Specially adapted filters may be needed for certain products (e.g., for antibiotics).

Table 2. Minimum Quantity to be Used for Each Medium

Quantity per Container	Minimum Quantity to be Used (unless otherwise justified and authorized)
Liquids (other than antibiotics)	
Less than 1 mL	The whole contents of each container
1–40 mL	Half the contents of each container, but not less than 1 mL
Greater than 40 mL, and not greater than 100 mL	20 mL
Greater than 100 mL	10% of the contents of the container, but not less than 20 mL
Antibiotic liquids	1 mL
Other preparations soluble in water or in isopropyl myristate	The whole contents of each container to provide not less than 200 mg
Insoluble preparations, creams, and ointments to be suspended or emulsified	Use the contents of each container to provide not less than 200 mg
Solids	
Less than 50 mg	The whole contents of each container
50 mg or more, but less than 300 mg	Half the contents of each container, but not less than 50 mg
300 mg–5 g	150 mg
Greater than 5 g	500 mg
Devices	
Catgut and other surgical sutures for veterinary use	3 sections of a strand (each 30-cm long)
◆Surgical dressing/cotton/gauze (in packages)	100 mg per package
Sutures and other individually packaged single-use material	The whole device
Other medical devices	The whole device, cut into pieces or disassembled◆

Table 3. Minimum Number of Articles to be Tested in Relation to the Number of Articles in the Batch

Number of Items in the Batch	Minimum Number of Items to be Tested for Each Medium (unless otherwise justified and authorized)*
Parenteral preparations	
Not more than 100 containers	10% or 4 containers, whichever is the greater
More than 100 but not more than 500 containers	10 containers
More than 500 containers	2% or 20 containers, whichever is less
◆For large-volume parenterals	2% or 10 containers, whichever is less
Antibiotic solids	
Pharmacy bulk packages (<5 g)	20 containers
Pharmacy bulk packages (≥5 g)	6 containers
Bulks and blends	See *Bulk solid products*◆
Ophthalmic and other noninjectable preparations	
Not more than 200 containers	5% or 2 containers, whichever is the greater
More than 200 containers	10 containers
If the product is presented in the form of single-dose containers, apply the scheme shown above for preparations for parenteral use.	

* If the contents of one container are enough to inoculate the two media, this column gives the number of containers needed for both the media together.

Table 3. Minimum Number of Articles to be Tested in Relation to the Number of Articles in the Batch (*Continued*)

Number of Items in the Batch	Minimum Number of Items to be Tested for Each Medium (unless otherwise justified and authorized)*
Devices	
Catgut and other surgical sutures for veterinary use	2 % or 5 packages, whichever is the greater, up to a maximum total of 20 packages
◆Not more than 100 articles	10% or 4 articles, whichever is greater
More than 100, but not more than 500 articles	10 articles
More than 500 articles	2% or 20 articles, whichever is less.◆
Bulk solid products	
Up to 4 containers	Each container
More than 4 containers, but not more than 50 containers	20% or 4 containers, whichever is greater
More than 50 containers	2% or 10 containers, whichever is greater

The technique described below assumes that membranes about 50 mm in diameter will be used. If filters of a different diameter are used, the volumes of the dilutions and the washings should be adjusted accordingly. The filtration apparatus and membrane are sterilized by appropriate means. The apparatus is designed so that the solution to be examined can be introduced and filtered under aseptic conditions: it permits the aseptic removal of the membrane for transfer to the medium, or it is suitable for carrying out the incubation after adding the medium to the apparatus itself.

AQUEOUS SOLUTIONS

If appropriate, transfer a small quantity of a suitable, sterile diluent such as ◆*Fluid A* (see *Diluting and Rinsing Fluids for Membrane Filtration*).◆ onto the membrane in the apparatus and filter. The diluent may contain suitable neutralizing substances and/or appropriate inactivating substances, for example, in the case of antibiotics.

Transfer the contents of the container or containers to be tested to the membrane or membranes, if necessary, after diluting to the volume used in the *Validation Test* with the chosen sterile diluent, but using not less than the quantities of the product to be examined prescribed in *Tables 2* and *3*. Filter immediately. If the product has antimicrobial properties, wash the membrane not less than three times by filtering through it each time the volume of the chosen sterile diluent used in the *Validation Test*. Do not exceed a washing cycle of 5 times 200 mL, even if during validation it has been demonstrated that such a cycle does not fully eliminate the antimicrobial activity. Transfer the whole membrane to the culture medium or cut it aseptically into two equal parts, and transfer one half to each of two suitable media. Use the same volume of each medium as in the *Validation Test*. Alternatively, transfer the medium onto the membrane in the apparatus. Incubate the media for not less than 14 days.

SOLUBLE SOLIDS (OTHER THAN ANTIBIOTICS)

Use for each medium not less than the quantity prescribed in *Tables 2* and *3* of the product dissolved in a suitable solvent, such as ◆*Fluid A* (*Diluting and Rinsing Fluids for Membrane Filtration*),◆ and proceed with the test as described above for *Aqueous Solutions* using a membrane appropriate to the chosen solvent.

OILS AND OILY SOLUTIONS

Use for each medium not less than the quantity of the product prescribed in *Tables 2* and *3*. Oils and oily solutions of sufficiently low viscosity may be filtered without dilution through a dry membrane. Viscous oils may be diluted as necessary with a suitable sterile diluent such as isopropyl myristate shown not to have antimicrobial activity in the conditions of the test. Allow the

oil to penetrate the membrane by its own weight, and then filter, applying the pressure or suction gradually. Wash the membrane at least three times by filtering through it each time about 100 mL of a suitable sterile solution such as ◆*Fluid A* (see *Diluting and Rinsing Fluids for Membrane Filtration*),◆ containing a suitable emulsifying agent at a concentration shown to be appropriate in the validation of the test, for example polysorbate 80 at a concentration of 10 g per liter ◆(*Fluid K*).◆ Transfer the membrane or membranes to the culture medium or media, or vice versa, as described above for *Aqueous Solutions*, and incubate at the same temperatures and for the same times.

OINTMENTS AND CREAMS

Use for each medium not less than the quantities of the product prescribed in *Tables 2* and *3*. Ointments in a fatty base and emulsions of the water-in-oil type may be diluted to 1% in isopropyl myristate as described above, by heating, if necessary, to not more than 40°. In exceptional cases it may be necessary to heat to not more than 44°. Filter as rapidly as possible, and proceed as described above for *Oils and Oily Solutions*.

◆PREFILLED SYRINGES

For prefilled syringes without attached sterile needles, expel the contents of each syringe into one or two separate membrane filter funnels or into separate pooling vessels prior to transfer. If a separate sterile needle is attached, directly expel the syringe contents as indicated above, and proceed as directed for *Aqueous Solutions*. Test the sterility of the needle, using *Direct Inoculation* under *Validation Test*.

SOLIDS FOR INJECTION OTHER THAN ANTIBIOTICS

Constitute the test articles as directed on the label, and proceed as directed for *Aqueous Solutions* or *Oils and Oily Solutions*, whichever applies. [NOTE—If necessary, excess diluent can be added to aid in the constitution and filtration of the constituted test article.]

ANTIBIOTIC SOLIDS FOR INJECTION

Pharmacy Bulk Packages, < 5 g—From each of 20 containers, aseptically transfer about 300 mg of solids, into a sterile 500-mL conical flask, dissolve in about 200 mL of *Fluid A* (see *Diluting and Rinsing Fluids for Membrane Filtration*), and mix; or constitute, as directed in the labeling, each of 20 containers and transfer a quantity of liquid or suspension, equivalent to about 300 mg of solids, into a sterile 500-mL conical flask, dissolve in about 200 mL of *Fluid A*, and mix. Proceed as directed for *Aqueous Solutions* or *Oils and Oily Solutions*, whichever applies.

Pharmacy Bulk Packages, ≥5 g—From each of 6 containers, aseptically transfer about 1 g of solids into a sterile 500-mL conical flask, dissolve in about 200 mL of *Fluid A*, and mix; or constitute, as directed in the labeling, each of 6 containers and transfer a quantity of liquid, equivalent to about 1 g of solids, into a sterile 500-mL conical flask, dissolve in about 200 mL of *Fluid A*, and mix. Proceed as directed for *Aqueous Solutions*.

ANTIBIOTIC SOLIDS, BULKS, AND BLENDS

Aseptically remove a sufficient quantity of solids from the appropriate amount of containers (see *Table 2*), mix to obtain a composite, equivalent to about 6 g of solids, and transfer to a sterile 500-mL conical flask. Dissolve in about 200 mL of *Fluid A*, and mix. Proceed as directed for *Aqueous Solutions*.

STERILE AEROSOL PRODUCTS

For fluid products in pressurized aerosol form, freeze the containers in an alcohol-dry ice mixture at least at –20° for about 1 hour. If feasible, allow the propellant to escape before aseptically opening the container, and transfer the contents to a sterile pooling vessel. Add 100 mL of *Fluid D* to the pooling vessel, and mix gently. Proceed as directed for *Aqueous Solutions* or *Oils and Oily Solutions*, whichever applies.

DEVICES WITH PATHWAYS LABELED STERILE

Aseptically pass not less than 10 pathway volumes of *Fluid D* through each device tested. Collect the fluids in an appropriate sterile vessel, and proceed as directed for *Aqueous Solutions* or *Oils and Oily Solutions*, whichever applies.

In the case of sterile, empty syringes, draw sterile diluent into the barrel through the sterile needle, if attached, or through a sterile needle attached for the purpose of the test, and express the contents into a sterile pooling vessel. Proceed as directed above.♦

Direct Inoculation of the Culture Medium

Transfer the quantity of the preparation to be examined prescribed in *Tables 2* and *3* directly into the culture medium so that the volume of the product is not more than 10% of the volume of the medium, unless otherwise prescribed.

If the product to be examined has antimicrobial activity, carry out the test after neutralizing this with a suitable neutralizing substance or by dilution in a sufficient quantity of culture medium. When it is necessary to use a large volume of the product, it may be preferable to use a concentrated culture medium prepared in such a way that it takes into account the subsequent dilution. Where appropriate, the concentrated medium may be added directly to the product in its container.

OILY LIQUIDS

Use media to which have been added a suitable emulsifying agent at a concentration shown to be appropriate in the validation of the test, for example polysorbate 80 at a concentration of 10 g per liter.

OINTMENTS AND CREAMS

Prepare by diluting to about 1 in 10 by emulsifying with the chosen emulsifying agent in a suitable sterile diluent such as ♦*Fluid A* (see *Diluting and Rinsing Fluids for Membrane Filtration*).♦ Transfer the diluted product to a medium not containing an emulsifying agent.

Incubate the inoculated media for not less than 14 days. Observe the cultures several times during the incubation period. Shake cultures containing oily products gently each day. However, when thioglycollate medium or other similar medium is used for the detection of anaerobic microorganisms, keep shaking or mixing to a minimum in order to maintain anaerobic conditions.

CATGUT AND OTHER SURGICAL SUTURES FOR VETERINARIAN USE

Use for each medium not less than the quantities of the product prescribed in *Tables 2* and *3*. Open the sealed package using aseptic precautions, and remove three sections of the strand for each culture medium. Carry out the test on three sections, each 30-cm long, which have been cut off from the beginning, the center, and the end of the strand. Use whole strands from freshly opened cassette packs. Transfer each section of the strand to the selected medium. Use sufficient medium to cover adequately the material to be tested (20 mL to 150 mL).

♦SOLIDS

Transfer a quantity of the product in the form of a dry solid (or prepare a suspension of the product by adding sterile diluent to the immediate container), corresponding to not less than the quantity indicated in *Tables 2* and *3*. Transfer the material so obtained to 200 mL of *Fluid Thioglycollate Medium*, and mix. Similarly, transfer the same quantity to 200 mL of *Soybean-Casein Digest Medium*, and mix. Proceed as directed above.

PURIFIED COTTON, GAUZE, SURGICAL DRESSINGS, AND RELATED ARTICLES

From each package of cotton, rolled gauze bandage, or large surgical dressings being tested, aseptically remove two or more portions of 100- to 500-mg each from the innermost part of the sample. From individually packaged, single-use materials, aseptically remove the entire article. Immerse the portions or article in each medium, and proceed as directed above.

STERILE DEVICES

Articles can be immersed intact or disassembled. To ensure that device pathways are also in contact with the media, immerse the appropriate number of units per medium in a volume of medium sufficient to immerse the device completely, and proceed as directed above. For extremely large devices, immerse those portions of the device that are to come into contact with the patient in a volume of medium sufficient to achieve complete immersion of those portions.

For catheters where the inside lumen and outside are required to be sterile, either cut them into pieces such that the medium is in contact with the entire lumen or fill the lumen with medium, and then immerse the intact unit.♦

OBSERVATION AND INTERPRETATION OF RESULTS

At intervals during the incubation period and at its conclusion, examine the media for macroscopic evidence of microbial growth. If the material being tested renders the medium turbid so that the presence or absence of microbial growth cannot be readily determined by visual examination, 14 days after the beginning of incubation transfer portions (each not less than 1 mL) of the medium to fresh vessels of the same medium, and then incubate the original and transfer vessels for not less than 4 days.

If no evidence of microbial growth is found, the product to be examined complies with the test for sterility. If evidence of microbial growth is found, the product to be examined does not comply with the test for sterility, unless it can be clearly demonstrated that the test was invalid for causes unrelated to the product to be examined. The test may be considered invalid only if one or more of the following conditions are fulfilled:

a. The data of the microbiological monitoring of the sterility testing facility show a fault.
b. A review of the testing procedure used during the test in question reveals a fault.
c. Microbial growth is found in the negative controls.
d. After determination of the identity of the microorganisms isolated from the test, the growth of this species (or these species) may be ascribed unequivocally to faults with respect to the material and or the technique used in conducting the sterility test procedure.

If the test is declared to be invalid, it is repeated with the same number of units as in the original test. If no evidence of microbial growth is found in the repeat test, the product examined complies with the test for sterility. If microbial growth is found in the repeat test, the product examined does not comply with the test for sterility.

APPLICATION OF THE TEST TO PARENTERAL PREPARATIONS, OPHTHALMIC, AND OTHER NONINJECTABLE PREPARATIONS REQUIRED TO COMPLY WITH THE TEST FOR STERILITY

When using the technique of membrane filtration, use, whenever possible, the whole contents of the container, but not less than the quantities indicated in *Tables 2* and *3*, diluting where necessary to about 100 mL with a suitable sterile solution, such as ◆*Fluid A* (see *Diluting and Rinsing Fluids for Membrane Filtration*).◆

When using the technique of direct inoculation of media, use the quantities shown in *Tables 2* and *3*, unless otherwise justified and authorized. The tests for bacterial and fungal sterility are carried out on the same sample of the product to be examined. When the volume or the quantity in a single container is insufficient to carry out the tests, the contents of two or more containers are used to inoculate the different media.▲USP27

⟨85⟩ BACTERIAL ENDOTOXINS TEST

◆Portions of this general chapter have been harmonized with the corresponding texts of the European Pharmacopeia and/or the Japanese Pharmacopeia. Those portions that are not harmonized are marked with symbols (◆◆) to specify this fact.◆

This chapter provides a test to detect or quantify bacterial endotoxins that may be present in or on the sample of the article(s) to which the test is applied. It uses Limulus Amebocyte Lysate (LAL) obtained from the aqueous extracts of circulating amebocytes of horseshoe crab (*Limulus polyphemus* or *Tachypleus tridentatus*) which has been prepared and characterized for use as an LAL Reagent.◆1

There are two types of techniques for this test: the gel-clot techniques, which are based on gel formation, and the photometric techniques. The latter include a turbidimetric method, which is based on the development of turbidity after cleavage of an endogenous substrate, and a chromogenic method, which is based on the development of color after cleavage of a synthetic peptide-chromogen complex. Proceed by any one of these techniques, unless otherwise indicated in the monograph. In case of dispute, the final decision is based on the gel-clot techniques, unless otherwise indicated in the monograph.

In the gel-clot techniques, the reaction endpoint is determined from dilutions of the material under test in direct comparison with parallel dilutions of a reference endotoxin, and quantities of endotoxin are expressed in USP Endotoxin Units (USP-EU). [NOTE—One USP-EU is equal to one IU of endotoxin.]

Since LAL Reagents have been formulated to be used also for turbidimetric or colorimetric tests, such tests may be used to comply with the requirements. These tests require the establishment of a standard regression curve; the endotoxin content of the test material is determined by interpolation from the curve. The procedures include incubation for a preselected time of reacting endotoxin and control solutions with LAL Reagent and reading of the spectrophotometric light absorbance at suitable wavelengths. In the endpoint turbidimetric procedure the reading is made immediately at the end of the incubation period. In the endpoint colorimetric procedure the reaction is arrested at the end of the preselected time by the addition of an enzyme reaction-terminating agent prior to the readings. In the turbidimetric and colorimetric kinetic assays the absorbance is measured throughout the reaction period and rate values are determined from those readings.

APPARATUS AND GLASSWARE

Depyrogenate all glassware and other heat-stable materials in a hot-air oven using a validated process.◆2 Commonly used minimum time and temperature settings are 30 minutes at 250°. If employing plastic apparatus, such as microplates and pipet tips for automatic pipetters, use only that which has been shown to be free of detectable endotoxin and not to interfere with the test. [NOTE—In this chapter, the term "tube" includes any other receptacle such as a micro-titer well.]

PREPARATION OF THE STANDARD ENDOTOXIN STOCK SOLUTION AND STANDARD SOLUTIONS

The USP Endotoxin RS has a defined potency of 10,000 USP Endotoxin Units (EU) per vial. Constitute the entire contents of 1 vial of the RSE with 5 mL of LAL Reagent Water◆3, mix intermittently for 30 minutes, using a vortex mixer, and use this concentrate for making appropriate serial dilutions. Preserve the concentrate in a refrigerator for making subsequent dilutions for not more than 14 days. Mix vigorously, using a vortex mixer, for not less than 3 minutes before use. Mix each dilution for not less than 30 seconds before proceeding to make the next dilution. Do not store dilutions, because of loss of activity by adsorption, in the absence of supporting data to the contrary.

◆1 LAL Reagent reacts with some β-glucans in addition to endotoxins. Some preparations that are treated will not react with β-glucans and must be used for samples that contain glucans.◆

◆2 For a validity test of the procedure for inactivating endotoxins, see *Dry-Heat Sterilization* under *Sterilization and Sterility Assurance of Compendial Articles* ⟨1211⟩. Use an LAL Reagent having a sensitivity of not less than 0.15 Endotoxin Unit per mL.◆

◆3 *Sterile Water for Injection* or other water that shows no reaction with the specific LAL Reagent with which it is to be used, at the limit of sensitivity of such reagent.◆

Preparatory Testing

Use an LAL Reagent of confirmed label sensitivity.

The validity of test results for bacterial endotoxins requires an adequate demonstration that specimens of the article or of solutions, washings, or extracts thereof to which the test is to be applied do not of themselves inhibit or enhance the reaction or otherwise interfere with the test. Validation is accomplished by performing the inhibition or enhancement test described under each of the three techniques indicated. Appropriate negative controls are included. Validation must be repeated if the LAL Reagent source or the method of manufacture or formulation of the article is changed.

Preparation of Sample Solutions

Prepare sample solutions by dissolving or diluting drugs or extracting medical devices using LAL Reagent Water. Some substances or preparations may be more appropriately dissolved, diluted, or extracted in other aqueous solutions. If necessary, adjust the pH of the solution (or dilution thereof) to be examined so that the pH of the mixture of the LAL Reagent and sample falls within the pH range specified by the LAL Reagent manufacturer. This usually applies to a product with a pH in the range of 6.0 to 8.0. The pH may be adjusted using an acid, base, or suitable buffer as recommended by the LAL Reagent manufacturer. Acids and bases may be prepared from concentrates or solids with LAL Reagent Water in containers free of detectable endotoxin. Buffers must be validated to be free of detectable endotoxin and interfering factors.

DETERMINATION OF MAXIMUM VALID DILUTION (MVD)

The Maximum Valid Dilution is the maximum allowable dilution of a specimen at which the endotoxin limit can be determined. It applies to injections or to solutions for parenteral administration in the form constituted or diluted for administration, or, where applicable, to the amount of drug by weight if the volume of the dosage form for administration could be varied. The general equation to determine MVD is:

MVD = (Endotoxin limit × Concentration of sample solution) / (λ)

where the concentration of sample solution and λ are as defined below. Where the endotoxin limit concentration is specified in the individual monograph in terms of volume (in EU per mL), divide the limit by λ, which is the labeled sensitivity (in EU per mL) of the LAL Reagent, to obtain the MVD factor. Where the endotoxin limit concentration is specified in the individual monograph in terms of weight or Units of active drug (in EU per mg or in EU per Unit), multiply the limit by the concentration (in mg per mL or in Units per mL) of the drug in the solution tested or of the drug constituted according to the label instructions, whichever is applicable, and divide the product of the multiplication by λ, to obtain the MVD factor. The MVD factor so obtained is the limit dilution factor for the preparation for the test to be valid.

ESTABLISHMENT OF ENDOTOXIN LIMITS

The endotoxin limit for parenteral drugs, defined on the basis of dose, is equal to K/M,[4] where K is the threshold human pyrogenic dose of endotoxin per kg of body weight, and M is equal to the maximum recommended human dose of product per kg of body weight in a single hour period.

The endotoxin limit for parenteral drugs is specified in individual monographs in units such as EU/mL, EU/mg, or EU/Unit of biological activity.

GEL-CLOT TECHNIQUES

The gel-clot techniques detect or quantify endotoxins based on clotting of the LAL Reagent in the presence of endotoxin. The concentration of endotoxin required to cause the lysate to clot under standard conditions is the labeled sensitivity of the LAL Reagent. To ensure both the precision and validity of the test, tests for confirming the labeled LAL Reagent sensitivity and for interfering factors are described under *Preparatory Testing for the Gel-Clot Techniques*.

Preparatory Testing for the Gel-Clot Techniques

Test for Confirmation of Labeled LAL Reagent Sensitivity—Confirm the labeled sensitivity using at least 1 vial of the LAL Reagent lot. Prepare a series of two-fold dilutions of the USP Endotoxin RS in LAL Reagent Water to give concentrations of 2λ, λ, 0.5λ, and 0.25λ, where λ is as defined above. Perform the test on the four standard concentrations in quadruplicate and include negative controls. The test for confirmation of lysate sensitivity is to be carried out when a new batch of LAL Reagent is used or when there is any change in the experimental conditions that may affect the outcome of the test.

Mix a volume of the LAL Reagent with an equal volume (such as 0.1-mL aliquots) of one of the standard solutions in each test tube. When single test vials or ampuls containing lyophilized LAL Reagent are used, add solutions directly to the vial or ampul. Incubate the reaction mixture for a constant period according to directions of the LAL Reagent manufacturer (usually at 37 ± 1° for 60 ± 2 minutes), avoiding vibration. To test the integrity of the gel, take each tube in turn directly from the incubator and invert it through about 180° in one smooth motion. If a firm gel has formed that remains in place upon inversion, record the result as positive. A result is negative if an intact gel is not formed. The test is not valid unless the lowest concentration of the standard solutions shows a negative result in all replicate tests.

The endpoint is the last positive test in the series of decreasing concentrations of endotoxin. Calculate the mean value of the logarithms of the endpoint concentration and then the antilogarithm of the mean value using the following equation:

Geometric Mean Endpoint Concentration = antilog ($\Sigma e/f$),

where Σe is the sum of the log endpoint concentrations of the dilution series used, and f is the number of replicate test tubes. The geometric mean endpoint concentration is the measured sensitivity of the LAL Reagent (in EU/mL). If this is not less than 0.5λ and not more than 2λ, the labeled sensitivity is confirmed and is used in tests performed with this lysate.

---

[4] K is 5 USP-EU/kg for any route of administration other than intrathecal (for which K is 0.2 USP-EU/kg body weight). For radiopharmaceutical products not administered intrathecally the endotoxin limit is calculated as $175/V$, where V is the maximum recommended dose in mL. For intrathecally administered radiopharmaceuticals, the endotoxin limit is obtained by the formula $14/V$. For formulations (usually anticancer products) administered on a per square meter of body surface, the formula is K/M, where $K = 5$ EU/kg and M is the (maximum dose/m² /hour × 1.80 m²)/70 Kg. ◆

Interfering Factors Test for the Gel-Clot Techniques— Prepare solutions A, B, C, and D as shown in *Table 1*, and perform the inhibition/enhancement test on the sample solutions at a dilution less than the MVD, not containing any detectable endotoxins, following the procedure in the *Test for Confirmation of Labeled LAL Reagent Sensitivity* above. The geometric mean endpoint concentrations of solutions B and C are determined using the equation in that test.

Table 1. Preparation of Solutions for the Inhibition/Enhancement Test for Gel-Clot Techniques

Solution	Endotoxin Concentration/Solution to which Endotoxin is Added	Diluent	Dilution Factor	Initial Endotoxin Concentration	Number of Replicates
A[a]	none/sample solution	—	—	—	4
B[b]	2λ/sample solution	sample solution	1	2λ	4
			2	1λ	4
			4	0.5λ	4
			8	0.25λ	4
C[c]	2λ/water for BET	LAL Reagent Water	1	2λ	2
			2	1λ	2
			4	0.5λ	2
			8	0.25λ	2
D[d]	none/LAL Reagent Water	—	—	—	2

* Prepare Solution A and positive product control Solution B using a dilution not greater than the MVD and treatments as directed in the *Interfering Factors Test for the Gel-Clot Techniques* under *Preparatory Testing for the Gel-Clot Techniques*. Positive control Solutions B and C contain the standard endotoxin preparation at a concentration corresponding to twice the labeled LAL Reagent sensitivity. The negative control Solution D is LAL Reagent Water.

This test must be repeated when any condition that is likely to influence the test results changes. The test is not valid unless Solutions A and D show no reaction and the result of Solution C confirms the labeled sensitivity.

If the sensitivity of the lysate determined in the presence of the sample solution under test of Solution B is not less than 0.5λ and not greater than 2λ, the sample solution does not contain factors which interfere under the experimental conditions used. Otherwise, the sample solution to be examined interferes with the test.

If the sample under test does not comply with the test at a dilution less than the MVD, repeat the test using a greater dilution, not exceeding the MVD. The use of a more sensitive lysate permits a greater dilution of the sample to be examined and this may contribute to the elimination of interference.

Interference may be overcome by suitable treatment, such as filtration, neutralization, dialysis, or heating. To establish that the chosen treatment effectively eliminates interference without loss of endotoxins, perform the assay described below using the preparation to be examined to which USP Endotoxin RS has been added and which has been subjected to the selected treatment.

Gel-Clot Limit Test

This test is used when a monograph contains a requirement for endotoxin limits.

Procedure— Prepare Solutions A, B, C, and D as shown in *Table 2*, and perform the test on these solutions following the procedure in the *Test for Confirmation of Labeled LAL Reagent Sensitivity* under *Preparatory Testing for the Gel-Clot Techniques*.

Table 2. Preparation of Solutions for the Gel-Clot Limit Test

Solution[*]	Endotoxin Concentration/Solution to which Endotoxin is Added	Number of Replicates
A	none/diluted sample solution	2
B	2λ/diluted sample solution	2
C	2λ/LAL Reagent Water	2
D	none/LAL Reagent Water	2

* Prepare Solution A and positive product control Solution B using a dilution not greater than the MVD and treatments as directed in the *Interfering Factors Test for the Gel-Clot Techniques* under *Preparatory Testing for the Gel-Clot Techniques*. Positive control Solutions B and C contain the standard endotoxin preparation at a concentration corresponding to twice the labeled LAL Reagent sensitivity. The negative control Solution D is LAL Reagent Water.

Interpretation— The test is not valid unless both replicates of positive control Solutions B and C are positive and those of negative control Solution D are negative. The preparation under test complies with the test when a negative result is found for both tubes containing Solution A. The preparation under test does not comply with the test when a positive result is found for both tubes containing Solution A.

Repeat the test when a positive result is found for 1 tube containing Solution A and a negative result for the other one. The preparation under test complies with the test when a negative result is found for both tubes containing Solution A in the repeat result. If the test is positive for the preparation under test at a dilution less than the MVD, the test may be repeated at a dilution not greater than the MVD.

Gel-Clot Assay

This assay quantifies bacterial endotoxins in sample solutions by titration to an endpoint.

Procedure—Prepare Solutions A, B, C, and D as shown in *Table 3*, and test these solutions by following the procedure in the *Test for Confirmation of Labeled LAL Reagent Sensitivity* under *Preparatory Testing for the Gel-Clot Techniques.*

Calculation and Interpretation—The test is not valid unless the following conditions are met: (1) both replicates of negative control Solution D are negative; (2) both replicates of positive product control Solution B are positive; and (3) the geometric mean endpoint concentration of Solution C is in the range of 0.5λ to 2λ.

Table 3. Preparation of Solutions for the Gel-Clot Assay

Solution	Endotoxin Concentration/Solution to which Endotoxin is Added	Diluent	Dilution Factor	Initial Endotoxin Concentration	Number of Replicates
A[a]	none/sample solution	LAL Reagent Water	1	—	2
			2	—	2
			4	—	2
			8	—	2
B[b]	2λ/sample solution	—	1	2λ	2
C[c]	2λ/LAL Reagent Water	LAL Reagent Water	1	2λ	2
			2	1λ	2
			4	0.5λ	2
			8	0.25λ	2
D[d]	none/LAL Reagent Water	—	—	—	2

[a] Solution A: a sample solution under test at the dilution, not to exceed the MVD, with which the *Interfering Factors Test for the Gel-Clot Techniques* was completed. Subsequent dilution of the sample solution must not exceed the MVD. Use LAL Reagent Water to make dilution series of four tubes containing the sample solution under test at concentrations of 1, , , and $\frac{1}{8}$ relative to the dilution with which the *Interfering Factors Test for the Gel-Clot Techniques* was completed. Other dilutions may be used as appropriate.
[b] Solution B: Solution A containing standard endotoxin at a concentration of 2λ (positive product control).
[c] Solution C: two series of 4 tubes of LAL Reagent Water containing the standard endotoxin at a concentration of 2λ, λ, 0.5λ, and 0.25λ, respectively.
[d] Solution D: LAL Reagent Water (negative control).

To determine the endotoxin concentration of Solution A, calculate the endpoint concentration for each replicate series of dilutions by multiplying each endpoint dilution factor by λ. The endotoxin concentration in the sample is the geometric mean endpoint concentration of the replicates (see the formula given in the *Test for Confirmation of Labeled LAL Reagent Sensitivity* under *Preparatory Testing for the Gel-Clot Techniques*). If the test is conducted with a diluted sample solution, calculate the concentration of endotoxin in the original sample solution by multiplying by the dilution factor. If none of the dilutions of the sample solution is positive in a valid assay, report the endotoxin concentration as less than λ (if the diluted sample was tested, less than λ times the lowest dilution factor of the sample.) If all dilutions are positive, the endotoxin concentration is reported as equal to or greater than the greatest dilution factor multiplied by λ (e.g., initial dilution factor times 8 times λ in *Table 3*).

The article meets the requirements of the test if the concentration of endotoxin is less than that specified in the individual monograph.

PHOTOMETRIC TECHNIQUES

The turbidimetric method measures increases in turbidity. Depending on the test principle used, this technique is classified as either endpoint-turbidimetric or kinetic-turbidimetric. The endpoint-turbidimetric technique is based on the quantitative relationship between the concentration of endotoxins and the turbidity (absorbance or transmission) of the reaction mixture at the end of an incubation period. The kinetic-turbidimetric technique is a method to measure either the onset time needed to reach a predetermined absorbance of the reaction mixture or the rate of turbidity development.

The chromogenic method measures the chromophore released from a suitable chromogenic peptide by the reaction of endotoxins with the LAL Reagent. Depending on the test principle employed, this technique is classified as either endpoint-chromogenic or kinetic-chromogenic. The endpoint-chromogenic technique is based on the quantitative relationship between the concentration of endotoxins and the release of chromophore at the end of an incubation period. The kinetic-chromogenic technique is a method to measure either the onset time needed to reach a predetermined absorbance of the reaction mixture or the rate of color development.

All photometric tests are carried out at the incubation temperature recommended by the LAL Reagent manufacturer, which is usually $37 \pm 1°$.

Preparatory Testing for the Photometric Techniques

To assure the precision or validity of the turbidimetric and chromogenic techniques, preparatory tests are conducted to verify that the criteria for the standard curve are valid and that the sample solution does not inhibit or enhance the reaction. Revalidation for the test method is required when conditions that are likely to influence the test result change.

Verification of Criteria for the Standard Curve—Using the Standard Endotoxin Solution, prepare at least three endotoxin concentrations to generate the standard curve. Perform the test using at least three replicates of each standard endotoxin concentration according to the manufacturer's instructions for the LAL Reagent (with regard to volume ratios, incubation time, temperature, pH, etc.). If the desired range in the kinetic methods is greater than two logs, additional standards should be included to bracket each log increase within the range of the standard curve. The absolute value of the correlation coefficient, $|r|$, must be greater than or equal to 0.980 for the range of endotoxin concentrations indicated by the manufacturer of the LAL Reagent.

Interfering Factors Test for the Photometric Techniques— Select an endotoxin concentration at or near the middle of the endotoxin standard curve. Prepare Solutions A, B, C, and D as shown in *Table 4*. Perform the test on Solutions A, B, C, and D at least in duplicate following the instructions for the LAL Reagent used (with regard to volume of sample and LAL Reagent, volume ratio of sample to LAL Reagent, incubation time, etc.).

Table 4. Preparation of Solutions for the Inhibition/Enhancement Test for Photometric Techniques

Solution	Endotoxin Concentration	Solution to which Endotoxin is Added	Number of Replicates
A[a]	none	sample solution	not less than 2
B[b]	middle concentration of the standard curve	sample solution	not less than 2
C[c]	at least 3 concentrations (lowest concentration is designated λ)	LAL Reagent Water	each not less than 2
D[d]	none	LAL Reagent Water	not less than 2

[a] Solution A: the sample solution may be diluted not to exceed MVD.
[b] Solution B: the preparation under test at the same dilution as Solution A, containing added endotoxin at a concentration equal to or near the middle of the standard curve.
[c] Solution C: the standard endotoxin at the concentrations used in the validation of the method described in *Verification of Criteria for the Standard Curve* under *Preparatory Testing for the Photometric Techniques* (positive control series).
[d] Solution D: LAL Reagent Water (negative control).

Calculate the mean recovery of the added endotoxin by subtracting the mean endotoxin concentration in the solution (if any) from that containing the added endotoxin. In order to be considered free of interfering factors under the conditions of the test, the measured concentration of the endotoxin added to the sample solution must be within 50% to 200% of the known added endotoxin concentration after subtraction of any endotoxin detected in the solution without added endotoxin.

When the endotoxin recovery is out of the specified ranges, the interfering factors must be removed as described in the *Interfering Factors Test for the Gel-Clot Techniques* under *Preparatory Testing for the Gel-Clot Techniques*. Repeating the *Interfering Factors Test for the Gel-Clot Techniques* validates the treatment.

Procedure for the Photometric Techniques

Follow the procedure described in the *Interfering Factors Test for the Photometric Techniques* under *Preparatory Testing for the Photometric Techniques*.

Calculation for the Photometric Techniques

Calculate the endotoxin concentration of each of the replicates of test Solution A using the standard curve generated by positive control series C. The test is not valid unless the following conditions are met: (1) the results of control series C comply with the requirements for validation defined under *Verification of Criteria for the Standard Curve* under *Preparatory Testing for the Photometric Techniques;* (2) the endotoxin recovery, calculated from the concentration found in Solution B after subtracting the endotoxin concentration found in Solution A is within 50 to 200%; and (3) the result of negative control series D does not exceed the limit of the blank value required in the description of the LAL Reagent used.

Interpretation of Results from the Photometric Techniques

In photometric assays, the preparation under test complies with the test if the mean endotoxin concentration of the replicates of Solution A, after correction for dilution and concentration, is less than the endotoxin limit for the product.

⟨661⟩ CONTAINERS

Many Pharmacopeial articles are of such nature as to require the greatest attention to the containers in which they are stored or maintained even for short periods of time. While the needs vary widely and some of them are not fully met by the containers available, objective standards are essential. It is the purpose of this chapter to provide such standards as have been developed for the materials of which pharmaceutical containers principally are made, i.e., glass and plastic.

A container intended to provide protection from light or offered as a "light-resistant" container meets the requirements for *Light Transmission*, where such protection or resistance is by virtue of the specific properties of the material of which the container is composed, including any coating applied thereto. A clear and colorless or a translucent container that is made light-resistant by means of an opaque enclosure (see *General Notices*) is exempt from the requirements for *Light Transmission*.

Containers composed of glass meet the requirements for *Chemical Resistance—Glass Containers*, and containers composed of plastic and intended for packaging products prepared for parenteral use meet the requirements under *Biological Tests—Plastics* and *Physicochemical Tests—Plastics*.

Where dry oral dosage forms, not meant for constitution into solution, are intended to be packaged in a container defined in the section *Polyethylene Containers*, the requirements given in that section are to be met.

Guidelines and requirements under *Single-Unit Containers and Unit-Dose Containers for Non-Sterile Solid and Liquid Dosage Forms* apply to official dosage forms that are repackaged into single-unit or unit-dose containers or mnemonic packs for dispensing pursuant to prescription.

LIGHT TRANSMISSION

Apparatus[1]—Use a spectrophotometer of suitable sensitivity and accuracy, adapted for measuring the amount of light transmitted by either transparent or translucent glass or plastic materials used for pharmaceutical containers. For transparent glass or plastic pharmaceutical containers, use a spectrophotometer of suitable sensitivity and accuracy for measuring and recording the amount of light transmitted. For translucent glass or plastic pharmaceutical containers, use a spectrophotometer as described above that, in addition, is capable of measuring and recording light transmitted in diffused as well as parallel rays.

---

[1] For further detail regarding apparatus and procedures, reference may be made to the following publications of the American Society for Testing and Materials, 100 Barr Harbor Drive, West Conshohocken, PA 19428-2959: "Standard Method of Test for Haze and Luminous Transmittance of Transparent Plastics," ASTM Designation D-1003-61; "Tentative Method of Test for Luminous Reflectance, Transmittance, and Color of Materials," ASTM E 308-66.

Preparation of Specimen—

Glass—Break the container or cut it with a circular saw fitted with a wet abrasive wheel, such as a carborundum or a bonded diamond wheel. Select sections to represent the average wall thickness in the case of blown glass containers, and trim them as necessary to give segments of a size convenient for mounting in the spectrophotometer. After cutting, wash and dry each specimen, taking care to avoid scratching the surfaces. If the specimen is too small to cover the opening in the specimen holder, mask the uncovered portion of the opening with opaque paper or masking tape, provided that the length of the specimen is greater than that of the slit in the spectrophotometer. Immediately before mounting in the specimen holder, wipe the specimen with lens tissue. Mount the specimen with the aid of a tacky wax, or by other convenient means, taking care to avoid leaving fingerprints or other marks on the surfaces through which light must pass.

Plastic—Cut circular sections from two or more areas of the container, and wash and dry them, taking care to avoid scratching the surfaces. Mount in the apparatus as described for *Glass*.

Procedure—Place the section in the spectrophotometer with its cylindrical axis parallel to the plane of the slit and approximately centered with respect to the slit. When properly placed, the light beam is normal to the surface of the section and reflection losses are at a minimum.

Measure the transmittance of the section with reference to air in the spectral region of interest, continuously with a recording instrument or at intervals of about 20 nm with a manual instrument, in the region of 290 to 450 nm.

Limits—The observed light transmission does not exceed the limits given in *Table 1* for containers intended for parenteral use.

Table 1.   Limits for Glass Types I, II, and III and Plastic Classes I–VI

Nominal Size (in mL)	Maximum Percentage of Light Transmission at Any Wavelength Between 290 and 450 nm	
	Flame-sealed Containers	Closure-sealed Containers
1	50	25
2	45	20
5	40	15
10	35	13
20	30	12
50	15	10

NOTE—Any container of a size intermediate to those listed above exhibits a transmission not greater than that of the next larger size container listed in the table. For containers larger than 50 mL, the limits for 50 mL apply.

The observed light transmission for containers of Type NP glass and for plastic containers for products intended for oral or topical administration does not exceed 10% at any wavelength in the range from 290 to 450 nm.

CHEMICAL RESISTANCE—GLASS CONTAINERS

The following tests are designed to determine the resistance to water attack of new (not previously used) glass containers. The degree of attack is determined by the amount of alkali released from the glass under the influence of the attacking medium under the conditions specified. This quantity of alkali is extremely small in the case of the more resistant glasses, thus calling for particular attention to all details of the tests and the use of apparatus of high quality and precision. The tests should be conducted in an area relatively free from fumes and excessive dust.

Glass Types—Glass containers suitable for packaging Pharmacopeial preparations may be classified as in *Table 2* on the basis of the tests set forth in this section. Containers of Type I borosilicate glass are generally used for preparations that are intended for parenteral administration. Containers of Type I glass, or of Type II glass (i.e., soda-lime glass that is suitably dealkalized) are usually used for packaging acidic and neutral parenteral preparations. Type I glass containers, or Type II glass containers (where stability data demonstrate their suitability), are used for alkaline parenteral preparations. Type III soda-lime glass containers usually are not used for parenteral preparations, except where suitable stability test data indicate that Type III glass is satisfactory for the parenteral preparations that are packaged therein. Containers of Type NP glass are intended for packaging nonparenteral articles, i.e., those intended for oral or topical use.

Table 2.   Glass Types and Test Limits

Type	General Description[1]	Type of Test	Size,[2] mL	mL of 0.020 N Acid
			Limits	
I	Highly resistant, borosilicate glass	*Powdered Glass*	All	1.0
II	Treated soda-lime glass		100 or less	0.7
		Water Attack	Over 100	0.2
III	Soda-lime glass	*Powdered Glass*	All	8.5
NP	General-purpose soda-lime glass	*Powdered Glass*	All	15.0

[1] The description applies to containers of this type of glass usually available.
[2] Size indicates the overflow capacity of the container.

Apparatus—

Autoclave—For these tests, use an autoclave capable of maintaining a temperature of $121 \pm 2.0°$, equipped with a thermometer, a pressure gauge, a vent cock, and a rack adequate to accommodate at least 12 test containers above the water level.

Mortar and Pestle—Use a hardened-steel mortar and pestle, made according to the specifications in the accompanying illustration.

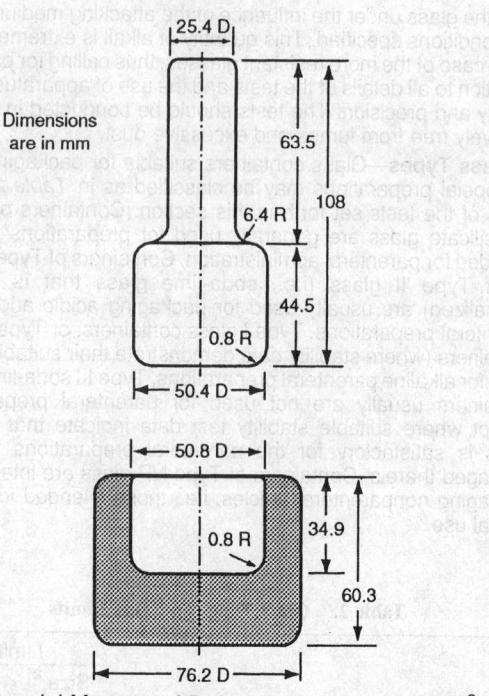

Dimensions are in mm

Special Mortar and Pestle for Pulverizing Glass²

Other Equipment—Also required are 20.3-cm (8-inch) sieves made of stainless steel including the Nos. 20, 40, and 50 sieves along with the pan and cover (see *Sizes of Standard Sieve Series in Range of Interest* under *Particle Size Distribution Estimation by Analytical Sieving* ⟨786⟩), 250-mL conical flasks made of resistant glass aged as specified, a 900-g (2-lb) hammer, a permanent magnet, a desiccator, and adequate volumetric apparatus.

Reagents—

High-Purity Water—The water used in these tests has a conductivity at 25°, as measured in an in-line cell just prior to dispensing, of not greater than 0.15 µS per cm (6.67 Megohm-cm). There must also be an assurance that this water is not contaminated by copper or its products (e.g., copper pipes, stills, or receivers). The water may be prepared by passing distilled water through a deionizer cartridge packed with a mixed bed of nuclear-grade resin, then through a cellulose ester membrane having openings not exceeding 0.45 µm.³ Do not use copper tubing. Flush the discharge lines before water is dispensed into test vessels. When the low conductivity specification can no longer be met, replace the deionizer cartridge.

Methyl Red Solution—Dissolve 24 mg of methyl red sodium in *Purified Water* to make 100 mL. If necessary, neutralize the solution with 0.02 N sodium hydroxide or acidify it with 0.02 N sulfuric acid so that the titration of 100 mL of *High-Purity Water*, containing 5 drops of indicator, does not require more than 0.020 mL of 0.020 N sodium hydroxide to effect the color change of the indicator, which should occur at a pH of 5.6.

---

² A suitable mortar and pestle is available (catalog No. H-17280) from Humboldt Manufacturing Co., 7300 West Agatite, Norridge, Chicago, IL 60656.

³ A suitable nuclear-grade resin mixture of the strong acid cation exchanger in the hydrogen form and the strong base anion exchanger in the hydroxide form, with a one-to-one cation to anion equivalence ratio, is available from the Millipore Corp., Bedford, MA 01730; Barnstead Co., 225 Rivermoor St., Boston, MA 02132; Illinois Water Treatment Co., 840 Cedar St., Rockford, IL 61105; and Vaponics, Inc., 200 Cordage Park, Plymouth, MA 02360.

A suitable in-line filter is available from the Millipore Corp.; Gelman Instrument Co., 600 S. Wagner Rd., Ann Arbor, MI 48106; and Schleicher and Schuell, Inc., 540 Washington St., Keene, NH 10003.

Powdered Glass Test

Rinse thoroughly with *Purified Water* 6 or more containers selected at random, and dry them with a current of clean, dry air. Crush the containers into fragments about 25 mm in size, divide about 100 g of the coarsely crushed glass into three approximately equal portions, and place one of the portions in the special mortar. With the pestle in place, crush the glass further by striking 3 or 4 blows with the hammer. Nest the sieves, and empty the mortar into the No. 20 sieve. Repeat the operation on each of the two remaining portions of glass, emptying the mortar each time into the No. 20 sieve. Shake the sieves for a short time, then remove the glass from the Nos. 20 and 40 sieves, and again crush and sieve as before. Repeat again this crushing and sieving operation. Empty the receiving pan, reassemble the nest of sieves, and shake by mechanical means for 5 minutes or by hand for an equivalent length of time. Transfer the portion retained on the No. 50 sieve, which should weigh in excess of 10 g, to a closed container, and store in a desiccator until used for the test.

Spread the specimen on a piece of glazed paper, and pass a magnet through it to remove particles of iron that may be introduced during the crushing. Transfer the specimen to a 250-mL conical flask of resistant glass, and wash it with six 30-mL portions of acetone, swirling each time for about 30 seconds and carefully decanting the acetone. After washing, the specimen should be free from agglomerations of glass powder, and the surface of the grains should be practically free from adhering fine particles. Dry the flask and contents for 20 minutes at 140°, transfer the grains to a weighing bottle, and cool in a desiccator. Use the test specimen within 48 hours after drying.

Procedure—Transfer 10.00 g of the prepared specimen, accurately weighed, to a 250-mL conical flask that has been digested (aged) previously with *High-Purity Water* in a bath at 90° for at least 24 hours or at 121° for 1 hour. Add 50.0 mL of *High-Purity Water* to this flask and to one similarly prepared to provide a blank. Cap all flasks with borosilicate glass beakers that previously have been treated as described for the flasks and that are of such size that the bottoms of the beakers fit snugly down on the top rims of the containers. Place the containers in the autoclave, and close it securely, leaving the vent cock open. Heat until steam issues vigorously from the vent cock, and continue heating for 10 minutes. Close the vent cock, and adjust the temperature to 121°, taking 19 to 23 minutes to reach the desired temperature. Hold the temperature at 121 ± 2.0° for 30 minutes, counting from the time this temperature is reached. Reduce the heat so that the autoclave cools and comes to atmospheric pressure in 38 to 46 minutes, being vented as necessary to prevent the formation of a vacuum. Cool the flask at once in running water, decant the water from the flask into a suitably cleansed vessel, and wash the residual powdered glass with four 15-mL portions of *High-Purity Water*, adding the decanted washings to the main portion. Add 5 drops of *Methyl Red Solution*, and titrate immediately with 0.020 N sulfuric acid. If the volume of titrating solution is expected to be less than 10 mL, use a microburet. Record the volume of 0.020 N sulfuric acid used to neutralize the extract from 10 g of the prepared specimen of glass, corrected for a blank. The volume does not exceed that indicated in *Table 2* for the type of glass concerned.

Water Attack at 121°

Rinse thoroughly 3 or more containers, selected at random, twice with *High-Purity Water*.

Procedure—Fill each container to 90% of its overflow capacity with *High-Purity Water*, and proceed as directed for *Procedure* under *Powdered Glass Test*, beginning with "Cap all flasks," except that the time of autoclaving shall be 60 minutes instead of 30 minutes, and ending with "to prevent the formation of a vacuum." Empty the contents from 1 or more containers into a 100-mL graduated cylinder, combining, in the case of smaller containers, the contents of several containers to obtain a volume of 100 mL. Place the pooled specimen in a 250-mL conical flask

of resistant glass, add 5 drops of *Methyl Red Solution*, and titrate, while warm, with 0.020 N sulfuric acid. Complete the titration within 60 minutes after opening the autoclave. Record the volume of 0.020 N sulfuric acid used, corrected for a blank obtained by titrating 100 mL of *High-Purity Water* at the same temperature and with the same amount of indicator. The volume does not exceed that indicated in *Table 2* for the type of glass concerned.

Arsenic

Arsenic ⟨211⟩—Use as the *Test Preparation* 35 mL of the water from one Type I glass container or, in the case of smaller containers, 35 mL of the combined contents of several Type I glass containers, prepared as directed for *Procedure* under *Water Attack at 121°*: the limit is 0.1 μg per g.

BIOLOGICAL TESTS—PLASTICS AND OTHER POLYMERS

Perform the in vitro biological tests according to the procedures set forth under *Biological Reactivity Tests, In Vitro* ⟨87⟩. Materials that meet the requirements of the in vitro tests are not required to undergo further testing. No plastic class designation is assigned to these materials. Materials that do not meet the requirements of the in vitro tests are not suitable for containers for drug products.

If a plastic class designation is needed for plastics and other polymers that meet the requirements under *Biological Reactivity Tests, In Vitro* ⟨87⟩, perform the appropriate in vivo tests specified for *Classification of Plastics* under *Biological Reactivity Tests, In Vivo* ⟨88⟩.

PHYSICOCHEMICAL TESTS—PLASTICS

The following tests, designed to determine physical and chemical properties of plastics and their extracts, are based on the extraction of the plastic material, and it is essential that the designated amount of the plastic be used. Also, the specified surface area must be available for extraction at the designated temperature.

Extracting Medium—Unless otherwise directed in a specific test below, use *Purified Water* (see monograph) as the extracting medium, maintained at a temperature of 70° during the extraction of the prepared *Sample*.

Apparatus—Use a water bath and the *Extraction Containers* as described under *Biological Reactivity Tests, In Vivo* ⟨88⟩.

Preparation of Apparatus—Proceed as directed in the first paragraph of *Preparation of Apparatus* under *Biological Reactivity Tests, In Vivo* ⟨88⟩. [NOTE—The containers and equipment need not be sterile.]

Procedure—

Preparation of Sample—From a homogeneous plastic specimen, use a portion, for each 20.0 mL of extracting medium, equivalent to 120 cm² total surface area (both sides combined), and subdivide into strips approximately 3 mm in width and as near to 5 cm in length as is practical. Transfer the subdivided *Sample* to a glass-stoppered, 250-mL graduated cylinder of Type I glass, and add about 150 mL of Purified Water. Agitate for about 30 seconds, drain off and discard the liquid, and repeat with a second washing.

Transfer the prepared *Sample* to a suitable extraction flask, and add the required amount of *Extracting Medium*. Extract by heating in a water bath at the temperature specified for the *Extracting Medium* for 24 hours. Cool, but not below 20°. Pipet 20 mL of the extract of the prepared *Sample* into a suitable container. Use this portion in the test for *Buffering Capacity*. Immediately decant the remaining extract into a suitably cleansed container, and seal.

Blank—Use *Purified Water* where a blank is specified in the following tests.

NONVOLATILE RESIDUE—Transfer, in suitable portions, 50.0 mL of the extract of the prepared *Sample* to a suitable, tared crucible (preferably a fused-silica crucible that has been acid-cleaned), and evaporate the volatile matter on a steam bath. Similarly evaporate 50.0 mL of the *Blank* in a second crucible. [NOTE—If an oily residue is expected, inspect the crucible repeatedly during the evaporation and drying period, and reduce the amount of heat if the oil tends to creep along the walls of the crucible.] Dry at 105° for 1 hour: the difference between the amounts obtained from the *Sample* and the *Blank* does not exceed 15 mg.

RESIDUE ON IGNITION ⟨281⟩—[NOTE—It is not necessary to perform this test when the *Nonvolatile Residue* test result does not exceed 5 mg.] Proceed with the *Nonvolatile Residue* obtained from the *Sample* and from the *Blank*, using, if necessary, additional sulfuric acid but adding the same amount of sulfuric acid to each crucible: the difference between the amounts of residue on ignition obtained from the *Sample* and the *Blank* does not exceed 5 mg.

HEAVY METALS—Pipet 20 mL of the extract of the prepared *Sample*, filtered if necessary, into one of two matched 50-mL color-comparison tubes. Adjust with 1 N acetic acid or 6 N ammonium hydroxide to a pH between 3.0 and 4.0, using short-range pH paper as external indicator, dilute with water to about 35 mL, and mix.

Into the second color-comparison tube pipet 2 mL of *Standard Lead Solution* (see *Heavy Metals* ⟨231⟩), and add 20 mL of the *Blank*. Adjust with 1 N acetic acid or 6 N ammonium hydroxide to a pH between 3.0 and 4.0, using short-range pH paper as external indicator, dilute with water to about 35 mL, and mix. To each tube add 1.2 mL of thioacetamide-glycerin base TS and 2 mL of *pH 3.5 Acetate Buffer* (see *Heavy Metals* ⟨231⟩), dilute with water to 50 mL, and mix: any brown color produced within 10 minutes in the tube containing the extract of the prepared *Sample* does not exceed that in the tube containing the *Standard Lead Solution*, both tubes being viewed downward over a white surface (1 ppm in extract).

BUFFERING CAPACITY—Titrate the previously collected 20-mL portion of the extract of the prepared *Sample* potentiometrically to a pH of 7.0, using either 0.010 N hydrochloric acid or 0.010 N sodium hydroxide, as required. Treat a 20.0-mL portion of the *Blank* similarly: if the same titrant was required for both *Sample* and *Blank*, the difference between the two volumes is not greater than 10.0 mL; and if acid was required for either the *Sample* or the *Blank* and alkali for the other, the total of the two volumes required is not greater than 10.0 mL.

CONTAINERS FOR OPHTHALMICS— PLASTICS

Plastics for ophthalmics are composed of a mixture of homologous compounds, having a range of molecular weights. Such plastics frequently contain other substances such as residues from the polymerization process, plasticizers, stabilizers, antioxidants, pigments, and lubricants. Factors such as plastic composition, processing and cleaning procedures, contacting media, inks, adhesives, absorption, adsorption and permeability of preservatives, and conditions of storage may also affect the suitability of a plastic for a specific use.

Definition—For the purposes of this chapter, a *container* is that which holds the drug and is or may be in direct contact with the drug.

Biological Tests—Plastics and other polymers used for containers for ophthalmics meet the requirements set forth in the section *Biological Tests—Plastics and Other Polymers*.

POLYETHYLENE CONTAINERS

The standards and tests provided in this section characterize high-density and low-density polyethylene containers that are interchangeably suitable for packaging dry oral dosage forms not meant for constitution into solution.

Where stability studies have been performed to establish the expiration date of a particular dry oral dosage form not meant for constitution into solution in a container meeting the requirements set forth herein for either high- or low-density polyethylene containers, then any other polyethylene container meeting the same sections of these requirements may be similarly used to package such dosage form, provided that the appropriate stability programs are expanded to include the alternative container, in order to assure that the identity, strength, quality, and purity of the dosage form are maintained throughout the expiration period.

Both high- and low-density polyethylene are long-chain polymers synthesized under controlled conditions of heat and pressure, with the aid of catalysts from not less than 85.0% ethylene and not less than 95.0% total olefins. The other olefin ingredients most frequently used are butene, hexene, and propylene. The ingredients used to manufacture the polyethylene, and those used in the fabrication of the containers, conform to the requirements in the applicable sections of the *Code of Federal Regulations*, Title 21.

High-density polyethylene and low-density polyethylene both have an IR absorption spectrum that is distinctive for polyethylene, and each possesses characteristic thermal properties. High-density polyethylene has a density between 0.941 and 0.965 g per cm³. Low-density polyethylene has a density between 0.850 and 0.940 g per cm³. The permeation properties of molded polyethylene containers may be altered when re-ground polymer is incorporated, depending upon the proportion of re-ground material in the final product. Other properties that may affect the suitability of polyethylene used in containers for packaging drugs are: oxygen and moisture permeability, modulus of elasticity, melt index, environmental stress crack resistance, and degree of crystallinity after molding. The requirements in this section are to be met when dry oral dosage forms, not meant for constitution into solution, are intended to be packaged in a container defined by this section.

Multiple Internal Reflectance—
APPARATUS—Use an IR spectrophotometer capable of correcting for the blank spectrum and equipped with a multiple internal reflectance accessory and a KRS-5 internal reflection plate.[4] A KRS-5 crystal 2 mm thick having an angle of incidence of 45° provides a sufficient number of reflections.

PREPARATION OF SPECIMEN—Cut 2 flat sections representative of the average wall thickness of the container, and trim them as necessary to obtain segments that are convenient for mounting in the multiple internal reflectance accessory. Taking care to avoid scratching the surfaces, wipe the specimens with dry paper or, if necessary, clean them with a soft cloth dampened with methanol, and permit them to dry. Securely mount the specimens on both sides of the KRS-5 internal reflection plate, ensuring adequate surface contact. Prior to mounting the specimens on the plate, they may be compressed to thin uniform films by exposing them to temperatures of about 177° under high pressures (15,000 psi or more).

PROCEDURE—Place the mounted specimen sections within the multiple internal reflectance accessory, and place the assembly in the specimen beam of the IR spectrophotometer. Adjust the specimen position and mirrors within the accessory to permit maximum light transmission of the unattenuated reference beam. (For a double-beam instrument, upon completing the adjustments in the accessory, attenuate the reference beam to permit full-scale deflection during the scanning of the specimen.) Determine the IR spectrum from 3500 to 600 cm⁻¹: the corrected spectrum of the specimen exhibits major absorption bands only at the same wavelengths as the spectrum of USP High-density Polyethylene RS or USP Low-density Polyethylene RS, similarly determined.

Thermal Analysis—Cut a section weighing about 12 mg, and place it in the test-specimen pan. Determine the thermogram under nitrogen at temperatures between 40° and 200° at a heating rate between 2° and 10° per minute followed by cooling at a rate between 2° and 10° per minute to 40°, using equipment capable of performing the determinations described under *Thermal Analysis* ⟨891⟩.

High-Density Polyethylene—The thermogram of the specimen is similar to the thermogram of USP High-Density Polyethylene RS, similarly determined, and the temperatures of the endotherms and exotherms in the thermogram of the specimen do not differ from those of the standard by more than 6.0°.

Low-Density Polyethylene—The thermogram of the specimen is similar to the thermogram of USP Low-Density Polyethylene RS, similarly determined, and the temperatures of the endotherms and exotherms in the thermogram of the specimen do not differ from those of the standard by more than 8.0°.

Light Transmission—Polyethylene containers intended to provide protection from light meet the requirements under *Light Transmission*.

Water Vapor Permeation—Fit the containers with impervious seals obtained by heat-sealing the bottles with an aluminum foil-polyethylene laminate or other suitable seal.[5] Test the containers as described under *Containers—Permeation* ⟨671⟩: the high-density polyethylene containers so tested meet the requirements if the moisture permeability exceeds 10 mg per day per liter in not more than 1 of the 10 test containers and exceeds 25 mg per day per liter in none of them. The low-density polyethylene containers so tested meet the requirements if the moisture permeability exceeds 20 mg per day per liter in not more than 1 of the 10 test containers and exceeds 30 mg per day per liter in none of them.

Heavy Metals and Nonvolatile Residue—Prepare extracts of specimens for these tests as directed for *Preparation of Sample* in the *Procedure* under *Physicochemical Tests—Plastics*, except that for each 20.0 mL of *Extracting Medium* the portion shall be 60 cm², regardless of thickness.

HEAVY METALS—Containers meet the requirements for *Heavy Metals* under *Physicochemical Tests—Plastics*.

NONVOLATILE RESIDUE—Proceed as directed for *Nonvolatile Residue* under *Physicochemical Tests—Plastics*, except that the blank shall be the same solvent used in each of the tests set forth below. The difference between the amounts obtained from the specimen and the blank does not exceed 12.0 mg when water maintained at a temperature of 70° is used as the extracting medium; does not exceed 75.0 mg when alcohol maintained at a temperature of 70° is used as the extracting medium; and does not exceed 100.0 mg for high-density polyethylene and does not exceed 350.0 mg for low-density polyethylene when hexanes maintained at a temperature of 50° are used as the extracting medium. Containers meet these requirements for *Nonvolatile Residue* for all of the above extracting media. [NOTE—Hexanes and alcohol are flammable. When evaporating these solvents, use a current of air with the water bath; when drying the residue, use an explosion-proof oven.]

---

[4] The multiple internal reflectance accessory and KRS-5 plate are available from several sources, including Beckman Instruments, Inc., 2500 Harbor Blvd., Fullerton, CA 92634, and from Perkin Elmer Corp., Main Ave., Norwalk, CT 06856.

[5] A suitable laminate for sealing has as the container contact layer polyethylene of not less than 0.025 mm (0.001 inch) and a second layer of aluminum foil of not less than 0.018 mm (0.0007 inch), with additional layers of suitable backing materials. A suitable seal can be obtained also by using glass plates and a sealing wax consisting of 60% of refined amorphous wax and 40% of refined crystalline paraffin wax.

POLYETHYLENE TEREPHTHALATE BOTTLES AND POLYETHYLENE TEREPHTHALATE G BOTTLES

The standards and tests provided in this section characterize polyethylene terephthalate (PET) and polyethylene terephthalate G (PETG) bottles that are interchangeably suitable for packaging liquid oral dosage forms.

Where stability studies have been performed to establish the expiration date of a particular liquid oral dosage form in a bottle meeting the requirements set forth herein for either PET or PETG bottles, any other PET or PETG bottle meeting these requirements may be similarly used to package such dosage form, provided that the appropriate stability programs are expanded to include the alternative bottle in order to assure that the identity, strength, quality, and purity of the dosage form are maintained throughout the expiration period.

The suitability of a specific PET or PETG bottle for use in the dispensing of a particular pharmaceutical liquid oral dosage form must be established by appropriate testing.

PET resins are long-chain crystalline polymers prepared by the condensation of ethylene glycol with dimethyl terephthalate or terephthalic acid. PET copolymer resins are prepared in a similar way, except that they may also contain a small amount of either isophthalic acid (not more than 3 mole percent) or 1,4-cyclohexanedimethanol (not more than 5 mole percent). Polymerization is conducted under controlled conditions of heat and vacuum, with the aid of catalysts and stabilizers.

PET copolymer resins have physical and spectral properties similar to PET and for practical purposes are treated as PET. The tests and specifications provided in this section to characterize PET resins and bottles apply also to PET copolymer resins and to bottles fabricated from them.

PET and PET copolymer resins generally exhibit a large degree of order in their molecular structure. As a result, they exhibit characteristic composition-dependent thermal behavior, including a glass transition temperature of about 76° and a melting temperature of about 250°. These resins have a distinctive IR absorption spectrum that allows them to be distinguished from other plastic materials (e.g., polycarbonate, polystyrene, polyethylene, and PETG resins). PET and PET copolymer resins have a density between 1.3 and 1.4 g per cm³ and a minimum intrinsic viscosity of 0.7 dL per g, which corresponds to a number average molecular weight of about 23,000 daltons.

PETG resins are high molecular weight polymers prepared by the condensation of ethylene glycol with dimethyl terephthalate or terephthalic acid and 15 to 34 mole percent of 1,4-cyclohexanedimethanol. PETG resins are clear, amorphous polymers, having a glass transition temperature of about 81° and no crystalline melting point, as determined by differential scanning calorimetry. PETG resins have a distinctive IR absorption spectrum that allows them to be distinguished from other plastic materials, including PET. PETG resins have a density of approximately 1.27 g per cm³ and a minimum instrinsic viscosity of 0.65 dL per g, which corresponds to a number average molecular weight of about 16,000 daltons.

PET and PETG resins, and other ingredients used in the fabrication of these bottles, conform to the requirements in the applicable sections of the Code of Federal Regulations, Title 21, regarding use in contact with food and alcoholic beverages. PET and PETG resins do not contain any plasticizers, processing aids, or antioxidants. Colorants, if used in the manufacture of PET and PETG bottles, do not migrate into the contained liquid.

Multiple Internal Reflectance—
APPARATUS—Use an IR spectrophotometer capable of correcting for the blank spectrum and equipped with a multiple internal reflectance accessory and a KRS-5 internal reflection plate.[6] A KRS-5 crystal having a thickness of 2 mm and an angle of incidence of 45° provides a sufficient number of reflections.

PREPARATION OF SPECIMEN—Cut 2 flat sections representative of the average wall thickness of the bottle, and trim them as necessary to obtain segments that are convenient for mounting in the multiple internal reflectance accessory. Taking care to avoid scratching the surfaces, wipe the specimens with dry paper or, if necessary, clean them with a soft cloth dampened with methanol, and permit them to dry. Securely mount the specimens on both sides of the KRS-5 internal reflection plate, ensuring adequate surface contact.

PROCEDURE—Place the mounted specimen sections within the multiple internal reflectance accessory, and place the assembly in the specimen beam of the IR spectrophotometer. Adjust the specimen position and mirrors within the accessory to permit maximum light transmission of the unattenuated beams. (For a double-beam instrument, upon completing the adjustments in the accessory, attenuate the reference beam to permit full-scale deflection during the scanning of the specimen.) Determine the IR spectrum from 4000 to 400 cm⁻¹. The corrected spectrum of the specimen exhibits major absorption bands only at the same wavelengths as the spectrum of the USP Polyethylene Terephthalate RS, or the USP Polyethylene Terephthalate G RS, similarly determined.

Thermal Analysis—Cut a section weighing about 12 mg from the bottle, and place it in the test-specimen pan. Determine the thermogram under nitrogen, using the heating and cooling conditions as specified for the resin type and using equipment capable of performing the determinations as described under *Thermal Analysis* ⟨891⟩.

*Polyethylene Terephthalate—*Heat the specimen from room temperature to 280° at a heating rate of about 20° per minute. Hold the specimen at 280° for 1 minute. Quickly cool the specimen to room temperature, and reheat it to 280° at a heating rate of about 5° per minute. The thermogram of the specimen is similar to the thermogram of USP Polyethylene Terephthalate RS, similarly determined: the melting point (T_m) of the specimen does not differ from that of the Standard by more than 9.0°, and the glass transition temperature (T_g) of the specimen does not differ from that of the Standard by more than 4.0°.

*Polyethylene Terephthalate G—*Heat the specimen from room temperature to 120° at a heating rate of about 20° per minute. Hold the specimen at 120° for 1 minute. Quickly cool the specimen to room temperature, and reheat it to 120° at a heating rate of about 10° per minute. The thermogram of the specimen is similar to the thermogram of USP Polyethylene Terephthalate G RS, similarly determined: the glass transition temperature (T_g) of the specimen does not differ from that of the Standard by more than 6.0°.

Light Transmission—PET and PETG bottles intended to provide protection from light meet the requirements under *Light Transmission*.

Water Vapor Permeation—[NOTE—Throughout the following procedure, determine the weights of bottles and closures, both as tare weights and weights of filled bottles, to the nearest 0.1 mg if the bottle volume is less than 200 mL; to the nearest mg if the bottle volume is 200 mL or more but less than 1000 mL; or to the nearest centigram (10 mg) if the bottle volume is 1000 mL or more.] Select 10 bottles of a uniform size and type, clean the sealing surfaces with a lint-free cloth, and close and open each bottle 30 times. Apply the closure firmly and uniformly each time the bottle is closed. Close screw-capped bottles with a torque that is within the range of tightness specified in the table provided under *Containers—Permeation* ⟨671⟩. Weigh each empty bottle

---

[6] The multiple internal reflectance accessory and KRS-5 plate are available from several sources, including Beckman Instruments, Inc., 2500 Harbor Boulevard, Fullerton, CA 92634, and from Perkin Elmer Corporation, 761 Main Ave., Norwalk, CT 06859-01560.

and its closure. Fill ten bottles with water at $25 \pm 2°$ until the meniscus is tangent to the top of the bottle opening. Record the weight of each bottle and its closure, and determine the average bottle volume, in liters, taken by the following formula:

$$\sum_{i=1}^{10}(W_{oi} - W_{ti})/9970,$$

where W_{oi} is the total weight, in g, of bottle i and its closure, W_{ti} is the tare weight, in g, of bottle i and its closure, and 9970 is the density of water at 25° times 10,000 (the number of bottles tested times the conversion factor for converting milliliters to liters).

Using a pipet, adjust the water level in the bottles to the fill point. Apply the closures using a torque that is within the range specified in the table provided under *Containers—Permeation* ⟨671⟩, and store the bottles at a temperature of $25 \pm 2°$ and a relative humidity of $50 \pm 2\%$. After 168 ± 1 hours (7 days), record the weight of the individual bottles. Return the bottles to storage for another 168 ± 1 hours. After the second 168 ± 1 hours, remove the bottles, record the weights of the individual bottles, and calculate the water vapor permeation rate, in mg per day per liter, for each bottle taken by the formula:

$$(W_{li} - W_{fi})/7V_a,$$

in which W_{li} is the weight, in mg, of bottle i at 14 days, W_{fi} is the weight, in mg, of bottle i at 7 days, 7 is the test time, in days, after the 7-day equilibration period, and V_a is the average bottle volume, in liters.

The bottles so tested meet the requirements and are *tight containers* if the water vapor permeation rate exceeds 100 mg per day per liter in not more than 1 of the 10 test bottles and exceeds 200 mg per day per liter in none of them.

Colorant Extraction—Select 3 test bottles. Cut a relatively flat portion from the side wall of one bottle, and trim it as necessary to fit the sample holder of the spectrophotometer. Obtain the visible spectrum of the side wall by scanning the portion of the visible spectrum from 350 to 700 nm. Determine, to the nearest 2 nm, the wavelength of maximum absorbance. Fill the remaining two test bottles, using 50% alcohol for PET bottles and 25% alcohol for PETG bottles. Fit the bottles with impervious seals, such as aluminum foil, and apply closures. Fill a glass bottle having the same capacity as that of the test bottles with the corresponding solvent, fit the bottle with an impervious seal, such as aluminum foil, and apply a closure. Incubate the test bottles and the glass bottle in a constant temperature room or in an oven at 49° for ten days. Remove the bottles, and allow them to equilibrate to room temperature. Concomitantly determine the absorbances of the test solutions in 5-cm cells at the wavelength of maximum absorbance (see *Spectrophotometry and Light-Scattering* ⟨851⟩), using the corresponding solvent from the glass bottle as the blank. The absorbance values so obtained are less than 0.01 for both test solutions.

Heavy Metals, Total Terephthaloyl Moieties, and Ethylene Glycol—

EXTRACTING MEDIA—

Purified Water—(see monograph).

50 Percent Alcohol—Dilute 125 mL of alcohol with water to 238 mL, and mix.

25 Percent Alcohol—Dilute 125 mL of *50 Percent Alcohol* with water to 250 mL, and mix.

n-Heptane.

PROCEDURE—[NOTE—Use the *50 Percent Alcohol Extracting Medium* with PET bottles. Use the *25 Percent Alcohol Extracting Medium* with PETG bottles.] For each *Extracting Medium*, fill a

sufficient number of test bottles to 90% of their nominal capacity to obtain not less than 30 mL of extract. Fill a corresponding number of glass bottles with *Purified Water Extracting Medium*, a corresponding number of glass bottles with *50 Percent Alcohol Extracting Medium* or *25 Percent Alcohol Extracting Medium*, and a corresponding number of glass bottles with *n-Heptane Extracting Medium* for use as *Extracting Media* blanks. Fit the bottles with impervious seals, such as aluminum foil, and apply closures. Incubate the test bottles and the glass bottles in a constant temperature room or in an oven at 49° for ten days. Remove the test bottles with the *Extracting Media* samples and the glass bottles with the *Extracting Media* blanks, and store them at room temperature. Do not transfer the *Extracting Media* samples to alternative storage vessels.

HEAVY METALS—Pipet 20 mL of the *Purified Water* extract of the test bottles, filtered if necessary, into one of two matched 50-mL color-comparison tubes, and retain the remaining *Purified Water* extract in the test bottles for use in the test for *Ethylene Glycol*. Adjust the extract with 1 N acetic acid or 6 N ammonium hydroxide to a pH between 3.0 and 4.0, using short-range pH paper as an external indicator. Dilute with water to about 35 mL, and mix.

Into the second color-comparison tube, pipet 2 mL of freshly prepared (on day of use) *Standard Lead Solution* (see *Heavy Metals* ⟨231⟩), and add 20 mL of *Purified Water*. Adjust with 1 N acetic acid or 6 N ammonium hydroxide to a pH between 3.0 and 4.0, using short-range pH paper as an external indicator. Dilute with water to about 35 mL, and mix.

To each tube add 1.2 mL of thioacetamide-glycerin base TS and 2 mL of *pH 3.5 Acetate Buffer* (see *Heavy Metals* ⟨231⟩), dilute with water to 50 mL, and mix: any color produced within 10 minutes in the tube containing the *Purified Water* extract of the test bottles does not exceed that in the tube containing the *Standard Lead Solution*, both tubes being viewed downward over a white surface (1 ppm in extract).

Total Terephthaloyl Moieties—Determine the absorbance of the *50 Percent Alcohol* or *25 Percent Alcohol* extract in a 1-cm cell at the wavelength of maximum absorbance at about 244 nm (see *Spectrophotometry and Light-Scattering* ⟨851⟩), using the corresponding *Extracting Medium* as the blank: the absorbance of the extract does not exceed 0.150, corresponding to not more than 1 ppm of total terephthaloyl moieties.

Determine the absorbance of the *n-Heptane* extract in a 1-cm cell at the wavelength of maximum absorbance at about 240 nm (see *Spectrophotometry and Light-Scattering* ⟨851⟩), using the *n-Heptane Extracting Medium* blank as the blank: the absorbance of the extract does not exceed 0.150, corresponding to not more than 1 ppm of total terephthaloyl moieties.

ETHYLENE GLYCOL—

Periodic Acid Solution—Dissolve 125 mg of periodic acid in 10 mL of water.

Dilute Sulfuric Acid—To 50 mL of water add slowly and with constant stirring 50 mL of sulfuric acid, and allow to cool to room temperature.

Sodium Bisulfite Solution—Dissolve 0.1 g of sodium bisulfite in 10 mL of water. Use this solution within seven days.

Disodium Chromotropate Solution—Dissolve 100 mg of disodium chromotropate in 100 mL of sulfuric acid. Protect this solution from light, and use within seven days.

Standard Solution—Dissolve an accurately weighed quantity of ethylene glycol in water, and dilute quantitatively, and stepwise if necessary, to obtain a solution having a known concentration of about 1 μg per mL.

Test Solution—Use the *Purified Water* extract.

Blank—Use the *Purified Water Extracting Medium* blank.

Procedure—Transfer 1.0 mL of *Standard Solution* to a 10-mL volumetric flask. Transfer 1.0 mL of *Test Solution* to a second 10-mL volumetric flask. Transfer 1.0 mL of *Purified Water Extracting Medium* blank to a third 10-mL volumetric flask. To each of the three flasks, add 100 μL of *Periodic Acid Solution*, swirl to mix, and allow to stand for 60 minutes. Add 1.0 mL of *Sodium Bisulfite Solution* to each flask, and mix. Add 100 μL of *Disodium*

Chromotrope Solution to each flask, and mix. [NOTE—All solutions should be analyzed within one hour after addition of the Disodium Chromotrope Solution.] Cautiously add 6 mL of sulfuric acid to each flask, mix, and allow the solutions to cool to room temperature. [Caution—Dilution of sulfuric acid produces substantial heat and can cause the solution to boil. Perform this addition carefully. Sulfur dioxide gas will be evolved. Use of a fume hood is recommended.] Dilute each solution with Dilute sulfuric acid to volume, and mix. Concomitantly determine the absorbances of the solutions from the Standard Solution and the Test Solution in 1-cm cells at the wavelength of maximum absorbance at about 575 nm (see Spectrophotometry and Light-Scattering ⟨851⟩), using the solution from the Purified Water Extracting Medium blank as the blank: the absorbance of the solution from the Test solution does not exceed that of the solution from the Standard solution, corresponding to not more than 1 ppm of ethylene glycol.

Add the following:

▲POLYPROPYLENE CONTAINERS

The standards and tests provided in this section characterize polypropylene containers, produced from either homopolymers or copolymers, that are interchangeably suitable for packaging dry solid and liquid oral dosage forms.

Where suitable stability studies have been performed to establish the expiration date of a particular dosage form in the appropriate polypropylene container, then any other polypropylene container meeting these requirements may be similarly used to package such dosage form, provided that the appropriate stability programs are expanded to include the alternative container, in order to assure that the potency, identity, strength, quality, and purity of the dosage form are maintained throughout the expiration period.

Propylene polymers are long-chain polymers synthesized from propylene or propylene and other olefins under controlled conditions of heat and pressure, with the aid of catalysts. Examples of other olefins most commonly used include ethylene and butene. The propylene polymers, the ingredients used to manufacture the propylene polymers, and the ingredients used in the fabrication of the containers conform to the applicable sections of the Code of Federal Regulations, Title 21.

Factors such as plastics composition, processing and cleaning procedures, contacting media, inks, adhesives, absorption, adsorption and permeability of preservatives, and conditions of storage may also affect the suitability of a plastic for a specific use. The suitability of a specific polypropylene must be established by appropriate testing.

Polypropylene has a distinctive IR spectrum and possesses characteristic thermal properties. It has a density between 0.880 and 0.913 g per cm³. The permeation properties of molded polypropylene containers may be altered when reground polymer is incorporated, depending on the proportion of reground material in the final product. Other properties that may affect the suitability of polypropylene used in containers for packaging drugs are the following: oxygen and moisture permeability, modulus of elasticity, melt flow index, environmental stress crack resistance, and degree of crystallinity after molding. The requirements in this section are to be met when dry solid and liquid oral dosage forms are to be packaged in a container defined by this section.

Multiple Internal Reflectance—

APPARATUS—Use an IR spectrophotometer capable of correcting for the blank spectrum and equipped with a multiple internal reflectance accessory and a KRS-5 internal reflection plate. A KRS-5 crystal 2-mm thick having an angle of incidence of 45° provides a sufficient number of reflections.

PREPARATION OF SPECIMEN—Cut 2 flat sections, representative of the average wall thickness of the container, and trim them as necessary to obtain segments that are convenient for mounting in the internal reflectance accessory. Taking care to avoid scratch-

ing the surfaces, wipe the specimens with dry paper, or if necessary with a soft cloth dampened with methanol, and permit them to dry. Securely mount the specimens on both sides of the KRS-5 internal reflection plate, ensuring adequate surface contact. Prior to mounting the specimens on the plate, they may be compressed to flat uniform films by exposure to temperatures between 220° and 240°. The specimen's time/temperature history during this operation should be limited to that necessary to mold the films.

PROCEDURE—Place the mounted specimen sections within the multiple internal reflectance accessory, and place the assembly in the specimen beam of the IR spectrophotometer. Adjust the specimen position and mirrors within the accessory to permit maximum light transmission of the unattenuated reference beam. (For a double beam instrument, upon completing the adjustment in the accessory, attenuate the reference beam to permit full-scale deflection during the scanning of the specimen.) Determine the IR spectrum from 3500 to 600 cm⁻¹. The corrected spectrum of the specimen exhibits major absorption bands only at the same wavelengths as the spectrum of the USP Reference Standard for either a polypropylene homopolymer or copolymer, similarly determined.

Thermal Analysis—Cut a section weighing about 12 mg, and place it in the test specimen pan. Intimate contact between the pan and the thermocouple is essential for reproducible results. Determine the thermogram under nitrogen at temperatures ranging from ambient to 30° above the melting point. Maintain the temperature for 10 minutes, then cool to 50° below the peak crystallization temperature at a rate of 10° to 20° per minute, using equipment capable of performing the determinations as described under Thermal Analysis ⟨891⟩. The thermogram of the specimen is similar to the thermogram of the appropriate USP Reference Standard for polypropylene. The temperatures of the endotherms and exotherms in the thermogram do not differ from those of the USP Reference Standard for homopolymers by more than 12.0° or from those of the USP Reference Standard for copolymers by more than 6.0°.

Light Transmission—Polypropylene containers intended to provide protection from light meet the requirements under Light Transmission.

Water Vapor Permeation—Fit the containers with impervious seals obtained by heat-sealing the bottles with an aluminum foil-polyethylene laminate or other suitable seal. Test the containers as described under Containers—Permeation ⟨671⟩. The containers meet the requirements if the moisture permeability exceeds 15 mg per day per liter in not more than one of the 10 test containers and exceeds 25 mg per day per liter in none of them.

Heavy Metals and Nonvolatile Residue—Prepare extracts of specimens for these tests as directed for Procedure under Physicochemical Tests—Plastics, except that for each 20 mL of Extracting Medium the portion shall be 60 cm², regardless of thickness.

HEAVY METALS—Containers meet the requirements for Heavy Metals under Physicochemical Tests—Plastics.

NONVOLATILE RESIDUE—Proceed as directed for Nonvolatile Residue under Physicochemical Tests—Plastics, except that the blank shall be the same solvent used in each of the tests set forth below. The difference between the amounts obtained from the specimen and the blank does not exceed 10.0 mg when water maintained at a temperature of 70° is used as the extracting medium, does not exceed 60.0 mg when alcohol maintained at a temperature of 70° is used as the extracting medium, and does not exceed 225.0 mg when hexanes maintained at a temperature of 50° is used as the extracting medium. Containers meet these requirements for Nonvolatile Residue for all of the above extracting media. [NOTE—Hexanes and alcohol are flammable. When evaporating these solvents, use a current of air with the water bath; when drying the residue, use an explosion-proof oven.]

Buffering Capacity—Prepare extracts of the specimen as described for *Procedure* under *Physicochemical Tests—Plastics*. Containers meet the requirements for *Buffering Capacity* under *Physicochemical Tests—Plastics*.▲USP27

REPACKAGING INTO SINGLE-UNIT CONTAINERS AND UNIT-DOSE CONTAINERS FOR NONSTERILE SOLID AND LIQUID DOSAGE FORMS

An official dosage form is required to bear on its label an expiration date assigned for the particular formulation and package of the article. This date limits the time during which the product may be dispensed or used. Because the expiration date stated on the manufacturer's or distributor's package has been determined for the drug in that particular package and is not intended to be applicable to the product where it has been repackaged in a different container, repackaged drugs dispensed pursuant to a prescription are exempt from this expiration date labeling requirement. It is necessary, therefore, that other precautions be taken by the dispenser to preserve the strength, quality, and purity of drugs that are repackaged for ultimate distribution or sale to patients.

The following guidelines and requirements are applicable where official dosage forms are repackaged into single-unit or unit-dose containers or mnemonic packs for dispensing pursuant to prescription.

Labeling—It is the responsibility of the dispenser, taking into account the nature of the drug repackaged, any packaging and beyond-use dating information in the manufacturer's product labeling, the characteristics of the containers, and the storage conditions to which the article may be subjected, to place a suitable beyond-use date on the label. Repackaged dosage forms must bear on their labels beyond-use dates as determined from information in the product labeling. Each single-unit or unit-dose container bears a separate label, unless the device holding the unit-dose form does not allow for the removal or separation of the intact single-unit or unit-dose container therefrom.

Storage—Store the repackaged article in a humidity-controlled environment and at the temperature specified in the individual monograph or in the product labeling. Where no temperature or humidity is specified in the monograph or in the labeling of the product, controlled room temperature and a relative humidity corresponding to 75% at 23° are not to be exceeded during repackaging or storage.

A refrigerator or freezer shall not be considered to be a humidity-controlled environment, and drugs that are to be stored at a cold temperature in a refrigerator or freezer shall be placed within an outer container that meets the monograph requirements for the drug contained therein.

Reprocessing—Reprocessing of repackaged unit-dose containers (i.e., removing dosage unit from one unit-dose container and placing dosage unit into another unit-dose container) shall not be done. However, reprocessing of the secondary package (e.g., removing the blister card from the cardboard carrier and placing the blister card into another cardboard carrier) is allowed provided that the original beyond-use date is maintained.

CUSTOMIZED PATIENT MEDICATION PACKAGES

In lieu of dispensing two or more prescribed drug products in separate containers, a pharmacist may, with the consent of the patient, the patient's caregiver, or a prescriber, provide a customized patient medication package (patient med pak).[7]

A patient med pak is a package prepared by a pharmacist for a specific patient comprising a series of containers and containing two or more prescribed solid oral dosage forms. The patient med pak is so designed or each container is so labeled as to indicate the day and time, or period of time, that the contents within each container are to be taken.

It is the responsibility of the dispenser to instruct the patient or caregiver on the use of the patient med pak.

Label—The patient med pak shall bear a label stating:
(1) the name of the patient;
(2) a serial number for the patient med pak itself and a separate identifying serial number for each of the prescription orders for each of the drug products contained therein;
(3) the name, strength, physical description or identification, and total quantity of each drug product contained therein;
(4) the directions for use and cautionary statements, if any, contained in the prescription order for each drug product therein;
(5) any storage instructions or cautionary statements required by the official compendia;
(6) the name of the prescriber of each drug product;
(7) the date of preparation of the patient med pak and the beyond-use date or period of time assigned to the patient med pak (such beyond-use date or period of time shall be not longer than the shortest recommended beyond-use date for any dosage form included therein or not longer than 60 days from the date of preparation of the patient med pak and shall not exceed the shortest expiration date on the original manufacturer's bulk containers for the dosage forms included therein); alternatively, the package label shall state the date of the prescription(s) or the date of preparation of the patient med pak, provided the package is accompanied by a record indicating the start date and the beyond-use date;
(8) the name, address, and telephone number of the dispenser (and the dispenser's registration number where necessary); and
(9) any other information, statements, or warnings required for any of the drug products contained therein.

If the patient med pak allows for the removal or separation of the intact containers therefrom, each individual container shall bear a label identifying each of the drug products contained therein.

Labeling—The patient med pak shall be accompanied by a patient package insert, in the event that any medication therein is required to be dispensed with such insert as accompanying labeling. Alternatively, such required information may be incorporated into a single, overall educational insert provided by the pharmacist for the total patient med pak.

Packaging—In the absence of more stringent packaging requirements for any of the drug products contained therein, each container of the patient med pak shall comply with the moisture permeation requirements for a Class B single-unit or unit-dose container (see *Containers—Permeation* ⟨671⟩). Each container shall be either not reclosable or so designed as to show evidence of having been opened.

Guidelines—It is the responsibility of the dispenser, when preparing a patient med pak, to take into account any applicable compendial requirements or guidelines and the physical and

---

[7] It should be noted that there is no special exemption for patient med paks from the requirements of the Poison Prevention Packaging Act. Thus the patient med pak, if it does not meet child-resistant standards, shall be placed in an outer package that does comply, or the necessary consent of the purchaser or physician, to dispense in a container not intended to be child-resistant, shall be obtained.

chemical compatibility of the dosage forms placed within each container, as well as any therapeutic incompatibilities that may attend the simultaneous administration of the medications. In this regard, pharmacists are encouraged to report to USP headquarters any observed or reported incompatibilities. Once a medication has been placed in a patient med pak with another solid dosage form, it may not be returned to stock, redistributed, or resold if unused.

Recordkeeping—In addition to any individual prescription filing requirements, a record of each patient med pak shall be made and filed. Each record shall contain, as a minimum:

(1) the name and address of the patient;
(2) the serial number of the prescription order for each drug product contained therein;
(3) the name of the manufacturer or labeler and lot number for each drug product contained therein;
(4) information identifying or describing the design, characteristics, or specifications of the patient med pak sufficient to allow subsequent preparation of an identical patient med pak for the patient;
(5) the date of preparation of the patient med pak and the beyond-use date that was assigned;
(6) any special labeling instructions; and
(7) the name or initials of the pharmacist who prepared the patient med pak.

⟨671⟩ CONTAINERS—PERMEATION

The tests that follow are provided to determine the moisture permeability of containers utilized for drugs being dispensed on prescription. The section *Multiple-Unit Containers for Capsules and Tablets* applies to multiple-unit containers (see *Preservation, Packaging, Storage, and Labeling* under *General Notices and Requirements*). The section *Single-Unit Containers and Unit-Dose Containers for Capsules and Tablets* applies to single-unit and unit-dose containers (see *Single-Unit Containers and Unit-Dose Containers for Nonsterile Solid and Liquid Dosage Forms* under *Containers* ⟨661⟩). As used herein, the term "container" refers to the entire system comprising, usually, the container itself, the liner (if used), the closure in the case of multiple-unit containers, and the lidding and blister in the case of single-unit and unit-dose containers.

Where the manufacturer's unopened multiple-unit, single-unit, or unit-dose packages are used for dispensing the drug, such containers are exempt from the requirements of this test.

MULTIPLE-UNIT CONTAINERS FOR CAPSULES AND TABLETS

Desiccant—Place a quantity of 4- to 8-mesh, anhydrous calcium chloride[1] in a shallow container, taking care to exclude any fine powder, then dry at 110° for 1 hour, and cool in a desiccator.

Procedure—Select 12 containers of a uniform size and type, clean the sealing surfaces with a lint-free cloth, and close and open each container 30 times. Apply the closure firmly and uniformly each time the container is closed. Close screw-capped containers with a torque that is within the range of tightness specified in the accompanying table. Add *Desiccant* to 10 of the containers, designated *test containers*, filling each to within 13 mm of the closure if the container volume is 20 mL or more, or filling each to two-thirds of capacity if the container volume is less than 20 mL. If the interior of the container is more than 63 mm in depth, an inert filler or spacer may be placed in the bottom to minimize the total weight of the container and *Desiccant*; the layer of *Desiccant* in such a container shall be not less than 5 cm in depth. Close each immediately after adding *Desiccant*, applying the torque designated in the accompanying table when closing screw-capped containers. To each of the remaining 2 containers, designated *controls*, add a sufficient number of glass beads to attain a weight approximately equal to that of each of the *test containers*, and close, applying the torque designated in the accompanying table when closing screw-capped containers. Record the weight of the individual containers so prepared to the nearest 0.1 mg if the container volume is less than 20 mL; to the nearest mg if the container volume is 20 mL or more but less than 200 mL; or to the nearest centigram (10 mg) if the container volume is 200 mL or more; and store at 75 ± 3% relative humidity and a temperature of 23 ± 2°. [NOTE—A saturated system of 35 g of sodium chloride with each 100 mL of water placed in the bottom of a desiccator maintains the specified humidity. Other methods may be employed to maintain these conditions.] After 336 ± 1 hours (14 days), record the weight of the individual containers in the same manner. Completely fill 5 empty containers of the same size and type as the containers under test with water or a noncompressible, free-flowing solid such as well-tamped fine glass beads, to the level indicated by the closure surface when in place. Transfer the contents of each to a graduated cylinder, and determine the average container volume, in mL. Calculate the rate of moisture permeability, in mg per day per liter, by the formula:

$$(1000 / 14 V)[(T_f - T_i) - (C_f - C_i)],$$

in which V is the volume, in mL, of the container, $(T_f - T_i)$ is the difference, in mg, between the final and initial weights of each *test container*, and $(C_f - C_i)$ is the difference, in mg, between the average final and average initial weights of the 2 *controls*. For containers used for drugs being dispensed on prescription, the containers so tested are *tight containers* if not more than one of the 10 *test containers* exceeds 100 mg per day per liter in moisture permeability, and none exceeds 200 mg per day per liter.

For containers used for drugs being dispensed on prescription, the containers are *well-closed containers* if not more than one of the 10 *test containers* exceeds 2000 mg per day per liter in moisture permeability, and none exceeds 3000 mg per day per liter.

Torque Applicable to Screw-Type Container

Closure Diameter[1] (mm)	Suggested Tightness Range with Manually Applied Torque;[2] (inch-pounds)
8	5
10	6
13	8
15	5–9
18	7–10
20	8–12
22	9–14
24	10–18
28	12–21
30	13–23
33	15–25
38	17–26
43	17–27
48	19–30
53	21–36
58	23–40
63	25–43
66	26–45
70	28–50
83	32–65
86	40–65
89	40–70
100	45–70

[1] Suitable 4- to 8-mesh, anhydrous calcium chloride is available commercially as Item JT1313-1 from VWR Scientific. Consult the VWR Scientific catalog for ordering information or call 1-800-234-9300.

Torque Applicable to Screw-Type Container *(Continued)*

Closure Diameter[1] (mm)	Suggested Tightness Range with Manually Applied Torque;[2] (inch-pounds)
110	45–70
120	55–95
132	60–95

[1] The torque designated for the next larger closure diameter is to be applied in testing containers having a closure diameter intermediate to the diameters listed.

[2] A suitable apparatus is available from Owens-Illinois, Toledo, OH 43666. (Model 25 torque tester is used for testing between 0 and 25; Model 50 for testing between 0 and 50; and Model 100 for testing between 0 and 100 inch-pounds of torque.) The torque values refer to application, not removal, of the closure. For further detail regarding instructions, reference may be made to "Standard Test Method for Application and Removal Torque of Threaded or Lug-Style Closures" ASTM Method D3198-97, published by the American Society for Testing and Materials, 1916 Race St., Philadelphia, PA 19103.

SINGLE-UNIT CONTAINERS AND UNIT-DOSE CONTAINERS FOR CAPSULES AND TABLETS

To permit an informed judgment regarding the suitability of the packaging for a particular type of product, the following procedure and classification scheme are provided for evaluating the moisture-permeation characteristics of single-unit and unit-dose containers. Inasmuch as equipment and operator performance may affect the moisture permeation of a container formed or closed, the moisture-permeation characteristics of the packaging system being utilized shall be determined.

Desiccant—Dry suitable desiccant pellets[2] at 110° for 1 hour prior to use. Use pellets weighing approximately 400 mg each and having a diameter of approximately 8 mm. [NOTE—If necessary due to limited unit-dose container size, pellets weighing less than 400 mg each and having a diameter of less than 8 mm may be used.]

Procedure—

Method I—Seal not less than 10 unit-dose containers with 1 pellet in each, and seal 10 additional, empty unit-dose containers to provide the controls, using finger cots or padded forceps to handle the sealed containers. Number the containers, and record the individual weights[3] to the nearest mg. Weigh the controls as a unit, and divide the total weight by the number of controls to obtain the average. Store all of the containers at $75 \pm 3\%$ relative humidity and at a temperature of $23 \pm 2°$. [NOTE—A saturated system of 35 g of sodium chloride with each 100 mL of water placed in the bottom of a desiccator maintains the specified humidity. Other methods may be employed to maintain these conditions.] After a 24-hour interval, and at each multiple thereof (see *Results*), remove the containers from the chamber, and allow them to equilibrate for 15 to 60 minutes in the weighing area. Again record the weight of the individual containers and the combined controls in the same manner. [NOTE—If any indicating pellets turn pink during this procedure, or if the pellet weight increase exceeds 10%, terminate the test, and regard only earlier

[2] Suitable moisture-indicating desiccant pellets are available commercially from sources such as Medical Packaging, Inc., 470 Route 31, Ringoes, NJ 08551-1409 [Telephone 800-257-5282; in NJ, 609-466-8991; FAX 609-466-3775], as Indicating Desiccant Pellets, Item No. TK-1002.

[3] Accurate comparisons of *Class A* containers may require test periods in excess of 28 days if weighings are performed on a *Class A* prescription balance (see *Prescription Balances and Volumetric Apparatus* ⟨1176⟩). The use of an analytical balance on which weights can be recorded to 4 or 5 decimal places may permit more precise characterization between containers and/or shorter test periods.

determinations as valid.] Return the containers to the humidity chamber. Calculate the rate of moisture permeation, in mg per day, of each container taken by the formula:

$$(1/N)[(W_F - W_I) - (C_F - C_I)],$$

in which N is the number of days expired in the test period (beginning after the initial 24-hour equilibration period); $(W_F - W_I)$ is the difference, in mg, between the final and initial weights of each test container; and $(C_F - C_I)$ is the difference, in mg, between the average final and average initial weights of the controls, the data being calculated to two significant figures. [NOTE—Where the permeations measured are less than 5 mg per day, and where the controls are observed to reach equilibrium within 7 days, the individual permeations may be determined more accurately by using the 7-day test container and control container weights as W_I and C_I, respectively, in the calculation. In this case, a suitable test interval for *Class A* (see *Results*) would be not less than 28 days following the initial 7-day equilibration period (a total of 35 days).]

Method II—Use this procedure for packs (e.g., punch-out cards) that incorporate a number of separately sealed unit-dose containers or blisters. Seal a sufficient number of packs, such that not less than 4 packs and a total of not less than 10 unit-dose containers or blisters filled with 1 pellet in each unit are tested. Seal a corresponding number of empty packs, each pack containing the same number of unit-dose containers or blisters as used in the test packs, to provide the controls. Store all of the containers at $75 \pm 3\%$ relative humidity and at a temperature of $23 \pm 2°$. [NOTE—A saturated system of 35 g of sodium chloride with each 100 mL of water placed in the bottom of a desiccator maintains the specified humidity. Other methods may be employed to maintain these conditions.] After 24 hours, and at each multiple thereof (see *Results*), remove the packs from the chamber, and allow them to equilibrate for about 45 minutes. Record the weights of the individual packs, and return them to the chamber. Weigh the control packs as a unit, and divide the total weight by the number of control packs to obtain the average empty pack weight. [NOTE—If any indicating pellets turn pink during the procedure, or if the average pellet weight increase in any pack exceeds 10%, terminate the test, and regard only earlier determinations as valid.] Calculate the average rate of moisture permeation, in mg per day, for each unit-dose container or blister in each pack taken by the formula:

$$(1/NX)[(W_F - W_I) - (C_F - C_I)],$$

in which N is the number of days expired in the test period (beginning after the initial 24-hour equilibration period); X is the number of separately sealed units per pack; $(W_F - W_I)$ is the difference, in mg, between the final and initial weights of each test pack; and $(C_F - C_I)$ is the difference, in mg, between the average final and average initial weights of the control packs, the rates being calculated to two significant figures.

Results—The individual unit-dose containers as tested in *Method I* are designated *Class A* if not more than 1 of 10 containers tested exceeds 0.5 mg per day in moisture permeation rate and none exceeds 1 mg per day; they are designated *Class B* if not more than 1 of 10 containers tested exceeds 5 mg per day and none exceeds 10 mg per day; they are designated *Class C* if not more than 1 of 10 containers tested exceeds 20 mg per day and none exceeds 40 mg per day; and they are designated *Class D* if the containers tested meet none of the moisture permeation rate requirements.

The packs as tested in *Method II* are designated *Class A* if no pack tested exceeds 0.5 mg per day in average blister moisture permeation rate; they are designated *Class B* if no pack tested exceeds 5 mg per day in average blister moisture permeation rate; they are designated *Class C* if no pack tested exceeds 20 mg per day in average blister moisture permeation rate; and they are designated *Class D* if the packs tested meet none of the above average blister moisture permeation rate requirements.

With the use of the *Desiccant* described herein, as stated for *Method I* and *Method II*, after every 24 hours, the test and control containers or packs are weighed; and suitable test intervals for the final weighings, W_F and C_F, are as follows: 24 hours for *Class D;* 48 hours for *Class C;* 7 days for *Class B;* and not less than 28 days for *Class A.*

⟨751⟩ METAL PARTICLES IN OPHTHALMIC OINTMENTS

The following test is designed to limit to a level considered to be unobjectionable the number and size of discrete metal particles that may occur in ophthalmic ointments.

Procedure—Extrude, as completely as practicable, the contents of 10 tubes individually into separate, clear, flat-bottom, 60-mm Petri dishes that are free from scratches. Cover the dishes, and heat at 85° for 2 hours, increasing the temperature slightly if necessary to ensure that a fully fluid state is obtained. Taking precautions against disturbing the melted sample, allow each to cool to room temperature and solidify.

Remove the covers, and invert each Petri dish on the stage of a suitable microscope adjusted to furnish 30 times magnification and equipped with an eye-piece micrometer disk that has been calibrated at the magnification being used. In addition to the usual source of light, direct an illuminator from above the ointment at a 45° angle. Examine the entire bottom of the Petri dish for metal particles. Varying the intensity of the illuminator from above allows such metal particles to be recognized by their characteristic reflection of light.

Count the number of metal particles that are 50 μm or larger in any dimension: the requirements are met if the total number of such particles in all 10 tubes does not exceed 50, and if not more than 1 tube is found to contain more than 8 such particles. If these results are not obtained, repeat the test on 20 additional tubes: the requirements are met if the total number of metal particles that are 50 μm or larger in any dimension does not exceed 150 in all 30 tubes tested, and if not more than 3 of the tubes are found to contain more than 8 such particles each.

⟨771⟩ OPHTHALMIC OINTMENTS

Added Substances—Suitable substances may be added to ophthalmic ointments to increase stability or usefulness, unless proscribed in the individual monograph, provided they are harmless in the amounts administered and do not interfere with the therapeutic efficacy or with the responses to the specified assays and tests. No coloring agent may be added, solely for the purpose of coloring the finished preparation, to an article intended for ophthalmic use (see also *Added Substances* under *General Notices* and under *Antimicrobial Effectiveness Testing* ⟨51⟩).

A suitable substance or mixture of substances to prevent the growth of microorganisms must be added to ophthalmic ointments that are packaged in multiple-use containers, regardless of the method of sterilization employed, unless otherwise directed in the individual monograph, or unless the formula itself is bacteriostatic. Such substances are used in concentrations that will prevent the growth of or kill microorganisms in the ophthalmic ointments (see also *Antimicrobial Effectiveness Testing* ⟨51⟩ and *Antimicrobial Agents—Content* ⟨341⟩). Sterilization processes are employed for the finished ointment or for all ingredients, if the ointment is manufactured under rigidly aseptic conditions, even though such substances are used (see also *Parenteral and Topical Preparations* in the section *Added Substances,* under *General Notices,* and *Sterilization and Sterility Assurance of Compendial Articles* ⟨1211⟩). Ophthalmic ointments that are packaged in single-use containers are not required to contain antibacterial agents; however, they meet the requirements for *Sterility Tests* ⟨71⟩.

Containers—Containers, including the closures, for ophthalmic ointments do not interact physically or chemically with the preparation in any manner to alter the strength, quality, or purity beyond the official requirements under the ordinary or customary conditions of handling, shipment, storage, sale, and use.

Metal Particles—Follow the *Procedure* set forth under *Metal Particles in Ophthalmic Ointments* ⟨751⟩.

Leakage—Select 10 tubes of the Ointment, with seals applied when specified. Thoroughly clean and dry the exterior surfaces of each tube with an absorbent cloth. Place the tubes in a horizontal position on a sheet of absorbent blotting paper in an oven maintained at a temperature of 60 ± 3° for 8 hours. No significant leakage occurs during or at the completion of the test (disregard traces of ointment presumed to originate externally from within the crimp of the tube or from the thread of the cap). If leakage is observed from one, but not more than one, of the tubes, repeat the test with 20 additional tubes of the Ointment. The requirement is met if no leakage is observed from the first 10 tubes tested, or if leakage is observed from not more than one of 30 tubes tested.

⟨785⟩ OSMOLARITY

Osmotic pressure is fundamentally related to all biological processes that involve diffusion of solutes or transfer of fluids through membranes. Thus, knowledge of the osmolar concentrations of parenteral fluids is essential. The labels of Pharmacopeial solutions that provide intravenous replenishment of fluid, nutrient(s), or electrolyte(s), as well as of the osmotic diuretic Mannitol Injection, are required to state the osmolar concentration.

The declaration of osmolar concentration on the label of a parenteral solution serves primarily to inform the practitioner whether the solution is hypo-osmotic, iso-osmotic, or hyper-osmotic. A quantitative statement facilitates calculation of the dilution required to render a hyper-osmotic solution iso-osmotic. It also simplifies many calculations involved in peritoneal dialysis and hemodialysis procedures. The osmolar concentration of an extemporaneously compounded intravenous solution prepared in the pharmacy (e.g., a hyperalimentation solution) from osmolar-labeled solutions also can be obtained simply by summing the osmoles contributed by each constituent.

The units of osmolar concentration are usually expressed as milliosmoles (abbreviation: mOsmol) of solute per liter of solution. In general terms, the weight of an osmole is the gram molecular weight of a substance divided by the number of ions or chemical species (n) formed upon dissolution. In ideal solutions, for example, $n = 1$ for glucose, $n = 2$ for sodium chloride or magnesium sulfate, $n = 3$ for calcium chloride, and $n = 4$ for sodium citrate.

The ideal osmolar concentration may be determined according to the formula:

$$\text{osmolar concentration (mOsmol/liter)} = \text{mOsM}$$

$$= \frac{\text{wt. of substance (g/liter)}}{\text{mol. wt. (g)}} \times \text{number of species} \times 1000.$$

As the concentration of the solute increases, interaction among solute particles increases, and actual osmolar values decrease when compared to ideal values. Deviation from ideal conditions is usually slight in solutions within the physiologic range and for more dilute solutions, but for highly concentrated solutions the actual osmolarities may be appreciably lower than ideal values. For example, the ideal osmolarity of 0.9% Sodium Chloride Injection is $9/58.4 \times 2 \times 1000 = 308$ mOsmol per liter. In fact, however, n is slightly less than 2 for solutions of sodium chloride at this concentration, and the actual measured osmolarity of 0.9% Sodium Chloride Injection is about 286 mOsmol per liter.

The theoretical osmolarity of a complex mixture, such as Protein Hydrolysate Injection, cannot be readily calculated. In such instances, actual values of osmolar concentration are to be used to meet the labeling requirement set forth in the individual monograph. They are determined by calculating the osmolarity from measured values of osmolal concentration and water content. Each osmole of solute added to 1 kg of water lowers the freezing point approximately 1.86° and lowers the vapor pressure approximately 0.3 mm of mercury (at 25°). These physical changes are measurable, and they permit accurate estimations of osmolal concentrations.

Where osmometers that measure the freezing-point depression are employed, a measured volume of solution (usually 2 mL) is placed in a glass tube immersed in a temperature-controlled bath. A thermistor and a vibrator are lowered into the mixture, and the temperature of the bath is decreased until the mixture is super-cooled. The vibrator is activated to induce crystallization of the water in the test solution, and the released heat of fusion raises the temperature of the mixture to its freezing point. By means of a Wheatstone bridge, the recorded freezing point is converted to a measurement in terms of milliosmolality, or its near equivalent for dilute solutions, milliosmolarity. The instrument is calibrated by using two standard solutions of sodium chloride that span the expected range of osmolarities.

Osmometers that measure the vapor pressures of solutions are less frequently employed. They require a smaller volume of specimen (generally about 5 μL), but the accuracy and precision of the resulting osmolality determination are comparable to those obtained by the use of osmometers that depend upon the observed freezing points of solutions.

Labeling—Where an osmolarity declaration is required in the individual monograph, the label states the total osmolar concentration in milliosmoles per liter. Where the contents are less than 100 mL, or where the label states that the article is not for direct injection but is to be diluted before use, the label alternatively may state the total osmolar concentration in milliosmoles per milliliter.

Change to read:

⟨795⟩ ▲PHARMACEUTICAL COMPOUNDING—NONSTERILE PREPARATIONS▲USP27

Change to read:

▲For the purposes of this chapter, the pharmacist or other licensed health care professional responsible for preparing the compounded preparations is referred to as "compounder".▲USP27

Compounding is an integral part of pharmacy practice and is essential to the provision of health care. The purpose of this chapter and applicable monographs on formulation is to help define what constitutes good ▲compounding▲USP27 practices and to provide general information to enhance the ▲compounder's▲USP27 ability in the ▲compounding facility▲USP27 to extemporaneously compound preparations that are of acceptable strength, quality, and purity.

Compounding is different from manufacturing, which is guided by GMPs (see *Good Manufacturing Practices for Bulk Pharmaceutical Excipients* ⟨1078⟩). ▲▲USP27 Some of the characteristics or criteria that differentiate compounding from manufacturing include the existence of specific ▲practitioner–patient–compounder▲USP27 relationships; the quantity of medication prepared in anticipation of receiving a prescription or a prescription order; and the conditions of sale, which are limited to specific prescription orders.

The pharmacist's responsibilities in compounding drug preparations are to dispense the finished preparation in accordance with a prescription or a prescriber's order or intent and to dispense those preparations in compliance with the requirements established by the Boards of Pharmacy and other regulatory agencies. ▲Compounders▲USP27 must be familiar with statutes and regulations that govern compounding because these requirements vary from state to state.

The ▲compounder▲USP27 is responsible for compounding preparations of acceptable strength, quality, and purity with appropriate packaging and labeling in accordance with good ▲compound-ing▲USP27 practices (see *Good Compounding Practices* ⟨1075⟩), official standards, and relevant scientific data and information. ▲Compounders▲USP27 engaging in compounding should ▲have to▲USP27 continually expand their compounding knowledge by participating in seminars, studying appropriate literature, and consulting colleagues.

Add the following:

▲RESPONSIBILITY OF THE COMPOUNDER

The compounder is responsible for ensuring that the quality is built into the compounded preparations of products, with key factors including at least the following general principles. (See also *Good Compounding Practices* ⟨1075⟩.)
(1) Personnel are capable and qualified to perform their assigned duties.
(2) Ingredients used in compounding have their expected identity, quality, and purity.
(3) Compounded preparations are of acceptable strength, quality, and purity, with appropriate packaging and labeling, and prepared in accordance with good compounding practices, official standards, and relevant scientific data and information.
(4) Critical processes are validated to ensure that procedures, when used, will consistently result in the expected qualities in the finished preparation.
(5) The compounding environment is suitable for its intended purpose.
(6) Appropriate stability evaluation is performed or determined from the literature for establishing reliable beyond-use dating to ensure that the finished preparations have their expected potency, purity, quality, and characteristics, at least until the labeled beyond-use date.
(7) There is assurance that processes are always carried out as intended or specified and are under control.
(8) Compounding conditions and procedures are adequate for preventing errors.
(9) Adequate procedures and records exist for investigating and correcting failures or problems in compounding, testing, or in the preparation itself.
▲USP27

Change to read:

COMPOUNDING ENVIRONMENT

Facilities

▲▲USP27 Areas designated for compounding have adequate space for the orderly placement of equipment and materials to prevent mixups between ingredients, containers, labels, in-process materials, and finished preparations. The compounding area is also to be designed, arranged, used, and maintained to prevent adventitious cross-contamination. Areas used for sterile preparations are to be separate and distinct from the nonsterile compounding area (see ▲*Environmental Quality and Control* under *Pharmaceutical Compounding—Sterile Preparations* ⟨797⟩).▲USP27 The entire compounding area is to be well-lighted.

Heating, ventilation, and air conditioning systems are to be controlled to avoid decomposition of chemicals (see *Storage Temperature* under *Preservation, Packaging, Storage, and Labeling* in the *General Notices and Requirements* and the manufacturers' labeled storage conditions). Storage areas provide an environment suitably controlled to ensure quality and stability of bulk chemicals and finished preparations.

Potable water is to be supplied for hand and equipment washing. This water meets the standards prescribed in the EPA's National Primary Drinking Water Regulations (40 CFR Part 141). *Purified Water* must be used for compounding nonsterile drug preparations when formulations indicate the inclusion of water. *Purified Water* must also be used for rinsing equipment and utensils. In those cases when a water is used to prepare a sterile preparation, *Water for Injection, Sterile Water for Injection,* or *Bacteriostatic Water for Injection* must be used (see *Water for Pharmaceutical Purposes* ⟨1231⟩ and ▲*Pharmaceutical Compounding—Sterile Preparations* ⟨797⟩).▲*USP27*

Compounding areas are to be maintained in a clean and sanitary condition. Adequate washing facilities are to be provided, including hot and cold water, soap or detergent, and air driers or single-service towels. Sewage, trash, and other refuse in the compounding area is to be disposed of in a safe, sanitary, and timely manner. Equipment is to be thoroughly cleaned promptly after use to avoid cross-contamination of ingredients and preparations. Special precautions are to be taken to clean equipment and compounding areas meticulously after compounding preparations that contain allergenic ingredients (e.g., sulfonamides or penicillins).

Equipment

Equipment is to be of appropriate design and size for compounding and suitable for the intended uses. The types and sizes of equipment will depend on the dosage forms and the quantities compounded (see *Weights and Balances* ⟨41⟩, *Prescription Balances and Volumetric Apparatus* ⟨1176⟩, and equipment manufacturers' instruction manuals). All equipment is to be constructed so that surfaces that contact pharmaceutical components, in-process materials, or finished preparations are not reactive, additive, or adsorptive to avoid altering the safety, identity, strength, quality, or purity of the preparation. ▲The use of micropipets, electronic or analytical balances, or triturations or dilutions shall be considered when needed quantities are too small to accurately measure with standard equipment required by a state Board of Pharmacy. Equipment and accessories used in compounding are to be inspected, maintained, cleaned, and validated at appropriate intervals to ensure the accuracy and reliability of their performance.▲*USP27*

Change to read:

STABILITY OF COMPOUNDED PREPARATIONS

"Stability" is defined as the extent to which a preparation retains, within specified limits, and throughout its period of storage and use, the same properties and characteristics that it possessed at the time of compounding. See the table *Criteria for Acceptable Levels of Stability* under *Stability Considerations in Dispensing Practice* ⟨1191⟩.

The ▲compounder▲*USP27* must avoid formulation ingredients and processing conditions that would result in a potentially toxic or ineffective preparation. The ▲compounder's▲*USP27* knowledge of the chemical reactions by which drugs degrade provides a means for establishing conditions under which the rate of degradation is minimized. The factors that influence the stability of ▲compounded preparations▲*USP27* are generally the same as

those for manufactured drug products (see *Factors Affecting Product Stability* and *Responsibility of the Pharmacist* under *Stability Considerations in Dispensing Practice* ⟨1191⟩).

Primary Packaging

Compounded preparations should be packaged in containers meeting USP standards (see *Containers* under *Preservation, Packaging, Storage, and Labeling* in the *General Notices and Requirements, Containers* ⟨661⟩, and *Containers—Permeation* ⟨671⟩). The container used depends on the physical and chemical properties of the compounded preparation. Container–drug interaction is to be considered with substances such as phenolic compounds and sorptive materials (e.g., polypeptides and proteins).

Sterility

Assurance of sterility in a compounded sterile preparation is mandatory. Compounding and packaging of sterile drugs, such as ophthalmic solutions, will require strict adherence to guidelines presented in the general ▲test▲*USP27* chapter ▲*Pharmaceutical Compounding—Sterile Preparations* ⟨797⟩▲*USP27* and in the manufacturers' labeling instructions.

Stability Criteria and Beyond-Use Dating

The beyond-use date is the date after which a compounded preparation is not to be used and is determined from the date the preparation is compounded. Because compounded preparations are intended for administration immediately or following short-term storage, their beyond-use dates may be assigned based on criteria different from those applied to assigning expiration dates to manufactured drug products.

▲Compounders▲*USP27* are to consult and apply drug-specific and general stability documentation and literature when available, and are to consider the nature of the drug and its degradation mechanism, the container in which it is packaged, the expected storage conditions, and the intended duration of therapy when assigning a beyond-use date (see *Expiration Date and Beyond-Use Date* under*Labeling* in the *General Notices and Requirements*). Beyond-use dates are to be assigned conservatively. When using manufactured solid dosage forms to prepare a solution or aqueous suspension, the ▲compounder▲*USP27* is also to consider factors such as hydrolysis and the freeze-thaw property of the final preparation before assigning a beyond-use date. In assigning a beyond-use date for a compounded drug preparation, in addition to using all available stability information, the ▲compounder▲*USP27* is also to use his or her pharmaceutical education and experience.

When a manufactured product is used as the source of active ingredient for a nonsterile compounded preparation, the product expiration date cannot be used to extrapolate directly a beyond-use date for the compounded preparation. However, a ▲compounder▲*USP27* may refer to the literature or to the manufacturer for stability information. The ▲compounder▲*USP27* may also refer to applicable publications to obtain stability, compatibility, and degradation information on ingredients. All stability data must be carefully interpreted in relation to the actual compounded formulation.

At all steps in the compounding, dispensing, and storage process, the ▲compounder▲*USP27* is to observe the compounded drug preparation for signs of instability. For more specific details of some of the common physical signs of deterioration, see *Observing Products for Evidence of Instability* under *Stability Considerations in Dispensing Practice* ⟨1191⟩. However, excessive chemical degradation and other drug concentration loss due to reactions may be invisible more often than they are visible.

In the absence of stability information that is applicable to a specific drug and preparation, the following maximum beyond-use dates are recommended for nonsterile compounded drug preparations[1] that are packaged in tight, light-resistant containers and stored at controlled room temperature unless otherwise indicated ▲(see *Preservation, Packaging, Storage, and Labeling* in the *General Notices and Requirements*).▲*USP27*

For Nonaqueous Liquids and Solid Formulations—
Where the Manufactured Drug Product is the Source of Active Ingredient—The beyond-use date is not later than 25% of the time remaining until the product's expiration date or 6 months, whichever is earlier.

Where a USP or NF Substance is the Source of Active Ingredient—The beyond-use date is not later than 6 months.

For Water-Containing Formulations (prepared from ingredients in solid form)—The beyond-use date is not later than 14 days ▲for liquid preparations▲*USP27* when stored at cold temperatures ▲between 2° and 8° (36° and 46° F).▲*USP27*

For All Other Formulations—The beyond-use date is not later than the intended duration of therapy or 30 days, whichever is earlier. These beyond-use date limits may be exceeded when there is supporting valid scientific stability information that is directly applicable to the specific preparation (i.e., the same drug concentration range, pH, excipients, vehicle, water content, etc.). See also the beyond-use dating information in the *Labeling* section under *Repackaging Into Single-Unit Containers and Unit-Dose Containers for Nonsterile Solid and Liquid Dosage Forms* under *Containers* ⟨661⟩.

Beyond-Use Labeling

Federal law requires that manufactured drug products be labeled with an expiration date. Some state laws may require a beyond-use date. The label on the container or package of an official compounded preparation must bear a beyond-use date. Good ▲compounding▲*USP27* practice dictates beyond-use labeling for all compounded preparations.

Change to read:

DEFINITIONS

For purposes of this chapter, the following terms shall have these meanings.

PREPARATION is a drug ▲dosage form,▲*USP27* a dietary supplement, or a finished device. It is the finished or partially finished preparation of one or more ▲▲*USP27* substances formulated for use on or for the patient or consumer (see *General Notices and Requirements*).

OFFICIAL SUBSTANCE includes an active drug entity, a dietary supplement, or a pharmaceutic ingredient (see also ▲*NF 22*)▲*USP27* or a component of a finished device.

ACTIVE INGREDIENT usually refers to chemicals, substances, or other components of articles intended for use in the diagnosis, cure, mitigation, treatment, or prevention of diseases in humans or other animals or for use as dietary supplements.

ADDED SUBSTANCES are ingredients that are necessary to prepare the preparation but are not intended or expected to cause a human pharmacologic response if administered alone in the amount or concentration contained in a single dose of the compounded preparation. The term added substances is usually used synonymously with the terms *inactive ingredients, excipients,* and *pharmaceutic ingredients.*

---

[1] For guidelines applicable to dating sterile compounded preparations, see ▲*Storage and Beyond-Use Dating* under *Pharmaceutical Compounding—Sterile Preparations* ⟨797⟩.▲*USP27*

Change to read:

INGREDIENT SELECTION ▲▲*USP27*

Sources

Official compounded preparations are prepared from ingredients that meet requirements of the compendial monograph for those individual ingredients for which monographs are provided.

A USP or an NF grade substance is the preferred source of ingredients for compounding all other preparations. If that is not available, or when food, cosmetics, or other substances are or must be used, then the use of another high-quality source, such as analytical reagent (AR), certified American Chemical Society (ACS), or Food Chemicals Codex (FCC) grade, is an option for professional judgment. For any substance used in compounding not purchased from a registered drug manufacturer, the ▲compounder▲*USP27* must establish purity and safety by reasonable means, which may include lot analysis, manufacturer reputation, or reliability of source.

A manufactured drug product may be a source of active ingredient. Only manufactured drugs from containers labeled with a batch control number and a future expiration date are acceptable as a potential source of active ingredients. When compounding with manufactured drug products, the ▲compounder▲*USP27* must consider all ingredients present in the drug product relative to the intended use of the compounded preparation.

▲▲*USP27* A ▲compounder▲*USP27* may not compound a drug ▲preparation▲*USP27* that appears on ▲the FDA list of drug products withdrawn or removed from the market for safety reasons.▲*USP27*

Compounding Nondrug Requirements

If the ▲preparation▲*USP27* is intended for use as a dietary ▲or nutritional▲*USP27* supplement (to supplement the diet) or cosmetic (e.g., to beautify), then the ▲compounder▲*USP27* must adhere to ▲*Good Compounding Practices* ⟨1075⟩ and to this chapter, and must comply with any federal and state requirements.▲*USP27*

Change to read:

CHECKLIST FOR ACCEPTABLE STRENGTH, QUALITY, AND PURITY

The following questions are to be considered carefully before compounding.
1. Have the physical and chemical properties and medicinal, dietary, and pharmaceutical uses of the drug substances been reviewed?
2. Is the quantity and quality of each active ingredient identifiable?
3. Will the active ingredients be effectively absorbed, locally or systemically according to the prescribed purpose, from the preparation and route of administration?
4. Are there added substances ▲(see *Definitions*),▲*USP27* confirmed or potentially present from manufactured products that may be expected to cause an allergic reaction, irritation, toxicity, or undesirable organoleptic response from the patient? Are there added substances ▲(see *Definitions*),▲*USP27* confirmed or potentially present that may be unfavorable (e.g., unsuitable pH or inadequate solubility)?
5. Were all calculations and measurements confirmed to ensure that the preparation will be compounded accurately ▲(see *Pharmaceutical Calculations in Prescription Compounding* ⟨1160⟩).▲*USP27*

Change to read:

COMPOUNDED PREPARATIONS

The term *compounded preparations* includes the terms *compounded dosage forms*, *compounded drugs*, and *compounded formulations*, and means finished forms that are prepared by or under the direct supervision of a licensed ▲compounder.▲*USP27*

When controlled substances are used, check with state and federal authorities concerning their policies. ▲Unless otherwise indicated or appropriate, compounded preparations are to be prepared to ensure that each preparation shall contain not less than 90.0 percent and not more than 110.0 percent of the theoretically calculated and labeled quantity of active ingredient per unit weight or volume and not less than 90.0 percent and not more than 110.0 percent of the theoretically calculated weight or volume per unit of the preparation.▲*USP27* Compounded preparations include, but are not restricted to, the following pharmaceutical dosage forms described under *Pharmaceutical Dosage Forms* ⟨1151⟩.

Capsules, Powders, Lozenges, and Tablets

When compounding these dosage forms, the ▲compounder▲*USP27* is to prepare an amount of the total formulation sufficient to allow the prescribed amount or quantity to be accurately dispensed. Selected practices and precautions for compounding these dosage forms include the following:

- reducing solid ingredients to the smallest reasonable particle size;
- implementing appropriate checks to ensure that all ingredients are blended to achieve a homogeneous mixture;
- monitoring humidity if moisture might cause hydrolysis, dosage form adhesion to containers, or softening or partial dissolution of capsule shells;
- accurately performing weighings to ensure that each unit shall be not less than 90% and not more than 110% of the theoretically calculated weight for each unit [NOTE—Preparations classified as dietary supplements are required by the U.S. Food and Drug regulations to be not less than 100% of the declared potency.]; and
- packaging dosage units according to container specifications for capsules and tablets of the specific active ingredient unless specified otherwise in individual monographs (see *Containers* ⟨661⟩).

Emulsions, Solutions, and Suspensions

When compounding these dosage forms, the ▲compounder▲*USP27* is to prepare a 2% to 3% excess amount of the total formulation to allow the prescribed amount to be accurately dispensed. Selected practices and precautions for compounding these dosage forms include the following.

- For single-unit containers, the weight of each filled container, corrected for tare weight, shall be the equivalent of not less than 100% and not more than 110% of the labeled volume.
- Aqueous suspensions are prepared by levigating the powder mixture to a smooth paste with an appropriate wetting agent. This paste is converted to a free-flowing fluid by adding adequate vehicle. Successive portions of the vehicle are used to wash the mortar, or other vessel, to transfer the suspension quantitatively to a calibrated dispensing bottle or graduate. The preparation may be homogenized to ensure a uniform final dispersion.
- Reducing solid ingredients to the smallest reasonable particle size.

- Solutions shall contain no visible undissolved matter when dispensed. [NOTE—An exception may occur with supersaturated solutions such as *Potassium Iodide Oral Solution*.]
- Emulsions and suspensions are labeled, "Shake well before using."

Suppositories

When compounding suppositories, the ▲compounder▲*USP27* is to prepare an excess amount of total formulation to allow the prescribed quantity to be accurately dispensed. Selected practices and precautions for compounding these dosage forms include the following:

- not using ingredients that are caustic or irritating, and thoroughly comminute solids that are abrasive to the mucous membranes;
- selecting a base that allows active ingredients to provide the intended local or systemic therapeutic effect;
- reducing solid ingredients to the smallest reasonable particle size; and
- weighing a representative number of suppositories to ensure that each is not less than 90% and not more than 110% of the average weight of all suppositories in the batch.

Creams, Topical Gels, Ointments, and Pastes

When compounding semisolid dosage forms, the ▲compounder▲*USP27* is to prepare an excess amount of total formulation to allow the prescribed quantity to be accurately dispensed. Selected practices and precautions for compounding these dosage forms include the following:

- not using ingredients that are caustic, irritating, or allergenic to the skin or other application sites unless they are necessary for a treatment;
- selecting a base or vehicle that allows active ingredients to provide the intended local or systemic therapeutic effect;
- reducing solid ingredients to the smallest reasonable particle size;
- geometrically incorporating the active ingredients with the added substances to achieve a uniform liquid or solid dispersion in the dosage form; and
- observing the uniformity of the dispersion by spreading a thin film of finished formulation on a flat transparent surface (e.g., clear glass ointment slab).

Change to read:

COMPOUNDING PROCESS

The ▲compounders▲*USP27* are to consider using the following steps to minimize error and maximize the prescriber's intent.

1. Judge the suitability of the prescription to be compounded in terms of its safety and intended use. Determine what legal limitations, if any, are applicable.
2. Perform necessary calculations to establish the amounts of ingredients needed (see ▲*Pharmaceutical Calculations in Prescription Compounding* ⟨1160⟩).▲*USP27*
3. Identify equipment needed.
4. Don the proper attire and wash hands.
5. Clean the compounding area and needed equipment.
6. Only one prescription should be compounded at one time in a specified compounding area.
7. Assemble all necessary materials to compound the prescription.
8. Compound the preparation following the formulation record or prescription (see *Compounding Records and Documents* below), according to the art and science of pharmacy.

9. Assess weight variation, adequacy of mixing, clarity, odor, color, consistency, and pH as appropriate.
10. Annotate the compounding log and describe the appearance of the formulation.
11. Label the prescription containers to include the following items: a) the name of the preparation; b) the internal identification number; c) the beyond-use date (see *Beyond-Use Labeling*); d) the initials of the ▲compounder▲USP27 who prepared the label; e) any storage requirements; and f) any other statements required by law.
12. Sign and date the prescription affirming that all procedures were carried out to ensure uniformity, identity, strength, quantity, and purity.
13. Thoroughly and promptly clean all equipment, and store properly.

Change to read:

COMPOUNDING RECORDS AND DOCUMENTS

All ▲compounders▲USP27 who dispense prescriptions must comply with the record keeping requirements of their individual states. If the ▲compounder▲USP27 compounds a preparation according to the manufacturer's labeling instructions, then further documentation is not required. All other compounded preparations require further documentation. Such compounding documents are to list the ingredients and the quantity of each in the order of the compounding process.

The objective of the documentation is to allow another ▲compounder▲USP27 to reproduce the identical prescription at a future date. The formulation record provides a consistent source document for preparing the preparation (recipe), and the compounding record documents the actual ingredients in the preparation and the person responsible for the compounding activity. These records are to be retained for the same period of time that is required for any prescription under state law. The record may be a copy of the prescription in written or machine readable form that includes a formulation record, a compounding record, and a Material Safety Data Sheets (MSDS) file.

Formulation Record

The formulation record is a file of individually compounded preparations. This record must list the name, strength, and dosage form of the preparation compounded, all ingredients and their quantities, equipment needed to prepare the preparation, when appropriate, and mixing instructions. Mixing instructions should include the order of mixing, mixing temperatures or other environmental controls, such as the duration of mixing, and other factors pertinent to the replication of the preparation as compounded. The formulation record must include an assigned beyond-use date, the container used in dispensing, the storage requirements, and any quality control procedures.

Compounding Record

The compounding record contains documentation of the name and strength of the compounded preparation, the formulation record reference for the preparation, and the sources and lot numbers of ingredients. The compounding record also includes information on the total number of dosage units compounded, the name of the person who prepared the preparation and the name of the ▲compounder▲USP27 who approved the preparation, the date of preparation, the assigned internal identification number or the prescription number and an assigned beyond-use date, and the prescription number. For all compounded preparations, results of quality control procedures are to be recorded (e.g., weight range of filled capsules). ▲When compounding problems

occur with preparations prepared according to USP compounding monographs, the compounder must complete a USP Monograph Experience Reporting Form, and submit the form to USP for evaluation.▲USP27

MSDS File

▲MSDS are to be readily accessible to all employees working with drug substances or bulk chemicals located on the compounding facility premises. Employees are to be instructed on how to retrieve and interpret needed information.▲USP27

Change to read:

QUALITY CONTROL

The safety, quality, and performance of compounded preparations depend on correct ingredients and calculations, accurate and precise measurements, appropriate formulation conditions and procedures, and prudent pharmaceutical judgment. As a final check, the ▲compounder▲USP27 is to review each procedure in the compounding process. To ensure accuracy and completeness, the ▲compounder▲USP27 is to observe the finished preparation to ensure that it appears as expected and is to investigate any discrepancies and take appropriate corrective action before the prescription is dispensed to the patient (see the *Checklist for Acceptable Strength, Quality, and Purity*, the appropriate pharmaceutical dosage form under *Compounded Preparations*, and the steps under *Compounding Process*).

Add the following:

▲VERIFICATION

Compounding procedures that are routinely performed, including batch compounding, shall be completed and verified according to written procedures. The act of verification of a compounding procedure involves checking to ensure that calculations, weighing and measuring, order of mixing, and compounding techniques were appropriate and accurately performed.▲USP27

PATIENT COUNSELING

The patient or the patient's agent should be counseled about proper use, storage, and evidence of instability in the compounded preparation at the time of dispensing (see *Responsibility of the Pharmacist* under *Stability Considerations in Dispensing Practice* ⟨1191⟩).

Change to read:

▲⟨797⟩ PHARMACEUTICAL COMPOUNDING—STERILE PREPARATIONS▲USP27

Change to read:

▲INTRODUCTION

This chapter provides procedures and requirements for compounding sterile preparations.

Sterile compounding differs from nonsterile compounding (see *Pharmaceutical Compounding—Nonsterile Preparations* ⟨795⟩ and *Good Compounding Practices* ⟨1075⟩) primarily by requiring

a test for sterility. Sterile compounding also requires cleaner facilities; specific training and testing of personnel in principles and practices of aseptic manipulations; air quality evaluation and maintenance; and sound knowledge of sterilization and solution stability principles and practices. Greater care is required for aqueous injections that are compounded sterile preparations (CSPs)—the most common CSPs used in therapy. Aqueous injections for administration into the vascular and central nervous systems pose the greatest risk of harm to patients if there are issues of nonsterility and large errors in ingredients.

The intent of this chapter is to prevent harm and fatality to patients that could result from microbial contamination (nonsterility), excessive bacterial endotoxins, large content errors in the strength of correct ingredients, and incorrect ingredients in CSPs. The quality control and testing for CSPs in this chapter are appropriate and necessary. The content of this chapter applies to health care institutions, pharmacies, physician practice facilities, and other facilities in which CSPs are prepared, stored, and dispensed. For the purposes of this chapter, CSPs include any of the following:

a. Preparations prepared according to the maufacturer's labeled instructions and other manipulations when manufacturing sterile products that expose the original contents to potential contamination.
b. Preparations containing nonsterile ingredients or employing nonsterile components and devices that must be sterilized before administration.
c. Biologics, diagnostics, drugs, nutrients, and radiopharmaceuticals that possess either of the above two characteristics, and which include, but are not limited to, baths and soaks for live organs and tissues, implants, inhalations, injections, powders for injection, irrigations, metered sprays, and ophthalmic and otic preparations.

The sections in this chapter are organized to facilitate practitioners' understanding of the fundamental accuracy and quality practices of CSPs. They provide a foundation for the development and implementation of essential procedures for the safe preparation of CSP's in the three risk levels, which are classified according to the potential for microbial, chemical, and physical contamination. The chapter is divided into the following main sections:
• Responsibilities of all compounding personnel
• The basis for the classification of a CSP into a low-, medium-, and high-risk level, with examples of CSPs and their quality assurance practices in each of these risk levels
• Verification of compounding accuracy and sterilization
• Personnel training and evaluation in aseptic manipulation skills, including representative sterile microbial culture medium transfer and fill challenges
• Environmental quality and control during the processing of CSPs
• Equipment used in the preparation of CSPs
• Verification of automated compounding devices for parenteral nutrition compounding
• Finished preparation release checks and tests
• Storage and beyond-use dating
• Maintaining product quality and control after CSPs leave the compounding facility, including education and training of personnel
• Packing, handling, storage, and transport of CSPs
• Patient or caregiver training
• Patient monitoring and adverse events reporting
• A quality assurance program for CSPs

It is the ultimate responsibility of all personnel who prepare CSPs to understand these fundamental practices and precautions, to develop and implement appropriate procedures, and to continually evaluate these procedures and the quality of final CSPs to prevent harm and fatality to patients who are treated with CSPs.▲*USP27*

Delete the following:

▲RESPONSIBILITY OF THE DISPENSING PHARMACIST

A pharmacist dispensing any SP is responsible for ensuring that the product has been prepared, labeled, controlled, stored, dispensed, and distributed properly. This includes the responsibility for ensuring that the SP is kept under appropriate controlled conditions at the location of use and that it is administered properly through adequate labeling and verbal or written instructions. The dispensing pharmacist is also responsible for ensuring that the SP retains its quality attributes within acceptable limits through a written quality assurance program. This program should ensure that for the entire labeled life of the product, or until manipulated by the clinician, patient, or caregiver, the potency, pH, sterility, freedom from pyrogens, particulate limits, container integrity, appearance, and other qualities or characteristics that the SP is expected to have do exist. The quality assurance program should encompass every SP under the pharmacy's control and includes all phases of its preparation, distribution, storage, administration, and use. The dispensing pharmacy should employ proper analytical testing, where appropriate, to ensure the microbiological, chemical, and physical quality of all SPs. These responsibilities apply equally to commercially available injectable drug products that are dispensed to patients without compounding or other manipulation and to SPs that have been repackaged, reconstituted, diluted, admixed, blended, or otherwise manipulated (collectively referred to as "Compounded") in any way prior to dispensing. The pharmacist is responsible for ensuring that quality is built into the preparation of products, with key factors including at least the following general principles:
(1) Personnel are capable and qualified to perform their assigned duties.
(2) Ingredients used in compounding have their expected identity, quality, and purity.
(3) Critical processes are validated to ensure that procedures, when used, will consistently result in the expected qualities in the finished product.
(4) The production environment is suitable for its intended purpose (addressing such matters as environmental cleanliness, control, monitoring, and the setting of action limits, as appropriate).
(5) Appropriate release checks or testing procedures are performed to ensure that finished products have their expected potency, purity, quality, and characteristics at the time of release.
(6) Appropriate stability evaluation is performed or determined from the literature for establishing reliable beyond-use dating to ensure that finished products have their expected potency, purity, quality, and characteristics at least until the labeled beyond-use date.
(7) There is assurance that processes are always carried out as intended or specified and are under control.
(8) Preparation conditions and procedures are adequate for preventing mixups.
(9) There are adequate procedures and records for investigating and correcting failures or problems in preparation, testing, or in the product itself.
(10) There is adequate separation of quality control functions and decisions from those of production.

Emphasis in this chapter is placed upon the quality and the control of the processes utilized, personnel performance, and the environmental conditions under which the processes are performed. Other factors, such as testing and stability, are addressed to the extent necessary for the limited quantities of products with relatively short beyond-use dating periods normally associated with home care pharmacy practice. This chapter is not intended to address issues concerning the manufacture of sterile drug products.▲*USP27*

Add the following:

▲RESPONSIBILITY OF COMPOUNDING PERSONNEL

Compounding personnel are responsible for ensuring that CSPs are accurately identified, measured, diluted, and mixed; and are correctly purified, sterilized, packaged, sealed, labeled, stored, dispensed, and distributed. These performance responsibilities include maintaining appropriate cleanliness conditions and providing labeling and supplementary instructions for the proper clinical administration of CSPs.

Compounding supervisors shall ensure through either direct measurement or appropriate information sources that specific CSPs maintain their labeled strength within monograph limits for USP articles, or within 10% if not specified, until their beyond-use dates. All CSPs are prepared in a manner that maintains sterility and minimizes the introduction of particulate matter.

A written quality assurance procedure includes the following in-process checks that are applied, as is appropriate, to specific CSPs: accuracy and precision of measuring and weighing; the requirement for sterility; methods of sterilization and purification; safe limits and ranges for strength of ingredients, bacterial endotoxins, particulate matter, and pH; labeling accuracy and completeness; beyond-use date assignment; and packaging and storage requirements. The dispenser shall, when appropriate and practicable, obtain and evaluate results of testing for identity, strength, purity, and sterility before a CSP is dispensed. Qualified licensed health care professionals who supervise compounding and dispensing of CSPs shall ensure that the following objectives are achieved.

1. Compounding personnel are adequately skilled, educated, instructed, and trained to correctly perform and document the following activities in their sterile compounding duties:
   a. Perform antiseptic hand cleansing and disinfection of nonsterile compounding surfaces;
   b. Select and appropriately don protective gloves, goggles, gowns, masks, and hair and shoe covers;
   c. Use laminar flow clean-air hoods, barrier isolators, and other contamination control devices that are appropriate for the risk level;
   d. Identify, weigh, and measure ingredients; and
   e. Manipulate sterile products aseptically, sterilize high-risk level CSPs, and label and quality inspect CSPs.
2. Ingredients have their correct identity, quality, and purity.
3. Opened or partially used packages of ingredients for subsequent use in CSPs are properly stored under restricted access conditions in the compounding facility. Such packages cannot be used when visual inspection detects unauthorized breaks in the container, closure, and seal; when the contents do not possess the expected appearance, aroma, and texture; when the contents do not pass identification tests specified by the compounding facility; and when either the beyond-use or expiration date has been exceeded.
4. To minimize the generation of bacterial endotoxins, water-containing CSPs that are nonsterile during any phase of the compounding procedure are sterilized within 6 hours after completing the preparation.
5. Sterilization methods achieve sterility of CSPs while maintaining the labeled strength of active ingredients and the physical integrity of packaging.
6. Measuring, mixing, sterilizing, and purifying devices are clean, appropriately accurate, and effective for their intended uses.
7. Potential harm from added substances and differences in rate and extent of bioavailability of active ingredients for other than oral route of administration are carefully evaluated before such CSPs are dispensed and administered.
8. Packaging selected for CSPs is appropriate to preserve the sterility and strength until the beyond-use date.
9. While being used, the compounding environment maintains the sterility or the presterilization purity, whichever is appropriate, of the CSP.
10. Labels on CSPs list the names and amounts or concentrations of all ingredients. Before being dispensed, and or administered, the clarity of solutions are visually confirmed; also the identity and amounts of ingredients, procedures to prepare and sterilize CSPs, and specific release criteria are reviewed to assure their accuracy and completeness.
11. Beyond-use dates are assigned based on direct testing or extrapolation from reliable literature sources and other documentation (see *Stability Criteria* and *Beyond-Use Dating* under *Pharmaceutical Compounding—Nonsterile Preparations* ⟨795⟩).
12. Procedures for measuring, mixing, dilution, purification, sterilization, packaging, and labeling conform to the correct sequence and quality established for the specified CSP.
13. Deficiencies in compounding, labeling, packaging, and quality testing and inspection can be rapidly identified and corrected.
14. When time and personnel availability so permit, compounding manipulations and procedures are separated from postcompounding quality inspection and review before CSPs are dispensed and administered.

This chapter emphasizes the need to maintain high standards for the quality and control of processes, components, and environments; and for the skill and knowledge of personnel who prepare CSPs. The rigor of in-process quality-control checks and of postcompounding quality inspection and testing increases corresponding to the potential hazard of the route of administration. For example, nonsterility, excessive bacterial endotoxin contamination, large errors in strength of correct ingredients, and incorrect ingredients in CSPs are potentially more dangerous to patients when the CSPs are administered into the vascular and central nervous systems than when administered by most other routes.▲*USP27*

Delete the following:

▲RISK LEVELS

With reference to the microbiological quality (i.e., sterility) of the finished drug product, an SP, in general, is compounded under either relatively *low-risk* or *high-risk* conditions, as determined by the potential for the introduction of microbial contamination. This contamination may result from the use of nonsterile components; novel, complex, or prolonged aseptic processes; or open exposure of the drug product or product containment devices to the atmosphere. In addition, long storage time between compounding and initiation of administration may affect the microbiological quality of the finished drug product.

The characteristics itemized below to distinguish between the high-risk and low-risk levels are intended to provide conceptual guidance and are not intended to be prescriptive. The pharmacist is expected to exercise professional judgment on a case-by-case basis when determining the risk level that would be appropriate for a particular process.

Low-Risk

An SP is considered to be aseptically processed under low-risk conditions when all of the following conditions prevail:
(1) The finished product is compounded with commercially available, sterile drug products.
(2) Compounding involves only basic, and relatively few, aseptic manipulations that are promptly executed.
(3) "Closed system" transfers are used: the container-closure system remains essentially intact throughout the aseptic process, compromised only by the penetration of a sterile, pyrogen-free needle or cannula through the designated stopper or port to affect transfer, withdrawal, or delivery in accordance with the labeled instructions for the pertinent,

commercially available devices. Opened ampuls should be regarded as if they are closed systems for purposes of this chapter.

Examples of low-risk processes include the following:

(1) Transferring sterile drug products from vials or ampuls into sterile final containers using a sterile needle and syringe.
(2) Transferring sterile drug products into sterile elastomeric infusion containers with the aid of a mechanical pump and an appropriate sterile transfer tubing device, with or without the subsequent addition of sterile drug products to the infusion container with a sterile needle and syringe.
(3) Compounding sterile nutritional solutions by combining *Dextrose Injection* and *Amino Acids Injection* via gravity transfer into sterile empty containers, with or without the subsequent addition of sterile drug products to the final container with a sterile needle and syringe.

High-Risk

Category I—A high-risk SP may fall into either of two subclassifications. High-risk SPs in *Category I* are those prepared from commercially available, sterile components where one or more of the following conditions prevail:

(1) Compounding involves the intermediate closed system pooling of sterile drug products. Pooling of additives is defined as a higher risk process than performing multiple single additives because contamination of the pool could result in contamination of units filled from the pool, thus potentially causing epidemic infection.
(2) Compounding includes complex and/or numerous aseptic manipulations executed over a prolonged period.
(3) An individual finished product is administered as a multi-day infusion via a portable pump or reservoir.

Examples of high-risk category I processes include the following:

(1) Compounding sterile nutritional solutions using an automated compounding device involving repeated attachment of fluid containers to proximal openings of the compounder tubing set and of empty final containers to the distal opening. The process concludes with the transfer of additives into the filled final container from individual drug product containers or from a pooled additive solution.
(2) Preparing ambulatory pump reservoirs by adding more than one drug product with the evacuation of air from the reservoir prior to dispensing.
(3) Preparing ambulatory pump reservoirs for multi-day (i.e., ambient temperature) administration.

Category II—High-risk SPs in *Category II* are those involving either of the following:

(1) A nonsterile drug substance or an injectable drug product prepared in-house from a nonsterile substance is used to compound the SP.
(2) "Open systems" are used, for example, when combining ingredients in a nonsealed reservoir before filling or when fluid passes through the atmosphere during a fill-seal operation.

Examples of high-risk category II processes include the following:

(1) Compounding injectable morphine solutions from nonsterile morphine substance and suitable vehicles.
(2) Compounding sterile nutritional solutions from nonsterile ingredients with initial mixing in a nonsealed or nonsterile reservoir.▲*USP27*

Add the following:

▲CSP MICROBIAL CONTAMINATION RISK LEVELS

The appropriate risk level—low, medium, or high—is assigned according to the corresponding probability of contaminating a CSP with (1) microbial contamination (microbial organisms, spores, and endotoxins) and (2) chemical and physical contamination (foreign chemicals and physical matter). Potential sources of contamination include, but are not limited to, solid and liquid matter from compounding personnel and objects; nonsterile components employed and incorporated before terminal sterilization; inappropriate conditions within the restricted compounding environment; prolonged presterilization procedures with aqueous preparations; and nonsterile dosage forms used to compound CSPs.

The characteristics described below for low-risk, medium-risk, and high-risk CSPs are intended as a guide to the breadth and depth of care necessary in compounding, but they are neither exhaustive nor prescriptive. The licensed health care professionals who supervise compounding are responsible for determining the procedural and environmental quality practices and attributes that are necessary for the risk level they assign to specific CSPs.

These risk levels apply to the quality of CSPs immediately after the final aseptic mixing or filling or immediately after the final sterilization, unless precluded by the specific characteristics of the preparation, such as lipid-based emulsions where administration must be completed within 12 hours of preparation. Upon subsequent storage and shipping of freshly finished CSPs, an increase in the risks of chemical degradation of ingredients, contamination from physical damage to packaging, and permeability of plastic and elastomeric packaging is expected. In such cases, compounding personnel consider the potential additional risks to the integrity of CSPs when assigning beyond-use dates. The pre-administration exposure duration and temperature limits specified in the following low-risk, medium-risk, and high-risk level sections apply in the absence of direct testing results or appropriate information sources that justify different limits for specific CSPs. For a summary of the criteria according to risk levels, please see the *Appendix*.

Low-Risk Level CSPs

CSPs compounded under all of the following conditions are at a low risk of contamination.

Low-Risk Conditions—

1. The CSPs are compounded with aseptic manipulations entirely within ISO Class 5 (see *Table 1*) or better air quality using only sterile ingredients, products, components, and devices.
2. The compounding involves only transfer, measuring, and mixing manipulations with closed or sealed packaging systems that are performed promptly and attentively.
3. Manipulations are limited to aseptically opening ampuls, penetrating sterile stoppers on vials with sterile needles and syringes, and transferring sterile liquids in sterile syringes to sterile administration devices and packages of other sterile products.
4. For a low-risk preparation, in the absence of passing a sterility test, the storage periods cannot exceed the following time periods: before administration, the CSPs are properly stored and are exposed for not more than 48 hours at controlled room temperature (see *General Notices and Requirements*), for not more than 14 days at a cold temperature (see *General Notices and Requirements*), and for 45 days in solid frozen state at −20° or colder.

Examples of Low-Risk Compounding—
1. Single transfers of sterile dosage forms from ampuls, bottles, bags, and vials using sterile syringes with sterile needles, other administration devices, and other sterile containers. The contents of ampuls require sterile filtration to remove any glass particles.
2. Manually measuring and mixing no more than three manufactured products to compound drug admixtures and nutritional solutions.

Quality Assurance—Quality assurance practices include, but are not limited to, the following:
1. Routine disinfection and air quality testing of the direct compounding environment to minimize microbial surface contamination and maintain ISO Class 5 air quality (see *Table 1*).
2. Visual confirmation that compounding personnel are properly donning and wearing appropriate items and types of protective garments and goggles.
3. Review of all orders and packages of ingredients to assure the correct identity and amounts of ingredients were compounded.
4. Visual inspection of CSPs to ensure the absence of particulate matter in solutions, the absence of leakage from vials and bags, and the accuracy and thoroughness of labeling.

Example of a Media-Fill Test Procedure—This, or an equivalent test, is performed at least annually by each person authorized to compound in a low-risk level under conditions that closely simulate the most challenging or stressful conditions encountered during compounding of low-risk level CSPs. Once begun, this test is completed without interruption. Within an ISO Class 5 air quality environment, (see *Table 1*) three sets of four 5-mL aliquots of sterile Soybean–Casein Digest Medium are transferred with the same sterile 10-mL syringe and vented needle combination into separate sealed empty sterile 30-mL clear vials (i.e., four 5-mL aliquots into each of three 30-mL vials). Sterile adhesive seals are aseptically affixed to the rubber closures on the three filled vials, then the vials are incubated as described in the *Personnel Training and Evaluation in Aseptic Manipulation Skills* section.

Medium-Risk Level CSPs

When CSPs are compounded aseptically under *Low-Risk Conditions*, and one or more of the following conditions exists, such CSPs are at a medium risk of contamination.

Medium-Risk Conditions—
1. Multiple individual or small doses of sterile products are combined or pooled to prepare a CSP that will be administered either to multiple patients or to one patient on multiple occasions.
2. The compounding process includes complex aseptic manipulations other than the single-volume transfer.
3. The compounding process requires unusually long duration, such as that required to complete dissolution or homogeneous mixing.
4. The sterile CSPs do not contain broad-spectrum bacteriostatic substances, and they are administered over several days (e.g., an externally worn or implanted infusion device).
5. For a medium-risk preparation, in the absence of passing a sterility test, the storage periods cannot exceed the following time periods: before administration, the CSPs are properly stored and are exposed for not more than 30 hours at controlled room temperature (see *General Notices and Requirements*), for not more than 7 days at a cold temperature (see *General Notices and Requirements*), and for 45 days in solid frozen state at −20° or colder.

Examples of Medium-Risk Compounding—
1. Compounding of total parenteral nutrition fluids using manual or automated devices during which there are multiple injections, detachments, and attachments of nutrient source products to the device or machine to deliver all nutritional components to a final sterile container.
2. Filling of reservoirs of injection and infusion devices with multiple sterile drug products and evacuation of air from those reservoirs before the filled device is dispensed.
3. Filling of reservoirs of injection and infusion devices with volumes of sterile drug solutions that will be administered over several days at ambient temperatures between 25° and 40°.
4. Transfer of volumes from multiple ampuls or vials into a single, final sterile container or product.

Quality Assurance—Quality assurance procedures for medium-risk level CSPs include all those for low-risk level CSPs, as well as a more challenging media-fill test passed annually, or more frequently.

Example of a Media-Fill Test Procedure—This, or an equivalent test, is performed under conditions that closely simulate the most challenging or stressful conditions encountered during compounding. This test is completed without interruption within an ISO Class 5 air quality environment (see *Table 1*). Six 100-mL aliquots of sterile Soybean–Casein Digest Medium are aseptically transferred by gravity through separate tubing sets into separate evacuated sterile containers. The six containers are then arranged as three pairs, and a sterile 10-mL syringe and 18-gauge needle combination is used to exchange two 5-mL aliquots of medium from one container to the other container in the pair. For example, after a 5-mL aliquot from the first container is added to the second container in the pair, the second container is agitated for 10 seconds, then a 5-mL aliquot is removed and returned to the first container in the pair. The first container is then agitated for 10 seconds, and the next 5-mL aliquot is transferred from it back to the second container in the pair. Following the two 5-mL aliquot exchanges in each pair of containers, a 5-mL aliquot of medium from each container is aseptically injected into a sealed empty sterile 10-mL clear vial using a sterile 10-mL syringe and vented needle. Sterile adhesive seals are aseptically affixed to the rubber closures on the three filled vials, then the vials are incubated as described in the *Personnel Training and Evaluation in Aseptic Manipulation Skills* section.

High-Risk Level CSPs

CSPs compounded under any of the following conditions are either contaminated or at a high risk to become contaminated with infectious microorganisms.

High-Risk Conditions—
1. Nonsterile ingredients, including manufactured products for routes of administration—other than those listed under *c.* in the *Introduction*—are incorporated or a nonsterile device is employed before terminal sterilization.
2. Sterile ingredients, components, devices, and mixtures are exposed to air quality inferior to ISO Class 5 (see *Table 1*). This includes storage in environments inferior to ISO Class 5 of opened or partially used packages of manufactured sterile products that lack antimicrobial preservatives.
3. Nonsterile preparations are exposed for at least 6 hours before being sterilized.
4. It is assumed, and not verified by examination of labeling and documentation from suppliers or by direct determination, that the chemical purity and content strength of ingredients meet their original or compendial specifications in unopened or in opened packages of bulk ingredients (see *Ingredient Selection* under *Pharmaceutical Compounding—Nonsterile Preparations* ⟨795⟩).
5. For a high-risk preparation, in the absence of passing a sterility test, the storage periods cannot exceed the following time periods: before administration, the CSPs are properly stored and are exposed for not more than 24 hours at

USP DI

Selected USP General Notices and Chapters   VI/47

controlled room temperature (see *General Notices and Requirements*), for not more than 3 days at a cold temperature (see *General Notices and Requirements*), and for 45 days in solid frozen state at –20° or colder.

All nonsterile measuring, mixing, and purifying devices are rinsed thoroughly with sterile, pyrogen-free water, and then thoroughly drained or dried immediately before use for high-risk compounding. All high-risk CSP solutions subjected to terminal steam sterilization are passed through a filter with a nominal porosity not larger than 1.2 μm preceding or during filling into their final containers. Sterilization of high-risk level CSPs by filtration is conducted entirely with an ISO Class 5 or superior air quality environment (see *Table 1*).

Examples of High-Risk Compounding—
1. Dissolving nonsterile bulk drug and nutrient powders to make solutions, which will be terminally sterilized.
2. Sterile ingredients, components, devices, and mixtures are exposed to air quality inferior to ISO Class 5 (see *Table 1*). This includes storage in environments inferior to ISO Class 5 of opened or partially used packages of manufactured sterile products that lack antimicrobial preservatives.
3. Measuring and mixing sterile ingredients in nonsterile devices before sterilization is performed.
4. Assuming, without appropriate evidence or direct determination, that packages of bulk ingredients contain at least 95% by weight of their active chemical moiety and have not been contaminated or adulterated between uses.

Quality Assurance—Quality assurance procedures for high-risk level CSPs include all those for low-risk level CSPs. In addition, a media-fill test that represents high-risk level compounding is performed semi-annually by each person authorized to compound high-risk level CSPs.

Example of a Media-Fill Test Procedure—This, or an equivalent test, is performed under conditions that closely simulate the most challenging or stressful conditions encountered when compounding high-risk level CSPs. This test is completed without interruption in the following sequence:

1. Dissolve 3 g of nonsterile commercially available Soybean–Casein Digest Medium in 100 mL of nonbacteriostatic water to make a 3% solution.
2. Draw 25 mL of the medium into each of three 30-mL sterile syringes. Transfer 5 mL from each syringe into separate sterile 10-mL vials. These vials are the controls, and they generate exponential microbial growth, indicated by visible turbidity upon incubation.
3. Under aseptic conditions and using aseptic techniques, affix a sterile 0.2-μm porosity filter unit and a 20-gauge needle to each syringe. Inject the next 10 mL from each syringe into three separate 10-mL sterile vials. Repeat the process into three more vials. Label all vials, affix sterile adhesive seals to the closure of the nine vials, and incubate them at 25° to 35°. Inspect for microbial growth over 14 days as described in the *Personnel Training and Evaluation in Aseptic Manipulation Skills* section.▲*USP27*

Delete the following:

▲VALIDATION

The sterilization or aseptic processing of an SP should be in accordance with properly designed and validated written procedures. The act of validation of a sterilization or aseptic process involves planned testing designed to demonstrate that microorganisms will be effectively destroyed, removed, or prevented from inadvertently being introduced by personnel or by process-related activities.

Sterilization Processes

A high-risk SP prepared from nonsterile ingredients or components should be sterilized using an appropriate sterilization process, such as filtration or heat sterilization. In general, each sterilization process should be validated to demonstrate suitability for its intended purpose and specific manner of intended uses.

STERILIZATION BY FILTRATION

A sterilizing filtration process should be capable of removing microorganisms from the liquid SP. Commercially available presterilized filtration devices should be certified to be appropriate for human use in sterile pharmaceutical applications, have a pore size of 0.2 μm or smaller (generally recognized as a sterilizing filter), and have been lot tested for retention of *Pseudomonas diminuta* at a minimum concentration of 10^7 organisms per cm^2 under specified operating parameters. The individual devices should be tested for membrane and housing integrity, nonpyrogenicity, and extractables by the manufacturer. Such devices should be capable of sterilizing an SP (see *Sterilization and Sterility Assurance of Compendial Articles* ⟨1211⟩). Before using such devices, the pharmacist should thoroughly evaluate their suitability for the intended SP and conditions of use.

The size and configuration of filtration devices should accommodate the volume being filtered to permit complete filtration within a reasonable period of time and without clogging to the point where mid-process filter changes would be required.

Filters and associated devices and apparatus (housing, gaskets, etc.) should be physically and chemically compatible with the product to be filtered and should be capable of withstanding the temperatures, pressures, and hydrostatic stresses imposed on the system. These capabilities are to be established through appropriate product-specific testing. To establish compatibility, the pharmacy may rely on vendor certification or on definitive evidence, specific to product and filter, obtained from a critical review of the literature or from reliable unpublished research.

Validation should be established experimentally for all filtration apparatus involving assembly in the pharmacy of the membrane (filtration medium) into its housing or holder. The pharmacy may rely on vendor certification of validation for commercially available presterilized ready-to-use filter devices or for pharmacy-assembled apparatus. (The sterilization process used for pharmacy-assembled apparatus must be properly validated.) When initially selecting a commercially available, sterile, pre-assembled filter device, the pharmacist should ensure that the vendor has validated the filter for the intended conditions of use and that an adequate challenge was used (minimum concentration of 10^7 organisms *Pseudomonas diminuta* per cm^2 of filter surface). Validation should encompass the filtration apparatus and configuration, duration of filtration, filtration operating conditions (filtration rate and temperature), and the critical product formulation parameters (pH, viscosity, ionic strength, and osmolarity) used to generate the supplied data are representative of the pharmacy's product, apparatus, specified operating parameters, etc., in regard to the factors that might physically or chemically alter filter integrity, affect microbial capture mechanisms, or shrink the microorganism during filtration.

Each filter device used for product sterilization should be checked for integrity at the time of use. Integrity testing of commercially available, sterile, self-contained filter devices requiring no preuse assembly may be performed at the conclusion of the filtration process. Filter integrity test kits suitable for pharmacy use (for example, those consisting of a small gauge and a three-way stopcock assembly) are commercially available for testing the bubble point of small disk-type filters. For pharmacy-assembled apparatus, as defined above, prefiltration integrity testing is recommended in addition to postfiltration testing. Quantitative integrity testing, such as the bubble-point or forward flow tests (see *Sterilization and Sterility Assurance of*

Compendial Articles ⟨1211⟩) should be used, as appropriate for larger filtration devices or when *Category II* high-risk SPs are sterilized.

Filtration should be performed in accordance with written procedures that list those filters determined to be acceptable for the various SPs to be filtered in the pharmacy or in accordance with master batch formulas that include definitive filter specifications. Filtration procedures and master batch formulas should also describe acceptable techniques for using and for checking the integrity of all listed filters. Fluid-filter compatibility must be established prior to the filtration of any SP not included in the procedure.

HEAT STERILIZATION

Terminal sterilization should be used when sterilizing *Category II* high-risk SPs. Sterilization may be accomplished in the final sealed container as a validated, controlled moist heat process (see *Sterilization and Sterility Assurance of Compendial Articles* ⟨1211⟩). In the absence of heat sterilization capabilities, or where heat labile drug products or container-closure systems preclude heat sterilization, an SP may be sterilized by filtration and aseptically processed and controlled in accordance with the standards set forth in this chapter.

Heat sterilization processes should be validated to ensure that the likelihood of survival of the most resistant microorganisms likely to constitute product bioburden is no greater than 10^{-6} under the specified operating conditions and parameters, such as sterilization time and temperature, size and nature of load, and chamber loading configuration. The validation and monitoring of heat sterilization processes should be in writing with all critical parameters specified, should be followed each time of use, and should be supervised by a pharmacist knowledgeable of the technology involved in the sterilization of drug products. Monitoring data should be recorded properly to ensure, retrospectively, that the processes were carried out as specified and that all critical parameters were within specified limits during processing.[1] ▲*USP27*

Add the following:

▲VERIFICATION OF COMPOUNDING ACCURACY AND STERILIZATION

The compounding procedures and sterilization methods for CSPs correspond to correctly designed and verified written documentation in the compounding facility. Verification requires planned testing designed to demonstrate effectiveness of all procedures critical to the accuracy and purity of finished CSPs. For example, sterility testing (see *Test for Sterility of the Product to be Examined* under *Sterility Tests* ⟨71⟩) may be applied to specimens of low- and medium-risk CSPs, and standard nonpathogenic bacterial cultures may be added to nondispensable specimens of high-risk CSPs before terminal sterilization for subsequent evaluation by sterility testing. Packaged and labeled CSPs are visually inspected for physical integrity and expected appearance, including final fill amount. To ensure that the identities and concentrations of ingredients are accurate, and in the absence of reliable observations and data to confirm and extrapolate those parameters, samples of CSPs are assayed.

Delete the following:

▲[1] PDA Technical Monograph No. 1, Validation of Steam Sterilization Cycles, 1978. ▲*USP27*

Sterilization Methods

The licensed health care professionals who supervise compounding are responsible for determining that the selected sterilization method (see *Methods of Sterilization* under *Sterilization and Sterility Assurance of Compendial Articles* ⟨1211⟩) both sterilizes and maintains the strength, purity, quality, and packaging integrity of CSPs. The selected sterilization process is expected from experience and appropriate information sources— and, preferably, verified wherever possible—to achieve sterility in the particular CSPs. General guidelines for matching CSPs and components to appropriate sterilization methods include the following:

1. CSPs have been ascertained to remain physically and chemically stable when subjected to the selected sterilization method.
2. Glass and metal devices may be covered tightly with aluminum foil, then exposed to dry heat in an oven at a mean temperature of 250° for 2 hours to achieve sterility and depyrogenation (see *Dry-Heat Sterilization* under *Sterilization and Sterility Assurance of Compendial Articles* ⟨1211⟩). Such items are either used immediately or stored until use in an environment suitable for compounding low- and medium-risk CSPs.
3. Personnel ascertain from appropriate information sources that the sterile microporous membrane filter used to sterilize CSP solutions, either during compounding or administration, is chemically and physically compatible with the CSP.

STERILIZATION BY FILTRATION

Commercially available sterile filters must be approved for human-use applications in sterilizing pharmaceutical fluids. Both filters that must be sterilized before processing CSPs and those filters that are commercially available, disposable, sterile, and pyrogen-free have a nominal porosity of 0.2 µm, which includes 0.22-µm porosity. They should be certified by the manufacturer to retain at least 10^7 microorganisms of a strain of *Brevundimonas* (*Pseudomonas*) *diminuta* on each cm² of upstream filter surface under conditions similar to those in which the CSPs will be sterilized. In emergency situations when sterile 0.2-µm porosity membranes are not available, filters of the same composition and 0.45-µm nominal porosity may be used. Sterilizing filters with 0.2-µm and 0.45-µm nominal porosities will not remove bacterial endotoxins and viruses by physical retention.

The supervising health care professional must ensure, directly or from appropriate documentation, that the filters are chemically and physically stable at the pressure and temperature conditions to be used, and that the filters will achieve sterility and maintain prefiltration pharmaceutical quality of the specific CSP. The filter dimensions and material must permit the sterilization process to be completed rapidly without the replacement of the filter during the process. When CSPs are known to contain excessive particulate matter, a prefilter or larger porosity membrane is placed upstream from the sterilizing filter to remove gross particulate contaminants in order to maximize the efficiency of the sterilizing filter.

When filter devices are assembled from separate nonsterile components by compounding personnel, such devices shall be identified to be sterile and ascertained to be effective under relevant conditions before they are used to sterilize CSPs. For example, sterility can be identified using biological indicators (see *Biological Indicators* ⟨1035⟩). Filter units used to sterilize CSPs can also be subjected to the manufacturer's recommended integrity test, such as the bubble point test.

When commercially available sterile disposable filter devices are used, the compounding personnel may accept the written certification from suppliers that the filters retain at least 10^7 cfu, of *Brevundimonas* (*Pseudomonas*) *diminuta* on each cm² of filter surface. Compounding personnel must ascertain that selected filters will achieve sterilization of the particular CSPs being

sterilized. Large deviations from usual or expected chemical and physical properties of CSPs may cause undetectable damage to filter integrity and shrinkage of microorganisms to sizes smaller than filter porosity.

Sterile, commercially available sterilizing filter devices for use on handheld syringes may be checked by feeling for greater resistance on the plunger when filtering air after an aqueous fluid has been filtered.

STEAM STERILIZATION

The process of thermal sterilization employing saturated steam under pressure, or autoclaving, is the preferred method to terminally sterilize aqueous preparations that have been verified to maintain their full chemical and physical stability under the conditions employed (see *Steam Sterilization* under *Sterilization and Sterility Assurance of Compendial Articles* ⟨1211⟩). To achieve sterility, it is necessary that all materials be exposed to steam at 121°, under a pressure of about one atmosphere or 15 psi, for the duration verified by testing to achieve sterility of the items, which is usually 20 to 60 minutes for CSPs. An allowance must be made for the time required for the material to reach 121° before the sterilization exposure duration is timed.

Items that are not directly exposed to pressurized steam may result in survival of microbial organisms and spores. Before their sterilization, plastic, glass, and metal devices are tightly wrapped in low particle shedding paper or fabrics, or sealed in envelopes that prevent poststerilization microbial penetration. Immediately before filling ampuls and vials that will be steam sterilized, solutions are passed through a filter having a porosity not larger than 1.2 μm for removal of particulate matter. Sealed containers must be able to generate steam internally; thus, stoppered and crimped empty vials must contain a small amount of moisture to generate steam.

The description of steam sterilization conditions and duration for specific CSPs is included in written documentation in the compounding facility. The effectiveness of steam sterilization is verified using appropriate biological indicators (see *Biological Indicators* ⟨1035⟩) or other confirmation methods (see *Sterilization and Sterility Assurance of Compendial Articles* ⟨1211⟩ or *Sterility Tests* ⟨71⟩).▲USP27

Delete the following:

▲ASEPTIC PROCESSING

All aseptic processing operations and configurations should be adequately established by media-fill validation.[2] Media fills should simulate as closely as possible actual aseptic operations. All manipulations, handling, environmental conditions, and other factors likely to influence the risk of process-associated contamination should be represented by the media-fill simulations. The intensity of such challenges should represent the greatest risk that would be expected during normal production. Media-fill validations should be repeated with sufficient frequency to ensure the ongoing capability of performing properly each aseptic processing operation used in the authorized facility. The frequency and results of media-fill runs should be documented.

The culture medium selected should be capable of supporting the growth of a broad spectrum of microorganisms likely to be production-associated contaminants in the authorized facility. Commercially available media can be obtained that, when reconstituted as directed by the manufacturer, are certified to have growth-promoting properties. Soybean–Casein Digest Medium is acceptable (see *Sterility Tests* ⟨71⟩). Incubation of medium-filled units should take at least 14 days and may be at

Delete the following:

▲[2] FDA Guideline on Sterile Drug Products Produced by Aseptic Processing, June 1987, pp. 20-27; PDA Technical Monograph No. 2, Validation of Aseptic Filling for Solution Drug Products, 1980.▲USP27

room temperature for 14 days or may be at room temperature for the first 7 days, with the final 1 to 7 days at 30° to 35°. Alternate suitable incubation schedules may be used as determined by the pharmacy to ensure enough growth of any potential contaminating microorganisms to be visually detectable. Microorganisms in all medium-filled units showing visible evidence of microbial growth should be promptly identified, and if this growth exceeds the action limits, an immediate investigation should be made with prompt correction of any identifiable causes of the failure. Review of environmental monitoring data obtained during the media fill should be included in the investigation, as well as a review of the cleaning, sanitizing, disinfection, production procedures, aseptic technique, personnel practices, and other factors as appropriate. Revalidation should occur after all media-fill failures (see *Table 1*).

Table 1. Media-Fill Validation of Aseptic Processing

Validation Purpose	Minimum Validation Requirements	
	Low- and Medium-Risk CSPs	High Risk CSPs[*]
General Initial	Personnel validation 3 consecutive media-fill runs without contamination	Process validation 3 consecutive media-fill runs without contamination
Revalidation	1 media-fill run quarterly without contamination	annual media-fill run without contamination
Failure Revalidation	3 consecutive media-fill runs without contamination	3 consecutive media-fill runs without contamination

[*] NOTE—Personnel should have first passed low- and medium-risk validation.▲USP27

Delete the following:

▲LOW-RISK OPERATIONS

A quality assurance program should include a system that incorporates validation and monitoring processes that ensure a compounded sterile preparation meets predetermined, specific criteria of quality. The primary objective of the validation of aseptic processing involving low-risk operations is to ensure that personnel are capable of using effective aseptic technique to compound an SP successfully under the most rigorous conditions encountered during normal work assignments. The validation program should include a system of proofs that show that processes and operators are appropriate for achieving predefined product-quality conditions and personnel have skills to perform those compounding activities reproducibly and repeatedly. The validation of the process includes media fills consisting of a planned repetitive sequence of compounded or repackaged units. The number of manipulations of each unit and the number of units in each media fill should reflect the most complex and prolonged aseptic manipulations likely to be encountered by an operator as a normal workload requirement. The number of units per media-fill run should be enough to ensure that the operator is capable of replicating acceptable aseptic procedures. A sampling plan and validation requirements are defined in written procedures. Media transfers could be used to represent procedures such as syringe transfers, use of automated compounding devices, multiple additive procedures, and various aseptic assemblies and connections. An example of a validation procedure for low-risk operations is as follows.

Scenario—A pharmacy prepares antibiotics, hydration solutions, and parenteral nutrition solutions. Low-risk CSP processing would include the reconstitution and preparation of antibiotics for administration of single units at set intervals. Many of these products are prepared in batches and stored in anticipation of future use. Operators should be trained and their techniques validated using a sterile culture medium to simulate the syringe

transfer of diluent to reconstitute lyophilized antibiotics, the transfer of that product to an empty sterile bag, bottle, or syringe; and any other manipulations that may be routine in the admixture processes.

Example of a Validation Procedure—Six 25-mL aliquots of sterile Soy–Casein Digest Medium are aseptically transferred to separate, empty 30-mL sterile vials. Ten milliliters of sterile Soy–Casein Digest Medium is removed from one of the vials and added to a vial of sterile, lyophilized Polyethylene Glycol. Four 2.5-mL aliquots of the resulting solution are added to 30-mL vials already containing 25-mL sterile Soy–Casein Digest Medium, and the vials are labeled. The six 30-mL vials are incubated at room temperature for a total of 14 days, with frequent checks for growth.

Media fills should be representative of peak periods of fatigue, stress, and pacing demands. For example, media fills could be scheduled immediately after normal production activity has ended. Media fills should not be performed during normal production.

Operators should pass an initial validation, performing three media fills with no contamination, before they are allowed to compound CSPs for patients. Subsequently, each operator should perform at least one media fill involving low-risk operations quarterly. If one contaminated unit results from a media fill, the operator should be retrained and then perform three consecutive media fills with no evidence of contamination before resuming preparation of CSPs for patients. Operators should also be revalidated if the nature of their aseptic compounding assignments changes to the extent that their previous media fills are not representative of their revised assignments.

Quality assurance programs for low-risk CSPs also include a system that employs routine methods to ensure that the finished products are reviewed for compounding accuracy and potential hazards, such as particulate matter, microorganisms, pyrogens, allergens, and cross-contamination from other drugs that may have been introduced into the compounding environment. Final products are inspected for particulate matter and leakage before release. A predetermined percentage of compounded products could be sequestered for routine sterility and pyrogen testing. Allergens and cross-contamination are best controlled through the strict adherence to proper procedures, which limit or eliminate the introduction of the allergens, and to frequent cleaning to reduce the potential of lingering drug residues in the work area. Personnel are trained in the proper methods of eliminating allergens and cleaning and disinfecting the workstation. That training is reviewed periodically.▲*USP27*

Delete the following:

▲HIGH-RISK OPERATIONS

In the case of high-risk operations, the focus of validation is on the process as well as personnel capability. Thus, the primary objective of the validation of aseptic processing for high-risk CSP operations is to ensure that the aseptic process is capable of being carried out consistently under control by any qualified operator, before the process is utilized for production of units intended for administration to patients. Accordingly, each type of high-risk operation is validated independently, rather than having operators perform representative sets of aseptic activities, as is the case with low-risk and medium-risk aseptic operations.

Personnel assigned to high-risk aseptic operations should be validated for low-risk and medium-risk operations as described above. In addition, this personnel should participate, at least annually, in the validation of each high-risk aseptic operation to which they are assigned.

For example, for high-risk operations involving nonsterile components, the media-fill run should simulate as closely as possible the most intensive conditions likely to be encountered during the normal production activities. The number of units in a media-fill run should be no less than the largest number of units

encountered during production involving the process being validated. However, the fill volume of media-fill units need not equal the fill volume of finished product units.

A media-fill run should be performed at least annually for each unique high-risk batch processing procedure and configuration. A media-fill failure for most operations (less than 1000 units) is one or more contaminated units after incubation. For batches equal to or greater than 1000 units, a media-fill failure is greater than one contaminated unit. When a media-fill failure occurs, three consecutive successful media fills should occur before the process failing the media fill may be used for the preparation of a CSP for patients. An example of a validation procedure for a high-risk operation is as follows:

Scenario—A pharmacy prepares individual cassettes of morphine for epidural use from morphine powder. The nonsterile powder is weighed, and then placed in the barrel of a 60-mL syringe. After replacing the syringe plunger, sterile 5% dextrose solution is drawn into the syringe to make a total volume of 50 mL. After shaking to dissolve the powder, a 0.22-µm disk filter is placed on the syringe, and the solution is pushed through the filter into a drug reservoir cassette for an ambulatory infusion pump. Typically, the pharmacy prepares a week's supply of two to three cassettes at one time.

Example of a Validation Procedure—A small quantity of an inert powder (for example, lactose or sugar) is placed in the barrel of a 60-mL syringe. After replacing the syringe plunger, sterile 5% dextrose solution is withdrawn into the syringe to make a total volume of 50 mL. A sterile 0.22-µm filter is connected to the syringe tip. After shaking to dissolve the powder, the solution is pushed through the filter: the first 5 mL are aseptically introduced into a test tube containing 10 mL of sterile Soybean–Casein Digest Medium; the next 40 mL are discarded in a sterile container; and the last 5 mL are aseptically introduced into another tube containing 10 mL of sterile Soybean–Casein Digest Medium. At least three syringes should be evaluated in this manner. The inoculated tubes of Medium should be incubated at 20° to 25° for 14 days, with frequent visual observations made for growth of microorganisms.▲*USP27*

Add the following:

▲PERSONNEL TRAINING AND EVALUATION IN ASEPTIC MANIPULATION SKILLS

Personnel who prepare CSPs must be provided with appropriate training from expert personnel, audio–video instructional sources, and professional publications in the theoretical principles and practical skills of aseptic manipulations before they begin to prepare CSPs. Compounding personnel shall perform didactic review, and pass written and media-fill testing of aseptic manipulative skills initially; at least annually thereafter for low- and medium-risk level compounding; and semi-anually for high-risk level compounding. Compounding personnel who fail written tests, or whose media-fill test vials result in gross microbial colonization, must be immediately re-instructed and re-evaluated by expert compounding personnel to assure correction of all aseptic practice deficiencies.

Media-Fill Challenge Testing—The skill of personnel to aseptically prepare CSPs may be evaluated using sterile fluid bacterial culture media-fill validation,[1] (i.e., sterile bacterial culture medium transfer via a sterile syringe and needle). Media-fill testing is used to assess the quality of the aseptic skill of compounding personnel. Media-fill tests represent the most challenging or stressful conditions actually encountered by the personnel being evaluated when they prepare particular risk level CSPs and when sterilizing high-risk level CSPs.

Commercially available sterile fluid culture media, such as Soybean–Casein Digest Medium (see *Sterility Tests* ⟨71⟩), shall be able to promote exponential colonization of bacteria that are

---

[1] FDA Guideline on Sterile Drug Products Produced by Aseptic Processing, June 1987, pp. 20-27; PDA Technical Monograph No. 2, Validation of Aseptic Filling for Solution Drug Products, 1980.

most likely to be transmitted to CSPs from the compounding personnel and environment. Media-filled vials are incubated at 25° to 35° for 14 days. Failure is indicated by visible turbidity in the medium on or before 14 days.

Example of a Media-Fill Test Procedure—Perform the test as directed in the section *Quality Assurance of Low-Risk Level CSPs*.▲*USP27*

Change to read:

ENVIRONMENTAL QUALITY AND CONTROL

Achieving and maintaining sterility and overall freedom from contamination of a pharmaceutical product is dependent upon the quality status of the components incorporated, the process utilized, personnel performance, and the environmental conditions under which the process is performed. The standards required for the environmental conditions depend upon the amount of exposure of the CSP to the immediate environment anticipated during processing. The quality and control of environmental conditions for ▲each risk level of operation▲*USP27* is explained in this section. In addition, operations using nonsterile components require the use of a method of preparation designed to produce a sterile product.

Critical Site Exposure

The degree of exposure of the product during processing will be affected by the length of time of exposure, the size of the critical site exposed, and the nature of the critical site.

A critical site is any opening providing a direct pathway between a sterile product and the environment or any surface coming in direct contact with the product and the environment. The risk of such a site picking up contamination from the environment increases with time of exposure. Therefore, the processing plan and the intent of the operator should give due consideration to organization, efficiency, and speed in order to keep such exposure time to a minimum. For example, an ampul should not be opened unnecessarily in advance of use.

The size of the critical site affects the risk of contamination entering the product: the greater the exposed area, the greater the risk. An open vial or bottle exposes to contamination a critical site of much larger area than the tip of a 26-gauge needle. Therefore, the risk of contamination when entering an open vial or bottle is much greater than during the momentary exposure of a needle tip.

The nature of a critical site also affects the risk of contamination. The relatively rough, permeable surface of ▲an elastomeric▲*USP27* closure retains microorganisms and other contaminants, after swabbing with an alcohol pad, more readily than does the smooth glass surface of the neck of an ampul. Therefore, the surface disinfection can be expected to be more effective for an ampul. ▲Once the ampul is open, the critical site of exposure is greatly increased, creating a pathway with the potential for introduction of glass, fiber, and dust into the fluid contained in the ampul.▲*USP27*

The prevention or elimination of airborne particles must be given high priority. ▲▲*USP27* Airborne contaminants are much more likely to reach critical sites than contaminants that are adhering to the floor or other surfaces below the work level. Further, particles that are relatively large or of high density settle from the airspace more quickly and thus can be removed from the vicinity of critical sites.

▲Clean Rooms and Barrier Isolators

In general, sterile product preparation facilities utilize laminar airflow workbenches (LAFWs) to provide an adequate critical site environment. A discussion of the necessary facilities and proper procedures for preparing sterile products using LAFWs in clean rooms is presented below. The use of alternative systems in clean rooms that have been verified to achieve the same or better level of environmental quality as that achieved by properly operated LAFWs may also be utilized. An emerging alternative technology utilizes barrier isolator systems to minimize the extent of personnel contact and interaction, to separate the external environment from the critical site, and to provide an ISO Class 5 environment (see *Table 1*) for preparing CSPs. A well-designed positive pressure barrier isolator, supported by adequate procedures for its maintenance, monitoring, and control, may offer an acceptable alternative to the use of conventional LAFWs in clean rooms for aseptic processing. An example of the arrangement of a clean-room floor plan for low- and medium-risk level CSPs is illustrated in the first drawing in Figure 1. The second drawing in Figure 1 depicts an appropriate multicompartment clean-room floor plan for high-risk level CSPs.

Environmental Controls

Engineering controls reduce the potential for airborne contamination in workspaces by limiting the amount and size of contaminants in the CSP processing environment. Primary engineering controls are used and generally include horizontal flow clean benches, vertical flow clean benches, biological safety cabinets, and barrier isolators. Primary environmental control must provide at least ISO Class 5 quality of air (see *Table 1*) to which sterile ingredients and components of CSPs are directly exposed. Secondary engineering controls generally provide a buffer zone or buffer room as a core for the location of the workbenches or isolators.

Table 1. International Organization of Standardization (ISO) Classification of Particulate Matter in Room Air
[Limits are in particles 0.5 µm and larger per cubic meter (current ISO) and cubic feet (former Federal Standard No. 209E, FS209E).]*

ISO Class	U.S. FS 209E	ISO, m³	FS 209E, ft.³
3	Class 1	35.2	1
4	Class 10	352	10
5	Class 100	3520	100
6	Class 1000	35,200	1000
7	Class 10,000	352,000	10,000
8	Class 100,000	3,520,000	100,000

Header spanning: Class Name (ISO Class, U.S. FS 209E), Particle Size (ISO, m³; FS 209E, ft.³)

* Adapted from the Federal Standard No. 209E, General Services Administration, Washington, DC, 20407 (September 11, 1992) and ISO [4644-1 : 1999 Clean rooms and associated controlled environments—Part 1: Classification of air cleanliness. For example, 3520 particles of 0.5 µm per m³ or larger (ISO Class 5) is equivalent to 100 particles per ft³ (Class 100) (1 m³ = 34.314 ft.³).

**EXAMPLE OF CLEAN ROOM FLOOR PLAN SUITABLE
FOR LOW AND MEDIUM RISK-LEVEL CSPs**

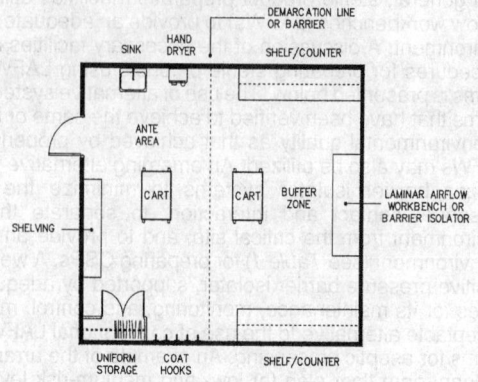

**EXAMPLE OF CLEAN ROOM FLOOR PLAN SUITABLE
FOR HIGH RISK-LEVEL CSPs**

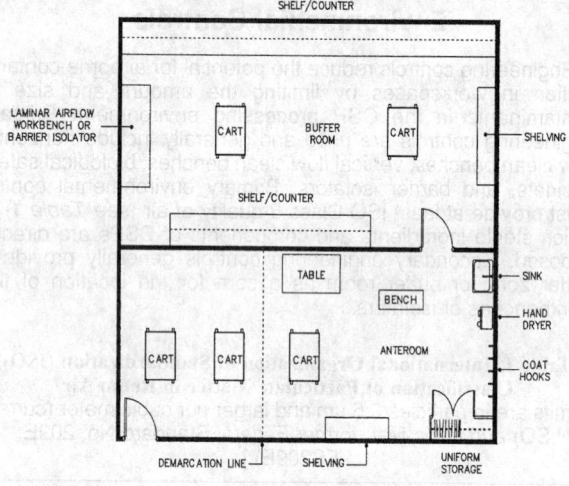

Fig. 1

Airflow through high-efficiency particulate air (HEPA) filters is unidirectional or columnar, and because of the pore size of the filter the "first air" at the face of the filter is, for the purposes of aseptic compounding, free from airborne particulate contamination. Barrier isolators provide a suitable environment by restricting any ambient air from the work chamber. These systems are not as sensitive to external environments as the HEPA-filtered unidirectional airflow units.

Several aspects of barrier isolation and filtered unidirectional airflow in work environment must be understood and practiced in the compounding process. Policies and procedures for maintaining and working in the prescribed conditions for aseptic processing must be prepared, updated, maintained, and implemented and are determined by the scope and risk levels of the activities undertaken in the SP compounding operation.

In general, the CSP work environment is designed to have the cleanest work surfaces (horizontal or vertical clean benches, biological safety cabinets, or isolators) located in a buffer area, which is preceded by an anteroom that provides a clean area for donning personnel barriers, such as hair covers, gloves, gowns, or full clean-room attire. The class limit of the buffer or core room has to be demonstrably better than that of ambient air to reduce the risk of contaminants being blown, dragged, or otherwise introduced into the filtered unidirectional airflow environment. For example, strong air currents from opened doors, personnel traffic, or air streams from the heating, ventilating, and air-conditioning

systems can easily disrupt the unidirectional, columnar airflow in the open-faced workbenches. The operators may also introduce disruptions in flow by their own movements and by the placement of objects onto the work surface.

Buffer or clean-room areas in which LAFWs are located are to provide at least ISO Class 8 air quality (see *Table 1*). Measuring, weighing, mixing, and other manipulations of nonsterile in-process CSPs are also performed in air quality of at least ISO Class 8 (see *Table 1*). Appropriate air conditioning and humidity controls must be in place for the buffer area.▲*USP27*

Tasks carried out within the buffer area should be limited to those for which a controlled environment is necessary. Only the furniture, equipment, supplies, and other goods required for the tasks to be performed may be brought into this room, and they should be nonpermeable, nonshedding, and resistant to disinfectants. Whenever such items are brought into the room, they should first be cleaned and sanitized. Whenever possible, equipment and other items used in the buffer area should not be taken from the room except for calibration, servicing, or other activity associated with the proper maintenance of the item.

The surfaces of ceilings, walls, floors, fixtures, shelving, counters, and cabinets in the buffer area should be smooth, impervious, free from cracks and crevices, and nonshedding, thereby promoting cleanability and minimizing spaces in which microorganisms and other contaminants may accumulate. The surfaces should be resistant to damage by sanitizing agents. Junctures of ceilings to walls should be coved or caulked to avoid cracks and crevices where dirt can accumulate. If ceilings consist of inlaid panels, the panels should be impregnated with a polymer to render them impervious and hydrophobic, and they should be caulked around each perimeter to seal them to the support frame. Walls may be of panels locked together and sealed or of epoxy-coated gypsum board. Preferably, floors are overlaid with wide sheet vinyl flooring with heat-welded seams and coving to the sidewall. Dust-collecting overhangs, such as ceiling utility pipes, or ledges, such as windowsills, should be avoided. The exterior lens surface of ceiling lighting fixtures should be smooth, mounted flush, and sealed. Any other penetrations through the ceiling or walls should be sealed.

The buffer area should contain no sinks or floor drains. Work surfaces should be constructed of smooth, impervious materials, such as stainless steel or molded plastic, so that they are readily cleanable and sanitizable. Carts should be of stainless steel wire or sheet metal construction with good quality, cleanable casters to promote mobility. Storage shelving, counters, and cabinets should be smooth, impervious, free from cracks and crevices, nonshedding, cleanable, and sanitizable. Their number, design, and manner of installation should promote effective cleaning and sanitizing.

▲CSP Environment

The contamination reduction conditions and procedures in this section include LAFWs being located within buffer or clean-room areas that maintain at least an ISO Class 8 (see *Table 1*). It is preferred, but not necessary, to locate barrier isolators within such a buffer air quality area. The frequency and amount of personnel access to buffer air quality areas is restricted to minimize contaminants, while allowing delivery of essential materials for CSPs. Food, drinks, and materials exposed in patient care and treatment areas must never be introduced into areas where components and ingredients for CSPs are present.

In an area near, but physically isolated from the buffer room area—the anteroom area—supplies, such as needles, syringes, ampuls, bags, vials of parenteral fluids, and packages of transfer tubing sets for large-volume fluids are uncartoned and disinfected.

Hand sanitizing and gowning activities also occur in the anteroom area adjacent to the buffer area. Faucet handles are designed to be hands-free. Before processing CSPs, hands are resanitized after donning all appropriate garb, except for gloves. A demarcation line or barrier identifies the separation of the buffer

area from the anteroom area. Compounding personnel must be capable of accessing the buffer area without use of their hands. Anteroom areas adjacent to buffer areas are intended to minimize the introduction of contaminants into buffer areas._▲USP27_

Cleaning and Sanitizing the Workspaces

The cleaning, sanitizing, and organizing of the ▲direct and contiguous compounding areas (DCCA) is_▲USP27_ the responsibility of trained operators (pharmacists and technicians) following written procedures and ▲is_▲USP27_ performed at the beginning of each shift. ▲Before compounding is performed, all items are_▲USP27_ removed from the ▲DCCA and all surfaces are cleaned of loose material and residue from spills, followed by an application of a residue-free sanitizing agent[2] that is left on for a time sufficient to exert its antimicrobial effect._▲USP27_

Work surfaces near the ▲DCCA in the buffer or clean area are_▲USP27_ cleaned in a similar manner, including counter tops and supply carts. Storage shelving ▲is_▲USP27_ emptied of all supplies and then cleaned and sanitized at least weekly, using approved agents.

Floors in the ▲buffer or clean area are_▲USP27_ cleaned by mopping once daily when no aseptic operations are in progress. Mopping may be performed by trained and supervised custodial personnel using approved agents described in the written procedures. Only approved cleaning and sanitizing agents ▲are used_▲USP27_ with careful consideration of compatibilities, effectiveness, and inappropriate or toxic residues. Their schedules of use and methods of application ▲are_▲USP27_ in accord with written procedures. All cleaning tools, such as wipers, sponges, and mops, ▲are_▲USP27_ nonshedding and dedicated to use in the ▲buffer or clean area._▲USP27_ Floor mops may be used in both the ▲buffer or clean area and anteroom area,_▲USP27_ but only in that order. Most wipers ▲are_▲USP27_ discarded after one use. If cleaning tools are reused, their cleanliness ▲is_▲USP27_ maintained by thorough rinsing and sanitization after use and by storing in a clean environment between uses. Trash ▲is_▲USP27_ collected in suitable plastic bags and removed with minimal agitation.

In the ▲anteroom area,_▲USP27_ supplies and equipment removed from shipping cartons ▲are_▲USP27_ wiped with a sanitizing agent, such as sterile 70% isopropyl alcohol (IPA)[3], which is checked periodically for contamination. Alternatively, if supplies are planned to be received in sealed pouches, the pouches can be removed as the supplies are introduced into the ▲buffer or clean area_▲USP27_ without the need to sanitize the individual supply items. No shipping or other external cartons may be taken into the ▲buffer or clean area._▲USP27_ Cleaning and sanitizing of the ▲anteroom area is_▲USP27_ performed at least weekly by trained and supervised custodial personnel, in accordance with written procedures. However, floors are cleaned and sanitized daily, always proceeding from the ▲buffer or clean area to the anteroom area._▲USP27_ Storage shelving ▲is_▲USP27_ emptied of all supplies and cleaned and sanitized at planned intervals, preferably monthly.

These cleaning and sanitizing procedures apply to both low-risk and high-risk operations.

Personnel ▲Cleansing_▲USP27_ and Gowning

Personnel are critical keys to the maintenance of asepsis when carrying out their assigned responsibilities. They must be thoroughly trained in aseptic techniques and be highly motivated to maintain these standards each time they prepare a sterile product.

Prior to entering the ▲buffer or clean area,_▲USP27_ operators should remove outer lab jackets or the like, makeup, and jewelry and should thoroughly scrub hands and arms to the elbow. After drying hands and arms they should properly don clean, nonshedding uniform components, including hair covers, shoe covers, knee-length coats or coveralls, and ▲appropriate protective_▲USP27_ gloves, in that order. The coats should fit snugly at the wrists and be zipped or snapped closed in the front. Shoe covers should be donned so that feet then touch the floor only on the clean side of the bench or other demarcation. Face masks should be donned just ▲before beginning activities in the DCCA to minimize airborne contaminants from coughing, sneezing, and talking.

When preparing CSPs in a vertical flow LAFW with a transparent shield between the face of the operator and sterile components, or when using an isolator, wearing a face mask is optional, but head and facial hair must be covered.

Appropriate powder-free protective gloves are sterile or, if nonsterile, are sanitized with an appropriate antimicrobial cleaner such as 70% alcohol before use. Protective gloves are put on as the last uniform component. When nonsterile gloves, chosen for their chemically protective composition, are used, they are disinfected with sterile 70% isopropyl alcohol or an antimicrobial agent that is allowed to evaporate before beginning compounding procedures. Sterile and sanitized gloves do not remain sterile and clean during compounding activities because they come in contact with nonsterile surfaces and air. Therefore, compounding personnel must be trained to avoid touching sterile surfaces of packages, transfer devices, and components within ISO Class 5 or superior environments (see *Table 1*). During protracted compounding activities, personnel should intermittently resanitize their gloves with sterile 70% isopropyl alcohol._▲USP27_

Proper scrubbing and gowning immediately prior to entry into the ▲buffer or clean area_▲USP27_ is required of all personnel, without exception. Should the operator find it necessary to leave the room, the coat may be carefully removed at the entrance and hung inside out for redonning upon re-entry, but only during the same shift. However, hair covers, masks, shoe covers, and gloves should be discarded and new ones donned prior to re-entry.

For high-risk operations, it is especially critical to minimize the risk of contamination on lab coats, coveralls, and other garb to be worn in the ▲buffer or clean area._▲USP27_ Preferably, fresh clean garb should be donned upon each entry into the ▲buffer or clean area_▲USP27_ to avoid liberating contaminants from previously worn garb. Alternatively, garb that has been worn may be removed with the intention of regarbing for re-entry into the ▲buffer or clean area_▲USP27_ and stored during the interim under proper control and protection in the ▲anteroom area._▲USP27_ Garb worn or taken outside the confines of the ▲anteroom area cannot be worn in the buffer or clean area._▲USP27_

Dispersion of particles from body surfaces, such as from skin rashes, sunburn, or cosmetics, increases the risk of contamination of critical sites and ▲must_▲USP27_ be appropriately controlled or minimized. If severe, the operator ▲must be excluded from the buffer or clean area_▲USP27_ until the condition is remedied, especially for high-risk operations.

---

[2] Approved by the pharmacist in charge.
[3] [NOTE—70% isopropyl alcohol (IPA) may harbor resistant microbial spores. Therefore, IPA used in aseptic areas should always be filtered through a 0.2-μm hydrophobic filter to render it sterile.]

Suggested Standard Operating Procedures

The pharmacy should have written, properly approved standard operating procedures (SOPs) designed to ensure the quality of the environment in which a CSP is prepared. The following procedures are recommended:

(1) Access to the ▲buffer or clean area is▲USP27 restricted to qualified personnel with specific responsibilities or assigned tasks in the area.

(2) All cartoned supplies ▲are decontaminated in the anteroom area▲USP27 by removing them from shipping cartons and wiping ▲or spraying▲USP27 with a disinfecting agent, such as sterile IPA, while being transferred to a clean, sanitized cart or other conveyance for introduction into the ▲buffer or clean area.▲USP27 Individual pouched supplies need not be wiped because the pouches can be removed as these supplies are introduced into the ▲buffer or clean area.▲USP27

(3) Supplies required frequently or otherwise needed close at hand but not necessarily needed for the scheduled operations of the shift ▲are▲USP27 decontaminated and stored on the shelving in the ▲anteroom area.▲USP27

(4) Carts used to bring supplies from the storeroom ▲cannot▲USP27 be rolled beyond the demarcation line in the ▲anteroom area,▲USP27 and carts used in the ▲buffer or clean area cannot▲USP27 be rolled outward beyond the demarcation line unless cleaned and sanitized before returning.

(5) Generally, supplies required for the scheduled operations of the shift ▲are▲USP27 prepared and brought into the ▲buffer or clean area,▲USP27 preferably on one or more movable carts. Supplies that are required for back-up or general support of operations may be stored on the designated shelving in the ▲buffer or clean area,▲USP27 but ▲avoid▲USP27 excessive accumulation of supplies. ▲▲USP27

(6) Objects that shed particles ▲cannot▲USP27 be brought into the ▲buffer or clean area,▲USP27 including pencils, cardboard cartons, paper towels, and cotton items. ▲Only nonshedding paper-related products (boxes, work records, and so forth) can be brought into the buffer or clean area.▲USP27

(7) Traffic flow in and out of the ▲buffer or clean area must be▲USP27 minimized.

(8) Personnel preparing to enter the ▲buffer or clean area must▲USP27 remove all jewelry from hands and arms.

(9) Personnel entering the ▲buffer or clean area must▲USP27 first scrub hands and arms with soap, including using a scrub brush on the fingers and nails. An air dryer or disposable nonshedding towels ▲are▲USP27 used to dry hands and arms after washing.

(10) Personnel entering the ▲buffer or clean area,▲USP27 after scrubbing, should don attire as described under ▲Personnel Cleansing and Gowning.▲USP27

(11) No chewing gum, candy, or food items may be brought into the ▲buffer or clean area or anteroom area.

(12) At the beginning of each compounding activity session, and after liquids are spilled, the surfaces of the direct compounding environment are first cleaned with Purified Water to remove water soluble residues. Immediately thereafter, the same surfaces are sanitized with sterile 70% isopropyl alcohol, or other effective antimicrobial agents, using a nonlinting wipe.

(13) When LAFWs or barrier isolators are used as the ISO Class 5 air quality environment (see Table 1), their blowers must be operated continuously during compounding activity, including during interruptions of less than 8 hours. When the blower is turned off and before other personnel enter to perform compounding activities, only one person can enter the contiguous buffer area for the purposes of turning on the blower (for at least 30 minutes) and of sanitizing the work surfaces.▲USP27

(14) Traffic in the area of the ▲DCCA is▲USP27 minimized and controlled. The ▲DCCA is▲USP27 shielded from all less clean air currents that are of higher velocity than the clean laminar airflow.

(15) Supplies to be utilized in the ▲DCCA▲USP27 for the planned procedures ▲are▲USP27 accumulated and then decontaminated by wiping ▲or spraying▲USP27 the outer surface with IPA or removing the outer wrap at the edge of the ▲DCCA▲USP27 as the item is introduced into the aseptic work area.

(16) After proper introduction into the ▲DCCA▲USP27 of supply items required for and limited to the assigned operations, they ▲are▲USP27 so arranged that a clear, uninterrupted path of HEPA-filtered air will bathe all critical sites at all times during the planned procedures. That is, no objects may be placed behind an exposed critical site in a horizontal position or above in the vertical laminar flow workbench.

(17) All supply items ▲are arranged in the DCCA so as▲USP27 to reduce clutter and to provide maximum efficiency and order for the flow of work.

(18) All procedures ▲are▲USP27 performed in a manner designed to minimize the risk of touch contamination. Gloves ▲are▲USP27 sanitized with adequate frequency ▲with an approved disinfectant.▲USP27

(19) All rubber stoppers of vials and bottles and the neck of ampuls ▲are▲USP27 sanitized with IPA prior to the introduction of a needle or spike for the removal of product.

(20) After the preparation of every admixture, the contents of the container ▲are▲USP27 thoroughly mixed and then inspected for the presence of particulate matter, evidence of incompatibility, or other defects.

(21) After procedures are completed, used syringes, bottles, vials, and other supplies ▲are▲USP27 removed, but with a minimum of exit and re-entry into the ▲DCCA▲USP27 to minimize the risk of introducing contamination into the aseptic workspace.

▲Environmental Monitoring

In addition to the evaluation and verification of personnel aseptic techniques and of the adequacy of compounding processes and procedures (see Personnel Training and Evaluation in Aseptic Manipulation Skills section), assessment and verification of the adequacy of the sterile compounding environment is essential, especially for preparing high-risk preparations. Evaluation of environmental quality is performed by measuring both the total number of particles and the number of viable microorganisms in the controlled air environments of the compounding area.

Certification that each LAFW and barrier isolator is functioning properly and meets the air quality requirement of ISO Class 5 (refer to Clean Rooms and Barrier Isolators and Table 1 in the Environmental Quality and Control section) is performed by a qualified operator(s) using current, state-of-the-art electronic air sampling at least every six months and whenever the LAFW or barrier isolator is relocated. Similarly, the air quality of the buffer or clean area and anteroom area is evaluated by a qualified operator(s) for conformance to ISO Class 7 and ISO Class 8 requirements, as appropriate, at least every six months and when renovations occur. These records are maintained and reviewed by the supervising pharmacist or other designated employee.

Evaluation of airborne microorganisms in the controlled air environments (LAFW, barrier isolators, buffer or clean area, and anteroom area) is performed by properly trained individuals using suitable electric air samplers or by exposing sterile nutrient agar plates for a suitable time frame. For either approach, the air

sampling is performed at locations judged by compounding personnel to be the most prone to contamination during compounding activities: this includes zones of air backwash turbulence within LAFWs and other areas where air backwash turbulence may enter the compounding area. Such evaluations are performed as a regular and ongoing process at least monthly for sterile compounding areas used for low- and medium-risk preparations and at least weekly for areas used for high-risk preparations.

For electric air samplers that actively collect volumes of air for evaluation, the instructions for verification and use of these devices must be followed. When using the passive exposure of sterile nutrient agar settling plates, the covers are removed and the media is exposed for a period usually lasting 1 hour or longer to collect viable microorganisms as they fall from the environment. At the end of the designated exposure period, the plates are recovered and incubated at a temperature and for a time period conducive to multiplication of microorganisms on the nutrient agar—usually at 30° to 35° for a minimum of 48 hours. The number of discrete colonies of microorganisms are then counted and reported as colony forming units (cfu). This provides a measurement of the level of microbial contamination in the air within the tested environment.

The greatest value of viable microorganism monitored in the air of the compounding environment is realized when normal baseline cfu counts are determined over a period of time. Determining the baseline cfu counts permits identification of a trend toward increasing microbial cfu counts. A sufficiently increasing trend in cfu counts over time must prompt a re-evaluation of the adequacy of cleaning procedures, operational procedures, and air filtration efficiency within the sterile compounding location. Action may be warranted when an increasing trend to 50% above the baseline for areas used for high- and medium- risk preparations or to 100% above baseline for areas used for low-risk preparations is found.

A written plan and schedule for the environmental monitoring procedures for airborne microorganisms must be established and followed. The plan must be adequate to evaluate the various controlled air environment areas (LAFW, barrier isolator, buffer or clean area, and anteroom area) of the sterile compounding facility. All compounding personnel are trained in and educated about the importance of this environmental monitoring process. For sterile compounding areas used for low- and medium-risk preparations, a minimum of monthly evaluation is appropriate. For sterile compounding areas used for high-risk preparations, at least weekly evaluation is appropriate. ▲*USP27*

Change to read:

PROCESSING

▲A written description of specific training and performance evaluation program for individuals involved in the use of aseptic techniques for the preparation of sterile products must be developed for each site. This program equips the personnel with the appropriate knowledge and trains them in the required skills necessary to perform the assigned tasks. Each person assigned to the aseptic area in the preparation of sterile products must successfully complete specialized training in aseptic techniques and aseptic area practices prior to preparing CSPs (see *Personnel Training and Evaluation in Aseptic Manipulation Skills* section).

Aseptic Technique

Critical operations are carried out by appropriately trained and qualified personnel in a DCCA using proper aseptic techniques described in a written procedure (see *Suggested Standard Operating Procedures*). Aseptic technique is equally applicable to the preparation of sterile sensitizing and chemotoxic agents. However, it is essential to recognize that additional precautions

must be utilized to protect the personnel and the compounding environment from the potential adverse effects of these chemotoxic products. The minimum requirements for this process include the following: working and verified vertical laminar airflow work bench, barrier isolator, or other environmental containment and control device with biohazard control capabilities; the protective capabilities of gowns, masks, bouffants, and gloves; sprayback and spill control techniques and equipment; the use specialized compounding devices and equipment; and proper disposal.▲*USP27*

Components

▲Compounding personnel ascertain that ingredients for CSPs are of the correct identity and appropriate quality using the following information: vendors' labels, labeling, certificates of analysis, direct chemical analysis, and knowledge of compounding facility storage conditions.▲*USP27*

STERILE ▲INGREDIENTS AND▲*USP27* COMPONENTS

Commercially available sterile drug products, sterile ready-to-use containers and devices are examples of sterile components. A written procedure for unit-by-unit physical inspection preparatory to use ▲is▲*USP27* followed to ensure that these components are sterile, free from defects, and otherwise suitable for their intended use.

NONSTERILE ▲INGREDIENTS AND▲*USP27* COMPONENTS

▲If any nonsterile components, including containers, devices, and ingredients are used to make a CSP, such CSPs must be compounded at a high-risk level. Nonsterile active ingredients and added substances, or excipients, for CSPs should preferably be official *USP* or *NF* articles. When nonofficial ingredients are used, they must be accompanied by certificates of analysis from their suppliers to aid compounding personnel in judging the identity, quality, and purity in relation to the intended use in a particular CSP. Physical inspection of a package of ingredients is necessary in order to detect breaks in the container, looseness in the cap or closure, and deviation from the expected appearance, aroma, and texture of the contents.

Bulk, or unformulated, drug substances and added substances, or excipients, must be stored in tightly closed containers under temperature, humidity, and lighting conditions that are either indicated in official monographs or approved by suppliers; also the date of receipt in the compounding facility must be clearly and indelibly marked on each package of ingredient. After receipt by the compounding facility, packages of ingredients that lack a supplier's expiration date cannot be used after one year, unless either appropriate inspection or testing indicates that the ingredient has retained its purity and quality for use in CSPs.

Careful consideration and evaluation of nonsterile ingredient sources is especially warranted when the CSP will be administered into the vascular, central nervous system, and eyes.

Upon receipt of each lot of the bulk drug substance or excipient used for CSPs, the individual compounding the preparation performs a visual inspection of the lot for evidence of deterioration, other types of unacceptable quality, and wrong identification. The bulk drug substance or excipient visual inspection is performed on a routine basis as described in the written protocol.▲*USP27*

Equipment

▲It is necessary that equipment, apparatus, and devices used to compound a CSP are consistently capable of operating properly and within acceptable tolerance limits. Written procedures outlining required equipment calibration, annual maintenance, monitoring for proper function, controlled procedures for use of the equipment and specified time frames for these activities are established and followed. Routine maintenance and time intervals are also outlined in these written procedures. Results from the equipment calibration, annual maintenance reports, and routine maintenance are kept on file for the lifetime of the equipment. Personnel is prepared through an appropriate combination of specific training and experience to operate or manipulate any piece of equipment, apparatus, or device they may use when preparing CSPs. Training includes gaining the ability to determine whether any item of equipment is operating properly or is malfunctioning.▲*USP27*

Add the following:

▲VERIFICATION OF AUTOMATED COMPOUNDING DEVICES FOR PARENTERAL NUTRITION COMPOUNDING

Automated compounding devices (ACDs) for the preparation of parenteral nutrition admixtures are widely used by pharmacists in hospitals and other health care settings. They are designed to streamline the labor-intensive processes involved in the compounding of these multiple-component formulations by automatically delivering the individual nutritional components in a predetermined sequence under computerized control. Parenteral nutrition admixtures often contain 20 or more individual additives representing as many as 50 or more individual components (e.g., 15 to 20 crystalline amino acids, dextrose monohydrate, and lipids; 10 to 12 electrolyte salts; 5 to 7 trace minerals; and 12 vitamins). Thus, the ACDs can improve the accuracy and precision of the compounding process compared to the traditional, manual compounding methods. Pharmacists should consult the general information chapter *Validation of Compendial Methods* ⟨1225⟩ for verification parameters to be considered when evaluating an ACD.

Accuracy

The accuracy of an ACD can be determined in various ways to ensure that the correct quantities of nutrients, electrolytes, or other nutritional components are delivered to the final infusion container. Initially, the ACD is tested for its volume and weight accuracy. For volume accuracy, a suitable volume of *Sterile Water for Injection*, which represents a typical additive volume (e.g., 40 mL for small-volume range of 1 to 100 mL; or 300 mL for large-volume range of 100 to 1000 mL), is programmed into the ACD and delivered to the appropriate volumetric container. The pharmacist then consults *Volumetric Apparatus* ⟨31⟩ for appropriate parameters to assess the volumetric performance of the ACD. For gravimetric accuracy, the balance used in conjunction with the ACD is tested using various weight sizes that represent the amounts typically used to deliver the various additives. The pharmacist consults *Weights and Balances* ⟨41⟩ for acceptable tolerances of the weights used. In addition, the same volume of *Sterile Water for Injection* used to assess volumetric accuracy is then weighed on the balance used in conjunction with the ACD. For example, if 40 mL of water was used in the volumetric assessment, its corresponding weight should be about 40 g (assuming the relative density of water is 1.0). In addition, during the use of the ACD, certain additives, such as potassium chloride (corrected for density differences) can also be tested in the same manner as an in-process test.

Finally, additional tests of accuracy may be employed that determine the content of certain ingredients in the final volume of the parenteral nutrition admixture. Generally, pharmacy departments do not have the capability to routinely perform chemical analyses such as analyses of dextrose or electrolyte concentrations. Consequently, hospital or institutional laboratories may be called upon to perform these quality assurance tests. However, the methods in such laboratories are often designed for biological, not pharmaceutical, systems. Thus, their testing procedures must be verified to meet the *USP* requirements stated in the individual monograph for the component being tested. For example, under *Dextrose Injection*, the following is stated: It contains not less than 95.0 percent and not more than 105.0 percent of the labeled amount of $C_6H_{12}O_6 \cdot H_2O$. The hospital or institutional chemistry laboratories have to validate their methods to apply to this range and correct for their typical measurement of anhydrous dextrose versus dextrose monohydrate. Similar ranges and issues exist, for example, for injections of calcium gluconate, magnesium sulfate, potassium chloride, and so forth. The critical point is the use of *USP* references and possible laboratory procedural differences.

Precision

The intermediate precision of the ACD can be determined on the basis of the day-to-day variations in performance of the accuracy measures. Thus, the pharmacist must keep a daily record of the above-described accuracy assessments and review the results over time. This review must occur at least at weekly intervals to avoid potentially clinically significant cumulative errors over time. This is especially true for additives with a narrow therapeutic index, such as potassium chloride.▲*USP27*

Change to read:

FINISHED ▲PREPARATION▲*USP27* RELEASE CHECKS AND TESTS

All ▲high-risk level CSPs for administration by injection into the vascular and central nervous systems that are prepared in groups of more than 25 identical individual single-dose packages (such as ampuls, bags, syringes, and vials), or in multiple dose vials for administration to multiple patients, or are exposed longer than 12 hours at 2° to 8° and longer than 6 hours at warmer than 8° before they are sterilized are tested to ensure that they are sterile (see *Sterility Tests* ⟨71⟩) and do not contain excessive bacterial endotoxins (see *Bacterial Endotoxins Test* ⟨85⟩). All CSPs that are intended to be solutions must be visually examined for the presence of particulate matter and not administered or dispensed when such matter is observed. The prescription orders, written compounding procedure, preparation records, and expended materials used to make CSPs in all contamination risk levels are inspected for accuracy of correct identities and amounts of ingredients, aseptic mixing and sterilization, packaging, labeling, and expected physical appearance before they are administered or dispensed.▲*USP27*

Physical Inspection

▲Finished CSPs are individually inspected in accordance with written procedures after compounding. If not distributed promptly, these products are individually inspected just prior to leaving the storage area. Those products that are not immediately distributed are stored in an appropriate location as described in the written procedures.▲*USP27* Immediately after compounding and as a condition of release, each product unit, where possible, should be inspected against lighted white ▲or black background or both▲*USP27* for evidence of visible particulates or other foreign matter. Pre-release inspection ▲also includes▲*USP27* container–

closure integrity and any other apparent visual defect. Products with observed defects should be immediately discarded or marked and segregated from acceptable products in a manner that prevents their administration. When products are not distributed promptly after preparation, a predistribution inspection ▲is▲USP27 conducted to ensure that a CSP with defects, such as precipitation, cloudiness, and leakage, which may develop between the time of release and the time of distribution, is not released.

Compounding Accuracy Checks

Written procedures for double-checking compounding accuracy ▲must be followed for every CSP during preparation and immediately▲USP27 prior to release. The double check system should meet state regulations and include label accuracy and accuracy of the addition of all drug products or ingredients used to prepare the finished product and their volumes or quantities. The used additive containers and, for those additives for which the entire container was not expended, the syringes used to measure the additive, should be quarantined with the final products until the final product check is completed. ▲Compounding personnel must visually confirm that ingredients measured in syringes match the written order being compounded. Preferably, a person other than the compounder can verify that correct volumes of correct ingredients were measured to make each CSP. For example, compounding personnel would pull the syringe plunger back to the volume measured.

When practical, confirm accuracy of measurements by weighing a volume of the measured fluid, then calculating that volume by dividing the weight by the accurate value of the density, or specific gravity, of the measured fluid. Correct density or specific gravity values programmed in automated compounding devices, which measure by weight using the quotient of the programmed volume divided by the density or specific gravity, must be confirmed to be accurate before and after delivering volumes of the liquids assigned to each channel or port. These volume accuracy checks and the following additional safety and accuracy checks in this section must be included in the standard operating procedures manual of the CSP facility.▲USP27

Sterility Testing

▲All high-risk level CSPs for administration by injection into the vascular and central nervous systems that are prepared in groups of more than 25 identical individual single-dose packages (such as ampuls, bags, syringes, vials), or in multiple dose vials for administration to multiple patients, or exposed longer than 12 hours at 2° to 8° and longer than 6 hours at warmer than 8° before they are sterilized must be tested to ensure that they are sterile (see *Sterility Tests* ⟨71⟩) before they are dispensed or administered. The *Membrane Filtration* method is the method of choice where feasible (e.g., components are compatible with the membrane). A method not described in the USP may be used if verification results demonstrate that the alternative is at least as effective and reliable as the USP *Membrane Filtration* method or the USP *Direct Inoculation of the Culture Medium* method where the membrane filtration method is not feasible.

In such a case, a written procedure requiring daily observation of the media and requiring an immediate recall if there is any evidence of microbial growth must be available. In addition, the patient and the physician of the patient to whom a potentially contaminated CSP was administered is notified of the potential risk. Positive sterility test results should prompt a rapid and systematic investigation of aseptic technique, environmental control, and other sterility assurance controls to identify sources of contamination and correct problems in the methods or processes.

Bacterial Endotoxin (Pyrogen) Testing

All high-risk level CSPs for administration by injection into the vascular and central nervous systems that are prepared in groups of more than 25 identical individual single-dose packages (such as ampuls, bags, syringes, vials), or in multiple dose vials for administration to multiple patients, or exposed longer than 12 hours at 2° to 8° and longer than 6 hours at warmer than 8° before they are sterilized must be tested to ensure that they do not contain excessive bacterial endotoxins (see *Bacterial Endotoxins Test* ⟨85⟩). In the absence of a bacterial endotoxins limit in the official monograph or other CSP formula source, the CSP must not exceed the amount of USP Endotoxin Units (EU per hour per kg of body weight or m² of body surface area) specified in the above chapter for the appropriate route of administration.

Identity and Strength Verification of Ingredients

Compounding facilities must have at least the following written procedures for verifying the correct identity and quality of CSPs before they are dispensed and administered:
1. That labels of CSPs bear correct names and amounts or concentrations of ingredients; the total volume; the beyond-use date; the appropriate route(s) of administration; the storage conditions; and other information for safe use.
2. That there are correct identities, purities, and amounts of ingredients by comparing the original written order to the written compounding record for the CSP.
3. That correct fill volumes in CSPs and correct quantities of filled units of the CSPs were obtained. When the strength of finished CSPs cannot be confirmed to be accurate, based on the above three inspections, the CSPs must be assayed by methods that are specific for the active ingredients.

To inhibit microbial growth from undetected contamination, finished CSPs that will not be immediately dispensed and administered must be refrigerated at 2° to 8°, unless their chemical and physical stability are known to be adversely affected by cold temperatures. When CSPs are filled into patient-worn infusion devices that are likely to attain temperatures exceeding 30° for more than 24 hours, the chemical and physical stability at such temperatures and durations must be confirmed from either appropriate literature sources or direct testing.▲USP27

Change to read:

STORAGE AND BEYOND-USE DATING

▲Beyond-use dates for compounded preparations are usually assigned based on professional experience, which should include careful interpretation of appropriate information sources for the same or similar formulations (see *Stability Criteria and Beyond-Use Dating* in the general test chapter *Pharmaceutical Compounding—Nonsterile Preparations* ⟨795⟩). Beyond-use dates for CSPs are rarely based on preparation-specific chemical assay results, which are used with the Arrhenius equation to determine expiration dates (see *General Notices and Requirements*) for manufactured products. The majority of CSPs are aqueous solutions in which hydrolysis of dissolved ingredients is the most common chemical degradation reaction. The extent of hydrolysis and other heat-catalyzed degradation reactions at any particular time point in the life of a CSP represents the thermodynamic sum of exposure temperatures and durations. Such lifetime stability exposure is represented in the mean kinetic temperature calculation (see *Pharmaceutical Calculations in Prescription Compounding* ⟨1160⟩). Drug hydrolysis rates increase exponentially with arithmetic temperature increase; thus, exposure of a beta-lactam antibiotic solution for one day at controlled room temperature (see *General Notices and Require-*

ments) will have an equivalent effect on the extent of hydrolysis of approximately 3 to 5 days in cold temperatures (see *General Notices and Requirements*).

Personnel who prepare, dispense, and administer CSPs must store them strictly in accordance with the conditions stated on the label of ingredient products and finished CSPs. When CSPs are known to have been exposed to temperatures warmer than the warmest labeled limit, but not exceeding 40° (see *General Notices and Requirements*) for more than 4 hours, such CSPs should be discarded, unless appropriate documentation or direct assay data confirms their continued stability.▲*USP27*

Determining Beyond-Use Dates

▲When CSPs deviate from conditions in the approved labeling of manufactured products contained in CSPs, compounding personnel may consult the manufacturer of particular products for advice on assigning beyond-use dates based on chemical and physical stability parameters. Beyond-use dates for CSPs that are prepared strictly in accordance with manufacturers' product labeling must be those specified in that labeling, or from appropriate literature sources or direct testing. Beyond-use dates for CSPs that lack justification from either appropriate literature sources or by direct testing evidence must be assigned as described in the section *Stability Criteria and Beyond-Use Dating* in the general test chapter *Pharmaceutical Compounding—Nonsterile Preparations* ⟨795⟩.

In addition, the pharmacist may refer to applicable publications to obtain relevant stability, compatibility, and degradation information regarding the drug or its congeners. When assigning a beyond-use date, pharmacists should consult and apply drug-specific and general stability documentation and literature where available, and they should consider the nature of drug and its degradation mechanism, the container in which it is packaged, the expected storage conditions, and the intended duration of therapy (see *Expiration Date and Beyond-Use Date* under *Labeling* in the *General Notices and Requirements*). Stability information must be carefully interpreted in relation to the actual compounded formulation and conditions for storage and use. Predictions based on other evidence, such as publications, charts, tables, and so forth would result in theoretical beyond-use dates. Theoretically predicted beyond-use dating introduces varying degrees of assumptions, and hence a likelihood of error or at least inaccuracy. The degree of error or inaccuracy would be dependent on the extent of differences between the CSP's characteristics (such as composition, concentration of ingredients, fill volume, or container type and material) and the characteristics of the products from which stability data or information are to be extrapolated. The greater the doubt of the accuracy of theoretically predicted beyond-use dating, the greater the need to determine dating periods experimentally. Theoretically predicted beyond-use dating periods should be carefully considered for CSPs prepared from nonsterile bulk active ingredients having therapeutic activity, especially where these CSPs are expected to be compounded routinely. When CSPs will be distributed to and administered in residential locations other than health care facilities, the effect of potentially uncontrolled and unmonitored temperature conditions must be considered when assigning beyond-use dates. It must be ascertained that CSPs will not be exposed to warm temperatures (see *General Notices and Requirements*) unless the compounding facility has evidence to justify stability of CSPs during such exposure.

It should be recognized that the truly valid evidence of stability for predicting beyond-use dating can be obtained only through product-specific experimental studies. Semi-quantitative procedures, such as thin-layer chromatography (TLC), may be acceptable for many CSPs. However, quantitative stability-indicating assays, such as high performance liquid chromatographic (HPLC) assays, would be more appropriate for certain CSPs. Examples include CSPs with a narrow therapeutic index, where close monitoring or dose titration is required to ensure therapeutic effectiveness and to avoid toxicity; where a theoret-

ically established beyond-use dating period is supported by only marginal evidence; or where a significant margin of safety cannot be verified for the proposed beyond-use dating period. In short, because beyond-use dating periods established from product-specific data acquired from the appropriate instrumental analyses are clearly more reliable than those predicted theoretically, the former approach is strongly urged to support dating periods exceeding 30 days.

To ensure consistent practices in determining and assigning beyond-use dates, the pharmacy should have written policies and procedures governing the determination of the beyond-use dates for all compounded products. When attempting to predict a theoretical beyond-use date, a compounded or an admixed product should be considered as a unique system that has physical and chemical properties and stability characteristics that differ from its components. For example, antioxidant, buffering, or antimicrobial properties of a sterile vial for injection (SVI) might be lost upon its dilution, with the potential of seriously compromising the chemical stability of the SVI's active ingredient or the physical or microbiological stability of the SVI formulation in general. Thus, the properties stabilized in the SVI formulation usually cannot be expected to be carried over to the compounded or admixed product. Product-specific, experimentally determined stability data evaluation protocols are preferable to published stability information. Pharmacists should consult the general information chapter *Stability* under *Pharmaceutical Dosage Forms* ⟨1151⟩ for the appropriate stability parameters to be considered when initiating or evaluating a product-specific stability study.

Compounding personnel who assign beyond-use dates to CSPs when lacking direct chemical assay results must critically interpret and evaluate the most appropriate available information sources to decide a conservative and safe beyond-use date. The standard operating procedures manual of the compounding facility and each specific CSP formula record must describe the general basis used to assign the beyond-use date and storage conditions.

If multiple-dose parenteral medication vials (MDVs) are used, refrigerate the MDVs after they are opened unless otherwise specified by the manufacturer. Discard the MDVs when empty, when suspected or visible contamination occurs, or when the manufacturer's stated expiration date is reached, provided the manufacturer's storage conditions have been adhered to. Expiration dating not specifically referenced in the package insert should not exceed 30 days once the vial has been opened.▲*USP27*

Monitoring Controlled Storage Areas

To ensure that product potency is retained through the manufacturer's labeled expiration date, pharmacists must monitor the drug storage areas within the pharmacy. Controlled temperature storage areas in the pharmacy (refrigerators, 2° to 8°; freezers, −20° to −10°; and incubators, 30° to 35°; etc.) should be monitored at least once daily and the results documented on a temperature log. Additionally, pharmacy personnel should note the storage temperature when placing the product into or removing the product from the storage unit in order to monitor any temperature aberrations. Suitable temperature recording devices may include a calibrated continuous recording device or an NBS calibrated thermometer that has adequate accuracy and sensitivity for the intended purpose and should be properly calibrated at suitable intervals. If the pharmacy uses a continuous temperature recording device, pharmacy personnel should verify at least once daily that the recording device itself is functioning properly.

The temperature sensing mechanisms should be suitably placed in the controlled temperature storage space to reflect accurately its true temperature. In addition, the pharmacy should adhere to appropriate procedures of all controlled storage spaces to ensure that such spaces are not subject to significantly prolonged temperature fluctuations as may occur, for example, by leaving a refrigerator door open too long.

Change to read:

MAINTAINING PRODUCT QUALITY AND CONTROL AFTER ▲THE CSP▲*USP27* LEAVES THE PHARMACY

▲Sterile Preparations for Institutional Use

This section pertains to the responsibilities of the pharmacy for maintaining product quality and control after the CSP leaves the pharmacy for distribution and use within the organized health care system to which the pharmacy belongs. The pharmacy is responsible for the quality of all CSPs prepared by or dispensed from the pharmacy, throughout the life cycle of the CSP, regardless of where the CSP exists physically within the organized health care system. In fulfilling this general responsibility, the pharmacy is responsible for the proper packaging, handling, transport, and storage of CSPs prepared by or dispensed from it, including the appropriate education, training, and supervision of pharmacy personnel assigned to these functions. The pharmacy should assist in the education and training of nonpharmacy personnel responsible for carrying out any aspect of these functions.

Establishing, maintaining, and assuring compliance with comprehensive written policies and procedures encompassing these responsibilities is a further responsibility of the pharmacy. Where nonpharmacy personnel are assigned tasks involving any of these responsibilities, the policies and procedures encompassing those tasks should be developed by the pharmacy in consultation with other institutional departments as appropriate. Activities or concerns that should be addressed as the pharmacy fulfills these responsibilities are as follows.

PACKAGING, HANDLING, AND TRANSPORT

Inappropriate processes or techniques involved with packaging, handling, and transport can adversely affect product quality and package integrity. While pharmacy personnel routinely perform many of the tasks associated with these functions, some tasks, such as transport, handling, and placement into storage, may be fulfilled by nonpharmacy personnel who are not under the direct administrative control of the pharmacy. Under these circumstances, appropriate written policies and procedures are established by the pharmacy with the involvement of other departments or services whose personnel are responsible for carrying out those CSP-related functions for which the pharmacy has a direct interest. The performance of the nonpharmacy personnel is monitored for compliance to established policies and procedures.

The critical requirements that are unique to CSPs and that are necessary to ensure product quality and packaging integrity must be addressed in written procedures. For example, techniques should be specified to prevent the depression of syringe plungers or dislodging of syringe tips during handling and transport. Additionally, disconnection of system components (for example, where CSPs are dispensed with administration sets attached to them) must be prevented throughout the life cycle of the product. Foam padding or inserts are particularly useful where CSPs are transported by pneumatic tube systems. Regardless of the methods used, the pharmacy has to evaluate their effectiveness and the reliability of the intended protection. Evaluation should be continuous, for example, through a surveillance system, including a system of problem reporting to the pharmacy.

Inappropriate transport and handling can adversely affect the quality of certain CSPs having unique stability concerns. For example, the physical shaking that might occur during pneumatic tube transport, or undue exposure to heat or light, have to be addressed on a product-specific basis. Alternate transport modes or special packaging measures might be needed for the proper assurance of quality of these CSPs. The use of tamper-proof closures and seals on CSP ports can add an additional measure of security to ensure product integrity regardless of transport method used.

Chemotoxic and other hazardous CSPs require safeguards to maintain the integrity of the CSP and to minimize the exposure potential of these products to the environment and to personnel who may come in contact with them. Special requirements associated with the packaging, transport, and handling of these agents include the prevention of accidental exposures or spills and the training of personnel in the event of an exposure or spill. Examples of special requirements of these agents also include exposure-reducing strategies such as the use of Luer lock syringes and connections, syringe caps, the capping of container ports, sealed plastic bags, impact-resistant containers, and cautionary labeling. Appropriate cushioning for pneumatic tube transport should be selected and evaluated to ensure that the products so conveyed can withstand the stresses induced by the system. Pneumatic transport of nonevaluated packaging alternatives should be avoided. Additional references should be consulted as necessary for further information on handling chemotoxic and other hazardous drugs.

USE AND STORAGE

The pharmacy is responsible for ensuring that CSPs in the patient-care setting maintain their quality until administered. The immediate labeling of the CSP container will display prominently and understandably the requirements for proper storage and expiration dating. Delivery and patient-care-setting personnel must be properly trained to deliver the CSP to the appropriate storage location. Outdated and unused CSPs must be returned to the pharmacy for disposal or possible reuse.

Written procedures have to exist to ensure that storage conditions in the patient-care setting are suitable for the CSP-specific storage requirements. Procedures include daily monitoring and documentation of drug storage refrigerators to ensure temperatures between $2°$ and $8°$ and the monthly inspection of all drug storage locations by pharmacy personnel. Inspections must confirm compliance with appropriate storage conditions, separation of drugs and food, proper use of multiple-dose containers, and the avoidance of using single-dose products as multiple-dose containers. CSPs, as well as all other drug products, must be stored in the patient-care area in such a way as to secure them from unauthorized personnel, visitors, and patients.

ADMINISTRATION

Procedures essential for generally ensuring product quality, especially sterility assurance, when readying a CSP for its subsequent administration include proper hand-washing, aseptic technique, site care, and change of administration sets. Additional procedures may also be essential for certain products, devices, or techniques. Examples where such special procedures are needed include in-line filtration, the operation of automated infusion control devices, and the replenishment of drug products into the reservoirs of implantable or portable infusion pumps.

REDISPENSED CSPS

The pharmacy must have the sole authority for determining whether a CSP not administered as originally intended can be used for an alternate patient or under alternate conditions. All CSPs that are not used as originally intended must be returned to the pharmacy for appropriate disposition, which may include redispensing, but only if adequate continuing quality can be fully ensured. The following may provide such assurance: the CSP was maintained under continuous refrigeration and protected from light, if required; no evidence of tampering or any readying for use outside the pharmacy exists; and there is sufficient time remaining until the originally assigned beyond-use time and date

will be reached. Thus, initial preparation and thaw times should be documented and reliable measures should have been taken to prevent and detect tampering. Compliance with all procedures associated with maintaining product quality is essential. The CSP must not be redispensed if there is not adequate assurance that product quality and packaging integrity (including the connections of devices, where applicable) were continuously maintained between the time the CSP left and the time that it was returned to the pharmacy. Additionally, CSPs must not be redispensed if redispensing cannot be supported by the originally assigned beyond-use time.

EDUCATION AND TRAINING

The assurance of CSP quality and packaging integrity is highly dependent upon the proper adherence of all personnel to the pertinent written procedures. The pharmacy must design, implement, and maintain a formal education, training, and competency assessment program that encompasses all the functions and tasks addressed in the foregoing sections and all personnel to whom such functions and tasks are assigned. This program includes the assessment and documentation of procedural breaches, administration mishaps, side effects, allergic reactions, and complications associated with dosage or administration, such as extravasation. This program should be coordinated with the institution's adverse-event and incident reporting programs.

Packing and Transporting CSPs

The following sections on *Packing CSPs for Transit* and *Transit of CSPs* describe how to maintain sterility and stability of CSPs until they are delivered to patient care locations for administration.

PACKING CSPS FOR TRANSIT

When CSPs are distributed to locations outside the premises in which they are compounded, compounding personnel select packing containers and materials that are expected to maintain physical integrity, sterility, and stability of CSPs during transit. Packing is selected that simultaneously protects CSPs from damage, leakage, contamination, and degradation; and protects personnel who transport packed CSPs from harm. The standard operating procedures manual of the compounding facility specifically describes appropriate packing containers and insulating and stuffing materials, based on information from product specifications, vendors, and experience of compounding personnel. Written instructions that clearly explain how to safely open containers of packed CSPs are provided to patients and other recipients.

TRANSIT OF CSPS

Compounding facilities that ship CSPs to locations outside their own premises must select modes of transport that are expected to deliver properly packed CSPs in undamaged, sterile, and stable condition to recipients.

Compounding personnel should ascertain that temperatures of CSPs during transit by the selected mode will not exceed the warmest temperature specified on the storage temperature range on CSPs labels. It is recommended that compounding personnel communicate directly with the couriers to learn shipping durations and exposure conditions that CSPs may encounter.

Compounding personnel must include specific handling and exposure instructions on the exteriors of containers packed with CSPs to be transported and obtain reasonable assurance of compliance therewith from transporters. Compounding personnel

must periodically review the delivery performance of couriers to ascertain that CSPs are being efficiently and properly transported.

STORAGE IN LOCATIONS OUTSIDE CSP FACILITIES

Compounding facilities that ship CSPs to patients and other recipients outside their own premises must ascertain or provide, whichever is the appropriate case, the following assurances:
1. Labels and accessory labeling for CSPs include clearly readable beyond-use dates, storage instructions, and disposal instructions for out-of-date units.
2. Each patient or other recipient is able to store the CSPs properly, including the use of a properly functioning refrigerator and freezer if CSPs are labeled for such storage.▲*USP27*

Change to read:

PATIENT OR CAREGIVER TRAINING

A formal training program ▲is▲*USP27* provided as a means to ensure understanding and compliance with the many special and complex responsibilities placed upon the patient or caregiver for the storage, handling, and administration of ▲CSPs.▲*USP27* The instructional objectives for the training program ▲includes▲*USP27* all home care responsibilities expected of the patient or caregiver and ▲is▲*USP27* specified in terms of patient or caregiver competencies.

Upon the conclusion of the training program, the patient or caregiver should, correctly and consistently, be able to do the following:
(1) Describe the therapy involved, including the disease or condition for which the ▲CSP▲*USP27* is prescribed, goals of therapy, expected therapeutic outcome, and potential side effects of the ▲CSP.▲*USP27*
(2) Inspect all drug products, devices, equipment, and supplies on receipt to ensure that proper temperatures were maintained during transport and that goods received show no evidence of deterioration or defects.
(3) Handle, store, and monitor all drug products and related supplies and equipment in the home, including all special requirements related to same.
(4) Visually inspect all drug products, devices, and other items the patient or caregiver is required to use immediately prior to administration in a manner to ensure that all items are acceptable for use. For example, ▲CSPs must▲*USP27* be free from leakage, container cracks, particulates, precipitate, haziness, discoloration, or other deviations from the normal expected appearance, and the immediate packages of sterile devices ▲must be▲*USP27* completely sealed with no evidence of loss of package integrity.
(5) Check labels immediately prior to administration to ensure the right drug, dose, patient, and time of administration.
(6) Clean the in-home preparation area, scrub hands, use proper aseptic technique, and manipulate all containers, equipment, apparatus, devices, and supplies used in conjunction with administration.
(7) Employ all techniques and precautions associated with ▲CSP▲*USP27* administration, for example, preparing supplies and equipment, handling of devices, priming the tubing, and discontinuing an infusion.
(8) Care for catheters, change dressings, and maintain site patency as indicated.
(9) Monitor for and detect occurrences of therapeutic complications such as infection, phlebitis, electrolyte imbalance, and catheter misplacement.
(10) Respond immediately to emergency or critical situations such as catheter breakage or displacement, tubing discon-

nection, clot formation, flow blockage, and equipment malfunction.

(11) Know when to seek and how to obtain professional emergency services or professional advice.

(12) Handle, contain, and dispose of wastes, such as needles, syringes, devices, biohazardous spills or residuals, and infectious substances.

Training programs ▲include a▲*USP27* hands-on demonstration and practice with actual items that the patient or caregiver is expected to use, such as ▲CSP▲*USP27* containers, devices, and equipment. The patient or caregiver ▲practices▲*USP27* aseptic and injection technique under the direct observation of a health professional.

The pharmacy, in conjunction with nursing or medical personnel, is responsible for ensuring initially and on an ongoing basis that the patient or caregiver understands, has mastered, and is capable of and willing to comply with all of these home care responsibilities. This ▲is▲*USP27* achieved through a formal, written assessment program. All specified competencies in the patient or caregiver's training program ▲are▲*USP27* formally assessed. The patient or caregiver ▲is▲*USP27* expected to demonstrate to appropriate health care personnel their mastery of their assigned activities before being allowed to administer ▲CSPs▲*USP27* unsupervised by a health professional.

Printed material such as checklists or instructions provided during training may serve as continuing post-training reinforcement of learning or as reminders of specific patient or caregiver responsibilities. Post-training verbal counseling ▲can▲*USP27* also be used periodically, as appropriate, to reinforce training and to ensure continuing correct and complete fulfillment of responsibilities.

Delete the following:

▲PATIENT MONITORING AND COMPLAINT SYSTEM

The pharmacy must have written policies and procedures describing the monitoring of patients using CSPs and the handling of reports of adverse events.

Outcome Monitoring

The pharmacy is responsible for developing a patient monitoring plan, which includes written outcome measures and systems for routine patient assessment. The outcome monitoring system should provide information suitable for the evaluation of the quality of patient care and of pharmaceutical services. Examples of assessment parameters include infection rates, rehospitalization rates, incidence of adverse drug reactions, catheter complications, and other variables that may serve as meaningful indicators of the effectiveness and suitability of the home use of CSPs. In selecting suitable outcome measures, the focus should be on high-risk, high-volume, or problem-prone factors.

Reports

The pharmacy should have policies and procedures for the receipt, documentation, handling, and disposition of reports of patient problems, complaints, adverse drug reactions, drug product or device defects, and other adverse events reported by patients, caregivers, family members, pharmacists, or other health professionals. The pharmacy should have a procedure to ensure that the patient receives prompt and appropriate medical attention as necessary in response to all adverse incidents from CSPs or devices. When a complaint or problem prompts a suspicion that a CSP or a device may be defective, the pharmacy should also be able to identify and recall the potentially defective item to the patient level whenever appropriate.

Procedures should also include a mechanism for periodic review of reports received to determine any need for correction of underlying systems problems. All reports received should be maintained for a reasonable period of time in a log, file, or binder dedicated for this purpose and readily retrievable as needed for subsequent analysis, legal or regulatory inquiry, or quality assurance audit. Standardized forms or formats for the reporting and recording of incidents, complaints, and so forth should be used. Reports should be completed and signed by the individual receiving it or by the individual involved in the situation. Procedures should depict the classification, documentation, investigation, and resolution of all reports and should provide a mechanism for participation in various federal and state reporting programs such as USP or FDA programs for reporting reaction problems, or defects with drug products or medical devices.▲*USP27*

Add the following:

▲PATIENT MONITORING AND ADVERSE EVENTS REPORTING

Compounding facilities must clinically monitor patients treated with CSPs according to the regulations and guidelines of their respective state health care practitioner licensure boards or of accepted standards of practice. Compounding facilities must provide patients and other recipients of CSPs with a way to address their questions and report any concerns that they may have with CSPs and their administration devices.

The standard operating procedures manuals of compounding facilities must describe specific instructions for receiving, acknowledging, and dating receipts; and for recording, or filing, and evaluating reports of adverse events and of the quality of preparation claimed to be associated with CSPs. Reports of adverse events with CSPs must be reviewed promptly and thoroughly by compounding supervisors to correct and prevent future occurrences. Compounding personnel are encouraged to participate in adverse event reporting and product defects programs of the Food and Drug Administration (FDA) and United States Pharmacopeia (USP).▲*USP27*

Change to read:

THE QUALITY ASSURANCE PROGRAM

A provider of ▲CSPs must▲*USP27* have in place a formal Quality Assurance (QA) Program[4] intended to provide a mechanism for monitoring, evaluating, correcting, and improving the activities and processes described in this chapter. Emphasis in the QA Program ▲is▲*USP27* placed on maintaining and improving the

---

[4] Other accepted terms that describe activities aimed at assessing and improving the quality of care rendered include Continuous Quality Improvement, Quality Assessment and Improvement, and Total Quality Management.

quality of systems and the provision of patient care. In addition, the QA program ▲ensures▲*USP27* that any plan aimed at correcting identified problems also includes appropriate follow-up to make certain that effective corrective actions were performed.[5]

Characteristics of a QA plan include the following:
(1) Formalization in writing;
(2) Consideration of all aspects of the preparation and dispensing of products as described in this chapter, including environmental testing, validation results, etc.;
(3) Description of specific monitoring and evaluation activities;
(4) Specification of how results are to be reported and evaluated;
(5) Identification of appropriate follow-up mechanisms when action limits or thresholds are exceeded; and
(6) Delineation of the individuals responsible for each aspect of the QA program.

In developing a specific plan, focus ▲is▲*USP27* on establishing objective, measurable indicators for monitoring activities and processes that are deemed high-risk, high-volume, or problem-prone. Appropriate evaluation of environmental monitoring might include, for example, the trending of an indicator such as settling plate counts. In general, the selection of indicators and the effectiveness of the overall QA plan ▲is▲*USP27* reassessed on an annual basis.

---

[5] The use of additional resources, such as the Accreditation Manual for Home Care from the Joint Commission on Accreditation of Healthcare Organizations, may prove helpful in the development of a QA plan.

USP DI

Add the following:

▲APPENDIX

CRITERIA	LOW-RISK LEVEL	MEDIUM-RISK LEVEL	HIGH-RISK LEVEL
Compounding Conditions	• Compounded entirely under ISO Class 5 (Class 100) conditions • Compounding involves only transfer, measuring, and mixing manipulations with closed or sealed packaging systems that are performed promptly and attentively • Manipulations are limited to aseptically opening ampuls, penetrating sterile stoppers on vials with sterile needles and syringes and transferring sterile liquids in sterile syringes to sterile administration devices and packages of other sterile products	• All conditions listed under low-risk level • Multiple individual or small doses of sterile products are combined or pooled to prepare a CSP that will be administered either to multiple patients or to one patient on multiple conditions • Compounding process includes complex aseptic manipulations other than the single-volume transfer • Compounding process requires unusually long duration • The sterile CSPs do not contain broad-spectrum bacteriostatic agents, and are administered over several days	• Nonsterile ingredients are incorporated or a nonsterile device is employed before terminal sterilization • Sterile ingredients, components, devices and mixtures are exposed to air quality inferior to ISO Class 5 (Class 100) • Nonsterile preparations are exposed for not more than 6 hours before being sterilized • Nonsterile preparations are terminally sterilized but are not tested for bacterial endotoxins • It is assumed that the chemical purity and content strength of ingredients meet their original or compendial specifications in unopened or in opened packages of bulk ingredients
QA Program	• Formalized in writing • Describes specific monitoring and evaluation activities • Reporting and evaluation of results • Identification of follow-up activities when thresholds are exceeded • Delineation of individual responsibilities for each aspect of the program	See low-risk level.	See low-risk level.
QA Practices	• Routine disinfection and quality testing of direct compounding environment • Visual confirmation of personnel processes regarding gowning, etc. • Review of orders and packages of ingredients to assure correct identity and amounts of ingredients • Visual inspection of CSP • Media-fill test procedure performed at least annually for each person	See low-risk level.	See low-risk level.
Outcome Monitoring	Yes	Yes	Yes

APPENDIX (Continued)

CRITERIA	LOW-RISK LEVEL	MEDIUM-RISK LEVEL	HIGH-RISK LEVEL
Reports/Documents	• Written policies and procedures • Adverse event reporting • Complaint procedures • Periodic review of quality control documents	See low-risk level.	See low-risk level.
Patient and Caregiver Training	• Formalized program that includes — Understanding of the therapy provided — Handling and storage of the CSP — Appropriate administration techniques — Use and maintenance of any infusion device involved — Use of printed material — Appropriate follow-up	See low-risk level.	See low-risk level.
Maintaining Product Quality and Control once the CSP leaves the Pharmacy (both institutional based and NICPs)	• Packaging, handling, and transport — Written policies and procedures including the packaging, handling, and transport of chemotoxic/hazardous CSPs • Use and storage — Written policies and procedures • Administration — Written polices and procedures dealing with such issues as handwashing, aseptic technique, site care, etc. • Education/Training — Written policies and procedures dealing with proper education of patients and caregivers ensuring all of the above	See low-risk level.	See low-risk level.
Storage and Beyond-Use Dating	• Specific labeling requirements • Specific beyond-use dating policies, procedures, and requirements • Policies regarding storage	See low-risk level.	See low-risk level.
Storage Conditions and Beyond-Use Dating for completed CSP	In the absence of sterility testing, storage periods (before administration) shall not exceed the following: Room temperature ≤48 hours 2°–8° ≤14 days ≤20 ° ≤45 days	Room temperature ≤30 hours 2°–8° ≤7 days ≤20 ° ≤45 days	Room temperature ≤24 hours 2°–8° ≤3 days ≤20 ° ≤45 days

APPENDIX *(Continued)*

CRITERIA	LOW-RISK LEVEL	MEDIUM-RISK LEVEL	HIGH-RISK LEVEL
Finished Product-Release Checks and Tests	• Written policies and procedures that address — Physical inspections — Compounding accuracy checks	See low-risk level.	See low-risk level.
Finished Product-Release Checks and Tests	• Written policies and procedures that address — Sterility testing — Pyrogen testing — Potency testing	See low-risk level.	See low-risk level.
CSP Work Environment	• Appropriate solid surfaces • Limited (but necessary) furniture, fixtures, etc. • Anteroom area • Buffer zone	See low-risk level.	See low-risk level.
Equipment	• Written policies and procedures that address calibration, routine maintenance, personnel training	See low-risk level.	See low-risk level.
Components	• Written policies and procedures that address Sterile components	See low-risk level.	Sterile and nonsterile drug components must meet the compendial standards if available • Written policies and procedures that address — Sterile components — Nonsterile components
Processing: Aseptic Technique	• Written policies and procedures that address specific training and performance evaluation • Critical operations are carried out in a Direct Compounding Common Area (DCCA)	See low-risk level.	See low-risk level.
Environmental Control	• Policies and procedures that address — Cleaning and sanitizing the workspaces (DCCA) — Personnel and gowning — Standard operating procedures	See low-risk level.	See low-risk level.

APPENDIX (*Continued*)

CRITERIA	LOW-RISK LEVEL	MEDIUM-RISK LEVEL	HIGH-RISK LEVEL
Verification Procedures • Sterility Testing	Not required	Not required	Yes, recommended
Verification Procedures • Environmental Monitoring	• Certification of LAFW and barrier isolates every six (6) months • Certification of the buffer room/zone and anteroom/zone every six (6) months • Bacterial monitoring using an appropriate manner at least monthly	See low-risk level.	See low-risk level.
Verification Procedures • Personnel Training and Education	Initially and annually thereafter • Didactic review • Written testing • Media-fill testing	See low-risk level.	See low-risk level.

▲*USP27*

⟨1091⟩ LABELING OF INACTIVE INGREDIENTS

This informational chapter provides guidelines for labeling of inactive ingredients present in dosage forms.

Within the past few years a number of trade associations representing pharmaceutical manufacturers have adopted voluntary guidelines for the disclosure and labeling of inactive ingredients. This is helpful to individuals who are sensitive to particular substances and who wish to identify the presence or confirm the absence of such substances in drug products. Because of the actions of these associations, the labeling of therapeutically inactive ingredients currently is deemed to constitute good pharmaceutical practice.

Although the manufacturers represented by these associations produce most of the products sold in this country, not all manufacturers, repackagers, or labelers here or abroad are members of these associations. Further, there are some differences in association guidelines. The guidelines presented here are designed to help promote consistency in labeling.

In accordance with good pharmaceutical practice, all dosage forms [NOTE—for requirements on parenteral and topical preparations, see the General Notices] should be labeled to state the identity of all added substances (therapeutically inactive ingredients) present therein, including colors, except that flavors and fragrances may be listed by the general term "flavor" or "fragrance." Such listing should be in alphabetical order by name and be distinguished from the identification statement of the active ingredient(s).

The name of an inactive ingredient should be taken from the current edition of one of the following reference works (in the following order of precedence): (1) the *United States Pharmacopeia* or the *National Formulary;* (2) *USAN and the USP Dictionary of Drug Names;* (3) CTFA *Cosmetic Ingredient Dictionary;* (4) *Food Chemicals Codex.* An ingredient not listed in any of the aforementioned reference works should be identified by its common or usual name (the name generally recognized by consumers or health-care professionals) or, if no common or usual name is available, by its chemical or other technical name.

An ingredient that may be, but not always is, present in a product should be qualified by words such as "or" or "may also contain."

The name of an ingredient whose identity is a trade secret may be omitted from the list if the list states "and other ingredients." For the purposes of this guideline, an ingredient is considered to be a trade secret only if its presence confers a significant competitive advantage upon its manufacturer and if its identity cannot be ascertained by the use of modern analytical technology.

An incidental trace ingredient having no functional or technical effect on the product need not be listed unless it has been demonstrated to cause sensitivity reactions or allergic responses.

Inactive ingredients should be listed on the label of a container of a product intended for sale without prescription, except that in the case of a container that is too small, such information may be contained in other labeling on or within the package.

⟨1101⟩ MEDICINE DROPPER

The Pharmacopeial medicine dropper consists of a tube made of glass or other suitable transparent material that generally is fitted with a collapsible bulb and, while varying in capacity, is constricted at the delivery end to a round opening having an external diameter of about 3 mm. The dropper, when held vertically, delivers water in drops each of which weighs between 45 mg and 55 mg.

In using a medicine dropper, one should keep in mind that few medicinal liquids have the same surface and flow characteristics as water, and therefore the size of drops varies materially from one preparation to another.

Where accuracy of dosage is important, a dropper that has been calibrated especially for the preparation with which it is supplied should be employed. The volume error incurred in measuring any liquid by means of a calibrated dropper should not exceed 15%, under normal use conditions.

⟨1121⟩ NOMENCLATURE

The USP (or NF) titles are legally recognized as the designations for use in labeling the articles to which they apply.

The value of designating each drug by one and only one nonproprietary[1] name is obvious, in terms of achieving simplicity and uniformity in drug nomenclature. In support of the U.S. Adopted Names program (see *Preface*), of which the U.S. Pharmacopeial Convention is a co-sponsor, the USP Committee of Revision gives consideration to the adoption of the U.S. Adopted Name, if any, as the official title for any compound that attains compendial recognition.

A compilation of the U.S. Adopted Names (USAN) published from the start of the USAN program in 1961, as well as other names for drugs, both current and retrospective, is provided in *USAN and the USP Dictionary of Drug Names.* This publication is intended to serve as a book of names useful for identifying and distinguishing all kinds of names for drugs, whether public or proprietary or chemical or code-designated names.[2]

A nonproprietary name of a drug serves numerous and varied purposes, its principal function being to identify the substance to which it applies by means of a designation that may be used by the professional and lay public free from the restrictions associated with registered trademarks. Teaching in pharmacy and medicine requires a common designation, especially for a drug that is available from several sources or is incorporated into a combination drug product; nonproprietary names facilitate communication among physicians; nonproprietary names must be used as the titles of the articles recognized by official drug compendia; a nonproprietary name is essential to the pharmaceutical manufacturer as a means of protecting trademark rights in the brand name for the article concerned; and, finally, the manufacturer is obligated by federal law to include the established nonproprietary name in advertising and labeling.

Under the terms of the Drug Amendments of 1962 to the Federal Food, Drug, and Cosmetic Act, which became law October 10, 1962, the Secretary of Health and Human Services is authorized to designate an official name for any drug wherever deemed "necessary or desirable in the interest of usefulness and simplicity."[3]

The Commissioner of Food and Drugs and the Secretary of Health and Human Services published in the *Federal Register* regulations effective November 26, 1984, which state, in part:

Sec. 299.4 Established names of drugs.

(e) "The Food and Drug Administration will not routinely designate official names under section 508 of the act. As a result, the established name under section 502(e) of the act will ordinarily be either the compendial name of the drug or, if there is no compendial name, the common or usual name of the drug. Interested persons, in the absence of the designation by the Food and Drug Administration of an official name, may rely on as the established name for any drug the current compendial name or the USAN adopted name listed in *USAN and the USP Dictionary of Drug Names.*[4]

It will be noted that the monographs on the biologics, which are produced under licenses issued by the Secretary of the U.S. Department of Health and Human Services, represent a special

---

[1] The term "generic" has been widely used in place of the more accurate and descriptive term "nonproprietary," with reference to drug nomenclature.

[2] *USAN and the USP Dictionary of Drug Names* is obtainable on order from the USAN Division, USP Convention, Inc., 12601 Twinbrook Parkway, Rockville, MD 20852.

[3] F.D.&C. Act, Sec. 508 [358].

[4] 53 Fed. Reg. 5369 (1988) amending 21 CFR § 299.4.

case. Although efforts continue toward achieving uniformity, there may be a difference between the respective title required by federal law and the USP title. Such differences are fewer than in past revisions of the Pharmacopeia. The USP title, where different from the FDA Bureau of Biologics title, does not constitute a synonym for labeling purposes; the conditions of licensing the biologic concerned require that each such article be designated by the name appearing in the product license issued to the manufacturer. Where a USP title differs from the title in the federal regulations, the former has been adopted with a view to usefulness and simplicity and conformity with the principles governing the selection of monograph titles generally.

⟨1146⟩ PACKAGING PRACTICE— REPACKAGING A SINGLE SOLID ORAL DRUG PRODUCT INTO A UNIT-DOSE CONTAINER

INTRODUCTION

Repackaging of solid oral drug products, such as tablets and capsules, into unit-dose configurations is common practice both for the pharmacy that is dispensing drugs pursuant to a prescription and for the pharmaceutical repackaging firm. This general chapter contains minimum standards to be used as a guideline for repackaging practices. This guideline is not intended to replace or supplant the requirements of regulatory agencies.

Repackaging preparations into unit-dose configurations is an important aspect of pharmaceutical care and of optimization of patient compliance. For purposes of this chapter, there are two types of repackaging: the first involves pharmacies that dispense prescription drugs; the second concerns commercial pharmaceutical repackaging firms.

NOMENCLATURE AND DEFINITIONS

DISPENSER—A dispenser is a licensed or registered practitioner who is legally responsible for providing a preparation for patient use, with a specific patient label, pursuant to a prescription or a medication order. In addition, dispensers may prepare limited quantities in anticipation of a prescription or medication order from a physician. Dispensers are governed by the board of pharmacy of the individual state.

PACKAGE—The term "package" is synonymous with the term "container." See *Containers* under *Preservation, Packaging, Storage, and Labeling* in the *General Notices and Requirements*.

PHARMACY—A pharmacy is an establishment that is legally responsible for providing the drug preparation for patient use, with a specific patient label, pursuant to a prescription or a medication order. The terms dispenser and pharmacy are used interchangeably.

REPACKAGING—Repackaging is the act of removing a preparation from its original primary container and placing it into another primary container, usually of smaller size.

REPACKAGER—A repackager is an establishment that repackages drugs and sends them to a second location in anticipation of a need. Repackaging firms repackage preparations for distribution (e.g., for resale to distributors, hospitals, or other pharmacies), a function that is beyond the regular practice of a pharmacy. Distribution is not patient specific in that there are no prescriptions. Unlike dispensers, repackaging firms are required to register with the FDA and to comply with the Current Good Manufacturing Practice regulations in 21 CFR 210 and 211.

MATERIALS

Blister packages offer a wide array of designs of both functionality and appearance. Various packaging materials are utilized to create blisters that are tailored to provide optimum performance. The blister container consists of two components: the blister, which is the formed cavity that holds the product, and the lid stock, which is the material that seals to the blister, as shown below. Because of the variety of blister films available, film selection should be based upon the degree of protection required. The choice of lid stock depends on how the blister is to be used, but generally the lid stock is made of aluminum foil. The material used to form the cavity is typically a plastic, which can be designed to protect the dosage form from moisture. There are widely varying degrees of moisture protection now available. For purposes of this general chapter, they are referred to as nominal, medium, high, and extreme moisture barrier properties.

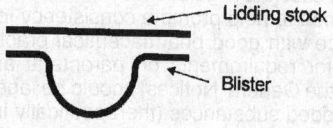

Schematic Presentation of a Typical Blister Pack

Polyvinyl Chloride—The most commonly used blister material is polyvinyl chloride (PVC). This material, which provides a nominal or zero barrier to moisture, is used when the product does not require effective moisture protection. PVC is available in a range of gauges and can be made opaque or can be tinted with pigments to block out specific light wavelengths.

The thickness of the PVC used is determined by the depth and size of the cavity to be formed. Because the plastic thins during the blister-forming process, care should be taken to ensure that the finished blister provides sufficient protection from light (if required) and that it is strong enough to adequately protect the dosage form. Common gauges of PVC used in the pharmaceutical industry range from 7.5 to 15 mil (0.0075 to 0.015 inch).

Barrier Films—Many drug preparations are extremely sensitive to moisture and therefore require high barrier films. Several materials may be used to provide moisture protection. Barrier films commonly used in the pharmaceutical industry are described below.

PVC/PCTFE Laminations—Polychlorotrifluoroethylene (PCTFE) film[1] is a thermoplastic film made from polychlorotrifluoroethylene fluoropolymer. The PCTFE film is laminated to the PVC by an adhesive layer between the PVC and the PCTFE film (duplex structure) or by a layer of polyethylene between the PVC-adhesive and the PCTFE-adhesive layers (triplex structure). By using various gauges of the PCTFE film, *medium* to *extreme* moisture barriers can be obtained.

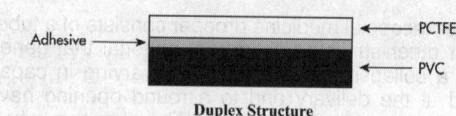

Duplex Structure

---

[1] PCTFE film is available from Allied Signal (as Aclar) and from other sources.

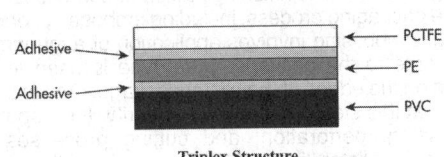

Triplex Structure

PVC/PVdC Laminations—PVC/PVdC is a film in which the PVC is coated with an emulsion of polyvinylidene chloride (PVdC). The PVdC layer is specified in g per m² and can be constructed to provide *medium* to *high* barrier protection. The coating weights commonly used in the pharmaceutical industry are 40, 60, and 90 g per m², and the film is offered with or without a middle layer of polyethylene. The polyethylene is used with heavier coating weights, such as 60 and 90 g per m², to improve the thermoforming characteristics of the blister cavity.

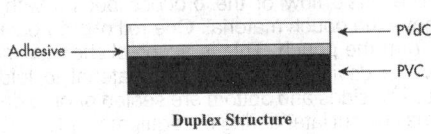

Duplex Structure

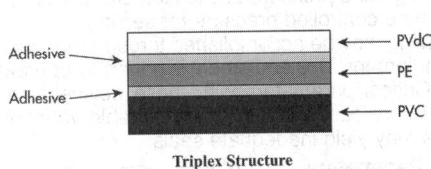

Triplex Structure

Polypropylene—Because of its morphology, polypropylene (PP) serves as a good moisture barrier, its spherulitic structure creating an arduous path for water molecules to traverse. Although not commonly used as a pharmaceutical blister film in the U.S., PP provides an economical alternative to medium barrier materials and is used in Europe as an alternative to PVC.

Cold Form Foil—This material is used for products that are extremely hygroscopic or light sensitive. It is an extreme moisture barrier and consists of three layers: PVC, aluminum foil, and nylon.

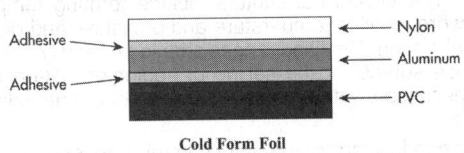

Cold Form Foil

Lid Stock—Lid stock is sealed to the molded blister as described above. Different designs of lid stocks are available, and selection of a particular design depends on how the package will be used. Standard designs—peelable, push-through, and child-resistant—are described below. The primary component of lid stock is typically aluminum and its gauge varies from 18 to 25 μm (0.0078 to 0.001 inch). The side of the aluminum foil laminate in contact with the product provides the heat-sealable layer that forms the seal to the blister material. The heat-seal coating should

be capable of forming an adequate seal with the blister film to which it is intended to seal. The materials used in the makeup of the heat-seal layer meet 21 CFR 175 and 177.

Peelable—Peelable foil, commonly used in an institutional setting, consists of several layers, as shown below, and can be peeled away from the blister. [NOTE—For child-resistant peelable foil, a layer of polyester with the appropriate adhesives would be added.] With the peelable foil lid stock, which is used in conjunction with blister tooling, a three-step process is required to open the blister.

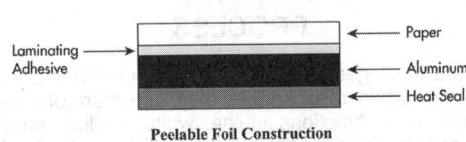

Peelable Foil Construction

First, the blister cavity must be separated from the rest of the blister card. Next, the paper and polyester layers are pulled back from an unsealed area. Finally, the product is pushed through the remaining aluminum foil. It is important to note that use of this type of foil structure helps make the package more child resistant. However, if child-resistant packaging is required, the package design should be tested in accordance with the protocol described in 16 CFR 1700, the Poison Prevention Packaging Act.

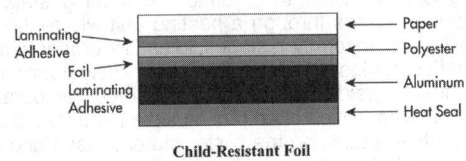

Child-Resistant Foil

Push-Through—There are two commonly used types of push-through foil: one with a paper outer layer separated from the aluminum by a layer of adhesive and one without paper (see diagrams below). The paper outer layer serves as an aesthetic and makes it possible to print on the back of the blister.

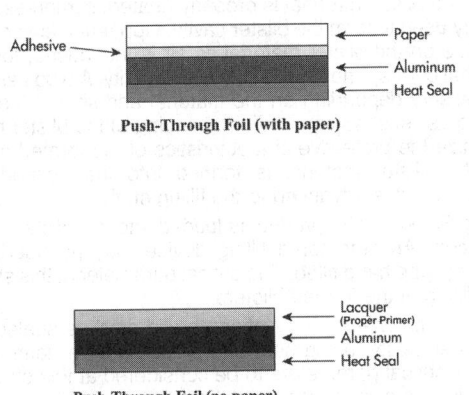

Push-Through Foil (with paper)

Push-Through Foil (no paper)

Other Package Styles—Other types of packages used for unit-dose packaging of solid dosage forms are strip packs, pouches, and sachets.

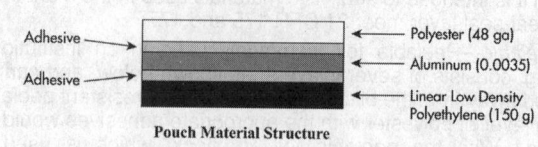

Pouch Material Structure

Adhesive → Polyester (48 ga)
Aluminum (0.0035)
Adhesive → Linear Low Density Polyethylene (150 g)

PROCESS

Unit-dose packages can be formed and sealed in a variety of ways. Larger scale repackagers may use thermoformers that accomplish these functions in-line, while smaller repackagers may purchase preformed blister material. This section begins with an overview of the process involved in thermoforming a blister, the fundamental process that also applies to other unit-dose package types such as pouches. The overview is not intended to be all encompassing, but it highlights the major operations along with their critical parameters.

Thermoforming a Blister Unit-Dose Package—The complete thermoforming process consists of four basic stations where the following operations occur: forming, filling, sealing, and finishing. Thermoforming requires the use of heat and air in forming the blister. The lid stock material is sealed to the blister cavity material for a defined time (the stroke of the machine) at the point where the heat plate closes on the two materials.

Forming Station—Prior to entering the forming station, the blister material passes through a heating unit where the blister material is heated uniformly in stages, to ensure proper formation. Because different plastics have different softening points, careful attention must be paid to determining the proper temperature of the heating station, which often has multiple temperature zones. The temperature, based on the blister material used and on the speed at which that material travels through the heating station, is a critical parameter for optimal performance. At the forming station the blister material is heated to the point where the plastic softens sufficiently to allow the cavity to be formed. The blister material is drawn from a reel-mounted roll (referred to as the web) and pulled through the machine. A splicing table is located at the reel unwind to provide room for a second roll of blister material to be readily available for splicing and resumption of the packaging process. An unwind device may be installed to aid in moving the blister material from the roll as adjusted for a specific index.

Once the blister material is properly heated, compressed air is generally used to form the blister cavity. Upper and lower forming dies close on the blister material as air is introduced, forming a blister that corresponds to the size of the cavity. A plug assist may be necessary depending on the material and size of the cavity. The plug assist ensures a uniform thinning of the blister material to optimize the protective characteristics of the formed material. Once the blister material is formed into the desired blister configuration, it is advanced to the filling station.

Filling Station—The product is loaded into the blister cavity at this station. An automated filling device may be used or the cavities may be hand filled. The critical parameter at this station is proper filling of the formed blisters.

Sealing Station—At this station, the lid stock is sealed to the filled blister cavity, using heat and pressure for a defined dwell time. The critical parameters to be considered at this station are temperature, pressure, and dwell time.

The lid stock material is staged on a roll above the blister cavity and may be preprinted or printed on-line. Lot numbers and expiration dates may be applied at this point. Preprinted lid stock materials will require a print registration system to control the position of the printing relative to the blister cavity. The critical parameters at this part of the station include legible and correct labeling.

Finishing Station—The finishing station encompasses all other steps in the packaging process, including embossing, perforation, and cutting. Embossing involves application of a lot number and expiration date to the package. Steel type is used to emboss information on the edges of the blister package. One of the critical parameters at this station is package integrity. It is important that the embossing, perforation, and cutting processes do not compromise the blister, lid, or seal. The quality of the embossing is another critical parameter in the process. The embossing must be legible, correct, and include all required information.

Pouch Unit-Dose Packages—The pouch process is also a form, fill, and seal operation, but it does not provide a defined, formed cavity as does the thermoforming process. Although the equipment used to form pouch unit-dose packages may function differently from that described for thermoforming a blister, the main operations (form, fill, and seal) and critical parameters at those stations are quite similar. [NOTE—See the aforementioned critical parameters defined in the section on thermoforming.]

The strip-pack process involves the drug product being dosed into a three-sided, formed pouch. Once filled with the drug, the machine seals the pouch, forming a strip of sealed unit-dose pouches. The basic flow of the process begins with the drug situated above the pouch material. One roll of strip-pack material is used to form the pouch. This is accomplished by moving the material over a device that forces the material to fold into two equal sides. The sides and bottom are sealed prior to dosing. The strip pack may be cut later during the equipment processing or roll continuously and be manually cut. Temperature and dwell time are the main critical factors for this equipment.

Preformed Unit-Dose Packages— Preformed containers are sealed either by heat or adhesion. Heat sealers may be manual units requiring hand pressure application or automated units that provide a more controlled pressure for sealing.

Heat sealing may be accomplished through the use of manual tabletop equipment. This equipment is generally operated at a set pressure. Critical parameters with these devices are pressure and temperature control because undesirable variation in these parameters may yield inadequate seals.

Critical Parameters—In order to ensure that the finished container performs as intended, qualification of critical parameters should be determined. Typically, validation of a packaging line consists of qualification of the installation, operation, and performance of a packaging system.

Installation Qualification—Equipment should be installed and found to be in proper working condition prior to use.

Operation Qualification—Operational qualification should be performed to establish that the equipment operates within the manufacturer's specified ranges. Incoming utilities for the equipment, such as air, electricity, etc., should be monitored and checked periodically.

Performance Qualification—Performance qualification should be done to ensure that the equipment is performing properly with the required materials to produce a container that functions as intended. The critical parameters include forming temperature and pressure, sealing temperature and pressure, and dwell time at the seal station. Qualified ranges should be readily available in a reference source for the set up of equipment. Re-evaluation may be necessary with changes to equipment, materials, or the process.

In-Process Inspections—Strict controls covering the packaging and labeling processes shall be in place. The final container should be evaluated for performance in each of the stations described above. Specifically, the formed container should be inspected visually to ensure that it is properly formed. Evaluation of the filling station should include a check to ensure that the unit-dose is properly filled (i.e., the correct product is present). The sealing station should be evaluated to ensure that a proper seal has been made and that the moisture permeation specifications of the sealed container have been met. A visual examination of the package should be performed to ensure that the final steps of the packaging process are acceptable.

Repackagers and dispensers should use a standard inspection plan to verify the adequacy of the package. A visual inspection should be performed to verify that the correct product is in the proper packaging materials with correct labeling. Seal integrity should be evaluated, using vacuum testing,[2] helium testing, tear testing, and other testing methods suitable to establish whether seal integrity is maintained.

PERFORMANCE

The primary purpose of the unit-dose package used in the packaging of a drug preparation is to ensure that throughout its intended expiration dating there is adequate protection from the environment as the dosage form is distributed and stored. It is also essential that the materials used do not interact with the dosage form.

When determining what type of package to use in the repackaging operation, consideration must be given to the dosage form's sensitivities (if any) to the storage and distribution environments (e.g., temperature, light, and moisture).

The materials used in constructing the unit-dose container as well as the process of forming and sealing the container all together define the properties of the finished container. As discussed in *Materials*, there is a wide variety of commercially available film structures that provide unit-dose containers with a range of moisture and light protection. Suppliers of these materials typically provide quantitative data obtained from well-established test methods, to highlight the protective properties of their material. These data are based on flat sheets of the film, not on the formed container.

It is critical to understand that once the film is formed, protective properties change because the overall thickness of the film decreases as the blister cavity is formed. Usually the change is a decrease, especially in the case of barrier properties. However, the extent of change will vary with the type of film structure used and is also highly dependent on the container-forming process used (see *Process*). Further, a suboptimal seal on the formed container will decrease the protective properties of the container. Insufficient temperature, time, or pressure during a heat-seal operation may enable the passage of moisture or oxygen through the seal area over time and may have an effect on the dosage form. In addition, if the seal area is designed with insufficient surface area, the same problem may occur. To ensure a good seal, a minimum sealing distance of 3 mm from the edge of the blister cavity to the nearest edge or perforation is recommended. Therefore, it is important to measure the performance of the formed and sealed container rather than the performance of the flat sheet.

Moisture is a critical factor in preparation integrity. *Containers—Permeation* ⟨671⟩ describes how to determine and classify moisture permeation rates. If the manufacturer's labeling includes "Protect From Moisture," the repackager shall utilize a high barrier film.

If light protection is required for a drug preparation, the repackager should follow the requirements for light transmission established under *Containers* ⟨661⟩. Again, this testing should be conducted on the formed container, because the light protective properties of the film are compromised once the film is thinned during the forming process. It is recommended that these tests, in conjunction with any guidance provided by the manufacturer, be considered appropriate for any container–closure system used in repackaging a drug preparation.

BEYOND-USE DATE

In the absence of stability data for the drug product in the repackaged container, the beyond-use dating period is one year or the time remaining of the expiration date, whichever is shorter. If current stability data are available for the drug product in the repackaged container, the length of time established by the stability study may be used to establish the beyond-use date but must not exceed the manufacturer's expiration date.

As stated in the *General Notices and Requirements*, the dispenser must maintain the facility where the dosage forms are packaged and stored at a temperature such that the mean kinetic temperature is not greater than 25°. The plastic material used in packaging the dosage forms must afford better protection than polyvinyl chloride, which does not provide adequate protection against moisture permeation. Records must be kept of the temperature of the facility where the dosage forms are stored, and of the plastic materials used in packaging.

MINIMUM REQUIREMENTS

The previous sections serve as a general introduction to repackaging by providing a basic understanding of materials selection, the form-fill-seal process, and the importance of performance of the sealed container. In this section, certain minimum requirements for repackaging, which must be met, are described in more detail.

Personnel—Each person with responsibility for the repackaging of a preparation shall have the education, training, and experience, or any combination thereof, to perform assigned functions in a manner such that the safety, identity, strength, quality, purity, potency, and pharmaceutical elegance of the drug dosage form are retained. Training should be documented.

Personnel engaged in the repackaging of a preparation shall wear clean clothing appropriate for the duties or processes performed.

Facility—The repackaging facility may require areas of low relative humidity, and temperature conditions should meet controlled room temperature requirements specified in the *General Notices*.

Equipment—Equipment used in the repackaging of a preparation shall be of appropriate design and suitably located to facilitate operations for its intended use. Its design should allow for cleaning to preclude cross-contamination as well as for maintenance to be performed. Equipment shall be constructed so those surfaces that contact components or a preparation are not reactive, additive, or absorptive.

Any substances required for operation, such as lubricants or coolants, shall not come into contact with components or a preparation.

Equipment and utensils shall be cleaned, maintained, and sanitized at appropriate intervals to prevent malfunctions or contamination. Preventive maintenance should be performed at appropriate intervals in accordance with the equipment manufacturer's recommendation. Any instruments used to monitor critical parameters should be calibrated on a defined schedule.

Process—Steps should be taken to determine the critical process parameters (e.g., seal temperature, dwell time, etc.) in operating the equipment. Set points for these parameters should be documented and procedures established to ensure that they are adhered to each time the equipment is operated.

Labeling—The labeling requirements for a commercial repackager and a pharmacist are different. For example, the commercial repackager must comply with 21 CFR 201.1, but the pharmacist or dispenser does not have to comply with this requirement. If stability data are unavailable, the dispenser shall repackage only

---

[2] Vacuum testing consists of placing samples from the packaging operation into a jar filled with water. A lid is placed over the samples to fully immerse them in the water. A container lid is applied to create a seal effective enough to create approximately 25 cm of vacuum. The vacuum pump is set and the samples are tested for approximately 1 minute, removed from the water, wiped down, and opened to determine if the inside of the unit-dose cavity or pouch is wet. This process should be adjusted until it is under control and additional testing may be performed to ensure that the seal integrity is consistently acceptable. Wetness indicates a defective seal and therefore the potential for the drug to degrade when exposed to the atmosphere. Defective packages must be removed from further use.

an amount of stock sufficient for a limited time and shall include product name and strength, lot number, manufacturer, and appropriate beyond-use date on the label. When quantities are repackaged in advance of immediate needs, each preparation must bear an identifying label, and the dispenser is required to maintain suitable repackaging records showing the name of the manufacturer, lot number, expiration date, date of repackaging, and designation of persons responsible for repackaging and for checking. The repackager or dispenser will use documented controls to prevent labeling errors.

Materials—The repackager or dispenser shall place an appropriate beyond-use date on the label and package in appropriate materials. Materials used by the repackager shall not be reactive, additive, or absorptive, and must meet the requirements described in 21 CFR 175 and 177.

Storage—The dispenser shall rotate and monitor stock closely to ensure that the dispensing of preparations is on a first-in–first-out (FIFO) basis. The repackager or dispenser shall store preparations under required environmental conditions (e.g., controlled room temperature with a mean kinetic temperature not higher than 25°).

Drug Product—The repackager or dispenser shall examine preparations for evidence of instability such as change in color or odor, and shall exercise professional judgment as to the acceptability of a package.

Complaints—The repackager or dispenser will maintain written procedures describing the handling of written and oral complaints regarding a drug product and will ensure that complaints are investigated and appropriately resolved.

Returned Goods—Policies and procedures relating to returned goods should be developed to ensure proper handling.

Reprocessing—Reprocessing of repackaged unit-dose containers (i.e., removal of medication from one unit-dose container and placing it into another unit-dose container) shall not be done. However, reprocessing of the secondary package (e.g., removing the blister card from the cardboard carrier and placing the blister card into another cardboard carrier) is allowed provided the original beyond-use date is maintained, and provided the integrity of the blister is ensured.

Special Considerations—If a product is known to be oxygen sensitive or if it exhibits extreme moisture or light sensitivity (e.g., cold form foil), it shall not be repackaged. If a product is refrigerated, it shall not be repackaged unless proper environmental conditions and suitable materials are available. Certain drug products (such as oncologic agents, hormones, or penicillin derivatives) require special handling because they are considered very potent or toxic, and because transfer of any portion of these products to another product could have deleterious effects.

⟨1151⟩ PHARMACEUTICAL DOSAGE FORMS

Dosage forms are provided for most of the Pharmacopeial drug substances, but the processes for the preparation of many of them are, in general, beyond the scope of the Pharmacopeia. In addition to defining the dosage forms, this section presents the general principles involved in the manufacture of some of them, particularly on a small scale. Other information that is given bears on the use of the Pharmacopeial substances in extemporaneous compounding of dosage forms.

BIOAVAILABILITY

Bioavailability, or the extent to which the therapeutic constituent of a pharmaceutical dosage form intended for oral or topical use is available for absorption, is influenced by a variety of factors. Among the inherent factors known to affect absorption are the method of manufacture or method of compounding; the

particle size and crystal form or polymorph of the drug substance; and the diluents and excipients used in formulating the dosage form, including fillers, binders, disintegrating agents, lubricants, coatings, solvents, suspending agents, and dyes. Lubricants and coatings are foremost among these. The maintenance of a demonstrably high degree of bioavailability requires particular attention to all aspects of production and quality control that may affect the nature of the finished dosage form.

STABILITY

The term "stability," with respect to a drug dosage form, refers to the chemical and physical integrity of the dosage unit, and, when appropriate, the ability of the dosage unit to maintain protection against microbiological contamination. The shelf life of the dosage form is the time lapse from initial preparation to the specified expiration date. The monograph specifications of identity, strength, quality, and purity apply throughout the shelf life of the product.

The stability parameters of a drug dosage form can be influenced by environmental conditions of storage (temperature, light, air, and humidity), as well as the package components. Pharmacopeial articles should include required storage conditions on their labeling. These are the conditions under which the expiration date shall apply. The storage requirements specified in the labeling for the article must be observed throughout the distribution of the article (i.e., beyond the time it leaves the manufacturer up to and including its handling by the dispenser or seller of the article to the consumer). Although labeling for the consumer should indicate proper storage conditions, it is recognized that control beyond the dispenser or seller is difficult. The beyond-use date shall be placed on the container label.

Stability Protocols—Stability of manufactured dosage forms must be demonstrated by the manufacturer by the use of methods adequate for the purpose. Monograph assays may be used for stability testing if they are stability-indicating (i.e., if they accurately differentiate between the intact drug molecules and their degradation products). Stability considerations should include not only the specific compendial requirements, but also changes in physical appearance of the product that would warn users that the product's continued integrity is questionable.

Stability studies on active substances and packaged dosage forms are conducted by means of "real-time," long-term tests at specific temperatures and relative humidities representing storage conditions experienced in the distribution chain of the climatic zone(s) of the country or region of the world concerned. Labeling of the packaged active substance or dosage form should reflect the effects of temperature, relative humidity, air, and light on its stability. Label temperature storage warnings will reflect both the results of the real-time storage tests and also allow for expected seasonal excursions of temperature.

Controlled room temperature (see the *Storage Temperature* section under *General Notices and Requirements—Preservation, Packaging, Storage, and Labeling*) delineates the allowable tolerance in storage circumstances at any location in the chain of distribution (e.g., pharmacies, hospitals, and warehouses). This terminology also allows patients or consumers to be counseled as to appropriate storage for the product. Products may be labeled either to store at "Controlled room temperature" or to store at temperatures "up to 25°" where labeling is supported by long-term stability studies at the designated storage condition of 25°. *Controlled room temperature* limits the permissible excursions to those consistent with the maintenance of a mean kinetic temperature calculated to be not more than 25°. See *Mean Kinetic Temperature*. The common international guideline for long-term stability studies specifies $25 \pm 2°$ at $60 \pm 5\%$ relative humidity. Accelerated studies are specified at $40 \pm 2°$ and at $75 \pm 5\%$ relative humidity. Accelerated studies also allow the interpretation of data and information on short-term spikes in storage conditions in addition to the excursions allowed for by controlled room temperature.

The term "room temperature" is used in different ways in different countries, and it is usually preferable for product labeling for products to be shipped outside the continental U.S. to refer to a maximum storage temperature or temperature range in degrees Celsius.

Mean Kinetic Temperature—Mean Kinetic Temperature (MKT) is defined as the single calculated temperature at which the total amount of degradation over a particular period is equal to the sum of the individual degradations that would occur at various temperatures. Thus, MKT may be considered as an isothermal storage temperature that simulates the nonisothermal effects of storage temperature variation. It is not a simple arithmetic mean. MKT is calculated from temperatures in a storage facility. It can be conveniently collected using electronic devices that measure temperatures at frequent intervals (e.g., every 15 minutes). MKT can be calculated directly or the data can be downloaded to a computer for processing. For dispensing sites, such as pharmacies and hospitals, where the use of such instruments may not be feasible, devices such as high-low thermometers capable of indicating weekly high and low temperatures over a 52-week period may be employed. The arithmetic mean of the weekly high and low temperatures is then used in the calculation of MKT. MKT is calculated by the following equation (derived from the Arrhenius equation):

$$T_k = \frac{\Delta H/R}{-ln\left(\dfrac{e^{-\Delta H/RT_1} + e^{-\Delta H/RT_2} + \ldots + e^{-\Delta H/RT_n}}{n}\right)},$$

in which T_k is the mean kinetic temperature; ΔH is the heat of activation, 83.144 kJ $\cdot$ mole^{-1} (unless more accurate information is available from experimental studies); R is the universal gas constant, 8.3144×10^{-3} kJ $\cdot$ mole^{-1} $\cdot$ degree^{-1}; T_1 is the value for the temperature recorded during the first time period, e.g., the first week; T_2 is the value for the temperature recorded during the second time period, e.g., second week; T_n is the value for the temperature recorded during the nth time period, e.g., nth week, n being the total number of storage temperatures recorded (minimum of 52 weekly entries) during the annual observation period; and all temperatures, T, being absolute temperatures in degrees Kelvin (K).

The following is an example of a typical storage and distribution temperature range in Kelvin degrees and the conversion factors used to convert this range into degrees Fahrenheit and Celsius.

Kelvin (K)	Fahrenheit (°F)	Celsius (°C)
288.1–303.1	59–86	15–30

Conversion Factors:
Fahrenheit to Kelvin = {[(°F − 32) × 5/9] + 273.1}
Celsius to Kelvin = 273.1 + °C
Fahrenheit to Celsius = [(°F − 32) × 5/9]

Climatic Zones—For convenience in planning for packaging and storage, and for stability studies, international practice identifies four climatic zones, which are described in *Table 1*. The United States, Europe, and Japan are characterized by zones I and II. The values in *Table 1* are based on observed temperatures and relative humidities, both outside and in rooms, from which mean kinetic temperatures and average humidity values are calculated.[1] Derived values are based on inspection of data from individual cities and on allowances for a margin of safety in assignment of these specified conditions.

Table 1. International Climatic Zones

Climatic Zone	Calculated Data				Derived Data		
	°C*	°C MKT**	% RH	mbar***	°C	% RH	mbar
I. *Temperate* United Kingdom Northern Europe Canada Russia	20.0	20.0	42	9.9	21	45	11.2
II *Mediterranean, Subtropical* United States Japan Southern Europe (Portugal-Greece)	21.6	22.0	52	13.5	25	60	19.0
III. *Hot, Dry* Iran Iraq Sudan	26.4	27.9	35	11.9	30	35	15.0
IV. *Hot, Humid* Brazil Ghana Indonesia Nicaragua Philippines	26.7	27.4	76	26.6	30	70	30.0

* Data recorded as <19° calculated as 19°.
** Calculated mean kinetic temperature.
*** Partial pressure of water vapor.

[1] The source of the data and information in *Table 1* is the International Conference on Harmonization sponsored by the International Federation of Pharmaceutical Manufacturers Associations.

A discussion of aspects of drug product stability that are of primary concern to the pharmacist in the dispensing of medications may be found under *Stability Considerations in Dispensing Practice* ⟨1191⟩.

Inasmuch as this chapter is for purposes of general information only, no statement herein is intended to modify or supplant any of the specific requirements pertinent to pharmaceutical preparations, which are given elsewhere in this Pharmacopeia.

TERMINOLOGY

Occasionally it is necessary to add solvent to the contents of a container just prior to use, usually because of instability of some drugs in the diluted form. Thus, a solid diluted to yield a suspension is called [*DRUG*] *for Suspension;* a solid dissolved and diluted to yield a solution is called [*DRUG*] *for Solution;* and a solution or suspension diluted to yield a more dilute form of the drug is called [*DRUG*] *Oral Concentrate.* After dilution, it is important that the drug be homogeneously dispersed before administration.

AEROSOLS

Pharmaceutical aerosols are products that are packaged under pressure and contain therapeutically active ingredients that are released upon activation of an appropriate valve system. They are intended for topical application to the skin as well as local application into the nose (nasal aerosols), mouth (lingual aerosols), or lungs (inhalation aerosols). These products may be fitted with valves enabling either continuous or metered-dose delivery; hence, the terms "[DRUG] Metered Topical Aerosols," "[DRUG] Metered Nasal Aerosols," etc.

The term "aerosol" refers to the fine mist of spray that results from most pressurized systems. However, the term has been broadly misapplied to all self-contained pressurized products, some of which deliver foams or semisolid fluids. In the case of *Inhalation Aerosols*, the particle size of the delivered medication must be carefully controlled and the average size of the particles should be under 5 μm. These products are also known as metered-dose inhalers (MDIs). Other aerosol sprays may contain particles up to several hundred micrometers in diameter.

The basic components of an aerosol system are the container, the propellant, the concentrate containing the active ingredient(s), the valve, and the actuator. The nature of these components determines such characteristics as particle size distribution, uniformity of dose for metered valves, delivery rate, wetness and temperature of the spray, spray pattern and velocity or plume geometry, foam density, and fluid viscosity.

Types of Aerosols

Aerosols consist of two-phase (gas and liquid) or three-phase (gas, liquid, and solid or liquid) systems. The two-phase aerosol consists of a solution of active ingredients in liquefied propellant and the vaporized propellant. The solvent is composed of the propellant or a mixture of the propellant and cosolvents such as alcohol, propylene glycol, and polyethylene glycols, which are often used to enhance the solubility of the active ingredients.

Three-phase systems consist of a suspension or emulsion of the active ingredient(s) in addition to the vaporized propellants. A suspension consists of the active ingredient(s) that may be dispersed in the propellant system with the aid of suitable excipients such as wetting agents and/or solid carriers such as talc or colloidal silicas.

A foam aerosol is an emulsion containing one or more active ingredients, surfactants, aqueous or nonaqueous liquids, and the propellants. If the propellant is in the internal (discontinuous) phase (i.e., of the oil-in-water type), a stable foam is discharged; and if the propellant is in the external (continuous) phase (i.e., of the water-in-oil type), a spray or a quick-breaking foam is discharged.

Propellants

The propellant supplies the necessary pressure within an aerosol system to expel material from the container and, in combination with other components, to convert the material into the desired physical form. Propellants may be broadly classified as liquefied or compressed gases having vapor pressures generally exceeding atmospheric pressure. Propellants within this definition include various hydrocarbons, especially halogenated derivatives of methane, ethane, and propane, low molecular weight hydrocarbons such as the butanes and pentanes, and compressed gases such as carbon dioxide, nitrogen, and nitrous oxide. Mixtures of propellants are frequently used to obtain desirable pressure, delivery, and spray characteristics. A good propellant system should have the proper vapor pressure characteristics consistent with the other aerosol components.

Valves

The primary function of the valve is to regulate the flow of the therapeutic agent and propellant from the container. The spray characteristics of the aerosol are influenced by orifice dimension, number, and location. Most aerosol valves provide for continuous spray operation and are used on most topical products. However, pharmaceutical products for oral or nasal inhalation often utilize metered-dose valves that must deliver a uniform quantity of spray upon each valve activation. The accuracy and reproducibility of the doses delivered from metering valves are generally good, comparing favorably to the uniformity of solid dosage forms such as tablets and capsules. However, when aerosol packages are stored improperly, or when they have not been used for long periods of time, valves must be primed before use. Materials used for the manufacture of valves should be inert to the formulations used. Plastic, rubber, aluminum, and stainless steel valve components are commonly used. Metered-dose valves must deliver an accurate dose within specified tolerances.

Actuators

An actuator is the fitting attached to an aerosol valve stem, which when depressed or moved, opens the valve, and directs the spray containing the drug preparation to the desired area. The actuator usually indicates the direction in which the preparation is dispensed and protects the hand or finger from the refrigerant effects of the propellant. Actuators incorporate an orifice which may vary widely in size and shape. The size of this orifice, the expansion chamber design, and the nature of the propellant and formulation influence the delivered dose as well as the physical characteristics of the spray, foam, or stream of solid particles dispensed. For inhalation aerosols, an actuator capable of delivering the medication in the proper particle size range and with the appropriate spray pattern and plume geometry is utilized.

Containers

Aerosol containers usually are made of glass, plastic, or metal, or a combination of these materials. Glass containers must be precisely engineered to provide the maximum in pressure safety and impact resistance. Plastics may be employed to coat glass containers for improved safety characteristics, or to coat metal containers to improve corrosion resistance and enhance stability of the formulation. Suitable metals include stainless steel,

aluminum, and tin-plated steel. Extractables or leachables (e.g., drawing oils, cleaning agents, etc.) and particulates on the internal surfaces of containers should be controlled.

Manufacture

Aerosols are usually prepared by one of two general processes. In the "cold-fill" process, the concentrate (generally cooled to a temperature below 0°) and the refrigerated propellant are measured into open containers (usually chilled). The valve-actuator assembly is then crimped onto the container to form a pressure-tight seal. During the interval between propellant addition and crimping, sufficient volatilization of propellant occurs to displace air from the container. In the "pressure-fill" method, the concentrate is placed in the container, and either the propellant is forced under pressure through the valve orifice after the valve is sealed, or the propellant is allowed to flow under the valve cap and then the valve assembly is sealed ("under-the-cap" filling). In both cases of the "pressure-fill" method, provision must be made for evacuation of air by means of vacuum or displacement with a small amount of propellant vapor. Manufacturing process controls usually include monitoring of proper formulation and propellant fill weight and pressure testing, leak testing, and valve function testing of the finished aerosol. Microbiological attributes should also be controlled.

Extractable Substances

Since pressurized inhalers and aerosols are normally formulated with organic solvents as the propellant or the vehicle, leaching of extractables from the elastomeric and plastic components into the formulation is a potentially serious problem. Thus, the composition and the quality of materials used in the manufacture of the valve components (e.g., stem, gaskets, housing, etc.) must be carefully selected and controlled. Their compatibility with formulation components should be well established so as to prevent distortion of the valve components and to minimize changes in the medication delivery, leak rate, and impurity profile of the drug product over time. The extractable profiles of a representative sample of each of the elastomeric and plastic components of the valve should be established under specified conditions and should be correlated to the extractable profile of the aged drug product or placebo, to ensure reproducible quality and purity of the drug product. Extractables, which may include polynuclear aromatics, nitrosamines, vulcanization accelerators, antioxidants, plasticizers, monomers, etc., should be identified and minimized wherever possible.

Specifications and limits for individual and total extractables from different valve components may require the use of different analytical methods. In addition, the standard USP biological testing (see the general test chapters *Biological Reactivity Tests, In Vitro* ⟨87⟩ and *Biological Reactivity Tests, In Vivo* ⟨88⟩) as well as other safety data may be needed.

Labeling

Medicinal aerosols should contain at least the following warning information on the label as in accordance with appropriate regulations.

Warning—Avoid inhaling. Avoid spraying into eyes or onto other mucous membranes.

NOTE—The statement "Avoid inhaling" is not necessary for preparations specifically designed for use by inhalation. The phrase "or other mucous membranes" is not necessary for preparations specifically designed for use on mucous membranes.

Warning—Contents under pressure. Do not puncture or incinerate container. Do not expose to heat or store at temperatures above 120° F (49° C). Keep out of reach of children.

In addition to the aforementioned warnings, the label of a drug packaged in an aerosol container in which the propellant consists in whole or in part of a halocarbon or hydrocarbon shall, where required under regulations of the FDA, bear either of the following warnings:

Warning—Do not inhale directly; deliberate inhalation of contents can cause death.

Warning—Use only as directed; intentional misuse by deliberately concentrating and inhaling the contents can be harmful or fatal.

BOLUSES

Boluses are large elongated tablets intended for administration to animals (see *Tablets*).

CAPSULES

Capsules are solid dosage forms in which the drug is enclosed within either a hard or soft soluble container or "shell." The shells are usually formed from gelatin; however, they also may be made from starch or other suitable substances. Hard-shell capsule sizes range from No. 5, the smallest, to No. 000, which is the largest, except for veterinary sizes. However, size No. 00 generally is the largest size acceptable to patients. Size 0 hard gelatin capsules having an elongated body (known as size OE) also are available, which provide greater fill capacity without an increase in diameter. Hard gelatin capsules consist of two, telescoping cap and body pieces. Generally, there are unique grooves or indentations molded into the cap and body portions to provide a positive closure when fully engaged, which helps prevent the accidental separation of the filled capsules during shipping and handling. Positive closure also may be affected by spot fusion ("welding") of the cap and body pieces together through direct thermal means or by application of ultrasonic energy. Factory-filled hard gelatin capsules may be completely sealed by banding, a process in which one or more layers of gelatin are applied over the seam of the cap and body, or by a liquid fusion process wherein the filled capsules are wetted with a hydroalcoholic solution that penetrates into the space where the cap overlaps the body, and then dried. Hard-shell capsules made from starch consist of two, fitted cap and body pieces. Since the two pieces do not telescope or interlock positively, they are sealed together at the time of filling to prevent their separation. Starch capsules are sealed by the application of a hydroalcoholic solution to the recessed section of the cap immediately prior to its being placed onto the body.

The banding of hard-shell gelatin capsules or the liquid sealing of hard-shell starch capsules enhances consumer safety by making the capsules difficult to open without causing visible, obvious damage, and may improve the stability of contents by limiting O_2 penetration. Industrially filled hard-shell capsules also are often of distinctive color and shape or are otherwise marked to identify them with the manufacturer. Additionally, such capsules may be printed axially or radially with strengths, product codes, etc. Pharmaceutical-grade printing inks are usually based on shellac and employ FDA-approved pigments and lake dyes.

In extemporaneous prescription practice, hard-shell capsules may be hand-filled; this permits the prescriber a latitude of choice in selecting either a single drug or a combination of drugs at the exact dosage level considered best for the individual patient. This flexibility gives hard-shell capsules an advantage over compressed tablets and soft-shell capsules as a dosage form. Hard-shell capsules are usually formed from gelatins having relatively high gel strength. Either type may be used, but blends of pork skin and bone gelatin are often used to optimize shell clarity and toughness. Hard-shell capsules also may be formed from starch or other suitable substances. Hard-shell capsules may also contain colorants, such as D&C and FD&C dyes or the various

iron oxides, opaquing agents such as titanium dioxide, dispersing agents, hardening agents such as sucrose, and preservatives. They normally contain between 10% and 15% water.

Hard gelatin capsules are made by a process that involves dipping shaped pins into gelatin solutions, after which the gelatin films are dried, trimmed, and removed from the pins, and the body and cap pieces are joined. Starch capsules are made by injection molding a mixture of starch and water, after which the capsules are dried. A separate mold is used for caps and bodies, and the two parts are supplied separately. The empty capsules should be stored in tight containers until they are filled. Since gelatin is of animal origin and starch is of vegetable origin, capsules made with these materials should be protected from potential sources of microbial contamination.

Hard-shell capsules typically are filled with powder, beads, or granules. Inert sugar beads (nonpareils) may be coated with active ingredients and coating compositions that provide extended-release profiles or enteric properties. Alternatively, larger-dose active ingredients themselves may be suitably formed into pellets and then coated. Semisolids or liquids also may be filled into hard-shell capsules; however, when the latter are encapsulated, one of the sealing techniques must be employed to prevent leakage.

In hard gelatin capsule filling operations, the body and cap of the shell are separated prior to dosing. In hard starch shell filling operations, the bodies and caps are supplied separately and are fed into separate hoppers of the filling machine. Machines employing various dosing principles may be employed to fill powders into hard-shell capsules; however, most fully automatic machines form powder plugs by compression and eject them into empty capsule bodies. Accessories to these machines generally are available for the other types of fills. Powder formulations often require adding fillers, lubricants, and glidants to the active ingredients to facilitate encapsulation. The formulation, as well as the method of filling, particularly the degree of compaction, may influence the rate of drug release. The addition of wetting agents to the powder mass is common where the active ingredient is hydrophobic. Disintegrants also may be included in powder formulations to facilitate deaggregation and dispersal of capsule plugs in the gut. Powder formulations often may be produced by dry blending; however, bulky formulations may require densification by roll compaction or other suitable granulation techniques.

Powder mixtures that tend to liquefy may be dispensed in hard-shell capsules if an absorbent such as magnesium carbonate, colloidal silicon dioxide, or other suitable substance is used. Potent drugs are often mixed with an inert diluent before being filled into capsules. Where two mutually incompatible drugs are prescribed together, it is sometimes possible to place one in a small capsule and then enclose it with the second drug in a larger capsule. Incompatible drugs also can be separated by placing coated pellets or tablets, or soft-shell capsules of one drug into the capsule shell before adding the second drug.

Thixotropic semisolids may be formed by gelling liquid drugs or vehicles with colloidal silicas or powdered high molecular weight polyethylene glycols. Various waxy or fatty compounds may be used to prepare semisolid matrices by fusion.

Soft-shell capsules made from gelatin (sometimes called softgels) or other suitable material require large-scale production methods. The soft gelatin shell is somewhat thicker than that of hard-shell capsules and may be plasticized by the addition of a polyol such as sorbitol or glycerin. The ratio of dry plasticizer to dry gelatin determines the "hardness" of the shell and may be varied to accommodate environmental conditions as well as the nature of the contents. Like hard shells, the shell composition may include approved dyes and pigments, opaquing agents such as titanium dioxide, and preservatives. Flavors may be added and up to 5% sucrose may be included for its sweetness and to produce a chewable shell. Soft gelatin shells normally contain 6% to 13% water. Soft-shell capsules also may be printed with a product code, strength, etc. In most cases, soft-shell capsules are filled with liquid contents. Typically, active ingredients are dissolved or suspended in a liquid vehicle. Classically, an oleaginous vehicle such as a vegetable oil was used; however,

nonaqueous, water-miscible liquid vehicles such as the lower-molecular-weight polyethylene glycols are more common today due to fewer bioavailability problems.

Available in a wide variety of sizes and shapes, soft-shell capsules are both formed, filled, and sealed in the same machine; typically, this is a rotary die process, although a plate process or reciprocating die process also may be employed. Soft-shell capsules also may be manufactured in a bubble process that forms seamless spherical capsules. With suitable equipment, powders and other dry solids also may be filled into soft-shell capsules.

Liquid-filled capsules of either type involve similar formulation technology and offer similar advantages and limitations. For instance, both may offer advantages over dry-filled capsules and tablets in content uniformity and drug dissolution. Greater homogeneity is possible in liquid systems, and liquids can be metered more accurately. Drug dissolution may benefit because the drug may already be in solution or at least suspended in a hydrophilic vehicle. However, the contact between the hard or soft shell and its liquid content is more intimate than exists with dry-filled capsules, and this may enhance the chances for undesired interactions. The liquid nature of capsule contents presents different technological problems than dry-filled capsules in regard to disintegration and dissolution testing. From formulation, technological, and biopharmaceutical points of view, liquid-filled capsules of either type have more in common than liquid-filled and dry-filled capsules having the same shell composition. Thus, for compendial purposes, standards and methods should be established based on capsule contents rather than on whether the contents are filled into hard- or soft-shell capsules.

DELAYED-RELEASE CAPSULES

Capsules may be coated, or, more commonly, encapsulated granules may be coated to resist releasing the drug in the gastric fluid of the stomach where a delay is important to alleviate potential problems of drug inactivation or gastric mucosal irritation. The term "delayed-release" is used for Pharmacopeial monographs on enteric coated capsules that are intended to delay the release of medicament until the capsule has passed through the stomach, and the individual monographs include tests and specifications for *Drug release* (see *Drug Release* ⟨724⟩) or *Disintegration* (see *Disintegration* ⟨701⟩).

EXTENDED-RELEASE CAPSULES

Extended-release capsules are formulated in such manner as to make the contained medicament available over an extended period of time following ingestion. Expressions such as "prolonged-action," "repeat-action," and "sustained-release" have also been used to describe such dosage forms. However, the term "extended-release" is used for Pharmacopeial purposes and requirements for *Drug release* (see *Drug Release* ⟨724⟩) typically are specified in the individual monographs.

CONCENTRATE FOR DIP

Concentrate for Dip is a preparation containing one or more active ingredients usually in the form of a paste or solution. It is used to prepare a diluted suspension, emulsion, or solution of the active ingredient(s) for the prevention and treatment of ectoparasitic infestations of animals. The diluted preparation (Dip) is applied by complete immersion of the animal or, where appropriate, by spraying. Concentrate for Dip may contain suitable antimicrobial preservatives.

CREAMS

Creams are semisolid dosage forms containing one or more drug substances dissolved or dispersed in a suitable base. This term has traditionally been applied to semisolids that possess a relatively fluid consistency formulated as either water-in-oil (e.g., *Cold Cream*) or oil-in-water (e.g., *Fluocinolone Acetonide Cream*) emulsions. However, more recently the term has been restricted to products consisting of oil-in-water emulsions or aqueous microcrystalline dispersions of long-chain fatty acids or alcohols that are water washable and more cosmetically and aesthetically acceptable. Creams can be used for administering drugs via the vaginal route (e.g., *Triple Sulfa Vaginal Cream*).

ELIXIRS

See *Solutions*.

EMULSIONS

Emulsions are two-phase systems in which one liquid is dispersed throughout another liquid in the form of small droplets. Where oil is the dispersed phase and an aqueous solution is the continuous phase, the system is designated as an oil-in-water emulsion. Conversely, where water or an aqueous solution is the dispersed phase and oil or oleaginous material is the continuous phase, the system is designated as a water-in-oil emulsion. Emulsions are stabilized by emulsifying agents that prevent coalescence, the merging of small droplets into larger droplets and, ultimately, into a single separated phase. Emulsifying agents (surfactants) do this by concentrating in the interface between the droplet and external phase and by providing a physical barrier around the particle to coalescence. Surfactants also reduce the interfacial tension between the phases, thus increasing the ease of emulsification upon mixing.

Natural, semisynthetic, and synthetic hydrophilic polymers may be used in conjunction with surfactants in oil-in-water emulsions as they accumulate at interfaces and also increase the viscosity of the aqueous phase, thereby decreasing the rate of formation of aggregates of droplets. Aggregation is generally accompanied by a relatively rapid separation of an emulsion into a droplet-rich and droplet-poor phase. Normally the density of an oil is lower than that of water, in which case the oil droplets and droplet aggregates rise, a process referred to as creaming. The greater the rate of aggregation, the greater the droplet size and the greater the rate of creaming. The water droplets in a water-in-oil emulsion generally sediment because of their greater density.

The consistency of emulsions varies widely, ranging from easily pourable liquids to semisolid creams. Generally oil-in-water creams are prepared at high temperature, where they are fluid, and cooled to room temperature, whereupon they solidify as a result of solidification of the internal phase. When this is the case, a high internal-phase volume to external-phase volume ratio is not necessary for semisolid character, and, for example, stearic acid creams or vanishing creams are semisolid with as little as 15% internal phase. Any semisolid character with water-in-oil emulsions generally is attributable to a semisolid external phase.

All emulsions require an antimicrobial agent because the aqueous phase is favorable to the growth of microorganisms. The presence of a preservative is particularly critical in oil-in-water emulsions where contamination of the external phase occurs readily. Since fungi and yeasts are found with greater frequency than bacteria, fungistatic as well as bacteriostatic properties are desirable. Bacteria have been shown to degrade nonionic and anionic emulsifying agents, glycerin, and many natural stabilizers such as tragacanth and guar gum.

Complications arise in preserving emulsion systems, as a result of partitioning of the antimicrobial agent out of the aqueous phase where it is most needed, or of complexation with emulsion ingredients that reduce effectiveness. Therefore, the effectiveness of the preservative system should always be tested in the final product. Preservatives commonly used in emulsions include methyl-, ethyl-, propyl-, and butyl-parabens, benzoic acid, and quaternary ammonium compounds.

See also *Creams* and *Ointments*.

EXTRACTS AND FLUIDEXTRACTS

Extracts are concentrated preparations of vegetable or animal drugs obtained by removal of the active constituents of the respective drugs with suitable menstrua, by evaporation of all or nearly all of the solvent, and by adjustment of the residual masses or powders to the prescribed standards.

In the manufacture of most extracts, the drugs are extracted by percolation. The entire percolates are concentrated, generally by distillation under reduced pressure in order to subject the drug principles to as little heat as possible.

Fluidextracts are liquid preparations of vegetable drugs, containing alcohol as a solvent or as a preservative, or both, and so made that, unless otherwise specified in an individual monograph, each mL contains the therapeutic constituents of 1 g of the standard drug that it represents.

A fluidextract that tends to deposit sediment may be aged and filtered or the clear portion decanted, provided the resulting clear liquid conforms to the Pharmacopeial standards.

Fluidextracts may be prepared from suitable extracts.

GELS

Gels (sometimes called Jellies) are semisolid systems consisting of either suspensions made up of small inorganic particles or large organic molecules interpenetrated by a liquid. Where the gel mass consists of a network of small discrete particles, the gel is classified as a two-phase system (e.g., *Aluminum Hydroxide Gel*). In a two-phase system, if the particle size of the dispersed phase is relatively large, the gel mass is sometimes referred to as a magma (e.g., *Bentonite Magma*). Both gels and magmas may be thixotropic, forming semisolids on standing and becoming liquid on agitation. They should be shaken before use to ensure homogeneity and should be labeled to that effect. (See *Suspensions*.)

Single-phase gels consist of organic macromolecules uniformly distributed throughout a liquid in such a manner that no apparent boundaries exist between the dispersed macromolecules and the liquid. Single-phase gels may be made from synthetic macromolecules (e.g., *Carbomer*) or from natural gums (e.g., *Tragacanth*). The latter preparations are also called mucilages. Although these gels are commonly aqueous, alcohols and oils may be used as the continuous phase. For example, mineral oil can be combined with a polyethylene resin to form an oleaginous ointment base.

Gels can be used to administer drugs topically or into body cavities (e.g., *Phenylephrine Hydrochloride Nasal Jelly*).

IMPLANTS (PELLETS)

Implants or pellets are small sterile solid masses consisting of a highly purified drug (with or without excipients) made by compression or molding. They are intended for implantation in the body (usually subcutaneously) for the purpose of providing continuous release of the drug over long periods of time. Implants are administered by means of a suitable special injector or surgical incision. This dosage form has been used to administer hormones such as testosterone or estradiol. They are packaged individually in sterile vials or foil strips.

INFUSIONS, INTRAMAMMARY

Intramammary infusions are suspensions of drugs in suitable oil vehicles. These preparations are intended for veterinary use only, and are administered by instillation via the teat canals into the udders of milk-producing animals.

INHALATIONS

Inhalations are drugs or solutions or suspensions of one or more drug substances administered by the nasal or oral respiratory route for local or systemic effect.

Solutions of drug substances in sterile water for inhalation or in sodium chloride inhalation solution may be nebulized by use of inert gases. Nebulizers are suitable for the administration of inhalation solutions only if they give droplets sufficiently fine and uniform in size so that the mist reaches the bronchioles. Nebulized solutions may be breathed directly from the nebulizer or the nebulizer may be attached to a plastic face mask, tent, or intermittent positive pressure breathing (IPPB) machine.

Another group of products, also known as metered-dose inhalers (MDIs) are propellant-driven drug suspensions or solutions in liquified gas propellant with or without a cosolvent and are intended for delivering metered doses of the drug to the respiratory tract. An MDI contains multiple doses, often exceeding several hundred. The most common single-dose volumes delivered are from 25 to 100 μL (also expressed as mg) per actuation.

Examples of MDIs containing drug solutions and suspensions in this pharmacopeia are *Epinephrine Inhalation Aerosol* and *Isoproterenol Hydrochloride and Phenylephrine Bitartrate Inhalation Aerosol*, respectively.

Powders may also be administered by mechanical devices that require manually produced pressure or a deep inhalation by the patient (e.g., *Cromolyn Sodium for Inhalation*).

A special class of inhalations termed inhalants consists of drugs or combination of drugs, that by virtue of their high vapor pressure, can be carried by an air current into the nasal passage where they exert their effect. The container from which the inhalant generally is administered is known as an inhaler.

INJECTIONS

An Injection is a preparation intended for parenteral administration or for constituting or diluting a parenteral article prior to administration (see *Injections* ⟨1⟩).

Each container of an Injection is filled with a volume in slight excess of the labeled "size" or that volume that is to be withdrawn. The excess volumes recommended in the accompanying table are usually sufficient to permit withdrawal and administration of the labeled volumes.

	Recommended Excess Volume	
Labeled Size	For Mobile Liquids	For Viscous Liquids
0.5 mL	0.10 mL	0.12 mL
1.0 mL	0.10 mL	0.15 mL
2.0 mL	0.15 mL	0.25 mL
5.0 mL	0.30 mL	0.50 mL
10.0 mL	0.50 mL	0.70 mL
20.0 mL	0.60 mL	0.90 mL
30.0 mL	0.80 mL	1.20 mL
50.0 mL or more	2%	3%

IRRIGATIONS

Irrigations are sterile solutions intended to bathe or flush open wounds or body cavities. They are used topically, never parenterally. They are labeled to indicate that they are not intended for injection.

LOTIONS

See *Solutions* or *Suspensions*.

LOZENGES

Lozenges are solid preparations, that are intended to dissolve or disintegrate slowly in the mouth. They contain one or more medicaments, usually in a flavored, sweetened base. They can be prepared by molding (gelatin and/or fused sucrose or sorbitol base) or by compression of sugar-based tablets. Molded lozenges are sometimes referred to as pastilles while compressed lozenges are often referred to as troches. They are usually intended for treatment of local irritation or infections of the mouth or throat but may contain active ingredients intended for systemic absorption after swallowing.

OINTMENTS

Ointments are semisolid preparations intended for external application to the skin or mucous membranes.

Ointment bases recognized for use as vehicles fall into four general classes: the hydrocarbon bases, the absorption bases, the water-removable bases, and the water-soluble bases. Each therapeutic ointment possesses as its base a representative of one of these four general classes.

Hydrocarbon Bases

These bases, which are known also as "oleaginous ointment bases," are represented by *White Petrolatum* and *White Ointment*. Only small amounts of an aqueous component can be incorporated into them. They serve to keep medicaments in prolonged contact with the skin and act as occlusive dressings. Hydrocarbon bases are used chiefly for their emollient effects, and are difficult to wash off. They do not "dry out" or change noticeably on aging.

Absorption Bases

This class of bases may be divided into two groups: the first group consisting of bases that permit the incorporation of aqueous solutions with the formation of a water-in-oil emulsion (*Hydrophilic Petrolatum* and *Lanolin*), and the second group consisting of water-in-oil emulsions that permit the incorporation of additional quantities of aqueous solutions (*Lanolin*). Absorption bases are useful also as emollients.

Water-Removable Bases

Such bases are oil-in-water emulsions, e.g., *Hydrophilic Ointment*, and are more correctly called "creams." (See *Creams*.) They are also described as "water-washable," since they may be readily washed from the skin or clothing with water, an attribute that makes them more acceptable for cosmetic reasons. Some medicaments may be more effective in these bases than in hydrocarbon bases. Other advantages of the water-removable bases are that they may be diluted with water and that they favor the absorption of serous discharges in dermatological conditions.

Water-Soluble Bases

This group of so-called "greaseless ointment bases" comprises water-soluble constituents. *Polyethylene Glycol Ointment* is the only Pharmacopeial preparation in this group. Bases of this type offer many of the advantages of the water-removable bases and, in addition, contain no water-insoluble substances such as petrolatum, anhydrous lanolin, or waxes. They are more correctly called "Gels." (See *Gels.*)

Choice of Base—The choice of an ointment base depends upon many factors, such as the action desired, the nature of the medicament to be incorporated and its bioavailability and stability, and the requisite shelf-life of the finished product. In some cases, it is necessary to use a base that is less than ideal in order to achieve the stability required. Drugs that hydrolyze rapidly, for example, are more stable in hydrocarbon bases than in bases containing water, even though they may be more effective in the latter.

OPHTHALMIC PREPARATIONS

Drugs are administered to the eyes in a wide variety of dosage forms, some of which require special consideration. They are discussed in the following paragraphs.

Ointments

Ophthalmic ointments are ointments for application to the eye. Special precautions must be taken in the preparation of ophthalmic ointments. They are manufactured from sterilized ingredients under rigidly aseptic conditions and meet the requirements under *Sterility Tests* ⟨71⟩. If the specific ingredients used in the formulation do not lend themselves to routine sterilization techniques, ingredients that meet the sterility requirements described under *Sterility Tests* ⟨71⟩, along with aseptic manufacture, may be employed. Ophthalmic ointments must contain a suitable substance or mixture of substances to prevent growth of, or to destroy, microorganisms accidentally introduced when the container is opened during use, unless otherwise directed in the individual monograph, or unless the formula itself is bacteriostatic (see *Added Substances* under *Ophthalmic Ointments* ⟨771⟩). The medicinal agent is added to the ointment base either as a solution or as a micronized powder. The finished ointment must be free from large particles and must meet the requirements for *Leakage* and for *Metal Particles* under *Ophthalmic Ointments* ⟨771⟩. The immediate containers for ophthalmic ointments shall be sterile at the time of filling and closing. It is mandatory that the immediate containers for ophthalmic ointments be sealed and tamper-proof so that sterility is assured at time of first use.

The ointment base that is selected must be nonirritating to the eye, permit diffusion of the drug throughout the secretions bathing the eye, and retain the activity of the medicament for a reasonable period under proper storage conditions.

Petrolatum is mainly used as a base for ophthalmic drugs. Some absorption bases, water-removable bases, and water-soluble bases may be desirable for water-soluble drugs. Such bases allow for better dispersion of water-soluble medicaments, but they must be nonirritating to the eye.

Solutions

Ophthalmic solutions are sterile solutions, essentially free from foreign particles, suitably compounded and packaged for instillation into the eye. Preparation of an ophthalmic solution requires careful consideration of such factors as the inherent toxicity of the drug itself, isotonicity value, the need for buffering agents, the need for a preservative (and, if needed, its selection), sterilization, and proper packaging. Similar considerations are also made for nasal and otic products.

ISOTONICITY VALUE

Lacrimal fluid is isotonic with blood, having an isotonicity value corresponding to that of a 0.9% sodium chloride solution. Ideally, an ophthalmic solution should have this isotonicity value; but the eye can tolerate isotonicity values as low as that of a 0.6% sodium chloride solution and as high as that of a 2.0% sodium chloride solution without marked discomfort.

Some ophthalmic solutions are necessarily hypertonic in order to enhance absorption and provide a concentration of the active ingredient(s) strong enough to exert a prompt and effective action. Where the amount of such solutions used is small, dilution with lacrimal fluid takes place rapidly so that discomfort from the hypertonicity is only temporary. However, any adjustment toward isotonicity by dilution with tears is negligible where large volumes of hypertonic solutions are used as collyria to wash the eyes; it is, therefore, important that solutions used for this purpose be approximately isotonic.

BUFFERING

Many drugs, notably alkaloidal salts, are most effective at pH levels that favor the undissociated free bases. At such pH levels, however, the drug may be unstable so that compromise levels must be found and held by means of buffers. One purpose of buffering some ophthalmic solutions is to prevent an increase in pH caused by the slow release of hydroxyl ions by glass. Such a rise in pH can affect both the solubility and the stability of the drug. The decision whether or not buffering agents should be added in preparing an ophthalmic solution must be based on several considerations. Normal tears have a pH of about 7.4 and possess some buffer capacity. The application of a solution to the eye stimulates the flow of tears and the rapid neutralization of any excess hydrogen or hydroxyl ions within the buffer capacity of the tears. Many ophthalmic drugs, such as alkaloidal salts, are weakly acidic and have only weak buffer capacity. Where only 1 or 2 drops of a solution containing them are added to the eye, the buffering action of the tears is usually adequate to raise the pH and prevent marked discomfort. In some cases pH may vary between 3.5 and 8.5. Some drugs, notably pilocarpine hydrochloride and epinephrine bitartrate, are more acid and overtax the buffer capacity of the lacrimal fluid. Ideally, an ophthalmic solution should have the same pH, as well as the same isotonicity value, as lacrimal fluid. This is not usually possible since, at pH 7.4, many drugs are not appreciably soluble in water. Most alkaloidal salts precipitate as the free alkaloid at this pH. Additionally, many drugs are chemically unstable at pH levels approaching 7.4. This instability is more marked at the high temperatures employed in heat sterilization. For this reason, the buffer system should be selected that is nearest to the physiological pH of 7.4 and does not cause precipitation of the drug or its rapid deterioration.

An ophthalmic preparation with a buffer system approaching the physiological pH can be obtained by mixing a sterile solution of the drug with a sterile buffer solution using aseptic technique. Even so, the possibility of a shorter shelf-life at the higher pH must be taken into consideration, and attention must be directed toward the attainment and maintenance of sterility throughout the manipulations.

Many drugs, when buffered to a therapeutically acceptable pH, would not be stable in solution for long periods of time. These products are lyophilized and are intended for reconstitution immediately before use (e.g., *Acetylcholine Chloride for Ophthalmic Solution*).

STERILIZATION

The sterility of solutions applied to an injured eye is of the greatest importance. Sterile preparations in special containers for individual use on one patient should be available in every hospital, office, or other installation where accidentally or surgically traumatized eyes are treated. The method of attaining sterility is determined primarily by the character of the particular product (see *Sterilization and Sterility Assurance of Compendial Articles* ⟨1211⟩).

Whenever possible, sterile membrane filtration under aseptic conditions is the preferred method. If it can be shown that product stability is not adversely affected, sterilization by autoclaving in the final container is also a preferred method.

Buffering certain drugs near the physiological pH range makes them quite unstable at high temperature.

Avoiding the use of heat by employing a bacteria-retaining filter is a valuable technique, provided caution is exercised in the selection, assembly, and use of the equipment. Single-filtration, presterilized disposable units are available and should be utilized wherever possible.

PRESERVATION

Ophthalmic solutions may be packaged in multiple-dose containers when intended for the individual use of one patient and where the ocular surfaces are intact. It is mandatory that the immediate containers for ophthalmic solutions be sealed and tamper-proof so that sterility is assured at time of first use. Each solution must contain a suitable substance or mixture of substances to prevent the growth of, or to destroy, microorganisms accidentally introduced when the container is opened during use.

Where intended for use in surgical procedures, ophthalmic solutions, although they must be sterile, should not contain antibacterial agents, since they may be irritating to the ocular tissues.

THICKENING AGENT

A pharmaceutical grade of methylcellulose (e.g., 1% if the viscosity is 25 centipoises, or 0.25% if 4000 centipoises) or other suitable thickening agents such as hydroxypropyl methylcellulose or polyvinyl alcohol occasionally are added to ophthalmic solutions to increase the viscosity and prolong contact of the drug with the tissue. The thickened ophthalmic solution must be free from visible particles.

Suspensions

Ophthalmic suspensions are sterile liquid preparations containing solid particles dispersed in a liquid vehicle intended for application to the eye (see *Suspensions*). It is imperative that such suspensions contain the drug in a micronized form to prevent irritation and/or scratching of the cornea. Ophthalmic suspensions should never be dispensed if there is evidence of caking or aggregation.

Strips

Fluorescein sodium solution should be dispensed in a sterile, single-use container or in the form of a sterile, impregnated paper strip. The strip releases a sufficient amount of the drug for diagnostic purposes when touched to the eye being examined for a foreign body or a corneal abrasion. Contact of the paper with the eye may be avoided by leaching the drug from the strip onto the eye with the aid of sterile water or sterile sodium chloride solution.

PASTES

Pastes are semisolid dosage forms that contain one or more drug substances intended for topical application. One class is made from a single-phase aqueous gel (e.g., *Carboxymethylcellulose Sodium Paste*). The other class, the fatty pastes (e.g., *Zinc Oxide Paste*), consists of thick, stiff ointments that do not ordinarily flow at body temperature, and therefore serve as protective coatings over the areas to which they are applied.

The fatty pastes appear less greasy and more absorptive than ointments by reason of a high proportion of drug substance(s) having an affinity for water. These pastes tend to absorb serous secretions, and are less penetrating and less macerating than ointments, so that they are preferred for acute lesions that have a tendency towards crusting, vesiculation, or oozing.

A dental paste is intended for adhesion to the mucous membrane for local effect (e.g., *Triamcinolone Acetonide Dental Paste*). Some paste preparations intended for administration to animals are applied orally. The paste is squeezed into the mouth of the animal, generally at the back of the tongue, or is spread inside the mouth.

PELLETS

See *Implants*.

POWDERS

Powders are intimate mixtures of dry, finely divided drugs and/ or chemicals that may be intended for internal (Oral Powders) or external (Topical Powders) use. Because of their greater specific surface area, powders disperse and dissolve more readily than compacted dosage forms. Children and those adults who experience difficulty in swallowing tablets or capsules may find powders more acceptable. Drugs that are too bulky to be formed into tablets or capsules of convenient size may be administered as powders. Immediately prior to use, oral powders are mixed in a beverage or apple sauce.

Often, stability problems encountered in liquid dosage forms are avoided in powdered dosage forms. Drugs that are unstable in aqueous suspensions or solutions may be prepared in the form of granules or powders. These are intended to be constituted by the pharmacist by the addition of a specified quantity of water just prior to dispensing. Because these constituted products have limited stability, they are required to have a specified expiration date after constitution and may require storage in a refrigerator.

Oral powders may be dispensed in doses premeasured by the pharmacist, i.e., divided powders, or in bulk. Traditionally, divided powders have been wrapped in materials such as bond paper and parchment. However, the pharmacist may provide greater protection from the environment by sealing individual doses in small cellophane or polyethylene envelopes.

Granules for veterinary use may be administered by sprinkling the dry powder on animal feed or by mixing it with animal food.

Bulk oral powders are limited to relatively nonpotent drugs such as laxatives, antacids, dietary supplements, and certain analgesics that the patient may safely measure by the teaspoonful or capful. Other bulky powders include douche powders, tooth powders, and dusting powders. Bulk powders are best dispensed in tight, wide-mouth glass containers to afford maximum protection from the atmosphere and to prevent the loss of volatile constituents.

Dusting powders are impalpable powders intended for topical application. They may be dispensed in sifter-top containers to facilitate dusting onto the skin. In general, dusting powders should be passed through at least a 100-mesh sieve to assure freedom from grit that could irritate traumatized areas (see *Powder Fineness* ⟨811⟩).

PREMIXES

Premixes are mixtures of one or more drug substances with suitable vehicles. Premixes are intended for admixture to animal feedstuffs before administration. They are used to facilitate dilution of the active drug components with animal feed. Premixes should be as homogeneous as possible. It is essential that materials of suitable fineness be used and that thorough mixing be achieved at all stages of premix preparation. Premixes may be prepared as powder, pellets, or in granulated form. The granulated form is free-flowing and free from aggregates.

SOLUTIONS

Solutions are liquid preparations that contain one or more chemical substances dissolved, i.e., molecularly dispersed, in a suitable solvent or mixture of mutually miscible solvents. Since molecules in solutions are uniformly dispersed, the use of solutions as dosage forms generally provides for the assurance of uniform dosage upon administration, and good accuracy when diluting or otherwise mixing solutions.

Substances in solutions, however, are more susceptible to chemical instability than the solid state and dose for dose, generally require more bulk and weight in packaging relative to solid dosage forms. For all solutions, but particularly those containing volatile solvents, tight containers, stored away from excessive heat, should be used. Consideration should also be given to the use of light-resistant containers when photolytic chemical degradation is a potential stability problem. Dosage forms categorized as "Solutions" are classified according to route of administration, such as "Oral Solutions" and "Topical Solutions," or by their solute and solvent systems, such as "Spirits," "Tinctures," and "Waters." Solutions intended for parenteral administration are officially entitled "Injections" (see *Injections* ⟨1⟩).

Oral Solutions

Oral Solutions are liquid preparations, intended for oral administration, that contain one or more substances with or without flavoring, sweetening, or coloring agents dissolved in water or cosolvent-water mixtures. Oral Solutions may be formulated for direct oral administration to the patient or they may be dispensed in a more concentrated form that must be diluted prior to administration. It is important to recognize that dilution with water of Oral Solutions containing cosolvents, such as alcohol, could lead to precipitation of some ingredients. Hence, great care must be taken in diluting concentrated solutions when cosolvents are present. Preparations dispensed as soluble solids or soluble mixtures of solids, with the intent of dissolving them in a solvent and administering them orally, are designated "for Oral Solution" (e.g., *Potassium Chloride for Oral Solution*).

Oral Solutions containing high concentrations of sucrose or other sugars traditionally have been designated as Syrups. A near-saturated solution of sucrose in purified water, for example, is known as Syrup or "Simple Syrup." Through common usage the term, syrup, also has been used to include any other liquid dosage form prepared in a sweet and viscid vehicle, including oral suspensions.

In addition to sucrose and other sugars, certain polyols such as sorbitol or glycerin may be present in Oral Solutions to inhibit crystallization and to modify solubility, taste, mouth-feel, and other vehicle properties. Antimicrobial agents to prevent the growth of bacteria, yeasts, and molds are generally also present. Some sugarless Oral Solutions contain sweetening agents such as sorbitol or aspartame, as well as thickening agents such as the cellulose gums. Such viscid sweetened solutions, containing no sugars, are occasionally prepared as vehicles for administration of drugs to diabetic patients.

Many oral solutions, that contain alcohol as a cosolvent, have been traditionally designated as Elixirs. However, many others designated as Oral Solutions also contain significant amounts of alcohol. Since high concentrations of alcohol can produce a pharmacologic effect when administered orally, other cosolvents, such as glycerin and propylene glycol, should be used to minimize the amount of alcohol required. To be designated as an Elixir, however, the solution must contain alcohol.

Topical Solutions

Topical Solutions are solutions, usually aqueous but often containing other solvents, such as alcohol and polyols, intended for topical application to the skin, or as in the case of Lidocaine Oral Topical Solution, to the oral mucosal surface. The term "lotion" is applied to solutions or suspensions applied topically.

Otic Solutions

Otic Solutions, intended for instillation in the outer ear, are aqueous, or they are solutions prepared with glycerin or other solvents and dispersing agents (e.g., *Antipyrine and Benzocaine Otic Solution* and *Neomycin and Polymyxin B Sulfates and Hydrocortisone Otic Solution*).

Ophthalmic Solutions

See *Ophthalmic Preparations*.

Spirits

Spirits are alcoholic or hydroalcoholic solutions of volatile substances prepared usually by simple solution or by admixture of the ingredients. Some spirits serve as flavoring agents while others have medicinal value. Reduction of the high alcoholic content of spirits by admixture with aqueous preparations often causes turbidity.

Spirits require storage in tight, light-resistant containers to prevent loss by evaporation and to limit oxidative changes.

Tinctures

Tinctures are alcoholic or hydroalcoholic solutions prepared from vegetable materials or from chemical substances.

The proportion of drug represented in the different chemical tinctures is not uniform but varies according to the established standards for each. Traditionally, tinctures of potent vegetable drugs essentially represent the activity of 10 g of the drug in each 100 mL of tincture, the potency being adjusted following assay. Most other vegetable tinctures represent 20 g of the respective vegetable material in each 100 mL of tincture.

PROCESS P

Carefully mix the ground drug or mixture of drugs with a sufficient quantity of the prescribed solvent or solvent mixture to render it evenly and distinctly damp, allow it to stand for 15 minutes, transfer it to a suitable percolator, and pack the drug firmly. Pour on enough of the prescribed solvent or solvent mixture to saturate the drug, cover the top of the percolator, and, when the liquid is about to drip from the percolator, close the lower orifice and allow the drug to macerate for 24 hours or for the time specified in the monograph. If no assay is directed, allow the percolation to proceed slowly, or at the specified rate, gradually adding sufficient solvent or solvent mixture to produce 1000 mL of tincture, and mix (for definitions of flow rates, see under *Fluidextracts*). If an assay is directed, collect only 950 mL of

percolate, mix this, and assay a portion of it as directed. Dilute the remainder with such quantity of the prescribed solvent or solvent mixture as calculation from the assay indicates is necessary to produce a tincture that conforms to the prescribed standard, and mix.

PROCESS M

Macerate the drug with 750 mL of the prescribed solvent or solvent mixture in a container that can be closed, and put in a warm place. Agitate it frequently during 3 days or until the soluble matter is dissolved. Transfer the mixture to a filter, and when most of the liquid has drained away, wash the residue on the filter with a sufficient quantity of the prescribed solvent or solvent mixture, combining the filtrates, to produce 1000 mL of tincture, and mix.

Tinctures require storage in tight, light-resistant containers, away from direct sunlight and excessive heat.

Waters, Aromatic

Aromatic waters are clear, saturated aqueous solutions (unless otherwise specified) of volatile oils or other aromatic or volatile substances. Their odors and tastes are similar, respectively, to those of the drugs or volatile substances from which they are prepared, and they are free from empyreumatic and other foreign odors. Aromatic waters may be prepared by distillation or solution of the aromatic substance, with or without the use of a dispersing agent.

Aromatic waters require protection from intense light and excessive heat.

SUPPOSITORIES

Suppositories are solid bodies of various weights and shapes, adapted for introduction into the rectal, vaginal, or urethral orifice of the human body. They usually melt, soften, or dissolve at body temperature. A suppository may act as a protectant or palliative to the local tissues at the point of introduction or as a carrier of therapeutic agents for systemic or local action. Suppository bases usually employed are cocoa butter, glycerinated gelatin, hydrogenated vegetable oils, mixtures of polyethylene glycols of various molecular weights, and fatty acid esters of polyethylene glycol.

The suppository base employed has a marked influence on the release of the active ingredient incorporated in it. While cocoa butter melts quickly at body temperature, it is immiscible with body fluids and this inhibits the diffusion of fat-soluble drugs to the affected sites. Polyethylene glycol is a suitable base for some antiseptics. In cases where systemic action is expected, it is preferable to incorporate the ionized rather than the nonionized form of the drug, in order to maximize bioavailability. Although nonionized drugs partition more readily out of water-miscible bases such as glycerinated gelatin and polyethylene glycol, the bases themselves tend to dissolve very slowly and thus retard release in this manner. Oleaginous vehicles such as cocoa butter are seldom used in vaginal preparations because of the nonabsorbable residue formed, while glycerinated gelatin is seldom used rectally because of its slow dissolution. Cocoa butter and its substitutes (Hard Fat) are superior for allaying irritation, as in preparations intended for treating internal hemorrhoids.

Cocoa Butter Suppositories

Suppositories having cocoa butter as the base may be made by means of incorporating the finely divided medicinal substance into the solid oil at room temperature and suitably shaping the resulting mass, or by working with the oil in the melted state and allowing the resulting suspension to cool in molds. A suitable quantity of hardening agents may be added to counteract the tendency of some medicaments such as chloral hydrate and phenol to soften the base. It is important that the finished suppository melt at body temperature.

The approximate weights of suppositories prepared with cocoa butter are given below. Suppositories prepared from other bases vary in weight and generally are heavier than the weights indicated here.

Rectal Suppositories for adults are tapered at one or both ends and usually weigh about 2 g each.

Vaginal Suppositories are usually globular or oviform and weigh about 5 g each. They are made from water-soluble or water-miscible vehicles such as polyethylene glycol or glycerinated gelatin.

Suppositories with cocoa butter base require storage in well-closed containers, preferably at a temperature below 30° (controlled room temperature).

Cocoa Butter Substitutes

Fat-type suppository bases can be produced from a variety of vegetable oils, such as coconut or palm kernel, which are modified by esterification, hydrogenation, and fractionation to obtain products of varying composition and melting temperatures (e.g., *Hydrogenated Vegetable Oil* and *Hard Fat*). These products can be so designed as to reduce rancidity. At the same time, desired characteristics such as narrow intervals between melting and solidification temperatures, and melting ranges to accommodate various formulation and climatic conditions, can be built in.

Glycerinated Gelatin Suppositories

Medicinal substances may be incorporated into glycerinated gelatin bases by addition of the prescribed quantities to a vehicle consisting of about 70 parts of glycerin, 20 parts of gelatin, and 10 parts of water.

Glycerinated gelatin suppositories require storage in tight containers, preferably at a temperature below 35°.

Polyethylene Glycol–Base Suppositories

Several combinations of polyethylene glycols having melting temperatures that are above body temperature have been used as suppository bases. Inasmuch as release from these bases depends on dissolution rather than on melting, there are significantly fewer problems in preparation and storage than exist with melting-type vehicles. However, high concentrations of higher-molecular-weight polyethylene glycols may lengthen dissolution time, resulting in problems with retention. Labels on polyethylene glycol suppositories should contain directions that they be moistened with water before inserting. Although they can be stored without refrigeration, they should be packaged in tightly closed containers.

Surfactant Suppository Bases

Several nonionic surface-active agents closely related chemically to the polyethylene glycols can be used as suppository vehicles. Examples of such surfactants are polyoxyethylene sorbitan fatty acid esters and the polyoxyethylene stearates. These surfactants are used alone or in combination with other suppository vehicles to yield a wide range of melting temperatures and consistencies. One of the major advantages of such vehicles is their water-dispersibility. However, care must be taken with the use of surfactants, because they may either increase the rate of drug absorption or interact with drug molecules, causing a decrease in therapeutic activity.

Tabled Suppositories or Inserts

Vaginal suppositories occasionally are prepared by the compression of powdered materials into a suitable shape. They are prepared also by encapsulation in soft gelatin.

SUSPENSIONS

Suspensions are liquid preparations that consist of solid particles dispersed throughout a liquid phase in which the particles are not soluble. Dosage forms officially categorized as "Suspensions" are designated as such if they are not included in other more specific categories of suspensions, such as Oral Suspensions, Topical Suspensions, etc. (see these other categories). Some suspensions are prepared and ready for use, while others are prepared as solid mixtures intended for constitution just before use with an appropriate vehicle. Such products are designated "for Oral Suspension", etc. The term "Milk" is sometimes used for suspensions in aqueous vehicles intended for oral administration (e.g., *Milk of Magnesia*). The term "Magma" is often used to describe suspensions of inorganic solids such as clays in water, where there is a tendency for strong hydration and aggregation of the solid, giving rise to gel-like consistency and thixotropic rheological behavior (e.g., *Bentonite Magma*). The term "Lotion" has been used to categorize many topical suspensions and emulsions intended for application to the skin (e.g., *Calamine Lotion*). Some suspensions are prepared in sterile form and are used as Injectables, as well as for ophthalmic and otic administration. These may be of two types, ready to use or intended for constitution with a prescribed amount of Water for Injection or other suitable diluent before use by the designated route. Suspensions should not be injected intravenously or intrathecally.

Suspensions intended for any route of administration should contain suitable antimicrobial agents to protect against bacteria, yeast, and mold contamination (see *Emulsions* for some consideration of antimicrobial preservative properties that apply also to Suspensions). By its very nature, the particular matter in a suspension may settle or sediment to the bottom of the container upon standing. Such sedimentation may also lead to caking and solidification of the sediment with a resulting difficulty in redispersing the suspension upon agitation. To prevent such problems, suitable ingredients that increase viscosity and the gel state of the suspension, such as clays, surfactants, polyols, polymers, or sugars, should be added. It is important that suspensions always be shaken well before use to ensure uniform distribution of the solid in the vehicle, thereby ensuring uniform and proper dosage. Suspensions require storage in tight containers.

Oral Suspensions

Oral Suspensions are liquid preparations containing solid particles dispersed in a liquid vehicle, with suitable flavoring agents, intended for oral administration. Some suspensions labeled as "Milks" or "Magmas" fall into this category.

Topical Suspensions

Topical Suspensions are liquid preparations containing solid particles dispersed in a liquid vehicle, intended for application to the skin. Some suspensions labeled as "Lotions" fall into this category.

Otic Suspensions

Otic Suspensions are liquid preparations containing micronized particles intended for instillation in the outer ear.

Ophthalmic Suspensions

See *Ophthalmic Preparations*.

SYRUPS

See *Solutions*.

SYSTEMS

In recent years, a number of dosage forms have been developed using modern technology that allows for the uniform release or targeting of drugs to the body. These products are commonly called delivery systems. The most widely used of these are Transdermal Systems.

Transdermal Systems

Transdermal drug delivery systems are self-contained, discrete dosage forms that, when applied to intact skin, are designed to deliver the drug(s) through the skin to the systemic circulation. Systems typically comprise an outer covering (barrier), a drug reservoir, which may have a rate-controlling membrane, a contact adhesive applied to some or all parts of the system and the system/skin interface, and a protective liner that is removed before applying the system. The activity of these systems is defined in terms of the release rate of the drug(s) from the system. The total duration of drug release from the system and the system surface area may also be stated.

Transdermal drug delivery systems work by diffusion: the drug diffuses from the drug reservoir, directly or through the rate-controlling membrane and/or contact adhesive if present, and then through the skin into the general circulation. Typically, modified-release systems are designed to provide drug delivery at a constant rate, such that a true steady-state blood concentration is achieved and maintained until the system is removed. At that time, blood concentration declines at a rate consistent with the pharmacokinetics of the drug.

Transdermal drug delivery systems are applied to body areas consistent with the labeling for the product(s). As long as drug concentration at the system/skin interface remains constant, the amount of drug in the dosage form does not influence plasma concentrations. The functional lifetime of the system is defined by the initial amount of drug in the reservoir and the release rate from the reservoir.

NOTE—Drugs for local rather than systemic effect are commonly applied to the skin embedded in glue on a cloth or plastic backing. These products are defined traditionally as plasters or tapes.

Ocular System

Another type of system is the ocular system, which is intended for placement in the lower conjunctival fornix from which the drug diffuses through a membrane at a constant rate (e.g., *Pilocarpine Ocular System*).

Intrauterine System

An intrauterine system, based on a similar principle but intended for release of drug over a much longer period of time, e.g., one year, is also available (e.g., *Progesterone Intrauterine Contraceptive System*).

TABLETS

Tablets are solid dosage forms containing medicinal substances with or without suitable diluents. They may be classed, according to the method of manufacture, as compressed tablets or molded tablets.

The vast majority of all tablets manufactured are made by compression, and compressed tablets are the most widely used dosage form in this country. Compressed tablets are prepared by the application of high pressures, utilizing steel punches and dies, to powders or granulations. Tablets can be produced in a wide variety of sizes, shapes, and surface markings, depending upon the design of the punches and dies. Capsule-shaped tablets are commonly referred to as caplets. Boluses are large tablets intended for veterinary use, usually for large animals.

Molded tablets are prepared by forcing dampened powders under low pressure into die cavities. Solidification depends upon crystal bridges built up during the subsequent drying process, and not upon the compaction force.

Tablet triturates are small, usually cylindrical, molded or compressed tablets. Tablet triturates were traditionally used as dispensing tablets in order to provide a convenient, measured quantity of a potent drug for compounding purposes. Such tablets are rarely used today. Hypodermic tablets are molded tablets made from completely and readily water-soluble ingredients and formerly were intended for use in making preparations for hypodermic injection. They are employed orally, or where rapid drug availability is required such as in the case of *Nitroglycerin Tablets*, sublingually.

Buccal tablets are intended to be inserted in the buccal pouch, and sublingual tablets are intended to be inserted beneath the tongue, where the active ingredient is absorbed directly through the oral mucosa. Few drugs are readily absorbed in this way, but for those that are (such as nitroglycerin and certain steroid hormones), a number of advantages may result.

Soluble, effervescent tablets are prepared by compression and contain, in addition to active ingredients, mixtures of acids (citric acid, tartaric acid) and sodium bicarbonate, which release carbon dioxide when dissolved in water. They are intended to be dissolved or dispersed in water before administration. Effervescent tablets should be stored in tightly closed containers or moisture-proof packs and labeled to indicate that they are not to be swallowed directly.

Chewable Tablets

Chewable tablets are formulated and manufactured so that they may be chewed, producing a pleasant tasting residue in the oral cavity that is easily swallowed and does not leave a bitter or unpleasant after-taste. These tablets have been used in tablet formulations for children, especially multivitamin formulations, and for the administration of antacids and selected antibiotics. Chewable tablets are prepared by compression, usually utilizing mannitol, sorbitol, or sucrose as binders and fillers, and containing colors and flavors to enhance their appearance and taste.

Preparation of Molded Tablets

Molded tablets are prepared from mixtures of medicinal substances and a diluent usually consisting of lactose and powdered sucrose in varying proportions. The powders are dampened with solutions containing high percentages of alcohol. The concentration of alcohol depends upon the solubility of the active ingredients and fillers in the solvent system and the desired degree of hardness of the finished tablets. The dampened powders are pressed into molds, removed, and allowed to dry. Molded tablets are quite friable and care must be taken in packaging and dispensing.

Formulation of Compressed Tablets

Most compressed tablets consist of the active ingredient and a diluent (filler), binder, disintegrating agent, and lubricant. Approved FD&C and D&C dyes or lakes (dyes adsorbed onto insoluble aluminum hydroxide), flavors, and sweetening agents may also be present. Diluents are added where the quantity of active ingredient is small or difficult to compress. Common tablet fillers include lactose, starch, dibasic calcium phosphate, and microcrystalline cellulose. Chewable tablets often contain sucrose, mannitol, or sorbitol as a filler. Where the amount of active ingredient is small, the overall tableting properties are in large measure determined by the filler. Because of problems encountered with bioavailability of hydrophobic drugs of low water-solubility, water-soluble diluents are used as fillers for these tablets.

Binders give adhesiveness to the powder during the preliminary granulation and to the compressed tablet. They add to the cohesive strength already available in the diluent. While binders may be added dry, they are more effective when added out of solution. Common binders include acacia, gelatin, sucrose, povidone, methylcellulose, carboxymethylcellulose, and hydrolyzed starch pastes. The most effective dry binder is microcrystalline cellulose, which is commonly used for this purpose in tablets prepared by direct compression.

A disintegrating agent serves to assist in the fragmentation of the tablet after administration. The most widely used tablet disintegrating agent is starch. Chemically modified starches and cellulose, alginic acid, microcrystalline cellulose, and cross-linked povidone, are also used for this purpose. Effervescent mixtures are used in soluble tablet systems as disintegrating agents. The concentration of the disintegrating agent, method of addition, and degree of compaction play a role in effectiveness.

Lubricants reduce friction during the compression and ejection cycle. In addition, they aid in preventing adherence of tablet material to the dies and punches. Metallic stearates, stearic acid, hydrogenated vegetable oils, and talc are used as lubricants. Because of the nature of this function, most lubricants are hydrophobic, and as such tend to reduce the rates of tablet disintegration and dissolution. Consequently, excessive concentrations of lubricant should be avoided. Polyethylene glycols and some lauryl sulfate salts have been used as soluble lubricants, but such agents generally do not possess optimal lubricating properties, and comparatively high concentrations are usually required.

Glidants are agents that improve powder fluidity, and they are commonly employed in direct compression where no granulation step is involved. The most effective glidants are the colloidal pyrogenic silicas.

Colorants are often added to tablet formulations for esthetic value or for product identification. Both D&C and FD&C dyes and lakes are used. Most dyes are photosensitive and they fade when exposed to light. The federal Food and Drug Administration regulates the colorants employed in drugs.

Manufacturing Methods

Tablets are prepared by three general methods: wet granulation, dry granulation (roll compaction or slugging), and direct compression. The purpose of both wet and dry granulation is to improve flow of the mixture and/or to enhance its compressibility.

Dry granulation (slugging) involves the compaction of powders at high pressures into large, often poorly formed tablet compacts. These compacts are then milled and screened to form a granulation of the desired particle size. The advantage of dry granulation is the elimination of both heat and moisture in the processing. Dry granulations can be produced also by extruding powders between hydraulically operated rollers to produce thin cakes which are subsequently screened or milled to give the desired granule size.

Excipients are available that allow production of tablets at high speeds without prior granulation steps. These directly compressible excipients consist of special physical forms of substances such as lactose, sucrose, dextrose, or cellulose, which possess the desirable properties of fluidity and compressibility. The most widely used direct-compaction fillers are microcrystalline cellulose, anhydrous lactose, spray-dried lactose, compressible sucrose, and some forms of modified starches. Direct compression avoids many of the problems associated with wet and dry granulations. However, the inherent physical properties of the individual filler materials are highly critical, and minor variations can alter flow and compression characteristics so as to make them unsuitable for direct compression.

Physical evidence of poor tablet quality is discussed under *Stability Considerations in Dispensing Practice* ⟨1191⟩.

WEIGHT VARIATION AND CONTENT UNIFORMITY

Tablets are required to meet a weight variation test (see *Uniformity of Dosage Units* ⟨905⟩) where the active ingredient comprises a major portion of the tablet and where control of weight may be presumed to be an adequate control of drug content uniformity. Weight variation is not an adequate indication of content uniformity where the drug substance comprises a relatively minor portion of the tablet, or where the tablet is sugar-coated. Thus, the Pharmacopeia generally requires that coated tablets and tablets containing 50 mg or less of active ingredient, comprising less than 50% by weight of the dosage-form unit, pass a content uniformity test (see *Uniformity of Dosage Units* ⟨905⟩), wherein individual tablets are assayed for actual drug content.

DISINTEGRATION AND DISSOLUTION

Disintegration is an essential attribute of tablets intended for administration by mouth, except for those intended to be chewed before being swallowed and for some types of extended-release tablets. A disintegration test is provided (see *Disintegration* ⟨701⟩), and limits on the times in which disintegration is to take place, appropriate for the types of tablets concerned, are given in the individual monographs.

For drugs of limited water-solubility, dissolution may be a more meaningful quality attribute than disintegration. A dissolution test (see *Dissolution* ⟨711⟩) is required in a number of monographs on tablets. In many cases, it is possible to correlate dissolution rates with biological availability of the active ingredient. However, such tests are useful mainly as a means of screening preliminary formulations and as a routine quality-control procedure.

Coatings

Tablets may be coated for a variety of reasons, including protection of the ingredients from air, moisture, or light, masking of unpleasant tastes and odors, improvement of appearance, and control of the site of drug release in the gastrointestinal tract.

PLAIN COATED TABLETS

Classically, tablets have been coated with sugar applied from aqueous suspensions containing insoluble powders such as starch, calcium carbonate, talc, or titanium dioxide, suspended by means of acacia or gelatin. For purposes of identification and esthetic value, the outside coatings may be colored. The finished coated tablets are polished by application of dilute solutions of wax in solvents such as chloroform or powdered mix. Water-protective coatings consisting of substances such as shellac or cellulose acetate phthalate are often applied out of nonaqueous solvents prior to application of sugar coats. Excessive quantities should be avoided. Drawbacks of sugar coating include the lengthy time necessary for application, the need for waterproof-

ing, which also adversely affects dissolution, and the increased bulk of the finished tablet. These factors have resulted in increased acceptance of film coatings. Film coatings consist of water-soluble or dispersible materials such as hydroxypropyl methylcellulose, methylcellulose, hydroxypropylcellulose, carboxymethylcellulose sodium, and mixtures of cellulose acetate phthalate and polyethylene glycols applied out of nonaqueous or aqueous solvents. Evaporation of the solvents leaves a thin film that adheres directly to the tablet and allows it to retain the original shape, including grooves or identification codes.

DELAYED-RELEASE TABLETS

Where the drug may be destroyed or inactivated by the gastric juice or where it may irritate the gastric mucosa, the use of "enteric" coatings is indicated. Such coatings are intended to delay the release of the medication until the tablet has passed through the stomach. The term "delayed-release" is used for Pharmacopeial purposes, and the individual monographs include tests and specifications for *Drug release* (see *Drug Release* ⟨724⟩) or *Disintegration* (see *Disintegration* ⟨701⟩).

EXTENDED-RELEASE TABLETS

Extended-release tablets are formulated in such manner as to make the contained medicament available over an extended period of time following ingestion. Expressions such as "prolonged-action," "repeat action," and "sustained-release" have also been used to describe such dosage forms. However, the term "extended-release" is used for Pharmacopeial purposes, and requirements for *Drug release* typically are specified in the individual monographs.

Add the following:

▲⟨1160⟩ PHARMACEUTICAL CALCULATIONS IN PRESCRIPTION COMPOUNDING

INTRODUCTION

The purpose of this chapter is to provide general information to guide and assist pharmacists in performing the necessary calculations when preparing or compounding any pharmaceutical article (see *Pharmaceutical Compounding—Nonsterile Preparations* ⟨795⟩, *Pharmaceutical Compounding—Sterile Preparations* ⟨797⟩, and *Good Compounding Practices* ⟨1075⟩) or when simply dispensing prescriptions (see *Stability Considerations in Dispensing Practice* ⟨1191⟩).

Correct pharmaceutical calculations can be accomplished by using, for example, proper conversions from one measurement system to another and properly placed decimal points, by understanding the arithmetical concepts, and by paying close attention to the details of the calculations. Before proceeding with any calculation, pharmacists should do the following: (a) read the entire formula or prescription carefully; (b) determine which materials are needed; and then (c) select the appropriate methods of preparation and the appropriate calculation.

There are often several ways to solve a given problem. Logical methods that require as few steps as possible should be selected in order to ensure that calculations are done correctly. The best approach is the one that yields results that are accurate and free of error. The pharmacist must double-check each calculation before proceeding with the preparation of the article or prescription order. One way of double-checking is by estimation.

This involves rounding off the quantities involved in the calculation, and comparing the estimated result with the calculated value.

Finally, the following steps should be taken: the dosage of each active ingredient in the prescription should be checked; all calculations should be doubly checked, preferably by another pharmacist; and where instruments are used in compounding, they should be carefully checked to ascertain that they will function properly. See *USP* general chapters *Aerosols, Metered-Dose Inhalers, and Dry Powder Inhalers* ⟨601⟩, *Deliverable Volume* ⟨698⟩, *Density of Solids* ⟨699⟩, *Osmolarity* ⟨785⟩, *pH* ⟨791⟩, *Pharmaceutical Com-pounding—Nonsterile Preparations* ⟨795⟩, *Pharmaceutical Compounding—Sterile Preparations* ⟨797⟩, *Viscosity* ⟨911⟩, *Specific Gravity* ⟨841⟩, *Cleaning Glass Apparatus* ⟨1051⟩, *Medicine Dropper* ⟨1101⟩, *Prescription Balances and Volumetric Apparatus* ⟨1176⟩, *Teaspoon* ⟨1221⟩, *Weighing on an Analytical Balance* ⟨1251⟩, and *Good Compounding Practices* ⟨1075⟩ for information on specific instruments.

BASIC MATHEMATICAL CONCEPTS

SIGNIFICANT FIGURES

Expressed values are considered significant to the last digit shown (see *Significant Figures and Tolerances* in the *General Notices*). Significant figures are digits with practical meaning. The accuracy of the determination is implied by the number of figures used in its expression. In some calculations zeros may not be significant. For example, for a measured weight of 0.0298 g, the zeros are not significant; they are used merely to locate the decimal point. In the example, 2980 g, the zero may also be used to indicate the decimal point, in which case the zero is not significant. Alternately, however, the zero may indicate that the weight is closer to 2981 g or 2979 g, in which case the zero is significant. In such a case, knowledge of the method of measurement would be required in order to indicate whether the zero is or is not significant. In the case of a volume measurement of 298 mL, all of the digits are significant. In a given result, the last significant figure written is approximate but all preceding figures are accurate. For example, a volume of 29.8 mL implies that 8 is approximate. The true volume falls between 29.75 and 29.85. Thus, 29.8 mL is accurate to the nearest 0.1 mL, which means that the measurement has been made within ±0.05 mL. Likewise, a value of 298 mL is accurate to the nearest 1 mL and implies a measurement falling between 297.5 and 298.5, which means that the measurement has been made within ±0.5 mL and is subject to a maximum error calculated as follows:

$$\frac{0.5\,mL}{298\,mL} \times 100\% = 0.17\%$$

A zero in a quantity such as 298.0 mL is a significant figure and implies that the measurement has been made within the limits of 297.95 and 298.05 with a possible error calculated as follows:

$$\frac{0.05\,mL}{298.0\,mL} \times 100\% = 0.017\%$$

EXAMPLES—

1. 29.8 mL = 29.8 ± 0.05 mL (accurate to the nearest 0.1 mL)
2. 29.80 mL = 29.80 ± 0.005 mL (accurate to the nearest 0.01 mL)
3. 29.800 mL = 29.800 ± 0.0005 mL (accurate to the nearest 0.001 mL)

The degree of accuracy in the last example is greatest. Thus, the number of significant figures provides an estimate both of true value and of accuracy.

EXAMPLES OF SIGNIFICANT FIGURES—

Measurement	Number of Significant Figures
2.98	3
2.980	4
0.0298	3
0.0029	2

Calculations—All figures should be retained until the calculations have been completed. Only the appropriate number of significant figures, however, should be retained in the final result.

Determining the number of significant figures—

Sums and Differences—When adding or subtracting, the number of decimal places in the result shall be the same as the number of decimal places in the component with the fewest decimal places.

EXAMPLE—

$$11.5 + 11.65 + 9.90 = 33.1$$

Products and Quotients—When multiplying or dividing, the result shall have no more significant figures than the measurement with the smallest number of significant figures entering into the calculation.

EXAMPLE—

$$4.266 \times 21 = 90$$

Rounding Off—For rules on rounding off measurements or calculated results, see *Interpretation of Requirements* under *Significant Figures and Tolerances* in the *General Notices*. Note, however, that in the example above, if 21 is an absolute number (e.g., the number of doses), then the answer, 89.586, is rounded off to 89.59 which has 4 significant figures.

LOGARITHMS

The logarithm of a number is the exponent or the power to which a given base must be raised in order to equal that number.

Definitions—

$$pH = -\log [H^+], \text{ and}$$

$$pKa = -\log Ka$$

pH = $-\log [H^+]$, and pKa = $-\log Ka$, where $[H^+]$ is the hydrogen ion concentration in an aqueous solution and Ka is the ionization constant of the acid in an aqueous solution. The $[H^+]$ = the antilogarithm of $(-pH)$, and the Ka = the antilogarithm of $(-pKa)$.

The pH of an aqueous solution containing a weak acid may be calculated using the Henderson-Hasselbalch equation:

$$pH = pKa + \log [salt]/[acid]$$

EXAMPLE—

A solution contains 0.020 moles per liter of sodium acetate and 0.010 mole per liter of acetic acid, which has a pKa value of 4.76. Calculate the pH and the $[H^+]$ of the solution. Substituting into the above equation, pH = 4.76 + log (0.020/0.010) = 5.06, and the $[H^+]$ = antilogarithm of (-5.06) = 8.69×10^{-6}.

BASIC PHARMACEUTICAL CALCULATIONS

The remainder of this chapter will focus on basic pharmaceutical calculations. It is important to recognize the rules involved when adding, subtracting, dividing, and multiplying values. The interrelationships between various units within the different weighing and measuring systems are also important and have to be understood.

CALCULATIONS IN COMPOUNDING

The pharmacist must be able to calculate the amount or concentration of drug substances in each unit or dosage portion of a compounded preparation at the time it is dispensed. Pharmacists must perform calculations and measurements to obtain, theoretically, 100% of the amount of each ingredient in compounded formulations. Calculations must account for the active ingredient, or active moiety, and water content of drug substances, which includes that in the chemical formulas of hydrates. Official drug substances and added substances must meet the requirements under *Loss on Drying* ⟨731⟩, which must be included in the calculations of amounts and concentrations of ingredients. The pharmacist should consider the effect of ambient humidity on the gain or loss of water from drugs and added substances in containers subjected to intermittent opening over prolonged storage. Each container should be opened for the shortest duration necessary and then closed tightly immediately after use.

The nature of the drug substance that is to be weighed and used in compounding a prescription must be known exactly. If the substance is a hydrate, its anhydrous equivalent weight may need to be calculated. On the other hand, if there is adsorbed moisture present that is either specified on a certificate of analysis or that is determined in the pharmacy immediately before the drug substance is used by the procedure under *Loss on Drying* ⟨731⟩, this information must be used when calculating the amount of drug substance that is to be weighed in order to determine the exact amount of anhydrous drug substance required.

There are cases in which the required amount of a dose is specified in terms of a cation [e.g., Li^+, netilmicin (n+)], an anion [e.g., F^-], or a molecule (e.g., theophylline in aminophylline). In these instances, the drug substance weighed is a salt or complex, a portion of which represents the pharmacologically active moiety. Thus, the exact amount of such substances weighed must be calculated on the basis of the required quantity of the pharmacological moiety.

The following formula may be used to calculate the exact theoretical weight of an ingredient in a compounded preparation:

$$W = ab/de,$$

in which W is the actual weighed amount; a is the prescribed or pharmacist-determined weight of the active or functional moiety of drug or added substance; b is the chemical formula weight of the ingredient, including waters of hydration for hydrous ingredients; d is the fraction of dry weight when the percent by weight of adsorbed moisture content is known from the loss on drying procedure (see *Loss on Drying* ⟨731⟩); and e is the formula weight of the active or functional moiety of a drug or added substance that is provided in the formula weight of the weighed ingredient.

Example 1: Triturate Morphine Sulfate USP and Lactose NF to obtain 10 g in which there are 30 mg of Morphine Sulfate USP for each 200 mg of the morphine-lactose mixture. [NOTE—Clinical dosages of morphine mean Morphine Sulfate USP, which is the pentahydrate.]

Equation Factor	Numerical Value
W	weight, in g, of Morphine Sulfate USP
a	1.5 g of morphine sulfate pentahydrate in the prescription
b	759 g/mole
d	1.0
e	759 g/mole

$$W = \frac{1.5\,g(759\,g/mole)}{1.0(759\,g/mole)} = 1.5\,g.$$

Example 2: Accurately weigh an amount of Aminophylline USP to obtain 250 mg of anhydrous theophylline. [NOTE—The powdered aminophylline dihydrate weighed contains 0.4% w/w adsorbed moisture as stated in the Certificate of Analysis.]

Equation Factor	Numerical Value
W	weight, in mg, of Aminophylline USP (dihydrate)
a	250 mg of theophylline
b	456 g/mole
d	0.996
e	360 g/mole

$$W = \frac{250\,mg\,(456\,g/mole)}{0.996\,(360\,g/mole)} = 318\,mg$$

Example 3: Accurately weigh an amount of Lithium Citrate USP (containing 2.5% moisture as stated in the Certificate of Analysis) to obtain 200 mEq of lithium (Li^+). [NOTE—One mEq of Li^+ is equivalent to 0.00694 g of Li^+.]

Equation Factor	Numerical Value
W	weight, in g, of Lithium Citrate USP (tetrahydrate)
a	200 mEq of Li^+ or 1.39 g of Li^+
b	282 g/mole
d	0.975
e	3 × 6.94 g/mole or 20.8 g/mole

$$W = \frac{1.39\,g(282\,g/mole)}{0.975\,(20.8\,g/mole)} = 19.3\,g.$$

Example 4: Accurately weigh an amount of Netilmicin Sulfate USP, equivalent to 2.5 g of netilmicin. [NOTE—Using the procedure under *Loss on Drying* ⟨731⟩, the Netilmicin Sulfate USP that was weighed lost 12% of its weight.]

Equation Factor	Numerical Value
W	weight, in g, of Netilmicin Sulfate USP
a	2.5 g
b	1442 g/mole
d	0.88
e	951 g/mole

$$W = \frac{2.5\,\mathrm{g}(1442\,\mathrm{g/mole})}{0.88\,(951\,\mathrm{g/mole})} = 4.31\,\mathrm{g}.$$

BUFFER SOLUTIONS

Definition—A buffer solution is an aqueous solution that resists a change in pH when small quantities of acid or base are added, when diluted with the solvent, or when the temperature changes. Most buffer solutions are mixtures of a weak acid and one of its salts or mixtures of a weak base and one of its salts. Water and solutions of a neutral salt such as sodium chloride have very little ability to resist the change of pH and are not capable of effective buffer action.

Preparation, Use, and Storage of Buffer Solutions—Buffer solutions for pharmacopeial tests should be prepared using freshly boiled and cooled water (see *Standard Buffer Solutions* under *Buffer Solutions in Reagents, Indicators, and Solutions*). They should be stored in containers such as Type I glass bottles and used within three months of preparation.

Buffers used in physiological systems are carefully chosen so as not to interfere with the pharmacological activity of the medicament or the normal function of the organism. Commonly used buffers in parenteral products for example are acetic, citric, glutamic, and phosphoric acids and their salts. Buffer solutions should be freshly prepared.

The Henderson-Hasselbalch equation, noted above, allows the pH of a buffer solution of a weak acid and its salt to be calculated. Appropriately modified, this equation may be applied to buffer solutions composed of a weak base and its salt.

Buffer Capacity—The buffer capacity of a solution is the measurement of the ability of that solution to resist a change in pH upon addition of small quantities of a strong acid or base. An aqueous solution has a buffer capacity of 1 when 1 liter of the buffer solution requires 1 gram equivalent of strong acid or base to change the pH by 1 unit. Therefore, the smaller the pH change upon the addition of a specified amount of acid or base, the greater the buffer capacity of the buffer solution. Usually, in analysis, much smaller volumes of buffer are used in order to determine the buffer capacity. An approximate formula for calculating the buffer capacity is gram equivalents of strong acid or base added per liter of buffer solution per unit of pH change, i.e., (Eq /L)/(pH change).

EXAMPLE—
The addition of 0.01 g equivalents of sodium hydroxide to 0.25 liter of a buffer solution produced a pH change of 0.50. The buffer capacity of the buffer solution is calculated as follows:

(0.01/0.25)/0.50 = 0.08(Eq/L)/(pH change)

DOSAGE CALCULATIONS

Special Dosage Regimens—Geriatric and pediatric patients require special consideration when designing dosage regimens. In geriatric patients, the organs are often not functioning efficiently as a result of age-related pharmacokinetic changes or disease. For these patients, modifications in dosing regimens are available in references such as *USP Drug Information*.

For pediatric patients, where organs are often not fully developed and functioning, careful consideration must be applied during dosing. Modifications in dosing regimens for pediatric patients are also available in references such as *USP Drug Information*. General rules for calculating doses for infants and children are available in pharmacy calculation textbooks. These rules are not drug-specific and should be used only in the absence of more complete information.

The usual method for calculating a dose for children is to use the information provided for children for the specific drug. The dose is frequently expressed as mg of drug per kg of body weight for a 24-hour period, and is then usually given in divided portions. The calculation may be made using the following equation:

(mg of drug per kg of body weight) × (kg of body weight) = dose for an individual for a 24-hour period

A less frequently used method of calculating the dose is based on the surface area of the individual's body. The dose is expressed as amount of drug per body surface area in m², as shown in the equation below:

(amount of drug per m² of body surface area) × (body surface area in m²) = dose for an individual for a 24-hour period.

The body surface area (BSA) may be determined from nomograms relating height and weight in dosage handbooks. The BSA for adult and pediatric patients may also be determined using the following equations:

BSA (m²) = square root of {[Height (in) × Weight (lb)] / 3131}

or

BSA (m²) = square root of {[Height (cm) × Weight (kg)]/ 3600}.

EXAMPLE—
Rx for Spironolactone Suspension 25 mg/tsp. Sig: 9 mg BID for an 18 month-old child who weighs 22 lbs.

The *USP DI 2002*, 22nd ed., states that the normal pediatric dosing regimen for Spironolactone is 1 to 3 mg per kg per day. In this case, the weight of the child is 22 lbs, which equals 22 lbs/(2.2 lbs/kg) = 10 kg. Therefore the normal dose for this child is 10 to 30 mg per day and the dose ordered is 18 mg per day as a single dose or divided into 2 to 4 doses. The dose is acceptable based on published dosing guidelines.

PERCENTAGE CONCENTRATIONS

Percentage concentrations of solutions are usually expressed in one of three common forms:

$$\text{Volume percent}\,(v/v) = \frac{\text{Volume of solute}}{\text{Volume of solution}} \times 100\%$$

$$\text{Weight percent}\,(w/w) = \frac{\text{Weight of solute} \times 100\%}{\text{Weight of solution}}$$

$$\text{Weight in volume percent}\,(w/v) = \frac{\text{Weight of solute (in g)}}{\text{Weight of solution (in mL)}} \times 100\%$$

See also *Percentage Measurements* under *Concentrations* in the *General Notices*. The above three equations may be used to calculate any one of the three values (i.e., weights, volumes, or percentages) in a given equation if the other two values are known.

Note that weights are always additive, i.e., 50 g plus 25 g = 75 g. Volumes of two different solvents or volumes of solvent plus a solid solute are not strictly additive. Thus 50 mL of water + 50 mL of pure alcohol do not produce a volume of 100 mL. Nevertheless, it is assumed that in some pharmaceutical calculations, volumes are additive, as discussed below under *Reconstitution of Drugs Using Volumes Other than Those on the Label.*

EXAMPLES—

1. Calculate the percentage concentrations (w/w) of the constituents of the solution prepared by dissolving 2.50 g of phenol in 10.00 g of glycerin. Using the weight percent equation above, the calculation is as follows.

   Total weight of the solution = 10.00 g + 2.50 g = 12.50 g.

   Weight percent of phenol = (2.50 g × 100%)/12.50 g = 20.0% of phenol.

   Weight percent of glycerin = (10 g × 100%)/12.50 g = 80.0% of glycerin.

2. A prescription order reads as follows:

   Eucalyptus Oil 3% (v/v) in Mineral Oil.

   Dispense 30.0 mL.

   What quantities should be used for this prescription? Using the volume percent equation above, the calculation is as follows.

   Amount of Eucalyptus Oil:

   $$3\% = (\text{Volume of oil in mL}/30.0 \text{ mL}) \times 100\%$$

   Solving the equation, the volume of oil = 0.90 mL

   Amount of Mineral Oil:

   To 0.90 mL of Eucalyptus Oil add sufficient Mineral Oil to prepare 30.0 mL.

3. A prescription order reads as follows:

Zinc oxide	7.5 g
Calamine	7.5 g
Starch	15 g
White petrolatum	30 g

   Calculate the percentage concentration for each of the four components. Using the weight percent equation above, the calculation is as follows.

   Total weight = 7.5 g + 7.5 g + 15 g + 30 g = 60.0 g.

   Weight percent of zinc oxide = (7.5 g zinc oxide/60 g ointment) × 100% = 12.5%.

   Weight percent of calamine = (7.5 g calamine/60 g ointment) × 100% = 12.5%.

   Weight percent of starch = (15 g starch/60 g ointment) × 100% = 25%.

   Weight percent of white petrolatum = (30 g white petrolatum/60 g ointment) × 100% = 50%.

SPECIFIC GRAVITY

The definition of Specific Gravity is usually based on the ratio of weight of a substance in air at 25° to that of the weight of an equal volume of water at the same temperature. The weight of 1 mL of water at 25° is approximately 1 g. The following equation may be used for calculations.

Specific Gravity = (Weight of the substance)/(Weight of an equal volume of water)

EXAMPLES—

1. A liquid weighs 125 g and has a volume of 110 mL. What is the specific gravity?

   The weight of an equal volume of water is 110 g.

   Using the above equation, specific gravity = 125 g/110 g = 1.14.

2. Hydrochloric Acid NF is approximately 37% (w/w) solution of hydrochloric acid (HCl) in water. How many grams of HCl are contained in 75.0 mL of HCl NF? (Specific gravity of Hydrochloric Acid NF is 1.18.)

   Calculate the weight of HCl NF using the above equation.

   The weight of an equal volume of water is 75 g.

   Specific Gravity 1.18 = weight of the HCl NF g /75.0 g.

   Solving the equation, the weight of HCl NF is 88.5 g.

   Now calculate the weight of HCl using the weight percent equation.

   37.0 % (w/w) = (weight of solute g/88.5 g) × 100.

   Solving the equation, the weight of the HCl is 32.7 g.

DILUTION AND CONCENTRATION

A concentrated solution can be diluted. Powders and other solid mixtures can be triturated or diluted to yield less concentrated forms. Because the amount of solute in the diluted solution or mixture is the same as the amount in the concentrated solution or mixture, the following relationship applies to dilution problems.

The quantity of *Solution 1* (Q_1) × concentration of *Solution 1* (C_1) = the quantity of *Solution 2* (Q_2) × concentration of *Solution 2* (C_2), or

$$(Q_1)(C_1) = (Q_2)(C_2).$$

Almost any quantity and concentration terms may be used. However, the units of the terms must be the same on both sides of the equation.

EXAMPLES—

1. Calculate the amount (Q_2), in g, of diluent that must be added to 60 g of a 10% (w/w) ointment to make a 5% (w/w) ointment.

   Let (Q_1) = 60 g, (C_1) = 10%, and (C_2) = 5%.

   Using the above equation,

   $$60 \text{ g} \times 10\% = (Q_2) \times 5\% \text{ (w/w)}$$

   Solving the above equation, the amount of product needed, Q_2, is 120 g. The initial amount of product added was 60 g, and therefore an additional 60 g of diluent must be added to the initial amount to give a total of 120 g.

2. How much diluent should be added to 10 g of a trituration (1 in 100) to make a mixture that contains 1 mg of drug in each 10 g of final mixture?

   Determine the final concentration by first converting mg to g. One mg of drug in 10 g of mixture is the same as 0.001g in 10 g.

   Let (Q_1) = 10 g, (C_1) = (1 in 100), and (C_2) = (0.001 in 10).

Using the equation for dilution, 10 g × (1/100) = (Q_2) g × (0.001/10).

Solving the above equation, (Q_2) = 1000 g.

Because 10 g of the final mixture contains all of the drug and some diluent, (1000 g − 10 g) or 990 g of diluent is required to prepare the mixture at a concentration of 0.001 g of drug in 10 g of final mixture.

3. Calculate the percentage strength of a solution obtained by diluting 400 mL of a 5.0% solution to 800 mL.

Let (Q_1) = 400 mL, (C_1) = 5%, and (Q_2) = 800 mL.

Using the equation for dilution, 400 mL × 5% = 800 mL × (C_2)%.

Solving the above equation, (C_2) = 2.5% (w/v).

USE OF POTENCY UNITS

See *Units of Potency* in the *General Notices*.

Because some substances may not be able to be defined by chemical and physical means, it may be necessary to express quantities of activity in biological units of potency.

EXAMPLES—

1. One mg of Pancreatin contains not less than 25 USP Units of amylase activity, 2.0 USP Units of lipase activity, and 25 USP Units of protease activity. If the patient takes 0.1 g (100 mg) per day, what is the daily amylase activity ingested?

    1 mg of Pancreatin corresponds to 25 USP Units of amylase activity.

    100 mg of Pancreatin corresponds to 100 × (25 USP Units of amylase activity) = 2500 Units.

2. A dose of penicillin G benzathine for streptococcal infection is 1.2 million units intramuscularly. If a specific product contains 1180 units per mg, how many milligrams would be in the dose?

    1180 units of penicillin G benzathine are contained in 1 mg.

    1 unit is contained in 1/1180 mg.

    1,200,000 units are contained in (1,200,000 × 1)/1180 units = 1017 mg.

BASE VS SALT OR ESTER FORMS OF DRUGS

Frequently the base form of a drug is administered in an altered form such as an ester or salt for stability or other reasons such as taste or solubility. This altered form of the drug usually has a different molecular weight (MW), and at times it may be useful to determine the amount of the base form of the drug in the altered form.

EXAMPLES—

1. Four hundred milligrams of erythromycin ethylsuccinate (molecular weight, 862.1) is administered. Determine the amount of erythromycin (molecular weight, 733.9) in this dose.

    862.1 g of erythromycin ethylsuccinate corresponds to 733.9 g of erythromycin.

    1 g of erythromycin ethylsuccinate corresponds to (733.9/862.1) g of erythromycin.

    0.400 g erythromycin ethylsuccinate corresponds to (733.9/862.1) × 0.400 g or 0.3405 g of erythromycin.

2. The molecular weight of testosterone cypionate is 412.6 and that of testosterone is 288.4. What is the dose of testosterone cypionate that would be equivalent to 60.0 mg of testosterone?

    288.4 g of testosterone corresponds to 412.6 g of testosterone cypionate.

1 g of testosterone corresponds to 412.6/288.4 g of testosterone cypionate.

60.0 mg or 0.0600 g of testosterone corresponds to (412.6/288.4) × 0.0600 = 0.0858 g or 85.8 mg of testosterone cypionate.

RECONSTITUTION OF DRUGS USING VOLUMES OTHER THAN THOSE ON THE LABEL

Occasionally it may be necessary to reconstitute a powder in order to provide a suitable drug concentration in the final product. This may be accomplished by estimating the volume of the powder and liquid medium required.

EXAMPLES—

1. If the volume of 250 mg of ceftriaxone sodium is 0.1 mL, how much diluent should be added to 500 mg of ceftriaxone sodium powder to make a suspension having a concentration of 250 mg per mL?

$$500 \text{ mg} \times \frac{1 \text{ mL}}{250 \text{ mg}} = 2 \text{ mL}.$$

2. Volume of 500 mg of ceftriaxone sodium =

$$500 \text{ mg} \times \frac{0.1 \text{ mL}}{250 \text{ mg}} = 0.2 \text{ mL}$$

3. Volume of the diluent required = (2 mL of suspension) − (0.2 mL of Ceftriaxone Sodium) = 1.8 mL.

4. What is the volume of dry powder cefonicid, if 2.50 mL of diluent is added to 1 g of powder to make a solution having a concentration of 325 mg per mL?

    Volume of solution containing 1 g of the powder =

$$1 \text{ g of cefonicid} \times \frac{1000 \text{ mg}}{1 \text{ g}} \times \frac{1 \text{ mL of solution}}{325 \text{ mg of cefonicid}} = 3.08 \text{ mL}$$

    Volume of dry powder cefonicid = 3.08 mL of solution − 2.50 mL of diluent = 0.58 mL.

ALLIGATION ALTERNATE AND ALGEBRA

Alligation—Alligation is a rapid method of determining the proportions in which substances of different strengths are mixed to yield a desired strength or concentration. Once the proportion is found, the calculation may be performed to find the exact amounts of substances required. Set up the problem as follows.

1. Place the desired percentage or concentration in the center.
2. Place the percentage of the substance with the lower strength on the lower left-hand side.
3. Place the percentage of the substance with the higher strength on the upper left-hand side.
4. Subtract the desired percentage from the lower percentage, and place the obtained difference on the upper right-hand side.
5. Subtract the higher percentage from the desired percentage, and place the obtained difference on the lower right-hand side.

The results obtained will determine how many parts of the two different percentage strengths should be mixed to produce the desired percentage strength of a drug mixture.

EXAMPLES—

1. How much ointment having a 12% drug concentration and how much ointment having a 16% drug concentration must be used to make 1 kg of a preparation containing a 12.5% drug concentration?

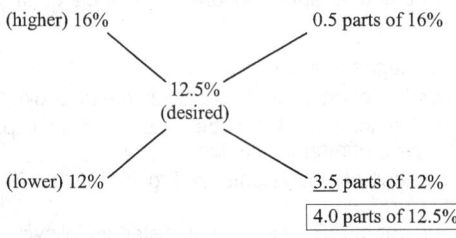

(higher) 16%   0.5 parts of 16%

12.5%
(desired)

(lower) 12%   3.5 parts of 12%
                     4.0 parts of 12.5%

In a total of 4.0 parts of 12.5% product, 3.5 parts of 12% ointment and 0.5 parts of 16% ointment are needed.

4 parts correspond to 1 kg or 1000 g.

1 part corresponds to 250 g.

3.5 parts correspond to 3.5×250 g or 875 g.

0.5 parts correspond to 0.5×250 g or 125 g.

2. How many mL of 20% dextrose in water and 50% dextrose in water are needed to make 750 mL of 35% dextrose in water?

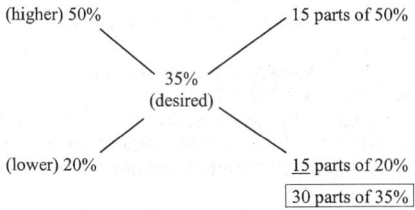

(higher) 50%   15 parts of 50%

35%
(desired)

(lower) 20%   15 parts of 20%
                     30 parts of 35%

In a total of 30 parts of 35% dextrose in water, 15 parts of 50% dextrose in water and 15 parts of 20% dextrose in water are required.

30 parts correspond to 750 mL.

15 parts correspond to 375 mL.

Thus use 375 mL of the 20% solution and 375 mL of the 50% solution to prepare the product.

Algebra—Instead of using alligation to solve the above problems, algebra may be used, following the scheme outlined below.

In order to represent the total amount (weights, parts, or volumes) of the final mixture or solution, 1 or a specified amount is used.

Let x be the amount of one portion and [1 (or the specified amount) − x] be the remaining portion. Set up the equation according to the statement below, and solve.

The amount in one part plus the amount in the other part equals the total amount in the final mixture or solution.

EXAMPLES—

1. How much ointment having a 12% drug concentration and how much ointment having a 16% drug concentration must

be used to make 1 kg of a preparation containing a 12.5% drug concentration?

Let 1 kg be the total amount of ointment to be prepared, let x be the quantity, in kg, of the 12% ointment, and let $(1 − x)$ be the quantity in kg of the 16% ointment. The equation is as follows:

$$(12/100)\ x + (16/100)(1 − x) = (12.5/100)(1).$$

Solving the equation, x equals 0.875 kg of the 12% ointment and $(1 − x)$ equals $(1 − 0.875)$ or 0.125 kg of the 16% ointment.

2. How many mL of 20% dextrose in water and 50% dextrose in water are needed to make 750 mL of 35% dextrose in water?

Let x be the volume, in mL, of the 20% solution, and let $(750 − x)$ be the volume in mL of the 50% solution. The equation is as follows:

$$(20/100)x + (50/100)(750 − x) = (35/100)(750).$$

Solving the equation, x equals 375 mL of the 20% solution and $(750 − x)$ equals $(750 − 375)$ or 375 mL of the 50% solution.

MOLAR, MOLAL, AND NORMAL CONCENTRATIONS

See *Concentrations* in the *General Notices*.

Molarity—The molar concentration, M, of the solution is the number of moles of the solute contained in one liter of solution.

Molality—The molal concentration, m, is the number of moles of the solute contained in one kilogram of solvent.

Normality—The normal concentration, N, of a solution expresses the number of milliequivalents (mEq) of solute contained in 1 mL of solution or the number of equivalents (Eq, gram-equivalent weight) of solute contained in 1 liter of solution. When using normality, the pharmacist must apply quantitative chemical analysis principles using molecular weight (MW). Normality depends on the reaction capacity of a chemical compound and therefore the reaction capacity must be known. For acids and bases, reaction capacity is the number of accessible protons available from, or the number of proton binding sites available on, each molecular aggregate. For electron transfer reactions, reaction capacity is the number of electrons gained or lost per molecular aggregate.

EXAMPLES—

1. How much sodium bicarbonate powder is needed to prepare 50.0 mL of a 0.07 N solution of sodium bicarbonate ($NaHCO_3$)? (MW of $NaHCO_3$ is 84.0 g per mol.)

In an acid or base reaction, because $NaHCO_3$ may act as an acid by giving up one proton, or as a base by accepting one proton, one Eq of $NaHCO_3$ is contained in each mole of $NaHCO_3$. Thus the equivalent weight of $NaHCO_3$ is 84 g. [NOTE—The volume, in liters, × normality of a solution equals the number of equivalents in the solution.]

The number of equivalents of $NaHCO_3$ required = (0.07 Eq/L)

(50.0 mL/1000 mL /L) = 0.0035 equivalents.

1 equivalent weight is 84.0 g.

0.0035 equivalents equals 84.0 g/Eq × 0.0035 Eq = 0.294 g.

2. A prescription calls for 250 mL of a 0.1 N hydrochloric acid (HCl) solution. How many mL of concentrated hydrochloric acid are needed to make this solution? [NOTE—The specific gravity of concentrated hydrochloric acid is 1.18, the molecular weight is 36.46 and the concentration is 37.5% (w/w). Because hydrochloric acid functions as an acid and reacts by giving up one proton in a chemical reaction, 1 Eq is contained in each mole of the compound. Thus the equivalent weight is 36.46 g.]

The number of equivalents of HCl required is 0.250 L × 0.1 N = 0.025 equivalents.

1 equivalent is 36.46 g.

0.025 equivalents correspond to 0.025 Eq × 36.46 g/Eq = 0.9115 g.

37.5 g of pure HCl are contained in 100 g of concentrated HCl.

Thus 1 g of pure HCl is contained in (100/37.5) g = 2.666 g of concentrated acid, and 0.9115 g is contained in (0.9115 × 2.666) g or 2.43 g of concentrated acid.

In order to determine the volume of the supplied acid required, use the definition for specific gravity as shown below.

Specific gravity = (weight of the substance)/(weight of an equal volume of water).

1.18 = 2.43 g/(weight of an equal volume of water).

The weight of an equal volume of water is 2.056 g or 2.06 g, which measures 2.06 mL. Thus, 2.06 mL of concentrated acid is required.

MILLIEQUIVALENTS AND MILLIMOLES

NOTE—This section addresses milliequivalents (mEq) and millimoles (mmol) as they apply to electrolytes for dosage calculations.

The quantities of electrolytes administered to patients are usually expressed in terms of mEq. This term must not be confused with a similar term used in quantitative chemical analysis as discussed above. Weight units such as mg or g are not often used for electrolytes because the electrical properties of ions are best expressed as mEq. An equivalent is the weight of a substance (equivalent weight) that supplies one unit of charge. An equivalent weight is the weight, in g, of an atom or radical divided by the valence of the atom or radical. A milliequivalent is one-thousandth of an equivalent (Eq). Because the ionization of phosphate depends on several factors, the concentration is usually expressed in millimoles, moles, or milliosmoles which are described below. [NOTE—Equivalent weight (Eq.wt) = wt. of an atom or radical (ion) in g/valence (or charge) of the atom or radical. Milliequivalent weight (mEq.wt) = Eq.wt. (g)/1000.]

EXAMPLES—

1. Potassium (K⁺) has a gram-atomic weight of 39.10. The valence of K⁺ is 1⁺. Calculate its milliequivalent weight (mEq wt).

    Eq wt = 39.10 g/1 = 39.10 g

    mEq wt = 39.10 g/1000 = 0.03910 g = 39.10 mg
2. Calcium (Ca²⁺) has a gram-atomic weight of 40.08. Calculate its milliequivalent weight (mEq wt).

    Eq wt = 40.08 g/2 = 20.04 g

    mEq wt. = 20.04 g/1000 = 0.02004 g = 20.04 mg

NOTE—The equivalent weight of a compound may be determined by dividing the molecular weight in g by the product of the valence of either relevant ion and the number of times this ion occurs in one molecule of the compound.

3. How many milliequivalents of potassium ion (K⁺) are there in a 250-mg Penicillin V Potassium Tablet? [NOTE—Molecular weight of penicillin V potassium is 388.48 g per mol; there is one potassium atom in the molecule; and the valence of K⁺ is 1.]

    Eq wt = 388.48 g/[1(valence) × 1(number of charges)] = 388.48 g.

    mEq wt = 388.48 g/1000 = 0.38848 g = 388.48 mg.

    (250 mg per Tablet)/(388.48 mg per mEq) = 0.644 mEq of K⁺ per Tablet.
4. How many equivalents of magnesium ion and sulfate ion are contained in 2 mL of a 50% Magnesium Sulfate Injection? (Molecular weight of MgSO₄ · 7H₂O is 246.48 g per mol.)

Amount of magnesium sulfate in 2 mL of 50% Magnesium Sulfate Injection =

$$2 \, \text{mL of Injection} \times \frac{50 \, \text{g of magnesium sulfate}}{100 \, \text{mL of Injection}} = 1 \, \text{g}.$$

Eq wt of MgSO₄.7H₂O = MW (g)/(valence of specified ion × number of specified ions in one mole of salt).

For the magnesium ion:

The number of equivalents is calculated as follows:

246.48/[2(valence) × 1 (number of ions in the compound)] = 123.24 g/Eq of magnesium ion.

The number of equivalents in 1 g is 1g/ 123.24 g/Eq = 0.008114 Eq.

The number of mEq may be calculated as follows.

The mEq wt = Eq wt (g)/1000 = (123.24 g/Eq)/1000 = 0.12324 g.

The number of milliequivalents of magnesium ion in 1 g is 1g/ 0.12324 g/mEq = 8.114 mEq.

For the sulfate ion:

The number of equivalents is calculated as follows:

246.48/[2(valence) × 1 (number of ions in the compound)] = 123.24 g/Eq of sulfate ion.

The number of equivalents in 1 g is 1g/123.24 g/Eq = 0.008114 Eq.

The number of mEq may be calculated as follows.

The mEq wt = Eq wt (g)/1000 = (123.24 g/Eq)/1000 = 0.12324 g.

The number of milliequivalents of sulfate ion in 1 g is 1g/ 0.12324 g/mEq = 8.114 mEq.
5. A vial of Sodium Chloride Injection contains 3 mEq of sodium chloride per mL. What is the percentage strength of this solution? (Molecular weight of sodium chloride is 58.44 g per mol.)

    1 mEq = 1 Eq/1000 = 58.44 g/1000 = 0.05844 g = 58.44 mg.

    Amount of sodium chloride in 3 mEq per mL = 58.44 mg per mEq × 3 mEq per mL = 175.32 mg per mL.

$$\frac{175.32 \, \text{mg}}{1 \, \text{mL}} = \frac{17532 \, \text{mg}}{100 \, \text{mL}} = \frac{17.532 \, \text{g}}{100 \, \text{mL}} = 17.5\%$$

Using mols and mmols—

A number of countries have adopted the International System of Units and no longer calculate doses using mEq as described above, but instead use the terms moles (mol) and millimoles (mmol). In *USP 27–NF 22*, the International System of Units is used except for the labeling of electrolytes.

Definitions—

A mole equals one gram atomic weight or gram molecular weight of a substance.

A millimole equals 1/1000 of a mole.

EXAMPLES—

1. Potassium (K) has a gram-atomic weight of 39.10. Calculate its weight in millimoles (mmol).

    The weight of one mole is 39.10 g and the weight in millimoles is 39.10 g/1000 =0.0391 g or 39.1 mg.
2. How many millimoles of Penicillin V are in a tablet that contains 250 mg of Penicillin V Potassium? (Molecular weight of penicillin V potassium is 388.48 g per mol.)

The weight of one mole is 388.48 and the weight in millimoles is 388.48/1000 = 0.3848 g or 388.48 mg. Thus there are 250 mg/388.48 mg/mmol = 0.644 mmol of Penicillin V ion per tablet.

ISOOSMOTIC SOLUTIONS

The following discussion and calculations have therapeutic implications in preparations of dosage forms intended for ophthalmic, subcutaneous, intravenous, intrathecal, and neonatal use.

Cells of the body, such as erythrocytes, will neither swell nor shrink when placed in a solution that is isotonic with the body fluids. However, the measurement of tonicity, a physiological property, is somewhat difficult. It is found that a 0.9% (w/v) solution of sodium chloride, which has a freezing point of − 0.52°, is isotonic with body fluids and is said to be isoosmotic with body fluids. In contrast to isotonicity, the freezing point depression is a physical property. Thus many solutions which are isoosmotic with body fluids are not necessarily isotonic with body fluids, e.g., a solution of urea. Nevertheless many pharmaceutical products are prepared using freezing point data or related sodium chloride data to prepare solutions that are isoosmotic with the body fluids. A closely related topic is osmolarity (see *Osmolarity* ⟨785⟩).

Freezing point data or sodium chloride equivalents of pharmaceuticals and excipients (see *Table 1* below) may be used to prepare isoosmotic solutions, as shown in the examples below.

Table 1. Sodium Chloride Equivalents (E) and Freezing Point (FP) Depressions for a 1% Solution of the Drug or Excipient

Drug or Excipient	E	FP Depression
Atropine sulfate	0.13	0.075
Sodium chloride	1.00	0.576

EXAMPLE—
Determine the amount of sodium chloride required to prepare 60 mL of an isoosmotic solution of atropine sulfate 0.5% using the sodium chloride equivalent values and also the freezing point depression values.
Using the sodium chloride equivalent values—
The total amount of substances equivalent to sodium chloride (for a 0.9% solution) = (0.9 g/100 mL) × 60 mL = 0.54 g.
The amount of atropine sulfate required = (0.5 g/100 mL) × 60 mL = 0.3 g.
1 g of atropine sulfate is equivalent to 0.13 g of sodium chloride.
0.3 g atropine sulfate is equivalent to 0.3 × 0.13 g = 0.039 g of sodium chloride.
Thus the required amount of sodium chloride is 0.54 − 0.039 = 0.501 g or 0.50 g.

Using freezing point depression values—
The freezing point depression required is 0.52°.
A 1% solution of atropine sulfate causes a freezing point depression of 0.075°.
A 0.5% solution of atropine sulfate causes a freezing point depression of 0.075° × 0.5 = 0.0375°.
The additional freezing point depression required is 0.52° − 0.0375° = 0.482°.
A 1% solution of sodium chloride causes a freezing point depression of 0.576°.
A (1%/ 0.576) solution of sodium chloride causes a freezing point depression of 1°.
A (1%/ 0.576) × 0.482 = 0.836% solution of sodium chloride causes a freezing point depression of 0.482°.
The required amount of sodium chloride is (0.836 g/100 mL) × 60 mL = 0.502 g or 0.50 g.

FLOW RATES IN INTRAVENOUS SETS

Some calculations concerning flow rates in intravenous sets are provided below. [NOTE—Examples below are *not* to be used for treatment purposes.]

EXAMPLES—
1. Sodium Heparin 8,000 units in 250 mL Sodium Chloride Injection 0.9% solution are to be infused over 4 hours. The administration set delivers 20 drops per mL.
   What is the flow rate in mL per hour?
   In 4 hours, 250 mL are to be delivered.
   In 1 hour, 250 mL/4 = 62.5 mL are delivered.
   What is the flow rate in drops per minute?
   In 60 minutes, 62.5 mL are delivered.
   In 1 minute, 62.5 mL/60 = 1.04 mL are delivered.
   1 mL = 20 drops.
   1.04 mL = 1.04 × 20 drops = 20.8 drops.
   Thus in 1 minute, 20.8 or 21 drops are administered.
2. A 14.5 kg patient is to receive 50 mg of Sodium Nitroprusside in 250 mL of dextrose 5% in water (D5W) at the rate of 1.3 µg per kg per minute. The set delivers 50 drops per mL.
   Calculate the flow rate in mL per hour.
   The dose for 1 kg is 1.3 µg per minute.
   The 14.5 kg patient should receive 14.5 × 1.3 µg = 18.85 µg per minute.
   50 mg or 50000 µg of drug are contained in 250 mL of D5W.
   18.85 µg are contained in 250 mL × 18.85/50000 = 0.09425 mL D5W, which is administered every minute.
   In 1 minute, 0.09425 mL are administered.
   In 1 hour or 60 minutes, 60 × 0.09425 mL = 5.655 or 5.7 mL are administered.
   Calculate the flow rate in drops per minute.
   1 mL corresponds to 50 drops per minute.
   0.09425 mL corresponds to 0.09425 × 50 = 4.712 or 4.7 drops per minute.

TEMPERATURE

The relationship between Celsius degrees (°C) and Fahrenheit degrees (°F) is expressed by the following equation:

$$9\,(°C) = 5\,(°F) - 160,$$

in which °C and °F are the numbers of Celsius degrees and Fahrenheit degrees, respectively.

EXAMPLES—
1. Convert 77 °F to Celsius degrees.
   9(°C) = 5(°F) − 160
   °C = [5(°F) − 160]/9 = [(5 × 77) − 160]/9 = 25 °C
2. Convert 30 °C to Fahrenheit degrees.
   9(°C) = 5(°F) − 160
   °F = [9(°C) + 160]/5 = [(9 × 30) + 160]/5 = 86 °F
The relationship between the Kelvin and the Celsius scales is expressed by the equation:

$$K = °C + 273.1,$$

in which K and °C are the numbers of Kelvin degrees and Celsius degrees, respectively.

APPLICATION OF MEAN KINETIC TEMPERATURE

See *Stability* under *Pharmaceutical Dosage Forms* ⟨1151⟩ for the definition of mean kinetic temperature (MKT). MKT is usually higher than the arithmetic mean temperature and is derived from the Arrhenius equation. MKT addresses temperature fluctuations during the storage period of the product. The mean kinetic temperature, T_K, is calculated by the following equation:

$$T_K = \frac{\dfrac{-\Delta H}{R}}{ln(\dfrac{e^{-\Delta H/RT_1} + e^{-\Delta H/RT_2} + ... + e^{-\Delta H/RT_n}}{n})},$$

in which ΔH is the heat of activation, which equals 83.144 kJ per mol (unless more accurate information is available from experimental studies); R is the universal gas constant, which equals 8.3144×10^{-3} kJ per degree per mol; T_1 is the average temperature, in degrees Kelvin, during the first time period, e.g., the first week; T_2 is the average temperature, in degrees Kelvin, during the second time period, e.g., second week; and T_n is the average temperature, in degrees Kelvin during the nth time period, e.g., nth week, n being the total number of temperatures recorded. The mean kinetic temperature is calculated from average storage temperatures recorded over a one-year period, with a minimum of twelve equally spaced average storage temperature observations being recorded (see *Pharmaceutical Dosage Forms* ⟨1151⟩. This calculation can be performed manually with a pocket calculator or electronically with computer software.

EXAMPLES—

1. The means of the highest and lowest temperatures for 52 weeks are 25 °C each. Calculate the MKT.

    $n = 52$
    $\Delta H/R = 10,000$ K
    $T_1, T_2, ..., T_n = 25\ °C = 273.1 + 25 = 298.1$ K
    $R = 0.0083144$ kJ K^{-1}mol^{-1}
    $\Delta H = 83.144$ kJ per mol

$$T_K = \frac{\dfrac{-\Delta H}{R}}{ln(\dfrac{e^{-\Delta H/RT_1} + e^{-\Delta H/RT_2} + ... + e^{-\Delta H/RT_n}}{n})}$$

$$= \frac{-10,000\text{K}}{ln(\dfrac{52 \times e^{-\Delta H/R \times 298.1}}{52})}$$

$$= \frac{-10,000\text{K}}{ln(\dfrac{52 \times e^{-33.515B}}{52})}$$

$$= \frac{-10,000\text{K}}{-33.5458} = 298.1\text{K} = 25.0°C$$

The calculated MKT is 25.0 °C. Therefore the controlled room temperature requirement is met by this pharmacy. [NOTE—If the averages of the highest and lowest weekly temperatures differed from each other and were in the allowed range of 15 °C to 30 °C (see *Controlled Room Temperature* under *Preservation, Packaging, Storage, and Labeling* in the *General Notices*), then each average would be substituted individually into the equation. The remaining two examples illustrate such calculations, except that the monthly averages are used]

2. A pharmacy recorded a yearly MKT on a monthly basis, starting in January and ending in December. Each month, the pharmacy recorded the monthly highest temperature and the monthly lowest temperature, and the average of the two was calculated and recorded for the MKT calculation at the end of the year. From these data the MKT may be estimated or it may be calculated. If more than half of the observed temperatures are lower than 25 °C and a mean lower than 23 °C is obtained, the MKT may be estimated without performing the actual calculation.

Table 2. Data for Calculation of MKT

n	Month	Lowest Temperature (in °C)	Highest Temperature (in °C)	Average Temperature (in °C)	Average Temperature (in K)	$\Delta H/RT$	$e^{-\Delta H/RT}$
1	Jan.	15	27	21	294.1	34.002	1.710×10^{-15}
2	Feb.	20	25	22.5	295.6	33.830	2.033×10^{-15}
3	Mar.	17	25	21	294.1	34.002	1.710×10^{-15}
4	Apr.	20	25	22.5	295.6	33.830	2.033×10^{-15}
5	May	22	27	24.5	297.6	33.602	2.551×10^{-15}
6	June	15	25	20	293.1	34.118	1.523×10^{-15}
7	July	20	26	23	296.1	33.772	2.152×10^{-15}
8	Aug.	22	26	24	297.1	33.659	2.411×10^{-15}
9	Sept.	23	27	25	298.1	33.546	2.699×10^{-15}
10	Oct.	20	28	24	297.1	33.659	2.411×10^{-15}
11	Nov.	20	24	22	295.1	33.887	1.919×10^{-15}
12	Dec.	22	28	25	298.1	33.546	2.699×10^{-15}

a. To estimate the MKT, the recorded temperatures are evaluated and the average is calculated. In this case, the calculated arithmetic mean is 22.9 °C. Therefore, the above requirements are met and it can be concluded that the mean kinetic temperature is lower than 25 °C. Therefore, the controlled room temperature requirement is met.

b. The second approach is to perform the actual calculation.

$$n = 12$$

$$T_K = \frac{\dfrac{-\Delta H}{R}}{ln(\dfrac{e^{-\Delta H/RT_1}+e^{-\Delta H/RT_2}+...+e^{-\Delta H/RT_n}}{n})}$$

$$= \frac{-10,000\text{K}}{ln(\dfrac{1.710\times10^{-15}+2.033\times10^{-15}+1.710\times10^{-15}+...+2.699\times10^{-15}}{12})}$$

$$= \frac{-10,000\text{K}}{ln(\dfrac{2.585 \times 10^{-14}}{12})}$$

$$= \frac{-10,000\text{K}}{-33.771} = 296.11\text{K} = 23.0 \text{ °C}$$

The calculated MKT is 23.0 °C, so the controlled room temperature requirement is met. [NOTE—These data and calculations are used only as an example.]

3. An article was stored for one year in a pharmacy where the observed monthly average of the highest and lowest temperatures was 25 °C (298.1 K), except for one month with an average of 28 °C (301.1 K). Calculate the MKT of the pharmacy.

$$n = 12$$

$$T_K = \frac{\dfrac{-\Delta H}{R}}{ln(\dfrac{e^{-\Delta H/RT_1}+e^{-\Delta H/RT_2}+...+e^{-\Delta H/RT_n}}{n})},$$

$$= \frac{\dfrac{-\Delta H}{R}}{ln(\dfrac{11 \times e^{-\Delta H/(R \times 298.1)}+1 \times e^{-\Delta H/(R \times 301.1)}}{12})}$$

$$= \frac{-10,000\text{K}}{ln(\dfrac{11 \times e^{-33.546}+1 \times e^{-33.212}}{12})}$$

$$= \frac{-10,000\text{K}}{ln(\dfrac{2.9692 \times 10^{-14}+3.7705 \times 10^{-15}}{12})}$$

$$= \frac{-10,000\text{K}}{ln(\dfrac{3.3463 \times 10^{-14}}{12})}$$

$$= \frac{-10,000\text{K}}{ln(2.7886 \times 10^{-15})}$$

$$= \frac{-10,000\text{K}}{-33.513} = 298.39\text{K} = 25.29° \text{ C}$$

The controlled room temperature requirement is not met because the calculated MKT exceeds 25 °C. (See *Note* in Example 2 above.)▲*USP27*

⟨1176⟩ PRESCRIPTION BALANCES AND VOLUMETRIC APPARATUS

Prescription Balances

NOTE—Balances other than the type described herein may be used provided these afford equivalent or better accuracy. This includes micro-, semimicro-, or electronic single-pan balances (see *Weights and Balances* ⟨41⟩). Some balances offer digital or direct-reading features. All balances should be calibrated and tested frequently using appropriate test weights, both singly and in combination.

Description—A prescription balance is a scale or balance adapted to weighing medicinal and other substances required in prescriptions or in other pharmaceutical compounding. It is constructed so as to support its full capacity without developing undue stresses, and its adjustment is not altered by repeated weighings of the capacity load. The removable pans or weighing

vessels should be of equal weight. The balance should have leveling feet or screws. The balance may feature dial-in weights and also a precision spring and dial instead of a weighbeam. A balance that has a graduated weighbeam must have a stop that halts the rider or poise at the "zero" reading. The reading edge of the rider is parallel to the graduations on the weighbeam. The distance from the face of the index plate to the indicator pointer or pointers should be not more than 1.0 mm, the points should be sharp, and when there are two, their ends should be separated by not more than 1.0 mm when the scale is in balance. The indicating elements and the lever system should be protected against drafts, and the balance lid should permit free movement of the loaded weighing pans when the lid is closed. The balance must have a mechanical arresting device.

Definitions—

Capacity—Maximum weight, including the weight of tares, to be placed on one pan. The *N.B.S. Handbook 44*, 4th ed., states: "*In the absence of information to the contrary*, the nominal capacity of a Class *A* balance shall be assumed to be 15.5 g (apothecaries' ounce)." Most of the commercially available Class *A* balances have a capacity of 120 g and bear a statement to that effect.

Weighbeam or Beam—A graduated bar equipped with a movable poise or rider. Metric graduations are in 0.01-g increments up to a maximum of 1.0 g.

Tare Bar—An auxiliary ungraduated weighbeam bar with a movable poise. This can be used to correct for variations in weighing-glasses or papers.

Balance Indicator—A combination of elements, one or both of which will oscillate with respect to the other, to indicate the equilibrium state of the balance during weighing.

Rest Point—The point on the index plate at which the indicator or pointer stops when the oscillations of the balance cease; or the index plate position of the indicator or pointer calculated from recorded consecutive oscillations in both directions past the "zero" of the index plate scale. If the balance has a two-pointer indicating mechanism, the position or the oscillations of only one of the pointers need be recorded or used to determine the rest point.

Sensitivity Requirements (SR)—The maximum change in load that will cause a specified change, one subdivision on the index plate, in the position of rest of the indicating element or elements of the balance.

Class A Prescription Balance—A balance that meets the tests for this type of balance has a sensitivity requirement of 6 mg or less with no load and with a load of 10 g on each pan. The Class *A* balance should be used for all of the weighing operations required in prescription compounding.

In order to avoid errors of 5% or more that might be due to the limit of sensitivity of the Class *A* prescription balance, do not weigh less than 120 mg of any material. If a smaller weight of dry material is required, mix a larger known weight of the ingredient with a known weight of dry diluent, and weigh an aliquot portion of the mixture for use.

Testing the Prescription Balance—A Class *A* prescription balance meets the following four basic tests. Use a set of test weights, and keep the rider on the weighbeam at zero unless directed to change its position.

1. *Sensitivity Requirement*—Level the balance, determine the rest point, and place a 6-mg weight on one of the empty pans. Repeat the operation with a 10-g weight in the center of each pan. The rest point is shifted not less than one division on the index plate each time the 6-mg weight is added.

2. *Arm Ratio Test*—This test is designed to check the equality of length of both arms of the balance. Determine the rest point of the balance with no weight on the pans. Place in the center of each pan a 30-g test weight, and determine the rest point. If the second rest point is not the same as the first, place a 20-mg weight on the lighter side; the rest point should move back to the original place on the index plate scale or farther.

3. *Shift Tests*—These tests are designed to check the arm and lever components of the balance.

A. Determine the rest point of the indicator without any weights on the pans.

B. Place one of the 10-g weights in the center of the left pan, and place the other 10-g weight successively toward the right, left, front, and back of the right pan, noting the rest point in each case. If in any case the rest point differs from the rest point determined in Step *A*, add a 10-mg weight to the lighter side; this should cause the rest point to shift back to the rest point determined in Step *A* or farther.

C. Place a 10-g weight in the center of the right pan, and place a 10-g weight successively toward the right, left, front, and back of the left pan, noting the rest point in each case. If in any case rest point is different from that obtained with no weights on the pans, this difference should be overcome by addition of the 10-mg weight to the lighter side.

D. Make a series of observations in which both weights are simultaneously shifted to off-center positions on their pans, both toward the outside, both toward the inside, one toward the outside, and the other toward the inside, both toward the back, and so on until all combinations have been checked. If in any case the rest point differs from that obtained with no weights on the pan, the addition of the 10-mg weight to the lighter side should overcome this difference.

A balance that does not meet the requirements of these tests must be adjusted.

4. *Rider and Graduated Beam Tests*—Determine the rest point for the balance with no weight on the pans. Place on the left pan the 500-mg test weight, move the rider to the 500-mg point on the beam, and determine the rest point. If it is different from the zero rest point, add a 6-mg weight to the lighter side. This should bring the rest point back to its original position or farther. Repeat this test, using the 1-g test weight and moving the rider to the 1-g division on the beam. If the rest point is different, it should be brought back at least to the zero rest point position by addition of 6 mg to the lighter pan. If the balance does not meet this test, the weighbeam graduations or the rider must be corrected.

Metric or apothecaries' weights for use with a prescription balance should be kept in a special rigid and compartmentalized box and handled with plastic or plastic-tipped forceps to prevent scratching or soiling. For prescription use, analytical weights (Class P or better) are recommended. However, Class Q weights have tolerances well within the limits of accuracy of the prescription balance, and they retain their accuracy for a long time with proper care. Coin-type (or disk-shaped) weights should not be used.

Test weights consisting of two 20-g or two 30-g, two 10-g, one 1-g, one 500-mg, one 20-mg, one 10-mg, and one 6-mg (or suitable combination totaling 6 mg) weights, adjusted to N.B.S. tolerances for analytical weights (Class P or better) should be used for testing the prescription balances. These weights should be kept in a tightly closed box and should be handled only with plastic or plastic-tipped forceps. The set of test weights should be used only for testing the balance or constantly used weights. If properly cared for, the set lasts indefinitely.

Volumetric Apparatus

Pharmaceutical devices for measuring volumes of liquids, including burets, pipets, and cylinders graduated either in metric or apothecary units meet the standard specifications for glass volumetric apparatus described in NTIS COM-73-10504 of the National Technical Information Service.[1] Conical graduates meet the standard specifications described in N.B.S. *Handbook 44*, 4th Edition, of the National Institute of Standards and Technology.[2] Graduated medicine droppers meet the specifications (see *Medicine Dropper* ⟨1101⟩). An acceptable ungraduated medicine

---

[1] NTIS COM-73-10504 is for sale by the National Technical Information Service, Springfield, VA 22151.
[2] N.B.S. Handbook 44, 4th ed. (1971) is for sale by the Superintendent of Documents, U. S. Government Printing Office, Washington, DC 20402.

dropper has a delivery end 3 mm in external diameter and delivers 20 drops of water, weighing 1 g at a temperature of 15°. A tolerance of ±10% of the delivery specification is reasonable.

Selection and Use of Graduates—

Capacity—The capacity of a graduate is the designated volume, at the maximum graduation, that the graduate will contain, or deliver, as indicated, at the specified temperature.

Cylindrical and Conical Graduates—The error in a measured volume caused by a deviation of ±1 mm, in reading the lower meniscus in a graduated cylinder remains constant along the height of the uniform column. The same deviation of ±1 mm causes a progressively larger error in a conical graduate, the extent of the error being further dependent upon the angle of the flared sides to the perpendicular of the upright graduate. A deviation of ±1 mm in the meniscus reading causes an error of approximately 0.5 mL in the measured volume at any mark on the uniform 100-mL cylinder graduate. The same deviation of ±1 mm can cause an error of 1.8 mL at the 100-mL mark on an acceptable conical graduate marked for 125 mL.

A general rule for selection of a graduate for use is to use the graduate with a capacity equal to or *just exceeding* the volume to be measured. Measurement of small volumes in large graduates tends to increase errors, because the larger diameter increases the volume error in a deviation of ±1 mm from the mark. The relation of the volume error to the internal diameters of graduated cylinders is based upon the equation $V = \pi r^2 h$. An acceptable 10-mL cylinder having an internal diameter of 1.18 cm holds 109 μL in 1 mm of the column. Reading 4.5 mL in this graduate with a deviation of ±1 mm from the mark causes an error of about ±2.5%, while the same deviation in a volume of 2.2 mL in the same graduate causes an error of about ±5%. Minimum volumes that can be measured within certain limits of error in graduated cylinders of different capacities are incorporated in the design details of graduates in N.B.S. *Handbook 44*, 4th ed., of the National Institute of Standards and Technology. Conical graduates having a capacity of less than 25 mL should not be used in prescription compounding.

⟨1191⟩ STABILITY CONSIDERATIONS IN DISPENSING PRACTICE

Note—Inasmuch as this chapter is for purposes of general information only, no statement in the chapter is intended to modify or supplant any of the specific requirements pertinent to Pharmacopeial articles, which are given elsewhere in this Pharmacopeia.

Aspects of drug product stability that are of primary concern to the pharmacist in the dispensing of medications are discussed herein.

Pharmacists should avoid ingredients and conditions that could result in excessive physical deterioration or chemical decomposition of drug preparations, especially when compounding (see *Pharmaceutical Compounding—Nonsterile Preparations* ⟨795⟩). The stability and clinical effect of manufactured dosage forms can be greatly compromised by seemingly negligible alterations or inappropriate prescription compounding. Pharmacists should establish and maintain compounding conditions that include the ensurance of drug stability to help prevent therapeutic failure and adverse responses.

STABILITY is defined as the extent to which a product retains, within specified limits, and throughout its period of storage and use (i.e., its shelf-life), the same properties and characteristics that it possessed at the time of its manufacture. Five types of stability generally recognized are shown in the accompanying table.

Criteria for Acceptable Levels of Stability

Type of Stability	Conditions Maintained Throughout the Shelf-Life of the Drug Product
Chemical	Each active ingredient retains its chemical integrity and labeled potency, within the specified limits.
Physical	The original physical properties, including appearance, palatability, uniformity, dissolution, and suspendability are retained.
Microbiological	Sterility or resistance to microbial growth is retained according to the specified requirements. Antimicrobial agents that are present retain effectiveness within the specified limits.
Therapeutic	The therapeutic effect remains unchanged.
Toxicological	No significant increase in toxicity occurs.

Factors Affecting Product Stability

Each ingredient, whether therapeutically active or pharmaceutically necessary, can affect the stability of drug substances and dosage forms. The primary environmental factors that can reduce stability include exposure to adverse temperatures, light, humidity, oxygen, and carbon dioxide. The major dosage form factors that influence drug stability include particle size (especially in emulsions and suspensions), pH, solvent system composition (i.e., percentage of "free" water and overall polarity), compatibility of anions and cations, solution ionic strength, primary container, specific chemical additives, and molecular binding and diffusion of drugs and excipients. In dosage forms, the following reactions usually cause loss of active drug content, and they usually do not provide obvious visual or olfactory evidence of their occurrence.

Hydrolysis—Esters and β-lactams are the chemical bonds that are most likely to hydrolyze in the presence of water. For example, the acetyl ester in aspirin is hydrolyzed to acetic acid and salicylic acid in the presence of moisture, but in a dry environment the hydrolysis of aspirin is negligible. The aspirin hydrolysis rate increases in direct proportion to the water vapor pressure in an environment.

The amide bond also hydrolyzes, though generally at a slower rate than comparable esters. For example, procaine (an ester) will hydrolyze upon autoclaving, but procainamide will not. The amide or peptide bond in peptides and proteins varies in the lability to hydrolysis.

The lactam and azomethine (or imine) bonds in benzodiazepines are also labile to hydrolysis. The major chemical accelerators or catalysts of hydrolysis are adverse pH and specific chemicals (e.g., dextrose and copper in the case of ampicillin hydrolysis).

Epimerization—Members of the tetracycline family are most likely to incur epimerization. This reaction occurs rapidly when the dissolved drug is exposed to a pH of an intermediate range (higher than 3), and it results in the steric rearrangement of the dimethylamino group. The epimer of tetracycline, epitetracycline, has little or no antibacterial activity.

Decarboxylation—Some dissolved carboxylic acids, such as p-aminosalicylic acid, lose carbon dioxide from the carboxyl group when heated. The resulting product has reduced pharmacological potency.

β-Keto decarboxylation can occur in some solid antibiotics that have a carbonyl group on the β-carbon of a carboxylic acid or a carboxylate anion. Such decarboxylations will occur in the following antibiotics: carbenicillin sodium, carbenicillin free acid, ticarcillin sodium, and ticarcillin free acid.

Dehydration—Acid-catalyzed dehydration of tetracycline forms epianhydrotetracycline, a product that both lacks antibacterial activity and causes toxicity.

Oxidation—The molecular structures most likely to oxidize are those with a hydroxyl group directly bonded to an aromatic ring (e.g., phenol derivatives such as catecholamines and morphine), conjugated dienes (e.g., vitamin A and unsaturated free fatty acids), heterocyclic aromatic rings, nitroso and nitrite derivatives, and aldehydes (e.g., flavorings). Products of oxidation usually lack therapeutic activity. Visual identification of oxidation, for example, the change from colorless epinephrine to its amber colored products, may not be visible in some dilutions or to some eyes.

Oxidation is catalyzed by pH values that are higher than optimum, polyvalent heavy metal ions (e.g., copper and iron), and exposure to oxygen and UV illumination. The latter two causes of oxidation justify the use of antioxidant chemicals, nitrogen atmospheres during ampul and vial filling, opaque external packaging, and transparent amber glass or plastic containers.

Photochemical Decomposition—Exposure to, primarily, UV illumination may cause oxidation (photo-oxidation) and scission (photolysis) of covalent bonds. Nifedipine, nitroprusside, riboflavin, and phenothiazines are very labile to photo-oxidation. In susceptible compounds, photochemical energy creates free radical intermediates, which can perpetuate chain reactions.

Ionic Strength—The effect of the total concentration of dissolved electrolytes on the rate of hydrolysis reactions results from the influence of ionic strength on interionic attraction. In general, the hydrolysis rate constant is inversely proportional to the ionic strength with oppositely-charged ions (e.g., drug cation and excipient anions) and directly proportional to the ionic strength with ions of like charge. A reaction that produces an ion of opposite charge to the original drug ion can increase the drug hydrolysis rate as the reaction proceeds, because of the increasing ionic strength. High ionic strength of inorganic salts can also reduce the solubility of some other drugs.

pH Effect—The degradation of many drugs in solution accelerates or decelerates exponentially as the pH is decreased or increased over a specific range of pH values. Improper pH ranks with exposure to elevated temperature as a factor most likely to cause a clinically significant loss of drug, resulting from hydrolysis and oxidation reactions. A drug solution or suspension, for example, may be stable for days, weeks, or even years in its original formulation, but when mixed with another liquid that changes the pH, it degrades in minutes or days. It is possible that a pH change of only one unit (e.g., from 4 to 3 or 8 to 9) could decrease drug stability by a factor of ten or greater.

A pH buffer system, which is usually a weak acid or base and its salt, is a common excipient used in liquid preparations to maintain the pH in a range that minimizes the drug degradation rate. The pH of drug solutions may also be either buffered or adjusted to achieve drug solubility. For example, pH in relation to pKa controls the fractions of the usually more soluble ionized and less soluble nonionized species of weak organic electrolytes.

The influence of pH on the physical stability of two phase systems, especially emulsions, is also important. For example, intravenous fat emulsion is destabilized by acidic pH.

Interionic (Ion^{N+}–Ion^{N-}) Compatibility—The compatibility or solubility of oppositely charged ions depends mainly on the number of charges per ion and the molecular size of the ions. In general, polyvalent ions of opposite charge are more likely to be incompatible. Thus, an incompatibility is likely to occur upon the addition of a large ion with a charge opposite to that of the drug.

Solid State Stability—Solid state reactions are relatively slow; thus, stability of drugs in the solid state is rarely a dispensing concern. The degradation rate of dry solids is usually characterized by first-order kinetics or a sigmoid curve. Therefore, solid drugs with lower melting point temperatures should not be combined with other chemicals that would form a eutectic mixture.

When moisture is present, the solid drug decomposition may change to zero-order chemical kinetics because the rate is controlled by the relatively small fraction of the drug that exists in a saturated solution, which is located (usually imperceptibly) at the surface or in the bulk of the solid drug product.

Temperature—In general, the rate of a chemical reaction increases exponentially for each 10° increase in temperature. This relationship has been observed for nearly all drug hydrolysis and some drug oxidation reactions. The actual factor of rate increase depends on the activation energy of the particular reaction. The activation energy is a function of the specific reactive bond and the drug formulation (e.g., solvent, pH, additives, etc.). As an example, consider a hydrolyzable drug that is exposed to a 20° increase in temperature, such as that from cold to controlled room temperature (see *General Notices and Requirements*). The shelf life of the drug at controlled room temperature should be expected to decrease to one-fourth to one-twenty-fifth of its shelf life under refrigeration.

The pharmacist should also be aware that inappropriately cold temperatures may cause harm. For example, refrigeration may cause extreme viscosity in some liquid drugs and cause supersaturation in others. Freezing may either break or cause a large increase in the droplet size of emulsions; it can denature proteins; and in rare cases, it can cause less soluble polymorphic states of some drugs to form.

Stability Studies in Manufacturing

The scope and design of a stability study vary according to the product and the manufacturer concerned. Ordinarily the formulator of a product first determines the effects of temperature, light, air, pH, moisture, and trace metals, and commonly used excipients or solvents on the active ingredient(s). From this information, one or more formulations of each dosage form are prepared, packaged in suitable containers, and stored under a variety of environmental conditions, both exaggerated and normal. See *Stability* under *Pharmaceutical Dosage Forms* ⟨1151⟩. At appropriate time intervals, samples of the product are assayed for potency by use of a stability-indicating method, observed for physical changes, and, where applicable, tested for sterility and/or for resistance to microbial growth and for toxicity and bioavailability. Such a study, in combination with clinical and toxicological results, enables the manufacturer to select the optimum formulation and container and to assign recommended storage conditions and an expiration date for each dosage form in its package.

Responsibility of the Pharmacist

The pharmacist helps to ensure that the products under his supervision meet acceptable criteria of stability by (1) dispensing oldest stock first and observing expiration dates; (2) storing products under the environmental conditions stated in the individual monographs and/or in the labeling; (3) observing products for evidence of instability; (4) properly treating and labeling products that are repackaged, diluted, or mixed with other products; (5) dispensing in the proper container with the proper closure; and (6) informing and educating patients concerning the proper storage and use of the products, including the disposition of outdated or excessively aged prescriptions.

Rotating Stock and Observance of Expiration Dates—Proper rotation of stock is necessary to ensure the dispensing of suitable products. A product that is dispensed on an infrequent basis should be closely monitored so that old stocks are given special attention, particularly with regard to expiration dates. The manufacturer can guarantee the quality of a product up to the time designated as its expiration date only if the product has been stored in the original container under recommended storage conditions.

Storage under Recommended Environmental Conditions—In most instances, the recommended storage conditions are stated on the label, in which case it is imperative to adhere to those conditions. They may include a specified temperature range or a designated storage place or condition (e.g., "refrigerator," or "controlled room temperature") as defined in the *General Notices*. Supplemental instructions, such as a

direction to protect the product from light, also should be followed carefully. Where a product is required to be protected from light and is in a clear or translucent container enclosed in an opaque outer covering, such outer covering is not to be removed and discarded until the contents have been used. In the absence of specific instructions, the product should be stored at controlled room temperature (see *Storage Temperature* in the *General Notices*). The product should be stored away from locations where excessive or variable heat, cold, or light prevails, such as near heating pipes or fluorescent lighting.

Observing Products for Evidence of Instability—Loss of potency usually results from a chemical change, the most common reactions being hydrolysis, oxidation-reduction, and photolysis. Chemical changes may occur also through interaction between ingredients within a product, or rarely between product and container. An apparent loss of potency in the active ingredient(s) may result from diffusion of the drug into or its combination with the surface of the container-closure system. An apparent gain in potency usually is caused by solvent evaporation or by leaching of materials from the container-closure system.

The chemical potency of the active ingredient(s) is required to remain within the limits specified in the monograph definition. Potency is determined by means of an assay procedure that differentiates between the intact molecule and its degradation products. Chemical stability data should be available from the manufacturer. Although chemical degradation ordinarily cannot be detected by the pharmacist, excessive chemical degradation sometimes is accompanied by observable physical changes. In addition, some physical changes not necessarily related to chemical potency, such as change in color and odor, or formation of a precipitate, or clouding of solution, may serve to alert the pharmacist to the possibility of a stability problem. It should be assumed that a product that has undergone a physical change not explained in the labeling may also have undergone a chemical change and such a product is never to be dispensed. Excessive microbial growth and/or contamination also may appear as a physical change. A gross change in a physical characteristic such as color or odor is a sign of instability in any product. Other common physical signs of deterioration of dosage forms include the following.

Solid Dosage Forms—Many solid dosage forms are designed for storage under low-moisture conditions. They require protection from environmental water, and therefore should be stored in tight containers (see *Containers* in the *General Notices*) or in the container supplied by the manufacturer. The appearance of fog or liquid droplets, or clumping of the product, inside the container signifies improper conditions. The presence of a desiccant inside the manufacturer's container indicates that special care should be taken in dispensing. Some degradation products, for example, salicylic acid from aspirin, may sublime and be deposited as crystals on the outside of the dosage form or on the walls of the container.

HARD AND SOFT GELATIN CAPSULES—Since the capsule formulation is encased in a gelatin shell, a change in gross physical appearance or consistency, including hardening or softening of the shell, is the primary evidence of instability. Evidence of release of gas, such as a distended paper seal, is another sign of instability.

UNCOATED TABLETS—Evidence of physical instability in uncoated tablets may be shown by excessive powder and/or pieces (i.e., crumbling as distinct from breakage) of tablet at the bottom of the container (from abraded, crushed, or broken tablets); cracks or chips in tablet surfaces; swelling; mottling; discoloration; fusion between tablets; or the appearance of crystals that obviously are not part of the tablet itself on the container walls or on the tablets.

COATED TABLETS—Evidence of physical instability in coated tablets is shown by cracks, mottling, or tackiness in the coating and the clumping of tablets.

DRY POWDERS AND GRANULES—Dry powders and granules that are not intended for constitution into a liquid form in the original container may cake into hard masses or change color, which may render them unacceptable.

POWDERS AND GRANULES INTENDED FOR CONSTITUTION AS SUSPENSIONS—Dry powders and granules intended for constitution into solutions or suspensions require special attention. Usually such forms are those antibiotics or vitamins that are particularly sensitive to moisture. Since they are always dispensed in the original container, they generally are not subject to contamination by moisture. However, an unusual caked appearance necessitates careful evaluation, and the presence of a fog or liquid droplets inside the container generally renders the preparation unfit for use. Presence of an objectionable odor also may be evidence of instability.

EFFERVESCENT TABLETS, GRANULES, AND POWDERS—Effervescent products are particularly sensitive to moisture. Swelling of the mass or development of gas pressure is a specific sign of instability, indicating that some of the effervescent action has occurred prematurely.

Liquid Dosage Forms—Of primary concern with respect to liquid dosage forms are homogeneity and freedom from excessive microbial contamination and growth. Instability may be indicated by cloudiness or precipitation in a solution, breaking of an emulsion, nonresuspendable caking of a suspension, or organoleptic changes. Microbial growth may be accompanied by discoloration, turbidity, or gas formation.

SOLUTIONS, ELIXIRS, AND SYRUPS—Precipitation and evidence of microbial or chemical gas formation are the two major signs of instability.

EMULSIONS—The breaking of an emulsion (i.e., separation of an oil phase that is not easily dispersed) is a characteristic sign of instability; this is not to be confused with creaming, an easily redispersible separation of the oil phase that is a common occurrence with stable emulsions.

SUSPENSIONS—A caked solid phase that cannot be resuspended by a reasonable amount of shaking is a primary indication of instability in a suspension. The presence of relatively large particles may mean that excessive crystal growth has occurred.

TINCTURES AND FLUIDEXTRACTS—Tinctures, fluidextracts, and similar preparations usually are dark in color because they are concentrated, and thus they should be scrutinized carefully for evidence of precipitation.

STERILE LIQUIDS—Maintenance of sterility is of course critical for sterile liquids. The presence of microbial contamination in sterile liquids usually cannot be detected visually, but any haze, color change, cloudiness, surface film, particulate or flocculent matter, or gas formation is sufficient reason to suspect possible contamination. Clarity of sterile solutions intended for ophthalmic or parenteral use is of utmost importance. Evidence that the integrity of the seal has been violated on such products should make them suspect.

Semisolids (Creams, Ointments, and Suppositories)—For creams, ointments, and suppositories, the primary indication of instability is often either discoloration or a noticeable change in consistency or odor.

CREAMS—Unlike ointments, creams usually are emulsions containing water and oil. Indications of instability in creams are emulsion breakage, crystal growth, shrinking due to evaporation of water, and gross microbial contamination.

OINTMENTS—Common signs of instability in ointments are a change in consistency and excessive "bleeding" (i.e., separation of excessive amounts of liquid) and formation of granules or grittiness.

SUPPOSITORIES—Excessive softening is the major indication of instability in suppositories, although some suppositories may dry out and harden or shrivel. Evidence of oil stains on packaging material should warn the pharmacist to examine individual suppositories more closely by removing any foil covering if necessary. As a general rule (although there are exceptions), suppositories should be stored in a refrigerator (see *Storage Temperature* in the *General Notices*).

Proper Treatment of Products Subjected to Additional Manipulations—In repackaging, diluting, or mixing a product with another product, the pharmacist may become responsible for its stability.

Repackaging—In general, repackaging is inadvisable. However, if repackaging is necessary, the manufacturer should be consulted concerning potential problems. In the filling of prescriptions, it is essential that suitable containers be used. Appropriate storage conditions and, where appropriate, an expiration date and beyond–use date should be indicated on the label of the prescription container. Single-unit packaging calls for care and judgment, and for strict observance of the following guidelines: (1) use appropriate packaging materials; (2) where stability data on the new package are not available, repackage at any one time only sufficient stock for a limited time; (3) include on the unit-dose label a lot number and an appropriate beyond-use date; (4) where a sterile product is repackaged from a multiple-dose vial into unit-dose (disposable) syringes, discard the latter if not used within 24 hours, unless data are available to support longer storage; (5) where quantities are repackaged in advance of immediate needs, maintain suitable repackaging records showing name of manufacturer, lot number, date, and designation of persons responsible for repackaging and for checking (see *General Notices*); (6) where safety closures are required, use container closure systems that ensure compliance with compendial and regulatory standards for storage.

Dilution or Mixing—Where a product is diluted, or where two products are mixed, the pharmacist should observe good professional and scientific procedures to guard against incompatibility and instability. For example, tinctures such as those of belladonna and digitalis contain high concentrations of alcohol to dissolve the active ingredient(s), and they may develop a precipitate if they are diluted or mixed with aqueous systems. Pertinent technical literature and labeling should be consulted routinely; it should be current literature, because at times formulas are changed by the manufacturer. If a particular combination is commonly used, consultation with the manufacturer(s) is advisable. Since the chemical stability of extemporaneously prepared mixtures is unknown, the use of such combinations should be discouraged; if such a mixture involved an incompatibility, the pharmacist might be responsible. Oral antibiotic preparations constituted from powder into liquid form should never be mixed with other products.

Combining parenteral products necessitates special care, particularly in the case of intravenous solutions, primarily because of the route of administration. This area of practice demands the utmost in care, aseptic technique, judgment, and diligence. Because of potential unobservable problems with respect to sterility and chemical stability, all extemporaneous parenteral preparations should be used within 24 hours unless data are available to support longer storage.

Informing and **Educating the Patient**—As a final step in meeting responsibility for the stability of drugs dispensed, the pharmacist is obligated to inform the patient regarding the proper storage conditions (for example, in a cool, dry place—not in the bathroom), for both prescription and nonprescription products, and to suggest a reasonable estimate of the time after which the medication should be discarded. Where beyond-use dates are applied, the pharmacist should emphasize to the patient that the dates are applicable only when proper storage conditions are used. Patients should be encouraged to clean out their drug storage cabinets periodically.

⟨1221⟩ TEASPOON

For household purposes, an American Standard Teaspoon has been established by the American National Standards Institute* as containing 4.93 ± 0.24 mL. In view of the almost universal practice of employing teaspoons ordinarily available in the household for the administration of medicine, the teaspoon may be regarded as representing 5 mL. Preparations intended for administration by teaspoon should be formulated on the basis of dosage in 5-mL units. Any dropper, syringe, medicine cup, special spoon, or other device used to administer liquids should deliver 5 mL wherever a teaspoon calibration is indicated. Under ideal conditions of use, the volume error incurred in measuring liquids for individual dose administration by means of such calibrated devices should be not greater than 10% of the indicated amount.

Household units are used often to inform the patient of the size of the dose. Fifteen milliliters should be considered 1 standard tablespoonful; 10 mL, 2 standard teaspoonfuls; and 5 mL, 1 standard teaspoonful. Doses of less than 5 mL are frequently stated as fractions of a teaspoonful or in drops.

Because of the difficulties involved in measuring liquids under normal conditions of use, patients should be cautioned that household spoons are not appropriate for measuring medicines. They should be directed to use the standard measures in the cooking-and-baking measuring spoon sets or, preferably, oral dosing devices that may be provided by the practitioner. It must be kept in mind that the actual volume of a spoonful of any given liquid is related to the latter's viscosity and surface tension, among other influencing factors. These factors can also cause variability in the true volumes contained in or delivered by medicine cups. Where accurate dosage is required, a calibrated syringe or dropper should be used.

⟨1211⟩ STERILIZATION AND STERILITY ASSURANCE OF COMPENDIAL ARTICLES

This informational chapter provides a general description of the concepts and principles involved in the quality control of articles that must be sterile. Any modifications or variations in sterility test procedures from those described under *Sterility Tests* ⟨71⟩ should be validated in the context of the entire sterility assurance program and are not intended to be alternative methods to those described in that chapter.

Within the strictest definition of sterility, a specimen would be deemed sterile only when there is complete absence of viable microorganisms from it. However, this absolute definition cannot currently be applied to an entire lot of finished compendial articles because of limitations in testing. Absolute sterility cannot be practically demonstrated without complete destruction of every finished article. The sterility of a lot purported to be sterile is therefore defined in probabilistic terms, where the likelihood of a contaminated unit or article is acceptably remote. Such a state of sterility assurance can be established only through the use of adequate sterilization cycles and subsequent aseptic processing, if any, under appropriate current good manufacturing practice, and not by reliance solely on sterility testing. The basic principles for validation and certification of a sterilizing process are enumerated as follows:

(1) Establish that the process equipment has capability of operating within the required parameters.

(2) Demonstrate that the critical control equipment and instrumentation are capable of operating within the prescribed parameters for the process equipment.

(3) Perform replicate cycles representing the required operational range of the equipment and employing actual or simulated product. Demonstrate that the processes have been carried out

---

* American National Standards Institute, 1430 Broadway, New York, NY 10018.

within the prescribed protocol limits and finally that the probability of microbial survival in the replicate processes completed is not greater than the prescribed limits.

(4) Monitor the validated process during routine operation. Periodically as needed, requalify and recertify the equipment.

(5) Complete the protocols, and document steps (1) through (4) above.

The principles and implementation of a program to validate an aseptic processing procedure are similar to the validation of a sterilization process. In aseptic processing, the components of the final dosage form are sterilized separately and the finished article is assembled in an aseptic manner.

Proper validation of the sterilization process or the aseptic process requires a high level of knowledge of the field of sterilization and clean room technology. In order to comply with currently acceptable and achievable limits in sterilization parameters, it is necessary to employ appropriate instrumentation and equipment to control the critical parameters such as temperature and time, humidity, and sterilizing gas concentration, or absorbed radiation. An important aspect of the validation program in many sterilization procedures involves the employment of biological indicators (see *Biological Indicators* ⟨1035⟩). The validated and certified process should be revalidated periodically; however, the revalidation program need not necessarily be as extensive as the original program.

A typical validation program, as outlined below, is one designed for the steam autoclave, but the principles are applicable to the other sterilization procedures discussed in this informational chapter. The program comprises several stages.

The *installation qualification* stage is intended to establish that controls and other instrumentation are properly designed and calibrated. Documentation should be on file demonstrating the quality of the required utilities such as steam, water, and air. The *operational qualification* stage is intended to confirm that the empty chamber functions within the parameters of temperature at all of the key chamber locations prescribed in the protocol. It is usually appropriate to develop heat profile records, i.e., simultaneous temperatures in the chamber employing multiple temperature-sensing devices. A typical acceptable range of temperature in the empty chamber is $\pm 1°$ when the chamber temperature is not less than 121°. The *confirmatory* stage of the validation program is the actual sterilization of materials or articles. This determination requires the employment of temperature-sensing devices inserted into samples of the articles as well as *either* samples of the articles to which appropriate concentrations of suitable test microorganisms have been added, *or* separate biological indicators in operationally fully loaded autoclave configurations. The effectiveness of heat delivery or penetration into the actual articles and the time of the exposure are the two main factors that determine the lethality of the sterilization process. The *final* stage of the validation program requires the documentation of the supporting data developed in executing the program.

It is generally accepted that terminally sterilized injectable articles or critical devices purporting to be sterile, when processed in the autoclave, attain a 10^{-6} microbial survivor probability, i.e., assurance of less than one chance in one million that viable microorganisms are present in the sterilized article or dosage form. With heat-stable articles, the approach often is to considerably exceed the critical time necessary to achieve the 10^{-6} microbial survivor probability (overkill). However, with an article where extensive heat exposure may have a damaging effect, it may not be feasible to employ this overkill approach. In this latter instance, the development of the sterilization cycle depends heavily on knowledge of the microbial burden of the product based on examination, over a suitable time period, of a substantial number of lots of the presterilized product.

The D value is the time (in minutes) required to reduce the microbial population by 90% or 1 log cycle (i.e., to a surviving fraction of 1/10), at a specific temperature. Therefore, where the D value of a biological indicator preparation of, for example, *Bacillus stearothermophilus* spores is 1.5 minutes under the total process parameters, e.g., at 121°, if it is treated for 12 minutes under the same conditions, it can be stated that the lethality input is 8D. The effect of applying this input to the product would depend on the initial microbial burden. Assuming that its resistance to sterilization is equivalent to that of the biological indicator, if the microbial burden of the product in question is 10^2 microorganisms, a lethality input of 2D yields a microbial burden of 1 (10^0 theoretical) and a further 6D yields a calculated microbial survivor probability of 10^{-6}. (Under the same conditions, a lethality input of 12D may be used in a typical "overkill" approach.) Generally, the survivor probability achieved for the article under the validated sterilization cycle is not completely correlated with what may occur with the biological indicator. For valid use, therefore, it is essential that the resistance of the biological indicator be greater than that of the natural microbial burden of the article sterilized. It is then appropriate to make a worst-case assumption and treat the microbial burden as though its heat resistance were equivalent to that of the biological indicator, although it is not likely that the most resistant of a typical microbial burden isolates will demonstrate a heat resistance of the magnitude shown by this species, frequently employed as a biological indicator for steam sterilization. In the above example, a 12-minute cycle is considered adequate for sterilization if the product had a microbial burden of 10^2 microorganisms. However, if the indicator originally had 10^6 microorganisms content, actually a 10^{-2} probability of survival could be expected; i.e., 1 in 100 biological indicators may yield positive results. This type of situation may be avoided by selection of the appropriate biological indicator. Alternatively, high content indicators may be used on the basis of a predetermined acceptable count reduction.

The D value for the *Bacillus stearothermophilus* preparation determined or verified for these conditions should be reestablished when a specific program of validation is changed. Determination of survival curves (see *Biological Indicators* ⟨1035⟩) or what has been called the fractional cycle approach may be employed to determine the D value of the biological indicator preferred for the specific sterilization procedure. The fractional cycle approach may also be used to evaluate the resistance of the microbial burden. Fractional cycles are studied either for microbial count-reduction or for fraction negative achievement. These numbers may be used to determine the lethality of the process under production conditions. The data can be used in qualified production equipment to establish appropriate sterilization cycles. A suitable biological indicator such as the *Bacillus stearothermophilus* preparation may be employed also during routine sterilization. Any microbial burden method for sterility assurance requires adequate surveillance of the microbial resistance of the article to detect any changes, in addition to periodic surveillance of other attributes.

Methods of Sterilization

In this informational chapter, five methods of terminal sterilization, including removal of microorganisms by filtration, and guidelines for aseptic processing are described. Modern technological developments, however, have led to the use of additional procedures. These include blow-molding (at high temperatures), forms of moist heat other than saturated steam and UV irradiation, as well as on-line continuous filling in aseptic processing. The choice of the appropriate process for a given dosage form or

component requires a high level of knowledge of sterilization techniques and information concerning any effects of the process on the material being sterilized.[1]

STEAM STERILIZATION

The process of thermal sterilization employing saturated steam under pressure is carried out in a chamber called an autoclave. It is probably the most widely employed sterilization process.[2] The basic principle of operation is that the air in the sterilizing chamber is displaced by the saturated steam, achieved by employing vents or traps. In order to displace air more effectively from the chamber and from within articles, the sterilization cycle may include air and steam evacuation stages. The design or choice of a cycle for given products or components depends on a number of factors, including the heat lability of the material, knowledge of heat penetration into the articles, and other factors described under the validation program (see above). Apart from that description of sterilization cycle parameters, using a temperature of 121°, the F_0 concept may be appropriate. The F_0, at a particular temperature other than 121°, is the time (in minutes) required to provide the lethality equivalent to that provided at 121° for a stated time. Modern autoclaves generally operate with a control system that is significantly more responsive than the steam reduction valve of older units that have been in service for many years. In order for these older units to achieve the precision and level of control of the cycle discussed in this chapter, it may be necessary to upgrade or modify the control equipment and instrumentation on these units. This modification is warranted only if the chamber and steam jacket are intact for continued safe use and if deposits that interfere with heat distribution can be removed.

DRY-HEAT STERILIZATION

The process of thermal sterilization of Pharmacopeial articles by dry heat is usually carried out by a batch process in an oven designed expressly for that purpose. A modern oven is supplied with heated, filtered air, distributed uniformly throughout the chamber by convection or radiation and employing a blower system with devices for sensing, monitoring, and controlling the critical parameters. The validation of a dry-heat sterilization facility is carried out in a manner similar to that for a steam sterilizer described earlier. Where the unit is employed for sterilizing components such as containers intended for intravenous solutions, care should be taken to avoid accumulation of

particulate matter in the chamber. A typical acceptable range in temperature in the empty chamber is ±15° when the unit is operating at not less than 250°.

In addition to the batch process described above, a continuous process is frequently employed to sterilize and depyrogenate glassware as part of an integrated continuous aseptic filling and sealing system. Heat distribution may be by convection or by direct transfer of heat from an open flame. The continuous system usually requires a much higher temperature than cited above for the batch process because of a much shorter dwell time. However, the total temperature input during the passage of the product should be equivalent to that achieved during the chamber process. The continuous process also usually necessitates a rapid cooling stage prior to the aseptic filling operation. In the qualification and validation program, in view of the short dwell time, parameters for uniformity of the temperature, and particularly the dwell time, should be established.

A microbial survival probability of 10^{-12} is considered achievable for heat-stable articles or components. An example of a biological indicator for validating and monitoring dry-heat sterilization is a preparation of *Bacillus subtilis* spores. Since dry heat is frequently employed to render glassware or containers free from pyrogens as well as viable microbes, a pyrogen challenge, where necessary, should be an integral part of the validation program, e.g., by inoculating one or more of the articles to be treated with 1000 or more USP Units of bacterial endotoxin. The test with *Limulus* lysate could be used to demonstrate that the endotoxic substance has been inactivated to not more than 1/1000 of the original amount (3 log cycle reduction). For the test to be valid, both the original amount and, after acceptable inactivation, the remaining amount of endotoxin should be measured. For additional information on the endotoxin assay, see *Bacterial Endotoxins Test* ⟨85⟩.

GAS STERILIZATION

The choice of gas sterilization as an alternative to heat is frequently made when the material to be sterilized cannot withstand the high temperatures obtained in the steam sterilization or dry-heat sterilization processes. The active agent generally employed in gaseous sterilization is ethylene oxide of acceptable sterilizing quality. Among the disadvantages of this sterilizing agent are its highly flammable nature unless mixed with suitable inert gases, its mutagenic properties, and the possibility of toxic residues in treated materials, particularly those containing chloride ions. The sterilization process is generally carried out in a pressurized chamber designed similarly to a steam autoclave but with the additional features (see below) unique to sterilizers employing this gas. Facilities employing this sterilizing agent should be designed to provide adequate post-sterilization degassing, to enable microbial survivor monitoring, and to minimize exposure of operators to the potentially harmful gas.[3]

Qualification of a sterilizing process employing ethylene oxide gas is accomplished along the lines discussed earlier. However, the program is more comprehensive than for the other sterilization procedures, since in addition to temperature, the humidity, vacuum/positive pressure, and ethylene oxide concentration also require rigid control. An important determination is to demonstrate that all critical process parameters in the chamber are adequate during the entire cycle. Since the sterilization parameters applied to the articles to be sterilized are critical variables, it is frequently advisable to precondition the load to achieve the required moisture content, to minimize the time of holding at the required temperature, prior to placement of the load

---

[1] A number of guidelines dealing particularly with the development and validation of sterilization cycles and related topics have been published. These include, of the Parenteral Drug Association, Inc. (PDA) *Validation of Steam Sterilization Cycles* (Technical Monograph No. 1), *Validation of Aseptic Filling for Solution Drug Products* (Technical Monograph No. 2) and *Validation of Dry Heat Processes Used for Sterilization and Depyrogenation* (Technical Monograph No. 3), and of the Pharmaceutical Manufacturers Association (PMA) *Validation of Sterilization of Large-Volume Parenterals—Current Concepts* (Science and Technology Publication No. 25). Other series of technical publications on these subjects of the Health Industry Manufacturers Association (HIMA) include *Validation of Sterilization Systems* (Report No. 78-4.1), *Sterilization Cycle Development* (Report No. 78-4.2), *Industrial Sterility: Medical Device Standards and Guidelines* (Document #9, Vol. 1) and *Operator Training ....* for *Ethylene Oxide Sterilization*, for *Steam Sterilization Equipment*, for *Dry Heat Sterilization Equipment* and for *Radiation Sterilization Equipment* Report Nos. 78-4.5 through 4.8). Recommended practice guidelines published by the Association for the Advancement of Medical Instrumentation (AAMI) include *Guideline for Industrial Ethylene Oxide Sterilization of Medical Devices—Process Design, Validation, Routine Sterilization* (No. OPEO-12/81) and *Process Control Guidelines for the Radiation Sterilization of Medical Devices* (No. RS-P 10/82). These detailed publications should be consulted for more extensive treatment of the principles and procedures described in this chapter.

[2] An autoclave cycle, where specified in the compendia for media or reagents, is a period of 15 minutes at 121°, unless otherwise indicated.

[3] See *Ethylene Oxide*, Encyclopedia of Industrial Chemical Analysis, 1971, *12*, 317-340, John Wiley & Sons, Inc., and *Use of Ethylene Oxide as a Sterilant in Medical Facilities*, NIOSH Special Occupational Hazard Review with Control Recommendations, August 1977, U. S. Department of Health and Human Services, Public Health Service, Centers for Disease Control and Prevention, National Institute for Occupational Safety and Health, Division of Criteria Documentation and Standards Development, Priorities and Research Analysis Branch, Rockville, MD.

in the ethylene oxide chamber. The validation process is generally made employing product inoculated with appropriate biological indicators such as spore preparations of *Bacillus subtilis*. For validation they may be used in full chamber loads of product, or simulated product. The monitoring of moisture and gas concentration requires the utilization of sophisticated instrumentation that only knowledgeable and experienced individuals can calibrate, operate, and maintain. The biological indicators may be employed also in monitoring routine runs.

As is indicated elsewhere in this chapter, the biological indicator may be employed in a fraction negative mode to establish the ultimate microbiological survivor probability in designing an ethylene oxide sterilization cycle using inoculated product or inoculated simulated product.

One of the principal limitations of the ethylene oxide sterilization process is the limited ability of the gas to diffuse to the innermost product areas that require sterilization. Package design and chamber loading patterns therefore must be determined so that there is minimal resistance to gas diffusion.

STERILIZATION BY IONIZING RADIATION

The rapid proliferation of medical devices unable to withstand heat sterilization and the concerns about the safety of ethylene oxide have resulted in increasing applications of radiation sterilization. It is, however, applicable also to drug substances and final dosage forms. The advantages of sterilization by irradiation include low chemical reactivity, low measurable residues, and the fact that there are fewer variables to control. In fact, radiation sterilization is unique in that the basis of control is essentially that of the absorbed radiation dose, which can be precisely measured. Because of this characteristic, new procedures have been developed to determine the sterilizing dose. These, however, are still under review and appraisal, particularly with regard to the need, or otherwise, for additional controls and safety measures. Irradiation causes only a minimal temperature rise, but can affect certain grades and types of plastics and glass.

The two types of ionizing radiation in use are radioisotope decay (gamma radiation) and electron-beam radiation. In either case the radiation dose to yield the required degree of sterility assurance should be established such that within the range of minimum and maximum doses set, the properties of the article being sterilized are acceptable.

For gamma irradiation, the validation of a procedure includes the establishment of article materials compatibility, establishment of product loading pattern and completion of dose mapping in the sterilization container (including identification of the minimum and maximum dose zones), establishment of timer setting, and demonstration of the delivery of the required sterilization dose. For electron-beam irradiation, in addition, the on-line control of voltage, current, conveyor speed, and electron beam scan dimension must be validated.

For gamma radiation sterilization, an effective sterilizing dose which is tolerated without damaging effect should be selected. Although 2.5 megarads (Mrad) of absorbed radiation was historically selected, it is desirable and acceptable in some cases to employ lower doses for devices, drug substances, and finished dosage forms. In other cases, however, higher doses are essential. In order to validate the efficacy particularly of the lower exposure levels, it is necessary to determine the magnitude (number and/or degree) of the natural radiation resistance of the microbial population of the product. Specific product loading patterns must be established and absorbed minimum and maximum dosage distribution must be determined by use of chemical dosimeters. (These dosimeters are usually dyed plastic cylinders, slides, or squares that show color intensification based directly on the amount of absorbed radiation energy; they require careful calibration.)

The setting of the preferred absorbed dose has been carried out on the basis of pure cultures of resistant microorganisms and employing inoculated product, e.g., with spores of *Bacillus pumilus* as biological indicators. A fractional experimental cycle approach provides the data to be utilized to determine the D_{10} value of the biological indicator. This information is then applied in extrapolating the amount of absorbed radiation to establish an appropriate microbial survivor probability. The most recent procedures for gamma radiation sterilization base the dose upon the radiation resistance of the natural heterogeneous microbial burden contained on the product to be sterilized. Such procedures are currently being refined but may provide a more representative assessment of radiation resistance, especially where significant numbers of radiation-resistant organisms are present.[4] These range from inoculation with standard resistant organisms such as *Bacillus pumilus* to subprocess (sublethal) dose exposure of finished product samples taken from production lines. Certain hypotheses are common to all of these methods. While the total microbial population present on an article generally consists of a mixture of microorganisms of differing sensitivity to radiation, the step of subjecting the article to a less than totally lethal sterilization dose eliminates the less resistant microbial fraction. This results in a residual relatively homogeneous population with respect to radiation resistance, and yields consistent and reproducible results of determinations with the residual population. The amount of laboratory manipulation required is dependent upon the particular procedure used.

One such procedure requires the enumeration of the microbial population on representative samples of independently manufactured lots of the article. The resistance of the microbial population is not determined and dose setting is based on a standard arbitrary radiation resistance assigned to the microbial population, derived from data obtained from manufacturers and from the literature. The assumption is made that the distribution of resistances chosen represents a more severe challenge than the natural microbial population on the product to be sterilized. This assumption, however, is verified by experiment. After verification, the appropriate radiation sterilization dose is read from a table.

Another, more elaborate, method does not require the enumeration of the microbial population but uses a series of incremental dose exposures to allow a dose to be established such that approximately one out of 100 samples irradiated at that dose will be nonsterile. This is not the ultimate sterilization dose, but provides the basis to determine the sterilization dose by extrapolation from the dose yielding one out of 100 nonsterile samples, using an appropriate resistance factor which characterizes the remaining microorganism-resistant population. A periodic audit is conducted to check that the findings continue to be operative.

More elaborate procedures, requiring more experimentation and including the isolation of microbial cultures, include one where, after determining the substerilization dose (yielding one out of 100 nonsterile samples), the resistance of the surviving microorganisms is used to determine the sterilizing dose. Another is based on different determinations, starting with a substerilization incremental dose which results in not more than 50% of the samples being nonsterile. After irradiation of sufficient samples at this dose, a number of microbial isolates are obtained. The radiation resistance of each of these is determined. The sterilization dose is then calculated using the resistance determinations and the 50% sterilizing dose initially determined. Audit procedures are required for these methods as for the others described.

Where the required minimum radiation dose has been determined and delivery of that dose has been confirmed (by chemical or physical dosimeters), release of the article being sterilized could be effected within the overall validation of sterility assurance (which may include such confirmation of applied dosage, the use of biological indicators, and other means).

---

[4] Detailed descriptions of these procedures have been published by the Association for the Advancement of Medical Instrumentation (AAMI) in the document entitled "*Process Control Guidelines for Radiation Sterilization of Medical Devices*" (No. AAMI RS-P 10/82).

STERILIZATION BY FILTRATION

Filtration through microbial retentive materials is frequently employed for the sterilization of heat-labile solutions by physical removal of the contained microorganisms. A filter assembly generally consists of a porous matrix sealed or clamped into an impermeable housing. The effectiveness of a filter medium or substrate depends upon the pore size of the porous material and may depend upon adsorption of bacteria on or in the filter matrix or upon a sieving mechanism. There is some evidence to indicate that sieving is the more important component of the mechanism. Fiber-shedding filters, particularly those containing asbestos, are to be avoided unless no alternative filtration procedures are possible. Where a fiber-shedding filter is required, it is obligatory that the process include a nonfiber-shedding filter introduced downstream or subsequent to the initial filtration step.

Filter rating—Rating the pore size of filter membranes is by a nominal rating that reflects the capability of the filter membrane to retain microorganisms of size represented by specified strains, not by determination of an average pore size and statement of distribution of sizes. Sterilizing filter membranes (those which are used for removing a majority of contaminating microorganisms) are membranes capable of retaining 100% of a culture of 10^7 microorganisms of a strain of *Pseudomonas diminuta* (ATCC 19146) per square centimeter of membrane surface under a pressure of not less than 30 psi (2.0 bar). Such filter membranes are nominally rated 0.22 μm or 0.2 μm, depending on the manufacturer's practice.[5] This rating of filter membranes is also specified for reagents or media that have to be sterilized by filtration (see treatment of Isopropyl Myristate under *Oils and Oily Solutions* or *Ointments and Creams* in the chapter *Sterility Tests* ⟨71⟩). Bacterial filter membranes (also known as analytical filter membranes), which are capable of retaining only larger microorganisms, are labeled with a nominal rating of 0.45 μm. No single authoritative method for rating 0.45-μm filters has been specified, and this rating depends on conventional practice among manufacturers; 0.45-μm filters are capable of retaining particular cultures of *Serratia marcescens* (ATCC 14756) or *Ps. diminuta*. Test pressures used vary from low (5 psi, 0.33 bar for *Serratia*, or 0.5 psi, 0.34 bar for *Ps. diminuta*) to high (50 psi, 3.4 bar). They are specified for sterility testing (see *Membrane Filtration* in the section *Test For Sterility of the Product to be Examined* under *Sterility Tests* ⟨71⟩), where less exhaustive microbial retention is required. There is a small probability of testing specimens contaminated solely with small microorganisms). Filter membranes with a very low nominal rating may be tested with a culture of *Acholeplasma laidlawii* or other strain of *Mycoplasma*, at a pressure of 7 psi (0.7 bar) and be nominally rated 0.1 μm. The nominal ratings based on microbial retention properties differ when rating is done by other means, e.g., by retention of latex spheres of various diameters. It is the user's responsibility to select a filter of correct rating for the particular purpose, depending on the nature of the product to be filtered. It is generally not feasible to repeat the tests of filtration capacity in the user's establishment. Microbial challenge tests are preferably performed under a manufacturer's conditions on each lot of manufactured filter membranes.

The user must determine whether filtration parameters employed in manufacturing will significantly influence microbial retention efficiency. Some of the other important concerns in the validation of the filtration process include product compatibility, sorption of drug, preservative and/or other additives, and initial effluent endotoxin content.

Since the effectiveness of the filtration process is also influenced by the microbial burden of the solution to be filtered, the determination of the microbiological quality of solutions prior to filtration is an important aspect of the validation of the filtration process in addition to establishment of the other parameters of the filtration procedure, such as pressures, flow rates, and filter unit characteristics. Hence, another method of describing filter-

retaining capability is by the log reduction value (LRV). For instance, a 0.2-μm filter that can retain 10^7 microorganisms of a specified strain will have an LRV of not less than 7, under the stated conditions.

The process of sterilization of solutions by filtration has recently achieved new levels of proficiency, largely as a result of the development and proliferation of membrane filter technology. This class of filter media lends itself to more effective standardization and quality control and also gives the user greater opportunity to confirm the characteristics or properties of the filter assembly before and after use. The fact that membrane filters are thin polymeric films offers many advantages but also some disadvantages when compared to depth filters such as porcelain or sintered material. Since much of the membrane surface is a void or open space, the properly assembled and sterilized filter offers the advantage of a high flow rate. A disadvantage is that since the membrane is usually fragile, it is essential to determine that the assembly was properly made and that the membrane was not ruptured during assembly, sterilization, or use. The housings and filter assemblies that are chosen to be used should first be validated for compatibility and integrity by the user. While it may be possible to mix assemblies and filter membranes produced by different manufacturers, the compatibility of these hybrid assemblies should first be validated. Additionally, there are other tests to be made by the manufacturer of the membrane filter, which are not usually repeated by the user. These include microbiological challenge tests. Results of these tests on each lot of manufactured filter membranes should be obtained from the manufacturer by the user for his records.

Filtration for sterilization purposes is usually carried out with assemblies having membranes of nominal pore size rating of 0.2 μm or less, based on the validated challenge of not less than 10^7 *Pseudomonas diminuta* (ATCC No. 19146) suspension per square centimeter of filter surface area. Membrane filter media which are now available include cellulose acetate, cellulose nitrate, fluorocarbonate, acrylic polymers, polycarbonate, polyester, polyvinyl chloride, vinyl, nylon, polytef, and even metal membranes, and they may be reinforced or supported by an internal fabric. A membrane filter assembly should be tested for initial integrity prior to use, provided that such test does not impair the validity of the system, and should be tested after the filtration process is completed to demonstrate that the filter assembly maintained its integrity throughout the entire filtration procedure. Typical use tests are the bubble point test, the diffusive airflow test, the pressure hold test, and the forward flow test. These tests should be correlated with microorganism retention.

ASEPTIC PROCESSING

While there is general agreement that sterilization of the final filled container as a dosage form or final packaged device is the preferred process for assuring the minimal risk of microbial contamination in a lot, there is a substantial class of products that are not terminally sterilized but are prepared by a series of aseptic steps. These are designed to prevent the introduction of viable microorganisms into components, where sterile, or once an intermediate process has rendered the bulk product or its components free from viable microorganisms. This section provides a review of the principles involved in producing aseptically processed products with a minimal risk of microbial contamination in the finished lot of final dosage forms.

A product defined as aseptically processed is likely to consist of components that have been sterilized by one of the processes described earlier in this chapter. For example, the bulk product, if a filterable liquid, may have been sterilized by filtration. The final empty container components would probably be sterilized by heat, dry heat being employed for glass vials and an autoclave being employed for rubber closures. The areas of critical concern are the immediate microbial environment where these presterilized components are exposed during assembly to produce the finished dosage form and the aseptic filling operation.

---

[5] Consult "Microbiological Evaluation of Filters for Sterilizing Liquids," Health Industry Manufacturers Association, Document No. 3, Vol. 4, 1982.

The requirements for a properly designed, validated and maintained filling or other aseptic processing facility are mainly directed to (i) an air environment free from viable microorganisms, of a proper design to permit effective maintenance of air supply units and (ii) the provision of trained operating personnel who are adequately equipped and gowned. The desired environment may be achieved through the high level of air filtration technology now available, which contributes to the delivery of air of the requisite microbiological quality.[6] The facilities include both primary (in the vicinity of the exposed article) and secondary (where the aseptic processing is carried out) barrier systems.

For a properly designed aseptic processing facility or aseptic filling area, consideration should be given to such features as nonporous and smooth surfaces, including walls and ceilings that can be sanitized frequently; gowning rooms with adequate space for personnel and storage of sterile garments; adequate separation of preparatory rooms for personnel from final aseptic processing rooms, with the availability where necessary of such devices as airlocks and/or air showers; proper pressure differentials between rooms, the most positive pressure being in the aseptic processing rooms or areas; the employment of laminar (unidirectional) airflow in the immediate vicinity of exposed product or components, and filtered air exposure thereto, with adequate air change frequency; appropriate humidity and temperature environmental controls; and a documented sanitization program. Proper training of personnel in hygienic and gowning techniques should be undertaken so that, for example, gowns, gloves, and other body coverings substantially cover exposed skin surfaces.

Certification and validation of the aseptic process and facility are achieved by establishing the efficiency of the filtration systems, by employing microbiological environmental monitoring procedures, and by processing of sterile culture medium as simulated product.

Monitoring of the aseptic facility should include periodic environmental filter examination as well as routine particulate and microbiological environmental monitoring, and may include periodic sterile culture medium processing.

Sterility Testing of Lots

It should be recognized that the referee sterility test might not detect microbial contamination if present in only a small percentage of the finished articles in the lot because the specified number of units to be taken imposes a significant statistical limitation on the utility of the test results. This inherent limitation, however, has to be accepted since current knowledge offers no nondestructive alternatives for ascertaining the microbiological quality of every finished article in the lot, and it is not a feasible option to increase the number of specimens significantly.

The primary means of supporting the claim that a lot of finished articles purporting to be sterile meets the specifications consist of the documentation of the actual production and sterilization record of the lot and of the additional validation records that the sterilization process possesses the capability of totally inactivating the established product microbial burden or a more resistant challenge. Further, it should be demonstrated that any processing steps involving exposed product following the sterilization procedure are performed in an aseptic manner, to prevent contamination. If data derived from the manufacturing process sterility assurance validation studies and from in-process controls are judged to provide greater assurance that the lot meets the required low probability of containing a contaminated unit (compared to sterility testing results from finished units drawn from that lot), any sterility test procedures adopted may be minimal, or dispensed with on a routine basis. However,

assuming that all of the above production criteria have been met, it may still be desirable to perform sterility testing on samples of the lot of finished articles. Such sterility testing is usually carried out directly after the lot is manufactured as a final product quality control test.[7] Sterility tests employed in this way in manufacturing control should not be confused with those described under *Sterility Tests* ⟨71⟩. The procedural details may be the same with regard to media, inocula and handling of specimens, but the number of units and/or incubation time(s) selected for testing may differ. The number should be chosen relative to the purpose to be served, i.e., according to whether greater or lesser reliance is placed on sterility testing in the context of all the measures for sterility assurance in manufacture. Also, longer times of incubation would make the test more sensitive to slow-growing microorganisms. In the growth promotion tests for media, such slow growers, particularly if isolated from the product microbial burden, should be included with the other test stains. Negative or satisfactory sterility test results serve only as further support of the existing evidence concerning the quality of the lot if all of the pertinent production records of the lot are in order and the sterilizing or aseptic process is known to be effective. Unsatisfactory test results, however, in manufacturing quality control indicate a need for further action (see *Performance, Observation, and Interpretation*).

DEFINITION OF A LOT AND SELECTION OF SPECIMENS FOR STERILITY TEST PURPOSES

Articles may be terminally sterilized either in a chamber or by a continuous process. In the chamber process, a number of articles are sterilized simultaneously under controlled conditions, for example, in a steam autoclave, so that for the purpose of sterility testing, the lot is considered to be the contents of a single chamber. In the continuous process, the articles are sterilized individually and consecutively, for example, by exposure to electron-beam radiation, so that the lot is considered to be not larger than the total number of similar items subjected to uniform sterilization for a period of not more than 24 hours.

For aseptic fills, the term "filling operation" describes a group of final containers, identical in all respects, that have been aseptically filled with the same product from the same bulk within a period of time not longer than 24 consecutive hours without an interruption or change that would affect the integrity of the filling assembly. The items tested should be representative of each filling assembly and should be selected at appropriate intervals throughout the entire filling operation. If more than three filling machines, each with either single or multiple filling stations, are used for filling a single lot, a minimum of 20 filled containers (not less than 10 per medium) should be tested for each filling machine, but the total number generally need not exceed 100 containers.

For small lots, in the case of either aseptic filling or terminal sterilization, if the number of final containers in the lot is between 20 and 200, about 10% of the containers should usually be tested. If the number of final containers in the lot is 20 or less, not fewer than 2 final containers should be tested.

Performance, Observation, and Interpretation

The facility for sterility testing should be such as to offer no greater a microbial challenge to the articles being tested than that of an aseptic processing production facility. The sterility testing

---

[6] Available published standards for such controlled work areas include the following: (1) Federal Standard No. 209B, Clean Room and Work Station Requirements for a Controlled Environment, Apr. 24, 1973. (2) NASA Standard for Clean Room and Work Stations for Microbially Controlled Environment, publication NHB5340.2, Aug. 1967. (3) Contamination Control of Aerospace Facilities, U. S. Air Force, T.O. 00-25-203 1 Dec. 1972, change 1-1 Oct. 1974.

[7] *Radioactive Pharmaceutical Products*—Because of rapid radioactive decay, it is not feasible to delay the release of some radioactive pharmaceutical products in order to complete sterility tests on them. In such cases, results of sterility tests provide only retrospective confirmatory evidence for sterility assurance, which therefore depends on the primary means thereto established in the manufacturing and validation/certification procedures.

procedure should be performed by individuals having a high level of aseptic technique proficiency. The test performance records of these individuals should be documented.

The extensive aseptic manipulations required to perform sterility testing may result in a probability of nonproduct-related contamination of the order of 10^{-3}, a level similar to the overall efficiency of an aseptic operation and comparable to the microbial survivor probability of aseptically processed articles. This level of probability is significantly greater than that usually attributed to a terminal sterilization process, namely, one in one million or 10^{-6} microbial survivor probability. Appropriate, known-to-be-sterile, finished articles should be employed periodically as negative controls as a check on the reliability of the test procedure. Preferably, the technicians performing the test should be unaware that they are testing negative controls. Of these tests, a false positive frequency not exceeding 2% is desirable.

For aseptically processed articles, these facts support the routine use of the test set forth under *Sterility Tests* ⟨71⟩ or a more elaborate one. The production and validation documentation should be acceptable and complete. For effectively terminally sterilized products, however, the lower microbial survivor probability may direct the use of a less extensive test than the compendial procedure specified under *Sterility Tests* ⟨71⟩, or even preclude the necessity altogether for performing one. This added reliability of sterility assurance of terminal sterilization depends upon a properly validated and documented sterilization process. Sterility testing alone is no substitute.

Interpretation of Quality Control Tests—The overall responsibility for the operation of the test unit and the interpretation of test results in relation to acceptance or rejection of a lot should be in the hands of those who have appropriate formal training in microbiology and have knowledge of industrial sterilization, aseptic processing, and the statistical concepts involved in sampling. These individuals should be knowledgeable also concerning the environmental control program in the test facility to assure that the microbiological quality of the air and critical work surfaces are consistently acceptable.

Quality control sterility tests (either according to the official referee test or modified tests) may be carried out in two separate stages in order to rule out false positive results. *First Stage.* Regardless of the sampling plan used, if no evidence of microbial growth is found, the results of the test may be taken as indicative of absence of intrinsic contamination of the lot.

If microbial growth is found, proceed to the *Second Stage* (unless the *First Stage* test can be invalidated). Evidence for invalidating a *First Stage* test in order to repeat it as a *First Stage* test may be obtained from a review of the testing environment and the relevant records thereto. Finding of microbial growth in negative controls need not be considered the sole grounds for invalidating a *First Stage* test. When proceeding to the *Second Stage*, particularly where depending on the results of the test for lot release, concurrently, initiate and document a complete review of all applicable production and control records. In this review, consideration should be paid to the following: (1) a check on monitoring records of the validated sterilization cycle applicable to the product; (2) sterility test history relating to the particular product for both finished and in-process samples, as well as sterilization records of supporting equipment, containers/closures, and sterile components, if any; and (3) environmental control data, including those obtained from media fills, exposure plates, filtering records, any sanitization records and microbial monitoring records of operators, gowns, gloves, and garbing practices.

Failing any lead from the above review, the current microbial profile of the product should be checked against the known historical profile for possible change. Records should be checked concomitantly for any changes in source of product components and/or in-processing procedures that might be contributory. Depending on the findings, and in extreme cases, consideration may have to be given to revalidation of the total manufacturing process. For the *Second Stage*, it is not possible to specify a particular number of specimens to be taken for testing. It is usual to select double the number specified for the *First Stage* under *Sterility Tests* ⟨71⟩, or other reasonable number. The minimum volumes tested from each specimen, the media, and the incubation periods are the same as those indicated for the *First Stage*.

If no microbial growth is found in the *Second Stage*, and the documented review of appropriate records and the indicated product investigation does not support the possibility of intrinsic contamination, the lot may meet the requirements of a test for sterility. If growth is found, the lot fails to meet the requirements of the test. As was indicated for the *First Stage* test, the *Second Stage* test may similarly be invalidated with appropriate evidence, and, if so done, repeated as a *Second Stage* test.

⟨1231⟩ WATER FOR PHARMACEUTICAL PURPOSES

Water is the most widely used substance, raw material, or ingredient in the production, processing, and formulation of compendial articles. Control of the microbiological quality of these waters is important because proliferation of microorganisms ubiquitous to water may occur during the purification, storage, and distribution of this substance. If water is used in the final product, these microorganisms or their metabolic products may eventually cause adverse consequences.

Water that is used in the early stages of the production of drug substances and that is the source or feed water for the preparation of the various types of purified waters must meet the requirements of the National Primary Drinking Water Regulations (NPDWR) (40 CFR 141) issued by the Environmental Protection Agency (EPA). Comparable regulations for drinking water of the European Union or Japan are acceptable. These requirements ensure the absence of coliforms, which, if determined to be of fecal origin, may portend or indicate the presence of other microorganisms of fecal origin, including viruses that may be pathogenic for humans. On the other hand, meeting these National Drinking Water Regulations would not rule out the presence of other microorganisms, which, while not considered a major public health concern, could, if present, constitute a hazard or be considered undesirable in a drug substance or formulated product. For this reason, there are many different grades of pharmaceutical waters.

TYPES OF WATER

Drinking Water—Drinking Water is not covered by a compendial monograph but must comply with the quality attributes of the EPA NPDWR or comparable regulations of the European Union or Japan. It may be derived from a variety of sources including a public water utility, a private water supply (e.g., a well), or a combination of more than one of these sources. Drinking Water may be used in the early stages of chemical synthesis and in the early stages of the cleaning of pharmaceutical manufacturing equipment. It is the prescribed source feed water for the production of pharmaceutical waters. As seasonal variations in the quality attributes of the drinking water supply can occur, processing steps in the production of pharmaceutical waters must be designed for this characteristic.

Purified Water—Purified Water (see *USP* monograph) is used as an excipient in the production of official preparations; in pharmaceutical applications, such as cleaning of certain equipment; and in the preparation of some bulk pharmaceutical chemicals. Purified Water must meet the requirements for ionic and organic chemical purity and must be protected from microbial proliferation. It is prepared using Drinking Water as a feed water and is purified using unit operations that include deionization, distillation, ion-exchange, reverse osmosis, filtration, or other suitable procedures. Purified Water systems must be validated.

Purified Water systems that produce, store, and circulate water under ambient conditions are susceptible to the establishment of tenacious biofilms of microorganisms, which can be the source of

undesirable levels of viable microorganisms or endotoxins in the effluent water. These systems require frequent sanitization and microbiological monitoring to ensure water of appropriate microbiological quality at the points of use.

Sterile Purified Water—Sterile Purified Water is *Purified Water* that is packaged and rendered sterile. It is used in the preparation of nonparenteral compendial dosage forms where a sterile form of *Purified Water* is required.

Water for Injection—Water for Injection (see *USP* monograph) is an excipient in the production of injections and for use in pharmaceutical applications, such as cleaning of certain equipment, and in the preparation of some bulk pharmaceutical chemicals. The source or feed water for this article is Drinking Water, which may have been preliminarily purified but which is finally subjected to distillation or reverse osmosis. It must meet all of the chemical requirements for *Purified Water* and in addition the requirements under *Bacterial Endotoxins Test* ⟨85⟩. It also must be protected from microbial contamination. The system used to produce, store, and distribute Water for Injection must be designed to prevent microbial contamination and the formation of microbial endotoxins, and it must be validated.

Sterile Water for Injection—Sterile Water for Injection (see *USP* monograph) is *Water for Injection* that is packaged and rendered sterile. Sterile Water for Injection is intended for extemporaneous prescription compounding and is distributed in sterile units. It is used as a diluent for parenteral products. It is packaged in single-dose containers not larger than 1 liter in size.

Bacteriostatic Water for Injection—Bacteriostatic Water for Injection (see *USP* monograph) is sterile *Water for Injection* to which has been added one or more suitable antimicrobial preservatives. It is intended to be used as a diluent in the preparation of parenteral products. It may be packaged in single-dose or multiple-dose containers not larger than 30 mL.

Sterile Water for Irrigation—Sterile Water for Irrigation (see *USP* monograph) is *Water for Injection*, packaged in single-dose containers of larger than 1 liter in size, that is intended to be delivered rapidly and is rendered sterile. It need not meet the requirement for small-volume injections under *Particulate Matter* ⟨788⟩.

Sterile Water for Inhalation—Sterile Water for Inhalation (see *USP* monograph) is *Water for Injection* that is packaged and rendered sterile and is intended for use in inhalators and in the preparation of inhalation solutions.

VALIDATION AND QUALIFICATION OF WATER PURIFICATION, STORAGE, AND DISTRIBUTION SYSTEMS

Establishing the dependability of pharmaceutical water purification, storage, and distribution systems requires an appropriate period of monitoring and observation. Ordinarily, few problems are encountered in maintaining the chemical purity of *Purified Water* and *Water for Injection*. However, it is more difficult to meet established microbiological quality criteria consistently. A typical program involves intensive daily sampling and testing of major process points for at least one month after operational criteria have been established for each sampling point.

Validation is the procedure whereby substantiation to a high level of assurance that a specific process will consistently produce a product conforming to an established set of quality attributes is acquired and documented. The validation defines the critical process parameters and their operating ranges. A validation program qualifies the design, installation, operation, and performance of equipment. It begins when the system is defined and moves through several stages: qualification of the installation (IQ), operational qualification (OQ), and performance qualification (PQ). A graphical representation of a typical water system validation life cycle is shown in Fig. 1. A validation plan for a water system typically includes the following steps:

(1) Establishing standards for quality attributes and operating parameters.

(2) Defining systems and subsystems suitable to produce the desired quality attributes from the available source water.

(3) Selecting equipment, controls, and monitoring technologies.

(4) Developing an IQ stage consisting of instrument calibrations, inspections to verify that the drawings accurately depict the as-built configuration of the water system and, where necessary, special tests to verify that the installation meets the design requirements.

(5) Developing an OQ stage consisting of tests and inspections to verify that the equipment, system alerts, and controls are operating reliably and that appropriate Alert and Action Levels are established. This phase of qualification may overlap with aspects of the next step.

(6) Developing a prospective PQ stage to confirm the appropriateness of critical process parameter operating ranges. A concurrent or retrospective PQ is performed to demonstrate system reproducibility over an appropriate time period. During this phase of validation, Alert and Action Levels for key quality attributes and operating parameters are verified.

(7) Supplementing a validation maintenance program (also called continuous validation life cycle) that includes a mechanism to control changes to the water system and establishes and carries out scheduled preventive maintenance including recalibration of instruments. In addition, validation maintenance includes a monitoring program for critical process parameters and a corrective action program.

(8) Instituting a schedule for periodic review of the system performance and requalification.

(9) Completing protocols and documenting Steps 1–8.

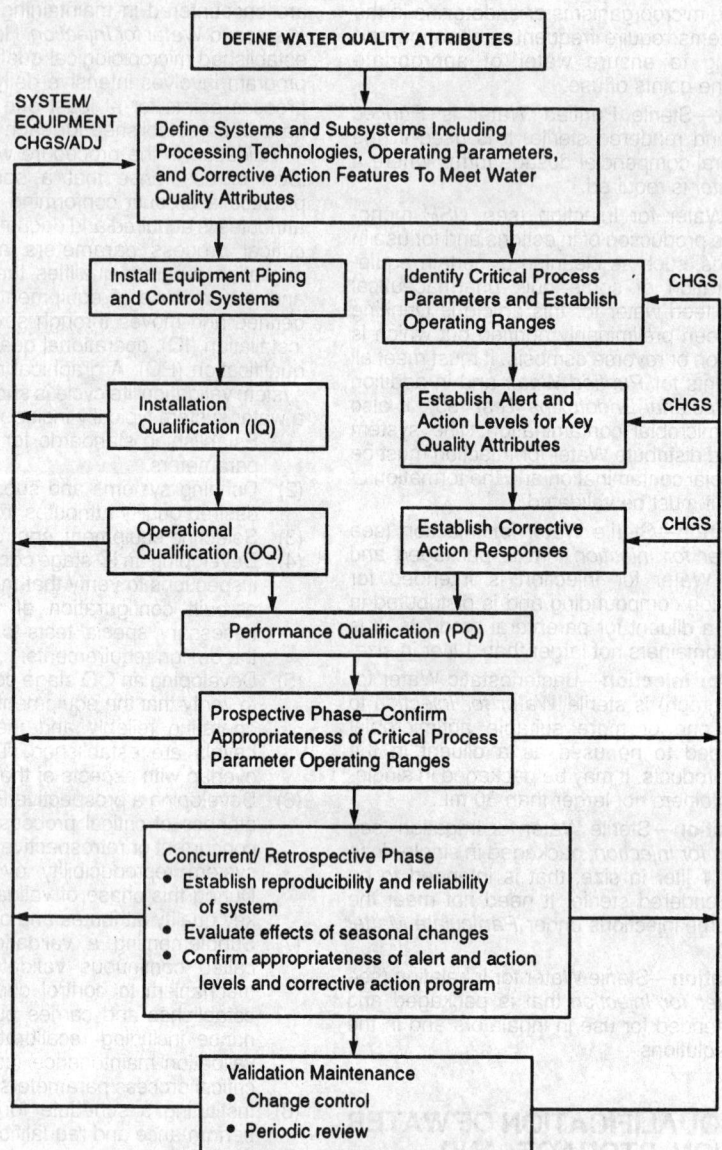

Fig. 1. Water system validation life cycle.

PHARMACEUTICAL WATER SYSTEMS

The quality attributes of water for a particular application are dictated by the requirements of its usage. Sequential processing steps that are used for treating water for different pharmaceutical purposes are shown in Fig. 2. A typical evaluation process to select an appropriate water quality for a particular pharmaceutical purpose is shown in the decision tree in Fig. 3. These diagrams may be used to assist in defining requirements for specific water uses and in the selection of unit operations.

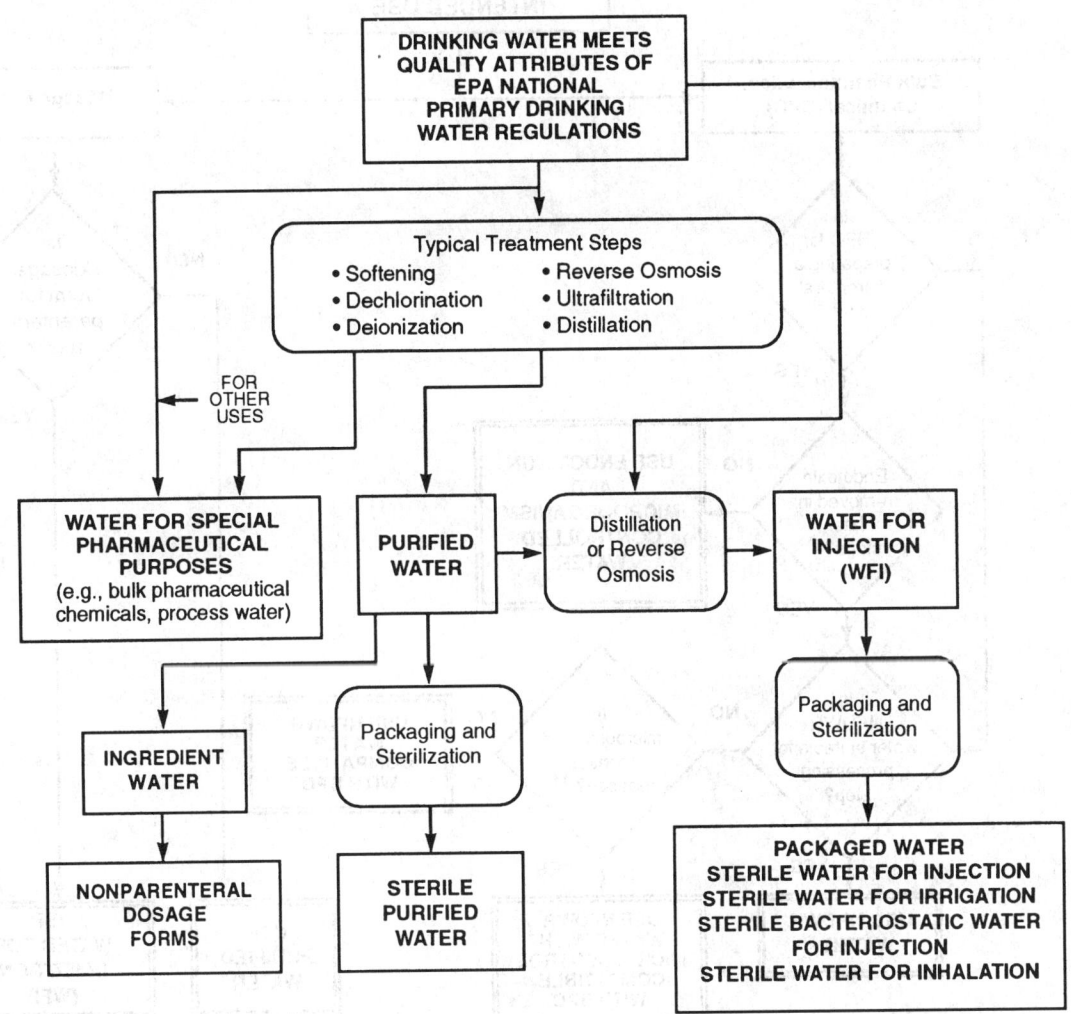

Fig. 2 Water for pharmaceutical purposes.

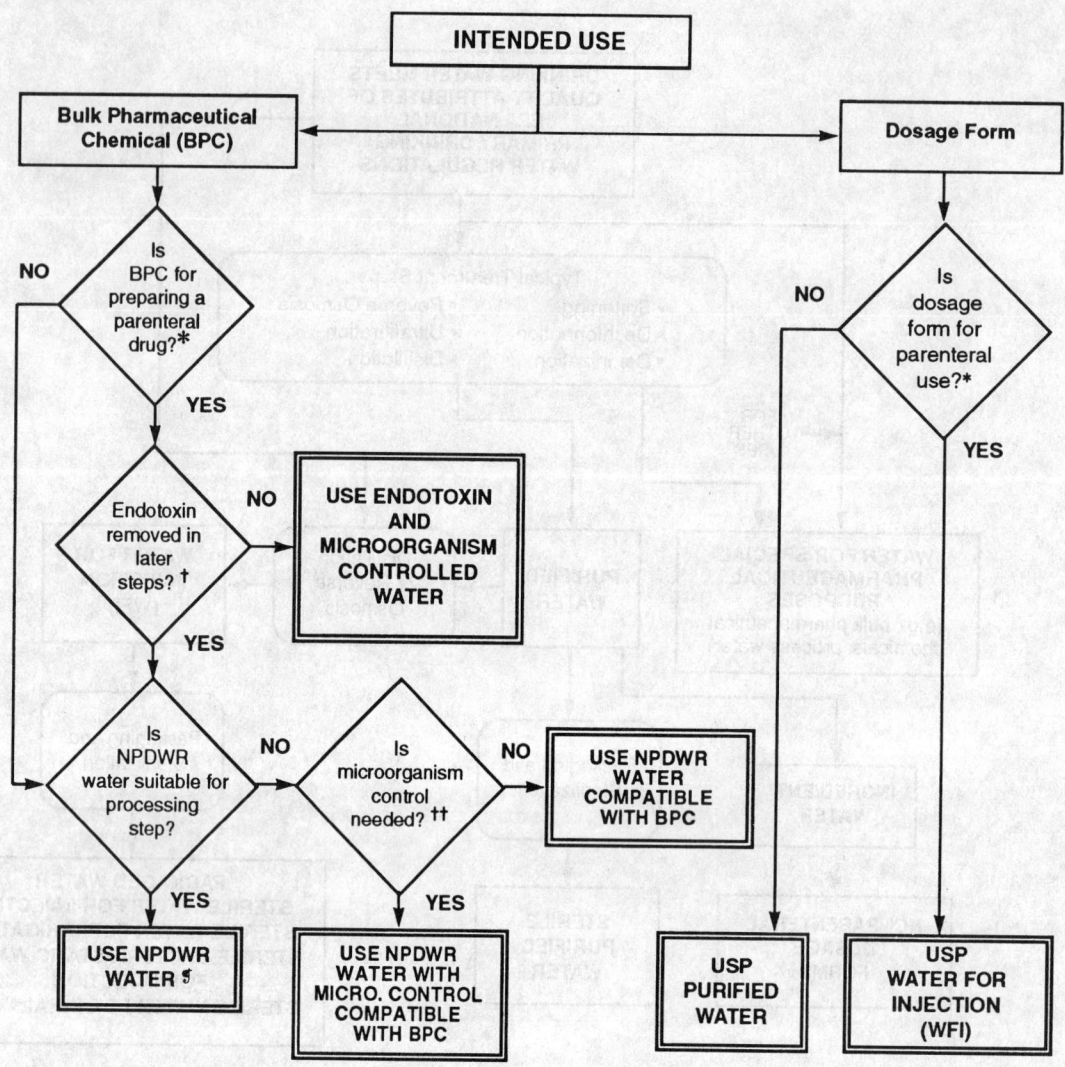

* Water for sterile BPC's or dosage forms must be rendered sterile if there is not a sterilization step following addition.

† Endotoxin removal can occur either in water treatment or in BPC process.

†† Microorganism control can occur either in water treatment or in BPC process.

¶ NPDWR Water—Water meeting EPA national primary drinking water regulations.

Fig. 3. Selection of water for pharmaceutical purposes.

PURIFIED WATER AND WATER FOR INJECTION SYSTEMS

The design, installation, and operation of systems to produce *Purified Water* and *Water for Injection* include similar components, control techniques, and procedures. The quality attributes of both waters differ only in the presence of a bacterial endotoxin requirement for *Water for Injection* and in their methods of preparation, at least at the last stage of preparation. The similarities in the quality attributes provide considerable common ground in the design of water systems to meet either requirement. The critical difference is the degree of control of the system and the final purification steps needed to ensure bacterial and bacterial endotoxin removal.

Production of pharmaceutical water employs sequential unit operations (processing steps) that address specific water quality attributes and protect the operation of subsequent treatment steps. The final unit operations used to produce *Water for Injection* have been limited to distillation and reverse osmosis.

Distillation has a long history of reliable performance and can be validated as a unit operation for the production of *Water for Injection*. Other technologies such as ultrafiltration may be suitable in the production of *Water for Injection*, but at this time experience with this process is not widespread.

The validation plan should be designed to establish the suitability of the system and to provide a thorough understanding of the purification mechanism, range of operating conditions, required pretreatment, and the most likely mode of failure. It is also necessary to demonstrate the effectiveness of the monitoring scheme and to establish the requirements for validation maintenance.

Trials conducted in a pilot installation can be valuable in defining the operating parameters and the expected water quality and in identifying failure modes. However, qualification of the specific unit operation can only be performed as part of the validation of the installed operational system.

The selection of specific unit operations and design characteristics for a water system should take into consideration the quality of the feed water, the technology chosen for subsequent processing steps, the extent and complexity of the water distribution system, and the appropriate compendial requirements. For example, in the design of a system for *Water for Injection*, the final process (distillation or reverse osmosis) must have effective bacterial endotoxin reduction capability and must be validated.

The following is a brief description of selected unit operations and the operation and validation concerns associated with them. This review is not comprehensive in that not all unit operations are discussed, nor are all potential problems addressed. The purpose is to highlight issues that focus on the design, installation, operation, maintenance, and monitoring parameters that facilitate water system validation.

Filtration technology plays an important role in water systems, and filtration units are available in a wide range of designs and for various applications. Removal efficiencies differ significantly from coarse filters, such as granular anthracite, quartz, or sand for larger water systems and depth cartridges for smaller water systems, to membrane filters for very small particle control. Unit and system configurations vary widely in type of filtering media and location in the process. (Use of membrane filters is discussed in a later paragraph.)

Granular or cartridge filters are used for prefiltration. They remove solid contaminants from the water supply and protect downstream system components from contamination that can inhibit equipment performance and shorten their effective life. Design and operational issues that may impact performance of depth filters include channeling of the filtering media, blockage from silt, microbial growth, and filtering-media loss. Control measures include pressure and flow monitoring, backwashing, sanitizing, and replacing filtering media. An important design concern is sizing of the filter to prevent channeling or media loss resulting from inappropriate water flow rates.

Activated carbon beds adsorb low-molecular-weight organic material and oxidizing additives, such as chlorine compounds, and remove them from the water. They are used to achieve certain quality attributes and to protect against reaction with downstream stainless steel surfaces, resins, and membranes. The chief operating concerns regarding activated carbon beds include the propensity to support bacteria growth, the potential for hydraulic channeling, the inability to be regenerated *in situ*, and the shedding of bacteria, endotoxins, organic chemicals, and fine carbon particles. Control measures include appropriate high water flow rates, sanitization with hot water or steam, backwashing, testing for adsorption capacity, and frequent replacement of the carbon bed. Alternative technologies such as chemical additives and regenerable organic scavenging devices can be used in place of activated carbon beds.

Chemical additives are used in water systems to control microorganisms by use of chlorine compounds and ozone, to enhance the removal of suspended solids by use of flocculating agents, to remove chlorine compounds, to adjust pH, and to remove carbonate compounds. Subsequent processing steps are required to remove the added chemicals. Control of additives and subsequent monitoring to ensure removal of additives and of any of their reaction products should be designed into the system and included in the monitoring program.

Organic scavenging devices use macroreticular anion-exchange resins capable of removing organic material and endotoxins from the water. They can be regenerated with appropriate biocidal caustic solutions. Operating concerns are associated with scavenging capacity and shedding of resin fragments. Control measures include testing of effluent, monitoring performance, and using downstream filters to remove resin fines.

Water softeners remove cations such as calcium and magnesium that interfere with the performance of downstream processing equipment such as reverse osmosis membranes, deionization columns, and distillation units. Water softener resin beds are regenerated with sodium chloride solution (brine). Concerns include microorganism proliferation, channeling due to inappropriate water flow rates, organic fouling of resin, fracture of the resin beads, and contamination from the brine solution used for regeneration. Control measures include recirculation of water during periods of low water use, periodic sanitization of the resin and brine system, use of microbial control devices (e.g., UV and chlorine), appropriate regeneration frequency, effluent monitoring (hardness), and downstream filtration to remove resin fines.

Deionization (DI), electrodeionization (EDI) and **Electrodialysis (EDR)** are effective methods of improving the chemical quality attributes of water by removing cations and anions.

DI systems have charged resins that require periodic regeneration with an acid and base. Typically, cationic resins are regenerated with either hydrochloric or sulfuric acid, which replace the captured positive ions with hydrogen ions. Anionic resins are regenerated with sodium or potassium hydroxide, which replace captured negative ions with hydroxide ions. Both regenerant chemicals are biocidal and offer a measure of microbial control. The system can be designed so that the cation and anion resins are separated or that they form a mixed bed. Rechargeable resin canisters can also be used for this purpose.

The EDI system uses a combination of mixed resin, selectively permeable membranes, and an electric charge to provide continuous flow (product and waste concentrate) and continuous regeneration. Water enters both the resin section and the waste (concentrate) section. As it passes through the resin, it is deionized to become product water. The resin acts as a conductor enabling the electrical potential to drive the captured cations and anions through the resin and appropriate membranes for concentration and removal in the waste water stream. The electrical potential also separates the water in the resin (product) section into hydrogen and hydroxide ions. This permits continuous regeneration of the resin without the need for regenerant additives.

Electrodialysis (EDR) is a similar process that uses only electricity and selectively permeable membranes to separate, concentrate, and flush the removed ions from the water stream. It, however, is less efficient than EDI because it contains no resin to enhance ion removal and current flow. Also, EDR units require periodic polarity reversal and flushing to maintain operating performance.

Concerns for all forms of deionization units include microbial and endotoxin control, chemical additive impact on resins and membranes, and loss, degradation, and fouling of resin. Issues of concern specific to DI units include regeneration frequency, channeling, complete resin separation for mixed bed regeneration, and mixing air contamination (mixed beds). Control measures vary but typically include recirculation loops, microbial control by UV light, conductivity monitoring, resin testing, microporous filtration of mixing air, microbial monitoring, frequent regeneration to minimize and control microorganism growth, sizing the equipment for suitable water flow, and use of elevated temperatures. Regeneration piping for mixed bed units should be configured to ensure that regeneration chemicals contact all internal surfaces and resins. Rechargeable canisters can be the source of contamination and should be carefully monitored. Full knowledge of previous resin use, minimum storage time between regeneration and use, and appropriate sanitizing procedures are critical factors ensuring proper performance.

Reverse osmosis (RO) units employ a semipermeable membrane and a substantial pressure differential to drive water through the membrane to achieve chemical, microbial, and endotoxin quality improvement. The process streams consist of supply water, product water (permeate), and waste water (reject). Pretreatment and system configuration variations may be necessary depending on source water to achieve desired performance and reliability. Concerns associated with the design and operation of RO units include membrane material sensitivity to bacteria and sanitizing agents, membrane fouling, membrane integrity, seal integrity, and the volume of waste water. Failure of membrane or seal integrity will result in product water

contamination. Methods of control consist of suitable pretreatment of the water stream, appropriate membrane material selection, integrity challenges, membrane design such as spiral wound to promote flushing action, periodic sanitization, monitoring of differential pressures, conductivity, microbial levels, and total organic carbon. The configuration of the RO unit offers control opportunities by expanding the single-pass scheme to parallel-staged, reject-staged, two-pass, and combination designs. An example would be the use of a two-pass design to improve reliability, quality, and efficiency. RO units can be used alone or in combination with DI and EDI units for operational and quality enhancements.

Ultrafiltration is another technology that uses a permeable membrane, but unlike RO it works by mechanical separation rather than osmosis. Due to the filtration ability of the membrane, macromolecular and microbial impurities, such as endotoxins, are reduced. This technology may be appropriate as an intermediate or final purification step. Similar to RO, successful performance is dependent upon other system unit operations and system configuration.

Issues of concern include compatibility of membrane material with sanitizing agents, membrane integrity, fouling by particles and microorganisms, cartridge contaminant retention, and seal integrity. Control measures include sanitization, designs capable of flushing the membrane surface, integrity challenges, regular cartridge changes, elevated feed water temperature, and monitoring total organic carbon and differential pressure. Additional flexibility in operation is possible based on the way units are arranged such as in a parallel or series configuration. Care should be taken to avoid stagnant water conditions that could promote microorganism growth in back-up or standby units.

Microbial retentive filters (membrane filters) prevent the passage of microorganisms and very small particles. They are used in tank air and inert gas vents and for filtration of compressed air gases used in the regeneration of mixed-bed deionization units. Areas of concern are blockage of tank vents by condensed water vapor, which can cause mechanical damage to the tank, and concentration of microorganisms on the surface of the membrane filter, creating the potential for contamination of the tank or deionizer contents. Control measures include the use of hydrophobic filters and heat tracing vent filter housings to prevent vapor condensation. Sterilization of the unit prior to initial use and periodically thereafter or regular filter changes are also recommended control methods. Microbial retentive filters are sometimes incorporated into purification systems or in water distribution piping. This application should be carefully controlled because as noted above, these units can become a source for microbial contamination. The potential exists for the release of microorganisms should the membrane filter rupture or as a result of microbial grow-through. Other means of controlling microorganisms and fine particles can be employed in place of membrane filters in the purification and distribution section of water systems. Filters that are intended to be microretentive should be sanitized and integrity tested prior to initial use and at appropriate intervals thereafter.

Positively charged filter media reduce endotoxin levels by electrostatic attraction and adsorption. Application may be unit operation or distribution system related depending upon the microbial control requirements. Filter media that are microbial retentive require the same concerns and controls as indicated in the previous paragraph. Concerns include flow rate, membrane and seal integrity, and retention capacity, which can be affected by the development of a finite charge potential on the filter. Control measures include monitoring differential pressure and endotoxin levels, proper sizing, testing membrane integrity, and configuring units in series to control break-through.

Distillation units provide chemical and microbial purification via thermal vaporization, mist elimination, and condensing. A variety of designs are available including single-effect, multiple-effect, and vapor compression. The latter two configurations are normally used in larger systems because of their generating capacity and efficiency. Distilled water systems may require less rigorous control of feed water quality than do membrane systems.

Areas of concern include carry-over of impurities, evaporator flooding, stagnant water, pump and compressor seal design, and conductivity (quality) variations during start-up and operation. Methods of control consist of reliable mist elimination, visual or automated high-water-level indication, use of sanitary pumps and compressors, proper drainage, blow down control, and use of on-line conductivity sensing with automated diversion of unacceptable quality water to the waste stream.

Storage tanks are included in water distribution systems to optimize processing equipment capacity. Storage also allows for routine maintenance while maintaining continuous supply to meet manufacturing needs. Design and operation considerations are needed to prevent the development of biofilm, to minimize corrosion, to aid in the use of chemical sanitization of the tanks, and to safeguard mechanical integrity. These considerations may include using closed tanks with smooth interiors and the ability to spray the tank head space. This minimizes corrosion and biofilm development and aids in sanitizing thermally or chemically.

Storage tanks require venting to compensate for the dynamics of changing water levels. This can be accomplished with a hydrophobic microbial retentive membrane filter fitted onto an atmospheric vent. Alternatively, an automatic membrane-filtered compressed gas pressurization and venting system may be used. Rupture disks equipped with a rupture alarm device serve as a further safeguard for the mechanical integrity of the tank.

Distribution configuration should allow for the continuous flow of water in the piping by means of recirculation or should provide for the periodic flushing of the system. Experience has shown that continuously recirculated systems are easier to maintain.

Pumps should be designed to deliver fully turbulent flow conditions to retard the development of biofilms. Components and distribution lines should be sloped and fitted with drain points so that the system can be completely drained. In distribution systems, where the water is circulated at a high temperature, dead legs and low-flow conditions should be avoided, and valved tie-in points should have length-to-diameter ratios of 6 or less. In ambient temperature distribution systems, particular care should be exercised to avoid pocket areas and provide for complete drainage. Water exiting from a loop should not be returned to the system. Distribution design should include the placement of sampling valves in the storage tank and at other locations such as in the return line of the recirculating water system. The primary sampling site for water should be the valves that deliver water to the point of use. Direct connections to processes or auxiliary equipment should be designed to prevent reverse flow into the controlled water system. The distribution system should permit sanitization for microorganism control. The system may be continuously operated at sanitizing conditions or sanitized periodically.

INSTALLATION AND MATERIALS OF CONSTRUCTION AND COMPONENT SELECTION

Installation techniques are important because they can affect the mechanical, corrosive, and sanitary integrity of the system. Valve installation attitude should promote gravity drainage. Pipe supports should provide appropriate slopes for drainage and should be designed to support the piping adequately under worst-case thermal conditions. Methods of connecting system components including units of operation, tanks, and distribution piping require careful attention to preclude potential problems.

Stainless steel welds should provide reliable joints that are internally smooth and corrosion-free. Low-carbon stainless steel, compatible wire filler, where necessary, inert gas, automatic welding machines, and regular inspection and documentation help to ensure acceptable weld quality. Follow-up cleaning and passivation are important for removing contamination and corrosion products and to reestablish the passive corrosion-resistant surface. Plastic materials can be fused (welded) in some cases and also require smooth, uniform internal surfaces.

Adhesives should be avoided due to the potential for voids and chemical reactions. Mechanical methods of joining, such as flange fittings, require care to avoid the creation of offsets, gaps, penetrations, and voids. Control measures include good alignment, properly sized gaskets, appropriate spacing, uniform sealing force, and the avoidance of threaded fittings.

Materials of construction should be selected to be compatible with control measures such as sanitizing, cleaning, and passivating. Temperature rating is a critical factor in choosing appropriate materials because surfaces may be required to handle elevated operating and sanitization temperatures. Should chemicals or additives be used to clean, control, or sanitize the system, materials resistant to these chemicals or additives must be utilized.

Materials should be capable of handling turbulent flow and elevated velocities without wear on the corrosive barrier impact, such as the passivation-related chromium oxide surface of stainless steel. The finish on metallic materials such as stainless steel, whether it be a refined mill finish, polished to a specific grit, or an electropolished treatment, should complement system design and provide satisfactory corrosion and microbial activity resistance. Auxiliary equipment and fittings that require seals, gaskets, diaphragms, filter media, and membranes should exclude materials that permit the possibility of extractables, shedding, and microbial activity.

Insulating materials exposed to stainless steel surfaces should be free of chlorides to avoid the phenomenon of stress corrosion cracking that can lead to system contamination and the destruction of tanks and critical system components.

Specifications are important to ensure proper selection of materials and to serve as a reference for system qualification and maintenance. Information such as mill reports for stainless steel and reports of composition, ratings, and material handling capabilities for nonmetallic substances should be reviewed for suitability and retained for reference.

Component (auxiliary equipment) selection should be made with assurance that it does not create a source for contamination intrusion. Heat exchangers should be double tube sheet or concentric tube design. They should include differential pressure monitoring or utilize heat transfer medium of equal or better quality to avoid problems should leaks develop. Pumps should be of sanitary design with seals that prevent contamination of the water. Valves should have smooth internal surfaces with the seat and closing device exposed to the flushing action of water, such as occurs in diaphragm valves. Valves with pocket areas or closing devices (e.g., ball, plug, gate, globe) that move into and out of a flow area should be avoided.

SANITIZATION

Microbial control in water systems is achieved primarily through sanitization practices. Systems can be sanitized using either thermal or chemical means. In-line UV light at a wavelength of 254 nm can also be used to "sanitize" water in the system continuously.

Thermal approaches to system sanitization include periodic or continuously circulating hot water and the use of steam. These techniques are limited to systems that are compatible with the higher temperatures needed to achieve sanitization, such as stainless steel and some polymer formulations. Although thermal methods control biofilm development, they are not effective in removing established biofilms.

Chemical methods, where compatible, can be used on a wider variety of construction materials. These methods typically employ oxidizing agents such as halogenated compounds, hydrogen peroxide, ozone, or peracetic acid. Halogenated compounds are effective sanitizers but are difficult to flush from the system and tend to leave biofilms intact. Compounds such as hydrogen peroxide, ozone, and peracetic acid oxidize bacteria and biofilms by forming reactive peroxides and free radicals (notably hydroxyl radicals). The short half-life of these compounds, particularly ozone, may require that it be added continuously during the sanitization process. Hydrogen peroxide and ozone rapidly degrade to water and oxygen; peracetic acid degrades to acetic acid in the presence of UV light.

UV light impacts on the development of biofilms by reducing the rate of new microbial colonization in the system; however, it is only partially effective against planktonic microorganisms. Alone, UV light is not an effective tool because it does not eliminate existing biofilm. However, when coupled with conventional thermal or chemical sanitization technologies, it is most effective and can prolong the interval between system sanitizations. The use of UV light also facilitates the degradation of hydrogen peroxide and ozone.

Sanitization steps require validation to demonstrate the capability of reducing and holding microbial contamination at acceptable levels. Validation of thermal methods should include a heat distribution study to demonstrate that sanitization temperatures are achieved throughout the system. Validation of chemical methods require a demonstration of adequate chemical concentrations throughout the system. In addition, when the sanitization process is completed, effective removal of chemical residues must be demonstrated.

The frequency of sanitization is generally dictated by the results of system monitoring. Conclusions derived from the trend analysis of the microbiological data should be used as the alert mechanism for maintenance. The frequency of sanitization should be established such that the system operates in a state of microbiological control and does not exceed Alert Levels.

OPERATION, MAINTENANCE, AND CONTROL

A preventive maintenance program should be established to ensure that the water system remains in a state of control. The program should include (1) procedures for operating the system, (2) monitoring programs for critical quality attributes and operating conditions including calibration of critical instruments, (3) schedule for periodic sanitization, (4) preventive maintenance of components, and (5) control of changes to the mechanical system and to operating conditions.

Operating Procedures—Procedures for operating the water system and performing routine maintenance and corrective action should be written, and they should also define the point when action is required. The procedures should be well documented, detail the function of each job, assign who is responsible for performing the work, and describe how the job is to be conducted.

Monitoring Program—Critical quality attributes and operating parameters should be documented and monitored. The program may include a combination of in-line sensors or recorders (e.g., a conductivity meter and recorder), manual documentation of operational parameters (such as carbon filter pressure drop) and laboratory tests (e.g., total microbial counts). The frequency of sampling, the requirement for evaluating test results, and the necessity for initiating corrective action should be included.

Sanitization—Depending on system design and the selected units of operation, routine periodic sanitization may be necessary to maintain the system in a state of microbial control. Technologies for sanitization are described above.

Preventive Maintenance—A preventive maintenance program should be in effect. The program should establish what preventive maintenance is to be performed, the frequency of maintenance work, and how the work should be documented.

Change Control—The mechanical configuration and operating conditions must be controlled. Proposed changes should be evaluated for their impact on the whole system. The need to requalify the system after changes are made should be determined. Following a decision to modify a water system, the affected drawings, manuals, and procedures should be revised.

SAMPLING CONSIDERATIONS

Water systems should be monitored at a frequency that is sufficient to ensure that the system is in control and continues to produce water of acceptable quality. Samples should be taken from representative locations within the processing and distribution system. Established sampling frequencies should be based on system validation data and should cover critical areas. Unit-operation sites might be sampled less frequently than point-of-use sites. The sampling plan should take into consideration the desired attributes of the water being sampled. For example, systems for *Water for Injection*, because of their more critical microbiological requirements, may require a more rigorous sampling frequency.

When sampling water systems, special care should be taken to ensure that the sample is representative. Sampling ports should be sanitized and thoroughly flushed before a sample is taken. Samples containing chemical sanitizing agents require neutralization prior to microbiological analysis. Samples for microbiological analysis should be tested immediately or suitably protected to preserve the sample until analysis can begin.

Samples of flowing water are only indicative of the concentration of planktonic (free-floating) microorganisms present in the system. Benthic (attached) microorganisms present as biofilms are generally present in greater numbers and are the source of the planktonic population. Microorganisms in biofilms represent a continuous source of contamination and are difficult to sample and quantify. Consequently, the planktonic population is used as an indicator of system contamination levels and is the basis for system Alert Levels. The consistent appearance of elevated planktonic levels is usually an indication of advanced biofilm development in need of remedial control. System control and sanitization are key in controlling biofilm formation and the consequent planktonic population.

MICROBIAL CONSIDERATIONS

The major exogenous source of microbial contamination is source or feed water. Feed water quality must, at a minimum, meet the quality attributes of drinking water for which the level of coliforms are regulated. A wide variety of other microorganisms, chiefly Gram-negative bacteria, may be present. These microorganisms may compromise subsequent purification steps.

Examples of other potential exogenous sources of microbial contamination include unprotected vents, faulty air filters, backflow from contaminated outlets, drain air-breaks, and replacement-activated carbon and deionizer resins. Sufficient care should be given to system design and maintenance in order to minimize microbial contamination from these sources.

Unit operations can be a major source of endogenous microbial contamination. Microorganisms present in feed water may adsorb to carbon beds, deionizer resins, filter membranes, and other unit operation surfaces and initiate the formation of a biofilm. Biofilm is an adaptive response by certain microorganisms to survive in a low-nutrient environment. Microorganisms in a biofilm are protected from the action of many biocides. Downstream colonization can occur when microorganisms are sloughed off and carried in other areas of the water system. Microorganisms may also attach to suspended particles such as carbon-bed fines and serve as a source of contamination to subsequent purification equipment and distribution systems.

Another source of endogenous microbial contamination is the distribution system. Microorganisms can colonize pipe surfaces, valves, and other areas. There they proliferate, forming a biofilm, which then provides a continuous source of microbial contamination.

Endotoxins are lipopolysaccharides from the cell envelope that is external to the cell wall of Gram-negative bacteria. Gram-negative bacteria readily form biofilms that can become a source of endotoxins. Endotoxins may either be associated with living microorganisms or fragments of dead microorganisms, or they may be free molecules. The free form of endotoxins may be released from cell surfaces or biofilms that colonize the water system, or they may enter the water system via the feed water. Endotoxin levels may be minimized by controlling the introduction of microorganisms and microbial proliferation in the system. This may be accomplished through the normal exclusion or removal action afforded by various unit operations within the treatment system as well as through system sanitization. Other control methods include the use of ultrafilters or charge-modified filters, either in-line or at the point of use. The presence of endotoxins may be monitored as described in the chapter *Bacterial Endotoxins Test* ⟨85⟩.

METHODOLOGICAL CONSIDERATIONS[*]

The objective of a water system microbiological monitoring program is to provide sufficient information to control the microbiological quality of the water produced. Product quality requirements should dictate water quality needs. An appropriate level of control may be maintained by using data trending techniques and limiting specific contraindicated microorganisms. Consequently, it may not be necessary to detect all of the microorganisms present. The monitoring program and methodology should indicate adverse trends and detect microorganisms that are potentially harmful to the finished product or consumer.

Final selection of method variables should be based on the individual requirements of the system being monitored. It should be recognized that there is no single method that is capable of detecting all of the potential microbial contaminants of a water system. Methods selected should be capable of isolating the numbers and types of organisms that have been deemed significant relative to system control and product impact for each individual system.

Several criteria should be considered when selecting a method to monitor the microbial content of a pharmaceutical water system. These include method sensitivity, range of organisms recovered, sample throughput, incubation period, cost, and technical complexity. An additional consideration is the use of the classical "culture" approaches vs. a sophisticated instrument approach.

THE CLASSICAL CULTURE APPROACH

Classical culture approaches for microbial testing of water include but are not limited to pour plates, spread plates, membrane filtration, and most-probable-number (MPN) tests. These methods are generally easy to perform, are less expensive, and provide excellent sample processing throughput. Method sensitivity can be increased via the use of larger sample sizes. This strategy is used in the membrane filtration method.

Culture approaches are further defined by the type of medium used in combination with the incubation temperature and duration. This combination should be selected according to the monitoring needs presented by a specific water system as well as its ability to recover microorganisms that could have a detrimental effect on the product or process.

There are two basic forms of media available for traditional microbiological analysis: "high" nutrient and "low" nutrient. High-nutrient media are intended as general media for the isolation and enumeration of heterotrophic bacteria. Low-nutrient media are beneficial for isolating slow-growing bacteria and bacteria that have been injured by previous exposure to disinfectants and sanitizers such as chlorine. Low-nutrient media may be compared to high-nutrient media, especially during the validation of a water system, in order to determine if any additional numbers or types of bacteria are present so that their impact on the end use may be

---

[*] For additional guidance concerning microbial-water testing methodology, consult *Standard Methods for the Examination of Water and Wastewater*, 18th Edition, American Public Health Association, Washington DC, 20005.

assessed. Additionally, the efficacy of system controls and sanitization on these slower-growing or impaired bacteria can also be assessed.

Duration and temperature of incubation are also critical aspects of a microbiological test method. Classical methodologies using high-nutrient media have required incubation at 30°C to 35°C for 48 to 72 hours. In certain water systems incubation at lower temperatures (e.g., 20°C to 25°C) and longer periods (e.g., 5 to 7 days) can produce higher counts when compared to classical methods. Whether or not a particular system needs to be monitored using lower incubation temperatures or longer incubation times should be determined during system validation.

The decision to use longer incubation periods should be made after considering the need for timely information and the type of corrective actions required when an Alert or Action Level is exceeded. The advantages gained by incubating for longer times, namely recovery of injured microorganisms, slow growers, or more fastidious microorganisms, should be balanced against the need to have a timely investigation and to take corrective action, as well as the ability of these microorganisms to detrimentally affect products or processes.

"INSTRUMENT" APPROACH

Examples of instrument approaches include microscopic direct counting techniques (e.g., epifluorescence and immunofluorescence), radiometric, impedometric, and biochemically based methodologies. These methods all possess a variety of advantages and disadvantages.

One advantage is their precision and accuracy. In general, instrument approaches often have a shorter lead time for obtaining results, which facilitates timely system control. This advantage, however, is often counterbalanced by limited sample processing throughput due to labor-intensive sample processing or other instrument limitations. In addition, instrumental approaches are destructive in that further isolate manipulation for characterization purposes are precluded. Generally, some form of microbial isolate characterization may be a required element of water system monitoring. Consequently, culturing approaches have traditionally been preferred over instrumental approaches because they offer a balance of desirable test attributes and post-test capabilities.

RECOMMENDED METHODOLOGIES

The following general methods obtained from *Standard Methods for the Examination of Water and Wastewater*, 18th Edition, American Public Health Association, Washington, DC 20005, are considered appropriate for establishing trends in the number of colony-forming units observed in the routine microbiological monitoring of ingredient water. It is recognized, however, that other combinations of media, time, and temperature of incubation may occasionally or even consistently result in higher numbers of colony-forming units being observed. The extended incubation periods that are usually required by some of the alternative methods available offer disadvantages that may outweigh the higher counts obtained. The somewhat higher baseline counts would not necessarily have greater utility in detecting an excursion or a trend.

Methodologies that can be recommended as generally satisfactory for monitoring pharmaceutical water systems are as follows:

Drinking Water:	POUR PLATE METHOD Minimum sample—1.0 mL Plate count agar Plate count agar 42 to 72 hours incubation at 30°C to 35°C
Purified Water:	POUR PLATE METHOD Minimum sample—1.0 mL Plate count agar 48 to 72 hours incubation at 30°C to 35°C
Water for Injection:	MEMBRANE FILTRATION METHOD Minimum sample—100 mL Plate count agar 48 to 72 hours incubation at 30°C to 35°C

Identification of Microorganisms

Identifying the isolates recovered from water-monitoring methods may be important in instances where specific waterborne microorganisms may be detrimental to the products or processes in which the water is used. Microorganism information such as this may also be useful when identifying the source of microbial contamination in a product or process.

Often a limited group of microorganisms are continuously recovered from a water system. After repeated characterization, an experienced microbiologist may become proficient at their identification based on only a few traits such as colonial morphology and staining characteristics. This level of characterization is adequate for most situations.

Alert and Action Levels

The individual monographs for *Purified Water* and *Water for Injection* do not include specific microbial limits. These were purposefully omitted since most current microbiological techniques available require at least 48 hours to obtain definitive results. By that time, the water from which the sample was taken has already been employed in the production process. Failure to meet a compendial specification would require rejecting the product lot involved, and this is not the intent of an alert or action guideline. The establishment of quantitative microbiological guidelines for water for pharmaceutical purposes is in order because such guidelines will establish procedures that are to be implemented in the event that significant excursions beyond these limits occur.

Water systems should be microbiologically monitored to confirm that they continue to operate within their design specifications and produce water of acceptable quality. Monitoring data may be compared to established process parameters or product specifications. A refinement to the use of process parameters and product specifications is the establishment of Alert and Action Levels, which signal a shift in process performance. Alert and Action Levels are distinct from process parameters and product specifications in that they are used for monitoring and control rather than accept or reject decisions.

Alert Levels are levels or ranges that, when exceeded, indicate that a process may have drifted from its normal operating condition. Alert Levels constitute a warning and do not necessarily require a corrective action.

Action Levels are levels or ranges that, when exceeded, indicate that a process has drifted from its normal operating range. Exceeding an Action Level indicates that corrective action should be taken to bring the process back into its normal operating range.

Alert and Action Levels are established within process and product specification tolerances and are based on a combination of technical and product-related considerations. Consequently, exceeding an Alert or Action Level does not imply that product quality has been compromised.

Technical considerations used to establish Alert and Action Levels should include a review of equipment design specifications to ensure that the purification equipment is capable of achieving the required level of purity. In addition, samples should be collected and analyzed over a period of time to develop data reflecting normal water quality trends. Historical or statistically based levels can be established using the above data. Levels established in this way measure process performance and are independent of product concerns.

Product-related Alert and Action Levels should represent both product-quality concerns and the ability to effectively manage the purification process. These levels are typically based on a review of process data and an assessment of product sensitivity to chemical and microbiological contamination. The assessment of product susceptibility might include preservative efficacy, water activity, pH, etc. The levels should be set such that, when exceeded, product quality is not compromised.

Monitoring data should be analyzed on an ongoing basis to ensure that the process continues to perform within acceptable limits. An analysis of data trends is often used to evaluate process performance. This information can be used to predict departures from established operating parameters, thereby signaling the need for appropriate preventative maintenance.

It should be recognized that the microbial Alert and Action Levels established for any pharmaceutical water system are necessarily linked to the monitoring method chosen. Using the recommended methodologies, generally considered appropriate Action Levels are 500 colony-forming units (cfu) per mL for *Drinking Water*, 100 cfu per mL for *Purified Water* and 10 cfu per 100 mL for *Water for Injection*.

It should be emphasized that the above action guidelines are not intended to be totally inclusive for every situation where ingredient waters are employed. For example, Gram-negative microorganisms are not excluded from ingredient waters, nor is the presence of Gram-negative microorganisms prohibited in *Drinking Water* in the Federal Regulations. The reason for this is that these microorganisms are ubiquitous to the aqueous environment and their exclusion would likely require a sterilization process that would not be appropriate or feasible in many manufacturing scenarios. However, there are situations where they might not be tolerated: in topical products and in some oral dosage forms. It is, therefore, incumbent upon the manufacturer to supplement the general action guidelines to fit each particular manufacturing situation.

Section VII

SELECTED LAWS AND REGULATIONS

FEDERAL FOOD, DRUG, AND COSMETIC ACT REQUIREMENTS RELATING TO DRUGS FOR HUMAN AND ANIMAL USE AND TO DIETARY SUPPLEMENTS

Former title: Federal Food, Drug, and Cosmetic Act Requirements Relating to Drugs for Human and Animal Use

Selected portions of the Federal Food, Drug, and Cosmetic Act as it relates to the regulation of drugs for human use are presented here as a service to practitioners and students of pharmacy and medicine. The complete text of the Act can be found in Title 21 of the United States Code §321 et al. The corresponding section number of the code appears in brackets after the section number of the Act.

In addition to federal requirements, statutes governing drugs and their quality have been enacted by various states. In many cases, state requirements parallel those of the federal law. However, this should not be assumed; and individual state laws and requirements also should be consulted.

It should be noted that many provisions of the Act make no distinction between drugs for animal use and drugs for human use, but simply refer to drugs. For ease of reference, those sections of the Act which specifically relate to drugs for animal use are indexed separately and appear at the end of this chapter.

Publication of these sections in the United States Pharmacopeia is for information purposes only and does not impart any legal effect.

INDEX TO SELECTED PORTIONS OF THE FEDERAL FOOD, DRUG, AND COSMETIC ACT RELATED TO DRUGS FOR HUMAN USE PRESENTED HEREIN

§ 1   **Title**

§ 201   **Definitions**
- (e)   person
- (g) (1)   drug
- (g) (2)   counterfeit drug
- (j)   official compendium
- (k)   label
- (l)   immediate container
- (m)   labeling
- (n)   misleading labeling or advertising
- (o)   antiseptic
- (p)   new drug
- (t) (1)   color additive
- (u)   safe
- (ff)   dietary supplement
- (ii)   compounded positron emission tomography drug

§ 301   **Prohibited Acts Regarding Adulterated and Misbranded Drugs**
- (a)   introduction into interstate commerce
- (b)   in interstate commerce
- (c)   receipt and delivery
- (d)   introduction into interstate commerce in violation of new drug and food requirements
- (e)   failure to permit access to or copying of any record
- (f)   refusal to permit inspection
- (g)   manufacture of adulterated or misbranded product
- (h)   giving a false guarantee
- (i)   forging, counterfeiting
- (k)   alteration of product while held for sale
- (o)   failure to provide to practitioners required labeling
- (p)   failure to register
- (t)   importing a drug in violation of 801(d)(1)

§ 303   **Penalties**
- (a)   fine or imprisonment; repeat offenders or violation with intent to defraud or mislead
- (b) (1)   fines and imprisonment for importing a drug in violation of 801(d)(1) or selling samples
- (b) (2)   fines or imprisonment for manufacturers and distributors of samples in violation of the law
- (b) (3)   failure to report
- (b) (4)   limits on manufacturer or distributor responsibility
- (b) (5)   informant rewards
- (b) (6)   penalties
- (c)   defenses
- (d)   misbranded food

§ 501   **Adulterated Drugs**
- (a)   filthy, putrid, decomposed substances insanitary conditions failure to conform to good manufacturing practices failure to conform to controls for positron emission tomography drug poisonous or deleterious container unsafe color additive
- (b)   failure to comply with compendial standards
- (c)   failure to comply with purported strength, quality, or purity
- (d)   other substance mixed with or substituted therefor

§ 502   **Misbranded Drugs**
- (a)   false and misleading labeling
- (b)   name and place of manufacturer, packer, or distributor quantity statement
- (c)   conspicuousness of statements
- (e)   established name and quantity requirements
- (f)   directions for use and adequate warnings
- (g)   compendial packaging and labeling requirements
- (h)   packaging requirements for drugs subject to deterioration
- (i)   misleading containers and imitations
- (j)   dangerous to health as labeled
- (m)   nonconforming color additive
- (n)   advertising requirements
- (o)   unregistered establishment or failure to bear identification symbol
- (p)   failure to comply with Poison Prevention Packaging Act

---

Inquiries regarding these requirements should be directed to the U.S. Food and Drug Administration, 5600 Fishers Lane, Rockville, MD 20857.

SELECTED PORTIONS OF THE FEDERAL FOOD, DRUG, AND COSMETIC ACT RELATED TO DRUGS FOR HUMAN USE

Short Title

§ 1 [301]   This Act may be cited as the Federal Food, Drug, and Cosmetic Act.

Definitions

§ 201 [321]   For the purposes of this Act—
(e)   The term "person" includes individual, partnership, corporation, and association.
(g) (1)   The term "drug" means (A) articles recognized in the official United States Pharmacopeia, official Homeopathic Pharmacopeia of the United States, or official National Formulatry, or any supplement to any of them; and (B) articles intended for use in the diagnosis, cure, mitigation, treatment, or prevention of disease in man or other animals; and (C) articles (other than food) intended to affect the structure or any function of the body of man or other animals; and (D) articles intended for use as a component of any articles specified in clause (A), (B), or (C). A food or dietary supplement for which a claim, subject to sections 403(r)(1)(B) and 403(r)(3) or sections 403(r)(1)(B) and 403(r)(5)(D), is made in accordance with the requirements of section 403(r) is not a drug solely because the label or the labeling contains such a claim. A food, dietary ingredient, or dietary sup-

plement for which a truthful and not misleading statement is made in accordance with section 403(r)(6) is not a drug under clause (C) solely because the label or the labeling contains such a statement.

(2)   The term "counterfeit drug" means a drug which, or the container or labeling of which, without authorization, bears the trademark, trade name, or other identifying mark, imprint, or device, or any likeness thereof, of a drug manufacturer, processor, packer, or distributor other than the person or persons who in fact manufactured, processed, packed, or distributed such drug and which thereby falsely purports or is represented to be the product of, or to have been packed or distributed by, such other drug manufacturer, processor, packer, or distributor.

(j)   The term "official compendium" means the official United States Pharmacopeia, official Homeopathic Pharmacopeia of the United States, official National Formulary, or any supplement to any of them.

(k)   The term "label" means a display of written, printed, or graphic matter upon the immediate container of any article; and a requirement made by or under authority of this Act that any word, statement, or other information appear on the label shall not be considered to be complied with unless such word, statement, or other information also appears on the outside container or wrapper, if any there be, of the retail package of such article, or is easily legible through the outside container or wrapper.

(l)   The term "immediate container" does not include package liners.

(m)   The term "labeling" means all labels and other written, printed, or graphic matter (1) upon any article or any of its containers or wrappers, or (2) accompanying such article.

(n)   If an article is alleged to be misbranded because the labeling or advertising is misleading, then in determining whether the labeling or advertising is misleading there shall be taken into account (among other things) not only representations made or suggested by statement, word, design, device, or any combination thereof, but also the extent to which the labeling or advertising fails to reveal facts material in the light of such representations or material with respect to consequences which may result from the use of the article to which the labeling or advertising relates under the conditions of use prescribed in the labeling or advertising thereof or under such conditions of use as are customary or usual.

(o)   The representation of a drug, in its labeling, as an antiseptic shall be considered to be a representation that it is a germicide, except in the case of a drug purporting to be, or represented as, an antiseptic for inhibitory use as a wet dressing, ointment, dusting powder, or such other use as involves prolonged contact with the body.

(p)   The term "new drug" means—

(1)   Any drug (except a new animal drug or an animal feed bearing or containing a new animal drug) the composition of which is such that such drug is not generally recognized, among experts qualified by scientific training and experience to evaluate the safety and effectiveness of drugs, as safe and effective for use under the conditions prescribed, recommended, or suggested in the labeling thereof, except that such a drug not so recognized shall not be deemed to be a "new drug" if at any time prior to the enactment of this Act it was subject to the Food and Drugs Act of June 30, 1906, as amended, and if at such time its labeling contained the same representations concerning the conditions of its use; or

(2)   Any drug (except a new animal drug or an animal feed bearing or containing a new animal drug) the composition of which is such that such drug, as a result of investigations to determine its safety and effectiveness for use under such conditions, has become so recognized, but which has not, otherwise than in such investigations, been used to a material extent or for a material time under such conditions.

(t) (1)   The term "color additive" means a material which—

(A)   is a dye, pigment, or other substance made by a process of synthesis or similar artifice, or extracted, isolated, or otherwise derived, with or without intermediate or final change of identity, from a vegetable, animal, mineral, or other source, and

(B)   when added or applied to a food, drug, or cosmetic, or to the human body or any part thereof, is capable (alone or through reaction with other substance) of imparting color thereto; except that such term does not include any material which the Secretary, by regulation, determines is used (or intended to be used) solely for a purpose or purposes other than coloring.

(2)   The term "color" includes black, white, and intermediate grays.

(u)   The term "safe," as used in paragraph(s) of this section and in sections 409, 512, and 721, has reference to the health of man or animal.

(ff)   The term "dietary supplement"—

(1)   means a product (other than tobacco) intended to supplement the diet that bears or contains one or more of the following dietary ingredients:

(A)   a vitamin;

(B)   a mineral;

(C)   an herb or other botanical;

(D)   an amino acid;

(E)   a dietary substance for use by man to supplement the diet by increasing the total dietary intake; or

(F)   a concentrate, metabolite, constituent, extract, or combination of any ingredients described in clause (A), (B), (C), (D), or (E);

(2)   means a product that—

(A)(i)   is intended for ingestion in a form described in section 350(c)(1)(B)(i) of this title; or

(ii)   complies with section 350(c)(1)(B)(ii) of this title;

(B)   is not represented for use as a conventional food or as a sole item of a meal or the diet; and

(C)   is labeled as a deitary supplement; and

(3)   does—

(A)   include an article that is approved as a new drug under section 355 of this title, or licensed as a biologic under section 262 of Title 42, and was, prior to such approval, certification, or license, marketed as a dietary supplement or as a food unless the Secretary has issued a regulation, after notice and comment, finding that the article, when used as or in a dietary supplement under the conditions of use and dosages set forth in the labeling for such dietary supplement, is unlawful under section 342(f) of this title; and

(B)   not include—

(i)   an article that is approved as a new drug under section 355 of this title, certified as an antibiotic under section 357 of this title, or licensed as a biologic under section 262 of Title 42, or

(ii)   an article authorized for investigation as a new drug, antibiotic, or biological for which substantial clinical investigations have been instituted and for which the existence of such investigations has been made public, which was not before such approval, certification, licensing, or authorization marketed as a dietary supplement or as a food unless the Secretary, in the Secretary's discretion, has issued a regulation, after notice and comment, finding that the article would be lawful under this chapter.

Except for purposes of paragraph (g), a dietary supplement shall be deemed to be a food within the meaning of this chapter.

(ii)   The term "compounded positron emission tomography drug"—

(1)   means a drug that—

(A)   exhibits spontaneous disintegration of unstable nuclei by the emission of positrons and is used for the purpose of providing dual photon positron emission tomographic diagnostic images; and

(B)   has been compounded by or on the order of a practitioner who is licensed by a State to compound or order compounding for a drug described in sub-paragraph (A), and is compounded in accordance with that State's law, for a patient or for research, teaching, or quality control; and (2) includes any nonradioactive reagent, reagent kit, ingredient, nuclide generator, accelerator, target material, electronic synthesizer, or other apparatus or computer program to be used in the preparation of such a drug.

(jj)   The term "antibiotic drug" means any drug (except drugs for use in animals other than humans) composed wholly or partly of any kind of penicillin, streptomycin, chlortetracycline,

chloramphenicol, bacitracin, or any other drug intended for human use containing any quantity of any chemical substance which is produced by a micro-organism and which has the capacity to inhibit or destroy micro-organisms in dilute solution (including a chemically synthesized equivalent of any such substance) or any derivative thereof.

Prohibited Acts

§ **301** [331]   The following acts and the causing thereof are prohibited:

(a)   The introduction or delivery for introduction into interstate commerce of any food, drug, device, or cosmetic that is adulterated or misbranded.

(b)   The adulteration or misbranding of any food, drug, device, or cosmetic in interstate commerce.

(c)   The receipt in interstate commerce of any food, drug, device, or cosmetic that is adulterated or misbranded, and the delivery or proffered delivery thereof for pay or otherwise.

(d)   The introduction or delivery for introduction into interstate commerce of any article in violation of section 404 or 505.

(e)   The refusal to permit access to or copying of any record as required by section 350a, 354, or 373 of this title; or the failure to establish or maintain any record, or make any report, required under section 350a, 354, 355(i) or (k), 360b(a)(4)(C), 360b(j), (l), or (m), 360e(f), or 360i of this title, or the refusal to permit access to or verification or copying of any such required record.

(f)   The refusal to permit entry or inspection as authorized by section 704.

(g)   The manufacture within any Territory of any food, drug, device, or cosmetic that is adulterated or misbranded.

(h)   The giving of a guaranty or undertaking referred to in section 333 (c) (2), which guaranty or undertaking is false, except by a person who relied upon a guaranty or undertaking to the same effect signed by, and containing the name and address of, the person residing in the United States from whom he received in good faith the food, drug, device, or cosmetic; or the giving of a guaranty or undertaking referred to in section 333 (c) (3), which guaranty or undertaking is false.

(i) (1)   Forging, counterfeiting, simulating, or falsely representing, or without proper authority using any mark, stamp, tag, label, or other identification device authorized or required by regulations promulgated under the provisions of section 404 or 721.

(2)   Making, selling, disposing of, or keeping in possession, control, or custody, or concealing any punch, die, plate, stone, or other thing designed to print, imprint, or reproduce the trademark, trade name, or other identifying mark, imprint, or device of another or any likeness of any of the foregoing upon any drug or container or labeling thereof so as to render such drugs a counterfeit drug.

(3)   The doing of any act which causes a drug to be a counterfeit drug, or the sale or dispensing, or the holding for sale or dispensing, of a counterfeit drug.

(k)   The alteration, mutilation, destruction, obliteration, or removal of the whole or any part of the labeling of, or the doing of any other act with respect to, a food, drug, device, or cosmetic, if such act is done while such article is held for sale (whether or not the first sale) after shipment in interstate commerce and results in such article being adulterated or misbranded.

(n)   The using, in labeling, advertising or other sales promotion of any reference to any report or analysis furnished in compliance with section 704.

(p)   The failure to register in accordance with section 510, the failure to provide any information required by section 510 (j) or 510 (k), or the failure to provide a notice required by section 510 (j) (2).

(t)   The importation of a drug in violation of section 801 (d) (1), the sale, purchase, or trade of a drug or drug sample or the offer to sell, purchase, or trade a drug or drug sample in violation of section 503 (c), the sale, purchase, or trade of a coupon, the offer to sell, purchase, or trade such a coupon, or the counterfeiting of such a coupon in violation of section 503 (c) (2), the distribution

of a drug sample in violation of section 503 (d) or the failure to otherwise comply with the requirements of section 503 (d), or the distribution of drugs in violation of section 503 (e) or the failure to otherwise comply with the requirements of section 503 (e).

(u)   The failure to comply with any requirements of the provisions of, or any regulations or orders of the Secretary, under section 512(a)(4)(A), 512(a)(4)(D), or 512(a)(5).

(v)   The introduction or delivery for introduction into interstate commerce of a dietary supplement that is unsafe under section 413.

Penalties

§ **303**[333]   (a) (1)   Any person who violates a provision of section 301 shall be imprisoned for not more than one year or fined not more than $1,000, or both.

(2)   Notwithstanding the provisions of paragraph (1) of this section, if any person commits such a violation after a conviction of him under this section has become final, or commits such a violation with the intent to defraud or mislead, such person shall be imprisoned for not more than three years or fined not more than $10,000, or both.

(b) (1)   Notwithstanding subsection (A), any person who violates section 301 (t) by (a) knowingly importing a drug in violation of section 801(d)(1), (B) knowingly selling, purchasing, or trading a drug or drug sample or knowingly offering to sell, purchase, or trade a drug or drug sample, in violation of section 503(c)(1), (C) knowingly selling, purchasing, or trading a coupon, knowingly offering to sell, purchase, or trade such a coupon, or knowingly counterfeiting such a coupon, in violation of section 503(c)(2), or (D) knowingly distributing drugs in violation of section 503(e)(2)(A), shall be imprisoned for not more than 10 years or fined not more than $250,000, or both.

(2)   Any manufacturer or distributor who distributes drug samples by means other than the mail or common carrier whose representative, during the course of the representative's employment or association with that manufacturer or distributor, violated section 301 (t) because of a violation of section 503 (c) (1) or violated any State law prohibiting the sale, purchase, or trade of a drug sample subject to section 503 (b) or the offer to sell, purchase, or trade such a drug sample shall, upon conviction of the representative for such violation, be subject to the following civil penalties:

(A)   A civil penalty of not more than $50,000 for each of the first two such violations resulting in a conviction of any representative of the manufacturer or distributor in any 10-year period.

(B)   A civil penalty of not more than $1,000,000 for each violation resulting in a conviction of any representative after the second conviction in any 10-year period.

For the purposes of this paragraph, multiple convictions of one or more persons arising out of the same event or transaction, or a related series of events or transactions, shall be considered as one violation.

(3)   Any manufacturer or distributor who violates section 301 (t) because of a failure to make a report required by section 503 (d) (E) shall be subject to a civil penalty of not more than $100,000.

(4) (A)   If a manufacturer or distributor or any representative of such manufacturer or distributor provides information leading to the institution of a criminal proceeding against, and conviction of, any representative of that manufacturer or distributor for a violation of section 301 (t) because of a sale, purchase, or trade or offer to purchase, sell, or trade a drug sample in violation of section 503 (c) (1) or for a violation of State law prohibiting the sale, purchase, or trade or offer to sell, purchase, or trade a drug sample, the conviction of such representative shall not be considered as a violation for purposes of paragraph (2).

(B) If, in an action brought under paragraph (2) against a manufacturer or distributor relating to the conviction of a representative of such manufacturer or distributor for the sale, purchase, or trade of a drug or the offer to sell, purchase, or trade a drug, it is shown, by clear and convincing evidence—

(i) that the manufacturer or distributor conducted, before the institution of a criminal proceeding against such representative for the violation which resulted in such conviction, an investigation of events or transactions which would have led to the reporting of information leading to the institution of a criminal proceeding against, and conviction of, such representative for such purchase, sale, or trade or offer to purchase, sell, or trade, or

(ii) that, except in the case of the conviction of a representative employed in a supervisory function, despite diligent implementation by the manufacturer or distributor of an independent audit and security system designed to detect such a violation, the manufacturer or distributor could not reasonably have been expected to have detected such violation, the conviction of such representative shall not be considered as a conviction for purposes of paragraph (2).

(5) If a person provides information leading to the institution of a criminal proceeding against, and conviction of, a person for a violation of section 301 (t) because of the sale, purchase, or trade of a drug sample or the offer to sell, purchase, or trade a drug sample in violation of section 503 (c) (1), such person shall be entitled to one-half of the criminal fine imposed and collected for such violation but not more than $125,000.

(6) Not withstanding subsection (a), any person who is a manufacturer or importer of a covered product pursuant to section 804(a) and knowingly fails to comply with a requirement of section 804(e) that is applicable to such manufacturer or importer, respectively, shall be imprisoned for not more than 10 years, or fined not more than $250,000, or both.

(c) No person shall be subject to the penalties of subsection (a) (1) of this section, (1) for having received in interstate commerce any article and delivered it or proffered delivery of it, if such delivery or proffer was made in good faith, unless he refuses to furnish on request of an officer or employee duly designated by the Secretary the name and address of the person from whom he purchased or received such article and copies of all documents, if any there be, pertaining to the delivery of the article to him; or (2) for having violated section 301 (a) or (d), if he establishes a guaranty or undertaking signed by, and containing the name and address of, the person residing in the United States from whom he received in good faith the article, to the effect, in case of an alleged violation of section 301 (a), that such article is not adulterated or misbranded, within the meaning of this Act, designating this Act, or to the effect, in case of an alleged violation of section 301 (d), that such article is not an article which may not, under the provisions of section 404 or 505, be introduced into interstate commerce; or (3) for having violated section 301 (a), where the violation exists because the article is adulterated by reason of containing a color additive not from a batch certified in accordance with regulations promulgated by the Secretary under this Act, if such person establishes a guaranty or undertaking signed by, and containing the name and address of, the manufacturer of the color additive, to the effect that such color additive was from a batch certified in accordance with the applicable regulations promulgated by the Secretary under this Act; or (4) for having violated section 301 (b), (c), or (k) by failure to comply with section 502 (f) in respect to an article received in interstate commerce to which neither section 503 (a) nor section 503 (b) (1) is applicable if the delivery or proffered delivery was made in good faith and the labeling at the time thereof contained the same directions for use and warning statements as were contained in the labeling at the time of such receipt of such article; or (5) for having violated section 301 (i) (2) if such person acted in good faith and had no reason to believe that use of the punch, die, plate, stone, or other thing involved would result in a drug being a counterfeit drug, or for having violated section 301 (i) (3) if the person doing the act or causing it to be done acted in good faith and had no reason to believe that the drug was a counterfeit drug.

Adulterated Drugs

§ **501**[351] A drug or device shall be deemed to be adulterated—

(a) (1) if it consists in whole or in part of any filthy, putrid, or decomposed substance; or (2) (A) if it has been prepared, packed, or held under insanitary conditions whereby it may have been contaminated with filth, or whereby it may have been rendered injurious to health; or (B) if it is a drug and the methods used in, or the facilities or controls used for, its manufacture, processing, packing, or holding do not conform to or are not operated or administered in conformity with current good manufacturing practice to assure that such drug meets the requirements of this Act as to safety and has the identity and strength, and meets the quality and purity characteristics, which it purports or is represented to possess; (C) if it is a compounded positron emission tomography drug and the methods used in, or the facilities and controls used for, its compounding, processing, packing, or holding do not conform to or are not operated or administered in conformity with the positron emission tomography compounding standards and the official monographs of the United States Pharmacopoeia to assure that such drug meets the requirements of this Act as to safety and has the identity and strength, and meets the quality and purity characteristics, that it purports or is represented to posses; or (3) if its container is composed, in whole or in part, of any poisonous or deleterious substance which may render the contents injurious to health; or (4) if (A) it bears or contains, for purposes of coloring only, a color additive which Is unsafe within the meaning of section 721 (a), or (B) it is a color additive the intended use of which in or on drugs or devices is for purposes of coloring only and is unsafe within the meaning of section 721 (a); or (5) if it is a new animal drug which is unsafe within the meaning of section 512; or (6) if it is an animal feed bearing or containing a new animal drug, and such feed is unsafe within the meaning of section 512.

(b) If it purports to be or is represented as a drug the name of which is recognized in an official compendium, and its strength differs from, or its quality or purity falls below, the standards set forth in such compendium. Such determination as to strength, quality, or purity shall be made in accordance with the tests or methods of assay set forth in such compendium, except that whenever tests or methods of assays have not been prescribed in such compendium, or such tests or methods of assay as are prescribed are, in the judgment of the Secretary, insufficient for the making of such determination, the Secretary shall bring such fact to the attention of the appropriate body charged with the revision of such compendium, and if such body fails within a reasonable time to prescribe tests or methods of assay which, in the judgment of the Secretary, are sufficient for purposes of this paragraph, then the Secretary shall promulgate regulations prescribing appropriate tests or methods of assay in accordance with which such determination as to strength, quality, or purity shall be made. No drug defined in an official compendium shall be deemed to be adulterated under this paragraph because it differs from the standard of strength, quality, or purity therefor set forth in such compendium, if its difference in strength, quality, or purity from such standards is plainly stated on its label. Whenever a drug is recognized in both the United States Pharmacopeia and the Homeopathic Pharmacopeia of the United States it shall be subject to the requirements of the United States Pharmacopeia unless it is labeled and offered for sale as a homeopathic drug, in which case it shall be subject to the provisions of the Homeopathic Pharmacopeia of the United States and not to those of the United States Pharmacopeia.

(c) If it is not subject to the provisions of paragraph (b) of this section and its strength differs from, or its purity or quality falls below, that which it purports or is represented to possess.

(d) If it is a drug and any substance has been (1) mixed or packed therewith so as to reduce its quality or strength or (2) substituted wholly or in part therefor.

Misbranded Drugs

§ **502**[352]   A drug or device shall be deemed to be misbranded—

(a)   If its labeling is false or misleading in any particular. Health care economic information provided to a formulary committee, or other similar entity, in the course of the committee or the entity carrying out its responsibilities for the selection of drugs for managed care or other similar organizations, shall not be considered to be false or misleading under this paragraph if the health care economic information directly relates to an indication approved under section 505 or under section 351(a) of the Public Health Service Act for such drug and is based on competent and reliable scientific evidence. The requirements set forth in section 505(a) or in section 351(a) of the Public Health Service Act shall not apply to health care economic information provided to such a committee or entity in accordance with the paragraph. Information that is relevant to the substantiation of the health care economic information presented pursuant to this paragraph shall be made available to the Secretary upon request. In this paragraph, the term "health care economic information" means any analysis that identifies, measures, or compares the economic consequences, including the costs of the represented health outcomes, of the use of a drug to the use of another drug, to another health care intervention, or to no intervention.

(b)   If in package form unless it bears a label containing (1) the name and place of business of the manufacturer, packer, or distributor; and (2) an accurate statement of the quantity of the contents in terms of weight, measure, or numerical count: *Provided*, That under clause (2) of this paragraph reasonable variations shall be permitted, and exemptions as to small packages shall be established, by regulations prescribed by the Secretary.

(c)   If any word, statement, or other information required by or under authority of this Act to appear on the label or labeling is not prominently placed thereon with such conspicuousness (as compared with other words, statements, designs, or devices, in the labeling) and in such terms as to render it likely to be read and understood by the ordinary individual under customary conditions of purchase and use.

(e) (1) (A)   If it is a drug, unless its label bears, to the exclusion of any other nonproprietary name (except the applicable systematic chemical name or the chemical formula)—

(i)   the established name (as defined in sunparagraph (3)) of the drug, if there is such a name;

(ii)   the established name and quantity or, if determined to be appropriate by the Secretary, the proportion of each active ingredient, including the quantity, kind, and proportion of any alcohol, and also including whether active or not the established name and quantity or if determined to be appropriate by the Secretary, the proportion of any bromides, ether, chloroform, acetanilide, acetophenetidin, amidopyrine, antipyrine, atropine, hyoscine, hyoscyamine, arsenic, digitalis, digitalis glucosides, mercury, ouabain, strophanthin, strychnine, thyroid, or any derivative or preparation of any such substances, contained therein, except that the requirement for stating the quantity of the active ingredients, other than the quantity of those specifically named in this subclause, shall not apply to nonprescription drugs not intended for human use; and

(iii)   the established name of each inactive ingredient listed in alphabetical order on the outside container of the retail package and, if determined to be appropriate by the Secretary, on the immediate container, as prescribed in regulation promulgated by the Secretary, except that nothing in this subclause shall be deemed to require that any trade secret be divulged, and except that the requirements of this subclause with respect to alphabetical order shall apply only to nonprescription drugs that are not also cosmetics and that this subclause shall not apply to nonprescription drugs not intended for human use.

(B)   For any prescription drug the established name of such drug or ingredient, as the case may be, on such label (and on any labeling on which a name for such drug or ingredient is used) shall be printed prominently and in type at least half as large as that used thereon for any proprietary name or designation for such drug or ingredient, except that to the extent that compliance with the requirements of subclause (ii) or (iii) of clause (A) or this clause is impracticable, exemptions shall be established by regulations promulgated by the Secretary.

(2)   If it is a device and it has an established name, unless its label bears, to the exclusion of any other nonproprietary name, its established name (as defined in sub-paragraph (4)) prominently printed in type at least half as large as that used thereon for any proprietary name or designation for such device, except that to the extent compliance with the requirements of this sub-paragraph is impracticable, exemptions shall be established by regulations promulgated by the Secretary.

(3)   As used in paragraph (l) the term "established name," with respect to a drug or ingredient thereof, means (A) the applicable official name designated pursuant to section 508, or (B) if there is no such name and such drug, or such ingredient, is an article recognized in an official compendium, then the official title thereof in such compendium, or (C) if neither clause (A) nor clause (B) of this sub-paragraph applies, then the common or usual name, if any, of such drug or of such ingredient: except that where clause (B) of this sub-paragraph applies to an article recognized in the United States Pharmacopeia and in the Homeopathic Pharmacopeia under different official titles, the official title used in the United States Pharmacopeia shall apply unless it is labeled and offered for sale as a homeopathic drug, in which case the official title used in the Homeopathic Pharmacopeia shall apply.

(f)   Unless its labeling bears (1) adequate directions for use; and (2) such adequate warnings against use in those pathological conditions or by children where its use may be dangerous to health, or against unsafe dosage or methods or duration of administration or application, in such manner and form, as are necessary for the protection of users, except that where any requirement of clause (1) of this paragraph, as applied to any drug or device, is not necessary for the protection of the public health, the Secretary shall promulgate regulations exempting such drug or device from such requirement.

(g)   If it purports to be a drug the name of which is recognized in an official compendium, unless it is packaged and labeled as prescribed therein. The method of packing may be modified with the consent of the Secretary. Whenever a drug is recognized in both the United States Pharmacopeia and the Homeopathic Pharmacopeia of the United States, it shall be subject to the requirements of the United States Pharmacopeia with respect to packaging, and labeling unless it is labeled and offered for sale as a homeopathic drug, in which case it shall be subject to the provisions of the Homeopathic Pharmacopeia of the United States, and not to those of the United States Pharmacopeia, except that in the event of inconsistency between the requirements of this paragraph and those of paragraph (e) as to the name by which the drug or its ingredients shall be designated, the requirements of paragraph (e) shall prevail.

(h)   If it has been found by the Secretary to be a drug liable to deterioration, unless it is packaged in such form and manner, and its label bears a statement of such precautions, as the Secretary shall by regulations require as necessary for the protection of the public health. No such regulation shall be established for any drug recognized in an official compendium until the Secretary shall have informed the appropriate body charged with the revision of such compendium of the need for such packaging or labeling requirements and such body shall have failed within a reasonable time to prescribe such requirements.

(i) (1)   If it is a drug and its container is so made, formed, or filled as to be misleading; or (2) if it is an imitation of another drug; or (3) if it is offered for sale under the name of another drug.

(j)   If it is dangerous to health when used in the dosage or manner, or with the frequency or duration prescribed, recommended, or suggested in the labeling thereof.

(m)   If it is a color additive the intended use of which is for the purpose of coloring only, unless its packaging and labeling are in conformity with such packaging and labeling requirements applicable to such color additive, as may be contained in regulations issued under section 721.

(n)   In the case of any prescription drug distributed or offered for sale in any State, unless the manufacturer, packer, or distributor thereof includes in all advertisements and other descriptive printed matter issued or caused to be issued by the manufacturer, packer, or distributor with respect to that drug a true statement of (1) the established name as defined in paragraph (e), printed prominently and in type at least half as large as that used for any trade or brand name thereof, (2) the formula showing quantitatively each ingredient of such drug to the extent required for labels under paragraph (e), and (3) such other information in brief summary relating to side effects, contraindications, and effectiveness as shall be required in regulations which shall be issued by the Secretary in accordance with the procedure specified in section 701 (e) of this Act: except that (A) except in extraordinary circumstances, no regulation issued under this paragraph shall require prior approval by the Secretary of the content of any advertisement, and (B) no advertisement of a prescription drug, published after the effective date of regulations issued under this paragraph applicable to advertisements of prescription drugs, shall, with respect to the matters specified in this paragraph or covered by such regulations, be subject to the provisions of sections 12 through 17 of the Federal Trade Commission Act, as amended (15 U.S.C. 52-57). This paragraph (n) shall not be applicable to any printed matter which the Secretary determines to be labeling as defined in section 201 (m) of this Act. Nothing in the Convention on Psychotropic Substances, signed at Vienna, Austria, on February 21, 1971, shall be construed to prevent drug price communications to consumers.

(o)   If it was manufactured, prepared, propagated, compounded, or processed in an establishment in any State not duly registered under section 510, if it was not included in a list required by section 510 (j), if a notice or other information respecting it was not provided as required by such section or section 510 (k), or if it does not bear such symbols from the uniform system for identification of devices prescribed under section 510 (e) as the Secretary by regulation requires.

(p)   If it is a drug and its packaging or labeling is in violation of an applicable regulation issued pursuant to section 3 or 4 of the Poison Prevention Packing Act of 1970.

Exemptions in Case of Drugs

§ **503**[353]   (a)   The Secretary is hereby directed to promulgate regulations exempting from any labeling or packaging requirement of this Act drugs and devices which are, in accordance with the practice of the trade, to be processed, labeled, or repacked in substantial quantities at establishments other than those where originally processed or packed, on condition that such drugs and devices are not adulterated or misbranded under the provisions of this Act upon removal from such processing, labeling, or repacking establishment.

(b) (1)   A drug intended for use by man which—

(A)   because of its toxicity or other potentiality for harmful effect, or the method of its use, or the collateral measures necessary to its use, is not safe for use except under the supervision of a practitioner licensed by law to administer such drug; or

(B)   is limited by an approved application under section 505 to use under the professional supervision of a practitioner licensed by law to administer such drug; shall be dispensed only (i) upon a written prescription of a practitioner licensed by law to administer such drug, or (ii) upon an oral prescription of such practitioner which is reduced promptly to writing and filed by the pharmacist, or (iii) by refilling any such written or oral prescription if such refilling is authorized by the prescriber either in the original prescription or by oral order which is reduced promptly to writing and filed by the pharmacist. The act of dispensing a drug contrary to the provisions of this paragraph shall be deemed to be an act which results in the drug being misbranded while held for sale.

(2)   Any drug dispensed by filling or refilling a written or oral prescription of a practitioner licensed by law to administer such drug shall be exempt from the requirements of section 502, ex-

cept paragraphs (a), (i) (2) and (3), (k), and (l), and the packaging requirements of paragraphs (g), (h), and (p), if the drug bears a label containing the name and address of the dispenser, the serial number and date of the prescription or of its filling, the name of the prescriber, and, if stated in the prescription, the name of the patient, and the directions for use and cautionary statements, if any, contained in such prescription. This exemption shall not apply to any drug dispensed in the course of the conduct of a business of dispensing drugs pursuant to diagnosis by mail, or to a drug dispensed in violation of paragraph (1) of this subsection.

(3)   The Secretary may by regulation remove drugs subject to section 505 from the requirements of paragraph (1) of this subsection when such requirements are not necessary for the protection of the public health.

(4) (A)   A drug that is subject to paragraph (1) shall be deemed to be misbranded if at any time prior to dispensing the label of the drug fails to bear, at a minimum, the symbol "Rx only.

(B)   A drug to which paragraph (1) does not apply shall be deemed to be misbranded if at any time prior to dispensing the label of the drug bears the symbol described in sub-paragraph (A).

(5)   Nothing in this subsection shall be construed to relieve any person from any requirement prescribed by or under authority of law with respect to drugs now included or which may hereafter be included within the classifications stated in section 3220 of the Internal Revenue Code (26 U.S.C. 3220), or to marijuana as defined in section 3238 (b) of the Internal Revenue Code (26 U.S.C. 3238 (b)).

(c) (1)   No person may sell, purchase, or trade or offer to sell, purchase, or trade any drug sample. For purpose of this paragraph and subsection (d), the term 'drug sample' means a unit of a drug, subject to subsection (b), which is not intended to be sold and is intended to promote the sale of the drug. Nothing in this paragraph shall subject an officer or executive of a drug manufacturer or distributor to criminal liability solely because of a sale, purchase, trade, or offer to sell, purchase, or trade in violation of this paragraph by other employees of the manufacturer or distributor.

(2)   No person may sell, purchase, or trade, offer to sell, purchase, or trade, or counterfeit any coupon. For purposes of this paragraph, the term 'coupon' means a form which may be redeemed, at no cost or at a reduced cost, for a drug which is prescribed in accordance with subsection (b).

(3) (A)   No person may sell, purchase, or trade, or offer to sell, purchase, or trade, any drug—

(i)   which is subject to subsection (b), and

(ii) (I)   which was purchased by a public or private hospital or other health care entity, or

(II)   which was donated or supplied at a reduced price to a charitable organization described in section 501 (c) (3) of the Internal Revenue Code of 1954.

(B)   Subparagraph (A) does not apply to—

(i)   the purchase or other acquisition by a hospital or other health care entity which is a member of a group purchasing organization of a drug for its own use from the group purchasing organization or from other hospitals or health care entities which are members of such organization,

(ii)   the sale, purchase, or trade of a drug or an offer to sell, purchase, or trade a drug by an organization described in sub-paragraph (A) (ii) (II) to a nonprofit affiliate of the organization to the extent otherwise permitted by law,

(iii)   a sale, purchase, or trade of a drug or an offer to sell, purchase, or trade a drug among hospitals or other health care entities which are under common control,

(iv)   a sale, purchase, or trade of a drug or an offer to sell, purchase, or trade a drug for emergency medical reasons, or

(v)   a sale, purchase, or trade of a drug, an offer to sell, purchase, or trade a drug, or the dispensing of a drug pursuant to a prescription executed in accordance with subsection (b).

For purposes of this paragraph, the term 'entity' does not include a wholesale distributor of drugs or a retail pharmacy licensed under State law and the term 'emergency medical reasons' includes transfers of a drug between health care entities

or from a health care entity to a retail pharmacy undertaken to alleviate temporary shortages of the drug arising from delays in or interruptions of regular distribution schedules.

(d) (1)   Except as provided in paragraphs (2) and (3), no person may distribute any drug sample. For purposes of this subsection, the term "distribute" does not include the providing of a drug sample to patient by a—

(A)   practitioner licensed to prescribe such drug,

(B)   health care professional acting at the direction and under the supervision of such a practitioner or

(C)   pharmacy of a hospital or of another health care entity that is acting at the direction of such a practitioner and that received such sample pursuant to paragraph (2) or (3).

(2) (A)   The manufacturer or authorized distributor of record of a drug subject to subsection (b) may, in accordance with this paragraph, distribute drug samples by mail or common carrier to practitioners licensed to prescribe such drugs, or, at the request of a licensed practitioner, to pharmacies of hospitals or other health care entities. Such a distribution of drug samples may only be made—

(i)   in response to a written request for drug samples made on a form which meets the requirements of sub-paragraph (B), and

(ii)   under a system which requires the recipient of the drug sample to execute a written receipt for the drug sample upon its delivery and the return of the receipt to the manufacturer or authorized distributor of record.

(B)   A written request for a drug sample required by sub-paragraph (A) (i) shall contain—

(i)   the name, address, professional designation, and signature of the practitioner making the request,

(ii)   the identity of the drug sample requested and the quantity requested,

(iii)   the name of the manufacturer of the drug sample requested, and

(iv)   the date of the request.

(C)   Each drug manufacturer or authorized distributor of record which makes distributions by mail or common carrier under this paragraph shall maintain, for a period of 3 years, the request forms submitted for such distributions and the receipts submitted for such distributions and shall maintain a record of distributions of drug samples which identifies the drugs distributed and the recipients of the distributions. Forms, receipts, and records required to be maintained under this sub-paragraph shall be made available by the drug manufacturer or authorized distributor to Federal and State officials engaged in the regulation of drugs and in the enforcement of laws applicable to drugs.

(3)   The manufacturer or authorized distributor of record of a drug subject to subsection (b) may, by means other than mail or common carrier, distribute drug samples only if the manufacturer or authorized distributor of record makes the distributions in accordance with sub-paragraph (A) and carries out the activities described in inline-paragraphs (B) through (F) as follows:

(A)   Drug samples may only be distributed—

(i)   to practitioners licensed to prescribe such drugs if they make a written request for the drug samples, or

(ii)   at the written request of such a licensed practitioner, to pharmacies of hospitals or other health care entities.

A written request for drug samples shall be made on a form which contains the practitioner's name, address, and professional designation, the identity of the drug sample requested, the quantity of drug samples requested, the name of the manufacturer or authorized distributor of record of the drug sample, the date of the request and signature of the practitioner making the request.

(B)   Drug manufacturers or authorized distributors of record shall store drug samples under conditions that will maintain their stability, integrity, and effectiveness and will assure that the drug samples will be free of contamination, deterioration, and adulteration.

(C)   Drug manufacturers or authorized distributors of record shall conduct, at least annually, a complete and accurate inventory of all drug samples in the possession of representatives of the manufacturer or authorized distributor of record. Drug manufacturers or authorized distributors of record shall maintain lists of the names and address of each of their representatives who distribute drug samples and of the sites where drug samples are stored. Drug manufacturers or authorized distributors of record shall maintain records for at least 3 years of all drug samples distributed, destroyed, or returned to the manufacturer or authorized distributor of record, of all inventories maintained under this sub-paragraph, of all thefts or significant losses of drug samples, and of all requests made under sub-paragraph (A) for drug samples. Records and lists maintained under this sub-paragraph shall be made available by the drug manufacturer or authorized distributor of record to the Secretary upon request.

(D)   Drug manufacturers or authorized distributors of record shall notify the Secretary of any significant loss of drug samples and any known theft of drug samples.

(E)   Drug manufacturers or authorized distributors of record shall report to the Secretary any conviction of their representatives for violations of subsection (c) (1) or a State law because of the sale, purchase, or trade of a drug sample or the offer to sell, purchase, or trade a drug sample.

(F)   Drug manufacturers or authorized distributors of record shall provide to the Secretary the name and telephone number of the individual responsible for responding to a request for information respecting drug samples.

(e) (1) (A)   Each person who is engaged in the wholesale distribution of a drug subject to subsection (b) and who is not the manufacturer or an authorized distributor of record of such drug shall, before each wholesale distribution of such drug (including each distribution to an authorized distributor of record or to a retail pharmacy), provide to the person who receives the drug a statement (in such form and containing such information as the Secretary may require) identifying each prior sale, purchase, or trade of such drug (including the date of the transaction and the names and addresses of all parties to the transaction).

(B)   Each manufacturer of a drug subject to subsection (b) shall maintain at its corporate offices a current list of the authorized distributors of record of such drug.

(2) (A)   No person may engage in the wholesale distribution in interstate commerce of drugs subject to subsection (b) in a State unless such person is licensed by the State in accordance with the guidelines issued under sub-paragraph (B).

(B)   The Secretary shall by regulation issue guidelines establishing minimum standards, terms, and conditions for the licensing of persons to make wholesale distributions in interstate commerce of drugs subject to subsection (b). Such guidelines shall prescribe requirements for the storage and handling of such drugs and for the establishment and maintenance of records of the distributions of such drugs.

New Drugs

§ 505[355]   (a)   No person shall introduce or deliver for introduction into interstate commerce any new drug, unless an approval of an application filed pursuant to subsection (b) or (j) is effective with respect to such drug.

(b) (1)   Any person may file with the Secretary an application with respect to any drug subject to the provisions of subsection (a). Such persons shall submit to the Secretary as a part of the application (A) full reports of investigations which have been made to show whether or not such drug is safe for use and whether such drug is effective in use; (B) a full list of the articles used as components of such drug; (C) a full statement of the composition of such drug; (D) a full description of the methods used in, and the facilities and controls used for, the manufacture, processing, and packing of such drug; (E) such samples of such drug and of the articles used as components thereof as the Secretary may require; and (F) specimens of the labeling proposed to be used for such drug. The applicant shall file with the application the patent number and the expiration date of any patent which claims the drug for which the applicant submitted the application or which claims a method of using such drug and with respect to which a claim of patent infringement could reasonably be as-

serted if a person not licensed by the owner engaged in the manufacture, use, or sale of the drug. If an application is filed under this subsection for a drug and a patent which claims such drug or a method of using such drug is issued after the filing date but before approval of the application, the applicant shall amend the application to include the information required by the preceding sentence. Upon approval of the application, the Secretary shall publish information submitted under the two preceding sentences. The Secretary shall, inconsultation with the Director of the National Institutes of Health and with representatives of the drug manufacturering industry, review and develop guidance, as appropriate, on the inclusion of women and minorities in clinical trials required by clause (A).

(2) An application submitted under paragraph (1) for a drug for which the investigations described in clause (A) of such paragraph and relied upon by the applicant for approval of the application were not conducted by or for the applicant and for which the applicant has not obtained a right of reference or use from the person by or for whom the investigations were conducted shall also include—

(A) a certification, in the opinion of the applicant and to the best of his knowledge, with respect to each patent which claims the drug for which such investigations were conducted or which claims a use for such drug for which the applicant is seeking approval under this subsection and for which information is required to be filed under paragraph (1) or subsection (c)—

(i)   that such patent information has not been filed,

(ii)   that such patent has expired,

(iii)   of the date on which such patent will expire, or

(iv)   that such patent is invalid or will not be infringed by the manufacture, use, or sale of the new drug for which the application is submitted; and

(B) if with respect to the drug for which investigations described in paragraph (1) (A) were conducted information was filed under paragraph (1) or subsection (c) for a method of use patent which does not claim a use for which the applicant is seeking approval under this subsection, a statement that the method of use patent does not claim such a use.

(3) (A) An applicant who makes a certification described in paragraph (2) (A) (iv) shall include in the application a statement that the applicant will give the notice required by sub-paragraph (B) to—

(i)   each owner of the patent which is the subject of the certification or the representative of such owner designated to receive such notice, and

(ii)   the holder of the approved application under subsection (b) for the drug which is claimed by the patent or a use of which is claimed by the patent or the representative of such holder designated to receive such notice.

(B) The notice referred to in sub-paragraph (A) shall state that an application has been submitted under this subsection for the drug with respect to which the certification is made to obtain approval to engage in the commercial manufacture, use, or sale of the drug before the expiration of the patent referred to in the certification. Such notice shall include a detailed statement of the factual and legal basis of the applicant's opinion that the patent is not valid or will not be infringed.

(C) If an application is amended to include a certification described in paragraph (2) (A) (iv), the notice required by sub-paragraph (B) shall be given when the amended application is submitted.

(4) (A) The Secretary shall issue guidance for the individuals who review applications submitted under paragraph (1) or under section 351 of the Public Health Service Act, which shall relate to promptness in conducting the review, technical excellence, lack of bias and conflict of interest, and knowledge of regulatory and scientific standards, and which shall apply equally to all individuals who review such applications.

(B) The Secretary shall meet with a sponsor of an investigation or an applicant for approval for a drug under this subsection or section 351 of the Public Health Service Act if the sponsor or applicant makes a reasonable written request for a meeting for the purpose of reaching agreement on the design and size of clinical trials intended to form the primary basis of an effectiveness claim. The sponsor or applicant shall provide information necessary for discussion and agreement on the design and size of the clinical trials. Minutes of any such meeting shall be prepared by the Secretary and made available to the sponsor or applicant upon request.

(C) Any agreement regarding the parameters of the design and size of clinical trials of a new drug under this paragraph that is reached between the Secretary and a sponsor or applicant shall be reduced to writing and made part of the administrative record by the Secretary. Such agreement shall not be changed after the testing begins, except—

(i)   with the written agreement of the sponsor or applicant; or

(ii)   pursuant to a decision, made in accordance with sub-paragraph (D) by the director of the reviewing division, that a substantial scientific issue essential to determining the safety or effectiveness of the drug has been identified after the testing has begun.

(D) A decision under sub-paragraph (C)(ii) by the director shall be in writing and the Secretary shall provide to the sponsor or applicant an opportunity for a meeting at which the director and the sponsor or applicant will be present and at which the director will document the scientific issue involved.

(E) The written decisions of the reviewing division shall be binding upon, and may not directly or indirectly be changed by, the field or compliance division personnel unless such field or compliance division personnel demonstrate to the reviewing division why such decision should be modified.

(F) No action by the reviewing division may be delayed because of the unavailability of information from or action by field personnel unless the reviewing division determines that a delay is necessary to assure the marketing of a safe and effective drug.

(G) For purposes of this paragraph, the reviewing division is the division responsible for the review of an application for approval of a drug under this subsection or section 351 of the Public Health Service Act (including all scientific and medical matters, chemistry manufacturing, and controls).

(c) (1) Within one hundred and eighty days after the filing of an application under subsection (b), or such additional period as may be agreed upon by the Secretary and the applicant, the Secretary shall either—

(A) Approve the application if he then finds that none of the grounds for denying approval specified in subsection (d) applies, or

(B) Give the applicant notice of an opportunity for a hearing before the Secretary under subsection (d) on the question whether such application is approvable. If the applicant elects to accept the opportunity for hearing by written request within thirty days after such notice, such hearing shall commence not more than ninety days after the expiration of such thirty days unless the Secretary and the applicant otherwise agree. Any such hearing shall thereafter be conducted on an expedited basis and the Secretary's order thereon shall be issued within ninety days after the date fixed by the Secretary for filing final briefs.

(2) If the patent information described in subsection (b) could not be filed with the submission of an application under subsection (b) because the application was filed before the patent information was required under subsection (b) or a patent was issued after the application was approved under such subsection, the holder of an approved application shall file with the Secretary the patent number and the expiration date of any patent which claims the drug for which the application was submitted or which claims a method of using such drug and with respect to which a claim of patent infringement could reasonably be asserted if a person not licensed by the owner engaged in the manufacture, use, or sale of the drug. If the holder of an approved application could not file patent information under subsection (b) because it was not required at the time the application was approved, the holder shall file such information under this subsection not later than thirty days after the date of the enactment of this sentence, and if the holder of an approved application could not file patent information under subsection (b) because no patent had been issued when an application was filed or approved, the holder shall file such information under this subsection not later than thirty

days after the date the patent involved is issued. Upon the submission of patent information under this subsection, the Secretary shall publish it.

(3)   The approval of an application filed under subsection (b) which contains a certification required by paragraph (2) of such subsection shall be made effective on the last applicable date determined under the following:

(A)   If the applicant only made a certification described in clause (i) or (ii) of subsection (b) (2) (A) or in both such clauses, the approval may be made effective immediately.

(B)   If the applicant made a certification described in clause (iii) of subsection (b) (2) (A), the approval may be made effective on the date certified under clause (iii).

(C)   If the applicant made a certification described in clause (iv) of subsection (b) (2) (A), the approval shall be made effective immediately unless an action is brought for infringement of a patent which is the subject of the certification before the expiration of forty-five days from the date the notice provided under paragraph (3) (B) is received. If such an action is brought before the expiration of such days, the approval may be made effective upon the expiration of the thirty-month period beginning on the date of the receipt of the notice provided under paragraph (3) (B) or such shorter or longer period as the court may order because either party to the action failed to reasonably cooperate in expediting the action, except that—

(i)   if before the expiration of such period the court decides that such patent is invalid or not infringed, the approval may be made effective on the date of the court decision,

(ii)   if before the expiration of such period the court decides that such patent has been infringed, the approval may be made effective on such date as the court orders under section 271 (e) (4) (A) of title 35, United States Code, or

(iii)   if before the expiration of such period the court grants a preliminary injunction prohibiting the applicant from engaging in the commercial manufacture or sale of the drug until the court decides the issues of patent validity and infringement and if the court decides that such patent is invalid or not infringed, the approval shall be made effective on the date of such court decision.

In such an action, each of the parties shall reasonably cooperate in expediting the action. Until the expiration of forty-five days from the date the notice made under paragraph (3) (B) is received, no action may be brought under section 2201 of title 28, United States Code, for a declaratory judgment with respect to the patent. Any action brought under such section 2201 shall be brought in the judicial district where the defendent has its principal place of business or a regular and established place of business.

(D) (i)   If an application (other than an abbreviated new drug application) submitted under subsection (b) for a drug, no active ingredient (including any ester or salt of the active ingredient) of which has been approved in any other application under subsection (b), was approved during the period beginning January 1, 1982, and ending on September 24, 1984, the Secretary may not make the approval of another application for a drug for which the investigations described in clause (A) of subsection (b) (1) and relied upon by the applicant for approval of the application were not conducted by or for the applicant and for which the applicant has not obtained a right of reference or use from the person by or for whom the investigations were conducted effective before the expiration of ten years from the date of the approval of the application previously approved under subsection (b).

(ii)   If an application submitted under subsection (b) for a drug, no active ingredient (including any ester or salt of the active ingredient) of which has been approved in any other application under subsection (b), is approved after September 24, 1984, no application which refers to the drug for which the subsection (b) application was submitted and for which the investigations described in clause (A) of subsection (b) (1) and relied upon by the applicant for approval of the application were not conducted by or for the applicant and for which the applicant has not obtained a right of reference or use from the person by or for whom the investigations were conducted may be submitted under subsection (b) before the expiration of five years from the date of the approval of the application under subsection (b), except that such an application may be submitted under subsection (b) after the

expiration of four years from the date of the approval of the subsection (b) application if it contains a certification of patent invalidity or noninfringement described in clause (iv) of subsection (b) (2) (A). The approval of such an application shall be made effective in accordance with this paragraph except that, if an action for patent infringement is commenced during the one-year period beginning forty-eight months after the date of the approval of the subsection (b) application, the thirty-month period referred to in sub-paragraph (C) shall be extended by such amount of time (if any) which is required for seven and one-half years to have elapsed from the date of approval of the subsection (b) application.

(iii)   If an application submitted under subsection (b) for a drug, which includes an active ingredient (including any ester or salt of the active ingredient) that has been approved in another application approved under subsection (b), is approved after September 24, 1984 and if such application contains reports of new clinical investigations (other than bioavailability studies) essential to the approval of the application and conducted or sponsored by the applicant, the Secretary may not make the approval of an application submitted under subsection (b) for the conditions of approval of such drug in the approved subsection (b) application effective before the expiration of three years from the date of the approval of the application under subsection (b) if the investigations described in clause (A) of subsection (b) (1) and relied upon by the applicant for approval of the application were not conducted by or for the applicant and if the applicant has not obtained a right of reference or use from the person by or for whom the investigations were conducted.

(iv)   If a supplement to an application approved under subsection (b) is approved after September 24, 1984 and the supplement contains reports of new clinical investigations (other than bioavailability studies) essential to the approval of the supplement and conducted or sponsored by the person submitting the supplement, the Secretary may not make the approval of an application submitted under subsection (b) for a change approved in the supplement effective before the expiration of three years from the date of the approval of the supplement under subsection (b) if the investigations described in clause (A) of subsection (b) (1) and relied upon by the applicant for approval of the application were not conducted by or for the applicant and if the applicant has not obtained a right of reference or use from the person by or for whom the investigations were conducted.

(v)   If an application (or supplement to an application) submitted under subsection (b) for a drug, which includes an active ingredient (including any ester or salt of the active ingredient) that has been approved in another application under subsection (b), was approved during the period beginning January 1, 1982, and ending on September 24, 1984, the Secretary may not make the approval of an application submitted under this subsection and for which the investigations described in clause (A) of subsection (b) (1) and relied upon by the applicant for approval of the application were not conducted by or for the applicant and for which the applicant has not obtained a right of reference or use from the person by or for whom the investigations were conducted and which refers to the drug for which the subsection (b) application was submitted effective before the expiration of two years from September 24, 1984.

(4)   A drug manufactured in a pilot or other small facility may be used to demonstrate the safety and effectiveness of the drug and to obtain approval for the drug prior to manufacture of the drug in a larger facility, unless the Secretary makes a determination that a full scale production facility is necessary to ensure the safety or effectiveness of the drug.

(d)   If the Secretary finds, after due notice to the applicant in accordance with subsection (c) and giving him an opportunity for a hearing, in accordance with said subsection, that (1) the investigations, reports of which are required to be submitted to the Secretary pursuant to subsection (b), do not include adequate tests by all methods reasonably applicable to show whether or not such drug is safe for use under the conditions prescribed, recommended, or suggested in the proposed labeling thereof; (2) the results of such tests show that such drug is unsafe for use under such conditions or do not show that such drug is safe for use un-

der such conditions; (3) the methods used in, and the facilities and controls used for, the manufacture, processing, and packing of such drug are inadequate to preserve its identity, strength, quality, and purity; (4) upon the basis of the information submitted to him as part of the application, or upon the basis of any other information before him with respect to such drug, he has insufficient information to determine whether such drug is safe for use under such conditions; or (5) evaluated on the basis of the information submitted to him as part of the application and any other information before him with respect to such drug, there is a lack of substantial evidence that the drug will have the effect it purports or is represented to have under the conditions of use prescribed, recommended, or suggested in the proposed labeling thereof; or

(6) the application failed to contain the patent information prescribed by subsection (b); or

(7) based on a fair evaluation of all material facts, such labeling is false or misleading in any particular; he shall issue an order refusing to approve the application. If, after such notice and opportunity for hearing, the Secretary finds that clauses (1) through (6) do not apply, he shall issue an order approving the application. As used in this subsection and subsection (e), the term "substantial evidence" means evidence consisting of adequate and well-controlled investigations, including clinical investigations, by experts qualified by scientific training and experience to evaluate the effectiveness of the drug involved, on the basis of which it could fairly and responsibly be concluded by such experts that the drug will have the effect it purports or is represented to have under the conditions of use prescribed, recommended, or suggested in the labeling or proposed labeling thereof. If the Secretary determines based on relevant science, that data from one adequate and well controlled clinical investigation and confirmatory evidence (obtained prior to or after such investigation) are sufficient to establish effectiveness, the Secretary may consider such data and evidence to constitute substantial evidence for purposes of the preceeding sentence.

(e) The Secretary shall, after due notice and opportunity for hearing to the applicant, withdraw approval of an application with respect to any drug under this section if the Secretary finds (1) that clinical or other experience, tests, or other scientific data show that such drug is unsafe for use under the conditions of use upon the basis of which the application was approved; (2) that new evidence of clinical experience, not contained in such application or not available to the Secretary until after such application was approved, or tests by new methods, or tests by methods not deemed reasonably applicable when such application was approved, evaluated together with the evidence available to the Secretary when the application was approved, shows that such drug is not shown to be safe for use under the conditions of use upon the basis of which the application was approved; or (3) on the basis of new information before him with respect to such drug, evaluated together with the evidence available to him when the application was approved, that there is a lack of substantial evidence that the drug will have the effect it purports or is represented to have under the conditions of use prescribed, recommended, or suggested in the labeling thereof; or

(4) the patent information prescribed by subsection (c) was not filed within thirty days after the receipt of written notice from the Secretary specifying the failure to file such information; or

(5) that the application contains any untrue statement of a material fact: *Provided,* That if the Secretary (or in his absence the officer acting as Secretary) finds that there is an imminent hazard to the public health, he may suspend the approval of such application immediately, and give the applicant prompt notice of his action and afford the applicant the opportunity for an expedited hearing under this subsection; but the authority conferred by this proviso to suspend the approval of an application shall not be delegated. The Secretary may also, after due notice and opportunity for hearing to the applicant, withdraw the approval of an application submitted under subsection (b) or (j) with respect to any drug under this section if the Secretary finds (1) that the applicant has failed to establish a system for maintaining required records, or has repeatedly or deliberately failed to maintain such records or to make required reports, in accordance with a regulation or order under subsection (k) or to comply with the notice re-

quirements of section 510 (k) (2), or the applicant has refused to permit access to, or copying or verification of, such records as required by paragraph (2) of such subsection; or (2) that on the basis of new information before him, evaluated together with the evidence before him when the application was approved, the methods used in, or the facilities and controls used for, the manufacture, processing, and packing of such drug are inadequate to assure and preserve its identity, strength, quality, and purity and were not made adequate within a reasonable time after receipt of written notice from the Secretary specifying the matter complained of; or (3) that on the basis of new information before him, evaluated together with the evidence before him when the application was approved, the labeling of such drug, based on a fair evaluation of all material facts, is false or misleading in any particular and was not corrected within a reasonable time after receipt of written notice from the Secretary specifying the matter complained of. Any order under this subsection shall state the findings upon which it is based.

(f) Whenever the Secretary finds that the facts so require, he shall revoke any previous order under subsection (d) or (e) refusing, withdrawing, or suspending approval of an application and shall approve such application or reinstate such approval, as may be appropriate.

(g) Orders of the Secretary issued under this section shall be served (1) in person by any officer or employee of the Department designated by the Secretary or (2) by mailing the order by registered mail or by certified mail addressed to the applicant or respondent at his last-known address in the records of the Secretary.

(h) An appeal may be taken by the applicant from an order of the Secretary refusing or withdrawing approval of an application under this section. Such appeal shall be taken by filing in the United States court of appeals for the circuit wherein such applicant resides or has his principal place of business, or in the United States Court of Appeals for the District of Columbia Circuit, within sixty days after the entry of such order, a written petition praying that the order of the Secretary be set aside. A copy of such petition shall be forthwith transmitted by the clerk of the court to the Secretary, or any officer designated by him for that purpose, and thereupon the Secretary shall certify and file in the court the record upon which the order complained of was entered, as provided in section 2112 of title 28, United States Code. Upon the filing of such petition such court shall have exclusive jurisdiction to affirm or set aside such order, except that until the filing of the record the Secretary may modify or set aside his order. No objection to the order of the Secretary shall be considered by the court unless such objection shall have been urged before the Secretary or unless there were reasonable grounds for failure so to do. The finding of the Secretary as to the facts, if supported by substantial evidence, shall be conclusive. If any person shall apply to the court for leave to adduce additional evidence, and shall show to the satisfaction of the court that such additional evidence is material and that there were reasonable grounds for failure to adduce such evidence in the proceeding before the Secretary, the court may order such additional evidence to be taken before the Secretary and to be adduced upon the hearing in such manner and upon such terms and conditions as to the court may seem proper. The Secretary may modify his findings as to the facts by reason of the additional evidence so taken, and he shall file with the court such modified findings which, if supported by substantial evidence, shall be conclusive, and his recommendation, if any, for the setting aside of the original order. The judgment of the court affirming or setting aside any such order of the Secretary shall be final, subject to review by the Supreme Court of the United States upon certiorari or certification as provided in section 1254 of title 28 of the United States Code. The commencement of proceedings under this subsection shall not, unless specifically ordered by the court to the contrary, operate as a stay of the Secretary's order.

(i) (1) The Secretary shall promulgate regulations for exempting from the operation of the foregoing subsections of this section drugs intended solely for investigational use by experts qualified by scientific training and experience to investigate the safety and effectiveness of drugs. Such regulations may, within the discre-

tion of the Secretary, among other conditions relating to the protection of the public health, provide for conditioning such exemption upon—

(A)   the submission to the Secretary, before any clinical testing of a new drug is undertaken, of reports, by the manufacturer or the sponsor of the investigation of such drug, or preclinical tests (including tests on animals) of such drug adequate to justify the proposed clinical testing;

(B)   the manufacturer or the sponsor of the investigation of a new drug proposed to be distributed to investigators for clinical testing obtaining a signed agreement from each of such investigators that patients to whom the drug is administered will be under his personal supervision, or under the supervision of investigators responsible to him, and that he will not supply such drug to any other investigator, or to clinics, for administration to human beings;

(C)   the establishment and maintenance of such records, and the making of such reports to the Secretary, by the manufacturer or the sponsor of the investigation of such drug, of data (including but not limited to analytical reports by investigators) obtained as the result of such investigational use of such drug, as the Secretary finds will enable him to evaluate the safety and effectiveness of such drug in the event of the filing of an application pursuant to subsection (b); and

(D)   the submission to the Secretary by the manufacturer or the sponsor of the investigation of a new drug of a statement of intent regarding whether the manufacturer or sponsor has plans for assessing pediatric safety and efficacy.

(2)   Subject to paragraph (3), a clinical investigation of a new drug may begin 30 days after the Secretary has received from the manufacturer or sponsor of the investigation a submission containing such information about the drug and the clinical investigation, including—

(A)   information on design of the investigation and adequate reports of basic information, certified by the applicant to be accurate reports, necessary to assess the safety of the drug for use in clinical investigation; and

(B)   adequate information on the chemistry and manufacturing of the drug, controls available for the drug, and primary data tabulations from animal or human studies.

(3) (A)   At any time, the Secretary may prohibit the sponsor of an investigation from conducting the investigation (referred to in this paragraph as a "clinical hold") if the Secretary makes a determination described in sub-paragraph (B). The Secretary shall specify the basis for the clinical hold, including the specific information available to the Secretary which served as the basis for such clinical hold, and confirm such determination in writing.

(B)   For purposes of sub-paragraph (A), a determination described in this sub-paragraph with respect to a clinical hold is that—

(i)   the drug involved represents an unreasonable risk to the safety of the persons who are the subjects of the clinical investigation, taking into account the qualifications of the clinical investigators, information about the drug, the design of the clinical investigation, the condition for which the drug is to be investigated, and the health status of the subjects involved; or

(ii)   the clinical hold should be issued for such other reasons as the Secretary may by regulation establish (including reasons established by regulation before November 21, 1997).

(C)   Any written request to the Secretary from the sponsor of an investigation that a clinical hold be removed shall receive a decision, in writing and specifying the reasons therefor, within 30 days after receipt of such request. Any such request shall include sufficient information to support the removal of such clinical hold.

(4)   Regulations under paragraph (1) shall provide that such exemption shall be conditioned upon the manufacturer, or the sponsor of the investigation, requiring that experts using such drugs for investigational purposes certify to such manufacturer or sponsor that they will inform any human beings to whom such drugs, or any controls used in connection therewith, are being administered, or their representatives, that such drugs are being used for investigational purposes and will obtain the consent of such human beings or their representatives, except where it is

not feasible or it is contrary to the best interests of such human beings. Nothing in this subsection shall be construed to require any clinical investigator to submit directly to the Secretary reports on the investigational use of drugs.

(j) (1)   Any person may file with the Secretary an abbreviated application for the approval of a new drug.

(2) (A)   An abbreviated application for a new drug shall contain—

(i)   information to show that the conditions of use prescribed, recommended, or suggested in the labeling proposed for the new drug have been previously approved for a drug listed under paragraph (7) (hereinafter in this subsection referred to as a "listed drug");

(ii) (I)   if the listed drug referred to in clause (i) has only one active ingredient, information to show that the active ingredient of the new drug is the same as that of the listed drug;

(II)   if the listed drug referred to in clause (i) has more than one active ingredient, information to show that the active ingredients of the new drug are the same as those of the listed drug, or

(III)   if the listed drug referred to in clause (i) has more than one active ingredient and if one of the active ingredients of the new drug is different and the application is filed pursuant to the approval of a petition filed under sub-paragraph (C), information to show that the other active ingredients of the new drug are the same as the active ingredients of the listed drug, information to show that the different active ingredient is an active ingredient of a listed drug or of a drug which does not meet the requirements of section 201 (p), and such other information respecting the different active ingredient with respect to which the petition was filed as the Secretary may require;

(iii)   information to show that the route of administration, the dosage form, and the strength of the new drug are the same as those of the listed drug referred to in clause (i) or, if the route of administration, the dosage form, or the strength of the new drug is different and the application is filed pursuant to the approval of a petition filed under sub-paragraph (C), such information respecting the route of administration, dosage form, or strength with respect to which the petition was filed as the Secretary may require;

(iv)   information to show that the new drug is bioequivalent to the listed drug referred to in clause (i), except that if the application is filed pursuant to the approval of a petition filed under sub-paragraph (C), information to show that the active ingredients of the new drug are of the same pharmacological or therapeutic class as those of the listed drug referred to in clause (i) and the new drug can be expected to have the same therapeutic effect as the listed drug when administered to patients for a condition of use referred to in clause (i);

(v)   information to show that the labeling proposed for the new drug is the same as the labeling approved for the listed drug referred to in clause (i) except for changes required because of differences approved under a petition filed under sub-paragraph (C) or because the new drug and the listed drug are produced or distributed by different manufacturers;

(vi)   the items specified in clauses (B) through (F) of subsection (b) (1);

(vii)   a certification, in the opinion of the applicant and to the best of his knowledge, with respect to each patent which claims the listed drug referred to in clause (i) or which claims a use for such listed drug for which the applicant is seeking approval under this subsection and for which information is required to be filed under subsection (b) or (c)—

(I)   that such patent information has not been filed,

(II)   that such patent has expired,

(III)   of the date on which such patent will expire, or

(IV)   that such patent is invalid or will not be infringed by the manufacture, use, or sale of the new drug for which the application is submitted; and

(viii)   if with respect to the listed drug referred to in clause (i) information was filed under subsection (b) or (c) for a method of use patent which does not claim a use for which the applicant is seeking approval under this subsection, a statement that the method of use patent does not claim such a use.

The Secretary may not require that an abbreviated application contain information in addition to that required by clauses (i) through (viii).

(B) (i) An applicant who makes a certification described in sub-paragraph (A) (vii) (IV) shall include in the application a statement that the applicant will give the notice required by clause (ii) to—

(I) each owner of the patent which is the subject of the certification or the representative of such owner designated to receive such notice, and

(II) the holder of the approved application under subsection (b) for the drug which is claimed by the patent or a use of which is claimed by the patent or the representative of such holder designated to receive such notice.

(ii) The notice referred to in clause (i) shall state that an application, which contains data from bioavailability or bioequivalence studies, has been submitted under this subsection for the drug with respect to which the certification is made to obtain approval to engage in the commercial manufacture, use, or sale of such drug before the expiration of the patent referred to in the certification. Such notice shall include a detailed statement of the factual and legal basis of the applicant's opinion that the patent is not valid or will not be infringed.

(iii) If an application is amended to include a certification described in sub-paragraph (A) (vii) (IV), the notice required by clause (ii) shall be given when the amended application is submitted.

(C) If a person wants to submit an abbreviated application for a new drug which has a different active ingredient or whose route of administration, dosage form, or strength differ from that of a listed drug, such person shall submit a petition to the Secretary seeking permission to file such an application. The Secretary shall approve or disapprove a petition submitted under this sub-paragraph within ninety days of the date the petition is submitted. The Secretary shall approve such a petition unless the Secretary finds—

(i) that investigations must be conducted to show the safety and effectiveness of the drug or of any of its active ingredients, the route of administration, the dosage form, or the strength, which differs from the listed drug; or

(ii) that any drug with a different active ingredient may not be adequately evaluated for approval as safe and effective on the basis of the information required to be submitted in an abbreviated application.

(3) (A) The Secretary shall issue guidance for the individuals who review applications submitted under paragraph (1), which shall relate to promptness in conducting the reivew, technical excellence, lack of bias and conflict of interest, and knowledge of regulatory and scientific standards, and which shall apply equally to all individuals who review such applications.

(B) The Secretary shall meet with a sponsor of an investigation or applicant for approval for a drug under this subsection if the sponsor or applicant makes a reasonable written request for a meeting for the purpose of reaching agreement on the design and size of bioavailability and bioequivalence studies needed for approval of such application. The sponsor or applicant shall provide information necessary for discussion and agreement on the design and size of such studies. Minutes of any such meeting shall be prepared by the Secretary and made available to the sponsor or applicant.

(C) Any agreement regarding the parameters of design and size of bioavailability and bioequivalence studies of a drug under this paragraph that is reached between the Secretary and a sponsor or applicant shall be reduced to writing and made part of the administrative record by the Secretary. Such agreement shall not be changed after the testing begins, except—

(i) with the written agreement of the sponsor or applicant; or

(ii) pursuant to a decision, made in accordance with sub-paragraph (D) by the director of the reviewing division, that a substantial scientific issue essential to determining the safety or effectiveness of the drug has been identified after the testing has begun.

(D) A decision under sub-paragraph (C)(ii) by the director shall be in writing and the Secretary shall provide to the sponsor or applicant an opportunity for a meeting at which the director and the sponsor or applicant will be present and at which the director will document the scientific issue involved.

(E) The written decisions of the reviewing division shall be binding upon, and may not directly or indirectly be changed by, the field or compliance office personnel unless such field or compliance office personnel demonstrate to the reviewing division why such decision should be modified.

(F) No action by the reviewing division may be delayed because of the unavailability of information from or action by field personnel unless the reviewing division determines that a delay is necessary to assure the marketing of a safe and effective drug.

(G) For purposes of this paragraph, the reviewing division is the division responsible for the review of an application for approval of a drug under this subsection (including scientific matters, chemistry, manufacturing, and controls).

(4) Subject to paragraph (5), the Secretary shall approve an application for a drug unless the Secretary finds that—

(A) the methods used in, or the facilities and controls used for, the manufacture, processing, and packing of the drug are inadequate to assure and preserve its identity, strength, quality, and purity;

(B) information submitted with the application is insufficient to show that each of the proposed conditions of use have been previously approved for the listed drug referred to in the application;

(C) (i) if the listed drug has only one active ingredient, information submitted with the application is insufficient to show that the active ingredient is the same as that of the listed drug;

(ii) if the listed drug has more than one active ingredient, information submitted with the application is insufficient to show that the active ingredients are the same as the active ingredients of the listed drug, or

(iii) if the listed drug has more than one active ingredient and if the application is for a drug which has an active ingredient different from the listed drug, information submitted with the application is insufficient to show—

(I) that the other active ingredients are the same as the active ingredients of the listed drug, or

(II) that the different active ingredient is an active ingredient of a listed drug or a drug which does not meet the requirements of section 201(p), or no petition to file an application for the drug with the different ingredient was approved under paragraph (2)(C);

(D) (i) if the application is for a drug whose route of administration, dosage form, or strength of the drug is the same as the route of administration, dosage form, or strength of the listed drug referred to in the application, information submitted in the application is insufficient to show that the route of administration, dosage form, or strength is the same as that of the listed drug, or

(ii) if the application is for a drug whose route of administration, dosage form, or strength of the drug is different from that of the listed drug referred to in the application, no petition to file an application for the drug with the different route of administration, dosage form, or strength was approved under paragraph (2)(C);

(E) if the application was filed pursuant to the approval of a petition under paragraph (2)(C), the application did not contain the information required by the Secretary respecting the active ingredient, route of administration, dosage form, or strength which is not the same;

(F) information submitted in the application is insufficient to show that the drug is bioequivalent to the listed drug referred to in the application or, if the application was filed pursuant to a petition approved under paragraph (2)(C) information submitted in the application is insufficient to show that the active ingredients of the new drug are of the same pharmacological or therapeutic class as those of the listed drug referred to in paragraph (2)(A)(i) and that the new drug can be expected to have the same therapeutic effect as the listed drug when administered to patients for a condition of use referred to in such paragraph;

(G)   information submitted in the application is insufficient to show that the labeling proposed for the drug is the same as the labeling approved for the listed drug referred to in the application except for changes required because of differences approved under a petition filed under paragraph (2)(C) or because the drug and the listed drug are produced or distributed by different manufacturers;

(H)   information submitted in the application or any other information available to the Secretary shows that (i) the inactive ingredients of the drug are unsafe for use under the conditions prescribed, recommended, or suggested in the labeling proposed for the drug, or (ii) the composition of the drug is unsafe under such conditions because of the type or quantity of inactive ingredients included or the manner in which the inactive ingredients are included;

(I)   the approval under subsection (c) of the listed drug referred to in the application under this subsection has been withdrawn or suspended for grounds described in the first sentence of subsection (e), the Secretary has published a notice of opportunity for hearing to withdraw approval of the listed drug under subsection (c) for grounds described in the first sentence of subsection (e), the approval under this subsection of the listed drug referred to in the application under this subsection has been withdrawn or suspended under paragraph (6), or the Secretary has determined that the listed drug has been withdrawn from sale for safety or effectiveness reasons;

(J)   the application does not meet any other requirement of paragraph (2)(A); or

(K)   the application contains an untrue statement of material fact.

(5) (A)   Within one hundred and eighty days of the initial receipt of an application under paragraph (2) or within such additional period as may be agreed upon by the Secretary and the applicant, the Secretary shall approve or disapprove the application.

(B)   The approval of an application submitted under paragraph (2) shall be made effective on the last applicable date determined under the following:

(i)   If the applicant only made a certification described in subclause (I) or (II) of paragraph (2) (A) (vii) or in both such subclauses, the approval may be made effective immediately.

(ii)   If the applicant made a certification described in subclause (III) of paragraph (2) (A) (vii), the approval may be made effective on the date certified under subclause (III).

(iii)   If the applicant made a certification described in subclause (IV) of paragraph (2) (A) (vii), the approval shall be made effective immediately unless an action is brought for infringement of a patent which is the subject of the certification before the expiration of forty-five days from the date the notice provided under paragraph (2) (B) (i) is received. If such an action is brought before the expiration of such days, the approval shall be made effective upon the expiration of the thirty-month period beginning on the date of the receipt of the notice provided under paragraph (2) (B) (i) or such shorter or longer period as the court may order because either party to the action failed to reasonably cooperate in expediting the action, except that—

(I)   if before the expiration of such period the court decides that such patent is invalid or not infringed, the approval shall be made effective on the date of the court decision,

(II)   if before the expiration of such period the court decides that such patent has been infringed, the approval shall be made effective on such date as the court orders under section 271 (e) (4) (A) of title 35, United States Code, or

(III)   if before the expiration of such period, the court grants a preliminary injunction prohibiting the applicant from engaging in the commercial manufacture or sale of the drug until the court decides the issues of patent validity and infringement, and if the court decides that such patent is invalid or not infringed, the approval shall be made effective on the date of such court decision.

In such an action, each of the parties shall reasonably cooperate in expediting the action. Until the expiration of forty-five days from the date the notice made under paragraph (2) (B) (i) is received, no action may be brought under section 2201 of title 28,

United States Code, for a declaratory judgment with respect to the patent. Any action brought under section 2201 shall be brought in the judicial district where the defendant has its principal place of business or a regular and established place of business.

(iv)   If the application contains a certification described in subclause (IV) of paragraph (2) (A) (vii) and is for a drug for which a previous application has been submitted under this subsection continuing such a certification, the application shall be made effective not earlier than one hundred and eighty days after—

(I)   the date the Secretary receives notice from the applicant under the previous application of the first commercial marketing of the drug under the previous application, or

(II)   the date of a decision of a court in an action described in clause (iii) holding the patent which is the subject of the certification to be invalid or not infringed, whichever is earlier.

(C)   If the Secretary decides to disapprove an application, the Secretary shall give the applicant notice of an opportunity for a hearing before the Secretary on the question of whether such application is approvable. If the applicant elects to accept the opportunity for hearing by written request within thirty days after such notice, such hearing shall commence not more than ninety days after the expiration of such thirty days unless the Secretary and the applicant otherwise agree. Any such hearing shall thereafter be conducted on an expedited basis and the Secretary's order thereon shall be issued within ninety days after the date fixed by the Secretary for filing final briefs.

(D) (i)   If an application (other than an abbreviated new drug application) submitted under subsection (b) for a drug, no active ingredient (including any ester or salt of the active ingredient) of which has been approved in any other application under subsection (b), was approved during the period beginning January 1, 1982, and ending on September 24, 1984, the Secretary may not make the approval of an application submitted under this subsection which refers to the drug for which the subsection (b) application was submitted effective before the expiration of ten years from the date of the approval of the application under subsection (b).

(ii)   If an application submitted under subsection (b) for a drug, no active ingredient (including any ester or salt of the active ingredient) of which has been approved in any other application under subsection (b), is approved after September 24, 1984, no application may be submitted under this subsection which refers to the drug for which the subsection (b) application was submitted before the expiration of five years from the date of the approval of the application under subsection (b), except that such an application may be submitted under this subsection after the expiration of four years from the date of the approval of the subsection (b) application if it contains a certification of patent invalidity or noninfringement described in subclause (IV) of paragraph (2) (A) (vii). The approval of such an application shall be made effective in accordance with sub-paragraph (B) except that, if an action for patent infringement is commenced during the one-year period beginning forty-eight months after the date of the approval of the subsection (b) application, the thirty-month period referred to in sub-paragraph (B) (iii) shall be extended by such amount of time (if any) which is required for seven and one-half years to have elapsed from the date of approval of the subsection (b) application.

(iii)   If an application submitted under subsection (b) for a drug, which includes an active ingredient (including any ester or salt of the active ingredient) that has been approved in another application approved under subsection (b), is approved after the date of enactment of this subsection and if such application contains reports of new clinical investigations (other than bioavailability studies) essential to the approval of the application and conducted or sponsored by the applicant, the Secretary may not make the approval of an application submitted under this subsection for the conditions of approval of such drug in the subsection (b) application effective before the expiration of three years from the date of the approval of the application under subsection (b) for such drug.

(iv)   If a supplement to an application approved under subsection (b) is approved after September 24, 1984 and the supplement contains reports of new clinical investigations (other than

bioavailability studies) essential to the approval of the supplement and conducted or sponsored by the person submitting the supplement, the Secretary may not make the approval of an application submitted under this subsection for a change approved in the supplement effective before the expiration of three years from the date of the approval of the supplement under subsection (b).

    (v) If an application (or supplement to an application) submitted under subsection (b) for a drug, which includes an active ingredient (including any ester or salt of the active ingredient) that has been approved in another application under subsection (b), was approved during the period beginning January 1, 1982, and ending on September 24, 1984, the Secretary may not make the approval of an application submitted under this subsection which refers to the drug for which the subsection (b) application was submitted or which refers to a change approved in a supplement to the subsection (b) application effective before the expiration of two years from September 24, 1984.

    (6) If a drug approved under this subsection refers in its approved application to a drug the approval of which was withdrawn or suspended for grounds described in the first sentence of subsection (e) or was withdrawn or suspended under this paragraph or which, as determined by the Secretary, has been withdrawn from sale for safety or effectiveness reasons, the approval of the drug under this subsection shall be withdrawn or suspended—

    (A) for the same period as the withdrawal or suspension under subsection (e), or this paragraph, or

    (B) if the listed drug has been withdrawn from sale, for the period of withdrawal from sale or, if earlier, the period ending on the date the Secretary determines that the withdrawal from sale is not for safety or effectiveness reasons.

    (7) (A) (i) Within sixty days of September 24, 1984, the Secretary shall publish and make available to the public—

    (I) a list in alphabetical order of the official and proprietary name of each drug which has been approved for safety and effectiveness under subsection (c) before the date of the enactment of this subsection;

    (II) the date of approval if the drug is approved after 1981 and the number of the application which was approved; and

    (III) whether in vitro or in vivo bioequivalence studies, or both such studies, are required for applications filed under this subsection which will refer to the drug published.

    (ii) Every thirty days after the publication of the first list under clause (i) the Secretary shall revise the list to include each drug which has been approved for safety and effectiveness under subsection (c) or approved under this subsection during the thirty-day period.

    (iii) When patent information submitted under subsection (b) or (c) respecting a drug included on the list is to be published by the Secretary the Secretary shall, in revisions made under clause (ii), include such information for such drug.

    (B) A drug approved for safety and effectiveness under subsection (c) or approved under this subsection shall, for purposes of this subsection, be considered to have been published under sub-paragraph (A) on the date of its approval or September 24, 1984, whichever is later.

    (C) If the approval of a drug was withdrawn or suspended for grounds described in the first sentence of subsection (e) or was withdrawn or suspended under paragraph (6) or if the Secretary determines that a drug has been withdrawn from sale for safety or effectiveness reasons, it may not be published in the list under inline-paragraph (A) or, if the withdrawal or suspension occurred after its publication in such list, it shall be immediately removed from such list—

    (i) for the same period as the withdrawal or suspension under subsection (e) or paragraph (6), or

    (ii) if the listed drug has been withdrawn from sale, for the period of withdrawal from sale or, if earlier, the period ending on the date the Secretary determines that the withdrawal from sale is not for safety or effectiveness reasons.

A notice of the removal shall be published in the Federal Register.

    (8) For purposes of this subsection:
    (A) The term 'bioavailability' means the rate and extent to which the active ingredient or therapeutic ingredient is absorbed from a drug and becomes available at the site of drug action.

    (B) A drug shall be considered to be bioequivalent to a listed drug if—

    (i) the rate and extent of absorption of the drug do not show a significant difference from the rate and extent of absorption of the listed drug when administered at the same molar dose of the therapeutic ingredient under similar experimental conditions in either a single dose or multiple doses; or

    (ii) the extent of absorption of the drug does not show a significant difference from the extent of absorption of the listed drug when administered at the same molar dose of the therapeutic ingredient under similar experimental conditions in either a single dose or multiple doses and the difference from the listed drug in the rate of absorption of the drug is intentional, is reflected in its proposed labeling, is not essential to the attainment of effective body drug concentrations on chronic use, and is considered medically insignificant for the drug.

    (9) The Secretary shall, with respect to each application submitted under this subsection, maintain a record of—

    (A) the name of the applicant,
    (B) the name of the drug covered by the application,
    (C) the name of each person to whom the review of the chemistry of the application was assigned and the date of such assignment, and
    (D) the name of each person to whom the bioequivalence review for such application was assigned and the date of such assignment.

The information the Secretary is required to maintain under this paragraph with respect to an application submitted under this subsection shall be made available to the public after the approval of such application.

    (k) (1) In the case of any drug for which an approval of an application filed under subsection (b) or (j) is in effect, the applicant shall establish and maintain such records, and make such reports to the Secretary, of data relating to clinical experience and other data or information, received or otherwise obtained by such applicant with respect to such drug, as the Secretary may by general regulation, or by order with respect to such application, prescribe on the basis of a finding that such records and reports are necessary in order to enable the Secretary to determine, or facilitate a determination, whether there is or may be ground for invoking subsection (e) of this section. Regulations and orders issued under subsection and under subsection (i) shall have due regard for the professional ethics of the medical profession and the interests of patients and shall provide, where the Secretary deems it to be appropriate, for the examination, upon request, by the persons to whom such regulations or orders are applicable, of similar information received or otherwise obtained by the Secretary.

    (2) Every person required under this section to maintain records, and every person in charge or custody thereof, shall, upon request of an officer or employee designated by the Secretary, permit such officer or employee at all reasonable times to have access to and copy and verify such records.

    (l) Safety and effectiveness data and information which has been submitted in an application under subsection (b) for a drug and which has not previously been disclosed to the public shall be made available to the public, upon request, unless extraordinary circumstances are shown—

    (1) if no work is being or will be undertaken to have the application approved,

    (2) if the Secretary has determined that the application is not approvable and all legal appeals have been exhausted,

    (3) if approval of the application under subsection (c) is withdrawn and all legal appeals have been exhausted,

    (4) if the Secretary has determined that such drug is not a new drug, or

    (5) upon the effective date of the approval of the first application under subsection (j) which refers to such drug or upon the date upon which the approval of an application under subsection (j) which refers to such drug could be made effective if such an application had been submitted.

(m)   For purposes of this section, the term 'patent' means a patent issued by the United States Patent and Trademark Office.

(n) (1)   For the purpose of providing expert scientific advice and recommendations to the Secretary regarding a clinical investigation or a drug or the approval for marketing of a drug under section 505 or section 351 of the Public Health Service Act, the Secretary shall establish panels of experts or use panels of experts established before the date of enactment of the Food and Drug Administration Modernization Act of 1997, or both.

(2)   The Secretary may delegate the appointment and oversight authority granted under section 904 to a director of a center or sucessor entity within the Food and Drug Administration.

(3)   The Secretary shall make appointments to each panel established under paragraph (1) so that each panel shall consist of—

(A)   members who are qualified by training and experience to evaluate the safety and effectiveness of the drugs to be referred to the panel and who, to the extent feasible, possess skill and experience in the development, manufacturer, or utilization of such drugs;

(B)   members with diverse expertise in such fields as clinical and administrative medicine, pharmacy, pharmacology, pharmacoeconomics, biological and physical sciences, and other related professions;

(C)   a representative of consumer interests, and a representative of interests of the drug manufacturing industry not directly affected by the matter to be brought before the panel; and

(D)   two or more members who are specialists or have other expertise in the particular disease or condition for which the drug under review is proposed to be indicated.

Scientific, trade, and consumer organizations shall be afforded an opportunity to nominate individuals for appointment to the panels. No individual who is in the regular full-time employ of the United States and engaged in the administration of this Act may be a voting member of any panel. The Secretary shall designate one of the members of each panel to serve as chairman thereof.

(4)   Each member of a panel shall publicly disclose all conflicts of interest that member of a panel shal publicly disclose all conflicts of interest that member may have with the work to be undertaken by the panel. No member of a panel may vote on any matter where the member or the immediate family of such member could gain financially from the advice given to the Secretary. The Secretary may grant a waiver of any conflict of interest requirement upon public disclosure of such conflict of interest if such waiver is necessary to afford the panel essential expertise, except that the Secretary may not grant a waiver for a member of a panel when the member's own scientific work is involved.

(5)   The Secretary shall, as appropriate, provide education and training to each new panel member before such member participates in a panel's activities, including education regarding requirements under this Act and related regulations of the Secretary, and the administrative processes and procedures related to panel meetings.

(6)   Panel members (other than officers or employees of the United States), while attending meetings or conferences of a panel or otherwise engaged in its business, shall be entitled to receive compensation for each day so engaged, including traveltime, at rates to be fixed by the Secretary, but not to exceed the daily equivalent of the rate in effect for positions classified above grade GS-15 of the General Schedule. While serving away from their homes or regular places of business, panel members may be allowed travel expenses (including per diem in lieu of subsistence) as authorized by section 5703 of title 5, United States Code, for persons in the Government service employed intermittently.

(7)   The Secretary shall ensure that scientific advisory panels meet regularly and at appropriate intervals so that any matter to be reviewed by such a panel can be presented to the panel not more than 60 days after the matter is ready for such review. Meetings of the panel may be held using electronic communication to convene the meetings.

(8)   Within 90 days after a scientific advisory panel makes recommendations on any matter under its review, the Food and Drug Administration official responsible for the matter shall review the conclusions and recommendations of the panel, and notify the affected persons of the final decision on the matter, or of the reasons that no such decision has been reached. Each such final decision shall be documented including the rationale for the decision.

§505A[355a]   PEDIATRIC STUDIES OF DRUGS

(a)   DEFINITIONS—As used in this section, the term "pediatric studies" or "studies" means at least one clinical investigation (that, at the Secretary's discretion, may include pharmacokinetic studies) in pediatric age groups (including neonates in appropriate cases) in which a drug is anticipated to be used.

(B)   MARKET EXCLUSIVITY FOR NEW DRUGS—If, prior to approval of an application that is submitted under section 505(b)(1), the Secretary determines that information relating to the use of a new drug in the pediatric population may produce health benefits in that population, the Secretary makes a written request for pediatric studies (which shall include a timeframe for completing such studies), and such studies are completed within any such timeframe and the reports thereof submitted in accordance with subsection (d)(2) or accepted in accordance with subsection (d)(3)—

(1) (A) (i)   the period referred to in subsection (c)(3)(D)(ii) of section 505, and in subsection (j)(5)(D)(ii) of such section, is deemed to be five years and six months rather than five years, and the references in subsections (c)(3)(D)(ii) and (j)(5)(D)(ii) of such section to four years, to forty-eight months, and to seven and one-half years are deemed to be four and one-half years, fifty-four months, and eight years, respectively; or

(ii)   the period referred to in clauses (iii) and (iv) of subsection (c)(3)(D) of such section, and in clauses (iii) and (iv) of subsection (j)(5)(D) of such section, is deemed to be three years and six months rather than three years; and

(B)   if the drug is designated under section 526 for a rare disease or condition, the period referred to in section 527(a) is deemed to be seven years and six months rather than seven years; and

(2) (A)   if the drug is the subject of—

(i)   a listed patent for which a certification has been submitted under subsection (b)(2)(A)(ii) or (j)(2)(A)(vii)(II) of section 505 and for which pediatric studies were submitted prior to the expiration of the patent (including any patent extensions); or

(ii)   a listed patent for which a certification has been submitted under subsections (b)(2)(A)(iii) or (j)(2)(A)(vii)(III) of section 505, the period during which an application may not be approved under section 505(c)(3) or section 505(j)(4)(B) shall be extended by a period of six months after the date the patent expires (including any patent extensions); or

(B)   if the drug is the subject of a listed patent for which a certification has been submitted under subsection (b)(2)(A)(iv) or (j)(2)(A)(vii)(IV) of section 505, and in the patent infringement litigation resulting from the certification the court determines that the patent is valid and would be infringed, the period during which an application may not be approved under section 505(c)(3) or section 505(j)(4)(B) shall be extended by a period of six months after the date the patent expires (including any patent extensions).

(c)   MARKET EXCLUSIVITY FOR ALREADY-MARKETED DRUGS—If the Secretary determines that information relating to the use of an approved drug in the pediatric population may produce health benefits in that population and makes a written request to the holder of an approved application under section 505(b)(1) [21 USC § 355(b)(1)] for pediatric studies (which shall include a timeframe for completing such studies), the holder agrees to the request, the studies are completed within any such timeframe, and the reports thereof are submitted in accordance with subsection (d)(2) or accepted in accordance with subsection (d)(3)—

(1) (A) (i)   the period referred to in subsection (c)(3)(D)(ii) of section 505 [21 USC § 355(c)(3)(D)(ii)], and in subsection (j)(5)(D)(ii) of such section, is deemed to be five years and six months rather than five years, and the references in subsections (c)(3)(D)(ii) and (j)(5)(D)(ii) of such section to four years, to forty-

eight months, and to seven and one-half years are deemed to be four and one-half years, fifty-four months, and eight years, respectively; or

(ii) the period referred to in clauses (iii) and (iv) of subsection (c)(3)(D) of such section, and in clauses (iii) and (iv) of subsection (j)(5)(D) of such section, is deemed to be three years and six months rather than three years; and

(B) if the drug is designated under section 526 [21 USC § 360bb] for a rare disease or condition, the period referred to in section 527(a) [21 USC § 360cc(a)] is deemed to be seven years and six months rather than seven years; and

(2) (A) if the drug is the subject of—

(i) a listed patent for which a certification has been submitted under subsection (b)(2)(A)(ii) or (j)(2)(A)(vii)(II) of section 505 [21 USC § 355 and for which pediatric studies were submitted prior to the expiration of the patent (including any patent extensions); or

(ii) a listed patent for which a certification has been submitted under subsection (b)(2)(A)(iii) or (j)(2)(A)(vii)(III) of section 505 [21 USC § 355 the period during which an application may not be approved under section 505(c)(3) or section 505(j)(4)(B) [21 USC § 355(c)(3) or (j)(4)(B)] shall be extended by a period of six months after the date the patent expires (including any patent extensions); or

(B) if the drug is the subject of a listed patent for which a certification has been submitted under subsection (b)(2)(A)(iv) or (j)(2)(A)(vii)(IV) of section 505 [21 USC § 355(b)(2)(A)(iv) or (j)(2)(A)(vii)(IV)], and in the patent infringement litigation resulting from the certification the court determines that the patent is valid and would be infringed, the period during which an application may not be approved under section 505(c)(3) or section 505(j)(4)(B) [21 USC § 355(c)(3) of (j)(4)(B)]shall be extended by a period of six months after the date the patent expires (including any patent extensions).

(c) MARKET EXCLUSIVITY FOR ALREADY-MARKETED DRUGS—If the Secretary determines that information relating to the use of an approved drug in the pediatric population may produce health benefits in that population and makes a written request to the holder of an approved application under section 505(b)(1) [21 USC § 355(b)(1)] for pediatric studies (which shall include a timeframe for completing such studies), the holder agrees to the request, the studies are completed within any such timeframe, and the reports thereof are submitted in accordance with subsection (d)(2) or accepted in accordance with subsection (d)(3)—

(1) (A) (i) the period referred to in subsection (c)(3)(D)(ii) of section 505 [21 USC § 355(c)(3)(D)(ii)], and in subsection (j)(5)(D)(ii) of such section, is deemed to be five years and six months rather than five years, and the references in subsections (c)(3)(D)(ii) and (j)(5)(D)(ii) of such section to four years, to forty-eight months, and to seven and one-half years are deemed to be four and one-half years, fifty-four months, and eight years, respectively; or

(ii) the period referred to in clauses (iii) and (iv) of subsection (c)(3)(D) of such section, and in clauses (iii) and (iv) of subsection (j)(5)(D) of such section, is deemed to be three years and six months rather than three years; and

(B) if the drug is designated under section 526 [21 USC § 360bb] for a rare disease or condition, the period referred to in section 527(a) [21 USC § 360cc(a)] is deemed to be seven years and six months rather than seven years; and

(2) (A) if the drug is the subject of—

(i) a listed patent for which a certification has been submitted under subsection (b)(2)(A)(ii) or (j)(2)(A)(vii)(II) of section 505 [21 USC § 355 and for which pediatric studies were submitted prior to the expiration of the patent (including any patent extensions); or

(ii) a listed patent for which a certification has been submitted under subsection (b)(2)(A)(iii) or (j)(2)(A)(vii)(III) of section 505 [21 USC § 355 the period during which an application may not be approved under section 505(c)(3) or section 505(j)(4)(B) [21 USC § 355(c)(3) or (j)(4)(B)] shall be extended by a period of six months after the date the patent expires (including any patent extensions); or

(B) if the drug is the subject of a listed patent for which a certification has been submitted under subsection (b)(2)(A)(iv) or (j)(2)(A)(vii)(IV) of section 505 [21 USC § 355(b)(2)(A)(iv) or (j)(2)(A)(vii)(IV)], and in the patent infringement litigation resulting from the certification the court determines that the patent is valid and would be infringed, the period during which an application may not be approved under section 505(c)(3) or section 505(j)(4)(B) [21 USC § 355(c)(3) of (j)(4)(B)]shall be extended by a period of six months after the date the patent expires (including any patent extensions).

(d) CONDUCT OF PEDIATRIC STUDIES

(1) Agreement for studies—The Secretary may, pursuant to a written request from the Secretary under subsection (b) or (c), after consultation with—

(A) the sponsor of an application for an investigational new drug under section 505(i) [21 USC § 355(i)];

(B) the sponsor of an application for a new drug under section 505(b)(1) [21 USC § 355(b)(1)]; or

(C) the holder of an approved application for a drug under section 505(b)(1) [21 USC § 355(b)(1)], agree with the sponsor or holder for the conduct of pediatric studies for such drug. Such agreement shall be in writing and shall include a timeframe for such studies.

(2) WRITTEN PROTOCOLS TO MEET THE STUDIES REQUIREMENT—If the sponsor or holder and the Secretary agree upon written protocols for the studies, the studies requirement of subsection (b) or (c) is satisfied upon the completion of the studies and submission of the reports thereof in accordance with the original written request and the written agreement referred to in paragraph (1). In reaching an agreement regarding written protocols, the Secretary shall take into account adequate representation of children of ethnic and racial minorities. Not later than 60 days after the submission of the report of the studies, the Secretary shall determine if such studies were or were not conducted in accordance with the original written request and the written agreement and reported in accordance with the requirements of the Secretary for filing and so notify the sponsor or holder.

(3) Other methods to meet the studies requirement. If the sponsor or holder and the Secretary have not agreed in writing on the protocols for the studies, the studies requirement of subsection (b) or (c) of this section is satisfied when such studies have been completed and the reports accepted by the Secretary. Not later than 90 days after the submission of the reports of the studies, the Secretary shall accept or reject such reports and so notify the sponsor or holder. The Secretary's only responsibility in accepting or rejecting the reports shall be to determine, within the 90 days, whether the studies fairly respond to the written request, have been conducted in accordance with commonly accepted scientific principles and protocols, and have been reported in accordance with the requirements of the Secretary for filing.

(4) WRITTEN REQUEST TO HOLDERS OF APPROVED APPLICATIONS FOR DRUGS THAT HAVE MARKET EXCLUSIVITY

(A) Request and response—If the Secretary makes a written request for pediatric studies (including neonates, as appropriate) under subsection (c) to the holder of an application approved under section 505(b)(1) [21 USC § 355 (b)(1)], the holder, not later than 180 days after receiving the written request, shall respond to the Secretary as to the intention of the holder to act on the request by—

(i) indicating when the pediatric studies will be initiated, if the holder agrees to the request; or

(ii) indicating that the holder does not agree to the request.

(B) No agreement to request.

(i) Referral—If the holder does not agree to a written request within the time period specified in subparagraph (A), and if the Secretary determines that there is a continuing need for information relating to the use of the drug in the pediatric population (including neonates, as appropriate), the Secretary shall refer the drug to the Foundation for the National Institutes of Health established under section 499 of the Public Health Service Act (42

U.S.C. 290b) (referred to in this paragraph as the "Foundation") for the conduct of the pediatric studies described in the written request.

(ii)   Public notice—The Secretary shall give public notice of the name of the drug, the name of the manufacturer, and the indications to be studied made in a referral under clause (i).

(C)   Lack of funds—On referral of a drug under subparagraph (B)(i), the Foundation shall issue a proposal to award a grant to conduct the requested studies unless the Foundation certifies to the Secretary, within a timeframe that the Secretary determines is appropriate through guidance, that the Foundation does not have funds available under section 499(j)(9)(B)(i) [42 USC § 290b(j)(9)(B)(i)] to conduct the requested studies. If the Foundation so certifies, the Secretary shall refer the drug for inclusion on the list established under section 409I of the Public Health Service Act [42 USC § 284m] for the conduct of the studies.

(D)   Effect of subsection—Nothing in this subsection (including with respect to referrals from the Secretary to the Foundation) alters or amends section 241(j) of title 420 or section 552 of title 5 or section 1905 of title 18, United States Code.

(E)   No requirement to refer—Nothing in this subsection shall be construed to require that every declined written request shall be referred to the Foundation.

(F)   Written requests under subsection (b)—For drugs under subsection (b) for which written requests have not been accepted, if the Secretary determines that there is a continuing need for information relating to the use of the drug in the pediatric population (including neonates, as appropriate), the Secretary shall issue a written request under subsection (c) after the date of approval of the drug.

(e)   DELAY OF EFFECTIVE DATE FOR CERTAIN APPLICATION—If the Secretary determines that the acceptance or approval of an application under section 505(b)(2) or 505(j) [21 USC § 355(b)(2) or (j)] for a new drug may occur after submission of reports of pediatric studies under this section, which were submitted prior to the expiration of the patent (including any patent extension) or the applicable period under clauses (ii) through (iv) of section 505(c)(3)(D) [21 USC § 355(c)(3)(D)] or clauses (ii) through (iv) of section 505(j)(5)(D) [21 USC § 355(j)(5)(D)], but before the Secretary has determined whether the requirements of subsection (d) have been satisfied, the Secretary shall delay the acceptance or approval under section 505(b)(2) or 505(j) [21 USC § 355 (b)(2) or (j)] until the determination under subsection (d) is made, but any such delay shall not exceed 90 days. In the event that requirements of this section are satisfied, the applicable six-month period under subsection (b) or (c) shall be deemed to have been running during the period of delay.

(f)   NOTICE OF DETERMINATIONS ON STUDIES REQUIREMENT—The Secretary shall publish a notice of any determination that the requirements of subsection (d) have been met and that submissions and approvals under subsection (b)(2) or (j) of section 505 [21 USC § 355(b)(2) or (j)] for a drug will be subject to the provisions of this section.

(g)   LIMITATIONS—A drug to which the six-month period under subsection (b) or (c) has already been applied—

(1)   may receive an additional six-month period under subsection (c)(1)(A)(ii) for a supplemental application if all other requirements under this section are satisfied, except that such a drug may not receive any additional such period under subsection (c)(2); and

(2)   may not receive any additional such period under subsection (c)(1)(B) of this section.

(h)   RELATIONSHIP TO REGULATIONS—Notwithstanding any other provision of law, if any pediatric study is required pursuant to regulations promulgated by the Secretary and such study meets the completeness, timeliness, and other requirements of this section, such study shall be deemed to satisfy the requirement for market exclusivity pursuant to this section.

(i)   LABELING SUPPLEMENTS

(1)   Priority status for pediatric supplements—Any supplement to an application under section 505 [21 USC § 355] proposing a labeling change pursuant to a report on a pediatric study under this section—

(A)   shall be considered to be a priority supplement; and

(B)   shall be subject to the performance goals established by the Commissioner for priority drugs.

(2)   Dispute resolution.

(A)   Request for labeling change and failure to agree—If the Commissioner determines that an application with respect to which a pediatric study is conducted under this section is approvable and that the only open issue for final action on the application is the reaching of an agreement between the sponsor of the application and the Commissioner on appropriate changes to the labeling for the drug that is the subject of the application, not later than 180 days after the date of submission of the application—

(i)   the Commissioner shall request that the sponsor of the application make any labeling change that the Commissioner determines to be appropriate; and

(ii)   if the sponsor of the application does not agree to make a labeling change requested by the Commissioner, the Commissioner shall refer the matter to the Pediatric Advisory Subcommittee of the Anti-Infective Drugs Advisory Committee.

(B)   Action by the Pediatric Advisory Subcommittee of the Anti-Infective Drugs Advisory Committee. Not later than 90 days after receiving a referral under subparagraph (A)(ii), the Pediatric Advisory Subcommittee of the Anti-Infective Drugs Advisory Committee shall—

(i)   review the pediatric study reports; and

(ii)   make a recommendation to the Commissioner concerning appropriate labeling changes, if any.

(C)   Consideration of recommendations. The Commissioner shall consider the recommendations of the Pediatric Advisory Subcommittee of the Anti-Infective Drugs Advisory Committee and, if appropriate, not later than 30 days after receiving the recommendation, make a request to the sponsor of the application to make any labeling change that the Commissioner determines to be appropriate.

(D)   Misbranding. If the sponsor of the application, within 30 days after receiving a request under subparagraph (C), does not agree to make a labeling change requested by the Commissioner, the Commissioner may deem the drug that is the subject of the application to be misbranded.

(E)   No effect on authority. Nothing in this subsection limits the authority of the United States to bring an enforcement action under this Act when a drug lacks appropriate pediatric labeling. Neither course of action (the Pediatric Advisory Subcommittee of the Anti-Infective Drugs Advisory Committee process or an enforcement action referred to in the preceding sentence) shall preclude, delay, or serve as the basis to stay the other course of action.

(j)   DISSEMINATION OF PEDIATRIC INFORMATION

(1)   In general—Not later than 180 days after the date of submission of a report on a pediatric study under this section, the Commissioner shall make available to the public a summary of the medical and clinical pharmacology reviews of pediatric studies conducted for the supplement, including by publication in the Federal Register.

(2)   Effect of subsection. Nothing in this subsection alters or amends section 301(j) of this Act [21 USC § 331(j)] or section 552 of Title 5 or section 1905 of Title 18, United States Code.

(k)   CLARIFICATION OF INTERACTION OF MARKET EXCLUSIVITY UNDER THIS SECTION AND MARKET EXCLUSIVITY AWARDED TO AN APPLICANT FOR APPROVAL OF A DRUG UNDER SECTION 505(j) of this title—If a 180-day period under section 505(j)(5)(B)(iv) [21 USC § 355 (j)(5)(B)(iv)] overlaps with a 6-month exclusivity period under this section, so that the applicant for approval of a drug under section 505(j) [21 USC § 355 (j)] entitled to

the 180-day period under that section loses a portion of the 180-day period to which the applicant is entitled for the drug, the 180-day period shall be extended from—

(1) the date on which the 180-day period would have expired by the number of days of the overlap, if the 180-day period would, but for the application of this subsection, expire after the 6-month exclusivity period; or

(2) the date on which the 6-month exclusivity period expires, by the number of days of the overlap if the 180-day period would, but for the application of this subsection, expire during the six-month exclusivity period.

(l) PROMPT APPROVAL OF DRUGS UNDER SECTION 505(J) WHEN PEDIATRIC INFORMATION IS ADDED TO LABELING

(1) General rule—A drug for which an application has been submitted or approved under section 505(j) [21 USC § 355(j)] shall not be considered ineligible for approval under that section or misbranded under section 502 [21 USC § 352] on the basis that the labeling of the drug omits a pediatric indication or any other aspect of labeling pertaining to pediatric use when the omitted indication or other aspect is protected by patent or by exclusivity under clause (iii) or (iv) of section 505(j)(5)(D) of this title [21 USC 355].

(2) Labeling—Notwithstanding clauses (iii) and (iv) of section 505(j)(5)(D) [21 USC § 355(j)(5)(D)], the Secretary may require that the labeling of a drug approved under section 505(j) [21 USC § 355(j)] that omits a pediatric indication or other aspect of labeling as described in paragraph (1) include—

(A) a statement that, because of marketing exclusivity for a manufacturer—

(i) the drug is not labeled for pediatric use; or

(ii) in the case of a drug for which there is an additional pediatric use not referred to in paragraph (1), the drug is not labeled for the pediatric use under paragraph (1); and

(B) a statement of any appropriate pediatric contraindications, warnings, or precautions that the Secretary considers necessary.

(3) Preservation of pediatric exclusivity and other provisions. This subsection does not affect—

(A) the availability or scope of exclusivity under this section;

(B) the availability or scope of exclusivity under section 505 [21 USC § 355] for pediatric formulations;

(C) the question of the eligibility for approval of any application under section 505(j) [21 USC § 355(j)] that omits any other conditions of approval entitled to exclusivity under clause (iii) or (iv) of section 505(j)(5)(D) [21 USC § 355(j)(5)(D)]; or

(D) except as expressly provided in paragraphs (1) and (2), the operation of section 355 of this title.

(m) REPORT—The Secretary shall conduct a study and report to Congress not later than January 1, 2001, based on the experience under the program established under this section. The study and report shall examine all relevant issues, including—

(1) the effectiveness of the program in improving information about important pediatric uses for approved drugs;

(2) the adequacy of the incentive provided under this section;

(3) the economic impact of the program on taxpayers and consumers, including the impact of the lack of lower cost generic drugs on patients, including on lower income patients; and

(4) any suggestions for modification that the Secretary determines to be appropriate.

(n) SUNSET—A drug may not receive any 6-month period under subsection (b) or (c) of this section unless—

(1) on or before October 1, 2007, the Secretary makes a written request for pediatric studies of the drug;

(2) on or before October 1, 2007, an application for the drug is accepted for filing under section 355(b) of this title; and

(3) all requirements of this section are met.

§**506** [356] FAST TRACK PRODUCTS

(a) DESIGNATION OF DRUG AS A FAST TRACK PRODUCT—

(1) IN GENERAL—The Secretary shall, at the request of the sponsor of a new drug, facilitate the development and expedite the review of such drug if it is intended for the treatment of a serious or life-threatening condition and it demonstrates the potential to address unmet medical needs for such a condition. (In this section, such a drug is referred to as a "fast track product".)

(2) REQUEST FOR DESIGNATION—The sponsor of a new drug may request the Secretary to designate the drug as a fast track product. A request for the designation may be made concurrently with, or at any time after, submission of an application for the investigation of the drug under section 505(i) or section 351(a)(3) of the Public Health Service Act.

(b) APPROVAL OF APPLICATION FOR A FAST TRACK PRODUCT—

(1) IN GENERAL—The Secretary may approve an application for approval of a fast track product under section 505(c) or section 351 of the Public Health Service Act upon a determination that the product has an effect on a clinical endpoint or on a surrogate endpoint that is reasonably likely to predict clinical benefit.

(2) LIMITATION—Approval of a fast track product under this subsection may be subject to the requirements—

(A) that the sponsor conduct appropriate post-approval studies to validate the surrogate endpoint or otherwise confirm the effect on the clinical endpoint; and

(B) that the sponsor submit copies of all promotional materials related to the fast track product during the preapproval review period and, following approval and for such period thereafter as the Secretary determines to be appropriate, at least 30 days prior to dissemination of the materials.

(3) EXPEDITED WITHDRAWAL OF APPROVAL—The Secretary may withdraw approval of a fast track product using expedited procedures (as prescribed by the Secretary in regulations which shall include an opportunity for an informal hearing) if—

(A) the sponsor fails to conduct any required post-approval study of the fast track drug with due diligence;

(B) a post-approval study of the fast track product fails to verify clinical benefit of the product;

(C) other evidence demonstrates that the fast track product is not safe or effective under the conditions of use; or

(D) the sponsor disseminates false or misleading promotional materials with respect to the product.

(c) REVIEW OF INCOMPLETE APPLICATIONS FOR APPROVAL OF A FAST TRACK PRODUCT—

(1) IN GENERAL—If the Secretary determines, after preliminary evaluation of clinical data submitted by the sponsor, that a fast track product may be effective, the Secretary shall evaluate for filing, and may commence review of portions of, an application for the approval of the product before the sponsor submits a complete application. The Secretary shall commence such review only if the applicant—

(A) provides a schedule for submission of information necessary to make the application complete; and

(B) pays any fee that may be required under section 736.

(2) EXCEPTION—Any time period for review of human drug applications that has been agreed to by the Secretary and that has been set forth in goals identified in letters of the Secretary (relating to the use of fees collected under section 736 to expedite the drug development process and the review of human drug applications) shall not apply to an application submitted under paragraph (1) until the date on which the application is complete.

(d) AWARENESS EFFORTS—The Secretary shall—

(1) develop and disseminate to physicians, patient organizations, pharmaceutical and biotechnology companies, and other appropriate persons a description of the provisions of this section applicable to fast track products; and

(2) establish a program to encourage the development of surrogate endpoints that are reasonably likely to predict clinical benefit for serious or life-threatening conditions for which there exist significant unmet medical needs.

Authority to Designate Official Names

§ **508**[358]   (a)   NECESSITY OR DESIRABILITY; USE IN OF-FICIAL COMPENDIUMS; INFRINGEMENT OF TRADE-MARKS   The Secretary may designate an official name for any drug or device if he determines that such action is necessary or desirable in the interest of usefulness and simplicity. Any official name designated under this section for any drug or device shall be the only official name of that drug or device used in any official compendium published after such name has been prescribed or for any other purpose of this Act. In no event, however, shall the Secretary establish an official name so as to infringe a valid trade-mark.

(b)   REVIEW OF NAMES IN OFFICIAL COMPENDIUMS   Within a reasonable time after October 10, 1962, and at such other times as he may deem necessary, the Secretary shall cause a review to be made of the official names by which drugs are identified in the official United States Pharmacopeia, the official Homeopathic Pharmacopeia of the United States, and the official National Formulary, and all supplements thereto and at such times as he may deem necessary shall cause a review to be made of the official names by which devices are identified in any official compendium (and all supplements thereto), to determine whether revision of any of those names is necessary or desirable in the interest of usefulness and simplicity.

(c)   DETERMINATIONS OF COMPLEXITY, USEFULNESS, MULTIPLICITY, OR LACK OF NAME; DESIGNATION BY SECRETARY   Whenever he determines after any such review that (1) any such official name is unduly complex or is not useful for any other reason, (2) two or more official names have been applied to a single drug or device, or to two or more drugs which are identical in chemical structure and pharmacological action and which are substantially identical in strength, quality, and purity or to two or more devices which are substantially equivalent in design and purpose, or (3) no official name has been applied to a medically useful drug or device, he shall transmit in writing to the compiler of each official compendium in which that drug or drugs or device are identified and recognized his request for the recommendation of a single official name for such drug or drugs or device which will have usefulness and simplicity. Whenever such a single official name has not been recommended within one hundred and eighty days after such request, or the Secretary determines that any name so recommended is not useful for any reason, he shall designate a single official name for such drug or drugs or device. Whenever he determines that the name so recommended is useful, he shall designate that name as the official name of such drug or drugs or device. Such designation shall be made as a regulation upon public notice and in accordance with the procedure set forth in section 553 of title 5, United States Code.

(d)   REVISED OFFICIAL NAMES; COMPILATION, PUBLICATION, AND PUBLIC DISTRIBUTION OF LISTINGS   After each such review, and at such other times as the Secretary may determine to be necessary or desirable, the Secretary shall cause to be compiled, published, and publicly distributed a list which shall list all revised official names of drugs or devices designated under this section and shall contain such descriptive and explanatory matter as the Secretary may determine to be required for the effective use of those names.

(e)   REQUEST BY COMPILER OF OFFICIAL COMPENDIUM FOR DISGNATION OF NAME   Upon a request in writing by any compiler of an official compendium that the Secretary exercise the authority granted to him under section 508 (a), he shall upon public notice and in accordance with the procedure set forth in section 553 of title 5, United States Code designate the official name of the drug or device for which the request is made.

Registration Requirements

§ **510**[360]   (a)   DEFINITIONS   As used in this section—

(1)   the term "manufacture, preparation, propagation, compounding, or processing" shall include repackaging or otherwise changing the container, wrapper, or labeling of any drug package or device package in furtherance of the distribution of the drug or device from the original place of manufacture to the person who makes final delivery or sale to the ultimate consumer or user; and

(2)   the term "name" shall include in the case of a partnership the name of each partner and, in the case of a corporation, the name of each corporate officer and director, and the State of incorporation.

(b)   ANNUAL REGISTRATION   On or before December 31 of each year every person who owns or operates any establishment in any State engaged in the manufacture, preparation, propagation, compounding, or processing of a drug or drugs or a device or devices shall register with the Secretary his name, places of business, and all such establishments.

(c)   NEW PRODUCERS   Every person upon first engaging in the manufacture, preparation, propagation, compounding, or processing of a drug or drugs or a device or devices in any establishment which he owns or operates in any State shall immediately register with the Secretary his name, place of business, and such establishment.

(d)   ADDITIONAL ESTABLISHMENTS   Every person duly registered in accordance with the foregoing subsections of this section shall immediately register with the Secretary any additional establishment which he owns or operates in any State and in which he begins the manufacture, preparation, propagation, compounding, or processing of a drug or drugs or a device or devices.

(e)   REGISTRATION NUMBER; UNIFORM SYSTEM OF IDENTIFICATION OF DEVICES INTENDED FOR HUMAN USE   The Secretary may assign a registration number to any person or any establishment registered in accordance with this section. The Secretary may also assign a listing number to each drug or class of drugs listed under subsection (j). Any number assigned pursuant to the preceding sentence shall be the same as that assigned pursuant to the National Drug Code. The Secretary may by regulation prescribe a uniform system for the identification of devices intended for human use and may require that persons who are required to list such devices pursuant to subsection (j) shall list such devices in accordance with such system.

(f)   AVAILABILITY OF REGISTRATIONS FOR INSPECTION   The Secretary shall make available for inspection, to any person so requesting, any registration filed pursuant to this section, except that any list submitted pursuant to paragraph (3) of subsection (j) and the information accompanying any list or notice filed under paragraph (1) or (2) of that subsection shall be exempt from such inspection unless the Secretary finds that such an exemption would be inconsistent with protection of the public health.

(g)   EXCLUSIONS FROM APPLICATION OF SECTION   The foregoing subsections of this section shall not apply to—

(1)   pharmacies which maintain establishments in conformance with any applicable local laws regulating the practice of pharmacy and medicine and which are regularly engaged in dispensing prescription drugs or devices, upon prescriptions of practitioners licensed to administer such drugs or devices to patients under the care of such practitioners in the course of their professional practice, and which do not manufacture, prepare, propagate, compound, or process drugs or devices for sale other than in the regular course of their business of dispensing or selling drugs or devices at retail;

(2)   practitioners licensed by law to prescribe or administer drugs or devices and who manufacture, prepare, propagate, compound, or process drugs or devices solely for use in the course of their professional practice;

(3)   persons who manufacture, prepare, propagate, compound, or process drugs or devices solely for use in research, teaching, or chemical analysis and not for sale;

(4) any distributor who acts as a wholesale distributor of devices, and who does not manufacture, repackage, process, or reliable a device; or

(5) such other classes of persons as the Secretary may by regulation exempt from the application of this section upon a finding that registration by such classes of persons in accordance with this section is not necessary for the protection of the public health.

In this subsection, the term "wholesale distributor" means any person (other than the manufacturer or the initial importer) who distributes a device from the original place of manufacture to the person who makes the final delivery or sale of the device to the ultimate consumer or user.

(h) INSPECTION OF PREMISES Every establishment in any State registered with the Secretary pursuant to this section shall be subject to inspection pursuant to section 704 and every such establishment engaged in the manufacture, propagation, compounding, or processing of a drug or drugs or of a device or devices classified in class II or III shall be so inspected by one or more officers or employees duly designated by the Secretary or by persons accredited to conduct inspections under § 374(g) at least once in the two-year period beginning with the date of registration of such establishment pursuant to this section and at least once in every successive two-year period thereafter.

(i) FOREIGN ESTABLISHMENTS (1) On or before Dec. 31 of each year, any establishment within any foreign country engaged in the manufacture, preparation, propagation, compounding, or processing of a drug or a device that is imported or offered for import into the United States shall through electronic means in accordance with the criteria of the Secretary, register with the Secretary the name and place of business of the establishment, the name of the United States agent for the establishment, the name of each importer of such drug or device in the US that is known to the establishment, and the name of each person who imports or offers for import such drug or device to the United States for purposes of importation.

(2) The establishment shall also provide the information required by subsection (j).

(3) The Secretary is authorized to enter into cooperative arrangements with officials of foreign countries to ensure that adequate and effective means are available for purposes of determing, from time to time, whether drugs or devices manufactured, prepared, propagated, compounded, or processed by an establishment described in paragraph (1), if imported or offered for import into the United States, shall be refused admission on any of the grounds set forth in section 801(a).

(j) FILING OF LISTS OF DRUGS AND DEVICES MANUFACTURES, PREPARED, PROPAGATED AND COMPOUNDED BY REGISTRANTS; STATEMENTS; ACCOMPANYING DISCLOSURES (1) Every person who registers with the Secretary under subsection (b), (c), (d), or (i) shall, at the time of registration under any such subsection, file with the Secretary a list of all drugs and a list of all devices and a brief statement of the basis for believing that each device included in the list is a device rather than a drug (with each drug and device in each list listed by its established name (as defined in section 502 (e)) and by any proprietary name) which are being manufactured, prepared, propagated, compounded, or processed by him for commercial distribution and which he has not included in any list of drugs or devices filed by him with the Secretary under this paragraph or paragraph (2) before such time of registration. Such list shall be prepared in such form and manner as the Secretary may prescribe and shall be accompanied by—

(A) in the case of a drug contained in the applicable list and subject to section 505 or 512, or a device intended for human use contained in the applicable list with respect to which a performance standard has been established under section 514 or which is subject to section 515, a reference to the authority for the marketing of such drug or device and a copy of all labeling for such drug or device;

(B) in the case of any other drug or device contained in an applicable list—

(i) which drug is subject to section 503 (b) (1), or which device is a restricted device, a copy of all labeling for such drug or device, a representative sampling of advertisements for such drug or device, and, upon request made by the Secretary for good cause, a copy of all advertisements for a particular drug product or device, or

(ii) which drug is not subject to section 503 (b) (1) or which device is not a restricted device, the label and package insert for such drug or device and a representative sampling of any other labeling for such drug or device;

(C) in the case of any drug contained in an applicable list which is described in inline-paragraph (B), a quantitative listing of its active ingredient or ingredients, except that with respect to a particular drug product the Secretary may require the submission of a quantitative listing of all ingredients if he finds that such submission is necessary to carry out the purposes of this Act; and

(D) if the registrant filing a list has determined that a particular drug product or device contained in such list is not subject to section 505 or 512, or the particular device contained in such list is not subject to a performance standard established under section 514 or to section 515 or is not a restricted device, a brief statement of the basis upon which the registrant made such determination if the Secretary requests such a statement with respect to that particular drug product or device.

(2) Each person who registers with the Secretary under this subsection shall report to the Secretary once during the month of June of each year and once during the month of December of each year the following information:

(A) A list of each drug or device introduced by the registrant for commercial distribution which has not been included in any list previously filed by him with the Secretary under this sub-paragraph or paragraph (1) of this subsection. A list under this sub-paragraph shall list a drug or device by its established name (as defined in section 502 (e)) and by any proprietary name it may have and shall be accompanied by the other information required by paragraph (1).

(B) If since the date the registrant last made a report under this paragraph (or if he has not made a report under this paragraph, since February 1, 1973) he has discontinued the manufacture, preparation, propagation, compounding, or processing for commercial distribution of a drug or device included in a list filed by him under sub-paragraph (A) or paragraph (1); notice of such discontinuance, the date of such discontinuance, and the identity (by established name (as defined in section 502 (e)) and by any proprietary name) of such drug or device.

(C) If since the date the registrant reported pursuant to sub-paragraph (B) a notice of discontinuance he has resumed the manufacture, preparation, propagation, compounding, or processing for commercial distribution of the drug or device with respect to which such notice of discontinuance was reported; notice of such resumption, the date of such resumption, the identity of such drug or device (each by established name (as defined in section 502 (e)) and by any proprietary name), and the other information required by paragraph (1), unless the registrant has previously reported such resumption to the Secretary pursuant to this inline-paragraph.

(D) Any material change in any information previously submitted pursuant to this paragraph or paragraph (1).

(3) The Secretary may also require each registrant under this section to submit a list of each drug product which (A) the registrant is manufacturing, preparing, propagating, compounding, or processing for commercial distribution, and (B) contains a particular ingredient. The Secretary may not require the submission of such a list unless he has made a finding that the submission of such a list is necessary to carry out the purposes of this Act.

Drugs for Rare Diseases or Conditions

RECOMMENDATIONS FOR INVESTIGATIONS OF DRUGS FOR RARE DISEASES OR CONDITIONS

§ **525** [360aa]   (a)   REQUEST BY SPONSOR; RESPONSE BY SECRETARY   The sponsor of a drug for a disease or condition which is rare in the States may request the Secretary to provide written recommendations for the non-clinical and clinical investigations which must be conducted with the drug before—

(1)   it may be approved for such disease or condition under section 505, or

(2)   if the drug is a biological product, it may be licensed for such disease or condition under section 351 of the Public Health Service Act.

(3) Redesignated (2)

If the Secretary has reason to believe that a drug for which a request is made under this section is a drug for a disease or condition which is rare in the States, the Secretary shall provide the person making the request written recommendations for the non-clinical and clinical investigations which the Secretary believes, on the basis of information available to the Secretary at the time of the request under this section, would be necessary for approval of such drug for such disease or condition under section 505 or licensing of such drug under section 351 of the Public Health Service Act for such disease or condition.

(b)   REGULATIONS   The Secretary shall by regulation promulgate procedures for the implementation of subsection (a).

DESIGNATION OF DRUGS FOR RARE DISEASES OR CONDITIONS

§ **526** [360bb]   (a)   REQUEST BY SPONSOR; PRECONDITIONS; "RARE DISEASE OR CONDITION" DEFINED   (1)   The manufacturer or the sponsor of a drug may request the Secretary to designate the drug as a drug for a rare disease or condition. A request for designation of a drug shall be made before the submission of an application under section 505(b) for the drug, or the submission of an application for licensing of the drug under section 351 of the Public Health Service Act. If the Secretary finds that a drug for which a request is submitted under this subsection is being or will be investigated for a rare disease or condition and—

(A)   if an application for such drug is approved under section 505, or

(B)   if a license for such drug is issued under section 351 of the Public Health Service Act, (C) Redesignated (B) the approval, certification or license would be for use for such disease or condition, the Secretary shall designate the drug as a drug for such disease or condition. A request for a designation of a drug under this subsection shall contain the consent of the applicant to notice being given by the Secretary under subsection (b) respecting the designation of the drug.

(2)   For purposes of paragraph (1), the term "rare disease or condition" means any disease or condition which (A) affects less than 200,000 persons in the U.S. or (B) affects more than 200,000 persons in the U.S. and for which there is no reasonable expectation that the cost of developing and making available in the United States a drug for such disease or condition will be recovered from sales in the United States of such drug. Determinations under the preceding sentence with respect to any drug shall be made on the basis of the facts and circumstances as of the date the request for designation of the drug under this subsection is made.

(b)   NOTIFICATION OF DISCONTINUACES OF DRUG OR APPLICATION AS CONDITION   A designation of a drug under subsection (a) shall be subject to the condition that—

(1)   if an application was approved for the drug under section 505(b) or a license was issued for the drug under section 351 of the Public Health Service Act, the manufacturer of the drug will notify the Secretary of any discontinuance of the production of the drug at least one year before discontinuance, and

(2)   if an application has not been approved for the drug under section 505(b) or a license has not been issued for the drug under section 351 of the Public Health Service Act and if preclinical investigations or investigations under section 505(i) are being conducted with the drug, the manufacturer or sponsor of the drug will notify the Secretary of any decision to discontinue active pursuit of approval of an application under section 505(b) or approval of a license under section 351 of the Public Health Service Act.

(c)   NOTICE TO PUBLIC   Notice respecting the designation of a drug under subsection (a) shall be made available to the public.

(d)   REGULATIONS   The Secretary shall by regulation promulgate procedures for the implementation of subsection (a).

PROTECTION FOR DRUGS FOR RARE DISEASES OR CONDITIONS

§ **527** [360cc]   (a)   EXCLUSIVE APPROVAL, CERTIFICATION, OR LICENSE   Except as provided in subsection (b) of this section, if the Secretary—

(1)   approves an application filed pursuant to section 505, or

(2)   issues a license under section 351 of the Public Health Service Act for a drug designated under section 526 for a rare disease or condition, the Secretary may not approve another application under section 505, or issue another license under section 351 of the Public Health Service Act for such drug for such disease or condition for a person who is not the holder of such approved application, of such certification, or of such license until the expiration of seven years from the date of the approval of the approved application, or the issuance of the license. Section 505 (c) (2) does not apply to the refusal to approve an application under the preceding sentence.

(3) Redesignated (2) (b)   EXCEPTIONS   If an application filed pursuant to section 505 is approved for a drug designated under section 526 for a rare disease or condition or if a license is issued under section 351 of the Public Health Service Act for such a drug, the Secretary may, during the seven-year period beginning on the date of the application approval, or of the issuance of the license, approve another application under section 505, or issue a license under section 351 of the Public Health Service Act, for such drug for such disease or condition for a person who is not the holder of such approved application, or of such license if—

(1)   the Secretary finds, after providing the holder notice and opportunity for the submission of views, that in such period the holder of the approved application, or of the license cannot assure the availability of sufficient quantities of the drug to meet the needs of persons with the disease or condition for which the drug was designated; or

(2)   such holder provides the Secretary in writing the consent of such holder for the approval of other applications, or the issuance of other licenses before the expiration of such seven-year period.

OPEN PROTOCOLS FOR INVESTIGATIONS OF DRUGS FOR RARE DISEASES OR CONDITIONS

§ **528** [360dd]   OPEN PROTOCOLS FOR INVESTIGATIONS OF DRUGS FOR RARE DISEASES OR CONDITIONS   If a drug is designated under section 526 as a drug for a rare disease or condition and if notice of a claimed exemption under section 505 (i) or regulations issued thereunder is filed for such drug, the Secretary shall encourage the sponsor of such drug to design protocols for clinical investigations of the drug which may be

conducted under the exemption to permit the addition to the investigations of persons with the disease or condition who need the drug to treat the disease or condition and who cannot be satisfactorily treated by available alternative drugs.

§ **551** [360aaa] REQUIREMENTS FOR DISSEMINATION OF TREATMENT INFORMATION ON DRUGS OR DEVICES

(a) IN GENERAL—Notwithstanding sections 301(d), 502(f), and 505, and section 351 of the Public Health Service Act (42 U.S.C. 262), a manufacturer may disseminate to—

(1) a health care practitioner;

(2) a pharmacy benefit manager;

(3) a health insurance issuer;

(4) a group health plan; or

(5) a Federal or State governmental agency;

written information concerning the safety, effectiveness, or benefit of a use not described in the approved labeling of a drug or device if the manufacturer meets the requirements of subsection (b) of this section.

(b) SPECIFIC REQUIREMENTS—A manufacturer may disseminate information under subsection (a) on a new use only if—

(1) (A) in the case of a drug, there is in effect for the drug an application filed under subsection (b) or (j) of section 505 or a biologics license issued under section 351 of the Public Health Service Act; or

(B) in the case of a device, the device is being commercially distribued in accordance with a regulation under subsection (d) or (e) of section 513, an order under subsection (f) of such section, or the approval of an application under section 515;

(2) the information meets the requirements of section 552;

(3) the information to be disseminated is not derived from clinical research conducted by another manufacturer or if it was derived from research conducted by another manufacturer, the manufacturer disseminating the information has the permission of such other manufacturer to make the dissemination;

(4) the manufacturer has, 60 days before such dissemination, submitted to the Secretary—

(A) a copy of the information to be disseminated; and

(B) any clinical trial information the manufacturer has relating to the safety or effectiveness of the new use, any reports of clinical experience pertinent to the safety of the new use, and a summary of such information;

(5) the manufacturer has complied with the requirements of section 554 (relating to a supplemental application for such use);

(6) the manufacturer includes along with the information to be disseminated under this subsection—

(A) a prominently displayed statement that discloses—

(i) that the information concerns a use of a drug or device that has not been approved or cleared by the Food and Drug Administration;

(ii) if applicable, that the information is being disseminated at the expense of the manufacturer;

(iii) if applicable, the name of any authors of the information who are employees of, consultants to, or have received compensation from, the manufacturer, or who have a significant financial interest in the manufacturer;

(iv) the official labeling for the drug or device and all updates with respect to the labeling;

(v) if applicable, a statement that there are products or treatments that have been approved or cleared for the use that is the subject of the information being disseminated pursuant to subsection (a)(1); and

(vi) the identification of any person that has provided funding for the conduct of a study relating to the new use of a drug or device for which such information is being disseminated; and

(B) a bibliography of other articles from a scientific reference publication of scientific or medical journal that have been previously published about the use of the drug or device covered by the information disseminated (unless the information already includes such bibliography).

(c) ADDITIONAL INFORMATION—If the Secretary determines, after providing notice of such determination and an opportunity for a meeting with respect to such determination, that the information submitted by a manufacturer under subsection (b)(3)(B), with respect to the use of a drug or device for which the manufacturer intends to disseminate information, fails to provide data, analyses, or other written matter that is objective and balanced, the Secretary may require the manufacturer to disseminate—

(1) additional objective and scientifically sound information that pertains to the safety or effectivess of the use and is necessary to provide objectivity and balance, including any information that the manufacturer has submitted to the Secretary or, where appropriate, a summary of such information or any other information that the Secretary has authority to make available to the public; and

(2) an objective statement of the Secretary, based on data or other scientifically sound information available to the Secretary, that bears on the safety or effectiveness of the new use of the drug or device.

§ **552** [360aaa-1] INFORMATION AUTHORIZED TO BE DISSEMINATED

(a) AUTHORIZED INFORMATION—A manufacturer may disseminate information under section 551 on a new use only if the information—

(1) is in the form of an unabridged—

(A) reprint or copy of an article, peer-reviewed by experts qualified by scientific training or experience to evaluate the safety or effectiveness of the drug or device involved, which was published in a scientific or medical journal (as defined in section 556 (5)), which is about a clinical investigation with respect to the drug or device, and which would be considered to be scientifically sound by such experts; or

(B) referencc publication, described in subsection (h), that includes information about a clinical investigation with respect to the drug or device that would be considered to be scientifically sound by experts qualified by scientific training or experience to evaluate the safety or effectivess of the drug or device that is the subject of such a clinical investigation; and

(2) is not false or misleading and would not pose a significiant risk to the public health.

(b) REFERENCE PUBLICATION—A reference publication referred to in subsection (a)(1)(B) is a publication that—

(1) has not been written, edited, excerpted, or published specifically for, or at the request of, a manufacturer of a drug or device;

(2) has not been edited or significantly influenced by such a manufacturer;

(3) is not solely distributed through such a manufacturer but is generally available in bookstores or other distribution channels where medical textbooks are sold;

(4) does not focus on any particular drug or device of a manufacturer that disseminates information under section 551 and does not have a primary focus on new uses of drugs or devices that are marketed or under investigation by a manufacturer supporting the dissemination or information; and

(5) presents materials that are not false or misleading.

§ **553** [360-aaa-2] ESTABLISHMENT OF LIST OF ARTICLES AND PUBLICATIONS DISSEMINATED AND LIST OF PROVIDERS THAT RECEIVED ARTICLES AND REFERENCE PUBLICATIONS

(a) IN GENERAL—A manufacturer may disseminate information under section 551 on a new use only if the manufacturer prepares and submits to the Secretary biannually—

(1) a list containing the titles of the articles and reference publications relating to the new use of drugs or devices that were disseminated by the manufacturer to a person described in section 551(a) for the 6-month period preceding the date on which the manufacturer submits the list to the Secretary; and

(2) a list that identifies the categories of providers (as described in section 551(a)) that received the articles and reference publications for the 6-month period described in paragraph (1).

(b) RECORDS—A manufacturer that disseminates information under section 551 shall keep records that may be used by the manufacturer when, pursuant to section 555, such manufacturer is required to take corrective action and shall be made available to the Secretary, upon request, for purposes of ensuring or

taking corrective action pursuant to such section. Such records, at the Secretary's discretion, may identify the recipient of information provided pursuant to section 551 or the categories of such recipients.

§ **554** [360aaa-3] REQUIREMENT REGARDING SUBMIS- SION OF SUPPLEMENTAL APPLICATION FOR NEW USE; EX- EMPTION FROM REQUIREMENT

(a)   IN GENERAL—A manufacturer may disseminate informa- tion under section 551 on a new use only if—

(1) (A)   the manufacturer has submitted to the Secretary a supplemental application for such use; or

(B)   the manufacturer meets the condition described in sub- section (b) or (c) (relating to a certification that the manufacturer will submit such as application); or

(2)   there is in effect for the manufacturer an exemption un- der subsection (d) from the requirement of paragraph (1).

(b)   CERTIFICATION ON SUPPLEMENTAL APPLICATION; CONDITION IN CASE OF COMPLETED STUDIES—For pur- poses of subsection (a)(1)(B), a manufacturer may disseminate information on a new use if the manufacturer has submitted to the Secretary an application containing a certification that—

(1)   the studies needed for the submission of a supplemen- tal application for the new use have been completed; and

(2)   the supplemental application will be submitted to the Secretary not later than 6 months after the date of the initial dis- semination of information under section 551.

(c)   CERTIFICATION ON SUPPLEMENTAL APPLICATION; CONDITION IN CASE OF PLANNED STUDIES—

(1)   IN GENERAL—For purposes of subsection (a)(1)(B), a manufacturer may disseminate information on a new use if—

(A)   the manufacturer has submitted to the Secretary an application containing—

(i)   a proposed protocol and schedule for conducting the studies needed for the submisstion of a supplemental applica- tion for the new use; and

(ii)   a certification that the supplemental application will be submitted to the Secretary not later than 36 months after the date of the initial dissemination of information under section 551 (or, as applicable, not later than such date as the Secretary may specify pursuant to an extension under paragraph (3)); and

(B)   the Secretary has determined that the proposed pro- tocol is adequate and that the schedule for completing such stu- dies is reasonable.

(2)   PROGRESS REPORTS ON STUDIES—A manufac- turer that submits to the Secretary an application under paragraph (1) shall submit to the Secretary periodic reports describing the status of the studies involved.

(3)   EXTENSION OF TIME REGARDING PLANNED STU- DIES—The period of 36 months authorized in paragraph (1)(A)(ii) for the completion of studies may be extended by the Secretary if—

(A)   the Secretary determines that the studies needed to submit such an application cannot be completed and submitted within 36 months; or

(B)   the manufacturer involved submits to the Secretary a written request for the extension and the Secretary determines that the manufacturer has acted with due diligence to conduct the studies in a timely manner, except that an extension under this inline-paragraph may not be provided for more than 24 addi- tional months.

(d)   EXEMPTION FROM REQUIREMENT OF SUPPLEMEN- TAL APPLICATION—

(1)   IN GENERAL—For purposes of subsection (a)(2), a manufacturer may disseminate information on a new use if—

(A)   the manufacturer has submitted to the Secretary an application for an exemption from meeting the requirement of subsection (a)(1); and

(B) (i)   the Secretary has approved the application in ac- cordance with paragraph (2); or

(ii)   the application is deemed under paragraph (3)(A) to have been approved (unless such approval is terminated pur- suant to paragraph (3)(B)).

(2)   CONDITIONS FOR APPROVAL—The Secretary may approve an application under paragraph (1) for an exemption if the Secretary makes a determination described in sub-paragraph (A) or (B), as follows:

(A)   The Secretary makes a determination that, for rea- sons defined by the Secretary, it would be economically prohibi- tive with respect to such drug or device for the manufacturer to incur the costs necessary for the submission of a supplemental application. In making such determination, the Secretary shall consider (in addition to any other considerations the Secretary finds appropriate)—

(i)   the lack of the availability under law of any period during which the manufacturer would have exclusive marketing rights with respect to the new use involved; and

(ii)   the size of the population expected to benefit from approval of the supplemental application.

(B)   The Secretary makes a determination that, for rea- sons defined by the Secretary, it would be unethical to conduct the studies necessary for the supplemental application. In making such determination, the Secretary shall consider (in addition to any other considerations the Secretary finds appropriate) whether the new use involved is the standard of medical care for a health condition.

(3)   TIME FOR CONSIDERATION OF APPLICATION; DEEMED APPROVAL—

(A)   IN GENERAL—The Secretary shall approve or deny an application under paragraph (1) for an exemption not later than 60 days after the recipt of the application. If the Secretary does not comply with the preceding sentence, the application is deemed to be approved.

(B)   TERMINATION OF DEEMED APPROVAL—If pur- suant to a deemed approval under sub-paragraph (A) a manufac- turer disseminates written information under section 551 on a new use, the Secretary may at any time terminate such approval and under section 555(b)(3) order the manufacturer to cease dissemi- nating the information.

(e)   REQUIREMENTS REGARDING APPLICATIONS—Ap- plications under this section shall be submitted in the form and manner prescribed by the Secretary.

Records of Interstate Shipment

§ 703[373]   For the purpose of enforcing the provisions of this Act, carriers engaged in interstate commerce, and persons re- ceiving foods, drugs, devices, or cosmetics in interstate com- merce or holding such articles so received, shall, upon the request of an officer or employee duly designated by the Secre- tary, permit such officer or employee, at reasonable times, to have access to and to copy all records showing the movement in interstate commerce of any food, drug, device, or cosmetic, or the holding thereof during or after such movement, and the quantity, shipper, and consignee thereof; and it shall be unlawful for any such carrier or person to fail to permit such access to and copying of any such record so requested when such request is accompanied by a statement in writing specifying the nature or kind of food, drug, device, or cosmetic to which such request re- lates, except that evidence obtained under this section, or any evidence which is directly or indirectly derived from such evi- dence, shall not be used in a criminal prosecution of the person from whom obtained, and except that carriers shall not be subject to the other provisions of this Act by reason of their receipt, car- riage, holding, or delivery of food, drugs, devices, or cosmetics in the usual course of business as carriers.

Inspections

§ **704**[374]   (a)   RIGHT OF AGENTS TO ENTER; SCOPE OF INSPECTION; NOTICE; PROMPTNESS; EXCLUSIONS   (1) For purposes of enforcement of this Act, officers or employees duly designated by the Secretary, upon presenting appropriate credentials and a written notice to the owner, operator, or agent in charge, are authorized (A) to enter, at reasonable times, any factory, warehouse, or establishment in which food, drugs, devices, or cosmetics are manufactured, processed, packed, or held, for introduction into interstate commerce or after such introduction, or to enter any vehicle being used to transport or hold such food, drugs, devices or cosmetics in interstate commerce; and (B) to inspect, at reasonable times and within reasonable limits and in a reasonable manner, such factory, warehouse, establishment, or vehicle and all pertinent equipment, finished and unfinished materials, containers, and labeling therein. In the case of any person (excluding farms and restaurants) who manufactures, processes, packs, transports, distributes, holds, or imports foods, the inspection shall extend to all records and other information described in section 350c of this title when the Secretary has a reasonable belief that an article of food is adulterated and presents a threat of serious adverse health consequences or death to humans or animals, subject to the limitations established in section 350c(d) of this title. In the case of any factory, warehouse, establishment, or consulting laboratory in which prescription drugs or restricted devices are manufactured, processed, packed, or held, inspection shall extend to all things therein (including records, files, papers, processes, controls, and facilities) bearing on whether prescription drugs, nonprescription drugs intended for human use, or restricted devices which are adulterated or misbranded within the meaning of this Act, or which may not be manufactured, introduced into interstate commerce, or sold, or offered for sale by reason of any provision of this Act, have been or are being manufactured, processed, packed, transported, or held in any such place, or otherwise bearing on violation of this Act. No inspection authorized by the preceding sentence or by paragraph (3) shall extend to financial data, sales data other than shipment data, pricing data, personnel data (other than data as to qualifications of technical and professional personnel performing functions subject to this Act), and research data (other than data relating to new drugs, antibiotic drugs, and devices and subject to reporting and inspection under regulations lawfully issued pursuant to section 505 (i) or (k), section 519, or 520 (g), and data relating to other drugs or devices which in the case of a new drug would be subject to reporting or inspection under lawful regulations issued pursuant to section 505 (j).) A separate notice shall be given for each such inspection, but a notice shall not be required for each entry made during the period covered by the inspection. Each such inspection shall be commenced and completed with reasonable promptness.

(2)   The provisions of the second sentence of this subsection shall not apply to—

(A)   pharmacies which maintain establishments in conformance with any applicable local laws regulating the practice of pharmacy and medicine and which are regularly engaged in dispensing prescription drugs or devices upon prescriptions of practitioners licensed to administer such drugs or devices to patients under the care of such practitioners in the course of their professional practice, and which do not, either through a subsidiary or otherwise, manufacture, prepare, propagate, compound, or process drugs or devices for sale other than in the regular course of their business of dispensing or selling drugs or devices at retail;

(B)   practitioners licensed by law to prescribe or administer drugs or prescribe or use devices, as the case may be, and who manufacture, prepare, propagate, compound, or process drugs or manufacture or process devices solely for use in the course of their professional practice;

(C)   persons who manufacture, prepare, propagate, compound, or process drugs or manufacture or process devices solely for use in research, teaching, or chemical analysis and not for sale;

(D)   such other classes of persons as the Secretary may by regulation exempt from the application of this section upon a finding that inspection as applied to such classes of persons in accordance with this section is not necessary for the protection of the public health.

(3)   An officer or employee making an inspection under paragraph (1) for purposes of enforcing the requirements of section 350a of this title applicable to infant formulas shall be permitted, at all reasonable times, to have access to and to copy and verify any records—

(A)   bearing on whether the infant formula manufactured or held in the facility inspected meets the requirements of section 350a of this title, or

(B)   required to be maintained under section 350a of this title.

(b)   WRITTEN REPORT TO OWNER; COPY TO SECRETARY   Upon completion of any such inspection of a factory, warehouse, consulting laboratory, or other establishment, and prior to leaving the premises, the officer or employee making the inspection shall give to the owner, operator, or agent in charge a report in writing setting forth any conditions or practices observed by him which, in his judgment, indicate that any food, drug, device, or cosmetic in such establishment (1) consists in whole or in part of any filthy, putrid, or decomposed substance, or (2) has been prepared, packed, or held under insanitary conditions whereby it may have become contaminated with filth, or whereby it may have been rendered injurious to health. A copy of such report shall be sent promptly to the Secretary.

(c)   RECEIPT FOR SAMPLES TAKEN   If the officer or employee making any such inspection of a factory, warehouse, or other establishment has obtained any sample in the course of the inspection, upon completion of the inspection and prior to leaving the premises he shall give to the owner, operator, or agent in charge a receipt describing the samples obtained.

Revision of United States Pharmacopeia; Development of Analysis and Mechanical and Physical Tests

Labor-Federal Security Appropriations Act

The Secretary, in carrying into effect the provisions of this chapter, is authorized hereafter to cooperate with associations and scientific societies in the revision of the United States Pharmacopeia and in the development of methods of analysis and mechanical and physical tests necessary to carry out the work of the Food and Drug Administration.

Definitions

§   **201** [321]   For the purposes of this Act—

(s)   The term "food additive" means any substance the intended use of which results or may reasonably be expected to result, directly or indirectly, in its becoming a component or otherwise affecting the characteristics of any food (including any substance intended for use in producing, manufacturing, packing, processing, preparing, treating, packaging, transporting, or holding food; and including any source of radiation intended for any such use), if such substance is not generally recognized, among experts qualified by scientific training and experience to evaluate its safety, as having been adequately shown through scientific procedures (or, in the case of a substance used in food prior to January 1, 1958, through either scientific procedures or experience based on common use in food) to be safe under the conditions of its intended use; except that such term does not include—

(1)   a pesticide chemical residue in or on a raw agricultural commodity or processed food; or

(2)   a pesticide chemical; or

(3)   a color additive; or

(4)   any substance used in accordance with a sanction or approval granted prior to September 6, 1958 pursuant to this Act, the Poultry Products Inspection Act (21 U.S.C. 451 and the following) or the Meat Inspection Act of March 4, 1907 (34 Stat. 1260), as amended and extended (21 USCA § 601 et seq);

(5)   a new animal drug; or

(6)   an ingredient described in paragraph (ff) in, or intended for use in, a dietary supplement.

(v)   The term "new animal drug" means any drug intended for use for animals other than man, including any drug intended for use in animal feed but not including such animal feed—

(1)   the composition of which is such that such drug is not generally recognized, among experts qualified by scientific training and experience to evaluate the safety and effectiveness of animal drugs, as safe and effective for use under the conditions prescribed, recommended, or suggested in the labeling thereof; except that such a drug not so recognized shall not be deemed to be a "new animal drug" if at any time prior to June 25, 1938, it was subject to the Food and Drug Act of June 30, 1906, as amended, and if at such time its labeling contained the same representations concerning the conditions of its use; or

(2)   the composition of which is such that such drug, as a result of investigations to determine its safety and effectiveness for use under such conditions, has become so recognized but which has not, otherwise than in such investigations, been used to a material extent or for a material time under such conditions.

(w)   The term "animal feed", as used in paragraph (w) of this section, in section 512, and in provisions of this Act referring to such paragraph or section, means an article which is intended for use for food for animals other than man and which is intended for use as a substantial source of nutrients in the diet of the animal, and is not limited to a mixture intended to be the sole ration of the animal.

(aa)   The term "abbreviated drug application" means an application submitted under section 505(j) for the approval of a drug that relies on the approved application of another drug with the same active ingredient to establish safety and efficacy, and

(1)   in the case of section 306, includes a supplement to such an application for a different or additional use of the drug but does not include a supplement to such an application for other than a different or additional use of the drug, and

(2)   in the case of sections 307 and 308, includes any supplement to such an application.

(dd)   For purposes of sections 306 and 307, the term "drug product" means a drug subject to regulation under section 505, 512, or 802 of this Act or under section 351 of the Public Health Service Act.

§   **501** [351]   A drug or device shall be deemed to be adulterated—

(a)   POISONOUS, INSANITARY, ETC., INGREDIENTS; ADEQUATE CONTROLS IN MANUFACTURE   (5)   if it is a new animal drug which is unsafe within the meaning of seciton 512; or (6) if it is an animal feed bearing or containing a new animal drug, and such animal feed is unsafe within the meaning of section 512.

§   **503** [353]

(f)   VETERINARY PRESCRIPTION DRUGS   (1) (A)   A drug intended for use by animals other than man, other than a veterinary feed directive drug intended for use in animal feed or an animal feed bearing or containing veterinary feed directive drug, which—

(i)   because of its toxicity or other potentiality for harmful effect, or the method of its use, or the collateral measures necessary for its use, is not safe for animal use except under the professional supervision of a licensed veterinarian, or

(ii)   is limited by an approved application under subsection (b) of section 512 to use under the professional supervision of a licensed veterinarian, shall be dispensed only by or upon the lawful written or oral order of a licensed veterinarian in the course of the veterinarian's professional practice.

(B)   For purposes of sub-paragraph (A), an order is lawful if the order—

(i)   is a prescription or other order authorized by law,

(ii)   is, if an oral order, promptly reduced to writing by the person lawfully filling the order, and filed by that person, and

(iii)   is refilled only if authorized in the original order or in a subsequent oral order promptly reduced to writing by the person lawfully filling the order, and filed by that person.

(C)   The act of dispensing a drug contrary to the provisions of this paragrpah shall be deemed to be an act which results in the drug being misbranded while held for sale.

(2)   Any drug when dispensed in accordance with paragraph (1) of this subsection—

(A)   shall be exempt from the requirements of section 502, except subsections (a), (g), (h), (i)(2), (i)(3), and (p) of such section, and

(B)   shall be exempt from the packaging requirements of subsections (g), (h), and (p) of such section if—

(i)   when dispensed by a licensed veterinarian, the drug bears a label containing the name and address of the practitioner and any directions for use and cautionary statements specified by the practitioner, or

(ii)   when dispensed by filling the lawful order of a licensed veterinarian, the drug bears a label containing the name and address of the dispenser, the serial number and date of the order or of its filling, the name of the licensed veterinarian, and the directions for use and cautionary statements, if any, contained in such order.

The preceding sentence shall not apply to any drug dispensed in the course of the conduct of a business of dispensing drugs pursuant to diagnosis by mail.

(3)   The Secretary may by regulation exempt drugs for animals other than man subject to section 512 from the requirements of paragraph (1) when such requirements are not necessary for the protection of the public health.

(4)   A drug which is subject to paragraph (1) shall be deemed to be misbranded if at any time prior to dispensing its label fails to bear the statement "Caution: Federal law restricts this drug to use by or on the order of a licensed veterinarian." A drug to which paragraph (1) does not apply shall be deemed to be misbranded if at any time prior to dispensing its label bears the statement specified in the preceding sentence.

New Animal Drugs

§   **512** [360b]   (a)   UNSAFE NEW ANIMAL DRUGS AND ANIMAL FEED CONTAINING SUCH DRUGS; CONDITIONS OF SAFETY; EXEMPTION OF DRUGS FOR RESEARCH; IMPORTANT TOLERANCES   (1)   A new animal drug shall, with respect to any particular use or intended use of such drug, be deemed unsafe for the purposes of section 501(a)(5) and section 402(a)(2)(D) unless—

(A)   there is in effect an approval of an application filed pursuant to subsection (b) of this section with respect to such use or intended use of such drug, and

(B)   such drug, its labeling, and such use conform to such approved application.

A new animal drug shall also be deemed unsafe for such purposes in the event of removal from the establishment of a manufacturer, packer, or distributor of such drug for use in the manufacture of animal feed in any State unless at the time of such removal such manufacturer, packer, or distributor has an unrevoked written statement from the consignee of such drug, or notice from the Secretary, to the effect that, with respect to the use of such drug in animal feed, such consignee (i) holds a license issued under subsection (m) and has in its possession current approved labeling for such drug in animal feed; or (ii) will, if the consignee is not a user of the drug, ship such drug only to a holder of a license issued under subsection (m).

(2)   An animal feed bearing or containing a new animal drug shall, with respect to any particular use or intended use of such animal feed, be deemed unsafe for the purposes of section 501(a)(6) unless—

(A)   there is in effect an approval of an application filed pursuant to subsection (b) of this section with respect to such drug, as used in such animal feed,

(B)   such animal feed is manufactured at a site for which there is in effect a license issued pursuant to subsection (m)(1) to manufacture such animal feed, and

(C)   such animal feed and its labeling, distribution, holding, and use conform to the conditions and indications of use published pursuant to subsection (i).

(3)   A new animal drug or an animal feed bearing or containing a new animal drug shall not be deemed unsafe for the purposes of section 501(a)(5) or (6) if such article is for investigational use and conforms to the terms of an exemption in effect with respect thereto under section 512(j).

(4) (A)   Except as provided in sub-paragraph (B), if an approval of an application filed under subsection (b) is in effect with respect to a particular use or intended use of a new animal drug, the drug shall not be deemed unsafe for the purposes of paragraph (1) and shall be exempt from the requirements of section 502(f) with respect to a different use or intended use of the drug, other than a use in or on animal feed, if such use or intended use—

(i)   is by or on the lawful written or oral order of a licensed veterinarian within the context of a veterinarian-client patient relationship, as defined by the Secretary; and

(ii)   is in compliance with regulations promulgated by the Secretary that establish the conditions for such different use or intended use. The regulations promulgated by the Secretary under clause (ii) may prohibit particular uses of an animal drug and shall not permit such different use of an animal drug if the labeling of another animal drug that contains the same active ingredient and which is in the same dosage form and concentration provides for such different use.

(B)   If the Secretary finds that there is a reasonable probability that a use of an animal drug authorized under sub-paragraph (A) may present a risk to the public health, the Secretary may—

(i)   establish a safe level for a residue of an animal drug when it is used for such different use authorized by sub-paragraph (A); and

(ii)   require the development of a practical, analytical method for the detection of residues of such drug above the safe level established under clause (i).

The use of an animal drug that results in residues exceeding a safe level established under clause (i) shall be considered an unsafe use of such drug under paragraph (1). Safe levels may be established under clause (i) either by regulation or order.

(C)   The Secretary may be general regulation provide access to the records of veterinarians to ascertain any use or intended use authorized under sub-paragraph (A) that the Secretary has determined may present a risk to the public health.

(D)   If the Secretary finds, after affording an opportunity for public comment, that a use of an animal drug authorized under sub-paragraph (A) presents a risk to the public health or that an analytical method required under sub-paragraph (B) has not been developed and submitted to the Secretary, the Secretary may, by order, prohibit any such use.

(5)   If the approval of an application filed under section 505 is in effect, the drug under such application shall not be deemed unsafe for purposes of paragraph (1) and shall be exempt from the requirements of section 502(f) with respect to a use or intended use of the drug in animals if such use of intended use—

(A)   is by or on the lawful written or oral order of a licensed veterinarian within the context of a veterinarian-client patient relationship, as defined by the Secretary; and

(B)   is in compliance with regulations promulgated by the Secretary that establish the conditions for the use or intended use of the drug in animals.

(6)   For purposes of section 402(a)(2)(D), a use or intended use of a new animal drug shall not be deemed unsafe under this section if the Secretary establishes a tolerance for such drug and any edible portion of any animal imported into the United States does not contain residues exceeding such tolerance. In establishing such tolerance, the Secretary shall rely on data sufficient to demonstrate that a proposed tolerance is safe based on similar food safety criteria used by the Secretary to establish tolerances for applications for new animal drugs filed under subsection (b)(1). The Secretary may consider and rely on data submitted by the drug manufacturer, including data submitted to appropriate regulatory authorities in any country where the new animal drug is lawfully used or data available from a relevant international organization, to the extent such data are not inconsistent with the criteria used by the Secretary to establish a tolerance for application for new animal drugs filed under subsection (b)(1). For purposes of this paragraph, "relevant international organization" means the Codex Alimenterius Commission or other international organization deemed appropriate by the Secretary. The Secretary may, under procedures specified by regulation, revoke a tolerance established under this paragraph if information demonstrates that the use of the new animal drug under actual use conditions results in food being imported into the United States with residues exceeding the tolerance or if scientific evidence shows the tolerance to be unsafe.

(b)   FILING APPLICATION FOR USES OF NEW ANIMAL DRUG; CONTENTS; PATENT INFORMATION; ABBREVIATED APPLICATION; PRESUBMISSION CONFERENCE   (1)   Any person may file with the Secretary an application with respect to any intended use or uses of a new animal drug. Such person shall submit to the Secretary as a part of the application (A) full reports of investigations which have been made to show whether or not such drug is safe and effective for use; (B) a full list of the articles used as components of such drug; (C) a full statement of the composition of such drug; (D) a full description of the methods used in, and the facilities and controls used for, the manufacture, processing, and packing of such drug; (E) such samples of such drug and of the articles used as components thereof, of any animal feed for use in or on which such drug is intended, and of the edible portions or products (before or after slaughter) of animals to which such drug (directly or in or on animal feed) is intended to be administered, as the Secretary may require; (F) specimens of the labeling proposed to be used for such drug, or in case such drug is intended for use in animal feed, proposed labeling appropriate for such use, and specimens of the labeling for the drug to be manufactured, packed, or distributed by the applicant; (G) a description of practicable methods for determining the quantity, if any, of such drug in or on food, and any substance formed in or on food, because of its use; and (H) the proposed tolerance or withdrawal period or other use restrictions for such drug if any tolerance or withdrawal period or other use restrictions are required in order to assure that the proposed use of such drug will be safe. The applicant shall file with the application the patent number and the expiration date of any patent which claims the new animal drug for which the applicant filed the application or which claims a method of using such drug and with respect to which a claim of patent infringement could reasonably be asserted if a person not licensed by the owner engaged in the manufacture, use, or sale of the drug. If an application is filed under this subsection for a drug and a patent which claims such drug or a method of using such drug is issued after the filing date but before approval of the application, the applicant shall amend the application to include the information required by the preceding sentence. Upon approval of the application, the Secretary shall publish information submitted under the two preceding sentences.

(2)   Any person may file with the Secretary an abbreviated application for the approval of a new animal drug. An abbreviated application shall contain the information required by subsection (n).

(3)   Any person intending to file an application under paragraph (1) or a request for an investigational exemption under subsection (j) shall be entitled to one or more conferences prior to such submission to reach an agreement acceptable to the Secretary establishing a submission or an investigational requirement,

which may include a requirement for a field investigation. A decision establishing a submission or an investigational requirement shall bind the Secretary and the applicant or requestor unless (A) the Secretary and the applicant or requestor mutually agree to modify the requirement, or (B) the Secretary by written order determines that a substantiated scientific requirement essential to the determination of safety or effectiveness of the animal drug involved has appeared after the conference. No later than 25 calendar days after each such conference, the Secretary shall provide a written order setting forth a scientific justification specific to the animal drug and intended uses under consideration if the agreement referred to in the first sentence requires more than one field investigation as being essential to provide substantial evidence of effectiveness for the intended uses of the drug. Nothing in this paragraph shall be construed as compelling the Secretary to require a field investigation.

(c)   PERIOD FOR SUBMISSION AND APPROVAL OF APPLICATION; PERIOD FOR NOTICE, AND EXPEDITION OF HEARING; PERIOD FOR ISSUANCE OF ORDER; ABBREVIATED APPLICATIONS; WITHDRAWAL PERIODS; EFFECTIVE DATE OF APPROVAL; RELATIONSHIP TO OTHER APPLICATIONS; WITHDRAWAL OR SUSPENSION OF APPROVAL; BIOEQUIVALENCE; FILING OF ADDITIONAL PATENT INFORMATION   (1)   Within one hundred and eighty days after the filing of an application pursuant to subsection (b), or such additional period as may be agreed upon by the Secretary and the applicant, the Secretary shall either (A) issue an order approving the application if he then finds that none of the grounds for denying approval specified in the subsection (d) applies, or (B) give the applicant notice of an opportunity for a hearing before the Secretary under subsection (d) on the question whether such application is approvable. If the applicant elects to accept the opportunity for a hearing by written request within thirty days after such notice, such hearing shall commence not more than ninety days after the expiration of such thirty days unless the Secretary and the applicant otherwise agree. Any such hearing shall thereafter be conducted on an expedited basis and the Secretary's order thereon shall be issued within ninety days after the date fixed by the Secretary for filing final briefs.

(2) (A)   Subject to sub-paragraph (C), the Secretary shall approve an abbreviated application for a drug unless the Secretary finds—

(i)   the methods used in, or the facilities and controls used for, the manufacture, processing, and packing of the drug are inadequate to assure and preserve its identity, strength, quality, and purity;

(ii)   the conditions of use prescribed, recommended, or suggested in the proposed labeling are not reasonably certain to be followed in practice or, except as provided in sub-paragraph (B), information submitted with the application is insufficient to show that each of the proposed conditions of use or similar limitations [whether in the labeling or published pursuant to subsection (i)] have been previously approved for the approved new animal drug referred to in the application;

(iii)   information submitted with the application is insufficient to show that the active ingredients are the same as those of the approved new animal drug referred to in the application;

(iv) (I)   if the application is for a drug whose active ingredients, route of administration, dosage form, strength, or use with other animal drugs in animal feed is the same as the active ingredients, route of administration, dosage form, strength, or use with other animal drugs in animal feed of the approved new animal drug referred to in the application, information submitted in the application is insufficient to show that the active ingredients, route of administration, dosage form, strength, or use with other animal drugs in animal feed is the same as that of the approved new animal drug, or

(II)   if the application is for a drug whose active ingredients, route of administration, dosage form, strength, or use with other animal drugs in animal feed is different from that of the approved new animal drug referred to in the application, no petition to file an application for the drug with the different active ingredi-

ents, route of administration, dosage form, strength, or use with other animal drugs in animal feed was approved under subsection (n)(3);

(v)   if the application was filed pursuant to the approval of a petition under subsection (n)(3), the application did not contain the information required by the Secretary respecting the active ingredients, route of administration, dosage form, strength, or use with other animal drugs in animal feed which is not the same;

(vi)   information submitted in the application is insufficient to show that the drug is bioequivalent to the approved new animal drug referred to in the application, or if the application is filed under a petition approved pursuant to subsection (n)(3), information submitted in the application is insufficient to show that the active ingredients of the new animal drug are of the same pharmacological or therapeutic class as the pharmacological or therapeutic class of the approved new animal drug and that the new animal drug can be expected to have the same therapeutic effect as the approved new animal drug when used in accordance with the labeling;

(vii)   information submitted in the application is insufficient to show that the labeling proposed for the drug is the same as the labeling approved for the approved new animal drug referred to in the application except for changes required because of differences approved under a petition filed under subsection (n)(3), because of a different withdrawal period, or because the drug and the approved new animal drug are produced or distributed by different manufacturers;

(viii)   information submitted in the application or any other information available to the Secretary shows that (I) the inactive ingredients of the drug are unsafe for use under the conditions prescribed, recommended, or suggested in the labeling proposed for the drug, (II) the composition of the drug is unsafe under such conditions because of the type or quantity of inactive ingredients included or the manner in which the inactive ingredients are included, or (III) in the case of a drug for food producing animals, the inactive ingredients of the drug or its composition may be unsafe with respect to human food safety;

(ix)   the approval under subsection (b)(1) of the approved new animal drug referred to in the application filed under subsection (b)(2) has been withdrawn or suspended for grounds described in paragraph (1) of subsection (e), the Secretary has published a notice of a hearing to withdraw approval of the approved new animal drug for such grounds, the approval under this paragraph of the new animal drug for which the application under subsection (b)(2) was filed has been withdrawn or suspended under inline-paragraph (G) for such grounds, or the Secretary has determined that the approved new animal drug has been withdrawn from sale for safety or effectiveness reasons;

(x)   the application does not meet any other requirement of subsection (n); or

(xi)   the application contains an untrue statement of material fact.

(B)   If the Secretary finds that a new animal drug for which an application is submitted under subsection (b)(2) is bioequivalent to the approved new animal drug referred to in such application and that residues of the new animal drug are consistent with the tolerances established for such approved new animal drug but at a withdrawal period which is different than the withdrawal period approved for such approved new animal drug, the Secretary may establish, on the basis of information submitted, such different withdrawal period as the withdrawal period for the new animal drug for purposes of the approval of such application for such drug.

(H)   For purposes of this paragraph:

(i)   The term "bioequivalence" means the rate and extent to which the active ingredient or therapeutic ingredient is absorbed from a new animal drug and becomes available at the site of drug action.

(ii)   A new animal drug shall be considered to be bioequivalent to the approved new animal drug referred to in its application under subsection (n) if—

(I)   the rate and extent of absorption of the drug do not show a significant difference from the rate and extent of absorption of the approved new animal drug referred to in the appli-

cation when administered at the same dose of the active ingredient under similar experimental conditions in either a single dose or multiple doses;

(II)   the extent of absorption of the drug does not show a significant difference from the extent of absorption of the approved new animal drug referred to in the application when administered at the same dose of the active ingredient under similar experimental conditions in either a single dose or multiple doses and the difference from the approved new animal drug in the rate of absorption of the drug is intentional, is reflected in its proposed labeling, is not essential to the attainment of effective drug concentrations in use, and is considered scientifically insignificant for the drug in attaining the intended purposes of its use and preserving human food safety or

(III)   in any case in which the Secretary determines that the measurement of the rate and extent of absorption or excretion of the new animal drug in biological fluids is inappropriate or impractical, an appropriate acute pharmacological effects test or other test of the new animal drug and, when deemed scientifically necessary, of the approved new animal drug referred to in the application in the species to be tested or in an appropriate animal model does not show a significant difference between the new animal drug and such approved new animal drug when administered at the same dose under similar experimental conditions.

If the approved new animal drug referred to in the application for a new animal drug under subsection (n) is approved for use in more than one animal species, the bioequivalency information described in subclause (I), (II), and (III) shall be obtained for one species, or if the Secretary deems appropriate based on scientific principles, shall be obtained for more than one species. The Secretary may prescribe the dose to be used in determining bioequivalency under subclauses (I), (II), or (III). To assure that the residues of the new animal drug will be consistent with the established tolerances for the approved new animal drug referred to in the application under subsection (b)(2) upon the expiration of the withdrawal period contained in the application for the new animal drug, the Secretary shall require bioequivalency data or residue depletion studies of the new animal drug or such other data or studies as the Secretary considers appropriate based on scientific principles. If the Secretary requires one or more residue studies under the preceding sentence, the Secretary may not require that the assay methodology used to determine the withdrawal period of the new animal drug be more rigorous than the methodology used to determined the withdrawal period for the approved new animal drug referred to in the application. If such studies are required and if the approved new animal drug, referred to in the application for the new animal drug for which such studies are required, is approved for use in more than one animal species, such studies shall be conducted for one species, or if the Secretary deems appropriate based on scientific principles, shall be conducted for more than one species.

(3)   If the patent information described in subsection (b)(1) could not be filed with the submission of an application under subsection (b)(1) because the application was filed before the patent information was required under subsection (b)(1) or a patent was issued after the application was approved under such subsection, the holder of an approved application shall file with the Secretary the patent number and the expiration date of any patent which claims the new animal drug for which the application was filed or which claims a method of using such drug and with respect to which a claim of patent infringement could reasonably be asserted if a person not licensed by the owner engaged in the manufacture, use, or sale of the drug. If the holder of an approved application could not file patent information under subsection (b)(1) because it was not required at the time the application was approved, the holder shall file such information under this subsection not later than 30 days after November 16, 1988, and if the holder of an approved application could not file patent information under subsection (b)(1) because no patent had been issued when an application was filed or approved, the holder shall file such information under this subsection not later than 30 days after the date the patent involved is issued. Upon the submission of patent information under this subsection, the Secretary shall publish it.

(4)   A drug manufactured in a pilot or other small facility may be used to demonstrate the safety and effectiveness of the drug and to obtain approval for the drug prior to manufacture of the drug in a larger facility, unless the Secretary makes a determination that a full scale production facility is necessary to ensure the safety or effectiveness of the drug.

(d)   GROUNDS FOR REFUSING APPLICATION; APPROVAL OF APPLICATION; FACTORS; "SUBSTANTIAL EVIDENCE" DEFINED; COMBINATION DRUGS   (1)   If the Secretary finds, after due notice to the applicant in accordance with subsection (c) and giving him an opportunity for a hearing, in accordance with said subsection, that —

(A)   the investigations, reports of which are required to be submitted to the Secretary pursuant to subsection (b), do not include adequate tests by all methods reasonably applicable to show whether or not such drug is safe for use under the conditions prescribed, recommended or suggested in the proposed labeling thereof;

(B)   the results of such tests show that such drug is unsafe for use under such conditions or do not show that such drug is safe for use under such conditions;

(C)   the methods used in, and the facilities and controls used for, the manufacture, processing, and packing of such drug are inadequate to preserve its identity, strength, quality, and purity;

(D)   upon the basis of the information submitted to him as part of the application, or upon the basis of any other information before him with respect to such drug, he has insufficient information to determine whether such drug is safe for use under such conditions;

(E)   evaluated on the basis of the information submitted to him as part of the application and any other information before him with respect to such drug, there is a lack of substantial evidence that the drug will have the effect it purports or is represented to have under the conditions of use prescribed, recommended, or suggested in the proposed labeling thereof;

(F)   upon the basis of the information submitted to the Secretary as part of the application or any other information before the Secretary with respect to such drug, any use prescribed, recommended, or suggested in labeling proposed for such drug will result in a residue of such drug in excess of a tolerance found by the Secretary to be safe for such drug.

(G)   the application failed to contain the patent information prescribed by subsection (b)(1);

(H)   based on a fair evaluation of all material facts, such labeling is false or misleading in any particular; or

(I)   such drug induces cancer when ingested by man or animal or, after tests which are appropriate for the evaluation for the safety of such drug, induces cancer in man or animal, except that the foregoing provisions of this sub-paragraph shall not apply with respect to such drug if the Secretary finds that, under the conditions of use specified in proposed labeling, and reasonably certain to be followed in practice (i) such drug will not adversely affect the animals, for which it is intended, and (ii) no residue of such drug will be found (by methods of examination prescribed or approved by the Secretary by regulations, which regulations shall not be subject to subsections (c), (d), and (h)), in any edible portion of such animals after slaughter or in any food yielded by or derived from the living animals;

he shall issue an order refusing to approve the application. If, after such notice and opportunity for hearing, the Secretary finds that sub-paragraphs (A) through (I) do not apply, he shall issue an order approving the application.

(2)   In determining whether such drug is safe for use under the conditions prescribed, recommended, or suggested in the proposed labeling thereof, the Secretary shall consider, among other relevant factors, (A) the probable consumption of such drug and of any substance formed in or on food because of the use of such drug, (B) the cumulative effect on man or animal of such drug, taking into account any chemically or pharmacologically related substance, (C) safety factors which in the opinion of experts, qualified by scientific training and experience to evaluate the safety of such drugs, are appropriate for the use of animal experimentation data, and (D) whether the conditions of use prescribed,

recommended, or suggested in the proposed labeling are reasonably certain to be followed in practice. Any order issued under this subsection refusing to approve an application shall state the findings upon which it is based.

(3)   As used in this section, the term "substantial evidence" means evidence consisting of one or more adequate and well controlled investigations, such as—

(A)   a study in a target species;

(B)   a study in laboratory animals;

(C)   any field investigation that may be required under this section and that meets the requirements of subsection (b)(3) if a presubmission conference is requested by the applicant;

(D)   a bioequivalence study; or

(E)   an in vitro study;

by experts qualified by scientific training and experience to evaluate the effectiveness of the drug involved, on the basis of which it could fairly and reasonably be concluded by such experts that the drug will have the effect it purports or is represented to have under the conditions of use prescribed, recommended, or suggested in the labeling or proposed labeling thereof.

(4)   In a case in which an animal drug contains more than one active ingredient, or the labeling of the drug prescribes, recommends, or suggests use of the drug in combination with one or more other animal drugs, and the active ingredients or drugs intended for use in the combination have previously been separately approved for particular uses and conditions of use for which they are intended for use in the combination—

(A)   the Secretary shall not issue an order under paragraph (1)(A), (1)(B), or (1)(D) refusing to approve the application for such combination on human food safety grounds unless the Secretary finds that the application fails to establish that—

(i)   none of the active ingredients or drugs intended for use in the combination, respectively, at the longest withdrawal time of any of the active ingredients or drugs in the combination, respectively, exceeds its established tolerance; or

(ii)   none of the active ingredients or drugs in the combination interferes with the methods of analysis for another of the active ingredients or drugs in the combination, respectively;

(B)   the Secretary shall not issue an order under paragraph (1)(A), (1)(B),or (1)(D) refusing to approve the application for such combination on target animal safety grounds unless the Secretary finds that—

(i) (I)   there is a substantiated scientific issue, specific to one or more of the active ingredients or animal drugs in the combination, that cannot adequately be evaluated based on information contained in the application for the combination (including any investigations, studies, or tests for which the applicant has a right of reference or use from the person by or for whom the investigations, studies, or tests were conducted); or

(II)   there is a scientific issue raised by target animal observations contained in studies submitted to the Secretary as part of the application; and

(ii)   based on the Secretary's evaluation of the information contained in the application with respect to the issues identified in clauses (i) (I) and (II), paragraph (1) (A), (B), or (D) apply;

(C)   except in the case of a combination that contains a nontopical antibacterial ingredient or animal drug, the Secretary shall not issue an order under paragraph (1)(E) refusing to approve an application for a combination animal drug intended for use other than in animal feed or drinking water unless the Secretary finds that the application fails to demonstrate that—

(i)   there is substantial evidence that any active ingredient or animal drug intended only for the same use as another active ingredient or animal drug in the combination makes a contribution to labeled effectiveness;

(ii)   each active ingredient or animal drug intended for at least one use that is different from all other active ingredients or animal drugs used in the combination provides appropriate concurrent use for the intended target population; or

(iii)   where based on scientific information the Secretary has reason to believe the active ingredients or animal drugs may be physically imcompatible or have disparate dosing regiments, such active ingredients or animal drugs are physically compatible or do not have disparate dosing regiments; and

(D)   the Secretary shall not issue an order under paragraph (1)(E) refusing to approve an application for a combination animal drug intended for use in animal feed or drinking water unless the Secretary finds that the application fails to demonstrate that—

(i)   there is substantial evidence that any active ingredient or animal drug intended only for the same use as another active ingredient or animal drug in the combination makes a contribution to the labeled effectiveness;

(ii)   each of the active ingredients or animal drugs intended for at least one use that is different from all other active ingredients or animal drugs used in the combination provides appropriate concurrent use for the intended target population;

(iii)   where a combination contains more than one nontopical antibacterial ingredient or animal drug, there is substantial evidence that each of the nontopical antibacterial ingredients or animal drugs makes a contribution to the labeled effectiveness except that for purposes of this clause, antibacterial ingredient or animal drug does not include the ionophore or arsenical classes of animal drugs; or

(iv)   where based on scientific information the Secretary has reason to belive the active ingredients or animal drugs intended for use in drinking water may be physically incompatible, such active ingredients or animal drugs intended for use in drinking water are physically compatible.

SELECTED PORTIONS OF THE FEDERAL FOOD, DRUG, AND COSMETIC ACT RELATED TO DIETARY SUPPLEMENTS

Definitions

§ **201**[321]   For purposes of this Act—

(f)   The term "food" means (1) articles used for food or drink for man or other animals, (2) chewing gum, and (3) articles used for components of any such article.

(g)   (1)   The term "drug" means (A) articles recognized in the official United States Pharmacopeia, official Homeopathic Pharmacopoeia of the United States, or official National Formulary, or any supplement to any of them; and (B) articles intended for use in the diagnosis, cure, mitigation, treatment or prevention of disease in man or other animals; and (C) articles (other than food) intended to affect the structure or any function of the body of man or other animals; and (D) articles intended for use as a component of any article specified in clause (A), (B), or (C). A food or dietary supplement for which a claim, subject to sections 403(r)(1)(B) and 403(r)(3) or sections 403(r)(1)(B) and 403(r)(5)(D), is made in accordance with the requirements of section 403(r) is not a drug solely because the label or the labeling contains such a claim. A food, dietary ingredient, or dietary supplement for which a truthful and not misleading statement is made in accordance with section 403(r)(6) is not a drug under clause (C) solely because the label or the labeling contains such a statement.

(j)   The term "official compendium" means the official United States Pharmacopoeia, official Homeopathic Pharmacopoeia of the United States, official National Formulary, or any supplement to any of them.

(k)   The term "label" means a display of written, printed, or graphic matter upon the immediate container of any article; and a requirement made by or under authority of this Act that any word, statement, or other information appear on the label shall not be considered to be complied with unless such word, statement, or other information also appears on the outside container or wrapper, if any there be, of the retail package of such article, or is easily legible through the outside container or wrapper.

(m)   The term "labeling" means all labels and other written, printed, or graphic matter (1) upon any article or any of its containers or wrappers, or (2) accompanying such article.

(n)   If an article is alleged to be misbranded because the labeling or advertising is misleading, then in determining whether the labeling or advertising is misleading there shall be taken into account (among other things) not only representations made or suggested by statement, word, design, device, or any combination thereof, but also the extent to which the labeling or advertising fails to reveal facts material in the light of such representations or material with respect to consequences which may result from the use of the article to which the labeling or advertising relates under the conditions of use prescribed in the labeling or advertising thereof or under such conditions of use as are customary or usual.

(s)   The term "food additive" means any substance the intended use of which results or may reasonably be expected to result, directly or indirectly, in its becoming a component or otherwise affecting the characteristics of any food (including any substance intended for use in producing, manufacturing, packing, processing, preparing, treating, packaging, transporting, or holding food; and including any source of radiation intended for any such use), if such substance is not generally recognized, among experts qualified by scientific training and experience to evaluate its safety, as having been adequately shown through scientific procedures (or, in the case of a substance used in food prior to January 1, 1958, through either scientific procedures or experience based on common use in food) to be safe under the conditions of its intended use; except that such term does not include

(1)   a pesticide chemical in or on a raw agricultural commodity or processed food; or

(2)   a pesticide chemical; or

(3)   a color additive; or

(4)   any substance used in accordance with a sanction or approval granted prior to September 6, 1958 pursuant to this Act, the Poultry Products Inspection Act (21 U.S.C. 451 and the following) or the Meat Inspection Act of March 4, 1907 (34 Stat. 1260), as amended and extended (21 U.S.C. 71 and the following);

(5)   a new animal drug; or

(6)   an ingredient described in paragraph (ff) in, or intended for use in, a dietary supplement.

(ff)   The term "dietary supplement"

(1)   means a product (other than tobacco) intended to supplement the diet that bears or contains one or more of the following dietary ingredients:

(A)   a vitamin;

(B)   a mineral;

(C)   an herb or other botanical;

(D)   an amino acid;

(E)   a dietary substance for use by man to supplement the diet by increasing the total dietary intake; or

(F)   a concentrate, metabolite, constituent, extract, or combination of any ingredient described in clause (A), (B), (C), (D), or (E);

(2)   means a product that

(A)   (i)   is intended for ingestion in a form described in section 411(c)(1)(B)(i); or

(ii)   complies with section 411 (c)(1)(B)(ii);

(B)   is not represented for use as a conventional food or as a sole item of a meal or the diet; and

(C)   is labeled as a dietary supplement; and

(3)   does

(A)   include an article that is approved as a new drug under section 505, or licensed as a biologic under section 351 of the Public Health Service Act (42 U.S.C. 262) and was, prior to such approval, certification, or license, marketed as a dietary supplement or as a food unless the Secretary has issued a regulation, after notice and comment, finding that the article, when used as or in a dietary supplement under the conditions of use and dosages set forth in the labeling for such dietary supplement, is unlawful under section 402(f); and

(B)   not include—

(i)   an article that is approved as a new drug under section 505, certified as an antibiotic under section 507, or licensed as a biologic under section 351 of the Public Health Service Act (42 U.S.C. 262), or;

(ii)   an article authorized for investigation as a new drug, antibiotic, or biological for which substantial clinical investigations have been instituted and for which the existence of such investigations has been made public, which was not before such approval, certification, licensing, or authorization marketed as a dietary supplement or as a food unless the Secretary, in the Secretary's discretion, has issued a regulation, after notice and comment, finding that the article would be lawful under this Act.

Except for purposes of paragraph (g), a dietary supplement shall be deemed to be a food within the meaning of this Act.

Adulterated Food

§   **402** [342]   A food shall be deemed to be adultered—
(a)   POISONOUS, INSANITARY, ETC. INGREDIENTS
(1)   If it bears or contains any poisonous or deleterious substance which may render it injurious to health; but in case the substance is not an added substance such food shall not be considered adultered under this clause if the quantity of such substance in such food does not ordinarily render it injurious to health; or (2)(A) if it bears or contains any added poisonous or added deleterious substance (other than a substance that is a pesticide chemical residue in or on a raw agricultural commodity or processed food, a food additive, a color additive, or a new animal drug) that is unsafe within the meaning of section 406; or (B) if it bears or contains a pesticide chemical residue that is unsafe within the meaning of section 408(a); or (C) if it is or if it bears or contains (i) any food additive that is unsafe within the meaning of section 409; or (ii) a new animal drug (or conversion product thereof) that is unsafe within the meaning of section 512; or (3) if it consists in whole or in part of any filthy, putrid, or decomposed substance, or if it is otherwise unfit for food; or (4) if it has been prepared, packed, or held under insanitary conditions whereby it may have become contaminated with filth, or whereby it may have been rendered injurious to health; or (5) if it is, in whole or in part, the product of a diseased animal or of an animal which has died otherwise than by slaughter; or (6) if its container is composed, in whole or in part, of any poisonous or deleterious substance which may render the contents injurious to health; or (7) if it has been intentionally subjected to radiation, unless the use of the radiation was in conformity with a regulation or exemption in effect pursuant to section 409.

(b)   ABSENCE, SUBSTITUTION, OR ADDITION OF CONSTITUENTS   (1)   If any valuable constituent has been in whole or in part omitted or abstracted therefrom; or (2) if any substance has been substituted wholly or in part therefore; or (3) if damage or inferiority has been concealed in any manner; or (4) if any substance has been added thereto or mixed or packed therewith so as to increase its bulk or weight, or reduce its quality or strength, or make it appear better or of greater value than it is.

(c)   COLOR ADDITIVES   If it is, or it bears or contains, a color additive which is unsafe within the meaning of section 721(a).

(d)   CONFECTIONERY CONTAINING ALCOHOL OR NONNUTRITIVE SUBSTANCE   If it is confectionery, and—

(1)   has partially or completely imbedded therein any nonnutritive object, except that this sub-paragraph shall not apply in the case of any nonnutritive object if, in the judgment of the Secretary as provided by regulations, such object is of practical functional value to the confectionery product and would not render the product injurious or hazardous to health;

(2)   bears or contains any alcohol other than alcohol not in excess of one-half of 1 per centum by volume derived solely from the use of flavoring extracts, except that this clause shall not apply to confectionery which is introduced or delivered for introduction into, or received or held for sale in, interstate commerce if the sale of such confectionery is permitted under the laws of the State in which such confectionery is intended to be offered for sale; or

(3)   bears or contains any nonnutritive substance, except that this paragraph shall not apply to a safe nonnutritive substance which is in or on confectionery by reason of its use for some practical functional purpose in the manufacture, packaging, or storage

of such confectionery if the use of the substance does not promote deception of the consumer or otherwise result in adulteration or misbranding in violation of any provision of this Act, except that the Secretary may, for the purpose of avoiding or resolving uncertainty as to the application of this inline-paragraph, issue regulations allowing or prohibiting the use of particular nonnutritive substances.

(e)   OLEOMARGARINE CONTAINING FILTHY, PUTRID, ETC., MATTER   If it is oleomargarine or margarine or butter and any of the raw material used therein consisted in whole or in part of any filthy, putrid, or decomposed substance, or such oleomargarine or margarine or butter is otherwise unfit for food.

(f)   DEITARY SUPPLEMENT OR INGREDIENT: SAFETY
(1)   If it is a dietary supplement or contains a dietary ingredient that—

(A)   presents a significant or unreasonable risk of illness or injury under—

(i)   conditions of use recommended or suggested in labeling, or

(ii)   if no conditions of use are suggested or recommended in the labeling, under ordinary conditions of use;

(B)   is a new dietary ingredient for which there is inadequate information to provide resonable assurance that such ingredient does not present a significant or unreasonable risk of illness or injury;

(C)   the Secretary declares to pose an imminent hazard to public health or safety, except that the authority to make such declaration shall not be delegated and the Secretary shall promptly after such a declaration initiate a proceeding in accordance with sections 554 and 556 of title 5, United States Code, to affirm or withdraw the declaration; or

(D)   is or contains a dietary ingredient that renders it adulterated under paragraph (a)(1) under the conditions of use recommended or suggested in the labeling of such dietary supplement.

In any proceeding under this inline-paragraph, the United States shall bear the burden of proof on each element to show that a dietary supplement is adultered. The court shall decide any issue under this paragraph on a de novo basis.

(2)   Before the Secretary may report to a United States attorney a violation of paragraph (1)(A) for a civil proceeding, the person against whom such proceeding would be initiated shall be given appropriate notice and the opportunity to present views, orally and in writing, at least 10 days before such notice, with regard to such proceeding.

(g)   DIETARY SUPPLEMENT: MANUFACTURING PRACTICES   (1)   If it is a dietary supplement and it has been prepared, packed, or held under conditions that do not meet current good manufacturing practice regulations, including regulations requiring, when necessary, expiration date labeling, issued by the Secretary under sub-paragraph (2).

(2)   The Secretary may by regulation prescribe good manufacturing practices for dietary supplements. Such regulations shall be modeled after current good manufacturing practice regulations for food and may not impose standards for which there is no current and generally available analytical methodology. No standard of current good manufacturing practice may be imposed unless such standard is included in a regulation promulgated after notice and opportunity for comment in accordance with chapter 5 of Title 5, United States Code.

Misbranded Food

§ 403 [343]   A food shall be deemed to be misbranded
(a)   FALSE OR MISLEADING LABEL   If
(1)   its labeling is false or misleading in any particular, or
(2)   in the case of a food to which section 411 applies, its advertising is false or misleading in a material respect or its labeling is in violation of section 411(b)(2).

(b)   OFFER FOR SALE UNDER ANOTHER NAME   If it is offered for sale under the name of another food.

(c)   IMITATION OF ANOTHER FOOD   If it is an imitation of another food, unless its label bears, in type of uniform size and prominence, the word "imitation" and, immediately thereafter, the name of the food imitated.

(d)   MISLEADING CONTAINER   If its container is so made, formed, or filled as to be misleading.

(e)   PACKAGE FORM   If in package form unless it bears a label containing

(1)   the name and place of business of the manufacturer, packer, or distributor; and

(2)   an accurate statement of the quantity of the contents in terms of weight, measure, or numerical count, except that under clause (2) of this paragraph reasonable variations shall be permitted, and exemptions as to small packages shall be established, by regulations prescribed by the Secretary.

(f)   PROMINENCE OF INFORMATION ON LABEL   If any word, statement, or other information required by or under authority of this Act to appear on the label or labeling is not prominently placed thereon with such conspicuousness (as compared with other words, statements, designs, or devices, in the labeling) and in such terms as to render it likely to be read and understood by the ordinary individual under customary conditions of purchase and use.

(g)   REPRESENTATION AS TO DEFINITION AND STANDARD OF IDENTITY   If it purports to be or is represented as a food for which a definition and standard of identity has been prescribed by regulations as provided by section 401, unless (1) it conforms to such definition and standard, and

(2)   its label bears the name of the food specified in the definition and standard, and, insofar as may be required by such regulations, the common names of optional ingredients (other than spices, flavoring, and coloring) present in such food.

(h)   REPRESENTATION AS TO STANDARDS OF QUALITY AND FILL OF CONTAINER   If it purports to be or is represented as

(1)   a food for which a standard of quality has been prescribed by regulations as provided by section 401, and its quality falls below such standard, unless its label bears, in such manner and form as such regulations specify, a statement that it falls below such standard; or

(2)   a food for which a standard or standards of fill of container have been prescribed by regulations as provided by section 401, and it falls below the standard of fill of container applicable thereto, unless its label bears, in such manner and form as such regulations specify, a statement that it falls below such standard; or

(3)   a food that is pasteurized unless—
(A)   such food has been subjected to a safe process or treatment that is prescribed as pasteurization for such food in a regulation promulgated under this chapter; or

(B)   (i)   such food has been subjected to a safe process or treatment that—

(I)   is reasonably certain to achieve destruction or elimination in the food of the most resistant microorganisms of public health significance that are likely to occur in the food;

(II)   is at least as protective of the public health as a process or treatment described in sub-paragraph (A);

(III)   is effective for a period that is at least as long as the shelf life of the food when stored under normal and moderate abuse conditions; and

(IV)   is the subject of a notification to the Secretary, including effectiveness data regarding the process or treatment; and

(ii)   at least 120 days have passed after the date of receipt of such notification by the Secretary without the Secretary making a determination that the process or treatment involved has not been shown to meet the requirements of subclauses (I) through (III) of clause (i).

For purposes of paragraph (3), a determination by the Secretary that a process or treatment has not been shown to meet the requirements fo subclauses (I) through (III) of sub-paragraph (B)(i) shall constitute final agency action under such subclauses.

(i)   LABEL WHERE NO REPRESENTATION AS TO DEFINI-TION AND STANDARD OF IDENTITY   Unless its label bears
(1)   the common or usual name of the food, if any there be, and
(2)   in case it is fabricated from two or more ingredients, the common or usual name of each such ingredient and if the food purports to be a beverage containing vegetable or fruit juice, a statement with appropriate prominence on the information panel of the total percentage of such fruit or vegetable juice contained in the food; except that spices, flavorings, and colors not required to be certified under section 721(c) unless sold as spices, flavorings, or such colors, may be designated as spices, flavorings, and colorings without naming each.
To the extent that compliance with the requirements of clause (2) of this paragraph is impracticable, or results in deception or unfair competition, exemptions shall be established by regulations promulgated by the Secretary.
(j)   REPRESENTATION FOR SPECIAL DIETARY USE   If it purports to be or is represented for special dietary uses, unless its label bears such information concerning its vitamin, mineral, and other dietary properties as the Secretary determines to be, and by regulations prescribes as, necessary in order fully to inform purchasers as to its value for such uses.
(k)   ARTIFICIAL FLAVORING, ARTIFICIAL COLORING, OR CHEMICAL PRESERVATIVES   If it bears or contains any artificial flavoring, artificial coloring, or chemical preservative, unless it bears labeling stating that fact, except that to the extent that compliance with the requirements of this paragraph is impracticable, exemptions shall be established by regulations promulgated by the Secretary. The provisions of this paragraph and paragraphs (g) and (i) with respect to artificial coloring shall not apply in the case of butter, cheese, or ice cream. The provisions of this paragraph with respect to chemical preservatives shall not apply to a pesticide chemical when used in or on a raw agricultural commodity which is the produce of the soil.
(l)   PESTICIDE CHEMICALS ON RAW AGRICULTURAL COMMODITIES   If it is a raw agricultural commodity which is the produce of the soil, bearing or containing a pesticide chemical applied after harvest, unless the shipping container of such commodity bears labeling which declares the presence of such chemical in or on such commodity and the common or usual name and the function of such chemical, except that no such declaration shall be required while such commodity, having been removed from the shipping container, is being held or displayed for sale at retail out of such container in accordance with the custom of the trade.
(m)   COLOR ADDITIVES   If it is a color additive, unless its packaging and labeling are in conformity with such packaging and labeling requirements, applicable to such color additive, as may be contained in regulations issued under section 721.
(n)   PACKAGING OR LABELING OF DRUGS IN VIOLATION OF REGULATIONS   If its packaging or labeling is in violation of an applicable regulation issued pursuant to section 3 or 4 of the Poison Prevention Packaging Act of 1970.
(q)   NUTRITION INFORMATION   (1)   Except as provided in sub-paragraphs (3), (4), and (5), if it is a food intended for human consumption and is offered for sale, unless its label or labeling bears nutrition information that provides
(A)   (i)   the serving size which is an amount customarily consumed and which is expressed in a common household measure that is appropriate to the food, or
(ii)   if the use of the food is not typically expressed in a serving size, the common household unit of measure that expresses the serving size of the food,
(B)   the number of servings or other units of measure per container,
(C)   the total number of calories
(i)   derived from any source, and
(ii)   derived from the total fat, in each serving size or other unit of measure of the food,

(D)   the amount of the following nutrients: Total fat, saturated fat, cholesterol, sodium, total carbohydrates, complex carbohydrates, sugars, dietary fiber, and total protein contained in each serving size or other unit of measure,
(E)   any vitamin, mineral, or other nutrient required to be placed on the label and labeling of food under this Act before October 1, 1990, if the Secretary determines that such information will assist consumers in maintaining healthy dietary practices.
The Secretary may by regulation require any information required to be placed on the label or labeling by this sub-paragraph or sub-paragraph (2)(A) to be highlighted on the label or labeling by larger type, bold type, or contrasting color if the Secretary determines that such highlighting will assist consumers in maintaining healthy dietary practices.
(2)   (A)   If the Secretary determines that a nutrient other than a nutrient required by sub-paragraph (1)(C), (1)(D), or (1)(E) should be included in the label or labeling of food subject to sub-paragraph (1) for purposes of providing information regarding the nutritional value of such food that will assist consumers in maintaining healthy dietary practices, the Secretary may by regulation require that information relating to such additional nutrient be included in the label or labeling of such food.
(B)   If the Secretary determines that the information relating to a nutrient required by sub-paragraph (1)(C), (1)(D), or (1)(E) or clause (A) of this inline-paragraph to be included in the label or labeling of food is not necessary to assist consumers in maintaining healthy dietary practices, the Secretary may by regulation remove information relating to such nutrient from such requirement.
(3)   For food that is received in bulk containers at a retail establishment, the Secretary may, by regulation, provide that the nutrition information required by sub-paragraphs (1) and (2) be displayed at the location in the retail establishment at which the food is offered for sale.
(4)   (A)   The Secretary shall provide for furnishing the nutrition information required by sub-paragraphs (1) and (2) with respect to raw agricultural commodities and raw fish by issuing voluntary nutrition guidelines, as provided by clause (B) or by issuing regulations that are mandatory as provided by clause (D).
(B)   (i)   Upon the expiration of 12 months after November 8, 1990, the Secretary, after providing an opportunity for comment, shall issue guidelines for food retailers offering raw agricultural commodities or raw fish to provide nutrition information specified in sub-paragraphs (1) and (2). Such guidelines shall take into account the actions taken by food retailers during such 12-month period to provide to consumers nutrition information on raw agricultural commodities and raw fish. Such guidelines shall only apply—
(I)   in the case of raw agricultural commodities, to the 20 varieties of vegetables most frequently consumed during a year and the 20 varieties of fruit most frequently consumed during a year, and
(II)   to the 20 varieties of raw fish most frequently consumed during a year.
The vegetables, fruits, and raw fish to which such guidelines apply shall be determined by the Secretary by regulation and the Secretary may apply such guidelines regionally.
(ii)   Upon the expiration of 12 months after November 8, 1990, the Secretary shall issue a final regulation defining the circumstances that constitute substantial compliance by food retailers with the guidelines issued under subclause (i). The regulation shall provide that there is not substantial compliance if a significant number of retailers have failed to comply with the guidelines. The size of the retailers and the portion of the market served by retailers in compliance with the guidelines shall be considered in determining whether the substantial-compliance standard has been met.
(C)   (i)   Upon the expiration of 30 months after November 8, 1990, the Secretary shall issue a report on actions taken by food retailers to provide consumers with nutrition information for raw agricultural commodities and raw fish under the guidelines issued under clause (A). Such report shall include a determination of whether there is substantial compliance with the guidelines.

(ii)   If the Secretary finds that there is substantial compliance with the guidelines, the Secretary shall issue a report and make a determination of the type required in subclause (i) every two years.

(5)(A)   Subparagraphs (1), (2), (3), and (4) shall not apply to food—

(i)   which is served in restaurants or other establishments in which food is served for immediate human consumption or which is sold for sale or use in such establishments,

(ii)   which is processed and prepared primarily in a retail establishment, which is ready for human consumption, which is of the type described in subclause (i), and which is offered for sale to consumers but not for immediate human consumption in such establishment and which is not offered for sale outside such establishment,

(iii)   which is an infant formula subject to section 412,

(iv)   which is a medical food as defined in section 5(b) of the Orphan Drug Act [21 U.S.C. 360ee(b)], or

(v)   which is described in section 405(2).

(B)   Subparagraphs (1) and (2) shall not apply to the label of a food if the Secretary determines by regulations that compliance with such sub-paragraphs is impracticable because the package of such food is too small to comply with the requirements of such sub-paragraphs and if the label of such food does not contain any nutrition information.

(C)   If a food contains insignificant amounts, as determined by the Secretary, of all the nutrients required by sub-paragraphs (1) and (2) to be listed in the label or labeling of food, the requirements of such inline-paragraphs shall not apply to such food if the label, labeling, or advertising of such food does not make any claim with respect to the nutritional value of such food. If a food contains insignificant amounts, as determined by the Secretary, of more than one-half the nutrients required by inline-paragraphs (1) and (2) to be in the label or labeling of the food, the Secretary shall require the amounts of such nutrients to be stated in a simplified form prescribed by the Secretary.

(D)   If a person offers food for sale and has annual gross sales made or business done in sales to consumers which is not more than $500,000 or has annual gross sales made or business done in sales of food to consumers which is not more than $50,000, the requirements of sub-paragraphs (1), (2), (3), and (4) shall not apply with respect to food sold by such person to consumers unless the label or labeling of food offered by such person provides nutrition information or makes a nutrition claim.

(E)   (i)   During the 12-month period for which an exemption from sub-paragraphs (1) and (2) is claimed pursuant to this subclause, the requirements of such sub-paragraphs shall not apply to any food product if—

(I)   the labeling for such product does not provide nutrition information or make a claim subject to paragraph (r),

(II)   the person who claims for such product an exemption from such sub-paragraphs employed fewer than an average of 100 full-time equivalent employees,

(III)   such person provided the notice described in subclause (iii), and

(IV)   in the case of a food product which was sold in the 12-month period preceding the period for which an exemption was claimed, fewer than 100,000 units of such product were sold in the United States during such preceding period, or in the case of a food product which was not sold in the 12-month period preceding the period for which such exemption is claimed, fewer than 100,000 units of such product are reasonably anticipated to be sold in the United States during the period from which such exemption is claimed.

(ii)   During the 12-month period after the applicable date referred to in this sentence, the requirements of sub-paragraphs (1) and (2) shall not apply to any food product which was first introduced into interstate commerce before May 8, 1994, if the labeling for such product does not provide nutrition in formation or make a claim subject to paragraph (r), if such person provided the notice described in subclause (iii), and if—

(I)   during the 12-month period preceding May 8, 1994, the person who claims for such product an exemption from such sub-paragraphs employed fewer than an average of 300 full-time equivalent employees and fewer than 600,000 units of such product were sold in the United States,

(II)   during the 12-month period preceding May 8, 1995, the person who claims for such product an exemption from such sub-paragraphs employed fewer than an average of 300 full-time equivalent employees and fewer than 400,000 units of such product were sold in the United States, or

(III)   during the 12-month period preceding May 8, 1996, the person who claims for such product an exemption from such sub-paragraphs employed fewer than an average of 200 full-time equivalent employees and fewer than 200,000 units of such product were sold in the United States.

(iii)   The notice referred to in subclauses (i) and (ii) shall be given to the Secretary prior to the beginning of the period during which the exemption under subclause (i) or (ii) is to be in effect, shall state that the person claiming such exemption for a food product has complied with the applicable requirements of subclause (i) or (ii), and shall—

(I)   state the average number of full-time equivalent employees such person employed during the 12 months preceding the date such person claims such exemption,

(II)   state the approximate number of units the person claiming the exemption sold in the United States,

(III)   if the exemption is claimed for a food product which was sold in the 12-month period preceding the period for which the exemption was claimed, state the approximate number of units of such product which were sold in the United States during such preceding period, and, if the exemption is claimed for a food product which was not sold in such preceding period, state the number of units of such product which such person reasonably anticipates will be sold in the United States during the period for which the exemption was claimed, and

(IV)   contain such information as the Secretary may require to verify the information required by the preceding provisions of this subclause if the Secretary has questioned the validity of such information.

If a person is not an importer, has fewer than 10 full-time equivalent employees, and sells fewer than 10,000 units of any food product in any year, such person is not required to file a notice for such product under this subclause for such year.

(iv)   In the case of a person who claimed an exemption under subclause (i) or (ii), if, during the period of such exemption, the number of full-time equivalent employees of such person exceeds the number in such subclause or if the number of food products sold in the United States exceeds the number in such subclause, such exemption shall extend to the expiration of 18 months after the date the number of full-time equivalent employees or food products sold exceeded the applicable number.

(v)   For any food product first introduced into interstate commerce after May 8, 2002, the Secretary may by regulation lower the employee or units of food products requirements of subclause (i) if the Secretary determines that the cost of compliance with such lower requirement will not place an undue burden on persons subject to such lower requirement.

(vi)   For purposes of subclauses (i), (ii), (iii), (iv), and (v)—

(I)   the term "unit" means the packaging or, if there is no packaging, the form in which a food product is offered for sale to consumers,

(II)   the term "food product" means food in any sized package which is manufactured by a single manufacturer or which bears the same brand name, which bears the same statement of identity, and which has similar preparation methods, and

(III)   the term "person" in the case of a corporation includes all domestic and foreign affiliates of the corporation.

(F)   A dietary supplement product (including a food to which section 411 applies) shall comply with the requirements of inline-paragraphs (1) and (2) in a manner which is appropriate for the product and which is specified in regulations of the Secretary which shall provide that

(i)   nutrition information shall first list those dietary ingredients that are present in the product in a significant amount and for which a recommendation for daily consumption has been established by the Secretary, except that a dietary ingredient shall not be required to be listed if it is not present in a significant amount, and shall list any other dietary ingredient present and identified as having no such recommendation;

(ii)   the listing of dietary ingredients shall include the quantity of each such ingredient (or of a proprietary blend of such ingredients) per serving;

(iii)   the listing of dietary ingredients may include the source of a dietary ingredient; and

(iv)   the nutrition information shall immediately precede the ingredient information required under subclause (i), except that no ingredient identified pursuant to subclause (i) shall be required to be identified a second time.

(G)   Subparagraphs (1), (2), (3), and (4) shall not apply to food which is sold by a food distributor if the food distributor principally sells food to restaurants or other establishments in which food is served for immediate human consumption and does not manufacture, process, or repackage the food it sells.

(r)   NUTRITION LEVELS AND HEALTH-RELATED CLAIMS

(1)   Except as provided in clauses (A) through (C) of sub-paragraph (5), if it is a food intended for human consumption which is offered for sale and for which a claim is made in the label or labeling of the food which expressly or by implication—

(A)   characterizes the level of any nutrient which is of the type required by paragraph (q)(1) or (q)(2) to be in the label or labeling of the food unless the claim is made in accordance with sub-paragraph (2), or

(B)   characterizes the relationship of any nutrient which is of the type required by paragraph (q)(1) or (q)(2) to be in the label or labeling of the food to a disease or a health-related condition unless the claim is made in accordance with sub-paragraph (3) or (5)(D).

A statement of the type required by paragraph (q) that appears as part of the nutrition information required or permitted by such paragraph is not a claim which is subject to this paragraph and a claim subject to clause (A) is not subject to clause (B).

(2)   (A)   Except as provided in inline-paragraphs (4)(A)(ii) and (4)(A)(iii) and clauses (A) through (C) of inline-paragraph (5), a claim described in sub-paragraph (1)(A)

(i)   may be made only if the characterization of the level made in the claim uses terms which are defined in regulations of the Secretary,

(ii)   may not state the absence of a nutrient unless—

(I)   the nutrient is usually present in the food or in a food which substitutes for the food as defined by the Secretary by regulation, or

(II)   the Secretary by regulation permits such a statement on the basis of a finding that such a statement would assist consumers in maintaining healthy dietary practices and the statement discloses that the nutrient is not usually present in the food,

(iii)   may not be made with respect to the level of cholesterol in the food if the food contains, as determined by the Secretary by regulation, fat or saturated fat in an amount which increases to persons in the general population the risk of disease or a health related condition which is diet related unless—

(I)   the Secretary finds by regulation that the level of cholesterol is substantially less than the level usually present in the food or in a food which substitutes for the food and which has a significant market share, or the Secretary by regulation permits a statement regarding the absence of cholesterol on the basis of a finding that cholesterol is not usually present in the food and that such a statement would assist consumers in maintaining healthy dietary practices and the regulation requires that the statement disclose that cholesterol is not usually present in the food, and

(II)   the label or labeling of the food discloses the level of such fat or saturated fat in immediate proximity to such claim and with appropriate prominence which shall be no less than one-half the size of the claim with respect to the level of cholesterol,

(iv)   may not be made with respect to the level of saturated fat in the food if the food contains cholesterol unless the label or labeling of the food discloses the level of cholesterol in the food in immediate proximity to such claim and with appropriate prominence which shall be no less than one-half the size of the claim with respect to the level of saturated fat,

(v)   may not state that a food is high in dietary fiber unless the food is low in total fat as defined by the Secretary or the label or labeling discloses the level of total fat in the food in immediate proximity to such statement and with appropriate prominence which shall be no less than one-half the size of the claim with respect to the level of dietary fiber, and

(vi)   may not be made if the Secretary by regulation prohibits the claim because the claim is misleading in light of the level of another nutrient in the food.

(B)   If a claim described in sub-paragraph (1)(A) is made with respect to a nutrient in a food and the Secretary makes a determination that the food contains a nutrient at a level that increases to persons in the general population the risk of a disease or health-related condition that is diet related, the label or labeling of such food shall contain, prominently and in immediate proximity to such claim, the following statement: "See nutrition information for _____ content." The blank shall identify the nutrient associated with the increased disease or health-related condition risk. In making the determination described in this clause, the Secretary shall take into account the significance of the food in the total daily diet.

(C)   Subparagraph (2)(A) does not apply to a claim described in sub-paragraph (1)(A) and contained in the label or labeling of a food if such claim is contained in the brand name of such food and such brand name was in use on such food before October 25, 1989, unless the brand name contains a term defined by the Secretary under inline-paragraph (2)(A)(i). Such a claim is subject to paragraph (a).

(D)   Subparagraph (2) does not apply to a claim described in inline-paragraph (1)(A) which uses the term "diet" and is contained in the label or labeling of a soft drink if (i) such claim is contained in the brand name of such soft drink, (ii) such brand name was in use on such soft drink before October 25, 1989, and (iii) the use of the term "diet" was in conformity with section 105.66 of title 21 of the Code of Federal Regulations. Such a claim is subject to paragraph (a).

(E)   Subclauses (i) through (v) of inline-paragraph (2)(A) do not apply to a statement in the label or labeling of food which describes the percentage of vitamins and minerals in the food in relation to the amount of such vitamins and minerals recommended for daily consumption by the Secretary.

(F)   Subclause (i) clause (A) does not apply to a statement in the labeling of a dietary supplement that characterizes the percentage level of a dietary ingredient for which the Secretary has not established a reference daily intake, daily recommended value, or other recommendation for daily consumption.

(G)   A claim of the type described in inline-paragraph (1)(A) for a nutrient, for which the Secretary has not promulgated a regulation under clause (A)(i), shall be authorized and may be made with respect to a food if—

(i)   a scientific body of the United States Government with official responsibility for public health protection or research directly relating to human nutrition (such as the National Institutes of Health or the Centers for Disease Control and Prevention) or the National Academy or Sciences or any of its subdivisions has published an authoritative statement, which is currently in effect, which identifies the nutrient level to which the claim refers;

(ii)   a person has submitted to the Secretary, at least 120 days (during which the Secretary may notify any person who is making a claim as authorized by clause (C) that such person has not submitted all the information required by such clause) before the first introduction into interstate commerce of the food with a label containing the claim, (I) a notice of the claim, which shall include the exact words used in the claim and shall include a concise description of the basis upon which such person relied for determining that the requirements of subclause (i) have been satisfied, (II) a copy of the statement referred to in subclause (i) upon which such person relied in making the claim, and (III) a balanced representation of the scientific literature relating to the nutrient level to which the claim refers;

VII/36 **Selected Laws and Regulations**

(iii)   the claim and the food for which the claim is made are in compliance with clauses (A) and (B), and are otherwise in compliance with paragraph (a) and section 201(n); and

(iv)   the claim is stated in a manner so that the claim is an accurate representation of the authoritative statement referred to in subclause (i) and so that the claim enables the public to comprehend the information provided in the claim and to understand the relative significance of such information in the context of a total daily diet.

For purposes of this clause, a statement shall be regarded as an authoritative statement of a scientific body described in subclause (i) only if the statement is published by the scientific body and shall not include a statement of an employee of the scientific body made in the individual capacity of the employee.

(H)   A claim submitted under the requirements of clause (G) may be made until—

(i)   such time as the Secretary issues a regulation—

(I)   prohibiting or modyifying the claim and the regulation has become effective, or

(II)   finding that the requirements of clause (G) have not been met, including finding that the petitioner had not submitted all the information required by such clause; or

(ii)   a district court of the United States in an enforcement proceeding under chapter III has determined that the requirements of clause (G) have not been met.

(3)   (A)   Except as provided in inline-paragraph (5), a claim described in sub-paragraph (1)(B) may only be made—

(i)   if the claim meets the requirements of the regulations of the Secretary promulgated under clause (B), and

(ii)   if the food for which the claim is made does not contain, as determined by the Secretary by regulation, any nutrient in an amount which increases to persons in the general population the risk of a disease or health-related condition which is diet related, taking into account the significance of the food in the total daily diet, except that the Secretary may by regulation permit such a claim based on a finding that such a claim would assist consumers in maintaining healthy dietary practices and based on a requirement that the label contain a disclosure of the type required by sub-paragraph (2)(B).

(B)   (i)   The Secretary shall promulgate regulations authorizing claims of the type described in inline-paragraph (1)(B) only if the Secretary determines, based on the totality of publicly available scientific evidence (including evidence from well-designed studies conducted in a manner which is consistent with generally recognized scientific procedures and principles), that there is significant scientific agreement, among experts qualified by scientific training and experience to evaluate such claims, that the claim is supported by such evidence.

(ii)   A regulation described in subclause (i) shall describe

(I)   the relationship between a nutrient of the type required in the label or labeling of food by paragraph (q)(1) or (q)(2) and a disease or health-related condition, and

(II)   the significance of each such nutrient in affecting such disease or health-related condition.

(iii)   A regulation described in subclause (i) shall require such claim to be stated in a manner so that the claim is an accurate representation of the matters set out in subclause (ii) and so that the claim enables the public to comprehend the information provided in the claim and to understand the relative significance of such information in the context of a total daily diet.

(C)   Notwithstanding the provision of clauses (A)(i) and (B), a claim of the type described in inline-paragraph (1)(B) which is not authorized by the Secretary in a regulation promulgated in accordance with clause (B) shall be authorized and may be made with respect to a food if—

(i)   a scientific body of the United States Government with official responsibility for public health protection or research directly relating to human nutrition (such as the national Institutes of Health or the Centers for Disease Control and Prevention) or the National Academy of Sciences or any of its subdivisions has published an authoritative statement, which is currently in effect, about the relationship between a nutrient and a disease or health-related condition to which the claim refers;

(ii)   a person has submitted to the Secretary, at least 120 days (during which the Secretary may notify any person who is making a claim as authorized by clause (C) that such person has not submitted all the information required by such clause) before the first introduction into interstate commerce of the food with a label containing the claim, (I) a notice of the claim, which shall include the exact words used in the claim and shall include a concise description of the basis upon which such person relied for determining that the requirements of subclause (i) have been satisfied, (II) a copy of the statement referred to in subclause (i) upon which such person relied in making the claim, and (III) a balanced representation of the scientific literature relating to the relationship to which the claim refers;

(iii)   the claim and the food for which the claim is made are in compliance with clause (A)(ii) and are otherwise in compliance with paragraph (a) and section 201(n); and

(iv)   the claim is stated in a manner so that the claim is an accurate representation of the authoritative statement referred to in subclause (i) and so that the claim enables the public to comprehend the information provided in the claim and to understand the relative significance of such information in the context of a total daily diet.

For purposes of this clause, a statement shall be regarded as an authoritative statement of a scientific body described in subclause (i) only if the statement is published by the scientific body and shall not include a statement of an employee of the scientific body made in the individual capacity of the employee.

(D)   A claim submitted under the requirements of clause (C) may be made until—

(i)   such time as the Secretary issues a regulation under the standard in clause (B)(i)—

(I)   prohibiting or modifying the claim and the regulation has become effective, or

(II)   finding that the requirements of clause (C) have not been met, including finding that the petitioner has not submitted all the information required by such clause; or

(ii)   a district court of the United States in an enforcement proceeding under chapter III has determined that the requirements of clause (C) have not been met.

(4) (A) (i)   Any person may petition the Secretary to issue a regulation under sub-paragraph (2)(A)(i) or (3)(B) relating to a claim described in inline-paragraph (1)(A) or (1)(B). Not later than 100 days after the petition is received by the Secretary, the Secretary shall issue a final decision denying the petition or file the petition for further action by the Secretary. If the Secretary does not act within such 100 days, the petition shall be deemed to be denied unless an extension is mutually agreed upon by the Secretary and the petitioner. If the Secretary denies the petition or the petition is deemed to be denied, the petition shall not be made available to the public. If the Secretary files the petition, the Secretary shall deny the petition or issue a proposed regulation to take the action requested in the petition not later than 90 days after the date of such decision. If the Secretary does not act within such 90 days, the petition shall be deemed to be denied unless an extension is mutually agreed upon by the Secretary and the petitioner. If the Secretary issues a proposed regulation, the rulemaking shall be completed within 540 days of the date the petition is received by the Secretary. If the the Secretary does not issue a regulation within such 540 days, the Secretary shall provide the Committee on Commerce of the House of Representatives and the Committee on Labor and Human Resources of the Senate the reasons action on the regulation did not occur within such 540 days.

(ii)   Any person may petition the Secretary for permission to use in a claim described in inline-paragraph (1)(A) terms that are consistent with the terms defined by the Secretary under inline-paragraph (2)(A)(i). Within 90 days of the submission of such a petition, the Secretary shall issue a final decision denying the petition or granting such permission.

(iii)   Any person may petition the Secretary for permission to use an implied claim described in inline-paragraph (1)(A) in a brand name. After publishing notice of an opportunity to comment on the petition in the Federal Register and making the petition available to the public, the Secretary shall grant the petition if

the Secretary finds that such claim is not misleading and is consistent with terms defined by the Secretary under inline-paragraph (2)(A)(i). The Secretary shall grant or deny the petition within 100 days of the date it is submitted to the Secretary and the petition shall be considered granted if the Secretary does not act on it within such 100 days.

(B)   A petition under clause (A)(i) respecting a claim described in sub-paragraph (1)(A) or (1)(B) shall include an explanation of the reasons why the claim meets the requirements of this paragraph and a summary of the scientific data which supports such reasons.

(C)   If a petition for a regulation under inline-paragraph (3)(B) relies on a report from an authoritative scientific body of the United States, the Secretary shall consider such report and shall justify any decision rejecting the conclusions of such report.

(5)   (A)   This paragraph does not apply to infant formulas subject to section 412(h) and medical foods as defined in section 5(b) of the Orphan Drug Act.

(B)   Subclauses (iii) through (v) of inline-paragraph (2)(A) and sub-paragraph (2)(B) do not apply to food which is served in restaurants or other establishments in which food is served for immediate human consumption or which is sold for sale or use in such establishments.

(C)   A inline-paragraph (1)(A) claim made with respect to a food which claim is required by a standard of identity issued under section 401 shall not be subject to inline-paragraph (2)(A)(i) or (2)(B).

(D)   A sub-paragraph (1)(B) claim made with respect to a dietary supplement of vitamins, minerals, herbs, or other similar nutritional substances shall not be subject to inline-paragraph (3) but shall be subject to a procedure and standard, respecting the validity of such claim, established by regulation of the Secretary.

(6)   For purposes of paragraph (r)(1)(B), a statement for a dietary supplement may be made if—

(A)   the statement claims a benefit related to a classical nutrient deficiency disease and discloses the prevalence of such disease in the United States, describes the role of a nutrient or dietary ingredient intended to affect the structure or function in humans, characterizes the documented mechanism by which a nutrient or dietary ingredient acts to maintain such structure or function, or describes general well-being from consumption of a nutrient or dietary ingredient,

(B)   the manufacturer of the dietary supplement has substantiation that such statement is truthful and not misleading, and

(C)   the statement contains, prominently displayed and in boldface type, the following:

"This statement has not been evaluated by the Food and Drug Administration. This product is not intended to diagnose, treat, cure, or prevent any disease."

A statement under this sub-paragraph may not claim to diagnose, mitigate, treat, cure, or prevent a specific disease or class of diseases. If the manufacturer of a dietary supplement proposes to make a statement described in the first sentence of this inline-paragraph in the labeling of the dietary supplement, the manufacturer shall notify the Secretary no later than 30 days after the first marketing of the dietary supplement with such statement that such a statement is being made.

(7)   The Secretary may make proposed regulations issued under this paragraph effective upon publication pending consideration of public comment and publication of a final regulation if the Secretary determines that such action is necessary—

(A)   to enable the Secretary to review and act promptly on petitions the Secretary determines provide for information necessary to—

(i)   enable consumers to develop and maintain healthy dietary practices;

(ii)   enable consumers to be informed promptly and effectively of important new knowledge regarding nutritional and health benefits of food; or

(iii)   ensure that scientifically sound nutritional and health information is provided to consumers as soon as possible; or

(B)   to enable the Secretary to act promptly to ban or modify a claim under this paragraph.

Such proposed regulations shall be deemed final agency action for purposes of judical review.

(s)   DIETARY SUPPLEMENTS   If—

(1)   it is a dietary supplement; and

(2)   (A)   the label or labeling of the supplement fails to list

(i)   the name of each ingredient of the supplement that is described in section 201(ff); and

(ii)(I)   the quantity of each such ingredient; or

(II)   with respect to a proprietary blend of such ingredients, the total quantity of all ingredients in the blend;

(B)   the label or labeling of the dietary supplement fails to identify the product by using the term "dietary supplement," which term may be modified with the name of such an ingredient;

(C)   the supplement contains an ingredient described in section 201(ff)(1)(C), and the label or labeling of the supplement fails to identify any part of the plant from which the ingredient is derived;

(D)   the supplement

(i)   is covered by the specifications of an official compendium;

(ii)   is represented as conforming to the specifications of an official compendium; and

(iii)   fails to so conform; or

(E)   the supplement

(i)   is not covered by the specifications of an official compendium; and

(ii)   (I)   fails to have the identity and strength that the supplement is represented to have; or

(II)   fails to meet the quality (including tablet or capsule disintegration), purity, or compositional specifications, based on validated assay or other appropriate methods, that the supplement is represented to meet.

A dietary supplement shall not be deemed misbranded solely because its label or labeling contains directions or conditions of use or warnings.

§   **403A**   (a) Except as provided in subsection (b), no State or political subdivision of a State may directly or indirectly establish under any authority or continue in effect as to any food in interstate commerce

(1)   any requirement for a food which is the subject of a standard of identity established under section 401 that is not identical to such standard of identity or that is not identical to the requirement of section 403(g), except that this paragraph does not apply to a standard of identity of a State or political subdivision of a State for maple syrup that is of the type required by sections 401 and 403(g),

(2)   any requirement for the labeling of food of the type required by section 403(c), 403(e), or 403(i)(2) that is not identical to the requirement of such section, except that this paragraph does not apply to a requirement of a State or political subdivision of a State that is of the type required by section 403(c) and that is applicable to maple syrup,

(3)   any requirement for the labeling of food of the type required by section 403(b), 403(d), 403(f), 403(h), 403(i)(1), or 403(k) that is not identical to the requirement of such section, except that this paragraph does not apply to a requirement of a State or political subdivision of a State that is of the type required by section 403(h)(1) and that is applicable to maple syrup,

(4)   any requirement for nutrition labeling of food that is not identical to the requirement of section 403(q), except a requirement for nutrition labeling of food which is exempt under subclause (i) or (ii) of section 403(q)(5)(A), or

(5)   any requirement respecting any claim of the type described in section 403(r)(1) made in the label or labeling of food that is not identical to the requirement of section 403(r), except a requirement respecting a claim made in the label or labeling of food which is exempt under section 403(r)(5)(B).

Paragraph (3) shall take effect in accordance with section 6(b) of the Nutrition Labeling and Education Act of 1990.

(b)   Upon petition of a State or a political subdivision of a State, the Secretary may exempt from subsection (a), under such conditions as may be prescribed by regulation, any State or local requirement that

(1)   would not cause any food to be in violation of any applicable requirement under Federal law,

(2)   would not unduly burden interstate commerce, and

(3)   is designed to address a particular need for information which need is not met by the requirements of the sections referred to in subsection (a).

DIETARY SUPPLEMENT LABELING EXEMPTIONS

§   **403B.**   (a) In General. A publication, including an article, a chapter in a book, or an official abstract of a peer-reviewed scientific publication that appears in an article and was prepared by the author or the editors of the publication, which is reprinted in its entirety, shall not be defined as labeling when used in connection with the sale of a dietary supplement to consumers when it

(1)   is not false or misleading;

(2)   does not promote a particular manufacturer or brand of a dietary supplement;

(3)   is displayed or presented, or is displayed or presented with other such items on the same subject matter, so as to present a balanced view of the available scientific information on a dietary supplement;

(4)   if displayed in an establishment, is physically separate from the dietary supplements; and

(5)   does not have appended to it any information by sticker or any other method.

(b)   Application. Subsection (a) shall not apply to or restrict a retailer or wholesaler of dietary supplements in any way whatsoever in the sale of books or other publications as a part of the business of such retailer or wholesaler.

(c)   Burden of Proof. In any proceeding brought under subsection (a), the burden of proof shall be on the United States to establish that an article or other such matter is false or misleading.

VITAMINS AND MINERALS

§   **411**   (a)(1)   Except as provided in paragraph (2)

(A)   the Secretary may not establish, under section 201(n), 401, or 403, maximum limits on the potency of any synthetic or natural vitamin or mineral within a food to which this section applies;

(B)   the Secretary may not classify any natural or synthetic vitamin or mineral (or combination thereof) as a drug solely because it exceeds the level of potency which the Secretary determines is nutritionally rational or useful;

(C)   the Secretary may not limit, under section 201(n), 401, or 403, the combination or number of any synthetic or natural

(i)   vitamin,

(ii)   mineral, or

(iii)   other ingredient of food, within a food to which this section applies.

(2)   Paragraph (1) shall not apply in the case of a vitamin, mineral, other ingredient of food, or food, which is represented for use by individuals in the treatment or management of specific diseases or disorders, by children, or by pregnant or lactating women. For purposes of this inline-paragraph, the term "children" means individuals who are under the age of twelve years.

(b)   (1)   A food to which this section applies shall not he deemed under section 403 to be misbranded solely because its label bears, in accordance with section 403(i)(2), all the ingredients in the food or its advertising contains references to ingredients in the food which are not vitamins or minerals.

(2)   The labeling for any food to which this section applies may not list its ingredients which are not dietary supplements ingredients described in section 201(ff)(i) except as a part of a list of all the ingredients of such food, and (ii) unless such ingredients are listed in accordance with applicable regulations under section 403. To the extent that compliance with clause (i) of this inline-

paragraph is impracticable or results in deception or unfair competition, exemptions shall be established by regulations promulgated by the Secretary.

(c)(1)   For purposes of this section, the term "food to which this section applies" means a food for humans which is a food for special dietary use

(A)   which is or contains any natural or synthetic vitamin or mineral, and

(B)   which

(i)   is intended for ingestion in tablet, capsule, powder, softgel, gelcap, or liquid form, or

(ii)   if not intended for ingestion in such a form, and is not represented as conventional food and is not represented for use as a sole item of a meal or of the diet.

(2)   For purposes of paragraph (1)(B)(i), a food shall be considered as intended for ingestion in liquid form only if it is formulated in a fluid carrier and it is intended for ingestion in daily quantities measured in drops or similar small units of measure.

(3)   For purposes of paragraph (1) and of section 403(j) insofar as that section is applicable to food to which this section applies, the term "special dietary use" as applied to food used by man means a particular use for which a food purports or is represented to be used, including but not limited to the following:

(A)   Supplying a special dietary need that exists by reason of a physical, physiological, pathological, or other condition, including but not limited to the condition of disease, convalescence, pregnancy, lactation, infancy, allergic hypersensitivity to food, underweight, overweight, or the need to control the intake of sodium.

(B)   Supplying a vitamin, mineral, or other ingredient for use by man to supplement his diet by increasing the total dietary intake.

(C)   Supplying a special dietary need by reason of being a food for use as the sole item of the diet.

NEW DIETARY INGREDIENTS

§   **413**   (a)   In General. A dietary supplement which contains a new dietary ingredient shall be deemed adulterated under section 402(f) unless it meets one of the following requirements:

(1)   The dietary supplement contains only dietary ingredients which have been present in the food supply as an article used for food in a form in which the food has not been chemically altered.

(2)   There is a history of use or other evidence of safety establishing that the dietary ingredient when used under the conditions recommended or suggested in the labeling of the dietary supplement will reasonably be expected to be safe and, at least 75 days before being introduced or delivered for introduction into interstate commerce, the manufacturer or distributor of the dietary ingredient or dietary supplement provides the Secretary with information, including any citation to published articles, which is the basis on which the manufacturer or distributor has concluded that a dietary supplement containing such dietary ingredient will reasonably be expected to be safe.

The Secretary shall keep confidential any information provided under paragraph (2) for 90 days following its receipt. After the expiration of such 90 days, the Secretary shall place such information on public display, except matters in the information which are trade secrets or otherwise confidential, commercial information.

(b)   Petition. Any person may file with the Secretary a petition proposing the issuance of an order prescribing the conditions under which a new dietary ingredient under its intended conditions of use will reasonably be expected to be safe. The Secretary shall make a decision on such petition within 180 days of the date the petition is filed with the Secretary. For purposes of chapter 7 of title 5, United States Code, the decision of the Secretary shall be considered final agency action.

(c)   Definition. For purposes of this section, the term "new dietary ingredient" means a dietary ingredient that was not marketed in the United States before October 15, 1994 and does not include any dietary ingredient which was marketed in the United States before October 15, 1994.

GOOD MANUFACTURING PRACTICES

As is indicated in the *General Notices*, tolerances stated in the *United States Pharmacopeia* and in the *National Formulary* are based upon the consideration that the article is produced under recognized principles of good manufacturing practice. In the United States, a drug not produced in accordance with current good manufacturing practices may be considered to be adulterated. The U. S. Food and Drug Administration has published regulations setting forth minimum current good manufacturing practices for the preparation of drug products. While the regulations are directed primarily to drug manufacturers, the principles embodied therein may be helpful to those engaged in the practice of pharmacy and it is for this reason that these regulations are reproduced here.

Publication of these regulations in this *Pharmacopeia* is for purposes of information and does not impart any legal effect under the Federal Food, Drug, and Cosmetic Act. For the complete regulations, please refer to the Code of Federal Regulations.

Part 210—Current Good Manufacturing Practices in Manufacturing, Processing, Packing, or Holding of Drugs: General

§ **210.1   Status of current good manufacturing practice regulations.**

(a)   The regulations set forth in this part and in Parts 211 through 226 of this chapter contain the minimum current good manufacturing practice for methods to be used in, and the facilities or controls to be used for, the manufacture, processing, packing, or holding of a drug to assure that such drug meets the requirements of the act as to safety, and has the identity and strength and meets the quality and purity characteristics that it purports or is represented to possess.

(b)   The failure to comply with any regulation set forth in this part and in Parts 211 through 226 of this chapter in the manufacture, processing, packing, or holding of a drug shall render such drug to be adulterated under section 501(a)(2)(B) of the act and such drug, as well as the person who is responsible for the failure to comply, shall be subject to regulatory action.

§ **210.2   Applicability of current good manufacturing practice regulations.**

(a)   The regulations in this part and in Parts 211 through 226 of this chapter as they may pertain to a drug and in Parts 600 through 680 of this chapter as they may pertain to a biological product for human use, shall be considered to supplement, not supersede, each other, unless the regulations explicitly provide otherwise. In the event that it is impossible to comply with all applicable regulations in these parts, the regulations specifically applicable to the drug in question shall supersede the more general.

(b)   If a person engages in only some operations subject to the regulations in this part and in Parts 211 through 226 and Parts 600 through 680 of this chapter, and not in others, that person need only comply with those regulations applicable to the operations in which he or she is engaged.

§ **210.3   Definitions.**

(a)   The definitions and interpretations contained in section 201 of the act shall be applicable to such terms when used in this part and in Parts 211 through 226 of this chapter.

(b)   The following definitions of terms apply to this part and to Parts 211 through 226 of this chapter.

(1)   "Act" means the Federal Food, Drug, and Cosmetic Act, as amended (21 U.S.C. 301 et seq.).

(2)   "Batch" means a specific quantity of a drug or other material that is intended to have uniform character and quality, within specified limits, and is produced according to a single manufacturing order during the same cycle of manufacture.

(3)   "Component" means any ingredient intended for use in the manufacture of a drug product, including those that may not appear in such drug product.

(4)   "Drug product" means a finished dosage form, for example, tablet, capsule, solution, etc., that contains an active drug ingredient generally, but not necessarily, in association with inactive ingredients. The term also includes a finished dosage form that does not contain an active ingredient but is intended to be used as a placebo.

(5)   "Fiber" means any particulate contaminant with a length at least three times greater than its width.

(6)   "Non-fiber-releasing filter" means any filter, which after any appropriate pretreatment such as washing or flushing, will not release fibers into the component or drug product that is being filtered. All filters composed of asbestos are deemed to be fiber-releasing filters.

(7)   "Active ingredient" means any component that is intended to furnish pharmacological activity or other direct effect in the diagnosis, cure, mitigation, treatment, or prevention of disease, or to affect the structure of any function of the body of man or other animals. The term includes those components that may undergo chemical change in the manufacture of the drug product and be present in the drug product in a modified form intended to furnish the specified activity or effect.

(8)   "Inactive ingredient" means any component other than an "active ingredient."

(9)   "In-process material" means any material fabricated, compounded, blended, or derived by chemical reaction that is produced for, and used in the preparation of the drug product.

(10)   "Lot" means a batch, or a specific identified portion of a batch, having uniform character and quality within specified limits; or, in the case of a drug product produced by continuous process, it is a specific identified amount produced in a unit of time or quantity in a manner that assures its having uniform character and quality within specified limits.

(11)   "Lot number, control number, or batch number" means any distinctive combination of letters, numbers, or symbols, or any combination of them, from which the complete history of the manufacture, processing, packing, holding, and distribution of a batch or lot of drug product or other material can be determined.

(12)   "Manufacture, processing, packing, or holding of a drug product" includes packaging and labeling operations, testing, and quality control of drug products.

(13)   "Quality control unit" means any person or organizational element designated by the firm to be responsible for the duties relating to quality control.

(14)   "Strength" means:
  (i)   The concentration of the drug substance (for example, weight/weight, weight/volume, or unit dose/volume basis), and/or
  (ii)   The potency, that is, the therapeutic activity of the drug product as indicated by appropriate laboratory tests or by adequately developed and controlled clinical data (expressed, for example, in terms of units by reference to a standard).

(15)   "Theoretical yield" means the quantity that would be produced at any appropriate phase of manufacture, processing, or packing of a particular drug product, based upon the quantity of components to be used, in the absence of any loss or error in actual production.

(16)   "Actual yield" means the quantity that is actually produced at any appropriate phase of manufacture, processing, or packing of a particular drug product.

(17)   "Percentage of theoretical yield" means the ratio of the actual yield (at any appropriate phase of manufacture, processing, or packing of a particular drug product) to the theoretical yield (at the same phase), stated as a percentage.

(18)   "Acceptance criteria" means the product specifications and acceptance/rejection criteria, such as acceptable quality level and unacceptable quality level, with an associated sam-

pling plan, that are necessary for making a decision to accept or reject a lot or batch (or any other convenient subgroups of manufactured units).

(19) "Representative sample" means a sample that consists of a number of units that are drawn based on rational criteria such as random sampling and intended to assure that the sample accurately portrays the material being sampled.

(20) Gang-printed labeling means labeling derived from a sheet of material on which more than one item of labeling is printed.

Part 211—Current Good Manufacturing Practice for Finished Pharmaceuticals

Subpart A—General Provisions

§ 211.1   Scope.
§ 211.3   Definitions.

Subpart B—Organization and Personnel

§ 211.22   Responsibilities of quality control unit.
§ 211.25   Personnel qualifications.
§ 211.28   Personnel responsibilities.
§ 211.34   Consultants.

Subpart C—Buildings and Facilities

§ 211.42   Design and construction features.
§ 211.44   Lighting.
§ 211.46   Ventilation, air filtration, air heating and cooling.
§ 211.48   Plumbing.
§ 211.50   Sewage and refuse.
§ 211.52   Washing and toilet facilities.
§ 211.56   Sanitation.
§ 211.58   Maintenance.

Subpart D—Equipment

§ 211.63   Equipment design, size, and location.
§ 211.65   Equipment construction.
§ 211.67   Equipment cleaning and maintenance.
§ 211.68   Automatic, mechanical, and electronic equipment.
§ 211.72   Filters.

Subpart E—Control of Components and Drug Product Containers and Closures

§ 211.80   General requirements.
§ 211.82   Receipt and storage of untested components, drug product containers, and closures.
§ 211.84   Testing and approval or rejection of components, drug product containers, and closures.
§ 211.86   Use of approved components, drug product containers, and closures.
§ 211.87   Retesting of approved components, drug product containers, and closures.
§ 211.89   Rejected components, drug product containers, and closures.
§ 211.94   Drug product containers and closures.

Subpart F—Production and Process Controls

§ 211.100   Written procedures; deviations.
§ 211.101   Charge-in of components.
§ 211.103   Calculation of yield.
§ 211.105   Equipment identification.
§ 211.110   Sampling and testing of in-process materials and drug products.
§ 211.111   Time limitations on production.
§ 211.113   Control of microbiological contamination.
§ 211.115   Reprocessing.

Subpart G—Packaging and Labeling Control

§ 211.122   Materials examination and usage criteria.
§ 211.125   Labeling issuance.
§ 211.130   Packaging and labeling operations.
§ 211.132   Tamper-evident packaging requirements for over-the-counter human drug products.
§ 211.134   Drug product inspection.
§ 211.137   Expiration dating.

Subpart H—Holding and Distribution

§ 211.142   Warehousing procedures.
§ 211.150   Distribution procedures.

Subpart I—Laboratory Controls

§ 211.160   General requirements.
§ 211.165   Testing and release for distribution.
§ 211.166   Stability testing.
§ 211.167   Special testing requirements.
§ 211.170   Reserve samples.
§ 211.173   Laboratory animals.
§ 211.176   Penicillin contamination.

Subpart J—Records and Reports

§ 211.180   General requirements.
§ 211.182   Equipment cleaning and use log.
§ 211.184   Component, drug product container, closure, and labeling records.
§ 211.186   Master production and control records.
§ 211.188   Batch production and control records.
§ 211.192   Production record review.
§ 211.194   Laboratory records.
§ 211.196   Distribution records.
§ 211.198   Complaint files.

Subpart K—Returned and Salvaged Drug Products

§ 211.204   Returned drug products.
§ 211.208   Drug product salvaging.

Subpart A—General Provisions

§ **211.1   Scope.**
(a)   The regulations in this part contain the minimum current good manufacturing practice for preparation of drug products for administration to humans or animals.

(b) The current good manufacturing practice regulations in this chapter, as they pertain to drug products, and in parts 600 through 680 of this chapter, as they pertain to biological products for human use, shall be considered to supplement, not supersede, the regulations in this part unless the regulations explicitly provide otherwise. In the event it is impossible to comply with applicable regulations both in this part and in other parts of this chapter or in parts 600 through 680 of this chapter, the regulation specifically applicable to the drug product in question shall supersede the regulation in this part.

(c) Pending consideration of a proposed exemption, published in the Federal Register of September 29, 1978, the requirements in this part shall not be enforced for OTC drug products if the products and all their ingredients are ordinarily marketed and consumed as human foods, and which products may also fall within the legal definition of drugs by virtue of their intended use. Therefore, until further notice, regulations under part 110 of this chapter, and where applicable, parts 113 to 129 of this chapter, shall be applied in determining whether these OTC drug products that are also foods are manufactured, processed, packed, or held under current good manufacturing practice.

§ 211.3 Definitions.

The definitions set forth in § 210.3 of this chapter apply in this part.

Subpart B—Organization and Personnel

§ 211.22 Responsibilities of quality control unit.

(a) There shall be a quality control unit that shall have the responsibility and authority to approve or reject all components, drug product containers, closures, in-process materials, packaging material, labeling, and drug products, and the authority to review production records to assure that no errors have occurred or, if errors have occurred, that they have been fully investigated. The quality control unit shall be responsible for approving or rejecting drug products manufactured, processed, packed, or held under contract by another company.

(b) Adequate laboratory facilities for the testing and approval (or rejection) of components, drug product containers, closures, packaging materials, in-process materials, and drug products shall be available to the quality control unit.

(c) The quality control unit shall have the responsibility for approving or rejecting all procedures or specifications impacting on the identity, strength, quality, and purity of the drug product.

(d) The responsibilities and procedures applicable to the quality control unit shall be in writing; such written procedures shall be followed.

§ 211.25 Personnel qualifications.

(a) Each person engaged in the manufacture, processing, packing, or holding of a drug product shall have education, training, and experience, or any combination thereof, to enable that person to perform the assigned functions. Training shall be in the particular operations that the employee performs and in current good manufacturing practice (including the current good manufacturing practice regulations in this chapter and written procedures required by these regulations) as they relate to the employee's functions. Training in current good manufacturing practice shall be conducted by qualified individuals on a continuing basis and with sufficient frequency to assure that employees remain familiar with CGMP requirements applicable to them.

(b) Each person responsible for supervising the manufacture, processing, packing, or holding of a drug product shall have the education, training, and experience, or any combination thereof, to perform assigned functions in such a manner as to provide assurance that the drug product has the safety, identity, strength, quality, and purity that it purports or is represented to possess.

(c) There shall be an adequate number of qualified personnel to perform and supervise the manufacture, processing, packing, or holding of each drug product.

§ 211.28 Personnel responsibilities.

(a) Personnel engaged in the manufacture, processing, packing, or holding of a drug product shall wear clean clothing appropriate for the duties they perform. Protective apparel, such as head, face, hand, and arm coverings, shall be worn as necessary to protect drug products from contamination.

(b) Personnel shall practice good sanitation and health habits.

(c) Only personnel authorized by supervisory personnel shall enter those areas of the buildings and facilities designated as limited-access areas.

(d) Any person shown at any time (either by medical examination or supervisory observation) to have an apparent illness or open lesions that may adversely affect the safety or quality of drug products shall be excluded from direct contact with components, drug product containers, closures, in-process materials, and drug products until the condition is corrected or determined by competent medical personnel not to jeopardize the safety or quality of drug products. All personnel shall be instructed to report to supervisory personnel any health conditions that may have an adverse effect on drug products.

§ 211.34 Consultants.

Consultants advising on the manufacture, processing, packing, or holding of drug products shall have sufficient education, training, and experience, or any combination thereof, to advise on the subject for which they are retained. Records shall be maintained stating the name, address, and qualifications of any consultants and the type of service they provide.

Subpart C—Buildings and Facilities

§ 211.42 Design and construction features.

(a) Any building or buildings used in the manufacture, processing, packing, or holding of a drug product shall be of suitable size, construction and location to facilitate cleaning, maintenance, and proper operations.

(b) Any such building shall have adequate space for the orderly placement of equipment and materials to prevent mixups between different components, drug product containers, closures, labeling, in-process materials, or drug products, and to prevent contamination. The flow of components, drug product containers, closures, labeling, in-process materials, and drug products through the building or buildings shall be designed to prevent contamination.

(c) Operations shall be performed within specifically defined areas of adequate size. There shall be separate or defined areas or such other control systems for the firm's operations as are necessary to prevent contamination or mixups during the course of the following procedures:

(1) Receipt, identification, storage, and withholding from use of components, drug product containers, closures, and labeling, pending the appropriate sampling, testing, or examination by the quality control unit before release for manufacturing or packaging;
(2) Holding rejected components, drug product containers, closures, and labeling before disposition;
(3) Storage of released components, drug product containers, closures, and labeling;
(4) Storage of in-process materials;
(5) Manufacturing and processing operations;
(6) Packaging and labeling operations;
(7) Quarantine storage before release of drug products;
(8) Storage of drug products after release;
(9) Control and laboratory operations;
(10) Aseptic processing, which includes as appropriate:
   (i) Floors, walls, and ceilings of smooth, hard surfaces that are easily cleanable;
   (ii) Temperature and humidity controls;
   (iii) An air supply filtered through high-efficiency particulate air filters under positive pressure, regardless of whether flow is laminar or nonlaminar;

(iv) A system for monitoring environmental conditions;
(v) A system for cleaning and disinfecting the room and equipment to produce aseptic conditions;
(vi) A system for maintaining any equipment used to control the aseptic conditions.
(11) Operations relating to the manufacture, processing, and packing of penicillin shall be performed in facilities separate from those used for other drug products for human use.

§ 211.44   Lighting.

Adequate lighting shall be provided in all areas.

§ 211.46   Ventilation, air filtration, air heating and cooling.

(a) Adequate ventilation shall be provided.
(b) Equipment for adequate control over air pressure, microorganisms, dust, humidity, and temperature shall be provided when appropriate for the manufacture, processing, packing, or holding of a drug product.
(c) Air filtration systems, including prefilters and particulate matter air filters, shall be used when appropriate on air supplies to production areas. If air is recirculated to production areas, measures shall be taken to control recirculation of dust from production. In areas where air contamination occurs during production, there shall be adequate exhaust systems or other systems adequate to control contaminants.
(d) Air-handling systems for the manufacture, processing, and packing of penicillin shall be completely separate from those for other drug products for human use.

§ 211.48   Plumbing.

(a) Potable water shall be supplied under continuous positive pressure in a plumbing system free of defects that could contribute contamination to any drug product. Potable water shall meet the standards prescribed in the Environmental Protection Agency's Primary Drinking Water Regulations set forth in 40 CFR part 141. Water not meeting such standards shall not be permitted in the potable water system.
(b) Drains shall be of adequate size and, where connected directly to a sewer, shall be provided with an air break or other mechanical device to prevent back-siphonage.

§ 211.50   Sewage and refuse.

Sewage, trash, and other refuse in and from the building and immediate premises shall be disposed of in a safe and sanitary manner.

§ 211.52   Washing and toilet facilities.

Adequate washing facilities shall be provided, including hot and cold water, soap or detergent, air driers or single-service towels, and clean toilet facilities easily accessible to working areas.

§ 211.56   Sanitation.

(a) Any building used in the manufacture, processing, packing, or holding of a drug product shall be maintained in a clean and sanitary condition. Any such building shall be free of infestation by rodents, birds, insects, and other vermin (other than laboratory animals). Trash and organic waste matter shall be held and disposed of in a timely and sanitary manner.
(b) There shall be written procedures assigning responsibility for sanitation and describing in sufficient detail the cleaning schedules, methods, equipment, and materials to be used in cleaning the buildings and facilities; such written procedures shall be followed.
(c) There shall be written procedures for use of suitable rodenticides, insecticides, fungicides, fumigating agents, and cleaning and sanitizing agents. Such written procedures shall be designed to prevent the contamination of equipment, components, drug product containers, closures, packaging, labeling materials, or drug products and shall be followed. Rodenticides, insecticides, and fungicides shall not be used unless registered and used in accordance with the Federal Insecticide, Fungicide, and Rodenticide Act (7 U.S.C. 135).

(d) Sanitation procedures shall apply to work performed by contractors or temporary employees as well as work performed by full-time employees during the ordinary course of operations.

§ 211.58   Maintenance.

Any building used in the manufacture, processing, packing, or holding of a drug product shall be maintained in a good state of repair.

Subpart D—Equipment

§ 211.63   Equipment design, size, and location.

Equipment used in the manufacture, processing, packing, or holding of a drug product shall be of appropriate design, adequate size, and suitably located to facilitate operations for its intended use and for its cleaning and maintenance.

§ 211.65   Equipment construction.

(a) Equipment shall be constructed so that surfaces that contact components, in-process materials, or drug products shall not be reactive, additive, or absorptive so as to alter the safety, identity, strength, quality, or purity of the drug product beyond the official or other established requirements.
(b) Any substances required for operation, such as lubricants or coolants, shall not come into contact with components, drug product containers, closures, in-process materials, or drug products so as to alter the safety, identity, strength, quality, or purity of the drug product beyond the official or other established requirements.

§ 211.67   Equipment cleaning and maintenance.

(a) Equipment and utensils shall be cleaned, maintained, and sanitized at appropriate intervals to prevent malfunctions or contamination that would alter the safety, identity, strength, quality, or purity of the drug product beyond the official or other established requirements.
(b) Written procedures shall be established and followed for cleaning and maintenance of equipment, including utensils, used in the manufacture, processing, packing, or holding of a drug product. These procedures shall include, but are not necessarily limited to, the following:
(1) Assignment of responsibility for cleaning and maintaining equipment;
(2) Maintenance and cleaning schedules, including, where appropriate, sanitizing schedules;
(3) A description in sufficient detail of the methods, equipment, and materials used in cleaning and maintenance operations, and the methods of disassembling and reassembling equipment as necessary to assure proper cleaning and maintenance;
(4) Removal or obliteration of previous batch identification;
(5) Protection of clean equipment from contamination prior to use;
(6) Inspection of equipment for cleanliness immediately before use.
(c) Records shall be kept of maintenance, cleaning, sanitizing, and inspection as specified in §§211.180 and 211.182.

§ 211.68   Automatic, mechanical, and electronic equipment.

(a) Automatic, mechanical, or electronic equipment or other types of equipment, including computers, or related systems that will perform a function satisfactorily, may be used in the manufacture, processing, packing, and holding of a drug product. If such equipment is so used, it shall be routinely calibrated, inspected, or checked according to a written program designed to assure proper performance. Written records of those calibration checks and inspections shall be maintained.

(b) Appropriate controls shall be exercised over computer or related systems to assure that changes in master production and control records or other records are instituted only by authorized personnel. Input to and output from the computer or related system of formulas or other records or data shall be checked for accuracy. The degree and frequency of input/output verification shall be based on the complexity and reliability of the computer or related system. A backup file of data entered into the computer or related system shall be maintained except where certain data, such as calculations performed in connection with laboratory analysis, are eliminated by computerization or other automated processes. In such instances a written record of the program shall be maintained along with appropriate validation data. Hard copy or alternative systems, such as duplicates, tapes, or microfilm, designed to assure that backup data are exact and complete and that it is secure from alteration, inadvertent erasures, or loss shall be maintained.

§ 211.72   Filters.

Filters for liquid filtration used in the manufacture, processing, or packing of injectable drug products intended for human use shall not release fibers into such products. Fiber-releasing filters may not be used in the manufacture, processing, or packing of these injectable drug products unless it is not possible to manufacture such drug products without the use of such filters. If use of a fiber-releasing filter is necessary, an additional non-fiber-releasing filter of 0.22 micron maximum mean porosity (0.45 micron if the manufacturing conditions so dictate) shall subsequently be used to reduce the content of particles in the injectable drug product. Use of an asbestos-containing filter, with or without subsequent use of a specific non-fiber-releasing filter, is permissible only upon submission of proof to the appropriate bureau of the Food and Drug Administration that use of a non-fiber-releasing filter will, or is likely to, compromise the safety or effectiveness of the injectable drug product.

Subpart E—Control of Components and Drug Product Containers and Closures

§ 211.80   General requirements.

(a) There shall be written procedures describing in sufficient detail the receipt, identification, storage, handling, sampling, testing, and approval or rejection of components and drug product containers and closures; such written procedures shall be followed.

(b) Components and drug product containers and closures shall at all times be handled and stored in a manner to prevent contamination.

(c) Bagged or boxed components of drug product containers, or closures shall be stored off the floor and suitably spaced to permit cleaning and inspection.

(d) Each container or grouping of containers for components or drug product containers, or closures shall be identified with a distinctive code for each lot in each shipment received. This code shall be used in recording the disposition of each lot. Each lot shall be appropriately identified as to its status (i.e., quarantine, approved, or rejected).

§ 211.82   Receipt and storage of untested components, drug product containers, and closures.

(a) Upon receipt and before acceptance, each container or grouping of containers of components, drug product containers, and closures shall be examined visually for appropriate labeling as to contents, container damage or broken seals, and contamination.

(b) Components, drug product containers, and closures shall be stored under quarantine until they have been tested or examined, as appropriate, and released. Storage within the area shall conform to the requirements of §211.80.

§ 211.84   Testing and approval or rejection of components, drug product containers, and closures.

(a) Each lot of components, drug product containers, and closures shall be withheld from use until the lot has been sampled, tested, or examined, as appropriate, and released for use by the quality control unit.

(b) Representative samples of each shipment of each lot shall be collected for testing or examination. The number of containers to be sampled, and the amount of material to be taken from each container, shall be based upon appropriate criteria such as statistical criteria for component variability, confidence levels, and degree of precision desired, the past quality history of the supplier, and the quantity needed for analysis and reserve where required by §211.170.

(c) Samples shall be collected in accordance with the following procedures:
(1) The containers of components selected shall be cleaned where necessary, by appropriate means.
(2) The containers shall be opened, sampled, and resealed in a manner designed to prevent contamination of their contents and contamination of other components, drug product containers, or closures.
(3) Sterile equipment and aseptic sampling techniques shall be used when necessary.
(4) If it is necessary to sample a component from the top, middle, and bottom of its container, such sample subdivisions shall not be composited for testing.
(5) Sample containers shall be identified so that the following information can be determined: name of the material sampled, the lot number, the container from which the sample was taken, the date on which the sample was taken, and the name of the person who collected the sample.
(6) Containers from which samples have been taken shall be marked to show that samples have been removed from them.

(d) Samples shall be examined and tested as follows:
(1) At least one test shall be conducted to verify the identity of each component of a drug product. Specific identity tests, if they exist, shall be used.
(2) Each component shall be tested for conformity with all appropriate written specifications for purity, strength, and quality. In lieu of such testing by the manufacturer, a report of analysis may be accepted from the supplier of a component, provided that at least one specific identity test is conducted on such component by the manufacturer, and provided that the manufacturer establishes the reliability of the supplier's analyses through appropriate validation of the supplier's test results at appropriate intervals.
(3) Containers and closures shall be tested for conformance with all appropriate written procedures. In lieu of such testing by the manufacturer, a certificate of testing may be accepted from the supplier, provided that at least a visual identification is conducted on such containers/closures by the manufacturer and provided that the manufacturer establishes the reliability of the supplier's test results through appropriate validation of the supplier's test results at appropriate intervals.

(4) When appropriate, components shall be microscopically examined.
(5) Each lot of a component, drug product container, or closure that is liable to contamination with filth, insect infestation, or other extraneous adulterant shall be examined against established specifications for such contamination.
(6) Each lot of a component, drug product container, or closure that is liable to microbiological contamination that is objectionable in view of its intended use shall be subjected to microbiological tests before use.

(e) Any lot of components, drug product containers, or closures that meets the appropriate written specifications of identity, strength, quality, and purity and related tests under paragraph (d) of this section may be approved and released for use. Any lot of such material that does not meet such specifications shall be rejected.

§ 211.86   Use of approved components, drug product containers, and closures.

Components, drug product containers, and closures approved for use shall be rotated so that the oldest approved stock is used first. Deviation from this requirement is permitted if such deviation is temporary and appropriate.

§ 211.87   Retesting of approved components, drug product containers, and closures.

Components, drug product containers, and closures shall be retested or reexamined, as appropriate, for identity, strength, quality, and purity and approved or rejected by the quality control unit in accordance with §211.84 as necessary, e.g., after storage for long periods or after exposure to air, heat or other conditions that might adversely affect the component, drug product container, or closure.

§ 211.89   Rejected components, drug product containers, and closures.

Rejected components, drug product containers, and closures shall be identified and controlled under a quarantine system designed to prevent their use in manufacturing or processing operations for which they are unsuitable.

§ 211.94   Drug product containers and closures.

(a) Drug product containers and closures shall not be reactive, additive, or absorptive so as to alter the safety, identity, strength, quality, or purity of the drug beyond the official or established requirements.
(b) Container closure systems shall provide adequate protection against foreseeable external factors in storage and use that can cause deterioration or contamination of the drug product.
(c) Drug product containers and closures shall be clean and, where indicated by the nature of the drug, sterilized and processed to remove pyrogenic properties to assure that they are suitable for their intended use.
(d) Standards or specifications, methods of testing, and, where indicated, methods of cleaning, sterilizing, and processing to remove pyrogenic properties shall be written and followed for drug product containers and closures.

Subpart F—Production and Process Controls

§ 211.100   Written procedures; deviations.

(a) There shall be written procedures for production and process control designed to assure that the drug products have the identity, strength, quality, and purity they purport or are represented to possess. Such procedures shall include all requirements in this subpart. These written procedures, including any changes, shall be drafted, reviewed, and approved by the appropriate organizational units and reviewed and approved by the quality control unit.
(b) Written production and process control procedures shall be followed in the execution of the various production and process control functions and shall be documented at the time of performance. Any deviation from the written procedures shall be recorded and justified.

§ 211.101   Charge-in of components.

Written production and control procedures shall include the following, which are designed to assure that the drug products produced have the identity, strength, quality, and purity they purport or are represented to possess:
(a) The batch shall be formulated with the intent to provide not less than 100 percent of the labeled or established amount of active ingredient.
(b) Components for drug product manufacturing shall be weighed, measured, or subdivided as appropriate. If a component is removed from the original container to another, the new container shall be identified with the following information:
(1) Component name or item code;
(2) Receiving or control number;
(3) Weight or measure in new container;
(4) Batch for which component was dispensed, including its product name, strength, and lot number.
(c) Weighing, measuring, or subdividing operations for components shall be adequately supervised. Each container of component dispensed to manufacturing shall be examined by a second person to assure that:
(1) The component was released by the quality control unit;
(2) The weight or measure is correct as stated in the batch production records;
(3) The containers are properly identified.
(d) Each component shall be added to the batch by one person and verified by a second person.

§ 211.103   Calculation of yield.

Actual yields and percentages of theoretical yield shall be determined at the conclusion of each appropriate phase of manufacturing, processing, packaging, or holding of the drug product. Such calculations shall be performed by one person and independently verified by a second person.

§ 211.105   Equipment identification.

(a) All compounding and storage containers, processing lines, and major equipment used using the production of a batch of a drug product shall be properly identified at all times to indicate their contents and, when necessary, the phase of processing of the batch.
(b) Major equipment shall be identified by a distinctive identification number or code that shall be recorded in the batch production record to show the specific equipment used in the manufacture of each batch of a drug product. In cases where only

one of a particular type of equipment exists in a manufacturing facility, the name of the equipment may be used in lieu of a distinctive identification number or code.

§ 211.110   Sampling and testing of in-process materials and drug products.

(a)   To assure batch uniformity and integrity of drug products, written procedures shall be established and followed that describe the in-process controls, and tests, or examinations to be conducted on appropriate samples of in-process materials of each batch. Such control procedures shall be established to monitor the output and to validate the performance of those manufacturing processes that may be responsible for causing variability in the characteristics of in-process material and the drug product. Such control procedures shall include, but are not limited to, the following, where appropriate:
(1)   Tablet or capsule weight variation;
(2)   Disintegration time;
(3)   Adequacy of mixing to assure uniformity and homogeneity;
(4)   Dissolution time and rate;
(5)   Clarity, completeness, or pH of solutions.
(b)   Valid in-process specifications for such characteristics shall be consistent with drug product final specifications and shall be derived from previous acceptable process average and process variability estimates where possible and determined by the application of suitable statistical procedures where appropriate. Examination and testing of samples shall assure that the drug product and in-process material conform to specifications.
(c)   In-process materials shall be tested for identity, strength, quality, and purity as appropriate, and approved or rejected by the quality control unit, during the production process, e.g., at commencement or completion of significant phases or after storage for long periods.
(d)   Rejected in-process materials shall be identified and controlled under a quarantine system designed to prevent their use in manufacturing or processing operations for which they are unsuitable.

§ 211.111   Time limitations on production.

When appropriate, time limits for the completion of each phase of production shall be established to assure the quality of the drug product. Deviation from established time limits may be acceptable if such deviation does not compromise the quality of the drug product. Such deviation shall be justified and documented.

§ 211.113   Control of microbiological contamination.

(a)   Appropriate written procedures, designed to prevent objectionable microorganisms in drug products not required to be sterile, shall be established and followed.
(b)   Appropriate written procedures, designed to prevent microbiological contamination of drug products purporting to be sterile, shall be established and followed. Such procedures shall include validation of any sterilization process.

§ 211.115   Reprocessing.

(a)   Written procedures shall be established and followed prescribing a system for reprocessing batches that do not conform to standards or specifications and the steps to be taken to insure that the reprocessed batches will conform with all established standards, specifications, and characteristics.
(b)   Reprocessing shall not be performed without the review and approval of the quality control unit.

Subpart G—Packaging and Labeling Control

§ 211.122   Materials examination and usage criteria.

(a)   There shall be written procedures describing in sufficient detail the receipt, identification, storage, handling, sampling, examination, and/or testing of labeling and packaging materials; such written procedures shall be followed. Labeling and packaging materials shall be representatively sampled, and examined or tested upon receipt and before use in packaging or labeling of a drug product.
(b)   Any labeling or packaging materials meeting appropriate written specifications may be approved and released for use. Any labeling or packaging materials that do not meet such specifications shall be rejected to prevent their use in operations for which they are unsuitable.
(c)   Records shall be maintained for each shipment received of each different labeling and packaging material indicating receipt, examination or testing, and whether accepted or rejected.
(d)   Labels and other labeling materials for each different drug product, strength, dosage form, or quantity of contents shall be stored separately with suitable identification. Access to the storage area shall be limited to authorized personnel.
(e)   Obsolete and outdated labels, labeling, and other packaging materials shall be destroyed.
(f)   Use of gang-printed labeling for different drug products, or different strengths or net contents of the same drug product, is prohibited unless the labeling from gang-printed sheets is adequately differentiated by size, shape, or color.
(g)   If cut labeling is used, packaging and labeling operations shall include one of the following special control procedures:
(1)   Dedication of labeling and packaging lines to each different strength of each different drug product;
(2)   Use of appropriate electronic or electromechanical equipment to conduct a 100-percent examination for correct labeling during or after completion of finishing operations; or
(3)   Use of visual inspection to conduct a 100-percent examination for correct labeling during or after completion of finishing operations for hand-applied labeling. Such examination shall be performed by one person and independently verified by a second person.
(h)   Printing devices on, or associated with, manufacturing lines used to imprint labeling upon the drug product unit label or case shall be monitored to assure that all imprinting conforms to the print specified in the batch production record.

§ 211.125   Labeling issuance.

(a)   Strict control shall be exercised over labeling issued for use in drug product labeling operations.
(b)   Labeling materials issued for a batch shall be carefully examined for identity and conformity to the labeling specified in the master or batch production records.
(c)   Procedures shall be used to reconcile the quantities of labeling issued, used, and returned, and shall require evaluation of discrepancies found between the quantity of drug product finished and the quantity of labeling issued when such discrepancies are outside narrow preset limits based on historical operating data. Such discrepancies shall be investigated in accordance with §211.192. Labeling reconciliation is waived for cut or roll labeling if a 100-percent examination for correct labeling is performed in accordance with §211.122(g)(2).
(d)   All excess labeling bearing lot or control numbers shall be destroyed.
(e)   Returned labeling shall be maintained and stored in a manner to prevent mixups and provide proper identification.
(f)   Procedures shall be written describing in sufficient detail the control procedures employed for the issuance of labeling; such written procedures shall be followed.

§ 211.130   Packaging and labeling operations.

There shall be written procedures designed to assure that correct labels, labeling, and packaging materials are used for drug products; such written procedures shall be followed. These procedures shall incorporate the following features:

(a)   Prevention of mixups and cross-contamination by physical or spatial separation from operations on other drug products.

(b)   Identification and handling of filled drug product containers that are set aside and held in unlabeled condition for future labeling operations to preclude mislabeling of individual containers, lots, or portions of lots. Identification need not be applied to each individual container but shall be sufficient to determine name, strength, quantity of contents, and lot or control number of each container.

(c)   Identification of the drug product with a lot or control number that permits determination of the history of the manufacture and control of the batch.

(d)   Examination of packaging and labeling materials for suitability and correctness before packaging operations, and documentation of such examination in the batch production record.

(e)   Inspection of the packaging and labeling facilities immediately before use to assure that all drug products have been removed from previous operations. Inspection shall also be made to assure that packaging and labeling materials not suitable for subsequent operations have been removed. Results of inspection shall be documented in the batch production records.

§ 211.132   Tamper-evident packaging requirements for over-the-counter (OTC) human drug products.

(a)   *General.* The Food and Drug Administration has the authority under the Federal Food, Drug, and Cosmetic Act (the act) to establish a uniform national requirement for tamper-resistant packaging of OTC drug products that will improve the security of OTC drug packaging and help assure the safety and effectiveness of OTC drug products. An OTC drug product (except a dermatological, dentifrice, insulin, or lozenge product) for retail sale that is not packaged in a tamper-resistant package or that is not properly labeled under this section is adulterated under section 501 of the act or misbranded under section 502 of the act, or both.

(b)   *Requirements for tamper-evident package.* (1) Each manufacturer and packer who packages an OTC drug product (except a dermatological, dentifrice, insulin, or lozenge product) for retail sale shall package the product in a tamper-evident package, if this product is accessible to the public while held for sale. A tamper-evident package is one having one or more indicators or barriers to entry which, if breached or missing, can reasonably be expected for provide visible evidence to consumers that tampering has occurred. To reduce the likelihood of successful tampering and to increase the likelihood that consumers will discover if a product has been tampered with, the package is required to be distinctive by design or by the use of one or more indicators or barriers to entry that employ an identifying characteristic (e.g., a pattern, name, registered trademark, logo, or picture). For purposes of this section, the term "distinctive by design" means the packaging cannot be duplicated with commonly available materials or through commonly available processes. A tamper-evident package may involve an immediate-container and closure system or secondary-container or carton system or any combination of systems intended to provide a visual indication of package integrity. The tamper-evident feature shall be designed to and shall remain intact when handled in a reasonable manner during manufacture, distribution, and retail display.

(2)   In addition to the tamper-evident packaging feature described in paragraph (b)(1) of this section, any two-piece, hard gelatin capsule covered by this section must be sealed using an acceptable tamper-evident technology.

(c)   *Labeling.* (1) In order to alert consumers to the specific tamper-evident feature(s) used, each retail package of an OTC drug product covered by this section (except ammonia inhalant in crushable glass ampules, containers of compressed medical oxygen, or aerosol products that depend upon the power of a liquefied or compressed gas to expel the contents from the container) is required to bear a statement that:

(i)   Identifies all tamper-evident feature(s) and any capsule sealing technologies used to comply with paragraph (b) of this section;

(ii)   Is prominently placed on the package; and

(iii)   Is so placed that it will be unaffected if the tamper-evident feature of the package is breached or missing.

(2)   If the tamper-evident feature chosen to meet the requirements in paragraph (b) of this section uses an identifying characteristic, that characteristic is required to be referred to in the labeling statement. For example, the labeling statement on a bottle with a shrink band could say "For your protection, this bottle has an imprinted seal around the neck."

(d)   *Request for exemptions from packaging and labeling requirements.* A manufacturer or packer may request an exemption from the packaging and labeling requirements of this section. A request for an exemption is required to be submitted in the form of a citizen petition under §10.30 of this chapter and should be clearly identified on the envelope as a "Request for Exemption from the Tamper-Evident Packaging Rule." The petition is required to contain the following:

(1)   The name of the drug product or, if the petition seeks an exemption for a drug class, the name of the drug class, and a list of products within that class.

(2)   The reasons that the drug product's compliance with the tamper-evident packaging or labeling requirements of this section is unnecessary or cannot be achieved.

(3)   A description of alternative steps that are available, or that the petitioner has already taken, to reduce the likelihood that the product or drug class will be the subject of malicious adulteration.

(4)   Other information justifying an exemption.

(e)   *OTC drug products subject to approved new drug applications.* Holders of approved new drug applications for OTC drug products are required under §314.70 of this chapter to provide the agency with notification of changes in packaging and labeling to comply with the requirements of this section. Changes in packaging and labeling required by this regulation may be made before FDA approval, as provided under §314.70(c) of this chapter. Manufacturing changes by which capsules are to be sealed require prior FDA approval under §314.70(b) of this chapter.

(f)   *Poison Prevention Packaging Act of 1970.* This section does not affect any requirements for "special packaging" as defined under § 310.3(1) of this chapter and required under the Poison Prevention Packaging Act of 1970.

§ 211.134   Drug product inspection.

(a)   Packaged and labeled products shall be examined during finishing operations to provide assurance that containers and packages in the lot have the correct label.

(b)   A representative sample of units shall be collected at the completion of finishing operations and shall be visually examined for correct labeling.

(c)   Results of these examinations shall be recorded in the batch production or control records.

§ 211.137   Expiration dating.

(a)   To assure that a drug product meets applicable standards of identity, strength, quality, and purity at the time of use, it shall bear an expiration date determined by appropriate stability testing described in §211.166.

(b)   Expiration dates shall be related to any storage conditions stated on the labeling, as determined by stability studies described in §211.166.

(c)   If the drug product is to be reconstituted at the time of dispensing, its labeling shall bear expiration information for both the reconstituted and unreconstituted drug products.

(d)   Expiration dates shall appear on labeling in accordance with the requirements of §201.17 of this chapter.

(e)   Homeopathic drug products shall be exempt from the requirements of this section.

(f)   Allergenic extracts that are labeled "No U.S. Standard of Potency" are exempt from the requirements of this section.

(g)   New drug products for investigational use are exempt from the requirements of this section, provided that they meet appropriate standards or specifications as demonstrated by stability studies during their use in clinical investigations. Where new drug products for investigational use are to be reconstituted at the time of dispensing, their labeling shall bear expiration information for the reconstituted drug product.

(h)   Pending consideration of a proposed exemption, published in the FEDERAL REGISTER of September 29, 1978, the requirements in this section shall not be enforced for human OTC drug products if their labeling does not bear dosage limitations and they are stable for at least 3 years as supported by appropriate stability data.

Subpart H—Holding and Distribution

§ 211.142   Warehousing procedures.

Written procedures describing the warehousing of drug products shall be established and followed. They shall include:

(a)   Quarantine of drug products before release by the quality control unit.

(b)   Storage of drug products under appropriate conditions of temperature, humidity, and light so that the identity, strength, quality, and purity of the drug products are not affected.

§ 211.150   Distribution procedures.

Written procedures shall be established, and followed, describing the distribution of drug products. They shall include:

(a)   A procedure whereby the oldest approved stock of a drug product is distributed first. Deviation from this requirement is permitted if such deviation is temporary and appropriate.

(b)   A system by which the distribution of each lot of drug product can be readily determined to facilitate its recall if necessary.

Subpart I—Laboratory Controls

§ 211.160   General requirements.

(a)   The establishment of any specifications, standards, sampling plans, test procedures, or other laboratory control mechanisms required by this subpart, including any change in such specifications, standards, sampling plans, test procedures, or other laboratory control mechanisms, shall be drafted by the appropriate organizational unit and reviewed and approved by the quality control unit. The requirements in this subpart shall be followed and shall be documented at the time of performance. Any deviation from the written specifications, standards, sampling plans, test procedures, or other laboratory control mechanisms shall be recorded and justified.

(b)   Laboratory controls shall include the establishment of scientifically sound and appropriate specifications, standards, sampling plans, and test procedures designed to assure that components, drug product containers, closures, in-process materials, labeling, and drug products conform to appropriate standards of identity, strength, quality, and purity. Laboratory controls shall include:

(1)   Determination of conformance to appropriate written specifications for the acceptance of each lot within each shipment of components, drug product containers, closures, and labeling used in the manufacture, processing, packing, or holding of drug products. The specifications shall include a descrip-

tion of the sampling and testing procedures used. Samples shall be representative and adequately identified. Such procedures shall also require appropriate retesting of any component, drug product container, or closure that is subject to deterioration.

(2)   Determination of conformance to written specifications and a description of sampling and testing procedures for in-process materials. Such samples shall be representative and properly identified.

(3)   Determination of conformance to written descriptions of sampling procedures and appropriate specifications for drug products. Such samples shall be representative and properly identified.

(4)   The calibration of instruments, apparatus, gauges, and recording devices at suitable intervals in accordance with an established written program containing specific directions, schedules, limits for accuracy and precision, and provisions for remedial action in the event accuracy and/or precision limits are not met. Instruments, apparatus, gauges, and recording devices not meeting established specifications shall not be used.

§ 211.165   Testing and release for distribution.

(a)   For each batch of drug product, there shall be appropriate laboratory determination of satisfactory conformance to final specifications for the drug product, including the identity and strength of each active ingredient, prior to release. Where sterility and/or pyrogen testing are conducted on specific batches of short lived radiopharmaceuticals, such batches may be released prior to completion of sterility and/or pyrogen testing, provided such testing is completed as soon as possible.

(b)   There shall be appropriate laboratory testing, as necessary, of each batch of drug product required to be free of objectionable microorganisms.

(c)   Any sampling and testing plans shall be described in written procedures that shall include the method of sampling and the number of units per batch to be tested; such written procedure shall be followed.

(d)   Acceptance criteria for the sampling and testing conducted by the quality control unit shall be adequate to assure that batches of drug products meet each appropriate specification and appropriate statistical quality control criteria as a condition for their approval and release. The statistical quality control criteria shall include appropriate acceptance levels and/or appropriate rejection levels.

(e)   The accuracy, sensitivity, specificity, and reproducibility of test methods employed by the firm shall be established and documented. Such validation and documentation may be accomplished in accordance with §211.194(a)(2).

(f)   Drug products failing to meet established standards or specifications and any other relevant quality control criteria shall be rejected. Reprocessing may be performed. Prior to acceptance and use, reprocessed material must meet appropriate standards, specifications, and any other relevant criteria.

§ 211.166   Stability testing.

(a)   There shall be a written testing program designed to assess the stability characteristics of drug products. The results of such stability testing shall be used in determining appropriate storage conditions and expiration dates. The written program shall be followed and shall include:

(1)   Sample size and test intervals based on statistical criteria for each attribute examined to assure valid estimates of stability;

(2)   Storage conditions for samples retained for testing;

(3)   Reliable, meaningful, and specific test methods;

(4)   Testing of the drug product in the same container-closure system as that in which the drug product is marketed;

(5) Testing of drug products for reconstitution at the time of dispensing (as directed in the labeling) as well as after they are reconstituted.

(b)   An adequate number of batches of each drug product shall be tested to determine an appropriate expiration date and a record of such data shall be maintained. Accelerated studies, combined with basic stability information on the components, drug products, and container-closure system, may be used to support tentative expiration dates provided full shelf life studies are not available and are being conducted. Where data from accelerated studies are used to project a tentative expiration date that is beyond a date supported by actual shelf life studies, there must be stability studies conducted, including drug product testing at appropriate intervals, until the tentative expiration date is verified or the appropriate expiration date determined.

(c)   For homeopathic drug products, the requirements of this section are as follows:

(1) There shall be a written assessment of stability based at least on testing or examination of the drug product for compatibility of the ingredients, and based on marketing experience with the drug product to indicate that there is no degradation of the product for the normal or expected period of use.

(2) Evaluation of stability shall be based on the same container-closure system in which the drug product is being marketed.

(d)   Allergenic extracts that are labeled "No U.S. Standard of Potency" are exempt from the requirements of this section.

§ 211.167   Special testing requirements.

(a)   For each batch of drug product purporting to be sterile and/or pyrogen-free, there shall be appropriate laboratory testing to determine conformance to such requirements. The test procedures shall be in writing and shall be followed.

(b)   For each batch of ophthalmic ointment, there shall be appropriate testing to determine conformance to specifications regarding the presence of foreign particles and harsh or abrasive substances. The test procedures shall be in writing and shall be followed.

(c)   For each batch of controlled-release dosage form, there shall be appropriate laboratory testing to determine conformance to the specifications for the rate of release of each active ingredient. The test procedures shall be in writing and shall be followed.

§ 211.170   Reserve samples.

(a)   An appropriately identified reserve sample that is representative of each lot in each shipment of each active ingredient shall be retained. The reserve sample consists of at least twice the quantity necessary for all tests required to determine whether the active ingredient meets its established specifications, except for sterility and pyrogen testing. The retention time is as follows:

(1) For an active ingredient in a drug product other than those described in paragraphs (a) (2) and (3) of this section, the reserve sample shall be retained for 1 year after the expiration date of the last lot of the drug product containing the active ingredient.

(2) For an active ingredient in a radioactive drug product, except for nonradioactive reagent kits, the reserve sample shall be retained for:

(i) Three months after the expiration date of the last lot of the drug product containing the active ingredient if the expiration dating period of the drug product is 30 days or less; or

(ii) Six months after the expiration date of the last lot of the drug product containing the active ingredient if the expiration dating period of the drug product is more than 30 days.

(3) For an active ingredient in an OTC drug product that is exempt from bearing an expiration date under §211.137, the

reserve sample shall be retained for 3 years after distribution of the last lot of the drug product containing the active ingredient.

(b)   An appropriately identified reserve sample that is representative of each lot or batch of drug product shall be retained and stored under conditions consistent with product labeling. The reserve sample shall be stored in the same immediate container-closure system in which the drug product is marketed or in one that has essentially the same characteristics. The reserve sample consists of at least twice the quantity necessary to perform all the required tests, except those for sterility and pyrogens. Except for those for drug products described in paragraph (b)(2) of this section, reserve samples from representative sample lots or batches selected by acceptable statistical procedures shall be examined visually at least once a year for evidence of deterioration unless visual examination would affect the integrity of the reserve samples. Any evidence of reserve sample deterioration shall be investigated in accordance with §211.192. The results of the examination shall be recorded and maintained with other stability data on the drug product. Reserve samples of compressed medical gases need not be retained. The retention time is as follows:

(1) For a drug product other than those described in paragraphs (b) (2) and (3) of this section, the reserve sample shall be retained for 1 year after the expiration date of the drug product.

(2) For a radioactive drug product, except for nonradioactive reagent kits, the reserve sample shall be retained for:

(i) Three months after the expiration date of the drug product if the expiration dating period of the drug product is 30 days or less; or

(ii) Six months after the expiration date of the drug product if the expiration dating period of the drug product is more than 30 days.

(3) For an OTC drug product that is exempt for bearing an expiration date under §211.137, the reserve sample must be retained for 3 years after the lot or batch of drug product is distributed.

§ 211.173   Laboratory animals.

Animals used in testing components, in-process materials, or drug products for compliance with established specifications shall be maintained and controlled in a manner that assures their suitability for their intended use. They shall be identified, and adequate records shall be maintained showing the history of their use.

§ 211.176   Penicillin contamination.

If a reasonable possibility exists that a non-penicillin drug product has been exposed to cross-contamination with penicillin, the non-penicillin drug product shall be tested for the presence of penicillin. Such drug product shall not be marketed if detectable levels are found when tested according to procedures specified in 'Procedures for Detecting and Measuring Penicillin Contamination in Drugs,' which is incorporated by reference. Copies are available from the Division of Research and Testing (HFD-470), Center for Drug Evaluation and Research, Food and Drug Administration, 5100 Paint Branch Pkwy., College Park, MD 20740, or available for inspection at the Office of the Federal Register, 800 North Capitol Street, NW suite 700, Washington, D.C. 20408.

Subpart J—Records and Reports

§ 211.180   General requirements.

(a)   Any production, control, or distribution record that is required to be maintained in compliance with this part and is specifically associated with a batch of a drug product shall be retained

for at least 1 year after the expiration date of the batch or, in the case of certain OTC drug products lacking expiration dating because they meet the criteria for exemption under §211.137, 3 years after distribution of the batch.

(b) Records shall be maintained for all components, drug product containers, closures, and labeling for at least 1 year after the expiration date or, in the case of certain OTC drug products lacking expiration dating because they meet the criteria for exemption under §211.137, 3 years after distribution of the last lot of drug product incorporating the component or using the container, closure, or labeling.

(c) All records required under this part, or copies of such records, shall be readily available for authorized inspection during the retention period at the establishment where the activities described in such records occurred. These records or copies thereof shall be subject to photocopying or other means of reproduction as part of such inspection. Records that can be immediately retrieved from another location by computer or other electronic means shall be considered as meeting the requirements of this paragraph.

(d) Records required under this part may be retained either as original records or as true copies such as photocopies, microfilm, microfiche, or other accurate reproductions of the original records. Where reduction techniques, such as microfilming, are used, suitable reader and photocopying equipment shall be readily available.

(e) Written records required by this part shall be maintained so that data therein can be used for evaluating, at least annually, the quality standards of each drug product to determine the need for changes in drug product specifications or manufacturing or control procedures. Written procedures shall be established and followed for such evaluations and shall include provisions for:
(1) A review of a representative number of batches, whether approved or rejected, and, where applicable, records associated with the batch.
(2) A review of complaints, recalls, returned or salvaged drug products, and investigations conducted under §211.192 for each drug product.

(f) Procedures shall be established to assure that the responsible officials of the firm, if they are not personally involved in or immediately aware of such actions, are notified in writing of any investigations conducted under §§211.198, 211.204, or 211.208 of these regulations, any recalls, reports of inspectional observations issued by the Food and Drug Administration, or any regulatory actions relating to good manufacturing practices brought by the Food and Drug Administration.

§ 211.182 Equipment cleaning and use log.

A written record of major equipment cleaning, maintenance (except routine maintenance such as lubrication and adjustments), and use shall be included in individual equipment logs that show the date, time, product, and lot number of each batch processed. If equipment is dedicated to manufacture of one product, then individual equipment logs are not required, provided that lots or batches of such product follow in numerical order and are manufactured in numerical sequence. In cases where dedicated equipment is employed, the records of cleaning, maintenance, and use shall be part of the batch record. The persons performing and double-checking the cleaning and maintenance shall date and sign or initial the log indicating that the work was performed. Entries in the log shall be in chronological order.

§ 211.184 Component, drug product container, closure, and labeling records.

These records shall include the following:
(a) The identity and quantity of each shipment of each lot of components, drug product containers, closures, and labeling; the name of the supplier; the supplier's lot number(s) if known; the

receiving code as specified in §211.80; and the date of receipt. The name and location of the prime manufacturer, if different from the supplier, shall be listed if known.

(b) The results of any test or examination performed (including those performed as required by §211.82(a), §211.84(d), or §211.122(a)) and the conclusions derived therefrom.

(c) An individual inventory record of each component, drug product container, and closure and, for each component, a reconciliation of the use of each lot of such component. The inventory record shall contain sufficient information to allow determination of any batch or lot of drug product associated with the use of each component, drug product container, and closure.

(d) Documentation of the examination and review of labels and labeling for conformity with established specifications in accord with §§211.122 (c) and 211.130 (c).

(e) The disposition of rejected components, drug product containers, closure, and labeling.

§ 211.186 Master production and control records.

(a) To assure uniformity from batch to batch, master production and control records for each drug product, including each batch size thereof, shall be prepared, dated, and signed (full signature, handwritten) by one person and independently checked, dated, and signed by a second person. The preparation of master production and control records shall be described in a written procedure and such written procedure shall be followed.

(b) Master production and control records shall include:
(1) The name and strength of the product and a description of the dosage form;
(2) The name and weight or measure of each active ingredient per dosage unit or per unit of weight or measure of the drug product, and a statement of the total weight or measure of any dosage unit;
(3) A complete list of components designated by names or codes sufficiently specific to indicate any special quality characteristic;
(4) An accurate statement of the weight or measure of each component, using the same weight system (metric, avoirdupois, or apothecary) for each component. Reasonable variations may be permitted, however, in the amount of components necessary for the preparation in the dosage form, provided they are justified in the master production and control records;
(5) A statement concerning any calculated excess of component;
(6) A statement of theoretical weight or measure at appropriate phases of processing;
(7) A statement of theoretical yield, including the maximum and minimum percentages of theoretical yield beyond which investigation according to §211.192 is required;
(8) A description of the drug product containers, closures, and packaging materials, including a specimen or copy of each label and all other labeling signed and dated by the person or persons responsible for approval of such labeling;
(9) Complete manufacturing and control instructions, sampling and testing procedures, specifications, special notations, and precautions to be followed.

§ 211.188 Batch production and control records.

Batch production and control records shall be prepared for each batch of drug product produced and shall include complete information relating to the production and control of each batch. These records shall include:
(a) An accurate reproduction of the appropriate master production or control record, checked for accuracy, dated, and signed;

(b) Documentation that each significant step in the manufacture, processing, packing, or holding of the batch was accomplished, including:

(1) Dates;
(2) Identity of individual major equipment and lines used;
(3) Specific identification of each batch of component or in-process material used;
(4) Weights and measures of components used in the course of processing;
(5) In-process and laboratory control results;
(6) Inspection of the packaging and labeling area before and after use;
(7) A statement of the actual yield and a statement of the percentage of theoretical yield at appropriate phases of processing;
(8) Complete labeling control records, including specimens or copies of all labeling used;
(9) Description of drug product containers and closures;
(10) Any sampling performed;
(11) Identification of the persons performing and directly supervising or checking each significant step in the operation;
(12) Any investigation made according to §211.192;
(13) Results of examinations made in accordance with §211.134.

§ 211.192   Production record review.

All drug product production and control records, including those for packaging and labeling, shall be reviewed and approved by the quality control unit to determine compliance with all established, approved written procedures before a batch is released or distributed. Any unexplained discrepancy (including a percentage of theoretical yield exceeding the maximum or minimum percentages established in master production and control records) or the failure of a batch or any of its components to meet any of its specifications shall be thoroughly investigated, whether or not the batch has already been distributed. The investigation shall extend to other batches of the same drug product and other drug products that may have been associated with the specific failure or discrepancy. A written record of the investigation shall be made and shall include the conclusions and followup.

§ 211.194   Laboratory records.

(a) Laboratory records shall include complete data derived from all tests necessary to assure compliance with established specifications and standards, including examinations and assays, as follows:

(1) A description of the sample received for testing with identification of source (that is, location from where sample was obtained), quantity, lot number or other distinctive code, date sample was taken, and date sample was received for testing.
(2) A statement of each method used in the testing of the sample. The statement shall indicate the location of data that establish that the methods used in the testing of the sample meet proper standards of accuracy and reliability as applied to the product tested. (If the method employed is in the current revision of the United States Pharmacopeia, National Formulary, Association of Official Analytical Chemists, Book of Methods,* or in other recognized standard references, or is detailed in an approved new drug application and the referenced method is not modified, a statement indicating the method and reference will suffice.) The suitability of all testing methods used shall be verified under actual conditions of use.
(3) A statement of the weight or measure of sample used for each test, where appropriate.

(4) A complete record of all data secured in the course of each test, including all graphs, charts, and spectra from laboratory instrumentation, properly identified to show the specific component, drug product container, closure, in-process material, or drug product, and lot tested.
(5) A record of all calculations performed in connection with the test, including units of measure, conversion factors, and equivalency factors.
(6) A statement of the results of tests and how the results compare with established standards of identity, strength, quality, and purity for the component, drug product container, closure, in-process material, or drug product tested.
(7) The initials or signature of the person who performs each test and the date(s) the tests were performed.
(8) The initials or signature of a second person showing that the original records have been reviewed for accuracy, completeness, and compliance with established standards.

(b) Complete records shall be maintained of any modification of an established method employed in testing. Such records shall include the reason for the modification and data to verify that the modification produced results that are at least as accurate and reliable for the material being tested as the established method.

(c) Complete records shall be maintained of any testing and standardization of laboratory reference standards, reagents, and standard solutions.

(d) Complete records shall be maintained of the periodic calibration of laboratory instruments, apparatus, gauges, and recording devices required by §211.160(b)(4).

(e) Complete records shall be maintained of all stability testing performed in accordance with §211.166.

§ 211.196   Distribution records.

Distribution records shall contain the name and strength of the product and description of the dosage form, name and address of the consignee, date and quantity shipped, and lot or control number of the drug product. For compressed medical gas products, distribution records are not required to contain lot or control numbers.

§ 211.198   Complaint files.

(a) Written procedures describing the handling of all written and oral complaints regarding a drug product shall be established and followed. Such procedures shall include provisions for review by the quality control unit, of any complaint involving the possible failure of a drug product to meet any of its specifications and, for such drug products, a determination as to the need for an investigation in accordance with §211.192. Such procedures shall include provisions for review to determine whether the complaint represents a serious and unexpected adverse drug experience which is required to be reported to the Food and Drug Administration in accordance with §310.305 of this chapter.

(b) A written record of each complaint shall be maintained in a file designated for drug product complaints. The file regarding such drug product complaints shall be maintained at the establishment where the drug product involved was manufactured, processed, or packed, or such file may be maintained at another facility if the written records in such files are readily available for inspection at that other facility. Written records involving a drug product shall be maintained until at least 1 year after the expiration date of the drug product, or 1 year after the date that the complaint was received, whichever is longer. In the case of certain OTC drug products lacking expiration dating because they meet the criteria for exemption under §211.137, such written records shall be maintained for 3 years after distribution of the drug product.

(1) The written record shall include the following information, where known: the name and strength of the drug product,

---

* Copies may be obtained from: Association of Official Analytical Chemists, 2200 Wilson Blvd., Suite 400, Arlington, VA   22201-3301.

lot number, name of complainant, nature of complaint, and reply to complainant.

(2) Where an investigation under §211.192 is conducted, the written record shall include the findings of the investigation and followup. The record or copy of the record of the investigation shall be maintained at the establishment where the investigation occurred in accordance with §211.180(c).

(3) Where an investigation under §211.192 is not conducted, the written record shall include the reason that an investigation was found not to be necessary and the name of the responsible person making such a determination.

Subpart K—Returned and Salvaged Drug Products

§ 211.204   Returned drug products.

Returned drug products shall be identified as such and held. If the conditions under which returned drug products have been held, stored, or shipped before or during their return, or if the condition of the drug product, its container, carton, or labeling, as a result of storage or shipping, casts doubt on the safety, identity, strength, quality or purity of the drug product, the returned drug product shall be destroyed unless examination, testing, or other investigations prove the drug product meets appropriate standards of safety, identity, strength, quality, or purity. A drug product may be reprocessed provided the subsequent drug product meets appropriate standards, specifications, and characteristics. Records of returned drug products shall be maintained and shall include the name and label potency of the drug product dosage form, lot number (or control number or batch number), reason for the return, quantity returned, date of disposition, and ultimate disposition of the returned drug product. If the reason for a drug product being returned implicates associated batches, an appropriate investigation shall be conducted in accordance with the requirements of §211.192. Procedures for the holding, testing, and reprocessing of returned drug products shall be in writing and shall be followed.

§ 211.208   Drug product salvaging.

Drug products that have been subjected to improper storage conditions including extremes in temperature, humidity, smoke, fumes, pressure, age, or radiation due to natural disasters, fires, accidents, or equipment failures shall not be salvaged and returned to the marketplace. Whenever there is a question whether drug products have been subjected to such conditions, salvaging operations may be conducted only if there is (a) evidence from laboratory tests and assays (including animal feeding studies where applicable) that the drug products meet all applicable standards of identity, strength, quality, and purity and (b) evidence from inspection of the premises that the drug products and their associated packaging were not subjected to improper storage conditions as a result of the disaster or accident. Organoleptic examinations shall be acceptable only as supplemental evidence that the drug products meet appropriate standards of identity, strength, quality, and purity. Records including name, lot number, and disposition shall be maintained for drug products subject to this section.

Section VIII

POISON CONTROL CENTER LISTING

The following is a list of emergency telephone numbers for United States and Canadian poison control centers.

UNITED STATES
American Association of Poison Control Centers
U.S. Poison Control Center Members
Updated May 2003
(Certified Centers are written in ***bold & italics***)

ALABAMA
Alabama Poison Center
2503 Phoenix Drive
Tuscaloosa, AL 35405
Emergency Phone: (800) 222-1222

Regional Poison Control Center
Children's Hospital
1600 7th Avenue South
Birmingham, AL 35233
Emergency Phone: (800) 222-1222

ALASKA
Oregon Poison Center
Oregon Health Sciences University
3181 SW Sam Jackson Park Road
CB550
Portland, OR 97201
Emergency Phone: (800) 222-1222

ARIZONA
Arizona Poison & Drug Info Center
Arizona Health Sciences Center
Room 1156
1501 North Campbell Avenue
Tucson, AZ 85724
Emergency Phone: (800) 222-1222

Banner Poison Control Center
Good Samaritan Regional Medical Center
1111 E. McDowell, Ancillary
Phoenix, AZ 85006
Emergency Phone: (800) 222-1222

ARKANSAS
Arkansas Poison & Drug Information Center
College of Pharmacy
University of Arkansas for Medical Sciences
4301 W. Markham
Mail Slot 522-2
Little Rock, AR 72205
Emergency Phone: (800) 222-1222

CALIFORNIA
***California Poison Control System -
Fresno/Madera Division***
Children's Hospital Central California
9300 Valley Children's Place, MB 15
Madera, CA 93638-8762
Emergency Phone: (800) 222-1222
TDD/TTY: (800) 972-3323

***California Poison Control System -
Sacramento Division***
UC Davis Medical Center
2315 Stockton Boulevard
Sacramento, CA 95817
Emergency Phone: (800) 222-1222
TDD/TTY: (800) 972-3323

***California Poison Control System - San
Diego Division***
University of California, San Diego, Medical
Center
200 West Arbor Drive
San Diego, CA 92103-8925
Emergency Phone: (800) 222-1222
TDD/TTY: (800) 972-3323

***California Poison Control System - San
Francisco Division***
UCSF Box 1369
San Francisco, CA 94143-1369
Emergency Phone: (800) 222-1222
TDD/TTY: (800) 972-3323

COLORADO
Rocky Mountain Poison & Drug Ctr
1001 Yosemite Street
Suite 200
Denver, CO 80230-6800
Emergency Phone: (800) 222-1222
TDD/TTY: (303) 739-1127

CONNECTICUT
Connecticut Poison Control Center
University of Connecticut Health Center
263 Farmington Avenue
Farmington, CT 06030-5365
Emergency Phone: (800) 222-1222
TDD/TTY: (866) 218-5372 (toll-free)

DELAWARE
The Poison Control Center
Children's Hospital of Philadelphia
3400 Civic Center Blvd
Philadelphia, PA 19104-4303
Emergency Phone: (800) 222-1222
TDD/TTY: (215) 590-8789

DISTRICT OF COLUMBIA
National Capital Poison Center
3201 New Mexico Avenue, NW
Suite 310
Washington, DC 20016
Emergency Phone & TDD/TTY: (800) 222-1222

FLORIDA
***Florida Poison Information Center -
Jacksonville***
655 West Eighth Street
Jacksonville, FL 32209
Emergency Phone: (800) 222-1222
TDD/TTY: (800) 282-3171 (FL only)

Florida Poison Information Center - Miami
University of Miami, Department of Pediatrics
P.O. Box 110626 (R-131)
Miami, FL 33101
Emergency Phone: (800) 222-1222

***Florida Poison Information Center -
Tampa***
Tampa General Hospital
P.O. Box 1289
Tampa, FL 33601
Emergency Phone: (800) 222-1222

GEORGIA
Georgia Poison Center
Hughes Spalding Children's Hospital
Grady Health System
80 Butler Street, SE
P.O. Box 26066
Atlanta, GA 30335-3801
Emergency Phone: (800) 222-1222
TDD/TTY: (404) 616-9287 (TDD)

HAWAII
Hawaii Poison Center
1319 Punahou Street
Honolulu, HI 96826
Emergency Phone: (808) 222-1222

Rocky Mountain Poison & Drug Ctr
1001 Yosemite Street
Suite 200
Denver, CO 80230-6800
Emergency Phone: (800) 222-1222
TDD/TYY: (303) 739-1127

IDAHO
Rocky Mountain Poison & Drug Center
1001 Yosemite Street
Suite 200
Denver, CO 80230-6800
Emergency Phone: (800) 222-1222
TDD/TTY: (303) 739-1127

ILLINOIS
Illinois Poison Center
222 S. Riverside Plaza, Suite 1900
Chicago, IL 60606
Emergency Phone: (800) 222-1222
TDD/TTY: (312) 906-6185

INDIANA
Indiana Poison Center
Methodist Hospital
Clarian Health Partners
I-65 at 21st Street
Indianapolis, IN 46206-1367
Emergency Phone: (800) 222-1222
TDD/TTY: (317) 962-2336 (TTY)

IOWA
Iowa Statewide Poison Control Center
St. Luke's Regional Medical Center
2720 Stone Park Boulevard
Sioux City, IA 51104
Emergency Phone: (800) 222-1222

KANSAS
Mid-America Poison Control Center
University of Kansas Medical Center
3901 Rainbow Blvd., Room B-400
Kansas City, KS 66160-7231
Emergency Phone: (800) 222-1222
TDD/TTY: (913) 588-6639 (TDD)

KENTUCKY
Kentucky Regional Poison Center
Medical Towers South, Suite 572
234 East Gray Street
Louisville, KY 40202
Emergency Phone: (800) 222-1222

LOUISIANA
Louisiana Drug and Poison Information Center
University of Louisiana at Monroe
College of Pharmacy
Sugar Hall
Monroe, LA 71209-6430
Emergency Phone: (800) 222-1222

MAINE
Northern New England Poison
22 Bramhall Street
Portland, ME 04102
Emergency Phone: (800) 222-1222
TDD/TTY: (877) 299-4447 (ME only)
        (207) 871-2879

MARYLAND
Maryland Poison Center
University of MD at Baltimore
School of Pharmacy
20 North Pine Street, PH 772
Baltimore, MD 21201
Emergency Phone: (800) 222-1222
TDD/TTY: (410) 706-1858 (TDD)

National Capital Poison Center
3201 New Mexico Avenue, NW
Suite 310
Washington, DC 20016
Emergency Phone & TDD/TTY: (800) 222-1222

MASSACHUSETTS
Regional Center for Poison Control and Prevention Serving Massachusetts & Rhode Island
300 Longwood Avenue
Boston, MA 02115
Emergency Phone: (800) 222-1222
TDD/TTY: (888) 244-5313

MICHIGAN
Children's Hospital of Michigan
Regional Poison Control Center
4160 John R Harper Professional Office Building
Suite 616
Detroit, MI 48201
Emergency Phone: (800) 222-1222
TDD/TTY: (800) 356-3232 (TDD)

DeVos Children's Hopsital Regional Poison Center
1300 Michigan, NE
Suite 203
Grand Rapids, MI 49506-2968
Emergency Phone: (800) 222-1222
TDD/TTY: (800) 356-3232 (TTY)

MINNESOTA
Hennepin Regional Poison Center
Hennepin County Medical Center
701 Park Avenue
Minneapolis, MN 55415
Emergency Phone: (800) 222-1222
TDD/TTY: (800) 222-1222

MISSISSIPPI
Mississippi Regional Poison Control Center
University of Mississippi Medical Center
2500 N. State Street
Jackson, MS 39216
Emergency Phone: (800) 222-1222

MISSOURI
Missouri Regional Poison Center
7980 Clayton Rd
Suite 200
St. Louis, MO 63117
Emergency Phone: (800) 222-1222
TDD/TTY: (314) 612-5705

MONTANA
Rocky Mountain Poison & Drug Ctr
1001 Yosemite Street
Suite 200
Denver, CO 80230-6800
Emergency Phone: (800) 222-1222
TDD/TTY: (303) 739-1127

NEBRASKA
The Poison Center
Children's Hospital
8200 Dodge Street
Omaha, NE 68114
Emergency Phone: (800) 222-1222

NEVADA
Oregon Poison Center
Oregon Health Sciences University
3181 SW Sam Jackson Park Road
CB550
Portland, OR 97201
Emergency Phone: (800) 222-1222

Rocky Mountain Poison & Drug Ctr
1001 Yosemite Street
Suite 200
Denver, CO 80230-6800
Emergency Phone: (800) 222-1222
TDD/TTY: (303) 739-1127

NEW HAMPSHIRE
New Hampshire Poison Information Center
Dartmouth-Hitchcock Medical Center
One Medical Center Drive
Lebanon, NH 03756
Emergency Phone: (800) 222-1222

NEW JERSEY
New Jersey Poison Information and Education System
located at Univ of Medicine and Dentistry at New Jersey
65 Bergen Street
Newark, NJ 07107-3001
Emergency Phone: (800) 222-1222
TDD/TTY: (973) 926-8008

NEW MEXICO
New Mexico Poison & Drug Information Center
MSC 09 5080
University of New Mexico
Albuquerque, NM 87131-0001
Emergency Phone: (800) 222-1222

NEW YORK
Central New York Poison Center
750 East Adams Street
Syracuse, NY 13210
Emergency Phone: (800) 222-1222

Finger Lakes Regional Poison & Drug Info Center
University of Rochester Medical Center
601 Elmwood Avenue
P.O. Box 321
Rochester, NY 14642
Emergency Phone: (800) 222-1222
TDD/TTY: (585) 273-3854

Long Island Regional Poison and Drug Information Center
Winthrop University Hospital
259 First Street
Mineola, NY 11501
Emergency Phone: (800) 222-1222
TDD/TTY: (516) 924-8811 (TDD Suffolk)
        (516) 747-3323 (TDD Nassau)

New York City Poison Control Center
NYC Bureau of Labs
455 First Avenue
Room 123, Box 81
New York, NY 10016
Emergency Phone: (800) 222-1222
TDD/TTY: (212) 689-9014 (TDD)

Western New York Regional Poison Control Center
Children's Hospital of Buffalo
219 Bryant Street
Buffalo, NY 14222
Emergency Phone: (800) 222-1222

NORTH CAROLINA
Carolinas Poison Center
Carolinas Medical Center
5000 Airport Center Parkway, Suite B
Charlotte, NC 28208
Emergency Phone: (800) 222-1222

NORTH DAKOTA
North Dakota Poison Information Center
Meritcare Medical Center
720 4th Street North
Fargo, ND 58122
Emergency Phone & TDD/TTY: (800) 222-1222

OHIO
Central Ohio Poison Center
700 Children's Drive, Room L032
Columbus, OH 43205
Emergency Phone: (800) 222-1222
TDD/TTY: (614) 228-2272 (TTY)

Cincinnati Drug & Poison Information Center
Regional Poison Control System
3333 Burnet Avenue
Vernon Place - 3rd Floor
Cincinnati, OH 45229
Emergency Phone: (800) 222-1222
TDD/TTY: (800) 253-7955

Greater Cleveland Poison Control Center
11100 Euclid Avenue
Cleveland, OH 44106-6010
Emergency Phone: (800) 222-1222

Access FREE monthly updates online at http://uspdi.micromedex.com

OKLAHOMA

Oklahoma Poison Control Center
Children's Hospital at OU Medical Center
940 N.E. 13th Street
Room 3510
Oklahoma City, OK 73104
Emergency Phone & TDD/TTY: (800) 222-1222

OREGON

Oregon Poison Center
Oregon Health Sciences University
3181 SW Sam Jackson Park Road
CB550
Portland, OR 97201
Emergency Phone: (800) 222-1222

PENNSYLVANIA

Penn State Poison Center
Pennsylvania State University
The Milton S. Hershey Medical Center
500 University Drive
MC H043, PO Box 850
Hershey, PA 17033-0850
Emergency Phone: (800) 222-1222
TDD/TTY: (717) 531-8335 (TTY)

Pittsburgh Poison Center
Children's Hospital of Pittsburgh
3705 Fifth Avenue
Pittsburgh, PA 15213
Emergency Phone: (800) 222-1222

The Poison Control Center
Children's Hospital of Philadelphia
3400 Civic Center Blvd
Philadelphia, PA 19104-4303
Emergency Phone: (800) 222-1222
TDD/TTY: (215) 590-8789

PUERTO RICO

San Jorge Children's Hospital Poison Center
Calle San Jorge #252
Santurce, Puerto Rico 00912
Emergency Phone: (800) 222-1222

RHODE ISLAND

*Regional Center for Poison Control and
Prevention*
Serving Massachusetts and Rhode Island
300 Longwood Avenue
Boston, MA 02115
Emergency Phone: (800) 222-1222
TDD/TTY: (888) 244-5313

SOUTH CAROLINA

Palmetto Poison Center
College of Pharmacy
University of South Carolina
Columbia, SC 29208
Emergency Phone: (800) 222-1222

SOUTH DAKOTA

Hennepin Regional Poison Center
Hennepin County Medical Center
701 Park Avenue
Minneapolis, MN 55415
Emergency Phone & TDD/TTY: (800) 222-1222

TENNESSEE

*Middle Tennessee Poison
Center*
501 Oxford House
1161 21st Avenue South
Nashville, TN 37232-4632
Emergency Phone: (800) 222-1222
TDD/TTY: (615) 936-2047 (TDD)

Southern Poison Center
University of Tennessee
875 Monroe Avenue
Suite 104
Memphis, TN 38163
Emergency Phone & TDD/TTY: (800) 222-1222

TEXAS

Central Texas Poison Center
Scott and White Memorial Hospital
2401 South 31st Street
Temple, TX 76508
Emergency Phone & TDD/TTY: (800) 222-1222

North Texas Poison Center
Parkland Memorial Hospital
5201 Harry Hines Blvd.
Dallas, TX 75235
Emergency Phone: (800) 222-1222

South Texas Poison Center
The Univ of Texas Health Science Ctr - San
Antonio
Department of Surgery
Mail Code 7849
7703 Floyd Curl Drive
San Antonio, TX 78229-3900
Emergency Phone & TDD/TTY: (800) 222-1222

Southeast Texas Poison Center
The University of Texas Medical Branch
3.112 Trauma Building
Galveston, TX 77555-1175
Emergency Phone & TDD/TTY: (800) 222-1222

Texas Panhandle Poison Center
1501 S. Coulter
Amarillo, TX 79106
Emergency Phone: (800) 222-1222

West Texas Regional Poison Center
Thomason Hospital
4815 Alameda Avenue
El Paso, TX 79905
Emergency Phone & TDD/TTY: (800) 222-1222

UTAH

Utah Poison Control Center
410 Chipeta Way, Suite 230
Salt Lake City, UT 84108
Emergency Phone: (800) 222-1222

VERMONT

Northern New England Poison Center
22 Bramhall Street
Portland, ME 04102
Emergency Phone: (800) 222-1222
TDD/TTY: (877) 299-4447 (ME only)
(207) 871-2879

VIRGINIA

Blue Ridge Poison Center
University of Virginia Health
System
PO Box 800774
Charlottesville, VA 22908-0774
Emergency Phone: (800) 222-1222

National Capital Poison Center
3201 New Mexico Avenue, NW
Suite 310
Washington, DC 20016
Emergency Phone & TDD/TTY: (800) 222-1222

Virginia Poison Center
Medical College of Virginia Hospitals
Virginia Commonwealth
University
P.O. Box 980522
Richmond, VA 23298-0522
Emergency Phone: (800) 222-1222

WASHINGTON

Washington Poison Center
155 NE 100th Street, Suite 400
Seattle, WA 98125-8012
Emergency Phone: (800) 222-1222
TDD/TTY: (206) 517-2394 (TDD)
(800) 572-0638 (TDD WA only)

WEST VIRGINIA

West Virginia Poison Center
3110 MacCorkle Ave, S.E.
Charleston, WV 25304
Emergency Phone & TDD/TTY: (800) 222-1222

WISCONSIN

Children's Hospital of Wisconsin Poison
Center
PO Box 1997, Mail Station 677A
Milwaukee, WI 53201-1997
Emergency Phone: (800) 222-1222
TDD/TTY: (414) 266-2542

WYOMING

The Poison Center
Children's Hospital
8200 Dodge Street
Omaha, NE 68114
Emergency Phone: (800) 222-1222

ANIMAL POISON CONTROL

ASPCA Animal Poison Control Center
Animal Poison Control Center
1717 South Philo Road, Suite 36
Urbana, IL 61802
Emergency Phone: (888) 426-4435

     Access FREE monthly updates online at http://uspdi.micromedex.com

CANADA
Source: Canadian Poison Control Centres.

ALBERTA AND SASKATCHEWAN
P.A.D.I.S.
Foothills General Hospital
1403 29th Street N.W.
Calgary, AB T2N 2T9
1-800-332-1414 toll-free
(403) 670-1414 local
(403) 670-1472 fax

BRITISH COLUMBIA
British Columbia Drug and Poison
 Information Centre
St. Paul's Hospital
1081 Burrard Street
Vancouver, B.C. V6Z 1Y6
1-800-567-8911 toll-free
(604) 682-5050 Greater Vancouver & lower
 mainland
(604) 631-5262 fax

NEW BRUNSWICK
Poison Information Centre
Clinidata
774 Main St. 6th floor
Moncton, NB
E1C 9Y3
(506) 867-3202
(506) 867-3259 fax

NEWFOUNDLAND
Poison Control Centre
The Janeway Child Health Centre
300 Prince Philip Dr.
St. John's, NF A1B 3V6
(709) 722-1110
(709) 726-0830 fax

NOVA SCOTIA / PEI
Poison Control Centre
The IWK/Grace Health Care
 Centre
5850 University Ave.
P.O. Box 3070
Halifax, NS B3J 3G9
1-800-565-8161
(902) 428-8161
(902) 428-3213 fax

ONTARIO
Ontario Regional Poison Information Centre
Children's Hospital of Eastern Ontario
401 Smyth Road
Ottawa, ON K1V 8L1
1-800-267-1373 toll-free
(613) 737-1100 local
(613) 738-4862 fax

Ontario Regional Poison Information Centre
The Hospital for Sick Children
555 University Avenue
Toronto, ON M5G 1X8
1-800-268-9017 toll-free
(416) 598-5900 local
(416) 813-7489 fax

QUEBEC
Centre Anti-Poison du Québec
1050 Chemin Ste-Foy, 1er étage
Quebec, QC G1S 4L8
1-800-463-5060 Toll-free
(418) 656-8090 local
(418) 654-2747 fax

Access FREE monthly updates online at http://uspdi.micromedex.com

Appendix IX

The USP Center for the Advancement of Patient Safety

Health care professionals are encouraged to report problems that they observe with the use of medications or medical devices. Without such input, manufacturers, government, the compendia, and colleagues may not be aware of problems that are experienced. This exchange of meaningful information is an integral part of improving the safety, efficacy, and quality of medical products. The individual practitioner is in the best position to recognize that a problem may exist and to report it.

The USP Center for the Advancement of Patient Safety (CAPS) oversees two separate reporting programs: the Medication Errors Reporting Program, and MEDMARX℠. USP CAPS publishes the *USP Quality Review*, an educational newsletter based on case reports received through the programs and for your convenience has current practitioner reporting news available on the Internet at http://www.usp.org/www.usp.org/patientSafety/index.html. USP CAPS also distributes, free of charge, on a monthly basis a news letter - CAPSLink - to 8,000 subscribers that provides analysis and recommendation on medication errors.

The USP Medication Errors Reporting (MER) Program: This nationwide program makes it possible for health professionals who encounter actual or potential medication errors to report confidentially to USP. By sharing these experiences, pharmacists, nurses, physicians, and other health care professionals can contribute to improved patient safety and to the development of valuable educational services for the prevention of future errors. The program encompasses a wide variety of problems such as misinterpretations, miscalculations, misadministrations, difficulty interpreting handwritten orders, or misunderstanding verbal orders. The MER Program is presented in cooperation with the Institute for Safe Medication Practices.

Through working with the (MER) Program, experience gained in the area of medication errors and managing national reporting databases, USP realized the need and value of creating a medication error reporting program for hospitals and building a national database. As a result of experience gained from the MER Program and feedback received from health care professionals USP utilized this knowledge to create MEDMARX, an Internet-accessible, anonymous reporting program. Introduced in July 1998, MEDMARX enables hospitals to report, track, and trend data. MEDMARX has grown today by more than 450,000 records from more than 700 hospitals.

Used as part of an internal quality improvement program MEDMARX allows a more thorough analysis of medication errors enabling hospitals to implement system wide strategies leading to error reduction and increased patient safety. In addition to focusing on internal quality improvement efforts hospitals can also search records entered anonymously by other users nationwide, generate comparison information, and learn from strategies implemented by other hospitals.

MEDMARX has incorporated nationally standardized data elements (i.e., definition and taxonomy) developed by the National Coordinating Council for Medication Error Reporting and Prevention (NCC MERP), and the American Society of Health-System Pharmacists (ASHP) allowing hospitals using MEDMARX to report and collect information utilizing a nationally standardized format. MEDMARX also supports the Joint Commission on the Accreditation of Healthcare Organizations (JCAHO) performance improvement and patient safety standards. The standards specify that a hospital should look outside their own facility, share information, consider other institutions' experiences and learn from their experiences to prevent the occurrence of errors.

To schedule a demonstration or for more information call 1-877-MEDMARX.

To receive information on USP's Patient Safety efforts call 800-487-7776. The USP reporting forms are now available on-line at:

www.usp.org/patientSafety/reporting/mer.html   Medication Errors Reporting Program

www.usp.org/patientSafety/reporting/medmarx/index.html   MEDMARX℠

USP is an active partner in MedWatch, the FDA's medical product reporting program. As a partner, USP supports the FDA's efforts to protect the public health by helping to identify serious adverse events.

MEDI-CATION ERRORS

REPORTING PROGRAM

USP MEDICATION ERRORS REPORTING PROGRAM

Presented in cooperation with the Institute for Safe Medication Practices

USP is an FDA MEDWATCH partner

Reporters should not provide any individually identifiable health information, including names of practitioners, names of patients, names of healthcare facilities, or dates of birth (age is acceptable).

Date and time of event:

Please describe the error. Include description/sequence of events, type of staff involved, and work environment (e.g., code situation, change of shift, short staffing, no 24-hr. pharmacy, floor stock). If more space is needed, please attach a separate page.

Did the error reach the patient? ☐ Yes ☐ No

Was the incorrect medication, dose, or dosage form administered to or taken by the patient? ☐ Yes ☐ No

Circle the appropriate Error Outcome Category (select one—see back for details): A   B   C   D   E   F   G   H   I

Describe the direct result of the error on the patient (e.g., death, type of harm, additional patient monitoring).

Indicate the possible error cause(s) and contributing factor(s) (e.g., abbreviation, similar names, distractions, etc.).

Indicate the location of the error (e.g., hospital, outpatient or community pharmacy, clinic, nursing home, patient's home, etc.).

What type of staff or healthcare practitioner made the initial error?

Indicate if other practitioner(s) were also involved in the error (type of staff perpetuating error).

What type of staff or healthcare practitioner discovered the error or recognized the potential for error?

How was the error (or potential for error) discovered/intercepted?

If available, provide patient age, gender, diagnosis. Do not provide any patient identifiers.

Please complete the following for the product(s) involved. (If more space is needed for additional products, please attach a separate page.)

	Product #1	Product #2
Brand/Product Name (If Applicable)		
Generic Name		
Manufacturer		
Labeler		
Dosage Form		
Strength/Concentration		
Type and Size of Container		

Reports are most useful when relevant materials such as product label, copy of prescription/order, etc., can be reviewed.
Can these materials be provided? ☐ Yes ☐ No   Please specify:

Suggest any recommendations to prevent recurrence of this error, or describe policies or procedures you instituted or plan to institute to prevent future similar errors.

Name and Title/Profession

Telephone Number (   )

Fax Number (   )

Facility/Address and Zip

E-mail

Address/Zip (where correspondence should be sent)

Your name, contact information, and a copy of this report are routinely shared with the Institute for Safe Medication Practices (ISMP). Copies of reports will be sent to third parties such as the manufacturer/labeler, and to the Food and Drug Administration (FDA). You have the option of including your name on these copies.

In addition to releasing my name and contact information to ISMP, USP may release my identity to these third parties as follows (check boxes that apply):

☐ The manufacturer and/or labeler as listed above   ☐ FDA   ☐ Other persons requesting a copy of this report   ☐ Anonymous to all third parties

Signature

Date

Date Received by USP

File Access Number

Return to:
USP CAPS
12601 Twinbrook Parkway
Rockville, MD 20852-1790

Submit via the Web at www.usp.org/mer
Call Toll Free: 800-23-ERROR (800-233-7767)
or FAX: 301-816-8532

PSF116G

USPDI
©USPC 2003

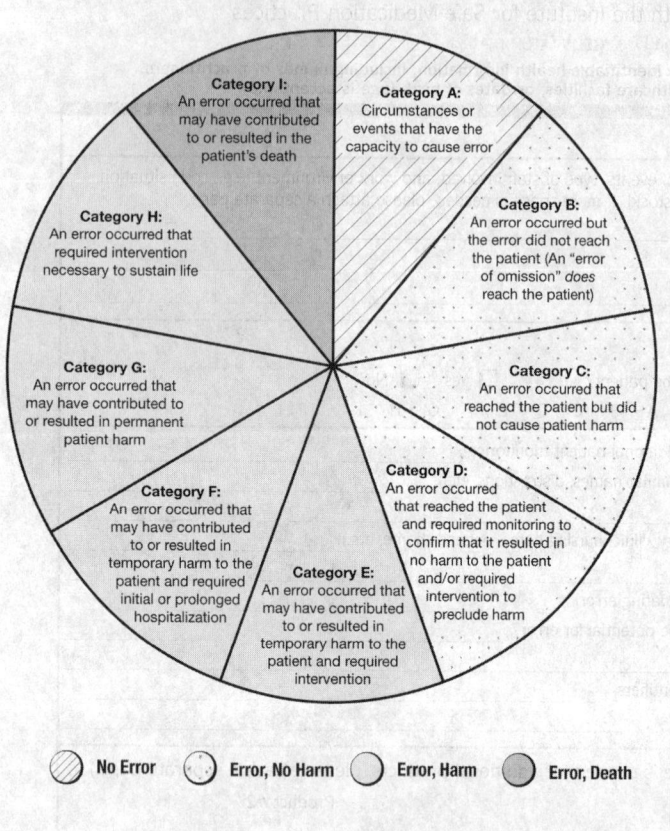

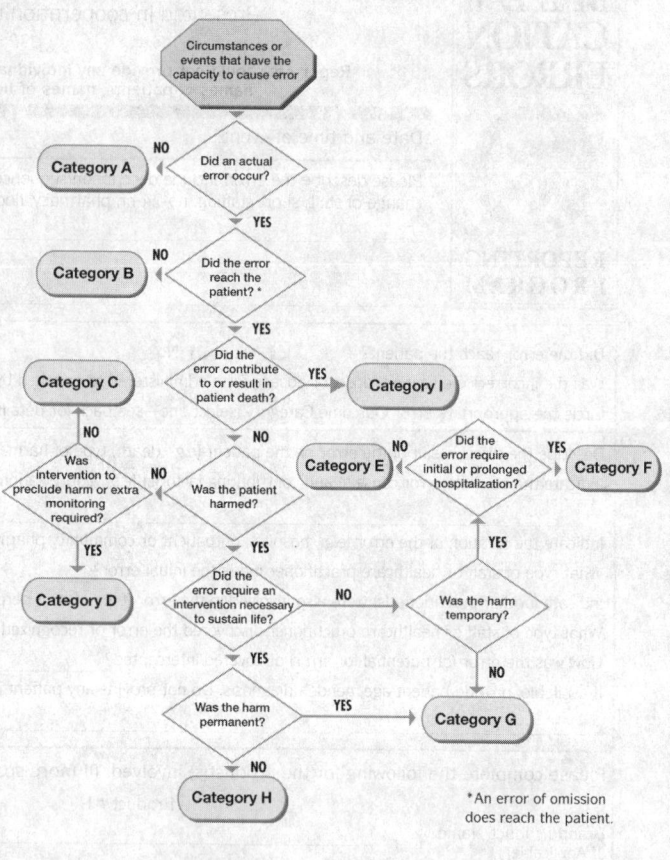

© 2003 National Coordinating Council for Medication Error Reporting and Prevention

Full-size copies are available: **INDEX**—www.nccmerp.org/pdf/indexColor2001-06-12.pdf; **ALGORITHM**—www.nccmerp.org/pdf/algorColor2001-06-12.pdf

National Coordinating Council for Medication Error Reporting and Prevention Definitions

Harm
Impairment of the physical, emotional, or psychological function or structure of the body and/or pain resulting therefrom.

Monitoring
To observe or record relevant physiological or psychological signs.

Intervention
May include change in therapy or active medical/surgical treatment.

Intervention Necessary to Sustain Life
Includes cardiovascular and respiratory support (e.g., CPR, defibrillation, intubation, etc.).

Return form to:

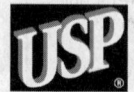

THE USP CENTER FOR THE ADVANCEMENT OF PATIENT SAFETY
12601 TWINBROOK PARKWAY
ROCKVILLE MD 20852-1790

MedWatch, the FDA Medical Products Reporting Program

For health care providers wishing to report serious adverse events or product problems directly to the FDA, a MedWatch form is provided.

Report experiences with:
* medications (drugs or biologics)
* medical devices (including *in vitro* diagnostics)
* special nutritional products (dietary supplements, medical foods, infant formulas)
* other products regulated by FDA

Report SERIOUS adverse events. An event is serious when the patient outcome is:
* death
* life-threatening (real risk of dying)
* hospitalization (initial or prolonged)
* disability (significant, persistent or permanent)
* congenital anomaly
* required intervention to prevent permanent impairment or damage

How to report:
* fill in the sections that apply to your report
* use section C for all products except medical devices
* attach additional blank pages if needed

* use a separate form for each patient
* report either to FDA or the manufacturer (or both)

Important numbers:
* 1-800-FDA-0178 to FAX report
* 1-800-FDA-1088 for more information or to report quality problems
* 1-800-822-7967 for a VAERS form for vaccines

If your report involves a serious adverse event with a device and it occurred in a facility outside a doctor's office, that facility may be legally required to report to FDA and/or the manufacturer. Please notify the person in that facility who would handle such reporting.

To report a medical device problem, you may submit an FDA MedWatch form.

Confidentiality: The patient's identity is held in strict confidence by FDA and protected to the fullest extent of the law. The reporter's identity may be shared with the manufacturer unless requested otherwise. However, FDA will not disclose the reporter's identity in response to a request from the public pursuant to the Freedom of Information Act.

MEDWATCH

The FDA Safety Information and Adverse Event Reporting Program

For **VOLUNTARY** reporting of adverse events and product problems

Form Approved: OMB No. 0910-0230 Expires: 09/03/05
See OMB statement on reverse

FDA Use Only

Triage unit sequence #

Page ____ of ____

PLEASE TYPE OR USE BLACK INK

A. Patient information

1. Patient identifier	2. Age at time of event:	3. Sex	4. Weight
	or	☐ female	____ lbs
	Date		or
In confidence	of birth:	☐ male	____ kgs

B. Adverse event or product problem

1. ☐ **Adverse event** and/or ☐ **Product problem** (e.g., defects/malfunctions)

2. **Outcomes attributed to adverse event**
(check all that apply)

☐ death _____ (mo/day/yr)
☐ life-threatening
☐ hospitalization - initial or prolonged

☐ disability
☐ congenital anomaly
☐ required intervention to prevent permanent impairment/damage
☐ other: _____

3. Date of event (mo/day/yr)	4. Date of this report (mo/day/yr)

5. **Describe event or problem**

6. **Relevant tests/laboratory data,** including dates

7. **Other relevant history, including preexisting medical conditions** (e.g., allergies, race, pregnancy, smoking and alcohol use, hepatic/renal dysfunction, etc.)

C. Suspect medication(s)

1. **Name** (give labeled strength & mfr/labeler, if known)
#1 _____
#2 _____

2. **Dose, frequency & route used**	3. **Therapy dates** (if unknown, give duration) from/to (or best estimate)
#1	#1
#2	#2

4. **Diagnosis for use** (indication)	5. **Event abated after use stopped or dose reduced**
#1	#1 ☐ yes ☐ no ☐ doesn't apply
#2	#2 ☐ yes ☐ no ☐ doesn't apply

6. **Lot #** (if known)	7. **Exp. date** (if known)	8. **Event reappeared after reintroduction**
#1	#1	#1 ☐ yes ☐ no ☐ doesn't apply
#2	#2	#2 ☐ yes ☐ no ☐ doesn't apply

9. **NDC #** (for product problems only)

10. **Concomitant medical products** and therapy dates (exclude treatment of event)

D. Suspect medical device

1. **Brand name**

2. **Type of device**

3. **Manufacturer name & address**	4. **Operator of device**
	☐ health professional
	☐ lay user/patient
	☐ other: _____
6. model # _____	5. **Expiration date** (mo/day/yr)
catalog # _____	7. **If implanted, give date** (mo/day/yr)
serial # _____	
lot # _____	8. **If explanted, give date** (mo/day/yr)
other # _____	

9. **Device available for evaluation?** (Do not send to FDA)
☐ yes ☐ no ☐ returned to manufacturer on _____ (mo/day/yr)

10. **Concomitant medical products** and therapy dates (exclude treatment of event)

E. Reporter (see confidentiality section on back)

1. **Name & address** | phone #

2. **Health professional?**	3. **Occupation**	4. **Also reported to**
☐ yes ☐ no		☐ manufacturer
		☐ user facility
5. If you do NOT want your identity disclosed to the manufacturer, place an " X " in this box. ☐		☐ distributor

FDA

Mail to: **MEDWATCH**
5600 Fishers Lane
Rockville, MD 20852-9787

or FAX to:
1-800-FDA-0178

FDA Form 3500

Submission of a report does not constitute an admission that medical personnel or the product caused or contributed to the event.

Section X

THE MEDICINE CHART

The Medicine Chart presents sample photographs of prescribed medicines in the United States. In general, commonly used brand name products and a representative sampling of generic products have been included. The pictorial listing is not intended to be inclusive and does not represent all products on the market. The inclusion of a product does not mean the authors have any particular knowledge that the product included has properties different from other products, nor should it be interpreted as an endorsement. Similarly, the fact that a particular product has not been included does not indicate that the product has been judged to be unsatisfactory or unacceptable.

The drug products in *The Medicine Chart* are listed alphabetically by generic name of active ingredient(s). In some instances, not all dosage forms and sizes are pictured. If others are available, a † symbol proceeds the products name. Letters or numbers representing the manufacturer's identification code are followed by an asterisk.

The size and color of the products shown are intended to match the actual product as closely as possible; however, there may be some differences due to variations caused by the photographic process. Also, manufacturers may occasionally change the color, imprinting, or shape of their products, and for a period of time both the "old" and the newly changed dosage forms may be on the market. Such changes may not occur uniformly throughout the different dosages of the product. When applicable these types of changes will be incorporated in the subsequent versions of *The Medicine Chart* as they are brought to our attention.

> Use of this chart is limited to serving as an initial guide in identifying drug products. The identity of a product should be verified further before any action is taken.

ABACAVIR

GX 623
300 mg

Ziagen®
GlaxoSmithKline

ABACAVIR, SULFATE, LAMIVUDINE, AND ZIDOVUDINE

GX LL1
300 mg/150 mg/300 mg

Trizivir®
GlaxoSmithKline

ACARBOSE

50 mg   100 mg

Precose®
Bayer Corporation
Pharmaceutical Division

ACITRETIN

10 mg

25 mg

Soriatane®
Roche

ACYCLOVIR

200 mg

400 mg

ZOVIRAX 300
800 mg

Zovirax®
GlaxoSmithKline

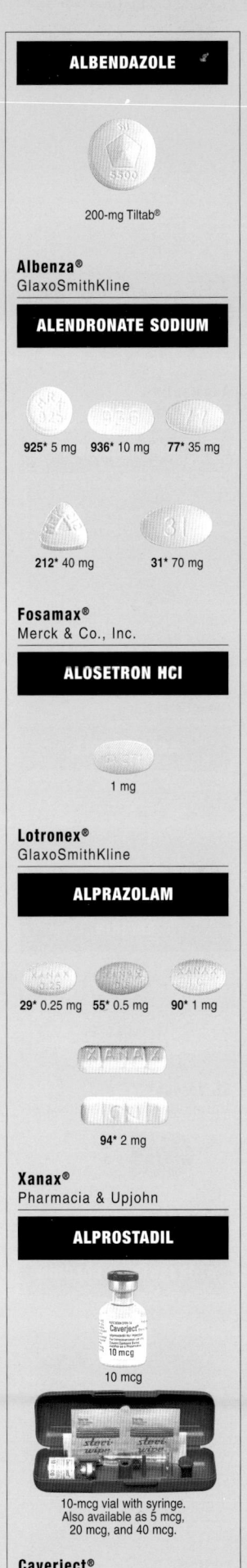

ALBENDAZOLE

200-mg Tiltab®

Albenza®
GlaxoSmithKline

ALENDRONATE SODIUM

925* 5 mg   **936*** 10 mg   **77*** 35 mg

212* 40 mg   **31*** 70 mg

Fosamax®
Merck & Co., Inc.

ALOSETRON HCl

1 mg

Lotronex®
GlaxoSmithKline

ALPRAZOLAM

29* 0.25 mg **55*** 0.5 mg **90*** 1 mg

XANAX

94* 2 mg

Xanax®
Pharmacia & Upjohn

ALPROSTADIL

Caverject
10 mcg

stevi wipe   stevi wipe

10-mcg vial with syringe.
Also available as 5 mcg,
20 mcg, and 40 mcg.

Caverject®
Pharmacia & Upjohn

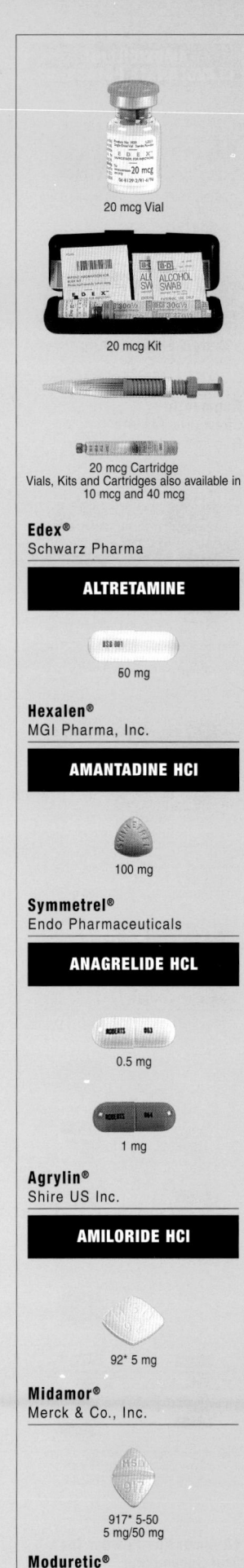

20 mcg Vial

20 mcg Kit

20 mcg Cartridge
Vials, Kits and Cartridges also available in
10 mcg and 40 mcg

Edex®
Schwarz Pharma

ALTRETAMINE

50 mg

Hexalen®
MGI Pharma, Inc.

AMANTADINE HCl

100 mg

Symmetrel®
Endo Pharmaceuticals

ANAGRELIDE HCl

0.5 mg

1 mg

Agrylin®
Shire US Inc.

AMILORIDE HCl

92* 5 mg

Midamor®
Merck & Co., Inc.

917* 5-50
5 mg/50 mg

Moduretic®
Merck & Co., Inc.

AMINOBENZOATE POTASSIUM

POTABA 54
500 mg

POTABA 51   POTABA 51
500 mg

Potaba®
Glenwood

POTABA
2 g/packet

Potaba Envules®
Glenwood

AMIODARONE HCL

200   WYETH 4188

4188* 200 mg

Cordarone®
Wyeth Pharmaceuticals

AMLODIPINE BESYLATE

2.5
152* 2.5 mg

5
153* 5 mg

NORVASC 10
154* 10 mg

Norvasc®
Pfizer Inc.

AMLODIPINE BESYLATE/ BENAZEPRIL HCl

BOCK   BOCK
2255* 2.5 mg/10 mg

LOTREL 2260
2260* 5 mg/10 mg

LOTREL 2265
2265* 5 mg/20 mg

10 mg/20 mg

Lotrel®
Novartis Pharmaceuticals

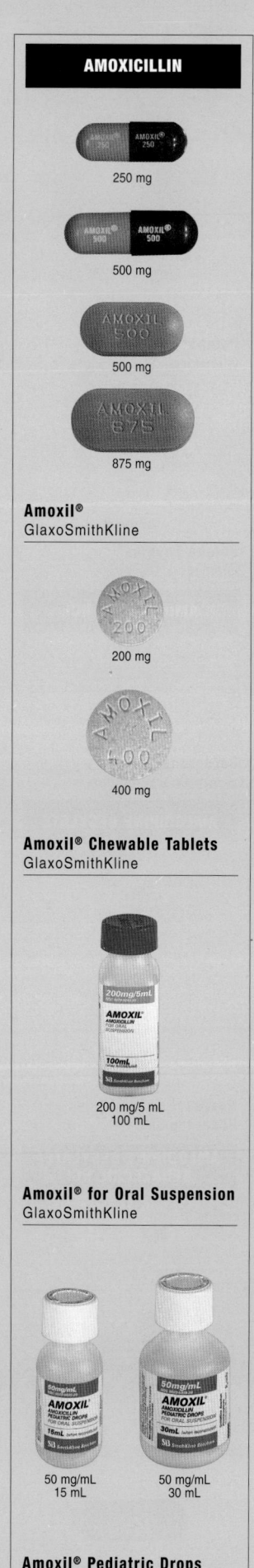

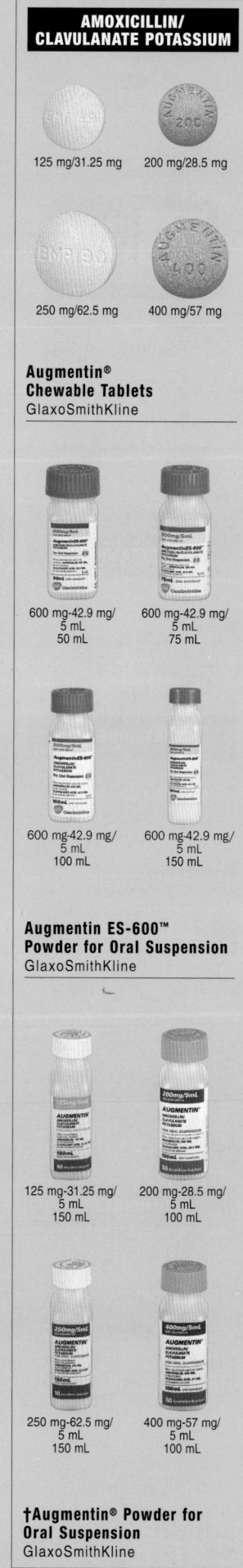

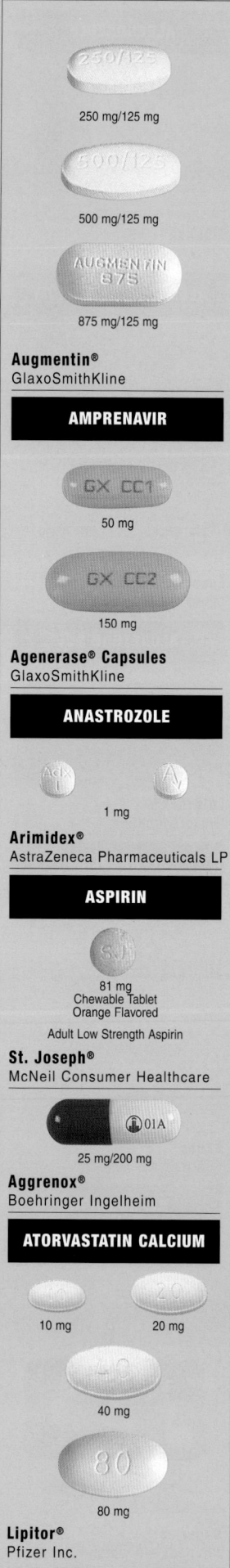

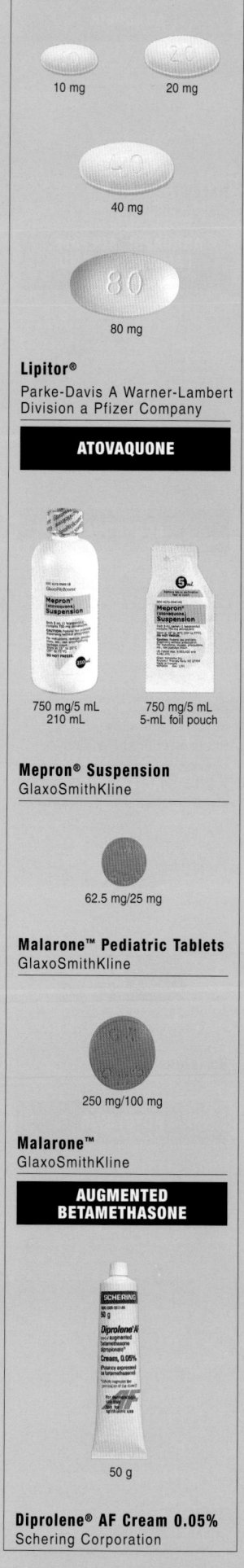

AMOXICILLIN

250 mg

500 mg

500 mg

875 mg

Amoxil®
GlaxoSmithKline

200 mg

400 mg

Amoxil® Chewable Tablets
GlaxoSmithKline

200 mg/5 mL
100 mL

Amoxil® for Oral Suspension
GlaxoSmithKline

50 mg/mL
15 mL

50 mg/mL
30 mL

**Amoxil® Pediatric Drops
for Oral Suspension**
GlaxoSmithKline

AMOXICILLIN/ CLAVULANATE POTASSIUM

125 mg/31.25 mg

200 mg/28.5 mg

250 mg/62.5 mg

400 mg/57 mg

**Augmentin®
Chewable Tablets**
GlaxoSmithKline

600 mg-42.9 mg/
5 mL
50 mL

600 mg-42.9 mg/
5 mL
75 mL

600 mg-42.9 mg/
5 mL
100 mL

600 mg-42.9 mg/
5 mL
150 mL

**Augmentin ES-600™
Powder for Oral Suspension**
GlaxoSmithKline

125 mg-31.25 mg/
5 mL
150 mL

200 mg-28.5 mg/
5 mL
100 mL

250 mg-62.5 mg/
5 mL
150 mL

400 mg-57 mg/
5 mL
100 mL

**†Augmentin® Powder for
Oral Suspension**
GlaxoSmithKline

250 mg/125 mg

500 mg/125 mg

875 mg/125 mg

Augmentin®
GlaxoSmithKline

AMPRENAVIR

50 mg

150 mg

Agenerase® Capsules
GlaxoSmithKline

ANASTROZOLE

1 mg

Arimidex®
AstraZeneca Pharmaceuticals LP

ASPIRIN

81 mg
Chewable Tablet
Orange Flavored

Adult Low Strength Aspirin

St. Joseph®
McNeil Consumer Healthcare

25 mg/200 mg

Aggrenox®
Boehringer Ingelheim

ATORVASTATIN CALCIUM

10 mg

20 mg

40 mg

80 mg

Lipitor®
Pfizer Inc.

10 mg

20 mg

40 mg

80 mg

Lipitor®
Parke-Davis A Warner-Lambert
Division a Pfizer Company

ATOVAQUONE

750 mg/5 mL
210 mL

750 mg/5 mL
5-mL foil pouch

Mepron® Suspension
GlaxoSmithKline

62.5 mg/25 mg

Malarone™ Pediatric Tablets
GlaxoSmithKline

250 mg/100 mg

Malarone™
GlaxoSmithKline

AUGMENTED BETAMETHASONE

50 g

Diprolene® AF Cream 0.05%
Schering Corporation

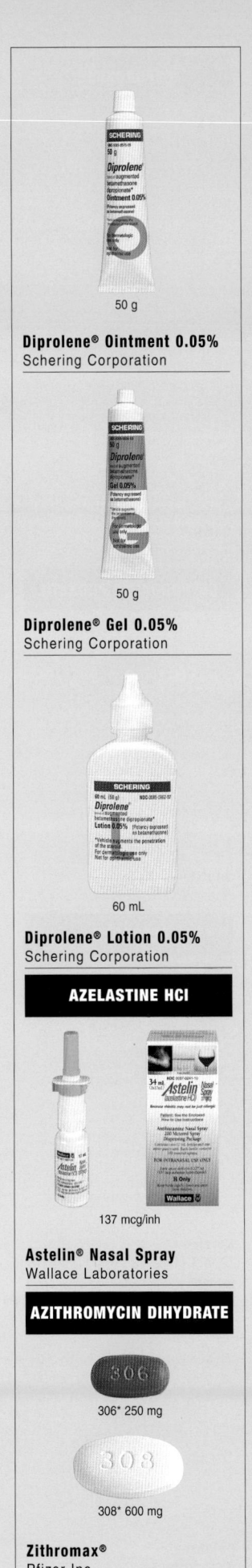

Diprolene® Ointment 0.05%
Schering Corporation

50 g

Diprolene® Gel 0.05%
Schering Corporation

50 g

Diprolene® Lotion 0.05%
Schering Corporation

60 mL

AZELASTINE HCl

137 mcg/inh

Astelin® Nasal Spray
Wallace Laboratories

AZITHROMYCIN DIHYDRATE

306* 250 mg

308* 600 mg

Zithromax®
Pfizer Inc.

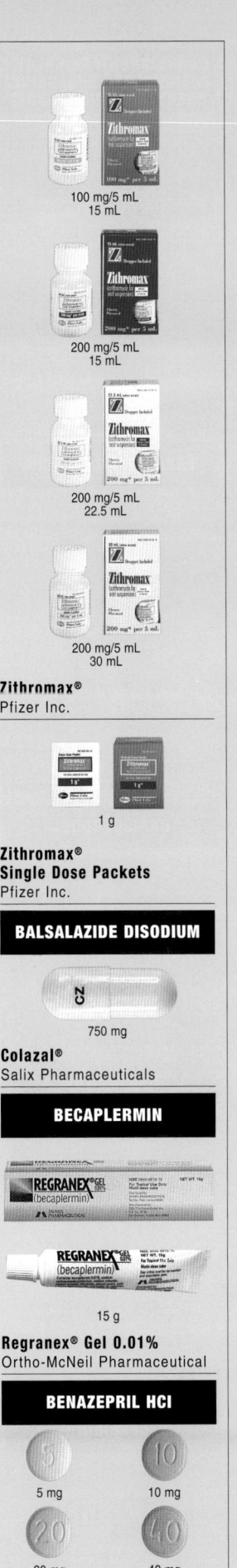

100 mg/5 mL
15 mL

200 mg/5 mL
15 mL

200 mg/5 mL
22.5 mL

200 mg/5 mL
30 mL

Zithromax®
Pfizer Inc.

1 g

**Zithromax®
Single Dose Packets**
Pfizer Inc.

BALSALAZIDE DISODIUM

750 mg

Colazal®
Salix Pharmaceuticals

BECAPLERMIN

15 g

Regranex® Gel 0.01%
Ortho-McNeil Pharmaceutical

BENAZEPRIL HCl

5 mg

10 mg

20 mg

40 mg

Lotensin®
Novartis Pharmaceuticals

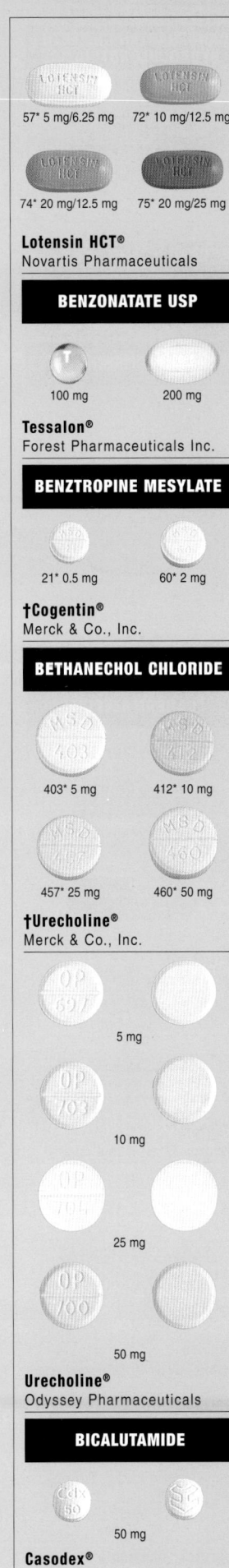

57* 5 mg/6.25 mg   72* 10 mg/12.5 mg

74* 20 mg/12.5 mg   75* 20 mg/25 mg

Lotensin HCT®
Novartis Pharmaceuticals

BENZONATATE USP

100 mg   200 mg

Tessalon®
Forest Pharmaceuticals Inc.

BENZTROPINE MESYLATE

21* 0.5 mg   60* 2 mg

†Cogentin®
Merck & Co., Inc.

BETHANECHOL CHLORIDE

403* 5 mg   412* 10 mg

457* 25 mg   460* 50 mg

†Urecholine®
Merck & Co., Inc.

5 mg

10 mg

25 mg

50 mg

Urecholine®
Odyssey Pharmaceuticals

BICALUTAMIDE

50 mg

Casodex®
AstraZeneca Pharmaceuticals LP

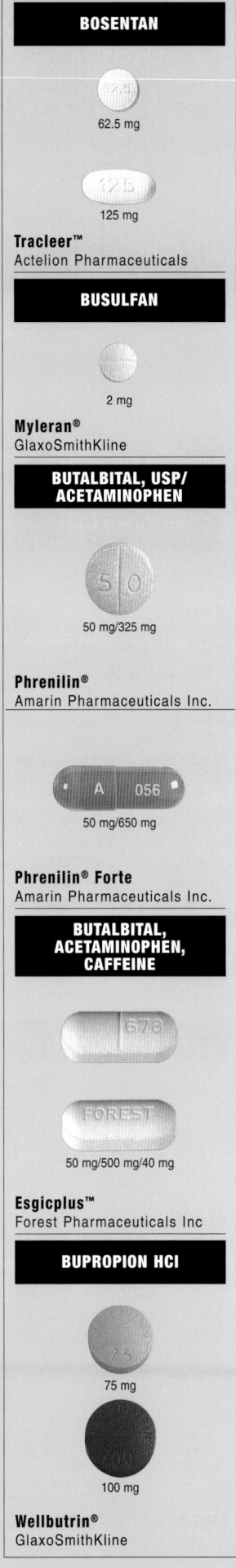

BOSENTAN

62.5 mg

125 mg

Tracleer™
Actelion Pharmaceuticals

BUSULFAN

2 mg

Myleran®
GlaxoSmithKline

BUTALBITAL, USP/ ACETAMINOPHEN

50 mg/325 mg

Phrenilin®
Amarin Pharmaceuticals Inc.

A 056

50 mg/650 mg

Phrenilin® Forte
Amarin Pharmaceuticals Inc.

BUTALBITAL, ACETAMINOPHEN, CAFFEINE

678

50 mg/500 mg/40 mg

Esgicplus™
Forest Pharmaceuticals Inc

BUPROPION HCl

75 mg

100 mg

Wellbutrin®
GlaxoSmithKline

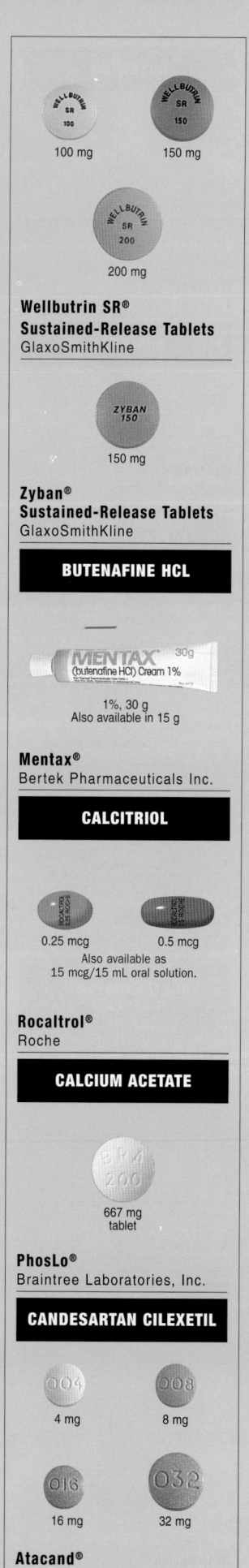

100 mg   150 mg

200 mg

Wellbutrin SR®
Sustained-Release Tablets
GlaxoSmithKline

150 mg

Zyban®
Sustained-Release Tablets
GlaxoSmithKline

BUTENAFINE HCL

1%, 30 g
Also available in 15 g

Mentax®
Bertek Pharmaceuticals Inc.

CALCITRIOL

0.25 mcg   0.5 mcg
Also available as
15 mcg/15 mL oral solution.

Rocaltrol®
Roche

CALCIUM ACETATE

667 mg
tablet

PhosLo®
Braintree Laboratories, Inc.

CANDESARTAN CILEXETIL

4 mg   8 mg

16 mg   32 mg

Atacand®
AstraZeneca LP

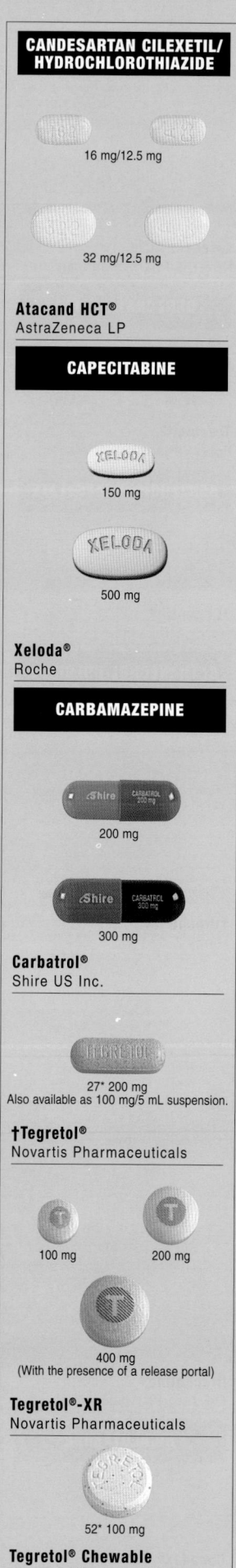

CANDESARTAN CILEXETIL/ HYDROCHLOROTHIAZIDE

16 mg/12.5 mg

32 mg/12.5 mg

Atacand HCT®
AstraZeneca LP

CAPECITABINE

150 mg

500 mg

Xeloda®
Roche

CARBAMAZEPINE

200 mg

300 mg

Carbatrol®
Shire US Inc.

27* 200 mg
Also available as 100 mg/5 mL suspension.

†Tegretol®
Novartis Pharmaceuticals

100 mg   200 mg

400 mg
(With the presence of a release portal)

Tegretol®-XR
Novartis Pharmaceuticals

52* 100 mg

Tegretol® Chewable
Novartis Pharmaceuticals

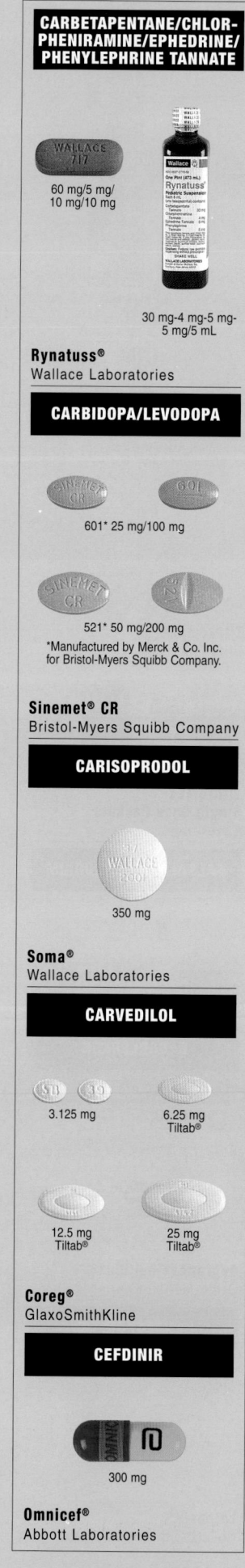

CARBETAPENTANE/CHLOR-PHENIRAMINE/EPHEDRINE/ PHENYLEPHRINE TANNATE

60 mg/5 mg/
10 mg/10 mg

30 mg-4 mg-5 mg-
5 mg/5 mL

Rynatuss®
Wallace Laboratories

CARBIDOPA/LEVODOPA

601* 25 mg/100 mg

521* 50 mg/200 mg
*Manufactured by Merck & Co. Inc.
for Bristol-Myers Squibb Company.

Sinemet® CR
Bristol-Myers Squibb Company

CARISOPRODOL

350 mg

Soma®
Wallace Laboratories

CARVEDILOL

3.125 mg   6.25 mg
Tiltab®

12.5 mg   25 mg
Tiltab®   Tiltab®

Coreg®
GlaxoSmithKline

CEFDINIR

300 mg

Omnicef®
Abbott Laboratories

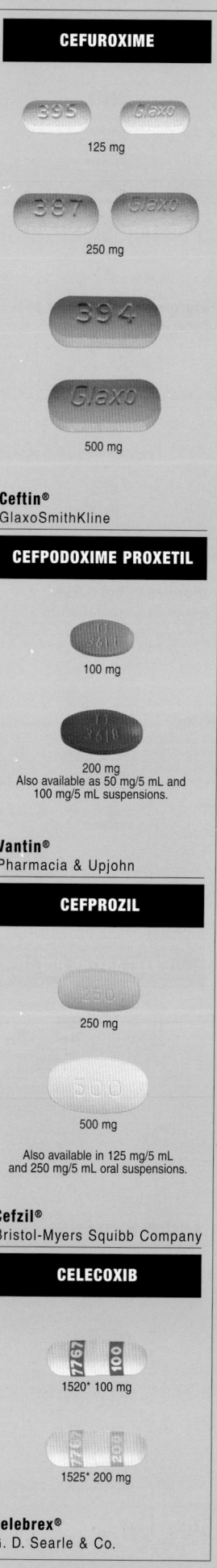

CEFUROXIME

125 mg

250 mg

500 mg

Ceftin®
GlaxoSmithKline

CEFPODOXIME PROXETIL

100 mg

200 mg
Also available as 50 mg/5 mL and
100 mg/5 mL suspensions.

Vantin®
Pharmacia & Upjohn

CEFPROZIL

250 mg

500 mg

Also available in 125 mg/5 mL
and 250 mg/5 mL oral suspensions.

Cefzil®
Bristol-Myers Squibb Company

CELECOXIB

1520* 100 mg

1525* 200 mg

Celebrex®
G. D. Searle & Co.

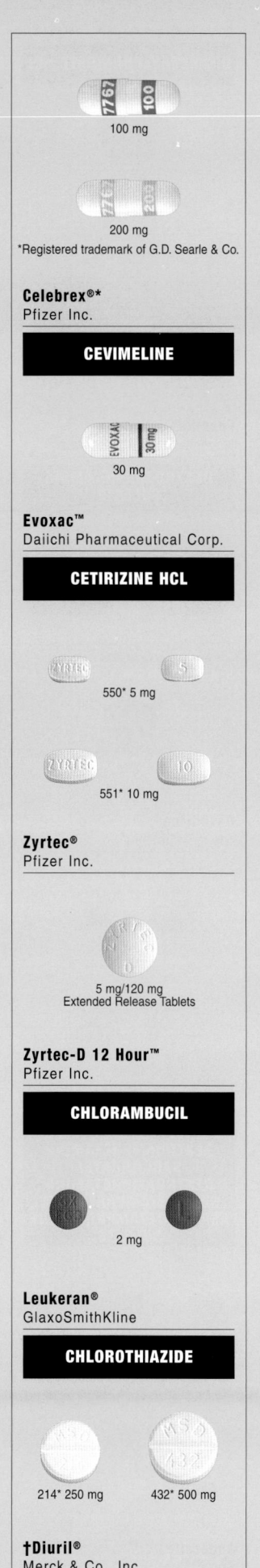

100 mg

200 mg

*Registered trademark of G.D. Searle & Co.

Celebrex®*
Pfizer Inc.

CEVIMELINE

30 mg

Evoxac™
Daiichi Pharmaceutical Corp.

CETIRIZINE HCL

550* 5 mg

551* 10 mg

Zyrtec®
Pfizer Inc.

5 mg/120 mg
Extended Release Tablets

Zyrtec-D 12 Hour™
Pfizer Inc.

CHLORAMBUCIL

2 mg

Leukeran®
GlaxoSmithKline

CHLOROTHIAZIDE

214* 250 mg   432* 500 mg

†Diuril®
Merck & Co., Inc.

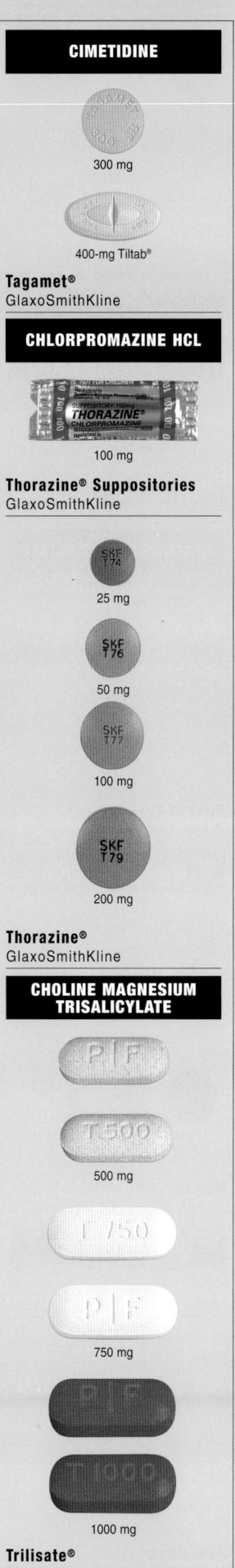

CIMETIDINE

300 mg

400-mg Tiltab®

Tagamet®
GlaxoSmithKline

CHLORPROMAZINE HCL

100 mg

Thorazine® Suppositories
GlaxoSmithKline

25 mg

50 mg

100 mg

200 mg

Thorazine®
GlaxoSmithKline

CHOLINE MAGNESIUM TRISALICYLATE

500 mg

750 mg

1000 mg

Trilisate®
The Purdue Frederick Co.

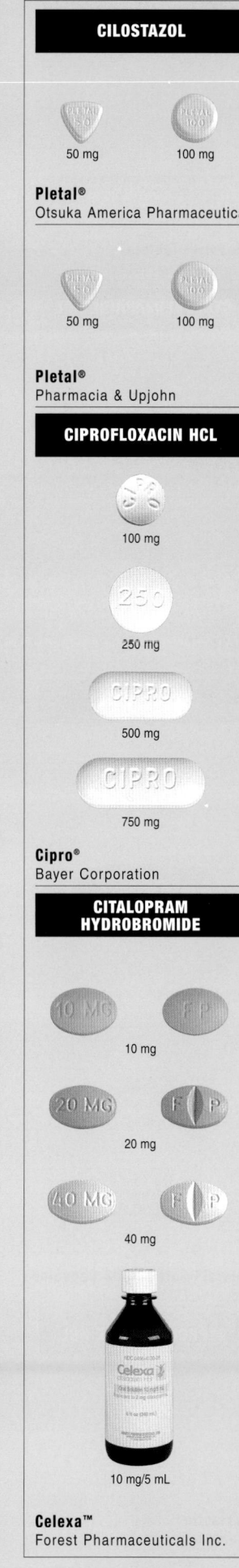

CILOSTAZOL

50 mg   100 mg

Pletal®
Otsuka America Pharmaceutical

50 mg   100 mg

Pletal®
Pharmacia & Upjohn

CIPROFLOXACIN HCL

100 mg

250 mg

500 mg

750 mg

Cipro®
Bayer Corporation

CITALOPRAM HYDROBROMIDE

10 mg

20 mg

40 mg

10 mg/5 mL

Celexa™
Forest Pharmaceuticals Inc.

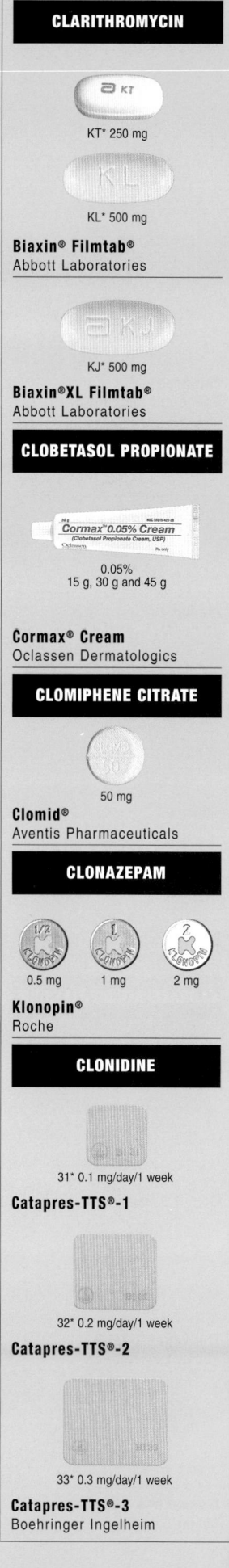

CLARITHROMYCIN

KT* 250 mg

KL* 500 mg

Biaxin® Filmtab®
Abbott Laboratories

KJ* 500 mg

Biaxin®XL Filmtab®
Abbott Laboratories

CLOBETASOL PROPIONATE

0.05%
15 g, 30 g and 45 g

Cormax® Cream
Oclassen Dermatologics

CLOMIPHENE CITRATE

50 mg

Clomid®
Aventis Pharmaceuticals

CLONAZEPAM

0.5 mg   1 mg   2 mg

Klonopin®
Roche

CLONIDINE

31* 0.1 mg/day/1 week

Catapres-TTS®-1

32* 0.2 mg/day/1 week

Catapres-TTS®-2

33* 0.3 mg/day/1 week

Catapres-TTS®-3
Boehringer Ingelheim

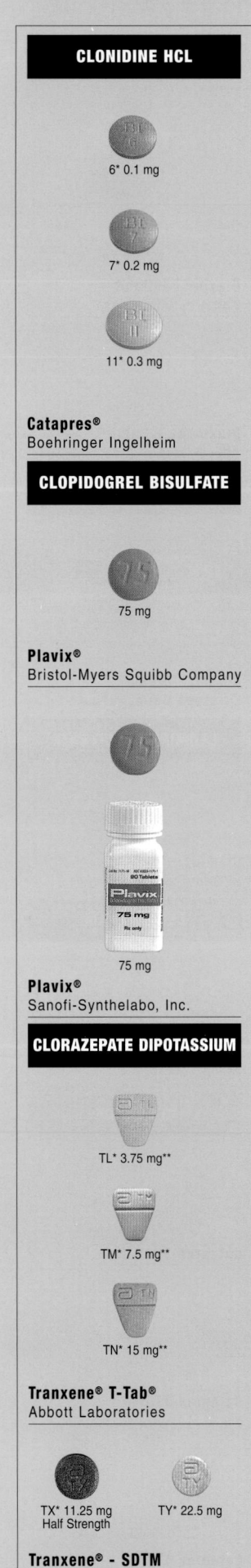

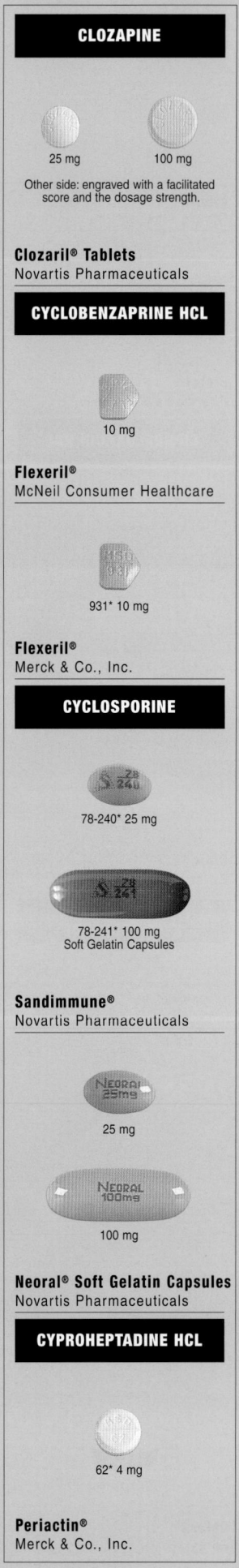

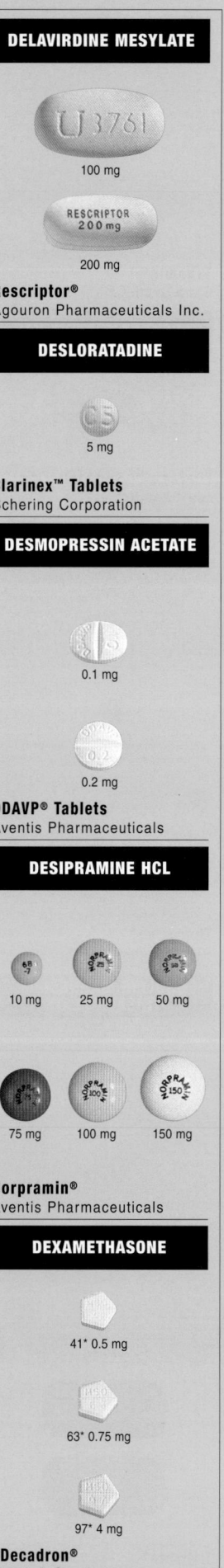

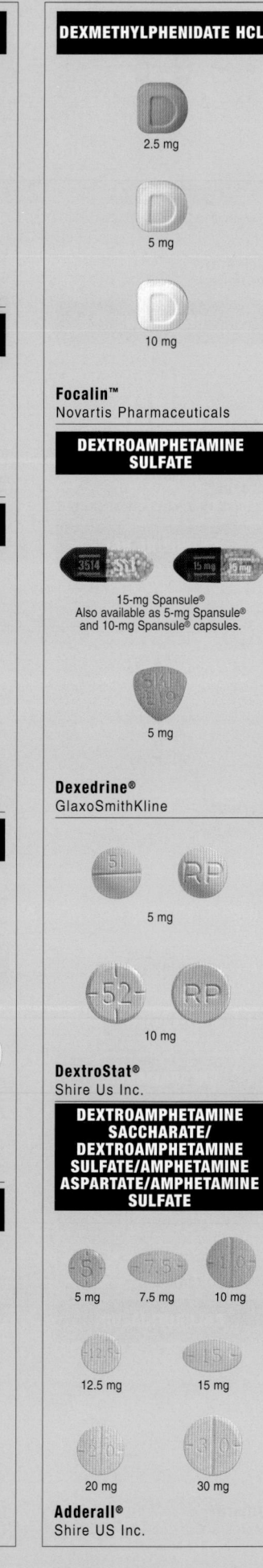

CLONIDINE HCL

6* 0.1 mg

7* 0.2 mg

11* 0.3 mg

Catapres®
Boehringer Ingelheim

CLOPIDOGREL BISULFATE

75 mg

Plavix®
Bristol-Myers Squibb Company

75 mg

75 mg

Plavix®
Sanofi-Synthelabo, Inc.

CLORAZEPATE DIPOTASSIUM

TL* 3.75 mg**

TM* 7.5 mg**

TN* 15 mg**

Tranxene® T-Tab®
Abbott Laboratories

TX* 11.25 mg
Half Strength   TY* 22.5 mg

Tranxene® - SDTM
Abbott Laboratories

CLOZAPINE

25 mg   100 mg

Other side: engraved with a facilitated
score and the dosage strength.

Clozaril® Tablets
Novartis Pharmaceuticals

CYCLOBENZAPRINE HCL

10 mg

Flexeril®
McNeil Consumer Healthcare

931* 10 mg

Flexeril®
Merck & Co., Inc.

CYCLOSPORINE

78-240* 25 mg

78-241* 100 mg
Soft Gelatin Capsules

Sandimmune®
Novartis Pharmaceuticals

25 mg

100 mg

Neoral® Soft Gelatin Capsules
Novartis Pharmaceuticals

CYPROHEPTADINE HCL

62* 4 mg

Periactin®
Merck & Co., Inc.

DELAVIRDINE MESYLATE

100 mg

RESCRIPTOR
200 mg

200 mg

Rescriptor®
Agouron Pharmaceuticals Inc.

DESLORATADINE

5 mg

Clarinex™ Tablets
Schering Corporation

DESMOPRESSIN ACETATE

0.1 mg

0.2 mg

DDAVP® Tablets
Aventis Pharmaceuticals

DESIPRAMINE HCL

10 mg   25 mg   50 mg

75 mg   100 mg   150 mg

Norpramin®
Aventis Pharmaceuticals

DEXAMETHASONE

41* 0.5 mg

63* 0.75 mg

97* 4 mg

†Decadron®
Merck & Co., Inc.

DEXMETHYLPHENIDATE HCL

2.5 mg

5 mg

10 mg

Focalin™
Novartis Pharmaceuticals

DEXTROAMPHETAMINE SULFATE

15-mg Spansule®
Also available as 5-mg Spansule®
and 10-mg Spansule® capsules.

5 mg

Dexedrine®
GlaxoSmithKline

5 mg

10 mg

DextroStat®
Shire Us Inc.

DEXTROAMPHETAMINE SACCHARATE/ DEXTROAMPHETAMINE SULFATE/AMPHETAMINE ASPARTATE/AMPHETAMINE SULFATE

5 mg   7.5 mg   10 mg

12.5 mg   15 mg

20 mg   30 mg

Adderall®
Shire US Inc.

DIAZEPAM

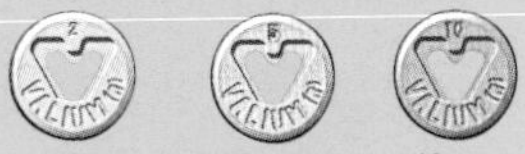

2 mg   5 mg   10 mg

†Valium®
Roche

DIBASIC SODIUM PHOSPHATE/MONOBASIC POTASSIUM PHOSPHATE/ MONOBASIC SODIUM PHOSPHATE

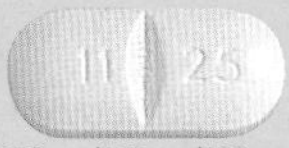

852 mg/155 mg/130 mg

K-Phos® Neutral
Beach Pharmaceuticals

DICLOFENAC POTASSIUM

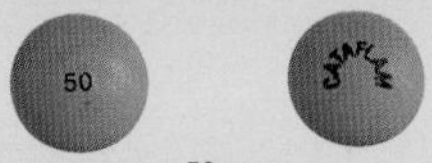

50   CATAFLAM

50 mg

Cataflam®
Novartis Pharmaceuticals

DICLOFENAC SODIUM

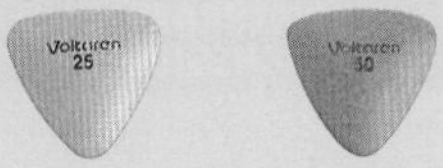

Voltaren 25   Voltaren 10

25 mg   50 mg

Voltaren 75

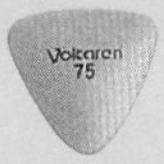

75 mg

Voltaren®
Novartis Pharmaceuticals

Voltaren XR

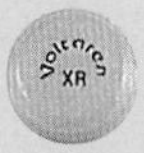

100 mg

Voltaren®-XR
Novartis Pharmaceuticals

DICLOFENAC SODIUM/ MISOPROSTOL

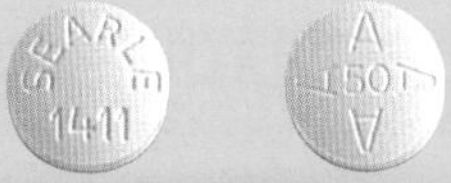

SEARLE 1411   A 50T

50 mg/200 mcg

SEARLE 1421   A 75T

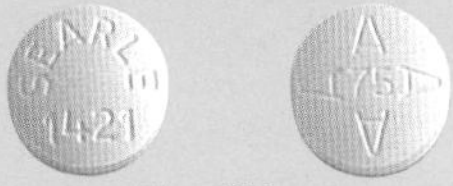

75 mg/200 mcg

Arthrotec®
G. D. Searle & Co.

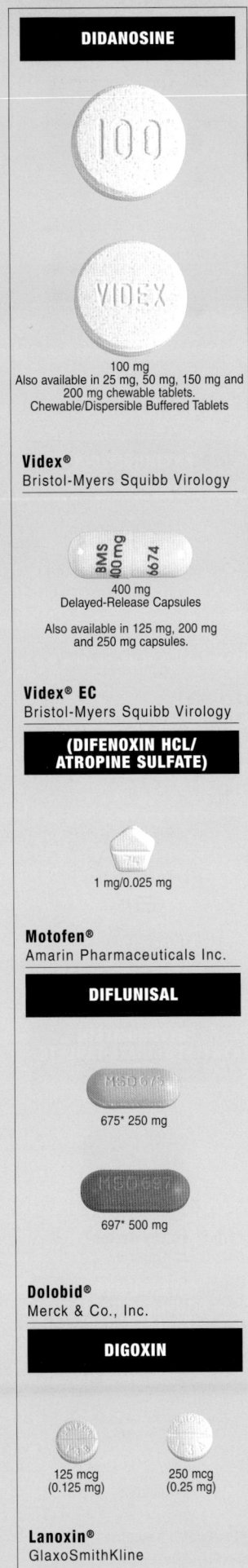

DIDANOSINE

100

VIDEX

100 mg
Also available in 25 mg, 50 mg, 150 mg and 200 mg chewable tablets.
Chewable/Dispersible Buffered Tablets

Videx®
Bristol-Myers Squibb Virology

BMS 400 mg 6674

400 mg
Delayed-Release Capsules

Also available in 125 mg, 200 mg
and 250 mg capsules.

Videx® EC
Bristol-Myers Squibb Virology

(DIFENOXIN HCL/ ATROPINE SULFATE)

1 mg/0.025 mg

Motofen®
Amarin Pharmaceuticals Inc.

DIFLUNISAL

MSD675   675* 250 mg

MSD697   697* 500 mg

Dolobid®
Merck & Co., Inc.

DIGOXIN

125 mcg
(0.125 mg)   250 mcg
(0.25 mg)

Lanoxin®
GlaxoSmithKline

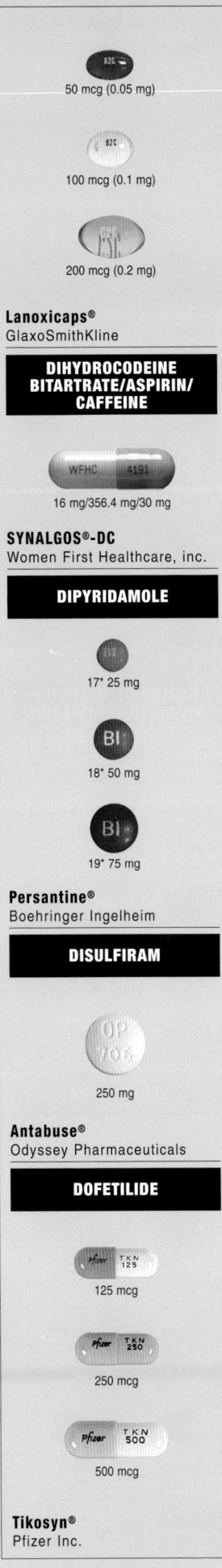

A2C

50 mcg (0.05 mg)

B2C

100 mcg (0.1 mg)

200 mcg (0.2 mg)

Lanoxicaps®
GlaxoSmithKline

DIHYDROCODEINE BITARTRATE/ASPIRIN/ CAFFEINE

WFHC   4191

16 mg/356.4 mg/30 mg

SYNALGOS®-DC
Women First Healthcare, inc.

DIPYRIDAMOLE

BI   17* 25 mg

BI   18* 50 mg

BI   19* 75 mg

Persantine®
Boehringer Ingelheim

DISULFIRAM

OP 706

250 mg

Antabuse®
Odyssey Pharmaceuticals

DOFETILIDE

Pfizer TKN 125

125 mcg

Pfizer TKN 250

250 mcg

Pfizer TKN 500

500 mcg

Tikosyn®
Pfizer Inc.

DOLASETRON MESYLATE

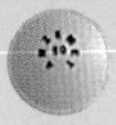

50 mg

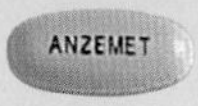

ANZEMET

100 mg

Anzemet® Tablets
Aventis Pharmaceuticals

DONEPEZIL HCL

5 mg   10 mg

Aricept®
Eisai inc.

DONEPEZIL HCL

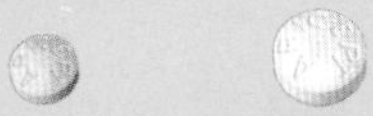

E245* 5 mg   E246* 10 mg

*Registered trademark of Eisai Co., Ltd,
Tokyo, Japan

Aricept®*
Pfizer Inc.

DOXAZOSIN MESYLATE

CARDURA   CARDURA

275* 1 mg   276* 2 mg

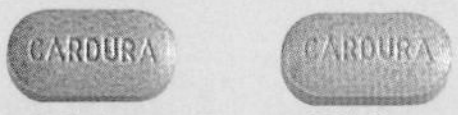

CARDURA   CARDURA

277* 4 mg   278* 8 mg

Cardura®
Pfizer Inc.

DOXEPIN HCl

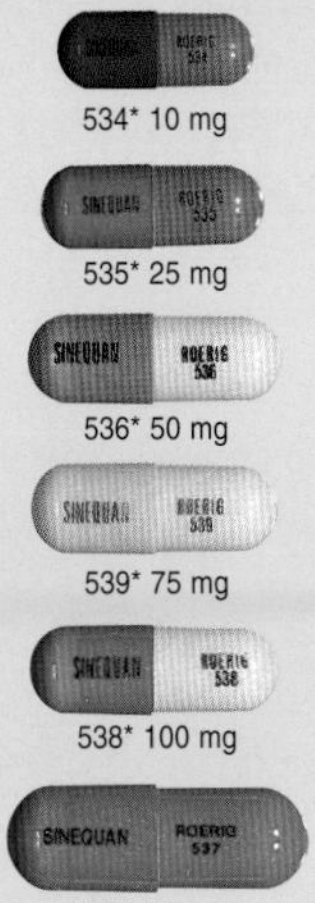

534* 10 mg

SINEQUAN   535* 25 mg

SINEQUAN   ROERIG 536
536* 50 mg

SINEQUAN   ROERIG 539
539* 75 mg

SINEQUAN   ROERIG 538
538* 100 mg

SINEQUAN   ROERIG 537
537* 150 mg

†Sinequan®
Pfizer Inc.

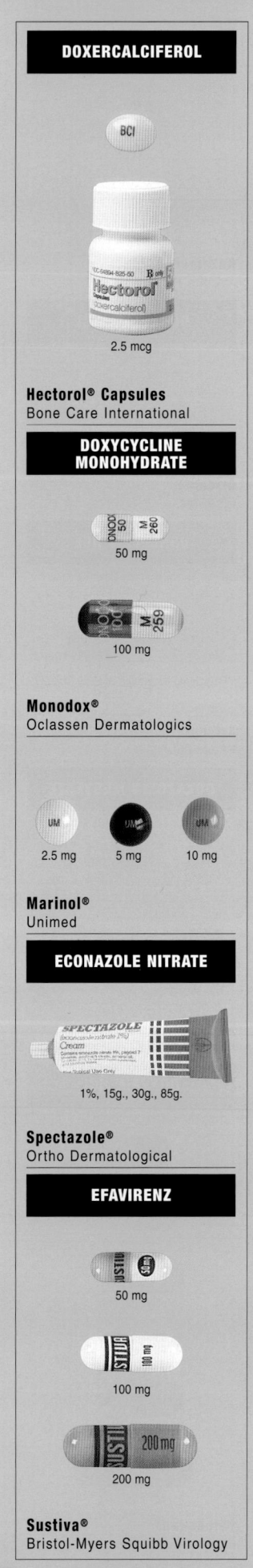

DOXERCALCIFEROL

BCl

2.5 mcg

Hectorol® Capsules
Bone Care International

DOXYCYCLINE MONOHYDRATE

50 mg

100 mg

Monodox®
Oclassen Dermatologics

2.5 mg   5 mg   10 mg

Marinol®
Unimed

ECONAZOLE NITRATE

1%, 15g., 30g., 85g.

Spectazole®
Ortho Dermatological

EFAVIRENZ

50 mg

100 mg

200 mg

Sustiva®
Bristol-Myers Squibb Virology

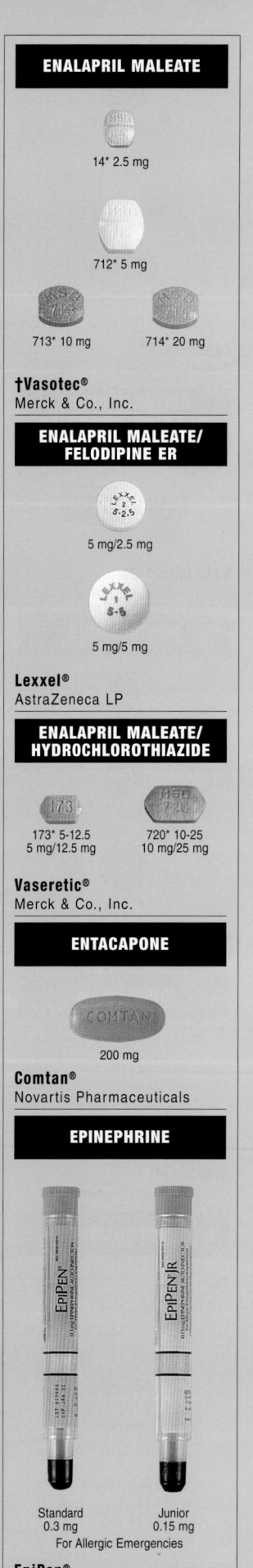

ENALAPRIL MALEATE

14* 2.5 mg

712* 5 mg

713* 10 mg   714* 20 mg

†Vasotec®
Merck & Co., Inc.

ENALAPRIL MALEATE/ FELODIPINE ER

5 mg/2.5 mg

5 mg/5 mg

Lexxel®
AstraZeneca LP

ENALAPRIL MALEATE/ HYDROCHLOROTHIAZIDE

173* 5-12.5   720* 10-25
5 mg/12.5 mg   10 mg/25 mg

Vaseretic®
Merck & Co., Inc.

ENTACAPONE

COMTAN

200 mg

Comtan®
Novartis Pharmaceuticals

EPINEPHRINE

Standard   Junior
0.3 mg   0.15 mg
For Allergic Emergencies

EpiPen®
Dey

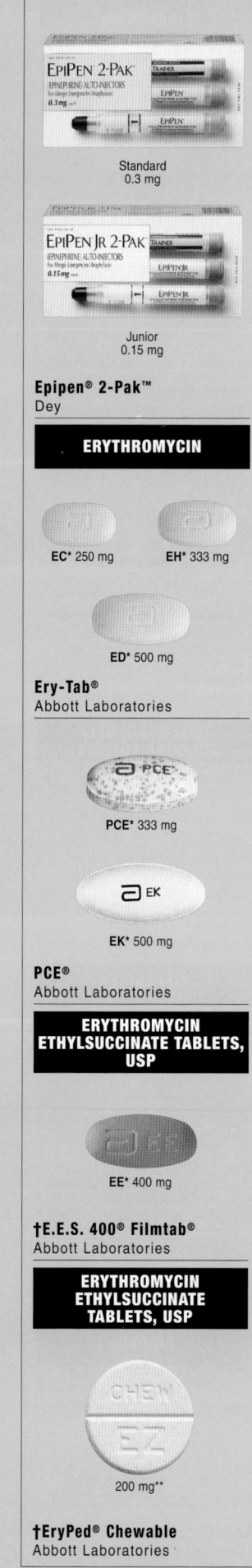

Standard
0.3 mg

Junior
0.15 mg

Epipen® 2-Pak™
Dey

ERYTHROMYCIN

EC* 250 mg   EH* 333 mg

ED* 500 mg

Ery-Tab®
Abbott Laboratories

PCE

PCE* 333 mg

EK

EK* 500 mg

PCE®
Abbott Laboratories

ERYTHROMYCIN ETHYLSUCCINATE TABLETS, USP

EE* 400 mg

†E.E.S. 400® Filmtab®
Abbott Laboratories

ERYTHROMYCIN ETHYLSUCCINATE TABLETS, USP

CHEW EZ

200 mg**

†EryPed® Chewable
Abbott Laboratories

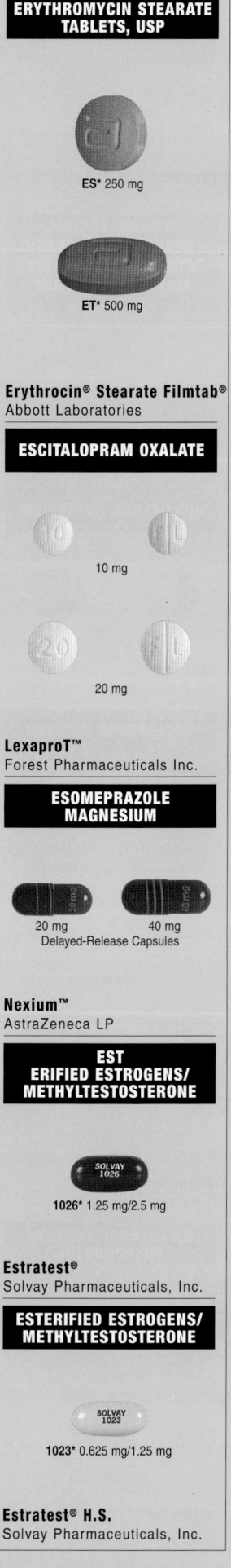

ERYTHROMYCIN STEARATE TABLETS, USP

ES* 250 mg

ET* 500 mg

Erythrocin® Stearate Filmtab®
Abbott Laboratories

ESCITALOPRAM OXALATE

10 mg

20 mg

LexaproT™
Forest Pharmaceuticals Inc.

ESOMEPRAZOLE MAGNESIUM

20 mg   40 mg
Delayed-Release Capsules

Nexium™
AstraZeneca LP

EST ERIFIED ESTROGENS/ METHYLTESTOSTERONE

SOLVAY 1026

1026* 1.25 mg/2.5 mg

Estratest®
Solvay Pharmaceuticals, Inc.

ESTERIFIED ESTROGENS/ METHYLTESTOSTERONE

SOLVAY 1023

1023* 0.625 mg/1.25 mg

Estratest® H.S.
Solvay Pharmaceuticals, Inc.

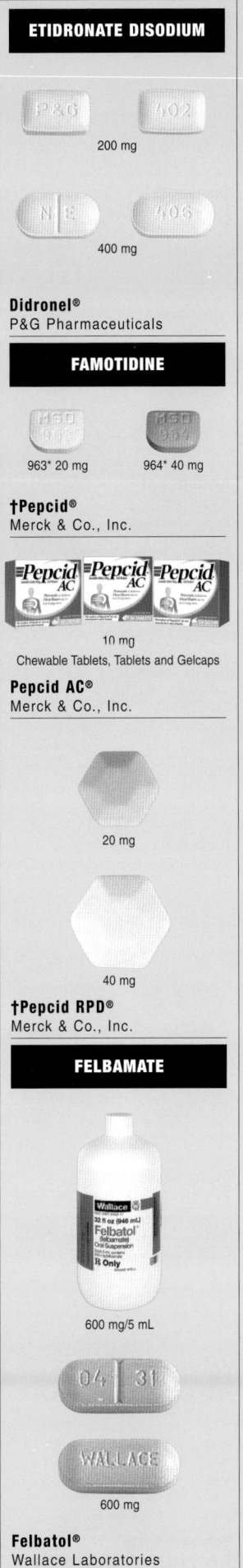
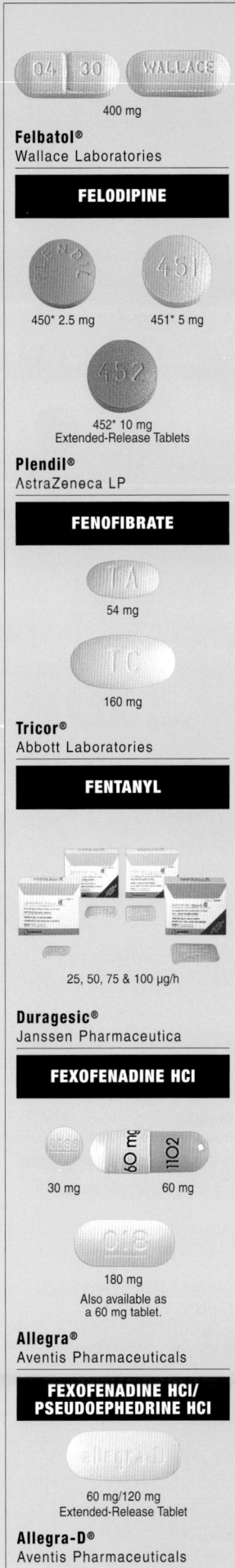
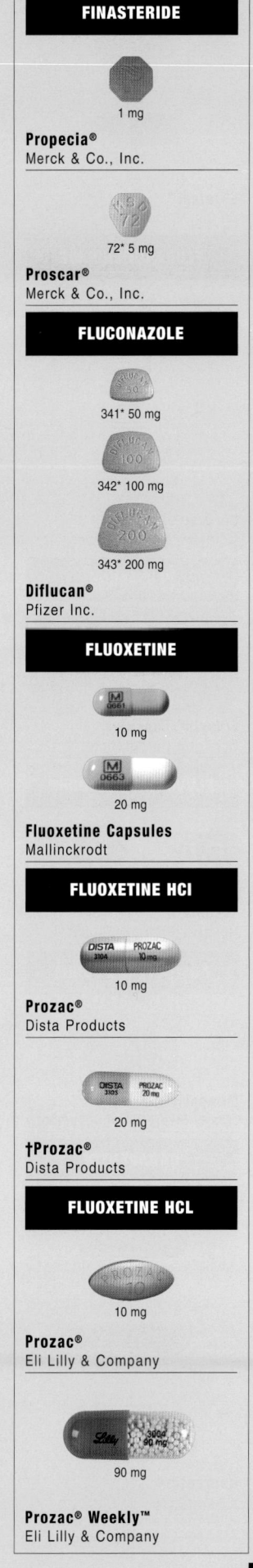

ESTROGENS, CONJUGATED

868* 0.3 mg   867* 0.625 mg

864* 0.9 mg   866* 1.25 mg

865* 2.5 mg

Premarin®
Wyeth Pharmaceuticals

ESTROGENS ESTERIFIE

0.3 mg

0.625 mg

1.25 mg

2.5 mg

Menest®
Monarch Pharmaceuticals

ESTROPIPATE

Ortho-Est 0.625
(0.75 mg)

Ortho-Est 1.25
(1.5 mg)

ORTHO-EST®
Women First Healthcare, Inc.

ETHACRYNIC ACID

65* 25 mg   90* 50 mg

†Edecrin®
Merck & Co., Inc.

ETHOSUXIMIDE

250 mg

Zarontin®
Parke-Davis A Warner-Lambert
Division a Pfizer Company

ETIDRONATE DISODIUM

200 mg

400 mg

Didronel®
P&G Pharmaceuticals

FAMOTIDINE

963* 20 mg   964* 40 mg

†Pepcid®
Merck & Co., Inc.

10 mg
Chewable Tablets, Tablets and Gelcaps

Pepcid AC®
Merck & Co., Inc.

20 mg

40 mg

†Pepcid RPD®
Merck & Co., Inc.

FELBAMATE

600 mg/5 mL

600 mg

Felbatol®
Wallace Laboratories

400 mg

Felbatol®
Wallace Laboratories

FELODIPINE

450* 2.5 mg   451* 5 mg

452* 10 mg
Extended-Release Tablets

Plendil®
AstraZeneca LP

FENOFIBRATE

54 mg

160 mg

Tricor®
Abbott Laboratories

FENTANYL

25, 50, 75 & 100 µg/h

Duragesic®
Janssen Pharmaceutica

FEXOFENADINE HCl

30 mg   60 mg

180 mg
Also available as
a 60 mg tablet.

Allegra®
Aventis Pharmaceuticals

FEXOFENADINE HCl/ PSEUDOEPHEDRINE HCl

60 mg/120 mg
Extended-Release Tablet

Allegra-D®
Aventis Pharmaceuticals

FINASTERIDE

1 mg

Propecia®
Merck & Co., Inc.

72* 5 mg

Proscar®
Merck & Co., Inc.

FLUCONAZOLE

341* 50 mg

342* 100 mg

343* 200 mg

Diflucan®
Pfizer Inc.

FLUOXETINE

10 mg

20 mg

Fluoxetine Capsules
Mallinckrodt

FLUOXETINE HCl

10 mg

Prozac®
Dista Products

20 mg

†Prozac®
Dista Products

FLUOXETINE HCL

10 mg

Prozac®
Eli Lilly & Company

90 mg

Prozac® Weekly™
Eli Lilly & Company

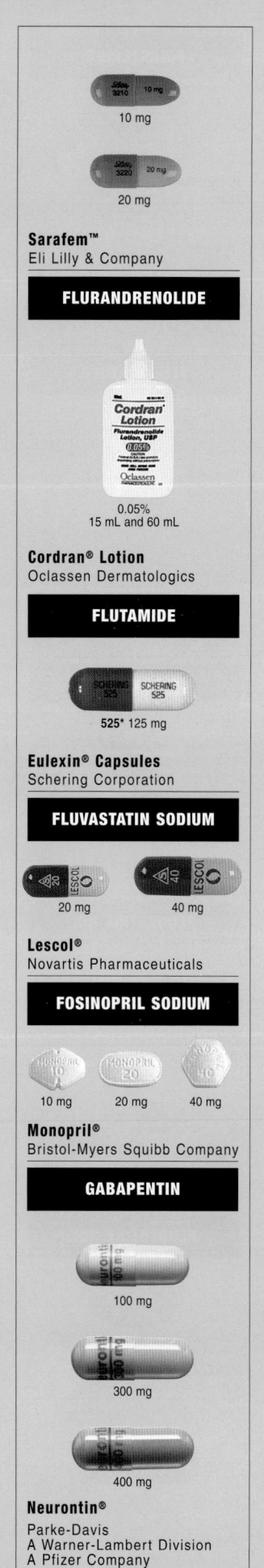

10 mg

20 mg

Sarafem™
Eli Lilly & Company

FLURANDRENOLIDE

0.05%
15 mL and 60 mL

Cordran® Lotion
Oclassen Dermatologics

FLUTAMIDE

525* 125 mg

Eulexin® Capsules
Schering Corporation

FLUVASTATIN SODIUM

20 mg   40 mg

Lescol®
Novartis Pharmaceuticals

FOSINOPRIL SODIUM

10 mg   20 mg   40 mg

Monopril®
Bristol-Myers Squibb Company

GABAPENTIN

100 mg

300 mg

400 mg

Neurontin®
Parke-Davis
A Warner-Lambert Division
A Pfizer Company

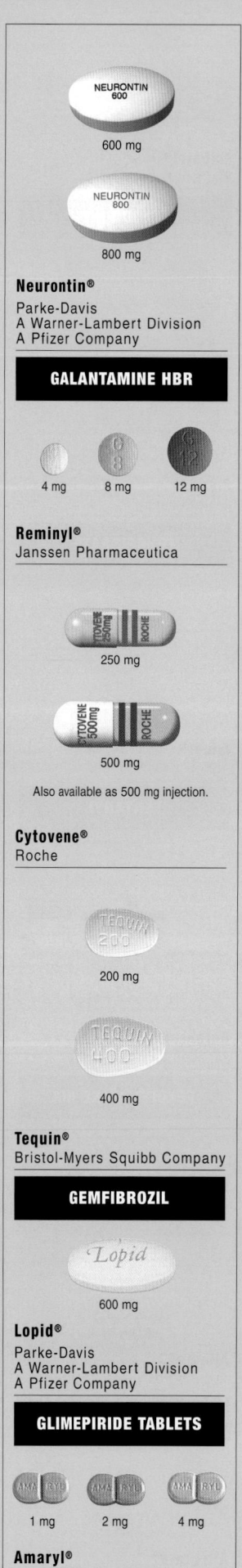

600 mg

800 mg

Neurontin®
Parke-Davis
A Warner-Lambert Division
A Pfizer Company

GALANTAMINE HBR

4 mg   8 mg   12 mg

Reminyl®
Janssen Pharmaceutica

250 mg

500 mg

Also available as 500 mg injection.

Cytovene®
Roche

200 mg

400 mg

Tequin®
Bristol-Myers Squibb Company

GEMFIBROZIL

600 mg

Lopid®
Parke-Davis
A Warner-Lambert Division
A Pfizer Company

GLIMEPIRIDE TABLETS

1 mg   2 mg   4 mg

Amaryl®
Aventis Pharmaceuticals

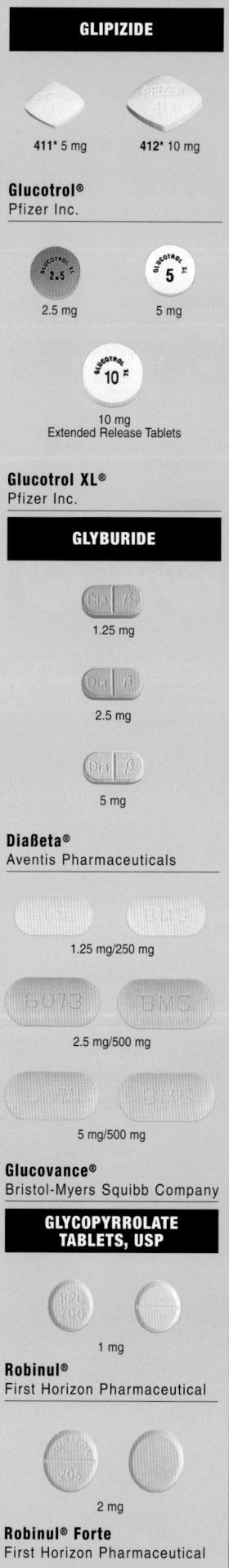

GLIPIZIDE

411* 5 mg   **412*** 10 mg

Glucotrol®
Pfizer Inc.

2.5 mg   5 mg

10 mg
Extended Release Tablets

Glucotrol XL®
Pfizer Inc.

GLYBURIDE

1.25 mg

2.5 mg

5 mg

Diaßeta®
Aventis Pharmaceuticals

1.25 mg/250 mg

2.5 mg/500 mg

5 mg/500 mg

Glucovance®
Bristol-Myers Squibb Company

GLYCOPYRROLATE TABLETS, USP

1 mg

Robinul®
First Horizon Pharmaceutical

2 mg

Robinul® Forte
First Horizon Pharmaceutical

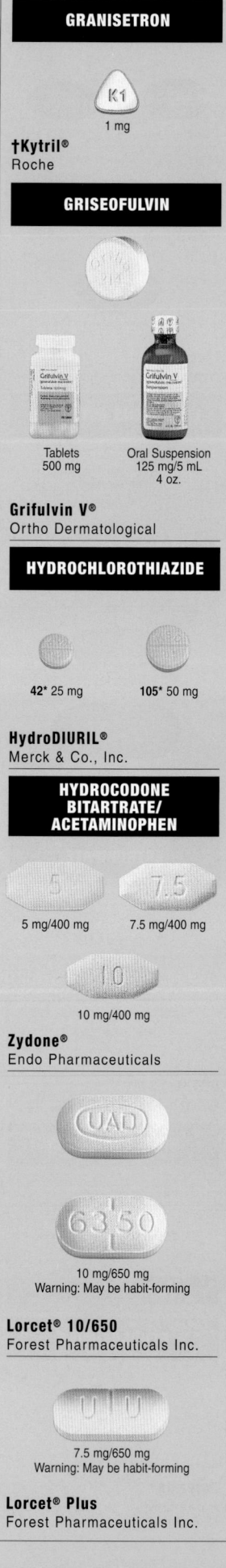

GRANISETRON

1 mg

†Kytril®
Roche

GRISEOFULVIN

Tablets
500 mg

Oral Suspension
125 mg/5 mL
4 oz.

Grifulvin V®
Ortho Dermatological

HYDROCHLOROTHIAZIDE

42* 25 mg   **105*** 50 mg

HydroDIURIL®
Merck & Co., Inc.

HYDROCODONE BITARTRATE/ ACETAMINOPHEN

5 mg/400 mg   7.5 mg/400 mg

10 mg/400 mg

Zydone®
Endo Pharmaceuticals

10 mg/650 mg
Warning: May be habit-forming

Lorcet® 10/650
Forest Pharmaceuticals Inc.

7.5 mg/650 mg
Warning: May be habit-forming

Lorcet® Plus
Forest Pharmaceuticals Inc.

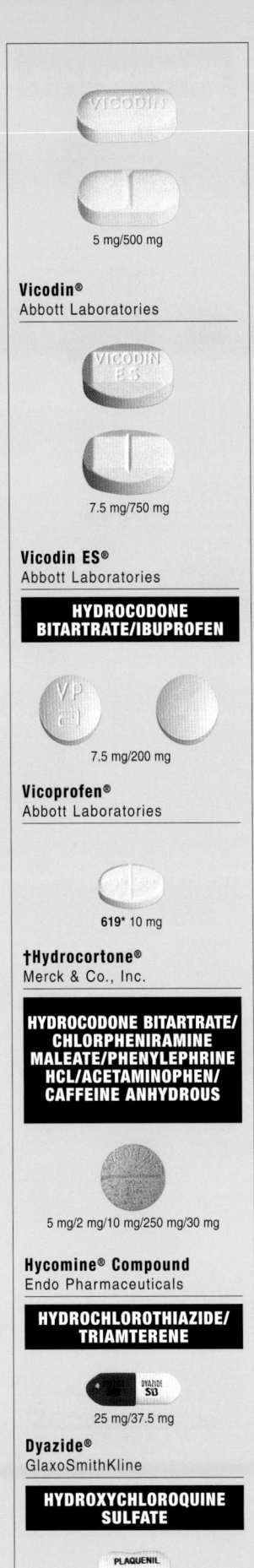

Vicodin®
Abbott Laboratories

5 mg/500 mg

Vicodin ES®
Abbott Laboratories

7.5 mg/750 mg

HYDROCODONE BITARTRATE/IBUPROFEN

7.5 mg/200 mg

Vicoprofen®
Abbott Laboratories

619* 10 mg

†Hydrocortone®
Merck & Co., Inc.

HYDROCODONE BITARTRATE/ CHLORPHENIRAMINE MALEATE/PHENYLEPHRINE HCL/ACETAMINOPHEN/ CAFFEINE ANHYDROUS

5 mg/2 mg/10 mg/250 mg/30 mg

Hycomine® Compound
Endo Pharmaceuticals

HYDROCHLOROTHIAZIDE/ TRIAMTERENE

25 mg/37.5 mg

Dyazide®
GlaxoSmithKline

HYDROXYCHLOROQUINE SULFATE

P62* 200 mg

Plaquenil®
Sanofi-Synthelabo, Inc.

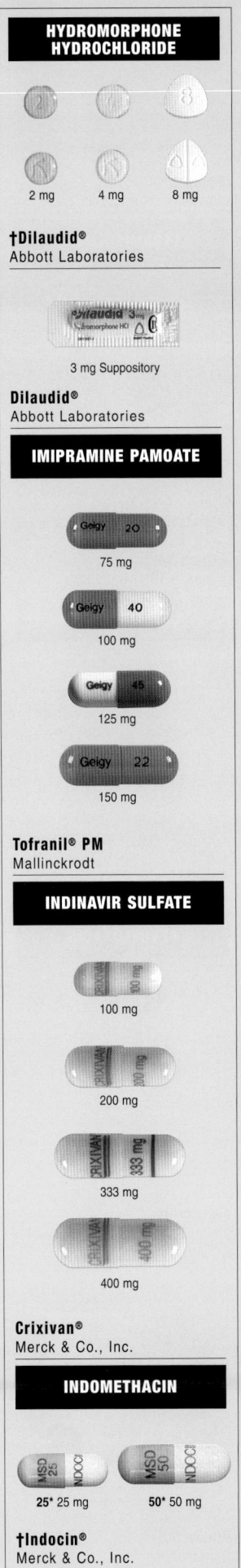

HYDROMORPHONE HYDROCHLORIDE

2 mg   4 mg   8 mg

†Dilaudid®
Abbott Laboratories

3 mg Suppository

Dilaudid®
Abbott Laboratories

IMIPRAMINE PAMOATE

75 mg

100 mg

125 mg

150 mg

Tofranil® PM
Mallinckrodt

INDINAVIR SULFATE

100 mg

200 mg

333 mg

400 mg

Crixivan®
Merck & Co., Inc.

INDOMETHACIN

25* 25 mg   **50*** 50 mg

†Indocin®
Merck & Co., Inc.

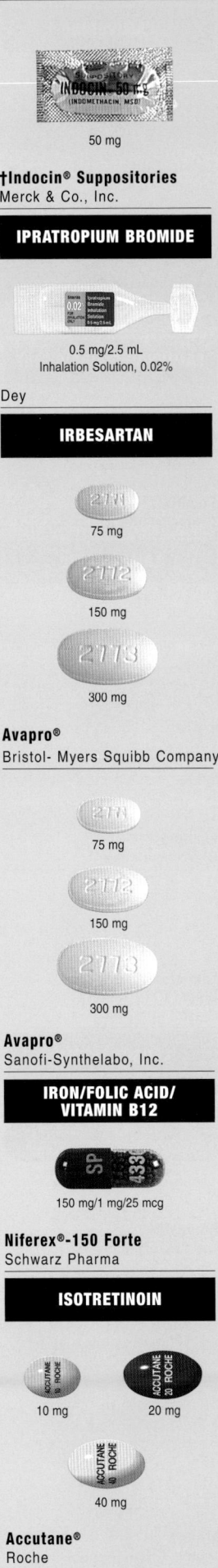

50 mg

†Indocin® Suppositories
Merck & Co., Inc.

IPRATROPIUM BROMIDE

0.5 mg/2.5 mL
Inhalation Solution, 0.02%

Dey

IRBESARTAN

75 mg

150 mg

300 mg

Avapro®
Bristol- Myers Squibb Company

75 mg

150 mg

300 mg

Avapro®
Sanofi-Synthelabo, Inc.

IRON/FOLIC ACID/ VITAMIN B12

150 mg/1 mg/25 mcg

Niferex®-150 Forte
Schwarz Pharma

ISOTRETINOIN

10 mg   20 mg

40 mg

Accutane®
Roche

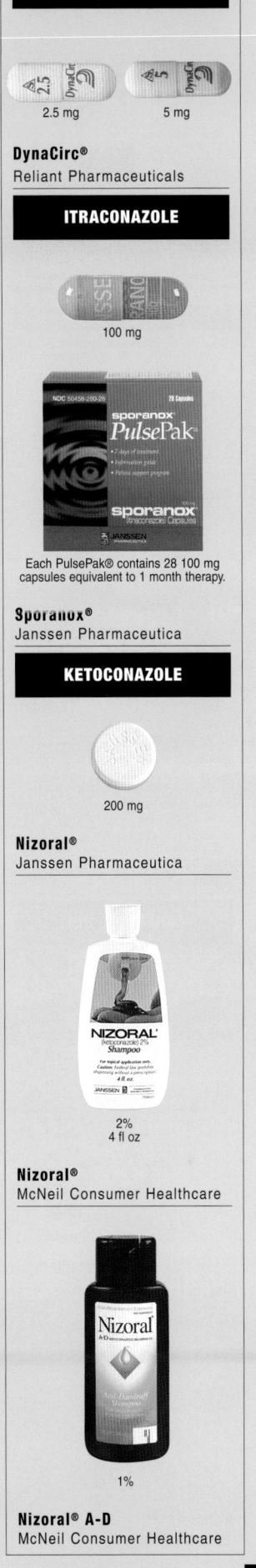

ISRADIPINE

2.5 mg   5 mg

DynaCirc®
Reliant Pharmaceuticals

ITRACONAZOLE

100 mg

Each PulsePak® contains 28 100 mg
capsules equivalent to 1 month therapy.

Sporanox®
Janssen Pharmaceutica

KETOCONAZOLE

200 mg

Nizoral®
Janssen Pharmaceutica

2%
4 fl oz

Nizoral®
McNeil Consumer Healthcare

1%

Nizoral® A-D
McNeil Consumer Healthcare

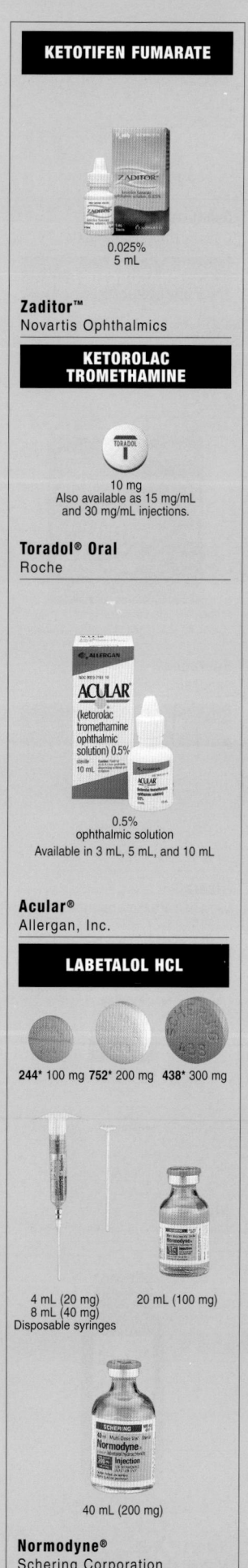

KETOTIFEN FUMARATE

0.025%
5 mL

Zaditor™
Novartis Ophthalmics

KETOROLAC TROMETHAMINE

10 mg
Also available as 15 mg/mL
and 30 mg/mL injections.

Toradol® Oral
Roche

0.5%
ophthalmic solution
Available in 3 mL, 5 mL, and 10 mL

Acular®
Allergan, Inc.

LABETALOL HCL

244* 100 mg **752*** 200 mg **438*** 300 mg

4 mL (20 mg)   20 mL (100 mg)
8 mL (40 mg)
Disposable syringes

40 mL (200 mg)

Normodyne®
Schering Corporation

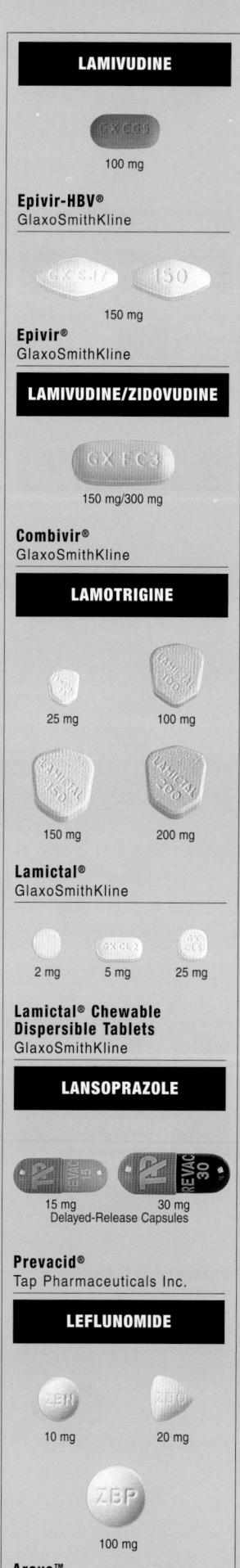

LAMIVUDINE

100 mg

Epivir-HBV®
GlaxoSmithKline

150 mg

Epivir®
GlaxoSmithKline

LAMIVUDINE/ZIDOVUDINE

150 mg/300 mg

Combivir®
GlaxoSmithKline

LAMOTRIGINE

25 mg   100 mg

150 mg   200 mg

Lamictal®
GlaxoSmithKline

2 mg   5 mg   25 mg

**Lamictal® Chewable
Dispersible Tablets**
GlaxoSmithKline

LANSOPRAZOLE

15 mg   30 mg
Delayed-Release Capsules

Prevacid®
Tap Pharmaceuticals Inc.

LEFLUNOMIDE

10 mg   20 mg

100 mg

Arava™
Aventis Pharmaceuticals

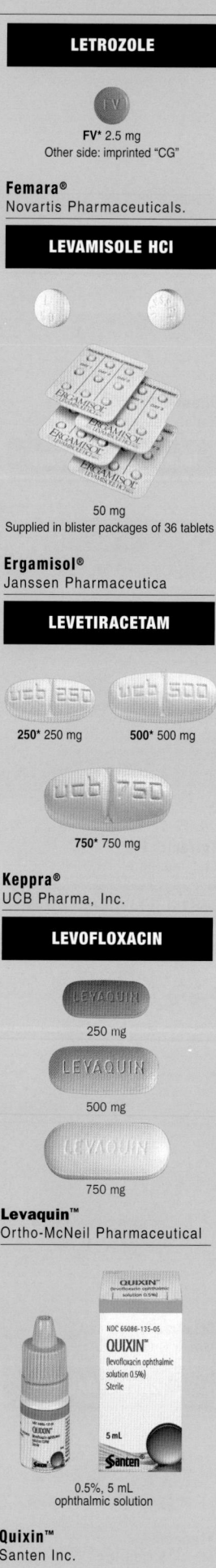

LETROZOLE

FV* 2.5 mg
Other side: imprinted "CG"

Femara®
Novartis Pharmaceuticals.

LEVAMISOLE HCl

50 mg
Supplied in blister packages of 36 tablets

Ergamisol®
Janssen Pharmaceutica

LEVETIRACETAM

250* 250 mg   **500*** 500 mg

750* 750 mg

Keppra®
UCB Pharma, Inc.

LEVOFLOXACIN

250 mg

500 mg

750 mg

Levaquin™
Ortho-McNeil Pharmaceutical

NDC 65086-135-05
QUIXIN™
(levofloxacin ophthalmic
solution 0.5%)
Sterile

5 mL
Santen

0.5%, 5 mL
ophthalmic solution

Quixin™
Santen Inc.

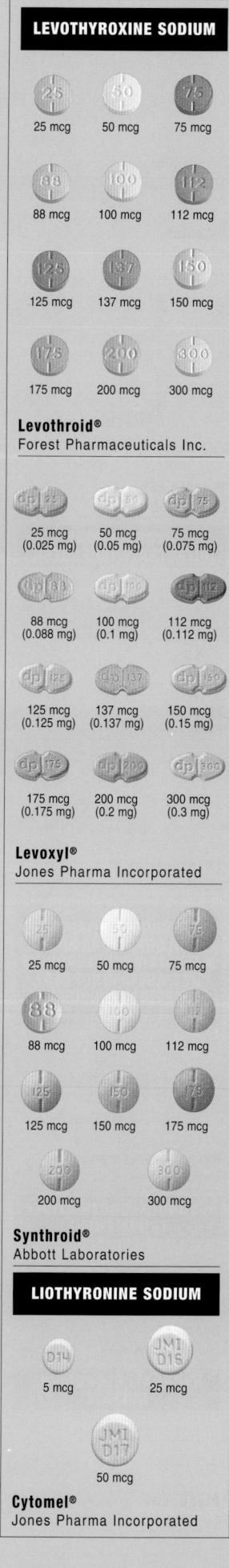

LEVOTHYROXINE SODIUM

25 mcg   50 mcg   75 mcg

88 mcg   100 mcg   112 mcg

125 mcg   137 mcg   150 mcg

175 mcg   200 mcg   300 mcg

Levothroid®
Forest Pharmaceuticals Inc.

25 mcg   50 mcg   75 mcg
(0.025 mg)   (0.05 mg)   (0.075 mg)

88 mcg   100 mcg   112 mcg
(0.088 mg)   (0.1 mg)   (0.112 mg)

125 mcg   137 mcg   150 mcg
(0.125 mg)   (0.137 mg)   (0.15 mg)

175 mcg   200 mcg   300 mcg
(0.175 mg)   (0.2 mg)   (0.3 mg)

Levoxyl®
Jones Pharma Incorporated

25 mcg   50 mcg   75 mcg

88 mcg   100 mcg   112 mcg

125 mcg   150 mcg   175 mcg

200 mcg   300 mcg

Synthroid®
Abbott Laboratories

LIOTHYRONINE SODIUM

5 mcg   25 mcg

50 mcg

Cytomel®
Jones Pharma Incorporated

LIOTRIX

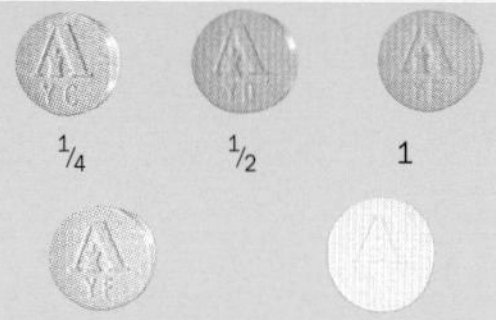

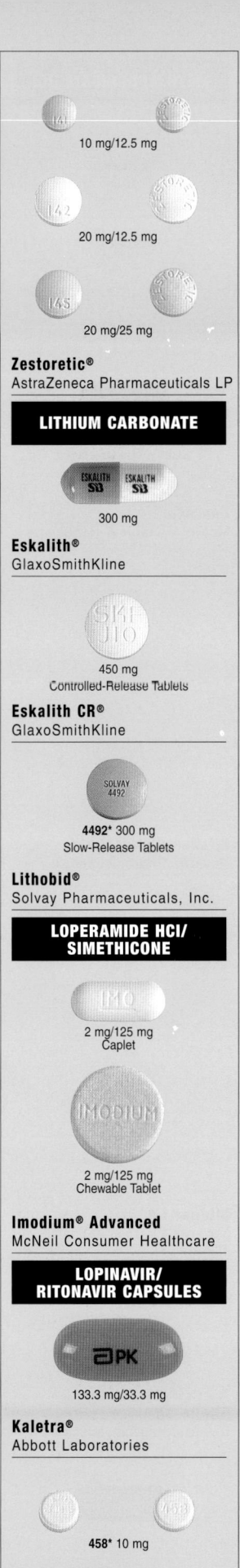

1/4 1/2 1

2 3

Thyrolar®
Forest Pharmaceuticals Inc.

(LISINOPRIL)

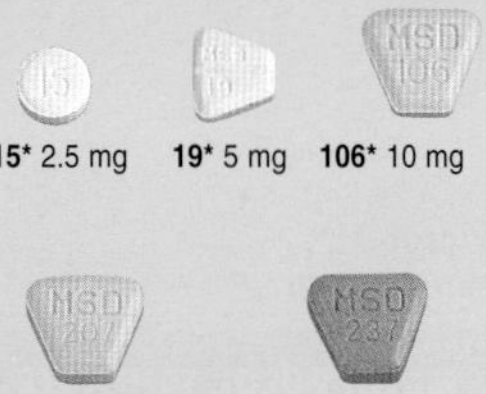

15* 2.5 mg **19*** 5 mg **106*** 10 mg

207* 20 mg **237*** 40 mg

Prinivil®
Merck & Co., Inc.

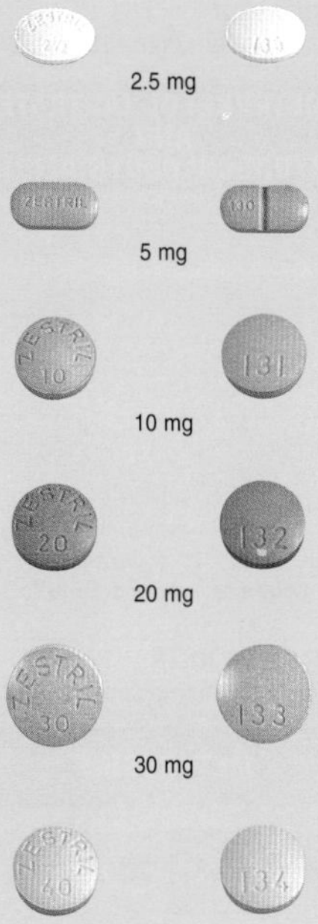

2.5 mg

5 mg

10 mg

20 mg

30 mg

40 mg

Zestril®
AstraZeneca Pharmaceuticals LP

LISINOPRIL/ HYDROCHLOROTHIAZIDE

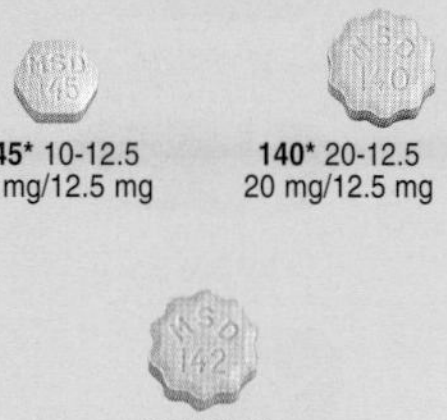

145* 10-12.5
10 mg/12.5 mg

140* 20-12.5
20 mg/12.5 mg

142* 20-25
20 mg/25 mg

Prinzide®
Merck & Co., Inc.

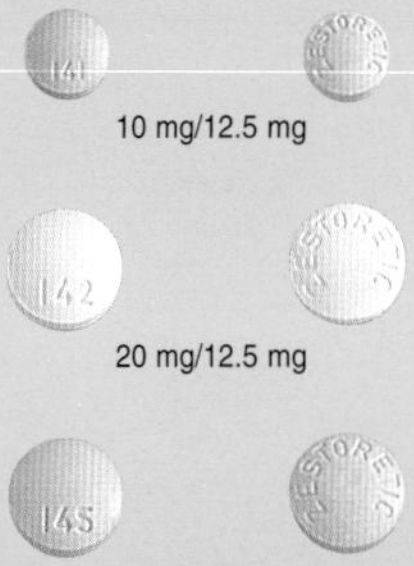

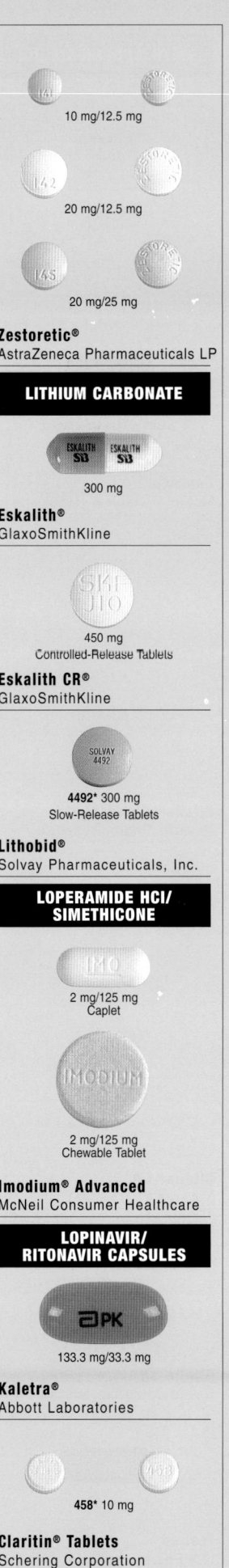

10 mg/12.5 mg

20 mg/12.5 mg

20 mg/25 mg

Zestoretic®
AstraZeneca Pharmaceuticals LP

LITHIUM CARBONATE

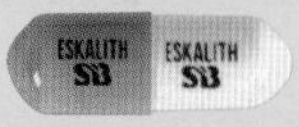

300 mg

Eskalith®
GlaxoSmithKline

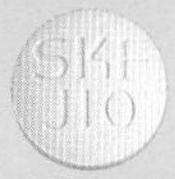

450 mg
Controlled-Release Tablets

Eskalith CR®
GlaxoSmithKline

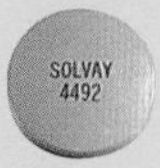

4492* 300 mg
Slow-Release Tablets

Lithobid®
Solvay Pharmaceuticals, Inc.

LOPERAMIDE HCl/ SIMETHICONE

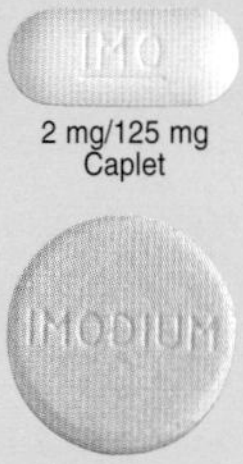

2 mg/125 mg
Caplet

2 mg/125 mg
Chewable Tablet

Imodium® Advanced
McNeil Consumer Healthcare

LOPINAVIR/ RITONAVIR CAPSULES

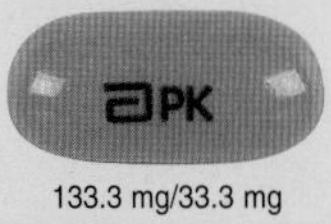

133.3 mg/33.3 mg

Kaletra®
Abbott Laboratories

458* 10 mg

Claritin® Tablets
Schering Corporation

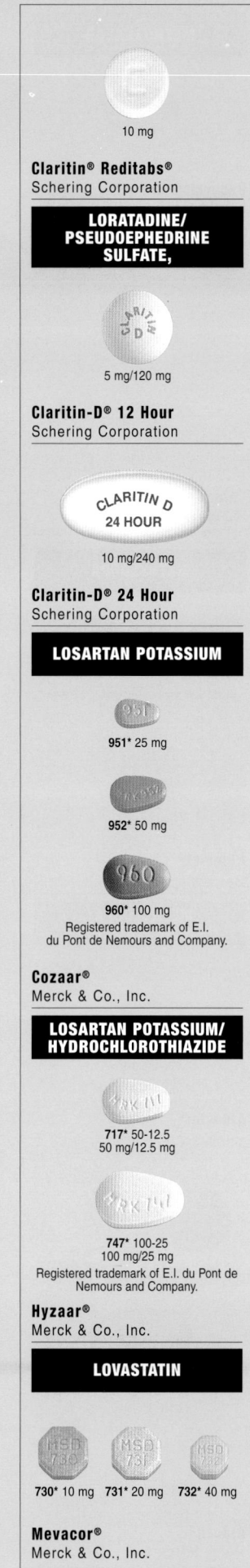

10 mg

Claritin® Reditabs®
Schering Corporation

LORATADINE/ PSEUDOEPHEDRINE SULFATE,

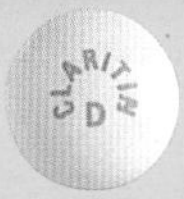

5 mg/120 mg

Claritin-D® 12 Hour
Schering Corporation

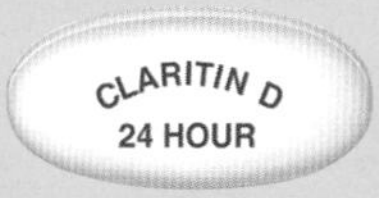

10 mg/240 mg

Claritin-D® 24 Hour
Schering Corporation

LOSARTAN POTASSIUM

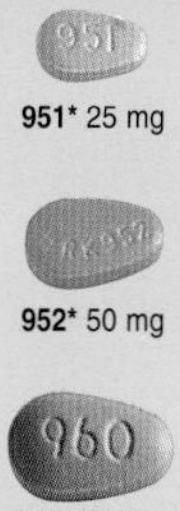

951* 25 mg

952* 50 mg

960* 100 mg
Registered trademark of E.I. du Pont de Nemours and Company.

Cozaar®
Merck & Co., Inc.

LOSARTAN POTASSIUM/ HYDROCHLOROTHIAZIDE

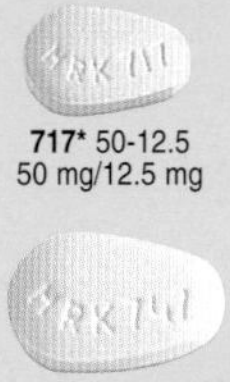

717* 50-12.5
50 mg/12.5 mg

747* 100-25
100 mg/25 mg
Registered trademark of E.I. du Pont de Nemours and Company.

Hyzaar®
Merck & Co., Inc.

LOVASTATIN

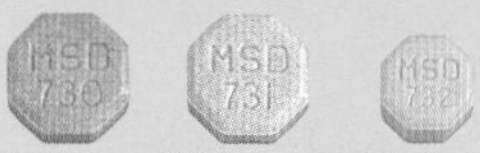

730* 10 mg **731*** 20 mg **732*** 40 mg

Mevacor®
Merck & Co., Inc.

MEBENDAZOLE

100 mg
Chewable Tablets

Vermox®
McNeil Consumer Healthcare

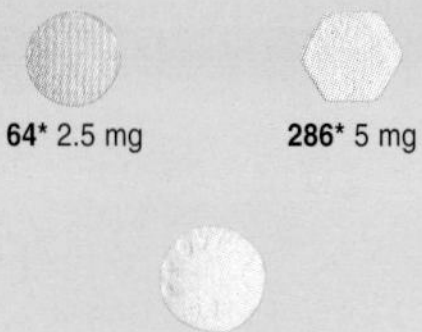

64* 2.5 mg **286*** 5 mg

50* 10 mg

Provera®
Pharmacia & Upjohn

MEFENAMIC ACID

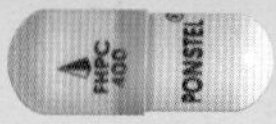

250 mg

Ponstel®
First Horizon Pharmaceutical

MEFLOQUINE HCl

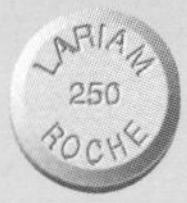

250 mg

Lariam®
Roche

MELOXICAM

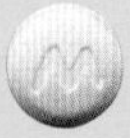

7.5 mg

Mobic®
Boehringer Ingelheim

MELPHALAN

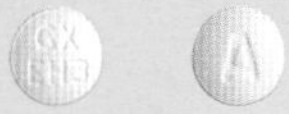

2 mg

Alkeran®
GlaxoSmithKline

MEPERIDINE HCL

D35* 50 mg
Scored tablet

D37* 100 mg

†Demerol®
Sanofi-Synthelabo, Inc.

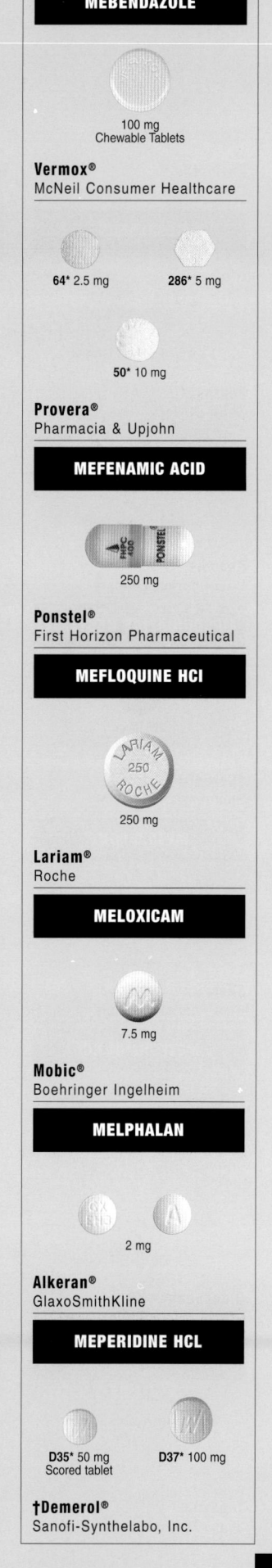

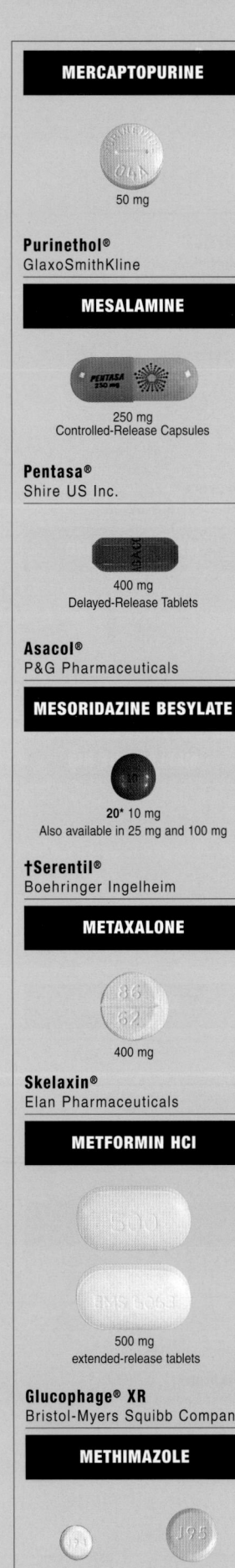

MERCAPTOPURINE

50 mg

Purinethol®
GlaxoSmithKline

MESALAMINE

250 mg
Controlled-Release Capsules

Pentasa®
Shire US Inc.

400 mg
Delayed-Release Tablets

Asacol®
P&G Pharmaceuticals

MESORIDAZINE BESYLATE

20* 10 mg
Also available in 25 mg and 100 mg

†Serentil®
Boehringer Ingelheim

METAXALONE

400 mg

Skelaxin®
Elan Pharmaceuticals

METFORMIN HCl

500 mg
extended-release tablets

Glucophage® XR
Bristol-Myers Squibb Company

METHIMAZOLE

5 mg   10 mg

Tapazole®
Jones Pharma Incorporated

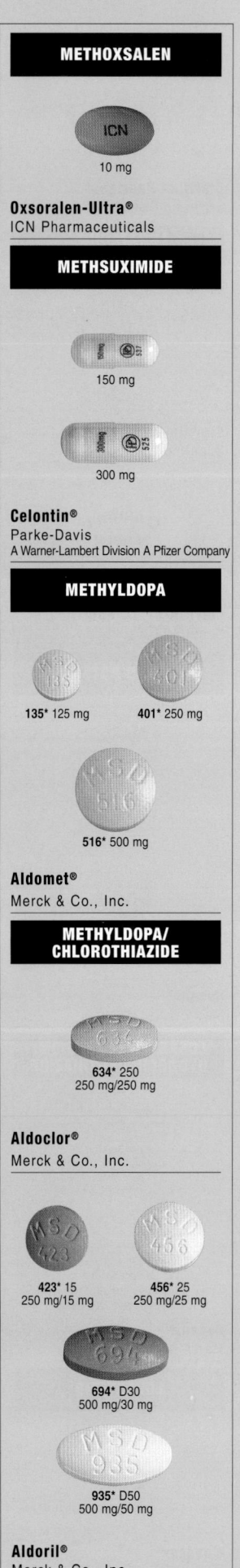

METHOXSALEN

10 mg

Oxsoralen-Ultra®
ICN Pharmaceuticals

METHSUXIMIDE

150 mg

300 mg

Celontin®
Parke-Davis
A Warner-Lambert Division A Pfizer Company

METHYLDOPA

135* 125 mg   **401*** 250 mg

516* 500 mg

Aldomet®
Merck & Co., Inc.

METHYLDOPA/ CHLOROTHIAZIDE

634* 250
250 mg/250 mg

Aldoclor®
Merck & Co., Inc.

423* 15   **456*** 25
250 mg/15 mg   250 mg/25 mg

694* D30
500 mg/30 mg

935* D50
500 mg/50 mg

Aldoril®
Merck & Co., Inc.

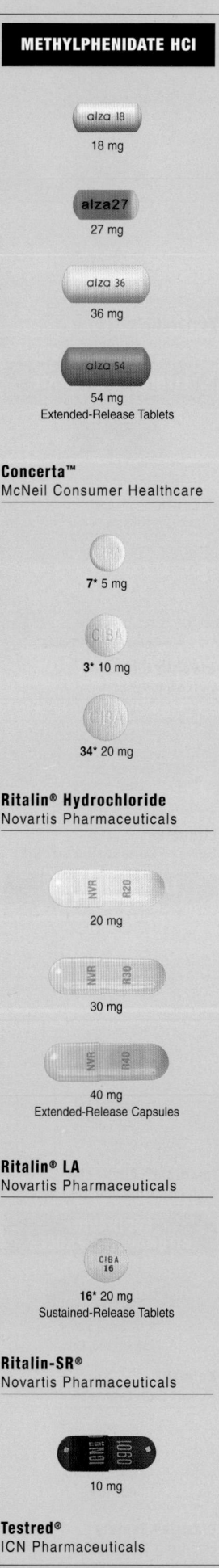

METHYLPHENIDATE HCl

alza 18
18 mg

alza27
27 mg

alza 36
36 mg

alza 54
54 mg
Extended-Release Tablets

Concerta™
McNeil Consumer Healthcare

7* 5 mg

3* 10 mg

34* 20 mg

Ritalin® Hydrochloride
Novartis Pharmaceuticals

20 mg

30 mg

40 mg
Extended-Release Capsules

Ritalin® LA
Novartis Pharmaceuticals

16* 20 mg
Sustained-Release Tablets

Ritalin-SR®
Novartis Pharmaceuticals

10 mg

Testred®
ICN Pharmaceuticals

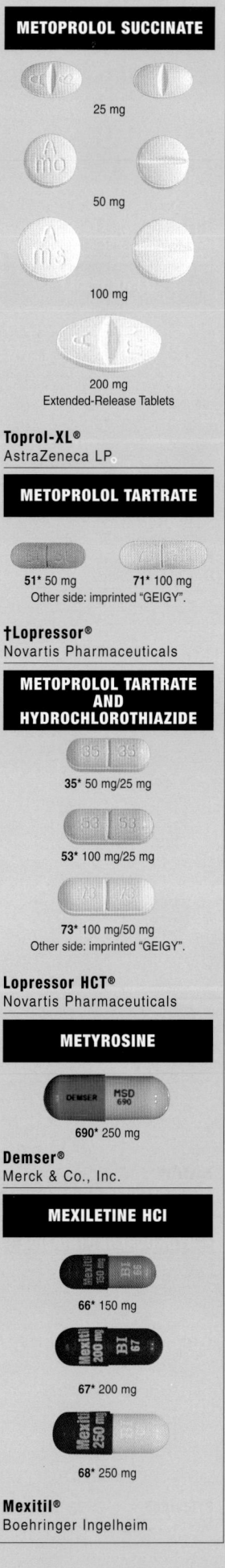

METOPROLOL SUCCINATE

25 mg

50 mg

100 mg

200 mg
Extended-Release Tablets

Toprol-XL®
AstraZeneca LP.

METOPROLOL TARTRATE

51* 50 mg   **71*** 100 mg
Other side: imprinted "GEIGY".

†Lopressor®
Novartis Pharmaceuticals

METOPROLOL TARTRATE AND HYDROCHLOROTHIAZIDE

35* 50 mg/25 mg

53* 100 mg/25 mg

73* 100 mg/50 mg
Other side: imprinted "GEIGY".

Lopressor HCT®
Novartis Pharmaceuticals

METYROSINE

690* 250 mg

Demser®
Merck & Co., Inc.

MEXILETINE HCl

66* 150 mg

67* 200 mg

68* 250 mg

Mexitil®
Boehringer Ingelheim

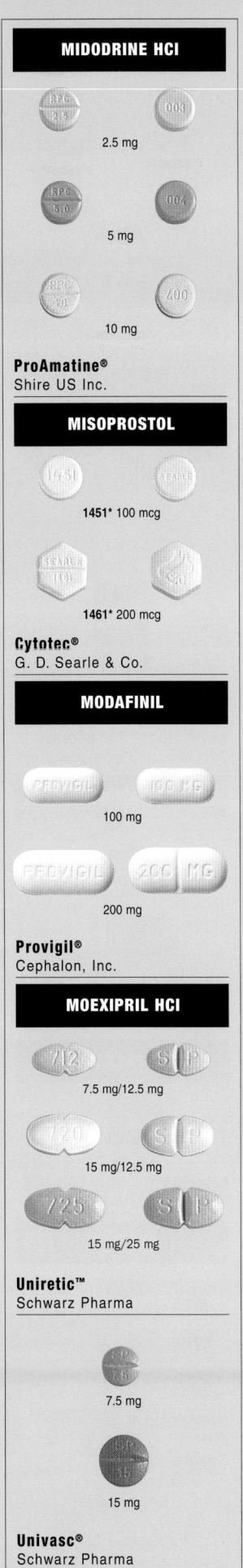

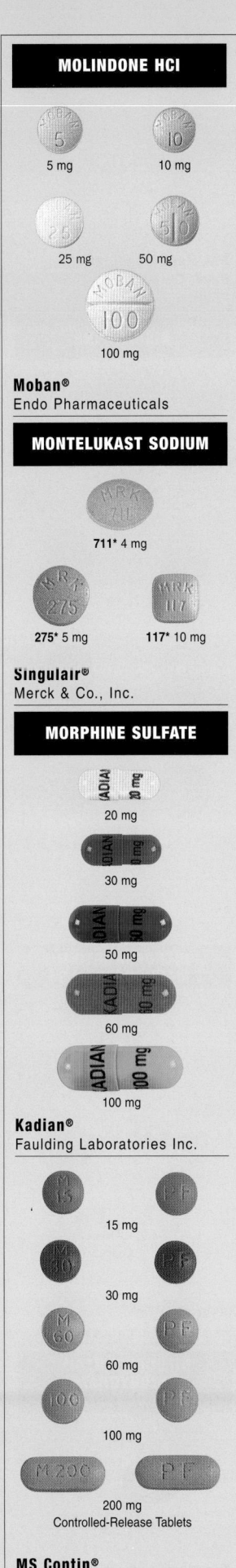

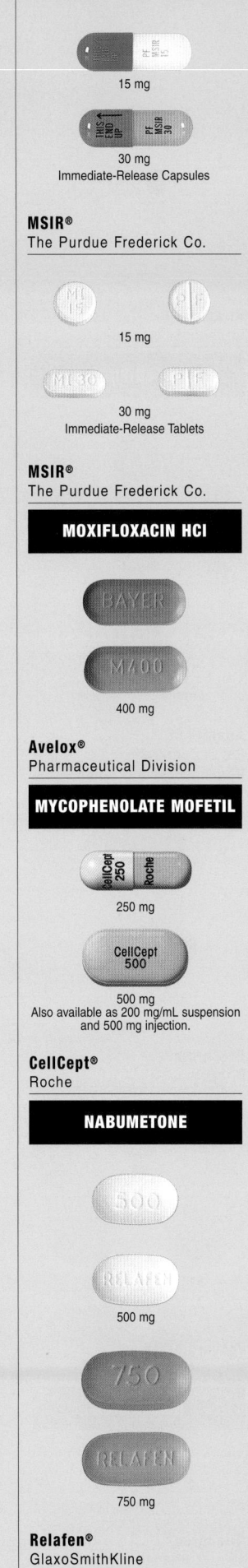

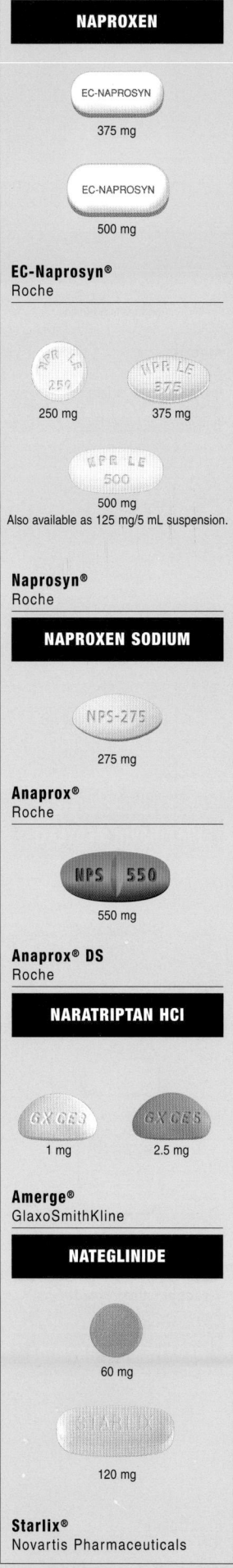

MIDODRINE HCl

2.5 mg

5 mg

10 mg

ProAmatine®
Shire US Inc.

MISOPROSTOL

1451* 100 mcg

1461* 200 mcg

Cytotec®
G. D. Searle & Co.

MODAFINIL

100 mg

200 mg

Provigil®
Cephalon, Inc.

MOEXIPRIL HCl

7.5 mg/12.5 mg

15 mg/12.5 mg

15 mg/25 mg

Uniretic™
Schwarz Pharma

7.5 mg

15 mg

Univasc®
Schwarz Pharma

MOLINDONE HCl

5 mg

10 mg

25 mg

50 mg

100 mg

Moban®
Endo Pharmaceuticals

MONTELUKAST SODIUM

711* 4 mg

275* 5 mg

117* 10 mg

Singulair®
Merck & Co., Inc.

MORPHINE SULFATE

20 mg

30 mg

50 mg

60 mg

100 mg

Kadian®
Faulding Laboratories Inc.

15 mg

30 mg

60 mg

100 mg

200 mg
Controlled-Release Tablets

MS Contin®
The Purdue Frederick Co.

15 mg

30 mg
Immediate-Release Capsules

MSIR®
The Purdue Frederick Co.

15 mg

30 mg
Immediate-Release Tablets

MSIR®
The Purdue Frederick Co.

MOXIFLOXACIN HCl

400 mg

Avelox®
Pharmaceutical Division

MYCOPHENOLATE MOFETIL

250 mg

500 mg
Also available as 200 mg/mL suspension
and 500 mg injection.

CellCept®
Roche

NABUMETONE

500 mg

750 mg

Relafen®
GlaxoSmithKline

NAPROXEN

375 mg

500 mg

EC-Naprosyn®
Roche

250 mg

375 mg

500 mg
Also available as 125 mg/5 mL suspension.

Naprosyn®
Roche

NAPROXEN SODIUM

275 mg

Anaprox®
Roche

550 mg

Anaprox® DS
Roche

NARATRIPTAN HCl

1 mg

2.5 mg

Amerge®
GlaxoSmithKline

NATEGLINIDE

60 mg

120 mg

Starlix®
Novartis Pharmaceuticals

MC 15

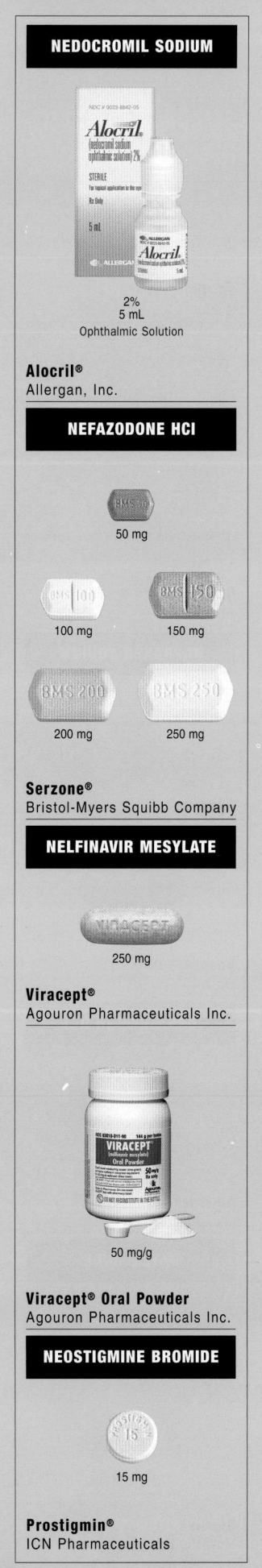

NEDOCROMIL SODIUM

2%
5 mL
Ophthalmic Solution

Alocril®
Allergan, Inc.

NEFAZODONE HCl

50 mg

100 mg

150 mg

200 mg

250 mg

Serzone®
Bristol-Myers Squibb Company

NELFINAVIR MESYLATE

250 mg

Viracept®
Agouron Pharmaceuticals Inc.

50 mg/g

Viracept® Oral Powder
Agouron Pharmaceuticals Inc.

NEOSTIGMINE BROMIDE

15 mg

Prostigmin®
ICN Pharmaceuticals

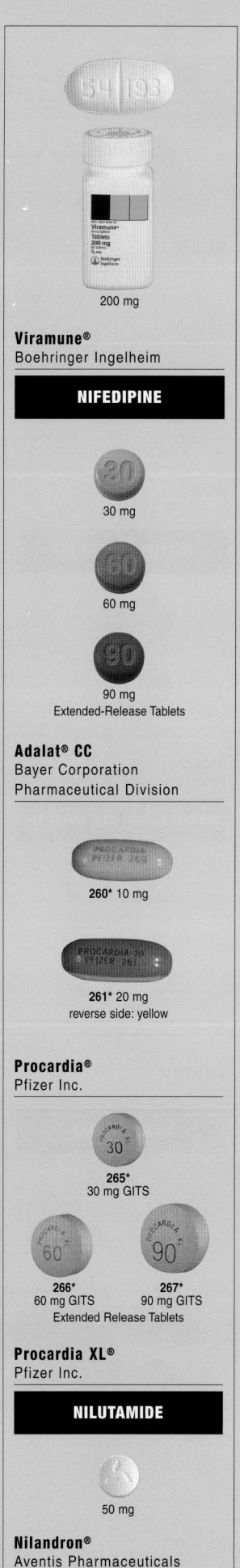

200 mg

Viramune®
Boehringer Ingelheim

NIFEDIPINE

30 mg

60 mg

90 mg
Extended-Release Tablets

Adalat® CC
Bayer Corporation
Pharmaceutical Division

260* 10 mg

261* 20 mg
reverse side: yellow

Procardia®
Pfizer Inc.

265*
30 mg GITS

266*
60 mg GITS

267*
90 mg GITS
Extended Release Tablets

Procardia XL®
Pfizer Inc.

NILUTAMIDE

50 mg

Nilandron®
Aventis Pharmaceuticals

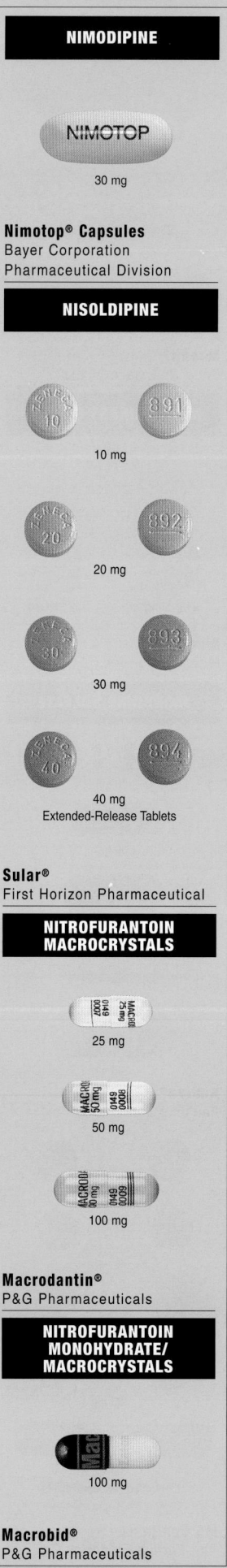

NIMODIPINE

NIMOTOP

30 mg

Nimotop® Capsules
Bayer Corporation
Pharmaceutical Division

NISOLDIPINE

10 mg

20 mg

30 mg

40 mg
Extended-Release Tablets

Sular®
First Horizon Pharmaceutical

NITROFURANTOIN MACROCRYSTALS

25 mg

50 mg

100 mg

Macrodantin®
P&G Pharmaceuticals

NITROFURANTOIN MONOHYDRATE/ MACROCRYSTALS

100 mg

Macrobid®
P&G Pharmaceuticals

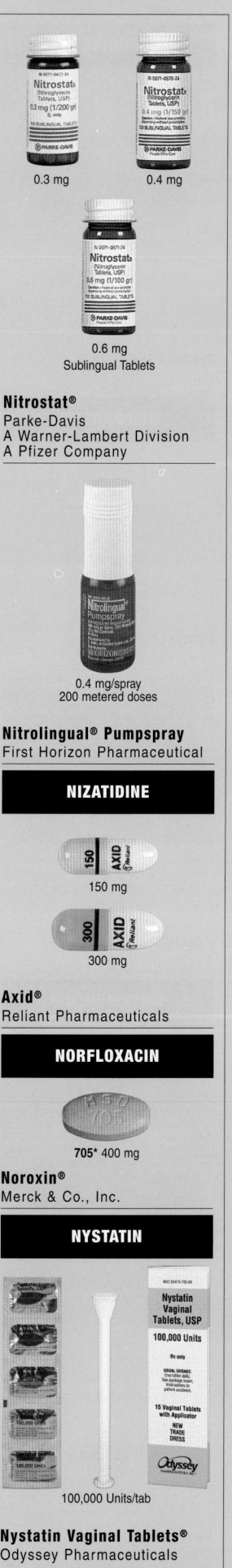

0.3 mg   0.4 mg

0.6 mg
Sublingual Tablets

Nitrostat®
Parke-Davis
A Warner-Lambert Division
A Pfizer Company

0.4 mg/spray
200 metered doses

Nitrolingual® Pumpspray
First Horizon Pharmaceutical

NIZATIDINE

150 mg

300 mg

Axid®
Reliant Pharmaceuticals

NORFLOXACIN

705* 400 mg

Noroxin®
Merck & Co., Inc.

NYSTATIN

100,000 Units/tab

Nystatin Vaginal Tablets®
Odyssey Pharmaceuticals

OFLOXACIN

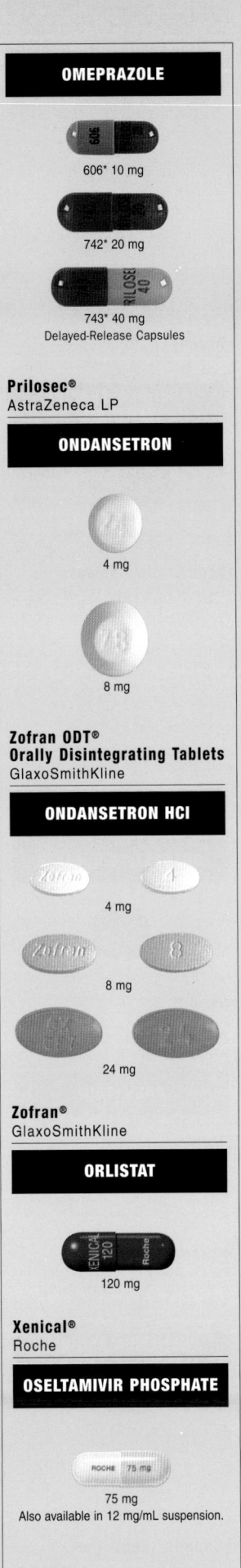

5 mL   10 mL
0.3%

Floxin® Otic
Daiichi Pharmaceutical Corp.

0.3%
5 mL
Also available in 10 mL

Ocuflox®
Allergan, Inc.

OLANZAPINE

15 mg

LILLY
4420
20 mg

Zyprexa®
Eli Lilly & Company

LILLY 4112 — 2.5 mg
LILLY 4115 — 5 mg
LILLY 4116 — 7.5 mg
LILLY 4117 — 10 mg

Zyprexa®
Eli Lilly & Company

OLMESARTAN MEDOXOMIL

5 mg   20 mg

SANKYO
40 mg

Benicar™
Sankyo Pharma, Inc.

OMEPRAZOLE

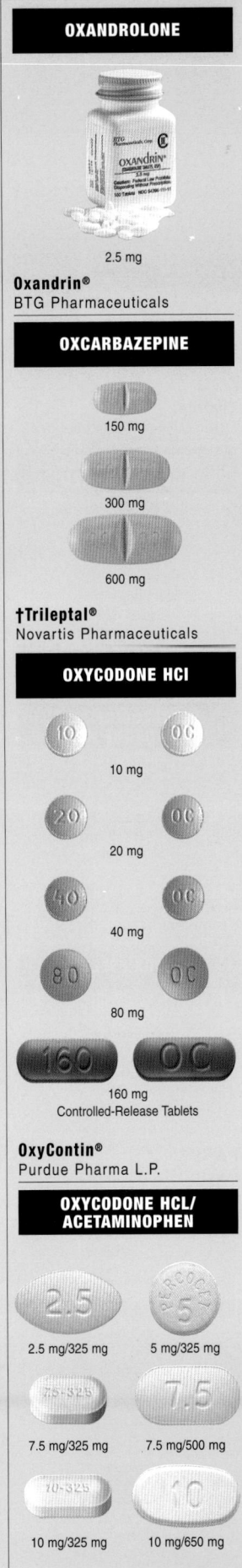

606* 10 mg

742* 20 mg

743* 40 mg
Delayed-Release Capsules

Prilosec®
AstraZeneca LP

ONDANSETRON

4 mg

8 mg

Zofran ODT®
Orally Disintegrating Tablets
GlaxoSmithKline

ONDANSETRON HCl

Zofran / 4
4 mg

Zofran / 8
8 mg

24 mg

Zofran®
GlaxoSmithKline

ORLISTAT

XENICAL 120
120 mg

Xenical®
Roche

OSELTAMIVIR PHOSPHATE

ROCHE 75 mg
75 mg
Also available in 12 mg/mL suspension.

Tamiflu™
Roche

OXANDROLONE

2.5 mg

Oxandrin®
BTG Pharmaceuticals

OXCARBAZEPINE

150 mg

300 mg

600 mg

†Trileptal®
Novartis Pharmaceuticals

OXYCODONE HCl

10   OC
10 mg

20   OC
20 mg

40   OC
40 mg

80   OC
80 mg

160   OC
160 mg
Controlled-Release Tablets

OxyContin®
Purdue Pharma L.P.

OXYCODONE HCl/
ACETAMINOPHEN

2.5 — 2.5 mg/325 mg
PERCOCET 5 — 5 mg/325 mg
75-325 — 7.5 mg/325 mg
7.5 — 7.5 mg/500 mg
10-325 — 10 mg/325 mg
10 — 10 mg/650 mg

Percocet®
Endo Pharmaceuticals

OXYCODONE HCl/
OXYCODONE
TEREPHTHALATE/ASPIRIN

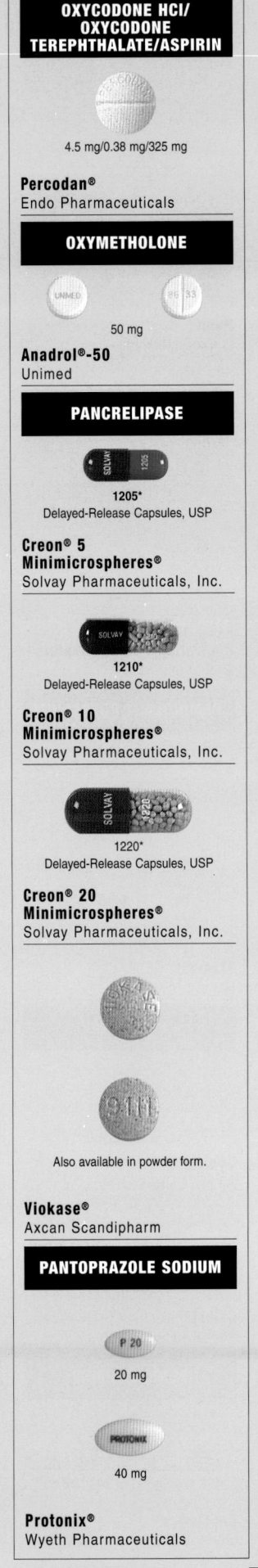

4.5 mg/0.38 mg/325 mg

Percodan®
Endo Pharmaceuticals

OXYMETHOLONE

UNIMED   85 33
50 mg

Anadrol®-50
Unimed

PANCRELIPASE

SOLVAY 1205
1205*
Delayed-Release Capsules, USP

Creon® 5
Minimicrospheres®
Solvay Pharmaceuticals, Inc.

SOLVAY
1210*
Delayed-Release Capsules, USP

Creon® 10
Minimicrospheres®
Solvay Pharmaceuticals, Inc.

SOLVAY 1220
1220*
Delayed-Release Capsules, USP

Creon® 20
Minimicrospheres®
Solvay Pharmaceuticals, Inc.

Also available in powder form.

Viokase®
Axcan Scandipharm

PANTOPRAZOLE SODIUM

P 20
20 mg

PROTONIX
40 mg

Protonix®
Wyeth Pharmaceuticals

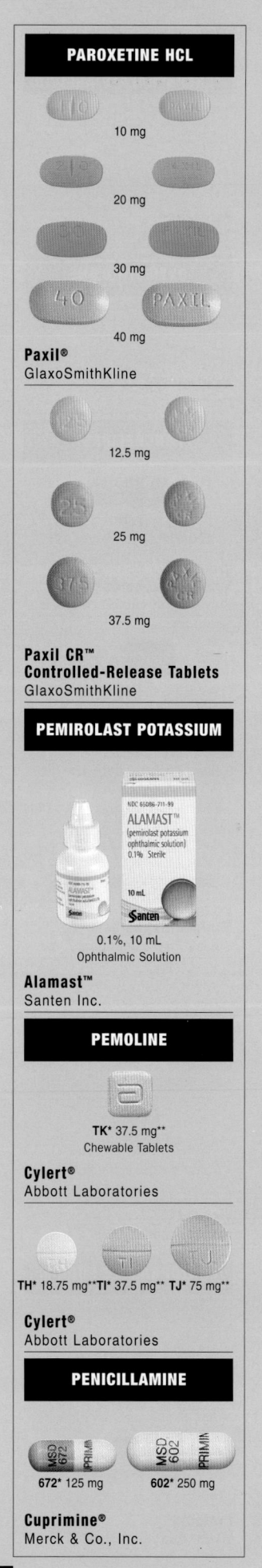

PAROXETINE HCL

10 mg

20 mg

30 mg

40 mg

Paxil®
GlaxoSmithKline

12.5 mg

25 mg

37.5 mg

Paxil CR™
Controlled-Release Tablets
GlaxoSmithKline

PEMIROLAST POTASSIUM

0.1%, 10 mL
Ophthalmic Solution

Alamast™
Santen Inc.

PEMOLINE

TK* 37.5 mg**
Chewable Tablets

Cylert®
Abbott Laboratories

TH* 18.75 mg** **TI*** 37.5 mg** **TJ*** 75 mg**

Cylert®
Abbott Laboratories

PENICILLAMINE

672* 125 mg   **602*** 250 mg

Cuprimine®
Merck & Co., Inc.

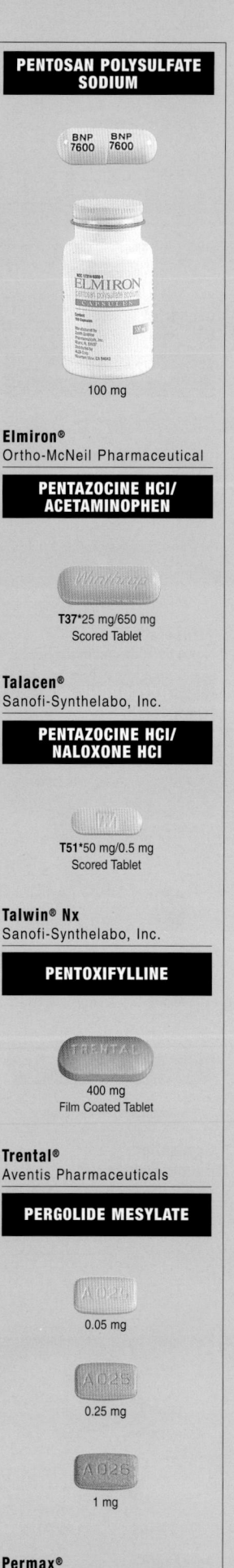

PENTOSAN POLYSULFATE
SODIUM

BNP 7600   BNP 7600

100 mg

Elmiron®
Ortho-McNeil Pharmaceutical

PENTAZOCINE HCl/
ACETAMINOPHEN

T37*25 mg/650 mg
Scored Tablet

Talacen®
Sanofi-Synthelabo, Inc.

PENTAZOCINE HCl/
NALOXONE HCl

T51*50 mg/0.5 mg
Scored Tablet

Talwin® Nx
Sanofi-Synthelabo, Inc.

PENTOXIFYLLINE

400 mg
Film Coated Tablet

Trental®
Aventis Pharmaceuticals

PERGOLIDE MESYLATE

0.05 mg

0.25 mg

1 mg

Permax®
Amarin Pharmaceuticals Inc.

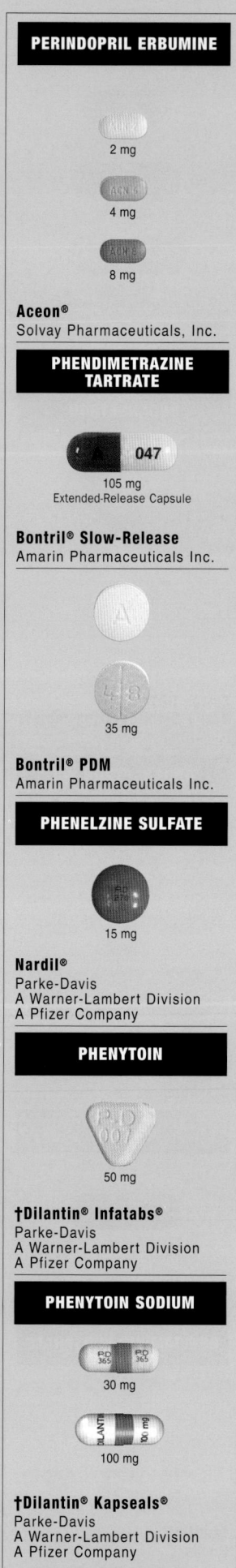

PERINDOPRIL ERBUMINE

2 mg

4 mg

8 mg

Aceon®
Solvay Pharmaceuticals, Inc.

PHENDIMETRAZINE
TARTRATE

047

105 mg
Extended-Release Capsule

Bontril® Slow-Release
Amarin Pharmaceuticals Inc.

35 mg

Bontril® PDM
Amarin Pharmaceuticals Inc.

PHENELZINE SULFATE

15 mg

Nardil®
Parke-Davis
A Warner-Lambert Division
A Pfizer Company

PHENYTOIN

50 mg

†Dilantin® Infatabs®
Parke-Davis
A Warner-Lambert Division
A Pfizer Company

PHENYTOIN SODIUM

30 mg

100 mg

†Dilantin® Kapseals®
Parke-Davis
A Warner-Lambert Erivision
A Pfizer Company

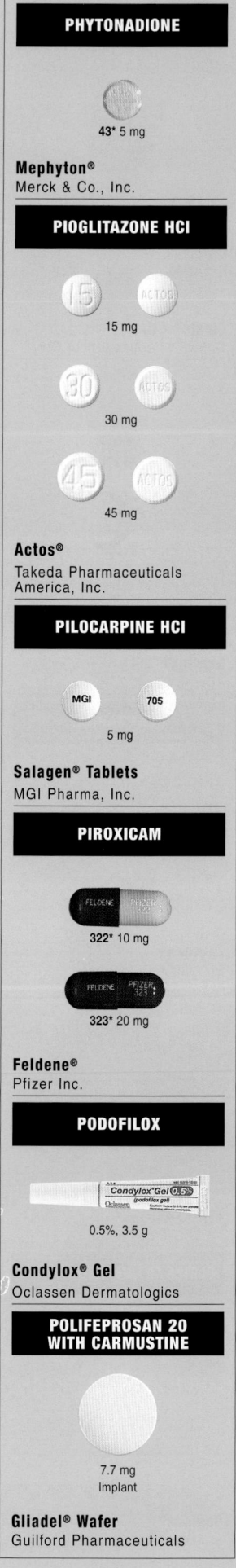

PHYTONADIONE

43* 5 mg

Mephyton®
Merck & Co., Inc.

PIOGLITAZONE HCl

15 mg

30 mg

45 mg

Actos®
Takeda Pharmaceuticals
America, Inc.

PILOCARPINE HCl

MGI   705

5 mg

Salagen® Tablets
MGI Pharma, Inc.

PIROXICAM

322* 10 mg

323* 20 mg

Feldene®
Pfizer Inc.

PODOFILOX

0.5%, 3.5 g

Condylox® Gel
Oclassen Dermatologics

POLIFEPROSAN 20
WITH CARMUSTINE

7.7 mg
Implant

Gliadel® Wafer
Guilford Pharmaceuticals

Section XI: Index

See Appendix A (p. **I/622**) and Appendix B (p. **I/668**) of the "Approved Drug Products with Therapeutic Equivalence Evaluations" section of this volume for listings of the products included in the Orange Book.

A

Fluoxymesterone
Fluoxymesterone USP, **IV**/256
Tablets USP, **IV**/256
Fluoxymesterone and Ethinyl Estradiol
Tablets, **IV**/256
Flupenthixol Decanoate
Injection, **IV**/256, 256
Flupenthixol Dihydrochloride
Tablets, **IV**/256
Fluphenazine Decanoate
Fluphenazine Decanoate USP, **IV**/257
Injection USP, **IV**/257
Fluphenazine Enanthate
Fluphenazine Enanthate USP, **IV**/257
Injection USP, **IV**/257
Fluphenazine Hydrochloride
Elixir USP, **IV**/257
Fluphenazine Hydrochloride USP, **IV**/257
Injection USP, **IV**/257
Solution, Oral, USP, **IV**/257
Tablets USP, **IV**/257
Flurandrenolide
Cream USP, **IV**/257
Flurandrenolide USP, **IV**/257
Lotion USP, **IV**/257
Ointment USP, **IV**/257
Tape USP, **IV**/257
Flurazepam Hydrochloride
Capsules USP, **IV**/258
Flurazepam Hydrochloride USP, **IV**/258
Flurazepam Monohydrochloride
Tablets, **IV**/258
Flurbiprofen
Capsules, Extended-release, **IV**/258
Flurbiprofen USP, **IV**/258
Tablets USP, **IV**/258
Flurbiprofen Sodium
Flurbiprofen Sodium USP, **IV**/258
Solution, Ophthalmic, USP, **IV**/258
Fluspirilene
Injection, **IV**/258
Flutamide
Capsules USP, **IV**/258
Flutamide USP, **IV**/258
Tablets, **IV**/258
Fluticasone Propionate
Aerosol, Inhalation, **IV**/259
Cream, **IV**/259
Ointment, **IV**/259
Powder for Inhalation, **IV**/259
Suspension, Nasal, **IV**/259
Fluvastatin Sodium
Capsules, **IV**/259
Fluvoxamine Maleate
Tablets, **IV**/259
Folic Acid
Folic Acid USP, **IV**/259
Injection USP, **IV**/259
Tablets USP, **IV**/259
Follitropin Alfa
for Injection, **IV**/259
Follitropin Beta
for Injection, **IV**/259
Fomepizole
Injection, **IV**/260
Fomivirsen Sodium
Injection, Intravitreal, **IV**/260
Fondaparinux Sodium
Injection, **IV**/260
Formaldehyde
Solution USP, **IV**/260
Formoterol Fumarate
Capsules for Inhalation, **IV**/260
Formoterol Fumarate Dihydrate
Powder for Inhalation, **IV**/260

Foscarnet Sodium
Injection, **IV**/261
Fosfomycin Tromethamine
for Solution, Oral, **IV**/261
Fosinopril Sodium
Tablets, **IV**/261
Fosphenytoin Sodium
Fosphenytoin Sodium USP, **IV**/261
Injection, **IV**/261
Framycetin Sulfate
Gauze, Impregnated, **IV**/261
Ointment, Ophthalmic, **IV**/261
Solution, Ophthalmic, **IV**/261
Framycetin Sulfate and Gramicidin
Ointment, **IV**/261
Framycetin Sulfate, Gramidicin, and Dexamethasone
Ointment, Ophthalmic, **IV**/261
Ointment, Otic, **IV**/261
Solution, Ophthalmic, **IV**/261
Solution, Otic, **IV**/261
Fructose
Fructose USP, **IV**/261
Injection USP, **IV**/262
Fructose, Dextrose, and Phosphoric Acid
Solution, Oral, **IV**/262
Fructose and Sodium Chloride
Injection USP, **IV**/262
Fuchsin, Basic
Basic Fuchsin USP, **IV**/262
Fulvestrant
Injection, **IV**/262
Fumaric Acid
Fumaric Acid NF, **IV**/262
Furazolidone
Furazolidone USP, **IV**/262
Suspension, Oral, USP, **IV**/262
Tablets USP, **IV**/262
Furosemide
Furosemide USP, **IV**/263
Injection USP, **IV**/263
Solution, Oral, USP, **IV**/263
Tablets USP, **IV**/263
Fusidic Acid
Cream, **IV**/263
Gauze, Impregnated, **IV**/263
for Injection, **IV**/263
Ointment, **IV**/263
Suspension, Hemihydrate, **IV**/263
Suspension, Oral, **IV**/263
Tablets, **IV**/263

G

Gabapentin
Capsules, **IV**/263
Gadodiamide
Gadodiamide USP, **IV**/263
Injection USP, **IV**/263
Gadopentetate Dimeglumine
Injection USP, **IV**/264
Gadoteridol
Gadoteridol USP, **IV**/264
Injection USP, **IV**/264
Gadoversetamide
Injection, **IV**/264
Galageenan
Galageenan NF, **IV**/264
Galantamine
Tablets, **IV**/264
Gallamine Triethiodide
Gallamine Triethiodide USP, **IV**/265
Injection USP, **IV**/265

Gallium Citrate Ga 67
Injection USP, **IV**/265
Gallium Nitrate
Injection, **IV**/265
Ganciclovir
Capsules, **IV**/265
Ganciclovir USP, **IV**/265
Implant, Intravitreal, **IV**/265
for Injection USP, **IV**/265
Ganciclovir Sodium, Sterile
Sterile Ganciclovir Sodium, **IV**/265
Ganirelix Acetate
Injection, **IV**/266
Garlic
Extract, Powdered, **IV**/266
Fluidextract NF, **IV**/266
Garlic NF, **IV**/266
Powdered NF, **IV**/266
Tablets, Delayed-release, NF, **IV**/266
Gatifloxacin
Solution, Intravenous, **IV**/266
Tablets, **IV**/266
Gauze, Absorbent
Absorbent Gauze USP, **IV**/266
Gauze, Petrolatum
Petrolatum Gauze USP, **IV**/267
Gelatin
Gelatin NF, **IV**/267
Gelatin, Absorbable
Film USP, **IV**/267
Sponge USP, **IV**/267
Gemcitabine
for Injection, **IV**/267
Gemcitabine Hydrochloride
for Injection, **IV**/267
Gemfibrozil
Capsules USP, **IV**/268
Gemfibrozil USP, **IV**/268
Tablets USP, **IV**/268
Gemtuzumab Ozogamicin
for Injection, **IV**/268
General Chapters, VI/3
Gentamicin
Infusion, Uterine, **IV**/268
Injection, Liposome, **IV**/268
Injection USP, **IV**/268
Gentamicin and Prednisolone Acetate
Ointment, Ophthalmic, USP, **IV**/269
Suspension, Ophthalmic, USP, **IV**/269
Gentamicin Sulfate
Cream USP, **IV**/268
Gentamicin Sulfate USP, **IV**/268
Ointment, Ophthalmic, USP, **IV**/268
Ointment USP, **IV**/268
Solution, Ophthalmic, USP, **IV**/268
Solution, Otic, **IV**/268
Gentamicin Sulfate and Betamethasone Acetate
Solution, Ophthalmic, USP, **IV**/268
Gentamicin Sulfate and Betamethasone Valerate
Solution, Otic, USP, **IV**/269
Solution, Topical, USP, **IV**/269
Ointment USP, **IV**/269
Gentamicin Sulfate in Sodium Chloride
Injection, **IV**/269
Gentian Violet
Cream USP, **IV**/269
Gentian Violet USP, **IV**/269
Solution, Topical, USP, **IV**/269
Tampons, Vaginal, **IV**/269
Gentisic Acid Ethanolamide
Gentisic Acid Ethanolamide NF, **IV**/269
Ginger
Ginger NF, **IV**/270
Powdered NF, **IV**/270

Ordering Information

Mail Order: Thomson MICROMEDEX USP DI Customer Service   **Phone Order:** (800) 877-6209
                        P.O. Box 187   **Fax Order:**   (201) 722-2680
                        Montvale, NJ 07645-0187 USA

International Phone Order: For international orders, please call +1 201 358-2233 for a distributor near you.

Payment: Required in advance in U.S. dollars drawn on a U.S. bank. Any bank fees, customs duties, tariffs, and taxes are the customer's responsibility. Errors in fax transmissions are the responsibility of the sender. Prices subject to change without notice.

Sales Tax: Add appropriate sales tax to product costs for orders according to the sales tax schedule below the order form.

Drug Information Publications

2004 USP DI® Volume I
Drug Information for the Health Care Professional   ***New Off-label Uses Indices***
Organized in a concise, outline format, *Drug Information for the Health Care Professional*
contains medically accepted uses—labeled and off label—of more than 11,000 generic and
brand-name drug products throughout the United States and Canada.
Item Number: U20041   **ISBN:** 1-56363-463-5   **Price:** $174.00 plus S&H ($9.95)

2004 USP DI® Volume II
Advice for the Patient®, Drug Information in Lay Language
Written in patient-friendly terms, *Advice for the Patient* is specifically designed to make
important drug information easy to grasp. Simplified monographs provide detailed information
on proper drug use, available dosage forms, precautions, side effects, and special consideration.
Item Number: U20042   **ISBN:** 1-56363-464-3   **Price:** $93.00 plus S&H ($9.95)

2004 USP DI® Volume III
Approved Drug Products and Legal Requirements
Contains important therapeutic equivalence information and selected federal requirements that
affect the prescribing and dispensing of prescription drugs and controlled substances.
Item Number: U20043   **ISBN:** 1-56363-465-1   **Price:** $145.00 plus S&H ($9.95)

> **FREE** monthly updates on-line with purchase of any USP DI book or CD-ROM product.

Drug Information Software

Trusted USP DI® Drug Information on the Internet

Access USP DI information on the Internet. Easily find and search complete USP DI monographs found in Volume I, Drug Information for the Health Care Professional and Volume II, Advice for the Patient. For instant access to the most up-to-date drug information in the industry, simply type in the drug you're researching to find the latest USP DI monograph.
USP DI Internet Subscription Price: $199.00

USP DI® Desktop Series CD-ROM

Using an integrated search engine, you get easy access to the specific information you need. Includes comprehensive coverage on all USP DI professional and patient monographs. Annual subscriptions includes quarterly updates sent via CD-ROM, plus free monthly online updates. Subscriptions may start at any point in the year.
Stand-alone Version: ISBN: 1-56363-466-X   **Price:** $199.00
Network Version (2+ users): Call (800) 877-6209 for pricing.

FREE USP DI Updates On-Line

USP DI Updates On-line keeps you on top of developments in the pharmaceutical industry with monographs for the newest drugs and major revisions for existing monographs. With your purchase of any USP DI print book or CD-ROM product, you have FREE access to the site during the length of your subscription. The monographs are provided as PDF files so they are easy to view, save on disk, or print.

To visit USP DI Updates On-line, log on to the MICROMEDEX Web site at http://uspdi.micromedex.com. Then enter the USER NAME and PASSWORD listed below.

USER NAME: usp2004   **PASSWORD: newinfo**

If you have questions regarding USP DI Updates On-line, please contact Thomson MICROMEDEX at (800) 877-6209.

THOMSON

MICROMEDEX

Change of Address Notification
If your address has changed, please send your new address with your latest mailing label to:
Thomson MICROMEDEX USP DI   P.O. Box 187   Montvale, NJ 07645-0187

To order, remove this form, fill out completely, and mail to Thomson MICROMEDEX Customer Service Department with payment or credit card information. For faster service order by phone or fax.

Mail Order
Thomson MICROMEDEX USP DI Customer Service Department
P.O. Box 187
Montvale, NJ 07645-0187

Phone Order (800) 877-6209
Fax Order (201) 722-2680
International Phone Order For international orders, please call +1 201 358-2233 for a distributor near you.

Ordered By:

Name _____

Title _____

Company _____

E-mail _____

Street Address _____

City _____ State _____ Zip _____ Country _____

Phone (_____) _____ Fax (_____) _____

Ship To (Only complete if different):

Name _____

Title _____

Company _____

Street Address _____

City _____ State _____ Zip _____ Country _____

Phone (_____) _____ Fax (_____) _____

Payment Method

☐ Enclosed is my check payable to Thomson MICROMEDEX.

☐ VISA   ☐ MasterCard   ☐ Amex   ☐ Discover

Card No. _____ Exp. Date_____

Signature _____

Payment is required in advance in U.S. dollars drawn on a U.S. bank. Any bank fees, customs duties, tariffs, and taxes are the customer's responsibility. Errors in fax transmissions are the responsibility of the sender. Prices subject to change without notice. Please allow 2-4 weeks for normal delivery. Inquire for faster delivery (additional charge).

Valid for 2004 editions only, prices and shipping & handling higher outside U.S.

Item #	Description	Price	Quantity	Total Price	Domestic Shipping	Shipping Quantity	Total Shipping
U20041	2004 USP DI® Volume I, Drug Information for the Health Care Professional ISBN 1-56363-463-5	$174.00			$9.95		
U20042	2004 USP DI® Volume II, Advice for the Patient® Drug Information in Lay Language ISBN 1-56363-464-3	$ 93.00			$9.95		
U20043	2004 USP DI® Volume III, Approved Drug Products and Legal Requirements ISBN 1-56363-465-1	$145.00			$9.95		
USPCD	USP DI® Desktop Series CD-ROM Stand-Alone Version ISBN 1-56363-466-X Network Version (2+ users) call (800) 877-6209 for pricing.	$199.00			$9.95		
USPIS	USP DI® Internet Subscription	$199.00			$0.00		

Total Price

Add Sales Tax
if in FL, IA, NJ

Subtotal

Shipping ← Shipping Total

GRAND TOTAL

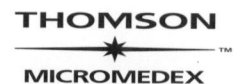

341M00A